Textbook of Neonatology

For Churchill Livingstone:

Project editors: Valerie Dearing, Barbara Simmons
Project controller: Nancy Arnott
Design direction: Sarah Cape

Textbook of Neonatology

Edited by

Janet M. Rennie MA MD FRCP FRCPCH DCH
Consultant and Senior Lecturer in Neonatal Medicine, King's College Hospital, London, UK

N. R. C. Roberton MA MB FRCP
Formerly Consultant Paediatrician and Neonatologist, Rosie Maternity Hospital, Cambridge, and Fellow, Fitzwilliam College, Cambridge, UK

THIRD EDITION

CHURCHILL LIVINGSTONE

EDINBURGH LONDON NEW YORK PHILADELPHIA SYDNEY TORONTO 1999

CHURCHILL LIVINGSTONE
A Division of Harcourt Brace and Company Limited

Churchill Livingstone, 1-3 Baxter's Place, Leith Walk, Edinburgh EH1 3AF

First edition 1986
Second edition 1992
Third edition 1999

ISBN 0443 055416

British Library of Cataloguing in Publication Data
A catalogue record for this book is available from the British Library.

Library of Congress Cataloging in Publication Data
A catalog record for this book is available from the Library of Congress.

Medical knowledge is constantly changing. As information becomes available, changes in treatment, procedures, equipment and the use of drugs become necessary. The author and publisher have, as far as it is possible, taken care to ensure that the information given in the text is accurate and up-to-date. However, readers are strongly advised to confirm that the information, especially with regard to drug usage, complies with current legislation and standard of practice.

The publisher's policy is to use **paper manufactured from sustainable forests**

Printed in China
SWTC/01

Preface

More than a decade has passed since the publication of the first edition, and seven years since the second. Much new knowledge has been gained, and the evaluation and organisation of neonatal intensive care has improved out of all recognition during this time. Nitric oxide treatment has made an unusually rapid transition from the laboratory to the cotside and is now established as an effective therapy for pulmonary hypertension in the term newborn. Exciting genetic advances continue, meaning that it is now essential for those of use who care for the newborn to be conversant with the techniques and terminology used in these laboratories. Antenatal diagnosis has changed the pattern of conditions which present to the neonatologist. Spina bifida is now rare but new management problems have been created by the increasing recognition of CNS, lung and renal malformations prenatally. These conditions present many dilemmas, not least because the natural history of many of these conditions remains to be defined. Intrapartum antibiotic prophylaxis against group B streptococcus is gaining acceptance but infection is still a killer in the neonatal period. Litigation has increased, and we have addressed this with two new chapters on the law as it relates to the neonate. Considerable challenges remain, not least the ethical and moral questions which are raised by the application of modern neonatal intensive care techniques to the very tiniest infants, whose long-term neurodevelopmental outcomes are being intensively studied around the world.

In the preparation of this book, the third edition, we have shared the editorial duties and we bear joint responsibility for any omissions. Many new authors have been recruited, often building on excellent chapters written by others for the first and second editions, whose contributions are gratefully acknowledged. We have worked hard with the chapter authors to introduce new material without losing that which was important, whilst striving to keep the overall length of the book the same. This task has been hard, but also enjoyable. We have learned much, and hope that all those who are involved in the diagnosis and treatment of sick newborn babies will find the book valuable as they strive to give the best possible care.

1999

Janet Rennie, London
Cliff Roberton, Isle of Skye

Acknowledgements

Any book of this size represents the hard work of an enormous number of people, first and foremost being the individual chapter authors. We convey our heartfelt thanks to them. Thanks are due to them not just for their own hard work but also to their secretaries, families and colleagues who have all borne an extra burden during the gestation of the chapters. As before, these long-suffering authors have put up with idiotic questions (now from both of us), nit-picking about the references, and ruthless editing of prose which had taken weeks to produce.

The staff at Churchill Livingstone (now Harcourt Brace) have cheerfully survived mergers and acquisitions so numerous that we have lost count. Sylvia Hull, of Churchill Livingstone, commissioned the first edition and is remembered with great affection. More recently, thanks are due in particular to Lucy Gardner (who got this edition going) and Antonia Seymour. Latterly Valerie Dearing, Barbara Simmons and Tim Horne have all made contributions.

On the rare occasions we have managed to emerge from our studies after battling with manuscripts or proofs, our spouses, Tricia Roberton and Ian Watts, have been remarkably tolerant, patient and supportive. Their good humour persisted even when dinner parties were interrupted by telephone conversations or the arrival of faxed spreadsheets bearing running totals of the latest word counts. To them, this book is dedicated.

Contributors

Nicholas Archer MA FRCP DCH
Consultant Paediatric Cardiologist, John Radcliffe Hospital, Oxford; Honorary Clinical Senior Lecturer, Department of Paediatrics, University of Oxford, Oxford, UK

Albert Aynsley-Green MA DPhil MB BS FRCP FRCPCH
Nuffield Professor of Child Health, Institute of Child Health and Great Ormond Street Hospital for Children NHS Trust, University of London, London, UK

Michael Baraitser MB ChB FRCP
Consultant Clinical Geneticist, Great Ormond Street Hospital for Sick Children, London, UK

Nicholas D. Barnes MA MB BChir FRCP FRCPCH
Consultant Paediatrician and Endocrinologist, Addenbrooke's Hospital, Cambridge, UK

P. J. Berry BA ChB BChir FRCP FRCPath
Professor of Paediatric Pathology, The Children's Hospital, Bristol, UK

Nicholas J. Bishop MB ChB MRCP MD FRCPCH
Senior Clinical Fellow, University of Sheffield, Division of Paediatrics, Sheffield, UK

Karen Brackley BMed Sci BM BS MRCOG DM
Lecturer in Fetal Medicine, Birmingham Women's Hospital, Birmingham, UK

A. Jeffrey L. Brain MS FRCS
Consultant Neonatal Surgeon, Addenbrooke's Hospital, Cambridge, UK

Valerie A. Broadbent MB BS FRCP MRCPCH
Consultant Paediatric Oncologist, Addenbrooke's Hospital, Cambridge, UK

Elizabeth M. Bryan MD FRCP DCH
Honorary Consultant Paediatrician and Director of the Multiple Births Foundation, Queen Charlotte's and Chelsea Hospital, London, UK

A. G. M. Campbell MB FRCP(Edin) Hon FRCPCH DCH
Emeritus Professor of Child Health, University of Aberdeen, Aberdeen, UK

Michael C. K. Chan MBE MD FRCP
Director, NHS Ethnic Health Unit, Leeds, UK

Radha Chari MD FRCSC
Assistant Professor, Department of Obstetrics and Gynecology, University of Alberta, Edmonton, Alberta, Canada

Tim Cheetham BSc MD MRCP
Senior Lecturer in Paediatric Endocrinology, Royal Victoria Infirmary, Newcastle-upon-Tyne, UK

T.J. Cole MA PhD
Senior Scientist, MRC Dunn Nutrition Centre, Cambridge, UK

Mark Davenport ChM FRCS(Paeds) FRCS(Eng) FRCPS(Glasgow)
Consultant Paediatric Surgeon, King's College Hospital, London, UK

Carl F. Davis MD MCh FRCS(Paeds)
Department of Surgical Paediatrics, Royal Hospital for Sick Children, Glasgow, UK

Linda S. de Vries MD FRCP
Consultant Neonatologist and Paediatric Neurologist, Wilhelmina Children's Hospital, Utrecht, The Netherlands

Peter R. F. Dear MD FRCP
Consultant and Senior Lecturer in Neonatal Medicine, St James's University Hospital, Leeds, UK

Nestor N. Demianczuk MD DES FRCSC ABOG
Associate Professor, Department of Obstetrics and Gynecology, University of Alberta; Director, Division of Maternal Fetal Medicine, Women's Health Program, Edmonton, Alberta, Canada

Sean P. Devane MD DCH FRCP(Irl) FRCPCH
Consultant Neonatologist, Children Nationwide Neonatal Unit, King's College Hospital, London, UK

Lex W. Doyle MD MSc FRACP
Associate Professor, Department of Obstetrics and Gynaecology, University of Melbourne and the Division of Paediatrics, the Royal Women's Hospital, Carlton, Australia

Richard E. J. Dyball ScD Vet MB
University Lecturer in Anatomy, University of Cambridge; Fellow and Tutor, Fitzwilliam College, Cambridge, UK

D. K. Edmonds FRACOG FRCOG
Consultant Obstetrician and Gynaecologist, Queen Charlotte's and Chelsea Hospital, London, UK

Philip C. Etches MA MB FRCP FRCPC FAAP DCH
Clinical Professor, Department of Pediatrics, University of Alberta; Head, Section of Newborn Medicine, Child Health Program; Director, Neonatal Intensive Care Unit, Royal Alexandra Hospital, Edmonton, Alberta, Canada

David J. Evans BM BCh MA MRCP
Research Fellow, Department of Paediatrics and Child Health, University of Leeds, Leeds, UK

Robert A. Evans MB BS FRCS
Consultant Otolaryngologist, Princess of Wales Hospital, Bridgend, Mid Glamorgan, Wales, UK

Mary S. Fewtrell BM BCh MA MRCP DCH
MRC Clinical Research Fellow and Honorary Consultant Paediatrician, Centre for Infant and Child Nutrition, Institute of Child Health, London, UK

David J. Field DM FRCP DCH
Professor of Neonatal Medicine, University of Leicester

Nicholas M. Fisk PhD FRACOG MRCOG DDU
Professor of Obstetrics and Gynaecology, Institute of Obstetrics and Gynaecology, Chelsea and Queen Charlotte's Hospital, London, UK

Gillian C. Forrest FRCPsych MRCGP
Consultant Child Psychiatrist, The Park Hospital for Children, Oxford, UK

Gillian M. Gandy MD MRCP
Consultant Emeritus, Rosie Maternity Hospital, Cambridge, UK

Roger F. Gray LRCP MRCS MB BS MA FRCS
Consultant ENT Surgeon, Cambridge University Teaching Hospital NHS Trust, Cambridge, UK

Andrew Green MB PhD MRCPI
Professor of Medical Genetics, National Centre for Medical Genetics, Our Lady's Hospital for Sick Children, Dublin, Eire

Anne Green PhD FRCPath FRSC
Consultant Clinical Biochemist; Head of Department of Clinical Chemistry (incorporating the West Midlands Regional Laboratory for Neonatal Screening and Inherited Metabolic Disorders), Birmingham Children's Hospital NHS Trust

Anne Greenough MD FRCP DCH
Professor of Clinical Respiratory Physiology, Department of Child Health, King's College Hospital, London, UK

Françoise H. D. Harlow BSc MB BS MRCOG
Specialist Registrar in Obstetrics and Gynaecology, Chelsea and Westminster Hospital, London, UK

J. M. Hawdon MA MB BS FRCP FRCPCH PhD
Consultant Neonatologist, University College London Hospitals, London, UK

Joanna T. Hawthorne PhD
Senior Research Associate, Centre for Family Research, University of Cambridge, Cambridge, UK

Robert N. Hensinger MD
Professor, Department of Surgery, University of Michigan, Ann Arbor, Michigan; Chief, Pediatric Orthopedics, Mott Children's Hospital (UM), Ann Arbor, Michigan USA

Alan Hill MD PhD FRCPC
Professor and Head, Division of Neurology, Department of Paediatrics, University of British Columbia, British Columbia Children's Hospital, Vancouver, Canada

N. Kevin Ives MA MB BChir DCH MRCP FRCPCH MD
Consultant Neonatologist and Honorary Senior Clinical Lecturer, University of Oxford Department of Paediatrics, John Radcliffe Hospital, Oxford, UK

Ann Johnson MD FRCP
Developmental Paediatrician, National Perinatal Epidemiology Unit, Oxford, UK

Eric T. Jones MD PhD
Clinical Professor of Orthopedic Surgery, Department of Orthopedic Surgery, West Virginia Medical Center, Morgantown, West Virginia, USA

Sue Keffler MA DipRCPath
Principal Biochemist, Department of Clinical Chemistry, Birmingham Children's Hospital, Birmingham, UK

A. W. R. Kelsall BSc(Hons) MB BChir MRCP FRCPCH
Consultant Paediatrician, Addenbrooke's NHS Trust Hospital, Cambridge, UK

Ashley King MA MB MRCPath
Research Fellow in Human Reproductive Immunobiology, University of Cambridge, Cambridge, UK

Phillipa M. Kyle MD MRCOG MRNZCOG
Consultant and Senior Clinical Lecturer in Fetal Medicine, St Michael's Hospital, Bristol, UK

Bertie Leigh Hon FRCPCH
Solicitor of the Supreme Court, Hempson's Solicitors, 33 Henrietta Street, London, UK

Elizabeth A. Letsky MB BS FRCPath FRCOG FRCPCH
Consultant Perinatal Haematologist and Honorary Senior Lecturer, Queen Charlotte's and Chelsea Hospital, London, UK

Malcolm I. Levene MD FRCP FRCPCH
Professor of Paediatrics and Child Health, University of Leeds, The General Infirmary at Leeds, Leeds, UK

Alan Lucas MA MD FRCP DCH
Professor of Infant and Child Nutrition, Centre for Infant and Child Nutrition, Institute of Child Health, London, UK

Alison Macfarlane BA DipStat
Medical Statistician, National Perinatal Epidemiology Unit, Radcliffe Hospital, Oxford, UK

Neil Marlow DM FRCP FRCPCH
Professor of Neonatal Medicine, University of Nottingham, Nottingham, UK

Giorgina Mieli-Vergani MD PhD FRCP
Professor of Paediatric Hepatology, Department of Child Health, King's College Hospital, London, UK

A. D. Milner MD FRCP DCH
Professor of Neonatology, United Medical and Dental Schools of Guy's and St Thomas' Hospitals, London, UK

Neena Modi MB ChB MD FRCPCH FRCP
Senior Lecturer and Consultant in Neonatal Paediatrics, Royal Postgraduate Medical School, Hammersmith Hospital, London, UK

A. T. Moore MA FRCS FRCOphth
Consultant Ophthalmologist, Addenbrooke's Hospital, Cambridge, and Moorfields Eye Hospital, London; Associate Lecturer, University of Cambridge Clinical Medical School, Cambridge, UK

Pierre D. E. Mouriquand MD FRCS FEBU
Professor of Paediatric Urology, Hopital Debrousse, Rue Soeur Bouvier, 69322 Lyon Cedex 05, France

The late Alex P. Mowat MB ChB FRCP DCH DObs RCOG
Consultant Paediatrician and Professor of Paediatric Hepatology, King's College Hospital, London, UK

Miranda Mugford BA(Hons) DPhil
Senior Lecturer (Health Services Research), School of Health Police and Practice, University of East Anglia, Norwich, UK

Visvan Navaratnam MB BS PhD
Director of Medical Studies, Christ's College, Cambridge, UK

Simon J. Newell MD FRCPH FRCP
Consultant and Senior Clinical Lecturer in Neonatal Medicine and Paediatric Gastroenterology, St James's University Hospital, Leeds, UK

Nan B. Okun MD FRCSC
Associate Professor, Department of Obstetrics and Gynecology, University of Alberta, Edmonton, Alberta, Canada

Janet M. Rennie MA MD FRCP FRCPCH DCH
Consultant and Senior Lecturer in Neonatal Medicine, King's College Hospital, London, UK

Martin P. M. Richards MA PhD
Director of the Centre for Family Research, University of Cambridge, Cambridge, UK

Sam Richmond MB BS FRCP FRCPCH
Consultant Neonatologist, Sunderland Royal Hospital, Sunderland, UK

Rodney R. A. Rivers FRCP
Reader in Paediatrics, Imperial College School of Medicine at St Mary's, London, UK

N. R. C. Roberton MA MB FRCP
Formerly Consultant Paediatrician and Neonatologist, Rosie Maternity Hospital, Cambridge, UK

Charles H. Rodeck BSc DSc FRCOG FRCPath
Professor of Obstetrics and Gynaecology, University College London Medical School, UK

Elke H. Roland MD FRCP(C)
Associate Professor, Division of Neurology, University of British Columbia, Vancouver, Canada

Simon Roth MB FRCP FRCPCH
Consultant Paediatrician, Wellhouse NHS Trust, Barnet General Hospital, Barnet, UK

Peter C. Rubin MA DM FRCP
Professor and Dean of the Faculty of Medicine and Health Sciences, University of Nottingham; Honorary Consultant Physician, Queen's Medical Centre, Nottingham, UK

Nicholas Rutter MD FRCP
Professor of Paediatric Medicine, University of Nottingham

John A. D. Spencer BSc MB BS FRCOG
Consultant Obstetrician and Gynaecologist, Northwick Park Hospital, Harrow, Middlesex, UK

G. Martin Steiner FRCP FRCR
Retired Consultant Paediatric Radiologist, The Children's Hospital, Sheffield, UK

Colin M. Stern FRCP FRCPCH PhD
Consultant Paediatrician, St Thomas's Hospital, London, UK

Ann L. Stewart MRCP FRCPCH
Honorary Senior Lecturer, Department of Paediatrics, University College, London and Department of Psychological Medicine, Institute of Psychiatry, London, UK

Patricia A. Tate MA MB BChir
General Practitioner, East Barnwell Health Centre, Cambridge, UK

Thomas L. Turner MB FRCP
Consultant Paediatrician, Queen Mother's Hospital, Glasgow, UK

Neil P. J. Walker MB FRCP
Honorary Consultant Dermatologist, Churchill Hospital, Oxford, UK

Duncan Wilcox MD FRCS(Paeds)
Consultant Paediatric Urologist, Great Ormond Street Children's Hospital and Guy's Hospital, London, UK

Robin Winter FRCP
Professor of Clinical Genetics and Dysmorphology, Mothercare Unit of Clinical Genetics and Fetal Medicine, Institute of Child Health, London, UK

Andrew R. Wolf MB BChir MD FRCA
Consultant in Paediatric Anaesthesia and Intensive Care, St Michael's Hospital, Bristol, UK

Ed Wraith MB ChB FRCP FRCPCH
Director, Willink Biochemical Genetics Unit, Royal Manchester Children's Hospital, Manchester

Daniel G. Young MB ChB FRCS(Edin and Glas) FRCPCH DTM&H
Head of Department of Surgical Paediatrics, University of Glasgow; Honorary Consultant Surgeon, Royal Hospital for Sick Children, Glasgow, UK

Victor Y. H. Yu MD MSc FRACP FRCP DCH
Professor of Neonatology, Monash University; Director of Neonatal Intensive Care, Monash Medical Centre, Melbourne, Australia

Abbreviations

A

α2M	Alpha-2-macroglobulin
A–aDO_2	Alveolar–arterial oxygen difference (of PaO_2)
a/A ratio	Arterial alveolar ratio (of PaO_2)
ABR	Auditory brainstem evoked responses
ACE	Angiotensin converting enzymes
ACT	Activated clotting time
ACTH	Adrenocorticotrophic hormone, corticotrophin
AD	Autosomal dominant
ADA	Adenosine deaminase
ADCC	Antibody dependent cytotoxicity
ADH	Antidiuretic hormone
ADP	Adenosine diphosphate
ADPKD	Autosomal dominant polycystic kidney disease
AFI	Amniotic fluid index
AFP	Alpha–feto protein
AGA	Appropriate for gestational age
AIDS	Aquired immune deficiency syndrome
AIHA	Autoimmune haemolytic anaemia
ALEC	Artificial lung expansing compound (Pumactant)
ALL	Acute lymphoblastic leukaemia
AMH	Anti-Mullerian hormone
AMP	Adenosine monophosphate
ANP	Atrial natriuretic peptide
AP	Aorto-pulmonary
APC	Activated protein C
APH	Antepartum haemorrhage
APTT	Activated partial thromboplastin time
AR	Aortic regurgitation Autosomal recessive
ARDS	Adult (acute) respiratory distress syndrome
ARM	Artificial rupture of the membranes
ARPKD	Autosomal recessive polycystic kidney disease
AS	Aortic stenosis
ASD	Atrial septal defect
ATP	Adenosine triphosphate
ATS	Anti-tetanus serum
AV	Atrio-ventricular
AVM	Arterio-venous malformation
AVP	Arginine vasopressin (i.e. ADH)
AVSD	Atrioventricular septal defect

B

BAL	Broncho–alveolar lavage
BAPM	British Association of Perinatal Medicine formerly BAPP – British Association of Perinatal Paediatrics
BBA	Born before arrival
BCG	Bacillus Calmette Guérin
BMC	Bone mineral content
BMR	Basal metabolic rate
BMT	Bone marrow transplant
BPA	British Paediatric Association
BP	Blood pressure
BPD	Broncho-pulmonary dysplasia (see page 608) Biparietal diameter
BPSU	British Paediatric Surveillance Unit
BT	Bleeding time

C

CaO_2	Arterial oxygen content
CA	Carbonic anhydrase
CAH	Congenital adrenal hyperplasia
c-AMP	Cylic adenosine monophosphate
CBF(V)	Cerebral blood flow (velocity)
CcO_2	Capillary oxygen content
CCAM	Congenital cystic adenomatoid malformation
CD	Cluster of differentiation
CDA	Congenital dyserythropoietic anaemia

CDG	Carbohydrate deficient glycoprotein
CDH	Congenital diaphramatic hernia
	Congenital dislocation of the hip (see DDH, p. 1069)
CDP	Cytidine choline diphosphate
CESDI	Confidential enquiry into stillbirths and deaths in infancy
CF	Cystic fibrosis
CFM	Cerebral function monitor
CFTR	Cystic fibrosis transmembrane regulator
cGMP	Cyclic Guanosine monophosphate
CHARGE	Coloboma, heart disease, choanal atresia, retardation, genital and ear anomalies
CHB	Complete heart block
CHD	Congenital heart disease
CHIPA	Chronic in utero partial asphyxia
CK	Creatine phosphokinase
CLAPA	Cleft lip and palate association
CLD	Chronic lung disease
CLSE	Calf lung surfactant extract
CMD	Congenital muscular dystrophy
CMV	Cytomegalovirus
CNEP	Continuous negative external pressure
CNS	Central nervous system
CONS	Coagulase negative staphylococci
COP	Colloid osmotic pressure
CP	Cerebral palsy
CPAP	Continuous positive airways pressure
CPC	Choroid plexus cysts
CPD(A)	Citrate phosphate dextrose (adenine)
CPR	Cardiopulmonary resuscitation
CRH	Corticotrophin releasing hormone
CRIB	Clinical risk index for babies
CRP	C reactive protein
CS	Caesarean section
CSAG	Clinical Standards Advisory Group
CSF	Cerebro-spinal fluid
CT	Computerized tomography
CTG	Cardiotocogram (cardiotocography)
CvO_2	Mixed venous oxygen content
CVB(S)	Chorionic villus biopsy (sampling)
CVP	Central venous pressure
CVS	Cardiovascular system
	Chorionic villus sample
CXR	Chest x-ray

D

2:3 DPG	2:3 diphosphoglycerate
DA	Ductus arteriosus
DAT	Direct antiglobulin (Coombs') test
DBM	Drip/donor breast milk
DCM	Dilated cardiomyopathy
DCT	Direct Coombs' test
DDAVP	Desmopressin: 1–deamino-8-D-arginine vasopressin
DDH	Developmental dysplasia of the hip
del	deletion
DHA	Docosahexanoic acid
DHSS	Department of Health and Social Security
DHT	Dihydrotestosterone
DIC	Disseminated intravascular coagulation
DIDMOAD	Diabetes insipidus, diabetes mellitus, optic atrophy, deafness
DILV	Double inlet left ventricle
DIV	Double inlet ventricle
DMSA	Dimercaptosuccinic acid
DNA	Deoxyribonucleic acid
DOH	Department of Health
DORV	Double outlet right ventricle
DOV	Double outlet ventricle
DPG	Diphosphoglycerate
DPPC	Dipalmitoyl phosphatidyl choline (Lecithin)
DQ	Development quotient
DRG	Diagnostic related groups
	Dorsal respiratory group
DTPA	Diethylenetriaminepentacetic acid
DVM	Delayed visual maturation
DZ	Dizygotic

E

EB	Epidermolysis bullosa
EBM	Expressed breast milk
EC	European Community
	Ejection click
ECF	Extracellular fluid
ECG	Electrocardiogram
ECM	External cardiac massage
ECMO	Extracorporeal membrane oxygenation
ECV	External cephalic version
EDD	Estimated date of delivery
EDFV	End–diastolic flow velocity
EDTA	Ethylenediamine tetracetic acid
EEG	Electroencephalogram
EFE	Endocardial fibroelastosis
EFM	Electronic fetal monitoring
EGF	Epithelial/epidermal growth factor
ELBW	Extremely low birthweight (< 1.0 kg birthweight)
ELISA	Enzyme linked immunosorbent assay
ELSO	Extracorporeal like support organisation
EMG	Electromyogram
EMLA	Eutectic mixture of local anaesthetic
ERG	Electroretinogram
ESPGAN	European Society for Paediatric Gastroenterology and Nutrition
ETT	Endotracheal tube
EVT	Extravillous trophoblast

F

FACS	Fluorescence activated cell sorting
FBC	Full blood count
FBM	Fetal breathing movements
FBS	Fetal blood sample
FDP	Fibrin degradation products
Fe_{H_2O}	Fractional excretion of water
Fe_{Na}	Fractional excretion of sodium
FEV_1	Forced expiratory volume in one minute
FEVR	Familial exudative vitreoretinopathy
FFP	Fresh frozen plasma
FFTS	Feto-fetal transfusion syndrome
FH	Family history
FHR	Fetal heart rate
FIGO	International Federation of Gynaecology & Obstetrics
F_IO_2	Fractional inspired oxygen concentration
FISH	Fluorescent in situ hybridisation
FRC	Functional residual capacity
FSE	Fetal scalp electrode
FSH	Follicle stimulating hormone
FTA-ABS	Fluorescent treponemal antibody absorption test
FUV	Fetal umbilical vein

G

GAD	Glutamic acid decarboxylase
GALT	Gut associated lymphoid tissue
γGT	Gamma glutamyl transferase
GABA	Gamma amino butyric acid
G6PD	Glucose-6-phosphate dehydrogenase
GBS	Group B beta haemolytic streptococcus
GCSF	Granulocyte colony stimulating factor
GDP	Gross domestic product
GFR	Glomerular filtration rate
GH	Growth hormone
GHRH	Growth hormone releasing hormone
GIFT	Gamete intrafallopian transfer
GI	Gastrointestinal
GIT	Gastrointestinal tract
GM-CSF	Granulocyte macrophage colony stimulating factor
GMH-IVH	Germinal matrix/intraventricular haemorrhage
GMP	Guanosine monophosphate
GnRH	Gonadotrophin releasing hormone
GOR	Gastro-oesophageal reflux
GP	General Practitioner
GSD	Glycogen storage disease
GSH	Reduced glutathione
GTP	Guanosine triphosphate
GTT	Glucose tolerance test
GU	Genitourinary
GVHD	Graft versus host disease

H

HAA	Hospital activity analysis
HAS	Human albumin solution
HBV	Hepatitis B virus
Hep A, B, C	Hepatitis A, B, C
HCG	Human chorionic gonadotrophin
HCM	Hypertrophic cardiomyopathy
HCV	Hepatitis C virus
HDL	High density lipoprotein
HDN	Haemolytic disease of the newborn Haemorrhagic disease of the newborn (VKDB)
HELLP	Haemolysis, elevated liver enzymes, low platelets
HES	Hospital episode system
HFFI	High frequency flow interruption
HFPPV	High frequency positive pressure ventilation
HFJV	High frequency jet ventilation
HFOV	High frequency oscillatory ventilation
HIE	Hypoxic ischaemic encephalopathy
HIV	Human immuno-deficiency virus
HLA	Human leucocyte antigen
HLHS	Hypoplastic left heart syndrome
HMD	Hyaline membrane disease
HMF	Human milk formula
HPA	Hypothalamic–pituitary–adrenal Human platelet antigen
HPI	Haemorrhagic parenchymal infarction
HRG	Health Resource Groupings
HVS	High vaginal swab
HPV	Human parvovirus
HS	Hereditary spherocytosis
HSV	Herpes simplex virus (I, II)
Hz	Hertz (cycles/second)

I

IAA	Interrupted aortic arch
ICAM	Intracellular adhesion molecule
ICD	International classification of disease
ICP	Intracranial pressure
IDA	Iminodiacetic acid
IDM	Infant of the diabetic mother
I:E	Inspiratory to expiratory ratio
IEM	Inborn error of metabolism
Ifn	Interferon
IgA, D, G, M	Immunoglobulins A, D, G, and M
IGF	Insulin like growth factor
IHV	Intra-hepatic venous (sampling)
IL	Interleukin
i.m.	Intramuscular
IMF	International Monetary Fund
INR	International normalized ratio
IPL	Intraparenchymal lesion

IPT	Intraperitoneal transfusion
IPPV	Inermittent positive pressure ventilation
IQ	Intelligence Quotient
IRT	Immunoreactive trypsin
ITP	Idiopathic thrombocytopenic purpura
IUGR	Intrauterine growth retardation/ restriction
i.v.	Intravenous
IVC	Inferior vena cava
IVF	In vitro fertilization
IVH	Intraventricular haemorrhage
IVIG	Intravenous immunoglobulin
IVS	Intact ventricular septum
IVT	Intravascular transfusion
IVU	Intravenous urogram

K

kPa	Kilopascal (= 7.5 mmHg)
KCCT	Kaolin cephalin clotting time
KIR	Killer inhibitory receptors

L

LAD	Left axis deviation
LBW	Low birthweight (< 2.50 kg)
LCAD	Long chain fatty acyl-CoA dehydrogenase
LCHAD	Long chain fatty 3-hydroxyacyl-CoA dehydrogenase
LCPUFA	Long chain polyunsaturated fatty acids
LCT	Long chain triglyceride
LGA	Large for gestational age
LH	Luteinising hormone
LLSE	Lower left sternal edge
LMP	Last menstrual period
LOS	Lower oesophageal sphincter
LP	Lumbar puncture
L:S	Lecithin to sphingomyelin ratio
LSCS	Lower segment caesarean section
LT	Leukotriene
LV	Left ventricle
LVH	Left ventricular hypertrophy
LVOT	Left ventricular outflow tract

M

MACS	Magnetically activated cell sorting
MAD	Multiple acyl–CoA dehydrogenase
MAG–3	Mercaptoacetyl triglycine
MAP	Mean airway pressure
MAPCA	Major aorto–pulmonary communicating arteries
MAS	Meconium aspiration syndrome
MCAD	Medium chain fatty acyl-CoA dehydrogenase deficiency
MCH	Mean corpuscular haemoglobin
MCHC	Mean corpuscular haemoglobin content
MCP	Major cationic protein
MCT	Medium chain triglycerides
MCUG	Micturating cysto–urethrogram
MCV	Mean corpuscular volume
meg CSF	Megakaryocyte colony stimulating factor
MHC	Major histocompatibility complex
MIC	Minimum inhibitory concentration
MIF	Migration inhibitory factor
MIP	Macrophage inflammatory protein
MMC	Meningomyelocele
mmHg	Millimetres of mercury
MMR	Mumps, measles and rubella vaccine
MOM	Multiples of the median
MPH	Massive pulmonary haemorrhage
MPI	Milk protein intolerance
MR	Magnetic resonance Mitral regurgitation
MRC	Medical Research Council
MRI	Magnetic resonance imaging
mRNA	Messenger ribonucleic acid
MRS	Magnetic resonance spectroscopy
MRSA	Methicillin resistant staphylococcus aureus
MS	Mitral stenosis
mt	Mitochondrial
MZ	Monozygotic

N

NADPH	Nicotinamide adenine dinucleotide phosphate
NAITP	Neonatal alloimmune thrombocytopenic purpura
NBAS	Neonatal behavioural assessment scale
NBT	Nitroblue tetrazolium
NCT	National Childbirth Trust
NEC	Necrotising enterocolitis
NG	Nasogastric
NGF	Nerve growth factor
NGT	Nasogastric tube
NHS	National Health Service
NICHHD	National Institute of Child Health and Human Development
NICU	Neonatal Intensive Care Unit
NIDCAP	Neonatal Individual Developmental Care and Assessment Programme
NIDDM	Non-insulin dependant diabetes mellitus
NIH	Non-immune hydrops
NIRS	Near infra red spectroscopy
NK	Natural killer (lympocytes)
NMDA	N-methyl-d-aspartate
NMR	Nuclear magnetic resonance Neonatal mortality risk
NO	Nitric oxide
NSAID	Non-steroidal anti-inflammatory drugs

NT	Nuchal translucency
NTD	Neural tube defect

O

17-OHP	17-hydroxyprogesterone
OCT	Ornithine carbamyl transferase
OFC	Occipito–frontal circumference
OI	Osteogenesis imperfecta
ONS	Office of National Statistics
OPCS	Office of Population, Censuses and Surveys
OR	Odds ratio

P

PA	Pulmonary artery
PABS	Pulmonary artery branch stenosis
$PaCO_2$	Partial pressure of CO_2 in arterial blood
$PACO_2$	Partial pressure of CO_2 in alveolar gas
PAF	Platelet activating factor
PAGE	Perfluorocarbon assisted gas exchange
PAH	Para-amino hippurate
PAI-1	Plasminogen activator inhibitor 1
PAIgG	Anti-platelet autoantibodies
PaO_2	Partial pressure of oxygen in arterial blood
PAO_2	Partial pressure of oxygen in alveolar gas
PAP	Pulmonary artery pressure
PAPP-A	Pregnancy associated protein A
PAPVC	Partial anomolous pulmonary venous connection
PC	Phosphatidylcholine
PCA	Post conceptional age
PCr	Phosphocreatine
PCR	Polymerase chain reaction
PCV	Packed cell volume
PDA	Patent ductus arteriosus
PE	Phosphatidylethanolamine
PEEP	Positive end expiratory pressure
PET	Pre-eclamptic toxaemia
PF 3	Platelet factor 3
PF 4	Platelet factor 4
PFC	Persistent fetal circulation Perfluorocarbon
PFK	Phosphofructokinase
PFO	Patent foramen ovale
PG	Phosphatidylglycerol
PGE, F, G, H	Prostaglandins E, F, G and H
PGI_2	Prostacyclin
PGSI	Prostaglandin synthetase inhibitor
pH	Hydrogen ion concentration
PHHI	Persistent hyperinsulinaemic hypoglycaemia of infancy (nesidioblastosis)
PHT	Pulmonary hypertension
PHVD	Post haemorrhagic ventricular dilatation
Pi	Inorganic orthophosphate
PI	Phosphatidylinositol
PIE	Pulmonary interstitial emphysema
PIP	Peak inflating pressure
PIVKA	Protein produced in Vitamin K absence
PK	Pyruvate kinase Prekallikrein
PKU	Phenylketonuria
PLV	Partial liquid ventilation
PNMR	Perinatal mortality rate
PNP	Purine nucleotide phosphorylase
PNW	Postnatal ward
POEMS	Programmable otoacoustic emissions
PP	Pancreatic polypeptide
PPF	Purified plasma fraction
PPHN	Persistent pulmonary hypertension of the newborn
PPROM	Preterm premature rupture of the membranes
PRA	Plasma renin activity
PRISM	Paediatric risk of mortality score
PRL	Prolactin
PROM	Preterm rupture of the membranes
PS	Pulmonary stenosis Phosphatidylserine
PSM	Pansystolic murmur
PT	Prothrombin time
PTH	Parathormone
PTL	Preterm labour
PTM	Preterm milk
PTT	Partial thromboplastin time
PTTK	PTT kaolin
PTV	Patient trigger ventilation
PUBS	Percutaneous umbilical blood sampling
PUFA	Polyunsaturated fatty acids
PUJ	Pyelo/pelvi ureteric junction
PUV	Posterior urethral valves
PVD	Pulmonary vascular disease
PVH	Periventricular haemorrhage
PVL	Periventricular leukomalacia
PVR	Pulmonary vascular resistance

Q

Qs	Proportion of the cardiac output which is shunted
Qt	Total cardiac output
q.v.	Quod vide = which see
QUALY	Quality adjusted life year

R

RA	Right atrium
RAAS	Renin angiotensin aldosterone system

RAH	Right atrial hypertrophy
RBC	Red blood cell
RBP	Retinol binding protein
RCOG	Royal College of Obstetricians and Gynaecologists
RCPCH	Royal College of Paediatrics and Child Health
RCT	Randomised controlled trial
RDA	Recommended dietary allowance
RDS	Respiratory distress syndrome
REM	Rapid eye movement (sleep)
RF	Risk factor
RFLP	Restriction fragment length polymorphism
RHA	Regional Health Authority
rHuEpo	Recombinant human erythropoietin
RIP	Respiratory inductance plethysmography Rest in Peace
RLF	Retrolental fibroplasia
RIS	Respiratory insufficiency syndrome
RNA	Ribonucleic acid
RNCE	Routine neonatal clinical examination
ROP	Retinopathy of prematurity
RSV	Respiratory syncytial virus
RV	Right ventricle Residual volume
RVET	Right ventricular ejection time
RVH	Right ventricular hypertrophy
RVOT	Right ventricular outflow tract
Rx	Recipe – prescribe for

S

SAH	s-adenosylhomocysteine
SANDS	Stillbirth and Neonatal Death Society
SaO_2	True arterial haemoglobin oxygen saturation
SB	Stillborn
SBR	Stillbirth rate
SBS	Short bowel syndrome
sc	Subcutaneously
SCBU	Special Care Baby Unit
SCID	Severe combined immunodeficiency
SD	Standard deviation (of the mean)
SEH	Subependymal haemorrhage
SEP(R)	Somatosensory evoked potential (response)
SFD	Small for dates
SGA	Small for gestational age
SH	Sulphydryl
SHO	Senior House Officer
SIADH	Syndrome of inappropriate ADH secretion
SIDS	Sudden infant death syndrome
SIMV	Synchronized intermittent mandatory ventilation
SLE	Systemic lupus erythematosus
SMS	Somatostatin
SNHL	Sensory neural hearing loss
SOD	Superoxide dismutase
SpA, B, C, D	Surfactant apoproteins A, B, C, D
SPA	Suprapubic aspiration (urine) Single protein absorptiometry
sPDA	Symptomatic patent ductus arteriosus
SpO_2	Transcutaneous haemoglobin oxygen saturation (from Oximeter)
SpR	Specialist Registrar
SSCA	Single stranded conformational assay
SVT	Supraventricular tachycardia

T

T_3	Tri-iodothyronine
T_4	Thyroxine
TAMBA	Twins and multiple births association
TAPVC/D	Total anomalous pulmonary venous connection/drainage
TAR	Thrombocytopenia and absent radius syndrome
TB	Tuberculosis
TBG	Thyroid binding globulin
$tcPCO_2$	Transcutaneous PCO_2
$tcPO_2$	Transcutaneous PO_2
TCT	Thrombin clotting time
TCU	Transitional care unit
T_E	Expiratory time
TEWL	Transepidermal water loss
TF	Tissue factor
TGA	Transposition of the great arteries
TGF	Tissue growth factor
TGV	Thoracic gas volume
THAM	Tris–hydroxymethylaminomethane
T_I	Inspiratory time
TI	Tricuspid incompetence
TLC	Total lung capacity
TLV	Total liquid ventilation
TNF α	Tumour necrosis factor alpha
TOE	Transoesophageal echocardiography
TOF	Tracheo-oesophageal fistula
TORCH	Toxoplasma, rubella, cytomegalovirus, herpes
tPa	Tissue plasminogen activator
TPFR	Total period fertility rate
TPHA	Treponema pallidum haemagglutination assay
TPN	Total parenteral nutrition
TPR	Temperature, pulse and respiration
TPV	Time to peak velocity
TR	Tricuspid regurgitation
TRH	Thyrotrophin releasing hormone
tRNA	Transfer RNA
TS	Tuberous sclerosis

TSH	Thyroid stimulating hormone (thyrotrophin)
TSI	Thyroid stimulating immunoglobulins
TT	Thrombin time
TTN	Transient tachypnoea of the newborn
TXA_2	Thromboxane A2

U

UAC	Umbilical artery catheter
UDPGT	Uridine diphosphoglucuronyl transferase
UFI	Urine flow impairment
URTI	Upper respiratory tract infection
US	Ultrasound
USS	Ultrasound scan
UTI	Urinary tract infection
UVC	Umbilical venous catheter

V

VACTERL	As for VATER with cardiac and limb defects
VATER	Vertebral defects, anal atresia, T–E fistula, radial and renal dysplasia
VC	Vital capacity
VDDR	Vitamin D dependant Rickets
VDRL	Veneral disease research laboratory (test for syphilis)
V_E	Minute volume
VE	Ventricular ectopics
VEGF	Vascular endothelial growth factor
VEP	Visual evoked potential
vi	Vide infra (see below in text)
viz	Videlicet = namely
VKDB	Vitamin K deficiency bleeding
VLBW	Very low birthweight (< 1.50 kg)
VRG	Ventral respiratory group
vs	Vide supra (see above in text)
VSD	Ventricular septal defect
V_T	Tidal volume
VT	Ventricular tachycardia
VUJ	Vesico-ureteric junction
vWF	von Willebrand factor
VZV	varicella zoster virus

W

WBC	White blood cell count
WHO	World Health Organization
WPW	Wolff–Parkinson–White syndrome

Z

ZIG	Zoster immune globulin

Contents

Section 4
General neonatal care

Section 5
Disorders of the newborn

Section 6
Pathology, radiology and biochemistry

Section 7
Ethics and the law

Section 8
Practical procedures

Section 9

Appendices

Section 1

Organization and delivery of neonatal care

1

Epidemiology

Alison Macfarlane Ann Johnson Miranda Mugford

BIRTHS AND BIRTH RATES

HOW BIRTH STATISTICS ARE COMPILED

There are three main routes through which data about births are collected. These have been described in considerable detail elsewhere,[84,88] but a brief description and update are given here.

The most frequently used source of data on a national scale is civil registration. In the United Kingdom parents are required by law to register a birth with the local Registrar of Births and Deaths. As well as issuing a certificate, the registrar passes the information to a central office, which compiles both national and local statistics. Scotland, Northern Ireland and the Republic of Ireland each have separate General Register Offices. In 1970, the General Register Office for England and Wales was merged with the Government Social Survey to form the Office of Population Censuses and Surveys. Then, in April 1996, OPCS merged with the Central Statistical Office and the Labour Market Statistics Group of the former Department of Employment to form the Office for National Statistics, which compiles and publishes a wide range of health, social and economic statistics.

In the UK, the law originally required all fetal deaths after 28 completed weeks of gestation to be registered as stillbirths. This limit was lowered to 24 weeks on 1 October 1992. All live births at any gestation have to be registered. In the Republic of Ireland there was no system for registering stillbirths before 1995, but they have been notified to Directors of Community Care since 1957. Statistics derived from this source and from birth and death registrations are then analysed centrally by the Irish Central Statistics Office. Perinatal statistics are also published separately by the Department of Health.

The second method of information collection is through birth notification. In the UK all births have to be notified to the local Director of Public Health. This is usually done by midwives immediately after the birth, and must be done within 36 hours. The system was devised so that a health visitor could be informed and then call to see the mother and baby.

Most health authorities now have child health computer systems which are used to administer vaccination and immunization programmes and to monitor developmental testing. In these systems the child's record is usually initiated by the birth notification, although some districts use a special Neonatal Discharge Record, devised in the late 1970s by the British Paediatric Association, now the Royal College of Paediatrics and Child Health.[43] In Wales these child health systems are being developed so that data from birth notifications can be used to produce national maternity statistics. In Northern Ireland, each of the four Health and Social Services Boards holds data from child health systems. Some of these are pooled to produce data for the province as a whole.

The third route for collecting data about births is through hospital-based systems. Traditionally these have collected data at discharge about hospital inpatient stays. More recently, systems have been developed that gather data about a person's episodes of care within a given trust. In the future, National Health Service districts should hold information about care given to their residents wherever this is provided, but they vary in the extent to which their computer systems enable them to capture information from provider units.

In England, information about inpatient stays in NHS hospitals is aggregated nationally through the Hospital Episode System. There is a separate Maternity Hospital Episode System to collect information about women delivering in and babies born in the maternity departments of NHS hospitals. MHES records include the standard admitted patient record plus a 'maternity tail', with a 'minimum dataset' and 'clinical options'. The items in the minimum datasets were specified by the Steering Group on Health Services Information,[131] chaired by Edith Körner. This was known as the Körner Committee, and the datasets it recommended are usually referred to as 'Körner minimum datasets'.

The Hospital Episode System started in April 1987

and Maternity HES finally got under way in September 1988, after a delay of 6 months. In the mid-1990s it was still very incomplete. By the financial year 1994–95 the system contained records for only 67% of deliveries in England.[63] Although the systems are working locally in some regions and districts, many of the data do not reach systems operating at national level. None of the records that reach national level contain data items from the 'clinical options'. Since the introduction of the NHS internal market a series of attempts has been made to revise the minimum dataset, but the proposed datasets contain few clinical data and the issue is yet to be resolved, at the time of writing. In Wales and Northern Ireland similar systems have been introduced. As these are mainly geared to contracting they also contain few clinical data, and this has led to the use of child health systems for collecting maternity data. In England data about episodes of care in neonatal intensive care units are collected, along with data about other episodes in paediatric departments, in the main part of HES. Unfortunately, these data cannot be linked, at national level at least, to the record of the baby's delivery. There is also a lack of consistency in recording levels of special and intensive care.

Scotland has had a maternity information system working nationally since the mid-1970s. Data about mothers are collected through the SMR2 Maternity Discharge Sheet, and data about babies through the SMR11 record. The system as a whole is now known as Core Patient Profile Information in Scottish Hospitals (COPPISH). Some of the data are published annually in *Scottish Health Statistics*, and others are used for ad hoc analyses. Data from these and other sources were brought together in a publication entitled *Births in Scotland 1976–1995*,[69] which appeared in 1997.

Scotland is the only country in the UK that makes a concerted attempt to collect data about babies admitted to neonatal units. The other three countries include them in statistics collected about activity in paediatric departments, but have not so far been able to identify them in separately published data. In England the intention was to code 'levels of care', but this has given rise to problems which are described later. Counts are published separately of the numbers of 'well babies' born in NHS hospitals but not admitted to neonatal units.

TRENDS AND VARIATIONS IN BIRTH RATES

The numbers of live births registered in recent years in each of the four countries of the UK and in the Republic of Ireland are shown in Table 1.1. This shows that in the late 1980s the numbers of births rose everywhere except in the Republic of Ireland, before falling again in the early 1990s. These figures are useful as a measure of the workload of the maternity and paediatric services, but they shed very little light on the reasons for the increases and decreases. These can arise either as a result of changes in the size and age structure of the child-bearing population, or as a consequence of changes in the birth rate within each age group.

One of the most long-standing measures of birth rate is the general fertility rate. In this the number of live births is expressed as a rate per 1000 women aged 15–44 or, in some cases, 15–49. Figure 1.1 shows the general fertility

Table 1.1 Live births in England, Wales, Scotland and Ireland 1975–1996

	England	Wales	England and Wales*	Scotland	Northern Ireland	Irish Republic
1975	568 900	38 030	603 445	67 943	26 130	67 178
1976	550 383	36 883	584 270	64 895	26 361	67 718
1977	536 953	31 765	569 259	62 342	25 437	68 892
1978	562 589	33 308	596 418	64 295	26 239	70 299
1979	601 316	36 174	638 028	68 366	28 178	72 539
1980	618 371	37 357	656 234	68 892	28 582	74 064
1981	598 126	35 842	634 492	69 054	27 302	72 158
1982	589 711	35 720	625 931	66 196	27 028	70 843
1983	593 255	35 494	629 134	65 078	27 255	67 117
1984	600 573	35 861	636 818	65 106	27 693	64 062
1985	619 301	36 771	656 417	66 676	27 635	62 388
1986	623 609	37 038	661 018	65 812	28 152	61 620
1987	643 330	37 816	681 511	66 241	27 865	58 433
1988	654 363	38 824	693 577	66 212	27 767	54 600
1989	649 357	38 019	687 725	63 480	26 080	52 018
1990	666 920	38 866	706 140	65 973	26 499	53 044
1991	660 806	38 079	699 217	67 024	26 265	52 718
1992	651 784	37 523	689 656	65 789	25 572	51 089
1993	636 461	36 578	673 467	63 337	24 909	49 304
1994	628 956	35 366	664 726	61 656	24 289	47 928+
1995	613 257	34 477	648 138	60 051	23 860	48 530+
1996	614 188	34 894	649 489	59 308	24 582	

Sources: ONS, General Register Offices for Scotland and Northern Ireland; Department of Health, Ireland
*Including births in England and Wales to women normally resident outside England and Wales
+Provisional

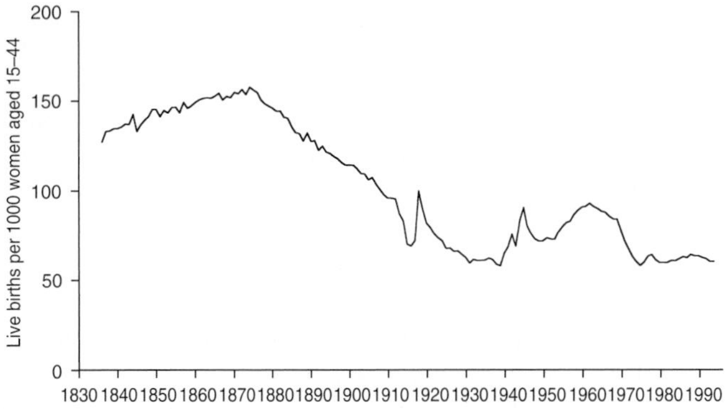

Fig. 1.1 General fertility rate, England and Wales 1938–1996. (Source: Office for National Statistics, Birth Statistics, Series FM1.)

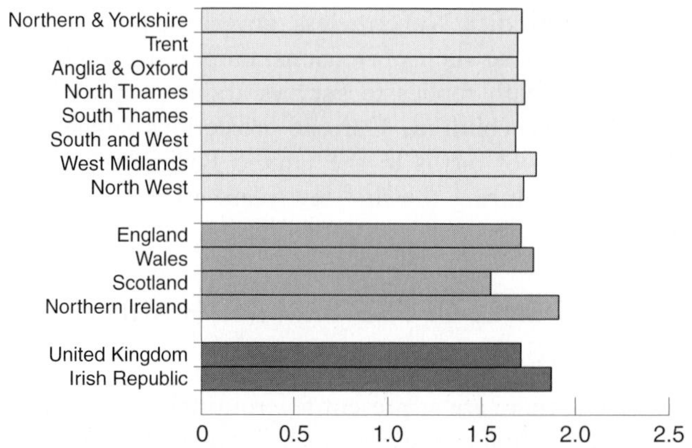

Fig. 1.2 Total period fertility rates, United Kingdom and Ireland, 1995. (Source: Birth Statistics, Series FM1.)

rate for England and Wales since 1838, the first full year after civil registration began in July 1837. The rates for the mid-19th century are probably an underestimate, as birth registration did not become compulsory in England and Wales until 1874. Shortly after this the fertility rate began to decline, a trend which continued steadily until the 1930s. This was interrupted only by a trough during World War I and a short-lived peak after the war ended. A similar peak followed World War II. After this there was longer term rise in the 1950s and 1960s, followed by a decline through most of the 1970s. Since the rate reached a minimum in 1977 it has fluctuated, gradually increasing in the late 1980s and decreasing in the early 1990s.

This overall rate masks changes since 1977 within age groups. These are set out in Table 1.2, which shows birth rates among women in their late teens and 20s rising slightly in the late 1980s as the 'bulge' of women born in the mid-1960s entered the child-bearing age range,[34] and then falling in the early 1990s. In contrast, rates among women in their 30s and 40s have risen consistently.

These age-specific rates can be summed up in a statistic called the 'total period fertility rate'. This is a standardized measure which gives the total number of children who would be born to each woman if she experienced the age-specific fertility rates for the year in question throughout her child-bearing life. As Table 1.2 shows, the rate rose gradually in the latter half of the 1980s, but has been falling in the 1990s. Figure 1.2 shows how TPFRs varied within England and between the countries of Britain and Ireland in 1995. The South and West region had the lowest rate, at 1.68, and the West Midlands had the highest at 1.79. Even this was considerably lower than the rates of 1.91 for Northern Ireland and 1.87 for the Irish Republic.

For planning services it would be useful to have some idea of future trends in births, but these are notoriously

Table 1.2 Age-specific fertility rates, England and Wales

Year	Live births, thousands	Live births per 1000 women in age group							TPFR
		15–44	Under 20	20–24	25–29	30–34	35–39	40 and over	
1964 (max)	876.0	92.9	42.5	181.6	187.3	107.7	49.8	13.7	2.93
1977 (min)	569.3	58.1	29.4	103.7	117.5	58.6	18.2	4.4	1.66
1979	638.0	63.3	30.3	111.3	131.2	69.0	21.3	4.7	1.84
1984	636.8	59.8	27.4	95.5	126.2	73.6	23.6	4.9	1.75
1985	656.4	61.0	29.5	94.5	127.6	76.4	24.1	5.0	1.78
1986	661.0	60.6	30.1	92.7	124.0	78.1	24.6	4.8	1.77
1987	681.5	62.0	30.9	93.4	125.1	81.3	26.5	5.1	1.81
1988	693.6	63.0	32.4	94.9	123.8	82.7	27.9	5.1	1.82
1989	687.7	62.5	31.9	92.2	120.0	83.7	29.4	5.2	1.80
1990	706.1	64.3	33.3	91.7	122.4	87.3	31.2	5.3	1.84
1991	699.2	63.8	33.1	89.6	119.9	87.0	32.1	5.3	1.82
1992	689.7	63.5	31.7	86.2	117.3	87.2	33.4	5.8	1.80
1993	673.5	62.6	31.0	82.7	114.1	87.0	34.1	6.2	1.76
1994	664.7	61.9	29.0	79.4	112.1	88.7	35.8	6.4	1.75
1995	648.1	60.4	28.5	76.8	108.6	87.3	36.2	6.8	1.72
1996	649.5	60.5	29.7	77.5	107.3	88.8	37.2	6.9	1.74

1. The rates for women of all ages, under 20, and 40 and over are based upon the female population aged 15–44, 15–19 and 40–44, respectively.
2. The 1996 rates are provisional and were calculated using 1994-based mid-1996 population projections.

Source: ONS Birth Statistics, Series FM1

difficult to predict. Nevertheless, government statisticians attempt to make such projections, combining analyses of past trends with replies to surveys about people's intentions to have children. Current projections suggest that the numbers of births in the United Kingdom will continue to fall during the first few years after 2000, before rising slightly.[34]

THE INCIDENCE OF PRETERM BIRTH AND LOW BIRTHWEIGHT

In the UK there are at present few routinely collected data about gestational age, except in Scotland.[69,87] In England, gestational age is one of the items included in the Körner maternity minimum dataset, so data should be available on a national basis, but for reasons described earlier they are incomplete and of poor quality.

In England and Wales, birthweight data have been collected since the mid-1950s through the birth notification system. From 1953 to 1973, each local authority, and from 1974 to 1986 each health authority, submitted a form to central government giving the numbers of low-weight births to women living in their area. Data from this source have been used in Figure 1.3, which shows that the percentage of liveborn babies weighing 2500 g and below remained at a similar level between 6% and 7% from the mid-1950s to the mid-1980s; 2500 g or less was the original definition of 'low birthweight'. The definition was changed in the ninth revision of the International Classification of Diseases[143] to 'under 2500 g'. Babies weighing under 1500 g at birth are now categorized as 'very low birthweight', and those weighing under 1000 g are described as 'extremely low birthweight'.[144]

These birthweight groups are used in Table 1.3, which shows recent trends in the incidence of low birthweight in England and Wales. Although the percentage of liveborn babies weighing under 2500 g has fluctuated since 1983, the general trend was upwards. There was a continuing increase in all groups of babies weighing under 2000 g. Between 1983 and 1988 there was no clear trend in the very small proportion of liveborn babies for whom birthweight was missing, and who are known to include a high proportion of small and immature babies.[4] In the middle of 1989, financial constraints in the OPCS led to a decline in the completeness of recording of birthweight on birth registration records. Birthweight was missing on up to 4% of records from 1989 to 1994, making the data for these years difficult to interpret. As shown later in Table 1.12, the mortality rate among babies with missing birthweights was well above the overall rate, suggesting that the group included a relatively high proportion of low-birthweight babies. By 1995, the numbers of missing birthweights had declined markedly and the data for 1995 onwards used in Tables 1.3, 1.4, 1.5 and 1.7 are much more reliable than those for the preceding years.

The reported incidence of low-weight births rose markedly in the mid-1990s, as Figure 1.3 shows. Analyses of birthweight data for both England and Wales and Scotland identified two separate trends, however. Although the percentages of low-weight births had increased, there had also been an increase in the proportion of heavier babies.[121]

An increase in the recording of very preterm births in Scotland can be seen in Figure 1.4, which is derived from information in the SMR2 system. This shows an increase since 1980 in the small proportion of births which occurred at 20–27 weeks of gestation, from around 0.25% of all live births in 1980 to around 0.30% in more recent years.[70] Earlier data had suggested a more extensive rise between 1975 and 1980, but the quality of the data for the 1970s has now been called into question.

The data for both England and Wales and Scotland suggest that there has been an increase in the reported incidence of very small and very preterm babies. It has been suggested that this is happening as a result of an increasing tendency to admit smaller and iller babies to neonatal nurseries. Although by law all live births should

Table 1.3 Low birthweight live births, England and Wales, 1983–95

Year	Total live births	Live births with stated birthweight	Percentage of live births with stated birthweight				
			Less than 1000 g	Less than 1500 g	1500–1999 g	2000–2499 g	Under 2500 g
1983	629 134	628 269	0.27	0.84	1.26	4.60	6.70
1984	636 818	636 006	0.29	0.87	1.28	4.55	6.70
1985	656 417	655 549	0.29	0.90	1.30	4.61	6.81
1986	661 018	660 394	0.31	0.92	1.35	4.66	6.92
1987	681 511	681 009	0.31	0.96	1.33	4.55	6.83
1988	693 577	692 746	0.32	0.94	1.30	4.36	6.59
1989	687 725	666 612	0.37	0.98	1.32	4.45	6.74
1990	706 140	678 374	0.34	0.96	1.32	4.51	6.79
1991	699 217	673 299	0.34	0.96	1.36	4.57	6.89
1992	689 656	663 689	0.36	1.00	1.30	4.51	6.82
1993	674 467	651 166	0.40	1.03	1.40	4.42	6.85
1994	664 726	646 914	0.44	1.12	1.41	4.44	6.98
1995	648 138	645 641	0.44	1.17	1.50	4.65	7.33
1996	649 485	647 948	0.49	1.22	1.45	4.61	7.28

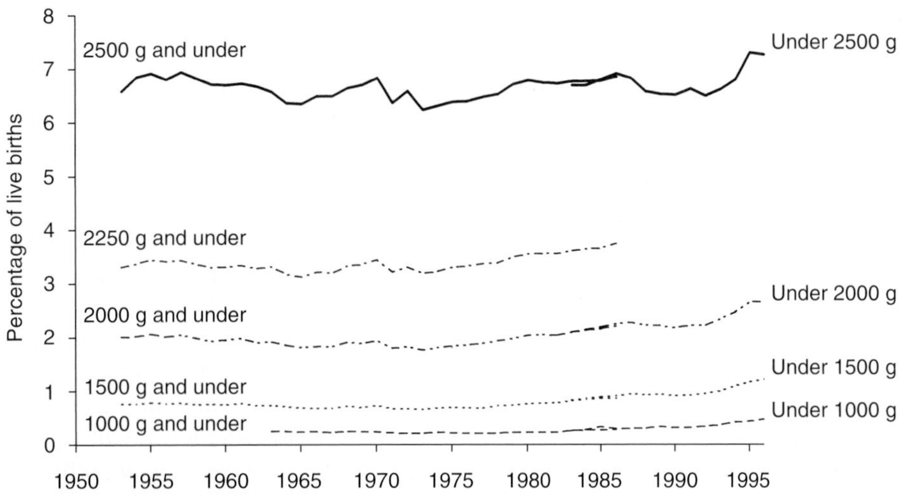

Fig. 1.3 Incidence of low birthweight, England and Wales 1953–96. (Source: LHS 27/1 low birthweight returns, 1955–86, and ONS Mortality Statistics, Series DH3 1983–1996. As these systems use different definitions these data are not continuous.)

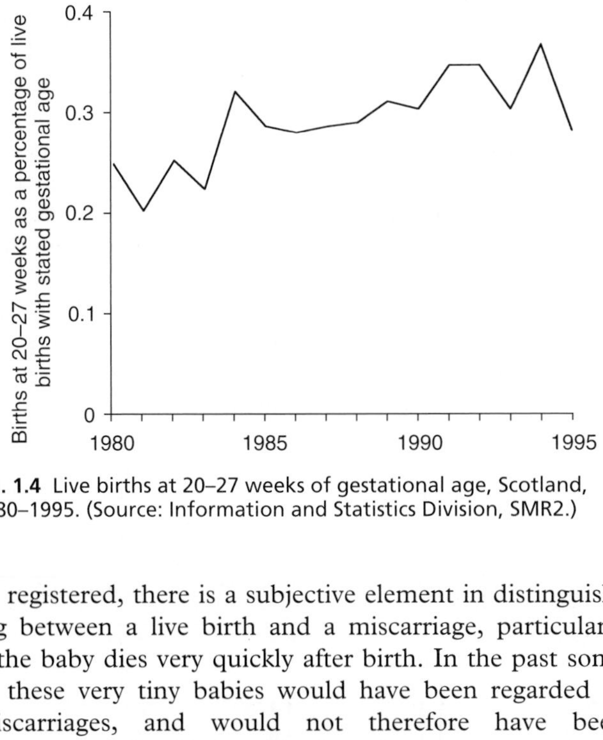

Fig. 1.4 Live births at 20–27 weeks of gestational age, Scotland, 1980–1995. (Source: Information and Statistics Division, SMR2.)

be registered, there is a subjective element in distinguishing between a live birth and a miscarriage, particularly if the baby dies very quickly after birth. In the past some of these very tiny babies would have been regarded as miscarriages, and would not therefore have been registered as live births. The lowering of the gestational age limit for registering fetal deaths as stillbirths in all countries of the United Kingdom in October 1992 may well have reinforced changes in people's perceptions of which events should be registered as live births. Another factor which may have contributed to the increase in registration is the growing recognition of parents' need to mourn an unsuccessful outcome of pregnancy (Chapter 6). The formalities of registration can sometimes form part of this, together with the process of holding a funeral.

The incidence of low birthweight varies between different geographical areas and different sectors of the population. Considerable differences were seen in the late 1980s between the countries and parts of countries which took part in the International Collaborative Effort on birthweight, plurality and perinatal and infant mortality.[59] This shows that Norway and Sweden had a much lower incidence of low birthweight than the other countries, whereas England and Wales, Scotland, Israel and the six states of the USA that took part in the study were among the places with the highest reported incidence.

Similar differences can be seen in the incidences of low birthweight in 1990 in European countries for which data are available. The data shown in Figure 1.5 are taken from a European study which used data collected routinely through the countries' vital statistics systems or medical birth registers.[90]

Although the overall incidence of low birthweight in a population tends to be a reflection of the health of that population in general, and of women of child-bearing age in particular, at the bottom end of the birthweight range it is affected by the country's criteria for birth registration.

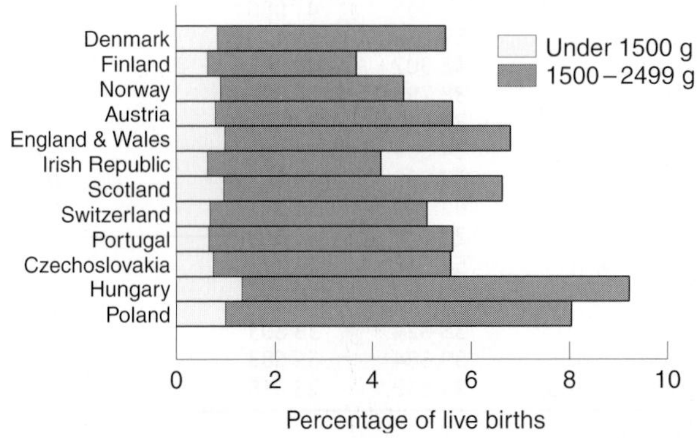

Fig. 1.5 Low birthweight among live births in selected European countries, 1990 (Source: Masuy-Stroobant[90])

In theory this should not affect live births, as in most countries a live birth is registrable regardless of gestational age or birthweight. There are, however, considerable variations in the criteria for the registration of late fetal deaths as stillbirths. This ranges from 12 weeks of gestational age in Japan to 24 weeks in the countries of the United Kingdom, to 28 weeks in many other European countries.[55,59] In the USA each state has its own registration system, and most use a gestational age of 20 weeks as a criterion for registering fetal deaths.[2]

Inevitably, these wide differences in the gestational age at which fetal deaths are registrable as stillbirths affect decisions about whether a very preterm birth should be regarded as a registrable live birth or as a miscarriage, although the extent to which they do so appears to vary from country to country. Thus, although in the years 1982–84 only 0.01% of live births registered in Norway weighed under 500 g, 0.14% of the births in the six US states were in this category.

A further factor which has to be taken into account is the extent to which data about gestational age and birthweight are missing, either because the information was not recorded initially, or because it was not passed on to population-based data collection systems. This is likely to have affected the trends shown in Figures 1.3 and 1.4, as well as comparisons between countries. Furthermore, where data are almost complete, birthweight is most likely to go unrecorded for babies who die very soon after birth.

Real differences in the low-birthweight rates within countries with the same or similar data collection systems are shown in Table 1.4. In 1995, the incidence of low-weight births in the former NHS regions of England ranged from 6.6% in the Oxford region to 8.0% in the West Midlands and North Western regions. Each of these regions includes a variety of different populations, and the differences between districts in the incidence of low birthweight are wider still. The Wessex and Oxford regions had the lowest reported incidence of very low-weight births, with 1.02% weighing under 1500 g, compared to 1.31% in the West Midlands region. Even though these make up a tiny proportion of all births, they make a considerable contribution to mortality rates. Comparing the countries of the UK, the incidences of low-weight and very low-weight births in Wales are slightly lower than those in England, and those for Scotland and Northern Ireland appear to be lower still.

Differences between geographical areas reflect, in their turn, differences in the characteristics of the populations and differences between groups within the population in the incidence of low birthweight. Table 1.5 shows differences in the incidence of low birthweight when live births are tabulated by the father's social class. The data are restricted to singleton births because the birthweight distribution for multiple births is different. For babies in each group, and for all birthweights under 2500 g combined, the table shows a clear gradient, with low birthweight being twice as common among babies with fathers in unskilled occupations than among those with fathers in professional occupations. Although since 1986 mothers have had the option of recording their occupation on their baby's birth certificate, legislation which would create a specific space for it has yet to be passed.[110] These data are as yet incomplete, so tabulations by mother's social class are not routinely published.

In Scotland, an analysis of births in the years 1980–84

Table 1.4 Incidence of low-weight live births in the former NHS regions of England and the other countries of the United Kingdom, 1995

Country or region	Number	Number with stated birthweight	Percentage weighing				
			Under 1000 g	1000–1499 g	1500–1999 g	2000–2499 g	Under 2500 g
Northern	34 103	34 071	0.39	0.75	1.5	4.9	7.5
Yorkshire	46 750	46 642	0.50	0.74	1.6	5.3	7.8
Trent	57 727	57 518	0.42	0.70	1.5	4.7	7.4
East Anglian	32 636	32 612	0.42	0.63	1.5	4.3	6.9
N W Thames	41 235	41 086	0.51	0.76	1.5	4.8	7.6
N E Thames	55 273	55 110	0.47	0.72	1.3	4.9	7.3
S E Thames	48 902	48 405	0.50	0.77	1.6	4.4	7.3
S W Thames	38 792	38 520	0.46	0.70	1.5	4.1	6.7
Wessex	37 510	37 451	0.34	0.68	1.4	4.2	6.7
Oxford	34 001	33 784	0.40	0.62	1.3	4.3	6.6
South Western	37 965	37 885	0.44	0.70	1.4	4.2	6.7
West Midlands	67 100	66 971	0.50	0.81	1.7	5.5	8.0
Mersey	28 645	28 548	0.40	0.82	1.4	4.3	7.0
North Western	52 618	52 335	0.42	0.72	1.6	5.3	8.0
England	613 257	610 938	0.45	0.73	1.5	4.7	7.3
Wales	38 824	38 803	0.39	0.74	1.5	4.3	7.0
Scotland	59 684	59 683	0.30	0.67	1.4	4.5	6.9
Northern Ireland	23 819	23 818	0.47	0.61	1.1	3.5	5.7

Source: ONS
Information and Statistics Division, Scottish Health Statistics
Health and Personal Social Services Statistics for Northern Ireland

Table 1.5 Low birthweight by social class of father for live singleton births, England and Wales, 1995

	Percentage weighing				
	Under 1000 g	1000–1499 g	1500–1999 g	2000–2499 g	Under 2500 g
Social class of father					
I Professional	0.23	0.39	0.71	2.56	3.88
II Managerial and technical	0.26	0.44	0.82	3.01	4.53
IIIn Skilled non-manual	0.32	0.61	1.02	3.52	5.47
IIIm Skilled manual	0.34	0.62	1.17	4.03	6.16
IV Partly skilled	0.46	0.62	1.26	4.72	7.06
V Unskilled	0.48	0.81	1.50	4.75	7.55
Other and not stated	0.43	0.52	1.44	4.65	7.04
Lone mother	0.45	0.85	1.68	5.52	8.50
Total	0.35	0.56	1.12	3.95	5.98

Source: ONS

showed a clear social class gradient in the incidence of preterm births at 20–27, 28–31 and 32–36 weeks.[68,83,87] In this case, the gestational ages of babies born within marriage were tabulated according to their father's social class, and births outside marriage were grouped into a single category. The data for 1990–95, shown in Table 1.6, were analysed in a different way and do not show such a clear gradient. By this time the proportion of births outside marriage had increased and the babies concerned were tabulated by their mother's social class. Women's occupations have a different distribution from those of men, with many being classified as IIIn, skilled non-manual, and they have a different association with mortality and morbidity. It is therefore difficult to interpret the data in Table 1.6 without a fuller analysis that tabulates births inside and outside marriage separately.

Birthweight distributions are known to differ between ethnic and racial groups.[88,116,123] At the time of writing ethnic origin is not recorded at birth registration, but it should be recorded in national NHS data collection systems. Although it has been recorded on most hospital notes and on some districts' birth notification forms for some years, the way it was recorded and classified varied widely. Now the definitions used in the 1991 census should be used universally.[100,101]

For the first time ever, in the population census that took place on 21 April 1991 people were asked to indicate how they described their ethnic origin. The categories used in the question were: White, Black-Caribbean, Black-African, Black-Other, Indian, Pakistani, Bangladeshi, Chinese, and any other ethnic group. People descended from more than one ethnic or racial group were asked to tick the one to which they considered they belonged, or to tick the 'Any other ethnic group' box and describe their ancestry.[111] This classification has been criticized on the grounds that it is more an indicator of skin colour than of cultural and social identity.[1] The Office for National Statistics has now published a series of books analysing the data collected through this question.[29]

In the case of data collected at birth and death registration, the closest approximation to ethnic origin is country of birth. This is increasingly unsatisfactory as a measure of ethnic origin, as many women in some ethnic groups having babies in the UK today were themselves born in the UK. Country of birth is more useful as an approximate measure of immigrant status.

Despite this, Table 1.7 gives some insight into the differences in the incidence of low birthweight in 1995. It was highest among babies with mothers from the 'New Commonwealth' countries of the Indian subcontinent and the Caribbean, and lowest among those with mothers from the 'Old Commonwealth' countries of Australia,

Table 1.6 Preterm births by social class for live singleton births, Scotland, 1990–95

Social class of father or mother	Total	Total with stated gestational age	Percentage born at each gestational age		
			20–27 weeks	28–31 weeks	32–36 weeks
I Professional	25 254	25 209	0.13	0.42	3.54
II Managerial and technical	70 721	70 546	0.20	0.49	3.97
IIIn Skilled non-manual	84 880	84 572	0.24	0.65	4.63
IIIm Skilled manual	50 454	50 265	0.25	0.59	4.87
IV Partly skilled	66 044	65 746	0.31	0.65	4.92
V Unskilled	30 482	30 350	0.24	0.71	4.88
Inadequate description	3 828	3 821	0.31	0.73	5.16
Not stated	39 979	39 834	1.15	1.74	7.03
Total	371 642	370 343	0.34	0.72	4.80

Source: Information and Statistics Division

Table 1.7 Low birthweight by mother's country of birth, 1995

Mother's country of birth	Live births		Percentage of stated birthweights				
	Total	Number with stated birthweight	Under 1000 g	1000–1499 g	1500–1999 g	2000–2500 g	Under 2500 g
All countries	648 001	645 784	0.45	0.73	1.50	4.66	7.33
United Kingdom	566 331	564 510	0.43	0.72	1.49	4.52	7.16
Irish Republic	5 166	5 145	0.47	0.76	1.55	4.28	7.06
Elsewhere in the European Union	8 026	7 993	0.33	0.53	1.08	4.22	6.14
Australia, Canada and New Zealand	3 052	3 037	0.36*	0.59*	0.99	3.06	5.00
'New Commonwealth'	47 337	47 117	0.68	0.90	1.87	6.79	10.25
Bangladesh	6 783	6 756	0.28	0.67	1.79	8.30	11.04
India	6 679	6 661	0.57	0.89	2.04	7.73	11.23
Pakistan	12 332	12 294	0.66	0.76	1.94	7.05	10.40
East Africa	5 122	5 102	0.67	0.96	2.27	8.31	12.21
Caribbean	2 910	2 890	1.42	1.63	2.28	6.33	11.66
Other and not stated	18 089	17 982	0.47	0.60	0.96	3.97	5.99

*Based on fewer than 20 births
Source: ONS

Canada and New Zealand, which in the past largely drew their immigrants from white European populations.

The highest rates were among babies of women from East Africa, a high proportion of whom are of Asian origin but were born in Kenya and Uganda. Although babies born to women from Bangladesh and Pakistan had similar incidences of birthweights under 2500 g, this was not the case for birthweights under 2000 g. These accounted for 3.4% of births to women from Pakistan, compared to only 2.7% of births to women from Bangladesh.

These data illustrate the considerable differences that exist between groups within the population in the incidence of low birthweight. The association between these and differences in mortality and morbidity will be discussed later, but it is important to remember when interpreting the data that being classified as low birthweight does not necessarily imply that the baby had clinical problems, particularly at the upper end of the low-birthweight range. On the other hand, the smaller the baby and the shorter its gestational age, the higher the risk of morbidity.

MULTIPLE BIRTHS

In England and Wales, multiple births account for just over a fifth of liveborn babies weighing under 1500 g, as Table 1.8 shows. After declining for many years, from the mid-1970s onwards, the incidence of multiple births, shown in Figure 1.6, started to increase. The increase continued through the 1980s, from 10.1 multiple births per 1000 maternities in 1982 to 11.4 in 1989 and 14.1 in 1995, with a slight drop to 13.8 in 1996. There are no data about multiple birth rates for England and Wales for 1981, as multiplicity was not recorded during this year because of industrial action by local registrars of births and deaths.

Table 1.8 Multiple births as a percentage of all births occurring in 1994, England and Wales

Birthweight (g)	Multiple births as a percentage of		
	Stillbirths	Live births	Infant deaths
Under 1500	13.7	22.3	23.2
1500–1999	10.1	26.2	13.0
2000–2499	8.9	17.0	11.0
2500 and over	2.1	1.3	3.3
All weights	9.1	2.6	13.7

Source: ONS

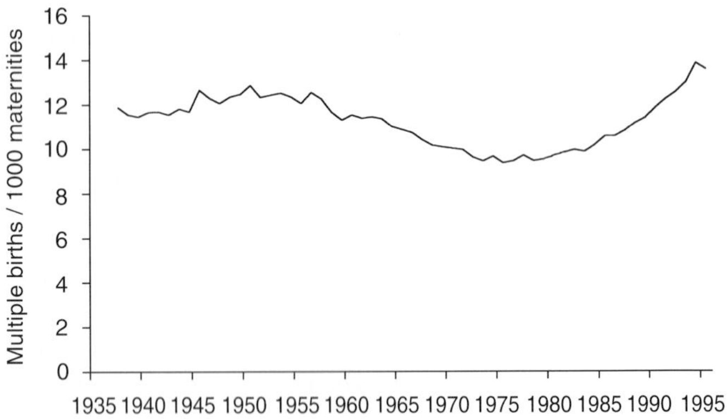

Fig. 1.6 Multiple birth rates, England and Wales, 1938–1996. (Source: ONS, Birth Statistics, Series FM1.)

Multiple birth rates for England and Wales are compared with those for Scotland and Ireland in Table 1.9. Trends in Scotland are similar to those for England and Wales, although rates are slightly lower. In Northern Ireland the twinning rate was already higher and did not

Table 1.9 Multiple birth rates, England and Wales, Scotland and Ireland

	England and Wales	Scotland	Northern Ireland	Irish Republic
Twins per 1000 maternities				
1971–75	9.9	10.0	10.7	12.3
1976–80	9.6	9.4	10.1	11.2
1981–85	10.1*	9.9	10.6	10.7
1986–90	10.9	11.0	10.7	11.2+
1991–95	12.6	12.3	12.2	11.9+
Triplet and higher-order births per 1000 maternities				
1971–75	0.11	0.08	0.08	0.12
1976–80	0.13	0.09	0.14	0.13
1981–85	0.14*	0.10	0.12	0.11
1986–90	0.25	0.19	0.14	0.14+
1991–95	0.37	0.31	0.31	0.26+

* Excluding 1981
\+ Provisional

Source: ONS
General Register Offices for Scotland and Northern Ireland
Central Statistics Office, Ireland

increase in the latter half of the 1980s, but rose considerably in the early 1990s. The statistics for the Irish Republic are not strictly comparable as they are based only on live births. The published rates increased steadily in the late 1980s and early 1990s.

The triplet and higher-order birth rates for England and Wales, shown in Figure 1.7, present a rather more dramatic picture than that for multiple births as a whole. After rising slightly during the 1970s, the proportion of triplet and higher-order births more than doubled during the 1980s, rising from 12 per 100 000 maternities in 1982 to 28 in 1989. After a slight pause it rose again sharply to 45.0 in 1995, before dropping slightly to 41.5 in 1996. Rates for Scotland, shown in Table 1.9, followed the same pattern but at a lower level. In Northern Ireland the rate rose in the late 1970s and then remained fairly level, before rising considerably in the 1990s, whereas in the Irish Republic there were signs of a slight rise in the latter half of the 1980s and a bigger rise in the early 1990s.

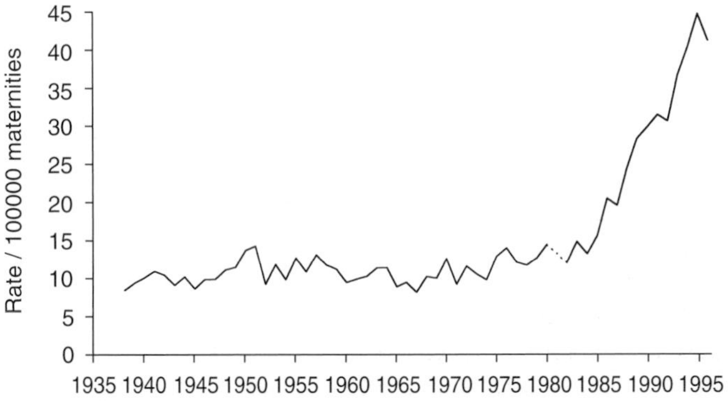

Fig. 1.7 Triplet and higher-order births, England and Wales, 1938–1996. (Source: ONS, Birth Statistics, Series FM1.)

Table 1.10 Incidence of triplet and higher-order deliveries in Europe, rates per 100 000 maternities, 1960–90

Country	1960	1965	1970	1975	1980	1985	1990
Denmark	10.5	14.4	9.9	20.9	10.5	13.1	28.7
Finland	6.1	15.4	17.1	13.8	16.0	22.5	38.4
Norway	12.9	15.1	9.3	5.3	7.9	17.7	38.1
Sweden	3.9	12.8	6.4	7.7	10.4	8.2	27.1
Austria	9.5	6.1	7.1	8.5	8.8	24.9	18.9
Belgium	5.0	10.9	8.4	10.0	16.9	24.7	57.9
England-Wales	9.7	9.1	12.9	13.5	15.0	16.5	30.6
France	9.4	8.2	9.5	12.6	18.8	24.6	43.3
F.R. Germany[3]	9.3	9.3	10.4	10.2	13.1	23.1	34.1
Ireland	–	–	–	–	16.2	11.2	15.2
Netherlands	10.4	8.1	7.5	15.8	13.8	17.8	60.1
Northern Ireland	9.5	8.8	6.2	0.0	14.0	10.9	19.0
Scotland	15.6	13.2	10.3	4.4	5.8	13.6	26.4
Switzerland[1]	13.1	9.8	10.1	14.9	23.2	35.5	37.2
Greece	14.6	11.8	12.4	14.7	8.1	–	–
Italy	12.1	9.8	10.4	7.1	13.3	15.3	37.8
Portugal	16.0	12.6	12.5	8.8	10.1	11.5	18.1
Spain	8.3	8.4	8.9	10.0	10.9	11.6	22.8
Bulgaria[2]	5.7	3.2	4.3	6.9	7.0	4.7	11.4
Czechoslovakia	5.5	7.4	10.5	9.4	9.7	10.7	11.5
D.R. Germany	7.5	8.5	8.4	6.1	9.0	11.3	–
Hungary	12.9	11.3	11.2	8.8	14.2	21.6	23.2
Poland	11.3	8.8	7.3	6.0	5.6	7.4	9.6

Source: Vital Registration data published in *Santé et mortalité en Europe*[90]

Notes:
[1]1961 instead of 1960
[2]1986 instead of 1985
[3]1989 instead of 1990
– not available

The rising triplet rate is a common feature in most European countries, as Table 1.10 shows. By 1990, the rates in Belgium and the Netherlands were the highest in Europe, followed by those in West Germany, Italy and France.[90] Despite its reputation for high rates of triplet and higher-order births, Australia's rate for 1994, 35.0 per 100 000 maternities, was no higher than some of these.[35]

The rise in the incidence of multiple births in general, and triplet and higher-order births in particular, is usually attributed to the increasing use of drugs for the medical management of subfertility and, since the mid-1980s, to techniques for assisted conception. The National Study of Triplet and Higher-Order Births estimated that 36% of mothers of triplets and 70% of mothers of quadruplet and higher-order births born in the years 1980 and 1982–85 had used drugs for the medical management of subfertility.[15]

The impact of IVF was negligible before 1985, but since then it has been considerable. Statistics produced by the Human Fertilization and Embryology Authority,[66] and its predecessor the Interim Licensing Authority for Human In Vitro Fertilization and Embryology,[71] show a clear association between the rise in triplet and higher-order births from 1985 onwards and the increasing use of IVF, gamete intrafallopian transfers and associated procedures. Research commissioned by the Medical Research Council[93] confirmed that multiple births often result from these procedures, as did a survey of triplet and higher-order births undertaken by the BAPM in 1989.[81] A more recent analysis of data for England and Wales showed rising rates of multiple births on the one hand and of assisted conception and prescriptions for drugs for the medical management of subfertility, but was unable to quantify the association as it was based solely on routinely collected data.[42] In Australia and New Zealand, twins occurred in 22.3% of GIFT pregnancies and 16.8% of IVF pregnancies in 1994, compared to only 1.36% of all pregnancies in Australia in 1994.[35,79]

MORTALITY IN THE FIRST YEAR OF LIFE

TRENDS IN MORTALITY RATES

The classic indicators of the outcome of pregnancy are stillbirth rates and death rates during the first year of life. These are defined in Figure 1.8. Trends since 1905 in neonatal and postneonatal mortality rates for England and Wales are illustrated in Figure 1.9. Although the series of infant mortality rates reaches back to the mid-19th century, the current subdivision of the first year of life into the first month and deaths at ages of at least 1 month but under a year, started in 1905. The publication of more detailed analyses started at a time when public concern about infant mortality, stemming from the unfitness of many potential recruits for the Boer War, led to a request to the General Register Office for more detailed statistics.[134]

Whereas neonatal mortality rates have decreased relatively steadily during the 20th century, postneonatal mortality, which was initially higher, shows a different pattern. It decreased very rapidly in the first half of the century with the decline in fatality from communicable diseases. It showed signs of levelling off between the mid-1970s and mid-1980s. After virtually halving in the late 1980s and early 1990s, the rate has levelled off again, accounting for under a half of infant deaths, as Figure 1.10 shows.

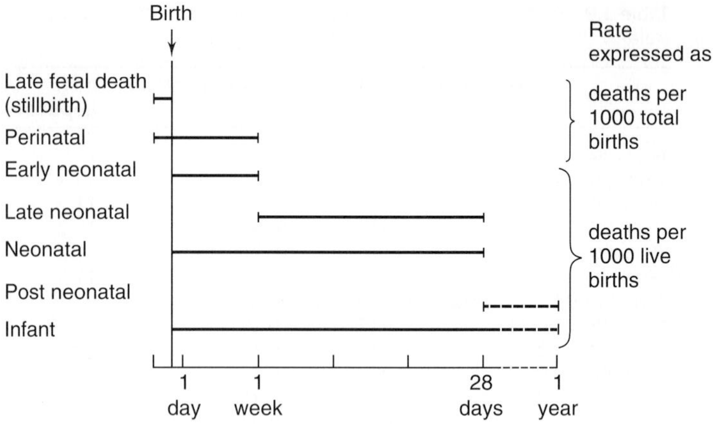

Fig. 1.8 Definitions of stillbirth and infant mortality rates.

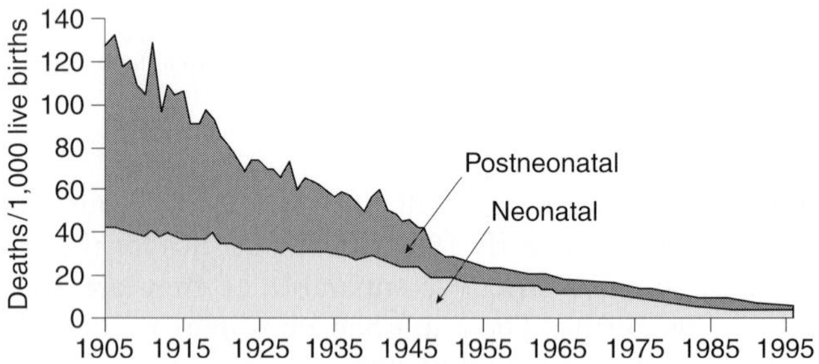

Fig. 1.9 Infant mortality, England and Wales, 1905–1996. (Source: ONS, Mortality Statistics, Series DH3.[107])

More recent trends in infant mortality are shown in Figure 1.11, which shows early and late neonatal mortality rates separately. The impact of the change in legislation about stillbirth registration on published stillbirth and perinatal mortality rates is illustrated in Figure 1.12. The published rates, shown with a dotted line from 1992 onwards, showed an apparent increase. Rates from which stillbirths at 24–27 weeks of gestation have been excluded are shown as a continuation of the solid line, and show an apparent halt in the downward trend seen in previous years.

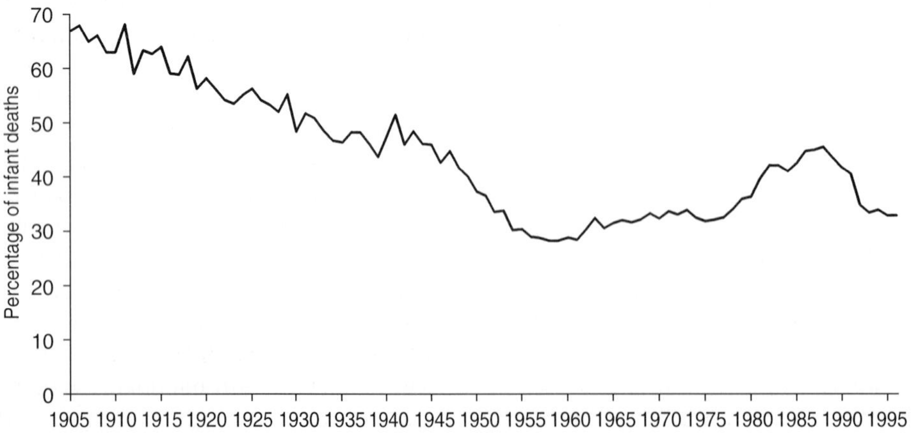

Fig. 1.10 Postneonatal mortality as a percentage of infant deaths England and Wales, 1905–1996. (Source: ONS, Mortality Statistics, Series DH3.)

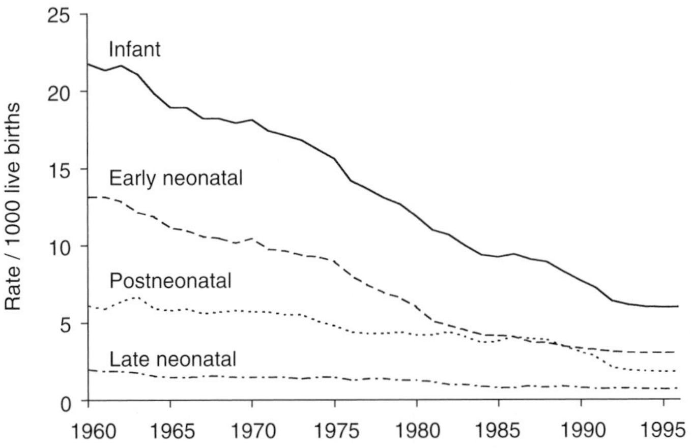

Fig. 1.11 Infant mortality rates, England and Wales, 1960–1996. (Source: ONS, Mortality Statistics, Series DH3.)

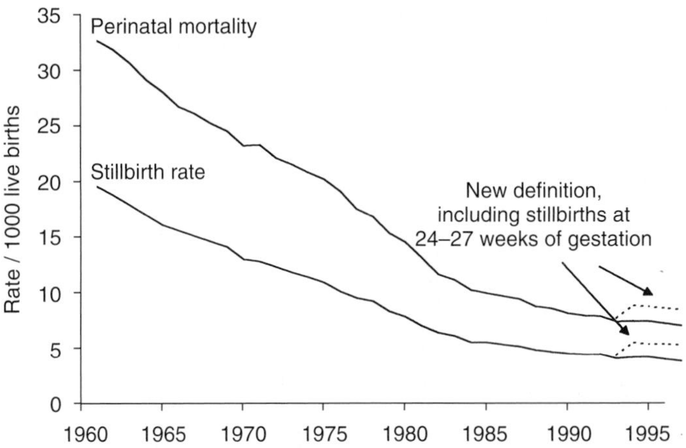

Fig. 1.12 Stillbirths and perinatal mortality rates, England and Wales, 1960–1996. (Source: ONS, Mortality Statistics, Series DH3.)

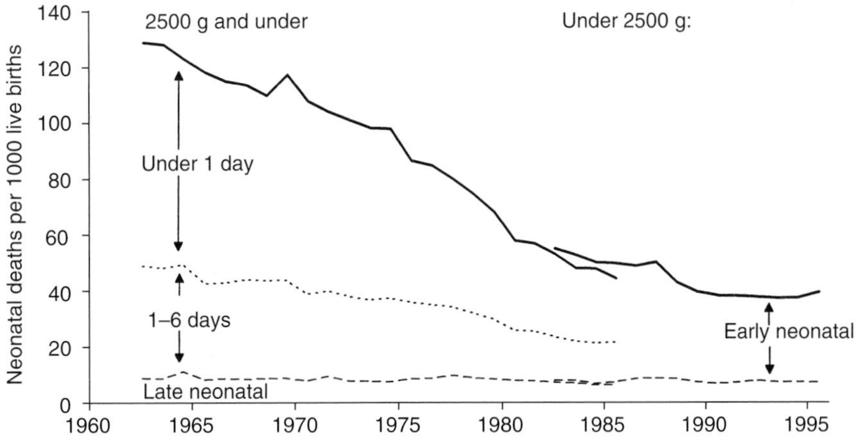

Fig. 1.13 Neonatal mortality among low-birthweight babies, England and Wales, 1963–1996. (Source: LHS 27/1 low birthweight returns 1955–1986, and ONS Mortality Statistics, Series DH3 1983–1996. These systems use different definitions, hence the breaks in the lines.)

Neonatal, postneonatal and infant mortality rates for England, Wales, Scotland and Ireland in the years since 1970 are shown in Table 1.11. These show continuing declines in neonatal mortality until the mid-1990s. As in England and Wales, there was a tendency for the postneonatal mortality rate to level off in the 1980s in each of the other countries, followed by a fall in the late 1980s and early 1990s. The trends in Scotland, Wales and both parts of Ireland are less clear than those in England and Wales, as they are based on smaller numbers of deaths. Similar trends were seen in the regions of England[88,89,119] and in other developed countries.[90] As a whole, however, infant mortality continues to decline in most countries, although it shows some signs of levelling off in the countries with the lowest rates, notably the Scandinavian countries, the Netherlands and Switzerland.

To what extent do trends in infant mortality in the UK reflect changes in the relative size of high-risk groups, and to what extent has mortality fallen within these groups? Figure 1.3 shows no increase in the incidence of low birthweight in England and Wales between the mid-1950s and mid-1980s but a rise in more recent years. Table 1.3 shows a similar picture, but with an increase in the reported incidence of babies in the lowest birthweight groups, who have the highest mortality. It has been suggested that the change in definition of stillbirth may have increased the tendency to register very preterm live births, rather than regarding them as miscarriages. Within birthweight groups, however, trends in mortality look different. A very marked fall between 1963 and 1986 in mortality in the first week after live birth among babies weighing 2500 g and under, followed by a further fall in the late 1980s, can be seen in Figure 1.13. A different pattern can be seen in Figure 1.14, which shows a more recent and very marked decline from the late 1970s onwards in mortality rates among babies weighing 1000 g and under, and subsequently among babies weighing under 1000 g.

The fuller data in Table 1.12 show that neonatal mortality continued to fall in England and Wales from

Table 1.11 Neonatal, postneonatal and infant mortality rates since 1970, England and Wales, Scotland and Ireland

	England	Wales	England and Wales	Scotland	Northern Ireland	Irish Republic
Neonatal mortality						
1970	12.3	12.8	12.3	12.8	15.8	12.8
1975	10.7	10.3	10.7	11.8	13.2	12.0
1980	7.6	7.9	7.7	7.8	8.0	6.7
1985	5.3	5.8	5.4	5.5	5.6	5.3
1986	5.2	5.0	5.3	5.2	6.0	5.0
1987	5.0	5.0	5.1	4.7	4.8	4.3
1988	4.9	4.7	4.9	4.5	5.4	5.3
1989	4.7	4.7	4.8	4.7	4.0	4.8
1990	4.6	3.9	4.6	4.4	4.0	4.8
1991	4.3	4.1	4.3	4.4	4.6	5.0
1992	4.3	3.8	4.3	4.6	4.1	4.3
1993	4.2	3.4	4.2	4.0	4.9	4.0
1994	4.0	4.1	4.1	4.0	4.2	4.0+
1995	4.2	3.9	4.2	4.0	5.5	4.7+
1996	4.1	3.6	4.1	3.9	3.7	
Postneonatal mortality						
1970	5.9	6.4	5.9	6.9	7.1	6.7
1975	5.3	4.2	5.0	5.4	7.2	5.6
1980	4.4	3.5	4.4	4.3	7.6	3.8
1985	3.9	4.0	4.0	3.9	4.0	3.6
1986	4.2	3.9	4.3	3.6	4.2	3.9
1987	4.0	4.5	4.1	3.8	3.8	3.6
1988	4.1	2.9	4.1	3.7	3.6	3.5
1989	3.7	3.3	3.7	4.0	2.9	3.3
1990	3.3	3.0	3.3	3.3	3.5	3.4
1991	3.0	2.4	3.0	2.7	2.8	2.6
1992	2.2	2.2	2.3	2.2	1.9	2.2
1993	2.1	2.1	2.1	2.5	2.1	2.1
1994	2.0	2.2	2.1	2.2	1.9	2.0+
1995	2.0	2.0	2.0	2.2	1.6	1.7+
1996	2.0	2.0	2.0	2.2	2.0	
Infant mortality						
1970	18.2	18.7	18.2	19.6	22.9	19.5
1975	15.7	14.5	15.7	17.2	20.4	17.5
1980	12.0	11.4	12.0	12.1	15.6	10.3
1985	9.2	9.8	9.4	9.4	9.6	8.8
1986	9.5	9.5	9.6	8.8	10.2	8.9
1987	9.1	9.5	9.2	8.5	8.7	7.9
1988	9.1	7.6	9.0	8.2	8.9	8.9
1989	8.4	8.0	8.4	8.7	6.9	8.1
1990	7.9	6.6	7.9	7.7	7.4	8.2
1991	7.3	6.6	7.4	7.1	7.4	7.6
1992	6.5	6.0	6.6	6.8	6.0	6.5
1993	6.3	5.5	6.3	6.5	7.1	6.1
1994	6.1	6.1	6.2	6.2	6.1	6.0
1995	6.1	5.8	6.1	6.2	7.1	6.4+
1996	6.1	5.6	6.1	6.2	5.8	

Source: ONS, General Register Offices for Scotland and Northern Ireland and Central Statistics Office, Ireland

the mid-1980s until the early 1990s, but from 1990 onwards the decline appeared to be confined to babies weighing under 2000 g. Trends for the larger babies are far from clear. Table 1.12 also illustrates the impact of the increase in 1989 of the numbers of birth records with missing birthweights. Between 1983 and 1988, when very few birthweights were missing, mortality in this group was very high, suggesting that the babies might not have been weighed because they were very ill or immature. Between 1989 and 1994 mortality in this group was lower than before, but still markedly higher than average. Thus, mortality in the groups under 2500 g is likely to have been artificially depleted over this period. In 1995, when the proportion of babies with missing birthweights was very much smaller, mortality among them rose, but not to its former level. This means that caution is needed when interpreting the trends in mortality among low-birthweight babies in the late 1980s and early 1990s, shown in Figures 1.13 and 1.14 and Table 1.12.

Table 1.13 shows neonatal mortality rates by birthweight for Scotland over the years 1984–95; these are tabulated by gestational age in Table 1.14. Neonatal

Table 1.12 Neonatal, postneonatal and infant mortality rates by birthweight, England and Wales, 1983–95

	Birthweight (g)							
	Under 1000	1000–1499	1500–1999	2000–2499	Under 2500	2500 and over	Not stated	All weights
Neonatal mortality								
1983	565.5	166.6	46.6	13.3	55.2	2.0	205.8	5.8
1984	539.0	146.5	44.3	12.0	52.9	1.9	204.4	5.5
1985	524.4	135.8	37.8	12.3	50.2	1.8	156.7	5.3
1986	514.3	132.7	40.1	10.7	49.9	1.7	163.5	5.2
1987	502.1	137.3	36.1	8.9	49.0	1.6	223.1	5.0
1988	506.1	134.4	34.6	9.6	50.3	1.5	113.1	4.9
1989	412.6	111.5	29.1	7.4	43.1	1.4	18.3	4.7
1990	451.2	88.6	25.0	6.5	40.0	1.3	17.4	4.6
1991	446.8	81.8	22.1	6.8	38.4	1.2	19.1	4.3
1992	399.5	80.6	23.7	6.7	37.4	1.2	15.9	4.2
1993	381.7	76.8	24.2	6.4	36.7	1.1	16.7	4.0
1994	367.8	71.6	18.5	5.7	37.6	1.2	19.9	4.1
1995	390.4	64.0	17.3	6.6	37.8	1.4	28.9	4.1
Postneonatal mortality								
1983	53.7	28.7	18.7	8.8	14.2	3.4	54.3	4.2
1984	46.4	31.5	16.6	8.7	13.9	3.1	16.0	3.8
1985	51.0	34.4	17.1	9.1	14.7	3.1	10.4	3.9
1986	59.1	30.4	20.9	9.0	15.4	3.3	17.6	4.2
1987	49.5	27.3	17.2	9.2	14.3	3.2	23.9	4.0
1988	54.8	34.9	18.6	10.3	16.4	3.2	7.2	4.0
1989	57.8	33.8	19.0	8.9	15.8	2.8	2.1	3.6
1990	59.6	28.7	16.0	7.7	13.9	2.4	3.9	3.2
1991	57.8	25.2	14.0	7.5	12.9	2.2	3.8	2.9
1992	71.7	23.4	11.9	6.1	12.2	1.5	2.5	2.2
1993	58.9	22.6	12.4	6.2	11.7	1.4	1.9	2.1
1994	54.3	18.7	9.8	4.5	10.1	1.4	2.2	2.0
1995	58.4	18.5	9.4	4.7	10.3	1.2	8.6	1.9
Infant mortality								
1983	620.2	195.3	65.3	22.1	69.4	5.4	260.1	10.0
1984	585.4	178.0	60.9	20.7	66.8	5.0	220.4	9.3
1985	575.4	170.2	54.8	21.4	64.9	4.9	302.2	9.2
1986	573.4	163.1	61.0	19.7	65.3	5.1	181.1	9.4
1987	551.6	164.6	53.3	18.1	63.3	4.9	247.0	9.0
1988	560.9	169.2	53.2	19.9	66.7	4.7	120.3	9.0
1989	470.5	145.3	48.2	16.3	58.9	4.2	20.4	8.3
1990	510.8	117.3	41.0	14.3	53.8	3.8	21.3	7.7
1991	504.6	107.0	36.0	14.3	51.3	3.3	22.8	7.2
1992	471.2	104.0	35.7	12.8	49.6	2.7	18.3	6.4
1993	440.6	99.3	36.6	12.5	48.4	2.5	18.6	6.2
1994	422.1	90.3	28.3	10.1	47.7	2.5	22.0	6.1
1995	448.8	82.5	26.7	11.3	48.1	2.6	37.4	6.0

Source: ONS Mortality Statistics, Series DH3
The rates given above for all weights differ slightly from the rates for England and Wales in Table 1.10, which are derived from unlinked data.

Table 1.13 Neonatal mortality rates by birthweight, Scotland, 1984–95

	Birthweight (g)									Total
	Under 1000	1000–1499	1500–1999	2000–2499	2500–2999	3000–3499	3500–3999	4000+	Not known	
1984	553.3	168.7	55.6	14.0	3.7	1.6	1.0	1.6	42.5	6.4
1985	585.6	163.5	48.1	10.0	3.2	1.4	1.0	1.6	19.4	5.5
1986	567.8	134.7	39.9	8.5	2.8	1.4	0.6	1.2	27.4	5.2
1987	578.3	145.0	25.8	10.1	2.7	1.2	0.7	1.4	14.7	4.7
1988	533.7	97.1	28.5	8.9	4.3	1.1	1.2	0.8	31.8	4.5
1989	505.0	139.9	34.3	12.0	2.4	1.2	0.6	0.9	71.8	4.7
1990	526.6	78.7	26.8	10.8	2.3	1.2	0.7	1.2	17.7	4.4
1991	469.8	101.6	21.4	10.0	2.5	1.2	1.1	2.0	8.6	4.4
1992	509.3	81.9	33.1	11.8	2.7	1.4	0.9	1.7	6.0	4.6
1993	386.7	92.8	31.0	7.7	2.9	1.5	0.7	1.1	8.8	4.0
1994	478.3	58.1	18.3	5.6	2.5	1.0	0.6	1.3	5.5	4.0
1995*	546.4	80.2	13.9	10.8	1.9	1.4	0.7	0.9	2.8	3.9

*Provisional

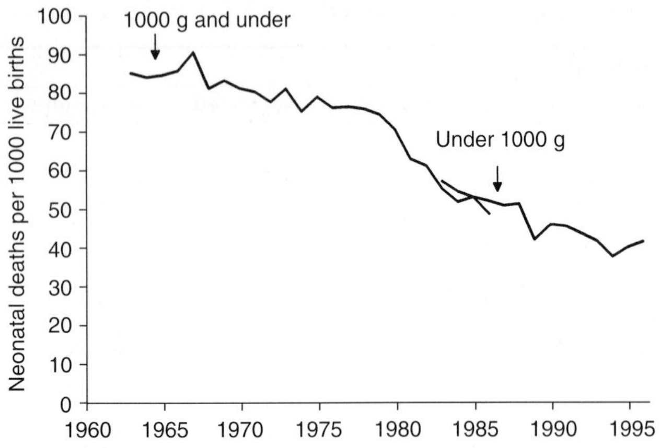

Fig. 1.14 Neonatal mortality among extremely low-birthweight babies, England and Wales, 1963–1996. (Source: LHS 271 low birthweight returns 1955–1986, and ONS Mortality Statistics, Series DH3 1983–1996. These systems use different definitions, hence the break in the lines.)

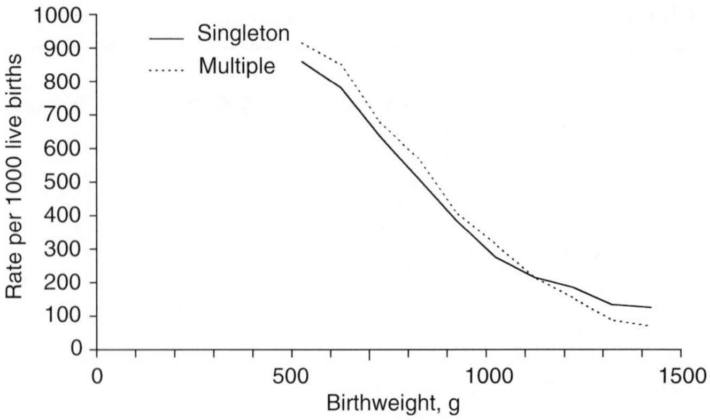

Fig. 1.15 Infant mortality and birthweights under 1500 g, singleton and multiple births, England and Wales, 1983–1987 combined.

mortality rates tended to decline, although there was considerable fluctuation because of the smaller numbers of babies involved. The exception was babies born before 26 weeks of gestational age, suggesting that the numbers of babies in this group may have risen with the increasing inclusion of babies with poor survival prospects.

Postneonatal mortality rates for England and Wales, given in Table 1.12, show no sign of a decline over the years 1983–88, particularly for babies with birthweights under 2500 g. Apart from a possible increase in the 2000–2499 g group, the picture was one of fluctuation, the extent of which is not surprising, given the relatively small numbers of deaths in each group. This was followed by a sharp decline between 1989 and 1992 in all groups, except for babies weighing under 1000 g.

Putting the neonatal and postneonatal mortality rates together to look at infant mortality as a whole, it can be seen that rates tended to decline up until 1985 and then started to level off. After a decline over the period from 1989 to 1993, they appear to be levelling off again.

There are considerable differences between the countries of Europe in their mortality rates for low and very low-birthweight babies. For example, although rates fell during the 1980s in all countries for which birthweight-specific early neonatal mortality rates were available, in 1990 rates for babies born weighing under 1500 g ranged from 175 per 1000 live births in Norway to 297 in Ireland and 398 in Hungary. Although the differences may reflect variations in the criteria for birth registration, the most marked differences are between the countries of eastern and western Europe.[90]

Although it is usual to present birthweight-specific mortality rates in 500 g groups, there is considerable variation within these groups, particularly at the bottom end of the scale. This can be seen in Figure 1.15, which is taken from a special analysis in which infant mortality rates for the years 1983–87 combined were analysed in 100-g groups.[4] It was necessary to combine 5 years' data to have sufficient numbers of deaths in each group to eliminate the effects of random variation. A similar picture emerges if infant mortality is analysed by single weeks of gestational age, with considerable variation before 30 weeks of gestational age.

Table 1.14 Neonatal mortality rates by gestational age, Scotland 1984–95

	Gestational age (weeks)							Total
	Less than 26	26–27	28–31	32–36	37–41	42 or more	Not known	
1984	793.1	472.4	165.6	20.0	2.0	2.2	16.0	6.4
1985	897.1	471.1	133.3	19.0	1.8	1.5	9.3	5.5
1986	763.2	454.5	128.9	15.5	1.7	2.3	9.9	5.2
1987	852.9	392.9	144.7	16.3	1.3	1.3	6.1	4.7
1988	700.0	384.6	89.6	13.9	1.6	1.0	13.4	4.5
1989	910.3	360.4	119.9	12.0	1.4	1.4	19.9	4.7
1990	802.3	283.2	102.3	11.7	1.5	0.8	7.5	4.4
1991	756.1	298.0	92.0	11.4	1.5	0.8	12.3	4.4
1992	666.7	382.8	60.2	14.4	1.7	0.9	4.5	4.6
1993	666.7	243.0	74.9	15.2	1.5	0.3	5.9	4.0
1994	710.5	292.0	59.7	9.1	1.1	3.1	2.7	4.0
1995*	823.5	355.6	63.8	10.5	1.3	0.7	0.0	3.9

*Provisional

Source: Scottish Stillbirth and Neonatal Death Reports, 1988, 1989, 1994 and ISD unpublished data

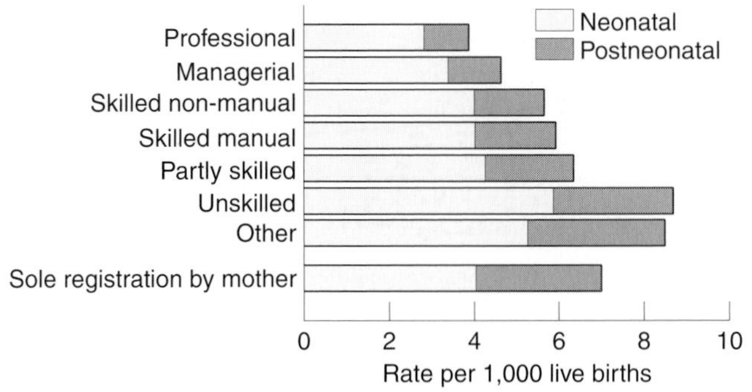

Fig. 1.16 Infant mortality by social class of father, England and Wales, 1996. (Source ONS Monitor DH3 97/3.)

Innumerable studies over the years have shown a social class gradient in stillbirth and infant mortality rates which mirrors the social class gradient in birthweight seen in Table 1.5.[41,86,88,105–109] Neonatal and postneonatal mortality rates for England and Wales, analysed by the social class of the baby's father, are shown in Figure 1.16. The analysis includes both births within marriage and those outside marriage registered jointly by both parents, who account for the majority of the rising proportion of births outside marriage. The very high mortality rates among babies registered by the mother on her own are also shown. The data are from the infant mortality-linked file of ONS.[106]

A notable feature in Figure 1.16 is the difference between neonatal and postneonatal mortality rates, with the latter showing much wider differences between classes. Deaths attributed to the sudden infant death syndrome show particularly marked social class differences, which contribute substantially to the social class differences in postneonatal mortality.[105]

Neonatal and postneonatal mortality rates by mothers' countries of birth are shown in Figure 1.17. The figure also shows that mortality rates for babies whose mothers were born in Pakistan are markedly higher than those with mothers born elsewhere in the Indian subcontinent, which are much closer to the overall level. Babies whose mothers came from Pakistan tend to have raised mortality rates associated with congenital malformations and relatively high mortality rates compared with other groups right across the birthweight range.[10] In recent years mortality rates have also been relatively high for babies born to women born in the Caribbean Commonwealth, but it should be borne in mind that this group of women is now relatively old, with 42% of those who had liveborn babies in 1995 being aged 35 or over. The 1991 census showed that well over half of women aged 16–44 who described their ethnic origin as Afro-Caribbean were born in the United Kingdom.

Multiple births account for over a fifth of infant deaths of babies weighing under 1500 g at birth and well over a tenth of all infant deaths, as Table 1.8 shows. Figure 1.15 shows how the relationship between mortality rates for singleton and multiple births changes with birthweight within the category below 1500 g. Overall infant mortality rates are higher for multiple than for singleton births. Not surprisingly, mortality is highest among babies born in triplet and higher-order births. This can be seen in Table 1.15, in which infant mortality rates for babies born in multiple births over the years 1975–94 are compared with those for singletons. Mortality among twins and among triplet and higher-order births fell markedly in the 1970s, but has not shown a consistent trend in more recent years. The increased survival of triplet and higher-order births, coupled with the rising incidence of these births, not only creates problems for the staff of neonatal units, but has meant that more and more parents are being faced with the problems of caring for three or more babies of the same age. These have considerable implications for families and for the health and social services.[15]

GEOGRAPHICAL VARIATIONS IN MORTALITY

Variations from district to district in perinatal and infant mortality rates have received considerable attention from

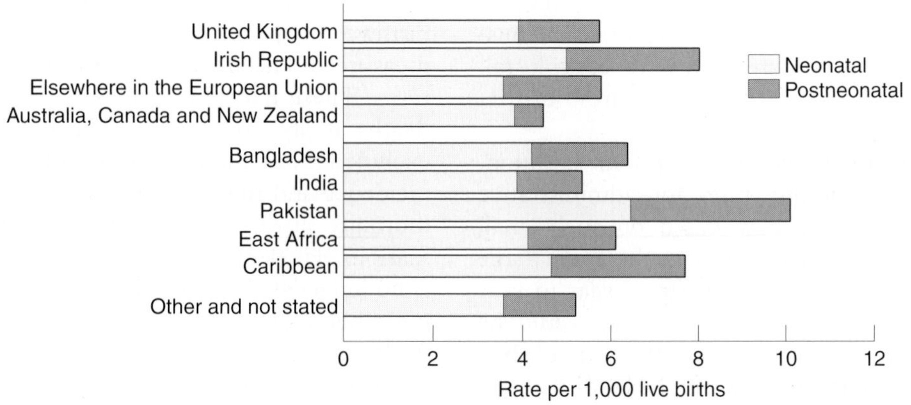

Fig. 1.17 Infant mortality by mother's country of birth, England and Wales, 1996. (Source: ONS Monitor DH3 97/3.)

Table 1.15 Infant mortality rates for singleton and multiple births by year of birth, England and Wales, 1975–94

	Singleton		Twins		Triplets and above	
	No.	Rate	No.	Rate	No.	Rate
1975	8438	14.3	824	71.8	56	249.3
1976	7459	13.0	665	61.8	42	169.4
1977	7697	12.7	586	55.3	26	133.3
1978	7172	12.2	648	56.9	52	248.8
1979	7395	11.8	621	52.3	41	167.3
1980	7057	11.0	583	47.4	43	154.7
1981	na		na		na	
1982	6089	9.9	496	40.8	19	82.6
1983	5786	9.4	492	39.9	21	75.8
1984	5318	8.5	492	39.6	35	138.9
1985	5642	8.8	504	38.3	25	79.4
1986	5508	8.5	611	44.7	38	92.5
1987	5573	8.4	574	40.6	46	113.0
1988	5384	7.9	593	40.4	52	101.2
1989	5065	7.5	562	37.6	58	98.6
1990	4740	6.9	565	36.1	45	71.9
1991	4168	6.1	531	33.0	67	101.4
1992	3858	5.7	473	28.8	49	77.3
1993	3604	5.5	481	29.6	55	75.1
1994	3444	5.3	494	29.8	51	64.4

Source: ONS Mortality Statistics, Series DH3

the press and parliament.[64,99] Politicians have sometimes assumed that these variations simply reflect differences in the quality of maternity care. As a result, they have tended to imply that districts and countries with the highest rates simply have to copy the practices of those with the lowest rates and the problem will be solved almost instantly.

Furthermore, infant mortality rates and their components are included in 'Public health common dataset', a set of public health indicators which are seen as proxy measures of the health of the population and which are used by Directors of Public Health in preparing their annual reports. They have also featured over the years in the Department of Health's 'health service indicators', which have been used as proxy measures of the quality of health care in a district. Closer inspection of the data shows that these interpretations are oversimplified and that the differences arise from a number of factors.

First, there is the question of which babies to register as births and deaths and which to categorize as miscarriages. Decisions about this are likely to reflect cultural, religious and social factors, which may vary from district to district.

Next, it is necessary to consider random variation. Neonatal and infant mortality rates for administrative districts within the UK are now based on such small numbers of events that what appear to be quite large differences from district to district, or from year to year within a district, are actually no larger than would be expected by chance. In the 1980s OPCS published perinatal and infant mortality rates for NHS districts in England and Wales based on 3 years' aggregated data in addition to rates for the most recent year. ONS was

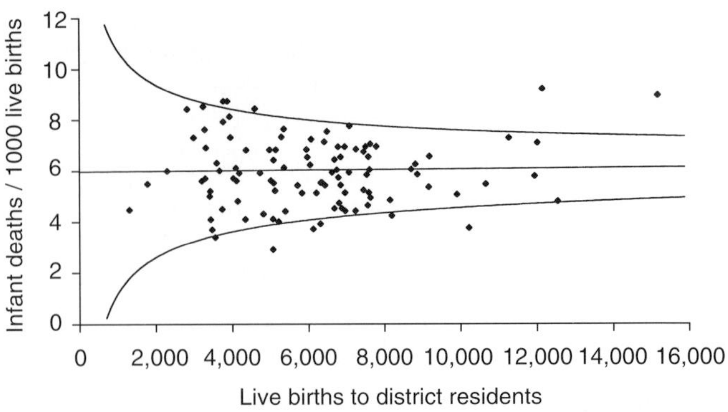

Fig. 1.18 Infant mortality rates for NHS districts, together with confidence limits for overall rate, based on numbers of live births, England and Wales, 1996. (Source: ONS, Monitor DH3 97/1.)

forced by the plethora of boundary changes to stop aggregating data in the 1990s. The data shown in Figure 1.18 are therefore based on data for a single year.[104] This shows the infant mortality rate for each district in the year 1996 plotted against the number of live births to district residents in this year. The horizontal line is the rate for England and Wales. The curved lines are its 95% confidence intervals for the relevant numbers of live births. It can be seen that in some of the smaller districts the rates differed considerably from that for England and Wales, without going outside the 95% confidence interval. In these instances, the difference between the district's rate and that for England and Wales is no greater than would be expected by chance.

A special analysis for the years 1983–85 found that the districts whose mortality rates fell below the lower 95% confidence limit tended to be those with high proportions of fathers in professional occupations and low proportions of mothers born in the 'New Commonwealth' or Pakistan.[14] Most analyses showed a high correlation between perinatal mortality rates and the proportion of low-weight births. This study showed that when mortality was analysed within birthweight groups, different districts had high and low rates.

These analyses lent support to earlier proposals that birthweight-specific mortality rates were a better proxy measure of the quality of services than crude mortality rates. These had also proposed that multiple births and deaths attributed to congenital malformations should be excluded. Now that, as a result of both decline in natural incidence and the introduction of screening programmes, mortality attributed to central nervous system malformations has declined to a much lower level, its inclusion is no longer such a critical factor. In any case, it would be more helpful to use birthweight-specific mortality rates as health service indicators than to continue the present practice of using crude rates. It is also a principle to consider when looking at trends over time and differences between countries.

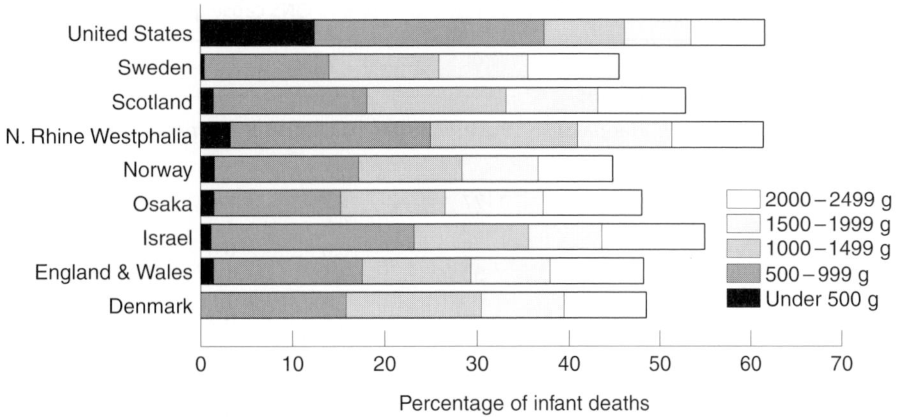

Fig. 1.19 The contribution of low birthweight to infant deaths in 'ICE' countries and regions, 1982–1984. (Source: International Collaborative Effort.)

The extent to which differences in the incidence and reporting of low birthweight can affect international comparisons of infant mortality rates is illustrated in Figure 1.19, which is based on data from the International Collaborative Effort referred to earlier. It shows the percentages of low-weight and very low-weight births among infant deaths in the same group of countries. In particular, it shows the impact of the inclusion of very small babies on reported infant mortality in the USA, where 12.3% of the babies who died had birthweights below 500 g, compared to 3.1% in North Rhine Westphalia and less than 1.5% elsewhere. Because of these differences, the World Health Organization has recommended that babies with birthweights below 1000 g should be excluded from comparisons between countries, and those weighing under 500 g should be excluded from comparisons within countries.[143]

CLASSIFICATION OF CLINICAL CAUSES OF DEATH

In publications based on death registration, information about causes of death is usually classified to a single 'underlying cause' using the International Classification of Diseases, which is revised approximately every 10 years by the World Health Organization. The version in use in England and Wales at the time of writing for coding data on death certificates is still the ninth revision,[143] but the tenth revision is now widely used for most other purposes.[144] The ICD is designed primarily for use in circumstances in which only limited amounts of clinical information, such as that given on death certificates, is available.

In the perinatal field, other classifications have been developed for use by people with access to the more detailed clinical information found in case notes and pathologists' reports. Perhaps the best known is the classification first developed in Aberdeen in the 1940s by Sir Dugald Baird.[8] This was revised in the early 1980s for use in stillbirth and neonatal mortality surveys in Scotland and the northern region of England, and has separate classifications for conditions in mothers[28] and babies.[60]

A further classification, designed by a pathologist, Jonathan Wigglesworth, is based on externally observable features, supplemented by information from the clinical history.[141] A modified version, produced for the International Collaborative Effort on Birthweight, Plurality, Perinatal and Infant Mortality, was designed for use by people who are further removed from clinical details, and is therefore based on the underlying cause of death coded using the ICD.[27] It also extended the classification to cover conditions associated with death in the postneonatal period. OPCS used this as a basis for a classification it developed for use on the new form of stillbirth and neonatal death certificate introduced in 1986.[5] These certificates have separate spaces to list conditions in the mother, the baby, and other factors relating to the death. The system was further developed for classifying stillbirths.[3] The classification is now used routinely by ONS in its published tabulations of cause of death, an example of which is shown in Table 1.16.

CONFIDENTIAL ENQUIRIES INTO STILLBIRTHS AND DEATHS IN INFANCY

As a result of public concern about levels of perinatal and infant mortality in the late 1970s, many special regional and local surveys and enquiries were set up. These varied in their format. Some were largely restricted to reviews of case notes, whereas others involved interviews with bereaved parents. Some took the form of 'confidential enquiries' based on the model of the Confidential Enquiries into Maternal Deaths. Some of these initiatives were for a single year or a limited period.[46] Others, notably those in Scotland and in the former Northern and South East Thames Regions of England, have been in existence for many years.

The rise in infant mortality in England and Wales in

Table 1.16 Stillbirths and infant deaths among babies born in 1994 by plurality and ONS cause groups, England and Wales

Cause and plurality	Numbers				Rates				
	Births		Deaths						
	Live	Still	Neonatal	Postneonatal	Stillbirth	Perinatal	Neonatal	Postneonatal	Infant
Singletons									
All causes	646 887	3468	2267	1177	5.3	8.0	3.5	1.8	5.3
Congenital anomalies	–	324	658	295	0.5	1.2	1.0	0.5	1.5
Antepartum infections	–	12	14	5	0.0	0.0	0.0	0.0	0.0
Immaturity related conditions	–	93	1070	93	0.1	1.5	1.7	0.1	1.8
Asphyxia, anoxia or trauma (intrapartum)	–	173	315	8	0.3	0.7	0.5	0.0	0.5
External conditions	–	–	7	69	–	0.0	0.0	0.1	0.1
Infections	–	15	81	178	0.0	0.1	0.1	0.3	0.4
Other specific conditions	–	110	19	41	0.2	0.2	0.0	0.1	0.1
Asphyxia, anoxia or trauma (antepartum)	–	1119	–	–	1.7	1.7	–	–	–
Remaining antepartum deaths	–	1568	–	–	2.4	2.4	–	–	–
Sudden infant deaths	–	–	39	319	–	0.0	0.1	0.5	0.6
Other conditions	–	54	64	169	0.1	0.2	0.1	0.3	0.4
All multiple births									
All causes	17 369	348	463	82	19.6	42.0	26.7	4.7	31.4
Congenital anomalies	–	37	74	12	2.1	5.6	4.3	0.7	5.0
Antepartum infections	–	1	2	–	0.1	0.1	0.1	–	0.1
Immaturity related conditions	–	15	319	15	0.9	17.3	18.4	0.9	19.2
Asphyxia, anoxia or trauma (intrapartum)	–	18	30	1	1.0	2.5	1.7	0.1	1.8
External conditions	–	–	–	2	–	–	–	0.1	0.1
Infections	–	1	14	17	0.1	0.4	0.8	1.0	1.8
Other specific conditions	–	16	6	1	0.9	1.2	0.3	0.1	0.4
Asphyxia, anoxia or trauma (antepartum)	–	85	–	–	4.9	4.9	–	–	–
Remaining antepartum deaths	–	169	–	–	9.6	9.6	–	–	–
Sudden infant deaths	–	–	2	18	–	–	0.1	1.0	1.2
Other conditions	–	6	16	16	0.3	1.1	0.9	0.9	1.8

Babies in this table were born in 1994 but may have died in 1994 or in 1995.
*Stillbirths and perinatal mortality rates per 1000 live and stillbirths
Neonatal, postneonatal and infant mortality rates per 1000 live births

1986 prompted a further enquiry into perinatal, neonatal and infant mortality by the backbench House of Commons Social Services Committee, as it was then called. This recommended 'a targeted programme to reduce perinatal and infant mortality rates, particularly in poorer families where rates are still unnecessarily high'.[64] In addition, it said: 'We recommend that all Regions introduce a regular system of confidential inquiries into all unexplained infant deaths and report to the Department of Health on a regular basis. We also recommend that Regions and the Department of Health set up a system for monitoring the results of such inquiries and making the lessons learned available to all health districts.'[64] In its reply, published in 1989, the government announced that it would be setting up a Confidential Enquiry into Stillbirths and Infant Deaths, and the Chief Medical Officer was setting up a working group to consider what form it might take.[37] Secondly, it acknowledged that many regions already conducted epidemiological surveys of stillbirths and neonatal deaths and it had asked the NHS Management Executive to ensure that all regions were doing them by April 1991. Instead of a targeted programme to reduce infant mortality, it stated that 'Targets need to be set to improve performance'.[37] The Chief Medical Officer's working group reported in 1990.[38] It recommended a national enquiry, with a regional and district reporting structure, into subsets of individual late fetal losses, stillbirths and infant deaths.

The Confidential Enquiry into Stillbirths and Deaths in Infancy was set up in 1992, with a budget of over £2 million per year for England,[62] Wales and Northern Ireland to conduct their own enquiries on the same lines, and the data for all three countries are combined. Scotland has been conducting its own enquiries over a much longer period. As the name suggests, the Enquiry's brief was to collect information on all late fetal losses at 20–23 weeks of gestation and all stillbirths and deaths in the first year of life, and to try to establish ways in which these deaths might be prevented. It was also to establish panels in each former NHS region to perform enquiries into a designated subset of the deaths.

One of its first priorities were 'sudden unexpected deaths in infancy', a category which went wider than the 'sudden infant death syndrome'. These were the focus of its 1994 report and of two papers in the *British Medical Journal* on smoking and sleeping position.[12,32,52] These distracted attention from the fuller data published in the CESDI report, which showed that a high proportion of the babies who died were in very deprived circumstances.[32,82,85] CESDI's other early priority was intrapartum-related deaths of normally formed mature babies. These were the subject of confidential enquiries from 1993 to 1995, the initial results of which were published in CESDI's report for 1995.[31–33] In 1996 and 1997 the deaths of a random sample of immature babies were the subject of confidential enquiries.

Ironically, since this considerable effort and expenditure started, stillbirth and infant mortality rates have been either levelling off, or falling more slowly than before, possibly for some of the reasons suggested earlier.

MORBIDITY IN CHILDHOOD IN RELATION TO CIRCUMSTANCES AT BIRTH

Although trends in mortality since the mid-1980s are somewhat uncertain, it is clear that over the preceding 20 years there was a dramatic decline in neonatal mortality, particularly among very small and immature babies. This raises the question of whether this fall in mortality has been associated with an increase, a decrease or no change in the rate of morbidity among the survivors.

Although there are a large number of follow-up studies in the medical and education literature, it has been difficult to answer this question. This is because information about long-term morbidity has not been collected in a standardized and comparable way, either in the countries of the UK or in most other countries.

There are few routine sources of information on morbidity available. Because of this, data about morbidity in children who were born with low birthweight or who needed neonatal intensive care for other reasons are available mostly from studies of cohorts of babies cared for in individual hospitals or, occasionally, born to residents in geographically defined populations. Comparisons between these studies and over time is difficult for a number of reasons, which will be outlined.

ROUTINELY COLLECTED MORBIDITY DATA

At present the routinely available sources of information on childhood morbidity in the UK include the censuses and surveys, hospital activity statistics, data from general practice systems, child health computer systems, the BD8 register of people with visual impairments, and registers of children with disabilities.

The General Household Survey, which interviews samples of households in Great Britain, asks people whether they have 'long-standing illness, disability or infirmity' and, if so, whether this restricts their activities in any way. In the case of children, this information is obtained from interviews with parents or other members of the household. In 1995, 5% of boys aged 0–4 years and 3% of girls were reported as having a limiting long-standing illness, compared with 3% and 2%, respectively, in 1975.[103]

For the first time since 1911, the population census taken in 1991 contained a question about health. It was similar but not identical to that in the General Household Survey, and asked whether people had 'any long-term illness, health problem or handicap which limits his/her daily activities or the work he/she can do'.[23,112] In the census, 2% of both boys and girls aged 0–4 years were stated to have a limiting long-term illness, which was lower than the 4% of boys and 3% of girls in the General Household Survey sample for 1991.[113] This may reflect the fact that census data are collected by a form completed by the 'head of household', whereas the General Household Survey uses interviewers.

Neither of these two involves clinical examinations or collecting detailed diagnostic data. Since the early 1990s this has been done in a series of health surveys which have been established in each of the four countries of the United Kingdom. Since 1995, the Health Survey for England has included children aged 2–15 and data about disability were collected for those aged 10 or over.[122] As only 72 children aged 10–15 years were found to have a disability, it is difficult to draw any firm conclusions about patterns of disability.

As has been mentioned earlier, information on inpatient stays in NHS hospitals is collected routinely in all four countries of the UK. This can be used to analyse trends in inpatient and day-case care for particular conditions or in particular specialties. In England, episodes of inpatient care in NHS hospitals, including those in neonatal units, are collected through the Hospital Episode System. The quality and completeness of the diagnostic data vary widely from district to district, making the picture incomplete at a national level. In Wales and Northern Ireland the data are collected through Hospital Activity Analysis; in Scotland, the SMR1 system deals with general hospital episodes and the SMR11 with neonatal stays.

In the past, records about successive hospital stays by the same person were not linked, but the potential for this now exists. There are now techniques that allow data about babies and children to be linked to data, such as birthweight, from birth records. If records are linked, as has been the case for some years in the Oxford Record Linkage Study, it then becomes possible, for example, to look at the impact of increasing survival of low-birthweight babies on hospital readmission rates in the early years of life.[97] In Scotland, record linkage at a national level is well developed. The other three countries of the UK lag far behind, but it is possible to do some linkage locally.

Since the mid-1930s visually impaired children and adults living in England and Wales have been able to register with local authorities as 'blind' or 'partially sighted', using a BD8 form. Although the registration system is used primarily for service planning, the new BD8 form introduced in 1990 also has a section which is anonymized and contains some epidemiological data.[49] This is used for monitoring the frequency and causes of blindness in the population, but some visually impaired people are not registered. Cross-checks with other sources suggest that the register is much more complete for people who are blind than for those who are partially sighted. As a result, the reported numbers and rates of visual impairment in England are probably underestimates.[50] Unless there are incentives for earlier reporting of children, it will continue to be difficult to monitor fluctuations in the prevalence of eye conditions such as ROP.

Under the 1989 Children Act, health authorities, educational authorities and social services are required to cooperate in maintaining registers of children with particular problems or conditions.[36] Such registers, which form a basis for service planning, may be part of the child health information systems held by community trusts, either as free-standing special needs registers[30] or as modules of an integrated computerized system which provides information on all children within an area.[142] The focus of these registers is primarily on service provision but, if appropriately compiled, they could also be used as a source of information on many aspects of health and development in childhood.

A further potential source of information on childhood morbidity in the UK is from the records of general practitioners. Until recently, most data about care given by general practitioners have come from four national surveys of people consulting GPs in sets of volunteer practices. Surveys took place in 1955–56, 1970–71, 1981–82 and 1991–92.[91] As well as background information about patients, diagnostic information was collected about each episode of illness and consultations within it.

Now that most general practices have computer systems, further developments are possible. Data from practices having computer systems provided by VAMP Health Ltd have been pooled for research or monitoring purposes in the General Practice Research Database.[61] More recently, the MIQUEST project has been attempting to aggregate anonymized data from a variety of systems used in general practice.[102] A major problem with all these initiatives is the lack of consistency in the way different practices record clinical and other information. Thus the potential of general practice systems to provide data about health service use and patterns of illness in young children in relation to birthweight and events occurring around the time of birth has yet to be realized.

SPECIAL STUDIES TO FOLLOW CHILDREN EXPOSED TO ADVERSE PERINATAL EVENTS

This section and the following one provide the epidemiological background to the studies reported in Chapter 7, and should be read in conjunction with it. There are two methods which are commonly used to investigate morbidity in specific groups of children. One is to survey a total population in order to detect impairments and disabilities. This may be done as a 'one-off' cross-sectional point prevalence survey, or alternatively by developing an ongoing register to which children are added when impairments or disabilities are identified. The contribution of the specific group of children to the total pool of impairment in the population can then be estimated and monitored over time.

Population registers of this sort have been set up to list children with particular impairments, such as cerebral palsy, sensorineural deafness and visual impairment.[76] Cerebral palsy registers based on geographically defined populations are now kept in several regions of England,[74,118] and in parts of other countries such as Sweden,[57] Western Australia,[130] California[56] and the Republic of Ireland.[40] These registers are based on populations defined by residence at the time of birth. Population movement across regional boundaries may result in under-ascertainment, particularly as diagnosis may be delayed in milder cases.

The other method of ascertaining the status of groups of children is to define a cohort or group of children for study and follow them longitudinally to monitor function and health status. This is known as a cohort study. Hundreds of such studies have been done over the past 20 years, but for a number of reasons difficulties are met when trying to interpret them, particularly in making comparisons between them.[7,48,98,114]

First, cohorts for study are defined in differing ways. Most are derived from individual hospitals or units, and are therefore subject to selection biases. Populations defined by geographical boundaries are more likely to be free of these biases and to reflect the care given to all babies born to residents in the area.

Other difficulties in interpretation arise when differing birthweight and gestational age groupings and diagnostic criteria are used. There are, for example, differences in the criteria for including children in diagnostic categories such as small for gestational age or chronic lung disease. Some standardization is possible by adopting WHO recommendations for grouping birthweight data,[144] and, when available, agreed classifications and definitions of neonatal conditions and diseases, such as RDS[80] and for intracranial ultrasound findings.[78]

Differences in denominators make it difficult to interpret the numbers and rates of impaired children within a specific cohort. Changes of practice, such as the increasing tendency to register very low-birthweight births, may alter survival rates independently of any changes in care.[47] Similarly, an increase in the number of children with impairments within a cohort can merely reflect an increased rate of survival with a constant rate of impairment. To improve comparability, the total number of births, the total number of live births, the total number of stillbirths and the number of survivors to hospital discharge within a cohort should all be reported.

A further problem in comparability results from the many different ways in which morbidity and health status may be ascertained and reported. The challenge is to reflect the complexity of the consequences of disease or organ damage in simple descriptive terms. This has often been attempted by considering separate domains or systems, such as neurodevelopmental state, sensory impairment, growth, behavioural attributes and learning abilities, and so on. Alternative measures of health service use, such as hospital admission, primary health care and ancillary services, can be used as a proxy measure of morbidity. These have additional important economic implications. Further measures could include family integrity and social adjustment.

In the past, a clear distinction between the concepts of impairment, disability and handicap, as defined in the International Classification of Impairments, Disabilities and Handicaps,[145] has made a useful basis for describing the effects of disease and illness on children.

There have been attempts to standardize systems for describing impairment in children; for example, a standard system for describing central motor deficit has been devised.[51] This allows pooling and comparison of data of children with cerebral palsy. A standard system has also been adopted for describing neurological impairment in 1-year-old and 4-year-old children, together with an assessment of the degree of disability.[6] Sensory impairment is perhaps more amenable to standardized description. ROP can be reported using a grading system which describes both the impairment and the degree of disability (Chapter 36).[72] Sensorineural deafness can be described using standard audiometric measures of frequency and intensity loss.[145] Growth parameters can also be expressed in consistent and comparable ways using standards appropriate for the population being described.[54]

Standard descriptions of disability are less easy to define, particularly the allocation of degrees of severity of the disability. Although a number of schemes have been suggested,[39,73,127] many studies have an arbitrary categorization of disability, usually into severe, moderate and mild. This means that pooling and cross-comparison of disability data is not often possible. Further difficulties arise in the presence of multiple system involvement. As part of the surveys of disability done by OPCS in the mid-1980s, objective measures of severity were derived by asking panels of judges to assign relative weightings to different abilities and disabilities, first within one domain and then within several together.[13]

In recent years, particularly with the emergence of international disability movements, this type of classification has been rejected in favour of a social model of disability, where the focus moves from the effects of disease and impairment on the person to society's response to that person. A model has been devised by the British Association for Community Child Health which retains the traditional concept of disease, impairment and disability but acknowledges the importance of environment in determining disadvantage and loss of social role.[67]

Another recent advance has been the development of quality of life measures. These focus on relating the impairments present to the quality of life experienced by the child and by the care-givers. Multiattribute health status descriptions, which were first developed for use in the cancer field, have been adapted. From these, a single value is estimated which reflects the global health-related quality of life for an individual.[126,136] The extent to which these will be used to inform parents confronted with treatment decisions or to inform those allocating limited resources to health care remains to be seen.

Finally, studies differ widely in the ages at which they measure morbidity. Discussions on the 'best' age for follow-up are usually non-productive, as at each age and developmental age the range of abilities and the impact of disabilities differ. Early ascertainment of morbidity allows rapid reporting back to the providers of neonatal intensive care, but the evaluation will inevitably be incomplete or perhaps inaccurate, and will be misleading for parents.[138] Later assessments allow a more detailed and accurate assessment of areas such as learning ability, social skills, language function and school performance, but mean that more children may be lost to follow-up.

Loss to follow-up is a concern if there is a difference in the characteristics of the children who are successfully followed and those who are lost. There is some evidence that in families who are difficult to locate, there is a higher frequency of disability among the children than in families who are easy to find.[139] If this occurs, there will be a selection bias resulting in an underestimate of the rate of disability in the cohort.

TRENDS IN MORBIDITY AMONG CHILDREN IN RELATION TO FACTORS AT BIRTH

Despite their problems, data from the various sources described above can give some insight into trends in morbidity among children in relation to their circumstances

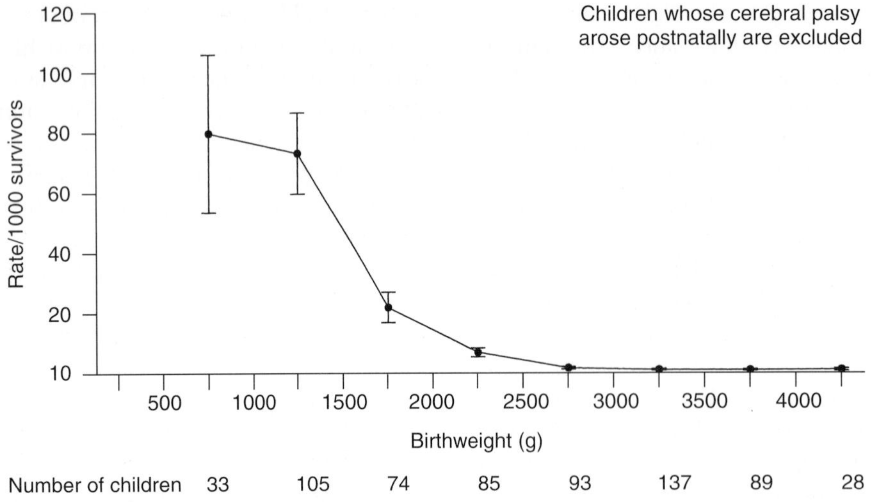

Fig. 1.20 Cerebral palsy rate, by birthweight with 95% confidence limits, among surviving children born in the former Oxford NHS Region, 1984–1991. Children whose cerebral palsy arose postnatally are excluded. (Source: Oxford Register of Early Childhood Impairment (ORECI) 1997.)

at birth (see also Chapter 7 for information on the outcome of preterm and high risk infants).

Cerebral palsy registers rely on multiple and differing sources of ascertainment, but all report prevalence rates close to 2 per 1000 liveborn children. Like the data from the former Oxford Region shown in Figure 1.20, they consistently show that the rate of cerebral palsy is highest among children with the lowest birthweights and the earliest gestational ages. Despite the higher rate of motor deficit associated with immaturity and low birthweight, half of the children on these population registers of cerebral palsy weighed more than 2500 g at birth.

Data from a number of registers show clearly that the birth-cohort prevalence rate of cerebral palsy among very low-birthweight babies increased during the 1980s.[57,118,130] There has also been an increase in the severity of cerebral palsy among VLBW babies during this time,[118] both in terms of the severity of the motor disability and in the presence of associated sensory and intellectual deficits.

In the areas where these population registers are held the rate of low-weight birth has remained steady, and birthweight-specific perinatal mortality has continued to fall during the 1980s and early 1990s. It is therefore likely that the increase in prevalence of cerebral palsy in preterm low-birthweight babies has resulted from higher survival rates of babies with a susceptibility to cerebral haemorrhage and ischaemia in the neonatal period. An alternative hypothesis is that the rise results from greater survival of babies who have had prenatal factors leading both to preterm birth and to later neurological deficit.[118]

By contrast, the birth-cohort prevalence rate of cerebral palsy among babies of normal birthweight has remained remarkably constant. Lesions of prenatal origin have been identified in many of these children born at term, emphasizing both the heterogeneity of the conditions included under the umbrella term of 'cerebral palsy' and the problems of relating perinatal events and later outcome.

Trends over time are less clearly seen in the many cohort studies done in the last 20 years, for the reasons already outlined. A review of 111 existing published studies of infants born between 1960 and the mid-1980s and weighing less than 1500 g at birth, highlighted some of these problems.[48] Of the 111 studies 98 were based on hospital populations, and the age of assessment and description of outcomes varied widely from study to study. Overall, it was concluded that the median cerebral palsy rate among babies weighing less than 1500 g at birth in all cohorts was 7.7%, with 95% confidence limits from 5.3 to 9.0%. There was little variation over the 20 years spanned by the review. The median handicap rate was 25%, with 95% confidence limits from 20.9 to 30.0%, although the way handicap was defined varied widely from study to study.

In recent years, the focus of attention has been on the later outcome of babies born before 28 weeks of gestation or weighing less than 1000 g at birth. It is generally agreed that disability rates are highest among the smallest and most preterm babies, so these groups of babies are particularly vulnerable. The numbers of such survivors are small, however, making it difficult to obtain an overall picture of trends in their outcome over time. This has been compounded by the changing perception of viability, a change in registration practice in the presence of transient signs of life, and more aggressive obstetric and neonatal management, which may have led to an increase in the numbers of live births and fewer fetal deaths in these groups. It is therefore useful to have concurrent information on stillbirths and late fetal deaths.

Table 1.17 Mortality and morbidity rates among extremely low-birthweight and very preterm children in geographically defined populations

Population				Survivors to discharge		Follow-up		Severe disability		
	Birth years	Birthweight, g or gestational age, weeks	Number of live births	Number	%	Age seen at follow-up, years	Number seen	Number	%	95% CI
Hamilton, Canada[127]	1977–80	501–1000 g	255	117	45.9	3	110	26	23.6	15.7–31.6
	1981–84	501–1000 g	266	129	48.4	3	122	15	12.3	6.5–18.1
Victoria, Australia[138]	1979–80	500–999 g	351	*89	25.3	2	89	20	22.5	14.3–32.6
	1985–87	500–999 g	560	217	38.8	2	212	27	12.7	8.3–17.2
Northern Region England[140]	1983	500–999 g	110	*43	39.1	2	43	5	13.9	3.9–25.1
Netherlands[137]	1983	<1000 g	292	*130	44.5	2	130	10	7.7	3.9–25.1
Scotland[128]	1984	<1000 g	204	64	31.4	4.5	60	8	13.3	5.9–24.6
Netherlands[137]	1983	<28 weeks	255	92	36.1	2	89	7	7.9	3.2–15.5
Northern Region England[135]	1983–86	<28 weeks	441	146	33.1	1	49	†9	18.4	8.8–32.0
	1987–90	<28 weeks	483	195	40.4	1	89	†25	28.1	19.1–38.6
	1991–94	<28 weeks	560	239	42.7	1	93	†25	26.9	18.2–37.1
Oxford[75]	1984–86	<28 weeks	240	90	37.5	4	81	24	29.6	20.0–40.1

* = survival to time of follow-up
† = sample of children followed

A further problem in assessing changing outcome over time has been the tendency to report the outcome of babies admitted to large regional centres, rather than all babies from a geographical area. Finally, among the studies of geographically defined populations of babies, some are defined by birthweight group and some by gestational age group. There is some evidence that both mortality and morbidity are more closely related to gestational age than birthweight, and information about prognosis by week of gestation is of more value to obstetricians than similar information by birthweight group.[124]

Table 1.17 shows the outcome in preschool years for geographically defined groups of babies born after 1980 at a gestational age of less than 28 weeks or with a birthweight of less than 1000 g. Studies that compare morbidity within a defined geographical area and in differing time periods provide the most reliable data for detecting morbidity trends over time in these tiny babies. Data from three large studies are now available, one from Canada,[127] one from Australia[138] and one from the UK.[135] Although both the Canadian and Australian studies show a fall in disability rate in the 1980s, the UK study showed no change in the rate of severe disability over a 12-year period (1983–1994) among babies born before 28 weeks of gestation.

Studies following children into the school years have shown that those who had low birthweights are more likely than average to have learning difficulties, adverse behavioural traits and motor difficulties.[58,114,117] Despite this, it is clear from studies of children of all birthweights that those who had a low birthweight make up a very small proportion of the total number of children who have special educational needs.[77,92]

Finally, babies who were born in the early 1980s and who were very preterm or with a very low birthweight are now reaching mid-adolescence. Early behavioural difficulties, such as attention deficit and hyperactivity disorders, may be associated with later adverse psychosocial outcomes in adolescence.[16] Growth patterns and sexual maturity may also have an impact on later psychological and physical health.

THE INCREASING DEMAND FOR NEONATAL CARE

The increase over the last quarter century in the proportion of babies that are born alive and that survive the first few days of life has led to a corresponding increase in the numbers requiring the normal level of neonatal care given by mothers, with the support of midwives, health visitors, general practitioners and paediatric staff. There has also been an increase in the numbers of babies likely to need additional care. The likelihood that a baby will need specialist neonatal care is highest among those with the lowest birthweights, and the proportion of babies of low or very low birthweight who survive birth has increased more quickly than the total numbers of live births.

TRENDS IN RESOURCES FOR NEONATAL CARE

Between 1976 and 1988, routine health service statistics presented a contradictory picture of neonatal resources. In 1992, the political debate about resources for neonatal care cited data about cots to make the case that the health service resources were being reduced, whereas the increasing number of whole-time equivalent midwives was quoted as evidence of health service expansion. As we show in the following paragraphs, the interpretation of the data was not correct in either case.

Nationally available data about the NHS include numbers of cots in neonatal units and their use, numbers of paediatric medical staff employed by health authorities, and numbers of midwifery and nursing staff working in maternity and neonatal units. So far there is little information about the resources needed from health and social services and families once babies leave neonatal units, although these cannot be assumed to be negligible.[94]

COTS FOR NEONATAL CARE

Cots for neonatal care are funded differently, depending on the type of care that is expected to be provided: the more intensive the nursing and the more equipment required, the greater the cost of providing the care. As techniques for care change continually, the definitions of levels of care need to change also, so the relevant professional bodies update these definitions from time to time. A working party set up jointly by the BPA and the RCOG published a report in 1978, in which it defined levels of care and the levels of staffing per cot it considered were necessary for each level.[21] There were revised by the BAPM in 1985,[20] 1992[18] and 1995.[19] Current recommendations are given in Chapter 3. Whereas details of definitions change at national level, data collected routinely at hospital level count staffed available cots for care of babies with relatively little additional evidence about the type of cot or level of care provided.

Data about neonatal cots in England up to 1986 are derived from the SH3 Hospital Return. Numbers of available cots were based on a daily count of staffed available cots in each neonatal unit or SCBU. Confusion can arise because the numbers of SCBU cots counted on the SH3 return were commonly referred to as 'special care cots', and levels of care within the neonatal units were not differentiated. As a result, the total number of cots included those designated for intensive care. The Steering Group on Health Services Information[131] drew on the reports of the professional bodies mentioned above when compiling the definitions of special and intensive care used in the definition of cots for hospital statistics to be collected from 1987 onwards. Such designation is at best artificial, as it is likely that care considered to be intensive often takes place other than in the intensive care area within a special-care nursery. Indeed, in many units such an area may not even be identifiable.

Table 1.18 shows that there has been a fall in the absolute numbers of cots in SCBUs in each of the four countries of the UK. This trend has been quoted as evidence of cuts in NHS spending, but such an interpretation does not take account of the changing definitions of cots and changing practice in neonatal care over the last three decades, described in Chapter 2. The basis for data collection changed in 1988, and in England the number and use of cots is measured in two different routine systems. Numbers of hospital cots are recorded in the KP70 hospital data system, and the use of cots is derived from the Hospital Episode System, both of which derive data from local health information systems and are administered centrally by the Department of Health. The numbers of cots for neonatal care appear to have continued to decline until 1990, with a levelling of the numbers and rates per 1000 births since then.

With increasing concern about the separation of babies from their mothers, policies of routine admission to special care for many babies have been changing. Evidence of this is found in Table 1.18, which shows falling admission rates to SCBUs, from a high point of about 20% of births in England in the mid-1970s to just over 10% in 1986. Since 1988 it is no longer the number of admissions but rather the number of 'finished consultant episodes' that is counted. Any baby who is admitted for neonatal care but receives care from different consultants during one admission will be described as receiving more than one FCE during that admission. This can happen if surgery or specialist diagnostic skills are required. Not surprisingly, therefore, numbers of finished consultant episodes for babies admitted, aged under 28 days and excluding healthy newborns, shown in Table 1.18 for 1989–90 until 1994–95, are much higher than the previous numbers of admissions to neonatal units.

Falling admission rates overall have not been accompanied by a significant fall in workload, as those babies who are admitted stay for longer. Table 1.18 also shows that the mean length of stay increased between 1980 and 1986. Data for 1989–90 and more recent years show that the mean duration of consultant episodes for babies admitted aged under 28 days has no clear trend, varying between 5.9 and 6.6 days. Data from this source cannot tell us how the casemix has changed, but there is evidence from local surveys that an increasing proportion of babies admitted receive intensive care.[22]

Although data about numbers of intensive care cots have not been routinely collected until recently, national surveys of cot provision have been conducted, and these give some idea of the changes over time, although methods and coverage differ. Table 1.19 summarizes data from three of these surveys. In 1980, the Department of Health and Social Security published data from the English NHS regions which showed that out of a total of 268 consultant units there were 42 with some intensive care cots, and that the total number of intensive care cots available was 173. By the end of 1986, a national survey of neonatal units[17] found that the number of cots available for intensive care in units where it is regularly practised had increased more than twofold since 1980, with 341 cots in 1986. In the 242 consultant obstetric units in England in 1986, 65 had at least three intensive care cots. The BAPM survey of transfers for neonatal

Table 1.18 Cots for neonatal care, England, Wales, Scotland and Northern Ireland, 1980–1988, 1998/9–1994/5

Year	Available cots[1]		Admissions[2]		Length of stay[3]
	Number	Rate[4]	Number	Rate[4]	Average days
England					
1980	3959	6.40	89 277	14.44	8.6
1981	3940	6.59	84 061	14.05	8.9
1982	3902	6.62	76 279	12.93	9.5
1983	3898	6.57	71 184	12.00	10.0
1984	3872	6.45	68 777	11.45	10.5
1985	3756	6.06	68 634	11.08	10.8
1986	3651	5.85	66 725	10.70	11.0
1987	3572	5.55	na	na	na
			Finished consultant episodes[5]		
1987–88	3625	5.63	na	na	na
1988–89	3581	5.47	na	na	na
1989–90	3496	5.38	60 743	9.35	9.6
1990–91	3375	5.06	75 545	11.33	8.7
1991–92	3412	5.16	77 301	11.70	9.4
1992–93	3403	5.22	75 018	11.51	10.0
1993–94	3286	5.04	83 307	13.09	9.9
1994–95	3341	5.25	80 229	12.76	10.6
1995–96	3220	5.12	75 736	12.35	11.1
Wales					
1980	237	6.34	5359	14.35	8.1
1981	238	6.64	4886	13.63	8.4
1982	236	6.61	4951	13.86	8.4
1983	231	6.51	4386	12.36	8.7
1984	229	6.39	4330	12.07	8.6
1985	223	6.06	4327	11.77	9.4
1986	221	5.97	4097	11.06	10.0
1987	218	5.76	4037	10.68	10.4
1988	219	5.64	3927	10.11	10.6
1987–88	218	5.76	4042	10.69	7.8
1988–89	219	5.64	3892	10.02	7.4
1989–90	219	5.76	4356	11.46	7.6
1990–91	194	4.99	3512	9.04	7.8
1991–92	223	5.86	3796	9.97	7.5
1992–93	210	5.60	3546	9.45	7.5
1993–94	213	5.82	3320	9.08	7.8
1994–95	213	5.81	3215	9.09	na
Scotland					
1980	626	9.10	20 202	29.30	6.2
1981	621	9.00	19 763	28.60	5.9
1982	619	9.40	17 824	26.90	6.1
1983	608	9.30	16 952	26.00	5.9
1984	597	9.20	15 869	24.40	6.5
1985	580	8.70	15 021	22.50	6.6
1986	na	na	na	na	na
1987	563	8.50	14 189	21.40	6.8
1988	552	8.30	14 500	21.90	6.9
1988–89	520	7.85	12 257	18.51	7.8
1989–90	497	7.83	11 597	18.27	8.3
1990–91	477	7.23	10 013	15.18	9.2
1991–92	465	6.94	10 020	14.95	8.8
1992–93	448	6.81	9339	14.20	9.1
1993–94	426	6.73	9144	14.44	9.4
1994–95	na	na	na	na	na
Northern Ireland					
1980	195	6.80	na	na	na
1981	198	7.30	3764	13.80	9.3
1982	na	na	na	na	na
1983	208	7.60	3657	13.40	9.0
1984	218	7.90	3856	13.90	9.1
1985	218	7.90	3667	13.30	9.6
1986	208	7.40	3570	12.70	10.0
1987	na	na	3729	na	9.9
1987–88	na	na	na	na	na
1988–89	176	6.34	3420	12.32	10.3
1989–90	171	6.54	3495	13.40	9.6
1990–91	171	6.45	3608	13.62	9.6
1991–92	170	6.48	3481	13.25	9.7
1992–93	169	6.61	3103	12.13	10.2
1993–94	168	6.74	2870	11.52	10.4
1994–95	na	na	na	na	na

[1]Up to 1986, staffed available cots in SCBU. After 1988, staffed cots available for neonatal care
[2]Up to 1986, numbers of babies admitted to SCBU
[3]Mean days of stay/episode
[4]Rate per 1000 live births
[5]After 1988, finished consultant episodes for admissions of babies under 28 days of age
Source: NHS Executive and DH Statistics Divisions 2&3

care was repeated for the years 1989–91 for a report on the access and availability of neonatal intensive care by a working party of the Clinical Standards Advisory Group.[25] Data from this source, which refer to the United Kingdom as a whole and are not identified separately for England, are also included in Table 1.19. These show that the rate of intensive care cot provision continued to increase relative to live births, from 0.22 cots per 1000 live births in England in 1980 to 0.74 per 1000 live births in the UK in 1991.

Table 1.19 Neonatal intensive care facilities in England, 1980, 1986, and United Kingdom, 1989–91

Year and country	Nurseries Number	Intensive care cots	
		Number	Rate per 1000 livebirths
England			
1980	42	173	0.22
1986	65	341	0.55
United Kingdom			
1989	na	514	0.66
1990	na	549	0.69
1991	257	584	0.74

Sources: Data for 1980 from Hansard
Data for 1986 from BAPM survey of neonatal referrals[17]
Data for 1989–90 from BAPM survey[25]

STAFF FOR NEONATAL CARE

The medical specialty of paediatrics has grown considerably, both in absolute numbers of 'whole-time equivalent' staff and in relation to the numbers of births, as Table 1.20 shows. Data about the division of work between neonatology and other paediatric work are not routinely collected, and so it is only possible to comment on the numbers in the specialty of paediatrics as a whole.

Recommendations for staffing of neonatal units have been made by successive committees. A report from the

Table 1.20 Paediatric medical staff in England, Wales, Scotland and Northern Ireland, 1980–94

Year	England		Wales		Scotland		Northern Ireland	
	wte[1]	rate[2]	wte[1]	rate[2]	wte[1]	rate[2]	wte[1]	rate[2]
Paediatrics and paediatric neurology								
1982	1745	2.96	110	3.08	214	3.23	na	na
1983	1780	3.00	117	3.30	216	3.32	62	2.27
1984	1821	3.03	119	3.32	217	3.33	66	2.38
1985	1837	2.97	122	3.32	223	3.34	65	2.35
1986	1933	3.10	125	3.37	226	3.43	69	2.45
1987	1994	3.10	na	na	229	3.46	72	2.58
1988	2322	3.55	124	3.19	238	3.59	77	2.77
1989	2222	3.42	135	3.55	246	3.88	77	2.95
1990	2339	3.51	145	3.73	260	3.94	78	2.94
1991	2410	3.65	159	4.18	272	4.06	79	3.01
1992	2559	3.93	160	4.26	267	4.06	94	3.68
1993	2833	4.45	188	5.14	271	4.28	na	na
1994	3070	4.88	216	6.11	289	na	na	na
Paediatric surgery								
1982	na	na	5	0.14	38	0.57	na	na
1983	na	na	5	0.14	36	0.55	11	0.40
1984	na	na	11	0.31	45	0.69	14	0.51
1985	100	0.16	4	0.11	43	0.64	14	0.51
1986	119	0.19	5	0.13	40	0.61	13	0.46
1987	131	0.20	na	na	45	0.68	12	0.43
1988	127	0.19	7	0.18	53	0.80	12	0.43
1989	141	0.22	7	0.18	54	0.85	13	0.50
1990	128	0.19	6	0.15	48	0.73	9	0.34
1991	155	0.23	4	0.11	33	0.49	11	0.42
1992	157	0.24	3	0.08	49	0.74	11	0.43
1993	163	0.26	3	0.08	44	0.69	na	na
1994	162	0.26	7	0.20	51	na	na	na

[1]Whole-time equivalent
[2]Rate per 1000 live births

Source: NHS Executive and Department of Health

Royal College of Physicians[125] made a range of recommendations depending on the size of units and whether they provide a regional referral service. The report concluded that 150 consultant neonatal paediatricians, 120 middle-grade medical staff and about 424 senior house officers would be needed in England and Wales to meet these recommendations. This represented about a third of the whole-time equivalent staff in the paediatric specialties at the time. The numbers of paediatric staff subsequently increased, and so the recommended staffing for neonatal care represents less than a quarter of the 1993 staffing for paediatrics in England and Wales. The staff numbers are expressed as whole-time equivalents, with each member of staff being counted as the proportion of the full contract hours worked. This avoids the problem of how to count part-time staff, but trends over time can be misleading when nationally agreed hours of work change. It is important to note that changes in the contractual hours of junior doctors during the last decade will have reduced the total medical time represented by the whole-time equivalent number of staff.

National data about midwives and nurses can be analysed to indicate how many of them work in neonatal areas. In many maternity units a certain amount of neonatal special care, such as phototherapy, is given in postnatal wards. Because of this blurring of the boundary between different levels of care, it is important to look at the total numbers of maternity unit staff available per birth, as well as the numbers of neonatal unit staff.

The total numbers of qualified hospital nurses and midwives working in the maternity area who were in post on 30 September in each of the years 1982–1994 in England are presented in Table 1.21. Data are shown only for England, as the other countries of the UK do not provide data in this form. In 1980 changes were made in the nationally agreed hours of work for nursing and midwifery staff in the UK. The change in weekly working hours from 40 to 37.5 had the effect of increasing the whole-time equivalents of part-time staff artificially by 6.7% with no actual increase in available staff. Since 1982 the numbers of whole-time equivalent midwives and nurses has not increased, and the rate per 1000 live births has fallen over the period. This trend is associated with a change in training for nurses under 'Project 2000'. Before 1989 student nurses and midwives were counted as part of the NHS workforce, but students are now supernumerary and are not recorded in staff numbers.

As staffing always has to be responsive to pressures in different parts of the maternity unit, the subdivision of midwives by place of work should not be seen as a rigid indication of staff available in the neonatal unit or elsewhere. All the same, in England the proportion of qualified

Table 1.21 Maternity, midwifery and nursing staff in England, 1982–94

	Midwives[1]		Nurses working in maternity care[2]	
	wte[3]	rate[4]	wte[3]	rate[4]
1982	20 250	34.34	10 670	18.09
1983	22 070	37.20	9 840	16.59
1984	22 570	37.58	9 520	15.85
1985	22 810	36.83	9 250	14.94
1986	23 030	36.93	9 100	14.59
1987	23 300	36.22	8 780	13.65
1988	23 310	35.62	8 590	13.13
1989	23 170	35.68	8 100	12.47
1990	23 980	35.96	7 930	11.89
1991	22 830	34.55	8 240	12.47
1992	22 800	34.98	8 160	12.52
1993	21 530	33.83	8 630	13.56
1994	20 740	32.98	8 030	12.77
1995	18 292	29.84	7 902	12.89
1996	18 548	30.20		

[1]Qualified midwives or students on NHS payroll, excludes 'Project 2000' students. Excludes agency staff.
[2]Includes registered, enrolled and unqualified, excludes 'Project 2000' students. Excludes agency staff.
[3]Whole-time equivalent
[4]Rate per 1000 live births

Source: NHS Executive and Department of Health Non-medical Staff Census

midwives working in hospital maternity units who were recorded as neonatal staff increased from under 3% in 1984 to nearly 8% in 1994. This rise must be interpreted with caution, as the numbers in the denominator have changed with the fall in numbers of student midwives on the payroll. Table 1.22 shows the numbers and rates per 1000 live births of nursing and midwifery staff in neonatal care, as analysed by the NHS executive from the staff census data. In parallel with the increased numbers of intensive care cots, rates of neonatal nursing and midwifery staff increased from 4 per 1000 live births in 1984 to over 6 per 1000 in 1994. Midwives form about a third of the neonatal nursing workforce.

Table 1.22 Nurses and midwives in neonatal care in hospital and community health services in England

	1984	1989	1993	1994
Numbers, wte[1]				
Nursing staff, excluding midwives				
Qualified[2]	1040	1740	2160	2170
Unqualified	710	360	370	330
Others	na	10	20	20
Total	1750	2110	2650	2520
Midwives Total	770	1100	1580	1650
Rate per 1000 live births				
Nursing staff, excluding midwives	2.91	3.25	4.16	4.01
Midwives	1.28	1.69	2.48	2.62

[1]NHS hospital and community health services qualified and unqualified nursing and midwifery staff working in neonatal areas, excluding agency staff and excluding 'Project 2000' students.
[2]Includes seniors 1–5.

Source: NHS Executive Department Stats(W)B Quarry House, Leeds

ORGANIZATION OF NEONATAL RESOURCES

Neonatal workload is to a large extent unpredictable. Fluctuations in workload mean that neonatal units are alternately underoccupied or overstretched, as has been shown in local surveys of neonatal unit activity.[22] In most NHS regions the problem of fluctuating demand is met by transfer of babies between units, so long as all units are not busy at the same time. The organization and success of such arrangements varies, as was shown in the BAPM surveys of referrals for neonatal medical care.[17,25] For more information on organization and transport see Chapter 2 and Appendix 15.

RELATIONSHIP BETWEEN RESOURCES FOR NEONATAL CARE AND OUTCOMES

It is clear from the above that over the past 20 years there has been a shift of resources towards neonatal intensive care, and this has coincided with a decline in neonatal and infant mortality. At the same time there have been changes in other factors known to be associated with neonatal mortality and other measures of the outcome of pregnancy. Because of the interrelationship between all of the variables, the relative contribution of care and other factors to the change in mortality and other outcomes is not easy to interpret. Some studies in the USA, Norway, Canada and England found a statistical association between increased amounts of 'care' and lower mortality for some groups of babies after taking account of pre-existing risk factors.[9,24,115,129,132]

Against this apparent trend, a series of papers from Sweden show that perinatal mortality was higher in the maternity hospitals with paediatric departments than in those without, even after taking account of differences in other factors likely to affect mortality.[44,45] Most of the studies quoted here were based on data from the late 1970s, when mortality was higher and resources for neonatal care less widespread.

More recent evidence is less clear. As there are fewer deaths, and as differences between the availability of resources become less pronounced, it becomes more likely that any statistical associations that do exist are masked by chance variation. In a replication[53] of the Norwegian study of access to care at the time of birth, the relationship between mortality and access to care was less strong for babies of different birthweights born between 1979 and 1981 than it had been for those born between 1967 and 1973.

A study in the West Midlands also showed that the inverse association between numbers of paediatricians and neonatal mortality was more marked in the earlier years of the study.[132] This study also illustrated the effect of including outcomes and resources beyond the hospital of birth, that is, where newborn babies are referred between hospitals. When this factor was taken into account, the apparent relationship between paediatric staffing and neonatal mortality almost disappeared.[96]

It is important to take into account not only the quantity of resources but how they are used. Several studies have attempted to adjust outcomes in terms of both mortality and morbidity to take account of predisposing factors, and then to assess the relationship between unexplained differences in outcome and aspects of care provision. With the purpose of such audit of practice in mind, several groups have developed risk scoring methods for admitted babies.[11,120,133]

The growing evidence from randomized controlled trials of particular aspects of perinatal care makes it clear that the choice of method of care can make a significant difference to mortality and morbidity.[26] In some cases this may mean that more resources are required to improve outcomes, but this is not necessarily the case. For example, giving inexpensive antenatal corticosteroids to women who are at high risk of preterm delivery can reduce the incidence of neonatal RDS and thus the cost of neonatal care.[95] In contrast, other types of care, such as neonatal ECMO for term babies with severe breathing difficulties, have been shown to reduce mortality and morbidity but can increase the cost of neonatal care.[65] Although the cost of care may be increased overall, research alongside the UK ECMO trial which is not published at the time of writing shows that the cost of additional healthy survival is comparable to other widely adopted life-extending technologies. Such data can help decisions about the use of resources have to take into account both the costs and the likely benefits.

REFERENCES

1. Ahmad W I U, Sheldon T 1992 'Race' and statistics. In: Ahmad W I U (ed) The politics of 'race' and health. University of Bradford and Ilkley Community College, Bradford
2. Alberman E, Bergsjo P, Cole S et al 1989 International collaborative effort (ICE) on birthweight, plurality and perinatal and infant mortality. Acta Obstetrica Gynecologica Scandinavica 68: 5–10
3. Alberman E, Blatchley N, Botting B, Schuman J, Dunn A 1997 Medical causes on stillbirth certificates in England and Wales: distribution and results of hierarchical classification tested by the Office for National Statistics. British Journal of Obstetrics and Gynaecology 104: 1043–1049
4. Alberman E, Botting B 1991 Trends in prevalence and survival of very low birthweight infants, England and Wales: 1983–7. Archives of Disease in Childhood 66: 1304–1308
5. Alberman E, Botting B, Blatchley N, Twidell A 1994 A new hierarchical classification of causes of infant deaths in England and Wales. Archives of Disease in Childhood 70: 403–409
6. Amiel-Tison C, Stewart A 1989 Follow-up studies during the first five years of life: a pervasive assessment of neurological function. Archives of Disease in Childhood 4: 496–502
7. Aylward G P, Pfeifer S I, Wright A, Verhuist S J 1989 Outcome of studies of low birth weight infants published in the last decade: a metaanalysis. Journal of Pediatrics 115: 515–520
8. Baird D, Wyper J F B 1941 High stillbirth and neonatal mortalities. Lancet ii: 657–659
9. Bakketeig L S, Hoffman H J, Sternthal P M 1978 Obstetric service and perinatal mortality in Norway. Acta Obstetrica Gynecologica Scandinavica 77 (Suppl): 3–19
10. Balarajan R, Raleigh V S 1990 Variations in perinatal, neonatal, postneonatal and infant mortality in England and Wales by mother's country of birth, 1982–85. In: Britton M(ed) Mortality and geography: a review in the mid-1980s in England and Wales. Series DS no 9. HMSO, London
11. Bard H 1993 Assessing neonatal risk: CRIB versus SNAP. Lancet 342: 449–450
12. Blair P S, Fleming P J, Bensley D 1996 Smoking and the sudden infant death syndrome: results from 1993–95 case-control study for confidential inquiry into stillbirths and deaths in infancy. British Medical Journal 313: 195–198
13. Bone M, Meltzer H 1989 OPCS survey of disability in Great Britain. Report No 3. HMSO, London
14. Botting B J, Macfarlane A J 1990 Geographic variations in infant mortality in relation to birthweight 1983–85. In: Britton M (ed) Mortality and geography: a review in the mid-1980s in England and Wales. Series DS no 9. HMSO, London
15. Botting B J, Macfarlane A J, Price F V (eds) 1990 Three, four and more: a study of triplet and higher order births. HMSO, London
16. Botting N, Powls A, Cooke R W I, Marlow N 1997 Attention deficit hyperactivity disorders and other psychiatric outcomes in very low birthweight children at age 12 years. Journal of Child Psychology and Psychiatry 38: 931–941
17. British Association of Perinatal Medicine 1989 Referrals for neonatal medical care in the United Kingdom over one year. British Medical Journal 298: 169–172
18. British Association of Perinatal Medicine 1992 Categories of babies requiring neonatal care. British Paediatric Association, London
19. British Association of Perinatal Medicine and Neonatal Nurses Association 1995 Standards for hospitals providing intensive care. BAPM, London
20. British Paediatric Association, British Association for Perinatal Paediatrics 1985 Categories of babies requiring neonatal care. Archives of Disease in Childhood 60: 599–600
21. British Paediatric Association/Royal College of Obstetricians and Gynaecologists Liaison Committee 1978 Recommendations for the improvement of infant care during the perinatal period in the UK. In: Second report from the Social Services Committee, Session 1979–80 HC 663 Vol 2. HMSO, London, pp 256–284
22. Catterson J 1996 Special care baby units study, 11th report 1995. Public Health Resource Unit, Oxford
23. Charlton J, Wallace M, White I 1994 Long-term illness: results from the 1991 census. Population Trends 75: 18–25
24. Chase H C 1973 A study of risks, medical care and infant mortality. American Journal of Public Health 63 (Suppl)
25. Clinical Standards Advisory Group 1993 Neonatal intensive care: access and availability of specialist services HMSO, London
26. Cochrane Library 1997 Issue 1 1997 Update Software, Oxford
27. Cole S K, Hartford R B, Bergsjo P, McCarthy B 1989 International Collaborative Effort (ICE) on birthweight, plurality, perinatal and infant mortality III: A method of grouping underlying causes of infant death to aid international comparisons. Acta Obstetrica Scandinavica 68: 113–117
28. Cole S K, Hey E N, Thomson A M 1986 Classifying perinatal death: an obstetric approach. British Journal of Obstetrics and Gynaecology 93: 1204–1212
29. Coleman D, Salt J (eds) 1996 Ethnicity in the 1991 census Vol 1. Demographic characteristics of ethnic minority populations. HMSO, London
30. Colver A F, Robinson A 1989 Establishing a register of children with special needs. Archives of Disease in Childhood 64: 1200–1203
31. Confidential Enquiry into Stillbirths and Deaths in Infancy 1995 Report, 1 January–31 December 1993. Department of Health, London
32. Confidential Enquiry into Stillbirths and Deaths in Infancy 1996 3rd Annual Report, 1 January–31 December 1994. Department of Health, London
33. Confidential Enquiry into Stillbirths and Deaths in Infancy 1997 4th Annual Report, 1 January–31 December 1995. Maternal and Child Health Research Consortium, London
34. Craig J 1997 Population review: (9) Summary of issues. Population Trends 88: 5–12
35. Day P, Lancaster P, Huang J 1997 Australia's mothers and babies 1994. Perinatal Statistics Series No 5. AIHW National Perinatal Statistics Unit, Sydney, Australia

36. Department of Health 1989 An introduction to the Children Act. HMSO, London
37. Department of Health 1989 Perinatal and neonatal mortality. Government reply to the first report from the Social Services Committee, Session 1988–89. Cm 741. HMSO, London
38. Department of Health 1990 Confidential Enquiry into Stillbirths and Deaths in Infancy. Report of a Working Group set up by the Chief Medical Officer. Department of Health, London
39. Disability and Perinatal Care 1994 Report of two working groups convened by National Perinatal Epidemiology Unit and Oxford Regional Health Authority
40. Dowding V M Barry C 1988 Cerebral palsy: changing patterns of birthweight and gestational age (1976/81). Irish Medical Journal 81: 25–29
41. Drever F, Whitehead M 1997 Inequalities in health. Series DS No 15. The Stationery Office, London
42. Dunn A, Macfarlane A J 1996 Recent trends in the incidence of multiple births and associated mortality in England and Wales. Archives of Disease in Childhood 75: F10–F19
43. Dunn P M 1980 A standard neonatal discharge record. In: Chalmers I G, McIlwaine G (eds) Perinatal audit and surveillance. RCOG, London
44. Eksmyr R 1985 Early neonatal deaths in geographically defined populations with different organisation of medical care. Acta Paediatrica Scandinavica 74: 848–854
45. Eksmyr R V 1985 Geographically defined populations with different organisation of medical care. Comparison of perinatal risks. Acta Paediatrica Scandinavica 74: 855–860
46. Enkin M, Chalmers I 1980 Inquiries into perinatal deaths at area health authority level: a status report winter 1979/80. Community Medicine 2: 219–224
47. Ens-Dokkum M, Johnson A, Schreuder A M et al 1994 Comparison of mortality and rates of cerebral palsy in two populations of very low birthweight infants. Archives of Disease in Childhood 70: F96–F100
48. Escobar G J, Littenberg B, Petitti D 1991 Outcome among surviving very low birth weight infants: a meta-analysis. Archives of Disease in Childhood 66: 204–211
49. Evans J R, Wormald R P 1993 Epidemiological functions of BD8 certification. Eye 7: 172–179
50. Evans J, Rooney C, Ashwood F, Dalton N, Wormald R 1996 Blindness and partial sight in England and Wales: April 1990–March 1991. Health Trends 28: 5–12
51. Evans P, Johnson A, Mutch L, Alberman E 1989 A standard form for recording clinical findings in children with a motor deficit of central origin. Developmental Medicine and Child Neurology 31: 119–127
52. Fleming P J, Blair P S, Bacon C et al 1996 Environment of infants during sleep and risk of the sudden infant death syndrome: results of 1993–95 case-control study for confidential enquiry into stillbirths and deaths in infancy. British Medical Journal 313: 191–195
53. Forbes J F, Larssen K, Bakketeig L S 1987 Access to intensive neonatal care for low birthweight infants: a population study in Norway. Paediatric and Perinatal Epidemiology 1: 33–42
54. Freeman J V, Cole T J, Chinn S, Jones P R M, White E M, Preece M A 1995 Cross sectional stature and weight reference curves for the UK, 1990. Archives of Disease in Childhood 73: 17–24
55. Gourbin C, Masuy-Stroobant G 1995 Registration of vital data: are live births and stillbirths comparable all over Europe? Bulletin of the World Health Organization 73: 449–460
56. Grether J K, Cummins S, Nelson K B 1992 The California Cerebral Palsy Project. Paediatric and Perinatal Epidemiology 6: 339–351
57. Hagberg B, Hagberg G, Olow I, Von Wendt L 1996 The changing panorama of cerebral palsy in Sweden VII Prevalence and origin in the birth period 1987–90. Acta Paediatrica Scandinavica 85: 954–960
58. Hall A, McLeod A, Counsell C, Thomson L, Mutch L 1995 School attainment, cognitive ability and motor function in a total Scottish very-low-birthweight population at eight years: a controlled study. Developmental Medicine and Child Neurology 37: 1037–1050
59. Hartford R B 1990 Definitions, standards, data quality and comparability. Paper given at the International Symposium on perinatal and infant mortality, Bethesda, Maryland, USA, 30 April–2 May
60. Hey E N, Lloyd D J, Wigglesworth J S 1986 Classifying perinatal death: fetal and neonatal factors. British Journal of Obstetrics and Gynaecology 93: 1213–1223
61. Hollowell J 1997 The General Practice Research Database: quality of morbidity data. Population Trends 87: 36–40
62. Horam J 1997 Reply to written question from Audrey Wise. Hansard, 20 March col 811. The Stationery Office, London
63. House of Commons Health Committee 1996 Public expenditure on health and personal social services. HC 698. The Stationery Office, London
64. House of Commons Social Services Committee 1988 Perinatal, neonatal and infant mortality. HC 54. HMSO, London
65. Howard S, Mugford M, Normand C et al 1996 A cost effectiveness analysis of neonatal ECMO using existing evidence. International Journal of Technology Assessment in Health Care 12: 80–92
66. Human Fertilisation and Embryology Authority 1994 Third Annual Report. HFEA, London
67. Hutchinson T 1995 The classification of disability. Archives of Disease in Childhood 73: 91–99
68. Information and Statistics Division 1987 Birthweight statistics 1980–84. Information and Statistics Division, Edinburgh
69. Information and Statistics Division 1997 Births in Scotland 1976–1995. Information and Statistics Division, Edinburgh
70. Information and Statistics Division, Edinburgh Unpublished data,
71. Interim Licensing Authority for Human In Vitro Fertilisation and Embryology 1990 Fifth report. Interim Licensing Authority, London
72. International Committee for the Classification of Retinopathy of Prematurity 1984 An international classification of retinopathy of prematurity. Paediatrics 74: 127–133
73. Jarvis S, Hey E 1984 Measuring disability and handicap due to cerebral palsy. In: Stanley F, Alberman A (eds) Epidemiology of the cerebral palsies. Spastics International Medical Publications, London
74. Jarvis S N, Holloway J S, Hey E N 1985 Increase in cerebral palsy in normal birthweight babies. Archives of Disease in Childhood 60: 1113–1121
75. Johnson A, Townshend P, Yudkin P, Bull D, Wilkinson A R 1993 Functional abilities at age 4 years of children born before 29 weeks of gestation. British Medical Journal 306: 1715–1718
76. Johnson M A, King R 1989 A regional register of early childhood impairments: a discussion paper. Community Medicine 11: 352–363
77. Kempley S T, Diffley F S, Ruiz G, Lowe D, Evans B G, Gamsu H R 1995 Birth weight and special educational need: effects of an increase in the survival of very low birthweight infants in London. Journal of Epidemiology and Community Health 49: 33–37
78. Kuban K, Teele R 1984 Rationale for grading intraventricular haemorrhage in premature infants. Paediatrics 74: 358–363
79. Lancaster P, Shafir E, Hurst T, Huang J 1997 Assisted conception in Australia and New Zealand, 1994 and 1995. Assisted conception series no 2. AIHW National Perinatal Statistics Unit, Sydney, Australia
80. Levene M I 1992 Development of audit measures and guidelines for good practice in the management of neonatal respiratory distress syndrome. Report of a Joint Working Group of the British Association of Perinatal Medicine and the Research Unit of the Royal College of Physicians. Archives of Disease in Childhood 67: 1221–1227
81. Levene M I, Wild J, Steer P 1992 Higher multiple births and the modern management of infertility in Britain. British Journal of Obstetrics and Gynaecology 99: 607–613
82. Logan S, Spencer N, Blackburn C 1996 Smoking is part of a causal chain, Letter. British Medical Journal 313: 1332–1333
83. Lumley J 1997 How important is social class a factor in preterm birth? Commentary. Lancet 49: 1040–1041
84. Macfarlane A J 1994 Sources of data. In: Maresh M (ed) Audit in obstetrics and gynaecology. Blackwell, Oxford, pp. 18–49
85. Macfarlane A J 1996 Sudden infant death syndrome: more attention should have been paid to socioeconomic factors, Letter. British Medical Journal 313: 1332
86. Macfarlane A J 1996 Inégalités en santé des enfants en Europe: une perspective épidémiologique. In: Santé et mortalité des enfants en Europe. Proceedings of the Chaire Quêtelet, 13–15 September 1994 Academia-Bruylant, Louvain-la-Neuve
87. Macfarlane A J, Cole S, Johnson A, Botting B 1988 Epidemiology of birth before 28 weeks of gestation. British Medical Bulletin 44: 861–893
88. Macfarlane A J, Mugford M 1984 Birth counts: statistics of pregnancy and childbirth. HMSO, London
89. Macfarlane A J, Prager K 1990 What is happening to postneonatal mortality? Paper given at International Symposium on perinatal and infant mortality, Bethesda, Maryland, USA 30 April–2 May

90. Masuy-Stroobant G 1996 Santé et mortalité infantile en Europe. Victoires d'hier et enjeux de demain. In: Masuy-Stroobant G, Gourbin C, Buekens P (eds) Santé et mortalité des enfants en Europe. Inégalités sociales d'hier et d' aujourd'hui, Chaire Quetelet 1994, Academia-Bruylant, Louvain-la-Neuve
91. McCormick A, Fleming D, Charlton J 1995 Morbidity statistics from general practice. Fourth national study 1991–92. Series MB5 no 3. HMSO, London
92. Middle C, Johnson A, Alderdice F, Petty T, Macfarlane A J 1996 Birthweight and health and development at the age of 7 years. Child Care, Health and Development 22 1: 55–72
93. MRC Working Party on children conceived by in-vitro fertilisation. 1990 Births in Great Britain resulting from assisted conception. British Medical Journal 300: 1229–1233
94. Mugford M 1990 The costs of a multiple birth. In: Botting B J, Macfarlane A J, Price F V (eds) Three four and more: a study of triplet and higher order births. HMSO, London, pp 205–217
95. Mugford M, Piercy J, Chalmers I 1991 Reducing the costs of neonatal care by effective prevention of respiratory distress syndrome. Archives of Disease in Childhood 66: 757–764
96. Mugford M, Szczepura A, Lodwick A, Stilwell J 1988 Factors affecting the outcome of maternity care II. Neonatal outcomes and resources beyond the hospital of birth. Journal of Epidemiology and Community Health 42: 170–175
97. Mutch L M, Ashurst A, Macfarlane A J 1992 Birthweight and hospital admission before the age of two years. Archives of Disease in Childhood 67: 900–904
98. Mutch L M, Johnson M A, Morley R 1989 Follow-up studies: design, organisation and analysis. Archives of Disease in Childhood 64: 1394–1402
99. National Audit Office Maternity Services 1990 Report by the Comptroller and Auditor General. HMSO, London
100. National Health Service, Department of Health 1990a Working Paper 11. Framework for information systems: overview. HMSO, London
101. National Health Service, Department of Health 1990b Framework for information systems: the next steps. HMSO, London
102. National Health Service Executive 1996 Collection of data from general practice: overview. NHS Executive, Leeds
103. Office for National Statistics 1997 Living in Britain. Results from the 1995 General Household Survey. The Stationery Office, London
104. Office for National Statistics 1997 Infant and perinatal mortality 1996: health authorities and regional offices. Monitor DH3 97/1. ONS, London
105. Office for National Statistics 1997 Sudden infant deaths, 1992–1996. Monitor DH3 97/2. ONS, London
106. Office for National Statistics 1997 Infant and perinatal mortality – social and biological factors, 1996. Monitor DH3 97/3. ONS, London
107. Office for National Statistics 1997 Mortality statistics: childhood, infant and perinatal, England and Wales, 1995. Series DH3 no 28. The Stationery Office, London
108. Office of Population Censuses and Surveys 1978 Occupational mortality 1970–72 England and Wales, decennial supplement. Series DS no 1. HMSO, London
109. Office of Population Censuses and Surveys 1988 Occupational mortality 1979–80, 1982–83 England and Wales, childhood supplement. Series DS no 8. HMSO, London
110. Office of Population Censuses and Surveys 1990 Registration: proposals for change. Cm 939. HMSO, London
111. Office of Population Censuses and Surveys, General Register Office, Scotland 1989 Publication of draft census order. Census newsletter No 11. OPCS, London
112. Office of Population Censuses and Surveys, General Register Office, Scotland 1993 1991 Census. Limiting long-term illness: Great Britain. HMSO, London
113. Office of Population Censuses and Surveys 1994 General Household Survey 1992. Series GHS no 23. HMSO, London
114. Ornstein M, Ohlsson A, Edmonds J, Asztalos E 1991 Neonatal follow-up of very low birthweight/extremely low birthweight infants to school age: a critical over-view. Acta Paediatrica Scandinavica 80: 741–748
115. Paneth N, Kiely J L, Wallenstein S, Marcus M, Pakter J, Susser M 1982 Newborn intensive care and neonatal mortality in low birthweight infants. New England Journal of Medicine 307: 149–155
116. Parsons L, Macfarlane A J, Golding J 1993 Pregnancy, birth and maternity care In: Ahmad WIU (ed) Race and health in contemporary Britain. Open University Press, Buckingham, pp 51–75
117. Pharaoh P O D, Stevenson C J, Cooke R W, Stevenson R C 1994 Clinical and subclinical deficits at 8 years in a geographically defined cohort of low birthweight infants. Archives of Disease in Childhood 70: 264–270
118. Pharaoh P O D, Platt M J, Cooke T 1996 The changing epidemiology of cerebral palsy. Archives of Disease in Childhood 75: F169–F173
119. Pharaoh P O D, Macfarlane A J 1982 Recent trends in postneonatal mortality. In: Studies in sudden infant deaths. Studies on Medical and Population Subjects No 45. HMSO, London
120. Pollack M M, Ruttiman U E, Getson P R 1988 The pediatric risk of mortality (PRISM) score. Critical Care Medicine 16: 1110–1116
121. Power C 1994 National trends in birth weight: implications for future adult disease. British Medical Journal 308: 1270–1271
122. Prescott-Clarke P, Primatesta P 1997 Health survey for England, 1995. Volume I: Findings. The Stationery Office, London
123. Raleigh V S, Balarajan R 1995 The health of infants and children among ethnic minorities. In: Botting B (ed) The health of our children. Series DS no 11. HMSO, London
124. Rennie J M 1996 Perinatal management at the lower margin of viability. Archives of Disease in Childhood 74: F214–F218
125. Royal College of Physicians 1988 Medical care of the newborn in England and Wales. Royal College of Physicians, London
126. Saigal S, Feeny D, Rosenbaum P, Furlong W, Burrows E, Stoskopf B 1996 Self-perceived health status and health-related quality of life of extremely low-birth-weight infants at adolescence. Journal of the American Medical Association 276: 453–459
127. Saigal S, Rosenbaum P, Hattersley B, Milner R 1989 Decreased disability rate among 3 year old survivors weighing 501 to 1000 g at birth and born to residents of a geographically defined region from 1981 to 1984 compared with 1977 to 1980. Journal of Paediatrics 114: 839–846
128. Scottish Low Birthweight Study Group 1992 The Scottish low birthweight study: I Survival, growth, neuromotor and sensory impairment. Archives of Disease in Childhood 67: 675–681
129. Sinclair J C, Torrance G W, Boyle M H, Horwood S P, Saigal S, Sackett D L 1981 Evaluation of neonatal intensive care programs. New England Journal of Medicine 305: 489–494
130. Stanley F J, Watson L 1992 Trends in perinatal mortality and cerebral palsy in Western Australia 1967–1985. British Medical Journal 304: 1658–1662
131. Steering Group on Health Services Information 1985 Supplement to first and fourth reports to the Secretary of State. HMSO, London
132. Stilwell J, Szczepura A, Mugford M 1988 Factors affecting the outcome of maternity care I. Relationship between staffing and perinatal deaths at the hospital of birth. Journal of Epidemiology and Community Health 42: 157–169
133. Tarnow-Mordi W O, Ogston S, Wilkinson A R et al 1990 Predicting death from initial disease severity in very low birthweight infants: a method for comparing the performance of neonatal units. British Medical Journal 300: 1611–1614
134. Tatham J 1907 Letter to the Registrar General. In: Sixty eighth report of the Registrar General of Births Marriages and Deaths in England and Wales 1905. Cd 3279. HMSO, London
135. Tin W, Wariyar U, Hey E for the Northern Neonatal Network 1997 Changing prognosis for babies of less than 28 weeks' gestation in the north of England between 1983 and 1994. British Medical Journal 314: 107–111
136. Tyson J E, Broyles R S 1996 Progress in assessing the long-term outcome of extremely low-birth-weight infants, Editorial. Journal of the American Medical Association 276: 492–493
137. Van Zeben van der Aa T M, Verloove-Vanhorick S P, Brand R, Ruys J H 1989 Morbidity of very low birthweight infants at corrected age of 2 years in a geographically defined population. Lancet i: 253–255
138. Victorian Infant Collaborative Study Group: L W Doyle (convenor), collaborators Callanan C, Carse E, Charlton M P et al 1995 Neurosensory outcome at 5 years and extremely low birthweight. Archives of Disease in Childhood 73: F143–F146
139. Wariyar U K, Richmond S 1989 Morbidity and preterm delivery: importance of 100% follow-up [letter] Lancet i: 387–388
140. Wariyar U, Richmond S, Hey E V 1989 Pregnancy outcome at 24–31 weeks' gestation: neonatal survivors. Archives of Disease in Childhood 64: 678–686

141. Wigglesworth J S 1980 Monitoring perinatal mortality – a pathophysiological approach. Lancet ii: 684–686
142. Woodruffe C, Abra A 1991 A special conditions register. Archives of Disease in Childhood 66: 927–930
143. World Health Organization 1977 Manual of the International statistical classification of diseases, injuries and causes of death, 9th revision. World Health Organization, Geneva
144. World Health Organization 1992 International statistical classification of diseases and related health problems, 10th revision. World Health Organization, Geneva
145. World Health Organization 1980 International classification of impairments, disabilities and handicaps. World Health Organization, Geneva

2

Organization of perinatal care

David Field

THREE-TIER STRUCTURE

Neonatology is a new specialty which has emerged over the last 30 years. During that time a variety of influences have helped shape the service in the UK and elsewhere. Initially it was the enthusiasm of a small number of individuals that led to the formation of a handful of units specializing in the care of sick newborn infants. However, pressure from the profession and the public[12,13,16,18,22,24,26] encouraged successive governments in the UK to develop a service with nationwide coverage. The rate of evolution varied around the country but, particularly during the 1980s, there was a steady move towards a three-tier service based on the 'health regions' (populations of 2–4 million) that existed at the time. The intention was that each of these geographical areas would be served by three types of neonatal unit:

- Level 1: hospitals which delivered infants expected to be well; resuscitation could be provided if necessary, but no ongoing care; infants requiring such support were transferred;
- Level 2: hospitals with higher delivery rates capable of providing resuscitation and limited ongoing care; infants with more complex problems were transferred;
- Level 3: regional centres, based largely on teaching hospitals, capable of providing a full range of neonatal services.

The rationale for this approach was:

- a reasonable geographical coverage was ensured;
- a high throughput for the level 3 units enabled maintenance of clinical skills;
- high levels of bed occupancy (in level 3 units) permitted efficient use of expensive resources.

The regional centres also had additional responsibilities, including specialist training for nurses and doctors and the provision of a transport service for sick babies born elsewhere. Although this structure, which had been adopted by a number of high-cost low-volume specialties, appeared a sensible approach for the delivery of neonatal intensive care, it was never fully established across the UK. Concerns that a centralized system of care was not appropriate centred on the following:

- Infants in outlying units were disadvantaged in terms of access and availability.
- A shortage of cots led to very long-distance transfers.
- There was possible deskilling in local units.
- There was disruption to family life following long-distance transfers.

TRANSFERS

In any service relying on treatment in a central unit patient transport becomes an essential element of the care package. In general families do not welcome the prospect of changing hospitals and teams at a time of anxiety, and if there are other children the move may cause additional worries and significant cost. Referring clinicians are therefore under particular pressure to achieve the best outcome while exposing mother and baby to the least possible risk and disruption.

Data comparing in utero and neonatal transfer from the perspective of mortality and morbidity must be viewed cautiously because of almost inevitable bias in the selection of patients. For example, some babies referred in utero are born relatively healthy and do not require intensive care, whereas babies who are referred after birth are selected because they are already ill. Among extremely preterm births selection bias operates in the opposite direction, because some of these babies die before they can be transferred to a referral centre.[15] The issue of variation in disease severity is discussed separately (p. 48).

There are data from the UK which indicate that mortality is increased where transfer is requested but is unavailable.[28] Similarly, infants moved between tertiary units to cope with peaks of demand have been reported to have a poorer outcome.[32] These findings are not surprising, as in both cases care is being determined by bed availability rather than the choice of the clinician. In fact, both represent a breakdown of the three-tier structure. More encouraging information is available from Australia and the USA, where specialist transport services, normally independent of the clinical units, have long been able to offer a more consistent service.[23,25] However, the most recent evidence from the UK suggests that infants are not jeopardized by well-planned transport.[5]

In utero transfers

Neonatal intensive care is unique in that it is possible to move the patient either before delivery or postnatally. There is no doubt that it is far easier, and in general safer for the infant, to move a baby in utero. However, there are risks for both mother and baby if delivery or some other unforeseen problem complicates the journey. Careful discussion between neonatal and obstetric teams at a senior level should precede any decision to transfer. Where there is a history of antepartum bleeding, uncontrolled pre-eclampsia or risk of impending delivery, in utero transfer should not take place. In utero transfer causes particular problems for the family when, after moving to another hospital, delivery is delayed, perhaps for several weeks.

Flying squad (postnatal) transfer

The same individual enthusiasm which marked the initial development of specialist neonatal units in the UK was also responsible for the provision of a transfer service. Units tended to construct their own equipment for this purpose, with medical and nursing staff culled from those on duty on the neonatal unit when transport was required. Recent events have highlighted the shortcomings in such arrangements.[29] More important is evidence which indicates that as overall demand for neonatal intensive care grew during the late 1980s, regional units were often unable to satisfy requests for flying squad transfers.[4]

OUTCOME AND PLACE OF DELIVERY

On first principles high throughput should be associated with the best outcomes irrespective of the specialty. This was certainly part of the rationale for regionalized care. However, evidence of this effect is sparse in neonatal care. Truly comparable data are difficult to derive since regional centres (by definition) attract infants at high risk of a poorer outcome, whereas the converse is true for other units. Despite these limitations there are reports that indicate that survival is higher among infants cared for entirely in tertiary centres.[10,20,30] Problems of differences in case mix when comparing units are common to other specialties with a centralized service. It was from adult intensive care that the idea of correcting for disease severity arose. The Clinical Risk Index for Babies[14] is a disease severity score for infants of 32 weeks' gestation or less. It has five components:

- Birthweight;
- Maximum base excess;
- Minimum appropriate F_iO_2 in the first 12 hours;
- Maximum appropriate F_iO_2 in the first 12 hours;
- Congenital anomaly.

Using this approach it is possible to assess hospitals in terms of actual mortality and a corrected (expected) mortality. Early use of CRIB comparing different methods of service delivery suggested poorer outcome for babies treated in units based in non-teaching hospitals as opposed to teaching centres. However, more recent studies by the CRIB investigators (personal communication) and elsewhere in the UK[5] have not confirmed this effect.

Given the limited data regarding differences in mortality between different size units, it is not surprising that information about morbidity arising from different methods of service delivery is even less convincing.[31,33] These reports have to be interpreted with care. For example, one report of neurodevelopmental outcome of infants born in 1979 and 1980 indicates a poorer outcome for babies cared for outside a 'regional centre'. At that time neonatal intensive care outside recognized centres was rudimentary, making comparisons with the present day of little value. Similarly, reports of outcome relating to the group of infants with birthweights 500–1000 g reflect not only clinical care but also decisions on, and hence personal attitudes to, viability. At present there are no convincing data which suggest that outcome (mortality or morbidity) varies significantly between properly run units of different size. If a difference does exist it is too small to be detected by current studies looking for such an effect.

Cost-effectiveness

Neonatal care is expensive, and it is therefore important that resources are not left idle. Similarly, given the limited number of professionals with the appropriate skills, it is important to maximize their potential for delivering neonatal care. Data do exist which support the concept that large units produce economies of scale.[11] However, the relationship is not linear, since increasing size brings additional, expensive, responsibilities, e.g. teaching, research etc. For smaller units, where joint cover of paediatric units often allows costs to be shared, the economic arguments are often similarly not straightforward. These issues are discussed more fully elsewhere (Chapter 4).

REFORMS OF THE 1990S

By the beginning of the 1990s rising demand for neonatal intensive care was generating increasing public disquiet over access to and availability of neonatal intensive care facilities. Both the UK government and health authorities were keen to respond to public demands for increased local services. The NHS reforms, introduced for other reasons, and an increase in the number of personnel with neonatal expertise available in district general hospitals, proved to be the vehicles for change.

By 1992 strategic planning and funding for neonatal care (in fact, for virtually all services) was reduced to health district level (average population 500 000). By 1996 any tendency towards increasing centralization had ceased, and a quarter of neonatal intensive care was delivered in small local units (i.e. less than three intensive care cots), whereas the old regional centres (at least six intensive care cots) retained approximately one half (Table 2.1).

On average the smaller units have no intensive care patients for 50% of the time. For an overwhelming majority of all units local demand was the main source of their throughput.[5] The move to more local care reduced the demand for urgent transfers (Table 2.2).

The changes which have taken place in the UK, in particular the desire of government to regulate expenditure on health care, have been mirrored in many other developed countries. For example, in the USA tighter financial controls have had a particular role in changing referral patterns. On the other hand, in Australia, despite financial restraint, the centralized pattern of service delivery continues, as the geography militates against any real change. For the developing world priorities have, quite rightly, been different.

THE CURRENT UK MODEL OF PERINATAL CARE

THE NORMAL BABY

The various changes described above have had an impact on the way medical care is provided for normal infants. In particular, early discharge has led to discussion about the value of, and who has the responsibility for, the routine examination (p. 269), which in the past has formed a central plank of the child health screening programme. The management of common early neonatal problems such as jaundice now falls into the remit of the community services.

Table 2.1 Data from British Association for Perinatal Medicine survey carried out in 1993–95

Number of cots	Number of units	Percentage of UK neonatal intensive care provided
1–3	102	25
4–5	52	30
6–14	54	45

Table 2.2 Annual totals of emergency transfers in Trent Region, UK

	1991	1992	1993	1994	1995
Number of babies transferred in utero or postnatally	618	563	600	496	454

THE SPECIAL-CARE INFANT

In the past any minor abnormality relating to pregnancy or delivery (e.g. delivery by caesarean section) was sufficient to lead to admission to the 'special care' unit. These infants were considered to be at increased risk of 'problems' and hence required observation. Time has shown that for most such infants admission was not only unnecessary but was harmful in terms of the mother–child relationship. It is now broadly accepted that neonatal units that admit more than 10% of births are admitting too many babies, 8% representing the national average. It is possible to lower the figure to 5% by having sufficient staff and expertise on postnatal wards to allow the least dependent babies to be nursed there.[6] Some units have achieved a reduction in admissions by having a 'low-tech' nursery based on one of their postnatal wards, and others have used staff with enhanced skills in neonatal care distributed across the postnatal wards. This type of transitional care is established in only a minority of UK units, as in general any expenditure is not offset by the reduction in special care admissions because the fixed costs of the service remain.

The development of community liaison programmes with neonatal unit staff available to visit newly discharged infants at home can reduce the time many infants need to spend as in-patients. However, there are few data to suggest that in this context the provision of 'hospital at home' is cost-effective. Similarly, increasing numbers of infants with disability who would, in the past, have remained in hospital are now discharged home to be cared for by their parents and other support workers. These include babies requiring oxygen, and babies needing tube or even intravenous feeding. It is likely that this approach, which avoids what would otherwise be prolonged hospital stay, is cost-effective but data at present are sparse. It is clear that an overwhelming majority of parents prefer approaches that lead to early discharge and, on occasions, they may press to take their child home when it is still inappropriate because he or she is too unstable.

THE INTENSIVE-CARE INFANT

As indicated in the introduction to this chapter, a majority of infants requiring intensive care in the UK now receive it in the hospital in which they are born. However, the need for subspecialist services (e.g. surgery, genetics or radiology) may still necessitate the involvement of a tertiary referral unit, almost certainly the old regional centre. Similarly, peaks in demand in the smaller units providing intensive care are generally met by the tertiary referral units. Therefore, despite the disappearance of the three-tier structure of the 1980s and a reduction in intensive care transfers, the position of the regional centres remains pivotal to the smooth running of the service.

Training, research and development all remain the responsibility of the tertiary centres. Whereas the old three-tier structure did go some considerable way towards safeguarding this function, the current system is struggling to ensure both workloads and finance for this to take place. Current methods of contracting, with all cases requiring ventilation being described as 'intensive care', are unhelpful in this regard.

The unique contribution of the larger neonatal centres relates to:

- involvement with a fetal medicine/high-risk obstetric service;
- care of complex cases requiring subspecialty input;
- care of the most immature infants requiring intensive care for prolonged periods;
- transport/acceptance of outside referrals;
- training;
- research.

It is these points that must find their way into contracts if the present service is to survive. For those with responsibility for allocation of resources a willingness among professionals to provide intensive care locally is not a sufficient criterion for going ahead. Careful consideration must be given to each of the following:

- Personnel: it is essential that specialist medical and nursing support can be provided throughout 24 hours;
- Equipment: must be both available and maintained adequately;
- Support services: appropriate support services (e.g. radiology, genetics) may be essential to the care of some infants;
- Environment: both the working environment for staff and facilities for other family members should be appropriate.

These issues are considered in more detail in Chapter 3, Standards and audit.

OUTSIDE ASSESSMENT

The NHS reforms of the early 1990s introduced a number of fundamental changes. In particular, responsibility for determining health care priorities (i.e. where and how health care funding should be spent) was moved from central government to a local level. These local 'purchasers' of care were separated managerially from the local organizations (in general hospitals) which provided care ('providers'). Although this was politically attractive it was recognized that these changes might adversely affect some aspects of healthcare provision. As a safeguard the Act which enabled the main reforms also established an independent body (the Clinical Standards Advisory Group, CSAG) with the remit to monitor all aspects of care delivered to patients. The CSAG, by commissioning research, is able to investigate, at its discretion, any branch of the NHS about which there is concern. There have been two reviews of neonatal intensive care.

1st CSAG report 1993[4]

There was anxiety that the introduction of local purchasing would rapidly distort patterns of service delivery.[21] It was felt that high-cost low-volume services would be most at risk, since purchasers might decide to constrain costs without due regard to the quality of care, encouraging local units to provide services previously delivered in specialist tertiary centres. Four services were investigated for evidence of such an effect 1 year after the introduction of the reforms, of which neonatal intensive care was one. The first report indicated the following:

- There was inadequate provision of neonatal intensive care cots nationally.
- Demand was still rising.
- The purchaser–provider system was little more than rudimentary, and hence quite unable to influence service provision at that stage.

2nd CSAG report 1996[5]

The neonatal service described in the first report was far from satisfactory, and the exercise was repeated 3 years later. Conclusions were as follows:

- Local purchasing had been a factor in increasing the number of local units offering intensive care.
- Demand appeared to have reached a plateau and was being met more readily.
- Purchasing arrangements were still largely rudimentary.
- The development of local services had not been subject to appraisal against recognized quality criteria.

The report also expressed a more non-specific concern that the structure that was emerging had no mechanism for adequately recognizing the additional clinical costs involved in training. As a result, units involved in training were financially unattractive to purchasers. In addition, the high workloads, necessary for junior doctors and nurses to gain experience, were falling in some teaching centres as outside referrals became less common.

The Audit Commission – 'Children First'[1]

The Audit Commission was established to oversee the financial management of local government. Its area of responsibility was widened in the late 1980s to include the NHS. The particular remit was to assess services in terms of whether they provided 'value for money'. The review of all hospital-based children's services in 1992 included neonatal care. Main points included:

- Few quality standards were in place (the gross variation (5%–25%) in the percentage of newborns admitted by individual hospitals for neonatal care was used as a particular example).
- Outcome data relating to later morbidity were sparse; a standardized national approach was recommended.
- The authors felt that there was adequate evidence to support the concept of centralized care (high throughput) being associated with better outcome in terms of survival.

Changing Childbirth 'Choice and Control'[8]

Public concern that childbirth had become too orientated towards hospital-based obstetrician-led delivery caused the government to carry out a review. The findings and recommendations were published in the above report. The central theme was that women should be offered greater choice in terms of both place of delivery and which professional groups provided that care. Although it was suggested that this policy change would herald an increase in the number of home births, there has been little to suggest that such an effect has taken place. However, the number of midwife-led delivery services, based in hospital maternity units, has increased.

TINA[29]

A serious road traffic accident involving an ambulance carrying a baby requiring intensive care[17] led to a formal review of neonatal transport arrangements in the UK by the Medical Devices Agency. The report – TINA – highlighted a number of problems:

- Wall clamps as a means of securing incubators in ambulances (in widespread use across the UK) are totally inadequate to provide restraint in the event of an accident. On closer consideration it became clear that even if the clamps were able to hold the trolley during an impact, the chassis of a standard ambulance was not.
- It was unreasonable to expect that any transport system weighing more than 200 lb could be carried safely in a standard ambulance (some of the systems examined weighed in excess of 700 lb). The validity of indemnity arrangements for staff injured in any accident and using such equipment seemed unclear, given that the situation was known to be unsafe.
- Existing Health and Safety legislation regarding manual handling was regularly breached by neonatal transport systems.
- Arrangements for staff training were patchy.
- The use of air transport was associated with many additional hazards, which appeared to have been fully addressed by only one transport service in the UK.

The report encouraged ambulance and hospital trusts to remedy these problems by issuing new official 'guidance'. Although Health and Safety legislation covered some areas of concern, measures to deal with the remaining deficiencies were left to the discretion of individual transport services.

DEFINITIONS

Traditionally the work of the neonatal service has been subdivided as follows:

- Normal care: that which could reasonably be expected to be given by the parents;
- Special care: for babies requiring some specialist medical or nursing input;
- Intensive care (sometimes divided into level 1 and level 2, or intensive care and high-dependency care): for babies requiring continuous medical and nursing support.

Within the UK a number of definitions exist relating to this broad structure (the most widely used is given in Table 3.7), and around the world there are further variations. These systems have been developed from clinical interest to allow the work of any one unit to be monitored over time and as an aid to audit. These classifications do not recognize complexity of care, multisystem failure or disease severity, i.e. they do not differentiate between the work of different types of unit.

In general the clinical classifications have not been validated as a marker of cost, although there are some notable exceptions.[9] Their inherent complexity has produced considerable confusion as greater priority has been given to cost in general. As a result, those interested in economics have looked at measures of activity more appropriate for their purposes, that is, simple to ascribe, easy to understand and related to cost. These have included diagnostic related groups, popular in the USA, which lump together patients likely to use similar amounts of 'resource', e.g. all those babies of a particular birthweight or gestation. More sophisticated versions of this type of system can go some way towards recognizing the complexity of care. Within the UK, health resource groupings have so far been the preferred approach. Here infants are banded together on the basis of their ICD code, predicting similar resource use. The use of HRGs is proving difficult, as many of the costs relating to neonatal care are determined by disease severity or interventions and not diagnosis.

It is important to understand that the two approaches to classification (clinical and for costing) are not the same. Within a service both are likely to be required, and ideally the routine collection of clinical data should allow cost codes to be derived automatically. Harmonization of classifications across wide geographical areas has obvious advantages for comparisons of both clinical practice and cost.

INTENSIVE-CARE COT PROVISION

Neonatal care is expensive and many of the costs remain fixed, even when the unit is operating below capacity. Therefore, although too few cots might deny access to those who could benefit, it is important that provision is not excessive. Over the last 20 years the intensive-care cot requirements for the UK have been variously estimated to be between 0.4 and 1.5 cots per 1000 births.[16,18,19,24,27] These exercises have been fraught with difficulty for a number of reasons:

- Definitions of intensive care changed.
- Demand for neonatal intensive care appeared to rise between 1970 and the early 1990s. The rate of rise and the point at which demand stabilized appeared to vary around the UK.
- Some estimates were derived from unit-based data, which were markedly affected by referral bias.
- Some estimates were based simply on opinion.

In general the situation now appears stable (Tables 2.3 and 2.4).

Two more recent studies have addressed this issue and have benefited from:

- population-based data;
- stable workload;
- consistent definitions over time.

Both reported figures of approximately 1.2 cots per 1000 births.[3,19] However, a number of other factors must also be taken into account when extrapolating these figures to other populations:

- Distribution of cots: for maximum efficiency cots should either be in a single unit or in a group of units that work cooperatively. If such arrangements do not exist a significant increase in provision will be required, as each unit will need to plan for random peaks in demand.
- Local geography: isolated communities face special problems and those responsible for planning health care may choose to make special provision outside a more general strategy.
- Variation in demand: there is evidence that the demand for neonatal intensive care is not uniform. Those responsible for local services must ensure that the 'norm' of intensive-care cot provision is appropriate for their community.
- Additional provision will need to be made for babies requiring neonatal surgery and/or cardiothoracic expertise.

Concern that improved survival among infants 'at the limit of viability' might lead to an increasing demand for neonatal intensive care cots does not seem justified on the basis of the above figures (Tables 2.3 and 2.4) or other published work.[2] Similar worries about infants with chronic lung disease are harder to interpret. This is because not only can these infants be defined in two separate ways, rates may be based on a variety of denominators (e.g. all births 32 weeks' gestation or less; births 32 weeks' gestation or less requiring ventilation; all births 32 weeks' gestation or less surviving 28 days, etc.). With these difficulties in mind it is fair to comment that the current incidence appears stable (Table 2.5).

OUTCOME

This topic is discussed in more detail elsewhere (Chapter 7); however, the measurement of outcome is important in determining that the organization of neonatal services is operating appropriately.

For clinicians involved in delivering the service, information relating to survival and late morbidity are the most important priorities to assess performance. Comparison of the crude survival rates achieved by different neonatal units is difficult because of potential variations in case mix. As discussed earlier, the introduction of the

Table 2.3 Data relating to old Oxford RHA. Definition of NIC up to and including 1992 based on BAPP recommendation 1984, data for 1993 and 1994 based on BAPM recommendation 1993

	1990	1991	1992	1993	1994
Average no. of babies receiving intensive care per day	20.4	20.2	19.2	21.6	22.8

Table 2.4 Trent RHA data 1991–94. Intensive-care definition based on BAPP recommendation 1984

Year	1991	1992	1993	1994
Days of ventilation	5752	5749	5839	5704
Days of ITC level 1	7789	7843	7702	7433
No. of babies < 32 weeks	863	823	902	882

Table 2.5 Incidence of chronic lung disease in Trent. Percentage and number (*n*) of ventilated babies 32 weeks' gestation or less developing chronic lung disease in Trent Health Region (UK). All babies involved in a transfer have been excluded. Chronic lung disease defined as oxygen/respiratory support dependent at 28 days of age. Denominator infants ≤ 32 weeks' gestation who required ventilation and survived at least 28 days.

	1992	1993	1994	1995
Percentage (*n*) with CLD	34 (85)	41 (101)	41 (101)	33 (74)

CRIB scoring system in 1990 provided a means of adjusting mortality rates by correcting for disease severity.[14]

Although CRIB has allowed the performance of neonatal units to be compared in terms of survival, no similar mechanism exists in relation to neurodevelopmental outcome. Individual neonatal units do perform regular neurodevelopmental examinations, but without standardization in terms of initial disease severity, nature and timing of review, these data are very difficult to interpret. A standardized approach for the UK has now been proposed which may overcome these difficulties.[7]

Those responsible for allocating resources at a local level will want to monitor survival and morbidity data, but they will also have a different agenda wanting to address broader issues of cost-effectiveness. For example, they will want to be reassured that length of stay (both in intensive care and overall) is comparable between units.

Where more than one unit provides services for a geographical area it will be important to look also at outcome data for the population, rather than by unit. This will allow the performance of the whole perinatal service to be monitored, taking account of interventions such as antenatal screening and intrapartum care.

TRAINING

Three different reforms/reorganizations are currently influencing the training of doctors and nurses in neonatal care:

- Specialist training is, at present, largely the responsibility of the old regional centres, as it is essential to have a high workload in order to provide the experience needed for training purposes. However, it may not be possible to maintain this situation if the remnants of the old regional structure are completely lost in the coming years. It is crucial that units of sufficient size to offer experience are protected if the service is to continue to develop.
- In keeping with other EU countries specialist medical training in the UK has become more structured. The proposed curriculum relies not only on the availability of a large patient base, but also on an adequate number of trained neonatologists to provide teaching. Current estimates of the numbers of neonatologists practising in the UK suggest that this target may be difficult to meet.
- Reforms of junior doctors' hours of work have considerably increased the number of senior house officers required to staff neonatal units. Some units have chosen to address this issue by using instead neonatal nurses with enhanced skills in intensive care of the newborn: nurse practitioners. Not all nurse practitioners work in this way, however, many having major roles in continuing education and service development. These individuals, who have undergone significant extra training, are certainly not a cheap way of providing medical cover. Nurse practitioners have been very important in allowing some smaller units to undertake neonatal care when this had not been possible before.

COST

The subject of cost is covered elsewhere (Chapter 4); however, there are important points that must be considered in relation to organization. As neonatal care has evolved in the UK a variety of very different units have emerged, all of which apparently provide neonatal intensive care. Approaches taken in contracts to identifying and describing intensive care activity (and hence the cost of what is provided) show marked variation, e.g.:

- Nothing: all neonatal activity being covered by a single block contract relating to, for example, all paediatric and or maternity activity;
- Consultant episodes: this approach measures all admissions to a neonatal service irrespective of gestation or disease severity; as a result, a 26-week gestation infant and a grunting term infant are equal in cost terms;
- Intensive care episode: similar to the above but only infants who receive intensive care of any duration are included;
- Intensive care activity: a minority of units base their costs on their measured intensive care activity, e.g. days of ventilation.

In theoretical terms large units should be able to provide neonatal care more cheaply than smaller units because of economies of scale.[11] The above costing/pricing mechanisms are largely too rudimentary to allow any such differences to emerge. Those who must decide where to allocate resources also have other pressures. A small local maternity unit has fixed costs which are not removed by moving all the babies that need intensive care to the regional centre. However, in local terms there may well be cost savings from carrying out limited intensive care on selected infants and transferring only babies identified as being more complex. As a result the case mix of referral centres includes a higher proportion of infants needing prolonged intensive care, but few of the current pricing structures recognize this fact.

THE FUTURE

The NHS reforms have initiated a process of evolution which is still ongoing. What has emerged is a more heterogeneous service, with intensive care provided by a wider range of professionals in a greater variety of hospitals. Most recent data indicate that this is without any detriment in terms of short-term outcome. The old regional units remain at the centre, taking more complex babies and coping with peaks in demand in smaller hospitals nearby. In addition, they continue to be responsible for education and research. However, whereas in the early days of neonatal care it was the enthusiasm of individuals that determined the nature of the service, now it is money and costs. Unfortunately, mechanisms for assessing cost-effectiveness and anything other than short-term outcome remain largely rudimentary. Therefore, in considering the future of the neonatal service it is essential that a balance is struck between a desire to deliver local services and the need to maintain specialist centres capable of developing the specialty. Unless the different contribution of the larger centres is recognized we are in danger of seeing the neonatal service threatened by:

- inefficiency: because of the need to replicate infrastructure on so many sites;
- lack of a training base: too few large services will remain;
- lack of a research base: insufficient units with a critical mass.

REFERENCES

1. Audit Commission 1992 Children first: a study of hospital services. Audit Commission services report No 7. London, HMSO
2. Bohin S, Mason E S, Clarke M, Field D J 1996 Outcome of extremely low birthweight infants/contribution to ITC workload made by very low birthweight infants. Archives of Disease in Childhood 74: F110–113
3. Burton P, Draper E, Fenton A, Field D 1995 Neonatal intensive care cots: estimating the requirements in Trent, UK. Journal of Epidemiology and Community Health 48: 617–628
4. Clinical Standards Advisory Group 1993 Access and availability of neonatal intensive care. London, HMSO
5. Clinical Standards Advisory Group 1996 Access and availability of neonatal intensive care. Second report. London, HMSO
6. Dear P R F, McLain B I 1987 Establishment of an intermediate care ward for babies and mothers. Archives of Disease in Childhood 62: 597–600
7. Disability and perinatal care: measurement at 2 years. A report of 2 working groups convened by the National Prenatal Epidemiology Unit and Oxford Regional Health Authority. Oxford, NPEU, 1994.
8. Expert Maternity Group. Changing Childbirth. Part 1. 1993 London HMSO
9. Field D, Hodges S, Mason E, Burton P 1989. The demand for neonatal intensive care. British Medical Journal 299: 1305–1308
10. Field D, Hodges S, Mason E, Burton P 1991 Survival and place of delivery. Archives of Disease in Childhood 66: 408–411
11. Fordham R, Field D, Hodges S, Normand C, Mason E, Burton P 1992 Cost of neonatal care across a regional health authority. Journal of Public Health Medicine 14: 127–130
12. House of Commons Committee of Public Accounts 1990 35th Report Maternity Services. London, HMSO
13. House of Commons Health Committee session 1991–1992. Second report: Maternity Services. London, HMSO
14. International Neonatal Network 1993 The CRIB (clinical risk index for babies) score: a tool for assessing initial neonatal risk and comparing performance of neonatal units. Lancet 342: 193–198
15. Lamont R F, Dunlop P D M, Crowley P 1983 Comparative mortality and morbidity of infants transferred in utero or postnatally. Journal of Perinatal Medicine 11: 200–203
16. Liaison Committee of the British Paediatric Association and the Royal College of Obstetricians and Gynaecologists 1977 Recommendations for the improvement of infant care during the perinatal period in the UK. London, BPA/RCOG
17. Madar R J, Milligan D W A 1994 Neonatal transport: safety and security. Archives of Disease in Childhood 71: F147–148
18. Medical care of the newborn in England and Wales. A report by the Royal College of Physicians. London, Royal College of Physicians, 1988
19. Morris D, Cottrell AJ, Hey EN 1993 Requirements for neonatal cots. A Northern Neonatal Network Study. Archives of Disease in Childhood 68: 544–599
20. Paneth N, Kiely J L, Wallenstein S, Marcus M, Parker J, Susser M 1982 Newborn intensive care and neonatal mortality in low birthweight babies. New England Journal of Medicine 307: 149–155
21. Pope C, Wild D 1992 Putting the clock back thirty years: neonatal services since the 1991 NHS reforms. Archives of Disease in Childhood 67: 879–881
22. Report by the Comptroller and Auditor General 1990 Maternity Services. London, HMSO
23. Roy R N, Kitchen W H 1977 NETS: a new system for neonatal transport. Medical Journal of Australia 2: 855–858
24. Sheldon Report 1974 Report of the expert group on the special care of babies. DHSS Report on Public Health and Medical Subjects, No 127. London, HMSO
25. Shenai J P, Major C W, Gaylord M S et al. 1991 A successful decade of regionalised perinatal care in Tennessee: the neonatal experience. Journal of Perinatology 11: 137–143
26. Short Report 1980 Perinatal and Neonatal Mortality. Second Report from the Social Services Committee. London, HMSO
27. Simpson H, Walker G 1981 Estimating the cots required for neonatal intensive care. Archives of Disease in Childhood. 56: 90–93
28. Sims D G, Wynn J, Chiswick M L 1982 Outcome for babies declined admission to a regional neonatal intensive care unit. Archives of Disease in Childhood 57: 334–337
29. Transport of neonates in ambulances (TINA). Medical Devices Agency. London 1995
30. Verloove-Vanhorick S P, Verwes R A, Ebeling M C A, Brand R, Ruys J H 1988 Mortality in very preterm and low birthweight infants according to place of delivery and level of care: results of a national collaborative survey of preterm and low birthweight infants in The Netherlands. Pediatrics 81: 404–411
31. Victorian Infant Study Group 1991 Eight year outcome in infants with birthweight of 500 to 999 grams: continuing regional study of 1979 and 1980 births. Journal of Pediatrics 118: 761–767
32. Wariyar U, Richmond S, Hey E 1989 Increased mortality of preterm infants transferred between perinatal centres. British Medical Journal 298: 318
33. Yu Y V, Wong P J, Bajuk B, Orgill A A, Astbury J 1986 Outcome of extremely low birthweight infants. British Journal of Obstetrics and Gynaecology 93: 162–170

3

Standards and clinical audit

Neil Marlow

WHAT IS AUDIT?

Clinical audit provides a framework for systematic review of the clinical process. In contrast to research, where an underlying hypothesis is formally tested, clinical audit is the process by which a clinical service is assessed against standards which may be set nationally or locally. Such a process must be distinguished from financial audit although clinical audit itself may have important financial consequences for the service.

In the UK, medical audit was promoted by the Government in 1989 as a means of protecting the interests of patients in the new health market, but it is clear that many services are based upon access and availability, or personal style directed by consultants, rather than pure evidence-based practice. Nonetheless, audit may assist us in uncovering ineffective interventions or processes and act as a stimulus to widening the evidence base to our practice, as part of continuing medical education. A well-administered audit programme should allow us to observe better outcomes and to be more cost-effective in our practice by ensuring the highest quality of clinical care.

As distinct from medical audit (which solely involves doctors and was the original spark to the establishment of formal audit within the UK health system), there is now consensus that all health care professional groups should contribute to the audit process from its conception to completion. Neonatal and perinatal care provide prime examples of areas of clinical practice which are truly multidisciplinary and where collaboration between medical staff across two major disciplines, together with midwives, neonatal nurses and practitioners and other health professionals, must occur if the service is to be adequately assessed. Indeed, audit and quality assurance are not recent developments and have been important aspects of many non-medical areas in the UK health system since well before emphasis was placed on medical audit in the Health Service reforms proposed in 1989. In one area of audit, perinatal medicine has led other areas of medical practice – the publishing of maternal and neonatal mortality statistics. These have now received international calibration through recommendations published by FIGO[26] and help to measure the effectiveness of each country's maternity services.

THE CLINICAL AUDIT PROCESS

Clinical audit may be carried out at a variety of levels. Most will be carried out within clinical directorates or units and this will form the base of most of this discussion. However, trusts/hospitals will need to audit activity which relates to cross-disciplinary practice, for example staff hours of work, clinic attendances, infection control practice. This will be part purchaser/government led within the contracting process and part trust/hospital led for reasons of finance or quality of care. Purchasers or governments may require (and should fund) health quality measures as part of their contract or as part of an external validation system, for example ISO 9000 standards[20] or the WHO 'baby friendly initiative'. It has been recommended that each neonatal intensive care unit produces a formal annual report, which is an audit of its activity, and that within this report activity relating to audit is identified.[13]

Audit may be undertaken of three areas of service:

- the structure of the service
- the process of care
- the outcome of care or the result of clinical intervention.

THE STRUCTURE OF THE SERVICE

This is concerned with the quantity and type of resources available and how they are used, for example the number and experience of medical, nursing or paramedical staff, the number of cots, the number of ventilators. These data are relatively simple to collect and are usually accurate. When related to population, deficiencies in service provision may be identified. Two structure-based audits of UK neonatal service provision have been performed since 1989[32] in order to evaluate changing resource availability since the NHS organizational changes. Many reports have defined which level of resources were required on a population basis for neonatal and neonatal intensive care services[22,42] and what were appropriate staffing levels for such services.[39] Because of a lack of research- or audit-based information these have been widely criticized. More recently the document 'Standards for Hospitals Providing Neonatal Intensive Care' has been published.[13] These standards provide clear recommendations for service structure, identifying the research basis for the recommendations wherever possible (see below). Such recommendations are able to form the basis for objective audit of neonatal care.[10]

Audit of structure by itself will only demonstrate potential areas where services may be inadequate and does not form a measure of quality of care until it is matched with patient-based information when it merges with the remaining two forms of audit. Structural deficiencies identified by audit may provide an explanation for poor results found during process or outcome audit.

THE PROCESS OF CARE

This may be considered in three areas:[18]

- the way patients progress through the system
- the way particular resources are used
- the way particular disorders are managed.

The way patients progress through the system

Examples of this would be admission and discharge procedures, recording of data in the clinical notes and the recording of communication with parents. Such audits form the backbone of clinical audit at the local level. Guidelines for the audit of clinical notes in paediatrics have been published and form a useful framework on which to base an audit, defining criteria which are both considered good practice and are simple to identify.[16]

The way particular resources are used

Examples would be attendance at delivery by paediatric SHOs, occupancy and casemix studies, use of transitional care facilities. This is an important group of topics which may have immense implications for the running of the service – for example we achieved a significant reduction in attendance at deliveries at our hospital by auditing which deliveries junior staff were being called to and the risk of resuscitation being required; we achieved a shorter stay in the NICU by freeing up beds on a transitional care ward by restricting admissions from other wards following audit and review of criteria for admission.

The way particular disorders are managed

Examples here relate to particular admission criteria (e.g. tachypnoea), to diagnostic groups (e.g. respiratory distress syndrome) or to therapeutic interventions (e.g. surfactant replacement therapy). In this area, evidence-based guidelines are becoming available covering the management of several neonatal conditions (see below). If an area is targeted that is not covered by such protocols, a formal literature search will be required to accompany the background work for the project.

THE OUTCOME OF CARE OR THE RESULT OF CLINICAL INTERVENTION

Audit of outcome provides the final arbiter of success for a service and addresses mortality or morbidity which accrue from medical intervention. Neonatal and perinatal mortality rates are clearly defined (Table 3.1), widely available and collated nationally, producing encouraging trends of improving mortality rates over recent years (Fig. 3.1). Although these offer the opportunity to set local targets and to review local performance, extreme care should be exercised in the interpretation of such data, which may be particularly susceptible to random variation due to small numbers (see below).

Table 3.1 Perinatal definitions[46]

Livebirth	Baby with signs of life observed after complete expulsion from the mother, irrespective of the duration of pregnancy (signs of life include breathing, heart beat, cord pulsation or voluntary movement)
Stillbirth (or late fetal death)	Fetal death prior to complete delivery of a baby born after the 24th week of pregnancy (168 days after the first day of the last menstrual period (LMP))
Abortion	A conceptus born without signs of life before the end of the 24th week of pregnancy (< 168 days from LMP)
Birthweight	The first weight of the fetus or newborn infant obtained after birth (preferably within the first hour)
Gestational age	The duration of gestation measured from the first day of the last menstrual period and expressed in complete weeks or days
Preterm	< 37 completed weeks (< 259 days)
Term	From 37 to less than 42 completed weeks' gestation (259–293 days)
Post-term	42 completed weeks or more (> 293 days)
The neonatal period	The first 28 days after delivery
Lethal congenital malformation	Death primarily due to congenital malformation

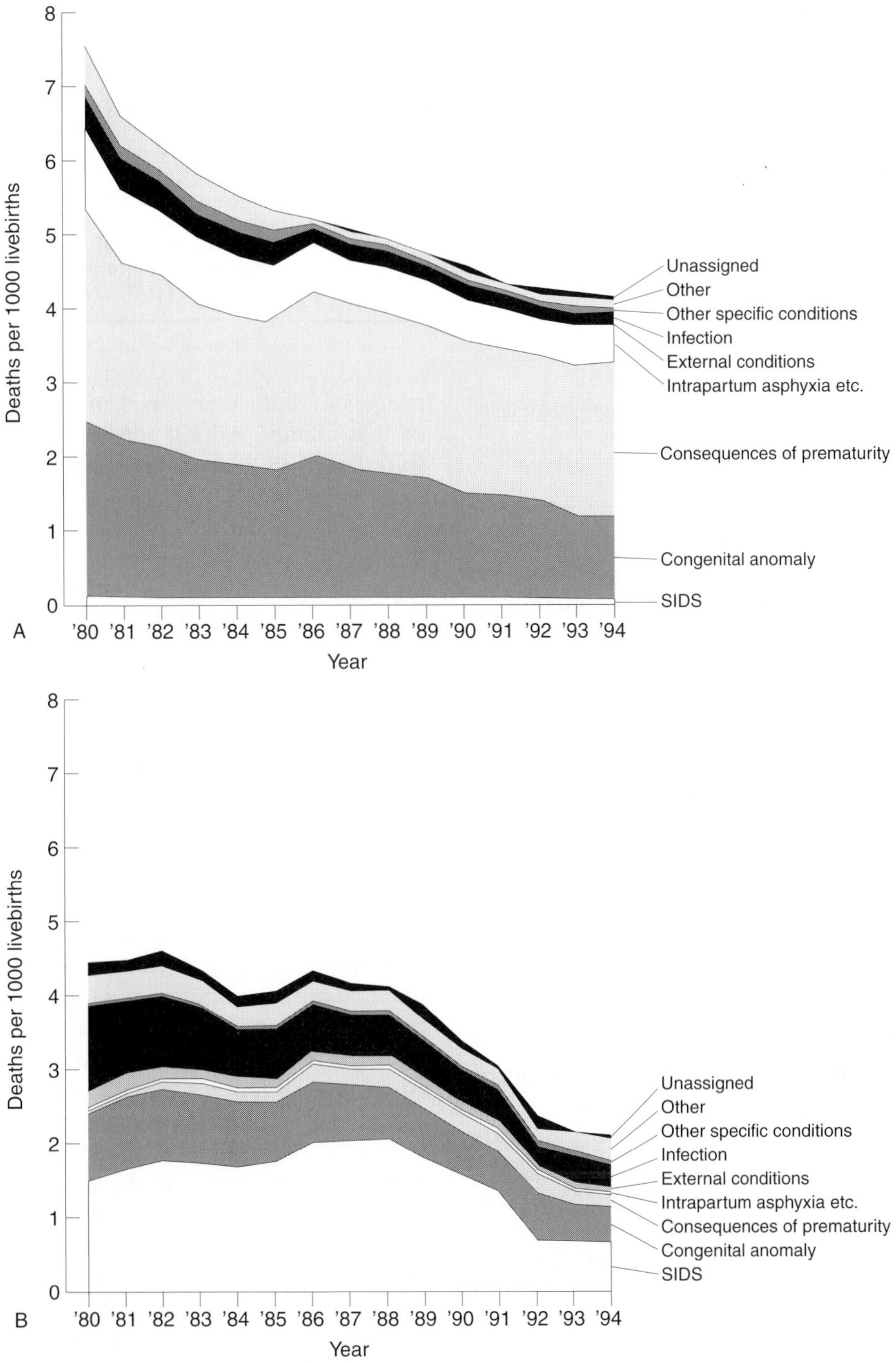

Fig. 3.1 Wigglesworth classification and neonatal/postneonatal mortality England and Wales 1980–1994: (A) neonatal mortality; (B) postneonatal mortality. (Source: OPCS)

Morbidity may be assessed within populations from individual units, geographic regions or nationally and may be sought for children who have been exposed to a particular intervention (e.g. a new ventilation strategy or medication). Rates may reflect short-term endpoints from the initial admission to a neonatal intensive care unit (e.g. rates of intraventricular haemorrhage, periventricular leukomalacia, chronic lung disease), medium-term outcomes (e.g. developmental outcomes at 2 years) or very long-term outcomes during school age. Care must be taken to control carefully for potential confounders, e.g. social factors and initial disease severity measures, which may have equal or greater roles in determining these latter outcomes.

Many units and districts have reported medium- and long-term morbidity rates for populations at risk of later disability, usually based on very low birthweight or very preterm populations. In contrast to mortality rates, which

Table 3.2 Health status and prematurity – definition of severe disability at 2 years[34]

Domain	Criterion
Motor	
Walking	Unable to walk
Sitting	Unable to sit without support
Hand use	Unable to feed self with either hand
Head control	Unable to control head without support
Communication	
Comprehension	Unable to understand five words or signs
Expression	Unable to express five words or signs
Vision	Sees light only or blind
Hearing	Hearing uncorrected even with aids
Cognitive function	Function below 50% of age-appropriate level
Malformation	
Other disabling condition	

Table 3.3 Components of the audit cycle

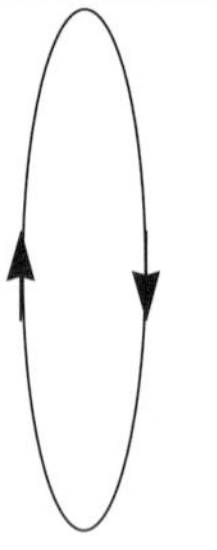

- Identification of audit subject (observation of practice)
- Setting of locally relevant standards of practice
- Definition of criteria for audit
- Comparison of practice against standard for defined criteria
- Implementation of changes based upon this comparison
- Re-observation of practice following changes
- Feedback of information to staff/consideration of the need for further audit cycle ('closing the loop')

are tightly defined both nationally and internationally, there is little agreement about measures of morbidity, making comparisons between studies very difficult. Where population-based studies have reported data based upon constant definitions there is a clear trend to increasing numbers of normal survivors.[45] In an attempt to standardize outcome studies, two working parties have produced clear statements on what data should be reported and how these might be collected nationally.[34] The combined reports recommended that an assessment of preterm populations at 2 years was most likely to produce results which would reflect current care practices and have recommended reporting outcomes in a series of health domains, in each of which criteria for severe disability are defined (see Table 3.2). These criteria require long-term validation, which is ongoing, but will facilitate interstudy comparisons, which can be furthered by the inclusion of key data points in publications.[33]

Professional and National Health Service indicators are currently being developed which may allow some comparison of different services, usually based on relatively few key outcome measures. However, within a high-cost and low-volume service, such as neonatal intensive care, the power of such comparisons may be so low as to make such practice potentially dangerous. Even within this development, audit tools are required to correct for casemix differences. The clinical risk index for babies is one such measure which has been developed specifically to facilitate such comparison,[30] although the power of even such compensated comparisons remains low.

THE AUDIT CYCLE

Whenever audit is effected there is a common series of processes which are required to complete the 'cycle' of audit. Completing this cycle is important and the weakest link is the process by which experience gained in the process of audit is returned to clinical care and the effect of that change is itself measured. The cycle of audit is well described and comprises a series of discrete steps as defined in Table 3.3.

The identification of topics for audit may be defined locally, be specified as part of a contract or as part of a regional or national initiative. For some time the American Academy of Pediatrics has issued statements of policy or guidelines in several neonatal topics which can also form the basis for audit. In the UK, the Royal College of Paediatrics and Child Health has established an audit group which selects, initiates and prioritizes topics for consideration for audit and formulates guidelines in these areas.

PROBLEMS WITH THE AUDIT PROCESS

Despite a huge investment, audit has not won the hearts and minds of many doctors. Part of this is the failure to understand the importance of a scientific base to collection, analysis and interpretation of audit data, which is as important in the audit process as it is in research. Appropriate support for audit, in terms of manpower and expertise, is critical for success, and is often not available. Correctly supported and executed, audit may make an important contribution to the success of a neonatal service.

Much audit is achieved by examining case records. Prospective collection of data is preferable but this usually demands excessive extra resources. Retrospective audit from case records is fraught with difficulty which must be acknowledged and investigated as part of the process. Problems that occur in retrospective reviews (and to some extent in prospective audits) are:[29]

1. bias due to poor diagnostic coding
2. bias in record retrieval (e.g. difficulty in identifying deaths)
3. bias related to sample size
4. reliability of audit data (e.g. variation in recording/definition between patients and errors in filing of data results in notes)
5. bias due to missing data
6. inadequate capture of 'non-routine' data to be used in audit

7. casemix and co-morbidity
8. inability to assess quality aspects of care: timeliness, coordination, continuity, empathic components and appropriateness.

A good audit project will address these deficiencies in the planning stage to avoid major errors. It is also important to decide how changes in management deemed necessary as a result of an audit are to be effected. The line of action and responsibility for implementation need to be carefully addressed; it is not adequate or acceptable to blame the notes retrieval service or managerial staff for inadequacies in a project if they are not involved at its inception. Financial consequences of audit must be identified and early managerial involvement is clearly crucial to the success of a project.

It is important that personnel in support services provided by the trust/hospital are therefore trained in wider aspects of audit to ensure that the above pitfalls may be avoided. Medical and nursing education must be expanded to include the assessment and processes involved in audit.

PERINATAL AUDIT TOOLS

PERINATAL MORTALITY

FIGO and the WHO have defined datasets which facilitate the international comparison of neonatal and perinatal morbidity (Table 3.4). In particular the definitions and methods of reporting data recommended by FIGO allow correction for major differences in neonatal service provision by presenting the information as totals, for babies without lethal malformations or greater than 1000 g birthweight or both

Table 3.4 International Federation of Gynecology and Obstetrics recommendations for the international collection of perinatal mortality statistics[26]

Data collection:
- Collect numbers of births ≥ 500 g birthweight, early and late neonatal deaths and identify stillbirths and neonatal deaths with lethal malformations and birthweight < 1000 g

Perinatal statistics:
- Lethal malformation rate per 1000 births
- Stillbirth rate per 1000 births (SBR)
- Neonatal mortality rate per 1000 livebirths (NMR)
- Perinatal mortality rate per 1000 births (PNMR)

Excluding lethal malformations (includes babies < 1000 g birthweight):
- SBR, NMR, PNMR

Excluding lethal malformations and births < 1000 g birthweight:
- SBR, NMR, PNMR

Excluding births < 1000 g birthweight (includes lethal malformations):
- SBR, NMR, PNMR

Table 3.5 WHO international classification of impairments disabilities and handicaps

Impairment:	Any loss or abnormality of psychological, physiological or anatomical structure or function
Disability:	Any restriction or lack (resulting from an impairment) of ability to perform an activity in the manner or within the range considered normal for a human being
Handicap:	A disadvantage for a given individual, resulting from an impairment or disability, that limits or prevents the fulfilment of a role that is normal (depending on age, sex and social and cultural factors) for that individual

MORBIDITY

Morbidity may be defined in terms of conditions, impairments, disabilities or handicaps (Table 3.5). Although conditions (e.g. cerebral palsy) and impairments (e.g. chronic oxygen dependency) may be useful outcomes for specific scenarios, the impact that these make upon the individual – or the disability produced – may be preferable as a measure of outcome as many children with cerebral palsy, for example, have relatively little disability.

Published criteria for the definition of severe disability at 2 years corrected for prematurity are described in Table 3.2. These are outcomes considered to be predictive of later dependency, although the veracity of this statement requires testing. It was considered that 2 years was better than 1 year in view of the inaccuracy in prediction of later gross developmental milestones at 1 year in the very preterm. Ideally, for complete ascertainment of impairment, children should also be assessed in school but this is beyond the resources of most neonatal services and requires careful analysis, allowing for confounding social and demographic variables. Again ideally, this information could be collected through routine systems, such as the Child Health Computer or the Disability Register to avoid duplication of effort, but linking to neonatal records or a system of 'flagging' high-risk children identified in the neonatal period is necessary. At present the locality disability registers are geared to service need rather than the definition of disability per se.

Data definition and essential information for the reporting of outcome studies are published[37] and should be followed when reporting such data, either in a local report or in the medical press.

NEONATAL DATA RECORDING

Population data. Registration of birth and perinatal death provides an opportunity for universal data collection. These data may be targeted at information gathering or to provide ongoing data for subsequent health care, e.g. child health systems. In the UK there are several methods of data collection, which were brought together

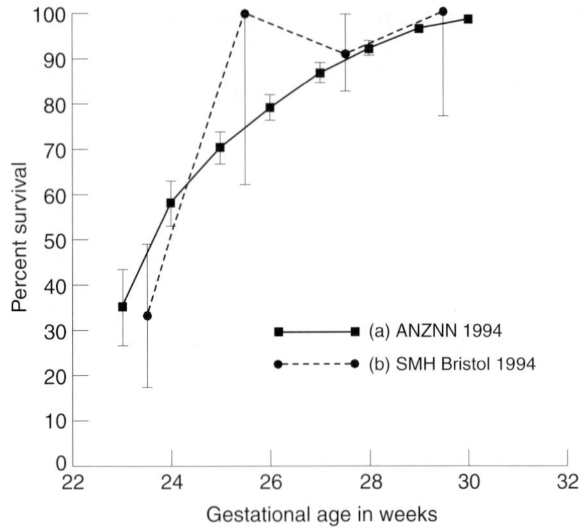

Fig. 3.2 Neonatal survival – effect of sample size (per cent survival; 95% CI).

in 1984 to provide a comprehensive picture of population variation and trends.[31] Standardization of collection of data has been attempted, e.g. DHSS Neonatal Discharge Form 1980, but local modifications to such documentation have reduced its value as a comparator. In Scotland birth data is collected in a standardized fashion (SMR11) and this provides an excellent source of population-based information. The national adoption of CESDI (confidential enquiry into stillbirths and deaths in infancy) has resulted in standardized reporting of perinatal death.

High-risk groups. In the UK there is no system for recording outcomes from neonatal intensive care and collating them on a national basis. Many NHS regions now collect such data but there is little attempt to standardize between regions. Even using regional data results in wide confidence intervals for estimates of important outcomes such as survival in very preterm children (Fig. 3.2).

As an example of good practice in this area, the Australian and New Zealand Neonatal Network have collated information from 22 NICUs from 1994 for babies <32 weeks' gestation or <1500 g birthweight. All units have a highly developed antenatal referral system with highly centralized care and well-organized neonatal retrieval services. In the first report of this collaboration[23] four main objectives were identified:

1. To provide a core dataset that will:
   a. identify trends and variations in mortality and morbidity which warrant further study
   b. enhance the ability to carry out multicentre studies and randomized trials
   c. provide information on neonatal outcomes adjusted for casemix and disease severity to assist with quality improvement
2. To monitor the use of new technologies
3. To develop and evaluate a risk score for babies in the network
4. To develop and assess clinical indicators for perinatal care through neonatal outcomes.

In the first year of data collection 2723 infants were registered and data in subsequent years will facilitate the achievement of these goals. An example of the power achieved using such a network is demonstrated by the narrow confidence intervals in Figure 3.2 plot (a) compared to a single UK teaching centre over 5 years (Fig. 3.2 plot (b)). In the USA, the Vermont-Oxford and SNAP networks are examples of similar initiatives.

CASEMIX CORRECTION

The clinical risk index for babies (CRIB score)[30]

The CRIB score, based upon a mix of patient-specific variables and markers of respiratory illness severity, is one of a range of tools which have been developed to adjust for casemix differences between units. Similar tools have been used to study outcomes in neonatal (SNAP) and paediatric[35,36] intensive care units in the USA in relation to unit staffing and structure. Other scoring systems have

Table 3.6 The CRIB score

Criterion	Allocated score
Birthweight (g)	
> 1350	0
851–1350	1
701–850	4
≤ 700	7
Gestation (weeks)	
> 24	0
≤ 24	1
Congenital malformations (excludes inevitably lethal malformations)	
None	0
Not acutely life threatening	1
Acutely life threatening	3
Maximum base excess in first 12 h (mmol/l)	
> −7.0	0
−7.0 to − 9.9	1
− 10 to − 14.9	2
≤ − 15	3
Minimum appropriate FiO_2 in first 12 h	
≤ 0.4	0
0.41–0.60	2
0.61–0.90	3
0.91–1.00	4
Maximum appropriate FiO_2 in first 12 h	
≤ 0.4	0
0.41–0.60	1
0.61–0.90	3
0.91–1.00	5

been designed to predict outcome based upon the intensity of therapeutic intervention.[27] The CRIB score (Table 3.6) comprises observations made at birth and after 12 hours, including birthweight, gestation, the presence of a malformation, lowest and highest oxygen concentrations and worst base deficit. One problem with such a score is that it reflects both the status of the child at birth, in terms of three measures, and also the severity of early illness in the child, which may be greatly modified by the quality of care. Adjusting outcomes using CRIB, therefore, may be used to compare the performance of units for babies more than 12 hours old; the components, and therefore the score, may also be considered to be outcomes.

CRIB predicts mortality in very low birthweight children more accurately than birthweight, gestation or other neonatal scoring systems (e.g. SNAP),[11] and may also be equally good at predicting poor outcome.[43] It was originally conceived that using CRIB would allow comparative performance of neonatal units to be assessed. Although some studies have demonstrated risk-adjusted outcomes to be better in larger units, others have failed to do so. At present there is no good evidence in the UK that outcome is different between large tertiary, teaching units and smaller district units, even allowing for casemix differences.

CRIB appears to be robust in that it has been used in studies of outcome in Australia, South Africa, Scotland, a

Table 3.7 Categories of babies requiring neonatal care[39]

Level 1 intensive care (maximal intensive care)
Care given in an intensive care nursery which provides continuous skill supervision by qualified and specially trained nursing and medical staff
Level 1 intensive care includes babies:
- receiving assisted ventilation (including continuous positive airway pressure) and in the first 24 h following withdrawal
- < 27 weeks' gestation for the first 48 h post-delivery
- < 1000 g for the first 48 h post-delivery
- requiring major surgery, for the preoperative period and postoperatively for 48 h
- on the day of death
- during transport by a team including medical and nursing staff
- receiving peritoneal dialysis
- requiring exchange transfusion complicated by other disease process
- with severe respiratory disease in the first 48 h of life requiring $FiO_2 > 0.6$
- who have recurrent apnoea needing frequent intervention, e.g. over five stimulations in 8 h or resuscitation with intermittent positive-pressure ventilation two or more times in 24 h
- who have a significant requirement for circulatory support, e.g. inotropes, three or more transfusions of colloid in 24 h, infusions of prostaglandins

Level 2 intensive care (high-dependency intensive care)
Care given in an intensive care nursery which provides continuous skill supervision by qualified and specially trained nursing staff who may care for more babies than in level 1 care. Medical supervision is not so immediate as in level 1 care
Level 2 intensive care includes babies:
- requiring parenteral nutrition
- who are having convulsions
- being transported by a trained skilled neonatal nurse alone
- with arterial line or chest drain
- with respiratory disease in the first 48 h of life requiring FiO_2 0.4–0.6
- with recurrent apnoea requiring stimulation up to five times in an 8-hour period or any resuscitation with IPPV
- who require an exchange transfusion alone
- more than 48 h post-operation and require complex nursing procedures
- with tracheostomy for the first 2 weeks

Special care
Care given in a special care nursery, transitional care ward, or postnatal ward which provides care and treatment exceeding normal routine care. Some aspects of special care may be undertaken by a mother supervised by qualified nursing staff
Special care should be provided for babies:
- requiring continuous monitoring of respiration, of heart rate or by transcutaneous transducers
- receiving additional oxygen
- with tracheostomy after the first 2 weeks
- being given intravenous glucose and electrolyte solutions
- who are being tube fed
- who have had minor surgery in the previous 24 h
- who require terminal care but not on the day of death
- being barrier nursed
- undergoing phototherapy
- receiving special monitoring (for example frequent glucose or bilirubin estimations)
- needing constant supervision (for example babies whose mothers are drug addicts)
- being treated with antibiotics

Normal care
Care given by the mother or mother substitute with medical or nursing advice if needed

Table 3.8 Summary of recommended staffing levels for neonatal intensive care units in the UK[13]

Nursing staff
- Senior nurse with management responsibility
- Designated nurse responsible for further education and in-service training
- One trained nurse per shift for each two neonatal intensive care cots (level 1 or level 2)
- One nurse per shift for each four special care cots
- One nurse per shift to provide one-to-one nursing when required (e.g. admission, transport) (plus sufficient staff on establishment to allow for leave, sickness, etc.)

Professional support staff
- Community support nurses and other roles not involved in direct patient care should be identified separately

Medical staff
- Named consultant responsible for the direction and management of the unit
- 24-h cover by consultants trained and experienced in the care of newborn babies (for referral units this should be by consultants whose principal duties are to neonatal care)
- 24-h cover by resident middle grade doctors with no *major* commitment to other clinical areas
- 24-h cover by senior house officer or more experienced professional with prime responsibility to the neonatal and maternity service

Table 3.9 Summary of two recommended minimum datasets to support annual reports for neonatal intensive care units[14]

Patient-based data	Unit-based data
*32 items and 8 optional data points**	*22 items to describe unit structure/staffing*
1. Name of hospital†	1. Name of hospital†
2. Mother's NHS number	2. Number of livebirths
3. Postcode of mother's residence at birth	3. Number of designated intensive care cots
4. Planned place of delivery at booking	4. Number of designated special care cots
5. Place of birth	**Nursing staff**:
6. Reason for change in place of birth	5. Funded nursing establishment by grade
7. Baby's NHS number	6. Nursing numbers in post by grade
8. Date of birth	7. Trained neonatal nursing numbers
9. Time of birth	8. Number of nurses in training
10. Source of admission to unit	9. Senior nurse with managerial responsibility
11. Reason for admission to unit	10. Nurse responsible for further education
12. Date of admission	**Medical staff:**
13. Date of discharge, transfer or death	11. Number of consultants with major involvement in neonatal care
14. Discharge or transfer destination	12. Consultant 24-hour cover
15. Reason for discharge or transfer	13. Resident middle grade 24-hour cover
16. Birthweight	14. Middle grade cover shared with paediatrics
17. Best estimate of gestation at delivery	15. Number of middle grade doctors providing cover
18. Plurality	16. Resident SHO 24-hour medical cover
19. Whether postmortem performed	17. Number of professionals contributing to 24-hour resident cover
20. Time of death	18. Number of advanced neonatal nurse practitioners
21. Early neonatal encephalopathy	19. Neonatal transport service
22. Retinopathy of prematurity examination	20. Babies receiving levels A and B care§
23. Retinopathy of prematurity stage	21. Babies receiving levels C & D care§
24. Therapy for retinopathy of prematurity	22. Transfer in requests refused
25. Cerebral ultrasound (as per policy)	
26. Hearing screening (as per policy)	
27. Days of endotracheal ventilation	
28. Days of CPAP	
29. Number of level 1 intensive care days‡	
30. Number of level 2 intensive care days‡	
31. Number of special care days	
32. Date of final added oxygen therapy	
• Gender	
• Air leak requiring drainage	
• Worst changes of intraventricular haemorrhage	
• Ventricular size	
• Cystic leukomalacia	
• Highest appropriate percentage inspired O_2	
• Lowest appropriate percentage inspired O_2	
• Worst base excess	

*These data points are defined in the dataset and comprise definitions for items which many units will collect, but do not form part of the minimum dataset.
†Variable common to both datasets.
‡British Association of Perinatal Medicine/Neonatal Nurses Association definition.
§Northern Neonatal Network definitions.

single UK region[11] and internationally, and has been shown to apply equally well to populations which include heavier infants and to more recent very low birthweight populations, born after the introduction of surfactant replacement therapy for RDS.

STANDARDS AND DATASETS FOR USE IN NEONATAL AUDIT

Several national and international standards for neonatal care have been published, including those for the reporting of mortality statistics noted above. Others include:

Standards for hospitals providing neonatal intensive care[13]

These are comprehensive standards for staffing, service size and management of neonatal intensive care services and represent best practice in the UK. They are based where possible on published evidence and cover service size, medical, nursing and paramedical staffing levels, equipment required, audit and continuing medical education within the neonatal intensive care unit. They complement previous attempts to define levels of care which can form the basis of the UK contracting process[39] (Table 3.7). In particular the levels of nurse staffing are based upon published reports from two UK services and represent the first attempt to make this evidence based (Table 3.8), whereas the levels of medical staffing are based upon Department of Health and British Paediatric Association guidelines. These have formed the basis for the review of neonatal services in the Audit Commission's 1997 report on maternity services.[10]

Minimum dataset for annual reports[14]

This document defines datapoints for collection of patient- and unit-based information for children admitted to a neonatal intensive care unit, which forms the basis for a unit annual report. It complements the similar, but more focused exercise published by the Australian and New Zealand Neonatal Network.[23] Individual datapoints (Table 3.9) are clearly and tightly defined and examples of how such a report should be presented are included. The aim of such recommendations is to bring neonatal unit data collection in line and facilitate comparison and the collection of information on a national level.

European Association of Perinatal Medicine report 'Perinatal Audit'[24]

This document describes methodology and suggests examples of criterion-based audit across the perinatal period for maternity and neonatal services. In it are defined many additional perinatal and outcome variables and it also contains suggested formats for tables and a suggested range of indicators (Table 3.10).

Table 3.10 Fetal and infant mortality and morbidity indicators proposed by the European Association of Perinatal Medicine working group on perinatal audit[24]

Death – including rates of:
- Fetal death
- Neonatal death
- Postneonatal death

Short-term outcome – five conditions:
- Respiratory distress syndrome
- Chronic lung disease
- Hypoxic/ischaemic encephalopathy
- Neonatal meningitis/encephalitis
- Spina bifida aperta

and three proxy indicators of conditions:
- Apgar score at 5 minutes after birth
- Number of days in a unit other than a 'well-baby' nursery
- Number of days of ventilatory assistance

Long-term outcome – seven conditions measured at 2 years of age and a measure of disability:
- Cerebral palsy
- Retinopathy of prematurity (stage 3 or worse)
- Cortical blindness
- Sensorineural deafness
- Severe developmental delay
- Growth disorder
- Congenital dislocation of the hip diagnosed after the age of 6 months

Severe disability at 2 years of age – any of:
- Is unable to sit unsupported
- Is unable to use hands for feeding
- Responds to light only or is blind
- Needs hearing aids
- Needs ongoing additional oxygen or ventilator support
- Needs special provision for feeding
- Has an overall developmental level of 1 year or less at 2 years

GUIDELINES FOR USE IN NEONATAL AUDIT

Perinatal care is one area of modern medicine which has embraced the concept of the controlled clinical trial. Thus in many areas it is possible to base good clinical practice on secure scientific evidence. The collation of these results for care in pregnancy and childbirth and for the care of the newborn,[44] for example as part of the Cochrane Collaboration,[25] has facilitated the dissemination of best practice and thus can facilitate audit. Although national bodies may publish guidelines for good practice from time to time (Table 3.11), clear information is needed for personnel at each unit and should be developed locally. Guidelines should give guidance and not comprise mandatory protocols. Care in the perinatal period should be tailored to the individual scenario and it may thus be necessary to deviate from unit guidelines if they are deemed inappropriate for a particular situation. However, default management plans are possible for many areas of care, and it is primarily for these that

Table 3.11 Examples of published guidelines for perinatal care

- Respiratory distress syndrome (BAPM 1992)[15]
- Neonatal resuscitation (BPA 1993)[38]
- Resuscitation of babies at birth (RCPCH/RCOG 1997)[41]
- Use of artificial surfactant (BAPM 1992)[12]
- Vitamin K administration to newborns (BPA 1992)[17]
- HIV guidelines (RCOG 1997)[40]
- Statements by the American Academy of Pediatrics:
  - Recording of the Apgar score (1996)[9]
  - Human milk, breastfeeding and transmission of human immunodeficiency virus (1995)[6]
  - Hospital stay for healthy term newborns (1995)[5]
  - The initiation or withdrawal of treatment for high-risk newborns (1995)[7,8]
  - The management of hyperbilirubinemia in the healthy term newborn (1994)[4]
  - Routine evaluation of blood pressure, hematocrit, and glucose in newborns (1993)[3]
  - Controversies concerning vitamin K and the newborn (1993)[2]
  - Guidelines for prevention of group B streptococcal infection by chemoprophylaxis (1992)[1]

guidelines make a valuable contribution to good practice. When guidelines are drawn up it is helpful to identify audit points and methods of audit so that prospective data collection may be made.

EXAMPLES OF AUDIT AT NATIONAL LEVEL

Structure audit – survey of neonatal intensive care facilities[32]

In 1989, before the NHS changes outlined in the UK Government White Paper 'Working for Patients' (1989) were enacted, the Standing Joint Committee of the BPA & Royal College of Obstetricians and Gynaecologists surveyed facilities which were available for sick newborn infants. Although not formally published, it was clear that there were major problems in data collection in many units for information other than basic structure (cots/staffing). Because of this, the exercise was repeated in 1994–5 and the results of this have been published. Changes in the designation of cots, consequent on the changing classification of neonatal intensive care,[19] have indicated that intensive care level 1 (maximal) and level 2 (high-dependency) cots have increased at the expense of special care cots. It is impossible without detailed research to determine the reasons for this shift, but some may have been a more appropriate recognition of work practices. Problems in data collection were identified and led to the development of the minimum dataset for annual reports (see above). This will become a regular review to identify demographic shifts in services and referral patterns.

Process audit – retinopathy of prematurity

In 1995 as part of a joint venture between the British Association of Perinatal Medicine, Royal College of Ophthalmologists and the RCPCH Research Unit an audit of the current policy and arrangements for screening and treatment of retinopathy of prematurity was undertaken. This was carried out to determine whether adequate services were available across the country for this disease which is potentially treatable by early intervention. As a result of this, a series of 'roadshows' have been established to raise the profile of services in this area across the country. To 'close the audit loop' the same survey will be undertaken after the education programme has been completed.

Outcome audit – Confidential Enquiry into Stillbirths and Deaths in Infancy

This national scheme for the investigation of perinatal and infant death was established in 1992 and began formal data collection and evaluation in 1993. The first report concentrates on intrapartum-related deaths, the second on sudden and unexplained deaths in infancy, and subsequent nested studies will evaluate other subgroups. The value of these data lies in their detailed appraisal by regionally convened expert panels and by the anonymous nature of the process, thereby facilitating objective assessment of clinical care. The first report,[21] which is of relevance to perinatal care, identified several common issues which require attention by relevant professional and managerial bodies, including:

- communication and record keeping – issues relating to training of staff in clear and sensitive communication with parents, audit of record keeping and standardization of case records
- the importance of professionally developed guidelines for all aspects of perinatal care
- the value of continuing training and education, including involvement in the CESDI process
- the need for particular regard with respect to standards and training in neonatal resuscitation
- recognition of the central position of the perinatal autopsy in clinical care.

Process and outcome – the British Paediatric Surveillance Unit

For conditions which are rare or infrequent, the BPSU scheme provides a system for the collation of national data. All consultant members are circulated monthly with a card requesting them to identify if they have encountered any of a group of index conditions. These may comprise up to 12 conditions over the paediatric age range. This is an ideal system for assembling cohorts of children with rare conditions (e.g. galactosaemia), identifying infrequent complications of new procedures (e.g. adverse outcome following waterbirth) or for monitoring the occurrence of well-recognized but infrequent conditions (e.g. necrotizing enterocolitis or neonatal meningitis). Once an individual has identified that he/she has seen one of the index conditions, detailed postal questionnaire responses are requested by the study coordinator. The rapid assembly of a national cohort can then be developed to monitor outcomes in these groups, as occurred with the cohort of children with galactosaemia.[28]

CONCLUSION

Audit of perinatal service structure, process and outcomes provides a mechanism by which care can be enhanced and the service monitored. The study of mortality still has much to teach us about the results and process of perinatal care but, increasingly, issues of neuromotor, cognitive and respiratory morbidity have assumed equal importance. The use of guidelines based upon published evidence, careful data collection and continuing audit at unit, regional and national level are critical to improved outcomes for newborn infants.

REFERENCES

1. Anonymous 1992 Guidelines for prevention of group B streptococcal (GBS) infection by chemoprophylaxis. Pediatrics 90: 775–778
2. Anonymous 1993 American Academy of Pediatrics Vitamin K Ad Hoc Task Force: controversies concerning vitamin K and the newborn. Pediatrics 91: 1001–1003
3. Anonymous 1993 Routine evaluation of blood pressure, hematocrit and glucose in newborns. Pediatrics 92: 474–476
4. Anonymous 1994 Practice parameter: management of hyperbilirubinemia in the healthy term newborn. Pediatrics 94: 558–565
5. Anonymous 1995 Hospital stay for healthy term newborns. Pediatrics 96: 788–790
6. Anonymous 1995 Human milk, breastfeeding and the transmission of human immunodeficiency virus in the United States. Pediatrics 96: 977–979
7. Anonymous 1995 Perinatal care at the threshold of viability. Pediatrics 96: 974–976
8. Anonymous 1995 The initiation or withdrawal of treatment for high-risk newborns. Pediatrics 96: 362–363
9. Anonymous 1996 Use and abuse of the Apgar score. Pediatrics 98: 141–142
10. Audit Commission 1997 Maternity services. HMSO, London
11. Bard H 1993 Assessing neonatal risk: CRIB vs SNAP. Lancet 342: 449–450
12. British Association of Perinatal Medicine 1994 The use of exogenous surfactant in newborn infants: report of a working party. BAPM, London
13. British Association of Perinatal Medicine 1996 Standards for hospitals providing neonatal intensive care. BAPM, London
14. British Association of Perinatal Medicine 1997 A minimum dataset to support annual reports from neonatal intensive care units: report of a working group. BAPM, London
15. British Association of Perinatal Medicine and the Research Unit of the Royal College of Physicians 1992 Report of a working group: development of audit measures and guidelines for good practice in the management of respiratory distress syndrome. Archives of Disease in Childhood 67: 1221–1227
16. British Paediatric Association 1990 Paediatric audit: report of a working group. BPA, London
17. British Paediatric Association 1992 Vitamin K administration to newborns: report of an expert working group. BPA, London
18. British Paediatric Association 1993 Paediatric medical audit. BPA, London
19. British Paediatric Association and British Association for Perinatal Paediatrics 1984 Categories of babies requiring intensive care. Archives of Disease in Childhood 60: 599–600
20. British Standards Institution 1994 BS.EN.ISO 9000. BSI, London
21. CESDI 1995 Annual report for 1 January – 31 December 1993. Department of Health, London
22. Clinical Standards Advisory Group 1993 Neonatal intensive care: access and availability of specialist services. HMSO, London
23. Donoghue D 1996 Australian and New Zealand Neonatal Network 1994. AIHW National Perinatal Statistics Unit, Sydney
24. Dunn P M, McIlwaine G 1996 Perinatal audit. Parthenon, London
25. Enkin M W, Keirse M J N C, Renfrew M et al 1997 Pregnancy and childbirth module, Cochrane Database of Systematic Reviews. Update Software, Oxford
26. FIGO Standing Committee on Perinatal Mortality and Morbidity 1982 Report of the committee following a workshop on monitoring and reporting perinatal mortality and morbidity. Chameleon Press, London
27. Gray J E, Richardson D K, McCormick M C, Workman-Daniels K, Goldmann D A 1992 Neonatal therapeutic intervention scoring system: a therapy-based severity-of-illness index. Pediatrics 90: 561–567
28. Honeyman M M, Green A, Holton J B, Leonard J V 1993 Galactosaemia: results of the British Paediatric Surveillance Unit study, 1988–90. Archives of Disease in Childhood 69: 339–341
29. Hopkins A 1996 Clinical audit: time for a reappraisal. Journal of the Royal College of Physicians of London 304: 15–25
30. International Neonatal Network 1993 The CRIB (clinical risk index for babies) score: a tool for assessing initial neonatal risk and comparing performance of neonatal units. Lancet 342: 193–198
31. MacFarlane A, Mugford M 1994 Health trends – the statistics of pregnancy and childbirth. HMSO, London
32. Milligan D W A 1997 Neonatal intensive care provision in the UK 1992–3. Archives of Disease in Childhood 76: F197–F200
33. Mutch L M, Johnson M A, Morley R 1989 Follow up studies: design, organisation and reporting. Archives of Disease in Childhood 641: 394–402
34. National Perinatal Epidemiology Unit/Oxford Health Authority 1994 Disability and perinatal care: measurement of health status at two years (report of two working groups). NPEU/Oxford HA, Oxford
35. Pollack M M, Ruttiman U E, Getson P R 1988 The pediatric risk of mortality (PRISM) score. Critical Care Medicine 16: 1110–1116
36. Pollack M M, Cuerdon T, Patel K M et al 1994 Impact of quality of care factors on paediatric intensive care unit mortality. Journal of the American Medical Association 272: 941–946
37. Redshaw M E, Harris A, Ingram J C 1994 The neonatal unit as a working environment: a survey of neonatal nursing – executive summary. HMSO, London
38. Report of a BPA Working Party 1993 Neonatal resuscitation. BPA, London
39. Report of the Working Group of the British Association of Perinatal Medicine and Neonatal Nurses Association 1992 Categories of babies requiring neonatal care. Archives of Disease in Childhood 67: 868–869
40. Royal College of Obstetricians and Gynaecologists 1997 HIV infection in maternity care and gynaecology: report of a working party. RCOG, London
41. Royal College of Paediatrics and Child Health and Royal College of Obstetricians and Gynaecologists 1997 Resuscitation of babies at birth. RCPCH, London
42. Royal College of Physicians 1988 Medical care of the newborn in England and Wales: a report by the Royal College of Physicians. RCP, London
43. Scottish Neonatal Consultants Collaborative Group and International Neonatal Network 1995 CRIB, mortality and impairment after neonatal intensive care. Lancet 345: 1020–1022
44. Sinclair J C, Bracken M B 1992 Effective care of the newborn. Oxford University Press, Oxford
45. Win Tin W 1994 The changing prognosis for babies born more than eight weeks early over the decade. Proceedings of the British Paediatric Association Annual Meeting 66: 24 (abstract P3)
46. World Health Organization 1980 International classification of impairments, disabilities and handicaps. WHO, Geneva, ch XIV

4

The cost of neonatal intensive care for tiny infants

Lex W. Doyle

Neonatal intensive care is expensive, particularly for the tiniest infants,[2,4,21] who are consuming more neonatal resources, especially assisted ventilation, as their survival rates increase over time.[6] Economic evaluations, in which costs and consequences of health care programmes are compared, can help to assess value for money spent on various health care programmes.

There are several reasons why economic evaluations of neonatal intensive care for tiny infants are vital.

Firstly, it is important to know that neonatal intensive care resources are being consumed efficiently. Others wanting to introduce neonatal intensive care would need to know if they could afford it, or whether they should spend the money on alternative health care programmes. Drummond et al[8] refer to the 'opportunity cost' of a health care programme, which relates to the health outcomes achievable by an alternative programme that is forgone because the resources are already committed to the first programme.

Secondly, it is possible that not all newborn infants will benefit equally from the increasing consumption of resources by tiny infants. Larger and more mature infants might suffer if attention to their care is diverted.[5] Other infants may be denied access to intensive care because the resources are fully occupied by tiny infants; their care may be jeopardized if they have to be transferred to other centres because the intensive care nursery in the hospital of birth is full.[1]

Thirdly, knowing only the costs of neonatal intensive care is not enough because the consequences of intensive care can last much longer for newborn infants than for older children or adults. Most adults admitted to intensive care units will die within a short time; in one study 73% of adults admitted to intensive care had died within 12 months.[3] Most neonates admitted to intensive care survive, and those survivors may well live for 70 or more years, in varying states of health.

METHODS OF ECONOMIC EVALUATION OF NEONATAL INTENSIVE CARE

The essential components of an economic evaluation of a health care programme involve both the costs (inputs) and consequences (outputs) of the programme (Table 4.1).[7] A target group for the health care programme is in an initial state of health. The group is then exposed to the manoeuvre of the health care programme, involving certain costs. The final state of the target group is subsequently determined, the consequences being expressed in health units, utilities, or economic benefits.

Depending on the question being asked, several different types of economic evaluations are possible

Table 4.1 Components of an economic evaluation (adapted from Drummond et al)[7]

Initial state ⇒	Manoeuvre ⇒ (health care programme)	Final state		
	Costs ⇒ (INPUTS)	Consequences (OUTPUTS)		
		Effects e.g. lives or life-years gained	Utilities e.g. quality-adjusted lives or life-years gained	Benefits e.g. economic benefits gained
	Direct costs Indirect costs Intangible costs			Direct benefits Indirect benefits Intangible benefits

Table 4.2 Characteristics of health care evaluations (adapted from Drummond et al)[9]

		Costs and consequences both examined		
		No		Yes
		Costs only	Consequences only	
Comparison of alternatives	No	PARTIAL EVALUATION Cost description	Outcome description	PARTIAL EVALUATION Cost–outcome description
	Yes	PARTIAL EVALUATION Cost analysis	Efficacy or effectiveness	FULL ECONOMIC EVALUATION Cost-minimization Cost–effectiveness Cost–utility Cost–benefit

(Table 4.2). A partial economic evaluation of a health care programme may examine only the costs, or the consequences, separately, with or without contrasting alternative courses of action. However, according to Drummond et al,[9] a full economic evaluation requires a contrast between alternative courses of action, in terms of both costs and consequences. Boyle et al[2] were the first to apply the methods of a full economic evaluation to neonatal intensive care, and described the calculation of cost–effectiveness, cost–utility, and cost–benefit ratios.

COST–EFFECTIVENESS ANALYSIS

In cost–effectiveness analysis the outcomes are measured in units of health (e.g. survival rates, life-years or days of morbidity). Cost–effectiveness analysis of any intervention or health care programme requires calculations of the change in costs divided by the change in outcome attributable to the intervention or health care programme; the results can be expressed as additional costs per life gained, or life-year gained. To calculate cost–effectiveness of neonatal intensive care the following data are required:

Change in costs. The best economic analysis will consider all costs, regardless of who has to pay – the patient, the hospital, the family, or the community at large. Costs can be direct, indirect, or intangible (Table 4.1). However, it is not always possible to measure all of these costs. With respect to direct costs, a distinction has to be made between charges and costs – only in some cases will the charge for a particular service equal the cost, and only under such circumstances can charges be substituted for costs. Costs have to be standardized to account for the effects of inflation if different eras are compared. When costs are compared between countries a further difficulty is the fluctuations over time in the currency rates relative to each other.

Change in survival rate or life-years gained. All livebirths must be accounted for in the denominator of any calculations of survival rate. They do not all have to be included in such calculations as long as the exclusion of certain infants, for example those with lethal malformations, does not bias the results. If the aim of the study is an economic evaluation of a regional programme, all livebirths in the region must be considered; if it is an economic evaluation of neonatal intensive care in one hospital then all livebirths in the hospital must be considered. To include outborn infants in an economic evaluation of one hospital will distort the analysis because outborn infants have a different prognosis and hence different costs. Moreover, the denominator of all outborn infants in the region or community is not included in the denominator. Compared with an economic evaluation involving a whole region, a disadvantage of an economic analysis in one hospital contrasting different eras may be that referral patterns have changed. This is especially true for very preterm infants transferred in utero because of pregnancy complications and who may have a different prognosis compared with those who were booked earlier in pregnancy for delivery at the hospital. When calculating life-years gained, it is usual to apply a discount rate to reflect the fact that future costs should not contribute so much to decisions being made in the present.[10] In other words, it is better to receive benefits earlier, or to defer costs, reflecting a 'time preference' in economic terms. A typical discount rate would be 5%.

COST–UTILITY ANALYSIS

In cost–utility analysis the social value of the outcomes is determined. Cost–utility analysis requires calculation of the change in costs divided by the change in outcome adjusted for the quality of life; the results can be expressed as additional costs per quality-adjusted life gained, or quality-adjusted life-year gained. To calculate the cost–utility of neonatal intensive care the following data are required:

Change in costs. As for cost–effectiveness.

Change in quality-adjusted survival rate, or quality-adjusted life-years gained. The previous comments regarding the denominator of any calculations of survival apply. Conventionally, an outcome with 'normal' health and quality of life is allotted a utility of 1, and death is allotted a utility of 0. Any outcome less than 'normal' health or quality of life has a value less than 1 and would be expected to range down to 0. However, in the study of Boyle et al[2] some outcomes with survival were rated worse than death; hence their utilities were as low as –0.39. The major difficulty in assigning utilities is the inability to define what constitutes a 'normal' quality of life and hence the variation that individuals, including the patient if consulted, would place on the same health state.

COST–BENEFIT ANALYSIS

In cost–benefit analysis outcomes are converted to dollars. Cost–benefit analysis requires the calculation of the additional costs per livebirth subtracted from the additional earnings per livebirth; the results can be expressed in units of currency and would be termed the net economic benefit (or net economic loss if negative). As with costs, benefits can be direct, indirect, or intangible (Table 4.1). To calculate the cost–benefit of neonatal intensive care the following data are required:

Change in costs. As for cost–effectiveness, but also other health-related costs over the infant's lifetime, which may be difficult to predict.

Change in earnings per additional survivor. The major difficulty is to estimate the lifetime earnings of a survivor, when such imponderables as life-expectancy, career choice (including the possibility of unemployment), and inflation have to be predicted so far into the future. As with costs, earnings have to be standardized to account for the effects of inflation if different eras are compared, and future costs, as well as benefits, should be discounted.[10]

RESULTS OF ECONOMIC EVALUATIONS OF NEONATAL INTENSIVE CARE FOR TINY INFANTS

There are numerous studies in the literature relating to the costs of neonatal intensive care over the past two decades, from North America,[2,12,15,16,23,24] the UK,[13,14,17,18] and Australia.[11,20–22,26] From these studies there is no doubt that neonatal intensive care is expensive, with high costs per survivor, particularly for infants of lower birthweight. There are limitations when comparing the reported studies, however. With only three exceptions[2,21,22] all of the other studies are only partial economic evaluations because they have not compared alternative courses of action. Some of the previous studies have not considered costs, but only charges.[12,16,23,24,26] Most studies have considered only admissions to their neonatal intensive care units,[11–18,20,23,26] and not all livebirths in their hospital or region. Some studies have implied that they are regional studies,[13,14,17,18] but the outcome for all livebirths of interest in the region has not been reported. Of those considering only admissions to their neonatal intensive care units, one had only outborn infants,[12] and of the others most have included outborn infants[11,13–18,20,23,24,26] who have a different prognosis and therefore different costs; some studies have reported costs and outcomes for inborn and outborn infants separately.[13,15] Some studies relate to the costs of neonatal intensive care shortly after the introduction of assisted ventilation in the 1970s;[7,12,15,16] others are related to costs in the 1980s when assisted ventilation had become more established.[11,13,14,17,18,20–24,26] Only one study[21] has considered both eras, and this study has now been extended to evaluate neonatal intensive care in the era after the introduction of exogenous surfactant.[22]

From the reported studies, the costs per survivor less than 1000 g (or 1001 g) birthweight were calculated where possible and then converted into Australian dollars for 1987[4] (Fig. 4.1). Generally, the costs per survivor for infants with birthweights under 1001 g are higher for the North American studies[2,12,15,16,23,24] than for the studies from the UK,[14,17,18] or Australia,[11,20–22,26] and the costs per survivor were higher for the Australian studies compared with the studies from the UK. The one Australian study[26] in which only charges were used resulted in lower costs per survivor compared with the Australian studies considering costs.[11,20–22] Such a discrepancy did not exist between the North American studies which considered charges,[12,16,23,24] and those which considered costs.[2,15] This occurred probably because the charges in the North American studies more closely reflected total costs than did charges in the Australian study. The costs per additional survivor from the earliest full economic evaluations[2,21] were higher than just the costs per survivor in those studies. This suggested that full economic evaluations, with a comparison between eras, might reveal costs per additional survivor even higher than expected, indicating that it is even more expensive to improve the survival rate of extremely tiny infants further. However, the more recent full economic evaluation from Victoria in the era after exogenous surfactant was introduced showed a reduction in the incremental costs per additional survivor.[22]

All studies have made certain assumptions in calculating costs (e.g. dollars per day for varying levels of care, discount rate) and determining consequences (life expectancy, utility values, outcome for children not followed). The estimates of costs per survivor, or cost–effectiveness or cost–utility ratios are therefore subject to variation in their underlying assumptions. However, in the full economic evaluations from Victoria the calculated cost–effectiveness and cost–utility ratios were quite robust to wide variations in the underlying assumptions.[21,22]

Future economic evaluations of neonatal intensive care will be needed continually as neonatal intensive care and other health care programmes change, and as economic circumstances alter.

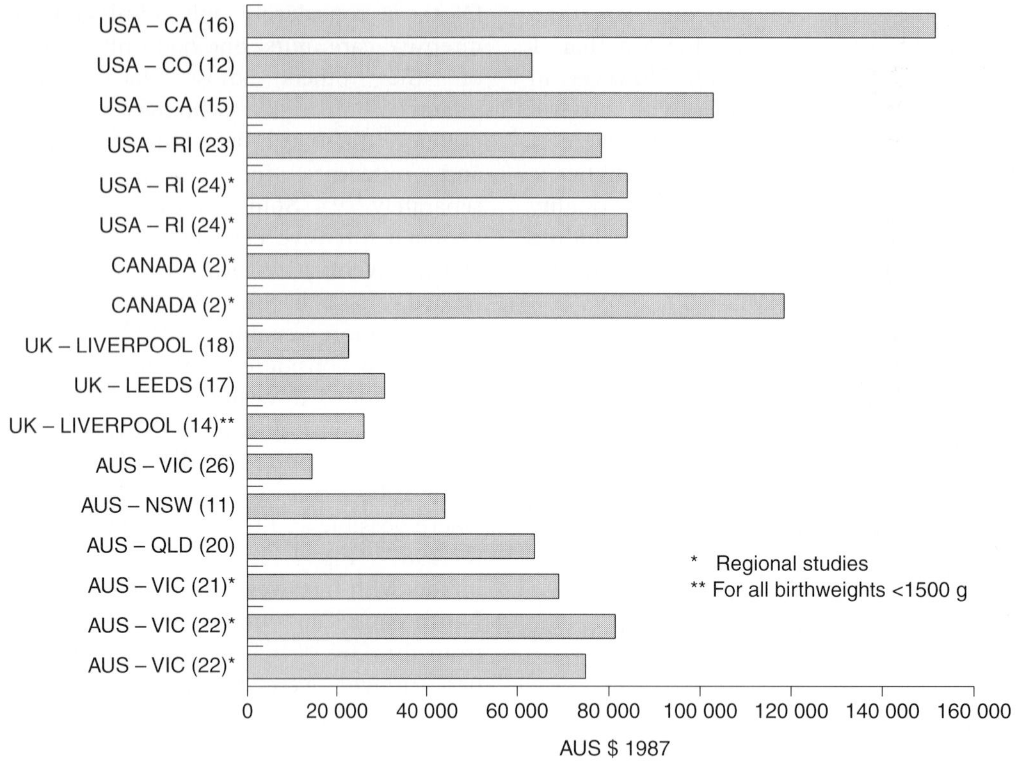

Fig. 4.1 Costs to hospital discharge per survivor (Aus $ 1987) for infants of birthweight < 1000 g (or 1001 g). (Reference numbers in brackets.)

COMPARISON OF THE ECONOMICS OF NEONATAL INTENSIVE CARE WITH OTHER HEALTH CARE PROGRAMMES

Torrance & Zipursky[19] in 1984 compared the cost–utility of various health care programmes, including neonatal intensive care, and showed that the cost per quality-adjusted life-year gained for infants 500–999 g birthweight in Canada ($52 300 – Aus $1987) was lower (i.e. cheaper) than some other health care programmes (Fig. 4.2), such as peritoneal dialysis ($81 790 – Aus $1987) or haemodialysis ($93 770 – Aus $1987), but was higher (i.e. more expensive) than others, such as coronary artery bypass for left coronary artery disease ($7290 – Aus $1987). Since that time, Welch & Larson[25] reported on the cost–effectiveness of some other health care programmes, including organ transplantation (liver $56 370 – Aus $1987 per life-year gained; heart $34 860 – Aus $1987 per lifeyear gained), and treatment of hyperlipidaemia ($193 070 – Aus $1987 per life-year gained) (Fig. 4.2). Neonatal intensive care in Victoria for infants of birthweight 500–999 g in the 1980s[21] ($5090 – Aus $1987 per quality-adjusted life-year gained) was much cheaper than in Canada, with costs approximately one-tenth that of the Canadian study[2] ($52 300 – Aus $1987 per quality-adjusted life-year gained). Subsequently, further reductions have been reported for infants 500–999 g birthweight in Victoria in the 1990s in the cost–utility ($4160 – Aus $1987 per quality-adjusted life-year gained) and cost–effectiveness ($3130 – Aus $1987 per life-year gained) ratios if only costs during the primary hospitalization were considered, but slightly higher ratios if long-term costs for severely disabled children were added[22] (cost–utility $8630 – Aus $1987 per quality-adjusted life-year gained; cost–effectiveness $7620 – Aus $1987 per life-year gained). Figure 4.2 shows that neonatal intensive care for extremely tiny infants compares favourably with many other health care programmes, even more so in Australia and since the introduction of exogenous surfactant and the increased use of antenatal steroid therapy in the 1990s. It should be noted that not all health care programmes cost money; some save money (e.g. screening for phenylketonuria, or postpartum anti-D prophylaxis) and have cost–utility or cost–effectiveness ratios less than zero.

In conclusion, despite fears to the contrary, the incremental costs of neonatal intensive care for tiny infants per quality-adjusted life-year gained have fallen (i.e. improved) rather than increased in the 1990s, with recent advances in technology and therapy. Neonatal intensive care for extremely tiny infants compares favourably with many other health care programmes in the community, not only with high-technology areas, such as dialysis and organ transplantation, but also with other low-technology interventions, such as the treatment of hyperlipidaemia or hypertension. All health care pro-

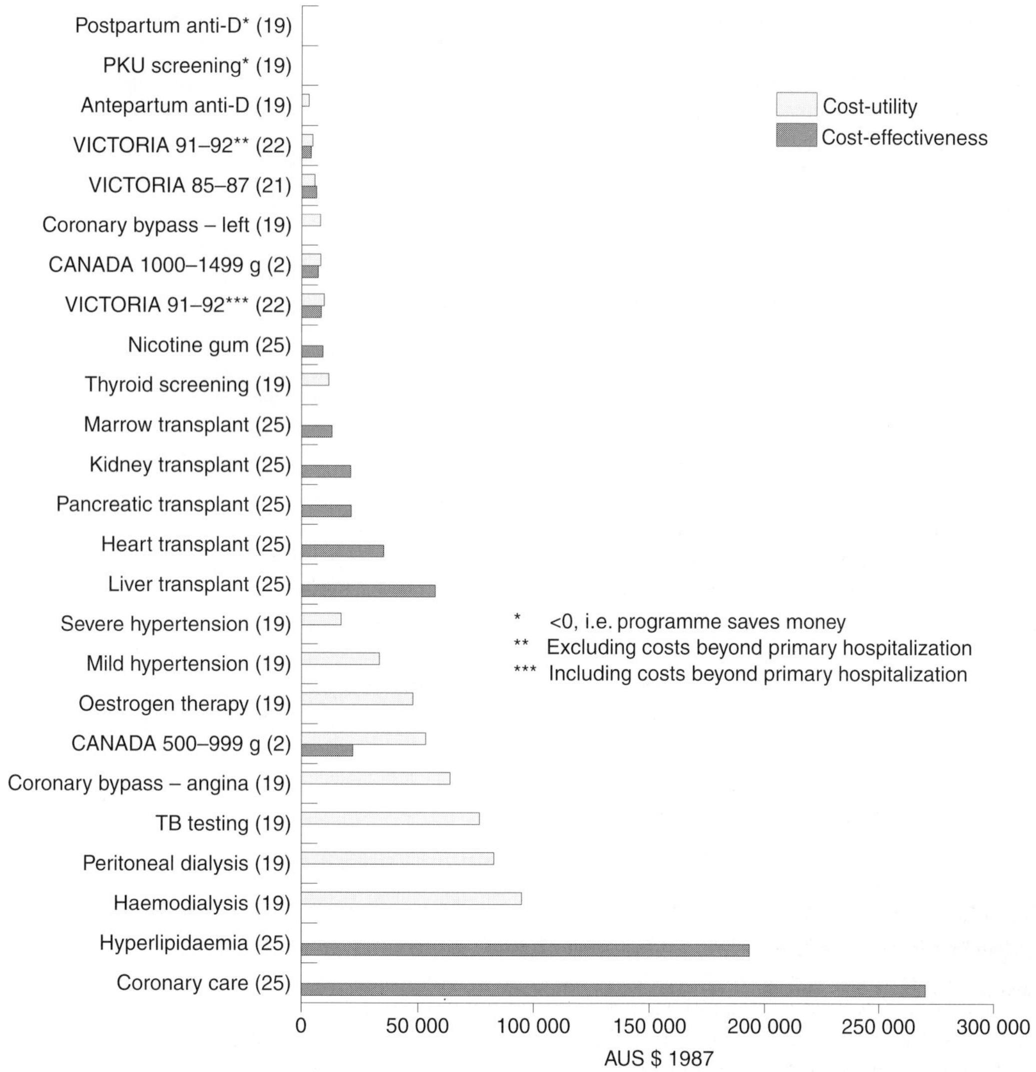

Fig. 4.2 Cost–effectiveness (Aus $1987 per life-year gained) and cost–utility ratios (Aus $1987 per quality-adjusted life-year gained) for various health care programmes. Lower cost–effectiveness and cost–utility ratios are more favourable economically. (Reference numbers in brackets.)

grammes should be continually evaluated economically in the future to ensure that funds available for health care are spent judiciously. To date, neonatal intensive care for extremely tiny infants seems a wise economic investment.

REFERENCES

1. Bowman E, Doyle L W, Murton L J, Roy R N D, Kitchen W H 1988 Increased mortality of preterm infants transferred between tertiary perinatal centres. British Medical Journal 297: 1098–1100
2. Boyle M H, Torrance G W, Sinclair J C, Horwood S P 1983 Economic evaluation of neonatal intensive care of very-low-birthweight infants. New England Journal of Medicine 308: 1330–1337
3. Cullen D J, Ferrara L C, Briggs B A, Walker P F, Gilbert J 1976 Survival, hospitalization charges and follow-up results in critically ill patients. New England Journal of Medicine 294: 982–987
4. Doyle L W 1996 Cost evaluation of intensive care for extremely tiny babies. Seminars in Neonatology 1: 289–296
5. Doyle L W, Murton L J, Kitchen W H 1989 Mortality with increasing assisted ventilation of very-low-birthweight infants. American Journal of Diseases of Children 143: 223–227
6. Doyle L W, Davis P, Dharmalingam A, Bowman E 1996 Assisted ventilation and survival of extremely low birthweight infants. Journal of Paediatrics and Child Health 32: 138–142
7. Drummond M F, Stoddart G L, Torrance G W 1987 Methods for the economic evaluation of health care programmes. Oxford University Press, Oxford, p 2
8. Drummond M F, Stoddart G L, Torrance G W 1987 Methods for the economic evaluation of health care programmes. Oxford University Press, Oxford, p 7
9. Drummond M F, Stoddart G L, Torrance G W 1987 Methods for the economic evaluation of health care programmes. Oxford University Press, Oxford, p 8
10. Drummond M F, Stoddart G L, Torrance G W 1987 Methods for the economic evaluation of health care programmes. Oxford University Press, Oxford, p 29
11. John E, Lee K, Li G M 1983 Cost of neonatal intensive care. Australian Paediatric Journal 19: 152–156
12. McCarthy J T, Koops B L, Honeyfield P R, Butterfield L J 1979 Who pays the bill for neonatal intensive care? Journal of Pediatrics 95: 755–761
13. Newns B, Drummond M F, Durbin G M, Culley P 1984 Costs and outcomes in a regional intensive care unit. Archives of Disease in Childhood 59: 1064–1067
14. Pharoah P O D, Stevenson R C, Cooke R W I, Sandu [sic] B 1988

Costs and benefits of neonatal intensive care. Archives of Disease in Childhood 63: 715–718
15. Phibbs C S, Williams R L, Phibbs R H 1981 Newborn risk factors and costs of neonatal intensive care. Pediatrics 68: 313–321
16. Pomerance J J, Ukrainski C T, Ukra T, Henderson D H, Nash A H, Meredith J L 1978 Cost of living for infants weighing 1,000 grams or less at birth. Pediatrics 61: 908–910
17. Ryan S, Sics A, Congdon P 1988 Cost of neonatal care. Archives of Disease in Childhood 63: 303–306
18. Sandhu B, Stevenson R C, Cooke R W I, Pharoah P O D 1986 Cost of neonatal intensive care for very-low-birthweight infants. Lancet i: 600–603
19. Torrance G W, Zipursky A 1984 Cost-effectiveness of antepartum prevention of Rh immunization. Clinical Perinatology 11: 267–281
20. Tudehope D I, Lee W, Harris F, Addison C 1989 Cost-analysis of neonatal intensive and special care. Australian Paediatric Journal 25: 61–65
21. Victorian Infant Collaborative Study Group 1993 The cost of improving the outcome for infants of birthweight 500–999 g in Victoria. Journal of Paediatrics and Child Health 29: 56–62
22. Victorian Infant Collaborative Study Group 1997 Economic outcome for intensive care of infants of birthweight 500–999 g born in Victoria in the post surfactant era. Journal of Paediatrics and Child Health 33: 202–208
23. Walker D B, Feldman A, Vohr B R, Oh W 1984 Cost-benefit analysis of neonatal intensive care for infants weighing less than 1,000 grams at birth. Pediatrics 74: 20–25
24. Walker D B, Vohr B R, Oh W 1985 Economic analysis of regionalized neonatal care for very low-birth-weight infants in the State of Rhode Island. Pediatrics 76: 69–74
25. Welch H G, Larson E B 1989 Cost-effectiveness of bone marrow transplantation in acute nonlymphocytic leukemia. New England Journal of Medicine 321: 807–812
26. Yu V Y H, Bajuk B 1981 Medical expenses of neonatal intensive care for very low birthweight infants. Australian Paediatric Journal 17: 183–185

5

Psychological aspects of neonatal care

Martin P. M. Richards   Joanna T. Hawthorne

INTRODUCTION

In this chapter we will review the research in psychology and the neighbouring social sciences which are relevant to the practice of neonatal paediatrics. Despite the large body of material, the coverage of relevant topics is patchy.

DEVELOPMENT IN A SOCIAL WORLD

BECOMING A PARENT

From the perspective of a neonatal ward, there may be a temptation to see parental behaviour as arising de novo in response to a new baby. But behaviour at this time develops from a long-drawn-out, social process that stretches back to the parents' own childhood.[172]

For some, there may be particular situations and experiences that create problems for them as new parents, and without knowledge of the origins of these difficulties it may be very difficult to provide effective support. However, it is important to see the process not simply in individual intrapsychic terms, but also as a cultural phenomenon which is formed by the common assumptions that are held in society about what is expected of a parent.

Links exist between a mother's own experience of mothering and her attitudes, feelings and behaviour as a parent, but these are indirect. The link is modified by more recent experience such as the change in many mothers' social status as they leave employment during pregnancy.[140] Brown & Harris[37] have presented a model of depression in women which embodies both longer-term factors, such as the loss of parents in childhood, and aspects of current situations such as the absence of a confiding relationship. This kind of analysis has begun to be extended to the experience of motherhood.[26,124]

Although there is a body of work which discusses men's involvement in child care,[15,106,118] there has been less discussion of fatherhood or of the sorts of factors that may account for individual differences in the child care practices of fathers.

Much work on bonding and the effects of separation of mother and infant in the neonatal period is based on the idea that mothers enter a 'sensitive period' at birth.[101] This notion of a sensitive period is based on analogies with the behaviour of animals which have been shown to be invalid;[168] there is no direct evidence for its existence in humans.[78] However, the neonatal period may have its own special psychological features. Winnicott[209] for example described what he called primary maternal preoccupation in the period after birth.

In considering a parent's actions and feelings in the neonatal period, it is important to recognize the influence of the social situation in which it usually occurs. Birth has become an event that occurs in public institutions under medical supervision and management.[51,184] The social and emotional aspects of the occasion are therefore usually muted. Not surprisingly, many mothers report that initially they felt indifferent to their babies and did not feel the babies to be their own until after they had left maternity hospital or a neonatal unit.[174] This has obvious implications for attempts to predict future parent–child relations from what can be seen in hospital.

The practice of medicine has had effects beyond changing the social situation at birth. It has helped to make the delivery of a healthy baby and the mother's survival more likely, which have probably had profound effects on parents' fears and fantasies during pregnancy and their expectations of the outcome.[153] Fears of an abnormal birth and/or baby seem to be fairly universal in our society,[81] but these are usually quickly dissipated after the arrival of a normal baby. However, they may take on great importance if all does not turn out well;[109] or the parents come to believe it has not turned out well, as for instance after a false positive identification in a neonatal screening test.[23,81] Given that long-standing and deep-seated unconscious processes may be involved, it is not surprising that simple reassurance is often not enough to resolve such fears.

Techniques that are in wide use during pregnancy may well have important effects on parents' feelings in the neonatal period. With the use of amniocentesis some parents now know the sex of their fetus, while many will have seen its image on an ultrasound screen. The least we can say about such techniques is that they are becoming part of the social processes that shape the experiences of parents and the attitudes and knowledge they bring to the social relationships with their children.[169] But they may create psychological problems. Screening for neural tube defects or triple testing for Down syndrome can cause considerable anxiety,[39,65,84,122] and this seems to be a general feature of prenatal screening.[81]

To these factors we must add the various courses, books, articles and films that are aimed at parents. In most cases these are explicitly intended to change the attitudes and actions of parents towards their children. Some specific programmes designed to alter maternal behaviour have been evaluated,[11,185] and are mentioned later in this chapter.

EFFECTS OF BIRTH ON MOTHERS AND THEIR BABIES

In the neonatal period a mother's (and, probably a father's) feelings, attitudes and physical state may influence her relationship with her baby.[31] These maternal attitudes can, in turn, be influenced by the nature of the labour and delivery.[167] After a caesarian section, some mothers describe motherhood in more negative terms, are less responsive towards their babies and generally less satisfied with their experiences of birth[41,100,112,141,205] than those who have had a normal delivery. Robson & Kumar[174] found that mothers were less likely to express positive feelings for their babies immediately after delivery if they had had their membranes artificially ruptured and, in addition, either had experienced a painful and unpleasant labour or had been given more than 125 mg of pethidine. In a later study Kumar & Robson[104] argue that childbirth per se can have a 'particular and deleterious effect' on the mental health of first-time mothers. When a mother feels badly informed and not in control of what is happening, her well-being may be reduced in the first postnatal weeks and she may feel ambivalent about her baby.[82]

There is also the possibility of associations between a mother's psychological characteristics and the likelihood that she will experience an obstetric complication. There are a number of somewhat inconsistent studies that set out to explore associations between measures such as anxiety in pregnancy and preterm delivery and other complications of birth.[97,116,196] Some of the studies indicate links between a mother's psychological state in pregnancy and the behaviour of the baby after birth. Mothers who are more anxious in pregnancy produce babies that cry more[147] and they themselves show less positive affect while feeding their babies.[64] Sadly, in this area, the sophistication of the research seldom matches the subtlety of the processes that require investigation.

The process of delivery and its management can also influence neonatal behaviour. Extensive use of techniques for induction of labour may increase the number of infants with lower birthweight[41] and hence increase the incidence of neonatal problems and admissions to neonatal units.[165] After elective and/or instrumental deliveries, babies are more often taken to professionals with feeding or sleeping difficulties, colic or infections than their 'normal' counterparts. Though these problems are often seen as 'minor' they can be of enormous significance to parents.[127] The most obvious link between obstetric technique and the behaviour of the neonate is the effect of analgesic and anaesthetic drugs in labour.[173,182] There is evidence that most of the widely used compounds depress respiration and the ability to organize sucking behaviour in infants.[4,59,167] A few studies suggest that narcotics, in particular, may have long-lasting effects on various psychological functions[30,59] but the significance of these effects is a matter of controversy.[95] Drugs given neonatally have a tendency to persist for longer than they do later in childhood. It may be that in optimal situations this is of little consequence, but, when a baby's health is damaged in other ways and the parent–child relationship is under stress, they become significant. In addition, early impressions may have long-term influences on parent–child interactions. A sleepy, unresponsive and difficult to feed baby makes a poor social partner, and even when the baby's behaviour has returned to more usual patterns a mother's response may remain negative.[33,133]

Other examples of the influence of medical practice on neonatal behaviour are provided by the practices of placing silver nitrate in the eyes of newborns and circumcision.[8,85,151,171]

EARLY SOCIAL INTERACTIONS

The behaviour of infant and caretaker are mutually interdependent – what each does influences the other.[146] This can be seen both in the patterning of behaviour on a short-term basis and in the growing knowledge and experience each has of the other. In the first hours after birth the latter process usually begins by the parent(s) actively exploring and examining the body of the infant, though the amount of social interaction may be quite low in an unsupportive hospital environment.[148] After a normal delivery when analgesics or anaesthetic drugs are not given to the mother, a newborn may remain in a quiet semi-alert state for some time.[33,62,101] It has been suggested that this is a behavioural adaptation facilitating the process of maternal exploration and the formation of the social relationship.

A baby who is unresponsive to his mother makes a

frustrating social partner, while a depressed, anxious or very tired mother is unlikely to be alert to an infant's behavioural state. In any of these cases, the interaction is unlikely to be mutually satisfying. If persisting interactional problems have arisen, it can be difficult to pinpoint their cause. This is best attempted by quiet observation of infant and mother together. Sometimes much can be learnt by holding a baby for a few minutes and trying to engage his attention.

Much physiological and behavioural research has been devoted to investigating the behavioural states of infants.[154,155] As responsiveness to stimulation is dependent on the state the baby is in, state changes are important to both parents and anyone doing a behavioural or neurological examination of a baby. The most widely used system for recording state includes two sleep states (REM and non-REM) and three awake states: quiet with regular respiration and no gross movements; gross movements; and crying and movement[156] (Ch. 44, Part 1). The organization of behavioural states is less predictable in preterm infants[5] and undergoes fairly rapid change in the first months of life.[9]

It is beyond the scope of the chapter to provide a general account of infant behaviour and its development, or of the many pre- or post-delivery influences. For further information the reader is directed elsewhere.[12,18,61,145,203]

THE CONCEPT OF BONDING

The development of specialized facilities for sick and preterm babies proceeded in the postwar years as neonatal physiology became better understood and the high mortality amongst low-birthweight babies was appreciated. In the early days, with the emphasis so strongly on the physiological, it was not surprising that the social and emotional needs of the babies and their parents were often neglected. It was assumed that sick babies should be cared for separately from their mothers – an assumption that persisted despite the growing appreciation of the need for the presence of parents on the paediatric ward. Visiting hours were often short and parents' separation from their children was emphasized by an insistence on their being gowned and masked. During their brief visits, parents were treated as spectators of their babies, were seldom allowed to touch them, and the idea that they should play any part in their care was often seen as inappropriate. Not surprisingly, many people, both parents and professionals, became uneasy and increasingly distressed by these arrangements. Then Klaus & Kennell began publishing papers about the ill-effects of early separation which they attributed to the prevention of a process they called 'bonding'. This they suggested would normally occur between mother and baby in the first postpartum hours. Quickly 'bonding' became the rallying cry for those whose efforts have now succeeded in changing practice and attitudes in neonatal units. Today, it is usual for high priority to be given to the need to maintain and encourage close parent–child relationships.

The concept of bonding has been subject to considerable experimental investigation and the theoretical ideas and evidence have been repeatedly reviewed.[77,105,166,168,175,181,185,197,206,214] While Klaus & Kennell[101] have reasserted their hypothesis in a slightly modified form, there is now a consensus that the original hypothesis is not supported by the evidence.

It is claimed that there is a sensitive period, initiated at birth and persisting for a number of days, during which a mother is particularly open to form a relationship with her baby. During this period separation leads to a disturbance of the mother–child relationship that is persistent. This disturbance includes, it has been suggested, failure to thrive and non-accidental injury. It has also been claimed that bonding failure leads to child abuse.[115] However, there is little evidence to link abuse with separation. Instead the indications are that reported abuse and neonatal problems share common factors such as low maternal age, lack of social support for mothers, abnormalities of pregnancy and delivery, and abnormalities in the child.[56,73,189]

Despite the criticisms of the concept of bonding, there is every reason to avoid early separation whenever possible, not least because it is something that most parents dislike. What seems a more helpful approach than the bonding hypothesis is to consider the needs of parents and their infants in the neonatal period and how these can best be met in the context of the hospital care of normal, sick and preterm babies.

NEEDS OF FAMILIES

The birth of a baby is an upheaval for parents.[32] Those for whom the event goes smoothly are probably those who have planned for the baby and whose pregnancy and delivery have been trouble free.[83] Increasingly, women's pregnancies are subjected to more testing. Most mothers view the prenatal scan at 18–20 weeks as a reassurance that all is well with their baby while staff see it as a way of detecting abnormalities. Parents value the photograph of their baby and view this as a social event and often the first time they feel that their pregnancy is real.

Anxiety in pregnancy may contribute to postnatal depression in women.[123,190] Several studies (see Green[81]) attribute some of this anxiety to screening tests, such as the triple test, or discovery of markers by ultrasound scanning of unpredictable meaning such as choroid plexus cysts or renal dilatation.[43,44,45,70] About 1% of the pregnant population will show these markers but they usually disappear during pregnancy. Those choroid plexus cysts that persist may be linked to chromosomal abnormalities and so some hospitals offer a late amniocentesis. Renal dilatation can diminish during pregnancy but show up later on as reflux[119,201] (see

Ch. 39, Part 2). Hospital policies vary about how to convey the findings of such tests to parents.

In the normal situation of birth, a mother quickly adjusts to the individual characteristics of her own baby. Conditions for a mother in the first postpartum days are special because, ideally at least, she should be able to spend as much of her time as possible attending to her baby. Her other concerns and responsibilities need to be reduced, if only for a few days. There is usually a degree of relief that the delivery is over and that the baby is normal and well. Both parents are pleased to be able to hold and see the baby that may have dominated their thoughts during the pregnancy.[144] While there may be great individual variation in all these reactions, there is generally a sense of continuity for parents as delivery follows pregnancy and the birth produces a healthy baby. This continuity has been stressed, particularly, by the more psychoanalytically oriented theorists.[55,71,210] Clearly, this continuity will be disrupted if parents are separated from their baby during the neonatal period, or if the baby is not normal.[94] When an abnormal baby is born, parents' worst fears may be realized and the fantasies of abnormality, which are so frequent in pregnancy, far from being dispelled by the reality of a normal baby, are fed and may grow. There may be guilt and depression at the failure to produce a normal child. The birth of a preterm baby often produces a severe emotional crisis.[21,40,98,117,161,192,195,215] However, when good support is provided for parents, and the children do not have persisting serious problems, Trause & Kramer[202] have shown that the feelings of the parents of premature infants may be similar to those with full-term infants within a month.

If any child is sick it is to be expected that parents will feel anxious. Curiously, however, some of the literature treats this anxiety as a side-effect that ought to be removed rather than a normal response to a worrying situation. Indeed, it should be a cause of considerable concern if parents show no anxiety. There are indications that levels of anxiety and contact with a baby in a neonatal unit may be positively associated,[88] but it is unclear whether this is because high levels of anxiety increase visiting or whether visiting provokes anxieties. In either case, this study showed that parents would have resisted any reduction in their contact and did not regret the time they had spent with their baby.

Neonatal problems can lead to maternal overprotectiveness[20,110] and it is possible that some of the high rates of hospital readmission for these babies may be explained by overanxiety by parents and professional staff, and not just the raised incidence of problems.[86] Parents have been found to perceive their preterm babies as weak.[19,161] Interviews with parents indicate that they often feel an unfulfilled need for information and time to discuss their baby's problems.[91] It seems plausible to suggest that overprotection may result if parents' emotional conflicts about the baby's condition are unresolved and the implications of the baby's problems have not been fully discussed.

Small-for-gestational age infants and their mothers have been found to be less interactive in comparison with appropriately grown infants and their mothers. SGA infants also had more unstable states than the AGA group but were more often in quiet-alert states, although SGA mothers were less vocal and more intrusive, irritable and less affectionate than mothers of AGA infants.[159] There are many studies that look at the outcome of preterm birth[213] (see Ch. 7).

Because parents bring their own cultural and personal experiences into their new relationship with their baby, each mother will react differently to a preterm baby.[139] It is the maternal perceptions of the baby (full- or preterm) that influence her interaction with the baby. Maternal perceptions and mothers' reports of infant characteristics, such as temperament, are partly reflections of expectations and maternal characteristics such as anxiety, depression or self-confidence. Similarly, the infant's sensitivity to and his motivation for human engagement mean that a certain pattern of interaction is being followed. Maternal perceptions of their relationship with their fetus during pregnancy can affect attachment of mother and infant at 1 year.[71]

The psychological effects on parents we have been discussing in this section are generally more or less transient. However, it should be remembered that more serious psychological and psychiatric problems may occur in the neonatal period.[35,68,103,134,176,217] Postnatal depression arises usually as a result of psychosocial variables[27] although excessive pain in labour has also been linked to depression. Postnatally depressed mothers may be unable to provide an appropriate environment for infant psychological development.[120] This can result in delay in expressive language, poor concentration, lack of shared affect and insecurity of attachment.[135] The incidence of postnatal depression which varies between 10% and 20%[51] has been rising and is a cause for concern.[47] Murray et al[135] and Sharp et al[183] have reported that boys of depressed mothers do worse intellectually than girls.

Some Btitish health visitors routinely use the Edinburgh Postnatal Depression Scale[46] as a screening device for newly delivered mothers. This scale can also be used during pregnancy[82] as an indicator of depression, which is more common prenatally than postnatally. Green et al[82] found that women who did not express positive feelings when their pregnancy was first confirmed were more likely to be depressed postpartum.

THE CONDITION OF THE INFANT

We have already discussed the mutual influence of parent and infant behaviour and some of the ways each of these may be influenced by obstetric and other factors. From the point of view of neonatal care, the effect of prematurity and sickness on infant behaviour and interaction with parents is of particular importance. A newborn preterm infant may be skinny, frail, unresponsive and ugly. Not only does he or she depart from the stereotype of the expected baby, but there is likely to be anxiety about survival and the baby's well-being.[96] Even calling a baby preterm may lead to it being viewed more negatively,[192] and there may be less support from the parents' families.[216] It is not surprising, therefore, that studies of preterm infants with their parents show that there may be less physical contact, less face-to-face interaction and less smiling. The general pattern of findings is for differences in social interaction to persist for a matter of weeks and then gradually to disappear.[49,76] In part, this probably reflects the growing similarity between the behaviour of preterm and full-term babies over the first year with the early reduced activity and general fussiness gradually approaching the norms for full-term babies[29,48] but the correspondence is not exact. Sometimes parents of preterm babies spend more time than those of full-term babies stimulating social responses and in affectionate exchanges, as if they were over-compensating for their own and their baby's earlier unresponsiveness.[48]

While the conceptional age of a baby is one determinant of behaviour – for instance, the unpredictable and uncoordinated state organization before 36 weeks in 'healthy' preterm babies[156] – the baby's health and physical condition are also important. The sicker baby is more likely to be held at arm's length on the lap and less likely to be nestled close in the arms, touched and talked to.[57,79] Overall measures of current morbidity may be associated with the baby's level of movements. Goldberg and Divitto concluded that long-term illness in a preterm infant has a more powerful effect on the mother's level of interaction than the otherwise important psychological variables in the mother's background. The explanation that mothers of the ill infants emotionally withdraw from them is supported by another study in which mothers interacted more with and preferred the less ill of pairs of same sex preterm twins.[131] Other research which has found a maternal overcompensation after a baby had been sick was probably dealing with less serious illness.[16,129] Several studies have pointed out the difficulties of interacting with irritable babies or sleepy babies[6,34,69,135,211] and indeed the baby's behaviour is seen as one of the main factors that affect parent–infant interaction.[170]

The Brazelton Neonatal Behavioural Assessment Scale is an interactive assessment designed to bring out the most organized behaviour of the baby.[33] The assessment can be used as an outcome measure, for example in studies looking at the effects of obstetric analgesia on the baby's behaviour[163,173,182,204] or as a baseline measure of a baby's behaviour.[208] The NBAS has also been used as an intervention with parents.[137,138] Fathers who had helped perform the assessment on their infants at birth were found to feel closer to them 1 month later.[136] Liptak and his colleagues[113] reported that mothers who had seen the NBAS demonstrated spent more time playing and talking with their infants at 1 and 3 months. The NBAS provides an opportunity to share with parents the numerous capabilities of their newborn and helps parents to identify the characteristics of the infant that may influence their caregiving. Keefer[99] has incorporated aspects of the NBAS into the regular pediatric examination of the newborn.

THE ENVIRONMENT OF THE NEONATAL UNIT

THE INFANT'S WORLD

The environment of the neonatal unit has many effects on infants and their parents.[54,162,211] For example, incubators provide a physical barrier and create a psychological distance for parents and staff.[92] A crying baby in an incubator is difficult to hear and this may partly account for the lack of relationship between an infant's behaviour and that of the caretakers which has been reported in neonatal units.[157] Another contributory factor is the traditional organization of work by regular routine which is still used in many hospitals. A large number of staff may deal with a particular baby, each paying brief visits. During a stay of 49 days in a Toronto nursery, a baby was attended by an average of 71 different nurses.[130] Clearly, in such a situation, it is very difficult for caretakers to learn anything of the individual character of a baby or for the baby to discover any consistency in the caretaking experience. While a few units have adopted policies whereby each nurse is assigned to the same baby on each shift to avoid this problem, it has been suggested that such schemes prevent flexible deployment of staff and may lead to what some see as an undesirably close relationship between staff and babies. Clearly, there is a conflict between the traditional bureaucratic style of organization in which there are roles that can be occupied by any one of a large number of people, and in which an emotional distance is maintained between staff and patient, and the characteristics of the usual parent–child relationship.

High levels of noise in some incubators[5,22] and the unvarying light through day and night that are sometimes experienced lead to further isolation for the baby from the normal social world.[80,164] Measurements of the physical environment suggest that levels of sensory stimulation are high but with little circadian variation or correlation between that experienced by the infant in the various sensory modalities.[108] Observations that a deterioration in clinical condition may follow the handling of a small or sick neonate and that handling can result in transient hypoxia have led to policies of minimal contact.[132,187] Premature infants can feel pain just as well as a healthy term infant.[28,193]

A wide range of stimulation programmes have been applied to preterm and sick babies, involving such things as rocking waterbeds, patterned sound and light, stroking, rubbing and touching, playing of baroque music and other forms of 'multimodal sensory enrichment'. In some cases, these interventions were combined with follow-up programmes in which mothers were given support and information postnatally.[178] Reviews of these studies[80,179] conclude that, despite their somewhat uneven methodological quality, there is evidence that scores from development tests and, in a few cases, growth are improved by these techniques. However, the fact that such a wide range of interventions based on such different rationales all had similar results suggests that the response is non-specific, perhaps mediated by greater nursing attention to babies in experimental groups.

Other interventions have been aimed at more specific features of the neonatal environment. Placing preterm babies on lambswool as compared with standard bedding seems to increase weight gain.[180] This effect is perhaps similar to that which has been demonstrated by swaddling, traditionally a very widespread practice outside the humid tropics.[42,114] Skin-to-skin care ('kangaroo') where mothers and fathers hold their preterm infants on their chest under protective clothing reduced crying, increased breast-feeding, weight gain and early discharge in one study.[10]

Some hospitals are now using the concept of developmental care. This was first developed by Heidi Als and colleagues,[7] who suggested that babies who were unable to maintain homeostasis needed physical containment in the fetal position, dimming of lights, protection from loud sounds and less handling. The Neonatal Individualized Developmental Care and Assessment Program may encourage staff to observe the baby's reaction to stimuli and then try to reduce the negative aspects of stimuli. Infants receiving developmental care spent less time on a respirator, less time in oxygen and performed better on development tests.[7]

THE SOCIAL WORLD OF THE NEONATAL UNIT FOR PARENTS AND STAFF

As neonatal units began to encourage parents to spend time with their infants, it became clear that more was involved than simply the absence of separation.[52] Were parents simply visitors and spectators or did they have a significant role in the care of their children? If they were to undertake caretaking tasks, how might this modify the traditional role of the nurse, doctor and midwife? As policies have changed, these questions have had to be settled and new working relationships developed. There seems wide agreement that parents should be encouraged to play their part in caretaking and that the nursing role should shift from one of undertaking all infant care to a more flexible position where priority is given to supporting parents in their role. Some tasks, like nasogastric tube feeding, which traditionally were always undertaken by nursing staff, are now taught to parents. But this transformation of role has not always been easy. It has sometimes been felt that there is an incompatibility between handing over some of the caretaking to parents and maintaining an overall responsibility for what happens. Rivalries occur over infants, and staff and parents can both feel excluded by each other. Specific problems arise over the need to cope with stressed and anxious parents.[51,87,199,215] There are also more straightforward matters of time pressures – it may be much quicker and simpler for an experienced nurse to tube feed a baby than for her to explain the technique to parents and stay with them while they do it inexpertly. Solving these kinds of problems depends on an appreciation of how things are seen from the parents' point of view. For parents, the period their baby is in a neonatal unit is likely to be a unique time in their lives, which they will always remember, but for staff these parents will be but one of the tens or hundreds they will deal with during the year. Many techniques have been evolved for sensitizing staff to these issues. The use of role-playing exercises and reading about the experiences of parents[194] both appear to be especially valuable.

A recent study of parents' experience of neonatal units in the UK found that: 'the words and actions of nursing and medical staff; the way a unit is run and organised; policies and how these are put into practice all contribute to the parents' sense of wellbeing, confidence and trust.'[162]

ADMISSION AND DISCHARGE POLICIES

Clinical and economic arguments may support the idea of centralized neonatal units, but centralization increases the likelihood of separation for parents and children. In a UK study,[164] 20% of babies in the sample had neonatal care in more than one unit and 6% had care in three or more hospitals. 13% of the mothers were moved to another hospital just before giving birth. The extent to which neonatal admissions are likely to disrupt parent–child relations will depend on the provision of facilities for the care of the mother beside her baby[74] and policies for joint admission. There should be sufficient rooms for parents and baby and they should be used only by the parents and not also by medical staff. Having these rooms available means that mothers or parents can come to stay at any time for the purposes of establishing breast-feeding, or when their baby is very ill and they live far away.

Criteria for admission and discharge are also crucial. Infants with relatively minor problems can be satisfactorily cared for in the general lying-in wards or transitional care wards where there is more specialized neonatal paediatric nursing and medical support. Different types of units tend to have a different casemix; Redshaw et al[162] state 'Regional centres cared for many of the smallest preterm babies and admitted most of the infants with suspected abnormalities; subregional and district units admitted twice as many babies with hypoglycemia and a fifth of admissions to district units were associated with feeding problems'.

VISITING

Though visiting a baby in a neonatal unit may not be sufficient to build a satisfactory parent–child relationship, some admissions are clearly unavoidable. However, even with open-door visiting policies, there are considerable psychological and practical obstacles to visiting. Parents may stay away for fear of what they may see, or feel that they do not want to risk becoming closely involved with their baby until they are reasonably confident that he will survive. More practical problems may include the costs of travel, the presence of other children requiring care at home, or the need for continuing medical care in another hospital for the mother.[92] Some parents will spend long hours every day, and perhaps night, in the neonatal unit, while others will come much less frequently. Parents' needs and wishes about such matters need to be respected, and visiting frequency should not be equated with the quality of the parent–child relationship. The importance of families using the social support they need from their extended family has been highlighted by McHaffie[117] and therefore allowing visits by grandparents and other family members or possibly close friends who are important to the baby's parents should be a priority. It should be part of the provision of adequate neonatal care to ensure that parents and other close relatives are not prevented from visiting either by practical barriers such as cost or by psychological ones. To ensure this, social work and counselling must be available as required in addition to sensitive nursing and medical support. Several units now have parent-run support groups but few units have counsellors as part of the team. Those that do have found that the staff on the units also need supportive help, although it may be difficult for them to admit it (Lewis, personal communication, 1995).

INFORMATION

Parents often receive insufficient information about the current medical problems of their baby or about prognosis.[163,164] This reflects both pressures on staff time and the characteristic of all medical consultations that space and time are required to absorb information and to reformulate it in understandable terms. A specialized worker to mediate between parents and nursing and medical staff may be desirable.[119] It is difficult to generalize about what should or should not be said to parents. It is inadequate simply to wait for parents to ask questions and inappropriate in most cases to convey all that may be found in the clinical notes. 'Be honest but not cruel'[24] would seem a reasonable motto, and experience gradually teaches how to respond to the varying needs parents may have for information. Full discussion and involvement in decision-making may be particularly important when it may become necessary to consider whether further treatment is appropriate.[13] Parents need to be given information in a variety of formats. In a study in Toronto[152] parents received detailed information in 77% of cases but only 39% of parents recalled this. Parents wanted most information about management.

It is clear from several studies that written information is a necessity but this is not always provided.[91,162] Carefully written information about what to expect in a neonatal unit and about some of the common problems should be given to parents so they can refer to it again and again. There is also a growing collection of books for parents about specific conditions and handicaps.[3,78,89] While publications are generally well received by parents, they should not be seen as a substitute for discussions.

When an abnormal baby is born, parents will want to know why and the chance of a recurrence of the problem in future pregnancies. Where genetic disorders are involved, this information may be best provided by specialized genetic counsellors. Follow-up studies show that genetic information is not always provided in a form that families can understand and that attitudes towards having further children may be more influenced by a sense of the burden created by the disease than knowledge of precise risk figures.[63,121]

PHOTOGRAPHS

A rather different kind of information is provided by the photographs of babies that many units give to parents. Particularly when visiting is impossible, these can provide a great comfort to parents to dispel fantasies about the baby's appearance. They may also serve as a tangible representation of the baby that parents can show to visiting friends and relatives. Photographs in or near the neonatal unit of babies who were in the unit and what they looked like when older also seem to be very helpful to parents.

SUPPORT FOR STAFF AND PARENTS

Neonatal units may be stressful for staff as well as parents, and there are increasing numbers of attempts to provide appropriate support.[142] A classic paper by Menzies[126] outlines sources of stress for nurses, and there has been much work on 'burn-out' of staff in intensive care units. Organization, staffing levels, education, training and emotional support are all areas in nursing where problems can arise. Lack of adequate provision in these areas can contribute to staff fatigue, sickness and stress levels, and reduce feelings of well-being.[143,164]

Acknowledgement of these pressures has led to the setting up of staff groups and other ways of providing opportunities for staff to deal with their feelings in safe situations.[149] Some units have appointed psychotherapists or counsellors, whose roles include the support of staff and parents. Indeed, even where the attempt has been to fill one or other of these roles, the boundaries soon become blurred.

Very few neonatal units in the UK have counsellors available for staff and/or parents. In a review of a counselling service offered by Lewis (personal communication, 1995), she reported that the service was equally utilized by parents and staff. She saw her work with the staff as vital, as, if their emotional needs were recognized, the atmosphere on the unit for all individuals, both parents and staff, became more open, communicative and supportive.

There is evidence that a team approach in neonatal units and postnatal care works well. The teams consist of psychologists, counsellors, social workers, medical and nursing staff, physical therapists and occupational therapists who are involved in developmental or family-centred care of the neonate and the family.[102,128] Neonatal staff are increasingly attempting to understand the parenting or 'maternal work' parents need to do in order to promote mother–infant attachment.[90,107,177,198]

Support for parents whose child dies is discussed elsewhere in this book, but it is equally important to recognize the grief and anxiety of parents whose children are handicapped or sick and where hopes and aspirations have been thwarted in other ways, such as by a multiple birth. Five stages of shock, denial, sadness and anger, adaptation and reorganization have been described as the evolution of parental responses to the birth of a baby with a congenital malformation,[58] while others have put more emphasis on the need to mourn the child who might have been.[186] The giving of bad news to parents is a demanding and distressing task. Mothers and fathers attach great importance to the approach and general attitude of the medical and nursing staff who first give the news[50] and in the initial period this may be more important than what is actually said about the condition. Many sessions will be required to allow the parents to make their own sense of the situation and gain the information they want. As Taylor[200] remarks, counselling is not a monologue, and despite the fraught situation the parents must be given the opportunity to talk until the problem is clearly understood. Where more than one professional is involved, it is vital that each recognizes what the other is doing[75,207] and good communication exists.

It is important when talking to parents to recognize the gap that may exist between a paediatric and a parental perspective. For instance, parents with healthy premature infants whose present or future problems are unlikely to be serious may sometimes require considerable counselling and reassurance. With multiple births, apart from any medical difficulty which any of the children may face, parents may feel acutely split in their attempts to divide their attention between their children and are simply overwhelmed by the task that faces them. Without help, these conflicts are sometimes resolved by giving most of the attention to one twin[67] (and see Botting et al[25] for triplets and higher multiples). This situation may be exacerbated by discharging siblings at different times.

A number of successful schemes tailored to local circumstances have been set up to provide continuing support to families with children at risk after discharge from neonatal units.[66,160] In some places parents have set up mutual support organizations.[111,158] There are also some areas where neonatal nurses work in the community, following up babies who are sent home tube-feeding or on oxygen. This has been a successful practice allowing babies to be discharged sooner, and helping parents gain confidence in looking after their babies themselves.[53]

PSYCHOSOCIAL INTERVENTIONS

In the last few years, there has been a growing interest in therapeutic interventions in the neonatal period to improve family relationships.[14,38,60,72,125] The new field of infancy research has exploded with programmes ranging from hospital-based to home-based interventions.[1,150,188] Although short-term benefits are often clearly seen, fewer studies have shown long-term effects of early intervention. It is clear from most recent studies on premature babies or babies with difficult sleeping, crying or feeding behaviours, that most parents need extra support, guidance and information about development.[213,217]

There are many issues surrounding the timing, length and type of these interventions. One study showed that there can be negative effects of early interventions for mothers who need little support.[2] If intervention programmes are introduced too late, caretaking patterns have already been established,[36,93] but starting interventions too early may be ineffective. It seems that future studies should focus on individualized intervention programmes that take the mother's needs and psychological status into account and focus on interactive work with the mother/infant dyad.[17,191,212,218]

REFERENCES

1. Achenbach T M, Howell C T, Aoki M F, Rauh V A 1993 Nine-year outcome of the Vermont intervention program for low birth weight infants. Pediatrics 91: 45–55
2. Affleck G, Tennen H, Rowe J, Roscher B, Walker L 1989 Effects of formal support on mother's adaptation to the hospital-to-home

transition of high-risk infants: the benefits and costs of helping. Child Development 60: 488–501
3. Alderson P 1983 Special care for babies in hospital. National Association for the Welfare of Children in Hospital, London
4. Aleksandrowicz M K 1974 The effects of pain relieving drugs administered during labour and delivery, on the behavior of the newborn: a review. Merrill Palmer Quarterly 20: 1, 121–141
5. Als H, Brazelton T B 1981 A new model for assessing the behavioural organization in preterm and full-term infants. Journal of American Academy of Child Psychiatry 20: 239–263
6. Als H, Duffy F 1983 The behaviour of the premature infant. In: Brazelton T B, Lester B M (eds) New approaches to developmental screening in infancy. Elsevier, New York, pp 153–173
7. Als H, Lawhon G, Brown E, Gibes R, Duffy F H, McAnutty G, Blickman J G 1986 Individualized behavioral and environmental care for the very low birthweight preterm infant at risk for bronchopulmonary dysplasia: neonatal intensive care and developmental outcome. Pediatrics 78: 1123–1132
8. Anders T F, Chalemian R J 1974 The effects of circumcision on sleep-wake states in human neonates. Psychosomatic Medicine 36: 174–179
9. Anders T, Keener M, Bowe R, Shoaff B 1982 A longitudinal study of night-time sleepwake patterns in infants from birth through one year. In: Call J, Galensen E (eds) Frontiers in infant psychiatry. Basic Books, New York, pp 152–170
10. Anderson G C 1991 Current knowledge about skin-to-skin (kangaroo) care for preterm infants (Review). Journal of Perinatology 11: 216–226
11. Andrews S R, Blumenthal J B, Johnson D L, Kahn A J, Ferguson C J, Lasater T M, Malone P E, Wallace D B 1982 The skills of mothering: a study of parent child development centers. Monograph of Society for Research in Child Development, No. 198, University of Chicago Press, Chicago, III
12. Appleton T, Clifton R, Goldberg S 1975 The development of behavioral competence in infancy. In: Horowitz F D (ed) Review of child development research. University of Chicago Press, Chicago, vol 6, pp 291–311
13. Arras J D 1987 Quality of life in neonatal ethics: beyond denial and evasion. In: Weil W B, Benjamin M (eds) Ethical issues at the onset of life. Blackwell Scientific Publications, Boston, pp 151–186
14. Barnard K E, Morisset C E, Spieker S 1993 Preventive interventions: enhancing parent–infant relationships. In: Zeanah C (ed) Handbook of infant mental health. Guildford Press, New York
15. Beail N, McGuire J (eds) 1982 Fathers: psychological perspectives. Junction Books, London
16. Beckwith L, Cohen S E 1978 Preterm birth: hazardous obstetrical and postnatal events as related to caregiver–infant behavior. Infant Behavior and Development 1: 403–411
17. Beckwith L, Sigman M 1995 Preventive interventions in infancy. Child and Adolescent Psychiatric Clinics of North America 4: 683–700
18. Bee H L 1995 The developing child. HarperCollins College, New York
19. Bidder R T, Crowe E A, Gray O P 1974 Mothers' attitudes to preterm infants. Archives of Disease in Childhood 49: 766–770
20. Bjerne I, Hanson E 1976 Psychomotor development and school adjustment of 7 year old children with low birth weight. Acta Paediatrica Scandinavica 65: 88–96
21. Blake A, Stewart A, Turean D 1975 Parents of babies of very low birthweight: longterm follow-up. Parent–infant interaction. Ciba Foundation Symposium 33. Elsevier, Amsterdam, pp 271–280
22. Blennow G, Svenningsen N W, Almquist M 1974 Noise levels in infant incubators (adverse effects?). Pediatrics 53: 29–33
23. Bodegard G, Fyro K, Larsson A 1984 Psychological reactions in 102 families with a newborn who has a falsely positive screening test for congenital hypothyroidism. Acta Paediatrica Scandinavica Supplement No. 304
24. Bogdan R, Brown M A, Foster S B 1982 Be honest but not cruel: staff–parent communication on a neonatal unit. Human Organisation 41: 6–16
25. Botting B, Macfarlane A, Price F 1990 Three, four or more. A national survey of triplets and higher order births. HMSO, London
26. Boulton M G 1983 On being a mother. Tavistock, London
27. Boyce P M, Stubbs J M 1994 The importance of postnatal depression. Medical Journal of Australia 151: 471–472
28. Bozzette M 1993 Observation of pain behavior in the NICU: an exploratory study. Journal of Perinatal and Neonatal Nursing 7: 76–87
29. Brachfeld S, Goldberg S, Sloman J 1980 Parent–infant interaction in free play at 8 and 12 months: effects of prematurity and immaturity. Infant Behavior and Development 3: 289–305
30. Brackbill Y 1979 Obstetrical medication and infant behavior. In: Osofsky J D (ed) Handbook of infant development. Wiley, New York, pp 76–125
31. Brazelton T B 1992 Touchpoints, your child's emotional and behavioural development. Penguin Books, London
32. Brazelton T B 1995 Working with families. Opportunities for early intervention. Pediatric Clinics of North America 42: 1–9
33. Brazelton T B, Nugent J K 1995 Neonatal Behavioral Assessment Scale, 3rd edn. MacKeith Press, London
34. Brazelton T B, Robey J S 1965 Observations of neonatal behavior. The effect of perinatal variables, in particular that of maternal medication. Journal of the American Academy of Child Psychiatry 4: 613
35. Brockington F, Kumar R (eds) 1982 Motherhood and mental illness. Academic Press, London
36. Bromwich R M, Parmalee A H 1979 An intervention programme for preterm infants. In: Field T M, Shuman H H (eds) Infants born at risk: behavior and development. SP Medical and Scientific Books, New York, pp 384–411
37. Brown G W, Harris J 1978 The social origins of depression. Tavistock, London
38. Brown J V, La Rossa M M, Aylward G P, Davis D J, Rutherford P K, Bakeman R 1980 Nursery-based intervention with prematurely born babies and their others: are there effects? Journal of Pediatrics 97: 487–491
39. Burton B K, Dillard R G, Clark E N 1985 Maternal serum alpha-fetoprotein screening: the effect of participation on anxiety and attitude toward pregnancy in women with normal results. American Journal of Obstetrics and Gynecology 152: 540–543
40. Caplan G, Mason E A, Kaplan D M 1965 Four studies of crisis in parents of prematures. Communications in Mental Health 1: 149–161
41. Chalmers I, Zlosnik J E, John D A, Campbell H 1976 Obstetric practice and outcome of pregnancy in Cardiff residents 1965–1973. British Medical Journal 1: 735–738
42. Chisholm J J, Richards M P M 1978 Swaddling, cradleboards and the development of children. Early Human Development 2: 255–275
43. Chitty L S, Hunt G H, Moore J, Lobb M O 1991 Effectiveness of routine ultrasonography in detecting fetal structural abnormalities in a low risk population. British Medical Journal 303: 1165–1169
44. Chudleigh P, Pearce J M, Campbell S 1984 The prenatal diagnosis of transient cysts of the fetal choroid plexus. Prenatal Diagnosis 4: 135–137
45. Clark S L, De Vore G R, Sabey P L 1988 Prenatal diagnosis of cysts of the fetal choroid plexus. Obstetrics and Gynecology 72: 585–587
46. Cox J L, Holden J, Sagovsky R 1987 Detection of postnatal depression: development of the 10-item Edinburgh Postnatal Depression Scale (EPDS). British Journal of Psychiatry 150: 782–786
47. Cox J L, Murray D, Chapman G 1993 A controlled study of the onset, duration and prevalence of postnatal depression. British Journal of Psychiatry 163: 27–31
48. Crawford W 1982 Mother–infant interaction in premature and full-term infants. Child Development 53: 957–962
49. Crnic K A, Ragozin A S, Greenberg M T, Robinson N M, Basham R B 1983 Social interaction and developmental competence of preterm and full-term infants during the first year of life. Child Development 54: 1119–1120
50. D'Arcy E 1968 Congenital defects: mothers' reactions to first information. British Medical Journal 3: 796–798
51. Davis J, Kitzinger S (eds) 1978 The place of birth. Oxford University Press, London
52. Davis J A, Richards M P M, Roberton N R C (eds) 1983 Parent–baby attachment in premature infants. Croom Helm, London
53. Dawson B 1994 'Special care' in the community role of the community neonatal liaison sister. Professional Nurse 10: 78–80
54. De Chateau P 1979 Effects of hospital practices on synchrony in the development of the infant–parent relationship. Seminars in Perinatology 3: 45–60
55. Deutch H 1947 The psychology of women. Vol. 2, motherhood. Research Books, London
56. Diamond L J, Jaudes P K 1983 Child abuse in a cerebral-palsied population. Developmental Medicine and Child Neurology 25: 169–174

57. Divitto B, Goldberg S 1979 The effects of newborn medical status on early parent–infant interaction. In: Field T M (ed) Infants born at risk: behavior and development. S P Medical Books, Jamaica, pp 311–332
58. Drotar D, Baskiewicz A, Irvin N, Kennell J, Klaus M 1975 The adaptation of parents to the birth of an infant with a congenital malformation: a hypothetical model. Pediatrics 56: 710–717
59. Dubowitz V 1975 Neurological fragility in the newborn – influence of medication in labour. British Journal of Anaesthetics 47: 1005–1010
60. Dudley M, Gyler L, Blinkhorn S, Barnett B 1993 Psychosocial interventions for very low birthweight infants: their scope and efficacy. Australian and New Zealand Journal of Psychiatry 27: 74–83
61. Durkin K 1995 (ed) Developmental social psychology: from infancy to old age. Blackwell, Cambridge, Mass
62. Emde R, Swedberg J, Suzuki B 1975 Human wakefulness and biological rhythm after birth. Archives of General Psychiatry 32: 780–786
63. Evers-Kiebooms G, van den Berghe H 1979 Impact of genetic counselling. a review of published follow-up studies. Clinical Genetics 15: 465–474
64. Farber E A, Vaughn B, Egeland B 1981 The relationship of prenatal maternal anxiety to infant behaviour and mother–infant interaction during the first six months of life. Early Human Development 5: 267–277
65. Fearn J, Hibbard B M, Lawrence K M, Roberts A, Robinson J O 1982 Screening for neural-tube defects and maternal anxiety. British Journal of Obstetrics and Gynaecology 89: 218–221
66. Ferrari L, Pelafigue A, Salbreux R 1988 Early and continuous action to prevent breakdown in the care of infants and their families after serious neonatal episodes. Infant Mental Health Journal 9: 82–92
67. Field R, Walden T, Widmayer S, Greenberg R 1982 The early development of preterm discordant twin pairs: bigger is not always better. In: Lipsitt L P, Field T M (eds) Infant behavior and development: perinatal risk and newborn behavior. Ablex, Norwood, pp 153–163
68. Field T M 1984 Early interactions between infants and their postpartum depressed mothers. Infant Behavior and Development 7: 517–522
69. Field T 1992 Interventions in early infancy. Infant Mental Health Journal 13: 329–336
70. Field T, Sandberg D, Quetel T A, Garcia R, Rosario M 1985 Effect of ultrasound feedback on pregnancy anxiety, fetal activity, and neonatal outcome. Obstetrics and Gynaecology 66: 525–528
71. Fonagy P, Steele H, Steele M 1991 Maternal representations of attachment during pregnancy predict the organization of infant–mother attachment at one year of age. Child Development 62: 891–905
72. Forrest G C 1993 Preterm labour and delivery: psychological sequelae. Baillière's Clinical Obstetrics and Gynaecology 7: 653–668
73. Gaines R, Sandgrund A, Green A H, Power E 1978 Etiological factors in child maltreatment: a multivariate study of abusing, neglecting and normal mothers. Journal for Abnormal Psychology 87: 531–540
74. Garrow D H 1983 Special care without separation: High Wycombe, England. In: Davis J A, Richards M P M, Roberton N R C (eds) Parent–baby attachment in premature infants. Croom Helm, London, pp 223–231
75. Gath A, Gumley D 1984 Down's syndrome and the family: follow-up of children first seen in infancy. Developmental Medicine and Child Neurology 26: 500–508
76. Goldberg S 1979 Premature birth: consequences for the parent–infant relationship. American Scientist 67: 214–220
77. Goldberg S 1983 Parent–infant bonding: another look. Child Development 54: 1355–1382
78. Goldberg S, Divitto B A 1983 Born too soon. Freeman, San Francisco
79. Goldberg S, Brackfield S, Divitto B 1980 Feeding, fussing and play: parent infant interaction in the first year as a function of prematurity and perinatal medical problems. In: Field T M (ed) High-risk infants and children: adults and peer reactions. Academic Press, New York, pp 54–67
80. Gottfried A W, Wallace-Lande P, Sherman-Brown S, King J, Coen C, Hodgmar J E 1981 Physical and social environment of newborn infants in special care units. Science 2145: 673–675
81. Green J 1990 Calming or harming. A critical review of the psychological effects of fetal diagnosis on pregnant women. Occasional paper. The Galton Society, London
82. Green J, Richards M P M, Kitzinger J V, Coupland V A 1991 Mothers' perceptions of their 6 week old babies: relationship with antenatal, intrapartum and postnatal factors. Irish Journal of Psychology 12: 133–144
83. Green J M, Coupland V A, Kitzinger J V 1991 Expectations, experiences and psychological outcomes of childbirth: a prospective study of 825 women. Birth 17: 15–24
84. Green J, Statham H, Snowdon C 1993 Women's knowledge of prenatal screening tests. Relationships with hospital screening policy and demographic factors. Journal of Reproductive and Infant Psychology 11: 11–20
85. Gunnar M R, Fisch R O, Malone S 1984 The effects of a pacifying stimulus on behavioral and adrenocortical responses to circumcision in the newborn. Journal of the American Academy of Child Psychiatry 23: 34–38
86. Hack M, De Monterice D, Merkatz I R, Jones P, Fanaroff A A 1981 Rehospitalization of the very low birthweight infant. American Journal of Diseases of Children 135: 263–266
87. Hancock E 1976 Crisis intervention in a newborn nursery intensive care unit. Social Work in Health Care 1: 421–432
88. Harper R G, Sia C, Sokal S, Sokal M 1976 Observations on unrestricted parental contact with infants in the neonatal intensive care unit. Journal of Pediatrics 89: 441–445
89. Harrison H 1983 The premature baby book. St Martin's Press, New York
90. Haut C, Peddicord K, O'Brien E 1994 Supporting parental bonding in the NICU: a care plan for nurses. Neonatal Network 13: 19–25
91. Hawthorne Amick J 1989 The effect of different routines in a special care baby unit on the mother–infant relationships (Great Britain). In: Nugent J K, Lester B M, Brazelton T B (eds) The cultural context of infancy. 1. Ablex, New Jersey
92. Hawthorne J T, Richards M P M, Callon M 1978 A study of parental visiting of babies in a special care unit. In: Brimblecombe F S W, Richards M P M, Roberton N R C (eds) Separation and special care baby units. Clinics in Developmental Medicine No. 68. Heinemann Medical Books, London, pp 33–54
93. Heinicke C, Beckwith L, Thompson A 1988 Early intervention in the family system: a framework and review. Infant Mental Health Journal 9: 111–141
94. Herzog J M 1979 Disturbance in parenting high-risk infants: clinical impressions and hypotheses. In: Field T M (ed) Infants born at risk. Spectrum, Jamaica, pp 102–129
95. Horowitz F D, Ashton J, Culp R, Gaddis E, Lewin S, Reichmann B 1977 The effects of obstetrical medication on the behaviour of Israeli newborn infants and some comparisons with Uruguayan and American Infants. Child Development 48: 1607–1623
96. Jeffcoate J A, Humphrey M E, Lloyd J K 1979 Role perception and response to stress in fathers and mothers following preterm delivery. Social Science and Medicine 13: 139–145
97. Joffe J M 1969 Prenatal determinants of behaviour. Pergamon, Oxford
98. Kaplan D M, Mason E A 1960 Maternal reactions to premature birth viewed as an acute emotional disorder. American Journal of Orthopsychiatry 30: 539–552
99. Keefer C H 1995 The combined physical and behavioural neonatal examination: A parent-centered approach to pediatric care. In: Brazelton T B, Nugent J K (eds) Neonatal Behavioural Assessment Scale, 3rd edn. MacKeith Press, London, pp 92–101
100. Kendall R E, Rennie D, Clarke J H, Dean C 1981 The social and obstetric correlates of psychiatric admissions in the puerperium. Psychological Medicine 11: 341–350
101. Klaus M H, Kennell H 1982 Parent–infant bonding, 2nd edn. Mosby, St Louis, MO
102. Korones S B 1983 The role of social workers in the neonatal intensive care unit. In: Davis J A, Richards M P M, Roberton N R C (eds) Parent baby attachment in premature infants. Croom Helm, London, pp 139–155
103. Kumar R, Brockington I F 1988 Motherhood and mental illness 2. Causes and consequences. John Wright, London
104. Kumar R, Robson K M 1984 A prospective study of emotional disorders in childbearing women. British Journal of Psychiatry 144: 35–47
105. Lamb M E 1983 Early mother–neonate contact and the mother–child relationship. Journal of Child Psychology and Psychiatry 24: 487–494
106. Lamb M E 1996 The role of the father in child development. Wiley, New York

107. Lasby K, Newton S, Sherrow T, Stainton M C, McNeil D 1994 Maternal work in the NICU: a case study of an 'NICU-experienced' mother. Issues in Comprehensive Pediatric Nursing 17: 147–160
108. Lawson K, Daum C, Turkewitz G 1977 Environmental characteristics of a neonatal intensive care unit. Child Development 48: 1633–1639
109. Lax R F 1972 Some aspects of the interaction between mother and impaired child: mothers' narcissistic trauma. International Journal of Psychoanalysis 53: 339–344
110. Levy D M 1966 Maternal overprotection. Norton, New York
111. Lindsay J K, Roman L, DeWys M, Eager M, Levick J, Quinn M 1993 Creative caring in the NICU: parent-to-parent support. Neonatal Network 12: 37–44
112. Lipson J G, Tilden V P 1980 Psychological integration of the Caesarean birth experience. American Journal of Orthopsychiatry 50: 598–609
113. Liptak G S, Keller B B, Feldman A W, Chamberlin R W 1983 Enhancing infant development and parent–practitioner interaction with the Brazelton Neonatal Assessment Scale. Pediatrics 72: 71–78
114. Lipton E L, Steinschneider A, Richmond J B 1965 Swaddling, a child practice: historical, cultural and experimental observations. Pediatrics 35: 521–567
115. Lynch M A, Roberts J, Gordon M 1976 Child abuse: early warning in the maternity hospital. Developmental Medicine and Child Neurology 18: 756–766
116. McDonald R L 1968 The role of the emotional factors in obstetric complications: a review. Psychosomatic Medicine 30: 222–237
117. McHaffie H E 1992 Social support in the neonatal intensive care unit. Journal of Advanced Nursing 17: 279–287
118. McKee L, O'Brien M (eds) 1982 The father figure. Tavistock, London
119. Malone P S J 1996 Antenatal diagnosis of renal tract anomalies: has it increased the sum of human happiness? Journal of the Royal Society of Medicine 89: 155–158
120. Malphurs J E, Field T M, Larraine C, Pickens J, Pelaez-Nogueras M, Yando R, Bendall D 1996 Alternating withdrawn and intrusive interaction behaviors of depressed mothers. Infant Mental Health Journal 17: 152–160
121. Marteau T, Richards M P M 1996 The troubled helix. Social and psychological implications of the new human genetics. Cambridge University Press, Cambridge
122. Marteau T, Cook R, Kidd J, Michie S, Johnston M, Slack J, Shaw R W 1992 Psychological effects of false positive results in prenatal screening for fetal abnormality: a prospective study. Prenatal Diagnosis 12: 205–214
123. Martin C J, Brown G W, Goldberg D P, Brockington I F 1989 Psychosocial stress and puerperal depression. Journal of Affective Disorders 16: 283–293
124. Mauthner N 1995 Postnatal depression: the significance of social contacts between mothers. Women's Studies International Forum 18: 311–323
125. Meisels S J, Shonkoff J P 1990 Handbook of early childhood intervention. Cambridge University Press, Cambridge
126. Menzies M 1960 The functioning of social systems as a defence against anxiety. Human Relations 13: 95–121
127. Messer D, Richards M P M 1993 The development of sleeping difficulties. In St James-Roberts I, Harris G, Messer D (eds) Infant crying, feeding and sleeping. Harvester Wheatsheaf, London
128. Meyer E C, Garcia Coll C T, Lester B M, Boukydis C F, McDonough S M 1994 Family-based intervention improves maternal psychological well-being and feeding interaction of preterm infants. Pediatrics 93: 241–246
129. Minde K 1993 Prematurity and serious medical illness in infancy: implications for development and intervention. In: Zeanah C (ed) Handbook of infant mental health. Guilford Press, New York
130. Minde K, Ford L, Celhoffer L, Boukydis C 1975 Interactions of mothers and nurses with premature infants. Canadian Medical Association Journal 113: 741–745
131. Minde K, Whitelaw A, Brown J, Fitzhardinge P 1983 Effect of neonatal complications in premature infants on early parent–infant interactions. Developmental Medicine and Child Neurology 25: 763–777
132. Murdoch D R, Darlow B A 1984 Handling during neonatal care. Archives of Disease in Childhood 59: 957–961
133. Murray A D, Thomas D B 1981 Effects of epidural anesthesia on newborns and their mothers. Child Development 52: 71–82
134. Murray D, Cox J L, Chapman G 1995 Childbirth: life event or start of a long term difficulty? British Journal of Psychiatry 166: 595–600
135. Murray L, Stanley C, Hooper R, King F, Fiori-Cowley A 1996 The role of infant factors in postnatal depression and mother–infant interactions. Developmental Medicine and Child Neurology 38: 109–119
136. Myers B J 1982 Early intervention using Brazelton training with middle-class mothers and fathers of newborns. Child Development 53: 462–471
137. Nugent J K 1985 Using the NBAS with infants and their families. March of Dimes, White Plains, NY
138. Nugent J K, Brazelton T B 1989 Preventive intervention with infants and families: the NBAS model. Infant Mental Health Journal 10: 84–99
139. Nugent J K, Lester B M, Brazelton T B 1989 The cultural context of infancy: 1 biology, culture and infant development. Ablex, New Jersey
140. Oakley A 1979 Becoming a mother. Martin Robertson, London
141. Oakley A, Richards M P M 1990. Elective delivery: attitudes and responses of parents and children. In: Garcia J, Kilpatrick R, Richards M P M (eds) The politics of maternity care. Oxford University Press, Oxford
142. Oates R K, Oates P 1995 Stress and mental health in neonatal intensive care units. Archives of Disease in Childhood: Fetal and Neonatal Edition 72: F107–F110
143. Oehler J M, Davidson M G, Starr L E, Lee D A 1991 Burnout, job stress, anxiety and perceived social support in neonatal nurses. Heart and Lung 20: 500–505
144. Osofsky H J, Osofsky J D 1980 Normal adaptation to pregnancy and new parenthood. In: Taylor P M (ed) Parent–infant relationships. Grune & Stratton, New York, pp 25–48
145. Osofsky J D (ed) 1979 Handbook of infant development. Wiley, New York
146. Osofsky J D, (ed) Danziger B 1974 Relationships between neonatal characteristics and mother-infant interaction. Developmental Psychology 10: 124–134
147. Ottinger D R, Simmons J E 1964 Behaviour of human neonates and prenatal maternal anxiety. Psychological Reports 14: 391–394
148. Packer M, Rosenblatt D 1979 Issues in the study of social behaviour in the first week of life. In: Schaffer D, Dunn J (eds) The first year of life. Wiley, Chichester, pp 7–36
149. Parente A S 1982 Psychological pressures in a neonatal ITU. British Journal of Hospital Medicine 27: 266–268
150. Parker S, Zahr L K, Cole J G 1992 Outcomes after developmental intervention in the neonatal intensive care unit for mothers of preterm infants with low socioeconomic status. Journal of Pediatrics 120: 780–785
151. Patel H 1966 The problem of routine circumcision. Canadian Medical Association Journal 95: 576–587
152. Perlman N B, Freedman J L, Abramovitch R 1991 Informational needs of parents of sick neonates. Pediatrics 88: 512–518
153. Pines D 1972 Pregnancy and motherhood: interaction between fantasy and reality. British Journal of Medical Psychology 45: 333–343
154. Prechtl H F R, Beintema D J 1991 The neurological examination of the fullterm newborn infant, 2nd edn. Clinics in Developmental Medicine No. 63. Heinemann Medical Books, London
155. Prechtl H F R, O'Brien M J 1982 Behavioural states of the fullterm newborn. The emergence of a concept. In: Stratton P (ed) Psychobiology of the human neonate. Wiley, Chichester, pp 53–74
156. Prechtl H F R, Fargel J W, Weinmann H M, Bakker H H 1979 Posture, motility and respiration of low risk infants. Developmental Medicine and Child Neurology 21: 3–27
157. Prince J, Firlej M, Harvey D 1978 Contact between babies in incubators and their caretakers. In: Brimblecombe F S W, Richards M P M, Roberton N R C (eds) Separation and special care baby units. Clinics in Developmental Medicine No. 68. Heinemann Medical Books, London, pp 55–63
158. Prudhoe C M, Peters D L 1995 Social support of parents and grandparents in the neonatal intensive care unit. Pediatric Nursing 21: 140–146
159. Pryor J 1996 Physical and behavioural correlates of twelve month development in small-for-gestational age and appropriately-grown infants. Journal of Infant and Reproductive Psychology 14: 233–242
160. Rauh V A, Achenbach T M, Nuvcombe B 1988 Minimising adverse effects of low birthweight: four year results of an early intervention program. Child Development 59: 544–553
161. Redshaw M E, Harris A 1995 Maternal perceptions of neonatal care. Acta Paediatrica 83: 593–598

162. Redshaw M E, Harris A, Ingram J C 1993 Nursing and medical staffing in neonatals. Journal of Nursing Management 1: 221–228
163. Redshaw M E, Rivers R P A, Rosenblatt D B 1985 Born too early. Oxford University Press, Oxford
164. Redshaw M, Harris A, Ingram J C 1996 Delivering neonatal care. The neonatal unit as a working environment: a survey of neonatal nursing. HMSO, London
165. Richards M P M 1977 The induction and acceleration of labour: some benefits and complications. Early Human Development 1: 3–17
166. Richards M P M 1979 Effects of development of medical interventions and the separation of newborns from their parents. In: Shaffer D, Dunn J (eds) The first year of life. Wiley, Chichester, pp 37–54
167. Richards M P M 1982 Effects of analgesics and anaesthetics given in childbirth on child development. Neuropharmacology 20: 1259–1265
168. Richards M P M 1984 The myth of bonding. In: Macfarlane J A (ed) Progress in child health. Churchill Livingstone, Edinburgh, pp 113–120
169. Richards M P M 1989 Social and ethical problems of fetal diagnosis and screening. Journal of Reproductive and Infant Psychology 7: 171–185
170. Richards M P M, Bernal J F 1972 An observational study of mother-infant interaction. In: Blurton-Jones N J (ed) Ethological studies of child behaviour. Cambridge University Press, London
171. Richards M P M, Bernal J F, Brackbill Y 1976 Early behavioral differences: gender or circumcision? Developmental Psychobiology 9: 89–95
172. Richards M P M, Dunn J F, Antonis B 1977 Caretaking in the first year of life: the role of fathers and mothers' social isolation. Child Care, Health and Development 3: 23–36
173. Richardson G A, Day N L, Taylor P M 1989 The effect of prenatal alcohol, marijuana and tobacco exposure on neonatal behavior. Infant Behavior and Development 12: 100–209
174. Robson K M, Kumar R 1980 Delayed onset of maternal affection after childbirth. British Journal of Psychiatry 136: 347–353
175. Ross G S 1980 Parental responses to infants in intensive care: the separation issue re-evaluated. Clinics in Perinatology 7: 47–60
176. Sandler M (ed) 1978 Mental illness in pregnancy and the puerperium. Oxford University Press, Oxford
177. Saunders A N 1994 Changing nurses' attitudes toward parenting in the NICU. Pediatric Nursing 20: 392–394
178. Scarr-Salapatek S, Williams M L 1973 The effects of early stimulation on low birthweight infants. Child Development 44: 94–101
179. Schaefer M, Hatcher R, Barglow P 1980 Prematurity and infant stimulation, a review of research. Child Psychiatry and Human Development 10: 199–212
180. Scott S, Lucas P, Cole T, Richards M P M 1983 Weight gain and movement patterns of very low birthweight babies nursed on lambswool. Lancet ii: 1014–1016
181. Seashore M J 1981 Mother–infant separation: Outcome assessment. In: Smeriglio V L, (ed) Newborns and parents. Erlbaum, Hillsdale, pp 45–88
182. Sepkoski C M 1986 Neonatal neurobehaviour 1. Development and its relation to obstetric medication. Clinics in Anaesthesiology 4: 209–217
183. Sharp D, Hay D F, Pawlby S, Schmucker G, Allen H, Kumar R 1995 The impact of postnatal depression on boy's intellectual development. Journal of Child Psychology and Psychiatry 36(8): 1315–1336
184. Simkin P, Enkin M 1989 Antenatal classes. In: Chalmers I, Enkin M, Keirse M J N C (eds) Effective care in pregnancy and childbirth. Oxford University Press, Oxford, vol 1, pp 318–334
185. Sluckin W, Herbert M, Sluckin A 1983 Maternal bonding. Blackwell Scientific Publications, Oxford
186. Solnit A J, Stark M H 1961 Mourning and the birth of a defective child. Psychoanalytic Study of Children 16: 523–534
187. Speidel B D 1978 Adverse effects of routine procedures on preterm infants. Lancet 1: 864–866
188. Spiker D, Ferguson J, Brooks-Gunn J 1993 Enhancing maternal interactive behavior and child social competence in low birthweight, premature infants. Child Development 64: 754–768
189. Starr R H 1988 Pre- and perinatal risk and physical abuse. Journal of Reproductive and Infant Psychology 6: 125–138
190. Stein A, Cooper P J, Campbell E A, Day A, Altham P M 1989 Social adversity and perinatal complications: their relationship to postnatal depression. British Medical Journal 298: 1073–1074
191. Stern D N 1995 The motherhood constellation: a unified view of mother–infant psychotherapy. Basic Books, New York
192. Stern M, Hildebrandt K A 1984 Prematurity stereotype: effects of labelling on adults' perceptions of infants. Developmental Psychology 20: 360–362
193. Stevens B J, Johnson C C, Horton L 1993 Multidimensional pain assessment in premature neonates: a pilot study. Journal of Obstetric, Gynecologic and Neonatal Nursing 22: 531–541
194. Stinson R, Stinson P 1983 The long dying of baby Andrew. Little Brown, Boston
195. Stjernqvist K 1992 Extremely low birth weight infants less than 901 g. Impact on the family during the first year. Scandinavian Journal of Social Medicine 20: 226–233
196. Stott D H 1971 The child's hazards in utero. In: Howells J G (ed) Modern perspectives in international child psychiatry. Bruner-Mazel, New York, pp 210–237
197. Svejda M J, Pannabeeker B J, Emde R N 1982 Parent-to-infant attachment: a critique of the early 'bonding' model. In: Emde R N, Harmon R J (eds) Attachment and affiliative systems. Plenum, New York, pp 83–94
198. Symanski M E 1992 Maternal–infant bonding. Practice issues for the 1990s (Review). Journal of Nurse–Midwifery 37(suppl 2): 67S–73S
199. Szur R, Freud W E, Elkan J, Eatnshaw A, Bender H 1981 Hospital care of the newborn: some aspects of personal stress. Journal of Child Psychotherapy 7: 3–28
200. Taylor D C 1982 Counselling the parents of handicapped children. British Medical Journal 284: 1027–1028
201. Thomas D F M, Madden N P, Irving H C, Arthur R J, Smith S E W 1994 Mild dilatation of the fetal kidney: a follow-up study. British Journal of Urology 74: 236–239
202. Trause M A, Kramer L I 1983 The effects of premature birth on parents and their relationship. Developmental Medicine and Child Neurology 25: 459–465
203. Trevarthen C, Murray L, Hubley P 1981 Psychology of infants. In: Davies J A, Dobbing J (eds) Scientific foundations of paediatrics, 2nd edn. Heinemann Medical Books, London, pp 211–273
204. Tronick E Z 1987 The neonatal behavioral assessment scale as a biomarker of the effects of environmental agents on the newborn. Environmental Health Perspective 74: 185–189
205. Trowell J 1982 Possible effects of emergency caesarian section on the mother–child relationship. Early Human Development 7: 41–52
206. Vietze P M, O'Connor S 1981 Mother-to-infant bonding: a review. In: Kretchmer N, Brasel J (eds) Biomedical and special bases of pediatrics. Masson, New York, pp 110–127
207. Walker J H, Thomas M, Russell I T 1971 Spina bifida – and the parents. Developmental Medicine and Child Neurology 13: 462–476
208. Widmayer S M, Field T M 1980 Effects of Brazelton demonstrations on early interactions of preterm infants and their teenage mothers. Infant Behavior and Development 3: 78–79
209. Winnicott D W 1958 Collected papers. Tavistock, London
210. Winnicott D W 1975 Through paediatrics to psychoanalysis. The Holgarth Press, London
211. Wolke D 1987 Environmental and developmental neonatology. Journal of Reproductive and Infant Psychology 5: 17–42
212. Wolke D 1991 Supporting the development of low-birthweight infants. Journal of Child Psychology and Psychiatry 32: 723–741
213. Wolke D, Meyer R, Ohrt B, Riegel K 1995 The incidence of sleeping problems in preterm and fullterm infants discharged from neonatal special care units: an epidemiological longitudinal study. Journal of Child Psychology and Psychiatry 36: 203–223
214. Yogman M W 1981 Parent–infant bonding: nature of intervention and inferences from data. In: Smeriglio V L (ed) Newborns and parents. Erlbaum, Hillsdale, pp 89–96
215. Yu V Y H, Jamieson J, Astbury J 1981 Parents' reaction to unrestricted parental contact with infants in the intensive care nursery. Medical Journal of Australia i: 294–296
216. Zarling C L, Hirsch B J, Landry S 1988 Maternal social networks and mother–infant interaction in full-term and very low birthweight preterm infants. Child Development 59: 178–185
217. Zeanah C H (ed) 1993 Handbook of infant mental health. The Guilford Press, New York
218. Zeanah C H, McDonough S 1989 Clinical approaches to families in early intervention. Seminars in Perinatology 13: 513–522

6

Handling perinatal death

Gillian C. Forrest

INTRODUCTION

Over the past 20 years, the fall in the perinatal mortality rate has been accompanied by a rise in our concern for the plight of parents whose baby is stillborn or dies shortly after birth. In 1994, in the UK alone, over 8000 couples were bereaved in this way, and many vivid accounts of their experiences are available.[1,7] However, there has been little systematic study of this area of grief, although by the mid-1960s Lindemann[10] and Parkes[13] had established the forms of typical and atypical bereavement reactions following the death of an adult. In 1970 Giles published one of the first accounts of grief reactions to perinatal death.[6] He studied 40 women during the first 3 days following the loss of their baby and this was followed by a study by Wolff et al of 50 women, 40 of whom were followed up for 3 years.[21] The results of these and other later studies have established that the grief reactions after perinatal death are no different qualitatively from those accompanying the death of an adult. They follow the same course: an initial period of numbness, shock and disbelief, which lasts a few hours or days; then intensive bouts of tearfulness, feelings of guilt, despair and anger (the 'pangs of grief'), searching for a cause of death, insomnia, anxiety and social withdrawal, which may last for months or years; finally, a stage of resolution with gradual return to emotional and social well-being. Not surprisingly, atypical grief reactions do occur, particularly after stillbirth, and these have been extensively described by Lewis & Page[9] and Mander.[11] They include prolonged and inhibited reactions, and severe relationship disturbance with husbands, existing children or the next baby, including child abuse. Lewis attributes the difficulty of successfully mourning a stillbirth to the 'painful emptiness' of such a birth. This may then be further heightened by the attitudes of doctors and midwives, and by the actual management of the delivery. The baby may be removed quickly, without ever being seen by the parents, the hospital making all the funeral arrangements and the mother being disharged home as soon as possible, with no follow-up. The experience can be very like that of relatives of persons 'missing, believed dead', who cannot get on with grieving because there is no object to mourn.

As far as the long-term effects of perinatal death are concerned, there is accumulating evidence that a significant proportion of families suffer ill-effects. Cullberg interviewed 56 women 1–2 years after perinatal death.[4] 19 were found to be suffering from serious maladaptive psychological symptoms. Nicol et al followed up 110 women for 6–36 months after a perinatal death.[12] They found 21% suffering from continuing severe psychological symptoms (depression, anxiety, tiredness, etc.), social adjustment problems, marital difficulties and a resolve to have no further children. Vance et al in a controlled, longitudinal study of families after perinatal death or sudden infant death, reported continuing high levels of psychological symptoms in 20% of bereaved mothers at 8 months compared with controls.[20]

To try to avoid these atypical bereavement reactions and promote recovery from the psychological effects of perinatal death, various authors and national groups have produced guidelines and recommendations for optimum care (e.g. Royal College of Obstetricians and Gynaecologists,[16] Stillbirth and Neonatal Death Society[17]). Their recommendations share certain key features: first, they emphasize the need to enhance the reality of the event by encouraging parents to see, hold and name their baby, take a photograph, be involved in the funeral arrangements and mark the grave; and, second, they stress the importance of good communication between well-trained and informed professionals and parents, with opportunities for discussions about the cause of death and the postmortem results, genetic and obstetric counselling, and sympathetic listening by professionals while parents express their grief.

The evaluation of the effectiveness of such care is clearly difficult. It is worth noting however that Parkes has reviewed bereavement counselling and concluded that bereavement counselling services 'are capable of reducing the risk of psychiatric and psychosomatic disorders resulting from bereavement'.[14] In addition, we have reported a study of support and counselling after perinatal death.[5] 50 women were randomly allocated to a group which received a planned programme of support, or to a group which received routine hospital care. At follow-up 6 months later, the supported group were showing significantly less psychiatric morbidity than the routine care group. This difference had disappeared by 14 months, when 80% of all women in the study had recovered from their symptoms.

There is, therefore, some evidence to support the subjective comments of many parents who have felt helped by compassionate and sympathetic care after their babies had died. The rest of this chapter will be devoted to a detailed account of the management of neonatal death and stillbirths and how the staff can help parents cope.

IN HOSPITAL

MANAGING A STILLBIRTH

The first confirmation of the death of the baby may be an ultrasound scan. It is important that the technicians are trained to manage these very difficult situations sympathetically, and with sensitivity. The mother will need the support of her partner or friend in the scanning room, and this should be allowed.

A woman whose baby has died in utero will be very fearful of the labour and delivery, and often has many unpleasant fantasies about what is happening to her dead baby. One woman wondered how it would be possible to give birth to a dead baby at all: 'decomposed, shapeless lump of cells'. If women express these uncertainties and fears, they are sometimes called 'morbid' or 'ghoulish' by staff. It is helpful to prepare parents for the delivery by giving accurate information about any abnormalities known to be present, including the skin changes to be expected, and reassuring them about the normal process of birth and pain relief. Husbands and partners should be encouraged to remain so that the couple can draw on their resources to help each other during labour. After the baby has been delivered, the midwife or the obstetrician should suggest that the parents see and hold their baby and bring him* to them. If any abnormalities are present, these can be described first, and then shown to the parents along with all the baby's normal parts. (In our study,[5] when describing this 6 and 14 months later, the parents of deformed babies all focused on these normally formed parts and none had found the experience of seeing their deformed baby horrifying or distressing.) If the parents do not wish to see the baby at all, a photograph, lock of hair, hand- or footprints should be taken and kept in the notes for possible use later. Many of the parents who decline to see the baby do, in fact, regret their decision weeks or even months later, and are then glad to have the photograph and any other mementoes. They should be encouraged to name their baby. Afterwards many parents like to be left alone to share their grief in private.

If a mother has been heavily sedated during labour, or had a caesarean section, she needs an opportunity to see her dead baby later when she has recovered sufficiently. One of the midwives could bring her baby to her room, or she and her partner could be taken to the room where the baby is laid out.

MANAGING A NEONATAL DEATH

When a woman is in premature labour, or where there is known to be fetal distress, it is very helpful if the paediatrician can see the parents before delivery, so that he or she is a familiar face and can prepare them by describing the special care unit and its procedures. If, even at this stage, it is clear that the baby's viability is marginal, the paediatrician can also discuss with the parents the baby's prognosis, and explain about resuscitation. In such circumstances, full cardiopulmonary resuscitation may not be appropriate, and it is very helpful if the paediatrician and parents can agree beforehand about how much should be attempted. The parents also need to be helped to understand that things may change rapidly during resuscitation attempts, and that if they hold their baby straight away after resuscitation has been abandoned, the baby may continue to make reflex gasps for some time. It is extremely important that all the staff handle the baby's body sensitively throughout this most traumatic time, not, for example, leaving the baby uncovered on a resuscitaire.

After the delivery the parents should be able to see their baby before he is taken to the special care unit even though this may have to be very rushed because of the baby's poor condition. A photograph of the baby taken as soon as possible for the mother to keep at her bedside and for the father to have at home can be a great comfort. Both parents should be encouraged to visit the unit as soon as possible to see and touch their baby and they value greatly being involved in the routine care of their baby such as nappy changing or tube feeding. The staff need to make every effort to keep them closely informed of the baby's progress.

Where a baby, usually born at term, has been irreparably damaged during delivery, or a baby of low birthweight suffers a fatal complication such as a massive cerebral haemorrhage, the parents have to adjust from a position of hope of recovery to one of accepting that their baby will inevitably die. This is a most painful transition for them (and the staff) to make, particularly with low-birthweight babies where an optimistic prognosis has

* Throughout this chapter, 'he' has been used to avoid the awkward use of he/she.

often been given and the parents' expectations of their baby's survival are correspondingly high. Whenever possible the news of the fatality or the baby's condition should be broken to parents in private so that they can release feelings without inhibitions. They will initially experience shock and numbness, followed sooner or later by intense feelings of grief and protest (anger).

At this time, or later, they will have many questions to ask about what has gone wrong, and the information may have to be repeated many times over before they can grasp it. In my experience, parents in these circumstances are seeking explanations and expressions of sympathy from the staff and a chance to ventilate their own feelings. It is when they are denied these that they may seek legal redress.

While the baby's condition is steadily deteriorating, parents may begin mourning before he has actually died and may find visiting him intolerably painful. In these circumstances, they will need a lot of support and understanding to maintain some contact. This situation may be difficult for the staff to accept, but if their attitudes to the parents are critical, it will only increase the parents' anger, guilt and despair, and make it harder still for them to visit.

When the baby is known to be dying the parents should be told, so that they can be with him. Some parents will want their other children to be present too. They may ask for a minister of religion to be called in to baptize the baby, or perform other important rituals. If at all possible, the family and baby should be placed in a separate single room with the minimum of equipment present. They can then be encouraged to hold the baby as he dies, and afterward, if the parents wish, they can help with the laying out. One mother said, 'No baby should die alone. It was all the comfort I could give him, to hold him in my arms as he died.'

THE POSTMORTEM EXAMINATION

The information provided by a careful postmortem examination or necropsy can clearly be important in establishing the cause of the baby's death and in identifying congenital abnormalities and any genetic implications. However, many parents, distraught at losing their baby, find consent for this examination very difficult. One mother put it like this: 'She's been through enough. Must she be cut up as well?' Parents can be helped to overcome this instinctive reluctance to consent by having a doctor explain to them that the examination is necessary to clarify what has gone wrong and if it is likely to happen again. Even so, there will be some parents who refuse, and these will include parents belonging to religious groups which forbid interference with a body after death. In these circumstances, it is important to assess the likelihood of the necropsy yielding vital information in each individual case, before pressing the parents to agree.

Pressure will make the parents feel torn between their protective feelings for their baby, even though he is dead, and their desire to comply with their doctor's wishes. For some of them the only way to resolve this conflict may be to leave the hospital altogether and withdraw from any further contact, thus increasing the likelihood of unresolved grief reactions.

Referral to the coroner should never be used simply in order to obtain more information about the exact medical cause of death when parents are refusing permission for a postmortem. It should only be made when the cause of death is unknown, or there were suspicious circumstances surrounding the death. It goes without saying that parents cannot be given a choice about referral to the coroner in these circumstances.

It follows from this discussion that the results of the postmortem examination will be very important to parents, and it is essential that they are given an opportunity later on to receive these (see below).

AFTER THE DEATH OR STILLBIRTH

The parents will be in a state of shock and numbness for a few hours or days before they can accept the reality of their baby's death. One woman, describing her reaction to her stillborn baby said, 'We looked at her in our arms, and I thought: she's asleep. Why doesn't she just wake up now?' Another: 'His mouth came open as we held him, and I thought he's coming alive!' Although it is important for medical staff to give explanations to the parents at this stage of what seems to have gone wrong, it is likely that these will have to be repeated later, perhaps several times. It may not be until the follow-up appointment several weeks later that parents are able to take in the information.

Wherever possible the mother should be given the choice of a single room or a return to her own ward. It is perhaps surprising that some women prefer to return to their own wards for the support of the friends they may have there. A few certainly wish to have contact with other babies straight away: 'I've got to face up to it, and I'd rather do it now than postpone it.'

Some parents like to have information written down, and obstetric units may have their own leaflets or use those produced by self-help organizations such as the Stillbirth and Neonatal Death Society. Parents also need the telephone number of the local contacts for the relevant voluntary organizations offering support to parents after the loss of a baby. The midwives should try to help parents express their feelings, and not hurry away if they come in and find them in tears. Lactation must be discussed – many women assume that they will not lactate if the baby has died – and help offered with the necessary registration and funeral arrangements (see below). Discharge should not be hurried, to allow time for contact with the unit's bereavement nurse, counsellor or social worker, who can offer support while mourning is being established and assess the couple's supportive network at home. The results of our study[5] and the work of Raphael in Australia[15] suggest that unsupported bereaved persons are more at risk of atypical reactions, so extra support needs to be mobilized for many couples in this situation, from ministers, health visitors, social workers or the local branch of SANDS. The community midwife and the general practitioner should be informed of all babies' deaths as soon as possible, so that they can arrange to visit the parents in the maternity unit before discharge or, failing this, immediately on the mother's return home.

FOLLOW-UP ARRANGEMENTS

These should be planned to ensure that the parents receive obstetric counselling, genetic counselling (where appropriate) and an opportunity to discuss the baby with his paediatrician. As has already been mentioned, the postmortem results are particularly important for the parents, as they frequently find it so difficult to give consent. These follow-up interviews are best arranged between 3 and 6 weeks after the baby's death or stillbirth – allowing time for the postmortem results to be available, and for the parents to have recovered from the initial numbing impact of the baby's loss. Although parents are usually willing to return to the hospital for the interview it tends to be distressing for them if they are given a routine appointment in the ordinary postnatal or paediatric clinic – particularly as this increases the possibility that some member of staff will not realize that their baby has died, and make distressing comments.

REGISTRATION AND FUNERAL ARRANGEMENTS

For most young couples this will be their first experience of bereavement, and they are bewildered by the complicated administrative procedure of registering the baby's death or stillbirth and arranging a funeral. By helping parents with these arrangements some of their distress can be relieved. These are described in detail elsewhere,[17] but a short account is given here.

REGISTRATION

In the UK all live births, irrespective of gestation, have to be registered by the Registrar of Births, Marriages and Deaths. All neonatal deaths (irrespective of gestation) and stillbirths (i.e. babies born dead after 24 weeks' gestation) also have to be registered. Such babies must then be properly buried or cremated. In some places a branch of the registrar's office is attached to the hospital, but in others parents have to travel to the central office in the town where the baby dies. They take the Medical Certificate of Cause of Death or Stillbirth provided by a doctor to the registrar, who then supplies a Certificate of Burial or Cremation which is required by the undertaker. In the past, parents of stillborn babies were often shocked to discover that they could not by law register a first name for their baby, but registration of a first name, if the parents request this, has been in practice from 1983.

FUNERAL ARRANGEMENTS

The funeral can be arranged either by the hospital (with a contracted firm of undertakers) or privately. The Department of Health has directed hospital administrators to meet the cost of any stillborn baby's funeral, unless the parents wish to pay for this themselves; in addition, some hospitals meet the cost of a funeral of a neonatal death. The exact details of hospital-arranged funerals vary up and down the country. In some areas the babies are cremated; in others they are buried in a local cemetery. In all cases, though, the babies should have their own coffins and a proper funeral should be held within a few days. The hospital administrators should be able to inform the parents of the time and place of the funeral, and the parents should be able to discuss arrangements with the funeral directors.

The advantages of the hospital-arranged funeral are that parents are relieved of the burden of making the arrangement, and the costs are minimal. The disadvantages are that it may prevent families from involvement in this important part of the mourning rituals. In some cases parents are told that they cannot attend the funeral, and this suggests that proper procedures are not being followed. They then often have great difficulty locating the site of the grave later (if the baby has been buried rather than cremated); and they usually find that they cannot mark the grave.

To improve the care of bereaved parents, it is clearly important for staff to be able to give them accurate information about the funeral arrangements applying locally, and discuss with them their needs and wishes. For parents of some religious faiths it is important that the funeral takes place quickly, usually within 24 hours. In these cases, hospital staff need to get the certification completed urgently.

Many units have produced leaflets for parents containing information about funeral arrangements. In Oxford, a member of the administrative staff has been specially designated as the 'Bereaved Persons' Welfare Officer' to help parents cope with these administrative issues.

Sometimes parents of babies under 24 weeks' gestation who are born dead ask if they can hold a funeral. This is particularly so where twins are delivered before 24 weeks' gestation, one of whom is born dead, while the other is liveborn but dies after a few hours or days. There are no legal requirements for registering the first twin or for holding a funeral. The second twin, however, will require a Birth Certificate, Death Certificate, Certificate of Burial or Cremation and a proper burial or cremation. It is clearly very upsetting and bewildering for the parents to come across such different administrative procedures for the two babies. There is, in fact, nothing to prevent parents of a baby born under 24 weeks' gestation from holding a funeral. In place of the Certificate of Burial or Cremation, the funeral director will require a note from the attending doctor stating the gestation of the baby and the (presumed) cause of death. This certificate 'in respect of a non-viable fetus' authorizes the undertaker to proceed with the burial or cremation. It is very important to help parents with this if they do feel the need to hold a funeral for their baby.

AT HOME

THE COURSE OF MOURNING A NEWBORN BABY

Grief is usually intense and constant initially, and then gradually the 'pangs of grief' described earlier occur with lessening frequency. They tend to be precipitated by reminders of the dead baby, e.g. the funeral, the expected date of delivery if he was premature, the onset of the mother's first period, the first Christmas or anniversary of his death; as well as by less-specific things – baby clothes, a piece of unfinished knitting, the baby counter in the chemist's shop.

Insomnia is very common but is best left to resolve spontaneously over the first few weeks. Ideas of guilt and self-blame may take over from the early searching for extraneous causes of the baby's death and intense guilt feelings may be experienced by women who have had a previous termination of pregnancy. (One women was convinced that the angry jealous spirit of her terminated baby had taken revenge on this much loved and wanted baby. She eventually 'appeased' the spirit by buying a set of baby clothes for him and placing them in the coffin.) Many couples experience difficulties relating with their friends and neighbours in the early weeks. They find themselves avoided by those who know that the baby died, and dread being asked about the 'new' baby by those who have not yet heard. Friends may not know that bereaved people need to rehearse the events around the death for a long time, and try to cheer the parents up by switching the conversation to a neutral topic. The parents then feel that they are being 'boring' and may withdraw socially for many months until the need passes. Many bereaved mothers experience destructive feelings towards other babies for a long time; these are frightening and upsetting and may lead them to withdraw from any contact with children. They are often reassured to find that these feelings occur very commonly, and pass with time.

Fathers tend to cope by plunging themselves into work activities as soon as possible. They appear to have shorter bereavement reactions than the mothers; in our study 86% of the fathers had recovered from the psychological symptoms of bereavement by 6 months, compared with only 50% of the mothers. For some couples this disparity in their grief reactions strains their relationship; for others it seems that the man readily takes on the supportive role, and they are drawn closer. Parents with other children at home often describe difficulties handling their questions about the baby; for example a 4-year-old asked, 'Why can't you go back to the hospital, Mummy, and fetch her when she is not dead any more?'; and a 3-year-old asked, 'What did I do? Hurt the baby so it went away?' The children's own grief reactions appear to be relatively brief, except when their parents, usually their mother, remain severely depressed, lethargic and withdrawn for several months. Then naughtiness at home or school, or withdrawal, sadness and preoccupation with death and coffins, may be seen.

TWINS

A particularly difficult set of circumstances arises if one twin dies and the other survives.[2] It is quite common for the parents and the staff to rejoice in the survival of the one baby and not mourn the other's death, even to the point of denying his existence at all. However, there have been many accounts of subsequent relationship problems between mothers and the surviving twin. He may have to take on the identity of his dead sibling as well as his own, which can be extremely onerous, or his mother may desperately overprotect him. In other cases, the mother may idealize the dead twin and make constant unfavourable comparisons between the survivor and him. These problems can be avoided if time and opportunity are given to the parents to grieve for their dead twin, for example encouraging the parents to name him, attend the funeral and have a marked grave. The Twins and Multiple Births Association offers support and help for these parents.

THE NEXT PREGNANCY

For many women, recovery is marked by embarking on another pregnancy. However, anxieties have been expressed that women may seek another 'replacement' baby before they have sufficiently mourned the dead baby.[3] It appears that pregnancy inhibits grief work and mourning[8] and so it seems important that women wait long enough to mourn one baby before conceiving again. In any case, they need to feel able to cope with the inevitable anxiety of the next pregnancy and delivery. The Stillbirth and Neonatal Death Society suggests this may take 9 months or more. It is likely to vary a great deal for the individual woman, but the more strongly and completely the identity of the dead baby has been established, the less likely it is that the 'replacement baby syndrome' will occur.

STAFF SUPPORT AND TRAINING

To help parents cope with the loss of their baby, staff need some training in the psychological, as well as the technical, aspects of care. Without acquiring skills in this area, junior medical and nursing staff will tend to withdraw from a situation which is painful and difficult. Apart from lectures and seminars, some units have found that discussion groups are helpful, enabling staff to discuss their own and their patients' attitudes to death and dying. Training packs for professionals and training videos are also available,[18,19] and can also play a useful role in training.

CONCLUSION

This chapter has outlined some of the problems associated with the loss of a baby in the perinatal period, and how medical and nursing staff can help parents cope. Medical care does not end with the death or stillbirth of the baby, and there is a great deal that can be done to alleviate parents' distress and facilitate their recovery from the loss.

USEFUL ADDRESSES

The Stillbirth and Neonatal Death Society
28 Portland Place
London W1N 4DE
Tel: 0171 436 5881

Twins and Multiple Births Association
PO Box 30
Little Sutton
South Wirral L66 1SB
Tel: 01732 868000

Miscarriage Association
c/o Clayton Hospital
Northgate
Wakefield
West Yorkshire WF1 3JS
Tel: 01924 200799

REFERENCES

1. Borg S, Lasker J 1982 When pregnancy fails. Routledge & Kegan Paul, London, pp 52–75
2. Bryan E 1992 Twins and higher multiple births. A guide to their nature and nurture. Edward Arnold, London
3. Cain A C, Cain B S 1964 On replacing a child. Journal of the American Academy of Child Psychiatry 3: 443–445
4. Cullberg J 1971 Mental reactions of women to perinatal death. Psychosomatic Medicine in Obstetrics and Gynaecology, 3rd International Congress. Karger, London, pp 326–329
5. Forrest G C, Standish E, Baum J D 1982 Support after perinatal death. British Medical Journal 285: 1475–1479
6. Giles P 1970 Reactions of women to perinatal death. Australia and New Zealand Journal of Obstetrics and Gynaecology 10: 207–210
7. Kohner N, Henley A 1995 When a baby dies. The experience of late miscarriage, stillbirth and neonatal death. Pandora Press, London
8. Lewis E 1979 Mourning by the family after a stillborn or neonatal death. Archives of Disease in Childhood 43: 303–306
9. Lewis E, Page A 1978 Failure to mourn a stillbirth: an overlooked catastrophe. British Journal of Medical Psychology 51: 237–241
10. Lindemann E 1944 Symptomatology and management of acute grief. American Journal of Psychiatry 101: 141–148
11. Mander R 1994 Loss and bereavement in childbearing. Blackwell Scientific Publications, Oxford
12. Nicol M T, Tompkins J R, Campbell N A, Syme G J 1986 Maternal grieving response after perinatal death. Medical Journal of Australia 144: 287–289
13. Parkes C M 1964 The effects of bereavement on physical and mental health. British Medical Journal 2: 274
14. Parkes C M 1980 Bereavement counselling: does it work? British Medical Journal 281: 3–6
15. Raphael B 1977 Preventive intervention with the recently bereaved. Archives of General Psychiatry 34: 1450–1454
16. Royal College of Obstetricians and Gynaecologists 1985 Report of the Royal College of Obstetricians and Gynaecologists working party on the management of perinatal deaths. Royal College of Obstetricians and Gynaecologists, London
17. Stillbirth and Neonatal Death Society 1995 Guidelines for professionals. SANDS, 28 Portland Place, London W1N 4DE
18. Training Pack – Pregnancy loss and the death of a baby; a training pack for professionals. National Extension College, 18 Brooklands Avenue, Cambridge CB2 2HN
19. Training Video – Death at birth. Miscarriage, stillbirth, neonatal death and termination for abnormality. Surrey Media Services
20. Vance J C, Najman J M, Thearle M J, Embleton G, Foster W J, Boyle F M 1995 Psychological changes in parents eight months after the loss of an infant from stillbirth, neonatal death, or sudden infant death syndrome – a longitudinal study. Pediatrics 96: 933–938
21. Wolff J R, Nielson P E, Schiller P 1970 The emotional reaction to a stillbirth. American Journal of Obstetrics and Gynecology 108: 73–77

7

Neurodevelopmental outcome

Part 1

Outcome

Ann L. Stewart Simon C. Roth

INTRODUCTION

In 1950 the World Health Organization called a conference to discuss perinatal mortality. The conference concluded that prematurity (defined as birth before 37 completed weeks of gestation or a birthweight of 2.5 kg or less) was the single most important cause of neonatal death. In addition, it was noted that there was virtually no information available concerning the reasons for premature birth and only very limited data on the long-term outcome of the few survivors. In response to these observations a number of studies were started to investigate the characteristics of preterm deliveries and the long-term outcome of the survivors. The results of the outcome studies published in the next decade were alarming. The findings confirmed the view of many workers that mortality figures alone should not be used as measures of standards in obstetrics and paediatrics – quality of life is of equal, or even greater, importance. Furthermore, these early outcome studies had a profound effect on the thinking of paediatricians and obstetricians. Attitudes to the management of sick or vulnerable newborn infants changed, and paediatricians began to apply the physiological principles that form the basis of clinical neonatology as it is now practised. Outcome study reports and the debates that surrounded their interpretation continue to affect attitudes to perinatal management and the provision of services.

HISTORICAL REVIEW: OUTCOME OF SPECIFIC HIGH-RISK NEONATAL GROUPS

BIRTH ASPHYXIA

The results of early follow-up studies of infants considered to have suffered birth asphyxia were confusing. Some indicated that survivors were rarely compromised, others that the majority had mental retardation, cerebral palsy or sensory neural hearing loss, or all three in combination.[19] Small and insignificant differences in IQ were noted by some authors[57] when mean values were compared with results from control groups, but none reported large discrepancies.

The majority of these early studies depended upon clinical descriptions and opinions for the diagnosis of birth asphyxia and hence the selection of cases. In some, the criteria for diagnosis were carefully described, in others they were not; but from consideration of all the studies it is obvious that a wide range of clinical conditions were included under the general heading of 'birth asphyxia' and that derangements in some of the infants were relatively trivial. Hence it is not surprising that the results were inconsistent. Apgar[15] attempted to introduce order into the chaos with a scoring system to be applied at 1 minute from birth and again at 5 minutes. The scheme was designed to describe the condition of the infant at birth and was not intended to be a measure of birth asphyxia. Several early studies showed that low (abnormal) scores at 1 and 5 minutes correlated well with neonatal death,[55] and there was a significant excess of infants with neurodevelopmental disorders among survivors who had low scores[56] but the proportion affected was not particularly large.

Data from one of the largest studies were reanalysed to include Apgar scores up to the age of 20 minutes. The proportion of term infants who had neurodevelopmental disorders increased very significantly when scores remained less than 4 for more than 15 minutes.[143] Shorter periods of observation apparently did not discriminate between different degrees of hypoxic insult or their potential for permanent damage. Steiner and Neligan[199] studied 14 cases of fresh stillbirth (cases in which no heartbeat could be heard immediately after delivery by an experienced observer, but in whom cardiopulmonary resuscitation was successful) and 11 cases of cardiac arrest occurring within the first 15 minutes after birth, all in term, externally normal, infants. Of these, 14 (56%) survived, but four (29%) were quadriplegic and mentally retarded, and there was a close relationship between the time taken to establish regular respirations after the return of the apex beat, and prognosis. This interval exceeded 30 minutes in all four abnormal infants, whereas all infants who established regular respirations less than 30 minutes after the return of the apex beat had satisfactory neurodevelopmental outcomes. In general, infants with satisfactory outcomes had acute hypoxic insults (e.g. shoulder dystocia), whereas infants who developed abnormally had suffered more prolonged asphyxia with evidence of fetal distress (e.g. during vaginal breech delivery).

Three other groups[31,190,215] reported the outcome of infants who were apparent stillbirths or who were considered to have suffered severe birth asphyxia as judged by Apgar scores or by the duration of active resuscitation required. All three came to the same conclusion, namely that if the infants survived the majority had a satisfactory neurodevelopmental outcome. D'Souza et al[61] concluded that even severe birth asphyxia was rarely associated with sensory neural hearing loss, although birth asphyxia is traditionally regarded as the cause of much sensory neural hearing loss in the community.[77] A similar conclusion was drawn from the analysis of data from very low-birthweight infants,[29] namely that the main predictor of SNHL was severe apnoea in the neonatal period, suggesting that if hypoxic damage was responsible it occurred after birth and not during the intrapartum period.

Because of the difficulties in defining birth asphyxia in the intrapartum period or at birth with clinical methods, additional neurological criteria were saught which might give a more accurate indication of the presence and extent of asphyxial damage. Amiel-Tison[6] showed in term infants that seizures, irritability, apathy or failure to suck feeds persisting for 10 days or more were almost invariably associated with an unfavourable outcome. Even grossly abnormal signs of this kind which resolved before 10 days of age did not appear to signify permanent damage. Several other groups have identified similar factors which appear to have prognostic significance, notably seizures, apathy, hypotonia or failure to suck feeds.[121,189] The sinister significance of the progression from hypotonia to extensor hypertonus has been described,[31] and persistent neck extensor hypertonus of more than 3 months' duration in term infants is frequently associated with adverse neurodevelopmental sequelae.[11]

There is evidence from continuous electroencephalographic (EEG) recordings[68] that seizures may often not be recognized clinically and that control may be very difficult to achieve in sick infants. In addition, therapeutic interventions including sedation and muscle paralysis may mask clinically recognized seizure activity. Other work questions whether seizures are symptoms or whether they are themselves the cause of any ensuing brain damage.[52] Thus, although clinically recognizable seizures carry an adverse prognosis, they should not be relied upon as a sole prognostic indicator. Continuous EEG recordings, especially using power spectral analysis techniques can detect seizure activity as well as provide prognostic information.[24]

From the early studies, Thomson et al[215] concluded that the available data did not support the hypothesis proposed by Lilienfeld and Pasamanick[127] of a spectrum of worsening outcomes according to the severity of the insult, described as 'the continuum of reproductive casualty'. By contrast, the evidence suggested 'an all or nothing' effect – in general infants who suffered birth asphyxia diagnosed on clinical criteria either died or survived intact. This 'all or nothing' effect is 'unphysiological' but it was the prevailing attitude for more than 10 years until the first objective measures of cerebral energy metabolism became available. Using magnetic resonance spectroscopy to measure cerebral oxidative phosphorylation in birth-asphyxiated infants, Azzopardi et al[18] compared the severity of the measured derangement to a range of outcomes at 1 year. The five outcome categories, ranging from unimpaired, neuromotor impaired without disability, neuromotor impaired with disability, multiple disabling impairments or dead, were associated with worsening neonatal measures of cerebral energetics, extending from normal to total energy failure; all infants with total energy failure died. This was the first study to use an objective measure of birth asphyxia and the first to demonstrate the continuum. Hence, it is very likely that previous 'all or nothing' results were due to the use of unsatisfactory definitions of birth asphyxia.[1,179] The recommendation by Bax and Nelson[21] that only precise, objective measures should be used to define birth asphyxia is to be welcomed. Only in that way will the true prognosis for birth asphyxia be established.

LOW-BIRTHWEIGHT STUDIES

The tiny frail infant has always been a source of public and professional interest. Couney, a pupil of the French paediatrician Boudin, exploited this and mounted exhibitions of very low-birthweight infants in their incubators in Europe and North America from the end of the last century until 1940.[192] Once these infants grew and became sufficiently robust to go home, it appears that interest waned, and no systematic documentation of their development or long-term prognosis was made, although Gesell studied some of Couney's 'incubator infants' in 1939.[192] There are a few reports in the literature concerning the growth and development of other prematurely born infants during this period. Hess and Lundeen[96] reported that only about half of a group of 212 infants weighing less than 1260 g at birth were of average physical and mental development but no details were given of the standards by which they were judged. Conversely, others reported that by school age the mental development of the prematurely born was normal,[53] and it was concluded that, by school age, premature infants had 'caught up with' their peers born at term.

Two important observations were reported simultaneously in 1956 by groups working independently. In Edinburgh, Drillien and Richmond[59] found that birthweight was not uniformly distributed among a group of surviving 'premature' infants weighing 2500 g or less at birth. Numbers decreased as birthweight fell, so that the majority of the infants in their sample weighed more than 2000 g. From this they predicted that outcome in a group of 'premature' infants would depend upon the relative proportions of birthweight subgroups within the sample studied. From Baltimore, USA, Knobloch et al[114] confirmed this prediction by reporting that the incidence of neurodevelopmental disorders diagnosed at 40 weeks of age (after correction for preterm birth) among premature infants was inversely proportional to birthweight. Hence for the next 30 years, studies concentrated on infants weighing less than 1501 g who were perceived as being the most vulnerable, usually described as very low-birthweight.

In 1958, another report from Edinburgh had an even greater impact on attitudes to the VLBW infant.[58] Drillien reported that in the second half of a 4-year study period the survival rate doubled among VLBW infants who weighed less than 1360 g, but all the additional survivors were abnormal. She warned that modernization of neonatal care for sick vulnerable infants aimed at improving survival might lead to increasing numbers of handicapped children entering the community, and that the price of reductions in mortality might be a very poor quality of life for the survivors. Implicit in these warnings was the belief that premature infants are usually born early because they are abnormal, and that postnatal interventions would merely salvage defective children.

Many studies of VLBW infants were reported in the next 10 years, all giving an equally gloomy prognosis, until Davies and Russell[49] reported the results of early feeding among 100 survivors of birthweight 1000–2000 g. Less than 10% of these infants had neurodevelopmental disorders at the age of 2 years. These authors attributed the apparent improvement to the avoidance of the potentially harmful effects of withholding feeding, including hypoglycaemia and hyperbilirubinaemia. Three years later, Rawlings et al[167] reported an equally low rate of neurodevelopmental disorders among even smaller infants who weighed less than 1501 g. The following year, Calâme and Prod'hom[32] reported similar results from infants in the same birthweight range. Both groups claimed that their results represented improvements due to the introduction of modern, physiologically based methods of care during the antenatal, intrapartum and neonatal periods, and the avoidance of potentially harmful methods, including the withholding of feeds or the indiscriminate use of oxygen. In due course, many other specialist centres reported similar results, and in general since the early 1970s the 'going rate' for serious neurodevelopmental disorders among infants weighing less than 1501 g in centres offering high standards of modern care has been about 10%.

In 1979 Kitchen et al[111] reported a controlled trial of certain aspects of neonatal care. Initially they tested the addition of intravenous dextrose solution to the basic routine of neonatal care among infants who weighed 1001–1500 g. Later, the correction of acid-base status with intravenous bicarbonate solutions was added to the management of the study group. Although all infants weighed more than 1000 g, no form of ventilatory assistance was used for either study or control infants. Considerable improvement in mortality was achieved in the study group in both stages of the trial, but the proportion of abnormal survivors more than doubled in the treated groups, just as it had in the early Edinburgh study in the 1950s.[58] In spite of a careful description of the methods of management used, given in an earlier report,[110] many failed to recognize that the care given to the infants in this trial was of a type which would be considered inadequate, even at the time of publication in the late 1970s (nearly 10 years after the study was completed), and was in fact little different from that employed in Edinburgh in the 1950s with similar disastrous consequences. This study should be regarded as a warning of what could happen if only incomplete routines of care are used. In particular, it highlights what may happen if interventions such as mechanical ventilation, are deliberately withheld from certain categories of infants, for example those weighing less than 800 g.

Two years after this report, Stewart et al[207] reviewed the literature on the outcome of the VLBW survivor. They drew attention to the difficulties of interpreting much of the information in the literature, usually because of lack of detail. They also pointed out that the majority of the reports which did include adequate information came from specialist centres and as a consequence were derived from selected groups of infants. Only three studies were of total communities.[33,145,182] Accepting these limitations, and the fact that such reports were the only available data, certain trends were distinguished. If the results of all studies were expressed as total deaths, 'handicapped' survivors and 'healthy' survivors and ranked according to the year of birth, the results within each succeeding 5-year period were similar, regardless of where the study was carried out. For example, the proportions of infants who died or who survived with or without disability in a study of 1080 infants born in 1976–77, after regionalization of care in the State of Florida, USA,[145] were identical to those among infants born in a specialist intensive care unit in the same 2 years.[207] An identical observation was reported from a large community-based study in North America,[115] which was interpreted as indicating that results depend upon prevailing expertise in general and not on any one aspect of intrapartum or neonatal management. Considering the whole 32-year period, mortality fell after 1960, while the proportions of healthy survivors increased. After a large reduction during the 1950s, the proportion of 'handicapped' survivors remained constant at 5–8% of the total livebirths. Subsequently there was no evidence of change in the proportion of 'handicapped' survivors, either among all very low-birthweight infants, who weighed 500–1500 g, or among the very smallest infants, who weighed less than 1000 g, in spite of continuing improvements in mortality.

The question of the net effect on the prevalence of morbidity in the community, of increasing survival with little or no change in the proportion of morbidity in survivors, has been investigated in two ways. Firstly, in a comparative study of infants of birthweight less than 2000 g born before and after modern methods of perinatal care began to be used in the UK, both mortality and morbidity fell.[4] The authors attributed these changes to modern methods of care. Because of the fall in morbidity among the LBW infants, they estimated that the prevalence of neurodevelopmental disability in the community as a whole had not increased as a consequence of increased survival. These conclusions are extremely important, but, as the authors themselves point out, their findings must be interpreted with caution because of the nature of the data. Nevertheless, these data show clearly that, although the prevalence of morbidity is much higher among LBW infants than among normal-weight term infants, because LBW infants account for less than 10% of livebirths the actual number affected is small; and they account for only a small proportion of the total neurodevelopmental disability in the population.[2] From consideration of available data for the UK, it was deduced that less than 2% of 'serious handicap' may be accounted for by very preterm delivery.[2] This proportion is, for example, less than half of that attributable to birth asphyxia (>5% of the total). Secondly, the concept of 'gains and losses' was applied to the question. Numbers were calculated for additional survivors due to prevailing improvements in mortality ('gains') and for the additional survivors who were expected to develop abnormally ('losses'). The results for various groups of infants born in Sweden, Western Australia and England and Wales are shown in Table 7.1 and clearly indicate that 'gains' far exceed 'losses'.[88,157,196] Others have argued that since such a small proportion (usually less than 2%) of births are VLBW, the incidence of morbidity would need to double in order to make a significant increase in the prevalence of morbidity in the community as a result of improvements in survival of VLBW infants.

Table 7.1 Estimated 'gains' and 'losses' per 1000 live births in Sweden, Western Australia and England and Wales

Birthweight	'Gains'	'Losses'	Condition
All, in Sweden 1971–75	3.8	0.1	Cerebral palsy
< 2000 g in Western Australia	101	5	Neurodevelopmental abnormality
< 2500 g in England and Wales, 1979	33	3.5	Neurodevelopmental abnormality
< 1500 g in England and Wales, 1979	168	21	Neurodevelopmental abnormality
< 1500 g in England and Wales, 1981	264	35	Neurodevelopmental abnormality

Sources: Stanley & Atkinson,[196] Hagberg et al,[88] Pharoah & Cooke,[157] Pharoah, personal communication 1983.

There have now been a large number of regional studies[70,129,163,228,229] and at least two national ones.[89,191,220] The results are the same; major morbidity ranges from 6% of survivors in the Netherlands study where only impairments causing serious disability were reported, to 13% in studies which included both moderate and severely affected survivors. Thus, the net gain of unimpaired survivors shown in Table 7.1 is still valid.

Outcome at school age

There are relatively few studies of school-aged subjects born since the widespread availability of modern methods of perinatal management, largely because long-term follow-up studies are difficult and extremely expensive. Some early studies indicated that VLBW children compared unfavourably on all measures with control groups of classmates or siblings.[35,60,130] Drillien et al[60] also reported an association between transient neurological signs detected in the first year of life and impaired performance on both educational and motor skill tests at 6–7 years. Subsequently, there have been several reports concerning preterm 4- and 8-year-olds in which similar associations were noted,[12,87,165,177,210,230] implying that poor school performance is of neurological origin.

In the majority of studies reported in the 1990s, school-aged VLBW subjects have group mean IQs well within the normal range but tend to perform less well in school than their peers.[48,89,139,158,173,233] Even in children without obvious functional disabilities, detailed testing reveals specific aspects of functioning with which VLBW children have difficulty. For example, as a group they perform less well than their peers on tests of fine motor and coordination skills[64,94] and visual–motor integration.[48,89] Poor concentration and an excess of attention deficits have been reported among VLBW children[79,86,94] and it has been suggested that these deficits may account for poor performance at school. It is equally likely that either they share a common neurological aetiology with the deficits which underlie the children's difficulties or they are a consequence of failure and frustration at lack of progress caused by these deficits.

School-aged VLBW children have been reported to have more behavioural and conduct disorders than their peers.[79,86,158] These data require cautious interpretation because the assessment methods differ and all are, to a certain extent, subjective. In the past, this was considered to be due to early mother–infant separation resulting from neonatal intensive care.[113] With increased understanding of the emotional consequences to the mother of giving birth to a sick and vulnerable VLBW infant,[238] management patterns changed dramatically, and for many years now mothers have been given both the opportunity and encouragement to handle their infants and participate in their care from the earliest stage.[26] However, behavioural disorders are still being reported, from which it may be inferred that they are not due solely to problems of interfamily interactions. Recently, it has been proposed that behavioural deviance may be associated with later psychotic illness in adult life in VLBW subjects, and both may be the result of perinatal brain damage.[62,95,234] Confirmation of this hypothesis is awaited.

THE EXTREMELY LOW-BIRTHWEIGHT INFANT (< 1000 g)

No infant whose birthweight was less than 1000 g survived in the first UK national study in 1946.[53,54] In a large study of 209 VLBW infants which began 1 year later in Denver, USA, just seven infants who weighed less than 1000 g survived, and all seven were grossly abnormal at follow-up.[132] After that date there was no mention of these tiniest infants described by the Melbourne group[146] as 'extremely low birthweight (ELBW)' for 10 years or more. The first study devoted entirely to the ELBW infant was that of Alden et al[5] and concerned infants born in 1965–70. Mortality was over 80% but less than one-third of the survivors had serious neurodevelopmental sequelae.

Since this first study, many other specialist centres have reported their experience with ELBW infants, including studies of those who weighed less than 801 g.[82,204] Mortality fell, healthy survival increased and serious morbidity remained constant at around 8% of total births or 15–25% of survivors. The results of regional studies of ELBW infants confirm that the outcome in community terms (where perinatal intensive care is available on a regional basis) is the same for these very tiny infants as that reported from specialist centres.[84,183,185,222]

Mortality (neonatal and postneonatal) rates of 50% or less are now being reported for ELBW infants both from specialist centres and in national data.[3,84,156,171,184] Initially, improvements in mortality mainly occurred among the heavier infants, who weighed more than 750 g, although improvements subsequently were reported in the tiniest infants also.[171,204] There is some evidence[156] that death in these tiny infants is merely being delayed, but neonatal (28-day) deaths are also decreasing and the absolute numbers of ELBW survivors in the UK, for example, have increased appreciably since 1983.[3] Originally, it was believed that morbidity as well as mortality increased with decreasing birthweight. However, close inspection of the data indicates that only mortality increases as birthweight decreases below 1000 g. Morbidity in ELBW survivors is greater than in VLBW (<1500 g) infants and is in the range 15–25% for serious, disabling impairments, but it does not increase as birthweight decreases below 1000 g.[185] Thus, just 10 years after the first report on the prognosis for the ELBW infant, Orgill et al[146] concluded 'we believe that a policy of benign neglect for these children is not justified in the present era of perinatal medicine'. There have now been three reports[155,184,223] showing an improvement in outcome among ELBW infants, which was greatest for infants weighing less than 750 g. However, the improvements were in very young subjects and were largely confined to serious neuromotor disabilities or to blindness due to retinopathy of prematurity.

ELBW at school age

There are several reports of studies of school-aged ELBW infants.[204] Recently, parents, school teachers and the ELBW survivors themselves have been asked to describe their perception of how they are functioning in all aspects of daily living, aged 8 and again at 14 years of age.[186,187]

Motor functioning. Few studies have examined motor skills specifically, but in general ELBW survivors do worse on tests of fine and higher motor performance and coordination[138] than their term peers, or even children with birthweights in the range 1000–1500 g. By contrast, the proportion of ELBW survivors with disabling neuromotor impairments is similar to their heavier peers weighing 1000–1500 g, at around 8–15%.[204]

Cognitive functioning. In all studies the group mean IQ is below 100,[204] and it is often as much as one standard deviation below the mean for the test, although the range may be very wide. Even half of one standard deviation is important in educational terms, but it is difficult to compare the school performance between studies because of the different criteria used to judge it. Some studies report numbers requiring special schooling; in others the numbers receiving some sort of extra educational provision are stated, but even these categories vary from country to country, or even within regions in the same country. In all case-controlled studies, the ELBW children have a lower mean IQ and a greater proportion with extra educational needs.[90] For example, in one UK group of ELBW 8-year-olds, the proportion receiving extra education provision was 33%,[204] compared to 18% in the general child population[162] and 15% in birthweight range 1000–1500 g. Unlike the overall impairment rate in the young ELBW survivors, the proportion failing in school appears to increase as birthweight falls below 800 g.[83] Thus, it appears that the ELBW survivor is at particular risk of difficulties with learning.[204] As these impairments cannot be recognized for certain until school age, it is important to continue close surveillance of these tiny subjects until they are well established in school, especially those with neonatal evidence of mild hypoxic–ischaemic brain damage (HIE) or subtle neurological signs persisting to 1 year of age (see p. 80). Hence, studies of very young ELBW children may seriously underestimate the extent of morbidity, especially deficits of school performance.[211]

THE EXTREMELY SHORT GESTATION INFANT

In almost all outcome studies of infants at the lower limit of viability, selection is by birthweight. There are few data concerning the long-term outcome of infants selected by gestation alone, although obstetricians are more likely to wish to make decisions on this basis than on estimated fetal weight. The usual reason given is uncertainty about the accuracy of measurements of gestation. Advances in ultrasound dating are overcoming this problem, and in future results should be reported according to both gestation and birthweight, particularly in view of reports,[217,228,229] including those concerning infants whose birthweight and gestation are discrepant (see p. 85), which imply that gestation may be the main determinant of neurodevelopmental outcome in survivors.

A far greater problem than the accuracy of measurement of gestation is the definition of the lower limit of viability and inconsistencies of recording and reporting which arise when this is inappropriate. For example, the lower limit of viability in the UK remained at 28 weeks long after survival at 26 weeks or less was possible. As a result, recording and reporting of pregnancies ending before 28 weeks depended on local circumstances and attitudes and, to an extent, on the outcome in individual cases. Thus, infants who survived long enough for transfer to a neonatal intensive care unit tended to be described as live births and those who did not as abortions.

In 1987–88 when the accepted lower limit of viability was still 28 weeks in the UK, large variations were found in the proportion of infants regarded as viable among those born at or before 27 weeks of gestation in 17 perinatal units in one UK region.[72] Viability rates ranged from 7.2 to 0 per 1000 live births, but no differences were noted among births from 28 to 32 weeks. The authors of this report concluded that local attitudes have the potential to affect perinatal mortality rates and a plea was made for a standard recording scheme for all infants weighing more than 500 g. This effect was clearly seen in the results reported for 1987–88 from the National Institute of Child Health and Human Developmental Neonatal Network, USA.[82] Intercentre variability of mortality rates of infants weighing less than 1000 g was about 35% whereas the variability for heavier infants (1000–1500 g) was less than 10%.

Two studies have attempted to overcome the problem of selection bias arising from inconsistent recording and reporting of extremely short-gestation pregnancies. Workers in Melbourne, where the local state laws defined the lower limit of viability at 26 weeks, believed that reporting was consistent at least down to 26 weeks.[240] Another group in the northeast of England[228,229] made a specific attempt to record the outcome of all pregnancies registering for antenatal care within the regional services, regardless of duration. Both came to the same conclusion: below 28 weeks, mortality depends upon week of gestation but early neurodevelopmental outcome does not. In both data sets, the prevalence of disabling neurodevelopmental impairments between 1 and 2 years only increased once, from 6 to 10% in the more mature infants to 20–25% below 26 weeks, and then remained constant. Table 7.2 shows a typical example.[17] Identical results have now been reported by several groups, including the Northern Neonatal Network in the UK[217] and the findings have been summarized by Rennie in a detailed review of the literature.[168] Table 7.3 shows the most recent survival figures according to week of ges-

Table 7.2 Outcome of infants born at 24 and 25 weeks

	Gestation (weeks)			
	24		25	
	n	%	*n*	%
Admitted	39	—	53	—
Died	27	69	31	58
Major impairment	3	8	4	8
Minor impairment	2	5	2	4
No. impairment	7	18	16	30
Total	39	100	53	100

Table 7.3 Summary of recent reports of survival by gestation; figures are given for survival to discharge for liveborn infants

Place	Year of birth	23 weeks	24 weeks	25 weeks	26 weeks	27 weeks
Minneapolis[73]	1986–90	13/32	28/75	54/90	72/113	
Copenhagen[97]	1987–90	7/13	13/26	24/36	41/55	
Detroit[98]	1988–91	5/27	17/29	17/26		
Cambridge[168]	1985–92	2/9	13/28	26/55	43/80	
Montreal[119]	1978–92	0/25	9/39	31/62	44/69	91/117
Cleveland[85]	1990–92	2/27	16/40	35/56	33/43	59/71
Trent[27]	1991–93	1/37	27/95	38/104	73/132	132/186
Northern Region[217]	1991–94	0/1	5/13	8/36	2/15	10/28
Melbourne[81]	1992–94	2/19	18/34	43/61	47/58	48/55
Wales[36]	1993–94	1/22	6/31	19/41	40/59	39/57
Totals		33/212	152/410	295/567	395/624	379/514
% survival (95% CI)		16% (12–22)	37% (33–42)	52% (46–54)	63% (61–69)	74% (72–80)

tation below 28 weeks.[27,36,73,81,85,97,98,119,168,217] Thus, if selection factors are operating, it appears that they are doing so in a similar fashion in all centres actively caring for very preterm infants.[168,217] However, even if these factors are ignored, interpretation of the data remains difficult because the numbers are still small.

There are very few reports on the older extremely preterm survivor. In one study, a group of infants born before 29 weeks of gestation to mothers living in a geographically defined region during a 3-year period were examined at 4 years of age.[102] Assessment methods included developmental testing as well as neurological examination and tests of hearing and vision. Overall, 23% were impaired with serious disability and only 35% were described as unimpaired, although that category included subtle neurological signs which the authors conceded are often associated with problems of learning. They interpreted their results as indicating a worsening prognosis with decreasing gestation. However, no age correction was made for preterm birth. As the children ranged from 12 to 16 weeks preterm, this factor alone might account for the apparent worsening of prognosis, at least that judged by developmental quotient.

The observation that outcome worsens around 26 weeks is interesting.[217,240] It implies that there may be an important change in brain maturation occurring at that particular stage in gestation, making those born at 25 weeks and less more vulnerable. Volpe[226] has proposed that damage to subplate neurons may play a role in the aetiology of difficulties with learning that lead to school failure, to which very preterm infants are so prone; and he proposes several approaches to testing the hypothesis. As a precaution, survivors born at gestations of 26 weeks or less should be kept under surveillance for several years after they enter school, at least until satisfactory predictors of school failures are identified. However, it must be emphasized that until more data are available it cannot not be assumed that long-term prognosis worsens for every gestational week below 26 weeks.

THE SMALL FOR GESTATIONAL AGE (SGA) INFANT

Clifford[41] first described the 'dysmature infant' in the late 1950s. Terminology has changed with time ('dysmature', 'light for dates', 'intrauterine growth retardation' and 'small for gestational age'), but the definition has remained constant. The infants have a birthweight which is either below the 10th centile or more than two standard deviations below the mean for their gestation according to standard charts.

Assessing the outcome of SGA infants has always presented investigators with special difficulties. These infants are a heterogeneous group with many causes for their poor growth. For example, growth retardation may be genetically determined, as in Down syndrome or other chromosome disorders, or it may be the consequence of an embryopathy as in rubella or cytomegalovirus infections. In one study[147] comparing 138 SGA and 138 appropriately grown (AGA) infants, although the rate of disability was greater in the SGA group (seven compared to two in the AGA group) six of the seven disabled SGA infants had severe congenital abnormalities to account for their disability. In these circumstances, the prognosis depends upon the underlying condition. Indeed, all the various factors associated with poor intrauterine growth can have an independent adverse effect on outcome.

Ever since Clifford[41] made his original description, there have been conflicting results from follow-up studies, with wide variations in outcome. Some reported that SGA infants had a much higher prevalence of serious impairments[42,78,135,194] than their AGA peers, while others found no difference.[34,69,93,172,206,212,236] The majority of these studies did not match the gestation of the SGA and AGA subjects nor take account of the differing complications in the two groups. Hence there may be a number of explanations for the findings, although these variations could alone be due to the aetiological mix of the infants studied.

Sample size is one of the main problems in assessing the outcome of SGA infants. By definition, these infants only constitute 10% of the newborn population, so in any one centre SGA infants with disabling impairments are rare. After reviewing the literature, Braert[30] suggested that most studies contain an inadequate number of subjects to show a significant effect.

Gestational age is probably the main determinant of outcome in all high-risk infants, including those who are SGA.[73,200,217] In an early study of a group of infants weighing less than 4 pounds at birth,[136] there was no difference in the prevalence of disability between those born prematurely (and presumably appropriately grown) and those born after 35 weeks of gestation. However, there was a difference in the type of impairment: the premature infants were more likely to have neuromotor impairments, usually spastic diplegia, hearing loss and retinopathy of prematurity, while mental retardation, cataracts and epilepsy were more common in the infants born after 35 weeks, and by inference, SGA.

An important consequence of the SGA infants' greater gestational age is that they rarely suffer hyaline membrane disease and the severe respiratory complications which may affect infants of comparable birthweight but of shorter gestation. In contrast, the complications suffered by SGA infants, including birth asphyxia and hypoglycaemia, may be less often lethal, but nevertheless are potentially damaging.[39,92] This probably explains the large differences in outcome among SGA and AGA infants reported in the past by the Toronto group.[42] All these infants were referred from other centres without special transport facilities or the facility to carry out ventilatory support in transit. Under these circumstances, AGA infants died from respiratory illness, whereas SGA infants lived in spite of quite severe biochemical derangements. It is possible, too, that some SGA infants may have suffered from their 'bad reputation'. Because it was genuinely believed that SGA infants were often severely impaired at follow-up, active resuscitation was not attempted and proper care was instituted only when it became obvious that the infant was going to survive. At this stage, the infants were probably hypoxic, cold and hypoglycaemic, and prophecy would be fulfilled at follow-up.

In a carefully documented but small study of SGA infants diagnosed on the basis of several different ultrasound measurements, neurodevelopmental outcome at 1–2 years appeared to be directly related to the period of gestation.[13] Others had come to the same conclusion from their own experience[34,71] and from a review of the literature, namely that morbidity in SGA survivors is largely determined by gestation. The only exceptions are infants whose birthweights are so profoundly discrepant for gestation that they fall below the third centile. These infants are usually born near to term. Their prognosis is poorer and they have an excess of serious neuromotor impairments and of deficits of cognitive functioning.[200] In a comparative study of the outcome of SGA infants resulting from pregnancies with and without maternal hypertension, the lighter infants of the hypertensive mothers had a better developmental outcome than SGA infants of normotensive mothers.[235] This was thought to indicate that earlier delivery of the sicker mothers removed these very tiny infants from a hostile intrauterine environment. An alternative explanation is the proposal originally made by Amiel-Tison[7] and later confirmed with brain-stem response studies[9] of 'advanced maturation' following intrauterine stress.

The importance of the stage in gestation at which growth retardation starts is clearly demonstrated in a study by Harvey et al.[91] They followed up a group of SGA infants whose growth retardation had been recognized in utero with serial ultrasound cephalometry. At the age of 5 years, the results of assessments of cognitive functioning were within the normal range and did not depend on the extent of the growth retardation judged from birthweight centile. There were, however, significant differences in test scores when the children were subdivided according to the age of onset of the growth retardation as recognized with ultrasound cephalometry. When the growth retardation was recognized before 26 weeks of gestation, the children scored worse than both controls and those whose growth retardation was first recognized after 26 weeks. In contrast, there was no difference between the scores of children with later onset of growth retardation and controls. Similarly, Villar et al[224] identified a group of SGA infants with postnatal catch-up growth and compared them with another group who remained small at follow-up. Neurodevelopmental assessment showed that the latter group had a less favourable outcome.

Birth asphyxia is one of the major confounding variables in SGA follow-up studies. Clifford,[41] in his original description, alluded to this problem by suggesting that 'dysmature infants' were poorly grown because of poor placental function and that they would tolerate the stresses of labour badly. Westwood[232] found that when birth asphyxia had been excluded the difference between AGA and SGA infants was considerably reduced. When SGA status is associated with poor placental function, the infant may suffer chronic hypoxia. Doppler flow studies of growth-retarded infants have shown that those with absent or reverse end-diastolic flow have a higher mortality and morbidity rate than those without this finding.[219]

Antenatal fetal haemodynamics have been used by Ley and colleagues[125,126] in an attempt to predict neurodevelopmental outcome in high-risk infants. These authors found that severe derangement of fetal aortic velocity waveform was associated with intellectual and neurological dysfunction at 7 years of age in both very preterm and SGA infants. Because no distinction was made between these two groups of infants, the results have to be interpreted with some caution but they do suggest a link between deranged fetal haemodynamics and subsequent poor neurodevelopmental performance in later life among SGA infants. The sensitivity and specificity in these studies is probably not high enough to make it a useful tool to guide clinicians without further confirmation.[174] Attempts have been made to predict neurodevelopmental outcome at 1 year according to different patterns of intrauterine growth in the third trimester. Although a rather higher than expected prevalence of subtle neurological impairment was found in the study group as a whole, no difference was detected between the infants who were small with a normal intrauterine growth velocity and those in whom growth velocity decreased during pregnancy.[178]

Interest is increasingly being shown in the relationship of poor intrauterine growth and other derangements of pregnancy with aspects of adult health. In particular, a relationship between poor intrauterine growth and cardiovascular disease in adults has been claimed. One of the earliest studies was based on records kept on 5600 men in Hertfordshire born between 1911 and 1930, in which it was found that underweight infants at 1 year of age had three times the risk of death from coronary artery disease than infants of normal weight.[20] Postulating that the link between vascular disease and poor intrauterine growth was insulin, which together with insulin-like growth factors is central to the regulation of intrauterine growth, these workers went on to look at insulin resistance. Since deficiency or resistance to insulin leads to non-insulin-dependent diabetis mellitus, which in turn is associated with an increased risk of cardiovascular disease, studies focused on control of glucose metabolism. Inverse relationships between 2-hour glucose level on glucose tolerance tests and birthweight and weight at 1 year were shown.[128] A subsequent study has supported the hypothesis,[198] although others have not.[66] Other end-points including blood pressure have been shown to have a relationship with intrauterine growth,[123,213] but these reports also demonstrate the complexity of the relationship as environmental factors start to play a role with increasing age.

These studies raise important hypotheses. However, there are problems with the interpretation of these data. For example, in several studies, the attrition rate was unacceptably high and no account was taken of subjects who may have died from the condition under investigation before the study took place. No distinction was made between intrauterine growth, measured by birthweight, and weight at 1 year which, at least in part, depends on growth velocity during the first year of life, although factors which influence growth after birth are very different from those operating in the intrauterine environment. In addition, the authors of the original reports did not consider the gestational age of the subjects. Between 1910 and 1930, any surviving low-birthweight infant was almost certain to have been SGA – and quite unlike even a moderately low-birthweight infant born in the past 10 years. Hence, extreme caution should be used in extrapolating these findings to future adults.

The concept of infant origins of adult disease is important, particularly the influence of events during pregnancy. If the responsible factors can be recognized, they could be prevented, or at least ameliorated. Although the hypotheses raised originally by the work of the Southampton Group[20] are very interesting, they are not yet proven. As Paneth and Susser[150] said in their critical review 'now test it'.

RHESUS INCOMPATIBILITY

Early follow-up studies of infants affected by Rhesus disease carried out shortly after the condition was recognized indicated a poor prognosis for the few survivors. Many of them developed hearing loss and neuromotor disability, and the neuromotor disability was usually severe and of the athetoid type. Cognitive functioning was obviously difficult to assess but was often estimated to be normal. Audiograms showed a very specific pattern of sensory neural hearing loss.[74] From a study of these children, Johnsen and Freiesleben[101] recognized the association between hyperbilirubinaemia and hearing loss which was subsequently shown to depend on the extent of hyperbilirubinaemia and was not specific to Rhesus disease.

More recently, since the introduction of intrauterine transfusions and planned early delivery by perinatal teams who are prepared to treat the infants with modern intensive care from birth, follow-up studies indicate an excellent prognosis.[159,170,206] Mortality among the most severely affected infants is still high. Such infants have to be delivered long before term and have all the usual hazards of preterm birth to contend with in addition to their Rhesus disease. However, if these infants do survive, their outcome depends on their intrapartum and neonatal condition and not on the number of intrauterine transfusions.[65,159]

RETINOPATHY OF PREMATURITY (ROP)

The history of ROP is an important lesson in the search for understanding of the aetiology of an impairment. It has been described colourfully and in considerable detail by Silverman.[193] An epidemic of blindness was noted in developed countries, particularly the USA, in the late 1940s. The affected infants had almost all been LBW and cared for in hospital centres where aggressive attempts were being made to improve the survival of sick and immature infants. In 1953–56, two groups reported studies associating ROP with the use of oxygen.[16,105] Following the publication of these reports, oxygen concentrations were restricted to 40% and the prevalence of ROP fell dramatically. However, although the condition became rare, it did not disappear completely.

Two other interesting observations were made in relation to changes in prevalence of ROP among VLBW infants. In a study of infants born in the 1950s, there was an apparently reciprocal relationship between the incidence of ROP and spastic diplegia.[137] Others noted that the decline in first-day deaths among VLBW infants in England and Wales stopped – and there may even have been an increase – coinciding with the fall in prevalence in ROP in the 1950s which appeared to follow the restriction of the use of oxygen.[28,46] Hence, it was concluded that although oxygen may be potentially harmful to the immature retina, it has a very important role in ensuring intact survival in VLBW infants. After arterial oxygen tension measurements and, later, continuous monitoring of arterial oxygen tension were introduced and widely used, it became clear that the relationship between ROP and oxygen therapy was complex. Initially, high arterial oxygen tensions in immature infants were thought to be responsible for ROP. Restriction of ambient oxygen levels to 40% or less appeared highly effective in preventing blindness. Once blood gas measurements were made, they indicated that the restriction of ambient oxygen concentrations did not prevent arterial oxygen tension levels in excess of 100 mmHg (13.3 kPa), yet levels above 100 mmHg (13.3 kPa) were not inevitably followed by visual abnormalities due to ROP. From clinical observations, no absolute level of arterial oxygen tension could be established[106] above which blindness due to ROP always ensued, and no critical time of exposure was recognized, so it was deduced that other factors were involved.[133] More recently, studies have demonstrated that fluctuations of transcutaneous oxygen tension measurements, even within conventional 'safe' limits, are strongly associated with the prevalence and severity of ROP.[47,76] The strongest associations were found with fluctuations in the first week of life.[47]

In general, affected infants weigh less than 1000 g,[75] and members of higher-order multiple births appear to be at particular risk.[201] Thus any apparent increase in prevalence may be due largely to improvements in survival of these tiniest infants, and possibly to the increasing numbers of higher-order births consequent on the greater use of assisted conception.[148] There is little information on the prevalence of the condition worldwide and even less on the proportion of infants with retinal changes in whom sight is affected. In one report,[116] based on the answers to questionnaires sent to major European neonatal intensive care units, the prevalence of visually impaired infants appeared to be low, although the proportion of infants in whom changes were detected had tended to increase. These findings did not depend on the introduction of treatment aimed at preventing retinal detachment. A strong association was noted in a study of very preterm infants, between changes of ROP and both periventricular haemorrhage and evidence of hypoxic–ischaemic brain injury diagnosed with ultrasound in the neonatal period. At follow-up, almost all the affected infants had neurodevelopmental impairments.[100] Strong associations of ROP with intraventricular haemorrhage[225] and with a diagnosis of neurodevelopmental impairment at school age[50] have been reported in other studies. All these data suggest that ROP and hypoxic–ischaemic brain injury may have a common aetiology. Animal experiments suggest that retinal vasoconstriction may be a normal physiological response to protect the immature retina.[166] Permanent damage may only occur if this response is abolished, as might be the case in the derangements of cerebral haemodynamics and fluctuations of arterial oxygen to which very immature, sick infants are particularly prone.

AETIOLOGY OF IMPAIRMENTS FOUND AT FOLLOW-UP

All prospective studies carried out since modern methods of management became available indicate that it was usually the sickest infants who had adverse sequelae. Several factors, including hyperbilirubinaemia, recurrent apnoeic spells and other respiratory illnesses, were associated with an excess risk of neurodevelopmental abnormality in VLBW survivors.[103,112,205] Interpretation of the results was complex, principally because it was difficult to discriminate between the effect of a treatment, for example mechanical ventilation, and the underlying condition for which it was used.

Because these data were inconclusive, some workers calculated relative risks for various conditions, such as low Apgar scores, low blood pH at or shortly after birth, neonatal seizures or apnoeic spells.[142,180] Others designed risk scores[152] or applied the optimality concept.[120,218] All these methods confirmed that the sickest infants were at highest risk of adverse sequelae, but none gave any conclusive information about the cause.

It was not possible to establish causal relationships between perinatal events and impaired development until the introduction of objective measures of brain structure and function, beginning with ultrasound in 1978,[151] gave access to the newborn brain during life. Although autopsy findings gave aetiological clues they proved to be misleading. For example, as large periventricular–intraventricular haemorrhages were a common finding at autopsy in VLBW infants, it was widely believed that smaller ones were the cause of impairments in survivors. Hence, when objective measures were introduced investigators tended to concentrate on haemorrhage and ignored other, less easily identified lesions. In the event, hypoxic–ischaemic lesions proved to be far more commonly associated with impaired survival, and causal relationships have been demonstrated.[176]

In term infants with clinical or biochemical evidence of birth asphyxia, deranged cerebral intracellular energy metabolism detected with magnetic resonance spectroscopy between 24 and 120 hours after birth has been shown to be very significantly related to either death or serious, disabling neurodevelopmental impairment detected at both 1[175] and 4 years.[179] These cerebral energetic measures were also significantly related to both cognitive scores at 4 years and to head growth velocity at 1 and 4 years. Because the distribution of occipitofrontal head circumference standard scores at or shortly after birth was normal in these birth-asphyxiated infants, it can be inferred that the critical brain insult occurred at or shortly before birth.

Recently, the findings on brain MRI have been compared with neurological outcome at 2 years in term infants with HIE, graded according to the criteria of Sarnat and Sarnat.[189] The first MRI was done within 4 weeks of birth and repeated at intervals to 2 years of age. There was a strong positive correlation between the site and extent of the MRI lesions and outcome.[181] No infant had a normal MRI, including those with mild HIE, and bilateral basal ganglia abnormalities were associated with serious disabilities.

The concept of 'secondary energy failure' has been proposed[169] to explain the delay in the maximum derangement of cerebral intracellular energy metabolism. The maximum fall in PCr/PI is consistently observed many hours after birth when the infant has been resuscitated and stabilized.[18,154,175,179] Indeed, this has been a consistent observation since the first animal experiments with magnetic resonance spectroscopy.[99] Recently, this pattern has been reproduced in a piglet model of hypoxic–ischaemic insult in which the acute derangement of cerebral energetics following the insult was reversed, only to be followed 24–48 hours later by a second one, the extent of which was directly related to the severity of the original insult.[131,153] It is now believed that the primary insult sets off a cascade of events, leading eventually to secondary energy failure in spite of adequate resuscitation. Hence, brain damage in infants is proportional to the extent of both the primary insult and the secondary energy failure.[195] Ideally, the primary insult should be avoided, but preventing the secondary energy failure may limit the damage. There is some evidence from the piglet model that moderate hypothermia may be effective.[216] Based on this knowledge, preventive strategies are being planned and some have been introduced already.

The timing of the injury leading to impairments is less certain. Two separate groups have estimated that just 10–11% of the hypoxic–ischaemic lesions identified with ultrasound brain imaging in very preterm infants occurred before the onset of labour, and the remainder occurred after the onset of labour.[23,202] There are reports, based on autopsy findings and brain scans, that antenatally acquired lesions are common in monozygotic twins of all gestations.[141] When one twin dies in utero, the surviving twin is at particular risk of brain damage. The lesions, most commonly in white matter, are either hypoxic–ischaemic or haemorrhagic, and the haemorrhagic lesions can be primary or secondary to hypoxic–ischaemic lesions. It is believed that acute haemodynamic changes, especially at the death of one twin, are responsible for a cascade of events leading to these lesions, and transchorionic embolization and coagulopathy are the probable mechanisms. These mechanisms may also be responsible for the increased risk of antenatal brain lesions following thromboembolic abnormalities or viral infections in pregnancy.[118,141]

NEUROLOGICAL SEQUELAE: NEUROMOTOR IMPAIRMENTS

Data on the aetiology of specific neuromotor conditions are confusing. There are a large number of reports, including large epidemiological studies,[164,197] of analyses which either antedate objective measures of brain structure or do not include them. The majority of the reports concern 'cerebral palsy', but the condition is either not defined (there appears to be an unjustified assumption that it is unnecessary) or the definition is subjective, imprecise and not based on objective and consistent observations. Diagnosis has been shown to depend critically on age, and variation of diagnosis over time in individual children has been described.[10,144] In addition, interobserver reliability has been shown to be poor.[25]

One group tried to overcome some of the deficiencies of the early studies.[44,164] They analysed data from a regional study carried out on children born in the 1980s to investigate separately the aetiology of symmetrical and asymmetrical spastic neuromotor impairments. They found that the asymmetrical group was strongly associated with intrapartum and neonatal complications, whereas the symmetrical group was not. Although the authors considered that the aetiology of the neuromotor impairments that they studied seemed to differ according to the type and distribution, they were unable to find convincing evidence of factors other than immaturity that might account for the aetiology of the symmetrical group, notably spastic diplegia.

Outcome studies of very preterm or low-birthweight infants who had ultrasound brain scans in the neonatal period show highly significant association of haemorrhagic parenchymal infarctions (HPI) or IPL (see p. 1253), formerly called intraparenchymal or grade IV haemorrhages, and hypoxic–ischaemic lesions with neuromotor impairments at 1, 4 and 8 years, especially impairments causing disability.[43,44,45,51,176,203,208] Although there is correspondence, the neurological impairment is almost always more extensive than would be expected for the size and site of the lesion seen on neonatal ultrasound. By contrast, germinal matrix (GLH) and intraventricular haemorrhages (IVH) are not associated with an increased risk of neuromotor impairment unless they are associated with other lesions, for example ventricular dilatation or frank loss of brain tissue (cysts).[43,45,51,149,176,203,208]

In a Swedish/German collaborative study, brain magnetic resonance imaging (MRI) was carried out on a group of 56 children with a diagnosis of bilateral spastic diplegia or tetraplegia.[117] Over half (30) were born preterm. Severity of the neuromotor impairment ranged from mild involvement of the legs to severe spasticity in all four limbs. All but three of these children had abnormal MRIs aged 5–17 years. The lesions were predominently hypoxic–ischaemic (PVL), presumed to have been present since birth.[117] This presumption is supported by the observation that HPI and hypoxic–ischaemic lesions identified with cranial ultrasound in the neonatal period in very preterm infants were still present on MRI at 14 years.[109] However, as only a small proportion of the hypoxic–ischaemic lesions seen on MRI in the same study were associated with frank neuromotor impairments, the relationship between clinical findings and brain MRI lesions in the Swedish/German study needs further proof.

There have been several reports of an association between GMH–IVH diagnosed in the neonatal period with cranial ultrasound in VLBW infants, and subtle neuromotor deficits.[122,138] For example, Marlow et al[138] reported poorer motor skills at 6 years associated with GMH–IVH in a group of infants without gross motor disabilities whose birthweight was less than 1250 g. These reports are difficult to interpret because the authors did not always distinguish between haemorrhage alone and that associated with minor hypoxic–ischaemic injury, as represented by non-progressive ventricular dilatation. In a large epidemiological study of 2-year-old VLBW infants,[160] there was a close association between 'cerebral palsy' and HPI or white matter lesions but no association between these lesions or GMH–IVH and what was termed 'non-disabling cerebral palsy', defined as frank neuromotor signs without functional deficits at the age of examination. The authors concluded that the aetiology of the two neuromotor disorders differed, and that only disabling neuromotor disorders were caused by white matter lesions. These findings[160] correspond with our own in very preterm (< 33 weeks) infants at 1, 4 and 8 years with both linear array apparatus[45,176,208] and high-resolution mechanical sector scanning.[203] HPI and white matter lesions were significantly associated with disabling neuromotor impairments, whereas non-progressive ventricular dilatation (linear array) or a combination of two or more of haemorrhage without parenchymal involvement (GMH–IVH), 'flares' or ventricular dilatation without cysts (sector scanning), were associated with neuromotor impairments without functional deficits at 8 years.

It has been proposed that chorioamnionitis plays a role in the pathogenesis of PVL and hence of neuromotor impairments.[124] This proposal is supported by the observation that newborn infants with sepsis or those born to mothers with proven infection are at increased risk of PVL.[221,239] Amniotic fluid concentrations of both interleukin-1 (IL-1) and interleukin-6 (IL-6) are higher in mothers whose newborns are subsequently found to have PVL than in those without this finding.[239] Intrauterine fetal infection may lead to activation of the cytokine network by stimulating the mononuclear cells to produce interleukin-1 (IL-1) and tumour necrosis factor (TNF) and thus increase the permeability of the blood–brain barrier.[124]

VISUAL IMPAIRMENT

A large proportion of visual impairment is caused by retinopathy of prematurity (ROP). In addition, VLBW and very preterm infants are at risk of cortical visual impairments (CVI) as a consequence of hypoxic–ischaemic brain damage (Chapter 44, Part 4). The prevalence of visual impairment in surviving low-birthweight infants is estimated to be about 5%.[161,191] A further 5% of these infants suffer from severe visual impairments, mainly due to high myopia, and at least 9% fail an eye test at school. There is also a very large prevalence of squint – maybe up to 20% – with a similar proportion having an acuity of worse than 6/12 in one eye.

Cortical visual impairment

Both term infants who have suffered a hypoxic–ischaemic insult and very preterm or very low-birthweight infants are prone to problems with visual development in the first years of life. The abnormality is due either to a field defect, which is very difficult to confirm in the young child, or a partial or complete absence of visual responses, currently described as cortical visual impairment, but previously referred to as cortical blindness or delayed visual maturation. This latter term is misleading as it implies that the problem will resolve, when in fact it is due not to delay but to actual damage to the visual cortex.

Miranda et al[140] first drew attention in 1977 to the association between cortical blindness assessed by pattern recognition in the first few weeks of life and cognitive functioning at 3–5 years. Some years later, Hungerford et al,[100] on the basis of brain ultrasound findings, implicated hypoxic–ischaemic brain injury in the aetiology of CVI. Stewart et al,[209] reporting the prediction of satisfactory progress at 1 year from a neurological examination at term, commented that absent or abnormal visual responses in very preterm infants was the only sign, on its own, that predicted a poor outcome at 1 year. These authors went on to report the outcome at 8 years of the children with absent or abnormal visual responses in their original study, and 90% were still impaired.[97] More recently, a direct association has been reported between CVI and MRI or ultrasound evidence of hypoxic–

ischaemic damage in the visual cortex and the optic radiations.[40,63]

HEARING DEFICITS

The prevalence of sensorineural hearing loss in VLBW and ELBW infants is probably less than visual impairment and is quoted between 1 and 3.5%.[214] Sensorineural hearing loss seems to be a particular problem in survivors of persistent pulmonary hypertension (PPHN), and large prevalences (4–21%) have been reported in this group whether or not extracorporeal membrane oxygenation was used.[38] This is probably because from 28 to 32 weeks of gestation the auditory nerve is particularly sensitive to hypoxia. Risk factors for hearing loss also include low birthweight, hypoxic–ischaemic encephalopathy, bacterial meningitis, hyperbilirubinaemia and a family history of deafness. Such infants should all be screened for hearing loss before they leave hospital, as early aiding and appropriate support can dramatically improve speech development.[214]

COGNITIVE DEFICITS

Very preterm subjects in whom hypoxic–ischaemic lesions were detected with ultrasound in the neonatal period, as represented by non-progressive ventricular dilatation, have been reported to have significantly lower IQ scores at 8 years than those without these lesions.[176,203] In the same subjects at 14–15 years, IQ scores were very significantly related to neurological impairments. Preliminary results of studies of brain intracellular oxidative phosphorylation metabolism, using magnetic resonance spectroscopy in term infants believed to have suffered birth asphyxia, have shown a strong association between deranged cerebral energy metabolism between 1 and 5 days of age and IQ at 4 years.[179] Extrapolating from an animal model, the extent of the cognitive deficit may be related to the degree of metabolic derangement identified as secondary energy failure, which in turn is related to the severity of the primary insult.[131,195]

These are very preliminary observations. However, it may be speculated that it is the hypoxic–ischaemic injury to which VLBW infants are particularly prone that affects cognitive development. This hypothesis is supported by the finding that a larger proportion of infants weighing less than 1000 g have non-progressive ventricular dilatation than their heavier peers weighing more than 1000 g at birth, which could possibly account for their lower IQ scores.[204]

SCHOOL PERFORMANCE

Although school performance is largely dependent on intact cognitive functioning, children can have IQ scores within the normal range but fail in school. In a cohort study of very preterm subjects with a mean IQ of 99 ± 16, large subscale differences were noted on cognitive testing at 8 years in almost half of the children tested.[176,177,203] These findings were interpreted as indicating poor interhemispheric interaction, with suboptimal right hemispheric function. Subsequent members of the cohort performed poorly on motor tests believed to indicate posterior corpus callosum function, and these scores were significantly related both to cognitive scores measuring right hemisphere function and to the need for extra educational provision.[107,109] Indeed, poor interhemispheric transfer efficiency may be a better predictor of school performance than IQ.

PLANNING FOLLOW-UP STUDIES

Planning, as in all studies, starts with defining the hypothesis to be tested. Only after that has been done can outcome meaures be chosen, and age and methods of ascertainment decided. The design of the study should be done in conjunction with biostatisticians or epidemiologists. The type of protocol will depend upon the hypothesis to be tested, the purpose of the study and, to a certain extent, the resources available. If a control group is necessary, the source and characteristics must be decided in advance, and the numbers of infants needed to give meaningful results should be calculated.

OUTCOME MEASURES

In outcome studies, as in any other study, outcome measures should be chosen primarily because they are appropriate to test the hypothesis under investigation, and they must be precisely defined. The age of the children at study, the assessment methods, the numbers to be enrolled and the interpretation all depend on these two factors. The use of inappropriate measures or vague, ill-defined terms and of subjective definitions of adverse outcomes has caused serious misunderstandings in the past, and will continue to do so if attention is not paid to the choice and definition of outcome measures.

HISTORY

The original follow-up studies were purely fact-finding and designed solely to discover the outcome for certain conditions such as low birthweight or birth asphyxia. The criteria used to judge outcome varied from study to study, but were mainly determined by perceptions of quality of life in general. No distinction was made between outcomes which might be a direct consequence of the condition under consideration or those which might be associated through common aetiological factors – or even associations which were obviously coincidental. For example, no distinction was made between adverse outcomes due to disability from neuromotor impairment and those solely due to social deprivation, and no attempts were made to assign causes when adverse outcomes were discovered.

Information concerning the cause of death among vulnerable infants came from autopsies, but establishing the causes of morbidity was much more difficult. Clinicians who examined the surviving infants and saw for themselves the predominantly neurological nature of the abnormalities in those infants with adverse sequelae described the infants as 'handicapped', as indeed they were, but the precise condition giving rise to the handicapped status was not always specified. Many different conditions were grouped together under the same general heading of 'handicap'. These same clinicians also knew the physiological and biochemical derangements which vulnerable infants had to overcome in order to survive; and they knew of the autopsy findings in the brains of comparable infants who died. Not surprisingly, deductions were made relating adverse sequelae in survivors to similar, albeit more extensive, brain lesions in dead infants. Thus, it was argued that if physiologically based interventions prevented infants from dying, sublethal damage also should be prevented. The cause and effect were deduced after such interventions were introduced, and were followed by a reduction in mortality and a much smaller proportion of morbidity among survivors, expressed as handicap, than had been reported in the original studies.

Workers with epidemiological or sociological backgrounds perceived the question in a different way. They[188] had reviewed the literature in the late 1960s and early 1970s and were unable to find satisfactory evidence for a causal relationship between perinatal events and long-term prognosis – as indeed there was not – neither from studies of LBW infants nor in studies of those who suffered intrapartum asphyxia. These analyses did not take account of the exclusion of all badly damaged children because they were unable to do the tests. Hence, the only correlates consistently reported were between socioeconomic factors and IQ. It was, therefore, suggested that any changes in morbidity were due to improvements in socioeconomic factors and owed little if anything to medical interventions. It was argued that development of specialist medical services for vulnerable infants was uneconomic and that resources should be invested in the improvement of social conditions.

These two apparently opposing views probably arose from the use of the word 'handicap'. Clinicians saw children with neurological or developmental disorders of varying severity. When the disorders interfered with function and were expected to continue to do so to such an extent that they would affect schooling and employment opportunities, they were described as 'handicaps'. The disorders themselves were clearly defined, usually in neurological terms, and central nervous system lesions were considered to be responsible. The clinicians did not consider that handicaps arising solely from environmental and emotional interactions, without any evidence of neurological impairment in the child, were relevant as indices of outcome of conditions arising during the perinatal period such as birth asphyxia, so they discounted them. They failed to recognize that the extent to which a child with a perinatally acquired neurological impairment would eventually be handicapped would depend on the interaction between the disorder, the child's own personality and his or her socioeconomic environment.

The epidemiologists and sociologists also failed to recognize two important deficiencies in their arguments. Firstly the interactional hypothesis, for which Sameroff and Chandler[188] proposed a model, was based on the lack of evidence relating perinatal events to outcome in studies of either birth asphyxia or low birthweight. The reports, from which this hypothesis was originally derived, were concerned with infants born and cared for before there was sufficient physiological or biochemical understanding or technical competence to make the measurements necessary to diagnose the conditions which might cause CNS sequelae. For example, micromethods for blood gas analysis were not generally available and there were no techniques for continuous intra-arterial or transcutaneous monitoring, far less objective measures of brain structure and function.

Secondly, cognitive functioning judged by IQ was universally used as the 'gold standard' for quality of survival. Obviously intact cognitive functioning is exceedingly important, but it is only one facet of a child's overall functioning. Conversely, ultimate IQ is affected by many factors which can and do operate independently at various stages in a child's development. IQ can only be measured accurately when the child is several years old. The minimum age is usually regarded as 3.5–4 years, and many observers consider 8–9 years as the first age at which a reliable estimate can be made. By this time environmental factors have had an important influence. In addition, the IQs of children with serious neuromotor or neurosensory impairments or deficits of cognitive functioning cannot be measured accurately, and the values from such children have often been omitted from the calculation of results, particularly where these were quoted as means. Children with moderate neuromotor impairments or sensory neural hearing losses often have IQs within the normal range. Hence mean IQ values alone are likely to be poor indices of outcome for perinatal events, particularly as information from infants with the most severe CNS damage will be excluded because they cannot be tested.

Thus, clinicians and epidemiologists have in the past had very different perceptions of the entity which they both called 'handicap'. Clinicians used the term to describe impairments that were predominantly neurodevelopmental and which caused or were considered likely to cause disability. Epidemiologists, on the other hand, considered a much wider definition to include the end result of interactions of many kinds, which did not necessarily include a physical impairment in the child. As a consequence, epidemiologists accused clinicians of making extravagant claims for medical interventions;[37] clinicians considered that epidemiologists did not understand the problem, and both failed to recognize their different perceptions of handicap.

THE FUTURE

In future, misunderstandings and errors of interpretation in follow-up studies will be avoided if the WHO recommendations contained in the manual of classification relating to the consequences of disease are followed[237] and outcome measures are chosen with care and defined precisely. In the WHO international classification, impairment is defined as 'any loss or abnormality of psychological, physiological, or anatomical structure or function'. Disability is defined as 'any restriction or lack (resulting from an impairment) of ability to perform an activity in the manner or within the range considered normal for a human being' and handicap as 'a disadvantage for a given individual, resulting from an impairment or a disability that limits or prevents the fulfilment of a role that is normal (depending on age, sex and social and cultural factors) for that individual'. Thus, impairments are outcome measures but not disabilities or handicaps, although the presence of disability gives an indication of severity for the affected individual at the age of assessment and, to an extent, can be used as a measure of severity when classifying outcomes for comparative purposes.

CHOICE

Impairments chosen as outcome measures must fulfil the following criteria:

- provide a measure of the hypothesis to be tested
- be detectable/measurable at the age chosen for study (or the age must be chosen because it is appropriate for detection of the impairment)
- be defined objectively, preferably by actual measurement, using age-appropriate standards
- include all affected children at the age under consideration.

Consider, for example, a study to examine the long-term effects of a perinatal intervention which is believed to reduce the likelihood of brain damage in a certain group of high-risk infants. The information is needed quickly before the procedure enters general use. Neurological impairment is the obvious choice of 'end-point'. Even subtle neuromotor and neurosensory impairments can be detected by the end of the first year of life. They can be defined objectively according to age-appropriate standards, using specific examination manoeuvres.[10,14] The analytical approach offers the best chance of good interobserver reliability, as all children can be categorized without the need to agree or interpret diagnostic definitions. By contrast, to use as an end-point a clinical diagnosis such as 'cerebral palsy' presents problems. All definitions are subjective: the diagnosis depends on the age of the child and may change over time in individual children, and the diagnosis will not be made in all children with neuromotor impairments, regardless of the definition employed. As a result there will be children whose neuromotor status is clearly not normal but who do not conform with the diagnostic criteria of cerebral palsy. Neuromotor impairments which may appear trivial at, say, 1–2 years may be associated with cognitive and other deficits which are only revealed when the children are older. These deficits, including those of fine motor coordination and control, are important as they are likely to interfere with school performance.[12,165,177,210]

AGE OF ASSESSMENT

The importance of the age of assessment cannot be emphasized enough. The type of impairment, the methods of assessment and the standards used to judge the findings all depend critically on age. The range of functions that can be assessed increases with age, and so therefore does the range of potential impairments. For example, in one study of very preterm infants,[45,210] the prevalence of neurodevelopmental impairments appeared to increase from 18% at 1 year to 30% at 4 years because of the emergence of deficits of cognitive functioning which could not be assessed in the younger children. Thus, it is impossible to interpret the results of follow-up studies with a large age span or to compare the findings of studies carried out at different ages, as has been demonstrated by a meta-analysis.[67]

Choosing the age for assessment in a follow-up study is perhaps the hardest decision to be made in planning. On the one hand the results are needed quickly, on the other hand all possible effects need to be explored, and that means that the children have to be in school long enough to show evidence of difficulties with school performance. Until more is known about the strengths and weaknesses of prediction, it is reasonable to compromise by taking the results of early assessments made at 12–18 months. At that age, disabling impairments are likely to be permanent and the subtle ones are probably markers for neurological damage which may interfere with function at a later age. Ideally, the children should be reassessed later when they are old enough for testing of cognitive and of fine and higher motor functioning, and of school performance. In the normal course of events, children with disabilities will be referred to the appropriate service agencies for ongoing management. However, children with subtle neurological impairments should also remain under surveillance, until they are well established in school.

AGE CORRECTION

For infants born preterm, ages must be corrected by subtracting the number of weeks that the infant was born preterm from the chronological age. Correction should be continued as long as the deficit is larger than the discrimination of the test, up to the age of 5 years.

MISSING VALUES

Outcome measures should be chosen to allow categorization of all subjects in a study. Failure to take this into account has been an important source of misinterpretation in the past. There are circumstances which may thwart even the best intentions, for example:

1. *Profoundly abnormal children:* there are children who are so seriously impaired that they cannot be tested with the study protocol. These children represent the extreme of abnormality and are thus of great importance. To exclude them is misleading. In descriptive studies such children are easily included but no score can be obtained on formal testing of, for example, cognitive functioning or higher motor skills. In some tests, including the McCarthy scale of children's abilities,[134] specific provision is made for this circumstance. When this has not been made, the problem may be overcome by assigning an arbitary low score. For tests with normally distributed scores, a value which is at or more than three standard deviations below the test mean may be used. In other circumstances, 'the worst case' value may be chosen.

2. *Test refusal:*

- Children themselves may refuse test items. This is usually because they know that they cannot do whatever is being asked of them. Indeed, they may say that they do not do it, meaning just that! Occasionally, a child may refuse to be tested because of disturbed behaviour. Excluding these children is just as misleading as excluding the profoundly abnormal children; they are not normal. One way of dealing with the problem is to assign arbitrary scores at the lower limit of the normal range. For example, the McCarthy scale of children's abilities describes scores ranging from 79 down to 70 (equivalent to 1.5–2 standard deviations below the mean) as 'suboptimal',[134] so children refusing to be tested can be assigned a score of 70.
- Parents may refuse to have their children tested or they may simply fail to cooperate by not keeping appointments. In studies where enormous efforts were made to examine such children, an excess of impairment was found.[227] Thus, there is good reason to keep their numbers to a minimum. When parents cannot be persuaded to allow testing or give any information, information should be sought from other sources, including local health care and education professionals who may be responsible for providing for the child's special needs.

3. *Children who cannot be traced:* every attempt must be made to achieve complete follow-up. In the original planning of a study, provision should be made to obtain key information which will allow tracing. For example, in the UK, National Health Service numbers may be recorded and 'flagging' of cases can be negotiated with the appropriate authorities. Even the simple expedient of taking the names and addresses of grandparents should be included in the original protocol.

The precise design of a follow-up study is always individual, depending primarily on the hypothesis to be tested and, to an extent, on the resources that are available. The following protocol provides an example for a study where outcome is to be judged according to neurodevelopmental status. It is designed to be carried out according to the proposals for standardized examination and recording made by Amiel-Tison and Stewart.[10,14] Assessment at 12 months, ideally with review of any suspicious findings at 18 months, gives an accurate estimate of serious impairments, and subtle neurological ones will also be identified. Level of cognitive functioning cannot be predicted on the basis of overall development at this young age. Developmental quotient (DQ) alone is a very poor predictor of performance, with low sensitivities for all important outcomes at 8 years.[177] Hence, reliance on DQs alone will seriously underestimate the prevalence of subsequent neurodevelopmental impairments.[211] Complete ascertainment depends on continuing follow-up until the children are established in school, aged at least 8 years, or even longer if psychotic illnesses are to be excluded.

Protocol

0–3 months:	Measurement of head circumference. Objective assessment of hearing, for example brain-stem testing (ABR). Ophthalmic examination to assess visual function as well as retinal condition.
9–12 months:	Measurement of height, weight and head circumference. Clinical examination, paying particular attention to physical defects including the eyes and heart. Standardized neurological examination.[10,14] Assessments of hearing and vision. Developmental testing using a standardized method which allows the calculation of a developmental quotient such as the Griffiths scales.[80] If at the 1-year assessment, a child (a) has no evidence that language development is

starting, (b) is not weight-bearing and cruising round the furniture, he or she should be reviewed at 15–18 months.

18 months: Review of language development. If this has not started, further investigation is needed including that of hearing.
Review of neuromotor function, including gross motor development, to exclude symmetrical spastic conditions including mild to moderate spastic diplegias.

4–5 years: Test of cognitive function, for example the McCarthy scale of children's abilities,[134] which includes a test of motor skills.
Standardized neurological examination[10,14] and head circumference.
Pure–tone audiogram with tympanogram and otoaudiological assessment when the result is abnormal, to distinguish sensory and conductive losses.
Test of visual acuity.
Assessment of behaviour.

8 years: As for 4 years, with, in addition:
Cognitive assessment, e.g. Weschler Intelligence Scale for Children[231] and the Kaufman Assessment Battery for Children (K-ABC)[104] which aims to assess processing.
Test of visual–motor integration.[22]

The measures in this protocol were chosen to assess as many aspects of the children's functioning as possible at each age. All are important and all must be considered when assigning outcome status. However, it must be emphasized that the protocol represents 'minimum requirements', and efficiency depends on the use of standardized examination and scoring schemes to which there is strict adherence.

REFERENCES

1. Adamson S J, Alessandri L M, Badawi N, Burton P R, Pemberton P J, Stanley F 1995 Predictors of neonatal encephalopathy in full term infants. British Medical Journal 311: 598–602
2. Alberman E 1982 The epidemiology of congenital defects: a pragmatic approach. In: Adinolfi M, Benson P, Giannelli F, Seller M (eds) Paediatric research: a genetic approach. Clinics in Developmental Medicine No. 83. Spastics International Medical Publications, Heinemann, London, p 1
3. Alberman E, Botting B 1991 Trends in prevalence and survival of very low birthweight infants, England and Wales: 1983–7. Archives of Disease in Childhood 66: 1304–1308
4. Alberman E, Benson J, McDonald A 1982 Cerebral palsy and severe educational subnormality in children with a birthweight of 4 lbs or less: a comparison of births in 1951–1953 and 1970–1973. Lancet ii: 606–608
5. Alden E R, Mandelkorn T, Woodrum D E, Wennberg R P, Parks C R, Hodson W A 1972 Morbidity and mortality of infants weighing less than 1000 g in an intensive care nursery. Pediatrics 50: 40–49
6. Amiel-Tison C 1969 Cerebral damage in full-term newborn: Aetiological factors, neonatal status and long term follow-up. Biologia Neonatorum 14: 234–250
7. Amiel-Tison C 1980 Possible acceleration of neurological maturation following high-risk pregnancy. American Journal of Obstetrics and Gynecology 138: 303–306
8. Amiel-Tison C, Grenier A 1986 Neurological assessment during the first year of life. Oxford University Press, New York
9. Amiel-Tison C, Pettigrew A 1991 Adaptive changes in the developing brain during intrauterine stress. Brain and Development 13: 67–76
10. Amiel-Tison C, Stewart A L 1989 Follow up studies during the first five years of life: a pervasive assessment of neurological function. Archives of Disease in Childhood 64: 496–502
11. Amiel-Tison C, Korobkin R, Esque-Vaucouloux M T 1977 Neck extensor hypertonia: a clinical sign of insult to the central nervous system of the newborn. Early Human Development 1: 181–190
12. Amiel-Tison C, Dubé R, Garel M, Jequier J C 1983 Outcome at age 5 years of full term infants with transient neurologic abnormalities in the first year of life. In: Stern L (ed) Intensive care IV. Masson, New York, pp 247–257
13. Amiel-Tison C, Llado J, Breart G, Tchobroutsky C 1988 Le prognostic vital et neuro-psychique évalué avant la naissance sur les caractéristiques du retard de croissance intra-uterin. In: Société Française de Médecine Perinatale: dixhuitièmés journées nationales (proceedings) pp 100–107.
14. Amiel-Tison C, Stewart A L, Tison A 1990 Neuromotor assessment in the first five years of life. Video made and obtainable from UCL Images, University College, London
15. Apgar V 1953 A proposal for a new method of evaluation of the newborn infant. Current Researches in Anesthesia and Analgesia 32: 260–267
16. Ashton N, Ward B, Serpell G 1953 Role of oxygen in the genesis of retrolental fibroplasia. A preliminary report. British Journal of Ophthalmology 37: 513–520
17. Azzopardi D, Stewart A L 1989 Outcome for infants born at 22–25 weeks of gestation. Pediatric Research 26: 519 (abstract)
18. Azzopardi D, Wyatt J S, Cady E B et al 1989 Prognosis of newborn infants with hypoxic–ischemic brain injury assessed by phosphorus magnetic resonance spectroscopy. Pediatric Research 25: 445–451.
19. Bailey J C 1968 Inter-relationship of asphyxia neonatorum, cerebral and mental retardation. In: Windle W F (ed) Neurological and psychological deficits of asphyxia neonatorum. Thomas, Springfield, IL.
20. Barker D J P, Winder P D, Osmond C, Margetts B, Simmonds J 1989 Weight in infancy and death from ischaemic heart disease. Lancet ii: 577–580
21. Bax M, Nelson K B 1993 Birth asphyxia: a statement. Developmental Medicine and Child Neurology 35: 1022–1024
22. Beery K E 1989 Developmental test of visual–motor integration. Modern Curriculum Press, Cleveland
23. Bejar R, Wozniek P, Allard M et al 1988 Antenatal origin of neurologic damage in newborn infants. I. Preterm infants. American Journal of Obstetrics and Gynecology 159: 357–363
24. Bell A H, McClure B G, Hicks E M 1990 Power spectral analysis of the EEG of term infants following birth asphyxia. Developmental Medicine and Child Neurology 32: 990–998
25. Blair E, Stanley F J 1985 Interobserver agreement in the classification of cerebral palsy. Developmental Medicine and Child Neurology 27: 615–622
26. Blake A, Stewart A, Turcan D 1975 Parents of babies of very low birth weight: long-term follow-up. In: Porter R, O'Connor M. (eds) Parent–infant interaction. Ciba Foundation Symposium no. 33 (new series), Elsevier, Amsterdam, pp 271–288
27. Bohin S, Draper E S, Field D J 1996 Impact of extremely immature infants on neonatal services. Archives of Disease in Childhood 74: F110–F113
28. Boulton D P G, Cross K W 1974 Further observations on cost of preventing retrolental fibroplasia. Lancet i: 445–448
29. Bradford B C, Baudin J, Conway M T, Hazell J W P, Stewart A L, Reynolds E O R 1985 Identification of hearing loss in very preterm infants by brainstem auditory evoked potentials. Archives of Disease in Childhood 60: 105–109
30. Braert G 1988 Available evidence relating intrauterine growth retardation to neuromotor dysfunction and mental handicap. In: Kubli F, Patel N, Schmidt W (eds) Perinatal events and brain damage in surviving infants. Springer-Verlag, Heidelberg, pp 92–98
31. Brown J K, Purvis R J, Forfar J O, Cockburn F 1974 Neurological

aspects of perinatal asphyxia. Developmental Medicine and Child Neurology 16: 567–580
32. Calâme A, Prod'hom L S 1972 Prognostic vital et qualité de survie des prématurés pesant 1500 g et moins à la naissance, soignés en 1966–1968. Schweirzerische Medizinische Wochenschrift 102: 65–70
33. Calâme A, Prod'hom L S, van Melle G 1977 Outcome of infants of very low birthweight treated in a neonatal intensive care unit. Revue d'Epidemiologie et de Santé Publique 25: 21–32
34. Calâme A, Ducret S, Jaunin L, Plancherel B 1983 High risk appropriate for gestational age (AGA) and small for gestational age (SGA) preterm infants. Helvetica Paediatrica Acta 38: 39–50
35. Calâme A, Fawer C L, Claeys V, Arrazola L, Ducret S, Jaunin L 1986 Neurodevelopmental outcome and school performance of very-low-birth-weight infants at 8 years of age. European Journal of Pediatrics 145: 461–466
36. Cartlidge P H T, Stewart J H 1997 survival of very low birthweight and very preterm infants in a geographically defined population. Acta Paediatrica 86: 105–110
37. Chalmers I, Mutch L 1981 Are current trends in perinatal practice associated with an increase or a decrease in handicapping conditions? Lancet i: 1415 (Letter)
38. Cheung P Y, Haluschak M M, Finer N N, Robertson C M T 1996 Sensorineural hearing loss in survivors of neonatal extracorporeal membrane oxygenation. Early Human Development 44: 225–233
39. Chiswick M L 1985 Intrauterine growth retardation. British Medical Journal 291: 845–847
40. Cioni G, Fazzi B, Ipata A E, Canapicchi R, van Hof-van Duin J 1996 Correlation between cerebral visual impairment and magnetic resonance imaging in children with neonatal encephalopathy. Developmental Medicine and Child Neurology 38: 120–132
41. Clifford S H 1957 Pediatric aspects of the placental dysfunction syndrome in postmaturity. Journal of the American Medical Association 165: 1663–1665
42. Commey J O O, Fitzhardinge P M 1979 Handicap in the preterm small-for-gestational age infant. Journal of Pediatrics 94: 779–786
43. Cooke R W I 1987 Early and late cranial ultrasonographic appearances and outcome in very low birthweight infants. Archives of Disease in Childhood 62: 931–937
44. Cooke R W I 1990 Cerebral palsy in very low birthweight infants. Archives of Disease in Childhood 65: 201–206
45. Costello A M de L, Hamilton P A, Baudin J et al 1988 Prediction of neurodevelopmental impairment at 4 years from brain ultrasound appearance in very preterm infants. Developmental Medicine and Child Neurology 30: 711–722
46. Cross K W 1973 Cost of preventing retrolental fibroplasia, Lancet ii: 954–956
47. Cunningham S, Fleck B W, Elton R A, McIntosh N 1995 Transcutaneous oxygen levels in retinopathy of prematurity. Lancet 346: 1464–1465
48. Dammann O, Walther H, Allers B et al 1996 Development of a regional cohort of very-low-birthweight children at six years: cognitive abilities are associated with neurological disability and social background. Development Medicine and Child Neurology 38: 97–108
49. Davies P A, Russell H 1968 Later progress of 100 infants weighing 1000 to 2000 g at birth fed immediately with breast milk. Developmental Medicine and Child Neurology 10: 725–735
50. Demant E, Nagahara N, Meyer G 1982 Effects of changes in systemic blood pressure on the electroretinogram of the cat: evidence for retinal autoregulation. Investigative Ophthalmology and Visual Science 23: 683–687
51. de Vries L S, Regev R, Pennock J M, Wigglesworth J S, Dubowitz L M S 1988 Ultrasound evolution and later outcome of infants with periventricular densities. Early Human Development 16: 225–233
52. Donselaar C A, Brouwer O F, Geerts A T, Arts W F M, Stroink H, Peters A C B 1997 Clinical course of untreated tonic–clonic seizures in childhood: prospective, hospital based study. British Medical Journal 314: 401–404
53. Douglas J W B 1965 Mental ability and school achievement of premature children at eight years of age. British Medical Journal ii: 1210–1212
54. Douglas J W B, Gear R 1976 Children of low birthweight in the 1946 national cohort. Archives of Disease in Childhood 51: 820–827
55. Drage J S, Kennedy C, Schwartz B K 1964 The Apgar score as an index of neonatal mortality. A report from the collaborative study of cerebral palsy. Obstetrics and Gynecology 24: 222–230
56. Drage J S, Kennedy C, Berendes H, Schwartz B K, Weiss L 1966 The Apgar score as an index of infant morbidity. Developmental Medicine and Child Neurology 8: 141–148
57. Drage J S, Berendes H W, Fisher D D 1969 Perinatal factors affecting human development. In: Scientific Publication No. 185, Pan-American Health Organization, Washington, p 222
58. Drillien C M 1958 Growth and development in a group of children of very low birth weight. Archives of Disease in Childhood 33: 10–18
59. Drillien C M, Richmond F 1956 Prematurity in Edinburgh. Archives of Disease in Childhood 31: 390–394
60. Drillien C M, Thomson A J M, Burgoyne K 1980 Low-birthweight children at early school age; a longitudinal study. Developmental Medicine and Child Neurology 22: 26–47
61. D'Souza S W, McCartney E, Nolan M, Taylor I G 1981 Hearing, speech and language in survivors of severe perinatal asphyxia. Archives of Disease in Childhood 56: 245–252
62. Dworkin R H, Cornblatt B A 1995 Predicting schizophrenia. Lancet 345: 139–140
63. Eken P, de Vries L S, van-Nieuwenhuizen O, Schalij-Delfos N E, Reits D, Spekreijse H 1996 Early predictors of cerebral visual impairment in infants with cystic leukomalacia. Neuropediatrics 27: 16–25
64. Elliman A M, Bryan E M, Elliman A D, Walker J, Harvey D R 1991 Coordination in low birthweight seven-year-olds. Acta Paediatrica 80: 316–322
65. Ellis M I 1980 Follow-up study of survivors after intra-uterine transfusion. Developmental Medicine and Child Neurology 22: 48–54
66. Eriksson M, Tibblin G, Cnattingrus S 1994 Low birthweight and ischaemic heart disease. Lancet 343: 731–732
67. Escobar G J, Littenberg B, Pettiti D B 1991 Outcome among surviving very low birthweight infants: a meta-analysis. Archives of Disease in Childhood 66: 204–211
68. Eyre J A, Oozeer R C, Wilkinson A R 1983 Diagnosis of neonatal seizure by continuous recording and rapid analysis of the electroencephalogram. Archives of Disease in Childhood 58: 785–790.
69. Fancourt R, Campbell S, Harvey D, Norman A P 1976 Follow-up of small-for-dates babies. British Medical Journal i: 1435–1437
70. Faneroff A A, Wright L L, Stevenson D K et al 1995 Very low birthweight outcomes of the National Institute of Child Health and Human Development Neonatal Research Network, May 1991 through December 1992. American Journal of Obstetrics and Gynecology 173: 1423–1431
71. Fawer C L, Calâme A 1988 Assessment of neurodevelopmental outcome. In: Levene M I, Bennett M J, Punt J (eds) Fetal and neonatal neurology and neurosurgery. Churchill Livingstone, Edinburgh, pp 71–88
72. Fenton A C, Field D J, Mason E, Clarke M 1990 Attitudes to viability of preterm infants and their effect on figures for perinatal mortality. British Medical Journal 300: 434–436
73. Ferrara T B, Hoekstra R E, Couser R J et al 1994 Survival and follow-up of infants born at 23 to 26 weeks of gestational age: effects of surfactant therapy. Journal of Pediatrics 124: 119–124
74. Fisch L, Osborn D A 1954 Congenital deafness and haemolytic disease of the newborn. Archives of Disease in Childhood 29: 309–316
75. Flynn J T, Phelps D L (eds) 1988 Retinopathy of prematurity: problem and challenge. March of Dimes Birth Defects Foundation: Birth Defects: Original Articles Series, Vol. 24, No. 1. Alan R Liss, New York
76. Flynn J, Bancalari E, Snyder E 1992 A cohort study of transcutaneous oxygen tension and the incidence and severity of retinopathy of prematurity. New England Journal of Medicine 326: 1050–1054
77. Fraser G R 1976 The causes of profound deafness in childhood. John Hopkins University Press, Baltimore, MD
78. Gherpelli J L D, Ferreira F, Costa H P F 1993 Neurological follow-up of small-for-gestational age newborn infants. A study of risk factors related to prognosis at one year of age. Arq Neuropsiquiatr 51: 50–58
79. Gillberg I C, Gillberg C 1989 Children with preschool minor neurodevelopmental disorders, IV: behaviour and school achievement at age 13. Developmental Medicine and Child Neurology 31: 3–13
80. Griffiths Mental Development Scales (1996 Revision) 1996 The Test Agency on behalf of the Association for Research in Infant and Child Development, Amersham
81. Gultom E, Doyle L W, Davis P, Dharmalingam A, Bowman E 1997

Changes over time in attitudes to treatment and survival rate, for extremely preterm infants (23–27 weeks' gestational age). Australian and New Zealand Journal of Obstetrics and Gynaecology 37: 56–58
82. Hack M, Horbar J D, Malloy M H, Tyson J E, Wright E, Wright L 1991 Very low birth weight outcomes of the National Institute of Child Health and Human Development Neonatal Network. Pediatrics 87: 587–597
83. Hack M, Taylor G, Klein N, Eiben R 1993 Outcome of <750 g birthweight children at school age. A regional study. Pediatric Research 33: 262 (Abstract)
84. Hack M, Wright L L, Shankaran S, Tyson J E, Horbar J D, Bauer C R, Younes N 1995 Very low birthweight outcomes of the National Institute of Child Health and Human Development Neonatal Network, November 1989 to October 1990. American Journal of Obstetrics and Gynecology 172: 457–464
85. Hack M, Friedman H, Faneroff A A 1996 Outcomes of extremely low birth weight infants. Pediatrics 98: 931–937
86. Hadders-Algra M, Huisjes H J, Touwen B C L 1988 Perinatal risk factors and minor neurological dysfunction: significance for behaviour and school achievement at nine years. Developmental Medicine and Child Neurology 30: 482–491
87. Hadders-Algra M, Touwen B C L, Huisjes H J 1988 Perinatal correlates of major and minor dysfunction at school age: a multivariate analysis. Developmental Medicine and Child Neurology 30: 472–481
88. Hagberg B, Hagberg G, Olow I 1982 Gains and hazards of intensive neonatal care: an analysis from Swedish cerebral palsy epidemiology. Developmental Medicine and Child Neurology 24: 13–19
89. Hall A, McLeod A, Counsell C, Thomson L, Mutch L 1995 School attainment, cognitive ability and motor function in a total Scottish very-low-birthweight population at eight years: a controlled study. Developmental Medicine and Child Neurology 37: 1037–1050
90. Halsey C L, Collin M F, Anderson C L 1993 Extremely low birth weight children and their peers: a comparison of preschool performance. Pediatrics 91: 807–811
91. Harvey D, Prince J, Bunton J, Parkinson C, Campbell S 1982 Abilities of children who were small-for-gestational-age babies. Pediatrics 69: 296–300
92. Hawdon J M, Ward-Platt M P 1993 Metabolic adaptation in small for gestational age infants. Archives of Disease in Childhood 68: 262–268
93. Hawdon J M, Hey E, Kolvin I, Fundudis T 1990 Born too small – is outcome still affected? Developmental Medicine and Child Neurology 32: 943–953
94. Hellgren L, Gillberg C, Gillberg I C, Enerskog I 1993 Children with deficits in attention, motor control and perception (DAMP) almost grown up: general health at 16 years. Developmental Medicine and Child Neurology 35: 881–892
95. Hendren R L, Hodde-Vargas J, Yeo R A, Vargas L A, Brooks W M, Ford C 1995 Neuropsychological study of children at risk for schizophrenia: a preliminary report. Journal of the American Academy of Child and Adolescent Psychiatry 34: 1284–1291
96. Hess J H, Lundeen E C 1949 The premature infant, 2nd Edn. W B Saunders, Philadelphia
97. Holmsgaard K W, Petersen S 1996 Infants with gestational age 28 weeks or less. Danish Medical Bulletin 43: 86–91
98. Holtrop P C, Ertzbischoff L M, Roberts C L, Batton D G, Lorenz R P 1994 Survival and short-term outcome in newborns of 23 to 25 weeks' gestation. American Journal of Obstetrics and Gynecology 170: 1266–1270
99. Hope P L, Reynolds E O R 1985 Investigation of cerebral energy metabolism in newborn infants by phosphorus nuclear magnetic resonance spectroscopy. Clinics in Perinatology 12: 261–275
100. Hungerford J, Stewart A, Hope P 1986 Ocular sequelae of preterm birth and their relation to ultrasound evidence of cerebral damage. British Journal of Ophthalmology 70: 463–468
101. Johnsen S, Freiesleben E 1952 The relation between erythroblastosis foetalis, kernicterus and impairment of hearing. Acta Otolaryngologica 42: 35–50
102. Johnson A, Townshend P, Yudkin P, Bull D, Wilkinson A R 1993 Functional abilities at age 4 years of children born before 29 weeks of gestation. British Medical Journal 306: 1715–1718
103. Jones R A K, Lukeman D 1982 Apnoea of immaturity 2. Mortality and handicap. Archives of Disease in Childhood 57: 766–768
104. Kaufman Assessment Battery for Children (K-ABC) 1983 American Guidance Inc., Circle Pines
105. Kinsey V E 1956 Retrolental fibroplasia. Cooperative study of retrolental fibroplasia and the use of oxygen. American Medical Association Archives of Ophthalmology 56: 481–543
106. Kinsey V E, Arnold H J, Kalina R E et al 1977 PaO_2 levels and retrolental fibroplasia: a report of the cooperative study. Pediatrics 60: 655–668
107. Kirkbride V, Baudin J, Lorek A et al 1994 Motor tests of interhemispheric control and cognitive function in very preterm infants at eight years. Pediatric Research 36: 20 (Abstract)
108. Kirkbride V, Baudin J, Townsend J et al 1994 Neonatal visual responses and neurodevelopmental outcomes at 8 years in very preterm infants. Pediatric Research 35: 274A
109. Kirkbride V, Rifkin L, Amess P, Townsend J, Stewart A 1996 Does neonatal ultrasound (US) predict MRI findings in adolescence? Pediatric Research 40: 536 (Abstract)
110. Kitchen W H, Campbell D G 1971 Controlled trial of intensive care for very low birth weight infants. Pediatrics 48: 711–714
111. Kitchen W H, Rickards A, Ryan M M et al 1979 A longitudinal study of very low-birthweight infants II. Developmental Medicine and Child Neurology 21: 582–589
112. Kitchen W H, Yu V Y H, Orgill A et al 1983 Collaborative study of very low-birthweight infants. American Journal of Diseases of Children 137: 555–559
113. Klaus M, Kennell J 1970 Mothers separated from their newborn infants. Pediatric Clinics of North America 17: 1015–1037
114. Knobloch H, Rider R, Harper P, Pasamanick B 1956 Neuropsychiatric sequelae of prematurity. Journal of the American Medical Association 171: 581–586
115. Koops B L, Morgan L J, Battaglia F C 1982 Neonatal mortality risk in relation to birth weight and gestational age: Update. Journal of Pediatrics 101: 969–977
116. Korner F, Bossi E, Meier-Gibbons F 1990 Visual morbidity of very low birthweight (VLBW) infants. In: Duc G, Huch A, Huch R (eds) The very low birthweight infant. Georg Thieme, Stuttgart, pp 25–40
117. Krägeloh-Mann I, Petersen D, Hagberg G, Vollmer B, Hagberg B, Michaelis R 1995 Bilateral spastic cerebral palsy – MRI pathology and origin analysis from a representative series of 56 cases. Developmental Medicine and Child Neurology 37: 379–397
118. Larroche J C 1995 Fetal cerebral pathology of circulatory origin. In: Levene M I, Lilford R J (eds) Fetal and neonatal neurology and neurosurgery, 2nd edn. Churchill Livingstone, London, pp 321–333
119. Lefebvre F, Glorieux J, St-Laurent-Gagnon T 1996 Neonatal survival and disability at age 18 months for infants born between 23 and 28 weeks of gestation. American Journal of Obstetrics and Gynecology 174: 833–838
120. Leijon I, Billström G, Lind I 1980 An 18-month follow-up study of growth-retarded neonates. Relation to biochemical tests of placental function in late pregnancy and neuro-behavourial condition in the newborn period. Early Human Development 4: 271–285
121. Levene M I, Grindulis H, Sands C, Moore J R 1986 Comparison of two methods of predicting outcome in perinatal asphyxia. Lancet i: 67–69
122. Levene M I, Dowling S, Graham M, Fogelman K, Galton M, Phillips M 1992 Impaired motor function (clumsiness) in 5 year old children: correlation with neonatal ultrasound. Archives of Disease in Childhood 67: 687–690
123. Levine R S, Hennekens H, Jesse M J 1994 Blood pressure in prospective population-based cohort of newborn and infant twins. British Medical Journal 308: 298–302
124. Leviton A 1993 Preterm birth and cerebral palsy: is tumour necrosis factor the missing link? Developmental Medicine and Child Neurology 35: 553–558
125. Ley D, Laurin J, Bjerre I, Marsal K 1996 Abnormal fetal aortic velocity waveform and minor neurological dysfunction at 7 years of age. Ultrasound in Obstetrics and Gynecology 8: 152–159
126. Ley D, Laurin J, Bjerre I, Marsal K 1996 Abnormal fetal aortic velocity waveform and intellectual function at 7 years of age. Ultrasound in Obstetrics and Gynecology 8: 160–165
127. Lilienfeld A M, Pasamanick B 1955 The association of maternal and fetal factors with the development of cerebral palsy and epilepsy. American Journal of Obstetrics and Gynecology 70: 93–101
128. Lithell H O, McKeigue P M, Berglund L, Mohsen R, Lithell U-B, Leon D A 1996 Relation of size at birth to non-insulin dependent diabetes and insulin concentrations in men aged 50–60 years. British Medical Journal 312: 406–410

129. Lloyd B W 1984. Outcome of very-low-birthweight babies from Wolverhampton. Lancet ii: 739–741
130. Lloyd B W, Wheldall K, Perks D 1988 Controlled study of intelligence and school performance of very low birthweight children from a defined geographical area. Developmental Medicine and Child Neurology 30: 36–42
131. Lorek A, Takei Y, Cady E B 1994 Delayed (secondary) cerebral energy failure after acute hypoxia–ischaemia in the newborn piglet: continuous 48 hour studies by phosphorus magnetic resonance spectroscopy. Pediatric Research 36: 699–706
132. Lubchenco L O, Horner F A, Reed L H et al 1963 Sequelae of premature birth. American Journal of Diseases of Children 106: 101–115
133. Lucey J F, Dangman B 1984 A re-examination of the role of oxygen in retrolental fibroplasia. Pediatrics 73: 82–96.
134. McCarthy P 1972 McCarthy scale of children's abilities. Psychological Corporation, New York
135. McCarton C M, Wallace I F, Divon M, Vaughan H G 1996 Cognitive and neurologic development of the premature, small for gestational age infant through age 6: comparison by birth weight and gestational age. Pediatrics 98: 1167–1178
136. McDonald A 1965 Retarded foetal growth. In: Dawkings M, MacGregor W G (eds) Gestational age, size and maturity. Clinics in Developmental Medicine No. 19. Spastics Society Medical Education and Information Unit, Heinemann, London, pp 14–27
137. McDonald A D 1967 Children of very low birthweight. Research Monograph No. 1. Medical Education and Information Unit of the Spastics Society, London
138. Marlow N, Roberts B L, Cooke R W I 1989 Motor skills in extremely low birthweight children at the age of six years. Archives of Disease in Childhood 64: 839–847
139. Marlow N, Roberts B L, Cooke R W I 1993 Outcome at 8 years for children with birth weights of 1250 g or less. Archives of Disease in Childhood 68 (suppl): 286–290
140. Miranda S, Hack M, Fantz R L, Faneroff A A, Klaus M H 1977 Neonatal pattern vision: a predictor of future mental performance. Journal of Pediatrics 91: 642–647
141. Murphy K W 1995 Intrauterine death in a twin: implications for the survivor. In: Ward R H, Whittle M (eds) Multiple pregnancy. RCOG Press, London, pp 218–230
142. Nelson K B, Broman S H 1977 Perinatal risk factors in children with serious motor and mental handicaps. Annals of Neurology 2: 371–377
143. Nelson K B, Ellenberg J H 1981 Apgar scores as predictors of chronic neurologic disability. Pediatrics 68: 36–44
144. Nelson K B, Ellenberg J H 1982 Children who 'outgrow' cerebral palsy. Pediatrics 69: 529–535
145. Nelson R M, Resnick M B, Eitzman V D 1979 Intensive care and the very low birthweight infant. Lancet ii 737 (Letter)
146. Orgill A A, Astbury J, Bajuk B, Yu V Y H 1982 Early development of infants 1000 g or less at birth. Archives of Disease in Childhood 57: 823–827
147. Ounsted M K, Moar V A, Scott A 1984 Children of deviant birthweight at the age of seven years: health, size and developmental status. Early Human Development 9: 323–340
148. Owen P, Patel N B 1995 Epidemiology of multiple pregnancy. In: Ward R H, Whittle M (eds) Multiple pregnancy. RCOG Press, London, pp 1–13
149. Palmer P, Dubowitz L M S, Levene M I, Dubowitz V 1982 Developmental and neurological progress of preterm infants with intraventricular haemorrhage and ventricular dilatation. Archives of Disease in Childhood 57: 748–753
150. Paneth N, Susser M 1995 Early origin of coronary heart disease (the 'Barker hypothesis'). British Medical Journal 310: 411–412
151. Pape K E, Blackwell R J, Cusick G et al 1979 Ultrasound detection of brain damage in pre-term infants. Lancet ii: 1261–1264
152. Parmelee A H, Harber A 1973 Who is the risk infant? Clinical Obstetrics and Gynecology 16: 376–387
153. Penrice J, Cady E B, Lorek A et al 1995 Proton MRS of the brain during hypoxia–ischaemia and delayed cerebral energy failure in the newborn piglet. Neuropediatrics 26: 341–342 (Abstract)
154. Penrice J, Cady E B, Lorek A et al 1996 Proton magnetic resonance spectroscopy of the brain in normal preterm and term infants, and early changes after perinatal hypoxia–ischaemia. Pediatric Research 40: 6–14
155. Perlman M, Claris O, Hao Y et al 1995 Secular changes in the outcomes to eighteen to twenty-four months of age of extremely low birth weight infants, with adjustment for changes in risk factors and severity of illness. Journal of Pediatrics 126: 75–87
156. Pharoah P O D, Alberman E D 1990 Annual statistical review. Archives of Disease in Childhood 65: 147–151
157. Pharoah P O D, Cooke R W I 1982 Impact of neonatal intensive care. Lancet ii: 281 (Letter)
158. Pharoah P O D, Stevenson C J, Cooke R W I, Stevenson R C 1994 Clinical and subclinical deficits at 8 years in a geographically defined cohort of low birthweight infants. Archives of Disease in Childhood 70: 264–270
159. Phibbs R H, Harvin D, Jones G et al 1971 Development of children who had received intrauterine transfusions. Pediatrics 47: 689–697
160. Pinto-Martin J A, Riolo S, Cnaan A, Holzman C, Susser M W, Paneth N 1995 Cranial ultrasound prediction of disabling and nondisabling cerebral palsy at age two in a low birth weight population. Pediatrics 95: 249–254
161. Pinto-Martin J A, Dobson V, Cnaan A, Zhao H, Paneth N S 1996 Vision outcome at 2 years in a low birthweight population. Pediatric Neurology 14: 281–287
162. Polnay L, Hull D 1993 Community paediatrics, 2nd edn. Churchill Livingstone, Edinburgh
163. Powell T G, Pharoah P O D, Cooke R W I 1986 Survival and morbidity in a geographically defined population of low birthweight infants. Lancet i: 539–543
164. Powell T G, Pharoah P O D, Cooke R W I, Rosenbloom L 1988 Cerebral palsy in low-birthweight infants. I. Spastic hemiplegia: associations with intrapartum stress. Developmental Medicine and Child Neurology 30: 11–18. II. Spastic diplegia: associations with fetal immatrity. Development Medicine and Child Neurology 30: 19–25
165. Praesse D P, Siewert J C, Ellison P H 1983 McCarthy performance and neurological functioning in children born 'at risk'. Journal of Psychoeducational Assessment 1: 273–283
166. Procianoy R S, Garcia-Prats J A, Hittner H M, Adams J M, Rudolph A J 1981 An association between retinopathy of prematurity and intraventricular haemorrhage in very low birth weight infants. Acta Paediatrica Scandinavica 70: 473–477
167. Rawlings G, Reynolds E O R, Stewart A L, Strang L B 1971 Changing prognosis for infants of very low birthweight. Lancet ii: 516–519
168. Rennie J M 1996 Perinatal management at the lower margin of viability. Archives of Disease in Childhood 74: F214–218
169. Reynolds E O R, Wyatt J S, Azzopardi D et al 1988 New non-invasive methods for assessing brain oxygenation and haemodynamics. British Medical Bulletin 44: 1052–1057
170. Richings J 1973 Later progress of infants who received transfusions in utero for severe rhesus haemolytic disease. Lancet i: 1220–1222
171. Roberton N R C 1993 Should we look after babies less than 800 g? Archives of Disease in Childhood 68: 326–329
172. Robertson C M T, Etches P C, Kyle J M 1990 Eight year school performance and growth of preterm small for gestational age infants: a comparative study with subjects matched for birthweight or gestational age. Journal of Pediatrics 116: 19–26
173. Ross G, Lipper E, Auld P 1991 Educational status and school related abilities of very low birth weight premature children. Pediatrics 88: 1125–1134
174. Roth S 1996 Small-for-gestational-age infants and antenatal prediction of outcome. Ultrasound in Obstetrics and Gynecology 8: 149–151
175. Roth S C, Edwards A D, Cady E B et al 1992 Relation between cerebral oxidative metabolism following birth asphyxia, and neurodevelopmental outcome and brain growth at one year. Developmental Medicine and Child Neurology 34: 285–295
176. Roth S C, Baudin J, McCormick D C et al 1993 Relation between ultrasound appearance of the brain in very preterm infants and neurodevelopmental impairment at eight years. Developmental Medicine and Child Neurology 35: 755–768
177. Roth S C, Baudin J, Pezzani-Goldsmith M, Townsend J, Reynolds E O R, Stewart A L 1994 Relation between neurodevelopmental status of very preterm infants at one and eight years. Developmental Medicine and Child Neurology 36: 1049–1062
178. Roth S, Chang T C, Robson S et al 1996 Neurodevelopmental outcome following different patterns of intrauterine growth (IUG). Pediatric Research 40: 549A
179. Roth S C, Azzopardi D, Baudin J et al 1997 Relation between cerebral oxidative metabolism following birth asphyxia, and

neurodevelopmental outcome and head circumference at four years. Developmental Medicine and Child Neurology 39: 718–725
180. Ruth V J, Raivio K O 1988 Perinatal brain damage: predictive value of metabolic acidosis and the Apgar score. British Medical Journal 297: 24–27
181. Rutherford M, Pennock J, Schwieso J, Cowan F, Dubowitz L 1996 Hypoxia–ischaemic encephalopathy: early and late magnetic resonance imaging findings in relation to outcome. Archives of Disease in Childhood 75: F145–151
182. Sabel K G, Olegard R, Victorin L 1976 Remaining sequelae with modern perinatal care. Pediatrics 57: 652–658
183. Saigal S, Rosenbaum P, Stoskopf B, Sinclair J C 1984 Outcome in infants 501–1000 gm birthweight delivered to residents of the McMaster health region. Journal of Pediatrics 105: 969–976
184. Saigal S, Rosenbaum P, Hattersley B, Milner R 1989 Decreased disability rate among 3-year-old survivors weighing 501 to 1000 grams at birth and born to residents of a geographically defined region from 1981 to 1984 compared with 1977 to 1980. Journal of Pediatrics 114: 839–846
185. Saigal S, Szatmari P, Rosenbaum P, Campbell D, King S 1991 Cognitive abilities and school performance of extremely low birth weight children and matched term control children at age 8 years: a regional study. Journal of Pediatrics 118: 751–760
186. Saigal S, Feeny D, Furlong W, Rosenbaum P, Burrows E, Torrance G 1994 Comparison of the health-related quality of life of extremely low birth weight children and a reference group at age eight years. Journal of Pediatrics 125: 418–425
187. Saigal S, Feeny D H, Furlong W J, Rosenbaum P 1995 How premature teens perceive their own health-related quality of life: comparison with controls. Pediatric Research 38: 453 (Abstract)
188. Sameroff A J, Chandler M J 1975 Reproductive risk and the continuum of caretaking casualty. In: Horowitz W D, Hetherington M, Scarr-Salapatek S, Siegal G (eds) Review of child development research. Vol. 4. University of Chicago Press, Chicago, p 187
189. Sarnat H B, Sarnat M S 1976 Neonatal encephalopathy following fetal distress. Archives of Neurology 33: 696–705
190. Scott H 1976 Outcome of very severe birth asphyxia. Archives of Disease in Childhood 51: 712–716
191. Scottish Low Birthweight Study Group 1992 The Scottish Low Birthweight Study. I: Survival, growth, neuromotor and sensory impairment at four years. Archives of Disease in Childhood 67: 675–681
192. Silverman W A 1979 Incubator-baby side shows. Pediatrics 64: 127–141
193. Silverman W A 1980 Retrolental fibroplasia: a modern parable. Grune & Stratton, New York
194. Spinillo A, Capuzzo E, Egbe T O, Fazzi E, Colonna L, Icola S 1995 Pregnancies complicated by idiopathic intrauterine growth retardation: severity of growth failure, neonatal morbidity and two-year infant neurodevelopmental outcome. Journal of Reproductive Medicine 40: 209–215
195. Springett R, Tyszczuk L, Penrice J et al 1996 Cytochrome oxidase redox state (Cû) correlates with the severity of delayed cerebral energy failure following transient hypoxia–ischaemia (HI) in the newborn piglet. Pediatric Research 40: 553 (Abstract)
196. Stanley F J, Atkinson S 1981 Impact of neonatal intensive care on cerebral palsy in infants of low birthweight. Lancet ii: 1162 (Letter)
197. Stanley F J, Watson L 1992 Trends in perinatal mortality and cerebral palsy in Western Australia, 1967–1985. British Medical Journal 304: 1658–1663
198. Stein C E, Fall C H D, Kumaran K, Osmond C, Coz V, Barker D J P 1996 Fetal growth and coronary heart disease in South India. Lancet ii: 1269–1273
199. Steiner H, Neligan G 1975 Perinatal cardiac arrest. Quality of the survivors. Archives of Disease in Childhood 50: 696–702
200. Stewart A L 1989 Fetal growth: mortality and morbidity. In: Sharp F, Fraser R B, Milner R D G (eds) Fetal growth, Royal College of Obstetricians and Gynaecologists, London, pp 403–412
201. Stewart A 1991 Higher order multiple births: the long term outcome. In: Harvey D, Bryan E (eds) The stress of multiple births. Multiple Births Foundation, London, pp 127–132
202. Stewart A L, Hope P L 1988 Outcome of very low birthweight or very preterm infants with special consideration of perinatal events. In: Kubli F, Patel N, Schmidt W, Linderkamp O (eds) Perinatal events and brain damage in surviving children. Springer-Verlag, Heidelberg, pp 257–264
203. Stewart A, Kirkbride V 1996 Very preterm infants at 14 years: relation with neonatal ultrasound brain scans and neurodevelopmental status at one year. Acta Paediatrica 416 (suppl): 44–47
204. Stewart A, Pezzani-Goldsmith M 1994 In: Amiel-Tison C, Stewart A (eds) The newborn infant: one brain for life. Les Editions INSERM, Paris, pp 151–166
205. Stewart A L, Reynolds E O R 1974 Improved prognosis for infants of very low birth weight. Pediatrics 54: 724–735
206. Stewart A L, Turcan D, Rawlings G, Hart S, Gregory S 1978 Outcome for infants at high risk of major handicap. In: Elliot K, O'Connor M (eds) Major mental handicap: methods and costs of prevention. Ciba Foundation Symposium 59 (New series). Elsevier, Amsterdam, p 151
207. Stewart A L, Reynolds E O R, Lipscomb A P 1981 Outcome for infants of very low birthweight: survey of world literature. Lancet i: 1038–1041
208. Stewart A L, Reynolds E O R, Hope P L et al 1987 Probability of neurodevelopmental disorders estimated from ultrasound appearance of brains of very preterm infants. Developmental Medicine and Child Neurology 29: 3–11
209. Stewart A L, Hope P L, Hamilton P A et al 1988 Prediction in very preterm infants of satisfactory neurodevelopmental progress at 12 months. Developmental Medicine and Child Neurology 30: 53–63
210. Stewart A L, Costello A M de L, Hamilton P A et al 1989 Relationship between neurodevelopmental status of very preterm infants at one and four years. Developmental Medicine and Child Neurology 31: 756–765
211. Stewart A L, Roth S C, Kirkbride V 1995 Follow-up by questionnaire? Early Human Development 41: 87–95
212. Sung I-K, Vohr B, Oh W 1993 Growth and neurodevelopmental outcome of very low birth weight infants with intrauterine growth retardation: comparison with control subjects matched by birth weight and gestational age. Journal of Pediatrics 123: 618–624
213. Taittonen L, Nuutinen M, Turtinen J, Uhari M 1996 Prenatal and postnatal factors in predicting later blood pressure among children: cardiovascular risk in young Finns. Pediatric Research 40: 627–632
214. Taylor M J, Saliba E, Laugier J 1996 Use of evoked potentials in preterm neonates. Archives of Disease in Childhood 74: F70–76
215. Thomson A J, Searle M, Russell G 1977 Quality of survival after severe birth asphyxia. Archives of Disease in Childhood 52: 620–626
216. Thoresen M, Penrice J, Lorek A et al 1995 Mild hypothermia after severe transient hypoxia–ischaemia ameliorates delayed cerebral energy failure in the newborn piglet. Pediatric Research 37: 667–670
217. Tin W, Wariyar U, Hey E for the Northern Neonatal Network 1997 Changing prognosis for babies of less than 28 weeks' gestation in the north of England between 1983 and 1994. British Medical Journal 314: 107–111
218. Touwen B C L, Huisjes H J, Jurgens-van der Zee Á D Bierman van Eendenburg M E C, Smrkovsky M, Olinga A A 1980 Obstetrical condition and neonatal neurological morbidity. An analysis with the help of the optimality concept. Early Human Development 4: 207–228
219. Valcamonico A, Danti L, Frusca T et al 1994 Absent end-diastolic velocity in umbilical artery: risk of neonatal morbidity and brain damage. American Journal of Obstetrics and Gynecology 170: 796–801
220. Van Zeban van der Aa T M, Verloove-Vanhorick S P, Brand R, Ruys J H 1989 Morbidity of very low birthweight infants at corrected age of two years in a geographically defined population. Lancet ii: 253–255
221. Verma U, Tejani N, Klein S et al 1994 Obstetrical antecedents of periventricular leukomalacia (PVL). American. Journal of Obstetrics and Gynecology 159: 357–363
222. Victorian Infant Collaborative Study Group 1991 Eight-year outcome in infants with birth weight of 500 to 999 grams: continuing regional study of 1979 and 1980 births. Journal of Pediatrics 118: 761–767
223. Victorian Infant Collaborative Study Group 1991 Improvement of outcome for infants of birth weight under 1000 g. Archives of Disease in Childhood 66: 765–769
224. Villar J, Smeriglio V, Martorell R, Brown C H, Klein R E 1984 Heterogeneous growth and mental development of intrauterine growth-retarded infants during the first 3 years of life. Pediatrics 74: 783–791
225. Vohr B R, Garcia-Coll C T 1985 Increased morbidity in low-birth weight survivors with severe retrolental fibroplasia. Journal of Pediatrics 106: 287–291
226. Volpe J J 1996 Subplate neurons – missing link in brain injury of the premature infant? Pediatrics 97: 112–113

227. Wariyar U, Richmond S 1989 Morbidity and preterm delivery: importance of 100% follow up. Lancet i: 387–388
228. Wariyar U, Richmond S, Hey E 1989 Pregnancy outcome at 24–31 weeks' gestation: mortality. Archives of Disease in Childhood 64: 670–677
229. Wariyar U, Richmond S, Hey E 1989 Pregnancy outcome at 24–31 weeks' gestation: neonatal survivors. Archives of Disease in Childhood 64: 678–686
230. Weisglas-Kuperus N, Baerts W, Fetter W P F et al 1994 Minor neurological dysfunction and quality of movement in relation to neonatal cerebral damage and subsequent development. Developmental Medicine and Child Neurology 36: 727–735
231. Weschler Intelligence Scale for Children (WISC-III) 1994 Psychological Corporation, New York
232. Westwood M, Kramer M S, Munz D, Lovett J M, Watters G V 1983 Growth and development of full-term non-asphyxiated small-for-gestational age newborns: follow-up through adolescence. Pediatrics 71: 367–382
233. Whitaker A H, Feldman J F, Van Rossem R et al 1996 Neonatal cranial ultrasound abnormalities in low birth weight infants: relation to cognitive outcomes at six years of age. Pediatrics 98: 719–729
234. Whitaker A H, Van Rossem R, Feldman J F et al 1997 Psychiatric outcomes in low-birth-weight children at age 6 years: relation to neonatal cranial ultrasound abnormalities. Archives of General Psychiatry 54: 847–856
235. Winer K E, Taguan N A, Outlawry V L, DiGuiseppe R, Borofdky L G 1982 Four to seven year evaluation in two groups of small for gestational age infants. American Journal of Obstetrics and Gynecology 143: 425–429
236. Wocadlo C, Rieger I 1994 Developmental outcome at 12 months corrected age for infants born less than 30 weeks gestation: influence of reduced intrauterine and postnatal growth. Early Human Development 39: 127–137
237. World Health Organization 1980 International classification of impairments, disabilities and handicaps. WHO, Geneva.
238. Yanyotti M 1994 When is it best to be born? A psychoanalyst's perspective: growing from a woman into a mother. In: Amiel-Tison C, Stewart A (eds) The newborn infant: one brain for life. Les Editions INSERM, Paris, pp 39–45
239. Yoon B H, Romero R, Yang S H et al 1996 Interleukin 6 concentrations in umbilical cord plasma are elevated in neonates with white matter lesions associated with periventricular leukomalacia. American Journal of Obstetrics and Gynecology 174: 1433–1440
240. Yu V Y H, Loke H L, Bajuk B, Szymonowicz W, Orgill A A, Astbury J 1986 Prognosis for infants born at 23 to 28 weeks' gestation. British Medical Journal 293: 1200–1203

Part 2

Predicting outcome using ultrasound imaging in the neonatal period

Janet M. Rennie

Parents whose baby is ill or premature initially fear that their child will die. Once this fear has been allayed their anxiety turns to the question 'will he be all right?' Assessing prognosis, and conveying the information in an understandable way to staff and parents, is an everyday challenge in neonatal medicine. The prognosis of conditions such as meningitis, specific congenital malformations, or hypoxic–ischaemic encephalopathy is given in the appropriate section of the book. Considerable endeavour has been directed at evaluating neonatal cranial ultrasound as a tool for the prediction of neurodevelopmental outcome in preterm infants and this literature will be summarized here. The intense interest in 'telling the future'[45] lies not only in the desire to provide early counselling for parents, but also because accurate identification of children destined to be handicapped at a time when the brain has unique plasticity, may allow intervention.[18,80] In future it may be possible to alter the programmed cell death which is part of normal brain development in order to allow more brain cells to survive.[26,37]

PROGNOSIS AFTER SPECIFIC CRANIAL ULTRASOUND DIAGNOSES

Ultrasound is a readily available, cheap and repeatable method with which to image the neonatal brain. Some training is required in order to be able to interpret ultrasound images correctly. The commonest errors occur in the misinterpretation of normal echoreflectant areas in the parieto-occipital cortex (the peritrigonal 'blush') as mild periventricular leukomalacia, and in overdiagnosis of germinal matrix haemorrhage because the choroid plexus is bulky and extends far anteriorly into the caudothalamic groove in preterm infants. Several atlases exist.[27,58] Chapter 47 gives examples of normal ultrasound images, and Table 44.16c in Chapter 44, Part 5 lists common abnormalities. Repeated imaging gives the best prognostic information. Abnormalities which persist are more likely to be genuine, and most conditions evolve over time in a characteristic way which makes the diagnosis more certain. A single poor-quality ultrasound image showing an indistinct bright patch in the parenchyma of the brain is not an indication for withdrawal of intensive care. The concept that cranial ultrasound can be used to 'pick the winners' from a cohort of preterm infants is misguided and wrong. However, used with caution, ultrasound can be a very useful prognostic tool, providing reassurance to a large number of parents and early warning of potential problems for an unfortunate few.

NORMAL CRANIAL ULTRASOUND IMAGE

A meta-analysis by Ng & Dear of the results of follow-up of 992 preterm babies with consistently normal cranial ultrasound scans revealed that 875 (88%) had a normal outcome.[49] The babies were studied in 10 centres throughout Europe, North America and Australia. Table 7.4 shows the numbers of infants and type of follow-up carried out and extends the observations of Ng & Dear with the results of more recent studies. The outcome of over 3500 preterm infants enrolled in 18 studies has now been reported: over 2000 of these infants had a normal

Table 7.4 Summary of reports containing information on outcome of preterm infants with normal cranial ultrasound scan

First author, year of publication, total cohort size	Year of cohort	No. with normal scan/no. seen	Gestation (weeks)	Birthweight (grams)	Follow-up details	Normal scan only			
						Normal outcome (*n*)	Normal outcome (% and 95% CI)	Major handicap (*n*)	Major handicap (% and 95% CI)
Palmer 1982,[50] not cohort study	1979–80	14/39	27–34	790–2500	12 months, Griffiths, 96% traced	14	93% (66–100)	0	0% (0–23)
Graziani 1985,[29] not cohort study	?	21/53	<33	<1501	20–30 months, Bayley, 100% traced	15	71% (48–89)	2	9% (1–30)
Catto-Smith[8] 1985, *n* = 56	1981	11/31	23–28	567–1378	24 months, Bayley, 95% traced	10	91% (59–100)	1	1% (0–41)
Kitchen 1985,[41] *n* = 227	1980–81	105/148	>23	<1500	24 months, Bayley, 95% traced	93	89% (82–95)	12	11% (5–17)
TeKolste 1985,[68] not cohort study	1980–81	43/72	<32	<1500	22 months, Bayley, 73% traced	29	67% (51–81)	5	12% (4–25)
Szymonowicz[67] 1986, *n* = 50	1982	16/32	24–32	430–1250	24 months, Bayley, 100% traced	16	100% (79–100)	0	0% (0–21)
Greisen 1986,[31] *n* = 121	?	57/114	30 ± 1.6 (SD)	<1500	24 months, Denver, clinical examination, 100%	51	90% (78–96)	5	9% (3–19)
Cooke 1987,[9] *n* = 798	1980–84	333/524		<1501	24–60 months, clinical examination, 100%	314	94% (91–96)	19	6% (3–9)
Fawer 1987,[20] 1991, *n* = 112	?	61/93	<34	1554 ± 384	18 months, Griffiths, 5 years, neurological examination, 82% traced	61	100% (94–100)	0	0% (0–6)
Graham 1987,[28] *n* = 200	?	64/156		<1501	18 months, Griffiths, 99% traced	61	95% (87–99)	3	5% (1–13)
Stewart 1987,[65] *n* = 485	1979–81	184/342	24–32	535–2500	12 months, Griffiths, 96% traced	166	90% (85–94)	8	4% (2–8)
Bozynski 1988,[6] *n* = 152	?	67/116	28.7	<1201	12–18 months, Milani, 66% traced	42	63% (50–74)	3	4% (1–12)
Tudehope 1989,[69] *n* = 218	1983–85	96/147	28	<1500	24 months, Griffiths, 99% traced	86	90% (82–95)	10	10% (5–18)
Fazzi 1992,[21] *n* = 203	?	53/148	24–36	<1501	1–3 years, clinical examination, Bayley, 83% seen	49	92% (82–98)	4	7% (2–18)
Weisglas-Kuperus 1992,[76] *n* = 114	1985–86	22/79	<36	<1500	90% seen at 3.5 years, neurological examination of Touwen	20	91% (71–99)	2	9% (1–29)
Van de Bor 1993,[72] *n* = 484	1983	234/304	<32	<1500	Questionnaire + examination, 100% follow-up	177	76% (70–81)	13	5% (3–9)
Pinto-Martin 1995,[56] *n* = 1105	1985–87	565/727		<2000	2 year clinical examination, 86% traced	531	94% (92–96)	0	0% (0–1)
Rennie 1997,[58] *n* = 658	1985–92	344/470	23–38	<1501	18 months, Bayley, 86% traced	303	88% (85–92)	41	12% (8–15)
Totals*		2290 with normal scan				2037	89% (88–90)	128	6% (5–7)

*NB The totals from the outcome columns and the total number of infants with the ultrasound appearance in column 2 do not add up in this or subsequent tables in this chapter. This is due to late deaths, and varying numbers of infants with minor handicaps who have not been included.

scan and of these 89% were normal at follow-up. Only 128 children with a normal scan had a major handicap (6%: 95% confidence intervals from 5 to 7). Not all the early researchers followed up an entire cohort.[29,50] In the research published since 1986, complete cohort studies have been usual. Studies in which there was only short-term follow-up or where follow-up was incomplete have been omitted from Table 7.4. Figure 7.1 shows the incidence of major handicap with 95% confidence intervals for each study.

The results of this 'meta-analysis' should be treated with caution as the original cohorts were not strictly comparable. In some of the handicapped cases the diagnosis was not cerebral palsy, but visual handicap or developmental delay. The numbers of infants in Table 7.4 do not add up because some died and some had minor handicaps which were not always reported.

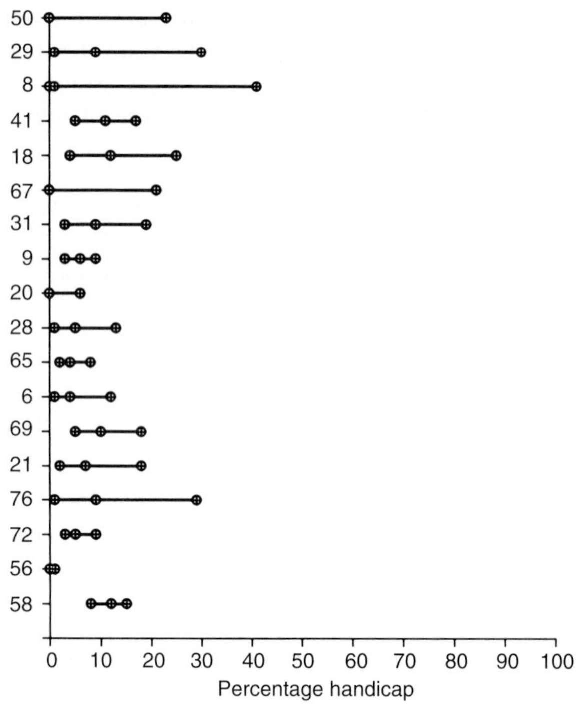

Fig. 7.1 Risk of major handicap shown as a percentage with bars representing 95% confidence intervals from Table 7.4. Reference no. on Y axis.

GERMINAL MATRIX HAEMORRHAGE (GMH)

There is general agreement that isolated germinal matrix haemorrhage which resolves is not associated with an increased risk of handicap (Table 7.5). Several studies report outcome of 'uncomplicated periventricular haemorrhage' where this is defined as increased echodensity within the lateral ventricle but without parenchymal echodensity or ventriculomegaly. Although there is a close correlation of CT/MRI and ultrasound with the findings at autopsy, it is not always possible to distinguish the germinal matrix bleeding from the intraventricular component in life. Several authorities[16,46] prefer to combine the two as a generic term GMH-IVH, and this is the term used in this book. The ultrasound finding of uncomplicated GMH-IVH is also associated with a good chance of normal outcome (Table 7.6). The recent large New Jersey study did suggest a small increased in risk of adverse outcome for GMH-IVH above the baseline risk.[56] Earlier work from Stanford also

Table 7.5 Summary of reports containing information on outcome of preterm infants with germinal matrix haemorrhage alone

First author, year of publication, cohort size	No. with GMH/ No. seen	Gestation (weeks)	Birthweight (grams)	Follow-up details	GMH alone (diagnosed with ultrasound)	
					Normal outcome (*n*)	Major handicap (*n*)
Palmer 1982,[50] not cohort study	12/39	27–34	790–2500	12 months, Griffiths, 96% traced	12	0
Catto-Smith 1985,[8] *n* = 56	14/31	23–28	567–1378	24 months, Bayley, 95% traced	12	2
Kitchen 1985,[41] *n* = 227	20/148	>23	500–1500	24 months, Bayley, 95% traced	17	3
TeKolste 1985,[68] not cohort study	14/72	<32	<1500	22 months, Bayley, 73% traced	12	6
Szymonowicz 1986,[67] *n* = 50	4/32	24–32	430–1250	24 months, Bayley, 100% traced	4	0
Cooke 1987,[9] *n* = 798	73/524		<1501	24–60 months, clinical examination, 100%	59	1
Tudehope 1989,[69] *n* = 218	31/162	28	<1500	24 months, Griffiths, 99% traced	31	0
Totals	168 with GMH				147 (88%; 95% CI 82–92)	12 (7%; 95% CI 4–12)

Table 7.6 Summary of reports containing information on outcome of preterm infants with uncomplicated GMH-IVH

First author, year of publication, total cohort size	No. with finding/ No. seen	Gestation (weeks)	Birthweight (grams)	Follow-up details	Uncomplicated GMH-IVH			
					Normal outcome (*n*)	Normal outcome (% and 95% CI)	Major handicap (*n*)	Major handicap (% and 95% CI)
Palmer 1982,[50] not cohort study	14/39	27–34	790–2500	12 months, Griffiths, 96% traced	14	100% (77–100)	0	0% (0–23)
Catto-Smith 1985,[8] *n* = 56	17/31	<28	567–1378	24 months, Bayley, 95% traced	9	53% (28–77)	8	47% (23–72)
TeKolste 1985,[68] not cohort study	27/72	<32	<1500	22 months, Bayley, 73% traced	16	59% (39–78)	8	30% (14–50)
Graziani 1985,[29] not cohort study	22/53	<33	<1501	20–30 months, Bayley, 100% traced	16	73% (50–89)	3	14% (3–35)
Greisen 1986,[31] *n* = 121	26/114	30 ± 1.6 (SD)	<1500	24 months, Denver, clinical examination, 100%	25	96% (80–100)	1	4% (0–20)
Stewart 1987,[65] *n* = 485	101/342	24–32	535–2500	12 months, Griffiths, 96% traced	97	96% (90–99)	4	4% (1–10)
Graham 1987,[28] *n* = 200	74/156		<1501	18 months, Griffiths, 99% traced	74	100% (95–100)	0	0% (0–5)
Tudehope 1989,[69] *n* = 218	38/162	28	<1500	24 months, Griffiths, 99% traced	26	68% (51–82)	2	5% (1–18)
Kitchen 1990,[42] *n* = 227	33/139	>23	500–1500	24 months, Bayley, 95% traced	31	94% (80–99)	2	6% (1–20)
Bozynski 1990,[7] *n* = 155	12/51	AGA	<1251	50% seen, Dubowitz neurological examination	5	42% (15–72)	6	50% (21–79)
Fawer 1991,[19] *n* = 112	17/93	<34	1554 ± 384	5 years, Touwen neurological examination, 82% traced	17	100% (80–100)	0	0% (0–20)
Weisglas-Kuperus 1992,[76] *n* = 114	20/79	<36	<1500	90% seen at 3.5 years, neurological examination of Touwen	19	95% (75–100)	1	5% (0–25)
Fazzi 1992,[21] *n* = 203	26/148	24–36	<1501	1–3 years clinical examination, Bayley, 83% seen	23	88% (70–98)	3	11% (2–30)
Van de Bor 1993,[72] *n* = 484	50/304	<32	<1500	Questionnaire + examination, 100% follow-up	45	90% (78–97)	5	10% (3–22)
Pinto-Martin 1995,[56] *n* = 1105	149/727		<2000	2 years, clinical examination 86% traced	102	69% (61–76)	37	25% (18–32)
Totals	626 cases				519	83% (80–86)	80	13% (10–15)

suggested that there was some increase in risk, with 7/26 surviving ELBW infants having a major handicap.[60] Early studies such as this report no detected PVL and this may account for the disparity in outcome compared to more recent work. Subependymal pseudocysts appear like strings of beads which lie along the floor of the lateral ventricle.[58] They are a congenital lesion which can be associated with other congenital abnormalities but which have a good prognosis.[57] Subependymal pseudocyts should not be confused with the cysts left behind after resolving GMH (see Table 44.16c, p. 1253).

ENLARGED CEREBRAL VENTRICLES

Enlargement of the lateral ventricles, often defined as a ventricular index above the 97th centile of Levene,[44] is a frequent finding in preterm neonates, particularly those with GMH-IVH. Enlargement can be rapidly progressive and due to post-haemorrhagic hydrocephalus with raised intracranial pressure, or non-progressive and largely due to atrophy. Both conditions can coexist. Definitions of ultrasound scan appearances of ventricular enlargement vary, inhibiting a composite analysis of the outcome studies. The large New Jersey study did not use any explicit criteria, classifying the ultrasound scan prior to discharge as showing ventricular enlargement if one ventricle had moderate enlargement.[78] The Ventriculomegaly Trial Group[73,74] classified ventriculomegaly as present if the ventricular index of the smallest ventricle was 4 mm above the 97th centile of Levene. The old Papile classification defined a grade II haemorrhage as bleeding into the ventricular space but not distending it, and a grade III as bleeding which did.[52] This system described the appearances of a single CT scan; using serial ultrasound imaging it is clear that the presence of even a small amount of blood within the ventricle causes enlargement in the vast majority of cases. It is true to say that a large GMH-IVH which forms a cast of the ventricles at the start is invariably followed by ventriculomegaly, usually progressive, and that all the original Papile grade III cases also developed hydrocephalus. The availability of serial ultrasound imaging has made the Papile classification less useful. Uncomplicated GMH-IVH, nearest to the old Papile Grade II, is now used to mean a GMH-IVH which resolves completely, without any degree of ventricular enlargement although there may be some haemosiderin on the inner ventricular wall or a germinal layer cyst. Complicated GMH-IVH means GMH-IVH associated with any degree of ventricular enlargement. See Chapter 44, Part 5 for more information on current classification of GMH-IVH.

Outcome studies do not always make clear the important distinction between ventricular dilatation due to cerebral atrophy and progressive hydrocephalus as a consequence of raised cerebrospinal fluid pressure. Cerebral atrophy is associated with an irregularly shaped (scalloped) ventricle and there may be evidence of loss of white matter in the parenchyma. The cerebral sulci abut directly onto the ventricular cavity instead of onto the periventricular white matter. These changes are easily seen with MR imaging, which can also demonstrate abnormal signal on T2-weighted scans indicative of a previous glial reaction. Head growth is normal or reduced, the fontanelle is lax and there are no symptoms of raised intracranial pressure. Six-year follow-up of the New Jersey cohort has shown an excess of mental retardation in the group with any ventriculomegaly or parenchymal lesions.[79] Half the cases of mental retardation in this cohort (birthweight less than 2 kg) could be accounted for by either form of white matter loss.

POSTHAEMORRHAGIC VENTRICULAR DILATATION PROGRESSING TO HYDROCEPHALUS

Progressive hydrocephalus tends to begin with trigonal enlargement and is associated with increased occipitofrontal circumference and split skull sutures. The cerebrospinal fluid pressure is raised, usually above 10 cm water, and there may be symptoms such as apnoea or vomiting. Pressure alone cannot be used to predict progression as some cases who eventually require surgical drainage have low pressure,[39] but there is a tendency for progressive hydrocephalus to be associated with a cerebrospinal fluid pressure above the upper limit of normal; about 7.8 cm cerebrospinal fluid (6 mmHg or 0.8 kPa). Persisting ventricular enlargement on ultrasound scan in cases of shunted hydrocephalus is usually indicative of some white matter loss in the periventricular region, and it is this loss of cerebral tissue which has the most adverse effect on prognosis. After shunting for hydrocephalus the cerebral mantle can reconstitute quite remarkably, and some of these children do very well.

The ventriculomegaly trial gave very useful follow up-information.[73,74] Babies who were enrolled into this study had ventricular widths 4 mm above the 97th centile of Levene. Only 11 of 112 were normal at 2 years. Table 7.7 summarizes the outcome for infants with ventriculomegaly who did not have associated parenchymal lesions, and Table 7.8 the outcome for those with shunted hydrocephalus. Cooke[10] and the Ventriculomegaly Trial Group[73,74] found that the outcome was worse for infants with fits or parenchymal echodensities. Shankaran et al[62] have pointed out the high revision rate of shunts in preterm infants; in their series, 18 children had 82 revisions between them and this worsened the prognosis.

PERIVENTRICULAR LEUKOMALACIA

There is no doubt that cystic periventricular leukomalacia is the most powerful predictor of cerebral palsy amongst the neonatal cranial ultrasound lesions so far described. In many cohort follow-up studies almost all the cases of cerebral palsy had bilateral occipital leukomalacia in the neonatal period.[28,53] Cysts involving more than one zone also have a poor prognosis.[63] The cysts of periventricular leukomalacia are transient, and eventually collapse leaving an irregular ventricular margin as described earlier. Older studies reporting an association between ventricular dilatation (and occasionally subependymal haemorrhage) and adverse outcome almost certainly included some undiagnosed cases of periventricular leukomalacia owing to poor resolution of 5 MHz scanheads.

Single cysts and cysts confined to the frontal region appear to have a better outcome than multiple bilateral occipital cysts, where the outlook is universally dismal. Too few studies have reported the outcome of anterior or central cysts to make it possible to give a confident prediction of a good outcome, although most of the reported survivors with single, small unilateral cysts or cysts confined to the frontal zone are normal at follow-up.[19,21,28,63] Some describe a good outcome in a subgroup of infants with frontal cysts present in the first week of life, although the example scans are more typical of subependymal pseudocysts (see above) on the floor of the frontal horn of the lateral ventricle.[40,66]

Table 7.7 Summary of reports containing information on outcome of infants with isolated, non-progressive ventriculomegaly alone

First author, year of publication, cohort size	No. with finding/ No. seen	Gestation (weeks)	Birthweight (grams)	Follow-up details	Isolated ventriculomegaly	
					Normal outcome (*n*)	Major handicap (*n*)
Palmer 1982,[50] not cohort study	9/39	27–34	790–2500	12 months, Griffiths, 96% traced	1	5
Allan 1984,[1] *n* = 268	14/268	<35		All traced, Denver	12	2
Graziani 1985,[29] n not given	6/53	<33	<1501	20–30 months, Bayley, 100% traced	6	0
Greisen 1986,[31] *n* = 121	21/114	30 ± 1.6 (SD)	<1500	24 months, Denver, clinical examination, 100%	15	6
Stewart 1987,[65] *n* = 485	41/342	24–32	535–2500	12 months, Griffiths, 96% traced	30	11
Cooke 1987,[9] *n* = 798	40/524		<1501	24–60 months, clinical examination, 100%	32	8
Shankaran 1989,[62] *n* = 111	10/111	<35	<1500	12–30 months, Bayley, all seen	7	3
Kitchen 1990,[42] *n* = 227	2/148	>23	500–1500	24 months, Bayley, 95% traced	1	1
Weisglas-Kuperus 1992,[76] *n* = 114	30/79	<36	<1500	90% seen at 3.5 years, Touwen examination	16	14
Ventriculomegaly trial 1994[74]	53	28 ± 3	<1500	Only 4 cases lost, 30 months, Griffiths	6	26
Totals	226 cases				128 (57%; 95% CI 50–63)	76 (34%; 95% CI 28–40)

Table 7.8 Summary of reports containing information on outcome of infants with shunted hydrocephalus

First author, year of publication	No. of cases	Gestation (weeks)	Birthweight (grams)	Follow-up details	Shunted hydrocephalus	
					Normal outcome (*n*)	Major handicap (*n*)
Palmer 1982[50]	1	27–34	790–2500	12 months, Griffiths	1	0
Leichty 1983[43]	9	34 ± 4.1	2100 ± 1090	12 months, Bayley	8	5
Allan 1984[1]	3	<35		Denver	0	3
Boynton 1986[5]	50	30 ± 2	1266 ± 303	Bayley	7	26
Cooke 1987[10]	54		<2500	24–60 months, clinical examination	13	37
Etches 1987[17]	29	25–37	<2000	18 months, Bayley	5	11
Hislop 1988[35]	19	25–39	<2740	Variable	4	12
Shankaran 1989[62]	23	<35	<1500	12–30 months, Bayley	8	11
Fazzi 1992[21]	6	24–36	<1501	1–3 years, clinical examination	3	3
Fernell 1990[24]	42	<34	<2500	Variable	7	32
Totals	236				56 24% (18–30)	140 59% (53–65)

There is little information about the ultrasound appearance of transient echodensity in the periventricular zone which does not progress to cystic change. Several groups have suggested that this appearance might indicate a minor degree of damage to the pre-myelin cells and have shown an increased incidence of neurological signs and/or clumsiness in later childhood.[2,13,14,38,47] Bennett et al[3] report Bayley scores at 12–24 months for 24 children who had ultrasound evidence of echodensity which did not progress to cysts: 12 were normal, 6 had minor abnormalities, and 4 had major abnormalities; 6/9 control children were classified as normal in this study. Caution is required when interpreting scans thought to show transient echodensity (see p. 1265), and Bennett et

Table 7.9 Cases of bilateral cystic periventricular leukomalacia and their outcome

Author, year	Cohort size, details	No. of cases	No. with cerebral palsy (CP)
Weindling 1985[75]	124, <1500 g or <34 weeks	8	8
De Vries 1987[12]	676, <34 weeks	12	4 died; 6 CP; 2 <9 months
Graham 1987[28]	*n* = 200, <1500 g	8	8
Fawer 1987[20]	*n* = 112, <1500 g	5	5
Cooke 1987[9]	*n* = 798, <1500 g	24	21
Monset-Couchard 1988[48]	*n* = 471, <1500 g	6	6
Hansen 1989[34]	*n* ≅ 1600, mostly <1500 g	16	16
Pidcock 1990[53]	*n* = 288	20	18
Weisglas-Kuperus 1992[76]	*n* = 79, <1500 g	2	1
Pierrat 1993[54]	Not given; 33 cases in 2 years	9	1 died; 8 CP
Fazzi 1994[22]	*n* = 299, <32 weeks	14	14
Rogers 1994[51]	*n* = 1239, <33 weeks	31	26 of 26 survivors
Total	>5600	155	137

al[3] underline this caution, pointing out that 81% of their study population were described as having periventricular echodense areas on at least one scan.

Table 7.9 summarizes the outcome for cases of bilateral cystic periventricular leukomalacia: 93% of the survivors are seriously handicapped. The predominant diagnosis at follow-up was cerebral palsy, either spastic quadriplegia or diplegia. Developmental delay was less often observed. Some large studies have been excluded because it was not possible to distinguish the outcome for different types of periventricular leukomalacia,[64] no late scan appearances were included[78] or because several conditions were lumped together.[7,31,56] Thirty-one of 45 cases from a cohort of 497 with cystic periventricular leukomalacia where the cysts were greater than 3 mm in size developed cerebral palsy but the location of the cysts was not further defined.[30] All the survivors with cysts greater than 2 cm developed cerebral palsy in a large series from Buffalo, New York.[59] These workers measured the extent of the cystic lesions in the newborn period, and if the anterioposterior extent was more than 2 cm in the parasagittal plane the outlook was particularly poor, with spastic quadriplegia developing in all eight cases.

There is overlap of cases in some series and where this occurs only the latest report is included in the table.[11,12,28,63] Fortunately periventricular leukomalacia of this severity is rare, occurring in only 2–4% of VLBW infants (p. 1264). The challenge for the next decade is to understand the factors which render the developing oligodendroglia vulnerable to injury in order to reduce this devastating complication of prematurity. White matter damage may be even more common than is suspected in preterm infants. 27 of 31 survivors (from a cohort of 51 VLBW infants) underwent MRI at a year, and abnormal myelination was found in 20 children.[23] Antenatal white matter damage was demonstrated with careful neuropathological examination in 20% of a series of perinatal autopsies.[25] There is an association with intrauterine growth retardation,[25,64] prolonged rupture of membranes and chorioamnionitis (p. 1263).

PORENCEPHALIC CYST SECONDARY TO PARENCHYMAL HAEMORRHAGE

The earlier literature reporting outcome of grade IV periventricular haemorrhage must now be reinterpreted, separating cases of periventricular leukomalacia involving extensive loss of myelin from those with single porencephalic cysts. Volpe's group were amongst the first to realize that all parenchymal lesions were not the same, although their classification did not illuminate the problem at the time.[33] Unilateral parenchymal echodensities which evolve into isolated single porencephalic cysts can be associated with no neurological signs at all.[3,4,11,42] These children are rare, but sufficiently frequently reported to make the outcome of porencephaly much less certain that that of periventricular leukomalacia. Complex pathology is a further confounder; there were only three survivors with porencephalic cysts from a cohort of 200 in Graham's study and all of them were handicapped, but they all had accompanying periventricular leukomalacia.[28] The wide spectrum of pathology which can result from a parenchymal echodensity seen in the first week of life makes it impossible to predict the degree of handicap with any accuracy at present.

CONCLUSION

GMH-IVH, unless followed by ventricular enlargement, has a good prognosis. Babies whose cranial ultrasound scan shows enlarged ventricles due to white matter loss have an intermediate prognosis. Shunted hydrocephalus in preterm children has a poor prognosis on the whole, although there are notable exceptions. Intraparenchymal brain lesions appearing early as echodense areas due to haemorrhage, venous infarction or oedema may disappear or evolve into single or multiple cysts. The prognosis depends on the type and extent of injury to white matter, and is particularly poor for extensive bilateral occipital cysts, or for areas of cystic periventricular leukomalacia contiguous for more than 2 cm. The information contained in the summary tables is presented in Figure 7.2.

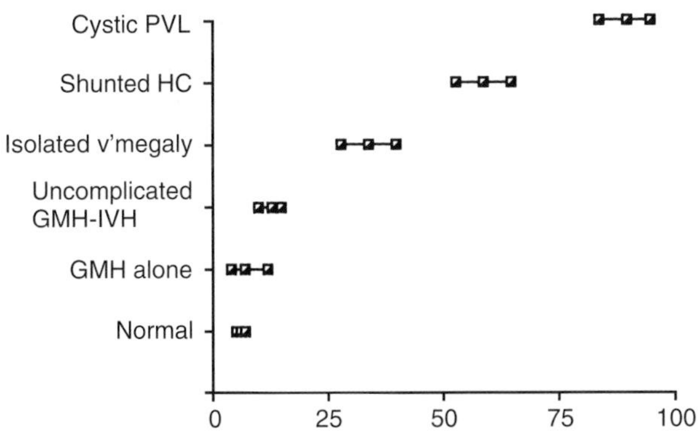

Fig. 7.2 Chance of major handicap after different cranial ultrasound diagnoses made in the neonatal period. Shown as percentage with 95% confidence intervals; data from the summary tables in this chapter.

LESIONS WHICH PREDICT DISABILITY

Cysts in the parenchyma and cerebral atrophy indicate loss of white matter and are the strongest predictors yet found for cerebral palsy.[51,56,59] Delayed myelination has been confirmed with later MRI studies, suggesting that the cysts are markers of even more diffuse injury to oligodendroglia.[14,23,32,70,71] Most studies are in remarkable agreement, showing a fivefold increase in the risk of cerebral palsy following ultrasound diagnosis of any parenchymal lesion, and a 15-fold increase in the presence of bilateral occipital periventricular leukomalacia.

Prediction of learning difficulties, which in some cases may be due to lesser degrees of white matter damage, is still imprecise.[47] Visual handicap can be accurately predicted from ultrasound abnormalities.[15,36,55,61,77]

White matter damage carries a high probability of cerebral palsy but by no means all cases in VLBW survivors have early ultrasound abnormalities. All but 7 of 45 children so afflicted had periventricular cysts or echodensity.[30] A normal scan is not therefore a guarantee of a normal outcome, although the chances are about 90%.[49]

REFERENCES

1. Allan W C, Dransfield D A, Tito A M 1984 Ventricular dilatation following periventricular–intraventricular hemorrhage: outcome at age 1 year. Pediatrics 73: 158–162
2. Appleton R E, Lee R E J, Hey E N 1990 Neurodevelopmental outcome of transient neonatal intracerebral echodensities. Archives of Disease in Childhood 69: 27–29
3. Bennett F C, Silver G, Leung E J, Mack L A 1990 Periventricular echodensities detected by cranial ultrasonography: usefulness in predicting neurodevelopmental outcome in low birthweight, preterm infants. Pediatrics 85: 400–404
4. Blackman J A, McGuiness G A, Bale J F, Smith W L 1991 Large postnatally acquired porencephalic cysts: unexpected developmental outcomes. Journal of Child Neurology 6: 58–64
5. Boynton B R, Boynton C A, Merritt T A, Vaucher Y E James H E, Bejar R F 1986 Ventriculoperitoneal shunts in low birthweight infants with intracranial hemorrhage: neurodevelopmental outcome. Neurosurgery 18: 141–145
6. Bozynski M E A, Nelson M N, Genaze D U et al 1988 Cranial ultrasonography and the prediction of cerebral palsy in infants weighing <1200 grams at birth. Developmental Medicine and Child Neurology 30: 342–348
7. Bozynski M E A, DiPietro M A, Meisels S J, Plunkett J W, Burpee B, Claflin C J 1990 Cranial sonography and neurological examination of extremely preterm infants. Developmental Medicine and Child Neurology 32: 575–581
8. Catto-Smith A G, Yu V Y H, Bajuk B, Orgill A A, Astbury J 1985 Effect of neonatal periventricular haemorrhage on neurodevelopmental outcome. Archives of Disease in Childhood 60: 8–11
9. Cooke R W I 1987 Early and late cranial ultrasonographic appearances and outcome in very low birthweight infants. Archives of Disease in Childhood 62: 931–937
10. Cooke R W I 1987 Determinants of major handicap in post haemorrhagic hydrocephalus. Archives of Disease in Childhood 62: 504–507
11. De Vries L S, Dubowitz L M S, Dubowitz V et al 1985 Predictive value of cranial ultrasound in the newborn baby: a reappraisal. Lancet ii: 137–140
12. De Vries L S, Connell J A, Dubowitz L M S, Oozeer R C, Dubowitz V 1987 Neurological, electrophysiological and MRI abnormalities in infants with extensive cystic leukomalacia. Neuropediatrics 18: 61–66
13. De Vries L S, Regev R, Pennock J M, Wigglesworth J S, Dubowitz L M S 1988 Ultrasound evolution and later outcome of infants with periventricular densities. Early Human Development 16: 225–233
14. De Vries L M S, Eken P, Groenendaal F, Van Haastert I C, Meiners L C 1993 Correlation between the degree of periventricular leukomalacia diagnosed using cranial ultrasound and MRI later in infancy in children with cerebral palsy. Neuropaediatrics 24: 263–268
15. Eken P, van Niuwenhuizen O, van der Graaf Y, Schalij-Delfos N E, de Vries L S 1994 Relation between neonatal cerebral ultrasound abnormalities and cerebral visual impairment. Developmental Medicine and Child Neurology 36: 3–15
16. Enzmann D R 1997 Imaging of neonatal hypoxic–ischaemic cerebral damage. In: Stevenson D K, Sunshine P (eds) Fetal and neonatal brain injury. Oxford Medical Publications, Oxford, ch 20, pp 302–355
17. Etches P C, Ward T F, Bhui P S, Peters K L, Robertson C M 1987 Outcome of shunted posthemorrhagic hydrocephalus in premature infants. Pediatric Neurology 3: 136–140
18. Farmer S F, Harrison L M 1991 Plasticity of central motor pathways in children with hemiplegic cerebral palsy. Neurology 41: 1505–1510
19. Fawer C-L, Calame A 1991 Significance of ultrasound appearances in the neurological development and cognitive abilities of preterm infants at 5 years. European Journal of Pediatrics 150: 515–520
20. Fawer C-L, Diebold P, Calame A 1987 Periventricular leucomalacia and neurodevelopmental outcome in preterm infants. Archives of Disease in Childhood 62: 30–36
21. Fazzi E, Lanzi G, Gerardo A, Ometto A, Orcesi S, Rondini G 1992 Neurodevelopmental outcome in very low birthweight infants with or without periventricular haemorrhage and/or leucomalacia. Acta Paediatrica Scandinavica 81: 808–811
22. Fazzi E, Orcesi S, Caffi L et al 1994 Neurodevelopmental outcome at 5–7 years in preterm infants with periventricular leukomalacia. Neuropediatrics 25: 134–139
23. Feldman H M, Scher M S, Kemp S S 1990 Neurodevelopmental outcome of children with evidence of periventricular leukomalacia on late MRI. Pediatric Neurology 6: 296–302
24. Fernell E, Hagberg G, Hagberg B 1990 Infantile hydrocephalus – the impact of enhanced preterm survival. Acta Paediatrica Scandinavica 79: 1080–1086
25. Gaffney G, Squier M V, Johnson A, Flavell V, Sellers S 1994 Clinical associations of prenatal ischaemic white matter injury. Archives of Disease in Childhood 70: F101–F106
26. Gluckman P D 1993 When and why do brain cells die? Developmental Medicine and Child Neurology 34: 1010–1021
27. Govaert P, de Vries L S 1997 An atlas of neonatal brain sonography. Clinics in Developmental Medicine No 141–142. MacKeith Press, London
28. Graham M, Levene M I, Trounce J Q, Rutter N 1987 Prediction of cerebral palsy in very low birthweight infants. Lancet ii: 593–596
29. Graziani L J, Pasto M, Stanley C et al 1985 Cranial ultrasound and clinical studies in preterm infants. Journal of Pediatrics 106: 269–276
30. Graziani L J, Mitchell D G, Kornhauser M et al 1992

Neurodevelopment of preterm infants: neonatal neurosonographic and serum bilirubin studies. Pediatrics 89: 229–234
31. Greisen G, Petersen M B, Pedersen S A, Baekgaard P 1986 Status at two years in 121 very low birthweight survivors related to neonatal intraventricular haemorrhage and mode of delivery. Acta Paediatrica Scandinavica 75: 24–30
32. Guit G L, Van De Bor M, Den Ouden L, Wondergem J H M 1990 Prediction of neurodevelopmental outcome in the preterm infant: MR staged myelination compared with cranial ultrasound. Pediatric Radiology 175: 107–109
33. Guzzetta F, Shackleford G D, Volpe S, Perlman J M, Volpe J J 1986 Periventricular intraparenchymal echodensities in the premature newborn: critical determinant of neurologic outcome. Pediatrics 78: 995–1006
34. Hansen N B, Kopechek J, Miller R R, Menke J A, Cordero L 1989 Prognostic significance of cystic intracranial lesions in neonates. Developmental and Behavioral Pediatrics 10: 129–133
35. Hislop J, Dubowitz L M S, Kaiser A, Singh M P, Whitelaw A 1988 Outcome of infants shunted for posthaemorrhagic ventricular dilatation. Developmental Medicine and Child Neurology 30: 451–456
36. Hungerford J, Stewart A, Hope P 1986 Ocular sequelae of preterm birth and their relation to ultrasound evidence of cerebral damage. British Journal of Ophthalmology 70: 463–468
37. Janowsky J S 1986 Outcome of perinatal brain damage. Developmental Medicine and Child Neurology 28: 375–389
38. Jongmans M, Henderson S, De Vries L S, Dubowitz L M S 1993 Duration of periventricular densities in preterm infants and neurological outcome at 6 years of age. Archives of Disease in Childhood 69: 9–13
39. Kaiser A, Whitelaw A 1985 Cerebrospinal fluid pressure during posthaemorrhagic ventriculomegaly in newborn infants. Archives of Disease in Childhood 60: 920–924
40. Keller M S, DiPietro M A, Teele R A 1987 Periventricular cavitations in the first week of life. American Journal of Neuroradiology 8: 291–295
41. Kitchen W H, Ford G W, Murton L J et al 1985 Mortality and two-year outcome of infants of birthweight 500–1500 g: relationship with neonatal cerebral ultrasound data. Australian Paediatric Journal 21: 253–259
42. Kitchen W H, Ford G W, Rickards A L, Doyle L W, Kelly E, Murton L J 1990 Five-year outcome of infants of birthweight 500–1500 grams: relationship with neonatal ultrasound data. American Journal of Perinatology 7: 60–65
43. Leichty E A, Gilmor R L, Bryson C Q, Bull M J 1983 Outcome of high-risk neonates with ventriculomegaly. Developmental Medicine and Child Neurology 25: 162–168
44. Levene M I 1981 Measurement of the growth of the lateral ventricles in preterm infants with real time ultrasound. Archives of Disease in Childhood 56: 900–940
45. Levene M I 1990 Cerebral ultrasound and neurological impairment: telling the future. Archives of Disease in Childhood 65: 469–471
46. Levene M I, de Vries L S 1995 Neonatal intracranial haemorrhage. In: Levene M I, Lilford R J (eds) Fetal and neonatal neurology and neurosurgery. Churchill Livingstone, Edinburgh, ch 21, pp 335–366
47. Levene M I, Dowling S, Graham M, Fogelman K, Galton M, Phillips M 1992 Impaired motor function (clumsiness) in five year old children: correlation with neonatal ultrasound scan. Archives of Disease in Childhood 67: 687–690
48. Monset-Couchard M, de Bethemann O, Radvanyi-Bouvet M-F, Papin C, Bordarier C, Relier J P 1988 Neurodevelopmental outcome in cystic periventricular leukomalacia : 30 cases. Neuropediatrics 19: 124–131
49. Ng P C, Dear P R F 1990 The predictive value of a normal ultrasound scan in the preterm baby – a meta-analysis. Acta Paediatrica Scandinavica 79: 286–291
50. Palmer P, Dubowitz L M S, Levene M I, Dubowitz V 1982 Developmental and neurological progress of preterm infants with intraventricular haemorrhage and ventricular dilatation. Archives of Disease in Childhood 57: 748–753
51. Paneth N, Rudelli R, Kazam E, Monte W 1994 Brain damage in the preterm infant. Clinics in Developmental Medicine No 131. MacKeith Press, London
52. Papile L-A, Burstein J, Burstein R, Koffler H 1978 Incidence and evolution of subependymal and intraventricular hemorrhage: a study of infants with birthweight <1500 g. Journal of Pediatrics 92: 529–534
53. Pidcock F S, Graziani L J, Stanley C, Mitchell D G, Merton D 1990 Neurosonographic features of periventricular echodensities associated with cerebral palsy in preterm infants. Journal of Pediatrics 116: 417–422
54. Pierrat V, Eken P, Duquennoy C, Rousseau S, De Vries L S 1993 Prognostic value of early somatosensory evoked potentials in neonates with cystic leukomalacia. Developmental Medicine and Child Neurology 35: 683–690
55. Pike M G, Holmstrom G, de Vries L S et al 1994 Patterns of visual impairment associated with lesions of the preterm infant brain. Developmental Medicine and Child Neurology 36: 849–862
56. Pinto-Martin J A, Riolo S, Cnaan A, Holzman C, Susser M, Paneth N 1995 Cranial ultrasound prediction of disabling and nondisabling cerebral palsy at age two in a low birthweight population. Pediatrics 95: 249–254
57. Rademaker K J, De Vries L S, Barth P G 1993 Subependymal pseudocysts: ultrasound diagnosis and findings at follow up. Acta Paediatrica Scandinavica 82: 394–399
58. Rennie J M 1997 Neonatal cerebral ultrasound. Cambridge University Press, Cambridge
59. Rogers B, Msall M, Owens T et al 1994 Cystic periventricular leukomalacia and type of cerebral palsy in preterm infants. Journal of Pediatrics 125: S1–S8
60. Salomon W L, Benitz W E, Enzmann D R, Bravo R H, Murphy-Irwin K, Stevenson D K 1987 Correlation of echoencephalographic findings and neurodevelopmental outcome: intracranial haemorrhage and ventriculomegaly in infants of birthweight 1,000 grams or less. Journal of Clinical Monitoring 3: 178–186
61. Scher M S, Dobson V, Carpenter N A, Guthrie R D 1989 Visual and neurological outcome of infants with periventricular leukomalacia. Developmental Medicine and Child Neurology 31: 353–365
62. Shankaran S, Keopke T, Woldt E et al 1989 Outcome after posthemorrhagic ventriculomegaly in comparison with mild hemorrhage without ventriculomegaly. Journal of Pediatrics 114: 109–114
63. Shortland D, Levene M I, Trounce J Q, Ng Y, Graham M 1988 The evolution and outcome of cavitating periventricular leukomalacia in infancy. A study of 46 cases. Journal of Perinatal Medicine 16: 241–247
64. Sinha S K, D'Souza S W, Rivlin E, Chiswick M L 1990 Ischaemic brain lesions diagnosed at birth in preterm infants: clinical events and developmental outcome. Archives of Disease in Childhood 65: 1017–1020
65. Stewart A L, Reynolds E O R, Hope P L et al 1987 Probability of neurodevelopmental disorders estimated from the ultrasound appearance of brains of very preterm infants. Developmental Medicine and Child Neurology 29: 3–11
66. Sudakoff G S, Mitchell D G, Stanley C, Graziani L J 1991 Frontal periventricular cavitations on the first day of life. Journal of Ultrasound Medicine 10: 25–30
67. Szymonowicz W, Yu V Y H, Bajuk B, Astbury J 1986 Neurodevelopmental outcome of periventricular haemorrhage and leukomalacia in infants 1250 g or less at birth. Early Human Development 14: 1–7
68. TeKolste K A, Bennett F C, Mack L A 1985 Follow up of infants receiving cranial ultrasound for intracranial hemorrhage. American Journal of Disease of Children 139: 299–303
69. Tudehope D I, Masel J, Mohay H et al 1989 Neonatal cranial ultrasonography as predictor of 2 year outcome of very low birthweight infants. Australian Paediatric Journal 25: 66–71
70. Van de Bor M, Guit G L, Schreuder A M, Wondergem J, Vielvoye G J 1989 Early detection of delayed myelination in preterm infants. Pediatrics 84: 407–411
71. Van de Bor M, den Ouden L, Guit G L 1992 Value of cranial ultrasound and magnetic resonance imaging in predicting neurodevelopmental outcome in preterm infants. Pediatrics 90: 196–199
72. Van de Bor M, Ens-Dokkum M, Schreuder A M, Veen S, Brand R, Veerlove-Vanhorick S P 1993 Outcome of periventricular–intraventricular haemorrhage at five years of age. Developmental Medicine and Child Neurology 35: 33–41
73. Ventriculomegaly Trial Group 1990 Randomised trial of early tapping in neonatal posthaemorrhagic ventricular dilatation. Archives of Disease in Childhood 65: 3–10
74. Ventriculomegaly Trial Group 1994 Randomised trial of early tapping in neonatal posthaemorrhagic ventricular dilatation: results at 30 months. Archives of Disease in Childhood 70: F129–F136
75. Weindling A M, Rochefort M J, Calvert S A, Fok T-F, Wilkinson A

1985 Development of cerebral palsy after ultrasonographic detection of periventricular cysts in the newborn. Developmental Medicine and Child Neurology 27: 800–806

76. Weisglas-Kuperus N, Baerts W, Fetter W P F, Sauer P J J 1992 Neonatal cerebral ultrasound, neonatal neurology and perinatal conditions as predictors of neurodevelopmental outcome in very low birthweight infants. Early Human Development 31: 131–148
77. Weisglas-Kuperus N, Heersema D J, Baerts W et al 1993 Visual functions in relation with neonatal cerebral ultrasound, neurology and cognitive development in very low birthweight children. Neuropaediatrics 24: 149–154
78. Whitaker A, Johnson J, Sebris S et al 1990 Neonatal cranial ultrasound abnormalities: association with developmental delay at age one in low birthweight infants. Developmental and Behavioural Pediatrics 11: 253–260
79. Whitaker A H, Feldman J F, Van Rossem R et al 1996 Neonatal cranial ultrasound abnormalities in low birthweight infants: relation to cognitive outcomes at six years of age. Pediatrics 98: 719–729
80. Wigglesworth J S 1989 Plasticity of the developing brain. In: Pape K E, Wigglesworth J S (eds) Perinatal brain lesions. Blackwell Scientific Publications, Cambridge, Massachusetts, pp 253–269

8

Specific problems in developing countries

Michael C. K. Chan

There are vast rural areas in the tropics where obstetric services are poorly developed or lacking. Women in these areas tend to be malnourished and during pregnancy continue to do hard manual work. Many babies are born to teenage mothers or to grand multiparae and are exposed to all the risks of pregnancy attendant on short birth intervals. Tens of millions of pregnant women are exposed to malaria, which is life-threatening to mother and baby and which contributes substantially to low birthweight. At parturition, mothers have to rely on attendants who lack facilities for simple resuscitation of asphyxiated babies or sterile handling of the umbilical cord and who may employ traditional practices that are injurious to the health of mother and baby.

In urban areas in developing countries, large numbers and many complicated deliveries associated with inadequate antenatal supervision create such pressure of work in the labour ward that little attention is given to the baby after birth. Often the mother's stay in the maternity hospital is measured in hours rather than days and discharge from the hospital ends her contact with the service until her next delivery. Neonates in need of special care interfere with this 'delivery'-oriented service and are given low priority for medical care and attention.

This unsatisfactory state of affairs has continued to deteriorate in the 1980s and the first half of the 1990s. The 1980s witnessed the biggest failure of development as developing countries were thrown into financial crisis through rising interest rates and falling commodity prices. The accumulation of massive national debts owed to industrialized countries led the International Monetary Fund and World Bank to introduce structural adjustment programmes into developing countries to improve economic growth and help poor people. Key features of these SAP were a reduction of government spending, currency devaluation and increasing local access for foreign and transnational corporations. Structural adjustment programmes have harmed health systems of sub-Saharan African countries, in particular. Their mothers and children have suffered poor dietary intake due to a fall in subsistence farming in favour of cash crops to boost exports.[24,26] In Zimbabwe investment in public health has fallen by 30% since SAP began in 1990.[16] An 'urban drift' of rural people who have become poor and dispossessed as a result of the fall in income from primary agricultural products has added to the problems of health care in cities that are growing at a phenomenal rate of thousands of new arrivals every week.

HIGH MATERNAL AND INFANT MORTALITY

Poverty was identified as the biggest single underlying cause of death, disease and suffering in developing countries in 1993 by the World Health Organization. The good news was that 80% of children had been vaccinated against five major childhood killer diseases – diphtheria, poliomyelitis, tetanus, tuberculosis and whooping cough, and infant mortality fell by 25% globally between 1980 and 1993.[40] However, infectious diseases, including resurgent malaria and tuberculosis have continued to increase and killed at least 17 million people out of an estimated 52 million deaths globally in 1995. Most deaths occurred in younger age groups including 9 million children killed by diarrhoea (3.1 m), acute respiratory infections (4.4 m), measles (>1 m) and whooping cough (0.355 m). The 47 least developed countries, of which 29 are in sub-Saharan Africa, suffered the highest mortality rates per 1000 live births: perinatal 80, neonatal 50, infant 100 and under 5 years 150.[41]

WHO now estimates that in 1990, 585 000 maternal deaths occurred globally. Most of these deaths (55%) occurred in Asia where 61% of the world's births take place. However, Africa, which has 20% of the world's births, accounted for 40% of all maternal deaths. By contrast, industrialized countries with 11% of all births had < 1% of total maternal deaths.[32] The main causes of maternal deaths are emergencies in women who do not receive antenatal care and present for the first time with bleeding, obstructed labour and puerperal sepsis. They have been unsupervised during labour which took place in unsanitary conditions at home. Their babies also have high death rates.

Neonatal morbidity and mortality in most tropical countries will not be influenced by recent advances in neonatology until basic obstetric services extend to most of the population to provide antenatal care that:

- improves nutrition, controls malaria and identifies mothers at risk
- affords facilities for clean deliveries and simple means of resuscitating the newborn and promotes breast-feeding
- identifies and cares for babies at special risk.

It is possible to achieve good survival in poor countries. In Kerala, a state in south India where the gross domestic product per person is US$200, the infant mortality rate is 17 per 1000 live births compared with 83 per 1000 for the whole of India where the GDP is US$225 per person. The key to Kerala's success is its commitment to progressive social policies, basic professional health care provided by trained birth attendants, midwives and doctors, and female education. In Kerala 87% of women are literate compared to only 24% in India.[19]

Recent attempts to improve neonatal care in the tropics have had variable success. Training traditional birth attendants to conduct clean deliveries, and in sterile handling of the umbilical cord, and providing them and all pregnant mothers with a WHO-recommended pack containing a sterile razor blade, sterile ligatures and antiseptic such as gentian violet, has been rewarded by an impressive decline in the incidence of neonatal tetanus. Between 1987 and 1995, annual deaths from neonatal tetanus declined from 800 000 to 500 000.[41] On the other hand, introduction of complex, sophisticated equipment into hospitals lacking reliable basic services, or nurses and doctors trained in its use, has had little discernible effect on perinatal mortality and has not been cost-effective. In consequence, reservations persist about the priority that should be accorded neonatal care in the overall provision of health services in some poor developing countries.

ORGANIZING HEALTH CARE DELIVERY

In 1993, it was the World Bank rather than the World Health Organization that addressed the growing disparities in the burden of disease, child mortality and complications of pregnancy and childbirth between the least developed countries and rich industrialized countries.[38] This initiative was probably a response to the criticisms of structural adjustment programmes. The Bank identified major problems of health systems which slowed the pace of progress in reducing the burden of death and disability. They included:

- misallocation of public resources by spending on health interventions with low cost-effectiveness while critical and highly effective programmes are underfunded
- inequity reflected in the disproportionate amount of government spending that benefits the affluent while the poor lack access to basic health services and receive low-quality care
- inefficiency in the choice of pharmaceuticals, in the development and supervision of health workers and in the use of hospital beds
- a cost explosion in some middle-income developing countries resulting from increasing numbers of physicians, new and expensive medical technologies and the link between expanding health insurance and fee-for-service payments to physicians.

In order to improve health, the World Bank recommended that governments pursue sound 'macro-economic' policies with a focus on the poor and expand basic schooling especially for girls. A high priority for government spending on health should be a limited package of public health measures and essential clinical interventions. The most cost-effective public health activities include immunization, school-based health services, information about family planning and nutrition, programmes to reduce tobacco and alcohol consumption, and AIDS prevention. Essential clinical care in all countries should involve at least prenatal and delivery care, family planning, basic care of the sick child and simple treatments for tuberculosis and sexually transmitted diseases.

This minimum health package recommended by the World Bank could cost as little as US$12 per person annually in low-income countries and reduce the current burden of disease by about 25%. Adoption of the package in all developing countries would require a quadrupling of expenditure on public health from US$5 billion in 1993 to US$20 billion annually. Spending on essential clinical services would increase from about US$20 billion to US$40 billion.

In reality, government health spending in the 47 least developed countries is between US$0.5 to US$4 per person annually and falls far short of the cost of the World Bank's minimum health package. Recognizing this huge economic gap, the World Bank report recommended that countries willing to undertake major reforms in health policy should be strong candidates for increased external assistance including donor finance of recurrent costs. Industrialized countries in the current climate of economic recession are unlikely to extend more aid to developing countries. There is, therefore, little prospect of the minimum health package of US$12 per person being realized in developing countries until the next millennium.

However, there are local examples of successful health systems for mothers and children in developing countries including some of the poorest in the world. They have included health care as part of a scheme of community development through health education, growing fruit and vegetables, rearing fish and chickens, and constructing pit latrines. These programmes of community-based health care have improved the health of mothers and children in Indonesia. In 1990 after a decade of the Indonesian government instituting community-based care, primary immunization coverage was more then 80%, deaths from diarrhoea fell from 400 000 to 58 000 and infant mortality per 1000 live births fell from 127 (1960) to 71.[34] In India and parts of sub-Saharan Africa, most successful community-based health care initiatives have been organized by voluntary, non-governmental organizations. As a result, the Indian government has encouraged its national health system to learn from and to collaborate with their 3000 voluntary charitable health organizations.

The aim of this chapter is to consider specific problems affecting the organization and delivery of neonatal care in tropical developing countries (Table 8.1) and explore simple, effective measures for managing them. Examples of good practice will be described. Attention will also be directed at diseases, including their prevention, that pose a threat to any newborn travelling to the tropics.

ESSENTIAL NEONATAL CARE

Neonatal care is essential not only to reduce mortality and improve the quality of survival by preventing disability but also to promote positive attitudes to family planning. Parents worldwide show increasing willingness to limit family size as confidence grows in their ability to produce healthy children with a normal life expectancy. In Latin America and the Caribbean where the mortality rate of children under age 5 fell from 158 per 1000 live births in 1960 to 47 in 1994, the number of children per mother fell from six in 1950 to three in 1990.[34]

Unsupervised, unskilled, delayed and complicated deliveries that characterize obstetrics in developing countries and the high frequency of low-birthweight babies contribute to a high prevalence of birth asphyxia and birth trauma. The problems associated with neonatal asphyxia emphasize the technological gap between developed and developing countries. Endotracheal intubation and ventilation cannot be applied in institutions where laryngoscopes and appropriate tubes are not available. The provision of simple mucus extractors and education in their use, together with instruction in bag-and-mask respiration, will do more to lessen the ill-effects of birth asphyxia in vast areas of the tropics than sophisticated technology. India produces a variety of mucus extractors made of plastic and hand-operated bag-and-mask resuscitators for a fraction of the price charged in industrialized countries. This equipment for neonatal resuscitation is now being made available in Indian primary health centres where there is a room set aside for delivering babies. Mouth-to-mouth respiration can no longer be recommended because of HIV in developing countries. Mouth-to-mask units with a one-way expiratory valve are a safe and appropriate alternative means of resuscitation.

Essential neonatal care for developing countries received a boost when a task force was set up in 1993 by the government of India to train physicians in skills to manage diarrhoea and acute respiratory infection and in neonatal care. The National Neonatology Forum established by Indian neonatal paediatricians in 1980 launched pilot initiatives in January 1994 with their government's Health Ministry in three districts of Rajasthan, Tamil Nadu and Madhya Pradesh. Nine districts in rural and urban settings were added in April 1994. The aim is to provide equipment (Table 8.2) and training of doctors and nurses for essential neonatal care at primary health centres, first referral units with 10–20 beds attended by a paediatrician and/or an obstetrician, and district hospitals. Essential neonatal care includes handwashing facilities, resuscitation of asphyxiated babies, provision of warmth, promotion of breast-feeding, care of low-birthweight babies and the identification and appropriate referral of sick neonates. This project is currently being evaluated. Lessons learnt

Table 8.1 Major problems affecting neonates in the tropics

Birth asphyxia and trauma
Low birthweight
Infections
Hepatitis B, herpes simplex,
Malaria, rubella, syphilis
Toxoplasmosis, trypanosomiasis
Tuberculosis, leprosy
Tetanus
Ophthalmia – *Chlamydia*, gonococcus
Amoebiasis
Strongyloides
HIV
Jaundice associated with glucose-6-phosphate dehydrogenase deficiency
Blood disorders
Haemorrhagic disease of the newborn
α-thalassaemia
Sickle cell anaemia
Urbanization and the decline in breast-feeding

Table 8.2 Equipment for district neonatal care in India

Primary health centre
- Bag resuscitator and mask (1)
- Mucus extractor (several)
- Weighing scale (1)

First referral unit
- Bag resuscitator and mask (2)
- Radiant warmer (2)
- Weighing scale (2)
- Mucus extractor (several)
- Oxygen hood (1)
- Phototherapy unit (1)

District hospital
Some as for first referral unit with additional radiant warmer and resuscitation equipment for caesarian section births in the operating room

will be of value to all developing countries seeking to provide essential neonatal care services.

LOW BIRTHWEIGHT

The 29th World Health Assembly (1976) defined low-birthweight infants as those weighing <2500 g at birth. Low-birthweight babies constitute 16% (20 million) of all live births worldwide. The vast majority are born in developing countries and of these, 7 million take place in India.

Low birthweight is a sensitive indicator of socio-economic development reflecting the nutritional status and health of mothers and the prospects of survival of newborn infants. There has been a rise in low-birthweight prevalence in some developing countries in the 1980s and 1990s. In Brazil low-birthweight births increased from 9.3% in 1978 to 14.5% in 1984, with a steep rise of 4% between 1982 and 1984. These statistics covered a population of 34 million in the north-east province and coincided with severe economic recession.[6] Between 1979 and 1990, the percentage of low-birthweight babies born in India rose from 31 to 33 and in Bangladesh from 31 to 50.

The proportion of low-birthweight babies born in 1990 varied from 6% in industrialized countries to 11% in Latin America, 16% in sub-Saharan Africa and 33% in South Asia.[34]

Perinatal mortality surveys published in the 1980s confirmed that birthweight and socioeconomic status are major determinants for neonatal survival. In a New Delhi hospital study of 27 394 consecutive singleton births, the perinatal mortality rate dropped from 340 in the 1501–2000 g birthweight group to 46.6 per 1000 births in the group 2001–2500 g; the lowest mortality rate of 16.7 was in the group 3001–3500 g.[25] Low-birthweight babies in a hospital in southern Brazil were 17 times more likely to die in the perinatal period than those weighing 2500 g or more; babies from the poorest families were three times more likely to die during the perinatal period than those in families with the highest incomes.[3] In this study low-birthweight babies comprised 71% of neonatal deaths, and they were 24 times more likely to die in the first month than normal-weight babies.[4]

INTRAUTERINE GROWTH RETARDATION

In developed countries the proportion of small for gestational age infants among babies of low birthweight ranges from 24% in Finland[22] to 37% in England and Wales and 45% in Sweden and the USA. In sub-Saharan Africa the proportion is 34% in Kenya,[29] 56% in Tanzania,[8] 62% in Nigeria[14] and 67% in South Africa.[37] The proportion is 58% in Brazil.[3] Much higher frequencies for small for gestational age infants are reported from India (77–90%).[7] These data were obtained using western centile charts. However, elite (wellnourished) mothers in these countries produce babies of similar weight to their western counterparts, from whom such charts are derived. Although the reliability of some of these estimates is suspect, they emphasize the need to institute early feeding of low-birthweight babies in developing countries to prevent hypoglycaemia. The low proportion of immature infants among low-birthweight babies in the tropics reduces the need for intensive care in this group.

The importance of the preponderance of intrauterine growth retarded infants among low-birthweight babies in developing countries is related to the observation that such infants grow into adults with an increased risk of death from ischaemic heart disease.[2] This association of low birthweight and heart disease may explain the 40% excess of deaths from cardiovascular disease observed in Bangladeshis, Pakistanis and Indians living in Great Britain. A collaborative study of birthweight and cardiovascular disease in adults is now being conducted in India with the participation of British epidemiologists to verify this hypothesis.

The factors contributing to low-birthweight births in developing countries are: maternal short stature, teenage pregnancy, short birth interval, maternal anaemia, maternal malnutrition, heavy manual work after mid-pregnancy, smoking and tobacco chewing during pregnancy, and malaria.

PREVENTION

The best management of low-weight births in developing countries would be their prevention by reducing teenage pregnancies, increasing the birth interval, improving maternal nutrition and treating anaemia, environment control and prompt treatment of tropical infections, and giving malarial chemoprophylaxis to pregnant women. These measures would promote significant increases in birthweight and break the cycle of growth-retarded female infants becoming stunted adults who will produce growth-retarded babies.

The percentage of married adolescents in many agricultural and traditional societies is high;[11] e.g. in 1971 it was 46% in Liberia and 60.1% in Nepal. Studies in Tanzania[1] and Nigeria[18] have reported high frequencies of low-birthweight infants in teenage mothers who tend to develop pre-eclamptic toxaemia and go into preterm labour. In Leicestershire second generation Asian Muslim women continue to marry in teenage; their babies were on average 76 g lighter than those of their first-generation counterparts.[15]

A substantial reduction in the proportion of babies born within 1 year of the previous one was identified as an important factor in heavier Pakistani newborns in Birmingham born in 1978 compared with those delivered in 1968.[13]

Heavy placental infections with *Plasmodium falciparum* occur more frequently in primiparous than multiparous indigenous women living in regions of stable (endemic) malaria. Infections usually take place during the wet season when malaria-carrying mosquitoes are abundant. The prevalence rate of placental malaria in tropical Africa is between 20 and 34%. There is abundant evidence that mean birthweights of infants born to women with infected placentae are lower when compared with birthweights of infants born to uninfected mothers. Mean differences, which are consistently in favour of infants born of uninfected placentae, range from 55 to 310 g.[28] Mean birthweight deficits are greater among infants of primiparae than among those of multiparae. Malaria is a contributory cause of low birthweight and accounts for 25–50% of the attributable risk in primigravidae in malarious areas of Africa.[9] Placental malaria influences birthweight by interfering with placental function and not by direct action of the malarial parasite on the fetus. Garnham, reviewing the morbid histological changes seen in malaria-infected placentae, found it difficult to understand how the fetus could be nourished by an organ showing evidence of such marked pathology which encroaches on and sometimes obliterates the intervillous spaces.[23] Control of malaria in pregnancy through prophylactic antimalarials, using permethrin-impregnated bed nets during the wet season, leads to an increase in mean birthweight in malaria-endemic areas and is recommended in antenatal care.

Other tropical diseases also have negative effects on birthweight. Neonates of mothers with leprosy weigh less than those of healthy mothers. Intrauterine growth retardation has been observed in babies of mothers with lepromatous leprosy as early as the 16th week of pregnancy. Pregnant women infected with African trypanosomiasis (*T. gambiense* and *T. rhodesiense*) are at high risk of abortion, hydramnios and preterm delivery. In Central and South American countries where Chagas' disease (*T. cruzi*) or American trypanosomiasis is endemic, between 0.5 and 2% of low-birthweight infants under 2000 g have congenital trypanosomiasis. Schistosomiasis can affect the placenta leading to abortions, preterm delivery and intrauterine growth retardation. Leishmaniasis in pregnancy has been observed to precipitate preterm deliveries. Women with onchocerciasis appear to have a higher than expected proportion of low-birthweight infants.

JAUNDICE

The significant increase of severe jaundice in newborn infants in the tropics during the past three decades has made it a major public health problem in parts of South-East Asia, tropical Africa, the Pacific islands and in some countries bordering the Mediterranean Sea. Neonatal jaundice received high priority at an informal Geneva consultation of senior paediatricians from these regions and WHO officials on the identification of serious diseases affecting child health not covered by WHO programmes in developing countries.[39] The regular use of phototherapy in jaundiced neonates has reduced the need for exchange transfusion with its attendant hazards of using blood which may not have been screened for HIV and hepatitis B.

There appear to be geographical and racial differences in the frequency of severe neonatal jaundice which reflect the interaction of genetic and environment factors. When compared with European babies, normal-term infants of Chinese and Malay origin tend to have higher maximum bilirubin levels that reach their peak at 4 or 5 days of life.[10] Neonatal jaundice is almost always due to a rise of unconjugated bilirubin in the blood, and it may be difficult to detect in dark-skinned babies. Kernicterus due to the deposition of unconjugated bilirubin in the basal ganglia had been observed as the main cause of death in the first postnatal week in Singapore before a screening programme for G6PD deficiency was instituted.[36] In the two large cities of Nigeria, Ibadan and Lagos, severe neonatal jaundice continues to be a major cause of admission for infants in the first 2 weeks of life, particularly of those born at home or discharged from hospital within 48 hours of birth.[17,30] Experience in Ibadan indicates that severe neonatal jaundice is important not only as a cause of cerebral palsy but also in the pathogenesis of deafness and speech retardation.[21]

CAUSES

The known causes of severe neonatal jaundice in the tropics are different from those found in temperate industrialized countries (Table 8.3). Glucose-6-phosphate dehydrogenase deficiency is an important cause of neonatal jaundice in South-East Asia and West Africa. Haemolysis from factors intrinsic and extrinsic to the red blood cells occurs in neonates with G6PD deficiency. Bacterial infections are frequent in a hot climate without a clean water supply and sanitation. The liver enzyme system for conjugating bilirubin is not functioning optimally in preterm babies. Trauma and asphyxia at birth occur when maternity services are inadequate. Extravasated blood in cephalhaematomata and in bruised tissues is resorbed with the production of bilirubin, which increases the load of unconjugated pigment to be removed by the neonate's liver. Studies in the USA have

Table 8.3 Common causes of neonatal hyperbilirubinaemia in the tropics

Glucose-6-phosphate dehydrogenase (G6PD) deficiency
Sepsis
Prematurity
Trauma and birth asphyxia
ABO haemolytic disease
Haemolytics agents – naphthalene

shown that the incidence of ABO haemolytic disease, based on a positive direct Coombs' test, is increased in black infants.[31] There is some evidence to suggest that the same occurs in African neonates.[12]

In addition, about 20% or 30% of newborn babies with unconjugated hyperbilirubinaemia in tropical countries have none of these causal factors to explain their jaundice. It is probable that environmental factors contribute to neonatal jaundice in the tropics. A report from Papua New Guinea showed the importance of environmental illumination of obstetric wards on the incidence of neonatal jaundice. Architectural modifications to prevent rain blowing into an obstetric ward were made by extending the roof overhangs to a width of several metres so that they excluded most of the daylight. An alarming increase in the incidence of severe neonatal jaundice from 0.5% to 17% was observed after the modifications. Other causes for the increase in neonatal jaundice were excluded.[5] This observation has implications for the design of obstetric wards and neonatal nurseries in the tropics, which should be built with windows facing north-south for coolness, and with roof overhangs limited to a width of 1 m to allow entry of adequate indirect sunlight to reduce neonatal jaundice. The use of natural illumination from indirect sunlight has been found to be of therapeutic value during the day in the tropics; if used with care it can reduce the need to use phototherapy units during daylight hours.

It has been suggested that the high incidence of severe neonatal jaundice in Nigerian babies could be a result of high exposure to infection and icterogenic drugs and chemicals in their homes.[20,30] Significant exposure to naphthalene, insecticides, mentholated balms and powders and traditional herbs was found in 65% of families studied by Familusi & Dawodu.[20] Although the incidence of jaundice did not differ significantly in neonates from households with or without a positive history of exposure, severe jaundice requiring exchange transfusion was significantly more frequent among neonates from families with exposure to naphthalene. Naphthalene can be inhaled or absorbed through the skin of an infant wearing clothes which have been stored in mothballs. It induces haemolysis, fragmentation and Heinz body formation in G6PD-deficient red cells through the oxidizing properties of α-naphthol. Even red cells with normal G6PD concentrations undergo haemolysis when exposed to naphthalene.[35] Preliminary analysis by high-performance liquid chromatography of some traditional Nigerian remedies for purging neonates of meconium and of mentholated balms has identified naphthalene as an ingredient. Naphthols were found in 6.9% of 625 Nigerian cord blood samples and aflatoxins in 14.6% indicating perinatal exposure.[27] There was, however, no significant difference in naphthol or aflatoxin exposure of neonates with and without jaundice. One in three with severe jaundice were G6PD deficient compared with 13.3% of controls ($p = 0.009$).[33]

Available evidence suggests that neonatal jaundice is common in some tropical communities because of a combination of genetic red cell disorders and exposure of infants to haemolytic environmental agents as a result of traditional practices during the perinatal period.

PROTECTION FOR NEWBORN TRAVELLERS TO THE TROPICS

Parents with young infants from temperate industrialized countries have become less apprehensive of travelling with them to the tropics. Provided certain measures are taken to protect their health, infants thrive as well in tropical countries as they would in Europe or North America.

Breast-feeding is usually more convenient than bottle-feeding and may be continued into the second year. If the infant is to be bottle-fed, powdered milk should be reconstituted with boiled water, and the milk should not be left to stand unrefrigerated for more than an hour. Bottles and utensils should be sterilized before use.

Cotton clothing is preferable to clothes made from synthetic fibres because it absorbs perspiration and prevents skin rashes. Although disposable nappies are convenient for travelling, the plastic covers used with them do not allow urine to evaporate and can lead to ammoniacal dermatitis.

Babies should not be exposed to direct tropical sunlight for fear of sunburn. Naked babies lying in the shade for a few hours can become sunburned, particularly on the beach. A bed net impregnated with permethrin should be placed over the cot to protect the baby from mosquito bites when asleep. Insect repellents may also be used on the skin.

IMMUNIZATION

BCG immunization is recommended for newborn infants living in cities of developing countries where tuberculosis is endemic. The vaccine prevents miliary and meningitic forms of tuberculosis. BCG vaccine stored in a refrigerator at 2–8°C should be reconstituted just before use. An intradermal injection of 0.1 ml of the vaccine is introduced into the skin of the left upper arm over the insertion of the left deltoid muscle, and this should produce a weal about 7 mm in diameter. No tuberculin test is necessary before immunization of a neonate. Between 3 and 6 weeks after immunization a small papule appears at the injection site, indicating the development of delayed hypersensitivity. The papule discharges pus, leaving a shallow ulcer that heals to form a scar. Immunity induced by a successful BCG vaccination provides protection for about 10 years. Immunocompromised infants should not be given this live-attenuated vaccine.

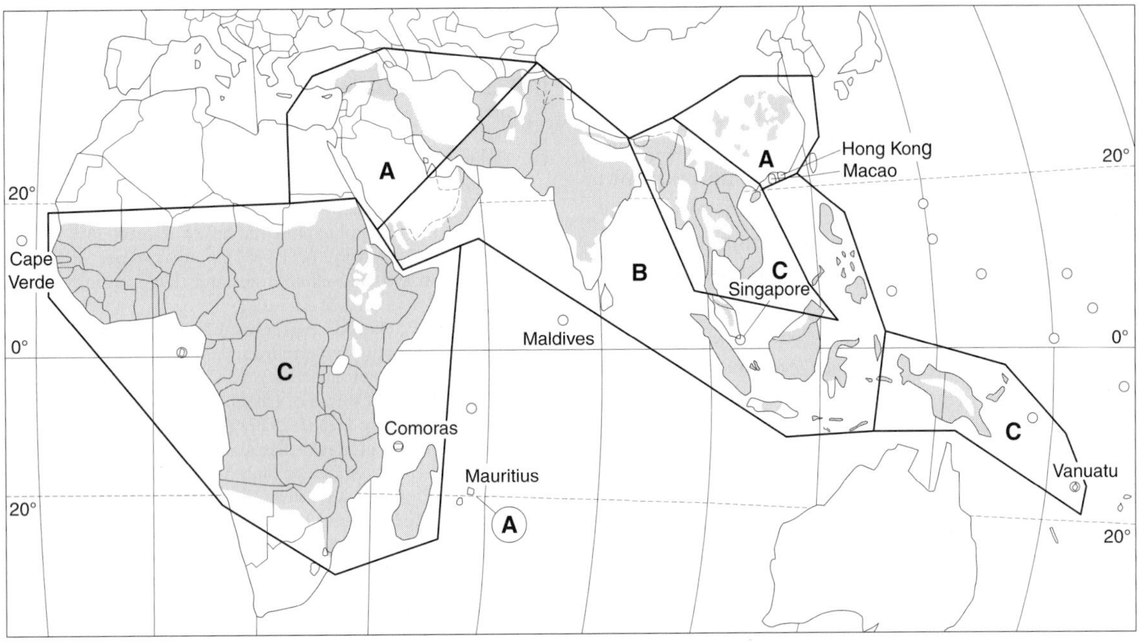

Fig. 8.1 WHO zones for malaria drug prophylaxis recommendations – 1996.[42] See text for descriptions of zones A, B and C.

The first dose of diphtheria, pertussis, tetanus and poliomyelitis vaccines should be administered in the second month of life. Parents should be reminded that two more doses should be given at monthly intervals and that a booster dose is recommended at about 18 months. Measles vaccine or MMR if available is recommended at 15 months.

Other vaccines, such as cholera, typhoid and yellow fever, are not recommended. Cholera vaccine is not efficient if given in a single dose. Two doses given 4 weeks apart can ensure protection for a maximum of only 6 months. This vaccine if given subcutaneously produces a severe local reaction and pain. The only useful vaccine against typhoid is the monovalent variety. The manufacturer does not recommend its use in infants. Both cholera and typhoid are diseases that can be avoided if mothers are willing to breast-feed their newborn infants. If they prefer bottle-feeding then they should be scrupulous in using boiled water for preparing milk and sterilized bottles and teats. Most parents who take their infants abroad live in good accommodation and should be able to take good care of their babies without these vaccines. Yellow fever vaccine is recommended only after infancy because of reports of encephalitis when used in younger children.

Pregnant women travelling to the tropics should be given protection against poliomyelitis, using the injectable killed Salk vaccine, and tetanus with two doses of toxoid administered 2 months apart during the last trimester. Yellow fever vaccine may be administered in the last trimester for travellers to endemic regions although it is a live-attenuated vaccine. No reliable reports of fetopathy have been recorded with yellow fever vaccination given as recommended here.

MALARIAL PROPHYLAXIS

All newborn infants (including those breast-fed) travelling to the tropics should be protected against malaria. In regions with no evidence of *P. falciparum* malarial parasites resistant to chloroquine (zone A Fig. 8.1), chloroquine 5 mg/kg once-weekly gives adequate protection. A liquid preparation of chloroquine is available. In zone B, chloroquine alone will protect against *P. vivax.* Chloroquine weekly and proguanil 5 mg/kg daily will give some protection against *P. falciparum* and may alleviate the disease if it occurs despite prophylaxis. Proguanil, in either dry or liquid form, is bitter and can be difficult to administer to babies with sensitive tastebuds. Zone C covers those parts of the world where drug-resistant malaria is commonplace. In Africa the risk of malaria is high in all except high-altitude areas. The risk is low in most areas of this zone in Asia and America, but high in parts of the Amazon basin (colonization and mining areas). Resistance to sulfadoxine-pyrimethamine is common in zone C in Asia, variable in zone C in Africa and America. The first choice for prophylaxis is mefloquine but recent reports of blood and skin complications have made it necessary for some travellers to take the second recommended choice combination of chloroquine weekly and proguanil daily. This combination is preferred even in parts of South-East Asia and Papua New Guinea where chloroquine resistance is common. In the border areas of Cambodia/ Myanmar/Thailand, doxycycline is recommended for prophylaxis in adults. As it is a tetracycline, it is not recommended for use in infants. It is not advisable to take infants to these remote and hazardous parts of the malaria-infested world.

Protection against mosquito bites is important in addition to chemoprophylaxis. Screening of the bedroom with fine netting will exclude flying insects but allow adequate ventilation. A bed net impregnated with permethrin 0.2 g/m^2 will repel mosquitoes even when there are tears and the net is not tucked under the mattress.

Advice should be obtained from specialists in tropical paediatrics if children are likely to live for more than 3 years in a malaria-endemic area. Complications from the long-term continuous use of chloroquine (retinal damage) have to be weighed against the acquisition of immunity from occasional natural infection treated promptly.

REFERENCES

1. Arkutu A A 1978 Pregnancy and labour in Tanzanian primigravidae aged 15 years and under. International Journal of Gynaecology and Obstetrics 16: 128–131
2. Barker D, Osmond C, Simmonds S, Wield G 1993 The relation of small head circumference and thinness at birth to death from cardiovascular disease in adult life. British Medical Journal 306: 422–426
3. Barros F C, Victora C G, Vaughan J P, Teixeira A M B, Ashworth A 1987b Infant mortality in southern Brazil; a population based study of causes of death. Archives of Disease in Childhood 62: 487–490
4. Barros F, C, Victora C G, Vaughan J P, Estanislau H J 1987a Perinatal mortality in southern Brazil; a population-based study of 7392 births. Bulletin of the World Health Organization 65: 95–104
5. Barss P, Comfort K 1985 Ward design and neonatal jaundice in the tropics: report of an epidemic. British Medical Journal 291: 400–401
6. Becker R A, Lechtig A 1986 Brazil; evolucao da mortalidade infantil no perioda 1977–84. Ministry of Health, Documentation Center, Brasilia, DF, Brazil
7. Bhargava S K, Sachdev H P S, Ramji S, Iyer P V 1987 Low birthweight: aetiology and prevention in India. Annals of Tropical Pediatrics 7: 59–65
8. Boersma E R, Mbise R K 1979 Intrauterine growth of live born Tanzanian infants. Tropical and Geographical Medicine 31: 7–19
9. Brabin B 1991 An assessment of low birthweight risk in primiparae as an indicator of malaria control in pregnancy. International Journal of Epidemiology 20: 276–283
10. Brown W R, Wong H B 1965 Ethnic group differences in bilirubinemia of Singapore newborns. Bulletin of the Kandang Kerbau Hospital Singapore 4: 35–43
11. Burr Hunt I I W 1976 Adolescent fertility – risks and consequences. Population Reports Series Journal 10: 157–175
12. Chintu C, Zipursky A, Blajchman M 1979 ABO haemolytic disease of the newborn. East African Medical Journal 56: 314–319
13. Clarson C L, Barker M J, Marshall T, Wharton B A 1982 Secular change in birth weight of Asian babies born in Birmingham. Archives of Disease in Childhood 57: 867–871
14. Dawodu A H, Laditan A A O 1985 Low birth weight in an urban community in Nigeria. Annals of Tropical Paediatrics 5: 61–66
15. Draper E S, Abrams K R, Clarke M 1995 Fall in birth weight of third generation Asian infants. British Medical Journal 311: 876
16. Editorial 1996 The World Bank, listening and learning. Lancet 347: 411
17. Effiong C E, Laditan A A O 1976 Neonatal jaundice in Ibadan: a study of cases seen in the out-patient clinic. Nigerian Journal of Paediatrics 3: 1–8
18. Effiong F, 1, Banjoka M O 1975 The obstetric performance of Nigerian primigravidae aged 16 and under. British Journal of Obstetrics and Gynaecology 82: 228–233
19. Evans I 1995 SAPping maternal health. Lancet 346: 1046
20. Familusi J B, Dawodu A H 1985 A survey of neonatal jaundice in association with household drugs and chemicals in Nigeria. Annals of Tropical Paediatrics 5: 219–222
21. Familusi J B, Dawodu A H, Owa J A 1982 Some epidemiological aspects of neonatal hyperbilirubinaemia in Nigeria. In: Fukuyama Y et al (eds) Child neurology. Excerpta Medica, Amsterdam, pp 272–280
22. Finland National Board of Health 1979 Health services year book of National Board of Health 1977–1978. Official Statistics of Finland, National Board of Health, Helsinki
23. Garnham P C C 1938 The placenta in malaria with special reference to reticuloendothelial immunity. Transactions of the Royal Society of Tropical Medicine and Hygiene 32: 13–34
24. George S 1992 The debt boomerang: how third world debt harms us all. Pluto Press, London
25. Ghosh S, Bhargava S K, Saxena H M K, Sagreiya K 1983 Perinatal mortality – report of a hospital based study. Annals of Tropical Paediatrics 3: 115–119
26. Logie D E, Woodroffe J 1993 Structural adjustment: the wrong prescription for Africa? British Medical Journal 307: 41–44
27. Maxwell S M, Familusi J B, Sodeinde O, Chan M C K, Hendrickse R G 1994 Detection of naphthols and aflatoxins in Nigerian cord blood. Annals of Tropical Paediatrics 14: 3–5
28. McGregor I A, Wilson M E, Billewicz W Z 1983 Malaria infection of the placenta in the Gambia, West Africa; its incidence and relationship to stillbirth, birthweight and placental weight. Transactions of the Royal Society of Tropical Medicine and Hygiene 77: 232–244
29. Meme J S 1978 A prospective study of neonatal deaths in Nairobi, Kenya. East Africa Medical Journal 55: 262–267
30. Olowe S A, Ransome-Kuti O 1980 The risk of jaundice in glucose-6-phosphate dehydrogenase deficient babies exposed to menthol. Acta Paediatrica Scandinavica 69: 341–345
31. Peevy K J, Wiseman H J 1978 ABO hemolytic disease of the newborn: evaluation of management and identification of racial and antigenic factors. Pediatrics 61: 475–478
32. Safe Motherhood 1995 Maternal mortality worse than we thought. WHO, Geneva
33. Sodeinde O, Chan M C K, Maxwell S M, Familusi J B, Hendrickse R G 1995 Neonatal jaundice, aflatoxins and naphthols: report of a study in Ibadan Nigeria. Annals of Tropical Paediatrics 15: 107–113
34. UNICEF 1996 State of the World's children, Oxford University Press, Oxford
35. Valaes T, Doxiadis S A, Fessas P H 1963 Acute haemolysis due to naphthalene inhalation. Journal of Pediatrics 63: 904–915
36. Wong H B 1966 Singapore kernicterus: a review and the present position. Bulletin of Kandang Kerbau Hospital, Singapore 5: 1–9
37. Woods D L, Malan A C 1979 Patterns of retarded fetal growth. Early Human Development 3: 257–262
38. World Development Report 1993 Investing in health. World Bank, New York
39. World Health Organization 1985 Serious childhood diseases: priority issues and possible actions at family, community and health centre levels. Report of an informal consultation. WHO MCH/85.3, Geneva
40. World Health Organization 1995 Bridging the gap. WHO, Geneva
41. World Health Organization 1996 World health report. WHO, Geneva
42. World Health Organization 1996 Health advice for international travel. WHO, Geneva

Section 2

Prenatal life

9

Basic embryology and the embryological basis of malformation syndromes

Richard E. J. Dyball   Visvan Navaratnam   Patricia A. Tate

INTRODUCTION

Despite its apparent protection, the mammalian embryo is very sensitive to the noxious influence of external teratogenic agents. It is probable that many seriously malformed embryos do not survive to full term. Nevertheless, 2–3% of liveborn infants show one or more congenital malformations at birth and, by the end of the first year of life, this figure may be doubled by discovery of abnormalities not noticed earlier. Congenital malformations are inevitably attended by disappointment and despair, and the parents will seek explanation, as well as information regarding the risk of recurrence in subsequent pregnancies.

Familiarity with the main events of organogenesis (Fig. 9.1) is of assistance to the clinician in identifying when and why a particular abnormality arose and could help with preventive action. It should be noted that the times indicated in Figure 9.1 refer to the time after fertilization and not that after the beginning of the last menstrual period. However, although a large number of birth defects have been described and attributed to specific factors, little is known as yet as to how an agent actually produces a defect, or how congenital abnormalities may be prevented. It is reasonable to assume that abnormal metabolic processes lead to abnormal cell death, retardation or acceleration of mitosis, persistence of cells destined to atrophy, or abnormal cell surface interactions, but basic embryological research has, as yet, not succeeded in explaining defective organogenesis at this level. At present, the clinical approach to the problem of defective organogenesis is either by postnatal repair or by the offer of termination of those embryos found (by ultrasound, amniocentesis, or chemical test) to be malformed in early pregnancy.

HOW DO TERATOGENS ACT?

While the details of the mechanisms of teratogenesis are not understood, it is clear that the nature of a teratogenic effect depends mainly on the timing of exposure and on the genetic constitution. Mammalian development starts with a rapid multiplication of cells showing little, if any, differentiation. A teratogen acting during this predifferentiation stage can damage most or all of the embryonic cells, resulting in embryonic death; or it may injure only a few cells, in which case the regulative potential of the embryo compensates and no abnormality results. Factors such as hypervitaminosis A and radiation, which are known to be very teratogenic in later stages of development, have no harmful effect in this early developmental phase. During the period of intense differentiation (3–8 weeks), most teratogens are highly effective and can produce serious malformations. As a rough guide to timing, gastrulation and the first appearance of somites (see Fig. 9.1) herald the onset of the vulnerable period. Any one of a number of extrinsic or intrinsic agents, disrupting homeostasis at such a crucial period, can result in similar abnormalities, though the nature of disruption may be very different. The same substance can produce different malformations if administered at different stages of morphogenesis and, when several organ primordia are developing simultaneously, it can bring about multiple malformations. During the fetal and neonatal periods (from 8 weeks to term) of development, which are characterized by growth of the organs, susceptibility to teratogenic agents rapidly decreases. A small number of organs, such as the cerebellum, cerebral cortex and some urogenital structures (including the gonads), do continue to differentiate and thus remain vulnerable.

NEURAL TUBE AND ASSOCIATED SKELETAL DEFECTS

The neural plate forms during the course of the third week by differentiation and thickening of ectoderm in the midline, induced by the underlying notochord and mesoderm. The plate then invaginates; its lateral margins (neural folds) rise up and fuse to establish the neural

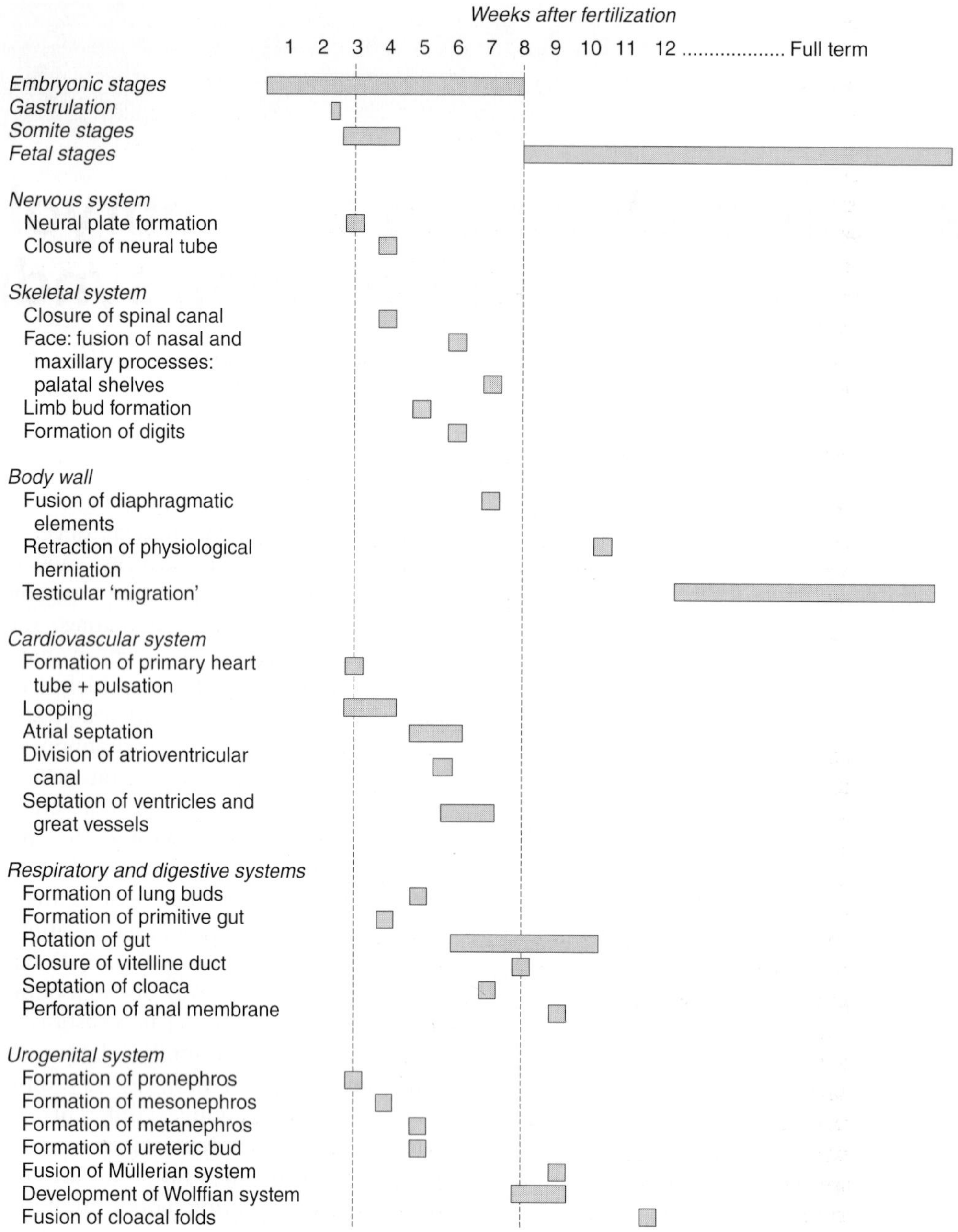

Fig. 9.1 Milestones in development.

tube. Fusion occurs between days 21 and 28, starting at midtrunk level and progressing to each end. Malformations of the spinal cord follow inadequate closure of the caudal part of the neural tube and are in turn the result of abnormalities of differential cell division and adhesiveness. Formation of the posterior arches of vertebrae normally follows that of the neural tube, so that anomalies of the tube lead to anomalies of the spine. The most frequent malformation is spina bifida, where the posterior arch of one or more vertebrae is not closed (Fig. 9.2). It is most often localized to the lumbosacral region but it may involve the entire length of the spinal cord. Spina bifida occulta, affecting 15–20% of the population and discovered only by chance, may be indicated by a small tuft of overlying hair; the skin and meninges are intact over the cord and only the posterior bony arch of the spine is missing. In meningocele, the meninges protrude through the bony defect, and in myelomeningocele, the cord itself also herniates. In severe forms of spina bifida, the spinal cord also lies open, the neural tube not having closed. Functional deficit in spinal bifida varies from negligible to severe dysfunction of the lower limbs with disturbances of pelvic physiology including micturition.

If the failure of neural tube closure is cranial, the abnormality is often associated with failure of ossification

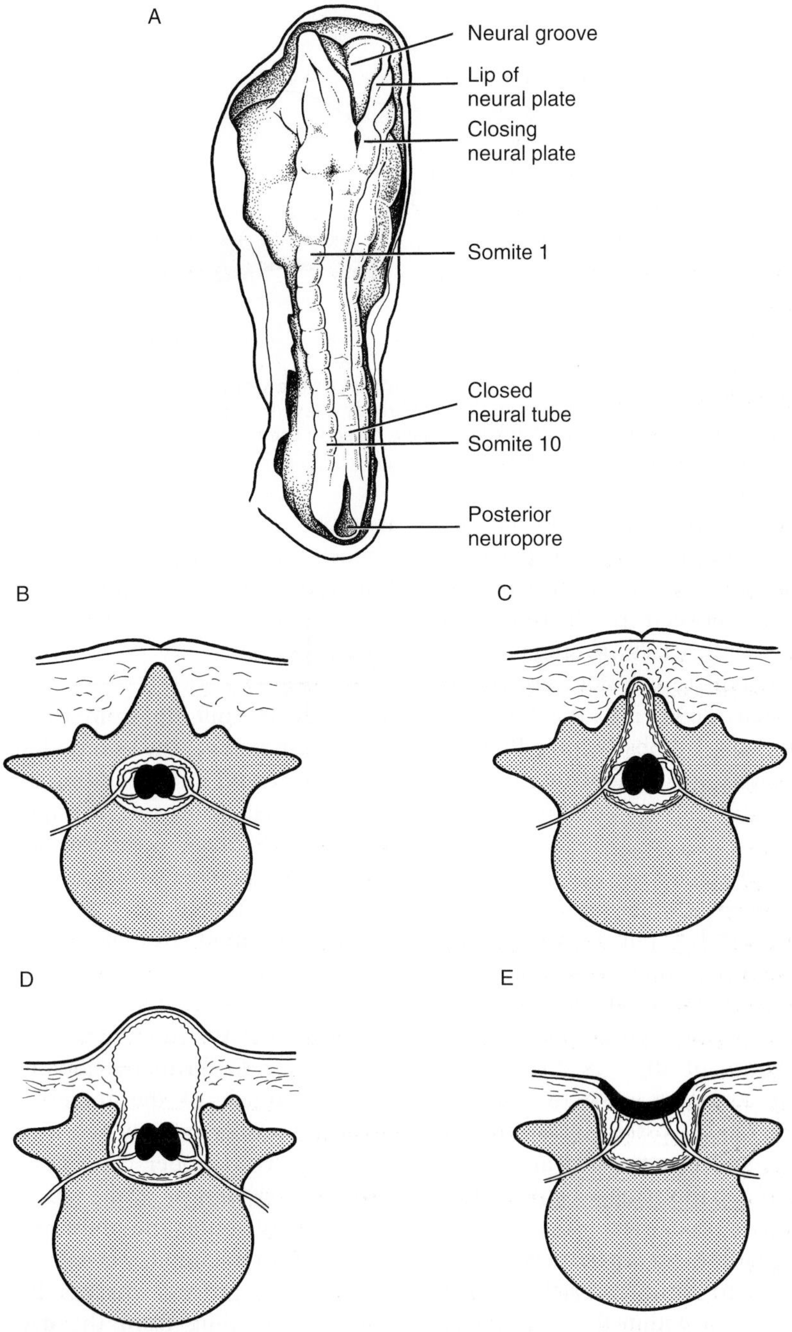

Fig. 9.2 (A) Embryo about day 23 with amnion removed to show somites on either side of the neural tube, which is closed except at the head and lumbar regions where neuropores are still present. (B, C, D, E) Cross-sections of neonatal lumbar vertebrae to show spinal cord (black) and meninges: (B) normal; (C) spina bifida occulta; (D) meningocele; (E) severe spina bifida with unclosed cord (meningomyelocele).

of the skull since the cranial vault bones, like the posterior arches of the vertebrae, differentiate under the influence of a normal neural tube. Meningocele can occur here as with spina bifida and can be treated surgically. In encephalocele, part of the brain herniates under the skin. If there is failure of closure of the neural tube in the cranial region, it is often associated with atrophy resulting in a condition known as anencephaly. Despite its name, such atrophy usually occurs after formation of the cranial nerves so that these nerves and the eyes are present in anencephalic fetuses despite the severe disruption of brain development. The brain stem and base of the cerebrum, including the pituitary, are also usually present. Congenital hydrocephalus is an anomaly characterized by

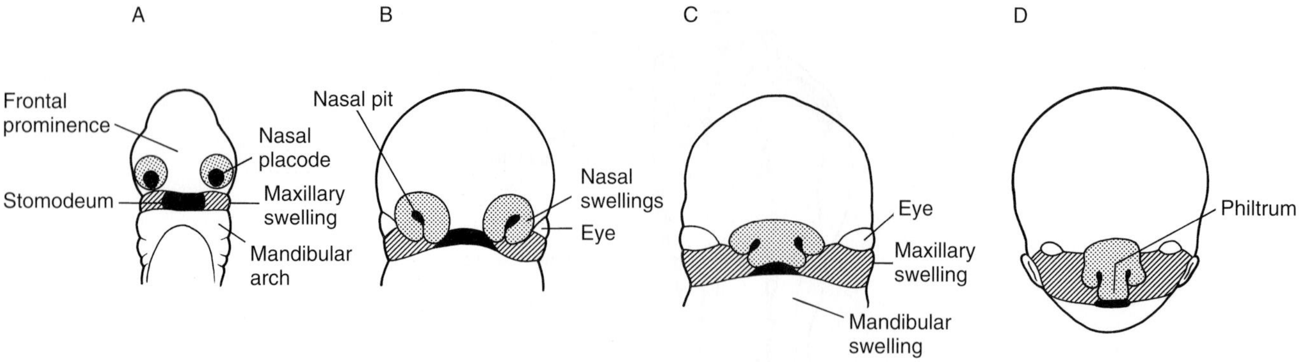

Fig. 9.3 (A) Frontal view of embryo in the fifth week to show the position of the stomodeum, nasal placodes, frontal prominence, maxillary swellings and mandibular arch. (B) By 6 weeks the nasal placodes have invaginated into pits surrounded by nasal swellings. (C) At 7 weeks the medial parts of the nasal swellings have fused in the midline and their lateral parts have fused with the maxillary swellings. (D) Facial appearance at 10 weeks.

abnormal accumulation of cerebrospinal fluid in the ventricles or subarachnoid space. It may be caused by obstruction of circulation, most commonly at the cerebral aqueduct, or by imbalance between production and absorption of the fluid. In some cases of spina bifida where the spinal cord is adherent to the skin, growth of the trunk pulls the brain stem down into the foramen magnum, causing hydrocephalus by obstructing flow of CSF from the fourth ventricle to the subarachnoid space (Arnold–Chiari syndrome).

EYE AND EAR

The eye develops as an outgrowth (optic vesicle) of the forebrain interacting with an ectodermal thickening (lens placode). The optic vesicle invaginates at its extremity, forming the optic cup from which are derived the layers of the retina and the inner layers of the iris and ciliary apparatus; the invagination continues onto the ventral aspect of the stalk allowing blood vessels access to the retina; non-closure of the ventral invagination in the iris region results in a radial defect (coloboma). Nerve fibres from the retina normally grow backwards towards the brain along the stalk and establish the optic nerve. The lens placode also invaginates to form a vesicle, which transforms into the lens lying just within the opening of the optic cup. The optic cup and lens become enclosed in mesoderm which contributes the outer coats of the eye, the anterior cover (cornea) becoming transparent. Occasionally, mesoderm in the pupillary region persists as an opaque membrane obscuring vision.

The ear is developed by the approximation of structures from different sources. A surface ectodermal thickening (otic placode) on the side of the neck invaginates to form the membranous labyrinth which becomes embedded in a mesodermal condensation comprising the bony labyrinth. The middle ear and auditory tube are derived from the first pharyngeal pouch, and the auditory ossicles arise from the mesoderm of the first and second pharyngeal arches. The external auditory meatus is an ectodermal invagination coming into apposition with the endodermal first pouch (middle ear) but separated by the tympanic membrane.

FACE

The face is built up from five swellings surrounding a deep depression, the stomodeum or primitive mouth (Fig. 9.3), and incorporating the special sense organs. These facial processes comprise mesodermal masses lifting the surface ectoderm and they are demarcated initially by grooves which become progressively filled as the swellings merge.

The unpaired frontal process is the largest facial swelling, forming the roof of the stomodeum. The other facial processes are derived from the first pharyngeal arch on each side; two mandibular swellings join ventrally in the midline to form the floor of the stomodeum (lower jaw and much of the tongue) and, laterally, the two maxillary processes grow below the eye towards the frontal process. The upper lip develops largely from the maxillary swellings, while an extension of the frontal process contributes the philtrum. Cleft lip, which may be unilateral or bilateral, occurs between the philtrum and the maxillary process whereas the rarer oblique facial cleft lesions, extending from the eye to the mouth, involve more extensive breakdown between the maxillary and frontal processes.

At the end of the fourth week, two ectodermal thickenings appear on the frontal prominence – these are the nasal placodes, which later form the nasal pits. Part of the frontal process juts inwards between the nasal pits and the mouth (primary palate) and this is joined by a pair of lateral palatal shelves growing inwards from the maxillary processes. These three elements normally fuse by 9–10 weeks but failure to do so leads to the different types of cleft palate, which may be independent or occur together with cleft lips.

Malformations in the face region occur in 1–2 per 1000 live births. The primary aetiological factor for such

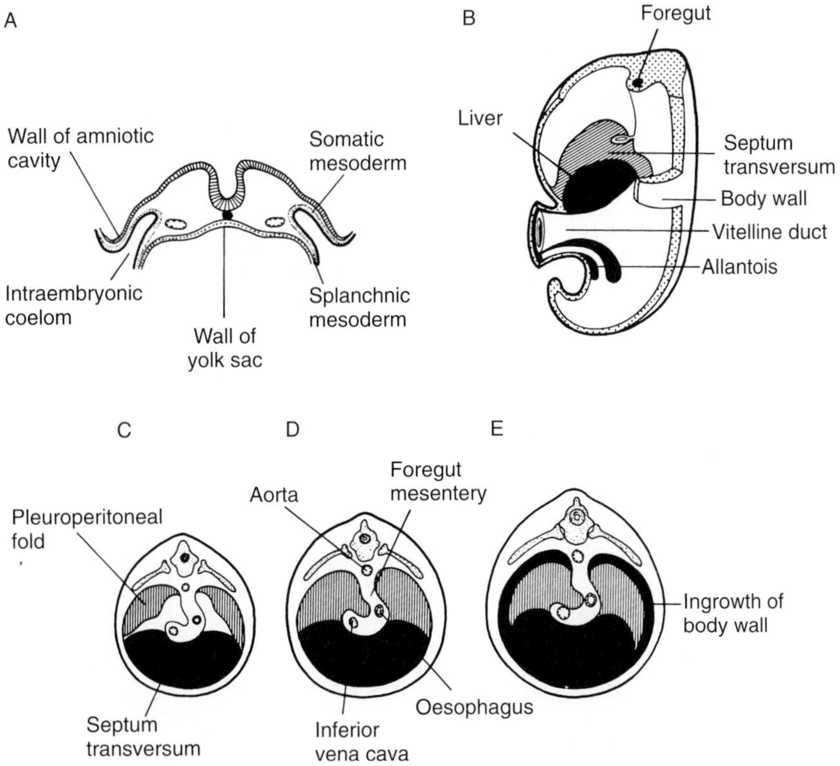

Fig. 9.4 (A) Transverse section at 3 weeks to show formation of somatic and splanchnic mesoderm. (B) Cutaway diagram at 5 weeks and (C, D, E) schematic cross-sections at 6, 7 and 10 weeks to show development of the diaphragm from the septum transversum, pleuroperitoneal folds, foregut mesentery and ingrowth of the body wall.

deformities is thought to be genetic, but various teratogens such as anticonvulsant drugs, hypervitaminosis A and alcohol have also been implicated.

The tongue is formed in the floor of the mouth by swellings contributed by the first and third pharyngeal arches which are demarcated by the sulcus terminalis. At this junction, an endodermal downgrowth (thyroglossal duct) establishes the main components of the thyroid gland in the neck; failure of this rudiment to descend results in a lingual thyroid or cyst.

LIMBS

Limb bud primordia appear at the end of the fourth week, the upper limb preceding the lower, formed by a series of reciprocal inductions of mesoderm and ectoderm. The essential constituents can be distinguished at 5 weeks in paddle-shaped limb buds, which subsequently undergo rotation. Programmed cell death (apoptosis) is important in the elimination of tissue along radial grooves in the flattened hand or foot plate to generate free digits. Total absence of limbs is known as amelia; meromelia (phocomelia) is the term applied to limbs where one or more of the long bones are missing, and the hand or foot bones are attached to the trunk. These abnormalities are rare and are usually of hereditary origin but, with other defects, were tragically associated with the use of the drug thalidomide. More frequently, unusual numbers of digits (polydactyly and syndactyly) are found, presumably as a result of atypical patterns of cell death.

BODY WALL

At the end of the third week, the intraembryonic mesoderm is divisible into:

- a paraxial portion on either side of the notochord and developing neural tube
- an intermediate portion
- a lateral plate. The lateral plate then cleaves into two layers:
  - — somatic mesoderm associated with the ectoderm, forming the skin and outer wall of the trunk
  - — splanchnic mesoderm associated with the yolk sac contributing to visceral coats.

The intraembryonic coelom lies between these two layers. Just caudal to the developing heart the diaphragm develops as a partition dividing the intraembryonic coelom into thoracic and abdominal compartments. It is derived from components of the septum transversum (which is a ventrally placed condensation of mesoderm), dorsolaterally placed pleuroperitoneal folds, the dorsal oesophageal mesentery and parts of the somatic mesoderm from the body wall (Fig. 9.4). Diaphragmatic hernias may

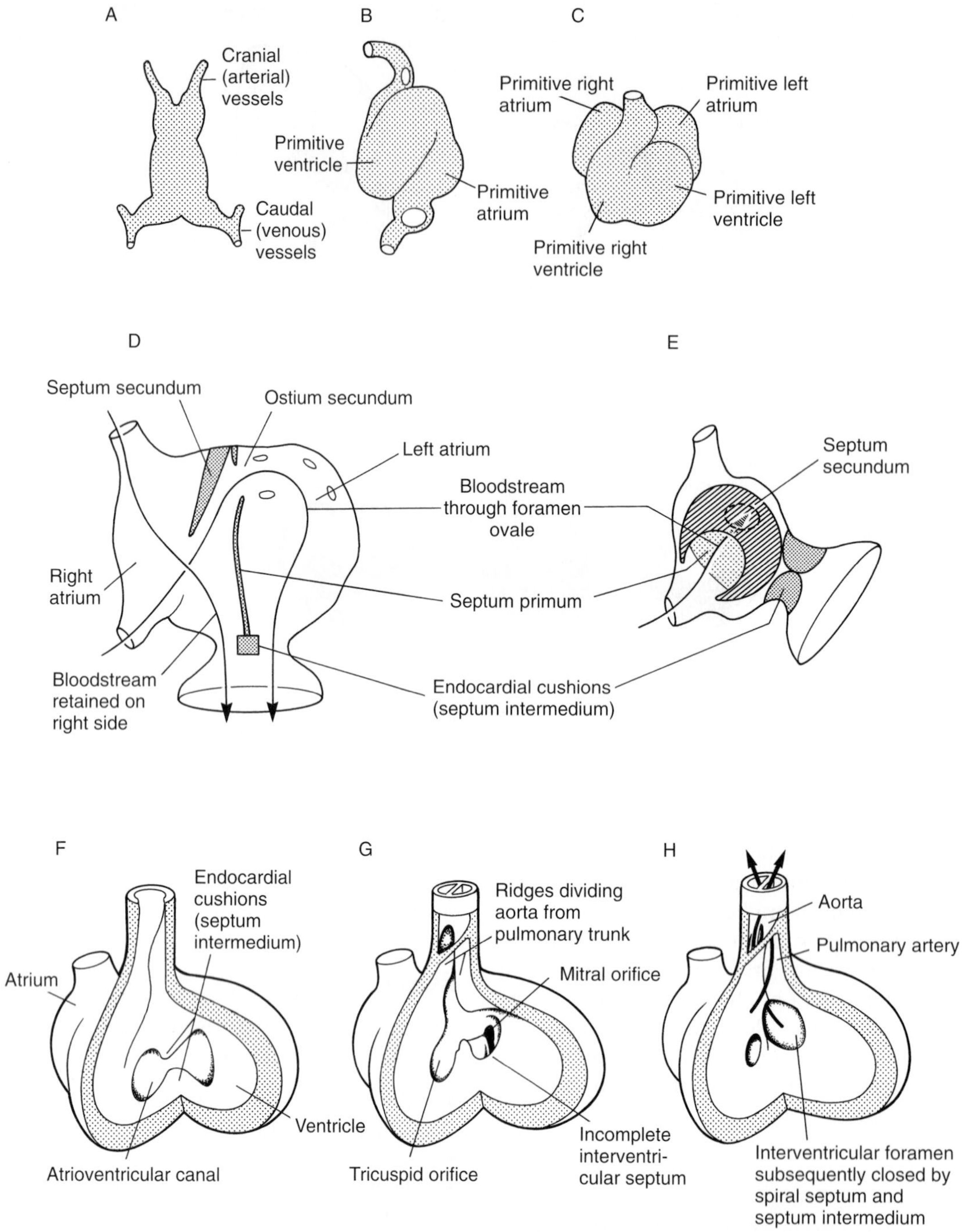

Fig. 9.5 (A) Anterior view of primitive linear heart tube at 21 days. (B,C) Over the next week the tube folds, with realignment of the atrial and ventricular regions. (D, E) During the fifth and sixth weeks, the atrioventricular canal becomes partitioned by endocardial cushions (septum intermedium) and the atrial region becomes divided by the growth of the septum primum and septum secundum. However, a deficiency (ostium secundum) appears in the septum primum which, though overlapped by the septum secundum, allows blood to flow from right to left through an oblique valve, the foramen ovale. (F, G, H) Septation of the ventricles, seen by removing the anterior walls: (F) the original atrioventricular canal has been divided into right (tricuspid) and left (mitral) channels; (G) in the fifth week, the almost vertical interventricular septum starts to form; (H) over the sixth to eighth weeks the interventricular foramen becomes obliterated by approximation of the interventricular septum with the septum intermedium and arterial spiral septum.

occur (at a frequency of 1 : 2000) when fusion of the different elements fails, allowing the stomach, spleen and intestinal loops to enter the thorax. Failure of a pleuroperitoneal fold to fuse with the septum transversum is the commonest site for such hernias and occurs more frequently on the left side.

Another developmental weak spot is the umbilicus. During the sixth week, rapid growth of the midgut causes it to extrude (physiological hernia) into the extra-embryonic coelom of the umbilical cord and normally this retracts before the end of the tenth week. After this, the principal contents of the cord are the umbilical vessels surrounded by Wharton's jelly. After birth, the umbilical vessels constrict and the mesoderm of the anterior abdominal wall closes round the vessels forming the umbilical cicatrix as the cord is cast off. Congenital umbilical herniation occurs if the muscle and skin of the anterior abdominal wall are absent or weak. In its most severe form (omphalocele), caused by failure of the physiologically herniated midgut to properly return at the tenth week, the defect is covered by peritoneum and amnion only; these coverings may break down during birth, leading to eventration of the abdominal viscera, often including the urinary bladder.

Between the third month and term, the testes 'descend', by virtue of differential growth, from their initially high lumbar position on the posterior body wall down to the scrotum (see Fig. 9.7). To allow this descent, bilateral prolongations of the coelomic cavity (the vaginal processes) protrude into the scrotum. They are open at first, but progressively narrow, until the proximal portion is entirely obliterated and the distal portion exists only as a double envelope around the testis (the tunica vaginalis). If the narrow canal connecting the lumen of the vaginal process with the peritoneum is not obliterated about the time of birth, loops of intestine may descend into the scrotum as a congenital inguinal hernia. The vaginal process runs parallel with the inferior ligament or gubernaculum of the testis; migration of the gland follows the line of this structure and is regulated by hormonal interactions between androgens and gonadotrophins. In some cases, possibly because of insufficient shortening of the gubernaculum, the testis may remain undescended within the abdomen, where it is unable to mature normally to fertility and is also at substantial risk of malignant change.

CARDIOVASCULAR SYSTEM

The cardiovascular system and blood cells are derived from mesoderm and they first appear at the beginning of the third week in relation to the yolk sac and, subsequently, at other sites. The heart develops initially as angiogenic clusters in the yolk sac mesoderm related to the pericardial coelom near the head end of the embryo. As the embryo grows, the primitive vascular tissue consolidates to form bilateral endocardial tubes which approach each other in the ventral midline and fuse to form a single linear heart tube. This acquires a myocardial mantle and begins to beat about the 21st day, driving blood from the caudal (venous) to the cranial (arterial) end of the tube. It transforms into a linear series of primitive chambers and constrictions to facilitate unidirectional blood flow. With growth in size, it undergoes complex looping during the fourth week so that the primitive chambers become realigned (Fig. 9.5A, B) to resemble the layout of the definitive chambers of the heart (Fig. 9.5C). Such realignment is an essential precursor to the internal partition into left and right chambers which begins during the fifth week. The partition is accomplished by a series of complementary septa within the atria, the ventricles and between the aorta and pulmonary trunks. As might be expected with such a complex process, abnormalities of septation are frequent.

Atrial septal defects are among the most common congenital heart abnormalities. Normally, interatrial septation results from a crescent-shaped downgrowth (septum primum) from the posterosuperior wall of the common atrium, which meets the septum intermedium in the atrioventricular canal, thus dividing the originally single atrium into right and left halves. Before the septum primum is complete, however, small openings appear in its upper portion, which merge to form the ostium secundum, thus maintaining free passage between the two atria. To the right of the septum primum, a thicker septum secundum develops (Fig. 9.5D, E) overlapping the former. This arrangement is necessary to generate a future complete septum which will nevertheless allow blood to pass from right to left atrium until birth (foramen ovale). After birth, increased left atrial pressure apposes the two septa and closes the foramen. If, however, either septum is excessively resorbed or inadequate, an atrial septal defect occurs.

Complementary to atrial septation, the atrioventricular canal becomes divided into right and left channels by subendocardial cushions of mesenchyme constituting the septum intermedium (Fig. 9.5F). At the same time, the bulboventricular chamber is partitioned into right and left ventricles by the formation of a more or less coronally placed interventricular septum. Concomitantly, spiral ridges develop at the arterial end of the heart so that the originally single arterial trunk becomes divided into pulmonary and aortic vessels (Fig. 9.5G, H), communicating respectively with the right and left ventricles. Interventricular septation is completed by the growing together of the spiral and interventricular septa with the septum intermedium.

Such a complex series of tissue interactions means that abnormalities may occur from excessive or inadequate fusion of the different elements. Retardation of the interventricular septum leads to ventricular septal defect, which is the commonest congenital heart malformation. If the endocardial cushions fail to fuse there is a persistent common atrioventricular canal and a septal defect of both atria and ventricles. Retardation of the spiral septum causes persistent common truncus arteriosus, whereas incorrect spiralling leads to transposition of the arterial trunks which are each connected to the inappropriate ventricle. Abnormal deviation of the spiral septum to the right results in VSD and pulmonary stenosis with overriding aorta which are the principal elements of Fallot's tetralogy.

Excessive fusion of septa or cushions at various levels could lead to valve atresia such as tricuspid or pulmonary atresia. Hypoplastic left heart is a rare but very serious condition where the left atrium and ventricle and ascending aorta are all vestigially small. Coarctation of the aorta is a commoner but milder manifestation of this condition.

Blood leaving the embryonic heart travels in a cranial direction through the truncus and ventral aorta from which it is carried by six pairs of pharyngeal arch arteries to the paired dorsal aortae. Segments of this system obliterate and disappear without trace, but the third arches contribute to the carotid circulation, and the fourth arch remains on the right as part of the right subclavian artery and on the left as the arch of the aorta. The sixth arch arteries become incorporated into the pulmonary arteries, and the ductus arteriosus is a persistence of the left sixth arch forming a shunt between the pulmonary artery and the dorsal aorta. Normally, this shunt closes down shortly after birth and fibroses to a ligament, but patency of the ductus arteriosus is among the commoner congenital malformations.

DIGESTIVE AND RESPIRATORY SYSTEMS

Toward the end of the first month, the process of body cylinder formation divides the yolk sac into an extraembryonic portion, which regresses early, and an intraembryonic portion, the primitive gut, which is the origin of the digestive and respiratory tubes (and their accessories such as the liver, pancreas and gall bladder). The lungs develop from a ventral midline laryngotracheal diverticulum from the foregut; the lung buds proliferate laterally into the mesenchyme of the primitive pleural cavities. Throughout prenatal and early postnatal life the bronchi continuously divide dichotomously and, after the seventh month, the terminal branches become primitive alveoli with squamous rather than cuboid epithelium in contact with capillary endothelium. They become capable of gas exchange and some alveolar cells secrete phospholipid surfactant which facilitates expansion after birth. Before birth the alveoli are filled with liquid, including secretion by the epithelium, but after birth the liquid is absorbed and replaced by air.

Gross abnormalities of lung structure (blind trachea, agenesis of one lung) are rare. More frequently, the bronchial tree may divide abnormally, to give supernumerary lobules. These are of little significance unless they are an anatomical embarrassment forming, for example, ectopic lung lobes arising (probably as separate buds) from the trachea or oesophagus. Congenital cysts of the lung (abnormal dilatation of bronchi) may be more important if they become the site of chronic infection, as a result of being poorly ventilated and having abnormal vascularization.

The development of the digestive system is characterized by extreme complexity in its rostral pharyngeal part where there is a series of paired pharyngeal pouches (which contribute to diverse structures such as the auditory tubes, palatine tonsils, thymus, and the parathyroid and thyroid glands), extensive elongation of the middle, abdominal part, and structural interaction with the urogenital system in the terminal or cloacal portion. Agenesis or complete absence of a segment may occur but, more commonly, a portion of the gut is constricted (atresia); this can occur at any level, because a feature of normal gut development is that its lumen becomes obliterated by mucosal growth and then recanalized. Atresia is more common at sites where development of the gut is complex, for example near the respiratory diverticulum where the oesophagus may be so affected. In such cases, the cranial part may end as a blind sac and the caudal part be attached to the trachea by a fistulous canal (tracheo-oesophageal fistula) or an uncanalized ligament (oesophageal atresia); more rarely, both cranial and caudal parts open into the trachea.

During normal development the primitive midgut rotates 270° counterclockwise on the axis of the superior mesenteric artery. If rotation is incomplete (90° only) or if there is reversed (clockwise) rotation, the viscera lie in abnormal positions and may not become properly anchored by their peritoneal attachments. As a result, the bowel may become twisted (volvulus) and there is danger of lumen obstruction or of strangulation of the blood supply. The vitelline duct, which connects the midgut to the yolk sac through the umbilicus, normally obliterates and disappears but may persist abnormally as a blind (Meckel's) diverticulum or, more rarely, as an umbilical fistula.

The hind end of the gut is termed the cloaca where its endodermal lining becomes continuous with surface ectoderm, the point of transition being marked originally by the presence of the cloacal membrane. A coronal ridge (urorectal septum) develops across the cloaca, dividing it into the urogenital sinus anteriorly and the primitive rectum posteriorly (see Fig. 9.6). The former which contributes to the urinary bladder and urethra communicates with the Wolffian and Müllerian duct systems. The Wolffian ducts contribute the genital ducts in the male whereas the Müllerian ducts form the uterus and vagina in the female (see below); an offshoot of each Wolffian duct forms the ureter in both sexes. An incomplete urorectal septum may result in a fistula between the rectum and the scrotum, vagina, bladder or urethra. In the primitive rectum the corresponding part of the cloacal membrane usually breaks down in the ninth week but failure to do so will result in an imperforate anus or rectal atresia.

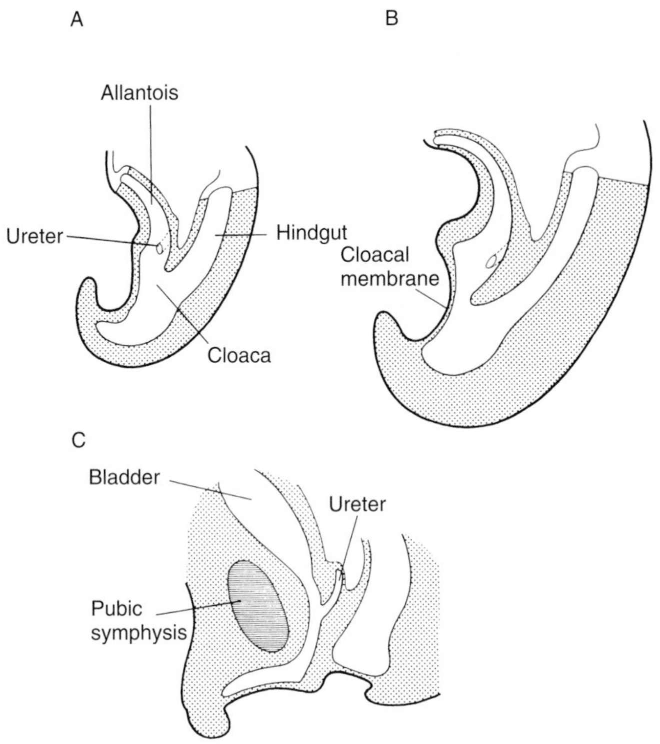

Fig. 9.6 Subdivision of the cloaca. (A) At the beginning of the fifth week, the cloaca is continuous with the allantois and hindgut. (B) By the seventh week, it becomes divided coronally by the urorectal septum into the urogenital sinus anteriorly and an anorectal canal posteriorly. (C) By 9 weeks the ureters have opened into the anterior chamber, which forms the bladder and urethra; the anal membrane breaks down thus opening the anorectal canal.

UROGENITAL SYSTEM

The urinary and genital systems both develop from the ridge of intermediate mesoderm on the posterior abdominal wall and both systems empty by ducts into the urogenital sinus section of the cloaca (Fig. 9.6). The nephrogenic part of the intermediate mesoderm differentiates successively into pronephros, mesonephros and metanephros. These three structures succeed each other not only in time but in space, in a cephalocaudal direction. The pronephros may be thought of as a rough draft and is rapidly replaced by the mesonephros, which attains functional capacity producing a dilute urine, but later regresses (Fig. 9.7); its remnants are incorporated into the urogenital system especially in the male. The metanephros forms the definitive kidney.

The mesonephric (Wolffian) duct receives the products of the mesonephric tubules and drains into the urogenital sinus. Differentiation of the metanephros begins in the sacral region at the start of the second month, when its blastema, contributing the glomeruli, proximal and distal tubules and loop of Henle, is penetrated by the ureteric bud (arising from the lower part of the Wolffian duct) which will constitute the collecting system. If differentiation of the ureteric bud or metanephric duct is defective, or junction between it and the metanephros fails, urine from the excretory portion of the kidney cannot be drained, leading to single or multiple congenital cysts.

Renal agenesis occurs in the absence of the ureteric bud, since the presence of the bud induces formation of the excretory parts of the kidney. Bilateral absence is rare, but unilateral agenesis occurs in about 1 : 1500 individuals. If the ureteric bud divides, the metanephric tissue may also divide, resulting in a double kidney or double ureter. Occasionally, ectopic ureters may open into the vagina or urethra rather than into the bladder.

Although the metanephros develops from the most caudal part of the urogenital mesodermal ridge, the adult kidney 'ascends' to the upper lumbar region as a result of diminution of body curvature and differential growth in the sacral and lumbar regions. Occasionally, a kidney fails to ascend and remains in the pelvis. If the lower poles of the two kidneys fuse, the result is a horseshoe kidney, the cranial progression of which is arrested at lower lumbar level by the inferior mesenteric artery.

The gonad differentiates from a ridge of intermediate mesoderm on the medial side of the middle of the mesonephros and, until the end of the sixth week, it has the same morphological appearance in both sexes despite underlying chromosomal differences which can be identified by tests such as analysis of amniotic smears. The first urogenital connection is established when the indifferent gonad anastomoses with the adjacent mesonephric tubules. Later, however, the chromosome constitution (in particular the SRY gene on the Y chromosome) determines differentiation of the genital gland into a testis or an ovary. Subsequent male differentiation is stimulated by testicular hormones, with development and differentiation of Wolffian structures and regression of Müllerian structures. Female differentiation is related to the absence of the SRY gene and androgens, Müllerian structures being promoted while Wolffian development is inhibited.

Until the seventh week of development, the genital tracts also have the same appearance in both sexes; they consist of the two Wolffian ducts and the two Müllerian or paramesonephric ducts, which form by invagination of coelomic epithelium lateral to the mesonephros. Caudally, the two Müllerian ducts approach each other and fuse to form a single median duct, which regresses in the male but becomes the uterovaginal canal in the female. The median septum should disappear at the end of the third month; lack of fusion of the ducts or non-elimination of the septum may lead to a double or bicornuate uterus and possibly to a double vagina. Partial or total atresia of the terminal portion of one or both Müllerian ducts may result in atresia of cervix or vagina. The mesonephric duct system largely disappears in the female, but parts may remain as cystic structures in the broad ligament (parovarian) or alongside the vagina.

In the male the mesonephric (Wolffian) duct becomes

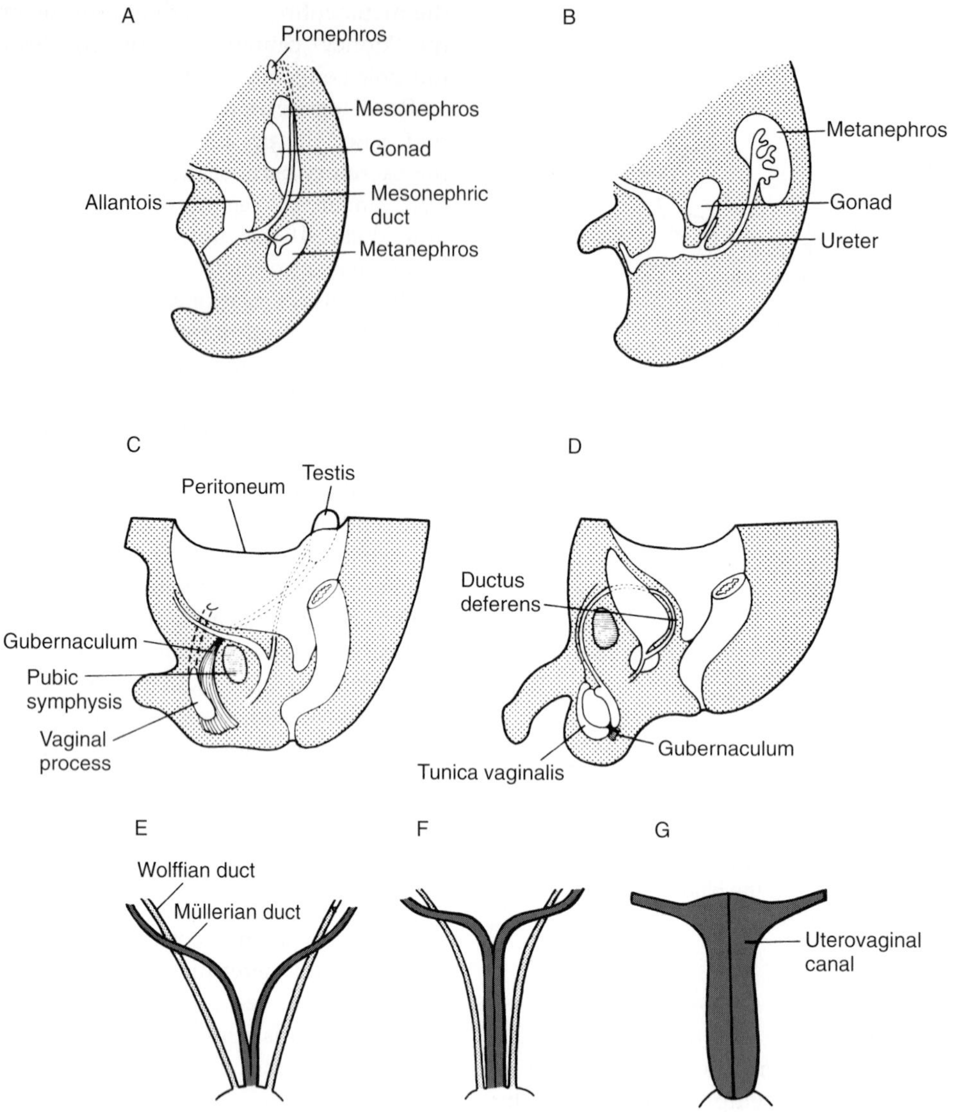

Fig. 9.7 (A) The intermediate mesoderm on the dorsal body wall differentiates between 21 and 28 days into pro-, meso- and metanephros in craniocaudal succession; the gonad differentiates medial to the mesonephros. (B) The metanephros develops at a sacral level but 'migrates' cranially. It is drained by the ureteric bud from the primitive mesonephric (Wolffian) duct. (C, D) Testicular descent; the testis migrates from its dorsal position (C, fifth month) to its definitive position in the scrotum (D, 8–9 months) guided by the gubernaculum. (E) By the seventh week, both Müllerian and Wolffian ducts are present. (F, G) the caudal ends of the Müllerian ducts fuse to form the uterus, the median septum disappearing in the third month.

the main genital duct; the connecting mesonephric tubules contribute the vasa efferentia and, possibly, a few blind aberrant tubules. The paramesonephric duct, if it is retained at all, contributes only small tubular remnants in the prostate or, rarely, near the upper pole of the testis.

Initially, the external genitalia also go through an indifferent stage. In both sexes, ridges (the cloacal folds) form on either side of the cloacal membrane with a genital (phallic) tubercle ventrally. The cloacal folds then divide into scrotal and urethral portions. In the male, the urethral folds fuse ventrally to enclose the penile urethra and the scrotal folds unite along a midline cutaneous raphe. Hypospadias occurs when fusion of the urethral folds is incomplete. More rarely, the genital tubercle also divides, so that its two components lie either side of the urethral groove. This results in epispadias and may occur with exstrophy of the bladder, in which the anterior abdominal wall and anterior bladder wall are both deficient.

In the female, the genital tubercle remains relatively smaller, as the clitoris; the urethral folds become the labia minora and the scrotal folds the labia majora.

FURTHER READING

In this chapter, the commonest congenital malformations have been used as broad foci for relevant descriptions of organogenesis, which of necessity have had to be synoptic. For more detailed and sequential accounts of human development, including correlation with experimental data, readers are advised to consult a specialized textbook of which a few recent examples are listed below.

Carlson B M 1994 Human embryology and developmental biology. Mosby Year Book, St Louis

Larsen W J 1997 Human embryology, 2nd edn. Churchill Livingstone, Edinburgh

McLachlan J 1994 Medical embryology. Addison Wesley, Wokingham

Moore K L, Persaud T V N 1993 The developing human, 5th edn. W B Saunders, Philadelphia

Williams P L 1995 Gray's anatomy, 38th edn. Churchill Livingstone, Edinburgh

10

Fetal growth, intrauterine growth retardation and small for gestational age babies

N. R. C. Roberton

INTRODUCTION

In the 1950s and 1960s there was a recognition that about one-third of babies included within the World Health Assembly's 1948 definition of prematurity – a birthweight less than 2500 g – were not truly premature (that is, less than 37 completed weeks of gestation) but were inappropriately small.[15] These were recognized as an at-risk group. The 1958 UK perinatal survey stated that 'in mature or prolonged pregnancies, premature [sic] babies have a mortality rate that is 8 times higher than for babies weighing over 2500 g'.[5]

Two contemporaneous papers established the norms for late fetal growth (Fig. 10.1), groups particularly at risk and what were then thought to be common clinical associations.[22,49]

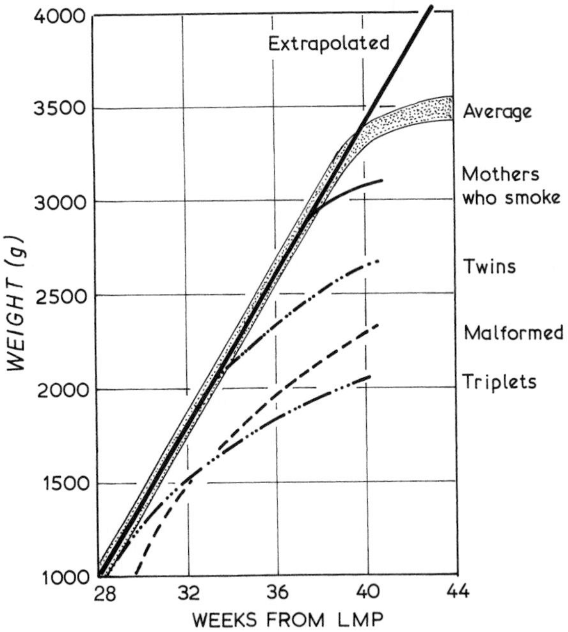

Fig. 10.1 Variation in fetal growth during the last trimester of pregnancy. The 'average' baby grows steadily until about 40 weeks of gestation, after which growth slows. Babies of mothers who smoke, and twins and triplets who have to share the nutrient supply from the placenta, start their slow growth sooner. The malformed baby has often grown slowly from early in the second trimester. (From Gruenwald[22] with permission.)

NOMENCLATURE AND DEFINITION

Various terms have been used to describe babies whose weight is low for their gestational age, including intrauterine growth retardation or restriction, fetal malnutrition, light for dates and small for dates. Although there is much to be said for the term light for dates, as many of these babies are of normal length and head circumference (see below) despite being of low birthweight, the term small for dates is now widely accepted and will be used here.

The definition of SFD varies with the purpose of the study in question. As with all biological phenomena, the 3rd centile, approximating to –2 standard deviations from the mean (strictly speaking –2 SD = 2.3rd centile) is the most mathematically acceptable definition. However, because of anxieties about morbidity, in particular from hypoglycaemia, in SFD babies, many neonatal units screen for this condition in all babies below the 5th or even 10th centile for birthweight. The validity of such practice is discussed below.

Even if the 3rd centile is taken as the cut-off, it has to be remembered that this is a mathematical concept which has been found useful in clinical practice to identify a population that is likely to include sufficient abnormal members to justify a screening procedure. However, the majority of the 3% of babies who, by definition, must fall below the 3rd centile will be the normal smallest members of a population who are not at risk from the problems of either fetal growth restriction in utero, or from the problems listed below, which occur in pathologically small for dates babies.[6]

FETAL GROWTH

Growth in the fetal period, usually defined as from the 12th week after the first day of the last menstrual period (i.e. 10 weeks from conception) has been assessed in two ways. First, morbid anatomists measured fetuses, stillbirths or neonatal deaths at autopsy and weighed their organs; secondly, in the last 20 years multiple ultrasound measurements of fetal growth have been made and translated into centile charts (Figs 10.2–10.7; Table 10.1).

The ultrasound data in Figures 10.2–10.6 are derived from British women,[8] those in Table 10.1 from Texan ones.[24] Small differences do exist, highlighting the fact that growth charts should be derived from studies of local populations.

In general, linear growth tends to be arithmetic (Figs 10.2–10.6) until close to the end of pregnancy, whereas organ growth, assessed from autopsy data, tends to be logarithmic (Fig. 10.7).

Brain growth (not shown in Fig. 10.7) normally follows the top organ growth trajectory, rising from about 25% of term weight at 24 weeks to 38% at 28 weeks and 68% at 34 weeks.[51] There is, therefore, a curious paradox that antenatal ultrasound measurements of head size, BPD and OFC (Figs 10.1, 10.3), are flattening off towards the end of the third trimester of pregnancy, whereas brain growth is actually accelerating. Furthermore, simple measurements such as weight disguise complex underlying changes in brain growth. By measuring brain DNA phosphorus[14] it is possible to show that fetal brain growth has two distinct phases (Fig. 10.8). The first, from 10 to 18 weeks, is associated with neuronal development; the second phase, from 18 weeks to term and beyond, is that of glial cell proliferation. The increasing weight of the brain through late fetal life, infancy and early childhood is due not only to glial cell development, but to a massive increase in the size of cells, dendritic proliferation and myelination.

TYPES OF SFD BABY

Table 10.2 gives a practical classification of SFD babies.

FETAL ABNORMALITY

There are many conditions that can blight the embryo and fetus early in gestation (Table 10.2).[26] The baby is usually ill at birth or has a recognizable dysmorphic syndrome. Taking a history from the mother may identify a teratogen. The problems from which these babies suffer are those of the primary condition considered elsewhere

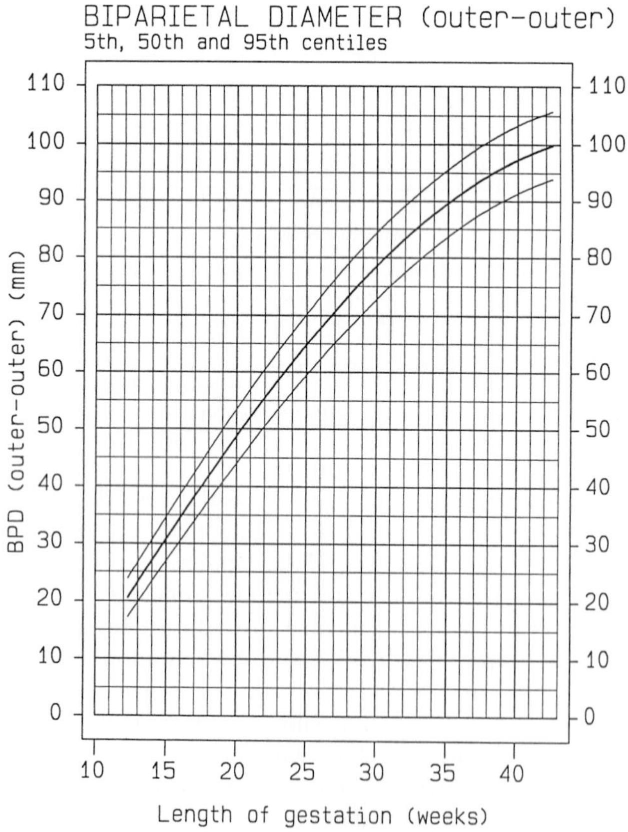

Fig. 10.2 Ultrasound measurement of fetal biparietal diameter. (From Chitty and Altman[8] with permission)

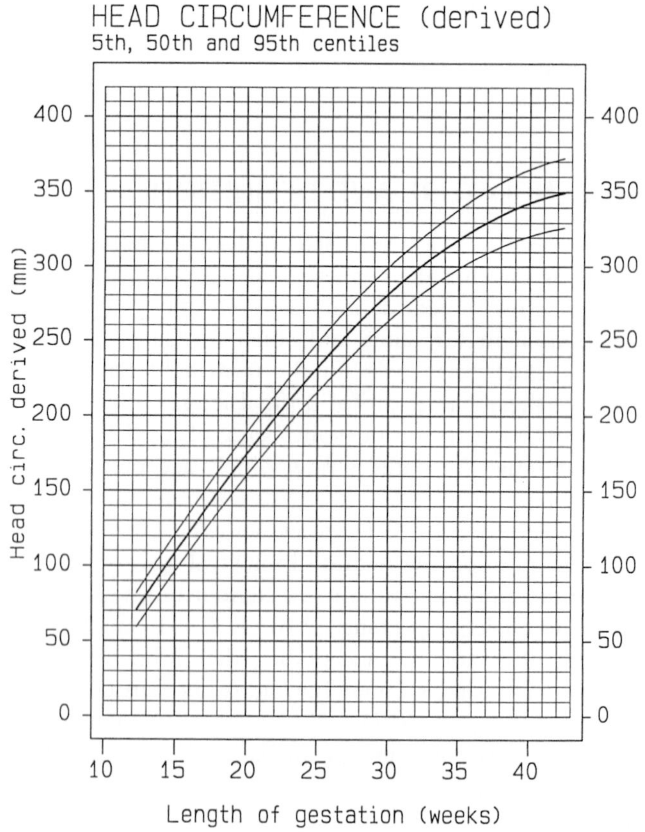

Fig. 10.3 Fetal head circumference during gestation. (From Chitty and Altman[8] with permission)

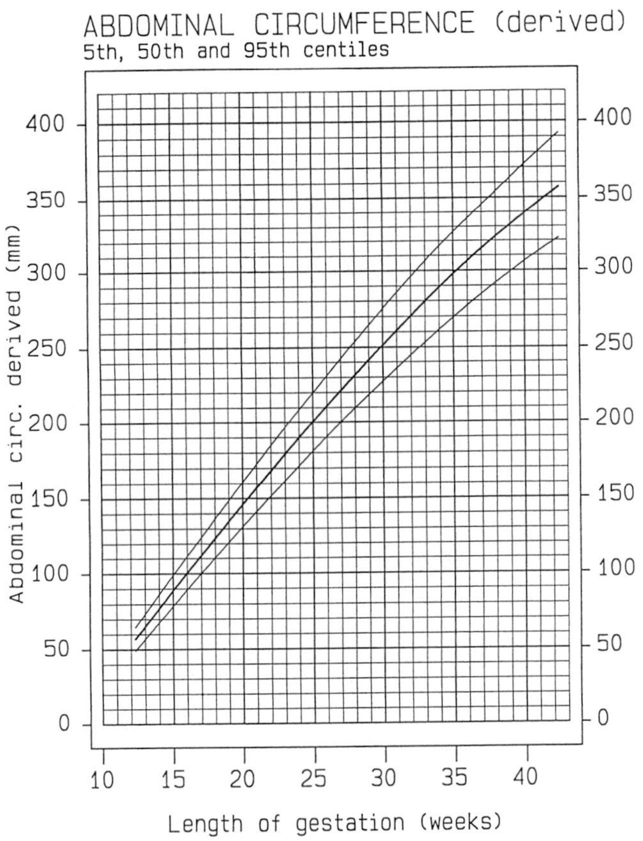

Fig. 10.4 Fetal abdominal circumference during gestation. (From Chitty and Altman[8] with permission)

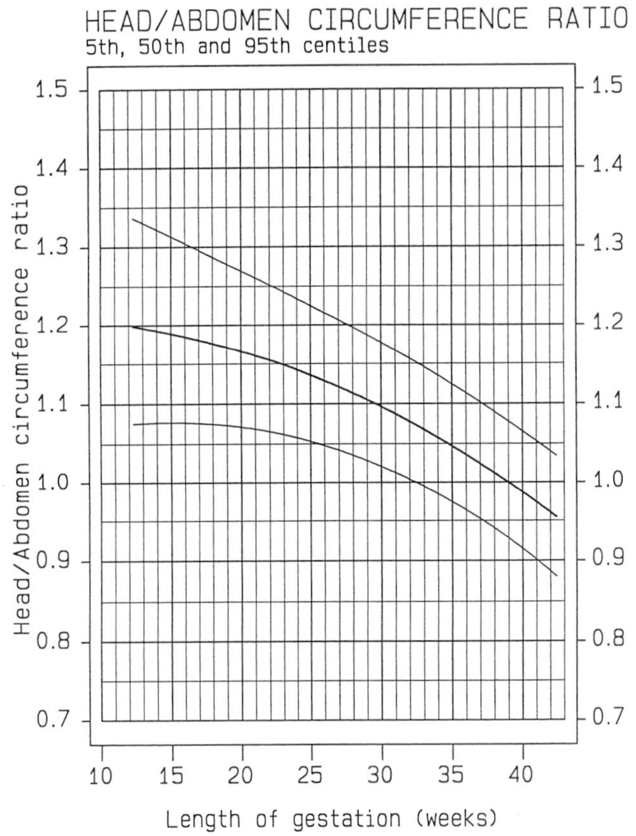

Fig. 10.5 Head/abdomen circumference ratio during gestation. (From Chitty and Altman[8] with permission)

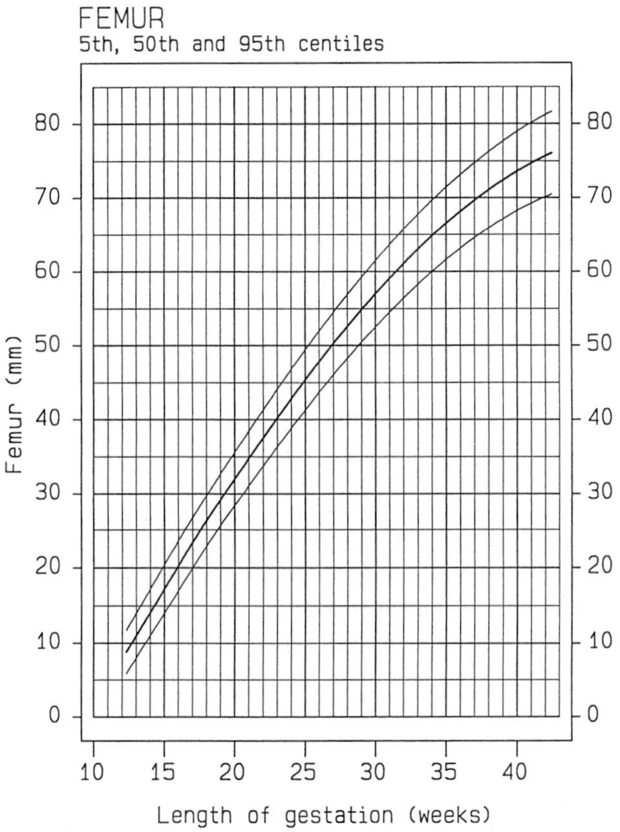

Fig. 10.6 Fetal femur length during gestation. (From Chitty and Altman[8] with permission)

Table 10.1 Relationship between selected fetal indices as measured by ultrasound and gestational age as determined by menstrual weeks (From Hadlock F P et al,[24] with permission)

Menstrual age (wk)	Biparietal diameter (cm)	Head circumference (cm)	Abdominal circumference (cm)	Femur length (cm)
12	2	7.1	5.6	0.8
13	2.3	8.4	6.9	1.1
14	2.7	9.8	8.1	1.5
15	3	11.1	9.3	1.8
16	3.3	12.4	10.5	2.1
17	3.7	13.7	11.7	2.4
18	4	15	12.9	2.7
19	4.3	16.3	14.1	3
20	4.6	17.5	15.2	3.3
21	5	18.7	16.4	3.6
22	5.3	19.9	17.5	3.9
23	5.6	21	18.6	4.2
24	5.8	22.1	19.7	4.4
25	6.1	23.2	20.8	4.7
26	6.4	24.2	21.9	4.9
27	6.7	25.2	22.9	5.2
28	7	26.2	24	5.4
29	7.2	27.1	25	5.6
30	7.5	28	26	5.8
31	7.7	28.9	27	6.1
32	7.9	29.7	28	6.3
33	8.2	30.4	29	6.5
34	8.4	31.2	30	6.6
35	8.6	31.8	30.9	6.8
36	8.8	32.5	31.8	7
37	9	33.1	32.7	7.2
38	9.1	33.6	33.6	7.3
39	9.3	34.1	34.5	7.5
40	9.5	34.5	35.4	7.6

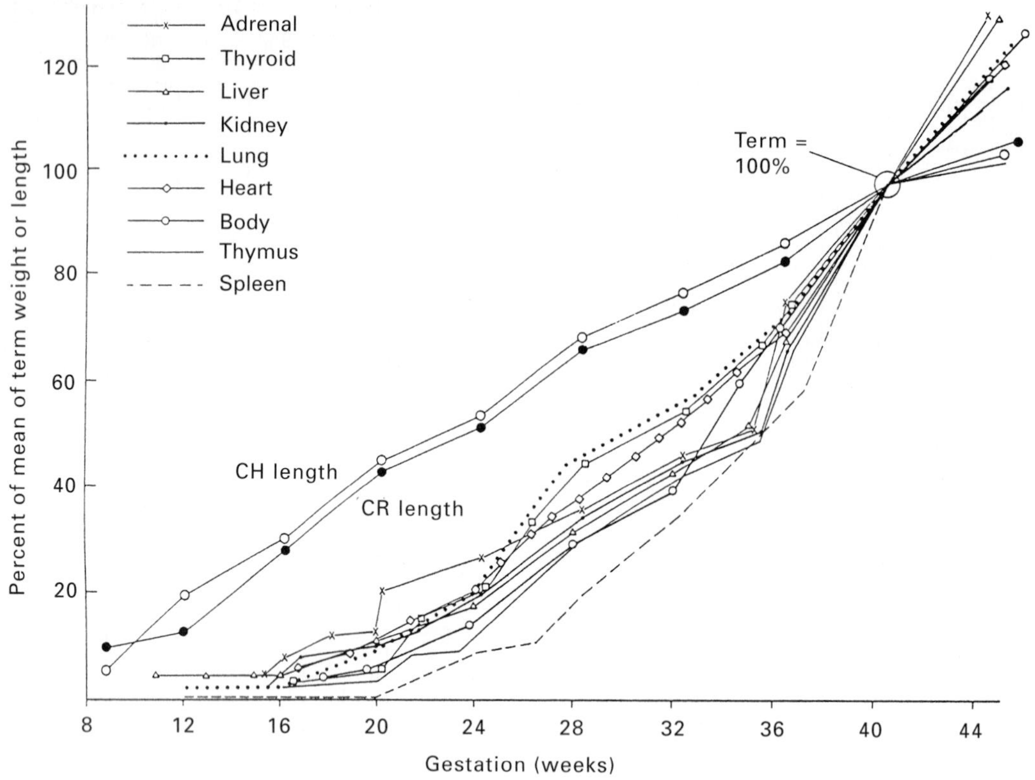

Fig. 10.7 Growth of fetal body length compared with body and organ weights. Linear growth tends to be arithmetic, while weights of the body and internal organs tend to increase geometrically. (From Singer et al[51] with permission) CH, crown–heel length; CR, crown–rump length.

Table 10.2 Classification of SFD

Fetal abnormality	Fetal poisoning	Constitutional	Reduced supply
Chromosomal e.g. Down, trisomy 18	Drugs: Recreational, therapeutic	Small parents	Socioeconomic
Congenital infection, e.g. rubella, CMV	Smoking	Ethnic	Altitude
	Alcohol		Malnutrition
Syndromes e.g. Silver	Ionizing radiation		Maternal ill health
			Illness in pregnancy
General Congenital malformation e.g. TOF, CHD, (Table 10.3)			Uteroplacental compromise
			Twinning

in this book, and are not those of the otherwise normal growth-retarded fetus described below.

Almost all congenital malformations, such as congenital heart disease, neural tube malformations and diaphragmatic hernia, that are compatible with long-term neurologically normal follow-up after corrective surgery in the neonatal period are likely to be associated with growth retardation at birth (Table 10.3).

FETAL POISONING

All forms of recreational drug abuse cause SFD babies. Mothers who drink alcohol to excess will have SFD babies with fetal alcohol syndrome. Mills et al[35] found that more than three standard drinks per day reduced birthweight by 100–150 g, and at least three to four drinks per day are necessary to cause the full fetal alcohol syndrome.[44] The mean birthweight of babies of women who drank heavily throughout pregnancy was 2.55 kg.[3] Although studies in Scotland and the Netherlands showed that normal social drinking in pregnancy has no ill effects,[19,56] Mills et al[35] showed that even the occasional drink resulted in a statistically significant reduction in birthweight of 14 g; whether this is clinically significant must be a matter of conjecture.

Smoking in pregnancy has long been known to cause fetal growth retardation,[11,17] reducing birthweight by 200–300 g. Alcohol plus smoking may be synergistic.[56]

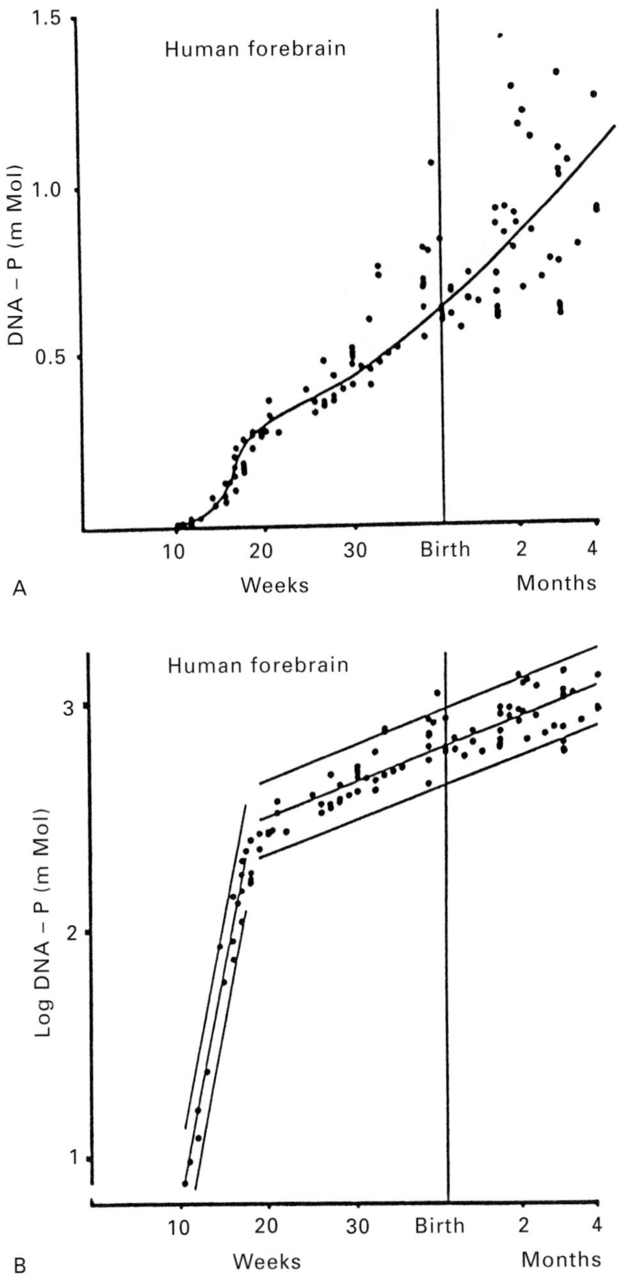

Fig. 10.8 Total DNA-P, equivalent to total cell number in the human forebrain from 10 gestational weeks to 4 postnatal months, showing the two-phase characteristics of prenatal cell multiplication. (B) A semilogarithmic plot of the same data that appear in (A) to show the sharp separation of the two phases at 18 gestational weeks. Regression lines with 95% confidence limits are added. (From Dobbing and Sands[14] with permission)

The deleterious effects of maternal smoking carry on into infancy: SFD infants of smoking women are readmitted to hospital more often than control SFD infants of non-smoking mothers.[57]

Addictive drugs, such as heroin (Chapter 28),[36] cocaine[7,64] and amphetamines,[32] but with the possible exception of cannabis,[13] also reduce birthweight but in such cases it is difficult to tease out the multiple social and medical factors that might compromise fetal growth in drug-abusing mothers.

Therapeutic drug use may also cause fetal malformations, and hence fetal growth restriction. The important teratogenic agents are listed in Chapters 9 and 26.

Table 10.3 Growth retardation and congenital malformation[26]

Disorder	% < 10th centile
Trisomy 18	83.7
Anencephaly	73.3
Gastroschisis	60.3
Oesophageal atresia	55.3
Renal agenesis	54.9
Trisomy 13	51.3
Omphalocoele	43.5
Intestinal atresia	42.7
Tetralogy of Fallot	33.6
Spina bifida	32.0
Cataract	31.5
Bladder exstrophy	31.2
Down syndrome	31.0
Choanal atresia	30.2
Cleft palate	30.2
ASD	29.8
Diaphragmatic hernia	29.5
Patent ductus arteriosus	29.5
Sex chromosome syndromes	28.2
Endocardial cushion defect	28.2
Coarctation	28.1
Hydrocephalus	27.9
VSD	27.4
Urinary tract obstruction	26.4
Hare lip, cleft palate	25.7
Cystic kidneys	25.5

CONSTITUTIONAL

At least half of all SFD babies in Britain have no known cause. They are proportionately small; that is, their weight, length and head circumference are all on the 3rd centile or below. In general these babies pose no obstetric or neonatal problems.[6]

Small women have small babies, what Ounsted and Ounsted[41] called the maternal constraint of fetal size, the most dramatic example of which is the different foal sizes in Shire horse–Shetland crosses (Fig. 10.9).[60] Some women were themselves SFD, though of normal weight in adult life, and produce SFD babies and thin babies[20,29,41] and go on producing SFD babies.[40]

Race is an important cause of this smallness for dates (Table 10.4),[34,50] having complex interrelationships with maternal nutrition (see below). A major practical implication of the ethnic differences in birthweight is the relevance of birthweight centiles derived from, for example, an indigenous sea-level Caucasian population to babies born in the same city or state to ethnic minorities with small mothers. Smallness for dates under such circumstances will be grossly overdiagnosed, leading to unwarranted, wasteful and potentially harmful intervention.

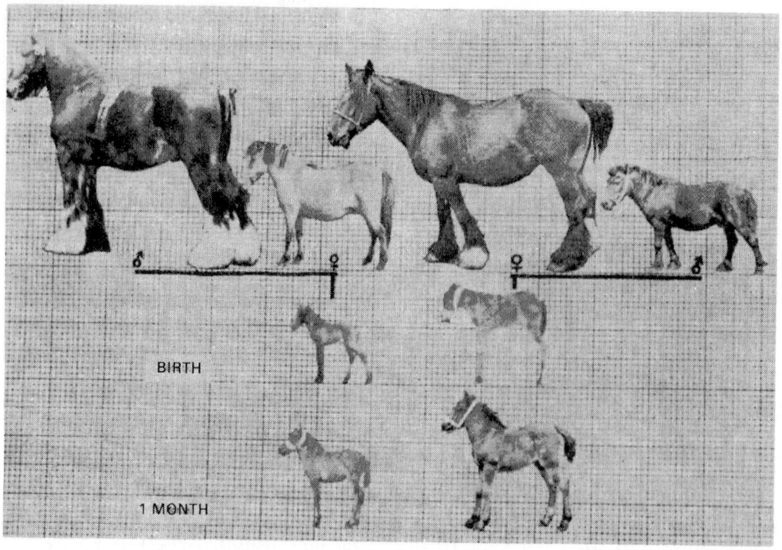

Fig. 10.9 Parents and offspring of reciprocal Shetland–Shire crosses. Note that where the mother was the Shetland pony, the foal was significantly smaller at birth and remained small at the age of 1 month. (From Walton and Hammond[60] with permission)

Table 10.4 Mean body weight at birth of different ethnic groups (From Meredith[34] with permission)

Group	Years studied	Weight in kg
Bambuti Pygmy	1956–59	2.64
Indian	1947–63	2.74
Ghanaian	1950–59	2.89
Malayan	1951–59	2.99
Japanese	1948–54	3.07
North Italian	1942–63	3.25
Swiss	1948–60	3.29
USA (White)	1962–65	3.32
British	1947–64	3.35
Norwegian	1955	3.45
USA (Amerindian)	1964–66	3.60

REDUCED SUPPLY (INTRAUTERINE GROWTH RETARDATION)

Many SFD babies were genetically and biologically intended to be of normal birthweight, but their growth in utero was compromised by maternal illness or defective function of the uteroplacental unit (Table 10.2). It is often said that such babies can be divided into two groups: those who are proportionally growth retarded, in which all measurements at birth fall below the 3rd centile, and those whose weight is below the 3rd centile but in whom length and head size are preserved. This concept is probably no longer tenable, as it is more likely that there is a continuum of growth abnormalities ranging between the two phenotypic extremes. The work of Fancourt et al[16] suggests that symmetrical growth retardation may well be the marker of more prolonged fetal compromise originating in the second trimester. The consequences of both of these types of IUGR are in general similar,[12,28] although the disproportionately SFD baby with a low ponderal index (weight (kg) × 100/length^3) is more prone to neonatal hypoglycaemia[59] and the proportionately SFD baby whose growth retardation started earlier in gestation during critical periods of brain growth may do less well on follow-up.[16]

The disproportionately small for dates babies were first clearly described by Gruenwald.[21] He described babies of normal length and head circumference who had some, but not complete, sparing of brain growth, but very small livers, lungs and thymuses at autopsy. These babies merge into a group of babies of similar scrawny appearance[10] whose weights are within the normal range, who were presumably programmed to be large babies until some cause of IUGR took over. These babies with Clifford syndrome are prone to the same complications as IUGR babies with weights below the 3rd centile.

This type of IUGR is the result of one of multiple causes of failure to deliver enough oxygen or nutrition to the fetus.[46,52] The end result, however, is the same: fetal hypoxia, hypoglycaemia and hypoaminoacidaemia with a fall-off in the level of many fetal growth-promoting hormones, including insulin, thyroxine and IGF. In response to this hostile in utero environment, growth of non-essential organs and tissues such as the adrenal, subcutaneous fat, the reticuloendothelial system and the liver is reduced; glycogen, as a nutritional reserve, is not laid down in liver or myocardium. Eventually brain growth, and thus head circumference, will be compromised, as will linear growth.

It is this group of SFD babies with IUGR resulting from reduced supply that are at risk from intrauterine fetal death and neonatal hypoglycaemia (p. 946). It is also the group that obstetricians put in a great deal of effort to detect antenatally. This is done initially by noting a fall-off in the ultrasound measurements of the fetal abdominal circumference, a poor rise in ultrasound-estimated fetal weight, and by a reduction in the rate of growth of the fetal skull (OFC/BPD). However, as Chard et al[6] emphasize, the majority of infants found antenatally to be small are normal: what matters is when fetal growth falls below the normal range (see Fig. 10.1).

CAUSES OF INTRAUTERINE GROWTH RETARDATION

Socioeconomic factors

It was originally thought that women who delivered IUGR babies came from depressed socioeconomic surroundings,[22,49] but more recent studies, once maternal size and race, drugs and smoking are allowed for, show that socioeconomic factors are much less significant.[1,2,4,27,42]

Altitude

Babies born at altitude in Colorado or Bolivia are smaller than those born at sea level.[31,54]

Malnutrition

Severe malnutrition imposed on a previously healthy well-grown population during the Nazi occupation of the Netherlands in 1944–45 resulted in a 300–400 g fall in birthweight and an increased neonatal morbidity, including malformations.[53,63]

In severely malnourished women in the developing world, where SFD babies are common (Table 10.4), nutritional supplements during pregnancy will also improve birthweight.[37,45,62] Nutritional supplements given to all pregnant women in these countries have little effect, but a prolonged period of adequate nutrition after emigration to a developed country, improvements in local nutrition over a period of years, or taking the food supplements for several pregnancies, all increase birthweight.[9,23,58] Wharton[61] studied low bodyweight Asian women living in England and divided them into those who were and were not malnourished, on the basis of skinfold thickness. Giving food supplements during pregnancy only increased the birthweight of babies born to malnourished women. In the poor, relatively malnourished black population of New York, caloric supplementation had no effect on birthweight and a high protein supplement increased the prematurity rate and neonatal mortality.[47,48] In Britain a low protein intake in late pregnancy and a high carbohydrate intake in early pregnancy produces thin though not necessarily small for dates babies.[20]

Maternal ill health

Almost every major illness in pregnancy will reduce fetal growth, important examples being serious maternal heart disease, chronic renal disease, collagen diseases and haemoglobinopathy. These are considered in greater detail in Chapter 13.

Proteinuric hypertension (pre-eclampsia)

This is probably the single largest cause of smallness for dates, as the result of changes produced in the placenta. It is discussed in detail in Chapter 15.

Placental factors

Abnormalities of placentation can cause IUGR babies. Circumvallate placentae and chorioangiomas have a particularly bad reputation, together with single umbilical arteries.[38]

Twins (Chapter 25)

Twins and higher multiples are often SFD; fetal growth tails off during the third trimester (see Fig. 10.1). Twins are very much at risk from the sequelae of being SFD, in particular intrapartum asphyxia and postnatal hypoglycaemia.

COMPLICATIONS IN SFD BABIES

The studies quoted at the beginning of this chapter imply an alarming increase in the morbidity and mortality of SFD babies. The problem for the obstetrician is intrauterine death and intrapartum asphyxia (Chapter 12). Postnatally the problems listed in Table 10.5 have, at various times, been said to be important, but in 1999 the only significant postnatal problem is hypoglycaemia, which is dealt with at length in Chapter 38, Part 1, and necrotizing enterocolitis in those with reduced fetal gut blood flow (p. 748).

SFD babies more often require resuscitation in the labour ward (Table 10.6),[28] have lower Apgar scores [33] and have more HIE.[18,30] Hypothermia is always preventable (p. 294), meconium aspiration is a disease of

Table 10.5 Problems in SFD

Hypoglycaemia
Birth asphyxia
Pulmonary disease
meconium aspiration
MPH
Hypothermia
Congenital malformation
Polycythaemia
Coagulopathy
Infection

Table 10.6 Incidence of birth asphyxia (requiring IPPV > 1 minute) in SFD and normal neonates (From MacDonald et al[33], with permission)

Gestation	SFD (%)	AFD (%)
≤36/52	36.6	6.2
>36/52	4.1	0.36

postmaturity (p. 538) and MPH no longer occurs in asphyxiated SFD babies (p. 550). With fetal screening (Chapter 14) significant malformations are now rare and were not a problem in the study of mature SFD babies in Cambridge.[25] SFD babies are often polycythaemic but this is rarely if ever a clinical problem, nor are problems with coagulation or infection frequent in our experience.[25]

THE PRETERM SFD BABY

It is now recognized that these babies are at increased risk from complications of prematurity compared to normally grown controls; in particular they develop more severe RDS (p. 485) and are at increased risk from NEC (p. 748).

A particular problem is the twin pair in which one twin is grossly small for dates – in the 500–750 g bracket compared to a normally grown sibling between 26 and 32 weeks. The prognosis for the growth-retarded twin, both in utero and after delivery, is poor.

FOLLOW-UP

This is dealt with in detail in Chapter 7. However, SFD babies do badly compared to normally grown controls, whether term or preterm. SFD babies have a much higher incidence of CP on follow-up than appropriately grown babies.[43,55] Even term SFD babies whose perinatal and neonatal course was completely normal do less well than normally grown controls, having IQ measurements 5–10 points lower on follow-up.[39] This is particularly true in those with reduced head growth from the time of the second trimester.[16]

REFERENCES

1. Abrams B, Newman V 1991 Small for gestational age birth. Maternal predictors and comparison with risk factors of spontaneous preterm delivery in the same cohort. American Journal of Obstetrics and Gynecology 164: 785–790
2. Arbuckle T E, Sherman G J 1989 Comparison of the risk factors for pre-term delivery and intrauterine growth retardation. Paediatric and Perinatal Epidemiology 3: 115–129
3. Autti-Ramo I, Korkman M, Hilakivi-Clark L et al 1992 Mental development of two year old children exposed to alcohol in utero. Journal of Pediatrics 120: 740–746
4. Brooke O G, Anderson H R, Bland J M et al 1989 Effects on birthweight of smoking, alcohol, caffeine, socioeconomic factors and psychosocial stress. British Medical Journal 298: 795–801
5. Butler N R, Bonham D G 1963 Perinatal mortality. E & S Livingstone, Edinburgh
6. Chard T, Yoong A, Maclntosh M 1993 The myth of fetal growth retardation at term. British Journal of Obstetrics and Gynaecology 100: 1076–1081
7. Chasnoff I J 1991 Cocaine and pregnancy: clinical and methodological issues. Clinics in Perinatology 18: 113–123
8. Chitty L, Altman D G 1993 Charts of fetal size. In: Dewbury K et al, eds. Ultrasound in obstetrics and gynaecology. Churchill Livingstone, Edinburgh,
9. Clarson C L, Barker M J, Marshall T, Wharton B A 1982 Secular changes in birthweight of Asian babies born in Birmingham. Archives of Disease in Childhood 57: 867–871
10. Clifford S H 1954 Post-maturity with placental dysfunction. Journal of Pediatrics 44: 1–13
11. Conter V, Cortinovis I, Rogari P. Riva L 1995 Weight growth in infants born to mothers who smoked during pregnancy. British Medical Journal 310: 768–771
12. Cuttini M, Cortinovis I, Bossi A, Vonderweid U de 1991 Proportionality of small for gestational age babies as a predictor of neonatal mortality and morbidity. Paediatric and Perinatal Epidemiology 5: 56–63
13. Day N L, Richardson G A 1991 Prenatal marijuana use: epidemiology, methodologic issues and infant outcome. Clinics in Perinatology 18: 77–91
14. Dobbing J, Sands J 1973 The quantitative growth and development of the human brain. Archives of Disease in Childhood 48: 757–767
15. Douglas J W B 1950 Some factors associated with prematurity. Journal of Obstetrics and Gynaecology of the British Empire 57: 143–170
16. Fancourt R, Campbell S, Harvey D, Norman A P 1976 Follow-up study of small for dates babies. British Medical Journal i: 1435–1437
17. Fielding J E 1978 Smoking and pregnancy. New England Journal of Medicine 298: 337–339
18. Finer N N, Robertson C M, Richards R T et al 1981 Hypoxic ischemic encephalopathy in term neonates: perinatal factors and outcome. Journal of Pediatrics 98: 112–117
19. Forrest F, Florey C du V, Taylor D et al 1991 Reported social alcohol consumption during pregnancy, and infant's development at 18 months. British Medical Journal 303: 22–26
20. Godfrey K M, Barker D J P, Robinson S, Osmond C 1997 Maternal birthweight and diet in pregnancy in relation to the infant's thinness at birth. British Journal of Obstetrics and Gynaecology 104: 663–667
21. Gruenwald P 1963 Chronic fetal distress and placental insufficiency. Biologia Neonatorum 5: 215–265
22. Gruenwald P 1966 Growth of the human fetus. I. Normal growth and its variation. American Journal of Obstetrics and Gynecology 94: 112–121
23. Gruenwald P, Funakawa H, Mitani S et al 1967 Influence of environmental factors on foetal growth in man. Lancet i: 1026–1029
24. Hadlock F P, Deter R L, Harrist R B, Park S K 1983 Computer assisted analysis of fetal age in the third trimester using multiple fetal growth parameters. Journal of Clinical Ultrasound 11: 313–316
25. Jones R A K, Roberton N R C 1986 Small for dates babies: are they really a problem? Archives of Disease in Childhood 61: 877–880
26. Khoury M J, Erickson J D, Cordero J F, McCarthy B J 1988 Congenital malformations and intrauterine growth retardation: a population study. Pediatrics 82: 83–90
27. Kramer M S, 1980 Intrauterine growth and gestational duration determinants. Pediatrics 80: 502–511
28. Kramer M S, Oliver M, McClean F H et al 1990 Impact of intrauterine growth retardation and body proportionality on fetal and neonatal outcome. Pediatrics 86: 707–713
29. Leff M, Orleans M, Haverkamp A D et al 1992 The association of maternal low birthweight and infant low birthweight in a racially mixed population. Pediatric and Perinatal Epidemiology 6: 51–61
30. Levene M I, Kornberg J, Williams T H C 1985 The incidence and severity of post-asphyxial encephalopathy in full term infants. Early Human Development 11: 21–26.
31. Lichty J A, Ting R Y, Bruns P D, Dyar E 1957 Studies of babies born at high altitudes. Relation of altitude to birthweight. American Journal of Diseases of Children 93: 666–669
32. Little B B, Snell L M, Gilstrap L C 1988 Methamphetamine abuse during pregnancy: outcome and fetal effects. Obstetrics and Gynecology 72: 541–544

33. MacDonald H M, Mulligan J C, Allen A C, Taylor P M 1980 Neonatal asphyxia: 1. Relationship of obstetric and neonatal complications to neonatal mortality in 405 consecutive deliveries. Journal of Pediatrics 96: 898–902
34. Meredith H V 1970 Bodyweight at birth of viable human infants. A worldwide comparative treatise. Human Biology 42: 217–264
35. Mills J L, Graubard B I, Harley E E, et al 1984 Maternal alcohol consumption and birthweight. Journal of the American Medical Association 252: 1875–1879
36. Naeye R L, Blanc W, Leblanc W, Khatamee M A 1973 Fetal complications of maternal heroin addiction: abnormal growth, infections, and episodes of stress. Journal of Pediatrics 83: 1055–1061
37. Naismith D J 1983 Maternal nutrition and fetal health. In: Chiswick M L ed. Recent advances in perinatal medicine. Churchill Livingstone, Edinburgh, pp. 21–39
38. Neerhof M G 1995 Causes of intrauterine growth restriction. Clinics in Perinatology 22: 375–385
39. Neligan G A, Scott D, Kolvin I, Garside R 1976 Born too soon or born too small. Spastics International Medical Publications no. 61. William Heinemann Medical Books, London
40. Ounsted M, Moar V A, Scott A 1985 Risk factors associated with small for dates and large for dates babies. British Journal of Obstetrics and Gynaecology 92: 226–232
41. Ounsted C, Ounsted M 1973 On fetal growth rate: its variation and its consequences. Clinics in Developmental Medicine, no. 46. Spastics International Medical Publications. William Heinemann Medical Books, London
42. Peacock J L, Bland J M, Anderson J R 1995 Preterm delivery: effects of socioeconomic factors, psychological stress, smoking, alcohol and caffeine. British Medical Journal 311: 531–536
43. Pharoah P O D, Cooke T, Rosenbloom L, Cooke R W I 1987 Effects of birthweight, gestational age and maternal obstetric history on birth prevalence of cerebal palsy. Archives of Disease in Childhood 62: 1035–1040
44. Pietrantoni M, Knuppel R A 1991 Alcohol use in pregnancy. Clinics in Perinatology 18: 93–111
45. Prentice A M, Whitehead R G, Watkinson M et al 1983 Prenatal dietary supplementation of African women and birthweight. Lancet i: 489–492
46. Robinson J S 1995 Fetal growth and development. In: Chamberlain GVP, ed. Turnbull's obstetrics, 2nd edn. Churchill Livingstone, Edinburgh, pp. 97–114
47. Rush D, Stein Z, Susser M 1980 Diet in pregnancy. A randomized controlled trial of nutritional supplements. Birth Defects: original article series. Vol. XVI. No. 3
48. Rush D, Stein Z, Susser M 1980 A randomized controlled trial of prenatal nutritional supplementation in New York City. Pediatrics 65: 683–697
49. Scott K E, Usher R, 1966 Fetal malnutrition: its incidence, causes and effects. American Journal of Obstetrics and Gynecology 94: 951–958
50. Shiono P H, Klebanoff M A, Graubard B I, et al 1986 Birthweight among women of different ethnic groups. Journal of the American Medical Association 255: 48–52
51. Singer D B, Sung C J, Wigglesworth J S 1991 Fetal growth and maturation with standards for body and organ development. In: Wigglesworth J S, Singer D B, eds. Textbook of fetal and perinatal pathology. Blackwell Scientific Publications, Oxford, pp. 11–47
52. Soothill P W, Nicoliades K H, Campbell S 1987 Prenatal asphyxia, hyperlacticaemia, hypoglycaemia and erythroblastosis in growth retarded fetuses. British Medical Journal 294: 1051–1053
53. Stein Z, Susser M, Rush D 1978 Prenatal nutrition and birthweight: experiments and quasi-experiments in the past decade. Journal of Reproductive Medicine 21: 287–299
54. Unger C, Weiser J K, McCullough R E 1988 Altitude, low birthweight and infant mortality in Colorado. Journal of the American Medical Association 259: 3427–3432
55. Uvebrant P, Hagberg G 1992 Intrauterine growth in children with cerebral palsy. Acta Paediatrica 81: 407–412
56. Verkerk P H, van Noord Zaadstra B M, Florey C du V et al 1993 The effect of moderate maternal alcohol consumption on birthweight and gestational age in a low risk population. Early Human Development 32: 121–129
57. Vik T, Vatten L, Markestad T et al 1996 Morbidity during the first year of life in small for gestational age infants. Archives of Disease in Childhood 75: F33–37
58. Villar J, Rivera J 1988 Nutritional supplementation during two consecutive pregnancies and the interim lactation period: effect on birthweight. Pediatrics 81: 51–57
59. Walther F J, Ramaekers L H J 1982 Neonatal morbidity of SGA infants in relation to their nutritional status at birth. Acta Paediatrica Scandinavica 71: 437–440
60. Walton A, Hammond S 1938 Maternal effects on growth and conformation in Shire horses–Shetland pony crosses. Proceedings of the Royal Society B 125: 311–335
61. Wharton B A 1982 Food, growth and the Asian fetus. In: Wharton B A ed. Topics in perinatal medicine 2. Pitman Books, London, pp. 7–19
62. Woods D L, Malan A F, Heese H de V 1979 Patterns of retarded fetal growth. Early Human Development 3: 237–262
63. Wynn M, Wynn A 1981 The importance of nutrition around the time of conception in the prevention of handicap. In Bateman E C, ed. Applied Nutrition. Libbey, London, p. 12
64. Zuckerman B, Frank D A, Hingson R et al 1989 Effects of maternal marijuana and cocaine use on fetal growth. New England Journal of Medicine 320: 726–728

11

Basic genetics

Andrew Green

THE NATURE AND STRUCTURE OF A GENE

Genetics is traditionally defined as the science of biological variation, and has been a scientific discipline for over 100 years. Human genetics makes up a large part of the field of genetics, but the principal laws of genetics are universal and apply equally to all species, including humans. Mendel's studies in the 19th century were originally felt to have no relevance to humans, and it is only in retrospect that their importance can be seen. Many of the principles of genetics were discovered through the study of smaller organisms, such as bacteria, yeast and fruit flies. The basic genetic mechanisms of cell division, development and differentiation happen in the same way in widely divergent species. Therefore, it is impossible to look at human genetics in isolation and there are large amounts of information from lower species which have bearing on human disorders. The study of the genetics of small organisms has had a profound impact on our understanding of human development, and of how human diseases develop. It is likely that such basic science will continue to contribute significantly to the understanding of human genetic disease. In this chapter I hope to outline the basic elements of genetics, and describe the types of genetic tests now available to help in neonatal diagnosis.

The basic unit of inheritance for any species is the *gene*. The original concept of a gene arose long before the relationship between genes and nucleic acids was ever understood. A gene was considered to be a stable heritable element which conferred a particular property or phenotype on an individual organism. This element was passed on to subsequent generations of a particular species, and the nature of the phenotype varied according to the nature of the gene. The concept of dominant and recessive traits, which will be discussed below, was derived from studies of inheritance patterns, long before the molecular basis of the gene was understood.

A gene can also be considered in another way, as a specific length of deoxyribonucleic acid which encodes a particular function, in most cases the synthesis of a protein. This also is a stable heritable unit. Each cell in an organism, regardless of its function, has the entire set of genes for that particular organism, but only a proportion of those genes will be active. DNA is found in the nucleus of every cell of an organism, as a double helix (Fig. 11.1).

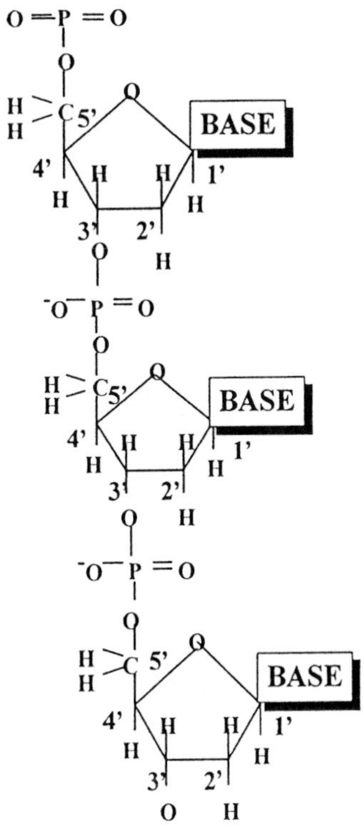

Fig. 11.1 Structure of a DNA chain. The deoxyribose and phosphate residues are linked to form the sugar–phosphate backbone.

Each strand of the double helix has a backbone of alternating phosphate and deoxyribose sugar molecules, with the sugars attached to the 5′ and 3′ hydroxyl groups of the phosphate group. Attached to the sugar molecule, lying within the helix, is one of four nitrogen-containing nucleic acid bases. Two of these bases, adenine (A) and guanine (G), are purines, and two are the smaller

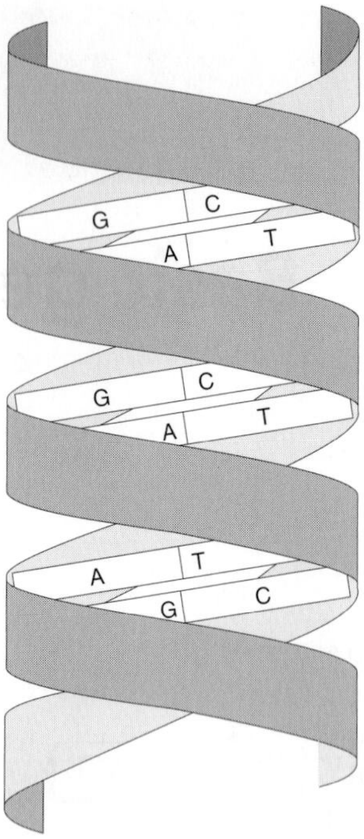

Fig. 11.2 Double helix structure of DNA. The double helix of deoxyribose and phosphate molecules is held together by paired purine and pyrimidine bonds.

pyrimidines cytosine (C) and thymine (T). The A and T bases pair together by hydrogen bonding, and the G and C bases similarly pair by hydrogen bonds (Fig. 11.2). The two strands of the double helix are held together by paired A–T or G–C bases of opposite strands of the double helix. The DNA strand can be read in only one direction, from 5′ (left hand) to 3′ (right hand). The two strands of DNA are complementary to each other, and the sequence of one strand can be predicted from its opposite. If one strand reads 5′-CAGCGTA-3′, then the opposite strand must read 5′-TACGCTG-3′. The double-stranded sequence would then be written as below:

5′-CAGCGTA-3′
3′-GTCGCAT-5′

The simplicity of the double helix structure allows for several important functions for DNA.

First, huge amounts of information can be stored in the DNA strand. If a molecule of DNA is 1 million bases long, then there are $4^{1\,000\,000}$ possible sequences for that stretch of DNA. A genome is the complete DNA sequence of an organism. In humans, the estimated genome size is 3×10^9 base pairs (bp). The human genome contains a huge amount of coded information, of which as yet only a small part is known.

Secondly, the double helix provides a framework for DNA replication. One strand of DNA acts as a template for the synthesis of a new strand. The double helix unwinds, allowing DNA replication enzymes access to the template strand of DNA. The replication system builds a

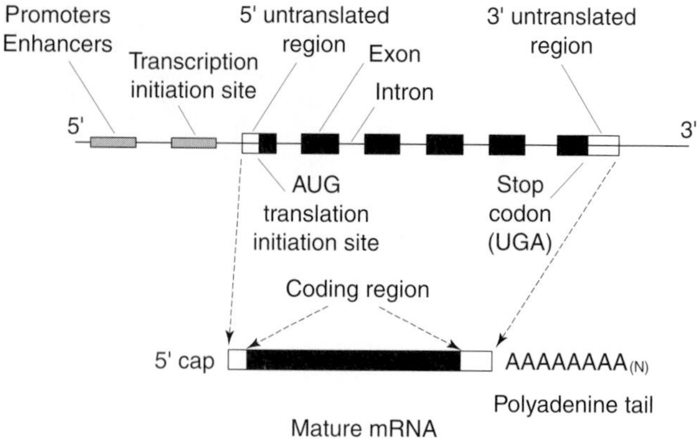

Fig. 11.3 An idealized gene.

new strand of DNA based on the template. The new double helix formed as a result will contain one original strand and a newly synthesized complementary second strand. This is the basic mechanism of DNA replication in all species.

Thirdly, the double helix provides a basis for repair of damaged DNA. A damaged base can be replaced, knowing its complementary base is present on the opposite strand. Damage to the sugar–phosphate backbone can also be repaired using the opposite strand as a template.

DECODING THE INFORMATION IN DNA

About 90% of the DNA in the human genome does not code for any specific property; only about 10% of the genome actually contains coding information in the form of a gene. In simple terms, the genetic code in DNA is transcribed into a molecule called messenger RNA. The mRNA is then translated into a protein, which carries out the function encoded by the specific DNA.

A gene has several distinct elements (Fig. 11.3). The major part of the gene is divided into coding regions, called exons, and non-coding regions called introns. Just before (5′) the first exon, there is a promoter which indicates where transcription of a gene should start. There can be several promoters for one gene, and different promoters can be used according to the tissue in which the gene is being expressed, in other words the promoter is tissue specific. Further 5′ of the promoter there can also be enhancers or suppressors, which can increase or decrease the level of transcription of the gene. Not all of the mRNA will code for protein, as some exons will code for mRNA that does not directly encode protein. These areas, known as untranslated regions, can be either at the start (5′) or the end (3′) of the mRNA.

To express the DNA code, mRNA is used. There are several different types of RNA, but mRNA is the most important in decoding DNA. There are three differences between RNA and DNA. First, the sugar backbone of

Table 11.1 The genetic code

First position	Second position								Third position
	U	Amino acid	C	Amino acid	A	Amino acid	G	Amino acid	
U	UUU	Phe	UCU	Ser	UAU	Tyr	UGU	Cys	U
	UUC	Phe	UCC	Ser	UAC	Tyr	UGC	Cys	C
	UUA	Leu	UCA	Ser	UAA	Stop	UGA	Stop	A
	UUG	Leu	UCG	Ser	UAG	Stop	UGG	Trp	G
C	CUU	Leu	CCU	Pro	CAU	His	CGU	Arg	U
	CUC	Leu	CCC	Pro	CAC	His	CGC	Arg	C
	CUA	Leu	CCA	Pro	CAA	Gln	CGA	Arg	A
	CUG	Leu	CCG	Pro	CAG	Gln	CGG	Arg	G
A	AUU	Ile	ACU	Thr	AAU	Asn	AGU	Ser	U
	AUC	Ile	ACC	Thr	AAC	Asn	AGC	Ser	C
	AUA	Ile	ACA	Thr	AAA	Lys	AGA	Arg	A
	AUG	Met	ACG	Thr	AAG	Lys	AGG	Arg	G
G	GUU	Val	GCU	Ala	GAU	Asp	GGU	Gly	U
	GUC	Val	GCC	Ala	GAC	Asp	GGC	Gly	C
	GUA	Val	GCA	Ala	GAA	Glu	GGA	Gly	A
	GUG	Val	GCG	Ala	GAG	Glu	GGG	Gly	G

RNA contains ribose rather than deoxyribose. Secondly, mRNA exists as a single strand, and remains more unstable. Thirdly, in RNA the base uracil (U) is used instead of thymine, whereas the other three nucleic acids remain the same.

The DNA code in most genes is expressed as a protein, which is a peptide made of the building blocks of individual amino acids. Each amino acid is coded for by a sequence of three DNA bases, known as a codon. For some amino acids there is more than one codon (Table 11.1). A long series of DNA codons in a gene will thus code for an entire protein. The mRNA codons coding for amino acids are identical to DNA codons, with the substitution of uracil (U) for thymine (T). There is a tightly controlled mechanism for the generation of protein from a DNA template.

To decode a gene into protein, the DNA is first transcribed into mRNA. A strand (the 'sense' strand) of the DNA double helix is used by the enzyme RNA polymerase to synthesize a complementary strand of mRNA. Transcription of mRNA starts from the 5′ end of the first exon of the gene, until the end of the most 3′ exon. The intervening introns are initially included, and the first molecule is known as pre-mRNA. The intronic RNA sequences are spliced out and a 3′ polyadenine tail is added, producing mature mRNA. The mature mRNA is then transferred from the nucleus to the ribosome to be used as a template for the production of protein. The mature mRNA has both 5′ and 3′ untranslated regions.

Protein synthesis does not begin at the 5′ end of the mRNA, but at the first 5′ AUG codon, which codes for the amino acid methionine. Protein translation stops at the first truncation codon (usually UGA) thereafter (see Fig. 11.3). In the ribosome, amino acid-specific transfer molecules, called transfer RNAs, bind a free molecule of

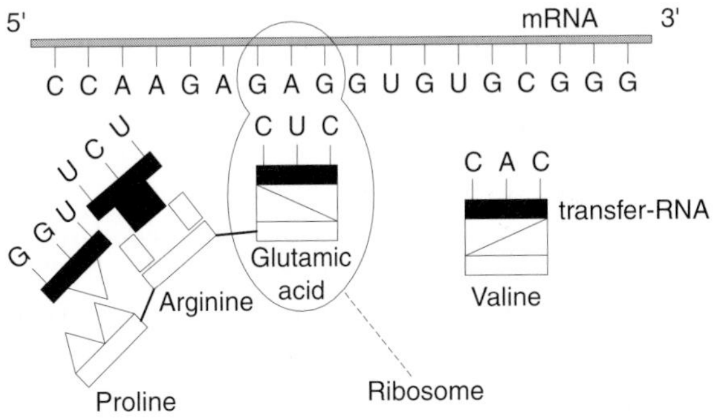

Fig. 11.4 Diagram of protein synthesis from mRNA.

their specific amino acid. The binding is carried out by an anticodon in the tRNA, which is complementary to the mRNA that codes for that specific amino acid. Using its anticodon, the tRNA binds the specific mRNA codon for its amino acid. By a complex machinery, the amino acid is then added to a growing peptide chain which will eventually form the mature protein (Fig. 11.4). The 5′ end of the mRNA corresponds to the NH_2 (amino terminus) of the protein, and the 3′ end of the mRNA corresponds to the COOH (carboxyl terminus) of the protein. Many proteins in higher species are modified after translation by the addition of phosphate or lipid groups.

CHROMOSOMES AND CELL DIVISION

The first coiling of DNA is in the form of the double helix. However, there are subsequent higher orders of coiling and packaging of DNA. The first order gives a loop of about 146 bp in size, wound around a histone protein. The complex is known as a nucleosome. The highest order of coiling of a large DNA molecule, with its

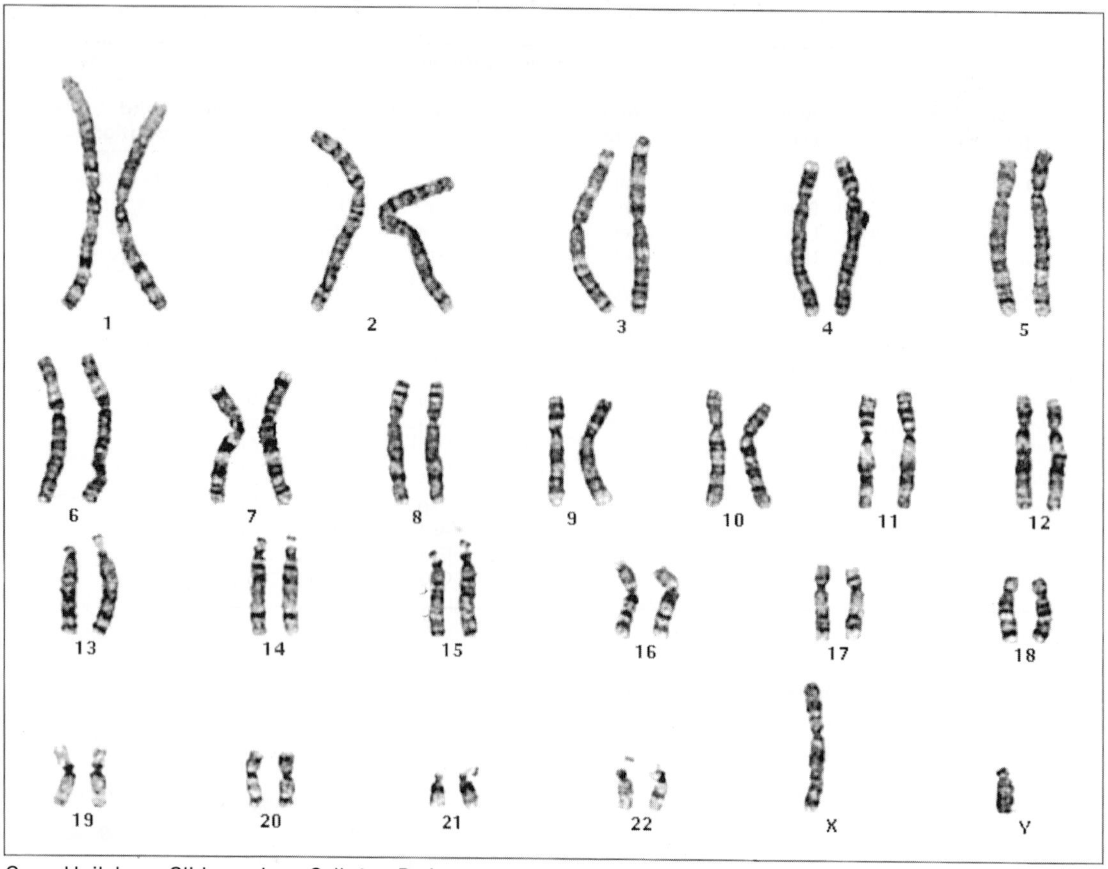

Case: Unilabs Slide: male Cell: 1 Patient:

Fig. 11.5 A normal human metaphase karyotype.

associated histones and other proteins, is known as a chromosome.

A chromosome consists of one very long double helix of DNA, containing very many genes in millions of base pairs. Humans are diploid; that is, they have two copies of every chromosome. The normal human chromosome complement is 46, made up of 22 pairs of autosomes (non-sex chromosomes) and two sex chromosomes, either X and Y in a male, or X and X in a female. Each member of a pair of autosomes contains the same genetic information. The pair of X chromosomes in a female will contain the same genetic information, but X and Y chromosomes in a male only have a small number of genes in common. A normal human metaphase karyotype is shown in Figure 11.5.

When cells divide, the genetic content must also be duplicated so that the daughter cells have the correct genetic material. Most cell division occurs as *mitosis*, where one cell divides to give two genetically identical cells. This is the process which allows the formation of a complete human being from one fertilized embryo, and is also the process by which the cells of many organs are constantly renewed. Mitosis is one short period during a carefully programmed cell cycle (Fig. 11.6). After mitosis the cell may enter a resting phase (G0), or go on to divide again (G1). A cell in G1 will then go on to synthesize new DNA as described above (S phase). There is then a second gap phase (G2) followed by mitosis (M).

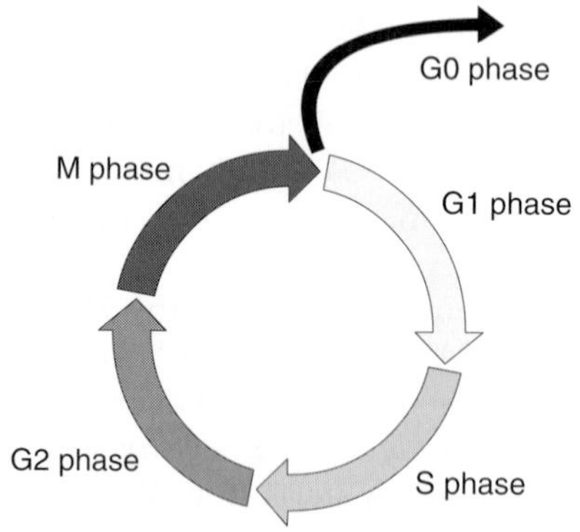

Fig. 11.6 Cell cycle.

Prior to mitosis the cell can be said to be in *interphase*, during which the chromosomes are very elongated. Just before mitosis, in S phase, the chromosomes are duplicated and begin to condense as two (sister) *chromatids* per chromosome. This condensation phase is known as *prophase*. In the next phase, *metaphase*, the condensed chromatids line up along the plane of the cell, and spindle fibres develop between the centromeres (narrow waist of each chromatid) and the polar centrioles. Standard analysis of human chromosomes is carried out in metaphase. The chromatids separate, starting from each centromere, and pass to the new daughter cell, in the step called *anaphase*. By the *telophase*, the chromatids have reached to opposite poles of the dividing cell, and division completes.

Meiosis is the form of division required to form gametes (sperm or oocyte). Gametes are *haploid*, with only one of each chromosome – 23 in the case of humans. This allows the formation of a new diploid organism from two haploid gametes. Meiosis occurs in two stages, meiosis I and meiosis II. The first phase of meiosis I, prophase I, is similar to that in mitosis, with the appearance of two condensed chromatids which have duplicated. At this stage, crossing over of genetic material from one chromatid to another can occur. It is estimated that one to two crossovers occur per chromosome in each meiosis. This introduces further genetic diversity, ensuring that the inherited chromosomes are different from the chromosomes of the parent. Metaphase I then occurs, where chromatids do not separate but go to the opposite ends of the cell in anaphase I and telophase I. The cells at this stage are still diploid.

The second meiotic division then occurs, where chromatids condense again in prophase II, and line up along the axis of the dividing cell in metaphase II. The chromatids then separate, passing to opposite ends of the cell in anaphase II. The new cells are then haploid, with 23 chromosomes, and the chromatids elongate into thin strands in telophase II.

CHROMOSOME ANALYSIS

To examine chromosomes from a patient (a karyotype), dividing cells in culture must be examined. These cells are usually lymphocytes, amniotic fluid cells or fibroblasts. Cells are arrested in the metaphase stage of mitosis, and stained in such a way that the chromosomes are easily visualized. The usual technique used is G-banding (using a Giemsa stain), which gives a characteristic positive and negative banding pattern to each chromosome. Each chromosome has a constriction, called a centromere, dividing the chromosome into a short arm (p) and a long arm (q). Each arm has a number of prominent bands, which can then be subdivided into smaller bands. The gene for the ABO blood group is localized to chromosome 9q34. The gene thus lies in the fourth subband from the centromere (q34) of the third band from the centromere (q34) on the long arm (q34) of chromosome 9 (9q34).

Chromosome abnormalities can be broadly classified into abnormalities of chromosome number, or a rearrangement of a normal number of chromosomes. The critical issue in most cases for determining the significance of a chromosome abnormality is whether the abnormality gives rise to an excess or deficiency of the normal diploid state (aneuploidy).

Abnormalities of chromosome number are relatively common, but many are not recognized as they may result in the early loss of a pregnancy. Triploidy (69 chromosomes) and tetraploidy (92 chromosomes) are relatively common causes of early pregnancy loss. Trisomy, the presence of a single extra chromosome (47 chromosomes), is also a common cause of miscarriage. Specific trisomies can give rise to an affected neonate, the commonest being trisomy 21 (Down syndrome), trisomy 13 (Patau syndrome) and trisomy 18 (Edward syndrome). All these trisomies usually occur as a result of autosomal non-dysjunction in meiotic division of the oocyte. In non-dysjunction the specific chromatids fail to separate, resulting in an extra chromosome in one oocyte and no chromosome in the opposite gamete. A fertilized embryo from the oocyte with an extra chromosome will therefore be trisomic. The fertilized oocyte with an absent chromosome will be monosomic, and be lost as an early miscarriage. Non-dysjunction tends to occur more frequently with increasing maternal age. Non-dysjunction can occur in the male germline, but rarely produces viable offspring.

There are numerous types of chromosome rearrangements, the commonest of which are shown in Figure 11.7. Pericentric and paracentric chromosome inversions are usually balanced, and inherited without any phenotypic effect. Paracentric inversions are usually associated with a low risk of producing a liveborn unbalanced karyotype, but pericentric inversions may carry a higher risk. Insertions, duplications, deletions, isochromosomes and ring chromosomes are all usually aneuploid and associated with significant clinical abnormalities. Reciprocal translocations occur where there is exchange of genetic material from one arm of a chromosome in return for genetic material from a different chromosome. Reciprocal translocations are usually balanced, without

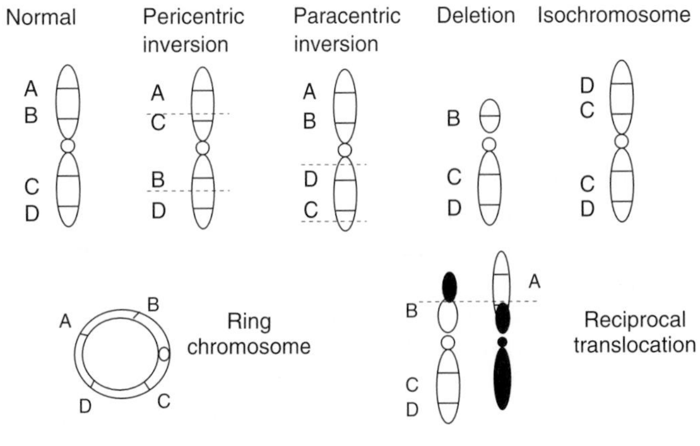

Fig. 11.7 Different types of chromosome anomaly. A–D represent notional chromosomal loci.

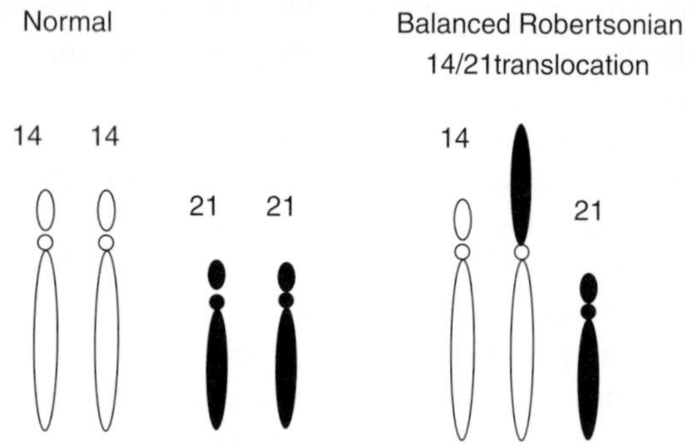

Fig. 11.8 Robertsonian translocation.

any clinical effect, but may carry a risk of having a child with problems due to an unbalanced karyotype.

Another type of translocation is between the acrocentric chromosomes (13–15, 21 and 22), where there is no appreciable coding material on a very small short (p) arm. This is known as a Robertsonian translocation. Robertsonian translocations are one of the commonest human chromosome translocations, and in the balanced form have no clinical effect. A Robertsonian translocation involving chromosomes 14 and 21 is shown in Figure 11.8. Those who carry a Robertsonian translocation involving chromosome 21 may be at significantly higher risk of having a child with Down syndrome as an unbalanced product of the translocation. The same applies to a lesser extent for those carrying a Robertsonian translocation involving chromosome 13, and a subsequent risk of a child with Patau syndrome.

The nomenclature for reporting a chromosome analysis is strict, and needs to be read carefully. A karyotype is reported initially as the number of chromosomes, regardless of whether or not those chromosomes are normal. The sex chromosomes are then described. If there is no further abnormality, the report is then complete. Any further abnormality is added after the sex chromosomes. A normal male karyotype is thus 46,XY. A male with nondysjunctional Down syndrome will have the karyotype 47,XY,+ 21, an extra unattached chromosome 21. A male with Down syndrome due to a Robertsonian translocation between chromosomes 14 and 21 will have the karyotype 46,XY,t(14;21), and his carrier mother will have a karyotype 45,XX,t(14;21).

A standard laboratory chromosome analysis will be performed on G-banded chromosomes, which will detect many common and less common chromosome abnormalities, and in most cases no further laboratory work is required. However, recombinant DNA technology has allowed new techniques for chromosome analysis, based on the hybridization of fluorescently labelled fragments of DNA to the DNA of chromosomes, prepared in a standard fashion, immobilized on a glass slide. The slides can then be visualized by eye using a fluorescent microscope, or indirectly by generating an image of the hybridization on computer. This technique is known as *FISH*, *f*luorescent *i*n *s*itu *h*ybridization. The information that can be gained from this technique depends on the origin of the fragments of DNA hybridized to the chromosome preparation. Labelled whole chromosome 'paints', consisting of DNA exclusively from one chromosome, are now commercially available. For example, whole chromosome paints can be used to identify the origin of extra chromosomal material which cannot be identified using G-banding techniques. Whole chromosome paints are also helpful in determining the origin of subtle complex translocations. It is also now technically possible to use a chromosome 21 paint on uncultured cells in interphase, to look for trisomy 21. A cell would show three fluorescent nuclear dots, representing three chromosomes 21, as opposed to two in the normal situation.

Fluorescently labelled small DNA fragments, corresponding to 40–50 kb of DNA from a specific chromosomal region, can also be hybridized to metaphase chromosomes. Chromosomal deletions which cannot be detected within the resolution of conventional cytogenetic analysis can be detected by this FISH method. A normal karyotype will give two hybridization signals, one from the same part of each chromosome. A karyotype containing a submicroscopic chromosomal deletion involving the segment of the chromosome corresponding to the 50 kb DNA fragment will only give one hybridization signal. An example would be the submicroscopic deletion of chromosome 22q11 which occurs in most cases of the Di George spectrum (see Chapters 30 and 34), which can only be seen by FISH analysis. FISH diagnosis of submicroscopic chromosomal deletions is likely to become available for a variety of specific clinical syndromes.

PATTERNS OF INHERITANCE

Single gene disorders have one of three principal modes of inheritance: autosomal dominant, autosomal recessive, and X-linked recessive. Other rare forms of inheritance include X-linked dominant, and mitochondrial disorders, as well as disorders due to abnormalities of genetic imprinting. Disorders caused by inheritance of unstable elements of DNA are now increasingly being recognized (see below).

AUTOSOMAL DOMINANT INHERITANCE

Autosomal dominant disorders are characterized by vertical transmission from parent to child, and the hallmark of these conditions is male to male transmission of the disease (Fig. 11.9).

Those affected with an autosomal dominant disorder have a fault in one or other copy of the two genes responsible for that condition. Each child of a person with an autosomal dominant disorder has a 50:50 chance of inheriting the gene responsible for the condition from

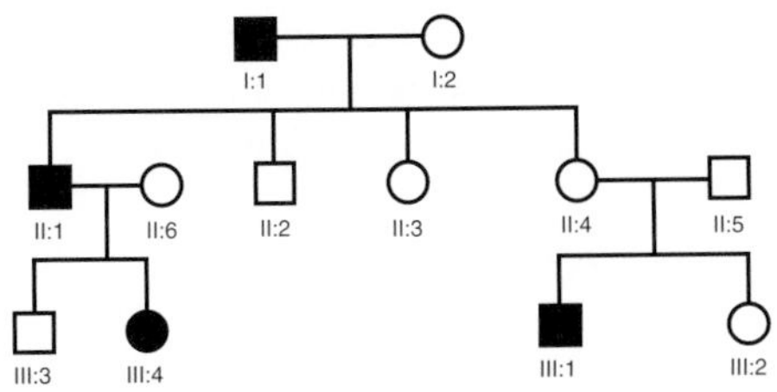

■ = affected

Fig. 11.9 Autosomal dominant inheritance. Note male to male transmission and non-penetrance in II:4. ■ = affected.

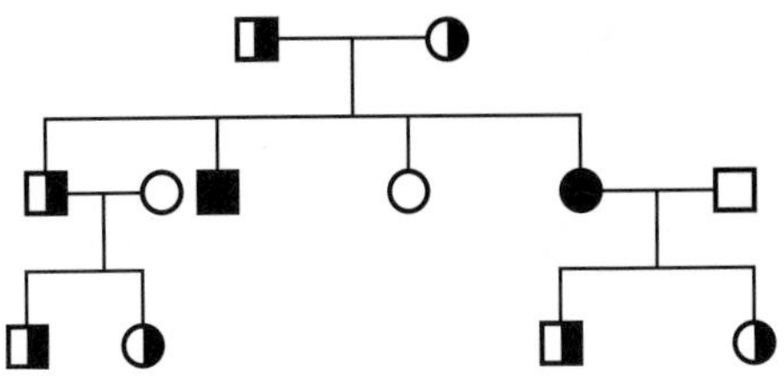

■ = affected

◧ = heterozygous carrier

Fig. 11.10 Autosomal recessive inheritance. ■ = affected; ◧ = heterozygous carrier.

its parent. There are many examples of autosomal dominant disorders, including neurofibromatosis 1 and 2, familial adenomatous polyposis coli, myotonic dystrophy and Huntington's disease. There can often be variability in both *expression* and *penetrance* of autosomal dominant disorders. For example, neurofibromatosis 1, an autosomal dominant condition, will almost always manifest in someone who has a neurofibromatosis 1 gene fault. This means that the condition has almost complete *penetrance*. However, different people can manifest the condition in different ways, some showing mild skin lesions and others with severe intracerebral complications. This means that the *expression* of the condition is very variable. In contrast, only 80% of those who have a single gene fault for the rare hereditary form of retinoblastoma will actually develop an eye tumour. The penetrance in this situation is 80%, but the expression of the gene fault is consistent, as manifested by a retinoblastoma.

Autosomal dominant disorders are not commonly seen in neonatal practice. A list of the more frequent conditions is outlined in Table 11.2.

AUTOSOMAL RECESSIVE INHERITANCE

When a child is diagnosed with an autosomal recessive disorder, then both copies of a particular gene responsible for the condition are faulty. Both his parents are therefore carriers for that condition, with one normal and one faulty gene. Two of the child's four grandparents are also carriers, and it is likely that many of the child's relatives are also unknowingly carriers (Fig. 11.10). In most cases, being a carrier for an autosomal recessive condition has no effect on that person. When both parents are carriers for a fault in the same gene, then there is a 25% chance of each of their children being affected by the condition. The risk of a healthy carrier sibling of having a child with the same condition depends on the chances of that sibling's partner also being a carrier. A child of a person with an autosomal recessive disorder will automatically be a carrier. The child's chances of being affected will depend upon whether its unaffected parent is a carrier for a fault in the same gene.

Autosomal recessive disorders are commonly encountered in neonatal practice, and the nature of the disorder depends on the population being seen. Each regional population has its own recessive disorder, where the frequency of carriers for that disorder is highest. For instance, cystic fibrosis is a very common autosomal recessive disorder in western Europe, whereas sickle cell anaemia is the commonest autosomal recessive disorder in West Africa. Common examples of autosomal recessive conditions include cystic fibrosis, sickle cell anaemia, several of the mucopolysaccharidoses, beta-thalassaemia, spinal muscular atrophy and congenital adrenal hyperplasia (Table 11.3). Prenatal diagnosis is available for many of these conditions.

Table 11.2 Autosomal dominant disorders in neonatal practice

System affected	Condition
Neurological	Congenital myotonic dystrophy Neurofibromatosis type 1
Ocular	Congenital cataract Retinoblastoma
Haematological	Spherocytosis
Skeletal	Stickler syndrome Craniosynostosis syndromes Achondroplasia Osteogenesis imperfecta
Other	Beckwith–Wiedemann syndrome Noonan syndrome

Table 11.3 Autosomal recessive disorders in neonatal practice

System affected	Condition
Neurological	Spinal muscular atrophy Congenital myopathies
Ocular	Congenital cataract Congenital glaucoma Albinism
Haematological	Thalassaemia Sickle cell anaemia
Skeletal	Short-rib polydactyly syndromes Jeune syndrome
Endocrine	Congenital adrenal hyperplasia
Metabolic	Cystic fibrosis Phenylketonuria Galactosaemia α_1-antitrypsin deficiency

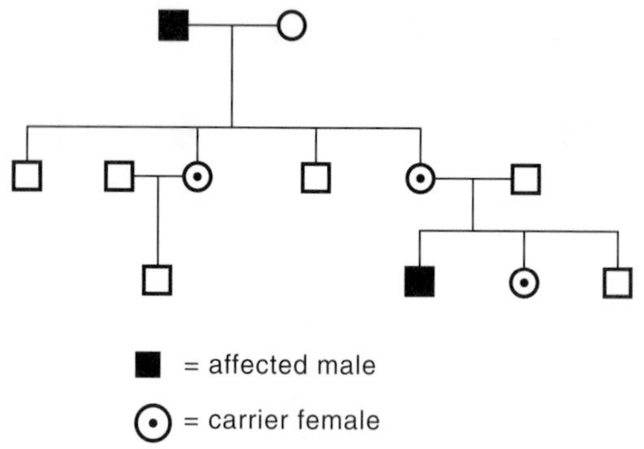

Fig. 11.11 X-linked recessive inheritance. ■ = affected male; ⊙ = carrier female.

X-LINKED RECESSIVE INHERITANCE

In X-linked recessive inheritance, the condition affects almost exclusively males; females can be carriers (Fig. 11.11). The classic examples of such conditions are haemophilia A and B, Duchenne and Becker muscular dystrophy, and Hunter syndrome.

The daughters of a man with an X-linked recessive condition are all obligate carriers. The sons of a man with an X-linked condition are all normal, as they inherit his Y chromosome and not his X chromosome. When a woman is a carrier of an X-linked condition, each of her sons has a 50:50 chance of being affected and each of her daughters has a 50:50 chance of being a carrier. There can be a relatively high mutation rate for some X-linked recessive conditions, and affected boys may have not family history of the condition. About one-third of occurrences of Duchenne muscular dystrophy are as a result of new mutations. Prenatal diagnosis is available for a wide range of X-linked recessive diseases. The more common X-linked disorders in neonatal practice are shown in Table 11.4.

POLYGENIC INHERITANCE

Many congenital conditions do not have a clear mode of inheritance and can be classed as polygenic or oligogenic, where a disease may arise as a result of the effects of several genes. A good example is cleft lip and palate, which usually occurs in the absence of a family history. However, monozygotic twins have a high concordance for cleft palate, suggesting a genetic influence.

Table 11.4 X-linked recessive disorders in neonatal practice

System affected	Condition
Neurological	Hunter syndrome
Ocular	Lowe syndrome
	Ocular albinism
Haematological	G6PD deficiency
	Haemophilia
Skeletal	Amelogenesis imperfecta
Endocrine	Androgen insensitivity syndrome
Metabolic	Adrenoleukodystrophy
	Fabry's disease
	Lesch–Nyhan syndrome
	Steroid sulphatase deficiency

OTHER FORMS OF INHERITANCE

There are also much rarer forms of inheritance, including X-linked dominant, which can be hard to distinguish from autosomal dominant, except that females will be more mildly affected and there is no male to male transmission. An example of an X-linked dominant condition is hypophosphataemic rickets.

Mitochondrially inherited diseases show a very unusual pattern of inheritance. Most of the proteins in the mitochondria are encoded for by nuclear genes, but the mitochondria also contain their own small genome of 18 kb, with many copies per cell. The mitochondrial genome replicates independently and far more frequently than the nuclear genome. Several important mitochondrial proteins are encoded by the mitochondrial genome. Mitochondria are only inherited via oocytes, and not sperm. Therefore, when a gene fault is in the mitochondrial genome it will pass exclusively down the female line, but both males and females can be affected. The children of an affected male will not inherit his mitochondrial gene fault. Children with mitochondrial disorders can present with many varied symptoms, including myoclonic seizures, acute acidoses, muscle weakness, deafness or diabetes. A number of mutations or deletions in the mitochondrial genome have been described in patients with a wide variety of conditions, including MELAS (myoclonic epilepsy with lactic acidosis and stroke-like episodes) or MERRF (myoclonic epilepsy with ragged red fibres on muscle biopsy). To complicate matters further, Leber's hereditary ophthalmopathy is a mitochondrially inherited condition with a characteristic mitochondrial mutation, but the expression appears to have an X-linked recessive influence.

Some conditions show a phenomenon known as genetic imprinting. An imprinted gene has been marked during meiosis, to indicate the parent from which it comes. For some genes it appears to be important not only to inherit two copies of that gene, but to inherit one from each parent. Some genes may be silenced, depending upon which parent has passed on that gene. A good example is the presence of a small deletion of chromosome 15q, which has a different effect depending upon which chromosome 15 is deleted. If the deletion occurs on the chromosome inherited from a child's normal father, the child will develop Prader–Willi syndrome. If the deletion occurs on the chromosome inherited from a child's normal mother, the child will develop a completely different clinical condition, Angelman syndrome. The genes in this area of chromosome 15 are therefore imprinted. In addition, if a child has two maternal copies of chromosome 15 (maternal disomy), but no paternal copy, he or she will also develop Prader–Willi syndrome. Other conditions that show imprinting effects include Russell–Silver syndrome, Beckwith–Wiedemann syndrome, and the rare condition of transient neonatal diabetes mellitus.

A new molecular mechanism for genetic disease has been described, that of inherited unstable triplet repeat expansions. At least nine different conditions are caused by this phenomenon. In one of these conditions a normal person has a stable number of a repetitive element of three bases of DNA (for example 20 copies of a CAG repeat) in a particular gene, that gene functions normally, and the children of that person have the same number of repeats in their gene. An affected person has an increased number of repeats (say 100 copies) in that gene, and the affected children of that person have more serious disease, with perhaps 200 repeats in the gene. The molecular genetic findings appear to be the genetic correlate of the phenomenon of anticipation, where a condition appears to worsen from generation to generation. The most extreme example is that of congenital myotonic dystrophy, where a minimally affected mother can have a profoundly affected infant. In this case there is a small repeat expansion of, say, 150 repeats in the mother, increasing to many hundreds of repeats in her affected infant.

This molecular mechanism is responsible for fragile X syndrome, Huntington's disease, Friedreich's ataxia, several forms of spinocerebellar ataxia, and probably several more conditions.

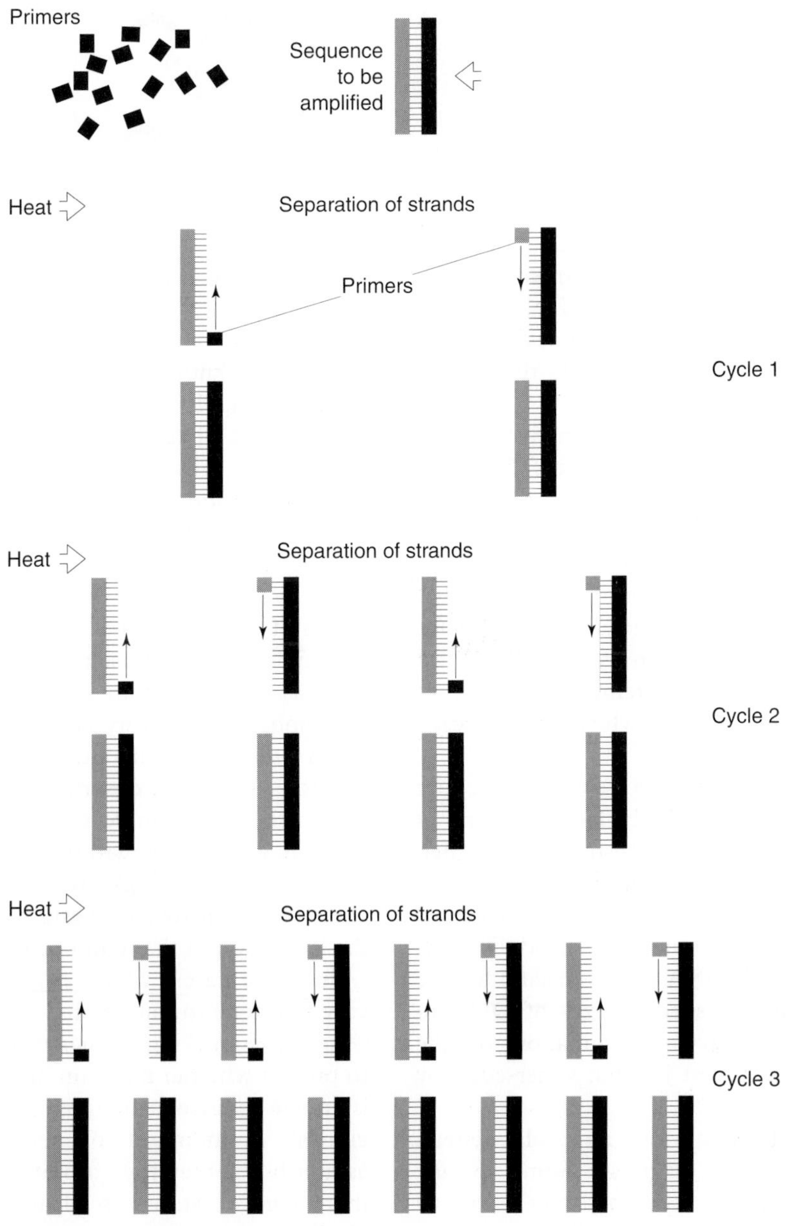

Fig. 11.12 Polymerase chain reaction (PCR).

MOLECULAR GENETIC ANALYSIS FOR SINGLE GENE DISORDERS

Laboratory tests for single gene disorders have been available for a considerable time. Haemoglobin electrophoresis for sickle cell anaemia and thalassaemia, and enzyme assays for Tay–Sachs disease are very effective in resolving clinical issues in individual families. However, an increasing number of specific DNA-based tests can now be used in the diagnosis and prediction of single gene disorders.

The two major techniques used in molecular genetic analysis are the polymerase chain reaction and Southern blotting. PCR is a technique which allows amplification of a specific genetic region in large quantities from a small amount of DNA template (Fig. 11.12). The DNA sequence of the region to be amplified must be known, so that synthetic pieces of single-stranded DNA (oligonucleotide primers) corresponding to the region can be designed and manufactured. The oligonucleotide primers are added in great excess to the DNA template, along with a thermostable DNA polymerase, and free nucleotides (A, C, T, G). The mixture is heated up to cause the two strands of template DNA to separate, and then cooled. As the DNA cools, the oligonucleotides bind to the template sequence and are extended by the polymerase. A new copy of the template DNA is thus produced. The cycle is repeated 30–40 times, with an exponential increase in the amount of the target sequence.

DNA generated by PCR can be used in many different ways to detect an abnormality in the sequence. There are numerous techniques which are used to screen PCR products for mutations, such as single-stranded conformational assay, or denaturing gradient gel electrophoresis. In some cases the complete sequence of the PCR product can be directly determined. Specific PCR assays for mutations have been developed, such as the ARMS test (amplification-resistant mutation system), or the use of a specific DNA restriction enzyme which recognizes a known mutant DNA sequence.

Southern blotting is a more protracted procedure involving the digestion of a relatively large amount of DNA by a restriction enzyme. The digested DNA is then electrophoresed through an agarose gel, giving a smear of DNA of different sizes. The DNA is then transferred (blotted) and fixed to a membrane. The fixed DNA is then hybridized to a labelled DNA probe specific for the gene to be analysed, and the specific sizes of DNA to which the probe binds allows determination of the 'genotype' (Fig. 11.13). This test is often superseded by PCR technology.

There are different degrees to which molecular genetic tests can contribute to clinical diagnosis. Some specific molecular genetic tests can be used to detect a known pathogenic DNA mutation and give a diagnosis, even without any knowledge of the patient's clinical status. For instance, the PCR detection of the ΔF508 deletion in both copies of a person's cystic fibrosis (CFTR) gene immediately gives a diagnosis of cystic fibrosis. Such direct mutation tests are possible where both the gene responsible for a condition has been isolated and specific pathogenic mutations have been identified. Similarly, a PCR test detects a deletion of exons 7 and 8 in both alleles of a gene called SMN on chromosome 5q in almost all children with spinal muscular atrophy. Southern blot analysis of DNA from infants with congenital myotonic dystrophy shows a very large expansion in a triplet repeat DNA sequence in the myotonin kinase gene on chromosome 19, as described earlier.

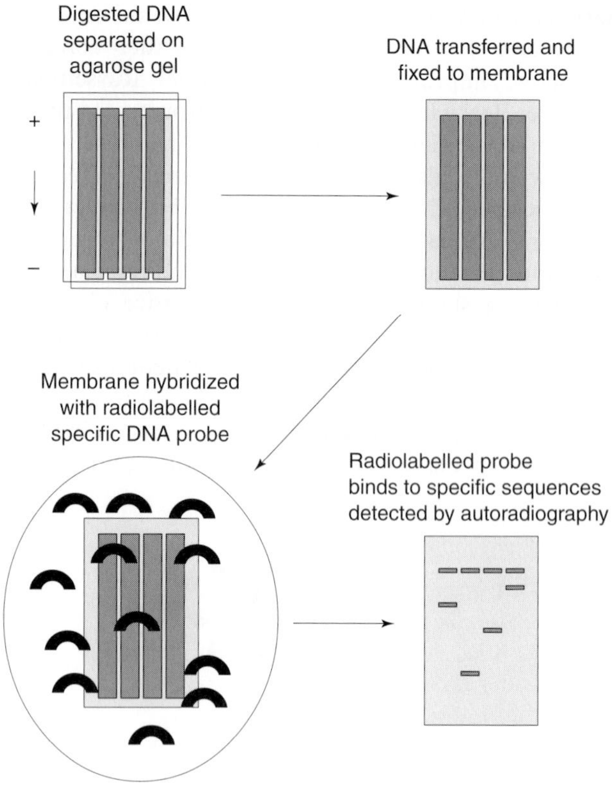

Fig. 11.13 Southern blotting and hybridization.

In other cases molecular genetic diagnosis can point towards a diagnosis without confirming it. For instance, the presence of a single ΔF508 CFTR gene mutation in a child with a history suggestive of cystic fibrosis increases the likelihood of that child being affected.

In some cases, where either a gene is not known or very few gene mutations have been identified in a known gene, gene tracking studies can be performed in a family to predict whether a person in that family is affected. This is known as linkage analysis. Such a study requires careful clinical examination of several family members, to establish whether they are affected or unaffected. When their clinical status is clear, DNA samples are then obtained.

Gene tracking analysis in the family uses the property of normal variations in a gene between different people. Some genetic areas show wide variation between individuals, and a DNA marker from such an area, which can detect many variations, is described as being polymorphic. Each variant of a polymorphic marker is known as an allele. There are now thousands of polymorphic markers covering most of the human genome, and such markers can be found very close to most known genes. There are several types of polymorphic DNA markers, including those characterized by different numbers of specific DNA-cutting enzymes recognition sites, or restriction fragment length polymorphisms. Other markers detect the variation in number of anonymous elements of repetitive DNA, and are called microsatellites or minisatellites.

If the two alleles of a polymorphic marker can be distinguished, to discriminate between the two copies of that particular chromosome from where the marker comes, then the marker is informative in that individual. Where a gene location is known, but the actual gene has yet to be found, the alleles of informative markers lying either side of the gene will be inherited along with each copy of the gene in question. This can be used to predict a child's clinical status.

If one set of alleles is found in the affected members of the family, but not in the unaffected, then the presence or absence of these alleles in the at-risk individual can be used to predict their chances of being affected. An example of linkage analysis for an autosomal recessive disorder is shown in Figure 11.14. This form of linkage analysis is often used in families with X-linked recessive conditions such as Duchenne muscular dystrophy, to predict whether a woman is a carrier. Such linkage analysis can also be used in prenatal diagnosis.

Because of its nature, linkage analysis is more prone to error than direct mutation testing. This can be due to difficulties in assessing a person's clinical status, and because of the possibility of recombination between the polymorphic markers. However, with the rapid advances in molecular genetics many more mutations are being found in many different genes, and linkage analysis is often superseded by direct mutation testing.

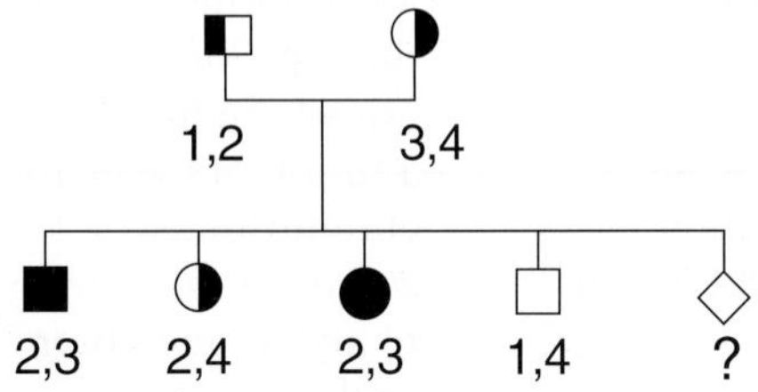

Fig. 11.14 Linkage analysis in an autosomal recessive disorder using an intragenic polymorphic marker. Alleles 2 and 3 are associated with a gene mutation and can be used to predict the status of another sibling. ■ = affected; ◧ = carrier.

There are many new molecular genetic tests being developed, and it is impossible to cover all such tests in the space available, but it is clear that new genetic tests will alter the clinical management of many infantile conditions.

FURTHER READING

1. Watson J D, Hopkins N H, Roberts J W, Steitz J A, Weiner A M 1993 Molecular biology of the gene. 5th edn. Benjamin Cummings, Menlo Park, California
2. Strachan T, Read A P 1996 Human molecular genetics. Bios, Oxford
3. Lewin B 1994 Genes V. Oxford University Press, Oxford
4. Connor M, Ferguson-Smith M Essential medical genetics. 5th edn. Blackwell Science, Oxford
5. Online Mendelian Inheritance in Man. A list of genetic disorders and the latest genetic developments for each condition. Website http://www3.ncbi.nlm.nih.gov:80/

GLOSSARY

3′	distal end of a gene, as indicated by the bond at the third hydroxyl group of the deoxyribose sugar
5′	proximal end of a gene, as indicated by the bond at the fifth hydroxyl group of the deoxyribose sugar
acrocentric	a chromosome with effectively only a long arm – chromosomes 13, 14, 15, 21 and 22
allele	a genetic variation of a gene or DNA marker
aneuploidy	an excess or deficiency of chromosomal material
anticodon	an element of transfer RNA which binds a specific amino acid
autosomal dominant	inheritance pattern characterized by transmission through several generations, male to male transmission, and a 50:50 risk to the children of an affected person
autosomal recessive	inheritance pattern characterized by several affected members of the same generation, with carrier parents and a 1:4 recurrence risk where both parents are carriers
base pair	unit of double-stranded DNA
centromere	element of chromosome involved in chromosome replication, found as a constriction in the chromosome
chromatid	condensed chromosome found just before mitosis
codon	3 bp element of DNA encoding an amino acid

diploid	a complement of two copies of each chromosome per cell
DNA marker	a piece of DNA corresponding to a specific gene or chromosomal segment
enhancers	elements of DNA which are involved in increasing gene transcription
exon	a part of a gene which is transcribed into mRNA
expression	the way in which a gene fault manifests clinically
FISH	fluorescent in situ hybridization, a new and powerful technique for studying specific chromosomes or regions of chromosomes
gamete	a germ cell – sperm or oocyte
genetic imprinting	the marking of a gene according to which parent has passed that gene to the child
haploid	a complement of one copy of each chromosome per cell (as in sperm or oocyte)
haplotype	a pattern of alleles of DNA markers representing one of the two copies of a chromosomal region
histone	a DNA-binding protein important in chromosomal folding
interphase	phase of mitosis in which the chromosomes are very elongated
intron	the part of a gene between the exons which is not transcribed into mRNA
isochromosome	an abnormal chromosome made up of two long or two short arms of a normal chromosome
karyotype	an analysis of the chromosome complement of a cell type
linkage analysis	the use of polymorphic DNA markers to perform gene tracking studies within a family
meiosis	the process of cell division to give haploid germ cells
metaphase	phase of mitosis in which the chromosomes are very condensed and easier to analyse
microsatellite marker	a DNA marker which detects variation in number of an anonymous small repetitive element of DNA
minisatellite marker	a DNA marker which detects variation in number of an anonymous medium repetitive element of DNA
mitosis	the normal process of cell division to give two diploid copies of a cell
non-dysjunction	a failure of meiosis, giving two copies of a chromosome in one gamete and no copy of a chromosome in the other gamete
nucleosome	the combination of a histone and its bound DNA
oligonucleotide primers	small lengths of synthetic single-stranded DNA of a specific sequence
paracentric inversion	a rearrangement of chromosomal material within one arm of a chromosome
PCR	polymerase chain reaction: a method of generating large amounts of specific DNA from a small amount of target sequence
penetrance	the number of people known to carry a gene mutation who manifest the condition
pericentric inversion	a rearrangement of chromosomal material around the centromere of a chromosome
promoter	element of a gene which is necessary to activate gene transcription
prophase	phase of the cell cycle where condensation of the chromosomes occurs, just before metaphase
reciprocal translocation	exchange of chromosomal segments between different chromosomes
restriction enzyme	an enzyme which cuts double-stranded DNA at a specific unique short DNA sequence
restriction fragment length polymorphism	a genetic variation between two copies of the same gene, where one gene may have one copy of a restriction enzyme recognition site, and the other two. This variation can be detected using PCR or Southern blotting
ribosome	area of the cell where mRNA is converted into protein
ring chromosome	an abnormal chromosome where the tips of the long and short arms have fused
Robertsonian translocation	a fusion of two acrocentric chromosomes
Southern blotting	a process of immobilizing DNA to nylon membrane for genetic analysis
suppressor	a DNA element which reduces the expression of a gene
telophase	the last phase of mitosis

telomere	the end of a chromosome
transcription	the process of converting DNA into mRNA
translation	the production of protein from a DNA sequence
triploidy	three of each chromosome, i.e. 69 chromosomes in man
trisomy	one extra chromosome, i.e. 47 chromosomes in man
X-linked recessive	inheritance characterized by affected males in several generations, and by female carriers.

12

Obstetrics for the neonatologist

Françoise H. D. Harlow   John A. D. Spencer

INTRODUCTION

Obstetrics is an ever-evolving specialty. In the earlier part of this century efforts were concentrated on reducing maternal mortality. The effects have been dramatic even in recent years. Between 1973–1975 and 1988–1990 the UK maternal mortality rate fell by 54%, from nine to four maternal deaths per million women aged 15–44.[37] During the 1960s to 1980s the focus widened to the fetus. Cardiotocographic monitoring and fetal scalp blood sampling were introduced in an attempt to decrease perinatal mortality. Early studies[83] showed that the introduction of continuous fetal heart rate monitoring was associated with a reduction in the incidence of intrapartum stillbirths in complicated labours. Consequently, the number of fetal monitors for use during labour in Great Britain increased by nearly 90% between 1977 and 1984.[163] However, subsequent analysis of pooled results[117,156] showed that continuous monitoring had no overall effect on perinatal mortality, but did significantly reduce the incidence of neonatal seizures. Despite this apparent advantage, follow-up of the largest study in Dublin[101] showed that the incidence of cerebral palsy was similar in both groups at 4 years of age, and only 22% of children with cerebral palsy had shown signs of birth asphyxia.[62] This study, however, recruited only uncomplicated pregnancies (with a normal volume of clear liquor) in whom the incidence of intrapartum stillbirth was already as low as 0.4 per 1000. Indeed, it seems increasingly likely that perinatal mortality and morbidity has reached its nadir in uncomplicated pregnancies in which placental function is normal at the onset of labour.

The focus of obstetric care is, therefore, changing once again. Identification of complicated pregnancies and abnormal placental function is increasingly the aim of modern obstetric management. This is reflected in the recent recommendations for the provision of maternity services.[36] This encourages midwives to manage the majority of low-risk pregnancies, with medical involvement concentrated on cases identified as being at increased risk of complications, or which subsequently deviate from the expected norm.

The aim of this chapter is to outline the antenatal and intrapartum assessment of fetal well-being determined by placental function, in the structurally and chromosomally normal fetus. Currently this is the best available predictor of neonatal outcome. Common complications and management strategies will be covered. Clearly this account cannot be exhaustive: the intention is to concentrate on aspects of obstetric care of relevance to the neonatologist.

ANTENATAL ASSESSMENT

This section covers the assessment of fetal growth and well-being and concludes with an overview of the management of antenatal complications which can adversely affect neonatal outcome.

FETAL GROWTH ASSESSMENT

An essential prerequisite of fetal growth assessment is knowledge of the true gestational age. The expected date of delivery is calculated from the date of the last menstrual period and assumes that the woman had a regular 28-day spontaneous menstrual cycle prior to conception. Ultrasonography in the first/early second trimester is used to confirm the gestational age. Only if the ultrasound date is more than 10 days different from the calculated date is the scan date subsequently used to derive the gestational age and gestational age and EDD. With the widespread introduction of anomaly scanning the need for postnatal clinical assessment of true gestational age, e.g. Dubowitz type scoring, has declined.

Uterine size is assessed clinically at each antenatal visit. After 20 weeks' gestation the symphysis–fundal height in centimetres approximates to the number of weeks' gestation. However, a single measurement of fundal height is merely a screening tool, comparing the individual against a population distribution. Its accuracy for the overall prediction of fetal growth abnormalities is acceptable, at the cost of a high false positive rate: for example, the reported figures for growth deficiency vary between 60–85% for sensitivity, 80–90% for specificity and 20–80% for positive predictive value. Serial fundal height measurements are the best available screening method and have been found to be as predictive of growth retardation as a single third trimester scan.[128] Abnormal fundal height measurements can also be due to reduced or excessive liquor volume surrounding the fetus. The significance of this will be discussed later.

If a discrepancy between the fundal height and gestational age is noted, an ultrasound scan is performed and the fetal biparietal diameter, head circumference and abdominal circumference are plotted on centile charts. Each of these measurements is taken in a standard way (British Medical Ultrasound Society Ultrasonic Fetal Measurement Survey recommendations), thereby limiting interobserver variability. The BPD is the maximum diameter of a transverse section of the fetal skull at the level of the parietal eminences. The correct section includes the cavum septum pellucidum, the thalami and the basal cisterns, and has a short midline. The BPD is then measured from outer to inner skull tables (Fig. 12.1(A)). The HC is measured on the same section using an ellipse which is matched to the outline of the fetal skull (Fig. 12.1(B)). The AC is measured with an ellipse on a section which is circular in outline and includes the stomach 'bubble' and a short length of umbilical vein (which is centrally placed between the lateral abdominal walls and a third of the way along an imaginary line from the anterior abdominal wall to the fetal spine) (Fig. 12.1(C)). Each measurement should be taken several times to obtain an average value.

The BPD, HC and AC measurements diagnose the fetal *size* at that point in time. If the measurements fall outside the normal range a second scan is performed 2 weeks later to determine fetal *growth* in relation to the centiles (Fig. 12.2). These centile charts are based on caucasian populations. Even in low-risk pregnancies, however, there is considerable variation in fetal growth velocity.[127] In addition, the pitfalls of applying the same ultrasound curves to different ethnic groups have been described[106] and separate ultrasound fetal growth curves have been proposed.[21]

The terms used to describe abnormal fundal height measurements are 'small for dates' or 'small for gestational age' and 'large for dates' or 'large for gestational age'. The possible ultrasound findings in each of these situations are described below.

Small for gestational age

The scan may show a fetus of normal size, i.e. a false positive clinical assessment (Fig. 12.2). The woman can be reassured and, provided the fundal height measure-

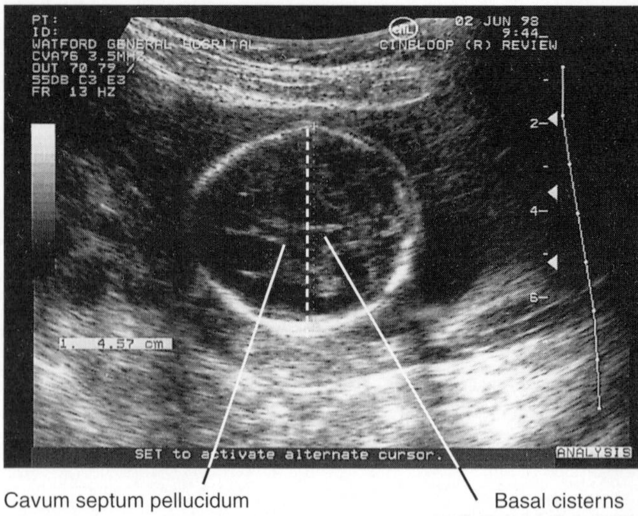

A

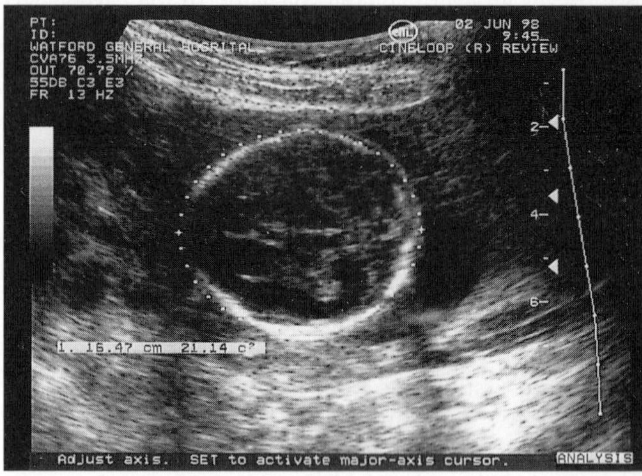

B

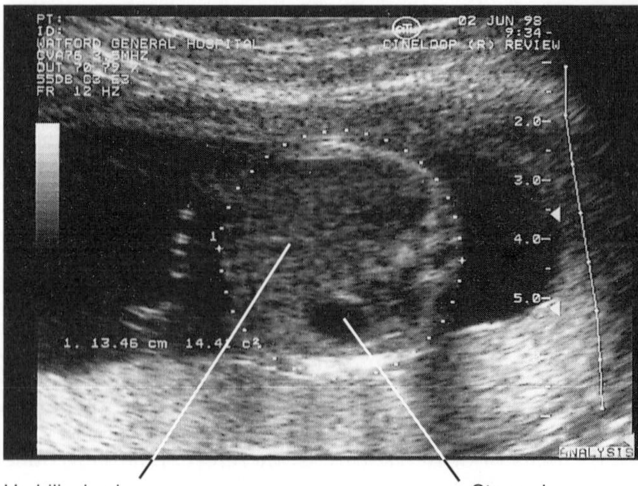

C

Fig. 12.1 (A) Transverse section of the fetal head from which the BPD should be measured. (B) Measurement of head circumference using the variable ellipse method (on the same transverse section as in (A). (C) Transverse section of the fetal abdomen on which the abdominal circumference should be measured.

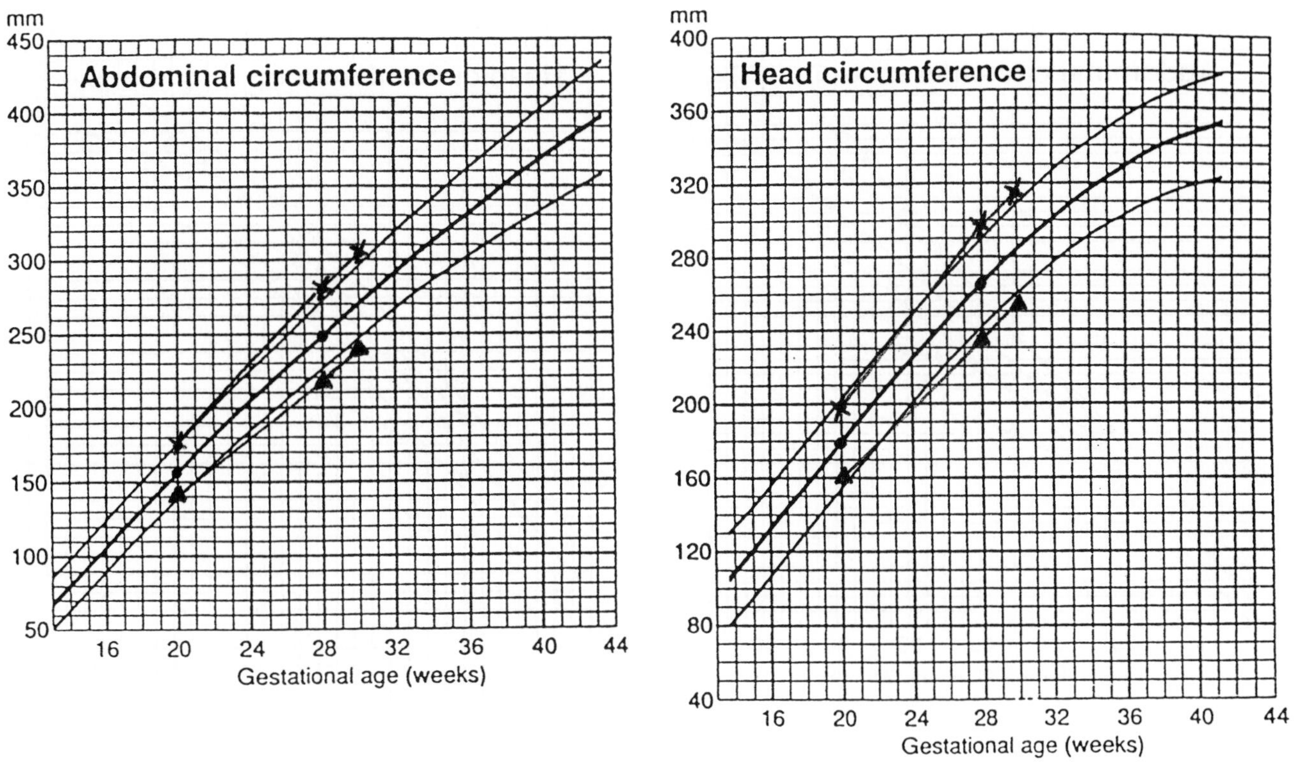

Fig. 12.2 Normal ultrasound fetal growth patterns (centile charts by Hadlock,[65,66] showing 10th, 50th and 90th percentile lines). The BPD growth pattern is usually similar to that of the HC for that fetus. The BPD measurement can be affected by fetal presentation particularly at later gestations e.g. breech fetuses have dolichocephalic (long thin) heads. The HC is a better measure of fetal head growth in such cases. • Normal fetal size; ▲–▲ 'constitutionally small' fetus; X–X 'constitutionally large' fetus.

ments continue to increase at an appropriate rate, no further scans are necessary.

The scan may confirm a small fetus which, when repeated 2 weeks later, shows growth parallel to but below the 10th centile (Fig. 12.2). This suggests a healthy SGA fetus with adequate placental function. This is a 'constitutionally small' fetus, which is no more at risk than the one shown as a false positive on clinical assessment.

Finally, repeated scans may show intrauterine growth restriction. This has been used to describe any fetus whose birthweight was below the 10th centile. Unfortunately, this led to much confusion in terminology as most of these fetuses are healthy, small for gestational age fetuses who have grown at a normal rate in utero (see above). A small proportion will have experienced 'true', progressive growth restriction in utero. The reported incidence of IUGR varies widely between different populations (1.8–23.1% of screened population[160]). Only some of this variation can be accounted for by different antenatal screening methods and postnatal definitions of IUGR. It is important that obstetricians try to identify true IUGR antenatally, as further investigation and intervention may be required.

True progressive IUGR can be detected antenatally on serial scans. Two patterns of abnormal growth are recognized, symmetrical and asymmetrical IUGR (Fig. 12.3). In the former the ultrasound measurements may initially seem similar to those for normal SGA fetuses, although usually presenting at earlier gestations and in a rather more severe form. At later gestations both the abdominal circumference and head measurements fall progressively away from the centiles, but in proportion to one another. This ultrasound growth pattern suggests a fundamental fetal problem, e.g. chromosomal abnormality or congenital infection, or maternal congenital uterine malformation, such as a bicornuate uterus, which globally restricts fetal growth. Referral to a fetal medicine unit for further investigation is merited.

In cases of asymmetrical IUGR the ultrasound growth pattern is quite different. Whereas the abdominal circumference measurements progressively tail off, the head measurements continue parallel to the centiles, often within the normal range (Fig. 12.3). This suggests reduced placental function, as this is the only supply of nutrition to the fetus in utero. As with starvation in children, the limited supply is diverted away from the abdomen and limbs to the brain, to maintain essential growth and function, and liver glycogen stores are consumed. Such an ultrasound growth pattern should prompt the obstetrician to instigate further investigation of fetal well-being related to placental insufficiency. If left unchecked, such fetuses can die in utero from chronic hypoxia, and this accounts for a significant proportion of antepartum

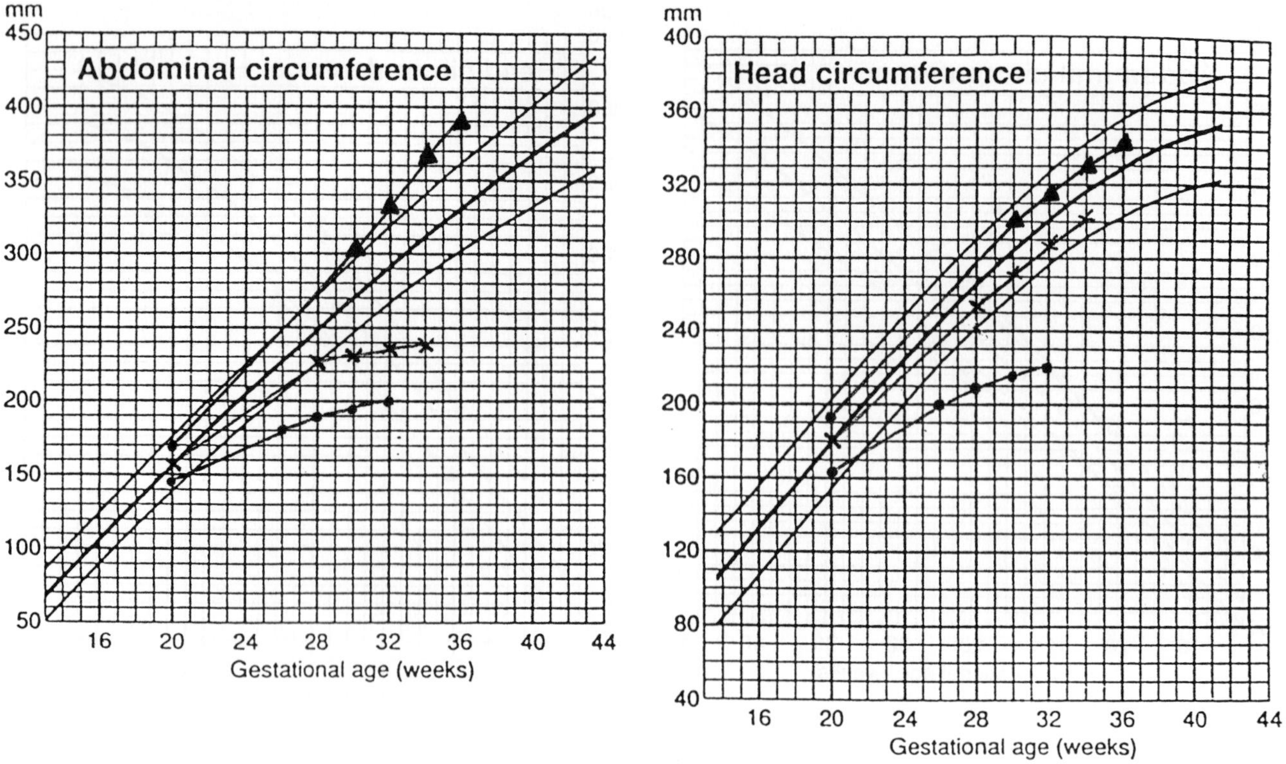

Fig. 12.3 Abnormal ultrasound fetal growth patterns (same centile charts as in Fig. 12.2). ●–● Symmetrical IUGR growth pattern; X–X asymmetrical IUGR growth pattern; ▲–▲ macrosomic fetal growth pattern.

stillbirths. Alternatively, the fetus may enter labour with unrecognized compromised placental reserve, such that it is unable to compensate for the most demanding period of its intrauterine existence. Clearly, the antenatal recognition of asymmetrical IUGR is of fundamental importance.

An example of the proportion of cases of severe IUGR (both symmetrical and asymmetrical) attributable to different causes is shown in Table 12.1.

Large for gestational age

The ultrasound scan may reveal that the fundal height measurement was a false positive or that the fetus is a large baby growing normally (Fig. 12.2) i.e. a 'constitutionally large' fetus.

Table 12.1 Aetiology of severe intrauterine growth deficiency, University of Iowa, 1984–1992

Diagnosis	*n*	%
Severe uteroplacental dysfunction	62	54.9
Chromosome abnormality	22	19.5
Associated structural malformations	13	11.5
Congenital infection	9	
proven	7	6.2
likely	2	1.8
Miscellaneous	7	6.2
Total	113	

Serial scans may indicate increasing growth velocity, particularly of the trunk (Fig. 12.3), suggestive of fetal macrosomia.[114] The most common cause is poorly controlled maternal diabetes, and this merits investigation. The fetus is exposed to abnormally high glucose concentrations and develops a typical cherubic appearance (Chapter 24). As the fetal bisacromial diameter is wider than the biparietal diameter, shoulder dystocia is more common.[109] Tight maternal diabetic control may limit this abnormal fetal growth pattern.

FETAL WELL-BEING

At each antenatal visit the woman is asked about fetal movements, the fetal heart is auscultated, the symphyseal–fundal height is measured and the liquor volume is clinically assessed. These are simple screening tests of fetal well-being related to placental function. Detected abnormalities require further investigation.

Fetal movements

Normal fetal movements are recognized to be an indicator of fetal well-being.[118] In 1973[146] it was first suggested that cessation of maternally perceived fetal movements may spell impending fetal asphyxia and death. Various attempts were then made to formalize fetal movement recording. The Cardiff 'count to 10' fetal activity chart[129] became particularly popular, the principle

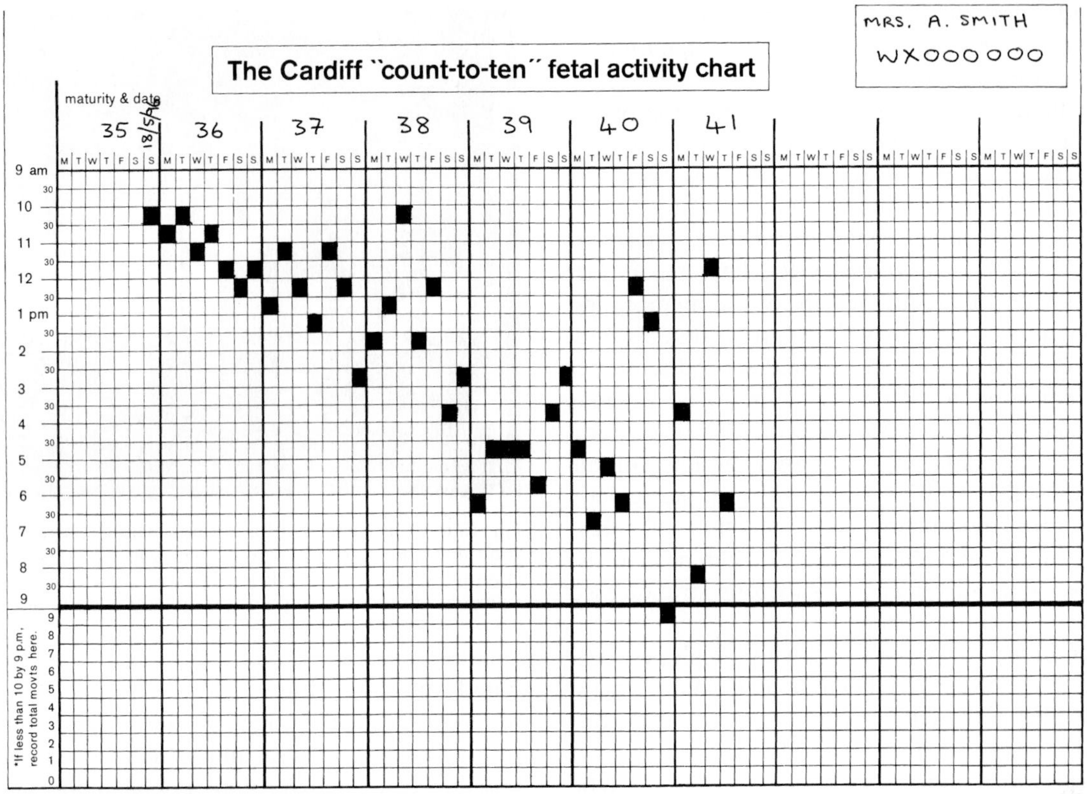

Fig. 12.4 Completed Cardiff 'count-to-10' fetal movement chart.

being to record the time taken each day to record 10 movements (Fig. 12.4). Prospective evaluation of these charts in high-risk pregnancies[97] showed that when there were fewer than 10 movements in 12 hours this was associated with a significant increase in perinatal mortality, fetal distress and fetal compromise. This led to the suggestion that whole population screening might be effective in reducing the perinatal mortality rate.

The definitive multicentre randomized controlled study of 68 654 women assessed routine use of the 'count to 10' method[61] and failed to show any overall benefit. However, all babies that died in utero were recognized promptly, and more CTGs were performed in the group using movement charts. It is likely that false reassurance about placental function resulted from a normal antepartum CTG (see later). It has also been appreciated that the absence or reduction in perceived fetal movements may only be significant if there are other indicators of placental compromise detected, e.g. asymmetrical IUGR or oligohydramnios.

The sequence of investigation of maternally reported decreased fetal movements which we use is schematically represented in Figure 12.5.

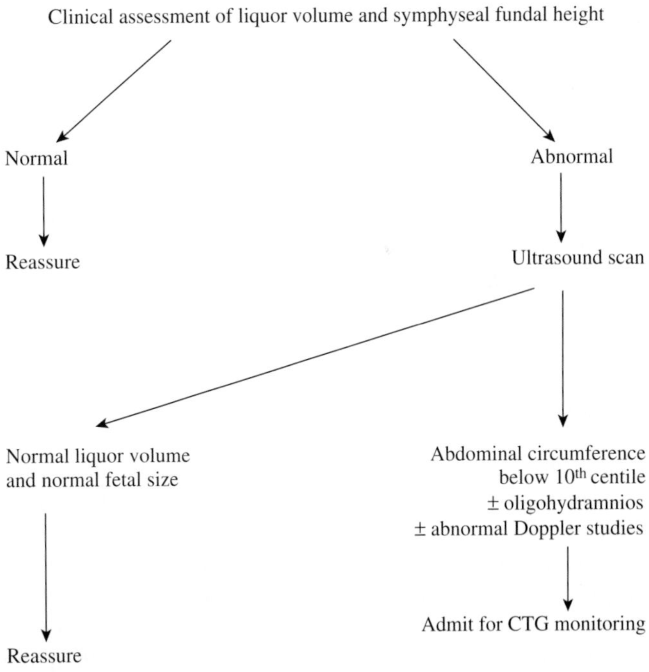

Fig. 12.5 Assessment of maternally reported decreased fetal movements.

Liquor volume assessment

Clinical assessment of liquor volume (by palpation) should be made at each antenatal visit, particularly if the symphyseal– fundal height is abnormal for the gestational age. If abnormal liquor volume is suspected, an ultrasound scan should be arranged to verify the situation. The measurements are recorded as either the depth of the deepest liquor pool (normal range 3–8 cm) or as an amniotic fluid index (the sum of the depths of the deepest pool of liquor in each of the four quadrants of the uterus). Normal ranges for gestational age are available.[111]

Amniotic fluid is produced partly by the amnion on the surface of the placenta, but fetal urine and lung fluid make a substantial contribution. In addition the fetus swallows appreciable amounts of liquor. Thus, oligohydramnios is a sign of placental insufficiency (particularly if this is associated with IUGR), fetal renal tract abnormalities and pre-labour rupture of the membranes, and these potential causes should be further investigated. Oligohydramnios presenting in the mid-second trimester or earlier predisposes to pulmonary hypoplasia, whereas prolonged oligohydramnios increases the risk of postural deformities.[145] In addition, decreased liquor volume enhances the likelihood of cord compression, particularly in labour.[39,134] Consequently, the detection of oligohydramnios should immediately alert the clinician to the need for closer fetal surveillance, as there is an increased perinatal mortality in this setting.

Polyhydramnios is also associated with a high perinatal loss rate. The aetiology is related to maternal diabetes (particularly likely if the fetus is large for gestational age), fetal central nervous system and gastrointestinal tract abnormalities (which impair fetal swallowing) and fetal hydrops. Each of these factors needs to be considered. In the diabetic mother the fetus has high blood glucose levels, causing an osmotic diuresis and fetal polyuria, leading to an abnormally high contribution of fetal urine to the liquor volume. Good maternal diabetic control can therefore be expected to reverse the process. The presence of polyhydramnios itself also increases the risk to the fetus as it predisposes to preterm pre-labour rupture of the membranes, preterm labour, cord prolapse and abruptio placentae.

In contrast, normal liquor volume on clinical assessment can be interpreted as a reassuring sign of fetal well-being.

Doppler studies

The combination of maternal risk factors, e.g. pre-eclampsia, with fundal height, amniotic fluid volume and fetal ultrasound measurements, are the features that best identify IUGR.[160] These are the fetuses most at risk of chronic hypoxia. Prior to 1977,[47] when Doppler ultrasound of the umbilical vessels was first reported, CTG was routinely used to monitor these, fetuses. When the two techniques were compared to identify fetal compromise[158] umbilical artery Doppler studies were found to have twice the sensitivity (60%), with a similar specificity of 85%, a positive predictive value of 64% and a false negative rate of 17%.

Umbilical artery Doppler studies give a measure of the resistance to blood flow by relating the peak systolic to the end-diastolic shifted frequencies, which both relate to

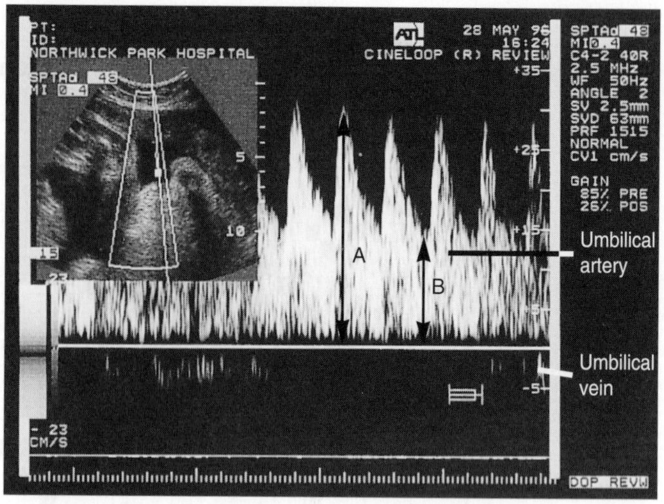

Fig. 12.6 Doppler study of a normal umbilical artery and vein in the third trimester of pregnancy The vein appears in the opposite channel to the artery as flow within it is away from the transducer. A, maximum systolic frequency; B, minimum end-diastolic frequency.

blood velocities (Fig. 12.6). A relative fall in the end-diastolic frequency suggests increased resistance to perfusion, consistent with impaired placental function and possible fetal hypoxia. Other fetal blood vessels can be studied to obtain more information. Hypoxaemic fetuses have a low middle cerebral artery blood flow resistance, whereas the reverse is true in the aorta.[8] This is thought to be indicative of a 'brain-sparing redistribution', which may help to explain why such infants are at increased risk of necrotizing enterocolitis.

Abnormal Doppler studies should alert the clinician to instigate vigilant fetal monitoring. They are not, in themselves, an indication for delivery, but form an important part of the emerging clinical picture.

Antenatal cardiotocography

Four randomized controlled trials have attempted to evaluate the use of routine weekly fetal heart rate records on outpatient high-risk pregnancies.[13,49,89,99] but none of these was large enough to demonstrate any potential clinical benefit.[60] Meta-analysis of the data, however, showed a reduction in admissions to hospital but a threefold increase in the stillbirth rate.[110] This suggests that a normal CTG in a high-risk pregnancy falsely reassures both clinician and mother of fetal well-being, when in reality it only assesses the situation at that point in time. Antenatal cardiotocography, therefore, has not been shown to be of value as a routine outpatient management test in high-risk pregnancies, though it is still widely used in this way.

There is evidence, however, that it is of considerable value in the antenatal management of identified fetal growth retardation. The characteristic changes associated with the progressive effects of chronic placental failure

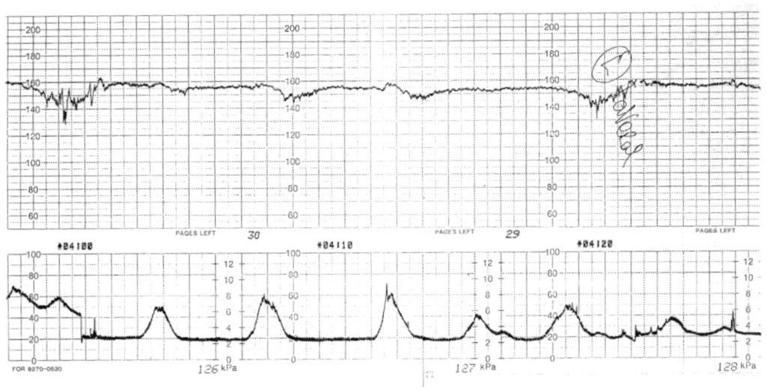

Fig. 12.7 Characteristic cardiotocograph changes associated with chronic uteroplacental insufficiency. The typical features are the reduced baseline variability, the lack of reassuring accelerations and the presence of recurrent, shallow, late decelerations. The tocograph trace shows uterine tightenings (Braxton Hicks), which can often be recorded antenatally.

include loss of accelerations (associated with a decrease in fetal movements), a reduced baseline variability and the onset of recurrent decelerations[45,48,88,142,161] (Fig. 12.7) (see later section for definitions of normal CTG patterns). Such evidence of 'critical fetal reserve' requires delivery. There is a significantly higher incidence of metabolic acidosis at delivery,[24,162] but if delivery is effected prior to such ominous CTG patterns then fetal decompensation into acidaemia is prevented.[71]

Thus, antenatal cardiotocography should be used in a restricted, purposeful way and probably in combination with other investigations, as a discriminating test of the effect of placental function on fetal well-being.

Biophysical profiles

The fetal heart rate record forms part of the 'biophysical profile', which also entails ultrasound scanning for assessment of fetal movements, fetal muscular tone, fetal breathing movements and amniotic fluid volume.[104] The combination of these variables into a single profile score, in selected high-risk pregnancies, significantly improved both the false positive and false negative rates for predicting fetal distress in labour, a low 5-minute Apgar score and perinatal mortality when compared with any of the variables used alone.[104] The sensitivity of the biophysical profile is around 50% and specificity is around 90% for both perinatal morbidity and mortality.[157] However, performing the full profile is time-consuming and, with the widespread introduction of Doppler studies, which have similar predictive values, the full biophysical profile is rarely performed nowadays.

ANTENATAL FETAL COMPLICATIONS AND THEIR MANAGEMENT

The fetus can be exposed to chronic hypoxia in utero owing to progressive placental insufficiency or to an acute hypoxic event as a result of sudden placental compromise. The placenta can also serve as a vehicle for the transmission of infections from the mother to the fetus. Alternatively, infections can ascend from the vagina to the fetus, especially if the amniotic membranes are breached. This is one of a number of causes of preterm labour. Each of these areas will be covered in more detail, with particular emphasis on antenatal interventions aimed to improve the subsequent neonatal course.

Intrauterine growth restriction

The antenatal diagnosis of chronic uteroplacental insufficiency and its importance has already been discussed. If the fetus shows sign of compromise antenatally, i.e. abnormal CTGs on a background of abnormal Doppler studies, delivery should be effected by caesarean section almost irrespective of the gestation. Such fetuses are unlikely to be able to compensate for the acute hypoxic stress of reduced placental perfusion with each uterine contraction for prolonged periods. If, however, the CTGs remain normal antenatally the management will be much more dependent on the gestational age. At term, induction of labour while the fetus remains uncompromised is logical. In the preterm situation, however, expectant management with daily CTGs, weekly scans to assess liquor volume and perform Doppler studies, and fortnightly fetal size measurements to assess growth are preferable as the risks of prematurity are appreciable. The aim is to quantify the rate of progression of the chronic placental problem. Rapid deterioration or abnormal CTGs should prompt delivery by caesarean section. Alternatively, if the fetus remains uncompromised, induction of labour at 38 weeks' gestation can be planned.

Prolonged pregnancy

This term denotes a pregnancy which has gone beyond 42 weeks from the date of the first day of the last menstrual period.[55] In places where women book in the first trimester and dating scans are performed, the incidence of prolonged pregnancy is less than 5%.[44,80] Though small, there is an increased risk of perinatal mortality after 42 weeks.[5,31] This is largely accounted for by an increased incidence of uteroplacental insufficiency and oligohydramnios. There is also an increased perinatal morbidity in prolonged pregnancies due to hypoxia, shoulder dystocia and birth injuries,[5] even when delivery is spontaneous rather than instrumental.

It is therefore usual to offer women induction of labour between 10 and 14 days after their expected date of delivery. If this is declined, an ultrasound scan should be performed to assess the amniotic fluid volume and fetal size. If there is oligohydramnios or IUGR, induction of labour while the fetus is healthy should be strongly advocated. If the scan is reassuring, it is customary to commence regular (at least twice weekly) CTG monitoring after 42 weeks. Provided there is prompt intervention when CTG abnormalities occur, the perinatal outcome in prolonged pregnancies is improved by such monitoring.[41,42]

Antepartum haemorrhage (APH)

This is the term used to describe any bleeding from the genital tract after the 24th week of pregnancy. It complicates 2–5% of all pregnancies.[20,63,73] Abruptio placentae and placenta praevia are the two most serious single causes; however, more frequently no specific aetiology for an APH is found.

Abruptio placentae, is premature separation of a normally situated placenta. It classically presents with abdominal pain, uterine contractions and a tense, tender, 'woody hard' uterus, with or without vaginal bleeding. Bleeding may be concealed in up to 35% of cases[51,92] and abdominal pain is not always a prominent feature.[123] Ultrasonography, though frequently performed in this setting, is not a sensitive method of diagnosis.[63] The fetal effects depend on the degree of placental separation and the condition of the placenta prior to the acute event. IUGR is said to be present in a substantial proportion of preterm cases requiring delivery.[73] Frequently fetal compromise precedes a deterioration in maternal condition, and over 50% of the perinatal deaths attributed to abruption are stillbirths.[72] The management of placental abruption is usually expectant unless there are signs of maternal or fetal compromise to prompt delivery. If there is evidence of fetal distress, the data suggest that the perinatal outcome is significantly improved by early caesarean section rather than attempted vaginal delivery.[72,78,91,125] In other cases the mode of delivery will depend on the severity of the maternal condition, and will be influenced by whether the woman is already in labour. Significant fetal bleeding[59] and transient neonatal coagulopathies[63] have been reported. The main risk to the fetus, however, is from acute hypoxia and asphyxia.

In contrast, it is uncommon for the fetus to become acutely hypoxic due to bleeding from a placenta praevia (a placenta attached partially or wholly to the lower uterine segment), unless the mother is so severely hypovolaemic that she can no longer perfuse the placental bed adequately. Usually, maternal haemodynamic instability indicates delivery by caesarean section at a much earlier point. Recurrent episodes of minor APH due to placenta praevia can lead to IUGR.[159] The main risk to the neonate, however, is from preterm delivery. This is not surprising, as a low-lying placenta is more common in earlier pregnancy, and with formation of the lower uterine segment in the third trimester an apparent change in placental position is frequently seen.[22,30,72] Fetal anaemia can occur, particularly at a difficult caesarean section when placental integrity has to be breached in order to reach the baby.

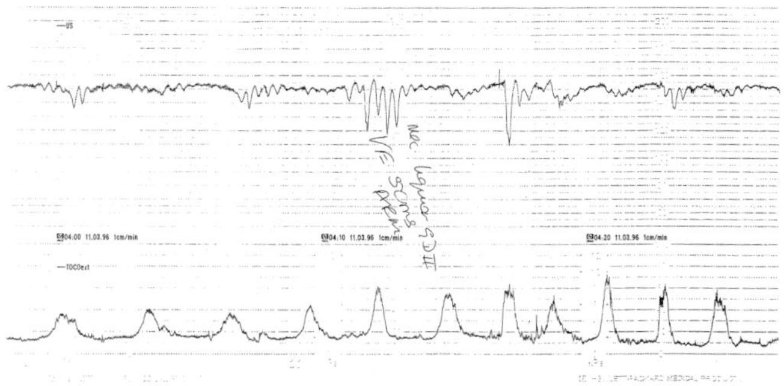

Fig. 12.8 Typical 'sinusoidal' cardiotocogram of severe fetal anaemia (see text for description of features).

Antepartum haemorrhage due to vasa praevia, i.e. umbilical vessels crossing the membranes, also leads to fetal anaemia. The typical CTG pattern in severe fetal anaemia (whatever the cause) is described as 'sinusoidal' (Fig. 12.8). This is a preterminal pattern which is rarely seen. Six rigid criteria must be fulfilled to make the diagnosis:[108]

- A stable baseline fetal heart rate of 120–160 beats per minute, with regular oscillations;
- An amplitude of 5–15 beats per minute;
- A frequency of 2–5 cycles per minute;
- Absent short-term variability;
- No areas of normal fetal heart rate variability or reactivity.

Pseudosinusoidal fetal heart rate patterns (vaguely defined as undulatory waveforms), in contrast, are common and usually innocuous. They are strongly associated with the use of pethidine and epidural analgesia and are also seen with fetal sucking movements. Such patterns will generally improve with time. There have been only occasional reports of major pseudosinusoidal fetal heart rate patterns (with amplitudes greater than 24 beats/minute) in association with preterminal fetal anaemia.[116]

Intrauterine infection

Maternal rubella, syphilis and hepatitis B serology will usually be routinely checked at the booking visit. Cytomegalovirus, however, is the most common cause of congenital infection in pregnancy. Evidence from controlled trials has not found routine maternal screening to be effective.[140] Toxoplasmosis screening is practised in France, where seropositivity is common. However, in the UK the incidence of primary infection in pregnancy is only 2 per 1000,[1] and only a very small percentage will have clinically affected infants.[38] A recent expert committee report did not recommend introducing such a service in the UK.[130] Screening for maternal HIV infection remains controversial. Recent evidence suggesting a significant reduction in the vertical transmission rate with antenatal and neonatal zidovudine treatment[29] may be influential. In addition, caesarean section delivery may offer some degree of protection to the baby.[119]

Maternal vaginal screening for potential pathogens has also been studied. Group B streptococcus can result in serious neonatal morbidity and is a cause of preterm labour. Intrapartum antibiotics have been shown to significantly decrease neonatal colonization, sepsis and death.[11,40,107,112,126] The problem is deciding which women should be treated. Studies have shown that transient and intermittent carriage is common[3] and that antenatal screening is a poor predictor of the intrapartum state.[10] Unfortunately, a rapid assay is not available. Bacterial vaginosis as a possible causal factor in preterm labour is also being investigated.[69]

Two other maternal infections merit discussion, herpes simplex and varicella zoster. Genital herpes simplex only poses a major risk to the fetus if vaginal delivery occurs in the presence of primary infection, which is often asymptomatic and therefore unrecognized. Symptomatic primary infection at term is an indication for delivery by caesarean section. Recurrent disease is now known to carry a low risk for the fetus[137] and caesarean section is only contemplated if there are active lesions in labour and the membranes have been ruptured for less than 4 hours. Maternal chickenpox in late pregnancy is associated with a high neonatal infection rate. If this occurs within 5 days of delivery the neonatal mortality may be as high as 30%.[56] Chickenpox contact near term in a susceptible mother is therefore an indication for zoster immunoglobulin to prevent maternal infection. However, if infection does occur, delaying delivery until the fetus has gained passive immunity from the mother is desirable. If delivery is unavoidable, the infant should be treated with both zoster immunoglobulin and acyclovir (p. 1158).

Preterm pre-labour rupture of the membranes (PPROM)

Term is defined as 37 completed weeks of gestation. PPROM is diagnosed on the basis of maternal history, liquor visualization and clinical or ultrasound evidence of oligohydramnios. The cause of PPROM is relevant to both the obstetrician and the neonatologist. Common aetiologies include polyhydramnios, chorioamnionitis, invasive testing, e.g. amniocentesis, maternal urinary tract infection and cervical incompetence. Underlying causes should be treated where possible. The management thereafter is usually conservative unless there is deterioration in the fetomaternal condition. The risks of prematurity are greater than those of the most common complication, chorioamnionitis.[87] Unfortunately, this is difficult to detect clinically in its early stages and conclusive tests are not currently available. Cord prolapse and placental abruption can also occur.

Preterm labour

PPROM predisposes to preterm labour, as does APH. Multiple pregnancies are at increased risk of almost every pregnancy complication, including preterm labour. Nonetheless, it is a frequently overdiagnosed entity, as cervical change in the presence of uterine contractions is necessary to fulfil the criteria for diagnosis. Indeed, in recent years interest has focused on methods of distinguishing those women in threatened preterm labour who will go on to deliver preterm, from those whose contractions will settle spontaneously. This would enable treatment to be targeted at the correct patients. Initial studies on fetal fibronectin detection in cervicovaginal secretions were promising.[54,115] More recent work,[94,103] however, has shown that the fetal fibronectin test has relatively poor positive predictive values for preterm delivery (36–50%) but good negative predictive values (91–98%). It has been suggested that fetal fibronectin is released in cases of subclinical chorioamnionitis. Thus, the role of fetal fibronectin testing is yet to be fully established and it is not currently in routine use.

Immediate delivery in cases of preterm labour is occasionally indicated for fetal or maternal reasons, e.g. placental abruption. Sometimes the woman is allowed to continue labouring irrespective of the gestational age, as the risks of continued intrauterine existence outweigh the disadvantages of prematurity, e.g. obvious chorioamnionitis. However, in the majority of cases the management is dependent on the gestational age. Previously, long-term tocolytic therapy was widely used. It has since become appreciated that tocolytics can have serious adverse effects and that only in certain situations is there a potential benefit. The neonatal morbidity following delivery between 34 and 37 weeks is unchanged whether or not attempts to arrest labour are successful,[50] and there is now no justification for tocolysis after 34 weeks. However, tocolytics do have a role between 25 and 34 weeks' gestation. Overall, the data of the 15 studies considered by Keirse et al[86] demonstrate that β-sympathomimetic drug therapy results in a lower incidence of preterm birth. The real value of tocolysis, however, is to enable sufficient time to enhance fetal lung maturity by the concomitant use of maternal corticosteroid therapy. Maternally administered corticosteroids have been in use since 1972[96] and have been extensively evaluated in the preterm labour setting. Data from 12 controlled trials reviewed by Crowley et al[35] demonstrated that corticosteroids reduce the occurrence of hyaline membrane disease overall, and this reduction in respiratory morbidity was also associated with reductions in the risk of GMH-IVH, NEC and neonatal death. A recent meta-analysis of all the randomized trials of antenatal corticosteroid therapy (1972–1994) has confirmed these benefits.[32] There has been no clear evidence of short- or long-term adverse effects on the mother or infant. This has led to their elective use in many other settings in which preterm delivery is anticipated, e.g. severe IUGR. The effects of steroids used for this purpose, however, have not been fully established. Indeed, the practice of weekly steroid therapy in higher-order multiple pregnancies has no scientific basis. Steroids are also frequently used outside the gestational age range for which they were originally clinically evaluated (28–34 weeks). The additional use of maternally administered TRH to further enhance lung maturity is still being evaluated, and this is not currently in routine use.

Tocolytic therapy in preterm labour should be continued if possible for 48 hours to try to maximize the effects of steroids. A variety of tocolytics are available, some of which have fetal side-effects relevant to the neonatologist. β-Sympathomimetic agents, e.g. ritodrine and salbutamol, cross the placenta and may cause fetal tachycardia and occasionally other adverse fetal cardiac effects, which may be significant in an already compromised fetus.[52,86] Maternal hyperglycaemia can result in troublesome neonatal hypoglycaemia, but long-term ill effects have not been recognized. Prostaglandin synthesis inhibitors, e.g. indomethacin, on the other hand, can have more serious neonatal consequences. The predominant problems are premature closure or constriction of the ductus arteriosus and reduced fetal urinary output, leading to oligohydramnios. Necrotizing enterocolitis, ileal perforation and neonatal GMH-IVH have also been reported.[4,102,122] Consequently, the use of indomethacin has been limited to short-term therapy (72 hours) before 32 weeks' gestation.

The role of antibiotic prophylaxis in PPROM and preterm labour is currently being studied in a large MRC trial (ORACLE: Overview of the Role of Antibiotics in Curtailing Labour and Early delivery). Meta-analysis of previous trials[33] has suggested a possible benefit. The ORACLE study results are eagerly awaited.

INTRAPARTUM ASSESSMENT AND MANAGEMENT

This section begins by discussing the mechanism of normal labour and methods of correcting slow progress. It then goes on to describe the fetal response to labour and ways of assessing intrapartum fetal well-being. Finally it covers methods of delivery: this is the time at which the neonatologist often becomes involved for the first time. We hope to have demonstrated, however, that the antenatal and intrapartum course leading up to this point should also be of interest to the attending paediatrician.

THE MECHANISM OF LABOUR

Recognition of the onset of labour determines all subsequent management objectives.

Diagnosis of labour

A diagnosis of labour is made when regular painful uterine activity effects a change in the cervix. Pain, however, is a subjective experience and is always important to the mother, especially when it is bad enough for her to ask for analgesia. Regularity – an objective observation – is usually accepted when contractions occur more frequently than once every 5 minutes. When regular contractions are considered painful by the mother the question of 'confirming' the diagnosis of labour is appropriate. If the cervix is 3 or more centimetres dilated then labour is usually diagnosed with certainty. If the cervix is less dilated, this is when conservative and active approaches differ in subsequent management.

Early graphical descriptions of labour[53] indicated that 'early' labour (defined as cervical dilatation of less than 3 cm) could last many hours. This led to the idea that there is a slow, or latent, phase of labour, followed by a faster, or active, phase. With a conservative approach, when the cervix is less than 3 cm dilated the woman would be told that she was not yet in 'established labour'. Usually a further examination is performed 4 hours later. 'Early' labour, however, may last for many hours and can lead to maternal exhaustion and reduced fetal reserve.

The philosophy of 'active management' of labour,[124] however, challenges the idea that prolonged labour is a normal and an inevitable consequence if women present 'early' in labour and have yet to get through the latent phase. In the National Maternity Hospital, Dublin, 98% of first labours deliver within 12 hours of the diagnosis of labour. Early and accurate diagnosis of labour is one key feature of the management. Effacement or dilatation of the cervix (by 1 cm), a 'show' and ruptured membranes are all features that are used to 'confirm' the onset of labour in such circumstances. The problem with this approach is that it inevitably leads to a rather low threshold for intervention such as oxytocin infusion.

Progress in labour

Once labour has been diagnosed then progress is expected within certain time limits. Regular examinations of the cervix are made, at least every 4 hours with conservative management, and every 1–2 hours with active management, so that the rate of dilatation can be plotted against time. The use of a composite graphical record of progress in labour, described as a 'partogram', was first reported from Africa[135] (Fig. 12.9). This was soon complemented by a nomogram of expected progress.[154] The most widespread expectation for progress in labour is a rate of at least 1 cm cervical dilatation per hour, which derives from the slowest 10% of women reported by Philpott.[135] With conservative management this expectation begins after the cervix has reached 3 cm dilatation; with active management it begins when labour is

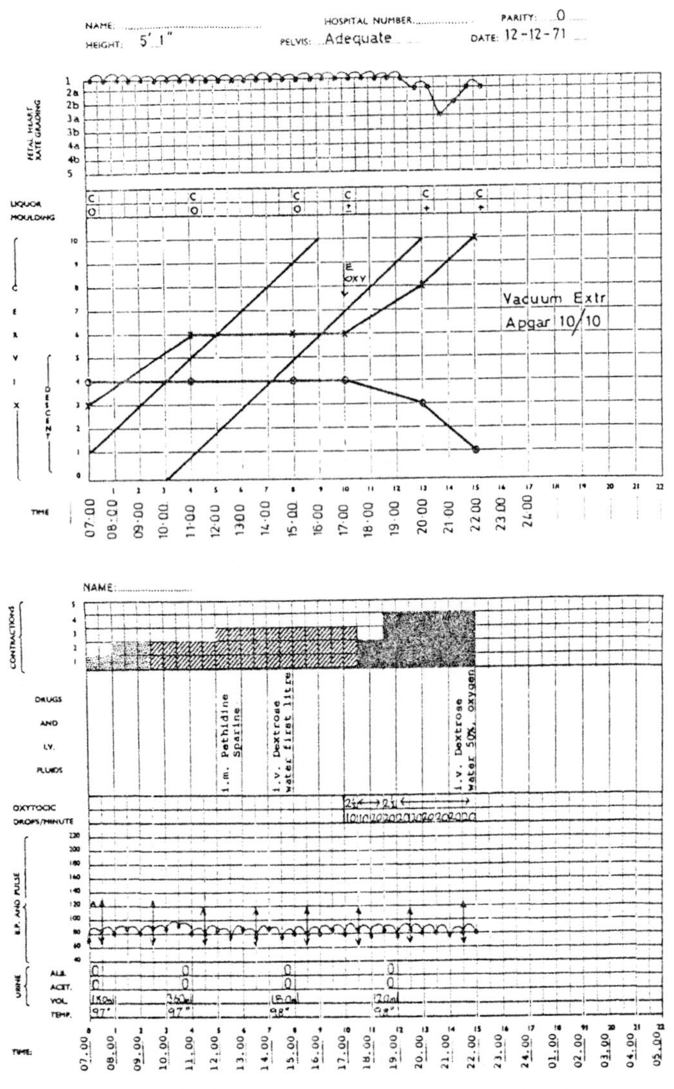

Fig. 12.9 The original example of a 'partogram' described by Philpott in 1972 (full size 25 × 40 cm). Various modifications have since been made, e.g. fetal heart rate grading is now obsolete and is replaced by simple, intermittent fetal heart rate measurement. A number of different partogram formats are now available. (Reproduced with permission from Philpott 1972[135].)

diagnosed. Interventions to augment progress are more frequent in active management. However, with active managment there is a reduction by almost 50% in the likelihood of a caesarean section due to dystocia, i.e. ineffective uterine activity.[98] Nonetheless, many midwives and pregnant women see active management of labour as unnecessary 'medical' intervention and prefer the conservative approach.

Management of the second stage of labour has undergone a change in recent years, particularly since the more widespread use of regional analgesia with epidurals. Once the cervix is fully dilated, progress is defined as descent of the presenting part through the birth canal. This is often judged by hourly vaginal examinations. As the fetus exerts pressure on the pelvic floor (levator ani muscles), the mother feels increasing rectal pressure and an irresistible urge to push. In multiparous women this sensation can occur before full dilatation is reached, and active pushing is then usually discouraged.

In the absence of an epidural, the usual limits of duration for pushing are 60–90 minutes for first labours and 30–60 minutes for multiparous women. These recommendations have some support, in that fetal hypoxia and acidaemia increase progressively during the second stage.[77] However, in recent years, with the increasing use of epidural analgesia, more time in the second stage before pushing has been shown to improve the chance of vaginal delivery[84] without a major deterioration in fetal pH.[105] Nevertheless, the need for operative assistance remains significantly increased[76] and many consider one additional hour sufficient to minimize this possibility.

Interventions during labour

There are two interventions designed to improve the rate of progress during spontaneous labour, amniotomy and intravenous infusion of oxytocin. Both can also be used to induce labour.

Rupture of the membranes

One of the aspects of active management is the use of amniotomy within 2 hours if cervical dilatation is not evident following the diagnosis of labour.[124] However, routine rupture of the membranes to prevent slow progress in labour has been criticized. A large collaborative study[16] showed that membranes ruptured spontaneously in only 66% of women before the second stage. Earlier amniotomy significantly shortened the duration of labour but was associated with a higher incidence of caput formation and moulding of the fetal head. In addition, there was an increased incidence of early uniform fetal heart rate decelerations and a significantly lower median umbilical artery pH at birth (albeit still within the normal range). These findings can be explained on the basis of increased uterine activity, greater head compression and cord compression. A more recent study[153] has suggested that the effect of amniotomy on the fetus is a balance between the adverse effects of augmentation and the benefits of reduced duration of labour.

Effects of oxytocin

Augmentation of spontaneous labour by oxytocin infusion aims to achieve optimal uterine activity with a maximum contraction frequency of once every 2 minutes. Uterine perfusion decreases during contractions, resulting in a decrease in blood flow to the intervillous space.[9] As long as the relaxation periods between contractions remain adequate, and sustained uterine tonus is avoided, fetal bradycardia is not seen[18] and fetal cerebral oxygenation remains unaffected.[131] Nevertheless, in clinical practice the use of oxytocin is associated with an increased incidence of fetal heart rate decelerations.[147]

INTRAPARTUM FETAL ASSESSMENT

The fetus responds to many aspects of labour and its management. Monitoring of fetal well-being requires an understanding of placental function and, in particular, knowledge of the influence of pregnancy complications and labour on maternal–fetal gas exchange. During labour, observations are made on the amount and colour of the amniotic fluid, but the mainstay of fetal monitoring is the recording, either intermittently or continuously, of the fetal heart rate. Optimal interpretation of some changes requires fetal blood sampling to determine the fetal acid–base level.

Amniotic fluid volume

A normal volume of amniotic fluid offers some degree of protection against the many effects of uterine contractions. The volume of the intervillous space is maintained and is not compressed against the fetus, and the umbilical cord is also less likely to be compressed. Oligohydramnios present before post-dates labour is a predictor for intrapartum fetal distress.[34] Thus, continuous fetal heart rate monitoring is advocated, and decelerations are more readily interpreted as an indication of clinically important fetal hypoxia. Likewise, reduced liquor volume in early labour, e.g. subsequent to amniotomy, is associated with an increased chance of subsequent fetal heart rate decelerations.[141] Infusion of saline into the amniotic cavity during labour has been shown to decrease the incidence of fetal heart rate decelerations, and may reduce the likelihood of caesarean section being considered necessary.

Meconium

The passage of meconium into the amniotic fluid during labour (fresh meconium) is one of the traditional indicators of fetal distress, and is associated with increased perinatal morbidity and mortality.[12] However, meconium-stained amniotic fluid before labour (old meconium) is found increasingly after 37 weeks' gestation, occurring in 15–20% of pregnancies reaching 41 weeks. It is often found at the time of caesarean section after prolonged labour in the absence of other evidence of fetal distress, yet it is rarely seen in situations of acute fetal distress, such as placental abruption and cord prolapse. The mechanism by which the fetal bowel is stimulated to pass meconium is unclear.

Meconium is sterile but its importance lies in the risk of neonatal meconium aspiration syndrome. This only occurs in about 1% of cases with meconium present. It is now believed that meconium aspiration can occur in utero prior to delivery. The precise aetiology remains obscure, although associated fetal distress predisposes to perinatal morbidity if meconium is present. The current view is that fetal hypoxia and acidaemia lead to an increase in fetal gasping and deep breathing movements, respectively. These are the breathing movements that cause inhalation of amniotic fluid, with meconium if present. Meconium aspiration is more common if the meconium is thick rather than thin.[144] Oligohydramnios leads to the meconium remaining thick and undiluted, and may be an important determinant of any subsequent fetal distress in such circumstances. The passage of prelabour meconium may represent a previous transient fetal stimulation, possibly hypoxic, although infection and thyrotoxicosis are rare causes.

Thus, meconium remains an indication for continuous monitoring of the fetal heart rate during labour, and the presence of meconium lowers the threshold for making a diagnosis of fetal distress if fetal heart rate abnormalities occur.

Fetal heart rate monitoring

The value of continuous electronic fetal heart rate monitoring (EFM) during labour remains controversial. Randomized trials have suggested that continuous EFM confers no outcome advantage over intermittent auscultation for normal, uncomplicated labours.[101] However, this may be a reflection of the rather simplistic interpretation advocated by early enthusiasts.[75] Simple 'pattern recognition' of changes in the fetal heart rate (FHR) has not been shown to be helpful, and it has since been realized that the FHR is a sophisticated reflection of fetal adaptation to changes in the intrauterine environment. The CTG must therefore be interpreted in the context of the clinical picture. The future of fetal heart rate monitoring requires further understanding and acceptance of a more physiological approach to interpretation.[151]

Despite its apparently limited value, EFM is still in widespread use. Continuous monitoring is considered mandatory in high-risk cases, e.g. in the presence of meconium or when there is recognized IUGR. It is therefore important that the attending paediatrician has a basic understanding of the implications of normal and abnormal FHR records.

FHR records are usually assessed with respect to four main features:[143]

- Baseline rate. This is the mean rate in beats per minute determined over a 5–10-minute interval, when stable in the absence of accelerations and decelerations.
- Baseline variability. This refers to oscillations of the recorded baseline FHR (previously described as long-term variability). Both amplitude and frequency may be important.

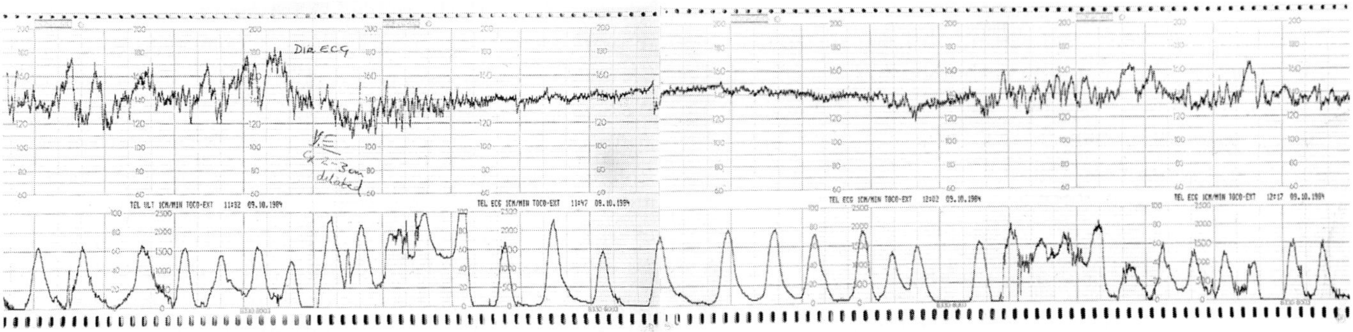

Fig. 12.10 Normal fetal rest–activity behavioural cycles. The trace begins and ends with periods of fetal activity, during which the baseline variability is greater than 5 bpm and there are plenty of accelerations of the fetal heart rate. In between is a physiological episode (lasting 14 minutes) of quiet fetal behaviour with low baseline variability and no accelerations.

- Accelerations. An acceleration is a transient rise in the FHR of at least 15 beats/minute, which lasts for more than 15 seconds. If the rate remains raised then this may be considered a tachycardia.
- Decelerations. A deceleration is a transient fall in the FHR. The commonly accepted classification of decelerations will be discussed later.

Normal intrapartum fetal heart rate patterns

The normal baseline FHR lies between 110 and 150 beats/minute at term (Fig. 12.10). During periods of fetal activity, baseline variability is usually greater than 5 beats/minute (and less than 25 beats/minute) and there should be two or more accelerations in a 20-minute period. It has been known for some time that acceleration is the only pattern not related to fetal acidaemia.[6] Recent interest in fetal stimulation has confirmed the absence of fetal acidaemia associated with a fetal response in the form of a FHR acceleration.[149] However, the absence of accelerations does not necessarily imply acidaemia: only about 2% will have a pH on a fetal blood sample (FBS) taken in labour <7.25.[6]

It was not until the 1980s that the influence of the fetal rest–activity behavioural cycle on intrapartum baseline FHR variability became widely recognized.[148] Episodes of low variability often less than 5 bpm are associated with the quiet fetal behavioural state and an absence of movement-related fetal heart rate accelerations. Such physiological episodes do not usually last more than 45 minutes. Further tests of fetal well-being are appropriate after this, as it may signify a previously unrecognized chronic placental problem. The typical FHR appearance of normal cyclical fetal behaviour is illustrated in Figure 12.10.

FHR decelerations (of any type) are not part of the normal CTG appearance in term fetuses. Early decelerations (synchronous with the contraction) are common, especially in the second stage of labour (Fig. 12.11). They are probably caused by a vagal reflex as a response to mild transient hypoxia as the mother bears down with contractions. Provided all the other aspects of the CTG are normal and the liquor is clear, early decelerations can be well tolerated by a healthy fetus.

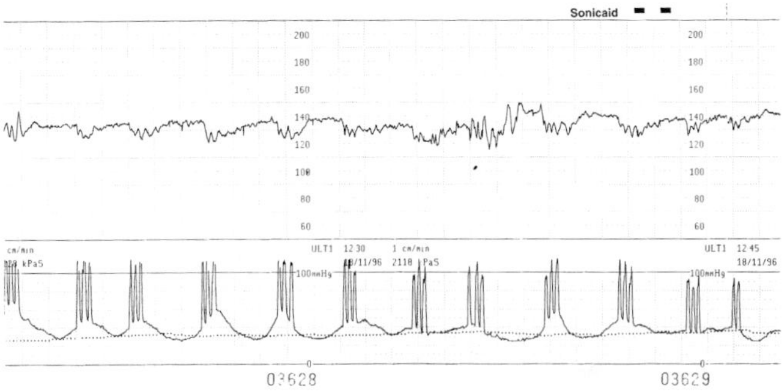

Fig. 12.11 Cardiotocogram in the active phase of the second stage of labour, showing early decelerations. The tocograph tracing shows spikes of activity during contractions, indicating that the mother is actively pushing. The baseline fetal heart rate is normal and a reassuring acceleration is seen (despite the currently low baseline variability). Small early decelerations occur with pushing. This is an acceptable feature of second-stage FHR records.

The interpretation of the FHR pattern of the preterm fetus in labour is similar to that of its term counterpart.[164] However, there are some subtle differences in the FHR pattern. The baseline rate is commonly faster and the variability is often rather less. Accelerations occur less frequently and are less marked. The differentiation between quiet and active sleep patterns may not be evident until 32 weeks' gestation. Small brief (<20 seconds) decelerations are often seen and are not considered significant.

Abnormalities of the fetal heart rate pattern

The significance of an abnormal pattern is much more difficult to judge. In general, the more of the four basic aspects of the FHR (baseline rate, baseline variability, accelerations, decelerations) that are abnormal, the more likely the fetus is to be acidotic. The role of the obstetrician is to seek a cause for the FHR abnormalities, as management will be influenced by the presumed aetiology. For example, repetitive early decelerations in a woman who has progressed from 2 to 10 cm dilation in half an hour will be considered much less sinister than a similar trace in a patient who is thought to have ruptured her previous caesarean section scar. Clearly, the management of these two situations will be quite different. For this reason it is difficult to give a comprehensive yet basic guide to CTG abnormalities in labour.

Abnormalities of the baseline FHR

Acute rises in FHR in labour probably reflect an increase in catecholamine secretion and indicate an early adaptive response to fetal hypoxia before the development of fetal acidaemia. Although chorioamnionitis should always be suspected, recent studies have shown that epidural analgesia is a benign cause of maternal fever and associated fetal tachycardia.[100] β-Mimetic tocolytic therapy frequently causes a maternal tachycardia and leads to a benign fetal tachycardia. Rarely a fetal tachyarrhythmia may be recognized for the first time in labour. Fetal tachycardia >180bpm has traditionally been regarded as a sign of fetal distress. Even in high-risk pregnancies, however, it is not particularly predictive of fetal acidaemia. If found in association with other abnormal FHR patterns the prognosis significantly worsens (Fig. 12.12). Fetal blood sampling or delivery then become more important.

Fetal bradycardia can also be benign. A persistent baseline FHR between 100 and 110 bpm can be seen normally in some post-dates pregnancies and in patients on β-blockers. Acute bradycardias <100 bpm can occur in a number of situations, including vaginal examination, suddenly reaching full dilatation and after epidural top-ups (even in the absence of maternal hypotension). An acute fall in FHR indicates an acute interruption of oxygen delivery, secondary to either maternal hypotension/aortocaval compression or umbilical cord compression. Acidaemia develops within 10–15 minutes and may continue to progress unless the situation is corrected. If the bradycardia fails to recover once appropriate treatment has been instigated, immediate delivery is necessary. However, if the baseline FHR returns to normal and there are no other abnormal FHR features, then conservative management is appropriate. If there is no obvious explanation for a recovered bradycardia then fetal blood sampling should be performed to assess fetal reserve in case there is previously unrecognized chronic placental insufficiency.

Again, fetal bradycardia in association with other abnormalities of the FHR is more sinister. The worst combination of FHR abnormalities described has been progressive bradycardia associated with absent FHR variability, which is regarded as a terminal response of a dying fetus[15,67] (Fig. 12.12).

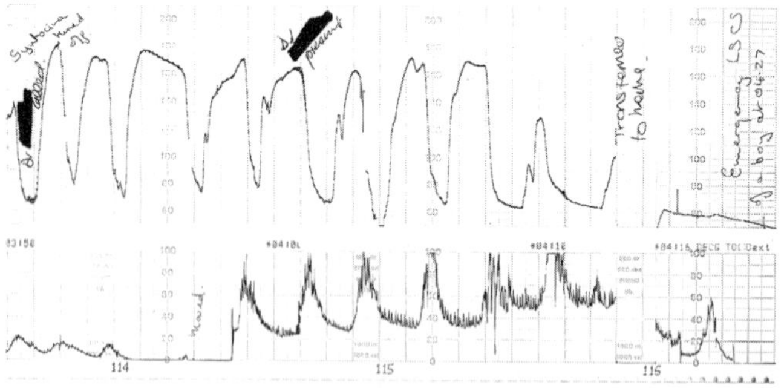

Fig. 12.12 Ominous cardiotocogram showing a complicated fetal tachycardia followed by a progressive bradycardia. The initial baseline fetal heart rate is tachycardic (170–180 bpm), complicated by absent baseline variability and recurrent deep late decelerations. There are no reassuring accelerations present. This is a severely abnormal pattern consistent with rapidly developing fetal acidosis. Prior to delivery the baseline fetal heart rate becomes progressively more bradycardic, with no baseline variability. This is a classic example of a terminal bradycardia. The infant (at term) weighed only 2.18 kg (IUGR) and has profound long-term neurological damage.

Abnormalities of the baseline variability

The significance of reduced baseline variability has already been discussed. Excessive variation (>25 bpm) is an early adaptive response to fetal hypoxia, and in isolation it has not been found to be particularly predictive of fetal acidaemia.[6] Commonly, however, abnormalities of the baseline variability are seen in conjunction with other FHR abnormalities. In such cases further tests of fetal well-being are appropriate.

Presence of decelerations

In general, decelerations should be considered transient bradycardias. FHR decelerations related to uterine contractions certainly represent interruption of maternal–fetal oxygen transfer. In a healthy fetus the most likely mechanism is chemoreceptor stimulation,[64] resulting in a vagal nerve response. Fetal acidaemia only occurs after a considerable reduction in fetal oxygen delivery.[81] Thus, FHR decelerations have a low predictive value for fetal acidaemia, particularly in the absence of associated complications or risk factors.

For example, epidural analgesia is recognized to have an association with late FHR decelerations: however, the outcome appears to be similar (in terms of mean umbilical artery pH and Apgar scores) to cases in which regional analgesia was not employed. Thus, FHR decelerations in this setting are probably more a reflection of adjustments of fetal cardiovascular control rather than an indication of the development of fetal acidaemia.[150] In contrast, however, late FHR decelerations may be the first signs of unrecognized placental insufficiency, and may be associated with a faster rate of development of acidaemia.[150] Again we return to the point that CTG interpretation is only one aspect of the emerging clinical picture. The obstetrician needs to work out why the fetus is mounting a response in the form of FHR decelerations. All decelerations indicate hypoxia, but acidaemia will be present in less than 50% of cases.

Various classifications of FHR decelerations have been proposed. The most widely used in the UK is early, variable and late.

Early decelerations. These are decelerations in which the trough of the decrease in the FHR is synchronous with the peak of the uterine contraction and does not fall below 90 bpm (Fig. 12.11). They are not particularly common. In the first stage of labour they are frequently secondary to treatable causes, such as supine hypotension, epidural analgesia, fetal manipulation etc. Correction of the apparent cause will allow the FHR to return to the baseline and the prognosis is unaffected. Of the three types of decelerations, early ones are the most benign. If the early decelerations persist or there are other abnormalities of the FHR, fetal blood sampling may become indicated.

Variable decelerations. A clear, concise definition of variable decelerations is difficult to find. They are either early in timing (synchronous with the peak of the contraction) but fall below 90 bpm, or they are variable in their shape and timing (Fig. 12.13). Variable decelerations usually represent fetal responses to umbilical cord compression. Fetal blood sampling or delivery (in the second stage of labour) are often performed, although the fetal prognosis is usually not affected unless the variable decelerations are 'atypical' or associated with other FHR abnormalities.

Late decelerations. These are decelerations in which the trough of the decrease in the FHR occurs after the peak of the uterine contraction (Figs 12.7 and 12.12). They are more likely to be associated with fetal acidaemia than other forms of decelerations,[6] but the correlation is still poor. Late decelerations, particularly in the setting of other FHR abnormalities, suggest fetal hypoxia secondary to uteroplacental insufficiency. Fetal blood sampling or delivery is therefore advisable.

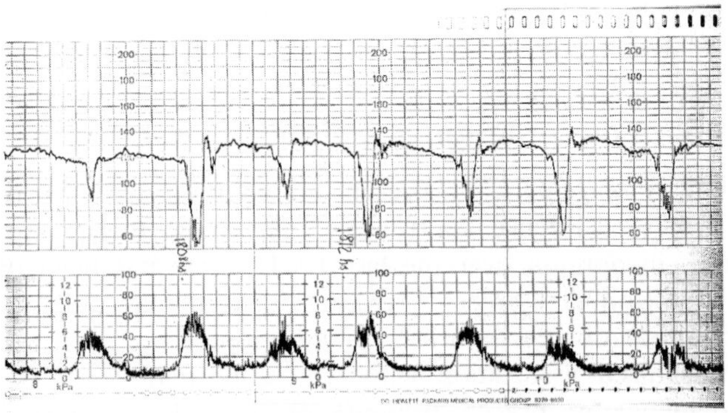

Fig. 12.13 Cardiotocogram illustrating variable fetal heart rate decelerations. The baseline fetal heart rate is normal (120–130 bpm). Although the baseline variability is reduced there are small accelerations after the decelerations, which are variable in shape and timing. The initial decelerations reach their nadir after the peak of the contraction, whereas the latter ones are synchronous with the contractions. The fetal heart rate often falls below 90 bpm during a deceleration. The umbilical cord was tightly round the baby's neck at delivery.

From the review of FHR patterns it is clear that no single abnormal pattern reliably predicts fetal outcome. Comprehensive evaluation of all the FHR characteristics previously mentioned is essential. This information must then be integrated into the clinical scenario before decisions can be made on management. Of most importance is the influence of pre-labour placental insufficiency on fetal tolerance to interruptions in oxygen delivery during labour. Acidaemia develops more rapidly in cases of IUGR.

Fetal scalp blood sampling

This was first described by Saling in Germany in 1962. Later it was suggested that fetal blood sampling could be deferred until an 'abnormal pattern' was seen on the fetal heart rate record.[6] Even then, most cases had a low risk of being associated with fetal acidaemia (always less than 50%). Moreover, clinical trials have clearly indicated that there is an increased risk of caesarean section if cardiotocography is used alone without fetal blood sampling. This has led the Royal College of Obstetricians and Gynaecologists to recommend that electronic monitoring should not be used without facilities for fetal blood sampling.[151]

A number of indications for fetal blood sampling (FBS) have already been mentioned. If the pH is ≤ 7.2 immediate delivery is indicated, providing the FBS was performed for a good reason and at the correct time. If the FBS pH is >7.2, it is usually appropriate to continue with the labour and repeat the sample 1 hour later, unless the situation deteriorates in the meantime, necessitating earlier intervention. The rate of fall of the fetal scalp pH is as important as each absolute value. This must be integrated into the clinical picture. For example, a rapidly falling pH (still above 7.2) in a woman who is soon going to be deliverable vaginally may be acceptable. In contrast, the same fetal scalp pH profile in a labour that is progressing slowly and is complicated by thick meconium is probably an indication for caesarean section.

Fetal pH falls more rapidly during pushing in the second stage.[77,151] The pH may decrease as fast as 0.1 units per 10 minutes during a prolonged bradycardia, and rapid delivery is essential to prevent acidaemia at birth.[85]

Umbilical cord blood sampling

Measurement of pH and blood gas values in blood from the umbilical cord immediately after delivery is an invaluable guide to the interaction between labour and the fetus. Umbilical venous blood values give an indication of the effects of placental gas transfer and correction of buffered arterial metabolic acids. Oxygen saturation and pH values are higher in venous blood, which is the best representation of cerebral blood oxygen content. Umbilical arterial blood gas analysis has shown that the fetal response to labour is a varying degree of acidaemia in the blood supplying the lower body.[151] The range of fetal adaptation to labour is wide. In a study[70] of over 15 000 term newborns with 5-minute Apgar scores ≥7, the median umbilical artery pH (UapH) was 7.26, with a 2.5th percentile value of 7.1. This defines the 'physiologic acidaemia' of the normal vigorous newborn. Indeed, umbilical artery pH values above 7.05 in term infants show no significant association with low Apgar scores[58] or adverse neurodevelopmental outcome.[46] Correction of such severe acidaemia after birth by healthy babies is rapid and correlates with a low $PaCO_2$ at 1 hour of age.[152]

The distribution of UapH values in preterm infants (<32 weeks' gestation) is skewed, with a median value of 7.25 (range 6.78–7.49) and mean (SD) of 7.23 (0.1).[7] There is a trend towards more infants having low UapH at lower gestations. After adjustment for other risk factors in preterm infants the UapH is not significantly associated with outcomes of neonatal death, cerebral palsy and developmental quotient at 1 year. Nonetheless, UapH measurement does provide useful information for the paediatrician attending the delivery.

DELIVERING THE INFANT

This section covers common medical interventions used to effect delivery, and the potential complications affecting the newborn infant.

Term infants

The majority of term infants will deliver spontaneously with the assistance of a midwife. Indications for an elective caesarean section are various, e.g. abnormal lie, placenta praevia and previous caesarean section. It is widely assumed that elective caesarean section ensures good condition at birth, but this is not always the case. Maternal hypotension due to regional anaesthesia, with or without aortocaval compression, can reduce placental perfusion and lead to acute fetal hypoxia.[90] There is also an increased incidence of fetal respiratory complications, such as transient tachypnoea of the newborn and hyaline membrane disease in the absence of the normal 'stress' of labour.

Emergency caesarean section (performed in labour) or instrumental vaginal delivery may be indicated either for fetal distress or failure to progress in labour. The urgency of the procedure will be determined by the presumed aetiology and severity of the problem. This information is usually available to the attending paediatrician. Instrumental vaginal delivery can be effected in most cases using either obstetric forceps or the vacuum extractor (ventouse). The trend is towards increased use of the ventouse, as recent studies[82,155] have suggested that maternal trauma and long-term morbidity are less than with forceps. Overall, the incidence of fetal complications is the same using either instrument; however, the nature of potential injuries varies according to the method used. Cephalhaematoma and superficial scalp trauma are significantly more likely with vacuum extraction, and one study has suggested an association with retinal haemorrhage.[43] Forceps, however, more commonly cause craniofacial injuries such as bruising, linear skull fractures, tentorial tears and facial nerve palsies. There is no significant difference in the number of jaundiced babies requiring phototherapy when forceps are compared with ventouse. Several long-term studies of term infants delivered by ventouse have shown no increase in mental retardation or cerebral palsy, nor any differences from infants delivered by forceps.[14,17,121,136] It must be stressed, however, that serious fetal injury is rare nowadays since heroic 'high' instrumental deliveries (using forceps or vacuum extraction) are no longer performed; caesarean section is the preferred mode for a potentially difficult delivery.

Instrumental delivery is more likely to be associated with shoulder dystocia, although this can occur with spontaneous vaginal delivery. Shoulder dystocia is an obstetric emergency in which acute fetal hypoxia rapidly develops. A number of manoeuvres can be employed to expedite delivery of the shoulders, including deliberate fracture of the baby's clavicles. There is an increased incidence of brachial plexus injuries, the majority of which recover spontaneously. Although aetiological factors such as fetal macrosomia are recognized, there is at present no reliable method for antenatal prediction of shoulder dystocia. Even if there were, caesarean section might not always circumvent the problem as 'shoulder dystocia' can also occur with delivery through a uterine incision.

Breech presentation

The management of breech presentation remains the subject of intense controversy. The most fundamental shift in opinion over the last 10–15 years has been the realization that breech presentation itself may well be a bad prognostic feature.[79] In addition, there is a well recognized association with fetal abnormality.[25,93] The incidence of breech presentation is higher preterm,[68] when it is usually the chance lie of a mobile fetus in a relatively large volume of amniotic fluid.

Many of the studies performed to assess the mortality and morbidity of the fetus undergoing vaginal breech delivery are poor. They are mostly retrospective reviews of practice and often simply compare babies delivered vaginally by the breech with those presenting head first.[28]

There has only been one small randomized controlled trial of the mode of delivery of breech presentation.[26] Despite the fact that many studies are of dubious quality, they are remarkably consistent in reporting minimal risk of long-term neurological damage after careful selection for vaginal delivery – the handicap rates are no higher than for infants born head first or by caesarean section.[132] The 'ideal' caesarean section rate with regard to breech presentation is not known, but it seems likely to be in the range of 30–65%. Vaginal delivery carries the risk of cord compression/prolapse and extended arms at delivery, as well as difficult delivery of the aftercoming head. This risk may be approximately 1–2%.[26,57] A variety of criteria for selection for vaginal breech delivery are proposed, but even these are controversial. An alternative management strategy for the breech fetus at term is to attempt to convert the presentation to cephalic by external manipulation prior to labour (external cephalic version, ECV). A meta-analysis of five randomized controlled trials on the use of ECV after 37 weeks[74] showed that the typical odds ratio for the reduction in breech births was 0.13 and for reduction in caesarean section 0.36. ECV does carry small risks to the fetus of bradycardia[138] and fetomaternal haemorrhage.[2]

Multiple pregnancy

The optimal mode of delivery in multiple pregnancies is also controversial. Elective caesarean section is frequently performed for triplets and higher-order multiples,[27,96,120] although no randomized studies are available to support this in preference to vaginal delivery. The planned mode of delivery of twins will be influenced by their presentations. The most common is vertex–vertex, and most obstetricians would advise vaginal delivery.[19,23,113,139] When the first twin presents as a breech delivery by caesarean section is often recommended,[23] although there are no data to suggest that vaginal delivery is inappropriate. For twins presenting as first twin vertex–second twin non-vertex, opinion is divided as to the optimal mode of delivery. A few would perform an elective caesarean section, believing that this reduces the neonatal mortality and morbidity of the second twin. However, this is not supported by the limited available data.[138] Vaginal delivery of the second, non-vertex, twin can be effected by external cephalic version or internal podalic version (grasping the feet and converting the lie to longitudinal) followed by breech extraction. Many would advocate that with careful fetal monitoring and recourse to caesarean section if necessary, the risks to the second twin can be minimized.

Preterm infants

The mode of delivery will be influenced by the gestational age, the fetal and maternal condition and whether the mother is already in spontaneous preterm labour. It is therefore difficult to make generalizations, and decisions need to be taken on an individual basis after discussion with the parents. Fetal blood sampling and vacuum extraction are usually avoided because of the increased risk of serious fetal trauma. Elective forceps delivery with episiotomy for preterm infants presenting by the vertex (previously thought to protect the fetal head), has not been shown to be of benefit,[86] and hence is normally only performed for standard obstetric reasons. The optimal management of breech presentations and multiple pregnancies preterm is even less well established than in the term setting. Caesarean section delivery for a very preterm infant may involve 'non-lower segment' uterine incisions, which are more susceptible to rupture in subsequent pregnancies.

CONCLUSION

The fetus spends many months in utero sustained by its placental 'lifeline'. Although many abrupt changes occur at the time of delivery, the baby's ability to adapt to extrauterine existence is inevitably influenced by antecedent events. It is of fundamental importance, therefore, that neonatologists in training gain some insight into our current understanding of fetal pathophysiology and its assessment and management. This chapter has covered the major areas of interest, but some issues remain unresolved.

REFERENCES

1. Ades A E 1992 Methods for estimating the incidence of primary infection in pregnancy: a reappraisal of toxoplasmosis and cytomegalovirus data. Epidemiology of Infections 108: 367–375
2. Alexander L, Newton J 1969 Acute renal failure after attempted external cephalic version. Journal of Obstetrics and Gynaecology of the British Commonwealth 76: 711–712
3. Anthony B F, Okada D M, Hobel C J 1978 Epidemiology of group B streptococcus: longitudinal observations during pregnancy. Journal of Infectious Diseases 137: 524–530
4. Bearts W, Fetter W P F, Hop W C J, Wallenburg H C S, Spritzer R, Sauer P J J 1990 Cerebral lesions in preterm infants after tocolytic indomethacin. Developmental Medicine and Child Neurology 32: 910–918
5. Bakketeig L, Bergsjo P 1989 Post-term pregnancy: magnitude of the problem. In: Chalmers I, Enkin M, Keirse M J N C (eds) Effective care in pregnancy and childbirth I. Oxford University Press, Oxford, pp 765–775
6. Beard R W, Filshie G M, Knight C A, Roberts G M 1971 The significance of the changes in the continuous fetal heart rate in the first stage of labour. Journal of Obstetrics and Gynaecology of the British Commonwealth 78: 865–881
7. Beeby P J, Elliott E J, Henderson-Smart D J, Rieger I D 1994 Predictive value of umbilical artery pH in preterm infants. Archives of Disease in Childhood 71: F93-F96
8. Bilardo C M, Nicolaides K H, Campbell S 1990 Doppler measurements of fetal and utero-placental circulations: relationship with umbilical venous blood gases measured at cordocentesis. American Journal of Obstetrics and Gynecology 162: 115–120
9. Borell U, Fernström I, Ohlson L, Wiqvist N 1965 Influence of uterine contractions on the uteroplacental blood flow at term. American Journal of Obstetrics and Gynecology 93: 44–57

10. Boyer K M, Gadzalla C A, Kelly P D, Burd L I, Gotoff S P 1983 Selective intrapartum chemoprophylaxis of neonatal group B streptococcal early-onset disease. II Predictive value of prenatal cultures. Journal of Infectious Diseases 148: 802–809
11. Boyer K M, Gotoff S P 1986 Prevention of early-onset neonatal group B streptococcal disease with selective intrapartum chemoprophylaxis. New England Journal of Medicine 314: 1665–1669
12. Boylan P C 1991 Liquor assessment: meconium and oligohydramnios. In: Spencer J A D (ed) Fetal monitoring. Oxford University Press, Oxford, pp 133–137
13. Brown V A, Sawers R S, Parsons R J, Duncan S L B, Cooke I D 1982 The value of antenatal cardiotocography in the management of high-risk pregnancy: a randomised controlled trial. British Journal of Obstetrics and Gynaecology 89: 716–722
14. Byre I, Dahlia K 1974 The long term development of children delivered by vacuum extraction. Developmental Medicine and Childhood Neurology 16: 378–381
15. Caldeyro-Barcia R, Mendez-Bauer C, Poseiro J J et al 1966 Control of human fetal heart rate during labor. In: Cassels D E (ed) The heart and circulation in the newborn and infant. Grune and Stratton, New York, pp 7–36
16. Caldeyro-Barcia R, Schwarcz R, Belizan J M et al 1974 Adverse perinatal effects of early amniotomy during labor. In: Gluck L (ed) Modern perinatal medicine. Mosby Yearbook, Chicago, pp 431–439
17. Carmody F, Grant A, Mutch M, Vacca A, Chalmers I 1986 Follow up of babies delivered in a randomized comparison of vacuum extraction and forceps delivery. Acta Obstetrica et Gynaecologica Scandinavica 65: 763–766
18. Cerevka J, Scheffs J S, Vasicka A 1970 Shape of uterine contractions (intra-amniotic pressure) and corresponding fetal heart rate. 1 Spontaneous and oxytocin induced labours. Obstetrics and Gynecology 35: 695–703
19. Cetrulo C L 1986 The controversy of mode of delivery in twins: the intrapartum management of twin gestation. Seminars in Perinatology (i) 10: 39–40
20. Chamberlain G V P, Phillip E, Howlett B, Masters K 1978 British births 1970 Heinemann, London
21. Chang T, Robson S, Spencer J, Gallivan S 1992 Ultrasonic fetal weight charts: a comparison between the Bangladeshi and Caucasian populations. 26th British Congress of Obstetrics and Gynaecology, Manchester (Abstract 102)
22. Chapman M G, Furness E T, Jones W R, Sheat J H 1989 Significance of the location of placenta site in early pregnancy. British Journal of Obstetrics and Gynaecology 86: 846–848
23. Chervenak F A, Johnson R E, Youcha S, Hobbins J C, Berkowitz R L 1985 Intrapartum management of twin gestation. Obstetrics and Gynecology 65: 119–124
24. Chew F T, Drew J H, Oats J N, Riley S F, Beischer N A 1985 Nonstressed antepartum cardiotocography in patients undergoing elective Cesarean Section – fetal outcome. American Journal of Obstetrics and Gynecology 151: 318–321
25. Collea J V, Rabin S C, Weghorst G R et al 1978 The randomised management of term frank breech presentation: vaginal delivery versus caesarean section. American Journal of Obstetrics and Gynecology 134: 186
26. Collea J V, Chien C, Quilligan E J 1980 The randomised management of term frank breech presentation: a study of 208 cases. American Journal of Obstetrics and Gynecology 137: 233–239
27. Collins M S, Bleyl J A 1990 Seventy one quadruplet pregnancies: management and outcome. American Journal of Obstetrics and Gynecology 162: 1384–1392
28. Confino E, Gleicher N, Elrad H, Ismajovich B, David M P 1985 The breech dilemma: a review. Obstetrics and Gynecology Survey 40: 330–337
29. Connor M 1994 AIDS Clinical Trial Group 076 study. Reduction of maternal–infant transmission of HIV type 1 with zidovudine treatment. New England Journal of Medicine 331: 1173–1179
30. Cotton D B, Read J A, Paul R H, Quilligan E J 1980 The conservative aggressive management of placenta praevia. American Journal of Obstetrics and Gynecology 137: 687–695
31. Crowley P 1989 Post-term pregnancy: induction or surveillance? In: Chalmers I, Enkin M, Keirse M J N C (eds) Effective care in pregnancy and childbirth 1. Oxford University Press, Oxford, pp 776–791
32. Crowley PA 1995 Antenatal corticosteroid therapy: a meta-analysis of the randomized trials, 1972 to 1994. American Journal of Obstetrics and Gynecology 173: 322–335
33. Crowley P 1995 Antibiotics for preterm prelabour rupture of the membranes. In: Enkin M W, Keirse M J N C, Renfrew M J, Neilson J P (eds) Pregnancy and childbirth module of the Cochrane Database of Systematic Reviews
34. Crowley P, O'Herlihy C, Boylan P 1984 The value of ultrasound measurement of amniotic fluid volume in the management of prolonged pregnancies. British Journal of Obstetrics and Gynaecology 91: 444–448
35. Crowley P, Chalmers I, Keirse M J N C 1990 The effects of corticosteroid administration before preterm delivery: an overview of the evidence from controlled trials. British Journal of Obstetrics and Gynaecology 97: 11–17
36. Department of Health 1993 Changing childbirth: Parts I and II. HMSO, London
37. Department of Health and Social Security 1994 Report on confidential enquiries into maternal deaths in the United Kingdom 1988–1990. HMSO, London
38. Desmonts G, Couvreur J 1974 Congenital toxoplasmosis: a prospective study of 378 pregnancies. New England Journal of Medicine 290: 1110–1116
39. Druzin M L, Gratacos J, Keegan K A, Paul R H 1981 Antepartum fetal heart rate testing. VII The significance of fetal bradycardia. American Journal of Obstetrics and Gynecology 139: 194–198
40. Easmon C S F, Hastings M J G, Deeley J, Bloxham B, Rivers R P A, Marwood R 1983 The effect of intrapartum chemoprophylaxis on the vertical transmission of group B streptococci. British Journal of Obstetrics and Gynaecology 90: 633–635
41. Eden R D, Gergely R Z, Schifrin B S, Wade M A 1982 Comparison of antepartum testing schemes for the management of postdate pregnancy. American Journal of Obstetrics and Gynecology 144: 683–692
42. Eden R D, Seifert L S, Kodack L D, Trofatter K F, Killam A P, Gall S A 1988 A modified biophysical profile for antenatal fetal surveillance. Obstetrics and Gynecology 71: 365–369
43. Ehlers N, Jensen I K, Hansen K B 1974 Retinal haemorrhages in the newborn – a comparison of delivery by forceps and by vacuum extractor. Acta Ophthalmologica 52: 73–82
44. Eik-Nes S H, Okland O, Aure J C, Ulstein M 1984 Ultrasound screening in pregnancy: a randomised controlled trial. Lancet i: 1347
45. Emmen L, Huisjes H J, Aarnoudse J G, Visser G H A, Okken A 1975 Antepartum diagnosis of the 'terminal' fetal state by cardiotocography. British Journal of Obstetrics and Gynaecology 82: 353–359
46. Fee S C, Malee K, Deddish R, Minogue J P, Socol M L 1990 Severe acidosis and subsequent neurological status. American Journal of Obstetrics and Gynecology 162: 802–806
47. FitzGerald D E, Drumm J E 1977 Non invasive measurement of human fetal circulation using ultrasound: a new method. British Medical Journal 2: 1450–1451
48. Flynn A M, Kelly J, O'Conor M 1979 Unstressed antepartum cardiotocography in the management of the fetus suspected of growth retardation. British Journal of Obstetrics and Gynaecology 86: 106–110
49. Flynn A M, Kelly J, Mansfield H, Needham P, O'Conor M, Viegas O 1982 A randomised controlled trial of non-stress antepartum cardiotocography. British Journal of Obstetrics and Gynaecology 89: 427–433
50. Fox J F, McCaul R W, Martin W E, Roberts W E, McLaughlin B, Morrison J C, 1992 Neonatal morbidity between 34–37 weeks gestation. American Journal of Obstetrics and Gynecology 166: 360–363
51. Fraser R, Watson R 1989 Bleeding during the latter half of pregnancy. In: Chalmers I (ed) Effective care in pregnancy and childbirth. Oxford University Press, Oxford
52. Friedman D M, Blackstone J, Hoskins I 1992 Adverse fetal cardiac effects of oral ritodrine tocolysis. 12th Annual SPO Meeting No 17. American Journal of Obstetrics and Gynecology 166: 326
53. Friedman E A 1954 The graphic analysis of labor. American Journal of Obstetrics and Gynecology 68: 1568–1575
54. Garite T J 1991 Oncofetal fibronectin in cervico-vaginal secretions is highly predictive of preterm delivery. American Journal of Obstetrics and Gynecology 164: 259–260
55. Gibb D 1984 Prolonged pregnancy. In: Studd J W W (ed) The management of labour. Blackwell Scientific, Oxford, pp 108–122

56. Gilbert G L 1993 Chickenpox during pregnancy. British Medical Journal 306: 1079–1080
57. Gimovsky M L, Petrie R H 1989 The intrapartum management of the breech presentation. Clinics in Perinatology 16: 976–986
58. Goldaber K G, Gilstrap L C, Leveno K J, Dax J S, McIntire D D 1991 Pathologic fetal acidemia. Obstetrics and Gynecology 78: 1103–1107
59. Golditch I A, Boyce N E 1970 Management of abruptio placenta. Journal of the American Medical Association 212: 288–293
60. Grant A, Mohide P 1982 Screening and diagnostic tests. In: Enkin M, Chalmers I (eds) Effectiveness and satisfaction in antenatal care. Heinemann, London, pp 22–59
61. Grant A, Elbourne D, Valentin L, Alexander S 1989 Routine formal fetal movement counting and risk of antepartum late death in normally formed singletons. Lancet i: 345–349
62. Grant A, O'Brien N, Joy M T, Hennessy E, MacDonald D 1989 Cerebral palsy among children born during the Dublin randomised trial of intrapartum monitoring. Lancet ii: 1233–1235
63. Green J R 1989 Placenta abnormalities: placenta praevia and abruptio placentae. In: Creasy R K, Resnik R (eds) Maternal–fetal medicine: principles and practice. W B Saunders, Philadelphia
64. Guissani D A, Spencer J A D, Moore P J, Bennet L, Hanson M A 1993 Afferent and efferent components of the cardiovascular reflex responses to acute hypoxia in term fetal sheep. Journal of Physiology 461: 431–449
65. Hadlock F P, Deter R L, Harrist R B, Park S K 1982 Fetal head circumference: relation to menstrual age. American Journal of Roentgenology 138: 649–653
66. Hadlock F P, Deter R L, Harrist R B, Park S K 1982 Fetal abdominal circumference as a predictor of menstrual age. American Journal of Roentgenology 139: 367–371
67. Hammacher K 1969 The clinical significance of cardiotokography. In: Huntingford P J, Hueter K A, Saling E (eds) Perinatal medicine. Thieme, Stuttgart, pp 80–85
68. Haughey M J 1985 Fetal position during pregnancy. American Journal of Obstetrics and Gynecology 153: 885–886
69. Hay P E, Lamont R F, Taylor-Robinson D, Morgan D J, Ison C, Pearson J 1994 Abnormal bacterial colonisation of the lower genital tract as a marker for subsequent preterm delivery and late miscarriage. British Medical Journal 308: 295–298
70. Helwig J T, Parer J T, Kilpatrick S J, Laros R K 1996 Umbilical cord blood acid–base state: What is normal? American Journal of Obstetrics and Gynecology 174: 1807–1814
71. Henson G L, Dawes G S, Redman C W G 1983 Antenatal fetal heart-rate variability in relation to fetal acid–base status at caesarean section. British Journal of Obstetrics and Gynaecology 90: 516–521
72. Hibbard B M 1988 Bleeding in late pregnancy. In: Hibbard B M (ed) Principles of obstetrics. Butterworths, London
73. Hibbard B M, Jeffcoate T N A 1966 Abruptio placentae. Obstetrics and Gynecology 27: 155–167
74. Hofmeyr G J 1991 ECV at term: How high the stakes? British Journal of Obstetrics and Gynaecology 98: 1–3
75. Hon E H 1968 An atlas of fetal heart rate patterns. Harty Press, Newhaven
76. Hoult I J, MacLennan A H, Carrie L E S 1977 Lumbar epidural analgesia in labour: relation to fetal malposition and instrumental delivery. British Medical Journal i: 14–16
77. Humphrey M D, Chang A, Wood E C, Morgan S, Hounslow D 1974 A decrease in fetal pH during the second stage of labour, when conducted in the dorsal position. Journal of Obstetrics and Gynaecology of the British Commonwealth 81: 600–602
78. Hurd W W, Miodovnik M, Lavin J P 1983 Selective management of abruptio placentae: a prospective study. Obstetrics and Gynecology 61: 467–473
79. Hytten F 1982 Breech presentation: Is it a bad omen? British Journal of Obstetrics and Gynaecology 60: 417–420
80. Ingemarsson I, Heden L 1989 Cervical score and onset of spontaneous labor in prolonged pregnancy dated by second-trimester ultrasonic scan. Obstetrics and Gynecology 74: 102–105
81. Itskovitz J, Goetzman B W, Rudolf A M 1982 The mechanism of late deceleration of the heart rate and its relationship to oxygenation in normoxemic and chronically hypoxemic fetal lambs. American Journal of Obstetrics and Gynecology 142: 66–73
82. Johanson R B 1994 Vacuum extraction versus forceps delivery. In: Pregnancy and childbirth module 'Cochrane database of systematic reviews' No 03256
83. Johnstone F D, Campbell D M, Hughes G J 1978 Has continuous intrapartum monitoring made any impact on fetal outcome? Lancet i: 1298–1300
84. Kadar N, Cruddas M, Campbell S 1986 Estimating the probability of spontaneous delivery conditional on time spent in the second stage. British Journal of Obstetrics and Gynaecology 93: 568–576
85. Katz M, Shani N, Meizner I, Insler V 1982 Is end-stage deceleration of the fetal heart ominous? British Journal of Obstetrics and Gynaecology 89: 186–189
86. Keirse M J N C, Grant A, King J F 1989 Preterm labour. In: Chalmers I, Enkin M, Keirse M I N C (eds) Effective care in pregnancy and childbirth I. Oxford University Press, Oxford, pp 694–745
87. Keirse M J N C, Ohlsson A, Treffers P E, Kanhai H H H 1989 Prelabour rupture of the membranes preterm. In: Chalmers I, Enkin M, Keirse M J N C (eds) Effective care in pregnancy and childbirth I. Oxford University Press, Oxford pp 666–692
88. Keirse M J N C, Trimbos J B 1980 Assessment of antepartum cardiotocograms in high risk pregnancy. British Journal of Obstetrics and Gynaecology 87: 261–269
89. Kidd L C, Patel N B, Smith R 1985 Non-stress antenatal cardiotocography – a prospective randomised clinical trial. British Journal of Obstetrics and Gynaecology 92: 1156–1159
90. Kinsella S M, Spencer J A D 1995 Maternal and fetal cardiovascular effects of epidural analgesia during labour. Contemporary Reviews in Obstetrics and Gynaecology 7: 145–150
91. Knab D R 1978 Abruptio placentae: an assessment of the time and method of delivery. Obstetrics and Gynecology 52: 625–629
92. Knuppel A R, Drukker J E 1986 Bleeding in late pregnancy: antepartum bleeding. In: Hayashi R H, Castillo M S (eds) High risk pregnancy: a team approach. W B Saunders, Philadelphia
93. Lamont R F, Dunlop P D M, Crowley P et al 1983 Spontaneous preterm labour and delivery at under 34 weeks gestation. British Medical Journal 286: 454–457
94. Leeson S C, Maresh M J A, Martindale E A et al 1996 Detection of fetal fibronectin as a predictor of preterm delivery in high risk asymptomatic pregnancies. British Journal of Obstetrics and Gynaecology 103: 48–53
95. Liggins G C, Howie R N 1972 A controlled trial of antepartum glucocorticoid treatment for prevention of the respiratory distress syndrome in premature infants. Pediatrics 50: 515–517
96. Lipitz S, Reichman B, Panet G et al 1989 The improving outcome of triplet pregnancies. American Journal of Obstetrics and Gynecology 161: 1279–1284
97. Liston R M, Cohen A W, Mennuti M T, Gabbe S G 1982 Antepartum fetal evaluation by maternal perception of fetal movement. Obstetrics and Gynecology 60: 424–426
98. Lopez-Zeno J A, Peaceman A M, Adashek J A, Socol M L 1992 A controlled trial of a program for the active management of labor. New England Journal of Medicine 326: 450–454
99. Lumley J, Lester A, Anderson I, Renou P, Wood C 1983 A randomised trial of weekly cardiotocography in high-risk obstetric patients. British Journal of Obstetrics and Gynaecology 90: 1018–1026
100. Macaulay J H, Randall N R, Bond K, Steer P J 1992 Continuous monitoring of fetal temperature by noninvasive probe and its relationship to maternal temperature, fetal heart rate, and cord arterial oxygen and pH. Obstetrics and Gynecology 79: 469–474
101. MacDonald D, Grant A, Sheridan-Pereira M, Boylan P, Chalmers I 1985 The Dublin randomised controlled trial of intrapartum fetal heart-rate monitoring. American Journal of Obstetrics and Gynecology 152: 524–539
102. Major C A, Lewis D F, Harding J A, Porto M A, Garite T J 1994 Tocolysis with indomethacin increases the incidence of necrotizing enterocolitis in the low-birth-weight neonate. American Journal of Obstetrics and Gynecology 170: 102–106
103. Malak T M, Sizmur F, Bell S C, Taylor D J 1996 Fetal fibronectin in cervicovaginal secretions as a predictor of preterm birth. British Journal of Obstetrics and Gynaecology 103: 648–653
104. Manning F A, Platt L D, Sipos L 1980 Antepartum fetal evaluation: development of a fetal biophysical profile. American Journal of Obstetrics and Gynecology 136: 787–795
105. Maresh M, Choong K-H, Beard R W 1983 Delayed pushing with lumbar epidural analgesia in labour. British Journal of Obstetrics and Gynaecology 90: 623–627
106. Meire H B, Farrant P 1981 Ultrasound demonstration of an unusual

fetal growth pattern in Indians. British Journal of Obstetrics and Gynaecology 88: 260–263
107. Merenstein G B, Todd W A, Brown G, Yost C C, Luzier T 1980 Group B beta-hemolytic streptococcus: randomised controlled treatment study at term. Obstetrics and Gynecology 55: 315–318
108. Modanlou H D, Freeman R K 1982 Sinusoidal fetal heart rate pattern: its definition and clinical significance. American Journal of Obstetrics and Gynecology 142: 1033–1038
109. Modanlou H D, Komatsu G 1982 Large for gestational neonates: anthropometric reason for shoulder dystocia. Obstetrics and Gynecology 60: 417–423
110. Mohide P, Keirse M J N C 1989 Biophysical assessment of fetal well-being. In: Chalmers 1, Enkin M, Keirse M J N C (eds) Effective care in pregnancy and childbirth 1. Oxford University Press, Oxford, pp 477–492
111. Moore T R, Cayle J E 1990 The amniotic fluid index in normal human pregnancy. American Journal of Obstetrics and Gynecology 162: 1168–1173
112. Morales W J, Lim D V, Walsh A F 1986 Prevention of neonatal group B streptococcal sepsis by the use of a rapid screening test and selective intrapartum chemoprophylaxis. American Journal of Obstetrics and Gynecology 155: 979–983
113. Morales W J, O'Brien W F, Knuppel R A, Gaylord S, Hayes P 1989 The effect of mode of delivery on the risk of intraventricular haemorrhage in non-discordant twin gestations under 1500 g. Obstetrics and Gynecology 73: 107–110
114. Naeye R L 1965 Infants of diabetic mothers: a quantitative morphologic study. Pediatrics 35: 980–988
115. Nageotte M P, Hollenback K A, Vanderwahl B A, Hutch K M 1992 Circulating cellular fibronectin in the prediction of preterm labor. American Journal of Obstetrics and Gynecology 166: 270–273
116. Neesham D E, Umstad M P, Cincotta R B, Johnston D L, McGrath G M 1993 Pseudosinusoidal fetal heart rate pattern and fetal anaemia: case report and review. Australian and New Zealand Journal of Obstetrics and Gynaecology 33: 386–388
117. Neilson J P 1994 Electronic fetal monitoring and scalp sampling versus intermittent auscultation in labour. In: Pregnancy and childbirth module 'Cochrane database of systematic reviews'. Update software, Oxford
118. Neldham S 1980 Fetal movements as an indicator of fetal wellbeing. Lancet i: 1222–1224
119. Newell M L 1994 Caesarean section and risk of vertical transmission of HIV I infection. Lancet 343: 1464–1467
120. Newman R B, Hamer C, Millar M C 1989 Outpatient triplet management: a contemporary review. American Journal of Obstetrics and Gynecology 161: 547–555
121. Ngan H, Miu P, Ko L, Ma H 1990 Long term neurological sequelae following vacuum extractor delivery. Australia and New Zealand Journal of Obstetrics and Gynaecology 30: 111–114
122. Norton M E, Merrill J, Cooper B A B, Kuller J A, Clyman R I 1993 Neonatal complications after the administration of indomethacin for preterm labor. New England Journal of Medicine 329: 1602–1607
123. Notelovitz M, Bottoms S F, Dase D F, Leichter P J 1979 Painless abruptio placentae. Obstetrics and Gynecology 53: 270–272
124. O'Driscoll K, Foley M, MacDonald D 1984 Active management of labor as an alternative to cesarean section for dystocia. Obstetrics and Gynecology 63: 485–490
125. Okonofua F E, Olatubosun O A 1985 Caesarean versus vaginal delivery in abruptio placentae associated with live fetuses. International Journal of Gynaecology and Obstetrics 23: 471–474
126. Omenaca Teres F, Matorras R, Garcia Perea A, Elorza M D 1987 Prevention of neonatal group B streptococcal sepsis (letter). Pediatric Infectious Diseases 6: 874
127. Owen P, Donnet M L, Ogston S A, Christie A D, Howie P W, Patel N B 1996 Standards for ultrasound fetal growth velocity. British Journal of Obstetrics and Gynaecology 103: 60–69
128. Pearce J M, Campbell S 1987 A comparison of symphysis–fundal height and ultrasound as screening tests for light-for-gestational age infants. British Journal of Obstetrics and Gynaecology 94: 100–104
129. Pearson J F 1977 Fetal movements – a new approach to antepartum care. Nursing Mirror 144: 49–51
130. Peckham C, Hall S, Patel N et al 1992 Prenatal screening for toxoplasmosis in the UK. Report of a working group. Royal College of Obstetricians and Gynaecologists, London
131. Peebles D M, Spencer J A D, Edwards A D et al 1993 Relation between frequency of uterine contractions and human fetal cerebral oxygen saturation studied during labour by near infrared spectroscopy. British Journal of Obstetrics and Gynaecology 101: 44–48
132. Penn Z J, Steer P J 1994 Breech Presentation. In: James D K, Steer P J, Weiner C P, Gonik B (eds) High risk pregnancy. Management options. W B Saunders, London, pp 173–198
133. Phelan J P, Stine L E, Mueller E, McCart D, Yeh S 1984 Observations of fetal heart rate characteristics related to external cephalic version and tocolysis. American Journal of Obstetrics and Gynecology 149: 658–661
134. Phelan J P, Platt L D, Yeh S Y, Broussard P, Paul R H 1985 The role of ultrasound assessment of amniotic fluid volume in the management of the postdate pregnancy. American Journal of Obstetrics and Gynecology 151: 304–308
135. Philpott R H 1972 Graphic records in labour. British Medical Journal 4: 163–165
136. Plena G, Svenningsen M, Gustafson B, Sunder B, Cronquist S 1977 Neonatal and prospective follow up study of infants delivered by vacuum extraction. Acta Obstetrica et Gynaecologia Scandinavica 56: 189–194
137. Prober C G, Sullender W M, Yasukawa L L, Au D S, Yeager A S, Arvin A M 1987 Low risk of herpes simplex virus infections in neonates exposed to the virus at the time of vaginal delivery by mothers with recurrent genital herpes simplex virus infections. New England Journal of Medicine 316: 240–244
138. Rabinovici J, Barhai G, Reichman B, Serr D M, Mashinach S 1988 Internal podalic version with unruptured membranes for the second twin in transverse lie. Obstetrics and Gynecology 71: 428–430
139. Rayburn W F, Lavin J P, Miodovnik M, Varner M W 1984 Multiple gestation: twin interval between delivery of the first and second twins. Obstetrics and Gynecology 63: 502–506
140. Report of the Committee on Infectious Diseases 1991 The Red Book, 22nd edn. American Academy of Pediatrics, Illinois
141. Robson S C, Crawford R A, Spencer J A D, Lee A 1992 Intrapartum amniotic fluid index and its relationship to fetal distress. American Journal of Obstetrics and Gynecology 166: 78–82
142. Rochard F, Schifrin B S, Goupil F, Legrand H, Blottiere J, Sureau C 1976 Non stressed fetal heart-rate monitoring in the antepartum period. American Journal of Obstetrics and Gynecology 126: 699–706
143. Rooth G, Hutch A, Hutch R, 1987 Guidelines for the use of fetal monitoring. International Journal of Gynaecology and Obstetrics 25: 159–167
144. Rossi E M, Philipson E H, Williams T G, Kalhan S C 1989 Meconium aspiration syndrome: intrapartum and neonatal attributes. American Journal of Obstetrics and Gynecology 161: 1106–1110
145. Rotschild A, Ling E W, Puterman M L, Farquharson D 1990 Neonatal outcome after prolonged preterm rupture of the membranes. American Journal of Obstetrics and Gynecology 162: 46–52
146. Sadovsky E, Yaffe H 1973 Daily fetal movement recording and fetal prognosis. Obstetrics and Gynecology 41: 845–850
147. Schwarcz R L, Belizan J M, Cifuentes J R, Cuadro J C, Marques M B, Caldeyro-Barcia R 1974 Fetal and maternal monitoring in spontaneous labors and in elective inductions. American Journal of Obstetrics and Gynecology 120: 356–362
148. Spencer J A D, Johnson P 1986 Fetal heart rate variability changes and fetal behavioural cycles during labour. British Journal of Obstetrics and Gynaecology 93: 314–321
149. Spencer J A D 1991 Predictive value of a fetal heart rate acceleration at the time of fetal blood sampling in labour. Journal of Perinatal Medicine 19: 207–215
150. Spencer J A D, Koutsoukis M, Lee A 1991 Fetal heart rate and neonatal condition related to epidural analgesia in women reaching the second stage of labour. European Journal of Obstetrics, Gynecology and Reproductive Biology 41: 173–178
151. Spencer J A D 1993 Fetal response to labour. In: Spencer J A D, Ward H R T (eds) Intrapartum fetal surveillance. Royal College of Obstetricians and Gynaecologists, London, pp 17–33
152. Spencer J A D, Robson S C, Karkas A 1993 Spontaneous recovery after severe metabolic acidaemia at birth. Early Human Development 32: 103–111
153. Stewart P, Kennedy J H, Calder A A 1982 Spontaneous labour: when should the membranes be ruptured? British Journal of Obstetrics and Gynaecology 89: 39–43
154. Studd J 1973 Partograms and nomograms of cervical dilatation in management of primigravid labour. British Medical Journal 4: 451–455

155. Sultan A H, Kamm M A, Bartram C I, Hudson C N 1994 Perineal damage at delivery. Contemporary Reviews in Obstetrics and Gynaecology 6: 18–24
156. Thacker S B 1989 Effectiveness and safety of intrapartum fetal monitoring. In: Spencer J A D (ed) Fetal monitoring. Castle House Publications, Tunbridge Wells
157. Thacker S B, Berkelman R L 1986 Assessing the diagnostic accuracy and efficacy of selected antepartum fetal surveillance techniques. Obstetrics and Gynecology Survey 41: 121–141
158. Trudinger B J, Cook C M, Jones L, Giles W B 1986 A comparison of fetal heart-rate monitoring and umbilical artery waveforms in the recognition of fetal compromise. British Journal of Obstetrics and Gynaecology 93: 171–175
159. Varma T R 1973 Fetal growth and placental function in patients with placenta praevia. Journal of Obstetrics and Gynaecology of the British Commonwealth 80: 311–315
160. Villar J, Belizan J M 1986 The evaluation of the methods used in the diagnosis of intrauterine growth retardation. Obstetrics and Gynecology Survey 41: 187–199
161. Visser G H A, Huisjes H J 1977 Diagnostic value of the unstressed antepartum cardiotocogram. British Journal of Obstetrics and Gynaecology 84: 321–326
162. Visser G H A, Redman C W G, Huisjes H J, Turnbull A C 1980 Nonstressed antepartum heart-rate monitoring: implications of decelerations after spontaneous contractions. American Journal of Obstetrics and Gynecology 138: 429–435
163. Wheble A M, Gillmer M D G, Spencer J A D, Sykes G S 1989 Changes in fetal monitoring practice in the UK. British Journal of Obstetrics and Gynaecology 96: 1140–1147
164. Zanini B, Paul R H, Huey J R 1980 Intrapartum fetal heart rate: correlation with scalp pH in the preterm fetus. American Journal of Obstetrics and Gynecology 136: 43–47

13

Maternal illness in pregnancy

Karen Brackley   Peter Rubin

CLINICAL PHARMACOLOGY IN PREGNANCY

Many women are prescribed drugs during their pregnancy, either by accident or by design. There are obvious legal and ethical constraints on systematically studying the effects of drugs on the developing human fetus, with the result that little is known about the use of drugs during human pregnancy. With very few exceptions (e.g. the studies on low-dose aspirin in the prevention of pre-eclampsia) information on drug use during pregnancy comes from anecdotal reports or very small series, which are often uncontrolled. A consideration of drug use during pregnancy can be divided into two broad aspects: the potential effect of drugs on pregnancy outcome and the effect of pregnancy on drug kinetics and effects.

DRUGS AND FETAL DEVELOPMENT

ORGANOGENESIS

In order to have a teratogenic effect it is necessary for a drug to be present during organogenesis, which takes place between 18 and 55 days following conception. It is very difficult, if not impossible, to say with certainty that a drug is safe during the first trimester. In the case of drugs that have been widely used for many years the weight of clinical experience can often be taken as reassurance. The list of teratogenic drugs in common usage is relatively short (Table 13.1). The use of a teratogenic drug during the first trimester does not mean that the woman will inevitably have an abnormal baby. The incidence of fetal abnormality when one of the drugs in Table 13.1 is used during the first trimester varies enormously. For example, the risk of abnormality when phenytoin or carbamazepine is used would normally be put at around 6%, whereas the risk with the retinoids is very high and probably exceeds 80%. The mechanisms of teratogenicity have not been worked out, but it is likely that the genetic make-up of the baby, as well as possibly the concentration of drug, will be important determining factors. The majority of drug-induced abnormalities can be identified by ultrasound scanning at 18–20 weeks' gestation. The effects of warfarin are an exception to this rule, as they largely involve cartilage and it is often not until birth or even later that it is known whether the baby has chondrodysplasia punctata (see below).

Table 13.1 Widely used drugs which are teratogenic

Anticonvulsants	carbamazepine, phenytoin and sodium valproate[1]
Antineoplastic drugs	
Danazol	
Lithium	
Retinoids[2]	
Warfarin	

[1]There is insufficient information about the newer anticonvulsants to take a position on whether they are teratogenic in humans or not.
[2]These drugs can remain in the body for up to 2 years following the last dose, and their prescription must be accompanied by very clear warnings about their high teratogenic potential and the need for effective contraception.

Table 13.2 Drugs which can influence fetal growth and development

Drug	Effect
Angiotensin-converting inhibitors	Impair fetal and neonatal renal function
Aspirin (analgesic doses)	Minor neonatal haemorrhage
β-blockers	Intrauterine growth retardation
Indomethacin	Necrotizing enterocolitis and intracranial haemorrhage; premature closure of the ductus arteriosus
Warfarin	Fetal intracranial haemorrhage

GROWTH AND DEVELOPMENT

Beyond the period of organogenesis several drugs can adversely influence the developing fetus (Table 13.2). The risk of intrauterine growth retardation with β-blockers is about 25%,[10] and is seen only when a β-blocker is given throughout pregnancy. The use of a β-blocker only in the third trimester is not associated with impairment of growth.[94] The use of a β-blocker in the third trimester will lead to neonatal bradycardia, but this rarely if ever needs pharmacological reversal. When used in the treatment of pregnancy hypertension a β-blocker is no more likely than placebo to be associated with neonatal hypoglycaemia.[95]

The haemorrhagic problems with aspirin are seen only when the drug is used in analgesic doses within 5 days before delivery.[106] A large study comparing low-dose aspirin with placebo in the prevention of pre-eclampsia failed to find any evidence of neonatal haemorrhage.[13] Indomethacin has been associated with necrotizing enterocolitis and intracranial haemorrhage when used in the management of preterm labour, in contrast to the effect on the ductus arteriosus which is seen at term.[75]

Anticoagulation in pregnancy is a particularly difficult problem (see below). Heparin can cause maternal osteoporosis in a manner which is dependent on the dose and duration of treatment. Warfarin is not only a teratogen but can also cause bleeding into the fetal brain, even though the mother's anticoagulation control is good. The most widely used approach to anticoagulation in pregnancy is to use small doses of low-dose heparin whenever possible, with warfarin reserved for a very small number of women where the risk of thrombosis is considered to be very high.

It is worth noting that steroids do not appear in the above text. There is no evidence that prednisolone is teratogenic in the human, or that it influences the fetal or neonatal endocrine system. Prednisolone is structurally different from the steroids such as dexamethasone or betamethasone, which are used to induce fetal lung maturity, in that it is largely metabolized in the placenta. Prednisolone has been used for many years in medical conditions such as asthma, inflammatory bowel disease, renal transplantation and autoimmune conditions, and has a very good safety record (see below).

THE EFFECTS OF PREGNANCY ON PHARMACOKINETICS

Several physiological changes of pregnancy combine to lower the plasma concentrations of some drugs. The volume of distribution can increase because of the substantial fluid retention that occurs during pregnancy. More importantly, certain liver metabolic pathways undergo induction as a result of the endocrine changes of pregnancy, and also renal blood flow increases by about 100%. Thus drugs which are metabolized by the relevant pathways, or drugs that undergo renal elimination, will have their clearance increased as a consequence of pregnancy. In some cases the resulting fall in drug level can be clinically significant, and this is the case with carbamazepine, phenytoin, lithium, digoxin and ampicillin. The dose of drug will often need to be increased, particularly in the third trimester, and where possible this is achieved with the help of therapeutic drug monitoring (see Further reading).

Table 13.3 Some drugs which have a good safety record in nursing mothers

Aminoglycosides
Antihypertensive drugs
Anticonvulsants (with exception of barbiturates)
Bronchodilator inhalers
Non-narcotic analgesics
Non-steroidal anti-inflammatory drugs
Penicillin antibiotics
Cephalosporin antibiotics
Prednisolone
Warfarin

Table 13.4 Some commonly used drugs that should be avoided by women who are breast-feeding. (*Reproduced with permission from Rubin[95a]*)

Drug	Effect
Amiodarone	Iodine content may cause neonatal hypothyroidism
Aspirin	Theoretical risk of Reye syndrome
Barbiturates	Drowsiness
Benzodiazepines	Lethargy
Carbimazole	Use of lowest effective dose to avoid hypothyroidism
Contraceptives	May diminish milk supply and reduce protein content
Cytotoxic drugs	Potential problems include immune suppression and neutropenia
Ephedrine	Irritability
Tetracyclines	Theoretical risk of tooth discoloration

BREAST-FEEDING

As the result of dilution in the mother, and also because of the volume of milk consumed by the baby, the dose of most drugs delivered by breast-feeding is insufficient to have any noticeable effect. Some of the more commonly used drugs which have a good safety record in this regard are listed in Table 13.3. Some drugs do reach the baby in sufficient quantities to have at least the potential for causing harm, and these are listed in Table 13.4.

MEDICAL DISORDERS IN PREGNANT WOMEN

DIABETES

The diagnosis and management of diabetes during pregnancy continues to pose a challenge. Broadly speaking, diabetic pregnancies can be divided into those where the woman has diabetes before conception and those where the condition develops during the pregnancy. Among the former, the vast majority will be insulin-dependent diabetics. The latter will largely have gestational diabetes, where the impairment of glucose tolerance comes on during the pregnancy and resolves following delivery. The diagnosis of gestational diabetes can only be made with certainty once the pregnancy is over and glucose tolerance has returned to normal. There will be some women in whom diabetes happens to be diagnosed for the first time during their pregnancy. The difference between a true gestational diabetic and someone whose glucose impairment will continue in the long term is of little practical importance with respect to management during pregnancy. What matters to the fetus is whether glucose tolerance is normal or not.

DIABETES AND THE FETUS

Congenital anomalies

The increase in congenital anomalies among the babies of women with pre-existing diabetes has been recognized for many years. Overall, the risk is two to three times that in the general population, and is directly related to the percentage of glycosylated haemoglobin at the time of conception.[105] The mechanism of this teratogenic effect is unknown, but it is related directly or indirectly to impaired glucose tolerance during the period of organogenesis, because the offspring of women with gestational diabetes do not show an excess of congenital abnormalities.

It is likely that poor diabetic control later in the pregnancy also has implications for the subsequent well-being of the baby. An inverse relationship has been found between the intellectual development of the offspring and ketone and free fatty acid levels in the second and third trimesters.[89]

Spontaneous miscarriage

There have been conflicting data published about the risk of spontaneous miscarriage in women with diabetes. One large prospective study in the USA found no excess of miscarriage rate in diabetic pregnancies,[64] but there was a suggestion in this study that poorly controlled diabetics may have been at increased risk of miscarriage.

Intrauterine fetal death

Despite advances in antenatal monitoring there is still a tendency for women with poorly controlled diabetes to have an increased incidence of intrauterine fetal death. The underlying mechanisms have not been elucidated.

Perinatal mortality

If deaths from congenital anomalies are excluded, women with pre-existing diabetes now have no greater risk of experiencing a perinatal death than does a woman without diabetes. There is still controversy as to whether gestational diabetes leads to an increased risk of perinatal mortality. Reliable data are surprisingly difficult to obtain, but if there is an increased perinatal mortality it appears only to be found in the most poorly controlled diabetic pregnancies.

Neonatal morbidity

In contrast to mortality, neonatal morbidity is still relatively common among the babies of diabetic women. The problems are described in Chapter 24.

SCREENING FOR GESTATIONAL DIABETES

There is really no consensus on screening for gestational diabetes, with substantial variations both between and within countries. At one extreme some authorities advocate an oral glucose tolerance test in every woman on her first attendance at the antenatal clinic, with the test being repeated at 28 weeks should she be considered at high risk: e.g. a previous baby weighing more than 4 kg, diabetes in a first-degree relative, maternal obesity or a previous abnormal glucose tolerance test.[78] At the other extreme is the pragmatic approach taken by many antenatal clinics in the UK, whereby women are screened for glycosuria and will have a random blood glucose estimation if glycosuria is present, and will go on to have a glucose tolerance test if the random glucose is abnormal. Whether screening influences outcome is still unresolved. There is inconsistency as to whether the glucose should be given intravenously or orally, and indeed whether the oral dose should be 50, 75 or 100 g. The most common approach to an oral GTT is to give a 75 g oral dose of glucose. The diagnostic criteria are then as shown in Table 13.5.

MANAGEMENT OF DIABETIC PREGNANCY

Organization of care is important and women should preferably be managed in a unit with special interests and expertise in the area. The optimum care of the diabetic pregnancy requires a multidisciplinary approach including not only the diabetologists and obstetrician but also dietitians, nurse specialists, neonatologists and ophthalmologists. It is particularly important for women to obtain preconception advice and for the control of the pregnancy to be optimized at that early stage. The aim of treatment is to maintain a normal blood glucose. Diet

Table 13.5 Diagnostic criteria for diabetes in pregnancy

	Venous plasma glucose (mmol/l)	
	Fasting	2 hours
Normal	<7.8	<7.8
Impaired glucose tolerance	<7.8	7.8–11.0
Diabetes	≥7.8 and/or	≥11.1

and insulin are the centrepiece of diabetes management. Oral hypoglycaemics are not used. Although there is no consistent evidence that oral hypoglycaemics are teratogenic, sulphonylureas cross the placenta and can cause fetal and neonatal hypoglycaemia.[2]

Diet

The aim is to provide sufficient energy for both mother and fetus, which amounts to 30–35 kcal/kg of non-pregnant ideal body weight. Daily carbohydrate consumption should be in the region of 220–240 g, providing at least 45% of the necessary calorie intake. Detailed and ongoing advice from an experienced dietitian is crucial to the success of dietary management.

Diet alone may be sufficient to control gestational diabetes, but if blood glucose exceeds 6 mmol/l in preprandial blood samples and those taken 2 hours after eating, then insulin should be introduced.

Insulin

Women with gestational diabetes who are not controlled by diet alone may achieve control using once-daily injections of an insulin formulation with intermediate duration of activity. With this exception, insulin during pregnancy would normally be given at least twice a day, as a mixture of short- and intermediate-duration insulins, or as multiple injections using a soluble insulin with each main meal and a longer-acting insulin at bedtime.

Monitoring of glucose

In order to achieve the aim of normoglycaemia throughout the day and night it is necessary for the diabetic woman to monitor her blood glucose at home, and this would normally be performed between two and six times each day. Well informed and experienced diabetic patients can then modify their insulin doses themselves. Longer-term control will be assessed by measuring glycosylated haemoglobin, which should ideally be in the middle of the normal range.

Labour and the puerperium

Insulin requirements fall once labour is established, and fall even further once the placenta has been delivered. During labour the most straightforward approach is to use 10% glucose at a constant rate of 1 litre every 8 hours, with human soluble insulin being given at 1 unit per hour and the dose adjusted according to hourly blood glucose monitoring. Once the baby is delivered the rate of insulin infusion should be reduced (or stopped if the woman has gestational diabetes), with the glucose being continued until the next meal, when prepregnancy insulin doses should be commenced. Careful dietary advice is needed in women who are going to breast-feed and they should be alert to the possibility of hypoglycaemia.

LIVER DISEASE

Liver disease is an uncommon complication of pregnancy but when it occurs can pose risks to mother and baby. The subject was recently reviewed.[32] Two forms of liver disease are specific to pregnancy, intrahepatic cholestasis and acute fatty liver. In addition, women may develop hepatitis while pregnant.

INTRAHEPATIC CHOLESTASIS OF PREGNANCY

The hallmark of this condition is pruritis affecting the limbs and trunk developing during the second half of pregnancy. The pruritis can come on several weeks before any abnormality of liver function tests. When liver function does become deranged this is in the form of modest elevations of transaminases, alkaline phosphatase and γ-GT. Jaundice is fairly uncommon. Total bile acid concentration is increased, mainly because of elevations in cholic acid and chenodeoxycholic acid. In more severe cases the prothrombin time may be abnormal. Delivery usually results in a rapid and extremely welcome resolution of the symptoms.

Intrahepatic cholestasis of pregnancy is a miserable condition for the mother to experience but poses little if any risk to her, with the exception of an increase in postpartum haemorrhage (probably related to vitamin K deficiency). In contrast, the fetus is at risk and both fetal distress and intrauterine death are more common in intrahepatic cholestasis of pregnancy through mechanisms which are not understood.[35]

Management of the mother's symptoms tends to be difficult, although recent small and open studies have suggested that ursodeoxycholic acid may be beneficial. However, this drug is not licensed for use in pregnancy and controlled trials are awaited. Vitamin K should be given to the mother to reduce the risk of bleeding and fetal monitoring is mandatory. It would be usual obstetric practice to deliver the baby at around 37/38 weeks to avoid the complications referred to above.

ACUTE FATTY LIVER OF PREGNANCY

This is another condition unique to pregnancy but is considerably more rare than intrahepatic cholestasis. Presentation is typically in the third trimester, with nausea and anorexia. There is often hypertension and proteinuria and the condition has some similarities to pre-eclampsia. Transaminases are elevated, but the biochemical findings that generally distinguish acute fatty liver from pre-eclampsia are a much higher elevation of uric acid and marked hypoglycaemia. Jaundice is a late feature of the disease. Magnetic resonance imaging or computerized tomography may help in the diagnosis. Once the condition is recognized the woman's condition must be stabilized (paying particular attention to any abnormalities in coagulation and blood glucose) and the baby should be delivered without further delay. Acute fatty liver of pregnancy carries a high mortality if not treated correctly.

HEPATITIS

Infection with hepatitis viruses A, B, C and D produces a clinical picture in the pregnant woman which is very similar to that outside pregnancy. Management of vertical transmission of hepatitis A, B and C to the neonate is described elsewhere (Chapter 31, Part 2). Hepatitis E differs in that this usually mild disease carries a significant risk of maternal death in pregnancy for reasons which are not understood. The high mortality makes it difficult to judge the frequency of vertical transmission, but one report suggests that this is very high.[51]

HEART DISEASE

In developed countries heart disease as a complication of pregnancy has become very rare. The success of paediatric cardiac surgery will lead to a progressive increase in the number of young women going through pregnancy with corrected defects, but preliminary information would suggest that these mothers cope well with the demands of pregnancy. Where a woman has herself had a congenital heart defect there is an increased risk that her baby will be similarly affected, although the probability varies with the type of defect.[72,73] Where a woman has had congenital aortic stenosis the risk in her baby is 18%, whereas with tetralogy of Fallot it is 3%. The situation in developing countries is very different and heart disease is still commonly encountered.

In our obstetric medical clinic the commonest reason for cardiological referral is the detection of a murmur, which proves to be an innocent flow murmur of pregnancy. The second most common reason is palpitations, which again almost invariably prove to be of no consequence. Among the 'real' cardiological problems that present in unselected obstetric populations the most common will be arrhythmias, which usually turn out to be supraventricular tachycardias. In most cases this is primary in origin, but it is always important to remember that this arrhythmia could be a manifestation of underlying cardiac disease, or indeed of pulmonary thromboembolism. The most effective pharmacological method for terminating an SVT is to use intravenous adenosine, and there have been reports of the safe use of this drug during pregnancy. Where the problem is recurrent the use of a cardioselective β-blocker such as atenolol is usually effective. Resistant supraventricular arrhythmias may be treated with amiodarone, although this is not by any means the drug of first choice even outside pregnancy. Amiodarone has a high iodine content (nearly 40% by weight of each dose) and there is obviously a risk of neonatal hypothyroidism. This has been reported although there are also case reports of the successful use of amiodarone to treat either maternal or fetal arrhythmias without untoward effects on the newborn. Nonetheless, the drug should be used only when other treatments have failed. Because of its high iodine content and very long half-life amiodarone is contraindicated in women who are breast-feeding.

Verapamil is a calcium antagonist with negative chronotropic effects. There is no evidence that the drug is teratogenic and it has been used in the treatment both of maternal and fetal arrhythmias. It appears to be safe in breast-feeding.

Digoxin is the treatment of choice for atrial fibrillation, which is a very uncommon complication of pregnancy in western countries. Digoxin has a long safety record during pregnancy and has been used to treat both maternal and fetal arrhythmias.

The remaining types of cardiac problem presenting in developed countries are extremely rare. Peripartum cardiomyopathy is a potentially life-threatening condition which presents during the third trimester or in the puerperium. Treatment is symptomatic and aimed at reducing heart failure and the risks of thromboembolism.

RENAL DISEASE

A comprehensive account of this complex and highly specialized subject is beyond the scope of this chapter and the reader should refer to Davison and Baylis 1995 for a recent review.[20]

PRE-EXISTING RENAL DISEASE

Whatever the underlying renal pathology three generalizations can be made about renal disease and pregnancy. The first is that the more severe the disease the less likely it is that pregnancy will end with a successful outcome. The second is that more severe renal disease increases the likelihood that pregnancy will result in a permanent deterioration in renal function. A third generalization is that if, in addition to renal impairment, there is hypertension of sufficient severity to require treatment, then again the prognosis both for the baby and for maternal renal function is worse than if hypertension is not present. In addition to these general principles the specific renal lesion may influence both the outcome of pregnancy and the subsequent course. Focal glomerulosclerosis, IgA nephropathy and reflux nephropathy in particular have been associated with worsening hypertension and renal function during pregnancy. In contrast, chronic glomerulonephritis may run a relatively benign course if hypertension is not present.

The management of chronic renal disease during pregnancy requires that a balance be maintained between prognosis for the baby and prognosis for the mother, the risks of permanent deterioration in maternal renal function being weighed against the risks of possibly fatal complications of prematurity in the baby. It is difficult to make generalizations and each case should be managed with close consultation between renal physicians, obstetricians and neonatalogists.

ASYMPTOMATIC BACTERIURIA

This condition is characterized by finding more than 100 000 organisms per ml of urine in two fresh, cleanly voided consecutive samples, with the same organism being implicated in each case. The most common organism by far is *Escherichia coli*. The incidence of asymptomatic bacteriuria in pregnancy is variously quoted between 2 and 10%, but most studies quote a figure in the region of 5%.[74]

The undisputed importance of identifying asymptomatic bacteriuria is that just under a half of these women go on to develop symptomatic urinary tract infections, and treatment at the asymptomatic stage will prevent this occurrence. Over the years there have been claims that asymptomatic bacteriuria is associated with a wide range of other pregnancy complications, but the evidence is lacking. The condition should be treated with an antibiotic to which the bacterium is sensitive, and most authorities would now recommend a 2-week course of treatment with subsequent urine cultures.

ACUTE PYELONEPHRITIS

This occurs in up to 2% of pregnancies and is one of the causes of preterm labour.[16] Treatment should be commenced in hospital, with intravenous antibiotics appropriate to the sensitivity of the organism and intravenous rehydration if appropriate.

ACUTE CYSTITIS

Acute cystitis occurs with a frequency approximately half that of pyelonephritis. Early and effective treatment will prevent progression to pyelonephritis.

RENAL TRANSPLANTATION AND PREGNANCY

Pregnancy is becoming increasingly common in women who have been the recipients of renal transplants. Current information suggests that pregnancy does not influence allograft survival one way or the other,[90] although it has been claimed that up to 9% of women have rejection episodes during pregnancy.[96] This is actually the same as for non-pregnant women during a similar period. These data are also now somewhat old, and it is likely that the use of newer immunosuppressive treatments will reduce the rejection rate still further.

Three drugs are the mainstay of immunosuppressive therapy.

- ***Prednisolone***. There is no evidence that prednisolone is teratogenic in the human. A surveillance study of Michigan Medicaid recipients identified 601 newborns who had been exposed during the first trimester to prednisolone, prednisone or methylprednisolone.[6] The number of birth defects observed in this population was no different from that expected. Although there have been anecdotal reports suggesting that prednisolone can lead to immunosuppression in the newborn, such observations are many years old and have not been repeated with the increasing use of prednisolone in the management of a wide variety of medical conditions. Similarly there is no persuasive evidence that prednisolone can influence the fetal or neonatal adrenal gland. This may be because prednisolone is significantly metabolized in the human placenta, with the result that very little will reach the fetus.
- ***Azathioprine***. Although azathioprine is teratogenic in rabbits the majority of reports in the human have not found it to be associated with congenital defects. There have been sporadic reports of chromosomal aberrations in infants who have been exposed in utero to azathioprine, but a cause and effect relationship has not been established. Azathioprine can cause leukopenia and thrombocytopenia in both mother and baby. There is a significant correlation between maternal leukocyte count in the third trimester and cord leukocyte count.[21] These authors recommended reducing the dose of azathioprine by 50% if the mother's white count fell more than one standard deviation below the normal for pregnancy. There have been several reports suggesting that azathioprine can cause intrauterine growth retardation, but the relevant contributions of drug and underlying disease are difficult to disentangle.
- ***Cyclosporin A***. This drug is not teratogenic in animals. Experience in humans has so far been very limited, but the current view is that it does not pose a major risk to the developing fetus. However, more information will become available as the drug is used more widely, and the information reported here may change in the light of new research.

Pregnancy in renal transplant recipients ends in preterm delivery in at least 40% of cases. The reasons are a mixture of obstetric intervention and spontaneous preterm labour. Intrauterine growth retardation is quoted at 20% and could be related either to drug treatment (see above) or to the underlying state of renal function.[81] In addition to the neonatal problems resulting from prematurity, the babies of renal transplant mothers will be at risk of becoming hepatitis B surface antigen carriers if the mother is also a carrier. Early administration of hyperimmunoglobulin (within a few hours of birth) has been reported to be 90% effective in reducing the carrier status in these infants, and is further described on pages 1161–1162.[5] Cytomegalovirus is an additional risk to both mother and baby. The newborn infants of renal transplant recipients can therefore be affected by the complications of prematurity, including respiratory distress syndrome, the risk of infection because of leukopenia, the complications of maternal hepatitis B surface antigen carrier status or CMV infection, and possibly chromosomal aberrations, although this has not been established.

The current view is that the proven benefits of using prednisolone, azathioprine and cyclosporin outweigh the potential difficulties, although the balance of benefits and risks may change as more information becomes available.

ANAEMIA AND PREGNANCY

IRON DEFICIENCY ANAEMIA

On a global basis iron deficiency anaemia is still a leading cause of maternal morbidity and mortality. In developed countries significant iron deficiency anaemia is uncommon, although most women are routinely prescribed supplements of iron and folic acid. There is really no consensus about the value of giving iron on a routine basis to a population which is largely well nourished. The opposing views are well described by Hibbard and Horn.[45] The only sure way of determining whether somebody needs iron supplementation is to check their serum ferritin, but this would be a very expensive exercise if carried out in all pregnant women. Routine administration of iron is cheaper but has the disadvantage that many women do not take the drug, and one advantage of knowing about the iron stores is that, if there is a definite reason to take iron, then perhaps compliance with therapy would be more likely.

THYROID DISEASE

HYPOTHYROIDISM

Severe hypothyroidism leads to difficulty in conceiving and so pregnancy is rare. Less severe forms, if untreated, lead to an increased risk of abortion and stillbirth through a mechanism which is not understood. It is unusual to diagnose hypothyroidism for the first time during pregnancy, and the majority of women present already on thyroxine replacement therapy. There is some evidence that it may be necessary to increase the thyroxine as the pregnancy proceeds,[61] but our own experience is that this is very rarely necessary. Nevertheless, TSH should be checked once during each trimester.

THYROTOXICOSIS

Both carbimazole (which is metabolized to methimazole) and propylthiouracil are used in the management of thyrotoxicosis during pregnancy. There are theoretical advantages to using propylthiouracil in that less crosses the placenta than with methimazole, and carbimazole has been associated with aplasia cutis, although the evidence is not strong. Propylthiouracil also crosses into breast milk in lower quantities than does carbimazole. However, in practice it is doubtful whether there is any material difference between these two drugs, and treatment should be at a dose which maintains the free T4 at the upper end of the normal range.

It has been reported that in up to 10% of women who have had Graves' disease TSH receptor-stimulating antibodies cross the placenta and produce a fetal tachycardia (heart rate >160 bpm) and a neonatal thyrotoxicosis.[85] Although the levels of these thyroid-stimulating antibodies can be measured in maternal blood, the assays are not readily available and measuring fetal heart rate in at-risk women is likely to be more useful. Treatment of fetal thyrotoxicosis is by increasing the maternal dose of antithyroid drugs until the fetal heart rate is in the normal range. The features and treatment of neonatal thyrotoxicosis are dealt with on page 964.

HYPERTENSIVE DISEASES IN PREGNANCY

Hypertension in pregnancy is a complication which can affect up to 15% of women, particularly in their first pregnancy. Despite reductions in the numbers dying from the hypertensive diseases of pregnancy in the United Kingdom they remain a major cause of maternal mortality, accounting for 15.5% of all direct maternal deaths.[1] Substandard care was evident in 80% of cases, despite previous recommendations by the Confidential Enquiry Report. High blood pressure in pregnancy is the reason behind many antenatal admissions and requires increased maternal and fetal surveillance during pregnancy. Pre-eclampsia is the main iatrogenic cause for preterm delivery and, together with the associated intrauterine growth restriction, leads to higher perinatal morbidity and mortality.[60]

Hypertension in pregnancy can be divided into two main categories: high blood pressure developing for the first time in pregnancy which subsequently settles after delivery, and high blood pressure which existed before the onset of pregnancy. An arbitrary level of blood pressure is used, i.e. 140/90 mmHg, although the actual rise from baseline blood pressure at the booking antenatal visit is also important. A dilemma may occur if a woman presents with hypertension in the second half of pregnancy and no record of blood pressure is available preconceptually or from early in pregnancy. The true diagnosis may only become evident some months postpartum.

Pre-eclampsia is often defined as a sustained blood pressure of 140/90 mmHg or more occurring after 20 weeks' gestation, including a rise of 30 mmHg in systolic and 15 mmHg in diastolic blood pressures from early pregnancy, together with significant proteinuria (>300 mg in 24 hours).[68] The term pregnancy-induced hypertension or gestational hypertension is used if there is no significant proteinuria, and is believed to represent a much milder form of the disease, often developing at a later stage in pregnancy. The occurrence of generalized seizures in a woman with pre-eclampsia heralds the onset of eclampsia, with considerably increased maternal morbidity and mortality.[29]

PRE-ECLAMPSIA

The exact cause of pre-eclampsia is still unclear and it remains a 'disease of theories'.[9] The concept that the problems originate in the placenta is becoming increasingly recognized. Defective implantation is thought to occur, with subsequent reduced uteroplacental perfusion and relative hypoxic conditions developing.[8,87] Pre-eclampsia is well established as a systemic disease affecting a variety of maternal organs, such as the brain, liver and kidneys, to different extents. Hypertension is just one of a number of features of the condition. There is evidence of generalized endothelial damage and dysfunction which leads to vasospasm and reduced perfusion of these organs.[92] Recent developments favour the release of some as yet unknown factor(s) into the maternal circulation from the hypoxic placenta which gives rise to this endothelial disruption.[91]

It was hoped that low-dose aspirin (60–75 mg/day) would be beneficial in terms of preventing or improving established pre-eclampsia, by altering the imbalance of vasoconstrictors and vasodilators that may lead to this vasospasm.[113] Unfortunately, the results of the CLASP trial involving nearly 10 000 women revealed no significant reduction in the incidence of pre-eclampsia in those who were considered to be at risk of developing the condition.[13] However, there was a possible benefit seen in those who had previously developed early-onset severe pre-eclampsia. In view of the apparent safety of low-dose aspirin in this large study, therapy is generally reserved for women who have chronic hypertension and are therefore at increased risk of early-onset pre-eclampsia, or for those who have previously experienced severe early disease in pregnancy. There is currently no other proven therapy to prevent pre-eclampsia.

Once pre-eclampsia has developed, it will progress at a variable rate until the fetus and placenta have been delivered. If a woman presents at term, labour should be induced to prevent serious deterioration in maternal and/or fetal condition. At earlier gestations the antenatal management aims to be conservative in order to prolong pregnancy and improve fetal maturity, but at the same time needs to avoid the development of severe maternal complications or fetal compromise. The complaint of symptoms such as headache, visual disturbances, epigastric pain or vomiting, or the presence of proteinuria in a pregnant woman with raised blood pressure, necessitates hospital admission for thorough assessment of the condition and possible delivery. Maternal investigations include blood tests to exclude renal or liver dysfunction, thrombocytopenia and other coagulation disturbances. The assessment of fetal well-being should involve growth scans, umbilical artery Doppler velocimetry and biophysical profiles. Antenatal steroids to improve fetal lung maturity are not contraindicated in pre-eclampsia. Interestingly, some women with pre-eclampsia have no evidence of fetal compromise, whereas others may have minimal maternal symptoms or signs but their fetuses are severely affected by placental disease.

The use of antihypertensive agents to control blood pressure should be considered if levels are consistently above 160/100 mmHg. Although these drugs will do nothing to prevent the disease, they will help to protect the maternal cerebral circulation from extremes of blood pressure and subsequent risks of intracerebral haemorrhage. In addition they may help to prolong the pregnancy for a clinically useful period in terms of neonatal outcome. The worry that antihypertensive agents may mask the deterioration in maternal disease as blood pressure is being artificially lowered should not be an issue, as constant vigilance for the development of other complications must always be maintained.

A variety of antihypertensive drugs are available which all act by different mechanisms. Methyldopa has a long safety history in pregnancy and is often used for chronic control of blood pressure in pregnant women.[14] There is evidence that β-blockers are associated with fetal growth retardation when used from early in pregnancy,[10] but this does not appear to be a problem when they are prescribed only in the third trimester.[94] Calcium channel blockers such as nifedipine are newer agents which can be useful for the rapid control of severe hypertension in the sublingual form, as well as a second-line agent for longer-term control in slow-release preparations. Angiotensin-converting enzyme (ACE) inhibitors should not be used in pregnancy as they have been associated with fetal renal failure.[93] Intravenous hydralazine or labetalol are useful for the acute control of severe hypertension prior to delivery or in the immediate postpartum period. The relationship between maternal blood pressure and fetal compromise is not entirely clear, except that prolongation of the pregnancy has obvious benefits for the neonate. The aim is to reduce maternal blood pressure gradually to safer levels, for example 135/85 mmHg in a usually normotensive woman. Hypotension is avoided as uteroplacental blood flow may be adversely affected and possibly precipitate fetal distress.

ANTICONVULSANT THERAPY

The incidence of eclampsia in the UK is 4.9/10 000 pregnancies.[29] Approximately half of the seizures occur antenatally or intrapartum. It is possible for eclampsia to occur with apparently normal blood pressures and no proteinuria. The pathophysiology of the seizures may involve cerebral vasospasm causing ischaemia, disruption of the blood–brain barrier and cerebral oedema.

Intravenous diazepam is the preferred drug to administer to control an established convulsion. There is now substantial evidence from a large multicentre randomized trial in 1680 women that magnesium sulphate is superior to either phenytoin or diazepam in preventing recurrent seizures, with reduced maternal morbidity and mortality.[31] The neonatal outcome was also better in the women who were prescribed magnesium sulphate rather than phenytoin, in terms of fewer admissions to the special care baby unit and less likelihood of being intubated at delivery. A systematic overview of several randomized trials suggests that magnesium sulphate is also better than phenytoin or diazepam at preventing convulsions in severe pre-eclampsia.[12]

If elective delivery is required before 32 weeks' gestation in a woman with pre-eclampsia, the chosen method would be caesarean section. After 34 weeks' gestation it may be possible to aim for vaginal delivery, especially with the use of prostaglandin gel to prime the cervix. Continual fetal heart rate monitoring is mandatory. Epidural analgesia, with improved control of maternal blood pressure, is recommended as long as the platelet count and clotting screen are normal. Ergometrine should be avoided in the third stage in view of its potential hypertensive side-effects. Following delivery close monitoring of the maternal condition should be carried out on the labour suite for at least 24 hours. Eclamptic fits may occur even over 1 week post-delivery.[29]

HELLP SYNDROME

This term was first used by Weinstein in 1982 to describe women whose pre-eclampsia was complicated by haemolysis, elevated liver enzymes and a low platelet count.[115] HELLP syndrome is uncommon, occurring in about 20% of cases of *severe* pre-eclampsia, with 30% of cases occurring postpartum.[102] Individual features of the HELLP syndrome are seen commonly in severe cases of pre-eclampsia. The importance of recognizing the syndrome rests largely on the need to place the woman in a very high-risk category. The occurrence of acute (adult) respiratory distress syndrome in association with HELLP carries a very grave prognosis with high maternal mortality.[62]

CHRONIC HYPERTENSION

This group includes pregnant women with essential hypertension (unknown aetiology) as well as those with underlying renal disease, systemic lupus erythematosus and other rarer diseases, such as Cushing syndrome, phaeochromocytoma and Conn syndrome. Women with essential hypertension tend to be older, parous and are more likely to have a family history of hypertension. The incidence of superimposed pre-eclampsia is five times greater in women with chronic hypertension. The problems associated with chronic hypertension in pregnancy are entirely due to the development of pre-eclampsia. Women who do not develop superimposed pre-eclampsia usually have uncomplicated pregnancies.

Blood pressure tends to decrease in the first half of pregnancy in normotensive individuals as well as in women with chronic hypertension. It may be necessary to reduce the dose of antihypertensive drug, or even to discontinue therapy at this stage. Methyldopa is probably the favoured antihypertensive agent for long-term use in pregnancy (see above). The early treatment of chronic hypertension does not prevent the later development of pre-eclampsia.[88]

The diagnosis of superimposed pre-eclampsia may be more difficult in a woman with established high blood pressure and proteinuria at the onset of pregnancy. The rise in blood pressure level is a useful guide, as well as increases in plasma urate levels, abnormal liver function tests and clotting disturbances.

SYSTEMIC LUPUS ERYTHEMATOSUS

SLE is not uncommon in pregnancy for the simple reason that young women both develop SLE and become pregnant. It seems unlikely that pregnancy influences the long-term prognosis in women with SLE, and even the traditional teaching that the condition tends to flare in the puerperium has been challenged recently.[26]

When women are in remission at the start of pregnancy recent experience suggests that in at least 80% the disease will remain inactive.[26] When the condition does relapse it will usually respond to prednisolone.

SLE can adversely affect pregnancy outcome in three ways. First, there is an increased risk of abortion, often in association with the antiphospholipid syndrome, which is discussed below. Secondly, there is a neonatal lupus syndrome, which can include haematological and cardiac abnormalities and is discussed in Chapter 30. Thirdly, maternal renal impairment and hypertension can adversely affect outcome for the fetus. As discussed above in the section on renal disease, the worse the impairment the more likely it is that there will be a fetal loss. One study suggested that fetal loss could be as high as 50% if serum creatinine was > 132 mmol/l.[44]

THROMBOEMBOLISM ASSOCIATED WITH PREGNANCY

Thromboembolic disease remains a major cause of maternal mortality, accounting for approximately one-quarter of all direct maternal deaths.[1] Over one-third of these cases occur in the antenatal period. There is also considerable morbidity associated with thromboembolism, related to the side-effects of treatment and the long-term complications such as chronic venous insufficiency after deep vein thrombosis. The risk of thromboembolism is increased approximately sixfold in pregnancy. This is attributed mainly to the higher levels of clotting factors and to the effects of venous stasis, secondary to increased venous tone in pregnancy and mechanical obstruction to the inferior vena cava caused by the gravid uterus. The incidence of thromboembolism has been estimated as occurring in between 0.3 and 1.2% of all pregnancies.[23] Particular risk factors in a pregnant woman include increasing maternal age, parity, obesity, bed rest, operative delivery, sickle cell disease, previous thromboembolism and the congenital or acquired thrombophilia syndromes. The importance of prophylaxis against thromboembolism post-caesarean section was highlighted in the latest Confidential Enquiry into maternal deaths,[1] as 76% of postpartum deaths occurred in women who had been delivered by caesarean section. The true recurrence risk of thromboembolism in pregnancy is not known. One study suggested the risk was as high as 12% in a woman with a past history of thromboembolism,[3] but this estimate was based on a postal survey with no confirmed diagnosis, and lower recurrence rates in the antenatal period are likely.

It is imperative that the diagnosis of a suspected deep vein thrombosis or pulmonary embolism in pregnancy is confirmed by an objective test to avoid unnecessary anticoagulation and because of the implications for future thromboprophylaxis in pregnancy. Non-invasive ultrasound techniques, including Doppler and colour flow imaging, are becoming increasingly popular to diagnose deep vein thrombosis in pregnancy. Unfortunately, these methods have limitations with isolated thromboses in the calf veins or for investigations above the inguinal ligament. The use of venography may be required and should not be withheld if clinically indicated. With adequate shielding of the uterus the direct radiation dose to the fetus is very small.

Chest X-ray, ECG and arterial blood gases should all be performed in a pregnant woman presenting with symptoms of a pulmonary embolus, but if normal do not exclude the diagnosis. Indeed, the classic ECG changes associated with pulmonary emboli (deep S waves in lead I, Q waves and inverted T waves in lead III) can be seen in normal pregnancy. A perfusion lung scan, with or without a ventilation scan, should therefore be arranged. The isotopes used have very short half-lives and the radiation to the fetus is negligible, being about 0.5 Sieverts (50 mrem – milli radiation equivalent man), which is approximately one-tenth of the maximum gestation exposure recommended in the USA.

ADVERSE EFFECTS OF ANTICOAGULANTS IN PREGNANCY

Heparin does not cross the placenta, whether in an unfractionated or low molecular weight form, and therefore has no direct adverse effects on the fetus. There are, however, potential risks to the mother from its use. Bleeding may occur, particularly with overdosage during acute full anticoagulation therapy, and it is important that close monitoring with activated partial thromboplastin times, anti-factor Xa assays or heparin levels is performed. Serious bleeding may require reversal of the anticoagulant effect using protamine. The use of prophylactic low doses of heparin, either unfractionated or low molecular weight, do not appear to be associated with a greater risk of haemorrhage in the antenatal period, and can be safely continued during the time of labour and delivery.[30,48,107]

Thrombocytopenia is a rare but potentially dangerous side-effect of heparin therapy. It is an antibody-mediated phenomenon, usually occurring between 6 and 10 days after heparin is commenced. Therapy should be discontinued as it may cause life-threatening venous or arterial thrombosis. Platelet counts should be monitored routinely during treatment with heparin. The risk of thrombocytopenia is believed to be lower with low molecular weight heparins.[69]

Heparin may also cause osteoporosis, and the risk appears to be related to the dose and duration of therapy. Daily doses in pregnancy of 20 000 units or more of unfractionated heparin for periods over 3 months are probably associated with the greatest risk.[46] Although symptomatic osteoporosis is reported to be rare, occurring in less than 5% of women receiving long-term prophylactic heparin,[17,37] subclinical disease may be more common.[24] Fortunately, heparin-induced osteoporosis does appear to be reversible on stopping treatment.[18] It is possible that the risk of osteoporosis is reduced by the use of low molecular weight heparins as the total dose is lower, but this requires further investigation in large clinical studies. The exact mechanism underlying the bone demineralization is not known.

Warfarin does cross the placenta and is associated with adverse fetal effects in terms of teratogenicity as well as fetal bleeding complications. The use of warfarin in the first trimester is associated with abnormal cartilage and bone formation (chondrodysplasia punctata), asplenia syndrome and diaphragmatic hernia. The risk of warfarin embryopathy has been quoted as 10% of live births in a retrospective study,[43] but estimates of approximately 5% are considered more accurate.[76] Warfarin exposure in the second and third trimester is not without risks to the fetus. Recurrent small intracerebral haemorrhages are thought to occur, leading to abnormalities such as optic atrophy, microcephaly and mental retardation. The risk is reduced by strict control of maternal anticoagulation, but fetal intraventricular haemorrhage has been reported in the presence of low therapeutic INR levels in the mother[112] because the fetal clotting system is so immature.

Warfarin should be avoided after 36 weeks' gestation because of potential fetal intracranial bleeding at the time of delivery. Warfarin has a relatively long half-life and should also be avoided for maternal reasons at this time, in view of possible haemorrhage when labour occurs.

MANAGEMENT OF THROMBOEMBOLISM IN PREGNANCY AND THE PUERPERIUM

High-dose intravenous heparin is used initially to treat deep vein thrombosis or pulmonary embolism to prevent further, potentially fatal, thromboembolism. Treatment should not be delayed until the results of investigations are available. A bolus dose of 5000 units of heparin is injected, followed by an intravenous infusion of between 24 000 and 40 000 units over 24 hours, aiming to keep the APTT ratio between 1.5 and 2.5. The acute use of thrombolytic agents such as streptokinase is reserved for life-threatening circumstances in pregnancy because of the possible bleeding complications.

After about 7 days the risks of further thromboembolism are lower, and some centres then advocate reducing the total dose of heparin. Twice-daily subcutaneous injections of 10 000 units of heparin would be standard therapy for the remainder of pregnancy.[22] This dosage would not be expected to alter the APTT ratio and monitoring can be performed using anti-Xa assays. Other authors recommend the maintenance of therapeutic levels of heparin throughout the entire antenatal period, using subcutaneous injection.[47] The antenatal use of warfarin in these circumstances is currently less popular because of the inherent fetal risks. Heparin doses are reduced to 7500 units 12-hourly at the onset of labour or for elective delivery. The insertion of an epidural is considered safe in these patients as long as the APTT and platelet count are normal.[86] Following delivery warfarin therapy is commenced for a period of 6–12 weeks postpartum. Heparin therapy is still required until full anticoagulation with warfarin is achieved, which may take at least 72 hours (INR 2.0–3.0). The introduction of warfarin in the puerperium reduces maternal exposure to heparin and therefore the risks of osteoporosis. However, following discussion, some women may decide to continue self-injection of heparin in the postnatal period for convenience. Warfarin does not cross into breast milk in any significant quantities, and breast-feeding is not contraindicated.

THROMBOPROPHYLAXIS IN PREGNANCY

The issue of thromboprophylaxis should preferably be discussed before conception or at least early in pregnancy, so that the associated risks and benefits are fully understood. The timing and duration of prophylactic therapy will depend on a number of variables, such as the severity of a previous thrombosis, recurrent events or the presence of a particular risk factor, such as a thrombophilia syndrome. Low-risk patients, such as those with a past history of deep vein thrombosis outside pregnancy and no additional risk factors, may only require prophylactic treatment during delivery and postpartum. High-risk patients, such as women with protein C or antithrombin III deficiency, will require prophylaxis throughout pregnancy and the puerperium. The management of women who have had a pregnancy-associated thromboembolism in the past is controversial, with some obstetricians starting prophylaxis during labour and others favouring an arbitrary number of weeks before the previous episode occurred in pregnancy.

Unfractionated heparin administered subcutaneously in 12-hourly doses of 7500–10 000 units is given antenatally. Low molecular weight heparins, such as enoxaparin, have been advocated for thromboprophylaxis in pregnancy.[69] The advantages of these preparations include once-daily dosage and possible, although as yet unproven, reduced risks of bleeding, thrombocytopenia and osteoporosis in pregnancy (see above). The disadvantages are associated with the costs, monitoring of anti-Xa activity and their longer half-life, causing more difficulty if rapid reversal of anticoagulant activity is required.

In 1995 the Royal College of Obstetricians and Gynaecologists[86] published guidelines concerning the recommended thromboprophylaxis in women undergoing caesarean section. Low-dose unfractionated heparin (5000 units b.d.) or a once-daily dose of low molecular weight drug should be continued for 5 days or until the patient is fully mobile.

Another clinical indication for warfarin during and after pregnancy is the presence of mechanical heart valves to prevent systemic embolization. High levels of anticoagulation with warfarin are required long term in these patients outside pregnancy. Low-dose heparin is not effective at preventing thromboembolism. Transfer to full anticoagulation with heparin is required as soon as the pregnancy test is positive in these women. Warfarin is recommended in the second and third trimesters until approximately 2 weeks prior to delivery. Heparin is then given until after delivery.

ANTIPHOSPHOLIPID SYNDROME

The antiphospholipid syndrome is an important condition in which the presence of specific antibodies is associated with a predisposition to both venous and arterial thrombosis. Other clinical features include mild thrombocytopenia, chorea, livedo reticularis and recurrent pregnancy loss. The detection of antiphospholipid antibodies, such as lupus anticoagulant and anticardiolipin antibodies, has been associated with early-onset pre-eclampsia, placental abruption and recurrent miscarriage (in the first and second trimesters). 15% of women with recurrent miscarriage (three or more consecutive losses) have positive tests for these antibodies.[84] If left untreated in pregnancy these women have an extremely high fetal loss rate.[83] Defective implantation and later thrombosis of the uteroplacental vasculature and placental infarction may be the cause of this adverse pregnancy outcome.[25,79] A recent randomized controlled trial found that the prognosis improved with low-dose aspirin, but the addition of low-dose heparin was of additional benefit.[82] 75 mg daily of aspirin and 5000 units 12-hourly of heparin were administered as soon as a fetal heartbeat was detected by transvaginal ultrasound, and continued until 34 weeks' gestation. Despite treatment, nearly one-quarter of the successful pregnancies delivered preterm (before 37 weeks' gestation), and therefore close monitoring is mandatory.

ASTHMA

Asthma affects approximately 3% of the child-bearing population[59] and it is therefore the most commonly encountered respiratory disease in pregnancy. Asthma is frequently underdiagnosed and undertreated, despite the availability of effective therapy. There is no consistent effect of pregnancy on asthma, with some individuals showing improvement, some deteriorating and some experiencing no change in symptoms. It is important to realize that poor control may reflect the woman's reluctance to take medication when pregnant because of fears of harmful drug effects on her unborn child, or even because of receiving incorrect advice from healthcare professionals. Health education is essential and the opportunity to screen pregnant women for previously unrecognized asthma and to improve longer-term control in asthmatics during routine antenatal care should be encouraged.[66]

THE EFFECT OF ASTHMA ON PREGNANCY

Studies in the literature vary in the reported incidence of complications in the pregnancies of asthmatic patients. Differences in study populations, such as severity of asthma, medication, race and smoking, are likely to explain some of this variation. In general, when asthma is severe, requiring chronic steroid therapy, there appears to be an increase in maternal and fetal morbidity, particularly if symptom control is poor.[40,111]. Perlow et al[80] reported an unexplained increased incidence of preterm delivery in women suffering with asthma, especially if they were dependent on steroids. A prospective study by Steenius-Aarniala et al[104] found a higher risk of pre-eclampsia and caesarean section in women with asthma than in non-asthmatic controls. A possible increased incidence of intrauterine growth restriction has been reported by some observers.[55,97,103] This may be explained by the combination of maternal hypoxaemia and respiratory alkalosis associated with acute asthma attacks causing reduced uteroplacental perfusion and fetal hypoxia.

However, the overall pregnancy outcome for a woman with well-managed asthma is comparable to the general population,[98] and an asthmatic patient contemplating pregnancy should be reassured accordingly but with emphasis on the importance of optimal disease control.

THE MANAGEMENT OF ASTHMA IN PREGNANCY

The management of asthma in pregnancy is essentially the same as in a non-pregnant woman. The avoidance of allergens and rapid control of infective exacerbations of disease are necessary. The recognition of asthma as a chronic inflammatory condition has led to major changes in the management of the condition over recent years. New guidelines have been published by the British Thoracic Society,[7] recommending a stepwise approach to care, with particular emphasis on the prevention of attacks with earlier introduction of steroids, rather than acute symptom control with regularly inhaled bronchodilators. Inhaled steroids are preferable to oral treatment because of the reduced incidence of maternal side-effects. However, oral prednisolone or prednisone should not be withheld from a pregnant patient if required to treat repeated severe asthma attacks.

There is no evidence of any teratogenic effects with the conventional drugs used to treat asthma, including β-agonists, oral or inhaled steroids, sodium cromoglycate and theophyllines. Earlier reports of cleft palate in the rodent fetus[33] exposed to corticosteroids have not been demonstrated in human studies.[6,108] The theoretical risk of suppression of the fetal hypothalamo–pituitary–adrenal axis by maternal steroid therapy has not been substantiated in clinical practice. β-Agonists do not delay the onset or slow the progress of normal labour.[103]

Women who have received chronic steroid therapy for their asthma should be prescribed intramuscular hydrocortisone during labour. Ergometrine should be avoided because it may cause bronchospasm.[101] Regional anaesthesia is preferable to general anaesthesia because of the increased risks of atelectasis and postoperative chest infection following intubation.

Women who suffer with asthma should be encouraged

to breast-feed, as there is some evidence that it may help to prevent atopic problems in their offspring.[49] None of the drugs used in the management of asthma (except tetracycline and iodides) are contraindicated in breast-feeding. The 4% background risk of a child developing asthma is increased approximately two- to threefold if one parent has asthma, particularly if they are atopic.

HYPEREMESIS GRAVIDARUM

Vomiting is a very common symptom of pregnancy, with over 50% of women reporting at least one episode by 16 weeks' gestation.[53] Hyperemesis gravidarum occurs when vomiting in early pregnancy becomes severe and prolonged, resulting in dehydration, ketosis and weight loss. Hospital admission is often required for intravenous hydration and electrolyte replacement. Most cases will then improve with no subsequent problems, but in some women the symptoms are intractable, necessitating frequent stays in hospital, and an increase in maternal and fetal complications is observed.

The mechanisms underlying hyperemesis gravidarum remain unclear. A variety of agents have been linked to the pathogenesis of the disorder. These include hormones such as hCG, free T4, progesterone, oestrogen and cortisol, mechanical factors such as delayed gastric emptying and lower oesophageal pressures, and psychological problems. The relationship between hCG and TSH is interesting as they share a common α-subunit and have similar receptors.[117] hCG may act as a thyroid stimulator in women with hyperemesis. Certainly levels of hCG and serum thyroxine are found to be proportional to the severity of vomiting and are inversely proportional to TSH.[39,109,117] A biochemical hyperthyroidism may be found in hyperemesis with no associated clinical features and with no detectable thyroid autoantibodies. These blood test abnormalities will usually return to normal as the vomiting improves.

Mild vomiting in pregnancy is appropriately regarded as a benign condition and, in fact, has been associated with a lower fetal loss rate and less likelihood of delivering preterm compared to pregnancies in which no vomiting occurs.[53] However, women with severe hyperemesis gravidarum associated with altered biochemistry and significant weight loss deliver infants with significantly lower birthweights than women with less severe disease who maintain their prepregnancy body weight.[41] In one study comparing women who required multiple hospital admissions for vomiting compared to single admissions, mean birthweight was significantly reduced and there was a tendency towards increased intrauterine growth restriction.[38] Consequently, increased fetal surveillance is mandatory in pregnancies complicated by severe hyperemesis gravidarum.

Severe hyperemesis is potentially dangerous for the mother as well as the fetus, with three maternal deaths being reported between 1991 and 1993.[1] Complications include Mallory–Weiss oesophageal tears, Mendelson syndrome, retinal haemorrhage and abnormal liver function. The finding of raised transaminase levels tend to resolve when maternal nutrition improves. Neurological problems may occur including Wernicke encephalopathy attributed to vitamin B_1 or thiamine deficiency, central pontine myelinosis, possibly due to overzealous correction of severe hyponatraemia, peripheral neuropathies and muscle wasting or weakness. The psychological morbidity associated with hyperemesis gravidarum can also be severe, and considerable upset to family life may occur, especially if repeated hospital admissions are required.

MANAGEMENT

A variety of medical disorders should be excluded when a woman presents with severe vomiting in pregnancy. Initially an ultrasound scan should be performed to exclude multiple pregnancy and the presence of a hydatidiform mole, in which the very high hCG levels may precipitate hyperemesis. A urinary tract infection should be excluded and a variety of gastrointestinal disorders non-specific to pregnancy should be considered, e.g. gastroenteritis, pancreatitis, gallstones and peptic ulcer disease. Endocrine disorders such as overt thyrotoxicosis, diabetic ketoacidosis and Addison's disease are included in the differential diagnosis, as well as vomiting secondary to drugs such as routine iron supplements.

The principles of treatment include adequate replacement of fluids and electrolytes with intravenous fluids, such as Hartmann's solution or normal saline (0.9%). Oral or intravenous thiamine supplements should be prescribed in women with persistent vomiting. Antiemetics should not be withheld, as none of the commonly prescribed drugs, including phenothiazines, cyclizine and dopamine antagonists, have been found to be teratogenic in human studies.[63] The treatment of gastritis or oesophageal reflux with histamine receptor antagonists such as ranitidine, the proton pump inhibitor omeprazole or antacids may be beneficial in some cases. More recently, the potential of corticosteroids to treat severe hyperemesis has been considered. Small uncontrolled studies have noted a dramatic rapid improvement in symptoms after oral prednisolone (40–60 mg daily) or intravenous hydrocortisone (50–100 mg b.d.).[70,71,110] The exact mechanism of action in these cases is unclear, but it may involve the central chemoreceptor trigger zone. Although steroids are known to be safe for the fetus, there remains some caution regarding maternal side-effects as long-term steroid therapy may occasionally be required to control symptoms throughout pregnancy. The results of a randomized double-blind placebo-controlled trial are awaited to clarify the future role of corticosteroids in this disorder.

In patients with very severe weight loss and malnutrition, total parenteral nutrition may even be needed.[11] Finally, it is important to provide constant psychological support and encouragement for the woman and her family.

NEUROLOGICAL DISORDERS IN PREGNANCY

EPILEPSY

Approximately 1 in 200 women of child-bearing age suffer with epilepsy. The new onset of fits during pregnancy should be thoroughly investigated. The diagnosis of eclampsia should always be considered even in the absence of hypertension. Other medical conditions such as meningitis, encephalitis, arteriovenous malformations, cerebral infarcts, tumours, metabolic disturbances and systemic lupus erythematosus are included in the differential diagnosis of seizures in pregnancy.

The effect of pregnancy on seizure rate in known epileptics is not consistent. Seizure frequency increases in approximately 30% of women during pregnancy. Several reasons for this observation have been proposed, including disturbed sleep and lowered antiepileptic drug levels owing to non-compliance with therapy, or vomiting, particularly in the first trimester.[99] Serum drug concentrations may also decrease as a result of increased drug metabolism, increased renal clearance and the larger maternal blood volume in pregnancy.[56] It is important to avoid fits in pregnancy because of the risks of aspiration, trauma and even death in the mother,[1] and because of the potential dangers to the fetus, especially if the fit is prolonged. The likelihood of hypoxia, hypoglycaemia and lactic acidosis increase with seizure duration. It has been reported that a fetal bradycardia lasted up to 20 minutes following an epileptic fit.[116] Status epilepticus has been associated with up to a 50% chance of fetal loss.

Monitoring serum anticonvulsant levels at monthly intervals during pregnancy can be useful, particularly in those women who are poorly controlled before pregnancy. In view of the above changes in drug metabolism and clearance during pregnancy, the dose of anticonvulsant will often need to be increased in order to maintain an effective serum concentration, aiming to maintain levels comparable to those prior to pregnancy. It should be noted that some difficulty in interpreting drug levels will be encountered if both bound and unbound drug concentrations are measured together in the laboratory, as decreased protein binding will occur in pregnancy, giving rise to higher levels of the more relevant unbound free drug. Salivary drug levels may be a more useful guide to the unbound plasma drug concentration in pregnancy.

All regularly used anticonvulsants are teratogenic, with up to a 10% risk of fetal abnormality reported with in utero exposure.[58] However, the incidence of congenital anomalies appears to be multifactorial, with some degree of genetic involvement which has not been clearly defined.[54] The risk of congenital malformations is increased in women with epilepsy even if they are not receiving any treatment. For example, compared to normal pregnancy the relative risk of facial clefts was reported as 4.7 in women on anticonvulsant therapy, and 2.7 if the mother had untreated epilepsy.[36]

Carbamazepine has been associated with craniofacial defects, spina bifida and fingernail hypoplasia. Phenytoin has been linked to the so-called 'hydantoin syndrome', in which affected infants suffer with microcephaly, mental retardation, growth deficiency, facial clefts, distal digital hypoplasia and hypertelorism. The use of sodium valproate carries a 1–2% risk of neural tube defects occurring in the fetus, with a relative risk being approximately 10.[77] Detailed ultrasound scanning at 20 weeks may detect a large proportion of these structural abnormalities, especially spina bifida, and should be routinely offered. A recent prospective case-control study investigated the effects of maternal carbamazepine and phenytoin monotherapy on subsequent neurobehavioural development in their children, assessed between 18 and 36 months of age.[100] There was a significantly higher risk of children having lower cognitive abilities if their mothers took phenytoin during pregnancy, independent of maternal or environmental factors. This effect was not seen with carbamazepine. Phenobarbitone or primidone therapy can be associated with neonatal withdrawal symptoms such as tremor, hyperexcitability, feeding problems and a high-pitched cry.

However, it is important to counsel epileptic women who are contemplating pregnancy that uncontrolled seizures are more hazardous to the fetus than the risks associated with anticonvulsants. The risk of congenital anomalies may be minimized by maintaining women on the lowest possible dose of drug that keeps them fit free, and by the use of monovalent rather than polyvalent therapy.[50,57] The importance of folic acid before conception and during the first 3 months of pregnancy should be particularly emphasized in these women, as the teratogenicity of certain drugs such as carbamazepine and phenytoin may be partly due to their action as folate antagonists.[19] The possibility of withdrawing anticonvulsant therapy in women who have been fit free for 2 years could also be considered in the prepregnancy counselling clinic. However, the implications of a further epileptic fit, particularly in terms of losing their driving licence, will be a common reason for unwillingness to follow this suggestion.

Another problem to be addressed in women taking anticonvulsants is the increased risk of vitamin K deficiency in the neonate, despite normal maternal levels of clotting factors.[15] To avoid haemorrhagic problems in the newborn, vitamin K supplements can be given to the mother in the last few weeks of pregnancy and/or to the neonate at birth.[67]

There are no particular problems to expect during labour in an epileptic woman, although it is important to ensure that normal doses of anticonvulsants are not missed. The possibility of fits may be increased because of hyperventilation, maternal exhaustion and lack of sleep. Caesarean section is only indicated for obstetric reasons. Serum drug concentrations may rise rapidly in the postpartum period if increased amounts were required during pregnancy. A reduction in dose of anticonvulsants should be made after delivery to avoid toxicity. None of the anticonvulsants are contraindicated in breast-feeding mothers.

STROKE

Although strokes are uncommon problems for obstetricians to encounter, with the gradually decreasing maternal mortality rates over the past 20 years or so strokes account for an increasing percentage of all deaths in pregnancy. For example, in the last Confidential Enquiry into maternal mortality between 1991 and 1993,[1] approximately 10% of the total number of maternal deaths were attributed to strokes. Strokes are defined as acute ischaemic or haemorrhagic events causing the onset of focal neurological symptoms. Ischaemic strokes may be secondary to arterial occlusion as a result of emboli from distant sources or local thrombosis within the vessel. Many studies also include cerebral venous thrombosis, a predominantly postpartum event, which is believed to be the cause of up to one-third of pregnancy-related cerebral infarcts. Haemorrhagic strokes can be classified as intracerebral or subarachnoid bleeds. Intracerebral haemorrhage may be due to severe hypertension or a result of congenital vascular anomalies such as aneurysms or arteriovenous malformations.

It is generally accepted that pregnancy and the puerperium are associated with an increased risk of stroke, but the exact increase is difficult to quantify owing to the unreliability of many of the available data.[42] For example, many of the published studies involve small numbers of patients, so that precise estimates of risk cannot be made. The classification of stroke tends to be suboptimal, especially in earlier series when accurate imaging techniques were not used. Referral bias will be present if studies are only conducted at regional referral centres. Lastly, follow-up studies to look at recurrence risks in future pregnancies have not been carried out. One large retrospective study looked at all women of child-bearing age discharged from various hospitals in central Maryland and Washington DC in 1988 and 1991 with a diagnosis of cerebral infarction or intracerebral haemorrhage (but not including subarachnoid haemorrhage).[52] The risks of both these conditions were found to be increased in the 6 weeks after delivery (by 8.7 for cerebral infarction and 28 for intracerebral haemorrhage), but not during pregnancy itself. The overall relative risk of stroke during or within 6 weeks after pregnancy was 2.4. However, these estimates are probably conservative and no adjustment was made for the lower frequency of risk factors for vascular disorders such as diabetes, ischaemic heart disease and hypertension in those women who present with stroke associated with pregnancy.

Any symptoms suggestive of stroke in a pregnant woman should be investigated promptly, as some causes are treatable. Neuroimaging techniques such as CT scanning and magnetic resonance imaging are safe in pregnancy with suitable screening of the fetus, and should not be withheld.

ISCHAEMIC STROKE

Strokes secondary to arterial occlusive disease are most common in the second and third trimesters of pregnancy or in the first week postpartum. The hypercoagulable state of pregnancy predisposes the mother to thrombus formation. Potential causes of local arterial abnormalities include atherosclerosis, vasculitis, homocystinuria, moya moya disease and Takayasu's disease. Cardiac disease in pregnancy can produce symptoms of focal cerebral ischaemia through a variety of mechanisms. Valve-related emboli may be associated with arrhythmias, infective endocarditis, mitral valve prolapse, prosthetic valves and rheumatic heart disease. Mural thrombus formation, e.g. in cardiomyopathy or post-myocardial infarction, may give rise to emboli. Paradoxical embolism may occur with a systemic venous thromboembolism in the presence of a cardiac defect such as an atrial septal defect or a patent foramen ovale. Haematological disease in pregnancy may also give rise to an increased risk of arterial stroke, e.g. sickle cell anaemia, thrombotic thrombocytopenic purpura and the thrombophilias. Interestingly, the hereditary and acquired thrombophilias are rarer causes of stroke than expected because of the associated poor obstetric history, with early pregnancy losses.

In ischaemic stroke the aim is to prevent progression or recurrence of the infarction. Interdisciplinary care is essential. General supportive measures are required and any cause or associated factors, e.g. an arrhythmia, should be treated. The role of anticoagulation is a dilemma even outside pregnancy, and certainly no prospective trials are available for guidance. The concern is the increased risk of catastrophic haemorrhagic transformation in healthy or infarcted brain tissue, but the risk of recurrent infarction is high if no anticoagulants are given. One possible plan is to anticoagulate in the presence of small infarcts with no evidence of haemorrhagic transformation on CT scan. However, if the infarct is large, the CT scan is repeated in approximately 3–5 days. If there are still no signs of haemorrhagic transformation, anticoagulant therapy can be commenced.

HAEMORRHAGIC STROKE

The incidence of haemorrhage from aneurysms and arteriovenous malformations increases in the second and third trimesters.[27] The overall maternal mortality from aneurysms is approximately 35%, which is consistent with the non-pregnant population, but the mortality associated with haemorrhage from AVMs is higher (28% in pregnancy compared to 10% outside pregnancy).[27] The initial neurological status of the patient following a bleed from an intracranial vascular anomaly correlates well with the mortality and neurological outcome. If there is profound alteration in consciousness at presentation, mortality rates reach 80–90% and operative mortality is also high (between 25 and 35%).

The differential diagnoses of intracranial haemorrhage include cerebral venous thrombosis, arterial occlusion, meningitis or encephalitis, eclampsia, intracranial tumour or abscess and demyelinating diseases. The sudden onset of symptoms, severity of headache, and the presence of meningism or photophobia favour the diagnosis of an intracranial bleed. A CT scan should be performed to confirm the diagnosis. If this is normal but the history is particularly suggestive of a subarachnoid haemorrhage, a lumbar puncture may be performed. If an intracerebral haemorrhage is confirmed, then cerebral angiography is required to identify the actual vascular anomaly.

The morbidity in the mother presenting with an intracranial haemorrhage includes seizures, hyponatraemia, raised intracranial pressure, rebleeding, vasospasm (particularly following a subarachnoid bleed) and subsequent permanent neurological deficit. Anticonvulsants may therefore be required, especially to prevent recurrent fits. Nimodipine has been shown to reduce posthaemorrhagic vasospasm in aneurysmal bleeding, and therefore lowers the risk of delayed ischaemic neurologic deficits and possible death. High-dose steroids may be needed to decrease intracranial oedema.

Regarding operative management, Dias and Sekhar[28] reported significant benefits in terms of maternal and fetal mortality in a study of 106 patients if aneurysms were treated surgically by clipping, compared to non-operative treatment. The surgical management of haemorrhage secondary to AVMs is more controversial in the general population, and therefore the decision to operate in pregnancy is less clear. Dias and Sekhar[28] found no significant differences in maternal or fetal mortality in 36 patients whether they underwent surgery or not, independent of other variables. The decision to operate on an AVM should be for the same reasons as in the non-pregnant patient, e.g. recurrent haemorrhage, intractable epilepsy, severe unrelenting headache or cerebrovascular ischaemia secondary to a steal phenomenon.

The obstetric management of women with intracranial haemorrhage has altered considerably over the years. The benefits of elective caesarean section to avoid the haemodynamic changes during labour have been questioned. The effect of mode of delivery on maternal and fetal mortality after intracranial haemorrhage secondary to untreated intracranial aneurysms or AVMs has also been reviewed.[28] No significant differences were found in mortality rates following vaginal or caesarean delivery. Caesarean section is indicated for obstetric reasons only or for delivery of the fetus when the mother is moribund. Life support may be needed until fetal maturity has been reached. The risk of recurrent haemorrhage during labour may be reduced by epidural anaesthesia, minimizing pushing in the second stage, and by performing a low forceps delivery if required.

MYASTHENIA GRAVIS

Myasthenia gravis is an uncommon autoimmune condition in which antibodies are directed against the acetylcholine receptors in motor end-plates of striated muscle. The clinical behaviour of myasthenia gravis in pregnancy is unpredictable, with approximately one-third of patients experiencing an improvement in symptoms, one-third noting a deterioration in their condition and one-third remaining stable. The effect of pregnancy on the disorder is not consistent between pregnancies and exacerbations may occur at any stage, but especially postpartum. Plasmapheresis has been used to treat myasthenic crises in pregnancy.[114] It has been suggested that patients who have undergone previous thymectomy have less risk of exacerbations in pregnancy, but this finding is not universal.[65]

Smooth muscle is not affected by the condition, so that the nature of contractions is unchanged and the duration of labour is not prolonged. The voluntary muscles used in the second stage may, however, be compromised, necessitating assisted vaginal delivery for maternal exhaustion. A variety of drugs often used in pregnancy should be used with caution as they may potentiate muscle weakness, e.g. narcotics, benzodiazepines and large doses of procaine local anaesthetic. Epidural anaesthesia is recommended. Magnesium sulphate should not be used as it may precipitate a myasthenic crisis.[4]

Transient neonatal myasthenia gravis may develop in the offspring of affected mothers in 10–12% of cases. Symptoms may be delayed up to 4 days after delivery, and are caused by passive transfer of IgG antibodies across the placenta. The condition usually lasts for 3 weeks. The neonate may present with poor sucking, a feeble cry, muscle weakness or respiratory distress secondary to aspiration and bronchial obstruction. The risk of this problem in the neonate is not predicted by maternal disease state or antibody titre levels.[34] Management includes close observation, supportive measures and possibly parenteral anticholinesterase therapy.

FURTHER READING

De Swiet M (ed) 1995 Medical disorders in obstetric practice, 3rd edn. Blackwell Science, Oxford

Rubin PC (ed) 1995 Prescribing in pregnancy. BMJ Publishing Group, London

REFERENCES

1. Department of Health, Welsh Office, Scottish Home and Health Department and Department of Health 1996 Confidential enquiries into maternal deaths in the United Kingdom 1991–93. HMSO, London
2. Adam P A J, Schwartz R 1968 Diagnosis and treatment: should oral hypoglycaemic agents be used in pediatric and pregnant patients? Pediatrics 42: 819–823
3. Badaracco M A, Vessey M 1974 Recurrence of venous thromboembolism disease and use of oral contraceptives. British Medical Journal i: 215–217
4. Bashuk R G, Krendel D A 1990 Myasthenia gravis presenting as weakness after magnesium administration. Muscle and Nerve 13: 708–712
5. Beasley R P, Hwang L-U, Lee G Y 1983 Prevention of perinatally transmitted hepatitis B virus infections with hepatitis B immune globulin and hepatitis B vaccine. Lancet ii: 1099–1102
6. Briggs G G, Freeman R K, Yaffe S J 1994 Drugs in pregnancy and lactation. Williams & Wilkins, Baltimore
7. British Thoracic Society 1993 Guidelines for the management of asthma. Thorax 48(suppl): S1–S24
8. Brosens I A 1977 Morphological changes in the utero-placental bed in pregnancy hypertension. Clinical Obstetrics and Gynecology 4: 573–593
9. Broughton Pipkin F, Rubin P C 1994 Pre-eclampsia – the 'disease of theories'. British Medical Bulletin 50: 381–396
10. Butters L, Kennedy S, Rubin P C 1990 Atenolol in the management of essential hypertension during pregnancy. British Medical Journal 301: 587–589
11. Charlin V, Borghesi L, Hasbun J, Von-Mulenbrock R, Moreno M I 1993 Parenteral nutrition in hyperemesis gravidarum. Nutrition 9: 29–32
12. Chien P F W, Khan K S, Arnott N 1996 Magnesium sulphate in the treatment of eclampsia and pre-eclampsia: an overview of the evidence from randomised trials. British Journal of Obstetrics and Gynaecology 103: 1085–1091
13. CLASP (Collaborative Low-dose Aspirin Study In Pregnancy) Collaborative Group 1994 CLASP: a randomized trial of low-dose aspirin for the prevention and treatment of pre-eclampsia among 9364 pregnant women. Lancet 343: 619–629
14. Cockburn J, Moar V A, Ounsted M et al 1986 Final report of study on hypertension during pregnancy: the effects of specific treatment on the growth and development of the children. Lancet i: 647–649
15. Cornelissen M, Steegers-Theunissen R, Kollee L et al 1993 Increasing incidence of neonatal vitamin K deficiency resulting from maternal anticonvulsant therapy. American Journal of Obstetrics and Gynecology 168: 923–928
16. Cunningham F G, Lucas M J 1994 Urinary tract infections complicating pregnancy. Clinical Obstetrics and Gynecology 8: 353–374
17. Dahlman T C 1993 Osteoporotic fractures and recurrence of thromboembolism during pregnancy and the puerperium in 184 women undergoing thromboprophylaxis with heparin. American Journal of Obstetrics and Gynecology 168: 1265–1270
18. Dahlman T C, Lindvall N, Hellgren M 1990 Osteopenia in pregnancy during longterm heparin treatment: a radiological study post partum. British Journal of Haematology 97: 221–228
19. Dansky L V, Rosenblatt D S, Andermann E 1992 Mechanisms of teratogenesis: folic acid and antiepileptic therapy. Neurology 42 (4 Suppl 5): 32–42
20. Davison J, Baylis C 1995 Renal disease. In: de Swiet M (ed) Medical disorders in obstetric practice, 3rd edn. Blackwell Science, Oxford, pp. 226–305
21. Davison J M, Dellagrammatikas H, Parkin J M 1985 Maternal azathioprine therapy and depressed haemopoiesis in the babies of renal allograft patients. British Journal of Obstetrics and Gynaecology 92: 233–239
22. de Swiet M 1991 Thromboembolism in obstetrics. Current Obstetrics and Gynaecology 1: 191–195
23. de Swiet M 1995 Thromboembolism. In de Swiet M (ed) Medical disorders in obstetric practice, 3rd edn. Blackwell Science, Oxford, pp. 116–142
24. de Swiet M, Dorrington Ward P, Fidler J et al 1983 Prolonged heparin therapy in pregnancy causes bone demineralization. British Journal of Obstetrics and Gynaecology 90: 1129–1134
25. De Wolf F, Carreras L O, Moerman P, Vermylen J, Van Assche A, Renaer M 1992 Decidual vasculopathy and extensive placental infarction in a patient with repeated thromboembolic accidents, recurrent fetal loss, and a lupus anticoagulant. American Journal of Obstetrics and Gynecology 142: 829–834
26. Derksen R H W M, Bruinse H W, de Groot PG and Kater L 1994. Pregnancy in systemic lupus erythematosus: a prospective study. Lupus 3: 149–155
27. Dias M S 1994 Neurovascular emergencies in pregnancy. Clinical Obstetrics and Gynecology 37: 337–354
28. Dias M S, Sekhar L N 1990 Intracranial hemorrhage from aneurysms and arteriovenous malformations during pregnancy and the puerperium. Neurosurgery 27: 855–865
29. Douglas K A, Redman C W G 1994 Eclampsia in the United Kingdom. British Medical Journal 309: 1395–1400
30. Dulitzki M, Pauzner R, Langevitz P et al 1996 Low molecular weight heparin during pregnancy and delivery: preliminary experience with 41 pregnancies. Obstetrics and Gynecology 87: 380–383
31. Eclampsia Trial Collaborative Group 1995 Which anticonvulsant for women with eclampsia? Evidence from the Collaborative Eclampsia Trial. Lancet 345: 1455–1463
32. Fagan E A 1994 Intrahepatic cholestasis of pregnancy. British Medical Journal 309: 1243–1244
33. Fainstalt T 1954 Cortisone-induced congenital cleft palate in rabbits. Endocrinology 55: 502
34. Fennell D F, Ringel S P 1987 Myasthenia gravis and pregnancy. Obstetrical and Gynecological Survey 41: 414–421
35. Fisk N M, Storey G N B 1988 Fetal outcome in obstetric cholestasis. British Journal of Obstetrics and Gynaecology 95: 1137–1143
36. Friis M L, Holm N V, Sindrup E H 1986 Facial clefts in sibs and children of epileptic patients. Neurology 36: 346–350
37. Ginsberg J S, Kowalchuck G, Hirsh J et al 1990 Heparin effect on bone density. Thrombosis and Haemostasis 64: 286–289
38. Godsey R K, Newman R B 1991 Hyperemesis gravidarum: a comparison of single and multiple admissions. Journal of Reproductive Medicine 36: 287–290
39. Goodwin T M, Montero M, Mestman J H, Pekary A E, Hershman J M 1992 The role of chorionic gonadotrophin in transient hyperthyroidism of hyperemesis gravidarum. Journal of Clinical Endocrinology and Metabolism 75: 1333–1337
40. Gordon M, Niswander K R, Berendes H, Kantor A G 1970 Fetal morbidity following potentially anoxigenic obstetric conditions. VII. Bronchial asthma. American Journal of Obstetrics and Gynecology 106: 421–429
41. Gross S, Librach C, Cecutti A 1989 Maternal weight loss associated with hyperemesis gravidarum: a predictor of fetal outcome. American Journal of Obstetrics and Gynecology 160: 906–909
42. Grosset D G, Ebrahim S 1995 Stroke in pregnancy and the puerperium: what magnitude of risk? Journal of Neurology, Neurosurgery and Psychiatry 58: 129–131
43. Hall J G, Pauli R M, Wilson K M 1980 Maternal and fetal sequelae of anticoagulation during pregnancy. American Journal of Medicine 68: 122–140
44. Hayslett J P and Lynn R I 1980 Effect of pregnancy in patients with lupus nephropathy. Kidney International 18: 207–210
45. Hibbard B, Horn E H 1988 Controversies in therapeutics series. Iron and folate supplements during pregnancy. British Medical Journal 297: 1325–1327
46. Hirsh J, Raschke R, Warkentin T E, Dalen J E, Deykin D, Poller L 1995 Heparin: mechanism of action, pharmacokinetics, dosing considerations, monitoring, efficacy, and safety. Chest 108: 258S–275S
47. Horn E H 1996 Anticoagulants in pregnancy. Current Obstetrics and Gynaecology 6: 111–118
48. Howell R, Fidler J, Letsky E, de Swiet M 1983 The risks of antenatal subcutaneous heparin prophylaxis: a controlled trial. British Journal of Obstetrics and Gynaecology 90: 1124–1128
49. Jellife D B, Jellife E F P 1977 'Breast is Best': modern meanings. New England Journal of Medicine 297: 912–915
50. Kaneko S, Otani K, Kondo T et al 1992 Malformation in infants of mothers with epilepsy receiving antiepileptic drugs. Neurology 42 (4 Suppl 5): 68–74

51. Khuroo M S, Kamili S, Jameel S 1995 Vertical transmission of hepatitis E virus. Lancet 345: 1025–1026
52. Kittner S J, Stern B J, Feeser B R et al 1996 Pregnancy and the risk of stroke. New England Journal of Medicine 335: 768–774
53. Klebanoff MA 1985 Epidemiology of vomiting in early pregnancy. Obstetrics and Gynecology 66: 612–616
54. Koch S, Losche G, Jager-Roman E et al 1992 Major and minor birth malformations and antiepileptic drugs. Neurology 42 (4 Suppl 5): 83–88
55. Lao T T, Huengsburg M 1990 Labour and delivery in mothers with asthma. European Journal of Obstetrics, Gynaecology and Reproductive Biology 35: 183–190
56. Leppik I E, Rask C A 1989 Pharmacokinetics of antiepileptic drugs during pregnancy. Seminars in Neurology 8: 240–246
57. Lindhout D 1992 Pharmacokinetics and drug interactions: role in antiepileptic-drug-induced teratogenesis. Neurology 42 (Suppl 5): 443–447
58. Lindhout D, Hoppener J E A, Meinardi H 1984 Teratogenicity of antiepileptic drug combinations with special emphasis on epoxidation (of carbamazepine). Epilepsia 25: 77–83
59. Littlejohns P, Ebrahim S, Anderson R 1989 Prevalence and diagnosis of chronic respiratory symptoms in adults. British Medical Journal 298: 1556–1560
60. Long P A, Abell D A, Beischer N A 1980 Fetal growth retardation and pre-eclampsia. British Journal of Obstetrics and Gynaecology 87: 13–18
61. Mandel S J, Larsen P R, Seely E W, Brent G A 1990 Increased need for thyroxine during pregnancy in women with primary hypothyroidism. New England Journal of Medicine 323: 91–96
62. Martin J N, Perry K G, Blake P G et al 1993 The presence of HELLP syndrome in the eclamptic parturient is a major maternal and perinatal risk indicator. American Journal of Obstetrics and Gynecology 168: 386
63. Milkovich L, Van Den Berg B J 1976 An evaluation of the teratogenicity of certain antinauseant drugs. American Journal of Obstetrics and Gynecology 125: 244–248
64. Mills J L, Simpson J L, Driscoll S G et al 1988 Incidence of spontaneous abortion among normal women and insulin-dependent diabetic women whose pregnancies were identified within 21 days of conception. New England Journal of Medicine 319: 1617–1623
65. Mitchell P J, Bebbington M 1992 Myasthenia gravis in pregnancy. Obstetrics and Gynecology 80: 178–181
66. Moore-Gillon J 1994 Asthma in pregnancy. British Journal of Obstetrics and Gynaecology 101: 658–660
67. Moslet U, Hansen E S 1992 A review of vitamin K, epilepsy and pregnancy. Acta Neurologica Scandinavica 85: 39–43
68. National High Blood Pressure Education Program 1990 Working group report on high blood pressure in pregnancy. American Journal of Obstetrics and Gynecology 163: 1691–1712
69. Nelson-Piercy C 1994 Low molecular weight heparin for obstetric thromboprophylaxis. British Journal of Obstetrics and Gynaecology 101: 6–8
70. Nelson-Piercy C, de Swiet M 1994 Corticosteroids for the treatment of hyperemesis gravidarum. British Journal of Obstetrics and Gynaecology 101: 1013–1015
71. Nelson-Piercy C, de Swiet M 1995 Complications of the use of corticosteroids for the treatment of hyperemesis gravidarum. British Journal of Obstetrics and Gynaecology 102: 507–509
72. Nora J J, Nora A H 1987 Maternal transmission of congenital heart diseases: new recurrent risk figures and the question of cytoplasmic inheritance and vulnerability to teratogens. American Journal of Cardiology 59: 459–463
73. Nora J J, Nora A H 1988 Update on counselling the family with a first degree relative with a congenital heart defect. American Journal of Medical Genetics 29: 137–142
74. Norden C W, Kass EH 1968 Bacteriuria of pregnancy – a critical reappraisal. Annual Review of Medicine 19: 431–470
75. Norton M E, Merrill J, Cooper B A B, Kuller J A, Clyman R I 1993 Neonatal complications after administration of indomethacin for preterm labor. New England Journal of Medicine 329: 1602–1607
76. Oakley C 1995 Anticoagulants in pregnancy. British Heart Journal 74: 107–111
77. Oakeshott P, Hunt G M 1989 Valproate and spina bifida. British Medical Journal 298: 1300–1301
78. O'Sullivan J B, Mahan C M, Charles D, Dandrow R V 1973 Screening criteria for high risk gestational diabetic patients. American Journal of Obstetrics and Gynecology 116: 895–900
79. Out H J, Kooijman C D, Bruinse H W, Derksen R H 1991 Histopathological findings in placentae from patients with intra-uterine fetal death and anti-phospholipid antibodies. European Journal of Obstetrics, Gynaecology and Reproductive Biology 41: 179–186
80. Perlow J H, Montgomery D, Morgan M A, Towers C V, Porto M 1992 Severity of asthma and perinatal outcome. American Journal of Obstetrics and Gynecology 167: 963–967
81. Pirson Y, Van Lierde M, Ghysen J, Squifflet J P, Alexandre G P J, Van Ypersele de Strihou C 1985 Retardation of fetal growth in patients receiving immunosuppressive therapy. New England Journal of Medicine 313: 328
82. Rai R, Cohen H, Dave M, Regan L 1997 Randomised controlled trial of aspirin and aspirin plus heparin in pregnant women with recurrent miscarriage associated with phospholipid antibodies (or antiphospholipid antibodies). British Medical Journal 314: 253–257
83. Rai R S, Clifford K, Cohen H, Regan L 1995 High prospective fetal loss rate in untreated pregnancies of women with recurrent miscarriage and antiphospholipid antibodies. Human Reproduction 10: 3301–3304
84. Rai R S, Regan L, Clifford K, Pickering W, Dave M, Mackie I 1995 Antiphospholipid antibodies and B-2 glycoprotein-I in 500 women with recurrent miscarriage: results of a comprehensive screening approach. Human Reproduction 10: 101–105
85. Ramsay I 1991 Fetal and neonatal hyperthyroidism. Contemporary Reviews in Obstetrics and Gynaecology 3: 74–78
86. RCOG Working Party 1995 Report of the RCOG working party on prophylaxis against thromboembolism in gynaecology and obstetrics. RCOG Press, London
87. Redman C W G 1991 Current topic: pre-eclampsia and the placenta. Placenta 12: 301–308
88. Redman C W G, Beilin L J, Bonnar J et al 1976 Fetal outcome in trial of antihypertensive treatment in pregnancy. Lancet ii: 753–756
89. Rizzo T, Metzger B E, Burns W J, Burns K 1991 Correlations between antepartum maternal metabolism and intelligence of offspring. New England Journal of Medicine 325: 9111–9116
90. Rizzoni G, Ehrich J H H et al 1992 Successful pregnancies in women on renal replacement therapy: report from the EDTA Registry. Nephrology, Dialysis and Transplantation 7: 1–9
91. Roberts J M, Redman C W G 1993 Pre-eclampsia: more than pregnancy-induced hypertension. Lancet 341: 1447–1451
92. Roberts J M, Taylor R N, Musci T J, Rodgers G M, Hubel C A, McLaughlin M K 1989 Pre-eclampsia: an endothelial cell disorder. American Journal of Obstetrics and Gynecology 161: 1200–1204
93. Rosa F W, Bosco L A, Graham C F, Milstien J B, Dreis M, Creamer J 1989 Neonatal anuria with maternal angiotensin-converting enzyme inhibition. Obstetrics and Gynecology 74: 371–374
94. Rubin P C, Butters L, Clark D M et al 1983 Placebo-controlled trial of atenolol treatment of pregnancy-associated hypertension. Lancet i: 431–434
95. Rubin P, Butters L, Reynolds B et al 1983 Atenolol elimination in the neonate. British Journal of Clinical Pharmacology 16: 659–662
95a. Rubin P C (ed) 1995 Prescribing in pregnancy, 2nd edn. BMJ Publishing, London
96. Rudolph J E, Shwihizir RT, Barius S A 1979 Pregnancy in renal transplant patients: a review. Transplantation 27: 26–29
97. Schatz M, Zeiger R S, Hoffman C P 1990 Intrauterine growth is related to gestational pulmonary function in pregnant asthmatic women. Chest 98: 389–392
98. Schatz M, Zeiger R S, Hoffman C P et al 1995 Perinatal outcomes in the pregnancies of asthmatic women: a prospective controlled analysis. American Journal of Respiratory and Critical Care Medicine 151: 1170–1174
99. Schmidt D, Canger R, Avanzini G et al 1983 Change of seizure frequency in pregnant epileptic women. Journal of Neurology, Neurosurgery and Psychiatry 46: 751–755
100. Scolnik D, Nulman I, Rovet J et al 1994 Neurodevelopment of children exposed in utero to phenytoin and carbamazepine monotherapy. Journal of the American Medical Association 271: 767–770
101. Sellers W F S, Long D R 1979 Bronchospasm following ergometrine. Anaesthesia 34: 909

102. Sibai B M, Ramadan M K, Usta I, Salama M, Mercer B M, Friedman S A 1993 Maternal morbidity and mortality in 442 pregnancies with hemolysis, elevated liver enzymes and low platelets (HELLP syndrome). American Journal of Obstetrics and Gynecology 169: 1000–1006
103. Sims C D, Chamberlain G V P, de Sweit M 1976 Lung function tests in bronchial asthma during and after pregnancy. British Journal of Obstetrics and Gynaecology 83: 434–437
104. Steenius-Aarniala B, Piirila P, Teramo K 1988 Asthma and pregnancy: a prospective study of 198 pregnancies. Thorax 43: 12–18
105. Stiete H, Stiete S, Petchaelis A et al 1994 Malformations in diabetic pregnancy. Diabetologia 37(suppl 1): A172
106. Stuart M J, Gross S J, Elrad H, Graeber J E 1982 Effects of acetyl salicylic acid ingestion on maternal and neonatal haemostasis. New England Journal of Medicine 307: 909–912
107. Sturridge F, Letsky E, de Swiet M 1994 The use of low molecular weight heparin for thromboprophylaxis. British Journal of Obstetrics and Gynaecology 101: 69–71
108. Taeusch H W 1975 Glucocorticoid prophylaxis for respiratory distress syndrome: a review of potential toxicity. Journal of Pediatrics 87: 617–623
109. Tareen A K, Baseer A, Jaffry H F, Shafiq M 1995 Thyroid hormone in hyperemesis gravidarum. Journal of Obstetrics and Gynaecology 21: 497–501
110. Taylor D J 1996 Successful management of hyperemesis gravidarum using steroid therapy. Quarterly Journal of Medicine 89: 103–107
111. Turner E S, Greenberger P A, Patterson R 1980 Management of the pregnant asthmatic patient. Annals of Internal Medicine 6: 905–918
112. Ville Y, Jenkins E, Shearer M J et al 1993 Fetal intraventricular haemorrhage and maternal warfarin. Lancet 341: 1211
113. Walsh S W 1985 Pre-eclampsia: An imbalance in placental prostacyclin and thromboxane production. American Journal of Obstetrics and Gynecology 152: 335–340
114. Watson W J, Katz V L, Bowes W A 1990 Plasmapheresis during pregnancy. Obstetrics and Gynecology 76: 451–457
115. Weinstein L 1982. Syndrome of hemolysis, elevated liver enzymes and low platelet count: a severe consequence of hypertension in pregnancy. American Journal of Obstetrics and Gynecology 142: 159–167
116. Yerby M S 1987 Problems and management of the pregnant woman with epilepsy. Epilepsia 28 (suppl 3): S29–S36
117. Yoshimura M, Hershman J M 1995 Thyrotropic action of human chorionic gonadotrophin. Thyroid 5: 425–434

14

Antenatal diagnosis and fetal medicine

Phillipa M. Kyle   Nicholas M. Fisk   Charles H. Rodeck

INTRODUCTION

In the 1980s there were major advances in prenatal diagnosis and fetal medicine. These have continued in the present decade, although the advances have been more in terms of scientific analysis and the understanding of results, rather than in ultrasound technology and invasive procedures. This is particularly evident in areas such as aneuploidy, Doppler assessment for fetal well-being, and the assessment of multiple pregnancy. The application of DNA analysis to prenatal diagnosis continues to escalate, so that an increasing number of single-gene disorders can be diagnosed on first-trimester fetal tissues. Aneuploidy risk calculation based on ultrasonic markers is being refined, incorporating maternal age into the calculation. First-trimester screening for aneuploidy now seems a reality, using nuchal translucency measurements, possibly combined with serum biochemical measurements. Invasive testing is still widely, performed although there has been a trend for the earlier-gestation tests such as chorionic villus sampling and amniocentesis to predominate. There has been a decline in the requirement for fetal blood sampling because of the availability of DNA testing on chorionic villi and amniotic fluid, and non-invasive assessment of IUGR.

Prenatal diagnosis is no longer the preserve of those at increased risk. All pregnant women worry whether their baby is normal, and in many countries nearly all women have an ultrasound scan. Fortunately, the vast majority can be reassured that no abnormality has been detected. In a few cases the fetus can be treated; others, with malformations detected in the third trimester, can be managed more rationally than in the past.

The access to the fetus offered by modern invasive procedures has not only provided considerable insight into fetal physiology, but has allowed the fetus to be considered as a patient in its own right. Samples for diagnosis can be obtained from the fetal circulation, urinary tract, liver and skin, and drugs or transfusions of red cells, platelets or bone marrow can be administered intravascularly or intraperitoneally. The results of fetal surgery have been largely disappointing, although a role may emerge for endoscopic interventions.

ANTENATAL DIAGNOSIS

STRUCTURAL MALFORMATIONS

Ultrasound is the chief method for detecting structural abnormalities. Since the first report of detection of a fetal anomaly leading to termination of pregnancy[65] a wide range of major malformations have been detected. With advances in ultrasound imaging the appearances of an increasing number of minor malformations have now been described, including subtle markers of chromosome abnormalities.

The standard of ultrasound achieved in practice has continued to improve dramatically and is available to an increasing proportion of the population. The assignation of 'levels' to various standards of ultrasound was previously used to indicate whether fetal anatomy was examined (level II and beyond), but has fallen into disuse now that visualization of common fetal structures is within the scope of all those performing obstetric scans.[121]

Routine ultrasound screening is recommended in the UK.[327] This examination is delayed until 18–20 weeks, when cardiac and renal structure becomes discernible. Routine screening detects 60–80% of major and 35% of minor congenital malformations,[80,222,230] in contrast to the 25% detected[180] under the indication-based system favoured in the USA.[268]

Only the main areas of ultrasound diagnoses are summarized below; exhaustive listings are available elsewhere.[357,418]

Neural tube defects

The diagnosis of anencephaly is straightforward: the cranial vault cannot be visualized in the standard view for

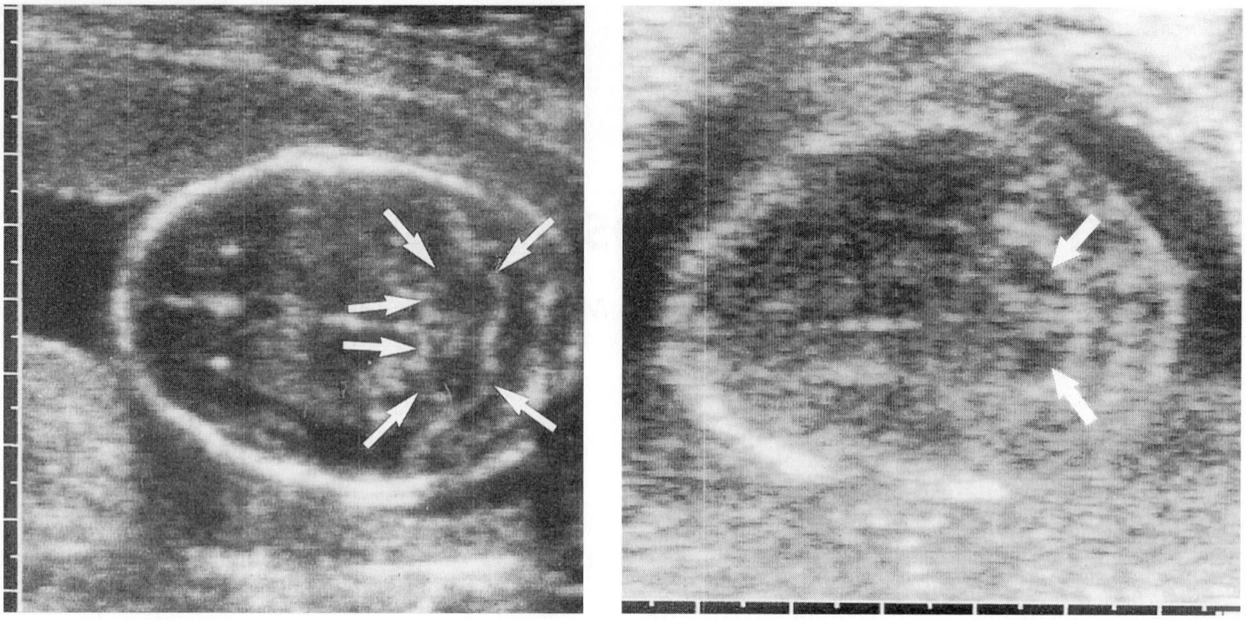

A B

Fig. 14.1 (A) The normal dumb-bell shape of the cerebellum (arrows) on ultrasound at 18 weeks. (B) Anterior curvature of the cerebellum, the 'banana' sign (arrows), in a fetus of similar gestation with open spina bifida.

biparietal diameter measurement. Detection of open myelomeningocoele is more complex. Although larger defects may be suggested by gross disruption in vertebral integrity in the longitudinal plane or by soft tissue signs, smaller defects will only be apparent in the horizontal planes of a few localized vertebrae, as subtle splaying in the lateral processes. These views can be difficult, especially if the fetal spine lies against the uterine wall, and in this context screening has been greatly facilitated by two cranial signs found in almost all fetuses with myelomeningocoele. Scalloping of the frontal bones gives the head a lemon-shaped appearance ('lemon' sign), whereas the normally dumbbell-shaped cerebellum appears either absent or banana shaped ('banana' sign; Fig. 14.1).[147,273,321] The latter results from downward herniation of posterior fossa contents and the former from the subsequent reduction in intracranial volume.

The initial approach to screening for NTDs comprised maternal serum α-feto protein estimation at 16 weeks, with investigation of positive results by amniocentesis for amniotic fluid AFP and acetylcholinesterase. However, only 88% of fetuses with anencephaly, and 79% with myelomeningocoele,[395] were so identified. The next advance was to introduce ultrasound at the time of blood collection. The reasons were, first, to exclude twins and death in utero, which raise AFP, and secondly the accuracy of AFP screening is increased when dating is based on biparietal diameter,[402] which is smaller in myelomeningocoele. Finally, the diagnosis of anencephaly is immediately obvious. Ultrasound also became the preferred investigation for a positive screen in view of reluctance to terminate a pregnancy solely on the basis of amniotic fluid biochemistry. Although the accuracy of AFP versus ultrasound has not been addressed in comparative trials, reports indicated that detection rates for myelomeningocoele of 80–100% with ultrasound exceed those with AFP alone.[11,213,336] Recent studies suggest that ultrasound sceening using the lemon and banana signs should theoretically detect 96–100% of myelomeningocoele.[67,396] It is important to recognize that ultrasound is both a screening and a diagnostic test, and that small spinal lesions in fetuses with suspicious cranial signs on screening may only be detected on detailed scanning by a very experienced operator. Most centres have dispensed with AFP screening for NTDs, although others have retained it either as a cautious 'belt and braces' approach or as a component of Down syndrome serum screening. With few exceptions myelomeningocoele is now essentially an ultrasonic diagnosis.

Other craniospinal malformations

Hydrocephalus is diagnosed in utero by elevated ratios of various measurements of the lateral ventricle to hemispheric width in the transverse plane,[66,134] or enlargement of the atrium of posterior horn of the lateral ventricle.[69] Unless there is progressive or gross dilatation, caution should be exercised in the interpretation of mild ventriculomegaly, especially in the mid-trimester. The level of obstruction is determined by examining the third and fourth ventricles and the aqueduct of Sylvius. Hydranencephaly is distinguished from severe hydrocephalus by the absence of midline structures and the lack of a residual cortical rim, but the distinction may be difficult in extreme cases. In holoprosencephaly the extent of midline ventricular fusion varies with the degree of failure of cleavage of the prosencephalon,[320] and there are often concomitant facial anomalies. The diagnosis of microcephaly should only be made in the presence of serial measurements of head circumference 3–4 standard deviations below the mean, so as to exclude growth retardation or incorrect dating. The ultrasonic appearances of encephalocoele, Dandy–Walker malformation, and intracranial cysts, tumours and haemorrhage are well described. Agenesis of the corpus callosum, increasingly recognized as separation of the lateral ventricles with upward displacement of the third ventricle, is more difficult to diagnose, and is often detected in association with other central nervous system abnormalities.[361]

Cardiac defects

Following characterization of the normal ultrasonic appearances of the fetal heart, a wide range of defects have been diagnosed. Inspection of the four-chamber view[103] in a transverse plane during the routine 18-week scan detects approximately 20–40% of severe congenital heart disease.[120,369] This view is abnormal with major defects such as hypoplastic ventricles, atrioventricular canal defects and tricuspid atresia, although minor lesions such as septal defects may be missed. Visualization of venoatrial and ventriculoarterial connections is more complex, but if it were introduced into routine screening it would theoretically increase the detection rate to greater than 80%.[384] Some cases are missed because the heart may be normal at the time of screening. Indications for fetal echocardiography include an abnormal four-chamber view, an affected sibling or family history, diabetes, exposure to cardiac teratogens, and monochorionic twin gestations. A high degree of accuracy can then be achieved for diagnosis of major vessel lesions such as pulmonary stenosis, truncus arteriosus, and transposition of the great vessels.[96] Colour and energy flow Doppler facilitates the demonstration of cardiac structure, and M-mode and pulsed wave Doppler provide an index of cardiac function, which is particularly useful in arrhythmias.

Intrathoracic defects

Most intrathoracic lesions identified prenatally are benign, but their significance is the association with pulmonary hypoplasia. Indirect indices of the severity of compression on the developing lung are the degree of mediastinal shift, the presence of polyhydramnios due to limited swallowing, and hydrops secondary to obstructed venous return. Left-sided diaphragmatic hernias are detected on ultrasound because of displacement of the heart to the right, fluid-filled bowel within the chest, and absence of the stomach intra-abdominally.[77,264] As herniated liver has the same echotexture as the lung right-sided lesions are more difficult to detect, especially in the absence of polyhydramnios or pleural effusion. Clues include derangement in the normal intra-abdominal course of the gall bladder and intrahepatic vein, although small lesions may go undetected. The appearances of CCAM of the lung vary from solitary large cysts to solid echogenic lesions with the worst prognosis.[4,383] The assessment of prognosis is difficult, although in recent series it appears good, other than a small minority (6%) in which both mediastinal shift and hydrops are present.[21,353] Some disappear, many get smaller and only a few stay the same or progress. Diagnosis cannot always be certain antenatally, and differentiation between CCAM, sequestrated lung, tracheal or bronchial atresia and congenital diaphragmatic hernia may be difficult.[205,240] Mediastinal teratomas have features on ultrasound similar to solid type III or microcystic CCAM lesions.[354]

Gastrointestinal defects

Although oesophageal atresia can be diagnosed when polyhydramnios occurs with non-visualization of the fetal stomach, these signs are not present in the common form associated with tracheo-oesophageal fistula.[118] Duodenal atresia produces polyhydramnios and a characteristic 'double-bubble' appearance, which may not be apparent until the third trimester.[269] Associated anomalies are common in the above two conditions, unlike in more distal obstructions. Small bowel obstructions are more likely to be associated with increased amniotic fluid volume than are large bowel obstructions such as anal atresia, which may go undetected in utero. Peristalsis may be seen[16] and bowel perforations may show up as ascites or, more commonly, hyperechogenicity from meconium peritonitis.[43] Caution must be exercised when gut echogenicity is detected as an isolated finding, as although this may be associated with cystic fibrosis[261] and aneuploidy, it may also occur in normal fetuses.[117] Meconium peritonitis can also produce pseudocysts, the differential diagnosis of which includes gastrointestinal duplications and choledochal, mesenteric and ovarian cysts (pp. 743, 1091).

The distinction of omphalocoele from gastroschisis is crucial, given the high incidence of cardiac and chromosomal abnormalities in the former.[152] Omphalocoele is characterized on ultrasound by its intimate relation to the umbilical vessels and its covering of omphaloperitoneal membrane. Aneuploidy seems largely confined to fetuses in which the herniated liver is not present within the omphalocoele.[28,304] More severe degrees of failure of fusion of the ectomesodermic folds, such as ectopia cordis, ectopia vesicae, pentalogy of Cantrell and the body stalk anomaly, are readily apparent. The incidence of gastroschisis is increasing in the UK, although the underlying reasons have not been determined.[387] Management of these babies after birth is discussed on pages 787–789.

Genitourinary defects

Renal and urinary tract abnormalities are common and comparatively easy to detect, largely because obstructive lesions manifest as cystic spaces, whereas those with poor urine output are characterized by oligohydramnios. Major anomalies such as renal agenesis or low obstructive uropathy will be detected on routine scan at 18–20 weeks, when urine output makes a major contribution to amniotic fluid volume, whereas more minor lesions, such as mild ureteropelvic junction obstruction, may not be obvious until later. As the lack of amniotic fluid in renal agenesis significantly impairs the ultrasound picture, it can be extremely difficult to demonstrate the absence of kidneys in the renal fossae. In these circumstances, referral for confirmation by transvaginal ultrasound and/or amnioinfusion has been recommended.[130] However, colour flow Doppler imaging of the renal arteries may be adequate to provide the diagnosis: the absence of renal artery colour image confirms no functioning tissue.[368] Multicystic kidneys are distinguished from hydronephrotic kidneys by their cystic spaces being more peripheral and variable in size, and their stroma more central.[31] The cysts of infantile polycystic kidneys are too small to be resolved by ultrasound, but the kidneys appear enlarged with abnormal echogenicity, associated with oligohydramnios. Occasionally with later-onset infantile polycystic kidney disease the kidneys may appear normal in utero.[355] The significance of mild pelvicalyceal dilatation remains controversial. Recent studies show that progressive enlargement, or an anteroposterior diameter of $\geq$ 10 mm in the third trimester, is more likely to be associated with pathology.[310] The ultrasound picture in low obstructive uropathy depends on the severity and duration of obstruction. The bladder is variably enlarged and thick walled, and careful scanning reveals dilatation of the upper urethra in those with posterior urethral valves.[184] Oligohydramnios, upper tract dilatation and hyperechogenic fetal kidneys may also be present. The subsequent management of these babies after birth is described in Chapter 39, Part 2.

Skeletal defects

Isolated malformations detected on routine scanning include kyphoscoliosis, hemivertebrae, limb reductions, sacral agenesis, polydactyly and flexion deformities. In addition, over 100 distinct skeletal dysplasias are amenable to prenatal diagnosis, both by serial measurement of long bones and by detection of abnormal skeletal shape or mineralization. Although severe limb shortening, abnormal head or chest shape, or polyhydramnios may alert the sonologist to their presence, determination of the exact type of skeletal dysplasia is difficult in the absence of a previous history, and requires detailed evaluation of hands and feet, thoracic dimensions, face and cranium, and measurement of all the long bones, before consulting comprehensive tables of diagnostic features.[357] In achondrogenesis, thanatophoric and diastrophic dwarfism, severe limb reduction will be obvious by 18 weeks,[122] whereas in the heterozygous form of achondroplasia this may not be observed until almost the third trimester.[123] If achondroplasia is suspected, amniocentesis can be performed for DNA testing on fibroblasts to detect or exclude the FGR3 receptor mutation known to cause achondroplasia.[45] Abnormal bone shape is a feature of camptomelic and thanatophoric dysplasia, whereas fractures, callus formation and hypomineralization may be seen in osteogenesis imperfecta types II–IV.[53] Hypomineralization is also seen in hypophosphatasia and achondrogenesis. Radial aplasia may be associated with trisomy 18, but also with rare genetic syndromes such as Fanconi's anaemia and the TAR syndrome.

Soft tissue abnormalities

Cleft lip, whether isolated or associated with cleft palate, can be detected by imaging the fetal face in coronal and transverse views.[359] Rarer midline clefts are often accompanied by other midline defects, such as holoprosencephaly, ethmocephaly or proboscis. The diagnosis of isolated cleft palate is extremely difficult.[319] These lesions are usually only detected on detailed scans of patients who have either other abnormalities or an at-risk history.

Cystic hygromas are readily apparent as multiseptate thin-walled cystic lesions, found most commonly around the dorsolateral region of the neck.[76] As they result from obstruction of the jugulolymphatic channels,[14] hygromas frequently progress in utero to hydrops and fetal demise,[1] although spontaneous resolution is possible.[81] They have a strong association with aneuploidy (50–80%), and therefore karyotyping is advised.

Hydrops is obvious as generalized skin oedema with ascites, and in many cases there will also be pericardial and pleural effusions, placentomegaly and polyhydramnios.

Subtle markers of aneuploidy

With advances in ultrasound resolution, many structures not previously visualized, such as the digits, feet and soft tissues of the neck, can now be demonstrated. Accordingly, the minor malformations and abnormal postures characteristic of aneuploid neonates may be seen in utero. Postaxial polydactyly is found more frequently in trisomy 13 than 18, but ventricular septal defects are common in both.[425] Profile of the trisomy 18 fetus reveals micrognathia and a protuberant upper lip.[25] The hands remain clenched in trisomy 18, with characteristic overlapping of the fingers, and the typical rocker bottom and equinovarus deformity are found in the feet. The sonographic features of trisomy 21 are more elusive.

These may include increased nuchal thickness (first or second trimester), mild renal pelvic dilatation, hyperechogenic bowel, brachycephaly, and hypoplasia of the middle phalanx of the fifth finger (clinodactyly).

Choroid plexus cysts are detected in approximately 1% of mid-trimester scans as sonolucent areas within echogenic choroid.[78] Soon after their appearance was described[83] they were found to be associated with trisomy 18.[146,274] Controversy has centred on whether karyotyping should be offered routinely to all fetuses with CPCs. The size, laterality and shape of the cysts are not helpful in predicting aneuploidy.[254] Choroid plexus cysts are now believed to be benign structures which usually disappear by 22–24 weeks. It has been estimated that the risk of aneuploidy with cysts unassociated with other anomalies lies between 1:350 and 1:500,[29,309] but this takes no account of the a priori risk. Current opinion is that if there are isolated CPCs on detailed anomaly scan, the risk of trisomy 18 is increased only marginally (i.e. relative risk 1.5) over that from maternal age alone.[375]

Transvaginal ultrasound

The greater resolution provided by high-frequency transvaginal transducers for structures within their 6–7 cm focal zone is ideal for visualization of the first-trimester fetus. The falx, vertebral column, kidneys, bladder, fingers and toes can all be identified with experience by 12 weeks' gestation.[392] This technique can be used at fortnightly intervals from 9–10 weeks in women at high risk. An increasing number of anomalies have now been detected,[2,54] including NTDs, cystic hygromas and skeletal anomalies. Indeed, some have proposed early anomaly screening at this gestation.[50] However, caution in diagnosing or excluding anomalies in the first trimester seems prudent; for example, it should be noted that midgut herniation ('omphalocoele') is physiological until 11 weeks,[393] and the calvarium may appear normal at 12 weeks in fetuses subsequently shown to be anencephalic.[159]

Transvaginal ultrasound has also been used to assess the uterine cervix during pregnancy for the prediction of preterm labour. A short cervix (< 2 cm) and/or widening of the internal os may indicate a higher risk. The efficiency of these measurements as a screening test for preterm labour is currently under assessment.[332]

INVASIVE PROCEDURES

Samples of fetal tissues suitable for karyotyping, biochemical analysis and DNA studies are simply obtained by CVS and amniocentesis. In many cases the choice of procedure is left to the patient, based on her informed perception of the relative advantages and disadvantages of each. Fetal blood sampling, a technically more difficult procedure, is performed after 18–20 weeks' gestation, not just for antenatal diagnosis, but for therapy. Each invasive procedure is associated with a small chance of procedure-related loss. In general, therefore, invasive procedures are offered rather than recommended to parents, who, after appropriate counselling, should be given time to consider the various risks of the condition being tested for against those of the procedure.

Amniocentesis

Amniocentesis is the comonest invasive procedure for prenatal diagnosis. Most are done at 14–16 weeks' gestation, when the amniotic cavity contains 150–200 ml of fluid allowing 20 ml to be withdrawn with impunity. A 22 G needle is inserted transabdominally and guided to a pool under ultrasound control. Simultaneous ultrasound monitoring reduces the number of dry and bloody taps[98,356] and obviates the rare risk of severe fetal trauma. It has thus replaced the older technique of 'semi-blind' insertion following ultrasound identification of a pool. Transplacental insertions have been linked with an increased abortion rate[202,386] and should be avoided. Even with an extensive anterior placenta, a small window avoiding the placenta can usually be found.

Patients are quoted a risk of spontaneous abortion attributable to the procedure of 1%, based on the results of the only randomized controlled trial.[386] Of the three major collaborative case-control studies, the Medical Research Council[242] reported an increased risk of spontaneous abortion of 1.3%, whereas lower rates were found in the other two.[267,373] As with all invasive procedures operator experience seems the most important variable, significantly lower miscarriage rates being found for operators with experience of more than 50 procedures.[242,398] The increased risk of respiratory distress identified in the MRC study has not been confirmed,[189] and it is not clear to what extent this was due to prolonged oligohydramnios following amniotic fluid leakage. This issue has not been entirely resolved, given evidence in humans[401] and animals[182] that removal of amniotic fluid on a single occasion may impair respiratory development.

Amniotic fluid contains cells desquamated from fetal skin, gastrointestinal, urogenital and respiratory tracts, and the amnion. In view of their small number, up to 2 weeks' cell culture is required prior to cytogenetic analysis, although with new techniques this period is shortening. A major disadvantage of amniocentesis is that termination of affected fetuses is not performed until well into the mid-trimester. Amniotic fluid can be satisfactorily obtained and cultured at 11–13 weeks,[27,168] but the safety of the early procedure has been questioned by a randomized trial showing a greater miscarriage rate than with CVS.[287]

Approximately 0.5% of amniotic cell cultures fail to grow, and maternal cell contamination leads to diagnostic difficulty in <0.2%.[326,390] Level 2 mosaicism (multiple cells with the same abnormality in a single flask) occurs in 0.7% of amniocenteses, and level 3 (multiple cells with the same abnormality in multiple flasks) in 0.2%,[55,187,426] but these are confirmed in the fetus in only 20 and 60% of cases, respectively.

Later in pregnancy amniocentesis is used in the assessment of haemolytic disease[417] and fetal pulmonary maturity, although improvements in neonatal care and early ultrasound dating have led to a considerable reduction in the latter indication.[195] In preterm premature rupture of the membranes, amniocentesis for bacteriological analysis of amniotic fluid has not attained general usage in view of concerns regarding the frequency of low-virulence microorganisms.[127] Amniocentesis is also used for infusing fluid (amnioinfusion) to visualize fetal anatomy in oligohydramnios, and for draining fluid (amnioreduction) in polyhydramnios secondary to structural problems or fetofetal transfusion syndrome.[130,132]

Chorionic villus sampling

Although obtaining chorionic tissue suitable for cytogenetic and biochemical analysis was first reported 30 years ago,[249] CVS was only introduced into clinical practice in the mid-1980s. CVS was originally performed transcervically, but is now commonly performed transabdominally. Not only do operators who perform other transabdominal procedures prefer this, but also it allows samples to be obtained in the second and third trimesters. Furthermore, it may reduce the chance of infection. Safety is at least comparable or better with the transabdominal route.[194,374] Initially CVS was performed between 8 and 12 weeks. However, concern was raised following a report of limb reduction defects, some in association with the oromandibular syndrome.[125,126] In all cases CVS was performed before 66 days' gestation, and by single-needle transabdominal aspiration. Subsequent population and case-control studies have been unable to confirm any link,[144] but theoretically it seens plausible that a procedure which may cause embolism, thrombosis or vasoconstriction at the time of limb bud formation, may be the cause of such malformations. Thus, it has been recommended that CVS is performed after 10 weeks' gestation.[210,343] In many centres the popularity of CVS declined after these reports, but now with the potential to test chorion villi for genetic syndromes together with first-trimester aneuploidy screening, the numbers of CVSs performed are again increasing.

Rapid cytogenetic results may be obtained from spontaneous mitoses in direct preparations from the chorionic villus cells[371] or after short-term culture for 12–24 hours. Long-term culture, of up to 2–3 weeks, ensures specimens of sufficient quality for banding studies, but may be complicated by maternal cell contamination in 10% of cases[372] and the possibility of culture artefact. Reports of false negative results on direct analysis[64,106] suggest that long-term culture provides a more accurate reflection of fetal karyotype. Most centres therefore perform both short and long-term cultures on each specimen. Culture is not needed for most of the enzyme deficiencies underlying inborn errors of metabolism, which can be assayed directly in villi. Villi are also an excellent source of DNA for molecular analysis. Results from CVS are thus available sooner than after amniocentesis, allowing women with abnormal results in the first trimester to undergo termination of pregnancy by suction curettage, which is both safer and less emotionally traumatic than second-trimester termination by either prostaglandin induction or dilatation and evacuation.

The CVS-related rate of fetal loss before 28 weeks above the background rate is 1–2% in centres with much experience.[287] One problem with CVS is a 1.0–1.5% incidence[52,64,220] of confined placental or pseudomosaicism,[198] where a discrepancy exists between chorionic and fetal karyotypes, necessitating further investigation by amniocentesis.[247] In most cases a bizarre aneuploid or polyploid mosaic is identified in the chorion, whereas the fetal karyotype, assessed from skin fibroblasts, is normal. Mosaicism confined to the placenta does not affect the fetal outcome, and this should be suspected when the direct preparation shows a few isolated abnormal cells. In this situation the cultured cell line result should be awaited, as this will usually be normal as the cells are obtained from the trophoblast and are more representative of the fetus. If the culture still shows mosaicism then an amniocentesis and a detailed anomaly scan are required. An amniocentesis cultures fibroblasts which truly represent the fetus, as they are sloughed skin cells.

Fetal blood sampling

Early attempts at fetal blood sampling via placentesis[200] were abandoned because of high fetal mortality and low success rates. Fetoscopy was the first satisfactory method of obtaining pure samples of fetal blood, from either chorionic plate vessels[183] or the umbilical cord.[344] There are now very few remaining indications for fetoscopy which, for FBS, has been replaced by the simpler and safer technique of direct ultrasound-guided needling of various fetal vessels. This is done as an outpatient procedure under local anaesthesia from 17 weeks' gestation. Sedation is rarely necessary. The most common approach, which involves inserting a 20 G needle transabdominally into the umbilical vein about 1 cm from the placental cord insertion,[88] yields an adequate sample in 97% of cases.[89] For anterior placentae the route is transplacental; for posterior, transamniotic. Maternal contamination from inadvertent intervillus sampling is ruled out before removal of the needle by comparing the sample's MCV distribution, determined rapidly on a

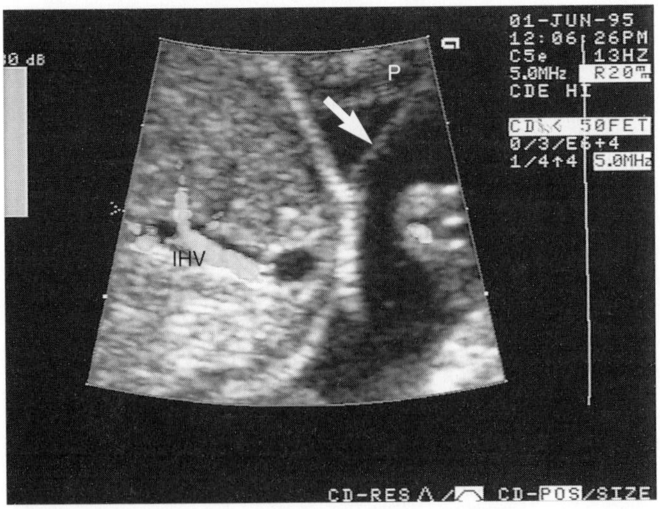

Fig. 14.2 Ultrasound view of needle (arrow) positioned within the intrahepatic vein for fetal blood sampling. IHV, intrahepatic vein; P, placenta.

particle size analyser, to that of the mother.[342] Even at term fetal MCV, which declines rapidly with gestation, remains significantly higher than that of healthy mothers.[131] The vein is the usual vessel sampled, being simpler and safer;[407] accidental sampling of the artery can be confirmed by ultrasonic observation of the direction of flow following injection of 200 μl of sterile saline.[275] When there is difficulty approaching the cord insertion because of obesity, oligo- or polyhydramnios, or fetal position, blood may be aspirated from the intrahepatic portion of the fetal umbilical vein (Fig. 14.2), as it may also after a failed attempt at the cord insertion.[209,289] Although FBS from the intrahepatic vein is more difficult than at the cord insertion, it obviates the need for laboratory confirmation of its source, and in multiple pregnancies the operator is certain as to which fetus is sampled. Alternative sites of sampling include a free loop of cord and the fetal heart.[18] Assessment of fetal loss rates from the last two methods is difficult to obtain as they are infrequently performed; the fetal loss rate after intrahepatic vein sampling may be as high as 6.2%, and 5% following intracardiac sampling, but these fetuses are often hydropic.

FBS was initially developed for the prenatal diagnosis of hereditary disease, particularly the haemoglobinopathies and haemophilias. These, however, are now done by DNA analysis on chorion villi or amniocytes. Standard cytogenetic and DNA studies may be done on fetal blood, and are especially useful when the mother presents too late for amniocentesis or CVS, or when these tests fail. As is evident from Table 14.1, FBS has also been used for assessment of fetal acid–base status in the latter half of pregnancy, but this information can now be inferred from non-invasive Doppler studies.[298] The main indications for FBS are now rapid karyotyping and assessment of potential anaemia or thrombocytopenia.

Table 14.1 Indications for fetal blood sampling

Prenatal diagnosis
Cytogenetic studies
late bookers, failed amniocentesis, mosaicism in chorion or amniotic fluid, ultrasound suspicion of aneuploidy
Genetic disease amenable to DNA diagnosis
late bookers, failed amniocentesis or CVS
Fetal assessment
Fetal malformations
karyotype, acid–base status
IUGR/fetal compromise
karyotype, acid–base status
Red cell alloimmunization
haematocrit, haemoglobin, Rh and Kell typing, acid–base status, transfusion
Hydrops fetalis
karyotype, haematology, virology, acid–base status, transfusion
Viral infections
specific: PCR, IgM, electron microscopy, inoculation
non-specific: platelets, liver function
Immune thrombocytopenic purpuras
platelet counts, antibody levels, PLA status, platelet transfusion
Poly-/oligohydramnios
karyotype, acid–base status, pressure measurement
Fetofetal transfusion syndrome
haemoglobins, acid–base, ?selective feticide

Determining the loss rate attributable to FBS is difficult, as fetal demise in the weeks after the procedure may instead be due to the underlying high-risk indication. This was clearly demonstrated in one series, which showed increased loss rates in procedures performed on sicker fetuses, i.e. prenatal diagnosis (2%), fetal structural abnormality (6%), assessment of severe IUGR (14%), and hydrops (25%).[238] Daffos et al[89] reported seven losses (1.2%) in 562 continuing pregnancies sampled predominantly for toxoplasmosis, and another group had losses in 0.9% of 469 continuing pregnancies sampled for prenatal diagnosis or karyotyping of minor malformations.[284] Many of these, however, were greater than 21 weeks, and loss rates seem higher earlier in gestation.[46,308] A reported summation of all the reported series shows an overall loss rate in procedures performed in low-risk cases of 2.7%,[151] although others more recently have reported a lower loss rate of 0.9%,[412] and this figure has been corroborated by the USA international registry (A Ludomirsky, personal communication). Such results are only achieved after considerable training and experience. Most losses are due to cord haematoma, cord tamponade or haemorrhage and, unlike losses after CVS or amniocentesis, are apparent at the time of the procedure. In late pregnancy emergency caesarean section is performed to salvage these infants, although some may be damaged. Intra-amniotic bleeding is observed ultrasonically after 40% of samplings,[89,407] and a histological study of cords within 48 hours of FBS showed that a degree of extravasation occurs in all cases.[196] This bleeding is almost always transient, owing to the abundance of thromboplastins in amniotic fluid.[270] Following intrahepatic vein FBS any bleeding is into the fetal peritoneal cavity, where it is reabsorbed within days.[298] Liver function is unaltered by intrahepatic vein FBS.[299] Cord tamponade caused by extravasation of transfused blood[366] and bradycardia due to vasospasm after arterial sampling[407] are rare complications of FBS at the placental cord insertion, which cannot occur with intrahepatic vein FBS because of the vein's lack of surrounding cord or arteries.[289] It may be that intrahepatic vein sampling is more appropriate in FBS for growth-retarded fetuses, which are more prone to bradycardia.[333]

Liver biopsy

In a small number of inborn errors of metabolism, such as the urea cycle disorders, the affected protein is not expressed in cultured fibroblasts and fetal liver may be the only tissue suitable for assay. Unlike in infancy, demonstration of abnormal metabolite accumulation is not possible in utero as these are rapidly cleared across the placenta. Fetal liver biopsy was first reported using fetoscopy,[348] and was then performed via an ultrasound-guided approach using a double-cannula aspiration technique at 17–19 weeks, with light-microscopic confirmation of the sample's hepatic source. To date, liver biopsy has been used in the prenatal diagnosis of four conditions: ornithine carbamyl transferase deficiency,[348] carbamyl phosphate synthetase deficiency,[318] glucose-6-phosphatase deficiency or Von Gierke's disease,[157] and primary hyperoxaluria.[94] However, because most of these defects are now known to be the result of a single gene defect, the diagnosis can instead be made from DNA analysis of chorion villi, so that liver biopsy is seldom required.

Skin biopsy

Prenatal diagnosis of many severe genodermatoses necessitates histological and ultrastructural examination of fetal skin, obtained at 18–22 weeks, initially by fetoscopy[345] but more recently by ultrasound-guided techniques.[19] The usual site chosen is the fetal buttock or leg. Epidermolysis bullosa letalis is characterized by separation of the epidermis from dermis at the lamina lucida on light microscopy, and a paucity of hemidesmosomes on electron microscopy.[345] The prenatal diagnostic features of epidermolysis bullosa dystrophica,[15] epidermolytic hyperkeratosis,[156] harlequin ichthyosis[108] and Sjögren–Larsson syndrome[212] have similarly been described. In oculocutaneous albinism, in which there is a lack of active melanin synthesis in hair bulb melanocytes, the biopsy must be taken from a hair-bearing area such as the scalp or an eyebrow.[105] The biopsy site is not detectable at birth, and in a series of 52 skin biopsies there were no procedure-related losses (Rodeck, unpublished observations). These disorders are increasingly being diagnosed by DNA technology.[241]

SCREENING STRATEGIES FOR DOWN SYNDROME

In the past, standard screening policy was to offer women over the age of 35 CVS or amniocentesis for karyotyping. As only 25–30% of trisomy 21 fetuses are born to 'older' mothers, and as utilization in this group rarely exceeds 50%, it is hardly surprising that the birth prevalence of Down syndrome only fell by 15% with this strategy.[406] Newer policies, which increase detection rates without increasing the numbers undergoing antenatal karyotyping, have been introduced into practice. The extent of Down syndrome screening in the UK in 1994 has been summarized.[405] All Scottish health boards offer multiple serum screening, but only 56% do so in England and Wales. In the others, 23% screen by maternal age alone and 21% by nuchal translucency.

Biochemical

The average maternal serum AFP value in Down pregnancies is 0.7–0.8 multiples of the median.[403] As this association is largely independent of maternal age, the two were then combined to give each woman a specific age- and AFP-adjusted risk.[87] Subsequently, raised hCG,[44] particularly the free β-hCG subunit, and low unconjugated oestriol[68] levels were found to be associated with trisomy 21. Again, in the absence of any relation to maternal age or each other, their levels and maternal age were next combined using an algorithm to predict fetal risk.[404] The reason for these biochemical changes is not yet understood, but is thought to relate to functional immaturity, producing a delay in the normal gestational rise or fall. Cutoffs of 1:250–1:300 have shown a sensitivity of up to 70%, with a false positive rate of 5%. Subsequent refinements using free-β-hCG[379] and a prior dating scan,[150] and confining the assay to 15–18 weeks' gestation, have increased the accuracy of the test. There continues to be controversy as to whether the double test (AFP + free-β-hCG) is more cost-effective than the triple test (AFP, hCG and oestriol) in large cumulative series for each strategy.[203,379] One thing that has been shown with serum screening is that detection rates are greater in older mothers (i.e. over 35), but this is at the cost of higher false positive rates.[166]

As biochemical screening takes place in the mid-trimester it does not allow susceptible women the option of first-trimester CVS for karyotyping. The drive now is to bring screening for aneuploidy into the first and early second trimester, to allow safer termination procedures to be performed. Hopefully the psychological effect of early diagnosis, and the privacy that this allows, will be improved. Two hormones may be useful for screening in the first trimester (10–13 weeks), as maternal serum pregnancy-associated plasma protein-A is reduced and free-β-hCG is raised in trisomy 21.[51]

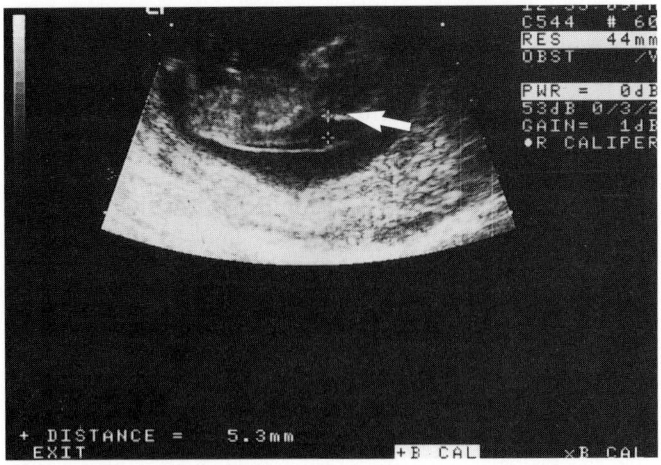

Fig. 14.3 Transabdominal ultrasound view of increased nuchal translucency in a fetus at 11 weeks' gestation.

Ultrasound

There have been major advances in ultrasound screening for aneuploidy. Initially second-trimester markers were identified in association with various trisomies, including choroid plexus cysts, echogenic bowel, renal pelvic dilatation and increased nuchal thickness. Women carrying fetuses with soft tissue markers of aneuploidy were informed of the increased risk and offered karyotyping. Increasingly, the risks of aneuploidy from these markers is being defined, particularly in relation to maternal age,[375] thus allowing more accurate information to be provided. The interpretation of soft markers is complex. Risk tables now exist, such that most centres use some form of computer program for risk adjustment based on maternal age and single or multiple markers/anomalies, as well as type of marker or anomaly.

The association between increased nuchal translucency in the first trimester (10–14 weeks) and aneuploidy has been confirmed in several studies[215,288,385] (Fig. 14.3). The association is with trisomies 21, 18 and 13 in particular. A test sensitivity, when related to crown–rump length and maternal age, of 80% with a false positive of 5% has been reported by one group in a low-risk population cohort of 20 000,[376] and these figures have been maintained as the recruitment rate has reached 60 000 (K. Nicolaides, personal communication). Other reports have not been so impressive, so that the feasibility and accuracy of NT as a method of population screening is still being assessed. Anxiety has been raised about the reproducibility of NT measurement,[337] and also that the majority of fetuses so detected miscarry spontaneously rather than continue to term.[39]

Other advantages of early ultrasound for screening include early diagnosis of pregnancy failure, better dating, detection of other abnormalities and, in multiple pregnancy, accurate determination of chorionicity. Test sensitivity may potentially be increased by incorporating free-β-hCG and/or PAPP-A measurement into the calculation,[303] and further evaluation of these tests is under way. CVS seems the most appropriate invasive test for those considered at high risk. Finally, those fetuses with an increased NT and normal karyotype are still at risk for cardiac[191] or syndromal defects,[190] and therefore follow-up of euploid nuchal translucency-positive fetuses is still recommended.

DETECTION OF SINGLE-GENE DISORDERS BY DNA ANALYSIS

Although DNA analysis for prenatal diagnosis was first used on amniotic cells,[199] it was its application to chorionic villi[307] that precipitated the recent expansion in DNA diagnoses in the first trimester. With the rapid progress being made in mapping disease-specific gene loci, the list of amenable conditions has increased exponentially such that advice should be sought with each new request for prenatal diagnosis. The molecular basis of virtually all the common monogenic diseases is now known, and in some cases, such as cystic fibrosis, population screening of prospective parents is a reality.

Direct oligonucleotide probes are suitable for the majority of conditions nowadays, where the particular point mutation or deletion characterizing the disease at the molecular level is known. Examples include sickle cell disease, α-thalassaemia and 21-hydroxylase deficiency. In rare cases in which the exact mutation is not yet known, indirect gene tracking is required using a series of informative intra- or extragenic markers around relevant loci, known as restriction fragment length polymorphisms. As this latter approach requires lengthy family studies, including analysis of DNA from a previously affected child, suitability for prenatal diagnosis is best assessed before conception. Recombination is a problem with indirect methods, the exact rate depending on the proximity of the markers used to the disease locus. Genetic heterogeneity and non-paternity are additional sources of error.

Prenatal diagnosis of late-onset autosomal dominant diseases such as Huntington's chorea and polycystic kidney disease poses counselling difficulties. A currently healthy parent with a 50% risk of having inherited the mutation may request prenatal diagnosis without wishing to know their own genetic status.

The polymerase chain reaction, in which target sequences are exponentially amplified from tiny amounts of DNA (p. 152), has several implications for prenatal diagnosis. First, results are available more rapidly and can be obtained on amniotic cells without culture. This has enabled prenatal typing of the Rh D, c, E, Kell and platelet type in the fetus who may be at risk for isoimmunization, early on in pregnancy without waiting for FBS.[30] For those fetuses not at risk, monitoring, both invasive and non-invasive, can be decreased or stopped. Secondly, DNA can be obtained for RFLP status from the Guthrie card of a deceased sibling.[420] Third, preimplantation diagnosis after in vitro fertilization seems feasible, and in this regard prenatal diagnosis of human embryos from a single cell biopsied at the 8-cell stage can be performed.[167]

MINIMALLY INVASIVE PRENATAL DIAGNOSIS

Currently all methods for fetal karyotyping or genotyping require invasive procedures to collect fetal cells and DNA. Amniocentesis, CVS and fetal blood sampling are each associated with a risk of fetal morbidity and mortality, and therefore a less invasive method of collecting such material would be welcomed. Two sources for the non-invasive isolation of fetal material have been investigated, namely cervical samples and maternal blood.

Enrichment of fetal cells in the maternal circulation

A variety of nucleated fetal cells have been demonstrated in the maternal circulation, including lymphocytes, erythrocytes and trophoblasts. Because the ratio of fetal to maternal nucleated cells is only $1{:}1 \times 10^{5-8}$ sorting procedures are needed to enrich sufficient cells for diagnosis.[323] Trophoblast cells are not ideal for several reasons. They are covered by a mucoprotein coat, making them difficult to enrich;[260] they have an extraembryonic origin, and thus placental mosaicism may confound the diagnosis; and finally many of the cells will be multinucleate, making chromosomal analysis by fluorescent in situ hybridization not possible. Lymphocytes have been enriched with variable accuracy by means of HLA antibody labelling, but have the disadvantages of requiring pre-enrichment paternal HLA typing, and persistence of lymphocytes from previous pregnancies can occur.[40] Nucleated red blood cells seem best suited for non-invasive prenatal diagnosis because (i) they are the predominant type of nucleated cells in early fetal blood; (ii) they are present in only minimal quantities in adult blood; and (iii) their restricted lifespan means they do not persist from previous pregnancies.

The first unequivocal demonstrations of fetal cells within the maternal circulation were independently reported in the early 1990s by three groups, two in the USA and one in Europe. Each identified and enriched nucleated RBC by monoclonal antibodies against the transferrin receptor and/or glycophorin A and performed FISH for genetic analysis. The two forms of sorting that can be used are fluorescence-activated cell sorting, and magnetically activated cell sorting. Male cells and fetal trisomies have been identified with specific probes.[149,323]

MACS has a number of advantages over FACS for cell sorting in that it is easier to operate, it is faster to perform, and finally it is much cheaper, requiring no expensive equipment. Nevertheless, this process is very labour intensive and thus the search is on for better sorting and cell identification techniques. Fetal DNA from unsorted maternal blood has been identified as early as 5 weeks,[391] and in a very limited series this has been used to predict fetal Rh type[226] and fetal gender.[227] However, this technique is only applicable to paternally derived autosomal dominant conditions, and therefore not to the majority of disorders.

Cervical sampling

One source for minimally invasive harvesting of fetal cells under evaluation is trophoblast cells shed into the uterine cervix. Despite a promising report that male DNA in cervical swabs successfully predicted fetal sex in 25 of 26 pregnancies,[163] experience with this technique has largely been limited to small series, with most workers unable to reproduce such accuracy. Fetal material undoubtedly can be sampled, but in only approximately 50% of cases,[3] and a recent report suggests it may be unreliable.[311] Both endocervical swabs and flushes have been used to collect the samples, and the cells have been analysed by FISH and/or PCR. Such a technique for prenatal diagnosis shares many of the problems of trophoblasts in the maternal circulation, and has other disadvantages, such as contamination by sperm DNA in the lower genital tract, and that vigorous sampling may indeed make it more an invasive rather than a non-invasive technique. A final assessment of the usefulness of this technique awaits further studies.

INBORN ERRORS OF METABOLISM

Since the first report of prenatal diagnosis by biochemical analysis of cultured amniotic fluid cells,[145] most of the 200 or so inborn errors of metabolism in which the enzymatic defect is known became amenable to biochemical detection in utero. The standard technique involved enzymatic analysis of fibroblasts from chorion villi or cultured amniotic fluid cells. However, the molecular basis of many of these diseases has now been identified, so that DNA analysis of chorion villi is now preferred.

FETAL PHYSIOLOGY

Our understanding of fetal physiology has for years been based on indirect sources. Observations in preterm neonates were first assumed to apply to the fetus of comparable gestation, and then extrapolated back to the mid-trimester. Non-invasive techniques such as cardiotocography, ultrasound and Doppler have provided

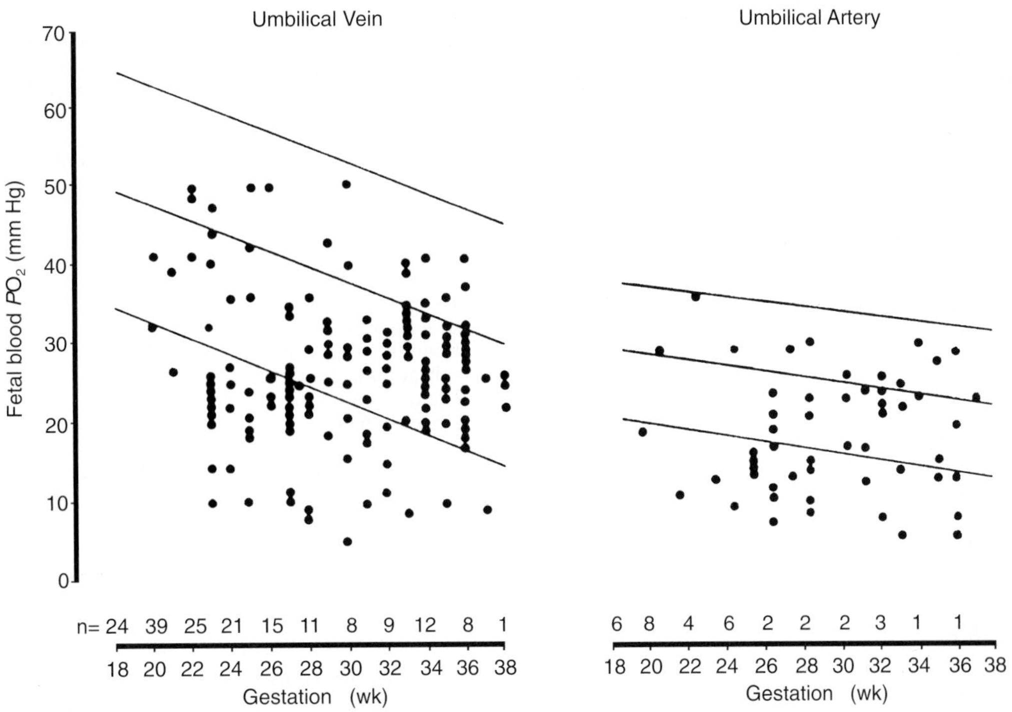

Fig. 14.4 Reference range (mean and 95% data intervals) for PO_2 in umbilical venous and arterial blood throughout gestation. (Reproduced with permission from Nicolaides et al[283])

information on fetal circulation, growth and behaviour. Amniotic fluid, being largely dependent on fetal urination, has been the traditional source for information about fetal biochemistry and endocrinology.[92] Access to the fetal circulation in the 1980s allowed fetal haematology and biochemistry to be evaluated directly in utero. Knowledge of normal values in the mid-trimester fetus is essential in the prenatal diagnosis of several fetal diseases and forms the basis for more effective treatment of maternal allo-immunization, better management of growth retardation, and is a prerequisite for other diagnostic and therapeutic approaches in the fetus. The main topics of clinical interest are summarized below, although more detailed listings are available elsewhere.[351]

HAEMATOLOGY

Haemoglobin, PCV and red cell mass increase, while MCV, reticulocytes and nucleated RBC decrease significantly with gestation,[140,248] reflecting the increase in fetal haemopoietic tissue, and the progressive change from hepatic to myeloid erythropoiesis. The normal range for haemoglobin increases from 9–13 g/dl at 17 weeks to 13–18 g/dl at term,[280] and haematocrit from 29–42% to 35–48% at 30 weeks.[140] The myeloid series does not change with gestation, nor do platelets, which normally exceed 150 × 10^9/l. Normal ranges are available for coagulation factors, which are reduced compared to the adult.[245]

ACID–BASE BALANCE

In normal pregnancies pH changes with gestational age, and ranges in the umbilical vein from 7.32 to 7.44. On the other hand, PO_2 decreases with gestational age, whereas PCO_2 and bicarbonate rise. The decrease in fetal PO_2 is compensated for by the rise in fetal haemoglobin, so that total oxygen content remains unchanged at 6–7 mmol/l. Normal ranges have been established for both umbilical venous and arterial samples[283] (Fig. 14.4).

CARDIOVASCULAR PHYSIOLOGY

Mean umbilical venous pressure is 4–5 mmHg between 20 and 33 weeks' gestation.[293] Blood volume has been measured in vivo, on the basis of the change in fetal haematocrit produced by transfusion of a known quantity of red cells. Fetoplacental blood volume rises from 25 ml at 18 weeks to 150 ml at 31 weeks, but during the same interval it decreases when expressed as a function of fetal weight from 117 to 93 ml/kg.[278]

BIOCHEMISTRY

Reference ranges are available for electrolytes and biochemical indices of renal, hepatic and bone function.[141,252] Fetal sodium and potassium are the same as maternal levels. Fetal glucose levels are lower than in the mother, and their maternofetal gradients have been used as an index of placental transfer.[294] Bilirubin is three times higher in the mid-trimester fetus than in the mother, but albumin levels are considerably lower, with values rising from 16 g/l at 15 weeks to 40 g/l at term.[252]

RENAL FUNCTION

Urea and creatinine levels in utero reflect the excretory function of the placenta and not that of the kidneys. Urinary sodium and phosphate decrease and creatinine increases with gestational age, consistent with progressive maturation of tubular function and an increase in glomerular filtration rate. Potassium and urea, however, do not change, suggesting that the changes in tubular reabsorption occur simultaneously with those in tubular secretion and glomerular filtration. Reference ranges related to gestation are used in the assessment of renal function in fetuses with obstructive uropathies.[302]

Table 14.2 Reported frequencies of chromosomal and other structural abnormalities in fetuses with malformations detected in utero. The risk of aneuploidy will be lower if the malformation is isolated, and for the softer markers the risk will vary with maternal age

Condition	Aneuploidy (%)	Structural malformations (%)
Hydrocephalus	10–15	30–60
Cystic hygroma	45–80	15–65
Non-immune hydrops	3–15	25
Cleft lip/palate	<1	15–50
Congenital heart disease	25–30	10–20
Diaphragmatic hernia	20–30	17–55
Tracheo-oesophageal fistula	15	50–60
Duodenal atresia	30–35	50–70
Exomphalos	50–65	60–75
Multicystic kidney	5–10	12–40
PUJ obstruction	1–2	20–27
Posterior urethral valves	6–24	25–40
Single umbilical artery	<1	20–45

FETAL MEDICINE

With the combination of ultrasound and invasive procedures several conditions can be managed more rationally than in the past, such as congenital malformations, maternal exposure to infectious agents, and IUGR. In others the fetus can be treated; intravascular transfusion has greatly improved the survival of alloimmunized fetuses, making it thus far the best model for fetal therapy.

NON-LETHAL MALFORMATIONS

Rapid karyotyping

Table 14.2 lists the risks of chromosomal and other structural malformations associated with common non-lethal congenital malformations. These are considerably higher for anomalies detected in utero than at birth. For example, in the literature the risk of an abnormal karyotype for infants with congenital heart disease is 5–10% and for exomphalos 10%, compared to risks of 32% and 66%, respectively, from antenatal studies.[84,274] Multiple malformations carry a 10 times higher risk of aneuploidy than isolated malformations.[375] The demonstration of any fetal anomaly on ultrasound therefore prompts a detailed search for other abnormalities. Rapid karyotyping by FBS, or transabdominal CVS is offered. This is recommended not only in the mid-trimester to allow termination of aneuploid pregnancies, but also in the third trimester, where knowledge of a serious chromosomal defect may alter antenatal and intrapartum management, including mode of delivery. Furthermore, termination of pregnancy after 24 weeks' gestation is legal in the UK if there is a substantial risk that the fetus has an abnormality that would result in the birth of a child with a serious handicap. Karyotyping should also be performed for conditions where the risk of intrauterine death is high, such as hydrops, because postmortem autolysis may jeopardize subsequent chromosomal studies and thus future genetic counselling. Indeed, post-mortem karyotyping following termination for fetal abnormality has a 27% failure rate, and therefore pretermination sampling is advised.[214] An association has been reported between fetal macrocytosis and chromosome abnormalities in the mid-trimester, especially triploidy.[131]

Management

The option of termination of pregnancy is offered for severe malformations and support given to those who wish to continue through to delivery despite a poor prognosis. Other malformations are suitable for early postnatal correction, such as certain cardiac defects, duodenal atresia and gastroschisis. Intrauterine surgery may have a role in a few situations, but less so than was originally hoped. The significance of antenatal detection of some conditions, such as PUJ obstruction or multicystic kidney, is not so much the alteration of perinatal management as the initiation of timely investigation and follow-up in infancy.

The worse prognosis for abnormalities diagnosed in utero rather than neonatally largely reflects the increased risks of aneuploidy, multiple malformations and intrauterine death. Whereas cystic hygroma at birth carries an excellent prognosis following surgical correction, the same lesion detected in utero leads to survival in less than 5%.[1,217] This high loss rate, which applies equally to euploid fetuses, reflects the frequency of hydrops and hypoxaemia in this condition.[388]

INTRAUTERINE GROWTH RETARDATION

Rapid karyotyping

The chance of a fetal chromosome abnormality in IUGR is as high as 6–16%,[116,284,299] although this risk is based on series of referred patients in which severe IUGR, often with oligohydramnios and malformations, was the indication for rapid karyoptyping. With severe IUGR and no structural malformations the risk is lower, 2–3%.[375] Clearly, the risk of aneuploidy remains remote in the milder forms of IUGR, which complicates 5–10% of all pregnancies in the late third trimester. Rapid karyotyping warrants consideration in severe IUGR, when associated with fetal malformations, or when diagnosed before 34 weeks.

Acid–base balance

During the 1980s, given the inaccuracy of conventional tests of fetal well-being, FBS was recommended in IUGR for fetal blood gas and acid–base determination.[276] Many data consequently exist on the biochemical status of fetuses with severe IUGR, indicating that many are hypercapnic, hyperlacticacidaemic, hypoglycaemic and hypoinsulinaemic, and have erythroblastosis, impaired placental transfer, and disturbed lipid and protein metabolism.[284,294,377] In view of these chronic and complex compensatory mechanisms, it seems unlikely that a single measurement of pH or PO_2 could accurately predict the stage at which decompensation occurs. In a series of 32 IUGR fetuses with absent end-diastolic flow velocity in the umbilical artery, we found that no measurement obtained at FBS was predictive of perinatal outcome, with similar pH, PO_2, PCO_2 and base excess levels in both survivors and perinatal deaths.[299] Thus the role of FBS in IUGR is the determination of karyotype rather than of acid–base status, so that unnecessary intervention can be avoided in non-viable fetuses.

Doppler ultrasound

Umbilical artery Doppler waveforms have been shown to discriminate between IUGR fetuses at high or low risk of perinatal death.[9,56] In particular, absent EDFV is associated with adverse perinatal outcome.[330,341] Although acidaemia and hypoxaemia are unlikely in the presence of EDFV, 45–80% of fetuses with absent EDFV are acidaemic (pH<7.31) and 79–100% hypoxaemic.[281,299] However, absent EDFV[341] and acidaemia/hypoxaemia[299] may persist for up to 5 weeks before fetal demise, rendering them too sensitive for use as indicators for preterm delivery. With knowledge of the fetal compensatory response to hypoxia by redistribution of blood flow, pulsed Doppler investigation of the involved fetal vessels provides more information about fetal condition. Redistribution of blood flow away from the kidneys, gut and skin towards the brain, adrenals and heart, can be demonstrated by increased flow velocity within the middle cerebral artery, and decreased flow velocity within the descending aorta. Alterations in the venous circulatory system may represent an end-stage response with cardiac decompensation, which can be measured at the level of the ductus venosus.[178] Increased pulsatility and reversed velocity at the time of atrial contraction may be found. Timing of delivery is currently based on combining Doppler studies with growth velocity, amniotic fluid levels and cardiotocography, although the accuracy of assessment of fetal condition warrants much further research.

RED CELL ALLOIMMUNIZATION

Despite a dramatic decline in incidence, maternal sensitization has not disappeared, for a variety of reasons, including antenatal sensitization, prophylaxis failure and antibodies other than anti-D. Untreated, 45–50% of affected infants will have no or only mild anaemia, and 25–30% moderate anaemia posing neonatal problems only. The remaining 20–25% develop hydrops and usually die in utero or neonatally; in half, the hydrops develops prior to 30 weeks.[49] The aim of antenatal management is to identify severely affected fetuses, to correct their anaemia by transfusion, and then deliver them at the optimal time. At each gestational age the risks of invasive monitoring are weighed against those of conservative management and delivery.

Antenatal screening

Routine serological testing of women is carried out:

- to identify pregnancies at risk of fetal and neonatal alloimmune disease (HDN);
- to identify RhD-negative women who require antenatal anti-D prophylaxis;
- to provide compatible blood swiftly in emergencies.

All women who have no antibodies at 10–16 weeks' gestation should be tested once again between 28 and 36 weeks. Some workers believe that RhD-negative women should have two tests, one at 28 weeks and one at 34–36 weeks, but sensitization late in pregnancy is unlikely to result in HDN requiring treatment.

Prophylaxis

Rhesus-negative women are at risk of sensitization from fetomaternal bleeding, not only at delivery but also in other situations, such as external cephalic version and

Table 14.3 Indications for giving anti-D immunoglobulin during pregnancy in rhesus-negative women

Abortion
Therapeutic termination
Spontaneous abortion and instrumentation
Spontaneous complete abortion >12 weeks
Threatened abortion >12 weeks
Repeat every 6 weeks if intermittent bleeding
Threatened abortion <12 weeks
Determine woman's RhD type
Anti-D immunoglobulin within 96 h if RhD negative
Episodes/procedures associated with FMH
Ectopic pregnancy
Chorionic villus sampling
Amniocentesis
Antepartum haemorrhage
External cephalic version
Falls and abdominal trauma
Dose
Before 20 weeks' gestation: 250 IU
After 20 weeks' gestation: 500 IU
+ Kleihauer test or other test to estimate volume of FMH (e.g. flow cytometry)

FMH, fetomaternal haemorrhage

amniocentesis. Table 14.3 gives a list of the current indications when anti-D immunoglobulin should be administered to rhesus-negative women. These are taken from the UK guidelines last updated in 1991.[266] Although the prevention programme has reduced neonatal deaths attributable to haemolytic disease of the newborn from 18.4/100 000 in 1977 to 1.3/100 000 in 1992, there remains a sensitization rate of around 1% among rhesus-negative women. A recent audit of the UK recommendations was carried out in Liverpool.[186] The results showed that although 95% of women received appropriate postnatal prophylaxis there were omissions in the antenatal treatment. In particular, the purpose of the Kleihauer test was ill understood, with a negative result often being interpreted as a reason not to give anti-D immunoglobulin. This test is meant to be used in conjunction with routine prophylaxis to ensure that sufficient anti-D is given. In addition to the indications in Table 14.3, the Royal College of Obstetricians and Gynaecologists supports routine antenatal prophylaxis, either a dose of 500 IU at 28 and 34 weeks, or a single larger dose early in the third trimester.[358] The rationale for this is that all rhesus-negative women are at risk from hidden bleeds. Where anti-D immunoglobulin is in short supply, primigravidae should have priority.

Assessment of severity

The detection of anti-D antibodies in the maternal circulation, or the delivery of a previously affected infant, alerts the clinician to a possible problem. Of more significance is whether the antibody level is rising, and therefore 2–4 weekly blood level measurements are required. In addition, the zygosity of the father and

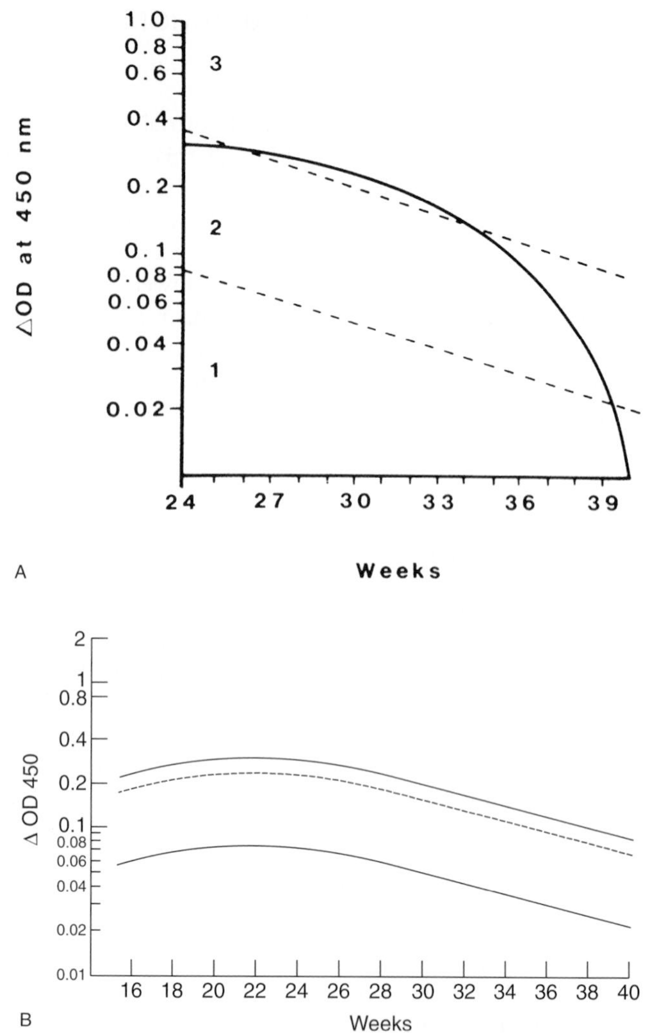

Fig. 14.5 Bilirubin is measured in liquor by the optical density at 450 nm. (A) This figure is plotted on this chart first described by Liley.[223] The Liley zones are (1) RhD-negative or mildly affected fetus, (2) indeterminate, usually moderately severe disease, and (3) severe disease, impending fetal death. (B) The Bowman graph, an extension of the original Liley chart (see text for more detail).

severity of previous history are important prognostic factors. Regular monitoring is indicated from 18 weeks, when the maternal antibody concentration exceeds 4 IU/ml.[47] Above this threshold antibody levels have a limited role as they correlate poorly with the degree of fetal anaemia,[271] although a rising level suggests an increase in severity. Non-invasive methods, such as sonographic measurement of placental thickness, umbilical vein diameter, spleen and liver size,[79,282,335] or Doppler assessment of velocities in the descending aorta, middle cerebral artery and ductus venosus,[85,285,305,306] are not entirely reliable in predicting the degree of anaemia. In general, all these non-invasive indices, when abnormal, have predictive value for fetal anaemia, but their clinical utility is weakened by the unacceptably high frequency of false negatives, i.e. normal results in the presence of severe anaemia. Demonstration of fetal ascites, however, indicates

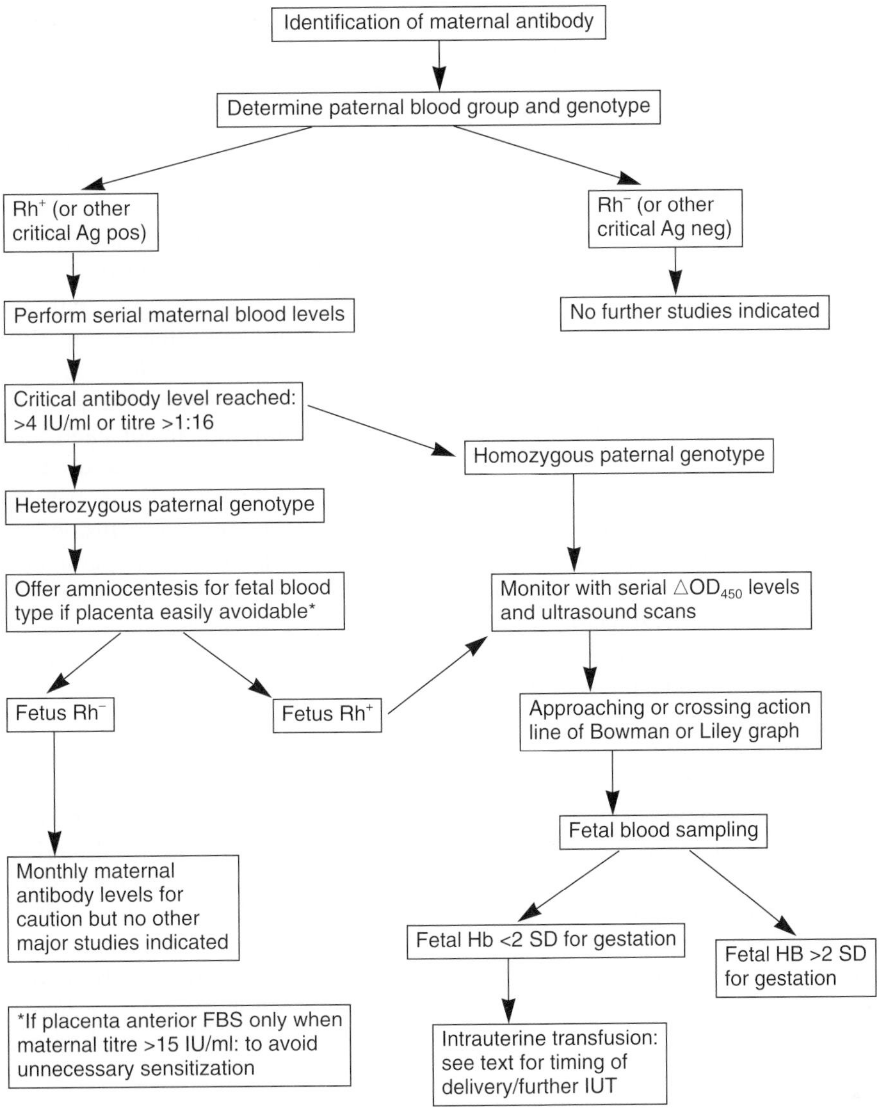

Fig. 14.6 Proposed algorithm for the management of alloimmune haemolytic disease.

severe anaemia (PCV <15%, Hb <4 g/dl) in the mid-trimester, although this threshold for ascites rises with advancing gestation.[79,280] Weekly sonographic surveillance for ascites is thus an integral part of monitoring in Rh disease, but cannot be relied upon as the sole method for two reasons. First, ascites is only found in two-thirds of fetuses with Hb <4 g/dl,[271] and secondly, anaemia of this degree is associated with hypoxaemia.[378]

Invasive monitoring necessitates amniocentesis or FBS. Severity has traditionally been assessed by spectrophotometric measurement of the deviation in optical density at 450 nm (ΔOD_{450}) caused by bilirubin in amniotic fluid[223] (Fig. 14.5(A)). Serial ΔOD_{450} s are plotted on Liley charts to give an indirect index of fetal red cell destruction, with delivery or transfusion indicated when the action line is reached.[417] Although this is reasonably reliable in the third trimester, amniocentesis has proved inaccurate in the mid-trimester, especially before 25 weeks.[277] However, new curves have recently been described extending back to 16 weeks' gestation, which were derived from more than 600 amniocenteses for alloimmunization[170] (Fig. 14.5(B)). This extended Liley chart is named the Bowman graph after the Winnipeg neonatologist who was involved with these cases. FBS, on the other hand, allows direct assessment of fetal PCV and Hb, permits transfusion to be performed at the same procedure if anaemia is detected, and yields additional information on fetal Rh and blood gas status. As FBS has a slightly greater loss rate, and provokes fetomaternal haemorrhage in 70% of procedures in which the placenta is transgressed, thereby increasing antibody levels,[290] amniocentesis remains the mainstay for monitoring mild/moderate disease in the late second and third trimester.[350] The ΔOD_{450} is unreliable in alloimmunization due to Kell antibodies,[32,397] which seem to suppress erythropoiesis rather than cause haemolysis. In this situation FBS is more appropriate.

Fetal blood group typing is now possible from

amniocytes using PCR to detect the RhD, c, E and Kell genes.[30,221] This has meant that when the partner is known to be heterozygous, typing can be performed early in gestation to decide whether the fetus is at risk or not, and in later gestation avoids the risks of serial amniocenteses where the fetus is Rh negative.[128] An algorithm for managing women with RBC antibodies is given in Figure 14.6.

Fetal blood transfusion

Intravascular transfusions were first administered fetoscopically,[347] but are now given by ultrasound-guided FBS.[20,33,276] The decision to administer an IVT is based on the PCV or Hb at FBS. Most use a haemoglobin of less than 2 SD for the gestation[280,281] as an indication for transfusion; some use an absolute haematocrit below 30%. The needle tip is kept within the umbilical vein and fresh Rh-negative packed cells compatible with the mother infused at 10–15 ml/min. The fetal heart rate and flow of infused blood are monitored on ultrasound to guard against inadvertent needle dislodgement and cord tamponade. Some centres advocate temporary immobilization of the fetus by intramuscular or intravascular curare or pancuronium.[99] The volume transfused is determined by consideration of the estimated fetoplacental volume and the fetal and donor PCVs[276] or Hbs,[280] according to published nomograms (Fig. 14.7). The PCV is rechecked after transfusion and, if less than the desired 40–45% a further increment is given. Exchange transfusion has been recommended to minimize circulatory overload[161] but is not widely used, as the more popular and quicker 'top-up' transfusion increases fetoplacental blood volume by up to 100% without adverse effects and with only minor changes in blood gases.[291]

The second transfusion should not be performed more than 2 weeks after the first because the rate of fall in PCV in each fetus at that stage is unpredictable.[295] Subsequent transfusions are timed at 2–4-week intervals when the PCV is estimated to have fallen to 20–25%, based on each fetus' calculated rate of fall in PCV/day, which is usually 1% per day (SD 0.3%).[295] Kleihauer testing of fetal samples indicates that erythropoiesis is usually completely suppressed after two to three transfusions.[295] As the donor blood in the fetal circulation is not susceptible to immune destruction, the rate of fall in PCV declines with increasing transfusions and thus the interval between procedures can be increased. The same principles are used in scheduling delivery between 36 and 38 weeks. Once an intrauterine transfusion has been performed, the timing of delivery will depend on when the last transfusion was performed and how many days it is likely to take for the haemoglobin to fall to a level about 2 SD below the mean. Intrauterine transfusions are not usually performed after 35 weeks. In a woman with no previous history but an antibody level above 4 IU/ml (or 1:16 titre) the delivery can be planned at 37–38 weeks of gestation. If the situation is more complicated and an amniocentesis has shown that at 35 weeks the ΔOD_{450} is soon to cross the action line, then we would induce labour soon after.

The direct intravascular route for transfusion is favoured over the older intraperitoneal route, as it yields direct information on the severity of the disease and corrects anaemia more physiologically. Intraperitoneal transfusion is ineffective in hydrops due to impaired absorption, and is associated with complications in 20%

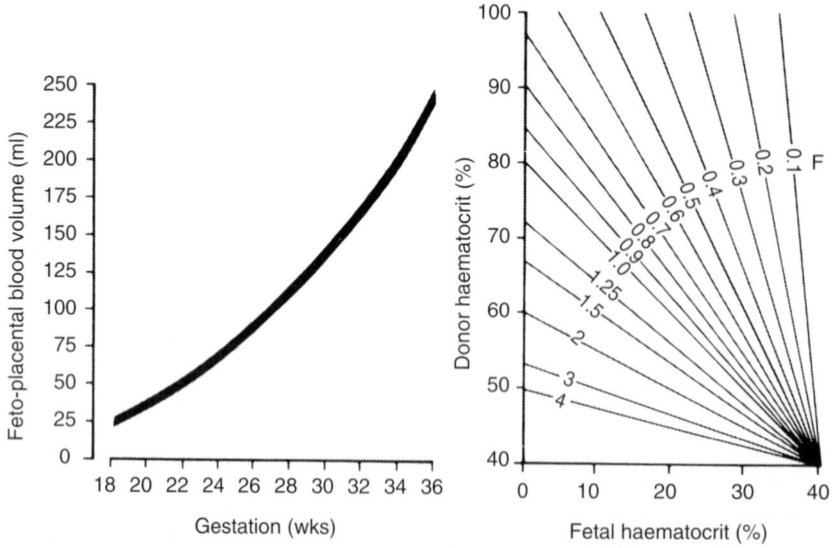

Fig. 14.7 Nomogram for calculating the volume of blood necessary to achieve a post-transfusion haematocrit of 40%. The mean fetoplacental blood volume at the relevant gestation (left) is multiplied by a ratio based on the fetal pretransfusion PCV and the donor Hct. (Reproduced with permission from Nicolaides et al[275])

of procedures.[338] Large rises in intraperitoneal pressure have been implicated in sudden death at the time of IPT.[293] However, a small IPT may be given in combination with IVT to increase the total volume administered while avoiding polycythaemia caused by the slower absorption of the intraperitoneal blood. Thus the interval between transfusions may be prolonged to 4–5 weeks and the total number of invasive procedures per pregnancy reduced.[295]

Survival

With serial intravascular transfusions survival rates of 78–95% have been achieved in severely affected fetuses.[276,322] One recent series has reported that in almost 600 intravascular transfusions, intact survival was 98% in those commenced in non-hydropic fetuses at greater than 24 weeks, and 70% in hydropic fetuses less than 24 weeks' gestation.[170] Therefore, the prognosis is now extremely optimistic. Fetal mortality correlates inversely with gestational age, and operator experience is undoubtedly also of importance.

FETAL THROMBOCYTOPENIA

Alloimmune thrombocytopenia

Perinatal alloimmune thrombocytopenia complicates 1:5000 births, with ICH affecting 10–20%.[263] Maternal antiplatelet antibodies cross the placenta, in a situation analagous to Rh disease. The consequent fetal thrombocytopenia may be profound, and there have been increasing reports in alloimmune thrombocytopenia of spontaneous ICH in utero, particularly in the third trimester,[104,142,257] but it may occur as early as 18 weeks' gestation. The human platelet-specific antigens are biallelic polymorphisms which involve the platelet surface glycoproteins. Recently, a nomenclature of human platelet antigens has been developed.[400] At present, HPAs 1–5 have been recognized. The genetic basis for these five HPAs has been identified, all involving a single point mutation in the DNA coding for the glycoproteins involved.[421] The most common is HPA1, which has a high-frequency (85%) or a low-frequency (15%) antigen. Only 2% of women will be homozygous for the low-frequency 'b' allele, and thus at risk for developing antibodies and alloimmunization. Fortunately, the actual occurrence of alloimmunization is much rarer than this (0.06%)[42] because the development of antibodies is dependent on the HLA type. HLA-Drw52a and HLA-Dr3 are most commonly associated with the development of HPA 1a antibodies.

Management of alloimmune thrombocytopenia

The most reliable method of assessing likely disease severity is by inference from previous pregnancies: usually a current pregnancy will be as severely or more affected than previous pregnancies.[331] This guides when investigation and treatment should begin, which may be as early as 18 weeks' gestation. Percutaneous FBS and estimation of fetal platelet count is the only way to determine whether a fetus is affected.[90] FBS can be undertaken safely in experienced hands in a fetus with a bleeding disorder, but compatible platelets should be available for transfusion if the fetus is affected, as otherwise exsanguination occurs in 10%.[312]

FBS should be considered in fetuses at high risk for alloimmune thrombocytopenia, and is carried out at 21–22 weeks' gestation, as the fetus may be thrombocytopenic at this stage. This allows for early diagnosis and therapy to increase the platelet count and thus prevent intracranial haemorrhage. A normal platelet count does not exclude the diagnosis, and therefore the procedure should be repeated at 28–32 weeks, unless from sampling amniotic fluid or fetal blood the fetal platelet type is found to be compatible.

If the fetus is thrombocytopenic, three treatment strategies have been proposed.

- Fetal platelet transfusions. These are used to cover the samplings and delivery, but may also be employed in a prophylactic manner, with weekly transfusions during the second and third trimesters and delivery once lung maturity is achieved. This prophylactic regimen is favoured in Europe, but it is arduous for the mother. In practice, transfusions are commenced at 26–28 weeks' gestation to the cover the time of greatest risk.[292]
- Intravenous gammaglobulin. Maternal infusion is less invasive and simpler than direct fetal sampling and is the preferred treatment option in the USA. However, it has proved less effective in the European experience and is extremely expensive. Reports of maternal IVIG raising the fetal platelet count are variable.[60,300] It may be that the IVIG may have a preventative effect on ICH, other than by increasing the fetal platelet count. In a series of 54 women with thrombocytopenic fetuses due to alloimmune thrombocytopenia given IVIG weekly, in whom 10 had a previous infant with ICH, no ICH occurred and yet 20% showed no increase in the platelet count with therapy.[61]
- Conservative. The final option is to follow the fetus regularly by ultrasound and, in countries where late termination is permitted, to offer termination if ICH is found. This may be suitable in cases in which there is no severe history and hence the risk of ICH versus a complication from recurrent sampling or transfusion is low. Sampling may be performed prior to delivery to assess whether a transfusion is required to cover this.[201]

There is no clear evidence to demonstrate that one strategy for treatment is superior to the other. Although prophylactic platelet transfusions may be the most effective, there is a not inconsiderable procedure-related loss secondary to the serial procedures,[413] and therefore this needs to be weighed against the overall risk of ICH with untreated disease.

Autoimmune thrombocytopenic purpura

Transplacental passage of antibodies in maternal immune thrombocytopenic purpura also produces fetal thrombocytopenia, albeit to a lesser degree. The older literature suggested that the 50% of infants with thrombocytopenia had a risk of intracranial haemorrhage during vaginal delivery,[179] and accordingly FBS for fetal platelet count determination prior to labour used to be performed in pregnancies complicated by ITP to decide on the mode of delivery.[250,365] More recent studies show a low incidence of severe fetal thrombocytopenia (5–20%) or infant morbidity with maternal ITP,[57,204,409] with no documented cases of antenatal ICH or ICH attributable to mode of delivery even in cases of severe thrombocytopenia. There is no correlation between maternal and fetal platelet counts,[314] the level of platelet-associated antibody does not correlate with fetal thrombocytopenia, but increased levels of free antiplatelet antibody are associated with fetal thrombocytopenia.[58,360] Platelet counts in affected infants may fall following delivery, but generally thrombocytopenia at this stage is not associated with significant morbidity.

Management

Treatment for maternal thrombocytopenia includes steroids, splenectomy (outside pregnancy) and IVIG to raise the platelet count prior to delivery. There is no evidence that these treatments affect fetal platelet count. The investigations required to detect fetal thrombocytopenia in this condition are controversial. The risk of severe fetal thrombocytopenia in a woman presenting with a documented fall in platelet count from normal in pregnancy and no history to suggest ITP is very low,[59,62] and does not justify FBS prior to labour. With a history of chronic ITP, the risk of severe thrombocytopenia ($<50 \times 10^9$/l) is between 5 and 20%, although it is difficult to determine whether mode of delivery affects the outcome. Recommendations have included FBS prior to delivery, and fetal scalp sampling to determine whether caesarean section should be performed. Fetal morbidity appears extremely low in this condition, so that opinion has moved away from fetal intervention unless there has been a strong history of a previous affected child with severe thrombocytopenia.

CONGENITAL INFECTIONS

Counselling a woman after perinatal exposure to teratogenic infectious agents previously involved quoting empirical risks. Now, direct serological investigation of the fetus and DNA analysis of fetoplacental tissues can be used to determine whether fetal infection has occurred. In rubella this may facilitate continuation of pregnancy, whereas in toxoplasmosis it determines the choice of antimicrobial therapy. FBS has no role in evaluating fetal status in maternal HIV infection, as the procedure itself could inoculate the fetus.

Rubella

Prenatal diagnosis of rubella infection is usually indicated following maternal exposure in the early second trimester, or where doubt exists as to whether exposure in the first trimester resulted from primary infection or reinfection. Rubella-specific IgM is detected in fetal serum by radioimmunoassay,[91,258] provided that FBS can be delayed until 21–22 weeks, when the fetal humoral response to infection becomes detectable. Even at 23 weeks occasional false negative IgMs have been reported.[111] To improve the accuracy of prenatal testing at this late gestation, fetal blood or other tissues are also tested by hybridization with a cDNA probe to rubella virus.[86] Earlier in pregnancy the same technique can be used on CVS specimens,[389] although concern remains that placental infection need not necessarily indicate fetal infection.[10]

Cytomegalovirus

The most severe congenital infections are due to primary maternal CMV infection. Primary infection is associated with a 40% transmission rate, although only 10% of those fetuses will develop long-term sequelae, mostly hearing and learning defects.[315] Of the 5–10% who are symptomatic at birth there will be a neonatal mortality of 30%, with long-term handicap in all survivors.

Prenatal diagnosis is based on ultrasound findings and the detection of viral particles in the amniotic fluid[97] or, less commonly, in fetal blood. Specific IgM in fetal sera may also be diagnostic.[216] Ultrasound findings include growth retardation, ascites or hydrops, intracranial calcification, ventriculomegaly or bowel echogenicity.

Prenatal diagnosis has been reported by virus isolation in amniotic fluid and by detection of specific IgM in fetal sera. Nevertheless, 90% of infants with congenital CMV infection remain neurologically and developmentally normal.

If primary CMV with transplacental transmission in pregnancy is confirmed there is a 5–10% chance of severe clinical disease, and therefore termination of pregnancy should be offered. Recurrent disease carries a much lower risk of handicap. Attempted treatment of an affected fetus with ganciclovir has been reported with equivocal results,[330] and although there is interest in this therapy, it is unlikely to be introduced until the results of neonatal treatment series are reported.

Toxoplasmosis

Although the risk of fetal infection increases the later in pregnancy that maternal infection occurs, severity is greatest with exposure in the first trimester. Termination of an infected fetus remains an option, although feto-placental infection is largely treatable.[102] The aim of fetal testing is to allow optimal transplacental therapy, initially with maternal spiramycin (3 g/day) to prevent transplacental transmission, with the addition of pyrimethamine and sulphonamide if fetal testing proves positive.[91] These two drugs are directly antiparasitic and have been shown to limit fetal damage. They are not used in the first instance when information about maternal infection is known, but rather only when fetal infection is proven, because of the potential hazards to mother and fetus. As no single test achieves suitable accuracy, prenatal diagnosis necessitates a combination of tests at 20–24 weeks, including:

- toxoplasmosis PCR in amniotic fluid;
- toxoplasmosis PCR in fetal serum;
- toxoplasmosis-specific IgA and IgM in fetal serum;
- non-specific indices of infection in fetal blood, such as abnormal liver function, thrombocytopenia and eosinophilia;
- culture of amniotic fluid and fetal blood after inoculation into mice;
- fortnightly ultrasound of the fetal brain to detect intracranial calcifications and ventriculomegaly.

Recently it was thought that PCR of amniotic fluid could reliably determine whether fetal infection had occurred or not.[185] However, this has not been confirmed and therefore the combination testing is still recommended. Serum IgA appears to confirm greater sensitivity than IgM for diagnosis of fetal and infant infection, and at present both are measured in fetal and infant serum if toxoplasmosis is suspected.[313] If fetal infection is proven the prognosis is still likely to be good, although vision may be affected later, unless intracranial signs of calcification and ventriculomegaly are detected on ultrasound.[37] At this stage termination would be offered.

Parvovirus

Human parvovirus (B19) infection is associated with increased risks of miscarriage, hydrops and intrauterine death.[13] HPV is best identified in fetal blood or other tissues by dot-blot hybridization, electron microscopy, or PCR of B19-specific DNA.[370] The mainstay of diagnosis, however, remains maternal serology in women with appropriate clinical symptoms. Anti-B19 IgM appears in the serum at the onset of illness and remains detectable for up to 3 months. IgG response begins after 7 days and persists, probably to confer lifelong immunity. FBS is not routinely indicated in pregnancies with maternal infection as at least 80% will result in livebirths, and as HPV does not seem to be teratogenic. An infective erythroid aplasia can cause profound fetal anaemia, and several cases of intrauterine transfusion have been reported leading to reversal of hydrops and intact survival.[316,364] As fetal anaemia may occur 1–11 weeks after maternal infection[352] weekly ultrasound examinations are recommended, with FBS and IVT indicated in the presence of hydrops. Hydrops without fetal anaemia has been documented and viral particles have been identified in the fetal myocardium, suggesting that a myocarditis may be contributory.

TACHYARRHYTHMIAS

Supraventricular tachycardia is the most common fetal tachyarrhythmia, with rates between 200 and 300 beats per minute (bpm). Atrial flutter and fibrillation also occur. As SVT is often intermittent, treatment is indicated only when SVT is sustained or associated with hydrops.[207a] In utero therapy seems preferable to delivery and neonatal treatment, as the fetus tolerates haemodynamic compromise better in utero, where gas exchange is not hindered by pulmonary oedema. Transplacental treatment by giving the mother digoxin leads to cardioversion in only 25–50% of non-hydropic cases[239,382] and is usually not effective in the presence of hydrops.[143] These poor results partly reflect difficulties in achieving therapeutic maternal levels owing to the increased intravascular volume and glomerular filtration rate of pregnancy. Whether digoxin actually crosses the placenta has been called into doubt by a report of similar digoxin-like immunoreactive substance levels in fetuses of treated and untreated mothers.[410] The addition of second-line drugs, such as flecainide and verapamil, results in eventual cardioversion in just over 50%,[239,382] and many consider flecainide as the first-line treatment for fetal SVT.[12,239] Reports of sudden death in adults with antiarrhythmics such as amiodarone have slowed their incorporation into fetal treatment. Direct fetal intravascular or intraperitoneal therapy may be useful in refractory cases or those with hydrops.[135] Adenosine has recently been reported to cause a chemical cardioversion when injected directly into the fetal circulation, and then sinus rhythm was maintained by transplacental digoxin therapy.[208] This needs to be explored further in cases resistant to initial maternal treatment. Doses required are much higher per kilogram estimated fetal body weight than in the neonate, presumably to allow for transplacental passage into maternal circulation, and to account for the enhanced fetoplacental blood volume.

CONGENITAL HEART BLOCK

Complete heart block in the fetus is rare, with an incidence of between 1:5000 and 1:22 000. The intrinsic ventricular rate is around 50–65 bpm and the heart usually enlarges and hypertrophies to compensate for the slow rate. Hydrops may occur as congestive heart failure develops.

Congenital heart block with a structurally abnormal heart carries a poor prognosis (85% mortality), whereas with a structurally normal heart the prognosis is good.[232] In 1966, the association between isolated CHB and maternal connective tissue disease was first described.[188] Anti-Ro and anti-La (SSA and SSB) antibodies are present in 60–80% of cases, often in mothers with subclinical disease. These antibodies are most frequently found in women with SLE or Sjögrens syndrome. Various therapeutic options based on maternal transplacental therapy are available, although none have shown proven efficacy. These include sympathomimetic agents to increase fetal heart rate and function[164] and maternal dexamethasone to suppress the fetal myocardial inflammation.[41,82]

ABNORMALITIES OF AMNIOTIC FLUID VOLUME

Oligohydramnios

Causes in the mid-trimester include urinary tract malformations, PPROM and IUGR. Although survival is less than 25% whatever the cause,[22,243] conditions with a hopeless prognosis, such as renal agenesis and lethal aneuploidies, should be ruled out. Absence of the acoustic window makes inspection of fetal anatomy difficult. Transvaginal ultrasound facilitates visualization of the renal fossae, as does colour Doppler of the renal arteries.[368] If still equivocal, invasive procedures may be required, including amnioinfusion and/or instillation of fluid into the fetal peritoneal cavity.[296] Amnioinfusion of a warmed physiological solution not only restores the acoustic window, but allows confirmation of PPROM, especially when a dye such as indigo carmine is added.[130] Amnioinfusion may unmask PPROM, which early in the mid-trimester would otherwise have gone undetected, the volume lost vaginally being too small to be noticed by the mother.[130]

Maternal[424] and even fetal administration of frusemide was previously advocated in cases of persistent nonvisualization of the fetal bladder, but is no longer recommended following reports of false negative diagnoses of renal agenesis,[169] and a study in sheep indicating that maternally administered frusemide does not produce a fetal diuresis or cross the placenta.[74] As 5–10% of fetuses in pregnancies with severe oligohydramnios will be chromosomally abnormal,[165] rapid karyotyping is carried out at the time of amnioinfusion.

In the rare case of a euploid fetus with oligohydramnios, intact membranes and an intact renal tract, there may be a role for serial amnioinfusions in the prevention of lethal pulmonary hypoplasia,[16] which otherwise complicates at least 60% of cases of severe mid-trimester oligohydramnios.[256]

Polyhydramnios

The more severe the polyhydramnios, the more likely that an underlying cause will be found. Using the MVP, mild and severe polyhydramnios have been arbitrarily defined as a deepest pool greater than 8 and 15 cm, respectively.[73] The amniotic fluid index definitions for mild and severe polyhydramnios are values outside the 97.5th centile for gestation, and an AFI greater than 40 cm, respectively.[255]

In one series of 102 cases 83% of mild polyhydramnios were idiopathic, whereas only 8% of severe polyhydramnios remained unexplained.[181] Maternal diabetes should be excluded and a detailed scan performed for structural malformations. In view of a 5–10% chance of chromosomal abnormality rapid karyotyping warrants consideration in moderate/severe polyhydramnios, which is often associated with a structural anomaly.[71]

The increased risks of preterm labour and PPROM in polyhydramnios seem mainly confined to those with severe polyhydramnios, i.e. an amniotic fluid index ≥ 40 cm or a deepest pool ≥ 15 cm.[71,132] These risks are almost universal in acute polyhydramnios, in which rapid accumulation of amniotic fluid occurs before 28 weeks in association with fetofetal transfusion syndrome.[414] Amnioreduction has been used with anecdotal success in severe polyhydramnios in order to prolong gestation and relieve maternal discomfort.[119,324] Removal of relatively small volumes of amniotic fluid can restore amniotic pressure to normal,[132] but usually larger volumes are removed to limit the number of procedures that may be required. Nevertheless, removal of volumes greater than 6 l at one time does carry the risk of precipitating abruption and/or preterm labour.[109]

Prostaglandin synthetase inhibitors have been used to reduce amniotic fluid. Indomethacin initially was described at a dose of 75–200 mg/day.[63,235] This acts by reducing fetal urine output[207] and hence amniotic fluid volume.[206] The amniotic cavity and fetal bladder are monitored daily on ultrasound so that the dose can be adjusted to ensure sufficient response without causing oligohydramnios. Concern has arisen about the potential deleterious effects of fetal ductal constriction secondary to indomethacin, and therefore monitoring of ductal patency by Doppler has been recommended[251] when exposure is for longer than 1 week. However, the risks of neonatal complications from premature closure of the ductus in utero seem remote, provided therapy is discontinued at 32 weeks. Sulindac, another prostaglandin synthetase inhibitor, has been shown to have less effect on the ductus arteriosus, but still reduces amniotic fluid volume.[70]

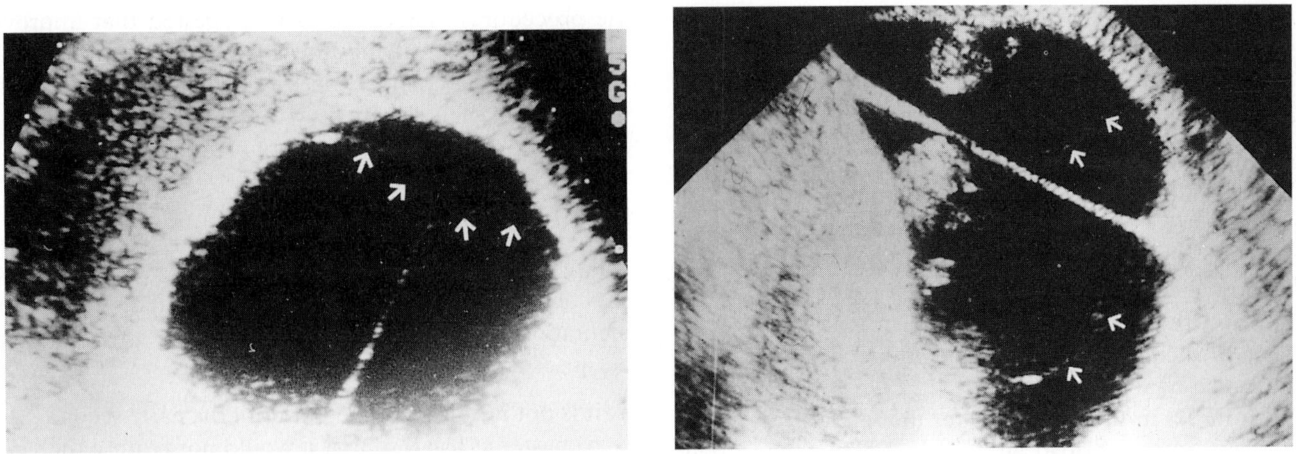

A B

Fig. 14.8 Transvaginal ultrasound view of first-trimester (A) monochorionic (B) dichorionic twin gestations, showing the amnions and chorions before fusion. (Reproduced with permission from the RCOG press)

MULTIPLE PREGNANCY

Selective feticide

In twin pregnancies discordant for fetal anomaly, selective termination of the affected fetus is an option. Initially, a variety of fetoscopic and then ultrasound-guided techniques have been described, including fetal exsanguination and intracardiac injection of air or potassium chloride.[158,349] KCl injection is now the recommended technique.[192] Selective feticide is contraindicated in monochorial pregnancies because of the risk of causing death in the normal twin, owing to vascular communications within the shared placenta.[158] In the 20% of cases concordant for fetal sex with a single placental mass on ultrasound, determination of chorionicity will require careful evaluation of the membranous septum. This requires evaluation of the septal thickness and the presence or absence of the twin peak or lambda sign[124] (Fig. 14.8). A thick septum > 2 mm, and/or containing three to four layers, strongly suggests dichorionic placentation,[23,93] although the reproducibility and hence the usefulness of this measurement has been shown to be poor.[380] A combination of all the signs should provide greater than 90% accuracy in chorionicity determination in the second trimester[362] but 100% accuracy in the first trimester.[253] The international experience in selective termination has been collected and shows that there is an overall pregnancy loss rate of 8.3%,[114] with procedures performed before 16 weeks' gestation carrying a lower risk (5.4%) of subsequent loss. Furthermore, recent data have shown that reduction at 20 weeks' gestation or later is associated with a worse perinatal outcome, with earlier delivery and lower birthweight.[231]

Rarely, selective feticide has been intentionally performed in monochorial twin pregnancies, not to terminate an anomalous fetus but to allow the survival of a fetus otherwise compromised by its co-twin. Robie et al[340] delivered an acardiac monster by sectio parva with successful outcome for the pump twin left in utero, and intrapericardial injection has been used to tamponade the donor's heart in two fetuses with fetofetal transfusion syndrome, allowing prolongation of the pregnancy and survival of the recipient.[408,423] Recently, cord ligation by endoscopic techniques has been reported,[325] and we have reported success with direct intravascular injection of pure alcohol.[101]

Multifetal pregnancy reduction

This procedure aims to obviate the daunting perinatal mortality in high-order multiple pregnancies (≥ 4) by reducing fetal numbers to a twin or triplet gestation with improved perinatal outcome. The initial approach, which involved transvaginal aspiration, has been abandoned in view of high loss rates,[193] and all are now done by transabdominal injection of KCl into the fetal thorax.[34,112] Most such pregnancies are the result of overzealous use of ovulation induction agents and are therefore usually multizygotic and multichorial, although not always in twins.[416] The procedure is best delayed until 10–12 weeks, when the risks of abortion and spontaneous regression have subsided and the nuchal translucency can be measured. The optimal number of fetuses to be left remains controversial, but most centres reduce to twins. The chief risk, that of complete abortion of all fetuses, varies around 8–16% and is influenced by the starting number and the finishing number after the reduction.[35,113] Furthermore, the international registry has shown that the loss rate has been reduced by half, i.e. to 8%, in a comparative study of the same centres 2 years later, indicating that operator experience is an important variable in determining loss rates.[115] In both series more than 80% of those reduced to twins or triplets delivered after 32 weeks' gestation, which is similar to spontaneous multiple pregnancies.[35,115]

Fetofetal transfusion syndrome

Although placental vascular communications are found in almost all monochorionic pregnancies, clinical signs of FFTS occur in only 4–26%.[148,339] FFTS is diagnosed in mid-trimester in the presence of acute discordance in amniotic fluid volume in monochorionic twins. The older neonatal criteria of a haemoglobin difference greater than 5 g/dl and birthweight difference of greater than 20% have now been discredited.[129] Their basis was never robust and they now have been shown to be frequently present in dichorionic twins or in monochorionic twins complicated by discordant IUGR.[95,415]

With FFTS in the mid-trimester the recipient develops acute circulatory overload and polyhydramnios, and may become hydropic, whereas the donor is growth retarded, oliguric, and has severe oligohydramnios. As perinatal mortality in FFTS diagnosed in the mid-trimester is 80–100%[160,414] aggressive therapeutic measures are warranted. Serial amnioreduction seems beneficial in prolonging gestation and improving survival, and is currently considered the treatment of choice. A randomized controlled trial would now be difficult to perform, as the empirical evidence from the above series shows that amnioreduction is of major benefit, with an overall survival rate of 63% in recent series. Amnioreduction also improves uterine perfusion compared to control needling procedures,[48] and may improve fetal blood gas status.[133] Aggressive amnioreduction may therefore not only prevent complications such as preterm labour, but also improve fetal condition and possibly ameliorate the disease process itself. For failures of amnioreduction more aggressive procedures may be required. Selective feticide of the donor has been used to allow survival of the recipient in seven cases, although this drastic procedure was performed primarily for prolongation of pregnancies threatened by gross polyhydramnios in the absence of hydrops or other fetal compromise.[408,423]

Fetoscopic laser ablation of placental vascular anastomoses has been attempted. Theoretically this technique should be the ideal treatment for FFTS if the condition is due to the presence of anastomoses and they can be selectively ablated. The results, however, have been disappointing. Perinatal survival was only 53% in each of the two large series,[100,399] which is lower than serial amnioreduction as above. The overall experience with laser is that in one-third of cases both babies survive, in another third one baby survives, and in the remaining third both babies die. Recently it has been shown that the communicating anastomoses in FFTS are both deep and limited in number.[17] In particular there is usually a paucity of superficial anastomoses, suggesting that the multiple anastomoses destroyed by laser are largely normal chorionic plate vessels. This would explain the extremely high procedure-related loss rate (50% of the pregnancies have an intrauterine death within 48 hours of the procedure). Therefore, it is suggested that improved methods for identifying the type and location of the communicating channels need to be available before laser therapy can be of benefit. Currently, the mainstay of treatment for FFTS remains serial amnioreduction.

FETAL STEM CELL THERAPY

A large number of haematological and genetic conditions are amenable to bone marrow or stem cell transplantation. The fetus is theoretically the ideal recipient because:

- it is not immunocompetent until the early second trimester at least, so that it would not require the immunosuppressive drugs that have to be used postnatally. Tolerance should therefore be achieved together with long-lasting chimaerism, which is the aim of this therapy;
- haematopoietic stem cells migrate from the liver to the bone marrow between 12 and 16 weeks of gestation, and therefore a virtual space should be available for the seeding of the graft, obviating the need for marrow ablation with toxic drugs, as in postnatal life.

Success has been achieved in various animal models[367,427] but has been more elusive in the human. The first attempt in the human fetus, using Rh alloimmunization as a model,[224] showed no evidence of chimaerism. So far, stem cell therapy has only worked in fetuses with immunodeficiency diseases.[139,394] It is to be hoped that this kind of treatment may become available for the haemoglobinopathies, the commonest genetic diseases in the world, but a great deal more experimental work is required. The subject has been recently reviewed.[137]

FETAL SURGERY

In several congenital malformations a satisfactory outcome is often achieved with postnatal surgical correction. In some, however, the uncorrected malformation results in progressive organ damage in utero, jeopardizing survival. There may be a role in such conditions for in utero intervention. Attempts at fetal surgery have taken one of two forms: open surgical correction at hysterotomy, or bypassing obstructive lesions by ultrasound-guided insertion of catheter shunts. These techniques should only be contemplated in centres with expertise, and for conditions in which animal models have demonstrated benefit from correction in utero. Unfortunately, the overall results for open fetal surgery have been disappointing. Despite being limited to a few very specialized centres, the problem of inexorable preterm labour subsequent to surgery has limited the enthusiasm for the approach. If fetal surgery is to be considered in the future, it is axiomatic that chromosomal and other structural malformations first be excluded. Moreover, reliable antenatal predictors are needed when selecting cases for intervention, so that fetal surgery is withheld from those which would otherwise have a satisfactory outcome, and from those in which the pathology is irreversible.

INTRATHORACIC LESIONS

Diaphragmatic hernia

The mortality rate from diaphragmatic hernia diagnosed in utero remains high at 75% despite optimal postnatal care.[5,177] The main determinant of outcome is the degree of pulmonary hypoplasia resulting from in utero lung compression, dependent on the timing and volume of visceral herniation through the diaphragm. Antenatal prediction of neonatal outcome is difficult, but some would say that polyhydramnios, mediastinal shift and a large volume of viscera within the chest are adverse indicators. Studies in an animal model have demonstrated that surgical correction in utero reverses the effects on fetal lung growth and allows survival at birth.[172] Harrison's San Francisco group demonstrated in non-human primates the safety and feasibility of fetal surgery,[6] but after a decade of developing appropriate techniques, and operating in the late mid-trimester on human fetuses, there have been significant problems. These include difficulty in reducing the herniated liver without kinking the umbilical vein, and the prevention of preterm labour. An alternative less invasive corrective approach to diaphragmatic hernia is tracheal ligation. The underlying theory is that preventing drainage of lung liquid will allow the lung to grow (PLUG – plug the lung until it grows), and animal experiments have confirmed this hypothesis.[171,422] Open tracheal ligation unfortunately still carries the risk of preterm labour, and may also result in tracheal stenosis. The recent development of endoscopic techniques for insertion of a temporary tracheal plug looks promising,[136] but much work needs to be done on the optimal timing, duration and method for PLUG before it can be introduced into clinical practice.

Fetal hydrothorax

Perinatal mortality in fetal hydrothorax exceeds 50%, and is higher when associated with hydrops than in isolation.[72,334] Compression of the lung during its canalicular phase (17–24 weeks) produces pulmonary hypoplasia, whereas large effusions cause hydrops by impairing swallowing and hydrops by vena caval obstruction and cardiac compression.[24,317] Chylothorax, the commonest cause in neonates, is diagnosed after alimentation by demonstrating chylomicrons in pleural fluid.[75] Although some claim to have made this diagnosis in the fetus by showing high mononuclear cell counts in aspirated pleural fluid,[26,110] chylothorax was not confirmed postnatally, given that these effusions often resolve soon after birth. We have been unable to detect any difference in lymphocyte counts or lipoprotein electrophoresis between fetuses confirmed neonatally to have chylothoraces and those with hydrothoraces from other causes (unpublished observations).

Ultrasound-guided aspiration of fetal hydrothoraces facilitates neonatal resuscitation if performed immediately prior to delivery.[363] Because the fluid reaccumulates within 6–48 hours,[272,317] long-term drainage is required. This is achieved by a plastic pleuroamniotic shunt, inserted under ultrasound guidance (Fig. 14.9) (Rocket of London, UK). In three series totalling 34 patients,[229,286,346] 17 (50%) resolved, of which 16 (94%) survived, with no respiratory complications. Only two infants survived when hydrops persisted (12%). A single aspiration is performed 1 week beforehand, as the effusion does not always reaccumulate,[24,26] especially with small or unilateral effusions. In fetal hydrothoraces unassociated with other abnormalities, shunting is indicated in the presence of hydrops, polyhydramnios, or if detected in mid-trimester. The catheters should be clamped immediately at delivery to prevent a pneumothorax; alternatively the neonate should be electively intubated and ventilated.

Cystic adenomatoid malformation of the lung

This rare malformation may result in pulmonary hypoplasia, hydrops and perinatal death in a small percentage of cases.[4] The solid type of lesion is more likely to be associated with a poor prognosis than the macrocystic lesion, where cysts can be visualized on ultrasound. In the macrocystic type of lesion long-term drainage of a solitary intrathoracic cyst can be performed, resulting in good outcome at birth.[279] The San Francisco group have also shown that with severe CCAM associated with hydrops, a combination that carries an extremely poor prognosis, open fetal surgical resection by lobectomy offers a good chance of survival. Lobectomy of the massively enlarged pulmonary lobe was performed between 21 and 27 weeks' gestation in eight fetuses, resulting in five survivors.[7] This is therefore one of the conditions where fetal surgery may have a role, although it should only be embarked upon in those cases which otherwise would have an extremely poor outlook.

OBSTRUCTIVE UROPATHY

Posterior urethral valves

In fetuses with PUV unassociated with other anomalies the two main factors determining perinatal outcome are pulmonary hypoplasia and renal dysplasia,[174,265] which seem related to the duration and severity of obstruction. Lack of a urinary contribution to amniotic fluid in the mid-trimester leads to pulmonary hypoplasia. Although

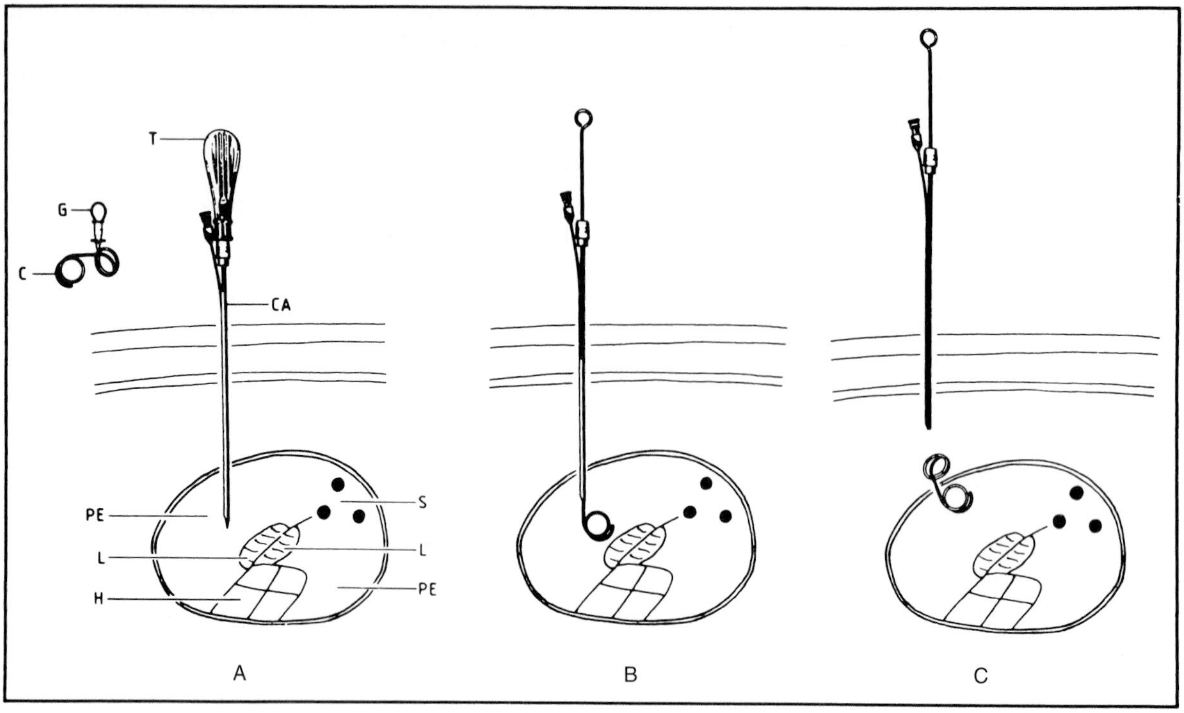

Fig. 14.9 Pleuroamniotic shunting. The trocar (T) and cannula (CA) are inserted transamniotically into the effusion (A). The guidewire (G) is then straightened, the double-pigtail catheter (C) inserted into the cannula, and the wire removed. A short introducer rod then deposits half the catheter within the hemithorax (B). The cannula is then withdrawn into the amniotic cavity, and a long introducer rod is inserted to position the other half of the shunt in the amniotic cavity (C). H, heart; S, spine; L, lungs. (Reproduced with permission from Rodeck et al[346])

its pathogenesis is not understood,[297] numerous animal and human studies indicate that lung hypoplasia is a consequence of oligohydramnios. Urethral obstruction has also been considered responsible for renal dysplasia, presumably mediated by raised urinary pressure.[173,211] However, intravesical pressure seems only marginally raised in fetuses with low obstructive uropathies.[301] There is an alternative embryological theory, which suggests that renal dysplasia is not secondary to PUV but results from the same early defect, resulting in abnormal interaction between the urethral bud and the metanephrogenic mesenchyme.[36,381]

As the surgical correction of PUV is relatively simple postnatally, a hypothesis emerged that bypass of the obstruction in utero would minimize renal dysplasia and would restore amniotic fluid, thereby preventing pulmonary hypoplasia and allowing survival at birth.[173] The basis for such intervention was rigorously tested in animals. Urinary obstruction in fetal lambs produces both renal dysplasia and lung hypoplasia,[153,176] whereas early decompression prevents these sequelae.[154,175]

The presence of a normal amniotic fluid volume indicates that lung hypoplasia will not occur, that the obstruction is incomplete and that the kidneys are producing adequate amounts of urine. Therefore, any benefit from bypass procedures needs to be restricted to those fetuses with severe oligohydramnios, in whom irreversible renal damage has not yet developed. Vesicoamniotic shunting of a fetus with severe renal dysplasia would not only fail to prevent neonatal renal failure, but would also fail to prevent pulmonary hypoplasia if the kidneys in utero were unable to restore amniotic fluid volume. Accordingly, accurate prediction of fetal renal function is important in selecting potential cases for intrauterine surgery. Although renal cysts are visualized in only 44% of dysplastic kidneys, their presence strongly suggests dysplasia.[234] Hyperechogenicity of the renal parenchyma predicts dysplasia with a sensitivity of 73% and a specificity of 80%.[234] In view of the inaccuracy of ultrasound in predicting renal function, other methods have been sought. Biochemical analysis of fetal urine for the prediction of later renal function has been thought to be useful by some,[155,162] but not by others.[411,419] Initially, threshold values to define an isotonic urine with probable poor outcome, Na^+>100 mEq/l, Cl^->90 mEq/l and osmolality >210 mmol/l, were used. Refinements have been made by providing normal values for electrolytes (Na^+ and Cl^-) with gestation between 16 and 33 weeks[302] (Fig 14.10) and by serial sampling, which may provide more accurate information.[197] Others have suggested that urinary microproteins may be useful indicators of renal damage, in particular urinary[225,236,262] and possibly fetal serum β_2 microglobulin.[38] In present practice a decision whether to shunt or not is based on a combination of urinary electrolytes, β_2 microglobulin, the appearance of the renal tract on ultrasound, and on bladder and liquor volumes.

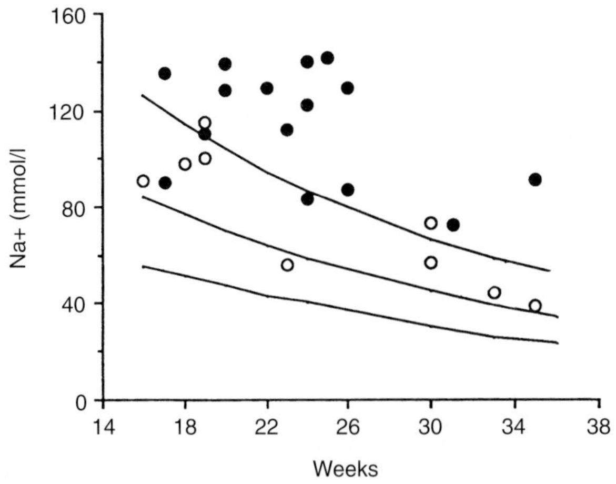

Fig. 14.10 Urinary sodium values in fetuses with lower urinary tract obstruction plotted against the reference range. •, fetuses with renal dysplasia; o, fetuses without renal dysplasia.

The standard method of vesicoamniotic shunting is by ultrasound-guided insertion of an indwelling plastic double-pigtail catheter (Rocket of London, UK),[174,237] as for pleuroamniotic shunting.

The results of 73 cases of shunting procedures for low obstructive uropathy reported to the International Registry were not encouraging, with only a 41% perinatal survival rate.[237] However, this included fetuses with pathologies other than PUV, with chromosomal and other abnormalities, and with normal amniotic fluid volume, and 70% of the contributing centres had had experience of only one case. Most of the scepticism about this procedure[107,328] can thus be attributed to poor case selection. Until the value of shunting procedures is established, selection criteria should be rigorously applied to restrict shunting to those few fetuses in whom it may be of benefit, i.e. otherwise normal male fetuses of normal karyotype with PUV, severe oligohydramnios and biochemical evidence of adequate renal function. Accordingly, only 2.5% of 200 fetuses referred with bilateral hydronephrosis in a recent series were considered suitable for shunting.[228]

OTHER SURGICAL CONDITIONS

Hydrocephalus

Obstruction of the aqueduct of Sylvius causes a rise in cerebrospinal fluid pressure, ventricular enlargement, cortical thinning and irreversible neurological damage. As ventricular shunting in the neonatal period dramatically improves outcome,[219] and as ventriculomegaly may progress in utero, the hypothesis emerged that intrauterine decompression of fetal hydrocephalus would prevent neurological damage. Although initial work in a primate model suggested that in utero shunting improved survival and outcome,[246] reports to the International Registry[237] showed that in utero shunting in human fetuses showed increased survival of severely handicapped infants, and therefore the technique has been abandoned.

Sacrococcygeal teratoma

Congenital sacrococcygeal teratomas are usually benign and in the neonatal period are associated with good outcome after surgical resection. When they are diagnosed in the mid-trimester, however, hydrops frequently develops secondary to cardiac failure from arteriovenous shunting, indicating impending fetal demise.[138] The San Francisco group have recently reported success with open surgical resection of the tumour,[8] although their previous more problematic experience had suggested that resection must take place before the initiation of end-stage cardiac failure in the fetus and the hydropic placenta leading to the maternal 'mirror syndrome'.[8,218]

FUTURE EXPERIMENTAL WORK

Ongoing animal experimental work suggests that fetal surgery may have some role in the correction of other fetal conditions in the future. An experimental model of spina bifida in the sheep suggests that in utero correction of the spinal defect can prevent the neurological dysfunction normally seen at birth.[244] Nevertheless, much more experimental work will need to be done to convince many that open fetal surgery, with all its attendant risks for the mother and the pregnancy, will be an appropriate and cost-effective option for this and other structural abnormalities.

REFERENCES

1. Abramowicz J S, Warsof S L, Doyle D L, Smith D, Levy D L 1989 Congenital cystic hygroma of the neck diagnosed prenatally: outcome with normal and abnormal karyotype. Prenatal Diagnosis 9: 321–327
2. Achiron R, Achiron A, Yagel S 1993 First trimester transvaginal sonographic diagnosis of Dandy–Walker malformation. Journal of Clinical Ultrasound 21: 62–64
3. Adinolfi M, Sherlock J, Soothill P, Rodeck C 1995 Molecular evidence of fetal-derived chromosome 21 markers (STRs) in transcervical samples. Prenatal Diagnosis 15: 35–39
4. Adzick N S, Harrison M R, Glick P L et al 1985 Fetal cystic adenomatoid malformation: prenatal diagnosis and natural history. Journal of Pediatric Surgery 20: 483–488
5. Adzick N S, Harrison M R, Glick P L, Nakayama D K, Manning F A 1985 Diaphragmatic hernia in the fetus: prenatal diagnosis and outcome in 94 cases. Journal of Pediatric Surgery 20: 357–361
6. Adzick N S, Harrison M R, Glick P L et al 1986 Fetal surgery in the primate. III Maternal outcome after fetal surgery. Journal of Pediatric Surgery 21: 477–480
7. Adzick N S, Harrison M R, Flake A W 1993 Fetal surgery for cystic adenomatoid malformation of the lung. Journal of Pediatric Surgery 28: 1–6
8. Adzick N S, Crombleholme T M, Morgan M A, Quinn T M 1997 A rapidly growing teratoma. Lancet 349: 538
9. Alfirevic Z, Neilson J P 1995. Doppler ultrasonography in high-risk pregnancies: systematic review with meta-analysis. American Journal of Obstetrics and Gynecology 172: 1379–1387
10. Alford C A, Neva F A, Weller T H 1964 Virologic and serologic studies on human products of conception after maternal rubella. New England Journal of Medicine 271: 1275–1281

11. Allen L C, Doran T A, Miskin M, Rudd N L, Benzie R J, Sheffield W 1982 Ultrasound and amniotic fluid alpha-fetoprotein in the prenatal diagnosis of spina bifida. Obstetrics and Gynecology 60: 169–173
12. Allan L D, Chita S K, Sharland G K, Maxwell D, Priestly K 1991 Flecainide in the treatment of fetal tachycardias. British Heart Journal 65: 46–48
13. Anand A, Gray E S, Brown T, Clewley J P, Cohen B J 1987 Human parvovirus infection in pregnancy and hydrops fetalis. New England Journal of Medicine 316: 183–186
14. Andres R L, Brace R A 1990 The development of hydrops fetalis in the ovine fetus after lymphatic ligation or lymphatic excision. American Journal of Obstetrics and Gynecology 162: 1331–1334
15. Anton-Lamprecht I, Jovanovich V, Arnold M L, Rauskolb R, Kern B, Schenck W 1981 Prenatal diagnosis of epidermolysis bullosa dystrophica Hallopeau Siemens with electron microscopy of fetal skin. Lancet ii: 1077–1079
16. Arulkumaran S, Nicolini U, Fisk N M, Rodeck C H 1990 Fetal vesicorectal fistula causing oligohydramnios in the second trimester. British Journal of Obstetrics and Gynaecology 97: 449–451
17. Bajoria R, Wigglesworth J, Fisk N 1995 Angioarchitecture of monochorionic placentas in relation to twin–twin transfusion syndrome. American Journal of Obstetrics and Gynecology 172: 856–863
18. Bang J 1983 Ultrasound guided fetal blood sampling. In. Albertini A, Crosignani P F (eds) Progress in perinatal medicine. Excerpta Medica, Amsterdam, p. 223
19. Bang J 1985 Intrauterine needle diagnosis. In: Holm HA, Kristensen JK (eds) Interventional ultrasound. Munksgaard, Copenhagen, pp 122–128
20. Bang J, Bock J E, Trolle D 1982 Ultrasound guided fetal intravenous transfusion for severe rhesus haemolytic disease. British Medical Journal 284: 373–374
21. Barret J, Chitayat D, Sermer M et al 1995 The prognostic factors in the prenatal diagnosis of the echogenic fetal lung. Prenatal Diagnosis 15: 849–853
22. Barss V A, Benacerraf B R, Frigoletto F D 1984 Second trimester oligohydramnios, a predictor of poor fetal outcome. Obstetrics and Gynecology 64: 608–610
23. Barss V A, Benacerraf B R, Frigoletto F D 1985 Ultrasonographic determination of chorion type in twin gestation. Obstetrics and Gynecology 66: 779–783
24. Benacerraf B R, Frigoletto F D 1985 Mid-trimester fetal thoracocentesis. Journal of Clinical Ultrasound 13: 202–204
25. Benacerraf B R, Frigoletto F D, Greene M F 1986 Abnormal facial features and extremities in human trisomy syndromes: prenatal ultrasound appearances. Radiology 159: 243–246
26. Benacerraf B R, Frigoletto F D, Wilson M 1986 Successful mid-trimester thoracocentesis with analysis of the lymphocyte subpopulation in the pleural effusion. Obstetrics and Gynecology 155: 398–399
27. Benacerraf B R, Greene M F, Saltzman D H et al 1988 Early amniocentesis for prenatal cytogenetic evaluation. Radiology 169: 709–710
28. Benacerraf B R, Saltzman D H, Estroff J A, Frigoletto F D 1990 Abnormal karyotype of fetuses with omphalocele: prediction based on omphalocele contents. Obstetrics and Gynecology 75: 317–319
29. Benaccerraf B R, Harlow B, Frigoletto F D 1990 Are choroid plexus cysts an indication for mid-trimester amniocentesis? American Journal of Obstetrics and Gynecology 162: 1001–1006
30. Bennett P R, Kim C L, Colin Y et al 1993 Prenatal determination of fetal RhD type by DNA amplification following chorion villus biopsy or amniocentesis. New England Journal of Medicine 329: 607–610
31. Beretsky L, Lankin D H, Rusoff J H, Phelan L 1984 Sonographic differentiation between the multicystic dysplastic kidney and the uretopelvic junction obstruction in utero using high resolution real time scanners employing digital detection. Journal of Clinical Ultrasound 11: 349–356
32. Berkowitz R L, Beyta Y, Sadovsky E 1982 Death in utero due to Kell sensitisation without excessive elevation of the Delta OD450 in amniotic fluid. Obstetrics and Gynecology 60: 746–749
33. Berkowitz R L, Chitkara U, Goldberg J D, Wilkins I, Chervenak F A, Lynch L 1986 Intrauterine intravascular transfusion for severe red blood cell iso-immunisation: ultrasound guided percutaneous approach. American Journal of Obstetrics and Gynecology 60: 746–749
34. Berkowitz R L, Lynch L, Chitkara U, Wilkins I A, Mehalek K E, Alvarez E 1988 Selective reduction of multifetal pregnancies in the first trimester. New England Journal of Medicine 318: 1043–1047
35. Berkowitz R L, Lynch L, Stone J, Alvarez M 1996 The current status of multifetal pregnancy reduction. American Journal of Obstetrics and Gynecology 174: 1265–1272
36. Berman D J, Maizels M 1982 The role of urinary obstruction in the genesis of renal dysplasia. A model in the chick embryo. Journal of Urology 128: 1091–1096
37. Berrebi A, Kobuch W E, Bessieres M H, Bloom M C, Rolland M, Sarramon M F 1994 Termination of pregnancy for maternal toxoplasmosis. Lancet 355: 36–39
38. Berry S, Lecolier B, Smith R S et al 1995 Predictive value of fetal serum β-microglobulin for neonatal renal function. Lancet 345: 1277–1278
39. Bewley S, Roberts L J, Mackinson A M, Rodeck C H 1995 First trimester nuchal translucency: problems with screening the general population 2. British Journal of Obstetrics and Gynaecology 102: 386–388
40. Bianchi D W, Zickwolf G K, Weil G J, Sylvester S, DeMaria M A 1996 Male fetal progenitor cells persist in maternal blood for as long as 27 years postpartum. Proceedings of the National Academy of Science USA 93: 705–708
41. Bierman F Z, Baxi L, Jaffe I, Driscoll I 1989 Fetal hydrops and congenital complete heart block: response to maternal steroid therapy. Journal of Pediatrics 112: 646–648
42. Blanchette V S, Chen L, Salmon de Freiberg S, Hoghan V A, Trudel E, Decary F 1990 Immunization to the Pl^{A1} antigen: results of a prospective study. British Journal of Haematology 74: 209–215
43. Blumenthal D H, Rushovich A M, Williams R K, Rochester D 1982 Prenatal sonographic findings of meconium peritonitis with pathological correlation. Journal of Clinical Ultrasound 10: 350–352
44. Bogart M H, Golbus M S, Sorg N D, Jones O W 1989 Human chorionic gonadotrophin levels in pregnancies with aneuploid fetuses. Prenatal Diagnosis 9: 379–384
45. Bonaventure J, Rousseau F, Legeani-Mallet L, le Merrer M, Munnich A, Maroteaux P 1996 Common mutations in fibroblast growth receptor 3 (FGR-3) gene account for achondroplasia, hypochondroplasia, and thanatophoric dwarfism. American Journal of Medical Genetics 63: 148–154
46. Bovicelli L, Orsini L F, Grannum P A T, Pittalis M C, Toffoli C, Dolcini B 1989 A new funipuncture technique: two needle ultrasound and needle biopsy guided procedure. Obstetrics and Gynecology 73: 428–431
47. Bowell P, Wainscoat J S, Peto T E et al 1982 Maternal anti-D concentrations and outcome in rhesus haemolytic disease of the newborn. British Medical Journal 285: 327–329
48. Bower S J, Flack N J, Sepulveda W, Talbert D, Fisk N M 1995 Uterine artery blood flow response to correction of amniotic fluid volume. American Journal of Obstetrics and Gynecology 173: 502–507
49. Bowman J M, Pollack J M 1965 Amniotic fluid spectrophotometry and early delivery in the management of erythroblastosis fetalis. Pediatrics 35: 815–835
50. Braithwaite J M, Armstrong M A, Economides D L 1996. Assessment of fetal anatomy at 12–13 weeks gestation by transabdominal and transvaginal sonography. British Journal of Obstetrics and Gynaecology 103: 82–85
51. Brambati B, MacIntosh M C M, Teisner B 1993 Low maternal serum levels of pregnancy associated plasma protein A (PAPP-A) in the first trimester in association with abnormal fetal karyotype. British Journal of Obstetrics and Gynaecology 100: 324–326
52. Breed A S, Mantingh A, Beekhuis H, Kloosterman M D, Bolscher H T, Anders GJ 1990 The predictive value of cytogenetic diagnosis after CVS: 1500 cases. Prenatal Diagnosis 10: 101–110
53. Brons J T J, Wladimiroff J W, Van Der Harten J J et al 1988 Prenatal ultrasonographic diagnosis of osteogenesis imperfecta. American Journal of Obstetrics and Gynecology 159: 176–181
54. Bronshtein M, Blumenfeld I, Kohn J, Blumenfeld Z 1994 Detection of cleft lip by early second-trimester transvaginal sonography. Obstetrics and Gynecology 84: 73–76
55. Bui T H, Iselius L, Lindsten J 1984 European collaborative study on prenatal diagnosis: mosaicism, pseudomosaicism and single abnormal cells in amniotic fluid cell cultures. Prenatal Diagnosis 4: 145–162

56. Burke G, Stuart B, Crowley P, Scanaill S N, Drumm J 1990 Is intrauterine growth retardation with normal umbilical artery blood flow a benign condition? British Medical Journal 300: 1044–1045
57. Burrows R F, Kelton J G 1993 Fetal thrombocytopenia and its relation to maternal thrombocytopenia. New England Journal of Medicine 329: 1463–1466
58. Burrows R F, Kelton J G 1990 Thrombocytopenia at delivery: a prospective survey of 6715 deliveries. American Journal of Obstetrics and Gynecology 163: 731–734
59. Burrows R F, Kelton J G 1990 Low fetal risks in pregnancies associated with idiopathic thrombocytopenic purpura. American Journal of Obstetrics and Gynecology 163: 1147–1150
60. Bussel J B, Berkowhitz R L, McFarland J G, Lynch L, Chitkara U 1988 Antenatal treatment of neonatal alloimmune thrombocytopenia. New England Journal of Medicine 319: 1372–1378
61. Bussel J B, Berkowitz R L, Lynch L et al 1996 Antenatal management of alloimmune thrombocytopenia with intravenous gamma-globulin: A randomized trial of the addition of low-dose steroid to intravenous gamma-globulin. American Journal of Obstetrics and Gynecology 174: 1414–1423
62. Bussel J B, McFarland J G, Kaplan C and Working Party 1991 Recommendations for the evaluation and treatment of neonatal autoimmune and alloimmune thrombocytopenia. Thrombosis and Haemostasis 65: 631–634
63. Cabrol D, Landesman R, Muller J, Uzan M, Sureau C, Saxena B B 1987 Treatment of polyhydramnios with prostaglandin synthetase inhibitor (indomethacin). American Journal of Obstetrics and Gynecology 157: 422–426
64. Callen D F, Korban G, Dawson G et al 1988 Extra embryonic/fetal karyotypic discordance during diagnostic chorionic villus sampling. Prenatal Diagnosis 8: 453–460
65. Campbell S, Johnstone F D, Holt E M et al 1972 Anencephaly: early ultrasonic diagnosis and active management. Lancet ii: 1226–1227
66. Campbell S, Pearce J M 1983 Ultrasound visualization of congenital malformations. British Medical Bulletin 39: 322–331
67. Campbell J, Gilbert W M, Nicolaides K H, Campbell S 1987 Ultrasound screening for spina bifida: cranial and cerebellar signs in a high-risk population. Obstetrics and Gynecology 70: 247–250
68. Canick J A, Knight G J, Palomaki G E, Haddow J E, Cuckle H S, Wald N J 1988 Maternal serum unconjugated oestriol as an antenatal screening test for Down's syndrome. British Journal of Obstetrics and Gynaecology 95: 330–333
69. Cardoza J D, Goldstein R B, Filly R A 1988 Exclusion of fetal ventriculomegaly with a single measurement: the width of the lateral ventricular atrium. Radiology 169: 711–714
70. Carlan S J, O'Brien W F, O'Leary T D, Mastrogiannis D 1992 Randomised comparative trial of indomethacin and sulindac for the treatment of refractory preterm labor. Obstetrics and Gynecology 79: 223–228
71. Carlson D E, Platt L D, Medearis A L, Horenstein J 1990 Quantifiable polyhydramnios: diagnosis and management. Obstetrics and Gynecology 75: 989–993
72. Castillo R A, Devoe L D, Falls G, Holzman G B, Hadi H A, Fadel H E 1987 Pleural effusions and pulmonary hypoplasia. American Journal of Obstetrics and Gynecology 157: 1252–1255
73. Chamberlain P F, Manning F A, Morrison I, Harman C R, Lange I R 1984 Ultrasound evaluation of AFV. II. The relationship of increased AFV to perinatal outcome. American Journal of Obstetrics and Gynecology 150: 250–254
74. Chamberlain P F, Cumming M, Tochia M G, Biehl D, Manning F A 1985 Ovine fetal urine production following maternal intravenous furosemide administration. American Journal of Obstetrics and Gynecology 151: 815–819
75. Chernick V, Reed M H 1970 Pneumothorax and chylothorax in the neonatal period. Journal of Pediatrics 76: 624–632
76. Chervenak F A, Isaacson G, Blakemore K J et al 1983 Fetal cystic hygroma. Causes and natural history. New England Journal of Medicine 309: 822–825
77. Chinn D H, Filly R A, Callen P W 1983 Congenital diaphragmatic hernia diagnosed prenatally by ultrasound. Radiology 148: 119–123
78. Chitkara U, Cogswell C, Norton K, Wilkins I A, Mehalek K, Berkowitz R L 1988 Choroid plexus cysts in the fetus: a benign anatomic variant or pathological entity? Report of 41 cases and review of the literature. Obstetrics and Gynecology 72: 185–189
79. Chitkara U, Wilkins I, Lynch L, Mehalek K, Berkowitz R L 1988 The role of sonography in assessing severity of fetal anemia in Rh and Kell iso-immunised pregnancies. Obstetrics and Gynecology 71: 393–398
80. Chitty L S, Hunt G H, Moore J, Lobb M O 1991 Effectiveness of routine ultrasonography in detecting fetal structural abnormalities in a low risk population. British Medical Journal 303: 1165–1169
81. Chodirker B N, Harman C R, Greenburg C R 1988 Spontaneous resolution of a cystic hygroma in a fetus with Turner syndrome. Prenatal Diagnosis 8: 291–296
82. Chua S, Ostman-Smith I, Sellers S, Redman C W G 1991 Congenital heart block with hydrops fetalis treated with high-dose dexamethasone: a case report. Journal of Obstetrics and Gynecology and Reproductive Biology 42: 155–158
83. Chudleigh P, Pearce M J, Campbell S 1984 The prenatal diagnosis of transient cysts of the fetal choroid plexus. Prenatal Diagnosis 4: 135–137
84. Copel J A, Cullen M, Green J J, Mahoney M J, Hobbins J C, Kleinman C S 1988 The frequency of aneuploidy in prenatally diagnosed congenital heart disease: an indication for fetal karyotyping. American Journal of Obstetrics and Gynecology 158: 409–413
85. Copel J A, Grannum P A, Belanger K, Green J, Hobbins J C 1988 Pulsed Doppler flow–velocity waveforms before and after intrauterine intravascular transfusion for severe erythroblastosis fetalis. American Journal of Obstetrics and Gynecology 158: 768–774
86. Cradock-Watson J E, Miller E, Ridehalgh M K S, Terry G M, Ho-Terry L 1989 Detection of rubella virus in fetal and placental tissues and in the throats of neonates after serologically confirmed rubella in pregnancy. Prenatal Diagnosis 9: 91–96
87. Cuckle H, Wald N J, Thompson N G 1987 Estimating a woman's risk of having a pregnancy associated with Down's syndrome using her age and maternal serum alpha-fetoprotein level. British Journal of Obstetrics and Gynaecology 94: 387–402
88. Daffos F, Capella-Pavlovsky M, Forestier F 1983 Fetal blood sampling via the umbilical cord using a needle guided by ultrasound. Report of 66 cases. Prenatal Diagnosis 3: 271–277
89. Daffos F, Capella-Pavlovsky M, Forestier F 1985 Fetal blood sampling during pregnancy with use of a needle guided by ultrasound: a study of 606 consecutive cases. American Journal of Obstetrics and Gynecology 153: 655–660
90. Daffos F, Forestier F, Kaplan C, Cox W 1988 Prenatal diagnosis and management of bleeding disorders with fetal blood sampling. American Journal of Obstetrics and Gynecology 158: 939–946
91. Daffos F, Forestier F, Capella-Pavlovsky M et al 1988 Prenatal management of 746 pregnancies at risk for congenital toxoplasmosis. New England Journal of Medicine 318: 271–275
92. Dallaire L, Potier M 1986 Amniotic fluid. In Milunsky A (ed) Genetic disorders and the fetus. Plenum Press, New York, pp 53–67
93. D'Alton M E, Dudley D K 1989 The ultrasonographic prediction of chorionicity in twin gestation. American Journal of Obstetrics and Gynecology 160: 557–561
94. Danpure C J, Jennings P J, Penketh R J, Wise P J, Rodeck C H 1989 Fetal liver alanine: glyoxalate aminotransferase and the prenatal diagnosis of primary hyperoxaluria Type I. Prenatal Diagnosis 9: 271–278
95. Danskin F H, Neilson J P 1989 Twin-to-twin transfusion syndrome: what are the appropriate diagnostic criteria? American Journal of Obstetrics and Gynecology 161: 365–369
96. Davis G K, Farquhar C M, Allan L D, Crawford D C, Chapman M G 1990 Structural cardiac abnormalities in the fetus: reliability of prenatal diagnosis and outcome. British Journal of Obstetrics and Gynaecology 97: 27–31
97. Davis L E, Tweed G V, Chin T D et al 1971 Intrauterine diagnosis of cytomegalovirus infection: viral recovery from amniocentesis fluid. American Journal of Obstetrics and Gynecology 109: 1217–1219
98. de Crespigny L, Robinson H P 1986 Amniocentesis: a comparison of 'monitored' versus 'blind' needle insertion technique. Australian and New Zealand Journal of Obstetrics and Gynaecology 26: 124–128
99. de Crespigny L C, Robinson H P, Quinn M, Doyle L, Ross A, Cauchi M 1985 Ultrasound guided fetal blood transfusion for severe rhesus iso-immunisation. Obstetrics and Gynecology 66: 529–532
100. De Lia J E, Kuhlmann R S, Harstad T W, Cruikshank D P 1995 Fetoscopic laser ablation of placental vessels in severe previable twin–twin transfusion syndrome. American Journal of Obstetrics and Gynecology 172: 1202–1211

101. Denbow M, Kyle P, Fogliani R, Johnson P, Fisk N 1997 Selective termination by intrahepatic vein alcohol injection of a monochorionic twin pregnancy discordant for fetal abnormality. British Journal of Obstetrics and Gynaecology 104: 626–627
102. Desmonts G, Couvreur J 1974 Congenital toxoplasmosis: a prospective study of 378 pregnancies. New England Journal of Medicine 290: 1110–1116
103. de Vore GR 1985 Prenatal diagnosis of congenital heart disease: a practical approach for the fetal ultrasonographer. Journal of Clinical Ultrasound 13: 229–235
104. de Vries L, Connell J, Bydder J M et al 1988 Recurrent intracranial haemorrhages in utero in an infant with alloimmune thrombocytopenia. British Journal of Obstetrics and Gynaecology 95: 299–302
105. Eady R A J, Gunner D B, Rodeck C H, Garner A 1983 Prenatal diagnosis of oculocutaneous albinism by electron microscopy of fetal skin. Journal of Investigative Dermatology 80: 210–212
106. Eichenbaum S Z, Krumins E J, Fortune D W, Duke J 1986 False negative finding on chorionic sampling (letter) Lancet ii: 391
107. Elder J S, Duckett J W, Snyder H M 1987 Intervention for fetal obstructive uropathy: has it been effective? Lancet ii: 1007–1010
108. Elias J, Mazur M, Sabbhaga R, Esterly J, Simpson J L 1980 Prenatal diagnosis of harlequin ichthyosis. Clinical Genetics 17: 275–279
109. Elliot J P, Sawyer S T, Radin T G, Strong R E 1994 Large-volume therapeutic amniocentesis in the treatment of hydramnios. Obstetrics and Gynecology 84: 1025–1027
110. Elser H, Borutto F, Schneider A, Schneider K 1983 Chylothorax in a twin pregnancy of 34 weeks – sonographically diagnosed. European Journal of Obstetrics, Gynaecology and Reproductive Biology 16: 205–211
111. Enders G, Jonatha W 1987 Prenatal diagnosis of intrauterine rubella. Infection 15: 162–164
112. Evans M, Fletcher J C, Zador I E, Newton B W, Quigg M H, Struyk C D 1988 Selective first-trimester termination in octuplet and quadruplet pregnancies: clinical and ethical issues. Obstetrics and Gynecology 71: 289–296
113. Evans M I, Dommergues M, Wapner R, Lynch L, Dumez Y, Goldberg I D 1993 Efficacy of transabdominal multifetal pregnancy reduction: collaborative experience amongst the world's largest centres. Obstetrics and Gynecology 82: 61–66
114. Evans M I, Goldberg J D, Dommergues M et al 1994 Efficacy of second-trimester selective termination for fetal abnormalities: international collaborative experience among the world's largest centers. American Journal of Obstetrics and Gynecology 171: 90–94
115. Evans M I, Dommergues M, Timor-Tritsch I et al 1994 Transabdominal versus transcervical and transvaginal multifetal pregnancy reduction: international collaborative experience of more than one thousand cases. American Journal of Obstetrics and Gynecology 170: 902–909
116. Eydoux P, Choiset A, Le Porrier N et al 1989 Chromosomal prenatal diagnosis: study of 936 cases of intrauterine abnormalities after ultrasound assessment. Prenatal Diagnosis 9: 255–268
117. Fakhry J, Reiser M, Shapiro L R, Schechter A, Pait L, Glennon A 1986 Increased echogenicity in the lower fetal abdomen: a common normal variant in the second trimester. Journal of Ultrasound in Medicine 5: 489–492
118. Farrant P T 1980 The antenatal diagnosis of oesophageal atresia by ultrasound. British Journal of Radiology 53: 1202–1203
119. Feingold M, Cetrulo C L, Newton E R, Weiss J, Shakr C, Shmoys S 1986 Serial amniocenteses in the treatment of twin–twin transfusion with acute polyhydramnios. Acta Genetica Medicina Gemellologica 35: 107–113
120. Fermont L, de Geeter B, Aubry M C, Kachener J, Sidi D 1985 A close collaboration between obstetricians and cardiologists allows antenatal detection of severe cardiac malformation by 2D echocardiography. In: Second World Congress of Paediatric Cardiology, Springer-Verlag, New York, p10
121. Filly R 1989 Level 1, level 2, level 3 obstetric sonography: I'll see your level and raise you one (letter). Radiology 172: 312
122. Filly R A, Golbus M S 1982 Ultrasonography of the normal and pathological fetal skeleton. Radiology Clinics of North America 20: 311–388
123. Filly R A, Golbus M S, Carey J C, Hall J G 1981 Short limbed dwarfism: ultrasonic diagnosis by mensuration of the fetal femoral length. Radiology 138: 653–656
124. Finberg H J 1992 The 'twin-peak' sign: reliable evidence of dichorionic twinning. Journal of Ultrasound Medicine 11: 571–577
125. Firth H V, Boyd P A, Chamberlain P F, MacKenzie I Z, Lindenbaum R H, Huson SM 1991 Severe limb abnormalities after chorion villus sampling at 56–66 days gestation. Lancet 337: 762–763
126. Firth H V, Boyd P A, Chamberlain P F, MacKenzie I Z, Morriss-Kay G M, Huson S M 1994 Analysis of limb reduction defects in babies exposed to chorion villus sampling. Lancet 343: 1069–1071
127. Fisk N M 1988 Modifications to selective conservative management in preterm premature rupture of the membranes. Obstetric and Gynecological Survey 43: 328–334
128. Fisk N M, Bennett P, Warwick R M et al 1994 Clinical utility of fetal RhD typing in alloimmunized pregnancies by means of polymerase chain reaction on amniocytes or chorionic villi. American Journal of Obstetrics and Gynecology 171: 50–54
129. Fisk N M, Borrell A, Hubinont C, Tannirandorn Y, Nicolini U, Rodeck C H 1990 Fetofetal transfusion syndrome: do the neonatal criteria apply in utero? Archives of Disease in Childhood 65: 657–661
130. Fisk N M, Ronderos-Dumit D, Soliani A, Nicolini U, Vaughan J I, Rodeck C H 1991. Diagnostic and therapeutic transabdominal amnioinfusion in oligohydramnios. Obstetrics and Gynecology 78: 270–278
131. Fisk N M, Tannirandorn Y, Santolaya J, Nicolini U, Letsky E A, Rodeck C H 1989 Fetal macrocytosis in association with chromosomal abnormalities. Obstetrics and Gynecology 74: 611–616
132. Fisk N M, Tannirandorn Y, Nicolini U, Talbert D G, Rodeck C H 1990 Amniotic pressure in disorders of amniotic fluid volume. Obstetrics and Gynecology 76: 210–214
133. Fisk N M, Vaughan J, Talbert D 1994 Impaired fetal blood gas status and polyhydramnios and its relation to raised amniotic pressure. Obstetrics and Gynecology 76: 210–214
134. Fiske C E, Filly R A, Callen P W 1981 Sonographic measurement of lateral ventricular width in early ventricular dilatation. Journal of Clinical Ultrasound 9: 303–307
135. Flack N J, Zosmer N, Bennett P R, Vaughan J, Fisk N M 1993 Amiodarone given by 3 routes to terminate fetal atrial flutter associated with severe hydrops. Obstetrics and Gynecology 82: 714–716
136. Flake A W 1996 Fetal tracheal ligation for right-sided congenital diaphragmatic hernia. (Abstract: Meeting, International Fetal Medicine and Surgery Society, Italy)
137. Flake A W 1998 In utero haematopoietic stem cell transplantation. In: Rodeck C H, Whittle M (eds) Fetal medicine: basic science and clinical practice. Churchill Livingstone, Edinburgh
138. Flake A W, Harrison M R, Adzick N S, Laberge J M, Warsof S L 1986 Fetal sacrococcygeal teratoma. Journal of Pediatric Surgery 21: 563–666
139. Flake A W, Roncarolo M G, Puck J M et al 1996 Treatment of X-linked severe combined immunodeficiency by in utero transplantation of paternal bone marrow. New England Journal of Medicine 335: 1806–1810
140. Forestier F, Daffos F, Galacteros F, Bardakjian J, Rainaut M, Beuzard Y 1986 Hematological values of 163 normal fetuses between 18 and 30 weeks of gestation. Pediatric Research 20: 342–346
141. Forestier F, Daffos F, Rainout M, Bruneau M, Trivin F 1987 Blood chemistry of normal human fetuses at mid-trimester of pregnancy. Pediatric Research 21: 579–583
142. Friedman J M, Aster R H 1985 Neonatal alloimmune thrombocytopenic purpura and congenital porencephaly in two siblings associated with a 'new' maternal antiplatelet antibody. Blood 65: 1412–1415
143. Frohn-Mulder I M, Stewart P A, Witsenburg M, Den Hollander N S, Wladimiroff J W, Hess J 1995 The efficacy of flecainide versus digoxin in the management of fetal supraventricular tachycardia. Prenatal Diagnosis 15: 1297–1302
144. Froster U G, Jackson L 1996 Limb defects and chorionic villus sampling: results from an international registry, 1992–94. Lancet 347: 489–494
145. Fujimoto W Y, Seegmiller J E, Uhlendorf B W, Jacobsen C B 1968 Biochemical diagnosis of an X-linked disease in utero. Lancet ii: 511–512
146. Furness M E 1987 Choroid plexus cysts and trisomy 18 (letter). Lancet ii: 693
147. Furness M E, Barbary J E, Verco P W 1987 Fetal head shape in spina

bifida in the second trimester. Journal of Clinical Ultrasound 15: 451–453
148. Galea P, Scott J M, Goel K M 1982 Feto-fetal transfusion syndrome. Archives of Disease in Childhood 57: 781–783
149. Ganshirt A D, Borjesson S R, Burschyk M et al 1993. Detection of fetal trisomies 21 and 18 from maternal blood using triple gradient and magnetic cell sorting. American Journal of Reproductive Immunology 30: 194–201
150. Gardosi J, Mongelli M 1993. Risk assessment adjusted for gestational age in maternal serum screening for Down's syndrome. British Medical Journal 306: 1509–1511
151. Ghidini A, Sepulveda W, Lockwood C, Romero R 1993 Complications of fetal blood sampling. American Journal of Obstetrics and Gynecology 168: 1339–1344
152. Gilbert W M, Nicolaides K H 1987 Fetal omphalocele: associated malformations and chromosomal defects. Obstetrics and Gynecology 70: 633–635
153. Glick P L, Harrison M R, Noall R A, Villa R L 1983 Correction of congenital hydronephrosis in utero III: early mid-trimester ureteral obstruction produces renal dysplasia. Journal of Pediatric Surgery 18: 681–687
154. Glick P L, Harrison M R, Adzick N S, Noall R A, Villa R L 1984 Correction of congenital hydronephrosis in utero. IV: In utero decompression prevents renal dysplasia. Journal of Pediatric Surgery 19: 649–657
155. Glick P L, Harrison M R, Golbus M S et al 1985 Management of the fetus with congenital hydronephrosis II: prognostic criteria and selection for treatment. Journal of Pediatric Surgery 20: 376–387
156. Golbus M S, Sagebiel R W, Filly R A, Gindhart T D, Hall J G 1980 Prenatal diagnosis of bullous ichthyosiform erythroderma (epidermolysis hyperkeratosis) by fetal skin biopsy. New England Journal of Medicine 302: 93–95
157. Golbus M S, Simpson T J, Koresawa M, Appelman Z, Alpers C E 1988 The prenatal determination of glucose 6 phosphatase activity by fetal liver biopsy. Prenatal Diagnosis 8: 401–404
158. Golbus M S, Cunningham N, Goldberg J D, Anderson R, Filly R, Callen P 1988 Selective termination of multiple gestation. American Journal of Medical Genetics 31: 339–348
159. Goldstein R B, Filly R B, Callen P W 1989 Sonography of anencephaly: pitfalls in early diagnosis. Journal of Clinical Ultrasound 17: 397–402
160. Gonsoulin W, Moise K J, Kirshon B, Cotton D B, Wheller J M, Carpenter R J 1990 Outcome of twin–twin transfusion syndrome diagnosed before 28 weeks of gestation. Obstetrics and Gynecology 75: 214–216
161. Grannum P A, Copel J, Plaxe S C, Scioscia A L, Hobbins J C 1986 In utero exchange transfusion by direct intravascular injection in severe erhythroblastosis fetalis. New England Journal of Medicine 314: 1431–1434
162. Grannum P A, Ghidini A, Scioscia A, Copel J A, Romero R, Hobbins J C 1989 Assessment of fetal renal reserve in low level obstructive uropathy. Lancet i: 281–282
163. Griffith-Jones M D, Miller D, Lilford R J, Scott J, Bulmer J 1992 Detection of fetal DNA in transcervical swabs from first trimester pregnancies by gene amplification: a new route to prenatal diagnosis? British Journal of Obstetrics and Gynaecology 99: 508–511
164. Groves A M, Allan L D, Rosenthal E 1993 Therapeutic use of inotropes in complete heart block in the fetus. British Heart Journal 69: 17 (Abstract)
165. Hackett G A, Nicolaides K H, Campbell S 1987 Doppler ultrasound assessment of fetal and uteroplacental circulations in severe second trimester oligohydramnios. British Journal of Obstetrics and Gynaecology 94: 1074–1077
166. Haddow J E, Palomaki G E, Knight G J, Cunningham G C, Lustig L S, Boyd PA 1994 Reducing the need for amniocentesis in women 35 years of age or older with serum markers for screening. New England Journal of Medicine 330: 1114–1118
167. Handyside A H, Lesko J G, Tarin J J, Winston R M, Hughes M R 1992 Birth of a normal girl after in vitro fertilization and preimplantation diagnostic testing for cystic fibrosis. New England Journal of Medicine 327: 905–909
168. Hanson F W, Zorn E M, Tennant F R, Marianos S, Samuels S 1987 Amniocentesis before 15 weeks gestation: outcome, risks and technical problems. American Journal of Obstetrics and Gynecology 156: 1524–1531
169. Harman C R 1984 Maternal furosemide may not provoke urine production in the compromised fetus. American Journal of Obstetrics and Gynecology 150: 322–323
170. Harman C R 1995 Invasive techniques in the management of alloimmune anaemia. In: Harman C R (ed) Invasive fetal testing and treatment. Blackwell Scientific, Boston pp. 107–192
171. Harrison M R, Adzick N S, Flake A W, Jennings R W 1993 The CDH two-step, a dance of necessity. Journal of Pediatric Surgery 28: 813–816
172. Harrison M R, Bressack M A, Churg A M, de Lorimier A A 1980 Correction of congenital diaphragmatic hernia in utero. II: Simulated correction permits fetal lung growth with survival at birth. Surgery 88: 260–268
173. Harrison M R, Filly R A, Parer J T, Faer M J, Jacobson J B, de Lorimier A A 1981 Management of the fetus with a urinary tract malformation. Journal of the American Medical Association 246: 635–639
174. Harrison M R, Golbus M S, Filly R A et al 1982 Management of the fetus with congenital hydronephrosis. Journal of Pediatric Surgery 17: 728–742
175. Harrison M R, Nakayama D K, Noall R, de Lorimier A A 1982 Correction of congenital hydronephrosis in utero II: Decompression reverses the effects of obstruction on the fetal lung and urinary tract. Journal of Pediatric Surgery 17: 965–974
176. Harrison M R, Ross N A, Noall R, de Lorimier A A 1983 Correction of congenital hydronephrosis in utero. I: The model: fetal urethral obstruction produces hydronephrosis and pulmonary hypoplasia in fetal lambs. Journal of Pediatric Surgery 18: 247–256
177. Harrison M R, Langer J C, Adzick N S et al 1990 Correction of congenital diaphragmatic hernia in utero. V: Initial clinical experience. Journal of Pediatric Surgery 25: 47–57
178. Hecher K, Campbell S, Doyle P, Harrington K, Nicolaides K 1995 Assessment of fetal compromise by Doppler ultrasound investigation of the fetal circulation. Arterial, intracardiac and venous blood flow studies. Circulation 91: 129–138
179. Hegde U M 1985 Immune thrombocytopenia in pregnancy and the newborn. British Journal of Obstetrics and Gynaecology 92: 657–659
180. Hegge F N, Franklin R W, Watson P T, Clahoun B C 1989 An evaluation of the time of discovery of fetal malformations by an indication-based system for ordering obstetric ultrasound. Obstetrics and Gynecology 74: 21–24
181. Hill L M, Breckle R, Thomas M L, Fries J K 1987 Polyhydramnios: ultrasonically detected prevalence and neonatal outcome. Obstetrics and Gynecology 69: 21–25
182. Hislop A, Fairweather D V I, Blackwell R J, Howard S 1984 The effect of amniocentesis and drainage of amniotic fluid on lung development in *Macaca fascicularis*. American Journal of Obstetrics and Gynecology 91: 835–842
183. Hobbins J C, Mahoney M J 1974 In utero diagnosis of haemoglobinopathies: technic for obtaining fetal blood. New England Journal of Medicine 290: 1065–1067
184. Hobbins J C, Romero R, Grannum P, Berkowitz T R L, Cullen M, Mahoney M J 1984 Antenatal diagnosis of renal anomalies with ultrasound. I. Obstructive uropathy. American Journal of Obstetrics and Gynecology 148: 868–877
185. Hohlfield P, Daffos F, Costa J, Thulliez P, Forestier F, Vidaud M 1994 Prenatal diagnosis of congenital toxoplasmosis with a polymerase-chain-reaction test on amniotic fluid. New England Journal of Medicine 331: 695–699
186. Howard H L, Martlew V J, McFadyen I R, Clarke C A 1997 Preventing rhesus haemolytic disease of the newborn by giving anti-D immunoglobulin: are the guidelines being followed? British Journal of Obstetrics and Gynaecology 104: 37–41
187. Hsu L Y F, Perlis T E 1984 The United States survey on chromosome mosaicism and pseudomosaicism in prenatal diagnosis. Prenatal Diagnosis 4: 97–130
188. Hull D, Binns B A, Joyce D 1966 Congenital heart block and widespread fibrosis due to maternal lupus erythematosus. Archives of Diseases of Childhood 41: 688–690
189. Hunter A G W 1987 Neonatal lung function following mid-trimester amniocentesis. Prenatal Diagnosis 7: 431–441
190. Hyett J A, Clayton P T, Moscoso G, Nicolaides K H 1995 Increased first trimester nuchal translucency as a prenatal manifestation of Smith–Lemli–Opitz syndrome. American Journal of Medical Genetics 58: 374–376

191. Hyett J, Moscoso G, Papapanagiotou G, Perdu M, Nicolaides K H 1996 Abnormalities of the heart and great arteries in chromosomally normal fetuses with increased nuchal translucency at 11–13 weeks gestation. Ultrasound in Obstetrics and Gynecology 7: 245–250
192. Isada N B, Pryde P G, Johnson M P, Hallak M, Blessed W B, Evans M I 1992 Fetal intracardiac potassium chloride injection to avoid the hopeless resuscitation of an abnormal abortus: I. Clinical issues. Obstetrics and Gynecology 80: 296–299
193. Itskowitz J, Boldes R, Thaler I et al 1989 Transvaginal ultrasonography-guided aspiration of gestational sacs for selective abortion in multiple pregnancy. American Journal of Obstetrics and Gynecology 160: 215–217
194. Jackson L G, Zachary J M, Fowler S E, Desnick R J, Golbus M S, Ledbetter D 1992 A randomized comparison of transcervical and transabdominal chorionic-villus sampling. New England Journal of Medicine 327: 594–598
195. James D J K, Tindall V R, Richardson T 1983 Is the lecithin–sphingomyelin ratio outdated? British Journal of Obstetrics and Gynaecology 90: 995–1000
196. Jauniaux E, Donner C, Simon P, Vanesse M, Hustin J, Rodesch F 1989 Pathological aspects of the umbilical cord after percutaneous umbilical blood sampling. Obstetrics and Gynecology 73: 215–218
197. Johnson M P, Bukowski T P, Reitleman C, Isada N B, Pryde P G, Eraus M I 1994 In utero surgical treatment of fetal obstructive uropathy: a new comprehensive approach to identify appropriate candidates for vesicoamniotic shunt therapy. American Journal of Obstetrics and Gynecology 170: 1770–1779
198. Kalousek D K, Dill F J 1983 Chromosomal mosaicism confined to the placenta in human conceptions. Science 221: 665–667
199. Kan Y W, Dozy Am 1978 Antenatal diagnosis of sickle cell anaemia by DNA analysis of amniotic-fluid cells. Lancet ii: 910
200. Kan Y W, Valenti C, Giudotti R, Carnazza V, Rieder RF 1974 Fetal blood sampling in utero. Lancet i: 79–80
201. Kaplan C, Daffos F, Forestier F et al 1988 Management of alloimmune thrombocytopenia: antenatal diagnosis and in utero transfusion of maternal platelets. Blood 72: 340–343
202. Kappel B, Nielsen J, Hansen K B, Mikklesen M, Therkelsen A A J 1987 Spontaneous abortion following mid-trimester amniocentesis. Clinical significance of placental perforation and blood stained amniotic fluid. British Journal of Obstetrics and Gynaecology 94: 50–54
203. Kellner L H, Weiner Z, Weiss R R et al 1995 Triple marker (α-fetoprotein, unconjugated estriol, human chorionic gonadotropin) versus α-fetoprotein plus free-β subunit in second-trimester maternal serum screening for fetal Down syndrome: a prospective comparison study. American Journal of Obstetrics and Gynecology 173: 1306–1309
204. Kelton J G, Inwood M J, Barr R M et al 1982 The prenatal prediction of thrombocytopenia in infants of mothers with clinically diagnosed immune thrombocytopenia. American Journal of Obstetrics and Gynecology 144: 449–454
205. King S J, Pilling D W, Walkinshaw S 1995 Fetal echogenic lung lesions: prenatal ultrasound diagnosis and outcome. Pediatric Radiology 25: 208–210
206. Kirshon B, Mari G, Moise K J 1990 Indomethacin therapy in the treatment of symptomatic polyhydramnios. Obstetrics and Gynecology 75: 202–205
207. Kirshon B, Moise K J, Wasserstrum N, Ou C, Huhta J C 1988 Influence of short term indomethacin therapy on fetal urine output. Obstetrics and Gynecology 72: 51–53
207a. Kleinman C S, Copel J A, Weinstein E M, Santulli T V, Hobbins J C 1985 In utero diagnosis and treatment of fetal supraventricular tachycardia. Seminars in Perinatology 9: 113–129
208. Kohl T, Tercanli S, Kececioglu D, Holzgreve W 1995 Direct fetal administration of adenosine for the termination of incessant supraventricular tachycardia. Obstetrics and Gynecology 85: 873–874
209. Koresawa M, Inaba J, Iwasaki H 1987 Fetal blood sampling by liver puncture. Acta Obstetrica Gyaecologica Japonica 39: 395–399
210. Kuliev A M, Modell B, Jackson L et al 1993 Risk evaluation of CVS. Prenatal Diagnosis 13: 197–209
211. Kurth K H, Alleman E R, Schroeder F H 1981 Major and minor complications of posterior urethral valves. Journal of Urology 126: 517–519
212. Kussef B G, Matsouka L Y, Stenn K S, Hobbins J C, Mahoney M J, Hashimoto K 1982 Prenatal diagnosis of Sjogren–Larsson syndrome. Journal of Pediatrics 101: 998–1001
213. Kyle P M, Harman C R, Evans J A et al 1994 Life without amniocentesis: elevated maternal serum α-fetoprotein in the Manitoba program 1986–91. Ultrasound in Obstetrics and Gynecology 4: 199–204
214. Kyle P M, Sepulveda W, Blunt S, Davies G, Cox P M, Fisk N M 1996 High failure rate of postmortem karyotyping after termination for fetal abnormality. Obstetrics and Gynecology 88: 859–862
215. Landwehr J B, Johnson M P, Hume R F, Yaron Y, Sokol R J, Evans M I 1996 Abnormal nuchal findings on screening ultrasonography: aneuploidy stratification on the basis of ultrasonographic anomaly and gestational age at detection. American Journal of Obstetrics and Gynecology 175: 995–999
216. Lange I, Rodeck C H, Morgan-Capner P et al 1982 Prenatal serological diagnosis of intrauterine cytomegalovirus infection. British Medical Journal 284: 1673–1674
217. Langer J C, Fitzgerald P G, Desa D et al 1990 Cervical cystic hygroma in the fetus: clinical spectrum and outcome. Journal of Pediatric Surgery 25: 58–62
218. Langer J C, Harrison M R, Scmidt K G et al 1989 Fetal hydrops and death from sacrococcygeal teratoma: rationale for fetal surgery. American Journal of Obstetrics and Gynecology 160: 1145–1150
219. Laurence K M, Coates S 1962 The natural history of hydrocephalus: detailed analysis of 182 unoperated cases. Archives of Disease in Childhood 37: 345–362
220. Ledbetter D H, Martin A O, Verlinsky Y et al 1990 Cytogenetic results of chorionic villus sampling: high success rate and diagnostic accuracy in the United States collaborative study. American Journal of Obstetrics and Gynecology 162: 495–501
221. Lee S, Bennett P, Overton T, Warwick R, Wu X, Redman C 1996 Prenatal diagnosis of Kell blood group genotypes: KEL1 and KEL2. American Journal of Obstetrics and Gynecology 175: 455–459
222. Levi S, Crouzet P, Schaaps J P et al 1989 Ultrasound screening for fetal malformations. Lancet i: 678
223. Liley A W 1961 Liquor amnii analysis in the management of the pregnancy complicated by rhesus sensitisation. American Journal of Obstetrics and Gynecology 82: 1359–1370
224. Linch D C, Rodeck C H, Nicolaides K H, Jones H M, Brent L 1986 Attempted bone marrow transplantation in a 17 week fetus. Lancet ii: 1453
225. Lipitz S, Ryan G, Samuell C et al 1993 Fetal urine analysis for the assessment of renal function in obstructive uropathy. American Journal of Obstetrics and Gynecology 168: 174–179
226. Lo Y, Bowell P, Selinger M et al 1993 Prenatal determination of fetal RhD status by analysis of peripheral blood of rhesus negative mothers. Lancet 341: 1147–1148
227. Lo Y, Patel P, Sampietro M, Gillmer M D G, Fleming K A, Wainscoat J S 1990 Detection of single-copy fetal DNA sequence from maternal blood. Lancet i: 1463–1464
228. Longaker M T, Adzick N S, Harrison M R 1989 Fetal obstructive uropathy. British Medical Journal 299: 325–326
229. Longaker M T, Laberge J, Dansereau J et al 1989 Primary fetal hydrothorax: natural history and management. Journal of Pediatric Surgery 24: 573–576
230. Luck C A 1992 Value of routine ultrasound scanning at 19 weeks: a four-year study of 8894 deliveries. British Medical Journal 304: 1474–1478
231. Lynch L, Berkowitz R L, Stone J, Alvarez M, Lapinski R 1996 Preterm delivery after selective termination in twin pregnancies. Obstetrics and Gynecology 87: 366–369
232. Machado, M V L, Tynan M J, Curry P V L, Allan L D 1988 Fetal complete heart block. British Heart Journal 60: 512–515
233. Macri J N, Kasturi R V, Krantz D A et al 1990 Maternal serum Down syndrome screening: free beta protein is a more effective marker than human chorionic gonadotropin. American Journal of Obstetrics and Gynecology 163: 1248–1253
234. Mahoney B S, Filly R A, Callen P W, Hricak H, Golbus M S, Harrison M R 1984 Fetal renal dysplasia: sonographic evaluation. Radiology 152: 143–146
235. Mamopoulos M, Assimakopoulos E, Reece E A, Andreou A, Zheng X, Mantelenakis S 1990 Maternal indomethacin therapy in the treatment of polyhydramnios. American Journal of Obstetrics and Gynecology 162: 1225–1229

236. Mandelbrot L, Dumez Y, Muller F, Dommergues M 1991 Prenatal prediction of renal function in fetal obstructive uropathies. Journal of Perinatal Medicine 19: 283–297
237. Manning F A, Harison M R, Rodeck C H and members of the International Fetal Medicine and Surgery Society 1986 Catheter shunts for fetal hydronephrosis and hydrocephalus. New England Journal of Medicine 315: 336–340
238. Maxwell D, Johnson P, Hurley P, Neales K, Allan L, Knott P 1991 Fetal blood sampling and pregnancy loss in relation to indication. British Journal of Obstetrics and Gynaecology 98: 892–897
239. Maxwell D J, Crawford D C, Curry P V, Tynan M J, Allan L D 1988 Obstetric importance, diagnosis and management of fetal tachycardias. British Medical Journal 297: 107–110
240. McCullagh M, MacConnachie I, Garvie D, Dykes E 1994 Accuracy of prenatal diagnosis in congenital cystic adenomatoid malformation. Archives of Disease in Childhood 71: F111–F113
241. McGrath J A, McMillan J R, Dunnill G S et al 1995 Genetic basis of lethal junctional epidermolysis in an affected fetus: implications for prenatal diagnosis in one family. Prenatal Diagnosis 15: 647–654
242. Medical Research Council Working Party on Amniocentesis 1978 An assessment of the hazards of amniocentesis. British Journal of Obstetrics and Gynaecology 85: suppl. 2
243. Mercer L J, Brown L G 1986 Fetal outcome with oligohydramnios in second trimester. Obstetrics and Gynecology 67: 840–842
244. Meuli M, Meuli-Simmen C, Hutchins G M, Yingling C D, Hoffman K D, Harrison M R, Adzick NS 1995 In utero surgery rescues neurological function at birth in sheep with spina bifida. Nature Medicine 1: 342–347
245. Mibashan R S, Rodeck C H 1984 Haemophilia and other genetic defects of haemostasis. In: Rodeck C H, Nicolaides K H (eds) Prenatal diagnosis. Proceedings of the eleventh study group of the Royal College of Obstetricians and Gynaecologists. RCOG, London, pp 179–194
246. Michejda M, Hodgen G D 1981 In utero diagnosis and treatment of non-human primate fetal skeletal anomalies. I: Hydrocephalus. Journal of the American Medical Association 246: 1093–1097
247. Mikkelsen M, Ayme S 1987 Chromosome findings in chorionic villi. A collaborative study. In: Vogel F, Sperling K (eds) Human genetics: Proceedings of the Seventh International Congress. Springer-Verlag, Berlin, pp 597–606
248. Millar D S, Davis L R, Rodeck C H, Nicolaides K H, Mibashan R S 1985 Normal blood cell values in the early mid-trimester fetus. Prenatal Diagnosis 5: 367–373
249. Mohr J 1968 Foetal genetic diagnosis: development of techniques for early sampling of foetal cells. Acta Pathologica, Microbiologica et Immunologica Scandinavica 73: 73–77
250. Moise K J, Carpenter R J, Cotton D B, Wasserstrum N, Kirshon B, Cano L 1988 Percutaneous umbilical cord blood sampling in the evaluation of fetal platelet counts in pregnant patients with autoimmune thrombocytopenic purpura. Obstetrics and Gynecology 72: 346–350
251. Moise K J, Huhta J C, Sharif D S et al 1988 Indomethacin in the treatment of premature labor. Effects on fetal ductus arteriosus. New England Journal of Medicine 319: 327–331
252. Moniz C F, Nicolaides K H, Bamforth F J, Rodeck C H 1985 Normal ranges for biochemical substances relating to renal, hepatic and bone function in fetal and maternal plasma throughout pregnancy. Journal of Clinical Pathology 38: 468–472
253. Monteagudo A, Timor-Tritsch I E, Sharma S 1994 Early and simple determination of chorionic and amniotic type in multifetal gestations in the first fourteen weeks by high-frequency transvaginal ultrasonography. American Journal of Obstetrics and Gynecology 170: 824–829
254. Montemagno R, Soothill P W, Scarcelli M, Rodeck C H 1995 Disappearance of fetal choroid plexus cysts during the second trimester in cases of chromosomal abnormality. British Journal of Obstetrics and Gynaecology 102: 752–753
255. Moore T R, Cayle J E 1990 The amniotic fluid index in normal human pregnancy. American Journal of Obstetrics and Gynecology 162: 1168–1173
256. Moore T R, Longo J, Leopold G R, Casola G, Gosnik B B 1989 The reliability and predictive value of an amniotic fluid scoring system in severe second trimester oligohydramnios. Obstetrics and Gynecology 73: 739–742
257. Morales W J, Stroup M 1985 Intracranial hemorrhage in utero due to isoimmune neonatal thrombocytopenia. Obstetrics and Gynecology 65: 20S–21S
258. Morgan-Capner P, Rodeck C H, Nicolaides K H, Cradock-Watson J A 1985 Prenatal detection of rubella-specific IgM in fetal sera. Prenatal Diagnosis 5: 21–26
259. Meuli M, Meuli-Simmen C, Hutchins G M et al 1995 In utero surgery rescues neurological function in sheep with spina bifida. Nature Medicine 1: 342–347
260. Mueller U W, Hawes C S, Wright A E 1990 Isolation of fetal trophoblast cells from peripheral blood of pregnant women. Lancet 336: 197–200
261. Muller F, Aubry M C, Gasser B, Duchatel F, Boue J, Boue A 1985 Prenatal diagnosis of cystic fibrosis. II. Meconium ileus in affected fetuses. Prenatal Diagnosis 5: 109–117
262. Muller F, Dommergues M, Mandelbrot L, Aubry M C, Fekete C, Dumez Y 1993 Fetal urinary biochemistry predicts postnatal renal function in children with bilateral obstructive uropathies. Obstetrics and Gynecology 82: 813–820
263. Muller-Eckhardt C, Grubert A, Weisheit M 1989 348 cases of suspected neonatal alloimmune thrombocytopenia. Lancet i: 363–366
264. Nakayama D K, Harrison M R, Chinn D H et al 1985 Prenatal diagnosis and natural history of the fetus with a congenital diaphragmatic hernia: initial clinical experience. Journal of Pediatric Surgery 20: 118–124
265. Nakayama D K, Harrison M R, de Lorimier A A 1986 Prognosis of posterior urethral valves presenting at birth. Journal of Pediatric Surgery 21: 43–45
266. National Blood Transfusion Service Immunoglobulin Working Party 1991 Recommendations for the use of anti-D immunoglobulin. Prescribers Journal 31: 137–145
267. National Institutes of Child Health and Human Development 1976 Mid-trimester amniocentesis for prenatal diagnosis. safety and accuracy. Journal of the American Medical Association 236: 1471–1476
268. National Institutes for Health Consensus Development Statement 1984 United States Department of Health and Human Services (NIH publication 84-667), Washington DC
269. Nelson L H, Clark C E, Fishburn J I, Urban R B, Penry M F 1982 Value of serial ultrasonography in the in utero detection of duodenal atresia. Obstetrics and Gynecology 59: 657–660
270. Ney J A, Fee S C, Dooley S L, Socol M L, Minogue J 1989 Factors influencing hemostasis after umbilical vein puncture in vitro. American Journal of Obstetrics and Gynecology 160: 424–426
271. Nicolaides K H, Rodeck C H, Mibashan R S 1985a Obstetric management and diagnosis of haematological disease in the fetus. In: Letsky E A (ed) Haematological disorders in pregnancy. Clinics in Haematology Vol 14, WB Saunders, London, pp 775–805
272. Nicolaides K H, Rodeck C H, Lange I et al 1985 Fetoscopy in the assessment of unexplained fetal hydrops. British Journal of Obstetrics and Gynaecology 92: 671–679
273. Nicolaides K H, Campbell S, Gabbe S G, Giudetti R 1986 Ultrasound screening for spina bifida: cranial and cerebellar signs. Lancet ii: 71–74
274. Nicolaides K H, Rodeck C H, Gosden C N 1986 Rapid karyotyping in non-lethal malformations. Lancet i: 283–287
275. Nicolaides K H, Soothill P W, Rodeck C H, Clewell W 1986 Rh disease: intravascular fetal blood transfusion by cordocentesis. Fetal Therapy 1: 185–192
276. Nicolaides K H, Soothill P W, Rodeck C H, Campbell S 1986 Ultrasound guided sampling of umbilical cord and placental blood to assess fetal well-being. Lancet i: 1065–1067
277. Nicolaides K H, Rodeck C H, Mibashan R S, Kemp J R 1986 Have Liley charts outlived their usefulness? American Journal of Obstetrics and Gynecology 15: 90–94
278. Nicolaides K H, Clewell W H, Rodeck C H 1987 Measurement of human fetoplacental blood volume in erythroblastosis fetalis. American Journal of Obstetrics and Gynecology 157: 50–53
279. Nicolaides K H, Blott M, Greenough M 1987 Chronic drainage of fetal pulmonary cyst (letter). Lancet i: 618
280. Nicolaides K H, Clewell W H, Mibashan R S, Soothill P W, Rodeck C H, Campbell S 1988 Fetal haemoglobin measurement in the assessment of red cell isoimmunization. Lancet i: 1073–1075
281. Nicolaides K H, Bilardo C M, Soothill P W, Campbell S 1988

Absence of end-diastolic frequencies in the umbilical artery: a sign of fetal hypoxia and acidosis. British Medical Journal 297: 1026–1027
282. Nicolaides K H, Fontanorosa M, Gabbe S G, Rodeck C H 1988 Failure of ultrasonographic parameters to predict the severity of fetal anemia in rhesus isoimmunisation. American Journal of Obstetrics and Gynecology 158: 920–926
283. Nicolaides K H, Economides D L, Soothill P W 1989 Blood gases, pH, and lactate in appropriate- and small-for-gestational-age fetuses. American Journal of Obstetrics and Gynecology 161: 996–1001
284. Nicolaides K H, Economides D L 1990 Cordocentesis of small-for-gestational age fetuses. In: Chamberlain G (ed) Modern antenatal care of the fetus. Blackwell Scientific, Oxford, pp 127–149
285. Nicolaides K H, Bilardo C M, Campbell S 1990 Prediction of fetal anemia by measurement of the mean blood velocity in the fetal aorta. American Journal of Obstetrics and Gynecology 162: 209–212
286. Nicolaides K H, Azar G B 1990 Thoraco-amniotic shunting. Fetal Diagnosis and Therapy 5: 153–164
287. Nicolaides K H, Brizot M, Patel F, Snijders R 1994 Comparison of chorionic villus sampling and amniocentesis for fetal karyotyping at 10–13 weeks gestation. Lancet 344: 435–439
288. Nicolaides K H, Brizot M L, Snijders R J M 1994 Fetal nuchal translucency: ultrasound screening for fetal trisomy in the first trimester of pregnancy. British Journal of Obstetrics and Gynaecology 101: 782–786
289. Nicolini U, Santolaya J, Ojo E et al 1988 The fetal intrahepatic vein as an alternative to cord needling for prenatal diagnosis and therapy. Prenatal Diagnosis 8: 665–671
290. Nicolini U, Kochenour N K, Greco P et al 1988 Consequences of fetomaternal haemorrhage after intrauterine transfusion. British Medical Journal 297: 1379–1381
291. Nicolini U, Santolaya J, Fisk N M et al 1988 Changes in fetal acid/base status during intravascular transfusion. Archives of Disease in Childhood 63: 710–714
292. Nicolini U, Rodeck C H, Kochenour N K et al 1988 In-utero platelet transfusion for alloimmune thrombocytopenia. Lancet ii: 506
293. Nicolini U, Talbert D G, Fisk N M, Rodeck C H 1989 Pathophysiology of pressure changes during intrauterine transfusion. American Journal of Obstetrics and Gynecology 160: 1139–1145
294. Nicolini U, Hubinont C, Santolaya J, Fisk N M, Coe A, Rodeck C H 1989 Maternal–fetal glucose gradient in normal pregnancies and in pregnancies complicated by alloimmunization and fetal growth retardation. American Journal of Obstetrics and Gynecology 161: 924–927
295. Nicolini U, Kochenour N K, Greco P, Letsky E, Rodeck C H 1989 When to perform the next intrauterine transfusion in patients with Rh allo-immunization: combined intravascular and intraperitoneal transfusion allows longer intervals. Fetal Therapy 4: 14–20
296. Nicolini U, Santolaya J, Hubinont C, Fisk N M, Maxwell D, Rodeck C H 1989 Visualization of fetal intra-abdominal organs in second trimester severe oligohydramnios by intraperitoneal infusion. Prenatal Diagnosis 9: 191–194
297. Nicolini U, Fisk N M, Rodeck C H, Talbert D G, Wigglesworth J S 1989 Low amniotic pressure in oligohydramnios–is this the cause of pulmonary hypoplasia? American Journal of Obstetrics and Gynecology 161: 1098–1101
298. Nicolini U, Nicolaidis P, Fisk NM et al 1990 Limited role of fetal blood sampling in predicting outcome in intrauterine growth retardation. Lancet ii: 768–772
299. Nicolini U, Nicolaidis P, Fisk N M, Tannirandorn Y, Rodeck C H 1990 Fetal blood sampling from the intrahepatic vein: analysis of safety and clinical experience with 214 procedures. Obstetrics and Gynecology 76: 47–53
300. Nicolini U, Tannirandorn Y, Gonzalez P et al 1990 Continuing controversy in alloimmune thrombocytopenia: fetal hyperimmunoglobulinemia fails to prevent thrombocytopenia. American Journal of Obstetrics and Gynecology 163: 1144–1146
301. Nicolini U, Tannirandorn Y, Vaughan J, Fisk N, Nicolaidis P, Rodeck C H 1991 Further predictors of renal dysplasia in fetal obstructive uropathy: bladder pressure and biochemistry of 'fresh urine'. Prenatal Diagnosis 11: 159–166
302. Nicolini U, Fisk N M, Rodeck C 1992 Fetal urine biochemistry: an index of renal maturation and dysfunction. British Journal of Obstetrics and Gynaecology 99: 46–50
303. Noble P L, Abraha H D, Snijders R J M, Sherwood R, Nicolaides K H 1995 Screening for fetal trisomy 21 in the first trimester of pregnancy: maternal serum free β-hCG and fetal nuchal translucency thickness. Ultrasound in Obstetrics and Gynecology 6: 390–395
304. Nyberg D, Fitzsimmons J, Mack L 1989 Chromosomal abnormalities in fetuses with omphalocele: significance of omphalocele contents. Journal of Ultrasound in Medicine 8: 299–308
305. Oepkes D, Brand R, Vandembusschel F P, Meerman R H, Kanhai H H 1994 The use of ultrasonography and Doppler in the prediction of fetal haemolytic anaemia: a multivariate study. British Journal of Obstetrics and Gynaecology 101: 680–684
306. Oepkes D, Vandenbussche F P, Van Bel F, Kanhai H H 1993 Fetal ductus venosus blood flow velocities before and after treatment of red cell alloimmunised pregnancies. Obstetrics and Gynecology 82: 237–241
307. Old J M, Ward R H T, Petrou M et al 1982 First trimester diagnosis of haemoglobinopathies: three cases. Lancet ii: 1413–1416
308. Orlandi F, Damiani G, Jakil C, Lauricella S, Bertolino O, Maggio A 1990 The risks of early cordocentesis (12–21 weeks): analysis of 500 procedures. Prenatal Diagnosis 10: 425–428
309. Ostlere S J, Irving H C, Lilford R J 1989 A prospective study of the incidence and significance of fetal choroid plexus cysts. Prenatal Diagnosis 9: 205–211
310. Ouzounian J G, Castro M A, Fresquez M, Al-Sulyman O M, Kovacs B W 1996 Prognostic significance of antenatally detected fetal pyelectasis. Ultrasound in Obstetrics and Gynecology 7: 424–428
311. Overton T G, Lighten A D, Fisk N M, Bennett P R 1996 Prenatal diagnosis by minimally invasive first trimester invasive transcervical sampling is unreliable. American Journal of Obstetrics and Gynecology 175: 382–387
312. Paidas M J, Berkowitz R L, Lynch L et al 1995 Alloimmune thrombocytopenia: fetal and neonatal losses related to thrombocytopenia. American Journal of Obstetrics and Gynecology 172: 475–479
313. Patel B, Young Y, Duffy K, Tanner R P, Johnson J, Holliman R E 1993 Immunoglobulin-A detection and the investigation of clinical toxoplasmosis. Journal of Medical Microbiology 38: 286–292
314. Payne S D, Resnik R, Moore T R, Hedriana H L, Kelly T F 1997 Maternal characteristics and risk of severe neonatal thrombocytopenia and intracranial haemorrhage in pregnancies complicated by autoimmune thrombocytopenia. American Journal of Obstetrics and Gynaecology 177: 149–155
315. Peckham C S, Johnson C, Ades A, Pearl K, Chin KS 1987 Early acquisition of cytomegalovirus infection. Archives of Disease in Childhood 62: 780–785
316. Peters M T, Nicolaides K H 1990 Cordocentesis for the diagnosis and treatment of human fetal parvovirus infection. Obstetrics and Gynecology 75: 501–504
317. Petres R E, Redwine F O, Cruickshank D P 1982 Congenital bilateral hydrothorax: antepartum diagnosis and successful intrauterine surgical management. Journal of the American Medical Association 248: 1360–1361
318. Piceni-Sereni L, Bachman C, Pfister U, Buscaglia M, Nicolini U 1988 Prenatal diagnosis of carbamoyl-phosphate synthetase deficiency by fetal liver biopsy. Prenatal Diagnosis 8: 307–309
319. Pilu G, Reece E A, Romero R, Bovicelli L, Hobbins J C 1986 Prenatal diagnosis of craniofacial malformations by ultrasound. American Journal of Obstetrics and Gynecology 155: 45–50
320. Pilu G, Romero R, Rizzo N, Jeanty P, Bovicelli L, Hobbins JC 1987 Criteria for the antenatal diagnosis of holoprosencephaly. American Journal of Perinatology 4: 41–49
321. Pilu G, Romero R, Reece A, Goldstein I, Hobbins J C, Bovicelli L 1988 Subnormal cerebellum in fetuses with spina bifida. American Journal of Obstetrics and Gynecology 158: 1052–1056
322. Poissonier M-H, Brossard Y, Demedeiros N et al 1989 Two hundred intrauterine exchange transfusions in severe blood incompatibilities. American Journal of Obstetrics and Gynecology 161: 709–713
323. Price J O, Elias S, Wachtel S S et al 1991 Prenatal diagnosis with fetal cells isolated from maternal blood by multiparameter flow cytometry. American Journal of Obstetrics and Gynecology 165: 1731–1737
324. Queenan J T 1970 Recurrent acute polyhydramnios. American Journal of Obstetrics and Gynecology 106: 625–626
325. Quintero R, Reich H, Bardicef M, Evans M, Cotton D B, Romero R 1994 Umbilical cord ligation of an acardiac twin by fetoscopy at 19 weeks gestation. New England Journal of Medicine 330: 469–471

326. Reid R S, Sepulveda W, Kyle P M, Davies G 1996 Amniotic fluid culture failure and clinical significance and association with aneuploidy. Obstetrics and Gynecology 87: 588–592
327. Report of the RCOG Working Party on Routine Ultrasound Examination in Pregnancy 1984 RCOG, London, pp 13–16
328. Reuss A, Wladimiroff J W, Stewart P A, Scholtmeijer R J 1988 Non-invasive management of fetal obstructive uropathy. Lancet ii: 949–951
329. Reuwer P J, Sijmons E A, Rietman G W, Van Tiel M W, Briunse H W 1987 Intrauterine growth retardation: prediction of perinatal distress by Doppler ultrasound. Lancet ii: 415–418
330. Revello M G, Percivalle E, Baldanti F 1993 Prenatal treatment of congenital human cytomegalovirus infection by fetal intravascular administration of ganciclovir. Clinical and Diagnosis Virology 1: 61–67
331. Reznikoff-Etievant M F 1988 Management of alloimmune neonatal thrombocytopenia and antenatal thrombocytopenia. Vox Sanguinis 55: 193–201
332. Rizzo G, Capponi A, Arduini D, Lorido C, Romanini C 1996 The value of fetal fibronectin in cervical and vaginal secretions and of ultrasonographic examination of the uterine cervix in predicting premature delivery for patients with perterm labor and intact membranes. American Journal of Obstetrics and Gynecology 175: 1146–1151
333. Rizzo G, Capponi A, Rinaldo D, Arduini D, Romanini C 1996 Release of vasoactive agents during cordocentesis: differences between normally grown and growth-restricted fetuses. American Journal of Obstetrics and Gynecology 175: 563–570
334. Roberts A B, Clarkson N S, Pattison M G, Mok P M 1986 Fetal hydrothorax in the second trimester of pregnancy: successful intrauterine treatment at 24 weeks gestation. Fetal Therapy 1: 203–209
335. Roberts A B, Mitchell J M, Pattison N S 1989 Fetal liver length in normal and isoimmunized pregnancies. American Journal of Obstetrics and Gynecology 161: 42–46
336. Roberts C J, Hibbard B M, Roberts E E, Evans K T, Laurence K M, Robertson I B 1983 Diagnostic effectiveness of ultrasound in the detection of neural tube defects. The South Wales experience of 2059 scans in high risk mothers. Lancet ii: 1068–1070
337. Roberts L J, Bewley S, Mackinson A M, Rodeck C H 1995 First trimester fetal nuchal translucency: problems with screening the general population 1. British Journal of Obstetrics and Gynaecology 102: 381–385
338. Robertson E G, Brown A, Ellis M O I, Walker W 1976 Intrauterine transfusion in the management of severe rhesus isoimmunization. British Journal of Obstetrics and Gynaecology 83: 694–697
339. Robertson E G, Neer K J 1983 Placental injection studies in twin gestation. American Journal of Obstetrics and Gynecology 147: 170–174
340. Robie G F, Payne G G, Morgan M A 1989 Selective delivery of an acardiac acephalic twin. New England Journal of Medicine 320: 512–513
341. Rochelson B, Schulman H, Farmakides G et al 1987 The significance of absent end-diastolic velocity in umbilical artery velocity waveforms. American Journal of Obstetrics and Gynecology 155: 1213–1218
342. Rodeck C H 1980 Fetoscopy guided by real time ultrasound for pure fetal blood samples, fetal skin samples, and examination of the fetus in utero. British Journal of Obstetrics and Gynaecology 87: 449–456
343. Rodeck C H 1993 Fetal development after chorionic villus sampling. Lancet 341: 468–469
344. Rodeck C H, Campbell S 1979 Umbilical cord insertion as a source of pure fetal blood for prenatal diagnosis. Lancet i: 1244–1245
345. Rodeck C H, Eady R A J, Gosden CM 1980 Prenatal diagnosis of epidermolysis bullosa letalis. Lancet i: 949–952
346. Rodeck C H, Fisk N M, Fraser D I, Nicolini U 1988 Long-term in utero drainage of fetal hydrothorax. New England Journal of Medicine 319: 1135–1138
347. Rodeck C H, Holman C A, Karnicki J, Kemp J, Whitmore D N, Austin M A 1981 Direct intravascular fetal blood transfusion by fetoscopy in severe rhesus isoimmunisation. Lancet i: 625–627
348. Rodeck C H, Patrick A D, Pembrey M E, Tzannatos C, Whitfield A E 1982 Fetal liver biopsy for prenatal diagnosis of ornithine carbamyl transferase deficiency. Lancet ii: 297–299
349. Rodeck C H, Mibashan R, Abramowitz J, Campbell S 1982 Selective feticide of the affected twin by fetoscopic air embolization. Prenatal Diagnosis 2: 189–194
350. Rodeck C H, Letsky E A 1989 How the management of erythroblastosis fetalis has changed. British Journal of Obstetrics and Gynaecology 96: 759–763
351. Rodeck C H, Nicolini U 1988 Physiology of the mid-trimester fetus. In: Whitelaw A, Cooke R W I (eds) The very immature infant less than 28 weeks gestation. British Medical Bulletin Vol 44, Churchill Livingstone, Edinburgh, pp 826–849
352. Rodis J , Hovick T J, Quinn D L, Rosengren S S, Tattersall P 1988 Human parvovirus infection in pregnancy. Obstetrics and Gynecology 72: 733–738
353. Roelofsen J, Oostendorp R, Volovics A, Hoogland H 1994 Prenatal diagnosis and fetal outcome of cystic adenomatoid malformation of the lung: case report and historical survey. Ultrasound in Obstetrics and Gynecology 4: 78–82
354. Romero R, Chervenak F A, Kotzen J, Berkowitz R L, Hobbins J C 1982 Antenatal sonographic findings of extralobar pulmonary sequestration. Journal of Ultrasound in Medicine 1: 131–132
355. Romero R, Cullen M, Jeanty P et al 1984 The diagnosis of congenital renal anomalies with ultrasound: II Infantile polycystic kidney disease. American Journal of Obstetrics and Gynecology 150: 259–262
356. Romero R, Jeanty P, Reece E A et al 1985 Sonographically monitored amniocentesis to decrease intraoperative complications. Obstetrics and Gynecology 65: 426–430
357. Romero R, Pilu G, Pilu G, Jeanty P, Ghidini A, Hobbins J 1988 Prenatal diagnosis of congenital anomalies. Appleton and Lange, Connecticut
358. Royal College of Physicians of Edinburgh/Royal College of Obstetricians and Gynaecologists 1997 Consensus Conference on Anti-D prophylaxis.
359. Salvodelli G, Schmid W, Schinzel A 1982 Prenatal diagnosis of cleft lip and palate by ultrasound. Prenatal Diagnosis 2: 313–317
360. Samuels P, Bussel JB, Braitman LE et al 1990 Estimation of the risk of thrombocytopenia in the offspring of pregnant women with presumed immune thrombocytopenic purpura. New England Journal of Medicine 323: 229–235
361. Sandri F, Pilu G, Cerisoli M, Bovicelli L, Alvisi C, Salvioli G P 1988 Sonographic diagnosis of agenesis of the corpus callosum in the fetus and newborn infant. American Journal of Perinatology 5: 226–231
362. Scardo J A, Ellings J M, Newman R B 1995 Prospective determination of chorionicity, amnionicity, and zygosity in twin gestations. American Journal of Obstetrics and Gynecology 173: 1376–1380
363. Schmidt W, Harms E, Wolf D 1985 Successful prenatal treatment of non-immune hydrops fetalis due to congenital chylothorax. British Journal of Obstetrics and Gynaecology 92: 671–679
364. Schwarz T F, Roggendorf M, Hottentrager B et al 1988 Human parvovirus B19 infection in pregnancy. Lancet ii: 566–567
365. Scioscia A L, Grannum P A T, Copel J A, Hobbins J C 1988 The use of percutaneous umbilical blood sampling in immune thrombocytopenic purpura. American Journal of Obstetrics and Gynecology 159: 1066–1068
366. Seeds J W, Bowes W A, Chescheir N C 1989 Echogenic venous turbulence is a critical feature of successful intravascular intrauterine transfusion. Obstetrics and Gynecology 73: 88–90
367. Seller M J, Polani P E 1986 Experimental chimaerism in a genetic defect in the house mouse *Mus musculus*. Nature 212: 80–86
368. Sepulveda W, Stagiannis K D, Flack N J, Fisk N M 1995 Prenatal diagnosis of renal agenesis using color flow imaging in severe second-trimester oligohydramnios. American Journal of Obstetrics and Gynecology 173: 1788–1792
369. Sharland G, Allan L 1992 Screening for congenital heart disease prenatally. Results of a $2\frac{1}{2}$-year study in the South East Thames Region. British Journal of Obstetrics and Gynaecology 99: 220–225
370. Sheikh A U, Ernest J M, O'Shea M 1992 Long-term outcome in fetal hydrops from parvovirus B19 infection. American Journal of Obstetrics and Gynecology 167: 337–341
371. Simoni G, Brambatti B, Danesino C 1983 Efficient direct chromosome analyses and enzyme determination from chorionic villi samples in the first trimester of pregnancy. Human Genetics 63: 349–357
372. Simoni G, Rosella F, Lalatta F, Fracarro M 1986 Maternal metaphases on direct preparation from chorionic villi and in cultures of villi cells. Human Genetics 72: 104
373. Simpson N E, Dallaire L, Miller J R, Siminovich L, Hamerton J L, Mckeen C 1976 Prenatal diagnosis of genetic disease in Canada:

report of a collaborative study. Canadian Medical Association Journal 115: 739–748
374. Smidt-Jensen S, Permin M, Philip J et al 1992 Randomised comparison of amniocentesis and transabdominal and transcervical chorionic villus sampling. Lancet 340: 1238–1244
375. Snijders R J M, Farrias M, von Kaisenberg C, Nicolaides K H 1996 Fetal abnormalities. In: Snijders R J M, Nicolaides K H (eds) Ultrasound markers for fetal chromosomal defects. Parthenon Publishing, London, pp. 1–62
376. Snijders R J M, Johnson S, Sebire N J, Noble P L, Nicolaides K H 1996 First-trimester ultrasound screening for chromosomal defects. Ultrasound in Obstetrics and Gynecology 7: 216–226
377. Soothill P W, Nicolaides K H, Campbell S 1987 Prenatal asphyxia, hyperlacticaemia, hypoglycaemia, and erythroblastosis in growth retarded fetuses. British Medical Journal 294: 1051–1053
378. Soothill P W, Nicolaides K H, Rodeck C H 1987 The effect of anaemia on fetal acid/base status. British Journal of Obstetrics and Gynaecology 94: 880–883
379. Spencer K, Carpenter P 1993 Prospective study of prenatal screening for Down's syndrome with free β-HCG. British Medical Journal 307: 764–769
380. Stagiannis K D, Sepulveda W, Southwell D, Price D, Fisk N M 1995 Ultrasonographic measurement of the dividing membrane during the second and third trimesters: a reproducibility study. American Journal of Obstetrics and Gynecology 173: 1546–1550
381. Stephens F D 1983 Congenital malformations of the urinary tract. Praeger, New York, pp 433–462
382. Stewart P A, Wladimiroff J W 1987 Cardiac tachyarrhythmias in the fetus: diagnosis, treatment and prognosis. Fetal Therapy 2: 7–16
383. Stocker J T, Madewell J E, Drake R M 1977 Congenital cystic adenomatoid malformation of the lung. classification and morphological spectrum. Human Pathology 8: 155–171
384. Stumpflen I, Stumpflen A, Wimmer M, Bernaschek G 1996 Effect of detailed fetal echocardiography as part of routine prenatal ultrasonographic screening on detection of congenital heart disease. Lancet 348: 854–857
385. Szabo J, Gellen J 1990 Nuchal fluid accumulation in trisomy 21 detected by vaginosonography in the first trimester. Lancet 336: 1133
386. Tabor A, Philip J, Madsen M, Bang J, Obel E B, Norgaard-Oedersen B 1986 Randomised controlled trial of genetic amniocentesis in 4606 low risk women. Lancet i: 1287–1293
387. Tan K H, Kilby M D, Whittle M J, Beattie B R, Booth I W, Botting B J 1996 Congenital anterior abdominal wall defects in England and Wales: retrospective analysis of OPCS data. British Medical Journal 313: 303–306
388. Tannirandorn Y, Nicolini U, Nicolaidis P C, Fisk N M, Arulkumaran S, Rodeck C H 1990 Fetal cystic hygromata: insights gained from fetal blood sampling. Prenatal Diagnosis 10: 189–193
389. Terry G M, Ho-Terry L, Warren R C, Rodeck C H, Cohen C H, Rees K R 1986 First trimester prenatal diagnosis of congenital rubella: a laboratory investigation. British Medical Journal 292: 930–933
390. Thirkelsen A J 1979 Cell culture and cytogenetic technique. In: Murken J-D, Stengel-Rutkowski S, Schwinger E N (eds) Prenatal diagnosis (Proceedings of the 3rd European Conference on Prenatal diagnosis of Genetic Disorders). Ferdinand Enke, Stuttgart, pp 258–270
391. Thomas M R, Tutschek B, Frost A et al 1995 The time of appearance and disappearance of fetal DNA from the maternal circulation. Prenatal Diagnosis 15: 641–646
392. Timor-Tritsch I E, Farine D, Rosen M 1988 A close look at early embryonic development with the high frequency transvaginal transducer. American Journal of Obstetrics and Gynecology 159: 676–681
393. Timor-Tritsch I E, Warren W P, Peisner D B, Pirrone E 1989 First-trimester midgut herniation: a high frequency transvaginal sonographic study. American Journal of Obstetrics and Gynecology 161: 831–833
394. Touraine J L, Raudrant D, Royo C et al 1989 In-utero transplantation of stem cells in bare lymphocyte syndrome. Lancet i: 1382
395. UK Collaborative Study on Alphafetoprotein in relation to Neural Tube Defects 1982 Fourth report. Estimating an individual's chance of having an open spina bifida and the value of repeat AFP testing. Journal of Epidemiology and Community Health 36: 87–92
396. Van den Hof M C, Nicolaides K H, Campbell J, Campbell S 1990 Evaluation of the lemon and banana signs in one hundred and thirty fetuses with open spina bifida. American Journal of Obstetrics and Gynecology 162: 322–327
397. Vaughan J I, Warwick R, Letsky E, Nicolini U, Rodeck C H, Fisk N M 1994 Erythropoietic suppression in fetal anemia because of Kell alloimmunization. American Journal of Obstetrics and Gynecology 171: 247–252
398. Verjaal M, Leschot N J 1981 Risk of amniocentesis and laboratory findings in a series of 1500 prenatal diagnoses. Prenatal diagnosis 1: 173–181
399. Ville Y, Hyett J, Hecher K, Nicolaides K H 1995 Preliminary experience with endoscopic laser surgery for severe twin–twin transfusion syndrome. New England Journal of Medicine 332: 224–227
400. von dem Borne A E G, Decary F 1990 Nomenclature of platelet-specific antigens. Human Immunology 29: 1–2
401. Vyas H, Milner A D, Hopkin I E 1982 Amniocentesis and fetal lung development. Archives of Disease in Childhood 57: 627–628
402. Wald N, Cuckle H, Boreham J, Stirrat G 1980 Small biparietal diameter of fetuses with spina bifida: implications for antenatal screening. British Journal of Obstetrics and Gynaecology 87: 219–221
403. Wald N J, Cuckle H S 1987 Screening for NTD's and Down syndrome. In: Rodeck CH (ed) Fetal diagnosis of genetic defects. Baillière's clinical obstetrics and gynaecology, Vol 1 (3). Baillière Tindall, London, pp 649–676
404. Wald N J, Cuckle H S, Densem J W et al 1988 Maternal serum screening for Down's syndrome in early pregnancy. British Medical Journal 297: 883–887
405. Wald N J, Huttly W, Wald K, Kennard A 1996 Down's syndrome screening in the UK (letter). Lancet 347: 330
406. Walker S, Howard P J 1986 Cytogenetic prenatal diagnosis and its relative effectiveness in the Mersey region and North Wales. Prenatal Diagnosis 6: 13–23
407. Weiner C P 1987 Cordocentesis for diagnostic indications: two years' experience. Obstetrics and Gynecology 70: 664–667
408. Weiner C P 1987 Diagnosis and treatment of twin to twin transfusion in the mid-second trimester of pregnancy. Fetal Therapy 2: 71–74
409. Weiner C P 1990 Use of cordocentesis in fetal hemolytic disease and autoimmune thrombocytopenia. American Journal of Obstetrics and Gynecology 162: 1126–1127
410. Weiner C P, Landas S, Personn T J 1987 Digoxin-like immunoreactive substance in fetuses with and without cardiac pathology. American Journal of Obstetrics and Gynecology 157: 368–371
411. Weiner C P, Williamson R, Bonsib S M et al 1986 In utero bladder diversion – problems with patient selection. Fetal Therapy 1: 196–202
412. Weiner C P, Okamura K 1996 Diagnostic fetal blood sampling – technique related losses. Fetal Diagnosis and Therapy 11: 169–175
413. Weiner E, Zosmer N, Bajoria R et al 1994 Direct fetal administration of immunoglobulins: another disappointing therapy in alloimmune thrombocytopenia. Fetal Diagnosis and Therapy 9: 159–164
414. Weir P E, Ratten G J, Beischer N A 1979 Acute polyhydramnios – a complication of monozygous twin pregnancy. British Journal of Obstetrics and Gynaecology 86: 849–853
415. Wenstrom K D, Tessen J A, Zlatnik F J, Sipes S L 1992 Frequency, distribution, and theoretical mechanisms of hematologic and weight discordance in monochorionic twins. Obstetrics and Gynecology 80: 257–261
416. Wenstrom K D, Syrop C H, Hammitt D G, Van Voorhis B J 1993 Increased risk of monochorionic twinning associated with assisted reproduction. Fertility and Sterility 60: 510–514
417. Whitfield C R 1970 A three year assessment of an action line method of timing intervention in rhesus iso-immunization. American Journal of Obstetrics and Gynecology 108: 1239–1244
418. Whittle M J, Connor J M 1994 Prenatal diagnosis in obstetric practice 2nd edn Blackwell Scientific, Oxford
419. Wilkins I A, Chitkara U, Lynch L, Goldberg J D, Mehalek K E, Berkowitz R L 1987 The nonpredictive value of fetal urinary electrolytes: preliminary report of outcomes and correlations with pathological diagnosis. American Journal of Obstetrics and Gynecology 157: 694–698

420. Williams C, Weber L, Williamson R, Hielm M 1988 Guthrie spots for DNA-based carrier testing in cystic fibrosis. Lancet ii: 693
421. Williamson L M, Bruce D, Lubenko A, Chana H J, Ouwehand W H 1992 Molecular biology for platelet alloantigen typing. Transfusion Medicine 2: 225–264
422. Wilson J M, Di Fiore J W, Peters C A 1993 Experimental fetal tracheal ligation prevents the pulmonary hypoplasia associated with fetal nephrectomy: possible application for congenital diaphragmatic hernia. Journal of Pediatric Surgery 28: 1433–1440
423. Wittman B K, Farquharson D F, Thomas W D, Baldwin V J, Wadsworth L D 1986 The role of feticide in the management of severe twin transfusion syndrome. American Journal of Obstetrics and Gynecology 155: 1023–1026
424. Wladimiroff J W 1975 Effect of frusemide on fetal urine production. British Journal of Obstetrics and Gynaecology 82: 221–224
425. Wladimiroff J W, Stewart P A, Reuss A, Sachs E S 1989 Cardiac and extracardiac anomalies as indicators for trisomies 13 and 18: a prenatal ultrasound study. Prenatal Diagnosis 9: 515–520
426. Worton R G, Stern R 1987 A Canadian collaborative study of mosaicism in amniotic fluid cell cultures. Prenatal Diagnosis 4: 131–144
427. Zanjani E D, Lim G, McGalve P B et al 1982 Adult haematopoietic cells transplanted to sheep fetuses continue to produce adult globins. Nature 295: 244–246

15

Immunobiology of placentation: implications for fetal growth and development

Ashley King

Normal growth and development of the fetus is dependent on placental function, of which the most important aspect is adequate transfer of oxygen and nutrients from the intervillous space to the fetal circulation until the end of gestation. To achieve this the placenta must reach an adequate size, but, in addition, considerable alterations in the structure of the placental villi are seen in the latter half of pregnancy which facilitate transport. The main period of placental growth is in early gestation when growth exceeds that of the fetus. Several observations indicate that early placental growth and the placental volume attained by mid-gestation are important determinants of fetal growth in late pregnancy.[9] Therefore, to understand fetal growth it is necessary to determine how the placenta develops in early gestation. Humans have evolved an unusually invasive and potentially dangerous form of placentation, and it is these intrusive placental cells which transform maternal uterine arteries resulting in the increased vascular conductance necessary for normal placental and fetal growth and development.[5]

TROPHOBLAST DIFFERENTIATION

By 7 days after initial contact with the surface epithelium, the blastocyst has become embedded into the uterine mucosal lining, the decidua. After this stage trophoblast differentiation in humans proceeds along two main pathways, villous and extravillous (Fig. 15.1). Villous trophoblast will eventually cover the villous tree, and will come into contact with those maternal cells circulating in the blood in the intervillous space. Functionally, villous trophoblast is primarily concerned with transport. Extravillous trophoblast is those placental cells which migrate into the uterine mucosa and arteries. These fetally-derived cells will therefore come into direct contact with maternal uterine tissues, and modify the maternal uterine spiral arteries to accommodate the required increase in blood flow.

The development of the placenta, unlike that of other organ systems, varies greatly between species. In humans, a discoid haemochorial placenta is formed attached to a

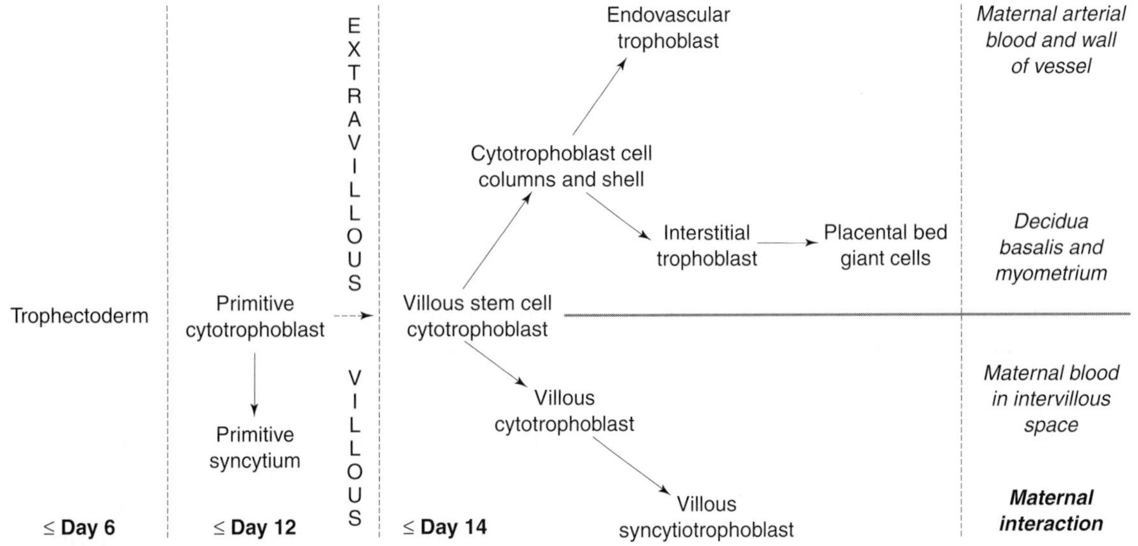

Fig. 15.1 Trophoblast differentiation at the implantation site.

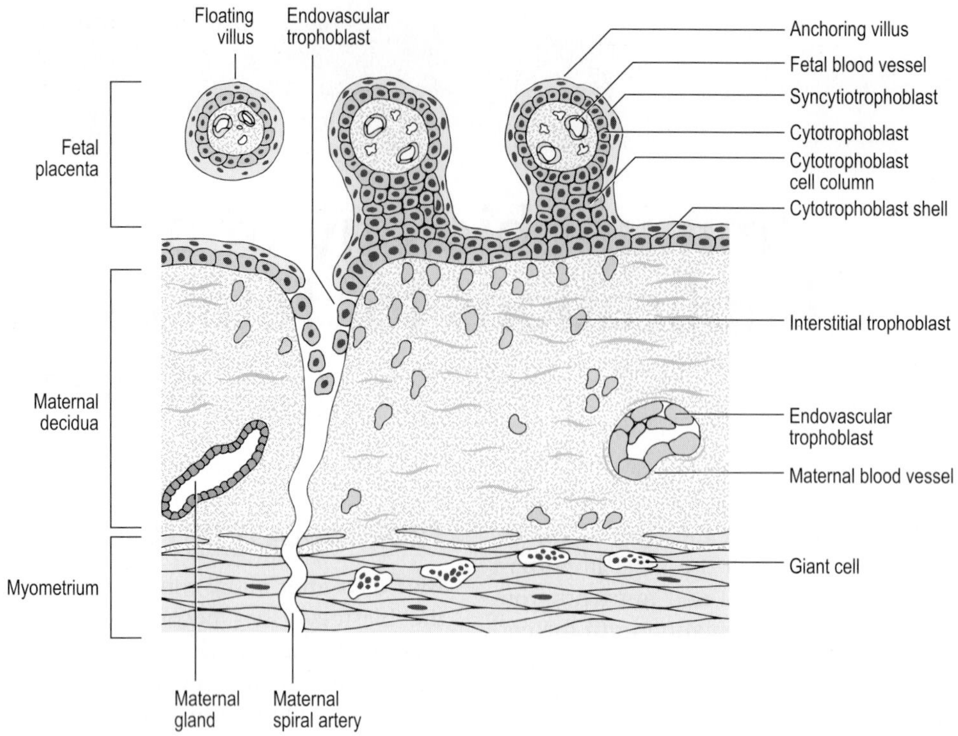

Fig. 15.2 Placental implantation site in humans.

circumscribed area of the uterine wall. Those uterine arteries subjacent to the implantation site are dramatically altered by the process whereby trophoblast cells infiltrate the decidua, surround the spiral arteries and destroy the muscular wall of the artery (Fig. 15.2). This is followed by retrograde migration of endovascular trophoblast down the arterial lumen away from the anchoring placental villi. The result is that the arterial wall is replaced by fibrinoid material in which trophoblast cells are impacted. Towards mid-gestation, trophoblast cells also move into the inner myometrium and similarly transform the arteries there. However, invasion does not proceed any further than this, and the deep-seated trophoblast cells are transformed into placental bed giant cells no longer capable of migration. This 'tapping' of uterine arteries by trophoblast results in dilated arteries no longer capable of vasoconstriction, and providing low resistance high flow delivered at low pressure to the intervillous space.[8] These anatomical changes resulting in increased vascular conductance can now be directly visualized using colour Doppler of the uterine arteries.[2]

Sheep have been the classical animal model used to study fetal growth. However, they have a diffuse epitheliochorial form of placentation which achieves the same end-point but by completely different means. There is no modification of the maternal arteries by trophoblast, nor even breaching of the surface epithelium. In contrast to humans, the whole uterine surface is used for the transfer of nutrients and the blood flow to the uterus remains much the same as in the non-pregnant animal.[7] Thus, humans and sheep have evolved two completely different systems of placentation, and great care must be taken in extrapolating data between them.

PATHOLOGY

The importance of extravillous trophoblast invasion can be appreciated by examining the placental bed of pathological pregnancies.[8] Meticulous histological studies have documented that in cases of intrauterine growth retardation, where no other aetiological factors such as viral infection have been found, and in pre-eclamptic toxaemia trophoblast invasion into arteries is inadequate. Both the number of vessels invaded in the placental bed and the extent of invasion into individual arteries can be deficient. There is suspicion that in these cases placental bed giant cells are prematurely formed and further invasion cannot then occur. The effect of this failure to invade the arteries means that the blood flow to the intervillous space is reduced and delivered at a higher pressure than normal. Obviously the effects will become increasingly apparent as the demands of both the fetus and placenta increase as pregnancy proceeds. The inadequate blood flow also disturbs the normal alterations in the villous structure which occur in the latter half of gestation, particularly the branching of the capillary tree. The direct effect of poor placental blood flow secondarily gives rise to defects in transport of oxygen and nutrients. These findings in pathological pregnancies emphasize the importance of trophoblast invasion in normal human fetal growth and development.

DECIDUA

When trophoblast fails to invade deeply enough into the uterus, it can be considered that the boundary drawn between mother and fetus is in the wrong place, either because of maternal factors limiting invasion or inherent failure of trophoblast to invade. That maternal uterine defensive systems normally operate to prevent over-invasion and uterine rupture can be seen from examining tubal pregnancies and cases of placenta percreta. Decidua is deficient in these pathological conditions of excessive trophoblast penetration. In contrast it seems probable that the decidual defence mechanisms are overzealous in IUGR and PET. The interaction of decidua with extravillous trophoblast must result in delineation of the correct territorial boundary with neither under- nor overinvasion by trophoblast.

Endometrium is transformed into decidua at the onset of pregnancy under the influence of progesterone. Decidua is composed of dilated glands interspersed with decidual stroma. The stroma is distinctive in at least two respects, both of which are likely to be important in the interaction of trophoblast with maternal tissues.[5] Firstly, the stromal cells become bloated and, unusually, secrete a rim of extracellular matrix material around each cell. Secondly, there is an influx of lymphocytes which phenotypically and functionally resemble natural killer cells.

TROPHOBLAST INTERACTION WITH MATERNAL EXTRACELLULAR MATRIX

The invasion and destruction of arterial walls is a feature of malignant cells, and its occurrence in placentation is a unique exception. The dramatic trophoblast infiltration into the uterus is therefore reminiscent of tumour invasion, but there are differences. Firstly, apart from the specific destruction of the arterial media and the thin Nitabuch's layer at the villous– decidual interface, little destructive necrosis such as accompanies malignant invasion is seen. Secondly, the extravillous trophoblast does not proliferate in the uterus, but differentiates from rounded cells of the anchoring villi to individual elongated pleomorphic interstitial trophoblast cells which finally merge to become giant cells. At present it is unknown what controls this differentiation process but, using the analogy with tumour invasion, interaction of trophoblast with the maternal extracellular matrix proteins such as laminin and fibronectin is likely to influence trophoblast migration and differentiation.

The cell surface adhesion molecules which bind cells to the surrounding ECM are integrins. As trophoblast moves from the villi into decidua there is a switch in the pattern of integrins expressed from those characteristic of binding to laminin in the basement membranes ($\alpha_6\beta_4$) to those which bind to fibronectin ($\alpha_5\beta_1$) and other forms of laminin ($\alpha_1\beta_1$). Trophoblast adhesion to and migration on these matrix proteins is mediated by these integrins, and adhesion can result in signal transduction in trophoblast cells.[1] Furthermore, there is some evidence that the normal switch in integrin expression does not occur in PET. Both the factors regulating integrin expression by trophoblast and the forms of matrix proteins produced by decidua are under active investigation.

TROPHOBLAST INTERACTION WITH MATERNAL DECIDUAL LYMPHOCYTES

Medawar was the first to draw attention to the paradox of reproduction when considered in comparison to transplantation of allograft.[6] As half the genetic component of trophoblast is paternal these cells are semi-allogeneic. The genes of most importance in initiating a maternal immune response to trophoblast would be those of the major histocompatibility complex, which in humans are known as human leukocyte antigens. Villous trophoblast expresses neither HLA class I nor class II genes, and is therefore presumably immunologically inert. In contrast, extravillous trophoblast does express the products of two HLA class I genes, HLA-G and HLA-C. Unlike classical class I genes (HLA-A, HLA-B), which present foreign peptides to T cells, HLA-G has a limited number of alleles and a very restricted pattern of expression limited to EVT early in gestation. HLA-C is also unusual in having low surface expression and few alleles with polymorphism not limited to the peptide-binding groove like HLA-A/B. Class I HLA molecules can act as target molecules for two types of lymphocytes, T cells and natural killer cells. The receptors used, the part of the HLA class I molecule recognized and the outcome of the interaction all differ between NK cells and T cells (Fig. 15.3).[3] Thus, in considering the local uterine maternal immune response to trophoblast, both the presence of decidual NK cells and T cells must be assessed.

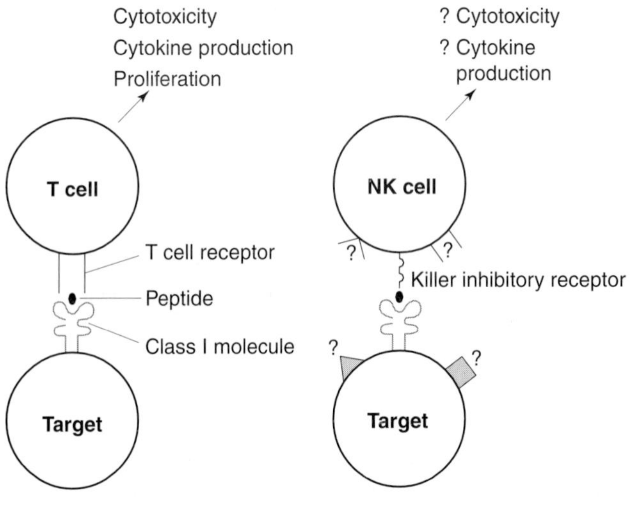

Fig. 15.3 Comparison of NK cell and T cell recognition systems.

Interestingly, the decidua in the first trimester contains very abundant lymphoid cells composed mostly of NK cells (70%) with only a few T cells (10%) and macrophages (20%). B cells are very sparse. Therefore, from the composition of decidual leukocytes, the potential to generate a classical allograft response to trophoblast would appear limited. Indeed, there is no convincing evidence in humans of either a local uterine B cell response resulting in the production of antitrophoblast antibodies or a T cell response as assessed by T cell proliferation in response to trophoblast. The uterine mucosa appears to be similar to other mucosal surfaces where tolerance to foreign antigens is the usual outcome.

The uterine NK cells ($CD56^{bright}$, $CD16^{-}$) are different in several respects from circulating NK cells in adults ($CD56^{dim}$, $CD16^{bright}$). The developmental relationship of these two NK cell populations is unknown. It is obvious that uterine NK cells are under the influence of progesterone and normally proliferate in the uterine mucosa in the luteal phase and in early pregnancy. The presence of these NK cells is temporally related to the period of trophoblast invasion as they disappear in mid-gestation. In addition, they are particularly dense around the infiltrating trophoblast cells in the decidua basalis compared to the decidua parietalis away from the implantation site. It is proposed that the maternal NK cells recognize and respond to the migrating EVT cells and then influence their invasive properties and differentiation into immotile giant cells.

It has recently become clear that NK cell function depends on a balance between activating and inhibitory signals delivered by different receptors.[3] Activating receptors (whose ligands are so far unknown) may trigger cytotoxicity or cytokine production. Killer inhibitory receptors are a new family of receptors which have recently been found on NK cells. KIR transduce a negative signal on recognition of HLA class I molecules on target cells. A particular KIR has specificity for a particular group of class I molecules. For example, HLA-C alleles can be divided into two groups on the basis of KIR recognition. Although it is not yet known how the repertoire of KIR varies on uterine NK cells between different women, there is variation in KIR expression on blood NK cells from different individuals.[4] There is therefore the potential for NK allorecognition of trophoblast, and the way this could operate differs completely from the paradigm of T cell allorecognition. The expression of a particular paternal HLA-C on trophoblast may stimulate the maternal NK cell population in different ways depending on the NK KIR repertoire. One possible scenario is that the cytokines produced by the NK cells may be altered, and these cytokines could modulate trophoblast integrin expression. The unravelling of the molecular basis for NK recognition of trophoblast and the delineation of subsequent NK effector functions which may affect trophoblast tapping of arteries are now major challenges.

REFERENCES

1. Burrows T D, King A, Loke Y W Trophoblast migration during human placental implantation. Human Reproduction Update 2: 307–321
2. Chan F Y, Pun T C, Lam C, Khoo J, Lee C P, Lam Y H 1995 Pregnancy screening by uterine artery Doppler velocimetry – which criterion performs best? Obstetrics and Gynecology 85: 596–602
3. Gumperz J E, Parham P 1995 The enigma of the natural killer cell. Nature 378: 245–248
4. Gumperz J E, Valiante N M, Parham P, Lanier L L, Tyan D 1996 Heterogeneous phenotypes of expression of the NKB1 natural killer cell class I receptor among individuals of different human histocompatibility leukocyte antigens types appear genetically regulated, but not linked to major histocompatibility complex haplotype. Journal of Experimental Medicine 183: 1817–1827
5. Loke Y W, King A 1995 Human implantation: cell biology and immunology. Cambridge University Press, Cambridge
6. Medawar P B 1953 Some immunological and endocrinological problems raised by the evolution of viviparity in vertebrates. In: Evolution 7. Society for Experimental Biology, Academic Press, New York, pp 320–338
7. Moll W 1985 Physiological aspects of placental ontogeny and phylogeny. Placenta 6: 141–154
8. Pijnenborg R 1994 Trophoblast invasion. Reproductive Medicine Review 3: 53–73
9. Schneider H 1996 Ontogenic changes in the nutritive function of the placenta. Placenta 17: 15–26

Section 3

Care around the time of birth

16

Resuscitation of the newborn

N. R. C. Roberton

Being born is stressful, particularly if it is by a vaginal delivery. During normal labour there is transient fetal hypoxia during each uterine contraction,[4,126] which results in the fetus becoming more and more acidaemic as the labour progresses. These changes have been followed by serial fetal scalp samples during the first and second stages of labour (Table 16.1).[16,124] Hormones associated with a stress response and biochemical markers of asphyxia (Table 16.2) are released by the fetus: in general, the greater the stress and trauma of the labour the higher the level of hormones released. Yet despite enduring this process for several hours, with modern obstetric care most newborn infants are pink, vigorous and howling lustily by 1–2 minutes of age. Reports spread over 20 years consistently report that about one neonate in 50–100 requires active resuscitation in the labour ward. Gupta and Tizard[70] reported that 5.7% of all deliveries were apnoeic at 1 minute of age, and that a quarter of these needed intubation in the delivery room. In the 1970 perinatal mortality survey, Chamberlain et al[36] reported that 4.7% of infants took more than 3 minutes to establish sustained respiration, and half of these required intubation. Milner and Vyas[104] reported that 2.1% of all newborn babies required intubation and IPPV. More recently, Palme-Kilander[121] found that only 1:100 babies needed active resuscitation and, unlike previous experience, only 20% of these (0.2% of the total) went on to need intubation and IPPV.

Table 16.2 Markers of hypoxia/stress in the neonate as a result of 'normal labour'

Catecholamines[69,141]
Arginine vasopressin[136,161]
Renin[136]
Angiotensin[110]
Endothelin I[85]
Cortisol[21,140]
↓Thyroid activity[21]
↓PaO_2[1]
Hypoxanthine[134]
Endorphins[2]
Plasma creatine kinase-BB[52]

Babies who require resuscitation fall into four groups: those who make no respiratory effort at all; those who make feeble and inadequate respiratory efforts, remain cyanosed and are often bradycardic; a third and uncommon group that remains cyanosed despite vigorous respiratory efforts; and, finally, the very small group in which neonatal apnoea is due to primary disorders in the muscles or the central nervous system (p. 262). The correct differential diagnosis and concurrent management of the acute respiratory failure in these four differing groups, in which minutes can mean the difference

Table 16.1 Changes in fetal blood gases in normal human labour (the standard deviation is given in parentheses)

	Stage of labour											
	Cervix 0–2 cm dilated		Cervix 3–5 cm dilated		Cervix 6 cm to fully dilated		FD(c)		FD(p)		Umbilical artery	
pH	7.29	(0.05)	7.30	(0.05)	7.29	(0.02)	7.28	(0.05)	7.23	(0.06)	7.23	(0.05)
BD (mmol/l)	−5.5	(2.4)	−5	(2.2)	−6.3	(2.1)	−6.7	(2.1)	−9.1	(3.5)	−7.4	(2.7)
PCO_2 (mmHg)	44	(6)	42	(6)	42	(6)	40	(5.5)	44	(9)	52	(10.5)
PO_2(mmHg)			23.7	(5.7)*					21.5	(4.3)†	17.2	(6.0)

Samples collected by fetal scalp sample except for cord arterial blood gas measurements.
Data of Beard and Morris[16] for pH, PCO_2 and base deficit, and of Paterson et al[124] for PO_2.
BD, base deficit; FD(c), full dilatation/head in mid-cavity; FD(p), full dilatation/head on perineum.
* Level taken some time during the first stage.
† Level taken some time during second stage.

Table 16.3 Perinatal complications requiring a paediatrician's presence at delivery

Caesarean section
Forceps
Breech
Ventouse (vacuum extraction)
Malpresentations
Multiple pregnancy
Meconium staining
Gestation < 36 weeks
Fetal distress
Known fetal complications
rhesus disease
congenital malformation

Table 16.4 The Apgar score

Clinical feature	Score		
	0	1	2
Heart rate	0	≤100	>100
Respiration	Absent	Gasping or irregular	Regular or crying lustily
Muscle tone	Limp	Diminished, or normal with no movements	Normal with active movements
Response to pharyngeal catheter	Nil	Grimace	Cough
Colour of trunk	White or or blue	Pink with blue extremities	Pink

Table 16.5 Mean pH and base deficit of infants with different Apgar scores[169]

	1-min Apgar score								
	1	2	3	4	5	6	7	8	9
No. of infants	5	12	17	11	22	30	62	147	589
Mean pH	7.17	7.12	7.10	7.22	7.18	7.17	7.19	7.20	7.21
SD	0.5	0.13	0.13	0.10	0.08	0.09	0.08	0.07	0.08
Mean BD	10.6	11.8	11.5	7.8	9.6	10.6	8.8	8.4	7.9
SD	4.0	5.9	6.3	5.5	4.3	3.2	4.1	3.7	3.6

BD, base deficit (mEq/1); SD, standard deviation.

between death, survival with cerebral palsy or neurologically intact survival, represent the pinnacle of the neonatal paediatrician's craft and skill. In no other area of medicine are the benefits of prompt and correct action more rewarding and more immediate.

Gupta and Tizard[70] estimated that 70% of infants requiring resuscitation come from predictably high-risk situations, and similar figures are given by Primhak et al[139] and Palme-Kilander.[121] For this reason skilled staff should attend the complicated deliveries listed in Table 16.3. The reasons for attending in the presence of meconium-stained liquor (p. 540) or prematurity (p. 493) are explained in detail elsewhere. Intubation is often needed in babies born by caesarean section (6.2%) and by the breech (8%).[104] Although a case can be made for not attending non-rotational forceps,[68] elective repeat caesarean section[137] or meconium-stained liquor in the absence of fetal distress (p. 168), quality perinatal care with rapid effective resuscitation needs skilled personnel attending up to 40% of all deliveries.[139] Furthermore, 30% of infants who need active resuscitation are delivered after an apparently normal labour in which there has been no evidence of fetal compromise.[70,139] Low et al[94] showed that careful assessment of antenatal risk factors failed to identify half of all babies with a base deficit > 12 mmol/l at birth. These data are compelling reasons for ensuring that someone capable of resuscitating a newborn baby, be it a midwife, a general practitioner, a paediatrician or an anaesthetist, is present or available within 2–3 minutes at every delivery.

It is increasingly recognised[56,123] that perinatal asphyxia is a relatively rare cause of permanent CNS damage (p. 1247). Nevertheless, intrapartum asphyxia is the cause of some cases of perinatally acquired brain damage, although the responsibility for preventing this lies primarily with the obstetrician and his conduct of labour. However, if a baby does not breathe after delivery, his PaO_2 falls immediately to close to zero and he rapidly becomes acidotic, that is, he develops the biochemical stigmata of asphyxia (p. 244), which can also cause brain damage or aggravate pre-existing CNS injury. It is the neonatologist's responsibility to prevent these postnatal problems by prompt adequate resuscitation, ensuring that there is no delay in the baby achieving adequate ventilation, normal blood gases and a normal cardiac output.

ASSESSMENT OF THE BABY AFTER DELIVERY

It is essential that the baby's condition is evaluated as quickly after delivery as possible. The response to resuscitation should be recorded as a narrative in the baby's notes, the account ending only when the baby is pink, breathing normally and active, or is at least pink and stable and connected if necessary to a ventilator.

APGAR SCORE

The traditional way of assessing the newborn is to use the Apgar score. This was devised by Virginia Apgar[12] and grades five clinical features with scores from 0 to 2 at 1 minute of age (Table 16.4). In recent years there has been a tendency to belittle the Apgar score[10] because it is a poor index of asphyxia (i.e. hypoxaemia plus acidaemia) and has little prognostic value.[50,128,158,162,169] (Table 16.5). Although these statements are undoubtedly true, particularly of term babies, deriding the score fails to understand its purpose:[101] it was never intended to be a marker of asphyxia, but rather a marker of a baby who has a problem,[7,12] and the sooner that problem is diagnosed and managed the better. Furthermore, in VLBW neonates the 1 and 5 minute Apgar scores are good early prognostic guides (see below). Components of the score do not, however, carry equivalent physiological weight. Heart rate and respiration are clearly more important than reflex responsiveness, and the so-called Sigtuna score, which rates just these two features, has been shown to be as effective as the Apgar as a means of scoring newborn babies.[5] Only tone represents higher cerebral function: the other components are scoring brain-stem reflex responses.

For these reasons the narrative description of the baby at birth and during resuscitation is important, and one should never just record that a baby had an Apgar of 5 at 1 minute, but should accurately describe the infant's condition: for instance, at 1 minute the infant was apnoeic, was pink with blue hands and feet, had a heart rate of 90 and normal tone; he grimaced when sucked out; or, at 1 minute the infant was pink with a heart rate of 120 and gasped twice, but he was limp and made no response to suction. In both these situations the Apgar score is 5, but clearly they have different clinical and physiological implications and require a different approach to resuscitation (see below). In addition to taking the Apgar score at 1 minute of age, the scores at 5 and 10 minutes, and at 15 and 20 minutes in babies who respond poorly to resuscitation, should also be noted. The 5-minute score is one component of the American Academy of Pediatrics criteria for the presence of perinatal asphyxia[34] and the 15–20-minute scores are more strongly correlated with subsequent neurological defects.[114] Furthermore, the improvement in the Apgar score from 0 to 20 minutes is an internationally understood and accepted shorthand for describing the success or otherwise of the resuscitative effort.

CORD BLOOD GAS ANALYSIS

In the heat of the moment in the labour ward this is usually the only other piece of information available to help diagnose the cause of a neonate's failure to breathe. It is the most satisfactory way of assessing whether or not asphyxia, rather than one of the other conditions listed in Table 16.6, is present.[172] Ideally, at all deliveries samples should be collected from both the umbilical artery and vein in a section of the cord double-clamped immediately after delivery.[87] In normal deliveries the umbilical arterial pH is lower than that of the umbilical vein (Table 16.7).[183] In the presence of cord compression the umbilical vein samples may still be normal and give a false impression of the fetal health, whereas the arterial sample, which is fetal blood, may show severe acidaemia. These blood gas data can be available within minutes, and can then be extremely useful in guiding the management of the baby's subsequent resuscitation. There is in general a poor relationship between Apgar score and pH,[63,162,169] although a statistical relationship may occur in well babies with only minimal reduction in the Apgar score.[103] Two per cent of babies with normal Apgar scores have a [H+] > 80 nmol/l (pH < 7.10), and most babies with a [H+] > 80 nmol/l (pH < 7.10) will have normal Apgar scores; if both are abnormal and no other problems are detected (Table 16.6) this is strongly suggestive of recent asphyxia.[63,165,172] However, it is only when umbilical artery [H+] values are > 100 nmo/l (pH < 7.0) that low Apgar scores are common or are still reduced at 5 minutes (Fig. 16.1),[63] and it is only in such neonates that the proportion with HIE or long-term neurological sequelae begins to rise. Even with such marked acidaemia the majority of babies do not develop HIE until the [H+] is > 150 mmol/l (pH < 6.80).[50,66,128]

Table 16.6 Factors other than asphyxia which may delay the onset of respiration after delivery

CNS injury prior to labour
Drugs depressing the CNS
Maternal hypocapnia
Trauma, especially to the CNS
Prematurity, in particular surfactant-deficient stiff lungs
Sepsis, especially group B streptococci
Muscle weakness due to prematurity or primary muscle disease
Anaemia
Congenital malformations
obstructing the airway or preventing lung expansion
neurological, impairing respiratory control

Table 16.7 Data on 1448 paired umbilical artery and umbilical venous cord blood gas analyses (in normal pregnancies[183] (mean + 2.5 and 97.5th centiles)

	UA	UV
pH	7.26 (7.05–7.38)	7.35 (7.17–7.48)
PCO_2	7.3 (4.9–10.7)	5.3 (3.5–7.9)
BD	2.4 (–2.5 to –9.7)	3.0 (–1.0 to –8.9)

OTHER MEASUREMENTS

Analysing blood for biochemical indicators of asphyxia, such as lactate, hypoxanthine or creatine kinase, may be useful as a research tool in assessing the management and outcome of antepartum events but is of no value in the care of the baby in the labour ward, or in the first 60 minutes of life. An important part of the early assessment of the baby who responds slowly to resuscitation is to measure his blood glucose (p. 946) and blood pressure (p. 504).

CAUSES OF DELAYED ONSET OF REGULAR RESPIRATION

A frequent misconception is that delayed onset of respiration at birth is always the result of intrapartum

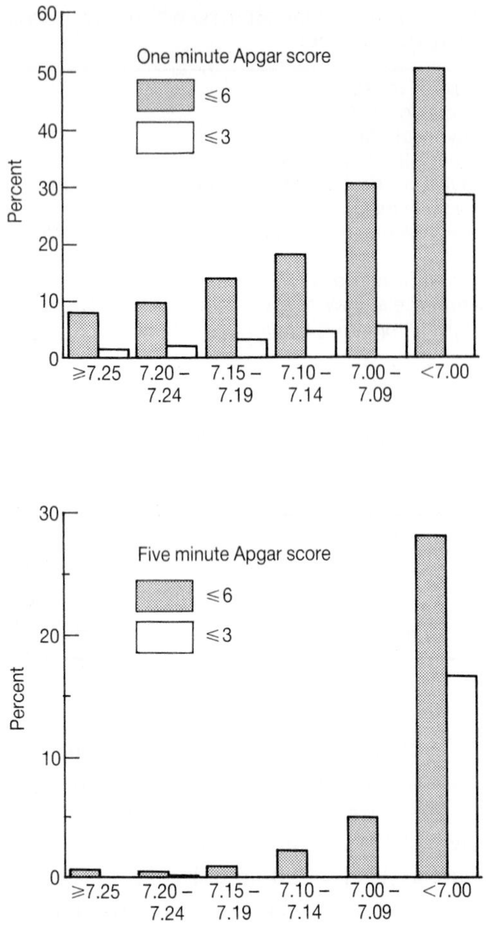

Fig. 16.1 Relationship between umbilical artery pH levels and Apgar scores at 1 (top) and 5 (bottom) minutes. (Reproduced with permission from Gilstrap et al[63])

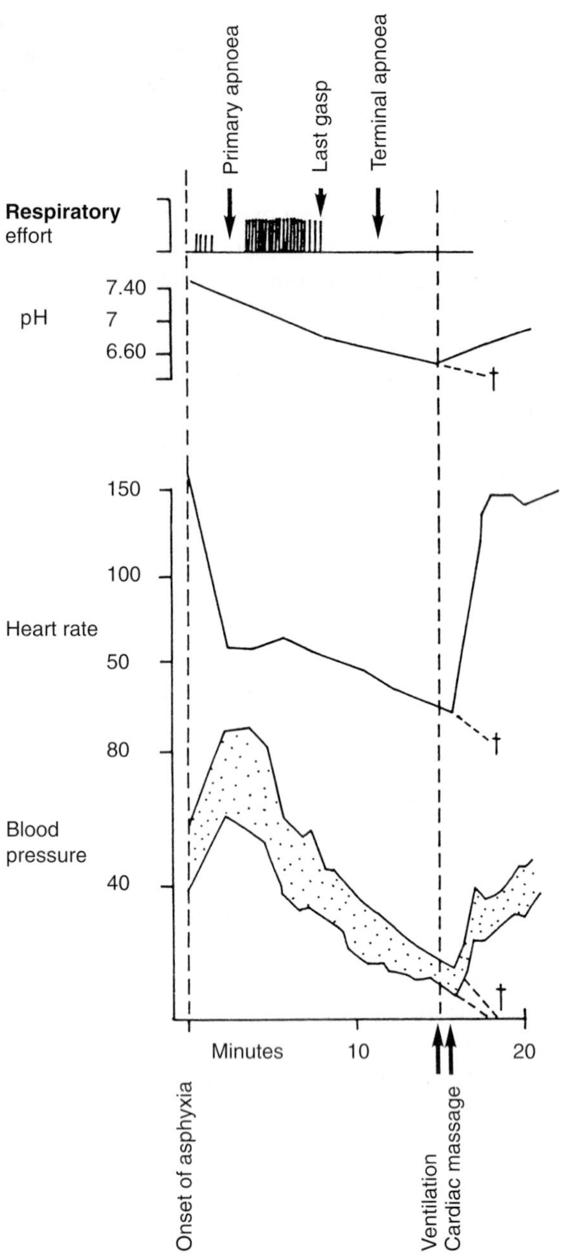

Fig. 16.2 Physiological changes during asphyxia and resuscitation of a newborn animal. (Adapted from Dawes et al[46])

asphyxia (see above), but many additional factors can delay the onset of respiration after delivery (Table 16.6). Several of these may be present in a single baby, yet each one needs to be recognized as quickly as possible and properly treated. In general, asphyxia and the conditions listed in Table 16.6 either prevent the onset of spontaneous respiration or cause a serious reduction in the baby's respiratory efforts. The baby who breathes vigorously but remains cyanosed, or the baby who fails to make any respiratory effort despite the absence of asphyxia, will be considered separately at the end of this chapter, under the heading of babies who fail to respond to resuscitation (p. 260).

ACUTE ASPHYXIA

This is the traditional cause of failure to breathe at delivery, and is probably the mechanism responsible for babies not breathing at birth after they have suffered some acute crisis, such as an antepartum haemorrhage or cord prolapse.

The animal model for acute neonatal asphyxia[44] has been of enormous value in explaining the physiological changes in the infant who is not breathing immediately after delivery, and in providing the theoretical basis for the management of his resuscitation. It will therefore be described in detail.

Acute postnatal asphyxia is induced in newborn animals by delivering them in good condition by caesarean section and then preventing them from breathing by immediately sealing their heads in a bag of saline. A very characteristic sequence of events then takes place (Fig. 16.2). After a few shallow breaths which, owing to the nature of the experiment, cannot result in any gas exchange, the animal stops 'breathing'. This early period of apnoea, so-called primary apnoea, may last for up to 10 minutes. However, after 1–2 minutes in primary apnoea the animal usually starts to gasp: the gasps occur with increasing frequency and vigour but then decreasing until the animal literally reaches the last gasp. The heart rate falls rapidly after the onset of asphyxia, plateaus or may rise slightly in primary apnoea and early in the phase of gasping, then begins to slow. Cardiac activity continues for 10 minutes or more after the last gasp. The period between the last gasp and cardiac arrest is known as secondary or terminal apnoea. The changes in blood pressure parallel those in heart rate. A severe mixed acidaemia develops. By the end of terminal apnoea the $PaCO_2$ may exceed 13.5 kPa (100 mmHg), the [H+] is usually greater than 300 nmol/l (pH < 6.5), and the PaO_2 is zero. The serum potassium rises to 15 mmol/l or more.

The neonatal primate is capable of surviving at least 20 minutes of complete oxygen deprivation, but in the latter part of this period brain damage is occurring. Survival is due to the existence of large stores of glycogen in the brain, liver and myocardium which can produce energy by anaerobic glycolysis during asphyxia,[156] and also to the ability of neonatal brain tissues to metabolize fuels such as lactate and ketones.[55,154,177] Reduction in the stores of glycogen for any reason, such as growth retardation (p. 138) or preceding partial asphyxia (see below), will reduce the fetus' ability to withstand an acute asphyxial insult.

Brain damage has been described in monkeys sacrificed towards the end of the phase of gasping, but as many human neonates clinically assessed to be in terminal apnoea when resuscitated survive without neurological sequelae (see below), it seems probable that brain damage following acute asphyxia is not inevitable unless it is very severe or was superimposed on preceding chronic partial asphyxia (see below).

The response to removing the bag of saline from the animal's head during the above experiment (Fig. 16.2) depends on the stage of asphyxia reached. If the animal is in primary apnoea it will remain apnoeic until the pH falls to a level which will provoke gasping, or until external stimuli have the same effect. As it will then inhale air or oxygen the animal's condition rapidly improves and the gasps soon change into regular respiration. If the animal is already making respiratory movements or gasping when the bag is removed, and air or oxygen enters its lungs, a regular respiratory pattern rapidly develops; if the bag is removed in terminal apnoea respiration will not occur. To resuscitate such an animal positive-pressure ventilation must be used, and if the heart rate is very slow (or is absent) external cardiac massage will be necessary.

Giving intravenous glucose and bicarbonate throughout the above experiment to combat the acidaemia and hypoglycaemia resulting from consumption of all the glycogen stores during asphyxia, prolongs the survival of the animal. If these agents are given during resuscitation by positive-pressure ventilation they will improve the cardiac output, expedite the onset of spontaneous respiration[3] and thereby minimize the likelihood of subsequent brain damage.[47]

RELEVANCE OF ACUTE EXPERIMENTS TO CLINICAL NEONATAL CARE

Because there is no reason to suppose that the response of a human neonate to acute asphyxia will be different from that observed in other mammals, it can be anticipated that the physiological responses of the human neonate immediately after delivery will depend on his pH: if his [H+] concentration is below 55 nmol/l (pH > 7.25) when delivered, he will behave as though in the phase of primary apnoea or gasping, and in the absence of other pathology (Table 16.6) regular respiration will soon start; if his [H+] concentration has risen to 80–100 nmol/l (pH 7–7.10) he may still breathe adequately but, particularly if there is some other complication such as heavy sedation or prematurity (see below), the primary apnoea may be prolonged,[32,108] or the gasping efforts may be too weak to establish alveolar ventilation. Still more severe intrapartum asphyxia will result in the delivery of an infant with a [H+] concentration above 100 nmol/l (pH < 7.0) who is limp, bradycardic and in terminal apnoea (see above).

The experiments on acute animal asphyxia have provided several other important pieces of information which help us to understand the behaviour and treatment of the human infant who is asphyxiated or apnoeic immediately after delivery. These include the following:

- The onset of gasping and therefore regular respiration can be expedited in primary apnoea by peripheral stimuli, including rubbing the baby with a warm towel or giving an intramuscular injection.
- Drugs administered to the mother, including all commonly used sedatives and analgesics, pass to the fetus and may prolong primary apnoea to such an extent that the acidaemia becomes severe and the phase of gasping may never occur. However, they also slow down the accumulation of carbon dioxide and lactic acid.
- A baby born in terminal apnoea will never establish spontaneous respiration unless he is actively resuscitated by intubation and IPPV. This crucial fact is the prime reason why, when confronted by an infant who is apnoeic at 2–3 minutes of age, there should be absolutely no delay in establishing effective ventilation.

In infants resuscitated from terminal apnoea the time from the onset of artificial ventilation to either the first gasp or regular respiration is proportional to the severity of the asphyxia before ventilation was started (Fig. 16.3).[3] If artificial ventilation started before the pH was

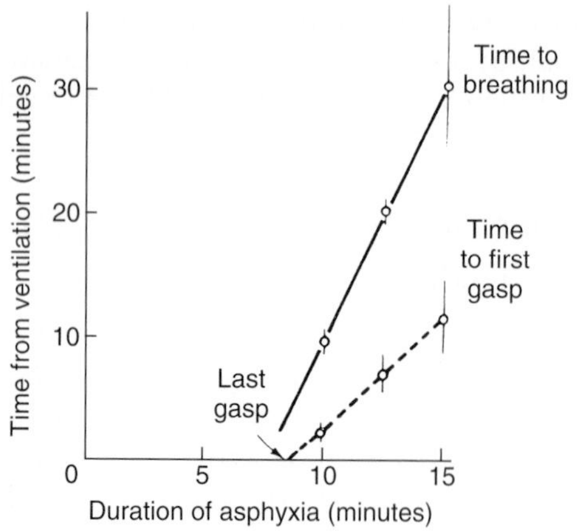

Fig. 16.3 Time from beginning positive-pressure ventilation with oxygen until the first gasp (- - - -) and until the establishment of regular breathing (——) in nearly newly delivered rhesus monkeys asphyxiated for 10, 12.5 or 15 minutes at 30°C. The vertical bars indicate the standard errors of the means in each group of five or six monkeys. (From Adamsons et al[3])

depressed too far, the infant may be expected to gasp (a Head's paradoxical reflex[70]) and start regular respiration after 3–4 minutes of IPPV, whereas if resuscitation was started well into terminal apnoea when the [H+] was probably greater than 150 nmol/l (pH < 6.8), gasping may be delayed for 20 minutes and regular respiration for over half an hour. Therefore, those infants who have not started to breathe spontaneously 4–5 minutes after starting IPPV should, in the absence of other causes of neonatal respiratory depression, be assumed to have a very low pH.

Injections of lobeline, nikethamide or vandid, or any other analeptic drug are not only valueless but dangerous. Like immersion of the newborn alternately in hot and cold water, sealing him in a hyperbaric oxygen chamber, or stuffing a raven's beak into his rectum, they are unnecessarily painful and physiologically unsound methods of initiating respiration in primary apnoea. In terminal apnoea they cause a more rapid fall in blood pressure and heart rate, and hence earlier death, than would have occurred if the infant had been treated by masterly inactivity.[44]

CHRONIC IN UTERO PARTIAL ASPHYXIA

Episodes of acute total asphyxia creating sudden total fetal anoxia as described above are rare in clinical practice. More common are events that lead to the gradual development of fetal hypoxia, acidaemia and chronic partial asphyxia. This can occur before or during labour. For example, some hours or even days before delivery a fetus may suffer an hypoxic/asphyxial insult which is not severe enough to kill him but which can cause neurological damage.[115,167] By the time the mother of such a baby goes into labour, he may have made a complete biochemical recovery and have normal blood gases.[160] As he has not suffered intrapartum asphyxia he may well show no signs of respiratory depression at birth, have a good Apgar score, and establish regular breathing without any apparent problems.

CHIPA in labour corresponds to animal experiments in which pregnant monkeys were given an excess of halothane to render them hypotensive, and their fetus thereby hypoxic and acidaemic, for periods of 4–6 hours. The animals were then delivered of newborns with widespread cortical, midbrain and cerebellar damage.[26] In clinical practice CHIPA can occur in apparently normal women merely as an exaggeration of the normal asphyxial stresses of labour, particularly if labour is prolonged or if there are additional problems, such as maternal supine hypotension, or simply the decline in uteroplacental function that occurs with postmaturity. Pathological causes of CHIPA in clinical practice include excessive use of oxytocic drugs, the growth-retarded fetus who already has reduced umbilical blood flow,[72] which falls even further during the normal uterine contractions of labour, or recurrent episodes of umbilical cord occlusion caused by entanglement around a fetal part or compression of the cord between the presenting part and the pelvis.

During such episodes the fetal blood pressure is normal or high to start with, and although the heart rate is commonly sustained there may be a bradycardia; the cardiac output is diverted primarily to the placenta, adrenals, brain and myocardium.[22,23,143] The fetal PO_2 and pH fall, and energy is produced by anaerobic metabolism of glycogen and glucose to lactate. Because the PCO_2 also rises, a combined metabolic and respiratory acidaemia develops. These changes may resolve rapidly if normal uteroplacental function is restored and the asphyxia is transient or treated.[125] However, if the heart rate and blood pressure fall the vital organs will eventually become ischaemic,[22,143] and the brain damage following perinatal CHIPA, as well as showing global neuronal loss, the so-called selective neuronal necrosis,[181] characteristically also shows damage in the watershed areas between the arteries supplying the cerebral cortex, with parasagittal cerebral injury (p. 1236).[181] These ischaemic lesions correspond to what is seen in the experimental animal model of partial asphyxia described by Brann and Myers.[26]

If episodes of partial antepartum asphyxia have been short-lived the fetus is unlikely to be seriously damaged; if delivered promptly, although his respiration may be depressed immediately after delivery and he may be acidaemic with a poor Apgar score, he usually responds quickly to resuscitation and is unlikely to suffer sequelae.

Sequelae are, however, more likely to occur if the CHIPA has been severe or prolonged.[26] If such asphyxia has persisted up to the time of delivery, and particularly if the heart, lungs or kidneys have been affected, the baby will be born in very poor condition, with a low Apgar score. If cord blood gas analysis is carried out he will have a marked metabolic, and in some cases respiratory, acidaemia with an [H+] > 100 nmol/l (pH < 7.0). However, how much brain damage has been suffered can only be assessed by his clinical condition in the next 12–24 hours, and by whether or not he develops HIE (p. 1238). Animal evidence also suggests that permanent neurological damage can occur with prolonged recurrent partial in utero asphyxia without the fetal pH falling. This is presumably because during transient episodes of asphyxia, if the blood pressure is not adequately sustained, cerebral oxygen delivery to watershed areas may fall below critical levels, despite the fact that at the same time there is not sufficient generalized oxygen lack to result in widespread anaerobic glycolysis, lactic acidaemia and a fall in pH. Despite the absence of systemic acidosis in these experiments, it is interesting that there were marked fetal heart rate changes during each episode of asphyxia.[39]

Finally, it is probably quite common for a fetus to recover from, or be resuscitated from, in utero asphyxia, and even for his acid–base status to recover in the presence of persisting hypoxia.[155,185] In such cases the fetus with a reasonable pH may make a satisfactory transition to extrauterine life (i.e. have a reasonable Apgar score), yet have suffered in utero asphyxia with damage to his central nervous system, which will manifest as HIE in the neonatal period. Similar in utero recovery can also occur after a single, acute, brain-damaging asphyxial insult.[100] This potential for 'in utero resuscitation' is yet another reason for the poor association between Apgar scores, cord blood gases and subsequent neurological disorders, and also explains why some babies who develop severe HIE cause few resuscitation problems in the labour ward.[54,77,82,128,148]

Although the various types of asphyxial insult described above do in their own right cause neuronal death at the time, there are now extensive data to show that a large amount of the long-term damage to the brain of babies who develop HIE is the result of the secondary energy failure that occurs postnatally, and which is described in detail in Chapter 44, Part 4.

The fact the prenatal asphyxia can evolve in these many different ways in the hours and days before and after delivery has important clinical and medicolegal implications, of which the three most important are:

- Most babies who have signs of fetal distress, a low Apgar score or acidaemia on cord blood gas analysis are normal in the neonatal period and on follow-up.
- Intrauterine problems days or weeks before labour can cause severe long-term neurological defects, yet the baby may show few if any neurological abnormalities in the neonatal period.
- In the absence of clinically apparent HIE in the neonatal period it is highly unlikely that intrapartum events are responsible for neurological sequelae.

PRE-EXISTING BRAIN DISEASE

Case reports in the past established that babies who had suffered a severe and clear insult some time before labour could show fetal distress, be neurologically abnormal in the neonatal period, and end up with cerebral palsy. A large and extremely important study from Oxford[58] showed that babies who were neonatal deaths following a labour characterized by marked CTG abnormalities had pathological changes in their brain that were old and must have antedated labour. Thus brain damage developing before labour can cause fetal distress in labour, a low Apgar score and neonatal death. Rarely, congenital malformations of the brain (see below,[27]) or congenital myopathies may also result in a baby being born with poor Apgar scores not due to perinatal asphyxia.

DEPRESSION OF THE RESPIRATORY CENTRE

Pharmacological

Almost all the drugs used as analgesics, sedatives or general anaesthetics during labour can cross the placenta and, in theory, depress the neonatal respiratory centre.[15] However, respiratory depression from drugs is likely to be important only in premature babies or those who have also suffered some degree of intrapartum asphyxia.[108] A drug-loaded full-term baby with an [H+] less than 55 nmol/l (pH > 7.25) will probably establish regular respiration unless the level of drug in the plasma is very high. If, however, respiration is depressed, as in animal experiments, this will take the form of prolongation of primary apnoea, and unless artifical ventilation is established the neonate will become progressively hypoxic and acidaemic, with all that this entails. Although sedative drugs do prolong survival in experimental asphyxia, this effect must never lull the paediatrician into believing that resuscitation is less urgent in the infant who is apnoeic because of drug depression than in the one who is apnoeic due to asphyxia.

Hypocapnia

The maternal $PaCO_2$ may be reduced voluntarily in women using to excess one of the breathing techniques associated with 'natural' childbirth or an inhalational analgesic such as Entonox. The hyperventilation may be involuntary during a general anaesthetic if there is exuberant bag squeezing by the anaesthetist. The fetal $PaCO_2$ is in equilibrium with that of the mother, and a fetus born with a $PaCO_2$ less than 4 kPa (30 mmHg) lacks the carbon dioxide drive to ventilation and may remain apnoeic until his $PaCO_2$ rises sufficiently to stimulate the respiratory centre.[111] Maternal hypocapnia may also reduce placental blood flow and thereby cause fetal hypoxia and acidaemia.[109]

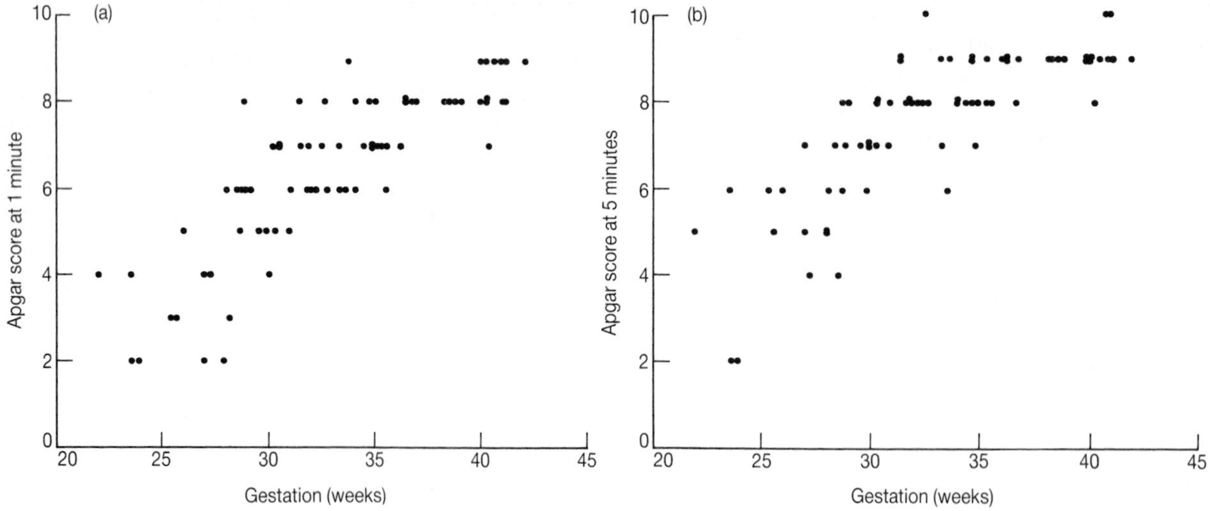

Fig. 16.4 Scattergram of 1-minute (a) and 5-minute (b) Apgar scores plotted against gestation. (Reproduced with permission from Catlin et al[35])

TRAUMA

In babies in poor condition at birth after a traumatic forceps or breech extraction it is difficult to separate the effects of trauma from the fetal asphyxia, which almost always coexists. Trauma alone is now very rare with improvements in obstetric practice,[41] but may, for example, cause a vault subdural haemorrhage in a baby who is in good condition at birth but who deteriorates during the first 12–24 hours as the haemorrhage increases in volume. It is important to remember, however, that subdural haemorrhage may occur after a spontaneous vaginal delivery.[67]

Endorphin levels are higher in the cord blood of infants exposed to the physical stresses of vaginal delivery[2] and, as these substances may depress the neonatal ventilation[74] it is possible that trauma can indirectly depress the central nervous system. Recent research which shows that the excitatory neurotransmitters responsible for the secondary energy failure of HIE are also released after traumic delivery[84] may provide a unifying mechanism for the interrelationship between birth trauma, birth asphyxia and subsequent neurological injury.

A rare traumatic cause of delayed onset of respiration at birth is injury or transection of the spinal cord in the cervical region. Depending on the level of the injury, both the intercostal muscles and the diaphragm will be paralysed and apnoea will result. Formerly common following extended breech presentations,[184] this type of injury now seems to be limited to babies delivered by rotational forceps.[98]

PREMATURITY

It is well recognized that the Apgar score is low in premature babies[35] (Fig. 16.4) and that active resuscitation is frequently required (Table 16.8). The score is an even poorer indicator of asphyxia, and correlates much better with gestation.[35,65,96,130] However, Goldenberg et al[65] did show that those preterm neonates who are asphyxiated (low pH) are more likely to have a low Apgar score. It is also clear that, whatever the cause of the low Apgar score in preterm babies, the score is a good marker of the neonate who is more likely to suffer sequelae or to die.[17,18,61,97] Against this background it is interesting to note that the antenatal administration of dexamethasone to induce lung maturity (p. 491) improves the Apgar score of treated preterm babies.[60]

Table 16.8 Percentage of infants requiring positive-pressure ventilation for resuscitation[97]

Gestation (weeks)	No. of births	Percentage requiring IPPV
≤28	173	49
29–32	288	18
33–34	415	8
35–36	1 340	2
37–38	5 895	0.7
≥39	24 726	0.4

The decision to intubate a VLBW infant for resuscitation in the labour ward is bound up with the controversies about the prophylactic administration of surfactant (p. 494 et seq.), the potentially damaging effects of hyperoxic reductions in cerebral blood flow,[95] and whether or not excess ventilation worsens the prognosis by increasing the risk of chronic lung disease.[13,135] It is difficult to understand how the latter problem is the result of a 30–60-minute period of IPPV following resuscitation rather than prolonged overventilation, perhaps resulting from an unjustified unwillingness to withdraw IPPV early, once it is clear that the baby has minimal lung disease.

The pendulum is swinging in favour of prophylactic surfactant for the baby below 28–29 weeks' gestation

(p. 509). Until modern prospective studies refute the older data that prompt resuscitation by IPPV is beneficial,[49,146] we believe that for all the reasons outlined on p. 493 it is important to stabilize and normalize the 'milieu intérieur' of babies below 30 weeks' gestation as soon after delivery as possible.

ANAEMIA

The infant who is severely anaemic may be in high-output heart failure. He lacks haemoglobin to deliver oxygen to the tissues, and this will make him more susceptible to asphyxia. Without haemoglobin he lacks one of the body's major buffers, and may therefore be more acidaemic.[163] As a result he may be in very poor condition at delivery, and may not only breathe inadequately but may respond poorly to resuscitation. Although severely asphyxiated infants are pale, coexisting anaemia must always be considered in a pale infant responding poorly to resuscitation. The two most likely causes of severe anaemia at birth are rhesus incompatibility and fetal haemorrhage; the delivery of a baby with the former is usually expected: unexpected severe anaemia at birth is, therefore, probably due to fetal haemorrhage; in addition to the normal resuscitation routines, such infants require urgent transfusion (pp. 814–815).

SEPSIS

Babies suffering from severe intrapartum infection, both preterm and at term, classically due to listeria[25] or group B streptococci,[99,127] can be born with very poor Apgar scores, though they are not asphyxiated. They are critically ill at the time of birth, with hypotension and septicaemia (i.e. a positive blood culture). Although the outlook for these babies is grave, the condition must be diagnosed and vigorous anti-infection therapy commenced (p. 1126), in addition to the management of their initial apnoea.

SUBSEQUENT EFFECTS OF ASPHYXIA (ACUTE OR CHRONIC) ON BODY SYSTEMS

The metabolism of all cells, including those in the central nervous system, is inhibited by a profound acidaemia, and myocardial performance and cardiac output fall as the $[H+]$ rises above 80 nmol/l ($pH < 7.10$).[19,48] Exposure to an $[H+]$ above 65 nmol/l ($pH < 7.25$) inhibits surfactant synthesis (p. 484), predisposing to RDS in premature infants (see below). These changes in organ function can be the result of asphyxia occurring before delivery, or of asphyxia secondary to inadequate resuscitation and care in the first few minutes of life in babies who were not asphyxiated at the moment of delivery, or both.

CENTRAL NERVOUS SYSTEM

The most serious impact of asphyxia is on the brain, not only because, by depressing the vital centres in the brain, it results in respiratory depression at birth, but also because asphyxia in term babies leading to HIE is a cause of perinatal brain damage and subsequent neurological handicap (p. 1246).

CARDIOVASCULAR SYSTEM

Heart failure follows severe birth asphyxia[30] (p. 696). Myers[112] noted that it could be one of the aetiological factors contributing to hypoxic–ischaemic encephalopathy, probably by reducing cerebral blood flow at a time when this is pressure passive.[175] The main cause of the heart failure is hypoxic and hypotensive myocardial ischaemia and necrosis,[31] with cardiac dilatation, stretching of the tricuspid valve ring and tricuspid incompetence.[29] It may be aggravated by hypoglycaemia,[6] hypervolaemia caused by injudicious volume expansion[144] or constriction of the placental vascular bed in response to asphyxia and hypoxia[116] or, conversely, by hypovolaemia if there has been partial umbilical artery obstruction.[176]

LUNG EFFECTS

The pulmonary blood flow falls during fetal asphyxia, but once the asphyxia is withdrawn there is a reactive hyperaemia[45] which, in the tissues damaged by asphyxia, causes fluid transudation and oedema. Preterm newborn animals delivered shortly after such an experiment develop pulmonary oedema and histological changes similar to those seen in human infants with RDS.[43] Intrapartum asphyxia therefore increases the incidence of RDS in short-gestation infants[93,170] (p. 484). The postasphyxial pulmonary oedema causes desquamation of the cells lining the terminal air spaces, which is one of the earliest histological changes seen in the lungs of human neonates dying from RDS,[59] the protein-rich oedema fluid inhibits surfactant,[83] the persisting acidaemia inhibits surfactant synthesis,[102] and the defective ventilatory excursion of the asphyxiated infant reduces the release on to the alveolar surface of whatever surfactant he does possess.[186] This is discussed in detail on page 484.

Asphyxiated term infants may gasp for a period after delivery. Alternatively they may be tachypnoeic, driven by the metabolic acidaemia (p. 555), or they may have apneoic pauses.[149] Severe asphyxia by the same mechanisms described above that damage preterm lungs – post-asphyxial hyperperfusion and protein exudation on to the alveolar surface – may also cause severe lung disease in term babies by a mechanism analogous to adult RDS (p. 555).

Evidence for the role of postnatal asphyxia in causing RDS comes from Drew,[49] who showed that efficient postnatal resuscitation of low-birthweight infants could reduce the severity of, and mortality from, RDS, presumably by preventing the deleterious effects of underventilation and acidaemia.

In term infants massive pulmonary haemorrhage (p. 550) is a rare pulmonary sequel of severe asphyxia.[51] Not only are the lungs damaged by the asphyxia, but myocardial ischaemia coupled with fluid overload during resuscitation may result in left ventricular failure.

RENAL EFFECTS

Whenever a neonate develops severe hypoxia or hypotension kidney damage may result. After birth asphyxia, proteinuria is common,[106] as is haematuria, and in severe cases renal failure develops (p. 1026). Myoglobinuria leading to acute tubular necrosis and renal failure can also occur.[89] Those with severe renal damage also tend to have severe neurological disease.[129]

TEMPERATURE HOMOEOSTASIS

Severely asphyxiated babies, particularly VLBW ones, are likely to get cold because it can be difficult to prevent heat loss during resuscitation in the labour ward. In addition, hypoxia is known to depress the thermogenic response to cold (Chapter 18),[152] and even in mildly asphyxiated babies the oxygen consumption is below normal in the first few hours.[150] Sedative drugs given intrapartum to the mother may also depress thermogenesis and result in a cold baby (p. 292).

OTHER ORGAN SYSTEMS

Intrapartum and postnatal asphyxia reduce gut motility in the neonatal period, causing feed intolerance,[20] and probably predispose the neonate to necrotizing enterocolitis.[147] They may also cause hypoglycaemia,[71] hypocalcaemia[174] and hyperammonaemia.[64] The pituitary gland may be affected. Inappropriate antidiuretic hormone production and hyponatraemia are common during the first few days in severely asphyxiated infants,[88] and growth hormone deficiency presenting later in childhood is more common in infants who were breech deliveries.[40] The liver may be damaged and become necrotic,[157] and liver enzymes are raised, though the increased incidence of neonatal jaundice following asphyxia is more likely to be the result of bruising than hepatic dysfunction.[33,57] Clotting factor deficiencies in asphyxiated infants are not reversed by vitamin K[73] and are usually the result of disseminated intravascular coagulation.[38] A recently recognized marker of intrapartum asphyxia is a rise in the nucleated RBC count in cord blood or in the first few hours postnatally.[171] More than 10 nucleated RBC/100 WBC or an absolute count $> 2 \times 10^9$/l strongly suggests fetal asphyxia,[113,132] and Naeye and Localio[113] suggest that this also helps to time the asphyxial insult to between 2 and 36 hours prior to the raised nucleated RBC count.

LABOUR WARD MANAGEMENT OF RESUSCITATION

PREPARATION

As we approach the millennium it is not acceptable for a baby to be born without facilities for adequate resuscitation being immediately available. A baby being born in poor condition is an unpredictable result of a proportion of apparently completely normal labours. Gupta and Tizard[70] found that 30% of babies needing intubation came from low-risk labours and 30 years later, despite all the improvements in perinatal care, an emergency 'crash' call for help in resuscitation was required following 1.5% of all deliveries.[90]

All delivery suites should therefore be equipped to deal with advanced resuscitation practices (see below) and, since blind drug or fluid therapy is no longer acceptable, this should include facilities for assessing whether the three most serious complications of asphyxia, acidaemia, hypotension and hypoglycaemia are present. Furthermore, as the labour ward resuscitation trolley is not the ideal site for complex resuscitation, modern maternity hospitals should be designed so that the delivery suite and the neonatal unit are adjacent to each other, so that the critically ill baby can be referred quickly to the NICU for treatment once he is pink and has an adequate heart rate. Under most circumstances (see below) treatment with drugs or volume expansion can and should wait until the baby is in the NICU and appropriate investigations have been carried out.

HISTORY

In an ideal world a paediatrician would attend all deliveries which are likely to produce an infant requiring resuscitation, having been fully briefed by the obstetrician about the mother's social, medical and obstetric history. However, the reality is that in many situations much of this history has to be obtained in a somewhat frenzied dialogue between the paediatrician and the birth attendants while resuscitation is under way.

If possible, the following information should always be readily available for the paediatrician:

- Maternal age, parity and marital status;
- Gestational age;
- Reasons for preterm delivery;
- Fetal growth during this pregnancy;
- The results of any diagnostic amniocenteses or ultrasound assessments which have been carried out;
- Illnesses in this pregnancy, e.g. diabetes, tuberculosis, malaria, rubella, HIV;

- Complications of this pregnancy, e.g. toxaemia, abruption;
- Important drugs taken during this pregnancy, e.g. anticonvulsants, anticoagulants;
- Previous perinatal morbidity and mortality, e.g. stillbirths, neonatal deaths or infants admitted to an NICU;
- Health of the surviving infants, e.g. cerebral palsy, chromosome abnormalities or hereditary disease such as haemophilia or muscular dystrophy;
- Maternal health during labour, e.g. temperature, evidence of infection;
- Course of labour, e.g. induction, duration of first and second stages, indications for intervention by forceps, caesarean section, CTG changes, fetal blood gases;
- Drugs administered during labour, e.g. uterine stimulants, steroids, antibiotics, opiates, tocolytics.

EQUIPMENT

Most neonatal resuscitation is now carried out on purpose-built resuscitation trolleys (Fig. 16.5), the essential components of which are:

• An adequate shelf on which to lie the infant. This should be at a comfortable height for the resuscitator, tiltable, and permit partial extension of the infant's neck. However, in general babies should lie flat[104] and there is no need to extend the neck during intubation (see below).

• A supply of oxygen for the face mask, bag and mask, T piece or endotracheal tube, capable of giving a flow of 5 l/min. Whichever method of administering oxygen is used, the gas must be passed through a variable-pressure blow-off valve which should normally be set at 30 cmH_2O.

Recent work suggests that using air for labour ward resuscitation is at least as effective as using oxygen[142] and may avoid a potentially damaging reduction in cerebral blood flow seen postnatally in preterm babies resuscitated with 80–100% oxygen.[95] However, it should be remembered that when using bag and mask systems without an attached oxygen reservoir (Fig. 16.6) at 5 l oxygen/min the baby receives only about 40% oxygen, and if the reservoir is attached this increases to 60–70%.[75]

• A mask for giving oxygen to the cyanosed but breathing baby.

• A suction tube with soft suction catheters sizes FG 8 and 10 to clear the airway, and FG 2/3 to suck through the ETT. The suction should not exceed 200 mmHg, and for routine use should be set at 100 mmHg (= 136 cmH_2O) to prevent damage to the oropharyngeal mucosa. Because of the risk of infection from the neonate, mouth-held mucus extractors should not be used.

• An overhead radiant heat source and sides to the resuscitation shelf to minimize the radiant and convective heat losses, respectively.

• A large stopclock with a sweep second hand, as time passes very quickly in any emergency procedure.

The equipment on the trolley must include:

• A bag and mask system for artificial ventilation. The easiest masks to use are those with a pneumatic rim to obtain a tight face seal connected to a self-inflating bag. The mask must be detachable from the bag unit, and replaceable with a connector for an endotracheal tube. Several bag and mask systems are commercially available (Fig. 16.6), but the Ambu bag and Paediatric Laerdal systems with soft face masks are preferable (see below). They must be squeezed gently in accordance with the manufacturer's instructions; if they are squeezed too

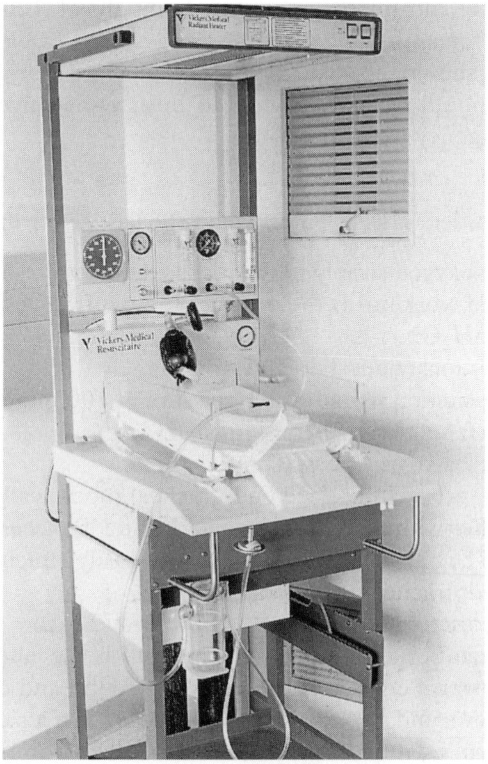

Fig. 16.5 Resuscitation trolley with overhead heater, large clock, adequate resuscitation area and appropriate storage space.

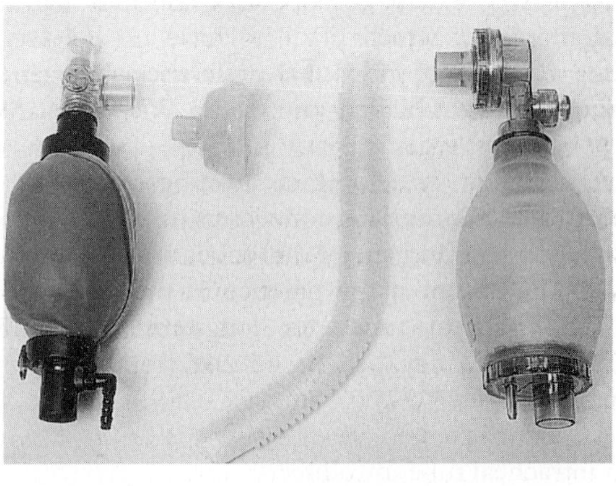

Fig. 16.6 Bag and mask systems appropriate for neonatal resuscitation. Ambu bag on the left; Paediatric Laerdal on the right. The hose should be connected to act as a reservoir if high oxygen concentrations are required.

violently they are capable of generating inflation pressures of 60–80 cmH_2O or greater. Various alternatives to these standard self-inflating bag and mask systems have been suggested. Some neonatologists prefer using an anaesthetic bag and mask system. These have the disadvantage that the bag is not self-inflating and the escape vent has to be held shut by the physician's fourth and fifth fingers while he is squeezing the bag with the other fingers. Its use therefore requires greater manual dexterity, but in skilled hands it is a safe and effective system.

A good alternative is simply to occlude a T piece connected to a face mask and to the gas supply via a pressure-limiting device,[80] but this has the disadvantage that unless the Resuscitaire is adapted, pure oxygen will be given. A T connector connected to the ETT is also an effective alternative to using a bag and mask system attached to the ETT in those babies for whom intubation is indicated, but has the same drawback of giving virtually pure oxygen. T-piece systems have many advantages, however: they are easy to sterilize and assemble, and they make it easier to monitor the inflation pressure and give a long inflation time, which is important to establish a FRC (see below).

More recently the laryngeal mask has been used successfully for neonatal resuscitation.[28]

Although there may be a place for alternative techniques, given the problems in training in neonatal resuscitation,[14] I believe that widespread uniformity in the use of proven and effective techniques has great merit, rather than each neonatal unit using its own gimmick. For this reason, residents and, if appropriate, nurses should be trained in the effective use of self-inflating bag and mask systems (Fig. 16.6), both for use in the labour ward and for subsequent resuscitation, and to resort promptly if necessary (Fig. 16.7) to endotracheal intubation and IPPV using either a T piece or the same bag and mask system to inflate the lungs.

- A selection of baby-sized oropharyngeal airways (sizes 00 and 000).
- At least two laryngoscopes (as one may fail at the crucial moment); which blade to have on the laryngoscope is a matter of individual preference, but generally speaking a straight-bladed one of the Wisconsin, Magill or Oxford Infant types is best.
- A selection of endotracheal tubes (2.5, 3.0 and 3.5 mm) and appropriate connectors from them to the resuscitation bag. In general oral tubes are easier to insert in emergencies, but if the practice of the unit is to use nasal endotracheal tubes for long-term ventilation a supply of these may be left on the trolley for use in appropriate cases.

- Endotracheal tube introducers.
- Magill forceps for nasal endotracheal tubes.
- Nasogastric tubes type FG 6 and 8 for emptying the stomach, particularly in meconium-affected babies.
- Disposable gloves.
- A selection of syringes, needles, specimen bottles and intravenous cannulae.
- Adhesive tape of a type that will not damage very fragile preterm skin.
- Cord clamps and ties.
- A large pair of scissors.
- A stethoscope.
- Equipment for emergency cannulation of the umbilical vessels (p. 1374) should be on the trolley, together with equipment for draining a pneumothorax (p. 1381).
- BM/Dextrostix.
- ECG monitor.
- An oximeter.
- A Dinamap blood pressure recorder.

The only drugs required on the trolley are:

- Sodium bicarbonate (4.2%, 7.5% or 8.4%), 10 ml ampoules;
- THAM 7%, 10 ml ampoules;
- Normal saline (for umbilical catheters), 10 ml ampoules;
- 10% dextrose, 10 ml ampoules;
- Albumin 4.5%, 100 ml bottle;
- Naloxone 0.4 mg/ml, 2 ml ampoules;
- Vitamin K, 1 mg ampoules.

A small box containing the following drugs, which are occasionally needed in emergencies, should be included: frusemide, calcium gluconate, 1:1000 and 1:10 000 adrenaline, atropine, glucagon. A supply of 1000 U/ml heparin for anticoagulation of syringes used in blood gas analysis should be kept in the labour ward refrigerator. There should be ready access to fresh O-negative blood for emergency transfusion.

Equipment checks on arrival in the labour ward:

- Is the oxygen supply to the resuscitation trolley turned on and working? Is the pressure blow-off valve set at 30 cmH_2O?
- Is the clock wound up and working?
- Is the suction working at a pressure of 100 mmHg and is a soft suction catheter attached?
- Is the laryngoscope working?
- Are appropriately-sized endotracheal tubes available, together with matching connectors and T pieces?
- Is the bag and mask unit there, and easily attached to an endotracheal tube connector?
- Is the thermal environment appropriate? Is the resuscitation unit heater switched on? Is the labour ward warm enough? If necessary go round and close windows and doors and turn off fans; when a sick preterm infant is expected his thermal environment takes priority over that of the obstetrician, the delivery ward staff and the parents. The room temperature

should be 70°F for a full-term infant, and least 75°F if a preterm baby is expected.

- Are there some warmed dry towels to wrap the baby in during resuscitation, and bonnets for preterm babies?

PERSONNEL

If twins or a VLBW infant or one requiring complex resuscitation, such as known hydrops or exomphalos, are anticipated, ensure that adequate staff are present: at least two neonatologists plus adequate nursing support are needed.

INITIAL CARE OF THE BABY AFTER DELIVERY

Start the clock on the resuscitation trolley the moment the baby is free from the mother's body (not when the cord is clamped). As soon as the baby (usually enclosed in a wet and bloody theatre towel) is placed on the trolley note his age (usually 30–40 seconds), and assess his heart rate, respiration, colour and tone. To check the heart rate it is essential to listen to the chest with a stethoscope: do not rely on feeling the umbilical arterial pulsation in the cord, as all you feel is your own heartbeat pounding away in your fingertips. Always dry the infant as soon as you receive him, discard the wet towel and cover him with prewarmed dry towels to minimize heat loss (p. 294).

It is then traditional to do the Apgar score (p. 242), ideally at 1 minute of age. What is much more important in the baby who does not breathe adequately is, by using his heart rate, respiratory activity and general clinical state set against the background of the maternal history and the course of the labour, to diagnose the cause of his poor transition to postnatal life (see above). Only by doing this rapidly and effectively in the first 60–90 seconds after the baby arrives on the resuscitation trolley can the neonatologist give appropriate care.

If the baby does not start to breathe, the crucial question is whether or not he is in primary or terminal apnoea (see above). Infants in primary apnoea are usually in reasonable clinical condition, with a heart rate > 80/min and good peripheral perfusion and body tone, although cyanosed and apnoeic (Apgar 4–7). Infants in terminal apnoea are more likely to be pale and apnoeic, with little or no body tone or reflex response, and their heart rate is usually less than 60/min (i.e. Apgar 1–3).

However, in many babies, particularly those born prematurely, this differentiation is not clear-cut, and if apnoea lasts longer than 2–3 minutes active resuscitation, usually with intubation and IPPV, is indicated.

CARE OF THE INFANT AFTER THE INITIAL ASSESSMENT

On the basis of the initial assessment, by 60–90 seconds of age most infants clearly fall into one of four groups:

- Fit, healthy, bawling lustily (90–95%);
- Blue and apnoeic, or not breathing too well; the pulse rate is 80–100; probably in primary apnoea or in the phase of gasping (5–6%);
- Obvious terminal apnoea, pale, limp and apnoeic, heart rate less than 60 (0.2–0.5%);
- Dead but resuscitatable (less than 0.1%).

Fit and healthy

Leave this baby alone; do not suck him out, as this may damage the pharyngeal mucosa and is a powerful vagal stimulus which may trigger a reflex bradycardia. Enthusiastic sucking is based on the frequently held misconception that what is coming out of the baby's mouth is inhaled amniotic fluid. It is not: it is fetal pulmonary fluid which has been in the lungs prior to birth, and it will do no harm if it stays there a few moments longer or is swallowed. If the upper airway is full of meconium, blood or some other extraneous material the infant should be laryngoscoped and his mouth, larynx and trachea meticulously cleared under direct vision.

This lusty breathing infant should be dried and wrapped in a warm blanket to minimize heat loss, his umbilical cord securely clamped or tied, given a dose of vitamin K and given to his mother, who, if she is intending to breast-feed, should be encouraged to put him to the breast. Snatching him away for some arcane medical ritual at this point is cruel and unnecessary – even the vitamin K can wait. In the first hour a baby is awake and alert, and this period is very important in establishing a close attachment between mother and baby (Chapter 5). Suckling at this time is also important in establishing long-term and successful lactation (p. 376). There is absolutely no need to bathe the infant immediately: it does not harm him to be covered in vernix or have some blood in his hair, whereas in many labour wards bathing is a very efficient way of dropping even a healthy baby's body temperature to less than 35°C.

Apnoeic or breathing inadequately, but with a good heart rate and tone (presumed primary apnoea)

Full-term infants

Follow the instructions in Fig. 16.7. Most of these babies respond to peripheral stimuli, such as rubbing with a warmed towel or flicking their toes (see above), plus giving oxygen by face mask, or to bag and mask ventilation.[121] However, a small percentage of such babies, despite apparently adequate bag and mask ventilation, will either remain cyanosed or will fail to establish regular respiration. In both these situations, by 2–3 minutes of age it is much safer to intubate the baby and establish pulmonary ventilation that way. The vast

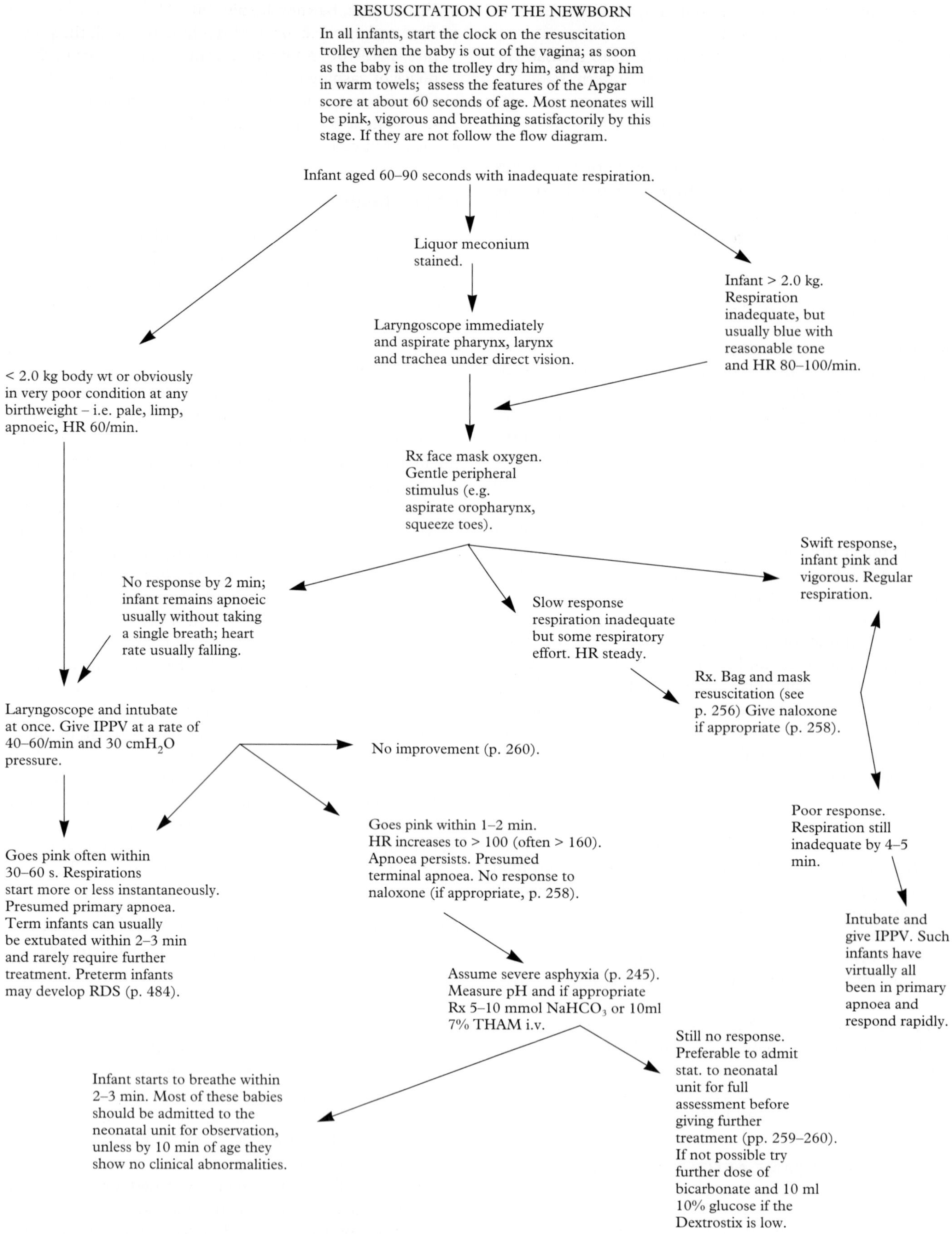
RESUSCITATION OF THE NEWBORN
In all infants, start the clock on the resuscitation trolley when the baby is out of the vagina; as soon as the baby is on the trolley dry him, and wrap him in warm towels; assess the features of the Apgar score at about 60 seconds of age. Most neonates will be pink, vigorous and breathing satisfactorily by this stage. If they are not follow the flow diagram.
Infant aged 60–90 seconds with inadequate respiration.
Liquor meconium stained.
Laryngoscope immediately and aspirate pharynx, larynx and trachea under direct vision.
Infant > 2.0 kg. Respiration inadequate, but usually blue with reasonable tone and HR 80–100/min.
< 2.0 kg body wt or obviously in very poor condition at any birthweight – i.e. pale, limp, apnoeic, HR 60/min.
Rx face mask oxygen. Gentle peripheral stimulus (e.g. aspirate oropharynx, squeeze toes).
Swift response, infant pink and vigorous. Regular respiration.
No response by 2 min; infant remains apnoeic usually without taking a single breath; heart rate usually falling.
Slow response respiration inadequate but some respiratory effort. HR steady.
Rx. Bag and mask resuscitation (see p. 256) Give naloxone if appropriate (p. 258).
Laryngoscope and intubate at once. Give IPPV at a rate of 40–60/min and 30 cmH_2O pressure.
No improvement (p. 260).
Poor response. Respiration still inadequate by 4–5 min.
Goes pink often within 30–60 s. Respirations start more or less instantaneously. Presumed primary apnoea. Term infants can usually be extubated within 2–3 min and rarely require further treatment. Preterm infants may develop RDS (p. 484).
Goes pink within 1–2 min. HR increases to > 100 (often > 160). Apnoea persists. Presumed terminal apnoea. No response to naloxone (if appropriate, p. 258).
Intubate and give IPPV. Such infants have virtually all been in primary apnoea and respond rapidly.
Assume severe asphyxia (p. 245). Measure pH and if appropriate Rx 5–10 mmol $NaHCO_3$ or 10ml 7% THAM i.v.
Still no response. Preferable to admit stat. to neonatal unit for full assessment before giving further treatment (pp. 259–260). If not possible try further dose of bicarbonate and 10 ml 10% glucose if the Dextrostix is low.
Infant starts to breathe within 2–3 min. Most of these babies should be admitted to the neonatal unit for observation, unless by 10 min of age they show no clinical abnormalities.

Fig. 16.7 Flow diagram for resuscitation of the newborn.

majority of infants in primary apnoea who require resuscitation by IPPV usually respond at once and will start to breathe very quickly, often gasping in response to lung inflation (Head's reflex), and then become pink. Such infants can usually be extubated within a further 2–3 minutes, rarely require further medical care, and can normally be transferred from the labour ward to the postnatal ward with their mother.

The clinical condition at birth (Apgar score of 4–7), combined with this prompt and characteristic response to resuscitation, enables a retrospective diagnosis of primary apnoea to be made with confidence (see above).

However, if, despite becoming pink on IPPV, the baby still does not make any respiratory effort it suggests that he was either in terminal apnoea or has some other cause for respiratory depression, such as drugs, congenital infection or primary neurological disease. The treatment of terminal apnoea is outlined below and, of the other possibilities, the only one which should be treated in the labour ward is opiate-induced ventilatory depression (see below).

Preterm infants

All preterm infants less than 30–32 weeks' gestation who do not go pink and establish regular normal respiration spontaneously immediately after delivery should be intubated and given IPPV at once, irrespective of whether they are diagnosed as being in primary or terminal apnoea. The disadvantages of delaying the onset of satisfactory ventilation and gas exchange are so great (p. 493) that no apnoeic preterm infant should ever be treated expectantly on the assumption that he is in primary apnoea and might start to breathe soon.

Babies in obvious terminal apnoea

These babies are usually pale and apnoeic, with a heart rate less than 60/min. About 0.2–0.5% of all deliveries result in this condition, and such babies represent about 5–10% of all infants apnoeic at 2 minutes of age. Such a baby is severely asphyxiated and will never breathe spontaneously unless he is resuscitated by positive-pressure ventilation. The longer intubation is delayed, the more profound the biochemical and physiological abnormalities and the greater the likelihood of permanent brain damage. Expeditious action is therefore essential (Fig. 16.7).

Most babies in terminal apnoea, following the first few inflations of the lungs with oxygen down the endotracheal tube, will become pink and their heart rate will rise, often to 160–180/min. If this does not happen despite adequate ventilation, it suggests either a technical error, poor myocardial function often compounded by profound metabolic acidaemia, hypoglycaemia, or severe lung disease (see below).

If there is a poor response and the heart rate is < 40 and falling, a short period of external cardiac massage (p. 257) plus some bicarbonate (p. 258) almost always results in the heart rate increasing and the baby becoming pink.

The pattern of the infant's response to ventilation should be noted carefully. If his heart rate increases and he becomes pink before the onset of respiration, it is characteristic and diagnostic of terminal apnoea (p. 245), in contrast to the infant who is resuscitated by IPPV in primary apnoea (see above). If the response suggests terminal apnoea it is then essential to note the time that elapses between starting IPPV and the first gasp, and between starting IPPV and the onset of regular respiration (p. 246) (Fig. 16.3), as these are excellent indicators of the severity of the asphyxia.

Of babies resuscitated from terminal apnoea the majority will respond within 4–5 minutes to the above management by starting to gasp and then breathing regularly (p. 245). If a baby does not start to breathe within this time it is very suggestive that he is suffering from either drug-induced respiratory depression or severe asphyxia and acidaemia (p. 259). Appropriate treatment for the first is to give naloxone (p. 258), but only to babies whose mothers received opiate drugs in the 6 hours prior to delivery. For other babies in terminal apnoea not breathing by 5–6 minutes of age, measure the pH and, if appropriate (see below), give bicarbonate or THAM.

Dead

If the obstetrician is certain that the fetal heart was heard up to 10 minutes prior to delivery it is always worth attempting to resuscitate the fresh stillbirth, i.e. the neonate with an Apgar score of 0.

Some such infants respond very quickly and dramatically to conventional cardiopulmonary resuscitation and are vigorous and active by 5–10 minutes of age. These were either not stillbirths (i.e. had very quiet and slow heart sounds not detected by the panicking paediatrician), or had undergone a sudden acute asphyxial stimulus that caused cardiac arrest just before delivery, without previous prolonged myocardium and brain-damaging asphyxia.

When confronted with a fresh stillbirth always send for help, as at any cardiac arrest more than one pair of expert hands is needed urgently. After starting the clock on the resuscitation trolley, an essential move, start the resuscitation by giving ECM (see below).

Next, laryngoscope the baby and aspirate any extraneous material in the airway, intubate him and give IPPV. Continue the ECM and IPPV simultaneously, as this may improve tissue perfusion.[131] For a prompt effect before vascular access is achieved, adrenaline (0.1–0.25 ml of 1:1000) can be given endotracheally at this stage[91] and rapidly reaches the systemic circulation (see below).

Insert an UVC as quickly as possible, as this is the quickest (and safest) way of guaranteeing vascular access. Sterile precautions can be reduced to a minimum since speed is of the essence. Once the UVC is inserted give 10–20 mmol of sodium bicarbonate intravenously, depending on the size of the neonate: this can be given over 2–3 minutes, in contrast to the slower rates at which this agent should be given to 'living' babies (p. 504).

By now the infant will be 4–5 minutes old. Assess the situation and attach the ECG monitor and oximeter. If there are no signs of cardiac activity consider drug therapy (see below), including intracardiac adrenaline.

If a heartbeat returns but cardiac output remains low, or bradycardia persists, the following drugs (see below) may be useful:

- atropine 0.1 mg i.v. for persisting bradycardia;
- lignocaine 1–2 mg/kg i.v. for ventricular tachycardia or fibrillation;
- calcium gluconate 1–2 ml 10% solution slowly i.v. under ECG control for hyperkalaemia and poor cardiac output;
- plasma/albumin 10 ml/kg for hypotension and poor cardiac output.

The baby should be admitted to a NICU, and his subsequent management is outlined on pages 259–260.

If by 10 minutes of age the Apgar score is still 0, and in particular if the oximeter or ECG shows persisting asystole without effective peripheral oxygenation from ECM and IPPV, then resuscitation should be withdrawn as neurologically intact survival is no longer possible.[86] For the baby who makes no respiratory effort by 25–30 minutes but is pink and well perfused, the outlook is also very poor. Such babies, however, should be transferred to the NICU for full evaluation, in particular to exclude non-asphyxial causes of failure to breathe which may have genetic implications (see below).

TECHNIQUES USED DURING RESUSCITATION

ARTIFICIAL VENTILATION

When resuscitating a baby by any method it is essential to make sure that the chest is moving and that the lungs are being inflated. If this is not happening you are doing something wrong, and if you are using bag and mask ventilation it is probably safest to proceed to intubation.

Bag and mask

This should be the first line of resuscitation after clearing the airway in all babies who make a poor transition to extrauterine life, unless they are very preterm (< 30/52 gestation), obviously in terminal apnoea (group 3 above) or stillborn (group 4 above), in which case they should be intubated immediately. All staff involved in neonatal resuscitation should be trained to carry out bag and mask resuscitation effectively, recognizing that it is not an easy technique. It is essential to have a tight seal where the mask is applied to the baby's face; to ensure an adequate airway the baby's neck should be slightly extended with his jaw held forward (an oropharyngeal airway may help). It is a common mistake either to overextend or overflex the neck during attempted bag and mask resuscitation (or for that matter during intubation); both these manoeuvres obstruct the airway at pharyngeal and laryngeal level.

Table 16.9 Efficacy of neonatal bag and mask systems in resuscitation[53]

System	Inflation pressure achieved (cmH_2O)	Inflation time achieved (secs)	Expiratory volume (ml)*
Neonatal Laerdal	20.2	1.11	5.5
Paediatric Laerdal	26.9	1.26	10.4
Penlon	19.2	0.8	8.3
Ambu Baby	30.3	1.8	15.4

* This volume gives a measure of the likely tidal gas exchange.

When using a bag and mask system, studies have shown that a soft-rimmed mask with a small dead space, such as the Bennett or Laerdal, is the easiest to use and gives the best face seal,[120] and that the Ambu bag and paediatric (but not neonatal) Laerdal bag and mask systems (Fig. 16.6) achieve the best respiratory exchange[53] (Table 16.9). In routine use, connected to 5 l oxygen/min, these give 40% oxygen, rising to 60–70% if the reservoir hose is used. It is clear from personal experience and the literature[122] that most babies requiring active intervention respond well to bag and mask resuscitation at birth. This is because most such babies are in primary apnoea, and the bag and mask system either augments their own spontaneous respiration when it occurs, or provokes a Head's reflex and thus spontaneous lung aeration.[122]

For the baby in terminal apnoea who has never drawn breath the situation is very different. The lungs of this baby contain fluid, and at the onset of respiration an air–liquid interface must be formed at the alveolar surface. Studies on the lungs of animals and human neonates[168] usually show that a pressure higher than that required for normal ventilation is necessary to expand such lungs artificially. When using a bag and mask on babies with unexpanded lungs, Milner et al[105] showed that a useful tidal exchange does not take place (Table 16.10) This matches perfectly with clinical experience. In a recent study about 1 in 500 term neonates did not respond to bag and mask ventilation,[121] and this is very close to the estimated incidence of babies born in terminal apnoea – and therefore with unexpanded lungs (see above), and also to the incidence of grades II and III hypoxic ischaemic encephalopathy (p. 1239). There is a great deal of overlap between these three groups.

Table 16.10 Expiratory volume achieved with first three breaths using bag and mask ventilation or endotracheal tubes. All babies were ventilated at pressures of approximately 30 cmH_2O. The expiratory volume gives a close estimate of the tidal exchange[105]

	Expiratory volume (ml)		
	Breath 1	Breath 2	Breath 3
Bag and mask	3.0	4.7	3.9
ETT and IPPV	14.3	10.5	17.0

For babies not responding to bag and mask resuscitation by 2–3 minutes of age, in particular if they are not being ventilated (no chest movement or air entry on auscultation), it is essential to progress at once to endotracheal intubation and IPPV.

Intubation and intermittent positive-pressure ventilation

This must be used in all babies who are not showing an adequate response to other forms of resuscitation by 2–3 minutes of age. It is not acceptable to advise continued attempts at bag and mask resuscitation because intubation could be difficult or dangerous. Apart from anything else, if it is really necessary to intubate it is never difficult in the presence of normal anatomy, and the dangers have been grossly overstated.

To intubate a baby (p. 1369), lie him with his head in the same plane as his body or only slightly extended; using your left hand insert the laryngoscope into his mouth and, with the tip of the blade in the vallecula, use it to pull the epiglottis forward and thus reveal the vocal cords. If an assistant presses lightly on the cricoid cartilage, or if you do it with the fifth finger of the hand holding the laryngoscope, the view of the larynx is improved.

Insert either a 3.0 or 3.5 mm external diameter tube. The former can be inserted into all but the smallest preterm infant (< 1.00 kg birthweight), and the latter should be used in full-term infants. A 2.5 mm tube has a high internal resistance and is often pushed in too far (see below). These tubes should only be used if it is not possible to insert a larger one.

Ideally a shouldered oral endotracheal tube should be used for resuscitation, as the shoulder makes it less likely that the tube will be pushed in too far. The operator must hold the tube firmly in place with the finger and thumb of his left hand.

Connect the tube to the bag system or to a T connector and ventilate the baby, ensuring both by observation of the chest (not the abdomen) and direct auscultation over both lung fields that the lungs are being ventilated.

Studies similar to those done with the bag and mask system have shown, perhaps surprisingly, that even IPPV down an endotracheal tube achieves poorer ventilation

Table 16.11 Tidal exchange and FRC established in term neonates taking a first spontaneous breath, and in the first inflation of those resuscitated with a 1-second and 2- to 5-second inflation time down an endotracheal tube. Mean values are given with range in parentheses[104]

	Spontaneous breath	1-second inflation of IPPV	2- to 5-second inflation of IPPV
Inspiratory/inflation pressure (cmH_2O)	33 (6.1–103)	30	30
Tidal exchange (ml)	40.3 (2.7–90)	18.6 (0–62.5)	33.6 (16.9–70)
FRC (ml)	18.7 (2.7–40)	7.5 (0–15.5)	15.9 (11.7–23.2)

than the baby's own spontaneous respirations[104] (Table 16.11). To achieve the optimal gas exchange, and at the same time establish an FRC, it is necessary to use a long inflation time. This is impossible to achieve using the commercial bag and mask systems; the most efficient way is to attach a simple T connector to the ETT and occlude the expiratory limb for at least 1–3 seconds, and preferably longer (Table 16.11).[24] When resuscitating preterm babies the tidal volume achieved is even less,[79] which is a further justification for early intubation and control of ventilation in such patients.

The IPPV should be at a pressure of 30 cmH_2O, and when using an inspiratory time of at least 1 second it is not usually possible (or necessary) to ventilate at an overall rate of more than 30–40/min. Occasionally, in neonates with severe underlying lung disease, such as early-onset RDS, or with severe meconium aspiration or diaphragmatic hernia, higher pressures and rates may be needed, and the resuscitation trolley should be designed in such a way that these alterations can be made rapidly and safely. Alternatively pure oxygen can be administered through a T piece rather than using bag and mask systems, which give less than 60–70% oxygen (see above).

EXTERNAL CARDIAC MASSAGE

This must be given properly. Unfortunately many authoritative sources give the wrong advice, namely to depress the sternum with two fingers. Several studies[42,173] have shown that this is ineffective. The baby must be held as shown in Fig. 16.8, with the fingers along the thoracolumbar spine and both thumbs placed over the lower sternum.[133] The sternum should be firmly depressed at a rate of 100–120/min, with sufficient vigour to obtain an acceptable pulse. The force required can be learned by practising during resuscitation of babies who have suffered cardiac arrest postnatally and have indwelling arterial cannulae connected to a pressure transducer.

ADMINISTERING DRUGS DURING RESUSCITATION

In the past drugs were commonly administered 'blind' during neonatal resuscitation because it was not possible

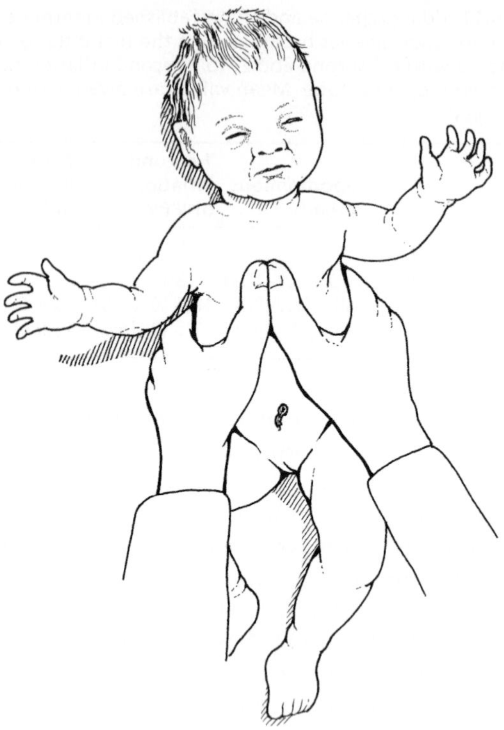

Fig. 16.8 Technique of chest compression for cardiopulmonary resuscitation.

to obtain more or less instantaneous clinical or biochemical assessment of whether the treatment was necessary. This is no longer the case, except perhaps in the resuscitation of the fresh stillbirth, since for three of the four most commonly used drugs a simple and instantly available test will answer whether they are needed or not. Before giving bicarbonate the pH and base deficit should be measured: before giving glucose hypoglycaemia should be confirmed by BM Stix; and the blood pressure should be checked by Dinamap before giving volume expansion with albumin. Naloxone, however, can be given on the basis of the history of administration of opiates to the mother.

If drugs have to be given during resuscitation to an apnoeic infant, particularly one who is in terminal apnoea or is stillborn, it is usually impossible to give them through a peripheral vein, because the infant is so underperfused that it is impossible to insert a drip.

It is also dangerous to inject drugs directly into the umbilical vein, as this may:

- swill an umbilical vein clot into the systemic circulation;
- result in the drug not reaching the systemic circulation when using small-volume infusions (e.g. naloxone, adrenaline);
- traumatize the umbilical artery, causing haemorrhage and making subsequent arterial catheterization difficult;
- go directly into the umbilical artery, causing spasm and ischaemia in the distribution of the iliac vessels (pp. 919–921);
- go down a patent urachus and into the bladder.

For these reasons an umbilical venous catheter should be inserted, and there should be appropriate provision for doing this on all resuscitation trolleys.

Naloxone

Naloxone is a pure antagonist of exogenous and endogenous opioids. Because of the surge of endorphins perinatally naloxone was tried as a general treatment for apnoea at birth, but this proved unsuccessful.[37] It is not without hazard, and its use in animals may increase the severity of asphyxial brain damage,[187] perhaps by causing a surge in catecholamines.[119] Care should be taken in administering naloxone to the newborn of narcotic addicts, as this may precipitate an acute withdrawal episode.[62]

Whatever the mechanism, the effects of intravenous naloxone are complex and potentially dangerous. It must therefore only be used if the mother of an apnoeic infant has received opiate analgesics in the 4–6 hours before delivery. Furthermore, it must only be given after respiration has been established, by IPPV if necessary, and the baby has become pink. Never give it to an apnoeic unventilated infant, although if an infant is pink but breathing irregularly it is perfectly safe to give intramuscular naloxone while watching the baby carefully until the drug begins to work and respiration becomes regular. A dose of 0.1 mg/kg should be given i.m. or i.v.[8] and may be repeated if necessary.

Sodium bicarbonate

The continuing sterile debate[76,81] about using base in neonatal resuscitation can only be perpetuated by those who have never seen the dramatic response in respiration, heart rate and cardiac output when a severely acidotic (pH < 7.0) pale, apnoeic, peripherally shutdown baby is given base at an appropriately safe rate of infusion. For every theoretical argument that says i.v. bicarbonate reduces CSF pH, that if it is given it results in a poorer outcome from cardiac arrest in animals or adults, the latter often with ventricular fibrillation,[11,188] or that it induces hypercapnia,[118] counter theoretical arguments can be mounted that it speeds the return of respiration,[3] increases tissue sensitivity to catecholamines[138] and in fact raises the intracellular pH of animal brains.[78,153]

Inappropriate therapy (e.g. with the pH > 7.0) at inappropriate rates (see p. 504) is wrong and potentially harmful, and the habit of giving babies who receive IPPV in the labour ward a homoeopathically useless 2–3 mmol of bicarbonate i.v. is also to be deprecated. However, if a neonate is not responding adequately to IPPV (persistent apnoea or bradycardia) and has a pH measured in cord blood or immediately after birth of < 7.0 ([H +] > 100 nmol/l) he should be given i.v. base, and since THAM does have the theoretical advantage of rapidly correcting CSF pH[145] it may be preferable.

Glucose

There has been some controversy in recent years about the use of glucose during neonatal resuscitation because glucose infusion during resuscitation in adults (animals) accentuates brain damage. However, this is not the case in neonates.[178] If, during resuscitation, a neonate is found to be hypoglycaemic on Dextrostix because he has used up his glycogen reserves during the preceding asphyxia, he should be given 1 g of glucose i.v. (10 ml of 10% dextrose) and his glucose homoeostasis maintained thereafter by an appropriate rate of infusion of i.v. dextrose (p. 948).

Adrenaline

This drug has a place in the resuscitation of the baby who is stillborn or extremely bradycardic, although the outcome in babies in whom it is used is extremely poor.[159] Initially it can be given intratracheally immediately after intubation,[91] and if adequate doses are given (0.25 ml 1:1000 adrenaline/kg; 250 μg/kg) adequate plasma levels are achieved.[151] If, after one or two doses of endotracheal or i.v. adrenaline, asystole persists, it is worth giving one or two doses of intracardiac adrenaline by 5–10 minutes of age, injecting at the 4–5th spaces at the left sternal edge. If conventional doses of 0.1–0.2 ml/kg 1:10 000 adrenaline do not produce electrical activity, there is some evidence that large doses (e.g. 1–200 μg/kg, 0.1–0.2 ml/kg 1:1000 adrenaline) should be given.[9,117,180]

Albumin/plasma expansion

It has become common practice to give large volumes of colloid 'blind' to babies with low Apgar scores without measuring blood pressure. This is bad practice[144] and infusions of albumin can be harmful.[39a] Most asphyxiated babies are hypervolaemic[92] and have a normal blood pressure once they are oxygenated[107] (Fig. 16.2). Those who are not, are likely to have ischaemic myocardial damage, and volume overload is therefore ill advised.

Only if an asphyxiated neonate is found to be hypotensive once adequately oxygenated and with a normal heart rate should volume replacement be considered, and if blood loss is likely (pp. 814–815) blood transfusion is the treatment of choice, rather than colloid. If there is nothing to suggest blood loss or cord entanglement which can cause fetal anaemia,[176] then inotropic therapy with dopamine and dobutamine is preferable[182] (p. 504), carefully adding volume replacement concurrently if the response to inotropes is poor.

Calcium

There is no point giving calcium to the asystolic neonate. However, if there is ECG evidence of ventricular activity, particularly with electromechanical dissociation, and poor cardiac output persists, because such babies are very likely to be hyperkalaemic (see above) the effect of a single dose of 0.2 ml/kg of 10% calcium gluconate should be tried.[9,179]

Analeptics

Drugs such as nikethamide or other analeptics are of no value in terminal apnoea, and in fact are positively dangerous (see above).

CONTINUING THERAPY FOLLOWING RESUSCITATION

The infant who has established regular respiration

Unless an infant, assessed as being in terminal apnoea, responds very rapidly to resuscitation, and is pink, vigorous and neurologically normal by 8–10 minutes of age, he should be admitted to the NICU. On admission, as well as carefully examining him and measuring his blood pressure, his PCV, blood glucose and blood gases should be measured. A chest X-ray is indicated if there is any evidence of cardiorespiratory distress. In most term babies these investigations are usually normal, no further treatment is required, and apart from looking slightly wide-eyed and overalert for a few hours (i.e. grade I HIE p. 1231), they make a very rapid recovery. Hypoglycaemia (glucose < 1.5 mmol/l) should always be corrected, but base deficits of 10–20 mmol/l usually correct spontaneously and rapidly,[164] and there is no need to give otherwise asymptomatic acidaemic term babies intravenous bicarbonate or THAM.

These babies can usually be transferred to their mothers on the postnatal ward by 24–36 hours of age.

If a preterm infant suffers this degree of asphyxia he will almost certainly develop RDS, and his subsequent management is described fully on pages 502–511. The treatment of the minority of term babies who develop grade I–III hypoxic–ischaemic encephalopathy with multiorgan involvement is given on pages 1242–1245.

The infant who does not start to breathe

If an infant has become pink with a good cardiac output, yet by 20 minutes of age has made no spontaneous respiratory effort despite adequate oxygenation and appropriate treatment with bicarbonate, glucose and naloxone, then further therapy should be delayed until further blood gas analysis, blood glucose measurements and a chest X-ray have been carried out. If these show some persisting abnormality appropriate therapy can be given, but if they are normal yet apnoea persists this is very suggestive of either profound neurological problems, with a grave prognosis, or, particularly if the evidence for asphyxia is minimal, some underlying neurological disorder (see below).

Despite controlling blood gases and biochemistry and achieving satisfactory cardiac, pulmonary and renal function, the occasional baby who has suffered from severe asphyxia may develop severe intractable cerebral oedema and may never establish spontaneous respiration. The prognosis for such babies is awful.[86,166] After making absolutely sure that the apnoea does not represent drug depression or an inherited neurological defect, and after discussion with the parents, it is appropriate to discontinue life-support procedures in a way and at a time that allows the parents to be with and to hold their baby as he dies.

THE INFANT WHO DOES NOT RESPOND TO IPPV AND RESUSCITATION

There are three main categories of baby who behave in this way:

- The baby who clinically is assessed as asphyxiated but, despite the procedures outlined in this chapter, is still cyanosed and often bradycardic at 5–10 minutes of age.
- The baby who is vigorous and active, makes good respiratory efforts, yet fails to go pink. This strongly suggests an unasphyxiated baby with a serious malformation in his respiratory tract or cardiovascular system.
- The baby born apnoeic or with very feeble respiratory efforts and no objective evidence of intrapartum complication who requires intubation and promptly goes pink with a good heart rate, but who remains hypotonic and with inadequate or absent respiration. This strongly suggests a primary neurological or myopathic disorder.

THE ASPHYXIATED BABY WHO DOES NOT RESPOND TO RESUSCITATION

There are five reasons for this state of affairs:

- There is some technical error in the resuscitation procedure.
- The infant is very ill with serious underlying lung disease.
- The infant has developed a pneumothorax.
- The asphyxial insult has been very severe.
- There is some congenital structural abnormality which prevents oxygenation.

The second, third and fifth conditions listed may also present as a baby who is breathing vigorously and, although not apparently asphyxiated, fails to go pink.

Technical error

In infants whose external appearance is normal, by far and away the most common reason for a poor response to resuscitation is a technical error. It is therefore essential to check as quickly as possible whether:

- The endotracheal tube is in the wrong place, either in the oesophagus or down one main stem bronchus, or even in some more distant part of the bronchial tree. This is very likely to occur if too small a tube is used or if the tube is not 'shouldered'. It is very easy to be misled by chest movement and breath sounds over the chest. The infant's chest may move if IPPV is applied to his stomach, and the conducted sounds of gas going in and out of the stomach may trap the unwary into thinking that it is going in and out of the lungs. Exactly the same problems can occur if only one lung or a section of it is being ventilated. If in doubt, check by auscultation that gas is not going into the abdomen and that air really does enter both sides of the chest equally. If necessary, relaryngoscope the baby to confirm that the endotracheal tube is in the larynx.
- An adequate inflation pressure (usually set to 30 cmH_2O) is being applied. The blow-off valve on the resuscitation trolley may become inadvertently set at a low pressure. Inadequate inflation is particularly common when using bag and mask ventilation (Table 16.10).
- Too small an endotracheal tube is being used – a common mistake. The 2.5 mm diameter tubes have a high internal resistance, allow a big airleak and are very easily pushed in too far, so that they lodge well down the bronchial tree. This not only results in very poor ventilation and oxygenation, but carries the risk of rupturing the lobe which is being ventilated, causing a pneumothorax.
- The oxygen has been disconnected.

As soon as these errors are recognized and remedied, the infant will rapidly pink up and become vigorous and active.

Severe illness

Some neonatal lung diseases may prevent adequate oxygenation of the neonate during and after resuscitation: obvious diagnostic clues are usually present.

RDS (p. 481). Is the infant very premature and likely to be developing severe RDS? In such infants the lungs feel very stiff during manual ventilation, and the excursion of the rib cage during inflation is poor. If this is the diagnosis, increase the F_IO_2, the inflating pressure to 35 cmH_2O if possible, and increase the rate at which ventilation is given. Give surfactant (p. 508). This almost always improves the infant sufficiently to allow him to be transferred to the NICU, where he can be connected to a ventilator.

Meconium aspiration (p. 537). The history will be obvious, and an integral part of the resuscitation of such infants is efficient and meticulous bronchial toilet. These babies have often suffered intrapartum asphyxia as well and may be delivered in terminal apnoea; appropriate treatment for this is also necessary. However, if the infant remains very difficult to ventilate and oxygenate, and his lungs 'feel' stiff and there is poor pulmonary expansion, one option available is to attempt further broncho-pulmonary lavage (p. 541). The only other short-term available treatment is raising the oxygen concentration, inflation pressures and ventilator rate until the baby turns pink.

Congenital pneumonia (p. 1142). Does the maternal history suggest systemic or genital infection? If it does, there is nothing that can be done in the short term other than increasing the oxygen, pressure and rate of ventilation, plus correcting acidaemia, hypoglycaemia and hypotension. In addition, the investigations and treatment appropriate for sepsis must be initiated as soon as possible.

Anaemia. As well as increasing the likelihood of an infant developing asphyxia (see above) the presence of anaemia may seriously compromise the baby's response to resuscitation. Treatment is by transfusion (pp. 814–815).

Pneumothorax

This should always be considered in any infant who responds poorly to resuscitation. Of all the medical conditions compromising the response to resuscitation this is not only the easiest to treat but is also the one in which successful treatment is most likely to result in a dramatic clinical improvement. A pneumothorax can occur spontaneously or as a result of some technical error during resuscitation (see above).

The clinical clues suggesting a pneumothorax are:

- a deviated mediastinum;
- a hyperresonant hemithorax;
- a distended abdomen;
- decreased air entry;
- odd vascular changes, e.g. pale lower half and cyanosed upper half.

There is rarely time to confirm the diagnosis radiologically, but a fibreoptic light source may help (p. 518).

In an infant who is deteriorating rapidly despite other resuscitative efforts, and in whom a pneumothorax is suspected clinically, insert a wide-bore needle into the second intercostal space in the midclavicular line. If you are wrong, surprisingly little harm is done: if you are right there will be a gratifying hiss of escaping air, the infant's condition will rapidly improve, and a chest drain can then be inserted (p. 520).

Table 16.12 Malformations causing persistent cyanosis or dyspnoea after delivery

Upper respiratory tract
Choanal atresia (p. 664)
Pierre–Robin syndrome (p. 768)
Laryngeal and tracheal malformations
atresia
webs
luminal tumours
clefts (p. 776)
Lung
Pulmonary hypoplasia
Potters syndrome (p. 641)
prolonged membrane rupture (p. 639)
idiopathic
Pleural effusions with or without hydrops (p. 557)
Congenital cystic adenomatoid malformation (p. 645)
Congenital lobar emphysema (p. 648)
Pulmonary lymphangiectasia (p. 647)
Extrapulmonary
Diaphragmatic hernia (p. 655)
Diaphragmatic eventration
Intrathoracic space-occupying tumours
Gross abdominal distension splinting the diaphragm
tumours
hepatosplenomegaly
ascites
dilated renal tract
Small chest
asphyxiating thoracic dystrophy
thanatophoric dwarfism

The vigorous, persistently cyanosed baby

Although babies with the rare disorders listed in Table 16.12 may behave like asphyxiated babies and breathe poorly after delivery, more often and more characteristically they cry and have vigorous respiratory efforts (because they are not asphyxiated), but fail to go pink because of their underlying lung or airway disorder. This pattern is so characteristic that when seen it should alert the physician to seek structural malformations, of which the commonest is the lung hypoplasia accompanying diaphragmatic hernia.

Initially many of the babies are not asphyxiated, but the underlying malformation results in defective oxygenation and inadequate ventilation, and the infant may rapidly develop the biochemical changes of asphyxia with secondary depression of ventilation.

Infants with laryngeal and tracheal malformations are usually unresuscitatable unless someone with extreme presence of mind not only recognizes the problem but can also perform an emergency tracheostomy (p. 669).

Table 16.13 Neurological causes of persisting hypoventilation and failure to respond to resuscitation. (Reproduced with permission from Brazy et al[27])

Structural CNS malformations
Severe antenatal brain damage (p. 247)
Fractured cervical spine with cord damage (p. 1081)
Dystrophia myotonica (p. 1292)
Congenital myopathies (p. 1293)
Werdnig–Hoffmann disease (p. 1289)
Brain tumour
Degenerative brain disorders (p. 1271 et. seq.)
Ondine's curse (central hypoventilation syndrome)

Infants with lung hypoplasia may have an instantly recognizable malformation such as thanatophoric dwarfism (p. 644) or Potter syndrome (p. 641), in which case active resuscitation can be withdrawn. In others, urgent transport to the NICU and X-ray is essential to establish the presence of potentially treatable conditions, such as diaphragmatic hernia (p. 655), pleural effusion (p. 557) adenomatoid malformation (p. 645), Pierre–Robin syndrome (p. 768) or choanal atresia (p. 664).

Persisting apnoea with hypotonia but good cardiovascular response

This can, of course, be due to severe terminal apnoea (see above), but if there is nothing in the maternal history to suggest either this or drug ingestion then some structural disorder of the CNS or a primary neuromuscular disease should be considered (Table 16.13). Clearly, it is inappropriate to infuse bicarbonate, glucose, naloxone or other drugs into these neonates, and this group is one of the reasons why these drugs should not be given blind without proper biochemical evaluation of the baby.

The many, individually rare, conditions which present in this way are reviewed by Brazy et al.[27]

REFERENCES

1. Aarnoudse M D, Huisjes H J, Gordon H, Oeseburg B, Zijlstra W G 1985 Fetal subcutaneous scalp PO_2 and abnormal heart rate during labour. American Journal of Obstetrics and Gynecology 153: 565–566
2. Abboud T K 1988 Maternal and fetal endorphins: effects of pregnancy and labour. Archives of Disease in Childhood 63: 707–709
3. Adamsons K, Behrman R, Dawes G S, James L S, Koford C 1964 Resuscitation by positive pressure ventilation and Tris-hydroxymethylaminomethane of rhesus monkeys asphyxiated at birth. Journal of Pediatrics 65: 807–818
4. Aldrich C J. D'Antona D, Wyatt J S et al 1994 Fetal cerebral oxygenation measured by near-infra red spectroscopy shortly before birth and acid base status at birth. Obstetrics and Gynecology 84: 861–866
5. Aksit S, Yaprak I, Bakiler R et al 1992 Sigtuna scores versus Apgar score: simple and practical evaluation of the newborn. Paediatric and Perinatal Epidemiology 6: 29–34
6. Amatayakul O, Cumming G R, Haworth J C 1970 Association of hypoglycaemia with cardiac enlargement and heart failure in newborn infants. Archives of Disease in Childhood 45: 717–720
7. American Academy of Pediatrics 1986 Use and abuse of the Apgar score. Pediatrics 78: 1148–1149
8. American Academy of Pediatrics 1990 Naloxone dosage and route of administration for infants and children: addendum to emergency procedures for infants and children. Pediatrics 86: 484–485
9. American Heart Association 1992 Guidelines for cardiopulmonary resuscitation and emergency cardiac care. Journal of the American Medical Association 268: 2171–2281
10. Anon 1989 Is the Apgar score outmoded? (editorial). Lancet i: 591–592
11. Arieff A I, Leach W, Park R, Lazarowitz V C 1982 Systemic effects of $NaHCO_3$ in experimental lactic acidosis in dogs. American Journal of Physiology 242: F586–591
12. Apgar V 1953 Proposal for a new method of evaluation of newborn infants. Anesthesia and Analgesia 32: 260–267
13. Avery M E, Tooley W H, Keller J B et al 1987 Is chronic lung disease in low birthweight infants preventable. A survey of eight centres. Pediatrics 79: 26–30
14. Barrie J R, Greenhalgh D L 1993 Training in neonatal resuscitation: the views of junior paediatricians. Journal of the Royal College of Physicians 27: 151–153
15. Barrier G, Sureau C 1982 Effects of drugs on labour, fetus and neonate. Clinics in Obstetrics and Gynaecology 9: 351–367
16. Beard R W, Morris E D 1965 Foetal and maternal acid base balance during normal labour. Journal of Obstetrics and Gynaecology of the British Commonwealth 72: 496–503
17. Beeby P J, Elliott E J, Henderson-Smart D et al 1994 Predictive value of umbilical artery pH in preterm infants. Archives of Disease in Childhood 71: F93–96
18. Behnke M, Carter R L, Hardt N S, Eyler F D, Cruz A C, Resnick M B 1987 The relationship of Apgar scores, gestational age and birthweight to survival of low birthweight infants. American Journal of Perinatology 4: 121–124
19. Beierholm E A, Grantham N, O'Keefe D D, Laver M B, Daggett W M 1975 Effects of acid-base changes, hypoxia and catecholamines on ventricular performance. American Journal of Physiology 228: 1555–1561
20. Berseth C L, McCoy H H 1992 Birth asphyxia alters neonatal intestinal mobility in term neonates. Pediatrics 90: 669–673
21. Bird J A, Spencer J A D, Mould T, Symonds M E 1996 Endocrine and metabolic adaptation following caesarean section or vaginal delivery. Archives of Disease in Childhood 74: F132–134
22. Block B S, Schlafer D H, Wentworth R A, Kreitzer L A, Nathanielsz P W 1990 Intrauterine asphyxia and the breakdown of the physiologic circulatory compensation in fetal sheep. American Journal of Obstetrics and Gynecology 162: 1325–1331
23. Bocking A D, Gagnon R, White S E, Homan J, Milne K M, Richardson B S 1988 Circulatory responses to prolonged hypoxemia in fetal sheep. American Journal of Obstetrics and Gynecology 159: 1418–1424
24. Boon A W, Milner A D, Hopkin I E 1979 Lung expansion, tidal exchange and formation of the functional residual capacity during resuscitation of asphyxiated neonates. Journal of Pediatrics 95: 1031–1036
25. Boucher M, Yonekura M L 1986 Perinatal listeriosis (early onset): correlation of antenatal manifestations and neonatal outcome. Obstetrics and Gynecology 68: 593–597
26. Brann A W, Myers R E 1975 Central nervous system findings in the newborn monkey following severe in utero partial asphyxia. Neurology 25: 327–330
27. Brazy J E, Kinney H C, Oakes W J 1987 Central nervous system structural lesions causing apnea at birth. Journal of Pediatrics 111: 163–175
28. Brimacombe J, Gandini D 1995 Resuscitation of neonates with the laryngeal mask airway. A caution. Pediatrics 95: 453–454
29. Bucciarelli R L, Nelson R M, Egan E A, Eitzman D V, Gessner I H 1977 Transient tricuspid insufficiency of the newborn. A form of myocardial dysfunction in stressed newborns. Pediatrics 59: 330–337
30. Burnard E D, James L S 1961 Failure of the heart after undue asphyxia at birth. Pediatrics 28: 545–565
31. Cabal L A, Devaskar U, Siassi B, Hodgman J E, Emmanouilides G 1980 Cardiogenic shock associated with perinatal asphyxia in term infants. Journal of Pediatrics 96: 705–710
32. Campbell A G M, Milligan J E, Talner J S 1968 The effect of pretreatment with phenobarbital, meperidine or hyperbaric oxygen on the response to anoxia and resuscitation in newborn rabbits. Journal of Pediatrics 72: 518–527

33. Campbell N, Harvey D R, Norman A P 1975 Increased frequency of neonatal jaundice in a maternity hospital. British Medical Journal ii: 548–552
34. Carter B S, Haverkamp A D, Merenstein G B 1993 The definition of acute perinatal asphyxia. Clinics in Perinatology 20: 287–304
35. Catlin E A, Carpenter M W, Brann B S et al 1986 The Apgar score revisited: influence of gestational age. Journal of Pediatrics 109: 865–868
36. Chamberlain R, Chamberlain G, Howlett B, Claireaux A 1975 British Births 1970, Vol. I The first week of life. Heinemann, London, Ch. 4
37. Chernick V, Manfreda J, DeBooy V, Davi M, Rigatto H, Seshia M 1988 Clinical trial of naloxone in birth asphyxia. Journal of Pediatrics 113: 519–525
38. Chessels J M, Wigglesworth J S 1971 Coagulation studies in severe birth asphyxia. Archives of Disease in Childhood 46: 253–256
39. Clapp J F III, Peress N S, Wesley M, Mann L I 1988 Brain damage after intermittent partial cord occlusion in the chronically instrumented fetal lamb. American Journal of Obstetrics and Gynecology 159: 504–509
39a. Cochrane Injuries Group Albumin Reviewers 1998 Human albumin administration in critically ill patiens: systematic review of randomised controlled trials. British Medical Journal 317: 235–240
40. Craft W H, Underwood L E, Van Wyk J J 1980 High incidence of perinatal insult in children with idiopathic hypopituitarism. Journal of Pediatrics 96: 397–402
41. Cyr R M, Usher R H, McLean F H 1984 Changing patterns of birth asphyxia and trauma over 20 years. American Journal of Obstetrics and Gynecology 148: 490–498
42. David R 1988 Closed chest cardiac massage in the newborn infant. Pediatrics 81: 552–554
43. Davis J A, Stafford A 1964 Respiratory distress in newborn rabbits. Biologia Neonatorum 7: 129–140
44. Dawes G S 1968 Fetal and neonatal physiology. Year Book, Chicago, pp 141–159
45. Dawes G S, Mott J C 1962 The vascular tone of the foetal lung. Journal of Physiology 164: 465–477
46. Dawes G S, Jacobson H N, Mott J C, Shelley H J, Stafford A 1963 Treatment of asphyxia in newborn lambs and monkeys. Journal of Physiology 169: 167–184
47. Dawes G S, Hibbard E, Windle W F 1964 The effect of alkali and glucose infusion on permanent brain damage in rhesus monkeys asphyxiated at birth. Journal of Pediatrics 65: 801–806
48. Downing S E, Talner N S, Gardner T H 1966 Influences of hypoxemia and acidemia on left ventricular function. American Journal of Physiology 210: 1327–1334
49. Drew J H 1982 Immediate intubation at birth of the very low birthweight infant. American Journal of Diseases of Children 136: 207–210
50. Fee S C, Malee K, Deddish R, Minogue J P, Socol M L 1990 Severe acidosis and subsequent neurologic status. American Journal of Obstetrics and Gynecology 162: 802–806
51. Fedrick J, Butler N R 1971 Certain causes of neonatal death. iv. Massive pulmonary haemorrhage. Biology of the Neonate 18: 243–262
52. Fernandez, F, Verdu A, Queso J, Perez-Higueras A 1987 Serum CPK-BB Isoenzyme in the assessment of brain damage in asphyctic term infants. Acta Paediatrica Scandinavica 76: 914–918
53. Field D, Milner A D, Hopkin I E 1986 Efficacy of manual resuscitation at birth. Archives of Disease in Childhood 61: 300–302
54. Finer N N, Robertson C M, Richards R T et al 1981 Hypoxic ischaemic encephalopathy in term neonates. Perinatal factors and outcome. Journal of Pediatrics 98: 112–117
55. Fisher D J, Heyman M A, Rudolph A M 1981 Myocardial consumption of oxygen and carbohydrates in newborn sheep. Pediatric Research 15: 843–846
56. Freeman J M, Nelson K B 1988 Intrapartum asphyxia and cerebral palsy. Pediatrics 82: 240–249
57. Friedman E A, Sachtleben M R 1976 Neonatal jaundice in association with oxytocin stimulation of labour and operative delivery. British Medical Journal i: 198–199
58. Gaffney G, Squier M V, Johnson A et al 1994 Clinical associations of prenatal ischaemic white matter injury. Archives of Disease in Childhood 70: F101–106
59. Gandy G M, Jacobson W, Gairdner D 1970 Hyaline membrane disease. I. Cellular changes. Archives of Disease in Childhood 45: 289–295
60. Gardner M O, Goldenberg R L, Gaudier F L et al 1995 Predicting low Apgar scores of infants weighing less than 1000 grams: the effect of corticosteroids. Obstetrics and Gynecology 85: 170–174
61. Gaudier F L, Goldenberg R L, Nelson K. G et al 1996 Infant's acid–base status at birth and Apgar scores on survival in 500–1000 g infants. Obstetrics and Gynecology 87: 175–180
62. Gibbs J, Newson T, Williams J, Davidson D C 1989 Naloxone hazard in infants of opioid abusers. Lancet ii: 159–160
63. Gilstrap L C, Leveno K J, Burris J, Williams M L, Little B B 1989 Diagnosis of birth asphyxia on the basis of fetal pH. Apgar score and newborn cerebral dysfunction. American Journal of Obstetrics and Gynecology 161: 825–830
64. Goldberg R N, Cabal L A, Sinatra F R, Plajstek C E, Hodgman J E 1979 Hyperammonemia associated with perinatal asphyxia. Pediatrics 64: 336–341
65. Goldenberg R L, Huddleston J F, Nelson K G 1984 Apgar scores and umbilical pH in preterm newborn infants. American Journal of Obstetrics and Gynecology 149: 651–654
66. Goodwin T M, Belai I, Hernandez P 1992 Asphyxial complications in the term newborn with severe umbilical acidaemia. American Journal of Obstetrics and Gynecology 162: 1506–1512
67. Govaert P 1993 Cranial haemorrhage in the term newborn infant. Cambridge University Press, Cambridge, pp 52–57
68. Gray L C, Grant H W 1984 Should a paediatrician be present at non-rotational forceps deliveries? British Journal of Obstetrics and Gynaecology 91: 899–900
69. Greenough A, Lagercranz H, Pool J, Dahlin I 1987 Plasma catecholamine levels in preterm infants. Acta Paediatrica Scandinavica 76: 54–59
70. Gupta J M, Tizard J P M 1967 The sequence of events in neonatal apnoea. Lancet ii: 55–59
71. Gutberlet R L, Cornblath M 1976 Neonatal hypoglycemia revisited 1975. Pediatrics 58: 10–17
72. Hackett G A, Campbell S, Gamsu H, Cohen-Overbeek T, Pearce J M F 1987 Doppler studies in the growth retarded fetus and prediction of neonatal necrotising enterocolitis, haemorrhage and neonatal morbidity. British Medical Journal 294: 13–16
73. Hambleton G, Appleyard W J 1973 Controlled trial of fresh frozen plasma in asphyxiated low birthweight infants. Archives of Disease in Childhood 48: 31–35
74. Hazinski T A, Grunstein M M, Schlueter M A, Tooley W H 1981 Effect of naloxone on ventilation in newborn rabbits. Journal of Applied Physiology 50: 713–717
75. Hermansen M C, Prior M M 1993 Oxygen concentrations from self inflating resuscitation bags. American Journal of Perinatology 10: 79–80
76. Hein H A 1993 The use of sodium bicarbonate in neonatal resuscitation: help or harm. Pediatrics 91: 496–497
77. Holden K R, Mellits E D, Freeman J M 1982 Neonatal seizures. 1. Correlation of prenatal and perinatal events with outcomes. Pediatrics 70: 165–176
78. Hope P L, Cady E B, Delpy D T et al 1988 Brain metabolism and intracellular pH during ischaemia: effects of systemic glucose and bicarbonate administration studied by 31P and 1 H nuclear magnetic resonance spectroscopy in vivo in the lamb. Journal of Neurochemistry 50: 1394–1402
79. Hoskyns E W, Milner A W, Boon A Q, Vyas H, Hopkin I E 1987 Endotracheal resuscitation of preterm infants at birth. Archives of Disease in Childhood 62: 663–666
80. Hoskyns E W, Milner A D, Hopkin I E 1987 A simple method of face mask resuscitation at birth. Archives of Disease in Childhood 62: 376–378
81. Howell J H 1987 Sodium bicarbonate in the perinatal setting revisited. Clinics in Perinatology 14: 807–816
82. Hull J, Dodd K L 1992 Falling incidence of hypoxic ischaemic encephalopathy in term infants. British Journal of Obstetrics and Gynaecology 99: 386–391
83. Ikegami M, Jacobs H, Jobe A 1983 Surfactant function in respiratory distress syndrome. Journal of Pediatrics 102: 443–447
84. Ikonomidou C, Qin Y, Labruyere J, Kirby C, Olney J W 1996 Prevention of trauma induced degeneration in infant rat-brain. Pediatric Research 39: 1020–1027

85. Isozaki-Fukuda Y, Kojima T, Hirata Y et al 1991 Plasma immunoreactive endothelin 1 concentration in human fetal blood: its relation to asphyxia. Pediatric Research 30: 244–247
86. Jain L, Ferre C, Vidyasagar D et al 1991 Cardiopulmonary resuscitation of apparently stillborn infants: survival and long term outcome. Journal of Pediatrics 118: 778–782
87. Johnson J W C, Ricards D S, Wagaman R A 1990 The case for routine umbilical acid-base studies at delivery. American Journal of Obstetrics and Gynecology 162: 621–625
88. Khare S K 1977 Neurohypophyseal dysfunction following perinatal asphyxia. Journal of Pediatrics 90: 628–629
89. Kojima T, Kobayashi T, Matsuzaki S, Iwase S, Kobayashi Y 1985 Effects of perinatal asphyxia and myoglobinuria on development of acute neonatal renal failure. Archives of Disease in Childhood 60: 908–912
90. Kroll L, Twohey L, Daubeny P et al 1994 Risk factors at delivery and the need for skilled resuscitation. European Journal of Obstetrics and Gynecology and Reproductive Biology 44: 175–177
91. Lindemann R 1984 Resuscitation of the newborn: endotracheal administration of adrenaline. Acta Paediatrica Scandinavica 73: 210–212
92. Linderkamp O, Versmold H T, Messow-Zahn K, Muller-Holve W, Riegel K P, Betke K 1978 The effect of intrapartum and intrauterine asphyxia on placental transfusion in premature full term infants. European Journal of Pediatrics 127: 91–99
93. Linderkamp O, Versmold H T, Fendel H, Riegel K P, Betke K 1978 Association of neonatal respiratory distress with birth asphyxia and deficiency of red cell mass in premature infants. European Journal of Pediatrics 129: 167–173
94. Low J A, Panagiotopoulos C, Derrick E J 1995 Newborn complications after intrapartum asphyxia with metabolic acidosis in the preterm fetus. American Journal of Obstetrics and Gynecology 172: 805–810
95. Lundstrom K E, Pryds O, Greisen G 1995 Oxygen at birth and prolonged cerebral vaso-constriction in preterm infants. Archives of Disease in Childhood 73: F81–86
96. Luthy D A, Shy K K, Strickland D et al 1987 State of infants at birth and risk for adverse neonatal events and long term sequelae. A study in low birthweight infants. American Journal of Obstetrics and Gynecology 157: 676–679
97. McDonald H M, Mulligan J C, Allen A C, Taylor P M 1980 Neonatal asphyxia. I. Relationship of obstetric and neonatal complications to neonatal mortality in 38 405 consecutive deliveries. Journal of Pediatrics 96: 898–902
98. MacKinnon J A, Perlman M, Kirpalani H et al 1993 Spinal cord injury at birth. Diagnostic and prognostic data in 22 patients. Journal of Pediatrics 122: 431–437
99. Maberry M C, Ramin S M, Gilstrap L C, Leveno K L, Dax J S 1990 Intrapartum asphyxia in pregnancies complicated by intra-amniotic infection. Obstetrics and Gynecology 76: 351–354
100. Mallard E C, Gunn A J, Williams C E et al 1992 Transient umbilical cord occlusion causes hippocampal damage in the fetal sheep. American Journal of Obstetrics and Gynecology 167: 1423–1430
101. Marlow N 1992 Do we need an Apgar score? Archives of Disease in Childhood 67: 765–769
102. Merritt T A, Farrell P M 1976 Diminished pulmonary lecithin synthesis in acidosis. Experimental findings as related to the respiratory distress syndrome. Pediatrics 57: 32–40
103. Miller J M, Bernard M, Brown H L, St Pierre J J, Gabert H A 1990 Umbilical cord blood gases for term healthy newborns. American Journal of Perinatology 7: 157–159
104. Milner A D, Vyas M 1985 Resuscitation of the newborn. In: Milner A D, Martin R J (eds) Neonatal and pediatric respiratory medicine. Butterworth, London, p 16
105. Milner A D, Vyas H, Hopkin I E 1984 Efficacy of face mask resuscitation at birth. British Medical Journal 289: 1563–1565
106. Miltényi M, Pohlandt F, Boka G, Kun E 1981 Tubular proteinuria after perinatal hypoxia. Acta Paediatrica Scandinavica 70: 399–403
107. Modanlou H, Yeh S Y, Siassi B, et al 1974 Direct monitoring of the arterial blood pressure in depressed and normal newborn infants during the first hour of life, Journal of Pediatrics 85: 553–559
108. Moore W M O, Davis J A 1966 Response of newborn rabbit to acute anoxia, and variations due to narcotic agents. British Journal of Anaesthesia 38: 787–793
109. Motoyama E K, Rivard G, Acheson F, Cook C D 1966 Adverse effects of maternal hyperventilation on the fetus. Lancet ii: 286–288
110. Mott J C 1975 The place of the renin-angiotensin system before and after birth. British Medical Bulletin 31: 44–50
111. Moya F, Morishima H O, Schnider S M, James L S 1965 Influence of maternal hyperventilation on the newborn infant. American Journal of Obstetrics and Gynecology 91: 76–84
112. Myers R E 1972 Two patterns of perinatal brain damage and their conditions of occurrence. American Journal of Obstetrics and Gynecology 112: 246–276
113. Naeye R L, Localio A R 1995 Determining the time before birth when ischemia and hypoxemia initiated cerebral palsy. Obstetrics and Gynecology 86: 713–719
114. Nelson K B, Ellenberg J H 1981 Apgar scores as predictors of chronic neurologic disability. Pediatrics 68: 36–44
115. Nijhuis J G, Kruyt N, Van Wijck J A M 1988 Fetal brain death. Two case reports. British Journal of Obstetrics and Gynaecology 95: 197–200
116. Oh W, Omori K, Emmanouilides G, Phelps D L 1975 Placenta to lamb fetus transfusion in utero during acute hypoxia. American Journal of Obstetrics and Gynecology 122: 316–322
117. O'Neil B J, Wilson R F 1994 The controversies in cardio-pulmonary resuscitation on high-dose epinephrine still continue. Critical Care Medicine 22: 194–195
118. Ostrea E M, O'Dell G B 1972 The influence of bicarbonate administration on blood pH in a closed system: clinical implications. Journal of Pediatrics 80: 671–680
119. Padbury J F, Agata Y, Polk D H, Wang D L, Callegari C C 1987 Neonatal adaptation: naloxone increases the catecholamine surge at birth. Pediatric Research 21: 590–593
120. Palme C, Nystrom B, Tunell R 1985 An evaluation of the efficiency of face masks in the resuscitation of newborn infants. Lancet ii: 207–210
121. Palme-Kilander C 1992 Methods of resuscitation in low Apgar score newborn infants – a national survey. Acta Paediatrica 81: 739–744
122. Palme-Kilander C, Tunell R 1993 Pulmonary gas exchange during face mask ventilation immediately after birth. Archives of Disease in Childhood 68: 11–16
123. Paneth N, Stark R I 1983 Cerebral palsy and mental retardation in relation to indicators of perinatal asphyxia. American Journal of Obstetrics and Gynecology 147: 960–966
124. Paterson P J, Dunstan M K, Trickey N R A, Beard R W 1970 A biochemical comparison of the mature and post-mature fetus and newborn infant. Journal of Obstetrics and Gynaecology of the British Commonwealth 77: 390–397
125. Patriarco M S, Viechnicki B M, Hutchinson T A, Klasko S K, Yeh S-Y 1987 A study on intrauterine fetal resuscitation with terbutaline. American Journal of Obstetrics and Gynecology 157: 384–387
126. Peebles D M, Spencer J A D, Edwards A D et al 1994 Relation between frequency of uterine contractions and human fetal cerebral oxygen saturation studied during labour by near infrared spectroscopy. British Journal of Obstetrics and Gynaecology 101: 44–48
127. Peevy K J, Chalhub E G 1983 Occult group B streptococcal infection: an important cause of intrauterine asphyxia. American Journal of Obstetrics and Gynecology 146: 989–990
128. Perlman J M, Risser R M 1996 Can asphyxiated infants at risk for neonatal seizures be rapidly identified by current high risk markers. Pediatrics 97: 456–462
129. Perlman J M, Tack E D 1988 Renal injury in the asphyxiated newborn infant: relationship to neurologic outcome. Journal of Pediatrics 113: 875–879
130. Perkins R P, Papile L A 1985 The very low birthweight infant: incidence and significance of low Apgar scores, 'asphyxia' and morbidity. American Journal of Perinatology 2: 108–113
131. Peters J, Ihle P 1990 Mechanics of the circulation during cardiopulmonary resuscitation, parts I and II. Intensive Care Medicine 16: 11–19, 20–27
132. Phelan J P, Ahn M O, Korst L M, Martin G I 1995 Nucleated red blood cells: a marker for fetal asphyxia? American Journal of Obstetrics and Gynecology 173: 1380–1384
133. Phillips G W L, Zideman D A 1986 Relation of infant heart to sternum: its significance in cardiopulmonary resuscitation. Lancet ii: 1024–1025
134. Pietz J, Guttenberg N, Gluck L 1988 Hypoxanthine: a marker of asphyxia. Obstetrics and Gynecology 72: 762–766
135. Poets C F, Sens B 1996 Changes in intubation rates and outcome of very low birthweight infants: a population based study. Pediatrics 98: 24–27

136. Pohjavuori M 1983 Obstetric determinants of plasma vasopressin concentrations and renin activity at birth. Journal of Pediatrics 103: 966–968
137. Press S, Tellechea C, Pregen S 1985 Caesarean delivery of full term infants: identification of those at high risk for requiring resuscitation. Journal of Pediatrics 106: 477–479
138. Preziosi M P, Roig J C, Hargrove N et al 1993 Metabolic acidaemia with hypoxia attenuates the haemodynamic responses to epinephrine during resuscitation in lambs. Critical Care Medicine 21: 1901–1907
139. Primhak R A, Herber S M, Whincup G, Milner R D G 1984 Which deliveries require paediatricians in attendance? British Medical Journal 289: 16–18
140. Procianoy R S, Cecin S K G 1985 The influence of labour and delivery on preterm fetal and renal function. Acta Paediatrica Scandinavica 74: 400–404
141. Puolakka J, Kauppila A, Tuimala R, Jouppila R, Vuori J 1983 The effect of parturition on umbilical blood plasma levels of norepinephrine. Obstetrics and Gynecology 61: 19–21
142. Ramji S, Ahuja S, Thirupuram S, et al 1993 Resuscitation of asphyxic newborn infants with room air or 100% oxygen. Pediatric Research 34: 809–812
143. Richardson B S 1989 Fetal adaptive responses to asphyxia. Clinics in Perinatology 16: 595–611
144. Roberton N R C 1997 Use of albumin in neonatal resuscitation. European Journal of Pediatrics 156: 428–431
145. Robin E D, Wilson R J, Bromberg P A 1961 Intracellular acid-base reactions and intracellular buffers. Annals of the New York Academy of Sciences 92: 539–544
146. Robson E, Hey E 1982 Resuscitation of preterm babies at birth reduces the risk of death from hyaline membrane disease. Archives of Disease in Childhood 57: 184–186
147. Ryder R W, Shelton J D, Guinan M E, The Committee on Necrotising Enterocolitis 1980 Necrotising enterocolitis. A prospective multicenter investigation. American Journal of Epidemiology 112: 113–124
148. Sarnat H B, Sarnat M S 1976 Neonatal encephalopathy following fetal distress. Archives of Neurology 33: 696–705
149. Sasidharan P 1992 Breathing pattern abnormalities in full term asphyxiated newborn infants. Archives of Disease in Childhood 67: 440–442
150. Schubring C 1986 Temperature regulation in healthy and resuscitated newborns immediately after birth. Journal of Perinatal Medicine 14: 27–33
151. Schwab K O, von Stockhausen H B 1994 Plasma catecholamines after endotracheal administration of adrenaline during postnatal resuscitation. Archives of Disease in Childhood 70: F213–217
152. Scopes J W, Ahmed I 1966 Minimal rates of oxygen consumption in sick and premature newborn infants. Archives of Disease in Childhood 41: 407–416
153. Sessler D, Mills P, Gregory G et al 1987 Effects of bicarbonate on arterial and brain intracellular pH in neonatal rabbits recovering from hypoxic lactic acidosis. Journal of Pediatrics 111: 817–823
154. Settergren G, Lindblad B S, Persson B 1976 Cerebral blood flow and exchange of oxygen, glucose, ketone bodies, lactate, pyruvate and amino acids in infants. Acta Paediatrica Scandinavica 65: 343–353
155. Shekarloo A, Mendez-Bauer C, Cook V, Freese U 1989 Terbutaline (intravenous bolus) for the treatment of acute intrapartum fetal distress. American Journal of Obstetrics and Gynecology 160: 615–618
156. Shelley H J 1961 Glycogen reserves and their changes at birth and in anoxia. British Medical Bulletin 17: 137–143
157. Shiraki K 1970 Hepatic cell necrosis in the newborn. American Journal of Diseases of Children 119: 395–400
158. Silverman F, Suidan J, Wasserman J, Antoine C, Young B K 1985 The Apgar score: is it enough? Obstetrics and Gynecology 66: 331–336
159. Sims D G, Heal C A, Bartle S M 1994 Use of adrenaline and atropine in neonatal resuscitation. Archives of Disease in Childhood 70: F3–10
160. Skillman C A, Plessinger M A, Woods J R, Clark K E 1985 Effect of graded reductions in uteroplacental blood flow in the fetal lamb. American Journal of Physiology 249: H1098–1105
161. Smith A, Prakash P, Nesbitt J et al 1990 The vasopressin response to severe birth asphyxia. Early Human Development 22: 119–129
162. Socol M L, Garcia P M, Riter S 1994 Depressed Apgar scores, acid base status, and neurologic outcome. American Journal of Obstetrics and Gynecology 170: 991–999
163. Soothill P W, Nicolaides K H, Rodeck C H 1987 Effect of anaemia on fetal acid-base status. British Journal of Obstetrics and Gynaecology 94: 880–883
164. Spencer J A D, Robson S C, Farakas A 1993 Spontaneous recovery after severe metabolic acidaemia at birth. Early Human Development 32: 103–112
165. Steer P J, Eigbe F, Lissauer T J, Beard R W 1989 Interrelationship among abnormal cardiotocograms in labour, meconium staining of the amniotic fluid, arterial cord blood pH and Apgar scores. Obstetrics and Gynecology 74: 715–721
166. Steiner H, Neligan G 1975 Perinatal cardiac arrest: quality of survivors. Archives of Disease in Childhood 50: 696–702
167. Stoddard R A, Clark S L, Minton S D 1988 In utero ischaemic injury: sonographic diagnosis and medicolegal implications. American Journal of Obstetrics and Gynecology 159: 23–25
168. Strang L B 1977 Neonatal respiration, physiological and clinical studies. Blackwell Scientific Publications, Oxford, p 71
169. Sykes G S, Molloy P M, Johnson P et al 1982 Do Apgar scores indicate asphyxia? Lancet ii: 494–496
170. Thibeault D W, Hobel C J 1974 The interrelationship of the foam stability test, immaturity and intrapartum complications in the respiratory distress syndrome. American Journal of Obstetrics and Gynecology 118: 56–61
171. Thilaganathan B, Athanasiou S, Ozmen S et al 1994 Umbilical cord blood erythroblast count as an index of intrauterine hypoxia. Archives of Disease in Childhood 70: F192–194
172. Thorp J A, Sampson J E, Parisi V M, Creasy R K 1989 Routine umbilical cord blood gas determinations. American Journal of Obstetrics and Gynecology 161: 600–605
173. Todres I D, Rogers M C 1975 Methods of external cardiac massage in the newborn infant. Journal of Pediatrics 86: 781–782
174. Tsang R C, Chen I, Hayes W, Atkinson W, Atherton H, Edwards N 1974 Neonatal hypocalcaemia in infants with birth asphyxia. Journal of Pediatrics 84: 428–433
175. Van Bel F, Walther F J 1990 Mycocardial dysfunction and cerebral blood flow velocity following birth asphyxia. Acta Paediatrica Scandinavica 79: 756–762
176. Van Haesbrouck P, Vanneste K, Pretere C et al 1987 Tight nuchal cord and neonatal hypovolaemic shock. Archives of Disease in Childhood 62: 1276–1277
177. Vannucci R C 1992 Perinatal brain metabolism. In: Polin R A, Fox W W (eds) Fetal and neonatal physiology. W B Saunders, Philadelphia, pp 1510–1519
178. Vannucci R C 1993 Mechanisms of perinatal hypoxic-ischaemic brain damage. Seminars in Perinatology 17: 330–337
179. Vincent J L 1987 Should we still administer calcium during cardiopulmonary resuscitation? Intensive Care Medicine 13: 369–370
180. Vincent J L 1989 Use of catecholamines in CPR. Intensive Care Medicine 15: 420–421
181. Volpe J J 1995 Neurology of the newborn. W B Saunders, Philadelphia, pp 279–313
182. Walther F J, Siassi B, Ramadan N A et al 1985 Cardiac output in newborn infants with transient myocardial dysfunction. Journal of Pediatrics 107: 781–785
183. Westgate J, Garibaldi J M, Greene K R 1994 Umbilical cord blood gas analysis at delivery: a time for quality data. British Journal of Obstetrics and Gynaecology 101: 1054–1063
184. Westgren M, Grundsell H, Ingemarsson I, Muhlow A, Svenningsen N W 1981 Hyperextension of the fetal head in breech presentation. A study with long term follow-up. British Journal of Obstetrics and Gynaecology 88: 101–104
185. Wilkenning R B, Doyle D W, Meschia G 1993 Fetal pH improvement after 24 hours of severe non-lethal hypoxia. Biology of the Neonate 63: 129–132
186. Wyszogrodski I, Kyei-Aboagye K, Taeusch H W, Avery M E 1975 Surfactant inactivation by hyperventilation: conservation by end expiratory pressure. Journal of Applied Physiology 38: 461–466
187. Young R S K, Hessert T R, Pritchard G A, Yagel S K 1984 Naloxone exacerbates hypoxic–ischaemic brain injury in the neonatal rat. American Journal of Obstetrics and Gynecology 150: 52–56
188. Zaritsky A 1995 Bicarbonate in cardiac arrest: the good, the bad and the puzzling. Critical Care Medicine 23: 429–430.

Section 4

General neonatal care

17

Examination of the newborn

Janet M. Rennie Gillian M. Gandy

INTRODUCTION

A thorough physical examination of every neonate is accepted as good practice and forms a core item of the child health surveillance programme in the UK[23] and that of many other developed countries. The aims of the programme are:

- diagnosis of congenital malformations;
- diagnosis of common neonatal problems, with advice about management or appropriate reassurance if no intervention is indicated;
- continuing screening, begun antenatally, to identify those babies who should be offered specific intervention, e.g. hepatitis vaccination;
- health education advice, e.g. regarding breast-feeding, cot death prevention, safe transport in cars;
- general parental reassurance.

Parents value reassurance about their baby and early diagnosis of problems even when the condition is not amenable to treatment. For some, early diagnosis may make all the difference to their child's subsequent health; examples are congenital cataract and urethral valves. Many first-time mothers lack confidence and need constant reassurance that all is well. The slightest variation from what the family considers to be normal may produce the most intense distress and anxiety at a stage when the mother is emotionally very labile. An all too frequent criticism of hospital-based perinatal care is that conflicting advice is given by too many would-be advisers. This early contact with health professionals offers an opportunity to give health education advice which should be unambiguous and supported by written information in simple English (translated where necessary). Good records must be kept and clear local guidelines agreed for referral arrangements; these protocols should be subject to regular audit. The problem of litigation arising from poor-quality screening programmes is increasing (Chapters 49 and 50). Although no screening test is perfect a successful action could easily be initiated by parents whose child became a carrier of hepatitis when the maternal carrier status was known; or by parents, deaf themselves since childhood, whose child's hearing aids were fitted late.

WHO SHOULD EXAMINE THE BABY?

Under ideal conditions babies should be examined by an experienced paediatrician who has the time to talk to and listen to the mother. This is seldom possible given current manpower levels, and the lot usually falls to the junior doctor. In some hospitals midwives are taking on the task of newborn examination, but their expertise remains to be evaluated. General practitioners usually take responsibility for infants born at home. Routine examination should be a valuable experience for juniors, who see the full range of normality, learn how to recognize and manage common neonatal problems, and develop their bedside communication skills. It is the aim of this chapter to help beginners to 'get it right' and to make the job as satisfying and rewarding as possible.

WHEN SHOULD BABIES BE EXAMINED?

Besides the routine check immediately after delivery, every newborn infant deserves at least one full examination before discharge home. For many years it was customary for a second examination to be carried out, but the value of this has been shown to be limited[30] and, with the current trend to short stay, a single examination should suffice. The timing for the full examination is not crucial and depends on the proposed length of stay. Whether other subsidiary examinations are performed will depend on the baby's condition at birth and his subsequent progress. Infants who remain in hospital for any length of time should be checked at least once a week.

EXAMINATION IN THE DELIVERY ROOM

All babies should be checked soon after birth; this will generally be done by the midwife following an uncomplicated full-term labour, but if called to the delivery the paediatrician should make a quick appraisal of the infant after any necessary resuscitation. This examination is usually confined to checking that the infant looks well and that there are no major abnormalities requiring immediate attention or explanation to the parents, such as hare lip/cleft palate, spina bifida, anal atresia or ambiguous genitalia. This is a most sensitive and important time for the parents to welcome the new arrival and they should be given the opportunity to be left alone with their baby. During the first few hours after birth a healthy newborn is often very alert and responsive, and this affords the best chance for successful mother/baby attachment and establishing breast-feeding. After the first few hours the infant usually sleeps for long periods and appears less responsive.

FULL ROUTINE EXAMINATION

As one of the most important functions of the examination is to answer any points about which the mother is concerned it should, if possible, always be done in her presence. The following general format is recommended:

- Check the maternal medical, obstetric and social history from the notes, the mother and the nursing staff.
- Introduce yourself to the mother, with an explanation about what you are doing.
- Examine the baby fully.
- Give reassurance and advice.

The time taken for a neonatal examination and the associated paperwork is very variable but it can be completed in 10–15 minutes if the infant is normal. The conscientious novice will take considerably longer.

HISTORY AND BACKGROUND KNOWLEDGE

Before approaching the mother and infant, read the baby notes to obtain basic information about the mother's previous obstetric and medical history as well as the type of delivery and the baby's condition at birth; note also the birthweight, gestational age and sex. If there are complicated medical or social problems it is helpful to discuss them with the nursing staff beforehand, and also to check the mother's notes for details.

It is useful to have a mental checklist of relevant background information to obtain before starting the examination. This should include:

- the baby's sex;
- the baby's birthweight and reputed gestational age, and whether these are mutually compatible;
- the mother's age and social background;
- whether there is any chronic maternal disease. If so, what treatment is the mother receiving?
- whether there is a history of recreational drug and/or alcohol use; is the mother a smoker?
- any possibly relevant family history;
- the outcome and dates of any previous pregnancies;
- whether the pregnancy was normal. Were there any complications?
- the results of pregnancy screening tests, e.g. 19-week ultrasound scan;
- any special diagnostic procedures, e.g. amniocentesis, performed;
- any discrepancy between the mother's dates and those derived by the obstetrician from clinical ultrasound assessments;
- any signs of fetal distress;
- drugs and/or anaesthesia given during labour;
- how the infant was delivered;
- his condition at birth (e.g. Apgar scores at 1 and 5 minutes);
- any resuscitation needed;
- length of time before sustained respiration was established;
- if the baby was in the neonatal unit, and if so, why?

INTRODUCTION TO THE MOTHER

The doctor should introduce herself and say what she has come for. To ask the baby's name and record it helps to establish a good relationship (it is also a useful ploy if one has started to talk to the parents about their baby without checking the sex). So many early worries are concerned with feeding that one should always enquire what method the mother is using and whether she is happy with it.

Enquiry about the health of any previous children may also provide useful background information, for instance if there have been any tragedies in the family, such as stillbirth, death or handicap, about which the mother may be extremely anxious. Often parents welcome the opportunity to discuss adverse past events. The paediatrician should also review and confirm any relevant items of background information previously gleaned from the notes. Always ask the mother whether she has any specific worries, when she is being discharged and what support she has at home. Knowledge of the father's and mother's occupations provides useful background information. By means of these preliminary pleasantries one can usually quickly establish a relationship and can gauge the level at which to discuss any problems. During these introductory minutes the examiner can not only make the mother and her baby feel like individuals rather than sausages on the unpopular conveyor belt, but can do two other very important parts of the examination:

- Observe the mother's attitude to her baby, whether she looks at him, and whether she is confident and happy or tense and withdrawn;
- Observe the baby, noting his colour, facies, breathing pattern, posture and movements.

An enormous amount can be learned by these simple observations while continuing to chat to the mother.

Table 17.1 Checklist for routine neonatal examination

Date	Neck	Legs
Examined by	Respiration	Hips
Head circumference	Heart	Feet
Head	Umbilicus	Back
Skull	Abdomen	Skin
Fontanelles	Genitalia	Posture
Face	Testes	Movements
Eyes	Herniae	Muscle tone
Ears	Femoral pulses	Feeding: breast–bottle
Nose	Arms	Urine
Mouth	Hands	Meconium

FORMAL EXAMINATION

For recording purposes it is useful to have a checklist printed or stamped in the baby's notes to serve as an aide memoire. Items are merely ticked if normal, but any abnormalities should be marked distinctively and a full description written out. The examination should be dated and signed. One such scheme is given in Table 17.1.

The examination can seldom be performed in a system-orientated manner because of crying and movement. Full advantage should be taken of any quiet or sleeping periods to feel the anterior fontanelle, look at the eyes, auscultate the heart and palpate the abdomen. These items should therefore be done first (assuming initial quietness), with as little disturbance as possible. Nothing, except perhaps examining the hips or mouth, is more likely to produce a wail of protest than undressing the baby. However, it is impossible to properly examine a newborn clothed, and the baby must be undressed down to the nappy for most of the examination time. Most parts of the examination can be performed in any behavioural state, and the order in which this is done is largely a matter of personal preference, but working from top to toe down the front and vice versa up the back is as good as any other. It is wise to leave the hips until nearly the end of the examination, even though this is arguably one of the most important items on the agenda and must be done with the infant quiet and relaxed, because it often does make the baby cry in the later stages of the procedure. Throughout the whole examination one is at first consciously, later almost subconsciously, observing such things as posture, muscle tone, movements and reaction to stimuli, so that finally there is very little need for a formal evaluation of the central nervous system unless suspicious signs have come to light. A suggested order for the examination is as follows: details of what one is looking for are given in the systematic review.

Order of examination

- Remove the baby's clothes except the nappy.
- Feel the anterior fontanelle for tension (leave until later if the baby is crying!).
- Look at the face for colour or any peculiarities.
- Listen to the heart and estimate heart rate. The lungs can also be auscultated but this is seldom informative.
- Palpate the abdomen.
- Return to the head and examine scalp and skull and measure head circumference and record it.
- Examine the eyes, ears, nose and mouth.
- Examine the neck, including the clavicles.
- Examine the arms, hands, legs and feet.
- Remove the nappy.
- Feel for the femoral pulses.
- Examine the genitalia and anus.
- Turn the baby to the prone position and examine his back and spine.
- Return the infant to the supine position and evaluate the central nervous system.
- Examine the hips.
- Make sure you have not omitted anything.

General observations to be made during the examination

- Note the skin texture and colour and the presence of naevi and rashes.
- Assess the nutritional state.
- Is the respiratory pattern and cry normal?
- Are posture, muscle tone and movements normal?
- Make a general evaluation of the neurological and behavioural state.
- Assess the gestational age (if indicated).
- Note the presence of any dysmorphic features or minor abnormalities.

At the conclusion of the examination one should always chat to the mother and reassure her that all is well. If any abnormalities have been revealed explain their nature, probable outcome and management, but remember that it may be necessary to return and repeat a full explanation all over again.

SYSTEMATIC REVIEW

SKIN

The skin of the neonate can produce such a vast spectrum of normal appearances that it is often the subject of much needless anxiety, both to the mother and to the nursing and medical staff. Occasionally, however, it is the skin that provides the first clue to an underlying illness. During the general examination the colour and texture of the skin should be noted as well as any birth marks or rashes.

Skin colour

Healthy warm babies should be reddish pink all over after the first few hours of life, but they can be covered with the normally white cheesy vernix; this can also be stained a golden yellow in postmaturity, or appear greenish if meconium has been passed before birth.

Cyanosis

Cyanosis is usually discernible when arterial blood is 80% saturated, but the ability to detect cyanosis varies between individuals and with different lighting conditions.[11] It can be difficult to evaluate in an infant who is very pale (anaemic or peripherally shut down) or racially pigmented. Plethoric infants (central packed-cell volume > 65%) can appear cyanosed because they have more than 5 g of reduced haemoglobin per 100 ml even when adequately oxygenated. Peripheral cyanosis of the hands and feet and circumoral cyanosis (acrocyanosis) is common during the first 48 hours. It is essential to ascertain that cyanosis is not central by noting whether or not the tongue is blue. Traumatic cyanosis or bruising of the presenting part, sometimes associated with petechiae, is also quite common, particularly over the face if there has been a nuchal cord. If there is any doubt check arterial oxygen saturation with a pulse oximeter (Chapter 21). Babies with confirmed central cyanosis should be admitted to the neonatal unit and investigated urgently, beginning with a blood gas estimation and a chest X-ray and proceeding to an early echocardiogram if there is no evidence of respiratory disease.

Cyanosis during crying early in postnatal life may be quite normal as a result of transient elevation of pulmonary vascular resistance with right-to-left shunting, but cyanotic attacks should always be taken seriously.

Pallor

Mature infants appear paler than preterm ones, because of their relatively thick skin. Generalized pallor may indicate anaemia, peripheral shutdown with shock, or both. The capillary filling time can be estimated by pressing on the skin, and should not be longer than 3 seconds if the skin is warm.

Jaundice

This is discussed in detail elsewhere (Chapter 31, Part 1) but will frequently be diagnosed first during the routine newborn examination. Icterus appearing in the first 24 hours requires investigation and treatment, and should at once raise the questions 'What is the mother's Rh and ABO group? Were there any antibodies and are there any signs indicating congenital infection?' Investigation should proceed immediately.

Jaundice appearing between 2 and 4 days is extremely common, with 65% of normal full-term infants acquiring a serum bilirubin of over 80 µmol/l, the level at which jaundice is visible. The peak level, reached on the third or fourth day, is around 220 µmol/l. Jaundice in preterm infants requires more careful evaluation, and if any jaundiced baby is ill in any other way, unduly lethargic, feeding poorly, vomiting, or has an unstable temperature, infection must be excluded. The degree of jaundice may be hard to judge clinically, but if in doubt the level must be measured, particularly in coloured babies in whom clinical assessment of jaundice is fraught with hazards. The threshold for measuring serum bilirubin rises rapidly with the experience of the examiner. Jaundice stains the skin in a cephalocaudal direction, so that any jaundice extending to the umbilicus in a term infant is likely to correspond to a bilirubin level of over 200 µmol/l, and should prompt collection of a serum sample. Most neonatologists would not treat jaundice in a healthy term infant until the bilirubin level was 350 µmol/l, and delay exchange until 450 µmol/l. Physiological jaundice rarely reaches these levels. Healthy infants are not immune from kernicterus, but levels of bilirubin above 550 µmol/l are probably required to produce it (Chapter 31, Part 1).

Skin texture

Note whether the skin is peeling (common in post-term infants), nice and firm (normal) or very loose (intrauterine growth retardation or dehydration). Oedema is uncommon in full-term infants and should always raise the question of hypoalbuminaemia. Pedal oedema and a low hairline in a baby girl should make the examiner think of Turner syndrome (p. 863).

Skin rashes

These are very common in newborn babies; most are benign and self-limiting, however alarming they may appear to the mother. Flat lesions may be described as macular (macules < 1 cm) or erythematous (blanch on pressure); petechial and ecchymotic lesions do not blanch on pressure. Raised lesions may be papular, vesicular (< 1 cm) or blistering (vesicles > 1 cm). Diagnosis of a petechial rash should prompt a platelet count. The most frequent skin disorder of newborn infants is erythema neonatorum (toxic erythema, p. 890). There is an eosinophilic infiltrate into the dermis and there can be an associated eosinophilia in the blood.

Other skin lesions seen in normal and abnormal babies are described in Chapter 35.

HEAD AND SKULL

Infant heads can be considerably distorted and moulded during labour and delivery: there may be a marked caput succedaneum (oedema caused by pressure over the presenting part) which subsides in 2–3 days, or the soft skull bones can be greatly moulded. Either or both of these factors can produce bizarre head shapes, which persist for the first few days and sometimes longer. It is important to distinguish deformation (the result of impact from mechanical forces on normal tissue) from malformation. Up to 20% of babies show effects of intrauterine constraint.[21] Babies who have been in the breech presentation for a long time in utero often have a 'breech head' with a prominent occipital shelf.[15]

Feel the anterior fontanelle for its tension and size; it can measure up to 4 × 4 cm at its widest points, though the size is very variable. Fullness may indicate raised intracranial pressure (cerebral oedema, hydrocephalus or meningitis). The posterior fontanelle is often open at this age, but is usually only fingertip size. Examine the cranial sutures for any undue separation, which is abnormal. Overriding of the bones of the vault is common in the first 48 hours, but ridging at the suture lines, as opposed to the 'step-up' feel of overriding, implies craniosynostosis (premature fusion of the sutures). The sagittal suture is the most commonly affected. Craniosynostosis occurs in about 0.4 per 1000 births and may require a neurosurgical procedure for cosmetic correction, or to allow brain growth if several sutures are fused.[25] Limb defects, particularly syndactyly, are the most common associated malformations, and it may be worth asking the parents if they have fused toes.

Palpate the skull bones: small areas of craniotabes caused by pressure on the maternal pelvis occur in 2% of normal newborns and are of no significance.[22] Cephalhaematomata (collections of blood between the periosteum and the skull bones) are felt as softish bumps over the affected bone, most commonly the parietal, and do not extend across the suture lines. Explain their benign nature to the mother and add that they may take 6 weeks or more to subside. There may be a chignon from the use of a vacuum extractor. Neonatal skull fractures are very rare. Elevation of the 'ping-pong' ball type of fracture, where the bone is depressed but not fractured, can be achieved with the application of a vacuum extractor. True skull fractures usually require no treatment but should be followed with a repeat X-ray, because if the dura has been torn a 'growing' fracture can develop.[37,39]

Inspect the scalp for any injury such as forceps marks or lacerations from scalp electrodes, fetal blood sampling or instrumental delivery. Look also for any bald patches or naevi over the scalp. A small defect of the scalp – cutis aplasia – might be confused with a scalp clip electrode scar.

Measure the OFC at its maximum and ensure that it falls within the normal range (approximately 33–37 cm at term). Compare the measurement against any pre-existing measurements: rapid enlargement of the head after birth, with boggy swelling crossing the suture lines, is caused by the rare and dangerous condition of subgaleal haemorrhage (p. 1230). There is a strong association with ventouse delivery. If the head is unduly small (below the 2nd centile) consider dysmorphic syndromes, congenital infections or isolated microcephaly. If the head is unduly large from the beginning consider familial megalencephaly or hydrocephalus. A large head in the presence of widely separated sutures or a full fontanelle requires immediate ultrasound evaluation. Remember that moulding of the skull can lead to an erroneously large OFC measurement, which returns to normal if repeated after the moulding has subsided.

FACE

Most babies' faces are unremarkable, apart from perhaps resembling one or other parent. Occasionally, however, the facial appearance is the first clue to an underlying disorder such as Down syndrome. The bloated face of infants born to mothers with poorly controlled diabetes is also characteristic. If unusual features are seen this should prompt a particularly diligent search for other dysmorphic manifestations, but if the baby is asymptomatic and otherwise normal it may well be familial and a look at the parents should confirm this.

EARS

Look at the general shape, size and position of the ears and feel the cartilage. Low-set ears are those in which the top of the pinna falls below a line drawn from the outer canthus of the eye at right angles to the facial profile (Fig. 17.1). Abnormally small or large floppy ears are characteristic of several syndromes. Overfolding of the helix can result from fetal constraint, and in mild cases resolves without treatment over the first weeks of life. Taping and splinting has now been shown to be remarkably successful, even in cases which previously would have required surgery.[7] Note any preauricular pits, skin tags or accessory auricles. Otoscopic examination does not usually form part of the routine examination.

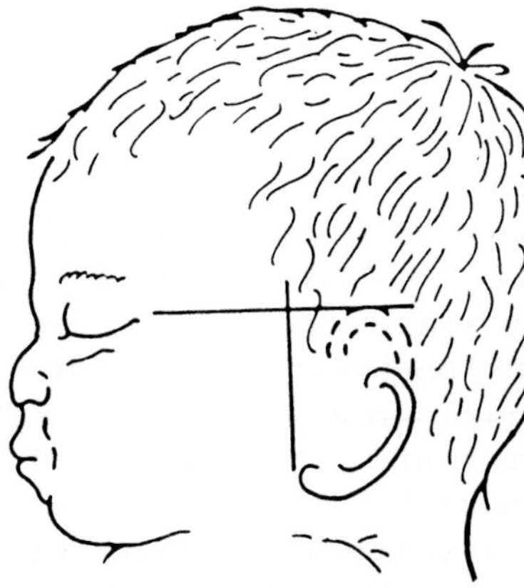

Fig. 17.1 In normal ears (dotted line) the top of the helix lies on a line drawn at right angles to the facial profile from the outer canthus of the eye. Low-set ears (solid line) are those in which the helix is set below the line.

NOSE

Inspect the nose for its general shape and the width of the bridge. If it appears abnormally wide, measure the distance between the inner canthi: this should not exceed about 2.5 cm in the term infant. The nose can appear quite squashed as a result of intrauterine compression. Occasionally the septal cartilage is dislocated, and this can be recognized by deviation of the columella. Compression of the tip of the nose causes collapse and increased deviation of the nostrils in this condition, which requires treatment by an ENT surgeon. Flaring of the alae nasi is not normal and its presence indicates some respiratory illness. Babies are obligate nose breathers and hence complete nasal obstruction (diagnosed by failure to mist a mirror) causes intense respiratory distress requiring immediate investigation. Snuffly noses are not too uncommon, but provided the baby can breathe normally during feeding serious problems are rarely present; if in doubt ensure that both nares are patent by passing a fine catheter through each nostril. The mother should be reassured that the symptom will disappear as the baby (and his nose) grows bigger.

EYES

The eyes should always be inspected for any gross abnormality, noting their size, dimensions and slant; check for any persistent strabismus or nystagmus. A third of newborns have an intermittent exotropia, but esotropia is not normal. Congenital cataract is the commonest form of preventable childhood blindness, and evaluating the red reflex is an essential part of the neonatal examination (see below), although it is not feasible to perform full fundoscopy on every child. Fundoscopy should of course be attempted if there is any question of abnormality. A mydriatic may be needed, and if there is any doubt the opinion of an ophthalmologist should be sought. Normally, the optic disc appears pale and the temporal side of the retina is less well vascularized than the nasal. Isolated retinal haemorrhages may be seen and have no significance.

Look for (and ask about) any discharge from the eyes. A slight mucoid discharge ('sticky eye') is very common in the first 2 days after birth, but later is likely to be due to failure of canalization of the the nasolacrimal duct. A membranous obstruction in this structure persists in 70% of neonates, but resolves spontaneously by 3 months of age in 70% and by a year in 96%.[46] After a year probing may be required; earlier in life simple cleaning of crusts is the best treatment. Referral is not required, but beware photophobia or conjunctivitis, which suggest another diagnosis. Occasionally congenital obstruction of the nasolacrimal duct combines with an obstruction to retrograde flow to produce a dacrocystocoele, a tense blue-grey swelling just beneath the medial canthus. These often become infected and an early ophthalmic opinion should be obtained. A frankly purulent discharge, particularly if accompanied by redness and swelling of the eyelids, should always be taken seriously and demands bacterial investigation and treatment (p. 1150). Subconjunctival haemorrhages are very common after birth (analogous to petechiae in the skin) and are harmless, although the mother may need reassurance. The sclerae provide a guide to jaundice, particularly in coloured infants.

Iris

The iris is normally blue or grey in the newborn. Look for colobomata (keyhole-shaped pupil): if present there could also be a defect in the retina, and this should prompt a search for other congenital malformations. Babies with aniridia often have a poor visual outcome.

Cornea

Check that the cornea does not appear abnormally large, especially if the baby has prominent eyes. The corneal diameter is normally about 10 mm; if it is greater than 13 mm, particularly if the cornea is also hazy, the baby might have congenital glaucoma (p. 906). The cornea should be bright and clear: corneal opacities deserve referral to an ophthalmologist as they can be due to herpetic ulceration, posterior corneal defects, endothelial dystrophies or abnormal metabolic infiltrations. Corneal haze after a forceps delivery usually resolves. Cataracts can be occasionally seen with the naked eye using a bright light shone tangentially. The lens should always be examined through an ophthalmoscope held 6–8 inches from the eye. If the lens is clear you should be able to see a red retinal reflex. If there is any doubt an ophthalmological opinion must be sought urgently, as the baby may have a congenital cataract. The best results are obtained after early treatment, before there is any chance of stimulus-deprivation amblyopia (p. 906). A dull red reflex can also be secondary to congenital melanoma or cytomegaloviral retinitis.

MOUTH

Note whether the mouth is of normal size or if there is micrognathia. Observe any asymmetry of the corners of the mouth and the nasolabial folds. Asymmetry due to facial palsy becomes more apparent when the baby cries.

Inspection of the inside of the mouth is best done either while the baby is crying lustily or by making him open it (pressing down on the chin sometimes does the trick). It is better not to use a tongue depressor. One should ensure that the palate is intact by seeing it directly: palpation is not enough. It is embarrassing, to say the least, to have missed a cleft in the soft palate which later turns up as a feeding problem or nasal regurgitation.

Minor variations of normal which may be seen include Epstein's pearls (white blobs on the palate or gums); natal teeth (which should be removed); short frenulum or 'tongue tie' (which almost never needs treatment); and bluish swellings (ranulae) on the floor of the mouth, which are mucus retention cysts and need no treatment. The mother may need reassurance as to the benign nature of these conditions.

NECK

The infant has a relatively short neck, which should be inspected for general shape and symmetry, palpated for any lumps or swellings and tested for its full range of movements. A webbed neck may suggest Turner syndrome (p. 863). A very short webbed neck with or without torticollis may indicate underlying abnormalities of the cervical spine (Klippel–Feil syndrome, pp. 876, 1079). Redundant skin posteriorly is one of the characteristics of Down syndrome (p. 859).

Cystic hygromas are soft fluctuant swellings, usually arising in the posterior triangle, which transilluminate readily. Sternomastoid 'tumours' are lesions in the sternomastoid muscle caused by haemorrhage or ischaemia, resulting in secondary fibrosis (p. 1078).

The clavicles should be palpated for fractures, especially if there is any suggestion of an Erb's palsy, if delivery was a difficult breech extraction or if there was shoulder dystocia.

CHEST AND CARDIORESPIRATORY SYSTEM

In the neonatal examination it is almost impossible to separate the cardiovascular and respiratory systems. Their postnatal adaptations are inextricably intertwined, and disorders of one can closely mimic or result from those of the other.

Start by inspecting the chest. Breast swelling is quite normal at this age and a few drops of 'witches' milk' may be expressed from them. These changes are of no significance unless there is obvious inflammation, but the mother may need reassurance.

Many deductions about the cardiorespiratory state can also be made by simple inspection. As well as noting the infant's colour, the single best clue to overall function, observe the respiratory rate and other signs of respiratory distress, such as retractions and grunting.

The respiratory rate is normally 40–60 breaths/minute, but remember that all infants, particularly preterm ones, can have pauses of 5–10 seconds interspersed with periods of regular breathing. True apnoeic attacks last longer than this and are extremely rare in the full-term neonate. Tachypnoea may be an indication of pulmonary pathology, but is also a most important sign of heart failure. Observe the respiratory pattern. When the infant is quiet there should be no flaring of the alae nasi, no grunting and no retractions. On crying, some babies, especially if premature, may exhibit mild sternal or subcostal retraction.

The lungs can be auscultated at the same time as the heart, but by and large this is an unrewarding exercise if there are no respiratory symptoms. Very occasionally one may hear bowel sounds in the chest, suggesting an asymptomatic diaphragmatic hernia.

Palpate the precordium for any thrills or a pronounced ventricular heave. The point of maximal impulse is usually found in the left fourth intercostal space inside the midclavicular line. Percussion of an asymptomatic infant's chest is a waste of time.

Check the peripheral pulses: a patent ductus arteriosus with a significant left-to-right shunt produces a bounding quality. Always palpate the femoral pulses: if they are absent or difficult to feel, suspect coarctation. Four-limb blood pressure may help by confirming a differential between the upper and lower limbs; however, normal newborns can have a difference of up to 20 ± 3.5 mmHg.[35] Femoral pulses vary with the state of the ductus. Counting the heart rate is most easily done when listening to the heart, and should be done preferably over a full minute because of its variability; this may be a counsel of perfection, as the infant is very likely to move under the tactile stimulus of the stethoscope. In practice, after a little experience one soon knows whether the rate is abnormally fast (> 160) or slow (< 100). Listen to both heart sounds: the second sound is often loud and single shortly after birth, but splitting can be detected in 75% of infants by 48 hours.

Innocent heart murmurs

An innocent murmur is one in which there is no cardiac disease: 60% of normal newborns have a systolic murmur at the age of 2 hours.[6] It is possible to make a positive diagnosis of an innocent murmur using clinical skills alone, and the following features were emphasized in a recent study from Oxford.[1]

- grade 1–2/6 murmur at the left sternal edge;
- no clicks on auscultation;
- normal pulses;
- otherwise normal clinical examination.

When a positive diagnosis of an innocent murmur was made in this way, no babies with cardiac disease were identified with subsequent echocardiography. The usual origin of an innocent murmur is the acute angle at the pulmonary artery bifurcation; a few cases have patent ductus arteriosus or tricuspid regurgitation, which resolves rapidly. McCrindle and colleagues[28] suggested six features to help non-cardiologists identify significant murmurs:

- pansystolic;
- grade 3/6 or more;

- best heard in the upper left sternal border;
- harsh quality;
- abnormal second heart sound;
- early or mid-systolic click.

Clinical examination was correct 98% of the time when similar criteria were applied to childhood murmurs, albeit by paediatric cardiologists.[28,41] Clinical evaluation without laboratory tests was equally effective in the hands of general paediatricians in Denmark.[24] In Israel 90 term infants with heart murmurs heard in the first 48 hours of life were evaluated using echocardiography; only one considered clinically to have an innocent murmur was reclassified after investigation because he was found to have a small muscular ventricular septal defect.[12] ECG and chest X-ray have traditionally been used to assist in the classification of murmurs as innocent, but the clinical diagnosis is rarely changed by ECG[31,41] or chest X-ray,[31,43] and in our view these tests should be abandoned for this purpose. An examination by an experienced colleague is a better aid to the identification of genuinely innocent murmurs. We agree with Hall[23] that the widespread availability of echocardiography now means that this investigation, with the accompanying expert consultation, should be offered early to babies whose neonatal murmur cannot confidently be classified as innocent. Babies who are then found to have an abnormality should have a chest X-ray and ECG performed as a baseline, and estimation of four-limb blood pressure performed.

Mention of 'heart murmurs' produces intense anxiety, and talking about 'holes in the heart' is guaranteed to produce a flood of tears; now that it is clear that many are due to pulmonary vessel 'kinking' *in a normal heart*, this is perhaps a less disturbing explanation. You can reassure the parents that 80–90% of murmurs found in the neonatal period will disappear during the first year, most of them within the first 3 months, and that if this is the case the baby will be discharged from outpatients. A practical guide to the action to be taken when a murmur is discovered is given in Table 17.2. Hopefully this approach will help to limit the problem of 'cardiac non-disease' – the restriction of activity in healthy children whose parents believe they have a heart problem.[47]

ABDOMEN

Inspection

Simple observation may yield quite a lot of information. Abdominal distension is easily appreciated, and because of the poorly developed abdominal musculature and scanty subcutaneous fat the intra-abdominal organs can sometimes be seen, particularly the bowel in premature infants. Look for any discharge or reddening of the skin around the umbilicus. The state of the cord stump will depend on the age of the baby. Shortly after birth the three vessels are easily seen. A single umbilical artery is present in 0.3% of newborns, and there is an association with renal abnormalities which was found in 7% of cases in one series.[5] A single umbilical artery in a baby with any other problem justifies further investigation of the renal tract. There is no need to investigate for isolated single umbilical artery in a well baby with no other problem.

Further investigation of the renal tract will also be required in infants who were found to have abnormalities on prenatal ultrasonography (p. 1040). Vesicoureteric reflux is now known to be a familial disease: 30% of infants screened because of a positive family history were found to have the condition.[40] In future this may emerge as a further important part of neonatal screening. A thick cord with profuse jelly is characteristic of infants of diabetic mothers, and a thin one is often seen in small-for-dates babies. Green discoloration indicates the passage of meconium before birth. The stump becomes dark and shrivelled and separates at about 10–14 days, longer if antibiotic prophylaxis is used. Persistent discharge should make one think of a patent urachus. Note whether there is an umbilical hernia and reassure the mother that no treatment is indicated. Record the time of first passage of meconium and urine.

Table 17.2 Action to be taken when a heart murmur is heard

Is there peripheral circulatory collapse?	If so immediate investigation is required
Is there central cyanosis?	Confirm with pulse oximeter. Urgent investigation
Is there any evidence of heart failure? (tachycardia, tachypnoea, enlarged liver)	If so immediate investigation is required
Can the femoral pulses be felt easily?	If not check four-limb blood pressure
Are there any dysmorphic features?	If so, investigation should be done
Is the murmur grade 1–2/6, systolic, not harsh, heard at the left sternal edge only in a well baby with normal pulses?	The murmur is innocent. If the baby is less than 48 hours old and remaining in hospital, listen again before discharge as the murmur may have gone. If mother and baby about to go home tell the parents the diagnosis and arrange follow up at 6 weeks. Some units offer echocardiography to these infants.
Is the murmur grade 3+ or more, running into diastole, or pansystolic, or is there a click, abnormal second heart sound or femoral pulses which are difficult to feel?	This murmur may be pathological. Even if the baby is well, ask a more senior colleague to listen. Watch the baby for signs of heart failure. Arrange echocardiography with the accompanying expert opinion as soon as possible. Carry out a chest X-ray and ECG as a baseline and to assist in differential diagnosis.

Palpation

It is essential for your hands to be warm and for the infant to be quiet and relaxed; if necessary have him suck on a dummy or a clean finger. Remember that a baby with a full stomach may well regurgitate milk if you press too hard – often to the distress of the mother, who may have just spent a lot of time in feeding and then cleaning up the baby!

Palpate the abdominal musculature: there is frequently a diastasis of the recti. Feel for the liver edge, which can be up to 2 cm below the right costal margin in normal infants. The kidneys are usually palpable with patience, and some observers have even gone so far as to state that failure to feel them indicates their absence. It is, however, probably much more important to detect any abnormally large renal masses. The spleen can often be 'tipped', but if more than 1 cm is palpable investigation is needed. Feel for an enlarged bladder; if present, try to express it and observe the urinary stream. Auscultation need not form part of the routine abdominal examination unless there is reason to suspect gastrointestinal abnormality (distension, bile-stained vomit, failure to pass meconium, or bloody stools).

GENITALIA

Male

Inspect the penis for length (normally about 3 cm); occasionally a penis looks deceptively short, but palpation will usually disclose a respectable organ buried in suprapubic fat. True micropenis is rare unless associated with other genital abnormalities. Phimosis is usual and needs no attention. Check the position of the urethral meatus, and if it is abnormally situated describe the hypospadias as glandular, coronal, midshaft or perineal; also inspect the shaft of the penis for curvature and compress it at its base to stimulate an erection, which may reveal a latent chordee. Glandular hypospadias without chordee usually needs no treatment, but in more severe degrees of hypospadias the baby will need corrective surgery at some time before school age. All cases should have the benefit of specialist advice.

Always ask about the urinary stream in boys. There may be a poor stream if there is meatal stenosis with hypospadias; constant dribbling of urine is nearly always abnormal and may indicate urethral valves.

Examine the scrotum for rugosity and feel for the testes. Pay particular attention if the scrotum appears to be underdeveloped. At full term both testes should be palpable, even if retractile. If one or both testes are undescended the mother should be told to ensure that the baby is re-examined later and that surgery will be needed by 5 years if descent has not occurred by 1 year of age. Neonatal testicular torsion is not unduly rare and has occurred some time before birth in almost all cases; the testis is hard and not tender. Urgent referral to a paediatric surgeon is indicated, although the testis is usually already infarcted.

Hydrocoeles can occur at this age but usually resolve spontaneously and do not require treatment. Examine the groins for indirect inguinal herniae: these are not uncommon, particularly in preterm infants, and can usually be reduced easily. If present, the mother should be warned about the symptoms and signs of incarceration/strangulation and an urgent surgical appointment arranged so that early surgery can be arranged.

Female

Inspect the vulva: the clitoris and labia minora are relatively prominent in preterm infants, but at full term the labia majora should cover the labia minora, although the clitoris may still appear relatively large. There is often a white mucoid vaginal discharge, which is occasionally bloodstained; this is normal and the mother should be reassured accordingly. Small hymenal skin tags or mucoid cysts which resolve spontaneously may occur around the vaginal opening. Inguinal herniae are rare in the female and their presence should raise the question of other abnormalities in the genital tract. For further advice see Chapter 42.

At this stage in the examination check the position of the anus and anal tone. A 'wink' can be produced by gently touching the anal margin.

SPINE

With the baby prone, inspect his back for any obvious curvature and look for any midline abnormality over the spine and base of the skull, such as a swelling, dimple, hairy patch or naevus. Any of these may indicate an underlying abnormality of the vertebral column or spinal cord. X-ray the relevant area and look very carefully for neurological deficit in the lower limbs and for abnormalities of bowel and bladder sphincter function. Ultrasound or MRI can be very helpful and should be performed if there is a midline abnormality above the sacrococcygeal region. Choice of investigation will vary according to local expertise and availability. Sacrococcygeal pits are common and harmless: in a study from St George's Hospital, London, no infant in a series of 75 with sacral dimple or pit alone was found to have a spinal abnormality.[18] Any midline lesion higher than this, i.e. any lesion other than those in or just above the natal cleft, should be investigated. Similarly, any lesion at any level with a fatty pad, hairy patch or an area of atretic skin deserves further investigation. See pages 1080 and 1304 for more information on spinal cord diastematomyelia and midline abnormalities.

UPPER LIMBS

Inspect the arms for shape, posture and symmetry and

size. In normal upper limbs the fingertips reach to mid-thigh when the arms are adducted to the body. Examine the hand for any flexion deformities of the fingers and inspect the palms for the arrangement of creases. Polydactyly (hands and feet) is sometimes a familial trait, but look carefully for any other dysmorphic features. All digital remnants should be surgically removed (p. 1077). In the past some were tied off with black silk and left to separate by dry gangrene, but this left a stump which produced an unsightly lump in many cases.

Observe spontaneous arm movements: stroking the hand or forearm is sometimes necessary to elicit active motion in the shoulder, elbow, wrist and hand. Test passive movements for muscle tone and range of motion. Owing to intrauterine restriction of space and activity the newborn may lack some elbow extension. Lack of active movement and pain on passive manoeuvres suggests a fracture or infection, whereas in brachial plexus or cervical spine injury passive motion is not restricted. A brachial plexus lesion is revealed by lack of movement in the arm; initially the arm is flaccid. After 48 hours an upper palsy can be distinguished from a complete palsy. In an upper root palsy (C5,6, sometimes C7) the arm is internally rotated and pronated and there is no active abduction or elbow flexion (Erb's palsy, the waiter's tip position, p. 1086). In a complete palsy of upper and lower roots the arm is flail; there may be a ptosis and a Horner syndrome owing to damage to the stellate ganglion adjacent to C8 and T1. Phrenic palsy should be considered in these cases. The hand may become clawed (Klumpke's paralysis). Although the prognosis of brachial plexus lesions is generally good, with most series reporting a recovery rate of 75–95%, the results of surgical repair have improved markedly since the early days, and babies who have no recovery in biceps function by 3 months should be referred to a specialist.[19]

LOWER LIMBS

Inspect the legs and feet for posture, symmetry, general size and shape, as well as for any obvious deformities. Observe spontaneous or stimulated active movements and test the range of passive movements.

The midpoint of the newborn baby's length is just above the umbilicus (*cf.* the symphysis pubis in the adult). Asymmetry in leg girth or length suggests one of the limb reduction defects (p. 880). Some restriction of joint motion is usual, secondary to limitation of intra-uterine space. Babies who were vertex presentations usually have fully flexed hips and knees, but in those who were extended breech presentations the knees may remain fully extended for a few days, so that the feet are somewhere near the mouth. The knees may lack up to 30° of full extension in the neonate. The tibiae are often laterally bowed and internally rotated. The feet should be inspected for their general configuration. They may provide confirmatory evidence of dysmorphic syndromes, such as the 'rocker-bottom' shape and short hallux in Edward syndrome. A convex 'rocker-bottom' sole and a rigid foot may also indicate congenital vertical talus (p. 1068), which will require surgery.[42] Puffy feet and hypoplastic nails are characteristic of Turner syndrome.

The feet and ankles may be found in many positions, most of which are related to intrauterine moulding (especially if there has been oligohydramnios); much more rarely there is an underlying neurological deficit. A calcaneovalgus position of the foot is almost invariably due to fetal position in utero and will correct in time, with or without simple manipulation. If there is an equinovarus position, without using undue force an attempt should be made to overcorrect it by abduction and dorsiflexion of the foot and ankle, so that the little toe touches the outside of the leg. If this manoeuvre is successful no treatment is indicated, but deformities that cannot be so corrected (true talipes equinovarus) require urgent orthopaedic attention (p. 1068). Simple metatarsus adductus (i.e. inturning of the forefoot) is not uncommon, 90% resolving with no treatment.

Overriding toes are common; syndactyly is often familial; neither usually needs treatment. It is most important to explain the nature and natural history of these minor deformities to the mother.

HIPS (see also pp. 1070–1072)

Screening for congenital dislocation of the hip, introduced in the 1950s, is one of the most important items in the newborn examination. A better term for this condition is developmental dysplasia of the hip, which is gradually gaining favour because it embraces all variants of this complex disorder. The incidence of all forms of DDH is 10.5 per 1000 births.[45] Expert management of DDH diagnosed in the neonatal period can be expected to produce a normal hip, whereas treatment initiated after the first year of life undoubtedly gives much worse results, even after prolonged and aggressive surgical treatment. Up to a quarter of adult hip osteoarthritis requiring surgery may be associated with DDH.[27] Sadly, despite initial confidence in the ability of the Ortolani and Barlow tests to detect DDH, the number of cases diagnosed late (0.2 per 1000) has not reduced and may even have increased.[38] It has been suggested that enthusiastic or repeated clinical examination may provoke harm.[29] Up to half the cases of DDH were 'missed' by a single neonatal examination in some series.[8] The yield can be increased with a second examination,[16] and this is the reason for recommending that the hips be examined by all medical practitioners who come into contact with a baby during the early months. There is no doubt that some completely irreducibly dislocated hips are not detectable with clinical examination in the newborn period and others may dislocate later, perhaps due to a

Table 17.3 Screening strategy for using ultrasound in the detection of DDH

Breech presentation (whether delivered by caesarean section or vaginally)
Family history of dysplastic hip
Any deformity suggesting intrauterine compression or oligohydramnios
Clicky hip on clinical examination, or one with restricted abduction
If sufficient manpower available, consider firstborn females

shallow acetabulum, which progresses to dislocation when weightbearing begins.

Ultrasonography can now be added to clinical examination as a further tool for detecting DDH.[20] Ultrasound can detect clinically stable but anatomically abnormal hips, and show normality in clinically suspect hips. Wholesale ultrasound screening is labour-intensive, produces a high number of false positive results and hence a high early treatment rate. Nevertheless, several large programmes are in place and if these are shown to reduce the considerable later morbidity of this condition there will be considerable pressure to adopt universal ultrasound screening. Developmental dysplasia of the hip is commoner following breech presentation, in females, if there is oligohydramnios, and in those with a positive family history.[9] The best current strategy is to use ultrasound selectively according to local service provision (Table 17.3). For example, screening all breech infants (4% of births) yields 22% of the cases of DDH, whereas adding firstborn females (18% of births) would uncover a further 29% of cases, bringing the total yield to 51%, at a 'cost' of screening 23% of births.[45] The risk factors in Table 17.3 should also be used to identify infants who need to be examined again at 6 weeks of age with extra care.

The cornerstone of the screening strategy for DDH remains a careful history and clinical examination. The Ortolani–Barlow manoeuvres must be performed in every newborn. Details follow, although these tests are hard to describe in words and are much better taught by demonstration. A teaching aid, the 'baby hippy', is also widely available. The timing of the examination is crucial: most unstable hips which are detected by clinical examination (or ultrasound) during the first day are false positive findings. There is a therapeutic dilemma between splinting all unstable hips immediately, risking avascular necrosis in otherwise normal hips, and delaying treatment, thereby risking a falsely reassuring second examination[10] and a poor result. This dilemma is likely to increase with the current trend to early discharge from maternity units.

Procedure

The infant should be lying supine on a flat firm surface, with the legs relaxed, pacified if necessary by sucking on a dummy or finger. The examination may well make the baby cry and interpretation is difficult if the thigh muscles are actively contracting.

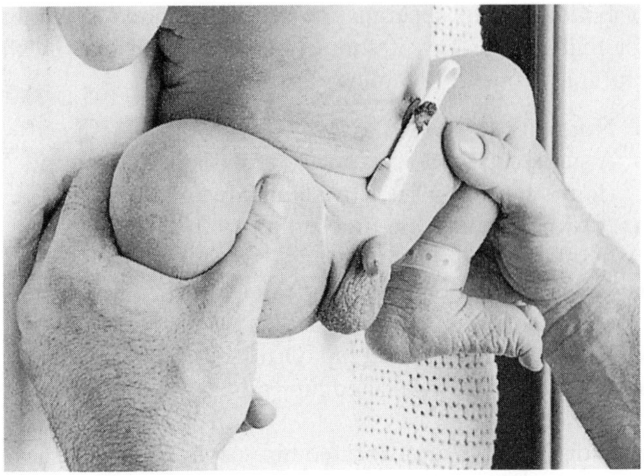

Fig. 17.2 Examination of the hips (see text for details).

First, straighten out the legs and look for any obvious inequality in length, and then carry out Ortolani's test.[32] This manoeuvre is designed to return a dislocated femoral head to the acetabulum. Fully flex the knees and flex the hips to a right-angle. Place the middle finger of each hand over the greater trochanters, thumbs over the internal aspect of the thighs, palms over the knees. Then, simultaneously, pull the leg away from the pelvis and slowly abduct and externally rotate the hips, pressing forwards and medially with the middle fingers (Fig. 17.2). A previously dislocated hip is indicated by a definite 'clunk' as the displaced femoral head slips forward into the acetabulum, rather like engaging the gear lever of a car. This is a quite different sensation from a ligamentous 'click', which is more common but may still be of significance.[26] It does, however, take some experience to tell the difference, the clue being whether there is any sensation of movement. In almost all normal babies it is possible to fully abduct the hips so that the knees almost touch the couch. Inability to do so may indicate a dislocated hip that cannot be reduced and is an indication for an ultrasound scan (Table 17.3).

The next stage of the examination is to do Barlow's test.[4] This is designed to 'dislocate' an unstable hip which is in joint. Some hips are 'loose' but cannot be completely dislocated using this clinical test. Hold the hips and knees as before. With the hips in about 70° abduction, test each hip in turn by pressing forwards and medially (i.e. towards the symphysis pubis) with the finger. Normally no movement is felt, but if the hip is dislocatable the femur is felt to move, again with a 'clunk' as it slips out of the acetabulum. The reverse procedure is then performed by pressing backwards and laterally with the thumb. Normally there is again no movement, but a dislocatable hip will 'clunk' out of the acetabulum and will return there when the pressure is released.

Following the examination and ultrasound screening for high-risk groups it should be possible to classify the hip(s) into one of the following categories:

- Normal;
- A stable hip with acetabular dysplasia on ultrasound (found because of positive family history, etc.);
- A clinically unstable ('loose') hip with acetabular dysplasia on ultrasound;
- A dislocatable hip (one that can be pushed out of the acetabulum and back again): Barlow positive;
- A reducible dislocated hip: Ortolani positive;
- An irreducible dislocated hip (this may easily be missed);
- A dislocatable or dislocated hip secondary to another problem, e.g. CNS disease.

For further information on the management of these types of DDH see Chapter 41.

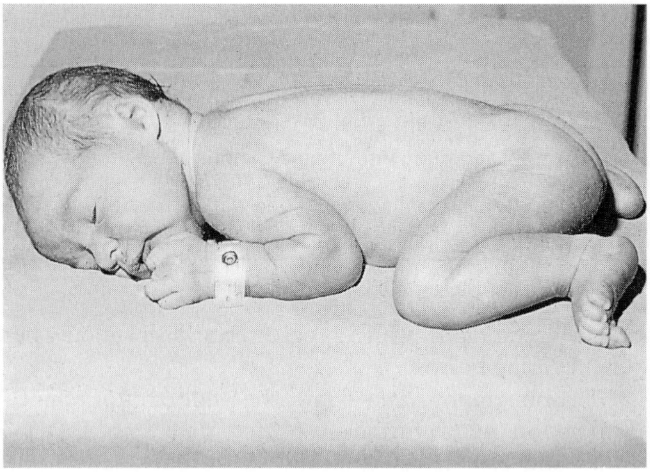

Fig. 17.3 Posture in prone position.

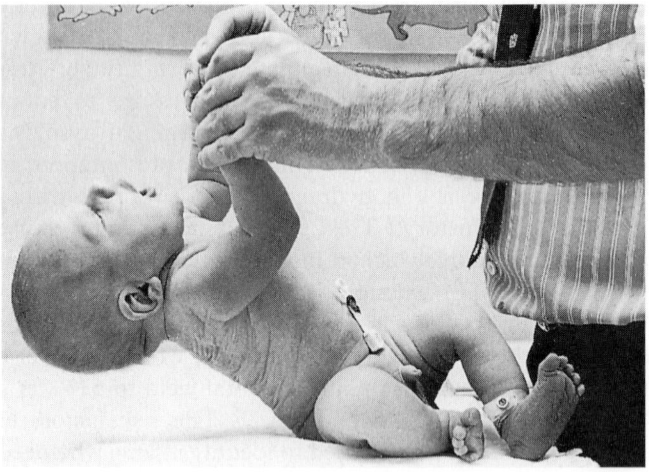

Fig. 17.4 Pull-to-sit manoeuvre. Note flexion of elbows and slight flexion of neck as the infant is pulled up by his wrists.

NEUROLOGICAL

Although much has been written about the neurological assessment of the neonate, formal testing is seldom needed during routine examination. More detail is contained in Chapter 44. Enough screening information can usually be gleaned from talking to the mother and from carefully watching, handling and listening to the baby throughout the examination.

The following general observations can act as a screening test, although one must take into account both gestational age (considered in more detail elsewhere) and postnatal age. The infant may be neurologically very labile during the first few days, and the most meaningful results are only obtained after this time. For a more comprehensive neurological assessment of both preterm and full-term neonates see Dubowitz and Dubowitz.[13]

Behavioural state

Healthy term infants should move between behavioural states, spending most time in quiet and active sleep.

Posture

The undisturbed normal neonate lies predominantly in a flexed position with no lateral preference (Fig. 17.3). When prone the knees are often tucked under the abdomen. The fists are clenched and the thumbs are intermittently furled. With the head in the midline the limbs are roughly symmetrical. Remember, however, that the presentation at birth can influence posture for several days.

Spontaneous motor activity

Normal infants move their limbs in an alternating fashion. Many babies may appear jittery. The prevalence of jittering was 44% in a sample of almost 1000 infants in Boston examined between 8 and 72 hours of age.[33] Half were jittery solely when crying, and the remainder were jittery during several behavioural states. How to distinguish jittering from fits is discussed in Chapter 44.

Muscle tone and strength

This is tested by:

- assessing resistance to passive movements;
- pull-to-sit manoeuvre (Fig. 17.4). Pull the baby up from the supine position by his wrists. In term infants there should be some elbow flexion and the head should come up almost in line with the body. When held sitting the head should remain erect for 2–3 seconds. The palmar grasp reflex may be tested at the same time;

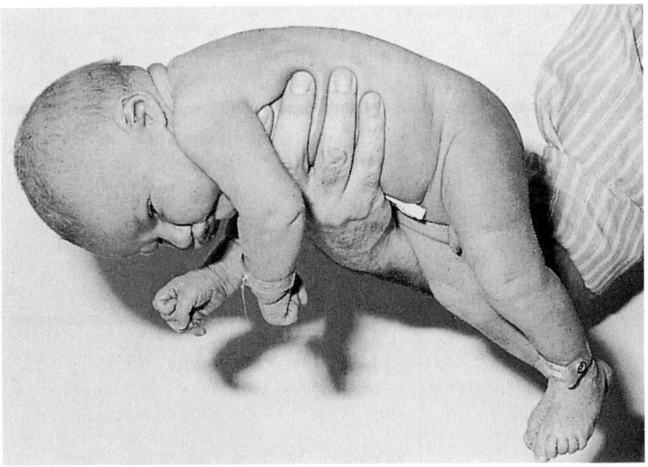

Fig. 17.5 Ventral suspension. Note the flexed arms and the head lying almost on a plane with the body.

- ventral suspension (Fig. 17.5) Hold the baby in the air with a hand under the chest: he should be able to hold his head in line with his body for a few seconds and he should be able to flex his limbs against gravity.

Other general observations

Crying will almost certainly be noted at some time during the examination. Pay particular attention if it is either high-pitched or very weak, or if the infant is reported to cry excessively. Feeding and sucking patterns will be obvious from the history. The eyes have already been discussed: they should lie in the mid-position in the orbit and move in a conjugate fashion; note any constant deviation, persistent strabismus and nystagmus.

Suspicious neurological signs

With practice and experience one is soon able to judge from the history and from handling an infant during the examination whether he is behaving normally. The purpose of such a screening procedure is to pick out those who merit more detailed study and follow-up. The features which should arouse suspicion and which need careful follow-up are:

- persistent failure to suck properly;
- a high-pitched cry;
- extreme irritability or 'staring-eyed' appearance;
- abnormal posturing, e.g. opisthotonus, excessive fisting, constantly fisted thumbs;
- generalized persistent hypertonia;
- 'frog' posture or generalized hypotonia. Paucity of spontaneous movements, including facial expressions;
- asymmetrical movements;
- a history of convulsions;
- midline lesions over the spine.

HEALTH EDUCATION

The normal newborn examination represents an opportunity to provide advice about well-baby care. Information is contained in the parent-held child health records, but a selection of leaflets on the following topics should be available, and the examining doctor needs to be up-to-date on government and local policies regarding them.

- **Cot death prevention** Babies should sleep on their backs, parents should not smoke, infant bedrooms should be kept at a comfortable temperature of about 18°C, and babies should be kept warm but not overclothed. There may be local initiatives in place for Care of the Next Infant – next siblings of infants who died of cot death.
- **Prevention of haemorrhagic disease of the newborn** If the parents chose oral vitamin K and the baby is to be breast-fed further oral doses of vitamin K are needed. Local policies may vary as to which babies are not considered suitable for oral vitamin K prophylaxis, i.e. who require intramuscular treatment because they are at high risk of vitamin K deficiency bleeding. Examples include preterm babies, babies whose mothers are taking antituberculous or anticonvulsant drugs, and babies with evidence of liver disease.
- **Breast-feeding promotion** The hospital should try to become a 'baby friendly' environment. The simple rules that have been shown to help promote breast-feeding (Chapter 19) should be followed. A breast-feeding counsellor should be on hand to provide advice and suitable literature.
- **Nutrition advice** Advice on weaning (no cow's milk until a year, to avoid iron deficiency) can begin in the maternity hospital.
- **Hygiene advice** Need for and methods of sterilizing bottles, dummies etc.
- **Hearing screening** Universal hearing screening is not yet generally available, but high-risk children, i.e. those with a family history of deafness in childhood in near relatives, those with a midline defect such as a cleft palate, and those who have required admission to the neonatal unit, should be referred for early hearing testing by whatever method is used locally. Advice on detecting deafness is contained in most parent-held child records. Further literature can be otained from the National Deaf Children's Society, whose standards are a suitable target for those auditing their service.
- **Sibling management** Many parents request literature on dealing with rivalry.
- **Screening for** those in need of immediate **vaccination**. This mainly refers to hepatitis and TB vaccination. For information see Chapter 31, Part 2.
- **HIV-positive mothers** Treatment of babies should begin immediately for the best results. In the UK HIV-positive mothers are advised against breast-feeding.
- **Advice on handling** How to deal with crying babies – no shaking. Advice on sleep problems.

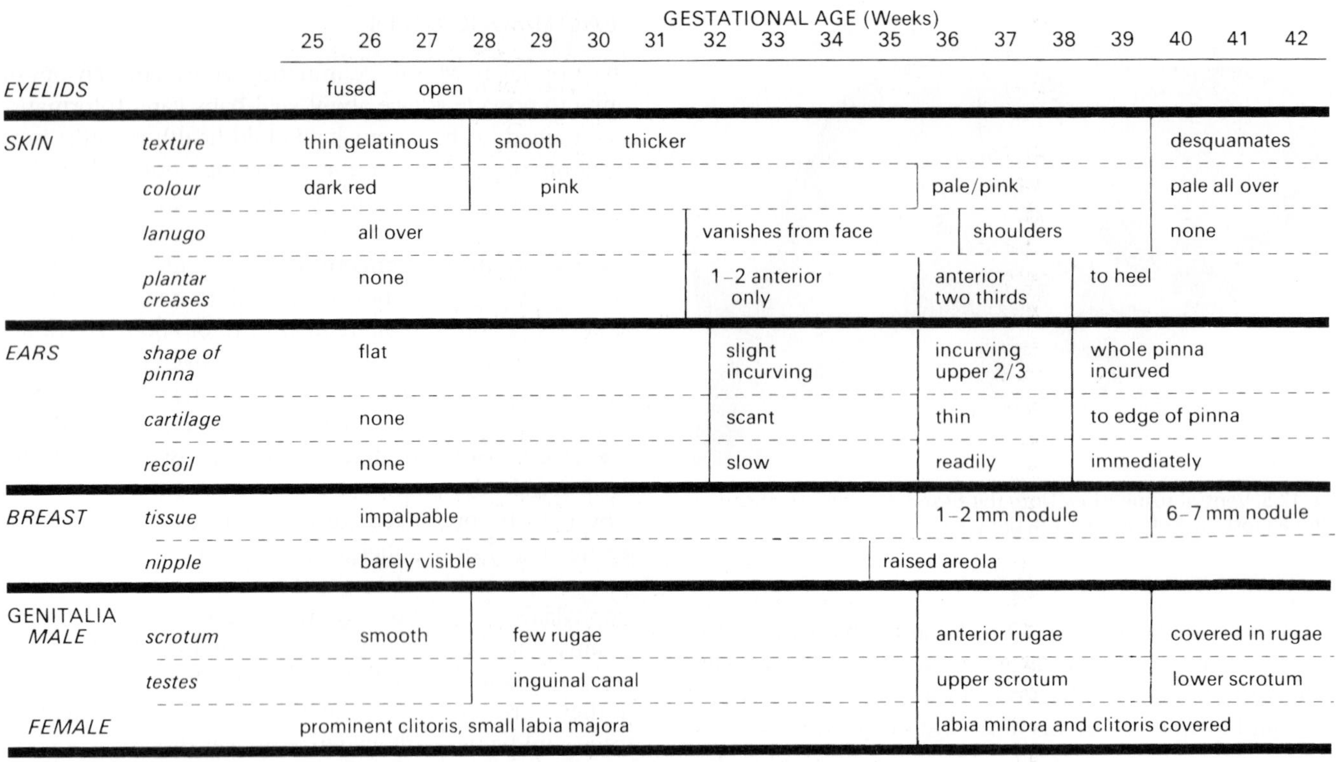
GESTATIONAL AGE (Weeks)
25 26 27 28 29 30 31 32 33 34 35 36 37 38 39 40 41 42
EYELIDS
fused
open
SKIN
texture
thin gelatinous
smooth
thicker
desquamates
colour
dark red
pink
pale/pink
pale all over
lanugo
all over
vanishes from face
shoulders
none
plantar creases
none
1–2 anterior only
anterior two thirds
to heel
EARS
shape of pinna
flat
slight incurving
incurving upper 2/3
whole pinna incurved
cartilage
none
scant
thin
to edge of pinna
recoil
none
slow
readily
immediately
BREAST
tissue
impalpable
1–2 mm nodule
6–7 mm nodule
nipple
barely visible
raised areola
GENITALIA MALE
scrotum
smooth
few rugae
anterior rugae
covered in rugae
testes
inguinal canal
upper scrotum
lower scrotum
FEMALE
prominent clitoris, small labia majora
labia minora and clitoris covered

Fig. 17.6 Approximate maturation of some physical characteristics used in the assessment of gestational age.

- **Safe transport in cars** The newborn period is a good time to give advice on the purchase of safe types of car seat and to encourage their use.
- **Maternal depression** Those working in a maternity hospital should be aware of the maternal depression scales and how to administer them. Literature informing mothers about this common and important problem and where to get help could help prevent tragedy.

GESTATIONAL AGE

The assessment of gestational age has become a veritable growth industry in recent years. Complex charts, graphs and tables have been produced, some of which purport to fix the maturity to within a week. The wise clinician will appreciate that this is an impossible goal and that formal assessment is unnecessary in the routine discharge examination of term infants (> 37 weeks) whose birthweight falls between the 10th and 90th centiles. This is not to deny the importance of trying to establish the gestational age of low-birthweight infants, or those who seem inappropriately grown according to their obstetric data. These babies are at risk from different conditions to appropriately grown infants. Furthermore, knowing the gestational age is of immense value in interpreting neurological behaviour in the neonatal period and in evaluating subsequent developmental progress.

The cornerstone for assigning gestational age should be an early obstetric ultrasound, as this, combined with mother's menstrual data, gives the best assessment. A recent evaluation of the clinical methods of assessing gestational age revealed that even the best were only half as accurate as estimates based on obstetric ultrasound at 15–19 weeks of gestation.[44] The clinical methods had 95% confidence intervals of 17 days, whereas the obstetric ultrasound had 95% confidence intervals of less than 7 days. One should be very wary of any maturity estimation based on ultrasound obtained only during the second half of pregnancy, and information from uterine size, date of quickening etc. is quite valueless.

The criteria used for estimating gestational age after birth may be divided into those based on physical maturation and those dependent on the development of the nervous system. Many such observations have been used to devise complex scoring systems. In theory this is a valid approach, but in practice it is too time-consuming and cumbersome to use routinely. Some criteria are more valuable than others, and little is lost by using only a few items.[34] The physical items proved more robust than the items assessing tone and posture in the evaluation of Wariyar et al,[44] and a retrospective assessment based on when the infant acquired the ability to suck and swallow reliably (34–35 weeks) was surprisingly accurate, provided the infant was not oxygen dependent.[44]

PHYSICAL CHARACTERISTICS

Many observations have been made on some of the

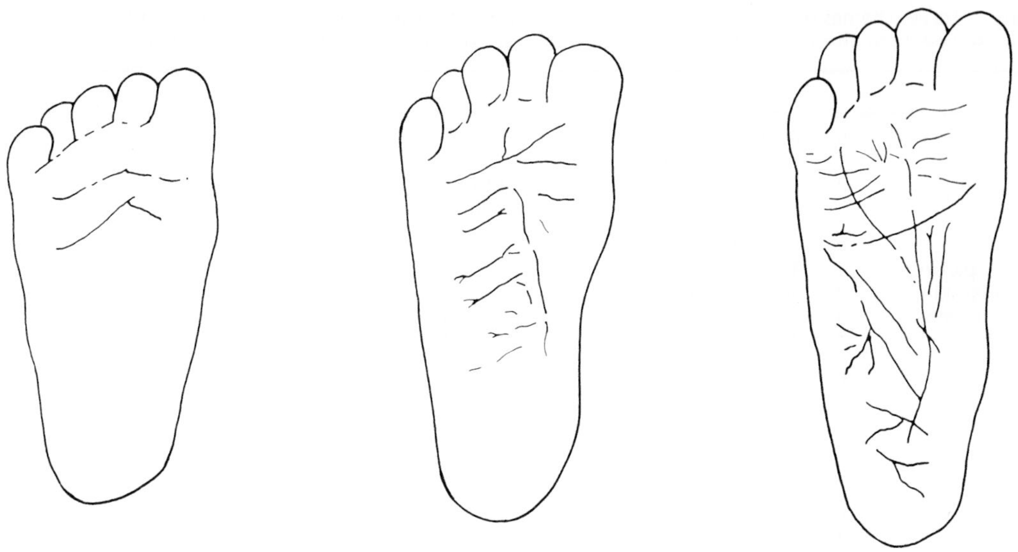

Fig. 17.7 Maturation of sole creases with increasing age. These are only of value if examined in the first few hours after birth: (A) 34–36 weeks, one or two anterior creases; (B) 37–38 weeks, creases over anterior two-thirds of sole; (C) 40 weeks, sole creases extend to heel.

visible and palpable characteristics of infants born at different gestational ages. As development is a smooth process and because maturation is inherently variable, it is impossible to give more than a rough idea of when certain changes take place. Figure 17.6 attempts to show when to expect some of the more important features.

The eyelids remain fused until about 25–26 weeks. The skin of the very immature infant (< 27 weeks) appears dark red in colour because it is so thin and fragile; it gradually thickens, and by full term is starting to desquamate. Blood vessels may at first be prominent and later disappear. Very fine lanugo hair is present initially and gradually vanishes by full term. The nails may reach the fingertips by 32 weeks, but extend beyond them at term. Plantar skin creases (Fig. 17.7), which are absent in immature infants, start to appear at around 32 weeks and gradually increase to cover the heel by full term; these, however, can only be adequately evaluated in the first few hours after birth. The ears (pinnae) are initially flat, have no cartilage, and remain in bizarre shapes after folding. From about 33 weeks some cartilage can be felt, the pinna starts incurving and recoils after folding, so that at term the ear is firm and fully shaped, with immediate recoil. The breasts of the very immature infant are non-existent, even the nipple being barely visible. A breast nodule is palpable by about 36 weeks. In the male the testes descend to the inguinal canal after about 29 weeks but may not be fully in the scrotum until term, the latter becoming progressively more rugose during this time. The immature female has a prominent clitoris with relatively small, widely separated labia majora. By full term both labia minora and clitoris are covered by the larger labia majora.

Various attempts have been made to quantify some of these changes by using scoring systems. A summary of three such schemes is given in Table 17.4. For interpretation of the data see Figure 17.8. Farr et al[17] used a system of 34 points derived from 11 criteria; Dubowitz et al[14] used the same physical criteria with a total of 35 points. Parkin et al[34] produced a much simpler scheme with 13 points derived from only four of the above criteria, details of which are given in Table 17.5. This simple system proved as accurate as the Dubowitz or expanded Ballard[2,3] score if half scores were allotted.[44]

Neurological criteria

The development of some reflexes and a gradual increase in muscle tone, combined with changes in the range of passive joint movements with advancing gestation, provide much information about maturity. Some of these items have been semiquantified into scoring systems for use in conjunction with physical characteristics.

The appearance times of four reflexes as described by Robinson[36] are probably most useful for premature infants less than 34 weeks. The items are not scored, but their presence or absence should give a reasonable idea of whether a given low-birthweight infant is compatible with his reputed gestational age (Fig. 17.6). To these can be added the ability to suck/swallow reliably at 34–35 weeks of gestation. The five reflexes are as follows:

- Pupil reaction to light appears between 29 and 31 weeks. The response can be extremely difficult to see in a tiny baby: one method is to look at the eye through the magnifying lens of an otoscope head, which is used as the light source.
- Glabellar tap: a blink in response to a tap on the glabella appears between 32 and 34 weeks.
- Traction response: flexion of the neck or arms when

Table 17.4 Summary of three schemes of assessing gestational age by physical criteria used in the assessment of gestational age. Includes the scoring systems used by three different authors. (Modified from Dubowitz et al[14] (D), Farr et al[17] (F), Parkin et al[34] (P))

			D	F	P
Skin colour	0	Dark red	0	0	0
	1	Uniformly pink	1	1	1
	2	Pale pink, variable over different parts of body	2	2	2
	3	Pale, only pink over ears, lips, palms or soles	3	3	3
Skin texture	0	Very thin and smooth, gelatinous feel	0	0	0
(by inspection and by picking	1	Thin and smooth	1	1	1
up a fold of abdominal skin	2	Medium thickness, smooth with or without rash and superficial peeling	2	2	2
between finger and thumb)	3	Slight thickening, stiff feeling, cracking and peeling hands and feet	3	3	3
	4	Thick parchment-like, superficial or deep cracking	4	4	4
Skin opacity	0	Numerous veins and venules, especially over abdomen	0	0	–
	1	Veins and tributaries seen	1	1	–
	2	A few large vessels clearly seen over abdomen	2	2	–
	3	A few large vessels indistinctly seen over abdomen	3	3	–
	4	No blood vessels seen	4	4	–
Lanugo hair	0	None	0	0	–
(over back)	1	Abundant, long and thick over whole back	1	1	–
	2	Thinning especially over lower back	2	2	–
	3	Small amount with bald areas	3	3	–
	4	At least one half of back devoid of lanugo	4	4	–
Plantar creases	0	None	0	0	–
(Skin stretched from toes to	1	Faint red marks over anterior half	1	1	–
heel) Only valid in first	2	Definite red marks over anterior half, indentations over less than anterior third	2	2	–
2–3 hours after birth	3	Indentations over more than anterior third	3	3	–
	4	Definite deep indentations over more than anterior third	4	4	–
Oedema	0	Obvious oedema of hands and feet, pitting over tibia	0	0	–
	1	No obvious oedema of hands and feet, pitting over tibia	1	1	–
	2	None	2	2	–
Ear form	0	Pinna flat and shapeless, little or no incurving of edge	0	0	–
(Inspect upper pinna above	1	Incurving of part of the edge	1	1	–
meatus)	2	Partial incurving of whole of upper part of pinna	2	2	–
	3	Well-defined incurving of whole of upper pinna	3	3	–
Ear firmness	0	Soft, easily folded, no recoil	0	0	0
(Palpate and fold upper	1	Soft, easily folded, slow recoil	1	1	1
pinna)	2	Cartilage to edge in places, ready recoil	2	2	2
	3	Firm, cartilage to edge, ready recoil	3	3	3
Breast size	0	No breast tissue palpable	0	0	0
(Pick up between finger and	1	Palpable on one or both sides but less than 0.5 cm	1	1	1
thumb)	2	Palpable on both sides, one or both 0.5–1 cm	2	2	2
	3	Palpable on both sides, one or both over 1 cm	3	3	3
Nipple formation	0	Barely visible, no areola	0	0	–
	1	Nipple well defined, areola smooth and flat, less than 0.75 cm	1	1	–
	2	Areola stippled, edge not raised, diameter less than 0.75 cm	2	1	–
	3	Areola stippled, raised edge, diameter over 0.75 cm	3	2	–
Genitalia					
Male	0	Scrotum empty	0	0	–
	1	At least one testis high in scrotum	1	1	–
	2	At least one testis completely descended	2	2	–
Female	0	Labia majora widely separated, labia minora protruding	0	0	–
	1	Labia majora almost cover labia minora	1	1	–
	2	Labia majora completely cover labia minora	2	2	–
Total scores			35	34	13

the baby is pulled up by the wrists from the supine position; appears between 33 and 36 weeks.

- Neck righting: the trunk follows the head when the neck is passively rotated in either direction from the supine; appears between 34 and 37 weeks.
- Ability to suck/swallow reliably. This matures with remarkable consistency between 34 and 35 weeks, and allows the infant to feed from breast or bottle provided he is not oxygen dependent.

The postnatal development of these reflexes can be used sequentially after birth so that an estimate of gestational age may be arrived at retrospectively.

Combination of the Robinson neurological assessment

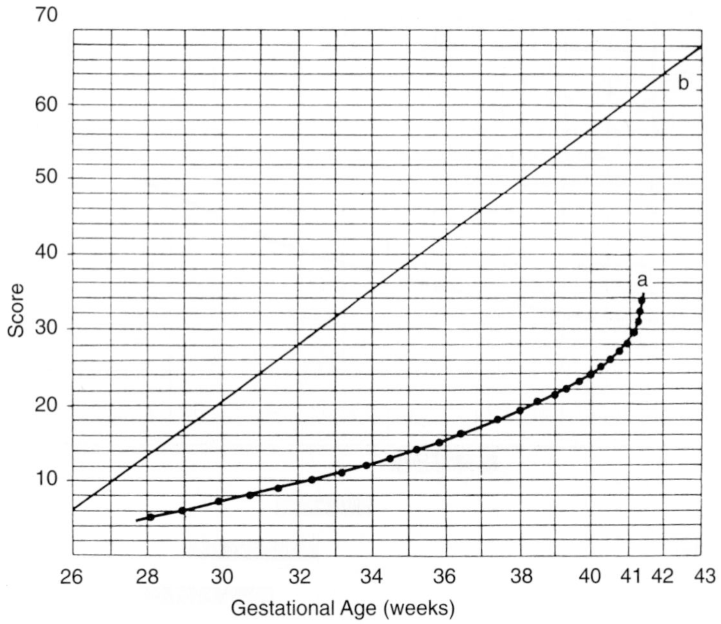

Fig. 17.8 Graph for calculating gestational age. See text and Table 17.4 for details. Curve (a) is based on scores derived from physical criteria.[17] Line (b) is based on combined total score of physical and neurological criteria as described by Dubowitz et al[14] (Fig. 17.10).

Table 17.5 Definition and scoring of the criteria used by Parkin et al[34]

Skin texture	
Tested by inspection and by picking up a fold of abdominal skin between finger and thumb	
0	Very thin with a gelatinous feel
1	Smooth and thin
2	Smooth, medium thickness, irritation rash and superficial peeling may be present
3	Slight thickening and stiff feeling, superficial cracking and peeling, especially on the hands and feet
4	Thick and parchment-like with superficial or deep cracking
Skin colour	
Estimated by inspection when the baby is quiet	
0	Dark red
1	Uniformly pink
2	Pale pink, though colour may vary to very pale over some parts of the body
3	Pale, nowhere really pink except ears, lips, palms and soles
Breast size	
Measured by picking up breast between finger and thumb	
0	No breast tissue palpable
1	Breast nodule palpable on one or both sides
2	Nodule palpable on both sides, one or both being 0.5–1 cm diameter
3	Nodules palpable on both sides, one or both being greater than 1 cm diameter
Ear firmness	
Tested by palpation and folding of the upper pinna	
0	Pinna soft and easily folded into bizarre positions, does not recoil spontaneously
1	Pinna soft along the edge and easily folded, recoils slowly spontaneously
2	Cartilage felt to edge of pinna though thin in places, pinna recoils readily
3	Firm pinna with definite cartilage extending to periphery, recoils immediately

for infants < 34 weeks' gestation and the Parkin modification of the Farr score for infants > 32–34 weeks is usually all that is required to assess a neonate's gestation (Fig. 17.9). However, the more complex scheme of Dubowitz et al[14] is widely used, though it is doubtful whether it adds to the accuracy of the simple schemes.

The Dubowitz score is based on a combination of physical criteria (Table 17.4) and others that are largely dependent on the assessment of muscle tone. The very immature infant is extremely floppy, with very little flexor tone in the neck, trunk or limbs. As gestation advances he gradually adopts a flexed posture and muscle tone increases, together with an ability to move against gravity.

Muscle tone can be assessed and graded by:

- observing the infant's posture in the supine position;
- assessing the head lag in response to traction on the wrists (pull-to-sit manoeuvre);
- observation in ventral suspension;
- manipulating the arms (scarf sign) and legs (heel-to-ear manoeuvre and popliteal angle);
- observing the flexion responses of the limbs following passive extension (arm and leg recoil);
- estimating the angles to which the wrist and ankle can be passively flexed (square window and ankle dorsiflexion). NB: this test is not one of muscle tone, as a greater degree of flexion can be obtained in the more mature infant; it must therefore represent an increase in the mobility of the joints concerned.

These items (35 points derived from 10 criteria) have been meticulously scored as shown in Figure 17.10. The

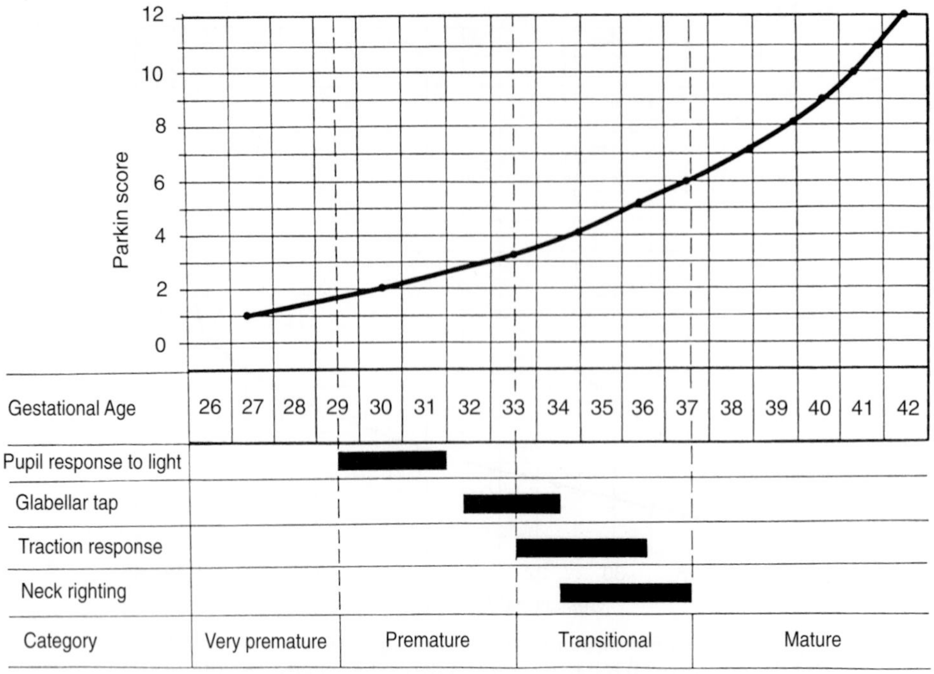

Fig. 17.9 Assessment of gestational age based on: (1) scoring four physical criteria (skin texture, skin colour, breast size and ear firmness) as described by Parkin et al[34], (2) the appearance times of four neurological reflexes.[36] See text for details of definitions.

total score so obtained is added to that derived from the Farr and Dubowitz physical criteria (Table 17.4). The gestational age is then estimated using the graph shown in Figure 17.8.

In summary, the estimation of gestational age from clinical observation of the infant is probably only accurate to within ±2 weeks, so that a more practical approach is first, to check whether a given infant is likely to be compatible with his reputed gestational age; secondly, in cases where the mother's dates are uncertain, or where there has been some confusion, one should attempt to assign the infant to a group, namely:

- Very premature, < 29 weeks;
- Premature, 29–32 weeks;
- Transitional, 33–36 weeks;
- Mature, 37–41 weeks;
- Postmature, > 41 weeks.

REFERENCES

1. Arlettaz R, Archer L N J, Wilkinson A R 1998 Natural history of innocent heart murmurs in newborn babies: a controlled echocardiographic study. Archives of Disease in Childhood 78: F166–F170
2. Ballard J L, Novak K K, Driver M A 1979 A simplified score of fetal maturation of newly born infants. Journal of Pediatrics 95: 769–774
3. Ballard J L, Khoury J C, Wedig K, Wang L, Eilers-Walsman B L, Lipp J R 1991 New Ballard score, expanded to include extremely premature infants. Journal of Pediatrics 119: 417–423
4. Barlow T G 1962 Early diagnosis and treatment of congenital dislocation of the hip. Journal of Bone and Joint Surgery 44: B292–B301
5. Bourke W G, Clarke T A, Mathews T G, O'Halpin D O, Donoghue V B 1993 Isolated single umbilical artery – the case for screening. Archives of Disease in Childhood 68: 600–601
6. Brando M, Rowe R D 1961 Auscultation of the heart in the early neonatal period. American Journal of Diseases in Children 101: 575–586
7. Brown F E, Cohen L B, Addante R R, Graham J M Jr 1986 Correction of congenital auricular deformities by splinting in the neonatal period. Pediatrics 78: 406–441
8. Catford J C, Bennet G C, Wilkinson J A 1982 Congenital hip dislocation: an increasing and still uncontrolled disability? British Medical Journal 285: 1527–1530
9. Chan A, McCaul K A, Cundy P J, Haan E A, Byron-Scott R 1997 Perinatal risk factors for developmental dysplasia of the hip. Archives of Disease in Childhood 76: F94–F100
10. Clarke N M P 1992 Diagnosing congenital dislocation of the hip. British Medical Journal 305: 435–436
11. Comroe J H 1965 Physiology of respiration. Year Book Medical Publishers, Chicago, p 208
12. Du Z-D, Rougin N, Barak M 1997 Clinical and echocardiographic evaluation of neonates with heart murmurs. Acta Paediatrica Scandinavica 86: 752–756
13. Dubowitz L, Dobowitz V 1981 The neurological assessment of the preterm and fullterm newborn infant. Clinics in Developmental Medicine No 79 SIMP/Heinemann, London
14. Dubowitz L M S, Dobowitz V, Goldberg C 1970 Clinical assessment of gestational age in the newborn infant. Journal of Pediatrics 77: 1–10
15. Dunn P M 1976 Congenital postural deformities. British Medical Bulletin 32: 71–76
16. Dunn P M, Evans R E, Thearle M J, Griffiths H E D, Witherow P J 1985 Congenital dislocation of the hip: early and late diagnosis and management compared. Archives of Disease in Childhood 60: 407–414
17. Farr V, Kerridge D F, Mitchell R G 1966 The value of some external characteristics in the assessment of gestational age. Developmental Medicine and Child Neurology 8: 657–660
18. Gibson P, Britton J, Hall DMB, Rowland Hill C 1995 Lumbosacral skin markers and identification of occult spinal dysraphism in neonates. Acta Paediatrica Scandinavica 84: 208–209
19. Gilbert A, Brockman R, Carlioz H 1991 Surgical treatment of brachial plexus palsy. Clinical Orthopaedics and Related Research 264: 39–47

SCORE		0	1	2	3	4	5
POSTURE Infant quiet, supine	arm flexion	none	none	none	slight	full	
	leg flexion	none	slight	more	flexed	full	
SQUARE WINDOW Flex hand on forearm. Estimate angle between forearm and hypothenar eminence.		90°	60°	45°	30°	0°	
ANKLE DORSIFLEXION Dorsiflex foot onto leg as fully as possible. Estimate angle between foot and leg.		90°	75°	45°	20°	0°	
ARM RECOIL Infant supine, flex forearms 5 seconds, then extend and release. Observe recoil at elbow		none 180°	sluggish 90°–180°	full recoil <90°			
LEG RECOIL Infant supine, flex hips and knees 5 seconds, then extend and release. Observe recoil at knee		none 180°	partial 90°–180°	full recoil <90°			
POPLITEAL ANGLE Infane supine, pelvis flat, thigh into knee-chest position, extend knee. Estimate angle		180°	160°	130°	110°	90°	<90°
HEEL-TO-EAR Infant supine, draw foot towards head, leave knee free. Observe distance between foot & head.							
SCARF SIGN Infant supine, pull arm to try to wrap it round the opposite shoulder. Note elbow position.		to opposite axilla	beyond midline	to midline	not to midline		
HEAD LAG Pull to sit from supine. Observe head in relation to trunk.		complete lag	partial control	in line with body	anterior to body		
VENTRAL SUSPENSON Suspend in prone position with one hand	head	floppy	slight ext'n	more ext'n	in body line	above body	
	back	flexed	slight ext'n	more ext'n	extended	extended	
	limbs	extended	slight flex'n	more flex'n	flexed	fully flexed	

Fig. 17.10 Definitions and scores for 10 neurological criteria used in gestational age assessment. (Modified from Dubowitz et al[14])

20. Graf R, Wilson B 1995 Sonography of the infant hip and its therapeutic implications. Chapman & Hall, Weinheim, Germany.
21. Graham J M Jr 1994 When is it best to be born? A morphological perspective – craniofacial deformation. In: Amiel-Tison C, Stewart A (eds) The newborn infant: one brain for life. INSERM, Paris, pp 23–38
22. Graham J M Jr, Smith D W 1979 Parietal craniotabes in the neonate: its origin and significance. Journal of Pediatrics 95: 114–116
23. Hall D M B 1996 Health for all children, 3rd edn. Oxford University Press, Oxford, pp 90–108
24. Hansen L K, Birkebaek N H, Oxhoj H 1995 Initial evaluation of children with heart murmurs by the non-specialised paediatricians. European Journal of Pediatrics 154: 15–17
25. Hunter A G W, Rudd N L 1977 Craniosynostosis II: its familial characteristics and associated clinical findings in 109 patients lacking bilateral polysyndactyly or syndactyly. Teratology 15: 301–310
26. Jones D A 1989 Importance of the clicking hip in screening for congenital dislocation of the hip. Lancet 1: 599–601
27. Lloyd-Roberts G C 1955 Osteoarthritis of the hip: a study of clinical pathology. Journal of Bone and Joint Surgery 37: 8–47
28. McCrindle B W, Shaffer K M, Kan J S, Zahka K G, Rowe S A, Kidd L 1996 Cardinal clinical signs in the differentiation of heart murmurs in children. Archives of Paediatric and Adolescent Medicine 150: 169–174
29. Moore F H 1989 Examining infants' hips – can it do harm? Journal of Bone and Joint Surgery 71: 4–5
30. Moss G D, Cartlidge P H T, Speidel B D, Chambers T L 1991 Routine examination in the newborn period. British Medical Journal 302: 878–879
31. Newburger J W, Rosenthal A, Williams R G, Fellows K, Miettinen O S 1983 Noninvasive tests in the initial evaluation of heart murmurs in children. New England Journal of Medicine 308: 61–64
32. Ortolani M 1937 Un segno poco noto e sua importanza per la diagnosi precoce di prelussazione congenita dell'anca. Pediatrica (Napoli) 45: 129–136
33. Parker S, Zuckerman B, Bauchner H, Frank D, Vinci R, Cabral H 1990 Jitteriness in full term neonates: prevalence and correlates. Pediatrics 85: 17–23
34. Parkin J M, Hey E N, Clowes J S 1976 Rapid assessment of gestational age at birth. Archives of Disease in Childhood 51: 259–263
35. Piazza S F, Chandra M, Harper R G, Sia C G, McVicar M, Huang H 1985 Upper versus lower systolic blood pressure in full term normal newborn. American Journal of Disease in Children 139: 797–799
36. Robinson R J 1966 Assessment of gestational age by neurological examination. Archives of Disease in Childhood 41: 437–447
37. Rothman L, Rose J S, Laster D W, Quaker R, Tenner M 1976 The spectrum of growing skull fracture. Pediatrics 57: 26–31
38. Sanfridson J, Redland-Johnell I, Uden A, 1991 Why is congenital dislocation of the hip still missed? Analysis of 96,891 infants screened in Malmo, 1956–1987. Acta Orthopedica Scandinavica 62: 87–91
39. Scarfo G B, Mariotti A, Tomaccini D, Palma L 1989 Growing skull fracture. Child's Nervous System 5: 163–167
40. Scott J E S, Swallow V, Coulthard M G, Lambert H J, Lee R E J 1997 Screening newborn babies for familial ureteric reflux. Lancet 350: 396–400
41. Smythe J F, Teixeira O H, Vlad P, Demers P P, Feldman W 1990 Initial evaluation of heart murmurs: are laboratory tests necessary? Pediatrics 86: 497–500
42. Staheli L T 1993 Shoes and common lower limb problems. In: David T J (ed) Recent advances in paediatrics vol 11. Churchill Livingstone, Edinburgh, pp 161–173
43. Temmerman A M, Mooyaart E L, Taverne P P 1991 The value of the routine chest roentgenogram in the cardiological evaluation of infants and children: a prospective study. European Journal of Pediatrics 150: 623–636
44. Wariyar U, Tin W, Hey E 1997 Gestational assessment assessed. Archives of Disease in Childhood 77: F216–F220
45. Yiv B C, Saidin R, Cundy P J et al 1997 Developmental dysplasia of the hip in South Australia in 1991: prevalence and risk factors. Journal of Pediatrics and Child Health 33: 151–156
46. Young J D H, Mac Ewen C J 1997 Managing congenital lacrimal obstruction in general practice. British Medical Journal 315: 293–296
47. Young P C 1993 The morbidity of cardiac nondisease revisited. Is there lingering concern associated with an innocent murmur? American Journal of Disease in Children 147: 975–977

18

Temperature control and its disorders

Nicholas Rutter

Children and adults can control their body temperature over a wide range of ambient conditions. They achieve this by making physiological or behavioural adjustments which affect the rate at which they produce or lose heat. The newborn infant is similarly homoeothermic but there are differences, mainly of degree, which make it more difficult for him to maintain a constant body temperature. A low bodyweight to surface area ratio means that heat production is low relative to heat loss. The physiological and behavioural responses to a warm or cold environment are less well developed than in older infants or children. The part played by the mother in the thermoregulation of newborn animals is vital, maternal body heat being used to warm the young as before delivery. However, routine care of the preterm newborn human often demands that the infant is removed from his mother, stripped naked and nursed in dry, draughty surroundings, conditions which may produce severe thermal stress.

An appropriate thermal environment with maintenance of a normal body temperature is important to the newborn, particularly if ill or small. Several studies in the past have shown that if such infants are allowed to become cold their chances of survival are considerably reduced,[22,28,59,93,96,97] their incidence of illness is increased and their rate of growth is diminished.[37–39] Although these studies were made when mortality rates were high and the infants were severely cold stressed, the implication is that cold stress is harmful and should be avoided. To these important reasons for choosing an infant's thermal environment carefully should be added thermal comfort, a concept that is well defined in children and adults.[2,3,51] There is no reason to suppose that infants do not feel uncomfortably cold or hot because their neurological development is too immature for them to express their feelings.

Those who care for newborn infants take responsibility for selecting an appropriate physical environment. This is not instinctive, and thought needs to be given to those factors which determine the thermal environment so that suitable conditions can be provided. Obsessive attention to detail, particularly in the management of the preterm infant, is important.

PHYSICAL, PHYSIOLOGICAL AND BEHAVIOURAL ASPECTS OF THERMOREGULATION

HEAT BALANCE

The law of conservation of energy demands that under equilibrium conditions heat losses balance heat production. If production exceeds loss, the body temperature rises until a new equilibrium is reached; if losses exceed production body temperature falls.

Heat production = heat loss by (convection + radiation + evaporation)

The amount of heat that a newborn infant loses by conduction is small and can be ignored.

HEAT PRODUCTION

The newborn infant produces heat by metabolic activity in all body tissues. Basal metabolic rate is difficult to measure since the newborn is rarely awake, quiet and starved, but resting levels can be measured. The resting metabolic rate (usually measured indirectly as the resting oxygen consumption) describes the metabolism of an infant who is lying still, asleep, more than an hour after the previous feed, and in neutral thermal surroundings (for definition see later). Under these conditions the heat production of a healthy term newborn infant is similar to that of an adult when expressed per unit weight, but almost half that of an adult when expressed per unit surface area. As it is surface area that determines a subject's heat loss, this relatively low heat production per unit area explains why the newborn requires a much warmer environment than an adult. Resting metabolic rate is similar in term and preterm infants when expressed per unit weight, but considerably lower in preterm infants

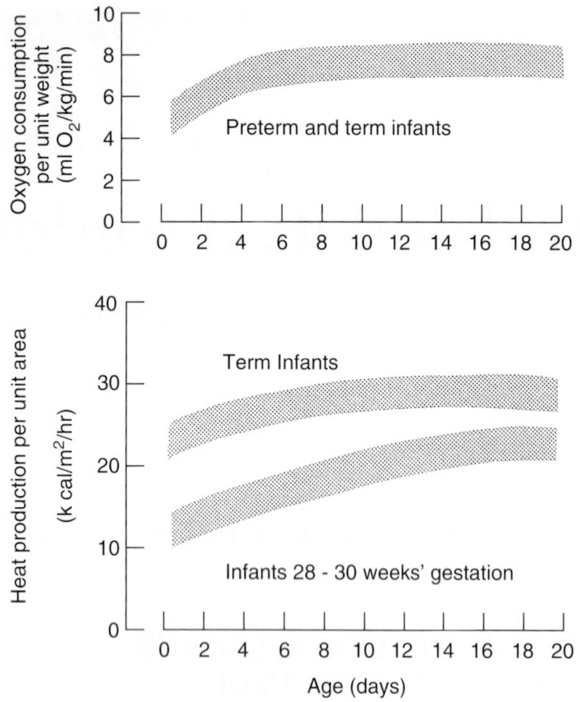

Fig. 18.1 Resting metabolic rate in the newborn period when expressed per unit weight (upper) and per unit surface area (lower). The ranges shown are the mean values ± 1 standard deviation. (Derived from data of Hey 1969[49])

when expressed per unit surface area (Fig. 18.1). Preterm infants thus require higher ambient temperatures than term infants.[54] Resting metabolic rate rises in the immediate newborn period.[49,57,92] The maximum rate of approximately 50 kcal/m²/h is reached by the age of 3–6 months, and thereafter remains constant through childhood into adult life.[62,69]

Many factors influence an infant's heat production (Table 18.1). It is higher in rapid eye movement sleep than deep sleep, suggesting that the brain is metabolically highly active.[100] The newborn infant is also able to increase heat production in response to cold stress (see below). There is considerable individual variation, particularly in small babies.[88]

Table 18.1 Factors affecting a newborn infant's heat production

Heat production is increased	Heat production is decreased
In infants who are awake	In infants who are in deep sleep[100]
In infants who are active	In infants who are ill, particularly following asphyxia or with hypoxia
Following ingestion of food[101]	In starved infants[104]
When growth is rapid[19]	In malnutrition[20]
In neonatal thyrotoxicosis	In infants with hypothyroidism
In infants in cardiac failure with a left-to-right shunt[63]	In infants with cyanotic congenital heart disease[63]
Following drug administration e.g. theophylline[36]	Following drug administration e.g. chlorpromazine

HEAT LOSS

Convection

Heat is lost by convection from the exposed surface of the infant to the surrounding air, and is determined largely by the difference in temperature between the two. If the ambient temperature exceeds the surface temperature of the infant, heat will be gained by convection. Convective heat loss also depends on the air speed. If it is rapid, the insulating effect of still air close to the infant's surface is lost (forced convection) and convective heat loss increases. Convection is a major source of heat loss when newborn infants are exposed in cool, draughty rooms.

Radiation

Heat is lost by radiation from the exposed surface of the infant to the surrounding surfaces that directly overlook the infant. This is proportional to the difference between these surface temperatures but independent of the temperature and speed of the intervening air. It is an important channel of heat loss when infants are exposed naked in a delivery room or a single-walled incubator, but a source of heat gain when an infant is nursed under a radiant warmer.

Evaporation of water

As water evaporates from the infant heat is lost (each millilitre of water that evaporates removes 560 calories of heat). Under normal conditions, in a term infant, evaporative heat loss amounts to about a quarter of the resting heat production.[53] About a quarter of this loss is by evaporation of water from the respiratory tract, the remainder occurring by passive diffusion of water through the epidermis (transepidermal water loss). Evaporative heat loss is nevertheless not important in term infants, except at delivery, when the skin is wet with amniotic fluid. Mature infants have the ability to increase evaporative heat loss in response to a warm environment by sweating.

Preterm infants, however, have high evaporative heat losses. Their insensible water loss is high compared with term infants, particularly in the most immature in the early neonatal period.[31,82,111] This is the result of a high TEWL, which is up to six times higher per unit surface area in a newborn infant of 26 weeks' gestation than in a term infant (Fig. 18.2).[42,44,86] The high TEWL occurs because the immature infant's skin has a thin, poorly keratinized stratum corneum which offers little resistance to the diffusion of water. Postnatal existence rapidly hastens the development of an effective epidermal barrier, so that by about 2 weeks of age even the most immature infant has a TEWL comparable to that of a term infant. The high TEWL of preterm infants is further increased

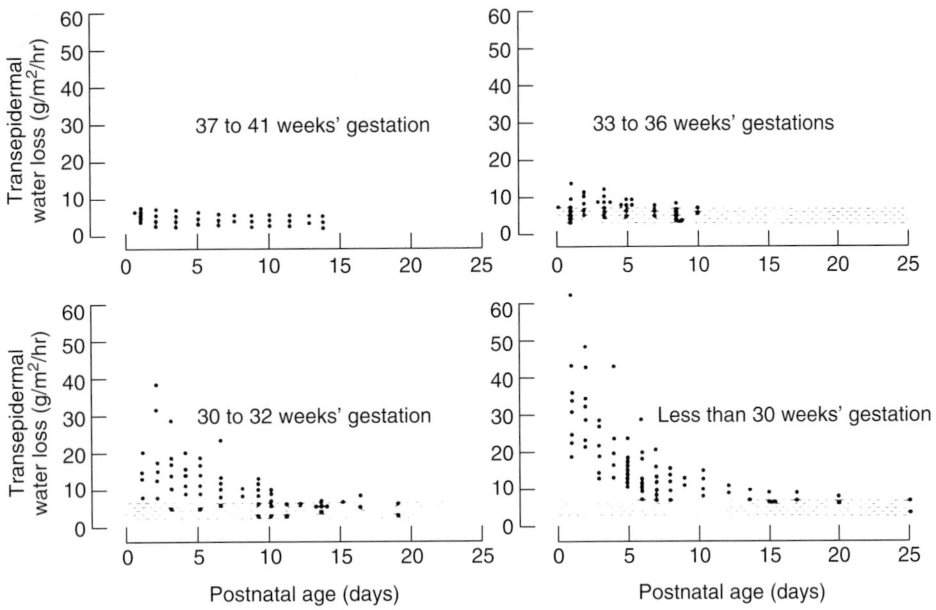

Fig. 18.2 Transepidermal water loss from the abdomen of newborn infants showing the separate influences of gestation and postnatal age. The shaded area is the range of water loss in term infants for comparison. (From data of Harpin & Rutter 1983[46])

by skin damage caused by monitoring probes or electrodes.[46]

Evaporative heat loss is increased in the newborn by exposure to radiant energy. Use of a radiant warmer increases evaporative heat loss by a factor of about 0.5–2.0[110,111] and phototherapy by 0.4–2.0.[80,111] The two together have an additive effect.[12] This increase is probably indirect and can be mainly explained by the higher surface temperatures, greater air speeds and lower local humidity when infants are exposed to radiant energy, as these three physical factors all increase evaporative heat loss. When these factors are allowed for, radiant warmers[65] and phototherapy[64] have little direct effect in increasing TEWL.

The high evaporative heat losses of infants of less than 30 weeks' gestation in the first week or so of life make their clinical management difficult. If nursed in dry incubators they readily become hypothermic, and if nursed under radiant warmers difficulties in management of fluid balance arise. Reduction of this high evaporative loss is necessary and can be achieved in a number of ways:

- By increasing the ambient humidity. Evaporative heat loss decreases linearly as humidity rises (Fig. 18.3), so that losses at high humidity are very low.[42,53,103]
- By protecting the infant from draughts. For example, an incubator with low air speeds can be used,[81,113] or the infant can be nursed under a perspex heat shield which is closed at one end.[31]
- By attempting to waterproof the infant. Plastic bubble blankets or clear plastic film draped over the preterm infant will reduce insensible water loss by 75%.[72] Topical application of soft paraffin grease may reduce TEWL in preterm infants by 50%.[87] A similar reduction in TEWL can be achieved by using a semipermeable polyurethane membrane as an artificial skin.[67,105]

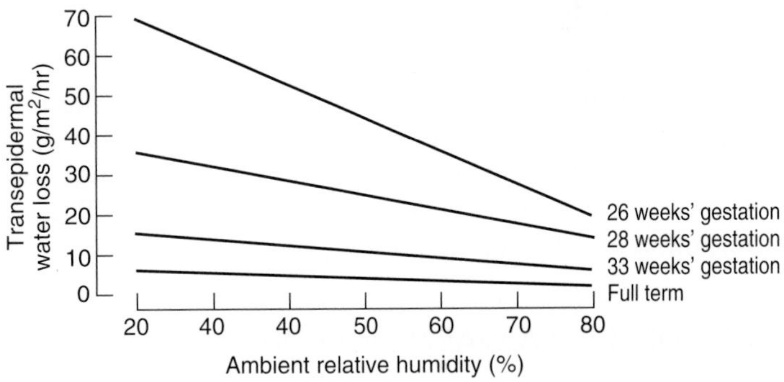

Fig. 18.3 The effect of ambient relative humidity on transepidermal water loss. It is most marked in the immature infant with a very high water loss. (Derived from data of Hammarlund and Sedin 1979[42])

RESPONSE TO A COLD ENVIRONMENT

As the environmental temperature falls the newborn infant makes physiological and behavioural responses in order to maintain a constant deep-body temperature. These responses are initiated by hypothalamic and cutaneous temperature receptors.

Physiological

The infant can increase heat production in response to cold stress without any increase in physical activity (shivering does not occur in the newborn). Non-shivering thermogenesis results from the metabolic activity of a specialized organ of heat production, brown adipose tissue.[58] This distinctive fat is found superficially (especially between the scapulae) and deep within the body (especially along the aorta) of the newborn infant. In response to cold, catecholamines are released which act directly on brown adipose tissue, stimulating oxidative phosphorylation and releasing energy as heat. A newborn infant can more than double his rate of heat production in this way.[49] Non-shivering thermogenesis is impaired in all newborn infants in the first 12 hours,[94] in ill infants especially following asphyxia or with hypoxia,[21,92] and after maternal sedative administration, especially diazepam.[25] Peripheral vasoconstriction also occurs in response to cold, diverting blood from the infant's surface to the core. This is well developed in term infants but limited in very immature infants in the immediate neonatal period.[23]

Behavioural

Whereas a child or adult will wake up and become restless when cold, the newborn infant may continue to sleep. Cold infants, however, do tend to be more active, sleep less and adopt a flexed posture in an attempt to increase heat production and decrease heat loss. These responses are also seen in preterm infants.

RESPONSE TO A WARM ENVIRONMENT

As the environmental temperature rises, the newborn infant attempts to prevent a rise in body temperature.

Physiological

Sweating in response to a warm environment occurs in term infants from birth.[45] The amount of water lost by sweating per unit area of skin is considerably lower than that lost by a heat-acclimatized adult, although the density of sweat glands is greater in the newborn. The amount of sweat which each gland can produce is therefore much lower in the newborn than the adult.[33] Sweating in the newborn is most marked on the forehead, temple and occiput, but occurs everywhere except the palms and the soles (which only sweat in response to emotional stress). It provides some measure of defence against overheating. In congenital anhidrotic ectodermal dysplasia, in which sweating is absent, the newborn infant is particularly susceptible to heat stress. Sweating is absent in infants below 36 weeks' gestation at birth but usually appears by about 2 weeks of age.[45,53] It occurs at fewer sites and is less marked than in term infants, providing poor defence against overheating. Infants born to mothers who have abused opiates during pregnancy have a well developed ability to sweat, even if born prematurely.

Vasodilatation in response to heat occurs in term and preterm infants, so that the skin of an overheated infant is warm and red.[48]

Behavioural

As the environmental temperature increases newborn infants become less active, sleep more and lie in an extended, sunbathing posture. Preterm infants also make these responses.[48,85]

BODY TEMPERATURE AND THERMAL NEUTRALITY

There is a zone of environmental temperature within which an infant's heat production is at a minimum, the body temperature is normal and there is no sweating. Fine thermoregulation is maintained by changes in skin blood flow, posture and activity.[51] This is termed the thermoneutral range (Fig. 18.4).

Infants are best nursed at an environmental temperature close to this range, probably around the lower end, since this is more comfortable for children and adults.[50]

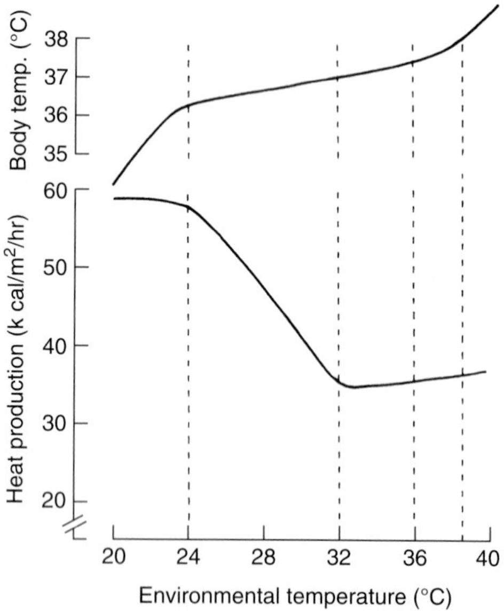

Fig. 18.4 The effect of environmental temperature on heat production and body temperature of a 1.9 kg infant of 34 weeks' gestation, nursed naked in surroundings of uniform temperature and moderate humidity. Between 32 and 36°C heat production is minimal, there is no sweating and body temperature is normal (neutral thermal range). When the environmental temperature exceeds 36°C the infant sweats, and above 38°C the body temperature rises rapidly. Below 32°C heat production increases by non-shivering thermogenesis, but below 24°C heat production has reached its maximum and body temperature rapidly falls.

The width and the absolute values of this neutral thermal range depend on the infant's resting heat production and insulation. In the term infant nursed naked, the range is wider and lower than in the preterm infant who has a low metabolic rate and poor tissue insulation because of lack of subcutaneous fat. Clothing and wrapping infants greatly widens and lowers the neutral thermal range.[55] Thus for a term infant in the first week the range is about 32–33.5°C when nursed naked, and 24–27°C when clothed. For a preterm infant of 30 weeks' gestation weighing 1.5 kg, the range is about 34–35°C when nursed naked and 28–30°C when clothed.

Body temperature falls substantially when an infant can no longer increase heat production in response to a cool environment, and it rises when sweating is insufficient as a means of heat loss. Between these extremes, a normal body temperature is maintained. Clearly a baby with a normal body temperature can be sweating or be markedly cold stressed, so that body temperature is an insensitive guide to the suitability of the thermal environment. Doctors and nurses commonly assume that if an infant has a normal body temperature the ambient temperature conditions must be satisfactory. In doing so they fail to distinguish between being cold and feeling cold. A careful observer can recognize that an infant is feeling cold before he actually becomes cold, by assessing his posture, activity, skin colour and peripheral skin temperature. However, the very low-birthweight infant is an exception. An infant of less than 1 kg has such a low heat production per surface area, limited metabolic response to cold and poor tissue insulation that he appears to be poikilothermic (i.e. his body temperature drifts up and down with the ambient temperature). Measurement of body temperature in such a baby is a convenient and reliable guide to the suitability of the thermal environment.

MEASUREMENT OF TEMPERATURE

Some measurement of core or surface temperature is useful in the newborn as a guide to the suitability of the thermal environment and in the detection of illness. The relative insensitivity of body temperature as a guide to the thermal environment of the mature neonate has been mentioned, but it is useful in very low-birthweight infants in the early neonatal period when they behave as if they were poikilothermic. In larger healthy infants considerable thermal stress is needed to raise or lower body temperature outside the normal range. Surface temperature measurements change readily, but normal values are less well defined and the measuring devices themselves alter temperature, so that a composite measurement influenced by both environmental and skin temperature is recorded.

Mayfield et al[77] have shown that in both term and preterm infants measurements of rectal, axillary and between skin and mattress temperatures all correlate well with core temperature as recorded by an electronic thermometer inserted 5 cm beyond the anus. In particular, they showed a close correlation between axillary and rectal temperature measurements when measured with the usual mercury-in-glass thermometer.

RECTAL TEMPERATURE

This can be measured using a flexible thermocouple or thermistor inserted 5 cm from the anal margin. There is little increase in temperature if the probe is inserted more deeply, but there is a considerable gradient in the first 5 cm,[23] most of which occurs in the first 3 cm. A flexible probe can be left in situ for continuous monitoring but is easily pushed out by the straining infant. The mercury-in-glass thermometer is commonly used: it should be lubricated with soft paraffin and inserted in a downwards and backwards direction (at an angle of 30° to the horizontal) to a depth of 3 cm from the anal margin (2 cm in a preterm infant).[114] Shallower insertion gives a falsely low recording because blood from the surface of the legs may return via venous plexuses around the anus. Most equilibration has occurred by a minute after insertion. The dangers of using a glass thermometer for rectal temperature measurement are haemorrhage and perforation of the rectum,[32,34,41,95] which are particularly likely to occur if the infant is struggling. Rectal temperature measurement is contraindicated if there is bowel disease, especially necrotizing enterocolitis.

Because of the small risk associated with rectal temperature measurement its routine use is becoming less common and axillary measurements are preferred. This is the current recommendation of the American Academy of Pediatrics. However, a single rectal temperature measurement in all newborn infants soon after delivery is an effective method for the early detection of imperforate anus. The normal range in infants is 36.5–37.5°C regardless of weight or gestation.

AXILLARY TEMPERATURE

This is measured using a mercury-in-glass thermometer, with the bulb placed firmly in the roof of the axilla and the infant's upper arm held tightly against the side of the chest wall. Equilibration takes longer (substantial changes in the measured temperature occur for up to 3 minutes) but it is safe. The normal range in infants of all weights and gestation is 35.6–37.3°C. On average it is about 0.5°C lower than rectal temperature, but the difference in an individual infant is unpredictable.

SKIN TEMPERATURE

A thermocouple or thermistor lightly taped to the infant's skin can be left there for repeated or continuous measurements. The upper abdomen is a convenient site, as changes with environmental temperature are not as great as at a peripheral site and the skin is conveniently flat. The normal range depends on the tissue insulation and therefore on the infant's size. In term infants the range is 35.5–36.5°C, in a preterm infant 36.2–37.2°C. The infant below 1 kg birthweight has an abdominal skin temperature which is very close to the rectal or axillary temperature.

If an electronic thermometer is placed between the infant's back and the underlying mattress and then allowed to equilibrate, the final measured temperature is similar to core, rectal or axillary measurements.[77]

PRACTICAL MANAGEMENT OF THE THERMAL ENVIRONMENT

AT DELIVERY

The rectal temperature of the newborn infant at delivery averages 37.8°C (range 37–39°C), about 1°C higher than the maternal temperature.[70] The placenta is an efficient heat exchanger in pregnancy, removing the heat produced by the fetus, but this is impaired during labour. The infant's body temperature falls immediately after delivery and can easily reach subnormal levels if steps are not taken to conserve heat. Heat losses in a newly born baby are very high.[43] Most delivery rooms and operating theatres have ambient air temperatures which are comfortable for clothed adults but cold for exposed infants. Heat losses by convection and radiation are high, and evaporative heat losses from the wet skin far exceed the infant's metabolic heat production. Furthermore, the ability of the infant to increase his metabolic rate immediately after birth is impaired,[94] particularly in the presence of birth asphyxia or maternal sedation. As ever, the very low-birthweight infant is at greater risk of cold stress because of his unfavourable weight to surface area ratio. The body temperature of an exposed 1 kg infant can fall at the rate of 1°C every 5 minutes.

There is no evidence that a marked fall in body temperature is an advantage to the infant. Indeed, there is good reason to believe that it is harmful. Preterm infants who become cold at delivery have a greater chance of dying, particularly of hyaline membrane disease.[96,97] Cold stress is associated with acidosis and hypoxia,[35] factors which impair surfactant production in the preterm newborn. It is difficult to examine the effects of cold itself in the preterm infant separately from birth asphyxia, hypoxia and the need for resuscitation, which in turn cause a fall in body temperature. However, the poor outcome of preterm infants who become cold after delivery justifies strenuous efforts to keep them warm. By contrast, the healthy term infant is less susceptible to cold stress at delivery and more resistant to the effects. Acidosis and hypoxia may occur, but transient grunting is the usual clinical effect. With care, this can be prevented without separating mother and infant.

The ideal temperature of a delivery room (or operating theatre, in cases of operative delivery) is about 25°C, not too hot for the mother and her attendants and not too cold for the infant. Draughts should be kept to a minimum at the moment of delivery. The infant should be dried at once with a warm dry towel and then given to the mother. Direct physical contact between the mother and the infant is a mode of thermoregulation much used in the animal world and is most effective when there are no intervening clothes or blankets. Unless the room temperature is in excess of 25°C or there is supplementary heating from a radiant source, the exposed parts of the infant should be dry and covered. Weighing, cleaning, bathing, care of the umbilical cord and the fixing of namebands not only interrupt contact between the mother and her infant, but cause cold stress and are best postponed.[94] If resuscitation is necessary this should be carried out after the infant has been dried. Supplementary heat is essential during resuscitation and can conveniently be provided by placing a fixed-output radiant heat source of about 400 W about 60 cm above the infant. The exposed trunk and legs of an infant born by breech delivery should be dried and wrapped before the head is delivered.

The delivery room or operating theatre is always too cold for a very low-birthweight infant. The infant should be thoroughly dried, wrapped, resuscitated and removed to a warmer environment as soon as possible.

NURSING CARE OF THE NEWBORN INFANT

A newborn infant when dressed, wrapped up, placed in a cot and nursed in a warm room is in a neutral thermal environment (see above). Heat production is at its minimum and energy intake is therefore available for growth. Mothers prefer to see their infant dressed rather than naked, and the clothed newborn seems more contented and less restless. A naked infant is poorly insulated and heat losses are high even in a warm room. Clothing a naked infant more than doubles the insulation, and bedding (a sheet and two blankets) further increases it, so that the resistance to heat loss of a clothed, wrapped infant is three times greater than that of a naked one (Table 18.2).[52,56] The head is a large part of the total surface area of the newborn infant and has a higher surface temperature because of the brain's high rate of metabolism. A woollen bonnet is an effective method of increasing thermal insulation, and is especially useful in low-birthweight infants, who have relatively larger heads and whose trunk may need to be exposed.[99]

The following recommendations are made for nursing healthy infants in the newborn period:[50]

- 2–2.5 kg: clothed, with bedding, in a room temperature of about 24°C;

Table 18.2 Resistance to heat loss (insulation) in an infant weighing 2.5 kg lying on a foam mattress in a cool, draught-free room. Insulation is measured in clo units (1 clo unit = 0.155°C m² W⁻¹ or 0.18°C m² kcal⁻¹). (Reproduced with permission from Hey 1983[52])

Resistance due to	Completely naked	Wearing bonnet and wrapped in one sheet	Fully clothed under blankets in a cot
One flannelette sheet and two blankets around a clothed baby	–	–	0.61
One flannelette swaddling sheet around an unclothed baby	–	0.81	–
Thick gauze bonnet over head	–	0.22	0.22
Vest, napkin and long nightdress	–	–	1.25
Boundary layer of still air around the skin	0.78	0.78	0.78
Body tissues (when vasoconstricted)	0.29	0.29	0.29
Total resistance	1.07	2.10	3.15

- 1.5–2 kg: clothed, with a bonnet and bedding, in a room temperature of about 26°C;
- <1.5 kg: clothed, with a bonnet, in an incubator temperature of about 30–32°C.

Babies weighing more than about 1.80 kg are commonly nursed in an environment 1–2°C cooler than this. They will have a minor and clinically unimportant increase in oxygen consumption as a result. Large term infants who are wrapped and covered with a sheet and blanket have a wide neutral thermal range and can tolerate cooler environments with little increase in metabolic rate. A newborn infant should be nursed clothed, even in an incubator, unless he needs to be exposed for observation or access.

INCUBATOR CARE

An incubator provides an infant with a high ambient temperature but at the same time allows his attendants to work at a lower, more comfortable temperature. Most incubators work by forced convection: air is heated and then circulated by a fan within the canopy of the incubator at an air speed of about 20 cm/s. There are two means of controlling the heater output:

- Air mode. The air temperature is set to a desired level and a thermostat in the air flow maintains this temperature. The control is proportional, i.e. the heater output is proportional to the difference between the set temperature and the actual temperature. If the incubator air temperature is just below the set temperature the heater output will be low; if it is substantially below the set temperature the heater will be on full power. This means that fluctuations in air temperature due to cycling of the thermostat are very small (Fig. 18.5).
- Servo mode. The output of the heater is controlled by the baby's skin temperature, and is set to a desired level. A thermistor or thermocouple is taped to the skin, preferably the upper abdomen, and the heater cycles to keep the skin temperature at that site constant. In practice, air temperature fluctuations are greater in servo mode than air mode, especially when the infant is handled (Fig. 18.5).

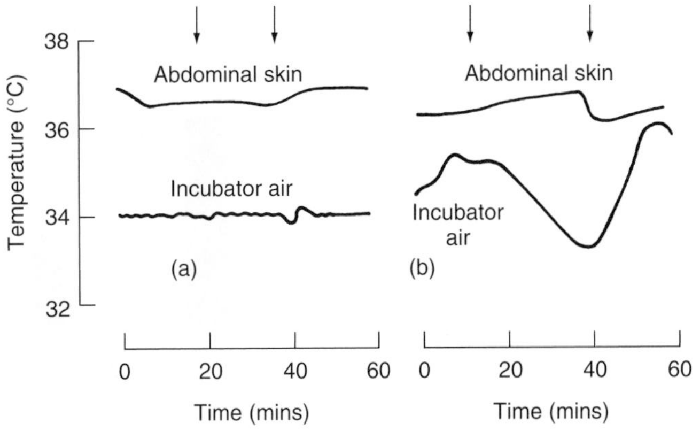

Fig. 18.5 Fluctuations in incubator air temperature when used (a) in air mode and (b) in servo mode. In air mode the set temperature (air) is 34°C and in servo mode the set temperature (skin) is 36.3°C. Handling for brief spells for routine nursing procedures is indicated (↓).

Air mode is probably satisfactory for nursing most newborn infants.[11] Servo mode has the disadvantages of wide fluctuations in air temperature,[30] particularly during nursing procedures, of providing an inappropriately low ambient temperature when the infant is febrile, and of lack of control when an infant with very high insensible water loss is nursed in a dry incubator.[9] The probe may also easily become detached, resulting in an inappropriate air temperature. A naked infant in an incubator loses heat predominantly by radiation, less by convection and evaporation (Fig. 18.6). Heat loss by radiation can be reduced by covering or clothing the baby (which is often impractical), or by placing a perspex heat shield over the baby, shielding him from the cooler inside walls of the incubator (which makes the baby less accessible). In practice, the radiant losses can be compensated for by using a higher air temperature setting. Some incubators have a double wall so that radiant losses are reduced.[74] Others use natural rather than forced convection, so that the air speed in the canopy is low (about 5 cm/s), reducing convective and evaporative heat loss.[81,113]

Incubators are useful for nursing small infants who can be clothed but need a very warm ambient temperature, and for naked or sick infants who need to be observed and who need intervention. They allow added oxygen

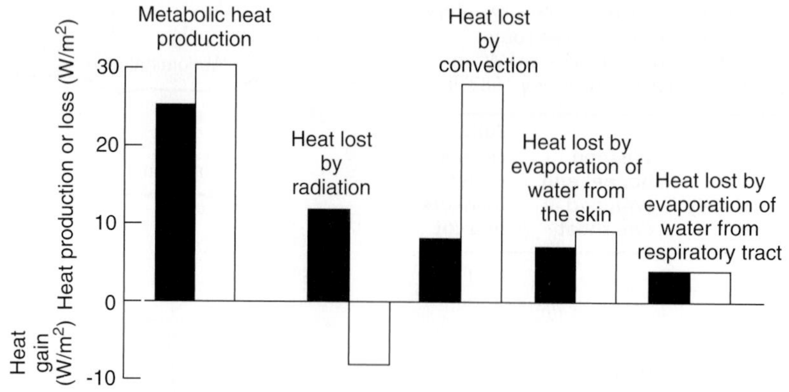

Fig. 18.6 Heat production, losses and gains of 11 preterm infants (mean birthweight 1.58 kg, gestation 32 weeks, age 7 days) nursed naked in an incubator (black bars) and under a radiant warmer (white bars) in presumed neutral thermal conditions. (Redrawn from Wheldon & Rutter 1982[109])

Table 18.3 Average incubator air temperatures needed to provide a suitable thermal environment for naked, healthy infants (From Hey 1975[51])

	Environmental temperature			
Birthweight (kg)	**35°C**	**34°C**	**33°C**	**32°C**
1.0–1.5	For 10 days	After 10 days	After 3 weeks	After 5 weeks
1.5–2.0		For 10 days	After 10 days	After 4 weeks
2.0–2.5		For 2 days	After 2 days	After 3 weeks
> 2.5			For 2 days	After 2 days

Note: a. In a single walled incubator the environmental temperature needs to be increased by 1°C for every 7°C difference between room and incubator temperature.
b. Very low birthweight infants (< 1 kg) need higher air temperatures and a humidified incubator in the first week.[91,108]
c. The values are averages but there is considerable individual variation.

and humidity to be given. Nursing and medical procedures disrupt the environmental temperature control, resulting in temperature instability.[79]

Temperature settings depend on whether the infant is clothed or naked, on the weight and the postnatal age. The values shown in Table 18.3 are those which have been estimated to provide an environmental temperature at the lower end of the neutral thermal range under conditions of low air speed (below 10 cm/s), moderate relative humidity (50%), and where the temperature of the inner wall is the same as the air temperature (i.e. when a radiant heat shield is being used or the incubator is double-walled).[51] When used in the servo mode the required set skin temperatures are the same as those recommended for infants nursed under radiant warmers (Table 18.4).

Table 18.4 Suggested abdominal skin temperature settings for infants nursed under radiant warmers or in servo-mode incubators

Weight (kg)	Abdominal skin temperature (°C)
< 1.0	36.9
1.0–1.5	36.7
1.5–2.0	36.5
2.0–2.5	36.3
> 2.5	36.0

There is a complex relationship between the water content of the air (absolute humidity), the water content of the air expressed as a percentage of the maximum possible water content (relative humidity), and air temperature. It has been well reviewed by Hey.[50] Room air at 20°C in the British Isles has a relative humidity of about 50%. In a warm neonatal intensive care unit at 30°C the same room air is only about 30% saturated, whereas in an unhumidified incubator at 37°C the relative humidity may be as low as 25%. An infant of less than 30 weeks' gestation, a day or so old, nursed in an unhumidified incubator, may have an evaporative heat loss that exceeds metabolic heat production (Fig. 18.7). The infant may therefore remain cold, even in an air temperature of 37°C. Humidification is an effective way of reducing this evaporative heat loss and maintaining a normal body temperature in such infants (Fig. 18.8). Its routine use is recommended in incubator-nursed infants below 30 weeks' gestation for the first week of life.[47] Modern incubator humidifiers are sophisticated devices with good humidity control: the maximum setting should be used, producing a relative humidity of 80–90% at the maximum air temperature. There is no simple, accurate method of measuring incubator humidity. Humidification itself is probably of no advantage to the more mature infant. The disadvantages of humidification are con-

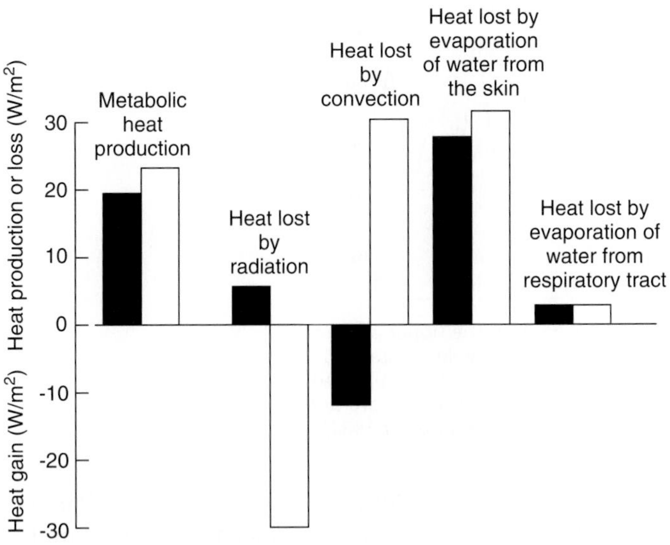

Fig. 18.7 Heat production, losses and gains of an infant of 28 weeks' gestation, birthweight 1.08 kg, on the 3rd day. When nursed naked in a dry incubator (black bars), air temperature 37.7°C, rectal temperature fell to 36.4°C. This is because her high skin evaporative heat loss exceeded the metabolic heat production. When nursed under a radiant warmer (white bars), set to provide a skin temperature of 36.8°C, rectal temperature rapidly rose to 36.8°C because of the high radiant heat gain. (Redrawn from Wheldon & Rutter 1982[109])

densation of moisture on the inner wall of the incubator and infection. The condensation can be reduced by using a high room temperature or a double-walled incubator. Infection is a possibility which has perhaps been exaggerated. *Pseudomonas* spp. flourish in a damp setting but the organism is rarely found in the incubator humidification system if this is regularly drained and refilled with sterile water. Alternative methods of reducing high evaporative heat losses, such as plastic covering or paraffin grease, are less effective (see earlier).

Incubators are generally safe devices. Overheating of the infant is rare unless the incubator is subjected to an additional source of heat such as direct sunlight. Cold stress is more common than heat stress. The perspex canopy provides a welcome barrier between the ill infant and his attendant, except when access is necessary for practical procedures, but parents often dislike this barrier and are relieved when their infant is transferred to a cot.

CARE UNDER RADIANT WARMERS

This is an alternative device for nursing naked infants who are either sick or small and need to be observed closely. The infant lies on an open cradle over which is suspended a heat source emitting radiant energy in the frequency spectrum 700–300 000 nm. The heater is placed approximately 90 cm from the infant's surface and the maximum output does not usually exceed 500 W/m^2, being controlled in a proportional way by the infant's skin temperature. A thermistor is lightly taped to the upper abdomen and the desired temperature selected. The

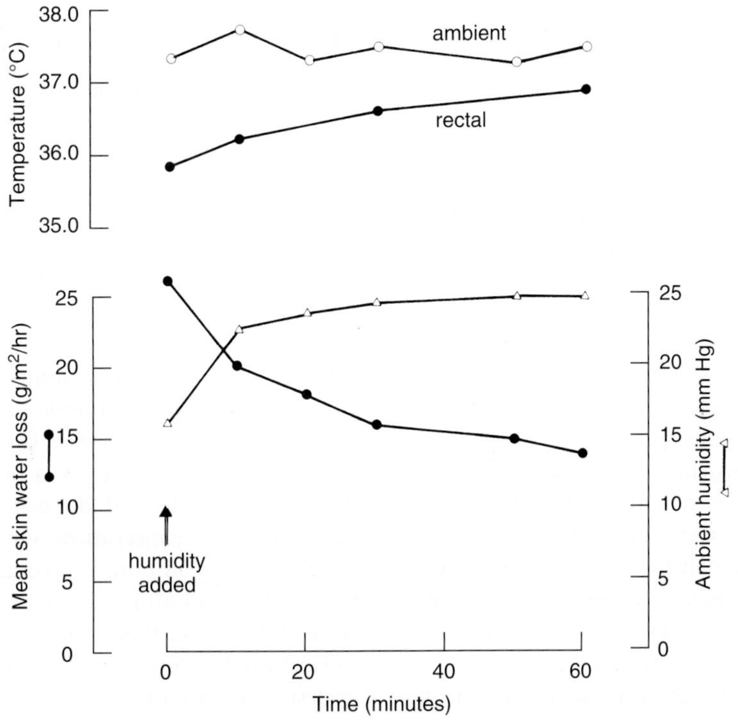

Fig. 18.8 The effect of humidifying an incubator. The baby (30 weeks' gestation, 1 day old) has a rectal temperature of 35.8°C in spite of an incubator temperature of 37.3°C. When humidity is added, skin water loss falls and the rectal temperature steadily increases to 37.0°C

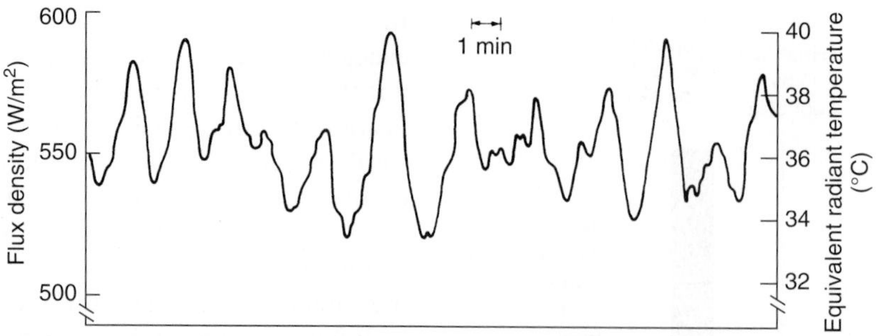

Fig. 18.9 Typical recording of radiant flux density incident on the upper abdomen of an infant nursed under a radiant warmer. The infant is 32 weeks' gestation, birthweight 1.42 kg, age 9 days: the room temperature is 28.5°C. The estimated mean radiant temperature is shown on the right-hand axis. Fluctuations are due to cycling of the servo-control system. (Redrawn from Wheldon & Rutter 1982[109])

recommended set temperatures depend on the infant's size (see Table 18.4). Fixed-output low-power heaters are only suitable for keeping infants warm during brief procedures such as resuscitation.

The thermal environment is obviously different from that provided by an incubator.[6,109] The infant is exposed to cool, dry, draughty air and a markedly fluctuating radiant heat source (Fig. 18.9). Heat loss by convection is therefore high, but heat is gained by radiation (see Fig. 18.6). Several studies have shown that infants nursed under radiant warmers have higher resting levels of oxygen consumption than those nursed in incubators:[68,73,75,109] the increase is about 10–20%. Evaporative heat loss is consistently higher in infants nursed under radiant warmers[12,60,110,111] and is due to an increase in water loss from the skin rather than the respiratory tract.[109] This increase, compared with incubator-nursed infants, varies from 25 to 150%, although problems of measuring insensible water loss may partly account for the higher values.[27] Surface temperature distribution is more uneven in infants nursed under radiant warmers: the peripheries are cooler than in infants nursed in incubators with the same mean skin temperature. Cardiovascular changes have been noted in preterm infants nursed under radiant warmers compared with incubators. Skin and limb blood flow is increased by 50% and there is a small (5%) increase in cardiac output caused by an increase in heart rate.[107] Radiant warmers therefore produce a fluctuating, asymmetrical thermal environment compared to the constant even temperature provided by an incubator.

No study has shown that either method is superior to the other in terms of the mortality, morbidity and growth of infants nursed in them. Radiant warmers are, however, potentially more dangerous than incubators. Overheating from probe detachment or interference can occur quickly: it is important, therefore, that the infant's surface or deep-body temperature is monitored frequently by means of an independent thermometer. The increased evaporative water loss may result in hypernatraemic dehydration[60] or, if overenthusiastically replaced, in an increased incidence of patent ductus arteriosus.[13] The infant's fluid intake needs to be carefully assessed (Chapter 39, Part 1). Insensible water loss can be reduced in infants under radiant warmers by covering them with a rigid perspex box.[14,112] This impairs the radiant heat exchange between infant and warmer, producing an indeterminate thermal environment which is a hybrid of a warmer and an incubator. A more acceptable measure is to cover the infant in a clear plastic film.[7,8] This results in a lower oxygen consumption and less demand for radiant heat.[5]

The advantages of using a radiant warmer are threefold: it is the most effective way of keeping a very small baby warm (see Fig. 18.7); it is the most effective way of warming cold infants; and it allows the parents and the staff easy access to the baby.

THE HEATED WATER-FILLED MATTRESS

This was developed because of the need to provide an alternative method of keeping small babies warm which is suitable for use in developing countries. Compared to the incubator or radiant warmer it is cheap, simple, readily acceptable to mothers and infants, and is not dependent on a continuous supply of electricity. The mattress is a polyvinyl bag filled with 10 litres of water and heated by a foil pad. This has a high thermal capacity and will therefore continue to provide warmth after the power source is interrupted. The water temperature is thermostatically controlled and can be regulated from 35 to 38°C. Sarman and Tunell[89] have shown that preterm infants can be safely nursed in a cot on a heated water-filled mattress if they are stable and do not have to be undressed for observation. Temperature control, metabolic rate and weight gain compared favourably with similar infants nursed in incubators. They also showed that the heated water-filled mattress is an excellent method for rewarming hypothermic preterm intants, being safer than and superior to an incubator.[90] Greenabate et al[40] found that preterm infants nursed on a water-filled mattress suffered less cold stress and grew better than those nursed in a space-heated room, but incubator nursing was superior to either.

THERMAL ENVIRONMENT DURING TRANSPORT

Transporting a small sick infant from one hospital to another for intensive care is a considerable challenge. Such infants are often cold to start with, their heat losses are great and their heat production is small. Furthermore, the environmental temperature during transport may be very low, sometimes below 0°C. The transport incubators which are used to keep babies warm during transit are generally less satisfactory in terms of performance than nursing incubators. The essentials of keeping a small sick infant warm during transport are as follows:

- To reduce the enormous radiant heat losses which occur if the infant is nursed naked. This can be achieved by covering the infant with a sheet, a blanket or a silver swaddler – this must not be too thick or else the already cold infant will still be insulated from the warm air of the incubator. The silver swaddler protects an infant against heat loss by radiation and convection, but no more so than an ordinary blanket.
- To reduce the high evaporative heat loss. The infant should be covered in a plastic film or bubble blanket after he has been thoroughly dried.
- To observe the infant by remote means. Heart rate, respiratory rate, temperature and transcutaneous oxygen tension or saturation can be measured without touching the infant.
- To maintain a high air temperature. In infants of 1 kg or below, the required air temperature will be close to 37°C.

A portable incubator with double walls or a radiant heat source in the wall will substantially reduce an infant's heat loss in very cold environments. Added humidity greatly assists maintenance of a normal body temperature in the very immature infant.

SURGERY

The newborn infant undergoing surgery is at particular risk of cold stress. The operating theatre air and wall temperatures are often low and the room is draughty. The baby is usually starved and drugged, so that his response to cold stress is blunted. Furthermore, exposed organs lose water and therefore heat by evaporation.

Cold stress can be minimized by the following measures:

- The air temperature in the theatre should be raised to 28–30°C.
- The infant should be well insulated before being taken to theatre. This is effectively achieved by wrapping the limbs, trunk and scalp with cotton-wool lagging.
- The area of the infant exposed for surgery should be kept to a minimum.
- Some supplementary source of heat should be provided: an electric warming pad below, or a radiant heater above the infant can be used.

DISORDERS OF TEMPERATURE CONTROL

THE INFANT WITH A LOW BODY TEMPERATURE (BELOW 36°C RECTAL)

Mild degrees of hypothermia are common, particularly following delivery. More severe hypothermia (below 34°C rectal) is less common and usually due to overwhelming cold stress. In hospital it is typically seen in small, sick preterm infants in the early neonatal period, when they are nursed in incubators and handled frequently. The use of a radiant warmer avoids this early hypothermia. Outside hospital, accidental hypothermia is liable to occur when an infant is born unexpectedly or when the birth is concealed. Hypothermia may occur in the first few weeks of life, particularly if the infant is nursed in an unheated room and the outside temperature drops below freezing on a cold winter night.[1,17,71] Infection (particularly pneumonia and septicaemia), serious congenital abnormality (particularly cyanotic heart disease or severe cardiac failure) and low birthweight are predisposing factors. Malnutrition also predisposes to hypothermia by reducing tissue insulation and the metabolic response to cold.[18,104] Intentional hypothermia is successfully used with cardiopulmonary bypass in infant cardiac surgery, body temperature being lowered by surface cooling to about 28°C.

Infants with moderate or severe hypothermia are lethargic, feed poorly, have a weak cry and reduced movements. Peripheral oedema is common and areas of sclerema may occur in severe cases. Marked facial erythema may give a false impression of a healthy infant, but the skin always feels strikingly cold. The diagnosis will be made when the rectal temperature is measured with a low-reading thermometer, but will be missed if the usual clinical thermometer with a minimum reading of 35°C is used. In very severe cases (rectal temperature below 28°C) the infant may appear virtually dead, with profound cardiorespiratory depression. There are anecdotal reports of such infants being left for dead but eventually making a full recovery.

There is limited information available about the safest and most effective method of rewarming cold infants. Very slow rewarming over several days has been advocated, particularly in infants with chronic cold exposure who have developed cold injury. Increasingly, though, it appears that it is safe to rewarm cold infants more rapidly, at a rate of 1–2°C/h. In an incubator this can be achieved using the maximum air temperature setting, or by setting the air temperature to a level which is 1–2°C higher than body temperature, and increasing it in a stepwise fashion until the infant is warm. Radiant warmers have been effectively used to treat hypothermic infants. Kaplan and Eidelman[61] rewarmed 16 severely hypothermic infants over 4 hours by radiant warmer, using a set skin temperature of 37°C. Sarman et al[90] found that a heated water-filled mattress was superior to an incubator in rewarming 53 hypothermic preterm infants admitted to an Istanbul hospital.

Complications may occur during rewarming. If rapid rewarming of the infant's surface diverts blood from the core, hypotension can result. It has been suggested that use of a plasma expander during rewarming may improve survival.[102] Hypoglycaemia should be looked for and prevented by a slow intravenous infusion of 10% dextrose. Care should be taken in interpreting blood gas results, as pH is temperature dependent,[24] rising by 0.016 pH unit for every 1°C fall in temperature, so that blood with a pH of 6.94 at 37°C will have a pH of 7.10 at 27°C. Because pH is always measured at 37°C it is easy to overestimate and therefore overtreat a metabolic acidosis in a hypothermic infant. Abdominal distension is common and necrotizing enterocolitis may occur. Feeding should not start until a normal body temperature has been achieved. Haemorrhagic pulmonary oedema is a sinister sign and a common autopsy finding in infants who die from hypothermia. The reported mortality rate in severe hypothermia is 20–50%, but this includes infants with congenital abnormalities or serious infection which contributed to the hypothermia. Most survivors develop normally.

If the cause of the hypothermia is obvious, as for example in a small baby born unattended at home or an infant abandoned in the cold, further investigation is not necessary as a routine. If, however, a young baby is admitted to hospital and found to be hypothermic, with a recent history of being unwell, then an infective cause should be looked for. A full infection screen, including a chest X-ray and a lumbar puncture, will be necessary. Respiratory syncytial virus infection, especially pneumonia or bronchiolitis, is particularly associated with hypothermia in very young infants. If accidental cold exposure and infection have been eliminated as the cause of hypothermia, thyroid function should be measured in case the infant has hypothyroidism.

THE INFANT WITH A RAISED BODY TEMPERATURE (ABOVE 38°C RECTAL)

There are two explanations for a raised body temperature: the infant may have an increased set-point temperature, or he may be overheated. In a study of a large number of term infants a raised body temperature was found in 1% in the early neonatal period.[106] Of these, 10% had a bacterial infection and 90% were overheated. Infants with a raised set-point temperature behave as if they are cold. Heat production is increased, probably by non-shivering thermogenesis, and heat loss is reduced by cutaneous vasoconstriction.[76] An increase in set-point temperature is a common finding in an infected newborn, although this is a less reliable and less marked sign than in older infants and children with infection. Of 371 infants aged up to 30 days, the rates of serious bacterial infection were 4.4% for those with a rectal temperature of 38.1–39°C, 7.6% for the range 39.1–39.9°C and 18% above 39.9°C, but only 6% of febrile infants had a temperature in the latter range.[16] An increased set-point temperature is also seen in infants with a serious congenital abnormality of the brain, especially hydranencephaly, encephalocoele, holoprosencephaly and trisomy 13, and following severe birth asphyxia, where it is a poor prognostic sign. Such infants have an instability of thermoregulation as a result of hypothalamic damage.[26]

Overheating is the commonest cause of a raised temperature and almost always the cause of hyperpyrexia (above 41°C rectal). It is common in restless, active infants and in overwrapped babies left in a warm room. It is also seen in an infant born to a pyrexial mother, regardless of whether the infant is infected. Hyperpyrexia is rare in the newborn and usually results from mechanical or electrical failure of a warming device. An incubator in direct sunlight behaves like a greenhouse: short-wave radiation passes directly through the perspex canopy and long-wave radiation heats the perspex, which in turn radiates to the infant. Serious overheating may occur if the servo probe becomes detached from an infant under a powerful radiant warmer. In early infancy overheating occurs with excessive wrapping, during heatwaves and when infants are left in closed cars exposed to sunlight. A mild fever of abrupt onset and short duration on the 3rd or 4th day of life is described in babies who are otherwise well and show no signs of infection. It tends to correspond with the nadir of the usual early neonatal weight loss, and as the latter is the result of extracellular fluid loss it is sometimes referred to as dehydration fever.

Mild overheating is not dangerous. It may be associated with an increase in the incidence of apnoeic spells in preterm infants,[10,83] although this is perhaps overemphasized. An increased set-point temperature is possibly beneficial to an infant with an infection.[66] However, hyperpyrexia from overheating is dangerous. Shock, protracted fits, diarrhoea, disseminated intravascular coagulation and renal and hepatic failure occur in overheated infants,[4] but the few who have appeared to die from overheating in the newborn period have done so suddenly, without prior symptoms. It is interesting that sudden death in infancy has been linked with overheating,[98] and that it is described in families with a history of malignant hyperpyrexia[29] and anhidrotic ectodermal dysplasia.[15]

The distinction between an overheated baby and one with an increased set-point temperature is important.[48,84] The overheated baby needs a cooler environment, not a series of painful investigations to find an infective cause for the 'fever'. There are several important differences (Table 18.5). A history of symptoms of infection and an

Table 18.5 Differences between a healthy infant who is overheated and a febrile infant with a raised set-point

Overheated infant	Febrile infant
High rectal temperature	High rectal temperature
Warm hands and feet	Cool hands and feet
Abdominal exceeds hand skin temperature by less than 2°C	Abdominal exceeds hand skin temperature by more than 3°C
Pink skin	Pale skin
Extended posture	Lethargic
Healthy appearance	Looks unwell

immediate assessment of the thermal environment are important. A useful physical sign is the degree of difference in skin temperature between the abdomen and the hand: the abdomen is always warmer than the hand; in the overheated infant the difference is less than 2°C (often less than 1°C), but in the infected infant it usually exceeds 3.5°C. The same applies to the difference between the rectal temperature and the sole temperature.[78]

REFERENCES

1. Arneil G C, Kerr M M 1963 Severe hypothermia in Glasgow infants in winter. Lancet ii: 756–759
2. Auliciems A 1972 Classroom performance as a function of thermal comfort. International Journal of Biometerology 16: 233–246
3. Auliciems A 1972 Some observed relationships between the atmospheric environment and mental work. Environmental Research 5: 217–240
4. Bacon C, Scott D, Jones P 1979 Heat stroke in well-wrapped infants. Lancet i: 422–425
5. Baumgart S 1984 Reduction of oxygen consumption, insensible water loss and radiant heat demand with use of a plastic blanket for low birthweight infants under radiant warmers. Journal of Pediatrics 100: 787–790
6. Baumgart S 1985 Partitioning of heat losses and gains in premature newborn infants under radiant warmers. Pediatrics 75: 89–99
7. Baumgart S, Fox W W, Polin R A 1982 Physiologic implications of two different heat shields for infants under radiant warmers. Journal of Pediatrics 100: 787–790
8. Baumgart S, Engle W D, Fox W W, Polin R A 1981 Effect of heat shielding on convective and evaporative heat losses and on radiant heat transfer in the premature infant. Journal of Pediatrics 99: 948–956
9. Belgaumkar T K, Scott K E 1975 Effects of low humidity on small premature infants in servocontrol incubators. I. Decrease in rectal temperature. Biology of the Neonate 26: 337–347
10. Belgaumkar T K, Scott K E 1975 Effects of low humidity on small premature infants in servocontrol incubators. II. Increased severity of apnoea. Biology of the Neonate 26: 348–352
11. Bell E F, Rios G R 1983 Air versus skin temperature servocontrol of infant incubators. Journal of Pediatrics 103: 954–959
12. Bell E F, Neidrich G A, Cashore W J, Oh W 1979 Combined effect of radiant warmer and phototherapy on insensible water loss in low birthweight infants. Journal of Pediatrics 94: 810–813
13. Bell E F, Warburton D, Stonestreet B S, Oh W 1980 Effect of fluid administration on the development of symptomatic patent ductus arteriosus and congestive heart failure in premature infants. New England Journal of Medicine 302: 598–604
14. Bell E F, Weinstein M R, Oh W 1980 Heat balance in premature infants: comparative effect of convectively incubated and radiant warmer, with and without plastic heat shield. Journal of Pediatrics 96: 460–465
15. Bernstein R, Hatchuel I, Jenkins T 1980 Hypohidrotic ectodermal dysplasia and sudden infant death syndrome. Lancet ii: 1024
16. Bonadio W A, Romine K, Gyuro J 1990 Relationship of fever magnitude to rate of serious bacterial infections in neonates. Journal of Pediatrics 116: 733–735
17. Bower B D, Jones L F, Weeks M N 1960 Cold injury in the newborn. British Medical Journal i: 303–309
18. Brooke O G 1972 Hypothermia in malnourished Jamaican children. Archives of Disease in Childhood 47: 525–530
19. Brooke O G 1980 Energy balance and metabolic rate in preterm infants fed with standard and high-energy formulas. British Journal of Nutrition 44: 13–23
20. Brooke O G, Ashworth A 1972 The influence of malnutrition on the postprandial metabolic rate and respiratory quotient. British Journal of Nutrition 27: 404–415
21. Bruck K, Adams F H, Bruck M 1962 Temperature regulation in infants with chronic hypoxemia. Pediatrics 30: 350–360
22. Buetow K C, Klein S W 1964 Effects of maintenance of 'normal' skin temperature on survival of infants of low birth weight. Pediatrics 34: 163–170
23. Chellapah G 1980 Aspects of thermoregulation in term and preterm newborn babies. PhD Thesis, University of Nottingham
24. Cohen J J, Kassirer J P 1982 Acid–base. Little Brown, Boston, pp 396–397, 466–469
25. Cree J E, Meyer J, Hailey D M 1973 Diazepam in labour: its metabolism and effect on the clinical condition and thermogenesis of the newborn. British Medical Journal iv: 251–255
26. Cross K W, Hey E N, Kennaird D L, Lewis S R, Urich H 1971 Lack of temperature control in infants with abnormalities of the central nervous system. Archives of Disease in Childhood 46: 437–443
27. Darnall R A 1981 Insensible weight loss measurements in newborn infants: possible overestimation with the Potter baby scale. Journal of Pediatrics 99: 795–797
28. Day R L, Caliguiri L, Kamenski C, Ehrlich F 1964 Body temperature and survival of premature infants. Pediatrics 34: 171–181
29. Denborough M A, Galloway G J, Hopkinson K C 1982 Malignant hyperpyrexia and sudden infant death. Lancet ii: 1068–1069
30. Ducker D A, Lyon A J, Ross Russell R, Bass C A, McIntosh N 1985 Incubator temperature control: effects on the very low birthweight infant. Archives of Disease in Childhood 60: 902–907
31. Fanaroff A A, Wald M, Gruber H S, Klaus M H 1972 Insensible water loss in low birth weight infants. Pediatrics 50: 236–245
32. Fonkalsrud E W, Chatsworthy H W 1965 Accidental perforation of the colon and rectum in newborn infants. New England Journal of Medicine 272: 1097–1100
33. Foster K G, Hey E N, Katz G 1969 The response of the sweat glands of the newborn baby to thermal stimuli and to intradermal acetylcholine. Journal of Physiology 203: 13–29
34. Frank J D, Brown S 1978 Thermometers and rectal perforations in the neonates. Archives of Disease in Childhood 53: 284–285
35. Gandy G M, Adamsons K, Cunningham N, Silverman W A, James L S 1964 Thermal environment and acid–base homeostasis in human infants during the first few hours of life. Journal of Clinical Investigation 43: 751–758
36. Gerhardt T, McCarthy J, Bancalari E 1979 Effect of aminophylline on respiratory centre activity and metabolic rate in premature infants with idiopathic apnea. Pediatrics 63: 537–542
37. Glass L, Silverman W A, Sinclair J C 1968 Effect of the thermal environment and cold resistance and growth of small infants after the first week of life. Pediatrics 41: 1033–1046
38. Glass L, Silverman W A, Sinclair J C 1969 Relationship of thermal environment and calorie intake to growth and resting metabolism in the late neonatal period. Biology of the Neonate 14: 324–340
39. Glass L, Lala R V, Jaiswal V, Nigam S K 1975 Effect of thermal environment and calorie intake on head growth of low birthweight infants during late neonatal period. Archives of Disease in Childhood 50: 541–542
40. Greenabate C, Tafari N, Rao M R, Yu K F, Clemens J D 1994 Comparison of heated water-filled mattress and space-heated room with infant incubator in providing warmth to low birthweight newborns. International Journal of Epidemiology 23: 1226–1233
41. Greenbaum E I, Carson M, Kincannan W N, O'Loughlin B J 1969 Rectal thermometer-induced pneumoperitoneum in the newborn. Pediatrics 44: 539–542
42. Hammarlund K, Sedin G 1979 Transepidermal water loss in newborn infants. III. Relation to gestational age. Acta Paediatrica Scandinavica 68: 795–801

43. Hammarlund K, Nilsson G E, Oberg P A, Sedin G 1980 Transepidermal water loss in newborn infants. V. Evaporation from the skin and heat exchange during the first hours of life. Acta Paediatrica Scandinavica 69: 385–392
44. Hammarlund K, Sedin G, Stromberg B 1983 Transepidermal water loss in newborn infants. VIII. Relation to gestational age and postnatal age in appropriate and small for gestational age infants. Acta Paediatrica Scandinavica 72: 721–728
45. Harpin V A, Rutter N 1982 Sweating in preterm babies. Journal of Pediatrics 100: 614–618
46. Harpin V A, Rutter N 1983 Barrier properties of the newborn infant's skin. Journal of Pediatrics 102: 419–425
47. Harpin V A, Rutter N 1985 Humidification of incubators. Archives of Disease in Childhood 60: 219–224
48. Harpin V A, Chellapah G, Rutter N 1983 The responses of the newborn infant to overheating. Biology of the Neonate 44: 65–75
49. Hey E N 1969 The relation between environmental temperature and oxygen consumption in the new-born baby. Journal of Physiology 200: 589–603
50. Hey E N 1971 The care of babies in incubators. In: Gairdner D, Hull D (eds) Recent advances in paediatrics, 4th edn. J & A Churchill, London, pp 171–216
51. Hey E N 1975 Thermal neutrality. British Medical Bulletin 31: 69–74
52. Hey E N 1983 Temperature regulation in sick infants. In: Tinker J, Rapin M (eds) Care of the critically ill patient. Springer, Berlin, pp 1013–1029
53. Hey E N, Katz G 1969 Evaporative water loss in the new-born baby. Journal of Physiology 200: 605–619
54. Hey E N, Katz G 1970 The optimum thermal environment for naked babies. Archives of Disease in Childhood 45: 328–334
55. Hey E N, O'Connell B 1970 Oxygen consumption and heat balance in the cot-nursed baby. Archives of Disease in Childhood 45: 335–343
56. Hey E N, Katz G, O'Connell B 1970 The total thermal insulation of the newborn baby. Journal of Physiology 207: 683–698
57. Hill J R, Rahimtulla K A 1965 Heat balance and the metabolic rate of new-born babies in relation to environmental temperature, and the effect of age and of weight on basal metabolic rate. Journal of Physiology 280: 239–265
58. Hull D 1966 The structure and function of brown adipose tissue. British Medical Bulletin 22: 92–96
59. Jolly H, Molyneaux P, Newell D J 1962 A controlled study of the effect of temperature on premature babies. Journal of Pediatrics 60: 889–894
60. Jones R W A, Rochefort M J, Baum J D 1976 Increased insensible water loss in newborn infants nursed under radiant heaters. British Medical Journal ii: 1347–1350
61. Kaplan M, Eidelman A I 1984 Improved prognosis in severely hypothermic newborn infants treated by rapid rewarming. Journal of Pediatrics 105: 470–474
62. Karlberg P 1952 Determination of standard energy metabolism (basal metabolism) in normal infants. Acta Paediatrica Scandinavica 41 (suppl. 89)
63. Kennaird D L 1976 Oxygen consumption and evaporative water loss in infants with congenital heart disease. Archives of Disease in Childhood 51: 34–41
64. Kjartansson S, Hammarlund K, Sedin G 1992 Insensible water loss from the skin during phototherapy in term and preterm infants. Acta Paediatrica 81: 764–768
65. Kjartansson S, Arsan S, Hammarlund K, Sjors G, Sedin G 1995 Water loss from the skin of term and preterm infants nursed under a radiant heater. Pediatric Research 37: 233–238
66. Kluger M J 1980 Fever. Pediatrics 66: 720–724
67. Knauth A, Gordin M, McNelis W, Baumgart S 1989 Semipermeable polyurethane membrane as an artificial skin for the premature neonate. Pediatrics 83: 945–950
68. LeBlanc M H 1982 Relative efficacy of an incubator and an open warmer in producing thermoneutrality for the small premature infant. Pediatrics 69: 439–445
69. Lee V A, Iliff A 1956 The energy metabolism of infants and young children during postprandial sleep. Pediatrics 18: 739–749
70. Mann T P 1968 Observations on temperatures of mothers and babies in the perinatal period. Journal of Obstetrics and Gynaecology of the British Commonwealth 75: 316–321
71. Mann T P, Elliott R I K 1957 Neonatal cold injury due to accidental exposure to cold. Lancet i: 229–234
72. Marks K H, Friedman Z, Maisels M J 1977 A simple device for reducing insensible water loss in low birth weight babies. Pediatrics 60: 223–226
73. Marks K H, Gunther R C, Rossi J A, Maisels M J 1980 Oxygen consumption and insensible water loss in premature infants under radiant heaters. Pediatrics 66: 228–232
74. Marks K H,Lee C, Bolan C D, Maisels M J 1981 Oxygen consumption and temperature control of premature infants in a double-wall incubator. Pediatrics 68: 93–98
75. Marks K H, Nardis E E, Momin M N 1986 Energy metabolism and substrate utilization in low birth weight neonates under radiant warmers. Pediatrics 78: 465–472
76. Matsaniotis N, Pastelis V, Agathopoulos A, Constantsas N 1971 Fever and biochemical thermogenesis. Pediatrics 68: 93–98
77. Mayfield S R, Bhatia J, Nakamura K T, Rios G R, Bell E F 1984 Temperature measurement in term and preterm infants. Journal of Pediatrics 104: 271–275
78. Messaritakis J, Anagnostakis D, Laskari H, Katerelos C 1990 Rectal–skin temperature difference in septicaemic newborn infants. Archives of Disease in Childhood 65: 380–382
79. Mok Q, Bass C A, Ducker D A, McIntosh N 1991 Temperature instability during nursing procedures in preterm neonates. Archives of Disease in Childhood 66: 783–786
80. Oh W, Karecki H 1972 Phototherapy and insensible water loss in the newborn infant. American Journal of Diseases of Children 124: 230–232
81. Okken A, Blijam C, Franz W, Bohn E 1982 Effects of forced convection of heated air on insensible water loss and heat loss in preterm infants in incubators. Journal of Pediatrics 101: 108–112
82. Okken A, Jonxis J H P, Rispens P, Zijlstra W G 1979 Insensible water loss and metabolic growth rate in low birth weight newborn babies. Pediatric Research 13: 1072–1075
83. Perlstein P H, Edwards N K, Sutherland J M 1970 Apnoea in premature infants and incubator air temperature changes. New England Journal of Medicine 282: 461–466
84. Pomerance J J, Brand R J, Meredith J L 1981 Differentiating environmental from disease-related fevers in the term newborn. Pediatrics 67: 485–487
85. Rutter N, Hull D 1979 Response of term babies to a warm environment. Archives of Disease in Childhood 54: 178–183
86. Rutter N, Hull D 1979 Water loss from the skin of term and preterm babies. Archives of Disease in Childhood 54: 858–868
87. Rutter N, Hull D 1981 Reduction of skin water loss in the newborn. I. Effect of applying topical agents. Archives of Disease in Childhood 56: 669–672
88. Rutter N, Brown S M, Hull D 1978 Variation in the resting oxygen consumption of small babies. Archives of Disease in Childhood 51: 34–41
89. Sarman I, Tunell R 1989 Providing warmth for preterm babies by a heated, water filled mattress. Archives of Disease in Childhood 64: 29–33
90. Sarman I, Can G, Tunell R 1989 Rewarming preterm infants on a heated, water filled mattress. Archives of Disease in Childhood 64: 687–692
91. Sauer P J J, Dane H J, Visser H K 1984 New standards for neutral thermal environment of healthy very low birthweight infants in week one of life. Archives of Disease in Childhood 59: 18–22
92. Scopes J W, Ahmed I 1966 Minimal rates of oxygen consumption in sick and premature newborn infants. Archives of Disease in Childhood 41: 407–416
93. Silverman W A, Fertig J W, Berger A P 1958 The influence of the thermal environment upon the survival of newly born premature infants. Pediatrics 22: 876–885
94. Smales O R C, Kime R 1978 Thermoregulation in babies immediately after birth. Archives of Disease in Childhood 53: 58–61
95. Smiddy F G, Benson E A 1969 Rectal perforation by thermometer. Lancet ii: 805–806
96. Stanley F J, Alberman E D 1978 Infants of very low birthweight. I. Perinatal factors affecting survival. Developmental Medicine and Child Neurology 20: 300–312
97. Stanley F J, Alberman E D 1978 Infants of very low birthweight. II. Perinatal factors in conditions associated with respiratory distress syndrome. Developmental Medicine and Child Neurology 20: 313–322
98. Stanton A N, Scott D J, Downham M P S 1980 Is overheating a factor in some unexpected infant deaths? Lancet i: 1054–1057

99. Stothers J K 1981 Head insulation and heat loss in the newborn. Archives of Disease in Childhood 56: 530–534
100 Stothers J K, Warner R M 1978 Oxygen consumption and neonatal sleep states. Journal of Physiology 278: 435–440
101. Stothers J K, Warner R M 1979 Effect of feeding on neonatal oxygen consumption. Archives of Disease in Childhood 54: 415–420
102. Tafari N, Gentz J 1974 Aspects of rewarming newborn infants with severe accidental hypothermia. Acta Paediatrica Scandinavica 63: 595–600
103. Thompson M H, Stothers J K, McLellan N J 1984 Weight and water loss in the neonate in natural and forced convection. Archives of Disease in Childhood 59: 951–956
104. Varga F 1959 The respective effect of starvation and changed body composition on energy metabolism in malnourished infants. Pediatrics 23: 1085–1090
105. Vernon H J, Lane A T, Wischerath L J, Davis J M, Menegus M A 1990 Semipermeable dressing and transepidermal water loss in premature infants. Pediatrics 86: 357–362
106. Voora S, Srinivasan G, Lilien L D, Yeh T F, Pildes R S 1982 Fever in full-term newborns in the first four days of life. Pediatrics 69: 40–44
107. Walther F J, Wu P Y K, Siassi B 1987 Cardiovascular changes in preterm infants nursed under radiant warmers. Pediatrics 80: 235–239
108. Wheldon A E, Hull D 1983 Incubation of very immature infants. Archives of Disease in Childhood 58: 504–508
109. Wheldon A E, Rutter N 1982 The heat balance of small babies nursed in incubators and under radiant warmers. Early Human Development 6: 131–143
110. Williams P R, Oh W 1974 Effects of radiant warmer on insensible water loss in newborn infants. American Journal of Diseases of Children 128: 511–514
111. Wu P Y K, Hodgman J 1974 Insensible water loss in preterm infants: changes with postnatal development and non-ionizing radiant energy. Pediatrics 54: 504–512
112. Yeh T F, Amma P, Lilien L D, Baccaro M, Matwynschyn J, Pyati S, Pildes R S 1979 Reduction of insensible water loss in premature infants under the radiant warmer. Journal of Pediatrics 94: 651–653
113. Yeh R F, Voora S, Lilien L D, Matwynschyn J, Srinivasan G, Pildes R S 1980 Oxygen consumption and insensible water loss in premature infants in single-space vs double-walled incubators. Journal of Pediatrics 97: 967–997
114. Young D G 1965 'Spontaneous' rupture of the rectum. Proceedings of the Royal Society of Medicine 58: 615–616

19

Infant feeding

Part 1

Nutritional physiology: dietary requirements of term and preterm infants

Mary Fewtrell Alan Lucas

FETAL NUTRITION

It has often been argued that an important objective in feeding low-birthweight infants is to attempt to reproduce postnatally the pattern of nutrient accretion and tissue composition that would have occurred in utero at a corresponding postconceptional age. It could be counter-argued that the optimal pattern of nutrient accretion after birth is not necessarily that seen in utero, but one that results in the most successful adaptation to extrauterine life, a concept which is readily accepted for the respiratory and cardiovascular systems. Nevertheless, an understanding of fetal nutritional physiology is relevant to clinical practice.

From analysis of 'reference fetuses' of different gestational ages, it is possible to calculate the daily fetal nutrient accretion rates[40,121,129] and to use these as a basis for studying postnatal nutrition and its disorders. For example, the intrauterine accretion of calcium and phosphorus is substantially higher than could be supplied by a standard formula or mature breast milk to premature infants. Coupled with the fact that at 28 weeks' gestation estimated calcium and phosphorus stores in bone are only 20% of those at term, these observations underpin our understanding of bone disease in infants born preterm.

Several other nutrients are laid down late in gestation, so that the preterm infant has low body stores. One example is body fat. By mid-gestation body fat content is less than 1% of body weight; at 28 weeks 3.5%; at 34 weeks 7.8%; and at term 15%. During the last month of intrauterine life the fetus lays down about 7 g of fat per day.[121]

Carbohydrate stores are also laid down relatively late. Shelley[103] estimated liver glycogen to be about 1 g/100 g of tissue at 31 weeks and 4 g/100 g at term. Widdowson[121] calculated total body carbohydrate at 9 g at 33 weeks and 34 g at term. These data have been used to calculate the ability of infants of different gestations to withstand starvation and maintain glucose homoeostasis after birth.

Total body water falls progressively from over 95% of body weight in the first trimester to around 75% at term[43] and continues to fall throughout infancy.

Lipid-soluble vitamins are transferred across the placenta by simple or facilitated diffusion,[76,84] hence fetal blood concentration of such vitamins correlates well with those in the mother, with the exception of vitamin E, for which fetal blood levels are around 30% of maternal values.[78] These vitamins accumulate in fetal tissues throughout pregnancy. Blood concentrations, and perhaps body stores, are reduced in preterm infants and those of poorly nourished mothers. Water-soluble vitamins are transported against concentration gradients, mostly by active transport: fetal blood levels of vitamins B_1, B_2, B_6, B_{12}, folate and vitamin C are two- to fourfold higher than those in maternal blood. Preterm infants and babies of undernourished mothers have lower blood levels of water-soluble vitamins at birth.[8]

'BIOLOGICAL CLOCK' OF FETAL DEVELOPMENT

Intermediary metabolism

Throughout fetal life there is a progressively changing picture of enzymatic differentiation.[51] Certain enzymes of amino acid metabolism develop late, including those concerned with the synthesis of cysteine from methionine, taurine from cysteine and tyrosine from phenylalanine, with degradation of tyrosine[88] and production of urea.[14] Low-birthweight infants might therefore be expected to have increased dietary requirements for certain amino acids (such as cysteine and taurine; p. 310) and be at risk for possibly deleterious accumulation of others (such as phenylalanine, tyrosine and methionine; p. 310).

Key enzymes in gluconeogenic pathways (e.g. phosphoenolpyruvate carboxykinase) may not develop until near or even just after term delivery.[51] A constant transplacental glucose infusion renders gluconeogenesis relatively unimportant in utero, and the fetal liver is more concerned with the storage of glucose as glycogen; phosphorylase and glucose 6-phosphatase ensure immediate glucose release after birth and defer the need for gluconeogenesis until around 24–48 hours of age; in contrast, the preterm neonate, born with low stores of liver glycogen[121] and reduced gluconeogenic ability, is at risk of hypoglycemia (p. 947).

Gastrointestinal tract (see Chapter 31)

ADAPTATIONS TO EXTRAUTERINE NUTRITION

Adaptation to feeding after birth involves major postnatal changes in gut structure and function and in intermediary metabolism. Although the fetal intestine is structurally mature by 25 weeks' gestation and capable of digesting and absorbing milk feeds, motor activity develops more slowly, and may limit the tolerance to enteral feeds.

Postnatally, enteral feeding appears to play a key part in triggering gut development. Studies on piglets and rats show marked structural and functional changes in the gastrointestinal tract and its adnexae following feeding – changes not seen in unfed animals. These effects are not confined to the gut: for example, enteral feeding may cause increased responsiveness to glucose by pancreatic β cells. Enteral feeding is not an entirely new experience for the newborn infant: by the end of pregnancy the fetus is swallowing about 500 ml of amniotic fluid daily, providing up to 3 g of protein[43] which may contribute to fetal nutrition. Thus in the last trimester the fetus has a similar fluid intake and about 25–50% of the protein intake of the breast-fed infant at term, although fat and carbohydrate intakes are much less. Enteral feeding in utero may help to prepare the gut for extrauterine feeding.

The following factors are important in regulating the adaptation of the intestine to extrauterine nutrition:

- Endocrine secretion. Corticosteroids and thyroxine are critical triggers for gut development.[65] Adrenalectomy, hypophysectomy and thyroidectomy in animals delay gut maturation, whereas administration of glucocorticoids or thyroxine prior to delivery causes elongation of microvilli, increases the activities of the brush border enzymes, sucrase, enteropeptidase and alkaline phosphatase, and induces pancreatic enzyme secretion postnatally.
- Intraluminal factors. These may be endogenous (secreted by the gastrointestinal tract) or exogenous (dietary nutrients), and act either directly on the cells of the GI tract, or indirectly via effects on hormone secretion. For example, in neonatal rats, enteral feeding with sucrose increases intestinal sucrase and isomaltase, whereas lactose increases gut lactase,[65] a finding consistent with the observed tolerance of preterm infants to lactose despite the late development of lactase in infants born at term. Surges in plasma levels of gut hormones can be induced by small, nutritionally insignificant volumes of milk, leading to the concept of minimal enteral feeding, where small volumes of milk are used to promote intestinal maturation and adaptation even when the infant is too sick to tolerate full enteral nutrition. Minimal enteral feeding has been demonstrated to produce more ordered patterns of gut motility[11] and results in improved growth, reduced requirements for phototherapy, and earlier achievement of full feeds taken by breast or bottle.[36,106] However, although intraluminal factors undoubtedly influence GI development, they do not provide the sole trigger for ontogenetic changes, as normal maturational patterns of enzymes may occur in surgically bypassed segments of gut.[114]
- Breast milk hormones and growth factors (Chapter 19, Part 2, p. 325). A large number of substances present in human milk have been demonstrated to play a role in regulating the adaptive changes that accompany the transition to enteral feeding. These include bombesin, somatostatin, epidermal growth factor, IGF-1 and IGF-2, and nucleotides. In many cases these substances undergo only limited degradation in the stomach and appear to retain bioactivity in the intestine. Although they may not be essential for survival, the higher incidence of gastrointestinal disease in infants fed formula suggests that these compounds may contribute to the protective effect of human milk.
- Bacteria. Studies on the GI flora of infants fed human milk or formula suggest that the indigenous microflora are an important factor in GI development and function, altering the activities of various enzymes.[111]

BIOLOGICAL CONSEQUENCES OF DEPRIVING INFANTS OF ENTERAL FEEDS AFTER BIRTH

Exclusive intravenous feeding in rats results in decreased weight of the small intestine, pancreas and oxyntic area of the stomach, associated with a significant reduction in small intestinal DNA and a dramatic reduction in antral gastrin content; in contrast, animal studies have shown that other organs not directly concerned with nutrition, such as spleen and testes, remain unaffected,[61] and

Heird[55] has demonstrated intestinal mucosal atrophy during parenteral nutrition, with concomitant reduction in brush border enzyme activities. These effects may be related to the very low concentrations of circulating gut hormones found in human infants deprived of enteral feeding.

Although after short periods of parenteral nutrition in neonates tolerance to enteral feeds usually increases rapidly (in the absence of structural anomaly of the gut), it remains to be established whether prolonged avoidance of enteral feeding could deprive the neonate of critical signals for gut development.

NON-NUTRITIONAL CONSEQUENCES OF ENTERAL FEEDING

When a neonate is fed, dynamic alterations occur in splanchnic blood flow, with a significant increase in velocity which is 35% greater in formula-fed term infants than in breast-fed infants. Fasting velocities are also higher in formula-fed infants.[28] Changes may also occur in pulmonary function, with decreased tidal volume, minute ventilation and compliance in VLBW infants randomized to intermittent versus continuous feeds.[13] However, a recent randomized controlled trial of continuous versus 3-hourly intermittent feeds in VLBW infants showed similar growth and macronutrient retention rates, and no significant difference in the time required to achieve full enteral feeds between the two groups.[105]

INDIVIDUAL NUTRIENTS: PHYSIOLOGY AND DIETARY NEEDS OF TERM AND PRETERM INFANTS

Calculation of the nutrient requirements for term infants has traditionally been based on the composition of breast milk. However, the precise dietary intake of breast-fed babies is unknown, and there is uncertainty over what

Table 19.1 Composition of mature human milk and nutritional guidelines for the composition of artificial feeds for full-term infants per 100 ml. (EC Directive Guidelines, 1991[27])

	Mean values for pooled samples of expressed mature human milk	Guidelines for infant formulas	
		Minimum	Maximum
Energy			
kJ	293	250	315
kcal	70	60	75
Protein (g)	1.3		
casein dominant infant formula		1.35	2.25
whey dominant infant formula		1.08	2.25
Lactose (g)	7	2.1	NS
Total carbohydrate (g)		4.2	10.5
Fat (g)	4.2	2.0	4.9
Vitamins			
A (μg)	60	36	135
D (μg)	0.01	0.6	1.9
E (μg)	0.35	0.3	NS
K (μg)	0.21	2.4	NS
Thiamin (μg)	16	24	NS
Riboflavin (μg)	30	36	NS
Nicotinic acid (μg)	230	150	NS
Pyridoxine (μg)	6	21	NS
B_{12} (μg)	0.01	0.06	NS
Folic acid (μg)	5.2	2.4	NS
Biotin (μg)	0.76	0.9	NS
C (μg)	3.8	4.8	NS
Minerals			
Sodium (mg)	15	12	45
Potassium (mg)	60	36	109
Chloride (mg)	43	30	94
Calcium (mg)	35	30	NS
Phosphorus (mg)	15	15	67.5
Magnesium (mg)	2.3	3.0	11.25
Iron (μg)	76	600	1500
Iodine (μg)	7	3.0	NS
Zinc (mg)	0.295	0.45	1.8
Copper (μg)	39	12	60

NS, not specified

should be regarded as an ideal pattern of growth during infancy. Recently in the west there have been marked changes in the growth performance of infants, which may be related to the changing eating habits of families as a whole. Animal studies and some human data indicate that early diet might have long-term consequences for future growth, development and morbidity, but optimal nutrient intakes for neonates have never been assessed in these terms. Thus appropriate dietary goals continue to be disputed. The EC Directive on Infant Formulae[27] recommendations for the nutrient content of the diet of formula-fed babies are shown in Table 19.1; under the Infant Formula and Follow-On Formula Regulations[57] of 1995, all infant formula manufacturers in the UK are required by law to comply with these.

Low-birthweight babies are not a homogeneous population: their requirements and tolerance of individual nutrients are influenced by gestation, postnatal age and concomitant illness. Nevertheless, there is now some international consensus on the advisable intakes for each nutrient. This field was comprehensively reviewed by the Committee on Nutrition of the European Society for Pediatric Gastroenterology and Nutrition[37], and more recently by a panel of international experts[113] who considered separately the needs of infants above or below 1000 g; a summary of the recommendations by this panel for intakes of individual nutrients is shown in Table 19.2. The scientific and clinical basis for current recommendations for the desirable nutrient intakes in preterm infants is illustrated below.

Table 19.2 Recommended intakes of individual nutrients for (formula-fed) stable/growing preterm infants. (International Consensus Recommendation, Tsang et al 1993[113])

	<1000 g			>1000 g		
	Per kg per day SI units	**Per kg per day mass units**	**Per 100 kcal mass units**	**Per kg per day SI units**	**Per kg per day mass units**	**Per 100 kcal mass units**
Energy kcal	110–120	110–120	100	110–120	110–120	100
kJ	460–502	460–502	419	460–502	460–502	419
Protein (g)	3.6–3.8	3.6–3.8	3.0–3.16	3.0–3.6	3.0–3.6	2.5–3.0
Fat (g)						
linoleic (g)	4–15% cal	4–15% cal	0.44–1.7 g	4–15% cal	4–15% cal	0.44–1.7 g
linolenic (g)	1–4% cal	1–4% cal	0.11–0.44 g	1–4% cal	1–4% cal	0.11–0.44 g
C18:2/C18:3	≥5	≥5	≥5	≥5	≥5	≥5
Carbohydrate (g)						
lactose (g)	3.8–11.4	3.8–11.4	3.16–9.5	3.8–11.8	3.8–11.8	3.16–9.8
oligomers (g)	0–8.4	0–8.4	0–7.0	0–8.4	0–8.4	0–7.0
Sodium (mmol/mg)	2–3	46–69	38–58	2–3	46–69	1.66–2.5
Potassium (mmol/mg)	2–3	78–120	65–100	2–3	78–120	1.66–2.5
Chloride (mmol/mg)	2–3	70–105	59–89	2–3	70–105	1.66–2.5
Calcium (mmol/mg)	2–3	120–230	100–192	2–3	120–230	1.66–2.5
Phosphorus (mmol/mg)	1.94–4.52	60–140	50–117	1.94–4.52	60–140	1.61–3.77
Magnesium (mmol/mg)	0.33–0.63	7.9–15	6.6–12.5	0.33–0.63	7.9–15	0.275–0.53
Iron (μmol/mg))	36	2	1.67	36	2	30
Zinc (μmol/μg)	15	1000	833	15	1000	12.7
Copper (μmol/μg)	1.9–2.4	120–150	100–125	1.9–2.4	120–150	1.6–2.0
Selenium (nmol/μg)	16–38	1.3–3.0	1.08–1.25	16–38	1.3–3.0	14–32
Manganese (nmol/μg)	136	7.5	6.3	136	7.5	115
Iodine (nmol/μg)	236–472	30–60	25–50	236–472	30–60	197–394
Vitamin A (IU)	700–1500	700–1500	583–1250	700–1500	700–1500	583–1250
Vitamin D (IU)	150–400*	150–400	125–333	150–400*	150–400	125–333
Vitamin E (IU)	6–12⁺	6–12	5–10	6–12⁺	6–12	5–10
Vitamin K (nmol/μg)	18–22	8–10	6.66–8.33	18–22	8–10	15–18.5
Vitamin C (mmol/mg)	102–136	18–24	15.20	102–136	18–24	85–114
Thiamin (μmol/μg)	0.53–0.71	180–240	150–200	0.53–0.71	180–240	0.45–0.59
Riboflavin (μmol/μg)	0.66–0.96	250–360	200–300	0.66–0.96	250–360	0.53–0.8
Pyridoxine (μmol/μg)	0.73–1.02	150–210	125–175	0.73–1.02	150–210	0.61–0.85
Niacin (mmol/mg)	30–39	3.6–4.8	3–4	30–39	3.6–4.8	25–33
B_{12} (nmol/μg)	0.22	0.3	0.25	0.22	0.3	0.18
Folate (nmol/μg)	56–113	25–50	21–42	56–113	25–50	48–95
Taurine (μmol/mg)	36–72	4.5–9.0	3.75–7.5	36–72	4.5–9.0	30–60
Carnitine (μmol/mg)	~18	~2.9	~2.4	~18	~2.9	~15
Inositol (mmol/mg)	0.18–0.45	32–81	27–67.5	0.18–0.45	32–81	0.15–0.375
Choline (μmol/mg)	138–270	14.4–28	12–23.4	138–270	14.4–28	115–225

*aim for 400 iu per day
⁺ max = 25 iu

PROTEINS AND AMINO ACIDS

The protein intake per kilogram bodyweight for the human infant is greater than for adults. In mammals, the protein content of milk correlates highly with postnatal growth rate. Nine amino acids are considered essential in human nutrition: arginine, lysine, leucine, isoleucine, valine, methionine, phenylalanine, threonine and tryptophan. However, because of the late development of certain enzymes of amino acid metabolism, the newborn infant may have an temporarily increased requirement for cysteine and histidine, and perhaps for taurine (see below).

Digestion and absorption

Luminal hydrolysis results in the breakdown of most large molecular weight proteins into peptides and amino acids. Most peptides are then hydrolysed by peptidases on the microvillus membrane prior to transport through the membrane, but some are absorbed intact. Although pepsin secretion is lower in preterm than term infants at birth, it is unaffected by the type of diet.[53] The activity of brush-border peptidases is also low in preterm infants at birth, but increases rapidly.

Protein requirements for term babies

These are discussed further on pages 325–328. The EC Directive guidelines[27] recommend that formulas containing unmodified cow's milk protein should contain 1.35–2.25 g of protein per 100 ml of reconstituted feed, whereas if the casein/whey ratio is adjusted to be closer to human milk (2:3), a minimum of 1.1 g of protein per 100 ml of feed is suggested. This implies that cow's milk whey has a higher biological value for human infants than cow's milk casein, but this has never been proven. As growth velocity falls during infancy there is a progressively decreased need for protein intake per kilogram of bodyweight.

Estimating the protein requirements for the preterm baby

That the rapid growth in preterm babies might greatly increase the need for dietary protein has been appreciated for over 40 years. The principles used to assess protein needs serve as a model for the investigation of requirements for other nutrients.

Relation of protein intake to growth

Weight gain and linear growth are the traditional measures of nutritional status. Gordon et al[48] demonstrated in 1947 that preterm infants gained weight more rapidly on high protein-containing formulas than on human milk, and Davidson et al[31] showed that weight gain was greater in preterm infants fed a formula supplying 4 g/kg/24 h rather than 2 g/kg/24 h. High intakes of protein may also result in an increase in linear growth and a greater rate of increase in head circumference.[16,70]

A factorial approach

Protein requirements may be derived using a combination of values for body composition[130] and for nitrogen retention derived from balance studies. The results from a number of such studies show that protein gain increases linearly with intakes between approximately 2 and 4 g/kg/24 h.[77] These calculations involve making assumptions about desirable postnatal growth performance, but the results emphasize that, in order to achieve the accretion of nitrogen at the same rate as seen in utero during the third trimester, the preterm infant requires substantially greater intakes of protein than would be obtained by a term infant fed on breast milk.

There is less certainty about the optimal protein intake for *sick* preterm infants. Such infants frequently fail to grow even when provided with a theoretically adequate nutrient supply, and the goal of nutritional management is effectively to maintain the status quo and prevent catabolism. Theoretically, a protein intake of 0.5 g/kg/24 h will result in a reduction of protein turnover to the point of equilibrium (that is, zero gain and zero loss), and from a pragmatic point of view this should be the minimum acceptable daily intake.

Assessment of protein undernutrition

A low concentration of plasma protein is a traditional index of protein malnutrition. Preterm infants fed on human milk (banked or own mother's) may develop hypoproteinaemia after the second month of postnatal life, and this is prevented by protein supplementation.[95] Using traditional nitrogen balance studies the protein deposition in new tissue can be estimated. In one such study of infants fed on a preterm formula providing 3.6 g protein per kilogram per day, the percentage of protein in new tissue (12.8%) was within the range described in utero (11–14%); in contrast, those fed on mature donor breast milk, providing around 2.2 g protein per kilogram per day, had only 8.7% protein in new tissue, suggesting a low protein content in lean body mass, as seen in experimental malnutrition.[92]

Assessment of protein 'overload'

The Committee of Nutrition of the American Academy of Pediatrics[3] stated in 1977 that 'the optimal diet for the low-birthweight infant may be defined as one that supports a rate of growth approximating that of the third trimester of intrauterine life, without imposing stress on the developing metabolic and excretory system'. Although the first part of this statement could be disputed, the second part is a matter of general agreement. Schultz et al[99] showed that compared with a breast-fed control group of infants receiving 2.0 g protein per kilogram per day, a formula-fed group receiving 4.4 g protein per kilogram per day demonstrated azotaemia, a lower blood glucose, hyperaminoacidaemia (especially phenylalanine) and metabolic acidosis, and regained birthweight more slowly. However, balance and stable isotope studies[128] have emphasized that the amount of energy absorbed is critical for the rate of protein synthesis. If energy intake is low, high protein intakes cannot be utilized and the infants' metabolic machinery is stressed; in contrast, diets with high available energy and large protein intakes, of at least 4 g/kg/24 h, result in increased nitrogen retention and growth, without metabolic strain. For this reason it is conventional to express protein (and indeed other nutrient requirements) in relation to energy intake (Table 19.2) as well as in absolute terms.

Long-term outcome studies

Most important is whether early nutrition could have long-term consequences, either adverse or beneficial. Using an experimental approach, Goldman et al[47] studied 304 infants below 2000 g who had been randomized to 2% or 4% protein diets providing, respectively, 3.0–3.6 g and 6.0–7.2 g protein per kilogram per day. Infants below 1300 g in the high protein intake group had a markedly higher incidence of low IQs (below 90) by Stanford–Binet score at 5 years of age. The incidence of strabismus in infants below 1700 g fed on a high protein intake was also increased. It has been suggested that transient hyperaminoacidaemia (especially tyrosine) on high protein intakes might have been responsible for these adverse outcomes, but currently the explanation is uncertain. Indeed, in a more recent study Lucas et al[68] looked at a group of preterm infants who had elevated plasma phenylalanine levels during the neonatal period, associated with the use of intravenous Vamin 9. Despite phenylalanine levels in the range reported to produce long-term cognitive deficits in infants with phenylketonuria, neurodevelopmental testing at 18 months post-term showed no difference between infants who had neonatal hyperphenylalaninaemia and those who did not. This study also noted that infants who developed hyperphenylalaninaemia had typically received total parenteral nutrition with a low energy protein ratio, emphasizing the importance of considering protein and energy intakes together.

On the positive side, there is evidence suggesting that long-term outcome may be improved by meeting the increased protein requirements of certain groups of infants, for example those born prematurely. Preterm infants randomized to receive a preterm formula containing 2 g/100 ml protein showed both better short-term growth than those fed a standard term formula containing 1.45 g/100 ml[70] and improved neurodevelopment 7.5–8 years later (Lucas et al, unpublished data).

Protein quality

Whey proteins have a lower concentration of aromatic amino acids (tyrosine and phenylalanine) than are found in caseins; the studies by Goldman[47] were performed with high-casein formulas (like cow's milk), but most modern formulas are whey predominant, reducing the possibility of hypertyrosinaemia and hyperphenylalaninaemia.[88] Whey is also a good source of cysteine, a potentially essential amino acid in the newborn period (see above). However, a high whey intake is associated with plasma threonine concentrations which are three times those of the breast milk-fed infant. In fact, plasma threonine (and other amino acid) concentrations are higher in the fetus than they are postnatally,[7] raising the possibility that high values in babies born preterm are not necessarily toxic.

Amino acid composition

The evidence that taurine is essential in the diet of formula-fed preterm infants is inconclusive, although breast-fed infants do have higher plasma and urine taurine concentrations and a higher rate of synthesis of bile acids than those fed on formula; the latter may partially explain the better fat absorption of infants fed human milk rather than formulas.[45,118] Rhesus monkeys fed a taurine-deficient formula for the first 6 or 12 months of life show abnormal retinal structure, although the abnormalities show some degree of spontaneous regression by 12 months even when the animals remain on the deficient diet.[56] A randomized trial of taurine supplementation in formula-fed preterm infants[115] showed no effect on growth, behaviour or electroretinograms, but some evidence of more rapid auditory maturation in the supplemented group at the equivalent of term (as assessed by brain-stem evoked response). Although there is no evidence that taurine deficiency is associated with adverse long-term clinical effects in human infants, it seems prudent to add taurine to low-birthweight formulas to achieve concentrations similar to those of breast milk.

Glutamine is used as a fuel by the small intestine and a precursor for the synthesis of purine and pyrimidine bases. Numerous studies in animals and adult humans have demonstrated that it has beneficial effects on the gastrointestinal tract, including the maintenance of structure and function during parenteral nutrition. These findings have led to the suggestion that glutamine may be particularly important for the stressed preterm infant. A recent small study showed that low birthweight infants who received a glutamine-supplemented formula from 3 to 30 days of age had lower rates of hospital-acquired infection[94] and showed better enteral feed tolerance.[79] However, further work is required before firm recommendations about glutamine supplementation of infant formulas can be made.

FAT

Digestion and absorption[53]

Fat provides about half the energy for infants fed human milk, and its digestion commences in the stomach, catalysed by lingual lipase[41] and gastric lipase. Gastric lipolysis is quantitatively greater in the infant than in the adult, and the output and activity of lipases in the preterm infant are equal to those of adults maintained on a high-fat diet. Although gastric function and the production of lipase are unaffected by infant diet, the extent of fat digestion is greater in infants fed human milk (25%) than formula (14%), probably because of the structural differences between triglyceride in human milk fat globules and that in formula fat particles. Both lingual and gastric lipases are able to penetrate the milk fat globule membrane and digest triglyceride without disrupting its structure. The contribution of pancreatic lipases is relatively lower in infants than in adults. However, the bile salt-dependent lipase present in human milk may contribute significantly to fat digestion. BSDL is present in high quantities even in the milk of mothers who deliver prematurely, and its concentration is independent of milk volume. Unlike gastric and pancreatic lipases, BSDL shows no positional or fatty acid specificity and is able to produce free fatty acids which are more easily absorbed than mono- or diglycerides at the low bile-salt concentration seen in newborn infants.

The products of fat digestion are absorbed, resynthesized as triglycerides and secreted mainly into the lymphatic system as chylomicrons, and thence into the blood via the great veins. The foregoing applies to long-chain triglycerides, which are best absorbed if they are unsaturated. In contrast, medium-chain triglycerides (8–10 carbon atoms to the chain) are handled quite differently: their digestion is largely independent of bile salts; they are well absorbed, hydrolysed or intact, and pass to the liver via the portal system. Faecal fat excretion in newborn infants is greater in infants fed on cow's milk than in those fed on human milk or vegetable fats.

Most modern formulas contain a mixture of animal and vegetable oils, adjusted to mimic the pattern of fatty acid saturation and chain lengths found in breast milk. When compared with human milk, such fat mixtures have a reduced content of fatty acids esterified to glycerol in the 2 position and an increase in those esterified in the 1 and 3 positions. The latter undergo hydrolysis in the gut, releasing palmitic acid, which is poorly absorbed and tends to form calcium soaps; this may be partly responsible for the harder stools seen in formula-fed infants, and could influence calcium absorption. Studies are currently under way in both term and preterm infants using a new fat blend (Betapol) containing a high proportion of fatty acids esterified in the 2 position to mimic that found in human milk.[87] Carnielli[21] showed increased absorption of palmitic acid in preterm infants fed a formula containing Betapol, and our own (unpublished) data using Betapol in preterm infants show increased calcium absorption (measured by stable isotope) and fat absorption.

Fat requirements

Because there are clinical and physiological ceilings on the amount of dietary energy that it is desirable to supply as carbohydrate or protein, a minimum of around 30% of dietary energy needs to be supplied as fat. Linoleic and α-linolenic acids are essential fatty acids for the development of the brain and for prostaglandin synthesis. Essential fatty acid deficiency is also associated with skin lesions and retarded growth.

Two other dietary factors are important for lipid metabolism. Carnitine[85,120] plays a key role by facilitating transport of long-chain fatty acids across the mitochondrial membrane prior to their oxidation. Preterm and SGA infants may have impaired endogenous carnitine synthesis, and if carnitine intake is deficient (as in total parenteral nutrition) plasma and tissue concentrations fall. Nevertheless, whether such infants are put at clinical risk from a low-carnitine diet requires exploration; a recent study of formula-fed term SGA infants randomly assigned a carnitine supplement or placebo showed no significant effect of supplementation on growth up to 1 year of age (Lucas et al, unpublished). Standard formulas usually contain similar concentrations of carnitine to those in breast milk, but some preterm formulas have additional carnitine.

Choline[54,120] is required for phospholipid and acetylcholine synthesis. About half the choline requirement is derived from the diet. Human and cow's milk-based diets provide a sufficient intake.

Inositol, a six-carbon cyclic polyalcohol sugar, is a component of membrane phospholipids, and compounds containing inositol are important in signal transduction. Breast milk, particularly colostrum, contains high concentrations, whereas the levels in infant formulas are lower and intravenous feeding solutions have none. A randomized double-blind placebo-controlled trial of inositol supplementation in intravenously fed preterm infants with respiratory distress syndrome[52] showed an increased rate of survival without CLD at 28 days, and a lower rate of stage 4 retinopathy of prematurity in supplemented infants; the effect on survival without CLD was not seen in those infants who had also received surfactant, and it was suggested that this lack of an additive effect sup-

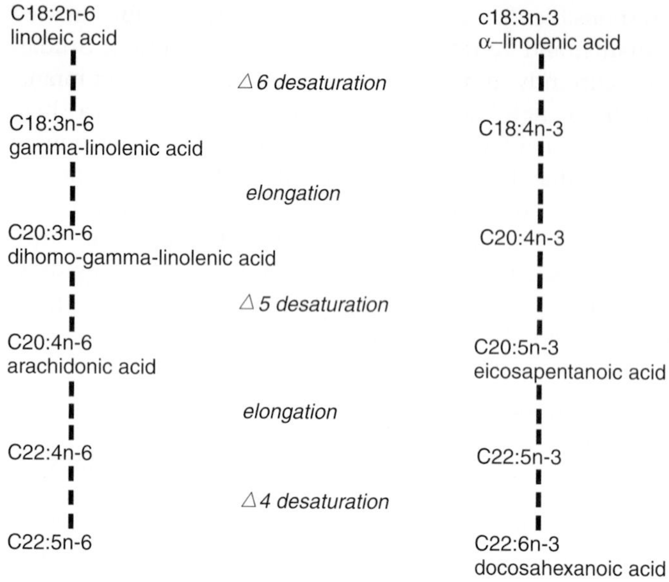

Fig. 19.1 Major steps in the formation of long chain polyunsaturated fatty acids (LCPs) from the C:18 essential fatty acids. Unsaturated fatty acids contain at least one double bond between adjacent carbon atoms: the number of double bonds is represented by 1n, 2n, 3n etc. LCPs are further classified by the position of the first double bond from the methyl or omega end of the hydrocarbon chain, represented as –3, –6, –9 or ω-3, ω-6, ω-9. Linoleic acid (C18: 2n-6) thus has a chain length of 18 carbons with two double bonds, the first of which is at the sixth carbon atom from the omega end.

ported the possibility that inositol increases endogenous surfactant synthesis. At present, it is recommended that all preterm infants receive supplementation based upon the level of inositol in human milk.

Essential fatty acid requirements

Two groups of long-chain polyunsaturated fatty acids, i.e. polyunsaturated fatty acids with greater than 18-carbon chain length) have received increasing interest recently: these are homologues of linoleic acid of the n-6 series (dihomogammalinolenic acid, arachidonic acid) and of α-linolenic acid of the n-3 series (eicosapentanoic acid, docosahexanoic acid). The LCPUFAs are synthesized from the precursor essential fatty acids by a process of chain elongation and desaturation (Fig. 19.1). They are found in high concentrations in the phospholipids of cell membranes, notably in the central nervous system.[82] In addition, arachidonic acid, dihomogammalinolenic acid and eicosapentanoic acid are precursors for eicosanoids – important modulators and mediators of a variety of essential biological processes.

Rapid accumulation of LCPUFA in the brain, particularly docosahexanoic acid, occurs from the third trimester to 18 months postpartum.[24] Human milk contains both the precursor essential fatty acids *and* adequate LCPUFA for structural lipid accretion.[25] However, infant formulas have traditionally contained only the parent essential fatty acids, the assumption being that the infant could synthesize LCPUFA from these. Recently, term and preterm infants fed on formulas which contain minimal LCPUFA have been shown to have lower red cell LCPUFA, and lower LCPUFA in the phospholipids of the cerebral cortex and subcutaneous tissues than infants fed breast milk.[18,38,39,74] Whether this biochemical deficiency in formula-fed infants has clinical relevance in terms of long-term growth or neurodevelopment remains controversial, and is the subject of a number of ongoing studies. At present, although there is evidence that supplementing infant formulas with LCPUFA results in *biochemical* improvement, there are relatively few published data relating to long term *clinical* outcome (see below). However, largely on the basis of the biochemical data supporting the view that preterm infants may have a reduced ability to synthesize LCPUFA from the parent essential fatty acids, ESPGAN[37] recommended that formulas for LBW infants should be enriched with metabolites of both linoleic and linolenic acids approximating the levels typical of human milk.

LCPUFA and clinical outcome in preterm infants

Uauy et al[117] showed that deficiency of DHA (docosahexanoic acid) in preterm infants fed unsupplemented formulas was associated with impaired visual function assessed by electroretinogams at 36 weeks' post conceptional age compared to infants fed human milk or formulas with added DHA. However, the differences had disappeared by 4 months post-term. Birch et al[12] showed deficits in visual acuity persisting up to 17 weeks post-term in unsupplemented preterm infants, and Carlson[20] found significantly poorer visual acuity in unsupplemented infants at 2 and 4 months post-term, but not at 6.5, 9 or 12 months. Taken together, these findings support the concept that LCPUFA supplementation may promote more rapid visual maturation; however, whether this has long-term effects on visual performance requires further investigation.

The suggestion that LCPUFA might have a beneficial effect on neurodevelopment in preterm infants gained support from the finding that those fed human milk have better developmental outcome than those fed unsupplemented formulas.[69] However, such comparisons are obviously confounded by socioeconomic factors, and there are many other differences between breast milk and formula which might explain the differences in outcome. In a small randomized study of standard preterm formula versus DHA-supplemented formula, Carlson[19] found that supplemented infants had a higher Bayley mental development index at 12 months post-term: these infants had scores similar to those seen in breast-fed infants. This was a small study (43 infants) and the results could reflect confounding from social and demographic factors, or a type-1 error due to the small sample size. Further studies are in progress.

LCPUFA and clinical outcome in term infants

The situation regarding the need for LCPUFA supplementation of term infant formulas is even more controversial. One randomized trial of docosahexanoic acid supplementation in term infants showed better visual acuity at both 16 and 30 weeks of age in the supplemented group[75], and Birch et al[12a] showed that breast-fed infants have better dot stereo acuity and letter matching ability at 3 years of age than those fed standard unsupplemented formula. However, Innis et al[58] found no difference between breast- and formula-fed infants in visual acuity or recognition memory at 39 weeks of age.

There are as yet no conclusive data relating to LCPUFA supplementation and neurodevelopmental outcome in term infants. Agostoni[1] reported a 10-point advantage in developmental quotient at 4 months of age in infants receiving an LCPUFA-supplemented formula, but this advantage had disappeared at 12- and 24-month follow-up. The ESPGAN committee[37] concluded that although supplementation might be beneficial, further data are required prior to a definite recommendation. A further important consideration is whether the addition of selected LCPUFAs is safe. Various strategies have been used, and they have not been without problems. There is a fine balance between the relative amounts of linoleic and linolenic acids and their longer-chain products, with inhibition of linoleic acid desaturation by long-chain n-3 fatty acids, and competition between arachidonic acid and eicosapentanoic acid for incorporation into membrane lipids. Early attempts at LCPUFA supplementation using fish oils alone as a source of DHA actually resulted in a growth disadvantage,[20] possibly due to a reduction in arachidonic acid formation. In a more recent study looking at LCPUFA supplementation in term infants, Janowsky[60] reported a negative correlation between plasma or red blood cell DHA levels at 4 months of age and subsequent vocabulary production and comprehension at 14 months of age; this was observed for both breast-fed and formula-fed infants. The optimum ratio of n-3 to n-6 LCPUFA, and different sources of LCPUFA, are areas currently under investigation.

Term babies

The EC Directive guidelines recommend that the fat content of infant formulas should lie between 2.0 and 4.9 g per 100 ml of feed.

Preterm babies

The main problem with dietary fat in preterm infants is the increased tendency to steatorrhoea. Reduced fat absorption in low-birthweight infants relates to:[91]

- reduced pancreatic lipase and carboxylic ester hydrolase activity;
- reduced bile acid pool size and secretion rate: the duodenal bile acid concentration may well be below the critical level for micelle formation;
- possible reduction in activity or excretion of lingual lipase.

Fat absorption from fresh breast milk is approximately 90%, but the observed range is enormous. Williamson et al[123] found that fat absorption from expressed breast milk dropped to 55% in very low-birthweight infants fed pasteurized milk, and to around 45% when the milk was boiled. These data may reflect loss, due to heat treatment, of the bile salt-stimulated lipase found in human milk. Unfortunately, there is little information on fat digestion in sick preterm infants.

A controversial issue is the addition of large quantities of medium-chain triglycerides to specially designed preterm infant formulas, largely because such babies absorb palmitic acid (n-16) poorly. The MCT content of human milk is low (less than 2% total fatty acids), whereas modern preterm formulas may contain up to 40% of the fat in this form. MCTs may spare dietary nitrogen and enhance calcium and magnesium absorption.[110] However, recent studies have failed to show improved energy or nitrogen balance, or better weight gain in preterm infants fed MCTs. Indeed, Okatmoto et al[83] showed that although better fat absorption occurred with a high-MCT diet, the infants had a higher incidence of abdominal distension, loose stools, vomiting and increased gastric aspirates. The availability of new fat blends such as Betapol may present an alternative solution in the future.

CARBOHYDRATE

Physiology[62]

The carbohydrate in human milk is almost entirely lactose, which provides 40% of ingested energy. Other carbohydrates, e.g. sucrose and maltodextrins, may be hydrolysed efficiently by active brush-border sucrase, maltase and isomaltase, even in preterm infants, and starch or glucose polymers can be digested by salivary and pancreatic amylase, by amylase present in human milk, and by intestinal mucosal hydrolases.

Dietary lactose undergoes one of two processes: hydrolysis into glucose and galactose by the intestinal brush-border lactase followed by absorption of glucose and galactose, or fermentation in the colon, with production of various gases and short-chain fatty acids.[6] The latter may be important in the nutrition and function of the intestine and colon. For example, short-chain fatty acids administered into the colon have been shown to stimulate intestinal growth following gut resection in animal models, and prevent mucosal atrophy after resection and TPN. There is controversy over the possible role of lactose fermentation in the development of necrotizing enterocolitis. However, although there are some experimental data linking excessive carbohydrate fermentation in the small intestine with an inflammatory condition resembling NEC, there is little evidence that *colonic* lactose fermentation is a primary factor.

Galactose and glucose are absorbed by the same carrier mechanism, and more than 90% reaches the portal vein. Most galactose is removed by the liver on first pass, and appears to be preferentially used for glycogen synthesis rather than conversion to glucose.

Term infants' requirements

The EC Directive recommendation[27] for carbohydrate intake is that it should be between 4.2 and 10.5 g/100 ml of reconstituted feed, and that the lactose content should be above 2.1 g/100 ml (Table 19.1). Other carbohydrate sources that are used (successfully) in modern formulas are maltodextrin and amylose. Although sucrose is well digested by human infants, it renders formulas significantly 'sweeter' than human milk: it is not incorporated in formulas used in the UK, but is present in certain soy-based formulas in the USA.

Preterm infants' requirements

It is difficult to infer from physiological studies which carbohydrate is optimal for low-birthweight infants. Lactose enhances gut absorption of calcium and magnesium and may encourage a favourable gut flora;[17] excessive intakes may result in diarrhoea and metabolic acidosis,[6] yet in practice a high lactose intake in preterm infants is usually well tolerated.

One approach in the design of preterm formulas is to use lactose as the principal carbohydrate source, but to replace a proportion of the carbohydrate with glucose polymers in order to prevent excess osmolality (see Table 19.2 for recommended intakes).

There has been interest recently in the provision of lower-carbohydrate high-fat formulas to preterm infants with chronic lung disease; the aim of the reduced carbohydrate is to lower the respiratory quotient and thereby reduce carbon dioxide production. Such formulas have been demonstrated to support adequate growth while reducing arterial carbon dioxide levels, but their role remains to be defined.[86]

ENERGY

The fundamental energy (E) equation is:

$$E_{intake} = E_{stored} + E_{expended} + E_{excreted} \qquad \text{Eqn. (1)}$$

Energy expended may be subdivided further:

$$E_{expended} = E_{BMR} + E_{activity} + E_{synthesis} + E_{thermoreg} \qquad \text{Eqn (2)}$$

where E_{stored} is the energy deposited during growth, E_{BMR} is the basal energy requirement, $E_{activity}$ is the additional cost of muscular activity, $E_{synthesis}$ is the metabolic cost of growing (excluding energy actually stored in new tissue) and $E_{thermoreg}$ is the energy cost of maintaining body temperature.

Table 19.3 Conventional Atwater conversion factors

	kcal/g	kJ/g
Carbohydrate (expressed as monosaccharide or lactose monohydrate)	3.75	16
Protein (total N × 6.38)	4	17
Fat	9	37

Traditionally the tools used to derive these values have been energy balances and indirect calorimetry (energy expenditure calculated from oxygen consumption and carbon dioxide production) performed under different experimental conditions during rest. More recently the 'doubly labelled water method' has been used to measure total energy expenditure over periods of several days. (The method depends on monitoring the differential disappearance from the body of two stable isotopes, ^{18}O and deuterium, both administered orally as labelled water.)

There has been dispute over which conversion factors should be used for either human or cow's milk to derive the metabolizable energy content (the gross energy of the food from bomb calorimetry minus the energy lost in the stools and urine) from macronutrient concentrations. Although not entirely appropriate to the milk-fed neonate, the conventional Atwater conversion factors derived by Southgate and Durnin[107] are commonly used (Table 19.3).

Term infants' requirements

The EC Directive guidelines recommend that formula should contain similar energy contents to those reported in human milk, i.e. 60–75 kcal/100 ml of reconstituted feed. However, from studies employing the doubly labelled water method, Lucas et al[71] suggested that infants fed on human milk may receive lower energy intakes than those commonly reported and those employed in modern formulas – the values obtained were 53 and 58 kcal/100 ml at 6 weeks and 3 months, respectively; this may explain why modern formula-fed term infants grow faster than their breast-fed counterparts.

Term SGA infants have been reported to have energy expenditures 5–10% higher than AGA infants, and may therefore benefit from increased energy to promote catch-up growth. In one study, a high-energy formula resulted in a marginal increase in weight gain and head growth.[15] However, it is likely that both extra energy and protein are required simultaneously, and this is currently under investigation.

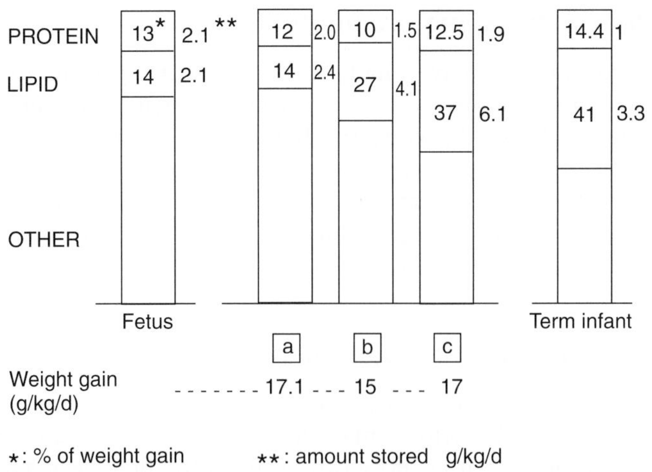

Fig. 19.2 Weight gain composition of the fetus (32–36 weeks) and of the term infant (0–4 months), compared with that of preterm infants fed different diets. (a) Protein-supplemented pooled human milk. (b) Pooled human milk. (c) Preterm formula. Figures represent the percentage of weight gain as protein or fat.

Preterm infants' requirements

The energy requirements for preterm infants cannot be calculated without some consideration of the desired composition of weight gain, as the deposition of different types of tissue incurs different energy costs. For example, 9 kcal are stored in each gram of fat, compared to 4 kcal per gram of protein. Thus, a weight gain high in fat will require more energy to be stored than one high in protein. As previously mentioned (p. 314), the ratio of energy to protein is important in determining the relative amount of lean tissue versus fat which is deposited. These considerations are not just theoretical, as the different diets used for preterm infants do result in variations in the composition of tissue deposited (Fig. 19.2). At present it is not known whether it is best to aim for a weight gain with 15% fat (as in the fetus) or nearer 40% fat (as in a term infant), and unless this can be shown to have implications for future health, one might argue that it is academic. The results to date have been conflicting: DeGamarra[34] and Cooper[29] both found no differences in growth at 2 or 3 years of age in preterm infants who had shown wide differences in adiposity as infants. However, Agras et al[2] reported that greater adiposity at birth was a predictor of greater fatness at 6 years of age. Further studies are obviously required.

All the components of the energy equation have been either measured or estimated in preterm infants, in order to calculate the optimal energy intake. The daily energy cost of activity is around 10 kcal/kg, the cost of thermogenesis 10 kcal/kg/24 h (depending on thermal environment) and, at growth rates of 15 g/kg/24 h, the cost of tissue synthesis is about 10–20 kcal/kg.[89,120] The remaining component of energy expenditure, basal metabolic rate, cannot be measured in preterm infants as it requires at least a 12-hour fast. However, total energy expenditure, which includes all four of these components, has been measured over 5 days with both the doubly labelled water method and indirect calorimetry in four preterm infants[93] growing at a mean rate of 15 g/kg/24 h, and was 58 kcal/kg/24 h (range 57–60). Other studies making measurements over 24-hour periods have produced similar figures, in the range 50–70 kcal/kg/24 h. If these figures are entered into Equation (2):

$$E_{expended} = E_{BMR} + E_{activity} + E_{synthesis} + E_{thermoreg}$$

57–70 ? 10 10–20 10

a value for BMR of between 17 and 40 g kg^{-1} 24 h^{-1} is obtained.

In order to estimate energy requirements, it is necessary to consider both energy stored and energy excreted. In the study by Roberts et al[93], energy stored was 59 kcal/kg/24 h (which is about twice the figure for in utero energy deposition and substantially higher than ideal estimates for preterm infants, owing to the increased fat deposition seen postnatally). Energy losses in the stools have been estimated to be around 10–30 kcal/kg bodyweight, but massive losses may occur (well in excess of 50% of intake) in sick babies with an immature gut. If these figures are entered into Equation (1):

$$E_{intake} = E_{stored} + E_{expended} + E_{excreted}$$

59 57–70 10–30

the required intake would be between 126 and 159 kcal/kg/24 h. This is in the middle of the range recommended by ESPGAN of 110–165 kcal/kg/24 h, and slightly above the 120 kcal/kg/24 h recommended by the recent international panel of experts for the stable preterm infant.

For logistic reasons, very few data are available on the specific energy requirements of sick (as opposed to stable) preterm infants; the techniques used to estimate energy expenditure are not easily applied in such cases. There are no definite data showing an advantage from increasing the energy intake above that recommended for stable preterm infants, and in practice the challenge is usually to provide the desired intake in the face of fluid restriction or feed intolerance associated with the prevailing illness. There are some data on infants with chronic lung disease demonstrating an increase in energy expenditure of 15–30%, particularly in those who are failing to thrive.[33,64,119,127] However, the poor growth in these infants may more often reflect suboptimal nutrient intake, since in most studies energy intakes fail to reach the estimated requirements for stable preterm infants, let alone those who might have higher requirements.[124]

WATER (Chapter 39, Part 1)

Water is a major nutrient (for review, see Wharton[120]). However, the quantity deposited in growth (around

10 ml/kg/24 h by preterm infants, for instance) is minute compared with water turnover. Clearly in sick babies it would be impossible to allow nutrient intakes to vary in parallel with water requirement, and water must be treated as an 'independent variable'.

NUCLEOTIDES

There has been increasing interest over the last decade in the role of nucleotides in infant nutrition. Breast milk contains at least 13 different nucleotides, accounting for 5% of non-protein nitrogen.[59] Cow's milk has lower levels and a different nucleotide profile. Until recently, no infant formula in the UK contained additional nucleotides, although supplemented formulas have been available in Spain and Japan for some years. Nucleotides are important in cell-mediated immunity, and it has been suggested that they are one of the anti-infective agents in breast milk, responsible for the lower levels of infection reported in breast-fed infants. However, although there is good evidence for the role of dietary nucleotides in animals (for example enhancing T-cell function,[96] improving intestinal growth and maturation in weanling rats[116]), the evidence for a clinical benefit in human infants is less convincing. A variety of short-term effects have been reported for nucleotide-supplemented formulas, including an alteration in the plasma lipoprotein profile during the first month of life with increased HDL-cholesterol in supplemented infants similar to the levels seen in breast-fed infants,[98] and alteration in the bowel flora following nucleotide supplementation, with a predominance of lactobacilli as seen in the breast-fed infant[46] (although this latter finding could not be reproduced by Balmer et al[9]). Also of interest is the report of increased killer T-cell function and increased production of interleukin-2 reported in infants fed a nucleotide-supplemented formula, compared to those fed a standard formula.[22] These changes persisted up to 6 months of age, but were not associated with any detectable change in the incidence or severity of infection. Thus, although there are potential advantages for the addition of nucleotides to infant formulas, further clinical outcome studies are required.

Nucleotides have been added to formulas in Spain and Japan for up to 7 years without apparent adverse side-effects, and they have also been used as flavour enhancers in foods for many years; thus safety is not thought to be a problem.

MACROMINERALS (Tables 19.1, 19.2, 19.4)

Sodium, potassium and chloride

Calculation of desirable intakes of sodium, potassium and chloride requires a knowledge of renal function (Chapter 39, Part 1).

Term infants' requirements

Two factors have had an important bearing on recommendations for dietary sodium intake in young infants. First, the concern that high salt intake might result in dangerous hypernatraemia at times of excessive water loss (e.g. diarrhoea), and secondly the theoretical, though unconvincing, evidence that early salt intake might predispose to later high blood pressure.

Preterm infants' requirements

Sodium. Major adjustments in body sodium occur in the neonatal period: massive renal losses of up to 10 mmol/kg/24 h or more can occur in the first week and may be independent of intake. It is impossible accurately to predict sodium needs in the early neonatal period, and in very small and sick infants, regardless of diet, plasma sodium should be monitored and hyponatraemia of < 133 mmol/l – and certainly < 130 mmol/l – should be corrected.

Preterm breast milk has a higher sodium content (10–20 mmol/l or more during the early weeks of lactation) than mature donor milk (about 6 mmol/l or less). Hyponatraemia has been noted in human milk-fed preterm infants; it is more severe in those fed donor milk. Intakes from donor milk and preterm milk, providing around 1 mmol and 2 mmol/kg/24 h, respectively, during the first month, are often inadequate, and Aperia et al[4] have recommended 3 mmol/kg/24 h.

The high sodium content of modern preterm formulas is usually only required in the early neonatal period. After that the excess sodium needs to be excreted. However, in a large randomized study[72], preterm neonates fed on a formula providing 3.6 mmol/l did not have an increased risk of hypernatraemia, compared to those fed standard formula or breast milk (providing under half the sodium intake), and 18 months later did not show any elevation in blood pressure.

Potassium and chloride. In general human milk and the available adapted formulas provided adequate potassium and chloride to meet intrauterine accretion rates of 0.9 and 0.7 mmol/kg/24 h.[120]

Calcium and phosphorus (Table 19.4)

Term infants

Calcium is less well absorbed from cow's milk than from human milk. However, in spite of the high levels of calcium and phosphorus in cow's milk, the relatively higher phosphorus intake has in the past resulted in hyperphosphataemia, hypocalcaemia with convulsions (see below), and other complications such as dental hypoplasia.[109] Moreover, the high phosphorus content in unmodified cow's milk may also induce hypo-

Table 19.4 Digestion, physiological role and deficiency states of calcium, phosphorus and magnesium

	Digestion	Physiological role	Deficiency states
Calcium	Absorption by both passive and active transport: Ca, Mg-ATPase facilitates uptake into the mucosal cells, where a calcium-binding protein is induced by vitamin D. 20–60% retention, according to diet (better with human milk) but increased by vitamin D and parathormone and reduced by complexing with dietary fat, phosphate and phytates. Part bound, e.g. to protein, part free in plasma	Bones are major stores. Also required for cell membrane function, neuromuscular activity, clotting and a wide variety of cellular functions	Tetany, bone demineralization, arrhythmias, paralytic ileus, fits
Phosphorus	70–95% absorption, increased by vitamin D, reduced by insoluble intraluminal complex formation, e.g. with phytate or if excessive calcium salts added. Commonly elevated in plasma in neonatal period in cow's milk formula-fed term infants; nadir in preterm infants at 1–2 weeks	Bone mineralization, ATP, DNA, RNA, phospholipids and many other biological roles	Rickets is rare in full term newborns. Phosphate deficiency syndrome may arise, particularly in infants fed by total parenteral nutrition: listlessness, poor feeding, rapid shallow breathing, muscle weakness, impaired oxygen release from haemoglobin, bone disease, nephrocalcinosis
Magnesium	Some transport mechanisms may be shared with calcium: absorption increased by vitamin D and parathormone and decreased by steatorrhoea and phytates. High fetal plasma levels, which may fall after birth	Stored in bone. Important intracellular cation, muscle contraction, cofactor for carbohydrate, protein and energy metabolism	Weakness, poor feeding, failure to thrive, paralytic ileus, calcium-resistant tetany, fits, apnoea

magnesaemia and, in some cases of neonatal tetany, convulsions can be alleviated only by administration of magnesium.[26] Current recommendations for calcium and phosphorus are shown in Table 19.1

Preterm infants' requirements

Considerable attention has been focused on the calcium and phosphorus requirements of low-birthweight infants,[120] stimulated by the high incidence of metabolic bone disease seen in this population (Chapter 38, Part 4).

Magnesium

The recommended intake for term infants is given in Table 19.1, and the physiology outlined in Table 19.5. Body magnesium content, largely in bone, rises rapidly in the third trimester so that preterm infants are born with low reserves.[30] In preterm infants, net magnesium absorption in the first week is about 50% and is largely independent of vitamin D. Magnesium deficiency may impair calcium homoeostasis. Atkinson et al[5] showed that infants fed on preterm milk (2.5–3.0 mg magnesium per 100 ml) failed to retain this element at intrauterine accretion rates, and showed evidence of falling reserves; in contrast, a formula-fed group receiving 2–3 times more magnesium retained it at a somewhat greater rate than in utero. In human milk-fed infants dietary supplementation with phosphorus improves magnesium retention by reducing urine losses.[63]

Iron

Term infants

Iron stores at birth are influenced by gestation, birthweight and the extent of the placental transfusion at delivery. Healthy breast-fed infants absorb iron well from human milk and usually maintain normal iron stores during the first 4–6 months (p. 329). However, the bioavailability of iron in cow's milk (especially) and cow's milk formulas is much less than in human milk. The EC Directive recommended that formulas used from birth should, if iron is added, contain 0.5–1. 5 mg/100 kcal, and follow-on milks should contain 1–2 mg/100 kcal (Table 19.1). The recommended daily intake in infancy is 6 mg, but in the USA 10–15 mg/day is recommended.

Preterm infants' requirements

A 1.0 kg fetus contains 64 mg iron,[122] and this increases subsequently in utero at a rate of 1.8 mg/kg/24 h. About 25% of iron is stored in the liver as ferritin, and most of the rest is present in haemoglobin. After birth, therefore, a 1.0 kg infant only has sufficient iron to synthesize about 18.0 g of haemoglobin (3.4 mg iron per gram haemoglobin), and since the iron content of human milk is 40 µg per 100 ml or less (providing 80 µg/kg/24 h fed at 200 ml/kg/24 h) human milk-fed preterm infants will eventually develop an iron deficiency anaemia without supplementation.

Iron stores usually remain adequate during the first 6–8 weeks, and iron supplementation at this stage has

Table 19.5 Trace metals

	Physiology	Deficiency states
Iodine	Well absorbed, concentrated in thyroid gland, incorporated in thyroxine and tri-iodothyronine. Excess is excreted in urine	Endemic goitre in areas where human milk is deficient; soy formulas are iodine-deficient and are usually supplemented
Zinc	Present in a large number of metalloenzymes, including alkaline phosphatase and carbonic anhydrase. Required for insulin activity. Absorption partly by active transport. Bioavailability influenced by diet: poor absorption from diets of plant origin. Nadir in plasma zinc at around 2–3 months. Infants fed by total parenteral nutrition and those with gut disease are especially liable to clinical deficiency	Acrodermatitis syndrome (see p. 895). Delayed diagnosis if signs mistaken for 'nappy rash' of another aetiology. (NB May be inherited as a rare autosomal recessive disorder). Also mild deficiency in infancy, or later, may be associated with reduced growth, loss of appetite, impaired taste acuity and perhaps pica. Impaired immune responses, poor wound healing
Copper	Copper-containing enzymes include cytochrome oxidase, tyrosinase and uricase; required for iron utilization, myelinization and connective tissue formation. Absorption: stomach and small intestine. Stored in liver and muscle, attached to caeruloplasmin	See text
Manganese	Role: found in mitochondria, required for carbohydrate metabolism; actively absorbed in duodenum. Transport protein: transmanganin, a specific β-globulin. Excretion is largely biliary	No deficiency state described in human infants
Chromium	Role: potentiates insulin-induced glucose uptake. Poorly absorbed. Transported by transferrin. Body stores: low	In one study, diabetic glucose tolerance tests were corrected in infants with kwashiorkor
Fluoride	Enters bone and teeth, increasing their hardness. Supplementation is not recommended currently during the first 6 months	Dental caries. Excess: fluorosis, including rotting of teeth
Molybdenum	Present in xanthine oxidase. Active transfer across the placenta	No deficiency disease clearly recognized in human infants
Selenium	Role: antioxidant – cofactor for vitamin E	Deficiency not defined in neonates but described in children and adults living in the Keshan province of China: generalized myopathy with cardiac failure and haemolytic anaemia. Possibly occurs in preterm infants on unsupplemented long-term parenteral nutrition
Cobalt	Cobalt is a component of vitamin B_{12} and may not be needed independently of B_{12} requirement	

no influence on anaemia of prematurity. By 12 weeks iron stores become depleted in unsupplemented infants, and iron deficiency anaemia develops.[50] Intakes of 2.0–3.0 mg/kg/24 h have been shown by several groups to prevent such anaemia.

It is recommended that preterm infants receive a supplement of no more than 2.5 mg/kg/24 h of iron, starting between 6 and 8 weeks of age and continuing until 12 months, or until full mixed feeding provides an adequate iron intake. Although there is no definite evidence that giving iron-fortified formulas from birth is harmful, some have argued that formulas designed for preterm infants should contain no additional iron.

Recently there has been increasing interest in the use of recombinant human erythropoietin in preterm infants to reduce the requirement for blood transfusion. Studies have demonstrated[100] that infants treated with r-HuEPO require higher amounts of iron – up to 6 mg/kg/24 h – and that this should be initiated at the same time as the r-HuEPO.

TRACE METALS

Summaries of physiological roles and the consequences of deficiency are shown in Table 19.5 and recommended intakes for term infants in Table 19.1.

Zinc

Zinc has been found in over 70 metalloproteins, mostly enzymes, including both DNA and RNA polymerase; it plays a critical role in cell replication and growth.[101,120]

Zinc accumulates in the fetus during the last trimester at around 250 μg/kg/24 h. The amount of zinc provided by 200 ml of human milk per kilogram per day falls from 1650 μg on the first day of lactation to 160 μg after 4 months. Therefore, human milk collected during the early (but not later) months of lactation theoretically provides enough zinc to meet 'in utero' accretion rates. Zinc in banked donor milk would be adequate. However, Dauncey et al[30] found that human milk-fed preterm infants did not achieve positive zinc balance until after 40 days of age.

Zinc deficiency has been described as a late sequel (2–4 months) of preterm birth:[90] these infants develop a syndrome very similar to acrodermatitis enteropathica, with growth arrest, irritability, anorexia, alopecia, diarrhoea, vesiculopustular lesions of the hands and feet, and the characteristic perioral, facial and perineal dermatitis; plasma zinc levels, though not necessarily helpful, are usually <35 μg/100 ml (5.4 mmol/l) (normal above 70 μg/100 ml). Infants respond rapidly to oral zinc sulphate (providing 1.0–3.5 mg zinc per day).

Although there is some evidence that plasma zinc levels are lower in healthy formula-fed term infants than breast-fed ones,[66] this does not appear to be reflected in any differences in growth; indeed, in another study[97] zinc supplementation of formula had no effect on growth velocity. However, the situation may be different in more vulnerable groups. For example, a randomized study in preterm infants fed either a zinc-supplemented or a placebo-supplemented term formula for 6 months from the time at which they attained 1.8 kg, showed higher plasma zinc levels, significantly greater linear growth velocity and higher maximum motor development scores in the supplemented group.[42] More recently, a randomized study of zinc supplementation in formula-fed SGA infants in Chile showed greater catch-up growth over the first 6 months of life in the supplemented group.[23]

The EC Directive guidelines[27] recommend a zinc concentration of 300–750 μg/100 ml formula for term infants, and the international consensus committee[113] recommended 490 μg/100 ml of formula for preterm infants. The value of zinc supplementation for the long-term growth and development of infants born preterm or small for gestational age requires further study.

Copper

Copper accumulates in the fetus during the last trimester at about 50 μg/kg/24 h; 200 ml per kilogram per day of human milk provides about 60–80 μg/kg/24 h. Nevertheless, Dauncey et al[30] found that preterm infants fed human milk were in negative balance during the first 12 days of life, and 1 out of 6 infants were still in negative balance at 40 days.[101,120]

Several cases of copper deficiency have been described in infants born prematurely and fed on cow's milk-based formulas or copper-free parenteral nutrition solutions.[101] The features of copper deficiency are:

- psychomotor retardation
- hypotonia
- pallor and hypopigmentation
- prominent scalp veins in periosteal depressions
- hepatosplenomegaly
- X-ray changes of osteoporosis, blurring and cupping of metaphyses, subperiosteal new bone formation, fractures
- sideroblastic anaemia, resistant to iron therapy
- Bone marrow shows vacuolated erythroid and myeloid cells, with iron deposition in the vacuoles
- neutropenia $<1.0 \times 10^9$/l (< 1000/mm^3)
- plasma copper usually < 30 mg/100 ml and caeruloplasmin 2–10 mg/100 ml.

Several features are liable to develop when plasma copper falls below 20 mg/100 ml and caeruloplasmin below 5 mg/100 ml. Treatment with copper 0.6–0.8 mg/kg/24 h, given as 1% copper sulphate solution, is effective.

There is no evidence that human milk-fed preterm infants require additional copper.

Iodine

Iodine is found almost entirely in the thyroid, where it is incorporated into thyroglobulin and thyroid hormones. It is possible that a syndrome of transient hypothyroidism, seen in preterm infants, could be due to lack of iodine in iodine-deficient areas.[35] The iodine content of breast milk is affected by maternal diet[80] but is usually sufficient. The EC directive guidelines suggest a minimum of 8 μg/100 ml of formula.

Other trace minerals

Manganese, selenium, chromium and molybdenum are all essential elements, but no definite deficiency states have been described in preterm infants fed human milk or cow's milk-based formulas;[120] quantitative recommendations cannot be made on strong grounds. Manganese is found in very large unphysiological quantities in some formulas (especially soy-based ones), with values up to 100–1000 times those in human milk. It is not known whether these intakes are toxic, but there seems no basis for giving more than 5 μg/100 ml of formula (human milk contains around 0.5–2.5 μg/100 ml).

Aluminium

Aluminium is not a nutrient – it has not been found in any metalloprotein, yet it has been added to drinking water (as a clarifying agent); it contaminates artificial formulas, especially soy formulas, which may contain 100 times the aluminium level of breast milk, and is present in massive concentrations in some components of intravenous feeding solutions, notably calcium and phosphorus preparations.[73] In patients on renal dialysis, with limited ability to excrete aluminium, toxicity is well described, with dementia, anaemia and bone disease. Preterm infants have immature kidney function and their intake of aluminium from parenteral nutrition solutions – and to a lesser extent from formulas – may be much higher than from breast milk. Studies are in progress to assess whether infants are at risk of aluminium toxicity.

VITAMINS

Clinical vitamin deficiency is rare in the neonatal period in the west, but a variety of circumstances predispose to deficiencies that may become apparent in infancy: these include maternal vitamin depletion, with reduced placental transport and low vitamin concentrations in breast milk, unsupplemented formulas (current formulas in the west are vitamin supplemented), total parenteral nutrition, the use of unconventional non-milk based diets, parasitic infestation, neonatal gut and biliary disease, and prematurity.

Optimal intake levels for many vitamins have not been determined in human infants. Broadly, vitamin intakes from breast milk have been taken as a guide (Table 19.1), but excess supplementation in formulas is usually employed in order to compensate for losses during preparation and storage and lower bioavailability. There is no clear evidence showing detrimental effects of excess vitamin supplementation, except for vitamins A and D, though it has been suggested that excessive vitamin E intake may interfere with wound healing and iron 'status'.

The physiological roles of vitamins and clinical consequences of deficiency are summarized in Table 19.6.

Term infants

Current recommended levels for formula-fed infants are shown in Table 19.1.

Preterm infants' requirements (Table 19.2)

Preterm infants may have special needs for some vitamins because:

- They are born with low body stores, especially of the fat-soluble vitamins which normally accumulate during the third trimester;
- they may have reduced absorptive capacities for some vitamins (e.g. vitamin E);
- they might benefit from 'pharmacological doses' of certain vitamins, e.g. vitamin E.

In what follows a brief account is given of selected vitamins that have been of particular interest in the dietary management of preterm infants.[112,120]

Vitamin A

Vitamin A is required for the synthesis of retinal pigments and for the development and maintenance of epithelial membranes. The active form, retinol, is transported in plasma, bound to retinol-binding protein. Synthesis of RBP usually occurs late in gestation, and plasma retinol and RBP concentrations are lower in preterm than in term infants.[104] RBP also has a lower level of saturation in premature neonates. These data suggest that preterm infants have low body stores of vitamin A and are therefore at risk of deficiency (see p. 619).

In view of these observations, vitamin A supplementation of human milk-fed preterm infants seems wise (see below). Vitamin A can be obtained from the diet in two forms: preformed vitamin A (largely retinol) and carotenoids (chiefly β-carotene). Although β-carotene is potentially a good, non-toxic source of vitamin A, its use in preterm infants is relatively unexplored. Vitamin A is light degraded: 70% can be lost from human milk during a 3-hour enteral infusion into an infant under phototherapy lighting.[10] Care must be taken to ensure that the principal source of vitamin A given to preterm infants is not light exposed.

Vitamin D

The term 'vitamin D' is often used to refer to both vitamin D_2, originating from the plant sterol ergosterol, and vitamin D_3, the natural vitamin synthesized in the skin from 7-dehydrocholesterol. Vitamin D_2 (or D_3) is converted to 25-hydroxyvitamin D (25-OHD, calcidiol) in the liver, and thence into the active metabolite 1,25-dihydroxyvitamin D (1,25-$(OH)_2$D), calcitriol, in the kidney. A major function of 1,25-$(OH)_2$D is to increase calcium and phosphorus absorption from the intestine, but it also conserves these two elements by its action on the kidney.

Preterm infants may have greater requirements for vitamin D than infants born at term; they have lower stores at birth and greater demands for skeletal mineralization, and although the vitamin D pathway is intact, it may not be fully developed at very low gestation. The dose normally recommended for full-term infants, 400 iu per day, is probably well in excess of requirements for normal babies. However, in preterm infants doses of up to 800–2000 iu per day have been given. Although these high doses have been shown to increase calcium absorption, vitamin D is no substitute for calcium and phosphorus supplementation in the prevention of bone disease (Chapter 38, Part 4). If intake of these minerals is adequate there seems no justification in giving more than 400–600 iu vitamin D per day. The use of 25-OHD rather than vitamin D may seem logical, as in very small preterm infants absorption of vitamin D may be impaired by a small bile-salt pool size and fat malabsorption. Nevertheless, the use of such active metabolites of vitamin D, and especially the more potent ones (for example 1-$_{\alpha}$-OHD), is experimental and potentially dangerous.

Table 19.6 Vitamins: physiology and diseases caused by deficiency (or excess)

	Physiology	Deficiency (or excess)
Vitamin A	Retinyl esters are the main contributor to vitamin A activity in milk, though both cow's and human milk contain the retinol precursor beta-carotene. Partly emulsified by bile salts, partly hydrolysed by lipase and re-esterified to retinyl palmitate in gut mucosa. One-sixth of dietary carotene is converted into active vitamin A. Stored in liver. Secreted by liver into the bloodstream in association with retinol-binding protein: secretion of vitamin A is tightly regulated, like that of a hormone. Required for the synthesis of rhodopsin and other retinal pigments: important for the development of epithelial cells (and therefore the maintenance of epithelial membranes). Degraded by light	Xerophthalmia, susceptibility to infection, keratinization of mucous membranes, blindness Excess, e.g. 18 000 iu/day or above: raised intracranial pressure, dry skin, loss of hair, brittle bones, irritability
Vitamin E	Placental transfer low. Liver stores may be low. Iron may interfere with absorption and activity. Polyunsaturated fatty acids increase E requirement. Role: antioxidant, prevents oxidation of unsaturated fats thereby increasing stability of cell membranes	Clinical disease states poorly defined. Reduces postnatal red cell haemolysis
Vitamin D	Absorptive mechanisms not fully investigated in human infant: bile salts may be required – absorbed into lymphatic system. Stored in adipose tissue and muscle with small amounts in skin and liver. Sunlight-induced synthesis in the skin from 7-dehydrocholesterol will be minimal in many neonates; active metabolites are 25- and 1,25-hydroxyvitamin D (25-OHD and 1,25-$(OH)_2D$): these act as steroid hormones. Principal role: the enhancement of calcium and phosphate absorption from gut and renal conservation of these elements. Also important for the normal mineralization of bones and teeth	Rickets, tetany. Maternal vitamin D deficiency may rarely result in neonatal rickets. Very small amounts of vitamin D in breast milk – occasionally insufficient, especially if light exposure minimal Excess: intakes of over 4000 iu/day may result in hypercalcaemia. At intakes greater than 10 000 iu/kg per day: ectopic calcification, failure to thrive
Vitamin K	Emulsified by bile salts. Synthesis by gut flora is much debated. Stores in liver are relatively small. Maternal deficiency predisposes to neonatal deficiency. Role: manufacture of clotting factors (including II, VII, IX and X) and bone metabolism	Haemorrhagic disease of newborn Excess: haemolytic anaemia can be caused by the water-soluble analogue
Thiamine (B_1)	Role: coenzyme in many enzyme systems: pathways involving acetyl CoA	Anorexia, irritability, fatigue, oedema, heart failure, constipation, peripheral neuropathy
Riboflavin (B_2)	Component of flavoenzymes: involved in electron transport processes, e.g. in energy metabolism, fatty acid oxidation. Degraded by light	Cheilosis, angular stomatitis, impaired fatty acid oxidation and iron economy
Niacin	Part of NAD–NADP system of Krebs cycle; involved in protein and fat synthesis. Dietary tryptophan will supply niacin: 60 mg tryptophan = 1 mg niacin	Diarrhoea, dermatitis, neurological disturbance
Pyridoxine (B_6)	Role: modification of functional groups, especially in amino acid metabolism (decarboxylation, transamination, oxidation, desulphurylation)	Convulsions, dermatitis, weakness, anaemia
Vitamin B_{12}	Coenzyme for methionine synthesis and indirectly for DNA synthesis, folic acid metabolism, conversion of methylmalonic to succinic acid	Pernicious anaemia, central nervous system damage
Folic acid	Role: enzyme systems taking part in one-carbon transfers in DNA, RNA, methionine and serine synthesis, needed for histidine utilization. Synthesized by gut flora	Megaloblastic anaemia, retarded growth, gastrointestinal disturbance
Pantothenic acid	Roles: part of coenzyme A system, involved in energy and fat metabolism. Synthesized by gut flora	No dietary deficiency state described in man
Biotin	Role: carboxylation reactions, especially concerned with fatty acid synthesis. Produced by gut flora	Possibly skin rashes
Vitamin C	Water-soluble. Absorbed in upper intestine. Not stored: excess excreted in urine. Maternal deficiency may result in neonatal deficiency. Intake from unsupplemented pasteurized cow's milk is minimal. Role: involved in collagen synthesis and in several aspects of amino acid metabolism: protects against hypertyrosinaemia and hyperphenylalaninaemia in newborn period; promotes conversion of folic acid to folinic acid, catecholamine synthesis, carnitine synthesis, iron absorption	Biochemical deficiency may arise in newborn period – overt scurvy rare below 3 months of age

Vitamin E

Increased intakes of vitamin E, which is a powerful antioxidant, may be required to prevent haemolytic anaemia in preterm infants, especially those receiving a diet rich in PUFA or iron. (Polyunsaturated lipids in cell membranes are liable to oxidative damage, which may be enhanced by iron.) There has been much interest in the use of pharmacological doses of vitamin E in preterm infants, but current evidence suggests that it is of no proven benefit in preventing or treating clinically significant retinopathy of prematurity (Chapter 36), and has no role in bronchopulmonary dysplasia (Chapter 29, Part 3) or in the prevention of intraventricular haemorrhage (Chapter 44, Part 3). Against giving high (pharmacological) doses of vitamin E is its potential toxicity; local reactions may occur at the site of intramuscular injection, and high plasma levels have been associated with sepsis and necrotizing enterocolitis in preterm infants.

Vitamin E requirements must be related to the amount of PUFA in the diet. Human milk contains adequate vitamin E in relation to its PUFA content. Additional supplements are of dubious benefit, but 5 mg/24 h is safe if the objective is to attempt to reduce anaemia. The better-absorbed water-soluble form should be used. High pharmacological doses (25–100 mg/24 h) require concomitant monitoring of plasma levels, which should not exceed 4 mg/100 ml.

Vitamin K

Despite recent controversy over the optimum route for administration and the dose required, vitamin K should be routinely given to full-term infants as a prophylaxis against haemorrhagic disease (p. 798). When given orally to breast-fed infants it is recommended that repeat doses are given at around 1 and 6 weeks, to avoid the risk of intracranial bleeding from late haemorrhagic disease. The effectiveness of multiple oral doses is still unevaluated, but the Danish experience over the last 3 years is that 12 weekly oral doses are completely effective, even in infants with liver disease.[81] The situation in sick term or preterm infants is not controversial: all such infants should receive 0.5–1.0 mg of vitamin K parenterally on the first day.

Folic acid

Folic acid dosages for preterm infants very considerably. Gandy and Jacobson[44] showed a major benefit of high-dose folic acid supplementation on the growth of erythroblastotic infants. In a large randomized study Stevens et al[108] were unable to demonstrate differences in growth between low-birthweight infants given either a supplement of 100 µg of folic acid per day (from 3 weeks to 12 months) or a formula containing only 3.5 µg folic acid per 100 ml (similar to human milk), and no infant became anaemic. More recently, however, Worthington-White et al[125] showed that formula-fed preterm infants who received supplemental folate for the first 6 months (100 µg/24 h) had higher serum folate concentrations and a significantly reduced fall in haemoglobin over the study period. An intake of at least 100 µg/24 h seems prudent for all low-birthweight infants until 40 weeks post-conceptional age.

Vitamin C and pyridoxal phosphate (B_6)

Vitamin C has been shown to prevent hypertyrosinaemia and hyperphenylalaninaemia in low-birthweight infants, especially those on high protein intakes. In view of this and the low vitamin C levels of unsupplemented preterm infants, a supplement is recommended (see below).

Supplementary B_6 might also be expected to improve protein utilization, in view of its role as a cofactor in amino acid metabolic pathways.

Riboflavin (B_2)

The requirement of preterm infants for riboflavin is currently under review. Most human milk-fed preterm infants develop biochemical evidence of riboflavin deficiency if they have received no supplement after the first week.[67] This problem is compounded by the massive destruction of riboflavin by light when milk is handled in neonatal units. Early biochemical riboflavin deficiency has been shown to be prevented using a preterm formula containing 180 µg of riboflavin per 100 ml, or by using a riboflavin-containing multivitamin preparation.[67]

REFERENCES

1. Agostoni C, Trojan S, Bellu R, Riva E, Giovannini M 1995 Neurodevelopmental quotient of healthy term infants at 4 months and feeding practice: the role of long chain polyunsaturated fatty acids. Pediatric Research 38: 262–266
2. Agras W S, Kraemer H C, Berkowitz R I, Hommer L D 1990 Influence of early feeding style on adiposity at 6 years of age. Journal of Pediatrics 116: 805–809
3. American Academy of Paediatrics Committee on Nutrition 1977 Nutritional needs of low-birth-weight infants. Pediatrics 60: 519–530
4. Aperia A, Broberger O, Zetterstrom R 1982 Implications of limitation of renal function for the nutrition of low birthweight infants. Acta Paediatrica Scandinavica Suppl. 296: 49–52
5. Atkinson S A, Radde I C, Anderson G H 1983 Macromineral balances in premature infants fed their own mother's milk or formula. Journal of Pediatrics 102: 96–106
6. Aurichio S, Rubino A, Murset G 1965 Intestinal glycosidase activities in the human embryo, fetus and newborn. Pediatrics 35: 944–954
7. Aynsley-Green A 1985 Metabolic and endocrine interrelations in the human fetus and neonate. American Journal of Clinical Nutrition 41: 399–418
8. Baker H, Frank O, Thompson A D et al 1975 Vitamin profile of 174 mothers and newborn at parturition. American Journal of Clinical Nutrition 28: 59–65
9. Balmer S E, Hanvey L S, Wharton B A 1994 Diet and faecal flora in the newborn: nucleotides. Archives of Disease in Childhood 70: F137–140
10. Bates C J, Liu D-S, Fuller N J, Lucas A 1985 Susceptibility of riboflavin and vitamin A in breast milk to photodegradation and its implications for the use of banked breast milk in infant feeding. Acta Paediatrica Scandinavica 74: 40–44
11. Berseth C L, Nordyke C 1993 Enteral nutrients promote postnatal maturation of intestinal motor activity in preterm infants. American Journal of Physiology 264:1046–1051
12. Birch D, Birch E, Hoffman D R, Uauy R 1992 Retinal development in very low birth weight infants fed diets differing in omega-3 fatty acids. Investigative Ophthalmology and Visual Science 33: 2365–2376

12a. Birch E, Birch D, Hoffman D, Hale L, Everett M, Uauy R 1993 Breast feeding and optimal visual development. Journal of Pediatric Ophthalmology and Strabismus 30: 33–38

13. Blondheim O, Abbasi S, Fox W W, Bhutani V K 1993 Effect of enteral gavage feeding rate on pulmonary functions of very low birth weight infants. Journal of Pediatrics 122: 751–755
14. Boehm G, Muller DM Beyreiss K, Raiha N C 1988 Evidence for functional immaturity of the ornithine-urea cycle in very-low-birth-weight infants. Biology of the Neonate 54: 121–125
15. Brooke O G, Kinzey J M 1985 High energy feeding in small for gestation neonates. Archives of Disease in Childhood 60: 42–46
16. Brooke O G, Wood C, Barley J 1982 Energy balance, nitrogen balance and growth in preterm infants fed expressed breast milk, a premature infant formula and two low-solute adapted formulae. Archives of Disease in Childhood 57: 898–904
17. Bullen C L, Willis A T 1971 Resistance of the breast fed infant to gastroenteritis. British Medical Journal iii: 338–343
18. Carlson S E, Rhodes P G, Ferguson M G 1986 Docosahexaenoic acid status of preterm infants at birth and following feeding with milk or formula. American Journal of Clinical Nutrition 44: 798–804
19. Carlson S E, Werkman S H, Peeples J M, Wilson W M 1994 Long chain fatty acids and early visual and cognitive development of preterm infants. European Journal of Clinical Nutrition 48: S27–30
20. Carlson S E, Werkman S H, Peeples J M et al 1992 Growth and development of very low birth weight infants in relation to n-3 and n-6 essential fatty acids. In: Sinclair A, Gibson R (eds) Essential fatty acids and eicosanoids: Invited papers from the Third International Congress. American Oil Chemists Society, Champaign, IL: 192–196
21. Carnielli V P, Luijendijk I H T, van Beek R H T, Boerma G J M, Degenhart H J, Sauer P J J 1995 Effect of dietary triacylglycerol fatty acid positional distribution on plasma lipid classes and their fatty acid composition in preterm infants. American Journal of Clinical Nutrition 62: 776–781
22. Carver J D, Pimentel B, Cox W I, Barness L A 1991 Dietary nucleotide effects upon immune function in infants. Pediatrics 88: 359–363
23. Castillo-Duran C, Rodriguez A, Venegas G, Alvarez P, Icaza G 1995 Zinc supplementation and growth of infants born small for gestational age. Journal of Pediatrics 127: 206–211
24. Clandinin M T, Chappell J E, Leong S, Heim T, Swyer P R, Chance G W 1980 Extrauterine fatty acid accretion in infant brain: implications for fatty acid requirements. Early Human Development 4: 131–138
25. Clandinin M T, Chappell J E, Heim T, Swyer P R, Chance G W 1981 Fatty acid utilization in perinatal de novo synthesis of tissues. Early Human Development 5: 355–366
26. Cockburn F, Brown J K, Belton N R, Forfar J O 1973 Neonatal convulsions associated with primary disturbance of calcium, phosphorus and magnesium. Archives of Disease in Childhood 48: 99–103
27. Commission Directive on Infant Formulae and Follow-on Formula (91/321/EC) 1996 O.J.No. L 175/35.
28. Coombs R C, Morgan M E, Durbin G M, Booth I W, McNeish A S 1992 Doppler assessment of human neonatal gut blood flow velocities: postnatal adaptation and response to feeds. Journal of Pediatric Gastroenterology and Nutrition 15: 6–12
29. Cooper P A, Rothberg A, Davies V A, Horn J, Vogelman L 1989 Three-year growth and developmental follow-up of very low birth weight infants fed own mother's milk, a premature formula, or one of two standard formulas. Journal of Paediatric Gastroenterology and Nutrition 8: 348–354
30. Dauncey M J, Shaw J C, Urman J 1977 The absorption and retention of magnesium, zinc and copper by low birthweight infants fed pasteurized human breast milk. Pediatric Research 11: 1033–1039
31. Davidson M, Levine S, Bauer C, Dann M 1967 Feeding studies in low birthweight infants. Journal of Pediatrics 70: 695–713
32. Dear PRF 1980 Effect of feeding on jugular venous blood flow in the normal newborn infant. Archives of Disease in Childhood 55: 365–370
33. De Gamarra E 1992 Energy expenditure in premature newborns with bronchopulmonary dysplasia. Biology of the Neonate 61: 337–344
34. De Gamarra M E, Schutz Y, Catzeflis C et al 1987 Composition of weight gain during the neonatal period and longitudinal growth follow-up in premature babies. Biology of the Neonate 52: 181–187
35. Delange F, Bourdoux P, Ketelbant-Balasse P, Van Humskerken A, Glinoer D, Ermans A M 1983 Transient primary hypothyroidism in the newborn. In: Dussault J H, Walker P (eds) Congenital hypothyroidism. Marcel Dekker, New York, pp 275–301
36. Dunn L, Hulman S, Weiner J, Kliegman R 1988 Beneficial effects of early hypocaloric enteral feeding on neonatal gastrointestinal function: preliminary report of a randomised controlled trial. Journal of Pediatrics 112: 622–629
37. ESPGAN 1987 Committee on Nutrition of preterm infant, European Society of Paediatric Gastroenterology and Nutrition. Nutrition and feeding of preterm infants. Acta Paediatrica Scandinavica 336: 1–14
38. Farquharson J, Cockburn F, Patrick W A, Jamieson E C, Logan R W 1992 Infant cerebral cortex phospholipid fatty acid composition and diet. Lancet 340: 810–813
39. Farquharson J, Jamieson E C, Abbasi K A, Patrick W J A, Logan R W, Cockburn F 1995 Effect of diet on the fatty acid composition of the major phospholipids of infant cerebral cortex. Archives of Disease in Childhood 72: 198–203
40. Fomon S J, Kaschke F, Ziegler E E, Nelson S E 1982 Body composition of reference children from birth to age 10 years. American Journal of Clinical Nutrition 35:1169–1175
41. Fredrikzon B, Hernell O, Blackberg L 1982 Lingual lipase: role in lipid digestion in infants with low birthweight and/or pancreatic insufficiency. Acta Paediatrica Scandinavica suppl. 296: 75–80
42. Friel J K, Andrews W L, Matthew J D et al 1993 Zinc supplementation in very low birth weight infants. Journal of Pediatric Gastroenterology and Nutrition 17: 97–104
43. Friis-Hansen B 1982 Body water metabolism in early infancy. Acta Paediatrica Scandinavica suppl. 296: 44–48
44. Gandy G M, Jacobson W 1977 Influence of folic acid on birth-weight and growth of the erythroblastotic infant. Archives of Disease in Childhood 52: 7–15, 16–21
45. Gaull G E, Rassin D K, Raiha N C R, Heinonen K 1977 Milk protein quantity and quality in low-birth-weight infants. III. Effects on sulfur amino acids in plasma and urine. Journal of Pediatrics 90: 348–355
46. Gil A, Corral E, Martinez A et al 1986 Effects of the addition of dietary nucleotides to an adapted milk formula on the microbial pattern of faeces in at term newborn infants. Journal of Clinical Nutrition and Gastroenterology 1: 127–131
47. Goldman H I, Goldman J S, Kaufman I 1974 Late effects of early dietary protein intake on low birthweight infants. Journal of Pediatrics 84: 764–769
48. Gordon H, Levine S, McNamara H 1947 Feeding of premature infants. American Journal of Diseases of Children 73: 442–452
49. Gorton M K, Cross E R 1964 Iron metabolism in premature infants. II. Prevention of iron deficiency. Journal of Pediatrics 64: 509–520
50. Graham G C, Placko R P, Moralls E, Acevedo G, Cordaus A 1970 Dietary protein quality in infants and children. American Journal of Diseases of Children 120: 419–423
51. Greengard O 1977 Enzymic differentiation of human liver: comparison with the rat model. Pediatric Research 11: 669–676
52. Hallman M, Bry K, Hoppu K, Lappi M, Pohjavouri M 1992 Inositol supplementation in premature infants with respiratory distress syndrome. New England Journal of Medicine 326: 1233–1239
53. Hamosh M 1996 Digestion in the newborn. Clinics in Perinatology 23: 191–210
54. Hanin I, Schuberth J 1974 Labelling of acetylcholine in the brain of mice fed on a diet containing deuterium labelled choline. Journal of Neurochemistry 23: 819–824
55. Heird W C 1977 Effects of total parenteral alimentation on intestinal function. In: Sunshine P (ed) Gastrointestinal function and neonatal nutrition, Ross Laboratories, Columbus, O H, p 16
56. Imaki H, Jacobson S G, Kemp C M, Knighton R W, Neuringer M, Sturman J 1993 Retinal morphology and visual pigment levels in 6- and 12-month-old rhesus monkeys fed a taurine-free human infant formula. Journal of Neuroscience Research 36: 290–304
57. Infant formula and follow-on formula regulations 1995 Statutory Instrument No. 77. HMSO, London
58. Innis S M, Nelson C M, Rioux F M, Waslen P, Lwanga D 1995 Visual acuity, cognitive development and nutrition in term infants. Pediatric Research 38: 310A
59. Janas L M, Picciano M F 1982 The nucleotide profile of human milk. Pediatric Research 16: 659–662
60. Janowsky J S, Scott D T, Wheeler R E, Auestad N 1995 Fatty acids affect early language development. Pediatric Research 38: 310A
61. Johnson L R, Copeland E, Dudrick S J, Lichtenberger L M, Castro G A 1975 Structural and hormonal alterations in the gastrointestinal tract of parenterally fed rats. Gastroenterology 68: 1177–1183

62. Kien C L 1996 Digestion, absorption and fermentation of carbohydrates in the newborn. Clinics in Perinatology 23: 211–228
63. Koo W K K, Tsang R C 1993 In: Tsang R C, Lucas A, Uauy R, Zlotkin S (eds) Nutritional needs of the preterm infant. Scientific basis and practical guidelines. Caduceus Medical Publishers, New York, pp 135–156
64. Kurzner S I, Garg M, Bautista D B, Sargent C W, Bowman C M, Keens T G 1988 Growth failure in infants with bronchopulmonary dysplasia. Nutrition and elevated resting metabolic expenditure. Pediatrics 81: 379–384
65. Lebenthal E, Lee P C, Heitlinger L E 1983 Impact of development of the gastrointestinal tract on infant feeding. Journal of Pediatrics 102: 1–9
66. Lombeck I, Fuchs A 1994 Zinc and copper in infants fed breast-milk or different formula. European Journal of Pediatrics 153: 770–776
67. Lucas A, Bates C 1984 Transient riboflavin depletion in preterm infants. Archives of Disease in Childhood 59: 837–841
68. Lucas A, Baker B A, Morley R 1993 Hyperphenylalaninaemia and outcome in intravenously fed preterm neonates. Archives of Disease in Childhood 68: 579–583
69. Lucas A, Morley R, Cole T J, Lister G, Leeson-Payne C 1992 Breast milk and subsequent intelligence quotient in children born preterm. Lancet 339: 261–264
70. Lucas A, Gore S M, Cole T J et al 1984 A multicentre trial on the feeding of low birthweight infants: effects of diet on early growth. Archives of Disease in Childhood 59: 722–730
71. Lucas A, Ewing E, Roberts S B, Coward W A 1987 How much energy does the breast-fed infant consume and expend? British Medical Journal 295: 75–77
72. Lucas A, Morley R, Hudson G J et al 1988 Early sodium intake and later blood pressure in preterm infants. Archives of Disease in Childhood 63: 656–657
73. McGraw M, Bishop N, Jamieson R et al 1986 Aluminium content of milk formula and intravenous fluids used in infants. Lancet i: 157
74. Makrides M, Neumann M A, Byard R W, Simmer K, Gibson R A 1994 Fatty acid composition of brain, retina and erythrocytes in breast- and formula-fed infants. American Journal of Clinical Nutrition 60: 189–194
75. Makrides M, Neumann M A, Simmer K, Pater J, Gibson R 1995 Are long chain polyunsaturated fatty acids essential nutrients in infancy? Lancet 345: 1463–1468
76. Malone J L 1975 Vitamin passage across the placenta. Clinics in Perinatology 2: 295–307
77. Micheli J-L, Schutz Y 1993 In: eds. Tsang R C, Lucas A, Uauy R, Zlotkin S, eds. Caduceus Medical Publishers, New York, pp 31–32
78. Mino M, Nishino H 1973 Fetal and maternal relationship in serum vitamin E level. Journal of Nutritional Science and Vitaminology 19: 475–482
79. Neu J, Roig J C, Meetze W H, Auestad N 1995 Tolerance to preterm formula with added glutamine in VLBW infants (VLBW, < 1250 g). Pediatric Research 37: 226A
80. Nohr S B, Laurberg P, Borlum K-G et al 1994 Iodine status in neonates in Denmark: regional variations and dependency on maternal iodine supplementation. Acta Paediatrica 83: 578–582
81. Norgaard-Hansen K, Ebbesen F 1996 Neonatal vitamin K prophylaxis in Denmark: three years' experience with oral administration during the first three months of life compared with one oral administration at birth. Acta Paediatrica 85: 1137–1139
82. O'Brien J S, Fillerup D L, Mead J F 1964 Quantification and fatty acid and fatty aldehyde composition of ethanolamine, choline, and serine glycerophosphatides in human cerebral grey and white matter. Journal of Lipid Research 5: 329–338
83. Okatmoto G, Muttard C R, Sucker C L, Hierd W C 1982 Use of medium chain triglycerides in feeding the low birthweight infant. American Journal of Diseases of Children 136: 428–431
84. Orzalesi M 1987 Vitamins and premature infants. Biology of the Neonate 52 (suppl. 1): 97–112
85. Penn D, Schmidt-Sommerfeld E, Pascu F 1981 Decreased tissue carnitine concentrations in newborn infants receiving total parenteral nutrition. Journal of Pediatrics 98: 976–978
86. Pereira G R, Baumgart S, Bennett M J, Stallings V A, Georgieff M K, Hamosh M, Ellis L 1994 Use of high-fat formula for premature infants with bronchopulmonary dysplasia: metabolic, pulmonary, and nutritional studies. Journal of Pediatrics 124: 605–611
87. Quinlan P, Moore S 1993 Modification of triglycerides by lipases: process technology and its application to the production of nutritionally improved fats. Inform 4: 580–585
88. Raiha N C R 1981 Perinatal development of some enzymes of amino acid metabolism in the liver. In: Davis J A, Dobbing J (eds) Scientific foundations of pediatrics. Heinemann, London, pp 129–138
89. Reichman B L, Chessex P, Putet G et al 1982 Partition of energy metabolism and energy cost of growth in the very low-birthweight infant. Pediatrics 69: 443–451
90. Reifen R M, Zlotkin S 1993 In: Tsang R C, Lucas A, Uauy R, Zlotkin S (eds) Nutritional needs of the preterm infant. Scientific basis and practical guidelines. Caduceus Medical Publishers, New York, p 198
91. Rey J, Schuri Z L, Amedee-Manesme O 1982 Fat absorption in low birthweight infants. Acta Paediatrica Scandinavica suppl. 296: 81–84
92. Roberts S B, Lucas A 1985 The effects of two extremes of dietary intake on body composition in preterm infants. Early Human Development 12: 301–307
93. Roberts S B, Coward W A, Schlingenseipen K-H, Nohria V, Lucas A 1986 Comparison of doubly labelled water method with calorimetry and a nutrient balance study for assessing energy expenditure, water intake and metabolizable energy intake in preterm infants. American Journal of Clinical Nutrition 44: 315–322
94. Roig J C, Bowling D, Dallas M, Sleasman J, Auestad N, Neu J 1995 Enteral glutamine supplementation decreases nosocomial infection and alters T cell subset in the very low birth weight (VLBW) (< 1250 g) neonate. Pediatric Research 37: 285A
95. Ronnholm K A R, Sipila I, Siimes M A 1982 Human milk protein supplementation for the prevention of hypoproteinemia without metabolic imbalance in breast milk fed very low birthweight infants. Journal of Pediatrics 101: 243–247
96. Rudolph F B, Kulkarni A D 1984 Involvement of dietary nucleotides in T lymphocyte function. Advances in Experimental Medicine and Biology 165: 175–178
97. Salmenpera L, Perheentupa J, Pakerinen P, Siimes M A 1994 Zinc supplementation of infant formula. American Journal of Clinical Nutrition 59: 985–989
98. Sanchez-Pozo A, Pita M L, Martinez A et al 1986 Effects of dietary nucleotides upon lipoprotein pattern of newborn infants. Nutrition Research 6: 763–771
99. Schultz K, Soltesz G, Mestyan J 1980 The metabolic consequences of human milk and formula feeding in premature infants. Acta Paediatrica Scandinavica 69: 647–652
100. Shannon K 1995 Recombinant human erythropoetin in neonatal anaemia. Clinics in Perinatology 22: 627–640
101. Shaw J C L 1982 Trace metal requirements of preterm infants. Acta Paediatrica Scandinavica suppl. 296: 93–100
102. Shaw J C L 1983 Iron absorption by the preterm infant. The effect of transfusion and iron supplements on serum ferritin levels. Acta Paediatrica Scandinavica suppl. 299: 83–89
103. Shelley H J 1964 Carbohydrate reserves in the newborn infant. British Medical Journal i: 273–275
104. Shenai J P, Chytil F, Jhaveri A, Stahlman M T 1981 Plasma vitamin A and retinol binding protein in premature and term neonates. Journal of Pediatrics 99: 302–305
105. Silvestre M A A, Morbach C A, Brans Y W, Shankaran S 1996 A prospective randomised trial comparing continuous versus intermittent feeding in VLBW infants. Journal of Pediatrics 128: 748–752
106. Slagle T A, Gross S J 1989 Effect of early low-volume enteral substrate on subsequent feeding tolerance in very low birth weight infants. Journal of Pediatrics 113: 526–531
107. Southgate D A T, Durnin J V G A 1970 Calorie conversion factors. An experimental reassessment of the factors used in the calculation of the energy values of human diets. British Journal of Nutrition 24: 517–535
108. Stevens D, Burman D, Strelling K, Morris A 1979 Folic acid supplementation in low birthweight infants. Pediatrics 64: 333–335
109. Stimmler L, Snodgrass G J A I, Jaffe E 1973 Enamel hypoplasia of the teeth associated with neonatal tetany. Lancet i: 1085–1086
110. Tantibhedyangkul P, Hashim S A 1978 Medium chain triglyceride feeding in premature infants: effects on calcium and magnesium absorption. Pediatrics 61: 537–545
111. Thomson A B R, Keelen M 1986 The development of the small intestine. Canadian Journal of Physiology and Pharmacology 64: 13–29

112. Tsang R E 1985 Vitamin and mineral requirements in preterm infants. Marcel Dekker, New York
113. Tsang R C, Lucas A, Uauy R, Zlotkin S (eds) 1993 Nutritional needs of the preterm infant. Scientific basis and practical guidelines. Caduceus Medical Publishers, New York, pp 288–289
114. Tsuboi K K, Kwon L K, Ford W D A et al 1986 Delayed ontological development in the bypassed ileum of the infant rat. Gastroenterology 80: 1550–1556
115. Tyson J E, Lasky R, Flood D, Mize C, Picone T, Paule C L 1989 Randomized trial of taurine supplementation for infants ≤ 1300 gram birth weight: effect on auditory brainstem-evoked responses. Pediatrics 83: 406–415
116. Uauy R, Stringel G 1988 Effect of dietary nucleotides on growth and maturation of the developing gut in the rat. Pediatric Research 23: 494A
117. Uauy R, Birch D G, Birch E E, Tyson J E, Hoffman D R 1990 Effect of dietary omega-3 fatty acids on retinal function of very low birth weight neonates. Pediatric Research 28: 485–492
118. Watkins J B, Jarvenpaa A-L, Szczepanik Van-Leeuven P et al 1983 Feeding the low-birth-weight infant. V. Effects of human milk taurine and cholesterol on bile acid kinetics. Gastroenterology 85: 793–800
119. Weinstein M R, Oh W 1981 Oxygen consumption in infants with bronchopulmonary dysplasia. Journal of Pediatrics 99: 958–961
120. Wharton B A 1987 Nutrition and feeding of preterm infants. Blackwell Scientific Publications, Oxford
121. Widdowson E M 1981 Nutrition. In: Davis J A, Dobbing J (eds) Scientific foundations of pediatrics, 2nd edn. Heinemann, London, pp 41–43
122. Widdowson E M, Dickerson J W T 1964 Chemical composition of the body. In: Comar C L, Bronner F (eds) Mineral metabolism Vol. II, Part A. Academic Press, New York, pp 1–247
123. Williamson S, Finucaine E, Elliott J, Gamsu H R 1978 Effect of heat treatment of human milk on absorption of nitrogen, fat, sodium, calcium and phosphorus by preterm infants. Archives of Disease in Childhood 53: 555–563
124. Wilson D C, McClure G, Halliday H L, Reid MMcC, Dodge J A 1991 Nutrition and bronchopulmonary dysplasia. Archives of Disease in Childhood 66: 37–38
125. Worthington-White D A, Behnke M, Gross S 1994 Preterm infants require additional folate to reduce the severity of the anemia of prematurity. American Journal of Clinical Nutrition 60: 930–935
126. Yao A C, Wallgren C G, Sinha S N, Lind J 1971 Peripheral circulatory response to feeding in the newborn. Pediatrics 47: 378–383
127. Yeh T F, McClenan D A, Ajayi O A, Pildes R S 1989 Metabolic rate and energy balance in infants with bronchopulmonary dysplasia. Journal of Pediatrics 114: 448–451
128. Young V R 1981 Protein-energy interrelationships in the newborn: a brief consideration of some basic aspects. In: Lebenthal E (ed) Textbook of gastroenterology and nutrition in infancy Vol. 1. Raven Press, New York, pp 257–263
129. Ziegler E E 1986 Protein requirements of preterm infants. In: Fomon S J, Heird W C, (eds) Energy and protein needs during infancy. Academic Press, Orlando
130. Ziegler E E, Biga R L, Fomon S J 1981 Nutritional requirements of the premature infant. In: Suskind RM (ed) Textbook of pediatric nutrition. Raven Press, New York, pp 29–39

Part 2

Feeding the full-term infant

Mary Fewtrell Alan Lucas

BREAST-FEEDING

Breast-feeding is a complex physiological event: indeed the term itself could be regarded as a misnomer, since 'feeding' is only one of several physiological processes that occur when a newborn infant is put to the breast. These processes can be summarized as follows:

- Provision of nutrients;
- Provision of immunological and antimicrobial protection;
- Induction of adaptive events that equip the infant for extrauterine nutrition;
- The passage of non-nutritive factors (other than antimicrobial ones) from mother to infant, for example breast milk hormones and growth factors;
- Provision of digestive enzymes, e.g. milk lipases;
- Effects on the mother, e.g. contraceptive role;
- Facilitation of mother–infant bonding.

NUTRITIVE ASPECTS OF HUMAN MILK

Human milk does not have a constant composition, and significant changes take place during the course of lactation, diurnally and during each feed. Uncertainty over the precise dietary intake of breast-fed infants poses a major problem for nutritional science. In Tables 19.7 and 19.8, the composition of average mature human milk is tabulated[19] together with the composition of unmodified cow's milk.

Protein

The protein content of milks of mammalian species appears to be related to the postnatal growth rate of the infant.[8] Human infants have especially slow postnatal growth rates compared to many other mammals, and the protein content of human milk is correspondingly very low. Previously the protein content of mature human milk may have been overestimated, because of its high content of non-protein nitrogen: a realistic figure is 1.0 g/100 ml compared to 3.5 g/100 ml in cow's milk.

The two main classes of protein in milk are whey and casein. Human milk is whey predominant (around 60% of total protein), though the casein content is still debated. Cow's milk, however, is casein predominant, with only 20% whey. In human whey, α-lactalbumin is the dominant protein, followed by lactoferrin. In contrast, the major whey protein in cow's milk is β-lactoglobulin,

Table 19.7 Nutrient content of baby milks available in the UK (per 100 ml)

Composition per 100 ml	Mature human milk		Demineralized whey-based formulas				Demineralized whey formulas		Modified milk formulas				Modified milk formulas	
	DHSS[a]	Macy et al[b]	Aptamil with Milupan** (M)	Premium** (C&G)	Farley's First Milk (FHP)**	SMA Gold** (Wyeth)	Boots Formula 1	Sainsbury's First Menu 1st stage milk	Milumil** (M)	Plus** (C&G)	Farley's** Second Milk (FHP)	SMA White** (Wyeth)	Boots Formula 2	Sainsbury's First Menu 2nd stage milk
Macronutrients														
Protein* (g)	1.34	1.45	1.50	1.41	1.45	1.5	1.5	1.43	1.9	1.7	1.7	1.6	1.6	1.51
casein (%)	–	32	40	40	40	40	4.0	40	80	77	80	80	80	80
whey (%)	–	68	60	60	60	60	60	60	20	23	20	20	20	20
Fat (g)	4.2	3.8	3.6	3.6	3.82	3.6			3.1	3.4	2.9	3.6		
LCPUFA	+	+	+	–	+	–	+	NS	–	–	–	–	+	NS
Carbohydrate+							7.2	6.75					7.2	6.68
Total (g)	7.0	–	7.2	7.5	6.96	7.2	7.2	6.75	8.1	7.2	8.3	7.0	7.2	6.68
Energy														
kcal	70	68	67	67	68	67	67	66	68	66	66	67	68	66
kJ	293	285	281	281	284	280	280	276	285	277	277	280	284	276
Minerals														
Calcium (mg)	35	33	66	53.3	39	46	52	30	88	80	61	56	62	55
Chloride (mg)	43	43	53	43	45	43	45	45	59#	56	55	55	47	50
Magnesium (mg)	2.8	4.0	5.2	5.1	5.2	6.7	5.2	5.1	7.0	5.4	6.0	5.3	5.5	5.0
Phosphorus (mg)	15	15	42	26.7	27	33	36	28	57	47	48	44	51	45
Potassium (mg)	60	55	75	66.7	57	65	75	57	98	90	86	80	81	70
Sodium (mg)	15	15	23	19	17	16	19	18	26#	25	25	22	22	21
Trace elements														
Copper (μg)	39	40	40	40.6	42	33	47	42	32	40	40	33	29	39
Iodine (μg)	76	150	10	9.9	4.5	10	7.5	4.5	9.0	9.9	10	10	7.2	10
Iron (μg)	76	150	700	510	690	800	1000	640	700	500	660	800	1000	650
Manganese (μg)	ND	0.7	10	7.0	3.4	10	4.0	3.3	8.0	7.0	3.3	10	4.1	3.2
Zinc (μg)	295	530	500	500	340	600	470	340	500	400	330	600	470	300
Potential renal solute load^ (mosmol/l)	88	91	104	94	93	95.7	100	NS	129	118	116	109.6	108	NS
Vitamins														
A retinol (μg)	60	53	60	84	100	75	62	100	63	80	97	75	61	98
B_1 thiamin (μg)	16	16	40	40	42	100	52	40	40	40	39	100	39	37
B_2 riboflavin (μg)	31	42.6	NS	120	55	150	130	53	NS	100	53	150	130	48
B_6 pyridoxine (μg)	6	11	40	40	35	60	52	34	40	40	33	60	52	30
B_{12} cyanocobalamin (μg)	0.01	trace	0.2	0.22	0.14	0.2	0.26	0.14	0.2	0.2	0.13	0.2	0.26	0.12
Biotin (μg)	0.76	0.4	1.0	1.52	1.0	2.0	2.0	1.0	1.0	1.5	1.0	2.0	2.0	1.0
Folic acid (μg)	5.2	0.18	10.0	10.2	3.4	8.0	9.1	3.3	11.0	10.0	3.3	8.0	9.1	3.0
Niacin (μg)	230	172	700	750	690	900	910	670	800	800	660	900	910	600
C ascorbic acid (mg)	3.8	4.3	8.0	8	6.9	9.0	6.8	6.7	8.0	8.0	6.6	9.0	6.6	6.1
Vitamin D (μg)	0.01	0.01	1.0	1.4	1.0	1.1	1.0	1.0	1.1	1.1	1.0	1.1	1.0	1.0
Vitamin E (mg)	0.35	0.56	0.6	1.1	0.48	0.74	0.81	0.46	0.6	0.81	0.46	0.74	0.68	0.5
K phytomenadione (μg)	ND	1.7	3.0	5.1	2.7	6.7	6.8	2.7	3.0	5.0	2.6	6.17	6.6	2.7
Others														
Nucleotides	+	+	–	–	–	+	–	–	–	–	–	+	–	–

* total nitrogen × 6.138
\+ figures declared as disaccharide
\# liquid formulation-sodium 34, chloride 67
^ method of Ziegler & Fomon[86]: calculated values
M Milupa
C&G Cow & Gate Nutricia
a DHSS Reports on Health and Social Subjects[19,20]
b Macy, Kelly and Sloan[54a] and Mettler[56]
** manufacturer's information
NS not stated
FHP Farley Health Products

which is absent from human milk and may be antigenic when fed to human infants. α-Lactalbumin is present in cow's milk, but lactoferrin occurs in only small amounts. Whey proteins have a high nutritive value for human infants: their essential amino acid content is high. Some work has suggested that infants fed on modified whey-predominant formulas retain more nitrogen and grow faster than those fed on unmodified (casein-predominant) formulas, but this is debated and formulas marketed in the USA are often casein predominant. Caseins may precipitate at low pH, forming a 'curd' in the infant's stomach, and this has led to the widespread belief that casein-dominant formulas may be more satisfying for hungry infants. Human milk casein yields a softer, more flocculent curd than cow's milk casein.

Human milk has a cysteine content about twice that of cow's milk and a methionine/cysteine ratio content that is seven times less than cow's milk. In view of the late development of cystathionase (which converts methionine to cystine), cysteine may be an essential amino acid in the newborn, and it has been suggested that the high cysteine content of human milk is biologically advantageous. In

Table 19.8 Nutrient content of follow-up baby milks available in the UK (per 100 ml)

Composition per 100 ml	**Follow-on milks**					
	Cow's milk	**Step-up** (C&G)**	**Farley's Follow-on milk** (FHP)**	**SMA Progress** (Wyeth)**	**Boots Follow-on Milk**	**Sainsbury's First Menu Follow-on Milk**
Macronutrients						
Protein* (g)	3.4	1.8	2.1	2.2	2.15	2.2
casein (%)	77[a]	80	80	80	62	NS
whey (%)	23[a]	20	20	20	38	NS
Fat (g)	3.9	3.8	3.1	3.0	3.41	3.5
saturated (%)	63.2[a]	36	50	42.9	47	NS
unsaturated (%)	36.6[a]	64	50	57.1	53	NS
Carbohydrate+						
lactose (g)	4.6	7.2	5.3	7.8	6.04	
maltodextrin (g)	—	—	2.7	—	0.39	
amylose (g)	—	—	—	—		
glucose (g)	—	—	—	—		
Total (g)	4.6	7.2	8.0	7.8	6.43	6.5
Energy						
kcal	67	70	68	67	65	66
kJ	280	293	285	281	272	275
Minerals						
Calcium (mg)	124	88	72	90	69	71
Chloride (mg)	98	51	68	62	72	72
Magnesium (mg)	12	6	7.8	8.0	8.5	8.4
Phosphorus (mg)	98	50	55	62	58	55
Potassium (mg)	155	86	91	107	97	95
Sodium (mg)	52	23	31	33	29	27
Trace elements						
Copper (μg)	20	49	41	40	50	52
Iodine (μg)	ND	11	11	12	6.5	7.2
Iron (μg)	50	1300	1200	1300	1260	850
Manganese (μg)	ND	11	4.0	10	3.3	3.9
Zinc (μg)	360	700	400	600	410	460
Potential renal solute load^ (mosmol/l)	225	116	140	147	144	NS
Vitamins						
A retinol (μg)	40	60	80	75	110	110
B_1 thiamin (μg)	40	40	40	100	42	41
B_2 riboflavin (μg)	200	100	150	150	63	65
B_6 pyridoxine (μg)	40	40	40	60	33	34
B_{12} cyanocobalamin (μg)	0.3	0.2	0.15	0.2	0.16	0.16
Biotin (μg)	2.1	1.6	3.0	2.0	1.2	1.1
Folic acid (μg)	5	11	7.0	8.0	3.9	3.7
Niacin (μg)	80	800	650	900	770	780
C ascorbic acid (mg)	1.5	8	10	9.0	6.8	6.9
Vitamin D (μg)	0.02	1.8	1.1	1.2	1.3	1.3
Vitamin E (mg)	0.09	0.81	0.48	0.74	0.55	0.55
K phytomenadione (μg)	ND	5.6	2.7	6.7	3.7	3.7

*	total nitrogen × 6.38
+	figures declared as disaccharide
#	liquid formulation-sodium 34, chloride 67
^	method of Ziegler & Fomon[86]: calculated values
M	Milupa
C&G	Cow & Gate Nutricia
a	DHSS Reports on Health and Social Subjects[19,20]
b	Macy, Kelly and Sloan[54a] and Mettler[56]
**	manufacturer's information
NS	not stated
FHP	Farley Health Products

addition, the relatively low content of tyrosine and phenylalanine in human milk may be related to the newborn infant's limited capacity to metabolize them.

The non-protein nitrogen content in human milk is unusually high: about 25% of the total, compared to 6% in cow's milk. It consists of free amino acids, urea, creatinine, creatine, uric acid and ammonia. Clearly, free amino acids must be included with protein from a

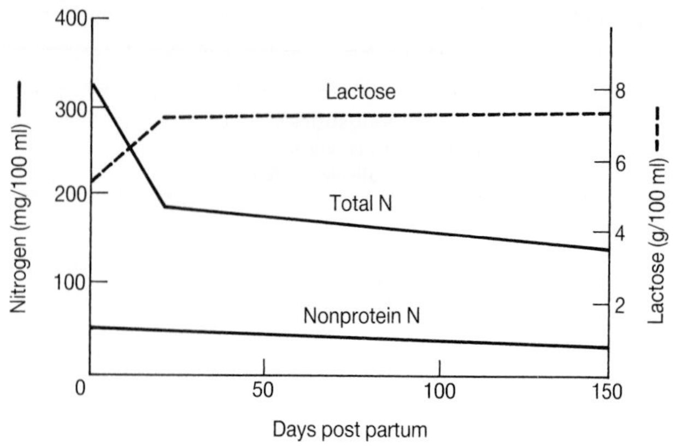

Fig. 19.3 Concentration of lactose, total nitrogen and non-protein nitrogen in human milk during the course of lactation. (After George & Lebenthal[27].)

Table 19.9 Fatty acid composition of mature human and cow's milk lipids (%, w/w)

Fatty acid	Human milk	Cow's milk
4:0	—	3.3
6:0	Trace	1.6
8:0	Trace	1.3
10:0	1.3	3.0
12:0	3.1	3.1
14:0	5.1	14.2
15:0	0.4	1.3
16:0	20.2	49.9
16:1	5.7	3.7
18:0	5.9	5.7
18:1	46.4	16.7
18:2	13.0	1.6
18:3	1.4	1.8

nutritional point of view; it is unknown whether other non-protein nitrogen fractions have nutritional value.[12] The free amino acids in human milk include taurine, which is present in significantly higher amounts than in cow's milk.

During early lactation milk protein content is much higher than in mature milk (Fig. 19.3). The falling protein content could represent an adaptation to the infant's decreasing protein requirements, or simply reflect the maturation of the mammary gland.[27]

Fat

The fat content of milk from different mothers is very variable, and in an individual usually increases during early lactation (1–2 weeks) and later declines. (Indeed, with the exception of lactose and lysozyme, most breast milk nutrients, including minerals and vitamins, decline after the first 2–3 months of lactation.) The fat concentration rises markedly during a feed, from around 2.1 g/100 ml to 4.1 g/100 ml.[52]

Cow's milk and human milk have similar fat contents and most of the lipid is triglyceride (98%); the principal difference is the pattern of fatty acids (Table 19.9). Human milk fatty acid profiles are, however, markedly influenced by diet. Vegetarians, for instance, consume more long-chain fatty acids than those on a mixed diet. Human milk has a higher proportion of unsaturated fatty acids than cow's milk and a greater concentration of the essential fatty acids. Unlike cow's milk, long-chain fatty acids in human milk are esterified to glycerol predominantly in the 1 position, which improves their absorption.

Breast milk lipids occur as globules ranging in size from 1 to 10 μm, emulsified in the aqueous phase of milk.[40] These globules consist of non-polar core lipids (such as triglycerides and cholesterol esters) covered with bipolar materials (including protein and phospholipids) which constitute the milk lipid globule membrane. The latter prevents the globules from coalescing and presents a large surface area for the action of lipolytic enzymes.

Carbohydrate

Lactose is present in higher concentrations in human milk (7 g/100 ml) than in cow's milk (4.7 g/100 ml). Lactose enhances calcium absorption from the gut, promotes the growth of lactobacilli, and may help to create a favourable gut flora that protects against gastroenteritis.[27]

Minerals

All major minerals are present in higher concentrations in cow's milk than in human milk (see Table 19.7); with the higher protein content of cow's milk, they account for its high renal solute load. The amount of sodium in cow's milk is regarded as excessive for the human infant. However, early human milk has a high sodium content which may be 10 times that seen in mature milk. The raised phosphate/calcium ratio in cow's milk has been implicated in neonatal hypocalcaemia (see below).

Trace metals

The major trace metal concentrations in mature human and cow's milk are shown in Table 19.8. Zinc concentrations in mature human milk are rather less than those in cow's milk, whereas the reverse is the case for copper; cow's milk has a substantially greater magnesium content. Copper, iron and zinc are present in higher concentrations in human colostrum than in later milk. However, the comparison of levels of trace nutrients in different milks is of less relevance than the bioavailability of these elements. There is good bioavailability of iron and other minerals from human milk. In cow's milk, iron and zinc are less available, the latter being bound to high molecular weight fractions.

Energy

Published values for the energy content of breast milk (obtained unphysiologically as expressed breast milk) of around 70 kcal/100 ml have been challenged. Using the doubly labelled water method, which avoids milk sampling, Lucas et al[51] suggest that a figure close to 60 kcal per 100 ml is realistic. Most formulas have significantly higher energy contents than this (see below).

ADEQUACY OF BREAST MILK FOR HEALTHY TERM INFANTS

From a biological viewpoint it seems likely that the diet of a breast-fed infant should not require supplementation in the first 4–6 months, yet there is continued debate on this issue.

Vitamins

In the west, vitamin deficiencies are generally rare in fully breast-fed infants when the mother is well nourished. Vitamins K and D, however, require special consideration.

Vitamin K

Levels are low in breast milk (0.4–2.8 μg/ml), though they are higher in colostrum (0.8–4.8 μg/ml). In contrast, non-supplemented formulas usually contain around 6–11 μg/ml and supplemented formulas up to 100 μg/ml. Parenteral prophylaxis at birth with 1 mg vitamin K is effective (p. 799). Recently oral vitamin K has been considered, because of concerns about a potential long-term carcinogenic effect of intramuscular vitamin K. However, it is doubtful whether a single oral dose provides sufficient vitamin K stores to protect breast-fed infants against haemorrhagic disease beyond the neonatal period.[82] Multiple oral doses are therefore recommended, with the consequent problems of ensuring that they are administered, and there have been reports of late haemorrhagic disease of the newborn in breast-fed infants who have received three oral doses, although 12 or more doses appear to be effective.[63]

Vitamin D

The need for vitamin D supplementation is controversial. In the human infant, cholecalciferol (vitamin D) is derived mainly from the skin, synthesized from 7-dehydrocholesterol under the influence of sunlight. Breast milk provides only about 10 iu of vitamin D daily in winter and 20 iu daily in the summer, and water-soluble vitamin D is present only in trace amounts that have negligible activity.[30] Healthy, exclusively breast-fed infants have adequate bone mineralization in the first 16 weeks of life[68] and maintain satisfactory serum levels of 25-hydroxycholecalciferol for at least 6 months,[9] suggesting that vitamin D supplements during this period are unnecessary. It would be reasonable, nevertheless, to give vitamin D supplements (400 iu/day) to those breast-fed infants who are unable to benefit from the effects of sunlight, such as dark-skinned racial groups[70] and those living in the inner city areas, where high-rise buildings occlude the sun and air pollution screens out ultraviolet light.[4]

Multivitamins

It has been recommended that in the UK children receive daily vitamin A (200 mg), vitamin C (200 mg) and vitamin D (7 mg) as a combined preparation (available under the Welfare Food Scheme; five-drop dosage) from 6 months to 5 years.[21] However, many professionals give multivitamins from 1 month to babies receiving breast milk. This is also supported,[21] especially when there is doubt about the mother's dietary status.

Iron

The breast-fed infant's requirement for supplemental iron is equally controversial. The low levels of iron in breast milk (compared with those in supplemented modern formulas) are very well absorbed (around 80%, compared to about 4–6% from fortified formulas). Nevertheless, a small proportion of breast-fed infants have lower iron stores at 6 months, and a greater proportion appear deficient at 9 months or later than those fed iron-supplemented formula.[26,34,71]

Iron deficiency may impair neurodevelopment and immunity. Its prevalence in the UK varies, depending on the socioeconomic and cultural group studied and the age of the infants or toddlers. The National Diet and Nutrition Survey found a prevalence of 12% in British children aged 18 months to $4\frac{1}{2}$ years,[61] but reported figures are higher in ethnic minority groups (particularly Asians) and in those from a deprived background.[14] This is a major community health concern. In bottle-fed infants, continued use of iron and vitamin C-fortified formulas during infancy is effective in preventing iron deficiency anaemia,[77] but in babies receiving breast milk plus weaning foods beyond 6 months, good nutritional advice is required. Iron from iron-fortified cereals may not be well absorbed. Haem iron, preferably from red meat, is ideal, though often not consumed in sufficient quantities. Other meats and vitamin C will enhance iron absorption from a meal. However, if there is any doubt about the sufficiency of iron intake it may be prudent to give supplemental iron drops;[17] careful instruction is required on the danger to the child and other siblings of accidental iron overdosage. Because iron stores are proportional to body mass at birth, small for gestational age babies may become iron-depleted well before 6 months.

Fluoride

Fluoride is not a nutrient, although epidemiological studies show its role in preventing dental caries. It has both systemic and topical actions. Systemically it acts on the teeth prior to eruption, being built into the structure of the enamel and making it resistant to decay. It also limits enamel demineralization. Fluoride also acts topically by promoting remineralization, possibly through antibacterial effects. The relative roles of systemic versus topical fluoride are still being debated. In areas where the water supply is fluoridated (fluoride ion > 0.3 ppm) infants consuming reconstituted formulas will have adequate intake, but in breast-fed babies intake will inevitably be low. The British Dental Association[23] and the American Academy of Pediatrics[1] have recommended that an intake of 0.25 mg of fluoride should be achieved from 2 weeks to 2 years of age (available as drops), but emphasize the dangers (fluorosis) of exceeding this dosage from all sources combined. When water becomes the principal part of the breast-fed infant's fluid intake, supplementation is no longer required if the water supply is fluoridated.

Protein and energy

Breast milk intake rises to a peak in the 3rd and 4th months, providing a mean of around 750–850 ml/24 h (more in boys than girls), the majority of exclusively breast-fed babies falling into the intake range of 500–1200 ml/24 h.[64] By the end of this period, at intakes of 150 ml/kg the infant would consume 1.5 g/kg/24 h of protein and 85–105 kcal/kg/24 h (according to which values for milk energy are accepted: see Lucas et al[51]). Beyond this age, protein and energy intakes per kilogram body weight will fall as the infant grows, and eventually, without the introduction of weaning foods, breast milk alone will no longer meet the infant's needs. The point at which this occurs is variable and difficult to define even for populations. The recommended dietary allowance (RDA) for protein, usually set near 2 g/kg/24 h for infancy, has an inbuilt safety margin, and it is now recognized that the RDA for energy (e.g. 116 kcal/kg/24 h at 3 months) is unrealistically high compared to the much lower intakes of breast-fed babies growing and developing normally.

The traditional approach to assessing the adequacy of the diet is to monitor growth and watch for centile crossing. However, healthy breast-fed babies being fed in accordance with present-day practices do not grow according to the accepted international National Center for Health Statistics growth standard, which was based largely on formula-fed infants. Data from several countries[83] show a marked secular trend in growth performance with the recent resurgence of breast-feeding. Typically in the first 3 months the breast-fed baby gains weight and length at a relatively fast rate, so that the centiles are above the NCHS values. However, beyond 4 months there is a progressive deceleration of growth, a process which persists throughout infancy, despite the introduction of weaning foods; indeed, Dewey et al[18] found that breast-fed infants remained leaner than their formula-fed peers up to 18 months of age, and preliminary data from Whitehead et al suggest that modern breast-fed babies remain lighter and shorter up to preschool age[83]. Skinfold thicknesses are also dramatically less in breast-fed babies than in previously reported studies, though interestingly head growth may be greater[83].

Whether these data should be treated as indicating that breast milk is an inadequate source of nutrition beyond 4 months (on average), or rather that new standards are required to accommodate the growth pattern of breast-fed babies, is a matter of considerable debate. The new British growth standards may go some way towards addressing this issue; the data covering the newborn period and infancy are based on a representative sample of infants including both breast and bottle feeders from the Cambridge area.[24] There are no specific growth standards for non-caucasian ethnic groups in the UK.

In the absence of long-term outcome data on the consequences of these different early growth patterns, most authorities take the view that exclusive breast-feeding provides adequate protein and energy for growth at least up to 4 months, and that sometime between 4 and 6 months weaning foods will need to be introduced. However, regardless of the deliberations of health professionals breast-fed babies themselves may play an important part in influencing the time of weaning.

ANTIBACTERIAL ASPECTS OF HUMAN MILK[29,47]

Grulee's studies in Chicago in the 1930s, based on a 9-month period of supervised follow-up of 20 061 babies, provided convincing evidence of the anti-infective advantages of breast-feeding in the preantibiotic era.[31] With overall improvements in public health and obstetric and paediatric care in western countries, these major differences in infection rates have diminished dramatically, though much less so in developing countries. In western society an increased morbidity (but not mortality) due to infection in bottle-fed babies is supported by recent evidence,[36] even when account has been taken of class differences in feeding preferences, but the major clinical importance of the protective properties of breast milk relates to infants in the developing world.

Immunoglobulins

The principal immunoglobulin in milk, secretory IgA, is

present in the highest concentrations in the first few days postpartum. There is little evidence that absorption of the relatively low concentrations of IgG in human milk occurs. Secretory IgA is relatively resistant to low pH and proteolytic enzymes, and can be recovered from the stools of breast-fed infants. It is likely that its protective effects are confined to the gut and perhaps to the respiratory tract. A wide variety of antibodies against viruses and bacteria and their toxins have been described in human milk, but their actions within the gut are not fully understood.

The antibodies produced in milk are directed against organisms to which the mother has been exposed via the gut and the respiratory tract, and which her infant might be more likely to meet in the same environment. Experimentally, the oral administration to lactating mothers of non-pathogenic *Escherichia coli* results in type-specific IgA, and IgA-secreting cells appearing in milk within a few days. This has led to the hypothesis that there is a selective transfer ('homing') of sensitized lymphocytes from the gut to the breast.

Other antimicrobial factors

Although all complement components have been demonstrated in human milk, their relatively low concentration, and the observation that heating milk up to 56°C for 30 minutes does not decrease its bacteriostatic action against *E. coli*, has cast doubt on the anti-infective role of milk complement. Human milk is one of the richest sources of lysozyme, which is present in about 3000 times the concentration reported in cow's milk. In vitro, it acts with IgA to lyse *E. coli* and some salmonellae, but its role in vivo is not established.

The iron-binding protein lactoferrin may deprive gut organisms of free iron as a growth factor, and has been shown to be bacteriostatic and bacteriocidal in vitro, although its protective role in vivo is uncertain. Lactoferrin increases markedly in milk during lactation, and has received recent attention as a possible growth factor.

Other factors present in human milk, for example oligonucleotides and glycoconjugates, may act as receptors and divert pathogens or toxins away from binding to the infant's pharynx or gut. Breast milk also contains nucleotides, which may promote cell-mediated immunity (see p. 1095). However, their role as anti-infective agents in vivo requires further investigation. Vitamin B_{12} and folate-binding proteins in milk might be antibacterial by depriving bacteria of these free vitamins as essential growth factors, but the antibacterial role in humans of these binding proteins is uncertain. Various other factors, such as protease inhibitors and anti-enterotoxin factor, have been demonstrated in milk, but their role in vivo remains speculative. The same applies to antiviral factors in breast milk, which include interferon synthesized by breast milk lymphocytes in response to viral change.

Nutritive aspects of antimicrobial factors

Previously it was believed that antimicrobial proteins, including IgA and lactoferrin, which comprise a significant proportion (30–40%) of milk protein, were not available for nutrition. Prentice et al[66] have challenged this view, suggesting that the great majority of these proteins are digested: by 6 weeks only 1% of lactoferrin and 17% of secretory IgA is detected in the stools, and 95% of total dietary protein (p. 325) could be regarded as nutritionally available.

Effects on gut flora

Breast-feeding promotes the growth of harmless lactobacilli (bifidobacteria) in the infant's gut, compared to the higher numbers of *E. coli* in formula-fed infants; this has been partly attributed to the presence of a growth factor ('bifidus factor') in human milk. More recent work suggests that factors that influence postnatal colonization of the gut are more complex; one group has observed that, whereas Nigerian breast-fed infants showed the expected predominance of bifidobacteria in their gut, UK infants, whether breast-fed or bottle-fed, had a predominance of *E. coli* and *Bacteroides* spp. in their gut flora.[76]

Cells in milk

Human milk is populated with macrophages, polymorphonuclear leukocytes and T and B lymphocytes; it has been calculated that the breast-fed infant ingests as many viable leukocytes each day as he has circulating at any one time. The B lymphocytes contain cell lines that have synthesized IgA in the breast, but whether these cells survive for long enough in the infant's gut to carry out any further useful biological role is unknown. There is evidence that T cells in milk may transfer tuberculin sensitivity from mother to infant,[75] presumably mediated through lymphokines, which might have been secreted before the infant ingested the milk. There is no evidence that T lymphocytes are transferred across the gut in humans or participate in 'graft versus host' disease.

Breast milk cells might protect against necrotizing enterocolitis, though this is disputed. In a neonatal rat model a disease resembling necrotizing enterocolitis, induced by hypoxia and an enteral challenge with *Klebsiella*, could be prevented by fresh breast milk.[65] Whatever the mechanism, necrotizing enterocolitis is less common in preterm infants fed breast milk than those fed formula.[50]

Table 19.10 Hormones reported in breast milk

Steroids	Prolactin
Thyroxine	Erythropoietin
Gonadotrophins	Melatonin
Luteinizing hormone-releasing hormone	Epidermal growth factor
Thyropin-releasing hormone	Prostaglandins
Thyroid-stimulating hormone	Calcitonin
Adrenocorticotrophic hormone	

BREAST MILK HORMONES

Possible 'messenger' substances in human milk

In recent years a wide variety of hormones and growth factors have been described in human milk.[72] A selection of these are listed in Table 19.10. In animals such factors may be absorbed from the gut, and data from preterm human neonates suggest that epidermal growth factor crosses the gut wall into the circulation.[25] It is an important question whether or not the lactating mother, in addition to providing nutrients and anti-infective factors, might also exert some control over neonatal metabolism and development through the mediation of 'chemical messengers' and trophic factor secreted into her milk.

ENZYMES IN HUMAN MILK[33]

The bile salt-stimulated lipase in human milk may play a significant part in intestinal lipolysis. Its presence may partly account for improved fat absorption from human milk compared to cow's milk, and for the observation that pasteurization results in lower fat absorption from breast milk in preterm infants.[84] Bile salt-stimulated lipase also has esterase activity, which may assist the digestion of breast milk retinyl esters.

Several other enzymes have been described in human milk. Breast milk amylase is identical in structure to the salivary enzyme, and probably compensates for the relatively slow postnatal development of the latter. Several proteases are also present, including trypsin, elastase and plasmin. However, it is doubtful whether they play an important role in the neonatal period because of the high antiprotease activity of human milk.

OTHER FACTORS IN BREAST MILK

Babies may consume from breast milk a variety of substances which have no physiological value to them. Maternal medications are discussed in Chapter 13. Addictive drugs cause increasing concern. Some recent evidence suggests a need for caution over the regular use of alcohol by breast-feeding mothers: Little et al[45] showed that one unit of alcohol or more each day for the first 3 months was associated with reduced motor development scores in the infant at 1 year. Pesticide residues are officially monitored. Organohalogens such as dioxins in breast milk are of current concern. These lipophilic chemicals are excreted in breast milk in 10–50 times the concentration in cow's milk or formulas, frequently exceeding accepted safety limits for cow's milk.[3] They accumulate in fat over long periods, and some are highly toxic to skin, liver and immune and nervous systems. They are also suspected carcinogens. Studies in infants to date have suggested that lactational exposure to these substances may be associated with decreased psychomotor function and abnormal thyroid function tests (decreased T3 and T4 with elevated TSH). The long-term significance of such findings is unknown, and further studies are under way (see Brouwer et al[11] for a review of this topic).

HUMAN IMMUNODEFICIENCY VIRUS AND OTHER VIRUSES IN BREAST MILK[48]

HIV has been found in breast milk in HIV-positive mothers, and there is now good evidence that transmission to the breast-fed baby occurs (p. 1117). A similar retrovirus, HTLVI, may be transmitted by breast-feeding, and bottle-feeding has been shown to be protective.[2] Whether HIV-positive mothers or those at high risk should avoid breast-feeding has evoked heated debate; in developing countries there may be no satisfactory alternative, but in many western countries, including the UK, it is recommended that such mothers be discouraged from breast-feeding their infants.

Both hepatitis B virus and hepatitis C virus may be found in the breast milk of seropositive mothers,[13,79] and transmission to the infant has been reported.[79] However, most evidence suggests that breast milk is an uncommon route of infection.[7,13,43,59] Mothers who wish to donate breast milk are now routinely screened for HBV, HCV and HIV, and excluded if positive.

Cytomegalovirus is commonly found in the milk of seropositive mothers, and the infants of such mothers who are breast-fed show a higher rate of seropositivity at 1 year of age (70%) than those who are bottle-fed (30%).[58]

MATERNAL ASPECTS OF BREAST-FEEDING

Advice and assistance

The practical management of breast-feeding is outlined on pages 381–383. Until recently, help and support for breast-feeding mothers has been provided largely by a number of support groups, including the National Childbirth Trust, La Lèche League, and the Association of Breastfeeding Mothers; the help available from healthcare professionals has been variable, depending on the interests and motivation of local personnel. However, in recognition of the increasing evidence that breast-feeding is beneficial to both infant and mother, the National Breast-feeding Working Group was set up by the Department of Health in 1992 to promote breast-feeding and provide information and education for mothers and healthcare workers; the aim is to increase the number of mothers who breast-feed for at least 3 months (the duration shown to provide protection against gastro-enteritis in a recent study); at present, although 60% breast-feed initially, only 40% are still doing so by 6 weeks. All district health authorities are required to implement policies that promote and protect breast-feeding, including the provision of comfortable surroundings in all hospitals and clinics where mothers can breast-feed their infants, and providing breast pumps for use when normal breast-feeding is not possible.

Breast-feeding and maternal health

Two recent studies have shown a reduced incidence of premenopausal breast cancer in women who have breast-fed their infants.[62,80]

'Adoptive lactation' and relactation

Women who adopt a child and wish to breast-feed may be successful, given motivation, persistence and appropriate help. Suckling may release sufficient prolactin to initiate lactation de novo. It is a prerequisite of lactogenesis that it is preceded by mammogenesis. Thus women who have had a previous pregnancy, or even a therapeutic or spontaneous abortion, are much more likely to succeed. Nevertheless, lactation has been achieved in mothers who have never been pregnant. Pharmacological assistance may be helpful. Schams[74] reported the use of thyroliberin to stimulate endogenous prolactin release after priming the breast with oestrogen to enhance mammogenesis. Dopamine-blocking agents, for example metaclopramide and sulpiride, which release prolactin, have also been used to stimulate milk production. During the period when lactation is becoming established the infant may be fed complementary feeds after suckling or by using a simple milk-containing device, worn on the mother's body (e.g.'Lactaid'), from which a tube passes into the infant's mouth while it is at the breast: thus feeding and breast stimulation occur concurrently. Using similar principles mothers may be helped to relactate if cessation of lactation has occurred, for instance due to illness of mother or infant.

CONTRAINDICATIONS TO BREAST-FEEDING

Many so-called contraindications to breast-feeding are relative rather than absolute: the parent's wishes should be explored and marginal cases may require collaborative discussion between obstetrician, paediatrician, physician, general practitioner, psychiatrist or pharmacologist.

Maternal drug treatment seldom constitutes an absolute contraindication, and few drugs have been demonstrated to have definite deleterious effects on the neonate (Chapter 13). Serious maternal illness or infection and psychiatric disorders may preclude breast-feeding, but each case needs to be reviewed individually.

In certain rare inborn errors of metabolism in the infant, breast-feeding can make safe nutritional management impossible: these include phenylketonuria, galactosaemia (p. 993) and alactasia (p. 756), although with skilled dietetic assistance breast-feeding may be achieved safely in some babies with PKU.

Structural defects of the palate do not necessarily prevent feeding, which can be successful once a plate has been fitted or the defect closed (p. 766).

ARTIFICIAL FEEDING FOR THE NORMAL TERM INFANT

GENERAL CONSIDERATIONS

The purpose of artificial feeding is to provide a satisfactory food for infants in situations where a substitute for breast milk is required. The 'ideal' artificial diet should:

- meet the nutrient needs of healthy infants;
- be well tolerated without inducing metabolic stress or biochemical disturbance;
- not result in short- or long-term morbidity.

Until recent years the artificial milks failed to meet any of these criteria – sometimes with serious consequences. Modern formulas come much closer to attaining these goals (Table 19.8).

RECOMMENDED DIETARY ALLOWANCES FOR FORMULA-FED INFANTS

From a teleological point of view breast milk should be the nutritional standard for formula-fed infants. Many of the current recommended dietary allowances are based on the concentrations of nutrients in human milk. However, in constructing a formula from non-human milk components account must be taken of (a) the bioavailability, (b) the digestibility and (c) the biological value of the nutrients, all of which may differ from those in human milk.

Milk volume

Based on human lactational studies, fluid intakes of around 150 ml/kg/24 h are satisfactory for the first 3–4 months in formula-fed infants. However, this is only an approximate guideline: healthy infants fed on formula ad libitum (as with breast-fed infants) will show considerable variations in intake in association with normal growth.

Artificial formula

Unmodified cow's milk

'Doorstep' milk should not be used for infants in the first 12 months.[17] Problems that may be encountered with cow's milk, or unmodified cow's milk formulas, include hyperosmolar dehydration associated with high renal solute load, hypocalcaemic fits associated with phosphate overload, casein curd obstruction, vitamin deficiency (e.g. rickets, scurvy) and iron deficiency anaemia. These problems are rarely seen in infants fed modern formulas. Skimmed and semi-skimmed milk should not be used because of their low energy and vitamin A contents. Indeed, the DHSS[21] recommends that fully skimmed milk should not be given before the age of 5.

Goat's milk

Goat's milk is not suitable for infant feeding because of its high solute load and low vitamin content. It is particularly deficient in folate, and severe megaloblastic anaemia may result if goat's milk is the sole feed.

Modern cow's milk-based formulas

Modern milk formulas have been extensively modified from their predecessors in their protein, lipid, electrolyte and trace nutrient composition. Table 19.7 shows the composition of the standard infant formulas available in Britain, and Table 19.8 the composition of follow-on formulas. There is no information on whether or not the more recent finer degrees of modification have resulted in significant benefits, but it seems reasonable on empirical grounds to manufacture products resembling human milk as closely as possible. The need for further 'humanization' of infant formulas is still actively under investigation. Topical issues include the possibility of lowering total protein content to, say, 1.2–1. 4 g/100 ml (cf. 1.5 g/100 ml currently; Table 19.7); the addition of fish oils or other sources of very long-chain lipids (C20 or greater) in view of their importance in the brain; and the addition of further factors found in human milk, including nucleotides (p. 316) and oligosaccharides.

Soya formulas

The problems encountered with earlier soya-based formulas have been largely overcome; formulas are now supplemented with methionine, taurine and carnitine, and contain adequate minerals to allow for losses due to phytate binding in the gut. They are able to support normal growth and bone mineralization when used as the sole diet.[35,57] However, some issues remain unresolved. Soya beans have a high aluminium content, but it is not known whether this has any clinical relevance.[6] More recently, attention has been drawn to the potentially large amounts of plant oestrogen (phytoestrogen) that may be ingested by infants who are fully fed on soya formulas:[38] studies are under way to assess the level of exposure and look for evidence of any biological effect from these weak oestrogenic substances.

In the UK, approximately 7% of formula-fed infants receive soya formulas. The main justification for using these should be to provide an alternative diet for infants with proven cow's milk allergy, although in practice most infants are started on soya formulas based on clinical suspicion (see below). A recent (unpublished) survey of infants in the Cambridge area receiving soya formula on prescription (estimated to represent 80% of soya formula sales) found that the main symptom leading to the introduction of soya formula was colic (present in 47% of the infants). Other symptoms reported were vomiting (22%), eczema (25%) and diarrhoea (28%); in 44% of the infants more than one symptom was present. The decision to start soya formula involved the GP in 44% of cases, the health visitor in 47% and the parents in 22%; a paediatrician was involved in only 3% of cases, suggesting that the majority of infants did not have strictly confirmed cow's milk allergy.

Soya protein is itself potentially allergenic. Double-blind placebo-controlled challenges with soya milk in infants with proven allergy to cow's milk protein have suggested that around 5% of these infants are also intolerant of soya protein.[16,73]

Practical aspects of formula feeding

Detailed instructions for the reconstitution of artificial feeds and the hygienic use of feeding utensils can be obtained from manufacturers, but the following points need emphasizing.

1. The safety of modern infant formulas is highly dependent on:

- correct reconstitution of feeds, with accurate use of the scoops provided by manufacturers;
- Attention to sterility.

Following the concern over the dangers of over- and underconcentration of infant feeds due to inaccurate reconstitution, measuring scoops are at least as wide as their depth, reducing error, and there has been widespread cooperation between manufacturers to produce scoops of standard size that dispense powder in the proportion of one scoopful for each 30 ml (1 fl oz) of water. Nevertheless, there are still inherent difficulties in accurately dispensing milk powder in this way,[39] and our own data[53] show significant deviations from recommended nutrient concentrations in milks made up by mothers.

2. Infant formulas may be provided in 'ready to feed' liquid form (commonly used by hospitals for convenience, and now beginning to gain popularity in the

community) or as powder (less expensive and most commonly used by parents). When powdered milk is used, the water added deserves attention:

- Water which has passed though a water softener will have an increased sodium content and should not be used.[21]
- Although water should be boiled before addition to powder formulas, repeated or prolonged boiling may raise the sodium content in the water to an undesirable extent.[21]
- Environmental contaminants, e.g. nitrates, lead, aluminium and agrochemicals,[21] continue to be a topic of public interest. High nitrate concentrations in the water supply have been associated with rare cases of methaemoglobinaemia (current recommended nitrate levels in water are < 50 mg/l).[21] Lead is still found in tap water in some pre-1976 houses with lead pipes. Soft water is particularly plumbosolvent. The 1993 WHO guidelines for the quality of drinking water recommended that the lead concentration of water used to make up formula feeds should not exceed 10 μg/l (48.3 nmol/l).[85]
- The poor microbiological standards of drinking water that may be found in developing countries, among other factors, makes formula feeding highly undesirable in this situation.
- It is the duty of the water authority to provide a safe water supply that fulfils international guidelines on chemical composition. Nevertheless, consumers have frequently wished to 'play safe'. Bottled water should be the same standard as water from the public supply, but some marketed waters are unsuitable for infants; for example, 'natural mineral water' may contain unacceptable levels of carbon dioxide, sodium, nitrate and fluoride.[21] Some water filter manufacturers do not recommend their product for preparing water for babies, because silver may leach from the filter.

BREAST VERSUS BOTTLE

The relevant question for the medical profession is whether or not there are clinical grounds for wishing to influence parental choice. In the developing world the evidence that breast-feeding has a major influence on infant mortality and morbidity is well established and the case for medical intervention is strong. In the west the situation is rather different: in spite of considerable speculation on the benefits of breast-feeding, it has been harder to prove major detrimental effects of bottle-feeding. The subject has been reviewed recently by the British Paediatric Association Standing Committee on Nutrition.[10]

Comparisons between breast- and bottle-fed infants are epidemiological, and as it is not possible to randomize infants to one feeding regimen or another it is difficult to be certain that observed differences are not due to social class, social circumstances or other factors, rather than to the selection of diet per se. For example, although it had been suggested that breast-feeding be promoted as protective against SIDS, a recent study found that after adjusting for confounding factors such as maternal smoking, unemployment and sleeping position, formula feeding was not an independent risk factor.[28] Such confounding has made it difficult to evaluate published data on the differences between breast- and bottle-fed babies in their subsequent health and development.

Despite these reservations, there is now convincing evidence from a large prospective study that infants who are breast-fed for at least 13 weeks have a lower incidence of gastroenteritis and respiratory tract infections than formula-fed infants; the benefit persists beyond the period of breast-feeding, up to 1 year of age, and is present in partially breast-fed as well as exclusively breast-fed infants.[36] In addition, epidemiological data have linked breast-feeding with a variety of potentially beneficial long-term outcomes: for example, a lower incidence of juvenile diabetes[55,81] and malignancies, notably lymphoma.[15] In the case of diabetes, the epidemiological observations are strengthened by the finding of antibodies to an amino acid sequence of bovine serum albumin in the serum of newly diagnosed diabetic children but not controls; these antibodies cross-react with an antigen on the surface of the pancreatic islet β cell.[41] In some studies babies previously breast-fed have had higher cognitive performance than those bottle-fed, even after attempts to adjust for confounding factors;[60,69] although a causal relationship has not been proven, recent understanding of breast milk lipid composition and brain development has provided a possible mechanism for these observations. The influence of early feeding practices on later obesity is unknown and the published evidence conflicting (see below).

It has been supposed by many authors that mother–infant interaction would be favourably affected by breast-feeding; however, in his review Levy[44] argued that there was no evidence to suggest that breast- and bottle-fed infants differed in this respect, and concluded that bottle-feeding per se could not be held responsible for disturbance in the mother–infant relationship in infancy or later. Levy also pointed out that during the early months the infant is not capable of clearly deciding that the bottle is not part of the mother's body, and that if a bottle is offered with love, warmth and sensitivity there is no evidence that the infant's chances of normal psychological development are impaired. A variety of emotional benefits to the mother have been put forward for breast-feeding, but these may cease to be benefits if the mother has set her mind against feeding her infant in this way.

Notwithstanding the above, the arguments presented suggest that there is now sufficient evidence of clinical benefit to promote breast-feeding as the 'ideal' for term infants in developed countries. To help achieve this goal better health education (starting at school) is required, and the National Breast-feeding Working Group was set up in 1992 in the UK in an attempt to increase the numbers of mothers who breast-feed for more than 3 months. In addition, steps have been taken to reduce public exposure to advertisements for infant formulas; under the Infant Formula and Follow-on Formula Regulations[37] it is an offence for formula manufacturers in the UK to provide free or discounted products to pregnant women, either directly or indirectly through the healthcare system.

OBESITY AND INFANT FEEDING

The overall incidence of obesity in infancy has declined in the past 20 years, perhaps related to a more general secular trend in the eating habits of families as a whole. Taitz observed that in 1971 79% of infants had weights greater than the 50th centile at 6 weeks of age, compared to 43% in 1976.[78] Previous reports of obesity in bottle-fed infants may have been due to feeding unmodified cow's milk, a tendency to overconcentrate artificial feeds during reconstitution, early introduction of cereals and excessive addition of sugar to bottle feeds.[20] However, there is evidence that, despite similar weight gains over the first 3 months of life, infants fed on modern formulas still become fatter than their breast-fed peers between 4 and 18 months.[18] Although several studies have shown a higher energy intake in formula- versus breast-fed infants, it is not clear whether this is because currently the RDA for energy is too high (see p. 308) or because errors occur during reconstitution of powdered formulas. A recent study showed that infants fed a powdered formula became fatter than those receiving a ready-to-feed formula with the same nutrient content; the volumes taken by the two groups of infants were identical, but the reconstituted powdered feeds were found to be more concentrated.[54]

Whether the early differences observed between breast- and formula-fed infants are reflected in long-term effects on body composition and risk of obesity is unknown. Kramer[42] reported that breast-feeding exerts a small though significant prophylactic effect against later obesity in 12- to 18-year-olds, but such studies need to be repeated in view of the changes in dietary practices over the past two decades. The majority of overweight infants do not remain so. Thus only about 10–20% of obese babies will be obese at 5–7 years.[67]

EARLY DIET AND LONG-TERM OUTCOME[49]

A fundamental question in infant nutrition is whether early diet has a long-term influence on health, growth and development. Such data are required to justify many of our current nutritional policies. Animal studies suggest that infancy may be a critical period during which dietary factors exert long-term 'programming' effects. Thus studies on rodents, and more recently primates, suggest that dietary manipulation in infancy may influence, in adult life, learning and memory; plasma insulin; cholesterol absorption, turnover and plasma levels; obesity and atherosclerosis. Corresponding formal studies have not been conducted in full-term infants and largely retrospective epidemiological data on the long-term consequence of such factors as early salt and lipid intake and of early malnutrition are inconclusive, mainly because of poor experimental design. Nevertheless, prospective data from studies on premature babies randomly assigned to diet (see Part 3) suggest that a very brief period of dietary manipulation (during the neonatal period) has significant effects on growth, development and allergic status in later infancy and early childhood. Barker and co-workers[5] have shown that birthweight, and weight at 1 year, is highly positively correlated with a reduced death rate from vascular disease in the 7 decade, and a reduction in the incidence of non-insulin dependent diabetes mellitus. These data suggest a possible link between fetal and infant nutrition and long-term morbidity. Further prospective studies are currently under way in this important field.

REFERENCES

1. American Academy of Pediatrics 1986 Committee on Nutrition. In: Forbes G B (ed) Pediatric nutrition handbook, pp. 170–173
2. Ando Y, Nakano S, Saito K et al 1987 Transmission of adult T cell leukaemia retrovirus (HTLV-1) from mother to child: comparison of bottle with breast fed babies. Japanese Journal of Cancer Research 78: 322–324
3. Astrup-Jensen A 1988 Environmental and occupational chemicals. In: Bennett P N (ed) Drugs and human lactation. Elsevier, Amsterdam, pp 551–573
4. Ankett M A, Parks Y A, Scott P H, Wharton B A 1986 Treatment with iron increases weight gain and psychomotor development. Archives of Disease in Childhood 61: 849–857
5. Barker D J P, Winter P D, Osmond C, Margetts B, Simmonds S J 1989 Weight in infancy and death from ischaemic heart disease. Lancet ii: 577–580
6. Baxter M J, Burrell J A, Crews H, Massey R C 1991 Aluminium levels in milk and infant formulae. Food Additives and Contaminants 8: 653–660
7. Beasley R P, Stevens C E, Shiao I S, Meng H C 1975 Evidence against breast-feeding as a mechanism for vertical transmission of hepatitis B. Lancet 7938: 740–741
8. Bernhart F W 1961 Correlation between growth-rate of the suckling of various species and the percentage of total calories from protein in the milk. Nature 191: 358–360
9. Birkbeck J A, Scott H F 1980 25-Hydroxycholecalciferol serum levels in breastfed infants. Archives of Disease in Childhood 55: 691–695
10. British Paediatric Association Standing Committee on Nutrition 1994 Is breast feeding beneficial in the UK? Archives of Disease in Childhood 71: 376–380
11. Brouwer A, Ahlborg U G, Van den Berg M et al 1995 Functional aspects of developmental toxicity of polyhalogenated aromatic hydrocarbons in experimental animals and human infants. European Journal of Pharmacology (Environmental Toxicology and Pharmaology Section) 293: 1–40
12. Carlson S E 1985 Human milk non-protein nitrogen: occurrence and possible functions. Advances in Pediatrics 32: 43–70

13. Chaudary R K 1983 Perinatal transmission of hepatitis B virus. Canadian Medical Association Journal 128: 664–666
14. Dallman P R 1986 Iron deficiency in the weanling: a nutritional problem on the way to resolution. Acta Paediatrica Scandinavica suppl. 323: 59–67
15. Davis M K, Savitz D A, Granbard B I 1988 Infant feeding and childhood cancer. Lancet ii: 365–8
16. Dean T P, Adler B R, Ruge F, Warner J O 1993 In vitro allergenicity of cow's milk substitutes. Clinical and Experimental Allergy 23: 205–210
17. Department of Health 1991 Weaning and the weaning diet. Report on Health and Social Subjects No 45. HMSO, London
18. Dewey K G, Heinig M J, Nommsen L A, Peerson J M, Lonnerdal B 1991 Growth of breast-fed and formula-fed infants from 0–18 months: the DARLING study. Pediatrics 89: 1035–1041
19. DHSS 1977 The composition of mature human milk. Report on Health and Social Subjects No. 12. HMSO, London
20. DHSS 1980 Artificial feeds for the young infant: Report on Health and Social Subjects No. 18. Report of the Committee on Medical Aspects of Food Policy. HMSO, London
21. DHSS 1988 Present day practice in infant feeding, third report. Report on Health and Social Subjects No. 32. HMSO, London
22. Dine M S, Gartside P S, Glueck C J, Rheines L, Greene G, Khoury P 1979 Where do the heaviest children come from? A prospective study of white children from birth to 5 years of age. Pediatrics 63: 1–7
23. Dowell T B, Joyston-Bechal S 1981 Fluoride supplements – age related dosage. British Dental Journal 150: 273–275
24. Freeman J V, Cole T J, Chinn S, Jones PRM, White E M, Preece M A 1995 Cross-sectional stature and weight reference curves for the UK. Archives of Disease in Childhood 73: 17–24
25. Gale S M, Read L C, George-Nascimento C, Wallace J C, Ballard F J 1989 Is dietary epidermal growth factor absorbed by premature human infants. Biology of the Neonate 55: 104–110
26. Garry P, Owen G M, Hooper E M, Gilbert B A 1981 Iron absorption from human milk and formula with and without iron supplementation. Pediatric Research 15: 822–828
27. George D E, Lebenthal E 1981 Human breast milk in comparison with cow's milk. In: Lebenthal E (ed) Textbook of gastroenterology and nutrition in infancy. Raven Press, New York, pp 295–320
28. Gilbert R E, Wigfield R E, Fleming P J, Berry P J, Rudd P T 1995 Bottle feeding and the sudden infant death syndrome. British Medical Journal 310: 88–90
29. Goldman A S, Thorpe L W, Goldblum R M, Hanson L A 1986 Review article. Anti-inflammatory properties of human milk. Acta Paediatrica 75: 689–695
30. Greer F R, Reeve L E, Chesney R W, DeLuca H F 1982 Water-soluble vitamin D in human milk: a myth. Pediatrics 69: 238
31. Grulee C G, Sanford H N, Herron P H 1935 Breast and artificial feeding. Journal of the American Medical Association 104: 1986–1988
32. Gyorgyi P 1971 The uniqueness of human milk. Biochemical aspects. American Journal of Clinical Nutrition 24: 970–975
33. Hamosh M 1996 Digestion in the newborn. Clinics in Perinatology 23: 191–210
34. Haschke F, Vanura H, Male C et al 1993 Iron nutrition and growth of breast- and formula-fed infants during the first 9 months of life. Journal of Pediatric Gastroenterology and Nutrition 16: 151–156
35. Hillman L S 1990 Mineral and vitamin D adequacy in infants fed human milk or formula between 6 and 12 months of age. Journal of Pediatrics 117: S134–142
36. Howie P W, Forsyth J S, Ogston S A, Clark A, Firey C du V 1990 Protective effect of breast feeding against infection. British Medical Journal 300: 11–16
37. Infant formula and follow-on formula regulations 1995. Statutory Instrument No. 77. HMSO, London
38. Irvine C, Fitzpatrick M, Robertson I, Woodhams D 1995 The potential adverse effects of soybean phytoestrogens in infant feeding (letter). New Zealand Medical Journal 25 May: 208–209
39. Jeffs S G 1989 Hazards of scoop measurements in infant feeding. Journal of the Royal College of General Practitioners 39: 113
40. Jensen R G 1996 The lipids in human milk. Progress in Lipid Research 35: 53–92
41. Karjalainen J, Martin J M, Knip M et al 1992 A bovine albumin peptide as a possible trigger of insulin-dependent diabetes. New England Journal of Medicine 327: 302–307
42. Kramer M S 1981. Do breast feeding and the delayed introduction of solid foods protect against subsequent obesity? Journal of Pediatrics 98: 883–887
43. Kurauchi O, Furui T, Itakura A et al 1993 Studies on transmission of hepatitis C virus from mother-to-child in the perinatal period. Archives of Gynecology and Obstetrics 253: 121–126
44. Levy R 1981 Mother–infant relations in the feeding situation. In: Lebenthal E (ed) Textbook of gastroenterology and nutrition in infancy. Raven Press, New York, pp 633–645
45. Little R E, Anderson K W, Ervin C H, Worthington-Roberts B, Clarren S K 1989 Maternal alcohol use during breast-feeding and infant mental and motor development at one year. New England Journal of Medicine 321: 425–430
46. Loomis W F 1970 Rickets. Scientific American 223: 76–91
47. Lucas A 1983 Human milk and infant feeding. In: Boyd R, Battaglia FC (eds) perinatal medicine. Butterworths, London, pp 172–200
48. Lucas A 1988 Aids and human milk banking. In: Hudson C N, Sharp F (eds) Proceedings of 19th RCOG Study Group: Aids in obstetrics and gynaecology, Royal College of Obstetricians and Gynaecologists, London, pp 271–281
49. Lucas A 1990 Does early diet program future outcome? Acta Paediatrica Scandinavica 365: 58–67
50. Lucas A, Cole T J 1990 Breast milk and neonatal necrotising enterocolitis. Lancet 336: 1519–1523
51. Lucas A, Ewing E, Roberts S B, Coward W A 1987 How much energy does the breast fed baby consume and expend? British Medical Journal 295: 75–77
52. Lucas A, Lucas P J, Baum J D 1980 The Nipple Shield Sampling System: a device for measuring the dietary intake of breast fed infants. Early Human Development 4: 365–372
53. Lucas A, Lockton S, Davies P S W 1991 Infant formula reconstitution errors. British Medical Journal 302: 350–351
54. Lucas A, Lockton S, Davies PSW 1992 Randomised trial of a ready-to-feed compared with powdered formula. Archives of Disease in Childhood 67: 935–939
54a. Macy I G, Kelly H J, Sloan R E 1953 The composition of bulks. National Academy of Science, National Research Council, Washington DC Publication 254
55. Mayer E J, Hamman R F, Gay E C, Lezotte D C, Savitz D A, Klingensmith G J 1988 Reduced risk of IDDM among breast-fed children. Diabetes 37: 1625–1632
56. Mettler A E 1976 Infant milk powder feeds compared on a common basis. Postgraduate Medical Journal 52: Supplement 8: 3–20
57. Mimouni F, Campaigne B, Neylan M, Tsang R C 1993 Bone mineralisation in the first year of life in infants fed human milk, cow-milk formula or soy-based formula. Journal of Pediatrics 122: 348
58. Minamishima I, Ueda K, Minematsu T et al 1994 Role of breast milk in aquisition of cytomegalovirus infection. Microbiology and Immunology 38: 549–552
59. Moriya T, Sasaki F, Mizui M et al 1995 Transmission of hepatitis C virus from mothers to infants: its frequency and risk factors revisited. Biomedicine and Pharmacotherapy 49: 59–64
60. Morrow-Tlucak M, Haude R H, Ernhart C B 1988 Breast-feeding and cognitive development in the first seven years of life. Social Science and Medicine 26: 635–639
61. National Diet and Nutrition Survey 1994 Children aged $1\frac{1}{2}$–$4\frac{1}{2}$ years. Gregory J, Collins D L, Davies P S W, Clark P L, Hughes J M. Volume I: Report of the Diet and Nutrition Survey. HMSO, London, 1994
62. Newcomb P A, Storer B E, Longnecker M P et al 1994 Lactation and a reduced risk of premenopausal breast cancer. New England Journal of Medicine 330: 81–87
63. Norgaard-Hansen K, Ebbesen F 1996 Neonatal vitamin K prophylaxis in Denmark: three years' experience with oral administration during the first three months of life compared with one oral administration at birth. Acta Paediatrica 85: 1137–1139
64. Paul A A, Black A E, Evans J, Cole T J, Whitehead R G 1985 Breastmilk intake and growth in infants from two to ten months. Journal of Human Nutrition and Dietetics 1: 437–450
65. Pitt J, Barlow B, Heird W C 1977 Protection against experimental necrotizing enterocolitis by maternal milk. I. Role of milk leucocytes. Pediatric Research 11: 906–909
66. Prentice A, Ewing G, Roberts S B, Lucas A, MacCarthy A, Jarjou C, Whitehead R G 1987 The nutrition role of breast-milk IgA and lactoferrin. Acta Paediatrica Scandinavica 76: 592–598

67. Poskitt E M E, Cole T J 1977 Do fat babies stay fat? British Medical Journal 1: 7–9
68. Roberts C C, Chan G M, Follard D, Rayburn C, Jackson R 1981 Adequate bone mineralization in breast fed infants. Journal of Pediatrics 99: 192–196
69. Rogers B 1978 Feeding in infancy and later ability and attainment: A longitudinal study. Developmental Medicine and Child Neurology 20: 421–426
70. Rudolf M, Arulantham K, Greenstein R M 1980 Unsuspected nutritional rickets. Pediatrics 66: 72–76
71. Saarinen U M, Siimes M A 1979 Iron absorption from breast milk, cow's milk and iron supplemented formula. Pediatric Research 13: 143–147
72. Sack J 1980 Hormones in milk. In: Firer S, Eidelman A I (eds) Human milk, its biological and social value. Excerpta Medica, Amsterdam, pp 56–61
73. Sampson H A 1988 The role of food hypersensitivity and mediator release in atopic dermatitis. Journal of Allergy and Clinical Immunology 81: 635–645
74. Schams D 1976 Hormonal control of lactation. In: Breast-feeding and the mother. Ciba Foundation Symposium 45. Elsevier/Exerpta Medica, Amsterdam, pp 27–48
75. Schlesinger J J, Covelli H D 1977 Evidence for transmission of lymphocyte responses to tuberculin by breast-feeding. Lancet 8037: 529–532
76. Simhon A, Douglas J R, Drasar B S, Soothill J F 1982 Effect of feeding on infants' faecal flora. Archives of Disease in Childhood 57: 54–58
77. Stekel A 1984 Prevention of iron deficiency. In: Stekel A (ed) Iron nutrition in infancy and childhood, Raven Press, New York, pp 179–92
78. Taitz L S 1977 Infantile obesity. Pediatric Clinics of North America 24: 107–115
79. Uehara S, Abe Y, Saito T et al 1993 The incidence of vertical transmission of hepatitis C virus. Tohoku Journal of Experimental Medicine 171: 195–202
80. United Kingdom National Case-Control study group 1993 Breast feeding and risk of breast cancer in young women. British Medical Journal 307: 17–20
81. Virtanen S M, Rasanen L, Aro A et al 1991 Infant feeding in children <7 years of age with newly diagnosed IDDM. Diabetes Care 14: 415–417
82. von Kries R, Shearer M J, Gobel U 1988 Vitamin K in infancy. European Journal of Pediatrics 147: 106–112
83. Whitehead R G, Paul A A, Cole T J 1989 Diet and the growth of healthy infants. Journal of Human Nutrition and Dietetics 2: 73–84
84. Williamson S, Finucaine E, Elliott J, Gamsu H R 1978 Effect of heat treatment of human milk on absorption of nitrogen, fat, sodium, calcium and phosphorus by preterm infants. Archives of Disease in Childhood 53: 555–563
85. World Health Organisation 1993 Guidelines for drinking-water quality. Vol 1. Recommendations. Geneva, WHO
86. Ziegler E E, Fomon S J 1971 Fluid intake, renal solute load and water balance in infancy. Journal of Pediatrics 78: 561–568

Part 3

Feeding low-birthweight infants

Mary Fewtrell Alan Lucas

GENERAL CONSIDERATIONS

The principal matters to be decided when planning enteral feeding in low-birthweight infants are which diet, which route of administration and what feeding schedule should be selected. Valuable short-term studies have been performed on preterm infant feeding, but only recently have investigators begun to explore how different dietary regimens influence short-term morbidity and mortality and, in the longer term, how they affect neurological development, growth and the incidence of subsequent illness. Information of this nature is critical in order to assess the value of current practice.

CHOICE OF DIET

A wide range of diets have been used for feeding low-birthweight infants, including the following:

- Human milk
  - Mother's own: 'preterm milk'
  - Banked donor milk (expressed breast milk or drip breast milk)
  - Fortified human milk
  - Human milk formulas (separated and reconstituted human milk);
- 'Term' infant formulas
  - Cow's milk based
  - Soya based;
- Special 'preterm' infant formulas.
- Parenteral feeding (Chapter 20)
  - Partial
  - Total.

HUMAN MILK

There has been major interest in human milk for feeding low-birthweight infants. The practice of encouraging mothers to provide milk for their own preterm infants has become widespread. Many centres throughout Europe and the USA set up human milk banks, though in more recent years concerns about the nutritional adequacy of donor milk and the theoretical risk of HIV transmission to recipients (p. 332) has resulted in numerous closures. The value of breast milk in neonatal intensive care needs critical appraisal.

NUTRITIONAL CONSIDERATIONS

Unmodified human milk may not always meet the theoretical requirements of low-birthweight infants for several nutrients, including:

- protein (especially when 'mature' donor milk is used, p. 309);
- energy (especially donor 'drip breast milk', p. 314);
- sodium (p. 316);
- calcium, phosphorus and magnesium (p. 317);
- trace elements, e.g. iron, zinc and copper (pp. 318–319);
- certain vitamins (e.g. B_2, B_6, folic acid, C, D, E and K, pp. 320–322).

However, human milk does have theoretical nutritional advantages compared with formulas, including the composition and easier absorption of its fats (p. 000), and the bioavailability of certain trace metals (p. 000). Formulas designed to meet the calculated nutrient needs of preterm infants result, inevitably, in a greater renal solute load imposed on the infant (p. 000) than that seen with human milk.

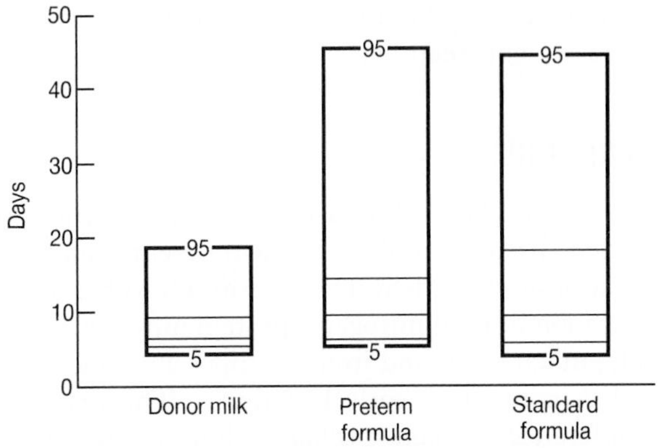

Fig. 19.4 Days to attain full enteral feeds according to diet in over 300 preterm infants under 1850 g birthweight. Data are represented in centiles; the horizontal lines in the data bar for each diet represent, from bottom to top, the 5th, 25th, 50th, 75th and 95th centiles for the number of postnatal days to reach an enteral intake of 150 ml/kg/24 h.

INFECTION AND NECROTIZING ENTEROCOLITIS

Information on the protective advantages in the west of human milk used for feeding low-birthweight infants is very scanty. However, in the developing world, where infection rates are high, the anti-infective role of human milk assumes much greater importance.[48]

Fresh breast milk might protect against NEC in a rat (p. 331), but similar effects in preterm babies have been debated. The principal problem in published studies on diet and NEC is small trial size. In a large study, with formal dietary assignments, Lucas and Cole[28] showed that babies fed exclusively on formula had six times more confirmed NEC than infants fed exclusively on breast milk (fresh or pasteurized), and three times the NEC rate of those fed formula in conjunction with breast milk. The authors suggested that using either raw maternal milk or pasteurized donor milk in the early diet of preterm infants might prevent about 500 cases of NEC each year in the UK; this is currently being explored in a national study.

ALLERGY

There is a theoretical possibility that feeding the preterm infant with cow's milk proteins at a time when gut permeability may be increased[50] could raise the chance of later cow's milk allergy. Indeed, Lucas et al[35] showed that preterm neonates rapidly developed latent sensitization to cow's milk. At the 18-month follow-up of a randomized trial of early nutrition Lucas et al[38] found no overall difference in allergic reactions between infants fed formula or donor breast milk, but in the subgroup of infants with atopy in one or more first-degree relatives, early formula feeding was associated with twice the incidence of subsequent allergic reactions compared to those in the exclusively human milk-fed group (for eczema the respective incidences were 41% and 16%).

GASTROINTESTINAL 'TOLERANCE'

Gastrointestinal 'tolerance' of human milk is greater than that of formulas. Cavell[9] has shown that human milk passes through the stomach faster than formula in preterm infants, and this observation is compatible with our own finding of increased vomiting and a higher residual intragastric volume in preterm infants fed either standard or special formulas. As a result, it may take substantially longer to establish full enteral feeding in infants fed formulas; in a five-centre study 95% of infants fed breast milk were on full feeds by 18 days, whereas the 95th centile for formula-fed babies was more than 40 days, owing to a proportion of infants in whom it was difficult to achieve feed tolerance (Fig. 19.4).[34] These data have implications for the design of feeding regimens (see below).

DEVELOPMENTAL SCORES

Preterm babies fed on their own mother's milk have been shown to have higher developmental scores at 18 months and higher IQs at 7.5–8 years than those fed on other diets, even after adjusting for a range of demographic, social and clinical factors that might confound this comparison.[41,47] Whether these findings reflect a failure to adjust for further (unknown) confounding factors, or whether fresh human milk has a beneficial effect on development, is an important question for investigation. The latter explanation is favoured by the observation that infants fed banked breast milk had higher developmental scores at 18 months than those fed term formulas, despite the lower macronutrient content of banked breast milk.[42]

TYPES OF BREAST MILK

The composition of breast milk depends on its source, the mode of its collection and on the postnatal and postconceptional age of the donor; it can be further modified by its subsequent treatment.

PRETERM MILK

The milk of mothers who have delivered preterm infants – so-called 'preterm milk' – has a different composition from that of mothers delivered at term. PTM has a higher concentration of total nitrogen,[2] protein nitrogen, sodium, chloride, magnesium and iron,[26] copper and zinc,[1] with a raised IgA content in early lactation.[22] The reasons for these differences remain speculative but may relate to the low volume often produced by PTM donors.[29]

PTM is thus more suitable than term donor milk for feeding preterm infants, particularly in view of its higher concentration of protein. However, protein intakes from PTM are very variable, and by the second month of PTM production protein concentrations often fall to values at which theoretical needs would be met only by very high volume intakes. PTM may be given raw to the mother's own infant, in which case antimicrobial components will remain intact. Neither microbiological examination nor pasteurization is necessary in this situation, provided that the collected milk is refrigerated adequately and fed to the infant within 48 hours, or at most 72 hours, or if it is frozen.

Many mothers who elect at the outset to provide milk for their own infants either totally or partially fail to do so. In over 600 mother's milk-fed infants from several centres studied between 1982 and 1985, maternal milk comprised less than 50% of total enteral intake. In a further study between 1988 and 1990, this figure had fallen below 40%. Factors contributing to lack of success in producing sufficient PTM include geographical separation of mother and child, inadequate support, the inherent difficulty of maintaining the milk supply by manual or mechanical expression, lack of motivation, and – not least – poor advice. Mothers need to be advised to express their milk at least as often as they would normally nurse a baby, that is, around 6–8 times a day (as a minimum).

EXPRESSED DONOR MILK

Expressed donor milk can be foremilk or hindmilk, obtained either before or after the donor's own infant has fed from the breast; these two types of milk will have, respectively, lower or higher fat and energy contents than milk received by the breast-fed infant. Mature donor milk will have a lower protein, sodium, zinc and copper content than that of milk produced in early lactation.

DRIP BREAST MILK

DBM is the milk that drips spontaneously from the contralateral breast during feeding in a proportion of lactating mothers – about 20% produce significant quantities. It can be collected during feeding into a presterilized glass or plastic shell worn over the contralateral nipple and areola. DBM has a similar composition to foremilk, with a low fat and energy content (often around 50 kcal/100 ml in pooled milk). Fat concentration and energy value correlate positively with the volume of DBM obtained, and negatively with the postnatal stage of the donor. Pools of donor breast milk may have energy contents as low as 45 kcal/100 ml compared to around 65 kcal/100 ml in mature expressed breast milk.[19,31]

Table 19.11 Major nutrient composition of breast milk fortifiers available in the UK (amounts given are what would be added to 100 ml of human milk)

	Cow & Gate Nutriprem	Milupa Eoprotein	Mead Johnson Enfamil	SMA Breast Milk Fortifier
Energy				
kJ	44	47	58	64
kcal	10	11	14	15
Protein (g)	0.7	0.6	0.7	1.0
Carbohydrate (g)	2.0	2.1	2.73	2.4
Fat (g)	nil	0.02	0.05	0.16
Sodium (mg)	6.0	20	7.0	18
Potassium (mg)	4.0	2.4	45	27
Calcium (mg)	60	38	90	90
Phosphorus (mg)	40	26	45	45
Magnesium (mg)	6.0	2.1	1.0	3.0
Vitamin A (μg)	130	30	234	270
Vitamin D (μg)	5.0	nil	6.5	7.6
Vitamin E (mg)	2.6	0.2	2.3	3.0
Vitamin K (μg)	6.3	0.2	9.1	11.0

(Manufacturers' data)

FORTIFIED HUMAN MILK

One solution to overcome the nutrient deficits in human milk for the preterm infant is to add a milk fortifier containing protein, energy, macrominerals, trace minerals and a comprehensive range of vitamins. Several are now commercially available (Table 19.11), usually in the form of a powder which is added to a fixed volume of milk. The addition of nutrients to a complex biological medium such as milk poses theoretical problems: breast milk varies greatly in composition, and the addition of a fixed supplement may result in some infants exceeding the upper recommended limit for certain nutrients while others remain below desirable intake levels. Fortification may also influence nutrient availability or alter the biological properties of human milk.

Despite these concerns, several studies have demonstrated improved short-term growth, nutrient retention and bone mineralization in infants receiving fortified rather than unfortified breast milk.[20,25,46,52] There are few long-term outcome data on these products as yet. In a recent study of 275 infants randomised to receive either a breast milk fortifier or control supplement containing only vitamins and phosphate, there was no significant difference in neurodevelopmental outcome at 18 months of age.[43] This study included infants who received preterm formula if insufficient breast milk was available. In the short term the fortifier was well tolerated, and there was an increased growth rate in infants who received more than 50% of their intake as breast milk. However, the study also produced findings of potential concern: infants who received the fortifier had a significant increase in the incidence of infection (proven plus suspected), and a trend towards an increase in the incidence of NEC (a much larger study would be needed to detect such an effect as significant). It remains to be established whether overall outcome in infants fed fortified breast milk is better than in infants fed a preterm formula when both diets provide similar nutrient intakes.

Although further research is required, the concept of human milk fortification, of both mother's own and donor milk, is promising and offers the potential benefits of human milk (discussed above) while avoiding the problem of nutrient deficits. At present, we would suggest that human milk should be fortified if the infant's weight gain is unsatisfactory.

HUMAN MILK FORMULA

This involves the addition of human milk protein and fat preparations (together with additional minerals) to whole human milk.[33] Rohnholm et al[51] have demonstrated that breast milk fortification with human milk protein improves growth and prevents hypoproteinaemia. However, the manufacture of HMF requires a large supply of donor milk and is impractical for most neonatal units.

HUMAN MILK BANKING

Units wishing to set up a human milk bank should consult the DHSS report[13] on the collection and storage of human milk, and the more recent review by Balmer and Wharton.[3] Problems that need to be considered are listed below.

- Funding and organizing the collection and transportation; creation of a milk kitchen and its staffing;
- Canvassing donors;
- Screening donors for HIV, HBV and HCV, with counselling;
- Selecting the type of donor milk to be used: drip or expressed;
- Monitoring and giving advice on milk storage facilities in the home;
- Issuing donors with apparatus for milk collection (pumps/collecting shells, sterilizing tanks, hypochlorite agents, collecting bottles and labels);
- Providing adequate advice and care for donors;
- Installing and running effective pasteurization equipment in the milk kitchen;
- Organizing milk storage and retrieval facilities (4°C refrigerator(s) and –20°C freezer(s) are required);
- Arranging bacteriological monitoring and developing criteria for milk rejection;
- Establishing the nutrient quality control of donor milk, either in collaboration with the biochemistry department or using simple analytical methods on the unit;
- Planning the preparation of individual feeds over a 24-hour period;
- Contingency planning for periods when milk bank staff are absent from the unit, or when supplies are low.

It is important to appreciate that once milk has been collected, bacterially decontaminated, stored, frozen and thawed, pasteurized, exposed to light, aliquoted and instilled into feeding apparatus, it may have undergone qualitative alterations that render it significantly different from milk obtained by an infant during normal suckling.[18] Freezing, thawing and heat treatment damage antimicrobial factors in milk and denature milk lipase; milk cells seldom survive the banking process. Evans et al[17] showed that accurate pasteurization for 30 minutes at 62.5°C destroyed 24% of the lysozyme, 57% of the lactoferrin, 34% of the IgG but little IgA (though loss of biological activity of IgA was not assessed), whereas after treatment at 73°C (as might occur with inaccurate pasteurization) only minimal quantities of these constituents remained intact. Heating milk may also reduce the vitamin C content. In addition, pasteurization may reduce fat absorption, perhaps by damaging milk lipase. The optimal time and temperature required to destroy bacteria reliably and preserve antimicrobial properties is under investigation: Wills et al[55] suggest that short-time, low-temperature pasteurization (56°C for 15 minutes) is effective, but milk should always be checked bacteriologically after pasteurization and before banking, although it does not require further checks after thawing. Some workers have argued that banked milk could be given raw, but others are concerned about bacteriological safety,[5] since the milk may contain potential pathogens, such as β haemolytic streptococci. Light exposure of breast milk results, within 3 hours, in a 50% reduction in riboflavin content and 70% loss of vitamin A.[4]

Screening of breast milk donors for HIV, hepatitis B and hepatitis C virus is now advised. The risk of acquiring HIV from donor breast milk is unknown (see above), but there have been no reported cases of preterm infants infected in this way. Published evidence suggests that pasteurization destroys HIV,[16] although some virologists continue to have doubts about this. Pasteurizers should be frequently calibrated to ensure their temperature control settings remain in the effective range (60–66°C).

Table 19.12 Nutrient content of low-birthweight formulas available in the UK (per 100 ml)

Composition per 100 ml	Mature human milk		Milupa Prematil with Milupan~** (M)	Nutriprem LBW** (C&G)	Osterprem (FHP)**	SMA LBW** (Wyeth)
	DHSSa	Macy				
Macronutrients						
Protein* (g)	1.34	1.45	2.4	2.4	2.0	2.0
Fat (g)	4.2	3.8	4.4	4.4	4.6	4.4
saturated (%)	50.1	52	79	43.4	42.3	48.2
unsaturated (%)	48.5	48	21	56.6	57.7	51.8
LCPUFA added	+	+	+	+	+	+
Carbohydrate+						
Total (g)	7.0	7.0	7.9	7.9	7.65	8.6
Energy						
kcal	70	68	80	80	80	82
kJ	293	285	336	336	336	335
Minerals						
Calcium (mg)	35	33	100	108	110	77
Chloride (mg)	43	43	48	48	60	74
Magnesium (mg)	2.8	4.0	10	10	5.0	7.0
Phosphorus (mg)	15	15	50	50	63	41
Potassium (mg)	60	55	80	80	72	33
Sodium (mg)	15	15	41	41	42	33
Trace elements						
Copper (μg)	39	40	80	80	96	74
Iodine (μg)	7	7	14	25	8	8.2
Iron (μg)	76	150	900	900	40	670
Manganese (μg)	ND	0.7	4.8	10.0	3.0	6.0
Zinc (μg)	295	530	700	700	880	820
Potential renal solute load^ (mosmol/l)	88	91	148	148	134	129
Vitamins						
A retinol (μg)	60	53	108	227	100	74
B_1 thiamin (μg)	16	16	140	140	95	82
B_2 riboflavin (μg)	31	42.6	200	200	180	131
B_6 pyridoxine (μg)	6	11	120	120	100	49
B_{12} cyanocobalamin (μg)	0.01	trace	0.2	0.2	0.2	0.25
Biotin (μg)	0.76	0.4	3.0	3.0	2.0	1.8
Folic acid (μg)	5.2	0.18	48	48	50	49
Niacin (μg)	230	172	3000	3000	1000	656
C ascorbic acid (mg)	3.8	4.3	16	16	28	7
Vitamin D (μg)	0.01	0.01	2.4	5.0	2.4	1.2
Vitamin E (mg)	0.35	0.56	3	3.0	10	1.1
K phytomenadione (μg)	ND	1.7	6.6	6.6	7.0	7.1
Other						
Carnitine (mg)	ND	ND	2	2	1.0	2.96
Choline (mg)	ND	9	10	10	5.6	13.1
Inositol (mg)	ND	39	ND	30	3.2	3.3
Taurine (mg)	4.8	ND	5.5	5.5	5.1	4.8
Osmolality (mmol/kg)			312	293	280	268

* total nitrogen × 6.38
\+ figures declared as disaccharide
\# liquid formulation – sodium 34, chloride 67
^ method of Ziegler & Fomon[57]: calculated values
~ Milupan is a lipid mixture containing LCPUFA

a DHSS Reports on Health and Social Subjects[11,12,14]
b Macy, Kelly and Sloan[44] and Mettler[45]
** manufacturer's information
NS not stated
LCPUFA long chain polyunsaturated fatty acids: + added, – not added

'TERM' INFANT FORMULAS

For many years formulas designed for full-term infants were used to feed low-birthweight infants, and some units still use them. Because modern formulas are based on the composition of mature breast milk, the theoretical arguments concerning the nutritional suitability of human milk for low-birthweight infants also apply to these formulas, yet 'term' formulas lack the non-nutrient factors present in breast milk. Such formulas (Table 19.7) contain around 1.5 g of protein/100 ml and 65–70 kcal/100 ml. Fed at 180–200 ml/kg they provide only 2.7–3.0 g/kg/24 h – below the limit recommended by the International Consensus Committee (Table 19.2). Sodium, calcium and phosphorus intakes, together with those of several trace nutrients, do not meet the calculated needs of low-birthweight infants. Data from a large multicentre trial show that infants fed standard formulas grow more slowly in the short term than those fed 'preterm' formulas, and have substantially lower motor and mental development scores at 18 months and lower IQs at 7.5–8 years[39] (Lucas et al unpublished data). In our view standard formulas have no place in the future management of preterm infants under 2 kg body weight, and preterm formulas should be used in their place. Soya formula should not be used for feeding low-birthweight infants.

SPECIAL PRETERM INFANT FORMULAS

In recent years a variety of formulas have been designed to meet the theoretical nutrient needs of low-birthweight infants (see Part 1). These formulas (Table 19.12) vary in their detailed composition, and continue to evolve.

The potential of preterm formulas for inducing 'metabolic strain' (e.g. renal solute and protein overload) is greater than with other available diets, particularly in very small and sick infants. However, clinical trials have shown that such formulas may carry a number of short-term advantages over unsupplemented human milk: they promote faster weight, length and head circumference gain, reduce hospital stay, and reduce the incidence of hyponatraemia, bone disease of prematurity, hypophosphataemia, hyperbilirubinaemia and some vitamin deficiencies.[8,21,37] More importantly, at follow-up infants previously fed preterm formulas are advantaged over those fed standard 'term' formula in linear growth,[37] developmental scores and IQ.[36,39]

DIETS FOR PRETERM INFANTS: OVERVIEW

In summary, recent evidence suggests that human milk has an important place in neonatal intensive care. Many infants tolerate human milk better than formula, and enteral feeds can be established faster, reducing the requirement for parenteral nutrition (which has known hazards: see Chapter 20). The use of breast milk is likely to be associated with a reduction in the incidence of necrotizing enterocolitis, and there is a strong possibility (p. 339) that it has a beneficial influence on developmental attainment.

Our policy is to use breast milk, preferably the mother's own, but donor milk if it is not available, to establish enteral feeds (up to 150 ml/kg) in infants of 28 weeks' gestation or less and in infants who have had prolonged intravenous feeding (when the gut may be atrophic) or prolonged respiratory disease. When mothers do not provide breast milk, preterm formula is used as a sole diet from after birth in larger, well babies and after the establishment of human milk feeds in smaller or ill babies. If no breast milk is available, either maternal or banked, preterm formula should be cautiously introduced. Although term formula is sometimes used to establish enteral feeds in infants who appear not to tolerate preterm formula, there is no scientific evidence to support this; a large randomized study of diet in preterm infants found no difference in the amount of vomiting, the time to tolerate full enteral feeds, or the incidence of NEC between infants receiving term formula versus preterm formula as their sole diet (Lucas et al, unpublished data). If term formula *is* used in this situation, it should be replaced by preterm formula as soon as possible. Preterm formula is also used as a supplement when mothers elect to provide their milk but do not have sufficient for the infant's requirements. Breast milk should be supplemented with phosphorus as a minimum, and a breast milk fortifier added as required to obtain satisfactory growth.

However, preterm infants are not a homogeneous population, and with the survival of extremely low-birthweight babies any single diet is now unlikely to be optimal from birth to discharge. For instance, from the calculations of Ziegler et al[56] a baby of 800–1200 g requires 15% more protein than one between 1200 and 1800 g. Furthermore, certain groups of babies appear more vulnerable than others to the effects of suboptimal nutrition. Lucas et al[36] showed that small for gestational age babies and males particularly were disadvantaged in terms of developmental scores in infancy if they were fed on mature pasteurized milk or standard term formula[39] rather than a nutrient-enriched preterm formula. Further work is required to explore how diets can be tailored to individual patients' needs.

ROUTE OF ADMINISTRATION OF FEEDS

Infants less than 34 weeks' gestation seldom have adequately developed reflexes to suck, so that feeding has to be intragastric, transpyloric or intravenous (Chapter 20). Short-term partial parenteral nutrition, accompanied by gradually increasing enteral feeding, often needs to be employed in immature infants.

INTRAGASTRIC FEEDING

Nasogastric or orogastric gavage feeding is the most commonly practised method of enteral feeding for preterm infants. A nasogastric tube is easier to fix in place than an orogastric one, but has the potential disadvantage of partially obstructing nasal air flow. In infants with nasal passages partially blocked by secretions it may be advisable to use the orogastric route. A 4-French gauge gavage tube is usually adequate for infants less than 1.3 kg; for bigger infants a 6-gauge tube may be used. The distance between the nares and the left hypochondrium should be measured and the tube passed to this distance and taped in place. Correct placing should be checked by testing the aspirate for acidity with litmus paper. As an additional check, a few millilitres of air may be syringed into the tube while listening with a stethoscope placed over the stomach.

An important pitfall to remember when giving human milk by tube is that significant loss of energy may occur from the adherence of fat to the feeding vessels.[7] This process may be accentuated by the change in physical characteristics of the fat induced by freezing for long periods. In addition, when a syringe pump is used to infuse human milk continuously the syringe should be positioned *below* the infant, otherwise the fat rises up the connecting tube towards the syringe and may never be received by the infant.

TRANSPYLORIC FEEDING

Transpyloric feeding (into the duodenum or jejunum) has been widely used in the past. There is no convincing evidence that it improves feed tolerance and growth or reduces aspiration, and a meta-analysis of studies comparing transpyloric with intragastric feeds found that the mortality rate was 15% higher in the transpyloric group.[53] Thus, current evidence does not support the routine use of this method.

FEEDING SCHEDULES

LARGE, WELL, PRETERM INFANTS

It is neither possible nor desirable to adhere to rigid feeding policies for low-birthweight infants: gastrointestinal 'tolerance' of enteral feeding is very variable and concomitant illness may impose additional constraints, and therefore feeding must be managed on an individual basis.

The following guidelines are suggested for infants less than 1500 g birthweight. Feeding, by nasogastric tube if necessary, should start early to prevent hypoglycaemia, at about 2 hours of age. A commonly employed schedule for increasing feed volumes is to give, on the first 4 successive days, 60, 90, 120 and 150 ml/kg/24 h, and for infants on diets requiring greater feed volumes than this to make further daily increments to 180 ml/kg/24 h by day 10, and 200 ml/kg/24 h by day 14. There are few data on the rate at which bolus feeds should be instilled down a tube: most units favour gravity feeding over 10–20 minutes, rather than by injection from a syringe.

Most infants weighing more than 1500 g will tolerate 3-hourly feeds; smaller infants will need to be fed every 1–2 hours. Initially, the nasogastric tube should be aspirated at least 4- to 6-hourly, just before a feed. If the volume of aspirate is small, e.g. up to 10% of the accumulated feed intake since the previous aspiration, it may be replaced without altering the feed schedule; if it is significantly more than this it is advisable to reduce the feed intake accordingly, especially in infants showing increased abdominal girth. In infants who develop increasing abdominal distension, constipation or very loose stools, with or without blood in the stools, enteral feeds should be stopped temporarily and NEC (pp. 747) considered. If feed volumes need to be reduced below the required total fluid for more than a few hours, an intravenous infusion must be considered.

SICK AND VERY IMMATURE PRETERM INFANTS

In infants who are sick or very immature it is both undesirable and often impossible to commence full enteral feeds after birth, and an intravenous infusion must be commenced. There are theoretical and clinical trial data[15] to support the idea of using small, subnutritional quantities of enteral food in babies who will not tolerate full feeds. Such 'minimal enteral nutrition' may provide a stimulus to gut development and promote growth and transition to later enteral feeding. In extremely immature infants (< 27 weeks), however, even minimal enteral feeds may not be tolerated initially.

In newborn infants who are receiving either minimal or no enteral nutrition the immediate aim of the intravenous infusion is to meet the infant's needs for water and electrolyte homoeostasis (pp. 1012–1013) and to prevent hypoglycaemia: the decision about when to add nutrients other than glucose to the infusion will depend on the patient's age, birthweight, the severity of his illness, and how well he tolerates enteral feeds.

The consequences of early deprivation of nutrients have received inadequate attention, but the calculated nutritional reserves of an infant weighing 1000 g would last for only 4–5 days in the unfed state. It is important to attend to early intravenous intake in such babies (Chapter 20) while enteral feeds are being established.

If after 48 hours an infant has only mild respiratory disease and there is no ileus, enteral feeds may be gradually introduced and increased at the rate of 10–20 ml/kg/24 h, taking several days to achieve full volumes. This should be accompanied by intravenous feeding. As enteral feeds become tolerated, the intravenous infusion may be reduced accordingly. If, however, enteral feeds are not tolerated (vomiting, large gastric aspirates or abdominal distension), full total parenteral nutrition is required.

When enteral feeding is commenced in very immature or sick infants it is advisable to use either a continuous infusion pump suitable for accurately administering volumes to the nearest 0.5 ml/h or less, or slowly infused hourly boluses. Subsequent increments in feed frequency are a matter for clinical judgement, together with careful monitoring of enteral tolerance.

ROUTINE NUTRITIONAL MONITORING

In very sick and immature infants plasma urea, sodium, potassium, calcium, albumin and acid–base status need to be measured daily (or more often), at least for the first few days. Even in well and growing preterm infants it is advisable to make these measurements weekly. Recording the daily intakes of each diet received by the infant, as opposed to that prescribed, is important as the two may be significantly different; if the desired intake cannot be achieved, consideration should be given to altering the type of feed or route of administration. The commonest cause of growth failure in preterm infants is poor nutrient intake. Protein intake is as important as energy intake, and the addition of energy alone to the diet will not promote satisfactory growth if protein intake is also deficient.

In healthy preterm neonates it is suggested that blood glucose should be monitored on admission (before 30 minutes in sick or asphyxiated neonates) and subsequently 4- to 6-hourly for the first 48 hours, more intensively if glucose concentrations are low. Accurate daily weights are important and, if at all possible, should be obtained in sick patients in order to calculate fluid needs. An electronic balance with digital display, and which rapidly averages a sequence of weights to reduce infant movement artefact, is ideal for use in neonatal intensive care units. Head circumference should be measured weekly using a paper tape measure. Although informative, length measurements are more difficult to perform accurately and require an appropriate stadiometer, preferably one that will fit into an incubator.

FEEDING PROBLEMS

Vomiting, large gastric aspirates, constipation and abdominal distension are common in very immature infants, and in infants under 28 weeks' gestation it often takes several weeks to establish full enteral feeding. Occasionally a switch from formula to human milk results in a dramatic improvement in feed tolerance; however, in intractable cases the possibility of an underlying structural anomaly of the gut or NEC should be considered. While enteral feeds are being increased and decreased repeatedly, several days may pass during which the nutrient intake is grossly deficient, and such cases should be identified early and parenteral nutrition commenced.

There have been a few cases of infants who have developed gut obstruction on preterm formula and required a laparotomy for surgical disimpaction of inspissated formula in the small intestine. This is an avoidable complication if enteral feeds are established using breast milk in small sick infants and preterm formulas are used with caution in the early days. A sudden drop in stool frequency in a baby on a preterm formula is an early sign, and should be acted upon by temporarily reducing or stopping the formula and returning to human milk or intravenous feeds.

PSYCHOSOCIAL ASPECTS

Practical involvement of parents in infant feeding during the period when suckling is not possible has considerable psychological benefits. For well infants, parents (under supervision) may be encouraged to measure out and give nasogastric tube feeds. Mothers who wish ultimately to breast-feed may start to put their infant to the breast from an early stage, even at 1000 g provided the infant is well. In our experience aspiration and choking does not occur. Randomized studies looking at the effects of non-nutritive sucking during the administration of tube-feeds have not shown consistent beneficial effects on growth or gastrointestinal function, although it may reduce hospital stay by up to 6 days.[53]

The difficulties for a mother who has delivered a 28-week infant and wishes eventually to fully breast-feed her baby should not be underestimated. Her chances of success are greatly influenced by the sympathetic attitude of the nursing staff, by skilled assistance and by frequent milk expression (at least 6–8 times a day). Even if a mother manages to maintain lactation for several weeks by mechanical expression, she may then be faced with problems in getting her infant to feed from the breast. One specific difficulty arises when the infant's mouth is too small to encompass a large nipple. It is important for attendant staff to explain that it requires patience and time to establish breast-feeding in this special situation.

POST-DISCHARGE NUTRITION

Preterm infants frequently leave hospital severely growth retarded and fulfilling the criteria for 'failure to thrive', yet until recently little attention has been paid to their subsequent nutrition. In our cohort of 926 preterm infants, 77% were below the 10th centile for weight at the time of hospital discharge, and the percentages remaining below this centile at 9 months, 18 months and 7.5–8 years were 38%, 34% and 19%, respectively. The figures were even higher for those infants weighing less than 1000 g at birth: 98%, 69%, 58% and 26% respectively.[27]

A study of formula-fed preterm infants after discharge from hospital demonstrated that, when fed ad libitum, these infants frequently consume volumes far in excess of those usually recommended by paediatricians: 16% took more than 350 ml/kg/24 h, 50% consumed more than 165 kcal/kg/24 h, and 35% more than 4 g/kg/24 h of protein.[32] Several studies have shown that the provision of increased nutrients, both in hospital and after discharge, can improve the short-term growth rate of preterm infants. Such studies emphasize that it is important to provide extra energy *and protein*; simply increasing the energy content by adding extra carbohydrate or fat is less likely to be effective, and may result in a higher percentage of body fat.[24] A small study of 32 infants randomized to receive either a standard 'term' formula or a nutrient-enriched post-discharge formula for 6 months after hospital discharge found that those on the post-discharge formula grew significantly faster in weight and length over the first 9 months[40] and had higher bone mineral content.[6] However, data are not yet available to indicate whether these outcomes are long-lasting. Further studies are under way to look at both the short- and long-term effects of different post-discharge nutrition regimens, including the use of preterm infant formulas and the comparative value of breast milk versus enriched formulas: there is, for example, no available information to indicate whether breast milk should be fortified post-discharge. The composition of post-discharge formulas currently available in the UK is shown in Table 19.13.

Table 19.13 Nutrient content of post-discharge formulas available in the UK (per 100 ml)

Composition per 100 ml	**Formula** **Nutriprem 2**** **(C&G)**	**Farley's** **Premcare****
Macronutrients		
Protein* (g)	1.8	1.85
casein (%)	40	40
whey (%)	60	60
Fat (g)	4.1	3.96
LCPUFA	+	+
Carbohydrate+		
lactose (g)	6.0	6.2
maltodextrin (g)	—	1.04
amylose (g)	—	—
glucose (g)	1.5	—
Total (g)	7.5	7.24
Energy		
kcal	74	72
kJ	310	301
Minerals		
Calcium (mg)	90	70
Chloride (mg)	45	45
Magnesium (mg)	6.1	5.2
Phosphorus (mg)	45	35
Potassium (mg)	71	78
Sodium (mg)	25	22
Trace elements		
Copper (μg)	62	57
Iodine (μg)	20	4.5
Iron (μg)	1100	650
Manganese (μg)	9	5
Zinc (μg)	700	600
Potential renal solute load^ (mosmol/l)	155	NS
Vitamins		
A retinol (μg)	99	100
B_1 thiamin (μg)	90	95
B_2 riboflavin (μg)	120	100
B_6 pyridoxine (μg)	80	80
B_{12} cyanocobalamin (μg)	0.44	0.2
Biotin (μg)	3	1.1
Folic acid (μg)	20	25
Niacin (μg)	1.6	1000
C ascorbic acid (mg)	16	15
Vitamin D (μg)	1.6	1.3
Vitamin E (mg)	1.6	1.5
K phytomenadione (μg)	5.9	6.0
Others		
Choline (mg)	7	
Inositol (mg)	30	
Taurine (mg)	5	
Osmolality (mmol/kg)	300	

* total nitrogen × 6.38
+ figures declared as disaccharide
# liquid formulation – sodium 34, chloride 67
^ method of Ziegler & Fomon[57]: calculated values
** manufacturer's information
LCPUFA long chain polyunsaturated fatty acids: + added, – not added

THE TERM GROWTH-RETARDED INFANT

Growth-retarded term infants are known to be at risk of continued growth failure[49,54] as well as learning and behavioural problems.[23] In addition, increasing epidemiological evidence suggests that early growth failure may 'programme' a number of adverse long-term outcomes, including ischaemic heart disease and type 2 diabetes mellitus. However, until recently relatively little attention has been paid to the nutritional requirements of such infants. Most data suggest that catch-up growth, if it occurs, is largely completed during the first 9 months of life. It is not clear at present why some growth-retarded infants fail to catch up, and to what extent this reflects their genetic potential. However, the possibility that catch-up growth might be influenced by early nutrition warrants investigation as a potential mechanism for reducing long-term morbidity.

Davies[10] found that increasing the protein and energy intake of growth-retarded infants did not improve catch-up growth, although protein with an unmodified casein/whey ratio was used, which may not be well utilized by these infants. More recently, in a study of 54 infants, those who were breast-fed showed significantly faster growth in weight, length and head circumference than those fed a standard term formula, even after adjusting for potential confounding factors. The differences persisted up to 1 year, beyond the period of exclusive breast-feeding.[30] Although similar in macronutrient content to term formula, breast milk contains a number of factors (nucleotides, LCPUFA, growth factors and hormones) which might be important in view of the known abnormalities in gut and pancreas morphology, structure and function seen in growth-retarded infants. Further studies are required to explore different dietary regimens in relation to long-term outcome.

REFERENCES

1. Atmmo T, Omololu A 1982 Trace element content of breast milk of mothers of preterm infants in Nigeria. Early Human Development 6: 309–313
2. Atkinson S A, Bryan M H, Anderson G H 1978 Human milk: difference in nitrogen concentration in milk from mothers of term and premature infants. Journal of Pediatrics 93: 67–69
3. Balmer S E, Wharton B A 1992 Human milk banking at Sorrento Maternity Hospital, Birmingham. Archives of Disease in Childhood 67: 556–559
4. Bates C J, Lui D S, Fuller N J, Lucas A 1985 Susceptibility of riboflavin and vitamin A in breast milk to photodegradation, and its implications for the use of banked breast milk in infant feeding. Acta Paediatrica Scandinavica 74: 40–44
5. Baum J D 1979 Raw breast milk for babies in neonatal units. Lancet ii: 898
6. Bishop N J, King F J, Lucas A 1993 Increased bone mineral content of preterm infants fed with a nutrient enriched formula after discharge from hospital. Archives of Disease in Childhood 68: 573–578
7. Brooke O G, Barley J 1978 Loss of energy during continuous infusions of breastmilk. Archives of Disease in Childhood 53: 344–345
8. Brooke O G, Wood C, Barley J 1982 Energy balance, nitrogen balance and growth in preterm infants fed expressed breast milk, a premature infant formula and two low-solute adapted formulae. Archives of Disease in Childhood 57: 898–904
9. Cavell B (1982) Reservoir and emptying function of the stomach of the premature infant. Acta Paediatrica Scandinavica, suppl. 296: 60–61
10. Davies D P 1981 Growth of 'small-for-dates' babies. Early Human Development 5: 95–105
11. DHHS 1977 The composition of mature human milk. Report on Health and Social Subjects No. 12 HMSO, London
12. DHSS 1980 Artificial feeds for the young infant. Report on Health and Social Subjects No. 12 Report of the Committee on Medical Aspects of Food Policy, HMSO, London
13. DHSS 1981 The collection and storage of human milk. Report on Health and Social Subjects No. 22. HMSO, London
14. DHSS 1983 Present day practice in infant feeding. Report on Health and Social Subjects No. 20 HMSO, London
15. Dunn L, Hulman S, Weiner J, Kliegman R 1988 Beneficial effects of early hypocaloric enteral feeding on neonatal gastrointestinal function: preliminary report of a randomized trial. Journal of Pediatrics 112: 622–629
16. Eglin R-P, Wilkinson A R 1987 HIV infection and pasteurisation of breast milk. Lancet i: 1093
17. Evans T J, Ryley J C, Neale L M 1978 Effects of storage and heat on antimicrobial proteins in human milk. Archives of Disease in Childhood 53: 239–241
18. Garza C, Johnson C A, Nichols B L 1982 Effects of methods of collection and storage on nutrients in human milk. Early Human Development 6: 295–303
19. Gibbs J A H, Fisher C, Bhattacharya S, Goddard P, Baum J D 1978 Drip breast milk: its composition, collection and pasteurisation. Early Human Development 1: 227–245
20. Greer F R, McCormick A 1988 Improved bone mineralisation and growth in premature infants fed fortified own mother's milk. Journal of Pediatrics 112: 961–969
21. Gross S J 1983 Growth and biochemical response of preterm infants fed human milk or modified infant formula. New England Journal of Medicine 308: 237–241
22. Gross S J, Buckley R H, Wakil S S, McAllister D C, David R J, Faix R G 1981 Elevated IgA concentration in milk produced by mothers delivered of preterm infants. Journal of Pediatrics 99: 389–393
23. Hadders-Algra M, Touwen BCL 1990 Body measurements, neurological and behavioural development in six-year-old children born preterm and/or small-for-gestational-age. Early Human Development 22: 1–13
24. Heird W C, Wu C 1996 Nutrition, growth and body composition. In: Posthospital nutrition in the preterm infant. Report of the 106th Ross Conference on Pediatric Research. Ross Products Division, Abbott Laboratories, Columbus, Ohio, pp 7–16
25. Kashyap S, Schulze K F, Forsyth M, Dell R B, Ramakrishnan R, Heird W C 1990 Growth, nutrient retention, and metabolic response of low-birth-weight infants fed supplemented and unsupplemented preterm human milk. American Journal of Clinical Nutrition 52: 254–262
26. Lemons J A, Moyle L, Hall D, Summons M 1982 Differences in the composition of preterm and term human milk during early lactation. Pediatric Research 16: 113–117
27. Lucas A 1996 Nutrition, growth and development of post-discharge preterm infants. In: Posthospital nutrition in the preterm infant. Report of the 106th Ross Conference on Pediatric Research. Ross Products Division, Abbott Laboratories, Columbus, Ohio, pp 81–90
28. Lucas A, Cole T J 1990 Breast milk and neonatal necrotising enterocolitis. Lancet 336: 1519–1523
29. Lucas A, Hudson G 1984 Preterm milk as a source of protein for low birthweight infants. Archives of Disease in Childhood 59: 831–836
30. Lucas A, Fewtrell M S, Davies P S W et al 1997 Breastfeeding and catch-up growth in infants born small for gestational age. Acta Paediatrica 86: 564–569
31. Lucas A, Gibbs J A H, Baum J D 1978 The biology of drip breast milk. Early Human Development 2: 351–361
32. Lucas A, King F J, Bishop N J 1992 Postdischarge formula consumption in infants born preterm. Archives of Disease in Childhood 67: 691–692
33. Lucas A, Lucas P J, Chavin S L, Lyster R L J and Baum D 1980 Human milk formula. Early Human Development 4: 15–21
34. Lucas A, Gore S M, Cole T J et al 1984 Multicentre trial on feeding low

birthweight infants: effect of diet on early growth. Archives of Disease in Childhood 59: 722–730
35. Lucas A, McLaughlan P, Coombs R R A 1984 Latent anaphylactic sensitisation of infants of low birthweight to cow's milk proteins. British Medical Journal 289: 1254–1256
36. Lucas A, Morley R, Cole T J et al 1989 Early diet in preterm babies and developmental status in infancy. Archives of Disease in Childhood 64: 1570–1578
37. Lucas A, Brooke O G, Barker B A, Bishop N, Morley R, 1989 High alkaline phosphatase activity and growth in preterm neonates. Archives of Disease in Childhood 64: 902–909
38. Lucas A, Brooke O G, Morley R, Cole T J, Bamford M F 1990 A randomised prospective study of early diet and later allergic or atopic disease. British Medical Journal 300: 837–840
39. Lucas A, Morley R, Cole T J et al 1990 Early diet in preterm babies and developmental status at 18 months. Lancet 335: 1477–1481
40. Lucas A, Bishop N J, King F J, Cole T J 1992 Randomised trial of nutrition for preterm infants after discharge. Archives of Disease in Childhood 67: 324–327
41. Lucas A, Morley R, Cole T J, Lister G, Leeson-Payne C 1992 Breast milk and subsequent intelligence quotient in children born preterm. Lancet 339: 261–264
42. Lucas A, Morley R, Cole T J, Gore S M 1994 A randomised multicentre study of human milk versus formula and later development in preterm infants. Archives of Disease in Childhood 70: F141–146
43. Lucas A, Fewtrell M S, Morley R et al 1996 Randomized outcome trial of human milk fortification in preterm infants. American Journal of Clinical nutrition 64: 142–151
44. Macy I G, Kelly H J, Sloan H E 1983 The composition of milks. National Academy of Science, National Research Council, Publication 254, Washington DC
45. Mettler A E 1976 Infant milk powder feeds compared on a common basis. Postgraduate Medical Journal 52: Supplement 8: 3–20
46. Modanlou H D, Lim M O, Hansen J W, Sickles V 1986 Growth, biochemical status, and mineral metabolism in very-low-birth-weight infants receiving fortified preterm human milk. Journal of Pediatric Gastroenterology and Nutrition 5: 762–767
47. Morley R, Cole T J, Lucas P J et al 1988 Mothers' choice to provide breast milk and developmental outcome. Archives of Disease in Childhood 63: 1382–1385
48. Narayanan I, Prakash K, Gujral V V 1982 The value of human milk in the prevention of infection in the high risk low birthweight infant. Journal of Pediatrics 99: 496–498
49. Ounsted M K, Moar V A, Scott A 1984 Children of deviant birthweight at the age of seven years: health, handicap, size and developmental status. Early Human Development 9: 323–340
50. Roberton D M, Paganelli R, Dinwiddie R, Levinski R J 1982 Milk antigen absorption in the neonate. Archives of Disease in Childhood 57: 369–372
51. Rohnholm K A R, Sipila I, Siimes M A 1982 Human milk protein supplementation for the prevention of hypoproteinaemia without metabolic imbalance in breast milk fed very low birthweight infants. Journal of Pediatrics 101: 243–247
52. Schanler R J, Abrams S A 1995 Postnatal attainment of intrauterine macromineral accretion rates in low birth weight infants fed fortified human milk. Journal of Pediatrics 126: 441–447
53. Steer P, Lucas A, Sinclair J C 1992 Feeding the low birth-weight infant. In: Sinclair J C, Bracken M B (eds) Effective care of the newborn infant. Oxford University Press, New York, pp 94–160
54. Walther F J 1988 Growth and development of term disproportionate small-for-gestational age infants at the age of 7 years. Early Human Development 18: 1–11
55. Wills M E, Han V E M, Harris D A, Baum J D 1982 Short time low temperature pasteurisation of human milk. Early Human Development 7: 71–80
56. Ziegler E E, Biga R L, Fomon S J 1981 Nutritional requirements of the premature infant. In: Suskind R M (ed) Textbook of pediatric nutrition. Raven Press, New York, pp 29–39
57. Ziegler E E, Fomon S J 1971 Fluid intake, renal solute load and water balance in infancy. Journal of Pediatrics 78: 561–568

20

Parenteral nutrition

Victor Y. H. Yu

The fetus is nourished parenterally during pregnancy through the regulatory function of the placenta. Extra-uterine adaptation depends on successful transition to the enteral route of nutrition. The parenteral route for maintaining nutritional integrity postnatally has been developed for infants whose gastrointestinal function is compromised and for whom adequate nutrition cannot be provided enterally.

INDICATIONS

Parenteral nutrition is indicated in the infant for whom feeding via the enteral route is impossible, inadequate or hazardous, because of malformation, disease or immaturity, and in whom this state is likely to be prolonged and pose a serious threat to life and health. It is used in infants with major anomalies such as intestinal atresia or omphalocoele, necrotizing enterocolitis (NEC) or protracted diarrhoea from a variety of causes. They may have had extensive intestinal resection or require multiple surgical procedures. In some, resting the gastrointestinal tract for a prolonged period is curative. In others, maintenance of adequate nutrition will permit corrective surgery to be carried out. Parenteral nutrition is also used in extremely preterm infants, especially those with respiratory distress, prior to enteral feeding or to supplement milk feeds which can then be increased slowly to avoid overtaxing the immature gastrointestinal tract while continuing to satisfy nutritional requirements.

In any clinical situation, however, parenteral nutrition is only justified if the benefits outweigh the hazards. As the safety of the technique depends on available resources and expertise, indications for parenteral nutrition necessarily vary between centres. If facilities for intensive medical and nursing care and frequent biochemical monitoring using microtechniques are unavailable, it seems wiser to transfer the infant to an appropriate centre for parenteral nutrition.

COMPOSITION OF INFUSATES

FLUIDS

The maturity of the infant, the type of incubator used, and the methods employed to curtail water loss will determine parenteral fluid requirements. Preterm infants adapt poorly to inadequate or excessive fluid intake compared with term infants. They have increased amounts of extracellular fluid, their kidneys have a poorer concentrating and diluting ability, they have a larger surface area in relation to weight, and their insensible water loss through the skin, especially in the first week, is significantly higher. Increased fluid loss occurs when the infant is placed under radiant warmers or phototherapy.[16] Fluid requirements are decreased with the use of double-walled incubators,[152] heat shields or plastic blankets[13] and high ambient humidity.[58]

The postnatal weight loss in infants born below 29 weeks' gestation averages 12–15% of birthweight.[48] A randomized clinical trial (RCT) was carried out in infants with a birthweight of 750–1500 g to compare two parenteral fluid regimes; one allowed 1–2% loss of birthweight per day to a maximum loss of 8–10% and another allowed 3–5% loss per day to a maximum of 13–15%.[81] No difference in neonatal mortality and morbidity was found between the two groups, suggesting that the gradual loss of 15% of birthweight in the first week after birth is safe. If extremely preterm infants are nursed in maximally humidified incubators, their fluid requirement should be no greater than that of more mature infants, that is, 60–80 ml/kg/d increasing to 100–120 ml/kg/d in the second week.[81] On the other hand, if measures to reduce insensible water loss are not taken, fluid requirements for some extremely preterm infants could be in excess of 150 ml/kg/d. Serial assessment of hydration status is mandatory, using clinical and laboratory parameters.

ENERGY

The estimation of energy requirement takes into account the components of total heat production (basal metabolic rate, physical activity, specific dynamic action of food, thermoregulatory heat production) and the energy cost of growth. In preterm infants, the basal metabolic rate is about 40 kcal/kg/d.[119] The energy cost of activity is 4 kcal/kg/d with minimal handling[119] and the specific dynamic action of parenteral nutrition is 13% of the basal heat production or 10% of the calories infused.[123] If an infant is nursed in a thermoneutral environment, an input of 50 kcal/kg/d is sufficient to match ongoing expenditure but it does not meet additional requirements of growth.[61]

Growth failure will result unless additional energy is provided. The energy cost of gaining 1 g of new tissue is 5 kcal.[119] To achieve the equivalent of third-trimester intrauterine weight gain of 14–15 g/kg/d, an additional 70 kcal/kg/d is required. Parenterally fed infants, compared to those enterally fed, begin to grow at a lower energy intake because of smaller faecal energy losses and reduced energy expenditure. Nevertheless, the goal energy intake for a rapidly growing preterm infant is theoretically about 120 kcal/kg/d, or even higher in long-term ventilated infants with chronic lung disease (CLD), whose energy requirements are increased by 25–30%.[147]

PROTEIN

In sick preterm infants, it is inadvisable to attempt to meet their energy needs immediately after birth with intravenous glucose as the sole energy source.[45] Randomized clinical trials in sick, preterm infants have shown that an intake of 1.5 g/kg/d amino amino acids from the day of birth resulted in a nitrogen retention rate of 9 mmol/kg/d and improved protein synthesis with no elevation of plasma amino acid levels.[93,120,121,125] In contrast, the control group had a negative nitrogen balance of about 10 mmol/kg/d, equivalent to a daily loss of 3% of the body's protein in the first 3 days after birth before amino acids were commenced. The energy intake should be at least 40–50 kcal/kg/d when amino acids are introduced, because with lower energy intakes, more of the infused amino acids are oxidized to meet endogenous energy needs and less remain for tissue synthesis. Energy from non-protein sources is essential for optimal nitrogen economy in parenteral nutrition; 150–200 non-protein calories per gram of nitrogen has been recommended.[158] Whether this non-protein energy is derived from glucose or fat makes no difference to the nitrogen-sparing effect (see below).

Parenteral protein requirements, as determined by a variety of methods, are in the range of 2.0–2.5 g/kg/d for term infants and 2.7–3.5 g/kg/d for preterm infants.[79] The intrauterine nitrogen accretion rate for a fetus is 24 mmol/kg/d at 24–36 weeks' gestation. The parenteral nitrogen required to achieve retention equal to the fetal accretion rate depends on a number of factors such as energy intake derived from glucose and fat, the quality of infused amino acids, vitamin and mineral co-factors, and the patient's clinical status. Crystalline amino acids in the form of L-sterioisomers are the preferred nitrogen source in parenteral nutrition as they have a high bioavailability resulting in a nitrogen retention of over 70% of the amount infused.[32,63] A parenteral nitrogen intake of 32 mmol/kg/d (equivalent to 3.3 g/kg/d of amino acids) can result in duplication of intrauterine nitrogen accretion rates. RCTs have shown that a parenteral intake of 4 g/kg/d compared to 2–3 g/kg/d resulted in higher nitrogen retention, net protein synthesis and weight gain.[40,158] As nitrogen retention has been shown to be reduced by more than 50% during dexamethasone therapy for CLD, it may be appropriate to provide additional amino acid intake during the treatment period.[127,146]

Preterm infants not only require more amino acids than term infants but also qualitatively different amino acids. Cysteine, taurine, tyrosine and histidine have been considered as conditionally essential amino acids in preterm infants.[77] Conversion of methionine to cysteine and taurine and conversion of phenylalanine to tyrosine are affected by enzyme immaturity. However, the addition of cysteine[87] and taurine[141] to parenteral nutrition solutions in preterm infants did not improve nitrogen retention or weight gain. Comparison of amino acid solutions based on the composition of egg protein and breast milk has shown that the latter results in a lower risk of high plasma phenylalanine levels but a higher risk of low tyrosine levels.[89,113] No adverse neuro-developmental outcome had been observed after hyper-phenylalaninaemia induced by parenteral nutrition.[85] Amino acid solutions designed for paediatric patients have been shown to result in a more favourable plasma aminogram, higher nitrogen retention and better weight gain in preterm infants.[66] Amino acid solutions have also been designed using the engineering technique of optimization, in which the composition is derived from calculations based on a large body of plasma amino acid data from patients who have received a variety of parenteral amino acid solutions. Studies have shown that preterm infants tolerate these 'designer' amino acid solutions well.[69]

CARBOHYDRATE

Neurophysiological and neurodevelopmental outcome data suggest that neonatal blood glucose concentration should be maintained above 2.6 mmol/l.[74,84] Parenteral glucose can reduce endogenous protein catabolism of preterm infants by about 80%.[8] The risks for hyperglycaemia and glycosuria increase with decreasing gestation and birthweight.[82] Hyperglycaemia during glucose infusion appears to be due primarily to persistent endogenous hepatic glucose production secondary to an insensitivity of hepatocytes to insulin.[38,110] If parenteral fluids are commenced at 60 ml/kg/d, 10% dextrose can be used to provide a glucose infusion rate of 6 g/kg/d (4 mg/kg/min). If over 80 ml/kg/d of fluid intake is prescribed in extremely preterm infants below 1000 g birthweight, it is advisable to use 5% dextrose to avoid hyperglycaemia. The initial response to hyperglycaemia (serum glucose of over 8 mmol/l) or glycosuria is to reduce the glucose infusion rate. Insulin can be infused in infants who remain hyperglycaemic at a glucose infusion rate of 8 g/kg/d (6 mg/kg/min),[98] commencing at 0.05 units/kg/h.[20] A RCT in infants of below 1000 g birthweight with glucose intolerance has shown that insulin therapy improved glucose intake and weight gain.[33] Since glucose tolerance improves with increasing postnatal age,[154] the glucose infusion rate can usually be progressively increased to 18–20 g/kg/d (12–14 mg/kg/min) in the second week after birth. It is necessary to limit the concentration of the dextrose solution infused into peripheral veins to about 12% because of the risks of subcutaneous tissue infiltration. Higher glucose infusion rates will require central venous access.

FAT

Nitrogen-sparing effects of carbohydrate and fat are similar in parenterally fed infants.[108,145] Essential fatty acid deficiency can be prevented by as little as 0.5 g/kg/d of Intralipid,[78] a fat emulsion derived from soybean oil containing 54% linoleic acid and 8% linolenic acid. Fat emulsions containing equal proportions of long- and medium-chain triglycerides (LCT/MCT) have been used in infants,[124] and one study showed greater nitrogen retention with LCT/MCT than with LCT emulsions.[142]

There is a diminished capacity to use exogenous fats in preterm[26] and in small-for-gestational-age infants,[7] due to deficient cellular uptake and utilization of free fatty acids rather than to low lipoprotein lipase activity.[122] Although heparin releases endothelial-bound lipoprotein lipase and hepatic lipase in the circulation,[157] it does not improve fat clearance in infants.[136] Carnitine plays an important role in the oxidation of fatty acids by facilitating their transport across mitochondrial membranes. Preterm infants fed parenterally with carnitine-free solutions develop low blood and tissue carnitine concentrations because of their small carnitine depots and limited capacity for carnitine biosynthesis. Some studies have shown improved fat clearance with carnitine supplementation,[21,37] and carnitine supplementation to enhance fatty acid oxidation has been recommended in those receiving total parenteral nutrition for over 1 month.[65]

Although it has been suggested that parenteral fat should be withheld in the first week after birth as early use of fat infusion might be associated with respiratory compromise (see 'Hazards' below), RCTs on parenteral fat commenced on the day of birth have shown that it was well tolerated with no increase in adverse effects,[29,47,93,134] although one of these four RCTs reported an increase in mortality rate associated with early fat infusion within the subgroup of infants who weighed 600–800 g at birth.[134] Free radicals generated when Intralipid undergoes peroxidation could be potentially damaging to preterm infants.[109] Phototherapy-induced formation of triglyceride hydroperoxides can be prevented by covering the Intralipid with aluminium foil.[96] Parenteral fat should be commenced in a dose not exceeding 1 g/kg/d increasing within a week to 3 g/kg/d,[67] although this should be reduced to 2 g/kg/d in preterm infants during acute sepsis because of their reduced fat oxidation rate.[99] Compared to 10% Intralipid, 20% Intralipid has a lower phospholipid/triglyceride ratio and liposomal content, and RCTs have shown that the 20% emulsion resulted in lower plasma triglyceride, cholesterol and phospholipid concentrations.[59,60] Two RCTs have shown that a continuous fat infusion regimen is better than an intermittent regimen, as reflected by less fluctuation in serum levels and a lower incidence of clinical and metabolic complications.[25,72] Plasma turbidity assessed by visual inspection or nephelometry does not reliably predict serum concentration.[128] When triglyceride levels exceed 1.7 mmol/l, it is necessary to reduce or interrupt fat infusion until normal values are regained.[34,101]

MINERALS AND TRACE ELEMENTS

Early hypernatraemia in preterm infants is caused mainly by their high insensible water loss, while early hyponatraemia is caused mainly by inappropriate arginine vasopressin release associated with periventricular haemorrhage, pneumothorax or hyaline membrane disease.[118] Late hyponatraemia in preterm infants is due to limited tubular sodium reabsorption.[3] A sodium supplement of 1 mmol/kg/d should suffice in the first week but 3–5 mmol/kg/d is recommended subsequently to prevent late hyponatraemia, further increased if the infant is receiving frusemide for CLD. Although a potassium intake of 1–2 mmol/kg/d is required for the growing preterm infant, it should be withheld in the first 3 days after birth in those who are extremely preterm because they are at risk of developing non-oliguric hyperkalaemia from immature distal tubular function.[27,53] Hypochloraemic alkalosis is prevented by a chloride intake of 2 mmol/kg/d. Chloride intakes in excess of 6 mmol/kg/d are inadvisable because of the risk of hyperchloraemic metabolic acidosis.[52]

Parenteral administration of calcium at 1 mmol/kg/d from birth can prevent early neonatal hypocalcaemia in preterm infants.[126] Requirements calculated to match intrauterine accretion rates in a rapidly growing preterm infant are, however, higher than that used to maintain

Table 20.1 Recommendations for intravenous minerals and trace elements in preterm infants (amount per kg per day)

Sodium	3–5 mmol	(70–120 mg)
Chloride	3–5 mmol	(110–180 mg)
Potassium	1–2 mmol	(40–80 mg)
Calcium*	1.5–2.2 mmol	(60–90 mg)
Phosphorus*	1.5–2.2 mmol	(50–70 mg)
Magnesium	0.3–0.4 mmol	(7–10 mg)
Zinc	6–8 μmol	(400–500 μg)
Copper	0.3–0.6 μmol	(20–40 μg)
Selenium	13–25 nmol	(1–2 μg)
Manganese	18–180 nmol	(1–10 μg)
Iodine	8 nmol	(1 μg)
Chromium	4–8 nmol	(0.2–0.4 μg)
Molybdenum	2–10 nmol	(0.2–1 μg)

*Based on a 120–150 ml/kg/d fluid intake of a solution which contains 1.3–1.5 mmol/dl of calcium and phosphorus (molar ratio 1 : 1) equivalent to 50–60 mg/dl of calcium and 40–45 mg/dl of phosphorus (weight ratio 1.3 : 1).

short-term homeostasis. Parenteral nutrition solutions should contain 1.3–1.5 mmol/100 ml calcium and phosphorus (molar ratio of 1 : 1 or a ratio of 1.3 : 1 by weight) and 0.2–0.3 mmol/100 ml of magnesium, administered with a fluid intake of 120–150 ml/kg/d.[51] These recommendations are described per unit volume to prevent administration of high concentrations of calcium and phosphorus resulting in precipitation of these minerals when fluid intake is restricted. Factors which affect solubility of calcium and phosphorus are discussed below (see 'Preparation'). High intakes of calcium and phosphorus should only be given through a central venous line.

Table 20.1 summarizes the recommendations on parenteral minerals and trace elements for preterm infants based on guidelines published by the American Society for Clinical Nutrition.[51] If parenteral nutrition is supplemental or is limited to 2 weeks, only zinc needs to be added to the infusate. Other trace elements are required if total parenteral nutrition continues for over 1 month. The risk of zinc deficiency is increased with excessive gastrointestinal fluid losses, as is the risk of copper deficiency when there are losses of copper-containing biliary secretion. Both copper and manganese supplementation should be withheld when cholestasis is present. Because selenium and chromium are excreted mainly through the kidneys, less should be given when renal function is impaired. Since destruction of erythrocytes postnatally provides the infant with 18 μmol/kg/d of iron, iron supplementation is unnecessary, especially if the infant is receiving repeated top-up transfusions. Molybdenum and fluoride supplements are recommended only with long-term (3–6 months) total parenteral nutrition. The aluminium content of parenteral nutrition infusates may be up to 1 μmol/dl as a result of aluminium contamination of the components used, such as calcium gluconate, which can contribute up to 80% of the total aluminium load. Although the consequences of aluminium accumulation and deposition in bone are unclear in infants receiving parenteral nutrition, it is advisable to minimize aluminium contamination in infusates.[91]

Table 20.2 Composition of Multivitamin Infusion Paediatric (amount per 5 ml vial)

Vitamin A	0.7 mg
Vitamin D	10 μg
Vitamin E	7 mg
Vitamin K	0.2 mg
Vitamin C	80 mg
Vitamin B_1	1.2 mg
Vitamin B_2	1.4 mg
Vitamin B_6	1 mg
Nicotinamide	17 mg
Panthenol	5 mg
Biotin	20 μg
Folic acid	140 μg
Vitamin B_{12}	1 μg

VITAMINS

The ideal parenteral vitamin preparation for use in infants is not yet available. One multivitamin infusion (M. V. I. Paediatric) is designed for paediatric use (Table 20.2). Term infants on this daily dose maintain serum vitamin levels within acceptable ranges.[90] Preterm infants should be given 40% of the standard dose (2 ml) per kilogram body weight, with a maximum not to exceed the term infant's dose of 5 ml, even though this dose results in low serum levels of vitamin A.[49] About 80% of vitamin A and 30% of vitamins D and E are lost during administration owing to adherence to tubing and photodegradation, especially during phototherapy.[49,132] By adding the vitamin preparation into the fat emulsion instead of the amino acid-glucose mixture, vitamin losses can be reduced and the risk of deficiency minimized.[10,39]

TECHNIQUES

PREPARATION

Computer programs are available which improve the efficiency of prescribing parenteral nutrition, reduce human error with automatic physiological safety and precipitation checks and increase the ease of nutritional data retrieval.[57,86,150,151] All preparations should be carried out under strict aseptic conditions using a laminar flow hood and terminal filtration with a 0.22-μm filter prior to delivery to the ward.

The solubility of calcium and phosphorus depends on other components within the infusate and the order in which they are mixed. Because of the low solubility product of these minerals, the one-bag system (amino acid, glucose and fat mixed into a single bag) is unable to deliver adequate amounts to prevent osteopenia and rickets in extremely preterm infants. The higher amino acid concentrations recommended for use in preterm infants do help to enhance their solubility by decreasing the pH of the solution. Phosphorus should be added before calcium to avoid the high concentrations of phosphorus causing immediate precipitation with calcium. Precipitation with phosphates is more likely with calcium chloride than with the gluconate salt. Glycerophosphate may allow greater delivery of calcium and phosphorus because they are stable in solution and have equivalent retention rates to standard salts.[56,117]

ADMINISTRATION

An infusion pump is required to maintain a constant rate of delivering the parenteral nutrition solution. A 0.22-µm bacterial filter is commonly used if terminal filtration is not carried out in the pharmacy. Distal to the filter, a second infusion pump delivers the fat emulsion close to the intravascular catheter. It is important to minimize mixing of the fat emulsion with calcium and heparin as this increases the risks of formation of calcium–phosphorus crystals and flocculation of Intralipid due to the destabilizing effect of divalent cations.[116]

Peripheral veins can be repeatedly cannulated using short 22- or 24-gauge catheters or scalp vein needles. Short catheters remain functional three times longer than steel needles, with no increase in complications.[12,106] When central venous catheters are used, the distal tip of the catheter is placed in the superior or inferior vena cava near the right atrium. Percutaneous central venous catheterization[31,94,95] is preferred over the surgical cut-down approach,[130] although the Broviac catheter which requires a cutdown has also been used successfully even in infants below 1000 g birthweight.[97,148] The addition of heparin (1 unit/ml) to the infusate further reduces significantly the incidence of phlebitis and thrombosis of both peripheral[5] and central venous catheters.[11,28] Infusion of lipid emulsions is known to prolong survival times of peripheral venous lines.[105] Parenteral nutrition has been administered routinely through umbilical arterial catheters in infants who require arterial access for blood gas and blood pressure monitoring in the first 2 weeks after birth.[155] This has been found to be comparable to central venous catheters in efficacy and safety.[71] The umbilical venous catheter has also been compared favourably with the use of peripheral veins in delivering parenteral nutrition.[104]

MONITORING

Investigations should be performed with discretion and a compromise must be made between the need for laboratory information and the risks and cost of repeated tests. As many preterm or postoperative infants requiring parenteral nutrition have metabolic problems associated with their primary condition, it is no easier to generalize on the frequency of laboratory monitoring than it is on the frequency of clinical examinations. Proposed guidelines for monitoring during parenteral nutrition are shown in Table 20.3.

Table 20.3 Monitoring during parenteral nutrition

- Daily body weight and weekly body length and head circumference
- Initially during grading up of parenteral nutrients or during periods of metabolic instability:
  - Strict fluid balance
  - 6- to 12-hourly urine/blood glucose
  - Daily plasma sodium, potassium, calcium, urea and acid–base
- When on full parenteral nutrition and during metabolic steady state:
  - Strict fluid balance
  - 12- to 24-hourly urine/blood glucose
  - Once/twice weekly plasma sodium, potassium, calcium, urea and acid–base
- Plasma magnesium, phosphorus, alkaline phosphatase, albumin, transaminases and bilirubin weekly
- Plasma triglycerides, amino acids, trace elements and ammonia not usually routinely monitored
- Screening for infection or coagulation defects as indicated

BENEFITS

RCTs have shown that infants on total[54,155] and supplemental[1,6,22,30,107] parenteral nutrition had significantly earlier and faster weight gain compared with those fed conventionally. Weight gain consistently at a rate above intrauterine growth rate can be achieved after 2 weeks of age for those born at 29 weeks' gestation.[48] It has been shown that total body water and extracellular fluid volume do not increase during parenteral nutrition but rather remain unchanged or decrease in spite of weight gain, thus supporting the hypothesis that the weight gain is due to tissue accretion rather than fluid retention.[36,111]

Apart from achieving nutritional adequacy and satisfactory postnatal growth, parenteral nutrition may also reduce the morbidity and mortality from specific diseases. Early introduction and excessive increases in oral feeding in preterm or sick infants increase the risk of aspiration pneumonia, cardiorespiratory disturbances and NEC. Parenteral nutrition, which allows the cautious and gradual establishment of oral feeding, is likely to minimize these risks in preterm or sick infants. A meta-analysis of the two RCTs of total parenteral nutrition[54,155] showed that the incidence of NEC was significantly reduced with parenteral nutrition.[62] The increased use and earlier initiation of parenteral nutrition have been associated with better tolerance of enteral feeds and a shorter convalescent period in preterm infants requiring prolonged assisted ventilation.[92]

HAZARDS

INFECTIONS AND TECHNICAL COMPLICATIONS

Infants on parenteral nutrition have an increased risk of bacterial sepsis caused by *Staphylococcus epidermidis* or

Table 20.4 Precautions taken to minimize the risk of sepsis

- Preparation of individual aliquots of parenteral nutrition solutions in the pharmacy
- Manipulations carried out in the ward to be avoided
- Silastic catheters instead of polyethylene/polyvinyl catheters to be used
- Central venous catheters must be placed under strict aseptic conditions
- Skin exit site for catheter placed in area which can be meticulously cleansed
- Proper care of the site and all the connectors and tubings essential
- Addition of heparin (1 unit/ml) to the infusate for peripheral/central venous catheters

S. aureus[15] and fungal sepsis caused by *Candida*.[149] The prevalence of catheter-related sepsis in infants ranges from 8% to 45%, with staff training playing a key role in its prevention.[114] The risk of polymicrobial bacteraemia is increased by manipulations of the parenteral infusate at the bedside.[44,70] Precautions which should be taken to minimize the risk of sepsis are listed in Table 20.4.

Uncommon but serious complications of central venous catheterization include superior or inferior vena cava obstruction, cardiac arrhythmia or tamponade, intracardiac thrombi, pleural effusion or chylothorax, pulmonary embolism, Budd–Chiari syndrome, and hydrocephalus secondary to jugular venous thrombosis. The success or failure of parenteral nutrition is obviously a function of careful technique. Many of these technical problems can be avoided with peripheral vein infusion, though this has the risks of excessive handling of the infant, localized necrosis tissue ulceration and subcutaneous calcium depositions.

METABOLIC COMPLICATIONS

The risks of abnormal plasma aminograms, hyperammonaemia, hyperchloraemic metabolic acidosis, rickets and trace element deficiencies are minimized with the careful choice of amino acid solutions and appropriate additives to the infusate. As septic infants are at risk for hyperammonaemia during parenteral nutrition,[140] their amino acid intake should be temporarily reduced or ceased when sepsis is first diagnosed.

RCTs have established the benefits and safety of parenteral fat commenced on the day of birth.[29,47,93,134] However, another RCT reported significantly prolonged oxygen and ventilatory therapy in infants commenced on parenteral fat on day 3 compared with controls.[55] Oxygenation and pulmonary haemodynamics in preterm infants with severe respiratory distress syndrome was not adversely affected when parenteral fat was infused at a dose of 1–4 g/kg/d[2,23,47] but deteriorated when the infusion rate exceeded an equivalent of 6–7 g/kg/d.[80,102] An association between parenteral fat administration and coagulase-negative staphylococcal bacteraemia in infants has been found[46] but there is no evidence that it impairs immune function in infants.[43,64,137,144] An increase in circulating free fatty acid levels can theoretically compete with bilirubin for binding to albumin. However, fat emulsion is also capable of binding unconjugated bilirubin[139] and infusions of 2–4 g/kg/d have been found to have no effect on total or unbound serum bilirubin.[24,136] Lipaemia does interfere with biochemical tests, leading to spurious conjugated hyperbilirubinaemia, hypercalcaemia and hyponatraemia. A transient increase in blood glucose occurs with parenteral fat infusion owing to altered glucose utilization.[156] Currently available parenteral fat emulsions do not contain long-chain polyunsaturated fatty acids of the n-6 and n-3 family which might be important for neurodevelopment. Infants are incapable of synthesizing these fatty acids and prolonged parenteral nutrition may result in a deficiency which is of potential importance.

Cholestatic jaundice occurs in 10–40% of infants on parenteral nutrition; it is very uncommon in those who receive it for less than 2 weeks, but 80% of those who require total parenteral nutrition for more than 2 months develop cholestasis.[14] Likely mechanisms include immaturity of the hepatobiliary system,[88] prolonged fasting,[115] impaired bile secretion and bile salt formation,[133] coexisting sepsis,[75] and underlying medical conditions associated with hypoxia or gastrointestinal conditions requiring surgery.[17] In the vast majority, cholestasis resolves when enteral feeding is initiated, but progression to biliary cirrhosis[103] and liver failure[112] can occur. Recovery from severe cholestasis following phenobarbitone therapy[135] and surgical biliary irrigation[35] has been reported. Rare hepatobiliary complications in infants following parenteral nutrition include cholelithiasis[138] and hepatocellular carcinoma.[100]

In view of the potential metabolic complications, parenteral nutrition is contraindicated in infants with fulminating sepsis, such as NEC or septicaemia prior to adequate clinical stabilization with antibiotic therapy. Acidosis must be corrected before parenteral nutrition is commenced. It should be withheld in infants with severe circulatory instability or acute renal failure.

TRANSITION TO ENTERAL NUTRITION

In spite of the adequacy of parenteral nutrition in meeting nutritional requirements for postnatal growth after birth, enteral feeding itself is vital for adaptation to extrauterine nutrition through its trophic effects on the gastrointestinal tract and its physiological effects on gastrointestinal exocrine and endocrine secretion and motility.[83] Milk feeds result in surges of secretion, glucagon, gastrin and motilin, all of which have trophic effects and mediate gastrointestinal secretion and motility. Parenterally fed young animals demonstrate not only a failure of growth of the stomach, small intestine and pancreas compared with those enterally fed, but also decreased disaccharidase activity in the atrophic proximal small intestine mucosa.[50] It has been shown in human infants that enteral feeding is necessary for normal gastric acid secretion.[68] Enteral feeding is associated with increases in blood gastrin and motilin levels[129] and intestinal motor activity.[19] Amino acid nitrogen flux, protein synthesis and breakdown are significantly higher during enteral than parenteral nutrition, reflecting the rapid growth and development of the gut in the enterally fed infant.[40] Glucagon, in addition to its role in gastrointestinal motility, stimulates bile flow.[9] Infants on total parenteral nutrition with no enteral intake secrete extremely dilute bile, a finding which may explain some of the adverse hepatobiliary changes associated with total parenteral nutrition.[4] Those who are parenterally fed also have significantly fewer immunoglobulin-containing intestinal plasma cells than those who are enterally fed.[73]

Instead of prolonged total parenteral nutrition, the early introduction of milk feeds prescribed even in subnutritional quantities is therefore beneficial for growth, development and maintenance of normal structure and function in the gastrointestinal and hepatobiliary systems.[18] Supplemental parenteral nutrition is becoming more widely accepted in neonatal practice with the realization that gastrointestinal function has a continuous spectrum ranging from normal to virtually nil, and that between these extremes there is an intermediate group in whom an adequate nutritional intake can be achieved using the enteral route to meet some nutritive requirements and the parenteral route to supply the remainder. Early introduction of enteral feeding is associated with a lower prevalence of severe feeding intolerance[76] and nosocomial infection.[143] RCTs have compared the effects of early (2–7 days) versus late (9–18 days) enteral feeding, both groups initially receiving the majority of their energy intake by the parenteral route.[42,131] Infants who received early low-volume enteral feeding had improved feeding tolerance, reached full enteral nutrition faster and had less indirect hyperbilirubinaemia, cholestatic jaundice and osteopenia of prematurity.

CONCLUSION

Parenteral nutrition, despite the many unanswered questions, represents a major breakthrough in the ability to provide adequate nutrition and to achieve normal growth in many preterm or sick infants who cannot tolerate or utilize enteral nutrients for long periods.[153] Because of its potential complications which can only be kept at an acceptable level by obsessional attention to detail, it should only be used in neonatal units where there are appropriate facilities and staff. Although its contribution towards improving the patient's short- and long-term outcomes compared with conventional feeding has not been definitely proven, it is life-saving in many instances of neonatal gastrointestinal failure. Therefore, its use in carefully selected infants who can be adequately cared for and monitored is recommended.

REFERENCES

1. Abitbol C L, Feldman D B, Ahmann P, Rudman D 1975 Plasma amino acid patterns during supplemental intravenous nutrition of low birthweight infants. Journal of Pediatrics 86: 766–772
2. Adamkin D H, Gelke K N, Wilkerson S A 1985 Clinical and laboratory observations: influence of intravenous fat therapy on tracheal effluent phospholipids and oxygenation in severe respiratory distress syndrome. Journal of Pediatrics 106: 122–124
3. Al-Dahhan J, Haycock G B, Chantler C, Stimmler L 1983 Sodium homeostasis in mature and immature neonates. I. Renal aspects. Archives of Disease in Childhood 58: 335–342
4. Al-Rabeeah A, Thurston O G, Walker K 1986 Effect of total parenteral nutrition on biliary lipids in neonates. Canadian Journal of Surgery 29: 289–291
5. Alpan G, Eyal F, Springer C, Glick B, Goder K, Armon J 1984 Heparinization of alimentation solutions administered through peripheral veins in premature infants: a controlled study. Pediatrics 74: 374–378
6. Anderson T L, Muttart C R, Bieber M A, Nicholson J F, Heird W C 1979 A controlled trial of glucose versus glucose and amino acids in premature infants. Journal of Pediatrics 94: 947–951
7. Andrew G, Chan G, Schiff D 1978 Lipid metabolism in the neonate. III. The ketogenic effect of Intralipid infusion in the neonate. Journal of Pediatrics 92: 995–997
8. Auld P A M, Bhanganada P, Mehta S 1966 The influence of an early caloric intake with I-V glucose on catabolism of premature infants. Pediatrics 37: 592–596
9. Aynsley-Green A 1983 Plasma hormone concentrations during enteral and parenteral nutrition in the human newborn. Journal of Pediatric Gastroenterology and Nutrition 2: 108–112
10. Baeckert P A, Greene H L, Fritz I, Oelberg D G, Adcock E W 1988 Vitamin concentrations in very low birth weight infants given vitamins intravenously in a lipid emulsion: measurement of vitamins A, D and E and riboflavin. Journal of Pediatrics 113: 1057–1063
11. Bailey M J 1979 Reduction of catheter-associated sepsis in parenteral nutrition using low-dose intravenous heparin. British Medical Journal i: 1671–1673
12. Batton D G, Maisels J, Appelbaum P 1982 Use of peripheral intravenous cannulas in premature infants: a controlled study. Pediatrics 70: 487–490
13. Baumgart S, Engle W D, Fox W W, Polin R A 1981 Effect of heat shielding on convective and evaporative heat loss and on radiant heat transfer in the premature infant. Journal of Pediatrics 99: 948–956
14. Beale E F, Nelson R M, Bucciarelli R L, Donnelly W H, Eitzman D V 1979 Intrahepatic cholestasis associated with parenteral nutrition in premature infants. Pediatrics 64: 342–347
15. Beganovic N, Verloove-Vanhorick S P, Brand R, Ruys J H 1988 Total parenteral nutrition and sepsis. Archives of Disease in Childhood 63: 66–69
16. Bell E F, Neidich G A, Cashore W J, Oh W1979 Combined effect of radiant warmer and phototherapy on insensible water loss in low-birth-weight infants, Journal of Pediatrics 94: 810–813
17. Bell R L, Ferry G D, Smith E O et al 1986 Total parenteral nutrition related cholestasis in infants. Journal of Parenteral and Enteral Nutrition 10: 356–359
18. Berseth C L 1995 Minimal enteral feedings. Clinical Perinatology 22: 195–204
19. Berseth C L, Nordyke C 1993 Enteral nutrients promote postnatal maturation of intestinal motor activity in preterm infants. American Journal of Physiology 264: G1046–1051
20. Binder N D, Raschko R K, Benda G I, Reynolds J W 1989 Insulin infusion with parenteral nutrition in extremely low birthweight infants with hyperglycemia. Journal of Pediatrics 114: 273–280
21. Bonner C M, DeBrie K L, Hug G, Landrigan E, Taylor B J 1995 Effects of parenteral L-carnitine supplementation on fat metabolism and nutrition in premature infants. Journal of Pediatrics 126: 287–292
22. Brans Y W, Sumners J E, Dweck H S, Cassady G 1974 Feeding the low birth weight infant: orally or parenterally? Preliminary results of a comparative study. Pediatrics 54: 15–22

23. Brans Y W, Dutton E B, Andrew D S, Menchaca E M, West D L 1986 Fat emulsion tolerance in very low birth weight neonates: effect on diffusion of oxygen in the lungs and on blood pH. Pediatrics 78: 79–84
24. Brans Y W, Ritter D A, Kenny J D, Andrew D S, Dutton E B, Carillo D W 1987 Influence of intravenous fat emulsion on serum bilirubin in very low birthweight infants. Archives of Disease in Childhood 62: 156–160
25. Brans Y W, Andrew D S, Carrillo D W, Dutton E P, Menchaca E M, Puleo-Schappke B A 1988 Tolerance of fat emulsions in very low birth weight neonates. American Journal of Diseases of Children 142: 145–152
26. Brans Y W, Andrew D S, Carillo D W, Dutton E B, Menchaca E M, Puleo-Scheppke B A 1990 Tolerance of fat emulsions in very low birthweight neonates: effect of birthweight on plasma lipid concentrations. American Journal of Perinatology 7: 114–117
27. Brion L P, Schwartz G J, Campbell D, Fleischman A R 1989 Early hyperkalaemia in very low birthweight infants in the absence of oliguria. Archives of Disease in Childhood 64: 270–282
28. Brismar B, Hardstedt C, Jacobson S, Kager L, Malmborg A 1982 Reduction of catheter-associated thrombosis in parenteral nutrition by intravenous heparin therapy. Archives of Surgery 117: 1196–1199
29. Brownlee K G, Kelly E J, Ng P C, Kendall-Smith S C, Dear P R 1993 Early or late parenteral nutrition for the sick preterm infant? Archives of Disease in Childhood 69: 281–283
30. Bryan M H, Wei P, Hamilton J R, Chance G W, Swyer P R 1973 Supplemental intravenous alimentation in low birth weight infants. Journal of Pediatrics 82: 940–944
31. Chathas M K, Paton J B, Fisher D E 1990 Percutaneous central venous catheterization. American Journal of Diseases of Children 144: 1246–1250
32. Chessex P, Zebiche H, Pineault M, Lopage D, Dallaire L 1985 Effect of aminoacid composition of parenteral solutions on nitrogen retention and metabolic response in very low birth weight infants. Journal of Pediatrics 106: 111–117
33. Collins J W Jr, Hoppe M, Brown K, Edidin D V, Padbury J, Ogata E S 1991 A controlled trial of insulin infusion and parenteral nutrition in extremely low birth weight infants with glucose intolerance. Journal of Pediatrics 118: 921–927
34. Cooke R J, Yeh Y, Gibson D, Debo D, Bell G L 1987 Soybean oil emulsion administration during parenteral nutrition in the preterm infant: effect on essential fatty acid, lipid and glucose metabolism. Journal of Pediatrics 111: 767–773
35. Cooper A, Ross A J III, O'Neil J A, Bishop H C, Templeton J M, Ziegler M M 1985 Resolution of intractable cholestasis associated with total parenteral nutrition following biliary irrigation. Journal of Pediatric Surgery 20: 772–774
36. Coran A G, Drongowski R A, Wesley J R 1984 Changes in total body water and extracellular fluid volume in infants receiving total parenteral nutrition. Journal of Pediatric Surgery 19: 771–776
37. Coran A G, Drongowski R A, Baker P J 1985 The metabolic effects of oral L-carnitine administration in infants receiving total parenteral nutrition with fat. Journal of Pediatric Surgery 20: 758–764
38. Cowett R M, Anderson G E, Maguire C A, Oh W 1988 Ontogeny of glucose homeostasis in low birth weight infants. Journal of Pediatrics 112: 462–465
39. Dahl G B, Svensson L, Kinnander N J G, Zander M, Berstrom U K 1994 Stability of vitamins in soybean oil fat emulsion under conditions simulating intravenous feeding of neonates and children. Journal of Parenteral and Enteral Nutrition 18: 234–239
40. Duffy B, Pencharz P 1986a The effect of feeding route (IV or oral) on the protein metabolism of the neonate. American Journal of Clinical Nutrition 43: 108–111
41. Duffy B, Pencharz P 1986b The effects of surgery on the nitrogen metabolism of parenterally fed human neonates. Pediatric Research 20: 32–35
42. Dunn L, Hulman S, Weiner J, Kliegman R 1988 Beneficial effects of early hypocaloric enteral feeding on neonatal gastrointestinal function: preliminary report of a randomized trial. Journal of Pediatrics 112: 622–629
43. English D, Roloff J S, Lukens J N, Parker P, Greene H L, Ghishan F K 1981 Intravenous lipid emulsions and human neutrophil function. Journal of Pediatrics 99: 913–916
44. Fleer A, Senders R C, Visser M R et al 1983 Septicemia due to coagulase-negative staphylococci in a neonatal intensive care unit: clinical and bacteriological features and contaminated parenteral fluids as a source of sepsis. Pediatric Infectious Diseases 2: 426–431
45. Forsyth J S, Crighton A 1995 Low birthweight infants and total parenteral nutrition immediately after birth. I. Energy expenditure and respiratory quotient of ventilated and non-ventilated infants. Archives of Disease in Childhood 73: F4–7
46. Freeman J, Goldman D A, Smith N E, Sidebottom D G, Epstein M F, Platt R 1990 Association of intravenous lipid emulsion and coagulase-negative staphylococcal bacteremia in neonatal intensive care units. New England Journal of Medicine 323: 301–308
47. Gilbertson N, Kovar I Z, Cox D J, Crowe L, Palmer N T 1991 Introduction of intravenous lipid administration on the first day of life in the low birth weight neonate. Journal of Pediatrics 119: 615–623
48. Gill A, Yu V Y H, Bajuk B, Astbury J 1986 Postnatal growth in infants born before 30 weeks' gestation. Archives of Disease in Childhood 61: 549–553
49. Gilles J, Jones G, Pencharz P 1983 Delivery of vitamins A, D and E in parenteral nutrition solutions. Journal of Parenteral and Enteral Nutrition 7: 11–14
50. Goldstein R M, Hebiguchi T, Luk G D, Taqi F, Franklin F A Jr, Niemiec P W, Dudgeon D L 1985 The effects of total parenteral nutrition on gastrointestinal growth and development. Journal of Pediatric Surgery 20: 785–791
51. Greene H L, Hambridge K M, Schanler R, Tsang R C 1988 Guidelines for the use of vitamins, trace elements, calcium, magnesium and phosphorus in infants and children receiving total parenteral nutrition: report of the Subcommittee on Pediatric Parenteral Nutrition Requirements from the Committee on Clinical Practice Issues of the American Society for Clinical Nutrition. American Journal of Clinical Nutrition 48: 1324–1342
52. Groh-Wargo S, Ciaccia A, Moore J 1988 Neonatal metabolic acidosis: effect of chloride from normal saline flushes. Journal of Parenteral and Enteral Nutrition 12: 159–161
53. Gruskay J, Costarino A T, Polin R A, Baumgart S 1988 Nonoliguric hyperkalemia in the premature infant weighing less than 1000 grams. Journal of Pediatrics 113: 381–386
54. Gunn T, Reaman G, Outerbridge E W, Cole E 1978 Peripheral total parenteral nutrition for premature infants with the respiratory distress syndrome: A controlled study. Journal of Pediatrics 92: 608–613
55. Hammerman C, Aramburo M J 1988 Decreased lipid intake reduces morbidity in sick premature neonates. Journal of Pediatrics 113: 1083–1088
56. Hanning R M, Atkinson S A, Whyte R K 1991 Efficacy of calcium glycerophosphate vs conventional mineral salts for total parenteral nutrition in low-birth-weight infants: a randomized clinical trial. American Journal of Clinical Nutrition 54: 903–908
57. Harper R G, Carrera E, Weiss S, Luongo M 1985 A complete computerized program for nutritional management in the neonatal intensive care nursery. American Journal of Perinatology 2: 161–162
58. Harpin V A, Rutter N 1985 Humidification of incubators. Archives of Disease in Childhood 60: 219–224
59. Haumont D, Deckelbaum R J, Richelle M et al 1989 Plasma lipid and plasma lipoprotein concentrations in low birth weight infants given parenteral nutrition with twenty or ten percent lipid emulsion. Journal of Pediatrics 115: 787–793
60. Haumont D, Richelle M, Deckelbaum R J, Coussaert E, Carpentier Y A 1992 Effect of liposomal content of lipid emulsions on plasma lipid concentrations in low birth weight infants receiving parenteral nutrition. Journal of Pediatrics 121: 759–763
61. Heimler R, Doumas B T, Jendrzejczak B M, Nemeth P B, Hoffman R G, Nelin L D 1993 Relationship between nutrition, weight change, and fluid compartments in preterm infants during the first week of life. Journal of Pediatrics 122: 110–114
62. Heird W C 1992 Parenteral feeding. In: Sinclair J C, Bracken M B (eds) Effective care of the newborn infant. Oxford: Oxford University Press, pp 141–160
63. Heird W C, Hay W, Helms R A, Storm M C, Kashyap S, Dell R B 1988 Pediatric parenteral amino acid mixture in low birth weight infants. Pediatrics 81: 41–50
64. Helms R A, Herrod H G, Burckart G J, Christensen M L 1983 E-rosette formation, total T-cells, and lymphocyte transformation in infants receiving intravenous safflower oil emulsion. Journal of Parenteral and Enteral Nutrition 7: 541–545

65. Helms R A, Whitington P F, Mauer E C, Catarau E M, Christensen M L, Borum P R 1986 Enhanced lipid utilisation in infants receiving oral L-carnitine during long-term parenteral nutrition. Journal of Pediatrics 109: 984–988
66. Helms R A, Christensen M L, Mauer E C, Storm M C 1987 Comparison of a pediatric versus standard amino acid formulation in preterm neonates requiring parenteral nutrition. Journal of Pediatrics 110: 466–470
67. Hilliard J L, Shannon D L, Hunter M A, Brans Y W 1983 Plasma lipid levels in preterm neonates receiving parenteral nutrition. Archives of Disease in Childhood 58: 29–33
68. Hyman P E, Feldman E J, Ament M E, Bryne W J, Euler A R 1983 Effect of enteral feeding on the maintenance of gastric acid secretory function. Gastroenterology 84: 341–345
69. Imura K, Okada A, Fukui Y et al 1988 Clinical studies on a newly devised amino acid solution for neonates. Journal of Parenteral and Enteral Nutrition 12: 496–504
70. Jarvis W R, Highsmith A K, Allen J R, Haley R W 1983 Polymicrobial bacteremia associated with lipid emulsion in a neonatal intensive care unit. Pediatr Infect Dis 2: 203–208
71. Kanarek K S, Kuznicki M B, Blair R C 1991 Infusion of total parenteral nutrition via the umbilical artery. Journal of Parenteral and Enteral Nutrition 15: 71–74
72. Kao L C, Cheng M H, Warburton D 1984 Triglycerides, free fatty acids, free fatty acids/albumin molar ratio, and cholesterol levels in serum of neonates receiving long-term lipid infusions: controlled trial of continuous and intermittent regimes. Journal of Pediatrics 104: 429–435
73. Knox W F 1986 Restricted feeding and human intestinal plasma cell development. Archives of Disease in Childhood 61: 744–749
74. Koh T H H G, Aynsley-Green A, Tarbit M, Eyre J A 1988 Neural dysfunction during hypoglycaemia. Archives of Disease in Childhood 63: 1353–1358
75. Kubota A, Okada A, Nezu R, Kamata S, Imura K, Takagi Y 1988 Hyperbilirubinemia in neonates associated with total parenteral nutrition. Journal of Parenteral and Enteral Nutrition 12: 602–606
76. LaGamma E F, Ostertag S G, Birenbaum H 1985 Failure of delayed oral feedings to prevent necrotizing enterocolitis. American Journal of Diseases of Children 139: 385–389
77. Laidlaw S A, Kopple J D 1987 Newer concepts of the indispensable amino acids. American Journal of Clinical Nutrition 46: 593–605
78. Lee E J, Simmer K, Gibson R A 1993 Essential fatty acid deficiency in parenterally fed preterm infants. Journal of Paediatrics and Child Health 29: 51–55
79. Lemons J A, Neal P, Ernst J 1986 Nitrogen sources for parenteral nutrition in the newborn infant. Clinical Perinatology 13: 91–109
80. Lloyd T R, Boucek M M 1986 Effect of Intralipid on the neonatal pulmonary bed: an echographic study. Journal of Pediatrics 108: 130–133
81. Lorenz J M, Kleinman L I, Kotagal U R, Reller M D 1982 Water balance in very low birth weight infants: relationship to water and sodium intake and effect on outcome. Journal of Pediatrics 101: 423–432
82. Louik C, Mitchell A A, Epstein M F, Shapiro S 1985 Risk factors for neonatal hyperglycemia associated with 10% dextrose infusion. American Journal of Diseases of Children 139: 783–786
83. Lucas A, Bloom S R, Aynsley-Green A 1983 Metabolic and endocrine effects of depriving preterm infants of enteral nutrition. Acta Paediatrica Scandinavica 72: 245–249
84. Lucas A, Morley R, Cole T J 1988 Adverse neurodevelopmental outcome of moderate neonatal hypoglycaemia. British Medical Journal 297: 1304–1308
85. Lucas A, Baker B A, Morley R M 1993 Hyperphenylalaninaemia and outcome in intravenously fed preterm infants. Archives of Disease in Childhood 68: 579–583
86. MacMahon P 1984 Prescribing and formulating neonatal intravenous feeding solutions by microcomputer. Archives of Disease in Childhood 59: 548–552
87. Malloy M H, Rassin D K, Richardson C J 1984 Total parenteral nutrition in sick preterm infants: effects of cysteine supplementation with nitrogen intakes of 240 and 400 mg/kg/day. Journal of Pediatric Gastroenterology and Nutrition 3: 239–244
88. Merritt R J 1986 Cholestasis associated with total parenteral nutrition. Journal of Pediatric Gastroenterology and Nutrition 5: 9–22
89. Mitton S G, Burston D, Brueton M J, Kovar I Z 1993 Plasma amino acid profiles in preterm infants receiving Vamin 9 glucose or Vamin Infant. Early Human Development 32: 71–78
90. Moore M C, Greene H L, Phillips B et al 1986 Evaluation of a pediatric multiple vitamin preparation for total parenteral nutrition in infants and children. Pediatrics 77: 530–538
91. Moreno A, Dominguez C, Ballabriga A 1994 Aluminium in the neonate related to parenteral nutrition. Acta Paediatrica 83: 25–29
92. Moyer-Mileur L, Chan G M 1986 Nutritional support of very low birth weight infants requiring prolonged assisted ventilation. American Journal of Diseases of Children 140: 929–932
93. Murdock N, Crighton A, Nelson L M, Forsyth J S 1995 Low birthweight infants and total parenteral nutrition immediately after birth. II. Randomised study of biochemical tolerance of intravenous glucose, amino acids, and lipids. Archives of Disease in Childhood 73: F8–12
94. Nakamura K T, Sato Y, Erenberg A 1990 Evaluation of a percutaneously placed 27-gauge central venous catheter in neonates weighing <1200 grams. Journal of Parenteral and Enteral Nutrition 14: 295–299
95. Neubauer A P 1995 Percutaneous central i.v. access in the neonate: experience with 535 Silastic catheters. Acta Paediatrica 84: 756–760
96. Neuzil J, Darlow B A, Inder T E, Sluis K B, Winterbourn C C, Stocker R 1995 Oxidation of parenteral lipid emulsion by ambient and phototherapy lights: potential toxicity of routine parenteral feeding. Journal of Pediatrics 126: 785–790
97. Ogata E S, Schulman S, Raffensperger J, Luck S, Rusnak M 1984 Caval catheterisation in the intensive care nursery: a useful means for providing parenteral nutrition to the extremely low birthweight infant. Journal of Pediatric Surgery 19: 258–262
98. Ostertag S G, Jovanovic L, Lewis B, Auld P A M 1986 Insulin pump therapy in the very low birth weight infant. Pediatrics 78: 625–630
99. Park W, Paust H, Brosicke H, Knoblack G, Helge H 1986 Impaired fat utilization in parenterally fed low birth weight infants suffering from sepsis. Journal of Parenteral and Enteral Nutrition 10: 627–630
100. Patterson K, Kapur S P, Chandra R S 1985 Hepatocellular carcinoma in a noncirrhotic infant after prolonged parenteral nutrition. Journal of Pediatrics 106: 797–800
101. Paust H, Schroder H, Park W, Jakobs C, Frauendienst G 1983 Fat elimination in parenterally fed low birthweight infants during the first two weeks of life. Journal of Parenteral and Enteral Nutrition 7: 557–559
102. Pereira G R, Fox W W, Stanley C A, Baker L, Schwartz J G 1980 Decreased oxygenation and hyperlipemia during intravenous fat infusions in premature infants. Pediatrics 66: 26–30
103. Pereira G R, Sherman M S, DiGiacomo J, Zieler M, Roth K, Jacobowski D 1981 Hyperalimentation induced cholestasis. American Journal of Diseases of Children 135: 842–845
104. Pereira G R, Lim B K, Ing C, Medeiros H F 1992 Umbilical vs peripheral vein catheterization for parenteral nutrition in sick premature neonates. Yonsei Medical Journal 33: 224–231
105. Phelps S J, Cochran E B 1989 Peripheral venous line infiltration in infants receiving 10% dextrose, 10% dextrose/amino acids, or 10% dextrose/amino acids/fat emulsion. Journal of Parenteral and Enteral Nutrition 13: 628–632
106. Phelps S J, Helms R A 1987 Risk factors affecting infiltration of peripheral venous lines in infants. Journal of Pediatrics 111: 384–389
107. Pildes R S, Ramamurthy R S, Cordero G V, Wong P W K 1973 Intravenous supplementation of L-amino acids and dextrose in low-birth-weight infants. Journal of Pediatrics 82: 945–950
108. Pineault M, Chessex P, Bisaillon S, Brisson G 1988 Total parenteral nutrition in the newborn: impact of the quality of infused energy on nitrogen metabolism. American Journal of Clinical Nutrition 47: 298–304
109. Pitkanen O, Hallman M, Anderson S 1991 Generation of free radicals in lipid emulsion used in parenteral nutrition. Pediatric Research 29: 56–59
110. Pollak A, Cowett R M, Schwartz R, Oh W 1978 Glucose disposal in low birth weight infants during steady state hyperglycemia: effects of exogenous insulin administration. Pediatrics 61: 546–549
111. Polley T Z, Benner J W, Rhodin A, Weintraub W H, Coran A G 1979 Changes in total body water in infants receiving total intravenous nutrition. Journal of Surgical Research 26: 555–559
112. Postuma R, Trevenen C L 1979 Liver disease in infants receiving total parenteral nutrition. Pediatrics 63: 110–115

113. Puntis J W, Ball P A, Preece M A, Green A, Brown G A, Booth I W 1989 Egg and breast milk based nitrogen sources compared. Archives of Disease in Childhood 64: 1472–1477
114. Puntis J W, Holden C E, Smallman S, Finkel Y, George R H, Booth I W 1991 Staff training: a key factor in reducing intravascular catheter sepsis. Archives of Disease in Childhood 66: 335–337
115. Rager R, Finegold M J 1975 Cholestasis in immature newborn infants: is parenteral alimentation responsible? Journal of Pediatrics 86: 264–269
116. Raupp P, von Kries R, Schmidt E, Pfahl H, Gunther O 1988 Incompatibility between fat emulsion and calcium plus heparin in parenteral nutrition of premature babies. Lancet I: 700
117. Raupp P, van Kries R, Pfahl H, Manz F 1991 Glycero- vs glucose phosphate in parenteral nutrition of premature infants: a comparative in vitro evaluation of calcium/phosphorus compatibility. Journal of Parenteral and Enteral Nutrition 15: 469–473
118. Rees L, Shaw J C L, Brook C G D, Forsling M L 1984 Hyponatraemia in the first week of life in preterm infants. II Sodium and water balance. Archives of Disease in Childhood 59: 423–429
119. Reichman B L, Chessex P, Putet G et al 1982 Partition of energy metabolism and energy cost of growth in the very low birth weight infant. Pediatrics 69: 446–451
120. Rivera A Jr, Bell E F, Stegink L D, Ziegler E E 1989 Plasma amino acid profiles during the first three days of life in infants with respiratory distress syndrome: effect of parenteral amino acid supplementation. Journal of Pediatrics 115: 465–468
121. Rivera A Jr, Bell E F, Bier D M 1993 Effect of intravenous amino acids on protein metabolism of preterm infants during the first three days of life. Pediatric Research 33: 106–111
122. Rovamo L M, Nikkila E A, Raivio K O 1988 Lipoprotein lipase, hepatic lipase, and carnitine in premature infants. Archives of Disease in Childhood 63: 140–147
123. Rubecz I, Mestyan J 1973 Energy metabolism and intravenous nutrition of premature infants. Biology of the Neonate 23: 45–58
124. Rubin M, Harell D, Naor N et al 1991 Lipid infusion with different triglyceride cores (long-chain vs medium-chain/long-chain triglycerides): effect on plasma lipids and bilirubin binding in premature infants. Journal of Parenteral and Enteral Nutrition 15: 642–646
125. Saini J, MacMahon P, Morgan J B, Kovar I Z 1989 Early parenteral feeding of amino acids. Archives of Disease in Childhood 64: 1362–1366
126. Salle B L, David L, Chopard J P, Grafmeyer D C, Renaud H 1977 Prevention of early neonatal hypocalcemia in low birth weight infants with continuous calcium infusion: effect on serum calcium, phosphorus, magnesium, and circulating immunoactive parathyroid hormone and calcitonin. Pediatric Research 11: 1180–1185
127. Schanler R J, Shulman R J, Prestridge L L 1994 Parenteral nutrient needs of very low birth weight infants. Journal of Pediatrics 125: 961–968
128. Schreiner R L, Glick M R, Nordschow C D, Gresham E L 1979 An evaluation of methods to monitor infants receiving intravenous lipids. Journal of Pediatrics 94: 197–200
129. Shulman D I, Kanarek K 1993 Gastrin, motilin, insulin, and insulin-like growth factor-I concentrations in very low birth weight infants receiving enteral or parenteral nutrition. Journal of Parenteral and Enteral Nutrition 17: 130–133
130. Shulman R J, Pokorny W J, Martin C G, Petitt R, Baldaia L, Roney D 1986 Comparison of percutaneous and surgical placement of central venous catheters in neonates. Journal of Pediatric Surgery 21: 348–350
131. Slagle T A, Gross S J 1988 Effect of early low-volume enteral substrate on subsequent feeding tolerance in very low birth weight infants. Journal of Pediatrics 13: 526–531
132. Smith J L, Canham J E, Wells P A 1988 Effect of phototherapy light, sodium bisulfite, and pH on vitamin stability in total parenteral nutrition and mixtures. Journal of Parenteral and Enteral Nutrition 12: 394–402
133. Sondheimer J M, Bryan H, Andrews W, Forster G G 1978 Cholestatic tendencies in premature infants on and off parenteral nutrition. Pediatrics 62: 984–989
134. Sosenko I R S, Rodriguez-Pierce M, Bancalari E 1993 Effect of early initiation of intravenous lipid administration on the incidence and severity of chronic lung disease in premature infants. Journal of Pediatrics 123: 975–982
135. South M, King A 1987 Parenteral nutrition associated cholestasis: recovery following phenobarbitone. Journal of Parenteral and Enteral Nutrition 11: 208–209
136. Spear M L, Stahl G E, Hamosh M, McNelis W G, Richardson L L, Spence V 1988 Effect of heparin dose and infusion rate on lipid clearance and bilirubin binding in premature infants receiving intravenous fat emulsions. Journal of Pediatrics 112: 94–98
137. Strunk R C, Murrow B W, Thilo E, Kunke K S, Johnson E G 1985 Normal macrophage function in infants receiving Intralipid by low-dose intermittent administration. Journal of Pediatrics 106: 640–645
138. Suita S, Ikeda K, Naito K, Doki T, Handa N 1984 Cholelithiasis in infants: association with parenteral nutrition. Journal of Parenteral and Enteral Nutrition 8: 568–570
139. Thaler M M, Wennberg R P 1977 Influence of intravenous nutrients on bilirubin transport. II Emulsified lipid solutions. Pediatric Research 11: 167–171
140. Thomas D W, Sinatra F R, Hack S L, Smith T M, Platzker A C G, Merritt R J 1982 Hyperammonemia in neonates receiving intravenous nutrition. Journal of Parenteral and Enteral Nutrition 6: 503–506
141. Thornton L, Griffin E 1991 Evaluation of a taurine containing amino acid solution in parenteral nutrition. Archives of Disease in Childhood 66: 21–25
142. Uhlemann M, Plath C, Heine W et al 1989 MCT fat emulsions enhance efficacy of whole-body protein metabolism in very small preterm neonates. Clinical Nutrition 8: 84
143. Unger A, Goetzman B W, Chan C, Lyons A B, Miller M F 1986 Nutritional practices and outcome of extremely premature infants. American Journal of Diseases of Children 140: 1027–1033
144. Usmani S S, Harper R G, Usmani S 1988F Effect of a lipid emulsion (Intralipid) on polymorphonuclear leukocyte functions in the neonate. Journal of Pediatrics 113: 132–136
145. Van Aerde J E, Sauer P J, Pencharz P B, Smith J M, Heim T, Swyer P R 1994 Metabolic consequences of increasing energy intake by adding lipid to parenteral nutrition in full-term infants. American Journal of Clinical Nutrition 59: 659–662
146. Van Goudoever J B, Wattimena J D L, Carnielli V P, Sulkers E J, Degenhart H J, Sauer P J J 1994 Effect of dexamethasone on protein metabolism in infants with bronchopulmonary dysplasia. Journal of Pediatrics 124: 112–118
147. Wahlig T M, Georgieff M K 1995 The effects of illness on neonatal metabolism and nutritional management. Clinical Perinatology 22: 77–96
148. Warner B W, Gorgone P, Schilling S, Farell M, Ghory M J 1987 Multiple purpose central venous access in infants less than 1000 grams. Journal of Pediatric Surgery 22: 820–822
149. Weese-Mayer D E, Fondriest D W, Brouilette R T, Shulman S T 1987 Risk factors associated with candidemia in the neonatal intensive care unit: a case control study. Pediatric Infectious Disease Journal 6: 190–196
150. Wilson F E, Yu V Y H, Hawgood S, Adamson T M, Wilkinson M H 1983 Computerised nutritional data management in neonatal intensive care. Archives of Disease in Childhood 58: 732–736
151. Yamamoto L G, Gainsley G J, Witek J E 1986 Pediatric Parenteral nutrition management using a comprehensive user-friendly computer program designed for personal computers. Journal of Parenteral and Enteral Nutrition 10: 535–539
152. Yeh T F, Voora S, Lilien L D, Matwynshyn J, Srinivasan G, Pildes R S 1980 Oxygen consumption and insensible water loss in premature infants in single-versus double-walled incubators. Journal of Pediatrics 97: 967–971
153. Yu V Y H, MacMahon R A (eds) 1992 Intravenous feeding of the neonate. Edward Arnold, London
154. Yu V Y H, James B E, Hendry P G, MacMahon R A 1979a Glucose tolerance in very low birthweight infants. Australian Paediatric Journal 15: 147–151
155. Yu V Y H, James B, Hendry P, MacMahon R A 1979b Total parenteral nutrition in very low birthweight infants: a controlled trial. Archives of Disease in Childhood 54: 653–661
156. Yunis K A, Oh W, Kalhan S, Cowett R M 1992 Glucose kinetics following administration of an intravenous fat emulsion to low birth weight neonates. American Journal of Physiology 263: E844–849
157. Zaidan H, Dhanireddy R, Hamosh M, Bengtsson-Olivecrona G, Hamosh P 1985 Lipid clearing in premature infants during continuous heparin infusion: role of circulating lipases. Pediatric Research 19: 23–25
158. Zlotkin S H, Bryan M H, Anderson G H 1981 Intravenous nitrogen and energy intakes required to duplicate in utero nitrogen accretion in prematurely born human infants. Journal of Pediatrics 99: 115–120

APPENDIX

NEONATAL PARENTERAL NUTRITION AT MONASH MEDICAL CENTRE, MELBOURNE

Indications

All neonates unlikely to establish full oral feeds within a week after birth or who subsequently are likely to have oral feeds withheld for more than 1 week receive parenteral nutrition. Categories of patients therefore include most neonates below 1500 g birthweight, those with necrotizing enterocolitis and those with gastrointestinal abnormalities. Contraindications are those described in the text.

Prescription

The amount of water, amino acids, glucose and fat are prescribed daily on a per kilogram basis by the medical staff (Table 20.5) These components of parenteral nutrition can be varied independently of each other.

Amino acids

If the neonate's blood urea is below 6 mmol/l, parenteral nutrition is started at 1.75 g/kg/24 h amino acids (using a Vamin-based formula). If the neonate's blood urea remains below 6 mmol/l, the amino acids are increased to 3.5 g/kg/24 h usually after 48 hours. Subsequent prescriptions are decided on the basis of the daily blood urea measurement.

Glucose

The neonate's glucose tolerance on the glucose-electrolyte solution, given on the day before parenteral nutrition started, is noted. If blood glucose is below 7 mmol/l and glycosuria is less than 1%, the same amount of glucose is given with the parenteral nutrition the following day. For example, if on the day before commencing parenteral nutrition the neonate tolerated 10% dextrose at 120 ml/kg/24 h, the glucose infusion on the first day of parenteral nutrition would be 12 g/kg/24 h. The amount of glucose given per day is then increased by 2 g/kg every day up to a level of 20 g/kg/24 h, unless hyperglycaemia (blood glucose >7 mmol/l) or glycosuria >1% develops.

Table 20.5 Prescribed amounts per kilogram per day

Volume (ml)		100–200	
Glucose (g)		6–20	
Fat (g)		1–3	
Amino acids (g)	1.75		3.50
Sodium (mmol)	2.00		4.00
Potassium (mmol)	1.00		2.00
Calcium (mmol)	0.90		1.80
Magnesium (mmol)	0.15		0.30
Phosphorus (mmol)	0.90		1.80
Chloride (mmol)	3.10		6.10
Acetate (mmol)	0.35		0.70
Zinc (μmol)	Background contamination in the solution		6.1
Copper (μmol)	Background contamination in the solution		0.3
Selenium (nmol)	Background contamination in the solution		25
Manganese (nmol)	Background contamination in the solution		18
Iodine (nmol)	Background contamination in the solution		8
Chromium (nmol)			4
M.V.I. Paediatric (ml)		2 (maximum 5 ml per 24 h)	

Fluid

The amount of fluid in which the prescribed nutrients are added may vary from 100 to 200 ml/kg/24 h (when less than 100 ml/kg/24 h is prescribed, the input of nutrients is reduced proportionally).

Minerals and trace elements

Minerals are added to the parenteral nutrition solution, making allowance for the amount already present in Vamin, up to the recommended amount for a growing preterm neonate when the neonate is receiving 3.5 g/kg/24 h of amino acids, and up to half that amount when the neonate is receiving 1.75 g/kg/24 h of amino acids. The pharmacist can modify the standard mineral content of the parenteral nutrition solution on request: either more sodium or potassium, or less sodium or calcium. Trace elements are added to the parenteral nutrition solution in the recommended amount for a growing preterm neonate when 3.5 g/kg/24 h of amino acids is given. Trace elements are not added when 1.75 g/kg/24 h amino acids is given, although the neonate does receive a small amount of trace elements present as background contamination of the parenteral nutrition solution.

Heparin

This is added to the above parenteral nutrition solution at a concentration of 1 unit/ml before water modification. The dose of heparin infused is equivalent to about 5 units/kg/h. A mixture of the prescribed amounts of amino acids, glucose, minerals and trace elements, with heparin added and volume adjusted to the prescribed fluid intake, is made up in a single bag in the pharmacy and delivered to the neonatal unit.

Fat

20% Intralipid is commenced at 1 g/kg/24 h and increased daily by 1 g/kg to 3 g/kg/24 h as tolerated. The Intralipid is run into the parenteral nutrition solution through a Y connection just proximal to the patient.

Vitamins

M.V.I. Paediatric, at a dose of 2 ml/kg/24 h up to a maximum of 5 ml per 24 hours, is added to the prescribed daily intake of 20% Intralipid.

21

Intensive care monitoring

N. R. C. Roberton Janet M. Rennie

INTRODUCTION

Even the most sophisticated monitor is no substitute for a good intensive care nurse. The equipment outlined in this chapter is there to help the expert nurse use minimal handling to care for the ill newborn baby. Any electronic monitor can only serve to augment the observational skills of the neonatal unit staff, as all laboratory, electronic and radiological investigations are subject to artefact on occasion (Chapters 46 and 47). Equipment can only achieve these aims if it is maintained and used properly, with a knowledge of how to set, choose and respond to alarms. This is possible without understanding the intricacies of the circuitry or exactly how the monitor works, although some understanding of the principles undoubtedly helps. The current level of complexity and of capital investment in electronic equipment entirely justifies a full-time medical physics technician in any sizeable neonatal unit. His or her many tasks include training new staff, carrying out routine maintenance repairs, maintaining an inventory and planning a logical purchasing strategy, including checking whether new items fulfil the appropriate national safety standards and regulations. The modern intensively monitored neonate has been likened to a person in a bath reaching for a faulty electrical device – all equipment attached to babies must be electrically isolated as they are in contact with the ground via the incubator.

PHYSIOLOGICAL MONITORING

RESPIRATION MONITORING

Apnoea

There are now five different systems in general use for monitoring respiration (see Fig. 29.89, p. 633). One consists of a ripple-type mattress with tubes leading from each section to a central manifold.[30] As the baby breathes in, weight distribution changes and small volumes of air pass up and down the tubes to equalize pressure, slightly cooling a heated thermistor situated in the manifold. If the baby stops breathing, an alarm is triggered after a preset interval, usually 15 seconds. The system is suitable for use with even the smallest babies. The disadvantages are that the mattress must be correctly inflated, as over- or underinflation will lead to false positive alarms.[53] Problems also arise if the sensitivity is set too high, as the baby's cardiac pulsation, which tends to slow and increase in volume during prolonged apnoea, may be sufficient to prevent the device alarming.[4] The device will also fail to alarm if the apnoea is of the obstructive type, when the baby continues to make occasional respiratory movements or gross body movements despite the apnoea. The main advantage of this type of monitor may be that the mattress limits the degree of head flattening which can occur in preterm infants[6] (p. 394).

An alternative to the mattress is the pressure-sensor pad,[60] which can be placed between the incubator or cot base and the infant's mattress (see Fig. 29.89). This also records the changes in weight distribution that occur with breathing. The alarm will again fail to sound during obstructive or mixed apnoea, and it too can be misled by increases in cardiac pulsation.

The third device[67] consists of a pressure-sensitive capsule which is attached to the baby's abdominal skin, close to the umbilicus or on the lower abdomen (see Fig. 29.89). The movements of the abdominal wall distort a membrane covering the capsule, producing pressure changes. This suffers the same disadvantages as the two previous devices, although it is affected less by gross body movements. The widely used Graesby respiration monitor is of this type.

The fourth technique is that of impedance.[39] Impedance monitors (see Fig. 29.89) detect respiration by using a high-frequency oscillator to send a small current across conventional ECG electrodes on the chest wall. The volume alterations during breathing produce small changes in electrical resistance, which are measured electronically. Such a system is not foolproof, particularly in small infants, as cardiac pulsations can also cause changes in resistance, producing a prominent artefact.[61] Unfortunately, impedance monitors may also fail to detect mixed and obstructive apnoeas.[68]

The final technique, respiratory inductive plethysmography is more recently described and, although not yet in routine clinical use, has proved a useful research tool (see Fig. 29.89). The underlying principle is that the magnetic field induced within a coil is proportional to the enclosed cross-sectional area. Therefore, if a coil, sewn into an elasticized band, is placed around the chest or abdomen, breathing can be detected by the changes in inductance.[14] Ideally, both chest and abdominal coils should be used. Originally this was an attempt to measure tidal volume non-invasively. However, two coils may also detect obstructive apnoea by analysing relative movement as well as being a 'failsafe' device.[5] RIP therefore has potential advantages over impedance in the detection of apnoea. Significant differences between apnoea detected by thoracic impedance and abdominal RIP have been shown,[66] which differences may be important when interpreting the results of trials into treatment for apnoea of prematurity.

Although RIP is promising in its ability to detect obstructive apnoea, the main challenge in respiratory monitoring lies in the non-invasive detection of airflow. Nasal thermistors[13] have been used for research but tend to be too precarious in their fixation for long-term use. The initial promise shown by acoustic detectors of airflow[33] has not been fulfilled. Electronic monitoring detects more apnoeic episodes than nursing staff, but the true value of this remains to be established. Some form of apnoea detector should be attached to all spontaneously breathing babies who either have apnoeic attacks or are suffering from a respiratory disease likely to be complicated by apnoea.

Dual monitoring of heart rate and oxygen saturation for apnoea

The best method to detect apnoea in the routine clinical setting may be by using a combination of heart rate, detected by ECG, and oxygen saturation by pulse oximetry. Although such a method is indirect, it allows detection of the two consequences of apnoea which may be harmful: bradycardia of less than 80 beats per minute and hypoxaemia, and as such is widely used in neonatal nurseries.

Respiratory pattern and waveform

The signals derived from the apparatus described above used to detect apnoea, no matter how simple, can be both transformed into a visual display of the respiratory waveform, and integrated to give a respiratory rate. A large number of devices are now commercially available which, in addition to being apnoea alarms, display the infant's respiratory rate and combine this with a visual display of the respiratory waveform and trend recording. These may be individual respiratory monitors or one module of a complex monitor which can display several measurements, including heart rate (and ECG), blood pressure, oxygen saturation and temperature.

From a research standpoint detailed recordings of respiratory waveform are useful in developing techniques of patient triggering for ventilators which involve accurately synchronizing inspiration and expiration (p. 568). At present equipment producing flow– volume loops and online pulmonary function tests remain research tools.[18]

BLOOD GASES

The target ranges for PaO_2, $PaCO_2$ and pH, and the physiological justification for the tight control required, are given in Chapter 29, Part 2. A wide variety of monitoring techniques and devices are available to assist in this meticulous control.

When blood gas analysis for PaO_2, $PaCO_2$, pH and base deficit became available on samples of 0.5 ml or less in the late 1960s, the practice evolved of drawing samples on a routine basis 4-hourly, or more frequently if there were problems.[52] This proved very successful, and seemed to strike an acceptable balance between exsanguinating the baby by removing too much blood and securing sufficiently tight control to prevent clinically inapparent changes in blood gases translating into clinically significant problems. Such a routine is still an acceptable way of managing babies in respiratory failure, but it does remove a lot of blood and, as in any intensive care situation, continuous monitoring has been found to give better information. Newer devices (Hellige Medical: Paratrend, Biomedical Sensors) promise to give the same information without the need to remove any blood from the infant. Experience with these devices is extremely limited at the time of writing. The first works via a sampling cartridge sited at the end of the arterial line into which blood is withdrawn and then replaced, the second via complex indwelling electrodes built into a wire passed through the catheter (see below).

To monitor blood gases adequately it is necessary to have an indwelling arterial line and some device for continuous PaO_2 (and occasionally $PaCO_2$) measurements. An indwelling arterial line enables the neonatologist to take frequent samples without contravening the minimal handling rule (p. 502) and, as outlined above, arterial blood gases should be measured at least 4–6-hourly during the acute phase of any respiratory illness, even in the presence of continuous PaO_2 monitoring. Arterial sampling is also done to calibrate the continuous PaO_2 device and to measure the $PaCO_2$ and acid–base status. If continuous recording devices are being used, have been found to be accurate, and the neonate is otherwise stable, the frequency of direct blood gas sampling can be

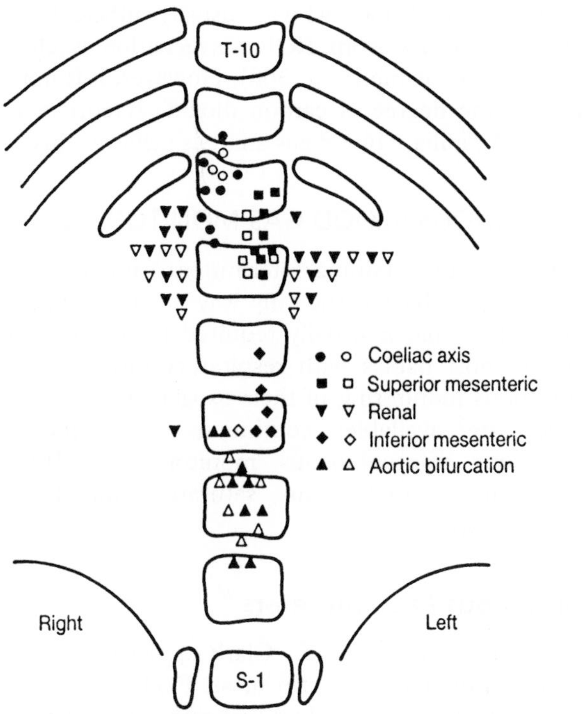

Fig. 21.1 Positions of important branches of the abdominal aorta which should be avoided by umbilical artery catheter tips. (Reproduced with permission from Phelps et al 1972[42])

reduced to 6–8-hourly after 4–5 days of age, or sooner if the infant is in less than 30% oxygen.

Umbilical arterial catheters

Umbilical artery catheterization was first described in 1960. The umbilical arteries are easily cannulated for 4–5 days after birth, either by inserting a catheter directly into the vessel on the cut surface of the cord (Chapter 51), or by using a side cannulation technique. The size of catheter should be 3.5 or 4.0 French gauge for a small preterm baby and 5.0 for a large term infant. In general end-hole catheters are preferred as they may cause less injury to the endothelium of the aorta wall[70] (p. 920). Where to position the catheter tip is a matter of controversy, but all agree that the area of D12–L3/4 should be avoided[42] (Fig. 21.1), as this is where the renal, coeliac and mesenteric vessels arise from the aorta. Positioning the catheter tip above this level still carries the theoretical risk of embolization, but avoids the considerable problems with arterial obstruction to the legs seen when the tip is in the lower aorta.[35] Kempley and Gamsu[26] found no difference in the complication rate in the first week between babies with a high or low UAC. In the second week babies with high catheters had more problems with abdominal distension and tenderness, although none developed NEC.

Once in situ, blood can be taken from the UAC as required for PaO_2 $PaCO_2$ and acid–base estimations, as well as other laboratory investigations; even blood cultures can be taken from them under appropriate circumstances.[47] Only coagulation studies present a problem: because of heparinization of the fluid infused through the catheter, more accurate and interpretable data are obtained from a peripheral venous sample. Blood pressure can be measured continuously via a transducer connected to the catheter. Umbilical artery catheters are widely used for intravenous fluid therapy, including antibiotics and TPN.[74] Other units reserve them for monitoring and sampling alone. The merits and demerits of these approaches remain to be established beyond doubt. One comparative audit of complication rates in a number of neonatal units with different practices in this regard showed no difference in adverse events.[16]

Peripheral arterial cannulae

If an umbilical artery catheter cannot be inserted (and the success rate is over 80% in experienced hands) then a peripheral site should be cannulated to allow for frequent arterial sampling without disturbing the baby. These cannulae can also be used for continuous measurement of blood pressure. They can also be used for withdrawing samples for biochemical and haematological monitoring; they must not be used for infusions, other than the 0.5–1 ml/h of heparinized saline used to keep them patent. The preferred arteries are the radial and posterior tibial, as they have good collateral supplies. The ulnar artery should not be cannulated unless the radial artery is patent (and vice-versa) (p. 925). The brachial and temporal arteries are end-arteries and should not be used (p. 1373). Cannulation of the temporal arteries has been associated with underlying brain damage attributed to reflex arterial spasm in the distribution of the ipsilateral internal carotid artery.[56]

Complications

Horrific complications have been reported from arterial cannulation (Chapter 37). The complication rate with UACs is no greater than that with peripheral arterial lines. Umbilical catheters can be left in situ for at least 2 weeks, whereas peripheral arterial lines rarely last for more than 6–7 days. The complications of either type of cannula can be reduced to a minimum if the following rules are observed:

- Heparinize all intra-arterial infusions with 0.5–1 unit per ml of heparin.
- Remove all arterial lines immediately if they show signs of partial or complete blockage (i.e. if there are any other than transient vascular changes in the area supplied).
- Remove all central lines (venous or arterial) if septicaemia is suspected.

Intermittent arterial puncture

If none of the available arteries can be cannulated but arterial blood is required, there is no alternative other than to use peripheral arterial puncture. Any artery can be used for this, and although in theory end-arteries should be avoided to prevent distal ischaemia secondary to spasm, in practice this is not only extremely rare but can probably always be reversed by vasodilators.[24,73]

Nevertheless, it must be emphasized that samples taken by direct puncture from a peripheral artery, albeit backed up by continuous transcutaneous blood gas or SpO_2 monitoring, is an unacceptable way of monitoring the ill, ventilated very low-birthweight neonate with RDS. There are two main drawbacks to using arterial puncture for controlling PaO_2. First, the number of available sites, and the number of times each can be used, is limited. Secondly, and more important, it contravenes the minimal handling rule in a way that is not only generally bad for the frequently disturbed and punctured baby, but is specifically bad in this situation as the disturbance lowers the baby's PaO_2. This makes the PaO_2 measurement on a sample obtained by direct puncture valueless for either calibrating a transcutaneous PaO_2 monitor or preventing ROP[19] (Fig. 21.3). However, in babies with mild disease who are too mature to be at high risk from ROP, an arterial stab done 3–4 times a day for 24–48 hours, backed up by $TcPO_2$ monitoring or oximetry, can be adequate.

In the extremely low-birthweight neonate who requires ventilation for months, peripheral arterial stabs may be all that is available after the sites for arterial cannulation have been rendered unusable. If one is forced into this situation in the neonate who is still at risk from ROP, great care should be taken to minimize the trauma of arterial puncture by, for instance, using local anaesthetic. Changes in the transcutaneous PO_2 monitors or oximeters should be watched carefully during the puncture attempt, and if there are significant falls the procedure should be abandoned and reattempted 20–30 minutes later under local anaesthetic after the baby has stabilized.

Capillary blood gases

These have no place in the early management of the critically ill low-birthweight baby at risk from ROP. Capillary PO_2 can never be relied on to detect hyperoxaemia,[17,32] and in the first few days after birth capillary acid–base values are also unreliable, tending to read high for PCO_2 and low for pH. However, after 48–72 hours of age capillary samples can be useful for monitoring pH and PCO_2. Traditionally the capillary sample is collected free from bubbles by pricking a warmed heel,[17] though more recently McLain et al[32] did not find the warming to be necessary. Capillary gas analysis is of greatest value in babies with chronic lung disease. In such babies, who are usually sufficiently mature not to be at risk from ROP, oxygenation is effectively monitored by oximetry (p. 368). However, it is important to know the degree of carbon dioxide retention in such cases and capillary blood gas analysis achieves this.

CONTINUOUS BLOOD GAS MONITORING

In addition to obtaining intermittent samples for blood gas analysis, which is the only way to monitor acid–base data and all that is usually required for $PaCO_2$ (but see below), most babies with respiratory disease now have continuous monitoring of their oxygenation. Three techniques are available: continuous PaO_2 monitoring, continuous transcutaneous monitoring ($TcPO_2$) and continuous transcutaneous saturation monitoring by oximetry (SpO_2).

Continuous PaO_2 catheters

These are miniaturized Clark polarographic PaO_2 electrodes built into the tip of an FG4 or FG5 double-lumen side-hole umbilical arterial catheter[19,62] (Fig. 21.2). One lumen contains the wiring for the electrode, and the other is a sampling lumen which can be used in exactly the same way as a normal UAC. The electrode tip is a silver/silver chloride electrode covered with potassium chloride and a gas permeable membrane. It generates a tiny current which is in proportion to the oxygen tension to which the tip is exposed. The readout unit is, in effect, a nano-ammeter. Our preference is to insert a continuously recording FG4 or FG5 PaO_2 catheter in the

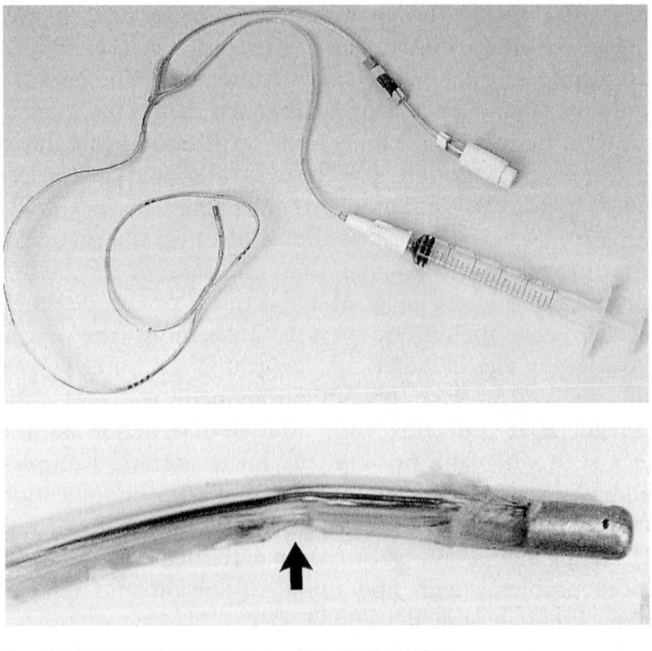

Fig. 21.2 A continuously recording PaO_2 catheter. ↑ – opening to sampling lumen.

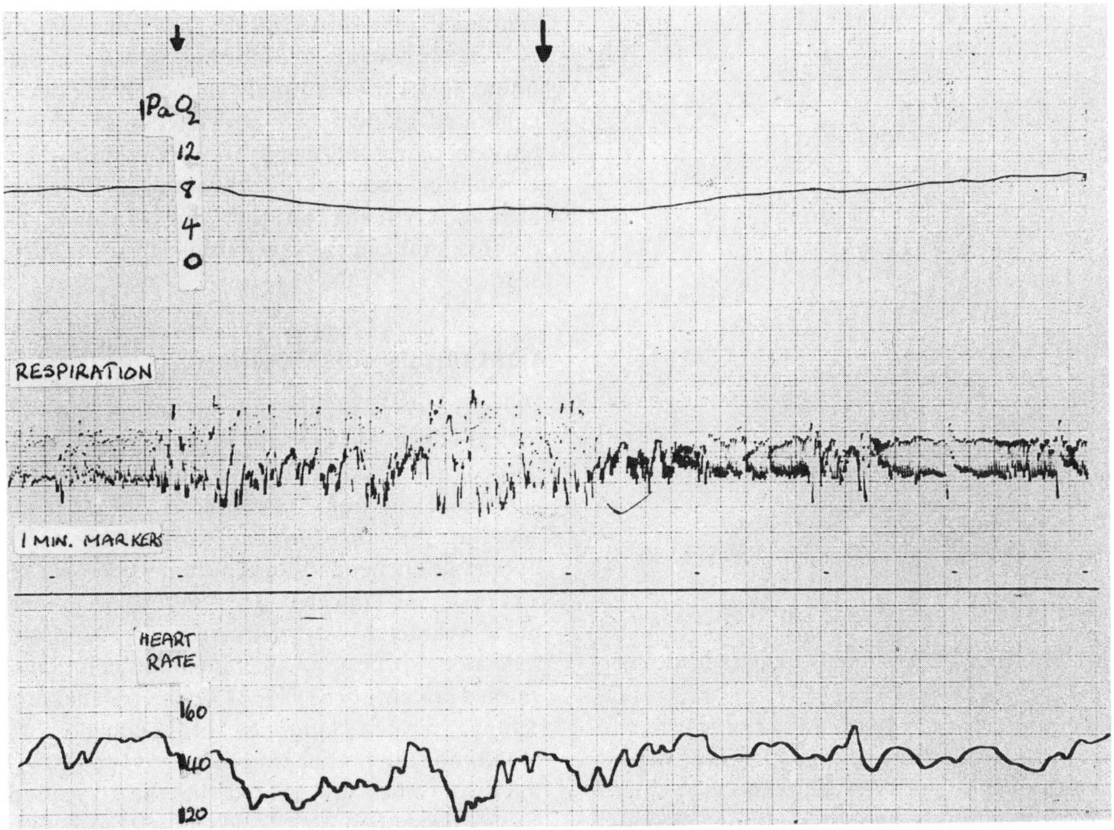

Fig. 21.3 Dip in PaO_2 brought on by crying during an attempt to calibrate an indwelling continuously recording PaO_2 device by obtaining a radial artery sample. (Reproduced with permission from Goddard et al[19])

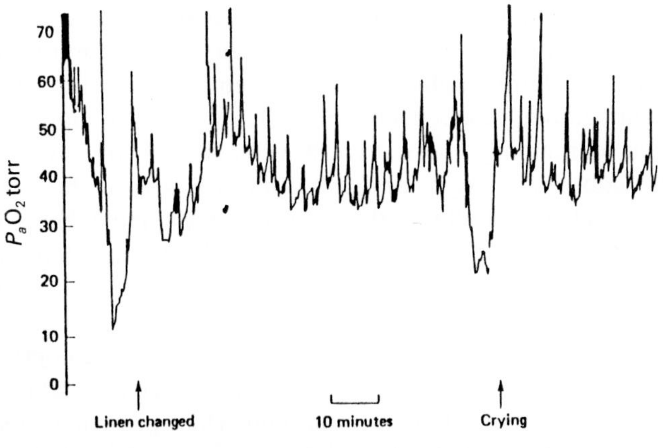

Fig. 21.4 A continuous record of PaO_2 from a large baby with moderate respiratory distress syndrome showing the marked fluctuations in PaO_2, most marked during nursing procedures. (Reproduced with permission from Roberton 1992[51])

first hour of life into all neonates with severe respiratory disease, especially very low-birthweight babies with RDS. These catheters are very reliable, reduce the number of blood gas analyses required by about half (thereby reducing the transfusion requirement), give instantaneous information on the baby's PaO_2, which provides prompt and early warning of deterioration in the baby's oxygenation and indicate when procedures are causing the baby an unacceptable degree of hypoxaemia (Figs 21.3, 21.4). In our hands such umbilical artery catheters continuously infused with a heparin solution containing 0.5–1 unit per ml can be left in situ for 2 weeks or more if necessary, with a very low incidence of complications. However, the accuracy of the PaO_2 transducer deteriorates over a period of days because of blood and protein coating the tip.[19,46] This means that the accuracy of the PaO_2 level must be checked every time an arterial blood sample is drawn.

Continuous transcutaneous monitoring

Transcutaneous monitoring for PO_2 and PCO_2 is possible using appropriately adapted electrodes accurately applied to the skin. The PO_2 electrode is a flat version of the Clark polarographic silver-platinum PO_2 sensitive electrode used in blood gas analysis.[57] Transcutaneous devices work on the principle that the partial pressure of oxygen and carbon dioxide diffusing from the capillaries through skin heated to 44°C is very close to true arterial PO_2 and PCO_2 Great care has to be taken with the in vitro calibration of these devices, and with how they are attached to the skin. To ensure accuracy, and to prevent skin damage from prolonged exposure to the temperature

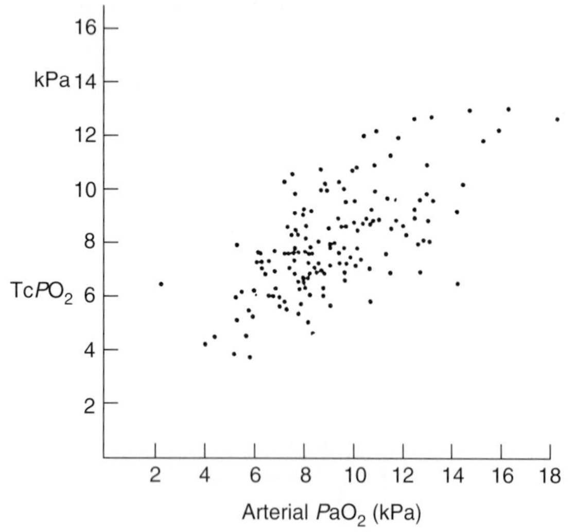

Fig. 21.5 Comparison of $TcPO_2$ readings and simultaneous PaO_2 readings.[11]

of 44°C, the electrode site should be changed every 4 hours (p. 931).

Transcutaneous devices give a very satisfactory instantaneous measure (±15%) of PaO_2 in most babies[2] and, if a continuous record is kept, provide useful information on trends in the baby's condition. Although in the hands of the original investigators these devices appeared to have a very close correlation with PaO_2[40] it must be emphasized that in routine clinical use they are not predictably accurate (Fig. 21.5) particularly at higher PaO_2 values.[72] $TcPO_2$ is inaccurate in ill hypotensive neonates following vasodilator therapy[29,40] and in mature babies with a thick skin.[20] $TcPO_2$ monitors are unpredictable in preterm babies with thin skin and protruding ribs. It is for these reasons that the accuracy of $TcPO_2$ monitors must always be checked by intermittent arterial blood gas analysis; initially this should be done 4 hourly but once the baby is stable this can reduce to 2–3 times per day.[2] In the absence of an indwelling continuously reading PaO_2 catheter continuous $TcPO_2$ monitoring, used in association with 3–4-hourly blood gas analyses on blood drawn from an indwelling arterial line, is an acceptable way of monitoring the critically ill neonate. However, the use of $TcPO_2$ monitors as the sole means of monitoring to prevent ROP is not safe.

$TcPCO_2$ monitors consistently overread by about a third: the true arterial value is 70–75% of the $TcPCO_2$.[49,72] The error is systematic and can be allowed for by deliberately calibrating the monitor to underread against the calibration gas. In addition, the method is subject to considerable drift over time. Because of their inherent inaccuracies $TcPCO_2$ monitors have not found favour in routine neonatal monitoring when 4-hourly analyses are available on blood drawn from arterial lines, although they can give early warning of tube blockage and pneumothorax. They are also useful when adjusting ventilator settings in critically ill ventilated babies.

Transcutaneous monitoring is now being used less often. To be used properly and safely the devices must be calibrated meticulously and fixed with great care. They have to be resited every 4 hours, with a relatively time-consuming recalibration procedure. The site leaves an area of erythema on the skin which is alarming for parents, and can cause a partial-thickness burn which can scar (p. 931).

Continuous pulse oximetry

Pulse oximetry is 'arguably the most significant technological advance ever made in [patient] monitoring',[55] yet 97% of doctors do not know how it works.[63] The correct shorthand for pulse oximetry is SpO_2. A good understanding of the principles involved is particularly important in neonatology, where hyperoxia and hypoxia are of equal concern. The first commercially available pulse oximeter was marketed in 1975, although the reflection spectra of haemoglobin solutions had been studied a century earlier.[37] Oximetry measures the percentage oxygen *saturation* of haemoglobin in arterial blood, not the partial *pressure* of oxygen (PaO_2), although the two values are related via the oxygen dissociation curve (see Appendix 12). Haemoglobin is fully saturated in the arterial blood of healthy individuals of any age. The normal value for SaO_2 is greater than 95%. Owing to the shape of the oxygen saturation curve values of SaO_2 below 90% can indicate critical hypoxia.

The technique of oximetry is dependent on the differential absorption of red (circa 660 nm) and infra-red (circa 940 nm) light by deoxyhaemoglobin and oxyhaemoglobin, respectively (Fig. 21.6). When a source of light containing these two wavelengths is transmitted through tissue, oxyhaemoglobin absorbs less of the light of wavelength 660 nm than does deoxygenated haemoglobin, and vice versa at 940 nm.[36] These wavelengths were chosen to be ideal for adult haemoglobin, but haemoglobin A and haemoglobin F have virtually identical extraction coefficients at these wavelengths. Fetal haemoglobin does, however, have a greater affinity for oxygen than adult haemoglobin when present in red cells, meaning that the calibration curve (see below) ought to be left shifted, which it is not. Sickle haemoglobins do not significantly alter the result. Other tissue structures and chemical compounds, particularly carboxyhaemoglobin and methaemoglobin, can absorb light of these wavelengths,[15,21] meaning that oximetry becomes inaccurate in their presence.

A breakthrough came when it was realised that if the absorption was compared at two different points on the pulse wave arterial blood could be separated from the other components. The probe of a pulse oximeter contains two light-emitting diodes which are placed across a suitable extremity to face a semiconductor photodetector.

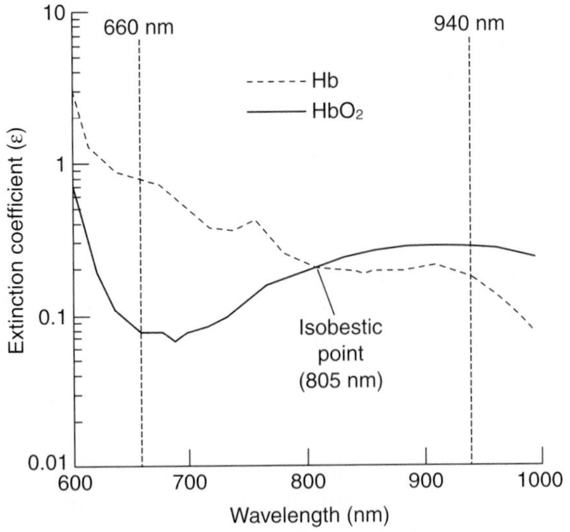

Fig. 21.6 Absorption spectra of oxygenated and deoxygenated haemoglobin, showing the two most commonly used wavelengths in oximetry. The extinction coefficient is a measure of absorption of light energy; the wavelengths are chosen at the point where the two species of haemoglobin have widely differing absorptions. (Reproduced with permission from Moyle et al[37])

This must be protected from extraneous light. A single detector suffices because the emitting diodes are switched rapidly on and off. The electrical signal from the photodetector is very small, and the pulsatile component less than 2% of the total. The cable must be screened from electrical interference and the signal requires amplification. A very small signal due to poor perfusion is one reason for an inaccurate result. The ratio of red/infra-red light is determined about 600 times per second and oxyhaemoglobin values derived from an algorithm within the device. The Nellcor pulse oximeter consistently reads 1.6 ± 2.7% higher than the Ohmeda,[64] largely because Ohmeda have chosen to subtract 2% to allow for dysfunctional haemoglobins. Furthermore, the manufacturers of both devices originally used healthy adult volunteers with normal levels of haemoglobin A (who could not be desaturated below 80% for ethical reasons) to calculate the calibration curves, which are therefore poorly validated at low levels. The result is then averaged over about 3–6 seconds before being displayed on the monitor, preferably in a way which allows confirmation of the pulsatile nature of the original signal. The fact that a reading should only be displayed if a pulsatile component is detected should prevent analysis of inadequate signals. Pulse oximeters have, however, produced pulsatile waveforms on the display even when completely detached from the infant.[44] The gold standard for calibration of a pulse oximeter is co-oximetry, but in routine clinical practice pulse oximetry is used without an in vivo calibration.

All pulse oximeters have an inaccuracy of 2–3% in the range of saturation between 70 and 100%; thus at a readout of 92% the true saturation could be anywhere

Table 21.1 Range of PaO_2 at different SaO_2 values using a continuous umbilical artery SaO_2 catheter (Muller, Gandy & Roberton, unpublished data)

	PaO_2 (kPa)	
SaO_2 (%)	Range	Average
94	5.33–12.67	9.6
95	6.67–15.07	10.13
96	6.93–13.33	10.4
97	6.93–15.73	11.33

between 88% and 96%.[65] Hay et al[23] have shown that at a saturation of 92% the arterial oxygen tension can be anywhere between 5.3 and 13 kPa. In part this is due to different manufacturers using different algorithms for analysing the light signal (see above). The errors get bigger with underperfusion,[7] or during dopamine infusion.[15] Anaemia and polycythaemia can also affect the result. The results are not affected by racial pigmentation of the skin or staining from bilirubin, but extraneous light can affect the reading. Bright room light has a red/infrared ratio of 1, which corresponds to an SpO_2 reading of 85%. When all these potential inaccuracies are translated into PaO_2 values the potential error is huge. Table 21.1 gives the very wide range of PaO_2 values obtained from a continuously recording SaO_2 umbilical artery catheter, a device which is inherently more accurate than a pulse oximeter.

Figure 21.7 shows the range of oximeter (SpO_2) readings recorded above and below the true SaO_2 recorded in one study.[7] This relative inaccuracy in the 90% range has major implications for neonatal intensive care, since it

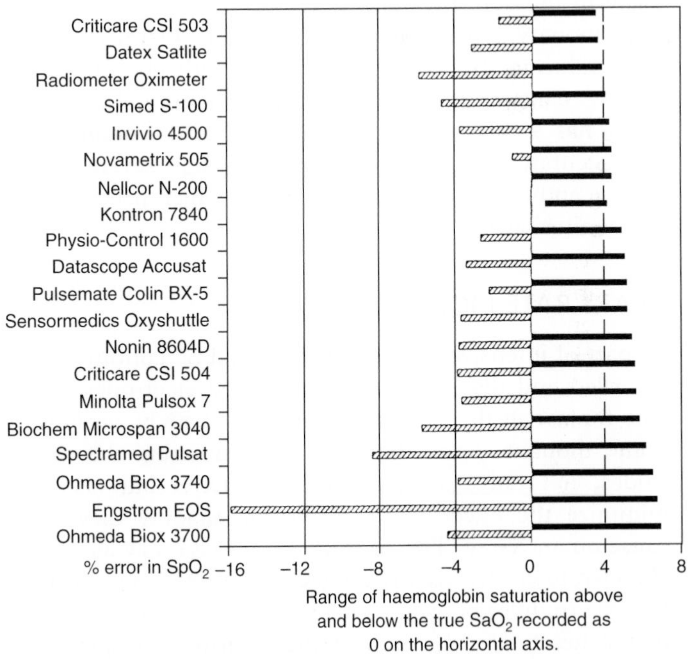

Fig. 21.7 Comparison of different oximeters. (Reproduced with permission from Clayton et al[7])

means that to avoid dangerous hyperoxaemia with the risk of ROP the target SpO_2 should be 90–91%, with the alarm set to go off at 95–96%.[15,45] The practical problem is that if the alarm is set at 95–96% babies who are normally oxygenated, with PaO_2 levels in the range 8–10 kPa, often have these saturation levels. This leads to a high number of nuisance alarms, with the possibly disastrous consequence that the alarm is switched off by nursing staff. Although a 95% upper alarm limit (using a Nellcor oximeter) detected 95% of instances of hyperoxaemia in one study of older children,[45] pulse oximetry must never be relied upon to prevent hyperoxaemia in at-risk babies,[9,36] as PaO_2 values may be unacceptably high at a saturation of 95%.

SpO_2 monitoring certainly has a place on the neonatal unit, but should not replace other means of measuring arterial oxygenation, for the reasons just discussed. Nor should oximetry be the sole means of estimating the heart rate, in view of the possibility of a pulsatile artefact from the diodes.[44] Babies in respiratory failure breathing high oxygen concentrations can be fully saturated but be about to collapse from dangerous hypercarbia. The devices are justifiably popular because they are the same price as $TcPO_2$ electrodes and are much easier to use. They do not require calibration, rarely injure the skin (p. 931), are not subject to drift and give virtually instantaneous results when properly attached. This latter feature is of benefit during resuscitation immediately after birth, during transport, and during the initial period of stabilization after admission to the neonatal unit. Oximetry can be very helpful in confirming or refuting hypoxia in infants suspected of having cyanotic congenital heart disease. The non-invasive sensors mean that two can be applied easily to measure pre- and postductal oxygen saturation in pulmonary hypertension (pp. 528–529). Oximetry is of great value in the long-term survivor with chronic lung disease (Chapter 29, Part 3) who is too mature to develop ROP, has a thick skin which makes $TcPO_2$ monitoring less accurate,[20] but who nevertheless has severe lung disease and a high oxygen requirement which needs careful monitoring.[48]

HEART RATE MONITORING

As part of intensive care an ECG should be continuously recorded and displayed. Small pregelled electrodes suitable for use in the preterm neonate are widely available. Some thought should be given to positioning the electrodes, not only to obtain a useful ECG but also to minimize the effect of the inevitable shadow they will cause on an X-ray. The pattern of the ECG may alert the clinician to electrolyte disturbances (p. 1024), myocardial hypoxia (p. 696) or even a pneumothorax.[34] The regularity of the heart rate is a sign of the severity of respiratory disease. A fixed slow heart rate is a sign of central nervous system depression. Tachycardia can be an early warning sign of haemorrhage or inadequate analgesia. Bradycardia can be an early sign of a blocked endotracheal tube or raised intracranial pressure.

BLOOD PRESSURE MONITORING

This is now an essential part of the care of ill neonates of all birthweights and gestations. Older methods, such as the flush method, have been superseded by invasive or oscillometric monitoring. For normal levels of blood pressure in newborn infants, see Appendix 4.

Oscillometry

Oscillometry detects movement (oscillations) within the limb caused by the inflow of blood. A small plastic sphygmomanometer-type cuff is inflated and automatically deflated at regular intervals. When the air pressure within the cuff is above systolic pressure no movement is detected; when the cuff pressure is reduced blood enters the limb, increasing the limb volume and compressing the cuff, thereby oscillating the pressure within it. When the oscillations are at a maximum the pressure corresponds to the mean arterial blood pressure, and most manufacturers make use of this by displaying the mean value in addition to the systolic and diastolic pressures. They are clearly motion sensitive, and to produce the most accurate result the cuff needs to be deflated at 3 mmHg per heartbeat, which is rather slow. These devices can only be relied upon if a suitably sized cuff is carefully applied, the baby weighs more than 1 kg and the blood pressure is reasonable. In the shocked low-birthweight baby these devices overestimate systolic blood pressures in the 35–45 mmHg range[12] by as much as 5–10 mmHg. A variation of oscillometry, using a pulse oximeter to detect the arrival of arterial blood in the peripheral limb, has been described and looks promising.[27]

Invasive blood pressure monitoring

Direct recording from an indwelling arterial cannula is the preferred method of monitoring blood pressure in sick very low-birthweight neonates. It is important to avoid common mistakes in using pressure transducers, in particular ensuring that the apparatus is at the same level as the baby's heart, and that there are no bubbles in the connecting lines. Any pressure-measuring system which is linked to a transducer via a fluid-filled pathway is susceptible to damping or resonance of the original signal. Suitable transducers must be able to respond rapidly in order to reproduce the rapidly changing pressures throughout the cardiac cycle: in technical terms they require a flat frequency response to at least 20 Hz. Having a visual display of the blood pressure waveform, which should show a good pulse pressure and a dichrotic notch, is a check on the presence of damping, as well as on the state of the cardiac output in the patient. Indwelling pressure transducers should be opened to the air (and closed to the baby) via a three-way tap so that the zero setting can be corrected once a day, and subjected to a two-point calibration using a conventional mercury sphygmomanometer when they are originally set up.

CENTRAL VENOUS PRESSURE MONITORING

Although widely used in infants and older children, CVP monitoring has not caught on in neonatology, yet it is clear that ventilated neonates with low CVP do badly.[58] If CVP monitoring is done in the neonate it is very difficult to pass a central line of sufficient diameter to give an undamped trace from a peripheral site. Umbilical venous catheterization has been used, passing the catheter through the ductus venosus into the right atrium. This may in part explain the paucity of data, as it is often impossible to get the catheter to pass through the ductus venosus, and leaving it in situ may result in serious venous thrombosis in the liver or air embolism (p. 924). However, the pressure in the IVC will also give clinically useful information.[31] To monitor CVP the transducer should be attached to the end of the UVC, and the techniques used are identical to those of blood pressure monitoring.

TEMPERATURE MONITORING

Temperature can be monitored either by 4-hourly use of a traditional mercury-in-glass rectal thermometer, or by the use of a rectal or skin thermistor left in place to minimize handling. The use of mercury in thermometers and sphygmomanometers is no longer permitted by many hospitals because of the risk of breakage and mercury contamination of the surrounding area. Measuring the central/peripheral temperature difference can provide useful information about the state of the circulation, particularly circulating blood volume.[3] Continuous skin or core temperature monitoring will need to be used if the incubator or radiant heat cradle is used in servo mode. The advantages, disadvantages and dangers of this type of control of the thermal environment compared to air control mode are outlined in Chapter 18.

CLINICAL AND LABORATORY MONITORING

FLUID BALANCE

A fluid balance chart is an integral part of the monitoring of all ill babies, although it is difficult to record accurately all the fluid infused, including that given as drugs or for flushing catheters after sampling.[38] Boluses of plasma, blood and bicarbonate must always be included. Urine output should be checked regularly. Critically ill neonates should have an absolute measure of urine output daily, together with urinalysis for protein, blood and electrolyte concentration (Chapter 39, Part 1). Because catheterization carries the risk of infection, and adhesive urine bags frequently damage the thin frail skin of preterm newborns, the most effective way of measuring urine output is to weigh disposable nappies (or cottonwool balls placed within them). These must be weighed as soon as possible to avoid evaporative loss.[8,25]

Weighing is the single most important investigation in assessing fluid balance in the critically ill neonate, and should be done at least once a day. In very preterm babies who have an enormous transepidermal water loss 12-hourly weighing is indicated.

It is possible to weigh the intubated ventilated neonate with an indwelling arterial catheter by transiently disconnecting the infusion and quickly putting him, still ventilated, on electronic scales by the incubator. Alternatively there are within-incubator scales on which the infant can be nursed.

BACTERIOLOGICAL MONITORING

As part of the work-up to exclude infection all neonates with respiratory distress will have a full set of swabs and a blood culture taken (pp. 502, 507). Thereafter, routine bacteriological assessment is not required except in the intubated neonate, in whom routine culture of endotracheal tube aspirates two or three times per week can be useful. Such surveillance enables identification of colonization of the respiratory tract with serious pathogens, and can help to target therapy should such infants develop a deteriorating chest X-ray or other symptoms suggestive of pneumonia.

Some studies[22,28] have reported a close correlation between organisms isolated from the trachea and those grown from blood cultures, but others have not.[59,69] Endotracheal cultures must be interpreted in the light of other clinical features of infection and the results of laboratory tests, such as the differential white count, CRP and blood culture. Organisms such as *Pseudomonas* and *Klebsiella* spp. grown from the aspirate can be regarded as commensals/contaminants provided the infant's condition is improving and there are no clinical signs of pneumonia. Deterioration in lung function and/or the chest radiograph appearance, accompanied by a rise in the CRP and WBC, suggests that the previous 'commensals' may have become pathogenic. Until more accurate data become available, for example from a positive blood culture, the endotracheal cultures should be used to guide the initial choice of antibiotics.

BIOCHEMICAL MONITORING

All ill neonates should have their plasma electrolytes, glucose, calcium and albumin measured at least daily. It is impossible to predict hypo- or hypernatraemia, hyperkalaemia, hypocalcaemia or hypoalbuminaemia in such babies, despite meticulous attention to the content and volume of the intravenous fluid therapy. The importance of glucose control is discussed in Chapter 38, Part 1.

In very ill neonates less than 0.80 kg in whom the management of fluid balance is fraught with difficulty (Chapter 39, Part 1), twice- or thrice-daily electrolyte measurement is necessary to complement the assessment of fluid balance by regularly weighing the baby and by clinical examination. If total parenteral nutrition is being used the appropriate biochemical monitoring must be instituted (p. 353). The severity of jaundice, if present, must always be assessed biochemically, several times per day if necessary, in view of the complex and potentially damaging synergy between severe illness and hyperbilirubinaemia in the aetiology of kernicterus (p. 722).

HAEMATOLOGICAL MONITORING

Ill babies, in particular those less than 1.50 kg, tolerate anaemia badly[1,50] and are also subject to large blood losses from monitoring. Such infants should have a daily haemoglobin and packed cell volume estimation, with more frequent tests if there are clinical indications such as pallor, a fall in blood pressure or known blood loss from haemorrhage. Examination of the blood film can be important: nucleated red cell counts can provide a clue to the duration of intrauterine hypoxia,[41] and in convalescent infants reticulocyte counts aid in decision making about blood transfusion.

The white cell count should always be checked as part of the initial evaluation when a neonate is admitted to the NICU. Thereafter daily white cell counts, with differential counts, in acutely ill infants can help in the detection of early sepsis, and in the evaluation of antibiotic therapy in established sepsis. Further white cell counts should be done at times of acute clinical deterioration.

Almost all preterm babies have abnormalities of the coagulation system, although not necessarily their platelet count unless sepsis is present, when thrombocytopenia may be a useful marker. The management of coagulation disturbances is outlined in Chapter 32, Part 1. When taking blood for coagulation study it is important to avoid contamination with the heparin used to keep peripheral arterial and umbilical arterial catheters patent. If possible, a peripheral venous sample should always be obtained.

MONITORING VENOUS AND ARTERIAL INFUSION PRESSURES

Modern infusion pumps are fitted with devices which continuously monitor the pressure required to deliver the infusion, and these can be set to alarm. Accuracy of delivery at small volumes is now taken for granted, but there is little information on which to base a decision regarding setting pressure alarm limits for infusions in neonatal intensive care units. The UK Department of Health standard of 300 mmHg is well above the operating pressure of most neonatal infusions.[10,43] Peripheral venous infusions operate at pressures up to 61 mmHg, so that one solution is to individualize the setting of the upper alarm limit to operating pressure plus 40 mmHg. An alternative approach is to choose 40 mmHg for general purposes. This provides an acceptable compromise between the number of nuisance alarms from self-clearing occlusions and detecting genuine blockages quickly. A suitable setting for umbilical arterial catheters is 100 mmHg.

X-RAY MONITORING

All babies with respiratory disease will have a chest X-ray as part of their assessment immediately after admission to the NICU, as unless this is done problems such as a pneumothorax, pleural effusion or diaphragmatic hernia, which need more than just oxygen, artificial ventilation and antibiotics, will not be recognized.

Thereafter chest X-rays should be done as indicated clinically. However, in the critically ill ventilated newborn, clinical signs and routine monitoring frequently fail to detect the development of pneumonia, small pneumothoraces and, in particular, PIE (pp. 511, 521), and misplaced endotracheal tubes, which predicate immediate alterations in therapy. For this reason we routinely perform CXRs daily in seriously ill ventilated babies, and of course if there is any deterioration, sudden or otherwise, which is not readily explained by clinical findings.

Another benefit of regular CXRs is that they form an excellent record of progress. Clearing of the CXR indicates that the lung disease is improving; conversely, if the early changes of CLD develop, appropriate changes in treatment can be made, including the early introduction of steroids (pp. 617–618).

Although there is justifiable anxiety about the irradiation dose received, the doses are small.[71] Fifty neonatal CXRs provide no more radiation than living for a year surrounded by the uranium-rich granite of Aberdeen.[54]

REFERENCES

1. Alverson D C 1995 The physiologic impact of anemia in the neonate. Clinics in Perinatology 22: 609–625
2. American Academy of Pediatrics 1989 Task force on transcutaneous oxygen monitors. Pediatrics 83: 122–126
3. Aynsley-Green A G, Pickering D 1974 Use of central and peripheral temperature measurements in care of the critically ill child. Archives of Disease in Childhood 49: 477–481
4. Blake A M, Collins, L M, Langham J, Reynolds EOR 1970. Clinical assessment of apnoea-alarm mattress for newborn infants. Lancet ii: 183–185
5. Brouillette R T, Morrow A S, Weese-Mayer, D E, Hunt C E 1987 Comparison of respiratory inductive plethysmography and thoracic impedance for apnea monitoring. Journal of Pediatrics 111: 377–383
6. Cartlidge P H T, Rutter N 1988 Reduction of head flattening in preterm infants. Archives of Disease in Childhood 63: 755–757

7. Clayton D G, Webb R K, Ralston A C, Duthie D, Runciman W B 1991 A comparison of the performance of 20 pulse oximeters under conditions of poor perfusion. Anaesthesia 46: 3–10
8. Cooke R J, Werkman S, Watson D 1989 Urine output measurements in premature infants. Pediatrics 83: 116–118
9. Dear P R F 1987 Monitoring oxygen in the newborn. Archives of Disease in Childhood 62: 879–891
10. Department of Health 1990 Evaluation of infusion pumps and controllers. Health Equipment Information No 198, Ninth report
11. Department of Health and Social Security 1981 Evaluation of transcutaneous oxygen monitors. Health Equipment Information No. 91. DHSS, London
12. Diprose G K, Evans D H, Archer L N J, Levene M I 1986 Dinamap fails to detect hypotension in very low birth weight infants. Archives of Disease in Childhood 61: 771–773
13. Dransfield D A, Fox W W 1980 A non-invasive method for recording central and obstructive apnea with bradycardia in infants. Critical Care Medicine 6: 663–666
14. Dufty P, Spriet L, Bryan M H, Bryan A C 1981 Respiratory induction plethysmography (Respitrace): an evaluation of its use in the infant. American Review of Respiratory Disease 123: 542–546
15. Dziedzic K, Vidyasagar D 1989 Pulse oximetry in neonatal intensive care. Clinics in Perinatology 16: 177–197
16. Fletcher M A, Brown D R, Landers S, Seguin J 1994 Umbilical arterial catheter use: report of an audit conducted by the study group for complications of perinatal care. American Journal of Perinatology 11: 94–99
17. Gandy G M, Grann L, Cunningham N 1964 The validity of pH and PCO_2 measurements in sick and healthy newborn infants. Pediatrics 34: 192–197
18. Gerhardt T O, Bancalari E 1991 Measurement and monitoring of pulmonary function. Clinics in Perinatology 18: 581–609
19. Goddard P, Keith I, Marcovitch H, Roberton N R C, Rolfe P, Scopes J W 1974 The use of a continuously recording intravascular oxygen electrode in the newborn. Archives of Disease in Childhood 49: 853–860
20. Hamilton P A, Whitehead M D, Reynolds E O R 1985 Under estimation of arterial oxygen tension by transcutaneous electrodes with increasing age of infants. Archives of Disease in Childhood 60: 1162–1165
21. Hanning C D, Alexander-Williams J M 1995 Pulse oximetry: a practical review. British Medical Journal 311: 367–370
22. Harris H, Wirtschafter D, Cassady G 1976. Endotracheal intubation and its relationship to bacterial colonisation and systemic infection in newborn infants. Pediatrics 58, 816–825
23. Hay W W, Brockway J M, Eyzaguirre M 1989 Neonatal pulse oximetry: accuracy and reliability. Pediatrics 83: 717–722
24. Heath R E 1986 Vasospasm in the neonate. Response to tolazoline infusion. Pediatrics 77: 405–408
25. Hermansen M C, Buches M 1988 Urine output determination from superabsorbent and regular diapers under radiant heat. Pediatrics 81: 428–431
26. Kempley S T, Gamsu H R 1992 Randomised trial of umbilical arterial catheter position: Doppler ultrasound findings. Archives of Disease in Childhood 67: 855–859
27. Langbaum M, Eyal F G 1994 A practical and reliable method of measuring blood pressure in the neonate by pulse oximetry. Journal of Pediatrics 125: 591–595
28. Lau Y L, Hey E N 1991 Sensitivity and specificity of daily tracheal aspirate cultures in providing organisms causing bacteremia in ventilated neonates. Pediatric Infectious Disease Journal 10: 290–294
29. Le Souef P N, Morgan A K, Soutter L P, Reynolds E O R, Parker D 1978 Comparison of transcutaneous oxygen tension with arterial oxygen tension in newborn infants with severe respiratory disease. Pediatrics 62: 692–697
30. Lewin J E 1969 An apnoea alarm mattress. Lancet ii: 667–668
31. Lloyd T R, Donnerstein R L Berg R A 1992 Accuracy of central venous pressure measurement from the abdominal inferior vena cava. Pediatrics 89: 506–508
32. McLain B I, Evans J, Dear P R F 1988 Comparison of capillary and arterial blood gas measurements in neonates. Archives of Disease in Childhood 63: 743–747
33. McLellan N J, Barnett T G 1983 Cardiorespiratory monitoring in infancy with an acoustic detector. Lancet ii: 1397–1398
34. Merenstein G B, Dougherty K, Lewis A 1972 Early detection of pneumothorax by oscilloscope monitor in the newborn infant. Journal of Pediatrics 80: 98–101
35. Mokrohisky S T, Levine R L, Blumhagen, J D, Wesenberg R C, Simmons M A 1978 Low positioning of umbilical artery catheters increases associated complications in newborn infants. New England Journal of Medicine 299: 561–564
36. Moyle J T B 1996 Uses and abuses of pulse oximetry. Archives of Disease in Childhood 74: 77–80
37. Moyle J T B, Hahn C E W, Adams A P 1994 Principles and practice series; pulse oximetry. BMJ Publishing, London
38. Noble-Jamieson C M, Kuzmin P, Airede K I 1986 Hidden sources of fluid and sodium intake in ill newborn infants. Archives of Disease in Childhood 61: 695–696
39. Pallett J E, Scopes J W 1965 Recording respirations in newborn babies by measuring impedance of the chest. Medical Electronics and Biological Engineering 31: 161–168
40. Peabody J L, Gregory G A, Willis M M, Tooley W M 1978 Transcutaneous oxygen tension in sick infants. American Review of Respiratory Disease 118: 83–87
41. Phelan J P, Ahn M O, Korst L M, Martin G L 1995 Nucleated red blood cells; a marker for fetal asphyxia. American Journal of Obstetrics and Gynecology 173: 1380–1384
42. Phelps D L, Lachman R S, Leake R D, Oh, W 1972. The radiologic localisation of the major aortic tributaries in the newborn infant. Journal of Pediatrics 81: 336–339
43. Pickstone M, Aulty B, Jacklin A, Langfield B, Wooton R 1994 Intravenous infusion of drugs – measuring and minimising the risk. British Journal of Intensive Care 4: 338–344
44. Poets C F, Wilken M, Seidenberg J, von der Hardt H 1993a Failure of pulse oximeter to detect sensor detachment. Lancet 341: 244
45. Poets C F, Wilken M, Seidenberg J, Southall D P, von der Hardt H 1993b Reliability of a pulse oximeter in the detection of hyperoxemia. Journal of Pediatrics 122: 87–90
46. Pollitzer M J, Soutter L P, Reynolds E O R 1980 Continuous monitoring of arterial oxygen tension in infants: four year experience with an intravascular oxygen electrode. Pediatrics 66: 31–36
47. Pourcyrous M, Korones S B, Bada H S, Patterson T, Baselski V 1988 Indwelling umbilical arterial catheter: a preferred sampling site for blood culture. Pediatrics 81: 821–825
48. Ramanathan R, Durand M, Larrazabal C 1987 Pulse oximetry in very low birthweight infants with acute and chronic lung disese. Pediatrics 79: 612–617
49. Rennie J M 1990 Transcutaneous carbon dioxide monitoring. Archives of Disease in Childhood 65: 345–346
50. Roberton N R C 1987 Top up transfusions in childhood. Archives of Disease in Childhood 62: 984–986
51. Roberton N R C 1993 A manual of neonatal intensive care. Edward Arnold, London p 111
52. Roberton N R C, Gupta J M, Dahlenburg G W, Tizard J P M 1968 Oxygen therapy in the newborn. Lancet i: 1323–1329
53. Rolfe P 1975. Monitoring in newborn intensive care. Medical and Biological Engineering and Computing 10/11: 399–401
54. Russell J G B 1988 Diagnostic radiography in children. Archives of Disease in Childhood 63: 1005–1006
55. Severinghaus J W, Astrup P B 1986 History of blood gas analysis VI: Oximetry. Journal of Clinical Monitoring 2: 270–288
56. Simmons M A, Levine R L, Lubchenko L O, Guggenheim M A 1978 Warning: serious sequelae of temporal artery catheterization? Journal of Pediatrics 92: 284
57. Simpson R M, Bryan H 1972 Transcutaneous oximetry. British Journal of Hospital Medicine 28: 269–272
58. Skinner J R, Milligan D W A, Hunter S, Hey E N 1992 Central venous pressure in the ventilated neonate. Archives of Disease in Childhood 67: 374–377
59. Slagle T A, Bifano E M, Wolf J W, Gross S J 1989 Routine endotracheal cultures for the prediction of sepsis in ventilated babies. Archives of Disease in Childhood 64: 34–38
60. Smith J E, Scopes J W 1972 A new apnoea alarm for babies. Lancet ii: 545–546
61. Southall D P, Richards J M, Lau, K C, Shinebourne E A 1980 An explanation for failure of impedance apnoea alarm systems. Archives of Disease in Childhood 55: 63–65
62. Soutter L P, Conway M J, Parker D 1975 A system for monitoring

arterial oxygen tension in sick newborn babies. Biomedical Engineering 10: 257–260
63. Stoneham M D, Saville G M, Wilson I H 1994 Knowledge about pulse oximetry among nursing and medical staff. Lancet 344: 1339–1342
64. Thilo E H, Andersen D, Wasserstein M L, Schmidt J, Luckey D 1993 Saturation by pulse oximetry: comparison of the results obtained by instruments of different brands. Journal of Pediatrics 122: 620–626
65. Tremper K K, Barker S J 1989. Pulse oximetry. Anaesthesiology 70: 98–108
66. Upton C J, Milner A D, Stokes G M 1990 Combined impedance and inductance for the detection of apnoea of prematurity. Early Human Development 24: 55–63
67. Valman H S, Wright B M, Lawrence C 1983 Measurement of respiratory rate in the newborn. British Medical Journal 286: 1783–1784
68. Warburton D, Stark A R, Taeusch H W 1977 Apnea monitor failure in infants with upper airway obstruction. Pediatrics 60: 742–744
69. Webber S, Wilkinson A R, Lindsell D et al 1990 Neonatal pneumonia. Archives of Disease in Childhood 68: 207–211
70. Wesstrom G, Finnström O, Stenport G 1979 Umbilical artery catheterisation in the newborn I. Thrombosis in relation to catheter type and position. Acta Paediatrica Scandinavica 68: 575–581
71. Wilson Costello D, Rad P S, Morrison S, Hack M 1996 Radiation exposure from diagnostic radiographs in extremely low birthweight infants. Pediatrics 97: 369–374
72. Wimberley P D, Frederiksen P S, Witt-Hanson J, Helberg S G, Friis-Hansen, B 1985 Evaluation of a transcutaneous oxygen and carbon dioxide monitor in a neonatal intensive care department. Acta Paediatrica Scandinavica 74: 352–359
73. Wong A F, McCulloch L M, Sola A 1992 Treatment of peripheral tissue ischemia with topical nitroglycerine ointment in neonates. Journal of Pediatrics 121: 980–983
74. Yu V Y H, James B, Hendry P, MacMahon R A 1979 Total parenteral nutrition in very low birth weight infants: a controlled trial. Archives of Disease in Childhood 54: 653–661

22

Care of the normal term newborn baby

N. R. C. Roberton

Much of what is in this chapter is dealt with in other parts of this book and covered in detail elsewhere.[75] However, by gathering all the information together in this chapter I hope to take the reader through the medical care of that much neglected neonate (except by his mother!), the one who is normal, healthy and full term. This baby nevertheless requires many routine procedures and, most important of all, he needs to be examined carefully and feeding has to be established. He is heir to multiple minor problems which can often cause considerable parental anxiety, though they are rarely of clinical importance.

ANTICIPATORY CARE

Many babies are normal at birth yet have a mother with a medical complication of pregnancy, such as pre-eclampsia, or a chronic illness such as asthma or diabetes (Table 22.1). The illness itself may have an effect on the newborn, as may the drugs required for treatment. However, with the exception of the important examples marked by an asterisk in Table 22.1, most maternal illnesses have no serious effects on the baby, who will be normal at birth, will stay normal thereafter, and should be cared for on a postnatal ward with his mother. Nevertheless, for all these illnesses it is essential to know of their existence so that appropriate action can be taken in time to prevent unnecessary sequelae, such as severe jaundice in babies with a family history of spherocytosis. Furthermore, it is only if the neonatologist is forewarned about these illnesses that he can deal adequately with questions that are likely to arise during the routine clinical examination (see below).

The effects of drugs passing to the fetus transplacentally and to the neonate in breast milk are discussed fully in Chapter 26.

CARE IN THE LABOUR WARD

RESUSCITATION (Chapter 16)

CORD CLAMPING[70]

Once a term baby is delivered there is no point delaying cord clamping: giving a large placental transfusion exposes the baby to the risks of polycythaemia (p. 835).

It is essential that there is a foolproof routine for clamping or ligating the umbilical cord in the labour ward, otherwise a fatal neonatal haemorrhage can ensue. Either two ligatures or one of the commercial cord clamps should be used.

CORD CARE

Correct umbilical care during the first week significantly reduces the incidence of infection, not only in the neonate but also in the mother.[19,29] The necrotic Wharton's jelly is readily colonized by organisms from the environment, which may spread to cause skin, conjunctival or systemic infection in the baby, or breast infection in the mother. Various techniques have been used to prevent this, of which the most popular is the use of a hexachlorophene-containing powder such as Sterzac. Spraying the umbilical cord with an antibiotic powder such as Polybactrin or Tribiotic gives better protection, a lower incidence of subsequent topical and superficial staphylococcal infections, and is completely safe.[7,27]

Spraying the umbilical cord with antibiotics is of particular importance in an infant in whom it is likely that umbilical vessel catheterization will be needed, as this lessens the likelihood of having to pass the catheter through a contaminated field. After applying antibiotic powder in the labour ward the cord should be cleaned daily with isopropyl alcohol.[27]

Table 22.1 Maternal illness: effect on normal neonatal care

Maternal illness	Effect on baby	Neonatal management
Cardiovascular disease		
Ischaemic heart disease	–	–
Rheumatic heart disease	–	–
Congenital heart disease		
acyanotic	–	Increased risk of congenital heart disease (p. 137)
cyanotic	IUGR	None for baby, but risk of maternal death if Eisenmenger
Hypertension	IUGR, may need to be delivered preterm	Neonatal hypotension from drug therapy
Respiratory disease		
Asthma	If severe IUGR	Increased incidence of asthma in child. No neonatal intervention of proven benefit to prevent this progression
Chronic bronchitis/smoker	IUGR	None, but increased respiratory morbidity and sudden infant death syndrome in infancy
Cystic fibrosis	–	None; breast-feeding safe. No hazard from maternal lung pathogens
Endocrine/metabolic disease		
Diabetes*	Infant of a diabetic mother (Ch. 24)	Usually no major problems but must be watched carefully (Ch. 24)
Thyrotoxicosis*	Neonatal thyrotoxicosis (p. 964)	Needs careful neonatal evaluation (pp. 964–965)
Hyperparathyroidism	Neonatal hypocalcaemia (p. 966)	Monitor neonatal calcium in first 7 days
Other endocrine disease, e.g. Addison's, hypothyroidism	–	–
Phenylketonuria*	Decreased development quotient and occipitofrontal circumference. Congenital heart disease	Nothing can be done in the neonatal period
Gastrointestinal disease		
Coeliac disease	–	–
Crohn's disease	If severe, prematurity or IUGR	–
Ulcerative colitis	If severe, prematurity or IUGR	–
Peptic ulceration	–	–
Stomas, colostomy etc.	–	–
Renal disease		
Chronic renal disease (nephrotic, renal failure etc.)	May be intrauterine growth retardation	Some forms of renal disease are hereditary, e.g. polycystic disease, Alport's syndrome, therefore check
Urinary infection	IUGR	–
Neurological disease		
Epilepsy	Teratogenic drug effects rare with common anticonvulsants (p. 192)	Sedation from maternal drugs if breast-fed (rare) Occasional haemorrhagic disease (pp. 799–800). Occasional withdrawal symptoms (p. 448)
Dystrophia myotonica*	Infant affected (usually more severely)	May be seriously ill in respiratory failure (p. 638)
Myasthenia*	Neonatal myasthenia (p. 1291)	Usually no problem but needs watching
Degenerative disease	–	–
multiple sclerosis	–	–
motor neuron disease	–	–
Infection in the mother		
Pyrexia of unknown origin	–	Watch baby for infection
Recognizable acute infection,	Usually nil (p. 1115)	See p. 1115, Table 43.6
Chronic maternal infection, carrier state*	Can be serious, e.g. human immunodeficiency virus, tuberculosis	See Chapter 13
Allergic disorders		
Hayfever, eczema etc.	–	Avoid early allergen exposure (e.g. cow's milk), particularly if mother herself has severe atopic disease

*Maternal illnesses that may have serious affects on the baby.

Table 22.1 Cont'd

Maternal illness	Effect on baby	Neonatal management
Haematological disorders		
Anaemia (iron, folate deficiency)	–	–
Autoimmune haemolytic anaemia	IgG transmitted to fetus	Neonatal haemolysis: watch for jaundice
Haemoglobinopathies	Most are β-chain defects (pp. 826–829), therefore few neonatal problems	–
Spherocytosis	50% of infants affected	Neonatal haemolysis and jaundice
Idiopathic thrombocytopenic purpura	Fetal haemorrhage can occur but is rare	Neonatal haemorrhage also rare but watch for bleeding and check platelets
Glucose-6-phosphate dehydrogenase deficiency	–	May get neonatal jaundice (p. 824) or have increased risk of infection (p. 1103)
Autoimmune disease		
Systemic lupus*	Congenital heart block	No treatment if heart rate normal: if heart block see page 709
Psychiatric disorders		
Drug dependency	IUGR	Watch for drug effects if neonate breast-fed and mother on treatment. Drug withdrawal (Ch. 28)
Malignant disease		
Current effect on baby	May need preterm delivery	
Previous – Rx chemotherapy Radiotherapy	Once pregnant no neonatal effects except IUGR after Wilms'	
Miscellaneous		
Abdominal trauma	Surprisingly few[20]	–
Malnutrition	IUGR (p. 139)	

EYE DISEASE PREVENTION

In many countries it is routine to instil one drop of 0.5–1.0% silver nitrate into each eye immediately after delivery to prevent gonococcal ophthalmia. The technique is effective, reduces the incidence of other types of conjuctivitis, and is free from side effects,[9] though other studies have reported that it caused an irritant chemical conjunctivitis in up to 90% of babies.[65] A 2.5% solution of povidone-iodine has been shown to be more effective[43] and protects against chlamydial conjunctivitis, which is otherwise more difficult to prevent even with the use of erythromycin ointment (p. 1151).

Whether or not prophylaxis is justified depends on the incidence and severity of neonatal conjunctivitis in the local population: it is not used in the UK.

VITAMIN K

Haemorrhagic disease of the newborn is potentially fatal, affecting as many as 1:100 births.[3] It exists in an early and late form (p. 799), and is primarily a risk in breast-fed babies. The condition can be prevented by giving 1mg of vitamin K intramuscularly after delivery to all babies. Considerable anxiety about this practice was generated by a series of papers from Bristol,[31] suggesting that it increased the risk of leukaemia in later childhood. Many studies from other parts of the world – Sweden,[26] the USA,48 Denmark,[67] Germany[85] and the UK5 – have failed to confirm the Bristol studies, which in any case had methodological flaws. If i.m. vitamin K is given haemorrhagic disease of any type is virtually unknown.[55] Various oral regimens have been used either to avoid giving injections or, more recently, to avoid the putative risk of malignancy. From these studies it is clear that a single oral dose at birth does not prevent the risk, particularly of late haemorrhagic disease,[36] which in one series was 13 times more common following oral vitamin K than after i.m. vitamin K prophylaxis.[55] Repeated doses of oral vitamin K of 0.5–1.0 mg given at birth and at the end of the first and fourth weeks have been suggested as an alternative to a single dose of the i.m. vitamin K. This routine is now widely practised in Britain8 but it is clear that it does not prevent late haemorrhagic disease of the newborn, particularly in breast-fed babies, only in part because of the failure to administer a complete course.[86] An oral dose of 2 mg at birth followed by 1mg weekly for 3 months is, however, effective, though clearly cumbersome.[36] I would therefore strongly endorse the views of Zipursky[97] that we should give all babies i.m. vitamin K1 at birth, and I would recommend a dose of 1.0mg.

For parents who refuse this, three doses of 2 mg of oral Konakion MM should be prescribed and they should be given at birth, at 1 week and at 1 month; the parents should be given a printed explanation that even this may fail to prevent serious haemorrhage in their baby.

TEMPERATURE CONTROL (Chapter 18)

The hazards of hypothermia are greatest in the labour ward immediately after delivery. It is not uncommon for the body temperature of a normal full-term baby to drop to 35–35.5°C by 15–30 minutes of age because of slipshod care. The labour ward may not have been warm enough, it may have been draughty, or those responsible for the baby's care may not have dried him or covered him quickly enough (p. 294). This problem is entirely preventable by attention to detail: close all doors and windows in the delivery room, and turn off all air circulation systems likely to cool the baby. The temperature of the room should be at least 20°C. The resuscitation trolley, with its overhead radiant heater switched on, should be put in the warmest and the least draughty part of the room. As soon as the infant is delivered he should be dried in prewarmed towels, and then wrapped in a warm dry blanket.

If the mother wants early skin–skin contact with her baby this should only take place in warm rooms (23–25°C) or under a heat source; if this is done the baby sustains his body temperature, cries less and has better blood glucose and base excess values than control cot-nursed babies.[15] He is also more likely to establish successful long-term lactation.[74]

BATHING

More harm comes from bathing babies on the labour ward than from not doing so[38]: it is one of the commonest causes of neonatal hypothermia and should be forbidden. Most blood, meconium and vernix is quickly and effectively removed by the initial drying in warm towels; thereafter, any surplus can be wiped clear with a tissue once the baby is on the ward.

MEASUREMENT

Babies should always be weighed after birth for social as well as medical reasons. If length measurements are to be taken they must be performed properly with an infant stadiometer, taking care to have the baby properly extended (Fig. 22.1). Stretching a tape measure alongside a supine infant or dangling one alongside the neonate held upside down by his ankles is valueless. Measure the head circumference at this stage, although it may be inaccurate in the presence of the caput succedaneum.

LABELLING

In hospital, as opposed to home confinements, it is essential to attach a name tag to the baby immediately after delivery to prevent ghastly incidents of confused parentage and identity. There seems to be little benefit, however, from the more complex procedure of foot-printing the baby.[81]

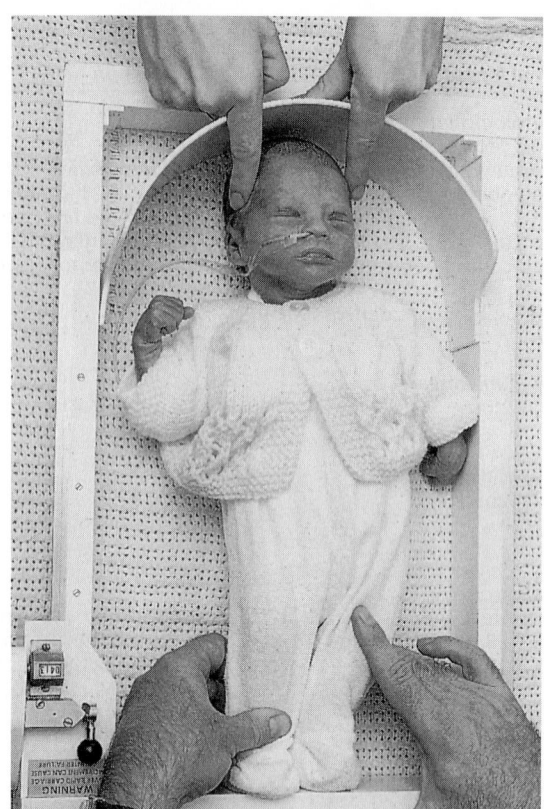

Fig. 22.1 Stadiometer in use for measuring newborn babies.

BONDING

The scientific basis of early mother–child interaction is outlined in detail in Chapter 5. In simple practical terms, both parents should be left alone with their baby immediately after birth, when he is particularly bright-eyed and attractive. Putting him to the breast early is one of the most important determinants of successful lactation[74,77] and, by releasing oxytocin, promotes uterine contraction, milk let-down and complex maternal behavioural responses.[83]

THE NORMAL NEONATE

CARDIORESPIRATORY FUNCTION

The normal term infant has a pulse rate of 120–160/min and a blood pressure of 50–55/30 to 80/50 mmHg (p. 1345); sinus arrhythmia is rare. His respiratory rate is 35–45/min without any apnoeic attacks, although during REM sleep his breathing is often irregular, with pauses of 3–5 seconds. In non-REM sleep his breathing is very regular and shallow.

TEMPERATURE CONTROL

The term baby maintains his temperature very accurately around 37°C, so that any departure from this always requires careful evaluation, in particular to exclude sepsis

(p. 1116). For the healthy clothed term baby who is in a cot, keeping the ward at a temperature of 20–22°C is adequate. If the room temperature falls below 20°C the baby should always wear a bonnet and be swaddled with one or two blankets. It is very important, however, not to overheat the baby by overwrapping him, lying him by a radiator, putting him in direct sunlight or putting an external heat source in the cot with him.

WEIGHT CHANGES

After weighing a baby at birth there is little point in weighing him again until the third or fourth day, as all babies lose weight during this time, primarily as a result of extracellular water loss. Thereafter, if he is still in hospital it is conventional to weigh him every other day to confirm that he is gaining weight adequately: this is the only check that breast-feeding is progressing satisfactorily (see below).

Weight loss in the first few days averages 4–7% and should not exceed 10–12% of the birthweight. It should always be assessed in relative terms, even though it means that a 4.50 kg baby may lose 450 g (i.e. 1 lb). In general breast-fed babies lose more weight (5–10%) than bottle-fed ones (2–6%),[56] but this difference may be less if the baby breast-feeds more frequently.[6] From 1 week of age the normal baby should gain weight at 20–30 g/day until the age of 6 months.[76]

URINE OUTPUT

Many neonates pass urine immediately after birth, and then, particularly if breast-fed with a poor fluid intake, may pass very little urine in the next 24–36 hours. Thereafter they pass 40–60 ml of urine/kg/24 hours, usually when they are fed or when their perineum is exposed! It is exceptionally unusual for any illness to present in an otherwise normal baby with just anuria or oliguria.

BOWEL ACTIVITY

Many babies defecate in the first 2 minutes, and usually regularly thereafter. Initially they pass meconium, a dark greenish compound which is composed of intestinal secretions, bile, including bilirubin, swallowed amniotic debris and the remains of desquamated intestinal mucosal cells.[37] By 2–3 days, 'changing' stools, a mixture of meconium and more normal stools, are passed. Once feeding is established, breast-fed babies pass very soft mustard-yellow stools, often with every feed. Their stools are acid (pH <6).[49] Bottle-fed babies pass a less acid (pH 6–7.5), firmer and paler stool, only once or twice a day.

The bacterial flora in the stools is described on page 1110.

NEUROLOGICAL ACTIVITY

The neurological capabilities of the neonate are outlined on pages 280–281. He can see and prefers a face to 'scrambled' shapes; he can hear and smell, and within the first few days and weeks of life he learns to recognize his mother by these senses.[54,82,84]

In the neonatal period a baby has irregular sleep–waking cycles: in the first few days he spends up to 18 hours asleep, with 50–60% of the sleep being REM.[79] He wakes up to feed or when uncomfortable, usually because he has passed urine or stool, but his sleep–wake pattern gradually becomes more regular[69] (Fig. 22.2).

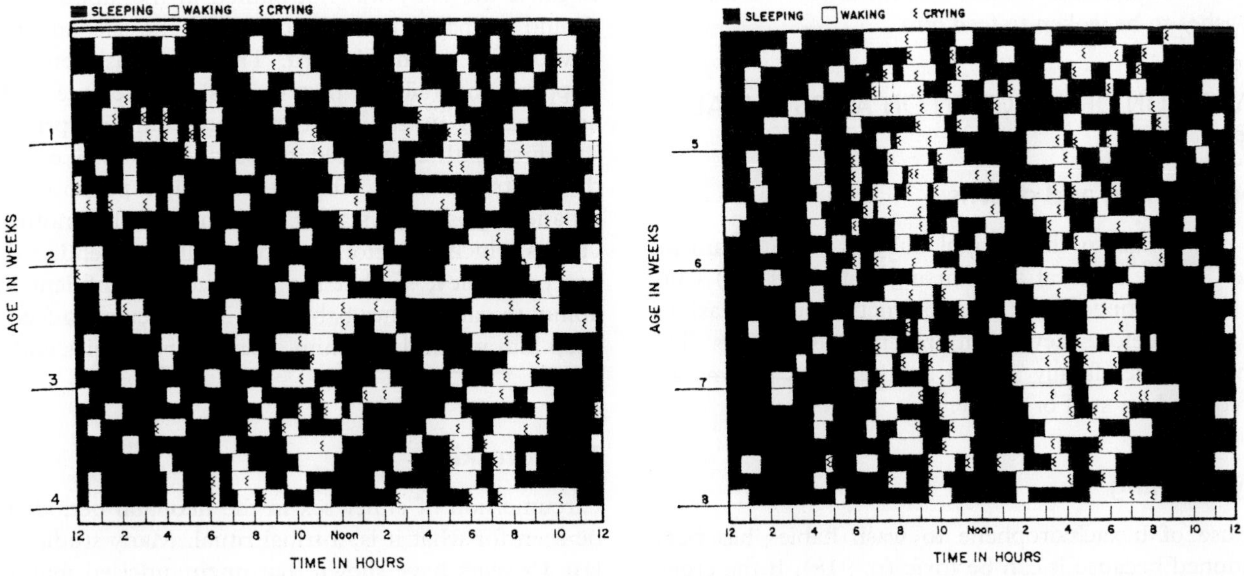

Fig. 22.2 Sleep–wake cycle in a normal baby during the first 2 months of life. (Reproduced with permission from Parmelee[69].)

Circadian rhythmicity is detectable in heart rate and body temperature by 1 month of age.[30]

POSTNATAL WARD CARE

ADMISSION ROUTINE

On arrival in the PNW from the labour ward the baby should have his temperature, pulse and respiration recorded. There is no need to check the blood pressure, haematocrit or blood glucose.[4] That he is in good condition should be confirmed. His identity should be checked, together with the security of his cord clamp, and whether or not he has received vitamin K_1.

ROUTINE OBSERVATION

Pulse and respiration should be recorded daily. It is doubtful whether there is any purpose in taking a full-term neonate's temperature if he is asymptomatic. However, detecting tachycardia and tachypnoea is important if cases of neonatal sepsis are to be recognized early[62] (p. 1116).

ROOMING IN

The standard management should be that the mother has her baby with her in a cot beside her bed throughout the 24 hours, i.e. the practice of rooming in. This is advantageous from the point of view of preventing cross-infection (p. 1112) and also promotes successful breast-feeding. Only if the mother has her baby with her can she learn to respond to and manage his every demand and need.

If she is ill, or if she requests it, the baby can go to the ward nursery overnight. However, if the baby is in the nursery overnight the mother should always be asked if she wishes to be woken to feed him.

PREVENTION OF INFECTION ON A POSTNATAL WARD

Hand washing and gowns

The major risk to the normal baby is from organisms carried by the medical and nursing staff (p. 1113) who, even on a routine PNW, must be meticulous in washing their hands before they touch or handle any babies. The mother and her family should do the same. Gowns are not required for staff or family.[10]

Baby washing

The use of hexachlorophene to wash babies has been abandoned because it can be toxic (p. 918). If the cross-infection techniques are good, and the baby rooms in so that he is colonized from his mother, all that is required is to wash him with any of the commercial baby soaps. If there is an outbreak of skin infection then chlorhexidine washing can be instituted.

Nursing routine

The nursing routines designed to prevent transmission of infection from staff to baby or from baby to baby are given on pages 1112–1114.

Visitors

Healthy visitors are not an infectious hazard, and the number a mother is allowed should be decided on a commonsense basis. There are no medical reasons why grandparents, husbands and siblings should not be allowed free access to the new family member.

Cord care

The early care of the cord with antibiotic spray and isopropyl alcohol is described above. Good care means that the cord stays dry and does not become necrotic, and does not drop off naturally for up to 3 weeks.[93] Redundant Wharton's jelly level may be cut off on the fourth or fifth day.

Skin care

No special skin care is given other than to protect the perianal area and genitalia with a liberal application of zinc and castor oil cream after every nappy change.

Well baby care

Because the baby was not bathed in the labour ward he should probably be washed during the second or third day on the postnatal ward. This first wash can be just 'topping and tailing', that is, washing the face and hair and cleaning up the groin and perineum. For primiparae this first bath may need to be a supervised or even a demonstrated affair. One of the major purposes of the inpatient postnatal stay is to reinforce the mothercraft classes which the mother – hopefully – attended during her pregnancy, so that she goes home confident in her ability to care for her baby, and in particular to feed him, keep him warm, bathe him, change his nappies and dress him.

The foreskin

Circumcision of either sex in the neonatal period should be seen for what it is, a tribal ritual. Many studies in the last 15 years have shown that uncircumcised males have an increased number of urinary tract infections, particularly under 1 year of age.[18,78,95] But as Winberg et al[94] pointed out, it is fundamentally illogical that mutilating someone might be beneficial. Furthermore, if the UTI is due to underlying reflux, with the potential for scarring and chronic pyelonephritis, the sooner this is unmasked the better. I do not believe, therefore, that the case has been made for routine neonatal male circumcision.

For those who elect to have their child treated in this way, they should be reminded that the parts in question are not bereft of nerve endings and contain blood vessels. Adequate analgesia and vitamin K_1 should therefore be provided.

All newborn males have 'phimosis'; the foreskin is not meant to be retractile at this age, and the parents must be told to leave it alone and not to try and retract it. Forcible retraction in infancy tears the tissues of the tip of the foreskin causing scarring, and is the commonest cause of genuine phimosis later in life.

IMMUNIZATIONS

Polio

In areas of the developing world where poliomyelitis is endemic there is a case for immunizing the neonate with oral polio vaccine, and there is a good antibody response to neonates given the vaccine at 7 days.[45] In developed countries routine polio vaccination is given at 2–3 months of age.

Hepatitis B

The American Academy of Pediatrics recommends universal immunization of all neonates against hepatitis B[2], and there is a great deal to recommend this approach where hepatitis B is endemic in the population. In the UK vaccination is only offered to infants of mothers who are seropositive for at least one of the hepatitis B antigens, although there is some local variation in practice. At birth, at-risk babies should receive 2 ml (200 μl) of the hepatitis B immunoglobulin and a first dose of one of the hepatitis B vaccines, ideally within the first 12 hours. Repeat doses of vaccine should be given at 1 and 6 months of age.[23]

Tuberculosis

In communities in which the prevalence of tuberculosis is high, BCG should be given at birth or in early infancy. In the UK this includes babies born into ethnic groups with a high incidence of close contact with a sputum-positive case (see also Table 22.1). The conversion rate to Mantoux positivity is nearly 100%.[68] It is estimated that this gives 60–80% protection against TB in childhood, with perhaps even greater protection against tuberculous meningitis.[16,17]

In the developed world BCG should not be given to the baby of an HIV-positive woman, but HIV screening is not justified in countries where universal neonatal BCG immunization is practised.[66]

ROUTINE NEONATAL CLINICAL EXAMINATION

TIMING AND PERSONNEL

All newborn babies should be examined carefully at least once in the first week.[64] The examination should be carried out by someone experienced in neonatal care, not so much because of what might otherwise be missed clinically, but because the examiner must know how to interpret a finding which is commonly trivial but which might be sinister, and how to answer the plethora of questions about all aspects of well-baby care that the mother is likely to ask.

It is essential for those carrying out the examination to have a clear understanding of what they are trying to achieve. They must remember that the patient is asymptomatic, that the midwives will usually have recognized a cleft palate or Down syndrome, and that the mother will have been over her new baby with a fine-tooth comb and will already know whether he has all his fingernails or whether his external genitalia are acceptable! There are, therefore, four main functions to the RNCE:

1. Detecting serious problems which would otherwise not have been detected and which merit early assessment and treatment. Basically there are only two common ones, congenital heart disease and developmental dysplasia of the hip.
2. Checking for many very rare but serious conditions which occur usually in less than 1:10 000 livebirths and which the average paediatrician will find once in a professional lifetime, e.g. the enlarged bladder of posterior urethral valves, the posterior abdominal mass of a congenital tumour, a cataract or a dermal sinus leading to the theca.
3. Noting and explaining to the mother the multitude of normal variations that may be present (Table 22.2).
4. Giving the mother a chance to ask about any aspects of the medical care of her baby.

Medically, the ideal time to carry out the examination is towards the end of the first week, as by that time transient abnormalities present on the first day, such as mumurs, slightly unstable hips and transient abnormalities in tone, will have cleared. By implication, therefore, a first-day examination is primarily for the reassurance of the mother, and if it is decided to offer such a service in a maternity unit it should be designed with this in mind. However, with the increasing practice of sending women home from the maternity hospital within 24–36 hours this first examination will be the only opportunity for

Table 22.2 Minor abnormalities which may cause maternal alarm

Skin lesions
strawberry naevi
'stork bite'
milia
erythema toxicum
innocent pigmented naevi
epithelial pearls in the mouth
Cephalhaematoma
Subconjunctival haemorrhage
Peripheral and traumatic cyanosis
Tongue tie
Diastasis recti
Protuberant xiphisternum
Hydrocoeles
Sacral dimple
Umbilical anomalies, e.g. hernia
Physiological jaundice
Snuffles
Periorbital oedema
Talipes calcaneovalgus
Vaginal skin tag
Breast enlargement
Hooded foreskin

professional paediatricians to check the baby, and this opportunity must be taken.

The physician has to be very careful that he does not overinterpret signs found on the first day in such a way that he subjects the infant to unnecessary investigation and treatment, and the parents to unnecessary anxiety: there is a serious risk that meddlesome interpretation of first-day physical signs can do much more harm than good. The details of the examination are given in Chapter 17.

GESTATIONAL AGE ASSESSMENT

This has become unnecessarily complex. If a baby is < 1.60 g he will be in a neonatal unit and his medical care will be in response to his clinical condition; assessing his gestational age, although of academic and perhaps sociological interest, will not influence his management. The same is true for the asymptomatic infant over 2.8–3.0 kg on a PNW. For the 5–10% of babies between these groups it is occasionally of clinical value to assess their gestational age postnatally, in that a small for dates 2.00 kg neonate will need to be cared for differently from an appropriate for dates term one (Chapter 23). However, in general, even for these babies all that is usually required is an assessment of whether or not the mother's dates are compatible with her infant's appearance, or whether they diverge by the duration of one menstrual cycle. Therefore, simplicity is of the essence and the examination and assessment outlined in Chapter 17 is recommended

BIOCHEMICAL SCREENING

Currently all newborn babies in the UK are screened for phenylketonuria and hypothyroidism. In addition, galactosaemia, cystic fibrosis, haemoglobinopathies and various aminoacidopathies are screened for in some parts of the country (pp. 993–994).

PHENYLKETONURIA

At 5–9 days of age all babies have a heel-prick blood sample analysed for phenylalanine using the Guthrie assay (p. 993) to exclude PKU. The baby should only be tested if his milk intake is normal. The blood is collected onto an absorbent card (Fig. 22.3), taking care to fill each of the circles with blood.

Approximately 1:2000 of all infants are positive on screening, about five times more than the prevalence of

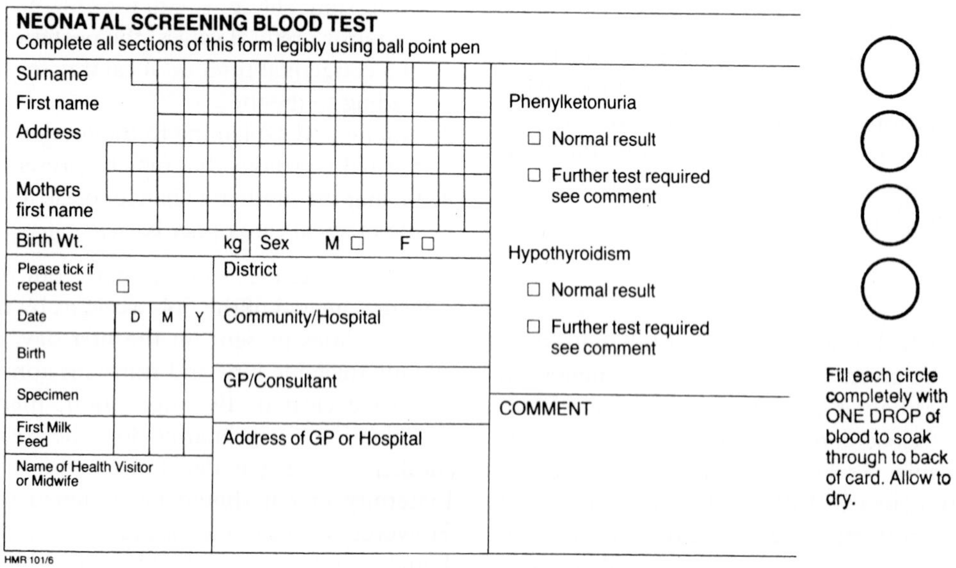
NEONATAL SCREENING BLOOD TEST
Complete all sections of this form legibly using ball point pen
Surname
First name
Address
Mothers first name
Birth Wt. kg Sex M ☐ F ☐
Please tick if repeat test ☐
District
Date D M Y
Community/Hospital
Birth
Specimen
GP/Consultant
First Milk Feed
Address of GP or Hospital
Name of Health Visitor or Midwife
Phenylketonuria
☐ Normal result
☐ Further test required see comment
Hypothyroidism
☐ Normal result
☐ Further test required see comment
COMMENT
Fill each circle completely with ONE DROP of blood to soak through to back of card. Allow to dry.
HMR 101/6

Fig. 22.3 Guthrie card in current use in East Anglia.

the disease (1:10 000). Those with positive tests are recalled and their plasma phenylalanine remeasured to determine whether or not they have PKU. If PKU or a variant is confirmed by a second high phenylalanine level the baby should be referred to a specialist centre for full investigation and stabilization on diet.

HYPOTHYROIDISM

Using another of the blood spots (Fig. 22.3) a radioimmunoassay is done for TSH; those with a high TSH are then recalled for further evaluation. This is required in about 0.2–0.3% of all infants tested. The incidence of hypothroidism detected in this way is about 1:3500 (p. 961). All infants identified should be treated and the diagnosis of hypothroidism confirmed later in the first year (p. 962).

OTHER METABOLIC ERRORS

The screening for these is described on pages 992–994.

HAEMOGLOBINOPATHIES

Babies from at-risk races can be screened for sickle cell disease and β-thalassaemia in the neonatal period (p. 827).

CYSTIC FIBROSIS (INCIDENCE 1:2000)

Blood spots from the Guthrie card (Fig. 22.3) can be analysed for IRT, which is markedly raised in most neonates with cystic fibrosis. The test is very specific, with a recall rate of only 0.5% and very few false positive or false negative results. The accuracy of the screening can be improved if positive IRT tests are combined with PCR analysis for the ΔF508 genotype in cystic fibrosis.[33,92] Screening for cystic fibrosis is not yet universally practised even in the UK, although preliminary studies show a definite benefit.[21,52,89]

FEEDING THE NORMAL TERM BABY

Every effort should be made to encourage a mother to breast-feed, and how to organize the maternity unit to facilitate this is well reviewed by Powers et al.[71] The key components are given in Table 22.3. However, for the normal term baby in the western world the disadvantages of bottle-feeding are few. It is therefore unjustifiable to pressurize a woman into breast-feeding. In the developing world, however, bottle-feeding should be avoided at all costs (p. 112). For a normally grown full-term infant the aim should be to establish the practice of 'demand' feeding: that is, the baby should be fed whenever he is hungry, even if this means a 2-hour or a 5-hour gap between feeds. The general principles of neonatal nutrition are outlined in Chapter 19.

Table 22.3 Hospital policies intended to promote breast-feeding (Adapted from Powers et al[71])

Antenatal education
Baby put to breast as soon after birth as possible
Establish rooming-in
Feed at least 8 times per day, up to 12 times if necessary
Do not have specific duration of feeds at the breast
Finish the first breast, going to the second if hungry
No supplementary/complementary feeds
No dummies
No discharge gift packs
Regular assessment of the mother's breasts

BREAST-FEEDING[34]

Preparation

A mother should be advised during the antenatal period that she should put the baby to the breast as soon after delivery as possible (p. 376). In the past great emphasis has been placed on procedures to prepare the nipples by using shells inside the bra or by manually stretching the nipples. These procedures are not of proven benefit.[1]

Position for feeding

The mother should be sitting in a suitable chair which keeps her upright and comfortable, or adopt a similar position in bed (Fig. 22.4). An alternative is for the baby to lie beside the mother in bed. If the mother is sitting up, the baby should be lying nearly horizontal and be facing her (i.e. front to front, not side to front). In this position

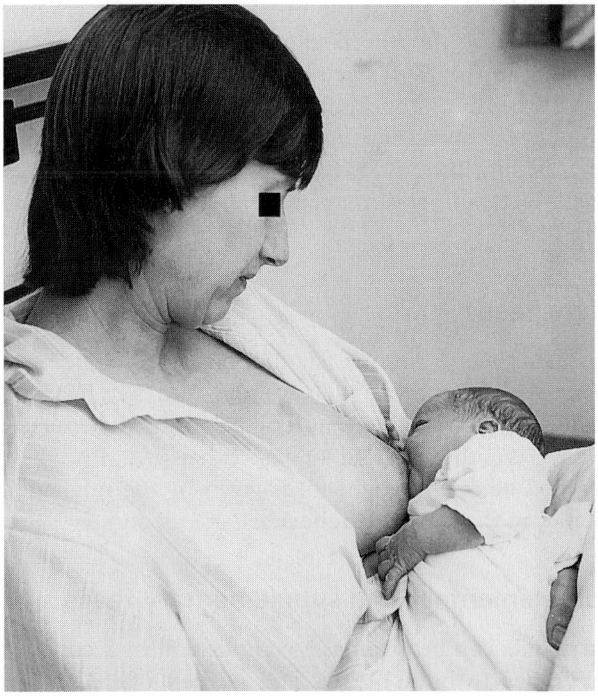

Fig. 22.4 Optimal position for breast-feeding a baby when the mother is in a sitting position.

the baby has to extend his neck slightly to feed, and his mother should then insert the whole of her nipple and most of the adjacent areola into his mouth.

During breast-feeding, sucking – that is, creating a vacuum in the mouth to draw milk out of the breast – is not an important mechanism. The baby obtains breast milk in two ways: first, the physical and psychological stimuli of putting the nipple into his mouth will evoke the let-down reflex in the mother so that her milk is actively squirted into his mouth. Secondly, in the feeding position outlined above, the baby's lower jaw is free and can compress the areola, squeezing milk through the nipple into his mouth.

When to start

There is no point in giving a baby a first feed of clear fluid (p. 549). The first breast-feed should be undertaken in the labour ward. If it cannot be given there, when the full-term baby is bright and alert (p. 376), then everyone can wait until the mother is safely ensconced in the postnatal ward.

Frequency of feeds

Left to their own devices, healthy infants in the first few days after delivery may feed 10 or more times a day.[12,13] In general, babies who feed frequently do better.[13,96] It is not essential for a baby to feed 10–12 times per day, but if he is awake and ready to feed he should not be prevented from doing so.

Breast-fed babies in general feed more frequently than bottle-fed ones, and in the first few days and weeks settle into a $2\frac{1}{2}$–$3\frac{1}{2}$ hourly feeding pattern. With the baby rooming in (p. 378), once he wakes and looks hungry he should be fed; imposing a 4-hourly schedule, and/or topping up breast-fed babies with clear fluid until the next feeding time is due, is one of the major causes of failed lactation and may actually increase the risk of jaundice.[50]

Night feeds

Postnatal ward routine should always assume that a breast-feeding mother will want to feed her baby overnight. Sometimes this may not be justified because the mother is either very ill or just exhausted. For reasons outlined below the night feeds given by the nursing staff should, in the short term, be 5 or 10% glucose.

Complementary and supplementary feeds

Extra milk can be given as a complementary feed (i.e. the baby goes to both breasts and is then offered a bottle until satisfied) or as a supplementary feed (i.e. an entire breast feed is omitted and replaced by an appropriate volume of formula). The decision to give such feeds to a breast-feeding baby is a major one, and probably the only genuine justifications are hypoglycaemia (p. 941) and persisting weight loss >10% of the birthweight (p. 386). Using these feeds significantly reduces the likelihood of establishing successful breast-feeding.[11,51,60]

Free samples

Giving free samples of formula to the mother at the time of discharge should be discouraged as it accelerates the postdischarge decline in breast-feeding.[25]

Duration of a feed

There is absolutely no scientific justification for the practice of starting the baby with 3 minutes at the breast on the first day, 5 minutes on the next day, increasing to 7 minutes and then 10 minutes. Even in the first day or two the baby should be put to the breast and left there until he has 'finished': that is, the breast is empty and/or he has lost interest in sucking. This will usually be after 7–10 minutes. Once lactation is established most of the milk a baby is going to get comes in the first 4–6 minutes. Sucking longer than this is therefore of nonutritive value.

One breast or two

In the first day or two, when only colostrum is being produced, the baby should go to both breasts during a feed. Thereafter, there is some evidence to show that prolonged feeding at one breast, ensuring that it is empty, reduces complications.[28] If, after this breast is empty, the baby has gone to sleep, the feed is over, but if he is still hungry the mother should give him some milk from the other breast. To ensure that one breast at a time is completely emptied the mother should always alternate which breast she offers first.

Volume of feed

No mention of volume of a breast feed is made here – deliberately. Women on average produce 700–800 ml of milk per day, with a wide range from 450 to 1200 ml, leaving about 100 ml in the breasts after each feed.[24] However, babies seem able to judge their own intake from the breast such that they grow and gain weight normally. Only if weight gain is unsatisfactory should some assessment of intake be attempted.

Nipple care

Frequent feeds or sucking for too long are not the cause of sore nipples.[80] Some women just have bad luck, and develop this complication despite careful antenatal breast preparation and good technique during feeding. The nipple may be oedematous and even have petechiae across the papillae: it becomes exquisitely tender and looks sore and inflamed. In all situations nipple soreness may progress to a crack or fissure, which is extremely painful and may take several days to heal. The management of sore nipples is outlined on page 384.

Monitoring breast-feeding in the PNW

The nurses (or the mother) should keep a record of when the baby goes to the breast. He should also be weighed routinely (p. 377), in the expectation that he will lose up to 10–12% of his birthweight (see above). Rarely, hypoglycaemia with fits may develop, even in term babies if they breast-feed very poorly in the first 48–72 hours (p. 946), and it is wise to monitor such babies using Dextrostix daily or twice daily from 48 hours of age until they are feeding well and gaining weight.

If weight gain is poor, or persistent weight loss occurs (p. 386), examine the baby carefully to ensure that he is well and perform a full blood count and take a urine sample to exclude infection (p. 1122). If these are normal the problem is almost certainly a poor intake, and in such babies the electrolytes should be checked as hypernatraemia may develop.

The only way to confirm a poor intake is by test weighing. In this, the baby is weighed on accurate scales just before and just after a feed, without changing his clothes or nappy. The technique is, however, none too accurate, and in particular may underestimate low intakes.[91] Several test weighings are necessary to get a feel for a baby's intake, which may vary considerably from feed to feed. Test weighing must be a last resort, and only in infants in whom failure to gain weight is becoming a serious problem. The anxiety provoked in a mother by the procedure can inhibit lactation[14] and may therefore make things worse.

BOTTLE-FEEDING

Starting feeds

If a mother has elected to bottle-feed her baby this should be started once the baby reaches the postnatal ward using one of the standard infant formulas (Chapter 19) which are, to all intents and purposes, identical. In most PNWs bottle-feeds are usually offered on a 4-hourly schedule. Although there is no biological justification for this, babies surprisingly often settle into such a regimen. The baby destined for bottle-feeds should be offered a bottle at the first scheduled feed after his admission to the PNW. If he is fast asleep there is no need to do anything, as a term neonate is designed on the assumption that he will be breast-fed and receive few calories during the first 24–48 hours. Leaving him for another 4 hours before his first bottle does him no harm at all. As with breast-fed neonates there is absolutely no justification for starting with clear fluids.

Technique of feeding

The baby should be swaddled and held closely and comfortably to the mother so that she can hold the bottle with her free hand. Touching the baby's mouth or lips with the teat will usually evoke the rooting reflex. He will open his mouth, the teat can then be popped in, and he will begin to suck. In bottle-feeding the mechanism is different from breast-feeding:[57] bottles do not have a 'let-down' reflex, so that in addition to compressing the teat with his gums and squeezing milk into his mouth as in breast-feeding, the baby has to generate a vacuum in his mouth to suck the milk out of the bottle. The amount obtained per suck can be varied by varying the size of the hole in the teat, but in general large holes should only be used in babies with sucking problems.

Temperature

Traditionally bottle milk is warmed to body temperature before feeding, but there is no need to do this, and babies take room-temperature milk perfectly satisfactorily.

Frequency of feeds

Demand feeding should be the routine, and bottle-fed babies usually settle into a $3\frac{1}{2}$–$4\frac{1}{2}$-hourly schedule, taking five to six feeds per day. The ward routine must adapt to these needs.

Volume of feeds

The traditional teaching about volumes is outlined in Table 22.4. For the healthy term baby this is only a guideline: he should be demand fed and allowed to take what he wants, which will usually be about 70–100 ml at each of six feeds, giving 150–180 ml/kg/24 hours.

FEEDING PROBLEMS

Feeding problems must be sorted out with the mother and baby together, ideally on the mother's PNW. Feeding problems are emphatically not an indication for transferring an otherwise normal baby to a neonatal intensive care unit.

Table 22.4 Volumes of bottle milk to feed to normal full-term babies

Day 1	60 ml/kg
Day 2	90 ml/kg
Day 3	120 ml/kg
Days 4–6	150 ml/kg
Days 7–10	180 ml/kg

Table 22.5 Factors contributing to sore nipples

Poor baby position at feeding
Sucking the nipple rather than the areola
Licking the nipple pre/post feeding
Poor hygiene – dried milk left on the nipple after a feed
Friction from clothing
Chemical irritation – soap, tincture of benzoin

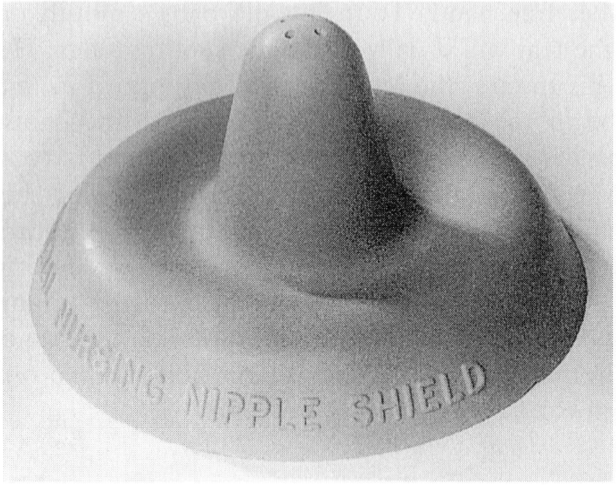

Fig. 22.5 Nipple shield for use in the presence of tender or cracked nipples.

MATERNAL

For obvious reasons these are limited to the breast-feeding mother.

Nipple problems (Table 22.5)

If the nipples do become sore the mother should be encouraged to persevere, while being meticulous with her feeding technique and with cleaning her nipples after a feed, in the justified expectation that things will rapidly improve within 2–3 days; alternatively, covering the sore nipple with a nipple shield can be helpful (Fig. 22.5).

If feeding is too painful, or if a fissure develops which is not healing, then there is no alternative but to abandon feeding from that breast until it has healed, but the baby can continue to feed from the other breast. The affected breast must be emptied 4-hourly by manual expression or with a breast pump, and the milk can be fed to the baby by bottle or tube (p. 396).

The inflamed nipple can be treated with an antiseptic cream such as Cetavlex,[34] and if inflammation becomes marked 0.5% hydrocortisone cream is helpful. Sprays, alcohols and tincture of benzoin are extremely painful and should never be used.

Breast engorgement

When the milk first comes in the breasts may become full very quickly and become so engorged that when a feed is due the nipple and areola cannot get into the baby's mouth. If this occurs, before each feed the mother should express 20–30 ml of milk to slacken her breasts sufficiently for the baby to fix satisfactorily. In most cases engorgement is transient and the milk supply settles down to meet demand within the first week or two. If it does not, a small amount of milk may always need to be expressed before the start of a feed.

The discomfort caused by engorgement may merit analgesia. In some women the engorgement results in extravasation of milk into a segment of the breast tissue itself. The mother may then become pyrexial, the breast red and tender, and a mass may be palpable in one lobule. This is the condition known as mastitis. The treatment is to give analgesics and regularly empty the breast 4-hourly. However, since manual expression is extremely painful, a breast pump is essential.

Breast abscess

This is usually secondary to mastitis, but can result from superficial staphylococcal infection if the cord care has been poor (p. 373). The mother is febrile and toxic, with an acutely tender inflamed breast lobule. She needs antibiotics, antipyretics and analgesics, and lactation will usually need to be suppressed.

Inadequate milk production

In most cases the mother's perception that she is not producing enough milk is incorrect.[39] However, if poor intake is documented (see above) the first thing to do is to increase the frequency of sucking to 2–3-hourly.[13] If this does not increase milk production, a trial of metoclopramide can be undertaken.[47] This drug increases prolactin production by the hypothalamus. If the baby is still not gaining weight, the mother should either give up breast-feeding or start regular complementary feeds (p. 386).

Too much milk

Milk may come out of the contralateral breast when the baby is sucking, it may drip out of both breasts between feeds, and/or the woman may have persisting problems with engorgement. Leaking milk can be absorbed with pads, and breast engorgement can be treated by emptying some milk out before the start of a feed. In general these problems settle down with the passage of time, as physiologically (see above) milk production is geared to consumption.

Taste

Babies would appear to be able to taste milk, as they take less if the milk contains lactic acid after vigorous maternal exercise[88] or it contains alcohol;[58] they take more if it contains garlic.[59]

Suppression of lactation

In most women, in the absence of sucking, prolactin secretion rapidly falls off and the milk production stops, with very little breast discomfort or engorgement. As bromocriptine is no longer available for this[73] simple analgesia is indicated.

Breast cancer

Breast-feeding does not influence the subsequent development of breast cancer.[61,87] The diagnosis of breast malignancy late in pregnancy or after delivery is a contra-indication to breast-feeding as immediate maternal treatment is imperative.

Rarities

Women with unilateral absence of a breast or who have had a mastectomy can try to feed from their single breast, though for obvious reasons the volume produced may be inadequate. Rare women, despite apparently normal breasts, fail to lactate, presumably owing to end-organ insensitivity to the hormonal stimuli.

Women who have had augmentation mammoplasty can breast-feed, as the augmentation procedure is carried out behind the normal breast tissue, which is left undamaged by the procedure. However, in general such women are less likely to be successful breast-feeders.[41]

Recently, anxiety has been expressed about whether the increased incidence of immune-mediated rheumatic disease in such women could be transmitted to the babies in breast milk.[53] However, an overview of the literature suggests that at present there is no contradiction to their breast-feeding.[46] Women who have had reduction mammoplasty, however, should not breast-feed, as the procedure disconnects the areola from the underlying structures.

BABY PROBLEMS

Baby problems are in general more common in breast-fed babies; however, they are not unknown in bottle-fed babies.

Baby not feeding

Some babies refuse to wake up and feed at the appropriate time; most are completely normal and just feel like having fewer feeds that day. If the baby is gaining weight normally he is getting enough to eat. However, if the feeds last for 2–3 minutes only, or are only demanded three or four times per day and the weight gain is poor, the first thing to do is to ensure that the baby is not ill. Examine him carefully to exclude dyspnoea, congenital heart disease, dysmorphic syndromes (e.g. Down syndrome) or some primary neuromuscular disorder (p. 1289), and to make sure that his mouth is normal: it is embarrassing to miss a cleft palate. Exclude hypoglycaemia (p. 942), and if there is any suspicion of infection (p. 1116) appropriate investigations should be carried out.

If all these are normal but the baby still feeds poorly the commonest causes are:

1. Prematurity (Chapter 23);
2. The aftermath of a difficult delivery, e.g. Kielland's forceps;
3. Sedation from intrapartum or antenatal drug therapy;
4. Sedation from drugs in the breast milk.

In groups 2 and 3 the baby will improve spontaneously within 24–48 hours. If he received a narcotic analgesic intrapartum, give a single dose of naloxone (p. 258). It may be necessary to give the baby one or two tube feeds before he sucks satisfactorily.

If 4 is the problem, unless the mother's therapy can be discontinued breast-feeding is contraindicated.

If neither 1, 2, 3 nor 4 is the case and the feeding problem persists, careful re-evaluation to exclude some underlying neurological or muscular disorder is indicated.

Crying

Persistent crying in the neonate is usually due to hunger. There are, however, many other causes for babies crying, notably pain, boredom and discomfort. If the diagnosis is hunger the appropriate treatment is food, even if the baby was only fed 2 hours previously (see above). If the crying baby shows no enthusiasm for feeding and is clean and dry, then he probably just needs a cuddle. If this does not work, one must exclude occult but painful conditions such as otitis media, intussusception, bone and joint sepsis and incarcerated hernia. It is commonly believed that crying in a baby is due to wind (see below) and/or can only be treated by a complementary feed of some non-maternal fluid such as water or Dextrose: neither of these assumptions is true!

Wind

The bottle-fed baby will always swallow some air with a feed, either because the mother has allowed the meniscus of the milk in the bottle to lie across the hole in the teat, or just because at the end of a bottle feed it is impossible to take the last few drops without taking some air as well. The breast-fed baby should swallow less air during a feed. However, after both sorts of feed the mother traditionally sits her baby upright, hopefully in such a position that the stomach gas bubble lies underneath the oesophageal hiatus and then, by rubbing or patting his back, induces the bubble to burst upwards. 'Winding' the baby in this way is supposed to prevent excess gas being propelled through the infant's small intestine where, by analogy with older patients, it is believed to cause abdominal pain and/or infantile colic (see below).

I would not dare to suggest that infants should not be 'winded', but if after a feed nothing comes up after 2–3 minutes of back patting the procedure should be abandoned and the baby allowed to sleep; if he is still restless and crying, another cause, specifically persisting hunger, should be considered.

Colic

Infantile colic can occur in the late neonatal period. Its aetiology remains a mystery, although food and lactose intolerance in the mother and baby have been investigated, with equivocal results.[42,44,63] Stressful psychosocial factors may play a part.[72] The treatment is to reassure the mother about the benign nature of the illness. Giving up breast-feeding or changing the bottle-fed formula is not justified, but antispasmodic drugs may help.[90]

Poor weight gain/persisting hunger

Because bottle-fed babies receive ad-libitum calories and fluid this problem is much commoner in breast-fed infants who, if denied adequate liquid and/or calories, will present with poor weight gain, persistent crying or both. If no other cause for these presenting features is found (see above), inadequate intake can be documented by test weighing. If, despite implementing all the tricks outlined above to improve milk intake, the breast-fed baby still fails to thrive, there comes a time when some extra source of liquid and/or calories is the only way to calm him, or get him to gain weight. This time has come when:

- there is persistent failure to settle a crying fractious breast-fed baby over a short period of time;
- the weight loss exceeds 10–12% (p. 377);
- there is a temperature (dehydration fever, see below), hypoglycaemia (p. 941), hypernatraemia or severe jaundice (but see p. 382);
- there is no weight gain by 6–7 days of age;
- there are sore nipples or engorgement, only one breast is being used, and the baby is hungry;
- the mother is demoralized by a crying baby – calming the baby with a few bottle feeds and giving her 8 hours' sleep may transform the situation and allow normal lactation to be established.

As one of the purported advantages of breast-feeding is a reduction in the incidence of cow's milk protein allergy,[40] and there is the possibility that this syndrome may be induced even by one or two cow's milk formula feeds in the neonatal period, the additional feeds should be given as 5–10% dextrose, which is non-allergenic, slakes thirst and does give some calories. However, there is no evidence that this practice decreases atopic disease in general.[35] In most cases no more than three or four such feeds will be required before normal breast-feeding can be resumed. However, if poor weight gain is still a problem, and expressed breast milk is not a feasible alternative, formula milk will have to be given.

Complementary and supplementary feeds

One may be forced into trying complementary and/or supplementary feeds in term babies with feeding problems, although the use of such feeds can make matters worse and cause lactation to fail completely. It may be, however, that the use of such feeds is the first objective marker of lactation that, for some reason or another, is inevitably going to prove inadequate.[32]

Dehydration fever

If a baby in the first week of life develops a fever, two likely and important causes are infection (p. 1116) or overheating due to some defect in the environmental control (p. 300). If these are excluded in a febrile baby who appears well but has an inadequate intake and has lost 10% or more of his birthweight, he may be suffering from dehydration. This can be confirmed clinically, and by measuring the plasma osmolality, which in dehydration fever will usually exceed 310 mOsmol/l.[22] Such a baby drinks clear fluids (or bottle milk) avidly, whereupon his temperature falls and he gains weight.

Gastroenterological symptoms

Vomiting (p. 745), diarrhoea (p. 746), abdominal distension (pp. 775–787) and jaundice (p. 722) all require evaluation in their own right: they are rarely due to feeding problems, although jaundice is frequently associated with breast-feeding (p. 718).

REFERENCES

1. Alexander J M, Grant A M, Campbell M J 1992. Randomised controlled trial of breast shells and Hoffman's exercises for inverted and non-protractile nipples. British Medical Journal 304: 1030–1032
2. American Academy of Pediatrics 1992 Universal hepatitis B immunization. Pediatrics 89: 795–800
3. American Academy of Pediatrics 1993 Controversies concerning vitamin K and the newborn. Pediatrics 91: 1001–1003
4. American Academy of Pediatrics 1993 Routine evaluation of blood pressure, hematocrit and glucose in newborns. Pediatrics 92: 474–476
5. Ansell P, Bull D, Roman E 1996. Childhood leukaemia and intramuscular vitamin K: findings from a case-control study. British Medical Journal 313: 204–205
6. Avoa A, Fischer P R 1990 The influence of prenatal instruction about breast feeding on neonatal weight loss. Pediatrics 86: 313–315
7. Barrett F F, Mason F O, Flemming D 1979 The effect of three cord care regimens on bacterial colonization of normal newborn infants. Journal of Pediatrics 94: 796–799
8. Barton J S, Tripp J H, McNinch A W 1995 Neonatal vitamin K prophylaxis in the British Isles: current practice and trends. British Medical Journal 310: 632–633
9. Bell T A, Grayson T J, Krohn M A et al 1993 Randomized trial of silver nitrate, erythromycin and no eye prophylaxis for the prevention of conjunctivitis among newborns not at risk for gonococcal ophthalmitis. Pediatrics 92: 755–760

10. Birenbaum H J, Glorioso L, Rosenberger C et al 1990 Gowning on a postpartum ward fails to decrease colonization in the newborn infant. American Journal of Diseases of Children 144: 1031–1033
11. Blomquist H K, Jonsbo F, Serenius F, Persson L A 1994 Supplementary feeding in the maternity ward shortens the duration of breast feeding. Acta Paediatrica 83: 1122–1126
12. Cable T A, Rothenberger L A 1984 Breast feeding behavioral patterns among La Leche league mothers. A descriptive study. Pediatrics 73: 830–835
13. de Carvalho M, Robertsen S, Friedman A, Klaus M 1983 Effect of frequent breast feeding on early milk production and infant weight gain. Pediatrics 72: 307–311
14. de Chateau P, Holmberg H, Jakobsson K, Winberg J 1977 A study of factors promoting and inhibiting lactation. Developmental Medicine and Child Neurology 19: 575–584
15. Christensson K, Siles C, Moreno L 1992 Temperature, metabolic adaptation and crying in healthy full term newborns cared for skin to skin or in a cot. Acta Paediatrica 81: 488–493
16. Clarke A, Rudd P 1992 Neonatal BCG immunization. Archives of Disease in Childhood 67: 473–474
17. Colditz G A, Berkey C S, Mosteller F et al 1995 The efficacy of Bacillus Calmette–Guerin vaccination of newborns and infants in the prevention of tuberculosis: meta-analysis of the published literature. Pediatrics 96: 29–35
18. Craig J C, Knight J F, Sureshkumar P et al 1996 Effect of circumcision on the incidence of urinary tract infection in pre-school boys. Journal of Pediatrics 128: 23–27
19. Cushing A H 1985 Omphalitis: a review. Pediatric Infectious Disease 4: 282–285
20. Dahmus M A, Sibai B M 1993 Blunt abdominal trauma: are there predictive factors for abruptio placentae or maternal fetal distress. American Journal of Obstetrics and Gynecology 169: 1054–1059
21. Dankert-Roelse J E, Te Meerman G J, Martijn A, Ten Kate L P, Knol K 1989 Survival and clinical outcome in patients with cystic fibrosis, with or without neonatal screening. Journal of Pediatrics 114: 362–367
22. Davis J A, Harvey D R, Stevens J F 1966 Osmolality as a measure of dehydration in the neonatal period. Archives of Disease in Childhood 41: 448–450
23. Delage G, Remy-Prince S, Ducic S, Pierri E, Montplaisir S 1988 Combined passive-active immunization against the hepatitis B virus of 132 newborns of chronic carrier mothers: long term results. Pediatric Infectious Disease Journal 7: 769–776
24. Dewey K G, Heinig M J, Nonunsen L A, Lonnerdal B 1991 Maternal versus infant factors related to breast milk intake and a residual milk volume: the DARLING Study. Pediatrics 87: 829–837
25. Dungy C I, Christensen-Szalansk J, Losch M, Russel D 1992 Effect of discharge samples on duration of breast feeding. Pediatrics 90: 233–237
26. Ekelund H, Finnstrom O, Gunnarskog J, Kallen B, Larsson Y 1993 Administration of vitamin K to newborn infants and childhood cancer. British Medical Journal 307: 89–91
27. Elias-Jones A C 1986 Triple antibiotic spray application to umbilical cord. Early Human Development 13: 299–302
28. Evans K, Evans R, Simmer K 1995 Effect of the method of breast feeding on breast engorgement, mastitis and infantile colic. Acta Paediatrica 84: 849–852
29. Gillespie W A, Simpson K, Tozer R C 1958 Staphylococcal infection in a maternity hospital: epidemiology and control. Lancet ii: 1075–1080
30. Glotzbach S F, Edgar D, Boeddiker M, Ariagno R L 1994 Biological rhythmicity in normal infants during the first 3 months of life. Pediatrics 94: 482–488
31. Golding J, Greenwood R, Birmingham K, Mott M 1992. Childhood cancer, intramuscular vitamin K and pethidine given during labour. British Medical Journal 305: 341–346
32. Gray-Donald K, Kramer M S, Munday S, Leduc D G 1985 Effect of formula supplementation in the hospital on the duration of breast feeding: a controlled clinical trial. Pediatrics 75: 514–518
33. Green M R, Weaver L T, Heeley A F et al 1993 Cystic fibrosis identified by neonatal screening: incidence, genotype and early natural history. Archives of Disease in Childhood 68: 464–467
34. Gunther M 1970 Infant feeding. Methuen, London
35. Gustafsson D, Lowhagen T, Andersson K 1992 Risk of developing atopic disease after early feeding with cows milk based formula. Archives of Disease in Childhood 67: 1008–1010
36. Hanson K N, Ebbesen F 1996 Neonatal vitamin K prophylaxis in Denmark: three years experience with oral administration during the first 3 months of life compared with one oral administration at birth. Acta Paediatrica 85: 1137–1139
37. Harries J T 1978 Meconium in health and disease. British Medical Bulletin 34: 75–78
38. Henningsson A, Nystrom B, Tunnell R 1981 Bathing or washing babies after birth. Lancet ii: 1401–1403
39. Hillervik-Lindquist C, Hofvander Y, Stolin S 1991 Studies on perceived breast milk insufficiency. Acta Paediatrica Scandinavica 80: 297–303
40. Host A, Husby S, Osterballe O 1988 A prospective study of cows milk allergy in exclusively breast fed infants. Acta Paediatrica Scandinavica 77: 663–670
41. Hurst N M 1996 Lactation after augmentation mammoplasty. Obstetrics and Gynecology 87: 30–34
42. Illingworth R S 1985 Infantile colic revisited. Archives of Disease in Childhood 60: 981–985
43. Isenberg S J, Apt L, Wood M 1995 A controlled trial of povidone iodine as prophylaxis against ophthalmia neonatorum. New England Journal of Medicine 332: 562–566
44. Jakobsson I, Linberg T 1983 Cow's milk proteins cause infantile colic in breast fed infants: A double blind crossover study. Pediatrics 71: 268–271
45. John T J 1984 Immune response of neonates to oral poliomyelitis vaccine. British Medical Journal 289: 881
46. Jordan M E, Blum R W M 1996 Should breast feeding by women with silicone implants be recommended? Archives of Pediatrics and Adolescent Medicine 150: 880–888
47. Kauppila A, Kivinen S, Ylikorkala D 1981 Metoclopramide increases prolactin release and milk secretion in puerperium with stimulating the secretion of thyrotropin and thyroid hormones. Journal of Clinical Endocrinology and Metabolism 52: 436–439
48. Klebanoff M A, Read J S, Mills J L, Shiono P H 1993 The risk of childhood cancer after neonatal exposure to vitamin K. New England Journal of Medicine 329: 905–908
49. Kleessem B, Bunke H, Tovar K et al 1995 Influence of two infant formulas and human milk on the development of the fecal flora in newborn infants. Acta Paediatrica 84: 1347–1356
50. Kuhr M, Paneth N 1982 Feeding practices and early neonatal jaundice. Journal of Pediatric Gastroenterology and Nutrition 1: 485–488
51. Kurinij N, Shiono P H 1991 Early formula supplementation of breast feeding. Pediatrics 88: 745–750
52. Kuzemko J A 1986 Screening, early neonatal diagnosis and prenatal diagnosis. Journal of the Royal Society of Medicine 79 (suppl. 12): 2–5
53. Levine J J, Lin H-C, Rowley M et al 1996 Lack of autoantibody expression in children born to mothers with silicone breast implants. Pediatrics 97: 243–245
54. McFarlane J A, Smith D M, Garrow D H 1978 The relationship between mother and neonate. In: Kitzinger S, Davis J A (eds) The place of birth. Oxford University Press, Oxford, pp 185–200
55. McNinch A W, Tripp J H 1991 Haemorrhagic disease of the newborn in the British Isles: 2 year prospective study. British Medical Journal 303: 1105–1109
56. Maisels M J, Gifford K, Antle C E, Leib G R 1988 Jaundice in the healthy newborn: a new approach to an old problem. Pediatrics 81: 505–511
57. Mathew O P 1991 Science of bottle feeding. Journal of Pediatrics 119: 511–519
58. Mennella J A, Beauchamp G K 1991 The transfer of alcohol to human milk. New England Journal of Medicine 325: 981–985
59. Mennella J A, Beauchamp G K 1993 The effects of repeated exposure to garlic flavoured milk on the nursling's behaviour. Pediatric Research 34: 805–808
60. Michaelsen K F, Larsen P S, Thomsen B L, Samuelson G 1994 The Copenhagen cohort study on infant nutrition and growth: duration of breast feeding and influencing factors. Acta Paediatrica 83: 565–571
61. Michaels K B, Willett W C, Rosner B A et al 1996 Prospective assessment of breast feeding and breast cancer among 89887 women. Lancet 347: 431–436
62. Mifsud A, Seal D, Wall R, Valman B 1988 Reduced neonatal mortality from infection after introduction of respiratory monitoring. British Medical Journal 296: 17–18
63. Moore D J, Robb T A, Davidson G P 1988 Breath hydrogen response to milk containing lactose in colicky and non-colicky infants. Journal of Pediatrics 113: 979–984

64. Moss G D, Cartlidge P H T, Speidel B D, Chambers T L 1991 Routine examination in the neonatal period. British Medical Journal 302: 878–879
65. Nishida H, Risenberg H M 1975 Silver nitrate ophthalmic solution and chemical conjunctivitis. Pediatrics 56: 368–373
66. O'Brien K L, Ruff A J, Louise M A et al 1995 Bacillus Calmette–Guerin complications in children born to HIV-1 infected women, with a review of the literature. Pediatrics 95: 414–418
67. Olsen J H, Hertz H, Blinkengerg K, Verder H 1994 Vitamin K regimens and incidence of childhood cancer in Denmark. British Medical Journal 308: 895–896
68. Ormerod L P, Garnett J M 1988 Tuberculin response after neonatal BCG vaccination. Archives of Disease in Childhood 63: 1491–1492
69. Parmelee A H 1961 Sleep patterns in infancy. Acta Paediatrica Scandinavica 50: 160–170
70. Peltonen T 1981 Placental transfusions–advantages and disadvantages European Journal of Pediatrics 137: 141–146
71. Powers N G, Naylor A J, Wester R A 1994 Hospital policies: crucial to breast feeding success. Seminars in Perinatology 18: 517–524
72. Rautava P, Helenius H, Lehtonen L 1993 Psychosocial predisposing factors for infantile colic. British Medical Journal 307: 600–604
73. Raybum W F 1996 Clinical commentary: The bromocriptine (Partodel) controversy and recommendations for lactation suppression. American Journal of Perinatology 13: 69–71
74. Righard L, Alade M O 1990 Effect of delivery room routines on success of first breast feed. Lancet 336: 1105–1107
75. Roberton N R C 1996 A manual of normal neonatal care, 2nd edn. Edward Arnold, London
76. Roche A F, Guo S, Moore W M 1989 Weight and recumbent length from 1–12 months of age: reference data for 1 month increments. American Journal of Clinical Nutrition 49: 599–607
77. Salariya E M, Easton P M, Cater J I 1978 Duration of breast feeding after early initiation of frequent feeding. Lancet ii: 1141–1143
78. Schoen E J 1993 Circumcision updated-indicated. Pediatrics 92: 860–861
79. Schulte F J 1981 Developmental neurophysiology. In Davis J A, Dobbing J (eds) Scientific foundation of paediatrics, 2nd Edn. Heinemann, London, pp 785–829
80. Slaven S, Harvey D R 1981 Unlimited suckling time improves breast feeding. Lancet i: 392–393
81. Thompson J E, Clark D A, Salisbury B, Cahill J 1981 Footprinting the newborn infant: not cost effective. Journal of Pediatrics 99: 797–798
82. Trevarthen C, Murray L, Hubley P 1981 Psychology of infants. In: Davis J A, Dobbing J Scientific foundation of paediatrics, 2nd Edn. Heinemann, London, pp 211–274
83. Unvas-Moberg K, Eriksson M 1996 Breast feeding: physiological endocrine and behavioural adaptations caused by oxytocin and local neurogenic activity in the nipple and mammary gland. Acta Paediatrica 85: 525–530
84. Varendi H, Porter R H, Winberg J 1994 Does the newborn baby find the nipple by smell? Lancet 344: 989–990
85. Von Kries R, Gobel U, Hachmeister A, Kaletsch U, Michaelis J 1996 Vitamin K and childhood cancer: a population based case-control study in Lower Saxony, Germany. British Medical Journal 313: 199–203
86. Von Kries R, Hachmeister A, Gobel U 1995 Repeated oral vitamin K prophylaxis in West Germany: acceptance and efficacy. British Medical Journal 310: 1097–1098
87. Vorherr H 1979 Pregnancy and lactation in relation to breast cancer risk. Seminars in Perinatology 3: 299–311
88. Wallace J P, Inbar G, Emsthausen K 1992 Infant acceptance of post exercise breast milk. Pediatrics 89: 1245–1247
89. Weaver L T, Green M R, Nicholson K et al 1994 Prognosis in cystic fibrosis treated with continuous flucloxacillin from the neonatal period. Archives of Disease in Childhood 70: 84–89
90. Weissbluth M D, Christoffel K K, Todd-Davis A 1984 Treatment of infantile colic with dicyclomine hydrochloride. Journal of Pediatrics 104: 951–955
91. Whitfield M F, Kay R, Stevens S 1981 Validity of routine clinical test weighing as a measure of the intake of a breast fed infant. Archives of Disease in Childhood 56: 919–921
92. Wilcken B, Wiley V, Sherry G et al 1995 Neonatal screening for cystic fibrosis: a comparison of two strategies for case detection in 1.2 million babies. Journal of Pediatrics 127: 965–970
93. Wilson C B, Ochs H D, Almquist J, Dassel S, Mauseth R, Ochs U H 1985 When is umbilical cord separation delayed? Journal of Pediatrics 107: 292–294
94. Winberg J, Bollgren I, Gothefors L et al 1989 The prepuce: a mistake of nature. Lancet i: 598–599
95. Wiswell T E, Enzenauer R W, Holton M E, Cornish J D, Hawkins C T 1987 Declining frequency of circumcision; implications for changes in the absolute incidence and male to female sex ratio of urinary tract infections in early infancy. Pediatrics 79: 338–342
96. Yamauchi Y, Yamanouchi I 1990 Breast feeding frequency during the first 24 hours after birth in full term neonates. Pediatrics 86: 171–175
97. Zipursky A 1996 Vitamin K at birth. British Medical Journal 313: 179–180

23

Care of the normal small baby and the convalescing NICU graduate

N. R. C. Roberton

INTRODUCTION

About 6–7% of babies born in the United Kingdom weigh less than 2.5 kg. One-third of these will be small for dates (Chapter 10), 70% of them will be in the birthweight bracket 2.0–2.5 kg, and the majority of these, and probably at least half of those weighing 1.5–2.0 kg, will have minimal or no illness in the neonatal period.

In the past it was recommended that all babies under 2.5 kg be admitted to special care baby units,[23] but in last 25 years it has been increasingly recognized that this is not necessary. This anxiety about babies weighing less than 2.5 kg came from a misinterpretation of the routinely collected data on such babies. There is no doubt that the incidence of illness is higher in babies between 1.75 and 2.50 kg, but for those who are asymptomatic at birth and subsequently, there is no evidence that caring for them on a postnatal ward with their mother causes any harm so long as certain basic monitoring procedures can be undertaken.[17] Furthermore, caring for these babies on a postnatal ward removes them from the greater hazard of nosocomial infection that occurs in neonatal intensive care units,[26,27,30] leaves the nurses on those units to look after the critically ill low-birthweight baby, and also, by keeping the baby with his mother, obviates the risks of mother–child separation (Chapter 5).

It is now generally accepted that there are only two criteria for admission to a NICU:

- Birthweight <1.70 kg;
- Illness.

For the asymptomatic baby weighing 1.7–2.50 kg postnatal ward care should now be the norm. In this chapter I will attempt to pull together the various aspects of the care of that baby, together with the care of the convalescent VLBW neonate still in the special care side of a NICU.

TRANSITIONAL CARE UNITS

Although babies weighing 1.70–2.50 kg can be managed safely on a postnatal ward with their mother they are at greater risk of complications in the neonatal period, and must therefore be supervised much more carefully than the entirely normal appropriate-for-dates full-term baby. To concentrate the skills necessary to do this, many hospitals in the late 1970s developed what became known as transitional care units. This also made it easier for the medical staff to visit the TCU on a daily basis and to check that all the babies were making acceptable progress, in addition to carrying out routine well-baby checks (Chapter 23).

The development of TCUs is easy and they are popular with both staff and patients in many centres.[22,50] One important aspect of their use is that, in addition to the care of small babies who never go into the neonatal unit, they can be used for other groups of babies who are better off out of the neonatal unit (Table 23.1).

Table 23.1 Patients in transitional care units other than small babies

Convalescent NICU graduates
e.g. babies finishing courses of antibiotics
Babies with specific feeding difficulties
e.g. hare lip/cleft palate
Malformed babies
e.g. Down syndrome
Terminal care
e.g. severe neural tube defects
trisomy 13, untreatable metabolic errors
Infants of diabetic mothers
Healthy term babies needing occasional intervention in the NICU
e.g. exchange transfusion in mild/moderate rhesus HDN
Babies who might develop complications and need careful supervision
e.g. infants of drug-addicted mothers
infants of mothers with thyrotoxicosis
Twins and triplets of appropriate weight and gestation

Another potential function if the unit has cubicles and/or isolation facilities is that it can be used for the care of big babies with infectious disorders, which in themselves are not necessarily very serious but which would pose a major risk of cross-infection if they were in a routine postnatal ward or in the neonatal unit. Examples would be mild gastroenteritis and gonococcal ophthalmia.

EQUIPMENT FOR TRANSITIONAL CARE

As well as having appropriately skilled nursing staff and regular neonatal medical input, TCUs should have better-equipped nurseries capable of being maintained at a temperature of 24°C at all times; the same should apply to single rooms which are being used as described above. In addition, the ward itself should be provided with overhead radiant heaters for cribs, phototherapy units, breast pumps, glucometers and accurate electronic scales. The ward should have a resuscitation area with piped oxygen, air and suction, where, should a baby suddenly deteriorate, prompt and efficient resuscitation can take place. The usual strict precautions to minimize nosocomial infection should apply (pp. 1112–1114); each baby should have his own stethoscope, baby bath, soap, Vaseline and tape measure. There is, however, no need for the staff to wear gowns or masks when dealing with the babies, but hand washing, as ever, is mandatory (p. 1113).

CARE OF MOTHERS IN TRANSITIONAL CARE

The 1.70–2.50 kg baby may well need to stay in hospital for 10–14 days before he is feeding and gaining weight satisfactorily and is safe to be discharged home. In our experience most mothers are prepared to stay in for this period of time. We find that if we tell her the truth, namely that it is in the best interests of both her and her baby to stay together in the hospital, she is usually happy to comply. We tell her that she will discharged as soon as possible, and we also have a liberal attitude to letting the mother go out for an hour or two to go home, to do some shopping, or to have a meal with her partner.

In the rare case where the mother does decide to go home, and in particular if the baby is only going to need to stay in hospital for a few more days, we would aim to keep him in the nursery of the TCU rather than admitting him to the NICU, for the same reasons that he was admitted to the TCU in the first place.

ROUTINE CARE OF SMALL BABIES ON A TCU

The care of these babies on the labour ward is identical to that described for term babies (Chapter 22). However, particular emphasis must be placed on keeping them warm (see below). They must also receive their vitamin K (pp. 375, 799). In the ward, umbilical cord care (p. 373), weighing (p. 377), clinical examination (p. 379), screening (p. 380) and family visiting (p. 378) are exactly the same as for term babies. It is also important to emphasize that rooming-in should be practised so long as the baby can maintain his body temperature in the environment of the open ward. Occasionally, for babies in the 1.70–2.00 kg birthweight range, the temperature at which the postnatal ward is comfortable for the mothers – say 20–21°C – may not be sufficient in the first 24–48 hours to sustain the babies' body temperature (p. 294), and thus care in the nursery, which is kept warmer (see above), may be necessary before rooming-in is started.

OBSERVATIONS

These babies are more at risk than normally grown term babies for developing illnesses in the neonatal period. They may, by 4–6 hours of age, develop mild transient tachypnoea, or develop infection at any stage in the neonatal period. They are also more prone to hypothermia. For these reasons they should have their temperature, pulse and respiration recorded on admission to the TCU and 6-hourly during the next 24–48 hours. Daily temperature, pulse and respiration observations therefter are probably acceptable. Apnoea monitoring is inappropriate in the TCU. If a baby is having apnoeic attacks this is a significant symptom for which transfer to the NICU is indicated.

TEMPERATURE CONTROL

Small babies, with a larger surface area to body mass ratio than term babies, are prone to hypothermia in both the labour ward and the TCU. The most effective way to prevent this is to keep the baby clothed and wearing a bonnet. He can and should be nursed in a cot, and I have no doubt at all that the normal 1.80 kg baby can be cot nursed. He may, however, need to be in a warmer than average ward: 22–24°C for the first few days, but by 10 days of age can usually be safely managed in a 21°C room. However, from the data of Azaz et al,[7] if the baby is in an ambient temperature below 22–23°C he is likely to be using the thermoregulatory mechanisms described in Chapter 18, which will place a metabolic demand on him. However, under normal circumstances this does not result in hypothermia nor in compromised weight gain.

If a small baby has a temperature of 35–35.5°C or less just after admission to the TCU from the labour ward, examine him and check that he is otherwise well. If he is, clothe him, including a bonnet, wrap him in a sheet and cover him in two blankets and place him in a warm environment under a radiant warmer or in a 25°C nursery, and check him and his temperature 30–60 minutes later. If his temperature rises to 37°C, as it usually does, no further treatment is required. If it does not, or if a baby who has been on a TCU for some time becomes cold, it is safer to admit him to the NICU for warming and for evaluation, in particular to exclude sepsis.

In general do not put cold babies on a hot water bottle or on heating pads in a cot, because if these are too hot the baby can be burned as he cannot wriggle free.

THE NORMAL PRETERM INFANT

It is now generally accepted that well babies at a gestation of 32–37 weeks with a birthweight of 1.70–2.50 kg can be cared for on a TCU by and with their mothers. In addition to babies who are admitted straight to the TCU direct from the labour ward, many babies of similar birthweight and gestation can be transferred to the unit after a 2–3-day spell in the NICU for some short-lived problem such as transient tachypnoea, the aftermath of mild birth depression or early hypothermia.

Weight changes

Babies of this birthweight and gestation, like term babies, lose up to 10% of their body weight in the first 4–5 days, after which they should gain weight at roughly 10–15 g/kg/24 hours. In the more premature babies nearer 32 weeks and 1.70 kg it may take 6–10 days before their weight begins to show a steady increase.

Prevention of infection

The more preterm babies, at gestations of 32–35 weeks, will have missed a considerable amount of the transplacental infusion of immunoglobulin which is received during the third trimester (p. 1096). They are therefore susceptible to infection, and symptoms suggesting infection in such babies should be meticulously assessed. Nevertheless, by being in the TCU they are less exposed to the risks of nosocomial infection (see above) and our experience is that infection rarely develops.[17,50]

Jaundice

Preterm babies are more likely to become jaundiced than term ones, particularly if they are not feeding well. Bilirubin levels should be measured if jaundice does appear, and phototherapy instituted as indicated using the guidelines appropriate for their gestation.

Hypoglycaemia

Preterm babies are more likely to develop hypoglycaemia (pp. 944, 946) than term babies, even if they are feeding well, though they are of course much less susceptible than small for dates babies (see below). They should therefore have Dextrostix/BM Stix measurements every 8 hours through the first 48 hours, and beyond that time if there are problems with feeding or weight gain. However, so long as these babies are taking adequate volumes of milk our experience is that they rarely become hypoglycaemic in the TCU.[50]

Table 23.2 Birthweight centiles to assess smallness for dates (Reproduced with permission from Yudkin et al[52])

Gestational age (weeks)	3rd	10th
Males		
34	1.69	1.91
35	1.85	2.10
36	2.01	2.28
37	2.17	2.45
38	2.31	2.60
39	2.45	2.75
40	2.58	2.87
41	2.70	2.97
42	2.70	2.98
Females		
34	1.67	1.87
35	1.81	2.03
36	1.96	2.20
37	2.12	2.36
38	2.26	2.51
39	2.38	2.65
40	2.49	2.76
41	2.59	2.86
42	2.60	2.87

SMALL FOR DATES BABIES

The fact that a baby is small for dates can be established using the data shown in Table 23.2. The individual clinician can decide whether or not to include babies below the 10th or the 3rd centile in his group of small-for-dates babies. It should be noted that even the 3rd centile in males goes up to 2.7 kg in babies who are postmature, and the 10th centile approaches 3.00 kg. Our experience is that babies between the 3rd and the 10th centiles rarely if ever have problems with hypoglycaemia so long as they are clinically well and feeding adequately.[31] We do not screen these babies with regular blood glucose measurements.

Scrawny babies (Clifford syndrome)

In addition to babies below the 3rd centile who are undoubtedly at risk from hypoglycaemia, it is important to recognize the baby with Clifford syndrome, who has a birthweight above the 3rd centile and indeed sometimes above even the 10th centile.[20] These babies have a normal length and head circumference for their gestation, have a characteristic scrawny, wide-eyed and alert appearance with little subcutaneous fat, and low liver glycogen stores, placing them at risk from hypoglycaemia. Their state of fetal malnutrition can be confirmed by measuring subcutaneous skinfold thickness.[38]

Clinical problems in small-for-dates babies

The conditions to which the small-for-dates baby is heir are outlined in Chapter 10. However, our experience is that if they escape perinatal asphyxia and do not get cold in the labour ward, the only significant problem is hypoglycaemia.[31]

Epidemiologically, small-for-dates babies have an increased incidence of congenital malformations. However, many of these are obvious at birth (Table 10.3, p. 137) and, for the SFD baby who is apparently normal on clinical examination, the chances of his having a significant congenital malformation are small.

SFD babies may be polycythaemic but do not need to be screened for it.[3] However, if a baby develops symptoms which could be interpreted as being due to polycythaemia (Chapter 32) he should be admitted to the NICU.

Hypoglycaemia in small-for-dates babies

This is the problem that raises major anxieties in the management of SFD babies, and was for many years the reason for separating them from their mothers and admitting them to neonatal ICUs for monitoring and appropriate feeding. However, for the healthy SFD baby weighing more than 1.70 kg the techniques of monitoring for hypoglycaemia, and appropriate prophylaxis to prevent hypoglycaemia by adequate feeding, can be administered safely on the TCU.

The definition and pathophysiology of hypoglycaemia in SFD babies are discussed in Chapter 35, Part 1. In general, within the first 24 hours every endeavour should be made to keep their blood glucose above 1.5 and thereafter above 2.0 mmol/l.

Monitoring for hypoglycaemia

Hypoglycaemia almost always appears in SFD babies within the first 48 hours, when the baby may have a poor caloric intake, especially if breast-fed, and before he has had a chance to lay down glycogen stores to replace those that were either never laid down or were depleted before delivery. The monitoring is based on the assumption that if a baby has an adequate blood glucose (>1.5–2.0 mmol/l) it is unlikely that he will develop hypoglycaemia (<1 mmol/l) in the next few hours, and even if he were to go transiently below 1.0 mmol/l there is no evidence that transient asymptomatic hypoglycaemia causes any long-term sequelae.

The tendency to become hypoglycaemic gets progressively less during the first 48 hours so long as the baby is retaining some milk. Babies whose weight is below the third centile (Table 23.2) should therefore have their blood glucose routinely monitored by Dextrostix or BM Stix at 2, 6, 12, 18, 24, 36 and 48 hours of age. The 18-hour estimation can probably be omitted safely in larger SFD babies as long as feeding is going well, either by nipple or by tube feeding.

Anxieties about the accuracy of Dextrostix/BM Stix estimations are reviewed on page 944. However, we have found them to be acceptable as, when inaccurate, they almost always underestimate true glucose.[41] Therefore, if the recorded value is below 1.5 mmol/l it is important to confirm that hypoglycaemia really is present by doing a true blood glucose estimation in the laboratory.

Prevention of hypoglycaemia

Because of the significant risk of symptomatic hypoglycaemia in small-for-dates babies the correct management is prevention. Babies who are identified as being below the 3rd centile should be fed as described below. If this is done, asymptomatic hypoglycaemia becomes very rare and symptomatic hypoglycaemia does not occur.[31,50]

Treatment of hypoglycaemia

The management of asymptomatic hypoglycaemia in the range 1.0–2.0 mmol/l by adjusting the feeds is described below. A baby with asymptomatic hypoglyaemia <1.0 mmol/l which does not promptly respond to a feed, or any symptomatic hypoglycaemia, should be admitted to the NICU and managed as described on page 747.

CARE OF THE INTENSIVE CARE GRADUATE

Most babies who survive neonatal intensive care have a period in their lives when they are asymptomatic but are still too small to go home, either because they are unable to bottle-feed satisfactorily, or because their small size places them at such risk of hypothermia that they need to stay, if not in an incubator, in the warm 25°C environment of the special care area of an NICU.

These babies in general remain well, but routines should be in place to detect any new problems that may arise before their discharge from the NICU. Serious complications of their initial illness, such as chronic lung disease (p. 613), posthaemorrhagic ventricular dilatation (pp.1258–1261), patent ductus arteriosus (p. 688) or problems to do with short bowel syndrome following resection for necrotizing enterocolitis (p. 755), are dealt with elsewhere in this book.

These patients range from the relatively large preterm baby of 1.5–1.6 kg who has suffered from mild surfactant-deficient RDS needing a short period of IPPV, to the ELBW baby weighing 0.60 kg who survived after a complicated neonatal course, but then has a prolonged stay in the neonatal unit until he is large enough and feeding well enough to be discharged home.

Environmental and emotional needs

The many studies dealing with the emotional needs of the convalescent preterm baby and his family are dealt with in detail in Chapter 5. Every effort should undoubtedly

WEEKLY EXAMINATION

Weight...............................	Age (days)............................
Head circumference...................	Feed......................................
CVS	Respiratory system.................
murmurs......................	Abdomen...............................
pulses..........................	Genitalia.................................
CNS..................................	Eyes......................................
Skin/umbilicus............	ENT: mouth...........................
Hips............................	Drugs.....................................
Other findings..............	....
....	....

Fig. 23.1 Routine 1-week examination.

be made to keep the baby as comfortable as possible (clothes/lambswool), out of noisy incubators[14] and with some attempt to impose a light–dark circadian cycle.[36] Non-nutritive sucking should probably be encouraged during tube feeds, though the benefits are small.[46] More extreme interventions, including kangaroo care, in which the baby spends prolonged periods snuggling in his mother's cleavage,[5] and complex sensory enrichments programmes, have also been described.[1] Trials suggest improved weight gain and earlier discharge; anxieties remain, however, about the designs of many of these studies[32] and the procedures they recommend have, as yet, not entered routine neonatal practice.

Routine surveillance

For the asymptomatic convalescent baby most neonatal units carry out a regular 1-week full clinical examination of the sort outlined in Figure 23.1. The baby's body weight and head circumference should be noted and plotted on an appropriate chart to ensure that normal progress is being made. He should be checked for the presence of clinical features which had not peviously been detected, such as murmurs or herniae. At these examinations conditions that would normally be looked for in the rouine neonatal clinical examination (p. 379), such as congenital dislocation of the hip, should be looked for. It is normal to do a weekly blood test to check for electrolyte disturbance and for anaemia.

Weight gain

The standard rules of neonatal weight gain apply. Babies should gain weight at 15 g/kg/24 hours; however, a not uncommon phenomenon is that, particularly towards the end of his convalescent phase in the neonatal unit, the baby feeds voraciously. If allowed ad libitum feeding many will take more than 180–200 ml/kg/24 hours, and will gain weight at a faster rate. This sort of catch-up growth is frequently seen once the baby goes home and the parents are much less rigid than the nursing staff, feeding volumes up to 300 ml/kg/24 hours.[35] In association with this the baby may develop some peripheral, rather firm oedema. This not uncommonly causes nursing alarm. However, if the baby is otherwise well and there is no evidence of any condition likely to cause peripheral oedema, in particular heart disease with heart failure, the condition is benign and requires no treatment. There is no need to reduce feeds, and in particular there is no need to give a speculative dose of diuretic in the hope of removing this oedema.

Table 23.3 Causes of poor weight gain

Inadequate caloric intake		
	EBM	
	Vomiting	
	Low-volume feeds (e.g. because of apnoea)	
Increased energy expenditure		
	Bronchopulmonary dysplasia	
	Hyperactivity	
		thyrotoxicosis
		cerebral irritability
		fits
		drug withdrawal
	Drug therapy	
		diuretic
		theophylline
	Cold stress	
		bathing, handling, inadequate clothing (supply bonnets)
	Misery	
		no non-nutritive sucking
		discomfort from sheets (lambswool better)
Insufficient supply of essentials other than energy		
	Sodium deficiency	
	Inadequate oxygen-carrying capacity – anaemia	
	Inadequate base – late metabolic acidosis	
Excessive nutrient losses (malabsorption)		
	Gastro-oesophageal reflux	
	Hypertrophic pyloric stenosis	
	Necrotizing enterocolitis	
	Gastroenteritis	
	Protein–energy malnutrition	
	Milk lactose and protein intolerance	
	Congenital enteropathies	
	Short bowel syndrome	

Poor weight gain (Table 23.3)

The commonest cause of poor weight gain, after obvious illness such as CLD and thyrotoxicosis has been excluded, is an inadequate caloric intake, usually because some form of breast milk is being used with a low protein and fat content. This should be dealt with by increasing the intake, if tolerated, or by adding fortifiers (p. 340). Various factors in the environment, such as non-nutritive sucking, lambswool and stimulation programmes, may also improve weight gain (see above).

Anaemia (p. 810), hyponatraemia[6] and metabolic

acidaemia may also be important causes. Hyponatraemia is again a problem of the EBM-fed baby and is one of the reasons for weekly checks of the electrolytes (see below). A metabolic acidaemia used to be seen when the formulae used for feeding preterm were casein rich;[49] since these have been withdrawn this problem rarely, if ever, occurs.

Finally, if weight gain remains poor, rare causes of failure to thrive should be considered (Table 23.3).

Murmurs

A not uncommon finding is that at about 4–6 weeks of age the <1.25 kg survivor develops a soft ejection mid-systolic murmur, maximal in the pulmonary area. Although it is tempting to attribute this to a patent ductus, echocardiographic studies show that this is rarely the case. The murmur arises from the pulmonary vessels, and is a benign flow murmur across the pulmonary valve or at the bifurcation of the pulmonary arteries.[24] It does not require further investigation, and resolves as the baby grows and gets bigger.

Head size and shape

Measuring head circumference is a crucial component of the weekly routine check. The hope is that the baby's head will grow normally, and that there will not be an acceleration in OFC due to underlying posthaemorrhagic ventricular dilatation, or a fall-off in the OFC due to ischaemic cerebral atrophy.

Many preterm babies characteristically develop a long thin dolichocephalic skull. This is the result of the thin, poorly supported skull bones adopting this formation under the influence of gravity while the baby is ill and lying on one side of his head or the other.[18] As geometrically the most efficient way of containing a given volume is within a circle, if the baby's brain growth is normal but is contained in an elliptical skull the head circumference may well be larger than would otherwise have been anticipated. However, this is a normal feature, and the skeletal abnormality can be minimized by nursing techniques in the early neonatal period that support the skull in an O-ring or on some other folded support,[18] but even without intervention the head shape normalizes spontaneously.[42]

Hernia

About 30% of babies under 1.00 kg develop an inguinal hernia during their convalescence,[28,40] with both males and females affected. In some cases it becomes huge. Under normal circumstances this can be repaired at some convenient time prior to the baby's discharge. However, both the literature[25] and our own experience suggest that repairing large hernias in babies with severe chronic lung disease can result in serious or even fatal deterioration. In such cases it is a matter of clinical judgement when to embark upon surgery. There is no need to rush into surgery for 'cosmetic' reasons.

Undescended testicles

As with hernias, delay in the descent of the testes in male ELBW babies is common. No specific treatment is indicated, but if the testes are still not descended by the time of discharge appropriate follow-up should be arranged with a paediatric surgeon.

Retinopathy of prematurity

As outlined on page 913, all babies below 32 weeks' gestation and below 1.50 kg birthweight who received additional oxygen should be routinely checked on a weekly or fortnightly basis for the development of retinopathy of prematurity. For those born at extremely short gestations, this screening programme should start at 32 weeks' postconceptional age. Care should be taken not to give a mydriatic that causes systemic side effects (Table 37.2, p. 918).

Biochemical abnormalities

Routinely each week, electrolytes, calcium, phosphorus and alkaline phosphatase should be measured. Particularly in preterm babies who are being fed with expressed breast milk, hyponatraemia is common owing to a combination of a low sodium intake and the relatively high fractional excretion of sodium (p. 1010). Sodium supplements should be given, ideally prophylactically in the form of breast milk fortifiers, but if these are not being used appropriate sodium supplements will need to be given. Some babies need up to 10 mmol/kg/24 hours as sodium chloride.

The same group of extremely low-birthweight babies are at risk from osteopenia of prematurity. This is discussed in detail in Chapter 38. It will manifest biochemically as hypophosphataemia, a rise in alkaline phosphatase, and occasionally, in severe cases, by hypercalcaemia. This condition should be prevented by appropriate use of supplements in breast-fed babies. However, if it does develop additional phosphate should be given in addition to the routine vitamin supplementation (p. 1005).

Anaemia of prematurity

The surviving VLBW baby becomes anaemic with a nadir of his haemoglobin at 6–8 weeks of age of 7–9 g/dl. The aetiology of the condition is multifactorial (p. 810). Deficiency of haematinics such as iron and folic acid may play a small part in certain groups of babies, but vitamin E deficiency is no longer important.[53] The anaemia is contributed to by iatrogenic blood loss (p. 839), and also by the fact that the rapidly expanding intravascular volume of the growing baby may outstrip the bone marrow's capacity to produce sufficient red cells.

In recent years it has become clear that most babies with the anaemia of prematurity and a low reticulocyte count have low levels of erythropoietin in the plasma (p. 810). The therapeutic use of erythropoietin in these babies is discussed in detail on pages 810–812, but given the cost of the preparation and the relatively trivial symptomatology that is found in association with the anaemia of prematurity, I do not believe that its use is justified on a routine basis. These babies can be allowed to drop their haemoglobin to 7–7.5 g/dl so long as they are not showing any symptoms of anaemia, such as tachycardia, tachypnoea or poor feeding.[2] If these do develop then the simplest form of management is a 10–15 ml/kg transfusion of packed red cells, which rarely needs to be repeated.

Eosinophilia

An interesting finding in many surviving low-birthweight babies is that they have a marked eosinophilia (1×10^9/l) by the age of 3–4 weeks. This often follows an episode of proven sepsis, but is otherwise a benign finding and should not trigger the neonatologist into a hunt for causes for eosinophilia such as parasitic infection.[39]

FEEDING LOW-BIRTHWEIGHT BABIES

THE CONVALESCENT PREMATURE BABY

It is now clear that many advantages flow from the early introduction of minimal enteral feeding to VLBW babies even while they are still very ill (p. 344). This results in their achieving full enteral nutrition sooner rather than later, and spares them the complications of long-term total parental nutrition (pp. 353–354). By the time the baby is convalescent from his acute neonatal illness he will usually be tolerating hourly feeds at a total daily volume of 180–200 ml/kg/24 hours.

In general, nasojejeunal tube feeds are no longer used as they have a high incidence of complications (p. 344), and the percentage of ingested calories absorbed is less if the gastric intraluminal phase of digestion is bypassed.

A large body of experience shows that, when introducing feeds, breast milk is better tolerated than formula. For this reason, if breast milk is not going to be used long term, many nurseries have instituted the practice of using half-strength formula feeds for the first few days until they are tolerated, when a switch to full-strength feeds with one of the preterm baby formulae (p. 343) causes no problem.

In the very small convalescent preterm baby weighing < 1.50 kg it is clear that intermittent bolus feeds are less well tolerated than a continuous milk infusion and cause apnoea, deteriorating respiratory mechanics and transient hypoxia,[15,29,51] complications which may be aggravated by the presence of a nasogastric tube blocking one nostril.[47] However, if these do not occur, continuous infusion or intermittent bolus feeds result in comparable weight gain and nutrient retention.[45]

Non-nutritive sucking using a pacifier during tube feeding may result in more rapid weight gain (see above).[46] It may also train the baby in the techniques of sucking. Once a baby is 30–32 weeks' gestation, so long as he is well enough he can be put to the mother's breast if she intends to breast-feed him.[13] It is unlikely that significant amounts of milk will be ingested in this way, but it can dramatically improve the mother's morale.

Once the baby is 33–34 weeks' gestation he should make a reasonable attempt at 'nipple' feeding, be it from a bottle or the breast, and by 35 weeks most neurologically normal convalescent ex-prematures should be able to nipple feed satisfactorily. For those whose mothers had always hoped to breast-feed, and who had maintained their lactation by expression, it is at these gestations (33–35 weeks) that every attempt should be made to encourage the baby to go to the breast, and if possible to have the mother living in the neonatal unit so that she can learn the technique of breast-feeding a low-birthweight survivor.

FEEDING THE BABY ON THE TCU

Breast-feeding

If the mother is intending to breast-feed her SFD or 32–36-week preterm baby he should always go to the breast in the labour ward (p. 376). Thereafter she should aim to put him to the breast 3-hourly through the next 48 hours, so that he obtains the colostrum and stimulates her lactation. The 3-hourly routine is recommended as these babies do better with small frequent feeds, and with the shorter interfeed interval hypoglycaemia is less likely. In babies of 32–33 weeks' gestation or 1.70–2.00 kg it is a matter of clinical judgement whether or not to give them complementary feeds by bottle or tube routinely during the first 48–72 hours, or indeed after this time. However, so long as the Dextrostix/BM Stix stay above 2.0 mmol/l there is probably no need to do this.

If a low blood glucose value is found (p. 947) a feed should be offered straight away and the rise in blood glucose checked 30–60 minutes later. Hypoglycaemia on a reagent strip must always be confirmed by a true glucose measured in the laboratory. Unless the baby is breast-feeding very well and the mother's lactation well established, this additional feed should be of formula, giving 15–20 ml/kg/feed. If the mother's own milk is available this is of course preferable, and can be given by bottle or tube. If the blood glucose has not risen above

Table 23.4 Volumes of milk to feed to normal 1.80–2.50 kg preterm and SFD neonates

Day	Volume/kg/24 h (ml)
1	60
2	90
3	120
4	150
7–10	180–200

1.5–2.0 mmol/l after the feed it may be safer to admit the baby to the NICU for i.v. glucose. If a breast-fed preterm or SFD baby has started complementary feeds for hypoglycaemia at any time in the first 24–48 hours, complementary feeds should probably be continued throughout the rest of that period and until the mother's milk comes in. Complements of 60 ml/kg should be given on day 1 and 90 ml/kg on day 2, divided into eight feeds (Table 23.4).

After the first 48–72 hours hypoglycaemia is unusual. A more relaxed attitude to demand feeding can then be taken, although babies weighing <2.00 kg normally need to breast-feed at least 3-hourly, and if they are not doing so a careful watch should be kept on the Dextrostix/BM Stix and weight gain. However, by the time they have reached 2.30–2.50 kg they are usually naturally stretching out the interfeed interval to 4 hours.

The management of breast-feeding problems in small babies is similar to that for term babies (p. 383) but, as might be expected, recourse to tube feeding is often necessary. Getting the 32–33-weeks baby to suckle successfully demands patience from the mother and skilled nursing support. Demoralization in all parties (nurse, mother, paediatrician and the baby) is not uncommon. It is rare, however, for healthy babies over 33 weeks' gestational age to require more than 3–4 days of complete tube feeding, plus a further 7–10 days when the occasional tube feed is needed.

Although 1.70–2.00 kg babies are less likely to establish breast-feeding than full-term ones the advantage of transitional ward care is that satisfactory breast-feeding is more likely to be achieved than if the mother and baby are separated by admitting the baby to a NICU.[50]

Bottle-feeding

Inevitably, feeding preterm and SFD babies is easier if the mother chooses to bottle-feed rather than breast-feed.

Bottle-fed babies <2.50 kg should also be demand fed, but aiming for a 3-hourly schedule or eight feeds per day, changing towards a 4-hourly schedule and six feeds per day by the time they are 2.50 kg. The babies should probably be offered one of the standard neonatal formulae (Table 19.7, Chapter 19), progressing after a few days to one of the newer preterm follow-up formulae (Table 19.13, Chapter 19); the volumes are given in Table 23.4. If most of this is taken and the baby is not becoming hypoglycaemic, nothing more needs to be done. One of the great advantages of bottle-feeding is that it is known how much milk the baby is taking, and if he is not taking enough and if there are problems with his weight, hypoglycaemia or jaundice, he should be topped up 3-hourly using a nasogastric tube.

Tube feeding

Indication

The decision to use tube feeds is usually based on several factors, including:

- the number of times a baby wakes for a feed – too often or too few;
- how well he suckles during a feed;
- how much milk he ultimately takes, despite apparent initial hunger and enthusiasm;
- the amount of weight lost, or the paucity of weight gain;
- Dextrostix/BM Stix readings.

Probably the most common indication for tube feeding is the small-for-dates baby in the first 24–48 hours whose dextrose is hovering around the 1.0 mmol/l level. This baby should immediately be fed, and as he is often unenthusiastic about it this should be given down the tube. Another clear indication for a tube feed is a 6-day-old baby, breast or bottle-fed, who has lost 8–10% of his birthweight and whose Dextrostix is only 1.0–1.5 mmol. Less dramatic is a bottle-fed baby who is falling 20–30% short of desired intake (Table 23.4) and whose weight gain is poor.

In these situations tube feeding should be considered. In many such babies often all that is required is one or two supplementary or complementary tube feeds before they settle into a satisfactory feeding pattern. In babies at 32–33 weeks' gestation whose attempts at breast-feeding or bottle-feeding are clearly hopeless, full tube feeding should be instituted and can be given on a TCU.

Technique

Oral tubes are marginally easier to pass and do not have the disadvantage that they partially obstruct the nasal airway. However, they cannot be left in situ, and if more than an occasional tube feed is likely to be necessary an indwelling 4 FG nasogastric feeding tube should be inserted. It is perfectly possible to breast- or bottle-feed with an indwelling NG tube, and the baby is spared the unpleasantness of repeated tube passage. The position of the tube should be confirmed by aspirating acid gastric contents or by auscultation over the stomach while blowing 5 ml of air down the tube. The tube should be aspirated before the start of each feed. This is not only essential to confirm that the tube is still in the stomach, but identifies those babies who are not tolerating oral feeds and have milk pooling in their stomach.

To give a tube feed under the influence of gravity the appropriate volume of milk should be allowed to run from some appropriate receptacle: a 20 ml syringe is very useful. It should never be syringed in, other than to overcome the surface tension of bubbles in the tube at the start of a feed. The milk should flow freely, usually over a period of 5–20 minutes, depending on the volume.

Volume and frequency

In general, in preterm and SFD babies the volume given (Table 23.4) should be divided into a 3-hourly feeding schedule. Two-hourly feeds can be given on a TCU for a day or two, but usually these babies and any needing hourly tube feeds are transferred to the NICU.

If the tube feed is complementing a bottle feed the deficit should be made up. If the tube feed is being given following a breast feed, in the first few days when only colostrum is likely to have been taken the full volume should be given (Table 23.4). Thereafter a smaller proportion can be given based on clinical assessment, the Dextrostix/BM Stix, the weight gain and hydration of the baby, and the result of any previous test weighing. If alternate tube and breast feeds are being given the appropriate volume due at that 3-hourly feed should be given by tube.

Complications of tube feeding

The physiological problems with tube feeds seen in the convalescent VLBW baby (see above) are not usually seen in TCU patients. Other complications from tube feeding include pharyngeal, oesphageal, gastric and duodenal perforation with pneumomediastinum and peritonitis.[11,43] Soft silicone tubes have been passed into the bronchus.[33] Gastric perforation can occur spontaneously in the neonatal period, possibly secondary to gut ischaemia around the time of delivery,[9] so that it is possible that in at least some of the reported cases the tube merely passed through a hole that was there anyway. Gastro-oesphageal reflux has been shown to be almost universal in tube-fed preterm infants, increasing the risk of aspiration pneumonia, and there appears to be an association between reflux and apnoea in some cases.[37]

NUTRITIONAL SUPPLEMENTS

Vitamin D

The convalescent ex-premature infant should be given vitamin D supplementation, 400–800 units daily. If this amount of vitamin D is given together with appropriate phosphate supplements, then osteopenia of prematurity should be extremely rare (p. 1005).

Folic acid

Preterm babies who are not folic acid supplemented may become folate deficient and develop a megaloblastic anaemia.[48] It is now routine practice to give folic acid to such babies. We give 1 mg orally weekly until the time of discharge.

Iron

VLBW babies are born before most of the body's stores of iron are laid down in the third trimester of pregnancy. Iron supplements in the past have made no significant difference to the severity of the anaemia of prematurity, but if the babies are being treated with erythropoietin, iron supplementation results in a better response to this drug (p. 811).

For the surviving convalescent premature baby who has received multiple transfusions and therefore multiple doses of intravenous iron, there is no need to rush into iron supplementation. There have been anxieties about iron increasing the susceptibility to infection, particularly as a result of studies in which parenteral iron was undoubtedly associated with this complication.[10] We therefore wait before starting ferrous citrate 2.5 ml/kg/24 hours at about 34 weeks' postconceptional age, shortly before the baby is due for discharge.

DISCHARGING SMALL BABIES

Whether it is the 32–36-week asymptomatic baby on a TCU, a normal small for-dates term baby, or the long-term survivor of neonatal intensive care, discharge can usually be considered if the baby is well and weighs between 1.8 and 2.0 kg. Under normal circumstances this corresponds in the convalescing baby to a postconceptional age of 36–38 weeks. For these babies the discharge must be carefully planned and only carried out when it is clear that it is safe to leave hospital, all the appropriate precautions have been taken, and the home environment and the parents are prepared.

The baby should only be considered for discharge when he is taking 3–4-hourly nipple feeds well and gaining weight at 15 g/kg/24 hours consistently, i.e. about 30 g per day. If he has had lung disease he should be able to feed without a fall in SpO_2 of more than 10%. He should not be having apnoeic attacks, and usually should not be receiving methylxanthines to prevent apnoea; the management of the baby with CLD still in oxygen and on drugs is discussed on page 618. He should be able to maintain his body temperature when normally clothed in a cool special care baby unit maintained at 20–22°C, or a transitional care ward maintained at the same temperature.

For the baby going home from the TCU the mother will have been responsible for most items of his care for the previous 10–14 days, and will, hopefully, now be confident in all aspects of feeding, bathing, changing and caring for him. The mother taking home the NICU graduate should live in the mother and baby suite of the unit for several days beforehand, particularly if she is primiparous, so that she can become skilled in all aspects of her baby's care. Ex-preterm babies are often difficult and fussy feeders, and the mother, the nursing and medical staff must be confident in her ability to cope with this problem prior to the baby's discharge.

IMMUNIZATIONS

It is now widely agreed that prematurity should make no difference to the immunization schedules, and that the baby should receive his first dose of vaccine at whatever postnatal age is recommended locally,[4] and that this results in a good antibody response to DTP, haemophilus and poliomyelitis.[12,21] Although there is a theoretical risk from using oral polio virus vaccine in the baby still in the NICU, no case of vaccine-transmitted polio has been reported from this environment.[19] Hepatitis B[34] and BCG[44] immunizations are, however, probably less effective in preterm babies, but should be given where appropriate (p. 379). In addition, we give influenza vaccine to NICU graduates who are discharged during the winter months.

If the routine immunizations are at 2 months of age with triple vaccine, Hib and polio this should be given at 2 months postdelivery age. This means that the 26-week premature baby should receive his first set of immunizations at 34 weeks postconception, when he will usually still be in the neonatal unit. This may provoke apneoic attacks and bradycardia; appropriate monitoring should therefore be started on the day of the immunization.[16] It will also cause a rise in CRP.[8]

There are very few contraindications to immunizing these babies, and most workers would feel that acquired neurological disease in the neonatal period is not a contraindication even to the pertussis component of the vaccine. It is particularly important that babies with chronic lung disease receive the pertussis component, as pertussis superimposed on the lung disease can be a devastating illness.

POST-DISCHARGE CARE

Vitamin supplements

The NICU graduate should receive iron and vitamin D supplementation from the time of discharge until he is at least 6 months old. For the preterm TCU graduate similar supplementation should be given if he is breast-fed, but as all formulae are now supplemented it is doubtful whether additional vitamins and iron are required for bottle-fed babies. SFD graduates from the TCU in general do not require supplements.

Table 23.5 Criteria for follow-up of NICU graduates

< 1.50 kg birthweight
Convulsions
HIE
Meningitis
Hyperbilirubinaemia requiring exchange transfusion
Intracranial lesion on ultrasound scan
Persisting murmurs
Persisting structural abnormalities, e.g. hernia, vesicoureteric reflux, undescended testicles
NEC survivors
Babies with CLD at discharge

Milk feeds

As outlined above, many neonatal intensive care unit graduates feed voraciously once discharged. To help manage this problem, special preterm follow-on milks have now been designed (p. 346).[35] For the larger preterm baby and the normal small-for-dates baby discharged from a TCU who is not breast-feeding, normal bottle feeds appropriate for their postconceptional age should be used (Table 19.8, p. 327).

Follow-up

For the TCU graduate who has had an uncomplicated course there is no need for the hospital to follow him up and see him again in outpatients. The postdischarge care of this baby should be part of the routine skills of the infant health surveillance system in the UK.

For the NICU graduate, however, follow-up is important, but it is important to be selective. There is no point in bringing back at frequent intervals to the well-baby clinic large numbers of neonatal intensive care graduates who had an uncomplicated course and who did not suffer any illness likely to result in neurological sequelae. This group of babies can be left to the routine surveillance programmes running in the community. However, hospital follow-up should be arranged for all babies who had the illnesses listed in Table 23.5.

REFERENCES

1. Als H, Lawhon G, Duffy F H et al 1994 Individualized developmental care for the very low-birth-weight preterm infant. Journal of the American Medical Association 272: 853–858
2. Alvarson D C 1995 The physiologic impact of anemia in the neonate. Clinics in Perinatology 22: 609–625
3. Americian Academy of Pediatrics 1993 Routine evaluation of blood pressure, hematocrit and glucose in newborns. Pediatrics 92: 474–476
4. American Academy of Pediatrics 1994 Red Book: report of the committee on infectious disease, 23rd edn. pp. 51–52
5. Anderson G C 1991 Current knowledge about skin-to-skin (kangaroo) care for preterm infants. Journal of Perinatology 11: 216–226
6. Arant B S 1993 Sodium chloride and potassium. In: Tsang R C, Lucas A, Uauy R, Zlotkin S (eds) Nutritional needs of the preterm infant. Williams & Wilkins, Baltimore, pp 157–175
7. Azaz Y, Fleming P J, Levine M, McCabe R, Stewart A, Johnson P 1992 The relationship between environmental temperature, metabolic rate,

and evaporative water loss in infants from birth to three months. Pediatric Research 32: 417–423
8. Balkundi D R, Nycyk J A, Cooke R W I 1994 Immunization and C reactive protein in infants on neonatal intensive care units. Archives of Disease in Childhood 71: 149
9. Bayatpour M, Bernard L, McCune F, Bariel W 1979 Spontaneous gastric rupture in the newborn. American Journal of Surgery 137: 267–269
10. Beecroft D M O, Dix M R, Farmer K 1977 Intramuscular iron-dextran and susceptibility of neonates to bacterial infections. Archives of Disease in Childhood 52: 778–781
11. Bell M J 1985 Perforation of the gastrointestinal tract and peritonitis in the neonate. Surgery, Gynecology and Obstetrics 160: 20–26
12. Bernbaum J C, Daft A, Anolik R et al 1985 Response of preterm infants to diphtheria-tetanus-pertussis immunizations. Journal of Pediatrics 107: 184–188
13. Bier J A B, Ferguson A, Anderson L et al 1993 Breast feeding of very low birthweight infants. Journal of Pediatrics 123: 773–778
14. Blennow G, Svenningsen N W, Almquist B 1974 Noise levels in incubators. Pediatrics 53: 29–33
15. Blondheim O, Abbasi S, Fox W W, Bhutani V K 1993 Effect of enteral gavage feeding rate on pulmonary functions of very low birthweight infants. Journal of Pediatrics 122: 751–755
16. Botham S J, Isaacs D 1994 Incidence of apnoea and bradycardia in preterm infants following triple antigen immunization. Journal of Paediatrics and Child Health 30: 533–535
17. Campbell D M, Gandy G M, Roberton N R C 1983 Which babies need admission to special care baby units? In: Davis J A, Richards M P M, Roberton N R C (eds). Parent baby attachment in premature infants. Croom Helm, London, pp 67–85
18. Cartlidge P H T, Rutter N 1988 Reduction of head flattening in preterm infants. Archives of Disease in Childhood 63: 755–757
19. Cherry J D, Enteroviruses. In: Remington J S, Klein J O (eds) Infectious diseases of the fetus and newborn infant, 4th edn. W B Saunders, Philadelphia, pp 404–446
20. Clifford S H 1954 Post-maturity with placental dysfunction. Journal of Pediatrics 44: 1–13
21. D'Angio C T, Maniscalco W M, Pichichero M E 1995 Immunologic response of extremely premature infants to tetanus, haemophilus influenzae and polio immunization. Pediatrics 96: 18–22
22. Dear P R F, McClain B I 1987 Establishment of an intermediate care ward for babies and mothers. Archives of Disease in Childhood 62: 597–600
23. Department of Health and Social Security 1971 Report of the expert group on special care for babies (Sheldon report). Reports on public health and medical subjects No. 127. HMSO, London
24. Dunkle L M, Rowe R D 1972 Transient murmurs stimulating pulmonary artery stenosis in premature infants. American Journal of Diseases of Children 124: 666–70
25. Emberton M, Patel L, Zideman D A et al 1996 Early repair of inguinal hernia in preterm infants with oxygen dependent bronchopulmonary dysplasia. Acta Paediatrica 85: 96–99
26. Gaynes R P, Edwards J R, Jarvis W R et al 1996 Nosocomial infections among neonates in high risk nurseries in the United States. Pediatrics 98: 357–361
27. Goldman D A, Leclair J, Malone A 1978 Bacterial colonization of neonates admitted to an intensive care environment. Journal of Pediatrics 63: 288–293
28. Harper R G, Garcia A, Sia C 1975 Inguinal hernia: a common problem of premature infants weighing 1000 grams or less at birth. Pediatrics 56: 112–115
29. Heldt G P 1988 The effect of gavage feeding on the mechanics of the lung, chest wall and diaphragm of preterm infants. Pediatric Research 24: 55–58.
30. Jarvis W R 1987 Epidemiology of nosocomial infections in pediatric patients. Pediatric Infectious Disease Journal 6: 344–351
31. Jones R A K, Roberton N R C 1986 Small for dates babies: are they really a problem? Archives of Disease in Childhood 61: 877–880
32. Lacy J B, Ohlsson A 1993 Behavioural outcomes of environmental or care giving hospital based interventions for preterm infants: a critical overview. Acta Paediatrica 82: 408–415
33. Laing I A, Lang M A, Callaghan O, Hume R 1986 Nasogastric compared with nasoduodenal feeding in low birthweight infants. Archives of Disease in Childhood 61: 138–141
34. Lau Y-L, Tam A Y C, Ng K W et al 1992 Response of preterm infants to hepatitis B vaccine. Journal of Pediatrics 121: 962–965
35. Lucas A, King F, Bishop N R 1992 Post-discharge formula consumption in infants born preterm. Archives of Disease in Childhood 67: 691–692
36. Mann N P, Haddow R, Stokes L et al 1986 Effect of night and day on preterm infants in a newborn nursery: randomized trial. British Medical Journal 293: 1265–1267
37. Newell S J, Booth I W, Morgan M E I, Durbin G M, McNeish A S 1989 Gastrooesophageal reflux in preterm infants. Archives of Disease in Childhood 64: 780–786
38. Oakley J R, Parsons R J, Whitelaw A G L 1977 Standards for skin fold thickness in British newborn infants. Archives of Disease in Childhood 52: 287–390
39. Patel L, Garvey B, Arnon S, Roberts I A G 1994 Eosinophilia in newborn infants. Acta Paediatrica 83: 797–801
40. Peevy K J, Speed F A, Hoff C J 1986 Epidemiology of inguinal hernia in pretern neonates. Pediatrics 77: 246–247
41. Reynolds G J, Davies S 1993 A clinical audit of cotside blood glucose measurement in the detection of neonatal hypoglycaemia. Journal of Paediatrics and Child Health 29: 289–291
42. Rutter N, Hinchcliffe W, Cartlidge P H T 1993 Do preterm infants always have flattened heads? Archives of Disease in Childhood 68: 606–607
43. Sands T, Glasson M, Berry A 1989 Hazards of nasogastric tube insertion in the newborn infant. Lancet ii: 680
44. Sedaghatian M R, Kardouni K 1993 Tuberculin reponse in preterm infants after BCG vaccination at birth. Archives of Disease in Childhood 69: F309–311
45. Silvestre M A A, Morbach C A, Brans Y W, Shankaran S 1996 A prospective randomized trial comparing continuous versus intermittent feeding methods in very low birthweight neonates. Journal of Pediatrics 128: 748–752
46. Steer P A, Lucas A, Sinclair J C 1992 Feeding the low birthweight infant. In: Sinclair J C, Bracken M B (eds) Effective care of the newborn infant. Oxford University Press, Oxford, pp 94–138
47. Stocks J 1980 Effect of nasogastric tubes on nasal resistance during infancy. Archives of Disease in Childhood 55: 17–21
48. Strelling M K, Blackledge D G, Goodall H B 1979. Diagnosis and management of folate deficiency in low birthweight infants. Archives of Disease in Childhood 54: 271–277
49. Svenningsen N W, Lindquist B 1973 Incidence of metabolic acidosis in term, preterm and small for gestational age infants in relation to dietary intake. Acta Paediatrica Scandinavica 62: 1–10
50. Whitby C, De Cates C, Roberton N R C 1982 Infants weighing 1.8 to 2.5 kg: should they be cared for in neonatal units or postnatal wards? Lancet i: 322–325
51. Wilkinson A, Yu V Y H 1974 Immediate effects of feeding on blood gases and some cardiorespiratory functions in ill newborn infants. Lancet i: 1083–1085
52. Yudkin P L, Aboualfa M, Eyre J et al 1987 New birthweight and head circumference centiles for gestational ages 24–42 weeks. Early Human Development 15: 45–52
53. Zipursky A 1984 Vitamin E deficiency anemia in newborn infants. Clinics in Perinatology 11: 393–402

24

The infant of a diabetic mother

J. M. Hawdon *Albert Aynsley-Green*

The fertility and well-being of diabetic women dramatically improved with the availability of insulin, but a high perinatal mortality rate of 20–25% persisted until the 1960s. In the last three decades perinatal mortality rates have fallen and rates below 3% have been achieved in some of the best centres.[22,45,71]

Pregnancy may occur either in an established diabetic or in one who develops transient or permanent diabetes during pregnancy. Gestational diabetes presents a special problem because the diagnosis may be unsuspected or missed unless pregnant women are routinely screened by urinalysis and by a subsequent oral glucose load, a process which has now been advocated for all pregnant women.[67] The pregnancy in established or gestational diabetes may be complicated by one or more of a wide variety of problems in the fetus and in the newborn. Before discussing each of these problems separately, it seems appropriate to start with Farquhar's[30] vivid and classic description of infants of poorly controlled diabetic mothers:

> they emerge at least alive from within the fiery metabolic furnace of diabetes mellitus, but they resemble one another so closely that they might well be related. They are plump, sleek, liberally coated with vernix caseosa, full-faced and plethoric. During their first two or more extrauterine hours they lie on their backs, bloated and flushed, their legs flexed and abducted, their lightly closed hands on each side of the head, the abdomen prominent and their respiration sighing. They convey a distinct impression of having such a surfeit of both food and fluid pressed upon them by an insistent hostess that they desire only peace so that they may recover from their excesses.

MACROSOMIA AND SMALLNESS FOR GESTATIONAL AGE

Macrosomia and organomegaly attributed to fetal hyperinsulinaemia are well known characteristics of the offspring of the poorly controlled diabetic woman. Glucose crosses the placenta by facilitated diffusion, therefore maternal hyperglycaemia imposes a carbohydrate surplus on the fetus. The fetus responds with increased secretion of insulin. Because insulin is an anabolic hormone the fetal hyperinsulinaemia stimulates protein, lipid and glycogen synthesis to cause macrosomia. Although this classic maternal hyperglycaemia– fetal hyperinsulinism theory of Pedersen[77] is widely accepted, the metabolic and endocrine disturbances are much more complex. For example, free amino acids also have a stimulatory effect on the development of the β cell, and the anabolic actions of insulin, in utero at least, could in part be mediated through the insulin-induced release of insulin-like growth factors.[26,59] Although body size 'normalizes' during infancy, these babies have an increased risk of obesity in adolescence.[5]

Rates of macrosomia vary between centres, for example from 20% with birthweights above the 97th centile in a Swedish study to only 8% with birthweights above the 90th centile in an Italian study of strict maternal diabetic control.[39,87] The relationship between overall maternal diabetes control and macrosomia is not close,[12] in that some infants may still be born with macrosomia after a pregnancy in which maternal blood glucose levels were apparently well controlled. This may be related to difficulties in defining the parameters describing optimal diabetic control in pregnancy.

The striking physical appearance (Fig. 24.1) of these infants has already been described. Much of the increased mass is fat.[107] The organomegaly is selective, the liver and heart are often enlarged and skeletal length is increased in proportion to weight, but the brain size is not increased relative to gestational age and so the head may appear disproportionately small.[72]

The clinical significance of macrosomia is the risk of the complications of delivery of a large infant, such as shoulder dystocia, obstructed labour and perinatal asphyxia.[1,62] In one study[1] 30% of the infants of diabetic mothers with a birthweight above 4000 g who were delivered vaginally developed shoulder dystocia, with frequent complications such as fractures and brachial plexus palsy.

Maternal diabetic vascular disease leading to placental

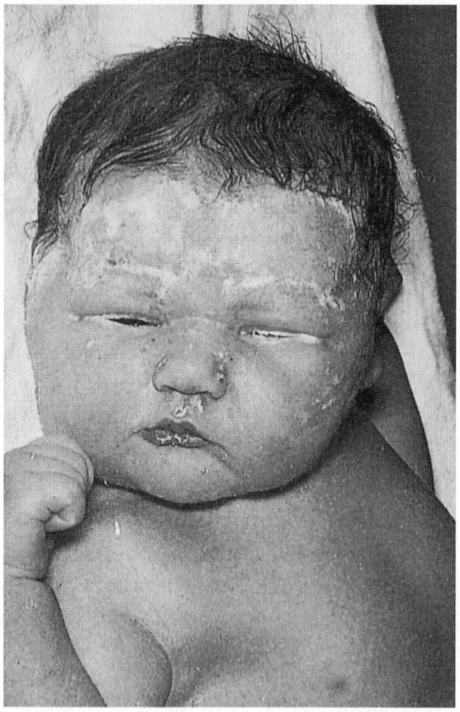

Fig. 24.1 An infant born to a poorly controlled diabetic mother. There is increased adiposity and facial plethora, together with respiratory distress.

insufficiency can impair fetal growth, so some of the infants will be born small for gestational age.[21] Overzealous diabetic control and maternal hypoglycaemia may have the same result.[50] The small for gestational age infant of the diabetic mother appears to be at even greater risk of adverse sequelae than the large obese infant, because the perinatal problems of the IDM are compounded by those of intrauterine malnutrition (Chapter 10).

RESPIRATORY COMPLICATIONS

Although the incidence of respiratory distress syndrome was previously reported to be 5–6 times higher in IDMs than in the normal population, this incidence is falling, in line with improved maternal diabetic control.[39,86] RDS appears to be secondary to the retarded maturation of various aspects of the pulmonary surfactant system, rather than simply to the reduced production of phospholipids. Infants of diabetic mothers may have typical RDS despite a normal lecithin–sphingomyelin ratio in the amniotic fluid. The structure and composition of surfactant phospholipids may be abnormal[73] (p. 484) and decreased concentrations of surfactant-associated protein, an important component of pulmonary surfactant, have been found in the amniotic fluid of diabetic pregnant women.[73] Animal studies have demonstrated that insulin inhibits cortisol-induced lecithin synthesis by pneumocytes, probably by inhibiting the production of fibroblast–pneumocyte factor, which promotes phosphatidylcholine synthesis, and that high glucose concentrations themselves inhibit the incorporation of choline into phosphatidylcholine and that butyrate inhibits the transcription of mRNA for surfactant proteins.[17,37,82,90] Infants of diabetic mothers are also at increased risk for transient tachypnoea of the newborn.[39] Finally, many diabetic women are delivered before term and/or by caesarean section, and the contribution of these factors to increased respiratory morbidity from RDS or TTN must be considered.[70] The management of these respiratory complications, should they occur, should not differ from each unit's standard policy.

HYPOCALCAEMIA AND HYPOMAGNESAEMIA

Neonatal hypocalcaemia has been reported in up to 50% of IDMs,[61,99] and both its incidence and severity appear to be related to the degree of maternal diabetes control.[27,99] Hypocalcaemia is usually associated with hyperphosphataemia and occasionally with hypomagnesaemia. The aetiology of the hypocalcaemia and hypomagnesaemia is not entirely clear, but most authors suggest functional hypoparathyroidism secondary to maternal magnesium loss.[27,64,74,100] Birth asphyxia may also exacerbate hypocalcaemia.

None of the studies that report hypocalcaemia have commented on whether the biochemical finding is of clinical significance. Usually no clinical signs are seen and no treatment is necessary. However, in the presence of signs of hypocalcaemia and hypomagnesaemia the deficit should be corrected as described elsewhere in this book (p. 352). Bone mineral content (measured by direct photon absorptiometry) has been reported to be significantly decreased in IDMs, but it is not known whether there are long-term consequences or whether early aggressive management is necessary.[68]

HYPERVISCOSITY, POLYCYTHAEMIA, JAUNDICE

Infants of diabetic mothers have an increased risk of being polycythaemic and developing the neonatal hyperviscosity syndrome.[61]

Normoblastaemia and extensive extramedullary erythropoiesis in the IDM were observed as early as 1944,[55] and the aetiology of the increased erythropoiesis has since been described.[84] Widness et al[108] found elevated umbilical plasma erythropoietin concentrations in IDMs, and these correlated directly with plasma insulin levels in both IDMs and controls. The raised erythropoietin levels are thought to be secondary to cellular hypoxia, which is the result of insulin-induced high glucose uptake and high metabolic rates causing relative cellular hypoxia. A more direct effect of insulin was shown in another study,[79] in which insulin stimulated growth in culture of late erythroid progenitors in cord blood from premature, term and IDM infants.

Lysis of this red cell load contributes to the prolonged unconjugated hyperbilirubinaemia often found in infants of diabetic mothers.[65,78,97,111] There may also be functional immaturity of hepatic enzymes.[93]

Renal vein thrombosis, which has been reported to occur with increased frequency in IDMs, is probably related to polycythaemia and hyperviscosity.[7,96]

Polycythaemia and hyperbilirubinaemia should be managed as described in Chapter 32, Part 3 and Chapter 31, Part 1.

HYPERTROPHIC CARDIOMYOPATHY

Cardiac enlargement and hypertrophy in IDMs was reported as early as 1944.[55] The condition has now been studied more extensively.[36a,101] Improved echocardiographic techniques have shown a generalized myocardial hypertrophy with a disproportionate thickening of the septum.[53,85,98] Symptomatic infants generally have severe hypertrophy and the hypertrophied septal muscles may bulge into the left ventricle, thereby narrowing the left ventricular outflow tract (Fig. 24.2). The cardiomyopathy may be related to maternal diabetes control[53,85] and to fetal and neonatal hyperinsulinaemia.[13]

If clinical signs occur the presentation is usually within the first weeks of postnatal life, with cardiorespiratory distress and congestive heart failure. Systolic ejection murmurs can be heard in most affected infants, and chest radiography reveals cardiomegaly.[38,106] The majority of the infants need supportive care only. If congestive heart failure develops, propranolol is recommended.[106] Digitalis and other positive inotropic agents are generally contraindicated because they increase systolic contraction and may exacerbate the outflow tract obstruction.[106]

The hypertrophic cardiomyopathy of the IDM is transient. Resolution of the signs can be expected in 2–4 weeks, and the septal hypertrophy regresses within 2–12 months.[85,106] (see also p. 698).

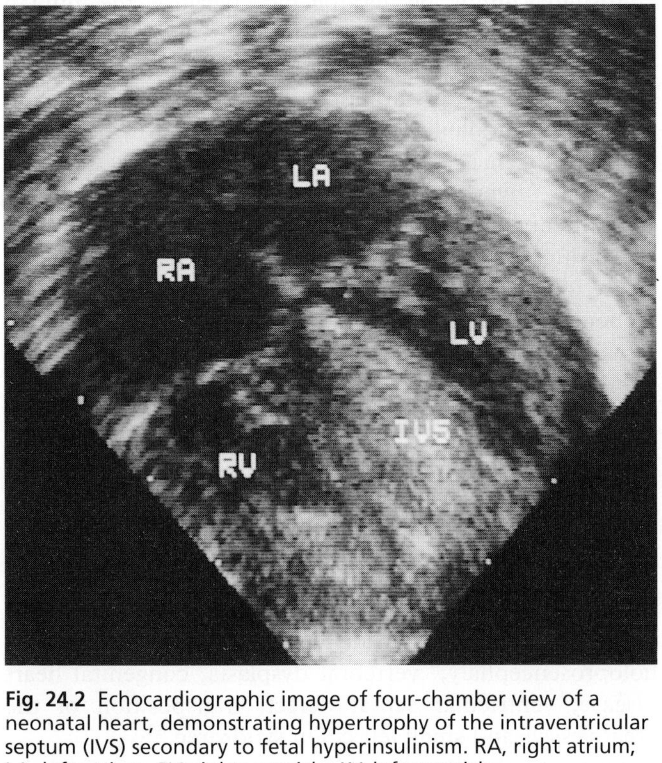

Fig. 24.2 Echocardiographic image of four-chamber view of a neonatal heart, demonstrating hypertrophy of the intraventricular septum (IVS) secondary to fetal hyperinsulinism. RA, right atrium; LA, left atrium; RV, right ventricle; LV, left ventricle.

HYPOGLYCAEMIA (see also Chapter 38, Part 1)

Most IDMs have transient (1–4 hours postnatally) asymptomatic hypoglycaemia before a spontaneous increase in blood glucose level occurs, a pattern also seen in newborn babies of non-diabetic mothers.[49] Others have a more prolonged period of severe symptomatic hypoglycaemia, and a minority develop late hypoglycaemia after an initial benign course. However, all regain normal blood glucose control within the first few days after birth. Recent data have shown that plasma insulin levels fall to normal within 12–24 hours of birth in all infants except those whose mothers' diabetes was poorly controlled.[40] For the full definition and symptoms of hypoglycaemia see page 942.

IDMs have hyperinsulinism at birth owing to increased placental transfer of glucose and other nutrients stimulating increased insulin secretion (see above).[10,46] The pancreas shows hyperplasia and hypertrophy of the islets of Langerhans[16,55,92] without evidence of nesidioblastosis. An increase of the glucagon and pancreatic polypeptide cell fractions in the pancreas has also been shown by modern immunocytochemical methods,[60] although it has been reported that some infants fail to develop the normal increase in plasma glucagon at 2–4 hours of age.[11] Other studies have demonstrated a counterregulatory hormone response which may curtail the period of hypoglycaemia.[6,14,43]

The effect of hyperinsulinism on the liver has been confirmed with stable isotope methods,[47] which demonstrated decreased glucose production. If raised insulin levels persist beyond the first postnatal day other metabolic fuels may be affected. For example, plasma free fatty acid and blood ketone body concentrations may be lower than in normal term infants, although recent studies have not confirmed this.[76] Plasma amino acid concentrations are less affected than in organic hyperinsulinism secondary to congenital pancreatic disorders such as islet cell dysregulation syndrome (p. 945). The characteristic low blood levels of branched-chain amino acids are a not invariable finding,[18,91,102] possibly because of other transient disturbances in postnatal metabolic adaptation, including the effects of concurrent asphyxia or hypoxia.

In relation to management, peripheral blood glucose values should be obtained from mother and cord at delivery and from the infant 3–4-hourly, before feeds, for 6–12 hours after birth. Frequency and duration of monitoring will depend upon antenatal diabetic control and cord blood glucose concentration: when control has been poor and cord blood glucose levels high monitoring should be more intensive. Blood glucose screening may be discontinued when at least two consecutive prefeed blood glucose levels are normal (Chapter 23). The fact that test strip reagents may underestimate blood glucose concentration if packed cell volume is high must be considered; plasma glucose concentration is not affected.[24] Therefore, in polycythaemic infants it is important to measure the plasma and not the whole blood concentration of glucose on test strips. Maternal blood glucose concentration at the time of delivery seems to be an important risk factor in the development of postnatal hypoglycaemia[3] in that mothers with high blood glucose levels are more likely to produce infants who develop hypoglycaemia.

Transient asymptomatic hypoglycaemia may be prevented by giving enteral feeds with milk within 1–2 hours after delivery, as it has been shown that a feed of 10 ml/kg human milk can cause an increase of blood glucose in the order of 1 mmol/l at this time.[8] Daily feed volumes of at least 100 ml/kg may be required to maintain normoglycaemia.

Sick infants unable to tolerate enteral feeding, or those who remain hypoglycaemic despite full enteral feeds, should receive an intravenous infusion of glucose at an initial rate of 4–8 mg/kg/min to prevent the development of hypoglycaemia. If enteral feeds have been tolerated these should not be reduced when intravenous glucose is commenced. Neurological signs of hypoglycaemia in any infant warrant immediate correction by a bolus injection of 200–400 mg/kg glucose followed by glucose infusion, the rate being adjusted as necessary to maintain normoglycaemia. Cortisol (5 mg/kg) has been recommended by others to be given intravenously or intramuscularly at 12-hour intervals. A single injection of glucagon (0.03–0.1 mg/kg), which has a temporary hyperglycaemic effect by releasing glucose from glycogen stores, is a useful measure in the event of delay in siting intravenous lines. Parenteral glucose may be decreased after blood glucose concentrations have been stable for 12 hours or so. Reactive hypoglycaemia may occur if the glucose infusion is decreased too quickly.

CONGENITAL ANOMALIES

Congenital anomalies in the offspring of a diabetic woman occur with a frequency approximately 2–4 times that observed in the general population.[52,69] Despite major improvements in the care of diabetic pregnancies and a fall in anomaly rates in centres where prepregnancy counselling occurs, there has been little overall change in the incidence of malformations. The problem has become even more compelling as the perinatal mortality has fallen, because malformations now account for a large proportion of perinatal losses and have replaced RDS as the leading cause of death in IDMs in many centres.[4,22,25,34,42,95]

The cause of diabetic embryopathy is not fully understood. Genetic factors (diabetes-related genes) are unlikely to play a role, as the incidence of birth defects is not increased in the newborn infants of diabetic fathers.[19] It is now generally accepted that congenital anomalies are related to the diabetic intrauterine environment during the period of organogenesis. As the organs most vulnerable to diabetic embryopathy are formed before the seventh week of gestation,[57] most malformations take place before the pregnancy is recognized and the intensified diabetes treatment is initiated. This explains the failure to decrease the incidence of diabetic embryopathy despite improvements in all other aspects of diabetic pregnancies, and suggests that good diabetic control before conception is mandatory.

The teratogenic effect of hyperglycaemia has been suggested by human studies[54,66,109] and has been confirmed in animal studies.[34,56] In one recent multicentre prospective study, however, there was no correlation between maternal glucose control and the likelihood of birth defects,[58] suggesting that maternal hyperglycaemia may not be the only teratogen. In rodent models hyperketonaemia[44,89] increased levels of somatomedin-inhibiting factors[88] and decreased myoinositol concentration in the neuroectoderm[94] have also been implicated.

Insulin cannot be teratogenic, because the human placenta is impermeable to insulin at early gestation[2] and fetal pancreatic β cells are not present before the 10th week.[51] However, disturbances in the secretion of relaxin, an insulin homologue, have been suggested to be potentially teratogenic.[29]

Finally, hypoglycaemia can also be embryotoxic in experimental animals,[15] but data from human studies are reassuring.[58,66] However, many diabetic patients are not aware of their hypoglycaemic episodes, particularly in diabetes of long duration when counterregulation is impaired.

Although infants of diabetic mothers are at risk for a wide variety of malformations, one syndrome seems to be particularly strongly associated with diabetes, with a relative risk of 212 compared to non-diabetics.[20] The syndrome of caudal regression is a condition in which agenesis or hypoplasia of the femora occurs in conjunction with agenesis of the lower vertebrae (sacral agenesis).[28,75] Other anomalies overrepresented in infants of diabetic mothers are anencephaly, meningomyelocele, holoprosencephaly,[9] vertebral dysplasia, congenital heart disease, ventricular septal defect, transposition of the great vessels and small left colon syndrome.[83]

Owing to the fact that the precise teratogen(s) and the

period(s) of greatest vulnerability[34] are not yet known, definite recommendations concerning the management of the diabetes during early pregnancy cannot be made. It seems prudent to say, however, that the prevention of birth defects should start before conception, with contraceptive advice offered so that every pregnancy can be planned in advance with optimum periconceptual metabolic control. Some reports suggest that early first-trimester improvement in glycaemic control,[35] combined with prenatal diagnosis of anomalies using serum α-fetoprotein determinations and ultrasound scanning,[68] could reduce the rate of congenital anomalies through early termination of affected fetuses.

OUTCOME

Some studies have indicated that one potential consequence of neonatal macrosomia is an increased risk of obesity in later life.[23,103] In other studies, however, the majority of children had normal weight for height and also had normal height for age.[31,81]

According to some studies, infants of poorly controlled diabetic mothers are at greater risk of brain damage and poor psychomotor development. This could be secondary to birth trauma, asphyxia, episodes of maternal ketosis or hypoglycaemia during pregnancy, and to neonatal hypoglycaemia.[41,110] However, other studies[33,80] show a more favourable outcome.

The risk of insulin-dependent diabetes developing by the age of 20 years in the offspring of diabetic women is at least seven times that for non-diabetic parents.[80,105] Interestingly, this is only one-third of the risk reported for the offspring of fathers with insulin-dependent diabetes,[104] and this is possibly because of a lower rate of DR4 allele transmission from mothers.[32]

Careful medical (strict glycaemic control) and obstetric care throughout pregnancy, in combination with appropriate neonatal care, greatly reduces the risk of the many complications discussed in this chapter. Perinatal mortality for IDM is now less than 3% in most major centres, and the vast majority of infants of strictly controlled euglycaemic mothers are of normal size; hypoglycaemia is rarely a problem, the C-peptide level in the cord blood is normal,[36] and the glucose production rate and the postnatal metabolic adjustment are also normal.[16,14,48]

REFERENCES

1. Acker D B, Sachs B P, Friedman E A 1985 Risk factors for shoulder dystocia. Obstetrics and Gynecology 66: 762–768
2. Adam P A J, Teramo K, Raiha N, Gitlin D, Schwartz R 1969 Human fetal insulin metabolism early in gestation. Response to acute elevation of the fetal glucose concentration and placental transfer of human insulin. Diabetes 18: 403–416
3. Anderson O, Hertel J, Schmolker L, Kuhl C 1985 Influence of the maternal plasma glucose concentration at delivery on the risk of hypoglycaemia in infants of insulin-dependent diabetic mothers. Acta Paediatrica Scandinavica 74: 268–273
4. Anon 1988 Congenital abnormalities in infants of diabetic mothers. Lancet i: 1313–1315
5. Anon 1990 Hyperinsulinaemia and macrosomia. New England Journal of Medicine 323: 340–342
6. Artal R, Doug N, Wu P, Sperling M A 1988 Circulating catecholamines and glucagon in infants of strictly controlled diabetic mothers. Biology of the Neonate 53: 121–125
7. Avery M E, Oppenheimer E H, Gordon H H 1957 Renal vein thrombosis in newborn infants of diabetic mothers. New England Journal of Medicine 256: 1134–1138
8. Aynsley-Green A 1982 The control of the adaptation to postnatal nutrition. In: Monographs in paediatrics, Vol. 16. Karger, Basle pp 53–87
9. Barr M, Hanson J W, Currey K et al 1983 Holoprosencephaly in infants of diabetic mothers. Journal of Pediatrics 102: 565–568
10. Block M B, Pildes R S, Mossabhoy N A, Steiner D F, Rubenstein A 1974 C-peptide immunoreactivity: a new method for studying infants of insulin-treated diabetic mothers. Pediatrics 53: 923–928
11. Bloom S R, Johnston D F 1972 Failure of glucagon release in infants of diabetic mothers. British Medical Journal iv: 453–454
12. Bradley R J, Nicolaides K H, Brudenell J M 1988 Are all infants of diabetic mothers 'macrosomic'? British Medical Journal 297: 1583–1584
13. Breitweser J A, Meyer R A, Sperling M A, Tsang R C, Kaplan S 1980 Cardiac septal hypertrophy in hyperinsulinaemic infants. Journal of Pediatrics 96: 535–539
14. Broberger U, Hansson U, Largercrantz H, Persson B 1984 Sympathoadrenal activity and metabolic adjustment during the first 12 hours after birth in infants of diabetic mothers. Acta Paediatrica Scandinavica 73: 620–625
15. Buchanan T A, Schemmer J K, Freinkel N 1986 Embryotoxic effects of brief maternal insulin hypoglycaemia during organogenesis in the rat. Journal of Clinical Investigation 78: 643–649
16. Cardell B S 1953 Hypertrophy and hyperplasia of the pancreatic islets in newborn infants. Pathology 66: 335–341
17. Carlson K S, Smith B T, Post M 1984 Insulin acts on the fibroblast to inhibit glucocorticoid stimulation of lung maturation. Journal of Applied Physiology 57: 1577–1579
18. Cockburn F, Glagden A, Michie E A, Forfar J C 1971 The influence of pre-eclampsia and diabetes mellitus on plasma free amino acids in maternal umbilical vein and infant blood. Journal of Obstetrics and Gynaecology of the British Commonwealth 78: 215–231
19. Comess L J, Bennett P H, Man M B et al 1969 Congenital anomalies and diabetes in the Pima Indians of Arizona. Diabetes 18: 471–477
20. Coombs C A, Kitzmuiller J C 1991 Spontaneous abortion and congenital malformation in diabetes. Clinical Obstetrics and Gynecology 5: 315–331
21. Cordero L, Landon M B 1993 Infant of the diabetic mother. Clinical Perinatology 20: 635–648
22. Coustan D R 1988 Pregnancy in diabetic women. New England Journal of Medicine 319: 1663–1665
23. Cummins M, Norrish M 1980 Follow-up of children of diabetic mothers. Archives of Disease in Childhood 55: 259–264
24. Dacombe C M, Dalton R G, Goldie D F, Osborne J P 1981 Effect of packed cell volume on blood glucose estimations. Archives of Disease in Childhood 56: 789–791
25. Damm P, Molsted-Pedersen L 1989 Significant decrease in congenital malformations in newborn infants of an unselected population of diabetic mothers. American Journal of Obstetics and Gynecology 161: 1163–1167
26. Delmis J, Drazaneic A, Ivanisevic M, Suchanek E 1992 Glucose, insulin, HGH and IGF-I levels in maternal serum, amniotic fluid and umbilical venous serum: a comparison between late normal pregnancy and pregnancies complicated with diabetes and fetal growth retardation. Journal of Perinatal Medicine 20: 47–56
27. Demaini S, Mimouni F, Tsang R C, Khoury J, Hertzberg V 1994 Impact of metabolic control of diabetes during pregnancy on neonatal hypocalcaemia: a randomized study. Obstetrics and Gynecology 83: 918–922
28. Duhamel B 1961 From the mermaid to anal imperforation: the syndrome of caudal regression. Archives of Disease in Childhood 36: 152–155

29. Edwards J R G, Newall D R 1988 Relaxin as an aetiological factor in diabetic embryopathy. Lancet i: 1428–1430
30. Farquhar J W 1959 The child of a diabetic woman. Archives of Disease in Childhood 34: 76–96
31. Farquhar J W 1963 Prognosis for babies born to diabetic mothers in Edinburgh. Archives of Disease in Childhood 44: 36–47
32. Field L L 1988 Insulin-dependent diabetes mellitus: a model for the study of multifactorial disorders. American Journal of Human Genetics 43: 793–798
33. Francois R, Picaud J J, Ruitton-Ugliengo A, David L, Cartal M Y, Bauer D 1974 The newborn of diabetic mothers. Biology of the Neonate 24: 1–3
34. Freinkel N 1988 Diabetic embryopathy and fuel-mediated organ teratogenesis: lessons from animal models. Hormone and Metabolic Research 20: 463–475
35. Fuhrmann K, Reicher H, Semmler K, Fisher F, Fisher M, Glockner E 1983 Prevention of congenital malformations in infants of insulin-dependent diabetic mothers. Diabetes Care 6: 213–223
36. Gerö L, Baranyi E, Bekefi D, Dimeny E, Szalay F 1982 Investigation on serum C-peptide concentrations in pregnant diabetic women and in newborns of diabetic mothers. Hormone and Metabolic Research 17: 516–520
36a. Gutgessell H P, Spur M E, Rosenberg H S 1980 Characterisation of the cardiomyopathy in infants of diabetic mothers. Circulation 61: 441–449
37. Gewolb I H 1993 High glucose causes delayed fetal lung maturation in vitro. Experimental Lung Research 19: 619–630
38. Halliday H L 1981 Hypertrophic cardiomyopathy in infants of poorly controlled diabetic mothers. Archives of Disease in Childhood 56: 258–263
39. Hanson U, Persson B 1993 Outcome of pregnancies complicated by type I insulin dependent diabetes in Sweden: acute pregnancy complications, neonatal mortality and morbidity. American Journal of Perinatology 10: 330–333
40. Hawdon J M, Aynsley-Green A 1996 Neonatal complications, including hypoglycaemia. In: Dornhorst A, Hadden D (eds) Diabetes and pregnancy: an international approach to diagnosis and management. Wiley, Chichester, (In press)
41. Haworth J C, McRae K N, Dilling L A 1976 Prognosis of infants of diabetic mothers in relation to neonatal hypoglycaemia. Developmental Medicine and Child Neurology 18: 471–479
42. Hawthorne G, Snodgrass A, Tunbridge M 1994 Outcome of diabetic pregnancy and glucose intolerance in pregnancy: an audit of fetal loss in Newcastle General Hospital 1977–1990. Diabetes Research and Clinical Practice 25: 183–190
43. Hertel J, Kuhl C 1986 Metabolic adaptation during the neonatal period in infants of diabetic mothers. Acid Endocrinologica 277 (suppl): 136–140
44. Horton W E Jr, Sadler T W 1983 Effects of maternal diabetes on early embryogenesis: alterations in morphogenesis produced by ketone body, beta-hydroxybutrate. Diabetes 32: 610–616
45. Hunter D J S 1992 Diabetes in pregnancy. In: Chalmers I, Enkin M, Keirse MJNC (eds) Effective care in pregnancy and childbirth. Oxford University Press, Oxford, pp 579–594
46. Jame P, Ktorza A, Bihoreau M T et al 1990 Impaired hepatic glycogenolysis related to hyperinsulinaemia in newborns from hyperglycaemic pregnant rats. Pediatric Research 28: 646–651
47. Kalhan S C, Savin S M, Adam P A F 1977 Attenuated glucose production rate in newborn infants of insulin dependent diabetic mothers. New England Journal of Medicine 296: 375–376
48. King C K, Tserng K, Kalhan S C 1982 Regulation of glucose production in newborn infants of diabetic mothers. Pediatric Research 16: 608–612
49. Komrower G M 1954 Blood sugar levels in babies born of diabetic mothers. Archives of Disease in Childhood 25: 28–33
50. Langer O, Levy J, Brustman C 1989 Glycemic control in gestational diabetes mellitus – how tight is tight enough: small for gestational age versus large for gestational age? American Journal of Obstetrics and Gynecology 161: 646–653
51. Like A, Orci L 1972 Embryogenesis of the human pancreatic islets. A light and electron microscopic study. Diabetes 21: 511–534
52. Lowy C, Beard R W, Goldschmidt J 1986 Congenital malformations in babies of diabetic mothers. Diabetic Medicine 3: 458–462
53. Mace S, Hirschfeld S S, Riggs T, Fanaroff A A, Merkatz I R 1979 Echocardiographic abnormalities in infants of diabetic mothers. Journal of Pediatrics 95: 1013–1019
54. Miller E M, Hare J W, Cloherty J R et al 1981 Major congenital anomalies and elevated hemoglobin A_{1c} in early weeks of diabetic pregnancy. New England Journal of Medicine 304: 1331–1334
55. Miller H C, Johnson R D, Durlacher S H 1944 A comparison of newborn infants with erythroblastosis fetalis with those born to diabetic mothers. Journal of Pediatrics 24: 603–615
56. Mills J L 1986 Malformations in infants of diabetic mothers. Teratogen update: environmentally induced birth defect risks. Alan R Liss, New York, pp 165–176
57. Mills J L, Baker L, Goldman A S 1979 Malformations in infants of diabetic mothers occur before the seventh gestational week. Diabetes 28: 292–293
58. Mills J L, Knopp R H, Simpson J L et al 1988 Lack of relation of increased malformation rates in infants of diabetic mothers to glycemic control during organogenesis. New England Journal of Medicine 318: 671–676
59. Milner R D G 1988 Endocrine control of fetal growth. In: Linblad B S (ed) Perinatal nutrition. Academic Press, New York, pp 45–62
60. Milner R D G, Wirdham P K, Tsanakas J 1981 Quantatitive morphology of B, A, D and PP cells in infants of diabetic mothers. Diabetes 30: 271–274
61. Mimouni F, Tsang R C, Hertzberg V S, Miodovnik M 1986 Polycythemia, hypomagnesemia and hypocalcemia in infants of diabetic mothers. American Journal of Diseases of Children 140: 798–800
62. Mimouni F, Miodovnik M, Siddiqi T A, Khoury J, Tsang R C 1988 Perinatal asphyxia in infants of insulin-dependent diabetic mothers. Journal of Pediatrics 113: 345–353
63. Mimouni F, Steichen J J, Tsang R C, Hertzberg V, Miodovnik M 1988 Decreased bone mineral content in infants of diabetic mothers. Americal Journal of Perinatology 5: 339–343
64. Mimouni F, Tsang R C, Hertzberg V S, Neumann V, Ellis K 1989 Parathyroid hormone and calcitriol changes in normal and insulin dependent diabetic pregnancies. Obstetrics and Gynecology 74: 49–54
65. Miodovnik M, Mimouni F, Tsang R C et al 1987 Management of the insulin-dependent diabetic during labour and delivery. Influence on neonatal outcome. Americal Journal of Perinatology 4: 106–114
66. Miodovnik M, Mimouni F, Dignan P S J et al 1988 Major malformations in infants of IDDM women. Vasculopathy and early first-trimester poor glycemic control. Diabetes Care 11: 713–718
67. Molsted-Pedersen L 1984 Detection of gestational diabetes. In Sutherland H M, Stowers J M (eds) Carbohydrate metabolism in pregnancy and the newborn. Churchill Livingstone, Edinburgh pp 209–210
68. Molsted-Pedersen L, Pedersen J F 1985 Congenital malformations in diabetic pregnancies. Acta Paediatrica Scandinavica suppl. 320: 79–84
69. Molsted-Pedersen L, Tygstrup I, Pedersen J 1964 Congenital malformations in newborn infants of diabetic women. Lancet i: 1124–1126
70. Morrison J J, Rennie J M, Milton P J D 1995 Neonatal respiratory morbidity and timing of elective caesarean section at term. British Journal of Obstetrics and Gynaecology 102: 101–106
71. Mountain K R 1991 The infant of the diabetic mother. Clinical Obstetrics and Gynecology 5: 413–442
72. Naeye R L 1965 Infants of diabetic mothers: a quantitive, morphologic study. Pediatrics 35: 980–988
73. Nogee L, McMahan M, Whitsett J A 1988 Hyaline membrane disease and surfactant protein, SAP-35, in diabetes in pregnancy. American Journal of Perinatology 5: 374–377
74. Noguchi A, Eren M, Tsang R C 1980 Parathyroid hormone in hypocalcemic and normocalcemic infants of diabetic mothers. Journal of Pediatrics 97: 112–114
75. Passarge E, Lenz W 1966 Syndrome of caudal regression in infants of diabetic mothers: observation of further cases. Pediatrics 37: 672–675
76. Patel D, Kalhan S 1992 Glycerol metabolism and triglyceride–fatty acid cycling in the human newborn: effect of maternal diabetes and intrauterine growth retardation. Pediatric Research 31: 52–58
77. Pedersen J 1954 Weight and length at birth of infants of diabetic mothers. Acta Endocrinologica 16: 330–341
78. Peevy K J, Landaw S A, Gross S J 1980 Hyperbilirubinemia in infants of diabetic mothers. Pediatrics 66: 417–419
79. Perrine S P, Greene M F, Lee P D K, Cohen R A, Faller D V 1986 Insulin stimulates cord blood erythroid progenitor growth: Evidence for

an aetiological role in neonatal polycythemia. British Journal of Haematology 64: 503–511
80. Persson B, Gentz J 1984 Follow-up of children of insulin-dependent and gestational diabetic mothers. Neuropsychological outcome. Acta Paediatrica Scandinavica 73: 343–358
81. Persson B, Gentz J, Möller E 1984 Follow up of children of insulin dependent (Type 1) and gestational diabetic mothers. Acta Paediatrica Scandinavica 73: 778–784
82. Peterec S M, Nichols K V, Dynia D W, Wilson C M, Cross I 1994 Butyrate modulates surfactant protein m RNA in fetal rat lung by altering mRNA transcription and stability. American Journal of Physiology 267: L9–15
83. Philippart A J, Reed O J, Georgeson K E 1975 Neonatal small left colon syndrome: intramural not intraluminal obstruction. Journal of Pediatric Surgery 10: 733–739
84. Phillips A F, Dubin J W, Malty P J, Raye J R 1982 Antenatal hypoxaemia and hyperinsulinaemia in the chronically hyperglycaemic fetal lamb. Pediatric Research 16: 653–658
85. Reller M D, Kaplan S 1988 Hypertrophic cardiomyopathy in infants of diabetic mothers: an update. American Journal of Perinatology 5: 353–358
86. Robert M, Neff R, Hubbel J, Taeusch H, Avery M 1976 Association between maternal diabetes and the respiratory distress syndrome in the newborn. New England Journal of Medicine 294: 357–360
87. Roversi G D, Garguilo M, Nicolini U et al 1979 A new approach to the treatment of diabetic pregnant women. American Journal of Obstetrics and Gynecology 135: 567–576
88. Sadler T W, Phillips L S, Balkan W, Goldstein S 1986 Somatostatin inhibitors from diabetic rat serum after birth and development of mouse embryos in culture. Diabetes 35: 861–865
89. Sadler T W, Hunter II E S, Wynn R E, Phillips L S 1989 Evidence for multifactorial origin of diabetes-induced embryopathies. Diabetes 38: 70–74
90. Smith B T, Giroud C J P, Robert M, Avery M E 1975 Insulin antagonism of cortisol action on lecithin synthesis by cultured fetal lung cells. Journal of Pediatrics 87: 953–955
91. Soltész G, Schultz K, Mestyan G, Horvath M 1978 Blood glucose and plasma free amino acid concentrations in infants of diabetic mothers. Pediatrics 61: 77–82
92. Steinke F, Driscoll S G 1965 The extractable insulin content of pancreas from fetuses and infants of diabetic and control mothers. Diabetes 17: 573–588
93. Stevenson D K, Ostrander C R, Hopper A O, Cohen R S, Johnson J D 1981 Pulmonary excretion of carbon monoxide as an index of bilirubin production. II a. Evidence for possible delayed clearance of bilirubin in infants of diabetic mothers. Journal of Pediatrics 98: 822–824
94. Sussman I, Matschinsky F M 1988 Diabetes affects sorbitol and myoinositol levels of neuroectodermal tissue during embryogenesis in rats. Diabetes 37: 974–981
95. Swenne I 1988 The fetus of the diabetic mother: growth and malformations. Archives of Disease in Childhood 63: 1119–1121
96. Takeuchi A, Benirschke K 1961 Renal venous thrombosis of the newborn and its relation to maternal diabetes. Biology of the Neonate 3: 237–256
97. Taylor P M, Wolfson J H, Bright N H, Birchard E L, Derinoz M N, Watson D W 1963 Hyperbilirubinemia in infants of diabetic mothers. Biology of the Neonate 5: 289–298
98. Trowitzsch E, Bigalke U, Gisbertz R, Kallfelz H C 1983 Echocardiographic profile of infants of diabetic mothers. European Journal of Pediatrics 140: 311–315
99. Tsang R C, Kleinman L I, Sutherland J M, Light J 1972 Hypocalcaemia in infants of diabetic mothers: studies in calcium, phosphorus and magnesium metabolism and parathormone responsiveness. Journal of Pediatrics 80: 384–395
100. Tsang R C, Chen I W, Friedman M A et al 1975 Parathyroid function in infants of diabetic mothers. Journal of Pediatrics 86: 399–404
101. Veille J-C, Sivakoff M, Hanson R, Fanaroff A A 1992 Interventricular septal thickness in fetuses of diabetic mothers. Obstetrics and Gynecology 79: 51–54
102. Vejtorp M, Pedersen F, Klebbe F G, Lund E 1977 Low concentration of plasma amino acids in newborn babies of diabetic mothers. Acta Paediatrica Scandinavica 66: 53–58
103. Vohr B R, Lipsitt L P, Oh W 1980 Somatic growth of children of diabetic mothers with reference to birth size. Journal of Pediatrics 97: 196–199
104. Warram J H, Krolewski A S, Gottlieb M S, Kahn C R 1984 Differences in risk of insulin dependent diabetes in offspring of diabetic mothers and diabetic fathers. New England Journal of Medicine 311: 149–152
105. Warram J H, Krolewski A S, Kahn C R 1988 Determinants of IDDM and perinatal mortality in children of diabetic mothers. Diabetes 37: 1328–1334
106. Way G L, Wolfe R R, Eshaghpour E, Bender R L, Jafe R B, Ruttenberg H D 1979 The natural history of hypertrophic cardiomyopathy in infants of diabetic mothers. Journal of Pediatrics 95: 1020–1026
107. Whitelaw A 1977 Subcutaneous fat in newborn infants of diabetic mothers: an indication of quality of diabetic control. Lancet i: 15–18
108. Widness J A, Susa J B, Garcia J F et al 1981 Increased erythropoiesis and elevated erythropoietin in infants born to diabetic mothers and in hyperinsulinemic rhesus fetuses. Journal of Clinical Investigation 67: 637–642
109. Ylinen K, Aula P, Stenman D-H, Kesäniemi-Kuokkanen T, Teramo K 1984 Risk of minor and major fetal malformations in diabetes with high haemoglobin A_{1c} values in early pregnancy. British Medical Journal 298: 345–346
110. Yssing M 1975 Long-term prognosis of children born to mothers diabetic when pregnant. In: Camerini-Davalos R A, Cole H S (eds) Early diabetes in early life. Academic Press, New York, pp 575–586
111. Zetterstrom R, Strindberg B, Arnhold R 1958 Hyperbilirubinaemia and ABO hemolytic disease in newborn infants of diabetic mothers. Acta Paediatrica Scandinavica 47: 238–250

25

Twins

Elizabeth M. Bryan

A special chapter on twins is justified by the disproportionate number of problems they present for the neonatologist.

TWINNING RATES

Estimates of the incidence of twins are hampered by the unknown number of abortions and early fetal deaths that occur in multiple pregnancies. Boklage[7] has estimated that for every twin pair born, at least 10 singletons are conceived as one of a twin pair. Ultrasound studies in early pregnancy frequently reveal the death and later reabsorption of one fetus in the first trimester – the vanishing twin syndrome.[77] Thus the prevalence of twins at a certain time is all that can be accurately estimated.

Furthermore some multiple births may not be recorded if a pair, one stillborn and one liveborn, are delivered before 24 weeks' gestation. The stillborn would be registered as an abortion and the liveborn would thus appear in the records as a single birth.

In the UK, as in the USA, and most European countries the proportion of twin births fell from about 1 in 80 maternities in the early 1950s to about 1 in 105 in 1980 (Fig. 1.6, p. 10). The cause of the decline is uncertain. Changes in parity and maternal age at conception may be contributory factors. Oral contraceptives, changing rates of spontaneous abortions and environmental agents affecting spermatozoa have also been suggested, but not proven.[8,30]

Since 1980, the twinning rate has been rising, and an earlier and more rapid rise has been seen amongst higher order births (Fig. 25.1). This is probably because of the more widespread use of infertility treatment, including ovulation-stimulation drugs, in vitro fertilization and gamete intrafallopian tube transfer.[29,52]

Twinning rates vary greatly in different parts of the world, and this is because of variations in dizygotic twinning. In general black Africans have the highest rates; the Far Eastern, mongolian, races the lowest; Asian Indians and Caucasians lie between. The prevalence of monozygotic twin births had been constant worldwide at 3.5 per 1000 maternities until very recently. A small and unexplained increase in the MZ twinning rate has been noted in the 1980s.[1]

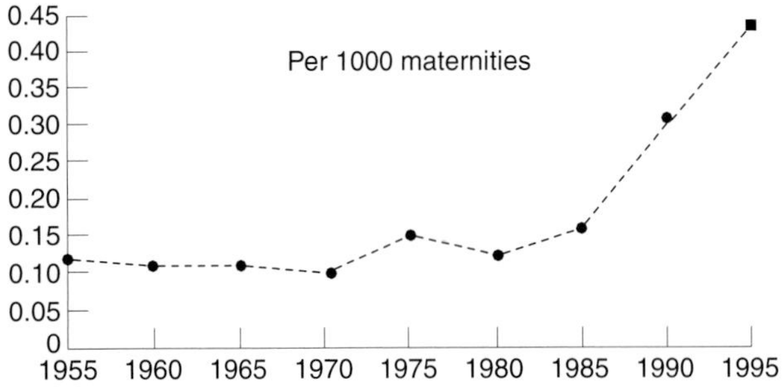

Fig. 25.1 Triplet rate in England and Wales 1955–1995 (Source OPCS).

TYPES OF TWINS

DZ twins arise when two ova are released and fertilized in one menstrual cycle, whereas MZ twins arise when one ova is fertilized and the resulting zygote divides into two. The ratio of MZ to DZ twins varies in different populations. In the UK approximately two-thirds are DZ, so in all, about one-third of the pairs will be of unlike sex, one-third both girls, and one-third both boys.

There are no known factors affecting the rate of MZ twinning, although there appear to be some extremely rare examples of MZ twinning occurring as an autosomal dominant.[81] It has also been suggested that there may be a higher rate of MZ twinning following ovulation stimulation whether or not fertilization took place in vitro.[28,89]

DZ twinning is known to be affected by a number of factors in addition to race, many of which appear to be related to differing maternal gonadotrophin levels. There are definite maternal genetic determinants but there is still uncertainty about paternal ones, if any. The rates are known to increase with maternal age, height, parity and

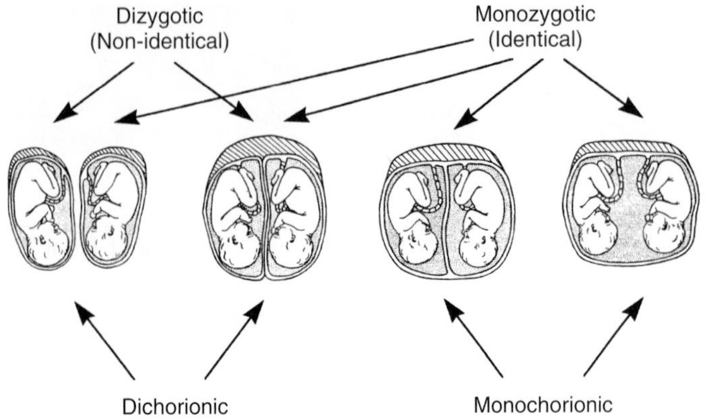

Fig. 25.2 Relationship between zygosity and chorionicity (reproduced by permission from MBF 1997).[62]

frequency of intercourse.[56] Many other factors have been suggested but most are as yet unconfirmed.

DETERMINATION OF ZYGOSITY

Information on zygosity in multiple births is of importance not only for epidemiological, genetic and obstetric reasons but also because of the difference in prognosis between MZ and DZ sets.[35] Furthermore, the parents themselves usually want to know about it, not least because their chances of having multiple births in future pregnancies will vary according to the zygosity. Too often, however, the zygosity is not considered at birth so that invaluable information from the placenta is lost and blood samples become harder to collect.

The zygosity of approximately half of Caucasian twins can be determined at birth either because the infants are of different sex and therefore DZ or because a monochorionic placenta conclusively demonstrates monozygosity. In other situations, however, many parents have been mistakenly told that their children are DZ on the evidence of a dichorionic placenta. It is now known that MZ twins whose zygote division occurs within the first 4 days or so of fertilization will also have two placental discs (separate or fused) and therefore two chorions (Fig. 25.2).

Like-sex DZ twins can only be distinguished reliably from the one-third of MZ twins who have dichorionic placentas by blood grouping, although the zygosity of many DZ pairs will later become evident from their differing physical features such as hair colour.

Blood groups provide useful genetic markers in that they have a simple mode of inheritance and commonly occurring variations. Tests are most practically done on cord blood samples but can of course be carried out at any age. More recently, other genetic markers such as red cell enzymes, serum proteins and tissue enzymes (in particular from the placenta) have been used. Monozygosity cannot be proven by genetic marker testing, but the probability increases with the number tested and the exact probability can be calculated; this is more precise if the parents' blood types and race are known.[19]

A highly reliable tool for zygosity testing is the mini-satellite DNA probe test.[27,46] An added advantage is that only small volumes of blood (or placental tissue) are needed.

FETAL GROWTH

The growth and development of the twin fetus is affected not only by the same intrauterine factors as the singleton fetus but by the interaction with the second fetus. At best it must compete for nutrition. At worst it may be severely, even lethally, damaged by the co-twin.[12]

The average weight of a newborn twin is about 800 g less than a singleton, but if allowance is made for differences in gestational age the discrepancy is reduced to 500 g.[45] Fetal growth is usually similar to that of a singleton until the end of the second trimester.[37,57] Corney et al[23] showed that DZ twins were heavier than both mono- and dichorionic MZ twins. In mixed sex pairs, boys tend to be heavier than girls, as in singletons.[70]

The typical pattern of intrauterine growth of twins is similar to that of a growth-retarded singleton in that the weight falls disproportionately more than the occipito-frontal circumference.[32] Birthweight and OFC centile charts for English twins are now available.[16]

INTRAPAIR DISCORDANCE

Birthweight discordance may be due to the different sites of implantation of two placentae, or of the umbilical cords, but the commonest cause of large discrepancies in fetal growth is probably haemodynamic imbalance in the chronic form of the fetofetal transfusion syndrome (Fig. 25.3).

FETOFETAL TRANSFUSION IN MONOCHORIONIC PREGNANCIES

All monochorionic placentae have vascular anastomoses between the two fetal circulations: inter-twin transfusion is therefore a normal event. It is only when this transfusion becomes unbalanced that problems arise.

The acute fetofetal transfusion syndrome results from an acute haemodynamic imbalance across the superficial arterio-arterial or venovenous anastomoses. It most commonly occurs during labour and may cause severe hypovolaemia in one twin and hypervolaemia in the other. An acute haemodynamic imbalance may also occur following the intrauterine death of one twin (see p. 220).

The chronic fetofetal transfusion syndrome results from a haemodynamic imbalance in the parenchymatous arteriovenous network and there is a conspicuous absence of superficial anastomoses.[2] It complicates, to a varying

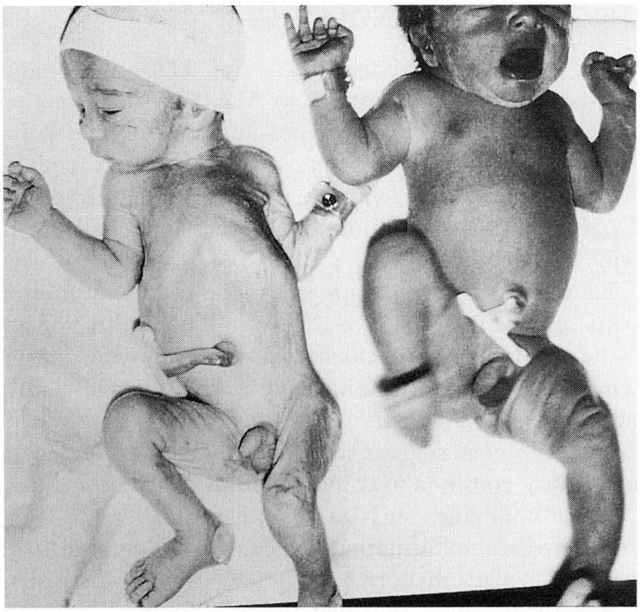

Fig. 25.3 The fetofetal transfusion syndrome showing intrauterine growth retardation and pallor of the donor (weight 1.6 kg, Hb 7.9 g/100 ml) and plethora of the recipient (weight 2.7 kg, Hb 21 g/100 ml).

degree, up to a third of monochorionic pregnancies and is the cause of up to 17% of perinatal mortality in twins. In the past, the diagnosis was made on the neonatal criteria of an intrapair cord blood haemoglobin difference of 5 g/l[74] and birthweight discrepancy. It is now recognized that in the more severe cases, presenting in the second trimester, these differences are usually absent and the main problems for the recipient fetus are severe polyhydramnios, cardiac complications and hydrops, and, for the donor, oligohydramnios.[34]

In the newborn, the recipient twin is characteristically heavier and polycythaemic and faces the complications of high blood viscosity, such as cardiac failure, hyperbilirubinaemia and intravascular thromboses, whereas the donor shows signs of intrauterine growth retardation, anaemia and hypoproteinaemia. Gross abnormalities of the donor's portion of the placenta may further reduce the nourishment available to him.[9] When anaemia is the presenting feature, care must be taken to distinguish from other causes of anaemia such as fetomaternal haemorrhage.

Prenatal treatment has included repeated amniocentesis, laser ablation of anastomoses, selective fetocide and transfusion of the donor with exsanguination of the recipient.[36] Amnioreduction is more successful if started before the onset of contractions; thus all monochorionic pregnancies should be closely monitored for early signs of the fetofetal transfusion syndrome. Postnatally, the treatment of the polycythaemic or anaemic twin is no different from that of singletons with the same problems (Ch. 32, Parts 2 and 3).

CONGENITAL ANOMALIES

In most, though not all, studies a higher prevalence of anomalies has been found amongst multiple births as compared with singletons.[54] Factors that may cause this apparent variation include the gestational criterion used for defining stillbirth, the range of anomalies studied, opportunities for and thoroughness of examination, twinship itself, maternal age and zygosity distribution.

The increase appears to be limited to twins of the same sex, and where zygosity has been determined it has been shown to be the MZ twins who are responsible for the increase.[21,24,64,65] Concordance rates vary considerably by type of anomaly, but in general discordance is more common even amongst MZ twins.[54] The less favourable environment of a monochorial placentation has been suggested as the explanation for the increase in anomalies in MZ twins.[17] However, this has not been confirmed.[24,59]

Congenital anomalies in twins pose new dilemmas. Not only may some conditions be treated antenatally but the possibility of selective fetocide, when one twin has an irremediable anomaly, provides a new and difficult choice for both obstetricians and parents.

ANOMALIES UNIQUE TO MULTIPLE CONCEPTION

Anomalies unique to the twinning process include conjoined twinning, fetus in fetu, acardia and fetus papyraceus.

Conjoined twinning

Conjoined twins occurs in approximately 1 in 50 000 pregnancies.[93] They are a form of MZ twinning in which the division of the zygote is incomplete. The increased incidence of additional unrelated malformations suggests that conjoined twinning may be associated with a fundamental disturbance of embryogenesis.[31]

There are no known predisposing factors to conjoined twinning but it is more common in females,[4,60,93] there is an increased frequency amongst triplet sets[79] and in parts of Africa,[5,93] and seasonal clustering has also been reported.[60]

The site and extent of the fusion is highly variable. Thoracopagus is the commonest form and accounts for about 70% of cases.[31,78]

Inevitably ethical dilemmas arise with conjoined twins, particularly when surgical separation means that the life of one is likely to be at the expense of the other.[75]

Acardia

Acardia or chorioangiopagus parasiticus, which occurs in about 1 in 30 000–35 000 deliveries,[42,67] varies in manifestations from a mass of amorphous tissues to an incomplete but otherwise well-formed fetus. An imbalance in the interfetal circulation resulting in atrophy of the heart or a primary failure of cardiac development have both been suggested as the aetiological mechanisms.

As survival of the acardiac fetus is dependent on a shared circulation with the (usually normal) co-twin, acardia occurs only in monochorionic, and therefore MZ, pregnancies. However, in one instance, a triploid twin acardiac with a 70 XXX + 15 karyotype was delivered with a co-twin with a normal male karyotype and a monochorionic placenta.[6] This sex discordance may be due to polar body twinning.

The male:female ratio in acardiac twins is lower than in twins in general.[49] The mean maternal age is high,[39] consistent with the finding that some acardiacs are trisomic.[50,80]

Relatively little attention has been paid to the pump twin. They appear to have a surprisingly high incidence of malformations[79] but, even when potentially normal, these infants have a high mortality rate, usually as a result of the combination of intrauterine cardiac failure and prematurity.[87] The size of the acardiac twin relative to the pump twin appears to strongly influence the perinatal outcome with a significantly higher rate of prematurity and therefore mortality amongst those with a higher birthweight ratio.[61] Their perinatal management should be greatly improved now that the problems can be foreseen by routine ultrasonic examination. Intrauterine treatment can be given for cardiac failure, and amniocentesis or indomethacin for polyhydramnios. Recently, various methods, including embolization and laser coagulation, have been used to cause fetocide.

DEATH OF ONE FETUS

The possible dangers of an intrauterine death to a surviving monochorionic twin are now well recognized. Many types of anomalies have been reported in the surviving twin[54] and the nature of these anomalies probably depends on the stage of gestation at which the co-twin dies.[48] Review of pooled data on 53 cases suggests that disruptions of the central nervous system are the most common complication (72%), followed by the gastrointestinal system (19%), kidneys (15%) and lungs (8%).[84] Cardiac malformations have also been reported,[3,25] as have cases of aplasia cutis.[58] It was originally thought that these anomalies were due to thromboplastin, released from the dead twin's tissues, crossing the placental anastomoses and causing disseminated intravascular coagulation (DIC) in the living twin. However, the current view is that these diverse lesions may all be the result of transient hypotension. As one fetus dies and the vascular resistance falls, the living twin may exsanguinate into the dead twin causing a damaging if not lethal hypoxic episode from the profound hypotension.

CHROMOSOMAL ANOMALIES

These are usually discordant in DZ twins and, surprisingly, also occasionally in MZ.[76,80] The twins are then known as heterokaryotypes and it is assumed that the maldistribution of chromosomes occurred at about the same time as the twinning process. Heterokaryotypes XY/XO are the explanation for the occasional pair of MZ twins of different sexes.[76]

Klinefelter syndrome appears to be more common in twins and in their relatives.[33,47,68,82] There also appears to be an increased incidence of Turner syndrome in twins[22,66,72] and of twinning among the (normal) family members of patients with Turner syndrome.[69] Carothers[22] et al.suggest that there may be a postzygotic mechanism common to twinning and X chromosome loss.

Some anomalies such as oesophageal atresia[38,88] and some cardiac malformations[18] occur more commonly in twins. Cardiac malformations are usually discordant in MZ twins, suggesting that the malformation develops as a result of some process peculiar to monozygotic twins. The fetofetal transfusion syndrome has been incriminated, but more recently it has been suggested that a disturbance in laterality may be the cause.[18]

The teratogenic effects of both drugs and intrauterine infections may have intrapair differences in expression.[15] This may be because of a difference in fetal susceptibility. In other instances where the teratogenic effect of the drug is sharply limited, as in the case of thalidomide, the discordance could be due to the insult acting at the very beginning or end of the sensitive period.[51] As DZ twins can be conceived several days apart, one embryo may be a few days retarded or accelerated in development and therefore escape unscathed.

PERINATAL MORTALITY

Twins account for about 2% of births but 9% of perinatal deaths.[30] Although there has been a steady fall in their perinatal mortality, the difference between multiple births and singletons still remains (Fig. 25.4). The increase amongst twins is largely due to their prematurity and low

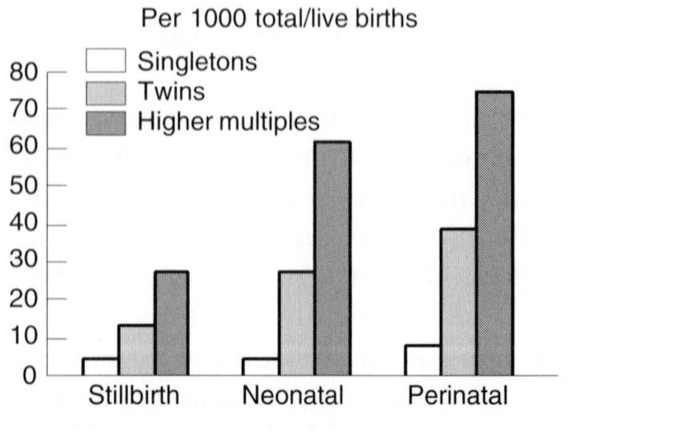

Fig. 25.4 Mortality in multiple births: England and Wales 1990 (Source OPCS DH3 No. 25).

Table 25.1 Mortality rates for singleton and multiple births in England and Wales in the years 1975–86 excluding 1981

Type of birth	Neonatal* (Number of total births live and still)	Stillbirths† Neonatal*	Perinatal† Infant*
Singleton	7.4 (4 845 382)	7.7 4.3	13.8 11.7
Twin	43.9 (95 312)	25.4 9.1	63.2 52.9
Triplet	135.0 (1812)	47.5 12.7	164.5 147.7
Quadruplet and higher order births	207.5 (164)	30.5 12.6	219.5 220.1

* Rate per 1000 live births.
† Rate per 100 total births.
Source: OPCS Series FHIDH3 Annual Reference Volumes.

birthweight. The average length of a twin pregnancy is about 20 days shorter than a singleton one. Between 20 and 30% of twins will be born preterm (less than 37 weeks' gestation). For the same reason, neonatal deaths are proportionately more common than fetal deaths. As expected, the perinatal mortality rate amongst higher order births is directly related to the number of fetuses[30] (Fig. 25.4, Table 25.1). Problems specific to multiple pregnancy contributing to the high mortality include the shared circulation of monochorionic twins, cord complications in monoamniotic twins[63,90] and the higher incidence of lethal malformations.[55]

54% of multiple births in 1982–84 weighed less than 2500 g compared with 6% of singletons.[30] Within each 500-g grouping under 2500 g, multiple births have a significantly lower perinatal mortality, presumably because they tend to be more mature for their birthweight.[71] Most, but not all, studies have shown the second-born baby to be at higher risk of death and morbidity.[20,44,86,92] Although the risk of birth asphyxia is now less, there is still an increased incidence and severity of respiratory distress syndrome in the second-born twin with a resultant higher neonatal mortality (p. 20).

The mortality rate is higher in MZ than DZ twins[63,73,86] mainly because of the complications of a monochorionic placenta[4,43], but even dichorionic MZ twins may be at a disadvantage when compared with DZ as their birthweights tend to be lower.[24]

Boys fare worse than girls, regardless of zygosity. The highest perinatal mortality rate occurs in male–male pairs,[40] and in unlike-sex pairs the male is at a significant disadvantage.[20]

SOCIAL

Parents of twins need particular understanding. Few are prepared for the emotional as well as practical and financial stresses involved in caring for two babies at once.[83,85] They are often faced not only with the problem of caring for and relating to two babies at once but two babies each of whom is more difficult because of the prematurity, low birthweight and other neonatal problems already described. Furthermore, many twins will be separated from their mother on intensive care neonatal wards. It may be particularly difficult for the mother if the two babies are on different wards; she may well forget the baby in a distant incubator.

If one baby is much more demanding, mothers may feel guilty that they are unable to give their twins equal attention. They should be reassured that sometimes that baby may need more attention.

A mother's relationship with her babies will be further impeded if she finds it difficult to tell them apart. The babies should always be clearly identifiable and called by their names. The cot should be made recognizable at a distance so that the parents can start relating to the particular baby as they approach.

Similarly, parents should be encouraged to dress the babies differently from the start despite pressures from friends and relatives. Twin names such as Joy and Jay or Robert and Roberta are also best avoided if the children's individuality is to be respected. The babies should preferably go home from hospital together, but if this is not practicable, because one needs a longer stay, parents should be encouraged and helped to visit the remaining baby. Facilities for the healthy child to attend with the parents must always be provided.

FEEDING

It is enormously important for a mother of twins to establish the easiest and most satisfactory feeding routine for both herself and her babies as soon as possible. For far too many, the feeding of their twins is remembered as a period of frustration, exhaustion and failure. Many who planned to breast-feed have been bitterly disappointed.

For some, the advantages of bottle-feeding so that others can feed their babies outweigh other considerations. But any mother who would like to breast-feed should be given every encouragement and practical help. Most mothers can fully breast-feed two babies but they will need informed prenatal preparation,[26] including demonstrations by mothers, as well as a lot of help during the neonatal period. No mother should be expected to feed her newborn twins simultaneously without an attendant.[10] There have been no studies which compare milk production for twins fed together with those fed separately, but the time saved by feeding them together is considerable.

PERINATAL BEREAVEMENT

Parents who lose one twin face particular problems.[14,53] They have to experience the joy of a new baby and the tragedy of bereavement simultaneously. Because they still have a live infant their loss is usually greatly underestimated, if acknowledged at all.

The parents are too often discouraged from talking about their dead baby. Yet concentration on the healthy baby to the exclusion of the stillbirth or neonatal death may encourage the mother to idealize the dead child (her angel baby) and hence alienate her from the survivor, especially if the surviving twin is difficult to handle because of illness or disturbed behaviour.

The pride involved in expecting twins is enormous, and failure is therefore deeply felt. Mothers inevitably feel shame and often some guilt. This guilt may be increased by any implication from friends or medical staff that the death was all for the best, even if logically this may seem so.[11] Twinship is also important to the survivor and this continues into adulthood. This has implications for the care of the surviving twin and his parents from birth onwards.[91]

Some parents have difficulty in distinguishing the two babies in their own minds. Some may feel that the dead one never existed – a fantasy baby. Substantive mementos, such as photographs or even an ultrasound scan showing the two babies together, can help to clear the emotional confusion. Naming the dead baby not only helps to distinguish the babies but later makes it much easier to talk to the survivor (who should always be told) about his twin.

Blood or placental samples should always be taken for zygosity determination. Even if one baby dies, parents usually want to know whether or not their twins were identical. The zygosity may also be important for reliable genetic counselling about congenital anomalies and the chances of further twin conceptions.

Where both babies are born alive but one baby is likely to die, the family should be encouraged to spend extra time with this one so that precious memories can be created and the parents may later find comfort in knowing that they have given this baby as much love and care as they could. A photograph of the two babies (together with their parents if they so wish) should be taken as quickly as possible.

If a twin is born dead before 24 completed weeks of the pregnancy (a miscarriage) and a sibling is liveborn, the legal paradox and ambiguity add to the parents' difficulties.[41]

An increasing number of parents are likely to face bereavement through choosing to lose a malformed twin fetus (or normal higher order fetuses) through selective fetocide. Their grief can be powerful but may be delayed until the delivery of the healthy baby. It is important that the fetus is respected and its loss recognized.[13]

Most, if not all, mothers continue to think of their surviving child as a twin even if the other baby was stillborn.[11] Many parents welcome the opportunity to reminisce about their lost baby, particularly with the medical staff, who may be the only people who knew him. Many years later they still appreciate an enquiry about their feelings towards the dead baby and any concerns about the survivor's feelings about his dead twin.

HIGHER ORDER BIRTHS

Any problems described for twins are increased with higher order births, and the number of triplets and more is likely to continue to increase with new methods for the treatment of infertility. The workload for neonatal units will be immense and worrying, and an increasing number of families will be competing for the much needed but inadequate help so far available.

REFERENCES

1. Allen G, Parisi P 1990 Trends in monozygotic and dizygotic twinning rates by maternal age and parity. Further analysis of Italian data, 1949–1985, and rediscussion of US data, 1964–1985. Acta Geneticae Medicae et Gemellologiae 39(3): 317–328
2. Bajoria R, Wigglesworth J, Fisk N 1995 Angioarchitecture of monochorionic placentas in relation to the twin twin transfusion syndrome. American Journal of Obstetrics and Gynecology 172: 856–863
3. Baker V V, Doering M C 1982 Fetus papyraceus: an unreported congenital anomaly of the surviving infant. American Journal of Obstetrics and Gynecology 143: 234
4. Benirschke K, Kim C K 1973 Multiple pregnancy. New England Journal of Medicine 288: 1329–1336
5. Bhettay G, Nelson M M, Beighton P 1975 Epidemic of conjoined twins in Southern Africa. Lancet ii: 741–743
6. Bieber F R, Nance W E, Morton C C, Brown J, Redwine F O, Jordan R L, Mohana Kumar T 1981 Genetic studies of an acardiac monster: evidence of polar body twinning in man. Science 214: 775–777
7. Boklage C 1990 Survival probability of human conceptions from fertilization to term. International Journal of Fertility 33: 75
8. Botting B, Macdonald Davies I, Macfarlane A J 1987 Recent trends in the incidence of multiple births and their mortality. Archives of Disease in Childhood 62: 941–950
9. Bryan E M 1977 IgG deficiency in association with placental oedema. Early Human Development 1: 133–143
10. Bryan E M 1983 Feeding twins. In: The nature and nurture of twins. Baillière Tindall, Eastbourne, ch 8, pp 101–111
11. Bryan E M 1986 The death of a newborn twin. How can support for parents be improved? Acta Geneticae Medicae et Gemellologiae 35: 115–118
12. Bryan E M 1986 The intrauterine hazards of twins. Archives of Disease in Childhood 61: 1044–1045
13. Bryan E M 1989 The response of mothers to selective feticide. Ethical Problems in Reproductive Medicine 1: 28–30
14. Bryan E M 1995 Perinatal bereavement after the loss of a twin. In: Ward H, Whittle M (eds) Multiple pregnancy RCOG Press, London, ch 19, pp 186–195
15. Bryan E M, Little J, Burn J 1987 Congenital anomalies in twins. Baillière's Clinical Obstetrics and Gynecology 1: 697–721
16. Buckler J M H, Green M 1994 Birth weight and head circumference standards for English twins. Archives of Disease in Childhood 71: 516
17. Bulmer M G 1970 The biology of twinning in man. Clarendon Press, Oxford
18. Burn J, Corney G 1984 Congenital heart defects and twinning. Acta Geneticae Medicae et Gemellologiae 33: 61–69
19. Burn J, Corney G 1988 Zygosity determination and the types of twinning. In: MacGillivray I, Campbell D M, Thompson B (eds) Twinning and twins. John Wiley, Chichester, pp 7–25
20. Butler N R, Alberman E D 1969 Perinatal problems – the second report of the 1958 British Perinatal Mortality Survey. Livingstone, Edinburgh, ch 7, p 122

21. Cameron A H, Edwards J H, Derom R, Thiery M, Boelaert R 1983 The value of twin surveys in the study of malformations. European Journal of Obstetrics and Gynecology 14: 347–356
22. Carothers A D, Frackiewicz A, deMey R et al 1980 A collaborative study of the aetiology of Turner syndrome. Annals of Human Genetics 43: 355–368
23. Corney G, Robson E B, Strong S J 1972 The effects of zygosity on the birthweight of twins. Annals of Human Genetics 36: 45–59
24. Corney G, MacGillivray I, Campbell D M, Thompson B, Little J 1983 Congenital anomalies in twins in Aberdeen and North-East Scotland. Acta Geneticae Medicae et Gemellologiae 28: 353–360
25. Daw E 1983 Fetus papyraceus – 11 cases. Postgraduate Medical Journal 59: 598–600
26. Denton J, Bryan E M 1995 Prenatal preparation for parenting twins, triplets or more: the social aspects. In: Ward H, Whittle M (eds) Multiple pregnancy. RCOG Press, London, ch 12, pp 119–128
27. Derom C, Bakker E, Vlietinck R, Derom R, Berghe H V D, Thiery M, Pearson P 1985 Zygosity determination in newborn twins using DNA variants. Journal of Medical Genetics 22: 279–282
28. Derom C, Derom R, Vlietinck R, Van den Berghe H, Thiery M 1987 Increased monozygotic twinning rate after ovulation induction. Lancet i: 1236–1238
29. Derom C, Derom R, Vlietinck R, Maes H, Van den Berghe H 1993 Iatrogenic multiple pregnancies in East Flanders, Belgium. Fertility and Sterility 60: 493–496
30. Dunn A, Macfarlane A 1996 Recent trends in the incidence of multiple births and associated mortality in England and Wales. Archives of Disease in Childhood 75: F10–F19
31. Edmonds D E, Layde P M 1982 Conjoined twins in the United States 1970–1977. Teratology 25: 301–308
32. Fenner A, Malm T, Kusserow V 1980 Intrauterine growth of twins. A retrospective analysis. European Journal of Pediatrics 133: 119–121
33. Ferguson-Smith M A 1966 Kleinfelter's syndrome and mental deficiency. In: Moore K L (ed) Sex chromatin. W B Saunders, Philadelphia, pp 277–315
34. Fisk N M 1995 The scientific basis of feto-fetal transfusion syndrome and its treatment. In: Ward H, Whittle M (eds) Multiple pregnancy. RCOG Press, London, pp 235–250
35. Fisk N, Bryan E 1993 Routine prenatal determination of chorionicity in multiple gestation: a plea to the obstetrician. British Journal of Obstetrics and Gynaecology 100: 975–977
36. Fisk N M, Borrell A, Hubinont C, Tannirandorn Y, Nicolini U, Rodeck C H 1990 Fetofetal transfusion syndrome; do the neonatal criteria apply in utero? Archives of Disease in Childhood 65: 657–661
37. Fliegner J R, Eggers T R 1984 The relationship between gestational age and birthweight in twin pregnancy. Australia and New Zealand Journal of Obstetrics and Gynecology 24: 192–197
38. Fraser F C, Nora J J 1975 Genetics of man. Lee & Febiger, Philadelphia, p 177
39. Frutiger P 1969 Zum Problem der Akardie. Acta Anatomica (Basle) 74: 505–531
40. Fujikura T, Froehlich L A 1971 Twin placentation and zygosity. Obstetrics and Gynecology 37: 34–43
41. Gabrielczyk M R 1987 Personal view. British Medical Journal 295: 209
42. Gillim D L, Hendricks C H 1953 Holoacardius: review of the literature and a case report. Obstetrics and Gynecology 2: 647–653
43. Gruenwald D P 1970 Environmental influences on twins apparent at birth, a preliminary study. Biology of the Neonate 15: 79–93
44. Guttmacher A F, Kohl S G 1958 The fetus of multiple gestation. Obstetrics and Gynecology 12: 528–541
45. Hemon D, Berger C, Lazer P 1982 Interaction between twinning and maternal factors associated with small for dateness. Presented at the International Workshop on Twins, Paris
46. Hill A V S, Jeffreys A J 1985 Use of minisatellite DNA probes for determination of twin zygosity at birth. Lancet ii: 1394–1395
47. Hoefnagel D, Benirschke K 1962 Twinning in Kleinfelter's syndrome. Lancet ii: 1282
48. Hoyme H E, Higginbottom M C, Jones K L 1981 Vascular etiology of disruptive structural defects in monozygotic twins. Pediatrics 67: 288–291
49. James W H 1978 A note on the epidemiology of acardiac monsters. Teratology 16: 211–216
50. Kerr M G, Rashad M N 1966 Autosomal trisomy in a discordant monozygotic twin. Nature 212: 726–727
51. Lenz W 1966 Malformations caused by drugs in pregnancy. American Journal of Diseases of Children 112: 99–106
52. Levene M I, Wild J, Steer P 1992 Higher multiple births and the modern management of infertility in Britain. British Journal of Obstetrics and Gynaecology 99: 607–613
53. Lewis E, Bryan E M 1988 Management of perinatal loss of a twin. British Medical Journal 297: 1321–1323
54. Little J, Bryan E M 1986 Congenital anomalies in twins. Seminars in Perinatology 10: 50–64
55. Little J, Bryan E M 1988 Congenital anomalies in twins. In: MacGillivray I, Campbell D, Thompson B (eds) Twinning and twins. John Wiley, Chichester, pp 207–240
56. MacGillivray I, Samphier M, Little J 1988 Factors affecting twinning. In: MacGillivray I, Campbell D M, Thompson B (eds) Twinning and twins. John Wiley, Chichester, pp 67–93
57. McKeown T, Record R G 1952 Observations on foetal growth in multiple pregnancy in man. Journal of Endocrinology 8: 386–401
58. Mannino F L, Jones K L, Benirschke K 1977 Congenital skin defects and fetus papyraceus. Journal of Pediatrics 91: 559–564
59. Melnick M, Myrianthopoulos N C 1979 The effects of chorion type on normal and abnormal developmental variation in monozygous twins. American Journal of Medical Genetics 4: 147–156
60. Milham S 1966 Symmetrical conjoined twins: an analysis of the birth records of 22 sets. Journal of Pediatrics 69: 643–647
61. Moore T R, Gale S, Benirschke K 1990 Perinatal outcome of forty-nine pregnancies complicated by acardiac twinning. American Journal of Obstetrics and Gynecology 163: 907–912
62. Multiple Births Foundation 1997 Are they identical? Zygosity determination for twins, triplets and more. MBF, London
63. Myrianthopoulos N C 1970 An epidemiologic survey of twins in a large, prospectively studied population. American Journal of Human Genetics 22: 611–629
64. Myrianthopoulos N C 1975 Congenital malformations in twins. Epidemiologic survey. Birth Defects Original Article Series XI, Vol. 8. National Foundation March of Dimes, New York. pp 1–29
65. Myrianthopoulos N C 1978 Congenital malformations. The contribution of twin studies. Birth Defects Original Article Series 14: 151–159
66. Nance W E, Uchida I 1964 Turner's syndrome, twinning and an unusual variant of glucose-6-phosphate dehydrogenase. American Journal of Human Genetics 16: 380–392
67. Napolitani F D, Schreiber I 1960 Acardiac monster. American Journal of Obstetrics and Gynecology 80: 582–589
68. Nielson J 1966 Twins in sibships with Klinefelter's syndrome. Journal of Medical Genetics 3: 114–116
69. Nielsen J, Dahl G 1976 Twins in the sibships and parental sibships of women with Turner's syndrome. Clinical Genetics 10: 93–96
70. Orlebeke J F, van-Baal G C, Boomsma D I, Neeleman D 1993 Birthweight in opposite sex twins as compared to same sex dizygotic twins. European Journal of Obstetrics and Gynecology and Reproductive Biology 50: 95–98
71. Patel N, Bowie W, Campbell D M et al 1984 Scottish twin study 1983 report. Social Paediatric and Obstetric Research Unit, University of Glasgow and Greater Glasgow Health Board
72. Pescia G, Ferrier P E, Wyss-Hutin D 1975 45,X Turner's syndrome in monozygotic twin sisters. Journal of Medical Genetics 12: 390–396
73. Potter E L 1963 Twin zygosity and placental form in relation to the outcome of pregnancy. American Journal of Obstetrics and Gynecology 87: 566–577
74. Rausen A R, Seki M, Strauss L 1965 Twin transfusion syndrome: review of 19 cases studed at one institution. Journal of Pediatrics 66: 613–628
75. Reijal A-L R, Nazer H M, Abu-Osba Y K, Rifai A, Ahmed S 1992 Conjoined twins: medical, surgical and ethical challenges. Australia and New Zealand Journal of Surgery 62: 287–291
76. Riekhof P L, Horton W A, Harris D J, Schimke R N 1972 Monozygotic twins with the Turner syndrome. American Journal of Obstetrics and Gynecology 112: 59–61
77. Robinson H P, Caines J S 1977 Sonar evidence of early pregnancy failure in patients with twin conceptions. British Journal of Obstetrics and Gynaecology 84: 22–25
78. Rudolph A J, Michaels J P, Nichols B L 1967 Obstetric management of conjoined twins. In: Bergsme D (ed) Conjoined twins. D Birth Defects Original Article Series III, National Foundation March of Dimes, New York

79. Schinzel A A G L, Smith D W, Miller J R 1979 Monozygotic twinning and structural defects. Journal of Pediatrics 95: 921–930
80. Scott J M, Ferguson-Smith M A 1973 Heterokaryotypic monozygotic twins and the acardiac monster. Journal of Obstetrics and Gynaecology of the British Commonwealth 80: 52–59
81. Segreti W D, Winter P M, Nance W E 1979 Familial studies of monozygotic twinning. In: Nance W E, Allens G, Parisi P (eds) Twin research. Biology and epidemiology. Allan R Liss, New York, pp 55–60
82. Soltan H C 1968 Genetic characteristics of families of XO and XXY patients, including evidence of source of X chromosomes in 7 aneuploid patients. Journal of Medical Genetics 5: 173–180
83. Spillman J R 1992 A study of maternity provision in the UK in response to the needs of families who have a multiple birth. Acta Geneticae Medicae et Gemellologiae 41: 353–364
84. Szymonowicz W, Preston H, Yu V Y H 1986 The surviving monozygotic twin. Archives of Disease in Childhood 61: 454–458
85. Taylor E M, Emery J L 1988 Maternal stress, family and health care of twins. Children and Society 4: 351–366
86. Thompson B, Pritchard C, Corney G 1983 Perinatal mortality in twins by zygosity and placentation. Paper presented at Fourth Congress of International Society for Twin Studies, London
87. Van Allen M I, Smith D W, Shepard T H 1983 Twin reversed arterial perfusion (TRAP) sequence: a study of 14 twin pregnancies with acardius. Seminars in Perinatology 7: 285–293
88. Van Staey M, De Bie S, Matton M, Th De Roose J 1984 Familial congenital esophageal atresia. Personal case report and review of the literature. Human Genetics 66: 260–266
89. Wenstrom K D, Syrop C H, Hammitt D G, Van Voorhis B J 1993 Increased risk of monochorionic twinning associated with assisted reproduction. Fertility and Sterility 60: 510–514
90. Wharton B, Edwards J H, Cameron A H 1968 Monoamniotic twins. Journal of Obstetrics and Gynecology 75: 158–163
91. Woodward J 1988 The bereaved twin. Acta Geneticae Medicae et Gemellologiae 37: 173–180
92. Wyshak G, White C 1963 Birth hazard of the second twin. Journal of the American Medical Association 186: 869–870
93. Zake E Z N 1984 Case reports of 16 sets of conjoined twins from a Uganda hospital. Acta Geneticae Medicae et Gemellologiae 33: 75–80

26

Pharmacology

George W. Rylance

INTRODUCTION

No other child offers greater challenges to the prescribing physician than the newborn. There are many reasons for this. Marked changes in maturation are seen throughout the period from 26 weeks' postconceptional age to 4 weeks post-term, and it is not surprising that significant differences in drug handling will be evident during this period. It is also likely that infants will react quite differently at the drug receptor site, and this is likely to be affected by gestational age, weight for dates and the general pathophysiological condition of the infant. The newborn infant is also at risk from diseases and problems that are not seen in older groups of children or in the adult population, and one cannot scale down information from the experience of using drugs in these groups.

Increasing amounts of information are becoming available on the disposition of drugs in newborns, and important differences in the drug-handling processes of absorption, distribution, metabolism and excretion have been observed between preterm newborns, full-term newborns and young infants. However, the information remains sketchy for many of the more commonly used drugs as the maturational process is not clearly predictable, and so monitoring of therapy by accurate observation and measurements of drug levels is particularly important. Appropriate prescribing practice and the achievement of optimum response to drug therapy requires the clinician to have knowledge of drug disposition and pharmacokinetics. In the period between 26 weeks' postconceptional age and 4 weeks post-term there are marked changes in maturation. These changes affect drug disposition and probably also the way infants react at the drug receptor sites, although there is less information on this latter aspect of neonatal pharmacology.

Drug disposition is the handling of a drug through the processes of absorption, distribution, metabolism and excretion. These processes are known to be affected by gestational age, weight for dates and the general pathophysiological condition of the infant.

Pharmacokinetics is the mathematical expression of these drug-handling processes, and this aspect of pharmacology relates to the time between the drug being administered and the processes taking place until the drug is either completely eliminated at cessation of therapy or, with continued therapy, reaches a steady state. Pharmacodynamics is the effects of the drug on the body, and might be considered to represent the processes and reactions relating a drug concentration to clinical effect at the receptor site. Knowledge of pharmacokinetics and pharmacodynamics allows the clinician to achieve optimum prescribing practice in demonstrating appropriate responses to questions such as Which drug to use? What dose? Which route? What dose interval? and How long should therapy be continued?

DRUG-HANDLING PROCESSES

ABSORPTION

Gastrointestinal

There are two major variables that affect the extent and rate of absorption, biopharmaceutical factors and individual patient factors. Most newborns are given drugs intravenously or as liquids, and the processes of disintegration of tablets and dissolution of drug are bypassed. Biopharmaceutical factors are therefore not of great importance at this age.

A number of pathophysiological factors affect gastrointestinal tract absorption, and these vary markedly throughout the newborn period as a result of constant change with maturation and the varying pathology.

Gastric emptying

The rate of gastric emptying is prolonged in the newborn period and older child values are reached at about 6 months of age.[45] The nature of the feed (infant formula or human milk) affects the rate of gastric emptying, as does gestational and postnatal age.[12,19] Preterm babies seem to have slower gastric emptying rates than more mature babies.[12] There is no evidence that this affects drug use, although theoretically it might have disadvantages for drugs such as penicillin, which are degraded in the stomach under acidic conditions. In such situations bioavailability (the amount of drug reaching the systemic circulation as a percentage or proportion of that given as dosage) will be reduced.

Gastrointestinal tract acidity

The pH of stomach juices varies in term babies over the course of the first few days of life. They have an initially neutral stomach juice, falling to a pH of 3 within 48 hours and then returning to neutral over the next 24 hours and for the next 10 days. These changes do not occur in premature infants, who seem to have little or no free acid during the first 14 days.[2,39] A typical acidic pH of 4 or 4.5 is reached at about 2 years of age.[49] Again it is not clear whether this has any real clinical relevance, although the theoretical benefit of reduced degradation of acid-labile drugs allowing more absorption during the early days of life is accepted.

The literature referring to studies of specific drugs gives no clear information to the practising clinician on the effects of these factors. Vitamin E has been shown to be absorbed as well in preterm babies as older term babies and infants.[8] Phenobarbitone has been shown to be more slowly absorbed in the first few days of life compared to later ages.[9] The reverse of this would be expected according to the theoretical basis of the pH partition hypothesis, which suggests that basic drugs should be absorbed more rapidly in an alkaline milieu.

Food

In older children food affects the absorption of drugs in different ways. Milk reduces the absorption of tetracyclines,[40] but food generally enhances the absorption of carbamazepine,[27] propranolol[31] and griseofulvin.[14] It is not known whether these drug–food interactions occur in the newborn period.

Disease factors

Little is known of the effects of specific disease on gastrointestinal absorption of drugs in the newborn. Hypoxic episodes and poor perfusion, both of which are common in ill newborns, might be expected to reduce the rate and amount of drug absorbed in such conditions. In older individuals severe cardiac insufficiency reduces the perfusion of the splanchnic area and so reduces and delays absorption.[46]

Drug metabolism by gastrointestinal microflora

The gastrointestinal tract becomes colonized with many different species of bacteria within the first hours of birth. This, or rather the content and type of intestinal flora, is a function of diet rather than age.[51] Whether these changes affect intestinal metabolism and hence the absorption of drugs has not been shown in the newborn period.

'First-pass' effects

This phenomenon, where passage through the gut wall and liver causes a decrease in the bioavailability of a drug as a result of metabolism at these sites, is not one which is likely to have great bearing on drug use in the newborn period. None of the relevant drugs known to have a high hepatic extraction on first passage through the liver is used to any extent by any route in the newborn period. Morphine is the only one that is sometimes used in this situation, and the effects of first-pass metabolism may account for some of the difficulties in appropriate dosing of children with this drug in early life.

Intramuscular absorption

The rate and extent of drug absorption from intramuscular sites depends primarily upon the area over which the solution spreads, blood flow through the area, and how easily the drug penetrates capillary walls. Factors which affect these variables, for example vasomotor instability, relative inefficiency of muscular contraction and relative change in blood flow to different muscles during maturation, might all be expected to affect the absorption of drugs in the newborn period. However, there are few data to demonstrate this in practice. Phenobarbitone administered intramuscularly at this age is more rapidly absorbed than at other ages,[9] although diazepam is more slowly absorbed.[34] The total amount of gentamicin and digoxin absorbed is less in preterm and term newborns than at other ages.[6,47]

It is likely that practical considerations will influence a clinician's choice of route of administration. The preterm neonate has a paucity of skeletal muscle mass, as well as subcutaneous fat. Intramuscular administration of drugs is therefore more difficult and problematic.

Rectal absorption

Absorption of drugs from the rectum does not follow a predictable pattern at any age. The surface area of the rectum, devoid of villi, is considerably smaller than that of the small intestine, and the amount absorbed probably depends mainly on the position of the main volume of drug in relation to the rectal veins. Defecation reflexes may expel suppositories and liquids, or move them to a inserted by means of rectal tubes or syringes, compared to suppositories. Rectally administered solutions of diazepam have been shown to be completely absorbed in older infants,[1] and commonly accepted effective anticonvulsant drug levels can be achieved within 5 minutes of an administered dose.[25]

Percutaneous absorption

The thickness of the keratinized stratum corneum and the degree of skin hydration determines the extent and rapidity of drug absorption following application to the skin. The preterm baby in particular has a thin, poorly keratinized skin which may afford a means of administering drugs in time-release formulations. Percutaneously administered theophylline is a means of treating preterm apnoea,[17] although the full possibilities and application of this approach have not yet been defined.

Conclusions

It is likely that practical considerations have much greater relevance to drug absorption than any theoretical factors. Although the amount and rate of drug delivery from absorption is a significant determinant of effect, spillage of part of an oral dose may have far greater effect. It should also be remembered that a slower rate of absorption does not of itself mean a decrease in total bioavailability, and for drugs whose elimination rate is rapid a slower absorption rate might be beneficial in reducing the fluctuation of drug levels between doses.

DISTRIBUTION

Distribution is the spread of drug throughout the body after it has entered the systemic circulation. The movement of drug between certain tissues and organs, commonly referred to as compartments, is reversible. The major determinants of the rate, extent and pattern of tissue distribution are listed in Table 26.1. Age and size affect all of these factors. Water and fat composition vary markedly between preterm, term and young infants. Total body water per unit body weight is high (87%) in the preterm baby, and considerably higher in the newborn (80%) than in older infants (p. 1016). The extra-

Table 26.1 Major determinants of drug disposition

Rate of absorption
Rates of penetration of biological membranes
Perfusion of organs and tissues
The volume and composition of tissue compartments
The extent of protein binding and binding to other tissues
The rates of biotransformation and excretion

influence water-soluble drugs, which are primarily distributed in this compartment and body water generally. Fat makes up only about one-fifth of body weight and is relatively scarce in the newborn period. Skeletal muscle mass is smaller in the newborn, representing 25% of body weight.[50] The factors that determine the volume and composition of tissue compartments and hence affect distribution according to drug affinity are primary determinants of drug dosage and its variability in the newborn period.

Distribution in blood

Vascular perfusion, diffusion of drugs and the extent of plasma protein binding are all further influences on the extent and rate of drug distribution. If a drug tends to concentrate in one type of tissue mass, as is the case with digoxin, there is a greater tendency for that drug to distribute fully in that tissue mass relatively slowly. This process of diffusion is greatly affected by the extent of perfusion which, if poor, will significantly reduce the time of distribution and hence the clinical effect of the drug at the receptor site. Drugs bind to plasma proteins and red cells in the vascular space. Most drugs bind to albumin, although this is particularly true of acidic drugs, and basic drugs more commonly bind to lipoproteins and α_1-acid glycoprotein.[38]

The process of drug binding to protein is reversible. Drug not bound to protein is free and the fractions of drug–protein complex and free drug are relatively constant; thus an increase in the concentration of protein, and hence the available binding sites, increases the rate and extent of formation of the drug–protein complex. Reduction in protein binding increases drug distribution; the extent of protein binding and the affinity of drug for protein and vice versa are affected by the pH of blood, its temperature and the presence of competitive binding substances.

The degree of binding to plasma proteins is probably the most important factor in determining the extent of whole blood drug distribution. As with other drug-handling processes there is continuing change in this throughout the newborn period. Concentrations of total protein, albumin and globulin are lower in the newborn period than at other ages in childhood.[45] Total protein levels and general binding percentages to protein do not reach adult values until the end of the first year.[16,32] There are also quantitative differences in albumin.[48] Fetal albumin is different in the newborn period than at other ages[33] and it also has a lower affinity for drugs. α_1-acid glycoprotein concentrations are also lower in the newborn.[52] When there is a reduced amount, or a decrease in the binding capacity, of plasma protein, the free (unbound) drug fraction is increased. In newborns, therefore, lower total plasma drug concentrations are infants and children, as a result of this free fraction for many drugs being greater in the newborn.

It is interesting to compare the clinical effects of two drugs, both of which are reported to have considerably lower plasma protein binding in newborns, and particularly preterm newborns, than in later infancy and childhood. Plasma protein binding of theophylline in children is approximately 55%, but in preterm infants it is 35–40%. The free fraction of theophylline is therefore $1\frac{1}{2}$ times greater in the preterm infant. This may account for the lower reported therapeutic range for reducing preterm apnoea as described in total plasma concentration compared to the reported therapeutic range for theophylline in asthma in older children. If the free fraction concentration at total plasma concentrations of 10–20 mg/l is approximately 4.5–9 mg/l in older children, then the same free fraction concentration range in neonates corresponds to a total plasma concentration range of approximately 6.5–13 mg/l, which is of the same order as the therapeutic range reported by Jones and Baillie[21] for the prevention of preterm apnoea. There is of course no reason why the therapeutic range for one effect of a drug should necessarily be the same as that for another effect, albeit one which is related to some extent through action on the respiratory system or centre. With regard to diazepam, the free fraction in preterm babies as a result of lower plasma protein binding is approximately 15–25%, compared to 10% in later infancy and childhood. One would therefore expect that if there is a relationship between the concentration of the free fraction and clinical effect, lower total concentrations of this drug might be as effective as the higher concentrations reportedly necessary for anticonvulsant effect in older children. Estimates of this range, which is not established, have been reported as 150–300 ng/l.[25] However, at these concentrations the clinical effect of diazepam in newborns seems to be less than that at other ages. The likely explanation is that there is not a close relationship between the concentration of total drug or the free fraction and the clinical effect for diazepam, but rather the critical influence is the affinity of drugs in binding to receptors at different ages. It may be supposed that diazepam binds less well at the receptor site in the newborn infant, although similar concentrations may be achieved in blood to those obtained in older infants. Values for the percentage protein binding of some of the more commonly used drugs in the newborn period are shown in Table 26.2.

Protein binding is also influenced by endogenous substances such as free fatty acids and bilirubin. These, as well as other drugs, competitively bind to the same plasma proteins and, depending on their respective affinities, affect the degree of plasma protein binding in newborns. If two drugs are used together and these competitively bind to plasma proteins, then the free fraction

Drug	Percentage bound to protein
Aspirin	95
Caffeine	25
Diazepam	75–90
Digoxin	16–30
Frusemide	95
Indomethacin	95
Penicillin	65
Phenobarbitone	20–35
Phenytoin	70
Theophylline	35–55

of one or both will be increased as a result of such combination therapy. Bilirubin and free fatty acids act in a similar way and both may displace drugs from albumin binding sites, increasing the free fraction. For bilirubin this phenomenon is particularly clinically important as it occurs in both directions. Displacement of unconjugated bilirubin from albumin-binding sites by sulphonamides is widely known as a cause of bilirubin toxicity (p. 720), although the problem has been reduced by the negligible use of sulphonamides in neonatal practice in recent years, and also the advances in obstetric and rhesus immunization practices.

It is only when plasma protein binding is about 90% or more that the majority of drug is in plasma, and it is only in this situation that clinically important effects of protein binding displacement of bilirubin or other drugs occur. This is because it is only within the plasma compartment that there is significant quantitative change in protein binding. By considering the drugs in Table 26.2 it can be seen that frusemide, indomethacin, diazepam, salicylates, phenytoin, sulphonamides (excluding sulphadiazine) and diazoxide will be important in competitive binding situations. In addition, all these drugs have lower plasma protein binding in newborn infants than older children, and the clinical effects of these drugs for similar total drug concentrations are likely to be greater in immature infants. Over 150 drugs have been reported to displace bilirubin from albumin in vitro,[11] but the true clinical risk of any one of these drugs is not easily assessed. Table 26.3 lists a number of these drugs according to the strength of their displacing properties, and the drugs listed are those most likely to be of clinical importance. The converse effect of bilirubin displacing drugs from binding sites has not been evaluated.

The blood–brain barrier, which is a determinant of distribution, is frequently considered to be more permeable in newborns than older children. However, there are no specific data to substantiate this and the impression is based on the reported easier penetration of certain substances into fetal animal brains than into adult brains and the higher concentration of protein in newborn human cerebrospinal fluid than in adults.

Table 26.3 Drugs which displace bilirubin

Potency of displacing property	Drug or drug group
Very strong	X-ray contrast media
Moderate to strong	Aspirin
	Indomethacin
	Other analgesic and anti-inflammatory agents
	Sulphonamides (excluding sulphadiazine)
Weak	Frusemide
	Sulphadiazine
Unlikely to displace	Antibiotics
	Antihistamines
	Narcotics
	Other diuretics
	Sedatives

Overall, the reduced plasma protein binding and the relatively large body water compartments found in newborns tend to give larger apparent volumes of distribution of drugs in babies than at other ages.

BIOTRANSFORMATION

Biotransformation is the process whereby lipid-soluble drug molecules are converted to more polar and more water-soluble products which can be efficiently removed from the body by excretion through the kidneys or other routes. Although these processes usually result in a lowering of biological activity of drugs as a result of a more rapid clearance than would otherwise be the case, this is not always so, as certain drugs produce intermediate or final products which are clinically active and therefore important in their therapeutic or toxic effects. Commonly used drugs which produce active metabolites are shown in Table 26.4. For most of these drugs, the parent drug effects are predominant and the metabolites are of little clinical relevance. However, this is not the case for theophylline or carbamazepine, for which a considerable part or even major part of the overall effect may be as a result of active metabolite.

The rate and route of converting a drug to metabolites in the body is the major determinant of the true course and intensity of its effect, the nature, frequency, time course and intensity of its adverse effects, and its usefulness and efficacy in therapeutics.

The major biotransformation processes are oxidation, reduction hydrolysis (phase I reactions) and conjugation (phase II reactions), carried out mainly in hepatic microsomes and by esterases.

Table 26.4 Drugs which produce active metabolites

Drug	Active metabolite(s)
Carbamazepine	Carbamazepine 10, 11-expoxide
Chloral hydrate	Trichloroethanol
Diazepam	Desmethyldiazepam
	Oxazepam
Theophylline	Caffeine

ESTERASE ACTIVITY

Esterases are primarily responsible for the hydrolysis of drugs and are found in plasma and other tissues, including the liver. A few commonly used drugs depend on this process for metabolism – pethidine, procaine and succinylcholine are the best-known examples. There is lower esterase activity in premature newborns than full-term babies.[13] Lower rates of hydrolysis of procaine, as well as low cholinesterase and arylesterase activity, have been described in newborns.[7,16,43]

HEPATIC MICROSOMAL ENZYME SYSTEM

This system, based on cytochrome P-450 and involving a large number of isoenzymes, is responsible for oxidation, reduction and conjugation reactions. Cytochrome P-450 and NADPH-cytochrome-C reductase activity in term babies is approximately half that found in adults in vitro.[3] However, more recent work demonstrates that the proportions of isoenzymes can change significantly as development proceeds.[23] In vivo, enzyme activity catalysing phase I reactions is generally reduced in newborns, and particularly in preterm babies. However, there is variability in the rates of different processes, suggesting differential maturation of this activity. Hydroxylation rates are reduced in the newborn for a number of drugs, including amylobarbitone, mepivacaine, nortriptyline, phenobarbitone and phenytoin, but dealkylation of mepivacaine and diazepam is less impaired.[35] The *N*-demethylation pathway is deficient for theophylline and caffeine[4,10] and the rate of maturation for this latter process appears to be slower with regard to theophylline than hydroxylation of phenytoin and phenobarbitone. Clearance rates of phenobarbitone exceed adult values before 3 weeks' postnatal age, but adult values are not achieved with theophylline until 2 months or more have elapsed. Interestingly, diazepam is demethylated to a reasonable extent, but is poorly hydroxylated and conjugated in preterms compared to full-term babies and older children.[30]

Sulphation and glycination phase II conjugation reactions proceed at similar rates to adults in newborns, although glucuronidation is significantly reduced.[26] In some cases the relatively poor conjugation with glucuronic acid may be compensated for by enhancement of sulphate conjugation,[28] as is the case for paracetamol, for which sulphate conjugation is more efficient than in older children and adults. There is no compensatory pathway for chloramphenicol. A dangerous situation can develop when plasma chloramphenicol levels rise on relatively low, weight-related doses as a result of this inefficient biotransformation process. The 'grey baby syndrome' results and may well be fatal. Some drugs which might be expected to have poor rates of conjugation in the liver may undergo glucuronidation in the intestine and β-glucuronidase activity may be seven times greater in the newborn intestine than in the adult.[53] Indomethacin undergoes enterohepatic recirculation, and this may be a factor in its conjugation.

The variation in efficiency of different metabolic pathways has not been clearly explained. Exposure to enzyme-inducing agents in utero may be one factor affecting some processes, and there may also be differential substrate specificity. However, the mechanisms that regulate biotransformation processes have still not been fully elucidated and it is likely that several factors are involved.

The effects of illness, nutritional status and other drug therapy on biotransformation process have not been defined, and although studies showing the effect of hypoxaemia on drug elimination through the kidney have been reported, no data on drugs which are hepatically metabolized are available.

It is important to realize that, although there are large gaps in knowledge and many of the mechanisms are poorly understood, drug elimination relating to hepatic biotransformation processes in the newborn, particularly preterm newborns, is generally slow in the first few weeks of life, and increases at varying rates according to the transformation process over the next few weeks. Some of these effects are not predictable, and therefore close monitoring in a clinical setting is important.

RENAL EXCRETION

Renal excretion is the main pathway for elimination of drugs and their metabolites from the body. It is dependent on three particular processes: glomerular filtration, tubular secretion and tubular reabsorption.

GLOMERULAR FILTRATION RATE

The effects of gestational age and postdelivery age on renal function are described in detail in Chapter 39. This variation in GFR with time, most of which cannot be defined for any drug or gestational age of child, has important consequences for therapy, particularly with those drugs which are potentially toxic and have a relatively low therapeutic index (narrow range of concentration between the achievement of clinical therapeutic activity and toxic effects).

TUBULAR SECRETION

This is reduced at birth, as expressed by the maximal tubular excretory capacity of PAH (TmPAH) per unit surface area. Adult values are reached after approximately 2–3 months.[18]

PASSIVE TUBULAR REABSORPTION

This depends on drug lipid solubility, pH of urine, tubular surface area and the rate of urine flow. Highly lipid-soluble drugs diffuse rapidly, whereas ionized acidic or basic drugs which are less lipid-soluble diffuse slowly.

The capacity to reabsorb drugs from the renal tubule in newborns seems to be reasonably developed, as drugs known to be reabsorbed in this way are excreted slowly in the first few days of life.[15] Glucose is actively reabsorbed by the tubule, and its slow elimination at this time provides further evidence of reasonable reabsorption capacity.

DRUGS AND THE FETUS

DRUG EXPOSURE

During pregnancy a mother is likely to take a number of drugs, to be exposed to chemicals in a social or work environment, and also to partake of some social/recreational chemicals such as alcohol. The fetus is therefore exposed to a wide range of drugs/chemicals considered advantageous to the mother but frequently undesirable and deleterious to the fetus itself. The main factors influencing the transfer of drugs across the placenta and their effects on the fetus are listed in Table 26.5.

DRUG HANDLING BY THE FETUS

In vitro studies have demonstrated that the fetus has considerable ability to metabolize some exogenous biological substances,[37,41,42] and cytochrome P-450 and hepatic microsomal enzymes capable of hydroxylation have been shown to be present.[54] However, the activity of

Table 26.5 Factors influencing placental transfer of drugs and effects on the fetus

Physiochemical properties	Water solubility Fat solubility Molecular weight
Drug-handling processes placenta fetus	 Distribution Elimination
Stage in pregnancy	Teratogenicity and death in first trimester Growth and developmental retardation in second and third trimesters
Drug load	Single high doses versus chronic low doses Interactions between drugs may enhance effects
Genetics	Specific enzyme deficiencies or relative delays in presence of enzymes due to genetic background

glucuronyl transferase is low. It is likely that there is greater interindividual variation in these processes during fetal life than at any other time postnatally, and the differences are probably a function of enzyme induction in utero and genetic variability. It is interesting that the fetal adrenal has higher concentrations of cytochrome P-450 than the liver.[22] This may suggest that the liver has a predominantly haemopoietic rather than detoxifying function during fetal life. Rates of glomerular filtration are extremely low prenatally, and tubular function seems to be even more poorly developed. It is unlikely that the fetal kidney plays an important role in drug elimination, as most drugs will be removed from fetal plasma via the placenta. However, there may be some recycling of drugs excreted in fetal urine as amniotic fluid, into which urine is passed, is swallowed.

Of major importance are the toxic and teratogenic effects of drugs on the fetus. Although biotransforming enzymes do not seem to be present in the first 3 months of fetal life, there are no specific data suggesting that teratogenicity at the time of organogenesis might be related to drug-handling problems. Because much larger contributions to drug disposition are made through the maternal unit via the mother's distribution, biotransformation and excretion processes, as well as transplacental exchange of drugs and their metabolites, it seems that the inability of the fetus to metabolize drugs will be only a small factor in overall drug disposition.

The most significant problem for the fetus will relate to repeated maternal dosing, because at this time maternal–fetal drug equilibrium will have been reached. Little drug will reach the fetus if a small number or single doses of rapidly cleared drugs are given to the mother.

There remains a possibility that wide variability in maturation of different elimination pathways in the newborn may cause some drugs to be converted to highly reactive metabolites which cannot be metabolized further. Such a block in what might postnatally be a long series of metabolic processes leading to the production of more polar metabolites could lead to toxicity in the fetus, and would produce an entirely different presentation to anything seen in postnatal life.

All drugs must be considered to be potentially harmful in the embryonic period, and the relative risks of benefit for the mother against potential toxicity in the fetus must always be assessed. In the first 2 weeks following conception it seems that there is probably an 'all or nothing' effect, in that either death may result or the fetus will be unaffected. For the remainder of the first trimester congenital malformations are the most likely drug effects, and subsequently, in the second and third trimesters, growth and developmental retardation are the likely effects. If drugs are administered to the mother shortly before delivery, a different spectrum of adverse effects is seen.

Drugs most likely to harm the fetus during pregnancy are listed in Table 26.6. Commonly used drugs which may produce adverse effects in newborns when administered shortly before delivery are shown in Table 26.7.

Table 26.6 Drugs most likely to harm the fetus

Period	Drug	Effect/comment
First trimester		
Proven	Cytotoxic drugs	Risk is greatest with alkylating agents
	Thalidomide	
	Vitamin A analogues	
Probable	Alcohol	Chronic use
	Anticonvulsants	
	Lithium	
	Warfarin	
	Live vaccines	Viraemia in fetus? Malformations
Possible	Chloroquine	
	Oestrogens	
	Progestogens	May produce virilization of the female fetus
	Trimethoprim (and cotrimoxazole)	
Second/third trimesters	Aminoglycosides	Auditory and vestibular nerve damage
	Antithyroids	Goitre and hypothyroidism
	Chloroquine	Choroidoretinitis
	Diazoxide	Fetal diabetes
	Lithium	Goitre
	Tetracyclines	Discoloration of primary and secondary dentition
	Thiazides	Thrombocytopenia

Table 26.7 Drugs which produce adverse effects in the newborn, if administered shortly before delivery

Drug	Effect
Alcohol	Withdrawal syndrome
Anaesthetics	Respiratory depression
Anticoagulants (oral)	Haemorrhage (fetus or newborn)
Antimalarials	Haemolytic anaemia
Aspirin	Haemorrhage (platelet function affected and hypoprothrombinaemia)
Barbiturates	Withdrawal syndrome if given for more than a few days
Benzodiazepines	Hypotonia/hypothermia
Chloramphenicol	'Grey baby syndrome'
Hypnotics/sedatives	Respiratory depression
Lithium	Hypotonia/cyanosis/bradycardia
Narcotic analgesics	Respiratory depression and withdrawal syndrome
Phenothiazines	Extrapyramidal effects
Propranolol	Hyperglycaemia
Sulphonamides	Displace unconjugated bilirubin from albumin (p. 420)

PHARMACOKINETICS AND CLINICAL RELEVANCE

Pharmacokinetics is the mathematical expression of the effects of drug-handling processes and relationships that occur between dose administration and drug concentrations in biological fluids. The relationships that describe 'what the body does to a drug' are usually considered in terms of model systems, rate constants of absorption and elimination, as well as of transfer, and apparent volumes of distribution. Although the terminology is somewhat baffling for clinicians on first consideration, many of the concepts are known already from an understanding of physiological principles. It is necessary for the clinician to have some knowledge of these principles and their application in the clinical setting. The basic units are derived from concentration–time data generated from studies when both single and repeat doses are given.

APPARENT VOLUME OF DISTRIBUTION (V_D)

This proportionality constant describes a conceptual volume into which drug is distributed and is an expression of the amount of drug in the body relative to that in plasma at any one time. When concentrations are higher in the tissue than in plasma for any drug, the volume of distribution of that drug will have a value greater than 1.0 l/kg. Conversely, volumes of distribution of less that 1.0 l/kg are associated with lower concentrations in tissue than in plasma. This relationship is described by the equation:

$$V_d(\text{l/kg}) = \frac{\text{Total drug in body (mg/kg)}}{\text{Plasma concentration (mg/l)}} \qquad (1)$$

The values for V_d vary according to drugs and individuals, although reported values will necessarily more usually describe values for any one drug in a group of subjects.

If a drug is distributed in total body water, the V_d will approximate to that volume. In the preterm newborn this value may be about 0.8 or 0.9 l/kg, whereas in the term newborn this would be slightly less, about 0.7–0.8 l/kg, so reflecting the usual total body water volume per unit body weight at these gestations. Highly protein-bound drugs tend to have smaller volumes of distribution than 0.7 l/kg in the early newborn period. Hence, the volume of distribution of the highly protein-bound sodium valproate is 0.28–0.43 l/kg.[20] However, some drugs which are highly protein bound in plasma may also bind strongly to tissues, and this is the case for both diazepam and phenytoin, each of which is 80–85% protein bound, with respective values for V_d of 1.8–2.0 l/kg and 0.7–2.0 l/kg in the first few days of life.

Apparent volumes of distribution in newborns are generally greater than in later infancy and childhood, and values for some of the more commonly used drugs are shown in Table 26.8.

The V_d is the major determinant of plasma concentration following a single dose, although the route by which the dose is given will influence how the volume of distribution expresses itself with regard to the concentration in a body fluid, usually plasma. Therefore, immediately following an intravenous dose, plasma concentration can be predicted using equation (1) above. In reality, the plasma concentration achieved immediately after an i.v. dose is affected by the time it takes to distribute drug to the various tissues in the body. In addition the initial concentration immediately begins to fall as a result of elimination processes. However, it is helpful to utilize the equation in clinical situations where immediate effect is necessary, and where a single dose or first loading dose prior to a repeating dose schedule is considered necessary.

Table 26.8 Approximate apparent volumes of distribution

Drug	V_d(l/kg)
Amikacin	0.55
Amoxycillin	1.10
Caffeine	0.90
Diazepam	1.90
Digoxin	10.00
Frusemide	0.30
Gentamicin	0.50
Indomethacin	5.50
Methicillin	0.45
Netilmicin	0.50
Phenobarbitone	0.85
Phenytoin	0.90
Theophylline	0.70
Ticarcillin	0.50

Example

The loading dose (D) of phenobarbitone (V_d = 0.8 l/kg) to achieve cessation of convulsions where the desired plasma concentration (C_p) is approximately 25 mg/l (range 15–30 mg/l) is obtained by rearranging equation (1), thus:

$$D = V_d \times C_p$$
$$D = 0.8\ \text{l/kg} \times 25\ \text{mg/l}$$
$$D = 20\ \text{mg/kg}$$

DRUG COMPARTMENTS AND RATE CONSTANTS (k)

Although a drug distributes into a number of tissues or compartments in the body following administration, most can be considered to distribute into a single compartment, as concentration–time data derived from studies in newborns and older children generally fit this simplest form of description. Following intravenous administration, concentration–time data will show a decline in concentration with time, with a peak concentration immediately or very soon after the dose has been completed. Following other forms of administration drug concentration will rise, reaching a peak before falling in a similar pattern to that seen following intravenous dosing. This single compartment of drug distribution and concentration change within the body is described simply in Figure 26.1.

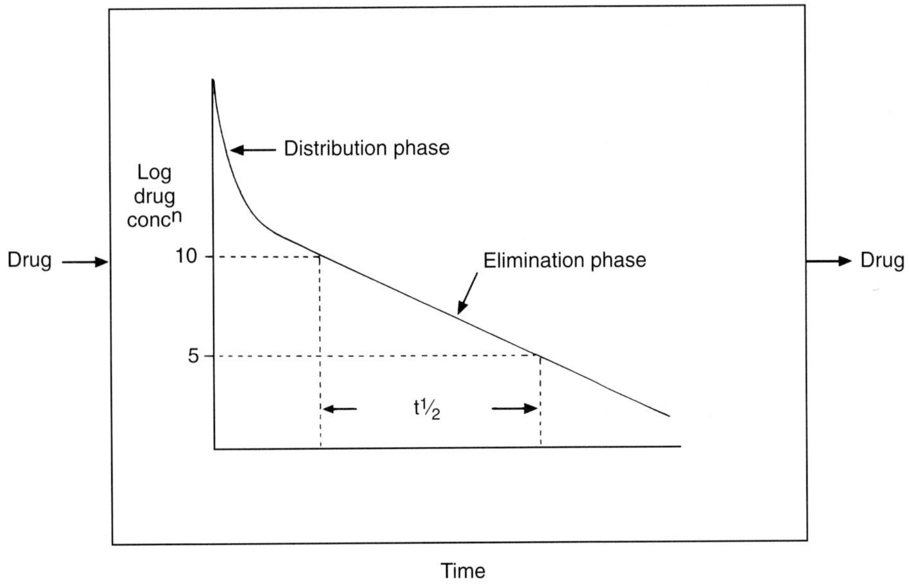

Fig. 26.1 Single-compartment drug distribution and blood concentration versus time.

In single-compartment kinetics, drug movement follows first-order kinetic principles in that the rate of change of drug concentration directly relates to the amount of drug present at any particular time. The more drug present, the faster will be the rate of removal. The fact that most drugs follow first-order kinetics for elimination means that it is possible to determine the amount of drug present at any one time, and also to describe rate constants (k) which are values for the fractional rate of drug elimination (k_e) or accumulation (absorption) (k_a). Rate constants are described in reciprocal units of time (h^{-1}) and, for elimination, will directly reflect the slope of the elimination phase of the concentration–time curve (Fig. 26.1).

Elimination half-life ($t_{\frac{1}{2}}$)

This is the usual term to describe the disappearance of drug from blood, although it can relate to disappearance from other compartments. It is the time taken for any given concentration of drug in blood to fall to one-half of its initial value. It is calculated from the elimination rate constant (k_e), representing the slope of the log concentration–time curve which is generated if blood drug concentration results following a single intravenous dose are plotted as in Figure 26.1.

The $t_{\frac{1}{2}}$ is then calculated from the relationship:

$$t_{\frac{1}{2}} = \frac{0.693}{k_e} \quad (2)$$

The elimination half-life describes only what is happening in blood and takes no account of distribution. This limits its application, as it does not represent a comprehensive index of drug removal from the body. However, it is frequently considered to be an indirect measure of drug elimination capacity and, for most drugs, it is inversely related to clearance rates, which are specific measures of drug elimination.

The values for elimination rate constant, elimination half-life and volume of distribution are independent of drug dose within any one individual, but each varies between individuals. Consideration of drug-handling processes in newborns, who have slower hepatic and renal clearance of most drugs, suggests that $t_{\frac{1}{2}}$ values at this age, and particularly in preterm babies, would be higher than in term newborns and older children. Comparative values for $t_{\frac{1}{2}}$ in newborns and children shown in Table 26.9 demonstrate this.

The elimination half-life is a major determinant of the extent of fluctuation in drug concentration between doses and also of the time taken before steady-state concentration is achieved following the institution of repeated dose regimens.

Table 26.9 Plasma elimination half-lives in hours for newborns and children (abstracted from literature)

Drug	Preterm infants	Term infants	Children
Caffeine*	31–132	26–231	2–4
Carbamazepine	–	–	6–18
Cefotaxime	3.0–5.7	2–3.5	–
Diazepam*	–	–	14–22
Digoxin	60–120	40–100	28–40
Gentamicin	3.5–16.1	2.3–5.9	1.2
Indomethacin*	12–51	–	–
Netilmicin	4–5.5	3.8–5.5	–
Phenobarbitone	60–200	41–120	37–73
Phenytoin*	60–130	10–100	2–30
Theophylline*	12–35	–	15–5

* Eliminated by 'dose-dependent' (Michaelis–Menten) kinetics at usual therapeutic concentration. Elimination half-life varies markedly.

For drugs for which there is good relationship between concentration in blood and clinical effect, fluctuation in concentration between doses is generally acceptable when the dose interval is less than or approximately equal to that of the $t_{\frac{1}{2}}$. This is particularly true for drugs given via the intravenous route. However, if drugs are given by other routes fluctuation will be affected by the rapidity of absorption from their sites of administration, and this is usually expressed as an absorption rate constant (k_a). Following administration by routes other than the intravenous there is a rise in blood drug concentration, indicating that absorption is proceeding more rapidly than elimination, and the absorption rate constant can be derived from the slope of this phase in the concentration–time graph, together with the slope of the elimination phase extrapolated back through the period when the concentration is increasing. Although the rate of absorption for most drugs commonly given by routes other than the intravenous is relatively slow, the absorption phases are generally considerably shorter than the elimination phases, and consequently the elimination half-life remains the primary determinant of fluctuation.

The combination of relatively slow absorption rates and long elimination half-lives for most drugs in the newborn period means that fluctuation in newborn plasma concentrations when dose intervals are similar to older infants and children is generally quite small, and indeed it allows drug doses to be given less frequently at this age than in later life.

The long half-life of drugs in the newborn period sometimes leads to certain problems. For example, renal toxicity of gentamicin relates to trough concentrations being above 3 mg/l for considerable periods of time, and yet appreciable peak levels of this drug in plasma need to be achieved in order to exceed the MIC of the organism. In order to allow time for the long elimination half-life to show sufficient fall-off in concentration to obtain values below 3 mg/l, the dose interval sometimes needs to be extended considerably, so that even once-daily dosing is appropriate. However, at this frequency there may not be sufficient peak concentrations exceeding the MICs of causative organisms per unit time within the treatment period. The risk–benefit consideration of this dosing process needs to be addressed, particularly in the newborn period. The elimination half-life also determines the time taken for a drug to reach *steady-state concentration* following the first dose or start of an infusion. A baby has a steady-state concentration when the amount of drug going into the body is equal to the amount being eliminated. It takes approximately 5–6 half-lives for a drug to reach a concentration very close to steady state, and this accumulation is represented in Table 26.10. It demonstrates in simple terms what happens to a drug concentration if doses are given as boluses by the intravenous route at intervals of the half-life. The percentages refer to the drug concentrations that would be obtained if the dose given were instantaneously distributed, and with values obtained as in equation (1) earlier. At the end of one half-life the concentration given by that equation will have fallen to half (50%) of the starting value. On giving further doses representing 100%, the concentration, when added to that remaining at the end of one half-life, becomes 150% and falls to 75% after two half-lives. The next dose gives 175%, falling to 87.5% at the eventual steady-state concentration after three half-lives have elapsed, and so on. The peaks of 100%, 150%, 175%, etc. are not reached if doses are given by intravenous infusion, and the concentration accumulation will then be described according to the interrupted line in Figure 26.2. In this case there is no fluctuation in eventual steady state. When doses are given via other routes, the build-up in drug concentration to steady state follows a pattern, as described in Figure 26.3. In this case, within each dose interval there is no instantaneous distribution (as indeed there never is following intravenous dosing), and the graph between dose intervals takes in the predominantly drug accumulation phase, in which absorption is taking place more rapidly than elimination, and the phase of fall-off in concentration, in which elimination proceeds more rapidly than absorption. Of course, elimination is occurring throughout the dose interval and influences the rate of rise of the concentration–time curve in the predominantly absorption phase.

Table 26.10 Theoretical plasma levels after half-life interval i.v. drug dosing as a percentage of mean steady-state concentration

Number of half-lives	Plasma level as a percentage of steady-state level (immediately post i.v. and before half-life stated)	Plasma level as a percentage of steady-state level (pre-dose and after half-life stated)
1	100	50
2	150	75
3	175	88
4	188	94
5	194	97
6	197	98
7	198	99

If an i.v. infusion is stopped, or if a repeated dose regimen is discontinued, there is a fall-off in drug concentration, usually according to first-order kinetics, with again about five or six half-lives elapsing before concentration returns to near zero. In both cases (i.v. infusion and repeated dose schedules), a single line describes the rate of decrease in drug concentration. As in the case of accumulation following the first dose, the major change in drug concentration occurs in the first one to three half-lives.

It is important in clinical practice to recognize these phases of accumulation and fall-off in concentration after starting and stopping therapy. In the first case, before five or six half-lives have elapsed the concentration in a baby's blood does not accurately reflect that which would be

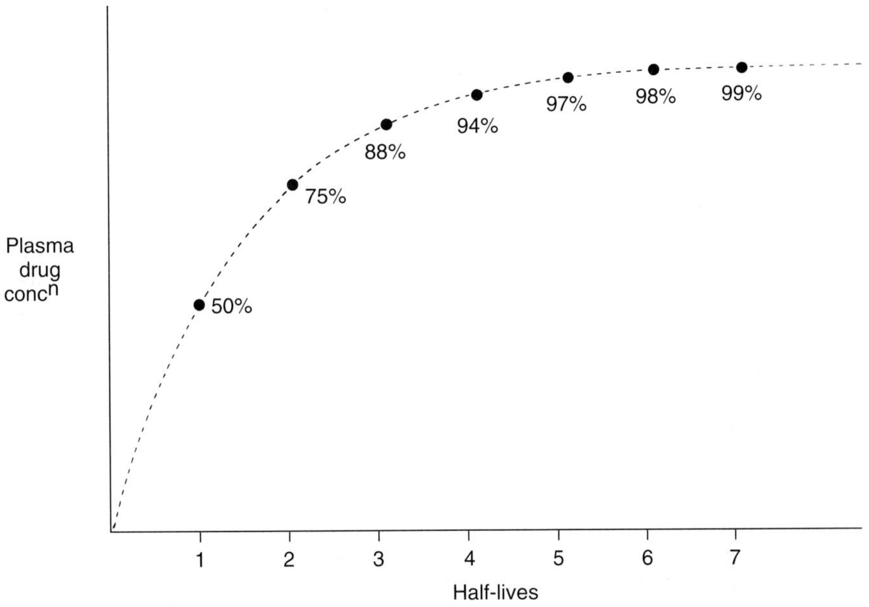

Fig. 26.2 Concentrations as a percentage of eventual steady-state concentrations with repeated doses without a loading dose and related to half-life intervals.

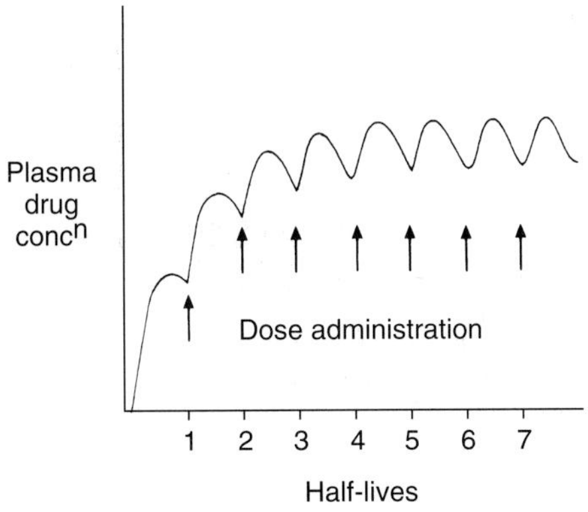

Fig. 26.3 Schematic representation of build-up in plasma drug concentration demonstrating achievement of steady-state after approximately five half-lives have elapsed (doses at half-life intervals for simplicity).

expected from the regular same-dose schedule which has been defined. Similarly, clinical effect will continue, albeit probably greatly reduced, for an appreciable period after the last dose is given. Where clinical effect needs to be rapidly achieved, and this is more frequent in newborn practice than at other ages, it is necessary to give a *loading dose* in order to reduce the time taken for a drug to reach steady state, that is, unless the half-life of a drug is particularly short. The loading dose necessary is determined as in equation (1), relating the desired concentration to the apparent volume of distribution for that drug. In some cases loading doses can prove toxic, particularly when there is slow distribution into tissues and particularly when certain tissues preferentially take up the drug. The large apparent volume of distribution is sometimes reflective of this position, and in the case of digoxin the loading or digitalizing dose is usually divided into three parts in order to reduce toxicity. Indeed, the finding by Krasula et al[24] that about one-quarter of children rapidly digitalized have electrocardiographic evidence of dysrhythmias has prompted many clinicians to reconsider whether such a loading dose is indicated for this drug.

Figure 26.4 describes, according to a mean concentration, what happens if a loading dose is not used when starting therapy with phenobarbitone, and compares the time taken to reach steady state in newborns, older infants and children, in whom the respective half-lives are approximately 5–7 days, 24–30 hours and 36–72 hours. The greater part of a month is required in preterm babies, who have phenobarbitone half-lives of approximately 100–120 hours before the steady-state concentration that reflects the dosing schedule is reached.

FIRST-ORDER AND ZERO-ORDER KINETICS

Most drugs are eliminated by first-order kinetics within the range of concentrations used for clinical effect in the newborn period. The exponential decline in drug concentration, as shown in Figure 26.5(A), where distribution is assumed to be instantaneous, demonstrates that the rate of decline of concentration in blood is proportional to the amount of drug or drug concentration present at any one time. This first-order elimination is graphically described when the logarithmic serum drug concentration is plotted against time, in which case a straight line decline is evident (Fig. 26.5(B)). Zero-order kinetics describes the elimination of a drug from a compartment (usually blood), which proceeds at a rate that is not proportionate to the concentration present or dose given. Pharmacokinetics are then frequently called dose-dependent or

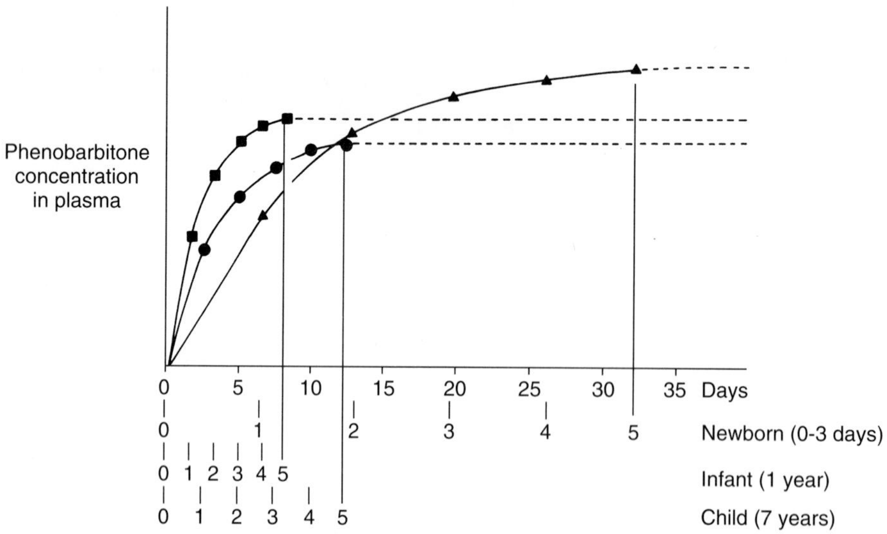

Fig. 26.4 Schematic representation of build-up in phenobarbitone concentration with repeated doses at different ages (different half-lives). ▲, newborn; ● Infant; ■, child.

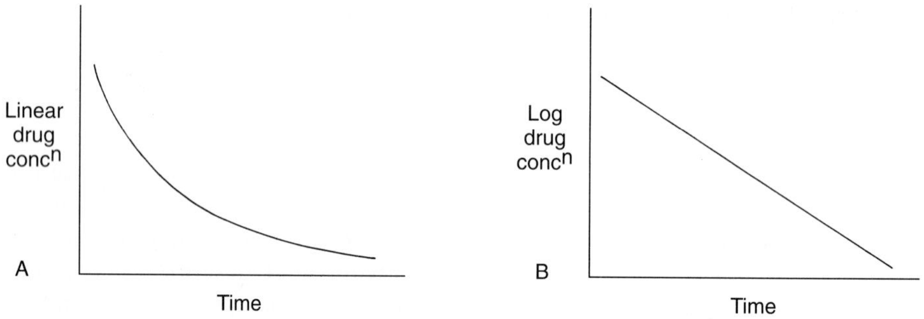

Fig. 26.5 First-order elimination kinetics on (A) linear scale drug concentration and (B) log scale drug concentration.

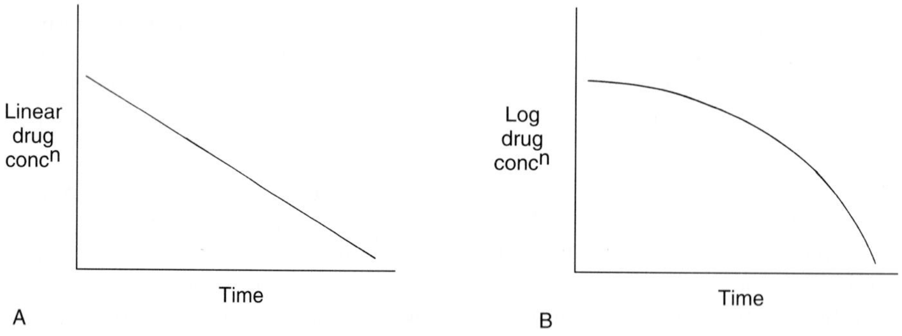

Fig. 26.6 Zero-order elimination kinetics on (A) linear scale drug concentration and (B) log scale drug concentration.

saturation kinetics, the latter term describing the situation obtaining when elimination processes become saturated and the rate of elimination cannot change with increasing concentrations, but proceeds at a constant rate (Fig. 26.6(A) and (B)).

It is likely that most drugs exhibit zero-order kinetics at certain concentrations, but these will usually be very high and much higher than those required to produce clinical effect. Most drugs might therefore be considered to exhibit first-order kinetics, both within and considerably above the range of concentration producing clinical effect, but for these drugs there will be a change to zero-order kinetics at some concentration well above a therapeutic range. The exhibition and change of kinetics from first-order to zero-order in drugs is usually described as Michaelis–Menten kinetics. Figure 26.7 describes the

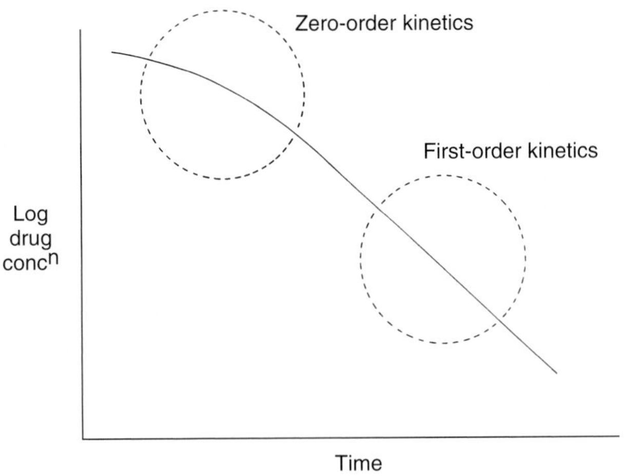

Fig. 26.7 Log concentration–time curve demonstrating Michaelis–Menten kinetics.

pattern and shape of the log concentration–time curve at high concentrations when zero-order kinetics are operative and the more usual first-order kinetics at lower concentrations, which for most drugs are more usually those of therapeutic activity.

A relatively greater number of drugs exhibit dose-dependent kinetics at the usual concentrations required for therapy in newborn practice than at older ages. The list of drugs exhibiting dose-dependent kinetics in Table 26.11 is therefore more extensive than would be the case in other ages of childhood or in adults.

The relevance to dosing situations is that doubling the daily dose or infusion rate for those drugs exhibiting first-order elimination kinetics will result in a twofold increase in drug concentration in blood. A knowledge of drug concentration in one situation therefore permits calculation of the appropriate dose to produce a different desired concentration. In the case of drugs exhibiting Michaelis–Menten kinetics, an increase in dose may result in a large and disproportionate increase in concentration at doses or concentrations within which zero-order kinetics are operable in any one individual. This dose and concentration will usually not be known to the clinician, nor can it be easily predicted. For those drugs listed in Table 26.11 it is appropriate to make only relatively small increases in doses when aiming to enhance the clinical effects. The problem of disproportionate change in drug concentration according to dose change, as in drugs demonstrating saturation kinetics, is diagrammatically expressed in Figure 26.8.

Table 26.11 Drugs which exhibit dose-dependent kinetics with usual therapeutic doses

Caffeine
Chloramphenicol
Diazepam
Frusemide
Indomethacin
Phenytoin
Salicylate
Theophylline

CLEARANCE

Clearance, rather than the elimination half-life, which is dependent upon the volume of distribution, is the true index of drug elimination. It therefore forms the basis of the effects and processes described above. The concept of clearance, reflecting the volume of blood from which drug is removed per unit time, is generally understood from its application in other instances of clinical practice, e.g. in consideration of renal function. Total body clearance (Cl_B) represents the sum total of several organ clearance mechanisms. Total body clearance is directly proportional to the apparent volume of distribution (V_d) and

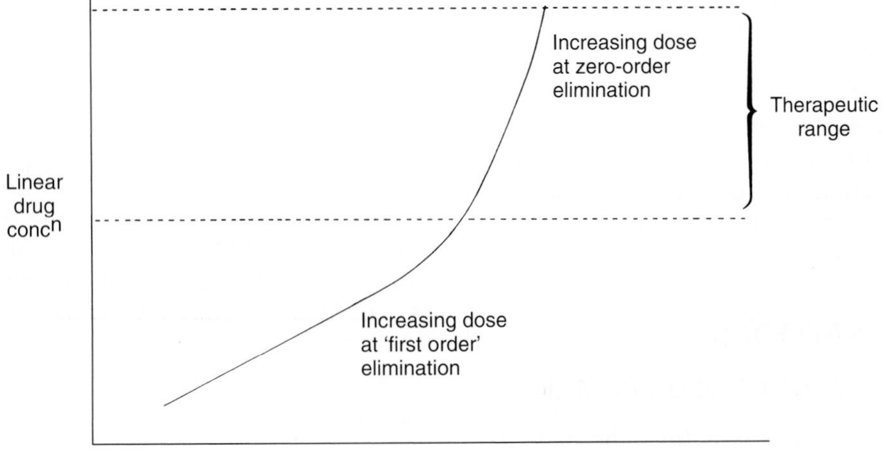

Fig. 26.8 Disproportionately large increase in concentration with increase in dose at concentrations when zero-order kinetics are operable.

inversely proportional to elimination half-life ($t_{\frac{1}{2}}$), as in the following equation:

$$Cl_B = \frac{0.693 \times V_d}{t_{\frac{1}{2}}} \quad \text{or} \quad k_c \times V_d \qquad (3)$$

In repeated dosing, clearance determines the dose required to produce a desired mean steady-state concentration (C_{ss}) according to the equation:

$$C_{ss} = \frac{FD}{V_d \times k_c \times \tau} \qquad (4)$$

where FD is the fraction of dose reaching the systemic circulation and τ is the dose interval. Rearrangement of this equation allows the daily dose of a drug (for which bioavailability values are known) that will produce a desired mean steady-state concentration to be calculated as:

Dose (mg/kg/24 h) = C_{ss}(mg/l) × clearance (1 kg/h) × 24 h

Example

To determine the daily maintenance dose of caffeine (clearance is 0.010 l/kg/h) to give a desired mean steady-state concentration of 20 mg/l (therapeutic range = 5–25 mg/l):

Dose = 20 mg/l × 0.010 l/kg/h × 24
Maintenance dose = 4.8 mg/kg/24 h

In the case of caffeine the elimination half-life is long (60–100 h) and doses can therefore be given once daily without significant fluctuation.

SUMMARY OF CLINICAL RELEVANCE OF PHARMACOKINETICS

- Apparent volumes of distribution are generally larger in the newborn, particularly preterm newborns, than at other ages. Larger weight-related single or loading doses are therefore required to achieve similar concentrations in blood as at other ages.
- Relatively lower degrees of plasma protein binding mean an increase in the free fraction of drug in the newborn, and pharmacological (free fraction) activity is achieved in newborns, compared to other ages, with lower total concentrations of drug in plasma. The relationship of preterm to term newborns is similar to that of newborns to older ages.

DRUGS AND BREAST-FEEDING

PREDICTING THE AMOUNT OF DRUG IN MILK

Almost all drugs and chemicals pass from the maternal blood to breast milk. The amount depends on a number of factors: lipid solubility, water solubility, degree of ionization at milk pH, and molecular weight. In general, transfer is least when drugs are water soluble, have a high molecular weight and are ionized at the usual pH of milk which is less than that of plasma (<7.40). For most drugs, about 1–2% of the maternal dose appears in breast milk. 'Basic' drugs which are ionized above pH 7.4 are found in slightly higher percentages than this.

The milk/plasma concentration ratio (M/P) for most drugs lies between 0.5 and 1.0, and with knowledge of reported M/P ratios and known or expected maternal drug concentrations it is possible to make a calculated prediction of the concentration of the drug in breast milk and therefore the likely concentration of the drug in the nursing infant after single and repeated doses.

Example

Phenobarbitone
M/P ratio = 0.45
Maternal concentration = 20 mg/l (2 mg/dl)
Baby is 5 kg at 6 weeks of age
Baby takes 150 ml each feed
Baby's body water is 0.7 l/kg

Amount of phenobarbitone received by the infant from each feed is:

$$\frac{150 \text{ [feed volume (ml)]}}{1000 \text{ (ml)}} \times 0.45 \text{ (M/P ratio)} \times 20 \text{ [maternal plasma concentration (mg/l)]}$$
$$= 1.35 \text{ mg } (0.27 \text{ mg/kg})$$

The maximum blood concentration after one feed is derived from:

$$\text{Concentration} = \frac{\text{Dose}}{\text{Volume of distribution}} = \frac{0.27 \text{ mg/kg}}{0.70 \text{ l/kg}} = 0.39 \text{ mg/l}$$

The eventual steady-state concentration of phenobarbitone is reached after five elimination half-lives have elapsed (approximately 10 days for this infant, where $t_{\frac{1}{2}}$ = 48 hours).

The steady-state (repeated dose) concentration in the infant's plasma (C_{ssp}) is calculated from

$$C_{ssp} = \frac{F \times D_{feed}}{V_d \times k_e \times \tau}$$

where F is the fraction of drug milk feed that is absorbed, assumed to be 100% or 1, D_{feed} is the drug dose in feed (mg/kg) = 0.27, k_e is the elimination rate constant (= $0.693/t_{\frac{1}{2}}$/h = 0.15/h), V_d is the volume of distribution (l/kg) = 0.70 and τ is the dose interval (hours) = 4.8 (mean of five feeds in 24 hours).

Then substituting:

$$C_{ssp} = \frac{0.027}{0.015 \times 0.7 \times 4.8} = 5.4 \text{ mg/l}$$

For most drugs, such theoretical calculations suggest that only very small amounts of drug are ingested by infants when breast-feeding. However, it should be remembered that milk is rich in fat and that it is known that there are active transport systems for some drugs. Higher milk/plasma ratios may therefore occur with some lipid-soluble drugs and those which have active transport or secretion systems.

EXTENT OF THE PROBLEM

The background theory suggests that most drugs cross from maternal plasma to milk, and that the levels in milk closely parallel those in plasma, with M/P ratios of 0.5–1.0. However, for most drugs there is little available information about the usual situation when repeated drug doses are taken by the mother. Generally, the problems associated with human milk drug excretion have been grossly overstated, and although most drugs are present in breast milk the amount is too small to cause harm to the baby. Only a few drugs are contraindicated in the breast-feeding mother, and these are listed in Table 26.12.

Special care should be taken with those drugs which are potentially toxic but unlikely or not known to cause problems. These are listed in Table 26.13, with reasonable monitoring practice. It is also necessary to consider that the effects of prolonged use of some drugs, for example psychoactive agents, may adversely affect the developing infant's brain, whereas short-course (1–2 weeks) therapy may not. Many of the more frequently expressed concerns about effects of drugs excreted in breast milk have no basis in practice or theory: for example, warfarin is not present in breast milk except in minuscule amounts.

PRINCIPLES OF PRACTICE FOR THE PAEDIATRICIAN

- Question the need for therapy. Develop good relationships in this area with the obstetrician and family physicians. Most routine therapy may not be necessary. Situations where therapy is contraindicated are rare (Table 26.12). Even special provision situations are uncommon (Table 26.13).
- Use the least potentially toxic drug compatible with appropriate care of the mother. An alternative (e.g. ibuprofen for aspirin; methylthiouracil for carbimazole) may be potentially safer and require less monitoring.
- Reduce the baby's exposure to the drug to a minimum by advising on feeding immediately before drug administration.
- Measure drug concentration in milk or baby's plasma where appropriate, and particularly in chronic therapy.
- Monitor therapy-related functions in the infant, e.g. blood film, thyroid function, heart rate and developmental progress, growth patterns, level of alertness, sleep.

Table 26.12 Drugs contraindicated in breast-feeding mothers

Amiodarone
Atenolol
Cytotoxics
Ergot alkaloids
Gold salts
Immunosuppressants
Phenindione

Table 26.13 Drugs that need special monitoring in breast-feeding infants

Drug (or group)	Monitoring requirement
Anticonvulsants } Antidepressants	Measure drug concentration in infant Monitor neurodevelopmental progress
	Measure lithium concentration
Antipsychotics	Monitor neurodevelopmental progress
Aspirin	Measure blood levels and acid–base, the latter weekly in infants <2 months
β-blockers	Measure infant heart rate
Carbimazole	Monitor free thyroxine and thyroid-stimulating hormone at 2-week intervals for first 2 months, then monthly
Chloramphenicol	Measure drug concentration Monitor blood film at 4-day intervals
Coffee/tea	Reduce intake if irritability occurs – unlikely unless > six cups per day
Metronidazole	Interrupt breast-feeding for 24 hours after single large dose. Use single daily dose rather than multiple in treatment courses
Radioisotopes	Measure radioactivity in milk for all isotopes
Gallium-67	Interrupt feeding until radioactivity clearance $\simeq$ 14 days
Iodine-125 and -131	Interrupt feeding until radioactivity clearance $\simeq$ 7–10 days
Technetium-99	Interrupt feeding for 24 hours, then resume

- Consult reference sources, regional paediatric clinical pharmacologist or drug information centre.

THERAPEUTIC DRUG MONITORING

The increased use of drugs in the fetus and newborn has been a natural accompaniment of the more aggressive diagnostic and therapeutic approaches in neonatal units over the past few years. Alongside the growth in technology allowing more detailed assessment and manipulation of pathophysiological processes, there has occurred the advent of sophisticated analytical techniques which have been adapted to micro samples for use in therapeutic drug monitoring.

In considering therapeutic drug monitoring, it is necessary to ask certain questions: Is drug level monitoring useful? Which drugs should be monitored? When should this be done?

IS DRUG LEVEL MONITORING USEFUL?

There is little information in the literature relating to this subject, particularly in newborn practice. The justification for its use to date has been based on the theoretical unpredictability of the newborn in terms of drug handling (see above). The lessons from past newborn therapeutic disasters must not be forgotten. Would the problem of 'grey baby syndrome' be as indelibly marked in paediatric experience if plasma chloramphenicol concentrations had been measured by clinicians of the past or present? For the present, it seems prudent to include some therapeutic drug monitoring in our newborn baby management.

WHICH DRUGS?

Certain conditions must be met before measurement of blood levels will be useful. There must clearly be a significant relationship between drug level and pharmacological effect, and the concentration of the unbound drug in plasma must be in equilibrium with the concentrations at the receptor site. In addition, tolerance should not occur and body function should return to normal when the drug is withdrawn.

Aranda et al[5] have suggested a number of therapeutic situations where monitoring drug levels should prove useful.

Old drugs, new uses

An increasing number of drugs which have been widely used in adult practice for years have more recently been used in different circumstances in newborn practice. Examples of these drugs and their indications are caffeine, theophylline (preterm apnoea); indomethacin (duct closure); tolazoline (persistent fetal circulation). Drug dosages in adults cannot be extrapolated for use in the newborn. New data are required based on the concentration of the drug in blood following different routes of administration. Specific dose guidelines should be available for drugs such as theophylline, which can be given i.v., orally or rectally. The usefulness of some drugs may be limited by the mode of deriving data for dosage guidelines. Early recommendations for indomethacin dosage in patent ductus arteriosus were based on studies relating effect to the dose given. A more appropriate course is to determine the relationship between plasma drug concentration and effect and then determine the relationship between the dose given and the concentration achieved.

New drugs

Although safety and benefit studies should first be carried out in adults and older children where possible, studies in newborns are necessary to confirm applicability.

Narrow therapeutic index drugs

Theophylline and gentamicin are examples of drugs for which the concentration necessary to produce effect is not considerably different from that which produces toxicity. Adjustment of dose to maintain plasma levels within a therapeutic window is possible with monitoring facilities and pharmacokinetic interpretation.

Inadequate effect or toxicity validation

An absence of the expected effect while on doses of drugs that clinicians assume to be relatively large is a feature of phenytoin use in the newborn. Loughnan et al[29] reported persistent seizures in newborns with low plasma concentrations of this drug while on daily maintenance doses of 8 mg/kg. Knowledge of drug level gives a ready answer to the clinician. Neonatal drug toxicity (hypotension, hypoglycaemia, renal inadequacy) may be difficult to separate from underlying disease problems. For central nervous system depression a measure of phenytoin or phenobarbitone levels is helpful in defining which mechanism is operable.

Drugs with active metabolites

Biotransformation of theophylline in the newborn produces caffeine. Although a therapeutic range of theophylline in preterm apnoea is accepted, reported ranges vary[21,44] and this may be because of the contribution of the active metabolite to overall effect.

The reported effectiveness of theophylline at levels approximating to 3 μg/ml (3 mg/l,[36]) takes no account of any contribution from caffeine. To offset these difficulties, clinicians seem to be opting more and more for the more predictable use of the active metabolite, when caffeine is administered itself. This is probably because of the wider therapeutic index of caffeine and the need for less frequent dosing, as much as for ease of interpretation and adjustment of the drug level itself.

PRACTICAL CONSIDERATIONS OF MONITORING LEVELS

The use of large volumes of blood and its repeated sampling have no place in modern newborn practice. Micromethods are mandatory and need to be highly sensitive and specific, but at the same time should afford simultaneous active metabolite measure. Rapidity is preferred, and good reproducibility within and without a laboratory, together with operator independence, is essential.

At present plasma sampling is the usual approach, although less invasive techniques, for example saliva sampling, may have a place, particularly as such fluid is protein free and salivary levels for certain drugs, e.g. theophylline, are likely to be representative of the free and pharmacologically active fraction. A peak–trough monitoring approach should prove most useful. For most drugs this will mean sampling at 1 hour post dose and immediately prior to the next dose. Such an approach gives an approximate estimate of individual plasma half-

Table 26.14 Drugs to monitor and their plasma therapeutic ranges

Drug	Sampling time	Range
Amikacin	1 h	15–20 μg/ml
	Pre-dose	< 4 μg/ml
Gentamicin	1 h	4–10 μg/ml
	Pre-dose	< 2 μg/ml
Tobramycin	1 h	4–8 μg/ml
	Pre-dose	< 2 μg/ml
Chloramphenicol	1 h	15–25 μg/ml
Caffeine	> 6 h	7–20 μg/ml
Theophylline	1 h	5–12 μg/ml
Phenobarbitone	> 6 h	15–30 μg/ml
Phenytoin	> 8 h	10–20 μg/ml

lives and of the fluctuations of concentration between doses, which are determined by the relationship between half-life and dose interval. Where serial information is available, an assessment of the extent and rate of maturational change in drug elimination is possible.

The present state of knowledge regarding efficacy and toxicity of drugs in the newborn suggests that although substantive data on the therapeutic ranges have not always been derived in the subjects to whom practice is directed, a strong case can be made for monitoring the drugs listed in Table 26.14 in all newborn units, and if levels are maintained within the described guidelines maximal efficacy with minimum toxicity in the majority may be expected.

REFERENCES

1. Agurell S, Berlin A, Ferngren H, Hellstrom B 1975 Plasma levels of diazepam after parenteral and rectal administration in children. Epilepsia 16: 277–283
2. Ames M D 1960 Gastric acidity in the first ten days of life of the prematurely born baby. American Journal of Diseases of Children 100: 252–256
3. Aranda J V, MacLeod S M, Renton K W, Eade N R 1974 Hepatic microsomal drug oxidation and electron transport in newborn infants. Journal of Pediatrics 85: 534–542
4. Aranda J V, Sitar D S, Parsons W D, Loughnan P M, Neims A H 1976 Pharmacokinetic aspects of theophylline in premature newborns. New England Journal of Medicine 295: 413–416
5. Aranda J V, Turmen T, Sasynuik B I 1980 Drug monitoring in the perinatal patient: uses and abuses. Therapeutic Drug Monitoring 2: 39–49
6. Assael B M, Gianni A, Marini A, Peneff P, Sereni F 1977 Gentamicin dosage in preterm and term neonates. Archives of Disease in Childhood 52: 883–886
7. Augustinsson R B, Brody S 1962 Plasma arylesterase activity in adults and newborn infants. Clinica Chimica Acta 7: 560–565
8. Bell E F, Brown E J, Milner R, Sinclair J C, Ziprusky A 1979 Vitamin E absorption in small premature infants. Pediatrics 63: 830–832
9. Boréus L O, Jalling B, Kallberg N 1975 Clinical pharmacology of phenobarbital in the neonate period. In: Morselli P L, Garattini S, Sereni F (eds) Basic and therapeutic aspects of perinatal pharmacology. Raven Press, New York, pp 331–340
10. Brazier J L, Renaud H, Ribon B, Salle B I 1979 Plasma xanthine levels in low birthweight infants treated or not treated with theophylline. Archives of Disease in Childhood 54: 194–199
11. Brodersen R 1978 Free bilirubin in blood plasma of the newborn: effects of albumin, fatty acids, pH, displacing drugs and phototherapy. In: Stern L, Oh W, Friis-Hansen B (eds) Intensive care of the newborn, Vol. II. Masson Publishing, New York, pp 177–184
12. Cavell B 1979 Gastric emptying in preterm infants. Acta Paediatrica Scandinavica 68: 725–730
13. Cook D R, Wingard I B, Taylor P H. 1976 Pharmacokinetics of succinylcholine in infants, children and adults. Clinical Pharmacology and Therapeutics 20: 493–498
14. Crounse R G 1961 Human pharmacology of griseofulvin: the effect of fat intake on gastrointestinal absorption. Journal of Investigative Dermatology 37: 529–533
15. Dost F H, Gladtke E 1969 Pharmacokinetics des 2-Sulfanilamido-3-methoxy-pyrazin beim Kinder. Arzneimittel-Forschung 19: 1304–1307
16. Ecobichon D J, Stephens D S 1973 Perinatal development of human blood esterases. Clinical Pharmacology and Therapeutics 14: 41–47
17. Evans N J, Rutter N, Hadgraft J, Parr G D 1985 Percutaneous administration of theophylline in the preterm infant. Journal of Pediatrics 107: 307–311
18. Gladtke E, Heimann G 1975 The rate of development of elimination function in kidney and liver of young infants. In: Morselli P L, Garattin S, Sereni F (eds) Basic and therapeutic aspects of perinatal pharmacology. Raven Press, New York, pp 393–403
19. Gupta M, Brans Y W 1978 Gastric retention in neonates. Pediatrics 62: 26–29
20. Irvine-Meek J M, Hall K W, Otten N H et al 1982 Pharmacokinetic study of valproic acid in a neonate. Pediatric Pharmacology 2: 317–321
21. Jones R A K, Baillie E 1979 Dosage schedule for intravenous aminophylline in apnoea of prematurity based on pharmacokinetic studies. Archives of Disease in Childhood 54: 190–193
22. Juchau M R, Pedersen M G 1973 Drug biotransformation reactions in the human fetal adrenal gland. Life Sciences 12 (Part II): 193–204
23. Kitigawa H, Fujitas, Suzuki T, Kitani K 1985 Disappearance of sex difference in rat liver drug metabolism in old age. Biochemical Pharmacology 34: 579–592
24. Krasula R, Yanagi R, Hastreiter A R, Levitsky, S Soyka L F 1974 Digoxin intoxication in infants and children: correlation with serum levels. Journal of Pediatrics 84: 265–269
25. Langslet A, Meberg A, Bredesen J E, Lunde P K M 1978 Plasma concentrations of diazepam and N-desmethyl diazepam in newborn infants after intravenous, intramuscular, rectal and oral administration. Acta Paediatrica Scandinavica 67: 699–704
26. Levy G, Garrettson E K 1974 Kinetics of salicylate elimination by newborn infants of mothers who ingested aspirin before delivery. Pediatrics 43: 201–210
27. Levy R H, Pitlick W H, Troupin A S, Green J R, Neal J M 1975a Pharmacokinetics of carbamazepine in normal man. Clinical Pharmacology and Therapeutics 17: 656–668
28. Levy G, Khanna N N, Soda D M, Tsuzuki O, Stern L 1975b Pharmacokinetics of acetaminophen in the human neonate: formation of acetaminophen glucuronide and sulfate in relation to plasma bilirubin concentration and D-glucaric acid excretion. Pediatrics 55: 818–825
29. Loughnan P M, Greenwald A, Purton W W, Aranda J V, Walters G, Neims A H 1977 Pharmacokinetic observations of phenytoin disposition in the newborn infant and young infant. Archives of Disease in Childhood 52: 302–309
30. Mandelli M, Morselli P L, Nordio S et al 1975 Placental transfer of diazepam and its disposition in the newborn. Clinical Pharmacology and Therapeutics 7: 564–572
31. Melander A, Danielson K, Scherstein B, Wahlin E 1977 Enhancement of the bioavailability of propranolol and metoprolol by food. Clinical Pharmacology and Therapeutics 22: 108–112
32. Metcoff J, Stare F 1947 The physiologic and clinical significance of plasma protein metabolites. New England Journal of Medicine 236: 26–35
33. Miyoshi K, Saijo K, Kotani Y, Kashiwagi T, Kawai H 1966 Characteristic properties of fetal human albumin on isomerisation equilibrium. Tokushima Journal of Experimental Medicine 13: 121–128
34. Morselli P L, Principi N, Tognoni G et al 1973 Diazepam elimination in premature and full term infants and children. Journal of Perinatal Medicine 1: 133–141
35. Morselli P L, Franco-Morselli R, Bossi L 1980 Clinical pharmacokinetics in newborns and infants. Clinical Pharmacokinetics 5: 485–527
36. Myers T, Milsap R, Krauss A N, Auld P A M, Reidenberg M N 1980 Low dose theophylline therapy in idiopathic apnea of prematurity. Journal of Pediatrics 96: 99–103
37. Pelkonen O, Kärki N T 1973 Drug metabolism in human fetal tissues. Life Sciences 13: 1163–1180

38. Piafsky K M, Woolner E A 1982 The binding of basic drugs to alpha-l-acid glycoprotein in cord serum. Journal of Pediatrics 100: 820–822
39. Polacek M A, Ellison R E 1966 Gastric acid secretion and parietal cell mass in the stomach of the newborn infant. American Journal of Surgery 111: 777–781
40. Price K E, Zolli Jr E, Atkinson J C, Luter H G 1957 Antibiotic inhibitors. Antibiotics and Chemotherapy 7: 672–688
41. Rane A, Tomson G 1980 Prenatal and neonatal drug metabolism in man. European Journal of Clinical Pharmacology 18: 9–15
42. Rane A, Sjoqvist F, Orrenius S 1973 Drugs and fetal metabolism. Clinical Pharmacology and Therapeutics 14: 662–672
43. Reidenberg M M, James M, Dring L G 1972 The rate of procaine hydrolysis in serum of normal subjects and disease patients. Clinical Pharmacology and Therapeutics 13: 279–284
44. Shannon D C, Gotay F, Stein I M, Rogers M C, Todres D, Moylan F M B 1975 Prevention of apnea and bradycardia in low birthweight infants. Pediatrics 55: 589–592
45. Smith C A 1951 The physiology of the newborn infant, 2nd edn. Charles C Thomas, Springfield, IL, pp 180–198
46. Sondheimer J M, Hamilton J R 1978 Intestinal function in infants with severe congenital heart disease. Journal of Pediatrics 92: 572–578
47. Szefler S J, Koup J R, Giacoia G P 1977 Paradoxical behaviour of serum digoxin concentrations in an anuric neonate. Journal of Pediatrics 91: 487–490
48. Wallace S 1977 Altered plasma albumin in the newborn infant. British Journal of Clinical Pharmacology 4: 82–85
49. Weber W W, Cohen S N 1975 Aging effects and drugs in man. In: Gillette J R, Mitchel J R (eds) Concepts in biochemical pharmacology. Springer, Berlin, pp 213–233
50. Widdowson E M 1974 Changes in body proportions and composition during growth. In: Davis J A, Dobbing J (eds) Scientific foundations of pediatrics. Heinemann, London, pp 153–163
51. Williams R F 1974 Colonisation of the developing body by bacteria. In: Davis J A, Dobbing J (eds) Scientific foundations of paediatrics. Heinemann, London, pp 789–801
52. Wood M, Wood A J J 1981 Changes in plasma drug binding and $\propto$ l-acid glycoprotein in mother and newborn infant. Clinical Pharmacology and Therapeutics 29: 522–526
53. Yaffe S J, Juchau M R 1974 Perinatal pharmacology. Annual Review of Pharmacology 14: 219–238
54. Yaffe S J, Rane A, Sjoqvist F, Boreus, L O, Orrenius S 1970 The presence of a monoxygenase system in human fetal liver microsomes. Life Sciences 9 (Part II): 1189–1200

27

Analgesia in the neonate

Andrew R. Wolf

INTRODUCTION

The provision of adequate analgesia in the neonate, an issue often ignored or relegated to secondary consideration, became topical in the mid 1980s when the landmark case of Baby Lawson reached the popular press in North America. Jeffery Lawson underwent thoracic surgery with an 'anaesthetic' consisting of pancuronium for paralysis without any analgesic or anaesthetic agent. Following media attention a national debate ensued,[13,61] prompting a re-evaluation of neonatal analgesia both in the operating room and in the neonatal nursery.[8,23] At the same time Anand and his colleagues at Oxford published data showing that infants undergoing surgery with inadequate analgesia mount a massive stress response which adversely affects postoperative recovery.[5,6] In the last decade, neurodevelopmental studies have shown that nociceptive pathways and their neurophysiological responses are present even in the very preterm. This leads to the uncomfortable conclusion that neonates subjected to multiple procedures (heel pricks, vascular access and intubation) without analgesia are being subjected to noxious stimuli that would not be tolerated in the older child.

At the outset, a distinction must be made between provision of analgesia for major surgery and the provision of analgesia for procedural pain or long-term sedation. While it is clear that opioids are well tolerated at high doses in the ventilated neonate and can be used acutely to reduce haemodynamic and stress responses to surgery, the inappropriate use of these drugs for longer-term sedation or for minor interventional procedures has resulted in the emergence of iatrogenic complications such as tolerance, withdrawal and delayed extubation due to chronic overdosage.

NOCICEPTION IN THE INFANT

As early as 6 weeks' gestation, dorsal horn cells in the spinal cord have formed synapses with the developing sensory neurons.[53,68] These sensory neurons grow peripherally to reach the skin of the limbs by 11 weeks, the rest of the trunk by 15 weeks and the remaining cutaneous and mucosal surfaces by 20 weeks.[35,66] At full term the density of nociceptive nerve endings in the newborn skin is at least as great as that of the adult.[27] Further organization of the laminar structure of the cells in the dorsal horn (Rexed's laminae) and their synapses together with the appearance of specific neurotransmitter vesicles begins at 13 weeks and is completed by 30 weeks.[59,60] By this time, nerve tracts associated with nociception are fully myelinated up to the thalamic level.[26] Synaptic connections of the thalamocortical tracts occur at 24 weeks' gestation,[41] and myelination of the nociceptive thalamocortical radiations is complete by 37 weeks.[26] Other nociceptive tracts may not be fully myelinated until much later,[3] but lack of myelination does not imply lack of function. Descending inhibitory tracts, which act via inputs into spinal cord cells to suppress the transmission of noxious stimuli, are probably formed anatomically but not fully functional at term.[19] The lack of descending inhibition from higher centres will tend to increase afferent nociceptive transmission in the spinal cord.

Few neurophysiological or cytochemical studies have been attempted in the human infant. Positron emission tomography has shown that glucose utilization and by inference cerebral metabolism is maximal in sensory areas of the neonatal brain[11] and that auditory- and visual-evoked potentials have developed by 30 weeks' gestation.[32,65] These data along with EEG data[65] imply a very complex level of integration and maturity within the cerebral cortex by this time. Somatosensory-evoked responses are present from 28 weeks' gestation although the latency is long, owing to slow peripheral and central transmission.

Neonates exhibit hypersensitivity and postinjury hyperalgesia similar to adults. Fitzgerald and colleagues studied the flexion withdrawal reflex in the lower limb and found it to be highly sensitive, with a low threshold in the preterm neonate.[20] They showed that the response is graded according to the stimulus and that repeated stimulation causes an exaggerated reflex.[21] Heel lancing also shows a similar sensitization response, which can be prevented by local anaesthetic applied to the heel.[21,22] The reflex is quite specific to the site of injury: if the heel lancing is confined to one heel alone then the protected side fails to show exaggerated flexion.[22]

Inadequate analgesia may also cause longer-term behavioural effects. Neonates given adequate anaesthesia and analgesia for circumcision are more attentive, better orientated, and less irritable than those not given analgesia, and this difference lasts for several days.[17] Furthermore, comforting interventions designed to reduce stress in preterm neonates in the intensive care unit are associated with improved clinical and developmental outcomes.[2] Therefore, while the effects of noxious stimuli in the young and very sick may not be easily apparent, the consequences may be profound.

MEASUREMENT OF PAIN IN THE NEONATE

The experience of pain belongs to each individual and its expression is dependent on the ability of that individual to communicate the experience. In the neonate, direct communication is impossible and observed behaviours to noxious stimuli change with maturation.[36] However, observational techniques have been developed that can give some measure of the quality of analgesia. The quality of analgesia can also be correlated with physiological and stress responses to pain.

Most of the early studies on infant pain measurement were based on a single painful stimulus such as a pin prick. This was a useful model because it provided a relatively consistent stimulus from which to identify and grade responses. However, the applicability of these data to postoperative pain in infants is limited because longer-lasting pain in this age group does not produce the easily identifiable and gross responses associated with pin-prick.[38] Heel-stick usually produces a reflex withdrawal of the lower limb which in its more exaggerated form consists of flexion and adduction of the upper and lower limbs, grimacing and crying.[22,58,62] These responses are specific, graded according to the stimulus and are associated with a measurable latency.[22,24] Swiping movements which have been interpreted as defensive motor activity have also been described.[24] Grunau & Craig have been able to categorize neonatal facial movements in response to a heel stab.[29] They found specific expressions to the noxious stimulus that were distinct from those to the non-noxious stimulus of heel rubbing. These were: eye squeezing, brow contraction, nasolabial furrowing, a taut tongue and mouth opening and are remarkably similar to adult responses. The Scandinavian cry group attempted to discriminate the cry of pain from other infant vocalizations using spectral analysis and harmonic structure of the cry.[67] Others have shown that the latency to the first cry and the duration of the first cry correlate with the intensity of the stimulus.[29] However, outside the initial pain response to heel-stick, cry analysis techniques are not discriminatory. Facial movements appear to be far more specific and can be applied across all age groups. Frank[24] has quantified body responses to acute pain using video techniques and a calibrated grid. She identified the velocity of leg movements, the number of leg movements and the movements towards the side affected by the pain. Collectively, these studies demonstrated that single behaviours are unreliable in the assessment of pain and that the interobserver correlation and specificity can be improved by a multidimensional approach which may also include physiological measurements.[39,55,67]

Unfortunately, the behavioural response to a standard noxious stimulus is inconsistent.[10,45,47] The state of consciousness at the time of stimulation affects the response: infants have reduced responses during quiet sleep with a longer latency to crying. Boys also respond more rapidly than girls[29] and medical conditions such as hyperbilirubinaemia or neurological impairment have also been shown to alter responses to noxious stimuli.[4] These observations emphasize the difficulty in using pain scales based on behavioural response alone as a tool for studies of analgesia in neonates.

The effects of painful stimuli on heart rate, blood pressure, sweating, ventilation, oxygen saturation, vagal tone and hormonal responses have all been investigated. Heart rate changes are the simplest to measure, but the responses are not consistent, even with a single heel-stab. Measurement of vagal tone using the amplitude of ventilatory sinus arrhythmia has produced encouraging data. Studies by Porter have shown that changes in vagal tone correlate with stimulus intensity, behavioural responses and variations in cry pitch.[57]

CLINICAL PAIN ASSESSMENT

Evaluation of pain and sedation can broadly be divided into three overlapping groups: assessment of instantaneous pain (heel-prick or procedural pain), assessment of longer-term postoperative pain, and assessment of sedation.

Instantaneous (procedural pain) in the neonate has been the most widely studied and can best be measured with the Neonatal Facial Coding System.[29] This tool has been extensively studied and validated.[14,30,37] In contrast, the measurement of postoperative pain in infants is difficult and becomes more so with decreasing age. Most postoperative pain tools for neonates are adapted versions of validated techniques used in older infants and children. These tools include the Objective Pain Scale (OPS)[51,52] and the Children's Hospital of Eastern Ontario Pain Scale.[44] The recently developed Pain Assessment Tool[34] combines many of the best features of the above tools. It incorporates both physiological measures (ventilation, oxygen saturation, heart rate, and blood pressure) and

Table 27.1 Combined infant pain and distress score (as used at Bristol Children's Hospital, PICU)

Modality	Undersedation	Ideal	Oversedation
Agitation	Major 2	Can be comforted 1	No movement 0
Facial expression	Brow/grimace/nasal flaring 2	Movement 1	No movement 0
Movement/posture	Flexed/tense 2	Appropriate 1	No movement 0
Ventilation			
On ventilator	Fighting ventilator 2	Comfortable 1	Apnoea/minimal effort 0
Self-ventilating	Crying/cannot be comforted	Not crying	Asleep/poor response to stimulation
Cardiovascular (heart rate or BP)	20% > baseline 2	+ or – 10% of baseline 1	10% < baseline 0
Totals			
Maximum	10		
Ideal	5		
Oversedation	< 2		
Increase analgesia/sedation if total	> 7		
Decrease analgesia/sedation if 2 or less			

This scoring tool – as used in the Bristol PICU – combines the OPS and NFCS tools. Scoring is carried out hourly by the nursing staff based on the previous hour's observations. Analgesia or sedation are adjusted accordingly from the summed score.

observational measures (posture, sleep pattern, facial expression, colour, cry, and overall perception). In the view of the author, practical assessment of pain and distress needs to use both physiological and observational criteria, yet must remain simple to be feasible. Trends in the hourly pain score give the best overall assessment, and the hourly score needs to be a summary score of that hour rather than a point assessment. At the Royal Hospital for Sick Children in Bristol, pain and distress is evaluated using a five-point scale that combines features of both the OPS and NFCS tools (Table 27.1).

In addition to pain assessment, it can be helpful to have guidelines for the expected duration of pain after different types of surgery. This then allows an appropriate analgesia plan for each individual. Data from pain studies in infancy using both systemic and local analgesia[69–72] have given insights into the different durations and intensities of pain after surgical procedures (Fig. 27.1). These studies have also shown that pain assessment tools measure sedation as much as analgesia, which can make comparison of sedating (opioid) and non-sedating (local analgesia) techniques difficult.

Assessment of comfort in the non-surgical ventilated infant is an area that has received limited attention, but the comfort scale[49] is an attempt to measure levels of sedation/comfort as opposed to analgesia and pain.

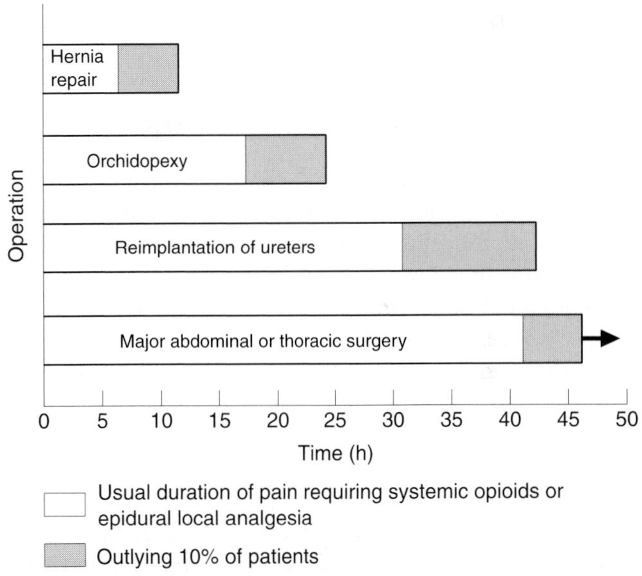

Fig. 27.1 Pain duration after common infant procedures. Values are derived from data on pain scores and analgesia requirements using local anaesthesia or opioids.[69–72] *Note:* 50% of patients undergoing hernia repair under general anaesthesia do not appear to suffer significant postoperative pain in the absence of perioperative local anaesthesia or opioids.

OPIOID ANALGESIA

The current interest in neonatal pain has encouraged much greater use of opioids in this age group. The two opioids most commonly used in the UK are morphine and fentanyl. Both drugs have a place in the neonatal nursery, but their clinical indications differ.

PHARMACODYNAMIC CONSIDERATIONS

Neonates are regarded as having a pharmacodynamic susceptibility to opioids which increases as gestational age falls. Opioid receptors change both in numbers and in receptor type during development[15,56] and in the rat this is associated with a large change in sensitivity,[56] but there are no comparable human data. However, it is difficult to separate true receptor-based or effector-based sensitivity from the effects due to selective distribution of the drug to the brain after administration. Lipid-soluble drugs, such as fentanyl, will redistribute rapidly out of the central compartment at a rate depending on the cardiac output, regional blood flow, the presence and absence of shunts, protein binding, sequestration within the peripheral compartments and the individual membrane permeability of the drug.[43] The brain forms 50% of the vessel-rich group of tissues in the neonate compared with only 25% in the adult. The cardiac index is high and the fraction of the cardiac output flowing to the brain is proportionately high compared to the adult. As a result, fat-soluble drugs are taken up rapidly by the infant brain and attain high peak concentrations at the effect site (biophase). Elimination of the drug from biophase is slow because of the limitations on peripheral uptake and drug elimination. Fat-soluble opioids such as fentanyl will therefore have a more rapid onset of effect, greater potency and slower offset than can be predicted by simply analysing pharmacokinetic data. Delivery of morphine into biophase may also be enhanced in the neonate and young infant owing to immaturity of the blood–brain barrier.[42]

PHARMACOKINETIC CONSIDERATIONS

Morphine pharmacokinetics change substantially in infancy. McRorie and colleagues showed that a fourfold reduction in the elimination half-life of morphine takes place in the first few years of life, with mean values of 7.2 hours below 1 month, compared to 1.7 hours in adults.[46] The prolonged half-life in the neonate is due primarily to the prolonged clearance of the drug. The data from Olkkola et al are similar but also demonstrated the large individual variability between subjects, particularly in the neonate. The mean elimination half-life in the newborn was measured at 13.9 hours with a standard deviation of 6.4 hours.[54] These data indicate that prediction of drug offset in an individual using averaged pharmacokinetic variables is not feasible. Active metabolites such as morphine-6-glucuronide, which are poorly excreted by the preterm infant's kidney, may further compound the unpredictability, but available data on mechanisms of morphine elimination and potency of the metabolic products remain limited in this age group.

Pharmacokinetic data for fentanyl show a similar pattern with even greater variability in the premature infant.[12,25,38] In the study by Gauntlett et al, two of the patients given a single dose of fentanyl had no clearance of the drug for 10 hours after abdominal surgery.[25] This phenomenon has been described in previous studies on infants undergoing abdominal surgery[38] and has been attributed to the effects of raised intra-abdominal pressure on liver blood flow.[48] The implications for infants undergoing abdominal surgery are clear: some infants will have a sustained effect from doses of opioid that would normally be expected to have a limited duration of action.

Fentanyl's main clinical use is to provide intense analgesia with ablation of the stress response for major surgery and to control pulmonary resistance in the patient with severe pulmonary hypertension.[33] The doses used in these patients (50–150 μg/kg as a single injection over several minutes) are well above the usual analgesic doses (0.5–10 μg/kg). Morphine has both slower onset and offset than fentanyl after a single dose, but its peripheral uptake is less and its elimination half-life is shorter than fentanyl, making it a much better choice for longer-term infusion. While initial doses of opioid infusions needed for analgesia and sedation are low, the dose requirements increase rapidly. Neonates undergoing ECMO require five times the initial opioid infusion rate by day 6 to achieve the same level of sedation owing to a combination of enhanced elimination[7] and true tolerance.[28] The use of long-term infusions of morphine for sedation alone is debatable: it is better to reserve analgesic drugs for pain relief or use low-dose infusions of morphine in conjunction with other long-acting sedatives such as chloral hydrate or promethazine.

CLINICAL USE OF OPIOIDS

The large individual variations of drug effect make effective opioid analgesia in infants difficult without individualized treatment, close supervision and modification of dosage based on behavioural effect (pain scores). Some form of nurse-controlled analgesia with formal noted assessments on a pain score sheet is the ideal. Even in the setting of an intensive care unit, chronic overdosage, severe ventilatory depression, apnoea and generalized seizures can occur.[16,40] Opioids may also delay the return of bowel function after abdominal surgery. Withdrawal from long-term opioid infusions can take days to weeks with overaggressive withdrawal causing severe agitation, disordered ventilatory patterns and abnormal limb movements. The use of formal comfort scores can be a useful guide to optimize the rate of withdrawal.

Fentanyl can be given by intermittent injection (0.5–10 μg/kg) during surgery to provide several hours of analgesia in the postoperative period. Higher doses (50–150 μg/kg) used for the control of haemodynamic and stress responses to major surgery necessitate postoperative ventilation. Infusions of fentanyl at 1–5 μg/kg/h will provide excellent analgesia after major surgery in ventilated neonates. A loading dose of 0.5–10 μg/kg may be needed if the infant has not already received a loading dose during surgery. Tolerance occurs rapidly with this drug.[7,28] High-dose infusions of fentanyl (5–15 μg/kg/h) are often given after neonatal cardiac surgery to stabilize systemic vascular resistance and prevent pulmonary hypertension, but prolonged infusions (greater than 48 h) result in drug accumulation and delayed extubation. Fentanyl should be used with extreme caution if at all in the spontaneously breathing neonate. The potency (100 times that of morphine) and the rapid uptake into biophase (high lipid solubility) prohibits its use by bolus injection in the non-ventilated patient.

Morphine remains the most popular drug for analgesia in the neonate and infant. In older infants, infusion rates between 5 and 40 µg/kg/h usually provide effective analgesia and sedation. Additional intravenous loading doses (50–150 µg/kg) should be given slowly owing to the lag time between delivery of the drug and its effect. Subcutaneous or intramuscular morphine should never be used in the sick infant as it may not be absorbed centrally until adequate peripheral perfusion is restored.[74] 'Nurse-controlled analgesia' is an emerging and useful technique for control of infant pain. The patient usually receives a background morphine infusion (2.5–10 µg/kg/h) topped up at appropriate intervals by 'nurse-controlled' doses according to formal pain assessment. The incremental doses used for NCA vary from about 2.5 to 10 µg/kg. In addition to direct observation pulse oximetry and a ventilatory monitoring with appropriate alarms should be used. Neonates and infants under 6 months should stay in a high-dependency unit.

Morphine can be used in the spontaneously breathing neonate but the doses required are usually far less than in older infants. It is the view of this author that in the postoperative neonate, single intermittent intravenous doses given slowly provide the safest and most effective delivery route. Loading doses of 10–50 µg/kg morphine can be given by slow infusion over 15 minutes in conjunction with sedation scores at 5-minute intervals. Once the desired level of comfort has been achieved, the infusion is discontinued even if the full dose has not been delivered. Additional doses are then given in the same fashion according to regular documented pain scores. The advantage of this technique is that once the appropriate therapeutic level has been reached, it can be maintained on an individual basis rather than using a recipe approach which cannot take into account the huge variation in pharmacokinetics in this age group.[54] Other methods of NCA in this age group also use low background morphine infusions (1–5 µg/kg/h).

LOCAL ANALGESIA[50]

High-dose opioid techniques may be beneficial to the sick neonate undergoing major surgery requiring postoperative ventilation, but may not be ideal if postoperative ventilation is not mandatory. Epidural analgesia with infusions of local anaesthetics (bupivacaine or lignocaine) can provide complete analgesia for thoracic and abdominal surgery (Fig. 27.2).

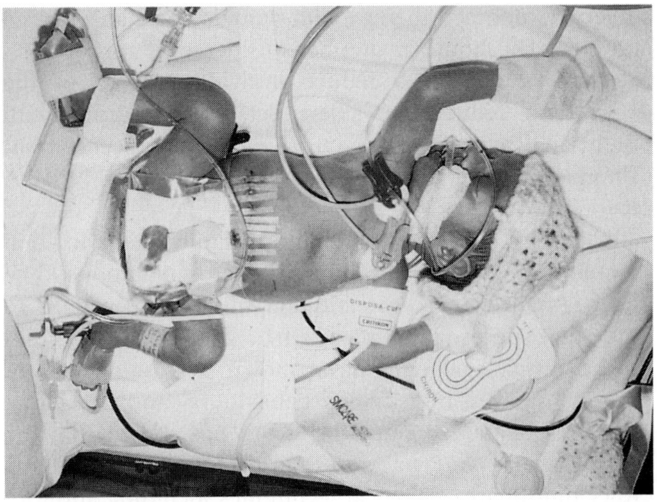

Fig. 27.2 This preterm neonate has had major abdominal surgery using epidural local analgesia combined with light general anaesthesia. Analgesia is maintained with a continuous epidural infusion of bupivacaine given via a thoracic epidural catheter. No opioids are required, to avoid sedation and ventilatory depression. If the infant cries it can be difficult to tell if this is due to pain, hunger, tiredness or other needs. Careful observation and measurement are needed to diagnose pain and the need for additional analgesia.

It has been shown to be as effective as morphine infusions, without causing sedation or ventilatory depression:[69] epidural infusions are associated with a rise in the slope of the carbon dioxide response curve because of a systemic effect of the local anaesthetic.[64] Epidural techniques also reduce the stress responses to major surgery better than low-dose opioid techniques.[73] The problems with the technique lie in the lack of sedation which can be misinterpreted as pain, the potential for toxicity due to systemic absorption and the abrupt offset of analgesia when nerve transmission returns. This technique is being used increasingly in major paediatric centres.

Local infiltration with lignocaine (maximum dose 3 mg/kg) or the longer-acting bupivacaine (maximum dose 2 mg/kg) should be used liberally for minor procedures such as chest drain insertion, but care must be taken to avoid overdosage owing to the increased risk of systemic toxicity in the neonate.[50]

The use of EMLA or amethocaine patches in the newborn is controversial. However, despite the fear of toxicity from systemic absorption, studies documenting levels in infants under 3 months old are encouraging. Prilocaine can produce methaemoglobinaemia, but the only case reported is in a 12-week-old boy in which 5 g of EMLA cream was left on for 5 hours. EMLA, while effective, remains underused in the neonatal nursery.[50]

ALTERNATIVE APPROACHES

Paracetamol and other NSAIDs can provide useful co-analgesia which can reduce opioid requirements after surgery. Combined therapy with opioids, local anaesthesia and NSAIDs should always be considered, if appropriate, to improve analgesia, reduce individual doses of the drugs, and reduce the side-effects. Other drugs with potent analgesic effects which have received recent attention in infants are $alpha_2$-agonists (clonidine) and NMDA receptor antagonists (ketamine).

In the rat, responses to pain are diminished with oral stimulation or orally administered sucrose solutions. The effect is naltrexone reversible and this has been used to argue that sucrose is acting as a true analgesic.[9,63] Studies in the human neonate have shown a dose-dependent effect of sucrose in reducing behavioural and heart rate responses to pain,[31] but other work has shown that the cardiovascular and stress responses are not reduced.[18] Other non-pharmacological techniques including auditory and tactile stimuli or massage can reduce heart rate, alter baseline cortisol levels and reduce behavioural responses to pain.[1] These are all comforting procedures with merit and may improve longer-term behavioural responses and even outcome.[2] However, they should be viewed as neonatal coping strategies which can modulate 'pain experience' rather than true analgesics.

REFERENCES

1. Acolet D, Modi N, Giannakoulopoulos X, Bond C, Weg W, Clow A, Glover V 1993 Changes in plasma cortisol and catecholamine concentrations in response to massage in preterm infants. Archives of Disease in Childhood 68: 29–31
2. Als H, Lawhon G, Brown E et al 1986 Individualized behavioral and environmental care for the very low birthweight preterm infant at high risk for bronchopulmonary dysplasia: neonatal intensive care unit and developmental outcome. Pediatrics 78: 1123–1132
3. Anand K J S, Carr D B 1989 The neuroanatomy, neurophysiology, neurochemistry of pain, stress and analgesia in newborns and children. Pediatric Clinics of North America 36: 795–822
4. Anand K J S, Hickey P R 1987 Pain and its effects in the human neonate and fetus. New England Journal of Medicine 317: 1321–1329
5. Anand K J S, Sippell W G, Aynsley-Green A 1987 Randomised trial of fentanyl anaesthesia in preterm babies undergoing surgery: Effects on the stress response. Lancet 1: 243–247
6. Anand K J S, Sippell W G, Schofield N M et al 1988 Does halothane anaesthesia decrease the stress response of newborn infants undergoing operation? British Medical Journal 296: 668–672
7. Arnold J H, Truog R D, Scavone J M et al 1991 Changes in the pharmacodynamic response to fentanyl in neonates during continuous infusion. Journal of Pediatrics 119: 639–643
8. Berry F, Gregory G 1987 Do premature infants require anesthesia for surgery? Anesthesiology 67: 291–293
9. Blass E M, Fitzgerald E 1988 Milk induced analgesia and comforting in 10 day old rats: opioid mediation. Pharmacology, Biochemistry and Behavior 29: 9–13
10. Burton I F, Derbyshire A J 1958 'Sleeping fit' caused by excruciating pain in an infant. Journal of Diseases of Children 96: 258–260
11. Chugani H T, Phelps M E 1986 Maturational changes in cerebral function in infants determined by 18-FDG positron emission tomography. Science 231: 840–844
12. Collins C, Koren G, Crean P, et al 1985 Fentanyl pharmacokinetics and hemodynamic effects in preterm infants during ligation of patent ductus arteriosus. Anesthesia and Analgesia 64: 1078–1080
13. Committee on Fetus and Newborn, Committee on Drugs, Section on Anesthesiology, Section on Surgery 1987 Neonatal anesthesia. Pediatrics 80: 446–448
14. Craig K D, Grunau R V E 1991 Neonatal pain perception and behavioral measurement. In: Anand K J S, McGrath P S (eds) Neonatal pain and distress. Elsevier, Amsterdam
15. De la Baume S, Patey G, Gros C, et al 1980 Ontogenesis of enkephalinergic systems in the rat brain. In: Way E L (ed) Endogenous and exogenous opioid agonists and antagonists. Pergamon Press, New York, pp 179–189
16. Dilworth N M, MacKellar A 1987 Pain relief for the pediatric surgical patient. Journal of Pediatric Surgery 22: 264–266
17. Dixon S, Snyder J, Holve R et al 1984 Behavioral effects of circumcision with and without anesthesia. Developmental and Behavioral Pediatrics 5: 246–250
18. Editorial 1992 Pacifiers, passive behavior and pain. Lancet 339: 275–276
19. Fitzgerald M, Koltzenburg 1986 The functional development of descending inhibitory pathways in dorsolateral funiculus of the newborn rat spinal cord. Developmental Brain Research 24: 261–270
20. Fitzgerald M, Shaw A, MacIntosh N 1987 The postnatal development of the flexor reflex: a comparative study in premature infants and newborn rat pups. Developmental Medicine and Child Neurology 30: 520–526
21. Fitzgerald M, Millard C, MacIntosh N 1988 Hyperalgesia in premature infants. Lancet 1: 292
22. Fitzgerald M, Millard C, MacIntosh N 1989 Cutaneous hypersensitivity following peripheral tissue damage in newborn infants and its reversal with topical anaesthesia. Pain 39: 31–36
23. Fletcher A 1987 Pain in the neonate. New England Journal of Medicine 317: 1347–1354
24. Frank L S 1986 A new method to quantitatively describe pain behavior in infants. Nursing Research 35: 28–31
25. Gauntlett I S, Fisher D M, Hertzka R E et al 1988 Pharmacokinetics of fentanyl in neonatal humans and lambs: effects of age. Anesthesiology 69: 683–687
26. Gilles F J, Shankle W, Dooling E C 1983 Myelinated tracts: growth patterns. In: Gilles F J, Leviton A, Dooling E C (eds) The developing human brain: growth and epidemiologic neuropathy. John Wright, Boston, pp 117–183
27. Gleiss J, Stuttgen G 1970 Morphologic and functional development of the skin. In: Stave U (ed) Physiology of the perinatal period. Appleton-Century-Crofts, New York, vol 2, pp 889–906
28. Greeley W J, Debruijn N P 1988 Changes in sufentanil pharmacokinetics within the neonatal period. Anesthesia and Analgesia 67: 86–90
29. Grunau R V E, Craig K D 1987 Pain expression in neonates: facial action and cry. Pain 28: 395–410
30. Grunau R V E, Johnston C C, Craig K D 1990 Neonatal facial and cry responses to invasive and non invasive procedures. Pain 32: 295–305
31. Haouari N, Wood C, Griffiths G, Levene M 1995 The analgesic effect of sucrose in full term infants: a randomised controlled trial. British Medical Journal 310: 1498–1500
32. Henderson-Smart D J, Pettigrew A G, Campbell D J 1983 Clinical apnea and brain-stem neural function in preterm neonates. New England Journal of Medicine 308: 353–357
33. Hickey P R 1985 Blunting of the stress response in the pulmonary circulation of infants with fentanyl. Anesthesia and Analgesia 64: 1137–1141
34. Hodkinson K, Bear M, Thorn J, Van Blaricum S 1994 Measuring pain in neonates: evaluating an instrument and developing a common language. Australian Journal of Advanced Nursing 12: 17–22
35. Humphrey T 1964 Some correlations between the appearance of human fetal reflexes and the development of the nervous system. Progress in Brain Research 4: 93–135
36. Izard C E, Hembree E A, Dougherty L M et al 1983 Changes in facial expression of 2 to 19 month old infants following acute pain. Developmental Psychology 19: 418–426
37. Johnston C C, Strada M E 1986 Acute pain responses in infants: a multidimensional description. Pain 24: 373–382
38. Johnston C C, Stevens B, Craig K D, Grunau R V E 1993 Developmental changes in pain expression in premature, full term, two and four month old infants. Pain 52: 201–208
39. Koehntop D E, Rodman J H, Brundage D M et al 1986 Pharmacokinetics of fentanyl in neonates. Anesthesia and Analgesia. 65: 227–232
40. Koren G, Butt W, Chinyanga H et al 1985 Postoperative morphine infusion in newborn infants: assessment of distribution characteristics and safety. Journal of Pediatrics 107: 963–967

41. Kostovic I, Rakie P 1984 Development of prestriate visual projections in the monkey and human fetal cerebrum revealed by transient cholinesterase staining. Journal of Neuroscience 4: 25–42
42. Kupfererberg H J, Way E L 1963 Pharmacologic basis for increased sensitivity of the newborn rat to morphine. Journal of Pharmacology and Experimental Therapeutics 141: 105–112
43. Macleod S M, Radde I C (eds) 1985 Textbook of paediatric clinical pharmacology. PSG Publishing, Littletown, Massachusetts
44. McGrath P J, Johnson G, Goodman J T et al 1985 CHEOPS: a behavioral scale for rating postoperative pain in children. In: Fields H L, Dubner R, Cervero F (eds) Advances in pain research and therapy. Raven Press, New York, vol 9, pp 395–402
45. McGraw M B 1941 Neural maturation as exemplified in the changing reactions of the infant to pinprick. Child Development 12: 31–42
46. McRorie T I, Lynn A M, Nespeca M K et al 1992 The maturation of morphine clearance and metabolism. American Journal of Diseases of Children 146: 972–976
47. Marshall R E, Stratton W C, Moore J A et al 1980 Circumcision 1. Effects upon newborn behavior. Infant Behavior and Development 3: 1–9
48. Masey S A, Koehler R C, Buck J R et al 1985 Effect of abdominal distention on central and regional hemodynamics in neonatal lambs. Pediatric Research 19: 1244–1249
49. Marx C M, Smith P G, Lowrie L H, Hamlett K W, Ambuel B A, Yamashita T S, Blumer J L 1994 Optimal sedation in mechanically ventilated pediatric critical care patients. Critical Care Medicine 22: 163–170
50. Murat I 1996 Regional anaesthesia in the newborn. In: Hughes D G, Mather S J, Wolf A R (eds) Handbook of neonatal anaesthesia. W B Saunders, London
51. Norden J, Hannallah R, Getson P et al 1991 Reliability of an objective pain scale in children. Anesthesia and Analgesia 72: S199
52. Norden J, Hannallah R, Getson P et al 1992 Concurrent validation of an objective pain scale for infants and children. Anesthesiology 75: A934
53. Okado N 1981 Onset of synapse formation in the human spinal cord. Journal of Comparative Neurology 201: 211–219
54. Olkkolo K T, Maunuksela E L, Korpela R et al 1988 Kinetics and dynamics of postoperative morphine in children. Clinical Pharmacology and Therapeutics 44: 123–136
55. Owens M E 1984 Pain in infancy: conceptual and methodological issues. Pain 20: 213–230
56. Pasternak G W, Zhang A Z, Tecoff L 1980 Developmental differences between high and low affinity opioid binding sites: their relationship to analgesia and ventilatory depression. Life Sciences 27: 1185–1190
57. Porter F 1989 Pain in the newborn. Clinics in Perinatology 16: 549–565
58. Rich E C, Marshall R E, Volpe J J 1974 The normal neonatal response to pinprick. Developmental Medicine and Child Neurology 16: 432–434
59. Rizvi T A, Wadha S, Mehra R D 1986 Ultrastructure of the marginal zone during prenatal development of the human cord. Experimental Brain Research 64: 483–490
60. Rizvi T A, Wasdwa S, Bijlani V 1987 Development of spinal substrate for nociception. Pain 4(suppl): 195
61. Rovner S 1987 Surgery without anesthesia: Can premies feel pain? Washington Post, August 13
62. Sherman M, Sherman I C 1925 Sensori-motor responses in infants. Journal of Comparative Psychology 5: 53–68
63. Shide D J, Blass E M 1989 Opioid effects of intraoral infusions of corn oil and polycose on stress reactions in 10 day old rats. Behavioral Neuroscience 103: 1168–1175
64. Takasaki M 1988 Ventilation and ventilatory response to carbon dioxide during caudal anaesthesia with lidocaine or bupivacaine in sedated children. Acta Anaesthesiologica Scandinavica 32: 218–221
65. Torres F, Anderson C 1985 The normal EEG of the human newborn. Journal of Clinical Neurophysiology 2: 89–103
66. Valman H B, Pearson J F 1980 What the fetus feels. British Medical Journal 280: 233–234
67. Wasz-Hockert O, Lind J, Vuorenkoski V 1968 The infant cry: a spectrographic and auditory analysis. Clinics in Developmental Medicine 2: 9–42
68. Williamson P S, Williamson M L 1983 Physiologic stress reduction by a local anesthetic during newborn circumcision. Pediatrics 71: 36–40
69. Wolf A R, Hughes D G 1993 Pain relief for infants undergoing abdominal surgery: comparison of infusions of IV morphine and extradural bupivacaine. British Journal of Anaesthesia 70: 10–16
70. Wolf A R, Valley R D, Fear D W et al 1988 Bupivacaine for caudal analgesia in infants and children: the optimal effective concentration. Anesthesiology 69: 102–106
71. Wolf A R, Hobbs A J, Wade A et al 1990 Post-operative analgesia after orchidopexy: the evaluation of a bupivacaine/morphine mixture. British Journal of Anaesthesia. 64: 430–435
72. Wolf A R, Hughes D, Hobbs A J et al 1991 Combined morphine/bupivacaine caudals for reconstructive penile surgery in children: systemic absorption of morphine and post-operative analgesia. Anaesthesia Intensive Care 19: 17–21
73. Wolf A R, Eyres R L, Laussen P C et al 1993 Effect of extradural analgesia on stress responses to abdominal surgery in infants. British Journal of Anaesthesia 70: 654–660
74. Wolf A R, Lawson R, Fisher S 1995 Ventilatory arrest after a fluid challenge in a neonate receiving subcutaneous morphine: British Journal of Anaesthesia 75: 787–789

28

Infants of drug-addicted mothers

Rodney Rivers

INTRODUCTION

The spread of illicit drug use from the developed to many of the developing countries is resulting in a worldwide increase in drug abuse.[84] In the UK, figures based on notifications to the Home Office[39] reveal an increase in registered adult addicts of 21% between 1993 and 1994. In 1994 heroin (66%), methadone (46%) and cocaine (9%) were the preferred substances of abuse, intravenous use (54%) being associated with HIV infection. A survey carried out in 1995 revealed a concerning level of involvement by the young.[55] Because of associated poly-drug use, including alcohol, the attribution of a causal relationship between fetal drug exposure and a neonatal outcome measure becomes difficult; self-reporting in pregnancy is also unreliable.[86] Attribution of long-term outcome measures to fetal drug exposure becomes even more problematic because of the difficulty of controlling for complications arising in pregnancy, including abruptio placentae, poor health, squalid accommodation, unemployment and poverty on a background of unsatisfactory relationships, periods of imprisonment and social instability. Chronic pelvic infection, HIV and hepatitis B, C and D may further contribute to the inability of a mother to provide appropriate child care. Finally, the selection of positive associations rather than negative ones for publication influences the readership's perception of the effects of drugs on the fetus and child.[49] Can one ever be certain that so-called normal controls have not been exposed to any 'recreational' drugs during pregnancy? The use of neuroactive drugs in pregnancy may result in a withdrawal syndrome in the newborn consequent upon the deprivation following birth. The hallmark of neonatal withdrawal, as highlighted by Volpe, is the dramatic movement disorder, jitteriness.[81] Drugs that have been associated with neonatal withdrawal syndromes are listed in Table 28.1 and those associated with withdrawal seizures in Table 28.2.

Table 28.1 Drugs described as being associated with a neonatal withdrawal syndome

Drug	Time of onset of withdrawal	
Heroin	0–96 h	peak 12–24 h
Methadone	12– > 72 h (may be up to 1–2 weeks)	peak 24–48 h
Barbiturates		
shorter acting	0–24 h	
longer acting	≥ 7 days	
Diazepam	2–6 h	
Chlordiazepoxide	3 weeks	
Tricyclic antidepressants	0–12 h	
Propoxyphene	< 24 h	
Pentazocine	< 24 h	
Codeine	< 24 h	
Dihydrocodeine (DF 118)	< 48 h	
Alcohol	< 24 h	

Table 28.2 Neonatal seizures following passive addiction

Opiates
Opioids
Barbiturates:
shorter acting
Tricyclic antidepressants
Propoxyphene

NARCOTICS

OPIATES

Heroin has high lipid and membrane solubility and is hydrolysed to morphine.[6] Morphine itself, the component of the opium poppy with most analgesic activity, is principally metabolized to 3- and 6-morphine glucuronides and to codeine. Following morphine dosing, the ratio of M3G to M6G is similar in the plasma of both newborns and older children.[12] However, as M3G is larger and more polar than morphine, placental transfer of fetally formed metabolite to the maternal circulation is likely to be restricted and fetal accumulation will occur.[61] M6G has some 37 times the analgesic effect of morphine sulphate, but M3G has excitatory effects. In the newborn, although M3G excitation may be blocked by receptor occupancy by morphine,[43] as the morphine level falls M3G becomes a potential cause of seizures.[62] This may partly explain why morphine is the drug of choice in heroin abstinence withdrawal seizures.[83]

Chronic opiate exposure in animals[70] and primates[29] results in changes in the cells of the major noradrenergic nucleus of the brain stem, the locus coeruleus. Upregulation of cyclic adenosine monophosphate, protein phosphorylation and enhanced nuclear c-*fos* proto-oncogene expression[34] result in alterations in neuronal metabolism and excitability, and have recently been reviewed.[59] Increased sensitivity at postsynaptic and β-adrenergic receptors innervated by the LC in the thalamus, hypothalamus, spinal cord and cerebral cortex is reported. On opiate withdrawal or inhibition by an opiate antagonist, increased LC neuron firing causes adrenaline depletion at 48–72 hours in the dog,[31] and is associated with hypertension, a fall in heart rate, pH, PaO_2, and with defaecation in the fetal sheep.[13] The increased firing of LC neurons in the rat is paralleled by the behavioural signs of withdrawal[70] and the syndrome, deriving from LC neuronal representation throughout the neuraxis, can be suppressed by the action of the α_2 agonist clonidine.[1] Clonidine also abolishes the signs of withdrawal in man[27] and in the neonate.[37]

The problems posed by narcotic use in pregnancy have recently been considered.[38] The aim must be to reduce fetal exposure to fluctuating drug levels and repeated episodes of 'withdrawal' by replacing heroin, with its short half-life, with the cross-tolerant synthetic drug methadone. Randomized trials of methadone maintenance programmes have been shown to reduce heroin use, mortality and criminality,[82] and in pregnancy to result in higher mean birthweights and head circumferences. Taken orally methadone has high bioavailability and a long half-life (20–30 hours), being metabolized in the liver. However, the higher the fetal plasma level at birth, the more rapid the initial fall and the more severe the neonatal withdrawal.[22] In a study in which babies were grouped by severity of withdrawal, the plasma half-life of methadone was 16 hours in the severe group and 23 hours in the mild withdrawing group; signs of withdrawal did not develop while methadone levels were above 0.06 μg/ml.[75] Maternal dose at delivery does not always correlate with withdrawal severity.[21,75,81] When attempts are made to achieve a maternal methadone dose of under 20 mg/day, signs of withdrawal in the neonatal period are likely to be mild or even absent.[75] This has the obvious advantage of shortening the period of hospital supervision. Some success has been achieved with discontinuation of methadone in pregnancy,[52] but this must always be balanced against the risk of a resumption of illicit drug use and fetal instability, with signs of withdrawal including fetal hyperactivity, tachycardia on CTG, and stillbirth.

Infants born to mothers abusing heroin tend to be of low birthweight and to demonstrate a withdrawal syndrome. Some 50% will be less than 2500 g at birth and 45–70% are below the 10th percentile for gestational age. The intrauterine growth retardation is frequently symmetrical, implying a disturbance of brain growth, with as many as 40% having head circumference measurements below the 10th percentile; causation, as indicated above, is likely to be multifactorial.[81]

METHADONE

Substitution programmes in the UK may account for much of the usage of methadone. Babies born to mothers on methadone may be below 2500 g at birth (10–35%), with up to 40% being small for gestational age. The neonatal withdrawal syndrome can be particularly severe and occurs in 60–95%.[46,81] Withdrawal signs occur later (days 2 and 3) than with heroin, with some only becoming severe by 10–14 days. Delayed withdrawal may relate to maternal use of benzodiazepines or other drugs.[79] Duration of withdrawal is longer and seizures more frequent with methadone than with heroin, occurring in 8% of one series (10 of 127) at a mean age of onset of 10 days.[36] EEG paroxysmal activity may precede or accompany observed seizures[36] and nutritive sucking is profoundly affected.[50]

OPIATE WITHDRAWAL SYNDROME

This occurs in 60–90% of babies in reported series, although it is highly probable that many mildly affected infants go unrecognized. Clinically evident withdrawal is more likely in the term than the preterm infant.[21] In both rats and humans it would seem that the gestationally related behavioural repertoire may affect the apparent incidence of withdrawal[45] (Table 28.3). Withdrawal is more likely when the mother is a long-standing addict on a high dose, with the last dose being taken within 24 hours of delivery. Some 63% of neonates present in the first 24 hours of life.[85]

Initial signs relate to central nervous system disturbance, being dominated by a very stimulus-sensitive rhythmic tremulousness, which is stopped by passive

Table 28.3 Neonatal heroin withdrawal syndrome. Severity of withdrawal in relation to gestational age in 178 infants. (From Doberczak, Kandall and Wilets[21], with permission)

	Moderate (%)	Severe (%)	Convulsions (%)
Term	50	16	7.3
Preterm	21	0	2.9

flexion of the part involved. In contrast to seizures, as emphasized by Volpe,[81] these movements are not accompanied by clonic jerks or abnormalities of gaze or eye deviation. Excessive alertness, agitation, activity and hypertonia become evident, with frantic sucking of fingers and hands. This is in contrast to the reduced level of consciousness associated with the jitteriness of hypoxic–ischaemic injury, of hypoglycaemia and of polycythaemia. In spite of the sucking behaviour, coordination of sucking and swallowing is disorganized, regurgitation and vomiting are common, and diarrhoea may develop by days 4–6. Seizures occur in some 1–2% of cases but may relate to accompanying conditions or even to treatment, e.g. chlorpromazine. Their occurrence demands full investigation.

Differential diagnosis

Withdrawal signs are non-specific; infections, metabolic, electrolyte and focal CNS pathology must be sought and polycythaemia excluded. Infection with syphilis, gonorrhoea or chlamydia may become manifest. Vigilance is required if other diagnoses are not to be missed.

Management

When opiate use is revealed, the constellation of withdrawal signs in the baby is readily recognized. (Table 28.4). The appearance of this range of signs in a young infant should always alert carers to the possibility of drug withdrawal as a cause, even in the face of maternal denial. Analysis of both urine and meconium may reveal evidence of in utero drug exposure.[66]

Several scoring systems have been developed in the United States and have been recently reviewed.[2] On the basis that the central nervous system excitation provokes the most undesirable features of withdrawal for the baby, and that signs of this precede the more peripheral disturbances of stuffy nose, sneezing, diarrhoea and sweating, a scoring system has been developed[51,73] which is weighted towards the neurologically based signs, treatment being commenced with a score of 6 or more on two successive occasions, 2–4 hours apart (Fig. 28.1).

Table 28.4 Signs of opiate withdrawal

Central nervous system	Gastrointestinal	Other
Jitteriness Irritability Shrill cry Hyperactivity Hypertonia Decreased sleep Excessive sucking Poor feeding Seizures	Regurgitation Vomiting Diarrhoea	Snuffles Sneezing Salivation Tachypnoea Yawning Hiccoughs Sweating Fever

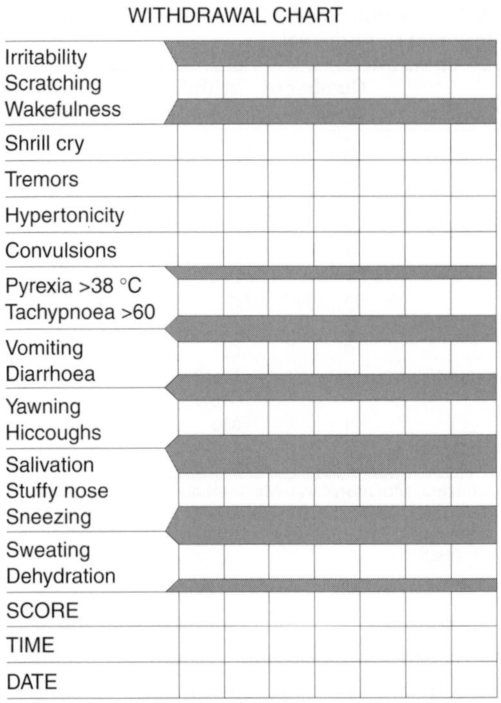

Fig. 28.1 Severity of drug withdrawal score chart based on clinical observations. At the time a baby is assessed each square may receive a score of 0 or 1. Only one item in any of the groups of items needs to be present for a score of 1 to be awarded. The maximum total score at a given time is therefore 10. Scores are recorded 2–4-hourly.

General care of the infant

These babies are at risk of meconium aspiration and the consequences of preterm delivery and poor intrauterine growth, in addition to withdrawal itself.[65] At delivery, naloxone is contraindicated as it may be capable of precipitating acute withdrawal and seizures, as seen in animals.[72] Because studies on the efficacy of stimulus reduction have shown little beneficial effect on withdrawal,[71] appropriate drug therapy, hydration and provision of nutrients are the cornerstones of management. Additional considerations are the provision of antenatal and postnatal therapy to reduce HIV acquisition when a mother is positive, along with prophylaxis against *Pneumocystis carinii* and hepatitis B protection.

Drug treatment

The introduction of an opiate when signs of significant central neurological disturbance develop will usually prevent the emergence of the later signs described above. Although the four drugs most used in treatment have been paregoric, phenobarbitone, diazepam and chlorpromazine,[14] these are now being superseded by the intravenous formulation of methadone given orally.[38] Methadone prevents withdrawal seizures, unlike phenobarbitone and diazepam, which ironically were often ineffectual.

Table 28.5 Seizure outcome by year in neonates requiring drug therapy for opiate withdrawal

Year	Number of cases	Withdrawal therapy	Seizures (cases)	Seizure therapy
1987	10	C	1	Mo
1988	9	C	3	↑C
			2	Mo
1989	8	C	1	Mo
1990	2	C	0	–
1991	7	C	2	D
1992	2	C	1	Mo
1993	4	C	2	Mo
1994	6	C:2	2	Mo
		Me:3	0	–
		Mo:1	0	–
1995	4	Me	0	–
1996 (1st 6 months)	5	Me	0	

C: chlorpromazine; Mo: morphine, Me: methadone; D: diazepam.
Of 44 treated with chlorpromazine, 14 developed seizures; of 12 treated with methadone and 1 treated with morphine, none developed seizures ($P = 0.057$ (χ^2 test)).

The reasons for the replacement of the above drugs by oral methadone include unpredictable or undesirable pharmacokinetics (variable absorption – oral morphine; delayed excretion – diazepam and chlorpromazine), polypharmacy (paregoric), side-effects, including depression of feeding and oversedation (phenobarbitone, diazepam, chlorpromazine), lack of efficacy in blocking aspects of the withdrawal syndrome (gastrointestinal – phenobarbitone; seizures – phenobarbitone and diazepam), possible toxicity (increased seizure risk – chlorpromazine) and potential side-effects from other components in the formulations used, including alcohol, benzoic acid (interference with albumin/bilirubin binding), phenol, sodium bisulphite (anaphylaxis in older patients), and propylene glycol (hyperosmolality in the newborn).

One unit's experience of the occurrence of seizures in term babies on chlorpromazine therapy for opiate withdrawal is shown in Table 28.5. Since converting from chlorpromazine to methadone, 12 term babies have been treated for withdrawal with methadone under the author's supervision and no opiate withdrawal-related seizures have been encountered. In the period 1987–1993 all babies with seizures on chlorpromazine that were treated with morphine had immediate cessation of seizures; control of seizures with diazepam was less satisfactory. It is noteworthy that at the time of seizure occurrence other signs of withdrawal were minimal; interestingly, the three infants with seizures in 1988 that were treated by an increase in chlorpromazine dosage did not have further seizures.

Treatment regimen

A proposed algorithm is shown in Figure 28.2. With repeated withdrawal scores of 6 and above, methadone is commenced at 6-hourly intervals until control is achieved (score 5 or less), commencing at 0.1 mg/kg/dose orally and increasing stepwise every 6 hours by 0.05 mg/kg/dose.

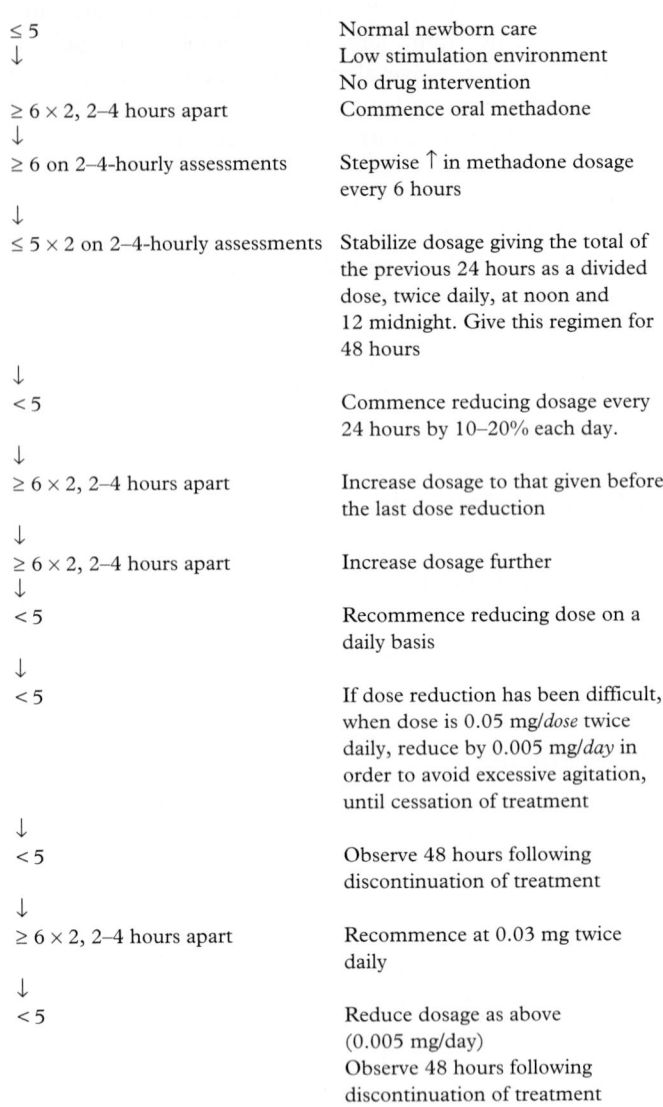

Withdrawal score/monitoring	Intervention
≤ 5	Normal newborn care
↓	Low stimulation environment
	No drug intervention
≥ 6 × 2, 2–4 hours apart	Commence oral methadone
↓	
≥ 6 on 2–4-hourly assessments	Stepwise ↑ in methadone dosage every 6 hours
↓	
≤ 5 × 2 on 2–4-hourly assessments	Stabilize dosage giving the total of the previous 24 hours as a divided dose, twice daily, at noon and 12 midnight. Give this regimen for 48 hours
↓	
< 5	Commence reducing dosage every 24 hours by 10–20% each day.
↓	
≥ 6 × 2, 2–4 hours apart	Increase dosage to that given before the last dose reduction
↓	
≥ 6 × 2, 2–4 hours apart	Increase dosage further
↓	
< 5	Recommence reducing dose on a daily basis
↓	
< 5	If dose reduction has been difficult, when dose is 0.05 mg/*dose* twice daily, reduce by 0.005 mg/*day* in order to avoid excessive agitation, until cessation of treatment
↓	
< 5	Observe 48 hours following discontinuation of treatment
↓	
≥ 6 × 2, 2–4 hours apart	Recommence at 0.03 mg twice daily
↓	
< 5	Reduce dosage as above (0.005 mg/day)
	Observe 48 hours following discontinuation of treatment

Fig. 28.2 Oral methadone regimen for opiate/methadone withdrawal.

With control, the total administered over the preceding 24 hours is divided twice daily for the succeeding 24 hours (doses at noon and midnight) and, provided control remains satisfactory (score < 5), dose reductions are made by 10–20% each day until a dose of 0.05 mg has been reached. Dose reduction has then often to be reduced to 0.005 mg/day if excessive agitation is to be avoided; on cessation of treatment the baby is observed for any significant relapse (score ≥ 5) for a further 48 hours. Administering a dose twice daily rather than once appears to reduce undesirable oversedation as well as preventing the emergence of agitation before the next dose is due. Seizures would be best treated by a single dose of parenteral methadone (0.25 mg/kg) or morphine (0.15 mg/kg) followed by maintenance therapy, but have not been observed with the above regimen. A failure of opiate to control seizures could result from other drug withdrawal (e.g. barbiturates, alcohol) or other causes, and uncontrolled seizures should be further investigated and treated with phenobarbitone. Monitoring for apnoea should be maintained until cessation of treatment.

These recommendations are based on the observation that a score of 6 achieved as a 'one-off': may sometimes be recorded on a single occasion only, and such babies may go on to avoid drug treatment altogether. However, two scores of 6 or a rising score > 6 is indicative of severe withdrawal. Recordings of withdrawal status tend to be made more frequently during obvious withdrawal because these babies are not easily ignored; to ensure a score of 6 is not a 'one-off': further assessment 2–4 hours later is recommended before commencing drug treatment. Because of the sequential nature of the development of signs of withdrawal, a baby scoring 6 or more on sequential occasions would inevitably be manifesting significant neurobehavioural disturbance. A reduction in treatment dosage should not be commenced until withdrawal is under control (score < 5). Dosing at 12 pm and 12 am allows adjustments in dosage to be made on the morning ward round against the knowledge of the withdrawal scores following previous dose reduction or dose increase instigated at noon the day before.

Outcome

If withdrawal is recognized for what it is, babies should no longer die from it. In one of the more dramatic case descriptions[68] a woman with two normal children, who had acquired the 'opium habit' having been prescribed opium to prevent a miscarriage in her third pregnancy, went on to have 15 neonatal deaths, all occurring within 3 days of birth from opiate withdrawal. Only with her 18th pregnancy was paregoric prescribed to protect the infant from the 'shock' of withdrawal. The baby survived. Among more recent reports of neonatal death, the mortality does not appear to be necessarily related to withdrawal.[26,28,64,85] A subacute withdrawal syndrome is recognized which, if it occurs after discharge home, may tax the parents to the limits of their tolerance; this is especially likely if the baby fails to sleep, is difficult to feed or makes excessive apparent demands for milk, suffering severe colic and vomiting. In some, these features may persist for several months and a small dose of diazepam may be prescribed with benefit, initially under supervision following rehospitalization.

Breast-feeding

This is not usually recommended for mothers on heroin as high peak blood levels of heroin are reflected in breast milk. However, mothers on methadone, codeine or morphine, when appropriately prescribed, may be recommended to take their medication after completion of a breast-feed. Provided that a mother's dose of methadone is not more than 20 mg/24 hours, breast-feeding has been thought to be reasonable.[15]

Sudden infant death syndrome

A number of studies have reported an increased risk of this, particularly following moderate or severe withdrawal.[47] It may be difficult to differentiate true SIDS from babies dying from neglect relative to their needs or from unrecognized infections.

Neurodevelopment

In spite of recently reviewed animal studies pointing to disordered neuronal and glial proliferation following in utero opiate exposure,[81] published human follow-up studies, with all their methodological difficulties,[33] suggest that by 2 years of age and at school entry age there may be no delay; however, intrauterine growth retardation, toxic compounds in street drug preparations, alcohol exposure, postnatal undernutrition and lack of social stimulation may all have additional subtle effects on the final intellectual performance and social integration of surviving infants.

Cocaine

Cocaine use in pregnancy has become a major concern.[35] The effects on the fetus and neonate have been extensively discussed,[80,87] although the scientific validity of some of the reported associations has been questioned owing to inadequate recruitment of controls.[53] Causal relationships can be difficult to prove,[60,69] but from the increasing body of available data it seems probable that disruption of brain architecture and possibly of long-term functioning could result from human fetal exposure. Disentangling the interrelationships between the biological and social factors remains a target for future research.[76,87]

The extent of cocaine usage during pregnancy in the UK remains unknown. The unreliability of interviewing techniques and of maternal urine testing[86] (positive only for 24 hours following administration), mitigate against the acquisition of firm data both on the number of fetuses being exposed and on the severity of individual exposure. Neonatally derived urine is positive for cocaine between 12 and 24 hours from the time of last fetal exposure, with the metabolite benzoylecgonine being detectable for up to 7 days.[63] Although results of screening by analysis of meconium have been reported,[66,67] if it is exposure to high concentrations that poses the most risk mere detection will not help predict outcome.[41] Hair analysis can be informative as to duration of exposure.[7] Reduced activity of plasma cholinesterase in the fetus and during infancy delays the metabolism of cocaine.[78]

Cocaine as water-soluble cocaine hydrochloride is taken by nasal insufflation, by mouth or intravenously;

Table 28.6 Effects of cocaine on fetus and newborn

Observation	Putative mechanisms
Uterine stimulation Placental abruption Preterm birth[32]	1. Catecholamines[42] 2. Direct effect on myometrium[57]
Fetal hypoxia, death Intrauterine growth retardation Low birthweight[48]	3. Catecholamine-induced vasoconstriction of maternofetal unit 4. Increased fetal metabolic rate
Diminished head circumference for gestation[5] Abnormalities of CNS development	3&4 above Impaired neuronal proliferation, migration and differentiation[80]
Intraventricular and parenchymal haemorrhage/ infarction[9,19,41,63]	Disturbed autoregulation Hypertensive episodes Ischaemic, vasoconstrictive episodes
Meconium staining of liquor[32] Necrotizing enterocolitis[23] Limb reduction defects[41] Gut atresias Myocardial ischaemia[54]	Sympathetic activation Vasoconstrictive episodes[44]

following alkali extraction, as heat-stable cocaine alkaloid (crack), it is inhaled as vapour on heating. Cocaine's pharmacological effects arise from blockading catecholamine, dopamine and tryptophan uptake, leading to prolonged sympathetic nervous stimulation with hypertension and vasoconstriction. Reduced serotonin synthesis may explain the alterations in sleep–wake cycling and reduced sleep requirements of affected babies.[25] A plasma catecholamine precursor[56] and CSF catecholamine levels[58] are raised in cocaine-exposed newborns. Some of the described clinical associations of cocaine use in pregnancy and their possible mechanisms are shown in Table 28.6. The confounding effects of other drugs, alcohol exposure and smoking are difficult to determine. Morphological changes in neuronal differentiation have been found in adult rats exposed to cocaine in utero,[30] and exaggeration of the deleterious effects of hypoxia by the presence of cocaine have been reported.[77]

Cocaine may be present at birth or may be derived postnatally in breast milk,[10] or from a nipple if topically applied as an analgesic.[8] Although the excessive sympathetic pathway activity of *opiate* withdrawal occurs as the opiate levels decline, with cocaine maximal sympathetic activity is seen at around its peak level. Abnormal sleep patterns are noted, with tremors and hypertonia being particularly prominent, together with long dull-alert periods of poor visual responsiveness but with the eyes open.[63] Seizures caused by cocaine are well recognized in adults and have been seen in exposed toddlers and infants.[3,74] Abnormalities of the EEG have been recorded.[20] Persisting hypertension was found in one small study.[40] The problems of small studies and confounding variables occur repeatedly in the literature.

Management

Usually no intervention is required; as breast-feeding shortly after crack use can cause seizures[10] it would seem prudent to discourage breast-feeding in known crack users.

Outcome

Variable increases in sudden infant death syndrome, with an overall risk of 8.5/1000, have been calculated from available reports;[4] these reports have, however, been challenged.[53] Impaired respiratory and arousal responses have been cited as being of possible relevance;[16] heart rate variability is also increased.[71] As regards the more global effects of cocaine on the fetal brain, a correlation between small head size, cocaine exposure and developmental scores has been reported,[11] although many of the cases were lost to follow-up. If the establishment of interneuronal connections is dependent on grouped repetitious patterns of neuronal stimulation,[24] then attention span, social stimulation and the child's own directed motivation will all have an impact upon brain development. Deficits leading to impulsiveness, deviant behaviour and inability to respond to normal educative techniques will only be discernible by appropriate longitudinal long-term testing. The best hope for any fetus must be preceding population-based school-age and preconceptional education concerning the wide-ranging potential effects of cocaine, together with comprehensive prenatal and postnatal support programmes.

OTHER DRUGS OF ADDICTION

Many drug-exposed infants must escape detection owing to the mildness and non-specificity of withdrawal signs, early discharge from hospital and slow elimination of many sedative/hypnotic/anxiolytic drugs. Most withdrawal signs are similar in content to those of opiate withdrawal, although there are exceptions. Short-acting barbiturates are associated with withdrawal seizures following jitteriness and hyperactivity, and longer-acting barbiturates cause a withdrawal syndrome which may last for months.[18] Seizures in the first 12 hours of life are a particular feature of tricyclic withdrawal and, in alcohol withdrawal, occur following the development of tremulousness; seizures of either origin are best controlled with phenobarbitone. Marijuana has not been consistently shown to be associated with neonatal or developmental abnormalities.[17]

ADDITIONAL MANAGEMENT ISSUES

A plan of management applicable to the UK support agencies has previously been described[51] (Fig. 28.3). This involves an antenatal planning meeting for all agencies

Shared antenatal care
Midwife/obstetrician/drug dependency unit

Booking scan/
HIV counselling

↓

20 weeks abnormality scan

↓

Between 24 + 30 weeks: discussion with paediatrician re postnatal management

↓

Predelivery multidisciplinary planning meeting
Midwife/obstetrician/GP/paediatrician/social services
DDU representative ± legal adviser ± probation officer

↓

Delivery

↓

Baby and mother cared for on postnatal ward
Monitor for withdrawal

↓

Cranial ultrasound
± eye examination (cocaine)

↓

Admit to neonatal unit if score becomes ≥ 5

↓

Commence drug intervention with score ≥ 6 × 2 occasions
2–4 hours apart

↓

Discharge multidisciplinary planning meeting
with neonatal nurse/paediatrician/GP/social services, health visitor ± legal adviser ± probation officer

↓

Discharge

↓

Follow-up

Fig. 28.3 Antenatal and postpartum plan.

involved in the care of the mother and baby, followed by postnatal monitoring in a transitional care facility on a postnatal ward, for up to 5 days in known cocaine exposure and for up to 14 days with moderate to high-dose methadone usage. Cranial ultrasound examinations are obtained and other focal lesions sought as indicated. A further planning meeting is held prior to discharge. Drug treatment, if required, is initiated on the special care baby unit (SCBU) and, unless they are going into foster care, babies are not transferred home on continuing withdrawal treatment. Some mothers will spend a period in a mother and baby home but, once at home, their health visitor and social worker are the principal sources of surveillance, in addition to paediatric follow-up. Facilitating parental involvement when their baby provides little positive behavioural return for their efforts is an essential part of the nursing support from birth onwards.

The disorganized social lifestyle and variable involvement in criminality to fund a continuing habit create a conflict of interests with the need of a developing child for social interaction and care. These children are often very demanding and may have disorganized sleep patterns for months. The inability to separate biological from social causes of impaired growth and developmental achievements does nothing to allay the fear that these children are often exposed to persistent disadvantage. A follow-up of 85 babies born at a London teaching hospital between 1968 and 1983, 2–13 years after discharge following treatment for opiate withdrawal, revealed that only 25% were living with both parents, 20% were with their mother and 12% were with their father. A further 36% were with relatives, had been adopted, fostered or were in other placements. Six parents and four children had died (Williams M J H, Cavanagh S 1986, personal communication). Not infrequently, the well-intentioned plans for providing family support have to be reversed and the children taken into care to avoid abuse or neglect.

REFERENCES

1. Aghajanian G K 1978 Tolerance of locus coeruleus neurons to morphine and suppression of withdrawal in response to clonidine. Nature 276: 186–188
2. Anand K J S, Arnold J H 1994 Opioid tolerance and dependence in infants and children. Critical Care Medicine 22: 334–342
3. Bateman D A, Heagarty M C 1989 Passive threebase cocaine ('crack') inhalation by infants and toddlers. American Journal of Diseases of Children 143: 25–27
4. Bauchner H, Zuckerman B 1990 Cocaine, sudden infant death syndrome, and home monitoring. Journal of Pediatrics 117: 904–906
5. Bingol N, Fuchs M, Diaz V, Stone R K, Gromisch D S 1987 Teratogenicity of cocaine in humans. Journal of Pediatrics 110: 93–96
6. Boerner U, Abbott S, Roe R L 1975 The metabolism of morphine and heroin in man. Drug Metabolism Review 4: 39–73
7. Callahan C M, Grant T M, Phipps P et al 1992 Measurement of gestational cocaine exposure: sensitivity of infants' hair, meconium and urine. Journal of Pediatrics 120: 763–768
8. Chaney N E, Franke J Wadlington W B 1988 Cocaine convulsions in a breast-feeding baby. Journal of Pediatrics 112: 134–135
9. Chasnoff I J, Bussey M E, Savich R, Stack C M 1986 Perinatal cerebral infarction and maternal cocaine use. Journal of Pediatrics 108: 456–459
10. Chasnoff I J, Lewis D E, Squires L 1987 Cocaine intoxication in a breast-fed infant. Pediatrics 80: 836–838
11. Chasnoff I J, Griffith D R, Freier C, Murray J 1992 Cocaine/polydrug use in pregnancy: two year follow up. Pediatrics 89: 284–289
12. Choonara I A, McKay P, Hain R, Rane A 1989 Morphine metabolism in children. British Journal of Clinical Pharmacology 28: 599–604
13. Cohen M S, Rudolph A M, Melmon K L 1980 Antagonism of morphine by naloxone in pregnant ewes and fetal lambs. Developmental Pharmacology and Therapeutics 1: 58–69
14. Committee on Drugs 1983 Neonatal drug withdrawal. Pediatrics 72: 895–902
15. Committee on Drugs, American Academy of Pediatrics 1989 Transfer of drugs and other chemicals into human milk. Pediatrics 84: 924–936
16. Davidson Ward S L, Bautista D, Chan L et al 1990 Sudden infant death

syndrome in infants of substance-abusing mothers. Journal of Pediatrics 117: 876–881
17. Day M L, Richardson G A 1991 Prenatal marijuana use: epidemiology, methodologic issues, and infant outcome. Clinical Perinatology 18: 77–91
18. Desmond M M, Schwanecke R R, Wilson G S, Yasunaga S, Burgdorff I 1972 Maternal barbiturate utilization and neonatal withdrawal symptomatology. Journal of Pediatrics 80: 192–197
19. Dixon S D, Bejar R 1989 Echocephalographic findings in neonates associated with maternal cocaine and methamphetamine use: incidence and clinical correlates. Journal of Pediatrics 115: 770–778
20. Doberczak T, Shonzer S, Senie R, Kandall S 1988 Neonatal neurologic and EEG effects of intrauterine cocaine exposure. Journal of Pediatrics 113: 354–359
21. Doberczak T M, Kandall S R, Wilets I 1991 Neonatal opiate abstinence syndrome in term and preterm infants. Journal of Pediatrics 118: 933–937
22. Doberczak T M, Kandall S R, Friedmann P 1993 Relationships between maternal methadone dosage, maternal–neonatal methadone levels, and neonatal withdrawal. Obstetrics and Gynecology 81: 936–940
23. Downing G J, Horner S R, Kilbride H W 1991 Characteristics of perinatal cocaine-exposed infants with necrotizing enterocolitis. American Journal of Diseases of Children 145: 26–27
24. Edelman G M 1987 Neural Darwinism. The theory of neuronal group selection. Basic Books, New York, pp 308–330
25. Farrar H C, Kearns G L 1989 Cocaine: clinical pharmacology and toxicology. Journal of Pediatrics 115: 665–675
26. Fricker H S Segal S 1978 Narcotic addiction, pregnancy, and the newborn. American Journal of Diseases of Children 132: 360–366
27. Gold M S, Redmond D E Jr, Klever H D 1978 Clonidine blocks acute opiate-withdrawal symptoms. Lancet ii: 599–602
28. Goodfriend M J, Shey I A, Milton D K 1956 The effects of maternal narcotic addiction on the newborn. American Journal of Obstetrics and Gynecology 71: 29–36
29. Grant S J, Huang Y H, Redmond D E Jr 1988 Behavior of monkeys during opiate withdrawal and locus coeruleus stimulation. Pharmacology Biochemistry and Behavior 30: 13–19
30. Gressens P, Kosofsky B E, Evard P 1992 Cocaine-induced disturbances of corticogenesis in the developing murine brain. Neuroscience Letters 140: 113–116
31. Gunne L-M 1962 Catecholamine metabolism in morphine withdrawal in the dog. Nature 195: 815–816
32. Hadeed A J, Siegel S R 1989 Maternal cocaine use during pregnancy: effect on the newborn infant. Pediatrics 84: 205–210
33. Hans S L, Marcus J, Jeremy R J, Auerbach J G 1984 Neurobehavioural development of children exposed in utero to opioid drugs. In: Yanai J (ed) Neurobehavioural teratology. Elsevier Science, Amsterdam, pp 245–273
34. Hayward M D, Duman R S, Nestler E J 1990 Induction of the c-*fos* proto-oncogene during opiate withdrawal in the locus coeruleus and other brain regions of rat brain. Brain Research 525: 256–266
35. Heagarty M C 1990 Crack cocaine. A new danger for children. American Journal of Diseases of Children 144: 756–757
36. Herzlinger R A, Kandall S R, Vaughan H G Jr 1977 Neonatal seizures associated with narcotic withdrawal. Journal of Pediatrics 91: 638–641
37. Hoder E L, Leckman J F, Ehrenkranz R, Klever H, Cohen D C, Poulsen, J A 1981 Clonidine in neonatal narcotic-abstinence syndrome. New England Journal of Medicine 305: 1284
38. Hoegerman G, Schnoll S 1991 Narcotic use in pregnancy. Clinical Perinatology 18: 51–76
39. Home Office Statistical Bulletin 1995 Statistics of drug addicts notified to the Home Office, United Kingdom 1994 17: 1–7
40. Horn P T 1992 Persisting hypertension after prenatal cocaine exposure. Journal of Pediatrics 121: 288–291
41. Hoyme H E, Jones K L, Dixon S D et al 1990 Prenatal cocaine exposure and fetal vascular disruption. Pediatrics 85: 743–747
42. Hurd W W, Smith A J, Gauvin J M, Hayashi R H 1991 Cocaine blocks extramural uptake of norepinephrine by the pregnant human uterus. Obstetrics and Gynecology 78: 249–253
43. Jacquet Y F, Klee W A, Rice K C, Iijima I, Minamikawa J 1977 Stereospecific and nonstereospecific effects of (+) and (–) morphine: evidence for a new class of receptors? Science 198: 842–845
44. Jones K L 1991 Developmental pathogenesis of defects associated with prenatal cocaine exposure: fetal vascular disruption. Clinical Perinatology 18: 139–146
45. Jones K L, Barr G A 1995 Ontogeny of morphine withdrawal in the rat. Behavioral Neuroscience 109: 1189–1198
46. Kandall S R, Albin S, Gartner L M, Lee K-S, Eidelman A, Lowinson J 1977 The narcotic-dependent mother: fetal and neonatal consequences. Early Human Development 1/2: 159–169
47. Kandall S R, Gaines J, Habel L, Davidson G, Jessop D 1993 Relationship of maternal substance abuse to subsequent sudden infant death syndrome in offspring. Journal of Pediatrics 123: 120–126
48. Kliegman R M, Madura D, Kiwi R, Eisenberg I 1994 Relation of maternal cocaine use to risks of prematurity and low birthweight. Journal of Pediatrics 124: 751–756
49. Koran G, Graham K, Shear H, Einarson T 1989 Bias against the null hypothesis: the reproductive hazards of cocaine. Lancet 2: 1440–1442
50. Kron R E, Litt M, Phoenix M D, Finnegan L P 1976 Neonatal narcotic abstinence: effect of pharmacotherapeutic agents and maternal drug usage on nutritive sucking behaviour. Journal of Pediatrics 88: 637–641
51. Lissauer T, Ghaus K, Rivers R P A 1994 Maternal drug abuse – effects on the child. Current Paediatrics 4: 235–239
52. Maas U, Kattner E, Weingart J B, Schafer A, Obladen M 1990 Infrequent neonatal opiate withdrawal following maternal methadone detoxification during pregnancy. Journal of Perinatal Medicine 18: 111–118
53. Mayes L C, Granger R H, Bornstein M H 1992 The problem of prenatal cocaine exposure. A rush to judgment. Journal of the American Medical Association 267: 406–408
54. Mehta S K, Finkelhor R S, Anderson R L, Harcar-sevcik R A, Vasser T E, Bahler R C 1993 Transient myocardial ischaemia in infants prenatally exposed to cocaine. Journal of Pediatrics 122: 945–949
55. Miller P M C, Plant, M 1996 Drinking, smoking, and illicit drug use among 15 and 16 year olds in the United Kingdom. British Medical Journal 313: 394–397
56. Mirochnick M, Meyer J, Cole J, Herren T, Zuckerman B 1991 Circulating catecholamine concentrations in cocaine-exposed neonates: a pilot study. Pediatrics 88: 481–485
57. Monga M, Weisbrodt M W, Andres R L, Sanborn B M 1993 The acute effect of cocaine exposure on pregnant human myometrial contractile activity. American Journal of Obstetrics and Gynecology 169: 782–785
58. Needlman R, Zuckerman B S, Anderson G, Mirochnick M, Cohen D J 1993 CSF monoamine precursors and metabolites in human neonates following in utero cocaine exposure. Pediatrics 92: 55–60
59. Nestler E J 1992 Molecular mechanisms of drug addiction. Journal of Neuroscience 12: 2439–2450
60. Newspiel D R 1992 Cocaine-associated abnormalities may not be causally related. American Journal of Diseases of Children 146: 278–279
61. Olsen G D, Gasser S R, Sommer K M, Grosso S M 1987 Placental permeability for morphine 3-glucuronide. In: Xth International Congress of Pharmacology, Proceedings, Sydney, Australia
62. Olsen G D, Sommer K M, Wheeler P L, Boyea S R, Michelson S P, Cheek D B C 1988 Accumulation and clearance of morphine 3-β-D glucuronide in fetal lambs. Journal of Pharmacology and Experimental Therapy 247: 576–584
63. Oro A S, Dixon S D 1987 Perinatal cocaine and methamphetamine exposure: maternal and neonatal correlates. Journal of Pediatrics 111: 571–578
64. Ostrea E M, Chavez C J, Strauss M E 1976 A study of factors that influence the severity of neonatal narcotic withdrawal. Journal of Pediatrics 88: 642–645
65. Ostrea E M, Chavez C J 1979 Perinatal problems (excluding neonatal withdrawal) in maternal drug addiction: a study of 830 cases. Journal of Pediatrics 94: 292–295
66. Ostrea E M, Brady M J, Parks P M, Asensio D C, Maluz A 1989 Drug screening of meconium in infants of drug-dependent mothers: an alternative to urine testing. Journal of Pediatrics 115: 474–477
67. Ostrea E M, Romero A, Knapp D K, Ostrea A R, Lucena J E, Utarnachitt R B 1994 Postmortem drug analysis of meconium in early-gestation human fetuses exposed to cocaine: clinical implications. Journal of Pediatrics 124: 477–479
68. Petty G E 1913 Narcotic drug disease and allied ailments. J.A. Davis Co, Tennessee

69. Potter S, Klein J, Valiante G et al 1994 Maternal cocaine use without evidence of fetal exposure. Journal of Pediatrics 125: 652–654
70. Rasmussen K, Beitner-Johnson D B, Krystal J H, Aghajanian G K, Nestler E J 1990 Opiate withdrawal and the rat locus coeruleus: behavioural, electrophysiological and biochemical correlates. Journal of Neuroscience 10: 2308–2317
71. Regalado M G, Schechtman V L, Del Angel A P, Bean X D 1996 Cardiac and respiratory patterns during sleep in cocaine-exposed neonates. Early Human Development 44: 187–200
72. Reynolds J E F (ed) 1993 Martindale: The extra pharmacopoeia, 30th edn. Pharmaceutical Press, London p. 685
73. Rivers R P A 1986 Neonatal opiate withdrawal. Archives of Disease in Childhood 61: 1236–1239
74. Rivkin M, Gilmore H E 1989 Generalized seizures in an infant due to environmentally acquired cocaine. Pediatrics 84: 1100–1102
75. Rosen T S, Pippenger C E 1976 Pharmacologic observations on the neonatal withdrawal syndrome. Journal of Pediatrics 88: 1044–1048
76. Singer L T, Yamashita T S, Hawkins S, Cairns D, Baley J, Kliegman R 1994 Increased incidence of intraventricular hemorrhage and developmental delay in cocaine-exposed very low birthweight infants. Journal of Pediatrics 124: 765–771
77. Spraggins Y R, Seidler F J, Slotkin T A 1994 Cocaine exacerbates hypoxia-induced cell damage in the developing brain: effects on ornithine decarboxylase activity and protein synthesis. Biology of the Neonate 66: 254–266
78. Stewart D J, Inaba T, Lucassen M, Kalow W 1979 Cocaine metabolism: cocaine and norcocaine hydrolysis by liver and serum esterases. Clinical Pharmacology and Therapy 25: 464–468
79. Sutton L R, Hinderliter S A 1990 Diazepam abuse in pregnant women on methadone maintenance. Implications for the neonate. Clinical Pediatrics (Philadelphia) 29: 108–111
80. Volpe J J 1992 Effect of cocaine use on the fetus. New England Journal of Medicine 327: 399–407
81. Volpe J J 1995 Teratogenic effects of drugs and passive addiction. In: Volpe JJ Neurology of the newborn, 3rd edn. W.B. Saunders, Philadelphia, pp. 824–842
82. Ward J, Mattick R P, Hall W 1992 Key issues in methadone maintenance treatment. University of New South Wales Press, Sydney
83. Wijburg F A, de Kleine M J K, Fleury P, Soepatmi S 1991 Morphine as an anti-epileptic drug in neonatal abstinence syndrome. Acta Paediatrica Scandinavica 80: 875–877
84. Wodak A 1994 Managing illicit drug use. A practical guide. Drugs 47: 446–457
85. Zelson C, Rubio E, Wasserman E 1971 Neonatal narcotic addiction: 10 year observation. Pediatrics 48: 178–189
86. Zuckerman B, Frank D A, Hingson R et al 1989 Effects of maternal marijuana and cocaine use on fetal growth. New England Journal of Medicine 320: 762–768
87. Zuckerman B, Frank D A 1994 Prenatal cocaine exposure: 9 years later. Journal of Pediatrics 124: 731–733

Section 5

Disorders of the newborn

29

Pulmonary diseases of the newborn

Part 1

Neonatal pulmonary physiology

Anne Greenough

FACTORS INFLUENCING MORPHOLOGICAL DEVELOPMENT OF THE LUNG

The human fetal lung originates in the 3-week-old embryo as a ventral diverticulum that arises from the caudal end of the laryngotracheal groove of the foregut. There are four major stages of lung development based on its microscopic appearance: embryonic 3–6 weeks; pseudoglandular 6–17 weeks; canalicular 17–26 weeks; and alveolar 27 weeks to term. The bronchial tree is developed by the 16th week of gestation. During the canalicular stage of development there is continued branching of respiratory bronchioles, vascularization of the terminal tubules and thinning of the airway epithelium. Towards the end of this stage (24 weeks) pulmonary gas exchange becomes theoretically possible. By 20–22 weeks of gestation both type I and type II pneumocytes can be identified. Type I cells are flattened and form over 90% of the gas-exchanging surface of the mature lung. The cuboidal type II cells have a secretory function and, from 24 weeks, osmiophilic lamellar bodies containing surfactant can be identified.

From 24 weeks to term further terminal branching occurs, with the development of saccules which become the alveolar ducts. Although alveoli begin to appear as shallow indentations at about 32 weeks of gestation, most alveolar development occurs post-term. The lung grows postnatally mainly by an increase in alveolar numbers, and by 4 years of age the adult number of alveoli are present.[212] The subsequent increase in lung volume and surface area is due to an increase in alveolar size. In the first 5 years there is little elastin in the alveolar walls, which only extends around the alveolar walls by 18 years;[138] the early 'relative' deficiency of elastin may facilitate the increase in size of the alveoli in the growing lung. There is a two- to threefold increase in the diameter and length of airways between birth and adulthood.[103] The amount of bronchial smooth muscle relative to airway size increases between birth and adulthood, the increase in the first weeks after birth being particularly rapid.

Abnormal lung growth can be the result of inadequate space, or of a reduction in either fetal breathing or amniotic fluid volume (p. 638). Space restriction can be due to an abnormality extrinsic to the lung, for example congenital diaphragmatic hernia, pleural effusion or asphyxiating thoracic dystrophy; or intrinsic to the lung, for example cystic adenomatoid malformation. The time of onset of the insult determines which structures are affected. Prior to 16 weeks of gestation branching of the airways is permanently impaired, which will also reduce the potential for the number of alveoli. An insult occurring later affects the number of alveoli.

FETAL BREATHING MOVEMENTS

Phrenic nerve or cervical cord resection, which abolishes FBMs, is associated with arrest of lung growth. Fetal breathing is dependent on normal diaphragmatic function, and pulmonary hypoplasia in newborns occurs with generalized neuromuscular disorders, isolated phrenic nerve agenesis and diaphragmatic amyoplasia. During periods of FBM rhythmical contractions of the diaphragm retard the loss of lung liquid and help to maintain lung expansion when the upper airway resistance is reduced;[106] this may be the mechanism by which FBMs preserve lung growth.

FETAL LUNG LIQUID

In fetal life the lung is filled with liquid, increasing from 4 to 6 ml/kg body weight at mid-gestation to about 20 ml/kg near term. The hourly rate of production is initially

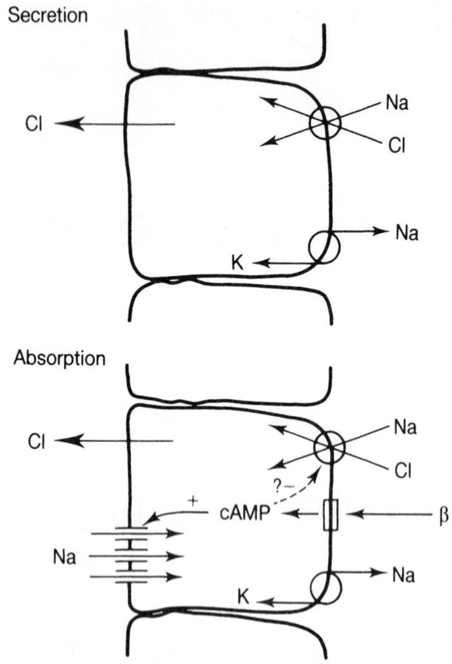

Fig. 29.1 Schematic model to explain the secretory and absorptive states of the lung. Na^+/K^+ ATP ase (K Na) generates a gradient for Na^+ which enters the intracellular space across the basolateral membrane linked to Cl^- (Na Cl). β receptor; Sodium channel in apical membrane; cAMP cyclic AMP. Reproduced with permission.[223]

2 ml/kg, increasing to 5 ml/kg. Compared to either amniotic fluid or plasma, lung liquid has a high chloride but low bicarbonate and protein concentration. The dominant force mediating lung liquid secretion is a chloride flux[165] (Fig. 29.1). The volume is principally regulated by the resistance to lung liquid efflux through the upper airway and by the presence of diaphragmatic activity associated with FBMs.[106] During labour and delivery, lung liquid secretion ceases and resorption begins (p. 457). The presence of lung liquid is important for normal lung development: chronic drainage results in pulmonary hypoplasia;[64] lung fluid restriction in the embryonic rat lung affects growth but not airway branching.[202]

AMNIOTIC FLUID VOLUME

Pulmonary hypoplasia is associated with oligohydramnios following, for example, prolonged rupture of the membranes or chronic drainage following amniocentesis. It appears to be due to the increased efflux of lung liquid from the intrapulmonary space. This is not as a result of external compression of the fetal thorax squeezing out lung liquid, as the amniotic fluid pressure under such circumstances is at or below the normal range.[160] Rather, prolonged oligohydramnios is associated with a decrease in lung liquid volume and the rate of both lung liquid secretion and tracheal fluid flow.[51] Tracheal ligation increases fetal intrathoracic pressure and causes lung hyperplasia; this can reverse the experimental pulmonary hypoplasia of clinically relevant entities such as oligohydramnios and CDH (p. 659).[52,88] There is, however, concern that although tracheal ligation increases cell proliferation it may be associated with decreased surfactant production.[23]

PULMONARY CIRCULATION

The pulmonary blood vessels and lymphatics develop from the mesenchyme of the splanchnic mesoderm of the foregut, which surrounds the lung buds as they push out from the laryngeal floor. Adjacent blood vessels fuse to form a rudimentary vasculature. The vascular plexus within each lung bud becomes supported by paired segmental arteries arising from the dorsal aorta, cranial to the coeliac arteries. At 32 days of gestation the sixth branchial arches appear, which give off the pulmonary arteries, and the segmental arteries cease to supply the lung. By 50 days of age the adult blood supply pattern is achieved. Occasionally an early segmental artery persists, captured within a lobe or lung segment (see sequestered lobe p. 646).[91] The arteries and airways develop together. There is progressive dichotomous branching of the pulmonary arteries during lung growth: 70% of the preacinar arteries are formed between the 10th and 14th weeks of gestation. Additional branching in the canalicular phase and in the last trimester around the developing saccules greatly increases the vascular supply to the area of gas exchange.

During fetal life the arterial walls contain a greater proportion of smooth muscle than in adult life. Postnatally there is rapid thinning in the first 2 weeks due to distension, and over the next year due to a slow reduction in the number of muscle fibres.[104] If such remodelling does not occur, but the infant has a structurally normal heart, this leads to persistent pulmonary hypertension (p. 529). Abnormal remodelling alters the pulmonary vascular reactivity and the response to pharmacological agents. Normal postnatal development can be divided into three overlapping phases.[81,91] Stage 1 starts from birth and lasts for about 4 days and represents adaptation to extrauterine life. Initially the endothelial cells are squat, have a low surface to volume ratio and many surface projections, but within 5 minutes after birth the endothelial cells become thinner, with less cell-to-cell contact, and fewer projections are evident as their surface membrane material is donated to allow the cells to spread rapidly (Fig. 29.2). The vessel walls become thinner.[92] Some of the changes are due to lung expansion, as prostacyclin so released dilates the pulmonary arteries. During stage 2, when the cells have taken up their definitive positions, they deposit connective tissue and fix the wall structure. In stage 3 there is growth of the pulmonary vasculature, which lasts until adulthood. The vascular smooth muscle develops less than the increase in

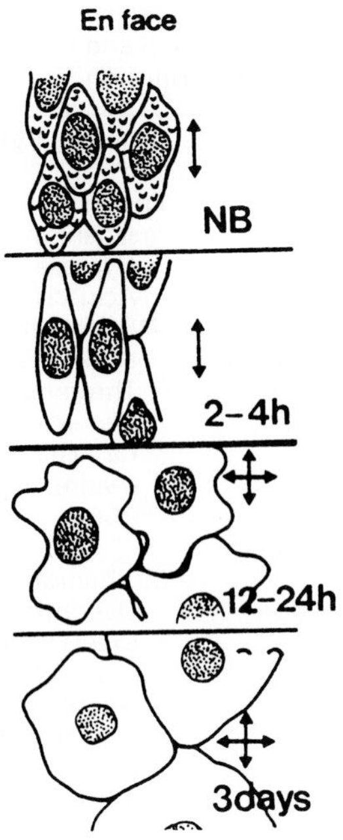

Fig. 29.2 Illustration of en face shape changes – the spreading of endothelial cells from birth to 3 days. Reproduced with permission.[91]

size of the respiratory arteries.[102] At birth almost the entire pulmonary vasculature is innervated. The majority of nerves identified to date contain the vasoconstrictor neuropeptides tyrosine and tyrosine hydroxylase.[91] Both nerve density and the immunoreactive expression of the neurotransmitters increase particularly rapidly in the first 2 weeks.[228]

CARDIORESPIRATORY ADAPTATION AT BIRTH

AERATION OF THE LUNGS

In fetal life the respiratory system is fluid filled. The replacement of lung liquid by air is largely accomplished within a few minutes of birth. Lung liquid production (p. 456) ceases during labour, and this effect is mediated by catecholamines[131,222] and AVP.[107] The fetal lung becomes increasingly sensitive to adrenaline with maturation: this is dependent on hormonal influences, particularly T_3 and glucocorticoids.[10] Some liquid is squeezed out under the high vaginal pressure during the second stage of delivery,[121] but the majority is absorbed into the pulmonary lymphatics and capillaries.[205] The transpulmonary pressure which inflates the lungs displaces liquid from the terminal respiratory units into the perivascular spaces. Air entry into the lung displaces liquid and reduces the hydraulic pressure in the pulmonary circulation, increasing blood flow. This increases the effective vascular surface area for fluid exchange, facilitating water absorption into the pulmonary vascular bed.

Stimulus for the first breath

Fetal breathing activity ceases during labour. Following birth, one of the most important stimuli to the onset of breathing is cooling. Audiovisual, proprioceptive and touch stimuli recruit central neurons and increase central arousal.[38,90] Hypoxia detected by central chemoreceptors is important, but peripheral chemoreceptor activity is not critical to the onset of respiration (p. 464).

The median time for the onset of respiratory activity is 10 seconds.[221] An 'opening pressure' is required to overcome the high flow resistance and inertia of liquid in the airways, as well as the surface tension at the air–liquid interface.[121] Both Karlberg et al[121] and Milner and Saunders[150] recorded inspiratory pressures during the first breath of greater than 20 cmH_2O, but not in all infants. Subsequently, using a dual-pressure tip transducer, Vyas et al[220] demonstrated that pressures greater than 20 cmH_2O were the norm. Expiration is also active for the first few breaths, with pressures ranging from 18 to 115 cmH_2O; this may aid the distribution of ventilation and facilitate further fluid clearance from the lungs.

CHANGES IN LUNG MECHANICS AFTER BIRTH

There is a fall in airways resistance and a rise in functional residual capacity, which is most rapid in the first 2 hours. Compliance, however, progressively increases over the 24-hour period as lung liquid is gradually absorbed. The changes in lung mechanics occur at a slower rate following elective caesarean section, when there is a delay in lung fluid absorption.

CIRCULATORY CHANGES AT BIRTH

In the fetus only about 12% of the right ventricular output enters the pulmonary circulation.[67] This is because of the high pulmonary vascular resistance, the presence of a patent ductus arteriosus and the low-resistance placental component of the systemic circulation. At birth, clamping of the umbilical cord and removal of the placenta from the circulation reduces venous return through the inferior vena cava to the right atrium. The foramen ovale closes because of the resultant lower right atrial pressure and the increase in left atrial pressure which occurs with the increased pulmonary venous return. The loss of the umbilical venous return also means diminished flow through the ductus venosus, and passive closure occurs usually within 3–7 days after birth.

Lung aeration results in opening up of the pulmonary capillary bed, acute lowering of pulmonary vascular resistance and an increase in pulmonary blood flow. This is due both to a mechanical effect and to oxygenation of the blood passing through the pulmonary circulation. In fetal lambs, mechanical expansion of the lungs with a non-oxygenated gas caused a decrease in pulmonary vascular resistance and a fourfold increase in pulmonary blood flow; a further increase resulted when oxygen was used as the ventilatory gas.[213] Inflation of the lungs also stimulates pulmonary stretch receptors, which leads to reflex vasodilatation of the pulmonary vascular bed. Mechanical expansion also creates surface forces at the gas–liquid interface within the alveoli, which physically expand small blood vessels and decrease perivascular pressure.[224] Approximately one-third of the pulmonary vasodilatation is due to the mechanical effects of ventilation, a third to raised arterial oxygen tensions, and a further third to lowering arterial carbon dioxide tensions or elevation of pH.

Pulmonary vascular resistance falls rapidly in the first minutes after birth, then more gradually over the next days and weeks of life. The pulmonary artery pressure is about 60 mmHg at birth and 30 mmHg at 24 hours of age. This change is associated with a rapid reduction in pulmonary artery wall thickness, which is due not to a loss of muscle cells but to a reorganization of the shape and orientation of the endothelial cells[80] (p. 456). During early neonatal life the pulmonary circulation remains unstable, and in certain disease states, particularly those associated with asphyxia or chronic hypoxia, the pulmonary vascular resistance increases or remains at the high fetal levels – PPHN (p. 527).

Colour Doppler imaging[224] demonstrated that in healthy infants the majority of measurable changes in cardiopulmonary haemodynamics occur by 8 hours, although some degree of right to left ductal shunting may be found up to 12 hours after birth. In most infants the ductus had closed or was closing by 24 hours of age. The increase in cardiac output immediately after birth reported by others[2] was found to be only temporary, and by 4 hours stroke volume and heart rate had decreased and cardiac output approximated to normal values for older term newborn infants. Measurements at 8, 12 and 24 hours showed a significant delay in ductal closure in infants with respiratory failure and pulmonary hypertension.

Endothelial-derived products, endothelin and NO are important in regulating fetal and transitional pulmonary vascular tone[198,242] (Table 29.1). Prostaglandins are also involved in the circulatory transition from fetal to postnatal life. PGI_2 production increases soon after birth and falls 2–5 hours later. Its production and release are related to pulmonary tissue stretch. PGI_2 participates in the reduction of pulmonary vascular resistance accompanying ventilation, but is not essential for maintaining low pulmonary vascular resistance once it has been established.[137] PGD_2 lowers pulmonary artery pressure in the fetus and newborn during the first 2–3 days, but in older animals it is a primary vasoconstrictor; this difference is related to the availability of the 11-ketoreductase enzyme system, which converts PGD_2 to the vasoconstrictor $PGF_{2\alpha}$. Bradykinin production is increased

Table 29.1 Factors that modulate pulmonary vascular resistance in the near-term and term transitional and neonatal pulmonary circulation. Reproduced with permission[122]

Lowers PVR	Increases PVR
Endogenous mediators and mechanisms	Endogenous mediators and mechanisms
Oxygen	Hypoxia
Nitric oxide	Acidosis
PGI_2, E_2, D_2	Endothelin-1
Adenosine, ATP, Magnesium	Leukotrienes
Bradykinin	Thromboxanes
Atrial natriuretic factor	Platelet-activating factor
Alkalosis	Ca^{2+} channel activation
K^+ channel activation	α-adrenergic stimulation
Histamine	$PGF_{2\alpha}$
Vagal nerve stimulation	
Acetylcholine	Mechanical factors
β-adrenergic stimulation	Overinflation or underinflation
	Excessive muscularization, vascular remodelling
Mechanical factors	Altered mechanical properties of smooth muscle
Lung inflation	Pulmonary hypoplasia
Vascular cell structural changes	Alveolar capillary dysplasia
Interstitial fluid and pressure changes	Pulmonary thromboemboli
Shear stress	Main pulmonary artery distension
	Ventricular dysfunction, venous hypertension

by ventilation with oxygen, but not with nitrogen.[100] Bradykinin increases PGI_2 production, and in addition results in the release of NO.[4] NO is generated in the endothelial cells by the effects of NO synthetase on L-arginine, forming citrulline and NO. The NO then diffuses into the smooth muscle cells, resulting in an increase in GMP and smooth muscle relaxation. Pharmacological NO blockage inhibits endothelium-dependent pulmonary vasodilatation and attenuates the rise in pulmonary blood flow after birth. Increased fetal oxygen tension augments endogenous NO release (Fig. 29.3). Pulmonary vasodilatation occurs in two phases, a rapid one due to mechanical ventilation, and a slow one due to vasodilator agents. Bradykinin may stimulate the release of NO during the rapid phase, and PGI_2 production during the slow one. Decreased production of endogenous vasoconstrictors, such as thromboxane and endothelin-1, which are considered as potentially contributing to the high pulmonary vascular resistance in utero, may also participate in the decrease in PVR at birth.

POSTNATAL FUNCTION

THE AIRWAYS

The nasal portion of the airway is firmly supported by its larger bony and smaller cartilaginous portions. Nasal resistance to airflow, which comprises approximately one-third of the total pulmonary resistance, is determined by the physical dimensions in a given individual, which are related to ethnic origin[163] and the state of the mucous

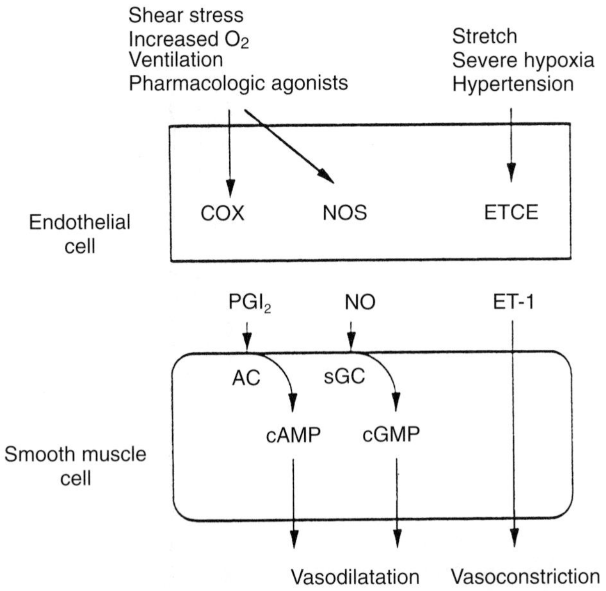

Fig. 29.3 Role of endothelium-derived products in the regulation of pulmonary vascular tone in the perinatal lung. AC, adrenylate cyclase; COX, cyclo-oxygenase; ETCE, endothelin-converting enzyme; NOS, NO synthase; PGI_2, prostacyclin; sGC, soluble guanylate cyclase. Reproduced with permission.[1]

membranes lining the airway. The prime function of the nose is to act as an entry port for respiration, humidifying and warming inspired gas and trapping extraneous particles. Infants are not necessarily obligate nose breathers, and full-term infants can establish oral breathing in the presence of nasal occlusion.[189] The pharyngeal portion of the airway is very compliant. In the absence of active muscle contraction there is apposition of the soft palate and tongue against the posterior pharyngeal wall, which is accentuated by neck flexion and negative pressures during inspiration, leading to collapse and obstruction of the airway. This is usually prevented, however, by the splinting and dilating actions of pharyngeal muscles. In the fetus and newborn infant there is increased flexibility of the epiglottis and the hyoid, thyroid and cricoid cartilages. In term infants the region is stabilized by a fat-laden superficial fascia which covers the neck and face; this is absent in the premature infant, as fat accumulation occurs in the final third of gestation.

Chemoreceptors in the larynx serve to prevent the entry of foreign material by triggering reflex apnoea. Changes in laryngeal diameter modulate airway resistance, and lung volume can be maintained by expiratory adduction of the vocal cords[58]. Laryngeal resistance can be varied by active abduction of the vocal cords during inspiration, and by passive as well as active adduction during expiration. Inspiratory abduction and expiratory adduction of the vocal cords occur during fetal breathing movements.[42]

The trachea and main bronchi are supported by cartilaginous rings; nevertheless, smooth muscle contraction can cause narrowing and markedly increase resistance, at least in the adult. In the newborn the small airways are more compliant, and expiratory collapse tends to lead to air trapping.

THE THORAX

In the newborn the thorax is round rather than dorsoventrally flattened, as in the adult, and the rib orientation is horizontal rather than caudal; thus the expansion potential of the thorax is limited. The neonatal thoracic cage has relatively soft and flexible bony elements, which makes the chest wall subject to collapse during increased inspiratory efforts and the lungs rather collapsed at rest. To compensate, the infant attempts to elevate the lung volume at end expiration by a rapid breathing rate, a short expiratory time, intercostal activity and grunting (expiratory laryngeal adduction). Grunting disappears in REM sleep[86] and is inhibited by intubation. The latter is associated with a fall in oxygenation,[89] which emphasizes the importance of expiratory laryngeal adductor activity in maintaining lung volume and hence a store of oxygen at a higher partial pressure than in the tissues. Instability of end-expiratory lung volume, particularly in the premature neonate, may explain fluctuations in arterial oxygen levels.[6]

THE RESPIRATORY MUSCLES (Fig. 29.4)

The main inspiratory muscle is the diaphragm, a dome-shaped muscle attached to the ribs. Diaphragmatic contraction results in the abdominal contents moving downwards, increasing the vertical dimension of the thoracic cavity. If the dome's descent is impeded by abdominal pressure, then the lower ribs are pulled up. This increases the rib cage diameter by virtue of the linkages between ribs, provided by the intercostal muscles and by the articulations of the ribs that lead to a 'pump and bucket handle action'. The configuration of the adult and neonatal diaphragm differs, the latter being relatively flat following birth, the dome shape developing with the physical growth of the thorax and internal organs.[49] There is an exaggerated asymmetrical movement of the newborn diaphragm during respiration. These differences mean the diaphragm is less efficient in the neonate than in the adult. The number of skeletal muscle fibres in the diaphragm is, however, fixed at the time of birth and the subsequent increase in muscle weight is due to hypertrophy. The respiratory muscle fibre composition of the diaphragm does change with age. The fibres are distinguished into several categories by histochemical and functional characteristics. Type I fibres are oxidative with a slow twitch, and fatigue resistant; types IIa and IIc are oxidative– glycolytic with a fast twitch, but also fatigue resistant. Type IIb, in contrast, are glycolytic with a fast twitch, and are fatiguable.[236] The proportion of type I fibres is low at birth and increases until 6 months of age;

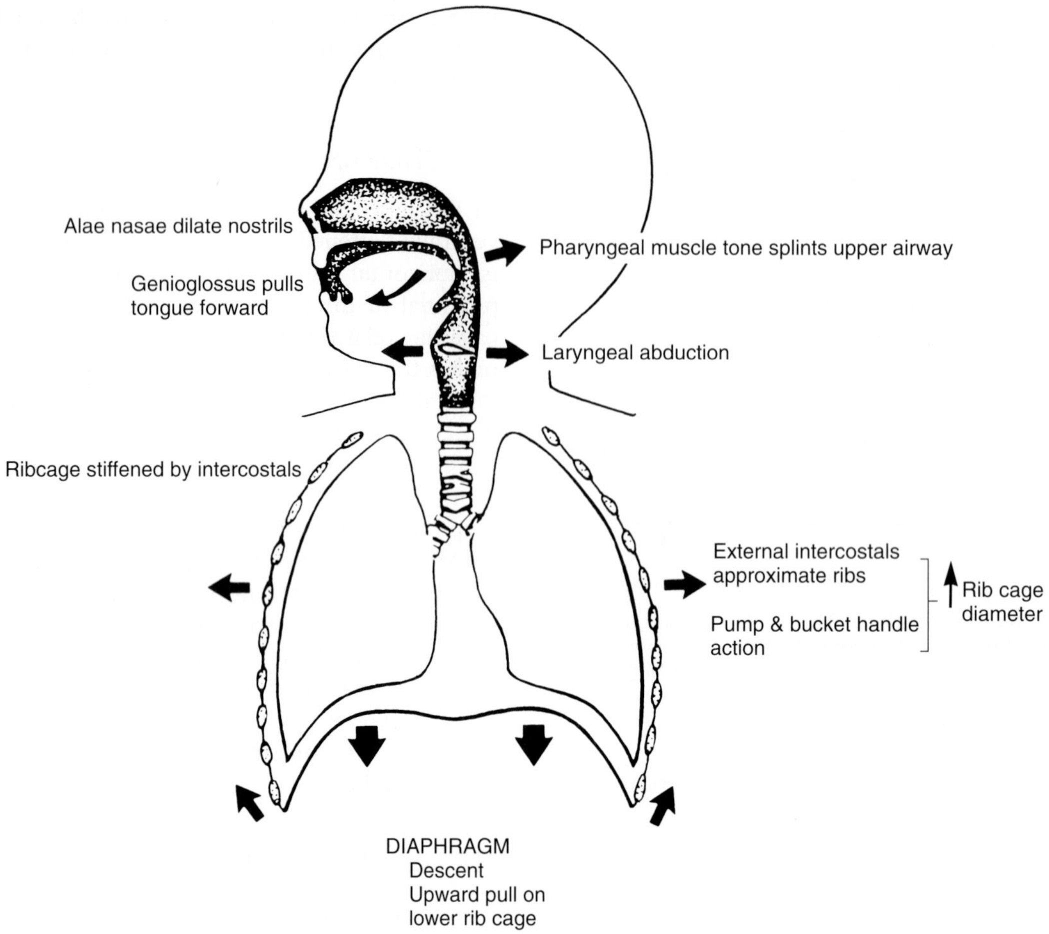

Fig. 29.4 Diagrammatic representation of the respiratory pump showing the various muscles and actions that make up inspiration. Although the diaphragm is the main muscle, many others act to optimize its function by opening the airways and splinting the floppy rib cage.

there is an associated increase in type IIb, but a decrease in type IIa fibres. Type IIc fibres, which are present at birth, disappear completely by 6 months.[147] This means that at birth the diaphragm has a relatively high percentage of oxidative fibres (types I, IIa and IIc) which are fatigue resistant. The proportion of type I fibres, however, may be particularly low in preterm infants, putting them at risk of diaphragmatic muscle fatigue. Optimal function of the diaphragm is dependent on rib cage stability and adequate abdominal muscle tone. This is particularly important when the system is loaded, as with stiff lungs or obstructed airways. The rib cage is more compliant in the newborn, who is therefore more dependent on intercostal muscle activity (see below).[97]

The internal and external intercostal muscles are components of the chest wall. It was previously thought that the external intercostals were primarily inspiratory, and the internal intercostals expiratory muscles. It is now appreciated that their actions are similar and depend on the volume of the rib cage: elevating the ribs at low lung volumes, but lowering them at high lung volumes.[48] The intercostal muscles also maintain the stability of the chest wall during inspiration and limit volume reduction during expiration. This tonic activity is abolished in REM sleep,[215] resulting in a reduction in end-expiratory lung volume and, more importantly, destabilization of the chest wall and out-of-phase movements of the abdomen and rib cage.[42] These problems particularly compromise the premature newborn because of the soft thoracic skeleton. During REM sleep such infants rely on diaphragmatic activity to compensate for the inefficiency of the chest wall, and thus diaphragmatic fatigue can result in a reduction in tidal volume and much of the increased diaphragmatic work being dissipated in 'sucking in ribs instead of air'.[22] Abdominal muscle tone may also be important in stabilizing the rib cage in REM sleep. Respiratory function is improved when the neonate is placed in the prone position.[54,144]

GAS EXCHANGE IN THE NEONATAL LUNG

At rest, oxygen consumption in the newborn (7 ml/min/kg) is approximately twice that of adults. Minute ventilation is proportionally increased and is achieved largely by an increased breathing rate. The increased rate, rather than depth, of breathing observed in the newborn presumably results from the constraints on increasing tidal volume imposed by the relatively stiff lungs and unstable rib cage. The disadvantage is that this increases the amount of dead space ventilation, although this is minimized by the relatively low volume of the proximal airways.[155] In addition, overventilation or underperfusion of some lung units contributes to the wasted ventilation. The contribution of ventilation–perfusion mismatch, as estimated from the a-ADO_2 is most marked in preterm infants in the first hours of life.

A major difference between the blood gases of newborn babies and older infants is the lower PaO_2 in relation to the inspired oxygen tension. This is largely because of right-to-left shunting of blood, either through areas of the lung with very low ventilation–perfusion ratios or, less commonly, through persisting fetal vascular channels (foramen ovale and ductus arteriosus). The total right-to-left shunt is estimated from the a-ADO_2. Estimates of the total shunt in healthy infants are 24% of the cardiac output in the first hour after birth and 10% at 1 week of age. Shunting through fetal vascular channels is only important immediately after birth in immature infants, or in sick infants with raised pulmonary vascular resistance. The contribution of lung units with a low ventilation–perfusion ratio to the shunt is significant in preterm infants[168] and babies with respiratory distress syndrome (p. 489). The low PaO_2 caused by right-to-left shunting (through cardiac shunts and perfused but non-ventilated lung units) cannot be overcome by administering 100% oxygen, because the blood that is being ventilated soon becomes fully saturated and increasing the oxygen tension adds little further oxygen. On the other hand, carbon dioxide accumulation from partial right-to-left shunting can be compensated for by increased ventilation of functioning lung units. Thus, provided respiratory efforts are maintained $PaCO_2$ will be normal or even low, despite right-to-left shunting.

GAS TRANSPORT IN THE BLOOD[45]

Oxygen

The majority of oxygen in whole blood is transported as oxyhaemoglobin (HbO_2) and only a small proportion is dissolved in solution. Haemoglobin increases the oxygen transport capacity of the blood 70-fold over that simply transported in the plasma. The haemoglobin concentration is regulated by a renal sensing mechanism which operates to maintain a balance between the oxygen supply and the requirement of the renal tissues. A decrease in the concentration or arterial oxygen saturation of haemoglobin, or an increase in haemoglobin affinity for oxygen, increases erythropoietin production (p. 810). The effect of erythropoietin on the bone marrow is usually limited by the amount of available iron. Under basal conditions, in the adult 4 ml of oxygen per minute per kilogram of body mass are loaded on to haemoglobin, but this rate can be increased 15-fold. Haemoglobin is a tetramer made up of four subunits, each of which contains a haem moiety (porphyrin and one atom of ferrous iron) attached to a polypeptide (globin) chain. Each of the four iron atoms can combine with an oxygen molecule; these remain in the ferrous state, hence the reaction is oxygenation rather than oxidation. In adult haemoglobin the four globin chains are predominantly $\alpha_2\beta_2$ (HbA) but in the fetus $\alpha_2\gamma_2$ (HbF) (see below). The quaternary structure of haemoglobin determines its affinity for oxygen: uptake of oxygen by haemoglobin results in a change of position of the haem moieties, facilitating further oxygen binding. The result is that the oxyhaemoglobin dissociation curve (the relationship of the percentage oxygen saturation of haemoglobin to the PO_2) has a characteristic sigmoid shape (Appendix 12). The oxyhaemoglobin dissociation curve is affected by the pH, temperature and concentration of 2,3-DPG. A rise in temperature or fall in pH (Bohr shift) shifts the curve to the right, which means that a higher PO_2 is required for haemoglobin to bind to a given amount of oxygen. This is quantified as the P_{50}, the PO_2 at which the haemoglobin is half saturated with oxygen. The higher the P_{50} the lower the affinity of haemoglobin for oxygen. 2,3-DPG is formed from a product of glycolysis, and therefore its concentration falls when the pH is low. 2,3-DPG binds preferentially to the β chains of deoxygenated haemoglobin. An increase in 2,3-DPG causes more oxygen to be liberated; that is, the oxygen dissociation curve is shifted to the right.

The fetus and newborn

Fetal erythrocytes are larger than, have a shorter half-life than and differ in ultrastructure from adult erythrocytes (p. 807). They also vary with regard to their mechanical, osmotic, thermal and acidic fragility. In addition they contain different haemoglobin (HbF), which is less easily denatured in alkaline or acidic solutions than adult haemoglobin. The γ chains of HbF have the same number of amino acids as the β chains, but differ in sequence by 39 amino acids. The γ chains of HbF have poorer binding to 2,3-DPG. The effect of 2,3-DPG on the P_{50} of fetal haemoglobin is approximately 40% of the effect on the P_{50} of adult haemoglobin (Appendix 12). The oxygen tension of fetal blood is one-fifth to one-fourth that of the adult, but the fetal arterial blood oxygen content and oxyhaemoglobin saturation are similar to those of the adult. This results from the high oxygen-carrying capacity and the increased oxygen affinity of HbF. The latter facilitates the movement of oxygen from mother to fetus; oxygen delivery to the fetal tissues is, however, sustained by the steep fetal oxygen dissociation curve, which means that a small decrease in oxygen tension results in a major change in oxyhaemoglobin saturation and unloading of oxygen.

In the newborn 75–84% of the haemoglobin is HbF. Neither birth, intrauterine hypoxia nor haemolytic disease of the newborn causes a change in the proportions of HbA and HbF at any given gestational age. Near term, however, a demand for accelerated erythropoiesis leads preferentially to synthesis of HbA. During the first year HbF decreases from 75 to 7% of the total haemoglobin.

The high oxygen affinity of HbF has disadvantages in postnatal life. In particular, the low P_{50} decreases the driving potential for oxygen diffusion, limiting the rate at which oxygen can be unloaded.[45] The oxygen consumption of the newborn at minimal activity, even in a thermally neutral environment, increases by 100–150% in the first few days. To meet these demands the infant's blood oxygen affinity decreases rapidly over the first 5 days and then more gradually, reaching adult values by 6 months.[46] During the first 5 days the 2,3-DPG levels rise to above those found in the adult; this decreases blood oxygen affinity by lowering intercellular pH. Prematurely born infants have a lower 2,3-DPG content, lower P_{50} and higher fetal haemoglobin concentration. They have a smaller oxygen unloading capacity and do not catch up until 3 months of age.[79]

Carbon dioxide

The relationship between CO_2 content and PCO_2 is essentially linear. Carbon dioxide is carried in the blood by three mechanisms: dissolved, secondly as bicarbonate (85%), and thirdly in combination with proteins as carbamino compounds (10%). Carbon dioxide is 20 times more soluble in water than oxygen. Bicarbonate is formed very rapidly in RBCs because of the presence of carbonic anhydrase, which catalyses the first part of the following reactions:

$$CO_2 + H_2O \overset{(CA)}{=} H_2CO_3 = HCO^-_3 + H^+$$

Ionic dissociation of H_2CO_3 is fast. HCO^-_3 then diffuses out of the RBC down a concentration gradient, but H^+ cannot follow and binds to haemoglobin. This is facilitated by the presence of reduced haemoglobin, which is a weaker acid than oxyhaemoglobin, and thus deoxygenation of the blood increases its ability to carry CO_2 (the Haldane effect). To maintain electrical neutrality, as HCO^-_3 diffuses out, Cl^- diffuses into the RBC (the chloride shift). These events increase the osmolar content of the RBC; thus the PCV is higher on the venous than on the arterial side of the circulation. Carbon dioxide also combines with the N terminals of amino acids of proteins, particularly haemoglobin, to form carbamino compounds:

$$CO_2 + R_2 + NH_2 = RNHCOO^- + H^+$$

Neonatal blood has a greater carbon dioxide transport capacity than adult blood because of its high haemoglobin level. In addition, carbon dioxide competes with 2,3-DPG for the haemoglobin binding site and, as 2,3-DPG binds less avidly with HbF than with adult haemoglobin, more carbon dioxide can be taken up. RBC carbonic anhydrase levels, however, are reduced by 25% in the neonate, and are even lower in those born prematurely.[124]

REGULATION OF BREATHING

The rhythmic transition from the inspiratory to the expiratory phase of the respiratory cycle is ordered by a centrally generated respiratory rhythm, which consists of three neural phases:[20]

- inspiration, corresponding to inspiratory muscle contraction;
- phase 1 expiration, corresponding to post-inspiration or passive expiration, when inspiratory muscles cease to contract progressively;
- phase 2 expiration, corresponding to active exhalation with expiratory muscle contraction.

RESPIRATORY 'CENTRES'

The respiratory neurons that take part in the respiratory rhythm are concentrated into two distinct medullary regions, the dorsal and ventral respiratory groups. The central respiratory rhythm generator is located within the subregions of the VRG. A variety of models of the central respiratory rhythm generator have been proposed, but a common assumption is that chemical neurotransmission is required to mediate synaptic interactions, which play a role in the generation of transmission and expression of the respiratory rhythm (Fig. 29.5).[20] As rhythm is generated it is ultimately transmitted synaptically to the spinal motorneurons and cranial pre-motor neurons; the latter control the activity of airway muscles.[20] Afferents from the forebrain, hypothalamus, central and peripheral chemoreceptors, muscles, joints and pain receptors are integrated into the DRG and VRG. The number of intersynaptic connections reaches a peak towards the end of fetal life.

NEUROTRANSMITTERS

Excitatory

The excitatory neurotransmitters include glutamate, which excites NMDA and non-NMDA receptors; the latter are involved in generating and transmitting respiratory rhythms to spinal and cranial respiratory neurons.[68] The transmission of inspiratory drive is further fine-tuned

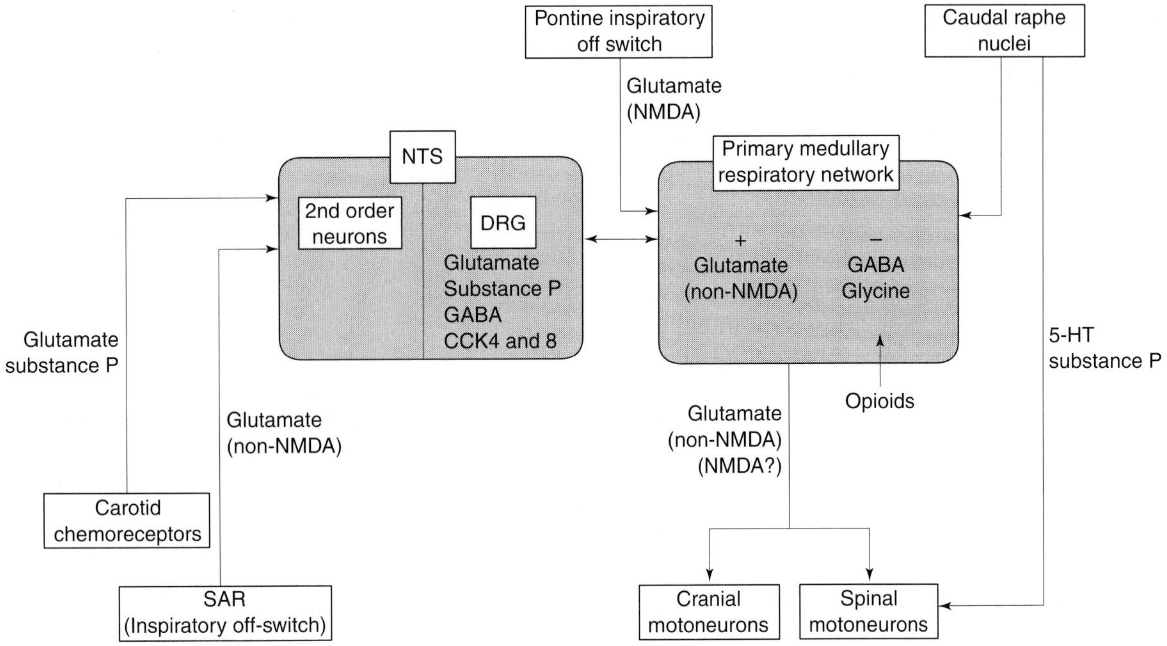

Fig. 29.5 Schematic representation of neurotransmitters and other neuroactive agents involved in CNS control of respiration. Reproduced with permission.[20]

by presynaptic glutaminergic modulation at the level of the spinal cord. Serotonin has diverse effects on respiratory neuronal activity, but the most consistent effect is to restore a normal breathing pattern in metabolic states such as hypoxia or ischaemia, which cause apneustic breathing.[134] Substance P is largely excitatory and may stimulate respiration by effects within the primary medullary respiratory network;[239] there may be endogenous release from projections from the caudal raphe nuclei to the inspiratory neurons.[105] It is likely that substance P is the mediator of the hypoxic drive from the peripheral chemoreceptors.[178] Around the time of birth there is an elevation of noradrenergic activity leading to activation of the locus coeruleus, which may be important for the forebrain drive of breathing.[132] If rabbit pups are put into a hypoxic or cold environment the increase in noradrenaline is significantly higher than in those nursed in a 'control' environment.[133] However, the stimulatory effect on breathing of cooling is not mediated by a noradrenergic mechanism.[73]

Inhibitory

Both GABA and glycine are essential for generating respiratory rhythm in the primary network. These inhibitory amino acids provide phasic waves of inhibitory postsynaptic potentials, which are received by the medullary respiratory neurons during their silent periods.[183] GABA and glycine are released by late and postinspiratory neurons to turn off inspiratory neurons and so facilitate the transition from inspiration to expiration. Synaptic inputs from peripheral sensory receptors and brain regions outside the primary medullary respiratory network input affect the full expression of the respiratory rhythm.[63] Phasic transition is modulated by two sources of synaptic input from outside the primary network: the slowly adapting pulmonary stretch receptors, and pontine neurons. Suppression of either of these prolongs inspiration (apneusis). Opioids (endorphins and exogenous drugs) decrease respiration by peripheral[16] and central action; the latter are due to a decrease in spontaneous respiratory unit activity and the suppression of recurrent excitation by glutaminergic inputs within the primary respiratory network.[47] There may be endogenous endorphinergic tonic inhibition of breathing in the neonate, which vanishes after the neonatal period.[131] Adenosine is ubiquitously formed in the body and has both central and peripheral effects. When administered centrally it depresses ventilation; this effect is most pronounced in young full-term and preterm models. If adenosine is given systemically, however, it stimulates breathing, probably by stimulating peripheral chemoreceptors; this effect may be more important in the adult. Adenosine antagonists (theophylline and caffeine) stimulate breathing and also block hypoxia-induced respiratory depression but not in humans.[194] Adenosine may mediate the secondary apnoea seen after birth asphyxia; removal of an inhibitory substance might explain why it is often necessary to ventilate an infant artificially for a period two or three times longer than the duration of asphyxia.[149] Prostaglandins E_1 and E_2 depress ventilation. Plasma concentrations of PGE_2 decrease at birth, and it has been suggested this may be important for the onset of respiration.

CHEMORECEPTORS

Both central and peripheral chemoreceptors are involved in the modification of respiratory activity in response to changes in blood gases. The central chemoreceptors are situated near the ventral surface of the medulla and respond to changes in carbon dioxide/pH and oxygen supply. The peripheral chemoreceptors are situated at the bifurcation of the common carotid arteries (carotid bodies) and in the aortic bodies above and below the aortic arch, the former being more important in humans.

In the fetus the arterial chemoreceptors are active in utero, but virtually silenced when the arterial PO_2 rises at birth.[17] Resetting of the carotid chemoreceptors to hypoxia then occurs, probably triggered by the rise in blood oxygen levels. The resetting of the chemoreceptors to hypoxia is essentially complete within 24–48 hours of birth,[25] and may be due to a change in dopamine levels. Dopamine inhibits chemoreceptor discharge in both newborn and adult. If rat pups are delivered into a hypoxic environment (12%) they maintain both their low sensitivity to hypoxia, with persistence of the immature inhibitory response to hypoxia,[59] and a high dopamine turnover.[99] In the lamb, hyperoxia induced by mechanical ventilation of the fetus for a few days before birth causes premature resetting.[18]

At birth, blood gas measurements indicate that there should be a powerful chemoreceptor drive to breathe. The carotid chemoreceptors, however, do not appear to be essential for the initiation of air breathing, and are probably quickly silenced by the rise in the PaO_2 that occurs. The relative inactivity of the chemoreceptors during this period is indicated by the reduced immediate ventilatory responses to hypoxia and hyperoxia in humans and an inability to detect chemoreceptor afferent activity in the lamb carotid sinus nerve. Presumably other drives maintain breathing efforts at this time.

Although the peripheral chemoreceptors are not essential for initiation of respiration, they are important in the development of breathing control, as their denervation increases the neonatal mortality of newborn animals.[57] The carotid chemoreceptor responses to both oxygen and carbon dioxide, however, are weak in the newborn and increase during postnatal development.[26,140] In the cat, the speed of maturation of O_2 and CO_2 responses differed, the response to hypoxia being weakest at 1 week and at nearly adult levels by 4 weeks, whereas CO_2 sensitivity continued to develop between 8 weeks and adulthood.[26] The mechanisms of carotid body maturation are unknown, but are unlikely to be due to changes in dopamine secretion, which takes place over days rather than weeks.[99]

Responses to changes in oxygen tension (Fig. 29.6)

The fetus. Fetuses respond to hypoxia with a suppression of ventilation, mediated by the lateral part of the lower pons. In response to hypoxia there are also cardiovascular reflexes, which include bradycardia and redistribution of the circulation to favour the heart, brain and adrenals[116] and which minimise oxygen consumption and conserve oxygen supplies for vital organs. Hyperoxia stimulates continuous fetal breathing.

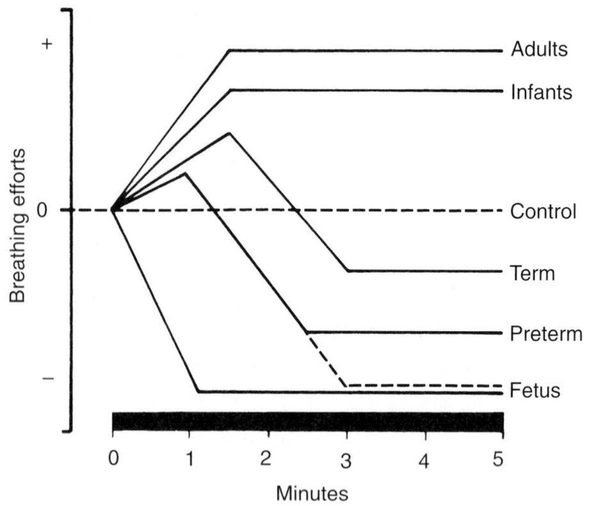

Fig. 29.6 Diagrammatic representation of the age-related responses to hypoxia, induced by breathing hypoxic gases for 5 minutes (solid bar). Breathing efforts assessed by diaphragmatic EMG in the fetus and by ventilatory responses in others. Dashed interrupted line indicates that apnoea may occur in preterm infants, resembling a fetal response. Reproduced with permission.[96]

The newborn. The newborn's response to hypoxia in the perinatal period is biphasic, a transient increase in minute ventilation followed by a decrease to or below baseline levels. The initial increase in ventilation is probably due to activation of peripheral chemoreceptors, as it is abolished by carotid sinus nerve section.[24] The subsequent reduction in ventilation may result from a fall in $PaCO_2$ following the initial hyperventilation, and may be due to a depression of central respiratory neurons.[186] It may also be explained by the suppressant effect of hypoxia in the fetal state persisting into the neonatal period. The biphasic response to hypoxia disappears at 12–14 days and the adult pattern is then seen, that is, stimulation without depression (Fig. 29.6). Very immature infants respond to hypoxia in a similar fashion to fetuses, that is, with apnoea. This inhibition of breathing is at a suprapontine level. More mature preterm infants have an initial increase (but less than in term infants) and then a more dramatic fall in ventilation in response to hypoxia.[185] In non-REM sleep the decrease in ventilation is the predominating response. The response to hypoxia is also modified by the temperature of the environment in which the infant is nursed: transient hyperventilation on exposure to 12% O_2 is not seen if the infant is in a cold rather than a warm environment. The decrease in ventilation and return to control levels after 21% O_2 was reinstituted, however, occurred in both thermal environments, and the ventilatory response to

3% CO_2 inhalation was unaffected by temperature.[29]

A hyperoxic gas causes a temporary suppression of breathing, which is attributed to the withdrawal of peripheral chemoreceptor drive. During the first few days the reduction in ventilation with 100% oxygen is less, consistent with inactivity of the carotid afferents during this resetting period. After a few minutes of hyperoxia ventilation increases to above control levels. In adults a similar but less marked hyperventilation has been attributed to hyperoxic cerebral vasoconstriction, which leads to increased brain tissue carbon dioxide.

The response to hyperoxia is slower in more immature infants. Prolonged exposure to supplemental oxygen also reduces the response to hyperoxia.

Response to carbon dioxide/acidosis

The fetus. Fetal breathing was initially thought to depend only on behavioural reflexes, as it was only observed during REM sleep. It is now known that fetal breathing is modified by chemical stimuli: the fetus responds to an increase in $PaCO_2$ with an increase in breathing, both elevated frequency and diaphragmatic activity. It is probably the hydrogen ion concentration, rather than carbon dioxide per se, that is the major stimulus to respiratory activity, although there is some evidence that carbon dioxide may have an effect independent of pH.[148] During non-REM sleep, however, only very high $PaCO_2$ levels (> 100 mmHg) can initiate breathing activity.[186] Lesions in the ventrolateral pons eliminate the hypoxic inhibition of breathing, and are associated with a lower threshold for carbon dioxide drive-augmented breathing through all states.[116]

The newborn. Inhalation of CO_2 increases ventilation in the newborn in both REM and quiet sleep. The slope of minute ventilation versus $PaCO_2$ levels is similar in the newborn to that in adults, but the response is shifted to the left because of lower resting carbon dioxide levels.[22,184] The tidal volume component of the ventilatory response assumes greater importance with postnatal development. The percentage of inhaled CO_2 influences the pattern of breathing: a low percentage (< 2%) primarily stimulates an increase in tidal volume,[118] whereas a higher percentage provokes an increase in respiratory frequency and tidal volume.[152] Periodic breathing is abolished with a small increase in inhaled CO_2.[118] Sleep state also influences the response to carbon dioxide, both in adults[173] and in the newborn.[22] In term infants the slope of ventilatory response is less during active than during quiet sleep (Fig. 29.7). This may be due to the mechanical instability associated with rib cage distortion in active sleep, as the diaphragmatic response is intact. In preterm infants[187] the slope of the ventilatory response is less, but increases with postnatal growth. As diaphragm EMG responses to CO_2 inhalation are also reduced in the preterm infant, this is probably due to the immaturity of the central chemoreceptors rather than mechanical differences in the respiratory pump.[184]

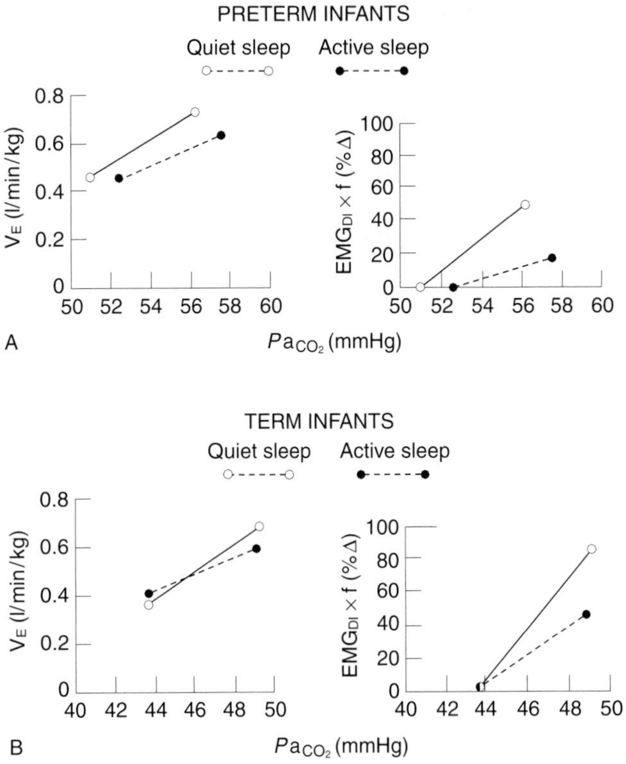

Fig. 29.7 The ventilatory response to CO_2 re-breathing in neonates. Note that (A) preterm and (B) term infants showed a decreased response to CO_2 in 'phasic' REM sleep as compared with quiet sleep. The vertical axis on the figures on the right is a measure of EMG activity multiplied by the change in respiratory rate. Reproduced with permission.[185]

RESPIRATORY REFLEXES

Hering–Breuer

Hering and Breuer[98] demonstrated that inflation of the lung resulted in cessation of respiratory activity (the Hering–Breuer inflation reflex). This is generated by stretch receptors within the airway and has an afferent pathway lying within the vagi. In the newborn the reflex produces a pattern of rapid, shallow tidal breathing and operates within the tidal volume range, whereas in older subjects it prevents excessive volume exchange, and can only be stimulated if the inflating volume is increased above a critical threshold.[36,76] The reflex is increased in infants with non-compliant lungs, and by the administration of theophylline. The reflex may be stronger in preterm than in term infants,[123] but this is controversial.[66] In the first 4–6 weeks of life there appears to be no change in the reflex,[30] but its strength then declines over the first year.[180]

If inhalation is prolonged, this stimulates expiratory muscle contraction (the Hering–Breuer expiratory reflex). The active expiration seen in infants ventilated at slow rates and over long inflation times may be a manifestation of this reflex.[75]

In animal models a prolonged inspiratory response can be generated by deflating the lung rapidly, either by attaching the endotracheal tube to a suction source or by creating a pneumothorax, or following an unusually vigorous expiratory effort which takes the lung below its end-expiratory level (the Hering–Breuer deflation reflex). This response does occur in the newborn[142] and may have a role in maintaining the FRC.

Head's paradoxical reflex

Head[95] noted that if vagal conduction was blocked, rapid inflation, instead of producing apnoea, resulted in a stronger and more pronounced diaphragmatic contraction, Head's paradoxical reflex. This has subsequently been termed the inspiratory augmenting reflex or provoked augmented inspiration, and is the underlying mechanism of the first breath and sighing. This reflex improves compliance and reopens partially collapsed airways. Its frequency is increased by low compliance, hypercapnia and hypoxia.[31]

The intercostal phrenic inhibitory reflex

Rapid chest wall distortion results in a shortening of inspiratory efforts. This reflex response is inhibited by an increase in FRC or by applying CPAP; the mechanism may be improved chest wall stability.[143]

Irritant reflexes

Subepithelial chemoreceptors in the trachea, bronchi and bronchioles detect insults to the epithelial surfaces; inhalation of toxic gases therefore causes a change in the frequency and depth of respiration. The response is less in REM sleep and in the premature infant,[65] who has fewer small myelinated vagal fibres and poorly developed receptors.

Upper airway reflexes

Breathing is stimulated by cold via the trigeminal afferents of the facial skin, whereas irritant stimuli to the nasal mucosa cause inhibition of breathing and cardiovascular reflex responses resembling those in diving mammals. The latter response is enhanced under anaesthesia and in the newborn,[225] when cortical dampening of the responses is reduced. Vigorous suctioning of the nasopharynx can stimulate apnoea and bradycardia via these reflexes.[39]

The laryngeal chemoreceptors defend the lower airway from inhalation. Introduction of water into the interarytenoid notch induces apnoea.[174] In active sleep laryngeal stimulation is more likely to induce apnoea and less likely to cause arousal.[173] This is of potential clinical significance, since gastro-oesophageal reflux is more common during active sleep.[112] There may be 'chemically selective' responses, as apnoea is more common if water rather than saline is used,[43] but differences in response to species-specific and other milks has not been demonstrated in humans.

Table 29.2 The tidal flow and volume were measured by a type 00 Fleisch pneumotachograph, and intrathoracic pressure with a 4 cm oesophageal balloon. Babies supine and in quiet sleep. Dead space eliminated by a bias flow of air

Measurement	No of infants studied	Mean	Standard deviation	Range
Tidal volume (ml/g)	266	4.8	1.0	2.9–7.9
Respiratory rate (bpm)	266	50.9	13.1	25.104
Minute volume (ml/min/kg)	266	232	3.6	78–144
Dynamic compliance (ml/cmH_2O/kg)	266	1.72	0.5	0.9–3.7
Total pulmonary resistance (cmH_2O/l/s)	266	42.5	1.6	3.1–171
Work of breathing (G.cm)	266	11.9	7.4	1.1–52.6
Expiratory time (s)	291	0.57	0.17	0.27–1.28
Inspiratory time (s)	291	0.51	0.10	0.28–0.87
Time to maximum expiratory flow/ total expiratory time (s)	291	0.51	0.12	0.18–0.83
Static compliance (ml/cmH_2O)	299	3.70	1.45	2.0–14.8
Respiratory system resistance (cmH_2O/l/s)	299	63.4	16.6	34.9–153.3
Time constant of respiratory system (s)	299	0.24	0.10	0.08–1.1
Thoracic gas volume (ml/kg)	271	29.8	6.2	14.5–15.6

Data of Milner and Marsh reproduced with their permission

LUNG MECHANICS (Table 29.2)[204]

LUNG VOLUMES

The tidal volume is the amount of gas entering or leaving the lung with each breath. Minute volume is calculated by multiplying the tidal volume by the respiratory rate over 1 minute. The volume exchanged following a maximum inspiratory and expiratory effort is called the vital capacity, and in the infant can be measured during crying (crying vital capacity). The residual volume remains after a maximum expiratory effort; RV plus vital capacity gives the total lung capacity. At end expiration the volume of gas remaining in the lung is referred to as the FRC and can be estimated by rebreathing an insoluble gas. Only areas of the lung in communication with the airways will be measured by such a method. Alternatively, the patient can be placed in a body plethysmograph and the TGV estimated by applying Boyle's law during airway occlusion; TGV is FRC plus trapped gas. The dead space is the part

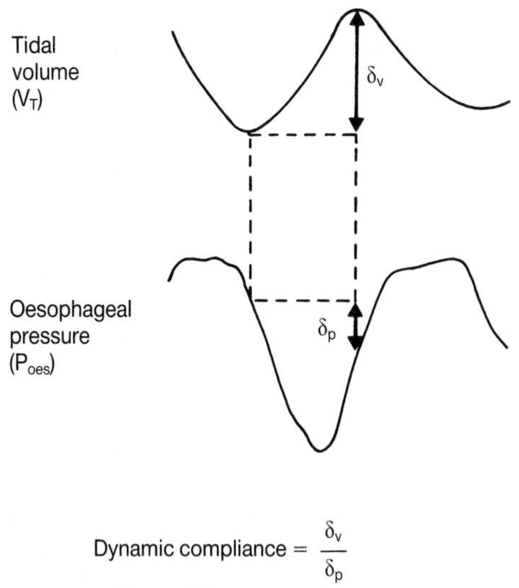

Fig. 29.8 Volume and oesophageal pressure traces during spontaneous breathing. The dynamic compliance is calculated by dividing the tidal volume (δV) by the pressure gradient between the beginning and end of inspiration (δP). Reproduced with permission.[77]

of the lung that does not take part in ventilation, and is made up of the anatomical dead space (the conducting airways) and the physiological dead space, which includes non-functioning alveoli. Alveolar ventilation can be estimated from the tidal volume minus the dead space.

In infants with respiratory distress, particularly transient tachypnoea of the newborn, the respiratory rate is increased and the tidal volume may be decreased (pp. 487, 515). In RDS and pneumonia the FRC is low (p. 487) and the physiological dead space increased.

COMPLIANCE

Compliance is a measure of the distensibility of the lungs and chest wall, i.e. the change in volume per unit pressure. Dynamic compliance is assessed during tidal breathing by measuring the change in volume (usually using the integrated signal of a flow measuring device, a pneumotachograph) divided by the change in pleural pressure (which under certain conditions is similar to the change in oesophageal pressure) between points of zero airflow (Fig. 29.8). In situations with a rapid respiratory rate and chest wall distortion dynamic compliance measurements can be inaccurate. Dynamic compliance is measured in ventilated infants by relating the volume change from a positive pressure inflation to the pressure drop, that is, peak inspiratory pressure to positive end-expiratory pressure, (PIP–PEEP) (Fig. 29.9), provided the infant is not making spontaneous respiratory efforts that interfere with volume delivery during inflation.

Static compliance requires the measurement of changes in lung volume over a larger range than the tidal volume, or an assumption has to be made that the end-expiratory transpulmonary pressure represents a static value, which is unlikely to be true in infants with lung disease.[199] Static compliance is usually measured in spontaneously breathing infants using an occlusion technique, which relies on occlusion during inspiration causing a transient inhibition of breathing by stimulation of the Hering–Breuer reflex. The airway pressure during the occlusion is related to the volume above end expiration at which the occlusion was made. This technique requires temporary cessation of breathing, which may be difficult to provoke in an infant with a rapid respiratory rate or a weak Hering–Breuer reflex. Static compliance measurements assess the compliance of both the lung and the chest wall. In the newborn chest wall compliance is very high, and so dynamic and static compliance values are essentially similar. Compliance is reduced in infants with RDS.

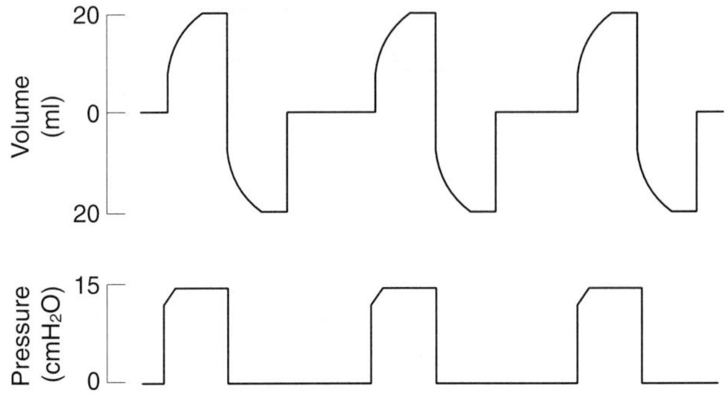

Fig. 29.9 Volume and pressure traces during mechanical ventilation. Compliance is calculated by dividing the change in volume by the difference in pressure from PIP to PEEP. Note that the positive pressure plateau has been maintained until volume delivery is complete.

Resistance

Resistance is a measure of the pressure necessary to generate airflow. Airway resistance can be assessed in a body plethysmograph, but after the first week the infant will usually require sedation and this technique is not applicable to oxygen-dependent patients.

Pulmonary resistance (Fig. 29.10), however, can be measured on the neonatal intensive care unit using an oesophageal balloon and pneumotachograph (see above); the pressure difference corresponding to the flow change between points of equal lung volume is measured. Resistance is increased in infants with meconium aspiration syndrome and, at follow-up, in those who required neonatal ventilation.[241]

SURFACTANT

ORIGINS

Alveolar type II cells

Alveolar type II cells produce surfactant.[177] These are compact cuboidal cells about 10 μm in diameter and

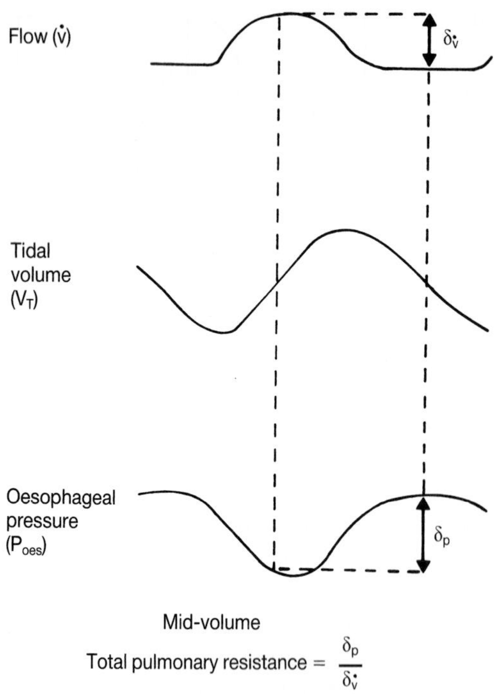

Fig. 29.10 Flow, volume and pressure traces during tidal breathing. The total pulmonary resistance is calculated by dividing the pressure gradient between mid-inspiration and mid-expiration (δP) by the simultaneous flow difference ($\delta \dot{V}$). Reproduced with permission.[77]

occur most often at the corners of the air spaces. They cover about 2% of the alveolar surface and account for about 15% of the cell numbers. They differentiate from the columnar epithelium during the canalicular phase of development (p. 455), but are not prominent until about 24 weeks' gestation, when they can be identified by their osmiophilic lamellar inclusion bodies.[127] Type II cells can now be isolated and cultured.[145] The biosynthesis of surfactant phosphatidylcholine occurs in the endoplasmic reticulum of the type II cell. The phospholipid then moves via intracellular pathways towards the lamellar bodies for secretion into the alveolus.

Lamellar bodies

The characteristic feature of the alveolar type II cell is the lamellar body, a storage granule of surfactant.[82] A mature lamellar body is about 1.5 µm in diameter and consists of a limiting membrane surrounding about 20–70 close-packed phospholipid bilayers, or lamellae, each with a width of 66 Å arranged in a hemisphere. The ends of these lamellae abut onto a baseplate, which is probably an extension of the limiting membrane. In the centre is a matrix core of proteinaceous material.[207,208] Lamellae can be isolated to a high degree of purity[71] and their lipid composition is very similar to that of surfactant obtained by bronchoalveolar lavage. Protein is probably not a major part of the lamellar structure, as no intra-membranous particles are seen in freeze fracture pictures.[233] Lamellar bodies develop from small multi-vesicular bodies and enlarge by accumulating lamellae; the largest lamellar bodies are found nearest to the cell's alveolar surface.[206]

Secretion of lamellar bodies

Surfactant is secreted as lamellar bodies from the type II cells by exocytosis[126] (Fig. 29.11). The control and regulation of this process is not clear. Lamellar bodies start to be released during late fetal life, and surfactant can be recovered from the tracheal effluent and amniotic fluid. The exocytosis process is stimulated by catecholamines, cAMP, ATP, Ca^{2+} and mechanical forces (stretch). Surfactant release is stimulated by adrenergic or prostaglandin stimulation,[141] labour or β-adrenergic drugs.[135,193] The most potent stimulus to release is gas entering the lung[193] and causing alveolar distension. Less surfactant is released in newborn animals who are stimulated to breathe but have tracheal occlusion.[136] A sigh increases surfactant release;[146,158] this is inhibited by parasympathetic block or vagotomy.[167] The protein SP-A is a potent inhibitor of phosphatidylcholine release from type II cells.[55]

The lamellar bodies unravel to tubular myelin, which forms the precursor to the surfactant monolayer at the air–liquid interface. The tubular myelin is a lattice of parallel lipid bilayers approximately 6.0 nm thick, with a regular spacing of approximately 50 nm. It is highly surface active, containing phospholipids and surfactant proteins in the presence of calcium (Fig. 29.12). The surface film is dynamic as a result of expansion and compression with ventilation. During this cycling, small vesicular forms of surfactant are generated: these have poor surfactant activity and are mainly taken up by type II cells, although some are degraded by macrophages or lost from the airways. The loss of surfactant into the airways is proportional to the rate and depth of respiration, and can be greatly reduced by the addition of CPAP during mechanical ventilation.[238] Surfactant lost in this way is swallowed or, in the case of the fetus, finds its way into the amniotic fluid (p. 475). The alveolar macrophages phagocytose some of the surfactant.[159]

Adsorption of surfactant to the surface

The air–fluid interface in the lungs rapidly expands with the onset of breathing; onto this a surface film is adsorbed which decreases the opening pressure of the distal bronchioles. Surfactant decreases the surface forces, facilitating fluid movement into the lung interstitium and preventing collapse of the aerated alveoli. The surfactant concentration in the hypophase increases as the fluid volume decreases and further surfactant secretion occurs.[113]

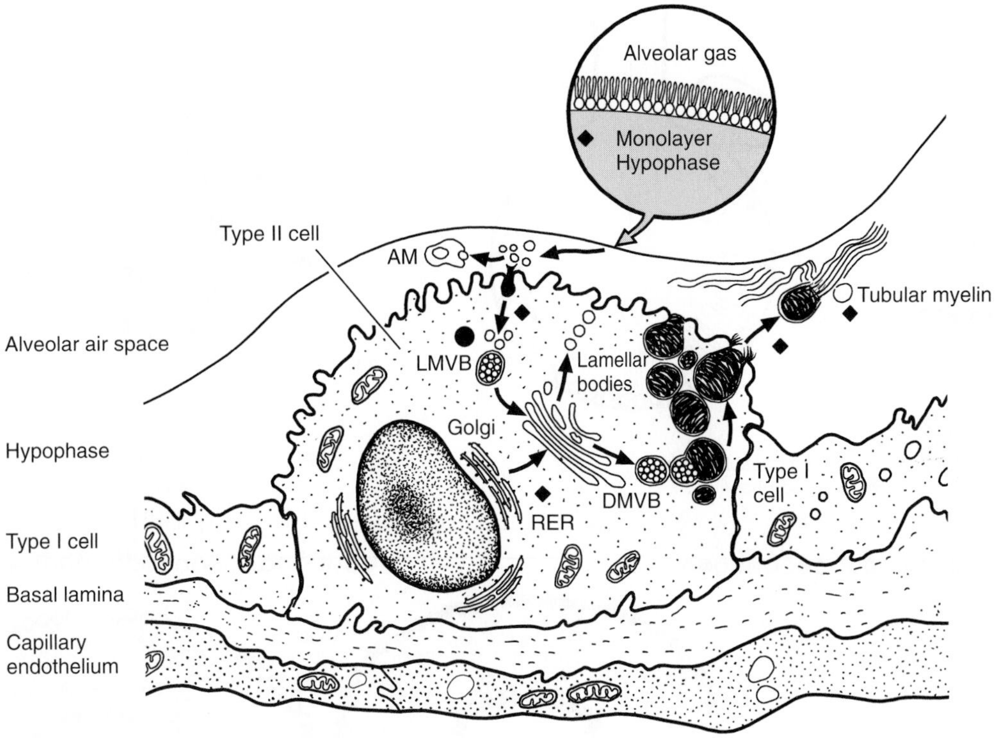

Fig. 29.11 An alveolar type II cell showing two surfactant release mechanisms: lamellar bodies and the constitutive release of surfactant protein-A. Surfactant is shown being both phagocytosed by an alveolar macrophage (AM; not to scale) and being taken back into the cell and reutilized. The inset illustrates the monolayer at low lung volume, comprising almost pure dipalmitoyl phosphatidylcholine which, in the gel (solid) phase, is able to withstand very large lateral forces, literally splinting open the alveolus. The thickness of the hypophase has been exaggerated, as it normally averages 0.14 μm over the flat sections and 0.89 μm at the wall junctions. RER = rough endoplasmic reticulum; LMVB = light multivesicular body; DMVB = dense multivesicular body. ♦ indicates possible sites of damage in ARDS; these include the synthesis, release and reuptake of surfactant, and the formation of tubular myelin and of the monomolecular layer. Reproduced with permission.[157]

Recycling of surfactant (Fig. 29.13)

Surfactant may be degraded locally in the alveoli and small airways. Enzymes that can degrade surfactant may be present in the alveolar fluid.[195] The breakdown products can then be absorbed and recycled by the alveolar cells. More than 90% of the phosphatidylcholine on the alveolar surface is reprocessed, conserving surfactant components as well as reactivating them to regenerate surfactant. The turnover time is approximately 10 hours.[203] The contribution to the alveolar surfactant pool from de novo synthesis is therefore modest. The disaturated phosphatidylglycerol and dipalmitoyl phosphatidylethanolamine are reused at an efficiency of 79%.[110] In adults the reuse of these substances may be different.[111] The molecules seem to be taken up by the type II cell intact, rather than broken down into their component parts. The surface of the type II cell that faces the alveolus is covered with microvilli and lectin receptors. Aerosolized DPPC and lectins can rapidly enter type II cells and become associated with multivesicular bodies and, subsequently, lamellar bodies.[234] These clearance pathways are much less active in the developing lung, and therefore have a longer turnover time for surfactant phophatidylcholine. In the preterm ventilated lamb the turnover time is approximately 13 hours, reprocessing the alveolar surfactant with little catabolic activity.[115] In the adult large amounts of surfactant phospholipid can be cleared in a dose-dependent fashion. The system is not overwhelmed by an exogenous dose 5–40 times greater than the size of the endogenous pool.

COMPOSITION

Surfactant is a complex mixture of substances, including phospholipids, neutral lipids and proteins.

Phosphatidylcholine and phosphatidylglycerol

Lipids are the major constituent of surfactant, and the most important are phosphatidylcholine and phosphatidylglycerol, representing 70–80% and 5–10% of the lipids, respectively. Another 10% of the lipids is made up of phosphatidylinositol, phosphatidylserine and phosphatidylethanolamine. Approximately 60% of the PC has both fatty acids saturated (i.e. disaturated) and, as the

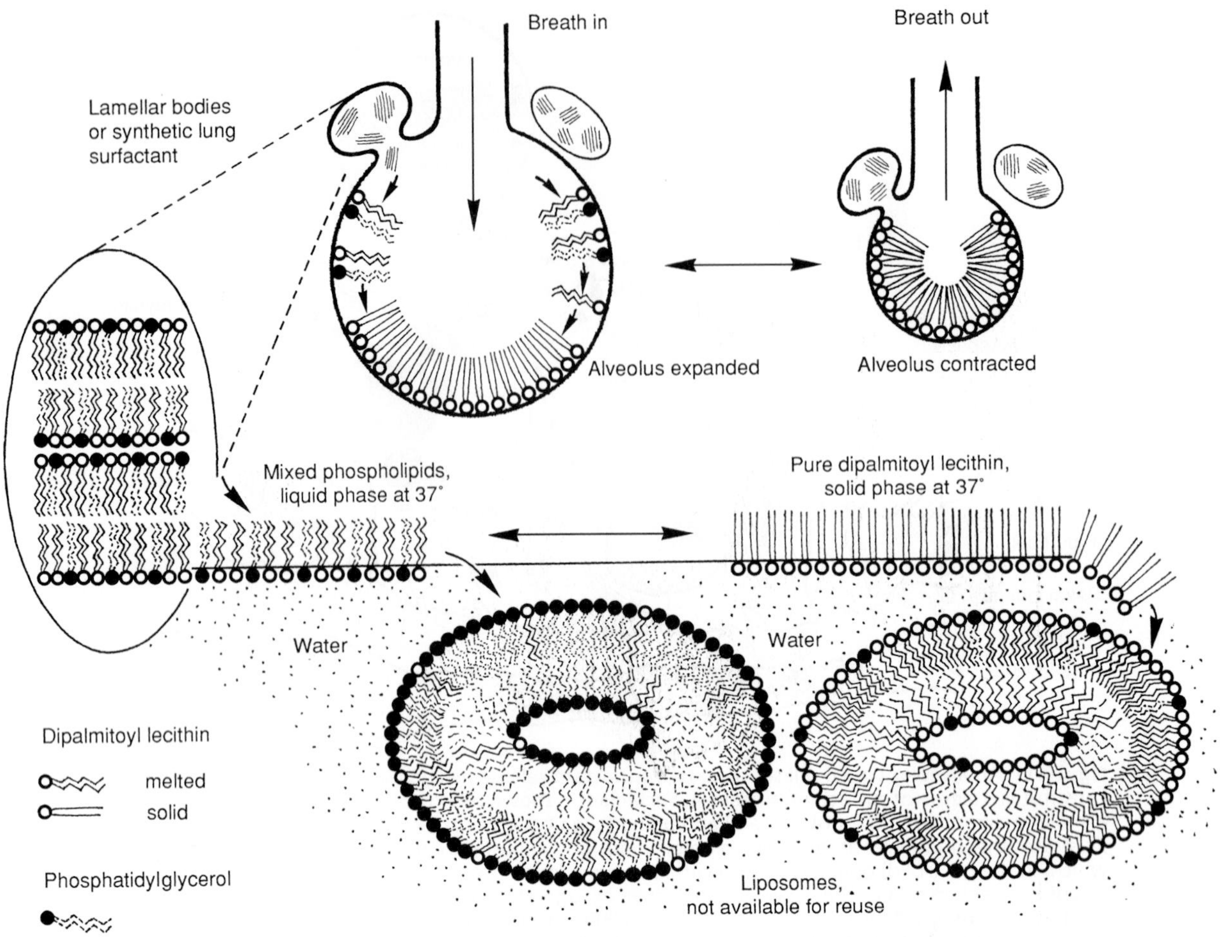

Fig. 29.12 Lipid molecules are arranged inside lamellar bodies (on the left) as closely packed bilayers. When the lamellar body releases these molecules they spread over the alveolar surface to form an oily monomolecular layer containing all the lipid species found in surfactant (left centre of diagram). This increases the surface pressure from zero of water to 25 mN/m. During inspiration the molecules spread out to cover the whole surface. During expiration the surfactant monolayer is compressed with such a force that many of the molecules are squeezed into the subphase (centre of diagram). Phospholipid molecules in water immediately form liposomes and cannot easily move back into the surface layer during its expansion. Repeated compression and expansion refines the surfactant monolayer. Those molecules retained in the surface are predominantly long, straight, disaturated phosphatidylcholine molecules. When these molecules are compressed they form a rigid layer with a high surface pressure and an apparent surface tension of zero. It is the rigidity of this layer which prevents alveolar collapse by splinting the alveoli open against compressing forces. Overcompression can result in loss of disaturated phosphatidylcholine from the surface. What happens in the alveolus is shown at the top of the diagram. Reproduced with permission.[9]

primary saturated fatty acid is palmitic acid, the major compound in surfactant is DPPC. The palmitic acid residues are non-polar and hydrophobic and orientate towards the air, whereas the phosphatidylcholine is polar and hydrophilic and associates with the liquid phase.[108] The shape and orientation of the DPPC means that it generates a stable monolayer and is able to maintain low surface pressures: during expiration the molecules become very closely packed as the palmitoyl moieties lack the C=C bonds that produce the kinks in the acyl chains (Fig. 29.12).[237]

DPPC is relatively rigid at body temperature, its phase transition (melt) being at approximately 41°C. Thus at body temperature DPPC cannot move rapidly enough to maintain a surface monolayer during the respiratory cycle, and a 'spreading' agent such as PG is required for normal surfactant function. Patients with RDS have low levels of DPPC and absent PG.[83] In poorly controlled diabetic pregnancies the fetus has low levels of PG even near term.

There is an increase in surfactant production towards the end of gestation: from 27 to 31 days (term) in rabbits there is a tenfold increase in surfactant; during a similar time period PC increases from 30 to 70% of the total phospholipids, whereas sphingomyelin decreases from 40 to 10%. This change is due to increased synthesis, whereas after birth there is increased secretion.

Other lipids

About 10% of the total lipids in surfactant are neutral. These are cholesterol, triacylglycerols and free fatty

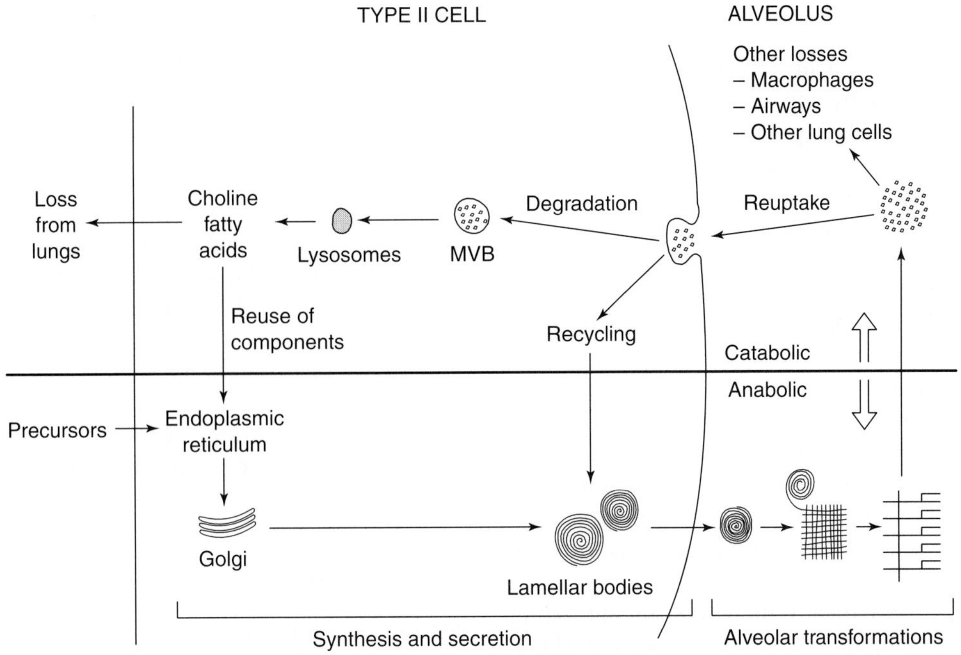

Fig. 29.13 Illustration of surfactant metabolism based on the saturated phosphatidylcholine component of surfactant. The anabolic pathway for synthesis and secretion links with alveolar transformations of the lamellar surfactant to tubular myelin and the monolayer. Catabolic pathways for phospholipid vesicles are minor pathways in the newborn lung but active in the adult lung. The majority of the surfactant is taken back into type II cells for recycling during the newborn period. Reproduced with permission.[114]

acids,[175] and they appear to be an integral part of the surfactant in lamellar bodies and on the alveolar surface. Cholesterol alters the fluidity and organization of lipid-rich membranes. Sphingomyelin represents less than 2% of surfactant lipid, and glycolipids and carbohydrates a very small fraction of the surfactant mass. The amount of sphingomyelin, a minor component of surfactant, remains unchanged through gestation, and thus the change in the amount of DPPC or lecithin can be assessed by comparing it to the amount of sphingomyelin. Lung maturity can therefore be assessed by measuring the ratio of lecithin to sphingomyelin, the L:S ratio (p. 475).

Surfactant proteins

Four surfactant-associated proteins – SP-A, SP-B, SP-C and SP-D – have been identified[226] comprising 5–10% of surfactant by weight.[56]

Surfactant protein A

SP-A is composed of approximately 248 amino acids.[14] There is considerable heterogeneity in its structure because of extensive post-translational modification. The human gene is located on chromosome 10; gene expression occurs exclusively in type II pneumocytes,[21] which appear to be the main site of synthesis.[7,235] Lamellar bodies are enriched with SP-A compared to lung homogenates.[166]

Synthesis of SP-A increases after 28 weeks of gestation.[13] Antibodies to this protein, however, are present in lung tissue at gestations as early as 16 weeks.[8] SP-A is developmentally regulated and induced in vivo by corticosteroids and TRH.[108] SP-A synthesis is enhanced by cAMP, β-adrenergic agents and epidermal growth factor. Dexamethasone increases the level of SP-A.[172,230,231] Insulin inhibits the accumulation of SP-A and SP-B mRNA, but has no effect on SP-C mRNA in vitro.[44] Insulin inhibits both SP-A and SP-B gene expression in vitro, and the levels of SP-A in the amniotic fluid of pregnancies complicated by diabetes mellitus are lower than in controls.

SP-A binds to and confers calcium-dependent aggregation on surfactant phospholipids.[93] It has an essential role in determining the structure of tubular myelin, and the stability and rapidity of spreading and recycling of phospholipids.[217,229] It regulates the synthesis and secretion of phospholipids, and enhances their uptake by type II cells by binding to specific high-affinity receptors on their apical surfaces. SP-A partially inhibits surfactant secretion from type II cells[55] and may prevent the accumulation of surfactant on the alveolar surface. Its major contribution towards surface activity is to enhance the effects of SP-B and/or SP-C.[94] SP-A may also have immune system-related functions. It also binds to alveolar macrophages.[130] Preincubation of alveolar macrophages with surfactant alone increased phagocytosis of *Staphylococcus aureus* by 70%.[216]

Surfactant protein B

The active 79 amino acid SP-B peptide (MW 7500–9000) is produced by the proteolytic cleavage of pro-SP-B, a 25–33 000 MW precursor protein.[41] The active SP-B peptide contains highly positively charged amino acids that form an amphipathic helix with the hydrophilic amino acid residues positioned near the phospholipid head groups at the membrane surface.[229]

SP-B is encoded by a single copy gene located on chromosome 2.[60] The mRNA for SP-B is detectable in human fetal lung tissue as early as 12–14 weeks' gestation, localized in the epithelial cells of bronchi and bronchioles. After 25 weeks it is localized in the type II cells. Glucocorticoids increase the expression of SP-B in fetal lung. Expression is restricted to type II pneumocytes and Clara cells. The active SP-B peptide is stored in lamellar bodies and secreted with phospholipids into the airway lumen.

SP-B, like SP-C, dramatically increases the spreading of surfactant phospholipids onto an aqueous surface. SP-B mixed with synthetic phospholipid mixtures can imitate some of the biophysical properties of natural surfactant.[182] In the presence of SP-A and calcium ions, SP-B contributes to the formation of tubular myelin. It enhances the uptake of phospholipids by type II cells in vitro. SP-B disrupts phospholipid vesicles and alters the ordering and packing of the phosphatidylcholine molecules. SP-B combined with lipid mixtures reconstitutes most of the surface activity of natural surfactant in vitro and increases lung compliance in vivo; SP-C and B together are even more effective. SP-C and B both stimulate lipid uptake in isolated cells. Natural surfactant containing SP-B is more effective when tested in preterm rabbits than a surfactant with low levels of SP-B.[151]

The absence of SP-B influences the composition of pulmonary surfactants. It is associated with absent or markedly decreased PG and an additional aberrant SP-C peptide.[219] SP-B deficiency is an inherited disease which leads to lethal respiratory failure within the first year of life (p. 648), and is refractory to mechanical ventilation, surfactant therapy, glucocorticoids and extracorporeal membrane oxygenation.[32,85] It can present as a congenital form of alveolar proteinosis, but not all cases have this feature; pulmonary hypertension is a prominent clinical finding. Lung transplantation is currently the only successful intervention (p. 648).

Surfactant protein C

This hydrophobic protein has a molecular weight of 3000–6000, depending on the separation system used. It contains 35 amino acids[117] and has a hydrophobic valine-rich region which is involved in the tight association of SP-C with phospholipids. The SP-C gene is located on chromosome 8.[72] It has been difficult to estimate levels of SP-C in biological samples because of difficulties in producing monospecific antisera, and interference by lipids in the assays.

SP-C alone can impart surface-like properties to phospholipids.[182] Concentrations as low as 1% can dramatically enhance surface adsorption and the spreading of phospholipids in vitro, but are less active in maintaining the morphological integrity of fetal rabbit lung in vivo. SP-C may play a role in enhancing the reuptake of phospholipids. Both SP-B and SP-C confer surfactant-like properties on mixtures of synthetic phospholipids, and may be useful in the preparation of synthetic surfactants for treatment.[209,210] Clinical experience has failed to demonstrate significant immune responses to SP-B and SP-C in response to treatment with bovine preparations.[161]

Surfactant protein D

SP-D has a molecular weight of 46 000 and is produced by type II and bronchiolar epithelial cells. Its expression increases with advancing gestation in association with differentiation of terminal airway cells.[40] SP-D does not have significant surfactant-like activities when mixed with phospholipids. It is, however, involved in the immune function of the lung,[125] binding to a variety of complex carbohydrates and glycolipids, and may have a role in host defence functions in the lung by interacting with the surfaces of bacteria and other micro-organisms.[229] SP-D alters SP-A dependent inhibition of surfactant secretion.[3]

SYNTHESIS

Phosphatidylcholine

Phosphatidylcholine is produced by the cytidine diphosphate choline pathway (Fig. 29.14).[190] Choline is taken up by the cell by facilitated transport and is then phosphorylated by choline kinase to phosphocholine, which in turn is converted to CDP choline (the rate-limiting step); this is then transferred to diacylglycerol to give PC. This produces molecules containing one saturated fatty acid, palmitic acid, and one unsaturated fatty acid, usually oleic acid. This molecule is then remodelled by deacylation to lysophosphatidylcholine, followed by reacylation with a palmitic acid derived from either palmitoyl CoA or a second molecule of lysophosphatidylcholine[12] to give DPPC. It has been suggested that only 50% of the DPPC is synthesized directly from saturated diacylglycerols as precursors,[176] and the rest by remodelling. Two remodelling mechanisms exist, both involving deacylation of de-novo synthesized 1-saturated-2-unsaturated PC to acyl-2-lysophosphatidylcholine. The latter is then either reacylated by reaction with a saturated acyl CoA, or transacylated in a reaction involving two molecules of

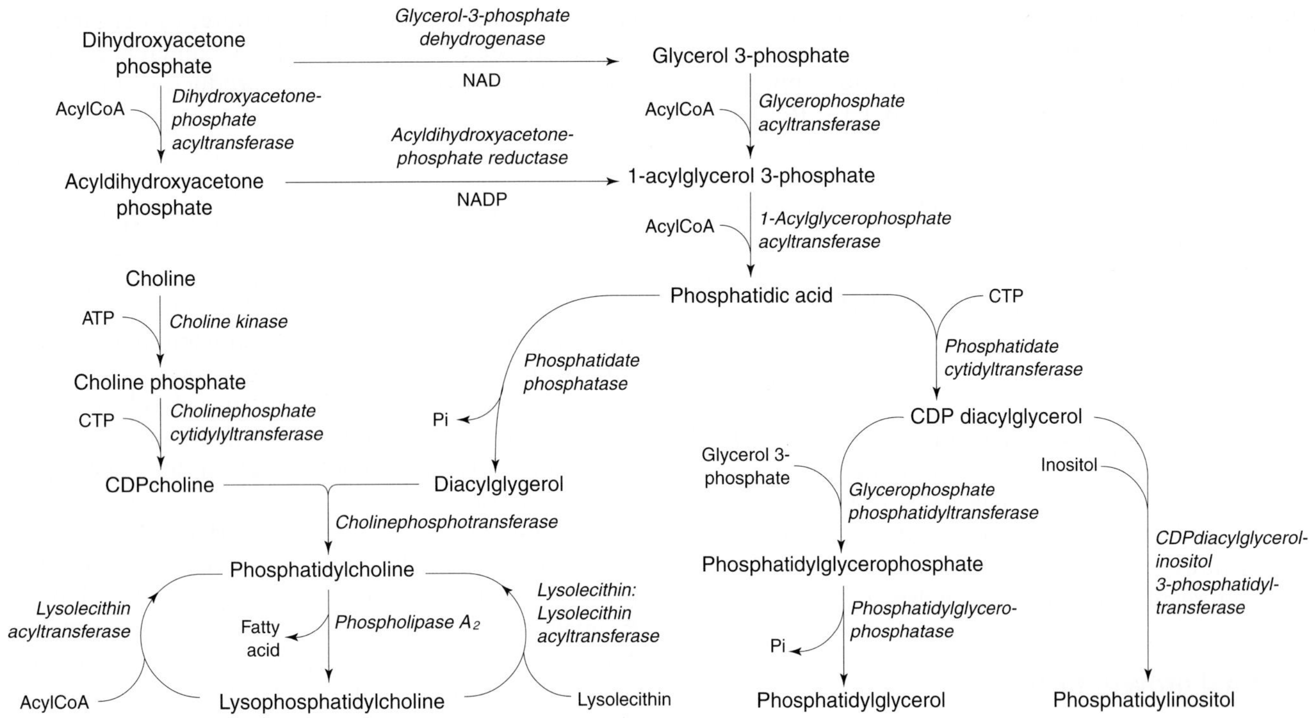

Fig. 29.14 Pathways in the biosynthesis of phosphatidylcholine, phosphatidylglycerol and phosphatidylinositol. Reproduced with permission.[190]

lysophosphatidylcholine.[191] Only the former mechanism is quantitatively important. Cholinephosphate cytidylyltransferase, which catalyses phosphocholine to CDP choline, is essentially inactive without lipids; CT activity is activated during fetal lung development and after corticosteroid administration. Several other hormones, including thyroid hormones, insulin and EGF, influence this sequence of events. PC synthesis via the methylation of PE is of minor importance,[62] except in conditions of choline deficiency.[240]

Phosphatidylglycerol synthesis

PG is synthesized together with the other acidic phospholipids, phosphatidylinositol and phosphatidylserine, from CDP-diacylglycerol, which is in turn derived from phosphatidic acid (Fig. 29.14). The subject is reviewed by Bleasdale and Johnston.[19]

FACTORS AFFECTING SURFACTANT MATURATION

Glucocorticoids

Endogenous cortisol is an important physiological stimulus to fetal lung maturation. In the fetal sheep there is a marked increase in plasma cortisol concentration at the end of gestation, and this is associated with an increase in DPPC in lung tissue and lung lavage fluid.[52] Administration of betamethasone to pregnant rabbits results in an increase in the total amount of phospholipid, as well as an increase in the percentage in PC of the total phospholipids.[192] CT is stimulated by glucocorticoids (p. 491). Cortisol induces fetal lung fibroblasts to produce fibroblast pneumocyte factor, which then stimulates surfactant production by the fetal type II pneumocytes.[200] In animal experiments glucocorticoids increase lung aeration, decrease the surface tension of the lung extract and increase the synthesis of both surfactant phospholipids and proteins.[120] In preterm infants, antenatal treatment with dexamethasone increases the surface activity of surfactant isolated from airway specimens and the ratio of Sp-A to phosphatidylcholine, but not in the offspring of mothers with severe hypertension.[120]

β-Adrenergic drugs

β-Adrenergic drugs stimulate adenylcyclase and inhibit phosphodiesterases, thereby increasing the amount of intracellular cAMP, which in turn increases the production[135] and secretion of surfactant. cAMP stimulates the synthesis of disaturated phospholipids and SP-A; it also mediates the effect of a number of hormones. Not all studies show benefit.[15]

Thyroid hormones

Thyroxine increases surfactant production and lung maturation. Infants who develop RDS have lower cord blood levels of T4 than those without. T4 does not easily cross the placenta, but T3 given to pregnant rats is associated with an increase in T3 in the fetal serum. T3 increases the type II cell receptors' response to fibroblast pneumocyte factor, which is necessary for appropriate surfactant production.[201] Unlike T4 and T3, TRH readily crosses the placenta; it increases the amount of surfactant phospholipid. The effects of TRH are not entirely mediated by thyroid hormone. TRH stimulates prolactin production and functions as a neurotransmitter in the CNS. It remains controversial whether antenatal administration of TRH reduces the incidence of RDS (p. 492).

Prolactin

Prolactin levels are lower in infants who develop RDS than in those who do not, and are also lower in immature versus mature infants and males versus females.[50] The effect of prolactin both in vivo and in cultured lung systems, however, is variable, and its role in surfactant production regulation remains speculative.

Epidermal growth factor

EGF may be important in the development of the pulmonary epithelium. Infusion of this substance into lambs prevents the development of hyaline membrane disease[28] and increases lung distensibility. There is a reduced amount of SP-A in the offspring of rats with EGF autoantibodies.[179] Müllerian inhibiting substance inhibits lung maturation by blocking the phosphorylation of EGF receptors:[27] this may be an explanation for the higher incidence of RDS in males. In non-human primate fetuses delivered at 78% of term, in utero treatment with EGF resulted in higher SP-A levels and L:S ratios in treated fetuses than in untreated fetuses.[74]

Fibroblast pneumocyte factor

Alveolar cells need fibroblasts and their pneumocyte factor to produce surfactant.[200] Glucocorticoids act on the fetal lung fibroblasts to induce the production of fibroblast pneumocyte factor, which in turn stimulates rapid surfactant synthesis by the alveolar type II cell.

Insulin

Insulin delays the maturation of alveolar type II cells and decreases the proportion of saturated PC.[78] In addition, the infants of diabetic mothers have delayed appearance of PG.[164] Hyperglycaemia also plays a role in the delay in lung maturation seen in these babies.[70]

Testosterone

Premature male infants are more prone to RDS than similarly immature female infants[171] (p. 483). Male lungs are approximately 1 week less mature, as determined by the disaturated PC content. These differences may be due to inhibition of surfactant production in males by androgens.[214]

SURFACTANT PHYSICAL PROPERTIES AND FUNCTIONS

Surfactant prevents atelectasis and thus reduces the work of breathing. This is achieved as in expiration it reduces surface tension and, in addition, becomes a 'solid' monolayer promoting stability of the alveoli. Surfactant also prevents the transudation of fluid: in conditions of high surface tension fluid is sucked into the alveolar spaces from the capillaries.

The presence of an insoluble surface film capable of maintaining a very low surface tension (or high surface pressure) in the air spaces was first inferred by Pattle.[170] A small bubble will normally diminish in size and disappear: the smaller it becomes the more rapidly its diameter decreases. This follows from the relationship described by the Laplace equation

$$P = \frac{2\gamma}{r}$$

where P = internal pressure, γ = surface tension and r = radius), that is, that the pressure difference across the bubble's wall is given by twice the tension in the wall divided by the radius. Thus, in the presence of a high surface tension and small radius, the high pressure difference causes gas to diffuse from the bubble into the surrounding liquid. In the lung, however, the presence of an insoluble surface film means that the surface tension is reduced as the radius decreases. The contribution of surface tension to the pressure volume behaviour of the lung was demonstrated by von Neergaard,[218] who showed that lungs inflated with saline have a higher compliance than those filled with air. Saline abolishes the surface tension forces, which are an important component of the static recoil force of the lung.

Surfactant lowers surface tension by forming an insoluble surface film. This opposes the surface tension of the underlying liquid by exerting surface pressure. The surface properties of surfactant result from its composition, that is, molecules with both a hydrophobic and a hydrophilic chain. When forming a film on water the polar group is attracted to the water, whereas the non-polar group is turned towards the gas phase. DPPC is a symmetrical molecule and the two straight hydrophobic fatty acid chains allow close packing of the monolayer. Compression of such a monolayer results in its being changed from a liquid to a condensed gel or solid state;[37,154] this is because the transition temperature of the refined mixture rises to above 37°C, so that in vivo the refined monolayer may be solid.[37] Immature surfactant is a mixture of saturated and unsaturated fatty acids, the latter disrupting the symmetry or rigidity of the monolayer. Compression of such a monolayer squeezes out the asymmetrical molecules. Repeated compression and expansion of the monolayer, as will occur during respiration, refines it to virtually pure phospholipids, mainly DPPC.[37]

In RDS the PC is both relatively unsaturated and less in quantity than in the mature species. This means an unstable monolayer is formed on compression in expiration, which buckles and does not reduce surface tension effectively. Even when the monolayer has been refined, there is so little DPPC available that the alveoli are small in size. Thus infants with RDS have a low FRC and an increased work of breathing (p. 487).

Inhibition of surfactant surface activity by proteins

The alveolar surfactant system may be altered by an inhibitory effect of proteins leaked from the intravascular or interstitial space due to an increased permeability of the capillary endothelial and/or alveolar–epithelial barrier.[197] In RDS the alveolar capillary membrane permeability is increased, and the hyaline membranes are a massive aggregation of fibrin. In addition proteinaceous material may be inhaled, for example as in meconium aspiration syndrome. There is a marked rank order of potency of proteins in interfering with surfactant function – fibrin monomer > fibrinogen > albumin > elastin > IgG > IgM – such that fibrin is 50 times more effective than albumin. Once the proteins are present in the surface monolayer they inhibit the ability of the compressed surfactant to lower surface tension. The leakage of protein on to the alveolar surface – at least in premature rabbits – can be inhibited by surfactant treatment[188] (p. 509) and treatment with antenatal steroids or TRH[109] (pp. 484, 491). In other conditions, such as meconium aspiration syndrome, the inhibitory effect of the proteins can be overcome by increasing the dose of surfactant (pp. 544–555). The currently available exogenous surfactants differ with regard to their inhibition by proteins: CLSE (calf lung surfactant extract) and Alveofact are only moderately inhibited by fibrinogen.[196] KL_4 surfactant, which has a synthetic peptide in lieu of SP-B, resists inhibition to serum proteins more than a natural surfactant (beractant).[139] KL_4 is a totally synthetic surfactant formulated with DPPC, palmitoyl-oleolyphosphatidylglycerol, palmitic acid and a 21 amino acid peptide of leucine/lysine that was designed to mimic the hydrophobic–hydrophilic domains of native SP-B and the protein/phospholipid interactions of natural surfactant. The KL_4 peptide is better able to inhibit disruption by exogenous proteins/peptides by increasing the lateral stability of the phospholipid layer.[139]

ASSESSMENT OF SURFACTANT MATURITY

Lecithin:sphingomyelin ratio

The fluid secreted by the fetal lung moves out into the amniotic fluid, carrying with it surfactant (p. 468). As the lung matures so the composition of the surfactant in the amniotic fluid changes. The proportion of surfactant (lecithin) in the amniotic fluid can be compared to that of sphingomyelin (L:S ratio). This is measured by thin-layer chromatography. An L:S ratio greater than 2.0 is usually associated with lung maturity, and in 95% of cases will predict the absence of RDS. A mature L:S ratio can be associated with RDS in the infants of diabetic mothers or those with rhesus disease: in these cases the abnormality is a deficiency of PG rather than a lack of DPPC. Relating the amniotic fluid surfactant to the albumin level provides a more reliable predictor of the absence of RDS in infants of diabetic mothers than does assessing the amount of DPPC.[211] Unfortunately, a low L:S ratio (< 2.0) predicts RDS with an accuracy of only 54%.[84] The lower the L:S ratio, the more likely the baby is to develop RDS: 21% of babies with an L:S ratio of 1.5–2.0 being affected, compared to 80% with an L:S ratio below 1.5.

The L:S ratio cannot necessarily be predicted by the fetal gestational age, as accelerated maturation can be seen in small-for-dates babies, whereas delayed maturation is associated with lung hypoplasia, mild diabetes and very small twins[162], and occasionally is familial.[84] Abnormal L:S ratios occur when the specimen is contaminated with blood, meconium or vaginal secretions. The predictive value of L:S ratios depends on amniotic fluid being sampled within 3 days of delivery. Once the patient is in labour the amniotic fluid L:S ratio is increased compared to that obtained at elective caesarean section.

The identification of phosphatidylglycerol in the amniotic fluid is helpful as babies with PG rarely develop RDS. A combination of a low L:S ratio with the absence of PG from amniotic fluid samples obtained within 3 days of delivery is a better predictor of the duration of respiratory support than either gestational age or birthweight, but only in pregnancies not complicated by premature rupture of the membranes.[87]

The L:S ratio can also be assessed in fluid from the pharynx[11,101,227] or stomach.[156] This can demonstrate retrospectively that a baby had mature lungs at birth, or provide further documentation on the course of a baby's illness.[119]

Other assessments of fetal lung maturity

Alternative methods which correlate highly to the L:S ratio are now available; these include fluorescence polarization[181] and assessment of lamellar body concentration. Such tests are less labour intensive and have a

Table 29.3 Predictors of lung maturity

Test	Reference
Lung profile	128
	129
DPPC:POPC ratio	5
Surfactant protein estimation	35
Shake test	153
Bubble test	69
	169
Oscillating bubble	61
Stable microbubble test	33
	34
Respiratory compliance	232

POPC, palmitoyl-oleoylphosphatidylcholine

turnaround time of 1 hour,[53] which may, if they prove accurate, mean they could be used to decide whether to give postnatal surfactant.

Analyses of other surfactant components are available (Table 29.3), as well as functional assessment of the surfactant or the lung itself (Table 29.3).

REFERENCES

1. Abman S H, Dunbar Ivy D, Ziegler J W, Kinsella J P 1996 Mechanisms of abnormal vasoreactivity in persistent pulmonary hypertension of the newborn infant. Journal of Perinatology 16: S18–S23
2. Agata Y, Hiraishi S, Oguchi K et al 1991 Changes in left ventricular output from fetal to early neonatal life. Journal of Pediatrics 119: 441–445
3. Akino T, Shiratori M, Tsuzuki A, Murata Y, Kuroki Y 1991 Native form of surfactant protein D (SP-D) which lipids are associated with, affects the acitivity of SP-A on type II cells. American Review of Respiratory Disease 143: A316
4. Altura B M, Chand N 1981 Bradykinin-induced relaxation of renal and pulmonary arteries is dependent upon intact endothelial cell. British Journal of Pharmacology 74: 10–11
5. Ashton M R, Postle A L D, Hall M A et al 1992 Phosphatidylcholine composition of endotracheal tube aspirates of neonates and subsequent respiratory distress. Archives of Disease in Childhood 67: 378–382
6. Asonye U O, Vidyasagar D 1981 Clinical applications of continuous transcutaneous PO_2 monitoring. In: Lauersen N H, Hochberg H M (eds) Clinical perinatal biochemical monitoring. Williams & Wilkins, Baltimore, pp 205–219
7. Balis J U, Paterson J F, Paciga J E et al 1985 Distribution and subcellular localisation of surfactant associated glycoproteins in human lung. Laboratory Investigation 52: 657–669
8. Ballard P L, Hawgood S, Liley H et al 1986 Regulation of pulmonary surfactant apoprotein SP 28–36 gene in fetal human lung. Proceedings of the National Academy of Science USA 83: 9527–9531
9. Bangham A D 1980 Breathing made easy. New Scientist 85: 408–410
10. Barker P M, Walters D V, Markiewicz M, Strang L B 1991 Development of the lung liquid reabsorptive mechanism in fetal sheep: synergism of triiodothyronine and hydrocortisone. Journal of Physiology 433:435–449
11. Barr P A, Jenkins P A, Baum J D 1975 L/S ratio in hypopharyngeal aspirate of newborn infants. Archives of Disease in Childhood 50: 856–861
12. Batenburg J J 1982 The phosphatidylcholine-lysophosphatidylcholine cycle. In: Farrell P M (ed) Lung development: biological and clinical perspectives Vol. 1. Academic Press, New York, Ch. 20, p 36
13. Batenburg J J, Hallman M 1990 Developmental biochemistry of alveoli. In: Scarpelli E M (ed) Pulmonary physiology: fetus, newborn, child and adolescent, 2nd edn. Lea & Febiger, Philadelphia, pp 106–139
14. Benson B, Hawgood S, Schilling J et al 1985 Structure of canine pulmonary surfactant apoproteins cDNA and complete amino-acid sequence. Proceedings of the National Academy of Science USA 82: 6379–6383
15. Bergman B, Hedner T, Lungborg 1980 Pressure volume relationship and fluid content in fetal rabbit lung after beta-adrenergic stimulating drugs. Pediatric Research 14: 1067–1070
16. Bianchi A L, Denavit-Saubié M, Champagnat J 1995 Central control of breathing in mammals: neuronal circuitry, membrane properties and neurotransmitters. Physiology Reviews 75: 1–45
17. Blanco C E, Dawes G S, Hanson M A, McCooke H B 1984 The response to hypoxia of arterial chemoreceptors in fetal sheep and newborn lambs. Journal of Applied Physiology 351: 25–37
18. Blanco C E, Hanson M A, McCooke H B, Williams B A 1987 Studies of chemoreceptor resetting after hyperoxic ventilation of the fetus in utero. In: Ribero J A, Pallot D J (eds) Chemoreceptors in respiratory control. Croom Helm, London, pp 221–227
19 Bleasdale J E, Johnston J M 1982 Phosphatidic acid production and utilisation. In: Farrell P M (ed) Lung development: biological and clinical perspectives, Vol. 1. Academic Press, New York, p 259
20. Bonham A C 1995 Neurotransmitters in the CNS control of breathing. Respiration Physiology 101: 219–230
21. Bruns G, Stroh H, Veldman G M, Latt S A, Floros J 1987 The 35 kd pulmonary surfactant associated protein is encoded on chromosome 10. Human Genetics 76: 58–62
22. Bryan A C, Bowes G, Maloney J E 1986 Control of breathing during sleep. In: Cherniack N S, Widdicombe J G (eds) Handbook of Physiology—the respiratory system Vol. II. American Physiological Society, Bethesda, MD, pp 529–579
23. Bullard K M, Sonne J, Hawgood S, Harrison M R, Adzick N S 1997 Tracheal ligation increases cell proliferation but decreases surfactant protein in fetal murine lungs in vitro. Journal of Pediatric Surgery 32: 207–211
24. Bureau M A, Lamarche J, Foulon P, Dalle D 1985 Postnatal maturation of respiration in intact and carotid body-chemodenervated lambs. Journal of Applied Physiology 59: 869–874
25. Calder N A, Williams B A, Kumar P, Hanson M A 1994 The respiratory response of healthy term infants to breath-to-breath alternations in inspired oxgyen at two postnatal ages. Pediatric Research 35: 321–324
26. Carroll J L, Bamford O S, Fitzgerald R S 1993 Postnatal maturation of carotid chemoreceptor responses to O_2 and CO_2 in the cat. Journal of Applied Physiology 75: 2383–2391
27. Catlin E A, Uitvlugt N D, Donahoe P K, Powerll D M, Hayashi M, MacLaughin D T 1991 Muellerian inhibiting substance blocks epidermal growth factor receptor phosphorylation in fetal rat lung membranes. Metabolism 40: 1178–1184
28. Catterton W Z, Escobedo M B, Sexson W R, Sundell H W, Stahlman M T 1979 Effect of epidermal growth factor on lung maturation in fetal rabbits. Pediatric Research 13: 104–108
29. Ceruti E 1966 Chemoreceptor reflexes in the newborn infant: effect of cooling on the response to hypoxia. Pediatrics 37: 556–564
30. Chan V, Greenough A 1992 Lung function and the Hering–Breuer reflex in the neonatal period. Early Human Development 28:111–118
31. Cherniack N S, von Euler C, Glogowska M, Homma J 1981 Characteristics and rate of occurrence of spontaneous and provoked augmented breaths. Acta Paediatrica Scandinavica 70: 349–360
32. Chetcuti P A J, Ball R J 1995 Surfactant aproprotein B deficiency. Archives of Disease in Childhood 73: F125–F127
33. Chida S, Fujiwara S 1993 Stable microbubble test for predicting the risk of respiratory distress syndrome. I. Comparisons with other predictors of fetal lung maturity. European Journal of Pediatrics 152: 148–151
34. Chida S, Fujiwara T, Konishi M et al 1993 Stable microbubble test for predicting the risk of respiratory distress syndrome. II. Prospective evaluation of the test on amniotic fluid and gastric aspirate. European Journal of Pediatrics 152: 152–156
35. Chida S, Phelps D, Cordle C, Soll R, Floros J, Taeusch W 1988 Surfactant associated proteins in tracheal aspirates of infants with respiratory distress syndrome after surfactant therapy. American Review of Respiratory Disease 137: 943–947
36. Clark F W, von Euler C 1972 On the regulation of depth and rate of breathing. Journal of Physiology 222: 267–295
37. Clements J A 1977 Functions of the alveolar lining layer. American Review of Respiratory Disease 115: 67–71
38. Condorelli S, Scarpelli E M 1975 Somatic–respiratory reflex and onset

of regular breathing movements in the lamb fetus in utero. Pediatric Research 9: 879–884
39. Cordero L, Hon E H 1971 Neonatal bradycardia following nasopharyngeal stimulation. Pediatrics 78: 441–447
40. Crouch E, Rust K, Mariencheck W, Parghi D, Chang D, Pearson A 1991 Developmental expression of pulmonary surfactant protein D (SP-D). American Journal of Respiratory Cell and Molecular Biology 5: 13–18
41. Curstedt T, Johansson J, Barros-Soderling J et al 1988 Low molecular mass surfactant protein type 1. The primary structure of hydrophobic 8-Kda polypeptide with eight half cysteine residues. European Journal of Biochemistry 172: 521–525
42. Curzi-Dascalova L 1978 Thoraco-abdominal respiratory correlations in infants: constancy and variability in different sleep states. Early Human Development 2: 25–38
43. Davies A M, Koenig J S, Thach B T 1988 Upper airway chemoreflex responses to saline and water in preterm infants. Journal of Applied Physiology 64: 1412–1420
44. Dekowski S A, Snyder J M 1992 Insulin regulation of messenger ribonucleic acid for the surfactant associated proteins in human fetal lung in vitro. Endocrinology 131: 669–676
45. Delivoria-Papadopoulos M, DiGiacomo J E 1992 Oxygen transport and delivery. In: Polin R A, Fox W W (eds) Fetal and neonatal physiology. W B Saunders, Philadelphia, pp. 801–813
46. Delivoria-Papadopoulos M, Roncervie N, Oski F I 1971 Postnatal changes in oxygen transport of term premature and sick infants: the role of red cell 2:3 diphosphoglycerate and adult hemoglobin. Pediatric Research 5: 235–245
47. Denavit-Saubié M, Champagnat J, Zieglgaensberger W 1978 Effects of opiates and methionine-enkephalin on pontine and bulbar respiratory neurones of the cat. Brain Research 155: 55–67
48. De Troyer A, Kelly S, Macklem P T, Zin W 1985 Mechanics of intercostal space and actions of external and internal intercostal muscles. Journal of Clinical Investigation 75: 850–857
49. Devlieger H 1987 The chest wall in the preterm infant. MD thesis, Université Catholique de Leuven, pp 136–140
50. Dhanireddy R, Smith Y F, Hamosh M, Mullon D K, Scanlon J W, Hamosh P 1983 Respiratory distress syndrome in the newborn: relationship to serum prolactin, thyroxine and sex. Biology of the Neonate 43: 9–15
51. Dickinson K A, Harding R 1987 Decline in lung liquid volume and secretion and tracheal flow rate in fetal lambs. Journal of Applied Physiology 62: 24–38
52. DiFiore J W, Wilson J M 1994 Lung development. Seminars in Pediatric Surgery 3: 221–232
53. Dilena B A, Ku F, Doyle I, Whiting M F 1997 Six alternative methods to the lecithin/sphingomyelin ratio in amniotic fluid for assessing fetal lung maturity. Annals of Clinical Biochemistry 34: 106–108
54. Dimitriou G, Greenough A, Castling D, Kavadia V 1996 A comparison of supine and prone positioning in oxygen-dependent and convalescent premature infants. British Journal of Intensive Care 6: 254–259
55. Dobbs D L, Wright J R, Hawgood S, Gonzalez R, Venstrom K, Nellenbogen J 1987 Pulmonary surfactant and its components inhibit secretion of phosphatidylcholine from cultured rat alveolar type II cells. Proceedings of the National Academy of Science USA 84: 1010–1014
56. Dobbs L G 1989 Pulmonary surfactant. Annual Review of Medicine 40: 431–446
57. Donnelly D F, Haddad G G 1990 Prolonged apnea and impaired survival in piglets after sinus and aortic nerve section. Journal of Applied Physiology 68: 1048–1052
58. Duara S 1992 Structure and function of the upper airway in neonates. In: Polin R A, Fox W W (eds) Fetal and neonatal physiology, Vol 1. W B Saunders, Philadelphia, pp. 823–828
59. Eden G J, Hanson M A 1987 Effects of chronic hypoxia on chemoreceptor function in the newborn. In: Ribero J A, Pallot D J (eds) Chemoreceptors in respiratory control. Croom Helm, London, pp 369–377
60. Emrie P A, Jones C, Hofmann T et al 1988 The coding sequence for the human 18,000 dalton hydrophobic pulmonary surfactant protein is located on chromosome 2 and identifies a restriction fragment length polymorphism. Somatic and Cellular Molecular Genetics 14: 105–110
61. Enhorning G 1977 A pulsating bubble technique for evaluating pulmonary surfactant. Journal of Applied Physiology 43: 198–201
62. Farrell P M, Hamosh M 1978 The biochemistry of fetal lung development. Clinics in Perinatology 5: 197–229
63. Feldman J L 1986 Neurophysiology of breathing in mammals. In: Bloom F E (ed) Handbook of physiology, Section 1: The nervous system, Vol IV: Intrinsic regulatory systems of the brain. American Physiological Society, Bethesda, pp 463–524
64. Fewell J E, Hislop A A, Kitterman J A, Johnson P 1983 Effect of tracheostomy on lung development in fetal lambs. Journal of Applied Physiology 55: 1103–1108
65. Fleming P J, Bryan A C, Bryan M H 1978 Functional immaturity of pulmonary irritant receptors and apnea in newborn preterm infants. Pediatrics 61: 515–518
66. Frantz I D, Alder S M, Abroms I F, Thach B T 1976 Respiratory response to airway occlusion in infants: sleep state and maturation. Journal of Applied Physiology 41: 634–635
67. Friedman A H, Fahey J T 1993 The transition from fetal to neonatal circulation: normal responses and implications for infants with heart disease. Seminars in Perinatology 17: 106–121
68. Funk G D, Smith J C, Feldman J L 1993 Generation and transmission of respiratory oscillations in medullary slices: role of excitatory amino acids. Journal of Neurophysiology 70: 1497–1515
69. Gandy G, Bradbrooke J G, Naidoo B T, Gairdner D 1968 Comparison of methods for evaluating surface properties of lung in the perinatal period. Archives of Disease in Childhood 43: 8–16
70. Gewolb I H, Rooney S A, Barrett C 1985 Delayed pulmonary maturation in the fetus of streptozotocin-diabetic rat. Experimental Lung Research 8: 141–151
71. Gill J, Reiss O K 1973 Isolation and characterisation of lamellar bodies and tubular myelin from rat lung homogenates. Journal of Cell Biology 58: 152–171
72. Glasser S W, Korfhagen T R, Perne C M et al 1988 Two genes encoding human pulmonary surfactant proteolipid SPL (pVal). Journal of Biological Chemistry 263: 10326–10331
73. Gluckman P D, Gunn T R, Johnston B M 1983 The effect of cooling on breathing and shivering unanaesthetized fetal lambs in utero. Journal of Physiology 343: 495–506
74. Goetzman B W, Read L C, Plopper C G et al 1994 Prenatal exposure to epidermal growth factor attenuates respiratory distress syndrome in rhesus infants. Pediatric Research 35: 30–36
75. Greenough A 1988 The premature infant's respiratory response to mechanical ventilation. Early Human Development 17: 1–5
76. Greenough A, Pool J 1991 Hering–Breuer reflex in young asthmatic children. Pediatric Pulmonology 11:345–349
77. Greenough A, Roberton N R C, Milner A D 1996 Neonatal respiratory disorders. Edward Arnold, London, p 105
78. Gross I, Walker-Smith G J, Wilson C M et al 1980 The influence of hormones on the biochemical development of fetal rat lung in organ culture. II insulin. Pediatric Research 14: 834–838
79. Guyton A C 1971 Regulation of cardiac output. Anaesthesiology 29: 314–326
80. Hall S M, Haworth S G 1986 Normal adaptation of pulmonary arterial intima to extrauterine life in the pig: ultrastructural studies. Journal of Pathology 149: 55–66
81. Hall S M, Haworth S G 1986 Conducting pulmonary arteries structural adaptation to extrauterine life. Cardiovascular Research 21: 208–216
82. Hallman M, Miyai K, Wagner R M 1976 Isolated lamellar bodies from rat lung; correlated ultrastructural and biochemical studies. Laboratory Investigation 35: 79–86
83. Hallman M, Feldman B H, Kirkpatrick E, Gluck L 1977 Absence of phosphatidylglycerol (PG) in RDS in the newborn. Pediatric Research 11: 714–720
84. Hallman M, Teramo K, Kankaanpaa K, Kulovich M V, Gluck L 1980 Prevention of respiratory distress syndrome: current view of lung maturity studies. Annals of Clinical Research 12: 36–44
85. Hamvas A, Nogee L M, deMello D E, Cole F S 1995 Pathophysiology and treatment of surfactant protein B deficiency. Biology of the Neonate 67: 18–31
86. Harding R 1986 The upper respiratory tract in perinatal life. In: Johnston B M, Gluckman P D (eds) Reproductive and perinatal medicine. Vol. III Respiratory control and lung development in the fetus and newborn. Perinatology Press, Ithaca, pp 331–376
87. Harper M A, Lorentz W B 1993 Immature lecithin:sphingomyelin ratios and neonatal respiratory course. American Journal of Obstetrics and Gynecology 168: 495–498

88. Harrison M R, Adzick N S, Flake A W et al 1996 Correction of congenital diaphragmatic hernia in utero. VIII: Response of the hypoplastic lung to tracheal occlusion. Journal of Pediatric Surgery 31: 1339–1348
89. Harrison V C, Heese H de V, Klein M 1968 The significance of grunting in hyaline membrane disease. Pediatrics 41: 549–559
90. Hasan S J, Rigaux A 1992 Effect of bilateral vagotomy on oxygenation, arousal and healthy movements in fetal sheep. Journal of Applied Physiology 73: 1402–1412
91. Haworth S G 1992 Development of the pulmonary circulation: Morphologic aspects. In: Polin R A, Fox W W (eds) Fetal and neonatal physiology, Vol 1. W B Saunders, Philadelphia, pp 671–682
92. Haworth S G, Hall S M, Chew M, Allen K 1987 Thinning of fetal pulmonary arterial wall and postnatal remodelling: ultrastructural studies on the respiratory unit arteries of the pig. Virchows Archiv 411: 161–171
93. Hawgood S, Benson B J, Hamilton R L 1985 Effects of surfactant associated protein and calcium ions on the structure and surface activity of lung surfactant lipids. Biochemistry 24: 185–190
94. Hawgood S, Benson B J, Schilling J, Damm D, Clements J, White R T 1987 Nucleotide and amino-acid sequences of pulmonary surfactant SP18 and evidence for cooperation between SP18 and SP 28–36 in surfactant lipid adsorption. Proceedings of the National Academy of Science USA 84: 66–70
95. Head H 1889 On the regulation of respiration. Journal of Physiology 10: 1–70
96. Henderson-Smart D J 1983 Regulation of breathing in the perinatal period. In: Saunders N A, Sulivan C E (eds) Sleeping and breathing: lung biology in health and disease, Vol 20. Marcel Dekker, New York
97. Henderson-Smart D J, Read D J C 1976 Depression of respiratory muscles and defective responses to nasal occlusion during active sleep in the newborn. Australian Paediatric Journal 12: 261–266
98. Hering B, Breuer J 1868 Die Selbsteuning der Athmung durch der nervus vagus. Sitzungsbericht der Kaiserlichen Akademie der Wissenschaften in Wien 57: 672–677
99. Hertzberg T, Hellstrom S, Holgert H, Lagercrantz H, Pequignot J M 1992 Ventilatory response to hypoxia in newborn rats born in hypoxia – possible relationship to carotid body dopamine. Journal of Physiology 456: 645–654
100. Heymann M A, Rudolph A M, Nies A S, Melmon K L 1969 Bradykinin production associated with oxygenation of fetal lamb. Circulation Research 25: 521–534
101. Hill C M 1976 The determination of the fatty acid profile of lecithin from human amniotic fluid and the pharyngeal aspirate of the newborn. Journal of Physiology 257: 15–17P
102. Hislop A, Reid L 1973 Pulmonary arterial development during childhood; branching pattern and structure. Thorax 28: 129–135
103. Hislop A, Haworth S G 1989 Airway size and structure in the normal fetal and infant lung and the effect on premature delivery and artificial ventilation. American Review of Respiratory Disease 140: 1717–1726
104. Hislop A, Reid L 1981 Growth and development of the respiratory system. Anatomical development. In: Davis J A, Dobbing J (eds) Scientific foundations of paediatrics, 2nd edn. Heinemann, London, pp 390–432
105. Holtman J R J, Speck D F 1994 Substance P immunoreactive projections to the ventral respiratory group in the rat. Peptides 15: 803–805
106. Hooper S B, Harding R 1995 Fetal lung liquid: a major determinant of the growth and functional development of the fetal lung. Clinical and Experimental Pharmacology and Physiology 22: 235–247
107. Hooper S B, Wallace M J, Harding R 1993 Amiloride blocks the inhibition of fetal lung liquid secretion caused by AVP but not by asphyxia. Journal of Applied Physiology 74: 111–115
108. Ikegami M, Jobe A H 1993 Surfactant metabolism. Seminars in Perinatology 17: 233–240
109. Ikegami M, Jobe A, Pettenazzo A, Seidner S, Berry D, Ruffini L 1987 Effects of maternal treatment with corticosteroids, T_3, TRH and their combinations on lung function of ventilated preterm rabbits with and without surfactant treatments. American Review of Respiratory Disease 136: 892–898
110. Jacobs H C, Jobe A H, Ikegami M, Jones S 1985 Reutilisation of phosphatidylglycerol and phosphatidylethanolamine by the pulmonary surfactant system in three day old rabbits. Biochimica et Biophysica Acta 834: 172–179
111. Jacobs H C, Ikegami M, Jobe A H, Berry D D 1985 Reutilisation of surfactant phosphatidylcholine in adult rabbits. Biochimica et Biophysica Acta 837: 77–82
112. Jeffery H E, Reid I, Rahilly P, Read D J C 1980 Gastro-esophageal reflux in 'near-miss' sudden infant death infants in active but not quiet sleep. Sleep 3: 393–399
113. Jobe AH 1992 Phospholipid metabolism and turnover. In: Polin R A, Fox W W (eds) Fetal and neonatal physiology, Vol 2. W B Saunders, Philadelphia, pp 986–995
114. Jobe A H, Ikegami M 1993 Surfactant metabolism. Clinics in Perinatology 20: 683–696
115. Jobe A, Ikegami M, Seidner S R, Pettenazzo A, Ruffini L 1989 Surfactant phosphatidylcholine metabolism and surfactant function in preterm ventilated lambs. American Review of Respiratory Disease 139: 352–359
116. Johnston B M, Bennet L, Gluckman P D 1989 In: Gluckman P D, Johnston B M, Nathanielsz P W (eds) Research in perinatal medicine, Vol. VIII Advances in fetal physiology. Perinatology Press, Ithaca, pp 77–193
117. Johansson J, Curstedt T, Robertson B et al 1988 Size and structure of the hydrophobic low molecular weight surfactant associated polypeptide. Biochemistry 27: 3544–3547
118. Kalapesi Z, Durand M, Leahy R N, Cates D B, MacCallum M, Rigatto H 1981 Effect of periodic or regular respiratory pattern on the ventilatory response to low inhaled CO_2 in preterm infants during sleep. American Review of Respiratory Disease 123: 8–11
119. Kanto W P, Borer R C, Barr M, Roloff D W 1976 Tracheal aspirate lecithin sphingomyelin ratios as predictors of recovery from RDS. Journal of Pediatrics 89: 612–616
120. Kari M A, Akino T, Hallman M 1995 Prenatal dexamethasone and exogenous surfactant therapy: surface activity and surfactant components in airway specimens. Pediatric Research 38: 678–684
121. Karlberg P, Cherry R B, Escardo F, Koch G 1962 Respiratory studies in newborn infants. II. Pulmonary ventilation and mechanics of breathing in the first minutes of life, including the onset of respiration. Acta Paediatrica Scandinavica 51: 121–136
122. Kinsella J, Abman S H 1995 Recent developments in the pathophysiology and treatment of persistent pulmonary hypertension of the newborn. Journal of Pediatrics 126: 853–864
123. Kirkpatrick S M L, Olinsky A, Bryan M H, Bryan A C 1976 Effect of premature delivery on the maturation of the Hering–Breuer inspiratory inhibitory reflex in human infants. Journal of Pediatrics 88: 1010–1014
124. Kleinmann L I, Petering H G, Sutherland J M 1967 Blood carbonic anhydrase activity and zinc concentration in infants with respiratory distress syndrome. New England Journal of Medicine 227: 1157–1161
125. Kuan S F, Rust K, Crouch E 1992 Interactions of surfactant protein D with bacterial lipopolysaccharides. Surfactant protein D is an *Escherichia coli*-binding protein in bronchoalveolar lavage. Journal of Clinical Investigation 90: 97–106
126. Kuhn C 1968 Cytochemistry of pulmonary alveolar epithelial cells. American Journal of Pathology 53: 809–833
127. Kuhn C 1982 The cytology of the lung: ultrastructure of the respiratory epithelium and extracellular lining layers. In: Farrell P M (ed) Lung development: biological and clinical perspectives, Vol. 1. Academic Press, New York, Ch. 3, p 27
128. Kulovich M V, Gluck L 1979 The lung profile. II. Complicated pregnancy. American Journal of Obstetrics and Gynecology 135: 64–70
129. Kulovich M V, Hallman M, Gluck L 1979 The lung profile. I. Normal pregnancy. American Journal of Obstetrics and Gynecology 135: 57–63
130. Kuroki Y, Mason R, Voelker D R 1988 Rat alveolar type II cells express a high affinity receptor for protein A. Proceedings of the National Academy of Science USA 85: 556–557
131. Lagercrantz H 1987 Neuromodulators and respiratory control in the infant. Clinics in Perinatology 14: 683–695
132. Lagercrantz H, Pequignot J M, Hertzberg T et al 1994 Birth related changes of expression and turnover of some neuroactive agents and respiratory control. Biology of the Neonate 65: 145–148
133. Lagercrantz H, Pequignot J, Pequignot J M, Peyrin L 1992 The first breaths of air stimulate noradrenaline turnover in the brain of the newborn rat. Acta Physiologica Scandinavica 144: 433–438
134. Lalley P M, Bischoff A M, Richter D W 1994 Serotonin 1-alpha-receptor activation suppresses respiratory apneusis in the cat. Neuroscience Letters 172: 59–62
135. Lawson E E, Brown E R, Torday J S, Madansky D L, Taeusch H W

1978 The effect of epinephrine on tracheal fluid flow and surfactant flux in fetal sheep. American Review of Respiratory Disease 118: 1023–1026
136. Lawson E E, Birdwell R L, Huang P S, Taeusch H W 1979 Augmentation of pulmonary surfactant secretion by lung expansion at birth. Pediatric Research 13: 611–614
137. Leffler C W, Hessler J R, Green RS 1984 The onset of breathing at birth stimulates pulmonary vascular prostacyclin synthesis. Pediatric Research 18: 938–942
138. Loosli C G, Potter E L 1959 Pre and postnatal development of the respiratory portion of the human lung. American Review of Respiratory Disease 80: 5–20
139. Manalo E, Merritt A, Kheiter A, Amirkhanian J, Cochrane C 1996 Comparative effects of some serum components and proteolytic products of fibrinogen on surface tension lowering abilities of beractant and a synthetic peptide containing surfactant KL_4. Pediatric Research 39: 947–952
140. Marchal F, Bairam A, Haouzi P et al 1992 Carotid chemoreceptor response to natural stimuli in the newborn kitten. Respiratory Physiology 87: 183–193
141. Marino P A, Rooney S A 1981 The effect of labour on surfactant secretion in newborn rabbit lung slices. Biochimica et Biophysica Acta 664: 389–396
142. Marsh M, Fox G, Ingram D, Milner A D 1994 The Hering–Breuer deflationary reflex in the newborn infant. Pediatric Pulmonology 18: 163–169
143. Martin R J, Nearman H S, Katona P G, Klaus M H 1977 The effect of a low continuous positive airway pressure on the reflex control of respiration in the preterm infant. Journal of Pediatrics 90: 976–981
144. Martin R J, Herrell N, Rubin D, Fanaroff A 1979 Effect of supine and prone positions on arterial oxygen tension in the preterm infant. Pediatrics 63: 528–531
145. Mason R J 1982 Isolation of alveolar type II cells. In: Farrell P M (ed) Lung development: biological and clinical perspectives Vol. 1. Academic Press, New York, Ch. 8, p 135
146. Massaro G D, Massaro D 1983 Morphological evidence that large inflations of the lung stimulate secretion of surfactant. American Review of Respiratory Disease 127: 235–236
147. Mayock D E, Hall J, Watchko J F, Standaert T V, Woodrum D E 1987 Diaphragmatic muscle fibre type development in swine. Pediatric Research 22: 449–454
148. Milhorn D E, Eldridge F L 1986 Role of ventrolateral medulla in regulation of respiratory and cardiovascular systems. Journal of Applied Physiology 61: 1249–1263
149. Milhorn D E, Eldridge F L, Kiley J P et al 1984 Prolonged inhibition of respiration following acute hypoxia in glomectomized cats. Respiration Physiology 57: 331–340
150. Milner A D, Saunders R A 1977 Pressure and volume changes during the first breath of human neonates. Archives of Disease in Childhood 52: 918–924
151. Mizuno K, Ikegami M, Chen C-M, Ueda T, Jobe A H 1995 Surfactant protein B supplementation improves in vivo function of modified natural surfactant. Pediatric Research 37: 271–276
152. Moriette G, van-Reempts P, Moore M, Cates D, Rigatto H 1985 The effect of rebreathing of CO_2 on ventilation and diaphragmatic electromyography in newborn infants. Respiratory Physiology 62: 387–397
153. Morley C J 1992 Surfactant. In: Roberton N R C (ed) Textbook of neonatology, 2nd edn. Churchill Livingstone, Edinburgh, pp 369–383
154. Morley C J, Bangham A D 1981 Physical properties of surfactant under compression. In: von Wichert (ed) Progress in respiration research 15. Clinical importance of surfactant defects. Karger, Basle, p 188
155. Mortola J P 1983 Body size–Respiratory function–Disease. Some functional mechanical implications of the structural design of the respiratory system in newborn mammals. American Review of Respiratory Disease 128: S69–S72
156. Motoyama E K, Namba Y, Rooney S A 1976 Phosphatidylcholine content and fatty acid composition of tracheal and gastric liquids from premature and fullterm newborn infants. Clinica Chimica Acta 70: 449–454
157. Nicholas T E, Doyle I R, Bersten A D 1997 Surfactant replacement therapy in ARDS: white knight or noise in the system? Thorax 52: 195–197
158. Nicholas T E, Barr H A 1983 The release of surfactant in rat lung by brief periods of hyperventilation. Respiration Physiology 52: 69–83
159. Nichols B 1976 Normal rabbit alveolar macrophages. I. The phagocytosis of tubular myelin. Journal of Experimental Medicine 144: 906–919
160. Nicolini U, Fisk N M, Talbert D G et al 1989 Intrauterine manometry: technique and application to fetal pathology. Prenatal Diagnosis 9: 243–254
161. Noack G, Berggren P, Curstedt T et al 1987 Severe neonatal respiratory distress syndrome treated with isolated phospholipid fraction of natural surfactant. Acta Paediatrica Scandinavica 76: 697–705
162. Obladen M, Gluck L 1977 RDS and tracheal phospholipid composition in twins: independent of gestational age. Journal of Pediatrics 90: 799–802
163. Ohki M, Naito K, Cole P 1991 Dimensions and resistances of the human nose: racial differences. Laryngoscope 101: 276–278
164. Ojomo E O, Coustan D R 1990 Absence of evidence of pulmonary maturity at amniocentesis in term infants of diabetic mothers. American Journal of Obstetrics and Gynecology 163: 954–957
165. Olver R E, Strang L B 1974 Ion fluxes across the pulmonary epithelium and the secretion of lung liquid in the fetal lamb. Journal of Physiology 241: 327–357
166. O'Reilly M A, Nogee L, Whitsett J A 1988 Requirement of the collagenous domain for carbohydrate processing and secretion of surfactant protein of M_r = 35,000. Biochimica et Biophysica Acta 969: 176–184
167. Oyarzun M J, Clements J A 1977 Ventilatory and cholinergic control of pulmonary surfactant in the rabbit. Journal of Applied Physiology 43: 39–45
168. Parks C R, Woodrum D E, Alden E R, Standaert T A, Hodson W A 1974 Gas exchange in the immature lung. I. Anatomical shunt in the premature infant. Journal of Applied Physiology 36: 103–107
169. Parkinson C M, Supramaniam G, Harvey D 1978 Bubble clicking in pharyngeal aspirate of newborn babies. British Medical Journal i: 758–759
170. Pattle R E 1955 Properties, function and origin of the alveolar lining layer. Nature 175: 1125–1126
171. Perelman R H, Palta M, Kirby R, Farrell P M 1986 Discordance between male and female deaths due to respiratory distress syndrome. Pediatrics 78: 238–244
172. Phelps D S, Church S, Kourembanas S et al 1987 Increases in the 35 kDa surfactant associated protein and its mRNA following in vivo dexamethasone treatment in fetal and neonatal rats. Electrophoresis 8: 235–238
173. Phillipson E A, Bowes G 1986 Control of breathing during sleep. In: Cherniack N S, Widdicombe J G (eds) Handbook of physiology – the respiratory system Vol. II. American Physiological Society, Bethesda, pp 649–690
174. Pickens D L, Schefft G L, Thach B T 1989 Pharyngeal fluid clearance and aspiration preventive mechanisms in sleeping infants. Journal of Applied Physiology 66: 1164–1171
175. Post M, Batenburg J, Schuurmans E, Laros C, Van Golde L 1982 Lamellar bodies isolated from adult human lung tissue. Experimental Lung Research 3: 17–28
176. Post M, Schuurmans E A, Batenburg J J, van Golde L M 1983 Mechanisms involved in the synthesis of disaturated phosphatidylcholine by alveolar type II cells isolated from adult rat lung. Biochimica et Biophysica Acta 750: 68–77
177. Post M, van Golde L M G 1988 Metabolic and developmental aspects of the pulmonary surfactant system. Biochimica et Biophysica Acta 947: 249–286
178. Prabhakar N, Runold M, Yamamoto Y et al 1984 Effect of substance P antagonist on the hypoxia-induced carotid chemoreceptor activity. Acta Physiologica Scandinavica 121: 301–303
179. Raaberg L, Nexo E, Jorgensen P E, Poulsen S S, Jakab M 1995 Fetal effects of epidermal growth factor deficiency induced in rats by auto antibodies against epidermal growth factor. Pediatric Research 37: 175–181
180. Rabbette P S, Dezateux C A, Fletcher M E, Stocks J 1991 The Hering–Breuer reflex declines during the first year of life. European Respiratory Journal 4: 533 (abstract)
181. Ragosch V, Juergens S, Lorenz U, Stolowsky C, Arabin B, Wietzel H-K 1992 Prediction of RDS by amniotic fluid analysis: a comparison of the prognostic value of traditional and recent methods. Journal of Perinatal Medicine 20: 351–360

182. Revak S D, Merritt T A, Degruse E et al 1988 Use of human surfactant low molecular weight apoproteins in the reconstitution of surfactant biological activity. Journal of Clinical Investigation 81: 826–833
183. Richter D W, Ballanyi K, Schwarzacher S 1992 Mechanisms of respiratory rhythm generation. Current Opinion in Neurobiology 2: 788–793
184. Rigatto H 1984 Control of ventilation in the newborn. Annual Review of Physiology 46: 661–674
185. Rigatto H 1992 Control of breathing in fetal life and onset and control of breathing in the neonate. In: Polin R A, Fox W W (eds) Fetal and neonatal physiology, Vol 1 W B Saunders, Philadelphia, pp 790–801
186. Rigatto H, Lee D, Davi M, Moore M, Rigatto E, Cates D 1988 Effect of increased arterial $PaCO_2$ on fetal breathing and behaviour in sheep. Journal of Applied Physiology 64: 892–897
187. Rigatto H, Kwiat Kouski K A, Hansan S U, Cates D B 1991 The ventilatory response to endogenous CO_2 in preterm infants. American Review of Respiratory Disease 143: 101–104
188. Robertson B, Berry D, Curstedt T et al 1985 Leakage of protein in the immature rabbit lung: effect of surfactant replacement. Respiratory Physiology 61: 265–276
189. Rodenstein D O, Perlmutter N, Stanescu D C 1985 Infants are not obligatory nasal breathers. American Review of Respiratory Disease 131: 343–347
190. Rooney S A 1985 The surfactant system and lung phospholipid biochemistry. American Review of Respiratory Disease 131: 439–460
191. Rooney S A 1992 Regulation of surfactant-associated phospholipid synthesis and secretion. In: Polin R A, Fox W W (eds) Fetal and neonatal physiology, Vol 2. W B Saunders, Philadelphia, pp 971–985
192. Rooney S A, Gobran L I, Marino P A, Maniscalco W M, Gross I 1979 Effects of betamethasone on phospholipid content composition and biosynthesis in fetal rabbit lung. Biochimica et Biophysica Acta 572: 64–76
193. Rooney S A, Gobran L I, Wai-Lee T S 1977 Stimulation of surfactant production by oxytocin-induced labour in the rabbit. Journal of Clinical Investigation 60: 754–759
194. Runold M, Lagercrantz H, Prabhakar N R, Fredholm B B 1989 Role of adenosine in hypoxic ventilatory depression. Journal of Applied Physiology 67: 541–546
195. Sahu S, Lynn W S, 1977 Phospholipase A in pulmonary secretions from patients with alveolar proteinosis. Biochimica et Biophysica Acta 487: 354–360
196. Seeger W, Grube C, Guenther A, Schmidt R 1993 Surfactant inhibition by plasma proteins: differential sensitivity of various surfactant proteins. European Respiratory Journal 6: 971–977
197. Seeger W, Stoehr G, Neuhof H 1985 Surfactant inhibitory plasma derived proteins. In: Walters D V, Strang L B, Geubelle F (eds) Physiology of the fetal and neonatal lung. Kluwer Academic Press, Lancaster, pp 225–240
198. Shaul P W 1995 Nitric oxide in the developing lung. Advances in Pediatrics 42: 367–414
199. Silverman M 1983 Respiratory function testing in infancy and childhood. In: Laszlo G, Sudlow M F (eds) Measurement in clinical respiratory physiology. Academic Press, London, pp 293–328
200. Smith B T 1978 Fibroplast pneumocyte factor: intercellular mediator of glucocorticoid effect on fetal lung. In: Stern L (ed) Neonatal intensive care. Mason, New York, pp 25–32
201. Smith B T 1979 Lung maturation in the fetal rat: acceleration by injection of fibroblast pneumocyte factor. Science 204: 1094–1095
202. Souza P, O'Brodovich H, Post M 1995 Lung fluid restriction affects growth but not airway branching of embryonic rat lung. International Journal of Developmental Biology 39: 629–637
203. Stevens P A, Wright J R, Clements J A 1989 Surfactant secretion and clearance in the newborn. Journal of Applied Physiology 67: 1595–1605
204. Stocks J, Sly P, Tepper R, Morgan W J 1996 Infant respiratory function testing. New York, Wiley Liss
205. Strang L B 1977 Neonatal respiration. Blackwell Scientific Publications, Oxford
206. Stratton C J 1975 Multilamellar body formation in mammalian lung: an ultrastructural study utilising three lipid retention procedures. Journal of Ultrastructure Research 52: 309–320
207. Stratton C J 1976 The three dimensional aspect of mammalian lung lamellar bodies. Tissue and Cell 8: 693–712
208. Stratton C J 1976 The high resolution ultrastructure of the periodicity and architecture of the lipid-retained and extracted lung multilamellar body laminations. Tissue and Cell 8: 713–728
209. Suzuki Y 1982 Effect of protein, cholesterol, and phosphatidylglycerol on the surface activity of the lipid–protein complex reconstituted from pig pulmonary surfactant. Journal of Lipid Research 23: 62–69
210. Takahashi A, Fujiwara T 1986 Proteolipid in bovine lung surfactant: its role in surfactant function. Biochemical and Biophysical Research Communications 135: 527–532
211. Tanasijevic M J, Winkelman J W, Wybenga D R, Richardson D K, Greene M F 1996 Prediction of fetal lung maturity in infants of diabetic mothers using the FLM S/A and disaturated phosphatidylcholine tests. American Journal of Clinical Pathology 105: 17–22
212. Thurlbeck W B 1982 Postnatal human lung growth. Thorax 34: 564–571
213. Tietel D F, Iwamoto H S, Rudolph A M 1987 Effects of birth related events on central blood flow patterns. Pediatric Research 22: 557–566
214. Torday J S 1985 Dihydrotesterone inhibits fibroblast pneumocyte factor-mediated synthesis of saturated phosphatidylcholine by fetal rat lung cells. Biochimica et Biophysica Acta 835: 23–28
215. Tusiewicz K, Moldfsky H, Bryan A C, Bryan M H 1977 Mechanics of the rib cage and the diaphragm during sleep. Journal of Applied Physiology 43: 600–602
216. Van Iwaarden F, Welmers B, Verhoef J, Haagsman H P, Van Golde L M G 1990 Pulmonary surfactant protein A enhances host defense mechanism of rat alveolar macrophage. American Journal of Respiratory and Cellular Molecular Biology 2: 91–98
217. Veldhuizen R A W, Yao L-J, Hearn S A, Possmayer F, Lewis J F 1996 Surfactant associated protein A is important for maintaining surfactant large-aggregate forms during surface-area cycling. Biochemistry 313: 835–840
218. von Neergaard K 1929 Neue Auffassungen ueber einen Grundbegriff der Atemmechanik. Die Retraktionskraft der Lunge abhaengig von der Oberflaechenspannung in den Alveolen. Zeitschrift fuer die Gesamte Experimentelle Medizin 66: 373–394
219. Vorbroker D K, Profitt S A, Nogee L M, Whitsett J A 1995 Aberrant processing of surfactant protein C in hereditary SP-B deficiency. American Journal of Physiology 268: L647–L656
220. Vyas H, Field D, Hopkin I E, Milner A D 1986 Determinants of the first inspiratory volume and functional residual capacity at birth. Pediatric Pulmonology 2: 189–193
221. Vyas H, Milner A D, Hopkin I E 1981 Comparison of intrathoracic pressure and volume changes during the spontaneous onset of respiration in babies born by caesarian section and by vaginal delivery. Journal of Pediatrics 99: 787–791
222. Walters D V, Olver R E 1978 The role of catecholamines in lung liquid absorption at birth. Pediatric Research 12: 239–242
223. Walters D V, Ramsden C A 1985 The secretion and absorption of fetal lung liquid. In: Walters D V, Strang L B , Geubelle F (eds) Physiology of the fetal and neonatal lung. Kluwer Academic Press, Lancaster, pp 61–74
224. Walther F J, Benders M J, Leighton J O 1993 Early changes in the neonatal circulatory transition. Journal of Pediatrics 123: 625–632
225. Wealthall S R 1975 Factors resulting in a failure to interrupt apnoea. In: Bosma J F, Showacre J (eds) Development of upper respiratory anatomy and function. US Government Printing Office, Washington DC, 212–225
226. Weaver T E, Whitsett J A 1991 Function and regulation of pulmonary surfactant-associated proteins. Biochemistry Journal 273: 249–264
227. Weller P H, Gupta J, Jenkins P A, Baum J D 1976 Pharyngeal L/S ratios in newborn infants. Lancet i: 12–16
228. Wharton J, Haworth S G, Polak J M 1988 Postnatal development of the innervation and paraganglia in the porcine pulmonary arterial bed. Journal of Pathology 154: 19–27
229. Whitsett J A, Nogee L M, Weaver T E, Horowitz A D 1995 Human surfactant protein B: structure, function, regulation and genetic disease. Physiological Reviews 75: 749–757
230. Whitsett J A, Pilot T, Clark J C et al 1987 Induction of surfactant protein in fetal lung: effects of cAMP and dexamethasone on SAP-35 RNA and synthesis. Journal of Biological Chemistry 262: 5256–5261
231. Whitsett J A, Weaver T E, Lieberman M A et al 1987 Differential effects of epidermal growth factor and transforming growth factor beta and synthesis of M_r = 35,000 surfactant associated proteins in fetal lung. Journal of Biological Chemistry 262: 7908–7913

232. Wilkie R A, Bryan M H, Tarnow-Mordi W O 1994 Static respiratory compliance in the newborn. II. Its potential for improving the selection of infants for early surfactant treatment. Archives of Disease in Childhood 70: F16–F18
233. Williams M C 1978 Freeze fracture studies of tubular myelin and lamellar bodies in fetal and adult rat lungs. Journal of Ultrastructure Research 64: 352–361
234. Williams M C 1987 Vesicles within vesicles: what role do multivesicular bodies play in alveolar type II cells? American Review of Respiratory Disease 135: 744–746
235. Williams M C, Benson B J 1981 Immunocytochemical localisation and identification of the major surfactant protein in adult rat lung. Journal of Histochemistry and Cytochemistry 29: 291–237
236. Woodrum D 1992 Respiratory muscles. In: Polin R A, Fox W W (eds) Fetal and neonatal physiology, Vol 1. W B Saunders, Philadelphia, pp 829–841
237. Wright J R, Clements J A 1987 Metabolism and turnover of lung surfactant. American Review of Respiratory Disease 136: 426–444
238. Wyszogrodski I, Kyei-Aboagye K, Taeusch H W, Avery M E 1975 Surfactant inactivation by hyperventilation: conservation by end-expiratory pressure. Journal of Applied Physiology 38: 461–466
239. Yamamoto M, Lagercrantz H, von Euler C 1981 Effects of substance P and TRH on ventilation and pattern of breathing in newborn rabbits. Acta Physiologica Scandinavica 113: 541–543
240. Yost R W, Chander A, Dodia C, Fisher A B 1986 Stimulation of the methylation pathway for phosphatidylcholine synthesis in rat lungs by choline deficiency. Biochimica et Biophysica Acta 875: 122–125
241. Yuksel B, Greenough A 1992 Neonatal respiratory support and lung function abnormalities at follow-up. Respiratory Medicine 86: 97–100
242. Ziegler J W, Ivy D D, Kinsella J P, Abman S H 1995 The role of nitric oxide, endothelin and prostaglandins in the transition of the pulmonary circulation. Clinics in Perinatology 22: 387–403

Part 2

Acute respiratory disease in the newborn

Anne Greenough N. R. C. Roberton

The largest single group of babies admitted to a neonatal unit are those suffering from some form of pulmonary disorder (Table 29.4), and this is the commonest diagnosis in neonates requiring IPPV (intermittent positive pressure ventilation) (Table 29.5). The importance of lung disease is further emphasized by the fact that respiratory disease, especially RDS (respiratory distress syndrome) and its complications, is the most common cause of death in the neonatal period, particularly when malformations are excluded from the analysis (Table 29.6).[166,1104]

RESPIRATORY DISTRESS SYNDROME

This is an acute illness,[929] usually of preterm infants (p. 482), characterized clinically by a respiratory rate ≥60/min, dyspnoea (intercostal, subcostal indrawing, sternal retraction) with a predominantly diaphragmatic breathing pattern and a characteristic expiratory grunt or moan, all presenting within 4–6 hours of delivery (p. 495). Oxygen administration is required to prevent cyanosis, and there is a reticulogranular chest X-ray appearance as a result of widespread atelectasis (p. 500).

Table 29.4 Major diagnoses in neonates admitted to the NICU at KCH, 1996

Lung disease	173
Premature <34 weeks, <1800 g without serious lung disease	164
Congenital malformation	44
Central nervous system disease	15
Infection (culture positive)	41
Haematological problems	14
Gut disorders	7
Maternal drug ingestion	14

Pathophysiologically the condition is characterized by non-compliant (stiff) lungs, which contain less surfactant than normal and become atelectatic at end-expiration (p. 488). Histologically, hyaline membranes occur lining

Table 29.5 Diagnoses in babies requiring IPPV, Cambridge Maternity Hospital

	1985–87	1990–94
Respiratory distress syndrome	270	524
Transient tachypnoea	7	59
CNS respiratory depression	6	41
Malformation	5	21
Sepsis	4	not recorded
Fetal haemorrhage	3	not recorded
Postoperatively	3	28*
Congenital heart disease	2	15
Miscellaneous	5	
Meconium aspiration	1	10
Rhesus disease		6

*Surgery alone (i.e. not RDS + NEC)

Table 29.6 Causes of neonatal death in Cambridge Maternity Hospital

	1982–89	1990–94
Respiratory distress syndrome	137*	38
Infection	24	13
Birth asphyxia	15	14
Extreme prematurity	14	44
Pulmonary hypoplasia	10	19
Miscellaneous	10	
Total non-malformed neonatal deaths	210	128
Malformations	84	46
Total neonatal deaths	294	174

*The majority of these babies had a large periventricular haemorrhage

Table 29.7 Incidence of neonatal respiratory disease in Nottingham[322] and Sweden[498]

	Sweden (Nov 76–Oct 77)	Nottingham (Apr 83–Mar 84)
Respiratory distress syndrome	105 (0.33%)	73 (0.96%)
Pulmonary maladaptation*	300 (0.93%)	27 (0.36%)
Infection	56 (0.17%)	4 (0.05%)
Meconium aspiration	29 (0.09%)	4 (0.05%)
Airleak (alone)	22 (0.07%)	— —
Persistent fetal circulation	19 (0.06%)	1 (0.01%)
Extreme immaturity	12 (0.04%)	12 (0.16%)
All disorders†	931 (2.90%)	158 (2.10%)
Total no. of neonates	32 281	7602

*This corresponds approximately to transient tachypnoea of the newborn (p. 514).
† This includes 350 babies (Sweden) and 19 babies (Nottingham) classified as having mild respiratory disturbance (p. 516).

the terminal airways. These give the condition its alternative name – hyaline membrane disease – which, to be semantically correct, should only be used in the presence of histological confirmation (that is, at autopsy); the term RDS is preferred.

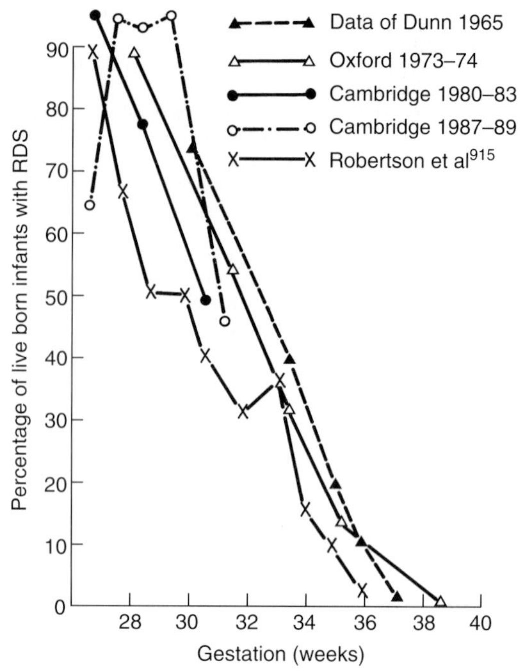

Fig. 29.15 Incidence of RDS at different gestations. Reproduced with permission from Greenough et al.[414]

INCIDENCE

The major determinant of the incidence of RDS is the proportion of deliveries which are preterm. Chamberlain et al[166] found that 2% of all babies and 20% of babies weighing <2.50 kg had some form of breathing difficulty, with twice as many boys affected as girls and three times as many boys dying. Hjalmarson[498] and Field et al[322] found a prevalence of lung disease in newborn babies of 2.9% and 2.1%, respectively (Table 29.7). In the Swedish study,[498] however, only 0.33% had RDS. This may be a reflection of the low incidence of prematurity, but as several of their cases of pulmonary maladaptation had a reticulogranular chest X-ray and died, they probably had RDS. The prevalence of RDS of 0.96% found in Nottingham[322] is representative of British diagnostic standards. In the USA, 1.72% of liveborn babies developed RDS in 1986–87.[72] On the basis of these data, it would appear that approximately 7000 British and 40 000 American babies develop RDS every year.

The prevalence at different gestations is given in Figure 29.15. There are small variations which may represent differences in diagnostic criteria, but in general there is a shift to the left in the graphs, suggesting a fall in incidence in recent years.

AETIOLOGY

The aetiology of RDS is immaturity of the lungs, in particular of the surfactant-synthesizing systems. Various factors contribute to this immaturity and interact with it to increase or decrease the incidence of the disorder.

Factors predisposing to RDS

Prematurity

RDS is very common in infants <30 weeks' gestation, and almost invariable in infants <28 weeks' gestation (Fig. 29.15), but remains a significant problem up to 34 weeks' gestation.[657] Some of the dyspnoea and hypoxaemia in very preterm babies, however, is due to their immature lung structure, with increased connective tissue and poorly developed alveoli. The maturation of surfactant synthesis is a mirror image of the incidence of RDS at different gestations (Fig. 29.16). Other factors may make the preterm neonate inherently susceptible to RDS. His

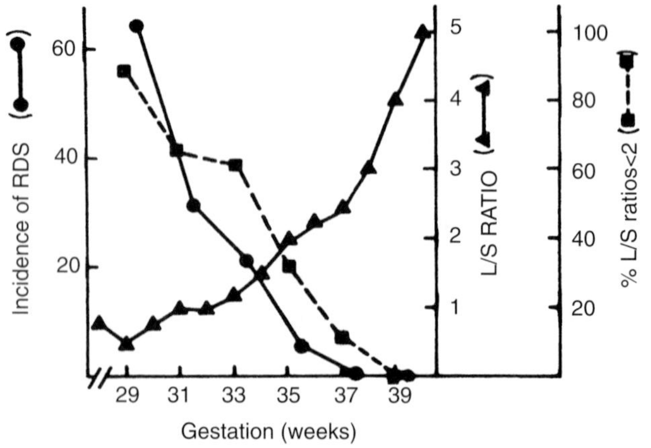

Fig. 29.16 Incidence of RDS at different gestations compared to L:S ratios. Reproduced with permission from Farrell and Avery.[312]

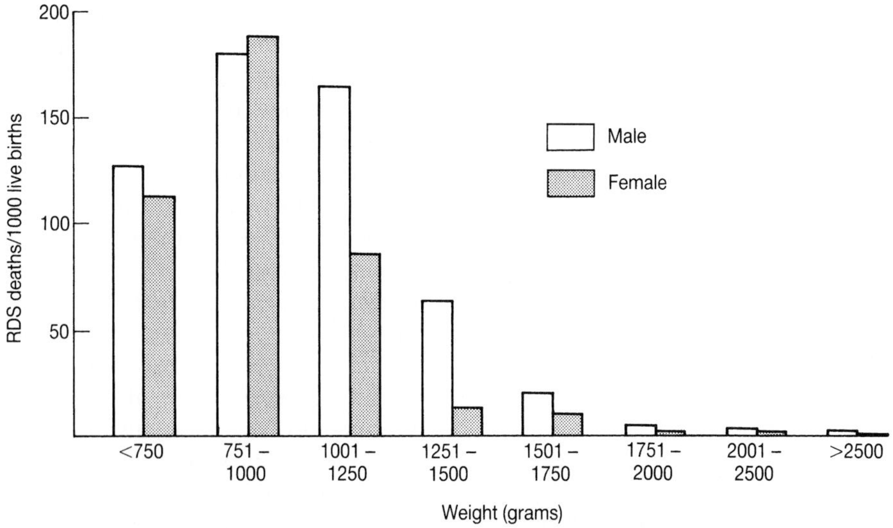

Fig. 29.17 Incidence of fatal RDS for males and females of different birthweights in Wisconsin 1979–82. The mortality in females is significantly less at birthweight 1.001–1.250 kg ($P < 0.005$) and 1.251–1.500 kg ($P < 0.001$). Reproduced with permission from Perelman et al.[834]

lung epithelia are more leaky than those of an infant born at term, increasing the likelihood of protein passing onto the alveolar surface, where it will inhibit surfactant function (see below). Fetal lung liquid is cleared slowly in the preterm neonate[519] and he is more prone to asphyxia (Chapter 16), hypoxia, hypotension and hypothermia, all of which are likely to impair surfactant synthesis (pp. 484–485) or increase alveolar capillary leakiness.

Gender

Boys are much more likely to develop RDS than girls, and are more likely to die from the disease[312] (Fig. 29.17). In male fetuses the delayed maturation of the L:S ratio and the late appearance of phosphatidylglycerol[327] are androgen induced.[610,1078]

Race

Black infants have a lower incidence of RDS, 60–70% of that of white infants of the same gestational age.[516] This is evident even in very immature infants, only 40% of African infants ≤32 weeks' gestational age developing RDS, compared to 75% of Caucasian infants.[568] No black baby with an L:S ratio >1.2 developed RDS, but white babies did develop the disease at these low ratios.[896] Allelic variation in the sufactant protein A gene has been reported between American whites and Nigerian blacks.[900]

Caesarean section

This remains controversial. Most studies done in the 1950s and 1960s,[313,1103,1104] but not all,[1037] suggested that caesarean section carried out before the mother went into labour increased the risk of the baby developing RDS. There are two physiological reasons for an association between caesarean section and RDS:

1. During labour there is a reduction in lung liquid production,[108,179] as the pulmonary epithelium changes from a chloride-excreting tissue (producing lung liquid) to a sodium-absorbing one. Adrenergic stimulation is important in controlling this switch[1136] and may also release surfactant,[555] but lung fluid production still falls in labour in the presence of adrenergic blockade.[108,179] Surfactant is released into the airways[149] and the pharyngeal L:S ratio is higher in babies born by caesarean section with, rather than without, labour.[1156] These factors may explain why babies born by caesarean section before labour have a larger residual volume of lung fluid and a smaller functional residual capacity to thoracic gas volume ratio in the hours immediately after delivery,[750] secrete less surfactant onto the alveolar surface,[632] and have more lung disease (see below).
2. About one-third of the fetal lung fluid is removed by squeezing of the baby's chest during vaginal delivery. This does not happen in delivery by caesarean section, either before or during labour. As babies born by caesarean section during labour do not, however, have an increased incidence of RDS, their improved lung function must be due to the adrenergic surge associated with labour (see above).

Data on gestations above 32–34 weeks tend to confirm the association of caesarean section before labour with both RDS and the less severe lung disease, TTN[31,205,768] (p. 514) (Fig. 29.18). This preventable disease[825] can be severe, as evidenced by the occasional infant who has required ECMO support.[578] The association between caesarean section and RDS in Cambridge for pregnancies

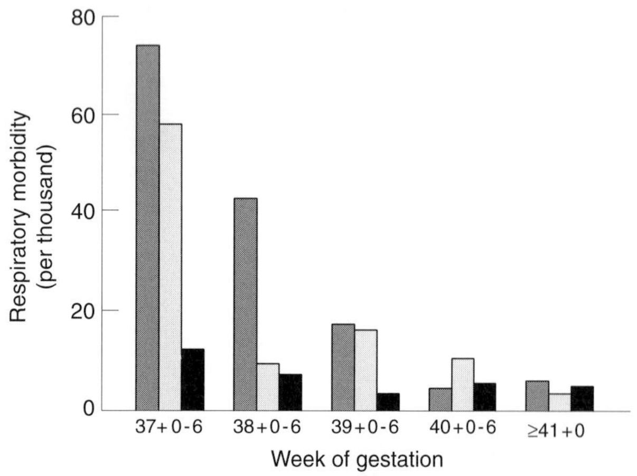

Fig. 29.18 Incidence of respiratory morbidity per 1000 livebirths, shown by each week of gestation and mode of delivery. Heavily shaded area = delivery by caesarean section before labour; medium shaded area = caesarean section during labour; black shaded area = vaginal delivery. Reproduced with permission from Morrison et al.[768]

Table 29.8 Incidence of respiratory distress syndrome by route of delivery, Cambridge Maternity Hospital 1987–1994

	Route of delivery*			
Gestational age (weeks)	**Spontaneous vertex delivery/ forceps**	**Breech**	**Caesarean section before labour**	**Caesarean section in labour**
24/25	83 (69)	28 (27)	30 (30)	24 (26)
26/27	185 (176)	80 (79)	103 (101)	97 (93)
28/29	238 (221)	98 (94)	153 (144)	129 (120)
30/31	285 (254)	118 (112)	190 (165)	156 (137)
Total	791 (620)	324 (312)	476 (440)	409 (376)
	78%†	96%	92%	92%

*Figures in parentheses are the number with RDS
† Incidence in SVD/forceps significantly less than caesarian section before or in labour ($P < 0.0001$)

<32 weeks' gestation is shown in Table 29.8. Although there is a statistically significant increase in RDS in babies delivered by caesarean section, this should not be used as an excuse for avoiding the operation where it is indicated in the interest of either maternal or fetal well-being.

Asphyxia/low Apgar score

Babies who are asphyxiated at birth are at increased risk of RDS.[665,1067] Worthington and Smith[1177] observed 81 babies between 25 and 37 weeks: 75% of those with an L:S ratio <2.0 who were asphyxiated developed RDS, compared with 40% of the non-asphyxiated babies. In those with L:S ratios above 2.0, 33% of the asphyxiated but none of the non-asphyxiated infants developed RDS. The incidence of RDS in premature babies with an Apgar score of 5 or less is twice as high as in those with a score above 5,[547] and in those less than 32 weeks' gestation the incidence is 54% in those with an Apgar <4, compared to 42% in babies with Apgars ≥4 ($P < 0.005$).[76]

During fetal asphyxia lung perfusion falls, resulting in ischaemic damage to pulmonary capillaries. When the fetus recovers from the acute asphyxia, pulmonary hyperperfusion occurs,[251] and if delivery occurs shortly afterwards a protein-rich fluid leaks out of the damaged pulmonary capillaries.[245,542] This leakage of proteins, which inhibits surfactant activity on the alveolar surface, is one of the key pathophysiological mechanisms in the development of RDS.[522,523,955] It explains the fall in lung surfactant during the first few hours of life in babies with RDS.[892] The protein leak can be prevented by exogenous surfactant,[525] but in babies who respond poorly to surfactant administration this benefit is probably overwhelmed by the large alveolar protein leak.[352,603] The surfactant apoprotein A (p. 471) is of specific benefit in minimizing the inhibitory effect of protein on either endogenous or exogenous surfactant.[1201] One of the beneficial effects of antenatal steroids (p. 491) may be that they considerably reduce this capillary leakiness,[524] the effects of which can be minimized by prompt and effective resuscitation.[91]

The association between asphyxia and RDS is also influenced by the fact that hypoxia and acidaemia (i.e. asphyxia) predispose to:

- pulmonary hypertension and hypoperfusion, with a right-to-left shunt (pp. 493, 530);
- a reduction in surfactant synthesis by inhibiting synthetic enzymes[740] (Fig. 29.19);
- Muscle hypotonia, which reduces the baby's respiratory efforts, resulting in a low FRC, diminished lung fluid removal and less surfactant secretion.

Maternal diabetes

The traditional,[901] though not universally accepted,[1104] view in the 1970s was that IDM had an increased incidence of RDS. Studies in the late 1970s showed that

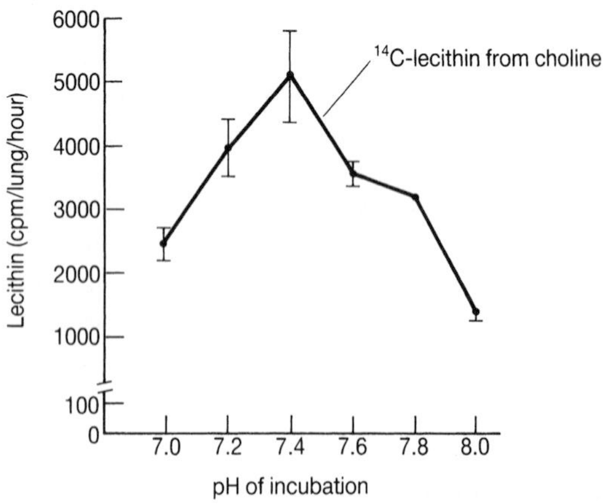

Fig. 29.19 Effect of pH on lecithin (effectively surfactant) synthesis in monkey lung slices. Note that both acidaemia and alkalemia compromise surfactant synthesis. Reproduced with permission from Merritt and Farrell.[740]

such fetuses had abnormal surfactant synthesis, in particular a delay in the appearance of PG (p. 474).[233,811] Gross et al[437] showed that insulin delayed the maturation of alveolar type II cells and decreased the proportion of saturated PC in the surfactant. Two reports have noted decreased levels of SP-A in amniotic fluid from diabetic women compared to non-diabetics.[566,998] In cultured human lung tissue, insulin inhibits the accumulation of SP-A and its mRNA during culture.[254,997]

The incidence of RDS in IDM was also increased by delivering diabetic mothers at 36–37 weeks by elective caesarean section before labour. Improvements in maternal diabetic control during pregnancy have now facilitated delays in delivery until the 39–40th weeks of gestation, and most studies report normal surfactant patterns in IDM. RDS now occurs in <1.0% of such babies,[23,307,593] even though in some the surfactant pattern at amniocentesis remains immature.[811]

Hypothyroidism

Thyroid activity is important in the prenatal development of the surfactant system (p. 473), and this may have therapeutic implications (p. 492). Most studies show that preterm babies who develop RDS have lower levels of thyroid hormones in their cord blood than controls.[231,260] The postnatal nadir in serum thyroxine concentration seen in preterm infants is very low in neonates with RDS.[1126] Although most term babies with congenital hypothyroidism detected by screening do not have RDS, some cases do occur.[204]

Familial predisposition

Families have been reported in which several relatively mature babies have developed RDS. The reason for this is unknown, but it is presumably because of an inherited abnormality in surfactant synthesis.[457] At preterm gestations, if a woman has one baby with RDS the risk of RDS in a subsequent LBW baby may be as high as 90%.[399] In a more recent study[785] the relative risk of RDS in a subsequent preterm infant was 3.3.

Surfactant protein B deficiency (p. 472) results in lethal respiratory failure,[799] which in some has been associated with histopathological features of congenital alveolar proteinosis (p. 648).[798] This abnormality has now been described in families[45,46,798,799] and the inheritance appears to be autosomal recessive.

Twins

Some reports suggest that surfactant synthesis is, if anything, accelerated in twin pregnancies, with faster surfactant maturation in the presenting twin.[1151] This may explain why the second twin is more likely to develop RDS,[803] as this is not always the result of asphyxia.[34] More recent data suggest that there is no difference between twins and singletons.[1166] There is a reasonable concordance in L:S ratios in twins, better in monozygotic than dizygotic pairs.[268,651]

Table 29.9 Neonatal mortality and temperature on admission to special care baby units[1018]

Admission temperature (°C)	Neonatal mortality per 1000 live births: Birthweight <1.5 kg	Birthweight 1.5–2.0 kg
≤32.9	864	636
33–34.9	415	153
≥35.0	373	38

Hypothermia

Postnatal hypothermia worsens the prognosis for preterm babies,[1018] (Table 29.9). There are multiple reasons for the increased mortality, including coagulation disturbances (p. 299). Surfactant function, however, is defective in cold babies;[380] the concomitant hypoxia and acidaemia impair surfactant synthesis;[740] hypothermia in animals induces pulmonary hypertension and a fall in PaO_2;[1163] similar mechanisms may apply to the neonate. In addition, below 34°C, even in the presence of adequate amounts of PG, DPPC cannot spread to form an adequately functioning monolayer.

Nutrition

In animal studies maternal malnutrition compromises fetal surfactant synthesis as well as lung growth.[639,663] Postnatally, although calorie deprivation does not appear to be important,[311] specific deficiencies in fatty acids or inositol may be relevant.[350,454] Inositol supplementation in babies with RDS improves the outcome.[455]

Intrauterine growth retardation

An appropriately grown infant of 28 weeks' gestational age is much more likely to develop severe RDS than a growth-retarded 32-week gestation infant of similar birthweight.[852] Some older studies suggested that at a given gestational age smallness for dates protected against RDS, but the reverse is now known to be the case, with severely growth-retarded infants having a higher incidence of the disease, which is more severe.[852,1069]

Haemolytic disease of the newborn

The development of pulmonary maturity may be delayed in severely affected HDN infants with or without hydrops.[868,1155] The presence of heart failure with proteinaceous pulmonary oedema fluid (p. 854) is very likely to aggravate any pre-existing surfactant deficiency due to prematurity.

Time of cord clamping

Mature babies receiving a placental transfusion do seem to have an increased respiratory morbidity in the first few days.[1186] Conversely, preterm neonates who have undergone early cord clamping and have a low red cell mass, particularly when combined with some degree of birth asphyxia, are also more prone to develop RDS.[295,665,1105] As a consequence, it has been recommended that following preterm delivery the cord should not be clamped until 1–1½ minutes after delivery.[1105] A recent small prospective study of babies less than 33 weeks' gestation showed that a 30-second delay in cord clamping had no effect on mortality, but that the late-clamped babies were easier to ventilate in the first few days and required fewer blood transfusions.[585]

Factors with equivocal effects on the incidence of RDS

Maternal hypertension

The incidence of RDS was reported to be higher in two series of preterm infants of hypertensive mothers than in controls.[1086,1173] This difference may be explained by delivery by caesarean section before labour in such infants (see above). In contrast, no effect of pre-eclampsia with or without growth retardation was demonstrated on the results of lung maturity tests, neonatal morbidity including RDS, or mortality.[349,948] A recent study found RDS in only 15% of babies of mothers with hypertensive pre-eclampsia, compared to 38% of non-hypertensive controls of similar weight and gestation.[967]

Prolonged rupture of membranes

Theoretically, prolonged rupture of the membranes may be advantageous in that it may be associated with preterm labour, which has primed the fetal lungs and it might expose the fetus to 'stress', increasing the hormones which induce surfactant synthesis. Part of this stress, however, could be infection. A review of prolonged rupture of membranes and RDS found that there were as many studies purporting to show benefit as there were demonstrating the reverse.[729] This lack of consistency persists in more recent studies.[448,1173]

Factors reducing the incidence of RDS

Maternal narcotic addiction,[378] smoking[659] and alcohol ingestion[529] all reduce the incidence of RDS, but obviously have no potential therapeutic implications. Heroin, like glucocorticoids, can mature the surfactant-synthesizing systems (p. 493), an effect that has been confirmed in animal studies. The effect of cocaine is as yet unclear,[78,465] although in animal work it induces surfactant synthesis.[1003]

PATHOLOGY OF RESPIRATORY DISTRESS SYNDROME

The initial histological finding[357] is alveolar epithelial cell necrosis, which develops within half an hour of birth. The epithelial cells become detached from the basement membrane and small patches of hyaline membranes form on the denuded areas. At the same time there is diffuse interstitial oedema. The lymphatics are dilated by the delayed clearance of fetal lung fluid, and the capillaries next to the membranes have a sludged appearance. There are very few osmiophilic granules in the type II cells (pp. 467–468), which in places contain vacuoles, suggesting that all the lamellar bodies have been discharged. In the early stages all these changes are rather patchy, but by 24 hours more extensive generalized membrane formation occurs in the transitional ducts and respiratory bronchioles (Figs 29.20, 29.21). Hyaline membranes line the overdistended terminal and respiratory bronchioles, particularly where the airways branch, and may extend into the putative alveolar ducts. The most distal components of the respiratory unit, the terminal sacs, although collapsed, are not lined by membrane. The hyaline membranes are eosinophilic on staining with haematoxylin and eosin, and contain nuclear debris from necrotic pneumocytes. Occasionally, when the infant has hyperbilirubinaemia the membranes are yellow, reflecting the presence of unconjugated bilirubin.[1091] The hyaline membranes are formed by the coagulation of plasma proteins which have leaked on to the lung surface through damaged capillaries and epithelial cells (p. 484); the fibrillary component of the membranes is derived from exuded fibrin.

After 24 hours a few inflammatory cells appear within the airway lumen; macrophages are usually the most prominent, although some polymorphs may also be present. Ingestion of the membrane by macrophages takes place over the next 2 or 3 days as the membrane separates. Macrophages are also present beneath the membrane

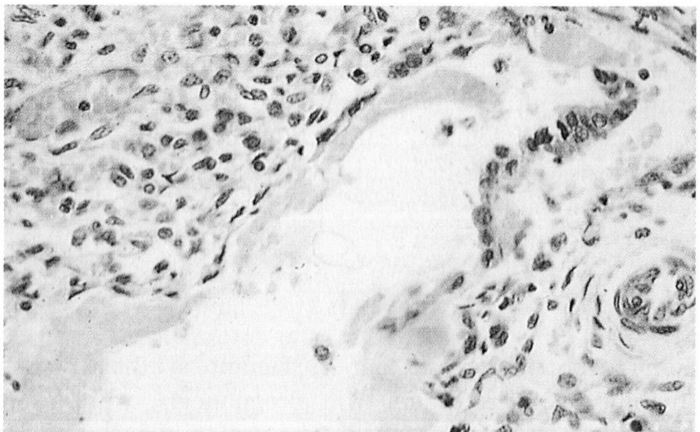

Fig. 29.20 Histology of RDS showing pink staining hyaline membranes lining a terminal bronchiole, with surrounding atelectasis.

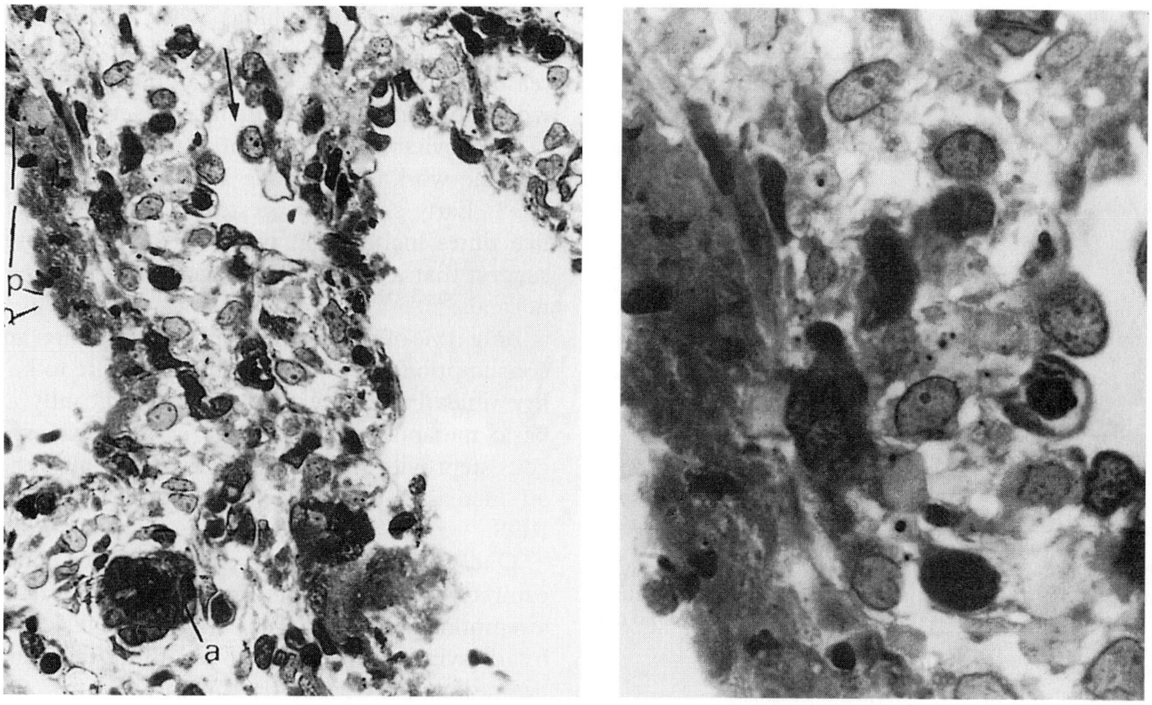

A B

Fig. 29.21 Histology of lung in a baby dying from HMD. (A) Hyaline membranes (h) with pyknotic nuclei (p) of desquamated epithelial cells embedded in it. An adjacent airspace (arrow) is unaffected. An arteriole (a) is very contracted. There is marked interstitial oedema and osmiophilic granules are absent (× 480). (B) Area of hyaline membrane in (A) under higher magnification (× 1100). Reproduced courtesy of Dr G M Gandy.

within the interstitium, which is usually oedematous and where there may be a mild fibroblastic response. Epithelial regeneration is detectable after 48 hours, usually beneath the separating membranes. Cuboidal cells from the unaffected transitional ducts become large and mitotic; they flatten out and spread beneath the hyaline membranes. Other cells produce lamellar bodies. Many of these reparative cells form abnormally thick epithelial squames and, with damaged capillaries, can present a considerable barrier to efficient gas exchange. During this stage of repair, surfactant can be detected in increasing quantities on the alveolar surface.[357]

By 7 days of age in an infant with uncomplicated RDS the hyaline membranes will have disappeared. In ventilated babies, however, the healing process is markedly altered and delayed. There is a hyperplastic healing process, with massive shedding of bronchiolar epithelial cells and type II pneumocytes. Hyaline membranes remain prominent. The terminal airways may be plugged with secretions, and there is progressive scarring and fibrosis of the alveoli and airways, leading to the full-blown picture of chronic lung disease (p. 613).

PATHOPHYSIOLOGY

Lung function

The lung function abnormalities in RDS are predictable from the structure of the immature lung, combined with congestion and atelectasis secondary to surfactant deficiency (Table 29.10). The lungs are non-compliant, approximately 0.3–0.5 ml/cmH_2O/kg when the disease is at its worst.[100,273] As surfactant begins to appear the compliance improves and has usually returned to values of 1–2 ml/cmH_2O/kg[214,744] by 6–7 days of age. Measurements of FRC and TGV show values below normal, ranging from FRC values as low as 3 ml/kg in severe disease[262] to normal values of 25–30 ml/kg in recovering babies.[897] Babies with RDS have a low tidal volume and a large physiological dead space. Minute ventilation may be markedly increased by an elevated respiratory rate in an attempt to sustain alveolar ventilation,[562] but this is usually unsuccessful, resulting in alveolar underventilation and carbon dioxide retention. A further sign of the reduction in lung volume is that the crying vital capacity is also low.[189]

Table 29.10 Values for lung mechanics in RDS (from various sources quoted in text)

Tidal volume (V_T)	4–6 ml/kg
Minute volume (V_E)	250–400 ml/kg/min
Alveolar ventilation (V_A)	50–90 ml/kg/min
Physiological dead space (V_D/V_T)	60–75%
Functional residual capacity (FRC)	3–20 ml/kg
Crying vital capacity	20–30 ml
Dynamic compliance (C_L)	0.0003–0.0005 l/cmH_2O/kg
Inspiratory resistance ($R_{aw\ Insp}$)	55–95 cmH_2O/l/s
Expiratory resistance ($R_{aw\ Exp}$)	140–200 cmH_2O/l/s
Work of breathing	800–3000 g.cm/min/kg

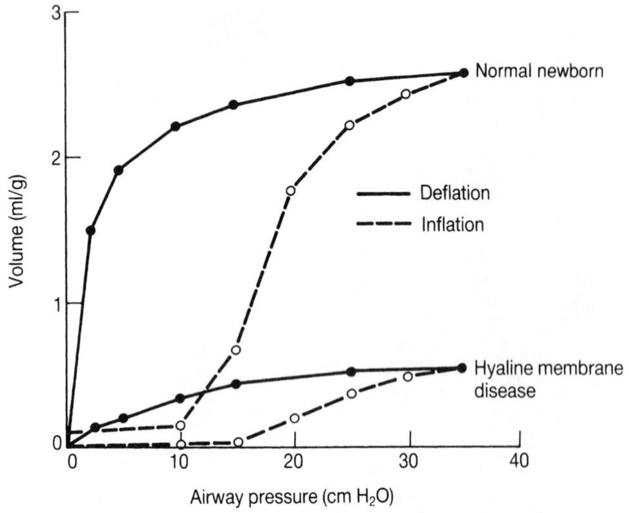

Fig. 29.22 Pressure–volume loops in excised lungs of neonates dying with and without HMD. In HMD the deflation curve closely follows the inflation curve and little air is retained at zero pressure. In normal lungs much more air is retained on the deflation limb of the loop (the phenomenon of hysteresis). Reproduced with permission from Gribetz et al.[432]

Pressure–volume loops on lungs excised at postmortem from babies dying of HMD have a characteristic pattern (Fig. 29.22). During inflation the volume change for a given increase in pressure is very small, and during deflation the change in volume follows a track almost similar to that seen during inflation, whereas in the normal lung air is retained until low volumes are reached (hysteresis). Furthermore, as the pressure drops to zero very little or no air is retained within the surfactant-less alveoli, corresponding to the very small FRC measured in vivo.

Inspiratory resistance is usually normal in RDS,[214,499] but expiratory resistance is increased, probably as a result of the closure of the airway prior to the expiratory grunt.[1033] It is also increased by the presence of an endotracheal tube.[288]

The time constant of the neonatal lung, measured in seconds, is the compliance (l/cmH_2O) multiplied by airways resistance (in cmH_2O/l/s). It is therefore very short in neonates with RDS because of the low compliance:

$$\text{Compliance } 0.001 \text{ l/cmH}_2\text{O} \times \text{resistance } 100 \text{ cmH}_2\text{O/l/s} = \text{time constant } 0.1 \text{ s}$$

The time constant gives a measure of the time available for gas to leave the lung during expiration, which is normally thought to take three time constants. Clinical studies[492,1008] have shown the respiratory rate of infants with RDS to be about 80–90/min, with an average inspiratory time of 0.25–0.35 seconds, which corresponds to a rate that requires minimal work. In infants with less stiff lungs, however, the time constant may not be short enough for those breathing at 80/min, who will still be retaining gas in their lungs when the next inspiration starts.[1033] Arguing teleologically, this may be one of the reasons why neonates breathe quickly, to retain gas within the lungs and maintain some level of FRC.

An inevitable sequel of the abnormal lung mechanics is that the work of breathing is increased in neonates with RDS. Early studies suggested that this was as much as five times higher than normal,[214] but more recent data suggest that it is usually not more than twice that seen in normals.[500,687] In healthy infants the work of breathing is only 1% of the total energy expenditure and oxygen consumption,[1050] so that even if this were to be increased five times in RDS it would not significantly add to the basic metabolic requirements of such patients. This is consistent with the fact that Levison et al[656] did not find an increased oxygen consumption in sick babies with RDS.

One very characteristic clinical feature of RDS is the expiratory grunt. This is the result of the infant attempting to sustain FRC (functional residual capacity) by delaying the escape of air from the lungs during expiration. He tries to do this in two ways: first, during expiration the diaphragm, a primarily inspiratory muscle, still contracts, trying to delay or brake the reduction in thoracic volume and thus retain gas within the alveoli;[244] secondly, by contracting the constrictor muscles of the larynx an attempt is made to close the upper airway, as in the Valsalva manouevre. As the abdominal muscles contract at the same time as the laryngeal muscles relax, there is an explosive exhalation of air, which is the characteristic 'grunt'. Bypassing this laryngeal component of expiratory braking by putting an endotracheal tube through the cords results in a fall in PaO_2 in babies with RDS.[469]

Surfactant

The preterm baby is born with poor reserves of surfactant (p. 482). Most babies, however, have some present in the first few hours of life,[892] and the deterioration so characteristic of the early clinical phase of RDS is due in part to the disappearance of these small quantities, compounded by fatigue as the neonate struggles to sustain ventilation in stiff, surfactant-deficient lungs. The disappearance of surfactant is primarily due to the inhibitory effect on surfactant of proteins (see above;[523]), which leak onto the alveolar surface in the early oedematous stage of lung damage. The deleterious effect of hypoxia and acidaemia on surfactant synthesis (p. 484) may also play a part, but patency of the ductus is not relevant.[20] The levels of surfactant proteins are also low in the first few hours of life in babies with RDS, and rise as the babies recover. The levels will also be increased by the use of exogenous natural surfactants which contain some SP-B and SP-C.[775]

The lungs remain non-compliant and atelectatic until

surfactant begins to reappear, from 36 to 48 hours of age, as detected in the L:S ratios of pharyngeal aspirates,[557] although more refined analysis of the surfactant shows that it may still have an unusual fatty acid composition for several more days.[971] Just because surfactant reappears, however, does not mean that clinical recovery is assured, as CLD (p. 608) can supervene if the lungs have been damaged by barotrauma or oxygen.

Pulmonary hypertension

Studies of pulmonary artery pressure, usually in large, non-ventilated, often diabetic babies with RDS,[773,933] showed it to be high but just below systemic levels, and higher in those with more severe disease. When sudden episodes of hypoxia occurred PAP could rise above systemic level,[537] increasing the right-to-left shunt, which could occur at foramen ovale or ductus level in RDS (see below).

PAP may now be estimated non-invasively using echocardiographic techniques. By measuring the ratio of the time to peak velocity and the right ventricular ejection time it is possible to obtain an indirect marker of PAP: the lower the ratio, the higher the PAP.[303] Alternatively, PAP can be estimated using the Bernoulli equation to measure the right ventricular–right atrial pressure difference and then adding 5 mmHg, which is the average right atrial pressure in RDS.[988] Using both approaches it has been found that PAP remains high throughout the first week, and even longer in some cases of RDS. The more severe the RDS, the higher the PAP, which may remain close to systemic levels in fatal cases[1137] (Fig. 29.23). Furthermore, at least during systole, PAP can be higher than systemic pressure, (Fig. 29.24) at which time there is likely to be right-to-left ductal shunting. In diastole the

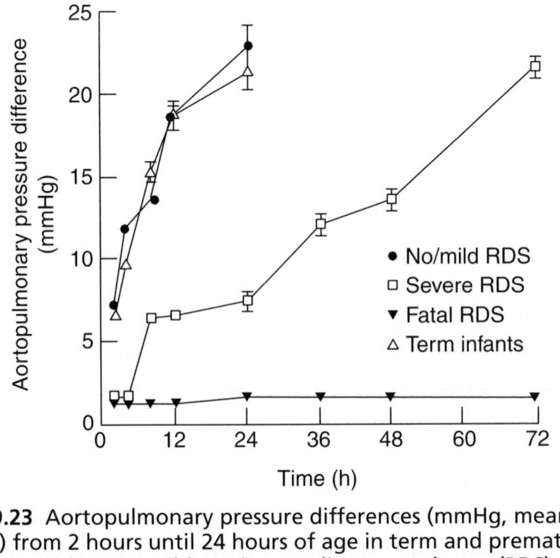

Fig. 29.23 Aortopulmonary pressure differences (mmHg, mean ± SEM) from 2 hours until 24 hours of age in term and premature neonates with no or mild respiratory distress syndrome (RDS) and until 72 hours of age in premature neonates with severe or fatal RDS. Reproduced with permission from Walther et al.[1137]

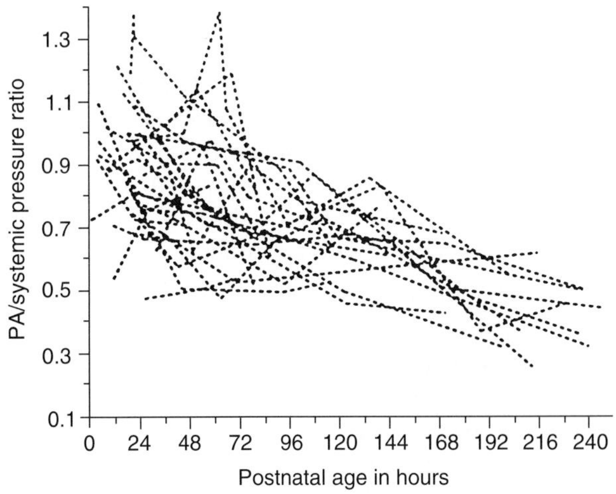

Fig. 29.24 Sequential pulmonary artery/systemic pressure ratios in babies with RDS. At a ratio >1.0, right-to-left shunting across the ductus is a possibility. Reproduced with permission from Skinner et al.[988]

systemic pressure is likely to be higher than the pulmonary pressure, and the overall effect is bidirectional ductal shunting; this is frequently detected echocardiographically in RDS.[303,304,988]

Mechanisms of hypoxia: right-to-left shunt with ventilation–perfusion imbalance

Hypoxaemia in RDS is caused by a large right–left shunt.[1036,1145] There are four main sites of right–left shunts.

1. Obligatory shunts caused by drainage of the veins of the myocardium directly into the left side of the heart, and also by anastomoses between the bronchial and pulmonary circulations. These are present in everyone, are small and of no haemodynamic or clinical significance.

2. Shunting through the foramen ovale occurs if right atrial pressure is higher than left atrial pressure. Interatrial right–left shunting does occur but is rare in neonates with RDS.[305,1016]

3. Shunting through a PDA: the ductus arteriosus is patent in most cases of RDS during the first 48–72 hours.[281,898] If PAP exceeds aortic pressure there will be a significant right–left shunt. Right–left shunts at ductal level are common in persistent pulmonary hypertension of the newborn (p. 527), but in uncomplicated RDS are small and constitute less than 10% of the total right–left shunt.[909,958] One clinically important facet of right–left ductal shunting is that blood drawn from an umbilical artery catheter can have a much lower PaO_2 than blood passing up the carotid arteries to the eyes (p. 503).

Colour Doppler studies of the vascular channels in babies with RDS have demonstrated that intravascular shunting at ductal or foramen ovale level is relatively unusual in uncomplicated RDS (as opposed to PPHN, pp. 527, 531), even though both channels stay potentially patent in the early neonatal period. In fact, the shunt through these channels is predominantly bidirectional or left–right in the first few days of life. This will have little effect on blood gas values, but will increase the cardiac output and the load on the right ventricle.[304,305,958]

4. The true intrapulmonary right–left shunt, when pulmonary capillary blood passes through the lung without coming into contact with a ventilated alveolus.

The combination of 1 to 4 is the true right-to-left shunt. There is another right–left shunt which contributes to the total right–left shunt or venous admixture seen in babies with RDS, and is the result of pulmonary blood flow passing partially ventilated alveoli – ventilation–perfusion imbalance. This large component of the right–left shunt in RDS can be eliminated by giving the baby 100% oxygen to breathe for 15 minutes: the hyperoxia or nitrogen washout test. This eliminates shunting resulting from partially oxygenated alveoli, and a shunt calculated at the end of a period of breathing 100% oxygen is the true shunt as outlined above.

In most babies with RDS the majority of the right-to-left shunt is the fourth component of the true shunt plus this ventilation–perfusion imbalance. The size of the total right–left shunt can be calculated from the following equation:

$$\frac{Qs}{Qt} = \frac{CcO_2 - CaO_2}{CcO_2 - CvO_2}$$

where Qs is the portion of the total cardiac output (Qt) which is shunted, CcO_2 is the end-pulmonary capillary oxygen content, CaO_2 is the arterial oxygen content and CvO_2 is the mixed venous oxygen content.

There are many inaccuracies inherent in this calculation, in particular the estimate of the mixed venous PO_2. Nevertheless, it can be used to derive charts from which the shunt can be read off knowing the infant's PaO_2 and the inspired oxygen concentration (Fig. 29.25).

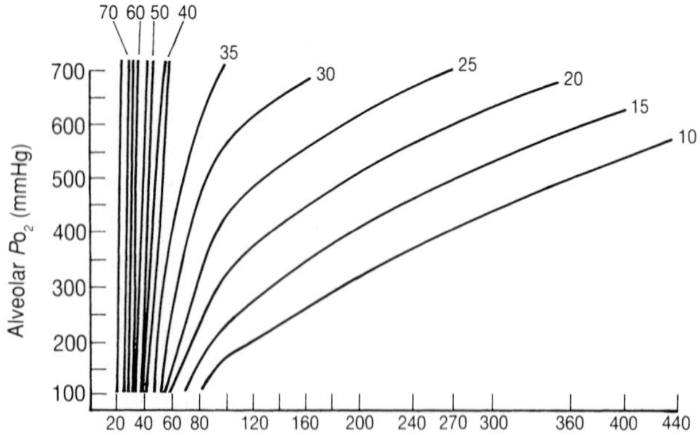

Fig. 29.25 Diagram showing the percentage shunt at different inspired oxygen concentrations and arterial PaO_2 values. The alveolar PO_2 is calculated using the alveolar air equation. Reproduced with permission from Gupta et al.[443]

Another way of estimating the severity of the lung disease is to measure the A–aDO_2, the alveolar–arterial oxygen difference; the higher this is, the more severe the disease. The only inaccuracies here are the calculation of the P_AO_2 from the alveolar air equation

$$P_AO_2 = P_IO_2 - \left[\frac{P_ACO_2}{R} + \left(P_ACO_2 \times F_IO_2 \times \frac{1-R}{R}\right)\right]$$

where P_IO_2 is the partial pressure of inspired oxygen (i.e. 100% oxygen = approximately 760 mmHg – water vapour pressure); P_ACO_2 is assumed to be the same as $PaCO_2$, though this is unlikely to be strictly true in severe cases of RDS; R is the respiratory quotient, assumed to be 0.8; and F_IO_2 is the fractional inspired oxygen concentration (100% oxygen = 1.0).

Carbon dioxide retention

The increased $PaCO_2$ in RDS is due to hypoventilation secondary to atelectasis, decreased tidal volume and increased dead space. Ventilation is also non-homogeneous, so that unlike the situation in patients with normal lungs, in whom end-tidal P_ACO_2 is a good measure of $PaCO_2$, in babies with RDS there is a risk that measurement of P_ACO_2 will seriously underestimate $PaCO_2$.[613]

Since the mixed venous $PvCO_2$ (normally 6.13 kPa, 46 mmHg) is usually only a fraction of a kilopascal above arterial or alveolar $PaCO_2$ (normally 5.33 kPa, 40 mmHg), the right–left shunt has to be enormous before the admixture of venous blood contributes significantly to hypercapnia in RDS.

PREVENTION OF RDS

Prevention of prematurity

The pathophysiology of preterm labour is as yet unsolved, and although some studies purport to have reduced the incidence of prematurity by manipulation of economic variables[821] the results are generally not convincing.[976,1123] Social improvements that reduce the incidence of prematurity are likely to be offset by the increased preparedness of obstetricians to deliver seriously ill women at gestations below 30 weeks, who in the past would have been allowed to abort or have an intrauterine death, and also by the increase in higher multiples delivering prematurely after ovulation induction or in-vitro fertilization (Chapter 25).

Tocolytic drugs to prevent preterm labour have in general proved disappointing,[583,644] although they may have a limited role in prolonging labour for 24–48 hours while dexamethasone (see below) is administered.[151] Nitric oxide donors such as glyceryl trinitrate, used in the form of patches, may prove effective and to date the only significant side-effect is headache, which affects 20% of patients.[641] There is clear evidence that genital tract infection is associated with preterm labour, and in women with preterm rupture of the membranes there is evidence that treatment with antibiotics reduces the prematurity rate.[386]

Antenatal steroid therapy

The serendipitous discovery by Liggins[661] that infusion of glucocorticoids to induce preterm labour in sheep produced preterm lambs with a reduced incidence of lung disease led to one of the most intensively investigated topics in neonatology in the last quarter century. It is now established that antenatal administration of dexamethasone or betamethasone to women in preterm labour significantly reduces the incidence of RDS, but also several other serious complications of prematurity, including GMH/IVH, NEC and PDA[230,1143] (Table 29.11). However, not all steroids cross the placenta: cortisol is largely inactivated, but degradation is resisted by synthetic steroids such as betamethasone and dexamethasone. Betamethasone has a maternal:fetal gradient of 3:1 and dexamethasone a gradient of 1:1.[49,80]

The effects of antenatal steroids are complex[48] (Table 29.11) and include inducing the enzymes for surfactant synthesis, the genes for the production of the surfactant proteins A, B, C and D,[734] and improving the quality of the surfactant produced.[1097] Glucocorticoids such as dexamethasone can cause substantial stimulation of SP-B gene expression to 2–3 times adult levels in fetal lung explants.[83] They mature the non-surfactant producing tissues of the lung,[142,626] and the septa become longer, thinner and less cellular, with larger air spaces and increased numbers of alveolar divisions.

The benefit is maximal in babies delivered between 24 and 168 hours of starting the maternal therapy[230] (Fig. 29.26). A smaller but probably useful benefit is also seen in women receiving less than 24 hours of therapy. No benefit accrues from repeated courses of therapy,[48] which may even be detrimental by suppressing the maternal and fetal hypothalamo–pituitary–adrenal axis,[50] as well as increasing the risk of maternal hyperglycaemia and infection. Neonatal Cushing syndrome has been reported after

Table 29.11 Some benefits of antenatal steroids

Improved Apgar scores	Gardner et al[359]
Maturation of lung structure	Bunton and Plopper[142] Lanteri et al[626]
Initiation of surfactant apoprotein synthesis	Mendelson et al[734]
Improved NO-mediated pulmonary venous relaxation	Zhou et al[1209]
Reduced pulmonary capillary leakiness	Ikegami et al[524]
Interaction with postnatal exogenous surfactant therapy	p. 492
Increased resistance to high oxygen exposure	Frank[339]
Better blood pressure in early neonatal period	Moise et al[755]
Higher neonatal white cell counts	Barak et al[59]
Less patent ductus arteriosus	Ward[1143] Eronen et al[299]
Less GMH/IVH	Ward[1143] Crowley[230] Garland et al[363] (Fig. 29.28)
Less NEC	Ward[1143] (Fig. 29.28)

repeated antenatal courses of steroids.[125] Conversely, they may depress the neonatal adrenal gland when used in conventional doses.[560]

The combination of steroids given prenatally with surfactant postnatally has been shown to be beneficial in animals[182] and there are data to show clinical benefit (Fig. 29.27),[543] although none of the human data come from prospective trials.

Gestational age

In the original study by Liggins and Howie[662] the greatest benefit was seen at gestations of 30–34 weeks, with a much smaller although statistically significant benefit below 30 weeks. Crowley's[230] meta-analysis (Fig. 29.26) demonstrated a benefit at less than 31 weeks, but evidence for benefit under 28 weeks is less strong.[271,360]

Preterm rupture of membranes

Although there has been concern that antenatal steroids may increase risk of infection, with appropriate clinical surveillance this did not seem to be a problem in the studies reviewed by Crowley[230] (Fig. 29.28).

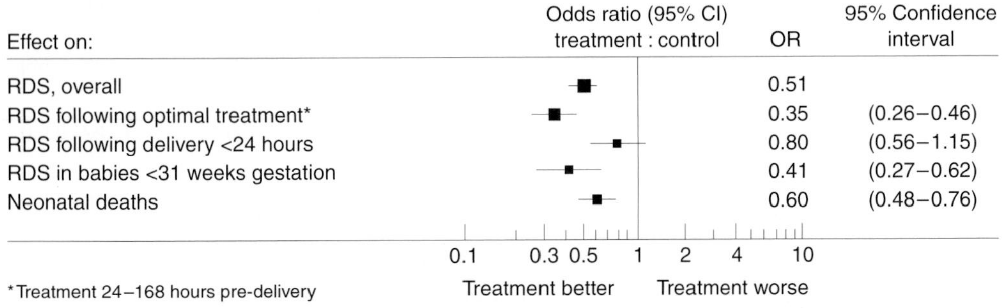

Fig. 29.26 Benefits of antenatal use of steroids. Adapted with permission from Crowley.[230]

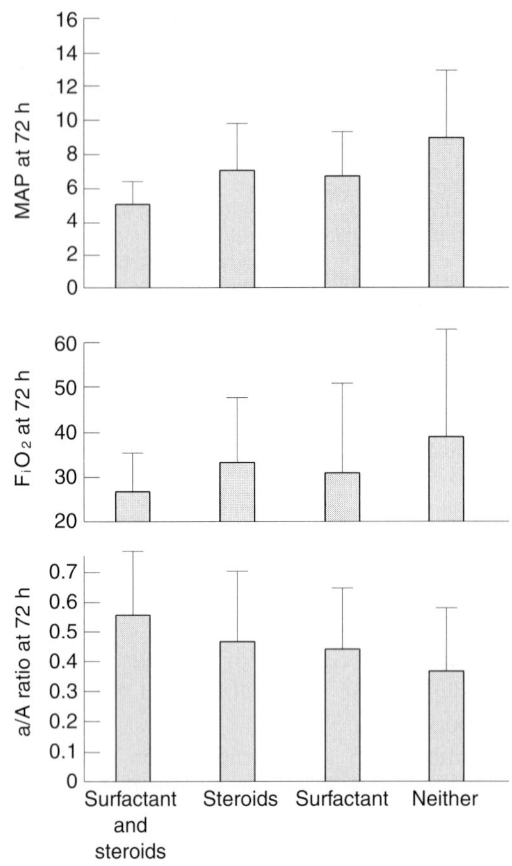

Fig. 29.27 Effects of maternal corticosteroids and surfactant on respiratory variables at 72 hours of age. Mean ±SD values are shown for MAP in cmH_2O, F_IO_2 as percentage of oxygen, and arterial-to-alveolar oxygenation ratio (a/A ratio). Infants ventilated at 72 hours and receiving both corticosteroids and surfactant required lower MAP than all other groups (P <0.006), whereas those receiving neither treatment had higher mean airway pressures than all other groups (P <0.006). Infants treated with both surfactant and corticosteroids had lower inspired concentrations than those receiving corticosteroid alone (P <0.05) or infants of either group not treated with corticosteroids (P <0.005). Similarly, the mean arterial-to-alveolar oxygenation ratio tended to be higher for the combined treatment groups than for corticosteroids alone (P =0.065), and the combined treatment group had a higher arterial-to-alveolar oxygenation ratio than the other groups not receiving corticosteroids (P <0.001). Corticosteroid treatment alone improved the arterial-to-alveolar oxygenation ratio relative to the infants receiving neither treatment (P <0.02). Reproduced with permission from Jobe et al.[543]

Maternal hypertension

Liggins and Howie[662] reported that steroid-treated hypertensive women had a significantly increased stillbirth rate and perinatal mortality. This resulted in many subsequent workers excluding such women from trials,[230] but clinical experience and observational studies suggest that steroids can be used safely in this situation.[624]

Diabetes

Glucocorticoids have been avoided in diabetic pregnancies because of their potential for causing hyperglycaemia, but nowadays the insulin regimen can be altered during the brief period of hyperglycaemia. Steroids switch on the surfactant protein-synthesizing systems in experimental diabetic rats.[753]

Twins

Where separate analysis has been done, dexamethasone has not benefited multiple pregnancies;[1094] whether this is a statistical artefact due to small numbers, or whether bigger doses of steroids should be given with multiple fetuses, remains speculative.

General effects

As well as the specific benefits for RDS outlined above, antenatal steroids appear to have a generally beneficial effect in preterm infants (Table 29.11). Some of these are as a consequence of reducing the incidence and severity of RDS, whereas others represent the maturing effect of steroids on many body systems. The interaction with the benefits of postnatal exogenous surfactant therapy is of particular importance (Fig. 29.27). Follow-up of steroid-treated babies shows no excess of handicap compared to controls.[272,686]

Thyroid preparations

Thyroid hormones are involved in the induction of surfactant synthesis.[47,387] There are reports of apparent

Study reference	No. events treatment	No. events control	Odds ratio (95% CI) treatment : control	OR	95% Confidence interval
RDS after steroids with premature membrane rupture	83/456	139/421		0.44	(0.32–0.66)
PVH in infants of treated mothers	19/999	50/998		0.38	(0.23–0.94)
NEC in infants of treated mothers	9/524	27/517		0.32	(0.16–0.64)

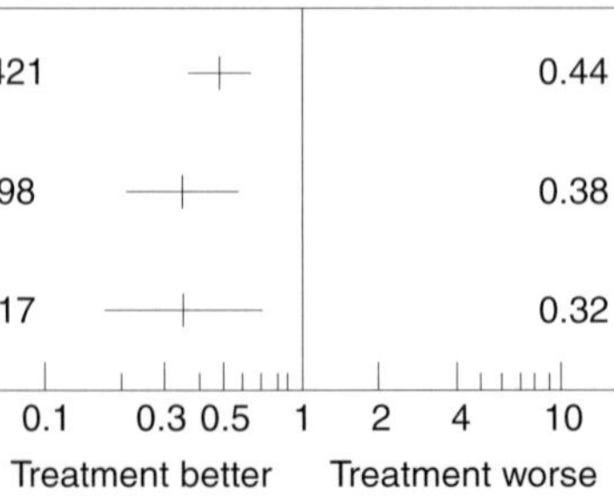

Fig. 29.28 Other benefits of antenatal steroids. Adapted with permission from Crowley.[230]

success with intra-amniotic therapy[922] as thyroid hormones and TSH do not cross the placenta, but most workers have studied the administration of TRH to the mother, usually in combination with dexamethasone. There is a consistent synergism between TRH and steroids in animal studies.[757,859] The result of an initial study in humans[758] was also promising. Subsequently a prospective study showed a significant reduction of RDS,[601] but in another study only the incidence of BPD in survivors was reduced, albeit significantly.[51] The most recent studies,[6,50a,212a] however, showed no benefit from TRH. It appears therefore that there is no benefit from the antenatal administration of TRH if antenatal steroids and postnatal surfactant are used.

Other antenatal drugs

Various drugs have been used in animal experiments to mature the surfactant synthetic pathways. These include opiates,[378] aminophylline[564] and ambroxol,[914] the last having been used with benefit in humans.[1147] Some,[1184] but not all,[317] animal experiments suggest that antenatal betamimetics may improve neonatal lung function. If there is an effect in the human neonate it appears to be small.[627]

Prevention of intrapartum asphyxia

Asphyxiated preterm neonates have an increased incidence of RDS (p. 484). If asphyxia is absent and the preterm neonate is presenting by the vertex, there is no need to proceed to caesarean section on a routine basis,[13] but if fetal distress develops delivery by caesarean section should be considered even at early gestations. During vaginal delivery of the preterm neonate a wide episiotomy is probably indicated and, although the routine use of forceps has been thought to be of no benefit,[62] recent data[969] suggest that in babies less than 1750 g it does reduce the incidence of GMH/IVH.

Routine caesarean section for preterm babies presenting by the breech is much more controversial. There are as yet no randomized controlled trials assessing the benefits or hazards of such a policy but, albeit at the expense of a considerably increased maternal morbidity, the current balance of opinion is in favour of caesarean section[511,581] for neonates less than 1500 g presenting by the breech, in particular to prevent problems of head entrapment.[113]

Prevention of postnatal asphyxia

After delivery, the neonatal paediatrician has a major responsibility to prevent postnatal asphyxia by prompt and vigorous resuscitation, to minimize those early neonatal events which are likely to increase the severity and complications of RDS. In theory there are three ways in which this effect is mediated.

1. By preventing postnatal hypoxic damage to lung capillaries, thereby minimizing the risk of pulmonary oedema and RDS. In both fetal and neonatal animals asphyxia can cause pulmonary oedema. This is the result of both an increase in filtration pressure in the microcirculation and hypoxic–ischaemic damage to the capillary and alveolar lining cells.[8,245,466] Oedema is an early histological feature of RDS (p. 486) and its presence on the alveolar surface inhibits surfactant activity (p. 484).[523] It is clear that these changes can be minimized or prevented by prompt, efficient resuscitation.[91]

2. By rapidly establishing normal blood gases and normal pulmonary perfusion. During resuscitation lowering $P\text{aCO}_2$ increasing $P\text{aO}_2$ and even ventilation itself all have an important role in maximizing perfusion and lowering pulmonary artery pressure.[161] At resuscitation, therefore, by using IPPV (p. 255) the baby's blood gases should be brought into the normal range as quickly as possible. Achieving normal blood gases is also important for sustaining surfactant synthesis. Merritt and Farrell,[740] in monkey lung tissue slices, showed that DPPC synthesis was pH sensitive, and that a fall in the pH of the tissue culture supernatant to just 7.20 was associated with reduced synthesis (Fig. 29.19).

3. By ensuring maximum surfactant release from the type II pneumocytes. The factors controlling surfactant release at birth are complex, but adequate expansion of the lungs is of considerable importance (pp. 248–249). Very low-birthweight neonates with a compliant, collapsible chest wall and weak muscles have great difficulty in achieving an adequate ventilatory excursion immediately after delivery, and there is, therefore, the potential for a vicious cycle being created (Fig. 29.29). Poor ventilation, leading to poor surfactant release, results in hypoxia, hypercapnia and acidaemia, which make things worse. These data led to the conclusion that unless a baby of <30 weeks' gestation and <1.50 kg birthweight is in excellent condition at 30 seconds of age, and is crying and vigorous, he should be actively resuscitated by

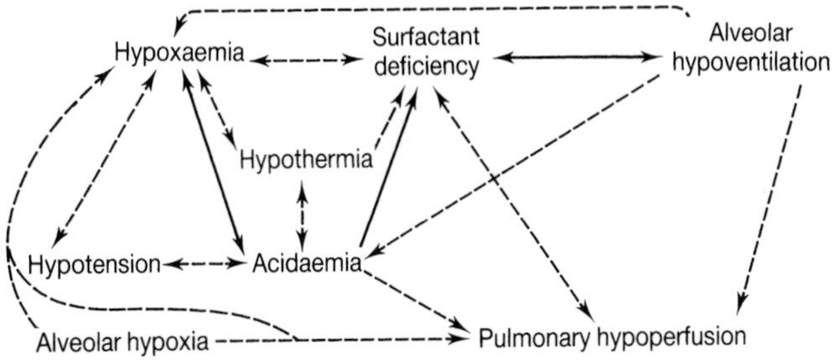

Fig. 29.29 Interrelationship of factors affecting surfactant and other components of lung function; solid lines indicate major effects. Reproduced with permission from Roberton.[907]

intubation and IPPV. This approach has been shown to reduce the morbidity and mortality from RDS.[274,918]

Avoiding drug depression

Many drugs given to the mother in preterm labour, including opiate analgesics, anaesthetic agents, benzodiazepines and the drugs used to control fulminating eclampsia, such as magnesium sulphate and chlormethiazole, can cause marked hypotonia and respiratory depression. The neonatologist must adapt care so that the impact of the drugs on the neonate is minimized or averted. In general, apart from using the specific opiate antagonist naloxone (p. 258) (except in infants of drug-addicted mothers, in whom naloxone will precipitate drug withdrawal signs in the neonate), this means ventilating the infant from the moment of birth until the drugs are excreted or metabolized, and is a further justification for the active policy of resuscitation outlined above.

Fetal hypocapnia

This can be secondary to maternal hypocapnia (p. 247) and may delay the spontaneous onset of respiration. Such infants require early intubation and sufficient ventilatory support to allow the $PaCO_2$ levels to rise into the normal range.

Maternal fluid overload

Excessive fluid administration to the mother in labour may result in neonatal hyponatraemia,[1058] which in turn seems to predispose to pneumothorax if the baby does develop RDS.[754]

Prophylactic surfactant

No new therapy in neonatal care has been subjected to such rigorous scrutiny; as stated by Lucey,[681] 'We now have a therapy which we know works and is safe'.

Many varieties of surfactant have been used (Table 29.12), of which Survanta, Curosurf and Exosurf are the most widely administered. Excellent reviews of their use have been published.[218,737,1001]

There are still controversies regarding the best surfactant, mechanism of action, dosage regimen, efficacy in babies weighing less than 0.75 kg and, in particular, whether it should be given prophylactically in the labour ward or as rescue therapy once the baby has clearly developed RDS. These topics are dealt with on page 508.

A large number of studies carried out using prophylactic surfactant – that is, administering surfactant within the first few minutes of life following intubation for resuscitation in the labour ward – have been submitted to

Table 29.12 Surfactants used in clinical studies

Type of surfactant	Animal source	Composition (or additives if animal derived)	Dose
Animal lung wash			
Surfactant TA	Cow	DPPC, palmitic acid triglyceride	120 mg/kg
Survanta	Cow	Similar to surfactant TA	100 mg/kg
Infasurf (CLSE)	Cow		100 mg/kg
Curosurf	Pig		100 mg/kg
Alveofact SF-RI 1	Cow		100 mg/kg
Human surfactant	Liquor amnii		
Artificial surfactant			
Belfast		DPPC+HDL	
ALEC (Pumactant)		70% DPPC 30% PG	100 mg/kg
Exosurf		DPPC+tyloxapol and hexadecanol	67.5 mg/kg
Surfactant KL_4	Cow	Synthetic SP-B analogue made of lysine+leucine	

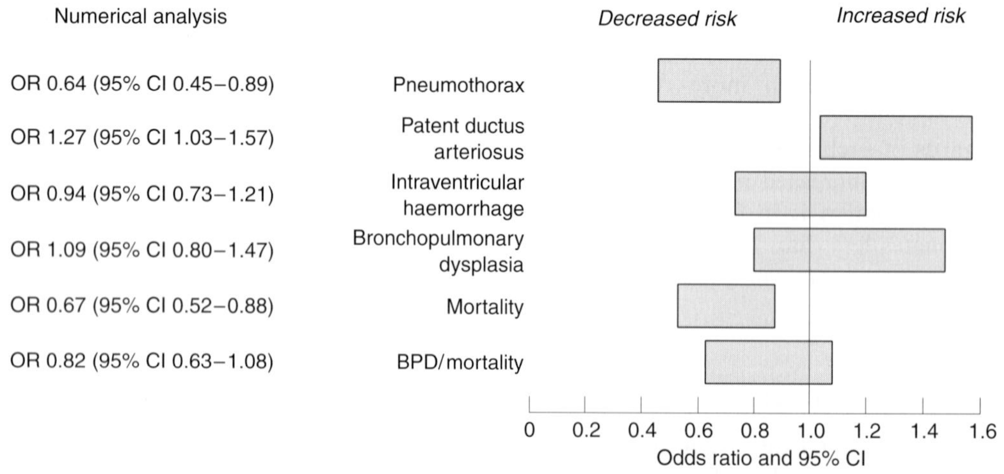

Fig. 29.30 Typical estimates of odds ratios for major complications associated with prematurity: overview from seven randomized controlled trials of prophylactic administration of synthetic surfactant.

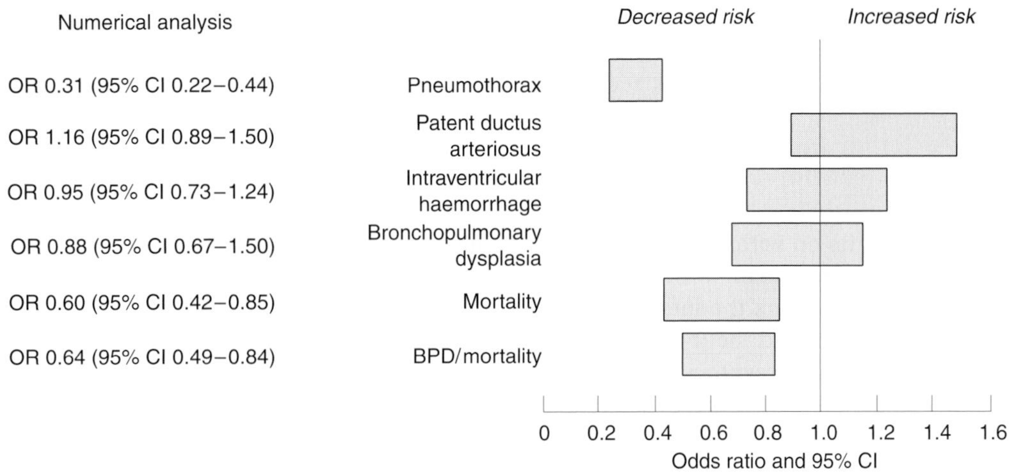

Fig. 29.31 Typical estimates of odds ratios for major complications associated with prematurity: overview from eight randomized controlled trials of prophylactic administration of natural surfactant extract.

meta-analysis and the outcomes are shown in Figures 29.30 and 29.31.[1001] The trials included were all subtly different: some gave only a single prophylactic dose; in others one or two extra doses were administered in the next 24 hours; the gestations studied varied, as did the dose of surfactant given. It can be seen, however, that prophylactic use of both synthetic and natural surfactants results in a significant reduction in pneumothorax, mortality and mortality + BPD; prophylactic synthetic surfactant causes a small but significant increase in the incidence of PDA. Disappointingly, there was no effect on the incidence of GMH/IVH or BPD alone.

All trials of surfactant therapy have shown a reduction in oxygen requirements. In five of the prophylactic trials there was a reduction in the oxygen requirement within an hour of birth, which increased at 24 hours; by 72 hours the effect was waning, except when ALEC was used.[763] Similar improvements in the ventilator pressures used have been reported, but only some trials report a reduction in the time on IPPV.[608] Technical problems have led to confusion regarding the effect of surfactant on compliance: the early improvements may not be detected by dynamic compliance measurements.[573] Surfactant also results in an elevation of lung volume[225] in association with increased oxygenation.[265]

CLINICAL FEATURES OF RDS

The diagnostic criteria for RDS were laid down before the era of neonatal intensive care.[929] These are:

- a respiratory rate above 60/min;
- grunting expiration;
- indrawing of the sternum, intercostal spaces and lower ribs during inspiration (Fig. 29.32);
- cyanosis without oxygen.

These signs must develop before the neonate is 4 hours old, and persist beyond 24 hours of age. Included in the definition, however, are those neonates whose lung disease is so severe that they have to be started on IPPV by 4 hours of age, or who die before 24 hours of age. A neonate who meets these diagnostic criteria is said to have respiratory distress, and the clinical features are present not only in the surfactant-deficient respiratory distress syndrome but in most of the other neonatal lung diseases (pp. 498–499).

General appearance (Fig. 29.32)

The baby in oxygen will be pink; pallor is an ominous feature and requires urgent investigation (p. 817). The capillary filling time should be rapid (<1 s); if it is not,

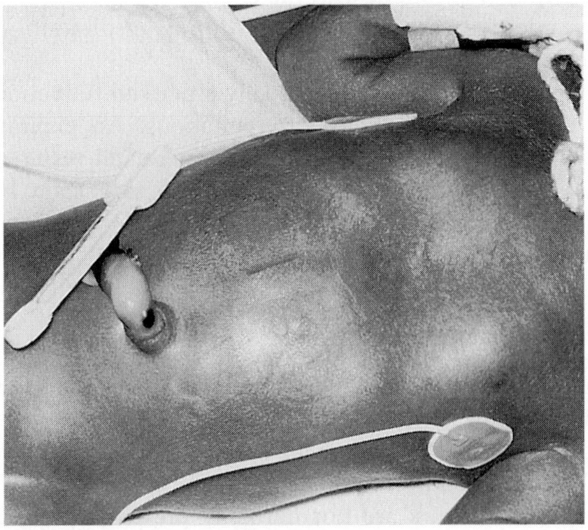

Fig. 29.32 Baby with RDS showing sternal and mild intercostal recession.

this abnormal sign is as ominous as pallor. The baby is usually hypotonic and lies in the frog position, with few spontaneous movements. Oedema is common, secondary to leaky capillaries.[528]

Natural history

By definition the disease comes on within the first 4 hours of life. In the absence of treatment with exogenous surfactant, over the next 24–36 hours the infant tires, the dyspnoea worsens (see below) and he becomes more oedematous. As he starts to resynthesize his own surfactant, the severity of the disease begins to abate from 36–48 hours of age, and this is often associated with a spontaneous diuresis (p. 506). If all goes well, the neonate who does not need ventilation will be asymptomatic with normal blood gases in room air by 7–10 days of age. If he has to be ventilated, however, the natural history may be much more prolonged; the earlier he is ventilated the shorter his gestation, and the harder he has to be ventilated the more prolonged his illness is likely to be.

Respiratory signs

The more mature baby with RDS may breathe at a fast rate, exceeding 100/min. This is more efficient in terms of the work of breathing. Some babies may alternate a breathing pattern of shallow tachypnoea, up to 100–120/min, with one in which they breathe comparatively slowly (say 40–60/min) with marked recession and grunting. The slow-breathing baby often has episodes of apnoea, and this is a sign that his respiration is beginning to fail.[244]

In addition to tachypnoea there is marked intercostal and sternal recession and flaring of the alae nasi. The respiration is primarily diaphragmatic, and with the compliant preterm rib cage this results in a marked see-saw pattern of respiration, with the chest moving inwards and the abdomen moving outwards during inspiration, and vice versa.

On auscultation there is usually a marked reduction in air entry, with a few sticky crepitations. An expiratory grunt is a feature of most forms of neonatal respiratory disease, and is an attempt by the baby to sustain FRC (p. 487). In uncomplicated RDS these clinical features gradually return to normal by 7 days.

Cardiovascular signs

The heart rate in mild to moderate cases of RDS is 140–160/min and shows normal variability. In infants with severe RDS it tends to be slower (120/min), with little beat-to-beat variation.[144,930] The heart sounds are normal. Murmurs are not normally present; if heard in the first 24–48 hours they suggest congenital heart disease or ischaemic myocardial injury, and require further investigation (p. 704). A murmur appearing after 3–4 days is usually due to a patent ductus (p. 512). Heart failure is not a feature of RDS; if present, it suggests cardiac disease.

Neonates with RDS are hypotensive,[787,933] and hypotension correlates with a poor prognosis.[353,447,456,633] It is less common, however, in those babies who receive antenatal steroids.[755]

There are many causes for the hypotension. Illness, hypoxia and acidaemia from any cause can depress the myocardium and reduce cardiac output. The baby may also have a low blood volume for many reasons: he may have missed his placental transfusion at birth;[1186] in the oedematous, ill neonate the plasma volume may have been further depleted by loss of fluid into the subcutaneous tissues or lungs; and all preterm neonates have a high transepidermal water loss (p. 290). All this can be compounded by two iatrogenic problems. The first is removing blood for biochemical, haematological and blood gas analysis; the second is IPPV which, when high pressures are used, can compromise venous return and reduce cardiac output (p. 574).

Hypotension and RDS have a complex interrelationship. Hypotension predisposes to acidaemia, which increases pulmonary vascular resistance,[932] which will also be increased by the release of angiotension II[133] in response to the systemic hypotension. The vicious cycles outlined in Figure 29.29 centre on acidaemia; hypotension also predisposes to GMH/IVH (pp. 1256–1257), renal failure (p. 1027) and NEC (p. 748). Hypotension present in the first hour can set all these adverse effects in train. It is therefore essential to measure the blood pressure and to correct hypotension as soon after admission to the neonatal unit as possible. Normal blood pressure values are given in Appendix 4.

The two other dramatic effects of RDS on the cardiovascular system are pulmonary hypertension (p. 489) and patency of the ductus arteriosus (p. 512).

Central nervous system

Even without RDS the preterm infant is hypotonic, inactive, and lies in the frog position. He spends 22–23 hours per day asleep. His fontanelle feels normal. He responds normally to pain or being disturbed, and his general neurological examination is normal, as are the neurological features used for gestational age assessment (p. 283). Abnormal neurological signs are often subtle (pp. 1209, 1257), but if present they are ominous, often suggesting a GMH/IVH.

Abdominal examination

Examination of the abdomen is usually unremarkable; the liver, spleen and kidneys are often palpable but are rarely significantly enlarged. Hepatosplenomegaly suggests heart failure or sepsis and should be dealt with accordingly. An easily felt liver in an infant with severe respiratory failure might suggest a right tension pneumothorax (p. 518).

Most babies with severe RDS have an ileus[284] and they do not pass meconium. An improvement in their general condition is often heralded by the appearance of bowel sounds and the passage of meconium, though gastric emptying may still be delayed.[1196] Jaundice is not uncommon and, if detected, the level of bilirubin must always be measured. Phototherapy and exchange transfusion are indicated in preterm infants at much lower levels than in the full-term neonate (p. 721).

DIFFERENTIAL DIAGNOSIS

The majority of severe neonatal lung disease presents within the first 4–6 hours of life (p. 495). After this age, as long as the baby has been adequately observed from 0 to 6 hours of age, the two major causes of respiratory illness are pneumonia and the dyspnoea of heart failure secondary to heart disease. Other conditions, such as aspiration and inhalation of the feed, some malformations, and occasionally a small pneumothorax, can present after 6 hours of age, but these are rare (Table 29.13). The differential diagnosis in the first 6 hours can usually be made on the basis of the history (including the gestation), the clinical examination, the blood gases and the chest X-ray (Table 29.13); the only difficulties arise with term babies who have persistent pulmonary hypertension and in neonates who are infected.

Pneumonia/septicaemia

Differentiating pneumonia – usually with septicaemia – from other forms of neonatal lung disease is to an extent a fruitless exercise, since confronted by a dyspnoeic infant in the first hour or two of life it is impossible on the basis of tests which give an answer within 60–90 minutes to exclude infection as the cause of the baby's symptoms. Furthermore, infection with GBS can coexist with RDS.[532] The features suggesting that sepsis is present in the first 6 hours are given on pages 1116 and 1128. However, a major effort should be made to establish whether infection is present within this period, since if it is confirmed more vigorous anti-infection therapy may be indicated, including higher dosages of antibiotics, immunoglobulin infusions or exchange transfusion (p. 1126).

Persistent pulmonary hypertension

Primary PPHN (p. 526) can be differentiated by the absence of significant parenchymal lung disease and the relevant echocardiographic findings (pp. 528, 531). Establishing with ultrasound those babies with RDS who also have marked PHT,[1137] although not identifying a separate clinical condition, may be of value if pulmonary vasodilator therapy, particularly with nitric oxide, is contemplated and available.

INVESTIGATION

Haematological

There are no unique haematological findings in RDS. The haemoglobin will vary with the local practice for cord clamping;[1186] neonates who develop RDS may be more anaemic.[665,1105] Anaemia may develop later due to GMH/IVH (p. 1257) or iatrogenic losses (p. 839).

Results of measurements of the coagulation system are often prolonged due to prematurity in infants with RDS, although DIC is rare. If present, it suggests complications such as birth asphyxia, septicaemia or a GMH-IVH.[186,715]

The white blood count will be normal for the baby's birthweight and gestation[712] (Appendix 1). Thrombocytopenia is not a feature of RDS unless there is DIC (p. 803) or the baby is ventilated.[53]

Biochemical

In the past, preterm babies with RDS were often hypernatraemic and had potassium values >7.0 mmol/l,[830,1101] and the treatment of RDS in the early 1960s by infusion of glucose and bicarbonate was in part designed to combat the hyperkalaemia.[1102] More recent biochemical surveillance, in which adequate standards of neonatal intensive care have been applied from the moment of delivery, has shown a more normal plasma electrolyte pattern, although marked early hyponatraemia can be seen if the mother has been overloaded with fluid during labour[1058] (p. 494). Hyperkalaemia of unknown cause is still occasionally seen in VLBW neonates with apparently normal renal function and urine output.[129,439] The plasma calcium is frequently low in the first 48–72 hours in ill LBW infants, reaching levels of 1.5–1.7 mmol/l in many cases.[910]

Although VLBW infants are prone to hypoglycaemia[223] (p. 942), when sick they are also susceptible to hyperglycaemia[849] (p. 950).

Infants with RDS have impaired renal function, with a reduced glomerular filtration rate and renal plasma flow and a correspondingly raised urea and creatinine;[441] they are also poor at excreting hydrogen ions.[15] If they are fluid restricted (p. 505) a mild to moderate elevation of plasma urea, creatinine and osmolarity is common, but this is an acceptable trade-off for the benefits of preventing the complications of fluid overload, particularly PDA (p. 512) and NEC (p. 748), and possibly reducing the incidence of chronic lung disease.[1053]

Serum albumin levels are often below 25–30 g/l in preterm infants,[158] and are lower in the cord blood of babies who develop RDS than in controls.[106] The albumin may remain below 25 g/l for days or even weeks

Table 29.13 Differential diagnosis of dyspnoea in the neonate

Condition	Gestational age	History	Examination[a]	Gases[b]	Presentation[c] <6 h	Presentation[c] >6 h	Chest radiograph	Comments
Respiratory distress syndrome	Prem				+++	N	Diagnostic but see pp. 500–501	Working diagnosis in all preterm neonates unless chest radiograph suggests alternative. Always consider infection (p. 497)
Transient tachypnoea	FT >prem[d]	Often CS delivery		Mild hypoxaemia needing 40% O_2	+++	R	Diagnostic but see p. 515	Commonest cause of breathlessness in term babies. By definition, a mild disease (p. 514)
Meconium aspiration	FT[e]	Meconium-stained liquor at resuscitation. Postmaturity	Meconium-stained baby. Meconium in larynx		+++	N	Streaky	Diagnosis obvious on history. Infection may co-exist
Pneumothorax or pneumediastinum	FT >prem	May be excessive resuscitation at birth			++	R[f]	Diagnostic	
Massive pulmonary haemorrhage	Prem >FT	Asphyxia or other cause of heart failure, bleeding tendency. Use of artificial surfactant	Crepitations; usually marked pallor. Blood up larynx or in endotracheal tube. PDA after presentation		+	+++	Unhelpful; usually a whiteout	Diagnosis based on clinical findings
After severe asphyxia	FT[g]	Severe asphyxia. Low Apgar	Other features of asphyxia (p. 1238)	Marked metabolic acidaemia	++	N	Unhelpful	Tachypnoea driven by acidaemia
Infection (pneumonia)	Any	May be helpful	Rarely differentiates this from other causes of dyspnoea	Often severe acidaemia and easy to reduce CO_2 without increasing PaO_2	++	+++	Unhelpful in most cases though may show patchy changes	Impossible to exclude in any baby (p. 497). This is the working diagnosis in the absence of specific chest radiograph findings in neonates >6 hours old with respiratory disease. WBC.CRP may be helpful (pp. 1124, 1143).
Congenital malformations	FT >prem	Usually normal delivery. May have been detected on antenatal ultrasound	Rarely helpful	May be profound hypoxaemia with raised CO_2	+++	+	Virtually always diagnostic	Diaphragmatic hernia, cysts, effusions, agenesis all present this way. TOF should not present this way (p. 771)
Congenital heart disease	FT >prem		Murmurs, heart size, signs of heart failure	CO_2 normal or reduced. In cyanotic CHD PaO_2 rarely >6–7 kPa even in oxygen with IPPV	R	+++	May be helpful or diagnostic	The alternative common diagnosis in infants presenting after 6 hours and particularly after 24 hours of age. ECG and echocardiogram usually diagnostic

Table 29.13 (Cont'd)

Condition	Gestational age	History	Examination[a]	Gases[b]	Presentation[c] <6 h	Presentation[c] >6 h	Chest radiograph	Comments
Pulmonary hypoplasia	Any	Prolonged rupture of membranes	Potter's features (p. 641). No kidneys palpable, amnion nodosum. Dwarf (p. 644)	Profound hypoxaemia and hypercapnia	+++	N	Diagnostic; very small lungs	Virtually always rapidly fatal
Persistent pulmonary hypertension	FT >prem	May have had mild asphyxia	May hear soft murmur of TI	Gases like cyanotic CHD, i.e. marked hypoxaemia with normal or reduced CO_2	+++	+	Usually normal or nearly so	Can be difficult to exclude cyanotic CHD unless echocardiogram available
Inhalation of feed	Any	Obvious			R	+++	Unhelpful	Should not happen to well run babies. Normal term babies rarely inhale, so always seek alternative diagnosis, especially infection
Inborn errors of metabolism	FT >prem	May be positive FH or history of unexplained NND in the past	No evidence of lung disease. Tachypnoea driven by acidaemia	Severe metabolic acidaemia, normal PaO_2 low $PaCO_2$	R ++	+++	Often normal	Diagnosis based on blood changes plus ketonaemia in many cases (pp. 688–690)
Primary neurological or muscle disease	FT >prem	May be positive FH or history of unexplained NND or infant death. Poly-hydramnios may occur	Marked hypotonia. Areflexia, odd face, deformities. No evidence of lung disease	Gases normal (unless apnoeic)	++	++	Often normal	Usually easy to identify as a group
Upper airway obstruction	FT >prem	May be typical in choanal atresia (p. 664)	Stridor present. Problems resolve on intubation. Laryngoscopy may be diagnostic	Gases normal when intubated; CO_2 may be raised beforehand	++	++	Often normal	

[a] Mentioning features other than cardinal features of respiratory disease (pp. 495–496).
[b] Most conditions cause hypoxaemia and hypercarbia; only if the blood gas patterns differ from this is it noted here.
[c] Frequency of presentation graded + to +++; N=never, R=rarely.
[d] Full term greater than premature. This means that the condition can occur at any gestation, but since full-term babies are more common than preterm ones, there are more cases in full-term neonates.
[e] If preterm consider listeria (p. 1149).
[f] Usually as a complication of pre-existing severe lung disease, especially RDS.
[g] Severely asphyxiated premature babies will develop RDS.

in critically ill babies on long-term IPPV. This is because of albumin leaking into the subcutaneous tissues,[528] the poor protein intake and impaired albumin synthesis in the liver of the seriously ill neonate. The low albumin level means that colloid osmotic pressure is also low, and often very close to the level at which tissue and pulmonary oedema develop.[96] Total complement levels are normal,[164] but anaphylatoxins are released if complications or RDS occur, such as pneumothorax or GMH/IVH.[298]

Blood gas measurements

Hypoxaemia is the hallmark of RDS and can be used to assess the severity of the lung disease (p. 501). The P_{50} in preterm infants is 2.9–3.1 kPa (22–23 mmHg) on the first day, rising to 3.3–3.5 kPa (25–26 mmHg) by term. It shows the expected variation with pH.[713] A mixed metabolic and respiratory acidaemia is found in most cases of RDS, with the $PaCO_2$ being raised in all but the mildest cases; indeed, the absence of hypercapnia or the presence of a low $PaCO_2$ should suggest a diagnosis other than RDS in a dyspnoeic neonate (p. 503).

Hormone levels

Older reports of bigger babies with RDS showed raised plasma levels of steroids,[39,515] as well as raised ADH (pp. 505, 1016), ANP (pp. 1012–1016) and angiotensin II (p. 496), but aldosterone levels are normal.[646] A recent report,[560] however, shows that the cortisol levels of ill 26-week-old babies are lower than healthy preterm babies, remain low for several days after birth, and are further depressed by prenatal therapy with dexamethasone. Levels of TSH, T_4 and T_3, although initially normal in cord blood,[596] drop below normal during the first week.[344] It is interesting, in view of the relationship between RDS and maternal diabetes, that insulin levels are raised in the cord blood of 'non-diabetic' neonates who go on to develop RDS[105] and subsequently may remain relatively high in response to persisting hyperglycaemia.[1206]

Prostaglandin I_2 (prostacyclin), prostaglandin E_2 and thromboxane A_2 levels are all markedly raised in the plasma of neonates with RDS. In those who go on to develop a PDA the levels in the first few days are no higher than in controls,[201,963] but are higher at 2 weeks of age in those who still have a patent ductus.[678]

ECG

Early studies done on large non-ventilated babies with RDS showed patterns of left ventricular loading, with large S waves in V_1 and V_2 compatible with a large left–right duct shunt[572] or changes compatible with hyperkalaemia (widening of the QRS interval, tall T waves) or hypoxia (wide QRS, flat T waves). More recently, ST segment depression as a sign of sub-endocardial ischaemia in the presence of large left–right ductal shunts has been described.[1148]

Echocardiography

Echocardiographic studies in neonates with RDS confirm the presence of a PDA in most cases (p. 512), but are otherwise normal in the absence of PPHN or severe depression of myocardial function.[546] Doppler echocardiography has been used more recently to investigate the degree of pulmonary hypertension in RDS (p. 489; see Figs 29.23, 29.24).

Measurements of surfactant

The diagnosis of RDS does not depend on one of the many measurements of surfactant in either amniotic fluid or gastric aspirate: apparently typical RDS can develop in the presence of L:S ratios (p. 475) greater than 2.0, even when PG is present[1158] or there is asphyxia (p. 484). Furthermore, surfactant-deficient RDS and congenital pneumonia, due in particular to GBS (p. 497), can coexist. There may be a role for rapid early assessment of neonatal surfactant levels in, say, gastric aspirate, to assess whether exogenous surfactant should be given,[188] but it should be remembered that RDS is a clinical diagnosis, and there are grounds for thinking that surfactant therapy will improve most forms of neonatal lung disease.

Chest X-ray

The chest X-ray is an essential part of the initial work-up of all dyspnoeic neonates. Not only is it important in the differential diagnosis (Table 29.13), but it should be used to identify thymic, cardiac and skeletal abnormalities as well as to check the position of indwelling cannulae (p. 363). Classically, in RDS the chest X-ray shows diffuse, fine granular opacification in both lung fields, with an air bronchogram where the air-filled bronchi stand out against the atelectatic lungs. The appearance can be very variable, from a slight granularity to lungs which are so opaque that it is impossible to distinguish between the lung field and the cardiac silhouette (Fig. 29.33). The

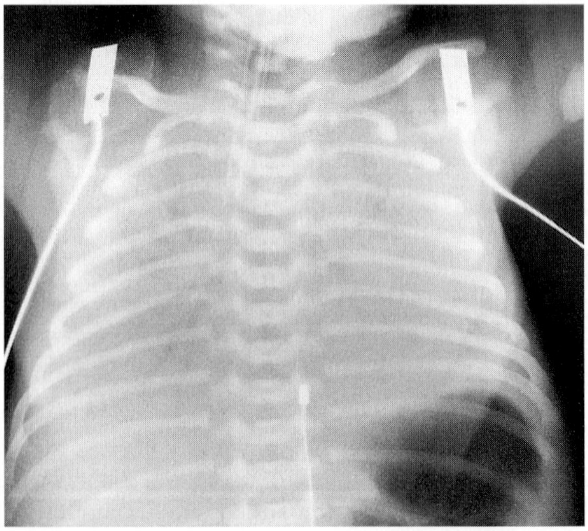

Fig. 29.33 Severe RDS. The lungs are totally opaque and cannot be separated from the heart border because of widespread atelectasis. An air bronchogram can be seen in the right lung.

more severe picture may take several hours to evolve, and an X-ray taken at 1 hour of age may show only comparatively mild changes, which deteriorate rapidly by 3–4 hours, despite impeccable therapy. Conversely, the 1-hour X-ray may show a 'white-out' yet the baby may only need mild respiratory support with CPAP or low-pressure IPPV, and by 4 hours of age, presumably as a result of clearance of fetal lung liquid, the X-ray may show marked improvement. The chest X-ray appearance also depends on the phase of the respiratory cycle: expiratory films look much worse than inspiratory ones. Positive-pressure support with both CPAP and IPPV can improve the X-ray appearance in a baby who had marked X-ray changes while breathing spontaneously, and surfactant treatment may have the same effect.[291] As a consequence of all these variables, the early chest X-ray appearance is a poor guide to both prognosis[558] and the response to exogenous surfactant therapy.[263]

As the respiratory disease worsens during the first 24–48 hours, the X-ray changes in general become more severe; as the baby recovers and surfactant reappears, the lung fields clear radiologically, and in uncomplicated cases the chest X-ray will have returned to normal by 7–10 days.

ASSESSING THE SEVERITY OF RDS

The initial methods of assessment were based on the respiratory rate, physical examination and other clinical features.[983] When blood gas measurements first became available it was found that neonates with RDS who within the first 6 hours of life could not achieve a $P\text{aO}_2$ of 13.3 kPa (100 mmHg) in 100% oxygen, had a much higher mortality (70–80%) than those who could (mortality 25–30%).[122,912] Subsequently this proved to be a poor discriminator, and the need for early ventilation identified a group with a very high mortality.[911] More recently there has been a reversal to scores based on blood gases in intubated neonates. Bartlett et al,[66] in their studies on ECMO, calculated the oxygenation index using the formula:

$$\text{OI} = \frac{\text{Mean airway pressure (cmH}_2\text{O)} \times \text{F}_\text{I}\text{O}_2 \times 100}{\text{Postductal } P\text{aO}_2 \text{ (mmHg)}}$$

Values over 25 defined a 50% mortality and over 40 an 80% mortality; however, Ortega et al[816] subsequently found that the score had to increase to 60 to predict an 80% mortality.

Tarnow-Mordi et al[1057] devised a complex mathematical formula for assessing the severity of RDS; more recently he and others have produced much more simple scoring systems, such as the CRIB score (p. 48),[203] which can be applied to all VLBW babies, including those without lung disease, as a means of comparing outcome between centres and countries.

TREATMENT OF RDS

This starts with the obstetrician, who must be encouraged to deliver the baby in optimal condition (pp. 484 and 493), and continues with the techniques described above under prevention.

Initial care

Transportation from labour ward to NICU

It is essential to ensure that there is no deterioration in a baby's lung disease due to slipshod care during this transfer. All VLBW neonates who are intubated after delivery (pp. 255, 493) should be ventilated in the transport incubator during transfer to the neonatal unit. In babies below 1.50 kg who look apparently well after resuscitation, any temptation to discontinue IPPV before transfer to the NICU should be strongly resisted; bigger babies who are clearly developing RDS by 10–15 minutes of age should be intubated and ventilated both before and during transfer.

Ventilator settings during transportation. The ventilator settings will have to be empirical, based on clinical assessment of the baby, and in particular whether there is adequate chest wall expansion. This usually means ventilator pressures of 20–25/5 cmH_2O and a rate of 60–80/min in 60–80% oxygen. SpO_2 measurements should also be employed if available (p. 366). There is a major risk of serious deterioration in the baby's condition if he is not properly ventilated during transfer and is allowed to become hypoxaemic, hypercapnic and acidaemic, as well as hypotensive and hypothermic.

Initial management in the NICU

The basic philosophy in the early care of VLBW neonates with RDS is to control the respiratory failure as soon as possible. As soon as the baby arrives in the NICU, still on IPPV, he must be put into an incubator prewarmed to 35–36°C (p. 295) or placed under a radiant heater.

In the next 30–60 minutes the following procedures should be carried out in all neonates with RDS:

- Examine carefully, including a rapid assessment of gestational age.
- Weigh (length and head circumference can wait till later).
- Connect to ECG and respiration monitors (pp. 361, 368).
- Connect to a pulse oximeter to obtain an immediate assessment of oxygenation (SpO_2).
- Measure the baby's temperature.
- Measure blood pressure using a Dinamap, and then subsequently using a continuously recording device once an arterial cannula is in situ.
- Insert a UAC (or, failing that, a peripheral arterial cannula) and measure $P\text{aO}_2$, $P\text{aCO}_2$ and pH.

- Treat abnormalities of blood gases (pp. 503–504), and blood pressure (pp. 504–505).
- Draw blood for haemoglobin and white blood cell count. Cross-match all ill neonates, as most eventually need transfusion.
- Do a chest X-ray, preferably after inserting the UAC (p. 363).
- Take a set of cultures, including a blood culture, but a lumbar puncture can usually be omitted (p. 1123). Blood culture can be taken from the UAC during the sterile insertion routine.
- Give surfactant, if it has not been given prophylactically in the labour ward (p. 494).
- Start antibiotics (p. 497).
- Send blood for electrolyte, calcium and albumin measurement. This establishes a baseline and identifies early abnormalities caused by problems with maternal fluid balance.
- Measure coagulation, especially in bruised babies <28 weeks' gestation.

When all this is done arrange to speak to the parents.

The only variation allowable in this routine is for bigger babies with apparently mild lung disease, in whom an initial peripheral arterial sample confirms that disease is only mild. In these babies arterial cannulation is not required, though an i.v. catheter will need to be inserted for antibiotics and parenteral fluids.

This protocol is not as invasive or dramatic as it sounds, and it must be remembered that it is much more dangerous to undertreat than overtreat at this stage. The old-fashioned attitude that the baby should be allowed to 'stabilize' or 'recover from the delivery' during this first hour is lethal, as it may result in disease passing unrecognized. This is particularly likely to occur:

- in the very preterm infant, in whom skin colour and respiratory pattern are notoriously misleading, the former because of transcutaneous oxygen absorption[306] and the latter because preterm infants can only breathe in a feeble fashion;
- in drug-depressed infants in whom, despite severe lung disease, respiratory drive is suppressed;
- in severely acidotic infants, in whom the acidaemia may depress respiration, have deleterious effects on surfactant synthesis (p. 484) and cause vasoconstriction and pallor, which makes assessment of cyanosis or 'pinkness' very difficult;
- in hypotensive infants, in whom peripheral vasoconstriction also makes assessment of colour difficult;
- in hypotensive infants, who may look surprisingly well with adequate blood gases before the hypotension adversely affects gas exchange (p. 496), myocardial function (p. 696), the brain (p. 1252) and the kidney (pp. 1026–1027);
- in infants with PPHN, in whom the signs of respiratory distress may be comparatively mild, despite severe hypoxaemia (p. 530).

General management of the baby with RDS

Minimal handling

It has been known for many years[778,1011] that when hypoxic babies are disturbed and handled their respiration may become very irregular or stop altogether, their right–left shunt increases and their PaO_2 falls rapidly (Fig. 29.34). Even apparently trivial acts, such as gently listening to the chest with a stethoscope or palpating the abdomen, may have this effect. Major disturbances such as sucking out an endotracheal tube, performing a lumbar puncture or taking a chest X-ray can cause catastrophic falls in PaO_2. The minimal handling maxim governs much of our approach to monitoring the sick preterm neonate. If procedures have to be carried out local anaesthetics seem to be relatively ineffective,[935] but systemic opiates[857] or even oral sucrose are beneficial.[875]

Physiotherapy

For the non-intubated baby with RDS secretions are not a problem unless infection develops, and in our view chest physiotherapy is contraindicated as it contravenes the minimal handling maxim and causes the baby's PaO_2

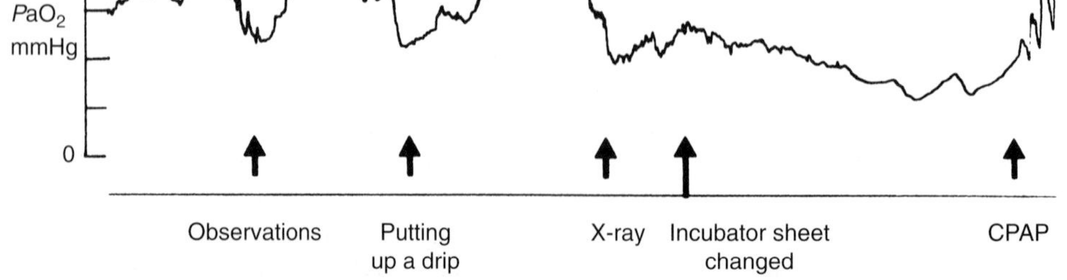

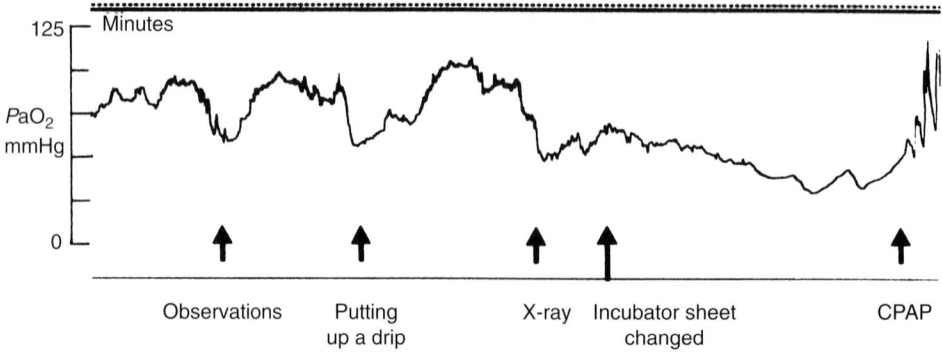

Fig. 29.34 Continuous recording of arterial oxygen tension. Reproduced from Speidel.[1011]

to fall. Similarly, there is no need to suction the endotracheal tube routinely in the first 24–48 hours. The use of physiotherapy in intubated neonates is discussed on page 577.

Posture

Babies with RDS should have their position changed every 2–3 hours. In general the prone position is preferable as blood gases tend to be better maintained[721] and lung function improved.[735] Keep the baby's neck slightly extended, for example by placing a small roll under it, as flexion, if marked,[1020] can obstruct the airways.

Temperature

The ill hypoxic neonate is frequently exposed to cold stress during long periods of exposure at resuscitation, or while umbilical artery catheters or peripheral intravenous infusions are being started. The deleterious effects of this are outlined on pages 299 and 485. The baby's thermal environment should be controlled as outlined in Chapter 18, and if he is exposed during any procedure he should be under a radiant heat source, with as much of him as possible covered up to minimize heat loss.

Blood gas management

Abnormalities of PaO_2, $PaCO_2$ and acid–base metabolism are characteristic of RDS, and keeping them within a reasonably normal range is the single most important component of the treatment. If this can be done the baby will almost certainly survive, unless he develops a complication such as a pneumothorax, GMH/IVH or infection. The detailed management of oxygen administration, CPAP and IPPV are covered on pages 561–579.

PaO_2. The traditional teaching is to maintain the PaO_2, measured in blood drawn from an umbilical artery catheter, distal to the ductus in the range 8–12 kPa (60–90 mmHg).[912] The lower level is still some way above that (approximately 5–6 kPa, 40 mmHg) at which cyanosis appears and the baby shows the effects of hypoxia, such as subtle EEG changes, a switch to anaerobic metabolism and a metabolic acidaemia. In very ill babies on high-pressure IPPV a PaO_2 in the range 5.6–8.0 kPa (40–60 mmHg) is an acceptable alternative to increasing the ventilator pressure, with all its attendant hazards (pp. 608–609).

The upper limit of 12 kPa (90 mmHg) was set to avoid the retinal hyperoxaemia which would cause ROP. This is a 'best-guess' figure based on studies of preductal versus postductal PaO_2 levels, the early controlled trials of oxygen and ROP, epidemiological data on patients with ROP, and estimates of preductal blood gases in babies breathing 40% oxygen. The initial studies of ROP showed that eye damage was rare in babies restricted to less than 40% oxygen, and subsequent studies on healthy asymptomatic LBW neonates showed that it is unusual to have a preductal PaO_2 > 20–22 kPa (150–160 mmHg) when breathing 40% oxygen.[595] Studies using postductal blood, i.e. an indwelling umbilical artery catheter, have shown that, because of an unpredictable right–left ductus shunt in neonates with RDS, to prevent the preductal (and hence ophthalmic) PaO_2 reaching 20 kPa (150 mmHg) the umbilical artery catheter PaO_2 should be less than 12 kPa (90 mmHg).[909] The wealth of clinical data[589] obtained subsequently has shown that ROP is exceptionally rare in preterm neonates in whom the PaO_2 in blood drawn from an umbilical catheter has never exceeded 12 kPa (90 mmHg). In the last decade, with the alarming incidence of ROP in neonates weighing <1.00 kg at birth (p. 911), anxiety has been expressed about the safety of an upper limit of 12 kPa (90 mmHg), and it is safer to maintain <1.00 kg babies below 10 kPa (75 mmHg).

$PaCO_2$. The $PaCO_2$ in a normal newborn baby is in the range 4.6–5.4 kPa (35–40 mmHg) (Appendix 7). Hypocapnia with lower levels than these is unlikely to be seen in spontaneously breathing neonates with RDS, but hypercapnia and respiratory acidaemia are common. Its importance depends on the relative role of a high $PaCO_2$ with a concomitant rise in cerebral blood flow in the genesis of GMH/IVH (p. 1256). Cerebral blood flow increases about 30% with each 1 kPa increase in $PaCO_2$. Some believe that in infants <1.50 kg no elevation of $PaCO_2$ should be allowed in the first 72–96 hours, when the development of a GMH/IVH is most likely.[1052] Others, however, argue for a degree of permissive hypercarbia, as such a policy has been associated with a reduced incidence of CLD.[362] If a VLBW baby in the first 6–12 hours cannot ventilate himself sufficiently well to keep his $PaCO_2$ below 6 kPa (45 mmHg), he should undoubtedly be intubated and ventilated (p. 563); however, once he is ventilated and has a satisfactory and stable $PaCO_2$, pH and clinical state, we would accept levels up to 7–7.5 kPa (52–56 mmHg) in severe disease, rather than put him at risk from increased ventilator pressures. We would accept even higher $PaCO_2$ levels in more mature neonates with RDS and in <1.50 kg infants more than a week old whom we are trying to wean off IPPV, so long as the baby was clinically stable and his PaO_2, pH and base excess were satisfactory. Hypocapnia ($PaCO_2$ <4 kPa (30 mmHg)) should be avoided because of its possible role in the genesis of PVL, (pp. 1263–1264) and CLD (p. 620).

Important information can be gained from measuring the rate of change in $PaCO_2$. A rapidly rising $PaCO_2$ is a sign of impending respiratory failure, usually associated with a fall in pH and therefore requiring IPPV irrespective of the postnatal age of the neonate, whereas more gradual changes, or a stable high $PaCO_2$ with an acceptable pH, can be managed conservatively.

pH. Metabolic alkalaemia is rare, is almost always iatrogenic as a result of excessive i.v. bicarbonate use, and requires no therapy; respiratory alkalaemia is also rare, and is usually due to a deliberate attempt to dilate the pulmonary vasculature in PPHN, but may also be due to excessive use of ventilator pressures (p. 575).

Acidaemia, however, is common in neonates with RDS. It is always essential to establish whether the acidaemia is respiratory, with a raised $PaCO_2$ (see above), or metabolic, with a normal $PaCO_2$ but a negative base excess, or a combination of both, which is, in fact, more likely.

The commonest cause of the metabolic acidaemia in a baby with RDS is a raised lactate from anaerobic metabolism. This in turn is secondary to hypoxaemia, hypotension, anaemia, infection, sepsis or strenuous respiratory muscle activity. When a metabolic acidaemia does develop, therefore, it is essential to identify the cause and so direct treatment: oxygen for hypoxia, antibiotics for infection, transfusion for anaemia and hypotension, or IPPV for exhaustion.

The use of intravenous alkali to correct metabolic acidaemia in preterm neonates remains controversial. There is evidence showing that inappropriately large or fast infusions of base may cause hypernatraemia or cerebral haemorrhage,[509] but this does not seem to be a convincing argument against using appropriate doses at safe rates. Acidaemia inhibits surfactant synthesis (p. 484) and increases pulmonary vascular resistance.[932] Once the pH falls below 7.15 other physiological functions, such as myocardial contractility[79] and diaphragmatic activity,[510] begin to deteriorate. The sick neonate has difficulty in excreting an acid load.[15] Our assessment, therefore, is that the ill VLBW neonate should have his pH kept ≥7.25 at all times. If the pH is <7.25 with a base deficit ≥10 mmol/l, intravenous alkali therapy is appropriate if other therapies such as blood transfusion, colloid infusion or increasing the PaO_2 are not immediately successful. Two alkalis have been used in neonatal therapy, sodium bicarbonate and THAM. Both are effective. The theoretical risk that following infusion of bicarbonate the cerebrospinal fluid might become even more acidotic does not seem to apply to the neonate,[505,961] in whom the medullary chemoreceptor drive is, in any case, less important.[143] THAM has the undoubted theoretical benefit of not giving a sodium load to ill VLBW babies. Because THAM infusions do not increase the $PaCO_2$, the use of this drug is theoretically preferable in the presence of a high $PaCO_2$. It may, however, cause apnoea,[902] and should only be given to ventilated neonates. The dose of base to be given is:

$$\text{Dose (mmol)} = \text{base deficit (mmol/l)} \times \text{body weight (kg)} \times 0.4$$

The rate of infusion should never exceed 0.5 mmol/min: 7% THAM solution contains approximately 0.5 mmol/ml.

Blood pressure

All neonates suffering from RDS must have their blood pressure monitored regularly. Those with a systolic pressure below 40–45 mmHg or a mean below 30–35 mmHg should be treated in the first instance by blood transfusion unless they are polycythaemic,[1149] in which case a volume load should be considered. A lower mean blood pressure limit of 30 mmHg should be regarded as roughly 2 standard deviations below the mean. Saline can be used if the neonate's haemoglobin is >15 g/dl (PCV >45%). The response to albumin is small and rarely sustained[103,294] and recent evidence suggests that albumin use can be harmful.[202a] In general, the first transfusion should be 15 ml/kg given by infusion over 10–15 minutes if the hypotension is severe in the hour or two after birth, but thereafter transfusions of blood are better given over a period of 30–120 minutes, guided by the condition of the neonate, his clinical response and the blood pressure rise during the transfusions. Transfusions should also be given to babies with features suggesting hypovolaemia which has not yet progressed to hypotension, such as poor capillary filling, peripheral vasoconstriction and a falling pH, often coupled with a record of large volumes of blood having been removed for analysis. There is, however, no place for routine plasma expanders soon after delivery.[784] If the hypotensive neonate is severely hypoxic or acidaemic, his cardiac function may be impaired and he will tolerate volume expansion badly, in which case dopamine is the preferred treatment.[377] Dopamine should also be used in those in whom volume expansion has failed to increase blood pressure: trials have shown it to be more effective than dobutamine.[293,594] The actions of dopamine are complex.[959] At 0.5–2.0 μg/kg/min dopaminergic actions dilate renal, mesenteric and coronary arteries; from 2 to 10 μg/kg/min myocardial contractility is increased directly by both α- and β-receptor-mediated actions, and also by the release of noradrenaline from cardiac adrenergic nerves. At doses above 10–15 μg/kg/min dopamine begins to show α-adrenergic activity and is a vasoconstrictor of all vascular beds. Initially, therefore, 2–4 μg/kg/min should be given,[960] increasing the dosage until the blood pressure is acceptable.

If plasma volume expansion plus dopamine does not reverse hypotension, four other sympathomimetic agents can be tried:

- Dobutamine. This is an isoprenaline analogue with a primarily β-adrenergic inotropic effect on the myocardium, with little peripheral vascular effect and no specific effect on the renal vascular bed.
- Isoprenaline. This betamimetic drug has a chronotropic and inotropic effect and is therefore of greatest benefit if hypotension is accompanied by bradycardia. It is not useful in shock because of its peripheral vasodilator effects.

- Adrenaline. This increases blood pressure by peripheral vasoconstriction plus increased myocardial contractility. Its vasoconstrictor effects on the renal vasculature are clearly undesirable.
- Dopexamine hydrochloride. A new synthetic catecholamine with predominant β_2-adrenergic and dopaminergic activity. In low doses (2–4 μg/kg/min) it can improve blood pressure and urine output,[569] but at higher doses it reduces systemic vascular resistance.

Finally, if catecholamines fail, treatment with hydrocortisone 1–2 mg may be successful.[479]

Maintenance of haemoglobin

There are many reasons for a preterm neonate to be anaemic (p. 814): there may have been an intrapartum haemorrhage, defective placental transfusion[1186] or a twin–twin or fetal–maternal haemorrhage. Blood loss after birth is iatrogenic, but a sudden drop in the haematocrit/haemoglobin level in a baby with RDS suggests that he has developed a GMH/IVH (p. 1257).

Experience has shown that ill neonates, in particular those who are premature, tolerate haemoglobin levels <13 g/dl (PCV <40%) badly.[906,1038] This is presumably because of the increase in cardiac output required to meet the oxygen demands of the tissues when, with a low haemoglobin, there is reduced blood oxygen carrying capacity. One policy is therefore to transfuse all ill neonates when their haemoglobin has fallen below 13 g/dl (PCV 40%).[536] This should be from a CMV-negative donor and be partially packed to a haemoglobin level appropriate for a premature baby (PCV 40–45%), but it does not need to be fresh, as the adverse metabolic features of 2- to 3-week-old CPDA donor blood are of no clinical significance when given as a 15 ml/kg transfusion over 30–120 minutes (Chapter 32, Part 4). If the baby has a clinically important patent ductus he should receive frusemide 1.0 mg/kg during the transfusion; otherwise there is no need to give diuretic cover. Transfusions may need to be given several times a week during the acute phase of the illness, and should be continued for as long as the baby is ventilated or has chronic lung disease requiring more than 30–40% oxygen (p. 614). With modern transfusion practice, donor exposure can be reduced to a minimum (p. 839).

Coagulation abnormalities

All preterm neonates have prolonged coagulation times (Appendix 2), but major abnormalities are usually only seen as a secondary phenomenon, particularly in babies who develop sepsis (p. 1117) or a GMH/IVH.[186,692] Although prospective studies of the benefits of routinely screening for and correcting coagulation abnormalities in ill VLBW neonates[94,1093] have yielded inconclusive results, many authorities (p. 805) feel that prophylactic factor replacement is justified. Routine administration of fresh frozen plasma soon after birth is of no benefit.[784]

If an overt coagulation disturbance occurs, such as DIC or thrombocytopenia, opinion is unanimous that this should be treated by factor replacement (p. 804), but it is also essential to control and reverse the underlying problem, such as hypoxaemia or sepsis, that caused the coagulopathy in the first place.

Exchange transfusion has no place in the routine management of RDS, but may be indicated in the presence of DIC or sepsis.

Fluid and electrolyte balance

Renal function is often impaired (p. 1018). Urine production may be no more than 1.0–1.5 ml/kg/h, close to the definition of oliguric renal failure (1 ml/kg/h) (pp. 1027–1028); however, peripheral oedema is usually due to leaky capillaries (see above).

Antidiuretic hormone levels are raised in babies with RDS, particularly when they are very ill[882] or after they develop a pneumothorax;[828,1167] conversely, others report a sodium and water loss after a (treated) pneumothorax.[647] Plasma levels of ANP are also high in the first few days of life in babies with RDS.[965] There is a complex and as yet not fully understood interrelationship between ANP levels, ductal shunting with atrial distension in RDS, and the postnatal natriuresis that appears to be an integral part of the recovery phase of RDS (p. 1016).[552] The increased capillary permeability in RDS (p. 496) results in fluid loss into all tissues, including the lungs, and this is worse when pancuronium is given (p. 576). If fluid balance is inadequately controlled the risks of PDA (p. 512), NEC (p. 748), CLD (p. 609), and probably GMH/IVH, are increased.[1077] Fluid balance, therefore, has to be very carefully designed for each baby (Chapter 32, Part 1).

Infants with RDS should start on 40–60 ml/kg/24 h of a 10% dextrose solution. The fluid intake should subsequently be guided by the baby's weight. The ill neonate loses about 1–3% of his body weight per day.[964] If he is losing more than that he is dehydrated; if his weight is static or he is gaining weight, he is having too much fluid.

Appropriate supplements of electrolytes can be given in the light of the serum electrolyte analyses. Sodium and potassium do not usually need to be added to the fluid intake for the first 36–48 hours, although the frequent presence of hypocalcaemia in such babies (pp. 497,966) means that calcium should usually be given (pp. 966–967).

Glucose infusion rates in excess of 6 mg/kg/min (p. 952) (approximately 85 ml of 10% dextrose per kilogram per 24 hours) are likely to cause hyperglycaemia, and hence glycosuria and an osmotic diuresis. If more than 80–100 ml/kg/24 h of fluid is necessary, it is essential to monitor the blood glucose regularly and change to 5% dextrose infusions if the blood glucose exceeds 7–8 mmol/l and/or there is glycosuria.

Characteristically a diuresis occurs when the baby's lung function improves,[296,402] concomitant with an improvement in the FRC and compliance.[224,475] Once this occurs it is a marker that the previous constraints on the fluid balance to 40–60 ml/kg/24 h will need to be relaxed to prevent dehydration, haemoconcentration and jaundice. Great care should then be taken to reduce the ventilator settings, to prevent barotrauma.[475]

Albumin

Hypoalbuminaemia, with a low colloid osmotic pressure predisposing to tissue oedema, is common in RDS. To try and prevent this, ill neonates have been given transfusions of albumin (0.5 g/kg of a preparation such as PPF) whenever the serum albumin falls below 20 g/l. As well as having a beneficial effect on colloid osmotic pressure and reducing the propensity to form oedema, the albumin infusions will usually, but not always, raise blood pressure and improve renal, but not respiratory, function (p. 504).[103,424,633] They may be harmful and should be used with care.[202a]

Nutrition in RDS

As the protein and calorie reserves of the VLBW neonate are so small (Chapter 19, Part 1), it is essential that some form of nutrition, including protein, is given as soon after birth as possible.

Most neonates with severe respiratory illness have an ileus[284] (p. 497) and delayed gastric emptying.[1196] Bowel sounds are absent and meconium is not passed. Anything put into the stomach will not pass the pylorus, and may be regurgitated and inhaled. Enteral feeding is, therefore, initially not feasible in the majority of ventilated babies <1.25 kg, as well as many larger sick neonates. Parenteral nutrition is therefore essential.[776] Initially aminoacids and glucose should be given, progressing to full TPN (Chapter 20), including the use of intravenous fat, until an adequate enteral intake of protein and calories has been achieved. There are anxieties regarding the use of intralipid in neonates with severe lung disease, in whom it may cause a fall in PaO_2[833] by increasing pulmonary vascular resistance.[862] Hammerman and Aramburo[460] and Sosenko et al[1006] demonstrated in randomized prospective trials that preterm neonates given intralipid were oxygen and ventilator dependent for longer than controls, and developed more CLD. Intralipid also predisposes the VLBW baby to *Staphylococcus epidermidis* sepsis (p. 1133). Pulmonary lipid emboli are more common in, but not exclusively limited to, neonates

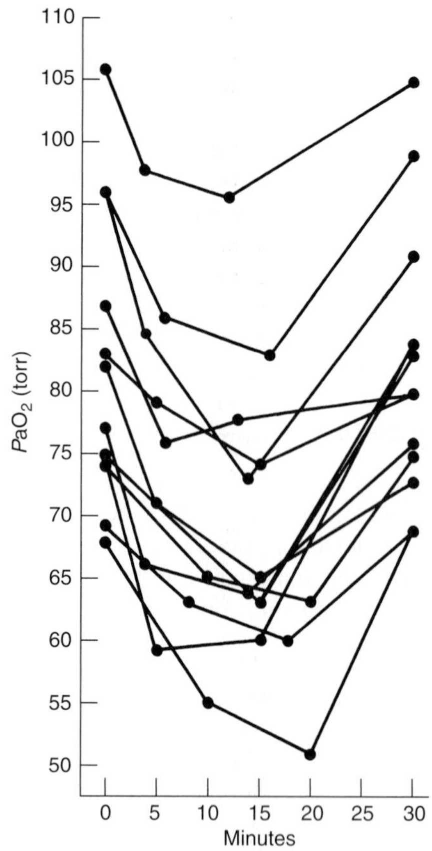

Fig. 29.35 Effect of small nasogastric tube feed of milk given between 0 and 5 minutes on the PaO_2 of babies recovering from RDS. Reproduced with permission from Wilkinson and Yu.[1162]

receiving intravenous fat.[982] Therefore, if lipid is to be used during the first week in ventilated neonates, the dose should not exceed 3 g/kg/24 h, or 2 g/kg/24 h if there is evidence of sepsis.

Once bowel sounds are present in a ventilated neonate, who is appropriately grown and has passed meconium irrespective of whether or not he has an indwelling UAC,[1082] enteral feeding can be started, if possible using his mother's own milk (pp. 343–344). Milk in the stomach, however, may compromise ventilation, increase the work of breathing,[480,827,853] lower the PaO_2[1162] (Fig. 29.35) and even cause apnoea (p. 631). In spontaneously breathing babies respiratory problems may be aggravated by the presence of a nasogastric tube obliterating one half of the upper airway.[427,1032] Another disadvantage of early enteral feeding is that it may predispose to gastro-oesophageal reflux[391,792,793] and NEC (p. 749).

Although this is an impressive theoretical body of evidence against early enteral feeding, neither gastro-oesophageal reflux, NEC, nor the physiological changes mentioned appear to be a major problem in VLBW neonates,[792,793] even when ventilated and with an indwelling UAC, provided that milk – ideally breast milk – is only given to those in whom it is clear that bowel activity is present. Furthermore, there are powerful reasons for attempting to introduce enteral feeds as soon as possible: the prolonged absence of enteral feeding compromises gut growth, the development of enzymes and normal peristaltic activity, and limits early weight gain, with the implications this may have for long-term neurological development (pp. 339, 343). The sooner enteral feeding is attempted in VLBW neonates, the sooner full enteral feeding is established.[282,680,1082]

Initially small volumes (0.5–1.0 ml every hour or every other hour) – so-called minimal enteral feeding[93] – should be given to preterm infants. The stomach should be aspirated through the nasogastric tube every 4–6 hours to confirm that the milk is passing through the pylorus; if it is not, and there is abdominal distension, the feeding should be discontinued for 24–48 hours before trying again. Feeds are more likely to be tolerated if the baby is prone.[1196] Once tolerated, the amount given can be steadily increased to the appropriate volume for the baby's postnatal age and weight (p. 395).

Drug therapy in RDS

Antibiotics

It is impossible to differentiate severe early-onset septicaemia from RDS, and the two conditions may coexist (pp. 497, 1128). Without antibiotic treatment early-onset septicaemia can be fatal within hours (p. 1128). For this reason, all dyspnoeic newborn babies, irrespective of their gestation or chest X-ray appearance, should have appropriate bacterial cultures taken and be treated with antibiotics from the earliest signs of respiratory illness. Penicillin and gentamicin are appropriate therapy as they act synergistically against group B streptococcus, and are also effective against virtually all the other organisms that can cause early-onset septicaemia and pneumonia (see Table 43.8, Chapter 43, Part 2). Treatment with immunoglobulin (p. 619) should also be considered in high-risk cases. The clinical features that make sepsis more likely in a dyspnoeic neonate are outlined on page 1128. In babies with RDS who are stable or improving, antibiotics should be stopped when negative culture results are notified at 48–72 hours. Some authorities recommend leaving the intubated baby on antibiotics, even if the endotracheal tube aspirate culture is negative, until anything up to 14 days of age, stopping earlier if weaning from IPPV and extubation is successful. This is influenced by reports that 25–30% of infants will develop pneumonia as a complication of being intubated and ventilated (p. 1144).[373,451] The diagnosis and management of pneumonia in neonates on long-term IPPV is discussed on pages 1144–1145.

Diuretics

The oliguria, peripheral and pulmonary oedema (p. 486) of early RDS, and the fact that a spontaneous diuresis is associated with an improvement in respiratory status (p. 506), have prompted several trials of the use of diuretics in preterm infants with RDS. The results are inconclusive: although some studies show a benefit, others do not;[403,945,1190] we prefer meticulous attention to fluid balance in such babies. For the oliguric baby with fluid retention and deteriorating lung function, the response to a dose of 1 mg/kg frusemide should be evaluated, especially if he is over 48 hours old.[1191] If this does not produce a diuresis, a combination of frusemide and dopamine may be effective.[1089]

Thyroxine

An improved prognosis in infants with RDS treated with thyroxine has been noted.[949] This interesting result needs confirmation, but has a sound theoretical basis as thyroxine is involved in surfactant synthesis, and neonates with RDS are relatively hypothyroid during the first week.[344]

Steroids

Shortly after the first report of the beneficial effects of antenatal steroids,[662] Baden et al[41] showed no benefits from a short postnatal course of hydrocortisone. In contrast, treatment by dexamethasone starting on the first day in ventilated babies with RDS reduced the incidence of CLD,[1192] but subsequent studies of the early use of steroids give conflicting results.[54,975,1044] Treatment started at 7–10 days, however, is beneficial[136,559] (pp. 617–618).

Vitamins

Vitamin K should be given to all neonates (p. 375). The purported benefits of vitamin E in GMH/IVH (p. 1262) or CLD (p. 619) and vitamin A in the prevention of CLD (p. 619) are not conclusive.

Pulmonary vasodilators

The various drugs, in particular inhaled nitric oxide to reduce PAP, are used primarily in babies with PPHN (pp. 533–535) or in those with severe lung disease on IPPV (pp. 577–579).[3]

Analgesia/sedation

Being ventilated is probably unpleasant and appropriate analgesia should be given (Chapter 27), as it should if a painful procedure is being undertaken. Sedation is rarely required in babies with RDS and is contraindicated in those who are breathing spontaneously, but may be useful in infants who remain chronically ventilator dependent because of CLD and in whom agitation interferes with the effectiveness of ventilation.

Methylxanthines

Methylxanthines are of proven benefit in apnoea of prematurity (p. 634) and in weaning babies from IPPV (p. 581). In spontaneously breathing babies with RDS apnoeic attacks are usually a sign of impending ventilatory exhaustion,[244] and are then an indication for IPPV rather than a methylxanthine.

Indomethacin

The use of indomethacin in preventing or treating PDA is discussed in detail on page 689, and its use to prevent GMH/IVH on page 1262.

Surfactant therapy

As with prophylactic surfactant, there is now a plethora of trials which show that surfactant given as 'rescue' therapy improves the outcome in babies with established RDS[1001] (Figs 29.36, 29.37). The results are strikingly similar to those with prophylactic surfactant, that is, a marked reduction in pneumothorax, mortality, and mortality plus BPD. There is a suggestion that with the rescue treatment using synthetic surfactant, there is also a significant reduction in PDA, GMH-IVH and BPD, but the number of studies included in the natural surfactant rescue meta-analysis is relatively small. As with the prophylactic studies, all the rescue studies show a marked reduction in oxygen requirements and intensity of ventilation, and an improvement in blood gases after the surfactant has been administered.

Method of administration. In general it is recommended that the surfactant preparation is injected over a period of a few seconds down an ETT followed, if necessary, by a period of hand ventilation using a bag. This can be done by disconnecting the baby from IPPV, or by using a side-hole injection device at the ETT connector. Slow infusion or nebulization may be less effective.[658,957,1098] The surfactant generally disseminates homogeneously,[248] particularly if large rather than small doses are used.[1112] As might be expected, deposition is influenced by gravity, with dependent parts of the lung

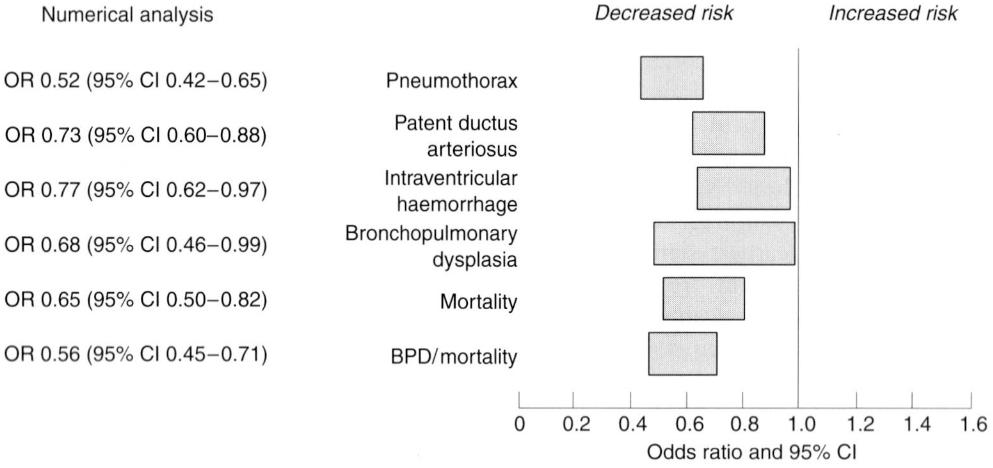

Fig. 29.36 Treatment with synthetic surfactant.

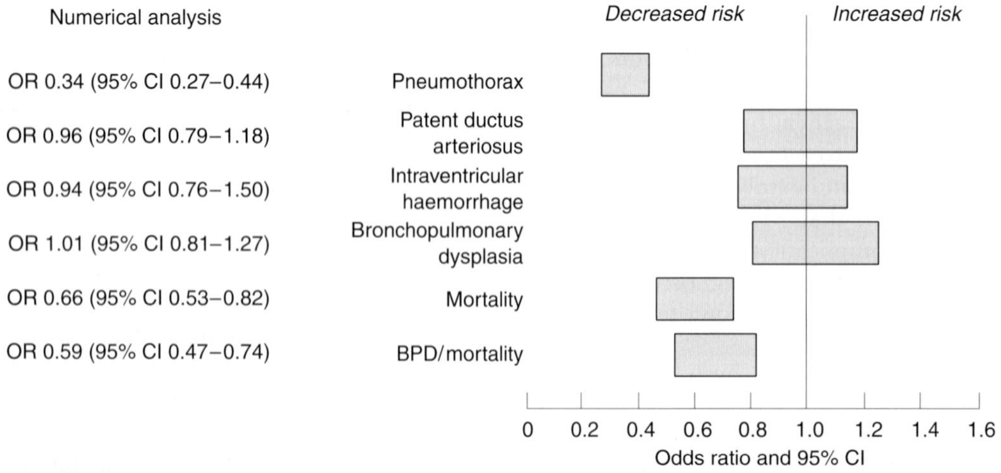

Fig. 29.37 Treatment with natural surfactant.

Table 29.14 Prophylaxis (P) versus rescue (R) (outcomes reported as percentages affected)

	No.		Mortality		CLD		PDA		Pneumothorax etc.		PVH		Surf. type
	P	R	P	R	P	R	P	R	P	R	P	R	
Kendig et al[577]	235	244	12	20[a]	36	36	40	40	7	12[a]	34	38	CLSE
Dunn et al[283]	62	60	15	13	58	29[a]	46	35	3	8	43	32	CLSE
Merritt et al[741]	49	51	42	35	12	8	69	75	20	8	41	47	Human
OSIRIS Collaborative Group[817]	1344	1346	26.7	30	36	37	27	26	12	17[a]	17	18	Exosurf
Egberts et al[292]	75	72	13	21	34	24	31	22	6	8	27	28	Curosurf
Kattwinkel et al[565]	627	621	0.5	1.8[a]	5	9[a]	21	26[a]	1.8	2.3	13.7	14.6	CLSE
Bevilacqua et al[95]	86	49	8	23[a]	9	10	33	25	6	14	37	47[b]	Curosurf
Walti et al[1140]	134	122	15	19	15	24	33	26	14	25	58	67[b]	Curosurf

[a]Significant reduction in prophylactically treated babies.
[b]There was a significant reduction in severe PVH in the prophylactic group.

receiving more of the dose.[130] There seems to be no benefit from manoeuvres aimed at trying to improve the distribution to different lobes.[1211]

Mechanism of action. Exogenous surfactants work in two ways. First, and most obviously, by coating the alveolar surface they improve lung function and hence pulmonary perfusion and oxygenation. The result of this spreading in both animals and man is complex.[749,1046] Lung histology undoubtedly improves.[851] All studies also agree that there is a rise in lung volume. In some studies a fall in compliance in the few hours after treatment has been reported, suggesting that surfactant-coated alveoli become overexpanded; only later, as expected, does the compliance rise.[98,225,385,765] Babies whose compliance falls may not have needed exogenous surfactant in the first place.[374] There is a fall in PAP, a rise in pulmonary blood flow and left-to-right ductal shunting in most studies,[458,958] but not all.[111] Prophylactic surfactant may also reduce pulmonary oedema formation.[155] The second effect of exogenous surfactants is that they are incorporated into the type II cells and either provide substrate for, or even stimulate, surfactant production.[805,851]

Number and size of doses. Early studies[608] suggested that at least 100 mg/kg of whichever surfactant was used should be given. Subsequent studies have confirmed that small doses are less effective, e.g. 2.5 ml/kg Exosurf compared with 5 ml/kg[92] and 50 mg/kg Alveofact compared with 100 mg/kg,[394] but that larger doses, e.g. 200 mg/kg tds Curosurf compared with 100 mg/kg tds,[452] confer no extra benefit.

Although beneficial effects, both clinically and physiologically, are seen after a single dose of surfactant, usually in the range of 100 mg/kg,[219,259] most studies show that better results are obtained with two or probably three doses, which is in fact what was used in the earlier studies.[297,608,1064] Speer et al,[1009] using Curosurf, and Corbet et al,[220] using Exosurf, both showed that three doses given at randomization, 12 and 24 hours of age gave better results than a single dose. The Osiris[817] trial, however, showed no benefit of three or four doses of Exosurf compared to two doses. Unlike the clinical

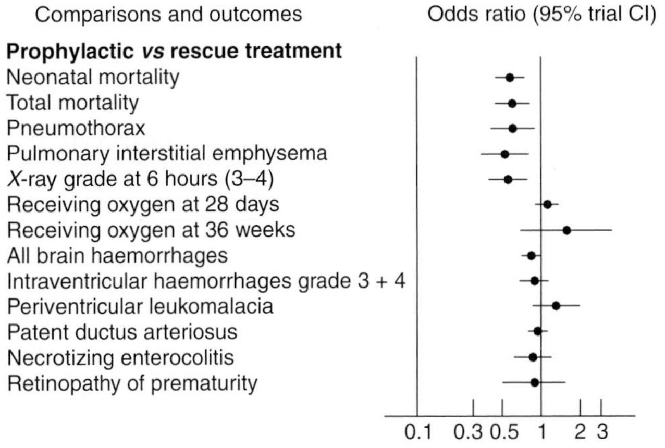

Fig. 29.38 Comparison of outcomes with prophylactic versus rescue treatment. Reproduced with permission from Morley.[764]

studies, respiratory physiological measurements show that multiple doses do not give a significant improvement in lung function compared to a single dose.[259]

Prophylactic versus rescue therapy. Kattwinkel et al[565] showed significant benefit from prophylactic therapy. Their study included babies of 29–32 weeks' gestation – hence the low mortality rate – but they attributed the statistical significance of their results mainly to babies of 29 weeks. Yet it was in such babies, and in those less than 29 weeks' gestation, that most of the other non-significant data were collected (Table 29.14). Subsequent studies have confirmed that prophylactic versus selective/rescue therapy not only reduces mortality but also other complications (Fig. 29.38).[764] The Osiris Study,[817] as well as showing a reduction in pneumothorax, also showed a significant reduction in death or oxygen dependence at 28 days.

In addition to the major outcome measures, several of the studies show a greater improvement in oxygenation and ease of ventilation in the first 24 hours in those receiving prophylactic treatment rather than rescue treatment.

Variation in individual response. Not all babies respond to surfactant, probably owing to a large protein

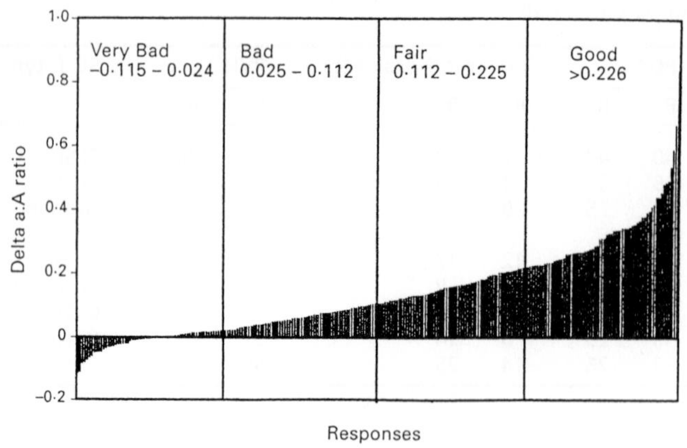

Fig. 29.39 Response to the first dose of surfactant treatment as measured by the Δ a:A ratio in 253 infants. Each column represents a single infant. Response was arbitrarily divided into quartiles and the range of values in each quartile is shown under the assigned name. Reproduced with permission from Kuint et al.[620]

Table 29.15 Mortality in relation to birthweight and response type as defined by the change in the a:A ratio (as shown in Fig. 29.39). Reproduced with permission from Kuint et al[620]

	Response				
Birthweight (g)	**Very bad *n* (%)**	**Bad *n* (%)**	**Fair *n* (%)**	**Good *n* (%)**	**Total *n* (%)**
<750	10/10 (100)	8/12 (67)	6/7 (86)	7/8 (88)	31/37 (84)
751–1000	15/25 (60)	8/14 (57)	4/11 (36)	4/10 (40)	31/60 (52)
1001–1500	8/20 (40)	3/15 (20)	2/23 (9)	0/15 (0)	13/73(18)
>1500	2/9 (22)	3/22 (14)	0/22 (0)	1/30 (3)	6/83 (7)
Total	35/64 (53)	22/63 (34)	12/63 (19)	12/63 (18)	81/253 (32)

leak onto the alveolar surface.[352,603] Fujiwara et al[354] and Charon et al[180] reported that, when observing the effect of surfactant TA on oxygenation, approximately two-thirds of babies had an immediate and sustained response, one-sixth relapsed and one-sixth had a poor or no response. They felt that the factors leading to an unsatisfactory response were the presence of a PDA, cardiogenic shock or PPHN and airleaks, which in some cases will lead to protein leaking onto the alveolar surface and there denaturing surfactant. This variation in response is well illustrated in the study by Kuint et al[620] (Fig. 29.39). A combination of the change in arterial–alveolar PO_2 ratio (Δa:A ratio) combined with birthweight provided a useful prognostic marker (Table 29.15). Failure to respond to surfactant indicates a poor prognosis.[462,620,987]

Different types of surfactant. From the data in Figures 29.30, 29.31, 29.36 and 29.37 the impression might be gained that there is little to choose between different types of surfactant. Animal studies suggest that species-specific natural surfactants were better than commercial 'natural' surfactants, which in turn were better than artificial surfactants, but this study was limited to short-term physiological variables.[232] The difference in response may well be due to the presence of

Table 29.16 Studies comparing different surfactants

Reference	Comparison	No difference	Difference
Horbar et al[506]	Exosurf vs. Survanta	Mortality BPD Airleak PVH	Reduced O_2 requirement with Survanta
Speer et al[1010]	Curosurf vs. Survanta	Mortality BPD Airleak PVH	Curosurf gave more rapid improvement than Survanta
Vermont-Oxford Network[1121]	Exosurf vs. Survanta	Mortality PVH	Less BPD and airleak in Survanta group. Reduced F_iO_2 and MAP requirement in Survanta group
Hudak et al[514]	Exosurf vs. Infasurf	Mortality BPD	More rapid improvement in first 72 hours with Infasurf. Reduced airleak with Infasurf
*Arnold et al[33]	Exosurf vs. Survanta	Time to extubation Time to no oxygen	Nil

*This trial was not a prospective randomized one.

the surfactant apoproteins.[807] Recently, several comparative studies have been published in neonates with RDS (Table 29.16). A meta-analysis of seven randomized controlled trials involving over 3000 infants demonstrated a decrease in the risk of pneumothorax and a trend towards improved survival with the use of a natural rather than an artificial surfactant[1000] (Fig. 29.40). As might be expected from earlier studies, natural surfactants containing a 'physiological' mixture of lipids and apoproteins have a more rapid effect on oxygenation, but other differences are minor.

A new synthetic surfactant containing a polypeptide KL_4 composed of lysine and leucine which mimics the effects of SP-B has now been produced;[202] this appears to be as resistant as natural surfactants to the inhibitory effects of proteins on the alveolar surface.[708] Attempts are also being made to produce SP-C analogues.[544]

Use in ELBW neonates. There is some controversy about whether surfactant should be administered to babies less than 750–800 g birthweight.[688] There is clear evidence, however, that it does work in such patients and improves survival without increasing handicap.[316,995,1030]

Infection. Swamping alveolar macrophages with instilled surfactant could, in theory, increase the baby's susceptibility to infection;[950] however, no clinical evidence has been found for such an association.

Cost. All preparations are expensive, but studies in the USA show that the use of surfactant, by reducing the duration and severity of RDS, decreased neonatal intensive care costs.[726,842,850]

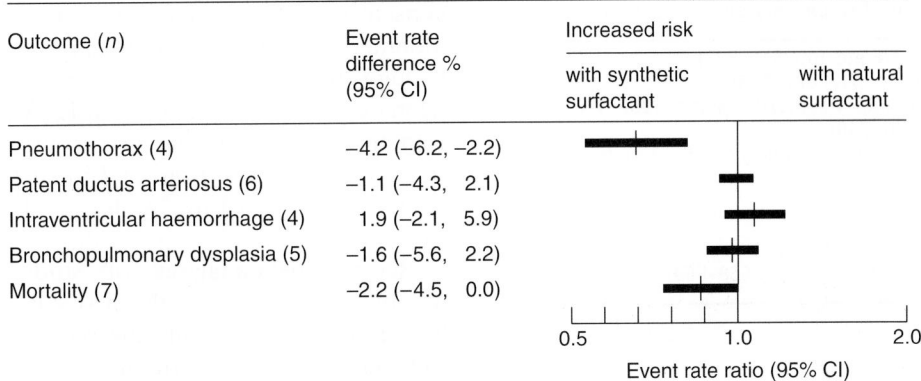

Outcome (*n*)	Event rate difference % (95% CI)
Pneumothorax (4)	−4.2 (−6.2, −2.2)
Patent ductus arteriosus (6)	−1.1 (−4.3, 2.1)
Intraventricular haemorrhage (4)	1.9 (−2.1, 5.9)
Bronchopulmonary dysplasia (5)	−1.6 (−5.6, 2.2)
Mortality (7)	−2.2 (−4.5, 0.0)

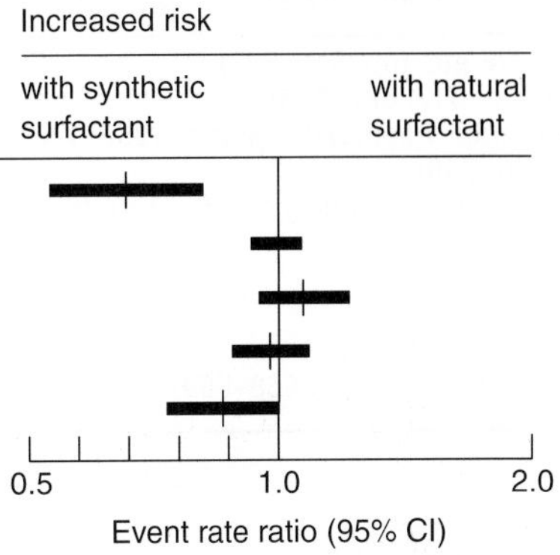

Fig. 29.40 Natural versus synthetic surfactant in the treatment of established RDS: overview of randomized controlled trials. Results are given as both the event rate difference and the event rate ratio with the 95% confidence interval. Treatment with natural surfactant extract leads to a significant decrease in the risk of pneumothorax and the risk of mortality. Reproduced with permission from Soll et al.[1002]

Side-effects of surfactants. During the administration of the surfactant there may be transient hypoxaemia and bradycardia.[660] It is recognized as being a particular problem with the large volume given as Exosurf,[817] but is not seen with ALEC.[10] Many anxieties have been expressed that immune responses to exogenous surfactant proteins instilled into the lung would cause short- or long-term problems. There are of course no data on the latter, and considerable data suggest that the former is not a problem,[1039] but is theoretically possible.[67] Surprisingly, antibodies to surfactant proteins are found in both treated infants and those given placebo,[187] and may, in both groups, be a marker for progression to CLD.[1040]

Massive pulmonary haemorrhage, particularly in ELBW neonates, has been noted and may be increased with the use of Exosurf. The overall incidence of MPH in these babies is approximately doubled.[873,1030,1115]

There were initial anxieties that following surfactant instillation there was either a fall[228] or a rise in cerebral blood flow velocity,[1110,1111] and even an increase in GMH/IVH.[212] Systemic hypotension and a transient flattening of the EEG were also reported.[228,481] More detailed studies have shown little more than a transient perturbation in cerebral haemodynamics, with no evidence of cerebral ischaemia if care is taken with the instillation,[81,290,684] and the pooled data show either no effect of surfactant on GMH/IVH incidence (Figs 29.30, 29.31, 29.37) or even a slight reduction (Fig. 29.36).

Long-term neurological follow-up shows no additional neurological deficits in surfactant-treated survivors,[671,766] nor any increase in severe ROP;[1065] surfactant-treated infants may have improved long-term lung function compared to untreated controls.[1,1205]

MONITORING

The general principles of monitoring the ill preterm neonate are laid out in Chapter 21, principles which were in many incidences worked up in babies with RDS. The important components of routine monitoring in RDS are given in Table 29.17.

Table 29.17 Application of monitoring principles to neonates with RDS

Respiratory	
PaO_2	Continuously; ideally from UAC, otherwise continuous SpO_2 always backed up by 4-hourly arterial samples from indwelling arterial cannula. Arterial stabs are the least favoured option. This should be continued until PO_2 stable in headbox oxygen
$PaCO_2$	4-hourly arterial until stable in headbox
pH	4-hourly arterial until stable in headbox
Chest X-ray	Daily during the acute phase while on IPPV
Respiratory rate	Apnoea monitor (if not on IPPV). Spontaneous respiratory rate hourly
Cardiological	Continuous display of ECG and heart rate, blood pressure; ideally continuous, recorded from arterial catheter, or hourly with Dinamap till level satisfactory, then 4-hourly
Temperature	4-hourly
Microbiology	On admission, then as indicated. Routine ETT aspirate cultured weekly
Fluid and electrolytes	Daily or twice daily weight, preferably by within incubator bed scales. Careful intake and output chart. Daily Na, K, Ca, albumin, bilirubin while ill
Haematology	Daily Hb, WBC, platelets while ill. PCV 3–4 times daily

COMPLICATIONS

The complications of RDS are listed in Table 29.18. Some of them are features of prematurity, others are genuine sequelae of surfactant-deficient RDS or the complications of the treatment given; most are combinations of all three. Many are dealt with in detail elsewhere in this book or in this chapter, in which case only the briefest of outlines will be given here.

Table 29.18 Complications of respiratory distress syndrome

Airleaks, pneumothorax, PIE etc. (pp. 516–527)
Patent ductus arteriosus (pp. 512, 687–688)
Germinal layer/intraventricular haemorrhage (pp. 1252–1262)
Necrotizing enterocolitis (p. 748)
Fluid and electrolyte imbalance, including renal failure (p. 1026)
Chronic lung disease (pp. 608–630)
Hypotension/anaemia (pp. 504–505)
Pneumonia/septicaemia (p. 1144)
Retinopathy of prematurity (pp. 909–913)
Complications related to intubation (pp. 668–669)

Airleaks, pneumothorax, pulmonary interstitial emphysema (pp. 516–527)

In the past some form of airleak was reported in about 5% of babies with RDS who were breathing spontaneously, an incidence which doubled with CPAP and rose to as high as 35–40% in babies treated with IPPV plus PEEP and inspiratory times exceeding 1 second. In recent years, with a change in IPPV patterns to faster rates and shorter inspiratory times (p. 517), and the use of surfactant (pp. 494, 508) there has been a gratifying reduction in the overall incidence of airleak syndromes to 5–10% in most ventilated infants. If, however, a pneumothorax does develop in a baby with RDS it must always be drained (p. 520).

Patent ductus arteriosus

It is arguable whether this should be regarded as a complication of RDS rather than an integral feature of the disease, as ultrasound studies show ductal patency in the first 24–48 hours in all preterm babies with RDS,[281,898] although in most cases the amount of shunt through the ductus is relatively small and usually bidirectional. The incidence of symptomatic PDA can be kept to a minimum by strict control of fluid intake in the first few days (p. 505, Table 29.19).[82]

The clinical presentation of a clinically significant ductus is a ventilated preterm baby aged 5–7 days who was beginning to recover from RDS, developing signs of heart failure and a loud precordial murmur filling systole, frequently extending into diastole. The oxygen and ventilatory requirements increase and a few infants develop MPH (p. 551). At this stage there is a wide consensus that fluids should be restricted and indomethacin given.[371] This approach results in a large enough reduction in the left–right shunt in 90% of neonates to allow weaning from IPPV over the next week, sometimes faster. If the first course is unsuccessful a second one can be given, and in such cases a prolonged course of say, 0.1 mg/kg for 6 days, may be more successful.[885,894]

Table 29.19 Prevalence of patent ductus arteriosus with different fluid regimens[82]

Fluid regimen*	No of neonates	PDA	Heart failure
High (169 ml/kg/24 h)	85	35	11
Low (122 ml/kg/24 h)	85	9	2
		$P < 0.001$	$P = 0.015$

*Average fluid intake per day on days 3–30

Recent meta-analyses of studies of prophylactic indomethacin given on the first day suggest that this is beneficial, with a significant reduction in symptomatic PDA in treated babies, though with no effect on neonatal mortality.[332] This tallies with animal studies which show that early ductus closure in baboons with RDS was of little physiological benefit.[770] However, given the beneficial effect of indomethacin on the incidence of GMH/IVH and MPH, as well as PDA, there is a case for prophylactic therapy in babies <28 weeks' gestational age with a high incidence of these complications.[200]

Ligation is only used in neonates who have not responded to this conservative management; failure to respond is most likely in patients with a large left atrial–aortic root ratio on echocardiography.[1085] The size of the infant should not be a deterrent to surgery, as it is in the extremely low-birthweight infant <1.00 kg in whom the ductus does not respond to indomethacin that successful weaning from the ventilator will not take place until the duct is ligated[217] (p. 689). Ligation is not indicated in the baby who is off the ventilator and thriving, even if he has a loud murmur causing heart failure, which in most cases is easy to control by fluid retention and frusemide.[683] In most such cases the ductus will close spontaneously while the baby is still on the neonatal unit, whereupon therapy for heart failure can be withdrawn.

Germinal layer–intraventricular haemorrhage (Chapter 44, Part 5)

This condition remains the commonest cause of death in the VLBW neonate ventilated for RDS (p. 481). The development of a large GMH/IVH is usually associated with clinical deterioration characterized by anaemia, increased ventilatory requirements and neurological signs, which can be very subtle (p. 1257). In many cases smaller GMH/IVHs are asymptomatic and detected only on routine ultrasound. Many aspects of the management of respiratory failure in the neonate are directed towards preventing GMH/IVH, including the use of prophylactic drugs (p. 1262), giving pancuronium to ventilated babies (p. 576), avoiding procedures that might provoke surges in cerebral blood flow (p. 1256), and correcting coagulation disturbances (p. 805). The relative efficacy of each of these procedures remains speculative.

Table 29.20 Survival in neonates with RDS

Birthweight (kg)	Oxford 1972–74		Cambridge 1980–83		Cambridge 1987–89		Cambridge 1990–94	
	RDS	Dead	RDS	Dead	RDS	Dead	RDS	Dead
1.00–1.50	41	13 (32%)	101	17(17%)	154	21 (14%)	239	27 (11%)
1.50–2.00	35	6 (17%)	44	1 (2%)	149	6 (4%)	158	3 (2%)

Infection (pp. 507, 1144)

Chronic lung disease

This has now become the single most important complication of RDS in terms of morbidity, duration of therapy and cost. It is described in detail in Part 3 of this chapter.

Necrotizing enterocolitis (p. 748)

Renal failure

One of the purposes of attempting early correction and maintenance of blood pressure, using dopamine to preserve renal perfusion and paying meticulous attention to the fluid balance in babies with RDS, is to sustain renal function. In some cases this is not successful, and in others an acute episode of collapse, such as may occur with bilateral tension pneumothoraces, results in acute tubular necrosis (p. 1027). If renal failure develops it should be treated as outlined on pages 1028–1029. If simple biochemical control cannot be achieved, there are no contraindications to either peritoneal dialysis or haemofiltration in ventilated VLBW babies with RDS. Although there is as yet little experience with haemofiltration, this procedure has much to recommend it as it avoids the major problem with peritoneal dialysis, which is the intraperitoneal fluid splinting the diaphragm and making oxygenation difficult in ventilated neonates. Venovenous ultrafiltration and haemodialysis using a manual syringe-driven technique has been successfully performed in two extremely low-birthweight infants.[226]

Complications of neonatal intensive care

Ill VLBW neonates with multiple tubes in situ are susceptible to all the iatrogenic complications described in Chapter 37, which should all be prevented if possible and treated on merit if they occur.

OUTCOME

Survival

If death does occur in a baby ≥26 weeks' gestation it is usually from one of the three major complications: infection, GMH/IVH or CLD. In babies of 22–25 weeks' gestation, hyaline membrane disease or one of the three major complications is often present at postmortem, but, particularly with deaths in the first 24 hours, it is often impossible to say whether the infant died from surfactant deficiency or respiratory failure due to the incompatibility of the canalicular stage of lung development (p. 455) with adequate postnatal gas exchange. Death from RDS in a baby weighing more than 1.5 kg is exceptionally rare (Table 29.20), and the overall mortality from the condition has now been reduced to between 5 and 10%,[412] although this may still be up to 15% of perinatal deaths.[72]

Sequelae

Up to 50% of babies surviving RDS whose birthweight was below 1.50 kg require readmission to a general paediatric ward within the first year after discharge from the neonatal unit,[760,782] and they continue to have a high incidence of readmission throughout childhood.[689] Amongst VLBW infants, those with birthweight <750 g and gestational age ≤28 weeks require the greatest number of admissions and the longest duration of stay; in the first year of life the duration of stay is inversely related to birthweight.[1203] This may be for further treatment of hydrocephalus secondary to a GMH/IVH, sequelae of surgery in NEC, for failure to thrive or for a repair of an inguinal hernia, which is very common in boys weighing <1.00 kg at birth. The major problems, however, are respiratory and neurological.

Respiratory

The most important respiratory sequel of RDS is CLD (pp. 608–630). Airway problems secondary to prolonged intubation may also occur (pp. 574, 668–669). After discharge, babies who have survived RDS in the neonatal period are more likely to have respiratory illness, particularly in the first year of life, than infants born at term or prematurely without respiratory problems. Although not all studies show an increased incidence of respiratory infection,[783] there is general agreement that lower respiratory tract infections in such infants are more severe.[666,783] In addition to more respiratory infections, surviving preterm babies also have persisting function abnormalities, with increased airway resistance and air trapping. Some studies find such changes in all preterm survivors,[177] but most report that these sequelae are more common in those neonates who required prolonged ventilation,[1202] often in high oxygen concentrations, and that they are particularly severe and frequent in infants with CLD (p. 621).

Long-term neurological sequelae (Chapter 7)

VLBW neonates who have been ventilated for RDS have a higher incidence of neurological sequelae than control infants. They are also at risk from ROP (p. 909). Whether or not a baby has a central nervous system handicap at follow-up seems to depend primarily on whether or not he develops GMH/IVH, or in particular PVL, in the neonatal period.[215,396] The relative importance of prenatal events (such as prenatal or intrapartum asphyxia) and postnatal events (such as hypotension or prolonged periods of hypoxia and acidaemia) in the genesis of GMH/IVH and PVL in critically ill neonates with RDS receiving ventilation is not clear, but if a neonate never had either of these brain abnormalities demonstrated by ultrasound, nor had seizures in the neonatal period, the risk from long-term sequelae would appear to be very small, except in those with CLD (p. 621).

TRANSIENT TACHYPNOEA OF THE NEWBORN

TTN was first described by Avery et al.[36] It has also been reported as wet lung,[1154] benign unexplained respiratory distress in the newborn,[1063] neonatal tachypnoea[704] or type 2 RDS.[866] The prevalence is controversial: several authors claim that it is underdiagnosed, and that as many as 71% of cases of RDS are due to TTN.[126] Tudehope and Smyth[1088] suggested that TTN is the commonest cause of neonatal respiratory distress and accounts for 41% of cases. In two major surveys of neonatal respiratory disease the prevalence of pulmonary maladaptation, which corresponds very largely to TTN, was 9.3/1000[498] and 3.6–4.5/1000,[322] and in Hjalmarson's[498] series comprised 32% of all neonatal lung disease (see Table 29.7).

AETIOLOGY

Avery et al[36] attributed TTN to a delay in fetal lung fluid clearance; newborn lambs with retained fetal lung fluid have similar clinical signs and radiographic appearances[328] to infants with this condition. Normal alveolar fluid has a very low protein content and can thus be absorbed into the circulation. Avery et al[36] postulated that the protein content could be increased during asphyxia, either by increased lung capillary permeability (p. 484) or by amniotic fluid inhalation; the resultant high protein-containing fluid would then be more slowly absorbed into the pulmonary circulation.[9] The protein may also interfere with surfactant function.[522,535]

TTN is more common following caesarean section before labour[768,1088] (see Fig. 29.18). In such infants who develop TTN noradrenaline levels are lower than in those delivered following labour.[409] In the absence of labour, anticipatory lung fluid clearance will not have occurred[1136] (pp. 457, 483) and the absence of vaginal squeeze may also delay lung liquid clearance (p. 483). Surfactant deficiency may be important in the pathogenesis of TTN.[149,535] Hallman and Teramo[453] estimated L:S ratios and phosphatidylglycerol in 506 amniotic fluid samples: seven infants had TTN and L:S ratios less than 2.0; unfortunately, it is not clear whether this was associated with the absence of PG.

TTN is also more common in babies born into families with a history of asthma.[947]

PRESENTATION

TTN is more frequent in term infants but can occur in preterm ones. The condition is associated with hypoproteinaemia, birth asphyxia, breech presentation and male gender.[1088]

The classic presentation is isolated tachypnoea with respiratory rates up to 100–120/min. The infant rarely grunts, which is a sign indicating atelectasis; retraction, a sign indicating non-compliant lungs, is minimal. The chest may be barrel-shaped as a result of hyperinflation, and the liver and spleen are palpable because of downward displacement of the diaphragm. Peripheral oedema is often present, and affected babies lose weight more slowly than controls.[878] On auscultation there may be added moist sounds, similar to those heard in heart failure. Tachycardia is common, but the blood pressure is usually normal.

TTN usually settles within 24 hours, but may persist for several days;[1015] in one study, 74% of babies had recovered by 48 hours.[1088] A more prolonged course was described in 19% of one series[126] and in 26% of another.[1088] In this second study, 25 infants with TTN had symptoms for less than 48 hours, but in nine symptoms persisted for a mean of 5.7 days. The majority of infants with prolonged TTN were male, marginally premature, born by caesarean section and mildly asphyxiated at birth, but their chest X-ray on the day of delivery was no different from that of the babies with transient symptoms: six of the nine required IPPV and PEEP. Halliday et al[450] reported six infants with severe TTN who required more than 60% oxygen in order to maintain a normal PaO_2. These six infants also had evidence of perinatal asphyxia, with both low Apgar scores and arterial pH immediately after birth.

Bucciarelli et al[139] noted an increased pulmonary vascular resistance in TTN, and attributed this to lung hyperinflation associated with retained fetal lung fluid. It could also be caused by perinatal asphyxia and acidosis. It has been questioned whether prolonged severe TTN in fact represents some other condition, such as post-

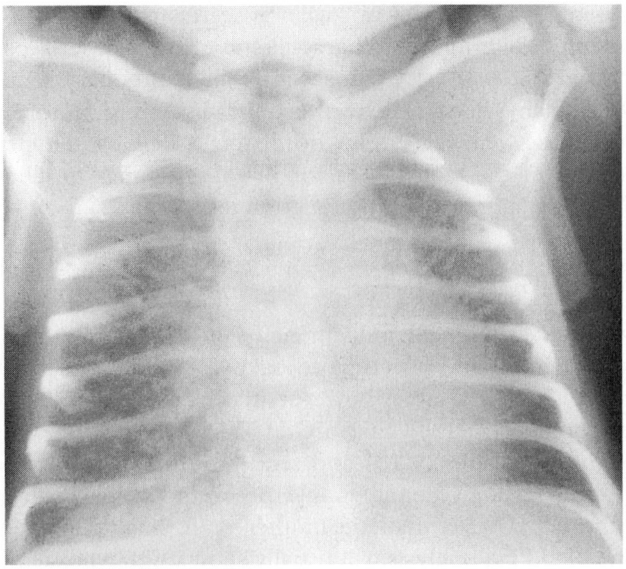

Fig. 29.41 Transient tachypnoea of the newborn. Fluid in the right horizontal fissure and pulmonary venous congestion.

asphyxial lung oedema or massive amniotic fluid aspiration.

INVESTIGATIONS

There are no specific haematological or biochemical features of TTN. Arterial blood gases usually show mild hypoxia; a marked respiratory or metabolic acidosis is unusual and, if present, makes a review of the diagnosis mandatory. The chest X-ray shows hyperinflation, sometimes with intercostal bulging of the pleura. There are prominent perihilar vascular markings, oedema of the interlobar septae and fluid present in the fissures[618] (Fig. 29.41). The prominent perihilar streaking is probably engorgement of the periarterial lymphatics, which participate in the clearance of lung fluid; fluid may also be present in the costophrenic angles. The chest X-ray usually clears by the next day, although complete resolution may take 3–7 days.

Echocardiography may have a role in identifying babies with severe TTN: Halliday et al[450] demonstrated that in the first 24 hours of life infants with mild or classic TTN had normal right ventricular function and pulmonary vascular resistance, with only mild left ventricular failure and mild abnormalities of left ventricular contractility. In contrast, in severe TTN there was generalized myocardial failure, pulmonary hypertension with right–left shunting, and abnormalities of systolic time intervals in both ventricles. The left ventricular pre-ejection period to ejection time ratio was increased for the first 3 days of life and correlated with the duration of treatment in oxygen.

Sandberg et al[943] found a reduced tidal volume but a raised minute volume due to the increased respiratory rate. Compliance was reduced, with raised airways resistance and FRC.

DIFFERENTIAL DIAGNOSIS

This disorder may be confused with many of the conditions in Table 29.13. The chest X-ray in RDS is often distinctive (p. 500), and RDS is rare in term babies. A rapid respiratory rate may be due to cerebral irritation resulting from asphyxia (p. 555), but these infants are distinguished by their history and the presence of a respiratory alkalaemia.

The chest X-ray appearance of TTN may be mimicked by heart failure. If this is due to asphyxia there will be a positive history, and the heart will usually be enlarged; if due to congenital heart disease a murmur may be present. The echocardiographic findings in severe TTN resemble those found in PPHN (pp. 528, 531), but the infants described by Halliday et al[450] all had the X-ray changes of TTN. It is not possible to differentiate TTN from early-onset sepsis (pp. 1116, 1128) when planning the initial treatment.

TREATMENT

Most infants with TTN require no form of respiratory support other than added oxygen, and rarely require an inspired oxygen concentration greater than 40% or support for more than 3 days. Intravenous penicillin should be administered until infection has been excluded (p. 507). Hydration should be maintained with intravenous glucose electrolyte solutions, and nasogastric tube feeds should be withheld for 24–48 hours until the respiratory rate settles. Fluid should be administered at 40–60 ml/kg/24 h during the acute illness.

As the proposed mechanism for TTN is a delay in fetal lung liquid reabsorption after birth, treatment with diuretics would seem logical. In a randomized prospective study, however, frusemide (2 mg/kg orally at the time of diagnosis and 1 mg/kg 12 h later if the symptoms persisted) made no significant difference to the duration of tachypnoea or of hospitalization.[1170]

Infants with the severe form of TTN may require up to 100% oxygen for several days,[139] and a few will need IPPV,[1088] though whether such patients genuinely have TTN is arguable.

MONITORING

The standard monitoring outlined in Chapter 21 should be applied. For those with mild disease oxygen therapy can be safely monitored by intermittent arterial stabs combined with $TcPO_2$ monitoring or oximetry. An umbilical arterial catheter should be inserted only if the infant is premature or requires more than 40% oxygen for more than 24 hours.

COMPLICATIONS

These are rare, though airleaks may occur, particularly if CPAP or IPPV is required.[438]

PROGNOSIS

The condition is self-limiting, although the symptoms may last up to 8 days,[1015] resulting in prolonged hospital admission.[878] Infants who have been followed up for as long as 1 year have had no recurrence of tachypnoea or other pulmonary disease.

MINIMAL RESPIRATORY DISEASE

In the epidemiological surveys of neonatal pulmonary disease (Table 29.7) this entity is usually defined as transient respiratory signs persisting for a mean of only 4 hours.[498] The prevalence in that study was 11/1000, but it is likely that many infants with mild transient TTN were included. In Nottingham the condition seemed to be rarer, with a prevalence of 2.5–3.4/1000 live births.[322]

AETIOLOGY

This is unclear. Some babies are hypothermic with a temperature of less than 35°C; surfactant function is temperature dependent,[380] and as these babies often improve within an hour or two when their temperature returns to normal, this may be the problem. Some babies have a low(ish) pH, at 7.20–7.25, and this may not only stimulate respiration (p. 555) but also transiently compromise surfactant synthesis[740] (p. 484). In other babies the tachypnoea may be the result of mild intrapartum asphyxia with or without minor degrees of aspiration of meconium or amniotic squames. In most cases the condition probably represents the very mild end of the spectrum of delayed clearance of lung liquid, which in the more marked form is diagnosed as TTN.

CLINICAL FEATURES

The baby, near or at term, presents within the first 2–3 hours, commonly after being transferred to the postnatal ward with his mother. He usually has an expiratory grunt or moan, which may be quite loud, there is mild sternal or intercostal recession, and he may have a respiratory rate up to 80–100/min. Cyanosis, if present, is relieved by giving 25–30% oxygen. There are no added sounds in the chest, and the rest of the clinical examination is normal.

DIFFERENTIAL DIAGNOSIS

This is always retrospective, made once the baby has recovered and shows no signs of infection or more serious pulmonary disease. The major anxiety when the baby first presents is whether or not what is seen is the first sign of the rapid deterioration characteristic of early-onset sepsis (p. 1128). In some infants with mild pulmonary hypoplasia tachypnoea can be the only presenting feature.[14] Such cases, however, can be distinguished by the persistence of the tachypnoea, small-volume lungs on chest X-ray, and abnormal lung function tests (p. 642).

INVESTIGATION

Experienced clinical judgement is of value in assessing these babies and electing to take a ‘watch and wait’ stance. It is advisable, however, to check a single blood gas (by arterial stab), take a chest X-ray to exclude other diagnoses (Table 29.13) and send off a blood count and culture. Hypoglycaemia should be excluded, particularly if the baby has a diabetic mother or is small for dates. The blood gas analysis will usually show mild hypoxaemia in air (PaO_2 6–8 kPa, 45–60 mmHg) which rapidly becomes normal in 25–30% oxygen; $PaCO_2$ and the pH will usually be normal or show a mild metabolic acidaemia, with a pH of 7.20–7.25 and a base deficit of 10 mmol/l. The haemoglobin and white count will be normal. The chest X-ray, particularly if taken within 1–2 hours of birth, often shows some streakiness or a rather non-specific haziness, both of which probably represent delayed clearing of the fetal lung liquid.

TREATMENT

By the time the results of these preliminary investigations are available the baby may be beginning to show signs more suggestive of sepsis, TTN or classic RDS. If he is not, and is already showing a marked improvement, all that needs to be done is to keep him in an appropriate inspired oxygen concentration. An intravenous infusion is rarely needed. Provided the blood gases are satisfactory and the respiratory distress remains minimal, nasogastric feeds of 60 ml/kg/24 h can be commenced by 6–10 hours of age. However, if there is anxiety about the presence of infection, antibiotics should be started. If the suspicion is mild the treatment can be limited to intravenous penicillin (p. 507), otherwise broad-spectrum cover should be given by adding an aminoglycoside.

PROGNOSIS

By definition this is excellent. Most babies are asymptomatic and in room air by 12 hours of age. The diagnosis is thus confirmed. If they do not behave in this way, they have another disorder.

PULMONARY AIR LEAKS

Pneumothorax and PIE are the most common forms of airleak in the newborn; pneumomediastinum, pneumopericardium and pneumoperitoneum also occur. Rarely, multiple airleaks may be complicated by subcutaneous emphysema and systemic air embolism.

PATHOPHYSIOLOGY

Pulmonary airleaks occur when there is uneven alveolar ventilation, air trapping and high transpulmonary pressure swings, the final common pathway being alveolar overdistension and rupture. Uneven ventilation is compounded by a lack of redistribution of pressure through the alveolar connecting channels, the pores of Kohn, which are reduced in number in the immature lung.[698] The rupture is thought to occur at the alveolar bases, in apposition to blood vessels. The gas tracks along the sheaths of pulmonary blood vessels to the mediastinum, where it accumulates in the roots of the lungs but not in the sheaths of the bronchi.[699] Air may then rupture into the pleura, mediastinum, pericardium or extrathoracic areas. This hypothesis[699] for the development of airleaks is not universally accepted, and an alternative is that interstitial air directly enters the pleural cavity after rupture of a subpleural bleb.[854] The existence of PIE supports Macklin's[699] hypothesis, as after alveolar rupture gas is trapped in the parenchyma by the extensive connective tissue matrix[883] and increased interstitial water in the preterm lung. This prevents decompression into the mediastinum,[1066] thereby splinting the lung and compressing the blood vessels[940] (see below).

PNEUMOTHORAX

Incidence

Older data suggested that spontaneous pneumothorax at birth was common: X-raying the chest of all newborns demonstrated that 1% have airleaks, but that only 10% of these were symptomatic.[1022] The prevalence was higher if there was lung disease or assisted ventilation: 4% of infants with lung disease develop airleaks, compared to 16% on CPAP[1198] and 34% of those being ventilated.[702]

In the last decade the incidence of pneumothorax has responded dramatically to the introduction of surfactant therapy, which has reduced the incidence of these complications by more than a half (pp. 494, 508), and to the use of pancuronium (p. 576) and faster ventilator rates (p. 565). As a result most units now report airleak rates of 5–10% in ventilated babies, only about double that reported in the past in spontaneously breathing neonates with RDS.

McIntosh[697] suggested that pneumothoraces were more common the more preterm the baby, but no such trend was found in those with RDS.[412] Fifteen to twenty per cent of pneumothoraces are bilateral; when unilateral the right lung is more frequently involved (two-thirds of cases).

Aetiology

Pneumothorax may occur immediately after birth[185] owing to the high transpulmonary pressure swings generated by the newborn during his first breaths[1127] or by active resuscitation (pp. 260–261). Thereafter, pneumothorax is usually a complication of respiratory disease, for example RDS or meconium aspiration syndrome, and congenital malformations, in all of which there may be alveolar overdistension and air trapping, made worse in many cases by IPPV. Pneumothorax may occasionally result from direct injury to the lung by causes other than mechanical ventilation, for example direct perforation by suction catheters passed through the endotracheal tube.[26,1119]

Four factors increase the incidence of airleaks:

- The addition of PEEP of 3–8 cmH_2O to IPPV may increase the incidence of airleaks to 34%, compared to 21% among infants ventilated without PEEP,[85] but these data have not been confirmed in a randomized study.
- Prolonged inspiratory time. The incidence of airleaks was reported to be 50% if an I:E ratio greater or equal to 1.0 was employed, but only 16% if the I:E ratio was less than or equal to 0.7.[1056] Primhak[864] reported that the only significant difference between ventilated babies with and without airleak was a longer inflation time in the former. A prolonged inspiratory time also results in babies actively expiring against the ventilator[405] (see below).
- High peak inspiratory pressures increase the risk of airleaks,[416,809] as does an elevated MAP; the prevalence of airleak is 17% if the MAP is below 12 cmH_2O but 39% if it is greater than 12 cmH_2O.[1056]
- Infants who breathe out of phase with the ventilator have an increased incidence of airleak.[1021] It was postulated that simultaneous inspiratory effort and inflation would generate large pressure and volume swings, rupturing the lung. It is now realized, however, that airleaks are virtually limited to babies whose inspiration has ceased and have started to exhale while the ventilator is still trying to inflate the lungs. This pattern of baby–ventilator interaction was called the 'active expiratory reflex' by Greenough et al.[415] It is most common in infants with stiff lungs and is not related to gestational age or birthweight.[405] It can be provoked by reducing the ventilator rate or increasing the inflation time.[320]

Clinical features

Small pneumothoraces may be asymptomatic, but when a large pneumothorax develops all of the clinical features of respiratory distress (p. 495) are present. In addition, with very large or tension pneumothoraces the infant's overall condition usually deteriorates, often dramatically, with pallor and shock: arterial blood pressure, heart rate and respiratory rate decreased in 77% of cases in one series.[806] Oxygenation frequently deteriorates, but the pH and $PaCO_2$ may not.[806] Physical findings may be difficult to elicit, but an increased resonance on percussion may be detected, and there is often a decrease in air entry on the affected side; a tension pneumothorax will result in a shift of the mediastinum and the position of the cardiac impulse. Abdominal distension, caused by displacement of the diaphragm, is another useful sign of a tension pneumothorax.

At the time of a pneumothorax there is a marked increase in cerebral blood flow velocity which correlates closely with the systemic haemodynamic changes.[490] In accordance with this, Lipscomb et al[668] demonstrated that pneumothorax causes and aggravates haemorrhage into the germinal layer and ventricles of preterm infants, 86% of infants with pneumothorax developing GMH-IVH compared to 42% without an airleak. Increased levels of ADH (antidiuretic hormone) may also occur, resulting in fluid retention (p. 505).

Diagnosis

Continuous monitoring of heart rate, blood pressure and PaO_2 will give instant warning of the baby's deterioration. The ECG trace may become low-amplitude,[738] and changes in transthoracic electrical impedance[797] and intraoesphageal pressure swings[609] have been used diagnostically.

Transillumination[619] with an intense beam from a fibreoptic light is of considerable help in the preterm baby with a thin chest wall: abnormal air collections cause increased transmission of light on the involved side; however, PIE can give a similar appearance.

The chest X-ray remains the gold standard for diagnosing pneumothorax and should be performed unless the infant's clinical condition makes emergency drainage mandatory. The diagnosis of a pneumothorax on the chest X-ray is usually obvious, but rarely the appearance of either lobar emphysema or cystic adenomatoid malformation of the lung may resemble a pneumothorax. A small pneumothorax may only be recognized by a difference in radiolucency between the two lung fields[1049] (Fig. 29.42). A large pneumothorax will have absent lung markings and a collapsed lung on the ipsilateral side (Fig. 29.43). A tension pneumothorax will be demonstrated by eversion of the diaphragm, bulging intercostal spaces and mediastinal shift (Fig. 29.43).

Ill, ventilated infants are usually nursed in the supine position and intrapleural air rises to lie retrosternally. Retrosternal air is best demonstrated by a horizontal-beam lateral-view chest X-ray (Fig. 29.44), which will also be useful in demonstrating the position of the chest drain tip[695] (see below; Fig. 29.45).

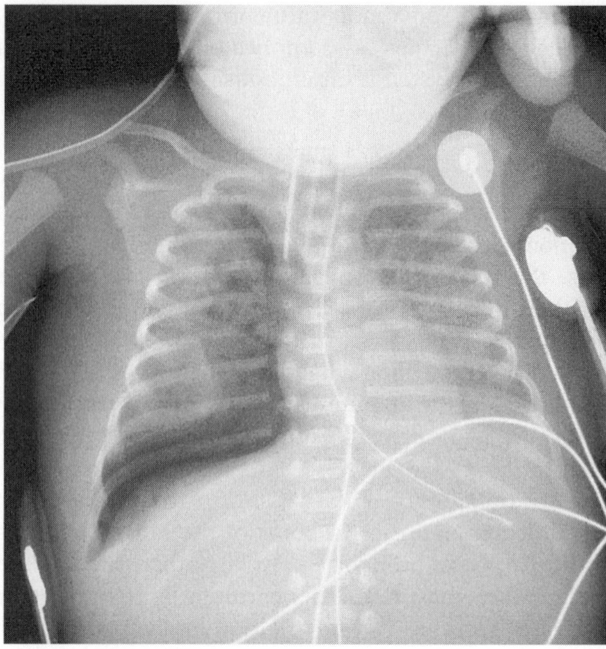

Fig. 29.42 Pneumothorax demonstrated by the difference in translucency of the two lung fields. There is also a small rim of paramediastinal and supradiaphragmatic gas.

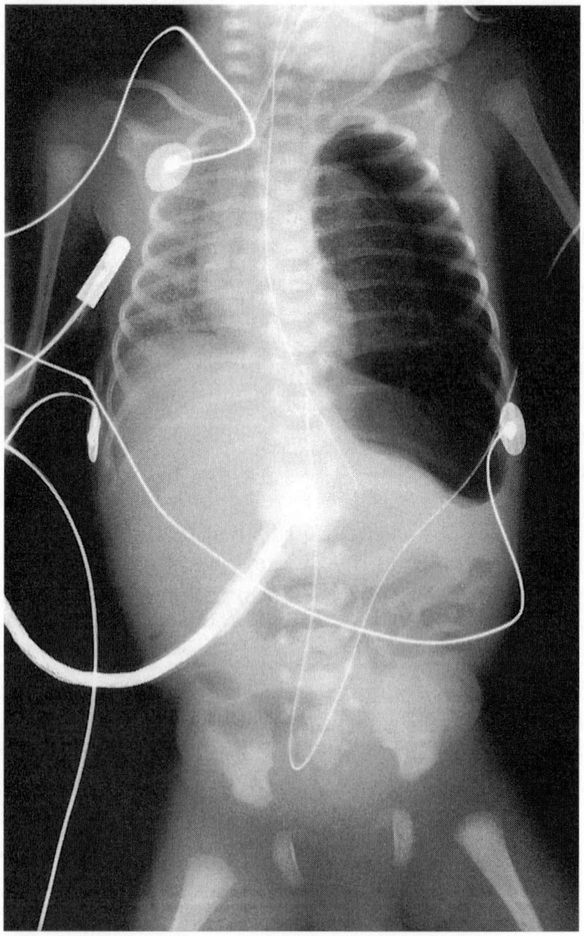

Fig. 29.43 Left tension pneumothorax, with displacement of left diaphragm downwards and mediastinum to the right. Note that the non-compliant left lung has only partially collapsed.

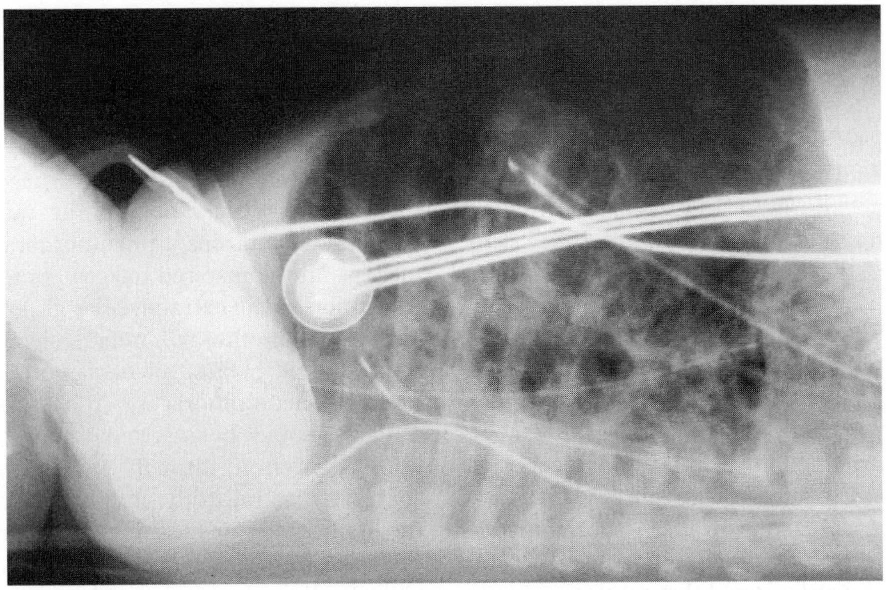

Fig. 29.44 Lateral chest X-ray with anterior collection of air – only one chest drain is positioned to lie anteriorly; the other tip lies posteriorly and the pneumothorax has been inadequately drained.

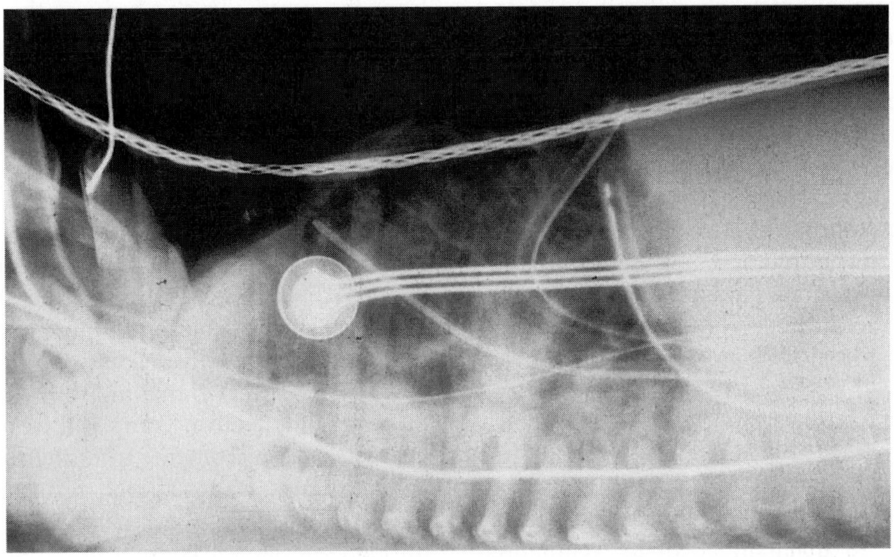

Fig. 29.45 Lateral chest X-ray to show position of chest drain tubes. All three tubes are correctly placed, i.e. restrosternally, resulting in drainage of the pneumothorax.

Investigation and monitoring

These routines are identical to those carried out in babies with RDS (pp. 497–501, Chapter 21).

Prevention

The risk of pneumothorax can be reduced in three ways:

- by administering surfactant (pp. 494, 508);
- by using the minimum ventilator pressure required (p. 565);
- by abolishing the baby's active expiratory efforts.

Abolishing active expiration

Ventilating babies at rates of 60/min or greater, rather than 30–40/min, reduces the incidence of airleaks. Bland et al[109] reported an 8% incidence of pneumothoraces in infants ventilated at rates between 60 and 110/min. Heicher et al[478] compared rates of 60/min with an inspiratory time of 0.5 seconds to rates of 20–40/min with an inspiratory time of 1.0 second. At peak pressures less than 25 cmH_2O only 14% of those ventilated at the faster rate had a pneumothorax, compared to 35% ventilated at the slower rate. Subsequently, two multicentre randomized studies also supported this observation.[804,856]

Physiological studies have demonstrated that spontaneous respiration synchronizes with the ventilator at fast rates;[419] infants actively expiring at a slow rate will breathe synchronously at rates ≥60/min, and this may be the mechanism by which pneumothoraces are reduced (p. 565). In a prospective trial HFOV also reduced the incidence of air leaks;[489] during HFOV very few infants' respiratory efforts are such that they interfere with effective ventilation;[176] this may also reduce the incidence of pneumothorax.

Paralysis/sedation. Breathing out of phase with the ventilator during IPPV increases the incidence of pneumothorax (see above). Early trials of paralysis, despite reducing mortality[484] and chronic lung disease,[860] were not associated with a reduction in airleaks. However, if pancuronium is given to infants who are showing the active expiration pattern (see above), there is a significant reduction in the incidence of pneumothoraces.[216,417] A recent randomized trial demonstrated that routine paralysis of all ventilated babies was no better at preventing pneumothorax than synchronized ventilation.[970] Paralysis should therefore be restricted to infants who are actively expiring. Active expiration may be difficult to detect clinically at slow rates; however, if oxygenation fails to improve, and obvious respiratory efforts continue as the ventilator rate is increased to 60–80/min, this identifies the majority of neonates with a persisting active respiratory pattern who are likely to benefit from paralysis[407] or the use of effective sedation/analgesia (pp. 576–577).

Patient-triggered ventilation. In theory, if inflation is always triggered by inspiration, by removing any adverse interaction between the patient and the ventilator PTV should reduce the incidence of airleaks,[199] but this has not been demonstrated in a prospective multicentre randomized trial.[90]

Bearing all these factors in mind, to minimize the incidence of pneumothoraces after giving surfactant, IPPV should be started at 60–80 breaths/min at the lowest peak pressure to maintain adequate ventilation, and an inspiratory time of 0.3–0.4 seconds (p. 567). If the baby makes obvious respiratory efforts, the ventilator rate should be increased to 70–100 breaths/min, maintaining a physiological I:E ratio (i.e. at least 1:1.2), with a tendency to use the faster rates in those who are more immature.[410] In the majority of infants increasing the ventilator rate will result in synchronous respiration.[419,421,1007] Approximately one-third of infants, however, will remain asynchronous despite rate manipulation, and should be either sedated or paralysed with vercuronium or pancuronium. If the former agent is used only small doses should be given because of the greater sensitivity of the end-plate in very immature infants, and only as boluses because of the slow recovery. Once the baby's ventilatory drive has been suppressed the ventilator rate should be reduced to 60–80 breaths/min, as gas trapping can occur at fast rates, particularly in relatively mature (>32 weeks' gestational age) paralysed infants.[494]

Treatment

Asymptomatic pneumothoraces need no treatment other than careful observation of the infant. In term infants with mild symptoms a pneumothorax may respond to an increase in the inspired oxygen content, which will favour resorption of the extra-alveolar gas.

A pneumothorax must always be drained in symptomatic babies, all babies on IPPV and those with tension pneumothoraces. A chest tube (French gauge 10–14) should be inserted under local anaesthesia, by blunt dissection through either the second intercostal space just lateral to the mid-clavicular line or, preferably, the sixth space in the midaxillary line. The latter site is preferred for cosmetic reasons, as any resultant scar is less obvious. If the lower site is chosen, turn the infant so that the affected side is uppermost and then aim the drain anteriorly. The drain should be positioned with the trocar removed and the infant very temporarily disconnected from the ventilator; this reduces the risk of inserting the drain into the lung, a complication which occurs in approximately 25% of cases.[752] This complication should be suspected if there is continuous drainage of air or the pneumothorax persists.

Once inserted, the tube should be connected to an underwater seal drain with suction of 5–10 cmH_2O. Heimlich valves are useful during transport, but can become blocked and so fail to operate if left in situ for any length of time. The tip of the chest tube should lie retrosternally to achieve the most effective drainage (Fig. 29.45). A retrospective review of 149 cases of chest drain placement[18] revealed that in 56% of cases posterior placement was ineffective, compared to only 4% for anterior (retrosternal) placement. Inserting the drain through the anterior chest wall achieved retrosternal positioning on 85% of occasions, compared to only 47% inserted through the lateral chest wall.[619] Anterior placement of the chest tube tip should be confirmed by an appropriate chest X-ray, a second drain only infrequently being required to ensure complete drainage (Figs 29.44, 29.45). If the infant is in extremis and there is no time for formal insertion of a drain, emergency drainage of a pneumothorax can be done by needle aspiration. A butterfly (18 gauge) should be used. This is then attached to a three-way tap which is held under water in a small sterile container. The needle is inserted through the skin in the second intercostal space anteriorly, and then the skin and needle are moved sideways before the needle is advanced through the underlying muscle; this reduces the likelihood of leaving an open track for the entry of air once the needle has been removed. Care must be taken not to remove too much air by needle aspiration, as this will tear the expanding lung. Following emergency drainage a chest tube must always be inserted. Percutaneous placement of small-bore pigtail catheters has been suggested as a possible alternative to the standard approach of thoracostomy tube placement in neonates.[1176]

Once a chest drain has been inserted it should be left in situ for at least 72–96 hours, or for 24 hours after it is no longer bubbling. The chest tubes should then be clamped for a further 24 hours and only removed if no pleural air accumulates. If the baby is still ventilator dependent the unclamped drain should be left in situ for longer before attempting to remove it.

After drainage of an uncomplicated pneumothorax a baby not on IPPV usually improves rapidly. In such babies the indications for antibiotics are those given on page 507. In ventilated babies the pneumothorax often precipitates a serious deterioration in their condition, the management of which is outlined on pages 579–580. The concurrent development of a large GMH/IVH may prove fatal.

Bronchopleural fistula

If there is a large tear in the pleural surface of the lung – a bronchopleural fistula – this may not close with conventional tube drainage of the pneumothorax. Alternative strategies are surgical closure at thoracotomy,[435] selective bronchial intubation[19,1187] (see below) or the instillation of fibrin glue into the pleural space.[87]

Prognosis

The mortality, though not the incidence, varies with the birthweight and is in general double that of babies who have RDS but no airleaks. Greenough and Roberton[412] found a mortality of 53% in infants <1.00 kg birthweight, compared to 33% in infants of 1.00–1.50 kg birthweight and only 8% for infants of 1.50–2.00 kg birthweight. Airleak (pneumothorax or PIE) increases the risk of death in the first 90 postnatal days; the strongest association with mortality, however, was if the leak occurred early (days 0 or 1) or particularly if it occurred late (days 4–27).[861] If a GMH/IVH occurs following a pneumothorax this will also have a detrimental effect on the neurological outcome.

PULMONARY INTERSTITIAL EMPHYSEMA

Aetiology

Pulmonary interstitial emphysema is gas trapped within the perivascular sheaths of the lung. It rarely occurs in term infants, whose easily expandable lung develops pneumothoraces. In the surfactant-deficient lung of the preterm infant[854,1066] rupture of the small airways occurs distal to the termination of their fascial sheath, and air dissects into the interstitium (p. 517). PIE therefore occurs mainly in neonates with RDS,[150] but has been noted (though much less frequently) in aspiration syndromes and sepsis. PIE is associated with positive-pressure ventilation, high peak inspiratory pressures and malpositioned endotracheal tubes.[416,470] It may be lobar in distribution, but more commonly involves both lungs. It frequently occurs with either a pneumothorax or pneumomediastinum.

Incidence

There is an inverse relationship between the incidence of PIE and birthweight. In one series 42% of infants with a birthweight less than 1.00 kg developed PIE, compared to 26% with birthweight over 1.00 kg.[470] Similar findings were reported by Yu et al:[1200] 32% and 22% respectively. As with pneumothorax (p. 519), the new ventilatory strategies and the use of surfactant have considerably reduced the incidence of PIE in the last 5–10 years.

Pathophysiology

In infants with interstitial emphysema the trapped gas reduces pulmonary perfusion by compressing the vessels and interfering with ventilation. As a result there is profound hypoxaemia combined with carbon dioxide retention (see above).

Presentation

Pulmonary interstitial emphysema virtually always presents radiologically; that is, it is found on the chest X-ray of a severely ill neonate carried out either on a routine basis or because his condition was deteriorating. Indeed, it is because of PIE and the changes in ventilator therapy it predicates that performing a chest X-ray is recommended as part of the routine monitoring of babies in respiratory failure (p. 370).

Diagnosis

Transillumination of the chest with diffuse PIE will give the same appearance as a large pneumothorax. The chest X-ray is, however, diagnostic, demonstrating hyperinflation and a characteristic cystic appearance; these may be diffuse, multiple, small, non-confluent, cystic radiolucencies (Figs 29.46, 29.47), and may be unilateral (Fig. 29.48); at a later stage large bullae may appear (Fig. 29.49). The appearance may be confused with lobar emphysema or with cystic adenomatoid malformation of the lung (pp. 645, 648).

Treatment

Affected babies usually have severe RDS and/or sepsis and require all the support described on pages 559–577, but their ventilator management is particularly difficult. For both generalized and localized disease the first thing

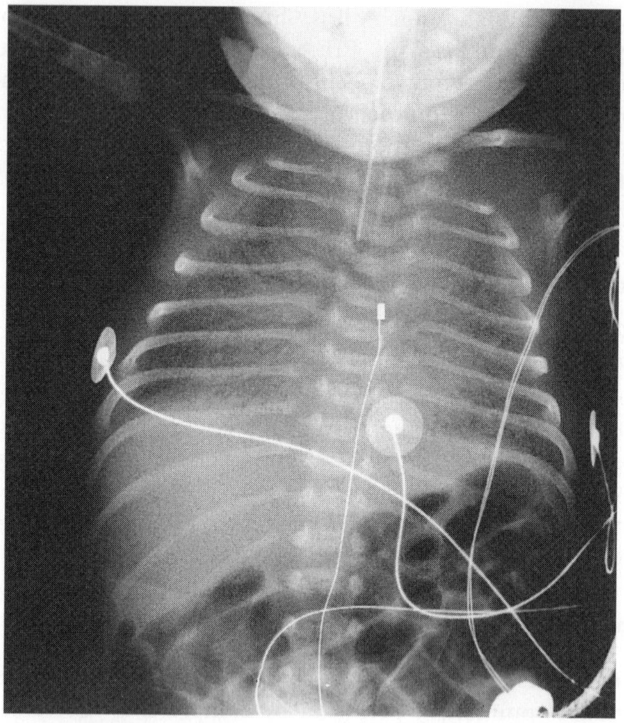

Fig. 29.46 Early PIE.

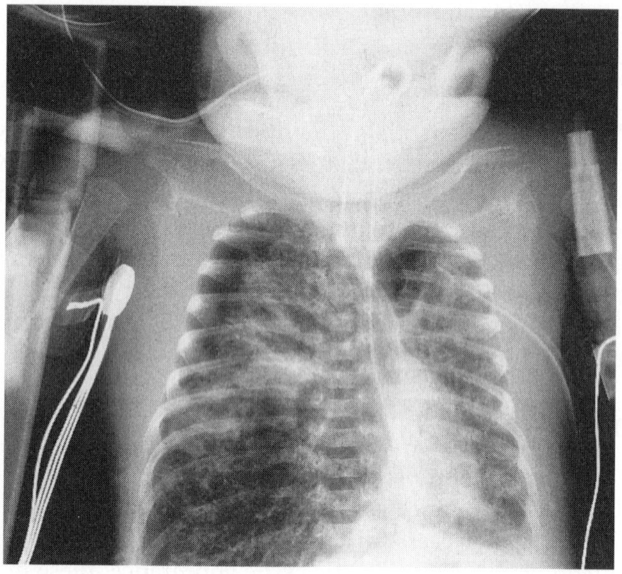

Fig. 29.47 Gross PIE of right lung with overdistension and downward displacement of diaphragm, and moderately severe PIE of left lung.

to do is to keep the ventilator pressures at the minimum compatible with acceptable gases (PaO_2 > 6–7 kPa (45–52 mmHg), pH > 7.25, $PaCO_2$ < 8 kPa (60 mmHg), and the baby should be paralysed to minimize the risk of extension of the airleaks. Withdrawal of PEEP may result in disappearance of the PIE.[645,676] With these comparatively conservative management routines generalized PIE will often suddenly disappear, and they should therefore be the first line of treatment.

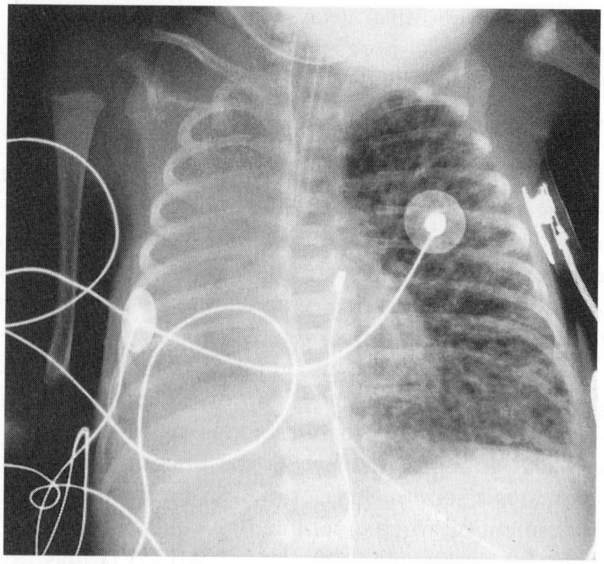

Fig. 29.48 Severe unilateral PIE.

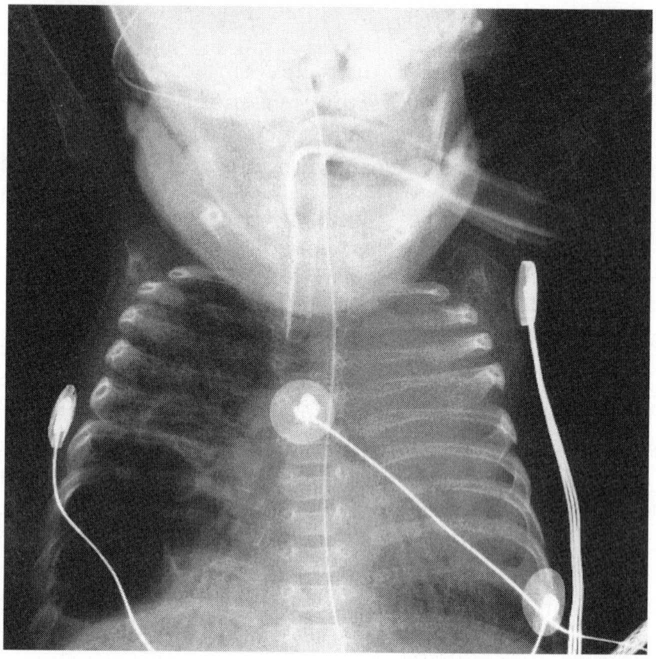

Fig. 29.49 PIE of right lung with gross cystic change in right middle lobe compressing right lower lobe and left lung.

Generalized PIE may respond to ventilator rates of 100–120/min.[794] Using such rates the number of babies who progress to pneumothorax may be reduced, but without any other advantage; indeed, in one series the severity of the PIE increased, possibly because of the absence of a pneumothorax decompressing the interstitial emphysema.[416]

Transfer from a conventional ventilator to HFJV,[121,858] HFFI[347] or HFOV[195] has improved oxygenation in some infants with severe respiratory failure due to PIE, but a randomized controlled trial of oscillation failed to show statistical benefit.[489] Keszler et al[579] reported a trial of

141 infants with PIE who were randomized to receive either HFJV or rapid-rate conventional ventilation with a short inspiratory time; 61% of infants on HFJV met with treatment success, compared to only 34% treated by conventional ventilation. Survival by original assignment was similar, as was the incidence of chronic lung disease, GMH/IVH, PDA, airway obstruction and airleak. In another study, 12 patients' oxygenation index improved following treatment with continuous negative pressure and intermittent mandatory ventilation.[238]

If the lungs do not decompress in response to different ventilator strategies an attempt can be made to achieve this by linear pleurotomy, thereby creating an artificial pneumothorax. This can be done by scarification of the lung using either a 21 G needle inserted through the chest wall[748] or by puncturing multiple blebs at thoracotomy.[1208]

With localized PIE the collections may not only persist but compress the adjacent normal lung parenchyma (Fig. 29.49), and sometimes cause a sudden deterioration in the infant's condition.

The conservative ventilatory management outlined above for generalized PIE should also be tried for localized disease, and is often successful.[676] In addition, in localized PIE, placing the infant with the hyperinflated lung dependent in the lateral decubitus position at all times will often result in partial or complete atelectasis of the desired segments.[206,1048] In this position the upper 'good' lung receives a greater proportion of the ventilation,[477] the affected dependent lung being underventilated and therefore decompressing.

Selective bronchial intubation may also be useful (Fig. 29.50). As soon as the affected lung is bypassed it becomes atelectatic; if selective intubation is maintained for 24–48 hours, when the affected lung is reventilated the PIE does not usually recur.[19,132,167] This technique is more useful if the left lung is affected, as selective intubation of the right main bronchus is easier to perform. It may be necessary to support the infant on HFOV to maintain adequate blood gases during selective intubation.[888] When using selective intubation of the right main bronchus, cutting an additional side hole in the endotracheal tube will reduce the problem of right upper lobe collapse.[700] Selective obstruction of one main bronchus has also been achieved by inserting a handmade latex oesophageal balloon under bronchoscopic control.[723] If selective bronchial intubation fails, alternatives include inserting a pneumothorax tube directly into the blebs[903] and leaving it there for 48 hours (Fig. 29.51), or carrying out multiple linear pleurotomies, as in generalized disease.[1208] If all else fails, surgical resection of the affected area may be required to alleviate the respiratory distress.[70,329] Two lobes may be resected successfully.[12]

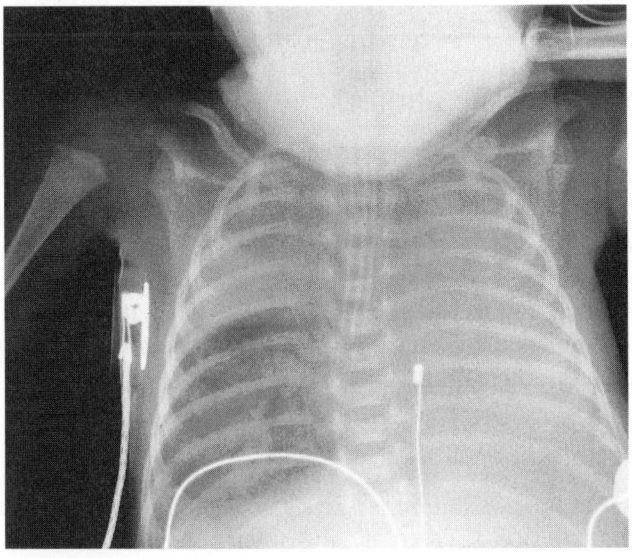

Fig. 29.50 Endotracheal tube inserted into right main bronchus, with resultant collapse of left lung and right upper lobe.

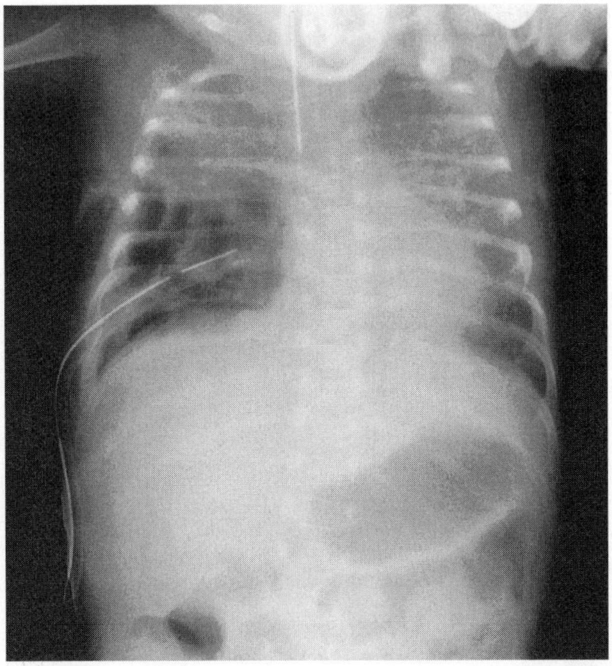

Fig. 29.51 Gross cystic changes in right middle lobe. Pneumothorax tube has been inserted directly into the blebs to drain them.

Prognosis

The incidence of CLD is greatly increased following diffuse PIE[1017,1199] (p. 609), and radiologically the changes of PIE may merge imperceptibly into those of CLD. Indeed, Stocker and Madewell[1031] have suggested that PIE may persist and cause a form of chronic lung disease, persistent interstitial pulmonary emphysema.

The mortality from diffuse PIE may be as high as 50%,[470,1200] although others have reported a much lower rate of 24%.[416] Gregoire et al[428] claimed that PIE appear-

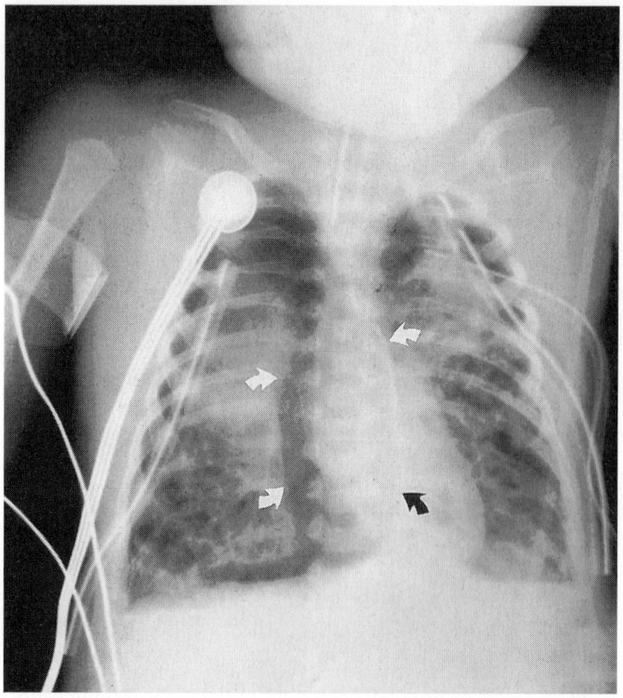

Fig. 29.52 Right lower lobe and left lung with gross cystic changes due to PIE. Bilateral pneumothorax and pneumomediastinum, including a posterior pneumomediastinum (outlined by arrows).

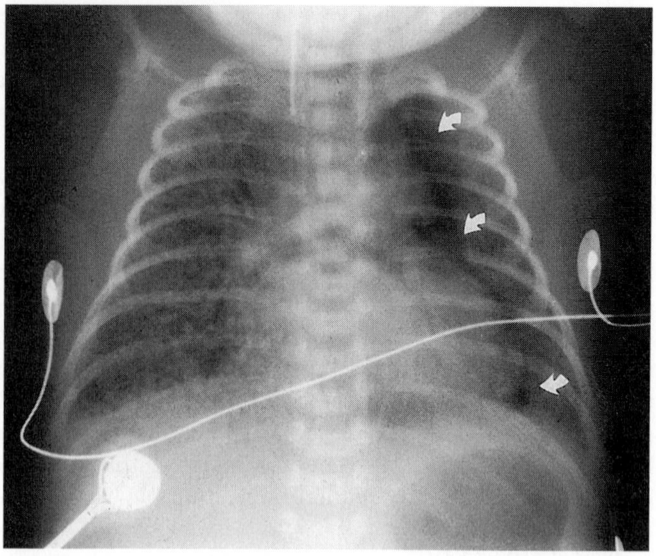

Fig. 29.53 Left-sided pneumomediastinum (between the arrows and the heart border).

ing on the first postnatal day always became bilateral and was invariably fatal. This was not confirmed,[416] although early-onset (<48 hours) PIE with an oxygen requirement greater than 60% was usually fatal.[762]

PNEUMOMEDIASTINUM

Incidence

Pneumomediastinum occurs in approximately 2.5 per 1000 live births.[769] Postmature infants are at increased risk, possibly because of the association with meconium aspiration.

Presentation

The infant with an isolated pneumomediastinum may be asymptomatic or have mild respiratory distress; only rarely does it cause severe symptoms. The sternum may appear bowed and the heart sounds muffled. Mediastinal shift rarely occurs. Air may track up into the soft tissues of the neck, but this is uncommon. Pneumomediastinum often coexists with multiple airleaks, including PIE and pneumothorax, in severely ill ventilated babies (Fig. 29.52).

Diagnosis

This is made on the chest X-ray (Fig. 29.53), as a halo of air adjacent to the borders of the heart; on lateral view it produces marked retrosternal hyperlucency. The mediastinal gas may elevate the thymus away from the pericardium, resulting in a crescentic configuration resembling a spinnaker sail.[771]

Treatment

An isolated pneumomediastinum is often asymptomatic and in general requires no treatment. It is very difficult to drain a pneumomediastinum, as the gas is collected in multiple independent lobules. Relatively successful attempts have been made, however, with multiple needling and tube drainage.[1062] In term infants the use of a high inspired oxygen concentration will be associated with resorption of the extra-alveolar air, but this should not be attempted in preterm infants at risk from ROP (p. 909).

PNEUMOPERICARDIUM

Pneumopericardium may be asymptomatic but usually causes cardiac tamponade, with sudden hypotension, bradycardia and cyanosis. The heart sounds are muffled, but a friction rub is rarely audible. The signs may be confused with those of a tension pneumothorax, but the chest X-ray is diagnostic (Fig. 29.54). It is usually accompanied by other major airleaks, such as pneumomediastinum, widespread PIE or tension pneumothorax.

Aetiology

Pneumopericardium may rarely occur spontaneously, but the majority of cases are in association with IPPV and barotrauma in the preterm infant. Its frequent association with PIE and pneumomediastinum suggests that the gas

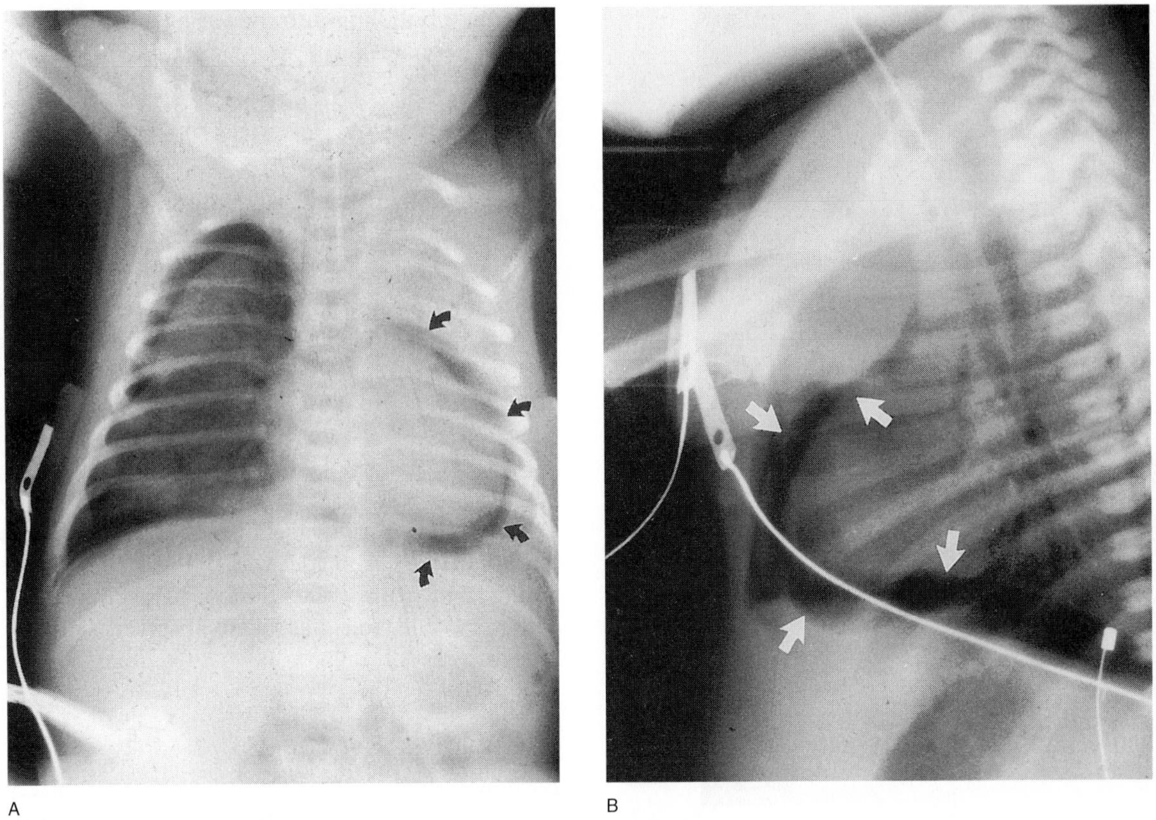

Fig. 29.54 Pneumopericardium (A. Anteroposterior view; B. lateral view). There is also a R. pneumothorax.

enters the pericardium through a defect in the pericardial sac, probably at the pericardial reflection near the ostia of the pulmonary veins. It has also been suggested that there is an anatomical predisposition to pneumopericardium.[1117] It occurred in 2% of infants weighing less than 1.50 kg.[503]

Diagnosis

The chest X-ray demonstrates gas completely surrounding the heart (Fig. 29.54), outlining the base of the great vessels and contained within the pericardium. Gas can be seen inferior to the diaphragmatic surface of the heart, differentiating this abnormality from a pneumomediastinum in which the mediastinal gas is limited inferiorly by the attachment of the mediastinal pleura to the central tendon of the diaphragm. In a haemodynamically significant pneumopericardium the transverse diameter of the heart is significantly reduced.

Treatment

A conservative approach can be adopted for small asymptomatic lesions. All symptomatic pneumopericardia should be drained immediately by direct pericardial tap via the subxiphoid route (p. 1382). The blood pressure should be monitored continuously, and the tap repeated if bradycardia or hypotension recurs. Catheter drainage may be necessary if the pericardial air reaccumulates.

Prognosis

The mortality for symptomatic pneumopericardium is between 80 and 90%,[503] and many survivors have neurological sequelae.

PNEUMOPERITONEUM

This may result from perforation of the gut (p. 751), but may also be caused by air dissecting from the chest through the diaphragmatic foramina into the peritoneum.[32] Pneumoperitoneum is therefore virtually always found in ventilated babies who already have a pneumothorax and a pneumomediastinum. In some cases the gas localizes in the connective tissue on the posterior wall of the abdomen – a pneumoretroperitoneum.[563]

Diagnosis

If the pneumoperitoneum is large the diagnosis can be made from the anteroposterior X-ray (Fig. 29.55). For smaller leaks a horizontal-beam lateral or right lateral X-ray is required (p. 751).

Rupture of the bowel, usually due to NEC (p. 751), can usually be excluded by the absence of a history of gastrointestinal disease, in particular bloody stools or intestinal obstruction, and a normal gut gas pattern on erect abdominal X-ray. If there is still doubt, differen-

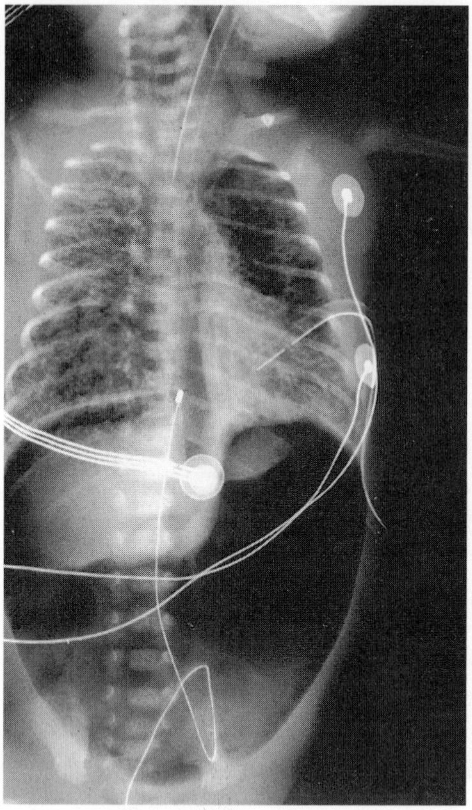

Fig. 29.55 Pneumoperitoneum associated with gross pulmonary interstitial emphysema.

tiating a pneumoperitoneum due to transdiaphragmatic air dissection from perforated bowel can be made by measuring the PO_2 of aspirated intraperitoneal gas.[1113] In ventilator-induced pneumoperitoneum the intraperitoneal PO_2 is very high, reflecting PAO_2, whereas the PO_2 of a surgical pneumoperitoneum is similar to room air or lower.

Treatment

If the abdomen is not under sufficient tension to cause respiratory embarassment, then no further treatment is necessary. If there is tension the peritoneum should be drained, either by needle aspiration or by inserting a drainage tube.

SYSTEMIC AIR EMBOLISM

This is a rare complication of IPPV: only 53 cases have been described. Affected infants are usually premature, have severe pulmonary insufficiency necessitating very high ventilator pressures (>40 cmH_2O), and the majority (94%) have other airleaks.[640] It is associated with a sudden and catastrophic deterioration in the baby's condition, with either pallor or cyanosis, hypotension and bizarre ECG irregularities. The situation in adults with ARDS on high-pressure IPPV who have chronic non-fatal low-grade bubbling into the vascular tree,[767] has not been seen in neonates.

Pathogenesis

Gas embolism results from alveolar–capillary or bronchovenous fistulae, which have been demonstrated by barium studies at autopsy.[123] Such communications are more likely to occur in airleak syndromes, but may also follow trauma to the lung. Laceration of lung tissue favours reversal of the intrabronchial pressure–pulmonary venous pressure gradient, thereby increasing the risk of pulmonary vascular air embolism.

Diagnosis

On the chest X-ray gas can be seen in the systemic and pulmonary arteries and veins (Fig. 29.56). Gas can be withdrawn from the umbilical venous or arterial catheters, and this has been observed in over half the reported cases.

Treatment

Early withdrawal of air from the umbilical artery catheter may be of benefit, particularly if the leak is small or has

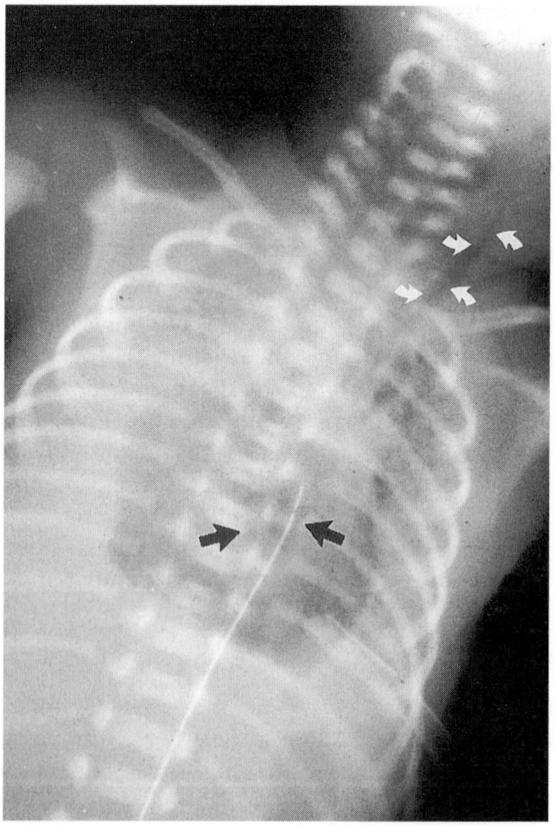

Fig. 29.56 Postmortem X-ray of a baby who died from systemic air embolism. Gas can be seen (black arrows) within the heart and in the great vessels in the neck (white arrows).

been introduced through an intravascular line. Placement of the infant in the Trendelenburg and left postero-anterior position may be helpful.[979]

Prognosis

This condition is usually fatal: only 4 of 53 reported cases survived.[640]

SUBCUTANEOUS EMPHYSEMA

This condition, with air tracking into the neck or other subcutaneous tissues, is usually associated with a pneumomediastinum. It requires no treatment. A localized subcutaneous collection of air under tension – a broncho-cutaneous fistula – has been described.[42]

PERSISTENT PULMONARY HYPERTENSION OF THE NEWBORN

This condition goes under several synonyms, of which the most common is persistent fetal circulation. This term should be avoided, as one of the characteristic features of the fetal circulation – the high-flow low-resistance circuit through the placenta – is missing. As the dominant pathophysiological feature of this condition is a high PAP, the descriptive term persistent pulmonary hypertension of the newborn is preferred.

DEFINITION AND CLASSIFICATION

This condition was first labelled the PFC syndrome by Gersony et al,[370] who described babies with a structurally normal heart but a large right–left shunt at atrial and ductus levels secondary to pulmonary hypertension. It is now understood that PPHN is the common endpoint of several very different pathophysiological mechanisms. By definition,[279,905] it is present when a baby has:

- severe hypoxaemia, usually a $PaO_2 < 5–6$ kPa (37.5–45 mmHg) in an F_IO_2 of 1.0 and IPPV if necessary;
- no severe lung disease (but see diaphragmatic hernia, p. 654). The neonate may have mild lung disease, but the hypoxaemia is disproportionately severe for the radiological, clinical and acid–base abnormalities;
- evidence of a right-to-left ductal shunt (usually a PaO_2 in the distal aortic (umbilical artery catheter) blood 1–2 kPa (7.5–15 mmHg) lower than simultaneous preductal (right radial artery) PaO_2 estimation). In the absence of a ductal shunt, a large shunt may be demonstrated echocardiographically at the foramen ovale.[1108]
- echocardiographic confirmation of a structurally normal heart.

It is important from both the theoretical and therapeutic points of view to separate this condition, which is a disease of the pulmonary vasculature, from diseases such as RDS (p. 489) and MAS (p. 540) which, although they can cause pulmonary hypertension in normal pulmonary vasculature in response to hypoxia and acidaemia, are nevertheless disorders of the lung parenchyma. There are at least eight distinct syndromes which can result in a baby developing PPHN.

1. Primary PPHN, or PPHN in the presence of mild neonatal lung disease. The babies with primary disease are those originally described by Gersony et al,[370] who are profoundly hypoxic but have no clinical or autopsy evidence of lung disease. This entity merges into PPHN in babies who have disproportionately severe hypoxaemia from what appears clinically, radiologically and on $PaCO_2$ measurements to be mild parenchymal lung disease. There is now considerable evidence to suggest that this entity is due to excessive muscularization of the pulmonary arterial system, starting in the antenatal period (see below), perhaps aggravated by intrapartum asphyxia[881] and iatrogenic overventilation in the early stages of mild disease[890] (see also 8 below).
2. PPHN secondary to severe intrapartum asphyxia. In these babies hypoxia and acidaemia, both of which are powerful pulmonary artery constrictors[685,932] and are present in severe asphyxia, prevent the normal postnatal changes in circulation. The tendency towards PPHN may be increased in such neonates by similar structural changes in the vasculature to those outlined above, and the large right–left shunt may be aggravated by systemic hypotension secondary to postasphyxial myocardial damage.[148]
3. PPHN secondary to infection. This particularly severe form of the disease, characteristically associated with GBS sepsis, is probably due to the release of vasoactive substances (p. 1128).
4. PPHN secondary to pulmonary hypoplasia. This is characteristic of neonates with diaphragmatic hernia, and is due to the abnormal development and reduced cross-sectional area of the pulmonary vasculature[367] (see Part 6, p. 654).
5. PPHN secondary to maternal drug therapy/fetal duct closure. This has been reported after the use of PGSIs before delivery, and a recent survey showed that mothers of inborn term babies with PPHN were 9.6 times more likely to have taken aspirin in pregnancy and 17.5 times more likely to have taken other PGSIs.[1116] These drugs, either by a direct effect on the pulmonary vasculature or by closing the fetal ductus, cause fetal pulmonary hypertension, which persists postnatally[655,1092] (Fig. 29.57). This is probably the result of changes in the pulmonary arterial musculature similar to those reported in primary PPHN.[654]
6. PPHN secondary to alveolar capillary dysplasia. Several reports have appeared of babies with clinical PPHN in whom, at postmortem, there appeared to be mis-alignment of the pulmonary vessels and poor apposition

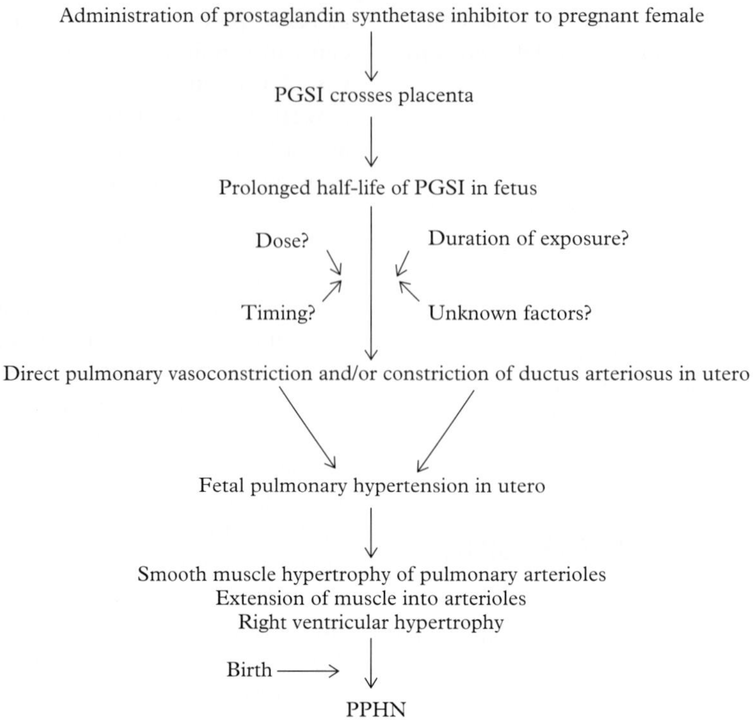

Fig. 29.57 Mechanism of drug-induced PPHN. Reproduced with permission from Turner and Levin.[1092]

of these vessels to the alveoli.[165] This condition is fatal and does not respond to ECMO.[181]

7. PPHN secondary to congenital heart disease. Conditions which obstruct the venous outflow from the lungs or cause myocardial failure can cause PHT and/or marked right–left shunting with hypoxaemia. These are considered in detail in Chapter 30, and are reviewed by Long.[672]

8. Iatrogenic PPHN secondary to overventilation (p. 575).

INCIDENCE

Brown and Pickering[135] found the prevalence of group 1 and 2 PPHN to be 1:1450 live births. In Cambridge, from 1985 to 1987, the prevalence excluding babies with septicaemia and diaphragmatic hernia was 1:1415 live births (a total of eight babies). Three cases were preterm with mild RDS, three were large term babies with apparently primary PPHN, one was secondary to meconium inhalation, and another fatal case was secondary to severe birth asphyxia in a term baby without meconium aspiration. Hjalmarson[498] found a prevalence of 1:1699, but in Nottingham there were no cases from 6870 live births in 1977 and an incidence of 1:7602 in 1983–84[322] (Table 29.7). The incidence in North America would appear to be much higher, as up to 2% of all NICU admissions required ECMO.[28] Similarly, Hageman et al[445] reported an incidence of 1:522 and Reece et al[881] an incidence of 1.5:1000. Pooling all the available data would suggest that the prevalence in North America is two to five times higher than that seen in the UK.

PATHOPHYSIOLOGY

The pathognomonic feature of this condition is the presence of PHT, producing right–left shunts at the level of the ductus arteriosus and the foramen ovale (p. 527). The comparatively small difference between pre- and postductal PaO_2 levels, rarely greater than 2–3 kPa (15–22 mmHg), suggests that only a small component of the shunt occurs at duct level, with the majority occurring through the foramen ovale.[1108]

Catheterization of the pulmonary artery has only been carried out in a small number of babies with PPHN, and they usually had meconium aspiration or were suffering from severe birth asphyxia.[336,831] These studies showed that the pulmonary artery pressure was at or above systemic levels.

Studies using contrast echocardiography have demonstrated significant right–left shunting at ductus and foramen ovale levels[279,990] and confirmed the PHT. Earlier studies using M-mode echocardiography showed functional changes in the right ventricle which often antedated the clinical deterioration in babies with both primary PPHN and PPHN secondary to lung disease.[899,1108] More recently, Skinner et al[990] have shown that a marked reduction in left ventricular function is the most significant marker of severe disease. These data on

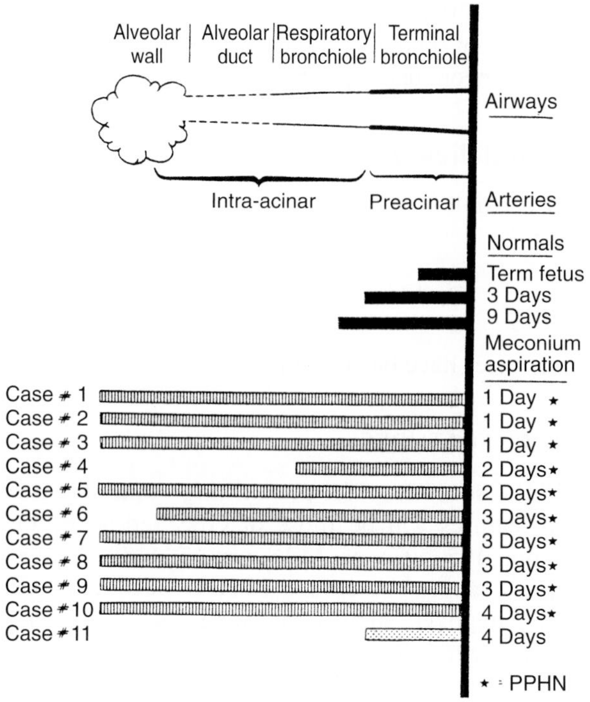

Fig. 29.58 Diagram of location of muscle in the walls of intra-acinar arteries in fatal cases of meconium aspiration. Even in normal neonates less than 7 days old no muscular arteries are found within the acinus. The 10 neonates with PPHN had extension of muscle into the small intra-acinar arteries, but in case 11 it was normal in distribution. Reproduced with permission from Murphy et al.[780]

PHT and different pre- and postductal PaO_2 levels in babies with PPHN are similar to those reported in severe surfactant-depleted RDS and MAS, where the primary disease is in the lung parenchyma (pp. 486, 539).[303,304,693,909,988,989,1137]

Abnormal pulmonary vasculature

In postmortem studies on babies with PPHN, virtually all secondary to meconium inhalation, the muscularity of the pulmonary arteries is markedly increased.[779,780] Not only is the amount of muscle in the vessel wall increased, it also extends into vessels surrounding the alveoli, whereas in the normal baby muscular pulmonary arteries rarely extend past the terminal bronchiole (Fig. 29.58). These data are supported by a series of experimental studies which, in addition to showing that antenatal therapy with prostaglandin synthetase inhibitors can cause PPHN,[1092] have suggested that fetal hypoxia[277,382] and fetal duct ligation[761,1161] can cause muscular hypertrophy of the fetal pulmonary arteries, an increase in the extracellular matrix around these vessels,[287] and then neonatal PPHN. Not all studies, however, support these views. Perlman et al[835] suggest that the human data (Fig. 29.58) are an artefact of the autopsy technique, and that the vasculature in babies with MAS is no different from that in normals. Furthermore, other meticulous animal studies on the morphometry of the fetal pulmonary vasculature after late fetal hypoxia have shown no significant pulmonary arterial abnormalities.[369,781] Postnatally, sustained pulmonary hypertension rapidly accelerates pulmonary vascular injury, with aggressive smooth muscle proliferation and remodelling. Initially the effects of hypertension are at least partially offset by the release of endogenous vasodilators, but this may not be sustained.[2]

Prenatal changes in the fetal pulmonary vasculature, priming it to overreact to factors known under normal circumstances to cause pulmonary artery vasoconstriction, such as hypoxia and acidaemia, would at least partially explain PPHN in groups 1, 2 and 5. It is also compatible with the fact that it is possible echocardiographically to identify early in their disease those babies with mild RDS and MAS who are likely to go on to develop PPHN.[899,1108]

Pulmonary microthrombi

Levin et al[652] described a group of babies at postmortem in whom they felt a significant component of the pulmonary obstruction was due to multiple platelet microthrombi. These occurred in babies with different causes of PPHN, including those with sepsis, MAS and primary PPHN.

Vasoactive agents

Many agents act on the pulmonary vasculature; these include nitric oxide, endothelins and various eicosanoids, including the prostaglandins, leukotrienes and thromboxane.[2] The role of other vasoactive agents, such as bradykinin and angiotensin, is uncertain.

Nitric oxide is a potent pulmonary vasodilator, probably active in the transition of the circulation at birth (p. 458). As yet there is no convincing evidence to suggest that decreased production of NO, or end-organ insensitivity to NO, is relevant in the aetiology of PPHN,[1023] although Castillo et al[162] showed a reduced conversion of L-arginine to NO in neonates with severe PPHN.

Endothelin-I is a potent pulmonary vasoconstrictor, the plasma level of which is raised in neonates with hypoxia[612] and severe PPHN;[622,923] its role in the aetiology of the condition and its interaction with NO production remains uncertain[1023] (p. 458).

Leukotriene inhibition increases pulmonary blood flow in fetal lambs,[638] and raised levels of the constrictor leukotrienes LTC_4 and LTD_4 have been found in the blood of some (but not all) neonates with PPHN compared to ventilated neonates without this complication; the levels fall with successful therapy.[269,461,617,1025]

In the PPHN that accompanies sepsis due to both GBS and other organisms,[376,968,1130] including viruses,[1074] there is initial severe arterial spasm followed by increased vascular permeability and an increased lung fluid content and lymph flow.[844,921,942] In these babies it is thought that thromboxane A_2[376,461,934] is the prostaglandin responsible, and that it has its effect without affecting the morphometry of the pulmonary vasculature.[60]

In animal experiments PPHN, but not the haematological features of group B streptococcal sepsis, can be prevented by treatment with drugs that inhibit thromboxane A_2 synthesis, such as indomethacin,[934] and can be reversed by intravenous infusion of the vasodilator prostaglandin PGE_2 and by isoprenaline.[127,229]

The increased capillary permeability in sepsis-induced PPHN appears to be due both to the action of bacterial endotoxins to sequester white cells in the lungs,[920,942] where they release vasoactive agents such as tumour necrosis factor, and to an additional effect of thromboxane A_2 since, as with the short-term effects on the pulmonary vasculature, long-term effects can be mitigated but not prevented by the use of indomethacin and dazmegrel. The role of thromboxane A_2 in the PPHN of non-infectious lung disease and asphyxia remains unresolved.[461,617]

Vascular hypoplasia

The PPHN of diaphragmatic hernia and other conditions associated with pulmonary hypoplasia is due to a reduction in the number of intralobar arteries, and to the fact that they are very muscular.[368]

Blood gas changes/asphyxia

A fall in pH causes pulmonary vasoconstriction in experimental animals,[931,932] and hypoxia is also a potent vasoconstrictor.[685] Neonatal pulmonary vasculature is extremely sensitive to changes in pH, $P\text{aO}_2$ and $P\text{aCO}_2$[161] Therefore, particularly in babies with prenatal pulmonary arterial muscular hypertrophy, perinatal and postnatal hypoxaemia and metabolic or respiratory acidaemia could cause marked pulmonary arterial spasm, pulmonary hypertension, a large right–left shunt, and the clinical entity of PPHN. This is entirely compatible with the epidemiological data linking PPHN with birth asphyxia, albeit mild,[485,881] and with the beneficial therapeutic effects of adequate oxygenation and alkalaemia (see below).

Polycythaemia

A rise in haematocrit in experimental animals causes PHT; however, the factors involved are far from clear, as a rise in PVR is not seen if fetal blood as opposed to adult blood is used to raise the haematocrit.[331] Polycythaemia is not a consistent feature of neonates with PPHN.[334]

Hypoglycaemia/hypocalcaemia

Although these factors are often mentioned in the aetiology of PPHN, the evidence that they are causally related, rather than merely an epiphenomenon in many critically ill neonates, is poor.

Mode of delivery

PPHN can follow inappropriately early repeat caesarean section.[578]

Heredity

Familial cases have been reported.[978]

CLINICAL FEATURES

In PPHN secondary to pre-existing lung disease the clinical features will be those of GBS sepsis (p. 1128), RDS (pp. 495–497) or MAS (pp. 541–542), together with the cyanosis of severe PPHN. Secondary effects from the hypoxia, such as acidaemia and hypotension, may be present. The age at diagnosis still depends on the underlying problem and its severity. In GBS infection (p. 1128), severe asphyxia (p. 555) and congenital diaphragmatic hernia (p. 655) PPHN will appear within 6 hours of birth in a critically ill neonate.

In babies with primary PPHN the presentation is often more subtle and may mimic that of cyanotic congenital heart disease. Babies with primary PPHN virtually always present within 12 hours of birth, and very rarely after 24 hours. A form presenting late in the neonatal period[871] may well be a variant of the rare primary pulmonary hypertension of later infancy and childhood.

The baby remains cyanosed even when high oxygen concentrations are administered by IPPV. Respiratory distress is, however, often mild. The respiratory rate is usually increased to 60–100/min, the higher rates being seen in term babies. Retraction is mild and grunting rare. The air entry is normal and there are rarely added sounds. The heart rate is normal or slightly increased. All pulses, including the femorals, are normal. The first heart sound is normal, but the second is commonly single and loud because of the rise in PAP. There is a right parasternal heave and a soft systolic murmur may be heard, signifying tricuspid incompetence or occasionally mitral incompetence. Heart failure is not usually present, but the infant may be hypotensive. Examination of the abdomen, genitourinary system and CNS is usually normal in the absence of predisposing factors such as sepsis or asphyxia. The clinical features of babies with diaphragmatic hernia are given on pages 655–656.

DIFFERENTIAL DIAGNOSIS (Table 29.13, pp. 498–499)

The differential diagnosis from cyanotic congenital heart disease is not usually too difficult in babies who present within the first 12 hours. Cyanotic congenital heart disease presenting this early is usually a severe form, with clear-cut clinical signs, heart failure, distinctive murmurs and obvious changes on the chest X-ray and ECG. In PPHN, however, the chest X-ray and ECG are often within the normal limits, and the findings on examination of the cardiovascular system are comparatively subtle (see above). If there is doubt, echocardiography will establish the normal cardiac anatomy in PPHN.

The response to manual hyperventilation up to 150/min with 100% oxygen may differentiate PPHN from cyanotic congenital heart disease.[334] In the former the PaO_2 will usually increase to >13 kPa (100 mmHg), whereas in cyanotic heart disease it will usually not rise above 5–6 kPa (37.5–45 mmHg). Not all neonates with PPHN, especially those with sepsis and diaphragmatic hernia, respond in this way, and in some forms of cyanotic congenital heart disease the PaO_2 may rise to 13–14 kPa (95–105 mmHg) in 100% oxygen.[549]

The features which suggest that the PPHN is secondary to sepsis are outlined on page 1128, but in their absence sepsis cannot be excluded.

INVESTIGATION

Haematological and biochemical

There are no specific abnormalities in babies with PPHN. However, thrombocytopenia has been reported in severe cases[956] and this may identify a group who respond poorly to vasodilators.[652] The thrombocytopenia may be a manifestation of abnormal prostaglandin activation (see above).

Blood gases

In both primary and secondary PPHN maximal PaO_2 values of 6 kPa (45 mmHg) are characteristic, often with a difference of at least 1–2 kPa (7.5–15 mmHg) between preductal and postductal PaO_2 (p. 527). At diagnosis there may be a metabolic acidaemia, but respiratory acidaemia, by definition, is unusual. Metabolic acidaemia is usually easy to control by an initial infusion of base followed by blood pressure support and maintaining the haematocrit above 40%. A resistant acidosis is either a feature of the terminal stages of PPHN or is due to some other underlying problem, in particular overwhelming sepsis.

Chest X-ray

In secondary PPHN the X-ray will be that of the underlying lung disease, though by definition the appearance will be less severe than anticipated for the severity of the hypoxaemia.

In primary PPHN the chest X-ray changes are often minimal; there may be a mild non-specific increase in lung markings, but little else is noted. In other cases, however, there will be cardiomegaly, pulmonary vascular congestion and even pleural effusions.[796]

Electrocardiogram

Various ECG changes have been reported in neonates with PPHN. The tracing may be normal, or more typically shows changes of right axis deviation, right atrial enlargement and right ventricular hypertrophy and overload.[483] In babies who develop PPHN following severe asphyxia, the ECG may show the changes of subendocardial ischaemia (p. 556).

Echocardiography

This is the single most useful investigation for establishing the diagnosis. First, and most importantly, it will exclude the various forms of cyanotic congenital heart disease by showing a normal cardiac anatomy. Secondly, pulmonary hypertension, right-to-left shunting at ductal and foramen ovale level, and ventricular function can be assessed (see above).[990]

Bacteriology

Because PPHN can be secondary to sepsis it is vital that, as in all neonates with respiratory disease, routine swabs and blood cultures are taken (pp. 502, 1118).

TREATMENT

The treatment of PPHN can be divided into two components: that of the coexisting lung disease, which is covered elsewhere in this chapter, and that of the PHT and the resistant hypoxaemia, in which the basic aim is to achieve and sustain pulmonary artery dilatation and hence a rise in PaO_2

Initial conservative management

Minimal handling

In no group of neonates is it more important to adhere to the 'minimal handling' maxim (p. 502). Slight disturbance, for example turning the baby or taking his temperature, may precipitate severe hypoxaemia, and major interventions such as endotracheal tube suctioning or arterial puncture can have devastating effects. Monitoring must therefore be continuous and electronic (Chapter 21), and interference with the baby reduced to an absolute minimum. Endotracheal tube suctioning should only be carried out when indicated; chest physiotherapy is contraindicated.

Blood pressure and blood volume

As the size of the right–left shunt is partly dependent on the systemic blood pressure (see above), the latter should be maintained at a mean of at least 35 mmHg (p. 504), with a systolic of 50 mmHg: values 5 mmHg lower are acceptable in preterm infants weighing less than 1.50 kg. Sustaining blood pressure is normally only difficult in infected babies, or after drugs such as tolazoline (see below).

As in all sick infants, the haemoglobin must be kept greater than 13 g/dl (PCV 40%) in order to maximize oxygen transport to the tissues. If polycythaemia (central PCV >70–75%) is present the existence of PPHN is one of the situations where a dilutional exchange transfusion is justified.

Coagulation disorders

If present, these should be corrected by appropriate factor replacement.

Fluid and electrolyte balance

The routine described on page 505 and in Chapter 39, Part 1 should be followed, usually starting with 40–60 ml/kg/24 h of 10% dextrose. An attempt should be made to keep all biochemical values normal. Electrolyte abnormalities, and hypoglycaemia in particular, must be corrected, and pH and base deficit must be kept within normal limits by the liberal use of THAM or bicarbonate as appropriate. Urine output must be carefully monitored, as hypotension is not uncommon, and tolazoline if used may cause renal failure (p. 634).

Antibiotics

Broad-spectrum antibiotic cover should be given to all these babies. Its use in ventilated neonates is described in detail on page 507, and the management of GBS sepsis on pages 1129–1130.

Nutrition

Enteral feeding should be avoided. If the baby, particularly if birthweight was less than 1.50 kg, is still ventilator dependent by days 3–4, he should be started on intravenous nutrition.

The effect of one or two doses of surfactant should always be considered in babies with PPHN secondary to any condition in which surfactant deficiency is likely, or in which it is likely that endogenous surfactant is being inhibited by a leak of plasma proteins on to the alveolar surface.

Ventilation

Initially IPPV should be used (p. 567) at rates of 60–80/min, pressures of 20–25/3 cmH_2O, and an inspiration time of 0.30–0.35 seconds, plus whatever oxygen concentration is required. A $PaCO_2$ of 5–5.5 kPa (37–40 mmHg), a pH > 7.30 and the best PaO_2 possible should be achieved. Only if this fails should one progress to the more aggressive management outlined below.

Occasionally pulmonary vasodilators may be effective in the unventilated, spontaneously breathing term neonate with PPHN. In general, however, once a baby's PaO_2 falls below 5–6 kPa (37–45 mmHg) in 95–100% oxygen, he should be ventilated. For the full-term baby prone to fight the ventilator, muscle paralysis should be used, and in this situation there are theoretical reasons for preferring D-tubocurarine to pancuronium.[520]

It is important to emphasize that the use of basic intensive care and ventilation as outlined above gives very good results in the treatment of PPHN,[1180] although in the USA a more aggressive approach is preferred.[1135]

PPHN unresponsive to conservative treatment

For babies with PPHN who do not respond to conventional treatment by having a sustained rise in their PaO_2, presumably with sustained relaxation of their pulmonary arteries, other techniques are required. These include hyperventilation, the use of vasodilator drugs and ECMO. Depending on the aetiology of the PPHN, different approaches should be tried.

Primary and drug-induced PPHN; PPHN secondary to mild lung disease

Hyperventilation. This was first described by Peckham and Fox.[831] Once the $PaCO_2$ is reduced to 2.5–3.5 kPa (19–26 mmHg) and the pH raised to 7.55–7.60 there may be a consistent and sustained rise in PaO_2 (Fig. 29.59). Both a low $PaCO_2$ and an alkalaemia are necessary: having one without the other does not seem to be successful.[1014] Base should therefore always be given to correct any metabolic acidaemia. Although a $PaCO_2$ of 2.5–3.5 kPa (19–26 mmHg) results in a 50% reduction of cerebral blood flow, which could cause cerebral ischaemia, there seems to be little substance for these fears in term babies,[137] but anxieties remain regarding the CNS effects of hypocapnia in preterm infants,[434,526] and marked hypocapnia (<2.5 kPa (19 mmHg) may reduce cardiac output.[160]

The main hazards of hyperventilation are, therefore, airleaks and subsequent CLD. Fox[333] reported that 50% of his patients developed some form of airleak during hyperventilation, and patients 'often' developed X-ray changes of chronic lung disease after 3 days' treatment.[334] Beck[73] reported that 50% of hyperventilated PPHN patients developed CLD. More importantly, animal work suggests that persisting hypocapnic alkalaemia markedly increases the hypoxic reactivity of the pulmonary vasculature, thereby tending to perpetuate the pathophysiology of PPHN.[392]

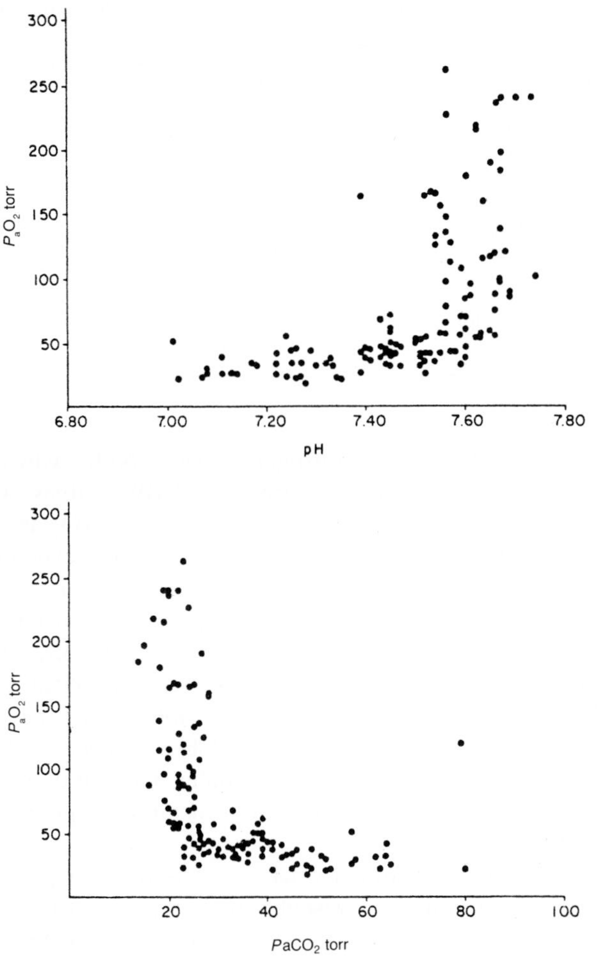

Fig. 29.59 Improvement in PaO_2 in neonates with PPHN when they were made markedly alkalaemic by hyperventilation (compare with Fig 29.77). Reproduced with permission from Drummond et al.[278]

The optimal ventilator rate for these babies would appear to be about 60–80/min. In paralysed babies faster rates may result in inadvertent PEEP (pp. 566–567) and slower rates may not sufficiently reduce the $PaCO_2$. The ventilator pressures should be the lowest compatible with a $PaCO_2$ of 4.7 kPa (35 mmHg), or in severe cases 4.0 kPa (30 mmHg).

High-frequency oscillation: jet ventilation. Anecdotally these forms of respiratory support have been associated with improvements in oxygenation,[604,1014,1118] but although many babies have been so treated, the data are uncontrolled.

Nitric oxide. Nitric oxide is the vasodilator substance which relaxes vascular smooth muscle, and was previously known as endothelial-derived relaxing factor. It is synthesized in the endothelial cells from L-arginine and oxygen.[289] Nitric oxide is a volatile gas and can therefore be administered as an inhalation. Since the preliminary studies of Kinsella et al[588] and Roberts et al[913] there have been a plethora of reports of the benefit of nitric oxide in PPHN. Its use has been reviewed by Steinhorn et al[1023] and Kinsella and Abman.[586] As experience is gained in its use concentrations above 20 parts per million (ppm) are rarely required[324,1207] (Fig. 29.60) except in very immature infants, particularly those with PIE.[629] In addition, the response time varies from baby to baby[586,1090] (Fig. 29.61). Infants with intra- and extrapulmonary shunts respond with a fall in PHT and a rise in pulmonary blood flow.[928] The efficacy of inhaled NO is improved if combined with a strategy to improve

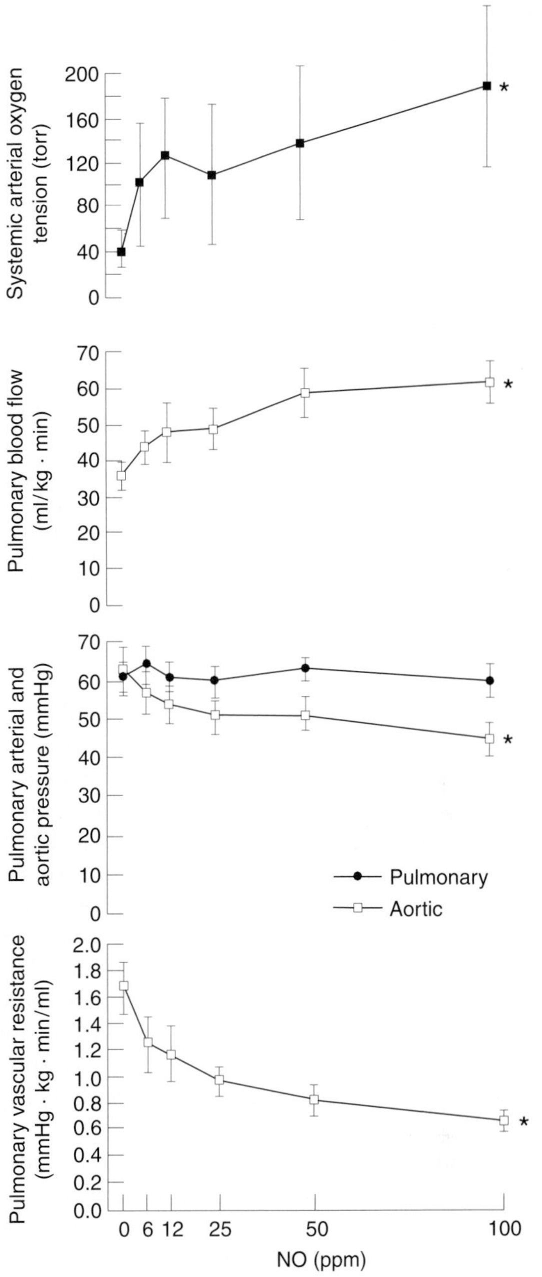

Fig. 29.60 Effect of 5-minute intervals of ventilation with nitric oxide at varying concentrations on pulmonary haemodynamics in six newborn lambs with persistent pulmonary hypertension. Values are mean ± SEM. *Variable changes significantly with increasing concentration of nitric oxide (P<0.002). Reproduced with permission from Zayek et al.[1207]

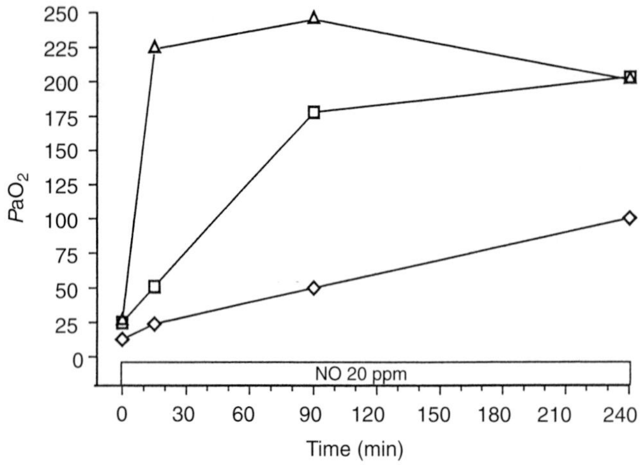

Fig. 29.61 Variability in time-dependent responses to inhaled NO in PPHN: change in PaO_2 for three patients with severe PPHN treated with inhaled NO. Note variability in responses and time-dependent improvement in oxygenation. All patients recovered without the need for ECMO. (Mean baseline PaO_2 = 19±3; F_IO_2 at 4-hour time point = 0.96). Reproduced with permission from Kinsella and Abman.[586]

lung volume.[586,1160] Where ECMO is practised NO inhalation can spare the baby exposure to this procedure.[324] Prospective randomized trials of NO inhalation are ongoing.[1019] Such studies have demonstrated benefits in oxygenation, but this has not yet been translated into improved survival, although the requirement for ECMO was reduced by 50% in one trial[791] (Table 29.21), and in a smaller trial transient improvements in oxygenation were not translated into a reduction in the incidence of infants meeting ECMO criteria.[61] ECMO may, however, be required for infants in whom the response to inhaled nitric oxide is poor or not sustained; in our experience and that of others adverse outcome is particularly likely in infants with dysplastic lungs, as in CDH.[383]

Nitric oxide binds rapidly to haemoglobin and, once bound, is inactivated and therefore produces no systemic effects. The nitrosylhaemoglobin so produced is rapidly converted to methaemoglobin, which is then reduced by methaemoglobin reductase in erythrocytes. Unfortunately, immature infants and those of certain ethnic groups have low levels of this enzyme. NO also reacts

Table 29.21 Results of NINO study[791]

	Control group	NO group	*P* value
Number	121	114	
Death by day 120 or ECMO *n* (%)	77 (63.6)	52 (45.6)	0.006
Death *n* (%)	20 (16.5)	16 (14.0)	0.600
ECMO *n* (%)	66 (54.4)	44 (38.6)	0.014
Change in OI	−0.8±21.1	−14.1±21.1	<0.001
Change in $AaDO_2$(mmHg)	−6.7±57.5	−60±85.1	<0.001
Length of hospitalization	29.5±22.6	36.4±44.8	0.17
Airleak after randomization	5 (5.1)	5 (5.2)	0.96
BPD	12 (11.9)	15 (15.3)	0.48

Table 29.22 Drugs that have been used to reduce pulmonary artery pressure in neonates

Drug	Reference
Tubocurarine	Hutchinson and Yu[520]
Chlorpromazine	Larsson et al[628]
Sodium nitroprusside	Benitz and Stevenson[82a]
Verapamil	Morett and Ortega[759]
Prostaglandin D_2	Soifer et al[999]
Acetylcholine, Isoprenaline, Morphine	Reviewed by Kulik and Lock[621]
Magnesium sulphate	Wu et al[1179]
Adenosine	Konduri et al[607]

rapidly with O_2 to form nitrogen dioxide (NO_2), which is toxic to the lung. Particularly in VLBW babies with RDS[777] care must therefore be taken that NO_2 is not being formed[747] and that the baby is not developing methaemoglobinaemia.[586,1133] These problems are more likely if high concentrations (80 ppm)[11] are used for prolonged periods in high inspired oxygen concentrations.[747] NO should only be administered if continuous NO and NO_2 monitoring is available and there is immediate access to methaemoglobin analysis.[1195] A small proportion of infants, usually with pulmonary hypoplasia and dysplasia, develop a sustained dependence on NO.[383]

In GBS sepsis, animal work suggests that early in the disease the pulmonary vasculature is sensitive to NO,[86] but other data show that the endogenous NO mechanism is fully active and that little benefit is likely to accrue from exogenous inhaled NO.[375,587,730]

Vasodilator drugs (Table 29.22). Until the advent of NO three drugs, tolazoline, prostacyclin and magnesium sulphate, were widely used. Other drugs have also been reported to be beneficial. All these agents share two problems: they lower systemic blood pressure as well as pulmonary artery pressure, and they have an impressive list of damaging side-effects.

Tolazoline (Fig. 29.62). This was the first vasodilator to be used[381] and has been the most widely used since.[621] Between 25 and 50% of babies with primary PPHN or PPHN secondary to mild RDS or MAS respond to this agent, but it often causes a profound drop in systemic blood pressure, especially in infected babies, and it is therefore contraindicated in this group. It may supplement the beneficial effects of nitric oxide.[236] The dose is 1–2 mg/kg by bolus, followed by an infusion of 1–2 mg/kg/h. Side-effects include renal failure and gastrointestinal haemorrhage.[1142] The systemic effects may be minimized by intratracheal therapy, which has been reported in lambs.[235]

Prostacyclin. This agent in doses of 5–40 ng/kg/min is an effective pulmonary vasodilator with a wide list of side-effects.[840] More recently, inhalation of prostacyclin in animals and babies has been shown to be at least as

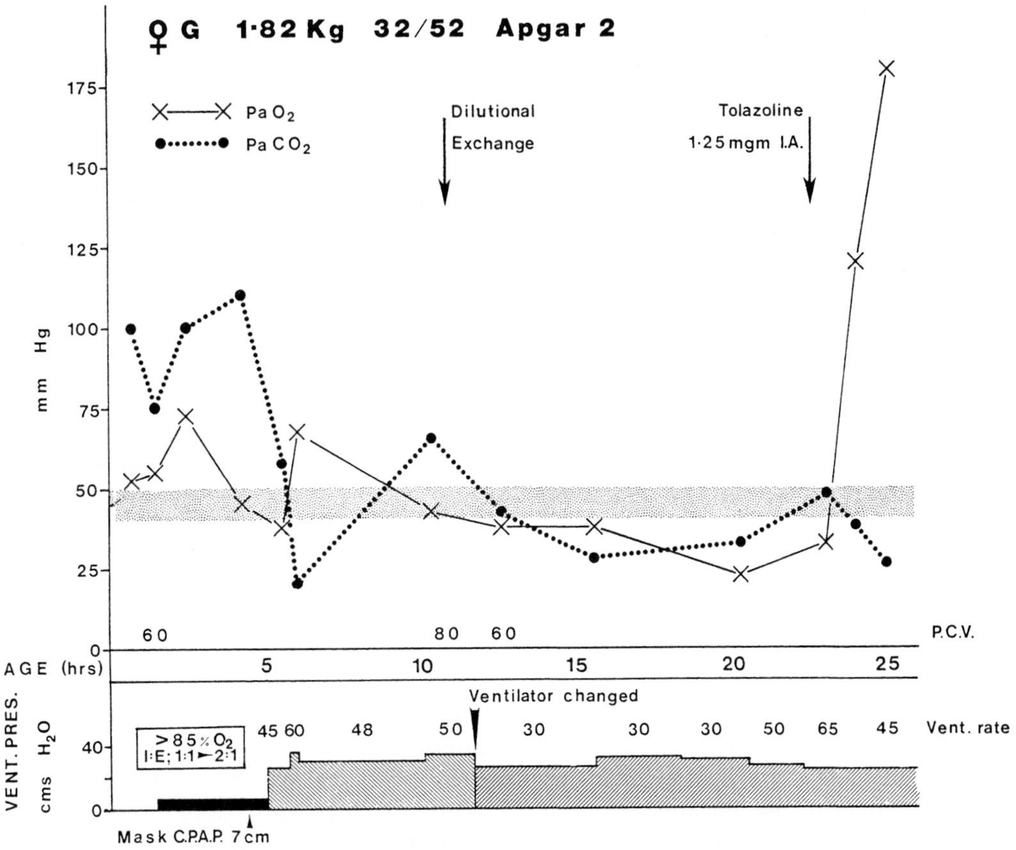

Fig. 29.62 Response to tolazoline in a baby with clinical RDS but comparatively mild X-ray changes. This was the first baby treated with tolazoline in the Cambridge Maternity Hospital. Subsequent use was often less dramatic!

effective as the parenteral preparation, with fewer side-effects, and causes an equivalent response to inhaled NO.[104,1210]

Magnesium sulphate. This drug was introduced into the treatment of PPHN by Abu-Osba et al in 1992.[4] As a loading dose of 200 mg/kg/h followed by an infusion of 20–100 mg/kg/h it is effective,[1076,1179] but less so and with more side-effects than NO.[938]

In general the drugs are more likely to succeed if they are given within the first 12–24 hours, to mature babies, to those with primary PPHN, and to neonates whose other biochemical and blood gas measurements are normal,[278] but particularly if the infant has been hyperventilated to a pH of 7.55–7.60 and a $PaCO_2$ of 3.0–3.5 kPa (23–26 mmHg). Babies with pulmonary microthrombi are less likely to respond.[652] Ventilated preterm babies who present with classic but mild RDS (p. 575), yet who by 6–10 hours, despite a surprisingly good chest radiograph, a normal pH and a low $PaCO_2$, remain profoundly hypoxaemic, often respond to a single bolus of tolazoline, and their requirement for oxygen and IPPV reduces dramatically in the next 24–48 hours (Fig. 29.62).

Whenever these drugs are used the baby's blood pressure must be carefully monitored. If hypotension occurs it should be corrected rapidly by volume expansion with albumin or blood, or with an infusion of dopamine. It has been suggested that tolazoline should only be given when the patient's systemic blood pressure is simultaneously being sustained by an infusion of dopamine, given in large enough doses for it to be a peripheral vasoconstrictor without acting on the pulmonary vasculature.[278,1071] To maximize the beneficial effects of pulmonary vasodilators they should be infused as close to the pulmonary circulation as possible, either using central lines in the right atrium or pulmonary artery, or into vessels draining into the superior vena cava. Blood draining into the inferior vena cava is likely to cross the foramen ovale (as part of the right-to-left shunt) and not pass through the pulmonary vasculature initially.

If no benefit is obtained after either a bolus injection or with 6–12 hours of an infusion, there is no point in persisting with these drugs.

PPHN secondary to sepsis

This is difficult to treat. The presence of sepsis and its complications, such as hypotension, hypoglycaemia and coagulation disturbances, makes most of the therapies for PPHN either impossible or very difficult to use. This is particularly a problem if there is oliguric renal failure, which limits the baby's ability to deal with the volume of the intravenous infusions of base, albumin, glucose, coagulation factors and inotropes that are necessary.

Severely affected babies are frequently hypocapnic and alkalaemic, yet despite aggressive ventilation this rarely achieves pulmonary vasodilatation and a rise in PaO_2. Vasodilator drugs, even in the presence of an adequate blood volume and systemic blood pressure support with dopamine and/or dobutamine, almost always cause profound hypotension in babies who are already tending to hypotension, and thus vasodilators are probably contraindicated in septic babies.

Recent animal data show that thromboxane A_2 and other prostaglandins are important mediators of PPHN in sepsis (p. 1128). Prostaglandin synthetase inhibitors or more specific thromboxane A_2 inhibitors have been used successfully in animals,[934,1061] but no reports of their use in humans have as yet appeared. On an anecdotal basis, a mixture of indomethacin blockade plus careful use of prostacyclin may be helpful.[886]

The small amount of animal data using NO suggests that this is likely to be of only marginal benefit if used early in the illness, as the endogenous system becomes maximally stimulated trying to relieve the PHT caused by the infection.[86,375] For all these reasons, the clinician is left with little alternative than to use the most vigorous therapy for neonatal sepsis (pp. 1129–1130) in the hope that the situation will gradually improve. ECMO has been used successfully in some affected term babies.

PPHN secondary to diaphragmatic hernia

(see pp. 657–658)

MONITORING BABIES WITH PPHN

The monitoring of these babies is outlined in Table 29.23. It must be both meticulous and continuous. Particular care must be taken to observe the minimal handling routines, as disturbing these babies can result in severe treatment-resistant hypoxaemia. Meticulous continuous PaO_2 monitoring is essential. Ideally, an indwelling continuously recording PaO_2 cannula should be placed in the lower aorta. To obtain some idea of the size of the ductal right–left shunt, and therefore indirectly of the level of PHT, the umbilical artery PaO_2 measurements should, if possible, be supplemented by a measure of the preductal PaO_2, using either a right radial artery catheter or a transcutaneous monitor placed on the right upper chest. Pre- (right hand) and postductal (either foot) SpO_2 measurements may also be helpful.[693]

Table 29.23 Monitoring for PPHN

PaO_2	Continuous monitoring essential: PaO_2, $tcPO_2$, SpO_2 all appropriate. In term babies no risk of ROP so PaO_2 can be high. Indwelling catheters should be used for sampling. Intermittent sampling by arterial puncture or capillary sampling contraindicated
$PaCO_2$	Monitor from an indwelling arterial catheter 3–4-hourly. If hypocapnia is being used $tcPCO_2$ may be helpful.
pH	As for $PaCO_2$
Chest X-ray	Daily, with minimal disturbance
Respiratory rate	Not really important: ventilation rates set at those demanded by the primary disorder
Cardiological	Continuous ECG and BP essential
Microbiology	Initial cultures always
Fluid and electrolytes	Not usually a problem unless associated with birth asphyxia. U and E, Ca^{2+} and albumin daily
Haematology	FBC daily, PCV 8-hourly
Temperature	Monitor continuously

WEANING THE BABY WITH PPHN OFF THERAPY

Once the neonate has acceptable blood gases, which may mean a PaO_2 of 16 kPa (120 mmHg) and a pH >7.55–7.60 (see above), and has been stable at these readings for 12–24 hours, weaning can begin. The rate at which this is done is dominated by the fear of recurrence, because even when a satisfactory PaO_2 has been obtained, implying pulmonary arterial vasodilatation, there is for some days afterwards a major risk that the pulmonary arteries will once more go into spasm, perhaps owing to the sensitizing effects of alkalaemia.[392] Reducing the ventilator pressures, drugs and oxygen concentrations should therefore be done extremely slowly. The general guidelines for weaning outlined on pages 580–582 should nevertheless be adhered to. First, bring down the ventilator pressure to <30 cmH_2O and then reduce the rate of infusion of the vasodilator drugs. In PPHN, however, ventilator pressures should never be reduced by more than 1–2 cmH_2O, oxygen by more than 3–5%, or the rate of vasodilator drugs by more than 20–25% at a time. Nitric oxide should be weaned by approximately 1 ppm, providing the methaemoglobin and NO_2 levels are below 2% and 5 ppm respectively. It is obviously essential to tailor the rate of NO reduction so that the infant's PaO_2 remains in the desired range (see above).

Fox and his group[280,334] introduced the concept of the 'transition phase' in the management of weaning. This occurs when the hypoxia in the baby is no longer due to PPHN, but to the chronic lung sequelae of hyperventilation in high oxygen concentrations. This usually occurs 3–4 days into the illness and can be identified by the fact that the PaO_2 becomes much less variable, implying that the pulmonary arterial tone is stabilizing. At this stage, although the chest X-ray is still showing pulmonary hyperaeration secondary to hyperventilation, rather than the changes of early CLD, the rate of weaning can usually be speeded up.

COMPLICATIONS

Pulmonary interstitial emphysema and pneumothorax are common, as is CLD (see above). If a pneumothorax occurs, irrespective of its size it must be drained. If one does occur during hyperventilation, the deterioration which it causes may so aggravate the pulmonary arterial vasocontriction that it pushes the baby into irreversible hypoxaemia, hypotension and bradycardia. PIE is particularly difficult to manage, as the only option (other than ECMO) is to try and reduce the ventilator pressure, which will almost inevitably result in a return to the PPHN as the $PaCO_2$ rises and the pH and PaO_2 fall. If a transition phase does not occur, or is not recognized, and hyperventilation has to be continued to sustain pulmonary vasodilatation and an acceptable PaO_2, 50% of babies are likely to develop CLD (p. 608).

The preterm baby with PPHN who is severely hypoxaemic and/or hypotensive is clearly a candidate for GMH/IVH and PVL, particularly if hypocapnia is used as treatment (p. 1264). Cerebral haemorrhage is unusual in term babies, except in those attached to ECMO,[625] but in those with PPHN secondary to severe birth asphyxia with or without meconium aspiration, major cerebral infarction can occur.[600]

All the drugs (Table 29.22) have side-effects, in particular the sequelae of systemic hypotension. NO may cause lung damage if nitrogen dioxide is formed, and methaemoglobinaemia is a risk, especially for the preterm baby.

NATURAL HISTORY AND PROGNOSIS

This varies with the aetiology, but is generally unpredictable. As the arterial muscularity of experimental pulmonary hypertension[348] can resolve within 2–3 days of normoxaemia, PPHN might be expected to have a short natural history, and indeed this seems to be the case, as Duara and Fox[279] found that after 3–4 days of hyperventilation the babies enter a transition phase with a more stable PaO_2. Many neonates respond promptly and rapidly to either conventional treatment[1180] or a short period of hyperventilation combined with NO, and the resulting mortality is low, in the 10–20% range, with most of the deaths being due to complications of prematurity, such as GMH/IVH or the neurological sequelae of severe birth asphyxia.

In many North American centres, however, an overall mortality of 30–40% is reported.[279] These see many severe cases who do not respond within 3–4 days to high ventilator pressures and vasodilators, and it is for these babies that ECMO is being used extensively,[74,400] whereas others employ high-frequency jet ventilation.[1014]

For those requiring ECMO with primary PPHN or PPHN complicating RDS or MAS, survival figures of 80–90% are reported, with slightly fewer infected babies surviving[556,815] (Table 29.36, p. 572).

In babies with group B streptococcal sepsis, the mortality rate ranges from 10 to 20% (p. 1130). Most of the babies die from either irreversible hypoxia secondary to the PPHN or from myocardial failure as bacterial toxins cause arrhythmias or profound hypotension. The results in diaphragmatic hernia are given on pages 658–659.

SEQUELAE

Full recovery is the aim: once the pulmonary arteries relax and the lungs are perfused, the normal progression of postnatal cardiopulmonary adaptation should take place, and the baby can be expected to make a complete recovery. Whether or not sequelae occur in survivors depends on whether the intensity of respiratory support caused CLD, and whether any neurological damage resulted from either severe hypoxia or techniques such as ECMO. The long-term follow-up of babies treated with tolazoline shows no excess of handicap compared to gestation-matched controls.[207]

Respiratory

No studies have been reported looking specifically at pulmonary sequelae in babies treated for PPHN. There is, however, no reason to suppose that the results would be any different from those seen in other infants who survived neonatal IPPV with or without CLD (pp. 513–514).

Neurological

There are no long-term sequelae in 60–70% of cases,[52,315,600,719,1079] with the poor results occurring in those who were hyperventilated the longest[102] or those who suffered a cerebral haemorrhage.[379] Right-sided cerebral lesions have been reported in 15% of ECMO survivors because of the ligation of the right common carotid artery, which is required after stopping ECMO.[952] Of the 30–40% with handicap, about a quarter have severe defects. A recent study reported an incidence of deafness of 53% in survivors of PPHN,[482] although no non-ECMO survivor was deaf in the series reported by Marron et al.[719]

MECONIUM ASPIRATION SYNDROME

DEFINITION

This illness follows the inhalation of meconium before, during or immediately after delivery. The baby will fulfil the standard criteria for respiratory distress (p. 495), with tachypnoea >60/min and dyspnoea, although grunting is rare. Additional oxygen therapy is required.

Incidence

In Europe the incidence is between 1:1000 and 1:5000 (Table 29.24), whereas in North America rates of

Table 29.24 Prevalence of meconium aspiration syndrome

Years	Rate 1000 live births	Mortality (%)	Country	Reference
1970–74*	2.4	28	USA	Carson et al[157]
1975*	0.6	0	USA	Carson et al[157]
1976–77	0.9	0	Sweden	Hjalmarson[498]
1978–80	3.4	NA	Canada	Cyr et al[240]
1977–81	3.2	40	USA	Davis et al[249]
1976–84	3.0	7.2	Lebanon	Mounla[774]
1981–86	1.9	8.3	UK	Coltart et al[213]
1983–84	0.5	0	UK	Field et al[322]
1984–88	3.4	NA	Saudi Arabia	N.R.C. Roberton, unpublished data
1985–89	1.8	4.5	UK	Cambridge unpublished data
1985–87	5.3	NA	USA	Sunoo et al[1043]
1973–87	6.5	4.2	USA	Wiswell et al[1171]
1990–94	0.2	0	UK	Cambridge unpublished data

*Before and after instituting a system of intrapartum airway toilet.
NA, not available.

2–5:1000 have recently been reported, although the disease seems to have been rare 30 years ago: Driscoll and Smith[276] reported only eight deaths from MAS out of nearly 300 neonatal deaths from lung disease. A high incidence of MAS is also reported from the Middle East (Table 29.24).

AETIOLOGY

To develop MAS a fetus must pass meconium, inhale it, and the inhaled material must damage the lungs. All these factors are inextricably interlinked with the presence of fetal asphyxia (see below, p. 168).

Passage of meconium

An overall prevalence of 8–22% is quoted,[270,431,602,732,876] again with the suggestion that the problem is more common in North America. In the large American National Institutes of Health perinatal study of more than 50 000 deliveries, the prevalence was 18.4%,[788] compared to 11.5% in the 1970 perinatal mortality survey in the UK.[166] Meconium aspiration is a disease of term or post-term pregnancy,[725,732] and this mirrors the fact that meconium staining of the liquor occurs in 5% or fewer of preterm pregnancies,[599,725,728,1152] when it suggests chorioamnionitis[449,728] (pp. 168, 1149). The prevalence increases to 10% or more after 38 weeks,[401] reaching 22% in patients at a gestational age of 42 weeks and 44% when these patients deliver 1–2 weeks later.[602] The babies may be somewhat small for dates, averaging 2.91 kg at 290 days,[431] but major growth retardation below the third centile is unusual.[548,1073]

Meconium staining before labour or during the second stage seems to be of little significance in the absence of other signs of fetal distress, such as fetal heart rate changes or acidaemia.[567,732,745,1193] Meconium staining, particularly if thick, appearing when the membranes rupture or early in the first stage of labour, is more often viewed with anxiety,[732] particularly if combined with abnormalities of fetal heart rate or fetal pH.[746,924]

The fetal passage of meconium may be due to a vagal reflex, but more convincing are the data showing that motilin, which is produced mainly by the jejunum and stimulates peristalsis, is very low in preterm infants and in unasphyxiated term infants, but is raised in asphyxiated term babies who pass meconium intrapartum.[679,703]

Inhalation

Inhalation can occur antenatally. During normal fetal breathing activity there is net movement of fluid out of the lung,[252] which will normally prevent meconium inhalation, but meconium inhalation can occur before delivery. Meconium has been found in the lungs of stillborn babies[134] and in those who die in the early neonatal period but could not have inhaled meconium intrapartum.[147,710,1043] Prolonged severe fetal hypoxia can stimulate fetal breathing, to the extent that amniotic fluid is inhaled,[504] and fetal gasping movements also draw intra-amniotic material into the alveoli.[112,711] Perinatally, meconium inhalation can occur if the baby breathes or gasps with his mouth, pharynx or larynx full of meconium-stained liquor. This may occur late in the second stage of labour, particularly if there is a severe mixed acidaemia to a fetal pH <7.0,[876] when the raised $PaCO_2$ may have provoked intrapartum gasping.

Postnatally any meconium in the upper airway can potentially cause MAS. However, the majority of babies with meconium below the vocal cords during resuscitation do not develop MAS,[309,924] or at worst have a variant of transient tachypnoea which lasts for only 24–48 hours. If meconium is inhaled, the development of severe MAS depends in part on whether there is coexisting asphyxia,[487,551,567] although respiratory disease can develop when cord blood gases are normal.[876]

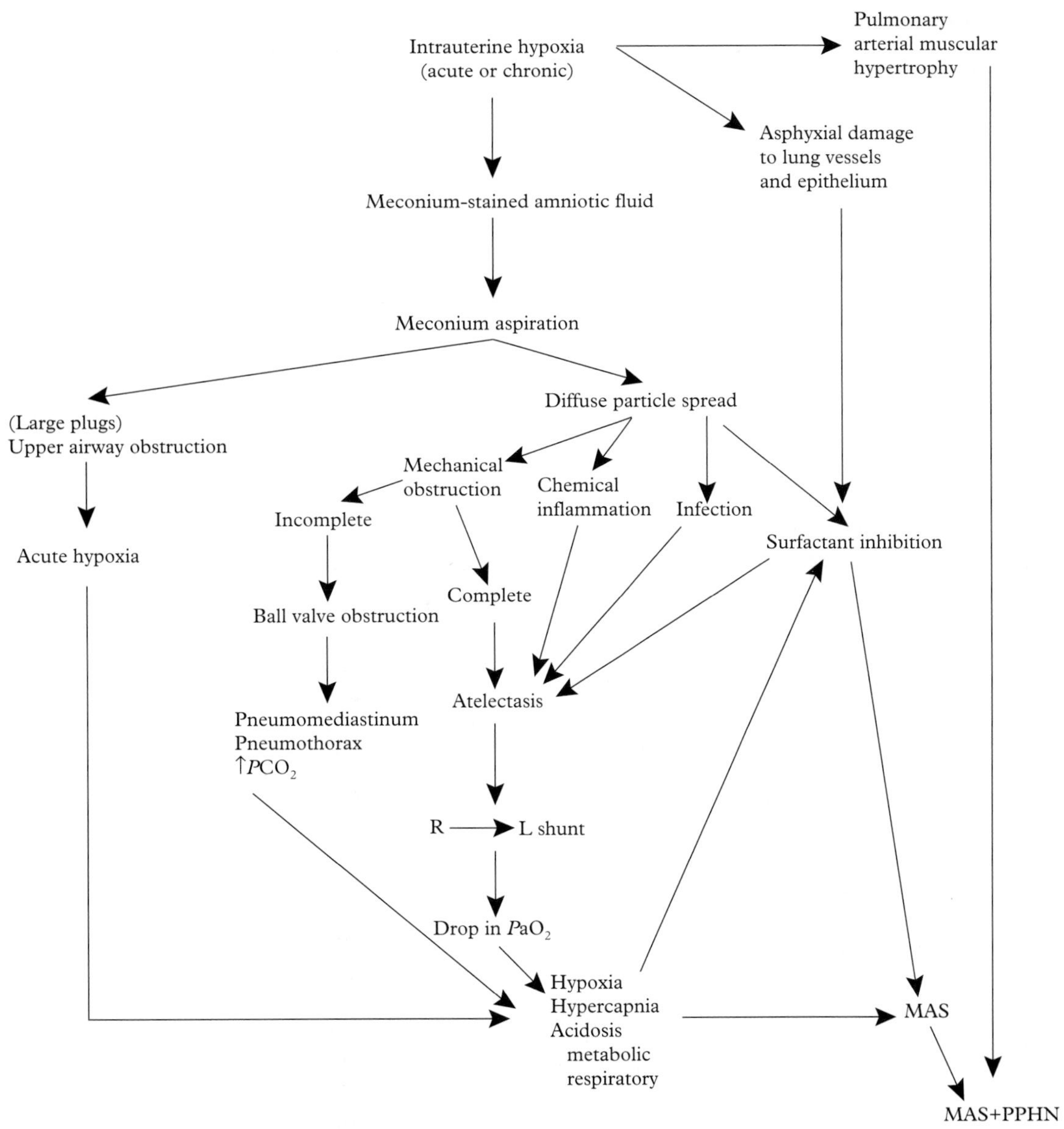

Fig. 29.63 Aetiology of MAS and its associated clinical syndromes.

Effect of meconium on the lungs[1096]

Meconium is a sticky, unpleasant material composed of inspissated fetal intestinal secretions.[467] When inhaled, it probably has at least four interacting deleterious effects on a neonatal lung (Fig. 29.63):

- It creates a ball valve mechanism in the airways, whereby air can be sucked past the plug but cannot be exhaled. This increases airway resistance, mainly in expiration,[1080,1096] causing gas trapping, pulmonary overexpansion and pneumothorax.
- It acts as a chemical irritant: 24–48 hours after inhalation there is an exudative and inflammatory pneumonitis with alveolar collapse and cellular necrosis; at this stage gas trapping is no longer a feature.[1096]
- The organic nature of the inhaled material, although initially sterile, may predispose the baby to pulmonary infection, particularly with *Escherichia coli.*[138] Meconium staining of the liquor may be a marker of chorioamnionitis predisposing the baby to 'congenital' penumonia,[728,1152] and meconium inhibits polymorph function.[194]
- Meconium inhibits surfactant at the alveolar surface,[191] as it does in vitro.[772,1042] This effect will combine with the deleterious effects on surfactant function of protein leaking on to the alveolar surface as a result of the coexisting perinatal asphyxia (p. 484).

These four factors combine to cause severe airway and alveolar disease, which is more likely to occur if there is coexisting asphyxial lung damage.[551,567,876]

Effect on pulmonary vasculature

A rise in pulmonary artery pressure occurs in all babies with hypoxia and acidaemia (pp. 489, 530). Tyler et al[1096] showed in animals that meconium in the lung increases pulmonary artery pressure, despite the blood gases being normal. Pulmonary hypertension has been reported in babies with MAS.[336] Furthermore, the clinical findings in babies who have inhaled meconium merge into those of PPHN (pp. 527–529), perhaps only in those who have increased muscularity of their pulmonary arteries.[780]

PATHOLOGY

The tracheal mucosa of stillborns may be stained green, but in neonates resuscitation will have removed meconium from the larger airways. The pleura may be normal, or petechial haemorrhages may be present on the lung surfaces due to acute hypoxaemia, particularly if death has occurred rapidly after birth. The lungs may be greenish yellow in colour. The cut surface can be normal or show congestion and haemorrhage. In some, meconium is expressible from the cut ends of the smaller bronchi. The pathognomonic histological feature is the presence of amniotic squames together with meconium in the terminal airways. Meconium itself appears as rather granular eosinophilic material, often containing small yellow 'meconium bodies'. Aspirated material will stimulate a macrophage reaction but, in the absence of an infective process, acute inflammation with neutrophils is not a feature. In addition to the meconium, hyaline membranes are frequently present. There may also be non-specific changes of an asphyxial insult to the lung, including interstitial oedema and haemorrhage. The changes of PPHN (p. 529) may be seen in the pulmonary vascular tree. Infants who die of MAS will have been ventilated at high pressures and rates, and thus the histological changes merge into those of CLD. In babies with MAS who die early in the neonatal period, severe asphyxial damage may be seen in other organs, in particular the brain, kidney and myocardium.

PREVENTION

Preventing or at least minimizing MAS antenatally or perinatally is still a matter of considerable controversy.

Antenatal

Meta-analyses suggest that the use of CTGs reduces the incidence of perinatal death from HIE and neonatal seizures (most likely due to grade II or III HIE), but at a cost of an increased intervention rate.[397,690,789,1122] If these aspects of intrapartum asphyxia can be avoided then presumably so can MAS.

In North America amnioinfusion is used. An inverse relationship has been found between amniotic fluid volume and fetal heart rate decelerations, a possible mechanism being either cord or head compression; amnioinfusion, by maintenance of amniotic fluid volume during labour, aims to stop this problem occurring and hence reduce the likelihood of MAS.[237] Amnioinfusion, using 1000 ml of saline 6 hourly until delivery, has been associated with better Apgar scores, less meconium below the cords and a lower rate of caesarean section,[1153] but not all studies have demonstrated positive effects.[1106,1153] A randomized trial[1041] involving women with oligohydramnios demonstrated that amnioinfusion starting in the latent phase of labour reduced meconium passage and operative deliveries for fetal distress. Possible adverse outcomes of amnioinfusion include an increased incidence of cord prolapse or infection; a longer duration of labour has also been experienced.[1041]

Suppression of fetal breathing movements by maternal narcotic administration, although successful in a baboon model, did not reduce the incidence of MAS in two clinical trials.[110,390]

Intrapartum/postpartum

Airway suctioning

Although it is clear that some meconium can be inhaled before labour, it is assumed that the majority of cases of MAS arise due to inhalation of meconium postnatally or during fetal gasping during the last few minutes of the second stage of labour. In uncontrolled studies, meticulous clearing of the airway at delivery was said to reduce considerably the incidence of MAS.[157,431,1073] These studies from the mid-1970s suggested that if suction was not carried out after crowning, or if meticulous tracheal toilet was not performed after intrapartum suction, MAS could still occur, although it was rare.[431]

Several recent studies have suggested that routine suctioning through the cords, or intubation with endotracheal toilet, is not justified, as these manoeuvres not only failed to reduce the incidence of MAS but were associated with increased morbidity.[309,664] However, many of the studies excluded babies who were most likely to be asphyxiated. Other studies[1169,1171] have confirmed that assiduous removal of meconium in the labour ward does reduce MAS, but that meticulous cleaning of the upper airway after delivery is all that is required and it is not necessary to start suctioning immediately after crowning. It is particularly important for an experienced paediatrician to attend deliveries where meconium staining is accompanied by fetal distress and low Apgar scores,[1194] as it is in these cases that MAS is particularly likely to be a problem. As soon as possible after delivery such a baby should be handed to the paediatrician who, irrespective of whether the baby is breathing or not, should gently insert a laryngoscope and carefully clear the upper airway of any meconium-stained material. If no meconium is seen below the cords it is not worth proceeding.[664] However, if meconium is seen, direct tracheal suction is indicated.[356,1169] Studies in kittens have demonstrated that inhaled meconium stayed in the trachea and major bronchial divisions for several minutes after the onset of respiration, and was therefore still in a site from which it could be aspirated.[841]

IPPV

The indications for resuscitation by IPPV (p. 254) are not affected by the presence of meconium, other than that it is always important to clear as much meconium from the airway as possible before applying positive pressure ventilation.

Compression of the neonatal thorax

This has been recommended but seems unlikely to prevent fetal gasping, which, apart from anything else, has a large diaphragmatic component. In addition, compression of the thorax can actually stimulate respiratory efforts.

Bronchial lavage

Instilling water or saline into the lower respiratory tract is controversial: an increase in wet lung has been noted following this procedure,[157] (p. 574) and repeated bronchial lavages can be harmful. In babies who are thought during the first 3–4 minutes to have inhaled large amounts of meconium, and in whom suctioning alone proves ineffective, 0.5–1.0 ml of saline should be instilled down the endotracheal tube, the baby hand-ventilated four or five times, and the endotracheal tube sucked out. If no meconium is obtained there is no need to persist. Only one or two lavages should be attempted. Once on IPPV, tracheal suction with saline lavage resulted in a 35% improvement (decrease) in airway resistance.[77]

Postnatal gastric aspiration

If the baby has inhaled meconium at delivery, it is likely that he has also swallowed some. His stomach should therefore be emptied as soon after delivery as possible.

SIGNS AND SYMPTOMS

General appearance

The baby is usually mature or postmature, with long fingernails and a dry skin which soon starts to flake. The skin, nails and umbilical cord are often stained greenish yellow. The baby is not usually febrile, unless he becomes secondarily infected. Peripheral oedema is not a feature, and if present it suggests either renal damage with renal failure (p. 1027) or iatrogenic fluid overload.

Table 29.25 Respiratory function in MAS[56]

	Mean values in MAS (1 SD)	Normal (expected values)
Birthweight (kg)	3.98	
Tidal volume (V_T) (ml)	16.3 (6.7)	24
Minute ventilation (V_E) (ml/min)	1647 (611)	800
Compliance (C_L) (ml/cmH_2O)	1.82 (0.76)	4–6
Inspiratory resistance (R_I) (cmH_2O/l/s)	100 (67)	15–30

Respiratory

The infant has tachypnoea, which may exceed 120/min (Table 29.25). Because he is mature with a firm rib cage, marked sternal retraction as seen in preterm neonates with RDS is rare, but intercostal and subcostal recession, the use of accessory muscles and flaring of the nostrils are usually present. An expiratory grunt may be heard. The meconium in the airways causes widespread sticky crepitations and occasional rhonchi, air trapping and an overdistended chest with an increased anteroposterior diameter. These are present whether or not early IPPV is given. The asphyxiated baby with neurological damage may be apnoeic but, when intubated and ventilated, the physical signs in the respiratory tract are identical to those in the spontaneously breathing neonate.

The baby may remain symptomatic for only 24 hours, or he may be very dyspnoeic for 7–10 days before recovery. Even in ventilated patients, however, the respiratory disease has usually abated to a resting tachypnoea of 50–70/min in room air by 14 days of age.

Cardiovascular

In the absence of asphyxial damage to the myocardium there are no specific cardiovascular features of MAS. Hypotension suggests myocardial damage, as do signs of congestive heart failure. In uncomplicated MAS the heart rate tends to be around 110–125/min, and the blood pressure is maintained within the normal range. If PPHN (p. 530) develops S2 may remain single, and there may be the murmur of tricuspid incompetence (p. 530).

Abdominal examination

The liver and spleen are often palpable because of downward displacement of the diaphragm caused by air trapping. In a severely affected infant bowel sounds may be absent, with delayed passage of meconium. The kidneys are not usually palpable, but there may be urinary retention and bladder distension in babies with severe neurological problems or those who receive pancuronium.

Central nervous system

Depending on the severity of the coexisting neurological insult, the baby may behave normally or show any of the neurological features of birth asphyxia, ranging from the common over-alert stage I HIE to the rare, flaccid unresponsive ventilated baby in stage III (p. 1239). Convulsions may occur and jitteriness persist for days.

DIFFERENTIAL DIAGNOSIS

This should rarely be a problem. A term baby who is dyspnoeic and has meconium-stained liquor in his trachea and larynx at delivery has MAS until proved otherwise, but it is always worth remembering that apparently feculent liquor may be due to yellow-green bilious vomiting secondary to upper gastrointestinal tract obstruction.[1182] It is important to exclude concurrent illness, in particular infection and PPHN.

PATHOPHYSIOLOGY

The respiratory failure and hypoxaemia in babies with MAS are due to stiff lungs, marked ventilation–perfusion imbalance and pulmonary hypertension precipitating extrapulmonary right–left shunts (Fig. 29.63).

Babies with MAS have a reduced compliance and tidal volume, and an increased airways resistance, but the tachypnoea increases the minute volume to twice normal[56] (Table 29.25). In the early stages of the disease, when the airways are plugged by meconium, as in the animal model[1096] there is a marked ventilation–perfusion abnormality which lessens as the lungs recover.[221,614] Later in the disease, shunting increases as the chemical pneumonitis becomes a dominant factor.[1096] In those who develop PPHN, the pulmonary artery pressure will be higher than the systemic,[336] with right–left shunting through the ductus arteriosus[653] and/or the foramen ovale.

INVESTIGATIONS

Haematological

The haemoglobin is normal but the white count is usually raised,[712,739] and is therefore of no help in evaluating the possibility of infection; neutropenia, as always, is of value (p. 1124). WBC function, however, is reduced.[194] Thrombocytopenia occurs in neonates with meconium aspiration who have PPHN,[956] are ventilated,[53] or who develop DIC secondary to severe asphyxia (p. 1243).

Biochemical

There are no characteristic biochemical features of MAS. If coexisting asphyxia is severe, there may be inappropriate ADH production and hyponatraemia (p. 1024). Renal failure secondary to acute tubular necrosis may cause hyperkalaemia and a raised urea. Hypocalcaemia may also occur, as in any critically ill neonate (p. 966).

Blood gases

Hypoxia is common, but in babies with mild to moderate disease who are mature, with an efficient respiratory pump (pp. 459–460), ventilation is not a problem and the $P\text{a}CO_2$ may even be low, normal or only slightly raised. A $P\text{a}CO_2$ >8 kPa (60 mmHg) is unusual, and is seen only in patients with severe lung disease who eventually need ventilation.

Changes in pH initially reflect the metabolic acidaemia of intrapartum asphyxia; mature babies commonly correct their acidaemia spontaneously from pH levels in the 7.10–7.15 range and base deficit values of 10–15 mmol/l.[1012] After the first hour or two persisting metabolic acidaemia indicates an underlying problem such as sepsis, hypotension or renal failure, which should be sought and remedied.

Urine analysis

Unless renal failure supervenes, the urinary output is normal (p. 1013). Many babies with MAS, although not in overt renal failure, have a raised urinary β_2-microglobulin, indicating that renal damage has occurred.[208] The urine may be greenish brown in colour as a result of the absorption of meconium pigments across the pulmonary epithelium and their excretion in the urine.[253]

ECG, echocardiography

In uncomplicated MAS the ECG and echocardiogram will be normal. If there has been severe intrapartum asphyxia there may be ECG changes suggesting subendocardial ischaemia, and the echocardiogram will show reduced cardiac contractility. In those who are going to develop PPHN, changes in the systolic time interval will be seen on M-mode echocardiography[1108] (p. 528).

Chest X-ray

A chest X-ray must be taken as part of the initial diagnostic work-up of the dyspnoeic baby. The common early change reported by Peterson and Pendelton[838] and Gooding and Gregory[389] was widespread patchy infiltration; they also reported that 20–30% of the patients had small pleural effusions. Overexpansion is also common in the early stage[1189] (Fig. 29.64) and is best seen on the lateral chest X-ray. In mild–moderate cases the changes resolve within 48 hours. In severe cases, as the disease progresses, by 72 hours of age with or without ventilation the appearance is often changed to that of

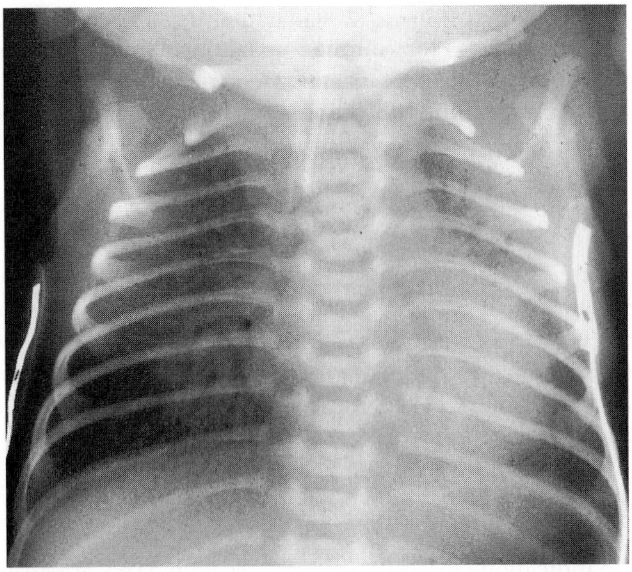

Fig. 29.64 Meconium aspiration syndrome showing overinflation, most marked in the right lung.

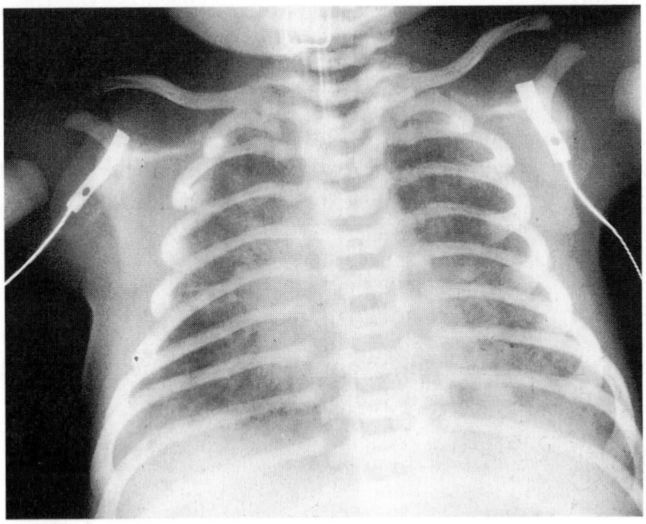

Fig. 29.65 Severe confluent pneumonitis in meconium aspiration syndrome.

diffuse and homogeneous opacification of both lung fields, presumably as a result of a pneumonitis and interstitial oedema secondary to the irritant effect of the inhaled meconium (see above, Fig. 29.65). These changes gradually resolve over the next week, but in severe cases the X-ray may still be abnormal at 14 days and merge into the pattern seen in CLD, although this is uncommon. Airleaks, in particular pneumothorax and pneumomediastinum, are very common in MAS (p. 517).

Microbiology

All babies suffering from MAS should have an infection screen as soon as possible after admission to the NICU. This is the only way to establish the coexistence of sepsis, and as antibiotics will be used in virtually all cases (p. 507), provides the essential baseline information upon which further antibiotic therapy can be planned. The value of routine superficial swabs in these babies, as in others (p. 1122), is doubtful.[301]

Table 29.26 Monitoring in MAS

PaO_2	Monitor continuously with $tcPO_2$ or SpO_2. In ventilated babies continuous PaO_2 catheter useful. Arterial line essential to avoid disturbance by sampling. Keep PaO_2 >6 kPa, SpO_2>90%. In term babies no risk of ROP so upper PO_2 cut-off point not critical
$PaCO_2$	Rarely required more than 4-hourly
pH	As for $PaCO_2$
Chest X-ray	Daily in acute phase
Respiratory rate	Monitor as indicated. Apnoeic attacks rare
Cardiological	HR/ECG/BP continuous in acute phase and on IPPV; BP 4-hourly thereafter until in <50–60% oxygen
Microbiology	Initial cultures. Others as indicated
Fluid and electrolytes	Daily weighing, fluid balance, daily urea, Na, K, calcium, albumin while in intensive care
Haematology	Daily PCV/Hb. Initial WBC and platelets repeated as indicated especially when on IPPV
Temperature	4-hourly

MONITORING (Table 29.26)

There is a temptation to undermonitor full-term babies with MAS because, despite marked tachypnoea and a very abnormal chest X-ray appearance, they often look surprisingly pink and vigorous. This temptation should be resisted, not only because of the importance of early detection of blood gas abnormalities, electrolyte disturbance or hypotension before secondary effects develop, but because the baby with MAS has a major risk of sudden deterioration due to a tension pneumothorax, sometimes bilateral.

TREATMENT

There is no specific treatment for MAS. The aim is to support the baby until his alveolar macrophages clear the debris and lung function returns to normal.

Initial management

It is easy to underestimate the severity of lung disease in mature babies. Only by doing the appropriate investigations can severe blood gas derangements, hypotension or radiological changes be detected early enough to minimize the undesirable sequelae of therapeutic delay.

Minimal handling

Term babies with serious lung disease of all types become very agitated when disturbed, and as a result hypoxic;

the philosophy of minimal handling therefore applies (p. 502).

Thermal environment

Term babies are much less prone to heat loss than preterm ones, but conversely can easily become overheated. They should be nursed naked for ease of observation, and their optimal thermal environment is an incubator set at 32–32.5°C (p. 296).

Respiratory failure

The relative efficiency of the respiratory system in mature babies will enable them to control their $PaCO_2$ unless the disease is severe or their respiration depressed by the neurological effects of asphyxia. Because these mature babies are not susceptible to ROP, the prime concern is preventing hypoxaemia.

Oxygen therapy

Most babies with MAS can be managed by giving an adequate concentration of warmed humidified oxygen into a headbox; this can be at a concentration of 80–90% if indicated, and may need to be sustained at this concentration for up to 2 weeks for those with severe disease. Unlike preterm babies with RDS there is no need to institute CPAP in the first 36–48 hours if the oxygen requirement exceeds 50–60% or the $PaCO_2$ rises to 6.0–6.5 kPa (45–50 mmHg) or greater.

In many mild cases oxygen therapy at 40% or less for 24–48 hours is all that is required, and in all cases, once the PaO_2 begins to rise, the F_IO_2 can be reduced. Many neonates with mild MAS have a normal PaO_2 in room air by 48 hours of age.

Acid–base homoeostasis

Carbon dioxide retention is only a problem in severe cases. A $PaCO_2$ of 7.5–8 kPa (55–60 mmHg) is acceptable so long as the pH is sustained above 7.25 and the blood pressure, peripheral blood flow, urinary output and clinical condition are acceptable. The $PaCO_2$ rising above 8 kPa (60 mmHg), particularly in the presence of a PaO_2 <6 kPa (45 mmHg), early in the disease, is usually an indication for intubation and ventilation.

The first blood gas analysis taken after birth may show a marked metabolic acidaemia. Provided that the baby is otherwise stable, with a normal PaO_2 and $PaCO_2$, and is passing urine, base deficits of 10–15 mmol/l can be left to correct spontaneously (p. 259). Once the base deficit has fallen to below 15 mmol/l or the pH below 7.10, it is prudent to correct the acidaemia (p. 484).

In babies who show features of HIE, more rigid control of the blood gases is required (pp. 1242–1244): hypoxia, hypercapnia and acidaemia are all undesirable. This indication for intubation and ventilation takes priority over the more conservative management of the blood gases outlined for babies with uncomplicated lung disease.

CPAP

CPAP at pressures of 4–7 cmH_2O may increase the PaO_2 in babies with MAS.[335] However, it is likely to increase the risk of pneuomothorax in a disease characterized by air trapping, and the use of a nasal prong in a term neonate usually makes him irritable and restless, with a fall in PaO_2.

IPPV

The indications for IPPV in neonates with MAS are given on page 563, and the initial ventilator settings on page 564. Theoretically, these babies should prefer a rate of 60–80/min, a long expiratory time and low levels of PEEP. Pancuronium is almost always required (p. 576).

When these large babies start to improve on IPPV weaning can usually be rapid. Once they are in 50–60% oxygen and on pressures <22/3 cmH_2O, pancuronium should be withheld. The rate can then be reduced quickly, and they can be extubated from low IMV rates without a period of CPAP.

High-frequency ventilation

HFJV used with surfactant, but not alone, has been reported to improve oxygenation in MAS.[247]

ECMO

ECMO has been demonstrated in a randomized trial to improve the survival of infants with an oxygenation index greater than 40, by 50%.[1099]

Pulmonary vasodilators

Drugs used to treat PHT can be effective in babies with MAS,[381,1029,1076] but their use has been superseded by inhalation of NO.[324,588]

Surfactant

Exogenous surfactant therapy has been used with anecdotal success.[35,580] Lavage with surfactant may be a particularly effective method of washing out meconium and improving gas exchange.[810] In a recent randomized prospective study surfactant-treated babies had fewer airleaks, were on IPPV and oxygen for shorter periods, and were much less likely to require ECMO;[323]

interestingly, the maximum effect on oxygenation was after three doses or more, suggesting that larger doses are required in non-RDS respiratory conditions. Surfactant was given within 6 hours of birth. Once on ECMO, the use of surfactant speeds recovery and the rate of weaning from ECMO.[677]

Antibiotics

The presence of organic and potentially infected material in the liquor and in the lung may predispose to pneumonia, and there are some data from animals to support this view.[138,330,1152] After taking a full set of cultures, but not doing a lumbar puncture, neonates diagnosed as having MAS should be put on broad-spectrum antibiotics, using penicillin and gentamicin. The antibiotics should be continued until the baby is in the convalescent stage of his illness and requiring less than 30–40% oxygen.

Blood volume and pressure

Anaemia is not usually a problem in babies with MAS, either immediately after delivery or as a result of blood sampling, but when the haemoglobin falls below 13 g/dl or the PCV below 40% the baby should be transfused. Blood pressure control is essential in all neonates with MAS, aiming to keep the pressure within the normal range (p. 504). Hypotension is usually only a problem in those who have suffered severe intrapartum asphyxia, with coexisting myocardial injury or after vasodilators (p. 534). If hypotension occurs it is managed in the usual way with volume expansion and inotropes (p. 504).

Physiotherapy[826]

In mild to moderate cases who are not ventilated and require less than 60% inspired oxygen concentration, chest physiotherapy is rarely necessary. In the severely affected neonate who is intubated and paralysed, chest percussion and endotracheal tube suction should be carried out (p. 577). Physiotherapy should only be continued as long as significant amounts of greenish material are produced, but should be abandoned if the neonate becomes irritable, restless and hypoxaemic.

Steroids

Steroids have been recommended; however, although in an animal model steroids reduced respiratory symptoms due to MAS the mortality rate was higher.[346] In a randomized trial involving 35 infants[1188] treated in the first 6 hours of life, no significant differences in the duration of ventilation or survival were noted and the steroid-treated group experienced an increased time to weaning.

Fluid and electrolyte balance

In uncomplicated MAS this is rarely a problem, and standard fluid therapy starting with 40–60 ml/kg/24 h on the first day and increasing thereafter can be used. When MAS has been accompanied by severe birth asphyxia, fluid restriction to 40 ml/kg/24 h at least is indicated. The initial fluid given should be 10% dextrose, with electrolytes added after 24–48 hours. If asphyxia has occurred hypoglycaemia is a possibility, and should always be sought and treated promptly.

Coagulation disturbances

DIC is not a feature of uncomplicated MAS but may be secondary to the concurrent birth asphyxia. Its management is outlined on page 804.

Nutrition

In the first day or two enteral feeding is not justified for the usual reasons (p. 506). Furthermore, as the the term baby has good caloric reserves there is no hurry. Mild–moderate cases of MAS have a short duration, so that some enteral feeding can be started by 2–3 days of age in most cases. For those still on IPPV at this stage, and the small number of non-ventilated cases who at 5–6 days cannot tolerate enteral feeding, intravenous nutrition can be started.

Neurological problems

MAS may be complicated by moderate to severe HIE, the management of which (pp. 1242–1245) takes precedence over the management of the MAS. If IPPV and stricter control of blood gases are indicated on neurological grounds this must be done, even though it is not necessary for treatment of the lung disease; the fluid balance must be that which is optimal for HIE. If large doses of drugs such as anticonvulsants are required, even though they may depress respiration, they must be given and the baby ventilated.

COMPLICATIONS

Babies with MAS may suffer from HIE (p. 1238) and renal failure (p. 1026). These are dealt with elsewhere.

Pneumothorax, airleaks

These are common complications, occurring in 15–20% of non-ventilated babies[389,838,1073] and 30–50% of those who require IPPV.[56,702,1124] PIE is rare, but pneumomediastinum, pneumopericardium and pneumoperitoneum can all occur.

Pneumothoraces may be both bilateral and under tension, and commonly cause acute deterioration in the baby's condition. It is therefore essential that babies with severe MAS are only cared for in units that have the capacity to respond instantaneously and effectively when a tension pneumothorax occurs (p. 520).

Persistent pulmonary hypertension

This is a common complication of severe MAS, and on histological and clinical grounds it would appear to be particularly frequent in fatal cases[780,1171] (p. 529). The incidence of this complication does seem to vary geographically,[956,1108] but this may be due to differences in definition. PPHN associated with MAS usually responds promptly to pulmonary vasodilators and conventional ventilation.

Chronic lung disease

This appears to be a rare complication of MAS,[207,727] although it may occur in any baby who survives after long-term high-pressure IPPV.

Other complications

The risk of infection in these babies is similar to that in all babies who are ventilated. They may be rather more prone to post-extubation problems[56] but, being mature, are not susceptible to problems with a patent ductus arteriosus. Their maturity also protects them from GMH/IVH and ROP, but severe neurological damage may occur secondary to the HIE.

MORTALITY

Few large series of MAS have been published in recent years. It appears from Table 29.24 that the mortality fell from up to 35–40% in series reported in the early 1970s, to virtually zero by the end of the 1980s. Some babies are still born with severe antenatal inhalation of meconium and, despite appropriate care, prove to be virtually unresuscitatable.[147,548] The majority of deaths subsequently are from respiratory failure, PPHN or airleaks,[1171] but some still die from the associated neurological or renal sequelae of severe asphyxia. Deaths from MAS should now be rare.

MORBIDITY

Neurological

The neurological sequelae in these babies are those of the coexisting HIE (pp. 1246–1247), but if this is absent and ECMO is avoided (p. 572) the outlook is good.

Pulmonary

MAS does predispose to long-term respiratory morbidity in infancy.[1204] Even at school age, although the majority of neonates who survived MAS were completely normal, 30–40% had problems with asthma and less than half had completely normal lung function tests.[696,1047] These results, and others which show airway dilatation in response to betamimetics,[611] suggest that meconium aspiration predisposed the infants to increased bronchial hyperreactivity. Yuksel et al[1204] demonstrated that lung function abnormalities at follow-up relate to the severity of MAS. Cordier et al[222] also demonstrated evidence of residual airways disease at 6–9 years of age in patients who had moderate to severe MAS, whereas 12 children who had had mild MAS had normal lung function.[1028]

ASPIRATION OF AMNIOTIC FLUID

Postmortem studies of stillbirths have revealed that amniotic squames can be inhaled by the fetus in utero, presumably as a result of 'terminal' gasping activity preceding intrauterine death.[1157] The importance of less severe manifestations of this entity, in the absence of meconium staining of the amniotic fluid, is speculative, but it is clear that there is a postnatal lung disease attributed to the inhalation of non-meconium stained amniotic squames.[946]

ASPIRATION SYNDROMES

In the neonatal period various respiratory problems can occur due to malfunction of the coordination of sucking, swallowing and breathing (Table 29.27). Meconium aspiration syndrome is considered above, and the aspiration seen in babies with copious bronchopulmonary secretions while still on IPPV[1175] or shortly after extubation (p. 581) is dealt with elsewhere.

INCIDENCE

The frequency of the conditions listed in Table 29.27 is not clear; they were not included in the surveys by Hjalmarson[498] or Field et al.[322] Nevertheless, the conditions are often found in term babies on a postnatal ward and in babies undergoing or recovering from neonatal intensive care.

Table 29.27 Types of aspiration syndrome in the newborn

1. Sucking/swallowing incoordination
   (a) Prematurity
   (b) Secondary to structural malformation or neurological disorders, cleft palate, Pierre-Robin syndrome, tracheo-oesophageal fistula, laryngeal cleft, hypoxic–ischaemic encephalopathy
   (c) Syndromes with poor sucking, e.g. Prader–Willi
2. Syndromes attributed to gastro-oesophageal reflux
   (a) In babies on IPPV – right upper lobe collapse
   (b) Wilson–Mikity syndrome
   (c) Apnoeic attacks
3. Massive regurgitation and inhalation of a feed

SWALLOWING INCOORDINATION

Pathophysiology

The anatomical structure of the pharynx and larynx is to a large extent responsible for protecting the airway from inhalation.[682] This function is aided by 'defensive' reflexes. The presence of any material in the pharynx initiates swallowing and reflex breath-holding.[1165] If the airway is still threatened, additional reflexes are provoked which are designed to protect the airway from the inhalation of unswallowed material. These include more prolonged apnoea, choking, laryngospasm and, of course, coughing.[243,846] These mechanisms provide a less effective shield over the airway in the neonatal period than they do in older children and adults. During sucking, the normal term neonate may have a reduction in ventilation,[21] PaO_2 and heart rate,[722] progressing to apnoea in some.[442,530,724,1024] This may be because of poor breathing/swallowing coordination or additional problems such as velopalatine insufficiency, with reflux into the nasopharynx.[855]

The preterm neonate has greater problems. He has immature sucking/swallowing coordination,[440,977] which may be overwhelmed by oral feeding; he has a high incidence of gastro-oesophageal reflux,[792] making him prone to massive regurgitation of stomach contents; and, if there has been brain damage, the neurological control of swallowing may be compromised. Even though his ability to protect his airway is as good as at term,[847] these frequent challenges mean that its integrity may eventually be breached[530] and inhalation of stomach contents will result. Even if the defence mechanisms are effective in preventing intrapulmonary inhalation, significant symptoms, especially apnoea,[243,716,792,846] may still result.

Coordinating sucking, swallowing and breathing becomes more difficult at all gestations if the neonate is sedated by, for example, the transplacental passage of opiates, or if he is tachypnoeic with RDS or TTN.[1072] In such situations it becomes virtually impossible to cope with anything other than normal oropharyngeal secretions.

Other common causes of breathing/swallowing incoordination in both preterm and term babies are structural malformations in the upper airway or gastrointestinal tract, or neurological problems which interfere with normal swallowing. Biochemical problems such as hypoglycaemia or hyponatraemia may occasionally have the same effect. Most causes of dysphagia and sucking/swallowing incoordination are extremely rare[527] (Table 29.28) and usually present with the primary disorder rather than with dysphagia.

Table 29.28 Dysphagia in the newborn[527]

Gross anatomical defects	
Palate	Cleft palate, submucous cleft
Tongue	Macroglossia, cysts, tumours, lymphangioma, ankyloglossia superior
Nose	Choanal atresia
Mandible	Micrognathia, Pierre-Robin syndrome
Temporomandibular joint	Ankylosis (congenital or infective), hypoplasia
Pharynx	Cyst, diverticulum, tumour
Larynx	Cleft, cyst
Oesophagus	Atresia, stenosis, short oesophagus, web, diverticulum, duplication, lung buds, TOF
Thorax	Vascular rings
Neuromuscular incoordination	
Delayed maturation	Prematurity, normal variant
Cerebral palsy	All types
Brain damage	Post-asphyxial, postinfection (prenatal or postnatal)
Abnormalities of the cranial nerve nuclei and their tracts	Bulbar and suprabulbar palsy Moebius syndrome Pharyngeal, cricopharyngeal incoordination (idiopathic, secondary to brain damage)
Congenital laryngeal stridor	
Myopathies	Myotonic dystrophy, myasthenia gravis
Hypotonia from any cause	Brain damage, Werdnig–Hoffman
Syndromes	
Infections	Tetanus, polio, stomatitis, oesophagitis

Clinical features

The commonest manifestation of swallowing/breathing incoordination is seen in the term baby who, during normal breast- or bottle-feeding in the first 48–72 hours, chokes, splutters, and may be transiently apnoeic and blue. The baby is often admitted to the NICU, but thereafter usually remains asymptomatic. Many of these babies are at the extreme end of the normal spectrum of the response to feeding[722] (see above). More serious examples are seen in babies who have survived severe birth asphyxia or have problems such as cleft palate. In these, even saliva may continually collect in the pharynx and the baby will be 'mucousy'. In more severe cases he may have saliva dribbling from his mouth, and may cough and splutter as he tries to clear his airways; cyanosis and bradycardia can occur.[442,530] Persistent retention of secretions in the pharynx and larynx, in addition to causing noisy breathing and upper respiratory tract symptoms, may result in tachypnoea and retraction, and on auscultation widespread conducted sounds are heard. The most striking symptom in such babies is reflex apnoea, which can be caused by a wide variety of foreign materials in the larynx.[63]

Investigation and differential diagnosis

When a baby has had an episode of the sort described above, and particularly if he is having them repeatedly, the physician has to do two things: first, identify the cause of the problem (Table 29.28), and secondly decide whether any material has been inhaled into the lungs (see p. 550).

On the basis of the history and clinical examination it should be possible to distinguish between those babies who have had a single, or at most two or three episodes, owing to immature mechanisms being overwhelmed, and who require observation only, and those with gastro-oesophageal reflux or a chronic neurological or structural problem. In the latter group the cause will usually be obvious, for example an infant with a cleft lip and palate, or one who is recovering from severe HIE. The clinical presentation of oesophageal atresia, with maternal polyhydramnios, followed by the baby having major problems with his secretions in the first 2–3 hours, is sufficiently classic that it should not be missed. Other babies may have covert gastro-oesophageal reflex, or may be refluxing into the nasopharynx during a feed, with subsequent reflex apnoea.[855] Appropriate pH[792] or contrast studies will demonstrate the abnormality. If one of the rare problems in Table 29.28 is suspected, appropriate studies by EMG, EEG, muscle biopsy, contrast radiography, pH probe, CT scan, laryngoscopy or bronchoscopy may be necessary to establish the final diagnosis.

In some babies with persisting problems no obvious cause may be found. Frank and Gatewood[343] described a group of such term babies who eventually developed adequate sucking and swallowing and were normal.

Treatment

In the term baby who has been admitted to the neonatal unit following such an episode on the postnatal ward, if no clinical abnormality is found (which is usually the case), breast- or bottle-feeding can be continued under careful supervision, proceeding to further investigation by endoscopy or contrast radiography only if choking persists. In convalescent low-birthweight neonates, or those with recognized neurological or structural problems, all that is usually necessary in the absence of signs of aspiration pneumonia is to omit one or two feeds before carefully restarting them, by nasogastric tube if necessary.

Babies with TOF or laryngeal cleft should be taken to theatre as soon as possible. Problems associated with palatal defects may be considerably improved by the use of a palatal prosthesis (pp. 768–769). In babies with Pierre-Robin syndrome, laryngomalacia or other surgical problems in which there is not only tongue/palate incoordination, but also a structural predisposition to inhalation, and in addition no prospect of immediate surgical correction, the airways should be meticulously suctioned and the baby laid prone. It may, however, occasionally be necessary to resort to tracheostomy in order to protect the lungs.

A small group of babies, typically those with severe neurological damage secondary to HIE, or those with a primary problem such as dystrophia myotonica, may have prolonged difficulties. Frequent suctioning of the mouth and pharynx will be required, and it may help to keep the babies lying prone or semiprone, allowing the mouth to empty by gravity. Persistence of problems is an ominous prognostic feature: despite suctioning and positioning and meticulous nursing care, inhalation of secretions will eventually result, progressing to aspiration pneumonia, which is a common terminal event in such cases.

GASTRO-OESOPHAGEAL REFLUX

This has been recognized with increasing frequency in the neonate (p. 757) and may occur in association with a hiatus hernia. It can be of great importance in sick, ventilated VLBW neonates, in whom the prevalence has been reported to be as high as 80%.[391] Hrabovsky and Mullett[512] found 22 cases in a 4-year period, most of whom had ventilator-dependent CLD. Newell et al[792] found an overall incidence of 85% in babies <1.50 kg but, unlike Goodwin et al,[391] found the incidence to be much lower during IPPV.[793] GOR is still present in many ex-premature infants at the time of discharge,[716] but less so than in term babies of the same postconceptional age.[541] The clinical relevance of these data remains speculative. Gastric contents refluxed to the larynx can trigger reflex apnoea (see above), and Hrabovsky and Mullett[512] clearly attributed some of the problems in their babies with CLD to reflux, as they resorted to fundoplication in 17 out of 22 cases. Strang[1034] attributed cases of Wilson–Mikity syndrome (p. 622) to gastric aspiration, and the radiological changes of that condition are more marked in the upper zones, into which milk tends to be aspirated in the recumbent preterm baby.

Diagnosis

This depends on a high level of clinical suspicion in all neonates with apparently inexplicable and recurrent respiratory problems, especially if there is recurrent apnoea unresponsive to theophylline,[792] a history suggesting reflux or recurrent vomiting, or right upper lobe collapse or consolidation on X-ray. To confirm the diagnosis, the demonstration of fat-laden macrophages in the tracheobronchial secretions is of value,[802] combined with radiological or pH probe demonstration of reflux.[512,792,813]

Treatment

If episodes of apnoea or recurrent pulmonary disease in a neonate are attributed to reflux, small frequent feeds or continuous milk infusion are advocated; nasojejunal feeds or thickened feeds may also be beneficial.[792] Lying a baby prone, as well as improving the blood gases (p. 503), reduces the amount of reflux[814] (p. 757), but the benefit of nursing an infant 'head up' is controversial. Whether neonates benefited from medical therapy of any form was questioned by Hrabovsky and Mullett[512] and, as a consequence, in their view, if problems from the GOR persist and are severe, fundoplication is recommended. In our experience this has rarely been necessary.

ASPIRATION PNEUMONIA

This may occur following one of the episodes of sucking/swallowing incoordination or reflux described above, and is most likely to occur in babies with neurological defects or structural malformations and in preterm infants. It may be covert due to reflux, or can follow an episode of massive regurgitation and vomiting (see Table 29.28), which is virtually limited to ill and convalescent babies of all gestations on the NICU. A common story is that the baby, often still tube-fed, is found covered in vomit, having activated his apnoea or heart rate alarm; he is usually cyanosed, apnoeic or gasping, and bradycardic. The nurses administer the standard first aid, suction and supplementary oxygen, and the infant usually makes a prompt recovery.

Incidence

No incidence figures are available for aspiration pneumonia, but about 5–10 cases per annum occur on a level 3 NICU.

Prevention

Most cases of aspiration pneumonia can and should be prevented by prompt clinical recognition and appropriate management of the disorders in which they are likely to occur (Table 29.28) and by careful attention to the feeding technique. This includes:

- not feeding babies with respiratory distress until their condition has stabilized and preferably begun to improve, they have bowel sounds and have passed meconium (pp. 506–507). Giving a tube feed (or worse, giving a full bottle feed), even to comparatively mature babies with mild to moderate oxygen-dependent lung disease, can have disastrous consequences;
- careful use of tube feeding in preterm babies (pp. 394–397), recovering dyspnoeic babies or those with hypoxic–ischaemic encephalopathy or structural malformations. Progress to bottle-feeding should be very carefully conducted on a trial basis, only when it is clear that the baby is biochemically and haematologically normal, tolerating nasogastric tubes well, has no problems with his secretions and is showing spontaneous sucking activity on his tube or on a dummy;
- aspirating the indwelling nasogastric tube every 4–6 hours to ensure that, even with minimal enteral feeds, milk has not pooled in the stomach, posing the threat of regurgitation;
- avoiding all enteral feeds (tube or oral) for 12–24 hours after extubation (p. 581).

Pathophysiology

The foreign material aspirated into the airway can have three effects: simple physical obstruction, chemical irritation and promotion of infection.[1183] The major problem is the irritant potential of the inhaled fluid. All fluids, including water (p. 574), are damaging, but gastric contents are particularly so because of their acidic pH.[534,1183] In the first few days of life, and by the end of of the first month, the pH of a neonate's stomach contents can be 2.5 or less if he has not been fed[37] or fed only clear fluids with no buffering capacity. We know of no evidence that dextrose, in particular the 10% solution which is hyperosmolar and acidic (pH 4–5), is any less damaging than gastric contents; gastric contents buffered with milk are probably less irritating. Inhaled curd is particulate and can obstruct airways, leading to lung collapse and/or consolidation, and may predispose to infection.

Differential diagnosis

There is no problem in recognizing the initial event or in identifying those babies with recurrent major problems in coordinating their sucking and swallowing. The conditions listed in Table 29.29 should always be considered for the baby who has had a massive vomit, remembering that reflux can only be diagnosed if there is a high level of clinical suspicion backed up by X-ray and pH studies (pp. 548, 747).

Clinical findings

In babies with sucking–swallowing incoordination the features of their primary diagnosis will be present (Table 29.28). In addition, if such infants have chronic pooling of secretions in their upper airway they will be mucousy, with rattling, noisy respiration, often coupled with some mild respiratory distress owing to obstruction of the airway by secretions. Widespread conducted sounds are therefore often heard on chest auscultation.

After a massive regurgitation or vomit which triggers an episode of apnoea, cyanosis and bradycardia, but which has been promptly and efficiently dealt with (see below), many neonates show no abnormal physical signs 10–15 minutes later. In these babies, and those with more

Table 29.29 Causes of massive vomiting leading to aspiration pneumonia

Paralytic ileus in association with any severe disease, including RDS and sepsis[284]
Apnoeic attacks leading to hypoxia
Fits
Intestinal obstruction, including necrotizing enterocolitis
Infection including gastroenteritis
Overfeeding (p. 397)
Gastro-oesophageal reflux

chronic problems, the clinical features suggesting that inhalation pneumonia has actually occurred are the non-specific ones of respiratory distress (p. 495). In a neonate with pre-existing lung disease, respiratory function deteriorates. In both, crepitations and rhonchi may be heard on auscultation.

Investigation

In the baby who rapidly reverts to normal and shows no signs of respiratory compromise 15–30 minutes after the episode, it is still advisable to carry out a chest X-ray. A new area of consolidation, particularly in the right upper lobe, is very suggestive of inhalation, but more generalized and non-specific changes may occur. In either the chronic situation or following a single severe episode, if the baby has the signs of respiratory disease he should be investigated for infection (pp. 502, 1118). Measurement of the electrolytes, blood sugar and calcium is indicated in all babies, and may identify a cause of a convulsion.

Treatment

The vomiting episode

When the baby is found, his mouth, nose and pharynx should be quickly and effectively sucked out; usually this will be a blind procedure. If the infant has become cyanosed, oxygen should be given by mask. Most babies respond briskly at this stage, and no further treatment is required other than the evaluation outlined above.

If the baby does not respond promptly, and a physician is available, the ideal way of clearing the airway is to use a laryngoscope and aspirate inhaled material under direct vision. This should always be done if the attack is so severe that the baby remains apnoeic or intubation is required for resuscitation. If the baby remains apnoeic and bradycardic after suctioning and face-mask oxygen, and no one is available for instant intubation, resuscitation should be by bag and mask, even though this carries the theoretical hazard of dispersing inhaled material into the distal branches of the bronchial tree. If this is necessary it may still be worth sucking out the trachea under direct vision at any time in the next 10–15 minutes. If milk is obtained this is not only beneficial, but also confirms the diagnosis. If oxygen is administered care must be taken not to expose preterm babies to the risk of hyperoxaemia and ROP (p. 909).

General management of aspiration pneumonia

If the neonate develops signs suggesting aspiration pneumonia, all the intensive care appropriate to his needs should be given (pp. 502–508). Electrolyte imbalance, hypoglycaemia and acidaemia must be corrected, hypotension treated, and coagulation disturbances remedied.

Oxygen. Sufficient oxygen should be given to keep the PaO_2 in the normal range. If the aspiration has been severe, or complicates pre-existing lung disease in a small preterm baby, the episode may trigger apnoea or cause such severe pneumonitis that the baby will require IPPV, which should be managed as outlined on pages 559–577.

Physiotherapy. If there are copious secretions following inhalation, or if the chest X-ray shows an area of consolidation, then 4-hourly physiotherapy should be given to encourage drainage from the affected region. The baby should also be nursed in the position that optimizes drainage from the affected lobe.

Feeding. In most babies it is wise to stop oral feeds for 24–48 hours after an episode of aspiration/inhalation. In the preterm neonate recourse to i.v. feeding may be necessary. In the term baby, once tachypnoea has settled, oral feeding can be restarted unless there is some chronic problem, in which case a period of nasogastric feeds will be necessary.

Antibiotics. Until the cultures are negative it is impossible to be sure that the whole episode was not triggered by infection. As a consequence broad-spectrum antibiotic cover should be given, usually flucloxacillin and an aminoglycoside (p. 1136). Antibiotics should be continued for at least 5–7 days, or until the baby is clinically much improved if there are marked chest X-ray changes or the neonate requires IPPV, even if the cultures are negative.

Morbidity and mortality

This is completely dependent on the underlying pathology, as the lung disease following inhalation on its own is rarely, if ever, fatal. Babies with persistent failure to suck or swallow secretions after severe birth asphyxia, or in the presence of congenital neurological problems, must have a guarded prognosis on the basis of their underlying defects. Most cases with a structural defect do well with appropriate surgery, but there remains an appreciable mortality with laryngotracheo-oesophageal cleft (p. 773) or Pierre-Robin syndrome (p. 768). For the baby whose problems are due to immaturity the outlook is excellent, as it can be anticipated that the lung disease will respond to the therapy outlined, although some infants may develop CLD and have a prolonged convalescence.

MASSIVE PULMONARY HAEMORRHAGE

DEFINITION

This condition is better named haemorrhagic pulmonary oedema, and is a form of fulminant lung oedema with leakage of red cells and capillary filtrate into the lungs.[1035] It must be clearly differentiated from the common occurrence of a small amount of bloodstained material

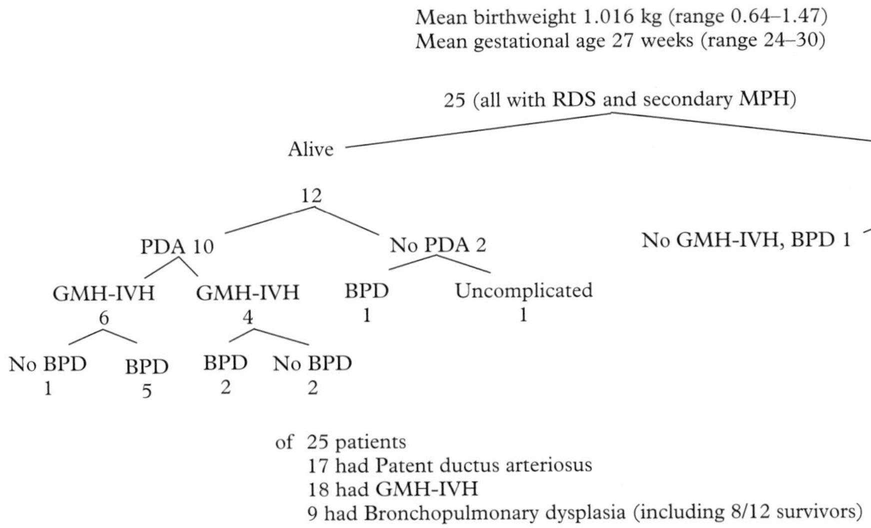

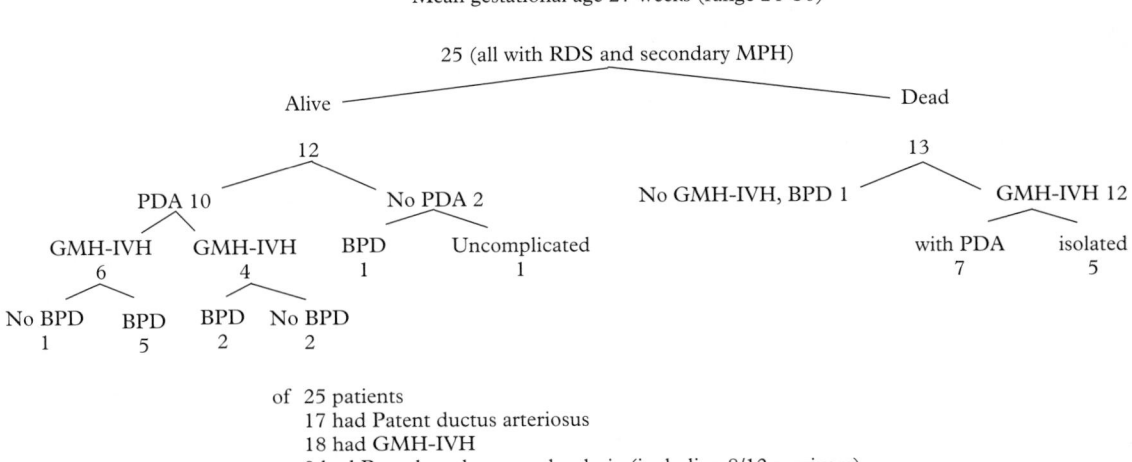

Fig. 29.66 Massive pulmonary haemorrhage, Cambridge Maternity Hospital, 1985–89.

Table 29.30 Causes of pulmonary oedema in the neonate. Reproduced with permission from Bland[107]

Increased pulmonary microvascular pressure	Reduced intravascular oncotic pressure	Reduced lymphatic drainage	Increased microvascular permeability
Heart failure Hypoxia Transfusions Intravenous fat Increased pulmonary blood flow Pulmonary hypoplasia	Prematurity Hydrops Fluid overload Hypoproteinaemia loss in gut loss from kidneys malnutrition	PIE Pulmonary fibrosis Raised CVP	Sepsis Endotoxaemia Emboli Oxygen toxicity

being periodically aspirated from the endotracheal tube of a ventilated baby; this is usually the result of trauma.

INCIDENCE

In the 1958 United Kingdom National Perinatal Mortality Survey[146] the prevalence of pulmonary haemorrhage was 0.93:1000, a figure similar to that seen in Oxford 10 years later[116] and to experience in Cambridge from 1985 to 1989 (Fig. 29.66), when the prevalence was 1.2:1000 live births. The lowest incidence of MPH reported was 0.1:1000 live births in the 1970 UK Perinatal Mortality Survey.[166] There has been a major change in the type of baby affected. In the earlier studies[146,314] it was primarily full-term babies, whereas now the disease occurs almost exclusively in babies weighing <1500 g who often have a patent ductus arteriosus[361] and have been treated with surfactant (p. 511).

AETIOLOGY

Massive pulmonary haemorrhage represents the extreme end of the spectrum of pulmonary oedema in the neonate. This has four main causes[107] (Table 29.30), which all increase fluid leak into the pulmonary interstitium and thus elevate pulmonary lymphatic flow. Although intra-alveolar fluid may appear at an early stage of interstitial oedema,[996] pulmonary oedema usually occurs as the antioedema systems become swamped, lung interstitial fluid rises, and fluid leaks into the alveoli because the alveolar epithelium has either been damaged or becomes leaky because of distension by the interstitial fluid.

Pulmonary oedema in the neonate seems to follow this general pattern. The first change is a rise in pulmonary capillary pressure, which causes an increase in interstitial fluid, which eventually leaks into the alveoli through holes in the epithelium initially only large enough to allow the passage of molecules such as albumin, but small enough to retain molecules such as IgG, IgM and fibrinogen and the majority of red cells.[8] As the changes become more marked, the holes in the endothelium and epithelium increase in size and larger molecules leak through. Adamson et al[7] and Cole et al[209] postulated that for massive pulmonary haemorrhage to develop, the holes must be so large as to allow capillary haemorrhage. In most cases the amount of blood lost is small and the haematocrit of the lung effluent is less than 10%.[209] The mechanisms listed in Table 29.30 and this final pathway to MPH are likely to be present in the clinical entities

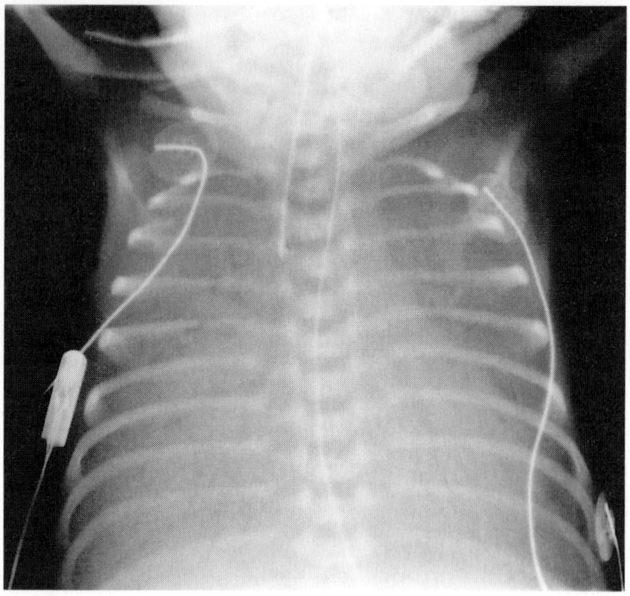

Fig. 29.67 Widespread homogeneous opacification of the lungs in a baby with massive pulmonary haemorrhage. Reproduced with permission from Greenough et al.[414]

which, in morbid anatomical studies,[300,926] correlate with the development of severe massive pulmonary haemorrhage. These include severe birth asphyxia, rhesus haemolytic disease with hydrops or near hydrops, left heart failure, congenital heart disease, sepsis, hypothermia,[709] fluid overload, oxygen toxicity and haemostatic failure.[314] They also apply in the situation which now has the highest incidence of MPH (Fig. 29.67), namely the neonate with severe RDS on IPPV in a high oxygen concentration and with heart failure secondary to a large pulmonary blood flow from a patent ductus arteriosus.[361] To this list must now be added the development of MPH as a complication of the use of exogenous surfactant replacement therapy, perhaps by increasing pulmonary blood flow as PaO_2 rises. Administration of the artificial surfactant Exosurf (p. 511) has been noted to increase the incidence of MPH.[670,1115] Results from 29 trials were examined in a meta-analysis to further explore the relationship of this treatment with pulmonary haemorrhage.[873] The study confirmed an association of MPH with synthetic, but not natural, surfactant use. The relative risk for MPH with artificial surfactant use was 2.44 ($P < 0.05$) compared with untreated controls. The incidence following use of Exosurf was 5–6%.[817] Surprisingly, despite clinical experience, PDA did not have an independent effect.

The role of coagulation disturbances in the aetiology of MPH is unclear. It is seen in babies with DIC, although this is rare, and it does not occur in thrombocytopenia, haemorrhagic disease of the newborn or haemophilia. Following the marked clinical deterioration with MPH it is not uncommon, however, for secondary DIC to develop.[209]

Another sequel of pulmonary haemorrhage is that the protein-rich fluid on the alveolar surface will inhibit surfactant function (p. 484), so that any pre-existing lung disease will deteriorate.

PATHOLOGY

The changes in the lungs are dependent on the stage of the illness reached by the time of death. In deaths before 48 hours of age and in stillbirths interstitial haemorrhage is common, but in deaths after 48 hours[300] and following surfactant administration[822] intra-alveolar bleeding dominates the clinical picture. The lungs are solid at postmortem and usually a deep reddish-purple colour. As the baby has usually received a high oxygen concentration before death, the lungs will be gasless and sink in water. Their pressure/volume characteristics will be those of low-compliance surfactant-less lungs (p. 488). Hyaline membranes will often be present, as MPH frequently complicates primary RDS. As in RDS, there will be necrosis and desquamation of the alveolar lining cells. In cases which come to autopsy more than 48 hours after the haemorrhage, and particularly if the neonate survives for several days on IPPV, usually in a high oxygen concentration and at high pressures, the changes merge into those seen in severe CLD (p. 612).

CLINICAL FEATURES

The two striking clinical features of MPH are a sudden deterioration and usually the simultaneous appearance of copious bloody secretions from the baby's airway – either up his endotracheal tube, or from his larynx and mouth if he is not already intubated.

The baby usually is hypotensive, pale and frequently limp and unresponsive, although term babies may occasionally be active and restless secondary to hypoxaemia, and 'fight' the ventilator. Occasionally collapse antedates the overt haemorrhage by an hour or two, and rarely the baby looks surprisingly well, despite the production of copious bloodstained pulmonary oedema.

Cardiac

As the condition is commonly secondary to heart failure, signs suggesting this may be present. A tachycardia greater than 160/min is not uncommon and the murmur of a PDA is frequently heard[361] (Fig. 29.66). Other signs of heart failure, including hepatosplenomegaly and a triple rhythm, can occur; peripheral oedema may indicate heart failure, hydrops, hypoalbuminaemia or fluid overload.

Hypotension is virtually always present, probably because of a combination of blood and fluid loss, heart failure and coexisting hypoxaemia and acidaemia.

Respiratory

Infants are dyspnoeic and cyanotic, and auscultation of the chest reveals widespread crepitations with some reduction in air entry.

DIFFERENTIAL DIAGNOSIS

Small amounts of blood coming up the endotracheal tube are usually due to trauma. A few babies may deteriorate clinically without apparent cause for an hour or two before the haemorrhage develops, but once copious bloodstained fluid appears from the airway the diagnosis is self-evident. The underlying cause, however, should be established if possible (Table 29.30), as this will influence subsequent treatment.

INVESTIGATIONS

Haematological

Although the haematocrit of the oedema fluid is usually ≤10%, considerable quantities of blood may be lost and the haemoglobin may fall to 10 g/dl or even lower. There are no specific white blood cell changes in MPH. Cole et al[209] found that coagulation disturbances were not a regular feature of their patients prior to the haemorrhage, but it is their and our experience that DIC is not uncommon afterwards.

Biochemical

Affected preterm babies usually have the same problems as those with severe RDS. In particular, hypoglycaemia, hypocalcaemia, hypoalbuminaemia and renal failure should be sought and remedied.

Chest X-ray

The chest X-ray in the baby who has had a large MPH shows a virtual 'white-out' (Fig. 29.67) with just an air bronchogram visible. As the condition improves on IPPV, the changes may clear or merge into those of CLD. Rarely, a lobar pattern of consolidation is found, suggesting that the haemorrhage has just occurred in part of the lung.

Bacteriology

The haemorrhage may be precipitated by sepsis. For this reason, an infection screen must always be taken immediately after the event. The infant's condition, however, will usually preclude lumbar puncture (p. 1123).

Blood gases

All components of arterial blood gas analysis deteriorate rapidly after the bleed. Hypoxia is severe, the $PaCO_2$ may increase to 10 kPa (75 mmHg) or more, and there is usually a marked metabolic acidosis with a base deficit of at least 10 mmol/l. The combined respiratory and metabolic acidaemia may result in a pH of 7.10 or less.

MONITORING

Monitoring in these babies is the same as that outlined under RDS (Chapter 21). The blood gases should be meticulously supervised in preterm babies susceptible to ROP. Clotting studies should be done daily until they normalize. A daily chest X-ray should be taken because of the high ventilator pressures that are frequently required, and the potential complications.

TREATMENT

Basic intensive care

This is identical to that described under RDS (pp. 502–508). Particular attention must be paid to maintaining the blood pressure with plasma and/or blood transfusion, progressing to inotropes as necessary (p. 504). The severe acidaemia should be corrected with intravenous base if IPPV and correction of the hypoxia and hypotension do not promptly return the pH and base deficit to an acceptable level. Underlying disorders must be treated. Heart failure due to anaemia in, for example, haemolytic disease should be treated by exchange transfusion with packed cells, aiming for a haemoglobin of 13–14 g/dl; asphyxial myocardial damage may need inotropic support (see below), and sepsis should be treated as outlined on pages 1126–1127.

Control of pulmonary oedema and heart failure

Fluid balance

There is often a conflict of interest between the fact that the baby is in congestive heart failure with pulmonary oedema, yet is hypotensive with low-volume pulses and poor peripheral perfusion. In general, however, fluid input should be restricted to 60–80 ml/kg/24 h, particularly if there is a coexisting patent ductus. The blood pressure can be sustained by judicious infusions of colloid or blood, and by the use of inotropes.

Diuretics

On the basis that these babies have left ventricular failure and pulmonary oedema, frusemide 1–1.5 mg/kg should be given as soon as possible after the bleed and repeated as necessary to treat fluid overload.

IPPV

All babies with MPH should be intubated and ventilated. They usually have severe lung disease, and peak inflating pressures above 30 cmH_2O may be necessary. For this reason (pp. 576–577) and, because mature babies in particular become very restless, pancuronium and sedation should be used routinely until the haemorrhage is controlled.

During IPPV a high PEEP (up to 6–7 cmH_2O) is employed, with initial settings for a preterm 'paralysed' baby of 50–60/min and an inspiration time of 0.4–0.5 s. Although in experimental studies this does not reduce the total lung water, it redistributes it back into the interstitial space, improving oxygenation and ventilation–perfusion balance.[705,824]

Surfactant

Paradoxically, although surfactant may precipitate MPH (p. 511) it is also therapeutically useful and, after stabilizing the baby on IPPV after the haemorrhage, a single dose of surfactant can improve oxygenation.[819]

Patent ductus arteriosus

PDA is common in preterm neonates who develop an MPH (see above); using prophylactic indomethacin may reduce both complications.[200] The first line of treatment is that outlined above for the pulmonary oedema and heart failure. While the baby is critically ill, acidaemic and bleeding, the use of indomethacin is contraindicated; 24–48 hours later, once the coagulopathy is controlled and the hypoxia and acid–base disorders corrected, the use of indomethacin should be reconsidered and surgical ligation may be necessary (p. 689).

Physiotherapy/suction

In the first few hours after the haemorrhage there may be copious bloody secretions and suction is required every 10–15 minutes in extreme cases, as there is a significant risk of the secretions clotting and blocking the airway or endotracheal tube. Physiotherapy, however, is not of proven value, and as these neonates are extremely fragile it should not be used as a routine in the early stages; adequate humidification should keep the secretions liquid enough to be sucked up the ETT.

Coagulopathy

In most cases the features of DIC are present. Transfusion of platelets, however, is rarely required, but infusions of fresh-frozen plasma are indicated and usually successful in promptly correcting the clotting deficiencies. After the first 24–48 hours, when the baby has become stable on IPPV, the acid–base disturbances have been corrected and the septicaemia (if present) treated, the coagulation problems usually remit and further factor replacement is not usually necessary.

Antibiotics

Sepsis is a recognized cause of MPH, and so antibiotics should be started after taking cultures. If the baby is already receiving antibiotics it is sensible to broaden the spectrum to cover infection by *Staphylococci* and *Pseudomonas* species.

Nutrition

This should be maintained as described under RDS (p. 506).

COMPLICATIONS

These babies are susceptible to all the major complications of respiratory failure. High-pressure ventilation predisposes them to airleaks and CLD is a common sequel (Fig. 29.66). At the time of their sudden collapse they are susceptible to neurological damage and GMH/IVH (p. 1257).

MORTALITY

For many years this was universally regarded as a fatal condition, but with modern intensive care at least 50% of babies can be expected to survive.[361,1083]

SEQUELAE

These are ill, low-birthweight babies, and they are subject to the same neurological and respiratory sequelae that occur in babies of the same gestation who have uncomplicated RDS (pp. 513–514).

ASPHYXIAL LUNG DISEASE

Many lung diseases may be the sequel of intrapartum asphyxia in the neonate, including surfactant-deficient RDS (p. 484), MAS (p. 538), PPHN (p. 527) and MPH (p. 552). Once these clear-cut clinical conditions have been excluded, intrapartum asphyxia affects the respiratory system in two ways: it may cause apnoea or irregular gasping respirations, or it may result in respiratory distress, which in its severe form produces a syndrome similar to 'adult' RDS (ARDS) or 'shock' lung.

APNOEA AND GASPING POST-ASPHYXIA

In the severely asphyxiated neonate respirations may be absent – prolonged terminal apnoea (p. 244) – or the only respiratory efforts may be large, juddering, gasping movements occurring 6–10 times per minute, occasionally interspersed with shallow irregular respirations. These respiratory patterns are all signs of severe asphyxia with concomitant neurological damage to the structures of the brain stem and above, which are responsible for the control of respiration. These babies require intubation and positive-pressure ventilation, and their management is that of neurological intensive care as outlined on pages 1242–1244.

POST-ASPHYXIAL LUNG DISEASE

Some babies who suffer intrapartum asphyxia remain tachypnoeic for 24–48 hours after delivery,[1067] and occasionally develop severe lung disease similar to adult RDS.[308] In some cases the syndrome is difficult to distinguish from TTN (p. 515), particularly the severe variant.[450] In the mildest cases, in whom tachypnoea lasts only for a few hours, the clinical features merge into minimal respiratory disease (p. 516), whereas in severe cases it merges into PPHN (p. 527).

Incidence

There are no figures available, but it is possible to estimate its frequency. Around 0.2–0.3% of liveborn babies are in terminal apnoea (Chapter 16); asphyxia with neurological features occurs in 0.6%.[650] In our experience, asphyxial lung disease occurs in a comparatively small proportion of the neonates drawn from these populations. In the series reported by Thibeault et al[1067] the incidence of the syndrome was approximately the same as that of MAS. These data suggest that about 1–2 babies per 1000 have asphyxia-induced neonatal respiratory distress.

Pathophysiology

The cause of post-asphyxial tachypnoea is multifactorial.

Aspiration

It is clear that intrauterine asphyxia can cause inhalation of amniotic fluid with (pp. 538, 546) or without meconium.[504] In the extreme form, non-meconium aspiration is seen at autopsy of stillbirths and early neonatal deaths following asphyxia.[1157] It is likely that lesser degrees of the same problem are present in neonates who survive milder degrees of asphyxia but who have, nevertheless, inhaled some amniotic debris and as a result become tachypnoeic.

Heart failure and pulmonary oedema

(Table 29.30)

Following birth asphyxia, cardiomegaly, heart failure and pulmonary oedema may occur as a result of asphyxial damage to the myocardium.[140,145,1139] In the absence of myocardial damage, severe metabolic acidaemia can also depress myocardial contractility, again leading to heart failure, pulmonary oedema and tachypnoea.[79,1146]

Asphyxia damages the pulmonary blood vessels, making them leaky, and this, plus the pulmonary oedema secondary to heart failure, may compromise surfactant function (p. 484). If the leak of protein-rich fluid on to the alveoli becomes large enough, ARDS will develop, with epithelial degeneration, surfactant inhibition, interstitital cellular infiltration, pulmonary hypertension and eventually alveolar fibrosis.[927] These mechanisms are likely to explain the severe lung disease seen occurring after asphyxia in full-term neonates.[308]

Metabolic acidaemia

Labour is an asphyxiating process and most babies will have a comparatively low pH at and after delivery[71,241] (pp. 241–242). Metabolic acidaemia stimulates hyperventilation.[539] In the neonate the chemoreceptors are sensitive to pH,[790,1131] and it would appear that an increase in respiration is more likely to be due to stimulation of peripheral chemoreceptors rather than medullary centres.[143]

Anaemia

Asphyxia caused by cord occlusion may trap blood in the placenta, causing fetal anaemia,[972,1114] and acute fetal haemorrhage from ruptured vasa praevia or following a large fetomaternal haemorrhage will result in the birth of a baby who is anaemic, shocked and acidotic.[879] Chronic fetal anaemia due to rhesus disease or fetomaternal haemorrhage also produces babies with acidaemia, anaemia and tachypnoea.[843] Anaemia from any cause predisposes to tachypnoea. Surviving preterm neonates who become anaemic around the second month are breathless as a manifestation of decreased oxygen delivery to the tissues,[1144] and in the few hours after birth similar mechanisms of tachypnoea probably apply. The lowered buffering capacity of blood with a low haemoglobin will also potentiate the effect of metabolic acidaemia on respiration (see above).

CNS effects

Damage to the CNS may stimulate tachypnoea in two ways. The neural control of respiration may be damaged such that it causes hyperventilation. This is well recognized in older patients,[643] but has not been reported in neonates. However, we have seen neurologically damaged babies who hyperventilate to $PaCO_2$ levels of 2.5–3.0 kPa (19–23 mmHg). These babies are usually several days old, but whether a similar mechanism can cause tachypnoea in the first 6–12 hours of life is unknown.

The second mechanism is the phenomenon of neurogenic pulmonary oedema, which may follow any rise in intracranial pressure or brain injury. It is primarily due to an increased pulmonary vascular permeability, leading to interstitial pulmonary oedema, hypoxia and tachypnoea.[211,718] The mechanism is probably active in the newborn, and explains, for example, the sudden deterioration in respiratory function following a GMH/IVH, but may also be of importance in babies with HIE or subdural haemorrhage following birth asphyxia.

Clinical features

This is primarily a disease of term babies who, within the first hour or two, usually present with tachypnoea of 100/min or more rather than with retraction and grunting, although in some babies the clinical picture may be dominated by the neurological sequelae of asphyxia, and apnoea may occur.[1067] The baby may be tachycardic and hypotensive with a triple rhythm, or have the systolic murmurs of tricuspid or mitral incompetence;[140,326] if there has been severe myocardial damage other signs of heart failure, crepitations and hepatomegaly may be found.[148] Other clinical findings are usually unremarkable unless there is coexisting brain or renal damage.

Irrespective of the aetiology, the cardiorespiratory features of the syndrome (as opposed to the neurological ones) usually settle in 24 hours, and virtually always within 48 hours of delivery.

Differential diagnosis

This is a diagnosis of exclusion in the neonate who has suffered intrapartum asphyxia. The chest X-ray excludes complications such as pneumothorax, and does not show the features of 'wet lung' seen in transient tachypnoea; other features differentiating post-asphyxial tachypnoea from TTN are given in Table 29.31; problems such as meconium aspiration, RDS and pulmonary haemorrhage are usually easy to exclude on the basis of the history and chest X-ray (Table 29.13). Excluding sepsis, as always, is important, as group B streptococcal infection may masquerade as asphyxia.[832] Evidence of myocardial damage should be sought by checking the chest X-ray and ECG; if it is present, much greater care must be taken regarding the use of bolus infusions.

Table 29.31 Differentiating asphyxial lung disease from transient tachypnoea

	Asphyxial lung disease	Transient tachypnoea
Signs of heart failure	±	–
Murmurs	±	–
Anaemia present	±	–
Neurological symptoms	±	–
History of birth asphyxia	++	±
Marked early metabolic acidaemia	++	±
'Wet lung' on chest X-ray	–	++

++ always present; ±, may be present; –, absent.

Investigation

The routine investigations of a neonate with respiratory distress should be carried out (pp. 497–501). The blood gases should be measured on an arterial sample; the usual picture is one of mild hypoxaemia which normalizes in 30–40% oxygen. Respiration is stimulated by the metabolic acidaemia (base deficit >20 mmol/l, with a corresponding low pH), damage to the CNS or by lung receptors stimulated by pulmonary oedema; the $PaCO_2$ is usually <4 kPa (30 mmHg). Severe hypoxaemia or the presence of a $PaCO_2$ above 5.5–6.0 kPa (42–45 mmHg) should suggest an alternative diagnosis.

Hypoglycaemia is common after asphyxia, as is DIC (p. 1243); both should be remedied promptly if found.

A chest X-ray is essential. In most cases it will be normal. If the tachypnoea is secondary to myocardial involvement and pulmonary oedema, there will be cardiomegaly[145] and mild pulmonary haziness. Severe changes suggest adult RDS.[308]

The ECG is also usually unremarkable, but it may show changes of ST-segment depression and T-wave inversion if there is severe asphyxia;[148,962] in lesser degrees of asphyxia there may only be slight flattening of the T wave.[540] The level of the myocardial isoenzyme creatine kinase may be raised.[865]

Treatment

Monitoring

An umbilical artery catheter is the preferred site for monitoring blood gases and blood pressure, as often the baby is peripherally shut down, making clinical assessment of oxygenation impossible and arterial puncture difficult; frequent samples may be needed until the pH returns to normal.

Blood gases

The baby should receive sufficient warmed humidified headbox oxygen to keep his PaO_2 above 8 kPa (60 mmHg); this does not usually require more than 30–40% oxygen and can be reduced within 24–48 hours. In a small number of patients, more severe but short-lived disease is present, for which IPPV is required.[1067] In those with ARDS, prolonged high-pressure ventilation similar to that used for neonatal RDS (pp. 563–567) may be necessary.[308]

Metabolic acidaemia

Term neonates are capable of surviving profound acidaemia.[355] Furthermore, the data of Daniel et al,[241] Sykes et al[1051] and Spencer et al[1012] suggest that they are capable of recovering spontaneously and quickly from pH levels of 7.10–7.15 and base deficits of >15 mmol/l. For this reason, expectant treatment of uncomplicated metabolic acidaemia immediately after delivery is justified if the pH is above 7.10, checking an arterial gas 30–60 minutes later to ensure that spontaneous correction is taking place. If the pH is below this value, or the infant has heart failure attributed to acidaemia, then the pH should be corrected to 7.30–7.40 using the standard formula (p. 504).

THAM has the theoretical advantage of rapidly correcting CSF pH,[916] but can cause apnoea in preterm neonates with RDS;[902] if used in term infants (infusion rate 0.5 mmol/kg/min or less[69]) careful monitoring must be undertaken.

Hypotension and heart failure

These are two of the most serious complications of severe asphyxia as they are associated with secondary ischaemic injury to the CNS, myocardium (endocardial ischaemia), kidneys (renal failure) and intestine (NEC). They must therefore be corrected urgently. The general approach to hypotension outlined on page 504 should be followed, taking great care with fluid balance if the myocardium is compromised. In general, the fluid intake should be restricted to 40 ml/kg/24 h until it is clear that the brain, myocardium and kidneys have not been damaged by asphyxia. If heart failure is present, frusemide should be given. IPPV with PEEP helps to control pulmonary oedema.

If hypovolaemia is a problem, in the absence of myocardial damage and heart failure, usually all that is required is a blood transfusion (or a volume infusion if the PCV is >45%), giving 15–20 ml/kg.

Anaemia

A haemoglobin <13 g/dl (PCV <40%) is an indication for transfusion in asphyxial lung disease, as in any dyspnoeic neonate.[906,1038] If there is coexisting myocardial asphyxial injury the transfusion should be given slowly and carefully under diuretic and/or inotrope support. In such a situation, if the haemoglobin level is <8–9 g/dl, the safest way of increasing it is with a single-volume exchange transfusion using packed red blood cells.

Hypoxic–ischaemic encephalopathy

The management of this is outlined in detail on pages 1242–1244; if severe anoxic brain damage has occurred its management will dominate the care of the dyspnoeic asphyxiated baby. If there is severe HIE it is essential to prevent the blood gas abnormalities (p. 1242).

Antibiotics

For the usual reasons (p. 507), after collecting the appropriate samples for culture, including blood, broad-spectrum antibiotics, usually with penicillin plus an aminoglycoside (p. 1129), should be administered.

Prognosis

The outlook is governed by the severity of the CNS injury. As far as the lung disease is concerned, provided massive pulmonary haemorrhage does not develop, the response to correction of the blood gases, a short period of IPPV and inotrope support is usually excellent. The typical baby is usually breathing room air and no longer requires any form of cardiorespiratory support by 48 hours of age, and often earlier.[1067] Even in those with adult-type RDS, survival is the rule.[308]

PLEURAL EFFUSIONS

ISOLATED

These are uncommon in the neonatal period. The incidence of primary fetal hydrothorax is estimated at one case per 15 000 pregnancies.[674]

Aetiology

Isolated effusions are usually a chylothorax (p. 558), but in one series[673] congenital heart disease was the commonest association. Approximately 9% of infants with MAS have pleural effusions.[1189] Rarer associations are TTN (p. 515), PPHN,[796] heart failure, congenital myotonic dystrophy[234] and trauma. Pleural effusions diagnosed antenatally are frequently associated with chromosomal or congenital abnormalities.[795] Intrauterine (CMV, toxoplasmosis, rubella), perinatal (GBS) and postnatal (*Staphylococcus*) infections can all result in pleural effusions.

Clinical signs

Infants with large effusions present at birth with failure to establish adequate respiration. They are frequently difficult to resuscitate, as antenatally the pleural effusion may have prevented normal lung growth.[163] On examination the trachea and mediastinum will be shifted to the contralateral side and the ipsilateral lung dull to percussion, with absent breath sounds. Small effusions may be asymptomatic and diagnosed incidentally on a chest radiogaph.

Diagnosis

Antenatally pleural effusions are detected by ultrasonography and should be suspected in fetuses whose mothers have polyhydramnios.[848] Postnatally, on the chest radiograph there may be a ‘whiteout’ on the affected side (Fig. 29.68), but if the effusion is small it is important to

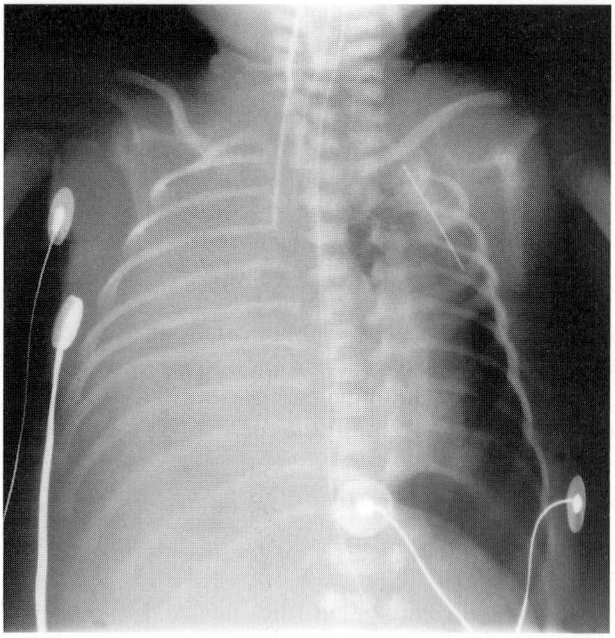

Fig. 29.68 Unilateral pleural effusion. Reproduced with permission from Greenough et al.[414]

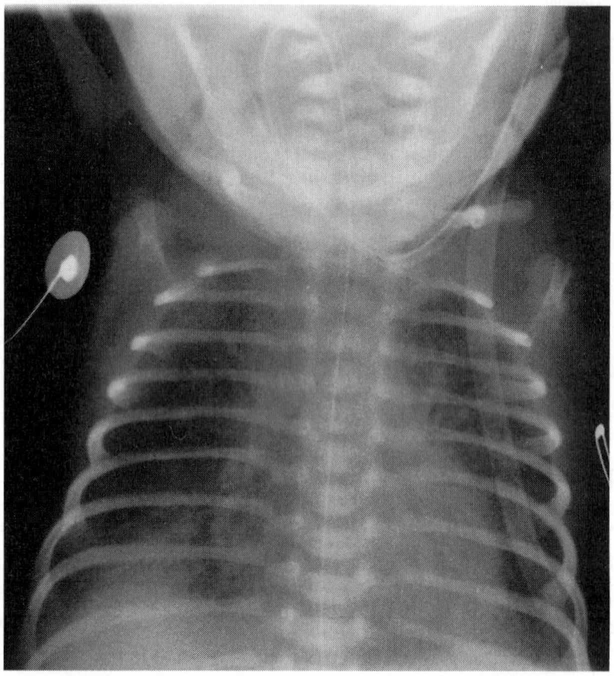

Fig. 29.69 Small pleural effusion. CXR in erect position: note obliteration of the right hemidiaphragm. Reproduced with permission from Greenough et al.[414]

remember that fluid will collect in the most dependent parts of the chest, around the lateral chest wall or the diaphragm (Figs 29.69, 29.70).

Differential diagnosis

At birth the presentation of a large effusion is similar to that of congenital diaphragmatic hernia (pp. 655–656),

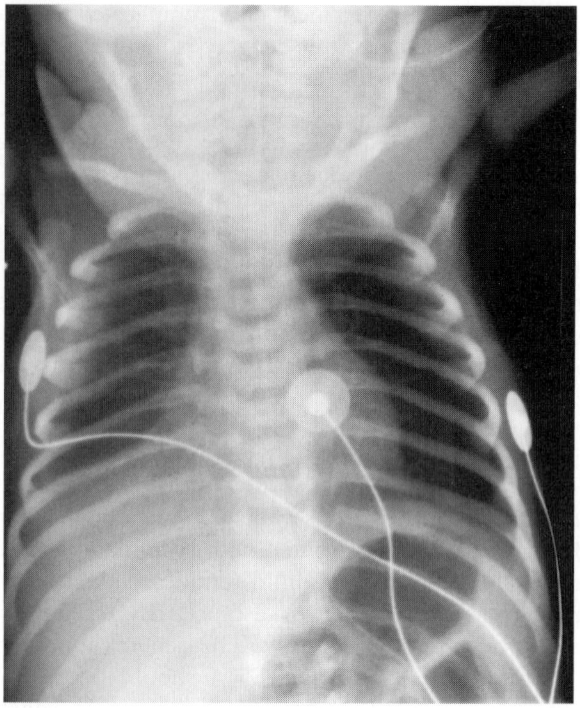

Fig. 29.70 Small pleural effusion. Supine X-ray showing a rim of fluid. Reproduced with permission from Greenough et al.[414]

but there are no bowel sounds in the chest. The chest X-ray appearance may be confused with an eventration or atelectasis.

Treatment

Antenatally pleural effusions are drained either intermittently by thoracocentesis[839] or continuously by a thoracoamniotic shunt.[115] At birth, infants with large pleural effusions require active resuscitation by intubation and positive pressure ventilation.[848] Thoracocentesis may also be required to achieve effective ventilation, and this may also be necessary later in the postnatal period. Aspirated fluid should always be sent for cytology to determine the lymphocyte count, and for biochemical and microbiological analysis.

Prognosis

Antenatally diagnosed pleural effusions, particularly if present prior to 32 weeks' gestation, carry a mortality as high as 55%.[444] Postnatally, effusions persisting for more than 3 days increase the risk of chronic oxygen dependency.[673]

CHYLOTHORAX

Incidence

One in 10 000 deliveries and one in 2000 neonatal admissions have a chylothorax.[1109]

Aetiology

Chylothorax may occur spontaneously or be associated with lymphoedema due to congenitally abnormal lymph vessels in conditions such as Turner syndrome or congenital lymphoedema. A congenital abnormality in the lymphatic system at the level of the thoracic duct below or above the fifth thoracic vertebra leads to a right- or left-sided chylothorax.[1109] It can be associated with foregut malformations and extralobar sequestration. Rarely, trauma to the thoracic duct at delivery by hyperexpansion of the spinal column in association with increased venous pressure during birth results in a chylothorax, but more commonly it is a complication of certain types of cardiac surgery (repair of coarctation of the aorta or ligation of a patent ductus arteriosus) or repair of a congenital posterolateral diaphragmatic hernia.[736] Another iatrogenic cause is superior vena caval obstruction in patients who have had venous catheterization for TPN.[22]

Clinical signs

Unusually chylothoraces result in hydrops, owing to impairment of venous return by cardiac and vena caval compression and/or loss of protein into the pleural space. In 50% of cases chylothoraces present in the first week, with symptoms as described under isolated pleural effusion. Chronic chylothorax may be associated with hypovolaemia, hypoalbuminaemia, hyponatraemia and weight loss. Such patients are immunocompromised owing to loss of lymphocytes and humoral antibodies.

Diagnosis

In an unfed infant the fluid obtained at thoracocentesis is clear, yellow, and contains large numbers of lymphocytes (20–50 per high-power field). Once the infant is milkfed the fluid will become chylous, clearing once an MCT formula is introduced.

Treatment

Chylothoraces may need to be drained antenatally (see above). Postnatally many cases respond to a single thoracocentesis, as this results in lung expansion tamponading the defect and preventing further pleural fluid formation. If the fluid reaccumulates, drainage is required and feeding with a milk containing fat only in the form of MCT. Pregestemil or Pepti junior can be tried, but a semielemental milk may be required and should be continued for at least 2 weeks after the effusion has disappeared.[131,471,867] Rarely in non-responsive cases total parenteral nutrition should be used. Pleural abrasion, ligation of the thoracic duct and pleurodesis are possible options for those chylothoraces that fail to respond to medical management.[25,867]

Prognosis

This condition usually resolves, but the mortality rate has been suggested to be as high as 60% for bilateral chylothoraces.[156] Our own experience is, however, more optimistic, with the majority surviving.

HAEMOTHORAX

Aetiology

Trauma, with damage to the arteries alongside the ribs from misplacement of a chest drain to drain a pneumothorax, rather than at thoracic surgery, is the commonest cause of a neonatal haemothorax. Rare causes include clotting abnormalities,[398] penetration of the fetal thorax at amniocentesis,[5] spontaneous rupture of a PDA, and arteriovenous malformations.

Diagnosis

The chest X-ray will demonstrate a whiteout, and a radioisotope lung scan can identify an underlying arteriovenous fistula.

Treatment

Resuscitation by urgent transfusion of blood and clotting factors may be required. Surgical intervention should be considered if a large blood vessel has been traumatized.

MANAGEMENT OF NEONATAL RESPIRATORY FAILURE

In recent years neonatologists have become confident in the use of ventilators. To prevent the sudden episodes of deterioration in VLBW neonates that often precede the appearance of a large GMH/IVH, we take control of the baby's vital functions from the moment of birth. As a result, IPPV is often started early in neonates with respiratory disease, and even from birth in very immature babies, regardless of their respiratory status. Some neonatologists,[533] however, advocate the so-called 'minitouch' technique, which incorporates prophylactic treatment with nasal CPAP and minimal handling.

OXYGEN THERAPY

Supplementary oxygen therapy

In mild-to-moderate respiratory disease all that is usually required to keep the baby's PaO_2 at 8–12 kPa (60–90 mmHg) (p. 503) is the administration of warmed humidified oxygen. Additional support by CPAP or IPPV is only indicated if a satisfactory PaO_2 cannot be achieved in 60–80% oxygen in a headbox, or at lower inspired oxygen concentrations if there are other features of respiratory failure (p. 563).

To avoid sudden changes in the inspired oxygen concentration, the oxygen should be given into a perspex box placed over the baby's head and shoulders (headbox). The concentration should be measured by an oxygen analyser placed near the baby's mouth. This form of therapy is frequently sufficient for preterm babies more than 30 weeks' gestation with RDS, all babies with minimal respiratory disease (p. 516), and most with TTN (p. 515). The occasional mature baby who develops RDS and most with MAS can also be managed with headbox oxygen, even though they may require concentrations of up to 80% for 72 hours or more, provided they do not develop other signs of respiratory failure. Headbox oxygen is often required for a prolonged period in low-birthweight infants who have required IPPV, and whose clinical features merge imperceptibly into those of CLD (p. 614).

Nasal oxygen

In babies requiring prolonged oxygen therapy for chronic lung disease, the administration of oxygen by nasal cannula allows the baby to be free from the incubator, to be picked up and cuddled, taken for walks, and bottle- or breast-fed. It is difficult to assess the oxygen concentration administered to such babies, but the data in Figure 29.71[1107] enable an approximation to be made.

Percutaneous oxygen

Oxygen can be absorbed through the thin skin of VLBW babies.[159] The average rise in PaO_2 when the babies were transferred from air to 95% oxygen was 1.2 kPa (9 mmHg).

Oxygen toxicity

Oxygen is toxic to tissues because it forms free radicals such as superoxide (O_2^-) and hydroxyl (OH^-).[574,1172]

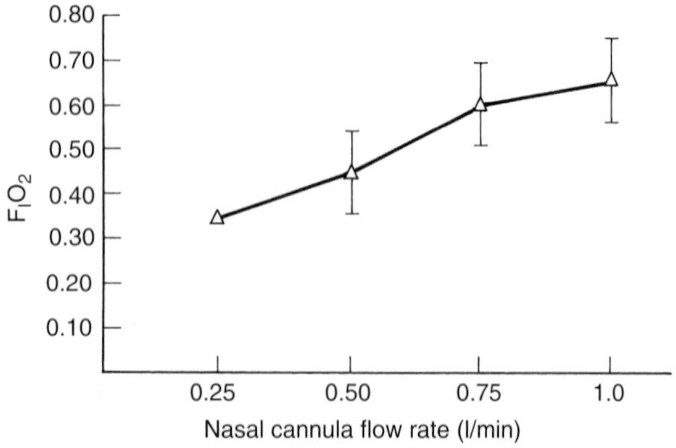

Fig. 29.71 Gas flow and oxygen concentration with nasal prong. Reproduced with permission from Vain et al.[1107]

The neonate is exposed to complex physiological and pharmacological stresses from these agents.[944,994]

The effects of oxygen on the lung are complex. If adults are exposed to even a few hours of pure oxygen they develop a tracheitis and reduced tracheal mucus velocity.[939] After about 16–24 hours they experience chest discomfort and cough. Dyspnoea develops after a further 24–48 hours.[531] During the first 24 hours there is a significant alveolar–capillary leak of protein.[250] If pure oxygen exposure is continued for 3–4 days, by IPPV if necessary, adult animals develop a fatal lung disease with oedematous alveolar walls, interstitial haemorrhage, atelectasis[192] and type II cell hyperplasia.[257] Surfactant is depleted in the early stages of oxygen exposure, with a reduction in both DPPC and PG,[584] and the levels continue to fall after the animal is removed from 100% oxygen.[255,501] In animals this loss can be prevented by treatment with vitamin E.[1141] Another deleterious effect of breathing pure oxygen is that all the nitrogen is washed out of the alveoli; as oxygen is much more rapidly taken up by pulmonary capillary blood than is nitrogen, this predisposes to atelectasis. Finally, pulmonary alveolar macrophage function is significantly reduced in animals by exposure to more than 80% oxygen for at least 3 days.[974]

Exposure of the neonatal lung to high F_IO_2 in the presence of lung disease also causes damage, probably because the oxygen free radicals interact with lung cell lipids. Neonates, however, seem to be more resistant to pulmonary oxygen toxicity than adults.[192] This resistance is dependent on the presence in the tissues of antioxidant enzymes such as superoxide dismutase, catalase and glutathione peroxidase, and an interaction with other components of neonatal intensive care, such as the use of intralipid, which may be protective.[1005] In the lungs of term babies the cells, including type II pneumocytes, are able rapidly to switch on antioxidant enzymes after birth,[342,570] an effect that may be stimulated by EGF[863] but this is less efficient in the preterm lung.[340,571,675]

The level of antioxidant enzymes and the resistance of the lung to hyperoxia are increased at term by prenatal maternal and postnatal treatment with dexamethasone.[246,339] This effect is less clear-cut in preterm animals, in whom the postnatal increase in enzymes and oxygen resistance may be absent.[571,1004] The effect of prenatal TRH varies between species and it may even decrease antioxidant levels,[184,919] but postnatally the levels of antioxidant enzymes do rise with improved survival[183,1138] in treated animals.

As might be anticipated, given the protective effect of drugs that induce surfactant, the administration of surfactant itself protects against oxygen toxicity.[513,845]

Although 100% oxygen clearly damages the lungs, the danger of lower oxygen concentrations to the human neonate is much less clear, as relevant data are difficult to find. In adult humans oxygen concentrations less than

60% rarely do harm, and exposure to between 50 and 90% results in limited damage.[597,786] In mature rabbits, exposure to 60% oxygen for 3 weeks does cause alveolar interstitial oedema, but increases surfactant production.[502] Rats in 60% oxygen for 2 weeks have small lungs with parenchymal thickening.[463] In the human neonate it should be remembered that it is only since positive pressure ventilation with 80–90% oxygen was used that changes attributed to oxygen toxicity have been described,[800] but studies in neonatal baboons suggest that exposure to a high oxygen concentration, even without IPPV, is damaging.[255]

Administration of 100% oxygen to babies is never justified, as with large shunts (p. 490) the increase in PaO_2 achieved by increasing from 90 to 100% oxygen is trivial and not worth the risks of both oxygen toxicity to the lung and the atelectasis that results from nitrogen washout. Several days in oxygen concentrations of 60–70% may cause some lung damage,[58] and is associated with antisurfactant and antimacrophage effects, but hypoxaemia must be avoided and this takes priority.

ASSISTED VENTILATION IN THE NEWBORN

CONTINUOUS POSITIVE AIRWAY PRESSURE

CPAP is a positive distending pressure, not usually exceeding 10 cmH_2O, applied continuously. The aim is to hold the alveoli and airways open and prevent them collapsing during expiration. The major benefit of CPAP is that it stabilizes the rib cage, reduces chest wall distortion during inspiration, and consequently increases the efficiency of the diaphragm.[446,966] It regularizes the respiratory rate – which usually falls – by stimulation of the Hering–Breuer reflex, and causes an increase in inspiratory time and tidal volume. There is an increase in FRC in proportion to the level of applied pressure; some alveoli will be overdistended, resulting in a fall in dynamic compliance.[756,895,1197] Administering CPAP, either in the larynx or in the nose, may increase the work of breathing if a small-diameter tube is used, as a result of the effort required to overcome the resistance of the tube.[384,648]

Indications

When it was first introduced, CPAP was applied to babies requiring 50–60% oxygen to keep their PaO_2 >8 kPa (60 mmHg). With increased familiarity the technique was used earlier in babies with RDS, often when they needed no more than 35–40% oxygen to maintain an acceptable PaO_2. Used in this way it improved blood gases and seemed to cause more rapid recovery.[17,68,118,286,430] In early randomized controlled trials, however, the benefits of CPAP seemed to be small[904] and problems were experienced. Babies over 2.0–2.5 kg birthweight become restless when the tube or face mask is applied, and as a result suffer hypoxia. Smaller babies tolerate the technique well, but in those below 1.20–1.50 kg intensive monitoring is required, so that such infants can be intubated and ventilated before critical respiratory failure results in collapse. Early CPAP has been used in some centres[38,533,554] and has been associated with a reduction in the requirement for mechanical ventilation and in its complications. The applicability of these results to other populations, particularly those with more severe disease, has been questioned[908] and the only prospective trials of CPAP in babies with relatively mild lung disease suggest that treated babies do less well than controls.[464,472]

Other uses

CPAP is useful to wean neonates from the ventilator (p. 580), although it may not reduce the need for reintubation.[30,170] It is helpful in the management of infants with recurrent apnoeic attacks (Chapter 29, Part 4), especially those who have chronic pulmonary insufficiency (p. 622). It is also sometimes useful in upper airways obstruction due to Pierre-Robin syndrome, congenital laryngeal stridor, or after extubation, when nasopharyngeal CPAP may be preferable, with the tip of the nasal cannula passing through the posterior choanae into the upper pharynx.[476]

Techniques of CPAP

CPAP was initially given through an endotracheal tube,[430] but in an attempt to avoid the hazards of intubation many other devices have been used, including Gregory's original headbox, face chambers and negative-pressure chambers. These devices have mostly been abandoned, and CPAP is now usually given by face mask or nasal prongs, the latter being preferable.

Nasal prongs

This is the simplest technique to use. CPAP is delivered to the baby through either a pair of tubes inserted into both nostrils, or a single tube into one nostril.[118] A prong, cut down from a soft, 3.0-mm, blue-line Portex endotracheal tube is inserted 1 cm into one nostril and connected to a lightweight T-piece circuit attached to a standard neonatal ventilator in CPAP mode. In this way the gas mixing, pressure measuring and humidification facilities of the ventilator circuit can be used. The tube is kept in place by a soft cord tied around it and fastened to both cheeks by lightweight sticky tape (Fig. 29.72). This allows easy access to the baby's head and mouth, and still enables him to be moved easily. The disadvantage is that the nostrils can occasionally become inflamed or even eroded from the pressure of the prong. Nasal CPAP can

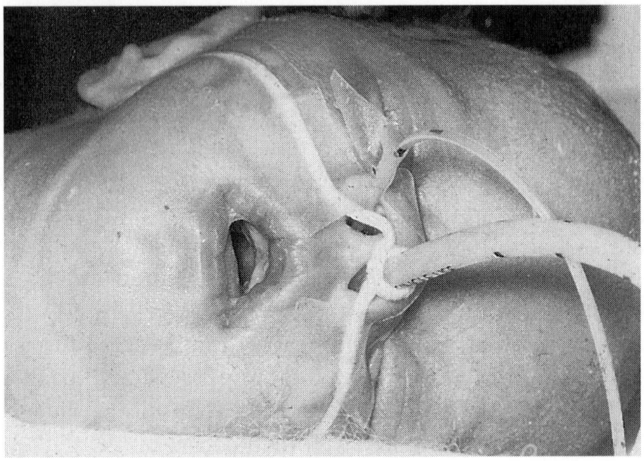

Fig. 29.72 Immobilization of endotracheal tube or single nasal prong.

effectively apply pressure to the airways, although some of the gas flow is lost through the mouth and the other nostril.[615]

An alternative device described by Benveniste et al[84] applies a jet of gas near to the exit of the curved attachment for the head prong in a way that mimics the actions of an expiratory valve, and thus applies CPAP at pressures of 3–22 cmH_2O at gas flows of 10–24 l/min. This device is widely used in the Scandinavian studies of CPAP in RDS.[533,554]

Face mask[17]

Although this was popular because it is easy to apply and avoids all the problems of nasal or endotracheal tubes, face mask CPAP has a number of disadvantages. The mask must be applied firmly to prevent gas leaks and maintain the pressure, and this can distort the baby's face. The apparatus holding the mask in place is strapped tightly around the back of the head, distorting its shape, causing pressure necrosis and even GMH/IVH or cerebellar haemorrhage.[820] It is difficult to use a nasogastric tube with face mask CPAP because this breaks the seal, yet without this tube the stomach cannot be easily aspirated and gaseous abdominal distension results. The presence of the mask also makes it difficult to attend to the baby's mouth and nose. The use of a face mask is the least successful of the techniques for CPAP, and is associated with the highest complication rate.[429]

CPAP settings

Various techniques[1054] have been described for ascertaining the optimal CPAP pressure, but are not helpful in clinical practice. In acute respiratory failure nasal CPAP is usually started at a pressure of 5 cmH_2O, at a gas flow of 5–10 l/min, depending on the size of the infant, and using the F_IO_2 that the neonate was breathing beforehand. The CPAP and F_IO_2 can then be adjusted on the basis of blood gas analysis. If the gases do not improve, it may be worth increasing the CPAP to 8–10 cmH_2O, although with nasal devices this may not be possible because of a leak through the mouth. If CPAP at 5–7 cmH_2O and 50–60% oxygen does not improve the blood gases, it is safer to resort to intubation and IPPV.

Hazards of CPAP

The most common complication is traumatic injuries to the nose and face from the prong or mask (p. 932). Although these can be minimized by good nursing technique, they are not completely avoidable. More serious complications are pneumothorax and GMH/IVH. The use of CPAP increases the risk of pneumothorax two- to threefold in babies with respiratory disease.[1198] For this reason CPAP should never be used in units without the facilities for both rapid recognition and drainage of a tension pneumothorax and the subsequent use of IPPV. The pneumothorax may precipitate a GMH/IVH (p. 1256), and the tight head bandages used to hold the face masks in place may cause intracerebellar haemorrhage.[820]

Management of the baby on CPAP

The monitoring necessary for a baby on CPAP in the acute phase of the disease is identical to that required for a baby on a ventilator (Chapter 21). There is a risk, with both prong and face mask CPAP, of gas distending the upper gastrointestinal tract. To minimize this, an open-ended nasogastric tube must always be in situ. In the acute period of a baby's illness enteral feeds should be withheld because of the risk of aspiration.

Weaning off CPAP

This is identical to the CPAP phase of weaning from IPPV (p. 580).

Continuous negative expanding pressure

This is an alternative way of providing distending pressure, in which the infant's body is placed in a negative pressure box from which his head protrudes and CNEP in the range –4 to –10 cmH_2O is applied.[941] In patients already ventilated, the peak and positive end-expiratory pressures are reduced by the level of negative pressure applied. To remove the infant from the chamber it is preferable to reduce the pressure over 15 minutes to prevent a sudden reduction in lung volume.

Early studies[818] demonstrated that CNEP was associated with improvements in oxygenation, the best results being experienced – not surprisingly – in infants with severe RDS. Improvements in blood gases have also been noted when CNEP is used in CLD.[941] In addition, respiratory rate decreases and, in infants with stiff lungs, compliance improves on CNEP.[358] Early attempts at CNEP were poorly tolerated, particularly in ELBW infants, because of difficulties in securing the infant and hypothermia. These problems have been overcome by newly designed neck seals[941] and providing a circulation of warm air. CNEP can, however, overdistend the lung and impair lung function in infants with CLD.

INTERMITTENT POSITIVE PRESSURE VENTILATION

Indications

It is now common practice to intubate and ventilate as an elective procedure in the early stages of most forms of severe neonatal respiratory disease. There are, however, only two absolute indications for starting IPPV; these are:

- a sudden collapse, with apnoea, bradycardia and failure to establish satisfactory ventilation after a short period of bag-and-mask ventilation;
- failure to establish adequate spontaneous ventilation in the labour ward after prompt and active resuscitation (pp. 259–260). The importance of this in the preterm baby at risk from RDS is outlined on page 493.

The relative indications for intubation and IPPV apply to babies who are breathing spontaneously, but are clinically, or on the basis of blood gas results, showing signs of impending respiratory failure. These indications vary with the gestational and postnatal age of the baby, the nature of the underlying disease, and whether the major feature of the respiratory failure is carbon dioxide retention, hypoxaemia or recurrent apnoeic spells. Most babies in impending respiratory failure fall into one of three clearly separate groups which require separate plans of action.

1. Very low-birthweight neonates <28 weeks' gestation and <1.00 kg. These babies are ventilated from the time of resuscitation in the labour ward (p. 255). This also applies to many babies between 28 and 32 weeks' gestation weighing 1.0–1.5 kg. However, a small number of these infants establish adequate regular respiration after birth, yet nevertheless develop signs of RDS. To prevent sudden collapse with its attendant complications (p. 579), and to give surfactant (p. 508), these babies should be ventilated once they need more than 35–40% oxygen to keep the PaO_2 >7–8 kPa (52–60 mmHg) and have a $PaCO_2$ >6–6.5 kPa (45–50 mmHg). The more of these criteria that are present, the sooner after birth they are met, or the more rapidly the neonate is deteriorating towards them, the sooner he should be intubated and ventilated.

2. Babies 1.50–2.25 kg at 32–35 weeks' gestation, usually with RDS. If these babies are deteriorating within the first 12–24 hours and are needing more than 40–60% oxygen they should be intubated and ventilated. Nasal CPAP may be sufficient support at 24–36 hours for infants whose $PaCO_2$ exceeds 6.5–7.0 kPa (50–52 mmHg), with maintenance of their pH >7.25, and whose oxygen requirements exceed 60%. However, if CPAP does not result in a prompt improvement such babies should be ventilated. Babies of this weight and gestation who are suffering from diseases other than RDS, for example pneumonia or septicaemia, rarely do well on CPAP, and should probably always be ventilated.

3. Mature babies >2.25–2.50 kg and >36–37 weeks' gestation. These babies have a comparatively rigid rib cage and well-developed respiratory muscles, and so can sustain vigorous respiratory efforts and tachypnoea >100–120/min for some days. They also tolerate CPAP badly, becoming distressed and irritable when the device is attached. They can be left in headbox oxygen at 80–90% for several days, with intubation and IPPV being used only if the $PaCO_2$ exceeds 8–9 kPa (60–67 mmHg), the PaO_2 is <6 kPa (45 mmHg) in 80–90% oxygen, or a metabolic acidaemia or hypotension are developing which do not respond to increasing the inspired oxygen concentration, plasma expansion or infusions of base.

Other indications for IPPV in the neonatal period are:

- PPHN. For the neonate with primary PPHN or PHT secondary to mild lung disease or drugs (p. 527), intubation and hyperventilation to lower the $PaCO_2$ to 3–3.5 kPa (23–26 mmHg) can be beneficial (p. 532);
- severe early-onset sepsis (p. 1129). The incidence of apnoea and PHT is high in this group of babies, who present within 6–12 hours of delivery. Early control of respiration and oxygenation is essential;
- massive pulmonary haemorrhage. This is an absolute indication for IPPV from the time of diagnosis (p. 553);
- diaphragmatic hernia. These babies should be ventilated and paralysed from birth (p. 657). Babies who present after birth should be routinely ventilated both pre- and postoperatively until their condition is stable (p. 657);
- severe birth asphyxia. Although hyperventilation to prevent cerebral oedema by keeping the $PaCO_2$ in the 3.0–3.5 kPa (22–25 mmHg) range (p. 1243) is no longer justified, the $PaCO_2$ in such babies should not be allowed to rise above 6 kPa (45 mmHg);
- apnoea. The small preterm baby with recurrent apnoea which is not controlled by methylxanthines or CPAP requires IPPV (p. 635).

Techniques of IPPV and ventilator settings

Most neonates are now ventilated using some form of positive pressure ventilation through an endotracheal tube. Negative pressure ventilators, though widely used 20 years ago,[818,1027] were less easy to use than positive pressure ventilators; as a consequence, although they avoid all the hazards of intubation and seem to be associated with a low incidence of CLD, they are not in general use.[941] Face mask ventilation[16] is now only used in a few units: not only is it difficult to employ, but holding the mask in place is associated with GMH/IVH (p. 562), and air entering the gastrointestinal tract may cause perforation.[363a] IPPV through nasal prongs has no advantages over nasal CPAP.[937]

Nevertheless, endotracheal intubation and positive pressure ventilation also have many drawbacks:

- Intubating small sick babies is difficult and may cause serious deterioration in the baby's condition (p. 573).
- The laryngoscope may damage the mouth, epiglottis or larynx.
- The presence of the endotracheal tube in the nose, trachea and larynx may cause local inflammation and damage such as erosions, ulcers and stenosis (pp. 574, 668–669).
- The tube in the pharynx may predispose to local infections, particularly otitis media.[44,258]
- The tube may be pushed too far down into the lungs (usually down the right main bronchus), causing overinflation of the right lung with the possibility of interstitial emphysema or pneumothorax[416] on the intubated side, and collapse and atelectasis of the contralateral lung.
- The tube hinders the clearance mechanisms of the lung, so that secretions are retained.
- The tube may be too small, increasing the airways resistance and thereby increasing the work of breathing for babies on low ventilator rates or CPAP.
- The haemodynamic effects of IPPV with PEEP may cause a fall in cardiac output (pp. 574–575).
- The two most serious complications of IPPV: pneumothorax (p. 517) and CLD (pp. 608–609).

Once a baby is on IPPV, apart from developing a GMH/IVH the most likely cause of death is one of the three major iatrogenic sequelae of intubation and IPPV: infection, pneumothorax and CLD.

There are seven techniques for treating respiratory failure in neonates:

1. pressure-limited time-controlled conventional-rate positive pressure ventilation;
2. volume-limited time-controlled conventional-rate positive pressure ventilation;
3. intermittent negative extrathoracic pressure and CNEP with IPPV;
4. patient-triggered ventilation;
5. high-frequency ventilation;
6. extracorporeal membrane oxygenation;
7. liquid ventilation.

The type of lung disease (Table 29.32) and the severity of the respiratory failure (Table 29.33) determine which technique is most useful and exactly how it is applied.

Table 29.32 Adjustments to conventional ventilation according to disease

Respiratory disease	Ventilator settings
RDS	low PEEP rates 60–100/min
MAS	low PEEP long expiratory time
Pulmonary hypoplasia Pulmonary airleak	low PEEP minimize PIP
Pulmonary haemorrhage Pulmonary oedema	high PEEP long inspiratory times

Table 29.33 Indications for 'newer' techniques of ventilation

Severe RDS ($F_IO_2 \geq 0.4$ despite surfactant)	HFO
Weaning	PTV
PPHN which does not respond to HFPPV and alkalinization	NO (+HFO if poor response to NO alone)
Severe respiratory failure (OI >40) in a term infant unresponsive to other techniques	ECMO

Table 29.34 Pressure-limited time-controlled ventilators (with triggered mode)

Ventilator	Triggering device (when fitted)	Response time in RDS (ms)
Sechrist IV	Impedance (SAVI)	40–80
Bearcub	Air flow	35–300
Draeger 8000*	Air flow	60–200
InfantStar	Body movement sensor (StarSync)	0–140
Bird VIP	Tidal volume	30–70
SLE 2000	Airway pressure	0–320
Neovent	–	
Healthdyne	–	
Bourns BP 200	–	

*Software subsequently modified to reduce trigger delay.
SAVI: Synchronized assisted ventilation in infants.

Pressure-limited time-controlled ventilation

This is given by machines (Table 29.34) which, by delivering a continuous flow of gas, distend the lung for a preset inspiratory time to a predetermined pressure. During expiration the ventilator gas flow continues to deliver PEEP if required.

Gas enters the lungs during the inspiratory time, and the amount that enters is determined by the peak pressures set on the ventilator and by the gas flow rate, which should always be large enough to ensure that the preset peak pressure can be reached during the available inspiratory time. At a fast flow the lungs are distended more quickly, and the peak pressure is reached sooner, thereby creating a relatively square-wave inspiratory gas flow.

When the desired pressure has been reached, the pressure-limiting valve opens and prevents any further rise; the longer the inspiratory time, the longer the lungs are held distended at this pressure. The higher the pressure is set, depending on the compliance of the lungs, the larger the volume of gas that enters the lungs, although this is limited in non-compliant lungs by the size of the leak around the endotracheal tube. This type of ventilator is the one most widely used in current neonatal practice (Table 29.34).

Peak inflating pressures. When starting a baby on IPPV the PIP should be adjusted to ensure adequate, but not excessive, chest wall expansion; in practice this usually equates to a delivered volume of approximately 6 ml/kg.[262] Sufficient pressure must be used to achieve acceptable blood gases. As high pressures are more likely to cause a pneumothorax (p. 517) or lead to CLD (p. 609), the lowest possible peak pressure compatible with normal blood gases should be used. In general, the starting pressures for a baby with respiratory disease, as opposed to central apnoea with normal lungs (p. 567), should be about 20–25 cmH_2O. The peak pressure can then be adjusted once blood gas analyses are available. Underventilation produces a high $PaCO_2$ and a low PaO_2, and overventilation a low $PaCO_2$ and sometimes an excessively high PaO_2.

Positive end-expiratory pressure. This acts like CPAP to hold the peripheral airways open during expiration. Except in severe PIE or cases with over-inflation, PEEP should always be used during ventilation as it conserves surfactant on the alveolar surface.[1185] Early studies demonstrated that a PEEP of about 5 cmH_2O improved oxygenation better than no PEEP or much higher levels,[486,733] the mechanism being via an increase in mean airway pressure. If too high a PEEP is applied, however, particularly if combined with a short expiratory time (p. 566), the lung cannot deflate properly. This causes hyperinflation, a reduced tidal volume and compromised gas exchange, the $PaCO_2$ rises[966] and the PaO_2 falls. Studies have suggested that the present population of infants with acute RDS or apnoea may not require more than 3 cmH_2O of PEEP;[318,413] however, in infants who have severe RDS even after surfactant, increasing PEEP up to 5 cmH_2O may result in a useful increase in lung volume.[242] Infants ventilated beyond the first week with type I CLD[521] have improved blood gases at 6 cmH_2O.[413]

Mean airway pressure. There is a good correlation between MAP and the degree of oxygenation,[119,486] such that PaO_2 may be improved by increasing the inspiratory time, the level of PEEP or the PIP, all three manoeuvres elevating MAP.

Most ventilators now used in neonatal intensive care display the mean airway pressure and the level can be calculated from the formula:

$$MAP = \left(\frac{T_I}{T_I + T_E}\right) PIP + \left(1 - \frac{1 - T_I}{T_I + T_E}\right) PEEP$$

where T_I and T_E are the inspiratory and expiratory times[261] or by using the formula:[319]

$$MAP = PEEP + \left(\frac{PIP - PEEP \times T_I}{T_I + T_E}\right)$$

Ventilator rates. When babies with RDS were first ventilated, the respiratory rate of the ill baby – about 80–100/min – was matched. Unfortunately, this resulted in a high incidence of CLD.[891] Studies in the 1970s[117,486,889] showed that with an I:E ratio of 1:2 (physiological ratio), the PaO_2 was lower at rates of 80/min than at 30/min. They also showed that at a rate of 30/min the PaO_2 was higher if the inspiratory time was longer than the expiratory time (reverse I:E ratio) and with 5 cmH_2O PEEP. These data were restricted to neonates with severe RDS. Nevertheless, by the late 1970s ventilator rates of 20–40/min with long inspiratory times were being widely used in neonates with all types of lung disease. The incidence of pneumothorax and other forms of airleak reached 35–40% (p. 517). Nowadays faster rates are again favoured. Heicher et al[478] found that they could ventilate babies at 60/min, with inspiratory times of 0.5 seconds at lower peak inspiratory pressures and with better blood gases and fewer pneumothoraces, than when rates of 30/min and inspiratory times of 1 second were used. In their study, however, there were few very sick infants requiring ventilator pressures more than 25 cmH_2O, and those who did were given pancuronium. Subsequently, Greenough et al[423] showed that when babies were kept at the same MAP, rates of 120/min in unparalysed neonates with RDS produced an improvement in PaO_2 over rates of 30 and 60/min. This improvement resulted from the neonates breathing in synchrony with the ventilator. By increasing the ventilator rate to 75–100/min most neonates can be induced to breathe in synchrony[419,1007] and thus have better blood gases,[421] but whether synchrony decreases the pneumothorax rate has not yet been investigated. Fast rates of 90–120/min may be beneficial in PIE (p. 522), where their use is associated with a lower incidence of pneumothorax,[416] and they have been reported to be of benefit in PPHN (p. 532), meconium aspiration (pp. 544, 564) and in the pulmonary hypoplasia of diaphragmatic hernia (p. 657). The benefits of rates faster than 100–120/min are few because most of the standard pressure-limited ventilators become mechanically inefficient at these rates.[120]

No studies have primarily assessed the effects of fast rates of ventilation on the incidence of chronic lung disease. Robinson et al[917] suggested that the incidence may be increased, but relatively few infants were studied and they were ventilated at a large range of rates. Greenough et al[426] showed that approximately half the infants surviving fast-rate IPPV are symptomatic during the first year of life, with persistent wheeze or cough, but this was not severe.

Inspiratory and expiratory times, inspiratory–expiratory ratios, inspiratory gas flow. In the 1970s studies, when rates of 20–40/min were being used, I:E ratios of 2:1 or even 3:1 were applied, giving inspiratory times as long as 1.5 seconds. This increased the MAP and improved oxygenation, but was one of the important factors correlating with the high pneumothorax rate[864,1059] (p. 517).

As part of studies on the use of faster rates, more attention has been paid to the importance of both inspiratory and expiratory times.[492] South and Morley[1008] found that the average inspiratory time in ventilated babies with RDS was 0.31 seconds (SD 0.06 s) and their average expiratory time was 0.42 seconds (SD 0.13 s), thus giving an I:E ratio of approximately 1:1.3. If such a ratio is employed with an appropriate rate for gestational age[423] a large number of babies with RDS will breathe in synchrony with the ventilator, with the attendant improvement in oxygenation.

Inspiratory flow rate has not been systematically studied. It will, however, influence the MAP by altering the time taken to reach the preset PIP. Calculations of MAP (see above) are based on the assumption that the peak inspiratory pressure is achieved throughout the inspiratory time, and that there is square-wave ventilation, assumptions that are only rarely justified (Fig. 29.73), because at the gas flows normally used only a fraction of the inspiratory time is spent at peak inspiratory pressure, particularly at the faster inspiratory rates. In practice, initial gas flows of 6–10 l/min are commonly used, but higher flows up to 20:l/min are sometimes needed when rates >100/min are being used in babies with severe lung disease who require a PIP exceeding 30 cmH_2O.

Problems with pressure-limited ventilators

Mechanical. Although the ventilators on the market (Table 29.34) purport to be versatile enough to meet all the possible setting permutations outlined above, this is not the case, particularly at rates >80–100/min. At these faster rates the ventilators have two main problems. First, although the other settings are kept identical at, say, 25/5cmH_2O with an inspiratory–expiratory ratio of 1:1, there is a change in the waveform with a loss of the positive-pressure plateau at faster rates (Fig. 29.73). This results in a reduction in tidal and minute volume and MAP, and thus a fall in PaO_2 and a rise in $PaCO_2$,[120] which can only be overcome by increasing the gas flow to make the waveform more square, or by increasing the peak inspiratory pressure.

Secondly, owing to the inertia of the moving parts of the ventilator, increasing the rate, particularly if combined with an increase in gas flow, makes it impossible to avoid an increase in PEEP, particularly in ventilators that

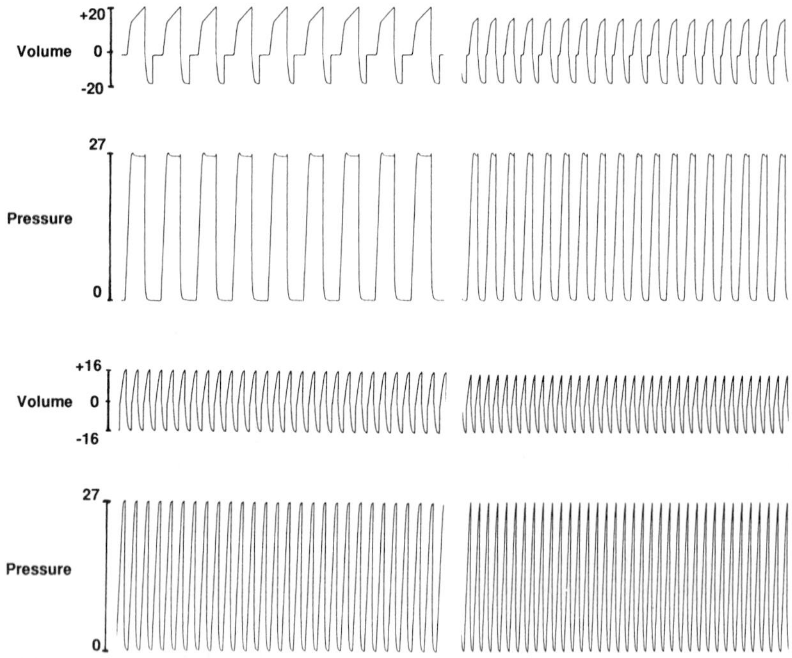

Fig. 29.73 Changes in airway pressure waveform and delivered volume as frequency increases. In each of the recordings the upper trace is the volume (inflation upwards, deflation downwards) and the lower trace is the airway pressure recording. A Sechrist ventilator was used: flow 10/min; peak pressure 30 cmH_2O; PEEP 3 cmH_2O; I:E 1:1. The ventilator rates are: upper right 30/min; upper left 60/min; lower right 90/min; lower left 120/min. Note the lower volume delivery at the higher rates, particularly in the lower two compared with the upper two traces.

incorporate non-assisted expiratory valves.[406] The increase in PEEP, sometimes called inadvertent PEEP, has the usual effects, a reduction in tidal volume and hence carbon dioxide retention,[406] and an increase in the risk of pneumothorax or PIE. In this situation prolongation of the expiratory time with respect to the inspiratory time is associated with an improvement in tidal volume, but this manoeuvre is limited by the need to maintain a minimum inspiratory time.[321] In an attempt to overcome this problem, Venturi systems or other types of assisted expiratory valves have been successfully incorporated into several ventilators.[406]

Another problem with pressure-limited ventilators at all rates is that the response of the pressure control valve is relatively slow, so that should the baby actively exhale during inspiration there may be a marked surge in airway pressure.[592]

Physiological. At faster rates the expiratory time of the ventilator may be shorter than the expiratory time constant of the neonate's lung, so that air is trapped, causing 2–3 cmH_2O inadvertent PEEP.[55,984] Gas trapping is a particular problem in paralysed infants,[494,984] but has only rarely been demonstrated in non-paralysed infants even at rates as high as 120/min.[494] Ventilator rates should be limited to 60/min (expiratory time = 0.5 s) if gas trapping and inadvertent PEEP are to be consistently prevented,[494] particularly in paralysed infants more than 31 weeks' gestation.

Ventilator settings with pressure-limited ventilators

Babies with abnormal lungs. Initially guided by the baby's colour and chest expansion, the following initial ventilator settings are appropriate provided the chest wall moves adequately, until the results of blood gas analyses are available (Table 29.35):

Pressure	20/3–25/5 cmH_2O
Rate	60/min
Inspiratory time	0.3–0.4 s
Oxygen	60–80%

The modifications that may be required in these settings are outlined on page 564 for meconium aspiration, page 522 for PIE, page 520 for pneumothorax, page 657 for diaphragmatic hernia, page 532 for PPHN and page 614 for babies with CLD.

Babies with normal lungs. There are three groups of neonates with normal lungs who may require IPPV:

- Babies with primary neurological or myopathic problems, e.g. congenital myopathy (p. 1284), fractured cervical spine (p. 1081);
- Babies with severe neurological depression due to birth asphyxia (pp. 1242–1244), drugs (p. 247) or an inborn error of metabolism (p. 991);
- Preterm babies with recurrent apnoea (p. 635).

Table 29.35 Adjustments to ventilator settings on the basis of blood gas changes

Low PaO_2	High $PaCO_2$	Increase peak pressure, which will also increase mean airway pressure: in spontaneously breathing babies $\uparrow$ rates may also work.
Low PaO_2	Normal $PaCO_2$	$\uparrow$ F_IO_2; $\uparrow$ MAP but maintain PIP (i.e. $\uparrow$ PEEP or $\uparrow$ T_I)
Low PaO_2	Low $PaCO_2$	Consider alternative diagnosis, e.g. PPHN, sepsis, overventilation. $\uparrow F_IO_2$; $\uparrow$ MAP; use vasodilators.
PaO_2 normal	High $PaCO_2$	$\downarrow$ PEEP, $\uparrow$ rate; keep MAP constant.
PaO_2 normal	Low $PaCO_2$	$\downarrow$ rate: maintain MAP.
PaO_2 high	$PaCO_2$ high	Rare: check for mechanical problems, e.g. blocked tube, $\downarrow$ PEEP, $\downarrow$ T_I: $\uparrow$ rate $\downarrow$ F_IO_2
PaO_2 high	$PaCO_2$ normal	$\downarrow$ MAP (usually $\downarrow$ PIP): $\downarrow$ F_IO_2
PaO_2 high	$PaCO_2$ low	$\downarrow$ pressure, $\downarrow$ rate, $\downarrow$ F_IO_2 (see text)
PaO_2 normal	$PaCO_2$ normal	Sit tight!

Their initial ventilator settings should be:

Pressure	15/3 cmH_2O
Rate	5–30/min
Inspiratory time	0.35–0.40 s
Oxygen concentration	21–30%

Subsequent management on IPPV: irrespective of the primary lung disease, once a baby has been established on a ventilator his blood gases should be measured. The ventilator setting should then be changed as outlined in Table 29.35 and the amount of ventilatory support adjusted to be the minimum compatible with acceptable blood gas status.

Volume-set, time-limited ventilation

These ventilators deliver a predetermined tidal volume to the baby irrespective of the pressure required to do so, unless a peak pressure safety valve is incorporated. During the time allowed for inspiration the ventilator delivers the preset tidal volume; some ventilators have the capacity then to hold the lung inflation for a defined pause before allowing passive expiration. They may also have the capability to provide PEEP during expiration.

The main problem with volume ventilation is that not all the tidal volume is delivered to the lungs. With the onset of inflation the pressure rises, compressing the gas in the ventilator circuit and the baby. Furthermore, unless cuffed endotracheal tubes are used, as the pressure rises there is a variable leak of gas around the tube. Because of these difficulties, the volume required to ventilate the baby cannot be calculated accurately, and often a tidal volume is used which is more than twice the baby's physiological tidal volume. Nevertheless, with the advent of new neonatal ventilators (for example the Bird VIP) specifically designed to deliver this ventilation mode, it has been reported in an anecdotal series to be superior to time-cycled pressure-limited ventilation.[57]

INTERMITTENT NEGATIVE EXTRATHORACIC PRESSURE AND CNEP WITH IPPV

Intermittent negative pressure ventilation was first introduced in the 1960s.[1027] More recently, infants have been exposed to CNEP with intermittent positive pressure ventilation; the peak and positive end expiratory pressures are reduced by the level of negative pressure applied. Successful use has been reported in infants with PPHN and PIE.[238] In a subsequent larger group,[239] the best effect was noted in infants with PPHN. A randomized trial has demonstrated benefits of CNEP and IPPV against IPPV alone.[872]

PATIENT-TRIGGERED VENTILATION (PTV)

PTV is a pressure-assist mode in which the patient's inspiratory effort 'triggers' a controlled positive pressure inflation. During PTV, synchronous intermittent positive pressure ventilation or assist control, all of the infant's respiratory efforts can trigger a positive pressure inflation (see below). During SIMV the maximum number of breaths that can be triggered is determined by the preset SIMV rate: for example, if the SIMV rate is 20 bpm only 20 of the infant's breaths can trigger the ventilator regardless of how fast he breathes. A further trigger mode is proportional assisted ventilation, in which the magnitude of ventilatory assistance is varied and is proportional to the patient's effort throughout the respiratory cycle.[951] PAV is not at present in routine use for neonates. Early attempts at PTV were with conventional ventilators modified to be triggered by a baby's respiratory efforts. Devices were developed to detect inspiratory activity in a variety of ways, including changes in abdominal expansion by a body movement sensor (Graseby capsule),[731] oesophageal pressure,[408] air flow,[411,751] airway pressure[491,493] and impedance.[1125] If a critical change in inspiratory activity is detected by any of these methods, the inspiratory control is triggered. There is some delay between the sensor being activated and the ventilator inflating the baby (the trigger delay or response time); the recently produced purpose-built ventilators (Table 29.34) have trigger sensors with improved function compared to the early devices, and in the majority of babies the trigger delay is usually less than 150 ms.[168] Comparison of triggering devices[89,168] suggests that airflow triggering systems perform least well in terms of delay, but are least prone to autocycling.[517] However, it is still important to limit the ventilator inflation time, otherwise it may extend into the baby's spontaneous expiration, resulting in asynchrony or even active expiration (p. 565).[491] However, if the inflation time is too short (<0.2 s), the volume delivered by the ventilator is compromised.[321] A prolonged inflation time has been show to reduce the triggering rate by stimulating the Hering–Breuer reflex.[1100] The optimum inflation time therefore appears to be between 0.2 and 0.4 s, being shorter in the less mature infant.[751]

Patient-triggered ventilators must incorporate an apnoea back-up so that if respiratory efforts are not sensed the infant is automatically switched to IPPV at the rate and pressure used prior to PTV.

Comparisons of triggered versus conventional ventilation in a series of physiological studies have demonstrated that the former is associated with a lower rate of asynchrony,[89] a higher tidal volume and improved blood gases.[198] Additional advantages were reduced fluctuations in both blood pressure[518] and cerebral blood flow velocity.[395]

PTV has been used successfully to shorten the duration of weaning,[169] and in a randomized controlled trial recruiting infants in the first 12 hours of life SIMV has been shown to reduce both the duration of ventilation in infants of birthweight greater than 2.0 kg (72 versus 93 hours) and the proportion of immature babies (birthweight <1.0 kg) oxygen dependent beyond 36 weeks' postconceptional age (47 versus 72%).[90] Triggered ventilation is not successful in all babies, particularly those less than 28 weeks' gestational age;[174] results in this group might, however, be improved if a body sensor rather than an airway trigger is used.[630] After 1 hour on PTV it is possible to predict those infants in whom it will ultimately fail; failure of oxygenation to improve and a relatively slow triggering rate compared to the predicted spontaneous respiratory rate for gestational age[751] are bad prognostic features. PTV and SIMV have been compared directly only in infants in the recovery stage of RDS. Three separate trials demonstrated no advantage to SIMV, and indeed if the maximum number of triggered breaths was reduced below 20 bpm this increased the duration of weaning, presumably by increasing the work of breathing.[171,264]

HIGH-FREQUENCY JET VENTILATION

HFJV is a modification of the technique initially developed to provide respiratory support during bronchoscopy. Frequencies between 60 and 600/min may be used. During HFJV a high-pressure source delivers gas in short bursts down a small-bore injector cannula, the tip of which usually lies within the endotracheal tube pointing towards the lung.[351] The bursts of gas entrain additional gas from areas surrounding the cannula down the endotracheal tube; expiration is passive. In most studies rates of 100–200/min have been used, although this can increase to 400–600/min. In an animal model[1150] it has been demonstrated that a relatively narrow range of inspiratory and expiratory times provides optimum HFJV. A significantly higher airway pressure gradient is necessary to maintain a constant tidal volume if the inspiratory time is shortened, and a reduction in expiratory time below 170 ms results in air trapping. Most jet ventilators operate like constant-flow time-cycled ventilators, and the pressure waveform is typically triangular, although pressure servocontrolled jet ventilators are available and produce a square pressure waveform.

HFJV may improve blood gas tensions when infants with respiratory failure are not responding to conventional ventilation,[858] and in such cases adequate blood gas tensions may be achieved with lower peak inflation pressures.[152] It has also been used with good results in babies with airleaks, in particular bronchopleural fistulae,[121,388] PPHN[154] and diaphragmatic hernia.[121] However, in a small trial it offered no benefit over conventional ventilation.[153]

Complications

Airleaks can occur with HFJV.[345,858] It has also been associated with a high incidence of necrotizing tracheobronchitis,[706] an ischaemic lesion resulting from intraluminal tracheal pressure compromising mucosal and submucosal blood flow. The lesions range from moderate erythema of the airway to severe necrotizing tracheobronchitis with total tracheal obstruction.[121] The high mean pressure and near constant intraluminal pressure may be important factors in the pathogenesis of this problem.[256] Although not all workers find a high incidence, perhaps because of meticulous humidification,[153] most studies find that HFJV does cause more tracheal damage than IPPV,[694,812] and that the longer the technique is applied the more likely it is that necrotizing tracheobronchitis will develop, with a prevalence ranging from 44 to 85%.[121,338] This serious complication suggests that HFJV should only be used for very short periods in babies with diaphragmatic hernia, PIE or severe airleak who are proving difficult to ventilate conventionally.[468]

HIGH-FREQUENCY FLOW INTERRUPTERS

These can best be classified as a subgroup of HFJV, but differ in that the intermittent high-pressure gas source is fed into a continuous positive airway pressure circuit immediately opposite the endotracheal tube connector. Small volumes of gas are delivered at high frequencies by interrupting a flow or high-pressure source. These devices can be used at frequencies up to 20 Hz (1200/min), and have been associated with improvements in blood gases in infants with PIE.[347,366] Significant improvements occurred over an 8-hour period, and this was associated with a reduction in mean airway pressure; PIE improved radiologically in seven of the nine infants studied.

Complications

Unlike HFOV (see below) HFFI does not incorporate an active expiratory phase and gas trapping may therefore be experienced, particularly at fast frequencies.

HIGH-FREQUENCY OSCILLATORY VENTILATION

During HFOV frequencies between 180 and 3000/min (3–50 Hz) may be used, but in practice 7–15 Hz is most commonly employed. During HFOV a volume generator feeds into a continuous positive airway pressure circuit close to the patient. The generator is either a piston, bellows or a loudspeaker driven by a generator and audio amplifier. Continuous flow is necessary to add fresh gas to the circuit and remove expired gas. HFOV may also be given at the same time as conventional ventilation (Fig. 29.74), but there are no data to suggest that such an approach is superior. HFOV can also be applied externally by means of a thoracoabdominal chamber connected to a vacuum source and a high-frequency oscillator.[474] During HFOV, two volume strategies have been pursued: a low-volume strategy, in which mean airway pressure is limited with the aim of preventing damage due to barotrauma, and a high-volume strategy in which mean airway pressure is elevated to promote optimum alveolar expansion and hence improve oxygenation. The high-volume strategy is successful in infants with homogeneous lung disease; in infants with severe atelectasis on conventional ventilation this approach means an increase in MAP on HFOV of 5–10 cmH_2O[262] compared to the MAP on IPPV. Nevertheless, using such a strategy, HFOV has been associated with a reduction in CLD,[196] which was not seen when a low-volume strategy was used.[488] The low-volume strategy is useful in infants with gas trapping, for example due to PIE. Severe lobar emphysema can resolve on HFOV if a low-volume strategy is pursued.[605] It may be applied only to the affected side if selective intubation is employed.[888]

Volume delivery during HFOV is proportional to the product of the frequency and the square of the oscillatory amplitude,[993] tidal volume delivery having an inverse relationship to frequency.[631] The oscillatory amplitude is increased until chest wall vibration is apparent, and then adjusted as needed to correct hypo- or hypercapnia. The oscillating volume entering and leaving the endotracheal tube depends on a number of factors, which include the comparative impedance of the respiratory tract and continuous positive airway pressure circuit. Early studies suggested that HFOV provided a tidal exchange considerably less than the baby's anatomical dead space.[351] It was suggested that gas exchange occurred additionally by mechanisms distinct from those operating during conventional ventilation; these include bulk flow by convection, convective mixing between lung units (Pendelluft) and augmented diffusion.[178] It has more recently been demonstrated that infants can be oscillated at a tidal volume of between 50 and 100% of their anatomical dead space when certain machines are

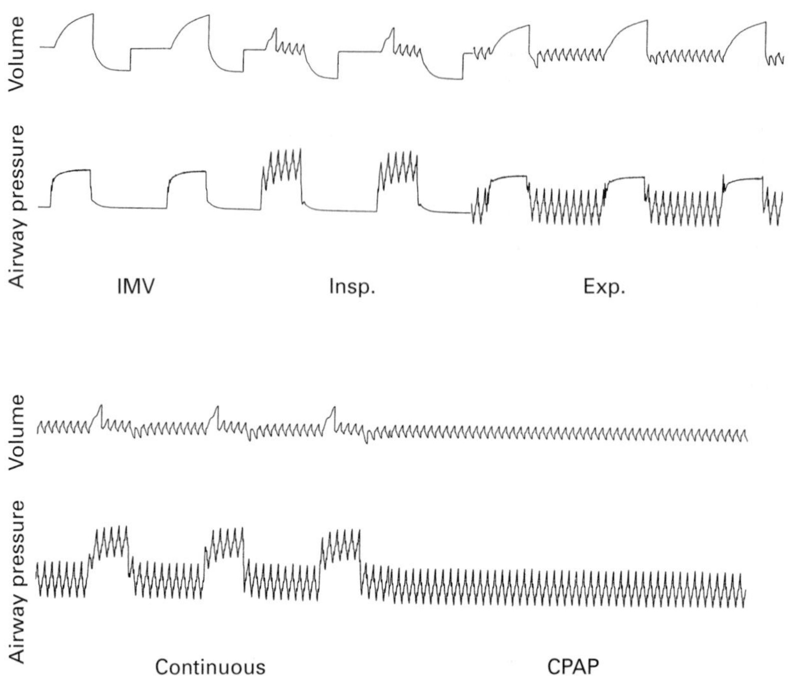

Fig. 29.74 HFOV with conventional ventilation. The upper trace demonstrates IMV, then a combination of IMV plus oscillation on the positive pressure plateau (Insp.) and on the right-hand part of the trace IMV plus oscillation on the expiratory pressure (Exp.). The lower two traces demonstrate oscillation throughout the ventilation cycle (continuous) and on top of constant mean airway pressure (CPAP). Reproduced with permission from Laubscher et al.[631]

used.[173] If an oscillator capable of delivering a constant volume is employed, however, oscillating at the resonant frequency of the respiratory system in RDS (between 12 and 24 Hz, 720–1440/min) is associated with an increased delivery to the infant.[507] Unfortunately, this does not apply to the majority of commercially available oscillators, whose performance is impaired at increased frequencies.[172,631]

HFOV in animals suppresses spontaneous respiration; although this is partly explained by changes in blood gas tensions, this effect also appears to be related to stimulation of pulmonary mechanoreceptors; vagal fibres are stimulated continuously and to a greater extent during HFOV than with static lung inflation.[707] In humans, however, perhaps due to the relatively small tidal volume delivered, spontaneous respiration is not inhibited, but rarely interferes with the effectiveness of respiratory support.[176,488]

Oxygenation improves as mean airway pressure increases in homogeneous lung disease[1070,1178] until the optimum lung volume is reached;[262] this is associated with improvements in pulmonary mechanics.[606,1132]

Carbon dioxide elimination is proportional to the oscillatory frequency and tidal volume.[993] In HFOV, carbon dioxide elimination may be improved by increasing oscillatory frequency and increasing the flow of gas.[1178] The position of the gas source is important,[925] carbon dioxide elimination being 50% greater when it is placed at the carinal end of the endotracheal tube. In clinical practice the impaired performance of commercially available oscillators at increased frequencies means that tidal volume, and hence carbon dioxide elimination, is higher at slow rates.[173]

There have been several anecdotal reports of benefit following HFOV[714] in babies with severe RDS,[175] hypoplastic lung, pneumonia, PPHN,[124] PIE[195] and diaphragmatic hernia.[561] The use of HFOV has enabled blood gas tensions to be maintained, with a lowering of mean airway pressure and resolution of PIE.[195] HFOV is not a successful form of rescue respiratory support in all infants; failure to improve oxygenation after 6 hours of treatment identifies non-responders.[175,823] It is, however, more successful in supporting infants ≥34 weeks' gestational age and birthweight ≥2.0 kg who had severe respiratory failure, as defined by a requirement for an F_IO_2 >0.5 and MAP >10 cmH_2O. In a randomized trial of such babies 60% of 40 infants assigned to conventional ventilation met treatment failure, compared to only 44% of 39 infants who received HFOV;[489] of the 24 patients in whom CMV failed, 15 responded to HFOV, but only four of 17 failing on HFOV responded to CMV (P = 0.03). A prospective randomized study,[488] however, failed to show benefit of HFOV over conventional IPPV. Infants of birthweight between 750 and 2000 g in respiratory failure due to RDS, pneumonia or PPHN were randomly assigned to either HFOV or IPPV during the first 24 hours of life. Over 600 infants were entered into the study. There was no difference in the mortality rate nor the incidence of airleak, PDA or CLD between infants ventilated conventionally or by HFOV. Worryingly, HFOV was associated with a significant increase in the incidence of grades 3 and 4 GMH/IVH and PVL. In that study,[488] however, a low-volume strategy was pursued, and two more recent studies,[197,808] which both adopted the high-volume strategy, did not show an increase of such complications during HFOV and one[197] reported that HFOV was associated with a reduction in CLD. Both these studies were relatively small. Interestingly, however, a subsequent larger study has confirmed this effect.[372] Using a lung recruitment stategy, randomization to HFOV after exogenous surfactant administration was associated with improved oxygenation, a lower incidence of chronic lung disease and reduced hospital costs compared to when conventional ventilation was used.[372] HFOV has also been shown to reduce the development of airleak in preterm infants who have severe respiratory failure but, unfortunately, the HFOV group again had an excess of intracerebral haemorrhage.[489]

Complications

Necrotizing tracheobronchitis has been described infrequently following HFOV,[591] and 4 hours of HFOV does not appear to affect lung morphology, surfactant, lymph flow, wet-to-dry weight ratios or pressure–volume curves.[341,459,1084] Inadvertent PEEP over 4 cmH_2O can occur when the oscillating frequency exceeds 20 Hz[508] and can reduce cardiac output.[256] The association of HFOV with an excess of GMH/IVH has been reported.[488,489]

EXTRACORPOREAL MEMBRANE OXYGENATION

ECMO provides a method of gas exchange in patients with respiratory failure without resorting to damaging patterns of ventilatory support, and allows the lungs a chance to recover. In adults experience with ECMO has been disappointing, but in the newborn ECMO has been associated with greater than 80% survival in infants with a predicted mortality of over 80%.[980] This method of respiratory support, however, cannot be used for infants less than 2.00 kg, in whom large GMH/IVHs develop.[190] ECMO has been used as a method of respiratory support in newborns suffering from RDS, MAS, sepsis, primary PPHN, congenital heart disease and diaphragmatic hernia. It is expensive, time-consuming and has many complications, yet over 70 centres now provide neonatal ECMO in the USA and there are five centres in the UK.

CRITERIA FOR INSTITUTING ECMO

These include:[28,65,74,669]

- severe but reversible cardiac or pulmonary disease unresponsive to optimal ventilation and pharmacological therapy. There should be no major ventilator-induced damage or chronic lung disease, and the baby must have had less than 10 days of aggressive IPPV;
- estimated mortality risk greater than 80% (p. 501);
- no GMH/IVH; low risk of spontaneous (or heparin-induced) GMH/IVH;
- birthweight >2.0 kg;
- absence of prolonged asphyxia predicted to cause brain damage;
- no chromosomal abnormality incompatible with quality of life.

TECHNIQUE

Venous blood is drained, usually from the right jugular vein; oxygen is then added and carbon dioxide removed by the membrane lung; oxygenated blood is then returned to the patient. Cannulation for ECMO is either venoarterial or venovenous.[27] For venoarterial bypass the right common carotid artery and right internal jugular vein are used. In venovenous bypass oxygenated blood is returned via the right femoral vein or umbilical vein, and the carotid artery is spared. More recently, venovenous ECMO is undertaken through a double-lumen catheter. Following decannulation the vessels are permanently ligated in the smallest infants.

Total respiratory support is provided by an extracorporeal blood flow of approximately 100 ml/kg/min, increasing up to 120 ml/kg/min.[64,669]

Infants are heparinized to achieve whole-blood ACT 2–3 times normal (an ACT of 160–200 seconds). Haematocrit and platelet count are maintained with transfusions of saline-washed packed red blood cells and platelet concentrates as necessary.

To allow the lung to rest inspired oxygen concentrations of 21–40%, ventilator rates of 10–20/min at pressures of 16–20 cmH_2O are used for the duration of the ECMO. The infant's blood gases are controlled by the membrane oxygenator and pump flow rate.

ECMO is maintained until pulmonary function recovers, usually within 10 days.[190,590,616]

When the infant starts to improve, as indicated by improving oxygenation, the ECMO circuit flow is reduced to 50 ml/min. When stable vital signs, adequate urine output and acceptable arterial blood gases are

Table 29.36 Survival related to disease of the first 7647 infants reported to the ELSO Registry. (Reproduced from Kanto[556] with permission)

Diagnosis	Survival rate
Meconium aspiration syndrome	93
Severe respiratory distress syndrome	83
Persistent pulmonary hypertension of the newborn	83
Sepsis	77
Congenital diaphragmatic hernia	59

achieved on this minimal flow for 4–5 hours, the ECMO cannulae are clamped and the baby is excluded from the ECMO circuit, which can be restarted if necessary.

RESULTS

Mortality associated with ECMO varies with the diagnosis. Redmond et al[880] claimed overall survival rates of 90% among neonates treated with ECMO, but only 38% of infants with diaphragmatic hernia recovered. Experience reported from the ELSO Registry is given in Table 29.36.[556]

Controversy exists as to whether the results with ECMO are better than would be achieved with conventional therapy. An initial randomized controlled study[65] was analysed by a statistical method called 'play the winner'. In that study, although ECMO was associated with a significant improvement in survival rate, only one of the 12 infants entered into the study was randomized to conventional therapy. More recently, O'Rourke et al[815] abandoned their prospective trial when four out of 10 conventionally treated babies had died, compared to none of mine treated with ECMO (P = 0.054). A multicentre trial performed in the UK involving 185 infants has recently been reported and demonstrated that ECMO reduced mortality by 50% in infants with PPHN or MAS.[1099]

COMPLICATIONS

Local vascular complications are common, including haemorrhage, vessel thrombosis and problems with wound healing. Renal failure has occurred as a result of aortic thrombosis. Following ligation of the carotid there is the potential for neurological sequelae, although brain circulation should be preserved through the circle of Willis. Studies by Towne et al[1079] showed the development of adequate collaterals and no evidence of consistent lateralizing lesions in 46 survivors.[379] These results are reassuring, but Schumacher et al[952] found varying degrees of right hemispheric brain injury in eight of 59 ECMO survivors. EEG abnormalities[29] and seizures have been reported in ECMO survivors.[1079] GMH/IVH and other haemorrhages, probably a consequence of anticoagulation, were a problem, occurring in 10 out of 35 neonates treated in early studies of neonatal ECMO.[190] Pulmonary haemorrhage can occur following successful completion of ECMO in infants who had prolonged acidosis, a high fluid requirement before ECMO, a need for blood pressure support during ECMO and evidence of renal and/or hepatic dysfunction.[393]

SEQUELAE

Neurological sequelae were not uncommon in infants treated with ECMO in the 1980s. Of the first 14 survivors of ECMO, seven (50%) were normal or near normal and 10 (71%) had normal mental ability at 1–3 years of age.[29] Short et al[980] reported that after 12 months of follow-up 69% of their patients were normal (DQ >90) on the mental index and 67% normal on the motor index of the Baley scales. Nevertheless, only approximately 10% of ECMO survivors suffer major morbidity, either significant developmental delay or neurological abnormality.[379,598] Infants with congenital diaphragmatic hernia, however, have significantly lower motor scores at 1 year of age than infants with other diagnoses.[88] In all studies poor outcomes were associated with major cerebral haemorrhage and chronic lung disease. Interim analysis of the UK multicentre trial does not demonstrate an excess of neurological sequelae in the ECMO-treated patients.[1099]

There have been few studies reported on the long-term respiratory status of ECMO survivors. Short et al[980] found a 15% prevalence of chronic lung disease, the risk factors being culture-proven streptococcal sepsis and being placed late (7–8 days of age) on ECMO. Other risk factors for CLD are lung hypoplasia and failure to respond to a trial of HFOV.[954] A comparison of nonrandomized infants, however, suggested that conventionally treated patients have a higher rate of CLD than those supported by ECMO with similar illness severity.[1133]

LIQUID VENTILATION

Liquid ventilation[193] is performed using perfluorocarbons, which have a low surface tension (25% of that of water) and a high solubility for respiratory gases, particularly oxygen. PFCs contain carbon and fluorine bonds, which are extremely strong and make them pharmacologically and chemically inert; they are also radio-opaque.

Liquid ventilation may be total, in which the PFC is preoxygenated and warmed as it is circulated to fill the lungs to the expected FRC.[495] The PFC is then moved backwards and forwards at a relatively slow rate and high tidal volume because of its higher viscosity.[495] TLV requires different circuitry than in current clinical practice. Partial liquid ventilation, or perfluorocarbon-associated gas exchange, however, has been used to support patients. During PLV, PFC again fills the lungs to FRC but the patient is then gas ventilated 'on top'. If no further PFC is given, that in the lung simply evaporates away. Throughout the period of PLV (usually less than 7 days) the PFC is topped up by adding sufficient via a side port in the endotracheal tube so that a meniscus remains visible there.[365,496,634]

In animal models, liquid ventilation has been demonstrated to reduce ventilation–perfusion mismatch and improve compliance and oxygenation, compared to gas.[1095] It also appears to be a less damaging form of respiratory support, particularly in very immature animals.[497,1174] It is compatible with both nitric oxide[1159] and surfactant.[635] Indeed, it appears to have several advantages over surfactant therapy, as it is not inactivated by proteins and has better spreading capability.[635] Clinical experience to date is limited to anecdotal series, the majority of patients receiving PLV while on ECMO. Under such circumstances, in adults,[496] children and neonates,[436,634] and premature infants,[636] PLV has been demonstrated to improve oxygenation and compliance. It has also improved oxygenation in premature infants with severe respiratory failure.[636] Randomized trials are currently under way to test the role of PLV in infants with mild respiratory failure (a/A ratio <0.2).

Toxicology studies suggest that PFCs are inert, but it is not known whether systemic absorption will limit the duration for which PLV is used. In one series two of the six children developed pneumothoraces,[365] but no other complications were experienced.

CARE OF BABIES ON VENTILATORS

Much of the medical care and monitoring of ventilated babies has been discussed under RDS (pp. 501–508), sepsis (pp. 1125–1127), birth asphyxia (pp. 1242–1244) and the various other respiratory disorders. There are, however, certain aspects which are unique to being ventilated.

INTUBATION

The technique of intubating babies and the choice of tubes is described on pages 1369–1371. Intubating small, sick babies can be difficult, and they become hypoxaemic, acidaemic and bradycardic during the procedure. During intubation stress hormones are released,[642,981] blood pressure and ICP rise,[874] and this, together with the blood gas changes, predisposes the neonate to GMH/IVH (p. 1257).[350a,575,720] For this reason it has been recommended[575] that intubation should only be carried out once the infant has received pancuronium and atropine, as this will mitigate the adverse physiological changes. Obviously such a policy should only be adopted by personnel who are confident of their ability to intubate successfully. Intubation may also cause bacteraemia.[267]

Type of endotracheal tube

There is no evidence that nasal tubes are superior to oral tubes for routine use,[701] and Spitzer and Fox[1013] reported an increased risk of postextubation atelectasis when nasal endotracheal tubes were used. Changing an oral endotracheal tube used for labour ward resuscitation to a nasal endotracheal tube on a routine basis is bad practice. For long-term intubation nasal endotracheal tubes can be easily fixed at the nose (Fig. 29.72), and greater stability may reduce laryngeal trauma.

Humidification

Inadequate warming and humidification of inspired gases will cool the baby and lead to dehydration of the bronchial secretions, with airway plugging and obstruction of the endotracheal tube. The gas from the ventilator should reach the tube adequately warmed and humidified. The British Standards Institution[128] recommends that the minimal accepted humidity is 33 mgH_2O per litre inspired gas, which is 75% of that obtained during normal breathing. Various humidifiers are available, but when tested they often fall short of the British Standard,[1060] providing air temperatures of 32–35°C and humidities in the range 29–32 mgH_2O/l. They do achieve some warming and humidification, and neonatal units using them report surprisingly few problems due to dry airway secretions or blocked endotracheal tubes.

Fixation

Many techniques for immobilizing endotracheal tubes have been described: one is to use a soft cord tied round the tube and stick it to the face with lightweight tape (Fig. 29.72), but each unit should devise its own system, steering a course between rigid immobilization which prevents accidental extubation but causes cosmetic deformity (p. 932) and the reverse – no deformity but frequently dislodged tubes.

Suctioning

Suctioning causes bradycardia, hypoxia, bacteraemia, pneumothorax and an increase in cerebral blood flow and ICP but a fall in cerebral oxygenation,[778,836,985,991,1055] although these effects are less in the paralysed baby.[310] The technique of endotracheal tube suction must allow oxygen administration throughout the procedure, and if the baby becomes bradycardic or the $tcPO_2$, continuous PaO_2 monitoring or oximetry demonstrates the oxygenation to have fallen below 6 kPa or the SpO_2 below 80%, the suction should be discontinued and the infant reconnected to the ventilator.

Inserting the suction catheter until a resistance is felt (when the catheter hits the carina) should be avoided

(p. 668): it should only be inserted far enough to reach just beyond the tip of the endotracheal tube.[43]

As a prelude to suction a small amount of water or saline is often put down the endotracheal tube. Both of these may damage the lungs and/or the surfactant system,[623] particularly if the fluid is not adequately warmed.[545] If some form of lubrication is deemed essential to enable the suction catheter to pass down the endotracheal tube, the smallest amount necessary, probably 0.3–0.5 ml, should be used.

Endotracheal suctioning during the acute respiratory illness should be minimized and tailored to the need of the individual. There is no evidence that suctioning is needed more often than every 12 hours in the routine care of babies ventilated for RDS.[1164]

Changing the tube

Given the stress of intubation (see above) endotracheal tubes should not be changed on a routine basis. If there are no signs to suggest obstruction, the tubes should be left in for as long as is necessary.

Duration of intubation

Nasal endotracheal tubes can be used for months with a surprisingly low incidence of complications (see below). A 'routine' change to a tracheostomy, as is practised in older children or adults on long-term IPPV, is contra-indicated in the neonate, who becomes very tracheostomy dependent and thus difficult to decannulate (p. 670).

Complications of intubation

Within a few hours of intubation the mucosa of the larynx and trachea shows deciliation, necrosis and desquamation.[364,550] Metaplastic change in the trachea of intubated neonates is common.[877] Nevertheless, remarkably few sequelae are seen and in adults at least re-epithelialization is the norm.[210] Many neonates have some hoarseness and/or mild stridor in the 24–48 hours after extubation. Nasal endotracheal tubes can be associated with ulceration and excoriation of the nostril, which results in stenosis, and oral tubes with dentition problems and a long narrow pressure-induced groove, or even cleft, in the palate[691] (pp. 932–933). Tracheomegaly, which looks alarming but seems to cause few functional problems, has also been seen after prolonged intubation.[99]

Serious damage to the larynx and trachea, such as granulomata or subglottic stenosis or cysts, occurs in about 1:100 intubated neonates (unpublished Cambridge data) (p. 932). These sequelae only occur in babies who have had prolonged and/or repeated intubations[973] and can be minimized by meticulous attention to endotracheal tube immobilization and by skilled and judicious timing of extubation. Severe, potentially fatal necrotizing tracheobronchitis may occur after a short period of intubation in some neonates for no apparent reason,[591] and is much more common after HFJV (p. 569).

TRACHEOSTOMY

Once a tracheostomy is placed in a neonate it is very difficult to remove. Because nasal endotracheal tubes can be used for 3–4 months or more if indicated in neonates, tracheostomy is only necessary when attempts to extubate have been persistently thwarted by laryngeal or tracheal problems (p. 669).

PREVENTION OF INFECTION

All infants who are started on ventilation should receive antibiotics. If, after 48 hours, there are no ongoing signs of infection and the cultures are negative, consideration should be given to stopping the drugs. The indications for restarting are given on page 1136.

FLUID AND ELECTROLYTE BALANCE

This is outlined in detail in Chapter 39, Part 1 and on page 505 (RDS). The application of PEEP may cause oliguria, but in adults at least this is the result of an adjustment of intrarenal blood flow distribution rather than inappropriate ADH secretion.[829]

MAINTENANCE OF BLOOD PRESSURE AND BLOOD VOLUME

Hypotension is seen in ventilated patients owing to the endotoxic shock of bacterial sepsis, the endocardial ischaemia of severe birth asphyxia, or the effect of severe illness in neonates with RDS. It should be managed in the usual way with transfusion and inotropes (p. 504). Anaemia commonly compounds the problem of hypotension, and ventilated babies should have their haemoglobin kept higher than 13–14 g/dl (PCV >40%).[536,1038]

An additional cause of hypotension in ventilated neonates is a reduction in cardiac output secondary to IPPV and PEEP. In adult patients with severe lung disease, and in experimental animals, high-pressure IPPV, particularly when accompanied by PEEP at levels of 10 cmH_2O or above, may compromise cardiac output in three ways:[538,1168]

- Reducing venous return;
- Obstructing the pulmonary vasculature, increasing right ventricular overload and hence the right ventricular volume, which in turn squashes the left ventricular cavity, reducing left ventricular output;
- Splinting the heart and pericardium between overinflated lungs (Fig. 29.75).

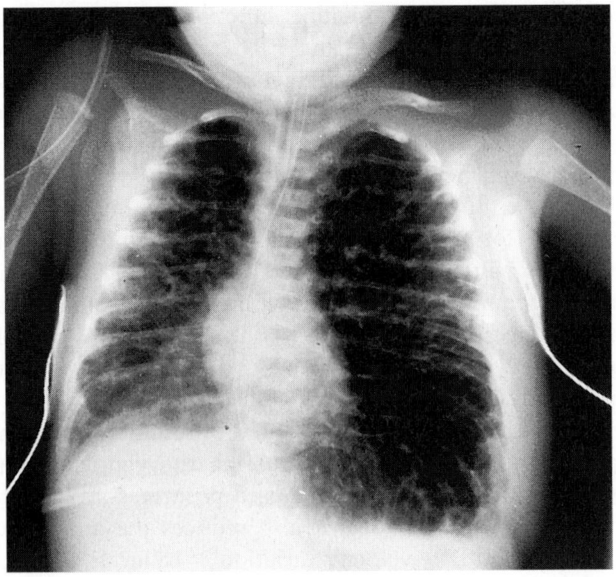

Fig. 29.75 Squashed heart with overventilation.

In ventilated babies with RDS Skinner et al[989] found that CVP ranged from 0 to 12 mmHg, but that when it fell to the 0–3 mmHg range the babies showed clinical evidence of hypovolaemia. Although not studied by Skinner et al,[989] by analogy with adult studies[870] one would anticipate that such babies would respond to volume expansion with colloid or blood.

In the very low-birthweight ventilated neonate PEEP above 4 cmH_2O reduces cardiac output,[473] and Trang et al[1081] suggest that at PEEP levels above 6 cmH_2O peripheral perfusion is reduced. Evans and Klukow[302] showed that output from both ventricles is lowest in the sickest babies, and that mean airway pressure is an important variable in reducing this output. Iatrogenic pulmonary hypertension causing profound hypoxia can certainly be caused by overventilation[75] (Fig. 29.76), which can also obstruct the bronchial circulation.[1129] Particularly when PIE is present, the chest X-ray in such babies shows that the heart is squashed and markedly reduced in volume (Fig. 29.75). Problems with hypotension and a low cardiac output can usually be overcome by transfusion; however, if the problem is left ventricular compression this can only be improved if it is possible to reduce the ventilator pressure.

CEREBRAL BLOOD FLOW

IPPV also influences the cerebral circulation in various ways, and thus may influence the incidence of GMH/IVH and PVL. Ventilated VLBW babies have a highly variable cerebral blood flow velocity, which can be reduced by the use of pancuronium[837] or by adequate volume replacement.[884]

Experimentally, hyperventilation reduces cerebral blood flow[637] and cerebral oxygenation,[553] and should be

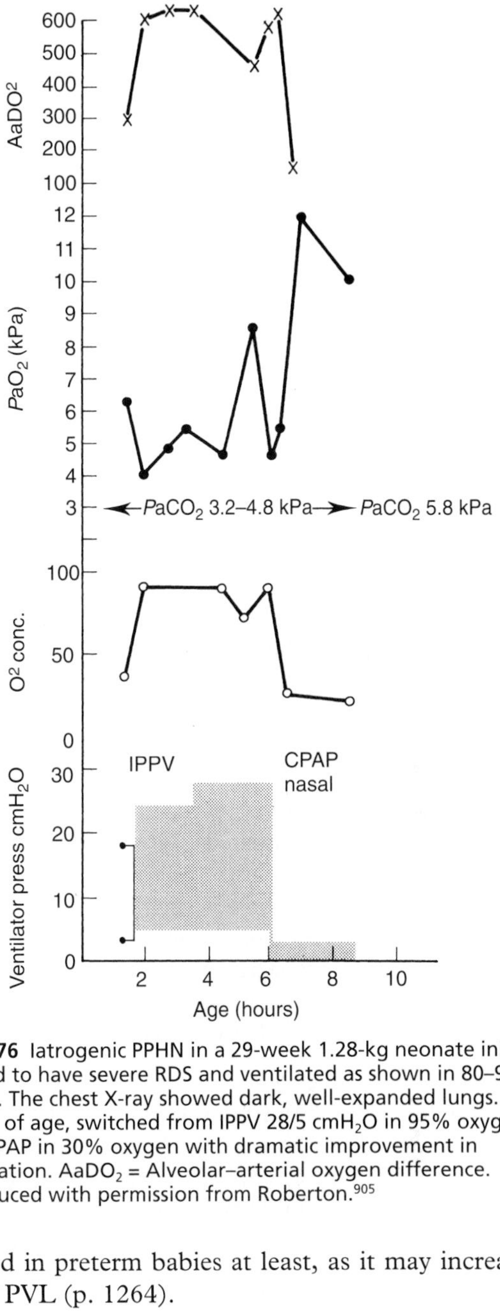

Fig. 29.76 Iatrogenic PPHN in a 29-week 1.28-kg neonate initially assessed to have severe RDS and ventilated as shown in 80–95% oxygen. The chest X-ray showed dark, well-expanded lungs. At 6 hours of age, switched from IPPV 28/5 cmH_2O in 95% oxygen to nasal CPAP in 30% oxygen with dramatic improvement in oxygenation. $AaDO_2$ = Alveolar–arterial oxygen difference. Reproduced with permission from Roberton.[905]

avoided in preterm babies at least, as it may increase the risk of PVL (p. 1264).

HAEMATOLOGICAL CARE

Ventilation per se has been claimed to result in thrombocytopenia,[53] but other than this there are no specific haematological features of being ventilated other than to maintain the haemoglobin at greater than 13 g/dl (p. 505).

NUTRITION

The nutritional management of the various diseases for which IPPV is required is outlined in the relevant sections. The ventilated neonate of all gestations can be fed enterally providing he has bowel sounds, has passed meconium, and there is nothing to suggest intra-abdominal sepsis or NEC (p. 506). Starting feeds should be delayed, however, if the infant is severely growth retarded and/or has compromised gastrointestinal blood flow antenatally.[576] The risk of reflux is not a contra-indication to enteral feeding, nor is the presence of an umbilical artery catheter. Furthermore, the earlier feeding is started, the sooner the neonate is likely to be established on full enteral feeds.[282,992] The alternative is parenteral nutrition, but this is not without hazard: for example, fat infusions may compromise lung function[460] (p. 354).

MONITORING

In addition to all the patient monitoring outlined in Chapter 21, the ventilator output should also be monitored. The inspired oxygen concentration should be checked, as should peak inspiratory and end-expiratory pressure, mean airway pressure and rate. Alarm systems must be included to identify disconnection or endotracheal tube blockage.

PARALYSING BABIES DURING VENTILATION

Following the lead of Thomas et al,[1068] who showed that neonates could be ventilated satisfactorily without paralysis, most neonatologists followed suit. It was recognized, however, that babies on IPPV often became hypoxic if they fought the ventilator and/or were restless, and that this improved when neuromuscular blocking agents such as pancuronium were given. The use of pancuronium is supported by three further lines of evidence.

- Greenough et al[415] showed that in the 25–30% of neonates with RDS who have the 'active expiratory reflex' (p. 517) there was an extremely high incidence of pneumothorax, and that the incidence of this and of GMH/IVH could be significantly reduced by the use of pancuronium.[417]
- The incidence of GMH/IVH is higher in those very low birthweight neonates with RDS who have a rapidly fluctuating cerebral blood flow velocity when they breathe out of phase with the ventilator. Paralysing such babies stabilizes the cerebral blood flow velocity and reduces the incidence of GMH/IVH.[835] A related benefit of pancuronium is that surges of intracranial pressure during nursing procedures are also minimized.[40,310]
- Pollitzer et al[860] showed that using pancuronium reduced CLD in ventilated neonates surviving RDS.

Pancuronium is not without its drawbacks. In babies with active respiration, albeit out of phase, abolition of spontaneous respiratory activity is associated with a fall in PaO_2 and a rise in $PaCO_2$;[934] following pancuronium or morphine administration lung function may deteriorate, with a fall in compliance and FRC and a rise in airways resistance, leading to a fall in oxygenation.[101] This can usually be overcome by increasing the peak inspiratory pressure by 4–6 cmH_2O immediately prior to giving the first dose of pancuronium.[420,425]

The use of pancuronium results in neonates being ventilated for a longer period and developing moderate oedema,[420] although this is not associated with a fall in plasma volume.[141] Prolonged use of pancuronium has been suggested to cause contractures or muscle atrophy,[936,986] but this can be avoided by appropriate passive physiotherapy.[404,425]

Alternative strategies to neuromuscular blocking agents have been sought. Increasing the ventilator rate reduces active expiration[320,419] and promotes synchrony, improving PaO_2 (p. 565); it also reduces the amount of cerebral blood flow velocity variation[887] to levels at which there is no association with GMH/IVH. Another increasingly popular alternative is to use narcotic analgesics,[743] in particular fentanyl[24] or alfentanil.[717] The pharmacokinetics of these drugs in preterm infants have not been fully explored, and their ability to suppress respiratory efforts and prevent pneumothoraces has not been subjected to a randomized study. Clinical experience suggests that intravenous infusion of these drugs frequently reduces adverse respiratory interactions with the ventilator, and in addition has the advantage of providing analgesia (Chapter 27). Chloral hydrate, which is also frequently administered, should probably not be used: absorption is uncertain in sick infants with RDS, clinically it appears relatively ineffective, and long-term use can produce toxic levels.

There is no place for routinely paralysing all ventilated neonates.[649] Comparison of routine paralysis with a policy of synchronized (fast-rate) ventilation and selective paralysis for those infants who, despite rate manipulation, consistently exhaled during the inspiratory cycle of the ventilator, demonstrated no advantage for routine paralysis in terms of mortality rate (16% versus 19%), pneumothorax rate (14% versus 14%) or oxygen dependency at 36 weeks postconceptional age (39% versus 32%).[970] Among infants with RDS pancuronium should be reserved for those who are actively expiring or fighting the ventilator despite appropriate changes in the rate (see above).[216,417] Paralysis, however, should be considered for:

- the mature term baby with MAS, PPHN or GBS sepsis who is chronically restless, hypoxic and impossible to maintain in synchrony with the ventilator, despite sedation and rate and inspiratory time manipulation. Infants with CDH should all be paralysed from birth (p. 657);
- any neonate, irrespective of gestation, who shows the 'active expiratory reflex' pattern and in whom this is not abolished by synchronous ventilation and sedation;

- any neonate who develops severe PIE, and infants who remain restless despite sedation following drainage of a pneumothorax.

Pancuronium is the most commonly used drug in this situation (100 μg/kg, given at intervals to suppress all respiratory activity, as it has fewer side-effects than curare, particularly histamine-releasing activity). Strict attention to fluid balance is mandatory, as fluid retention during paralysis is common.[420] The excretion of pancuronium in the neonate with kidney and liver problems is variable and this agent interacts with other drugs, in particular the aminoglycosides;[801] as a consequence very high plasma levels and prolonged paralysis may occur with infusions of the drug. This may worsen pulmonary mechanics,[101] and for these reasons infusions should be avoided and the drug given by boluses as required, although this does not necessarily avoid all the side-effects. Vecuronium and atracurium have been used as alternatives, particularly as the latter's metabolism is independent of renal activity. Variations in the sensitivity of the neuromuscular junction in neonates, however, mean that the initial dose of vecuronium given should be small (10–20 μg) and, as the duration of action and recovery time is longer in babies, maintenance doses should also be low and infusions avoided.

ANALGESIA (Chapter 27)

Neonates in pain show stress reactions that are clearly adverse and likely to increase the risk of serious side-effects such as GMH/IVH.[24] Being ventilated may be unpleasant and painful. For this reason, ventilated babies should initially at least receive some form of analgesic, which will reduce the levels of stress hormones but will probably have little effect on complications or morbidity.[869] Using opiate analgesics might also result in the baby breathing in synchrony with the ventilator, with all the benefit this produces.

PHYSIOTHERAPY IN VENTILATED NEONATES[826]

With adequate humidification of the ventilator gases, problems with retained sticky secretions or endotracheal tube blockage are rare in the first 3–4 days of IPPV. Studies on babies with RDS on IPPV have found that chest physiotherapy may cause serious hypoxia and considerable release of stress hormones,[433] and physiotherapy is therefore not warranted as a routine.[337,985,1164] Frequent endotracheal suction and/or regular chest physiotherapy may be needed, however, in:

- the neonate with pneumonia and increased secretions (p. 1144);
- babies with meconium aspiration (p. 545);
- massive pulmonary haemorrhage (p. 554);
- the phase of bronchorrhoea as infants develop CLD[742] (p. 611);
- postextubation (p. 581).

In these babies, except for those with MPH (p. 554), gentle percussion and postural drainage followed by endotracheal tube suction should probably be carried out 3- to 4-hourly for as long as they are intubated, and in the immediate postextubation period.

Optimal therapy is given in the conventional way by gentle manual percussion,[1087] rather than by more novel methods of vibrating the chest, e.g. using an electric toothbrush.

POSTURE

The position of ventilated neonates should be changed 2- to 3-hourly from the back to the right and then the left side, to aid the movement of airway secretions. The prone position (except in babies with UACs, p. 1374), with the baby's head turned to one side, should also be used, since, as in the unventilated neonate, in addition to draining secretions this will improve his blood gases.[266,1128]

With severe unilateral lung disease such as PIE the neonate should lie on the affected side, as this not only frequently improves oxygenation,[477] but also hastens the disappearance of interstitial gas,[953] (p. 523). In any posture, however, it is important to avoid excessive neck flexion or extension in the intubated neonate, as this can cause up to 2.5 cm of variation in the position of the endotracheal tube: flexion pushes the tube downwards into one bronchus, and extension pulls it upwards.[1075]

THE PROFOUNDLY HYPOXIC NEONATE

A small number of ventilated neonates, despite the management outlined above, fail to achieve an adequate PaO_2.

PROFOUND HYPOXIA WITH NORMOCAPNIA OR HYPOCAPNIA

The ventilated baby who has these blood gas abnormalities in the absence of severe lung disease, but in whom the diagnosis of mild RDS or meconium aspiration has been made, should be managed as described on pages 532–536 for PPHN. In the ventilated baby with severe clinical and radiological lung disease whose PaO_2 stays <5 kPa in 95% oxygen despite a normal or low $PaCO_2$, despite vigorous treatment of any underlying problems such as hypoglycaemia, acidaemia, sepsis, systemic hypotension or pneumothorax, there are only three therapeutic options left: increasing ventilation, using vasodilator drugs or starting ECMO. In some infants allowing the $PaCO_2$ to rise to 7–8 kPa[1180] (permissive hypercapnia) while making adjustments which are likely to increase the

*P*aO_2, plus the judicious use of pulmonary vasodilators, is often successful.

Use of sedation or paralysis

If such a baby is breathing out of synchrony with the ventilator, or worse is restless and actively fighting the ventilator, this must be stopped by the use of either sedative drugs or pancuronium; the latter is more likely to be successful.

Adjusting the ventilator

The first thing to do is to increase the mean airway pressure, although all such manoeuvres could reduce carbon dioxide elimination. There are three alternatives all designed to increase MAP: increase the PEEP, increase inspiratory time, and increase the I:E ratio while lowering ventilator rate. If one of these brings the *P*aO_2 into the acceptable range nothing more needs to be done. It should be remembered that, provided there is no evidence of a metabolic acidosis, relatively low levels of *P*aO_2 (6–7 kPa (45–52 mmHg)) can be tolerated, with good results.[893] If *P*aO_2 fails to rise above 5 kPa (37 mmHg), however, the next step should be to try and overventilate the baby to reduce the *P*aCO_2 to the 3–3.5 kPa (23–26 mmHg) range and achieve a pH >7.55 in the hope that this will cause pulmonary vasodilatation. This can sometimes be successful (Fig. 29.77). Whenever the inspiratory pressures are >25 cmH_2O, and certainly >30 cmH_2O, pancuronium should be given to try and reduce the severity of barotrauma from out-of-phase respiratory efforts. Using tubocurarine in this situation may be preferable, because this drug has some pulmonary vasodilator action of its own owing to its histamine-releasing activity.[520] If this still fails, pulmonary vasodilator drugs (pp. 533–535) should be tried.

IATROGENIC HYPOXAEMIA

If these manouevres fail to raise the *P*aO_2 in a profoundly hypoxic neonate, it is essential to check that he has not been overventilated to such an extent that his mean airway pressure is compromising pulmonary artery perfusion and causing iatrogenic PPHN. The diagnostic clues in such neonates, as well as the low *P*aO_2, are that they always have a very low *P*aCO_2, often less than 3–3.5 kPa (23–26 mmHg), a raised pH (>7.45–7.50) and their chest X-ray shows dark, overexpanded lungs. Reducing the ventilator settings dramatically improves oxygenation[75] (Fig. 29.76); occasionally a single dose of tolazoline may be required to cause the pulmonary artery pressure to fall. A similar situation may be seen with inadvertent PEEP in older neonates with CLD and increased airways resistance who require a long T_E; reducing the rate and hence increasing T_E will dramatically improve ventilation.[1026]

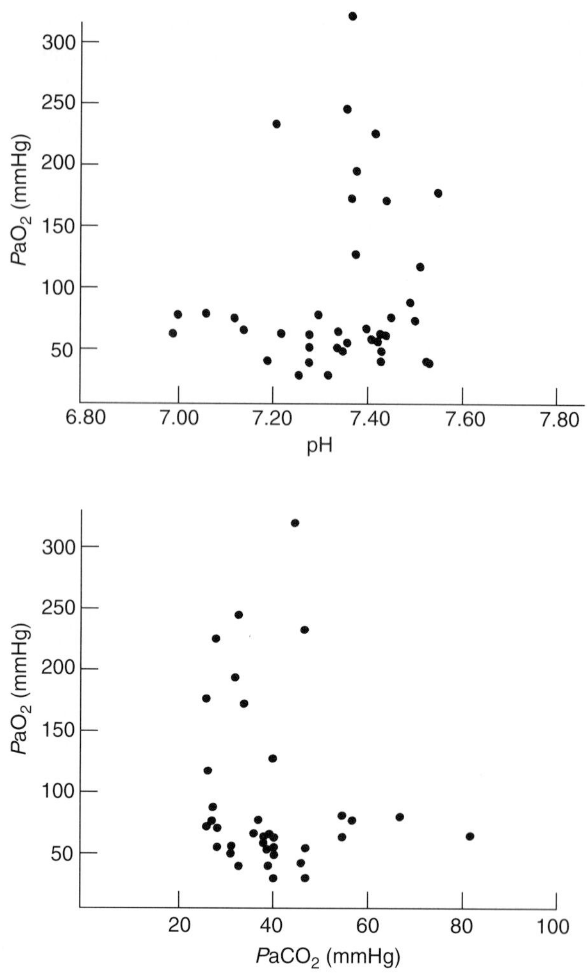

Fig. 29.77 Improvement in *P*aO_2 in neonates with RDS and secondary PPHN hyperventilated to *P*aCO_2 values <40 mmHg (5.3 kPa). Note less consistent response than in babies with primary PPHN (Fig. 29.59). To convert *P*aO_2 to kPa divide by 7.5. Reproduced with permission from Drummond et al.[278]

PROFOUND HYPOXAEMIA WITH CARBON DIOXIDE RETENTION

If severe hypoxaemia is combined with hypercapnia, particularly if this is >7–8 kPa (52–60 mmHg), and technical problems with the ventilator circuit and tube can be excluded, the correct therapy is to increase the ventilator pressure and/or rate (see Table 29.35) (p. 567). If necessary, in order to minimize the risks of barotrauma in a neonate who is clinically stable with an acceptable blood pressure, less than perfect blood gases can be tolerated, provided that the *P*aO_2 is >5.5–6.0 kPa (41–45 mmHg), the *P*aCO_2 <8 kPa (60 mmHg) and the pH >7.25.

The severe lung disease of such patients usually means that reducing their *P*aCO_2 to below 5 kPa (37 mmHg) is almost always impossible. Unfortunately, tolazoline is not only rarely effective in the preterm or infected patient with such problems, but also often causes profound hypotension, which is difficult to treat. Pulmonary vasodilators, however, may be helpful in the severe lung disease found in term babies with MAS (p. 544) or diaphragmatic hernia (p. 657). In such infants, particularly those with PIE and severe persistent pulmonary hypertension, fast ventilator rates of 100–150/min, oscillatory or jet ventilation have been suggested (see above) and are occasionally successful.

DETERIORATION ON IPPV

Not all babies who are stable on IPPV remain so: their condition may and often does worsen, and this can be a sudden collapse or a gradual deterioration.

SUDDEN COLLAPSE

Sudden spontaneous episodes of hypoxaemia are not uncommon in ventilated preterm babies. These may be due to episodes of active exhalation[114] and usually respond to short term increases in F_IO_2 or pressure. More prolonged deterioration is usually due to one of three things: a blocked or displaced endotracheal tube; an acute airleak, usually a pneumothorax; or the sudden development of a large GMH/IVH (p. 1257). If the third possibility is not present, prompt and efficient management of the other two is essential to prevent it developing. The management of this crisis is outlined in the algorithm in Figure 29.78.[907] First, it is important to establish that the endotracheal tube is in situ and patent. Using a portable battery-operated capnometer (Nellcor, UK) which detects exhaled carbon diagnosis may facilitate this. Sutherland et al[1045] were able to confirm all episodes of accidental extubation by the absence of intermittent changes in carbon dioxide in time with ventilation. While

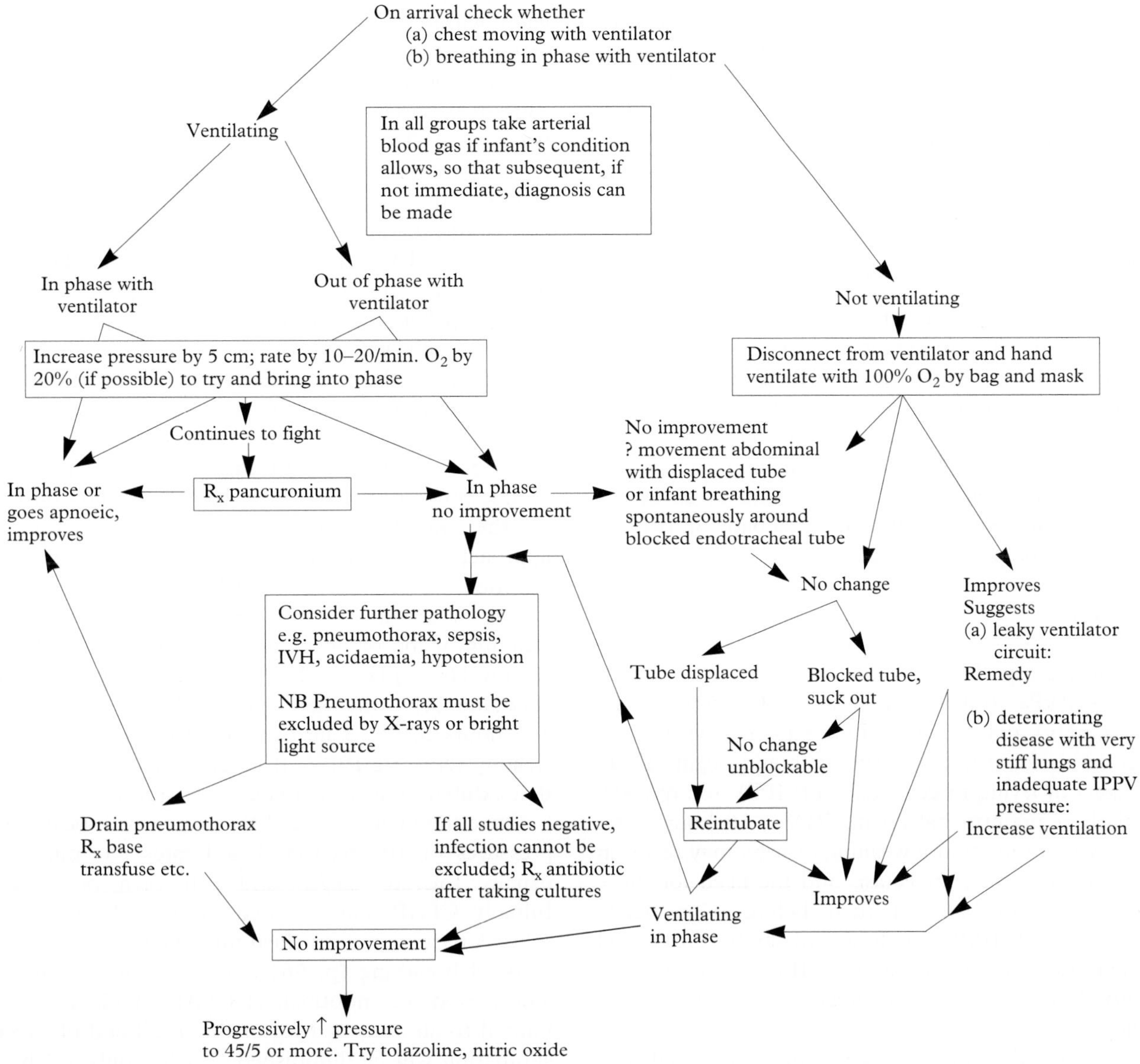

Fig. 29.78 Treatment of collapse while on IPPV. Reproduced with permission from Roberton.[907]

Table 29.37 Causes of gradual deterioration on IPPV

Infection	Especially pneumonia (p. 1144) but can also be septicaemia from, for example, a long line for i.v. feeding (p. 1134)
GMH/IVH	Gradual development of the bleed or an extension (p. 1257)
Anaemia/hypotension	From blood loss, infection or any other cause (pp. 814–815)
Airleak	Of any type: X-ray necessary (p. 514 et seq)
Pulmonary oedema	Particularly in association with a patent ductus (p. 512)
Electrolyte imbalance	Hyponatraemia or hypocalcaemia, hypo- or hyperkalaemia, renal failure
Hypoglycaemia	
Partial blockage of endotracheal tube	
Progression to chronic lung disease (Part 3)	

doing this, or if the CO_2 does vary with ventilation, increase the ventilation using either the ventilator or a bag and mask system. If this is effective, there is time to evaluate the baby more calmly; if it is not, exclude pneumothorax by either transillumination or chest X-ray; if the infant's condition is critical consider emergency chest aspiration (p. 520).

GRADUAL DETERIORATION

In addition to the natural tendency for diseases such as RDS untreated with surfactant to worsen over the first 24–48 hours, there are many reasons for a ventilated baby to gradually deteriorate (Table 29.37). Most of these conditions can be assessed quite quickly by clinical examination, chest X-ray, biochemical tests and cranial ultrasound if necessary. The real problem, as always, is infection. Assessment of pneumonia in a baby on IPPV is described in detail on page 1144.

WEANING

Once satisfactory blood gases have been achieved (PaO_2 8–12 kPa (60–90 mmHg), $PaCO_2$ 5.5–6.5 kPa (40–50 mmHg), pH >7.25) and the baby has been stable at these levels for 6 hours, weaning should begin. There are dangers in trying to get a baby off IPPV too quickly, particularly a preterm baby with RDS <36 hours after birth, in whom too rapid a weaning process may result in a recurrence of severe atelectasis and the need for more intensive ventilator support than before. Conversely, complications of IPPV, such as infection, CLD and airleak, are related to the duration of IPPV, and every opportunity should be taken to extubate the baby as soon as possible.

When weaning, reduce the most damaging modality of ventilation first, that is, the peak inspiratory pressure, as this is a major factor in the aetiology of pneumothorax and CLD (pp. 517, 609). This is relatively easy in babies with RDS or meconium aspiration, in whom pressures can be lowered as rapidly as the blood gases allow, but great care should be taken with babies with PPHN, in whom even modest changes can result in worsening of their blood gas status and precipitate pulmonary vasoconstriction (pp. 489, 530).

After reducing the peak pressures down to 25 cmH_2O at, say, rates of 60–80/min in 60% oxygen, oxygen and peak pressures can then be reduced simultaneously, dropping pressure if $PaCO_2$ is well controlled or if there is a respiratory alkalaemia. Pressure and oxygen are lowered if the PaO_2 is >8–9 kPa (60–70 mmHg). In general the settings should be reduced in small increments: 5–10% for oxygen and 2–3 cmH_2O for peak inspiratory pressure. If they are reduced too far and too quickly the baby may become hypercapnic or hypoxic to levels worse than those before the change. After each change, check the blood gases within 30–60 minutes to ensure that they are still satisfactory.

Pancuronium should not be discontinued until problems caused by airleaks (severe PIE or pneumothorax) have been controlled, and the ventilator settings have been reduced to 22–25 cmH_2O and 50–60% oxygen.

Once the baby is making spontaneous respiratory efforts and the peak pressures have been reduced to, say, 16–18/3 cmH_2O, the ventilator rate can be reduced initially in steps of 5–10/min, dropping to steps of 2–5/min when the rate is below 20, in the expectation that the baby will breathe spontaneously, although still supported by the occasional ventilator inflation. During this phase, using a short inspiratory time of ≤0.5 seconds results in a faster weaning process.[422] An alternative method of weaning is to transfer the infant to PTV and reduce pressure to 10–14 cmH_2O, depending on the size of the infant, before considering extubation. This approach has been shown to significantly shorten the duration of weaning.[170] SIMV is probably not suitable during weaning (p. 568). During the later stages of weaning, if the blood gases are acceptable (PaO_2 >8 kPa (60 mmHg), pH >7.25) and the baby is breathing spontaneously, the settings should be reduced every 4–6 hours to see if he can sustain normal gases on the steadily reducing IPPV. If he can, this is very suggestive that extubation is likely to be successful.

Once the neonate is in 40% oxygen with peak inflating pressures of 10–16 cmH_2O and rates <10/min, he will usually tolerate CPAP and can then be extubated. Initially CPAP may be tried through the endotracheal tube. A narrow endotracheal tube, however, increases the work of breathing (p. 561), so the baby can tire easily. The period on endotracheal CPAP should therefore be limited to an hour or two, or the likelihood of successful extubation will be diminished.[582] After only 1–2 hours of endotracheal tube CPAP with normal gases the infant should be extubated. It may sometimes be helpful to increase the inspired oxygen concentration by 5–10% (with meticulous PaO_2 monitoring) to help sustain oxygenation over the immediate postextubation period. There remains debate as to whether extubation onto nasal CPAP rather than into a headbox reduces the likelihood of reintubation.[97,170]

In most babies, if nasal CPAP is used it can be discontinued after 48–72 hours, putting the baby in a headbox in the same inspired oxygen concentration. Particularly in very preterm babies, however, the nasal CPAP may be required for several days or weeks to prevent recurrent apnoeic attacks (p. 634).

In babies >1.50 kg birthweight weaning can often be rapid, over a period of 12–24 hours, with no need for prolonged periods on low IMV rates or nasal CPAP. Conversely, in neonates <1.00 kg birthweight the later stages of weaning may take weeks (see below).

In babies <1.5 kg and <32 weeks' gestational age, aminophylline or oral theophylline (5 mg/kg/24 h) or caffeine citrate (5 mg/kg/24 h) should be administered at least 12 hours prior to extubation, for example once ventilator rate has been reduced to 40 bpm. In prospective controlled trials this has proved to shorten the duration of weaning, but only in babies <30 days of age.[285,418] The side-effects and monitoring of theophylline therapy are the same as when it is used for apnoea of prematurity (p. 634).

WEANING PROBLEMS

After any step in weaning the baby may deteriorate or the blood gases at the new setting be unacceptable. One finding which is common in VLBW neonates, and which suggests that the weaning procedure is not progressing smoothly, is the development over 6–12 hours of a metabolic acidaemia, a sign that the work of breathing at the new low ventilator setting is excessive. In this situation, after ensuring that some unrelated adverse event such as a blocked endotracheal tube or a pneumothorax has not occurred, all that is usually required is to revert to the previous ventilator setting. In some babies, however, following the deterioration much more vigorous ventilation may be necessary for 24–48 hours before the weaning process can once more be resumed. The criteria for reintubation after extubation are not materially different from the indications for ventilating the baby in the first place (p. 563).

EXTUBATION

Extubation carries the risk of severe hypoxia leading to GMH/IVH, inhalation of gastric contents and the need for reintubation, with the possibility of laryngeal trauma. It is essential, therefore, only to attempt extubation with the baby in the best possible condition, including normal electrolytes, a haemoglobin >13 g/dl and normal acid–base status. Feeding should be discontinued 6–12 hours before extubation and not restarted for a further 12 hours, so that the risks of regurgitation and milk inhalation are reduced to a minimum.

After extubation the neonate often has considerable difficulty clearing his secretions, as airway ciliary function has been compromised by the damage caused by the endotracheal tube. The inspired oxygen must therefore be humidified and warmed. Regular physiotherapy and oropharyngeal suction should be started,[325] as always, applied in such a way that it does not cause deterioration in the baby's blood gases or result in apnoea and bradycardia. In general, both physiotherapy and suction should be used 3- to 4-hourly, adapting the frequency on the basis of clinical findings or the chest X-ray (see below).

Nursing recently extubated babies in the prone position results in better blood gases.[667]

Extubation problems

Stridor

Minor degrees of stridor are not uncommon and usually only last for an hour or two, or at most 24 hours. If persistent the infant may benefit from higher-pressure nasopharyngeal CPAP (p. 561), using pressures up to 6–8 or 10 cmH_2O; whether or not this will work can only be assessed on a trial and error basis. Nebulized adrenaline can also be administered. If the stridor is marked and unresponsive with severe respiratory distress, and there is progressive deterioration of the blood gases, there is no alternative but to reintubate. In such patients the endotracheal tube should be left in place with the baby on CPAP or minimal ventilation for at least 2–3 days before a further attempt at extubation is made, and only after pretreating the baby with dexamethasone (0.5 mg/kg) over the previous 24 hours and continuing the drug for 24–48 hours afterwards. A recent prospective trial showed that this was beneficial.[227] The management of the baby in whom this does not work, and in whom some more serious laryngeal damage has occurred, is outlined on page 669.

Lobar collapse

Despite careful physiotherapy and suction postextubation (v.s.), up to 20% of neonates develop collapse consolidation of one lung or just one lobe, particularly the right upper, because of plugging of the bronchi with secretions.[1181] This complication seems to be more common after nasal intubation.[1013] It may cause such severe deterioration that reintubation and IPPV are necessary, but in other infants may be virtually asymptomatic. The milder cases can be treated by vigorous physiotherapy. Occasionally it is worth sucking out the airway of more severely affected neonates under direct vision at laryngoscopy. By turning the head away from the affected lung, the suction catheter can usually be directed into the appropriate main stem bronchus.

In order to detect areas of asymptomatic collapse, particularly in the right upper lobe, before they progress to total lung collapse, it is worth X-raying all neonates 24–36 hours after extubation, or whenever there is any deterioration in their clinical condition or blood gases.

Recurrent failure to wean or extubate

Repeated unsuccessful attempts to extubate a neonate over a period of a week is usually only a problem in extremely low birthweight neonates whose weight is not increasing and in whom the repeated episodes of extubation and deterioration make adequate nutrition even more difficult to achieve. Rarely it is due to laryngeal damage. Poor lung function is not usually responsible.[1120] Affected infants should be reintubated using a nasal endotracheal tube, restarted on IPPV at a rate of 5–10/min, and kept there until they are in a better condition and gaining weight consistently. Repeated failure to wean a neonate off IPPV is very suggestive of a neurological problem, either secondary to GMH/IVH or some primary muscular or neurological disorder, including, particularly in term babies, the congenital hypoventilation syndrome (Ondine's curse).

REFERENCES

1. Abbasi S, Bhutani V K, Gerdes J S 1993 Long term pulmonary consequences of respiratory distress syndrome in preterm infants treated with exogenous surfactant. Journal of Pediatrics 122: 446–452
2. Abman S H, Dunbar Ivy D, Ziegler J W, Kinsella J P 1996 Mechanisms of abnormal vasoreactivity in persistent pulmonary hypertension of the newborn infant. Journal of Perinatology 16: S18–S23
3. Abman S H, Kinsella J P, Schaffer M S, Wilkening R B 1993 Inhaled nitric oxide in the management of a premature newborn with severe respiratory distress and pulmonary hypertension. Pediatrics 92: 606–609
4. Abu-Osba Y K, Gala O, Manasra A, Rejjal A 1992 Treatment of severe persistent pulmonary hypertension of the newborn with magnesium sulphate. Archives of Disease in Childhood 67: 31–35
5. Achiron R, Zakut H 1986 Fetal haemothorax complicating amniocentesis. Acta Obstetrica Gynaecologica Scandinavica 65: 869–870
6. ACTOBAT Study Group 1995 Australian collaborative trial of antenatal thyrotropin releasing hormone (ACTOBAT) for prevention of neonatal respiratory disease. Lancet 345: 877–882
7. Adamson T M, Boyd R D H, Normand I C S, Reynolds E O R, Shaw J C L 1969 Haemorrhagic pulmonary oedema (massive pulmonary haemorrhage) in the newborn. Lancet i: 494–495
8. Adamson T M, Boyd R D H, Hill J R, Normand I C S, Reynolds E O R, Strang L B 1970 Effect of asphyxia due to umbilical cord occlusion in the foetal lamb on a leakage of liquid from the circulation and permeability of lung capillaries to albumin. Journal of Physiology 207: 493–505
9. Aherne W, Dawkins M J R 1964 The resorption of fluid from pulmonary airways in the rabbit, and the effect on this of prematurity and prenatal hypoxia. Biologia Neonatorum 7: 214–218
10. Ahluwalia J S, Morley C J 1995 Changes in oxygenation and heart rate after administration of artificial surfactant (ALEC) to preterm infants. Archives of Disease in Childhood 72: F121–122
11. Ahluwalia J S, Kelsall A W R, Raine J et al 1994 Safety of inhaled nitric oxide in premature neonates. Acta Paediatrica 83:347–348
12. Ahluwalia J S, Rennie J M, Wells F C 1996 Successful outcome of severe unilateral pulmonary interstitial emphysema after bi-lobectomy in a very low birthweight infant. Journal of the Royal Society of Medicine 89: 167–168
13. Ahn M O, Cha K Y, Phelan J P 1992 The low birthweight infant: is there a preferred route of delivery? Clinics in Perinatology 19: 411:423
14. Aiton N R, Fox G R, Hannam S, Stern C M M, Milner A D 1996 Pulmonary hypoplasia presenting as persistent tachypnoea in the first few months of life. British Medical Journal 312: 1149–1150
15. Allen A C, Usher R H 1971 Renal acid excretion in infants with respiratory distress syndrome. Pediatric Research 5: 345–355
16. Allen L P, Blake A M, Durbin G, Ingram D, Reynolds E O R, Wimberley P D 1975 Continuous positive airway pressure and mechanical ventilation by face mask in newborn infants. British Medical Journal iv: 137–139
17. Allen L P, Reynolds E O R, Rivers R P A, LeSouef P N, Wimberley P D 1977 Controlled trial of continuous positive airway pressure given by face mask for hyaline membrane disease. Archives of Disease in Childhood 52: 373–378
18. Allen R W, Jung A L, Lester P D 1981 Effectiveness of chest tube evacuation of pneumothorax in neonates. Journal of Pediatrics 99: 629–634
19. Al-Nishi N, Dyer D, Sharief N, Al-Alaiyan S 1994 Selective bronchial occlusion for treatment of bullous interstitial emphysema and bronchopleural fistula. Journal of Pediatric Surgery 29: 1545–1547
20. Alpan G, Mauray F, Clyman R I 1989 Effect of patent ductus arteriosus on water accumulation and protein permeability in the lungs of mechanically ventilated premature lambs. Pediatric Research 26: 570–575
21. Al-Sayed L, Schrank W, Thach BT 1994 Ventilatory sparing strategies and swallowing pattern during bottle feeding in human infants. Journal of Applied Physiology 77: 78–83
22. Amodio J, Abramson S, Berdon W et al 1987 Iatrogenic causes of large pleural fluid collections in the premature infant, ultrasonic radiographic findings. Pediatric Radiology 17: 104–108
23. Amon E, Lipshitz J, Sibai B M, Abdella T N, Whybrew D W, El-Nazer A 1986 Quantitative analysis of amniotic fluid phospholipids in diabetic pregnant women. Obstetrics and Gynecology 68: 373–378
24. Anand K J S, Sippell W G, Aynsley-Green A 1987 Randomised trial of fentanyl anaesthesia in preterm babies undergoing surgery: effects on the stress response. Lancet i: 243–248
25. Andersen E A, Hertel J, Pedersen S A, Sorensen J R 1984 Congenital chylothorax: management by ligature of the thoracic duct. Scandinavian Journal of Thoracic and Cardiovascular Surgery 18: 193–194
26. Anderson K D, Chandra R 1976 Pneumothorax secondary to perforation of segmental bronchi by suction catheters. Journal of Pediatric Surgery 11: 687–693
27. Andrews A F, Klein M D, Tommasian J M 1983 Venovenous ECMO in neonates with respiratory failure. Journal of Pediatric Surgery 18: 339–346
28. Andrews A F, Roloff D, Bartlett R H 1984 Use of extracorporeal membrane oxygenation in persistent pulmonary hypertension of the newborn. Clinics in Perinatology 11: 729–735
29. Andrews A F, Nixon C A, Cilley R E, Roloff D W, Bartlett R H 1986 One-to three-year outcome for 14 neonatal survivors of extracorporeal membrane oxygenation. Pediatrics 78: 692–698
30. Annibale D J, Hulsey T C, Engstrom P C, Wallin L A, Ohning B L 1994 Randomized, controlled trial of nasopharyngeal continuous positive airway pressure in the extubation of very low birth weight infants. Journal of Pediatrics. 124: 455–460
31. Annibale D J, Hulsey T C, Wagner C L et al 1995 Comparative neonatal morbidity of abdominal and vaginal deliveries after uncomplicated pregnancies. Archives of Pediatrics and Adolescent Medicine 149: 862–867
32. Aranda J V, Stern L, Dunbar J S 1972 Pneumothorax with pneumoperitoneum in a newborn infant. American Journal of Diseases of Children 123: 163–166

33. Arnold C, Adams E, Torres E, Sidebottom R 1996 Exosurf versus Survanta surfactant preparations: proportional-hazards regression analysis of time to successful extubation and discontinuation of oxygen therapy. Journal of Perinatology 16: 9–14
34. Arnold C, McClean F H, Kramer M S, Usher R H 1987 Respiratory distress syndrome in second-born versus first-born twins. New England Journal of Medicine 317: 1121–1124
35. Auten R L, Notter R H, Kendis J W, Southgate W M 1991 Surfactant treatment of full term newborns with respiratory failure. Pediatrics 87: 101–107
36. Avery M E, Gatewood O B, Brumley G 1966 Transient tachypnea of the newborn. American Journal of Diseases of Children 111: 380–385
37. Avery G B, Randolph J G, Weaver T 1966 Gastric acidity in the first day of life. Pediatrics 37: 1005–1007
38. Avery M E, Tooley W H, Keller J B et al 1987 Is chronic lung disease in low birthweight infants preventable? A survey of eight centres. Pediatrics 79: 26–30
39. Bacon G E, George R, Koeff S T, Howatt W F 1975 Plasma corticoids in the respiratory distress syndrome and in normal infants. Pediatrics 55: 500–502
40. Bada H S, Burnette T M, Arheart K L et al 1995 Pancuronium attenuates associated hemodynamic and transcutaneous oxygen tension changes during nursery procedures. Journal of Perinatology 15: 119–123
41. Baden M, Bauer C R, Colle E, Klein G, Taeusch H W, Stern L 1972 A controlled trial of hydrocortisone therapy in infants with respiratory distress syndrome. Pediatrics 50: 526–534
42. Baildam E M, Dady I M, Chiswick M L 1993 Bronchocutaneous fistula associated with mechanical ventilation. Archives of Disease in Childhood 69: 525–526
43. Bailey C, Kattwinkel J, Teja K, Buckley T 1988 Shallow versus deep endotracheal suctioning in young rabbits: pathological effects on the tracheal and bronchial wall. Pediatrics 82: 746–751
44. Balkany T, Berman S, Simmons M et al 1978 Middle ear effusions in neonates. Laryngoscope 88: 398–405
45. Ball R, Chetcuti P, Beverley D 1995 Fatal familial surfactant protein B deficiency. Archives of Disease in Childhood 73: F53 (letter)
46. Ball R, Chetcuti P, Primhak R 1995 Clinical aspects of familal surfactant protein B deficiency (abstract) Biology of the Neonate 67 (suppl 1): 81
47. Ballard P L, 1984 Combined hormonal treatment and lung maturation. Seminars in Perinatology 8: 283–292
48. Ballard P L, Ballard R A 1995 Scientific basis and therapeutic regimens for use of antenatal glucocorticoids. American Journal of Obstetrics and Gynecology 173: 254–262
49. Ballard P L, Granberg P L, Ballard R A 1975 Glucocorticoid levels in maternal and cord serum after prenatal betamethasone therapy to prevent respiratory distress syndrome. Journal of Clinical Investigation 56: 1548–1554
50. Ballard P L, Gluckman P D, Liggins G C, Kaplan S L, Grumbach M M 1980 Steroid and growth hormone levels in premature infants after prenatal betamethasone therapy to prevent respiratory distress syndrome. Pediatric Research 14: 122–127
50a. Ballard R A, Ballard P L, Cnaan A et al 1998 Antenatal thyrotropin-releasing hormone to prevent lung disease in preterm infants. New England Journal of Medicine 338: 493–498
51. Ballard R A, Ballard P L, Creasy R K et al 1992 Respiratory disease in very low birthweight infants after prenatal thyrotropin releasing hormone and glucocorticoids. Lancet 339: 510–515
52. Ballard R A, Leonard C H 1984 Developmental follow-up of infants with persistent pulmonary hypertension of the newborn. Clinics in Perinatology 11: 737–744
53. Ballin A, Koren G, Kohelet D et al 1987 Reduction in platelet counts induced by mechanical ventilation in newborn infants. Journal of Pediatrics 111: 445–449
54. Ballot D E, Rothberg A D, Gootlich E et al 1992 Early dexamethasone therapy in hyaline membrane disease: effects on the cytopathological changes of bronchial epithelium and ventilatory requirements. Pediatric Reviews and Communications 6: 221–229
55. Bancalari E, 1986 Inadvertent positive end expiratory pressure during mechanical ventilation. Journal of Pediatrics 108: 567–569
56. Bancalari E, Berlin J A 1978 Meconium aspiration and other asphyxial disorders. Clinics in Perinatology 5: 317–334
57. Bandy K P, Nicks J J, Donn S M 1992 Volume controlled ventilation for severe neonatal respiratory failure. Neonatal Intensive Care 5: 70–74
58. Banerjee C K, Girling D J, Wigglesworth J S 1972 Pulmonary fibroplasia in newborn babies treated with oxygen and artificial ventilation. Archives of Disease in Childhood 47: 509–518
59. Barak M, Cohen A, Herschikowitz S 1992 Total leucocyte and neutrophil count changes associated with antenatal betamethasone administration in premature infants. Acta Paediatrica 81: 760–763
60. Barefield E S, Hicks T P, Phillips J B 1994 Thromboxane and pulmonary morphometry in the development of the pulmonary hypertensive response to Group B streptococcus. Critical Care Medicine 22: 506–514
61. Barefield E S, Karle V A, Phillips J B, Carlo W A 1996 Inhaled nitric oxide in term infants with hypoxaemic respiratory failure. Journal of Pediatrics 129: 279–286
62. Barrett J M, Boehm F H, Vaughn W K 1983 The effect of type of delivery on neonatal outcome on singleton infants of birthweight of 1000G or less. Journal of the American Medical Association 250: 625–629
63. Bartlett D, 1985 Ventilatory and protective mechanisms of the infant larynx. American Review of Respiratory Disease 131: Suppl 49–50
64. Bartlett R H, Andrews A F, Toomasian J M, Haiduc N J, Gazzaniga A B 1982 ECMO for newborn respiratory failure, 45 cases. Surgery 92: 425–433
65. Bartlett R H, Roloff D W, Cornell R G, Andrews A F, Dillon P W Zwishenberger J B 1985 Extracorporeal circulation in neonatal respiratory failure. A prospective randomised study. Pediatrics 76: 479–487
66. Bartlett R H, Toomasian J, Roloff D, Gazzaniga A B, Corwin H G, Rucker R 1986 Extracorporeal membrane oxygenation (ECMO) in neonatal respiratory failure. Annals of Surgery 204: 236–245
67. Bartmann P, Bamberger U, Pohlandt F, Gortner L 1992 Immunogenicity and immunomodulatory activity of bovine surfactant (SF-RI 1). Acta Paediatrica 81: 383–388
68. Baum J D, Roberton N R C 1974 Distending pressure in infants with respiratory distress syndrome. Archives of Disease in Childhood 49: 771–781
69. Baum J D, Roberton N R C 1975 Immediate effects of alkaline infusion in infants with respiratory distress syndrome. Journal of Pediatrics 87: 255–261
70. Bauer B R, Brennan M J, Doyle C 1978 Surgical resection for pulmonary interstitial emphysema in the newborn infant. Journal of Pediatrics 93: 656–661
71. Beard R W, Morris E D 1965 Foetal and maternal acid-base balance during normal labour. Journal of Obstetrics and Gynaecology of the British Commonwealth 72: 496–506
72. Becerra J E, Rowley D L, Atrash H K 1992 Case fatality rates associated with conditions originating in the perinatal period: United States 1986 through 1987. Pediatrics 89: 1256–1259
73. Beck R 1985 Chronic lung disease following hypocapnic alkalosis for persistent pulmonary hypertension. Journal of Pediatrics 106: 527–528
74. Beck R, Anderson K D, Pearson G D, Cronin J, Miller M K, Short B L 1986 Criteria for extracorporeal membrane oxygenation in a population of infants with persistent pulmonary hypertension of the newborn. Journal of Pediatric Surgery 21: 297–302
75. Beddis I R, Silverman M 1980 Hypoxia in a neonate caused by intermittent positive pressure ventilation. Archives of Disease in Childhood 55: 403–405
76. Beeby P J, Elliott E J, Henderson-Smart D J, Rieger I D 1994 Predictive value of umbilical artery pH in preterm infants. Archives of Disease in Childhood 71: F93–F96
77. Beeram M R, Dhanireddy R 1992 Effects of saline instillation during tracheal suction on lung mechanics in newborn infants. Journal of Perinatology 12: 120–123
78. Beeram M R, Young M, Abedin M 1995 Effect of maternal illicit drug use on the mortality of very low birth weight infants. Journal of Perinatology 15: 546–460
79. Beierholm E A, Grantham N, O' Keefe D D, Laver M B, Daggett W M 1975 Effects of acid–base changes, hypoxia and catecholamines on ventricular performance. American Journal of Physiology 228: 1555–1561
80. Beitins I Z, Bayard F, Ances I G, Kowwarski A, Migeon C J 1972

The transplacental passage of prednisone and prednisolone in pregnancies near term. Journal of Pediatrics 81: 936–945
81. Bell A H, Skov L, Lundstrom K E, Saugstad O D, Griesen G 1994 Cerebral blood flow and plasma hypoxanthine in relation to surfactant treatment. Acta Paediatrica 83: 910–914
82. Bell E F, Warburton D, Stonestreet B S, Oh W 1980 Effect of fluid administration on the development of symptomatic patent ductus arteriosus and congestive heart failure in premature infants. New England Journal of Medicine 303: 598–604
82a. Benitz W B, Stevenson D K 1988 Refractory neonatal hypoxaemia: diagnostic evaluation and pharmacologic management. Resuscitation 16: 49–64
83. Benson B J 1993 Genetically engineered human pulmonary surfactant. Clinics in Perinatology 20: 791–811
84. Benveniste D, Berg O, Pederson J E P 1976 A technique for delivery of continuous positive pressure to the neonate. Journal of Pediatrics 88: 1015–1019
85. Berg T E, Pagtakhan R D, Reed M H, Langston C, Chernick V 1975 Bronchopulmonary dysplasia and lung rupture in hyaline membrane disease: influence of continuous distending pressure. Pediatrics 55: 51–53
86. Berger J I, Gibson R L, Redding G J 1993 Effect of inhaled nitric oxide during Group B streptococcal sepsis in piglets. American Review of Respiratory Disease 147: 1080–1086
87. Berger J T, Gilhooly J 1993 Fibrin glue treatment of persistent pneumothorax in a premature infant. Journal of Pediatrics 122: 958–960
88. Bernbaum J, Schwartz I P, Gerdes M, D'Agostino J A, Coburn C E, Polin R A 1995 Survivors of extracorporeal membrane oxygenation at 1 year of age: the relationship of primary diagnosis with health and neurodevelopmental sequelae. Pediatrics 96: 907–913
89. Bernstein G, Cleary J P, Heldt G P, Rossar F R, Shellemberg L D, Mannino F L 1993 Response time and reliability of three neonatal patient triggered ventilators. American Review of Respiratory Disease 148: 358–364
90. Bernstein G, Mannino F L, Heldt G P et al 1996 Randomized multicenter trial comparing synchronized and conventional intermittent mandatory ventilation in neonates. Journal of Pediatrics 128: 453–463
91. Berry D, Jobe A, Ikegami M, Seidner J, Pettenazzo A, Elkady T 1988 Pulmonary effects of acute prenatal asphyxia in ventilated premature lambs. Journal of Applied Physiology 65: 26–33
92. Berry D D, Pramanik A K, Phillips J E et al 1994 Comparison of the effect of three doses of a synthetic surfactant on the alveolar–arterial oxygen gradient in infants weighing ≥1250 grams with respiratory distress syndrome. Journal of Pediatrics 124: 294–301
93. Berseth C L 1995 Minimal enteral feedings. Clinics in Perinatology 22: 195–205
94. Beverley D W, Pitts-Tucker T J, Congdon P J, Arthur R J, Tate G 1985 Prevention of intraventricular haemorrhage by fresh frozen plasma. Archives of Disease in Childhood 60: 710–713
95. Bevilacqua G, Halliday H, Parmigiani S et al 1993 Randomized multicentre trial of treatment with porcine natural surfactant for moderately severe neonatal respiratory distress syndrome. Journal of Perinatal Medicine 21: 329–340
96. Bhat R, Malalis L, Shukla A, Vidyasagar D 1983 Colloid osmotic pressure in infants with hyaline membrane disease. Chest 83: 776–779
97. B-Horng So, Tamura M, Mishina J, Watanabe T, Kamoshita S 1995 Application of nasal continuous positive airway pressure to early extubation in very low birthweight infants. Archives of Disease in Childhood 72: F191–F193
98. Bhutani V, Abbasi S, Long W A, Gerdes J S 1992 Pulmonary mechanics and energetics in preterm infants who had respiratory distress syndrome treated with synthetic surfactant. Journal of Pediatrics 120: 518–524
99. Bhutani V K, Ritchie W G, Shaffer T H 1986 Acquired tracheomegaly in very preterm neonates. American Journal of Diseases of Children 140: 449–452
100. Bhutani V K, Sivieri E M, Abbasi S, Shaffer T H 1988 Evaluation of neonatal pulmonary mechanics and energetics. Pediatric Pulmonology 4: 150–158
101. Bhutani V K, Abbasi S, Silvieri E M 1988 Continuous skeletal muscle paralysis: effect on neonatal pulmonary mechanics. Pediatrics 81: 419–422
102. Bifano E M, Pfannenstiel A 1988 Duration of hyperventilation and outcome in infants with persistent pulmonary hypertension. Pediatrics 81: 657–661
103. Bignall S, Bailey P C, Bass C A, Cramb R, Rivers R P A, Wadsworth J 1989 The cardiovascular and oncotic effects of albumin infusion in premature infants. Early Human Development 20: 191–201
104. Bindl L, Fahnenstich H, Peukert U 1994 Aerosolized prostacyclin for pulmonary hypertension in neonates. Archives of Disease in Childhood 71: F214–F216
105. Bistritzer T, Hertzianu I, Lagstein R, Goldberg M, Lazebnik N, Aladjem M 1986 Cord blood insulin concentration in premature infants with respiratory distress syndrome. Journal of Pediatrics 108: 293–295
106. Bland R D 1972 Cord blood total protein level as a screening aid for the idiopathic respiratory distress syndrome. New England Journal of Medicine 287: 9–13
107. Bland R D 1982 Edema formation in the newborn lung. Clinics in Perinatology 9: 593–611
108. Bland R D 1992 Formation of fetal liquid and its removal near birth. In: Polin R A, Fox WW (eds) Fetal and neonatal physiology. W B Saunders Co, Philadelphia, pp. 782–789
109. Bland R D, Kim M H, Light M J, Woodson J L 1980 High frequency ventilation in severe hyaline membrane disease: an alternative therapy. Critical Care Medicine 8: 275–280
110. Block M R, Kallenberger D A, Kern J D, Nerveux D 1981 In utero meconium aspiration by the baboon fetus. Obstetrics and Gynecology 57: 37–40
111. Bloom M C, Roques-Gineste M, Fries F, Lelong-Tissier M C 1995 Pulmonary haemodynamics after surfactant replacement in severe neonatal respiratory distress syndrome. Archives of Disease in Childhood 73: F95–F98
112. Boddy K, Dawes G S 1975 Fetal breathing. British Medical Bulletin 31: 3–7
113. Bodmer B Benjamin A, McLean F, Usher R H 1986 Has the use of cesarean section reduced the risks of pregnancy in the preterm breech presentation? American Journal of Obstetrics and Gynecology 154: 244–250
114. Bolivar J M, Gerhardt T, Gonzalez A et al 1995 Mechanism for episodes of hypoxemia in preterm infants undergoing mechanical ventilation. Journal of Pediatrics 127: 767–773
115. Booth P, Nicolaides K H, Greenough A, Gamsu H R 1987 Pleuroamniotic shunting for fetal chylothorax. Early Human Development 15: 365–367
116. Boothby C B, de Sa D J 1973 Massive pulmonary haemorrhage in the newborn. Archives of Disease in Childhood 48: 21–30
117. Boros S J, Campbell K 1980 A comparison of the effects of high frequency–low tidal volume and low frequency–high tidal volume mechanical ventilation. Journal of Pediatrics 97: 108–112
118. Boros S J, Reynolds J W 1975 Hyaline membrane disease treated with early nasal end expiratory pressure: one year's experience. Pediatrics 56: 218–223
119. Boros S J, Matalon S, Ewald R, Leonard A, Hunt C 1977 The effect of independent variations in inspiratory expiratory ratio and expiratory pressure during mechanical ventilation in hyaline membrane disease. The significance of mean airway pressure. Journal of Pediatrics 91: 794–798
120. Boros S J, Bing D R, Mammel M C, Hagen E, Gordon M J 1984 Using conventional infant ventilators at unconventional rates. Pediatrics 74: 487–492
121. Boros S J, Mammel M C, Coleman J M et al 1985 Neonatal high frequency jet ventilation: four years' experience. Pediatrics 75: 657–663
122. Boston R W, Geller F, Smith C A 1966 Arterial blood gas tensions and acid base balance in management of respiratory distress syndrome. Journal of Pediatrics 68: 74–89
123. Bowen F W, Chandra R, Avery G B 1973 Pulmonary interstitial emphysema with gas embolism in hyaline membrane disease. American Journal of Diseases of Children 126: 117–118
124. Boynton B R, Mannino F L, Davis R F, Kopotic R J, Friedrichsen G 1984 Combined high-frequency oscillatory ventilation and intermittent mandatory ventilation in critically ill neonates. Journal of Pediatrics 105: 297–302
125. Bradley B S, Kumar S P, Mehta P N, Ezhuthachan S G 1994 Neonatal cushingoid syndrome resulting from serial courses of

antenatal betamethasone. American Journal of Obstetrics and Gynecology 83: 869–872
126. Brice J E, Walker C H 1977 Changing pattern of respiratory distress in the newborn. Lancet ii: 752–754
127. Brigham K L, Serafin W, Zadoff A, Blair I, Meyrick B, Oates J A 1988 Prostaglandin E_2 attenuation of sheep lung responses to endotoxin. Journal of Applied Physiology 64: 2568–2574
128. British Standards Institution 1970 Specifications for humidifiers for use with breathing machines. BS4494. London
129. Brion L P, Schwartz G J, Campbell D, Fleischman A R 1989 Early hyperkalaemia in very low birthweight infants in the absence of oliguria. Archives of Disease in Childhood 64: 270–272
130. Broadbent R, Fox T F, Dolovich M, et al 1995 Chest position and pulmonary deposition of surfactant in surfactant depleted rabbits. Archives of Disease in Childhood 72: F84–F89
131. Brodman R F, Zarelson T M, Schiebler G L 1974 Treatment of congenital chylothorax. Journal of Pediatrics 85: 516–520
132. Brooks J G, Bustamente S A, Koops B L 1977 Selective bronchial intubation for the treatment of severe localised pulmonary interstitial emphysema in newborn infants. Journal of Pediatrics 91: 648–652
133. Broughton Pipkin F, Smales O R C 1977 A study of factors affecting blood pressure and angiotensin II in newborn infants. Journal of Pediatrics 91: 113–119
134. Brown B L, Gleicher N 1981 Intrauterine meconium aspiration. Obstetrics and Gynecology 57: 26–29
135. Brown R, Pickering D 1974 Persistent transitional circulation. Archives of Disease in Childhood 49: 883–885
136. Brozanski B S, Jones J G, Gilmour C H et al 1995 Effect of pulse dexamethasone therapy on the incidence and severity of chronic lung disease in the very low birthweight infant. Journal of Pediatrics 126: 769–776
137. Bruce D A 1984 Effects of hyperventilation on cerebral blood flow and metabolism. Clinics in Perinatology 11: 673–680
138. Bryan C S 1967 Enhancement of bacterial infection by meconium. Johns Hopkins Medical Journal 121: 9–16
139. Bucciarelli R L, Egan E A, Gressner I H, Eitzman D V 1976 Persistence of fetal cardiopulmonary circulation. Manifestation of transient tachypnea of the newborn. Pediatrics 58: 192–197
140. Bucciarelli R L, Nelson R M, Egan E A, Eitzman M D, Gessner I H 1977 Transient tricuspid insufficiency of the newborn. A form of myocardial dysfunction in stressed newborns. Pediatrics 59: 330–337
141. Buckner P S, Todd D A, Lui K, John E 1991 Effect of short term muscle relaxation in neonatal plasma volume. Critical Care Medicine 19: 1357–1361
142. Bunton T E, Plopper C G 1984 Triamcinolone induced structural alterations in the development of the lung of the fetal rhesus Macaque. American Journal of Obstetrics and Gynecology 148: 203–215
143. Bureau M A, Begin R, Berthiaume Y 1979 Central chemical regulation of respiration in term newborn. Journal of Applied Physiology 47: 1212–1217
144. Burnard E D 1959 Changes in heart size in the dyspnoeic newborn infants. British Medical Journal i: 1495–1500
145. Burnard E D, James L S 1961 Failure of the heart after undue asphyxia at birth. Pediatrics 28: 545–565
146. Butler N R, Bonham D G 1963 Perinatal mortality. E & S Livingstone Edinburgh, p 197
147. Byrne D L, Gau G 1987 In utero meconium aspiration: an unpreventable cause of neonatal death. British Journal of Obstetrics and Gynaecology 94: 813–814
148. Cabal L A, Devaskar U, Siassi B, Hodgman J E, Emmanouilides G 1980 Cardiogenic shock associated with perinatal asphyxia in preterm infants. Journal of Pediatrics 96: 705–710
149. Callen P, Goldsworthy S, Graves I, Harvey D, Mellows H, Parkinson C 1979 Mode of delivery and the lecithin/sphingomyelin ratio. British Journal of Obstetrics and Gynaecology 86: 965–968
150. Campbell R E 1970 Intrapulmonary interstitial emphysema. A complication of hyaline membrane disease. American Journal of Radiology 110: 449–456
151. Canadian Preterm Labor Investigators Group 1992 Treatment of preterm labour with beta adrenergic agonist ritodrine. New England Journal of Medicine 327: 308–312
152. Carlo W A, Chatburn R L, Martin R J 1984 Decrease in airway pressure during high frequency jet ventilation versus conventional ventilation in infants with respiratory distress syndrome. Journal of Pediatrics 104: 101–107
153. Carlo W A, Chatburn R L, Martin R J 1987 Randomized trial of high frequency jet ventilation in respiratory distress syndrome. Journal of Pediatrics 110: 275–278
154. Carlo W A, Beoglos A, Chatburn R L, Walsh M C, Martin R J 1989 High frequency jet ventilation in neonatal pulmonary hypertension. American Journal of Diseases of Children 143: 233–238
155. Carlton D P, Cho S C, Davis P, Lont M, Bland R D 1995 Surfactant treatment at birth reduces lung vascular injury and edema in preterm lambs. Pediatric Research 37: 265–270
156. Carmant L, Le Guennec J-C 1989 Congenital chylothorax and persistent pulmonary hypertension of the newborn. Acta Paediatrica Scandinavica 78: 789–792
157. Carson B S, Losey R W, Bowes W W, Simmons M A 1976 Combined obstetric and pediatric approach to prevent meconium aspiration syndrome. American Journal of Obstetrics and Gynecology 126: 712–715
158. Cartlidge P H T, Rutter N 1986 Serum albumin concentrations and oedema in the newborn. Archives of Disease in Childhood 61: 657–660
159. Cartlidge P H T, Rutter N 1988 Percutaneous oxygen delivery to the preterm infant. Lancet i: 315–317
160. Cartwright D, Gregory G A, Lou H, Heyman M A 1984 The effect of hypocarbia on the cardiovascular system of puppies. Pediatric Research 18: 685–690
161. Cassin S, Dawes G S, Mott J C, Ross B B, Strang L B 1964 The vascular resistance of the fetal and newly ventilated lung of the lamb. Journal of Physiology 171: 61–79
162. Castillo L, de Rojas-Walker T, Yu YM et al 1995 Whole body arginine metabolism and nitric oxide synthesis in newborns with persistent pulmonary hypertension. Pediatric Research 38: 17–24
163. Castillo R A, Devoe L D, Falls G, Holzman G B, Hadi H A, Fadel H E 1987 Pleural effusions and pulmonary hypoplasia. American Journal of Obstetrics and Gynecology 157: 1252–1255
164. Cat R, Rosario N A, Taborda de Messias I 1993 Evaluation of complement activation in premature newborn infants with hyaline membrane disease. European Journal of Pediatrics 152: 205–208
165. Cater G, Thibeault D W, Beatty E C, Kilbride H W, Huntrakoon M 1989 Misalignment of lung vessels and alveolar capillary dysplasia: a cause of persistent pulmonary hypertension. Journal of Pediatrics 114: 293–300
166. Chamberlain R, Chamberlain G, Howlett B, Claireaux A 1975 British births 1970. Heinemann, London
167. Chan V, Greenough A 1992 Severe localized pulmonary interstitial emphysema – decompression by selective bronchial intubation. Journal of Perinatal Medicine 20: 313–316
168. Chan V, Greenough A 1993 Neonatal patient triggered ventilators. Performance in acute and chronic lung disease. British Journal of Intensive Care 3: 216–219
169. Chan V, Greenough A 1993 Randomised controlled trial of weaning by patient triggered ventilation or conventional ventilation. European Journal of Pediatrics 152: 51–54
170. Chan V, Greenough A 1993 Randomized trial of methods of extubation in acute and chronic respiratory distress. Archives of Disease in Childhood 68: 570–572
171. Chan V, Greenough A 1994 Comparison of weaning by patient triggered ventilation or synchronous mandatory intermittent ventilation. Acta Paediatrica 83: 335–337
172. Chan V, Greenough A 1994 The effect of frequency on carbon dioxide levels during high frequency oscillation. Journal of Perinatal Medicine 22: 103–106
173. Chan V, Greenough A, Milner A D 1993 The effect of frequency and mean airway pressure on volume delivery during high frequency oscillation. Pediatric Pulmonology 15: 183–186
174. Chan V, Greenough A, Muramatsu K 1994 Influence of lung function and reflex activity on the success of patient triggered ventilation. Early Human Development 37: 9–14
175. Chan V, Greenough A, Gamsu H R 1994 High frequency oscillation for preterm infants with severe respiratory failure. Archives of Disease in Childhood 70: F44–F46
176. Chan V, Greenough A, Dimitriou G 1995 High frequency oscillation, respiratory activity and changes in blood gases. Early Human Development 40: 87–94
177. Chan K N, Noble-Jamieson C M, Elliman A, Bryan E M, Silverman M 1989 Lung function in children of low birthweight. Archives of Disease in Childhood 64: 1284–1293

178. Chang H K 1984 Mechanisms of gas transport during ventilation by high frequency oscillation. Journal of Applied Physiology 56: 553–563
179. Chapman D L, Carlton D P, Neilson D W, Cummings J J, Poulain F R, Bland R D 1994 Changes in lung liquid during spontaneous labor in fetal sheep. Journal of Applied Physiology 76: 523–530
180. Charon A, Taeusch W, Fitzgibbon C, Smith G, Treves S, Phelps D 1989 Factors associated with surfactant treatment response in infants with severe respiratory distress syndrome. Pediatrics 83: 348–354
181. Chelliah B P, Brown D, Cohen M, Talleyrand A J, Shen-Schwarz S 1995 Alveolar capillary dysplasia – a cause of persistent pulmonary hypertension unresponsive to a second course of extracorporeal membrane oxygenation. Pediatrics 96: 1159–1161
182. Chen C M, Ikegami M, Ueda T, Polk D H, Jobe A H 1995 Fetal corticosteroid and T_4 treatment effects on lung function of surfactant treated preterm lambs. American Journal of Respiratory and Critical Care Medicine 151: 21–26
183. Chen Y, Sosenko I R S, Frank L 1995 Positive regulation of pulmonary antioxidant gene expression by prenatal thyrotropin releasing hormone plus dexamethasone treatment in premature rats exposed to hyperoxia. Pediatric Research 37: 611–616
184. Chen Y W, Whitney P L, Frank L 1993 Negative regulation of antioxidant gene expression in the developing fetal rat lung by prenatal hormonal treatments. Pediatric Research 33: 171–176
185. Chernick V, Avery M E 1963 Spontaneous alveolar rupture at birth. Pediatrics 32: 816–824
186. Chessels J M, Wigglesworth J S 1972 Coagulation studies in preterm infants with respiratory distress and intracranial haemorrhage. Archives of Disease in Childhood 47: 564–570
187. Chida S, Phelps D S, Soll R F, Taeusch H W 1991 Surfactant proteins and anti-surfactant antibodies in sera from infants with respiratory distress syndrome with and without surfactant treatment. Pediatrics 88: 84–89
188. Chida S, Tujiwara T, Konishi M et al 1993 Stable microbubble test for predicting the risk of respiratory distress syndrome. European Journal of Pediatrics 152: 152–156
189. Chiswick M L, Milner R D G 1976 Crying vital capacity measurement of neonatal lung function. Archives of Disease in Childhood 51: 22–27
190. Cilley R E, Zwischenberger J B, Andrews A F, Bowerman R A, Roloff D W, Bartlett R H 1986 Intracranial hemorrhage during extracorporeal membrane oxygenation in neonates. Pediatrics 78: 699–704
191. Clark D A, Nieman G F, Thompson J E, Paskanik A M, Rokhar J E, Bredenberg C E 1987 Surfactant displacement by meconium free fatty acids: an alternative explanation for atelectasis in meconium aspiration syndrome. Journal of Pediatrics 110: 765–770
192. Clark J M, Lambertsen C J 1971 Pulmonary oxygen toxicity. Pharmacology Review 23: 37–133
193. Clark L C, Gollan F 1966 Survival of mammals breathing organic liquids equilibrated with oxygen at atmospheric pressure. Science 152: 1756
194. Clark P, Duff P 1995 Inhibition of neutrophil oxidative burst and phagocytosis by meconium. American Journal of Obstetrics and Gynecology 173: 1301–1305
195. Clark R H, Gerstmann D R, Null D N et al 1986 Pulmonary interstitial emphysema treated by high frequency oscillatory ventilation. Critical Care Medicine 14: 926–930
196. Clark R H, Gerstmann D R, Null D M, deLemos R A 1992 Prospective randomized comparison of high frequency oscillatory and conventional ventilation in respiratory distress syndrome. Pediatrics 89: 5–12
197. Clark R H, Yoder B A, Sell M S 1994 Prospective randomized comparisons of high frequency oscillation and conventional ventilation in candidates for extracorporeal membrane oxygenation. Journal of Pediatrics 124: 447–454
198. Cleary J P, Bernstein G, Mannino F L, Heldt G P 1995 Improved oxygenation during synchronized intermittent mandatory ventilation in neonates with respiratory distress syndrome: a randomized crossover study. Journal of Pediatrics 126: 407–411
199. Clifford R D, Whincup G, Thomas R 1988 Patient triggered ventilation prevents pneumothoraces in premature babies. Lancet i: 529–530
200. Clyman R I 1996 Recommendations for the postnatal use of indomethacin: an analysis of four separate treatment strategies. Journal of Pediatrics 128: 601–607
201. Clyman R I, Brett C, Mauray F 1980 Circulating prostaglandin E_2 concentrations and incidence of patent ductus arteriosus in preterm infants with respiratory distress syndrome. Pediatrics 66: 725–729
202. Cochrane C G, Revak D S, Merritt T A et al 1996 The efficacy and safety of KL_4 surfactant in preterm infants with respiratory distress syndrome. American Journal of Respiratory and Critical Care Medicine 153: 404–410
202a. Cochrane Injuries Group Albumin Reviewers 1998 Human albumin administration in critically ill patients: systematic review of randomised controlled trials. British Medical Journal 317: 235–240
203. Cockburn F, Cooke R W I, Gamsu H R 1993 The CRIB (Clinical Risk Index for Babies) score: a tool for assessing initial neonatal risk and comparing performance of neonatal intensive care units. Lancet 342: 193–198
204. Cohen G R, Thorp J, Yeast J D, Meyer B A, O'Kell R, Macy C 1991 A markedly immature lecithin sphingomyelin ratio at term and congenital hypothyroidism. American Journal of Diseases of Children 145: 1227–1228
205. Cohen M, Carson B S 1985 Respiratory morbidity benefit of awaiting onset of labour after elective caesarean section. Obstetrics and Gynecology 65: 818–824
206. Cohen R S, Smith D W, Stevenson D K, Moskowitz P S, Graham C B 1984 Lateral decubitus position as therapy for persistent pulmonary interstitial emphysema in neonates: a preliminary report. Journal of Pediatrics 104: 441–443
207. Cohen R S, Stevenson D K, Malachowski N, Ariagno R L, Johnson J D, Sunshine P 1980 Late morbidity among survivors of respiratory failure treated with tolazoline. Journal of Pediatrics 97: 644–647
208. Cole J W, Portman R J, Lim Y, Perlman J M, Robson A M 1985 Urinary β_2-microglobulin in full term newborns: evidence for proximal tubular dysfunction in infants with meconium stained amniotic fluid. Pediatrics 76: 958–964
209. Cole V A, Normand I C S, Reynolds E O R et al 1973 Pathogenesis of hemorrhagic pulmonary edema and massive pulmonary hemorrhage in the newborn. Pediatrics 51: 175–187
210. Colice G L 1992 Resolution of laryngeal injury following translaryngeal intubation. American Review of Respiratory Disease 145: 361–364
211. Colice G L, Matthay M A, Bass E, Matthay R A 1984 Neurogenic pulmonary edema. American Review of Respiratory Disease 130: 941–948
212. Collaborative European Multicentre Study Group 1991 Factors influencing the clinical response to surfactant replacement therapy in babies with severe respiratory distress syndrome. European Journal of Pediatrics 150: 433–439
212a. Collaborative Santiago Surfactant Group 1998 Collaborative trial of prenatal thyrotropin-releasing hormone and corticosteroids for prevention of respiratory distress syndrome. American Journal of Obstetrics and Gynecology 178: 33–39
213. Coltart T M, Byrne D L, Bates S A 1989 Meconium aspiration syndrome: a 6 year retrospective study. British Journal of Obstetrics and Gynaecology 96: 411–414
214. Cook C D, Sutherland J M, Segal S et al 1957 Studies of respiratory physiology in the newborn infant. III. Measurements of the mechanics of respiration. Journal of Clinical Investigation 36: 440–448
215. Cooke R W I 1987 Early and late cranial ultrasonographic appearances and outcome in very low birthweight infants. Archives of Disease in Childhood 62: 931–937
216. Cooke R W I, Rennie J M 1984 Pancuronium and pneumothorax. Lancet i: 286–287
217. Cooke R W I, Gribbin B, Gunning A J, Pickering D 1978 Ligation of patent ductus arteriosus in the very low birthweight newborn infant. Archives of Disease in Childhood 53: 271–275
218. Corbet A 1993 Clinical trials of synthetic surfactant in the respiratory distress syndrome of premature infants. Clinics in Perinatology 20: 737–760
219. Corbet A, Bucciarelli R, Goldman S, Mammel M, Wold D, Long W 1991 Decreased mortality rate among small premature infants treated at birth with a single dose of synthetic surfactant. A multicenter controlled trial. Journal of Pediatrics 118: 277–284

220. Corbet A, Gerdes J, Long W et al 1995 Double-blind randomized trial of one versus three prophylactic doses of synthetic surfactant in 826 neonates weighing 700–1000 grams: effects on mortality rate. Journal of Pediatrics 126: 969–978
221. Corbet A J S, Burnard E D 1972 Changes of venous admixture with inspired oxygen in hyaline membrane disease and foetal aspiration pneumonia. Australian Paediatric Journal 9: 25–30
222. Cordier M P, Gaultier C L, Boule M 1984 Infants with meconium aspiration syndrome: follow-up study. American Review of Respiratory Disease 129: 218 (abstract)
223. Cornblath M, Schwartz R 1976 Disorders of carbohydrate metabolism in infancy. W B Saunders, Philadelphia, pp 82–83
224. Costarino A T, Baumgart S, Norman M E, Polin R A 1985 Renal adaptation to extrauterine life in patients with respiratory distress syndrome. American Journal of Diseases of Children 139: 1060–1063
225. Cotton R B, Olsson T, Law A B et al 1993 The physiological effects of surfactant treatment on gas exchange in newborn premature infants with hyaline membrane disease. Pediatric Research 34: 495–501
226. Coulthard M G, Sharp J 1995 Haemodialysis and ultrafiltration in babies weighing under 1000 g. Archives of Disease in Childhood 73: F162–F165
227. Couser R J, Ferrara T B, Falde B et al 1992 Effectiveness of dexamethasone in preventing extubation failure in preterm infants at increased risk for airway edema. Journal of Pediatrics 121: 591–596
228. Cowan F, Whitelaw A, Wertheim D, Silverman M 1991 Cerebral blood flow velocity changes after rapid administration of surfactant. Archives of Disease in Childhood 66: 1105–1109
229. Crowley M R, Fineman J R, Soier S J 1991 Effect of vasoactive drugs on thromboxane A_2 mimetic-induced pulmonary hypertension in newborn lambs. Pediatric Research 29: 167–172
230. Crowley P A 1995 Antenatal corticosteroid therapy. A meta-analysis of the randomized trials 1972–1994. American Journal of Obstetrics and Gynecology 173: 322–335
231. Cuestas R A, Lindall A, Engel R R 1976 Low thyroid hormones and respiratory distress syndrome of the newborn. New England Journal of Medicine 295: 297–302
232. Cummings J J, Holm B A, Hudak M L, Hudak B B, Ferguson W H, Egan E A 1992 A controlled clinical comparison of four different surfactant preparations in surfactant deficient preterm lambs. American Review of Respiratory Disease 145: 999–1004
233. Cunningham M D, Desai N S, Thompson S A, Greene J M 1978 Amniotic fluid phosphatidylglycerol in diabetic pregnancies. American Journal of Obstetrics and Gynecology 131: 719–724
234. Curry C J R, Chopra D, Finer N N 1988 Hydrops and pleural effusions in congenital myotonic dystrophy. Journal of Pediatrics 113: 555–557
235. Curtis J, O'Neill J J, Pettet G 1993 Endotracheal administration of tolazoline in hypoxia induced pulmonary hypertension. Pediatrics 92: 403–408
236. Curtis J, Palacino J J, O'Neil J J 1996 Production of pulmonary vasodilation by tolazoline, independent of nitric oxide production in neonatal lambs. Journal of Pediatrics 128: 118–124
237. Cusick W, Smulian J C, Vintzileos A M 1995 Intrapartum use of fetal heart rate monitoring, contraction monitoring and amnioinfusion. Clinics in Perinatology 22: 875–906
238. Cvetnic W G, Waffarn F, Martin J M 1989 Continuous negative pressure and intermittent mandatory ventilation in the management of pulmonary interstitial emphysema. Journal of Perinatology 9: 26–32
239. Cvetnic W G, Cunningham M D, Sills J H, Gluck L 1990 Reintroduction of continuous negative pressure ventilation in neonates: two-year experience. Pediatric Pulmonology 8: 245–253
240. Cyr R M, Usher R H, Mclean F H 1984 Changing patterns of birth asphyxia and trauma over 20 years. American Journal of Obstetrics and Gynecology 148: 490–498
241. Daniel S S, Adamsons K, James L S 1966 Lactate and pyruvate as an index of prenatal oxygen deprivation. Pediatrics 37: 942–953
242. da Silva W J, Abbasi S, Pereira G, Bhutani V K 1994 Role of positive end expiratory pressure changes on functional residual capacity in surfactant treated preterm infants. Pediatric Pulmonology 18: 89–92
243. Davies A M, Koenig J S, Thach B T 1989 Characteristics of upper airway chemoreflex prolonged apnea in human infants. American Review of Respiratory Disease 139: 668–673
244. Davis G M, Bureau M A 1987 Pulmonary and chest wall mechanics in the control of respiration in the newborn. Clinics in Perinatology 14: 551–579
245. Davis J A, Stafford A 1964 Respiratory distress in newborn rabbits. Biologia Neonatorum 7: 129–140
246. Davis J M, Whitin J 1992 Prophylactic effects of dexamethasone in lung injury caused by hyperoxia and hyperventilation. Journal of Applied Physiology 72: 1320–1325
247. Davis J M, Richter S E, Kendig J W, Notter R H 1992 High frequency jet ventilation and surfactant treatment of newborns with severe respiratory failure. Pediatric Pulmonology 13: 108–112
248. Davis J M, Russ G A, Metlay L, Dickerson B, Greenspan B S 1992 Short-term distribution kinetics of intratracheally administered exogenous lung surfactant. Pediatric Research 31: 445–450
249. Davis R O, Phillips J B, Harris B A, Wilson E R, Huddleston J F 1985 Fatal meconium aspiration syndrome occurring despite airway management considered appropriate. American Journal of Obstetrics and Gynecology 151: 731–736
250. Davis W B, Rennard S I, Bitterman P B, Crystal R G 1983 Early reversible changes in human alveolar structures induced by hyperoxia. New England Journal of Medicine 309: 878–883
251. Dawes G S, Mott J C 1962 The vascular tone of the fetal lung. Journal of Physiology 164: 465–477
252. Dawes G S, Fox H E, LeDuc B M, Liggins G C, Richards R T 1972 Respiratory movements and rapid eye movement in the fetal lamb. Journal of Physiology 220: 119–143
253. Dehan M, Francoual J, Lindenbaum A 1978 Diagnosis of meconium aspiration by spectrophotometric analysis of urine. Archives of Disease in Childhood 53: 74–76
254. Dekowski S A, Snyder J M 1992 Insulin regulation of messenger ribonucleic acid for the surfactant-associated protein in human fetal lung in vitro. Endocrinology 131: 669–676
255. DeLemos R A, Coalson J J, Gerstmann D R, Kuehl T J, Null D M 1987 Oxygen toxicity in the premature baboon with hyaline membrane disease. American Review of Respiratory Disease 136: 677–682
256. DeLemos R A, Gerstmann D R, Clark R H, Guajardo A, Null D M 1987 High frequency ventilation—the relationship between the ventilator design and clinical strategy in the treatment of hyaline membrane disease and its complications: a brief review. Pediatric Pulmonology 3: 370–372
257. De Los Santos R, Seidenfeld J J, Anzueto A et al 1987 One hundred percent oxygen lung injury in adult baboons. American Review of Respiratory Disease 136: 657–661
258. DeSa D J 1983 Mucosal metaplasia and chronic inflammation in the middle ear of infants receiving intensive care in the neonatal period. Archives of Disease in Childhood 58: 24–28
259. de Winter J P, Merth I T, van Bel F, Egberts J, Brand R, Quanjer P H 1994 Changes in respiratory system mechanics in ventilated lungs of preterm infants with two different schedules of treatment. Pediatric Research 35: 541–549
260. Dhanireddy R, Smith Y F, Hamosh M et al 1983 Respiratory distress syndrome in the newborn: relationship to serum prolactin, thyroxine and sex. Biology of the Neonate 43: 9–15
261. Dillard R G 1980 Mean airway pressure calculations. Journal of Pediatrics 97: 506–507
262. Dimitriou G, Greenough A 1995 Measurement of lung volume and optimization of oxygenation during high frequency oscillation. Archives of Disease in Childhood 72: F180–F183
263. Dimitriou G, Greenough A, Giffin F J, Karani J 1995 The appearance of early chest radiographs and the response to surfactant replacement therapy. British Journal of Radiology 68: 1177–1180
264. Dimitriou G, Greenough A, Giffin F, Chan V 1995 Synchronous intermittent mandatory ventilation modes versus patient triggered ventilation during weaning. Archives of Disease in Childhood 72: F188–F190
265. Dimitriou G, Greenough A, Kavadia V 1997 Changes in lung volume, compliance and oxygenation in the first 48 hours of life in infants given surfactant. Journal of Perinatal Medicine 25: 49–54
266. Dimitriou G, Greenough A, Castling D, Kavadia V 1996 A comparison of supine and prone positioning in oxygen dependent and convalescent premature infants. British Journal of Intensive Care 6: 254–259
267. Dinner M, Tjeuw M, Artusio J F 1987 Bacteremia as a complication of nasotracheal intubation. Anesthesia and Analgesia 66: 460–462

268. Dobbie H G, Whittle M J, Wilson A I, Whitfield C R 1983 Amniotic fluid phospholipid profile in multiple pregnancy and the effect of zygosity. British Journal of Obstetrics and Gynaecology 90: 1001–1006
269. Dobyns E L, Wescott J Y, Kennaugh J M, Ross M N, Stenmark K R 1994 Eicosanoids decrease with successful extracorporeal membrane oxygenation therapy in neonatal pulmonary hypertension. American Journal of Respiratory and Critical Care Medicine 149: 873–880
270. Dooley S L, Pesavento D J, Depp R, Socol M L, Tamura R K, Wiringa K S 1985 Meconium below the cords at delivery: correlation with intrapartum events. American Journal of Obstetrics and Gynecology 153: 767–770
271. Doyle L W, Kitchen W H, Ford G W, Rickards A L, Lissenden J V, Ryan M M 1986 Effects of antenatal steroid therapy on mortality and morbidity in very low birthweight infants. Journal of Pediatrics 108: 287–292
272. Doyle L W, Kitchen W H, Ford G W, Richards A L, Kelly E A 1989 Antenatal steroid therapy and 5 year outcome of extremely low birthweight infants. Obstetrics and Gynecology 73: 743–746
273. Dreizzen E, Migdal M, Praud J P et al 1988 Passive compliance of total respiratory system in preterm newborn infants with respiratory distress syndrome. Journal of Pediatrics 112: 778–781
274. Drew J H 1982 Immediate intubation at birth of the very low birthweight infant. American Journal of Diseases of Children 136: 207–210
275. Driscoll D J 1987 Use of inotropic and chronotropic agents in neonates. Clinics in Perinatology 14: 931–949
276. Driscoll S G, Smith C A 1962 Neonatal pulmonary disorders. Pediatric Clinics of North America 9: 325–352
277. Drummond W H, Bissonette J M 1978 Persistent pulmonary hypertension in the neonate. Development of an animal model. American Journal of Obstetrics and Gynecology 131: 761–763
278. Drummond W H, Gregory G A, Heyman M A, Phibbs R A 1981 The independent effects of hyperventilation, tolazoline and dopamine on infants with persistent pulmonary hypertension. Journal of Pediatrics 98: 603–611
279. Duara S, Fox W W 1986 Persistent pulmonary hypertension of the neonate. In Thibeault D W, Gregory G A (eds) Neonatal pulmonary care, 2nd Edn. Appleton Century Crofts, Norwalk, CT, pp 461–481
280. Duara S, Gewitz M H, Fox W W 1984 Use of mechanical ventilation for clinical management of persistent pulmonary hypertension of the newborn. Clinics in Perinatology 11: 641–652
281. Dudell G G, Gersony W M 1984 Patent ductus arteriosus in neonates with severe respiratory disease. Journal of Pediatrics 104: 915–920
282. Dunn L, Hulman S, Weiner J, Kliegman R 1988 Beneficial effects of early hypocaloric enteral feeding on neonatal gastrointestinal function. Journal of Pediatrics 112: 622–629
283. Dunn M S, Shennan A T, Zayack D, Possmayer F 1991 Bovine surfactant replacement therapy in neonates of less than 30 weeks' gestation: a randomized controlled trial of prophylaxis versus treatment. Pediatrics 87: 377–386
284. Dunn P M 1963 Intestinal obstruction in the newborn with special reference to transient functional ileus associated with respiratory distress syndrome. Archives of Disease in Childhood 38: 459–467
285. Durand D J, Goodman A, Ray P, Ballard R A, Clyman R I 1987 Theophylline treatment in the extubation of infants weighing less than 1250 grams. A controlled trial. Pediatrics 80: 684–688
286. Durbin G M, Hunter N J, McIntosh N, Reynolds E O R, Wimberley P D 1976 Controlled trial of continuous inflating pressure for hyaline membrane disease. Archives of Disease in Childhood 51: 163–169
287. Durmowicz A G, Stenmark K R 1996 Alterations in extracellular matrix protein expression in neonatal pulmonary hypertension: implications for vascular function. Journal of Perinatology 16: S11–S18
288. Edberg K E, Sandberg K, Silberberg A 1991 Lung volumes, gas mixing and mechanics of breathing in mechanically ventilated very low birth weight infants with idiopathic respiratory distress syndrome. Pediatric Research 30: 496–500
289. Edwards A D 1995 The pharmacology of inhaled nitric oxide. Archives of Disease in Childhood. 72: F127–F130
290. Edwards A D, McCormick D C, Roth S C et al 1992 Cerebral hemodynamic effects of treatment with modified natural surfactant investigated by near infrared spectroscopy. Pediatric Research 32: 532–536
291. Edwards D K, Hilton S V W, Merritt T A, Hallman M, Mannino F, Boynton B R 1985 Respiratory distress syndrome treated with human surfactant. Radiographic findings. Radiology 157: 329–334
292. Egberts J, de Winter J P, Sedin G 1993 Comparison of prophylaxis and rescue treatment with Curosurf in neonates less than 30 weeks' gestation: a randomized trial. Pediatrics 92: 768–774
293. Emery E F, Greenough A 1993 Randomized trial of two inotropes in preterm infants. European Journal of Pediatrics 152: 1–3
294. Emery E F, Greenough A, Gamsu H R 1992 Randomized controlled trial of colloid infusions in hypotensive preterm infants. Archives of Disease in Childhood 67: 1185–1188
295. Emmanouilides G C, Moss A J 1971 Respiratory distress in the newborn. Effects of cord clamping before and after onset of respiration. Biology of the Neonate 18: 363–368
296. Engle W D, Arant B S, Wiriyathian S, Rosenfeld C R 1983 Diuresis and respiratory distress syndrome. Journal of Pediatrics 103: 912–917
297. Enhorning G, Shennan A, Possmayer F, Dunn M, Chen C P, Milligan J 1985 Prevention of neonatal respiratory distress syndrome by tracheal instillation of surfactant. A randomized clinical trial. Pediatrics 76: 145–153
298. Enskog A, Bengtsson A, Bengtson J P, Heideman M, Andreasson S, Larsson L 1996 Complement anaphylatoxin C3a and C5a formation in premature children with respiratory distress. European Journal of Pediatrics 155: 41–45
299. Eronen M, Kari A, Pesonen E, Hallman M 1993 The effect of antenatal dexamethasone administration on the fetal and neonatal ductus arteriosus. American Journal of Diseases of Children 147: 187–192
300. Esterley J R, Oppenheimer E H 1966 Massive pulmonary hemorrhage in the newborn. I. Pathologic considerations. Journal of Pediatrics 69: 3–11
301. Evans M E, Schaffner W, Federspiel C F, Cotton R B, McKee K T, Stratton C W 1988 Sensitivity, specificity and predictive value of body surface cultures in a neonatal intensive care unit. Journal of the American Association 259: 248–252
302. Evans N, Kluckow M 1996 Early determinants of right and left ventricular output in ventilated preterm infants. Archives of Disease in Childhood 74: F88–F94
303. Evans N J, Archer L N J 1991 Doppler assessment of pulmonary artery pressure during recovery from hyaline membrane disease. Archives of Disease in Childhood 66: 802–804
304. Evans N J, Archer L N J 1991 Doppler measurement of pulmonary artery pressure and extrapulmonary shunting in the acute phase of hyaline membrane disease. Archives of Disease in Childhood 66: 6–11
305. Evans N J, Iyer P 1994 Incompetence of the foramen ovale in preterm infants supported by mechanical ventilation. Journal of Pediatrics 125: 786–792
306. Evans N J, Rutter N 1986 Percutaneous respiration in the newborn infant. Journal of Pediatrics 108: 282–286
307. Fadel H E, Saad S A, Nelson G H, Davis H C 1986 Effect of maternal fetal disorders on lung maturation. I. Diabetes mellitus. American Journal of Obstetrics and Gynecology 155: 544–553
308. Faix R G, Viscardi R M, Dipietro M A, Nicks J J 1989 Adult respiratory distress syndrome in full term newborns. Pediatrics 83: 171–176
309. Falciglia H S 1988 Failure to prevent meconium aspiration syndrome. Obstetrics and Gynecology 71: 249–253
310. Fanconi S, Duc G 1987 Intratracheal suction in sick preterm infants: prevention of intracranial hypertension and cerebral hypoperfusion by muscle paralysis. Pediatrics 79: 538–543
311. Farrell P M 1986 Nutrition and infant lung function. Pediatric Pulmonology 2: 44–59
312. Farrell P M, Avery M E 1975 State of the art. HMD. American Review of Respiratory Disease 111: 657–688
313. Fedrick J, Butler N R 1970 Certain causes of neonatal death. I. Hyaline membranes. Biology of the Neonate 15: 229–255
314. Fedrick J, Butler N R 1971 Certain causes of neonatal death. IV. Massive pulmonary haemorrhage. Biology of the Neonate 18: 243–262
315. Ferrara B, Johnson D E, Chang P N, Thompson T R 1984 Efficacy and neurological outcome of profound hypocapnic alkalosis for the treatment of persistent pulmonary hypertension in infancy. Journal of Pediatrics 105: 457–461

316. Ferrara T B, Hoekstra R E, Couser R J 1994 Survival and follow up of infants born at 23–26 weeks of gestational age: effects of surfactant therapy. Journal of Pediatrics 124: 119–124
317. Fiascone J M, Hu L-M, Vreeland P N 1992 Terbutaline does not improve lung function in preterm infants. American Journal of Obstetrics and Gynecology 167: 847–853
318. Field D, Milner A, Hopkin I E 1985 Effects of positive end expiratory pressure during ventilation of the preterm infant. Archives of Disease in Childhood 60: 843–847
319. Field D J, Milner A D, Hopkin I E 1985 Calculation of mean airway pressure during neonatal intermittent positive pressure ventilation. Pediatric Pulmonology 1: 141–144
320. Field D J, Milner A D, Hopkin I E 1985 Manipulation of ventilator settings to prevent active expiration against positive pressure inflation. Archives of Disease in Childhood 60: 1036–1040
321. Field D J, Milner A D, Hopkin I 1985 Inspiratory time and tidal volume during high frequency positive pressure ventilation. Archives of Disease in Childhood 60: 259–261
322. Field D J, Milner A D, Hopkin I E, Madeley R J 1987 Changing patterns in neonatal respiratory disease. Pediatric Pulmonology 3: 231–235
323. Findlay R D, Taeusch H W, Walther F J 1996 Surfactant replacement therapy for meconium aspiration syndrome. Pediatrics 97: 48–52
324. Finer N N, Etches P C, Kamstra B, Tierney A J, Peliowski A, Ryan C A 1994 Inhaled nitric oxide in infants referred for extracorporeal membrane oxygenation: dose response. Journal of Pediatrics 124: 302–308
325. Finer N N, Moriartey R R, Boyd J, Phillips H J, Stewart A R, Ulan O 1979 Post-extubation atelectasis: a retrospective review and prospective controlled study. Journal of Pediatrics 94: 110–113
326. Finley J P, Howwman-Giles R B, Gilday D L, Bloom K R, Rowe R D 1979 Transient myocardial ischemia of the newborn infant demonstrated by thallium myocardial imaging. Journal of Pediatrics 94: 263–270
327. Fleisher B, Kulovich M V, Hallman M, Gluck L 1985 Lung profile: sex difference in normal pregnancy. Obstetrics and Gynecology 66: 327–330
328. Fletcher B D, Sachs B F, Kotas R V 1970 Radiological demonstration of post-natal liquid in the lungs of newborn lambs. Pediatrics 46: 252–258
329. Fletcher D B, Outerbridge G E, Youssef S 1974 Pulmonary interstitial emphysema in a newborn infant treated by lobectomy. Pediatrics 54: 808–811
330. Florman A L, Teubner D 1969 Enhancement of bacterial growth in amniotic fluid by meconium. Journal of Pediatrics 74: 111–114
331. Fouron J C, Bard H, Riopel L, deMuylder X, van Ameringer M-R, Urfer F 1985 Circulatory changes in newborn lambs with experimental polycythemia: comparison between fetal and adult type blood. Pediatrics 75: 1054–1060
332. Fowlie P W 1996 Prophylactic indomethacin: systemic review and meta-analysis. Archives of Disease in Childhood 74: F81–F87
333. Fox W W 1982 Mechanical ventilation in the management of persistent pulmonary hypertension of the neonate (PPHN). 83rd Ross Conference on Paediatric Research: Cardiovascular Sequelae of Asphyxia in the Newborn. Columbus, OH, Ross Laboratories, p 102
334. Fox W W, Duara S 1983 Persistent pulmonary hypertension in the neonate. Diagnosis and management. Journal of Pediatrics 103: 505–514
335. Fox W W, Berman L S, Downes J J, Peckham G J 1975 The therapeutic application of end-expiratory pressure in the meconium aspiration syndrome. Pediatrics 56: 214–216
336. Fox W W, Gewitz M H, Dinwiddie R, Drummond W H, Peckham G J 1977 Pulmonary hypertension in the perinatal aspiration syndromes. Pediatrics 59: 205–211
337. Fox W W, Schwartz J G, Shaffer T H 1978 Pulmonary physiotherapy, in neonates: physiologic changes and respiratory management. Journal of Pediatrics 92: 977–981
338. Fox W W, Spiker A R, Musci M 1984 Tracheal secretion impaction during hyperventilation for persistent pulmonary hypertension of the neonate (abstract). Pediatric Research 18: 323
339. Frank L 1992 Prenatal dexamethasone treatment improves survival of newborn rats during prolonged high oxygen exposure. Pediatric Research 32: 215–221
340. Frank L, Sosenko IRS 1991 Failure of premature rabbits to increase antioxidant enzymes during hyperoxic exposure: increased susceptibility to pulmonary oxygen toxicity compared with term rabbits. Pediatric Research 29: 292–296
341. Frank L, Noack W, Lunkenheimer P P et al 1975 Light and electron microscopic investigations of pulmonary tissue after high frequency positive pressure ventilation (HFPPV). Anaesthetist 24: 171–176
342. Frank L, Bucher J R, Roberts R J 1978 Oxygen toxicity in neonatal and adult animals of various species. Journal of Applied Physiology 45: 699–704
343. Frank M M, Gatewood, O M B 1966 Transient pharyngeal incoordination in the newborn. American Journal of Diseases of Children 111: 178–181
344. Franklin R C, Purdie G L, O'Grady C M 1986 Neonatal thyroid function: prematurity, prenatal steroids and respiratory distress syndrome. Archives of Disease in Childhood 61: 589–592
345. Frantz I D, Close R H 1985 Elevated lung volume and alveolar pressure during jet ventilation of rabbits. American Review of Respiratory Disease 131: 134–138
346. Frantz I D, Wang N S, Thach B T 1975 Experimental meconium aspiration: effects of glucocorticoid treatment. Journal of Pediatrics 86: 434–441
347. Frantz I D, Werthammer J, Stark A R 1983 High frequency ventilation in premature infants with lung disease: adequate gas exchange at low tracheal pressure. Pediatrics 71: 483–488
348. Fried R, Reid L 1984 Early recovery from hypoxic pulmonary hypertension: a structural and functional study. Journal of Applied Physiology 57: 1247–1253
349. Friedman S A, Schiff E, Kao L, Sibai B M 1995 Neonatal outcome after preterm delivery for pre-eclampsia. American Journal of Obstetrics and Gynecology 172: 1785–1792
350. Friedman Z, Rosenberg A 1979 Abnormal lung surfactant related to essential fatty acid deficiency in a neonate. Pediatrics 63: 855–859
350a. Friesen R H, Honda A T, Thieme R E 1987 Changes in anterior fontanelle pressure in preterm neonates during tracheal intubation. Anesthesia and Analgesia 66: 874–878
351. Froese A B, Bryan A C 1987 High frequency ventilation. American Review of Respiratory Disease 135: 1363–1374
352. Fuchimukai T, Fujiwara T, Takahishi A, Enhorning G 1987 Artificial pulmonary surfactant inhibited by proteins. Journal of Applied Physiology 62: 429–437
353. Fujimura A, Salisbury D M, Robinson R O et al 1979 Clinical events relating to intraventricular haemorrhage in the newborn. Archives of Disease in Childhood 54: 409–414
354. Fujiwara T, Konishi M, Chida S, Maeta H 1988 Factors affecting the response to a postnatal single dose of a reconstituted bovine surfactant (surfactant T A) In: Lachmann B (ed) Surfactant replacement therapy. Springer, Berlin, pp 91–107
355. Fysh W J, Turner G M, Dunn P M 1982 Neurological normality after extreme birth asphyxia. Case report. British Journal of Obstetrics and Gynaecology 89: 24–26
356. Gage J E, Taeusch H W, Treves S, Caldicott W 1981 Suctioning of upper airway meconium in newborn infants. Journal of the American Medical Association 246: 2590–2592
357. Gandy G, Jacobson W, Gairdner D 1970 Hyaline membrane disease. I. Cellular changes. Archives of Disease in Childhood 45: 289–310
358. Gappa M, Costeloe K, Southall D P, Rabbette P S, Stocks J 1994 Effect of continuous negative extrathoracic pressure on respiratory mechanics and timing in infants recovering from neonatal respiratory distress syndrome. Pediatric Research 36: 364–372
359. Gardner M O, Goldenberg R L, Gaudier F L, Dubard M B, Nelson K G, Hauth J C 1995 Predicting low Apgar scores of infants weighing less than 1000 grams: the effect of corticosteroids. Obstetrics and Gynecology 85: 170–174
360. Garite J J, Rumney P J, Briggs G G et al 1992 A randomized placebo-controlled trial of betamethasone for the prevention of respiratory distress syndrome at 24–28 weeks' gestation. American Journal of Obstetrics and Gynecology 166: 646–651
361. Garland J, Buck R, Weinberg M 1994 Pulmonary hemorrhage risk in infants with a clinically diagnosed patent ductus arteriosus. A retrospective cohort study. Pediatrics 94: 719–723
362. Garland J S, Buck R K, Allred E N, Leviton A 1995 Hypocarbia before surfactant therapy appears to increase bronchopulmonary

dysplasia risk in infants with respiratory distress syndrome. Archives of Pediatrics and Adolescent Medicine 149: 617–622

363. Garland J S, Buck R, Leviton A 1995 Effect of maternal glucocorticoid exposure on risk of severe intraventricular hemorrhage in surfactant treated preterm infants. Journal of Pediatrics 126: 272–279

363a. Garland J S, Nelson D B, Rice T, Neu J 1985 Increased risk of gastrointestinal perforations in neonates mechanically ventilated with either face mask or nasal prongs. Pediatrics 76: 406–410

364. Gau G S, Ryder T A, Mobberley M A 1987 Iatrogenic epithelial change caused by endotracheal intubation of neonates. Early Human Development 15: 221–229

365. Gauger P G, Pranikoff T, Schreiner R J, Moler F W, Hirschl R B 1992 Initial experience with partial liquid ventilation in pediatric patients with the acute respiratory distress syndrome. Critical Care Medicine 24: 16–22

366. Gaylor M S, Quissell B J, Lair M E 1987 High frequency ventilation in the treatment of infants weighing less than 1500 grams with pulmonary interstitial emphysema. Pediatrics 79: 915–921

367. Geggel R L, Reid L M 1984 The structural basis for persistent pulmonary hypertension of the newborn. Clinics in Perinatology 11: 525–549

368. Geggel R L, Murphy J D, Langleben D, Crone R K, Vacanti J P, Reid L M 1985 Congenital diaphragmatic hernia: arterial structural changes and persistent pulmonary hypertension after surgical repair. Journal of Pediatrics 107: 457–464

369. Geggel R L, Aronovitz M J, Reid L M 1986 Effects of chronic in utero hypoxemia on rat neonatal pulmonary arterial structure. Journal of Pediatrics 108: 756–759

370. Gersony W M, Duc G V, Sinclair J C 1969 'PFC' syndrome (abstract). Circulation 40 (suppl. III): 87

371. Gersony W M, Peckham G J, Ellison R C, Meittenen O S, Nadas A S 1983 Effects of indomethacin in premature infants with PDA. Journal of Pediatrics 102: 895–906

372. Gerstmann D R, Minton S D, Stoddard R A et al 1996 The Provo multicentre early high frequency oscillatory ventilation trial improved pulmonary and clinical outcome in respiratory distress syndrome. Pediatrics 98: 1044–1057

373. Giacoia G P, Neter E, Ogra P 1981 Respiratory infections in infants on mechanical ventilators. The immune response as a diagnostic aid. Journal of Pediatrics 98: 691–695

374. Gibson A T, Primhak R A 1994 Early changes in lung function and response to surfactant replacement therapy. European Journal of Pediatrics 153: 495–500

375. Gibson R L, Berger J I, Redding G J, Standaert T A, Mayock D E, Truog W E 1994 Effect of nitric oxide synthase inhibition during group B streptococcal sepsis in neonatal piglets. Pediatric Research 36: 776–783

376. Gibson R L, Truog W E, Redding G J 1988 Thromboxane associated pulmonary hypertension during three types of Gram positive bacteremia in piglets. Pediatric Research 23: 553–556

377. Gill A B, Weindling A M 1993 Randomized controlled trial of plasma protein fraction versus dopamine in hypotensive very low birthweight infants. Archives of Disease in Childhood 69: 284–287

378. Glass L, Rajegowda B D, Evans H E 1971 Absence of respiratory distress syndrome in premature infants of heroin addicted mothers. Lancet i: 685–686

379. Glass P, Miller M, Short B 1989 Morbidity of survivors of extracorporeal membrane oxygenation: neurodevelopmental outcome at 1 year of age. Pediatrics 83: 72–78

380. Gluck L, Kulovich M V, Eidelman A I, Cordero L, Khazin A F 1972 Biochemical development of surfactant activity in mammalian lung. IV. Pulmonary lecithin synthesis in the human fetus and newborn and etiology of the respiratory distress syndrome. Pediatric Research 6: 81–99

381. Goetzman B W, Sunshine P, Johnson J D et al 1976 Neonatal hypoxia and pulmonary vasospasm: response to tolazoline. Journal of Pediatrics 89: 617–621

382. Goldberg S J, Levy R A, Siassi B, Betten J 1971 The effects of maternal hypoxia and hyperoxia upon the neonatal pulmonary vasculature. Pediatrics 48: 528–533

383. Goldman A P, Tasker R C, Haworth S G, Sigston P E, Macrae D J 1996 Four patterns of response to inhaled nitric oxide for persistent pulmonary hypertension of the newborn. Pediatrics 98: 708–713

384. Goldman S L, Brady J P, Dumpit F M 1979 Increased work of breathing associated with nasal prongs. Pediatrics 64: 160–164

385. Goldsmith L S, Greenspan J S, Rubenstein D, Wolfson M R, Shaffer T H 1991 Immediate improvement in lung volume after exogenous surfactant: alveolar recruitment after distension. Journal of Pediatrics 119: 424–428

386. Gomez R, Ghezzi F, Romero R, Munoz H, Tolosa J E, Rojas I 1995 Premature labor and intra-amniotic infection. Clinical aspects and role of the cytokines in diagnosis and pathophysiology. Clinics in Perinatology 22: 281–342

387. Gonzales L W, Ballard P L, Ertsey R, Williams M C 1986 Glucocorticoids and thyroid hormones stimulate biochemical and morphological differentiation of human fetal lung in organ culture. Journal of Clinical Endocrinology and Metabolism 62: 678–691

388. Gonzalez F, Harris T, Black P, Richardson P 1987 Decreased gas flow through pneumothoraces in neonates receiving high-frequency jet versus conventional ventilation. Journal of Pediatrics 110: 464–466

389. Gooding C A, Gregory G A 1971 Reoentgenographic analysis of meconium aspiration of the newborn. Radiology 110: 131–140

390. Goodlin R C 1970 Suppression of fetal breathing to prevent aspiration of meconium. Obstetrics and Gynecology 36: 944–947

391. Goodwin S R, Graves S A, Haberkern C M 1985 Aspiration in intubated premature infants. Pediatrics 75: 85–88

392. Gordon J B, Martinez F R, Keller P A, Tod M L, Madden J A 1993 Differing effects of acute and prolonged alkalosis on hypoxic pulmonary vasoconstriction. American Review of Respiratory Disease 148: 1651–1656

393. Goretsky M J, Martinasek D, Warner B W 1996 Pulmonary hemorrhage: a novel complication after extracorporeal life support. Journal of Pediatric Surgery. 31: 1276–1281

394. Gortner L, Pohlandt F, Bartmann P et al 1994 High dose versus low dose bovine surfactant treatment in very premature infants. Acta Paediatrica 83: 135–141

395. Govindaswami B, Heldt G P, Bernstein G, Beyar R 1993 Reduction in cerebral blood flow velocity (CBFV) variability in infants <1500 g during synchronized ventilation (SIMV). Pediatric Research 33: 1258 (abstract)

396. Graham M, Levene M, Trounce J Q, Rutter N 1987 Prediction of cerebral palsy in very low birthweight infants: prospective ultrasound study. Lancet i: 593–596

397. Grant A 1989 Monitoring the fetus during labour. In: Chalmers I, Enkin M, Kierse M J N C (eds) Effective care in pregnancy and childbirth. Oxford University Press, Oxford, pp 846–882

398. Grausz J P, Harvey D R 1967 Neonatal haemothorax: a report of two cases. Archives of Disease in Childhood 42: 675–676

399. Graven S N, Misenheimer H R 1965 Respiratory distress syndrome and the high risk mother. American Journal of Diseases of Children 109: 489–494

400. Graves E D, Redmond C R, Aronsman R M 1988 Persistent pulmonary hypertension in the neonate. Chest 93: 639–641

401. Green J N, Paul R H 1978 The value of amniocentesis in prolonged pregnancy. Obstetrics and Gynecology 51: 293–298

402. Green T P, Thompson T R, Johnson D E, Lock J E 1983 Diuresis and pulmonary function in premature infants with respiratory distress syndrome. Journal of Pediatrics 103: 618–623

403. Green T P, Johnson D E, Bass J L, Landrum B G, Ferrara T B, Thompson T R 1988 Prophylactic furosemide in severe respiratory distress syndrome: blinded prospective study. Journal of Pediatrics 112: 605–612

404. Greenough A 1984 Pancuronium bromide induced joint contractures in the newborn. Archives of Disease in Childhood 59: 390–391

405. Greenough A 1988 The premature infant's respiratory response to mechanical ventilation. Early Human Development 17: 1–5

406. Greenough A, Greenall F 1987 Performance of respirators at fast rates commonly used in neonatal intensive care units. Pediatric Pulmonology 3: 257–261

407. Greenough A, Greenall F 1988 Observation of spontaneous respiratory interaction with artificial ventilation. Archives of Disease in Childhood 63: 168–171

408. Greenough A, Greenall F 1988 Patient triggered ventilation in premature neonates. Archives of Disease in Childhood 63: 77–78

409. Greenough A, Lagercrantz H 1992 Catecholamine abnormalities in transient tachypnoea of the premature newborn. Journal of Perinatal Medicine 20: 223–226

410. Greenough A, Milner A D 1987 High frequency ventilation in the neonatal period. European Journal of Paediatrics 146: 446–449
411. Greenough A, Pool J 1988 Neonatal patient triggered ventilation. Archives of Disease in Childhood 63: 394–397
412. Greenough A, Roberton N R C 1985 Morbidity and survival in neonates ventilated for the respiratory distress syndrome. British Medical Journal 290: 597–600
413. Greenough A, Chan V, Hird M F 1992 Positive end expiratory pressure in acute and chronic neonatal respiratory distress. Archives of Disease in Childhood 67: 320–323
414. Greenough A, Milner A D, Roberton N R C 1996 Neonatal respiratory disorders. Edward Arnold, London
415. Greenough A, Morley C J, Davis J A 1983 The interaction of spontaneous respiration with artificial ventilation in preterm babies. Journal of Pediatrics 103: 769–773
416. Greenough A, Dixon A D, Roberton N R C 1984 Pulmonary interstitial emphysema. Archives of Disease in Childhood 59: 1046–1051
417. Greenough A, Morley C J, Wood S, Davis J A 1984 Pancuronium prevents pneumothoraces in ventilated premature babies who actively expire against positive pressure ventilation. Lancet i: 1–3
418. Greenough A, Elias Jones A, Pool J, Morley C J, Davis J A 1985 The therapeutic actions of theophylline in preterm ventilated infants. Early Human Development 12: 15–22
419. Greenough A, Morley C J, Pool J 1986 Fighting the ventilator: are fast rates an effective alternative to paralysis? Early Human Development 13: 189–194
420. Greenough A, Gamsu H R, Greenall F 1987 Investigation of the effects of paralysis by pancuronium on heart rate variability, blood pressure and fluid balance. Acta Paediatrica Scandinavica 78: 829–834
421. Greenough A, Greenall F, Gamsu H R 1987 Synchronous respiration – which ventilator rate is best? Acta Paediatrica Scandinavica 76: 713–718
422. Greenough A, Greenall F, Gamsu H R 1987 Inspiratory times when weaning from mechanical ventilation. Archives of Disease in Childhood 62: 1269–1270
423. Greenough A, Pool J, Greenall F, Morley C J, Gamsu H 1987 Comparison of different rates of artificial ventilation in premature neonates with respiratory distress syndrome. Acta Paediatrica Scandinavica 76: 706–712
424. Greenough A, Greenall F, Gamsu H R 1988 Immediate effects of albumin infusion in ill premature infants. Archives of Disease in Childhood 63: 307–308
425. Greenough A, Pool J B, Lagercrantz H 1988 Catecholamine and blood pressure levels in paralysed preterm ventilated infants. Early Human Development 16: 219–224
426. Greenough A, Maconochie I, Yuksel B 1990 Recurrent respiratory symptoms in the first year of life following preterm delivery. Journal of Perinatal Medicine 18: 489–494
427. Greenspan J S, Wolfson M R, Holt W J, Shaffer T H 1990 Neonatal gastric intubation: differential respiratory effects between nasogastric and orogastric tubes. Pediatric Pulmonology 8: 254–258
428. Gregoire R, Yulish B, Martin R, Fletcher B, Fanaroff A 1979 Natural history of pulmonary interstitial emphysema in the preterm infant (abstract). Pediatric Research 13: 495
429. Gregory G A 1986 Devices for applying continuous positive airway pressure. In: Thibeault D W, Gregory G A (eds) Neonatal pulmonary care, 2nd Edn. Appleton Century Crofts, Norwalk CT, pp 307–320
430. Gregory G A, Kitterman J A, Phibbs R H, Tooley W H, Hamilton W K 1971 Treatment of idiopathic respiratory distress syndrome with continuous positive pressure. New England Journal of Medicine 284: 1333–1340
431. Gregory G A, Gooding C A, Phibbs R H, Tooley W H 1974 Meconium aspiration in infants: a prospective study. Journal of Pediatrics 85: 848–852
432. Gribetz I, Frank N R, Avery M E 1959 Static volume pressure relations of excised lungs of infants with hyaline membrane disease; newborn and stillborn infants. Journal of Clinical Investigation 38: 2168–2175
433. Griesen G, Frederiksen P S, Hertel J, Christensen N J 1985 Catecholamine response to chest physiotherapy and endotracheal suctioning preterm infants. Acta Paediatrica Scandinavica 74: 525–529
434. Griesen G, Munck H, Lou H 1987 Severe hypocarbia in preterm infants and neurodevelopmental deficit. Acta Paediatrica Scandinavica 76: 401–404
435. Grosfeld J, Lemons J, Ballantine T V, Schreiner R L 1980 Emergency thoracotomy for acquired bronchopleural fistula in the premature infant with respiratory distress. Journal of Pediatric Surgery 15: 416–421
436. Gross G W, Greenspan J S, Fox W W, Rubenstein S D, Wolfson M R, Shaffer T H 1995 Use of liquid ventilation with perflubron during extracorporeal membrane oxygenation: chest radiographic appearances. Pediatric Radiology 194: 717–720
437. Gross I, Walker-Smith G J, Wilson C M et al 1980 The influence of hormones on the biochemical development of fetal rat lung in organ culture. II. Insulin. Pediatric Research 14: 834–838
438. Gross T L, Sokol R J, Kwong M S 1983 Transient tachypnea of the newborn. The relationship to preterm delivery and significant neonatal morbidity. American Journal of Obstetrics and Gynecology 14: 236–241
439. Gruskay J, Costarino A T, Polin R A, Baumgart S 1988 Non-oliguric hyperkalemia in the premature infant weighing less than 1000 grams. Journal of Pediatrics 113: 381–386
440. Gryboski J D 1969 Suck and swallow in the premature infant. Pediatrics 43: 96–101
441. Guignard J-P, Torrado A, Mazouni S M, Gautier E 1976 Renal function in respiratory distress syndrome. Journal of Pediatrics 88: 845–850
442. Guilleminault C, Coons S 1984 Apnea and bradycardia during feeding in infants weighing > 2000 gm. Journal of Pediatrics 104: 932–935
443. Gupta J M, Dahlenburg G W, Davis J A 1967 Changes in blood gas tensions following administration of the amine buffer THAM to infants with respiratory distress syndrome. Archives of Disease in Childhood 42: 416–427
444. Hagay Z, Reece A, Roberts A, Hobbins J C 1993 Isolated fetal pleural effusion: a prenatal management dilemma. Obstetrics and Gynecology 81: 174–152
445. Hageman J R, Adams A, Gardner T H 1984 Persistent pulmonary hypertension of the newborn. Trends in incidence, diagnosis and management. American Journal of Diseases of Children 138: 592–595
446. Hagen R, Bryan A C, Bryan M H, Gulston G 1976 The effects of stabilization of the rib cage on respiration in preterm infants (abstract). Pediatric Research 10: 461
447. Hall R T, Oliver T K 1971 Aortic blood pressure in infants admitted to a neonatal intensive care unit. American Journal of Diseases of Children 121: 145–147
448. Hallak M, Bottoms S F 1993 Accelerated pulmonary maturation from preterm premature rupture of membranes: a myth. American Journal of Obstetics and Gynecology 169: 1045–1049
449. Halliday H L, Hirata T 1979 Perinatal listeriosis—a review of twelve patients. American Journal of Obstetrics and Gynecology 133: 405–410
450. Halliday H L, McClure G, Reid M McC 1981 Transient tachypnoea of the newborn: two distinct clinical entities? Archives of Disease in Childhood 56: 322–325
451. Halliday H L, McClure G, Reid M M, Lappin T R, Meban C, Thomas P S 1984 Controlled trial of artificial surfactant to prevent respiratory distress syndrome. Lancet i: 476–478
452. Halliday H L, Tarnow-Mordi W O, Corcoran J D, Paterson C C 1993 Multicentre randomized trial comparing high and low dose surfactant regimens for the treatment of respiratory distress syndrome (Curosurf 4 trial). Archives of Disease in Childhood 69: 276–280
453. Hallman M, Teramo K 1981 Measurement of the lecithin/sphingomyelin ratio and phosphatidylglycerol in amniotic fluid: an accurate method for the assessment of fetal lung maturity. British Journal of Obstetrics and Gynaecology 88: 860–813
454. Hallman M, Arjomaa P, Hoppu K 1987 Inositol supplementation in respiratory distress syndrome: relationship between serum concentration, renal excretion and lung effluent phospholipids. Journal of Pediatrics 110: 604–610
455. Hallman M, Bry K, Hoppu K, Lappi M, Pohjavuori M 1992 Inositol supplementation in premature infants with respiratory distress syndrome. New England Journal of Medicine 326: 1233–1239
456. Hallman M, Merritt T A, Bry K, Berry C 1993 Association between neonatal care practices and efficacy of exogenous human surfactant: results of a bi-center randomized trial. Pediatrics 91: 552–560

457. Hallman M, Teramo K, Kankaanpaa K, Kulovich M V, Gluck L 1980 Prevention of respiratory distress syndrome: current view on lung maturity studies. Annals of Clinical Research 12: 36–44
458. Hamdan A H, Shaw N J 1995 Changes in pulmonary artery pressure in infants with respiratory distress syndrome following treatment with Exosurf. Archives of Disease in Childhood 72: F176–F179
459. Hamilton P P, Onayemi A, Smyth J A et al 1983 Comparison of conventional and high frequency ventilation: oxygenation and lung pathology. Journal of Applied Physiology 55: 131–138
460. Hammerman C, Aramburo M J 1988 Decreased lipid intake reduces morbidity in sick premature neonates. Journal of Pediatrics 113: 1083–1088
461. Hammerman C, Lass N, Strates E, Komar K, Bui K-C 1987 Prostanoids in neonates with persistent pulmonary hypertension. Journal of Pediatrics 110: 470–472
462. Hamvas A, Devine T, Cole FS 1993 Surfactant therapy failure identifies infants at risk for pulmonary mortality. American Journal of Diseases in Children 147: 665–668
463. Han R N N, Buch S, Tseu I et al 1996 Changes in structure, mechanics and insulin-like growth factor related gene expression in the lungs of newborn rats exposed to air or 60% oxygen. Pediatric Research 39: 921–929
464. Han V K M, Beverly D W, Clarson C et al 1987 Randomized controlled trial of very early continuous distending pressure in the management of preterm infants. Early Human Development 15: 21–32
465. Hanlon-Lundberg K, Williams M, Rhim T, Covert R F, Mittendorf R, Holt J A 1996 Accelerated fetal lung maturity profiles and maternal cocaine exposure. Obstetrics and Gynecology 87: 128–132
466. Hansen T I, Hazinski T A, Bland R D 1984 Effects of asphyxia on lung fluid balance in fetal lambs. Journal of Clinical Investigation 74: 370–376
467. Harries J T, 1978 Meconium in health and disease. British Medical Bulletin 34: 75–78
468. Harris J T, Chistensen R D 1984 High frequency jet ventilation treatment of pulmonary interstitial emphysema (abstract). Pediatric Research 18: 326
469. Harrison V C, Heese H deV, Klein M 1968 The significance of grunting in hyaline membrane disease. Pediatrics 41: 549–559
470. Hart S M, McNair M, Gamsu H R, Price J F 1983 Pulmonary interstitial emphysema in very low birthweight infants. Archives of Disease in Childhood 58: 612–615
471. Hashim S A, Roholt H B, Babayan V K, Van Itallie T B 1964 Treatment of chyluria and chylothorax with medium chain triglyceride. New England Journal of Medicine 270: 756–761
472. Hauer A C, Rosegger H, Haas J, Haxhija E Q 1996 Reaction of term newborns with prolonged postnatal dyspnoea to early oxygen, mask CPAP and volume expansion: a prospective randomized clinical trial. European Journal of Pediatrics 155: 805–810
473. Hausdorf G, Hellwege H H 1987 Influence of positive end expiratory pressure on cardiac performance in premature infants: a Doppler echocardiographic study. Critical Care Medicine 15: 661–664
474. Hayek Z, Peliowski A, Ryan C A, Jones R, Finer N N 1986 External high frequency oscillation in cats. Experience in the normal lung and after saline lung lavage. American Review of Respiratory Disease 133: 630–634
475. Heaf D P, Belik J, Spitzer A R, Gewitz M H, Fox W W 1982 Changes in pulmonary function during the diuretic phase of respiratory distress syndrome. Journal of Pediatrics 101: 103–107
476. Heaf D P, Helms P J, Dinwiddie R 1982 Nasopharyngeal airways in Pierre Robin syndrome. Journal of Pediatrics 100: 698–703
477. Heaf D P, Helms P, Gordon I, Turner H M 1983 Postural effects on gas exchange in infants. New England Journal of Medicine 308: 1505–1508
478. Heicher D A, Kasting D S, Richards J R 1981 Prospective clinical comparison of two methods of mechanical ventilation of neonates: rapid rate and short inspiratory time versus slow rate and long inspiratory time. Journal of Pediatrics 98: 957–961
479. Helbock H J, Insoft R M, Conte F A 1993 Glucocorticoid responsive hypotension in extremely low birthweight newborns. Pediatrics 92: 715–717
480. Heldt G P 1988 The effect of gavage feeding on the mechanics of the lung, chest wall and diaphragm in preterm infants. Pediatric Research 24: 55–58
481. Hellstrom-Westas L, Bell A H, Skov L, Greisen G, Svenningsen N W 1992 Cerebro-electrical depression following surfactant treatment in preterm neonates. Pediatrics 89: 643–647
482. Hendricks-Munoz K D, Walton J P 1988 Hearing loss in infants with persistent fetal circulation. Pediatrics 81: 650–656
483. Henry G W 1984 Non-invasive assessment of cardiac function and pulmonary hypertension in persistent pulmonary hypertension of the newborn. Clinics in Perinatology 11: 627–640
484. Henry G W, Stevens D S, Schreiner R L, Grosfield J L, Ballantine T V R 1979 Respiratory paralysis to improve oxygenation and mortality in large newborn infants with respiratory distress. Journal of Pediatric Surgery 14: 761–766
485. Heritage C K, Cunningham M D 1985 Association of elective repeat caesarean section delivery and persistent pulmonary hypertension of the newborn. American Journal of Obstetrics and Gynecology 152: 627–629
486. Herman S, Reynolds E O R 1973 Methods for improving oxygenation in infants mechanically ventilated for severe HMD. Archives of Disease in Childhood 48: 612–617
487. Hernandez C, Little B B, Dax J S, Gilstrap L C, Rosenfeld C R 1993 Prediction of the severity of meconium aspiration syndrome. American Journal of Obstetrics and Gynecology 169: 61–70
488. HIFI Study Group 1989 High frequency oscillatory ventilation compared with conventional mechanical ventilation in the treatment of respiratory failure in preterm infants. New England Journal of Medicine 320: 88–93
489. HIFO Study Group 1993 Randomized study of high frequency oscillatory ventilation in infants with severe respiratory distress syndrome. Journal of Pediatrics 122: 609–619
490. Hill A, Perlman J M, Volpe J J 1982 Relationship of pneumothorax to occurrence of intraventricular hemorrhage in the premature newborn. Pediatrics 69: 144–149
491. Hird M F, Greenough 1990 Causes of failure of neonatal patient triggered ventilation. Early Human Development 23: 101–108
492. Hird M F, Greenough A 1991 Inflation time in mechanical ventilation of preterm neonates. European Journal of Pediatrics 150: 440–443
493. Hird M F, Greenough A 1991 Comparison of triggering systems for neonatal patient triggered ventilation. Archives of Disease in Childhood 66: 426–428
494. Hird M, Greenough A, Gamsu H R 1990 Gas trapping during high frequency positive pressure ventilation using conventional ventilators. Early Human Development 22: 51–56
495. Hirschl R B, Merz S I, Montoya J P et al 1995 Development and application of a simplified liquid ventilator. Critical Care Medicine 23: 157–163
496. Hirschl R B, Pranikoff T, Gauger P, Schreiner R J, Dechert R, Bartlett R H 1995 Liquid ventilation in adults, children and full term neonates. Lancet 346: 1201–1202
497. Hirschl R B, Tooley R, Parent A C, Johnson K, Bartlett R H 1995 Improvement of gas exchange pulmonary function and lung injury with partial liquid ventilation. Chest 108: 500–508
498. Hjalmarson O 1981 Epidemiology and classification of acute neonatal respiratory disorders. Acta Paediatrica Scandinavica 70: 773–783
499. Hjalmarson O, Olsson T 1974a Mechanical and ventilatory parameters in healthy and diseased newborn infants. Acta Paediatrica Scandinavica Suppl. 247: 26–48
500. Hjalmarson O, Olsson T 1974b Work of breathing. Acta Paediatrica Scandinavica Suppl. 247: 49–60
501. Holm B A, Notter R H, Siegle J, Matalon S 1985 Pulmonary physiological and surfactant changes during injury and recovery from hypoxia. Journal of Applied Physiology 59: 1402–1409
502. Holm B A, Notter R H, Leary J F, Matalon S 1987 Alveolar epithelial changes in rabbits after a 21 day exposure to 60% oxygen. Journal of Applied Physiology 62: 2230–2236
503. Hook B, Hack M, Morrison S, Borawski-Clark E, Newman N S, Fanaroff A 1995 Pneumopericardium in very low birthweight infants. Journal of Perinatology 15: 27–31
504. Hooper S B, Harding R 1990 Changes in lung liquid dynamics induced by prolonged fetal hypoxemia. Journal of Applied Physiology 69: 127–135
505. Hope P L, Cady E B, Delpy D T, Ives N K, Gardner R M, Reynolds E O R 1988 Brain metabolism and intracellular pH during ischaemia: effects of systemic glucose and bicarbonate administration

studied by ^{31}P and ^{1}H nuclear magnetic resonance spectroscopy in vivo in the lamb. Journal of Neurochemistry 50: 1394–1402
506. Horbar J D, Wright L L, Soll R F 1993 A multicenter randomized trial comparing two surfactants for the treatment of neonatal respiratory distress syndrome. Journal of Pediatrics 123: 757–766
507. Hoskyns E N, Milner A D, Hopkin I E 1991 Combined conventional ventilation with high frequency oscillation in neonates. European Journal of Pediatrics 150: 357–361
508. Hoskyns E W, Milner A D, Hopkin I E 1987. Dynamic lung inflation during high frequency oscillation in respiratory distress syndrome. Early Human Development 15: 186–187
509. Howell J H 1987 Sodium bicarbonate in the perinatal setting—revisited. Clinics in Perinatology 14: 807–816
510. Howell S, Fitzgerald R S, Roussos C 1985 Effects of uncompensated and compensated metabolic acidosis on canine diaphragms. Journal of Applied Physiology 59: 1376–1382
511. Howie P W, Patel N B 1984 Obstetric management of preterm labour. Clinics in Obstetrics and Gynaecology 11: 373–390
512. Hrabovsky E E, Mullett M D 1986 Gastroesophageal reflux and the premature infant. Journal of Pediatric Surgery 21: 583–587
513. Huang Y-C T, Sane A C, Simonson S G 1995 Artificial surfactant attenuates hyperoxic lung injury in primates. I: Physiology and biochemistry. Journal of Applied Physiology 78: 1816–1822
514. Hudak M L, Farrell E E, Rosenberg A A et al 1996 A multicenter randomized masked comparison of natural versus synthetic surfactant for the treatment of respiratory distress syndrome. Journal of Pediatrics 128: 396–406
515. Hughes D, Murphy J F, Dyas J et al 1987 Blood spot glucocorticoid concentrations in ill preterm infants. Archives of Disease in Childhood 62: 1014–1018
516. Hulsey T C, Alexander G R, Robillard P Y, Annibale D J, Keenan A 1993 Hyaline membrane disease: the role of ethnicity and maternal risk characteristics. American Journal of Obstetrics and Gynecology 168: 572–576
517. Hummler H, Gerhardt T, Claure N, Everett R, Bancalari E 1994 Patient triggered ventilation (PTV) in neonates: comparison of air flow and an impedance triggered system. Pediatric Research 35: 337A
518. Hummler H, Gerhardt T, Claure N, Everett R, Bancalari E 1994 Influence of patient triggered ventilation (PTV) on ventilation and blood pressure fluctuations in neonates. Pediatric Research 35: 338A
519. Humphreys P W, Normand I C S, Reynolds E O R, Strang L B 1967 Pulmonary lymph flow and the uptake of liquid from the lungs of lambs at the start of breathing. Journal of Physiology 193: 1–29
520. Hutchinson A A, Yu V Y H 1980 Curare in the treatment of pulmonary hypertension as it occurs in the idiopathic respiratory distress syndrome. Australian Journal of Paediatrics 16: 94–100
521. Hyde I, English R E, Williams J A 1989 The changing pattern of chronic lung disease of prematurity. Archives of Disease in Childhood 64: 448–451
522. Ikegami M 1994 Surfactant inactivation. In: Boynton B R, Carlo W A, Jobe A H (eds) New therapies for neonatal respiratory failure. Cambridge University Press, Cambridge, pp 36–48
523. Ikegami M, Jacobs H, Jobe A 1983 Surfactant function in respiratory distress syndrome. Journal of Pediatrics 102: 443–447
524. Ikegami M, Berry D, Elkady T, Pettenazzo A, Seidner S, Jobe A 1987 Corticosteroids and surfactant change lung function and protein leaks in the lungs of ventilated premature rabbits. Journal of Clinical Investigation 79: 1371–1378
525. Ikegami M, Jobe A H, Tabor B L, Rider E D, Lewis J F 1992 Lung albumin recovery in surfactant treated preterm ventilated lambs. American Review of Respiratory Disease 145: 1005–1008
526. Ikonen R S, Janas M O, Koivikko M J, Laippala P, Kuusinen E J 1992 Hyperbilirubinaemia, hypocarbia and periventricular leucomalacia in preterm infants: relationship to cerebral palsy. Acta Paediatrica 81: 802–809
527. Illingworth R S 1969 Sucking and swallowing difficulties in infancy. Diagnostic problems of dysphagia. Archives of Disease in Childhood 44: 655–665
528. Ingomar C J, Klebe J G 1974 The transcapillary escape rate of T1824 in newborn infants of diabetic mothers and newborn infants with RDS or birth asphyxia. Acta Paediatrica Scandinavica 63: 565–570
529. Ioffe S, Chernick V 1987. Maternal alcohol ingestion and the incidence of respiratory distress syndrome. American Journal of Obstetrics and Gynecology 156: 1231–1235
530. Itani Y, Fujioka M, Nishimura G, Niitsu N, Oono T 1988 Upper G I examinations in older premature infants with persistent apnea: correlation with simultaneous cardiorespiratory monitoring. Pediatric Radiology 18: 464–467
531. Jackson R M 1985 Pulmonary oxygen toxicity. Chest 88: 900–905
532. Jacob J, Edwards D, Gluck L 1980 Early onset sepsis and pneumonia observed as respiratory distress syndrome. American Journal of Diseases of Children 134: 766–768
533. Jacobsen T, Gronvall J, Petersen S, Andersen G E 1993 Minitouch treatment of very low birthweight infants. Acta Paediatrica 82: 934–938
534. James C F, Modell J H, Gibbs C P, Kuck E J, Ruiz B C 1984 Pulmonary aspiration—effects of volume and pH in the rat. Anesthesia and Analgesia 63: 665–668
535. James D K, Chiswick M L, Harkes A, Williams M, Hallworth J 1984 Non-specificity of surfactant deficiency in neonatal respiratory disorders. British Medical Journal 288: 1635–1638
536. James L, Greenough A, Naik S 1997 The effect of blood transfusion on oxygenation in premature ventilated neonates. European Journal of Pediatrics 156: 139–141
537. James L S, Rowe R D 1957 The pattern of response of pulmonary and systemic arterial pressure in newborn and older infants to short periods of hypoxia. Journal of Pediatrics 57: 5–11
538. Jardin F, Farcot J C, Boisante L, Curien N, Margaraz A, Bourdarias J 1981 Influence of positive end expiratory pressure on left ventricular performance. New England Journal of Medicine 304: 387–392
539. Javaheri S, Herrera L, Kazemi H, 1979 Ventilatory drive in acute metabolic acidosis. Journal of Applied Physiology 45: 913–918
540. Jedeikin R, Primhak A, Shennan A T, Swyer P R, Rowe R D 1983 Serial electrocardiographic changes in healthy and stressed neonates. Archives of Disease in Childhood 58: 605–611
541. Jeffery H E, Page M 1995 Developmental inactivation of gastro-oesophageal reflux in preterm infants. Acta Paediatrica 84: 245–250
542. Jeffries A L, Coates G, O'Brodovich H, 1984 Pulmonary epithelial permeability in hyaline membrane disease. New England Journal of Medicine 311: 1075–1080
543. Jobe A H, Mitchell B R, Gankel J H 1993 Beneficial effects of the combined use of prenatal corticosteroids and postnatal surfactant on preterm infants. American Journal of Obstetrics and Gynecology 186: 508–513
544. Johansson J, Curstedt T, Robertson B 1996 Synthetic protein analogues in artificial surfactants. Acta Paediatrica 85: 642–646
545. John E, Ermocilla R, Golden J, Cash R, McDevitt M, Cassady G 1980 Effects of gas temperature and particulate water on rabbit lung during ventilation. Pediatric Research 14: 1186–1191
546. Johnson G L, Cunningham M D, Desai N S, Cottrill C M, Noonan J 1980 Echocardiography in hypoxemic neonatal pulmonary disease. Journal of Pediatrics 96: 716–720
547. Jones M D, Burd L I, Bowes W A, Battaglia F C, Lubchencho L O 1975 Premature rupture of membranes and the respiratory distress syndrome. New England Journal of Medicine 292: 1253–1257
548. Jones R A K, Roberton N R C 1984 Problems of the small for dates baby. Clinics in Obstetrics and Gynaecology 11: 499–524
549. Jones R W A, Baumer J H, Joseph M C, Shinebourne E A 1976 Arterial oxygen tension and response to oxygen breathing in differential diagnosis of congenital heart disease in infancy. Archives of Disease in Childhood 51: 667–673
550. Joshi V V, Mandavia S G, Stern L, Wigglesworth F W 1972 Acute lesions induced by endotracheal intubation. American Journal of Diseases of Children 124: 646–649
551. Jovanovic R, Nguyen H T 1989 Experimental meconium aspiration in guinea pigs. Obstetrics and Gynecology 73: 652–656
552. Kääpä P, Seppänen M, Kero P, Ekblad H, Arjamaa O, Vuolteenaho O 1995 Haemodynamic control of atrial natriuretic peptide plasma levels in neonatal respiratory distress syndrome. American Journal of Perinatology 12: 235–239
553. Kamei A, Ozaki T, Takashima S 1994 Monitoring of the intracranial hemodynamics and oxygenation during and after hyperventilation in newborn rabbits with near infrared spectroscopy. Pediatric Research 35: 334–338
554. Kamper J, Wulff K, Larsen C, Lindeqvist S 1993 Early treatment with nasal continuous positive airway pressure in very low birthweight infants. Acta Paediatrica 82: 193–197
555. Kanjanapone V, Hartig-Becken I, Epstein M F 1980 Effect of

isoxuprine on fetal lung surfactant in rabbits. Pediatric Research 14: 278–281
556. Kanto W P 1994 A decade of experience with neonatal extracorporeal membrane oxygenation. Journal of Pediatrics 124: 335–347
557. Kanto W P, Borer R C, Barr M, Roloff D W 1976 Tracheal aspirate lecithin-sphingomyelin ratios as predictors of recovery from respiratory distress syndrome. Journal of Pediatrics 89: 612–616
558. Kanto W P, Kuhns L P, Borer R C, Roloff D W 1978 Failure of serial chest radiographs to predict recovery from respiratory distress syndrome. American Journal of Obstetrics and Gynecology 131: 757–760
559. Kari M A, Heinonen K, Ikonen R S, Koivisto M, Raivio K O 1993 Dexamethasone treatment in preterm infants at risk for bronchopulmonary dysplasia. Archives of Disease in Childhood 68: 566–569
560. Kari M A, Raivio K O, Stenman U H, Voutilainen R 1996 Serum cortisol, dehydroepiandrosterone sulphate and steroid-binding globulins in preterm neonates: effect of gestational age and dexamethasone therapy. Pediatric Research 40: 319–324
561. Karl S R, Ballantine T V N, Schnides M T 1983 High frequency ventilation at rates of 375–1800 cycles/minute in 4 neonates with congenital diaphragmatic hernia. Journal of Pediatric Surgery 18: 822–828
562. Karlberg P, Cook C D, O'Brien D, Cherry R B, Smith C A 1954 Studies of respiratory physiology in the newborn infant. II. Observations during and after respiratory distress. Acta Paediatrica Scandinavica Suppl. 100: 397–411
563. Karlowicz M G 1994 Pneumoretroperitoneum and perirenal air associated with tension pneumothorax. American Journal of Perinatology 11: 63–64
564. Karotkin E H, Kido M, Cashore W J et al 1976 Acceleration of fetal lung maturation by aminophylline in fetal rabbits. Pediatric Research 10: 722–724
565. Kattwinkel J, Bloom B T, Delmore P et al 1993 Prophylactic administration of calf lung surfactant extract is more effective than early treatment of respiratory distress syndrome in neonates of 29 through 32 weeks' gestation. Pediatrics 92: 90–98
566. Katyal S L, Amenta J S, Singh G, Silverman J A 1984 Deficient lung surfactant apoproteins in amniotic fluid with mature phospholipid profile from diabetic pregnancies. American Journal of Obstetrics and Gynecology 184: 48
567. Katz V L, Bowes W A 1992 Meconium aspiration syndrome: reflections on a murky subject. American Journal of Obstetrics and Gynecology 166: 171–183
568. Kavvadia V, Greenough A 1998 Influence of ethnic origin on respiratory distress syndrome in very premature infants. Archives of Disease in Childhood 78: F25–F28
569. Kawczynski P, Piotrowski A 1996 Circulatory and diuretic effects of dopexamine infusion in low birthweight infants with respiratory failure. Intensive Care Medicine. 22: 65–70
570. Keeney S E, Cress S E, Brocon S E, Bidani A 1992 The effect of hyperoxic exposure on antioxidant enzyme activities of the alveolar type II cells in neonatal and adult rats. Pediatric Research 31: 441–444
571. Keeney S E, Mathews M J, Rassin D K 1993 Antioxidant enzyme responses to hyperoxia in preterm and term rats after prenatal dexamethasone administration. Pediatric Research 33: 177–180
572. Keith J D, Rose V, Braudo M, Rowe R D 1961 The electrocardiogram in the respiratory distress syndrome and related cardiovascular dynamics. Journal of Pediatrics 59: 167–187
573. Kelly E, Bryan H, Possmayer F, Findova H, Bryan C 1993 Compliance of the respiratory system in newborns pre and post surfactant replacement therapy. Pediatric Pulmonology 15: 225–230
574. Kelly F J, Lubec G 1995 Hyperoxic injury of immature guinea pig lung is mediated via hydroxyl radicals. Pediatric Research 38: 286–291
575. Kelly M A, Finer N N 1984 Nasotracheal intubation in the neonate: physiologic responses and effects of atropine and pancuronium. Journal of Pediatrics 105: 303–309
576. Kempley S T, Gamsu H R, Vyas S, Nicolaides K 1991 Effects of intrauterine growth retardation on postnatal visceral and cerebral blood flow velocity. Archives of Disease in Childhood 66: 1115–1118
577. Kendig J W, Notter R H, Cox C et al 1991 A comparison of surfactant as immediate prophylaxis and as rescue therapy in newborns of less than 30 weeks' gestation. New England Journal of Medicine 324: 865–871
578. Keszler M, Carbone M T, Cox C, Schumacher R E 1992 Severe respiratory failure after elective repeat cesarean delivery: a potentially preventable condition leading to extracorporeal membrane oxygenation. Pediatrics 89: 670–672
579. Keszler M, Donn S M, Bucciarelli R L et al 1991 Multicenter controlled trial comparing high frequency jet ventilation and conventional mechanical ventilation in patients with pulmonary interstitial emphysema. Journal of Pediatrics 119: 85–93
580. Khammash H, Perlman M, Wojtulewicz J, Dunn M 1993 Surfactant therapy in full term neonates with severe respiratory failure. Pediatrics 92: 135–139
581. Kiely J L 1991 Mode of delivery and neonatal death in 17587 infants presenting by the breech. British Journal of Obstetrics and Gynaecology 98: 898–904
582. Kim E H, Boutwell W C 1987 Successful direct extubation of very low birthweight infants from low intermittent mandatory ventilation rate. Pediatrics 80: 409–414
583. King J F, Grant A, Keirse M J N C, Chalmers I 1988 Betamimetics in preterm labour: an overview of the randomised controlled trials. British Journal of Obstetrics and Gynaecology 95: 211–222
584. King R J, Coalson J J, Seidenfeld J, Anzueto A R, Smith D B, Peters J I 1989 Oxygen and pneumonia induced lung injury. II. Properties of surfactant. Journal of Applied Physiology 67: 357–365
585. Kinmond S, Aitchison T C, Holland B M, Jones J G, Turner T L, Wardrop C A 1993 Umbilical cord clamping and preterm infants: a randomized trial. British Medical Journal 306: 172–175
586. Kinsella J P, Abman S H 1995 Recent developments in the pathophysiology and treatment of persistent pulmonary hypertension of the newborn. Journal of Pediatrics 126: 853–864
587. Kinsella J P, Abman S H 1996 Clinical pathophysiology of persistent pulmonary hypertension of the newborn and the role of nitric oxide therapy. Journal of Perinatology 16: 524–527
588. Kinsella J P, Neish S R, Shaffer E, Abman S H 1992 Low dose inhalational nitric oxide in persistent pulmonary hypertension of the newborn. Lancet 340: 819–820
589. Kinsey V E, Arnold H J, Kalinare R E et al 1977 PaO_2 levels and retrolental fibroplasia: a report of the co-operative study. Pediatrics 60: 655–668
590. Kirkpatrick B V, Krummel T M, Mueller D G, Ormazabal M A, Greenfield L J, Salzberg A M 1983 Use of ECMO for respiratory failure in term babies. Pediatrics 72: 872–876
591. Kirpalani H, Higa T, Perlman M, Friedberg J, Cutz E 1985 Diagnosis and therapy of necrotizing tracheobronchitis in ventilated neonates. Critical Care Medicine 13: 792–797
592. Kirpalani H, Santos-Lyn R, Roberts R 1988 Some infant ventilators do not develop peak inspiratory pressures reliably during active expiration. Critical Care Medicine 16: 880–883
593. Kjos S L, Walter F J, Montorom M, Paul R H, Diaz F, Stabiler M 1990 Prevalence and etiology of respiratory distress in infants of diabetic mothers: predictive value of lung maturation tests. American Journal of Obstetrics and Gynecology 163: 898–903
594. Klarr J M, Faix R G, Pryce C J E, Bhatt-Mehta V 1994 Randomized trial of dopamine versus dobutamine for treatment of hypotension in preterm infants with respiratory distress syndrome. Journal of Pediatrics 125: 117–122
595. Klaus M H, Meyer B P 1966 Oxygen therapy for the newborn. Pediatric Clinics of North America 13: 731–752
596. Klein A H, Foley B, Foley T P, MacDonald H M, Fisher D A 1981 Thyroid function studies in cord blood from premature infants with and without RDS. Journal of Pediatrics 98: 818–820
597. Klein J 1990 Normobaric pulmonary oxygen toxicity. Anesthesia and Analgesia 70: 195–207
598. Klein M D, Whittlesey G C 1994 Extracorporeal membrane oxygenation. Pediatric Clinics of North America. 41: 365–384
599. Klein V R, Cunningham F G 1986 Amniotic fluid: a source of fetal evaluation. Seminars in Perinatology 10: 125–135
600. Klesh K W, Murphy T F, Scher M S, Buchanan D E, Maxwell E P, Guthrie R D 1987 Cerebral infarction in persistent pulmonary hypertension of the newborn. American Journal of Diseases of Children 141: 852–857
601. Knight D B, Liggins G C, Wealthall SR 1994 A randomized

controlled trial of antepartum thyrotropin releasing hormone and betamethasone in the prevention of respiratory disease in preterm infants. American Journal of Obstetrics and Gynecology 171: 11–16
602. Knox G E, Huddleston J F, Flowers C E 1979 Management of prolonged pregnancy: results of a prospective randomized trial. American Journal of Obstetrics and Gynecology 134: 376–381
603. Kobayashi T, Nitta K, Ganzuka M, Inui S, Grossmann G, Robertson B 1991 Inactivation of exogenous surfactant by pulmonary edema fluid. Pediatric Research 29: 353–356
604. Kohelet D, Perlman M, Kirpalani H, Hanna G, Koren G 1988 High frequency oscillation in the rescue of infants with persistent pulmonary hypertension. Critical Care Medicine 16: 510–516
605. Kohlhauser C, Popow C, Helbich T, Hermon M, Weninger M, Herold C J 1995 Successful treatment of severe neonatal lobar emphysema by high frequency oscillatory ventilation. Pediatric Pulmonology 19: 52–55
606. Kolton M, Cattran C B, Kent G, Volgyesi G, Froese A B, Bryan A C 1982 Oxygenation during high-frequency ventilation compared with conventional mechanical ventilation in two models of lung injury. Anesthesia and Analgesia 61: 323–332
607. Konduri G, Garcia D C, Kazzi N J, Shankaran S 1996 Adenosine expression improves oxygenation in term infants with respiratory failure. Pediatrics 97: 295–300
608. Konishi M, Fujiwara T, Takeuki Y et al 1988 Surfactant replacement therapy in neonatal respiratory distress syndrome. European Journal of Pediatrics 144: 20–25
609. Korvenranta H, Kero P 1983 Intraesophageal pressure monitoring in infants with respiratory disorders. Critical Care Medicine 11: 276–279
610. Kotas R V, Avery M E 1971 Accelerated appearance of pulmonary surfactant in the fetal rabbit. Journal of Applied Physiology 30: 358–361
611. Koumbourlis A C, Mutich R L, Motoyama E S 1995 Contribution of airway hyperresponsiveness to lower airway obstruction after extracorporeal membrane oxygenation for meconium aspiration syndrome. Critical Care Medicine 23: 749–754
612. Kourembanas S, Marsden P A, McQuillan L P, Fuller D V 1991 Hypoxia induces endothelin gene expression and secretion in cultured human endothelium. Journal of Clinical Investigation 88: 1054–1057
613. Krauss A N, Auld P A M 1969 Ventilation perfusion abnormalities in the premature infant: triple gradient. Pediatric Research 3: 255–264
614. Krauss A N, Soodalter J A, Auld P A M 1971 Adjustment of ventilation and perfusion in the fullterm normal and distressed neonate as determined by urinary-alveolar nitrogen gradients. Pediatrics 47: 865–869
615. Krouskop R W, Brown E H, Sweet A Y 1975 The early use of continuous positive airways pressure in the treatment of idiopathic respiratory distress syndrome. Journal of Pediatrics 87: 263–267
616. Krummel T M, Greenfield L J, Kirkpatrick B V, Mueller D G, Ormazabal M, Salzberg A M 1982 Clinical use of an extracorporeal membrane oxygenator in neonatal pulmonary failure. Journal of Pediatric Surgery 17: 525–531
617. Kühl P G, Cotton R B, Schweer H, Seyberth H 1989 Endogenous formation of prostanoids in neonates with persistent pulmonary hypertension. Archives of Disease in Childhood 64: 949–952
618. Kuhn M P, Fletcher B D, de Lemos R A 1969 Roentgen findings in transient tachypnea of the newborn. Radiology 92: 751–757
619. Kuhns L R, Bednarek F J, Wyman M L, Roloff D W, Borer R C 1975 Diagnosis of pneumothorax or pneumomediastinum in the neonate by transillumination. Pediatrics 56: 355–360
620. Kuint J, Reichman B, Neumann L, Shinwell E S 1994 Prognostic response of the immediate response to surfactant. Archives of Disease in Childhood 71: F170–F173
621. Kulik T J, Lock J E 1984 Pulmonary vasodilator therapy in persistent pulmonary hypertension of the newborn. Clinics in Perinatology 11: 693–701
622. Kumar P, Kazzi N J, Shankaran S 1996 Plasma immunoreactive endothelin-1 concentrations in infants with persistent pulmonary hypertension of the newborn. American Journal of Perinatology 13: 335–341
623. Lachman B 1987 Combination of saline instillation with artificial ventilation damages bronchial surfactant. Lancet i: 1375
624. Lamont R F, Dunlop P D M, Levene M I, Elder M G 1983 Use of glucocorticoids in pregnancies complicated by severe hypertension and proteinuria. British Journal of Obstetrics and Gynaecology 90: 199–202
625. Langham M R, Krummel T M, Bartlett R H et al 1987 Mortality with extracorporeal membrane oxygenation following repair of congenital diaphragmatic hernia in 93 infants. Journal of Pediatric Surgery 22: 1150–1154
626. Lanteri C J, Willet K E, Kano S et al 1994 Time course in lung mechanics following fetal steroid treatment. American Journal of Respiratory and Critical Care Medicine 150: 759–765
627. Laros R K, Kitterman J A, Heilbron D C 1991 Outcome of very low birthweight infants exposed to beta sympathomimetics in utero. American Journal of Obstetrics and Gynecology 164: 1657–1665
628. Larsson L E, Ekstrom-Jodal B, Hjalmarson O 1982 The effect of chlorpromazine in severe hypoxia in newborn infants. Acta Paediatrica Scandinavica 71: 399–402
629. Laubscher B, Greenough A, Devane S P 1997 Response to nitric oxide: influence of gestational age. European Journal of Pediatrics 156: 639–642
630. Laubscher B Greenough A, Kavadia V 1997 Comparison of body surface and airway triggered ventilation in extremely premature infants. Acta Paediatrica 86: 102–104
631. Laubscher B, Greenough A, Costeloe K 1996 Performance of four neonatal high frequency oscillators. British Journal of Intensive Care 6: 148–152
632. Lawson E E, Birdwell R L, Huang P S, Taeusch H W 1977 Augmentation of pulmonary surfactant release by lung expansion at birth (abstract). Pediatric Research 11: 574
633. Lay K S, Bancalari E, Malkus H, Baker R, Strauss J 1980 Acute effects of albumin infusion on blood volume and renal functions in premature infants with the respiratory distress syndrome. Journal of Pediatrics 97: 619–623
634. Leach C L, Greenspan J S, Rubenstin S D et al 1995 Partial liquid ventilation with Liquivent: a pilot and safety and efficacy study in premature newborns with severe respiratory distress syndrome. Pediatric Research 37: 220 (abstract)
635. Leach C L, Holm B, Morin F C et al 1995 Partial liquid ventilation in premature lambs with respiratory distress syndrome: efficacy and compatibility with exogenous surfactant. Journal of Pediatrics 126: 412–420
636. Leach C L, Greenspan J S, Rubenstein S D et al 1996 Partial liquid ventilation with perfluorocarbon in premature infants with severe respiratory distress syndrome. New England Journal of Medicine 335: 761–767
637. Leahy F A N, Cates D, MacCallum M, Rigatto H 1980 Effect of CO_2 and 100% O_2 on cerebral blood flow in preterm infants. Journal of Applied Physiology 48: 468–472
638. Lebidois J, Soifer S J, Clyman R I, Heyman M A 1987 Piriprost—a putative leukotriene synthesis inhibitor—increases pulmonary blood flow in fetal lambs. Pediatric Research 22: 350–354
639. Lechner A J, Winson D C, Bauman J E 1986 Lung mechanics, cellularity and surfactant after prenatal starvation in guinea pigs. Journal of Applied Physiology 60: 1610–1614
640. Lee S K, Tanswell A K 1989 Pulmonary vascular air embolism in the newborn. Archives of Disease in Childhood 64: 507–510
641. Lees C, Campbell S, Jauniaux E et al 1994 Arrest of preterm labour and prolongation of gestation with glyceryl trinitrate, a nitric oxide donor. Lancet 343: 1325–1326
642. Lehtinen A-M, Hovorka J, Widholm O 1984 Modification of aspects of the endocrine response to tracheal intubation by lignocaine, halothane and thiopentone. British Journal of Anaesthesia 56: 239–246
643. Leigh R J, Shaw D A 1976. Rapid regular respiration in unconcious patients. Archives of Neurology 33: 356–361
644. Leonardi M R, Hankins G D V 1992 What's new in tocolytics. Clinics in Perinatology 19: 367–384
645. Leonidas J C, Hall R T, Rhodes P G 1975 Conservative management of unilateral pulmonary interstitial emphysema under tension. Journal of Pediatrics 87: 776–778
646. Leslie G I, Gallery E D M, Arnold J D, Nicholson E 1991 Hyaline membrane disease and early neonatal aldosterone metabolism in infants of less than 33 weeks gestation. Acta Paediatrica Scandinavica 80: 628–633
647. Leslie G I, Phillips J B, Work J, Cassady G 1985 Diuresis and

natriuresis following acute pneumothorax in very low birthweight infants. Australian Paediatric Journal 21: 269–272

648. Le Souef P, England S J, Bryan A C 1984 Total resistance of the respiratory system in preterm infants with and without an endotracheal tube. Journal of Pediatrics 104: 108–111
649. Levene M I, Quinn M W 1992 Use of sedatives and muscle relaxants in newborn babies receiving mechanical ventilation. Archives of Disease in Childhood 67: 870–873
650. Levene M I, Kornberg J, Williams T H C 1985 The incidence and severity of post asphyxial encephalopathy in full-term infants. Early Human Development 11: 21–28
651. Leveno K J, Quirk J G, Whalley P J, Herbert W N P, Trubey R 1984 Fetal lung maturation in twin gestations. American Journal of Obstetrics and Gynecology 148: 405–411
652. Levin D L, Weinberg A G, Perkin R M 1983 Pulmonary microthrombi syndrome in newborn infants with unresponsive persistent pulmonary hypertension. Journal of Pediatrics 102: 299–303
653. Levin D L, Heyman M, Kitterman J A, Gregory G A, Phibbs R H, Rudolph A M 1976 Persistent pulmonary hypertension in the newborn infant. Journal of Pediatrics 89: 626–630
654. Levin D L, Fixler D E, Morriss F C, Tyson J 1978 Morphologic analysis of the pulmonary vascular bed in infants exposed in utero to prostaglandin synthetase inhibitors. Journal of Pediatrics 92: 478–483
655. Levin D L, Mills L J, Parkey M, Garriott J, Campbell W 1979 Constriction of the fetal ductus arteriosus after administration of indomethacin to the pregnant ewe. Journal of Pediatrics 94: 647–650
656. Levison H, Delivoria-Papadopoulos M, Swyer P R 1964 Oxygen consumption in newly born infants with respiratory distress syndrome. Biologia Neonatorum 7: 255–269
657. Lewis D F, Futayyeh S, Towers C et al 1996 Preterm delivery from 34 to 37 weeks' gestation: is respiratory distress syndrome a problem? American Journal of Obstetrics and Gynecology 174: 525–528
658. Lewis J F, Ikegami M, Jobe A H et al 1993 Physiologic responses and distribution of aerosolized surfactant (Survanta) in a non-uniform pattern of lung injury. American Review of Respiratory Disease 147: 1364–1370
659. Lieberman E, Torday J, Barbieri R, Cohen A, Van Vunakis H, Weiss S T 1992 Association of intrauterine cigarette smoke exposure with indices of fetal lung maturation. Obstetrics and Gynecology 79: 564–570
660. Liechty E A, Donovan E, Purohit D et al 1991 Reduction of neonatal mortality after multiple doses of bovine surfactant in low birthweight neonates with respiratory distress syndrome. Pediatrics 88: 19–28
661. Liggins G C 1969 Premature delivery of fetal lambs infused with glucocorticoids. Journal of Endocrinology 45: 515–523
662. Liggins G C, Howie R N 1972 A controlled trial of antepartum glucocorticoid treatment for prevention of the respiratory distress syndrome in premature infants. Pediatrics 50: 515–525
663. Lin Y, Lechner A J 1991 Surfactant content and type II cell development in fetal guinea pig lungs during prenatal starvation. Pediatric Research 29: 288–291
664. Linder N, Aranda J V, Tsur M et al 1988 Need for endotracheal intubation and suction in meconium stained neonates. Journal of Pediatrics 112: 613–615
665. Linderkamp O, Versmold H T, Fendel H, Riegel K P, Betke K 1978 Association of neonatal respiratory distress with birth asphyxia and deficiency of red cell mass in premature infants. European Journal of Pediatrics 129: 167–173
666. Lindroth M, Jonson B, Svenningsen M W, Mortensson W 1980 Pulmonary mechanics, chest X-ray and lung disease after mechanical ventilation in low birthweight infants. Acta Paediatrica Scandinavica 69: 761–770
667. Lioy J, Manginello F P 1988 A comparison of prone and supine positioning in the immediate post-extubation period of neonates. Journal of Pediatrics 112: 982–984
668. Lipscomb A P, Reynolds E O R, Blackwell R J et al 1981 Pneumothorax and cerebral haemorrhage in preterm infants. Lancet i: 414–417
669. Loe E A, Graves E D, Ochsner J L, Falterman K W, Arensman R M 1985 ECMO for newborn respiratory failure. Journal of Pediatric Surgery 20: 684–688
670. Long W, Corbet A, Allen A et al 1992 Retrospective search for bleeding diathesis among premature newborn infants with pulmonary hemorrhage after synthetic surfactant treatment. Journal of Pediatrics 120: S45–S48
671. Long W, Zucker J A, Kraybill E N 1995 Symposium in synthetic surfactant. II. Health and developmental outcomes at one year. Journal of Pediatrics 126: S1–S80
672. Long W A 1984 Structural cardiovascular abnormalities presenting as persistent pulmonary hypertension of the newborn. Clinics in Perinatology 11: 601–626
673. Long W A, Lawson E E, Harned H S, Kraybill E N 1984 Pleural effusion in the first days of life. American Journal of Perinatology 1: 190–194
674. Longaker M T, Laberge J M, Dansereau J et al 1989 Primary fetal hydrothorax: natural history and management. Journal of Pediatric Surgery 24: 573–576
675. Loo C K, Smith G J, Lykke A W J 1989 Effects of hyperoxia on surfactant morphology and cell viability in organotypic cultures of fetal rat lungs. Experimental Lung Research 15: 597–617
676. Lopez J B, Campbell R E, Bishop H C 1977 Clinical note: non-operative resolution of prolonged localised intrapulmonary interstitial emphysema associated with hyaline membrane disease. Journal of Pediatrics 91: 653–654
677. Lotze A, Knight G, Martin G R 1993 Improved pulmonary outcome after exogenous surfactant for respiratory failure in term infants requiring extracorporeal membrane oxygenation. Journal of Pediatrics 121: 261–268
678. Lucas A, Mitchell M D 1978 Plasma prostaglandins in preterm neonates before and after treatment for patent ductus arteriosus. Lancet ii: 130–132
679. Lucas A, Christofides N D, Adrian T E, Bloom S R, Aynsley-Green A 1979 Fetal distress, meconium and motilin. Lancet i: 718
680. Lucas A, Bloom S R, Aynsley-Green A 1986 Gut hormones and minimal enteral feeding. Acta Paediatrica Scandinavica 75: 719–723
681. Lucey J F 1991 The surfactant era – starting off right! Pediatrics 88: 168
682. Lund W S 1976 Deglutition. In: Hinchcliffe R, Harrison D (eds) Scientific Foundations of Ortolaryngology. Heinemann, London, pp 591–598
683. Lundell B P W, Boreus L D 1983 Digoxin therapy and left ventricular performance in premature infants with patent ductus arteriosus. Acta Paediatrica Scandinavica 72: 339–343
684. Lundstrom K E, Greisen G 1996 Changes in EEG, systemic circulation and blood gas parameters following two or six aliquots of porcine surfactant. Acta Paediatrica 85: 708–712
685. Lyrene R K, Philips J B 1984 Control of pulmonary vascular resistance in the fetus and newborn. Clinics in Perinatology 11: 551–564
686. MacArthur B A, Howie R N, Dezcete J A, Elkins J 1981 Cognitive and psychosocial development of 4-year-old children whose mothers were treated antenatally with betamethasone. Pediatrics 68: 638–643
687. McCann E M, Goldman S L, Brady J P 1987 Pulmonary function in the sick newborn infant. Pediatric Research 21: 313–325
688. McClure G 1992 Surfactant therapy – time for thought. Archives of Disease in Childhood 67: 1228–1230
689. McCormick M D, Workman Daniels K, Grooks Gunn J et al 1993 Hospitalization of very low birthweight children at school age. Journal of Pediatrics 122: 360–365
690. MacDonald D, Grant A, Sherida-Pereira M, Boylan P, Chalmers I 1985 The Dublin randomized controlled trial of intrapartum fetal heart rate monitoring. American Journal of Obstetrics and Gynecology 152: 524–539
691. McDonald M G, Chou M M 1986. Preventing complications from lines and tubes. Seminars in Perinatology 10: 224–233
692. McDonald M M, Johnson M L, Rumack C M et al 1984 Role of coagulopathy in newborn intracranial hemorrhage. Pediatrics 74: 26–31
693. MacDonald P D, Yu V Y H 1992 Simultaneous measurement of preductal and postductal oxygen saturation by pulse oximetry in hyaline membrane disease. Archives of Disease in Childhood 67: 1166–1168
694. McEvoy R D, Davies N J, Hedenstierna G, Hartman M T, Spragg R G, Wagner P D 1982 Lung mucociliary transport during high frequency ventilation. American Review of Respiratory Disease 126: 452–456
695. MacEwan D W, Dunbar J S, Smith R D, Brown B St J 1971

Pneumothorax in young infants—recognition and evaluation. Journal of the Canadian Association of Radiology 22: 264–268
696. MacFarlane P I, Heaf D P 1988 Pulmonary function in children after neonatal meconium aspiration syndrome. Archives of Disease in Childhood 63: 368–372
697. McIntosh N 1983 Pulmonary air leaks in the newborn period. British Journal of Hospital Medicine 29: 512–517
698. Macklin C C 1936 Alveolar pores and their significance in the human lung. Archives of Pathology 21: 202–210
699. Macklin C C 1939 Transport of air along sheaths of pulmonic blood vessels from alveoli to mediastinum, clinical implications. Archives of Internal Medicine 64: 913–926
700. MacMahon P, Fleming P J, Thearle M J, Speidel B D 1982 An improved selective bronchial intubation technique for managing severe localized interstitial emphysema. Acta Paediatrica Scandinavica 71: 151–153
701. McMillan D D, Rademaker A W, Buchan K A, Reid A, Machin G, Sauve R S 1986 Benefits of orotracheal and nasotracheal intubation in neonates requiring ventilatory assistance. Pediatrics 7: 39–44
702. Madansky D L, Lawson E E, Chernick V, Taeusch H W 1979 Pneumothorax and other forms of pulmonary air leak in the newborn. American Review of Respiratory Disease 120: 729–737
703. Mahmoud E L, Benirschke K, Vaucher Y E, Poitras P 1988 Motilin levels in term neonates who have passed meconium prior to birth. Journal of Paediatric Gastroenterology and Nutrition 7: 95–99
704. Malan A F 1966 Neonatal tachypnoea. Australian Paediatric Journal 3: 159–163
705. Malo J, Ali J, Wood L D H 1984 How does positive end expiratory pressure reduce intrapulmonary shunt in canine pulmonary edema? Journal of Applied Physiology 57: 1002–1010
706. Mammel M C, Boros S J 1987 Airway damage and mechanical ventilation. Pediatric Pulmonology 3: 443–447
707. Man G C W, Man S F P, Kappagoda C T 1983 Effects of high frequency oscillatory ventilation on vagal and phrenic nerve activity. Journal of Applied Physiology 54: 502–507
708. Manalo E, Merritt T A, Kheiter A, Amirkhanian J, Cochrane C 1996 Comparative effects of some serum components and proteolytic products of fibrinogen in surface tension-lowering abilities of Beractant and a synthetic peptide containing surfactant KL_4. Pediatric Research 39: 947–952
709. Mann T P, Elliott R I K 1957 Neonatal cold injury due to accidental exposure to cold. Lancet i: 229–234
710. Manning F A, Schreiber F A, Turkel S B 1978 Fatal meconium aspiration 'in utero'. A case report. American Journal of Obstetrics and Gynecology 132: 111–113
711. Manning F A, Martin C B, Murata Y, Miyaki K, Danzier G 1979 Breathing movements before death in the primate fetus. American Journal of Obstetrics and Gynecology 135: 71–76
712. Manroe B L, Weinberg A G, Rosenfield C R, Browne R 1979 The neonatal blood count in health and disease. I. Reference value for neutrophil cells. Journal of Pediatrics 95: 89–98
713. Manzke H 1972 Relationship between extracellular and intracellular hydrogen ion concentrations and haemoglobin oxygen affinity in the blood of premature infants with RDS. Biology of the Neonate 20: 321–333
714. Marchak B E, Thompson W K, Duffty P 1981 Treatment of RDS by high frequency oscillatory ventilator. A preliminary report. Journal of Pediatrics 99: 287–292
715. Margolis C Z, Orzalesi M M, Schwartz A D 1973 Disseminated intravascular coagulation in the respiratory distress syndrome. American Journal of Diseases of Children 125: 324–326
716. Marino A J, Assing E, Carbone M T, Hiatt I M, Hegyi T, Graff M 1995 The incidence of gastroesophageal reflux in preterm infants. Journal of Perinatology 15: 369–371
717. Marlow N, Weindling A M, VanPeer A, Heykants J 1990 Alfentanil pharmacokinetics in preterm infants. Archives of Disease in Childhood 65: 349–351
718. Maron M B 1987 Analysis of airway fluid protein concentration in neurogenic pulmonary edema. Journal of Applied Physiology 62: 470–476
719. Marron M J, Crisafi M A, Driscoll J H et al 1992 Hearing and neurodevelopmental outcome in survivors of persistent pulmonary hypertension of the newborn. Pediatrics 90: 392–396
720. Marshall T A, Deeder R, Pai S, Berkowitz G P, Austin T L 1984 Physiological changes associated with endotracheal intubation in preterm infants. Critical Care Medicine 12: 501–503
721. Martin R J, Herrell N, Rubin D, Fanaroff A 1979 Effect of supine and prone positions on arterial oxygen tension in the preterm infant. Pediatrics 63: 528–531
722. Mathew O P 1991 The science of bottle feeding. Journal of Pediatrics 119: 511–519
723. Mathew O P, Thach B T 1980 Selective bronchial obstruction for treatment of bullous interstitial emphysema. Journal of Pediatrics 96: 475–477
724. Mathew O P, Clark M L, Pronske M L, Luna-Solarzano H G, Peterson M D 1985 Breathing pattern and ventilation during oral feeding in term newborn infants. Journal of Pediatrics 106: 810–813
725. Matthews T G, Warshaw J B 1979 Relevance of gestational age distribution of meconium passage in utero. Pediatrics 64: 30–31
726. Mauskopf J A, Backhouse M E, Jones D, Shoham-Vardi I, Cohen J, Ghezzi F 1995 Synthetic surfactant for rescue treatment of respiratory distress syndrome in premature infants weighing from 700–1350 g: impact on hospital resource use and charges. Journal of Pediatrics 126: 94–101
727. Mayes L, Perkett E, Stahlman M T 1983 Severe bronchopulmonary dysplasia: a retrospective review. Acta Paediatrica Scandinavica 72: 225–229
728. Mazor M, Furman B, Wiznitzer A, Hipps R 1995 Maternal and perinatal outcome of patients with preterm labour and meconium stained amniotic fluid. Obstetrics and Gynecology 86: 830–833
729. Mead P B 1980 Management of the patient with premature rupture of the membranes. Clinics in Perinatology 243–255
730. Meadow W, Rudinsky B, Bell A et al 1995 Effects of inhibition of endothelium derived relaxation factor on haemodynamics and oxygen utilization during group B streptococcal sepsis in piglets. Critical Care Medicine 23: 705–714
731. Mehta A, Callan K, Bright B M, Stacey T E 1986 Patient triggered ventilation in the newborn. Lancet ii: 706–712
732. Meis P J, Hall M, Marshall J R, Hobel C J 1978 Meconium passage: a new classification for risk assessment in labour. American Journal of Obstetrics and Gynecology 131: 509–513
733. Memon A, Dave R, Branca P A, Atkinson G W, Kagen J J 1979 Improved method of gas exchange in HMD (abstract). American Review of Respiratory Disease 119 (suppl.): 275
734. Mendelson C R, Alcorn J L, Gao E 1993 The pulmonary surfactant protein genes and their regulation in fetal lung. Seminars in Perinatology 17: 223–232
735. Mendoza J C, Roberts R L, Look L N 1991 Postural effects on pulmonary function and heart rate of preterm infants with lung disease. Journal of Pediatrics 118: 445–448
736. Mercer S 1986 Factors involved in chylothorax following repair of congenital posterolateral diaphragmatic hernia. Journal of Pediatric Surgery 21: 9–11
737. Mercier C E, Soll R F 1993 Clinical trials of natural surfactant extract in respiratory distress syndrome. Clinics in Perinatology 20: 711–736
738. Merenstein G B, Dougherty K, Lewis A 1972 Early detection of pneumothorax by oscilloscope monitor in the newborn infant. Journal of Pediatrics 80: 98–101
739. Merlob P, Amir J, Zaizov R, Reisner S H 1980 The differential leucocyte count in full term newborn infants with meconium aspiration and neonatal asphyxia. Acta Paediatrica Scandinavica 69: 779–780
740. Merritt T A, Farrell P M 1976 Diminished pulmonary lecithin synthesis in acidosis: experimental findings as related to the RDS. Pediatrics 57: 32–40
741. Merritt T A, Hallman M, Berry C et al 1991 Randomized placebo controlled trial of human surfactant given at birth versus rescue administration in very low birthweight infants with lung immaturity. Journal of Pediatrics 118: 581–594
742. Merritt T A, Stuard I D, Puccia J et al 1981 Newborn tracheal aspirate cytology: classification during respiratory distress syndrome and bronchopulmonary dysplasia. Journal of Pediatrics 98: 949–956
743. Miall-Allen V M, Whitelaw A G 1987 Effect of pancuronium and pethidine on heart rate and blood pressure in ventilated infants. Archives of Disease in Childhood 62: 1179–1180
744. Migdal M, Dreizzen E, Praud J P et al 1987 Compliance of the total respiratory system in healthy preterm and fullterm newborns. Pediatric Pulmonology 3: 214–218

745. Miller F C 1979 Meconium staining of the amniotic fluid. Clinics in Obstetrics and Gynaecology 6: 359–365
746. Miller F C, Sacks D A, Yeh S Y et al 1975 Significance of meconium during labour. American Journal of Obstetrics and Gynecology 122: 573–580
747. Miller O I, Celermajer D S, Deanfield J E, Macrae D J 1994 Guidelines for the safe administration of inhaled nitric oxide. Archives of Disease in Childhood 70: F47–49
748. Milligan D W A, Issler H, Massam M, Reynolds E O R 1984 Treatment of neonatal pulmonary interstitial emphysema by lung puncture. Lancet i: 1010–1011
749. Milner A D 1993 How does exogenous surfactant work? Archives of Disease in Childhood 68: 253–254
750. Milner A D, Vyas H 1982 Lung expansion at birth. Journal of Pediatrics 101: 879–886
751. Mitchell A, Greenough A, Hurd M 1989 Limitations of patient triggered ventilation in neonates. Archives of Disease in Childhood 64: 924–929
752. Moessinger A C, Driscoll J M Jr, Wigger H J 1978 High incidence of lung perforation by chest tube in neonatal pneumothorax. Journal of Pediatrics 92: 635–637
753. Moglia B B, Phelps D S 1996 Changes in surfactant protein A mRNA levels in a rat model of insulin-treated diabetic pregnancy. Pediatric Research 39: 241–247
754. Mohan P, Rojas J, Davidson K et al 1984 Pulmonary air leak associated with neonatal hyponatremia in premature infants. Journal of Pediatrics 105: 153–157
755. Moise A A, Wearden M E, Kozinetz C A, Gest A L, Welty S E, Hansen T N 1995 Antenatal steroids are associated with less need for blood pressure support in extremely premature infants. Pediatrics 95: 845–850
756. Moomjian A S, Schwartz J G, Shutack J-G, Rooklin A R, Shaffer T H, Fox W W 1981 Use of external expiratory resistance in intubated neonates to increase lung volume. Archives of Disease in Childhood 56: 869–873
757. Moraga F A, Riquelme R A, Lopez A A, Moya F R, Llanos A J 1994 Maternal administration of glucocorticoid and thyrotropin-releasing hormone enhances fetal lung maturation in undisturbed preterm lambs. American Journal of Obstetrics and Gynecology 171: 729–734
758. Morales W J, O'Brien W F, Angell J L, Knuppel R A, Sawai S 1989 Fetal lung maturation: the combined use of corticosteroids and thyrotropin-releasing hormone. Obstetrics and Gynecology 73: 111–116
759. Morett L A, Ortega R 1987 Pulmonary hypertension in the fetus, the newborn and the child. Clinics in Perinatology 14: 227–242
760. Morgan M E I 1985 Late morbidity of very low birthweight infants. British Medical Journal 29: 171–173
761. Morin F C 1989 Ligating the ductus arteriosus before birth causes persistent pulmonary hypertension in the newborn lamb. Pediatric Research 25: 245–250
762. Morisot C, Kacet N, Bouchez M C et al 1990 Risk factors for fatal pulmonary interstitial emphysema in neonates. European Journal of Pediatrics 149: 493–495
763. Morley C J 1987 The Cambridge experience of artificial surfactant. In: Walters D N, Strang L B, Geubelle F (eds) Physiology of the fetal and neonatal lung. MTP Press, Lancaster, pp 255–272
764. Morley C J 1997 Systematic review of prophylactic versus rescue surfactant. Archives of Disease in Childhood 77: 70–75
765. Morley C J, Greenough A 1991 Respiratory compliance in very premature babies treated with artificial surfactant (ALEC). Archives of Disease in Childhood 66: 467–471
766. Morley C J, Morley R 1990 Follow-up of premature babies treated with artificial surfactant (ALEC). Archives of Disease in Childhood 65: 667–669
767. Morris W P, Butler B D, Tonnesen A S, Allen S J 1993 Continuous venous air embolism in patients receiving positive end expiratory pressure. American Review of Respiratory Disease 147: 1034–1037
768. Morrison J J, Rennie J M, Milton P J 1995 Neonatal respiratory morbidity and mode of delivery at term: influence of timing of elective caesarean section. British Journal of Obstetrics and Gynaecology 102: 101–106
769. Morrow G, Hope J W, Boggs T R 1967 Pneumomediastinum, a silent lesion in the newborn. Journal of Pediatrics 70: 554–560
770. Morrow W R, Taylor AF, Kinsella J P, Lally K P, Gerstmann D R, deLemos R A 1995 Effect of ductal patency on organ blood flow and pulmonary function in the preterm baboon with hyaline membrane disease. Critical Care Medicine 23: 179–186
771. Moseley J E 1960 Loculated pneumomediastinum in the newborn. A thymic 'spinnaker' sign. Radiology 75: 788–790
772. Moses D, Holm B A, Spitale P, Liu M Y, Enhorning G 1991 Inhibition of pulmonary surfactant function by meconium. American Journal of Obstetrics and Gynecology 164: 477–481
773. Moss A J, Emmanouilides G C, Rettori O, Higashino S M, Adams F H 1965 Postnatal circulatory and metabolic adjustments in normal and distressed premature infants. Biologia Neonatorum 8: 177–197
774. Mounla N A 1987 Neonatal respiratory disorders. Acta Paediatrica Scandinavica 76: 159–160
775. Moya F R, Montes H F, Thomas V L, Mouzinho A M, Smith J F, Rosenfeld C R 1994 Surfactant protein A and saturated phosphatidylcholine in respiratory distress syndrome. American Journal of Respiratory and Critical Care Medicine 150: 1672–1677
776. Moyer-Miller L, Chan G M 1986 Nutritional support of very low birthweight infants requiring prolonged assisted ventilation. American Journal of Diseases of Children 140: 929–932
777. Mupanemunda R H, Edwards A D 1995 Treatment of newborn infants with inhaled nitric oxide. Archives of Disease in Childhood 72: F131–134
778. Murdoch D R, Darlow B A 1984 Handling during neonatal intensive care. Archives of Disease in Childhood 59: 957–961
779. Murphy J D, Rabinowitz M, Goldstein J D, Reid L M 1981 Structural basis of persistent pulmonary hypertension of the newborn infant. Journal of Pediatrics 98: 962–967
780. Murphy J D, Vawter G F, Reid L M 1984 Pulmonary vascular disease in fatal meconium aspiration. Journal of Pediatrics 104: 758–762
781. Murphy J D, Aronovitz M J, Reid L M 1986 Effects of chronic in utero hypoxia on the pulmonary vasculature of the newborn guinea pig. Pediatric Research 20: 292–295
782. Mutch L, Newdick M, Lodwick A, Chalmers I 1986 Secular changes in re-hospitalization of very low birthweight infants. Pediatrics 78: 164–171
783. Myers M G, McGuinness G A, Lachenbruch P A, Koontz F P, Hollingshead R, Olson D B 1986 Respiratory illness in survivors of infant respiratory distress syndrome. American Review of Respiratory Disease 133: 1011–1018
784. NNNI Trial Group (Northern Neonatal Nursing Initiative) 1996 A randomized trial comparing the effect of prophylactic intravenous fresh frozen plasma, gelatin or glucose on early mortality and morbidity in preterm babies. European Journal of Pediatrics 155: 580–588
785. Nagourney B A, Kramer M S, Klebanoff M A, Usher R H 1996 Recurrent respiratory distress syndrome in successive preterm pregnancies. Journal of Pediatrics. 129: 591–596
786. Nash G, Blennerhassett J B, Pontoppidan H 1967 Pulmonary lesions associated with oxygen therapy and artificial ventilation. New England Journal of Medicine 276: 368–374
787. Neligan G A, Smith C A 1960 The blood pressure of newborn infants in asphyxial states and hyaline membrane disease. Pediatrics 26: 735–744
788. Nelson K B, Ellenberg J H 1984 Obstetric complications as risk factors for cerebral palsy or seizure disorders. Journal of the American Medical Association 251: 1843–1848
789. Nelson K B, Dambrosia J M, Ting T Y, Grether J K 1996 Uncertain value of electronic fetal monitoring in predicting cerebral palsy. New England Journal of Medicine 334: 613–618
790. Nelson N M 1976 Respiration and circulation after birth. In: Smith C A, Nelson N M (eds) The physiology of the newborn infant, 4th Edn. Charles C Thomas, Springfield, IL, pp 210–214
791. Neonatal Inhaled Nitric Oxide Study Group 1997 Inhaled nitric oxide in full-term and nearly full-term infants with hypoxic respiratory failure. New England Journal of Medicine 336: 597–604
792. Newell S J, Booth I W, Morgan M E I, Durbin G M, McNeish A S 1989 Gastro-oesophageal reflux in preterm infants. Archives of Disease in Childhood 64: 780–786
793. Newell S J, Morgan M E I, Durbin G M, Booth I W, McNeish A S 1989 Does mechanical ventilation precipitate gastro-oesophageal reflux during enteral feeding? Archives of Disease in Childhood 64: 1352–1355

794. Ng K P K, Easa D 1979 Management of interstitial emphysema by high frequency low positive pressure hand ventilation in the neonate. Journal of Pediatrics 95: 117–118
795. Nicolaides K H, Azar G B 1990 Thoracoamniotic shunting. Fetal Diagnosis and Therapy 5: 153–164
796. Nielson H C, Riemenschneider T A, Jaffe R B 1976 Persistent transitional circulation. Radiology 120: 649–652
797. Noack G, Freyschuss U 1977 The early detection of pneumothorax with transthoracic impedance in newborn infants. Acta Paediatrica Scandinavica 66: 677–680
798. Nogee L, de Mello D, Dehner L, Colten H 1993 Pulmonary surfactant protein B deficiency in congenital pulmonary alveolar proteinosis. New England Journal of Medicine 328: 406–410
799. Nogee L, Garnier G, Singer L et al 1994 A mutation in the surfactant protein B gene responsible for fatal neonatal respiratory disease in multiple kindreds. Journal of Clinical Investigation 93: 1860–1863
800. Northway W H, Rosan R C, Porter D Y 1967 Pulmonary disease following respirator therapy of hyaline membrane disease. New England Journal of Medicine 276: 357–368
801. Nugent S K, Laravuso R, Rogers M C 1979 Pharmocology and use of muscle relaxants in infants and children. Journal of Pediatrics 94: 481–487
802. Nussbaum E, Maggi J C, Mathis R, Galant S P 1987 Association of lipid laden alveolar macrophages and gastro-oesophageal reflux in children. Journal of Pediatrics 110: 190–194
803. Obladen M, Gluck L 1977 RDS and tracheal phospholipid composition in twins: independent of gestational age. Journal of Pediatrics 90: 799–802
804. Octave Study Group 1991 Multicentre randomised controlled trial of high against low frequency positive pressure ventilation. Archives of Disease in Childhood 66: 770–778
805. Oetomo S B, Lewis J, Ikegami M, Jobe A H 1990 Surfactant treatments alter endogenous surfactant metabolism in rabbit lungs. Journal of Applied Physiology 68: 1590–1596
806. Ogata E S, Gregory G A, Kitterman J A, Phibbs R H, Tooley W H 1976 Pneumothorax in the respiratory distress syndrome: incidence and effect on vital signs, blood gases and pH. Pediatrics 58: 177–183
807. Ogawa A, Brown C L, Schlueter M A, Benson B J, Clements J A, Hawgood S 1994 Lung function, surfactant apoprotein content and level of PEEP in prematurely delivered rabbits. Journal of Applied Physiology 77: 1840–1849
808. Ogawa Y, Miyasaka K, Kawano T et al 1993 A multicentre randomized trial of high frequency oscillatory ventilation as compared with conventional mechanical ventilation in preterm infants with respiratory failure. Early Human Development 32: 1–10
809. Oh W, Stern L 1977 Diseases of the respiratory system. In: Behrman R E (ed) Neonatal and perinatal medicine: disease of the fetus and infant. C V Mosby, St Louis, p 558
810. Ohama Y, Itakura Y, Koyama N, Eguchi H, Ogawa Y 1994 Effect of surfactant lavage in a rabbit model of meconium aspiration syndrome. Acta Paediatrica Japonica 36: 236–238
811. Ojomo E O, Coustan D R 1990 Absence of evidence of pulmonary maturity at amniocentesis in term infants of diabetic mothers. American Journal of Obstetrics and Gynecology 163: 954–957
812. Ophoven J P, Mammel M C, Gardon M J 1984 Tracheobronchial histopathology associated with high frequency ventilation. Critical Care Medicine 12: 829–832
813. Orenstein S R, Orenstein D M 1988 Gastroesophageal reflux and respiratory disease in children. Journal of Pediatrics 112: 847–858
814. Orenstein S R, Whitington P F 1983 Positioning for prevention of infant gastroesophageal reflux. Journal of Pediatrics 103: 534–537
815. O'Rourke P P, Crone R K, Vacanti J P et al 1989 Extracorporeal membrane oxygenation and conventional medical therapy in neonates with persistent pulmonary hypertension of the newborn: a prospective randomized study. Pediatrics 84: 957–963
816. Ortega M, Ramos A D, Platzker A G, Atkinson J B, Bowman C M 1988 Early prediction of ultimate outcome in newborn infants with severe respiratory failure. Journal of Pediatrics 113: 744–747
817. Osiris Collaborative Group 1992 Early versus delayed neonatal administration of a synthetic surfactant – the judgement of Osiris. Lancet ii: 1363–1369
818. Outerbridge E 1979 The negative pressure ventilator. In: Thibeault G W, Gregory G A (eds) Neonatal pulmonary care. Addison-Wesley, CA, pp 168–177
819. Pandit P B, Dunn M S, Colucci E A 1995 Surfactant therapy in neonates with respiratory deterioration due to pulmonary hemorrhage. Pediatrics 95: 32–36
820. Pape K E, Armstrong D L, Fitzhardinge P M 1976 Central nervous system pathology associated with mask ventilation in the very low birthweight infant: a new etiology for intracerebellar hemorrhages. Pediatrics 58: 473–483
821. Papiernik E, Bouyer J, Dreyfus J et al 1985 Prevention of preterm births: a perinatal study in Hagenau, France. Pediatrics 76: 154–158
822. Pappin A, Shenker N, Hack M, Redline R W 1994 Extensive intraalveolar pulmonary hemorrhage in infants dying after surfactant therapy. Journal of Pediatrics 124: 621–626
823. Paranka M S, Clark R H, Yoder B A, Null D M 1995 Predictors of failure of high frequency oscillatory ventilation in term infants with severe respiratory failure. Pediatrics 95: 400–404
824. Pare P D, Warriner B, Baile E M, Hogg J C, 1983 Reduction of pulmonary extravascular water with positive end expiratory pressure in canine pulmonary edema. American Review of Respiratory Disease 127: 590–593
825. Parilla B V, Dooley S L, Jansen R D, Socol M L 1993 Iatrogenic respiratory distress syndrome following elective repeat cesarean delivery. Obstetrics and Gynecology 81: 392–395
826. Parker A 1995 Physiotherapy. In: Greenough A, Roberton N R C, Milner A D (eds) Neonatal respiratory disorders. Edward Arnold, London, pp 164–173
827. Patel B D, Dinwiddie R, Kumar S P, Fox W W 1977 The effects of feeding on arterial blood gases and lung mechanics in newborn infants recovering from respiratory disease. Journal of Pediatrics 90: 435–438
828. Paxson C L, Stoerner J W, Denson S E, Adcock E W, Morriss F H 1977 Syndrome of inappropriate antidiuretic hormone secretion in neonates with pneumothorax or atelectasis. Journal of Pediatrics 91: 459–463
829. Payen D M, Farge D, Beloucif S et al 1987 No involvement of antidiuretic hormone in acute antidiuresis during PEEP ventilation in humans. Anesthesiology 66: 17–23
830. Payne W W, Acharya P T 1965 The effect of abnormal birth on blood chemistry during the first 48 hours of life. Archives of Disease in Childhood 40: 436–441
831. Peckham G J, Fox W W 1978 Physiologic factors affecting pulmonary artery pressure in infants with persistent pulmonary hypertension. Journal of Pediatrics 93: 1005–1010
832. Peevy K J, Chalhub E G 1983 Occult Group B streptococcal infection: an important cause of intrauterine asphyxia. American Journal of Obstetrics and Gynecology 146: 989–990
833. Pereira G R, Fox W W, Stanley C A, Baker L, Schwartz J G 1980 Decreased oxygenation and hyperlipemia during intravenous fat infusions in premature infants. Pediatrics 66: 26–30
834. Perelman R H, Palta M, Kirby R, Farrell P M 1986 Discordance between male and female deaths due to the respiratory distress syndrome. Pediatrics 78: 238–244
835. Perlman E J, Moore G W, Hutchins G M 1989 The pulmonary vasculature in meconium aspiration. Human Pathology 20: 701–706
836. Perlman J M, Volpe J J 1983 Suctioning in the preterm infant: effects on cerebral blood flow velocity, intracranial pressure and arterial blood pressure. Pediatrics 72: 329–334
837. Perlman J M, Goodman S, Kreusser K L, Volpe J J 1985 Reduction in intraventricular hemorrhage by elimination of fluctuating cerebral blood flow velocity in preterm infants with respiratory distress syndrome. New England Journal of Medicine 312: 1352–1357
838. Peterson H G, Pendleton M E 1955 Contrasting roentgenographic pulmonary patterns of the hyaline membrane and fetal aspiration syndromes. American Journal of Roentgenology 74: 800–813
839. Petres R E, Redwine F O, Cruikshank D P 1982 Congenital bilateral chylothorax: antepartum diagnosis and successful intrauterine surgical management. Journal of the American Medical Association 248: 1360–1365
840. Petros A J 1995 Epoprostenol (prostacyclin) for the treatment of pulmonary hypertension. BPA Medicines Standing Committee, London
841. Pfenninger E, Dick W, Brecht-Krauss D, Bitter F, Hofmann H, Bowdler I 1984 Investigation of intrapartum clearance of the upper airway in the presence of meconium contaminated amniotic fluid using an animal model. Journal of Perinatal Medicine 12: 57–68

842. Phibbs C S, Phibbs R A, Wakeley A, Schlueter M A, Sniderman S, Tooley W H 1993 Cost effects of surfactant therapy for neonatal respiratory distress syndrome. Journal of Pediatrics 123: 953–962
843. Phibbs R H, Johnson P, Kitterman J A, Gregory G A, Tooley W H 1972 Cardiorespiratory status of erythroblastotic infants. Pediatrics 49: 5–14
844. Philips J B III, Lyrene R K, Godoy G et al 1988 Hemodynamic responses of chronically instrumented piglets to bolus injections of group B streptococcus. Pediatric Research 23: 81–85
845. Piantadosi C A, Fracicia P J, Duhaylongsod F G et al 1995 Artificial surfactant attenuates hyperoxic lung injury in primates. II: Morphometric analysis. Journal of Applied Physiology 78: 1823–1831
846. Pickens D L, Scheft G, Thach B T 1988 Prolonged apnea associated with upper airway protective reflexes in apnea of prematurity. American Review of Respiratory Disease 137: 113–118
847. Pickens D L, Scheft G, Thach B T 1989 Pharyngeal fluid clearance and aspiration: preventative mechanisms in sleeping infants. Journal of Applied Physiology 66: 1164–1171
848. Pijpers L, Reuss A, Stewart P A, Wladimiroff J W 1989 Non-invasive management of isolated bilateral fetal hydrothorax. American Journal of Obstetrics and Gynecology 161: 330–332
849. Pildes R S 1986 Neonatal hyperglycemia. Journal of Pediatrics 109: 905–907
850. Pinkerton K E, Lewis J, Mulder A M et al 1993 Cost effects of surfactant therapy for neonatal respiratory distress syndrome. Journal of Pediatrics 123: 953–962
851. Pinkerton K E, Lewis J E, Rider E D et al 1994 Lung parenchyma and type II cell morphometrics: effect of surfactant treatment on preterm ventilated lamb lungs. Journal of Applied Physiology 77: 1953–1960
852. Piper J M, Xenakis E M-J, McFarland M 1996 Do growth retarded premature infants have different rates of perinatal morbidity and mortality than appropriately grown premature infants. Obstetrics and Gynecology 87: 169–174
853. Pitcher-Wilmott R, Shutack J G, Fox W W 1979 Decreased lung volume after nasogastric feeding of neonates recovering from respiratory disease. Journal of Pediatrics 95: 119–121
854. Plenat F, Vert P, Didier F, Andre M 1978 Pulmonary interstitial emphysema. Clinics in Perinatology 5: 351–375
855. Plexico D T, Loughlin G M 1981 Nasopharyngeal reflux and neonatal apnea. American Journal of Diseases of Children 135: 793–794
856. Pohlandt F, Sayle H, Schroeder H et al 1992 Decreased incidence of extra-alveolar air leakage or death prior to air leakage in high versus low rate positive pressure ventilation: results of a seven centre randomized trial in preterm infants. European Journal of Pediatrics 151: 904–909
857. Pokela M L 1994 Pain relief can reduce hypoxemia in distressed neonates during routine treatment procedures. Pediatrics 93: 379–383
858. Pokora T, Bing D, Mammel M, Boros S 1983 Neonatal high frequency jet ventilation. Pediatrics 72: 27–32
859. Polk D H, Ikegami M, Jobe A H et al 1995 Postnatal lung function in preterm lambs: effects of a single exposure to betamethasone and thyroid hormones. American Journal of Obstetrics and Gynecology 172: 872–881
860. Pollitzer M J, Reynolds E O R, Shaw D G, Thomas R M 1981 Pancuronium during mechanical ventilation speeds recovery of lungs of infants with hyaline membrane disease. Lancet i: 346–348
861. Powers W F, Clemens J A 1993 Prognostic implications of age at detection of air leak in very low birthweight infants requiring ventilatory support. Journal of Pediatrics 123: 611–617
862. Prasertsom W, Phillipos E Z, van Aerde J E, Robertson M 1996 Pulmonary vascular resistance during lipid infusion in neonates. Archives of Disease in Childhood 74: F95–F98
863. Price L T, Chen Y, Frank L 1993 Epidermal growth factor increases antioxidant enzyme and surfactant system development during hyperoxia and protects fetal rat lungs in vitro from hyperoxic toxicity. Pediatric Research 34: 577–585
864. Primhak R A 1983 Factors associated with pulmonary airleak in premature infants receiving mechanical ventilation. Journal of Pediatrics 102: 764–767
865. Primhak R A, Jedeikin R, Ellis G et al 1985 Myocardial ischaemia in asphyxia neonatorum. Acta Paediatrica Scandinavica 74: 595–600
866. Prod'hom L S, Levison H, Cherry R B, Smith E A 1965 Adjustment of ventilation, intrapulmonary gas exchange and acid balance in the first day of life. Pediatrics 35: 662–676
867. Puntis J W L, Roberts K D, Handy D 1987 How should chlyothorax be managed? Archives of Disease in Childhood 62: 593–596
868. Quinlan R W, Buhi W C, Cruz A C 1984 Fetal pulmonary maturity in isoimmunized pregnancies. American Journal of Obstetrics and Gynecology 148: 787–789
869. Quinn M W, Wild J, Dean H G et al 1993 Randomized double-blind controlled trial of effect of morphine on catecholamine concentrations in ventilated preterm babies. Lancet 342: 324–327
870. Qvist J, Pontoppidan H, Wilson R S et al 1975 Hemodynamic responses to mechanical ventilation with PEEP: the effect of hypervolemia. Anesthesiology 42: 45–55
871. Raine J, Hislop A A, Redington A N, Haworth S G, Shinebourne E A 1991 Fatal persistent pulmonary hypertension presenting late in the neonatal period. Archives of Disease in Childhood 66: 398–402
872. Raine J, Cowan F, Samuels M P, Wertheim D, Southall D P 1994 Continuous negative extrathoracic pressure and cerebral blood flow velocity: a pilot study. Acta Paediatrica 83: 438–439
873. Raju T N K, Langenberg P 1993 Pulmonary hemorrhage and exogenous surfactant therapy: a meta-analysis. Journal of Pediatrics 123: 603–610
874. Raju T N K, Vidyasagar D, Torres C, Grundy D, Bennett E J 1980 Intracranial pressure during intubation and anesthesia in infants. Journal of Pediatrics 96: 860–862
875. Ramenghi L A, Wood C M, Griffith G C, Levene M I 1996 Reduction of pain response in premature infants using intraoral sucrose. Archives of Disease in Childhood 74: F126–F128
876. Ramin K D, Leveno K J, Kelly M A, Carmody T J 1996 Amniotic fluid meconium: a fetal environmental hazard. Obstetrics and Gynecology 87: 181–184
877. Rasche R F H, Kuhns L P 1972 Histopathologic changes in airway mucosa of infants after endotracheal intubation. Pediatrics 50: 632–637
878. Rawlings J S, Smith F R, Wiswell T E 1984 Transient tachypnea of the newborn. An analysis of neonatal and obstetric risk factors. American Journal of Diseases of Children 138: 869–871
879. Raye J R, Gutberlet R L, Stahlman M 1970 Symptomatic posthemorrhagic anemia in the newborn. Pediatric Clinics of North America 17: 402–413
880. Redmond C R, Graves E D, Falterman K W, Ochsner J L, Arensman R M 1987 ECMO for respiratory and cardiac failure in infants and children. Journal of Thoracic and Cardiovascular Surgery 93: 199–204
881. Reece E A, Moya F, Yakigi R, Holford T, Duncan C, Ehrenkranz R A 1987 Persistent pulmonary hypertension: assessment of perinatal risk factors. Obstetrics and Gynecology 70: 696–700
882. Rees L, Forsling M L, Brook C D G 1980 Vasopressin concentrations in the neonatal period. Clinical Endocrinology 12: 357–362
883. Reid L, Rubino L 1959 The connective tissue septa in the fetal human lung. Thorax 14: 35–45
884. Rennie J M 1989 Cerebral blood flow velocity variability after cardiovascular support in premature babies. Archives of Disease in Childhood 64: 897–901
885. Rennie J M, Cooke R W 1991 Prolonged low dose indomethacin for the persistent ductus arteriosus of prematurity. Archives of Disease in Childhood 66: 55–58
886. Rennie J M, Roberton N R C 1993 Manipulation of the prostaglandin pathways in the management of overwhelming GBS sepsis. European Journal of Pediatrics 15: 926 (abstract)
887. Rennie J M, South M, Morley C J 1987 Cerebral blood flow velocity variability in infants receiving assisted ventilation. Archives of Disease in Childhood 62: 1247–1251
888. Rettwitz-Volk W, Schloesser R, von Loewenich V 1993 One-sided high frequency oscillating ventilation in the treatment of unilateral pulmonary emphysema. Acta Paediatrica 82: 190–192
889. Reynolds E O R 1971 Effects of alterations in mechanical ventilation settings on pulmonary gas exchange in hyaline membrane disease Archives of Disease in Childhood 46: 152–159
890. Reynolds E O R 1994 Commentator on: Carlo WA, Greenough A, Chatburn R L. Advances on conventional mechanical ventilation. In: Boynton B R, Carlo W A, Jobe A H (eds). New therapies for neonatal respiratory failure. Cambridge University Press, Cambridge, p 138

891. Reynolds E O R, Taghizadeh A 1974 Improved prognosis of infants mechanically ventilated for hyaline membrane disease. Archives of Disease in Childhood 49: 505–515
892. Reynolds E O R, Roberton N R C, Wigglesworth J S 1968 Hyaline membrane disease, respiratory distress and surfactant deficiency. Pediatrics 42: 758–768
893. Rhodes P G, Graves G R, Patel D M, Campbell S B, Blumenthal B I 1983 Minimizing pneumothorax and bronchopulmonary dysplasia in ventilated infants with hyaline membrane disease. Journal of Pediatrics 103: 634–637
894. Rhodes P G, Ferguson M G, Reddy N S, Joransen J A, Gibson J 1988 Effects of prolonged versus acute indomethacin therapy in very low birth-weight infants with patent ductus arteriosus. European Journal of Pediatrics 147: 481–484
895. Richardson C P, Jung A L 1978 Effects of continuous positive airway pressure on pulmonary function and blood gases in infants with respiratory distress syndrome. Pediatric Research 12: 771–774
896. Richardson D K, Torday J S 1994 Racial differences in predictive value of the lecithin/sphingomyelin ratio. American Journal of Obstetrics and Gynecology 170: 1273–1278
897. Richardson P, Bowes C L, Carlstrom J R 1986 The functional residual capacity of infants with respiratory distress syndrome. Acta Paediatrica Scandinavica 75: 267–271
898. Rigby M L, Pickering D, Wilkinson A 1984 Cross sectional echocardiography in determining persistent patency of the ductus arteriosus in preterm infants. Archives of Disease in Childhood 59: 341–345
899. Riggs T, Hirschfeld S, Fanaroff A A, Liebman J, Fletcher B, Meyer R 1977 Persistence of the fetal circulation syndrome: an echocardiographic study. Journal of Pediatrics 91: 626–631
900. Rishi A, Hatzis D, McAlmon F, Floros J 1992 An allelic variant of the 6A gene for surfactant protein A. American Journal of Physiology 262: 2566–2573
901. Robert M, Neff R, Hubbell J, Taeusch W, Avery M 1976 Association between maternal diabetes and the respiratory distress syndrome in the newborn. New England Journal of Medicine 294: 357–360
902. Roberton N R C 1970 Apnoea after THAM administration in the newborn. Archives of Disease in Childhood 45: 206–214
903. Roberton N R C 1976 Treatment of cystic ventilator lung disease. Proceedings of the Royal Society of Medicine 69: 344–347
904. Roberton N R C 1976 CPAP or not CPAP. Archives of Disease in Childhood 51: 161–162
905. Roberton N R C 1985 Persistent fetal circulation. Chairman's Summary. In: Clinch J, Matthews T (eds) Perinatal medicine. MTP Press, Lancaster, pp 199–200
906. Roberton N R C 1987 Top-up transfusions in childhood. Archives of Disease in Childhood 62: 984–986
907. Roberton N R C 1992 A manual of neonatal intensive care, 3rd edn. Edward Arnold, London pp 128-129
908. Roberton NRC 1993 Does CPAP work when it really matters? Acta Paediatrica 82: 206–207
909. Roberton N R C, Dahlenberg G W 1969 Ductus arteriosus shunts in the respiratory distress syndrome. Pediatric Research 3: 149–159
910. Roberton N R C, Smith M A 1975 Early neonatal hypocalcaemia. Archives of Disease in Childhood 50: 604–609
911. Roberton N R C, Tizard J P M 1975 Prognosis for infants with idiopathic respiratory distress syndrome. British Medical Journal 3: 271–274
912. Roberton N R C, Gupta J M, Dahlenberg G W, Tizard J P M 1968 Oxygen therapy in the newborn. Lancet i: 1323–1329
913. Roberts J D, Polaner D M, Lang P, Zapol W M 1992 Inhaled nitric oxide in persistent pulmonary hypertension of the newborn. Lancet 340: 818–819
914. Robertson B 1981 Neonatal pulmonary mechanics and morphology after experimental therapeutic regimes. In: Scarpelli E M, Cosmi E V (eds) Reviews in perinatal medicine, Vol. 4. Raven Press, New York, pp 337–379
915. Robertson P A, Sniderman S H, Laros R K et al 1992 Neonatal morbidity according to gestational age and birthweight from five tertiary care centres in the United States 1983 through 1986. American Journal of Obstetrics and Gynecology 166: 1629–1645
916. Robin E D, Wilson R J, Bromberg P A 1961 Intracellular acid-base relations and intracellular buffers. Annals of the New York Academy of Sciences 92: 539–544
917. Robinson M J, Maayan C, Eyal F G, Armon Y, Bar-Yishay E, Godfrey S 1982 Does the pattern of ventilation determine the degree of lung damage following intensive care of the newborn? Israel Journal of Medical Science 18: 835–839
918. Robson E, Hey E 1982 Resuscitation of preterm babies at birth reduces the risk of death from hyaline membrane disease. Archives of Disease in Childhood 57: 184–186
919. Rodriguez M P, Sosenko I R S, Antigua M C, Frank L 1991 Prenatal hormone treatment with thyrotropin releasing hormone and with thyrotropin releasing hormone plus dexamethasone delays antioxidant enzyme maturation but does not inhibit a protective antioxidant enzyme response to hyperoxia in newborn rat lung. Pediatric Research 30: 522–527
920. Rojas J, Stahlman M 1984 The effects of group B streptoccocus and other organisms on the pulmonary vasculature. Clinics in Perinatology 11: 591–599
921. Rojas J, Larsson L E, Hellerqvist C G, Brigham K L, Gray M E, Stahlman M T 1983 Pulmonary hemodynamic and ultrastructural changes associated with group B streptococcal toxemia in adult sheep and newborn lambs. Pediatric Research 70: 1002–1008
922. Romaguera J, Ramirez M, Adamsons K 1993 Intra-amniotic thyroxine to accelerate fetal maturation. Seminars in Perinatology 17: 260–266
923. Rosenberg A A, Kennaugh J, Koppenhafer S L, Loomis M, Chatfield B A, Abman S H 1993 Elevated immunoreactive endothelin I levels in newborn infants with persistent pulmonary hypertension. Journal of Pediatrics 123: 109–114
924. Rossi E M, Philipson E, Williams T G, Calhan S C 1989 Meconium aspiration syndrome: intrapartum and neonatal attributes. American Journal of Obstetrics and Gynecology 161: 1106–1110
925. Rossing T H, Solway J, Saari A F et al 1984 Influence of the endotracheal tube on CO_2 transport during high frequency ventilation. American Review of Respiratory Disease 129: 54–56
926. Rowe S, Avery M E 1966 Massive pulmonary hemorrhage in the newborn. II. Clinical considerations. Journal of Pediatrics 69: 12–20
927. Royall J A, Levin D L 1988 Adult respiratory distress syndrome in pediatric patients. I. Clinical aspects, pathophysiology, pathology and mechanisms of lung injury. Journal of Pediatrics 112: 169–180
928. Roze J C, Storme L, Zupan V, Morville P, Dinh-Xuan A T, Mercier J C 1994 Echocardiographic investigation of inhaled nitric oxide in newborn babies with severe hypoxaemia. Lancet 344: 303–305
929. Rudolph A J, Smith C A 1960 Idiopathic respiratory distress syndrome of the newborn. Journal of Pediatrics 57: 905–921
930. Rudolph A J, Vallbona C, Desmond M M 1965 Cardiodynamic studies in the newborn. III. Heart rate pattern in infants with idiopathic respiratory distress syndrome. Pediatrics 36: 551–559
931. Rudolph A M 1977 Fetal and neonatal pulmonary circulation. American Review of Respiratory Disease 115 (suppl.): 11–18
932. Rudolph A M, Yuan S 1966 Response of the pulmonary vasculature to hypoxia and hydrogen ion changes. Journal of Clinical Investigation 45: 399–411
933. Rudolph A M, Drorbaugh J E, Auld P A M et al 1961 Studies on the circulation in the neonatal period: the circulation in the respiratory distress syndrome: Pediatrics 27: 551–566
934. Runkle B, Goldberg R N, Streitfeld M M et 1984 Cardiovascular changes in group B streptococcal sepsis in the piglet: response to indomethacin and the relationship to prostacyclin and thromboxane A_2. Pediatric Research 18: 874–878
935. Rushforth J A, Griffiths G, Thorpe H, Levene M I 1995 Can topical lignocaine reduce behavioural response to heel prick? Archives of Disease in Childhood 72: F49–F51
936. Rutledge M, Hawkins E, Langston C 1986 Skeletal muscle atrophy induced in infants by chronic pancuronium treatment. Journal of Pediatrics 109: 883–886
937. Ryan C A, Finer N N, Peters K L 1989 Nasal intermittent positive pressure ventilation offers no advantages over nasal continuous positive airway pressure in apnea of prematurity. American Journal of Diseases of Children 143: 1196–1198
938. Ryan C A, Finer N N, Barrington K J 1994 Effects of magnesium sulphate and nitric oxide in pulmonary hypertension induced by hypoxia in newborn piglets. Archives of Disease in Childhood 71: F151–155
939. Sackner M A, Landa J, Hirsch J, Zapata A 1975 Pulmonary effects of oxygen breathing. Annals of Internal Medicine 82: 40–43

940. Salmon G W, Forbes G B, Davenport H 1947 Air block in the newborn infant. Journal of Pediatrics 30: 260–265
941. Samuels M P, Southall D P 1989 Negative extrathoracic pressure in treatment of respiratory failure in infants and young children. British Medical Journal 299: 1253–1257
942. Sandberg K, Engelhardt B, Hellerqvist C, Sundell H 1987 Pulmonary response to group B streptococcal toxin in young lambs. Journal of Applied Physiology 63: 2024–2030
943. Sandberg K, Sjoqvist BA, Hjalmarson O, Olsson T 1987 Lung function in newborn infants with tachypnea of unknown cause. Pediatric Research 22: 581–586
944. Saugstad O D 1996 Mechanisms of tissue injury by oxygen radicals: implications for neonatal disease. Acta Paediatrica 85: 1–4
945. Savage M O, Wilkinson A R, Baum J D, Roberton N R C 1975 Frusemide in respiratory distress syndrome. Archives of Disease in Childhood 50: 709–713
946. Schaffer A J, Avery ME 1977 Aspiration pneumonia. In: Schaffer A J, Avery M E (eds) Disease of the newborn, 3rd edn. Philadelphia, W B Saunders, pp 116–126
947. Schatz M, Zeiger R S, Hoffman C P, Saunders B S, Harden K M, Forsythe A B 1991 Increased transient tachypnea of the newborn in infants of asthmatic mothers. American Journal of Disease of Children 145: 156–158
948. Schiff E, Friedman S A, Mercer B M, Sibai B M 1993 Fetal lung maturity is not accelerated in pre-eclamptic pregnancies. American Journal of Obstetrics and Gynecology 169: 1096–1101
949. Schonberger W, Grimm W, Emmrich P, Gempp J 1981 Reduction of mortality rate in premature infants by substitution of thyroid hormones. European Journal of Pediatrics 135: 245–253
950. Schrod L, Hornemann F, von Stockhausen H B 1996 Chemiluminescence activity of phagocytes from tracheal aspirates of premature infants after surfactant therapy. Acta Paediatrica 85: 719–723
951. Schulze A, Schaller P, Gerhardt B, Mildler H, Gruyrex D 1990 An infant ventilatory technique for resistive unloading during spontaneous breathing. Results in a rabbit model of airway obstruction. Pediatric Research 28: 79–82
952. Schumacher R E, Barks J D E, Johnston M V et al 1988 Right sided brain lesions in infants following extracorporeal membrane oxygenation. Pediatrics 82: 155–161
953. Schwartz A M, Graham C B 1986 Neonatal tension pulmonary interstitial emphysema in bronchopulmonary dysplasia: treatment with lateral decubitus positioning. Radiology 161: 351–354
954. Schwendeman C A, Clark R H, Yoder B A, Null D M, Gertsmann D R, De Lemos R A 1992 Frequency of chronic lung disease in infants with severe respiratory failure treated with high frequency ventilation and/or extracorporeal membrane oxygenation. Critical Care Medicine 20: 372–377
955. Seeger W, Stohr G, Wolf H R D, Neuhof H 1985 Alteration of surfactant function due to protein leakage: special interaction with fibrin monomer. Journal of Applied Physiology 58: 326–338
956. Segal M L, Goetzman B W, Schick J B 1980 Thrombocytopenia and pulmonary hypertension in the perinatal aspiration syndrome. Journal of Pediatrics 96: 727–730
957. Segerer H, van Gelder W, Angenent F W M 1993 Pulmonary distribution and efficacy of exogenous surfactant in lung lavaged rabbits are influenced by the instillation technique. Pediatric Research 34: 490–494
958. Seppänen M P, Kääpä P O, Kero P O, Saraste M 1994 Doppler derived systolic pulmonary artery pressure in acute neonatal respiratory distress syndrome. Pediatrics 93: 769–773
959. Seri I 1995 Cardiovascular, renal and endocrine actions of dopamine in neonates and children. Journal of Pediatrics 126: 333–344
960. Seri I, Rudas G, Bors Z, Kanyicska B, Tulassay T 1993 Effects of low dose dopamine infusion on cardiovascular and renal functions, cerebral blood flow and plasma catecholamine levels in sick preterm neonates. Pediatric Research 34: 742–749
961. Sessler D, Mills P, Gregory G, Litt L, James T 1987 Effects of bicarbonate on arterial and brain intracellular pH in neonatal rabbits recovering from hypoxic lactic acidosis. Journal of Pediatrics 111: 817–823
962. Setzer E, Ermocilla R, Tonkin I, John E, Sansa M, Cassady G 1980 Papillary muscle necrosis in a neonatal autopsy population. Incidence and associated clinical manifestations. Journal of Pediatrics 96: 289–294
963. Seyberth H W, Müller H, Ulmer H E, Wille L 1984 Urinary excretion rates of 6-keto-$PGF_{1\alpha}$ in preterm infants recovering from respiratory distress with and without patent ductus arteriosus. Pediatric Research 18: 520–524
964. Shaffer S G, Bradt S K, Hall R T 1986 Postnatal changes in total body water and extracellular volume in the preterm infant with respiratory distress syndrome. Journal of Pediatrics 109: 509–514
965. Shaffer S G, Geer P G, Goetz K L 1986 Elevated atrial natriuretic factor in neonates with respiratory distress syndrome. Journal of Pediatrics 109: 1028–1033
966. Shaffer T H, Koen P A, Moskowitz G D, Ferguson J D, Delivoria-Papadopoulos M 1978 Positive end expiratory pressure: effects on lung mechanics of premature lambs. Biology of the Neonate 34: 1–10
967. Shah DM, Shenai J P, Vaughn W K 1995 Neonatal outcome of mothers with pre-eclampsia. Journal of Perinatology 15: 264–267
968. Shankran S, Farooki Z Q, Desai R 1982 Hemolytic streptococcal infection appearing as persistent fetal circulation. American Journal of Diseases of Children 136: 725–727
969. Shaver D C, Bada H S, Korones S B, Anderson G D, Wong S P, Arheart K L 1992 Early and late intraventricular hemorrhage: the role of obstetric factors. Obstetrics and Gynecology 80: 831–837
970. Shaw N J, Cooke R W I, Gill A B, Shaw N J, Saaed M 1993 Randomised trial of routine versus selective paralysis during ventilation for neonatal respiratory distress syndrome. Archives of Disease in Childhood 69: 479–482
971. Shelley S A, Kovacevic M, Paciga J E, Balis J U 1979 Sequential changes of surfactant phosphatidylcholine in hyaline membrane disease of the newborn. New England Journal of Medicine 300: 112–116
972. Shepherd A J, Richardson C J, Brown J P 1985 Nuchal cord as a cause of neonatal anemia. American Journal of Diseases of Children 139: 71–73
973. Sherman J M, Lowitt S, Stephenson C, Ironson G 1986 Factors influencing aquired subglottic stenosis in infants. Journal of Pediatrics 109: 322–327
974. Sherman M P, Evans M J, Campbell L A 1988 Prevention of pulmonary alveolar macrophage proliferation in newborn rabbits by hyperoxia. Journal of Pediatrics 112: 782–786
975. Shinwell E S, Karplus M, Zmora E 1996 Failure of early postnatal dexamethasone to prevent chronic lung disease in infants with respiratory distress syndrome. Archives of Disease in Childhood 74: 33–37
976. Shiono P H, Klebanoff M A 1993 A review of risk scoring for premature birth. Clinics in Perinatology 20: 107–125
977. Shivpuri C R, Martin R J, Carlo W A, Fanaroff A S 1983 Decreased ventilation in preterm infants during oral feeding. Journal of Pediatrics 103: 285–289
978. Shohet I, Reichman B, Schibi G, Brish M 1984 Familial persistent pulmonary hypertension. Archives of Disease in Childhood 59: 783–785
979. Shook D R, Cram K B, Williams H J 1975 Pulmonary venous air embolism in hyaline membrane disease. American Journal of Radiology 125: 538–542
980. Short B L, Miller M K, Anderson K D 1987 Extracorporeal membrane oxygenation in the management of respiratory failure in the newborn. Clinics in Perinatology 14: 737–748
981. Shribman A J, Smith G, Achola K J 1987 Cardiovascular and catecholamine responses to laryngoscopy with and without intubation. British Journal of Anaesthesia 59: 295–299
982. Shulman R J, Langston C, Schanler R J 1987 Pulmonary vascular lipid deposition after administration of intravenous fat to infants. Pediatrics 79: 99–102
983. Silverman W A, Anderson D H 1956 A controlled clinical trial of effects of water mist on obstructive respiratory signs, death rate and necropsy findings in premature infants. Pediatrics 17: 1–9
984. Simbruner G 1986 Inadvertent positive end expiratory pressure in mechanically ventilated newborn infants: detection and effect on lung mechanics and gas exchange. Journal of Pediatrics 108: 589–595
985. Simbruner G, Coradello H, Foder M, Havelec L, Lubec G, Pollak A 1981 Effects of tracheal suction on oxygenation, circulation and lung mechanics in newborn infants. Archives of Disease in Childhood 54: 326–330
986. Sinha S K, Levene M I 1984 Pancuronium bromide induced joint

contractions in the newborn. Archives of Disease in Childhood 59: 73–75
987. Skelton R, Jeffery H E 1996 Factors affecting the neonatal response to artificial surfactant. Journal of Paediatrics and Child Health 32: 236–241
988. Skinner J R, Boys R J, Hunter S, Hey E N 1992 Pulmonary and systemic arterial pressure in hyaline membrane disease. Archives of Disease in Childhood 67: 366–373
989. Skinner J R, Milligan D W A, Hunter S, Hey E N 1992 Central venous pressure in the ventilated neonate. Archives of Disease in Childhood 67: 374–377
990. Skinner J R, Hunter S, Hey E N 1996 Haemodynamic features at presentation in persistent pulmonary hypertension of the newborn and outcome. Archives of Disease in Childhood 74: F26–F32
991. Skov L, Ryding J, Pryds D, Greisen G 1992 Changes in cerebral oxygenation and cerebral blood volume during endotracheal suctioning in ventilated neonates. Acta Paediatrica 81: 389–393
992. Slagle T A, Gross S J 1988 Effect of early volume enteral substrate on subsequent feeding tolerance in very low birthweight infants. Journal of Pediatrics 113: 526–531
993. Slutsky A S, Brown R, Lehr J et al 1981 High frequency ventilation: a promising new approach to mechanical ventilation. Medical Instrumentation 15: 228–233
994. Smith C V, Hansen T N, Martin N E et al 1993 Oxidant stress responses to premature infants during exposure to hyperoxia. Pediatric Research 34: 360–365
995. Smyth J, Allen M, MacMurray B 1995 Double blind randomized placebo controlled Canadian multicenter trial of two doses of synthetic surfactant or air placebo in 224 infants weighing 500–749 grams with respiratory distress syndrome. Journal of Pediatrics 126: 581–589
996. Snashall P D 1980 Pulmonary oedema. British Journal of Diseases of the Chest 74: 2–22
997. Snyder J M, Mendelson C R 1987 Insulin inhibits the accumulation of the major lung surfactant apoprotein in human fetal lung explants maintained in vitro. Endocrinology 120: 1250–1257
998. Snyder J M, Kwun J E, O'Brien J A, Rosenfeld C R, Odom M J 1988 The concentration of the 35-kDa surfactant apoprotein in amniotic fluid from normal and diabetic pregnancies. Pediatric Research 24: 728–734
999. Soifer S J, Clyman R I, Heymann M A 1988 Effects of prostaglandin D2 on pulmonary arterial pressure and oxygenation in newborn infants with persistent pulmonary hypertension. Journal of Pediatrics 112: 774–777
1000. Soll R F 1996 Appropriate surfactant usage. European Journal of Pediatrics 155: S8–S13
1001. Soll R F, Merritt T A, Hallman M 1994 Surfactant in the prevention and treatment of respiratory distress syndrome. In: Boynton B R, Carlo W A, Jobe A H (eds) New therapies for neonatal respiratory failure. Cambridge University Press, Cambridge, pp 49–80
1002. Soll R F, Sinclair J C, Bracken M B 1995 Natural surfactant extract vs synthetic surfactant: meta-analysis of randomized controlled trials. Pediatric Research 37: 274A
1003. Sosenko I R 1993 Antenatal cocaine exposure produces accelerated surfactant maturation without stimulation of antioxidant enzyme development in the late gestation rat. Pediatric Research 33: 327–331
1004. Sosenko I R S, Chen Y, Price L, Frank L 1995 Failure of premature rabbits to increase lung antioxidant enzyme activities after hyperoxic exposure: antioxidant enzyme gene expression and pharmacologic intervention with endotoxin and dexamethasone. Pediatric Research 37: 496–475
1005. Sosenko I R S, Innis S M, Frank L 1991 Intralipid increases lung polyunsaturated fatty acids and protects newborn rats from oxygen toxicity. Pediatric Research 30: 413–417
1006. Sosenko I R S, Rodriguez-Pierce M, Bancalari E 1993 Effect of early initiation of intravenous lipid administration on the incidence and severity of chronic lung disease in premature infants. Journal of Pediatrics 123: 975–982
1007. South M, Morley C J 1986 Synchronous mechanical ventilation of the neonate. Archives of Disease in Childhood 61: 1190–1195
1008. South M, Morley C J 1986 Spontaneous respiratory timing in intubated neonates with RDS (abstract). Early Human Development 14: 147–148
1009. Speer C P, Robertson B, Curstedt T et al 1992 Randomized European multicenter trial of surfactant replacement therapy for severe neonatal respiratory distress syndrome: single versus multiple doses of Curosurf. Pediatrics 89: 13–20
1010. Speer C P, Gefeller O, Gronek P 1995 Randomized clinical trial of two treatment regimens of natural surfactant preparations in neonatal respiratory distress syndrome. Archives of Disease in Childhood 72: F8–F13
1011. Speidel B D 1978 Adverse effects of routine procedures on preterm infants. Lancet i: 864–866
1012. Spencer J A D, Robson S C, Farkas A 1993 Spontaneous recovery after severe metabolic acidaemia at birth. Early Human Development 32: 103–112
1013. Spitzer A R, Fox W W 1982 Post-extubation atelectasis – the role of oral versus nasal endotracheal tubes. Journal of Pediatrics 100: 806–811
1014. Spitzer A R, Davis J, Clarke W T, Bernbaum J, Fox W W 1988 Pulmonary hypertension and persistent fetal circulation in the newborn. Clinics in Perinatology 15: 389–413
1015. Stahlman M T 1977 Respiratory disorders in the newborn: type II respiratory distress. In: Kendig E L (ed) Disorders of the respiratory tract in children. W B Saunders, Philadelphia, pp 290–292
1016. Stahlman M, Blankenship W J, Shepard F M, Gray J, Young W C, Malan A F 1972 Circulatory studies in clinical hyaline membrane disease. Biology of the Neonate 20: 300–320
1017. Stahlman M T, Cheatham W, Gray M E 1979 The role of air dissection in bronchopulmonary dysplasia. Journal of Pediatrics 95: 878–885
1018. Stanley F J, Alberman E D 1978 Infants of very low birthweight. I. Perinatal factors affecting survival. Developmental Medicine and Child Neurology 20: 300–312
1019. Stark A R, Davidson D 1995 Inhaled nitric oxide for persistent pulmonary hypertension of the newborn: implications and strategy for future 'high-tech' neonatal clinical trials. Pediatrics 96: 1147–1151
1020. Stark A R, Thach B T 1976 Mechanisms of airway obstruction leading to apnea in newborn infants. Journal of Pediatrics 89: 982–985
1021. Stark A R, Bascom R, Frantz I D 1979 Muscle relaxation in mechanically ventilated infants. Journal of Pediatrics 94: 439–444
1022. Steele R W, Metz J R, Bass J W, DuBois J J 1971 Pneumothorax and pneumomediastinum in the newborn. Radiology 98: 629–632
1023. Steinhorn R H, Millard S L, Morin F C 1995 Persistent pulmonary hypertension of the newborn: role of nitric oxide and endothelin in pathophysiology and treatment. Clinics in Perinatology 22: 405–428
1024. Steinschneider A, Weinstein S L, Diamond E 1982 The sudden infant death syndrome and apnea/obstruction during neonatal sleep and feeding. Pediatrics 70: 858–863
1025. Stenmark K R, James S L, Voelkel N F, Toews W H, Reeves J T, Murphy R C 1983 Leukotriene C_4 and D_4 in neonates with hypoxia and pulmonary hypertension. New England Journal of Medicine 309: 77–80
1026. Stenson B J, Glover R M, Wilkie R A et al 1995 Life-threatening inadvertent positive end expiratory pressure. American Journal of Perinatology 12: 336–338
1027. Stern L 1970 Description and utilization of the negative pressure apparatus. Biology of the Neonate 16: 24–29
1028. Stevens J C, Eigen H, Wysomierski D 1988 Absence of long term pulmonary sequelae after mild meconium aspiration syndrome. Pediatric Pulmonology 5: 74–81
1029. Stevenson D K, Kasting D S, Darnall R A et al 1979 Refractory hypoxemia associated with neonatal pulmonary disease. Journal of Pediatrics 95: 595–599
1030. Stevenson D, Walther F, Long W et al 1992 Controlled trial of a single dose of synthetic surfactant at birth in premature infants weighing 500–699 grams. Journal of Pediatrics 120: S3–S12
1031. Stocker T J, Madewell J E 1977 Persistent interstitial pulmonary emphysema: another complication of the respiratory distress syndrome. Pediatrics 59: 847–857
1032. Stocks J 1980 Effect of nasogastric tubes on nasal resistance during infancy. Archives of Disease in Childhood 5: 17–21
1033. Strang L B 1977 Neonatal respiration. Blackwell Scientific Publications, Oxford, p 207
1034. Strang L B 1977 Milk aspiration and Wilson–Mikity syndrome. In:

Strang L B (ed) Neonatal respiration. Blackwell Scientific Publications, Oxford, p 274

1035. Strang L B 1977 Haemorrhagic lung oedema and massive pulmonary haemorrhage. In: Strang L B (ed) Neonatal respiration. Blackwell Scientific Publications, Oxford, p 259
1036. Strang L B, McLeish M H 1961 Ventilatory failure and right-to-left shunt in newborn infants with respiratory distress. Pediatrics 28: 17–27
1037. Strang L B, Anderson G S, Platt J W 1957 Neonatal death and selective caesarean section. Lancet i: 954–956
1038. Strauss R G 1995 Red blood cell transfusion practices in the neonate. Clinics in Perinatology 22: 641–655
1039. Strayer D S, Robertson B 1992 Surfactant as an immunogen: implications for therapy of respiratory distress syndrome. Acta Paediatrica 81: 446–447
1040. Strayer D S, Merritt T A, Hallman M 1995 Levels of SP-A-anti-SP-A immune complexes in neonatal respiratory distress syndrome correlate with subsequent development of bronchopulmonary dysplasia. Acta Paediatrica 84: 128–131
1041. Strong T H, Hetzler G, Sarno A P, Paul R H 1990 Prophylactic intrapartum amnioinfusion: a randomized clinical trial. American Journal of Obstetrics and Gynecology 162: 1370–1375
1042. Sun B, Curstedt T, Robertson B 1993 Surfactant inhibition in experimental meconium aspiration. Acta Paediatrica 82: 182–189
1043. Sunoo C, Kosasa T S, Hale R W 1989 Meconium aspiration syndrome without evidence of fetal distress in early labour before elective caesarean delivery. Obstetrics and Gynecology 73: 707–709
1044. Suske G, Oestreich K, Varnholt V, Lasch P, Kachel W 1996 Influence of early postnatal dexamethasone therapy on ventilator-dependency in surfactant-substituted preterm infants. Acta Paediatrica 85: 713–718
1045. Sutherland P D, Quinn M 1993 Nellcor Stat Cap differentiates oesophageal from tracheal intubation. Archives of Disease in Childhood 73: F184–F186
1046. Svenningsen N W 1992 Pulmonary functional residual capacity and lung mechanics in surfactant treated infants. Seminars in Perinatology 16: 181–185
1047. Swaminathan S, Quinn J, Stabile M W, Bader D, Platzker A C G, Keens T G 1989 Long term pulmonary sequelae of meconium aspiration syndrome. Journal of Pediatrics 114: 356–361
1048. Swingle H M, Eggert L D, Bucciarelli R L 1984 New approach to management of unilateral tension pulmonary interstitial emphysema in premature infants. Pediatrics 74: 354–357
1049. Swischuk L E 1976 Two lesser known but useful signs of neonatal pneumothorax. American Journal of Roentgenology 127: 623–627
1050. Swyer P R, Reiman R C, Wright J J 1960. Ventilation and ventilatory mechanics in the newborn: methods and results in 15 infants. Journal of Pediatrics 56: 612–622
1051. Sykes G S, Molloy P M, Johnson P et al 1982 Do Apgar scores indicate asphyxia. Lancet i: 494–496
1052. Szymonowicz W, Yu V Y H, Walker A, Wilson F, 1986 Reduction in periventricular haemorrhage in preterm infants. Archives of Disease in Childhood 61: 661–665
1053. Tammela O K, Lanning F P, Koivisto M E 1992 The relationship of fluid restriction during the first month of life to the occurrence and severity of bronchopulmonary dysplasia in low birthweight infants: a 1-year radiological follow up. European Journal of Pediatrics 151: 367–371
1054. Tanswell A K, Clubb R A, Smith B T, Boston R W 1980 Individualised continuous distending pressure applied within 6 hours of delivery in neonates with respiratory distress syndrome. Archives of Disease in Childhood 55: 33–39
1055. Tarnow-Mordi W 1991 Is routine endotracheal suction justified? Archives of Disease in Childhood 66: 374–375
1056. Tarnow-Mordi W O, Wilkinson A R 1985 Inspiratory:expiratory ratio and pulmonary interstitial emphysema. Archives of Disease in Childhood 60: 496–497
1057. Tarnow-Mordi W, Ogston S, Wilkinson A R et al 1990 Predicting death from initial disease severity in very low birthweight infants: a method for comparing the performance of neonatal units. British Medical Journal 300: 1611–1614
1058. Tarnow-Mordi W O, Shaw J C L, Liu D, Gardner D A, Flynn F V 1981 Iatrogenic hyponatraemia of the newborn due to maternal fluid overload—a prospective study. British Medical Journal 283: 639–642
1059. Tarnow-Mordi W O, Narang A, Wilkinson A R 1985 Lack of association of barotrauma and airleak in hyaline membrane disease. Archives of Disease in Childhood 60: 555–560
1060. Tarnow-Mordi W O, Fletcher M, Sutton P, Wilkinson A R 1986 Evidence of inadequate humidification of inspired gas during artificial ventilation of newborn babies in the British Isles. Lancet ii: 909–910
1061. Tarpey M N, Gray G B, Lyrene R K et al 1987 Thromboxane synthesis inhibition reverses group B streptococcus induced pulmonary hypertension. Critical Care Medicine 15: 644–647
1062. Taylor J, Dibbins A, Sobel D B 1993 Neonatal pneumomediastinum: indications for and complications of treatment. Critical Care Medicine 21: 296–298
1063. Taylor P M, Allen A C, Stinson D A 1971 Benign unexplained respiratory distress of the newborn. Pediatric Clinics of North America 18: 975–1004
1064. Ten Centre Study Group 1987 Ten centre trial of artificial surfactant (artificial lung expanding compound) in very premature babies. British Medical Journal 294: 991–996
1065. Termote J U M, Schalij-Delfos N E, Wittebol-Post D et al 1994 Surfactant replacement therapy: a new risk factor in developing retinopathy of prematurity? European Journal of Pediatrics 153: 113–116
1066. Thibeault D W, Lachman R S, Laul V R, Kwong M S 1973 Pulmonary interstitial emphysema, pneumomediastinum and pneumothorax. Occurrence in the newborn infant. American Journal of Diseases of Children 126: 611–614
1067. Thibeault D W, Hall F K, Sheehan M B, Hall R T 1984 Postasphyxial lung disease in newborn infants with severe perinatal acidosis. American Journal of Obstetrics and Gynecology 150: 393–399
1068. Thomas V D, Fletcher G, Sunshine P, Shafer I A, Klaus M H 1965 Prolonged respirator use in pulmonary insufficiency of the newborn. Journal of the American Medical Association 193: 183–190
1069. Thompson P J, Greenough A, Gamsu H R, Nicolaides K H 1992 Ventilatory requirements for respiratory distress syndrome in small for gestational age infants. European Journal of Pediatrics 151: 528–531
1070. Thompson W K, Marchak B E, Froese A B, Bryan A C 1982 High frequency oscillation compared with standard ventilation in pulmonary injury model. Journal of Applied Physiology 52: 543–548
1071. Tiefenbrunn L J, Riemenschneider T A 1986 Persistent pulmonary hypertension of the newborn. American Heart Journal 111: 564–572
1072. Timms B J M, Di Fiore J M, Martin R J, Miller M J 1993 Increased respiratory drive as an inhibitor of oral feeding of preterm infants. Journal of Pediatrics 123: 127–131
1073. Ting P, Brady J P 1975 Tracheal suction in meconium aspiration. American Journal of Obstetrics and Gynecology 122: 767–770
1074. Toce S S, Keenan W J 1988 Congenital echovirus 11 pneumonia with pulmonary hypertension. Pediatric Infectious Disease 7: 360–361
1075. Todres I D, de Bros F, Kramer S S, Moylan F M B, Shannon D C 1976 Endotracheal tube displacement in the newborn infant. Journal of Pediatrics 89: 126–127
1076. Tolsa J F, Cotting J, Sekarski N, Payot M, Micheli J L, Calame A 1995 Magnesium sulphate as an alternative and safe treatment for severe persistent pulmonary hypertension of the newborn. Archives of Disease in Childhood 72: F184–F187
1077. Tooley W H 1979 Epidemiology of bronchopulmonary dysplasia. Journal of Pediatrics 95: 851–858
1078. Torday J 1992 Cellular timing of fetal lung development. Seminars in Perinatology 16: 130–139
1079. Towne B H, Lott I T, Hicks D A, Healey T 1985 Long term follow-up of infants and children treated with extracorporeal membrane oxygenation (ECMO)—a preliminary report. Journal of Pediatric Surgery 20: 410–414
1080. Tran N, Lowe C, Sivieri E M, Shaffer T H 1980 Sequential effects of acute meconium obstruction on pulmonary function. Pediatric Research 14: 34–38
1081. Trang T T, Tibballs J, Mercier J C, Beaufils F 1988 Optimization of oxygen transport in mechanically ventilated newborns using oximetry and pulsed Doppler-derived cardiac output. Critical Care Medicine 16: 1094–1097
1082. Troche B, Harvey-Wilkes K, Engle W D et al 1995 Early minimal

feedings promote growth in critically ill premature infants. Biology of the Neonate 67: 172–181
1083. Trompeter R, Yu V Y H, Aynsley-Green A, Roberton N R C 1975 Massive pulmonary haemorrhage in the newborn infant. Archives of Disease in Childhood 50: 123–127
1084. Truog W E, Standaert T A, Murphy J, Palmer S, Woodrum D E, Hodson W A 1983 Effect of high-frequency oscillation on the gas exchange and pulmonary phospholipids in experimental hyaline membrane disease. American Review of Respiratory Disease 127: 585–589
1085. Trus T, Winthrop A L, Pipe S, Shah J, Langer J C, Lau G Y P 1993 Optimal management of patent ductus arteriosus in the neonate weighing less than 800 g. Journal of Pediatric Surgery 28: 1137–1139
1086. Tubman T R J, Rollins M D, Patterson C, Halliday H L 1991 Increased incidence of respiratory distress syndrome in babies of hypertensive mothers. Archives of Disease in Childhood 66: 52–4
1087. Tudehope D I, Bagley C 1980 Techniques of physiotherapy in intubated babies with respiratory distress syndrome. Australian Paediatric Journal 16: 226–228
1088. Tudehope D I, Smyth M H 1979 Is transient tachypnoea of the newborn always a benign condition? Australian Paediatric Journal 15: 160–165
1089. Tulassay T, Seri I 1986 Acute oliguria in preterm infants with hyaline membrane disease. Interaction of dopamine and frusemide. Acta Paediatrica Scandinavica 75: 420–424
1090. Turbow R, Waffarn F, Yang L, Sills J, Hallman M 1995 Variable oxygenation response to inhaled nitric oxide in severe persistent pulmonary hypertension of the newborn. Acta Paediatrica 84: 1305–1308
1091. Turkel S P, Mapp J R 1983 A ten year retrospective study of pink and yellow neonatal hyaline membrane disease. Pediatrics 72: 170–175
1092. Turner G R, Levin D L 1984 Prostaglandin synthesis inhibition in persistent pulmonary hypertension of the newborn. Clinics in Perinatology 11: 581–589
1093. Turner T, Prowse C V, Precott R J, Cash J D 1981 A clinical trial on the early detection and correction of haemostatic defects in selected high risk neonates. British Journal of Haematology 47: 65–75
1094. Turrentine M A, Dupras-Wilson P, Wilkins I 1996 A retrospective analysis of the effect of antenatal steroid administration on the incidence of respiratory distress syndrome in preterm twin pregnancies. American Journal of Perinatology 13: 351–354
1095. Tütüncü A S, Faithfull N S, Lachmann B 1993 Comparison of ventilatory support with intratracheal perfluorocarbon administration and conventional mechanical ventilation in animals with acute respiratory failure. American Review of Respiratory Disease 148: 785–792
1096. Tyler D C, Murphy J, Cheney F W 1978 Mechanical and chemical damage to lung tissue caused by meconium aspiration. Pediatrics 62: 454–459
1097. Ueda T, Ikegami M, Polk D 1995 Effects of fetal corticosteroid treatment on postnatal surfactant function in preterm lambs. Journal of Applied Physiology 79: 846–851
1098. Ueda T, Ikegami M, Rider E D, Jobe A H 1994 Distribution of surfactant and ventilation in surfactant treated preterm lambs. Journal of Applied Physiology 76: 45–55
1099. UK Collaborative ECMO Trial Group 1996 UK collaborative randomised trial of neonatal extracorporeal membrane oxygenation. Lancet 348: 75–82
1100. Upton C J, Milner A D, Stokes G M 1990 The effect of changes in inspiratory time on neonatal triggered ventilation. European Journal of Pediatrics 149: 668–670
1101. Usher R H 1959 The respiratory distress syndrome of prematurity. I. Changes in potassium in the serum and ECG, and effects of therapy. Pediatrics 24: 562–576
1102. Usher R H 1963 Reduction of mortality from RDS of prematurity with early administration of intravenous glucose and sodium bicarbonate. Pediatrics 32: 966–975
1103. Usher R H, McLean F, Maughan G B 1964 Respiratory distress syndrome in infants delivered by caesarean section. American Journal of Obstetrics and Gynecology 88: 806–815
1104. Usher R H, Allen A C, McLean F H 1971 Risk of respiratory distress syndrome related to gestational age, route of delivery and maternal diabetes. American Journal of Obstetrics and Gynecology 111: 826–832
1105. Usher R H, Saigal S, O'Neill A, Surainder Y, Chua L-B 1975 Estimation of RBC volume in premature infants with and without respiratory distress syndrome. Biology of the Neonate 26: 241–248
1106. Usta I M, Mercer B M, Aswad N K, Sibai B M 1995 The impact of a policy of amnioinfusion for meconium stained amnotic fluid. Obstetrics and Gynecology 85: 237–241
1107. Vain N E, Prudent L M, Stevens D P, Weeter M M, Maisels M J 1989 Regulation of oxygen concentration delivered to infants via nasal cannulas. American Journal of Diseases of Children 143: 1458–1460
1108. Valdes-Cruz L M, Dudell G G, Ferrara A 1981 Utility of M-mode echocardiography for early identification of infants with persistent pulmonary hypertension of the newborn. Pediatrics 68: 515–525
1109. Van Aerde J, Campbell A N, Smyth J A, Lloyd D, Bryan M H 1984 Spontaneous chylothorax in newborns. American Journal of Diseases of Children 138: 961–964
1110. van Bel F, de Winter PJ, Wijnands HB, van de Bor M, Egberts J 1992 Cerebral and aortic blood flow velocity patterns in preterm infants receiving prophylactic surfactant treatment. Acta Paediatrica 81: 504–510
1111. van de Bor M, Ma E J, Walther F J 1991 Cerebral blood flow velocity after surfactant instillation in preterm infants. Journal of Pediatrics 118: 285–287
1112. van der Bleek J, Plötz F B, van Overbeek F M et al 1993 Distribution of exogenous surfactant in rabbits with severe respiratory failure: the effect of volume. Pediatric Research 34: 154–158
1113. Vanhaesebrouck P, Leroy J G, Depraeter C, Parijs M, Thiery M 1989 Simple test to distinguish between surgical and non-surgical pneumoperitoneum in ventilated neonates. Archives of Disease in Childhood 64: 48–49
1114. Vanhaesebrouck P, Vanneste K, Praeter C de, van Trapper Y, Thiery M 1987 Tight nuchal cord and neonatal hypovolaemic shock. Archives of Disease in Childhood 62: 1276–1277
1115. van Houten J, Long W, Mullett M 1992 Pulmonary hemorrhage in premature infants after treatment with synthetic surfactant. An autopsy evaluation. Journal of Pediatrics 120: S40–S44
1116. van Marter L, Leviton A, Allred EN et al 1996 Persistent pulmonary hypertension of the newborn and smoking and aspirin and non-steroidal anti-inflammatory drug consumption during pregnancy. Pediatrics 97: 658–663
1117. van Norstrand C, Beamish W E, Schiff D 1975 Neonatal pneumopericardium. Canadian Medical Association Journal 112: 186–192
1118. Varnholt V, Lasch P, Suske G, Kachel W, Brands W 1992 High frequency oscillatory ventilation and extracorporeal membrane oxygenation in severe persistent pulmonary hypertension of the newborn. European Journal of Pediatrics 151: 769–774
1119. Vaughan R S, Menke J A, Giacoia G P 1978 Pneumothorax: a complication of endotracheal tube suctioning. Journal of Pediatrics 92: 633–635
1120. Veness-Meeham K A, Richter S, Davis J M 1990 Pulmonary function testing prior to extubation in infants with respiratory distress syndrome. Pediatric Pulmonology 9: 2–6
1121. Vermont-Oxford Neonatal Network 1996 A multicenter randomized trial comparing synthetic surfactant with modified bovine surfactant in the treatment of neonatal respiratory distress syndrome. Pediatrics 97: 1–6
1122. Vidyasagar D, Yeh T F, Harris V, Pildes R S 1975 Assisted ventilation in infants with meconium aspiration syndrome. Pediatrics 56: 208–213
1123. Villar J, Farnot U, Barros F, Victora C, Langer A, Belizan J M 1992 A randomized trial of psychosocial support during high risk pregnancies. New England Journal of Medicine 237: 1266–1271
1124. Vintzileos A M, Nochimson D J, Guzman E R, Knuppel R A, Lake M, Schifrin B S 1995 Intrapartum electronic fetal heart rate monitoring versus intermittent auscultation: a meta-analysis. Obstetrics and Gynecology 85: 149–155
1125. Vishveshwara N, Freeman B, Peck M, Calwag N, Shock S, Rajani K B 1991 Patient triggered synchronized ventilation of newborns: report of a preliminary study and three years' experience. Journal of Perinatology 11: 347–354

1126. Vulsma T, Kok J H 1996 Prematurity-associated neurologic and developmental abnormalities and neonatal thyroid function. New England Journal of Medicine 334: 857–858
1127. Vyas H, Field D, Hopkin I E, Milner A D 1986 Determinants of the first inspiratory volume and functional residual capacity at birth. Pediatric Pulmonology 2: 189–193
1128. Wagaman M J, Shutack J G, Moomjian A S, Schwartz J G, Shaffer T H, Fox W W 1979 Improved oxygenation and lung compliance with prone positioning of the neonates. Journal of Pediatrics 94: 789–791
1129. Wagner E M, Mitzner W A, Bleecker E R 1987 Effects of airway volume on bronchial blood flow. Journal of Applied Physiology 62: 561–566
1130. Waites K B, Grouse D T, Philips J B, Canupp K C, Castle G H 1989 Ureaplasmal pneumonia and sepsis associated with persistent pulmonary hypertension of the newborn. Pediatrics 83: 79–85
1131. Walker D W 1984 Peripheral and central chemoreceptors in the fetus and newborn. Annual Review of Physiology 46: 687–703
1132. Walsh M C, Carlo W A 1988 Sustained inflation during HFOV improves pulmonary mechanics and oxygenation. Journal of Applied Physiology 65: 368–372
1133. Walsh-Sukys M C 1993 Persistent pulmonary hypertension of the newborn. Clinics in Perinatology 20: 127–143
1134. Walsh-Sukys M C, Bauer R E, Cornell D J, Friedman H G, Stork E K, Hack M 1994 Severe respiratory failure in neonates: mortality and morbidity rates and neurodevelopmental outcomes. Journal of Pediatrics 125: 104–110
1135. Walsh-Sukys M C, Cornell D J, Houston L N, Keszler M, Kanto W P 1994 Treatment of persistent pulmonary hypertension of the newborn with hyperventilation: an assessment of diffusion of innovation. Pediatrics 94: 303–306
1136. Walters D V, Olver R E 1978 The role of catecholamines in lung liquid absorption at birth. Pediatric Research 12: 239–242
1137. Walther F J, Benders M J, Leighton J O 1992 Persistent pulmonary hypertension in premature neonates with severe respiratory distress syndrome. Pediatrics 90: 899–904
1138. Walther F J, Ikegami M, Warburton D, Polk D H 1991 Corticosteroids, thyrotropin releasing hormone and antioxidant enzymes in preterm lamb lungs. Pediatric Research 30: 518–521
1139. Walther F J, Siassi B, Ramadan N A, Wu P Y K 1985 Cardiac output in newborn infants with transient myocardial dysfunction. Journal of Pediatrics 107: 781–785
1140. Walti H, Paris-Llado J, Breart G et al 1995 Porcine surfactant replacement therapy in newborns of 25–31 weeks' gestation: a randomized multicentre trial of prophylaxis versus rescue with multiple low doses. Acta Paediatrica 84: 913–921
1141. Ward J A, Roberts R J 1984 Vitamin E inhibition of the effects of hyperoxia on the pulmonary surfactant system of the newborn rabbit. Pediatric Research 18: 329–334
1142. Ward R M 1984 Pharmacology of tolazoline. Clinics in Perinatology 11: 703–713
1143. Ward R M 1994 Pharmacologic enhancement of fetal lung maturation. Clinics in Perinatology 21: 523–542
1144. Wardrop C A J, Holland B M, Veale K E A, Jones J G, Gray O P 1978 Non-physiological anaemia of prematurity. Archives of Disease in Childhood 53: 855–860
1145. Warley M A, Gairdner D 1962 Respiratory distress syndrome of the newborn—principles of treatment. Archives of Disease in Childhood 37: 455–465
1146. Watters T A, Weydland M F, Parmley W W et al 1987 Factors influencing myocardial response to metabolic acidosis in isolated rat hearts. American Journal of Physiology 253: H1261–H1270
1147. Wauer RR, Schmalisch G, Bohme B, Arand J, Lehmann D 1992 Randomized double blind trial of ambroxol for the treatment of respiratory distress syndrome. European Journal of Pediatrics 151: 357–363
1148. Way G L, Pierce J R, Wolfe R R, McGrath R, Wiggins J, Merenstein G B 1979 ST depression suggesting subendocardial ischemia in neonates with respiratory distress syndrome and patent ductus arteriosus. Journal of Pediatrics 95: 609–611
1149. Weindling AM 1989 Blood pressure monitoring in the newborn. Archives of Disease in Childhood 64: 444–447
1150. Weisberger S A, Carlo W A, Chatburn R L, Fouke J M, Martin R J 1986 Effect of varying inspiratory and expiratory times during high-frequency jet ventilation. Journal of Pediatrics 108: 596–600
1151. Weller P H, Jenkins P A, Gupta J, Baum J D 1976 Pharyngeal lecithin-sphingomyelin ratio in newborn infants. Lancet i: 12–15
1152. Wen T S, Eirksen N L, Blanco J D, Graham J M, Oshiro B T, Prieto J A 1993 Association of clinical intra-amniotic infection and meconium. American Journal of Perinatology 10: 438–440
1153. Wenstrom K D, Parsons M T 1989 The prevention of meconium aspiration in labour using amnioinfusion. Obstetrics and Gynecology 73: 647–651
1154. Wesenberg R L, Graven S N, McCabe E B 1971 Radiological findings in wet lung disease. Radiology 98: 69–74
1155. Whitfield C R, Chan W H, Sproule W B, Stewart A D 1972 Amniotic fluid lecithin-sphingomyelin ratio and fetal lung development. British Medical Journal ii: 85–86
1156. Whittle M J, Hill C M 1980 Relationship between amniotic lecithin-sphingomyelin ratio, fetal cord blood cortisol levels and duration of induced labour. British Journal of Obstetrics and Gynaecology 87: 38–42
1157. Wigglesworth J S 1984 Perinatal pathology. W B Saunders, Philadelphia, pp 106–107
1158. Wigton T R, Tamura R K, Wickstrom E, Atkins V, Deddish R, Socol M L 1993 Neonatal morbidity after preterm delivery in the presence of documented lung maturity. American Journal of Obstetrics and Gynecology 169: 951–955
1159. Wilcox D T, Glick P L, Karamanoukian H L, Leach C, Morin F C, Fuhrman B P 1995 Perfluorocarbon associated gas exchange improves pulmonary mechanics, oxygenation, ventilation and allows nitric oxide delivery in the hypoplastic lung congenital diaphragmatic hernia lung model. Critical Care Medicine 23: 1858–1063
1160. Wilcox D T, Glick P L, Karamanoukian H L, Morin F C, Fuhrman B P, Leach C L 1994 Perfluorocarbon associated gas exchange (PAGE) and nitric oxide in the lamb congenital diaphragmatic hernia model. Pediatric Research 35: 260A
1161. Wild L M, Nickerson P A, Morin F C 1989 Ligating the ductus arteriosus before birth remodels the pulmonary vasculature of the lamb. Pediatric Research 25: 251–257
1162. Wilkinson A R, Yu V Y H 1974 Immediate effects of feeding on blood gases and some cardiorespiratory functions in ill newborn infants. Lancet i: 1083–1085
1163. Will D H, McMurtry I F, Reeves J T, Grover R F 1978 Cold induced pulmonary hypertension in cattle. Journal of Applied Physiology 45: 469–473
1164. Wilson G, Hughes G, Rennie J, Morley C 1991 Evaluation of two endotracheal suction regimes in babies ventilated for respiratory distress syndrome. Early Human Development 25: 87–90
1165. Wilson S L, Thach B T, Brouilette R T, Abu-Osba Y K 1981 Coordination of breathing and swallowing in human infants. Journal of Applied Physiology 50: 851–858
1166. Winn H N, Romero R, Roberts A, Liu H, Hobbins J C 1992 Comparison of fetal lung maturation in preterm singleton and twin pregnancies. American Journal of Perinatology 9: 326–328
1167. Wiriyathan S, Rosenfield C R, Arant B S, Porter J C, Faucher D J, Engle W D 1986 Urinary arginine-vasopressin in the neonatal period. Pediatric Research 20: 103–108
1168. Wise R A, Robotham J L, Bromerger-Barnea B, Permutt S 1981 Effect of PEEP on left ventricular function in right heart bypassed dogs. Journal of Applied Physiology 51: 541–546
1169. Wiswell T E, Henley M A 1992 Intratracheal suctioning, systemic infection and the meconium aspiration syndrome. Pediatrics 89: 203–206
1170. Wiswell T E, Rawlings J S, Smith F R, Goo E D 1985 Effect of furosemide on the clinical course of transient tachypnea of the newborn. Pediatrics 75: 908–910
1171. Wiswell T E, Tuggle J M, Turner B S 1990 Meconium aspiration syndrome: have we made a difference? Pediatrics 85: 715–721
1172. Wispe J R, Roberts R J 1987 Molecular basis of pulmonary oxygen toxicity. Clinics in Perinatology 14: 651–666
1173. Wolf E J, Vintzileos A M, Rosenkrantz T S, Rodis J F, Salafia C M, Pezzullo J G 1993 Do survival and morbidity of very low birthweight infants vary according to the primary pregnancy complication that

results in preterm delivery? American Journal of Obstetrics and Gynecology 169: 1233–1239

1174. Wolfson M R, Greenspan J S, Deoras K S, Rubenstein S D, Shaffer T H 1992 Comparison of gas and liquid ventilation: clinical, physiological and histological correlates. Journal of Applied Physiology. 72: 1024–1031

1175. Wong Y C, Beardsmore C S, Meek J H, Stocks J, Silverman M 1982 Bronchial hypersecretion in preterm neonates. Archives of Disease in Childhood 57: 117–122

1176. Wood B, Dubik M 1995 A new device for pleural drainage in newborn infants. Pediatrics 96: 955–956

1177. Worthington D, Smith B T 1978 Relation of amniotic fluid lecithin/sphingomyelin ratio and fetal asphyxia to respiratory distress syndrome in premature infants. Canadian Medical Association Journal 118: 1384–1388

1178. Wright K, Lyrene R K, Truog W E, Standaert T A, Murphy J, Woodrum D E 1981. Ventilation by high-frequency oscillation in rabbits with oleic acid lung disease. Journal of Applied Physiology 50: 1056–1060

1179. Wu T J, Teng R J, Yau K I T 1995 Persistent pulmonary hypertension of the newborn treated with magnesium sulphate in premature neonates. Pediatrics 96: 472–474

1180. Wung J T, James L S, Kilchevsky E, James E, 1985 Management of infants with severe respiratory failure and persistence of the fetal circulation without hyperventilation. Pediatrics 76: 488–490

1181. Wyman M L, Kuhns L R 1977 Lobar opacification of the lung after tracheal extubation in neonates. Journal of Pediatrics 91: 109–112

1182. Wynn R J, Schreiner R L 1979 Spurious elevation of amniotic fluid bilirubin in acute hydramnios with fetal intestinal obstruction. American Journal of Obstetrics and Gynecology 134: 105–106

1183. Wynne J W, Modell J H 1977 Respiratory aspiration of stomach contents. Annals of Internal Medicine 87: 466–467

1184. Wyszogrodski J, Taeusch H W Jr, Avery M E 1974 Isoxuprine induced alterations of pulmonary pressure volume relationship in premature rabbits. American Journal of Obstetrics and Gynecology 119: 1107–1111

1185. Wyszogrodski J, Kyei-Aboagye N, Taeusch H W Jr 1975 Surfactant inactivation by hyperventilation: conservation by end-expiratory pressure. Journal of Applied Physiology 38: 461–466

1186. Yao A C, Lind J 1974 Placental transfusion American Journal of Diseases of Children 127: 128–141

1187. Yeh T, Pildes R, Salem M 1978 Treatment of persistent tension pneumothorax in a neonate by selective bronchial intubation. Anesthesiology 49: 37–38

1188. Yeh T F, Srinivasan G, Harris V, Pildes R S 1977 Hydrocortisone therapy in meconium aspiration syndrome: a controlled trial. Journal of Pediatrics 90: 140–143

1189. Yeh T F, Harris V, Srinivasan G, Lillien L, Pyati S, Pildes R S 1979 Roentgenographic findings in infants with meconium aspiration syndrome. Journal of the American Medical Association 242: 60–63

1190. Yeh T F, Shibli A, Leu S T, Admam M, Pildes R S 1984 Furosemide therapy in premature infants with respiratory distress syndrome: a randomized controlled study. Journal of Pediatrics 105: 603–609

1191. Yeh T F, Raval D, John E, Pildes R S 1985 Renal response to furosemide in preterm infants with respiratory distress syndrome during the first three postnatal days. Archives of Disease in Childhood 60: 621–626

1192. Yeh T F, Torre J A, Rastogi A, Anyebuno M A, Pildes R S 1990 Early postnatal dexamethasone therapy in premature infants with severe respiratory distress syndrome: a double-blind controlled study. Journal of Pediatrics 117: 273–282

1193. Yeomans E R, Gilstrap L C, Leveno K J, Burris J S 1989 Meconium in the amniotic fluid and fetal acid base status. Obstetrics and Gynecology 73: 175–178

1194. Yoder B A 1994 Meconium stained amniotic fluid and respiratory complications. Impact of selective tracheal suction. Obstetrics and Gynecology 83: 77–84

1195. Young J D, Dyar O J 1996 Delivery and monitoring of inhaled nitric oxide. Intensive Care Medicine 22: 77–86

1196. Yu V Y H 1975 Effect of body position on gastric emptying in the neonate. Archives of Disease in Childhood 50: 500–504

1197. Yu V Y H, Rolfe P 1977 Effect of continuous positive airway pressure breathing on cardiorespiratory function in infants with respiratory distress syndrome. Acta Paediatrica Scandinavica 66: 59–64

1198. Yu V Y H, Liew S W, Roberton N R C 1975 Pneumothorax in the newborn. Archives of Disease in Childhood 50: 449–453

1199. Yu V Y K, Orgill A A, Lim S B, Bajuk B, Astbury J 1983 Bronchopulmonary dysplasia in very low birthweight infants. Australian Paediatric Journal 19: 233–236

1200. Yu V Y K, Wong P Y, Bajuk B, Symonowicz W 1986 Pulmonary airleak in extremely low birthweight infants. Archives of Disease in Childhood 61: 239–241

1201. Yukitake K, Brown C L, Schlueter M A 1995 Surfactant apoprotein A modifies the inhibitory effect of plasma proteins on surfactant activity in vivo. Pediatric Research 37: 21–25

1202. Yuksel B, Greenough A 1992 Neonatal respiratory support and lung function abnormalities at follow-up. Respiratory Medicine 86: 97–100

1203. Yuksel B, Greenough A 1994 Birthweight and hospital re-admission of infants born prematurely. Archives of Pediatric and Adolescent Medicine 148: 384–388

1204. Yuksel B, Greenough A, Gamsu H R 1993 Neonatal meconium aspiration syndrome and respiratory morbidity during infancy. Pediatric Pulmonology 16: 358–361

1205. Yuksel B, Greenough A, Gamsu H R 1993 Respiratory function at follow-up after neonatal surfactant replacement therapy. Respiratory Medicine 87: 217–221

1206. Zarif M, Pildes R S, Vidyasagar D 1976 Insulin and growth hormone responses in neonatal hyperglycaemia. Diabetes 25: 428–433

1207. Zayek M, Cleveland D, Morin F C 1993 Treatment of persistent pulmonary hypertension in the newborn lamb by inhaled nitric oxide. Journal of Pediatrics 122: 743–750

1208. Zerella J T, Trump D S 1987 Surgical management of neonatal interstitial emphysema. Journal of Pediatric Surgery 22: 34–37

1209. Zhou H, Gao Y, Raj J U 1996 Antenatal betamethasone therapy augments nitric oxide mediated relaxation of preterm ovine pulmonary veins. Journal of Applied Physiology 80: 390–396

1210. Zobel G, Dacar D, Rodl S, Friehs I 1995 Inhaled nitric oxide versus inhaled prostacyclin and intravenous versus inhaled prostacyclin in acute respiratory failure in pulmonary hypertension in piglets. Pediatric Research 38: 198–204

1211. Zola E M, Gunkel J H, Chan R K, et al 1993 Comparison of three dosing procedures for administration of bovine surfactant to neonates with respiratory distress syndrome. Journal of Pediatrics 122: 453–459

Part 3

Chronic lung disease in the newborn

Anne Greenough

BRONCHOPULMONARY DYSPLASIA

Bronchopulmonary dysplasia, a severe chronic lung disease virtually confined to preterm infants who have been ventilated, was first described in 1967.[165] Northway described four stages of BPD, based on a sequence of X-ray changes (p. 611). These stages, however, do not occur consistently and it has become apparent that there are difficulties in staging and diagnosing BPD by radiographic pattern alone. As a consequence, clinical diagnostic criteria are now used. BPD has been defined as a requirement for mechanical ventilation for a variable period soon after birth, dependence on supplemental oxygen at 28 days and evidence of pulmonary insufficiency. A simpler definition was used by the HIFI Study Group:[104] a need for supplemental oxygen and evidence of an abnormal CXR at more than 28 days of life. It has been argued that oxygen dependency beyond 36 weeks PCA is a more useful definition, as this rather than oxygen dependence at 28 days correlates more closely with continuing respiratory morbidity after discharge.[218] The positive predictive value of these definitions for abnormal pulmonary findings at 2 years of age was 38% for a requirement for oxygen at 28 days, and 65% for oxygen dependency beyond 36 weeks' PCA.[218] Many infants who have prolonged oxygen dependence do not have the CXR appearance described by Northway et al.[165] Such infants are therefore diagnosed as suffering from CLD, and BPD is reserved for those who have cystic abnormalities on the CXR appearance (type IV BPD, p. 612).[81] Nevertheless, BPD is still used widely as an umbrella term and in this chapter will be used to refer to infants who meet the HIFI Study Group criteria.

INCIDENCE

Over the last two decades the incidence of BPD in VLBW neonates has increased from approximately 10% to 30%, most of the extra cases being explained by improved survival.[174] A UK study, however, has suggested the reverse trend from 1980 to 1990, with relative odds of 0.88 for each year of a reduction in BPD risk in infants of low birthweight.[47] This trend was explained by the use of lower maximum peak inspiratory pressures and oxygen concentrations. BPD is commonest in VLBW infants;[25,191] in one study almost 50% of infants weighing less than 1000 g developed BPD.[7] In ventilated infants the incidence varies from 4.2% to 40%.[12,61,82,190] Twenty-two per cent of ventilated, premature infants at King's College Hospital in 1995–1996 remained oxygen dependent beyond 28 days, and 14% beyond 36 weeks' PCA. The longer infants are ventilated the more likely they are to develop BPD; in one series 70% of infants ventilated for longer than 2 weeks developed BPD,[7] and in our institution 77 of 129 infants ventilated longer than 1 week were oxygen dependent beyond 28 days, compared to only 20 of 173 who were ventilated for less than a week ($P < 0.001$). The incidence varies according to the primary disorder: 18% in RDS,[264] 20% in apnoea[135] and 6% in persistent pulmonary hypertension.[95]

AETIOLOGY (Fig. 29.79)[89]

BPD may represent a delayed recovery stage of RDS, but also occurs after apnoea[102] and in infants born at term with meconium aspiration syndrome,[192] congenital heart disease,[14] and particularly those with severe lung disease, as evidenced by a requirement for ECMO.[124] In the latter group the risk of developing BPD was 11.5 times higher if ECMO was initiated at greater than 96 hours of age and 5.2 times higher if the primary diagnosis was RDS.[124] Epidemiological studies have revealed numerous associations, including oxygen toxicity, barotrauma and immaturity.[105] Other factors may be contributory: airleak, pulmonary oedema and PDA.[269]

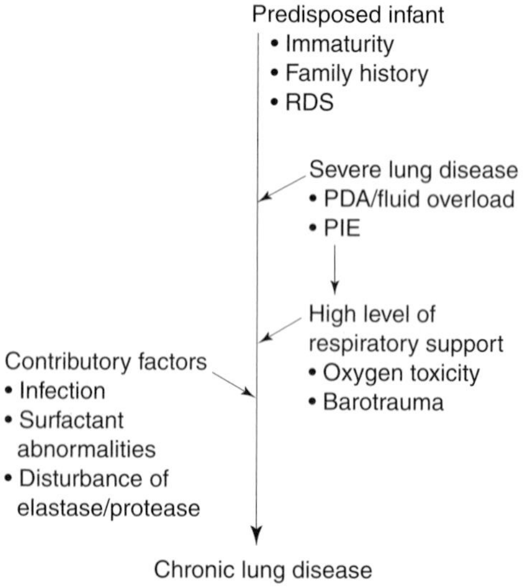

Fig. 29.79 Aetiological associations of CLD. Reproduced with permission from Greenough et al.[89]

Oxygen toxicity

Northway et al[165] originally ascribed BPD to oxygen toxicity, as the chronic phase was invariably associated with therapy in high oxygen concentrations for more than 150 hours. Prolonged exposure to high oxygen concentrations has complex biochemical, microscopic and gross anatomical effects on lung tissues (p. 560).[24,50,70]

Positive pressure support

BPD was first reported in infants who received oxygen concentrations of less than 60% when this was used in association with CPAP[248] or mechanical ventilation.[14] IPPV seemed particularly damaging if peak inflating pressures above 35 cmH_2O were used.[17,242] An inverse relationship has been demonstrated between hypocarbia and the subsequent development of BPD,[76,129] further incriminating baro- or volutrauma.

Stocks et al[239] and, more recently, Yuksel and Greenough[273] demonstrated that at follow-up, airways resistance was significantly increased in infants who had received IPPV compared to those who had required supplementary oxygen or no form of respiratory support. Stahlman et al[233] reported that CXR changes at 11 years correlated best with the use and duration of IPPV.

Immaturity

Wung et al[264] described two different types of BPD, the classic form following severe RDS and high-pressure ventilation, and a second form found in infants all less than 1.0 kg birthweight, who had no or only mild RDS and did not require mechanical ventilation. Edwards et al[61] reported that the smaller survivors among infants ventilated for RDS were most likely to develop BPD. However, certain agents that prolong pregnancy unfavourably affect the incidence of CLD. Antenatal administration of indomethacin significantly prolonged gestation in women threatened with preterm labour between 24 and 34 weeks, but its use was associated with an increased BPD rate, particularly in those infants who delivered within 120 hours of their mothers starting treatment.[68] It was postulated that indomethacin could have delayed the development of lamellar bodies and surfactant components.

PDA and fluid overload

PDA increases the incidence of BPD: in one series[26] 72% of infants with BPD had a PDA, and this increased to 84% if only infants weighing less than 1250 g were considered. Interestingly, however, although the prophylactic use of low-dose indomethacin, initiated in the first 24 hours of life, can decrease the incidence of left–right shunting and symptomatic PDA, it does not significantly reduce the incidence of BPD.[49,72] Infection, particularly if temporally related, potentiates the effect of PDA on the risk of CLD.[79] Fluid overload may explain the association of PDA and BPD, via congestive heart failure and deteriorating lung function.[248]

Infants with a delayed diuresis appear to be at significantly greater risk of BPD.[231] On average, infants with BPD had their postnatal diuresis approximately 48 hours later than those without. A retrospective review[249] demonstrated that, compared to control infants, those with BPD received greater quantities of total, crystalloid and colloid fluids per kg in the first days of life. Infants with BPD generally had a weight gain in the first 4 days, in contrast to the weight loss seen in the controls. Although trying to promote an early diuresis with diuretics[209] or albumin infusion[85] does not significantly improve respiratory status, fluid restriction may reduce the incidence of BPD.[243] In a prospective randomized study, fluid restriction during the first 4 weeks of life resulted in a significant increase in the number of patients alive without CLD at 4 weeks.[244] Earlier studies, although demonstrating fluid restriction to be associated with a lower incidence of NEC and PDA,[15] did not show a favourable impact on BPD, but in one[15] infants were only randomized on day 3 and in the other[137] fluid restriction was only maintained for 5 days. Withholding sodium supplementation in the first 3–5 days reduces BPD compared to a regimen that included daily maintenance sodium.[48] The likely mechanism is fluid overload, as the caregivers tended to prescribe daily increases in parenteral fluids for the salt-supplemented infants.[48]

Airleak

PIE has been associated with a high incidence of BPD,[156] particularly type II CLD (see later).[43] Respiratory function is compromised by air dissection into false air spaces, which creates a large dead space for ventilation; these spaces then increase in size with time and compress lung tissue.[232]

Infection

BPD is twice as common in infants who develop postnatal infection with cytomegalovirus as in non-infected infants[210] (p. 1162). The role of ureaplasma[33] in the aetiology of BPD is controversial: the association may simply reflect an increased occurrence of ureaplasma in extremely low birthweight infants. A review of four cohort studies demonstrated a combined estimate of relative risk of 1.91 (95% CI 1.54–2.37), but no significant association was found in infants who weighed >1250 g.[252]

Surfactant abnormalities

BPD may result from persisting surfactant abnormalities.[166] In infants with BPD the L:S ratio increases slowly,[99] and in those with lethal BPD phosphatidylglycerol appears several months later than in infants who survive. These findings could be secondary to the proliferative changes in BPD reducing the number of type II cells. Abnormalities related to surfactant proteins, particularly SP-A, have been associated with BPD. A deficiency of SP-A mRNA expression was demonstrated to persist following RDS in a model of chronic lung injury.[42] SP-A is important in blocking the surfactant-inactivating effects of serum proteins during oedema formation (p. 471). Almost all infants with RDS show detectable immune complexes between SP-A and antisurfactant protein-A antibodies (SAS).[240] Plasma levels of SAS immune complexes correlate significantly with the development of BPD, independent of gestational age and birthweight.[241] Infants with BPD may be characterized by a postsurfactant slump, that is, a respiratory deterioration following an initial response to surfactant.[225]

Disturbance of elastase/protease system

Lactosylceramide, which is a marker of destructive inflammation,[186] is strikingly elevated in lung effluent during the first neonatal week in infants who develop BPD.[99] It is released by white blood cells into the extracellular space and disturbs surfactant function.[186] The granulocytes commonly present in the tracheal aspirates of infants with BPD also release elastase,[147] collagenase and phospholipase A_2,[97] which destroy lung parenchyma and break down surfactant. Tracheal lavage studies have demonstrated that patients in whom BPD ultimately developed had early evidence of increased pulmonary inflammation and a significantly less favourable protease–antiprotease balance. They had similar amounts of secretory leukocyte protease inhibitor concentrations, but higher elastase activity than similarly aged infants without BPD.[254] Free elastase activity in tracheal aspirate fluid also increases the risk of PIE.[230] Elastase, however, was only detected in the tracheal aspirates of infants who had pneumonia or who required prolonged hyperoxic ventilation.[28] Further evidence that BPD may be associated with an unfavourable protease–antiprotease balance is that supplemental α-antitrypsin prevented the reduced lung compliance observed in untreated hyperoxia-exposed neonatal rats.[123]

Predisposition to BPD

Increased airways hyperreactivity may predispose to the development of BPD. The role of a family history of asthma, however, is controversial.[37,162] More infants weighing less than 1500 g with BPD are HLA-A_2 positive compared to controls.[38] Infants who are unable to secrete adequate amounts of cortisol in settings of increased stress injury may be at risk of continuing lung injury. At the end of the first week, infants who subsequently developed BPD had significantly lower cortisol secretion in response to ACTH than infants who recovered without BPD.[253]

PATHOPHYSIOLOGY

There is a significant influx of inflammatory cells into the airways of infants with RDS and BPD compared to controls.[147] RDS is associated with a significant pulmonary inflammatory reaction, and affected infants have an excess of neutrophils and alveolar macrophages in their lung effluent compared to healthy subjects. Ninety per cent of aspirates from days 1–4 contain neutrophils, but this usually declines. Immunohistochemical analysis of whole lung lobes demonstrated a rapid temporal increase from birth in the mucosal density of $CD68^+$ macrophages, polymorphonuclear neutrophils and TNFα immunoreactive cells, which was maximal in those dying at or after 72 hours. The inflammatory infiltration was seen to be associated with a striking loss of endothelial basement membrane and interstitial sulphated glycoaminoglycans, which was almost complete by 72 hours.[157] Barotrauma and oxygen toxicity induce an inflammatory reaction, and in infants who develop CLD it persists, with 95% of 11–15-day-old infants with BPD having neutrophils in their aspirates. The activated neutrophils mediate endothelial cytotoxicity and inhibit phosphatidylcholine synthesis[278] (Fig. 29.80). In older infants with BPD 90% of the recovered cells from BAL fluid are alveolar macrophages.[40] At all ages from birth, lavage supernatants demonstrated a highly significant increase over controls of the β-chemokine MIP-1-α. Significantly higher concentrations of MIP-1-α were associated with the later development of fibrosis.[158]

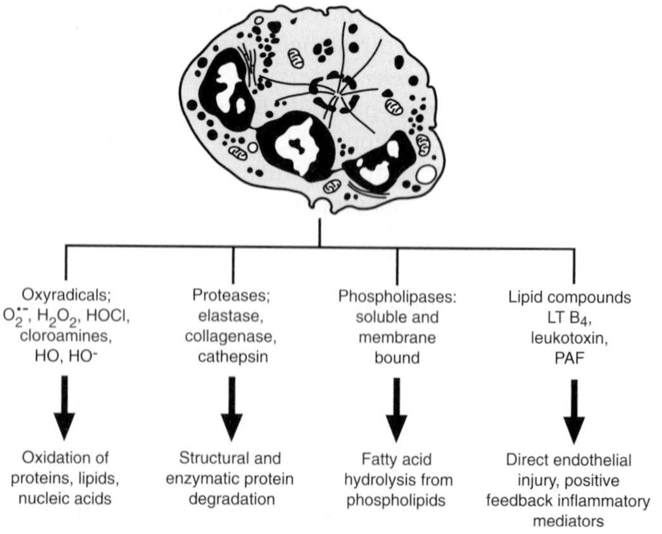

Fig. 29.80 Neutrophil constituents implicated in host autoinjury. Reproduced with permission from Zimmerman.[278]

Mediator release from the neutrophils may increase airway hyperreactivity. The BAL fluid of such patients contains elevated levels of lipid mediators, including leukotrienes,[92,151] which cause bronchoconstriction, vasoconstriction oedema, neutrophil chemotaxis and mucus production in the lung. Leukotriene B4, the anaphylatoxin C5a and IL-8, important chemoattractants for human neutrophils, have been detected in the BAL of infants with CLD.[91] Urinary leukotriene levels are high at 28 days[56] and remain elevated in such infants compared to healthy controls, even when studied at 6 months of age.[45] In addition to leukotriene C4, a potent bronchoconstrictor, eicosanoids and PAF, potent lipid mediators with known injurious effects on the lung,[236] are also found in large quantities in the tracheobronchial effluent of infants in whom BPD subsequently develops. Increased concentrations of the soluble form of ICAM-1, a glycoprotein that allows cell-to-cell contact, have been found in the tracheal aspirates of infants with early BPD.[120] It has been suggested that increased concentrations of IL-8 in BAL may represent a marker for the development of BPD.[139] C5a and IL-8, via activation of neutrophils and/or inducing PAF production, may contribute to the persistently abnormal lung permeability in early BPD.[90] Proinflammatory cytokines IL-1β and IL-6, which may have a role in initiating the inflammatory response, are increased in BAL fluid from infants who develop CLD compared to those with RDS and control groups; the IL-6 may be produced by cells within the air spaces.[126] In contrast to the early increase in IL-6 activity in lung lavage samples from infants with BPD, TNF increases late.[10] TNF is a potent inducer of IL-6 expression by inflammatory and structural cells and IL-6 inhibits the release of TNF by macrophages, forming a negative feedback loop. Bacchi et al therefore, proposed that early elevated IL-6 might be a response to severe lung injury and an early marker of BPD, whereas TNF may contribute to the chronic inflammation.[10] BAL-derived macrophages from preterm newborns with RDS may not contain IL-10 during the early stages of lung inflammation.[113] IL-10 can inhibit the production of proinflammatory cytokines by monocytes and macrophages, and thus the implication of Jones'[113] findings are that the macrophages in preterm lungs may not be able to control an inflammatory process as effectively as those in more mature hosts.

CLINICAL PRESENTATION

The majority of infants with CLD are born very prematurely and at 2–3 months of age are still dyspnoeic despite oxygen supplementation, and may gain weight poorly. A minority with type II CLD (v.i.) or BPD are oedematous and have obvious signs of right heart failure and bronchospasm. The latter group have retractions and other obvious abnormalities related to chronic increased work of breathing, such as a Harrison sulcus. These patients, despite increasing postnatal age, frequently fail to thrive and are at high risk of deterioration in their respiratory failure related to recurrent respiratory infections. Cor pulmonale develops in infants who are chronically hypoxaemic. Infants with BPD have ongoing respiratory support requirements – supplemental oxygen and IPPV – from the first week. Copious endotracheal secretions are common and there is chronic carbon dioxide retention. In infants with persistent pulmonary problems – persistent atelectasis, lobar hyperinflation, aspiration and unexplained respiratory distress – abnormalities of the trachea and/or bronchus are common. Bronchoscopy reveals tracheo- or bronchomalacia or inspissated secretions.[150] In addition, large airway collapse can be seen on the CXR as thinning or tapering of the airways, or alternatively demonstrated by cine-computed tomography.[140] Tracheo- and bronchomalacia usually improve as the infant grows, but in severe cases surgery may be necessary, the airway being held open by fixing the trachea to the aorta. Increasing oxygen requirements, hypoxic and hypercapnic episodes in association with radiological changes of fixed lobar emphysema, or recurrent atelectasis may be associated with tracheobronchial stenosis, which can be demonstrated by tracheobronchography with iopydol-iopydone. In some affected patients endoscopy and balloon dilatation may be successful.[20] Episodes of hypoxaemia occur because of apnoea and, in ventilated infants, extubation may be complicated by inspiratory stridor secondary to tracheal scarring (pp. 574, 668).

Feeding difficulties and aspiration are common owing to bulbar dysfunction, gastro-oesophageal reflux or rumination. Parenteral nutrition may be needed, although excessive infusions of lipid solutions may compromise pulmonary function[55] and have been implicated in increasing the risk of CLD;[46] this has been confirmed in a prospective trial in infants less than 800 g.[228] Growth failure is common. Osteopenia has been reported as a complication of BPD,[234] but Ryan et al[201] found no difference between infants with BPD and gestation-matched controls, although both groups were severely undermineralized compared to infants born at full term.

IMAGING

The progress of X-ray change in BPD varies in timing and specificity between patients.[62] Northway et al[165] described four distinct radiographic appearances:

- Stage 1: radiographically indistinguishable from severe RDS (1–3 days);
- Stage 2: marked radio-opacity of the lungs (4–10 days);
- Stage 3: clearing of the radio-opacity into a cystic, bubbly pattern (10–20 days) (Fig. 29.81);

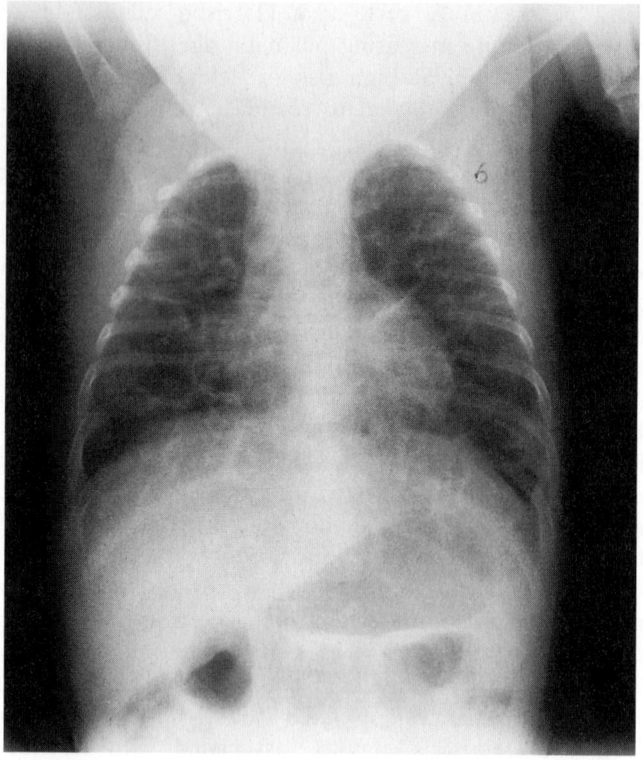

Fig. 29.81 Stage 3 BPD.

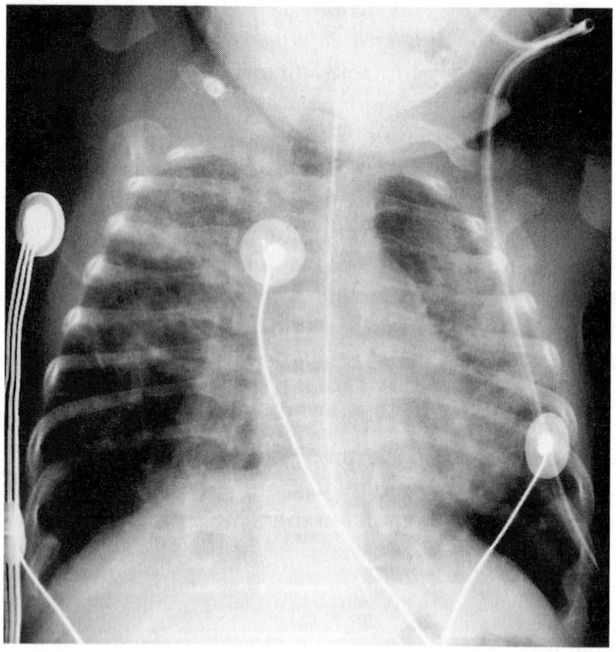

Fig. 29.82 Stage 4 BPD.

- Stage 4: hyperexpansion, streaks of abnormal density and areas of emphysema with variable cardiomegaly (from 1 month) (Figs 29.82, 29.83).

Hyde et al[108] suggested that infants with BPD who have an abnormal CXR on the 28th day of life can be divided into two groups. Those with type I disease have

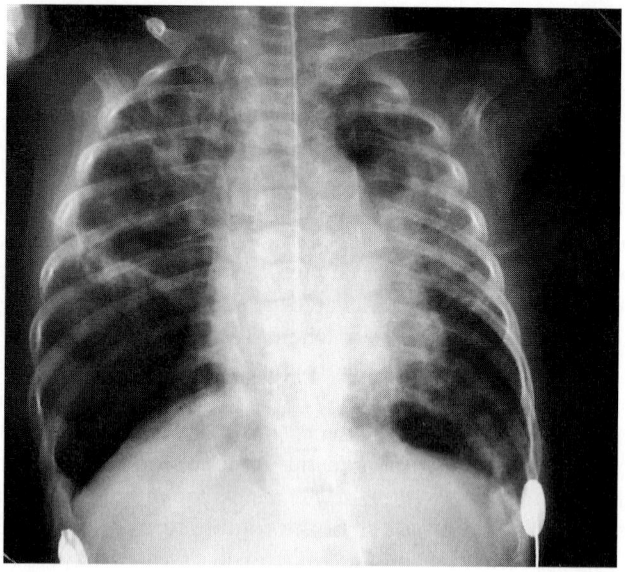

Fig. 29.83 Late stage 4 BPD with gross cystic overexpansion and compression of the mediastinum.

homogeneous or patchy ill-defined opacification in the lungs without coarse reticulation. Type II disease is characterized by classic coarse reticulation and streaky densities, interspersed with small cystic translucencies. Type I disease resolves and represents the typical CLD of premature infants; type II always follows PIE and has a poorer prognosis.

Alternative scoring systems have been developed. Toce et al[247] noted that the higher clinical scores correlated with the worst X-ray appearances, as quantified by their scoring system. Another system is based on assessing the volume of the lungs, the degree of hyperinflation, the presence and severity of interstitial changes and the presence and magnitude of cysts, but not cardiovascular abnormalities. Using this scoring system, the X-ray appearance at 1 month was used to predict oxygen dependency at a PCA equivalent to 36 weeks[141] and the most severe lung function abnormalities at 6 months of age.[275] The infants who had the highest chest radiograph scores, which predicted long-term abnormalities, were the only ones who had cystic elements and/or interstitial changes present on their CXR. An alternative scheme records the appearance and extent of linear opacities and cystic changes, which were found to correlate significantly with the respiratory support index.[257]

Rarely, abnormalities on the CXR consistent with BPD may be unilateral if complications such as atelectasis or tension pneumothorax protect the contralateral lung against the development of BPD.[221]

Lesions in survivors of BPD with chronic pulmonary dysfunction are visualized better on CT scan than on CXR (Fig. 29.84). Common findings in such patients are multifocal areas of hyperaeration, linear and triangular subpleural opacities, but not bronchiectasis.[169]

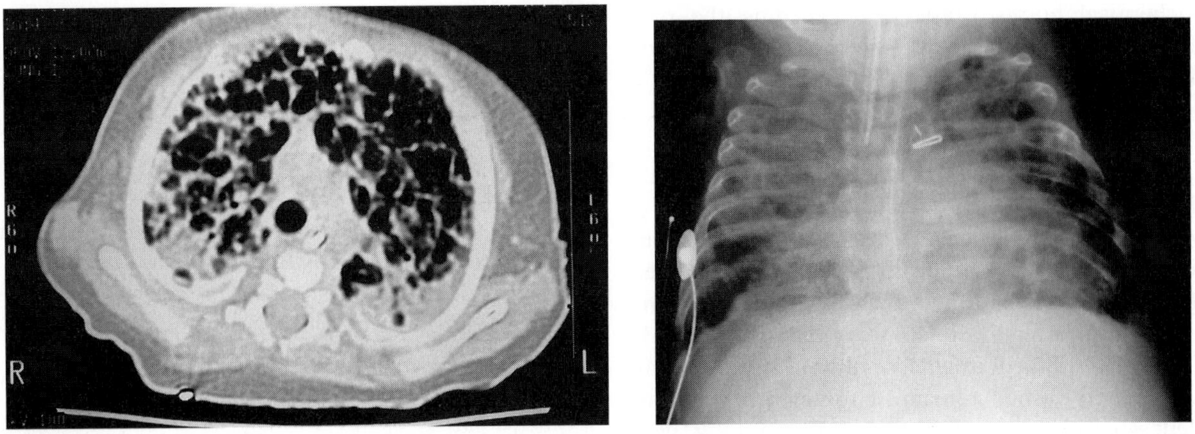

Fig. 29.84 Left: CT scan of a 7-month-old infant with stage 4 BPD reveals gross cystic abnormalities throughout the lung fields; the widespread distribution of the abnormalities is not so apparent on the infant's CXR (right).

PATHOLOGY

In BPD there is a progression from the initial exudative stage of diffuse alveolar damage in RDS (p. 486) to a regenerative and fibroproliferative reparative stage. In early BPD the lungs have a grossly abnormal appearance, being firm, heavy and darker than normal; the surface is irregular, with emphysematous areas alternating with areas of collapse. Histological examination demonstrates areas of emphysema which may coalesce into larger cystic areas, surrounded by areas of atelectasis. There is widespread bronchial and bronchiolar mucosal hyperplasia and metaplasia, which reduces the lumen of small airways, and in some cases excessive mucus secretion with exudation of alveolar macrophages. Hypertrophy of peribronchiolar smooth muscle and an increase in fibrous tissue with focal thickening of the basal membrane occur, together with the vascular changes of pulmonary hypertension. Later, normal conducting bronchi may be found, with marked uniform expansion of distal air spaces and little or no interstitial fibrosis. In long-standing healed BPD, seen in infants aged between 2 and 40 months, there is alveolar septal fibrosis, cardiomegaly and evidence of pulmonary hypertensive vascular disease.[237]

Cytology of tracheal aspirates

This may facilitate the early diagnosis of BPD as changes in aspiration cytology precede those on the CXR. Although neutrophils are present in 90% of aspirates from days 1 to 4, after that postnatal age they usually decline, being present on days 11–15 only in infants who go on to develop BPD. The initial changes show a destructive process (sloughed epithelial cells, fragments of hyaline membrane); this is replaced by regenerative changes with metaplastic epithelial cells and histiocytes, followed by a transitional stage with evidence of epithelial recovery but with dysplastic and metaplastic cells still present.[54] The most severe stage is the presence of histiocytes plus sheets of cells showing squamous metaplasia and dysplasia. The speed of progression from one stage to another is dependent on the oxygen dose, i.e. the product of oxygen concentration and hours of exposure.[196] In addition, surfactant replacement therapy can modify the progression of the usual cytological changes.[149]

DIFFERENTIAL DIAGNOSIS OF CLD

The diagnosis is made from the clinical history and the CXR and is rarely, if ever, difficult. Infants with BPD have usually been ventilated for RDS and have typical X-ray changes. Infants with Wilson–Mikity syndrome have a normal early CXR with an insidious development of radiographic abnormalities (p. 623). PIE resembles both conditions radiologically and can form cystic structures which suggest areas of focal emphysema as seen in BPD, but these are usually transient and disappear within 2 weeks.[101] A persistent form of PIE has been described[238] which merges into stages 3 and 4 BPD. Other rare conditions, such as viral pneumonia,[133] aspiration problems, lung infections associated with immune deficiency, cystic fibrosis and idiopathic pulmonary fibrosis (Hamman–Rich syndrome) can usually be differentiated on the history of associated clinical features. The changes due to both total anomalous pulmonary venous return (p. 695) and pulmonary lymphangiectasia (p. 647) are distinguished from CLD as they are present from birth.

MANAGEMENT

General

The management of babies with BPD is one of the most demanding and time-consuming areas of neonatal intensive care. The general aim is to maintain haematological and biochemical homoeostasis while keeping the baby free of infection and gradually weaning him off the ventilator and into progressively lower concentrations of oxygen.

A comprehensive care plan should include attention to the appropriate auditory, tactile and visual experiences and the opportunity to suckle. The provision of sleep–wake rhythms is also very important as the infant becomes older. Parental support is essential through these prolonged admissions, although with the advent of home oxygen therapy long hospital stays should only be necessary for ventilated infants or those failing to gain weight. Patients who remain chronically ventilator dependent should eventually be transferred to a ward more suited to older infants.

Ventilator management

Peak inspiratory pressure and inspired oxygen concentrations should be kept at the minimum compatible with achieving a PaO_2 of 6.7–9.3 kPa (50–70 mmHg) and oxygen saturations of at least 92% (preferably 95%) (p. 616). Ventilator rates over 60 bpm offer no advantage to this group of infants.[35] In infants with type I CLD (p. 611) increasing the PEEP level to 6 cmH_2O improves oxygenation without adversely affecting CO_2 elimination.[83] $PaCO_2$ may be allowed to rise after the first week of life, when the risk of GMH/IVH is reduced. Levels up to 13.3 kPa (100 mmHg) may be tolerated, provided there is no evidence of a respiratory acidosis (pH < 7.25).

Many infants with BPD require prolonged ventilation. Chronic use of either an oral or a nasal endotracheal tube is associated with cosmetic defects (p. 932). Tracheostomy avoids these problems and eases the nursing of an increasingly active infant, but they are often difficult to close in this population (p. 670). Their use should therefore be restricted to infants still fully ventilated after 3 months of age.

Patient-triggered ventilation (p. 568) is of limited use in infants with BPD, particularly as they may have difficulty in generating sufficient flow or pressure to exceed the critical trigger level (p. 568). Continuous negative pressure ventilation has recently been resurrected,[204] but its value has not been established. HFOV can be useful in infants with type I CLD who deteriorate, but we have not found it beneficial in those with type II CLD, in whom HFOV can emphasize the asymmetry of their lung disease. Both NO and surfactant therapy have been shown anecdotally acutely to improve gas exchange in infants with CLD (p. 618); randomized trials are required to assess whether there is any long-term benefit.

Sedation should be kept to a minimum, as the aim should be to promote the infant's respiratory efforts so that he can become independent of the ventilator.

Weaning

Frequent attempts should be made to wean the infant from the ventilator by reducing the rate. During weaning, a rise in $PaCO_2$ should be ignored unless the pH falls below 7.25. Arterial oxygen tension should be maintained between 6.7 and 9.3 kPa (50 and 70 mmHg) and arterial oxygen saturation at least 92%, to minimize pulmonary hypertension. Theophylline may be useful to hasten weaning, but has only been of proven value in infants less than 1 month old (p. 581). Steroids, particularly if started in the first 2 weeks, hasten weaning[53] as well as having many other beneficial effects (p. 617).

Extubation should initially be attempted after a short period of endotracheal CPAP to ensure adequate respiratory drive. Infants who subsequently require reventilation for apnoea should be extubated only after a sufficiently long period on endotracheal CPAP has demonstrated them to have adequate respiratory drive. Nasal CPAP is not well tolerated in these relatively mature infants,[34] although it may be useful for those who have acquired tracheobronchomalacia.[171]

Reintubation and ventilation should be avoided unless there is frequent or major apnoea, severe metabolic acidosis indicating respiratory fatigue, or a marked deterioration in the blood gases. Physiotherapy and increasing the inspired oxygen concentration should be the first line of treatment for worsening blood gases, which will usually be due to atelectasis associated with secretions.

Oxygen therapy

Once infants are off IPPV or CPAP, oxygen should be administered to keep the PaO_2 above 6.7 kPa or the saturation above 92%, preferably 95%. For older infants administration via nasal cannulae allows them to be sat in a chair, fed and cuddled (p. 560). The exact oxygen concentration given by nasal cannulae is difficult to monitor (p. 560), and they should not be used in immature infants who are young enough to be still at risk of retinopathy.

Haematology

While infants remain significantly oxygen dependent – that is, a requirement for an inspired oxygen concentration greater than 40% – at least weekly PCV estimations should be performed. Transfusions (15 ml/kg) should be given if the PCV falls below 40%. Once the infant no longer requires respiratory support a weekly haemoglobin check is advisable, and the infant should be transfused only if he is suffering from symptomatic anaemia, with a poor reticulocyte response (p. 839).

Fluid and electrolytes

In severe BPD excessive fluid intake should be avoided, giving a maximum of 150 ml/kg/24 h. If the infant is gaining weight in excess of 20 g/kg/24 h on such a regimen, this may indicate heart failure and regular diuretics should be considered. If the infant receives chronic diuretic therapy his acid–base balance, chloride and calcium levels must be carefully monitored; an appropriate supplement can then be administered if these become abnormal. Regular renal ultrasound should be performed to check for nephrocalcinosis.

Infection

Chest infections are a frequent complication[272] and should be treated promptly with physiotherapy, antibiotics or antiviral therapy as appropriate. The respiratory tract of an infant with BPD is frequently colonized with potentially pathogenic bacteria, and it is important to differentiate this from true infection. Routine white blood cell counts are too non-specific to be of value: culturing surface sites and C-reactive protein measurements and endotracheal tube aspirates may help (p. 1123). If there is any respiratory or radiological deterioration, however, endotracheal or nasopharyngeal secretions and blood should be cultured. The other routine investigations for infection must also be carried out (pp. 1118–1124).

The infants are also exposed to viral infections, and if lower respiratory infection develops nasopharyngeal secretions should be sent for immunofluorescence screening for RSV, adenovirus and influenza. If such infections are identified treatment with ribavirin should be considered[78] (p. 1145).

Once the infant reaches 2 months of age, even though he remains on the NICU, the routine immunizations should be given, but a killed polio vaccine used (p. 398). Immunization against influenza should also be considered, especially for infants receiving home oxygen therapy. Immunoprophylaxis against RSV should be considered for those infants less than 6 months of age at the start of the RSV season.[146]

Nutrition

An infant with BPD requires a calorie intake approximately 20–40% greater than age-matched infants without respiratory embarrassment. Energy requirements above 150 kcal/kg are rare, however, and are often associated with malabsorption.[188] Prolonged periods of TPN should be avoided because of the side-effects, particularly on the lungs: for example, intralipid may cause a fall in PaO_2 by increasing pulmonary vascular resistance[182] (pp. 354, 506). In any case, TPN for prolonged periods is usually not practical because of limited venous access. Large-volume enterally administered feeds are poorly tolerated and restriction to 120 ml/kg/day, using either a concentrated feed or calorie supplementation, is preferable. Whereas healthy premature infants can be weaned from 24 kcal/oz of a premature formula at 2 kg, most infants with CLD benefit from use of a premature formula until they reach approximately 3.0 kg. If the infant is receiving human milk a milk fortifier should be used. If these options fail to provide adequate calories for growth, because of fluid restriction or high calorie needs, then addition of modular components such as carbohydrate or fat or both can be used to concentrate the formula to 30 kcal/oz. Fats are available as LCT or MCT. LCT is available as a fat emulsion (4.5 kcal/ml), whereas MCT is not emulsified (8.3 kcal/ml). The standard supplemental dose is 1.0 or 0.5 ml/oz of formula respectively. MCT must be mixed thoroughly and added just prior to a bolus feed or it will separate out and adhere to the tubing. Fat should not provide more than 60% of the total calories to avoid the risk of developing ketosis; fat can also slow gastric emptying, and so is contraindicated in patients with reflux. Carbohydrate is available as readily digestible glucose polymers (powder 4–5 kcal/g or liquid 2 kcal/ml). A typical supplement is 1 g powder or 1–2 ml of liquid per ounce of formula. It is usually well tolerated, but occasionally can cause loose stools.[22] Weight gain in excess of 20 g/kg/day may indicate a need for diuretics, and certainly the infant should be examined for signs of heart failure.

The early provision of adequate protein/calorie support and specific antioxidant-related nutrients is important to try and limit the immature lung's susceptibility to oxygen-induced lung damage.[73] Recent evidence suggests that early lipid provision, especially in the form of PUFAs, is important in reducing endogenous CO_2 production, improving the bioavailability of fat-soluble vitamins and providing an alternative means of augmenting antioxidant defence.[73] In rats given a high-PUFA diet survival in >95% oxygen$_2$ was improved.[227] High-fat formula feeds, compared to high-carbohydrate formulae, were associated with similar adequate growth in infants with CLD, but lower carbon dioxide production.[176] Unfortunately infants with CLD may have limited fat absorption,[22] with lower duodenal lipase activity and a higher faecal fat excretion rate. This may be due to the longer duration of TPN to which infants with BPD are exposed; this is associated with lower stimulation of postnatal development of the liver and pancreas compared to enteral feeding. TPN also results in decreased secretion of enterohormones and choleostasis.

A number of infants with CLD suffer from aspiration (p. 548) and gastro-oesophageal reflux. This can be difficult to manage, but fundoplication is rarely required (p. 548). If feed thickeners are used and the infant is on a concentrated feed, the osmolality should be checked. Other feeding problems are common, and include refusal to feed, tiring on feeding, and vomiting. There are a number of possible causes (Table 29.38).

Table 29.38 Causes of CLD-associated feeding problems[188]

Hypoxaemia during feeding
Hypertonic electrolyte solutions inadequately mixed with the formula can alter gastrointestinal motility
Medication, e.g. theophylline
Gastro-oesophageal reflux
Delayed gastric emptying
Intercurrent infection
Oral hypersensitivity
repeated negative stimuli to the oral area
lack of development of appropriate feeding behaviour

Oxygen monitoring

Chronic intermittent hypoxia may result in increased pulmonary vascular resistance, pulmonary hypertension and right heart failure. Transcutaneous oxygen monitoring significantly underestimates arterial PO_2, in infants with BPD,[100,194] but over a wide range of PaO_2, $PaCO_2$, pH, heart rate, BP, haematocrit and fetal haemoglobin there is a close correlation between pulse oximeter values and arterial SaO_2 at saturations greater than 78%.[184,226]

Cardiovascular status

Approximately one-quarter of infants with BPD develop pulmonary hypertension. This is indicated clinically by a single heart sound and the murmur of tricuspid regurgitation (an enlarged liver may simply reflect hyper-expanded lungs). Although cardiac catheterization of infants with BPD is not routinely indicated and carries a mortality of 3%, it can be used to assess the responsiveness of the pulmonary vascular bed to changes in the oxygen tension.[2,18] If pulmonary artery pressure falls with a rise in oxygenation, continuous oxygen therapy by nasal cannula should be used. Pulmonary hypertension may also be detected non-invasively by echocardiography (p. 489).

A PDA should always be treated promptly by fluid restriction and indomethacin if the infant is less than 14 days of age (p. 689). If the PDA persists and the baby remains ventilator dependent, surgical ligation should be performed.

Forty per cent of infants with BPD develop systemic hypertension,[1] which may appear after discharge. The mechanism is unclear but could be due to renal damage following prolonged umbilical artery catheter usage or chronic diuretic therapy resulting in nephrocalcinosis. Although the hypertension is frequently transient and responds to antihypertensive medication,[65] it may result in left ventricular hypertrophy or cerebrovascular accident.

BPD spells

Certain infants, despite appropriate respiratory support, suddenly become grey, pale, sweaty and cyanosed, frequently associated with poor chest wall expansion. They are difficult to ventilate by bag and mask and may take many minutes to resuscitate. These episodes seem to occur in agitated infants. Simultaneous measurements of tidal flow, airway and oesophageal pressure and oxygen saturation have demonstrated that the episodes of hypoxaemia are preceded by an active exhalation. A mean decrease in end-expiratory lung volume of approximately 6 ml/kg was demonstrated, which could lead to small airway closure and the development of intrapulmonary shunts.[23] Adequate sedation can help, but it is often necessary to ventilate and paralyse such infants for up to a week until the episodes cease.

Drug therapy

Diuretics. Diuretics are useful in improving lung function in the short term. The administration of frusemide acutely increases lung compliance and reduces airway resistance.[116,160] It may also facilitate a reduction in ventilator requirements[138] and cause transient improvements in blood gases in both ventilated and non-ventilated babies.[116,117] Long-term improvement in lung function may be seen,[66,138] but, as the effect was seen after the diuresis had ceased it is likely that a non-diuretic effect is responsible.[160] Prolonged therapy with hydrochlorothiazide and spironolactone has been suggested to be useful in hypertensive infants with BPD[1] and to improve outcome in severe BPD.[4] Unfortunately, however, this was not confirmed in a randomized trial. Although giving orally administered spironolactone and chlorothiazide to oxygen-dependent infants with BPD was associated with improved pulmonary function and reduced fractional inspired oxygen requirement, the combination did not result in any long-term benefits, that is, a reduction in the number of days that the infants required supplementary oxygen, or maintained in the improvement in pulmonary function after the diuretic therapy was discontinued.[115]

Frusemide increases urinary excretion of sodium, chloride and potassium, and consequently may cause hypochloraemia, hyponatraemia and hypokalaemia in addition to hypocalcaemia.[138] It may also cause a metabolic alkalosis,[58] and in adults and animals compensatory hypoventilation and hypercarbia have been described;[103] these can be prevented by the provision of extra chloride. Other complications include secondary hyperparathyroidism, rickets and ototoxicity.[202] In adults the ototoxicity of frusemide is related to its plasma concentration, and there is a synergistic effect with aminoglycosides. Chronic diuretic therapy may cause hypercalciuria, renal calcification and nephrolithiasis,[107] leading to haematuria and urinary tract infections. Renal calcification is commonest in the most immature infants and those receiving the longest course of therapy or given it by the intravenous route.[220] Frusemide therapy should therefore be restricted to intermittent courses. Renal calcification resolves spontaneously if frusemide is stopped; chlorothiazide allows dissolution of calculi by reducing urinary calcium excretion.[107]

Digoxin. Infants with BPD may develop cor pulmonale and signs of left ventricular dysfunction and left-sided heart failure. Digoxin should not be used as it may increase pulmonary vascular resistance.

Theophylline. Intravenous aminophylline therapy improves lung function and hastens weaning from the ventilator in infants with BPD, but only in those less than 30 days old.[195] The lack of response in the older age group was explained by extensive pulmonary fibrosis resulting in irreversible airways obstruction. Oral theophylline over a 4-day period causes improvements in lung function; the addition of a diuretic results in a synergistic effect.[119] Theophylline has a number of effects which may be beneficial in BPD: decreasing the frequency and duration of respiratory pauses that occur in association with BPD, improving diaphragmatic function[159] and lowering pulmonary artery pressure, and acting as a weak diuretic. Theophylline has side-effects including vomiting and tachycardia; blood levels must therefore be measured regularly.

Bronchodilator therapy. The use of bronchodilators is controversial, as bronchiolar smooth muscles may only be feebly developed in preterm infants. There is, however, morphological evidence of peribronchiolar smooth muscle hypertrophy in infants with BPD who have been mechanically ventilated with high inspired oxygen concentrations.[24] To date, however, administration of inhaled bronchodilators on the NICU has only been associated with short-term improvements. Inhaled bronchodilator therapy has been shown to reduce airways resistance in infants with BPD at term[118,154,260] and improve pulmonary resistance, dynamic compliance, tidal volume and transcutaneous blood gases when administered to ventilated infants with CLD at approximately 1 month of age.[31] Salbutamol causes a dose-related improvement in lung mechanics in ventilator-dependent infants, the beneficial effects of 200 μg of salbutamol lasting 3 hours.[57] Inhaled ipratropium bromide gives similar short-term improvements in lung function.[260] Synergism occurs between ipratropium bromide and salbutamol in improving respiratory mechanics in ventilated infants for up to 1–2 hours after administration.[29]

After discharge, therapy with inhaled ipratropium bromide or terbutaline, utilizing a coffee cup spacer device, improves lung function and reduces symptoms in wheezy VLBW survivors.[271,274] In non-symptomatic infants a nebulized bronchodilator, however, may cause a deterioration in lung function, as evidenced by an increase in airways resistance;[276] this can be avoided by administering the bronchodilator by inhaler and spacer device.[271]

Disodium cromoglycate. Disodium cromoglycate both has an anti-inflammatory effect and reduces non-specific bronchial hyperreactivity; its use has been associated with a clinical improvement and a reduction in inspired oxygen concentration and ventilator pressures.[235] At follow-up it reduces symptoms and bronchodilator usage in VLBW infants.[273]

Steroids. Steroids have a number of possible beneficial actions, including stabilizing membranes and reducing pulmonary oedema, enhancing surfactant synthesis, suppressing collagen synthesis and reducing bronchospasm and inflammation in small airways, and leukotriene production. Dexamethasone given to ventilated infants reduces the pulmonary inflammatory response, microvascular permeability and release of inflammatory mediators and neutrophil influx into the airways.[92]

Short-term benefits regarding reduction in respiratory rate, peak inspiration pressure, fractional inspired oxygen concentration, alveolar oxygen gradient and improved rate of weaning have been shown in infants with severe BPD.[8,142] Neither study, however, nor the UK multicentre trial,[44] showed that steroid administration resulted in any difference in mortality or length of hospital stay. Follow-up at 3 years also failed to reveal any significant differences in outcome between steroid-treated and placebo-treated patients.[114] A longer course of therapy may be required to influence outcome. Cummings et al[53] compared a 42-day course of steroid therapy with one lasting 18 days, both starting at a dose of 0.5 mg dexamethasone per kilogram body weight. Infants in the 42-day, but not in the 18-day, group were weaned from mechanical ventilation and supplemental oxygen significantly faster than controls. No complications were noted and neurological outcome was better in the infants given the longer course. The efficacy of very early administration (<48 hours of age) of corticosteroids remains controversial. A shorter duration of ventilation and supplementary oxygen requirement has been demonstrated in two studies.[205,266] A third, however, reported only improved respiratory status at 72 hours of treatment.[219] The effectiveness of administering steroids in the first 12 hours of life may be determined by the infant's birthweight. Rastogi et al[185] demonstrated an improvement in ventilator variables at 5 and 14 days in infants who received a 12-day tapering course of steroids, starting at 0.5 mg/kg/day, compared to those who received placebo; the impact was more marked in babies with a birthweight of less than 1250 g. In that study dexamethasone administration was also associated with a higher proportion of infants being extubated by 14 days, and a reduced incidence of oxygen dependency at 28 days and 36 weeks' PCA.[185] The improved long-term outcome in this latter study may be explained by use of a 12-day course, rather than only two doses,[205] and that all of the infants had received postnatal surfactant.

Numerous side-effects have been reported following steroid therapy. These include pneumothorax, sepsis,

NEC, hyperglycaemia, hypertension, periventricular densities and leucomalacia, diabetic ketoacidosis, hypertrophic cardiomyopathy and greater weight loss.[94,109,163,181,185,187,229] Fitzhardinge et al[71] found no difference in the immune competence of infants given steroid or placebo in the first 24 hours of life, and Ng et al[161] documented a similar incidence and pattern of septicaemia in 24 infants given steroids and 18 not so treated. It remains important, however, to meticulously exclude sepsis before embarking on steroid therapy: some authorities recommend prophylactic antibiotics or anticandida agents to run concurrently. Rennie et al[189] found no evidence of adrenal suppression after 13 days of dexamethasone treatment; all except one of 12 infants had the expected twofold rise in serum cortisol in a short synacthen test, but others[51] have demonstrated that dexamethasone does cause secondary adrenal suppression at the hypothalamic–pituitary level.

To avoid the side-effects of systemically administered steroids, this therapy has been given by inhalation. A rare side-effect of beclomethasone inhalation therapy is tongue hypertrophy, which resolves after cessation of treatment.[134] Although anecdotal studies[41,132] suggested benefit, in a randomized controlled trial[59] this was not substantiated, as systemically administered steroids were associated with a greater positive effect on respiratory function and a faster onset of action than inhaled steroids. We would therefore not routinely recommend their use, although they may have a place for infants who have a continuing requirement for a relatively low inspired oxygen concentration (≤30%).

Steroid therapy should be commenced early, certainly at 2 rather than 4 weeks[53] in infants in whom reduction of ventilator therapy is not possible, provided a PDA and infection have been excluded. In practice we start at 1 week of age in infants whose respiratory failure is worsening or not improving. On present evidence usually only a single course is merited; we use a 10-day tapering course, 0.5 mg/kg/day for 3 days, then 0.3 mg/kg/day for 3 days, and finally 0.1 mg/kg/day. Although further courses may result in benefit they can be associated with important side-effects, particularly hypertension.[84] We would retreat an infant if the respiratory failure worsened and infection had been excluded or treated. In such patients a prolonged course (up to 6 weeks) can be required: frequently infants deteriorate if a second course is stopped too soon. Such infants require very careful monitoring to facilitate early detection of side-effects.

Surfactant. Surfactant dysfunction may persist and contribute to the continuing respiratory support required by neonates with CLD (pp. 609–610). In a pilot study, in infants between 7 and 30 days of age treatment with a single dose of a natural surfactant reduced the inspired oxygen concentration requirement.[170] A randomized trial is required to assess whether surfactant improves long-term outcome in this group of patients.

Helium. During heliox (helium–oxygen mixture) breathing a significant decrease in pulmonary resistance, resistive work of breathing and mechanical work of breathing is reported, although ventilation remains unchanged.[262] Heliox breathing may result in a caloric saving of 2 kcal/kg/24 h.

Nifedipine. In infants with BPD nifedipine may achieve a lower pulmonary vascular resistance and greater cardiac output.[27] Nifedipine may thus have a useful role in children with BPD whose pulmonary artery hypertension is unresponsive to oxygen. The long-term effects of calcium channel blockers, however, have not been investigated and adverse effects such as systemic arterial hypotension and tachycardia are reported.

Nitric oxide. Inhaled NO may be useful in infants with BPD or developing CLD. A reduction in the oxygenation index was seen in eight of nine patients, but the optimum dose ranged from 6 to 60 ppm and the magnitude of response was variable.[136]

Recommendations for drug therapy. At King's College Hospital diuretics are reserved to treat acute fluid overload; a single dose of frusemide is then administered. If infants have signs of incipient right failure or are poorly tolerant of a modest fluid volume regimen (120 ml/kg/day), then regular chlorothiazide and spironolactone are given. Theophylline, commenced to facilitate extubation, is continued to prevent apnoeic episodes but is stopped if the infant has signs of gastro-oesophageal reflux. On the NICU bronchodilators are rarely prescribed, and only if the infant has obvious wheezing on auscultation. Steroids are given to all infants who are likely to develop CLD: these are administered systemically as a 10-day course at least by 7 days, unless there are specific contraindications. Other drug therapies discussed would be used only on an individual basis or in the context of randomized trials.

HOME RESPIRATORY SUPPORT

Pinney and Cotton[178] first described a home care programme in 1976. Infants were sent home on oxygen if they were feeding well, gaining weight, and had an oxygen requirement of more than 25%. Oxygen was delivered from cylinders by a single feeding catheter inserted into one nostril. Since then other delivery systems have been used, including twin nasal cannulae. Recently oxygen concentrators have been introduced and are particularly useful for infants requiring high flow, which otherwise would necessitate frequent cylinder changes. Small portable oxygen cylinders should also be provided, whichever system is used, as they are necessary for transport related to social activities.

On discharge the infants should have no medical problem other than the increased inspired oxygen requirement, although some parents may cope with tube feeds. At regular intervals the infants should be seen either at home or in hospital, progress and weight checked and the need for continuing oxygen administration assessed. Monitoring of oxygen saturation is most reliable, and saturation should be maintained at least above 92% to ensure appropriate weight gain;[93] others have recommended a minimum SaO_2, of 95%[106,180]. Maintaining such an SaO_2 the mean weight percentile increased from less than the 5th to the 25th between discharge and last follow-up in one series.[106] In addition, in that study the readmission rate was only 30%, compared to 66% in a previous series.[1] At regular intervals PaO_2 should be checked and, once it is at least 7.3 kPa (55 mmHg) after a period in room air with a saturation greater than 92%, oxygen may be discontinued. Weaning should be gradual, beginning with short intervals in room air. The time spent in room air should be lengthened over several weeks if the oxygen saturation level is maintained. It is essential that the inspired oxygen concentration should not be reduced abruptly, as if this is sufficient to cause hypoxaemia it can lead to worsening pulmonary hypertension, changes consistent with increased airway constriction[246] and an increased incidence of apnoea, which responds to improving arterial oxygen saturation.[212] It is essential to ensure that patients maintain their oxygen saturation levels at all times, particularly after feeding, at which time desaturation is a common problem.[223] For the first month after oxygen is no longer needed, parents should be advised to keep the equipment at home in case of an increased need associated with minor respiratory infections.

Pinney and Cotton[178] reported that infants require on average 3 months of supplemental oxygen following discharge, and that early hospital discharge means a financial saving of $18 000 per infant. Hudak et al[106] reported a similar duration of home oxygen therapy – 4.5 months. Some infants, however, may require years of home oxygen.[86]

Only a very small number of infants with BPD have been discharged on home ventilation. The infant must have a tracheostomy. Home ventilation requires an enormous investment in equipment, community services and education for parents;[172] in one series[211] the average duration of home ventilation was 365 days.

PROPHYLAXIS

Antenatal therapy

Although meta-analysis has demonstrated that steroid treatment given to women at high risk of preterm delivery reduces the incidence of death and RDS by approximately 50% (p. 491),[52] even in combination with postnatal surfactant, it has failed to favourably affect the incidence of BPD (pp. 494, 508).[111] Preliminary data suggested that thyrotrophin-releasing hormone might reduce CLD by as much as 50%,[11] but unfortunately this was not confirmed by a large Australian study.[3]

Vitamin E

Vitamin E deficiency enhances the toxic effects of oxygen upon the lung; this is prevented by vitamin E treatment.[245] Healthy term and premature infants have a mean plasma vitamin E level of less than 0.25 mg/dl within the first 24 hours of life;[155] vitamin E inadequacy in adults is indicated by a level of less than 0.5 mg/dl. Daily vitamin E administration to infants with an inspired oxygen concentration greater than 40% was associated with an increase in vitamin E levels (3.2 mg/dl 24 hours after a third dose) and a reduction in the number of infants with a chest radiograph appearance compatible with BPD.[64] A randomized controlled trial from the same group and others,[63,203] however, has failed to confirm this effect. Although the failure of vitamin E to prevent BPD may have resulted from too low a dosage, the incidence of culture-proven neonatal sepsis and NEC is significantly higher in infants maintained at pharmacological levels of vitamin E for 8 days or more, compared to those placebo treated. Vitamin E decreases the oxygen-dependent intracellular killing ability of neutrophils, resulting in a decreased resistance to infection in preterm infants.[112]

Vitamin A

VLBW infants are frequently deficient in vitamin A because of deprivation of transplacental acquisition, and parenteral administration of vitamin A is inefficient[36] because of photodegradation and absorption of the vitamin to the intravenous tubing. VLBW neonates with BPD may have suboptimal plasma concentrations of vitamin A postnatally for extended periods.[216] Vitamin A supplementation, by influencing the normal differentiation of regenerating airways, could have a favourable effect on the healing processes and lessen BPD. Shenai et al[217] conducted a randomized controlled trial in oxygen-dependent infants: vitamin A (retinyl palmitate 2000 iu) or saline was given from day 4 as 14 intramuscular injections over a 28-day period. Vitamin A administration resulted in significantly higher mean plasma concentrations of vitamin A than placebo and less BPD; the need for supplemental oxygen, mechanical ventilation and intensive care was also reduced. This beneficial effect, however, has not been confirmed.[175] The precise requirement of vitamin A in VLBW infants and the optimal dosage,[110] mode and duration of its administration need further investigation. Vitamin A must be carefully monitored if side-effects, such as non-specific neurological signs secondary to raised intracranial pressure due to toxic levels, are to be avoided.

Antioxidant superoxide dismutase

Pretreatment of rats with superoxide dismutase prevents toxic changes in lung macrophages[222] and damage to lung cells[21] when exposed to hyperoxia. Human neonates appear to be deficient in SOD[199,267] (p. 560). Rosenfeld et al[197] determined that in preterm infants with severe RDS a dosage of 0.25 mg/kg given subcutaneously every 12 hours was not associated with any side-effects. A randomized trial[198] in infants with severe respiratory distress at 24 hours of age demonstrated that SOD-treated infants had less clinical and radiological evidence of BPD, with fewer CPAP requirements and less hospitalization for respiratory problems. In a rat model pretreatment with intratracheal SOD and catalase was associated with significantly longer survival in hyperoxia than saline pretreatment.[251] Although toxicity has not been reported, antioxidant therapy may affect the bactericidal activity of polymorphonuclear cells (see above).

Allopurinol

Allopurinol is a synthetic competitive inhibitor of xanthine oxidase and a free radical scavenger. Unfortunately, administration of 20 mg/ml for 7 days in a randomized placebo-controlled trial failed to significantly reduce the incidence of CLD.[200]

Surfactant

Exogenous surfactant replacement therapy, although significantly reducing the incidence of BPD and death, does not reduce the incidence of BPD alone (pp. 494, 508).[67,98,121,131,148,152,214]

Inositol

Inositol supplementation (80 mg/kg) during the first 5 days of life improved survival without CLD from 55 to 71%.[96]

Cromolyn sodium

Aerosolized cromolyn sodium (20 mg) given every 6 hours in a randomized placebo-controlled trial to infants ventilated for RDS in a pilot study failed to reduce the subsequent development of BPD by 50%.[255]

Ambroxol

Ambroxol given over the first 5 days has been associated with a 50% reduction in the incidence of BPD without adverse effect.[256]

Respiratory support

Avoiding the use of 'aggressive' respiratory suport may be associated with a reduction in BPD incidence. Avery et al[9] reported that one of eight centres caring for critically ill neonates with RDS not only had the best outcome for low birthweight infants, but also the lowest incidence of BPD. The institution's respiratory support policy was found to differ markedly from the other institutions: they used CPAP (5 cmH_2O via nasal prongs) soon after birth, in preference to ventilation for infants with respiratory distress. Hyperventilation was avoided and $PaCO_2$ allowed to rise as high as 60 mmHg (8 kPa) before endotracheal intubation was performed; muscle relaxants were not used. Unfortunately, the study was neither randomized nor controlled: differences in the patient population and other management policies might thus explain these results. Other centres, however, have also reported an association of a decrease in BPD incidence with a reduction in the proportion of patients intubated and mechanically ventilated.[179]

The efficacy of HFOV in reducing BPD remains controversial.[39,104,168]

PROGNOSIS

Mortality

Predischarge mortality is usually caused by intercurrent infection, cor pulmonale or respiratory failure. In one series[69] sepsis occurred in 77% of infants with BPD. The mortality of stage 4 BPD is 40%: infants usually die at about 3 months of age, between 67 and 80% of deaths occurring during the initial hospitalization. Requirement for support for mechanical ventilation of more than 50 days is associated with a poor prognosis, with no intact survivors in one series.[259]

The mortality in the first year of life of Northway grade IV BPD is between 20 and 40%.[7] Sauve and Singhal[208] reported a postdischarge death rate of 11.2%. SIDS was reported to be seven times higher in infants with BPD.[258] This result, however, has not been subsequently confirmed.[80,208]

Survival rate can be related to the length of hospital stay,[213] 47% of infants surviving if their stay was 3 months or less, but the survival rate falling to 17% in those requiring hospitalization of 5 months. The survival rates of infants with Northway grade IV BPD were 27% in infants oxygen dependent for 3 months, and 0% in infants who were oxygen dependent at 5 months. A comparison of surviving infants with BPD with those who died suggested that hypochloraemia (<80 mmol/l) might be an accurate predictor of poor outcome.[177] Chloride deficiency is known to be associated with poor weight gain, anorexia and hypertension; poor head growth has also been reported.[177] Other predictors of death in hospital include male gender and length of ventilatory support and supplementary oxygen.[215]

Morbidity

The mean duration of oxygen therapy and ventilation was 68 and 37 days, respectively, in infants with CLD,[270] which is increased in infants of birthweight less than 1000 g to an average of 84 days of added oxygen and 76 days of assisted ventilation.[268] The duration of hospital treatment ranges from 2.5 to 8 months. Prolonged hospital stay is associated with a mean developmental score of less than 85; chronically oxygen-dependent infants have a significantly poorer growth rate. Recent interventions have aimed at reducing the costs of care in BPD by decreasing the length of stay for high-risk neonates;[125] this has focused on early assessment of the home environment and avoiding the attainment of a preset weight as criteria for discharge.[125]

Rehospitalization is required in up to 50% of infants in the first year,[13,122,144,167] and 20% in the second year.[143] Infants with BPD are readmitted an average of five times during the first 2 years of life (range 1–13).[270]

Morbidity relating to growth

The average weight and height at term of infants with BPD is frequently at or below the third centile, growth failure being partially the result of increased metabolic demands from increased work of breathing;[130] growth accelerates as respiratory symptoms improve. Growth retardation is associated with severe and prolonged respiratory dysfunction.[143] Infants with BPD are at greater risk of growth retardation in their second year than infants with RDS.[145] Infants with BPD have a significantly lower energy intake but higher energy expenditure than control infants,[265] although they appear to absorb calorie intake as well as controls. At school age, however, children who had had BPD only, did not have poorer growth than controls.[250]

Central nervous system morbidity

Delays in development are common,[164] poor developmental outcome correlating positively with prolonged hospitalization and requirement for oxygen.[143,213] At 12 and 18 months infants with BPD perform significantly less well than infants with RDS at cognitive, sensorimotor and language tests.[143] Neurodevelopmental and hearing abnormalities occur more frequently in BPD survivors,[208] but tend to improve as the child gets older. At 3 years of age 29% of infants surviving with stage IV BPD have minor abnormalities, including right ventricular hypertrophy on the electrocardiogram, weight and height less than the third percentile, and an IQ in the 80–90 range. Thirty four per cent have a significant handicap, including one or more of the following: cerebral palsy, mental retardation, deafness or blindness. In general, the degree of handicap found at follow-up among infants with severe BPD does not differ from that of a group of infants with severe RDS ventilated for longer than 24 hours, but without BPD.[102,143,164] At 8 years of age, although the duration of pulmonary disease affects outcome, prematurity with or without BPD, along with adverse social factors, compromises the outcome of low birthweight infants with a history of BPD.[193]

Pulmonary morbidity

Northway[164] reported increased pulmonary dysfunction and recurrent lower respiratory tract infections in infants with BPD after discharge, but these abnormalities decreased with time, patients being clinically well by the age of 3–4 years.[143] Specific pulmonary function abnormalities reported in the first year of life include high airways resistance, low dynamic pulmonary compliance, FRC, abnormal gas exchange (hypercarbia, low oxygen saturation), elevated minute volume and lower mixing index. The most consistent finding in BPD has been increased pulmonary or airway resistance.[153,167,239,277]

Lung function usually improves with age,[77,153,263] and is often normal at 1 year. Severe lower airway obstruction, however, may persist in a small number of infants who have recurrent respiratory symptoms with bronchial hyperreactivity and abnormal blood gas levels.[224] Prospective follow-up of all inborn VLBW infants at King's College Hospital[87,88] revealed approximately twice as much wheezing among BPD survivors as in term infants from the same geographical area. Pulmonary function tests may still be abnormal, with reduced exercise tolerance, in school-aged children.[224] These infants also had positive metacholine challenge tests, indicating bronchial hyperreactivity, and there was a positive response to bronchodilator therapy. Andreasson et al[6] reported airways obstruction in 10 out of 11 8-year-olds with BPD, but only nine out of 24 controls who had had RDS only; hyperinflation was more common and FRC significantly higher in children with BPD. In addition, BPD patients seen at approximately 8 years of age may still have a mild degree of exercise intolerance,[173] even if pulmonary function at rest is only slightly impaired.[206]

Respiratory infection is also more common in survivors with BPD (p. 1145). In a small proportion of patients ongoing respiratory problems, even up to 5 years of age, may be due to aspiration, which can be demonstrated by the degree of lipid-laden macrophages in the BAL or by using a pH probe.[183]

Numerous chronic complications of BPD may be seen on the CXR,[60] including cor pulmonale, right ventricular hypertrophy and enlargement of the main pulmonary artery reflecting pulmonary hypertension. Absolute cardiomegaly is infrequently observed, probably because of the pulmonary hyperexpansion. Atelectasis and subsegmental or segmental collapse may occur, frequently affecting the left lower lobe. Rickets, caused by dietary or parenteral nutritional deficiency of calcium and vitamin D, or to the calciuric effect of frusemide, may manifest by rib fractures together with generalized demineralization and metaphyseal fraying, widening and cupping. The

CXR abnormalities of BPD may persist for some years. Mayes et al[144] have demonstrated radiological abnormalities at 6 months, and Harrod et al[102] reported abnormalities in all patients studied between 1 and 5 years. Smyth et al[224] found persistent atelectasis and hyperinflation in eight out of nine children studied between 7 and 9 years of age. Most patients, however, remain either radiologically stable or show a trend towards radiological improvement.

Cardiovascular morbidity

Cardiac catheterization of BPD survivors reveals persisting elevation of pulmonary artery pressure and a high pulmonary vascular resistance, cardiac index and intrapulmonary shunt fraction.[19] Pulmonary hypertension can be detected non-invasively by Doppler echocardiographic demonstration of tricuspid regurgitation, or by estimation of the pulmonary systolic time interval. Such measurements can be used to identify a response to elevation of the inspired oxygen concentration.[16] Systemic hypertension is also common in infants with severe BPD, affecting 13% of 87 patients who required home oxygen therapy (see above). In the survivors, however, it resolved prior to weaning from supplementary oxygen.[5]

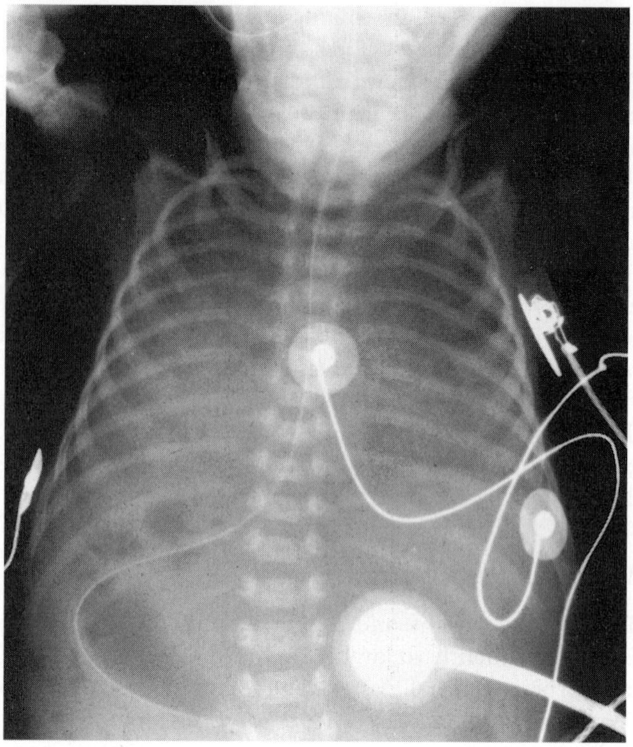

Fig. 29.85 Respiratory insufficiency syndrome – diffuse haziness, small-volume lung field.

OTHER FORMS OF CLD

RESPIRATORY INSUFFICIENCY SYNDROME

A form of CLD has been described in very immature infants, usually of birthweight less than 1000 g, who suffered from no or only mild RDS and had not required ventilation.[264] The illness was characterized by apnoea and bradycardia and the chest radiograph by diffuse haziness, streaky infiltrates with small cystic areas, and a small chest (Fig. 29.85). The prognosis is good, the disease usually resolving before discharge. This form of CLD is similar to RIS,[32] except that RIS is characterized by initial apnoea occurring 72 hours after delivery and more than 50% of the infants require ventilation; 76% survive.

Rhodes et al[192] described a group of nine out of 150 infants ventilated for idiopathic RDS who had a radiographic appearance of diffuse haziness with loss of identifiable lung marking. This occurred at 5–15 days, but was not associated with clinical signs or symptoms or increased oxygen needs; these changes disappeared in 1–5 days.

CHRONIC PULMONARY INSUFFICIENCY OF PREMATURITY

Krauss et al[128] described a series of infants who were previously healthy and presented with respiratory distress, frequent apnoea and a requirement for supplemental oxygen developing at age 4–7 days; the symptoms persisted for 2–4 weeks. This condition is now more usually seen in very immature infants who have made at least a partial recovery from RDS but who then go on to develop apnoea and increasing oxygen requirements.

Diagnosis

The CXR demonstrates small volume lungs with hazy lung fields (Fig. 29.86) and is distinct from that seen in BPD and Wilson–Mikity syndrome.

Management

The infants frequently require supplemental oxygen. CPAP is useful to treat worsening hypoxaemia and apnoea. Theophylline should be given, but antibiotics are only necessary to treat secondary infection.

Prognosis

The infants have slowly progressive atelectasis, hypoxaemia and hypercarbia, but recovery is usually complete by 6 weeks of age.

WILSON–MIKITY SYNDROME

Wilson–Mikity syndrome affects infants of less than

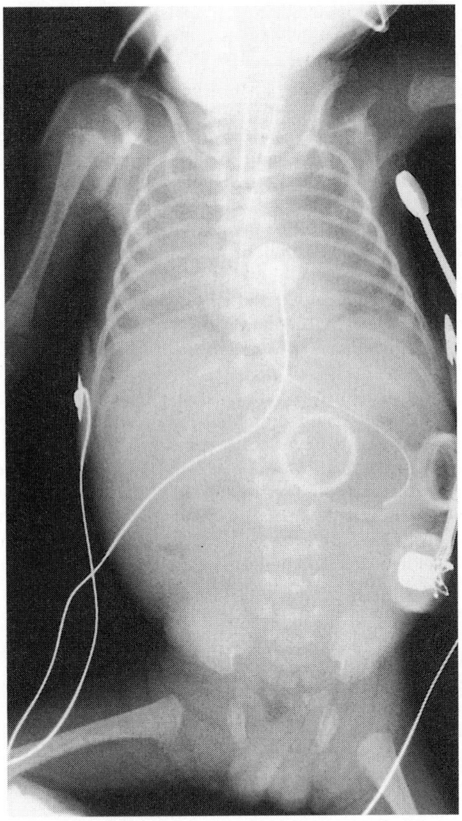

Fig. 29.86 Chronic pulmonary insufficiency syndrome.

32 weeks' gestation, with an equal male and female distribution. Infants classically have no respiratory problems in the first week of life and the diagnosis is made when progressive respiratory failure develops during the second week, in association with diffuse small bilateral cystic translucencies on the CXR.[261] There is an insidious onset of cyanosis, tachypnoea and retraction, which persists for several months. The infant has intrapulmonary shunting and maldistribution of ventilation and perfusion;[127] pulmonary hypertension can be detected at cardiac catheterization. The increased pulmonary vascular resistance is unresponsive to oxygen, suggesting damage to the pulmonary capillary bed. Longitudinal studies of pulmonary function have demonstrated a low compliance and a high resistance and thoracic gas volume, which return to normal only at or after the onset of clinical recovery.[207] Air trapping was demonstrated in these infants in association with episodes of clinical deterioration.

Symptoms

The clinical characteristics of the illness include a premature infant in the first month of life, insidious onset of hyperpnoea and cyanosis, and dyspnoea, especially on effort. The infant frequently has an overexpanded chest, wheezing and coughing, but no rales unless heart failure occurs and no fever unless infection intervenes. Cor pulmonale may develop and there is a variable effect on general growth.

Aetiology

Burnard[30] suggested that the only consistent aetiological association of this condition was low gestational age, typically less than 32 completed weeks of gestation. Others have suggested it represents a functional and anatomical immaturity of the airways[207] or repeated aspiration (p. 548). Fujimura et al[74] reported high plasma IgM levels on the first day of life in infants with Wilson–Mikity syndrome. The same group[75] found a high incidence of chorioamnionitis in mothers of infants with Wilson–Mikity syndrome, associated with a raised cord blood IgM, suggesting intrauterine infection. These findings were absent with other forms of CLD.

Diagnosis

The diagnosis is made from the characteristic clinical course and the CXR. The changes affect both lungs and initially, unlike BPD, are more marked in the upper zones. There is a diffuse fine reticular pattern infiltrating the lung fields, interspersed with areas of emphysematous cysts (Fig. 29.87). As the disease progresses the cysts coalesce, and marked hyperinflation is a prominent feature.

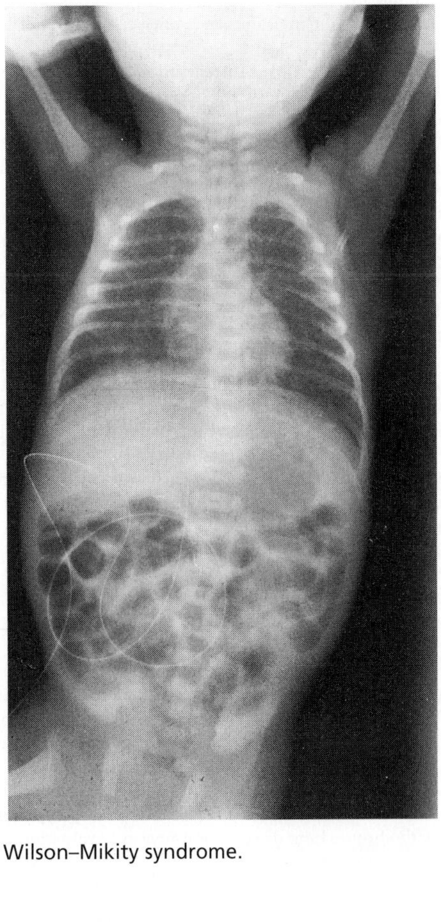

Fig. 29.87 Wilson–Mikity syndrome.

Management

An increased inspired oxygen concentration is frequently required, but not mechanical ventilation. Ventilation should be avoided if possible, as this, as in other forms of CLD, may result in a deterioration in the clinical course.

Prognosis

Symptoms may persist for many months. Respiratory infections are increased in the first year of life. Abnormal lung function, suggesting persistent small airway damage, has been found in survivors even at 8–10 years of age, but the usual tendency is for the pulmonary disease to resolve. Death may occur from cardiac failure, respiratory failure or infection.

REFERENCES

1. Abman S H, Accurso F J, Koops B L 1984 Experience with home oxygen in the management of infants with bronchopulmonary dysplasia. Journal of Pediatrics 23: 471–476
2. Abman S H, Wolfe R R, Accurso F J, Koops B L, Bowman C M, Wiggins J W 1985 Pulmonary vascular response to oxygen in infants with severe bronchopulmonary dysplasia. Pediatrics 75: 80–84
3. ACTOBAT Study Group 1995 Australian collaborative trial of antenatal thyrotropin releasing hormone (ACTOBAT) for prevention of neonatal respiratory disease. Lancet 345: 877–882
4. Albersheim S G, Solimano A J, Sharma A K et al 1989 Randomized double blind controlled trial of long term diuretic therapy for bronchopulmonary dysplasia. Journal of Pediatrics 115: 615–620
5. Anderson A H, Warady B A, Daily D K, Johnson J A, Thomas M K 1993 Systemic hypertension in infants with severe bronchopulmonary dysplasia: associated clinical factors. American Journal of Perinatology 10: 190–193
6. Andreasson B, Lindroth M, Mortensson W, Svenningsen N W, Jonson B 1989 Lung function eight years after neonatal ventilation. Archives of Disease in Childhood 64: 108–113
7. Ariagno R L 1988 Use of steroids. In: Merrit T A, Northway W H, Boynton B R (eds) Bronchopulmonary dysplasia. Blackwell Scientific Publications, Boston, pp 375–402
8. Avery G B, Fletcher A B, Kaplan M, Brudno D S 1985 Controlled trial of dexamethasone in respirator-dependent infants with BPD. Pediatrics 75: 106–111
9. Avery M E, Tooley W H, Keller J B et al 1987 Is chronic lung disease in low birth weight infants preventable? A survey of 8 centres. Pediatrics 79: 26–30
10. Bacchi A, Viscardi R M, Tacrak V, Ensor J E, McCrea K A, Hasday J D 1994 Increased activity of interleukin-6 but not tumour necrosis factor-alpha in lung lavage of premature infants is associated with the development of bronchopulmonary dysplasia. Pediatric Research 36: 244–252
11. Ballard R A, Ballard P L, Creasy R et al 1992 Respiratory disease in very low birthweight infants after prenatal thyrotropin releasing hormone and glucocorticoid. Lancet 339: 510–515
12. Bancalari E, Asdenour G E, Feller R, Gannon J 1979 Bronchopulmonary dysplasia: clinical presentation. Journal of Pediatrics 95: 819–823
13. Bancalari E, Gerhardt T 1986 Bronchopulmonary dysplasia. Pediatric Clinics of North America 33: 1–23
14. Barnes N D, Glover W J, Hull D, Milner A D 1969 Effects of prolonged positive pressure ventilation in infancy. Lancet ii: 1096–1099
15. Bell E F, Warburton D, Stonestreet B, Oh W 1980 Effect of fluid administration on the development of symptomatic patent ductus arteriosus and congestive heart failure in premature infants. New England Journal of Medicine 302: 598–604
16. Benatar A, Clarke J, Silverman M 1995 Pulmonary hypertension in infants with chronic lung disease: non-invasive evaluation and short term effect of oxygen treatment. Archives of Disease in Childhood 72: F14–F19
17. Berg T J, Pagtakhan R D, Reed M H, Langston C, Chernick V 1975 Bronchopulmonary dysplasia and lung rupture in hyaline membrane disease: influence of continuous distending pressure. Pediatrics 55: 51–53
18. Berman W, Yabek S M, Dillon T, Burstein R, Corlew S 1982 Evaluation of infants with bronchopulmonary dysplasia using cardiac catheterization. Pediatrics 70: 708–712
19. Berman W, Katz R, Yabek S M, Dillon T, Fripp R R, Papile L 1986 Long-term follow-up of bronchopulmonary dysplasia. Journal of Pediatrics 109: 45–50
20. Betremieux P, Treguier C, Pladys P, Bourdiniere J, Leclech G, Lefrancois C 1995 Tracheobronchography and balloon dilatation in acquired neonatal tracheal stenosis. Archives of Disease in Childhood 72: F3–F7
21. Block E R, Fisher A B 1977 Protection of hyperoxic induced depression of pulmonary serotonin by pretreatment with superoxide dismutase. American Review of Respiratory Disease 116: 441–446
22. Boehm G, Bierbach U, Moro G, Minoli I 1996 Limited fat digestion in infants with bronchopulmonary dysplasia. Journal of Pediatric Gastroenterology and Nutrition 22: 161–166
23. Bolivar J M, Gerhardt T, Gonzalez A et al 1995 Mechanisms for episodes of hypoxemia in preterm infants undergoing mechanical ventilation. Journal of Pediatrics 127: 767–773
24. Bonikos D S, Bensch K G, Northway W H Jr 1976 Oxygen toxicity in the newborn. The effect of chronic continuous 100 per cent oxygen exposure on the lungs of newborn mice. American Journal of Pathology 85: 623–650
25. Boynton B R, Mannino F L, Randel R C et al 1984 Minimizing bronchopulmonary dysplasia in VLBW infants (letter). Journal of Pediatrics 104: 962–963
26. Brown E R 1979 Increased risk of bronchopulmonary dysplasia in infants with patent ductus arteriosus. Journal of Pediatrics 95: 865–866
27. Brownlee J R, Beekman R H, Rosenthal A 1988 Acute hemodynamic effects of nifedipine in infants with bronchopulmonary dysplasia and pulmonary hypertension. Pediatric Research 24: 186–190
28. Bruce M C, Schuyler M, Martin R J, Starcher B C, Tomashefski J F, Wedig K E 1992 Risk factors for the degradation of lung elastic fibres in the ventilated neonate. American Review of Respiratory Disease 146: 204–212
29. Brundage K L, Mohsini K G, Froese A B, Fisher J T 1990 Bronchodilator response to ipratropium bromide in infants with bronchopulmonary dysplasia. American Review of Respiratory Disease 142: 1137–1142
30. Burnard E D 1966 The pulmonary syndrome of Wilson and Mikity and respiratory function in very small premature infants. Pediatric Clinics of North America 13: 999–1016
31. Cabal L A, Larrazabal C, Ramanathan R et al 1987 Effects of metaproterenol on pulmonary mechanics, oxygenation and ventilation in infants with chronic lung disease. Journal of Pediatrics 110: 116–119
32. Carlsson J, Svenningsen N W 1975 Respiratory insufficiency syndrome (RIS) in preterm infants with gestational age of 32 weeks and less. Acta Paediatrica Scandinavica 64: 813–821
33. Cassell G H, Waites K B, Crouse D T et al 1988 Association of *ureaplasma urealyticum* infection of the lower respiratory tract with chronic lung disease and death in very-low-birth-weight infants. Lancet ii: 240–244
34. Chan V, Greenough A 1993 Randomized trial of methods of extubation in acute and chronic respiratory distress. Archives of Disease in Childhood 68: 570–572
35. Chan V, Greenough A, Hird M F 1991 Comparison of different rates of artificial ventilation for preterm infants ventilated beyond the first week of life. Early Human Development 26: 177–183
36. Chan V, Greenough A, Cheeseman P, Gamsu H R 1993 Vitamin A levels and feeding practice of neonates with and without chronic lung disease. Journal of Perinatal Medicine 21: 205–210
37. Chan R N, Noble-Jamieson C M, Elliman A, Bryan E M, Aber U R, Silverman M 1988 Airway responsiveness in low birthweight children and their mothers. Archives of Disease in Childhood 63: 905–910
38. Clark D A, Pincus L G, Oliphant M, Hubbell C, Oates R P, Davey F R 1982 HLA-A2 and chronic lung disease in neonates. Journal of the American Medical Association 248: 1868–1869
39. Clark R H, Gerstmann D R, Null D M, deLemos R A 1992

Prospective randomized comparison of high frequency oscillatory and conventional ventilation in respiratory distress syndrome. Pediatrics 89: 5–12
40. Clement A, Chadelar K, Sardet A, Grimfeld A, Tournier G 1988 Alveolar macrophage status in bronchopulmonary dysplasia. Pediatric Research 23: 470–473
41. Cloutier M M, McLellan N 1993 Nebulized steroid therapy in bronchopulmonary dysplasia. Pediatric Pulmonology 15: 111–116
42. Coalson J J, King R J, Yang F et al 1995 SP-A deficiency in primate model of bronchopulmonary dysplasia with infection. American Journal of Respiratory and Critical Care Medicine 151: 854–866
43. Cochran D P, Pilling D W, Shaw N J 1994 The relationship of pulmonary interstitial emphysema to subsequent type of chronic lung disease. British Journal of Radiology 76: 1155–1157
44. Collaborative Dexamethasone Trial Group 1991 Dexamethasone therapy in neonatal chronic lung disease: an international placebo-controlled trial. Pediatrics 88: 421–427
45. Cook A J, Yuksel B, Sampson A P, Greenough A, Price J F 1996 Cysteinyl leukotriene involvement in chronic lung disease in premature infants. European Respiratory Journal 9: 1907–1912
46. Cooke R W I 1991 Factors associated with chronic lung disease in preterm infants. Archives of Disease in Childhood 66: 776–779
47. Corcoran J D, Patterson C C, Thomas P S, Halliday H L 1993 Reduction in the risk of bronchopulmonary dysplasia from 1980–1990: results of a multivariate logistic regression analysis. European Journal of Pediatrics 152: 677–681
48. Costarino A T, Gruskay J A, Corcoran L, Polin R A, Baumgart S 1992 Sodium restriction versus daily maintenance replacement in very low birthweight premature neonates: a randomized blind therapeutic trial. Journal of Pediatrics 120: 99–106
49. Couser R J, Ferrara B, Wright G B et al 1996 Prophylactic indomethacin therapy in the first 24 hours of life for the prevention of patent ductus arteriosus in preterm infants treated prophylactically in the delivery room. Journal of Pediatrics 128: 631–637
50. Crapo J D, Peters-Golden M, Marsh-Salin J, Shelburne J 1978 Pathologic changes in the lungs of oxygen-adapted rats. A morphometric analysis. Laboratory Investigation 39: 640–653
51. Cronin C M G, Dean H, MacDonald N T, Seshia M M K 1993 Basal and post-ACTH cortisol levels in preterm infants following treatment with dexamethasone. Clinical and Investigative Medicine 16: 8–14
52. Crowley P, Chalmers I, Keirse M 1990 The effects of corticosteroid administration before preterm delivery: an overview of the evidence from controlled trials. British Journal of Obstetrics and Gynaecology 97: 11–25
53. Cummings J J, D'Eugenio D B, Gross S J 1989 A controlled trial of dexamethasone in preterm infants at high risk for bronchopulmonary dysplasia. New England Journal of Medicine 320: 1505–1510
54. D'Ablang G, Bernard B, Zahavov I, Barton L, Kaplan B, Schwinn C P 1975 Neonatal pulmonary cytology and bronchopulmonary dysplasia. Acta Cytologica 19: 21–27
55. Dahms B B, Halpin T C 1980 Pulmonary arterial lipid deposit in infants receiving intravenous lipid infusion. Pediatrics 97: 800–805
56. Davidson D, Drafta D, Wilkens B A 1995 Elevated urinary leukotriene E4 in chronic lung disease of prematurity. American Journal of Respiratory and Critical Care Medicine 151: 841–845
57. Denjean A, Gulmaraes H, Migdal M, Miramand J L, Dehan M, Gaultier C 1992 Dose-related bronchodilator response to aerosolized salbutamol (albuterol) in ventilator-dependent premature infants. Journal of Pediatrics 120: 974–979
58. De Rubertis F R, Michelis M F, Beck N, Davis B B 1970 Complications of diuretic therapy: severe alkalosis and syndrome resembling inappropriate secretion of anti-diuretic hormone. Metabolism 19: 709–719
59. Dimitriou G, Greenough A, Giffin F J, Kavadia V 1996 Inhaled versus systemic steroids in chronic oxygen dependency of preterm infants. European Journal of Pediatrics 156: 51–55
60. Edwards D K 1979 Radiographic aspects of bronchopulmonary dysplasia. Journal of Pediatrics 95: 823–829
61. Edwards D K, Dyer W M, Northway W H 1977 Twelve years' experience with bronchopulmonary dysplasia. Pediatrics 59: 839–846
62. Edwards D K, Jacob J, Gluck L 1980 The immature lung: radiographic appearance, course and complications. American Journal of Radiology 135: 659–666
63. Ehrenkranz R A, Ablow R C, Warshaw J B 1979 Prevention of bronchopulmonary dysplasia with vitamin E administration during the acute stages of respiratory distress syndrome. Journal of Pediatrics 95: 873–878
64. Ehrenkranz R A, Bonta B W, Ablow R C 1978 Amelioration of bronchopulmonary dysplasia after vitamin E administration. New England Journal of Medicine 299: 564–570
65. Emery E F, Greenough A 1992 Effect of dexamethasone on blood pressure: relationship to postnatal age. European Journal of Pediatrics 151: 364–366
66. Engelhardt B, Elliott S, Hazinski T A 1986 Short-and long-term effects of furosemide on lung function in infants with bronchopulmonary dysplasia. Journal of Pediatrics 109: 1034–1039
67. Enhorning G, Shennau A, Possmaner F, Dunn M, Chen C, Million J 1985 Prevention of neonatal respiratory distress syndrome by tracheal instillation of surfactant: a randomised clinical trial. Pediatrics 76: 145–153
68. Eronen M, Pesonen E, Kurki T, Teramo K, Ylikorkala O, Hallman M 1994 Increased incidence of bronchopulmonary dysplasia after antenatal administration of indomethacin to prevent preterm labor. Journal of Pediatrics 124: 782–788
69. Escobedo M B, Gonzalez A 1986 Bronchopulmonary dysplasia in the tiny infant. Clinics in Perinatology 13: 315–326
70. Escobedo M B, Hilliard J L, Smith F et al 1982 A baboon model of bronchopulmonary dysplasia. Experimental and Molecular Pathology 37: 323–334
71. Fitzhardinge P M, Eisen A, Lejtenyi C, Metrakos K, Romsay M 1974 Sequelae of early steroid administration to the newborn infant. Pediatrics 53: 877–883
72. Fowlie P W 1996 Prophylactic indomethacin: systematic review and meta-analysis. Archives of Disease in Childhood 74: F81–F87
73. Frank L 1992 Antioxidants, nutrition and bronchopulmonary dysplasia. Clinics in Perinatology 19: 541–562
74. Fujimura M, Takeuchi T, Ando M et al 1983 Elevated immunoglobulin M levels in low birth-weight neonates with chronic respiratory insufficiency. Early Human Development 9: 27–32
75. Fujimura M, Takeuchi T, Kitajima H, Nakayama M 1989 Chorioamnionitis and serum IgM in Wilson-Mikity syndrome. Archives of Disease in Childhood 64: 1379–1383
76. Garland J S, Buck R K, Allred E N, Leviton A 1995 Hypocarbia before surfactant therapy appears to increase bronchopulmonary dysplasia risk in infants with respiratory distress syndrome. Archives of Pediatrics and Adolescent Medicine 149: 617–622
77. Gerhardt T, Hehre D, Feller R, Reifenberg L, Bancalari E 1987 Serial determination of pulmonary function in infants with chronic lung disease. Journal of Pediatrics 110: 448–456
78. Giffin F, Greenough A, Yuksel B 1995 Antiviral therapy in neonatal chronic lung disease. Early Human Development 42: 97–109
79. Gonzalez A, Sosenko I R S, Chandar J, Hummler H, Claure N, Bancalari E 1996 Influence of infection on patent ductus arteriosus and chronic lung disease in premature infants weighing 1000 g or less. Journal of Pediatrics 128: 470–478
80. Gray P H, Rogers Y 1994 Are infants with bronchopulmonary dysplasia at risk for sudden infant death syndrome? Pediatrics 93: 774–777
81. Greenough A, 1990 Personal practice—bronchopulmonary dysplasia Archives of Disease in Childhood 65: 1082–1088
82. Greenough A, Roberton N R C 1985 Morbidity and mortality in neonates ventilated for the respiratory distress syndrome. British Medical Journal 290: 597–600
83. Greenough A, Chan V, Hird M F 1992 Positive end expiratory pressure in acute and chronic neonatal respiratory distress. Archives of Disease in Childhood 67: 320–323
84. Greenough A, Emery E F, Gamsu H R 1992 Dexamethasone and hypertension in preterm infants. European Journal of Pediatrics 151: 134–135
85. Greenough A, Emery E F, Hird M F, Gamsu H R 1993 Randomised controlled trial of albumin infusion in ill preterm infants. European Journal of Pediatrics 152: 157–159
86. Greenough A, Hird M F, Gamsu H R 1991 Home oxygen therapy following neonatal intensive care. Early Human Development 26: 29–35
87. Greenough A, Maconochie I, Gamsu H R 1988 Do respiratory problems cease when preterm babies leave neonatal intensive care? (abstract). European Respiratory Journal 1: (suppl. 2): 227

88. Greenough A, Maconochie I, Yuksel B 1990 Recurrent respiratory symptoms in the first year of life following preterm delivery. Journal of Perinatal Medicine 18: 489–494
89. Greenough A, Milner A D, Roberton N R C 1995 Neonatal respiratory disorders. Edward Arnold, London, p 396
90. Groneck P, Speer C P 1995 Inflammatory mediators and bronchopulmonary dysplasia. Archives of Disease in Childhood 73: F1–F3
91. Groneck P, Goetze-Speer B, Oppermann M, Eiffert H, Speer C P 1994 Association of pulmonary inflammation and increased microvascular permeability during the development of bronchopulmonary dysplasia: a sequential analysis of inflammatory mediators in respiratory fluids of high risk preterm infants. Pediatrics 93: 712–718
92. Groneck P, Reuss D, Götze-Speer B, Speer C P 1993 Effects of dexamethasone on chemotactic activity and inflammatory mediators in tracheobronchial aspirates of preterm infants at risk for chronic lung disease. Journal of Pediatrics 122: 938–944
93. Groothuis J R, Rosenberg A A 1987 Home oxygen promotes weight gain in infants with bronchopulmonary dysplasia. American Journal of Diseases in Children 141: 992–995
94. Gunn T, Reece E R, Metrakos K, Cole E 1981 Depressed T cells following neonatal steroid treatment. Pediatrics 67: 61–67
95. Hageman J R, Adams M A, Gardner T H 1985 Pulmonary complications of hyperventilation therapy for persistent pulmonary hypertension. Critical Care Medicine 13: 1013–1014
96. Hallman M, Bry K, Hoppu K et al 1992 Inositol supplementation in premature infants with respiratory distress syndrome. New England Journal of Medicine 362: 1233–1239
97. Hallman M, Spragg R, Harrell J H, Moser K M, Gluck L 1982 Evidence of lung surfactant abnormality in respiratory failure. Journal of Clinical Investigation 70: 673–683
98. Hallman M, Merritt T A, Jarvenpaa A-L 1985 Exogenous human surfactant for treatment of severe respiratory distress syndrome: a randomized prospective clinical trial. Journal of Pediatrics 106: 963–969
99. Hallman M, Pitkanen O, Rauvala H, Merritt T A 1987 Glycolipid accumulation in lung effluent in bronchopulmonary dysplasia. Pediatric Research 21: 454A
100. Hamilton P A, Whitehead M D, Reynolds E O R 1985 Underestimation of arterial oxygen tension by transcutaneous electrode with increasing age in infants. Archives of Disease in Childhood 60: 145–153
101. Harris H 1977 Pulmonary pseudocysts in the newborn infant. Pediatrics 59: 199–202
102. Harrod J R, L'Heureux P, Wangensteen O D, Hunt C E 1974 Long term follow-up of severe respiratory distress syndrome treated with IPPB. Journal of Pediatrics 84: 277–286
103. Hazinski T A 1985 Furosemide decreases ventilation in young rabbits. Journal of Pediatrics 106: 81–85
104. HIFI Study Group 1989 High frequency oscillatory ventilation compared with conventional mechanical ventilation in the treatment of respiratory failure in preterm infants. New England Journal of Medicine 320: 88–93
105. Hodson W A, Truog W E, Mayock D E, Lyrene R, Woodrum D E 1979 Bronchopulmonary dysplasia: the need for epidemiologic studies. Journal of Pediatrics 95: 848–851
106. Hudak B B, Allen M C, Hudak M L, Loughlin G M 1989 Home oxygen therapy for chronic lung disease in extremely low birth weight infants. American Journal of Diseases of Children 143: 357–360
107. Hufnagle K G, Khan S N, Penn D, Cacciarelli A, Williams P 1982 Renal calcification: a complication of long term frusemide therapy in premature infants. Pediatrics 70: 360–363
108. Hyde I, English R E, Wilhams J A 1989 The changing pattern of chronic lung disease of prematurity. Archives of Disease in Childhood 64: 448–451
109. Israel B A, Sherman F S, Guthrie R D 1993 Hypertrophic cardiomyopathy associated with dexamethasone therapy for chronic lung disease in preterm infants. American Journal of Perinatology 10: 307–310
110. Italian Collaborative Group on Preterm Delivery 1993 Supplementation and plasma levels of vitamin A in premature newborns at risk for chronic lung disease. Developmental Pharmacology and Therapy 20: 144–151
111. Jobe A H, Mitchell B R, Harry Gunkel J 1993 Beneficial effects of the combined use of prenatal corticosteroids and postnatal surfactant on preterm infants. American Journal of Obstetrics and Gynecology 168: 508–513
112. Johnson L, Bowen F W, Abbasi S et al 1985 Relationship of prolonged pharmacologic serum levels of vitamin E to incidence of sepsis and necrotizing enterocolitis in infants with birth weight 1,500 grams or less. Pediatrics 75: 619–638
113. Jones C A, Cayabyab R G, Kwong K Y C et al 1996 Undetectable interleukin IL-10 and persistent IL-8 expression early in hyaline membrane disease: a possible developmental basis for the predisposition to chronic lung inflammation in preterm newborns. Pediatric Research 39: 966–975
114. Jones R, Wincott E, Elbourne D, Grant A 1995 Controlled trial of dexamethasone in neonatal chronic lung disease: a 3-year follow-up. Pediatrics 96: 897–906
115. Kao L C, Durand D J, McCrea R C, Birch M, Powers R J, Nickerson B G 1994 Randomized trial of long-term diuretic therapy for infants with oxygen-dependent bronchopulmonary dysplasia. Journal of Pediatrics 124: 772–781
116. Kao L C, Warburton D, Sargent C W, Platzker A C G, Keens T G 1983 Furosemide acutely decreases airway resistance in chronic bronchopulmonary dysplasia. Journal of Pediatrics 103: 624–629
117. Kao L C, Warburton D, Cheng M H, Cedeno C, Platzker A C G, Keens T G 1984 Effect of oral diuretics on pulmonary mechanics in infants with chronic bronchopulmonary dysplasia: results of a double-blind crossover sequential trial. Pediatrics 74: 37–44
118. Kao L C, Warburton D, Platzker A C G, Keens T G 1984 Effect of isoproterenol inhalation on airway resistance in chronic bronchopulmonary dysplasia. Pediatrics 73: 509–514
119. Kao L C, Durand D J, Dhillias B L, Nickerson B G 1987 Oral theophylline and diuretics improve pulmonary mechanics in infants with bronchopulmonary dysplasia. Journal of Pediatrics 111: 439–444
120. Kojima T, Sasai M, Kobayashi Y 1993 Increased soluble ICAM-1 in tracheal aspirates of infants with bronchopulmonary dysplasia. Lancet 342: 1023–1024
121. Konishi M, Fujiwara T, Naito N et al 1988 Surfactant replacement therapy in neonatal respiratory distress syndrome: a multi-centre, randomised clinical trial. Comparison of high vs low dose of surfactant TA. European Journal of Pediatrics 147: 20–25
122. Koops B L, Amban S H, Accurso F J 1984 Outpatient management and follow-up of bronchopulmonary dysplasia. Clinics in Perinatology 11: 101–122
123. Koppel R, Han R N N, Cox D, Tanswell K, Rabinovitch M 1994 Alpha-1-antitrypsin protects neonatal rats from pulmonary vascular and parenchymal effects of oxygen toxicity. Pediatric Research 36: 763–770
124. Kornhauser M S, Cullen J A, Baumgart S, McKee L J, Gross G W, Spitzer A R 1994 Risk factors for bronchopulmonary dysplasia after extracorporeal membrane oxygenation. Archives of Pediatrics and Adolescent Medicine 148: 820–825
125. Kotagal U R, Perlstein P H, Gamblian V, Donovan E F, Atherton H D 1995 Description and evaluation of a program for the early discharge of infants from an NICU. Journal of Pediatrics 127: 285–290
126. Kotecha S, Wilson L, Wangoo A, Silverman M, Shaw R J 1996 Increase in interleukin (IL)-1beta and IL-6 in BAL fluid obtained from infants with chronic lung disease of prematurity. Pediatric Research 40: 1250–1256
127. Krauss A N, Levin A R, Grossman H, Auld P A M 1970 Physiologic studies on infants with Wilson-Mikity syndrome. Journal of Pediatrics 77: 27–36
128. Krauss A N, Klain D B, Auld P A M 1975 Chronic pulmonary insufficiency of prematurity (CPIP). Pediatrics 55: 55–58
129. Kraybill E N, Runyan D K, Bose C L, Khan J H 1989 Risk factors for chronic lung disease in infants with birth weights of 751 to 1000 grams. Journal of Pediatrics 115: 115–120
130. Kurzner S I, Garg M, Bautista D B, Sargent C W, Bowmann C M, Keens T G 1988 Growth failure in bronchopulmonary dysplasia: elevated metabolic rates and pulmonary mechanics. Journal of Pediatrics 112: 73–80
131. Kwong M, Egan E, Notter R, Shapiro D 1985 Double-blind clinical trial of calf lung surfactant extract for the prevention of hyaline membrane disease in extremely premature infants. Pediatrics 76: 585–592
132. LaForce W R, Brudno D S 1993 Controlled trial of beclomethasone dipropionate by nebulization in oxygen- and ventilator-dependent infants. Journal of Pediatrics 122: 285–288

133. Lamarre A, Linsao L, Reilly B J, Swyer P R. Levison H 1973 Residual pulmonary abnormalities in survivors of idiopathic respiratory distress syndrome. American Review of Respiratory Disease 108: 56–61
134. Linder N, Kuint J, German B, Lubin D, Loewenthal R 1995 Hypertrophy of the tongue associated with inhaled corticosteroid therapy in premature infants. Journal of Pediatrics 127: 651–653
135. Lindroth M, Svenningsen N W, Ahlstrom H, Jonson B 1980 Evaluation of mechanical ventilation in newborn infants. II. Pulmonary and neurodevelopmental sequelae in relation to original diagnosis. Acta Paediatrica Scandinavica 69: 151–158
136. Lonnqvist P A, Jonsson B, Winberg P, Frostell C G 1995 Inhaled nitric oxide in infants with developing or established chronic lung disease. Acta Paediatrica 84;1188–1192
137. Lorenz J M, Kleinman LI, Kotagal UR, Reller MD 1982 Water balance in very low birthweight infants: relationship to water and sodium intake and effect on outcome. Journal of Pediatrics 101: 423–432
138. McCann E M, Lewis K, Deming D D, Donovan M J, Brady J P 1985 Controlled trial of furosemide therapy in infants with chronic lung disease. Journal of Pediatrics 106: 957–962
139. McColm J R, McIntosh N 1994 Interleukin 8 in bronchoalveolar lavage samples as predictor of chronic lung disease in premature infants. Lancet 343: 729 (letter)
140. McCubbin M, Frey E E, Wagener J S, Tribby R, Smith W L 1989 Large airway collapse in bronchopulmonary dysplasia. Journal of Pediatrics 114: 304–307
141. Maconochie I, Greenough A, Yuksel B, Page A, Karani J 1991 A chest radiograph scoring system to predict chronic oxygen dependency in low birth weight infants. Early Human Development 26: 37–43
142. Mammel M C, Green T P, Johnson D E, Thompson T R 1983 Controlled trial of dexamethasone therapy in infants with bronchopulmonary dysplasia. Lancet i: 1356–1358
143. Markestad T, Fitzhardinge P M 1981 Growth and development in children recovering from bronchopulmonary dysplasia. Journal of Pediatrics 98: 597–602
144. Mayes L, Perkett E, Stahlman M T 1983 Severe bronchopulmonary dysplasia: a retrospective review. Acta Paediatrica Scandinavica 72: 225–229
145. Meisels S J, Plunkett J W, Roloff D W, Pasick P L, Stiefel G S 1986 Growth and development of preterm infants wth respiratory distress syndrome and bronchopulmonary dysplasia. Pediatrics 77: 345–352
146. Meissner H C, Welliver R C, Chartrand S A, Fulton D R, Rodriguez W J A, Groothuis J R 1996 Prevention of respiratory syncytial virus infection in high risk infants: consensus opinion on the role of immunoprophylaxis with respiratory syncytial virus hyperimmune globulin. Pediatric Infectious Diseases Journal 15: 1059–1068
147. Merritt T A, Cochrane C G, Holcomb K et al 1983 Elastase and alpha-1-proteinase inhibitor activity in tracheal aspirates during respiratory distress syndrome. Journal of Clinical Investigation 72: 656–666
148. Merritt T A, Hallman M, Bloom B 1986 Prophylactic human surfactant: a randomised bicentre study demonstrating a reduction in mortality and bronchopulmonary dysplasia from respiratory distress syndrome in very preterm infants. New England Journal of Medicine 315: 785–790
149. Merritt T A, Hallman M, Holcomb K 1986 Human surfactant treatment of severe respiratory distress: pulmonary effluent indicators of lung inflammation. Journal of Pediatrics 108: 741–748
150. Miller R W, Woo P, Kellman R K, Slagle TS 1987 Tracheobronchial abnormalities in infants with bronchopulmonary dysplasia. Journal of Pediatrics 111: 779–782
151. Mirro R, Armstead W, Leffler C 1990 Increased airway leukotriene levels in infants with severe bronchopulmonary dysplasia. American Journal of Diseases of Children 144: 160–161
152. Morley C J, Greenough A, Gore S M 1988 Randomised trial of artificial surfactant (ALEC) given at birth to babies between 23 and 34 weeks' gestation. Early Human Development 17: 41–54
153. Morray J P, Fox W W, Kettrick R G, Downes J J 1982 Improvement in lung mechanics as a function of age in the infant with severe bronchopulmonary dysplasia. Pediatric Research 16: 290–294
154. Motoyama E K, Fort M D, Klesh K W, Mutich R L, Guthrie R D 1987 Early onset of airway reactivity in premature infants with bronchopulmonary dysplasia. American Review of Respiratory Disease 136: 50–57
155. Moyer W J 1950 Vitamin E levels in term and premature newborn infants. Pediatrics 6: 893–896
156. Moylan F M B, Walker A M, Kramer S S, Todres I D, Shannon D C 1978 Alveolar rupture as an independent predictor of bronchopulmonary dysplasia. Critical Care Medicine 6: 10–13
157. Murch S H, Costeloe K, Klein N J et al 1996 Mucosal tumour necrosis factor-alpha production and extensive disruption of sulfated glycosaminoglycans begins within hours of birth in neonatal respiratory distress syndrome. Pediatric Research 40: 484–489
158. Murch S H, Costeloe K, Klein N J, McDonald T T 1996 Early production of macrophage inflammatory protein-1-alpha occurs in respiratory distress syndrome and is associated with poor outcome. Pediatric Research 40: 490–497
159. Murciano D, Aubier M, Lecocguic Y, Pariente R 1984 Effects of theophylline on diaphragmatic strength and fatigue in patients with chronic obstructive pulmonary disease. New England Journal of Medicine 311: 349–353
160. Najak Z D, Harris E M, Lazzara A, Pruitt A W 1983 Pulmonary effects of furosemide in preterm infants with lung disease. Journal of Pediatrics 102: 758–763
161. Ng P C, Thomson M A, Dear P R F 1990 Dexamethasone and infection in preterm babies: a controlled study. Archives of Disease in Childhood 65: 54–58
162. Nickerson B G, Taussig L M 1980 Family history of asthma in infants with bronchopulmonary dysplasia. Pediatrics 65: 1140–1144
163. Noble-Jamieson C M, Regev R, Silverman M 1989 Dexamethasone in neonatal chronic lung disease: pulmonary effects and intracranial complications. European Journal of Pediatrics 148: 365–367
164. Northway W H Jr 1979 Observations on bronchopulmonary dysplasia. Journal of Pediatrics 95: 815–818
165. Northway W H Jr, Rosan R C, Porter D Y 1967 Pulmonary disease following respirator therapy of hyaline membrane disease: bronchopulmonary dysplasia. New England Journal of Medicine 276: 357–368
166. Obladen M 1988 Alterations in surfactant composition. In: Merrit A, Northway W H, Boynton B R (eds) Bronchopulmonary dysplasia. Blackwell Scientific Publications, Boston, pp 131–141
167. O'Brodovich H M, Mellins R B 1985 Bronchopulmonary dysplasia. American Review of Respiratory Disease 132: 694–709
168. Ogawa Y, Miyasaka K, Kawano T et al 1993 A multicentre randomized trial of high frequency oscillatory ventilation as compared with conventional mechanical ventilation in preterm infants with respiratory failure. Early Human Development 32: 1–10
169. Oppenheim C, Marmou-Mani T, Sayegh N, de Blic J, Scheinmann P, Lallemand D 1994 Bronchopulmonary dysplasia: value of CT in identifying pulmonary sequelae. American Journal of Roentgenology 163: 169–172
170. Pandit P B, Dunn M S, Kelly E N, Perlman M 1995 Surfactant replacement in neonates with early chronic lung disease. Pediatrics 95: 851–854
171. Panitch H B, Allen J L, Alpert B E, Schidlow D V 1994 Effects of CPAP on lung mechanics in infants with acquired tracheobronchomalacia. American Journal of Respiratory and Critical Care Medicine 150: 1341–1346
172. Panitch H B, Downes J J, Kennedy J S et al 1996 Guidelines for home care of children with chronic respiratory insufficiency. Pediatric Pulmonology 21: 52–56
173. Parat S, Moriette G, Delaperche M-F, Escourrou P, Denjean A, Gaultier C 1995 Long term pulmonary functional outcome of bronchopulmonary dysplasia and premature birth. Pediatric Pulmonology 20: 289–296
174. Parker R A, Lindstrom D P, Cotton R B 1992 Improved survival accounts for most, but not all, of the increase in bronchopulmonary dysplasia. Pediatrics 90: 663–668
175. Pearson E, Bose C, Snidow T et al 1992 Trial of vitamin A supplementation in very low birthweight infants at risk for bronchopulmonary dysplasia. Journal of Pediatrics 121: 420–427
176. Pereira G R, Baumgart S, Bennett M J et al 1994 Use of high fat formula for premature infants with bronchopulmonary dysplasia. Metabolic, pulmonary and nutritional studies. Journal of Pediatrics 124: 605–611
177. Perlman J M, Moore V, Siegel M J, Dawson J 1986 Is chloride depletion an important contributing cause of death in infants with bronchopulmonary dysplasia? Pediatrics 77: 212–216

178. Pinney M A, Cotton E K 1976 Home management of bronchopulmonary dysplasia. Pediatrics 58: 856–859
179. Poets C F, Sens B 1996 Changes in intubation rates and outcome of very low birth weight infants: a population-based study. Pediatrics 98: 24–27
180. Poets C F, Samuels M P, Southall D P 1993 Hypoxaemia in infants with bronchopulmonary dysplasia. Pediatrics 92: 186–187
181. Pomerance J J, Puri A P 1980 Treatment of neonatal bronchopulmonary dysplasia with steroids. Pediatric Research 14: 649A
182. Prasertsom W, Phillipos E Z, van Aerde J E, Robertson M 1996 Pulmonary vascular resistance during lipid infusion in neonates. Archives of Disease in Childhood 74: F95–F98
183. Radford P J, Stillwell P C, Blue B, Hertel G 1995 Aspiration complicating bronchopulmonary dysplasia. Chest 107: 185–188
184. Ramanathan R, Durand M, Larrazabal C 1987 Pulse oximetry in very low birth weight infants with acute and chronic lung disease. Pediatrics 79: 612–617
185. Rastogi A, Akintorin S M, Bez M L, Morales P, Pildes R S 1996 A controlled trial of dexamethasone to prevent bronchopulmonary dysplasia in surfactant-treated infants. Pediatrics 98: 204–210
186. Rauvala H, Hallman M 1984 Glycolipid accumulation in bronchoalveolar space in adult respiratory distress syndrome. Journal of Lipid Research 25: 1257–1262
187. Regev R, DeVries L S, Noble-Jamieson C M, Silverman M 1987 Dexamethasone and increased intracranial echogenicity. Lancet i: 632–633
188. Reimers K J, Carlson S J, Lombard K A 1992 Nutritional management of infants with bronchopulmonary dysplasia. Nutrition in Clinical Practice 7: 127–132
189. Rennie J M, Baker B, Lucas A 1989 Does dexamethasone suppress the ACTH response in preterm babies? Archives of Disease in Childhood 64: 612–613
190. Reynolds E O R, Taghizadeh A 1974 Improved prognosis of infants mechanically ventilated for hyaline membrane disease. Archives of Disease in Childhood 49: 505–515
191. Rhodes P G, Graves G R, Patel D M, Campbell S B, Blumenthal B I 1983 Minimizing pneumothorax and BPD in ventilated infants with hyaline membrane disease. Journal of Pediatrics 103: 634–637
192. Rhodes P G, Hall R T, Leonidas J C 1975 Chronic pulmonary disease in neonates with assisted ventilation. Pediatrics 55: 788–795
193. Robertson C M T, Etches P C, Goldson E, Kyle J M 1992 Eight-year school performance, neurodevelopmental and growth outcome of neonates with bronchopulmonary dysplasia: a comparative study. Pediatrics 89: 365–372
194. Rome E S, Stork E K, Carlo W A, Martin R J 1984 Limitations of transcutaneous PO_2 and PCO_2 monitoring in infants with bronchopulmonary dysplasia. Pediatrics 74: 217–220
195. Rooklin A R, Moomjiian A S, Fox W W 1979. Theophylline therapy in bronchopulmonary dysplasia. Journal of Pediatrics 95: 882–884
196. Rosan R C 1975 Hyaline membrane disease and a related spectrum of neonatal pneumopathies. Perspectives in Pediatric Pathology 2: 15–60
197. Rosenfeld W, Evans H, Jhaveri R 1982 Safety and plasma concentrations of bovine superoxide dismutase administered to human premature infants. Developmental Pharmacology and Therapeutics 5: 151–161
198. Rosenfeld W, Evans H, Concepcion L, Jhaveri R, Schaeffer M, Friedman A 1984 Prevention of bronchopulmonary dysplasia by administration of bovine superoxide dismutase in preterm infants with respiratory distress syndrome. Journal of Pediatrics 105: 781–785
199. Rosenfeld W, Sadhev S, Zabalera I, Jhaveri R 1986 Measurement of superoxide dismutase in neonates utilising polyclonal antibodies. Pediatric Research 20: 209A
200. Russell G A B and Cooke R W I 1995 Randomized controlled trial of allopurinol prophylaxis in very preterm infants. Archives of Disease in Childhood 73: F27–F31
201. Ryan S, Congdon P J, Horsman A, James J R, Truscott J, Arthur R 1987 Bone mineral content in bronchopulmonary dysplasia. Archives of Disease in Childhood 62: 889–894
202. Rybak L P 1982 Pathophysiology of frusemide toxicity. Journal of Otolaryngology 11: 127–135
203. Saldanha R L, Cepeda E E, Poland R L 1982 The effect of vitamin E prophylaxis on the incidence and severity of bronchopulmonary dysplasia. Journal of Pediatrics 101: 89–93
204. Samuels M P, Southall D P 1989 Negative extrathoracic pressure in treatment of respiratory failure in infants and young children. British Medical Journal 299: 1253–1257
205. Sanders R J, Cox C, Phelps D L, Sinkin R A 1994 Two doses of early intravenous dexamethasone for the prevention of bronchopulmonary dysplasia in babies with respiratory distress syndrome. Pediatric Research 36: 122–128
206. Santuz P, Baraldi E, Zaramella P, Filippone M, Zacchello F 1995 Factors limiting exercise performance in long term survivors of bronchopulmonary dysplasia. American Journal of Respiratory and Critical Care Medicine 152: 1284–1289
207. Saunders R A, Milner A D, Hopkin I E 1978 Longitudinal studies of infants with the Wilson–Mikity syndrome. Biology of the Neonate 33: 90–99
208. Sauve R S, Singhal N 1985 long-term morbidity in infants with bronchopulmonary dysplasia. Pediatrics 76: 725–733
209. Savage M O, Wilkinson A R, Baum J D, Roberton N R C 1975 Frusemide in respiratory distress syndrome. Archives of Disease in Childhood 50: 709–713
210. Sawyer M H, Edwards D K, Spector S A 1987 Cytomegalovirus infection and bronchopulmonary dysplasia in premature infants. American Journal of Diseases of Children 141: 303–305
211. Schreiner M S, Donar M E, Kettrick R G 1987 Pediatric home mechanical ventilation. Pediatric Clinics of North America 34: 47–60
212. Sekar K C, Duke J C 1991 Sleep apnea and hypoxemia in recently weaned premature infants with and without bronchopulmonary dysplasia. Pediatric Pulmonology 10: 112–116
213. Shankaran S, Szego E, Eizert D, Siegel P 1984 Severe bronchopulmonary dysplasia: predictors of survival and outcome. Chest 86: 607–610
214. Shapiro D, Notter R, Movin F 1985 Double-blind randomized trial of a calf lung surfactant extract administered at birth to very premature infants for prevention of respiratory distress syndrome. Pediatrics 76: 593–599
215. Shaw N J, Ruggins N, Cooke R W I 1993 Infants with chronic lung disease: predictors of mortality at Day 28. Journal of Perinatology 13: 464–467
216. Shenai J P, Chytil F, Stahlman M T 1985 Vitamin A status of neonates with bronchopulmonary dysplasia. Pediatric Research 19: 185–188
217. Shenai J P, Kennedy K A, Chytil F, Stahlman M T 1987 Clinical trial of vitamin A supplementation in infants susceptible to bronchopulmonary dysplasia. Journal of Pediatrics 111: 269–277
218. Shennan A T, Dunn M S, Ohlsson A, Lennox K, Hoskins E M 1988 Abnormal pulmonary outcomes in premature infants: prediction from oxygen requirement in the neonatal period. Pediatrics 82: 527–532
219. Shinwell E S, Karphis M, Zmora E et al 1996 Failure of early postnatal dexamethasone to prevent chronic lung disease in infants with respiratory distress syndrome. Archives of Disease in Childhood 74: F33–F37
220. Short A, Cooke R W I 1990 The incidence of renal calcification in preterm infants. Archives of Disease in Childhood 66: 412–417
221. Sickles E A, Gooding C A 1976 Asymmetric lung involvement in bronchopulmonary dysplasia. Radiology 118: 379–383
222. Simon L 1980 Protection against toxic effect of sustained hyperoxia on lung macrophages by superoxide dismutase. Clinical Research 28: 432A
223. Singer L, Martin R J, Hawkins S W, Benson-Szekely L J, Yamashita T S, Carlo W A 1992 Oxygen desaturation complicates feeding in infants with bronchopulmonary dysplasia after discharge. Pediatrics 90: 380–384
224. Smyth J A, Tabachnik E, Duncan W J, Reilly B J, Levison H 1981 Pulmonary function and bronchial hyperreactivity in long-term survivors of bronchopulmonary dysplasia. Pediatrics 68: 336–340
225. Sobel D B, Carroll A 1994 Postsurfactant slump: early prediction of neonatal chronic lung disease? Journal of Perinatology 14: 268–274
226. Solimano A J, Smyth J A, Mann T K, Albersheim S G, Lockitch G 1986 Pulse oximetry advantages in infants with bronchopulmonary dysplasia. Pediatrics 78: 844–849
227. Sosenko I R S, Frank L 1991 Oxidants and antioxidants. In: Cherniak N, Mellins R B (eds) Basic mechanisms of paediatric respiratory disease: cellular and integrative. BC Decker, Philadelphia, p 315
228. Sosenko I R S, Rodriguez-Pierce M, Bancalari E 1993 Effects of early initiation of intravenous lipid administration on the incidence and

severity of chronic lung disease in premature infants. Journal of Pediatrics 123: 975–982
229. Spear M L, Reeves G, Pearlman S A 1993 Diabetic ketoacidosis after steroid administration for bronchopulmonary dysplasia: a case report. Journal of Perinatology 13: 232–234
230. Speer C P, Ruess D, Harms K, Herting E, Gefeller O 1993 Neutrophil elastase and acute pulmonary damage in neonates with severe respiratory distress syndrome. Pediatrics 91: 794–799
231. Spitzer A R, Fox W W, Delivoria-Papadopoulos M 1981 Maximum diuresis—a factor in predicting recovery from respiratory distress syndrome and the development of bronchopulmonary dysplasia. Journal of Pediatrics 98: 476–479
232. Stahlman M T, Cheatham W, Gray M E 1979 The role of air dissection in bronchopulmonary dysplasia. Journal of Pediatrics 95: 878–885
233. Stahlman M, Hedvall G, Lindstrom D, Snell J 1982 Role of hyaline membrane disease in production of later childhood lung abnormalities. Pediatrics 69: 572–576
234. Steichen J J, Gratton T L, Tsang R C 1980 Osteopenia of prematurity: the cause and possible treatment. Journal of Pediatrics 96: 528–534
235. Stenmark K R, Eyzaguippe M, Remigio L, Secombe J, Henson P M 1985 Recovery of platelet activating factor and leukotrienes from infants with severe bronchopulmonary dysplasia: Clinical improvement with cromolyn treatment. American Review of Respiratory Disease 13: 236A
236. Stenmark K R, Eyzaguippe M, Westcott J Y, Henson P M, Murphy R C 1987 Potential role of eicosanoids and PAF in the pathophysiology of bronchopulmonary dysplasia. American Review of Respiratory Disease 136: 770–772
237. Stocker J T 1986 Pathologic features of long-standing 'healed' bronchopulmonary dysplasia: a study of 28 3- to 40-month-old infants. Human Pathology 17: 943–961
238. Stocker J T, Madewell J E 1977 Persistent interstitial pulmonary emphysema: another complication of the respiratory distress syndrome. Pediatrics 59: 847–857
239. Stocks J, Godfrey S, Reynolds E O R 1978 Airway resistance in infants after various treatments for hyaline membrane disease: Special emphasis on prolonged high levels of inspired oxygen. Pediatrics 61: 178–183
240. Strayer D S, Merritt T A, Lwebuga-Mukasa J, Hallman M 1986 Surfactant-anti-surfactant immune complexes in neonatal respiratory distress syndrome. American Journal of Pathology 122: 353–362
241. Strayer D S, Merritt T A, Hallman M 1995 Levels of SpA-anti-SpA immune complexes in neonatal respiratory distress syndrome correlated with subsequent development of bronchopulmonary dysplasia. Acta Paediatrica 84: 128–131
242. Taghizadeh A, Reynolds E O R 1976 Pathogenesis of bronchopulmonary dysplasia following hyaline membrane disease. American Journal of Pathology 82: 241–254
243. Tammela O K T 1995 Appropriate fluid regimens to prevent bronchopulmonary dysplasia. European Journal of Pediatrics 154 (Suppl 3): S15–S18
244. Tammela O K T, Lanning F P, Koivisto M E 1992 The relationship of fluid restriction during the first month of life to the occurrence and severity of bronchopulmonary dysplasia in low birthweight infants: a 1-year radiological follow-up. European Journal of Pediatrics 151: 367–371
245. Taylor D W 1956 The effects of vitamin E and of methylene blue on the manifestations of oxygen poisoning in the rat. Journal of Physiology 131: 200–207
246. Teague W G, Pian M S, Heldt G P, Tooley W H 1988 An acute reduction in the fraction of inspired oxygen increases airway constriction in infants with chronic lung disease. American Review of Respiratory Disease 137: 861–865
247. Toce S S, Farrell P M, Leavitt L A, Samuels D P, Edwards D K 1984 Clinical and roentgenographic scoring systems for assessing bronchopulmonary dysplasia. American Journal of Diseases of Children 138: 581–585
248. Tooley W H 1979 Epidemiology of bronchopulmonary dysplasia. Journal of Pediatrics 95: 851–855
249. van Marter L J, Leviton A, Allred E N, Pagano M, Kuban K C K 1990 Hydration during the first days of life and the risk of bronchopulmonary dysplasia in low birth weight infants. Journal of Pediatrics 116: 942–949
250. Vrlenich L A, Bozynski M E A, Shyr Y, Schork A, Roloff D W, McCormick M C 1995 The effect of bronchopulmonary dysplasia on growth at school age. Pediatrics 95: 855–859
251. Walther F J, Nunez F L, Remedios D-C, Hill K E 1993 Mitigation of pulmonary oxygen toxicity in rats by intratracheal instillation of polyethylene glycol-conjugated antioxidant enzymes. Pediatric Research 33: 332–335
252. Wang E E L, Cassell G H, Sanchez P J, Regan J A, Payne N R, Liu P P 1993 *Ureaplasma urealyticum* and chronic lung disease of prematurity: critical appraisal of the literature on causation. Clinical Infectious Diseases 17: S112–S116
253. Watterberg K L, Scott S M 1995 Evidence of early adrenal insufficiency in babies who develop bronchopulmonary dysplasia. Pediatrics 95: 120–125
254. Watterberg K L, Carmichael D F, Gerdes J S, Werner S, Backstrom C, Murphy S 1994 Secretory leukocyte protease inhibitor and lung inflammation in developing bronchopulmonary dysplasia. Journal of Pediatrics 125: 264–269
255. Watterberg KL, Murphy S, and the Neonatal Cromolyn Study Group 1993 Failure of cromolyn sodium to reduce the incidence of bronchopulmonary dysplasia: a pilot study. Pediatrics 91: 803–806
256. Wauer R R, Schmatisch G, Bohne B et al 1992 Randomized double blind trial of ambroxol for the treatment of respiratory distress syndrome. European Journal of Pediatrics 151: 357–363
257. Weinstein M R, Petters M E, Sadek M, Palta M for the newborn lung project 1994 A new radiographic scoring system for bronchopulmonary dysplasia. Pediatric Pulmonology 18: 284–289
258. Werthammer J, Brown E R, Neff R K, Taeusch H W 1982 Sudden infant death syndrome in infants with bronchopulmonary dysplasia Pediatrics 69: 301–304
259. Wheater M, Rennie J M 1994 Poor prognosis after prolonged ventilation for bronchopulmonary dysplasia. Archives of Disease in Childhood 71: F210–F211
260. Wilkie R A, Bryan M H 1987 Effect of bronchodilators on airway resistance in ventilator-dependent neonates with chronic lung disease. Journal of Pediatrics 111: 278–282
261. Wilson M G, Mikity V G 1960 A new form of respiratory disease in premature infants. American Journal of Diseases of Children 99: 489–499
262. Wolfson M R, Bhutani V K, Shaffer T H, Bowen F W J 1984 Mechanics and energetics of breathing helium in infants with bronchopulmonary dysplasia. Journal of Pediatrics 104: 752–757
263. Wong Y C, Beardsmore C S, Silverman M 1982 Pulmonary sequelae of neonatal respiratory distress in very low birthweight infants: clinical and physiological study. Archives of Disease in Childhood 57: 418–424
264. Wung J T, Koons A H, Driscoll J M, James L S 1979 Changing incidence of bronchopulmonary dysplasia. Journal of Pediatrics 95: 845–847
265. Yeh T F, McClenan D A, Ajayi O A, Pildes R S 1989 Metabolic and energy balance in infants with bronchopulmonary dysplasia. Journal of Pediatrics 114: 448–451
266. Yeh T F, Torre, J A, Rastogi A, Anyebuno M A, Pildes R S 1990 Early postnatal dexamethasone therapy in premature infants with severe respiratory distress syndrome: a double blind controlled study. Journal of Pediatrics 117: 273–282
267. Yoshioka T, Sugive A, Shimaola T 1979 Superoxide dismutase activity in the maternal and cord blood. Biology of the Neonate 36: 173–180
268. Yu V Y H, Hollingsworth E 1979 Respiratory failure in infants weighing 1000 g or less at birth. Australian Paediatric Journal 15: 152–159
269. Yu V Y H, Orgill A A, Lim S B, Bajuk B, Astbury J 1983 Bronchopulmonary dysplasia in very low birthweight infants. Australian Paediatric Journal 19: 233–236
270. Yu V Y H, Orgill A A, Lim S B, Bajuk B, Astbury J 1983 Growth development of very low birthweight infants recovering from bronchopulmonary dysplasia. Archives of Disease in Childhood 58: 791–794
271. Yuksel B, Greenough A 1991 Ipratropium bromide in symptomatic preterm infants. European Journal of Pediatrics 150: 854–857
272. Yuksel B, Greenough A 1992 Acute deteriorations in neonatal chronic lung disease. European Journal of Pediatrics 151: 697–700
273. Yuksel B, Greenough A 1992 Neonatal respiratory support and lung function abnormalities at follow-up. Respiratory Medicine 86: 97–100

274. Yuksel B, Greenough A, Maconochie I 1990 Effective bronchodilator therapy by a simple spacer device for wheezy premature infants in the first two years of life. Archives of Disease in Childhood 65: 782–785
275. Yuksel B, Greenough A, Karani J, Page A 1991 Chest radiograph scoring system for use in preterm infants. British Journal of Radiology 64: 1015–1018
276. Yuksel B, Greenough A, Green S 1991 Paradoxical response to nebulised ipratropium bromide in asymptomatic preterm infants. Respiratory Medicine 185: 189–194
277. Yuksel B, Greenough A, Green S 1991 Lung function abnormalities at six months of age following neonatal intensive care. Archives of Disease in Childhood 66: 472–476
278. Zimmerman J J 1995 Bronchoalveolar inflammatory pathophysiology of bronchopulmonary dysplasia. Clinics in Perinatology 22: 429–456

Part 4

Apnoea and bradycardia

A. D. Milner

Apnoea is one of the commonest problems encountered on the neonatal intensive care unit. It is difficult to quote a definitive prevalence of apnoeic attacks, as the definition used varies considerably from study to study, ranging from 2 to 60 seconds of absence of breathing. Using a definition of 20 seconds, Henderson-Smart[24] found that apnoeic attacks occurred in 78% of infants born at 26–27 weeks' gestation, 75% at 28–29 weeks, 54% at 30–31 weeks, 14% at 32–33 weeks and 7% at 34–35 weeks.

The physiology of the control of breathing is considered in detail elsewhere (Part 1 of this Chapter). Briefly, the control of breathing in the preterm infant differs from that in the term infant in a number of important ways. The response to a hypoxic mixture, e.g. 15% oxygen – probably a central effect – is strikingly different from the sustained stimulation seen in adults: both the fetus and the very low-birthweight infant have only a suppression of ventilation in response to hypoxia.[2]

The preterm infant also has a reduced ventilatory response to carbon dioxide which is related to gestational age.[34] Measurements of the ventilatory response to added respiratory dead space found that at 24–26 weeks' gestation the infants only made 70% of the appropriate response, but that total compensation occurred by 36 weeks.[74] There was no evidence of enhanced postnatal development; i.e. the maturation was purely related to postconceptional age.

PATHOPHYSIOLOGY OF APNOEA

Physiological studies have shown that apnoea can be divided into three types. The first, obstructive apnoea, arises typically in situations where the upper airway can become totally occluded while the baby continues to make regular, and ever-increasing, respiratory efforts in an attempt to overcome the obstruction. This is a frequent occurrence in babies born with the Pierre–Robin syndrome (p. 768), in which the tongue, mounted on a hypoplastic mandible, can fall back through the palatal defect to cause airflow obstruction. Obstructive apnoea may also occur in Down syndrome. It is also more common in infants with GMH/IVH and later abnormal neurological development.[10] Various studies in preterm infants have shown a very constant occurrence of obstructive apnoea of between 6 and 12% of total apnoeas.[15,16,75]

The second type is central apnoea, in which both airflow and respiratory effort cease. Apnoea then occurs at end expiration. Usually during central apnoea cardiac pulsation is transmitted up the airway and can be detected via a sensitive pressure transducer connected to a face mask, indicating the patency of the airway.[44] However, this cardiac pulsation is lost in some apparently central apnoeas, implying airway closure.[75]

The possibility that preterm infants with central apnoea have a central disturbance in the regulation of breathing and response to carbon dioxide is appealing. Preterm infants have a flatter response slope to carbon dioxide than term infants, but this improves with both increasing gestational and postnatal age.[57] This effect appears to be centrally mediated.[46] At a given gestational age, infants with apnoeic attacks also appear to have a flatter response to carbon dioxide than those without,[18,21,34] and the response seems to improve as apnoeic attacks resolve.[23] This theory is supported by the fact that preterm infants with apnoeic attacks show prolonged brain-stem conduction times compared to controls.[25] The more preterm infants often also show the fetal response to hypoxia, and become apnoeic.

Sometimes the attacks of apnoea occur repeatedly, mimicking periodic respiration. In these preterm infants the apnoea is related to oscillations in ventilatory drive, with apnoea occurring when there are wide variations in amplitude of breathing and long cycle-time breathing patterns.[78] In this situation it would appear that it is an exaggeration of the instability of respiratory control rather insensitivity that is responsible.

The third type of apnoea is described as 'mixed'. Superficially it resembles central apnoea initially, with cessation of respiration usually – but not always – at end expiration.[44] However, the baby then makes intermittent respiratory efforts without achieving any respiratory exchange, indicating that the airway is obstructed. Butcher-Puech et al[10] showed that the proportion of mixed apnoea was 9% at apnoea durations of 10–14 seconds, which increased to 60% in apnoeas of greater than 20 seconds. Upton et al[75] found that all apnoea persisting for more than 20 seconds fell into this category. This would support the idea of progressive airway closure, with initially central episodes becoming mixed owing to collapse of the soft tissues of the pharynx as apnoea continues. This has been demonstrated to be the commonest site of obstruction in mixed and obstructive apnoea,[41] and appears to be more common during spontaneous neck flexion.[68] Laryngeal closure has also been demonstrated by direct upper airways endoscopy during apnoeic attacks in preterm infants.[59]

During these observations it was noted that pooling of secretions in the arytenoid notch sometimes stimulated closure of the aryepiglottic folds, and that this was followed by a period of mixed apnoea. It is possible that the apnoea is then caused by the intercostal phrenic inhibitory reflex, i.e. the respiratory effort against a closed airway produces chest wall distortion.

However, central control is not the only important aetiological factor: upper airways reflexes may also be important in the onset of apnoea. Instillation of water into the larynx of fetal sheep has been shown to cause prolonged apnoea associated with swallowing.[63] Such a laryngeal chemoreflex has also been noted in a proportion of preterm infants with apnoeic attacks.[52] This reflex is mediated by low osmolality and does not occur with normal saline. However, apnoea can occur with upper airway protective reflexes, which may be induced by the instillation of saline.[55] This introduces the intriguing possibility that upper airway secretions may act as an endogenous stimulus to produce reflex apnoea. Regurgitation of gastric contents is also known to induce apnoea,[42] although the majority of apnoeic episodes are not associated with reflux. Newell et al,[50] however, did show that a number of infants with apnoea had severe gastro-oesophageal reflux and responded to antireflux measures rather than conventional treatment with methylxanthines.

It is common for apnoeic episodes to become more problematical once feeding has commenced. Rosen et al[58] demonstrated severe hypoxaemia and apnoeic attacks during oral feeds in a group of preterm infants. They postulated that pharyngeal incoordination was responsible, as the problem disappeared as the babies matured. Gastro-oesophageal reflux was excluded as a cause of these episodes. Anecdotally, nasogastric feeding may also precipitate an increase in apnoea frequency. Gastro-oesophageal reflux may be the mechanism by which this occurs.[40] It is also well documented that enteral feeding has adverse effects on PaO_2[81] and on breathing patterns in sick preterm infants, although not on lung mechanics.[82]

The effect of sleep state on the frequency of apnoeic attacks is confused by the fact that the periodic breathing pattern commonly seen in active sleep contains many short apnoeic episodes of no significance. Additionally, two studies looking at this question and using an identical definition of an apnoeic attack have given directly contradictory results.[20,33] Knill et al[31] did suggest that ribcage distortion in active sleep results in a reflex which may inhibit inspiration and result in a predisposition to apnoeic attacks in this sleep state. Davi et al,[13] however, showed that such ribcage distortion is common to all preterm infants, independent of sleep state. Although sleep state affects the periodicity of respiration, on balance it appears to have no major effect on the occurrence of significant apnoeic attacks. The supine position is associated with an increased incidence of apnoea.[35]

OTHER AETIOLOGICAL FACTORS

Apnoea of prematurity is associated with a number of other aetiological factors. Rising environmental temperature is well known to increase apnoea frequency,[54] and infants at risk should be nursed in a thermoneutral environment. Anaemia is often the precipitating factor in the onset of apnoea in the previously well, growing, preterm infant. This is presumably secondary to tissue hypoxia, and may respond to blood transfusion.[30,56] Minor surgery, particularly hernia repair, is now commonly required while preterm infants are still relatively immature. General anaesthesia may increase the incidence of apnoea,[36] particularly if there is associated anaemia[80] and all preterm and ex-preterm infants undergoing surgery, even minor procedures, require postoperative monitoring.[12] Other risk factors significantly associated with apnoea of prematurity are previous respiratory distress syndrome and mechanical ventilation, patency of the ductus arteriosus, and CLD.[70]

An important distinction should be made, however, between so-called 'primary' apnoea or apnoea of prematurity and apnoea secondary to other disorders. Hypoxia, previous asphyxia, hypoglycaemia, hypocalcaemia, GMH/IVH, maternal drug abuse, and septicaemia and other infections may all cause apnoea, even in mature infants. Convulsions may also present as apparent apnoeic episodes.[49]

BRADYCARDIA

Bradycardia commonly accompanies apnoea, although its definition has also been variable: usually less than 80–100 beats per minute, but occasionally defined as a percentage drop below baseline. Bradycardia has generally

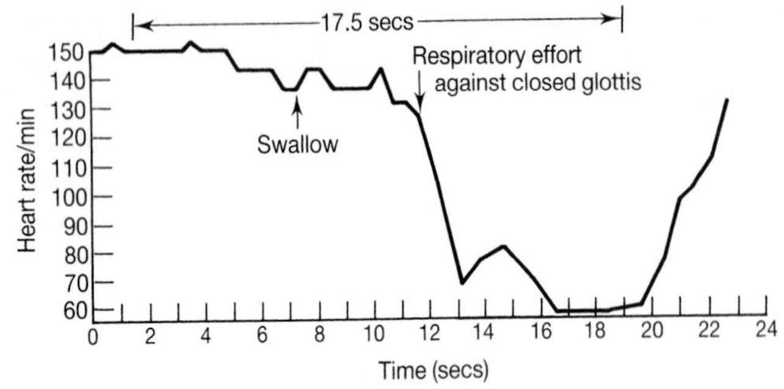

Fig. 29.88 Heart rate changes during and after a 17.5-second apnoeic episode. The heart rate falls over 2 seconds when the baby makes respiratory efforts against a closed airway.

been considered to occur with prolonged apnoea as a direct result of hypoxia. Recent studies have shown that this is not so. Deuel[14] noted that bradycardia could occur at any point during apnoea, and was commonly associated with very short apnoeas. Vyas et al[77] confirmed that bradycardia often occurred within 10 seconds of apnoea, and noted that it was particularly marked when respiratory efforts were made against a closed glottis during mixed apnoea (Fig. 29.88). This has been confirmed by Upton et al[73] who suggested that bradycardia occurs too early for central hypoxaemia to be the cause; this has also been confirmed by others.[27] Another postulated mechanism is that bradycardia occurs as a peripheral chemoreceptor reflex response to falling oxygen saturation when apnoea is present.[26] Although bradycardia may occur with nasopharyngeal suction,[11] defecation, crying and stretching, we have found that only 14% of bradycardias are not associated with apnoea.[73] Forty per cent of bradycardias are associated with apnoeas shorter than 10 seconds, and although some of these are of little clinical significance they may be associated with profound drops in oxygen saturation. Nevertheless, there is evidence of interaction between oxygen saturation and bradycardia. Henderson-Smart et al[26] demonstrated a close relationship between the onset in the fall in transcutaneous oxygen and bradycardia, and Upton et al[73] found an inverse relationship between the saturation at the onset of apnoea and the frequency of bradycardia.

The clinical significance of bradycardic episodes is at present unclear. It is well known that during bradycardia pulse pressure increases and stroke volume is maintained in all but the terminally ill.[22] It has also been shown that in such a situation the blood supply to the brain is selectively preserved, even in extremely preterm infants.[64] However, a progressive decrease in systolic flow velocity in the anterior cerebral artery has been observed as bradycardia drops below 80.[53] Therefore, in the absence of evidence to the contrary, it is best to treat bradycardia as a potentially serious condition, even in the apparent absence of apnoea.

MONITORING

As apnoea is extremely common in very low-birthweight infants, and a problem even in full-term babies who are sufficiently ill to require intensive care, all babies admitted to neonatal units should be monitored initially. There are now five different systems in general use for monitoring respiration. The ripple mattress used in the past[38] is now obsolete. One consists of a pressure-sensor pad,[60] which can be placed between the incubator or cot base and the infant's mattress (Fig. 29.89(A)) This records changes in the weight distribution that occur with breathing. The alarm will fail to sound during obstructive or mixed apnoea, as the infant will then still make respiratory efforts. During apnoea associated with bradycardia the cardiac impulse increases in intensity. This can prevent the alarm sounding if the sensitivity of the device is set too high.

The second device[76] consists of a pressure-sensitive capsule which is attached to the baby's abdominal skin, close to the umbilicus or on the lower abdomen (Fig. 29.89(B)). The movements of the abdominal wall distort a membrane which is covering the capsule, producing pressure changes. This suffers the same disadvantages as the previous device, although it is affected less by gross body movement.

As an alternative there is now a pressure sensor which is held in contact with the infant's abdominal wall by a belt. This has similar problems.

The fourth technique is that of impedance.[51] Impedance monitors (Fig. 29.89(C)) detect respiration by using a high-frequency oscillator to send a small current across conventional electrodes on the chest wall. The volume alterations during breathing produce small changes in resistance, which are measured electronically. Such a system is not foolproof, particularly in small infants, as cardiac pulsation can also cause a change in resistance and a prominent artefact.[61] Unfortunately, impedance monitors may also fail to detect mixed and obstructive apnoeas.[79]

The final technique, respiratory inductive plethysmography, is more recently described and, although not yet in routine clinical use, has proved a useful research tool (Fig. 29.89(D)). The underlying principle is that the magnetic field induced within a coil is proportional to the enclosed cross-sectional area. Therefore, if a coil sewn into an elasticated band is placed around the chest or abdomen, breathing can be detected by the changes in inductance.[17] Ideally, both chest and abdominal coils should be used. Originally this was an attempt to measure tidal volume non-invasively. However, two coils may also detect obstructive apnoea by analysing relative movement as well as being a 'failsafe' device.[8] RIP therefore has potential advantages over impedance in the detection of apnoea. We have shown significant differences between apnoea detected by thoracic impedance and abdominal

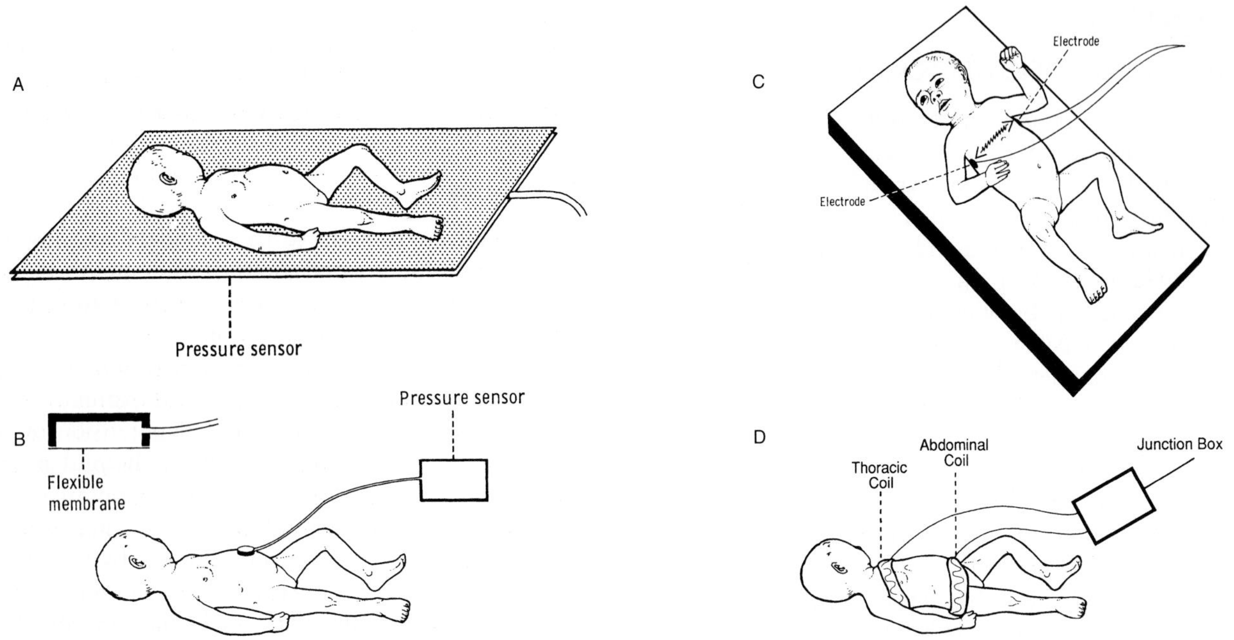

Fig. 29.89 Apnoea monitors: (A) pressure sensor, (B) pressure capsule, (C) impedance, (D) respiratory inductive plethysmography.

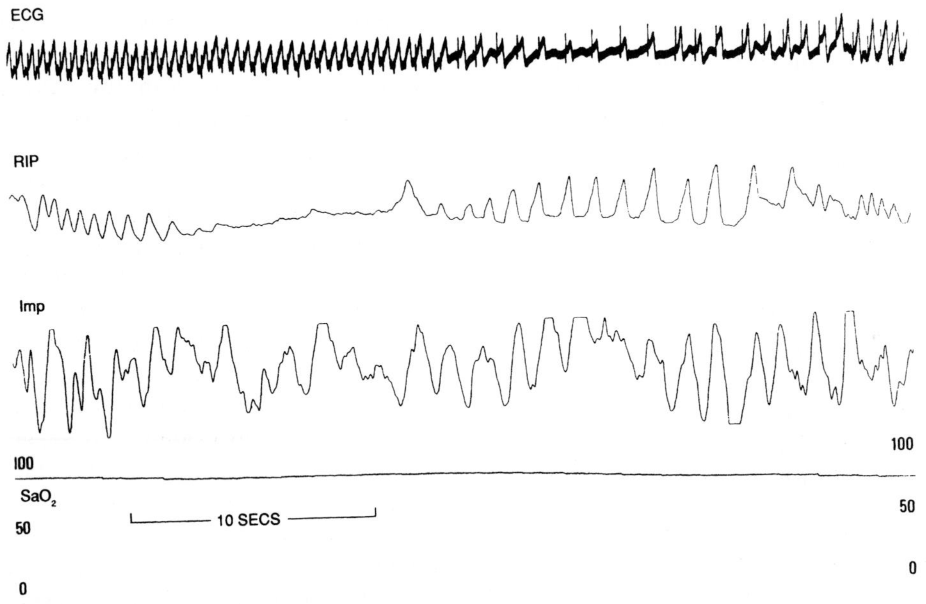

Fig. 29.90 Polygraphic recording from a preterm infant, showing a short apnoea evident on abdominal respiratory inductive plethysmography but not thoracic impedance (Imp). Note the bradycardia and profound drop in oxygen saturation (SaO_2).

RIP (Fig. 29.90).[72] These differences may be important when interpreting the results of trials on treatment for apnoea of prematurity.

Although RIP is promising in its ability to detect obstructive apnoea, the main challenge in monitoring lies in the detection of airflow non-invasively. Nasal thermistors[15] have been used for research but tend to be too precarious in their fixation for long-term use. The initial promise shown by acoustic airflow detectors[39] has not been fulfilled. There is increasing evidence that the best method of detecting apnoea in the routine clinical setting is by a combination of heart rate, detected by ECG, and oxygen saturation detected by pulse oximetry.[56] Although such a method is indirect, it allows detection of the two consequences of apnoea which may be harmful: bradycardia of less than 80 beats per minute, and hypoxaemia.

MANAGEMENT

INDIVIDUAL APNOEIC ATTACKS

The vast majority of apnoeic episodes lasting for up to 30 seconds will terminate spontaneously and require no intervention. If the baby is still apnoeic by the time the doctor or nurse observes the baby, attracted by the alarm, and the heart rate is beginning to fall, intervention is indicated. Gently flicking the sole of the foot is often sufficient to cause the baby to cry and re-establish regular respiration. It is sensible to monitor for hypoxaemia with either a pulse oximeter or transcutaneous monitor in infants with recurrent apnoea, to check for the level of desaturation during apnoea and to avoid hyperoxia during resuscitation. If such a measure is taken, facial oxygen may also be given during the recovery period following an apnoeic attack, as most attacks requiring stimulation are associated with a drop in oxygen saturation.[47] Gentle mouth suction may also help, as secretions or regurgitated milk may be present. This should not be overzealous or it may precipitate further deterioration.[11]

If the baby fails to respond within a minute to the above measures, bag and mask resuscitation is required. If the heart rate does not increase within 30 seconds, then intubation and IPPV are required. If possible, avoid using high oxygen concentrations as there is a very real chance of producing ROP in infants who have relatively normal lungs but require frequent resuscitation for recurrent apnoea. If the baby's condition allows it, an attempt to extubate soon after a quick response to resuscitation is advised, to try and avoid long-term ventilation. In practice this is often difficult.

Following resuscitation the baby should be carefully examined, with particular note being taken of general condition and tone, any respiratory distress, murmurs or abdominal distension. Temperature is not likely to be a reliable sign of sepsis at this time, as the infant may be cold following prolonged resuscitation.

INVESTIGATIONS

If apnoea presents in an otherwise well preterm infant, handling normally between attacks, the diagnosis is probably apnoea of prematurity and the only investigations required are a blood glucose to exclude hypoglycaemia (or hyperglycaemia, which may be a clue to the presence of sepsis) and a blood count to exclude anaemia and sepsis. If the infant is not premature, or is in any way unwell, further assessment is needed. This should include a full infection screen (including chest X-ray, lumbar puncture and urine culture) (pp. 1118–1124), electrolytes, calcium, blood gases and a cerebral ultrasound. If problems with unexplained apnoeic attacks remain severe, consideration should be given to performing a barium swallow or oesophageal pH monitoring (to exclude reflux), and cerebral function monitoring or EEG (to exclude convulsions). If PDA (p. 687) or NEC (p. 747) is suspected, they need to be investigated accordingly.

TREATMENT

If the apnoea is thought to be secondary, the underlying cause should be treated first. If the infant is unwell, broad-spectrum antibiotic cover should be given until the culture results are known. Babies with GMH/IVH or symptomatic anaemia[65] require transfusion to bring the haemoglobin up to at least 12 g/dl. If the infant is acidotic a cause should be sought, such as hypotension or sepsis. An infusion of 10–20 ml/kg plasma is helpful in such a situation, although bicarbonate is also sometimes needed. Although oxygen is helpful acutely during apnoea, it should not be given long term unless hypoxaemia has been demonstrated between episodes, in view of the risk of ROP in these infants, who usually have normal lungs.

Undoubtedly a small increase in ambient oxygen concentration is associated with a reduction in the incidence of apnoeic attacks. We have demonstrated that infants who are well oxygenated at the start of an episode have less profound drops in SpO_2 and are less likely to become bradycardic than those who are poorly oxygenated.[73] If oxygen is to be given in this way, however, stringent efforts must be made to avoid hyperoxaemia and possible retinopathy. Pulse oximetry is unreliable at excluding hyperoxaemia,[9] and so arterial PaO_2 should always be checked when such infants receive oxygen.

The incubator temperature should also be checked; if it is too high, reducing it by 1°C may help reduce the number of apnoeas (p. 300). In some babies the onset of apnoea coincides with the introduction of nasogastric feeding. If the apnoea is particularly troublesome, it may be advisable to continue i.v. feeding for a further few days. There is no evidence to suggest that intermittent passage of feeding tubes is superior to using indwelling ones.[67]

Having excluded or treated any underlying disorders, methylxanthines are the mainstay of treatment of apnoea. Kuzemko and Paala[37] first described the successful use of aminophylline suppositories in reducing apnoea. Such a route is no longer recommended because of unpredictable absorption. The approach was then to start infants with apnoea on intravenous aminophylline using a loading dose of 5 mg/kg followed by a maintenance dose of 4.4 mg/kg/24 h by infusion. Once oral feeding was tolerated the infants received oral theophylline at an initial daily dose of 5 mg/kg in three divided doses, but increasing up to 8 mg/kg/24 h as necessary. Levels should always be checked, with the therapeutic range being 5–15 mg/l (28–84 mmol/l). If the response was poor the upper end of the therapeutic range was selected, as further improvement may occur with increasing dosage.[48] Toxic effects such as vomiting and tachycardia may occur with theophylline, but should be limited by careful control of the blood levels.

Theophylline is methylated in the body to produce caffeine, which has fewer peripheral side-effects and is therefore commonly used as an alternative treatment.[3] Caffeine citrate is usually given orally or intravenously, with a loading dose of 20 mg/kg caffeine citrate (equivalent to 10 mg/kg of caffeine) and a once-daily maintenance of 5 mg/kg (2.5 mg/kg equivalent). The efficacy of theophylline and caffeine has been shown in a double-blind trial to be identical.[4] Reasons for preferring caffeine are the once-daily dosage and the greater safety, so that measuring blood levels is only necessary if response is poor.

Doxapram is a respiratory stimulant which has also been used when methylxanthine treatment has failed.[1] Side-effects, such as salivation, jitteriness, mild liver dysfunction and gastrointestinal irritation, have limited its use, but these may be minimized by starting at a low dose of 0.5 mg/kg/h and increasing slowly up to 2.5 mg/kg/h as necessary.[6,7] The equivalent oral dose is up to 24 mg/kg 6 hourly.[5] Doxapram has no advantage over aminophylline in the initial treatment of apnoea but can be helpful as an additional drug if the apnoea has failed to respond to aminophylline.[19] Its derivative, keto-doxapram, is thought to have fewer side-effects and has shown initial promise, although full results of clinical trials are awaited.

If drug treatment does not result in a significant improvement the baby should be started on CPAP of 3–5 cmH_2O via bilateral or single nasal prongs.[62] The prong should be cut so as to terminate at the level of the soft palate. CPAP mainly works by splinting the upper airway and selectively helps mixed and obstructive apnoea.[43] IPPV via a nasal prong has also been advocated in an attempt to avoid intubation of babies with intractable apnoea.[45]

As already stated, the role of gastro-oesophageal reflux in the aetiology of apnoea remains controversial. If the presence of reflux is confirmed either by contrast radiography or by oesophageal pH studies, and the apnoea is resistant to the above measures, agressive antireflux measures may be helpful.[50]

Various other physical treatments have been advocated to avoid ventilation. These include rocking beds[69] and oscillating water beds. The usefulness of such devices is not clear and evidence is contradictory.[28,32,66]

A depressingly large proportion of very immature babies, i.e. those less than 28 weeks' gestation, fail to respond to these measures and require intubation and ventilation. As these babies have relatively normal lungs, it is usually possible to achieve satisfactory blood gases with a low inflation pressure of 10–15 cmH_2O, an inspired oxygen concentration of less than 25% and a rate of 20–30/min with a physiological I:E ratio of 1:3 (p. 567). Efforts should be made at regular intervals to extubate such babies, by transferring them to nasal CPAP or IPPV. Otherwise, secretions build up, oxygen requirements increase and extubation becomes increasingly more difficult, with CLD the inevitable conclusion. All other forms of medical management discussed here should be used to the full in order to try to prevent this chain of events.

OUTCOME

The relationship between pure obstructive apnoea and poor neurological development has already been discussed.[10] However, it is possible that these infants had GMH/IVH leading to apnoea, rather than just apnoea of prematurity. Jones and Lukeman[29] did find a prevalence of major handicap of 24% in infants surviving recurrent apnoea. However, the majority of these infants had other adverse perinatal factors associated with poor outcome. The best evidence comes from a cohort of 164 infants with apnoea studied by Tudehope et al.[71] After correction for low birthweight, mechanical ventilation and CLD, apnoea per se had no adverse effect on intellectual performance. However, it may have contributed to functional handicap and was clearly associated with the development of CLD. These results re-emphasize the importance of early and effective treatment of apnoea and bradycardia, and the avoidance of prolonged ventilation.

REFERENCES

1. Alpan G, Eyal F, Sagi E, Springer C, Patz D, Goder K 1984 Doxapram in the treatment of idiopathic apnea of prematurity unresponsive to aminophylline. Journal of Pediatrics 104: 634–637
2. Alvaro R, Alvarez J, Kwiat Kowski K, Cates D, Rigatto H 1992 Small preterm infants (less than or equal to 1100 g) have only a sustained decrease in ventilation in response to hypoxia. Pediatric Research 32: 431–435
3. Aranda J V, Gorman W, Bergsteinsson H, Gunn T 1977 Efficacy of caffeine in treatment of apnea in the low-birth-weight infant. Journal of Pediatrics 90: 467–472
4. Bairam A, Boutroy M J, Badonnel Y, Vert P 1987 Theophylline versus caffeine: comparative effects in treatment of idiopathic apnea in the preterm infant. Journal of Pediatrics 110: 636–639
5. Bairam A, Akrahoff-Gershan L, Beharry K et al 1991 Gastrointestinal absorption of doxapram in neonates. American Journal of Perinatology 8: 636–639
6. Barrington K J, Finer N N, Torok-Both G, Jamali F, Coutts R T 1987 Dose-response relationship of doxapram in the therapy for refractory idiopathic apnea of prematurity. Pediatrics 80: 22–27
7. Brion L P, Vega-Rich C, Reinersman G, Roth P 1991 Low-dose doxapram for apnea unresponsive to aminophylline in very low birthweight infants. Journal of perinatology 11: 359–364
8. Brouillette R T, Morrow A S, Weese-Mayer D E, Hunt C E 1987 Comparison of respiratory inductive plethysmography and thoracic impedance for apnea monitoring. Journal of Pediatrics 111: 377–383
9. Bucher H U, Fanconi S, Baeckert P, Duc G 1989 Hyperoxaemia in newborn infants: detection by pulse oximetry. Pediatrics 84: 226–230
10. Butcher-Puech M C, Henderson-Smart D J, Holley D, Lacey J L, Edwards D A 1985 Relation between apnoea duration and type and neurological status of preterm infants. Archives of Disease in Childhood 60: 953–958
11. Cordero L, Hon E H 1971 Neonatal bradycardia following nasopharyngeal stimulation. Journal of Pediatrics 78: 441–447

12. Cote C J, Zaslavsky A, Downes J J et al 1995 Post-operative apnea in former pre-term infants after inguinal herniorraphy. A combined analysis. Anesthesiology 82: 809–822
13. Davi M, Sankaran K, MacCallum M, Cates D, Rigatto H 1979 Effect of sleep state on chest distortion and on the ventilatory response to CO_2 in neonates. Pediatric Research 13: 932–986
14. Deuel R K 1973 Polygraphic monitoring of apneic spells. Archives of Neurology 28: 71–76
15. Dransfield D A, Fox W W 1980 A non-invasive method for recording central and obstructive apnea with bradycardia in infants. Critical Care Medicine 8: 663–666
16. Dransfield D A, Spitzer A R, Fox W W 1983 Episodic airway obstruction in premature infants. American Journal of Diseases of Children 137: 441–443
17. Duffty P, Spriet L, Bryan M H, Bryan A C 1981 Respiratory induction plethysmography (Respitrace): an evaluation of its use in the infant. American Review of Respiratory Disease 123: 542–546
18. Durand M, Cabal L A, Gonzalez F et al 1985 Ventilatory control and carbon dioxide response in preterm infants with idiopathic apnea. American Journal of Diseases of Children 139: 717–720
19. Eyal F, Alpan G, Sagi E et al 1985 Aminophylline versus doxapram in idiopathic apnea of prematurity: a double-blind controlled study. Pediatrics 75: 709–713
20. Gabriel M, Albani M, Schulte F J 1976 Apneic spells and sleep states in preterm infants. Pediatrics 57: 142–147
21. Gerhardt T, Bancalari E 1984 Apnea of prematurity. I. Lung function and regulation of breathing. Pediatrics 74: 58–62
22. Girling D J 1972 Changes in heart rate, blood pressure and pulse pressure during apnoeic attacks in newborn babies. Archives of Disease in Childhood 47: 405–410
23. Hazinski T A, Severinghaus J W, Marin M S, Tooley W H 1984 Estimation of ventilatory response to carbon dioxide in newborn infants using skin surface blood gas electrodes. Journal of Pediatrics 105: 389–393
24. Henderson-Smart D J 1981 The effect of gestational age on the incidence and duration of recurrent apnoea in newborn babies. Australian Paediatric Journal 17: 273–276
25. Henderson-Smart D J, Pettigrew A G, Campbell D J 1983 Clinical apnea and brain-stem neural function in preterm infants. New England Journal of Medicine 308: 353–357
26. Henderson-Smart D J, Butcher-Puech M C, Edwards D A 1986 Incidence and mechanism of bradycardia during apnoea in preterm infants. Archives of Disease in Childhood 61: 227–232
27. Hiatt I M, Hegyi T, Indyk L, Dangman B C, James L S 1981 Continuous monitoring of PO_2 during apnea of prematurity. Journal of Pediatrics 98: 288–291
28. Jones R A K 1981 A controlled trial of a regularly cycled oscillating waterbed and a non-oscillating waterbed in the prevention of apnoea in the preterm infant. Archives of Disease in Childhood 56: 889–891
29. Jones R A K, Lukeman D 1982 Apnoea of immaturity. 2. Mortality and handicap. Archives of Disease in Childhood 57: 766–768
30. Joshi A, Gerhardt T, Shandloff P, Bancalari E 1987 Blood transfusion effect on the respiratory pattern of preterm infants. Pediatrics 80: 79–84
31. Knill R, Andrews W, Bryan A C, Bryan M H 1976 Respiratory load compensation in infants. Journal of Applied Physiology 40: 357–361
32. Korner A F, Guilleminault C, Van den Hoed J, Baldwin R B 1978 Reduction of sleep apnea and bradycardia in preterm infants on oscillating water beds: a controlled polygraphic study. Pediatrics 61: 528–533
33. Krauss A N, Solomon G E, Auld P A M 1977 Sleep state, apnea and bradycardia in preterm infants. Developmental Medicine and Child Neurology 19: 160–168
34. Krauss A N, Klein D B, Waldman S, Auld P A M 1975 Ventilatory response to carbon dioxide in newborn infants. Pediatric Research 9: 46–50
35. Kurlak LO, Ruggins NR, Stephenson TJ 1994 Effect of nursing position on incidence, type and duration of clinically significant apnoea in preterm infants. Archives of Disease in Childhood 71: F6–9
36. Kurth C D, Spitzer A R, Broennle A M, Downes J J 1987 Postoperative apnea in preterm infants. Anesthesiology 66: 483–488
37. Kuzemko J A, Paala J 1973 Apnoeic attacks in the newborn treated with aminophylline. Archives of Disease in Childhood 48: 404–406
38. Lewin J E 1969 An apnoea alarm mattress. Lancet ii: 667–668
39. McLellan N J, Barnett T G 1983 Cardiorespiratory monitoring in infancy with an acoustic detector. Lancet ii: 1397–1398
40. Marino A J, Asing E, Carbone M T, Hiatt I M, Hegyi T, Graff M 1995 The incidence of gastrooesophageal reflux in preterm infants. Journal of Perinatology 15: 369–371
41. Mathew O P, Roberts J L, Thach B T 1982 Pharyngeal airway obstruction in preterm infants during mixed and obstructive apnea. Journal of Pediatrics 100: 964–968
42. Menon A P, Schefft G L, Thach B T 1985 Apnea associated with regurgitation in infants. Journal of Pediatrics 106: 625–629
43. Miller M J, Carlo W A, Martin R J 1985 Continuous positive airway pressure selectively reduces obstructive apnea in preterm infants. Journal of Pediatrics 106: 91–94
44. Milner A D, Boon A W, Saunders R A, Hopkin I E 1980 Upper airways obstruction and apnoea in preterm babies. Archives of Disease in Childhood 55: 22–25
45. Moretti C, Marzetti G, Agostino R et al 1981 Prolonged intermittent positive pressure ventilation by nasal prongs in intractable apnoea of prematurity. Acta Paediatrica Scandinavica 70: 211–216
46. Moriette G, Van Reempts P, Moore M, Cates D, Rigatto H 1985 The effect of rebreathing CO_2 on ventilation and diaphragmatic electromyography in newborn infants. Respiration Physiology 62: 387–397
47. Muttitt S C, Finer N N, Tierney A J, Rossman J 1988 Neonatal apnea:diagnosis by nurse versus computer. Pediatrics 82: 713–720
48. Muttitt S C, Tierney A J, Finer N N 1988 The dose response of theophylline in the treatment of apnea of prematurity. Journal of Pediatrics 112: 115–121
49. Navelet Y, Wood C, Robieux I, Tardieu M 1989 Seizures presenting as apnoea. Archives of Disease in Childhood 64: 357–359
50. Newell S J, Booth I W, Morgan M E I, Durbin G M, McNeish A S 1989 Gastro-oesophageal reflux in preterm infants. Archives of Disease in Childhood 64: 780–786
51. Pallett J E, Scopes J W 1965 Recording respirations in newborn babies by measuring impedance of the chest. Medical Electronics and Biological Engineering 31: 161–168
52. Perkett E A, Vaughan R L 1982 Evidence for a laryngeal chemoreflex in some human preterm infants. Acta Paediatrica Scandinavica 71: 969–972
53. Perlman J M, Volpe J J 1985 Episodes of apnea and bradycardia in the preterm infant: impact on cerebral circulation. Pediatrics 76: 333–338
54. Perlstein P H, Edwards N K, Sutherland J M 1970 Apnea in premature infants and incubator-air-temperature changes. New England Journal of Medicine 282: 461–466
55. Pickens D L, Schefft G, Thach B T 1988 Prolonged apnea associated with upper airway protective reflexes in apnea of prematurity. American Review of Respiratory Disease 137: 113–118
56. Poets C F, Stebbens V A, Richard D, Southall D P 1995 Prolonged episodes of hypoxemia in preterm infants undetectable by cardiorespiratory monitors. Pediatrics 95: 860–863
57. Rigatto H, Brady J P, Verduzco R de la T 1975 Chemoreceptor reflexes in preterm infants. II. The effect of gestational and postnatal age on the ventilatory response to inhaled carbon dioxide. Pediatrics 55: 614–620
58. Rosen C L, Glaze D G, Frost J D 1984 Hypoxemia associated with feeding in the preterm infant and full-term neonate. American Journal of Diseases of Children 138: 623–628
59. Ruggins N R, Upton C J, Milner A D 1991 The site of airways obstruction in preterm infants with apnoea. Archives of Disease in Childhood 66: 787–792
60. Smith J E, Scopes J W 1972 A new apnoea alarm for babies. Lancet ii: 545–546
61. Southall D P, Richards J M, Lau K C, Shinebourne E A 1980 An explanation for failure of impedance apnoea alarm systems. Archives of Disease in Childhood 55: 63–65
62. Speidel B D, Dunn P M 1976 Use of nasal continuous positive airway pressure to treat severe recurrent apnoea in very preterm infants. Lancet ii: 658–660
63. Storey A T, Johnson P 1975 Laryngeal water receptors initiating apnea in the lamb. Experimental Neurology 47: 42–55
64. Storrs C N 1977 Cardiovascular effects of apnoea in preterm infants. Archives of Disease in Childhood 52: 534–540
65. Stute H, Greiner B, Linderkamp O 1995 Effect of blood transfusion on cardiorespiratory abnormalities in preterm infants. Archives of Disease in Childhood 72: F194–196

66. Svenningsen NW, Wittstrom C, Hellstrom-Westas L 1995 Oscillating air mattress in neonatal care of very preterm babies. Technology and Health Care 3: 43–46
67. Symington A, Ballantyne M, Pinelli J, Stevens B 1995 In-dwelling versus intermittent feeding tubes in premature neonates. Journal of Obstetric, Gynecologic, and Neonatal Nursing 24: 321–326
68. Thach B T, Stark A R 1979 Spontaneous neck flexion and airway obstruction during apneic spells in preterm infants. Journal of Pediatrics 94: 275–281
69. Tuck S J, Monin P, Duvivier C, May T, Vert P 1982 Effect of a rocking bed on apnoea of prematurity. Archives of Disease in Childhood 57: 475–477
70. Tudehope D I, Rogers Y 1984 Clinical spectrum of neonatal apnoea in very low birthweight infants. Australian Paediatric Journal 20: 131–135
71. Tudehope D I, Rogers Y M, Burns Y R, Mohay H, O'Callaghan M J 1986 Apnoea in very low birthweight infants: Outcome at 2 years. Australian Paediatric Journal 22: 131–134
72. Upton C J, Milner A D, Stokes G M 1990 Combined impedance and inductance for the detection of apnoea of prematurity. Early Human Development 24: 55–63
73. Upton C J, Milner A D, Stokes G M 1991 Apnoea, bradycardia and oxygen saturation in preterm infants. Archives of Disease in Childhood 66: 381–385
74. Upton C J, Milner A D, Stokes G M 1992 Response to tube breathing in preterm infants with apnea. Pediatric Pulmonology 12: 23–28
75. Upton C J, Milner A D, Stokes G M 1992 Upper airway patency during apnoea of prematurity. Archives of Disease in Childhood 67: 419–424
76. Valman H B, Wright B M, Lawrence C 1983 Measurement of respiratory rate in the newborn. British Medical Journal 286: 1783–1784
77. Vyas H, Milner A D, Hopkin I E 1981 Relationship between apnoea and bradycardia in preterm infants. Acta Paediatrica Scandinavica 70: 785–790
78. Waggener T B, Stark A R, Cohlan B A, Frantz I D 1984 Apnea duration is related to ventilatory oscillation characteristics in newborn infants. Journal of Applied Physiology 57: 536–544
79. Warburton D, Stark A R, Taeusch H W 1977 Apnea monitor failure in infants with upper airway obstruction. Pediatrics 60: 742–744
80. Welborn L G, Hannalah R S, Luban N L et al 1991 Anemia and postoperative apnea in former pre-term infants. Anesthesiology 74: 1003–1006
81. Yu V Y H 1976 Cardiorespiratory response to feeding in newborn infants. Archives of Disease in Childhood 51: 305–309
82. Yu V Y H, Rolfe P 1976 Effect of feeding on ventilation and respiratory mechanics in newborn infants. Archives of Disease in Childhood 51: 310–313

Part 5

Malformations of the lower respiratory tract

A. D. Milner A. Greenough

Although there is inevitably some overlap, congenital abnormalities of the lower respiratory tract can be considered under the following headings:

- Pulmonary hypoplasia and agenesis;
- Defects of the diaphragm;
- Defects of the chest wall (see Chapter 31, Part 4);
- Abnormal lung and airway development;
- Cilial abnormalities.

PULMONARY HYPOPLASIA AND AGENESIS

Pulmonary hypoplasia is defined as the incomplete development of the lung so that it is smaller in both weight and volume, with a reduction in the number of airway branches, alveoli, arteries and veins. Agenesis is associated with the failure of any respiratory development beyond the carina.

LUNG GROWTH

Lung development occurs in four distinct stages. During the embryonic phase, which lasts from 3 to 6 weeks after conception, the rudimentary tract first appears as a ventral diverticulum lined by epithelium of endodermal origin which arises from the foregut of the embryo. From this endoderm arises the lining epithelium of the whole of the respiratory system, including the airways and the alveoli. As the epithelium develops from the pharyngeal floor it is invested by the mesenchyme of the splanchnic mesoderm from the ventral surface of the foregut; this mesenchyme differentiates into cartilage, muscle, connective tissue and the pulmonary blood vessels and lymphatics and the alveoli. The groove between the oesophagus and the respiratory diverticulum deepens and then separates; the single bud quickly divides into two.

The second phase is the pseudoglandular stage, which lasts from 7 to 17 weeks. This is the active phase of development, with extensive branching of the respiratory tree, continuing until completion by about the 16th week. The airways are blind-ending tubes and respiratory exchange is not possible.

During the third, or canalicular, stage, between 18 and 24 weeks of gestation, there is a change in the cellular structure of the rudimentary acini and the respiratory portion of the lung becomes delineated. A capillary plexus begins to develop around the terminal bronchioles so that a rudimentary gas exchange system starts to form. At the end of the canalicular stage respiration is possible.

The last stage is the terminal sac phase, from 24 weeks to term. The terminal bronchioles now begin to subdivide and later alveoli appear in the terminal saccules, but most true alveolar development occurs post-term. This process increases rapidly after birth and continues until approximately 3 years of age.

Cartilage deposition begins at about 10 weeks and by 16 weeks the formation of the new bronchi is almost complete. Cartilage continues to increase until the 24th week.

Concurrent with airway branching there is progressive branching of the pulmonary arteries. During the canalicular and terminal sac phases there is branching of both the arteries and the arterioles, which increases the vascular supply to the area of gas exchange, and this further increases post-term. At approximately 24 weeks' gestation the capillary network, which arose from vascular structures in the mesenchyme, proliferates close to the developing airway. Towards the end of gestation there is a decrease in the muscle present in the arterial walls and an increase in the chemical reactivity of the vessels.

From approximately 24 weeks of gestation the alveolar lining cells differentiate into type I and type II pneumocytes. Type I cells are flattened and form over 90% of the gas exchange surface of the mature lung. The type II cells are secretory and are responsible for surfactant production and excretion. Typical osmiophilic inclusions and lamellar bodies may appear within the type II cells as early as 20 weeks of gestation. The lamellar bodies contain phospholipids, in particular dipalmitoyl phosphatidylcholine (Chapter 29, Part 1).

AETIOLOGY

Arrest of the single respiratory bud in the embyronic phase will lead to bilateral pulmonary agenesis. If the bud develops on one side only, unilateral lung agenesis will occur.

Pulmonary hypoplasia may be primary or secondary to conditions that impair lung growth.

PRIMARY PULMONARY HYPOPLASIA

This was diagnosed in eight of 1377 infants admitted to a neonatal intensive care unit in Texas.[145] It appears to represent a form of pulmonary hypoplasia in which no obvious cause of fetal compression is present and no other disease coexists. However, in six of the eight cases described intrauterine hypoxaemia had occurred, and this is known to inhibit fetal breathing movements. It is also possible that the infants had suffered from delayed development of the lungs, the anatomical development progressing at less than the normal rate such that morphological maturity was not present at the time of birth.

SECONDARY PULMONARY HYPOPLASIA

Reduction in intrathoracic space

In human infants conditions which restrict thoracic volume are frequently associated with pulmonary hypoplasia: these include asphyxiating thoracic dystrophy, pleural effusions,[33,34] tumours of the thorax including cystic adenomatoid malformation,[117] and congenital diaphragmatic hernia.[8] The mechanism, which has been studied most in diaphragmatic hernia, seems to be an overall reduction in bronchial and vascular branching and in alveolar development.[51] Abnormal lung growth can be produced experimentally by limiting the intrathoracic space by, for example, producing a diaphragmatic hernia[127] or placing a space-occupying balloon within the thorax.[67] Re-establishment of the normal amount of intrathoracic space antenatally induces the lungs to start growing again.[67] This fact has encouraged the concept of antenatal surgery to prevent the abnormal lung growth associated with such space-occupying lesions. There is also some evidence that anterior abdominal wall defects adversely affect antenatal lung growth.[151]

Reduction in fetal breathing movements

Pulmonary hypoplasia has been associated with neurological abnormalities or neuromuscular disease present in utero, for example Werdnig–Hoffman disease[45] and myotonic dystrophy.[158] In congenital myotonic dystrophy the fetus breathes poorly, and this results in pulmonary hypoplasia.[146]

Phrenic nerve agenesis and diaphragmatic amyoplasia are also associated with pulmonary hypoplasia.[63] The marked reduction in the number of bronchial branches found at postmortem in affected infants indicates interference with lung development before the 16th week of gestation. Diaphragmatic atrophy and pulmonary hypoplasia have also been reported in an infant presenting at birth with a unilateral cervical spinal cord lesion.[132] This suggests that normal diaphragmatic neuromuscular development is essential for permitting lung growth, even before the fetus is capable of regular respiratory movements.

Fetal breathing movements in the human can be recorded by ultrasound as early as 11 weeks of gestation.[25] Although these respiratory movements are insufficient to clear the tracheal dead space, they do produce significant changes in intrathoracic pressure, which could influence lung development. Selective destruction of the upper cervical cord resulting in cessation of fetal breathing movements[166] was associated with arrested lung growth and development. This occurred without atrophy of the diaphragm, thus excluding a thoracic compression mechanism. Liggins et al[88] demonstrated that the amplitude of pressure changes of the fetal breathing movements were an important determinant of normal lung growth.

Reduction in amniotic fluid volume

Pulmonary hypoplasia is common in infants born following pregnancies complicated by oligohydramnios. Oligohydramnios may result from reduced production of urine, with fetal renal abnormalities,[120] uteroplacental insufficiency or loss of amniotic fluid following premature membrane rupture.[11] Oligohydramnios produced experimentally by chronic drainage of amniotic fluid[101,108] or by urinary tract obstruction[68] is associated with the development of pulmonary hypoplasia. Subsequent infusion of saline in an attempt to restore a normal amniotic fluid volume after urinary tract obstruction[108] is associated with less hypoplasia of the lungs, further suggesting that adequate amniotic fluid volume is necessary for normal lung growth. This is now accepted to be a safe technique.[84]

Potter[125] reported a series of 49 cases of bilateral renal agenesis and pulmonary hypoplasia, now known eponymously as Potter syndrome. Associated with renal agenesis, there is a reduction in airway numbers, indicating interference with development between 12 and 16 weeks of gestation, and a reduction in the size and number of alveoli suggestive of a continuing disturbance to growth during later fetal life.[71]

Hislop et al[71] postulated that there are factors other than the oligohydramnios that interfere with lung growth, for example reduced hydroxyproline production by the kidney. Oligohydramnios may also have an independent effect on lung growth, as pulmonary hypoplasia associated with oligohydramnios can occur without renal agenesis and, furthermore, in such babies hydroxyproline levels can be high.[164] However, Perlman and Levin[120] studied the lung pathology in infants dying perinatally with urinary tract malformations and found pulmonary hypoplasia only if there had been both oligohydramnios and fetal anuria.

Chronic amniotic fluid leakage, owing to preterm premature rupture of the membranes, led to pulmonary hypoplasia in 28% in one series[121] and 23% in another.[19,20] The time of onset of oligohydramnios is an important factor. Pulmonary hypoplasia occurs in 23% of infants if the onset of oligohydramnios is prior to 26 weeks of gestation,[20,111] but not with premature membrane rupture after 26 weeks.

If the membranes rupture before 24 weeks' gestation, the risk of severe pulmonary hypoplasia is between 26 and 40%.[111,157] These latter authors reported that the presence of oligohydramnios had a 100% sensitivity but only a 38% specificity for predicting pulmonary hypoplasia. PPROM, however, does not lead to hypoplasia if the amniotic volume is preserved.[156]

The early removal of even small volumes of amniotic fluid, as occurs in amniocentesis, can impair lung growth and result in respiratory abnormalities. The Medical Research Council Working Party on Amniocentesis[98] documented an 8.2% prevalence of unexplained respiratory difficulties persisting for longer than 24 hours among infants born at 34–35 weeks' gestational age, compared to only 0.9% in controls. In support of this finding, studies have shown a reduced crying vital capacity[159] and a raised total pulmonary resistance[99] in the infants of mothers who had had mid-trimester amniocentesis. There are also recent reports indicating that first-trimester amniocentesis may also affect lung growth and development.[152]

Several mechanisms have been postulated for impairment of lung growth associated with oligohydramnios. Nakayama et al[108] suggested that thoracic compression had an important role; others have suggested that such prolonged thoracic compression may inhibit fetal breathing movements. Manning[94] reported a 60% reduction in fetal breathing movements up to 24 hours after amniocentesis. Adzick et al[2] investigated the relative contribution of reduction in fetal breathing movements and amniotic fluid volume in fetal rabbits. Both procedures resulted in lung hypoplasia, but the combination resulted in the most severe lung disease, suggesting that they have additive effects. In humans Blott et al[21] and Blott and Greenough[19] have demonstrated that sustained breathing activity was absent in fetuses who developed pulmonary hypoplasia with the oligohydramnios following PPROM, but in those in whom fetal breathing persisted despite a similar duration of PPROM and the development of oligohydramnios there was normal lung growth.[64] Roberts and Mitchell[131] came to similar conclusions. However, gasping and short bursts of respiration may occur in those developing pulmonary hypoplasia.[58,102,137]

In oligohydramnios, pulmonary hypoplasia may be caused by disturbance of the dynamics of fetal lung fluid. Fetal lung fluid is produced by an active process[114] and fills the lungs to a similar volume to the postnatal functional residual capacity. There is controversy regarding the mechanisms that maintain this fetal lung volume, in particular the role of fetal breathing movements, but the larynx and upper airway are important and act as a sphincter.[1] The importance of fetal lung liquid in normal lung growth was investigated by Alcorn et al;[6] chronic tracheal drainage was associated with a reduction in lung weight, whereas tracheal ligation stimulated the growth of lung tissue. It is possible that the insertion of fetal upper airway plugs may help lung development in high-risk situations (p. 659).

Rhesus disease

Hypoplastic lungs are found in association with rhesus isoimmunization, particularly in hydropic fetuses who have pleural effusions, and thus the mechanism may be thoracic compression. Chamberlain et al[34] demonstrated a significant positive correlation between the degree of fetal anaemia and the reduction in lung weight in a series of 96 infants. Detailed analysis of the lungs of six babies demonstrated that the variable reduction in lung volume is associated with a reduction in airway number. This suggested that an early immune mechanism affecting lung growth may operate in rhesus disease.

Drugs

Pulmonary hypoplasia has also been linked with the use of angiotensin-converting enzyme inhibitors, which have been used in the treatment of pregnancy-induced hypertension.[128]

INCIDENCE

Bilateral pulmonary agenesis is a rare abnormality, sometimes occurring in anencephalic infants.[126] Although unilateral hypoplasia occurs more frequently than unilateral agenesis, both are relatively rare compared to hypoplasia affecting both lungs. This is present in 15–20% of early neonatal deaths and is the commonest single abnormality found at postmortem.[165] Page and Stocker[118] found 77 infants with pulmonary hypoplasia of various aetiologies from a total of 756 autopsies. The incidence of pulmonary hypoplasia is difficult to estimate, as this condition is probably underreported in survivors, as the diagnosis may be masked by the other respiratory problems that are frequently concurrent.

CLINICAL PRESENTATION

Bilateral agenesis of the lungs is obviously not compatible with life. Those with unilateral hypoplasia, or even agenesis, are rarely symptomatic in the neonatal period but will have mediastinal shift towards the affected side (usually the right), which may be picked up clinically. Those with hypoplasia may have a single pulmonary artery, the affected lung being supplied by bronchial arteries alone. Unilateral pulmonary agenesis is often associated with other congenital defects affecting the heart and the gastrointestinal, genitourinary and skeletal systems.[141] These abnormalities are associated with a mortality rate of approximately 50% (Fig. 29.91).

Infants with severe bilateral pulmonary hypoplasia are often impossible to resuscitate at birth. They have small, non-compliant lungs which cannot be inflated despite the

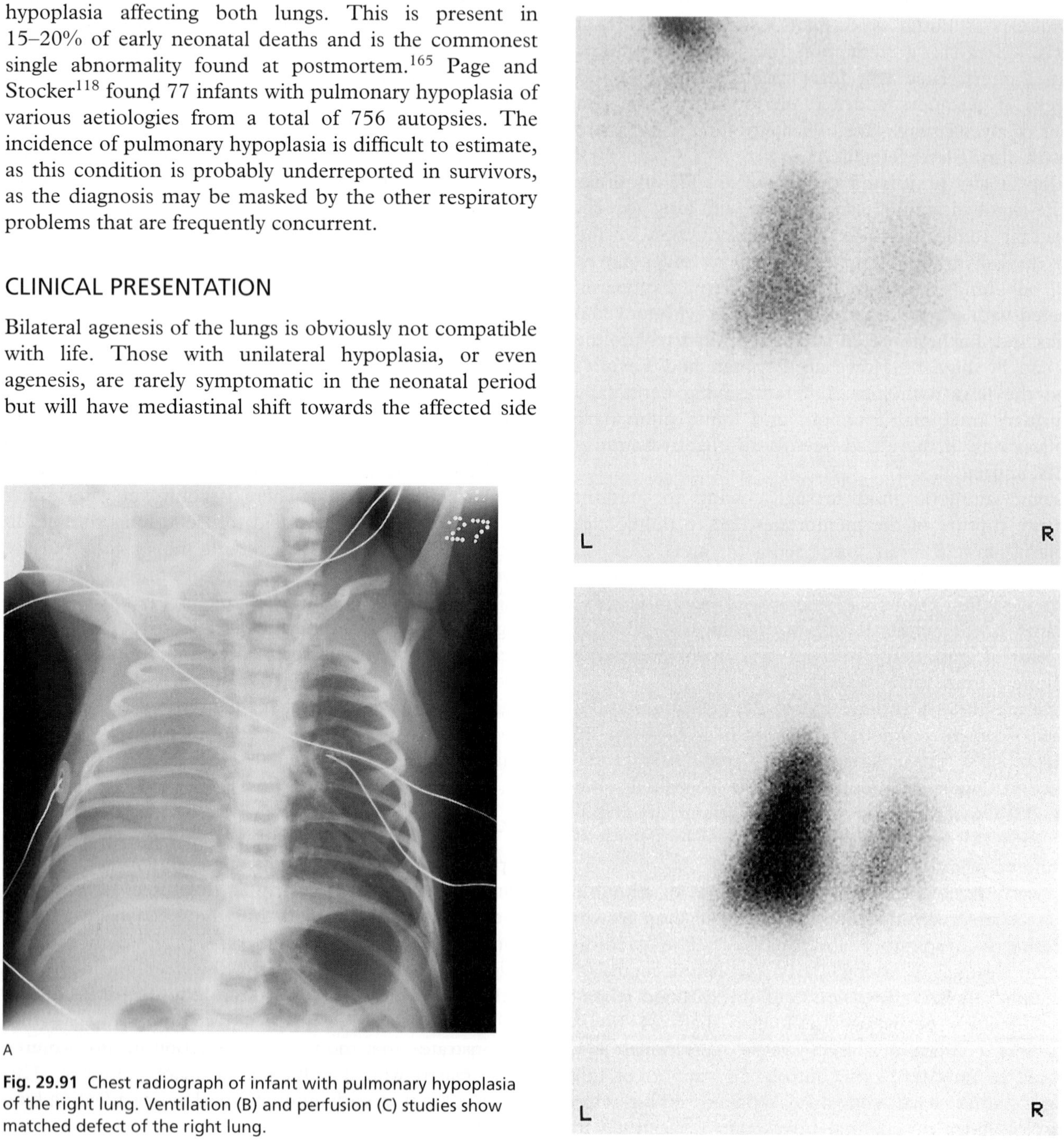

A B C

Fig. 29.91 Chest radiograph of infant with pulmonary hypoplasia of the right lung. Ventilation (B) and perfusion (C) studies show matched defect of the right lung.

use of very high pressures. Other infants less severely affected are still difficult to resuscitate, and may continue to need artificial ventilation in the neonatal period, with high pressures and inspired oxygen concentrations.[145] The clinical picture is often complicated by respiratory distress syndrome, as many infants with pulmonary hypoplasia are delivered preterm (see below). Hypoxia, acidosis and persistent fetal circulation are common features. Pneumothorax and pneumomediastinum frequently complicate pulmonary hypoplasia and occur very soon after birth.[146]

Pulmonary hypoplasia may result from a number of neurological diseases,[166] including Werdnig–Hoffman disease and congenital myotonic dystrophy.[133]

Infants severely affected by myotonic dystrophy are extremely floppy at birth, requiring respiratory support because of both pulmonary hypoplasia and poor respiratory effort. The respiratory embarrassment is further increased by diaphragmatic hypoplasia. Although this is usually bilateral, the right hemidiaphragm is raised much higher on the chest radiograph than the left.[38] The diaphragm is hypoplastic but there is also evidence of necrosis, which is worse on the right, caused by overstretching by intra-abdominal pressure and moulding by the right lobe of the liver.[136] The ribs may be hypoplastic, and this has been linked to a poor prognosis.[57,116] The baby has a characteristic myopathic facies (p. 1292) and talipes equinovarus is common. The condition has an inheritance pattern usually from the mother, which shows anticipation due to an increase in the number of trinucleotide repeats.[66] The mother may have only mild symptoms and thus be diagnosed only after the birth of the baby.[65] There is often a past history of stillbirths or neonatal deaths, and the pregnancy may be complicated by poor fetal movements[17] and polyhydramnios secondary to reduced fetal swallowing.[52]

Pulmonary hypoplasia is frequently associated with other anomalies, including[118] major diaphragmatic anomalies, renal anomalies, chromosomal disorders, extralobar pulmonary sequestration, severe musculoskeletal disorders and isolated right-sided cardiac lesions (hypoplastic right heart and pulmonary stenosis).

Pulmonary hypoplasia secondary to renal agenesis was first described by Potter[125] and subsequently referred to as Potter syndrome. In this condition the alveoli may be absent and the lungs poorly vascularized. Three-quarters of affected infants are male. As a consequence of the renal agenesis there is oligohydramnios, and this results in postural deformities; the infants also suffer from intrauterine growth retardation.[121] Postnatally the babies present with severe dyspnoea secondary to the pulmonary hypoplasia. They are difficult to resuscitate, and even on high-pressure IPPV and with an F_IO_2 of 1.0 it is impossible to achieve normal blood gases. The syndrome should be recognized at once on the basis of the classic 'Potter's' facies, that is, large low-set ears, prominent epicanthic folds and a flattened nose, together with the postural limb defects: large floppy hands and feet, often with fixed deformities at the wrist and ankle. Another syndrome associating pulmonary hypoplasia and facial abnormalities has been described by Pena and Shokeir;[119] in addition, this syndrome includes joint contractures and camptodactyly, but no renal malformations.

DIAGNOSIS

Those with severe lung hypoplasia usually present in the delivery suite. The diagnosis should be suspected in infants who are difficult to resuscitate. The clinical diagnosis of uncomplicated postnatal pulmonary hypoplasia is difficult in an infant born preterm, as RDS may complicate the picture. The diagnosis should be suspected in any infant in whom very high inflating pressures are necessary at resuscitation and during subsequent ventilation, particularly if this is associated with a 'positive' antenatal history, for example oligohydramnios. The chest radiograph demonstrates small-volume lungs, with a bell-shaped chest and clear lung fields[121] (Fig. 29.92).

If RDS coexists the chest X-ray will be opaque. Less severe degrees of bilateral pulmonary hypoplasia have tachypnoea and relatively mild recession, which may be misdiagnosed as transient tachypnoea but which persists for several weeks.[5]

The diagnosis of unilateral agenesis of the lung[93] should be suspected in a patient with marked deviation of

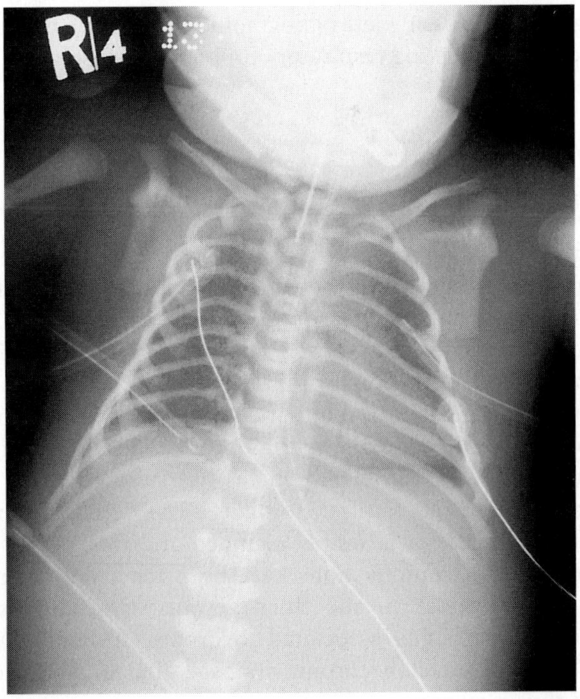

Fig. 29.92 Chest radiograph of an infant with bilateral pulmonary hypoplasia secondary to pleural effusions. The effusions have been drained.

the trachea to one side and rotation of the mediastinum, yet an otherwise symmetrical chest. Breath sounds may be heard over the portions of the affected chest into which the normal lung has herniated, but they are usually absent in the subaxillary area. The chest radiograph may document displacement of the mediastinum by the compensatory hypertrophy of the remaining lung; the affected hemithorax is opaque and filled with the mediastinal structures. The presence of another anomaly, such as a vertebral defect, is common and, if present, the thorax may be asymmetrical.

DIFFERENTIAL DIAGNOSIS

Pulmonary hypoplasia must be differentiated from other conditions in which the infant at birth is difficult to oxygenate, despite very high inflating pressures and inspired oxygen concentrations. Severe RDS, pulmonary haemorrhage resulting from perinatal asphyxia, septicaemia, particularly caused by GBS, congenital diaphragmatic hernia and PPHN should all be considered. Certain of these conditions may coexist, particularly if the infant is born preterm, but most can be differentiated on the basis of the history, clinical examination and chest X-ray (pp. 498–499). In uncomplicated pulmonary hypoplasia the small lungs on chest X-ray, the chronic nature of the infant's respiratory problems and his continuing need for vigorous respiratory support suggest the diagnosis, and merge into the clinical features of the preterm infant with CLD following severe surfactant-deficient RDS. The diagnosis can be confirmed by measuring the FRC using a gas dilution[5] or plethysmographic technique, but only once any coexisting respiratory problem has resolved.

MANAGEMENT

Antenatal

Early antenatal diagnosis by ultrasound examination has permitted the possibility of therapeutic intervention; this has been directed at relieving thoracic compression. One successful method has been thoracoamniotic shunting. Large cysts or effusions within the thoracic cavity can be drained,[26,110] into the amniotic cavity by insertion of a double-pigtail catheter, positioned under ultrasound guidance. The catheter remains in situ, resulting in chronic drainage until the infant is delivered at term, when the catheter is simply clamped and then removed. No antenatal complications have been reported,[22,23] and in certain cases chronic drainage was associated with resolution of the associated hydrops. Although this technique does allow chronic drainage of pleural effusions and thus may permit normal lung growth subsequently,[153] infants with antenatally diagnosed pleural effusions have a high incidence of other congenital abnormalities.

Postnatal

The eventual outcome of an infant with bilateral primary pulmonary hypoplasia depends on the severity of the lung underdevelopment, but in some recovery is possible with appropriate supportive care. It is important not to overdistend the lungs with aggressive mechanical ventilation, as refractory pneumothorax may easily be induced. Supportive care, oxygen therapy and closely monitored assisted ventilation will allow many of these infants to be sustained until the parenchymal development is adequate to allow survival.

Potter syndrome is a fatal condition; management is thus directed at making the correct diagnosis, preferably antenatally so that operative delivery may be avoided. Once a renal ultrasound has confirmed the absence of kidneys, the infant should be allowed to die with dignity.

PPROM with onset in the second trimester of pregnancy is also associated with a poor prognosis: in one series 36% of infants died.[20] The major cause of death is pulmonary hypoplasia, and such infants require high-pressure ventilation and inspired oxygen concentrations from birth; despite this, they frequently die within the first 48 hours of life. Another cause of mortality is sepsis, which may not have been suspected antenatally despite careful antenatal screening.[24] As a consequence all such infants, after the appropriate specimens have been taken, should be started on broad-spectrum antibiotics immediately after birth.

Following PPROM the infant may suffer from a number of respiratory problems in addition to abnormal lung growth. The majority are born preterm and develop RDS. In one series[20] 11 of 22 infants required mechanical ventilation, but this was not associated with high peak pressures (<30 cmH_2O) and was prolonged in only one infant, who had a patent ductus arteriosus. McIntosh[92] has suggested that some of these infants may suffer from a dry lung syndrome, and described four cases who required very high-pressure ventilation for resuscitation in the first 24 hours of life, but then made a rapid improvement on the second day and were spontaneously breathing air after a few days. McIntosh[92] postulated that this clinical course may be due to collapse of the airways resulting from the oligohydramnios, and that the resulting dry lungs would only respond to high inflation pressures. He further suggested that such infants be delivered electively, with paediatricians in attendance of sufficient seniority to assess immediately whether the normally accepted inflation pressures need to be overridden.

Prolonged compression by the uterus in the absence of the usual cushion of amniotic fluid in PPROM may result in aberrant limb development and flexion deformities.[121] In an attempt to limit both progressive pulmonary hypoplasia and limb deformity, elective delivery at 34 weeks has been recommended.[20] This seems successful as, although infants were born with compressive limb abnormalities, in all cases these responded to physiotherapy in the neonatal period, and lung disease was easily managed.

Regardless of aetiology, the management of pulmonary hypoplasia is directed at supporting the infant in the hope that postnatal lung growth will eventually allow him to lead an independent life. Infants with pulmonary hypoplasia often require supportive ventilation for many months. The combination of fast rates and low pressures is the least damaging to the small stiff lungs, but in practice these infants are often difficult to oxygenate and may require high peak inspiratory pressures and a reversed inspiratory–expiratory ratio. Newer forms of treatment, including inhaled nitric oxide[82] and high-frequency oscillation,[35] are worth trying if the infant remains hypoxic. Infants with pulmonary hypoplasia would not be considered for ECMO (extracorporeal membrane oxygenation) because of the chronic nature of their respiratory illness.

The most severely affected infants are at risk of developing right heart failure; fluids should therefore be restricted and diuretics given as necessary. It is vitally important, however, that sufficient calorie intake is given to ensure adequate growth, of both the infant and the lungs. The infant may be oxygen dependent for many months; steroids are unlikely to influence this and are contraindicated, as lung maturation may be achieved at the expense of further limiting lung growth. For such infants home oxygen therapy via nasal cannulae in appropriate circumstances, may allow earlier discharge. It is important that this is monitored carefully: inadequate oxygen saturations still further increase the chances of right heart failure by causing pulmonary hypertension. A home care team is also required, including at least a paediatrician, a physiotherapist and a dietitian (p. 618). Good communication between hospital and community services is essential. Such infants, and even those less severely affected, are at risk of deterioration from respiratory infections; they should therefore be fully immunized (p. 398).

PROGNOSIS

The mortality is increased in association with agenesis of the right lung, compared to the left. This is due to the greater distortion of the trachea and major vessels from increased mediastinal shift. The mortality of primary pulmonary hypoplasia is high, only two of eight infants surviving in one series.[145] Mortality is also increased by the associated anomalies, in particular renal agenesis (Potter syndrome) and congenital diaphragmatic hernia. Infants with the classic oligohydramnios syndrome (pulmonary hypoplasia, abnormal facies and limb abnormalities) are also reported to have a high mortality rate: 86% in one series[148] and 100% in another.[20]

Long-term lung function in infants with pulmonary hypoplasia is determined by the original diagnosis. Wohl et al[169] and Chatrath et al[36] have examined children at least 6 years after surgical repair of congenital diaphragmatic hernia and found no effect on lung growth (p. 659). Lung volume, as estimated by functional residual capacity, however, was reduced in five of 21 infants with PPROM occurring in the second trimester, measured at a mean age of 15 months.[150] The abnormality occurred in those with the longest duration of oligohydramnios and those born very preterm and ventilated in the neonatal period. Those with mild to moderate hypoplasia appear to have good compensatory growth in early infancy.[5]

SMALL CHEST SYNDROMES

There are a variety of conditions in which neonatal respiratory distress is primarily due to limited rib growth, so that the thoracic volume is strikingly reduced (Table 29.39). The most extensively documented is asphyxiating thoracic dystrophy, first described by Jeune et al in 1954.[78] It is inherited as an autosomal recessive and is a generalized chondrodystrophy which mainly affects the thoracic cage, producing short ribs with flared and irregular costochrondral junctions and a small bell-shaped thorax. The limbs tend to be a little shortened, with wide irregular metaphyses and often pyriform deformity of the epiphyses of the short tubular bones.[85] Associated anomalies include polydactyly, abnormal dentition, hypoplasia of the abdominal wall muscles and renal abnormalities.[69]

There is a further condition closely related to Jeune syndrome in which there is dysplasia of the thorax and pelvis, and a degree of laryngeal stenosis, leading to difficulties at intubation and respiratory problems in the neonatal period. This appears to be inherited as an autosomal dominant. In the cases described so far the mother has been affected, so that the babies have had to be delivered by caesarean section.[14,16,32]

Achondroplasia, which is inherited as an autosomal dominant, can also restrict rib growth to such an extent that the affected infant develops respiratory distress in the immediate neonatal period.[15,75]

It was originally considered that thanatophoric (death bringing) dwarfism, first described by Maroteaux and Savart,[96] represents a severe form of achondroplasia. This now seems unlikely, and there is dispute whether this represents a spontaneous mutation or a recessive condition. It is a chondrodystrophy in which the limbs are very short and the thorax very narrow, leading to death at delivery or within a few hours. The oldest survivor reported died at the age of 26 days.[115]

Respiratory symptoms may also develop from thoracic narrowing in three similar conditions, i.e. Majewski, Saldino–Noonan and Ellis van Creveld syndromes. These

Table 29.39 Congenital chest wall anomalies producing neonatal respiratory symptoms

Condition	Inheritance	Features	Prognosis
Asphyxiating thoracic dystrophy[113]	Recessive	Short ribs, bell-shaped chest, +/– short limbs, hypoplastic iliac wings	Death from neonatal respiratory failure or good survival
Chondroectodermal dysplasia	Recessive	Short ribs, medial polydactyly, CHD, hypoplastic nails	Respiratory distress but good outcome
Short rib, polydactyly syndromes[97]	Recessive	Short ribs, polydactyly/syndactyly, vertebral/pelvic abnormalities, CHD, renal, anal and genital abnormalities	Neonatal death from respiratory failure
Achondroplasia[75]	Dominant (80% new mutations)	Short ribs and limbs, short broad hands, large head, flat nose	Neonatal respiratory distress, upper airway obstruction. Good prognosis
Achondrogenesis[124]	Recessive	Short thin ribs, short limbs, unossified vertebrae, large head	Stillborn or early neonatal death
Thanatophoric dysplasia[103]	Sporadic mutation	Very short limbs, gross pulmonary hypoplasia, cardiac, renal, anal abnormalities. Hydrocephalus	Almost always death within hours from respiratory failure
Camptomelic dysplasia[139]	Recessive	Short limbs, bowed long bones, narrow thorax often with 11 ribs, large head, sometimes hydrocephalus	Early neonatal death from respiratory failure common
Osteogenesis imperfecta (types II, III)[41]	Recessive, some dominant	Multiple antenatal bone fractures, chest deformity	Type II, stillborn or neonatal death; type III, often childhood death
Hypophosphatasia (perinatal form)	Recessive	Short ribs and long bones multiple fractures, poor ossification, chest deformed	Death from respiratory failure in early infancy
Spondylothoracic dysostoses[79]	Recessive	Abnormal vertebrae, fused or absent ribs, chest wall deformity. Crablike vertebral defects on CXR	Death in first year from respiratory failure

conditions frequently have polydactyly in addition (Table 29.39). Further details are given elsewhere[140] (Chapter 34).

PATHOPHYSIOLOGY

Although the primary defect in these conditions is hypoplasia of the thoracic cavity, a proportion have an associated pulmonary hypoplasia. Thus of five children dying in early childhood from asphyxiating thoracic dystrophy[113] only one, who died at 12 hours of age, had associated pulmonary hypoplasia. Thorough quantitative morphometric techniques carried out on a baby who died at 4 months of age from asphyxiating thoracic dystrophy also failed to show any abnormality in the growth and development of the lung.[167]

CLINICAL PRESENTATION AND INVESTIGATIONS

The large majority of affected infants will show signs of respiratory distress, with tachypnoea, chest wall recession and cyanosis from birth. The small thoracic cage is relatively easy to identify in comparison to the abdomen, which tends to be distended by displacement of the liver and spleen out of the thoracic cage, a feature not seen in babies with primary pulmonary hypoplasia. The chest X-ray is sometimes initially misinterpreted as showing cardiomegaly, as the cardiac–transthoracic ratio will inevitably exceed 0.55. The lungs usually appear well expanded, but the chest deformity is easily identified when compared to the abdominal girth. It is obviously necessary to carry out a total body X-ray to define the underlying chondrodystrophy.

MANAGEMENT

Many of these babies require respiratory support from birth, often with relatively high inflation pressures and high respiratory rates, similar to those with pulmonary hypoplasia. Those severely affected are likely to die within hours of delivery, and it is probably not appropriate to embark on HFOV or ECMO in view of the structural problems, which will not resolve in the short term. In the past bone grafts were used to increase the size of the thoracic cage in one child, who was eventually weaned off the ventilator at the age of $2\frac{1}{2}$ years and then led a normal childhood with relatively few respiratory symptoms until she tragically died at the age of 16 years with encephalitis.[16] Acrylic prostheses have been used to expand the thoracic cage. This is claimed to be a relatively simple and effective technique.[155] An alternative approach is to divide the ribs and underlying tissues in a staggered fashion, so that either bone or periostium overlies the lung at the end of the operation.[47] Wiebicke and Pasterkamp[163] recommend the use of long-term continuous positive airway pressure via a tracheostomy. Their patient was still requiring this form of therapy at night at the age of 4 years.

LONG-TERM PROGNOSIS

Those less severely affected and surviving the immediate neonatal period often die in the first year of life from respiratory failure, often brought on by a relatively trivial respiratory infection. Although some die in early childhood, the long-term prognosis of those surviving the first year of life is strikingly better, provided there is no associated severe renal disease.[113]

ABNORMAL LUNG AND AIRWAY DEVELOPMENT

CONGENITAL LUNG CYSTS

Congenital lung cysts sometimes produce symptoms in the immediate neonatal period, although many are not apparent until later in infancy, when they become infected or are found by chance on a chest X-ray. One classification divides them into bronchogenic (i.e. derived from the trachea or main bronchi, and lying outside the lung), alveolar and combined forms.[43] They are thought to represent an anomalous development of the bronchopulmonary system. They may lie outside the normal lung structure (extrapulmonary), or within it (intrapulmonary). The cysts, whether single or multiple, tend to be limited to one lung and are not particularly associated with cystic disease elsewhere in the body. They affect males and females equally and do not show any familial tendency.

CLINICAL PRESENTATION

Bronchogenic cysts may produce symptoms in the neonatal period, owing to compression of the trachea or main bronchi, as the majority lie in the region of the carina and may produce congenital lobar emphysema[61] (p. 648). The airway compression will cause coughing and wheezing, particularly at times when the baby is crying, and if severe may produce respiratory distress at rest. Intrapulmonary cysts tend to produce symptoms as a result of distension of the cyst, as air gains free access on inspiration but is obstructed during expiration, either through the pores of Kohn or through a direct connection to the main airway. This will produce compression of the ipsilateral lung, mediastinal shift, and hence compression on the contralateral lung. Of the 51 cases reported in the series from Melbourne,[123] 14 presented in this manner. Although lung cysts can lead to pneumothorax this occurs later in life rather than in the immediate neonatal period. More detailed information can be obtained using ultrasound when the lesion is radio-opaque and CT when it is radiolucent.[44,70]

DIAGNOSIS

Diagnosis is usually established from the chest X-ray appearance. If the cyst is very large, it may be difficult to distinguish it from congenital lobar emphysema. Acquired cysts complicating PIE and CLD are increasingly being recognized in the neonatal period and early infancy.

TREATMENT

All extrapulmonary cysts should be removed, because even those that are apparently asymptomatic are likely to produce symptoms as a result of infection or compression later. This may require surgical excision, although some can be aspirated percutaneously or at bronchoscopy.[46] As, unlike acquired cysts, congenital intrapulmonary cysts do not show spontaneous regression, these too should be resected if the baby is symptomatic.

CONGENITAL CYSTIC ADENOMATOID MALFORMATION OF THE LUNG

This is a rare form of congenital cystic lung disease first described by Stoek in 1897,[143] consisting of a mass of cysts lined by proliferating bronchial or cuboidal epithelium with intervening normal portions of lung. Stocker et al[142] classified the malformation into three different pathological classes: type 1, multiple large thin-walled cysts, often confused with congenital emphysema (50%); type 2, multiple evenly spaced cysts, all less than 1–2 cm in diameter (40%); type 3, a bulky firm mass with evenly spaced small cysts. This is relatively rare, accounting for less than 10% of malformations. Sometimes more than one lobe is involved, but the defect is almost always restricted to one lung. Those stillborn or dying shortly after birth[117] often have hypoplasia of any remaining ipsilateral lobe and also the opposite lung. Males and females are equally affected and, although there are associated congenital anomalies in approximately 20%,[142] there is no evidence of a familial tendency.

CLINICAL FEATURES

Approximately 25% of affected infants are stillborn. These babies are often preterm, have hydrops fetalis and an increased incidence of solid (type 3) lesions.[12,154] Of those liveborn, approximately 50% are preterm. Some are hydropic and there is a history of polyhydramnios in approximately 25%. Of those diagnosed antenatally, up to 40% show regression in size as the pregnancy progresses.[28,31,91,109,130]

Symptoms of acute respiratory distress with tachypnoea and cyanosis usually develop immediately after birth, but may be absent or delayed for days or even weeks in those

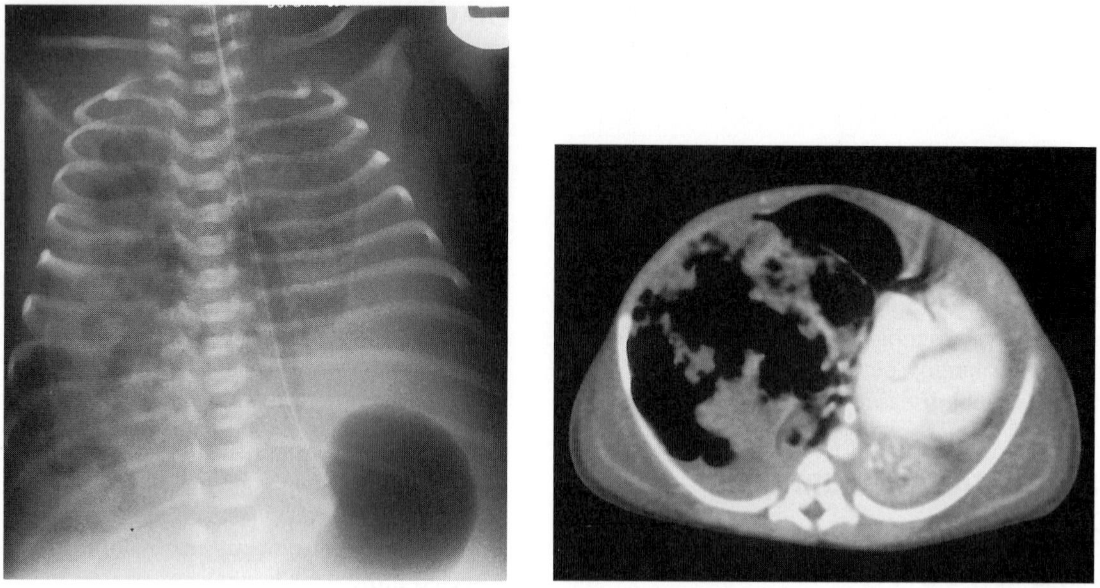

A B

Fig. 29.93 Chest radiograph (A) and CT scan (B) of an infant with cystic adenomatoid malformation of the right lung, causing mediastinal shift and compression of the left lung.

with less extensive lesions.[160] The cardiac apex tends to be shifted away from the affected side, and there are usually reduced breath sounds over the lesion.

DIAGNOSIS

Diagnosis is increasingly made antenatally on ultrasound screening, and can then be confused with congenital diaphragmatic hernia and sequestrated lung.[81] The presence of hydrops is associated with a much worse prognosis for fetal and neonatal death.[83,154] Postnatally, chest X-ray will show an expansile cystic mass causing mediastinal shift (Fig. 29.93). It is relatively easy to distinguish this condition from congenital diaphragmatic hernia, either by screening for diaphragmatic movement or, alternatively, by passing a nasogastric tube into the stomach prior to the chest X-ray.

MANAGEMENT

Fetal lobectomy, cystoamniotic shunting or repeated aspiration may have a role in the management of the fetus found to have non-immune hydrops.[4,29,83,130,147] Those who are symptomatic in the immediate neonatal period will require surgery, consisting of thoracotomy and excision of the affected lobe or lobes. This will prevent ongoing problems caused by compression of normal lung and infection in the lesion. Although CCAM may be associated with PPHN requiring therapy[9] (see pp. 531–535), recovery from surgery is usually relatively uneventful, provided the baby does not have associated pulmonary hypoplasia.

There is a claim that CCAM left in situ can undergo malignant change.[105] However, the current approach for those with lesions which are either small or only apparent on CT scan is to follow up and only operate if the lesion becomes infected, or the child develops respiratory symptoms due to the lesion.[109,130]

PROGNOSIS

Anecdotal experience suggests that babies surviving surgical intervention do well in the long term, and certainly the two children that we have followed up and two other children who developed symptoms within the first 24 hours[59] had normal lung function when studied 8 and 11 years postoperatively.

PULMONARY SEQUESTRATION

This is a congenital abnormality of the lung in which abnormal lung tissue develops which is not primarily connected to the tracheobronchial tree and which derives its arterial blood supply from the thoracic or abdominal aorta. Although the classification has recently been challenged as unhelpful,[39] the sequestrations are traditionally divided into intralobar, in which the lesion lies within the pleural cavity and in close contact with normal lung, and extralobar, when the affected segment is more distal and lies within a pleura of its own. It has been claimed that sequestration represents a secondary and more caudal development from the primitive foregut, the intralobar sequestrations separating early and the extralobar at a later stage. It has also been claimed that the intralobular sequestration may arise as an acquired lesion, possibly secondary to local infection.[72] In some there is a sequestrated hypoplastic right lung which, in addition, has an abnormal venous drainage into the inferior vena cava. This produces a characteristic chest X-ray appearance, from which the term scimitar syndrome has arisen.[60] There is also a related condition, known as the horseshoe lung.[53] In these infants the posteroinferior segments of both lungs are fused behind the heart but in front of the oesophagus. The hypoplastic right lung usually drains into the inferior vena cava and the isthmus of the lung tissue is supplied by the right pulmonary artery. This may produce cardiorespiratory symptoms in the neonatal period.

PATHOPHYSIOLOGY

The affected lobe is predominantly cystic, with airless alveoli and respiratory epithelium and cartilage supplied by a systemic artery. In a recent survey of the world literature,[161] 85% were found to involve the lower zone, with the majority on the left. Twenty-five per cent were homogeneous, 33% non-homogeneous and 37% cystic. Occasionally the sequestered lobe has the histological characteristics of type 1 CCAM.[10]

CLINICAL FEATURES

The large majority of intralobar sequestrations are asymptomatic in the neonatal period, awaiting the onset of infection and secondary aeration. In a series from Melbourne[123] only 20% produced respiratory distress in the neonatal period because of compression of normal lung tissue. Occasionally intralobar sequestration can lead to heart failure due to massive arteriovenous shunting.[134] More commonly, the lesion may produce a hydrothorax as a result of lymphatic obstruction.[27,30] Extralobar sequestration is otherwise rarely symptomatic in the neonatal period, unless very large, but does occur in association with diaphragmatic hernias, and may then be found at operation.

DIAGNOSIS

Chest X-ray of sequestration is that of a dense lesion in the posteromedial part of the left or, less commonly, right lower zone. Arteriography is necessary to define the systemic supply when the condition is suspected. The extralobar lesion is usually seen as a dense triangular or ball-like lesion close to the diaphragm. Ultrasound and CT scans are also useful in establishing the diagnosis.[48,138]

MANAGEMENT

Intralobar sequestration producing symptoms in the immediate neonatal period requires local excision, as it is likely to produce continuing problems due to infection and local compression, and may lead to heart failure due to arteriovenous shunting. This is a relatively simple procedure from which the infant recovers rapidly.

As the abnormal systemic venous drainage affects normal lung in the scimitar syndrome as well as the sequestrated area, it is important to identify the scimitar vein and implant this into the left atrium.[74] Failure to do this, or simply to ligate the scimitar vein, has led to massive and fatal haemorrhage from the affected lung.[7]

CONGENITAL PULMONARY LYMPHANGIECTASIS

Pulmonary lymphangiectasis is a condition in which there is cystic dilatation of pulmonary lymphatics and obstruction to their drainage. It is usually, though not always, bilateral. Noonan et al[112] reported three affected patients and reviewed the 45 described in the literature. They considered that this condition could be subdivided into three groups. First, infants in whom the pulmonary lymphangiectasis was part of a generalized lymphangiectasis. These babies usually presented with hydrops fetalis and, if they survived, developed malabsorption and hemihypertrophy. In the second and largest group the pulmonary lymphangiectasis occurred in babies who had associated congenital heart disease, particularly conditions such as total anomalous pulmonary venous drainage and hypoplastic left heart, in which there was an element of pulmonary venous obstruction. It has, however, also been described in patients with pulmonary stenosis and atrial septal defects[13] and ventricular septal defects. In the third group there was no such association, and it was considered that the generalized lymphangiectasis had arisen primarily as a developmental defect of the lung. This condition has been reported to occur in association with Noonan syndrome, and also sometimes with Turner syndrome. Some cases are familial, probably inherited as an autosomal recessive condition.[100]

PATHOPHYSIOLOGY

The lymphatic channels grow into the lung buds at 9 weeks of fetal life. These lymphatics originate as spaces within the lung bud and then fuse to form channels. Laurence[86] first suggested that this condition represents a failure of fusion to occur, leading to cystic dilatation. As a result of this, the lungs are large, firm and heavy and distend poorly. There are dilated lymphatics underneath the pleural surfaces, with fluid cystic dilatation of the lymphatics throughout the lung tissue. The condition is commoner in boys than in girls (1.8:1).

CLINICAL FEATURES

Most patients develop severe respiratory distress at birth or soon after. Intense cyanosis is present and, owing to the stiffness of the lungs, there is marked recession and grunting, with a clinical presentation not unlike that of RDS, except that most of the babies are born at term. On occasions the lymphatic distension leads to the development of pleural effusions[76] and has been recorded as a cause of neonatal pneumothorax occurring in full-term babies.[135] Unilateral localized pulmonary lymphangiectasis has also mimicked congenital lobar emphysema, owing to alveolar rupture and replacement of the fluid with air.[168]

DIAGNOSIS

Chest X-ray is rarely diagnostic, as it can appear normal or may show a fine reticular marking very similar to that occurring in transient tachypnoea, or a ground glass appearance in a hyperaerated lung. The diagnosis is usually only made at thoracotomy and lung biopsy.

MANAGEMENT

The bilateral form of the disorder, presenting with severe respiratory symptoms in the immediate neonatal period, is almost always fatal, although some babies have survived for a number of months.[77,122] The long-term outlook will obviously have to be considered before embarking on long-term respiratory support.

PULMONARY ALVEOLAR PROTEINOSIS

This is a rare condition in adults and older children which exceptionally can produce chronic respiratory symptoms in the neonatal period. The cause remains unknown but the progressive respiratory distress and cyanosis are due to the accumulation in the alveoli of material staining positively with periodic acid–Schiff. This material is a lipoprotein related to surfactant and probably derived from the proliferation and breakdown of type II pneumocytes. One suggestion is that the accumulation is due to defective clearance of lipoprotein derived from the normal breakdown of type II pneumocytes by alveolar macrophages. This condition can be familial, inherited as an autosomal recessive. The majority of these cases have apoprotein B deficiency.[37]

Whatever the cause, the collection of this material produces a lung that is stiff, with progressive impairment of respiratory exchange which can present at birth.[42] This accumulation is not associated with any inflammation or pulmonary fibrosis.

CLINICAL FEATURES AND DIAGNOSIS

Affected infants have onset of respiratory distress within 24 hours of birth, with tachypnoea, failure to thrive, often diarrhoea and vomiting and progressive cyanosis. Chest X-ray will show either a typical picture of RDS (p. 500) or a fine diffuse opacification, often radiating in a feathery manner from the hilar region, similar to that seen in pulmonary oedema but without any associated cardiomegaly. IgA levels may be reduced and, in some, alveolar macrophage activity is defective. The diagnosis is made at lung biopsy. Surfactant therapy may provide a temporary improvement and pulmonary lavage is sometimes helpful.[37] Only lung transplantation provides any hope of long-term survival.

CONGENITAL LOBAR EMPHYSEMA

Congenital lobar emphysema is a rare but well recognized cause of respiratory distress occurring in the neonatal period. The condition is probably more common than the 1:90 000 reported from Melbourne.[123] These authors found the left upper lobe to be involved most frequently, followed by the right upper. The right middle lobe is involved in 10%. In some babies both the left upper and right middle lobes were affected.[54] Male infants are affected more commonly than females and over 10% have associated congenital heart disease.

PATHOPHYSIOLOGY

Several mechanisms for the hyperinflation have been proposed. Several studies have described defective development of the cartilaginous plates in the large airways. This was claimed to be the cause in 32 of the 68 cases reported up to 1961,[18] and to be present in 22 of the 28 infants reported by Lincoln et al[89] It is, however, not clear how this abnormality could cause the gross hyperinflation that occurred.

Intraluminal mucus and inflammatory exudate have also been claimed to be responsible for the hyperinflation, as the result of a ball valve effect.[106,149] Isolated cases of extraluminal compression by bronchogenic cysts, teratomas, neuroblastomas and mediastinal cysts have also been reported as causes of congenital lobar emphysema presenting in the neonatal period. There is an increased incidence of congenital heart disease, possibly acting by the same mechanism. For example, hyperinflation of the right middle lobe has been associated with a persistent patent ductus,[87] and Fallot's tetralogy with a right aortic arch has been associated with right upper lobe emphysema.[80]

In a careful morphological study, 25% of the resected lobes were found to have an increase in the number of alveoli with apparently normal bronchial cartilage.

Whatever the cause of the condition, the affected lobe or lung is diffusely distended and pale in colour. The respiratory symptoms are a result of almost total collapse of unaffected lobes on the ipsilateral side and compression of the contralateral lung, due to gross mediastinal shift. The emphysematous lobes are virtually without perfusion or ventilation.

CLINICAL FEATURES

Symptoms may develop any time within the neonatal period, with increasing respiratory rate, hyperinflation which is particularly marked on the affected side, recession and intermittent cyanosis. An expiratory wheeze may be audible, but the most striking finding is a reduction in breath sounds over the affected side. There may also be clinically apparent signs of mediastinal shift, with displacement of the liver down into the abdomen.

DIAGNOSIS

A chest X-ray taken in the immediate neonatal period will often show delayed clearance of lung fluid from the affected lobe.[40] Subsequent pictures will show hyperinflation of the affected lobe with compression of ipsilateral unaffected lobes and gross mediastinal shift to the other side. Cursory inspection may suggest the presence of a pneumothorax, but a closer look will reveal that lung markings are still present. It can be more difficult to differentiate between congenital lobar emphysema and the presence of a large acquired lung cyst in a preterm baby who has developed PIE or CLD (pp. 521, 613). Congenital adenomatoid malformation can also produce large cystic lesions, but the cysts usually affect different lobes. Gross unilateral pulmonary hypoplasia or pulmonary agenesis can produce a similar picture with mediastinal shift, but these babies rarely have severe respiratory distress in the neonatal period and breath sounds will be most readily heard over the radiolucent area in these conditions. It may be necessary to proceed to ventilation–perfusion studies to resolve the diagnosis. In congenital lobar emphysema the affected area will have grossly reduced ventilation and perfusion compared to the unaffected lobes. CT has also been used to define the morphological abnormality more closely.[95]

TREATMENT

Although congenital lobar emphysema presenting with relatively mild symptoms, or found coincidentally on X-ray later in infancy, may be treated conservatively, those with significant respiratory distress in the neonatal period are very likely to become progressively worse, and the mortality rate is very high without treatment. Occasionally relief of symptoms follows bronchoscopy and removal of mucus or other debris from the airway. This is, however, a hazardous procedure in a baby who has severe respiratory distress and is cyanosed when not receiving additional oxygen. Selective intubation of the contralateral main stem bronchus has been attempted in this condition.[62] Although this led to temporary collapse of the lobe, deterioration followed removal of the endotracheal tube. The definitive treatment, therefore, remains that of lobectomy, which should be carried out without delay. In the absence of associated congenital heart disease this is associated with a mortality of less than 5%.

PROGNOSIS

Occasionally infants develop hyperinflation of a further lobe or segment in subsequent weeks. In a study by Phelan et al,[123] 12 of their series of 21 patients had attacks of coughing and wheezing over the next 12 months. Long-term studies have been very encouraging, although the information is limited. De Muth and Sloan[49] found a mild reduction in VC 5–14 years after resection. The eight patients followed up by Frenckner and Freyschuss[59] had a VC which was 90% of that predicted for height, indicating some compensatory growth of the remaining lung tissue. They also found that these children had a normal working capacity and normal alveolar gas exchange even during intense exercise. McBride et al[90] found similar results in 18 subjects investigated at the age of 8–30 years. TLC was within normal limits but there was evidence of abnormal airway obstruction, with a reduction in FEV_1, FEV_1/VC ratio, the maximum mid-expiratory flow rate and the specific conductance. Four of these showed some improvement after inhaled adrenaline. Radiospirometry showed that at TLC the operated lung was nearly normal in size compared to the contralateral lung, indicating good compensatory growth of the lung parenchyma but perhaps less effective compensatory growth of the airways.

CILIARY ABNORMALITIES

THE IMMOTILE CILIA SYNDROME

Although classically producing upper and lower respiratory symptoms later in infancy and early childhood, this condition is now increasingly recognized as a cause of secretion retention and pneumonia in the immediate neonatal period.[129,162] The overall incidence is in the region of 1 per 16 000 deliveries.

Pathophysiology

The primary defect in this condition is abnormal or absent ciliary function. Although cilia have been identified in the respiratory tract as early as the 7th week of gestation,[104] there is no evidence that the respiratory tract incurs damage during fetal life as a result of ciliary dysfunction. It has been conjectured that alignment of the heart and gastrointestinal tract is determined by ciliary function. This would explain the presence of dextrocardia and situs inversus in 50% of the cases in this condition. It was initially thought that ciliary dysfunction was always due to lack or partial lack of dynein arms on the outer microtubular doublets,[3] which can be recognized on electron microscopy. Since then, other defects have been found in association with this condition, including a defect in radial spoke linkages,[144] an absence of central tubules, and even the total absence of all cilia on the respiratory tract cells.[50] A further group of patients have been identified who have ciliary dysfunction and yet normal ciliary ultrastructure on electron microscopy.[107] It is now well established that all these conditions are inherited as autosomal recessives. It is interesting that the electron microscopy appearances seem always to be identical in affected subjects from any one family, indicating that this is a group of conditions with similar functional problems due to at least three separate genetic disorders.[107] The main pathological effect of ciliary dysfunction in the immediate neonatal period is sputum retention, leading to areas of atelectasis and pneumonia.

Clinical features

Although the majority of these babies will be asymptomatic in the immediate neonatal period, a proportion develop tachypnoea, recession, rales and rhonchi on auscultation, and often cyanosis. These symptoms often develop within the first 24 hours of life.[162] Mucoid nasal discharge has also been described as a feature in the immediate neonatal period.[73]

Diagnosis

This condition is unlikely to be suspected in infants in the absence of dextrocardia and situs inversus, unless there is an affected sibling or close relative. It is possible to assess nasociliary transport by inserting ^{99m}Tc-labelled serum albumin into the nares and scanning for transport.[55] However, diagnosis is confirmed by assessing ciliary function and ultrastructure. It is relatively easy to obtain a superficial epithelial biopsy by passing a bronchial biopsy brush via the nares to the nasopharyngeal space and then gently withdrawing and twisting the brush. The cells are then transferred to a small quantity of saline and examined under a light microscope with a stage which is heated to 37°C. It is relatively easy to see whether the cilia are immotile or have poorly coordinated beating. More subtle functional changes can only be identified if the ciliary beat rate is measured, either with electronic counting devices or by strobing techniques. Electron microscopic studies will provide further supportive evidence in the majority of cases.

Management and prognosis

These children will have recurrent upper respiratory tract infections, with sinusitis and otitis media, and at least a third acquire bronchiectasis secondary to lower respiratory tract infections and sputum retention in later childhood. The large majority thrive remarkably well, and so management should be vigorous. This should include antibiotics for acute infective episodes, accompanied by regular chest physiotherapy throughout the child's life. Symptoms presenting in the neonatal period usually respond to this therapy within a few days, but it is obviously essential that these children are provided with long-term follow-up. Respiratory function tests carried out on a group of patients aged 21–43 years showed evidence of small airway disease in most, with a tendency to hyperinflation but normal working capacity in all but one.[56]

REFERENCES

1. Adams F H, Desilets D T, Towers B 1967 Control of flow of fetal lung liquid at the laryngeal outlet. Respiratory Physiology 2: 302–309
2. Adzick N S, Harrison M R, Glick P L, Villa R L, Finkbeiner W 1984 Experimental pulmonary hypoplasia and oligohydramnios; relative contributions of lung fluid and fetal breathing movements. Journal of Pediatric Surgery 19: 658–663
3. Afzelius B A 1976 A human syndrome caused by immotile cilia. Science 193: 317–321
4. Adzick N S, Harrison M R, Flake A W, Howell L J, Golbus M S, Filly R A 1993 Fetal treatment for cystic adenomatoid malformation of the lung. Journal of Pediatric Surgery 28: 806–812
5. Aiton N R, Fox G F, Hannam S, Stern C M, Milner A D 1996 Pulmonary hypoplasia presenting as persistent tachypnoea in the first few months of life. British Medical Journal 312: 1149–1150
6. Alcorn D, Adamson T M, Lambert T F, Maloney J E, Ritchie B C, Robinson P M 1977 Effects of chronic tracheal ligation and drainage in the fetal lamb lung. Journal of Anatomy 123: 649–660
7. Alivizatos P, Cheatle T, de-Leval M, Stark J 1985 Pulmonary sequestration complicated by anomalies of pulmonary venous return. Journal of Pediatric Surgery 20: 76–99
8. Areechon W, Reid L 1963 Hypoplasia of lung with congenital diaphragmatic hernia. British Medical Journal i: 230–233
9. Atkinson J B, Ford E G, Kitagawa H, Lally K P, Humphries B 1992 Persistent pulmonary hypertension complicating cystic adenomatoid malformation in neonates. Journal of Pediatric Surgery 27: 54–56
10. Aulicino M R, Reis E D, Dolgin S E, Unger P D, Shah K D 1994 Intra-abdominal pulmonary sequestration exhibiting congenital cystic adenomatoid malformation. Report of a case and review of the literature. Archives of Pathology and Laboratory Medicine 118: 1034–1037
11. Bain A D, Smith I I, Gauld I K 1964 Newborn born after prolonged leakage of liquor amnii. British Medical Journal ii: 598–599
12. Bale P M 1979 Congenital cystic malformation of the lung. A form of congenital bronchiolar (adenomatoid) malformation. American Journal of Clinical Pathology 71: 411–420
13. Baltaxe H A, Lee J G, Ehlers K H, Engle M A 1975 Pulmonary lymphangiectasia demonstrated by lymphangiography in 2 patients with Noonan's Syndrome. Radiology 115: 149–154
14. Bankier A, Danks D M 1983 Thoracic–pelvic dysostosis: a new autosomal dominant form. Journal of Medical Genetics 20: 276–279
15. Barnes N D, Hull D, Symons J S 1969 Thoracic dystrophy. Archives of Disease in Childhood 44: 11–16
16. Barnes N D, Hull D, Milner A D, Waterson D J 1971 Chest reconstruction in thoracic dystrophy. Archives of Disease in Childhood 46: 833–837
17. Bell D B, Smith D W 1972 Myotonic dystrophy in the neonate. Journal of Pediatrics 81: 83–86
18. Binet J P, Wezelof C, Fredet J 1962 Five cases of lobar emphysema in infancy: importance of bronchial malformation and value of postoperative steroid therapy. Diseases of the Chest 41: 126–129
19. Blott M, Greenough A 1988 Dry lung syndrome after oligohydramnios (letter). Archives of Disease in Childhood 63: 683–684
20. Blott M, Greenough A 1988 Neonatal outcome after prolonged rupture of the membranes starting in the second trimester. Archives of Disease in Childhood 63: 1146–1150
21. Blott M, Greenough A, Nicolaides K H, Moscoso G, Gibb D,

Campbell S 1987 Fetal breathing movements as predictor of favourable pregnancy outcome after oligohydramnios due to membrane rupture in second trimester. Lancet ii: 129–131

22. Blott M, Nicolaides K H, Greenough A 1988 Postnatal respiratory function after chronic drainage of fetal pulmonary cyst. American Journal of Obstetrics and Gynecology 159: 858–859
23. Blott M, Nicolaides K H, Greenough A 1988 Pleuro-amniotic shunting for decompression of fetal pleural effusions. Obstetrics and Gynecology 71: 798–800
24. Blott M, Greenough A, Gibb D 1989 Premature membrane rupture in pregnancy of less than 34 weeks. Early Human Development 20: 125–133
25. Boddy K, Dawes G S 1975 Fetal breathing. British Medical Bulletin 31: 3–7
26. Booth P, Nicolaides K H, Greenough A, Gamsu H R 1987 Pleuroamniotic shunting for the fetal chylothorax. Early Human Development 15: 365–367
27. Boyer J, Dozor A, Brudnicki A, Slim M, Paliotta M, Kwark H E 1996 Extralobar pulmonary sequestration masquerading as a congenital pleural effusion. Pediatrics 97: 115–117
28. Bromley B, Parad R, Estroff J A, Benacerraf B R 1995 Fetal lung masses: prenatal course and outcome. Journal of Ultrasound in Medicine 14: 927–936
29. Brown M F, Lewis D, Brouillette R M, Hilman B, Brown E G 1995 Successful prenatal management of hydrops, caused by congenital cystic adenomatoid malformation, using serial aspirations. Journal of Pediatric Surgery 30: 1098–1099
30. Brus F, Nikkels P G, Van Loon A J, Okken A 1993 Non-immune hydrops fetalis and bilateral pulmonary hypoplasia in a newborn infant with extralobar pulmonary sequestration. Acta Paediatrica 82: 416–418
31. Budorick N E, Pretorius D H, Leopold G R, Stamm E R 1992 Spontaneous improvement of intrathoracic masses diagnosed in utero. Journal of Ultrasound in Medicine 11: 653–662
32. Burn J, Hall C, Marsden D, Matthew D J 1986 Autosomal dominant thoracolaryngopelvic dysplasia: Barnes Syndrome. Journal of Medical Genetics 23: 345–349
33. Castillo R A, Devoe L D, Falls G, Holzman G B, Hadi H A, Fadel H E 1987 Pleural effusions and pulmonary hypoplasia. American Journal of Obstetrics and Gynecology 157: 1252–1255
34. Chamberlain D, Hislop A, Hey E, Reid L 1977 Pulmonary hypoplasia in babies with severe rhesus isoimmunisation. Journal of Pathology 122: 43–51
35. Chan V, Greenough A, Gamsu H R 1994 High frequency oscillation for preterm infants with severe respiratory failure. Archives of Disease in Childhood 61: 1226–1228
36. Chatrath R R, El Shafie M, Jones R S 1971. Fate of hypoplastic lungs after repair of congenital diaphragmatic hernia. Archives of Disease in Childhood 46: 633–638
37. Checuti P A, Ball R J 1995 Surfactant apoprotein B deficiency. Archives of Disease in Childhood. 73: F125–127
38. Chudley A E, Barmada M A 1979 Diaphragmatic elevation in neonatal myotonic dystrophy. American Journal of Diseases of Children 133: 1182–1183
39. Clements B S, Warner J O 1987 Pulmonary sequestration and related congenital bronchopulmonary–vascular malformations: nomenclature and classification based on anatomical and embryological considerations. Thorax 42: 401–408
40. Cleveland R H, Weber B 1993 Retained fetal lung fluid in congenital lobar emphysema: a possible predictor of an alveolar lobe. Pediatric Radiology 23: 291–295
41. Cole W G, Campbell PE, Rogers J G, Bateman J F 1990 The clinical features of osteogenesis imperfecta resulting from a non-functional carboxy terminal pro alpha (I) propeptide of type I procollagen and a severe deficiency of normal type I collagen in tissues. Journal of Medical Genetics 27: 545–551
42. Coleman M, Dehner L P, Sibley R K, Burke P, Thompson T R 1980 Pulmonary alveolar proteinosis: an uncommon cause of chronic neonatal respiratory distress. American Review of Respiratory Disease 121: 583–586
43. Cooke F N, Blades B 1952 Cystic disease of the lung. Journal of Thoracic Surgery 23: 546–556
44. Coran AG, Drongowski R 1994 Congenital cystic disease of the tracheobronchial tree in infants and children. Experience with 44 consecutive cases. Archives of Surgery 129: 521–527
45. Cunningham M, Stocks J 1978 Werdnig-Hoffmann disease. Archives of Disease in Childhood 53: 921–925
46. Dab I, Malfroot A, Van de Velde A, Deneyer M 1994 Endoscopic unroofing of a bronchogenic cyst. Pediatric Pulmonology 18: 46–50
47. Davis J T, Ruberg R L, Leppink D M, McCoy K S, Wright C C 1995 Lateral thoracic expansion for Jeune's asphyxiating dystrophy: a new approach. Annals of Thoracic Surgery 60: 694–696
48. Deeg K H, Hoffbeck M, Singer H 1992 Diagnosis of intralobar lung sequestration by colour-coded Doppler sonography. European Journal of Pediatrics 151: 710–712
49. De Muth G R, Sloan H 1966 Congenital lobar emphysema: long term effects and sequelae in treated cases. Surgery 59: 601–607
50. de Santi M M, Gardi C, Marlocco G, Canciani M, Mastella G, Lungarella G 1988 Cilia lacking respiratory cells in ciliary aplasia. Biology of the Cell 64: 67–70
51. Dibbins A W, Weiner E S 1974 Mortality from neonatal diaphragmatic hernia. Journal of Pediatric Surgery 9: 653–657
52. Dunn L J, Derker L J 1973 Recurrent hydramnios in association with myotonia dystrophica. Obstetrics and Gynecology 42: 104–106
53. Dupuis C, Remy J, Remy-Jardin M, Coulomb M, Breviere G M, Ben Landen S 1994 The 'horseshoe' lung: six new cases. Pediatric Pulmonology 17: 124–130
54. Ekkelkamp S, Vos A 1987 Successful surgical treatment of a newborn with bilateral congenital lobar emphysema. Journal of Pediatric Surgery 22: 1001–1002
55. Escribano A, Armengot M, Marco V, Basterra J, Brines J 1993 An isotopic study of nasal mucociliary transport in newborns: preliminary investigation. Pediatric Pulmonology 16: 167–169
56. Evander E, Arborelius M, Jonson B, Simonsson B G, Svensson G 1983 Lung function and bronchial reactivity in six patients with immotile cilia syndrome. European Journal of Respiratory Diseases Suppl. 127: 137–143
57. Field K, Pajewski M, Mundel G, Caspi E, Spira R 1975 Thin ribs in neonatal myotonic dystrophy. Clinical Genetics 7: 417–420
58. Fox E E, Moessinger A C 1985 Fetal breathing movements and lung hypoplasia, preliminary human observations. American Journal of Obstetrics and Gynecology 151: 531–533
59. Frenckner B, Freyschuss V 1982 Pulmonary function after lobectomy for congenital lobar emphysema and congenital cystic adenomatoid malformation. Scandinavian Journal of Thoracic and Cardiovascular Surgery 16: 293–298
60. Gao Y A, Burrows P E, Benson L N, Rabinovitch M, Freedom R M 1993 Scimitar syndrome in infancy. Journal of the American College of Cardiology 22: 873–882
61. Gerami S, Richardson R, Harrington B, Pate J W 1969 Obstructive emphysema due to mediastinal bronchogenic cysts in infancy. Journal of Thoracic and Cardiovascular Surgery 58: 432–436
62. Glenski J A, Thibeault D W, Hall E W, Hall R T, Germann D R 1986 Selective bronchial intubation in infants with lobar emphysema: indications, complications and long term outcome. American Journal of Perinatology 3: 199–204
63. Goldstein J D, Reid L M 1980 Pulmonary hypoplasia resulting from phrenic nerve agenesis and diaphragmatic amyoplasia. Journal of Pediatrics 97: 282–287
64. Greenough A, Blott M, Nicolaides K, Campbell S 1988 Interpretation of fetal breathing movements in oligohydramnios due to membrane rupture. Lancet i: 182–183
65. Harper P S 1975 Congenital myotonic dystrophy in Britain. II. Genetic basis. Archives of Disease in Childhood 50: 514–521
66. Harper PS 1996 New genes for old diseases: the molecular basis of myotonic dystrophy and Huntington's disease. The Lumleian Lecture 1991. Journal of the Royal College of Physicians of London 30: 221–231
67. Harrison M R, Bressack M A, Chung A M, DeLorrimer A A 1980 Correction of congenital diaphragmatic hernia in utero. II. Simulated correction permits fetal lung growth with survival at birth. Surgery 88: 260–268
68. Harrison M R, Ross N, Noall R, DeLorrimer A A 1983 Correction of congenital hydronephrosis in utero. I. The model: fetal urethral obstruction produces hydronephrosis and pulmonary hypoplasia in lambs. Journal of Pediatric Surgery 18: 247–256
69. Herdman R C, Langer L O 1968 The thoracic asphyxiant dystrophy and renal disease. American Journal of Diseases of Children 116: 192–201

70. Hernanz-Schulman M 1993 Cysts and cyst-like lesions of the lung. Radiologic Clinics of North America 31: 631–649
71. Hislop A, Hey E, Reid L 1979 The lungs in congenital bilateral renal agenesis and dysplasia. Archives of Disease in Childhood 54: 32–38
72. Holder PD, Langston C 1986 Intralobular pulmonary sequestration (a nonentity?) Pediatric Pulmonology 2: 147–153
73. Holmes L B, Blennerhassett J B, Austen K F 1968 A reappraisal of Kartagener's Syndrome. American Journal of Medical Science 255: 13–28
74. Horcher E, Helmer F 1987 Scimitar syndrome and associated pulmonary sequestration: a report of a successfully corrected case. Progress in Pediatric Surgery 21: 107–111
75. Hull D, Barnes N D 1972 Children with small chests. Archives of Disease in Childhood 47: 12–19
76. Hunter W S, Becroft D M 1984 Congenital pulmonary lymphangiectasis associated with pleural effusions. Archives of Disease in Childhood 59: 278–279
77. Javett S N, Webster I, Braudo J L 1963 Congenital dilatation of the pulmonary lymphatics. Pediatrics 31: 416–419
78. Jeune M, Carron R, Bernard C, Loaec Y 1954 Polychondrodystrophie avec blocage thoracique d'évolution fatale. Pédiatrie 9: 390–397
79. Karnes P S, Day D, Berry S A, Pierpont M E 1991 Jarcho–Levin syndrome: four new cases and classification of subtypes. American Journal of Medical Genetics 40: 264–270
80. Keller M S 1983 Congenital lobar emphysema with tracheal bronchus. Journal of the Canadian Association of Radiologists 34: 306–307
81. King S J, Pilling D W, Walkinshaw S 1995 Fetal echogenic lung lesions: prenatal ultrasound diagnosis and outcome. Pediatric Radiology 25: 208–210
82. Kinsella J P, Neish S R, Dunbar I et al 1993 Clinical responses to prolonged treatment of persistent pulmonary hypertension of the newborn with low doses of inhaled nitric oxide. Journal of Pediatrics 123: 103–108
83. Kuller J A, Yankowitz J, Goldberg J D et al 1992 Outcome of antenatally diagnosed cystic adenomatoid malformations. American Journal of Obstetrics and Gynecology 167: 1038–1041
84. Lameier L N, Katz V L 1993 Amnio-infusion: a review. Obstetrical and Gynecological Survey 48: 829–837
85. Langer L O 1968 Thoracic-pelvic-phalangeal dystrophy. Radiology 91: 447–450
86. Laurence K M 1959 Congenital pulmonary lymphangiectasia. Journal of Clinical Pathology 12: 62–69
87. Leape L L, Longino L A 1964 Infantile lobar emphysema. Pediatrics 34: 246–251
88. Liggins G C, Vilos G A, Campos G A, Kitterman J A, Lee C H 1981 The effect of bilateral thoracoplasty on lung development in fetal sheep. Journal of Developmental Physiology 3: 275–282
89. Lincoln J C R, Stark J, Subramanian S 1971 Congenital lobar emphysema. Annals of Surgery 173: 55–59
90. McBride J T, Wohl M E B, Strieder D J 1980 Lung growth and airway function after lobectomy in infancy for congenital lobar emphysema. Journal of Clinical Investigation 66: 962–967
91. MacGillivray T E, Harrison M R, Goldstein R B, Adzick N S 1993 Disappearing fetal lung lesions. Journal of Pediatric Surgery 28: 1321–1324
92. McIntosh N 1988 Dry lung syndrome after oligohydramnios. Archives of Disease of Childhood 63: 190–193
93. Maltz D L, Nadas A S 1968 Agenesis of the lung: presentation of eight new cases and review of the literature. Pediatrics 42: 175–188
94. Manning F A 1977 Effects of amniocentesis on fetal breathing movements. British Medical Journal ii: 1582–1583
95. Markowitz R I, Mercurio M R, Vahjen G A, Gross I, Touloukian R J 1989 Congenital lobar emphysema. The role of CT and V/Q scan. Clinical Pediatrics 28: 19–23
96. Maroteaux P, Savart P 1964 La dystrophie thoracique asphyxiante. Etude radiologique et rapports avec le syndrome d'Ellis et Van Creveld. Annales de Radiologie 7: 332–339
97. Martinez-Frias M L, Bermejo E, Urioste M et al 1993 Lethal short rib-polydactyly syndromes: further evidence for their overlapping in a continuous spectrum. Journal of Medical Genetics. 30: 937–941
98. Medical Research Council Working Party on Amniocentesis. 1978 An assessment of hazards of amniocentesis. British Journal of Obstetrics and Gynaecology 85: 1–41
99. Milner A D, Hoskyns E W, Hopkin I E 1992 The effects of midtrimester amniocentesis on lung function in the neonatal period. European Journal of Pediatrics 151: 458–460
100. Moerman P, Vandenberghe K, Devlieger H, Van Hole C, Fryns J P, Lauweryns J M 1993 Congenital pulmonary lymphangiectasis with chylothorax: a heterogeneous lymphatic vessel abnormality. American Journal of Medical Genetics 47: 54–58
101. Moessinger A C, Fewell J E, Stark R I et al 1985 Lung hypoplasia and breathing movements following oligohydramnios in fetal lambs. In: Jones C T, Nathanielsz P W (eds) Physiological development of the fetus and newborn. Academic Press, London, pp 293–298
102. Moessinger A C, Fox H E, Higgins A, Rey H R, Al Haideri M 1987 Fetal breathing movements are not a reliable predictor of continued lung development in pregnancies complicated by oligohydramnios. Lancet ii: 1297–1300
103. Moir D H and Kowslowski K 1976 Survival in thanatophoric dwarfism. Pediatric Radiology 5: 123–125
104. Moscoso G J, Driver M, Codd J, Whimter W F 1988 The morphology of ciliogenesis in the developing fetal human respiratory epithelium. Pathology Research and Practice 183: 403–411
105. Murphy J J, Blair G K, Fraser C, Ashmore P G, et al 1993 Rhabdosarcoma arising within congenital pulmonary cysts: report of 3 cases. Journal of Pediatric Surgery 27: 1364–1367
106. Murray G F 1967 Congenital lobar emphysema. Surgery, Gynecology and Obstetrics 124: 611–615
107. Mygind N, Pedersen M, Nielsen M H 1983 Primary and secondary ciliary dyskinesia. Acta Otolaryngology 95: 688–694
108. Nakayama D K, Glick P L, Harrison M R, Villa R L, Noall R 1983 Experimental pulmonary hypoplasia due to oligohydramnios and its reversal by relieving thoracic compression. Journal of Pediatric Surgery 18: 347–353
109. Neilson I R, Russon P, Laberge J M et al 1991 Congenital adenomatoid malformation of the lung: current management and prognosis. Journal of Pediatric Surgery 26: 975–980
110. Nicolaides K H, Blott M, Greenough A 1987 Chronic drainage of fetal pulmonary cyst. Lancet i: 618
111. Nimrod C, Varela-Gittings F, Machin G, Campbell D, Wesenberg R 1984 The effect of very prolonged membrane rupture on fetal development. American Journal of Obstetrics and Gynecology 148: 540–545
112. Noonan J A, Walters L R, Reeves J T 1970 Congenital pulmonary lymphangiectasis. American Journal of Diseases of Children 120: 314–318
113. Oberklaid F, Danks D M, Mayne V, Campbell P 1970 Asphyxiating thoracic dysplasia. Archives of Disease of Childhood 52: 758–765
114. Olver R E, Strang L B 1974 Ion fluxes across the pulmonary epithelium and the secretion of lung liquid in the fetal lamb. Journal of Physiology 242: 327–337
115. O'Malley B P, Parker R, Saphyakhajon P, Oizilbash A H 1972 Thanatophoric dwarfs. Journal of the Canadian Association of Radiologists 23: 62–69
116. Osborne J P, Murphy E G, Hill A 1983 Thin ribs on chest X-ray a useful sign in the differential diagnosis of the floppy newborn. Developmental Medicine and Child Neurology 25: 343–345
117. Oster A G, Fortune D W 1987 Congenital cystic adenomatoid malformation of the lung. American Journal of Clinical Pathology 70: 595–604
118. Page D V, Stocker J T 1982 Anomalies associated with pulmonary hypoplasia. American Review of Respiratory Disease 125: 216–221
119. Pena S D J, Shokeir M H K 1974 Syndrome of camptodactyly, multiple ankyloses, facial anomalies and pulmonary hypoplasia: a lethal condition. Journal of Pediatrics 85: 373
120. Perlman M, Levin M 1974 Fetal pulmonary hypoplasia, anuria and oligohydramnios: clinicopathologic observations and review of the literature. American Journal of Obstetrics and Gynecology 118: 1119–1123
121. Perlman M, Williams J, Hirsch M 1976 Neonatal pulmonary hypoplasia after prolonged leakage of amniotic fluid. Archives of Disease in Childhood 51: 349–353
122. Pernot C, Bernard C, Hoeffel J C, Marcon F, Morali A 1984 Diffuse pulmonary lymphangiectasia of late disclosure associated with cardiomegaly. Archives Françaises de Pédiatrie 41: 617–622
123. Phelan P D, Landau L I, Olinsky A 1990 Respiratory illness in

children, 3rd edn. Blackwell Scientific Publications, Boston
124. Pilu G, Rizzio N, Perolo A 1983 Anomalies of the skeletal system. In: Chervanek F A, Isaacson G C, Campbell S (eds) Ultrasound in obstetrics and gynecology. Little, Brown and Company, Boston, pp 981–997
125. Potter E L 1946 Bilateral renal agenesis. Journal of Pediatrics 29: 68–76
126. Potter E L 1952 Pathology of the fetus and newborn. Year Book Medical Publishers, Chicago Inc.
127. Pringle K C, Turner J W, Schofield J C, Soper R J 1984 Creation and repair of diaphragmatic hernia in the fetal lamb: lung development and morphology. Journal of Pediatric Surgery 19: 131–140
128. Pryde P G, Sedman A B, Nugent C E, and Barr M Jr 1993 Angiotensin-converting enzyme inhibitor fetopathy. Journal of the American Society of Nephrology 3: 1575–1582
129. Ramet J, Byloos J, Delree M, Sacre L, Clement P 1986 Neonatal diagnosis of the immotile cilia syndrome. Chest 90: 138–140
130. Revillon Y, Jan D, Plattner V et al 1993 Congenital cystic adenomatoid malformation of the lung: prenatal management and prognosis. Journal of Pediatric Surgery 28: 1009–1011
131. Roberts A B, Mitchell J 1995 Pulmonary hypoplasia and fetal breathing in preterm premature rupture of membranes. Early Human Development 41: 27–37
132. Rothschild A, Ling E W, Wensley D F, Norman M F Thurlbeck W M 1994 Unilateral cervical spinal cord lesion in a term newborn, associated with ipsilateral diaphragmatic atrophy and pulmonary hypoplasia. Pediatric Pulmonology 18: 53–57
133. Rutherford M A, Heckmatt J Z, Dubowitz V 1989 Congenital myotonic dystrophy: respiratory function at birth determines survival. Archives of Disease in Childhood 64: 191–195
134. Sholler G F, Whight C M, Nunn G R 1985 Pulmonary sequestration in a newborn mimicking cardiac disease: a trap for diagnosis. Australian Paediatric Journal 21: 279–280
135. Siegal A, Katsenstein M, Wolach B 1985 Neonatal pneumothorax, a rare complication of pulmonary cystic lymphangiectasis. European Journal of Respiratory Disease 66: 153–157
136. Silver M M, Vilos G A, Silver M D, Shaheed W S, Turner K L 1983 Morphological and morphometric analysis of muscle in the neonatal myotonic dystrophy syndrome. Human Pathology 5: 1171–1187
137. Sival D A, Visser G H, Prechtl H F 1992 Fetal breathing movements are not a good indicator of lung development after premature rupture of membranes and oligohydamnios – a preliminary study. Early Human Development 28: 133–143
138. Spinetta G, Montrucchio E, Franchi M, Cerimele M, Moretti A, Sani L 1987 Computerized tomography in pulmonary sequestration. Acta Bio-Medica de L'Ateno Parmanse 58: 117–123
139. Spranger J, Langen L O, Maroteaux P 1970 Increasing frequency of a syndrome of multiple osseous defects. Lancet ii: 716
140. Spranger J, Langer L O, Weller M H, Herrmann J 1974 Skeletal dysplasia: short rib-polydactyly syndromes and related conditions. Birth Defect Series 10: 635–639
141. Steadland K M, Langham M R Jr, Greene M A, Bagwell CE, Kays D W, Talbert J L 1995 Unilateral pulmonary agenesis, esophageal atresia, and distal tracheo-esophageal fistula. Annals of Thoracic Surgery 59: 511–513
142. Stocker J T, Drake R M, Madewell J E 1978 Cystic and congenital lung disease in the newborn. Pediatric Pathology 4: 93–99
143. Stoek O 1897 Über Angeborene Blasige Missbildung der Lunge. Wiener Klinische Wochenschrift 10: 25–30
144. Sturgess J M, Thompson M W, Lzegledy-Nady E, Turner J A 1986 Genetic aspects of inmotile cilia syndrome. American Journal of Medical Genetics 25: 149–160
145. Swischuk L E 1979 Primary pulmonary hypoplasia in the neonate. Journal of Pediatrics 95: 573–578
146. Swischuk L E 1979 Bilateral pulmonary hypoplasia in the neonate. American Journal of Roentgenology 133: 1057–1063
147. Taguchi T, Suita S, Yamanouchi T et al 1995 Antenatal diagnosis and surgical management of congenital cystic adenomatoid malformation of the lung. Fetal Diagnosis and Therapy 10: 400–407
148. Thibeault D W 1985 Neonatal pulmonary hypoplasia with premature rupture of the fetal membranes and oligohydramnios. Journal of Pediatrics 107: 273–277
149. Thompson J, Forfar J O 1958 Regional obstructive emphysema in infancy. Archives of Disease in Childhood 33: 97–102
150. Thompson P, Greenough A, Blott M, Nicolaides K 1990 Chronic respiratory morbidity following PROM. Archives of Disease in Childhood 65: 878–880
151. Thompson P J, Greenough A, Dykes E, Nicolaides K H 1993 Impaired respiratory function in infants with anterior abdominal wall defects. Journal of Pediatric Surgery 28: 664–666.
152. Thompson P J, Greenough A, Nicolaides K H 1992 Lung volume measured by functional residual capacity in infants following first trimester amniocentesis or chorion villus sampling. British Journal of Obstetrics and Gynaecology 99: 479–482
153. Thompson P J, Greenough A, Nicolaides K H 1992 Respiratory function in infancy following pleuro-amniotic shunting. Fetal Diagnosis and Therapy 8: 79–83
154. Thorpe-Beeston J G, Nicolaides K H 1994 Cystic adenomatoid malformation of the lung: prenatal diagnosis and outcome. Prenatal Diagnosis 14: 677–688
155. Todd D W, Tinguely S J, Norberg W J 1986 A thoracic expansion technique for Jeune's asphyxiating thoracic dystrophy. Journal of Pediatric Surgery, 21: 161–163
156. Van Reempts P, Kegelaers B, Van Dam K, Van Overmeire B 1993 Neonatal outcome after very prolonged and premature rupture of membranes. American Journal of Perinatology 10: 288–291
157. Vergani P, Ghidini A, Locatelli A et al 1994 Risk factors for pulmonary hypoplasia in second-trimester premature rupture of membranes. American Journal of Obstetrics and Gynecology 170: 1359–1364
158. Vilos G A, McLeod W J, Carmichael L, Probert C, Harding P G R 1984 Absence or impaired response of fetal breathing movements to intravenous glucose is associated with pulmonary hypoplasia in congenital myotonic dystrophy. American Journal of Obstetrics and Gynecology 148: 558–562
159. Vyas H, Hopkin I E, Milner A D 1982 Amniocentesis and fetal lung development. Archives of Disease in Childhood 52: 627–628
160. Walker J, Cudmore R E 1990 Respiratory problems and cystic adenomatoid malformation of lung. Archives of Disease in Childhood 65: 649–650
161. Weinbaum P J, Bors-Koefoed R, Green K W, Prenatt L 1989 Antenatal sonographic findings in a case of intra-abdominal pulmonary sequestration. Obstetrics and Gynecology 73: 860–862
162. Whitelaw A, Evans A, Corrin B 1981 Immotile cilia syndrome: a new cause of neonatal respiratory distress. Archives of Disease in Childhood 56: 432–435
163. Wiebicke W, Pasterkamp H 1988 Long term continuous positive airway pressure in a child with asphyxiating thoracic dystrophy. Pediatric Pulmonology 4: 54–58
164. Wigglesworth J S, Desai R 1981 Use of DNA estimation for growth assessment in normal and hypoplastic fetal lungs. Archives of Disease in Childhood 56: 601–605
165. Wigglesworth J S, Desai R 1982 Is fetal respiratory function a major determinant of perinatal survival? Lancet i: 264–247
166. Wigglesworth J S, Winson R M L, Bartlett K 1977 Influence of the central nervous system on fetal lung development. Archives of Disease in Childhood 52: 965–967
167. Williams A J, Vawter G, Reid L M 1984 Lung structure in asphyxiating thoracic dystrophy. Archives of Pathology and Laboratory Medicine 108: 658–661
168. Wockel W, Heller K, Volmer I 1986 Congenital unilateral pulmonary lymphangiectasis. Deutsche Medzinische Wochenschrift 111: 264–267
169. Wohl M E B, Griscom N T, Schuster S R, Zwerdling R G, Strieder D 1973 Lung growth and function following repair of congenital diaphragmatic hernia. Pediatric Research 7: 424–430

Part 6

Diaphragmatic hernia

Mark Davenport

INTRODUCTION

A number of diaphragmatic abnormalities may present with respiratory problems during infancy, the most common being a posterolateral congenital diaphragmatic hernia. This is usually associated with severe lung hypoplasia and, despite many advances in its management, still has a high mortality. Anterior diaphragmatic hernias are smaller and tend to present later in infancy, often with gastrointestinal symptoms alone. Eventration of the diaphragm is a condition in which the cupola becomes thinned, stretched and immobile but yet is still intact. Some degree of respiratory impairment is seen in most of these cases.

CONGENITAL POSTEROLATERAL DIAPHRAGMATIC HERNIA

In 1848 the Czech anatomist Vincent Bochdalek described bowel herniation through the posterior part of the diaphragm, attributing it to the effects of an inverted fetus and rupture of the lumbocostal membrane.[9] Although such posterolateral hernias are still widely known by the eponym Bochdalek's hernia, he was certainly not the first to describe this type of diaphragmatic defect. Detailed reports of CDH in both children[39] and adults[11] had been published previously.

The embryological development of the diaphragm is complex (pp. 125–126): its mesenchyme is derived from the septum transversum and the dorsal mesentery of the oesophagus, and its muscular component from the innermost muscle layer of the thoracic cage and descending cervical myoblasts.[45] The nerve supply to this muscle is via the phrenic nerve (C3,4,5). There is a communication between the pleural and the peritoneal cavities (the pleuroperitoneal canal) up to the 8th week of gestation, and the most widely held view of the aetiology of CDH is that there is a failure to close this. Secondary migration of viscera then occurs into the hemithorax and interferes with the developing lung bud.

An important alternative hypothesis has also been advanced from observations using a nitrophen-induced model of CDH in animal embryos.[40,45] This suggests that lung hypoplasia is actually the primary problem in embryogenesis, and that the diaphragmatic defect and intrathoracic movement of viscera occur as a secondary event.

ANATOMY AND PATHOPHYSIOLOGY (Fig. 29.94)

The diaphragmatic defect occurs in the posterolateral segment, although it may range from a simple muscular slit to complete agenesis.[70] Left-sided hernias account for about 80% of most series.[18,29,61,69] Bilateral CDH occurs rarely and is associated with an awful prognosis.[7,14] In left-sided hernias the hemithorax contains herniated bowel, stomach, spleen, and often part of the left lobe of the liver. The herniated bowel is inevitably malrotated because of its abnormal development, although consequent duodenal obstruction is uncommon. A thin, almost translucent hernial sac occurs in about 20% of cases. Right-sided hernias usually contain the right lobe of the liver, and because of its volume this tends to plug the defect and may minimize herniation of other viscera.

Some degree of lung hypoplasia occurs with virtually all diaphragmatic hernias[15] (p. 638). This is most obvious on the ipsilateral side, where perhaps only a nubbin of tissue might remain, but it is also seen on the contralateral side. Compared to normal term lungs there is an absolute decrease in lung weight and volume and a decrease in compliance. The number of bronchial generations is reduced and true alveoli, which should start to be seen by 34 weeks' gestation, are uncommon. Most terminal air spaces are therefore still in the saccular phase of development. Along with an absolute decrease in lung tissue there is a reduction in the total number of preacinar pulmonary vessels, although the ratio of capillaries per alveolus is retained. The pulmonary and

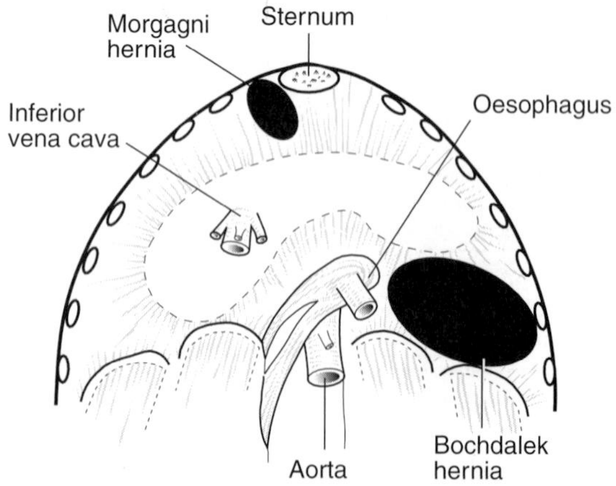

Fig. 29.94 Schematic illustration of the anatomy of congenital diaphragmatic hernia: posterolateral hernia of Bochdalek and anterior hernia of Morgagni.

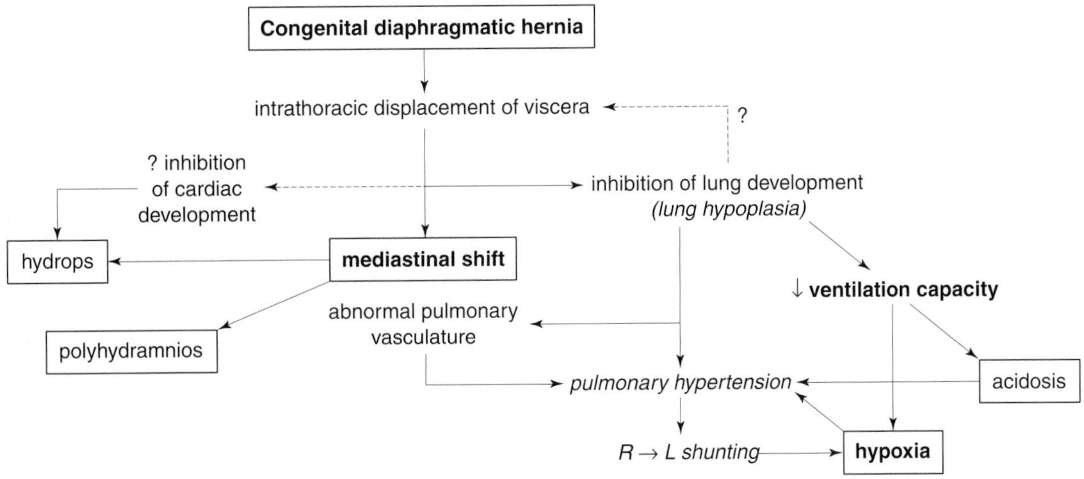

Fig. 29.95 Pathophysiology of congenital diaphragmatic hernia. Pulmonary hypertension, R–L shunting and hypoxia are the characteristic features of PPHN.

intra-acinar arteries have an abnormally high smooth muscle content, although it is unclear why this should be so. A CDH may also cause changes in the developing cardiovascular system. For instance, the left ventricle, interventricular septum and atria have all been shown to be smaller, both in age-matched human controls and in the experimental CDH lamb model.[42,67] This may simply be due to direct compression by herniated viscera, as right-sided hernias have been shown to cause diminution of the right rather than the left ventricle.

The pathophysiological sequence that explains some of the clinical features of a CDH is illustrated in Figure 29.95. There is also an exaggerated response of the abnormally muscularized arterial resistance vessels to hypoxia, acidosis and hypercarbia, which causes in turn pulmonary hypertension and shunting of blood at several different levels from the right to the left side of the heart – PPHN (p. 527).

DEMOGRAPHY

The prevalence of CDH at birth has been estimated from 1 in 2000 to 1 in 5000, and does not appear to have any predilection for race or geographical area.[14,60,73] The sex ratio is equal, although right-sided defects may be more common in males.[7] Although most CDHs are sporadic, with no known cause, there may be a genetic component in a small number as there are reports of CDH in twins and families.[20,51]

ASSOCIATIONS

Although CDH was once thought of as an isolated anomaly, more accurate studies (which include stillbirths and intrauterine deaths) and the advent of widespread prenatal ultrasound have shown this to be incorrect.[7,33,69,73] About 30–50% of diagnosed fetuses will have a further anomaly,[73] although because of intrauterine deaths, terminations and stillbirths this falls to about 20–30% in liveborn infants.

Various anomalies may be found, including chromosomal anomalies (e.g. Turner syndrome and trisomies 13, 18 and 21), major CNS malformations (e.g. anencephaly, neural tube defects) and most types of congenital cardiac defects (e.g. VSD, aortic coarctation, tetralogy of Fallot, hypoplastic left heart and transposition of the great vessels).[7,33,73] Similarly, there is also a wide range of renal anomalies (e.g. agenesis and hydronephrosis) and, in males, undescended testes.[7]

Fryns syndrome is characterized by a diaphragmatic hernia in an infant with an abnormal facies, distal limb anomalies, undescended testes in males and various gut and genitourinary anomalies.[25,48]

CLINICAL FEATURES

Antenatal ultrasound diagnosis of a diaphragmatic hernia has been possible for well over a decade now.[20] The specific features include bowel loops, and liver or, more usually, stomach seen in the transverse four-chamber view within the thorax. Secondary features include mediastinal shift, hydrops fetalis and, most commonly, polyhydramnios. Right-sided defects are more difficult to diagnose as the herniated fetal liver has a similar echogenicity to fetal lung.

The typical postnatal presentation is of increasing respiratory distress and cyanosis shortly after birth in a term infant. There are decreased breath sounds and air entry on the side of the hernia, with a shift of the trachea and cardiac impulse to the opposite side. The abdomen has a flat or even scaphoid appearance, as much of the viscera have already been displaced to the chest cavity.

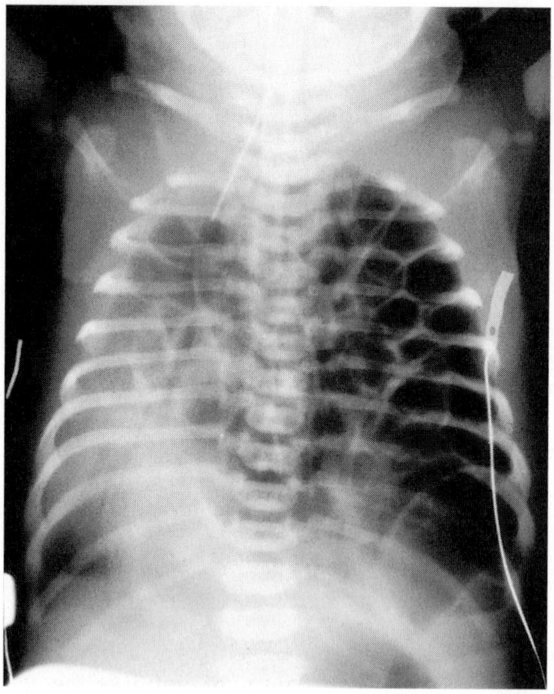

Fig. 29.96 Chest radiograph of infant at 1 hour of life, showing left diaphragmatic hernia, displacement of air-filled viscera into the hemithorax, and a marked shift of mediastinum and heart.

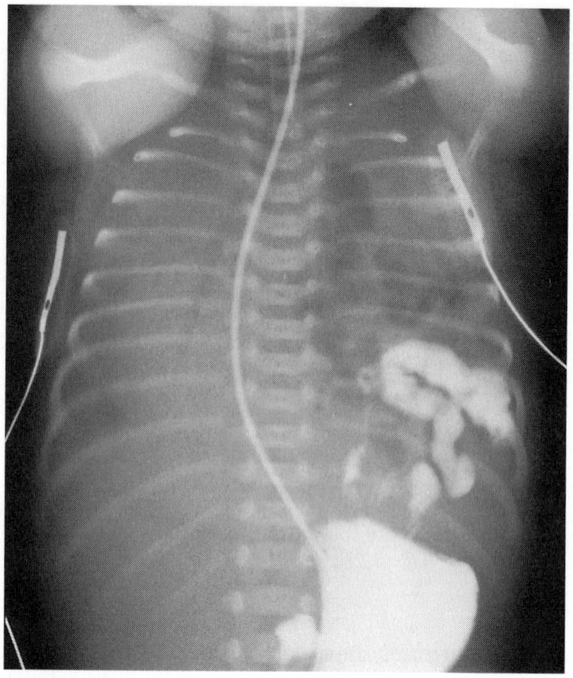

Fig. 29.97 Chest radiograph of infant with contrast medium in the stomach and small intestine, the latter lying within the left hemithorax.

A chest radiograph is diagnostic in most infants and will show air-filled loops of bowel within the hemithorax, often with severe mediastinal displacement (Fig. 29.96). Occasionally there may be confusion with the radiographic appearance of a cystic adenomatoid malformation of the lung, which may also present with respiratory distress. This can be distinguished on the plain film by noting the normal abdominal gas pattern and diaphragmatic integrity, or more accurately by introducing radio-opaque contrast material into the stomach and proximal gastrointestinal tract (Fig. 29.97). An ultrasound scan can also differentiate these conditions. Occasionally, air does not enter the proximal bowel because of rapid intubation and resuscitation in the delivery room, especially if there has been an antenatal diagnosis. The usual radiographic appearance is then of complete opacification on the side of the hernia – a 'whiteout' (Fig. 29.98).

About 5% of infants with CDH will present beyond the first 24 hours of life with failure to thrive, recurrent chest infections, a pleural effusion, or even as an incidental finding on a chest X-ray.[49] It is important to note that a previously normal chest X-ray does not exclude a CDH. There is an interesting association between the delayed presentation of a right-sided diaphragmatic hernia and GBS septicaemia.[4,59] Such infants present with respiratory distress and opacification of the right lung. Visceral herniation only occurs in the recovery phase of the illness, being diagnosed on a chest X-ray or by CT.

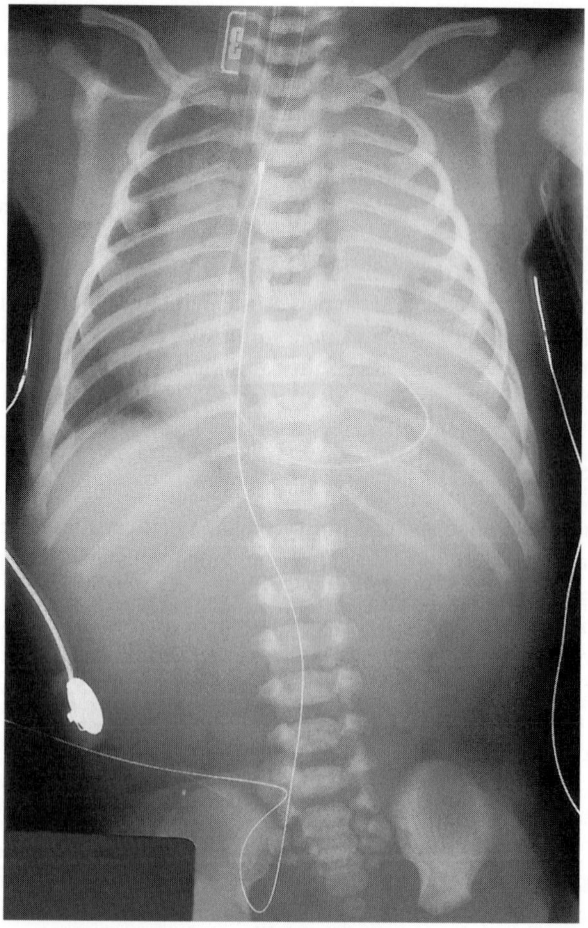

Fig. 29.98 Chest radiograph of early appearance of diaphragmatic hernia, with a 'whiteout' on the left side.

MANAGEMENT

Antenatal

An increasing proportion of infants with CDH are diagnosed in utero by screening ultrasonography during the second trimester. An amniocentesis should be offered, and if a chromosomal anomaly is found most obstetricians would recommend termination as this is an invariably lethal combination.

It is important that these infants are delivered in regional centres where there are the necessary obstetric, intensive care and neonatal surgical facilities. We tend to induce vaginal delivery at about 38 weeks' gestation to minimize the risks of unintended early labour and delivery in a peripheral unit.

Medical

Infants with CDH presenting within 24 hours of birth are at a considerable risk of death and should be endotracheally intubated, paralysed and ventilated. Prolonged attempts at bagging using a facemask can be dangerous and should be avoided, specifically because of the detrimental effects of intestinal distension. A large-bore nasogastric tube (e.g. 8 French gauge) should also be passed to decompress the stomach and small bowel. Neonatal resuscitation should then proceed on conventional lines. Initially, the main problem is hypoventilation due to lung hypoplasia, and there will be a proportion of infants in whom this is so extreme as to be incompatible with life, and who will die in the delivery room. Initial peak inflation pressures should be limited to 25 cmH_2O (to reduce barotrauma in small, stiff lungs), with rates of 60–80 per minute. PEEP is kept low to achieve maximum alveolar ventilation. These infants should be paralysed (e.g. vecuronium 0.1–1.3 mg kg^{-1} h^{-1}) and have analgesia (e.g. fentanyl 2–8 mg kg^{-1} h^{-1}).

Most infants will respond to medical measures and achieve acceptable blood gases. This has been described as the 'honeymoon' phase, as these infants can be deceptively well for a period before becoming increasingly unstable, often with severe hypoxic episodes, hypercarbia and an uncorrectable acidosis. The dominant pathophysiological problem in this phase is pulmonary hypertension and right-to-left shunting. Such PPHN can be diagnosed clinically by the typical rapid swings in oxygenation, and confirmed by measuring pre- and post-ductal arterial oxygen levels. Echocardiography during this period will show an enlarged right heart with pulmonary and tricuspid regurgitation and a right–left shunt at the foramen ovale and ductus arteriosus.

Newer ventilation techniques, such as HFOV and HFJV, have been used in infants with diaphragmatic hernia.[12,43] There is also a range of pharmacological agents which have been used to treat the PPHN associated with a CDH, including tolazoline,[68] prostacyclin,[13] nitroprusside and, most recently, nitric oxide.[24,44] These options are discussed fully on pages 532–535 and pages 568–572. There is also a functional surfactant deficit in infants with CDH, and benefit has been shown from using exogenous surfactant both in experimental models and when administered to high-risk neonates prior to the first breath.[27,28]

Surgical

Nowadays there is no role for early (within 24 hours of birth) surgical repair. Abdominal replacement of the viscera and repair of the hernial defect causes a marked reduction in lung compliance and detrimental fluid shifts,[63] and should therefore be carried out only when the infant has achieved a period of cardiorespiratory stability (of at least 24 hours) with acceptable blood gases on conventional ventilation (e.g. $F_IO_2 < 0.5$, $PO_2 > 8$ kPa [60 mmHg]).[18]

European paediatric surgical centres were the first to delay surgical repair, during the early 1980s,[13,17,18,64] and this seems to be prevailing in North America.[47,56] Although early reports did not show a clear survival advantage, probably because of the small numbers involved, they did show that the concept was not harmful. The largest single-centre experience with delayed surgery was reported from Manchester, where 86 high-risk infants had a survival rate of just over 70%.[18]

The surgical repair of a CDH is performed through a subcostal incision. The displaced viscera are removed from the hemithorax and returned to the abdomen. A hernial sac, if found, should be excised to allow a tension-free musculoaponeurotic closure. The posterior margin of the defect may not be apparent initially and most have to be developed from the posterior abdominal wall. Primary closure is possible in about 75% of cases, but in those where this is impossible because of excessive tension or agenesis then other techniques have to be used. A patch of artificial material or a rotation flap from an adjacent muscle group can be used to repair the defect.[8] A chest tube left in the empty hemithorax is not necessary, and may be dangerous if used with suction as the hypoplastic lung may overexpand and rupture.

The role of extracorporeal membrane oxygenation

Extracorporeal membrane oxygenation is now an option for infants with CDH if conventional methods of medical therapy are failing. The concept behind this technique is simple: near-total cardiopulmonary support for a prolonged period of time (in practice up to 10–14 days). ECMO was developed in the USA in the 1970s,[26] but has only recently become available in the UK because of the perceived lack of controlled data from its early trials.[5,58] Unfortunately, even the recent UK Collaborative ECMO trial[71] failed to recruit enough infants in the CDH subgroup for the differences in survival to be statistically significant. The North American ECMO experience suggests that a survival rate of about 40–60% will be found in infants with CDH, which is significantly worse than for other indications in neonates (e.g. MAS, p. 572).[36,46,65]

The indications,[46,55] technique[5] and morbidity[53] associated with ECMO are fully discussed in Part 2 (pp. 571–572). Surgical repair of the hernia may be performed while on ECMO but should be deferred until the infant has improved enough to be ready for decannulation and cessation of heparinization.[78]

PREDICTION OF PROGNOSIS

It is logical to try and find specific or measurable features which will predict outcome in diaphragmatic hernia because of the high mortality of this disease and the range of possible treatment options. A number of studies have assessed various factors as being of prognostic value, and can be divided into antenatal and postnatal.

Antenatal

In general, the earlier in gestation the diagnosis is made the worse the outcome. For instance, only 42% survived from a cohort of 83 fetuses with isolated CDH diagnosed before 24 weeks' gestation, compared to all of a cohort of 10 fetuses diagnosed after 24 weeks.[33] The development of polyhydramnios has also been a poor prognostic feature in some series,[3] although not in all.[21,66] The fetal stomach is found in the chest in most cases, but if it is found within the abdomen this seems to be a good prognostic feature.[21]

Associated congenital cardiac anomalies are of course indicative of a very poor outcome,[69] but a number of groups have also looked at echocardiographic features of the fetal heart as a measure of lung hypoplasia or pulmonary vascular anomalies. The ratio of left-to-right ventricular internal measurements[21,66] and the ratio of aortic to pulmonary artery diameters[21] have both been put forward as valuable prognostic features in isolated diaphragmatic hernias. Both these indices reflect left ventricular underdevelopment.

Postnatal

For those infants who are not diagnosed antenatally, the age at presentation is important. The minority who present after 24 hours of life should have the prospect of a 100% survival. The earlier the symptoms, the worse the outcome. Survival is also worse in premature infants and those of low birthweight.[36,46]

Achieving normal blood gases is the final result of an effective pulmonary system, and the degree to which this is successful has been used as a prognostic factor. Thus, if a postductal $PaCO_2$ of < 5.5 kPa (40 mmHg)[10] or a postductal PaO_2 of > 13 kPa (100 mmHg)[57,76] can be achieved with conventional ventilation, this suggests adequate lung tissue for survival and a good prognosis. In one recent series there was a survival of 91% in those infants who had achieved a postductal PaO_2 of > 13 kPa (100 mmHg), compared to only 7% survival in those who did not.[76] The amount of ventilation required to achieve such blood gases can also be incorporated into a variety of ventilation indices (Table 29.40).[10,37,74,76]

Table 29.40 Indices of ventilation

oxygenation index (OI) =

$$\frac{\text{mean airway pressure (cmH}_2\text{O)} \times F_IO_2 \times 100}{PaO_2\ \text{(mmHg)}}$$

ventilation index (VI) =

$$\text{respiratory rate (bpm)} \times \text{mean airway pressure (cmH}_2\text{O)}$$

At present it is not possible to measure the critical lung mass in neonates directly, although there have been attempts to measure some indirect indices of lung function (e.g. compliance and functional residual capacity) early in the postnatal period in these infants.[23,63] One group has shown that a preoperative compliance lower than 0.18 ml cmH_2O^{-1} kg^{-1} was associated with a poor outcome.[23]

Echocardiography has been used to assess the degree of PPHN.[34,35] Some echocardiographic variables may also have value when performed sequentially to show the improvement in pulmonary vascular stability and, perhaps, the most appropriate physiological time for surgery.[61]

The size of the diaphragm defect itself has been related to prognosis. Diaphragmatic agenesis[46,70] particularly, and all those where a patch is needed to repair the defect,[74] have been associated with a poorer outcome.

OUTCOME IN CONGENITAL DIAPHRAGMATIC HERNIA

No surgical series of diaphragmatic hernias has ever been able to emulate Robert Gross's first report of 100% survival in seven infants and children in 1946.[30] This paradox is of course entirely due to preselection, as only the less affected infants used to survive to reach paediatric surgical centres. Table 29.41 illustrates recent survival statistics from a number of different centres throughout the world.

Surviving infants have usually required a prolonged stay in intensive care, often with periods of hypoxia, hypercarbia and acidosis. Although early studies suggested that long-term complications in survivors were minimal, this was probably because of selection of a smaller but better-'quality' cohort. Currently, more

Table 29.41 Surgical outcome in infants with high-risk congenital diaphragmatic hernia

Author Centre	*n*	Period of study	Options available	Survival (%)
Heiss et al[36]	16	1974–81	–	50
(Ann Arbor, USA)	34	1982–87	ECMO	76
Charlton et al[18]	56	1976–83	Immediate repair	55
(Manchester, UK)	86	1983–89	delayed	71
Goh et al[29] (London, UK)	69	1987–90	Delayed repair	66
West et al[74]	65	1975–87	–	43
(Indianapolis, USA)	46	1987–92	ECMO & delayed repair	67
Bos et al[13] (Rotterdam, Holland)	46	1986–89	Delayed repair	43
Sweed et al[69] (Dublin, Ireland)	116*	1973–90		23

*Unselected, includes infants not reaching surgical centres.

marginal survival is possible and the incidence of long-term problems is higher.[54]

Pulmonary function

Dramatic changes occur in lung structure after surgical repair, although not immediately. Lung weight and volumes do increase measurably after about 3 weeks, but only after an early decrease in compliance in the early postoperative period.[63] Histologically there is an increase in the number of alveoli, and a decrease in muscularization of the interacinar arteries, although there is no actual change in bronchiolar airway generation.[6] The radiographic appearance of the chest does return to normal, although there are persisting anomalies in tested lung function (typically FEV_1 and FVC).[19] The progressive improvement in ventilation can be assessed using ventilation–perfusion scans, and such studies show particularly a long-term persistence of ipsilateral perfusion defects.[41]

Gastrointestinal function

The principal gastrointestinal problem is one of acid reflux caused by distortion of the gastro-oesophageal junction and crura; this may occur in up to 40% of survivors.[46] Intensive medical treatment (e.g. antacids, H_2 receptor blockers and cisapride) should be tried, although because of the anatomical basis for reflux, surgical correction (e.g. a Nissen antireflux procedure) may be necessary.

Neurological

There is a long-term worry of neurological impairment in survivors, which is presumed to be due to neonatal hypoxia and periods of cardiovascular instability. One study of selected high-risk long-term survivors found a major neurological handicap in two of 23 children, although there was no clear relationship between poor outcome and measured indices of hypoxia and acidosis during the neonatal period.[22]

INNOVATIONS IN THERAPY

Antenatal surgery

Antenatal repair of in-utero CDH is a controversial technique offered at the Fetal Treatment Center at the University of California, San Francisco.[1,32] In one recent report of its experience between 1989 and 1991, 61 antenatally diagnosed fetuses were referred for consideration of surgery.[33] Second-trimester surgery was attempted in 14 fetuses, and of these five died during the operation: three shortly after closure of the hysterotomy, with two being born prematurely but dying. Only four survived to term and eventually to leave hospital. The technical problems of intrauterine surgery and repair of a CDH are formidable, with a high risk of inducing preterm labour. For this concept to be at all successful, the fetus must be returned to an intrauterine environment until near term to allow reversal of lung hypoplasia.

A rather more elegant technique of antenatal therapy has recently been proposed: intrauterine tracheal occlusion, or PLUG (plug the lung until it grows).[1,38] This concept arose from the clinical observation that the lungs in congenital laryngeal atresia are grossly hyperplastic and even cause inversion of the domes of the diaphragm – the very opposite to the lungs in CDH.[75] Such pulmonary hyperplasia arises because fetal lungs are net fluid producers, and occlusion therefore results in lung fluid retention. Experimental ligation of the trachea can mimic laryngeal atresia and has been studied in a variety of animal models of diaphragmatic hernia[2,38] and lung hypoplasia.[77] In the human fetus intrauterine endoscopy is envisaged to allow placement of an occlusion plug within the trachea, and hence gradual reduction of the herniated viscera and, hopefully, reversibility of pulmonary hypoplasia.

Lung transplantation

This is an obvious therapeutic concept for irreversible lung hypoplasia which has been reported in a ventilated infant with a right-sided CDH.[72] The upper and lower lobes of a right lung from a 6-week-old donor were successfully transplanted; successful weaning and survival were achieved.

ANTERIOR DIAPHRAGMATIC HERNIAS

The Italian anatomist Giovanni Morgagni first described a hernia occurring between the costal and the sternal

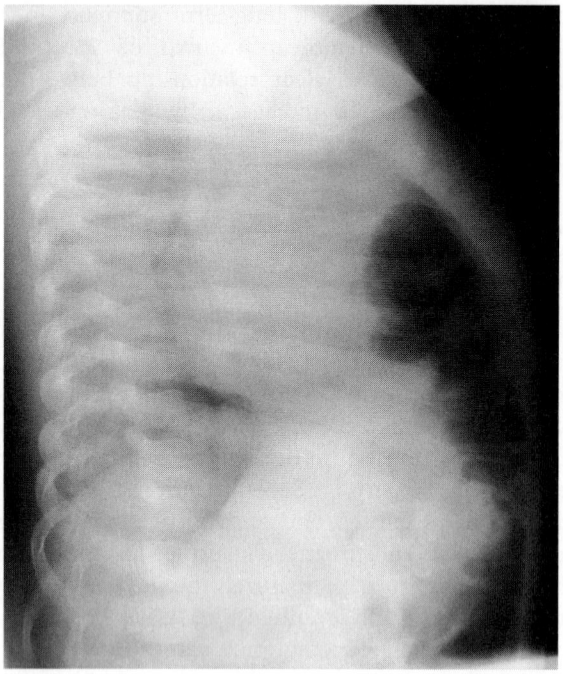

Fig. 29.99 Lateral chest radiograph of infant who presented with intermittent vomiting, showing anterior Morgagni hernia.

muscle origins of the diaphragm in a series published in 1769.[52] There is usually a hernial sac, and over 90% occur on the right side (Fig. 29.99). Compared to posterolateral defects there is seldom any associated lung hypoplasia, and consequently symptoms are mild. There may be other anomalies in a minority of cases, including extralobar lung sequestrations and congenital cardiac defects. Morgagni hernias have also been described in Down syndrome.[31]

Most of the clinical features are due to incarceration of part of the bowel (commonly the transverse colon) and include vomiting, failure to thrive and intestinal obstruction. Some may be found incidentally on a chest radiograph. Surgical repair is performed through an upper abdominal approach and is usually straightforward.

The pentalogy of Cantrell is a rare syndrome of an anterior diaphragmatic defect with pericardial defects, a short sternum, exomphalos and major intracardiac anomalies.[16,50] The defect itself differs anatomically from a Morgagni hernia and has been attributed to a defective septum transversum.

DIAPHRAGMATIC EVENTRATION

Eventration can be congenital or acquired. Congenital absence of anterior horn cells may be responsible (Werdnig–Hoffman disease), with others being due to intrauterine infection (e.g. rubella, cytomegalovirus) or as part of a more generalized chromosomal anomaly (e.g. trisomies 13–15 or 18). These anomalies are usually left-sided and may even be bilateral.[62] Diaphragmatic denervation due to phrenic nerve injury may be related to birth injury (when it is often associated with brachial plexus injury) or thoracic surgery (e.g. patent ductus arteriosus ligation).

Eventration may be asymptomatic, but most present in infancy with respiratory distress, recurrent chest infections or bronchiectasis. Paradoxical movement of the hemidiaphragm causes mediastinal shift, basal atelectasis and futile movement of air from the ipsilateral to the contralateral lung.

Chest radiography (PA and lateral views), and fluoroscopic screening should establish the diagnosis, and radionuclide ventilation scans may allow assessment of the degree of ventilatory impairment. The management of eventration depends on the symptoms; if asymptomatic an expectant course should be pursued. If there is respiratory distress, however, then a more aggressive approach should be followed. Positive-pressure endotracheal ventilation overcomes any immediate problems, and once the infant is stable he should undergo definitive surgical correction. This is achieved by radial plication of the diaphragm by either an abdominal or a thoracic approach. The taut plicated diaphragm increases breathing capacity and tidal volume.

REFERENCES

1. Adzick N S, Harrison M R 1994 Fetal surgical therapy. Lancet 343: 897–901
2. Adzick N S, Harrison M R, Glick P L 1984 Experimental pulmonary hypoplasia and oligohydramnios: relative contributions of lung fluid and breathing movements. Journal of Pediatric Surgery 19: 658–665
3. Adzick N S, Harrison M R, Glick P L, Nakayama D K, Manning F A, de Lorimier A A 1985 Diaphragmatic hernia in the fetus: prenatal diagnosis and outcome in 94 cases. Journal of Pediatric Surgery 20: 357–361
4. Banagale R C, Watters J H 1983 Delayed right-sided diaphragmatic hernia following group B streptococcal infection. Human Pathology 14: 67–69
5. Bartlett R H, Roloff D W, Cornell R G, Andrews A F, Dillon P W, Zwischenberger J B 1985 Extracorporeal circulation in neonatal respiratory failure: a prospective randomised study. Pediatrics 76: 479–487
6. Beals D A, Schloo B L, Vacanti J P, Reid L M, Wilson J M 1992 Pulmonary growth and remodelling in infants with high-risk congenital diaphragmatic hernia. Journal of Pediatric Surgery 27: 997–1002
7. Benjamin D R, Juul S, Siebert J R 1988 Congenital posterolateral diaphragmatic hernia: associated malformations. Journal of Pediatric Surgery 23; 899–903
8. Bianchi A, Doig C M, Cohen S J 1983 The reverse latissimus dorsi flap for congenital diaphragmatic hernia. Journal of Pediatric Surgery 18: 560–563
9. Bochdalek V A 1848 Einige Betrachtungen uber die Entstehung des angeborenen Zwerchfellbruches. Als Betrag zur pathologischen Anatomie der Hernien. Vierteljahrschrift fur die praktische Heilkunde. 19: 89
10. Bohn D, Tamura M, Perrin D, Barker G, Rabinovitch M 1987 Ventilatory predictors of pulmonary hypoplasia in congenital diaphragmatic hernia, confirmed by morphological assessment. Journal of Pediatrics 111: 423–431
11. Bonet T 1679 De Suffocatione Observatio XLI. Suffocatio excitata a tenium intestorum vulnus diaphragmatis, in thoracem ingrestu. Sepuhuchretum sive anatomia procteia et cadaveribus morbo denatus. Geneva

12. Boros S J, Mammel M C, Coleman J M et al 1985 Neonatal high frequency ventilation: four years' outcome. Pediatrics 75: 657–663
13. Bos A P, Tibboel D, Koot V C M, Hazebroek F W J, Molenaar J C 1993 Persistent pulmonary hypertension in high risk congenital diaphragmatic patients: incidence and vasodilator therapy. Journal of Pediatric Surgery 28: 1463–1465
14. Butler N, Claireaux A E 1962 Congenital diaphragmatic hernia as a cause of perinatal mortality. Lancet i: 659–663
15. Campanale R P, Rowland R H 1955 Hypoplasia of the lung associated with congenital diaphragmatic hernia. Annals of Surgery 142: 176–189
16. Cantrell J R, Haller J A, Ravitch M M 1958 A syndrome of congenital defects involving the abdominal wall, sternum, diaphragm, pericardium and heart. Surgery Gynecology and Obstetrics 107: 602–614
17. Cartlidge P H T, Mann N P, Kapilla L 1986 Preoperative stabilisation in congenital diaphragmatic hernia. Archives of Disease in Childhood 61: 1226–1228
18. Charlton A, Bruce J B, Davenport M 1991 Timing of surgery in congenital diaphragmatic hernia: low mortality after pre-operative stabilisation. Anaesthesia 46: 820–823
19. Chatrath R R, E I Shafie M, Jones R S 1971 Fate of hypoplastic lungs after repair of congenital diaphragmatic hernia. Archives of Disease in Childhood 46: 633–635
20. Crane J P 1979 Familial diaphragmatic hernia: prenatal diagnostic approach and analysis of twelve families. Clinical Genetics 16: 244–252
21. Crawford D C, Wright V M, Drake D P, Allan L D 1989 Fetal diaphragmatic hernia: the value of fetal echocardiography in the prediction of postnatal outcome. British Journal of Obstetrics and Gynaecology 96: 705–710
22. Davenport M, Rivlin E, D'Souza S W, Bianchi A 1992 Neurodevelopmental outcome following delayed surgery for congenital diaphragmatic hernia. Archives of Disease in Childhood 67: 1353–1356
23. Dimitriou G, Greenough A, Chan V, Gamsu H R, Howard E R, Nicolaides K H 1995 Prognostic indicators in congenital diaphragmatic hernia. Journal of Pediatric Surgery 30: 1694–1697
24. Finer N N, Etches P C, Kamstra B, Tierney A J, Peliowski A, Ryan C A 1994 Inhaled nitric oxide in infants referred for extracorporeal membrane oxygenation: dose response. Journal of Pediatrics 124: 302–308
25. Fryns J P, Moerman F, Goddeeris P et al 1979 A new lethal syndrome with cloudy corneae, diaphagmatic defects and distal limb deformities. Human Genetics 50: 65–70
26. German J C, Gazzaniga A B, Ragnar A 1977 Management of pulmonary insufficiency in diaphragmatic hernia using extracorporeal circulation with a membrane oxygenator. Journal of Pediatric Surgery 12: 905–912
27. Glick P L, Leach C L, Besner G E et al 1992 Pathophysiology of congenital diaphragmatic hernia III: exogenous surfactant therapy for the high-risk neonate with CDH. Journal of Pediatric Surgery 27: 866–869
28. Glick P L, Stannard V, Leach C L et al 1992 The fetal lamb CDH model is surfactant deficient. Journal of Pediatric Surgery 27: 382–388
29. Goh D W, Drake D P, Brereton R J, Kiely E M, Spitz L 1992 Delayed surgery for congenital diaphragmatic hernia. British Journal of Surgery 79: 644–646
30. Gross R E 1946 Congenital hernia of the diaphragm. American Journal of Diseases of Children 71: 580–592
31. Harris G J, Soper R T, Kimura K K 1993 Foramen of Morgagni hernia in identical twins: is this an inheritable defect? Journal of Pediatric Surgery 28: 177–178
32. Harrison M R, Adzick N S, Flake A W et al 1993 Correction of congenital diaphragmatic hernia in utero: VI. Hard earned lessons. Journal of Pediatric Surgery 28: 1411–1418
33. Harrison M R, Adzick N S, Estes J M, Howell L J 1994 A prospective study of the outcome for fetuses with diaphragmatic hernia. Journal of the American Medical Association 271: 382–384
34. Hasegawa S, Kohno S, Sugiyama T et al 1994 Usefulness of echocardiographic measurement of bilateral pulmonary artery dimensions in congenital diaphragmatic hernia. Journal of Pediatric Surgery 29: 622–624
35. Haugen S, Linker D, Eik-Nes S et al 1991 Congenital diaphragmatic hernia: determination of the optimal time for operation by echocardiographic monitoring of the pulmonary artery pressure. Journal of Pediatric Surgery 26: 560–562
36. Heiss K F, Clark R H 1995 Prediction of mortality in neonates with congenital diaphragmatic hernia treated with extracorporeal membrane oxygenation. Critical Care Medicine 23: 1915–1919
37. Heiss K, Manning P, Oldham K T et al 1989 Reversal of mortality for congenital diaphragmatic hernia. Annals of Surgery 209: 225–230
38. Hedrick M H, Estes K M, Sullivan K M et al 1994 Plug the Lung Until it Grows (PLUG): a new method to treat congenital diaphragmatic hernia in utero. Journal of Pediatric Surgery 29: 612–617
39. Holt C 1701 Child that lived two months with congenital diaphragmatic hernia. Philosophical Transactions 22: 992
40. Iritani I 1984 Experimental study on pathogenesis and embryogenesis of congenital diaphragmatic hernia. Anatomy and Embryology 169: 133–139
41. Jeandot R, Lambert B, Brendel A J, Guyot M, Demarquez J L 1989 Lung ventilation and perfusion scintigraphy in the follow up of repaired congenital diaphragmatic hernia. European Journal of Nuclear Medicine 15: 591–596
42. Karamanoukian H L, Glick P L, Wilcox D, O'Toole S J, Rosman J E, Azizkhan RG 1995 Pathophysiology of congenital diaphragmatic hernia XI: anatomic and biochemical characterisation of the heart in the fetal lamb CDH model. Journal of Pediatric Surgery 30: 925–929
43. Karl S R, Ballantine T V N, Snider M T 1983 High frequency ventilation at rates of 375 to 1800 cycles per minute in four neonates with congenital diaphragmatic hernia. Journal of Pediatric Surgery 18: 822–828
44. Kinsella J P, Neish S R, Ivy D, Shaffer E, Abman S H 1993 Clinical responses to prolonged treatment of persistent pulmonary hypertension of the newborn with low doses of inhaled nitric oxide. Journal of Pediatrics 123: 103–108
45. Kluth D, Tenbrick R, Ekesparre M V et al 1993 The natural history of congenital diaphragmatic hernia and pulmonary hypoplasia in the embryo. Journal of Pediatric Surgery 28: 456–463
46. Lally K P, Paranka M S, Roden J et al 1992 Congenital diaphragmatic hernia, stabilisation and repair on ECMO. Annals of Surgery 216: 569–573
47. Langer J C, Filler R M, Bohn D J et al 1988 Timing of surgery for congenital diaphragmatic hernia: is emergency operation necessary? Journal of Pediatric Surgery 23: 731–734
48. Langer J C, Winthrop A L, Whelan D 1994 Fryns syndrome: a rare familial cause of congenital diaphragmatic hernia. Journal of Pediatric Surgery 29: 1266–1267
49. Malone P S, Brain A J, Kiely S M, Spitz L 1989 Congenital diaphragmatic defects that present late. Archives of Disease in Childhood 64: 1542–1544
50. Milne L W, Moroson A M, Campbell J R, Harrison M W 1984 Pars sternalis diaphragmatic hernia with omphalocele: a report of 2 cases. Journal of Pediatric Surgery 19: 394–397
51. Mishalany H, Gordo J 1986 Congenital diaphragmatic hernia in monozygotic twins. Journal of Pediatric Surgery 21: 372–374
52. Morgagni G B 1769 Seats and causes of disease investigated by anatomy, Vol 3. Translated by B Alexander. Millere and Cadell, London, p 205
53. Nagaraj H S, Mitchell K A, Fallat M E, Groff D B, Cook L N 1992 Surgical complications and procedures in neonates on extracorporeal membrane oxygenation. Journal of Pediatric Surgery 27: 1106–1109
54. Naik S, Greenough A, Zhang Y-X, Davenport M 1996 Prediction of morbidity following congenital diaphragmatic hernia repair. Journal of Pediatric Surgery 31: 1651–1654
55. Newman K D, Anderson K D, Meurs K V et al 1990 Extracorporeal membrane oxygenation and congenital diaphragmatic hernia: should any infant be excluded? Journal of Pediatric Surgery 25: 1048–1053
56. Nio M, Haase G, Kennaugh J, Bui K, Atkinson J B 1994 A prospective randomised trial of delayed versus immediate repair of congenital diaphragmatic hernia. Journal of Pediatric Surgery 29: 618–621
57. O'Rourke P P, Vacanti J P, Crone R K, Fellows K, Lillehei C, Hougen T J 1989 Use of postductal PaO_2 as a predictor of pulmonary vascular hypoplasia in infants with congenital diaphragmatic hernia. Journal of Pediatric Surgery 23: 904–907
58. O'Rourke P P, Crone R K, Vacanti J P et al 1989 Extracorporeal membrane oxygenation and conventional medical therapy in neonates with persistent pulmonary hypertension of the newborn: a prospective randomised study. Pediatrics 84: 957–963
59. Philips A F, Bierny J-P, Crowe CP 1995 Perinatal/neonatal casebooks. Journal of Perinatology 15: 160–162
60. Puri P, Gorman W A 1987 Natural history of congenital diaphragmatic hernia. Implications for early intrauterine surgery. Pediatric Surgery International 2: 327–330

61. Reynolds M, Luck S R, Lappen R 1984 The 'critical' neonate with diaphragmatic hernia: a 21-year perspective. Journal of Pediatric Surgery 19: 364–369
62. Rodgers B M, Hawks P 1986 Bilateral congenital eventration of the diaphragm. Successful management. Journal of Pediatric Surgery 21: 858–864
63. Sakai H, Tamura M, Hosokawa Y, Bryan A C, Barker G A, Bohn D J 1987 The effect of surgical repair on respiratory mechanics in congenital diaphragmatic hernia. Journal of Pediatrics 111: 432–458
64. Shanbhogue L K R, Tam P K H, Ninan G, Lloyd D A 1990 Preoperative stabilisation in congenital diaphragmatic hernia. Archives of Disease in Childhood 65: 1043–1044
65. Shanley C J, Hirschl R B, Schumacher R E et al 1994 Extracorporeal life support for neonatal respiratory failure – a 20 year experience. Annals of Surgery 220: 269–282
66. Sharland G K, Lochhart S M, Heward A J, Allan L D 1992 Prognosis in fetal diaphragmatic hernia. American Journal of Obstetrics and Gynecology 166: 9–13
67. Siebert J R, Haas J E, Beckwith J B 1984 Left ventricular hypoplasia in congenital diaphragmatic hernia. Journal of Pediatric Surgery 19: 567–571
68. Stevens D C, Screiner R L, Bull M J et al 1980 An analysis of tolazoline therapy in the critically ill neonate. Journal of Pediatric Surgery 15: 964–970
69. Sweed Y, Puri P 1993 Congenital diaphragmatic hernia: influence of associated malformations on survival. Archives of Disease in Childhood 69: 68–70
70. Tsang T M, Tam P K H, Dudley N E, Stevens J 1995 Diaphragmatic agenesis as a distinct clinical entity. Journal of Pediatric Surgery 30: 16–18
71. UK Collaborative ECMO Trial Group 1996 UK collaborative randomised trial of neonatal extracorporeal membrane oxygenation. Lancet 248: 75–82
72. Van Meurs K P, Rhine W D, Benitz W E et al 1994 Lobar lung transplantation as a treatment for congenital diaphragmatic hernia. Journal of Pediatric Surgery 29: 1557–1560
73. Wenstrom K D, Weiner C P, Hanson J W 1991 A five year statewide experience with congenital diaphragmatic hernia. American Journal of Obstetrics and Gynecology 165: 838–842
74. West K W, Bengstrom K, Rescorla F J, Engle W A, Grosfeld J L 1992 Delayed surgical repair and ECMO improves survival in congenital diaphragmatic hernia. Annals of Surgery 216: 454–462
75. Wigglesworth J, Hislop A 1987 Fetal lung growth in congenital larnygeal atresia. Pediatric Pathology 7: 515–525
76. Wilson J M, Lund D P, Lillehei C W, Vacanti J P 1991 Congenital diaphragmatic hernia: predictors of severity in the ECMO era. Journal of Pediatric Surgery 26: 1028–1034
77. Wilson J M, DiFiore J W, Peters C A 1993 Experimental fetal tracheal ligation prevents the pulmonary hypoplasia associated with fetal nephrectomy: possible application for congenital diaphragmatic hernia. Journal of Pediatric Surgery 28: 1433–1440
78. Wilson J M, Bower L K, Lund D P 1994 Evolution of the technique of congenital diaphragmatic hernia repair on ECMO. Journal of Pediatric Surgery 29: 1109–1112

Part 7

Airways problems

Roger F. Gray Robert A. Evans

INTRODUCTION

The neonatal mortality rate has fallen dramatically in the last two decades, particularly for infants weighing less than 1500 g (Chapter 1). The idea that newborn babies who fail to breathe should be offered more active treatment than cutaneous stimulation is surprisingly recent. Most contemporary hospital consultants must have breathed spontaneously at birth, because endotracheal intubation and oxygen insufflation was a daring innovation requiring rare skill in the 1950s.

Reviving the newborn with a tube and a few puffs of oxygen was so effective that it led in the 1960s to the desire to maintain respiration in the immature for long periods. Once it was understood how to prevent retrolental fibroplasia there was no constraint on the numbers of infants 'tubed'. To the small numbers of infants with congenital deformities of the airways were added problems acquired as a result of protracted endotracheal intubation. This chapter discusses the congenital deformities and shows how acquired subglottic stenosis may be minimized or, if the worst happens, treated surgically.

DEVELOPMENT OF THE LARYNX AND TRACHEA

At the 28th day of intrauterine life (Fig. 29.100(A)) a groove appears (Fig. 29.100(B)) running from the primitive pharynx to the foregut, where it branches into the lung buds next to the primitive stomach. The groove first doubles itself (Fig. 29.100(C)) and then closes over from the caudal end (Fig. 29.100(D)) to form two tubes (Fig. 29.100(E)). One tube is the developing trachea and the other the oesophagus. Incomplete separation of the passages results in a fistula between the two (p. 771).

By 32 days the 6 mm embryo has a swelling at the cranial end of the groove (the hypobranchial eminence), in which the larynx develops. The epiglottis, arytenoid, thyroid and cricoid cartilages become visible between the 41st and 44th days. These are formed from the cartilage of the fourth, fifth and sixth branchial arches. A cleft larynx (p. 773) is the result of incomplete fusion of the lips of the tracheo-oesophageal wall, and may be viewed as the most superior variety of TOF.

The left and right cartilages of the fourth arch, due to become the arytenoids, adhere to each other until the

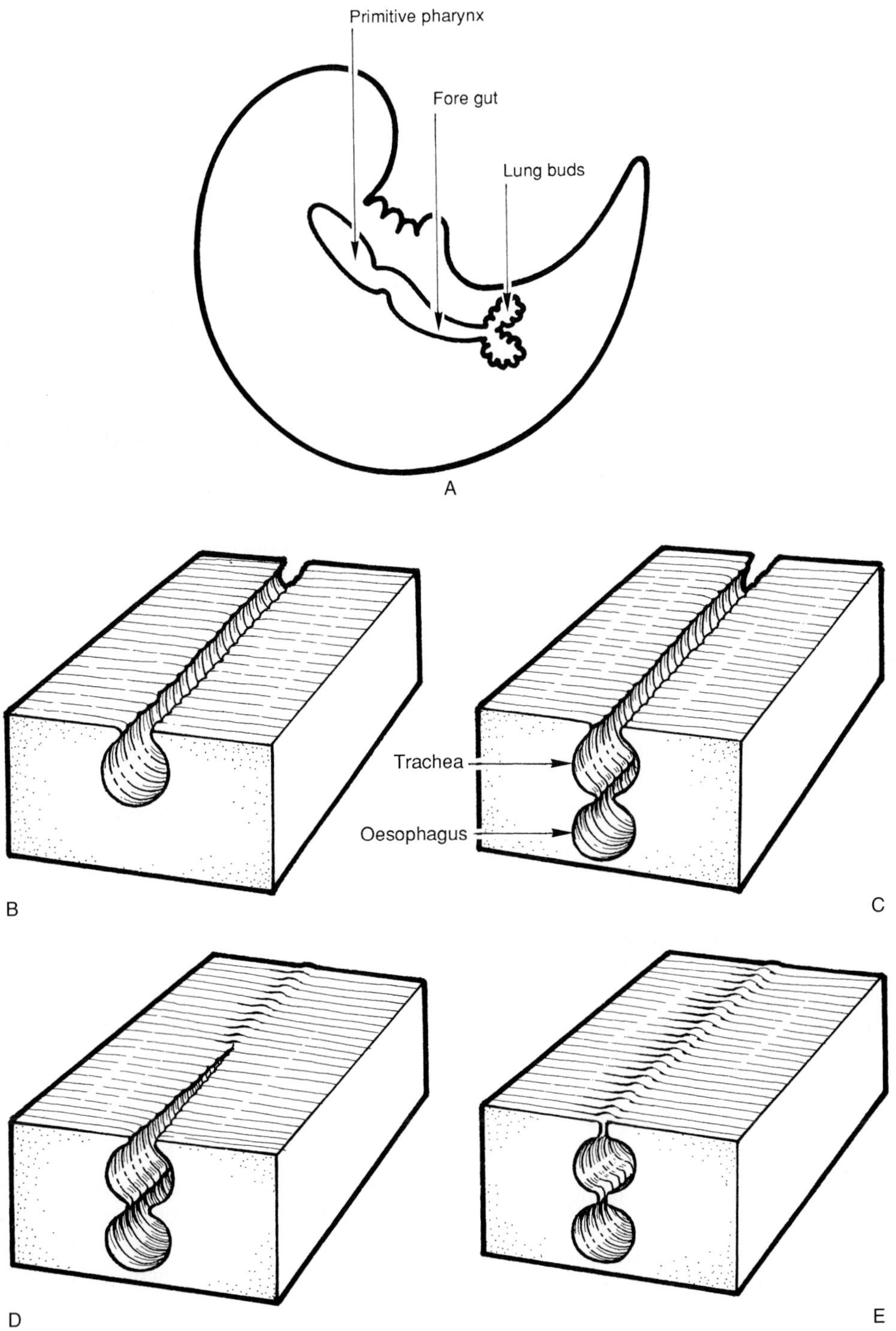

Fig. 29.100 (A) The 28th day of interuterine life. (B) A groove appears in the floor of the primitive pharynx. (C) The groove doubles itself. (D) Closing over from the tail end. (E) Trachea and oesophagus form.

12th week and the larynx is occluded. Perhaps this will limit early admission to the NICU.

Laryngeal webs are the result of incomplete separation of the arytenoid cartilages. The cricoid forms from the sixth arch cartilages, and these unite first anteriorly then posteriorly, as expected from the pattern of closure of the tracheo-oesophageal groove. A cleft in the cricoid is therefore usually in its posterior surface.

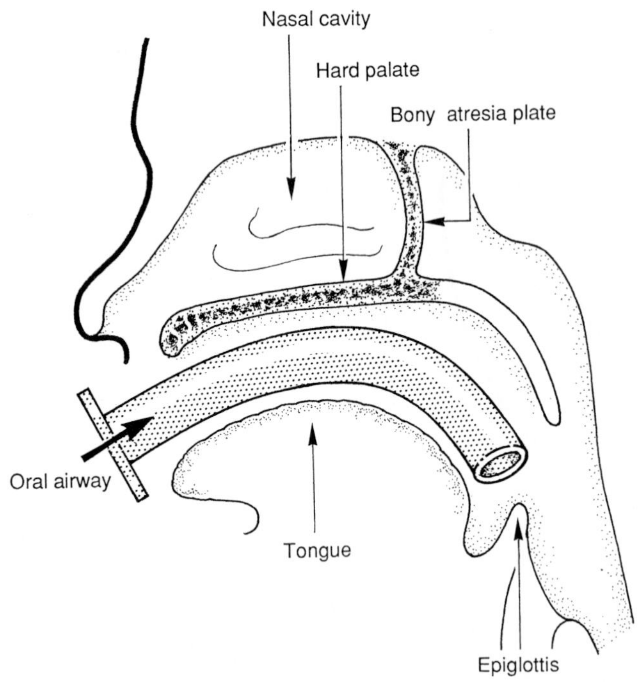

Fig. 29.101 Choanal atresia. A bony plate blocks the nose.

STRUCTURAL ABNORMALITIES IN THE NOSE

CHOANAL ATRESIA

One in 25 000 liveborn babies presents with respiratory obstruction caused by this condition, which is temporarily relieved by inserting an oral airway. Nasal obstruction is shown in Figure 29.101, and when bilateral is a surgical emergency. Babies are obliged to breathe through the nose, and asphyxiate if the obstruction is not relieved. Choanal atresia is part of the CHARGE syndrome (p. 870), but may exist in isolation.

Investigation

The diagnosis can be confirmed in the labour suite by looking for steam on a mirror held under the baby's nose, and nasal catheters will not pass into the pharynx. An oropharyngeal airway should be taped in place and the otolaryngologist contacted with a view to surgery the next day. CT is preferred to plain films with contrast, because CT shows the thickness of the atresia plate.[5]

Surgery and postoperative care

The obstruction is dealt with by drilling away the bony plate. A Hopkins rod-lens telescope is useful.[25] The new passages are kept open for 6 weeks by fixing 4 mm tubes in the nose with a continuous suture. The tubes need to be irrigated with 5 ml of saline each side as often as required, and sucked clear to keep an airway.

Most babies do well and may be sent home if the mother is capable of keeping the tubes patent. Breast-feeding is possible, but painful if the ends of the tubes are sharp. After the tubes have been removed the airways generally remain patent. An upper respiratory infection will readily block the narrow nasal passages, and vasoconstrictor drops (paediatric otrivine) will be needed. The mother can check the airway by looking for steamy patches on a handbag mirror held under the nose. A proportion of babies (about 10–20%) reblock and have to have the passages dilated or redrilled under general anaesthesia.

LARYNGEAL AND TRACHEAL DEFECTS

Congenital abnormalities are rare, estimated at between 1 in 10 000 and 1 in 50 000.[39] The leading symptoms are stridor and hoarseness, which always require investigation in the newborn. Analysis of the sound spectrum of the stridor to localize the source is promising but not yet reliable.[19]

LARYNGEAL ATRESIA AND TRACHEAL AGENESIS

Rarely the fourth arch cartilages, which are due to form the arytenoids, fail to separate at the 12th week of intra-uterine life or, worse, the tracheo-oesophageal groove fails to develop. Either of these forms an almost insuperable obstacle to resuscitation. The few infants that survive labour and delivery asphyxiate in the first 20 minutes of independent life. Immediate cardiopulmonary bypass, followed by reconstruction or transplantation of the trachea, would be necessary. The bronchi are reported to arise from the oesophagus in some cases, causing further difficulties.[23]

LARYNGOMALACIA

This is the commonest cause of inspiratory stridor and the least serious. The baby makes a crowing sound when breathing in. This is worst when lying on the back and least when lying face downwards.

Investigation

Fibreoptic laryngoscopy in the ward on the conscious baby allows the laryngeal inlet to be seen in action.

Pathology

The floppy parts of the laryngeal inlet, the aryepiglottic folds and the laryngeal surface of the epiglottis, are drawn inwards by each inspiration and partially obstruct the airway even though the vocal cords are wide apart. Breathing out is easier than breathing in.

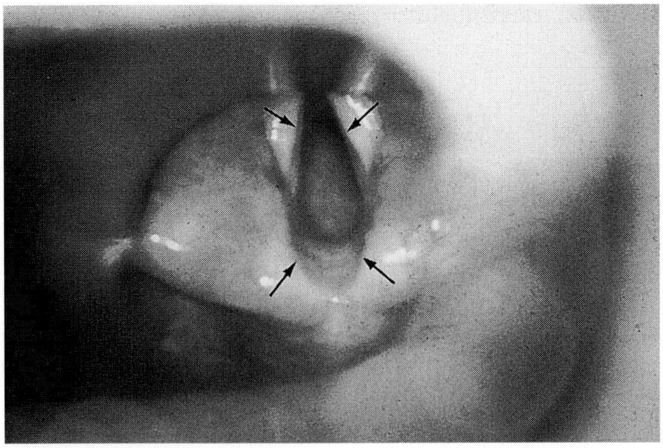

Fig. 29.102 A haemangioma (arrows) just below the vocal cords. (Courtesy of Mr Martin Bailey.)

Management

Mild cases are managed conservatively; severe cases should be assessed with a pulse oximeter. If saturation levels drop to less than 80% when stridor is present, surgery must be considered. Solomons and Prescott[36] recommend excision of the lax mucosa over the arytenoids, which they call supraglottic trimming. Seid et al[35] advocate laser division of the aryepiglottic mucosa, and either would be a better option than tracheostomy with its attendant risks and complications. If the baby survives 2 years the problem disappears as the larynx grows and stiffens. Rarely the whole trachea is floppy as well, and collapses on inspiration (tracheomalacia). Diseases which soften cartilage, such as polychondritis and rickets, should be treated, but tracheostomy is often needed.

SUBGLOTTIC HAEMANGIOMA

This is the next most common cause of stridor. The noise lies in the inspiratory phase of breathing, but is equally bad in all body positions (Fig. 29.102).

Investigation

Microlaryngoscopy under general anaesthesia is needed, because most haemangiomas are subglottic and may be missed when the larynx is viewed with a flexible laryngoscope in the ward. When the anaesthetist is satisfied the endotracheal tube is withdrawn and the cords are gently parted to see each side of the subglottis in turn.

Management

Small haemangiomas are watched, middle-sized ones excised with a carbon dioxide laser, and large ones require tracheostomy.[28] Haemangiomas sometimes resolve spontaneously with time and growth. Surgical intervention can be postponed in favourable cases by using systemic prednisolone. Occasionally the emergency has passed by the time the steroids have to be reduced.

A large capillary haemangioma of the skin of the neck or face may have a counterpart around the larynx. A long wait for spontaneous resolution with or without steroids or a tracheostomy, if necessary, is usually required.

VASCULAR RINGS

Variations in the vascular anatomy in the mediastinum and neck occur when branchial arch arteries persist into neonatal life. A double aorta encircling the trachea and oesophagus is one of the commonest (Fig. 29.103), followed by the pinching of trachea and oesphagus between an ectopic aorta and the ligamentum arteriosum (Fig. 29.104). One of the least common is a left-sided origin to the right brachiocephalic artery which indents the trachea (Fig. 29.105). All three present as stridor, which is independent of posture and may be two-way, i.e. present on expiration as well as inspiration. Feeding is sometimes difficult (dysphagia lusoria), although the main cause for this is that the infant has little time to swallow between breaths.

Investigations

Desnos et al[13] reviewed vascular strictures and found that discrete laryngoscopy and tracheoscopy to see the impression of the vessel upon the trachea was the most useful investigation. A barium swallow often helped to

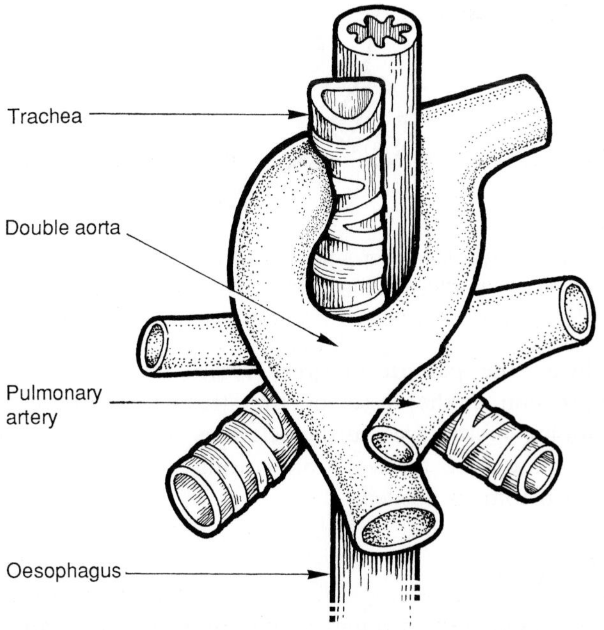

Fig. 29.103 Vascular ring. The double aorta.

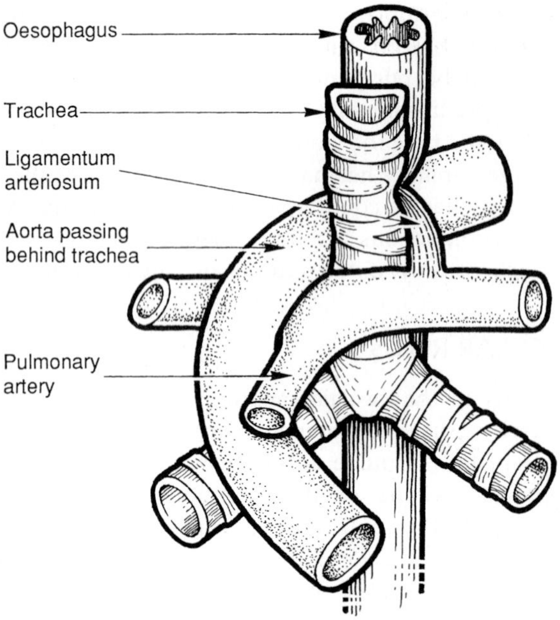

Fig. 29.104 Vascular ring. Trachea pinched between aorta and ligamentum arteriosum.

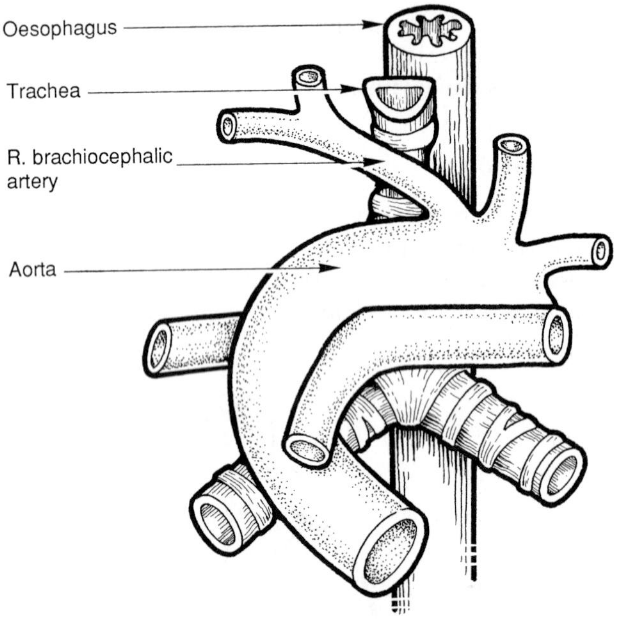

Fig. 29.105 Vascular ring. Trachea pinched by left subclavian or brachiocephalic artery arising anomalously from the aorta.

indicate the pattern of great vessels by showing the impression of the vessel on the stream of barium. CT scanning of the area further clarifies the anatomy, and will show how to avoid puncturing a major vessel if tracheostomy is needed.

Management

The anomalous vessel may require resection or rearrangement by a paediatric thoracic surgeon. If a tracheostomy has been unavoidable, vascular surgery may allow the tube to be removed.

LARYNGEAL CLEFT

This is a rare congenital deformity[18] and is the highest type of TOF.[8] In type I the defect is between the arytenoids and the cricoid ring is intact. In type 2 the cricoid is cleft, in type 3 there is a common trachea and oesophagus,[22] and type 4 extends into the bronchi. A type I cleft is often mistaken for laryngomalacia.

Investigation

Direct laryngoscopy is required, and even then the condition may be missed. To look specifically for a posterior cleft the tube should be taken out and the space between the arytenoids gently probed.[1]

Management

When a baby fails to thrive because of stridor and overspill, surgical repair of the cleft is indicated.

INVESTIGATION OF STRIDOR

Stridor is noisy breathing. When a baby makes a loud crowing sound on inspiration, pathological narrowing of the upper airway is the cause. The importance of stridor is that the narrow airway it represents demands hard work from a neonate to satisfy the needs of gas exchange. The work involved may be equivalent to jogging in an adult. In the short term this further embarrasses the respiratory system, possibly to the extreme of respiratory arrest. In the long term the obligatory energy output causes failure to thrive.

External examination

A mildly stridulous baby may have no physical signs except for the noise. If this is louder when the baby is on his back and relieved by turning him over, the condition is most likely to be a floppy larynx – laryngomalacia (p. 664). Severe stridor is unaffected by posture and shows intercostal, sternal and tracheal recession as evidence of negative intrathoracic pressure, and strong action of all the muscles of respiration. A rising pulse rate warns that respiratory collapse is imminent and investigation must be postponed until after the baby has been intubated.

X-rays

Plain films of the chest and neck may show distortion of the column of air in the trachea. A common pitfall is that the part of the film of most interest is just off the top of the picture or covered by the patient's hospital number! A barium swallow is most useful if external compression of the trachea by abnormalities of the great vessels is suspected. An excellent review of these conditions is found in Desnos et al.[13]

Endoscopy

Problems above the vocal cords are more frequent causes of stridor, but those below the vocal cords are generally the most serious.

The Mackintosh (anaesthetist's) laryngoscope

A view of the larynx is obtained at intubation but it is fleeting, uses one eye, and only the supraglottis is in view. Worse still, the physician's mind and other eye are on the pulse oximeter display.

The fibreoptic laryngoscope

The 3.5 mm paediatric laryngoscope gives an excellent view of the larynx in the neonate when passed just over the back of the tongue.[21] No anaesthesia is required. It is ideal for confirming a diagnosis of laryngomalacia or vocal cord palsy, as the lively actions of the supraglottis are close to the tip of the scope. No reliable view of the subglottis or trachea is obtained. Passing the endoscope through the cords blocks the airway, and this is why flexible scopes in special care baby units will not replace rigid endoscopy.

Microlaryngoscopy

The best view is down the eyepieces of an operating microscope when there is no tube between the vocal cords and the baby is completely still. This makes heavy demands on the anaesthetist but can be achieved with patience and skill. To see beyond the vocal cords it is simple to push a slim rigid fibreoptic telescope into the trachea.

Indication for tracheostomy

This should be done if there is a fixed obstruction to respiration, the resolution of which requires specialized surgery or a long period of poor growth. The baby who cannot be extubated is considered on page 668.

BRONCHOSCOPY FOR ATELECTASIS

Neonates suffer atelactasis because of inspissated mucus. When a mucus plug fails to respond to physiotherapy and suction, close cooperation between the neonatologist and the laryngologist may solve the problem. A rigid Stortz ventilating 2.5 mm broncoscope is used in the neonatal unit without anaesthesia. The bronchoscope replaces the endotracheal tube until the obstruction is found and relieved. A second chest X-ray will show whether the procedure has been successful, and whether excessive pressure or rupture of a bulla has caused a pneumothorax.[16]

CARE OF THE INTUBATED BABY

Babies must be intubated with speed and skill. It is the maintenance of the tube and the techniques of suction that may be improved to minimize injury to larynx, trachea and bronchi. Pashley[30] reviewed the risk factors and predictors of stenosis in 37 children who developed severe subglottic stenosis. He proposed a risk factor equal to number of intubations × number of days intubated × number of days ventilated. The child with an RF figure greater than 3000 was at great risk of severe stenosis.

TUBE DESIGN AND SIZE

The tube should be of a non-irritant silicone rubber, which means no free monomers, and all radicals properly polymerized and inert. The Coles shouldered tube may be accidentally forced through a larynx too small for it.

TUBE SIZE

A small leak of air past the tube is desirable. A 3 mm internal diameter tube in a baby under 1500 g is likely to be rather tight and not leak. However, a 2.5 mm internal diameter tube is often inadequate as an airway, and the larger size has to be tolerated. Loss of cilia where the tube lies against the tracheal wall is inevitable (Fig. 29.106).

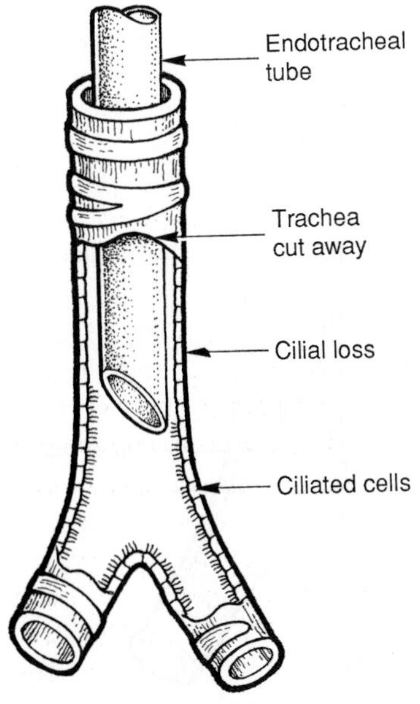

Fig. 29.106 Cilia are lost where the tube lies. The mucociliary escalator stops here and mechanical suction is needed.

TUBE MOVEMENT

An oral tube is easier to insert but harder to stabilize. A baby tends to suck and chew on an oral tube. A nasal tube requires additional skill but, once in place, can be fixed rigidly to the baby's face.[24] There are risks, however (pp. 932–933): nasal tubes occasionally cause damage to the nasal septum or notch the alae of the nose; oral tubes may cause the palatal arch to become too high, or damage the alveolar ridge.[16] Many techniques have been used successfully to immobilize endotracheal tubes (p. 573). Avoid fixing the tube with its tip in the right main bronchus or allowing it to bear down upon the carina when the neck is flexed. The management of the endotracheal tube in ventilated neonates is discussed in greater detail on pages 573–574.

SUCTION CATHETER TIPS

These should be soft and rounded. Faceted, bevelled and roughly cut tips are to be avoided. Look at the catheter under magnification and see if you would consider it fit to enter your own trachea.

DEPTH OF SUCTION

A sterile endotracheal tube suction technique taught to nurses and followed correctly will introduce no new organisms to the airway. However, evidence is emerging of mechanical trauma (pp. 932–933). Bronchial ulceration results from repeated deep suction.[4] Granulations, polyps and stenoses have been described in severe cases of overzealous suction.[17] The same authors recommend that the person performing suction should hold the catheter so that the tip does not go beyond the distal end of the endotracheal tube. This is best done by measuring the catheter against a spare tube which has been cut and taped to the side of the cot. The depth of suction required is then obvious (Fig. 29.107).

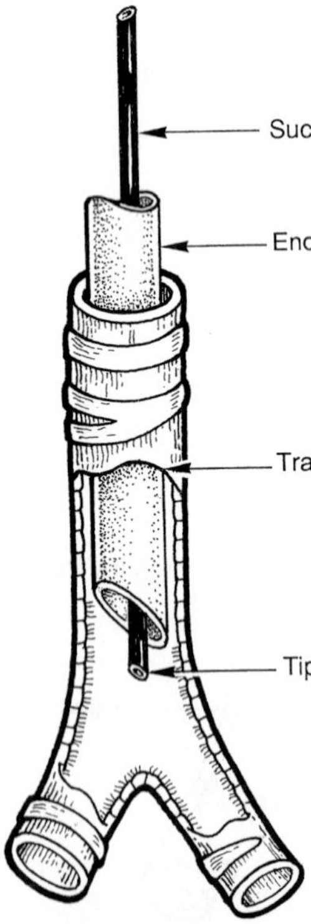

Fig. 29.107 The sucker needs to go only just beyond the tube tip. The mucociliary escalator brings the mucus this far.

SUBGLOTTIC STENOSIS

At University College Hospital, London, between 1981 and 1983, 2.6% of surviving intubated babies suffered subglottic stenosis.[31] Stenosis is the most important cause of failure of extubation. Holinger et al[20] reported that all but one of 39 cases of acquired subglottic stenosis could not be extubated, whereas 66% of a similar series of congenital subglottic stenosis could be extubated. In both groups the worst cases required tracheostomy. Unfortunately, the acquired condition is more common and occurs at a rate of 2.5–8.5% in infants requiring prolonged intubation.[26,29]

ACQUIRED SUBGLOTTIC STENOSIS

A full-term baby has a subglottis 5 mm in diameter. A 3.5 mm endotracheal tube has an external diameter of 4.8 mm, so that in the smaller preterm baby there is a risk of trauma in the emergency intubation of such a baby with RDS. No direct measurements of preterm babies' airways have been made, but sizes may be inferred from the external diameters given in Table 29.42.

Pathology

The larynx and trachea suffer changes as a consequence of irritation and pressure from the tube: it is a retained foreign body! Tracheal epithelium is initially shed where the tube touches. Quiney and Gould[31] showed that, in 43 infants who died while intubated, damage occurring in the first week was followed by re-epithelialization with the tube still in place. (It was noted that the shoulder of a Coles tube entering the subglottis was probably the cause of damage in two of the series.) However, this new epithelium is relatively devoid of cilia and is thickened by inflammatory cells and oedema. Where the tube is too

Table 29.42 Preterm endotracheal tube diameters

	Internal (mm)	External (mm)
25 weeks' gestation	2.5	3.4
30 weeks' gestation	3.0	4.2
35 weeks' gestation	3.5	4.8

tight, or oedema renders it so, persistent ulceration is seen with exposure of mesoderm. If re-epithelialization is frustrated, mesoderm heals by second intention, that is, by granulation and contracture.

Perichondritis of the cricoid may result in collapse of the ring, and the arytenoids may become fibrosed to the cricoid. These are then lifelong structural changes.

Clinical features

Extubation is usually followed by mild stridor before the inflammatory oedema in the larnyx and trachea settles. It is to be expected that the infant will need to cough collections of mucus past patches of trachea denuded of cilia. Rattling respiration bears witness to localized interruptions in the mucociliary stream.

Weaning a baby off IPPV by substituting CPAP is helpful. Disconnecting the endotracheal tube from CPAP as the next stage leaves the baby breathing unassisted. This causes the PaO_2 to fall to a lower level than it would if the baby was extubated, and is to be avoided. The baby should be extubated in combination with nasal CPAP at the same pressure and inspired oxygen level[14] (p. 561).

Increasing stridor and secretions suggest swelling of the mucosa and granulations previously held in check by pressure from the tube. The pulse and respiration rate rise as the baby brings more muscular energy to the task of gas exchange. Effective at first, this is partly self-defeating because the muscular work itself increases the need for respiration. All is well until the baby tires of the effort, and then respiratory collapse occurs. Nasopharyngeal CPAP or a headbox with humidified oxygen will postpone the collapse for a period. A falling oxygen saturation associated with increasing stridor and sternal recession is an indication for reintubation.

Duration of intubation

Reintubation, even gently performed, results in further loss of epithelium, which is unlikely to heal in less than a week. Two weeks with the tube held as still as possible is a reasonable trial period. Systemic steroids reduce inflammatory oedema around the tube (p. 581), and the benefit is most helpful 24 hours before and after the second extubation.

Diagnosis and endoscopy (Fig. 29.108)

Plain X-rays of the airway are unhelpful, but CT or MRI will show the stricture nicely. Rigid endoscopy to measure the width and length of the stricture is required. The lumen is assessed by measuring the external diameter of the largest bronchoscope or endotracheal tube that will pass. Tubes are sized by their internal diameter, which in this case is misleading.

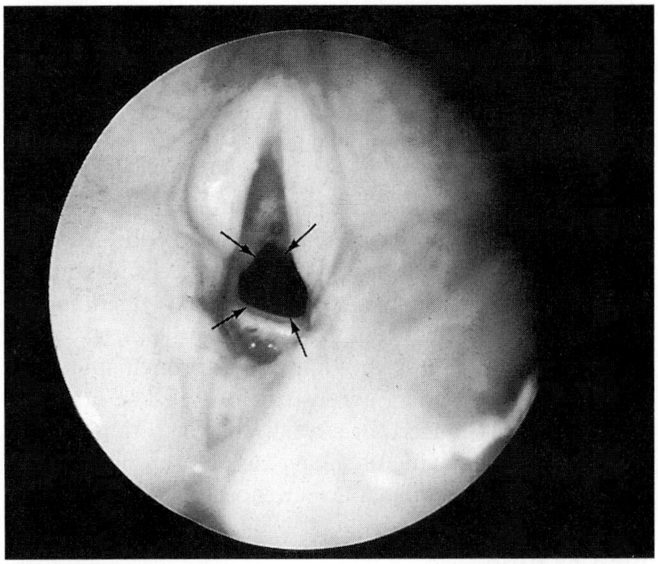

Fig. 29.108 Stenosis (arrows) just below the vocal cords due to protracted intubation. (Courtesy of Mr Martin Bailey.)

Management

Mild cases respond to added oxygen and a waiting policy. In severe cases oxygen, humidification, CPAP and steroids all fail, and protracted intubation makes the larynx worse. Tracheostomy is indicated unless an anterior cricoid split (p. 670) is successful.

GRANULOMAS AND CYSTS

Endotracheal intubation causes granulations in the posterior larynx (p. 932). With the continued irritation of tube movement, tongues of chronic inflammatory tissue form and may encircle the tube, causing an adhesion. The laryngoscopic view is then of two passages into the trachea. Subglottic cysts[38] and anterior subglottic granulomas[34] also occur. These may be removed with cup forceps or vaporized with the carbon dioxide laser.

TRACHEOSTOMY

This is an alternative airway used while awaiting correction of laryngeal stenosis or its resolution by natural growth. The operation in an infant differs from that in an adult only in that the incision in the tracheal wall is a vertical slit rather than a circular window. Compared with an endotracheal tube the cannula is short, with a wider lumen which, by reducing dead space and resistance, facilitates disconnection from a ventilator.

Postoperative care

The tube must not come out, and tapes are tied with reef knots while flexing the neck. For additional security the tube is sutured to the skin. When exposed to room air and a foreign body (the tube), the tracheal mucosal glands go into overdrive and a tremendous outpouring of mucus occurs.

To prevent blockage with leathery green crusts, humidified air, and suction about every 20 minutes are required for the first 3 days. The baby should be nursed in a paediatric intensive care unit with staff and facilities for immediate reinsertion of a displaced tube. A chest X-ray to check the position of the tube is needed: this will also show an accidental pneumothorax, pneumopericardium or surgical emphysema of the neck. The technique of suction is very important: bronchial damage results from deep and vigorous suction.[4,17] The first tube should not be changed for a week, by which time a track has developed, making changing easier. The first change should be performed by an experienced doctor.

Type of tube

A plastic tracheostomy tube of the Great Ormond Street (Franklin) pattern is recommended. Portex and Shiley paediatric tubes are also satisfactory. Flexible tubes cause less trauma and granulations within the trachea than metal tubes. In the past silver tracheostomy tubes with an inner section that could be removed for easy cleaning were widely used, but there is no evidence that this reduced the mortality from tube obstruction.

Tracheostomy fatalities

Because the tube is now the baby's airway anything that obstructs the tube may prove fatal. Despite all precautions neonatal tracheostomy still carries a mortality of about 5%.[33] Granulations and crusts may block the tube and accidental decannulation may be fatal. Severe haemorrhage may occur from ulceration and penetration of the innominate artery, which is an anterior relation of the tracheal wall where the tube tip may bear. Even with strict attention to aseptic technique there is an increased incidence of chest infection.

Tracheostomy at home

Sooner or later the infant with a tracheostomy will be allowed home. It is essential that the child's parents are able and willing to change the tube and have had practice under the ward sister's eye. Tracheal dilators and portable suction will have to be supplied by the hospital. A speaking valve must be available before the age of 2 if the child is to learn to talk.

Duration of tracheostomy

The length of time tracheostomy will be required varies from child to child, but is a matter of months and years rather than days and weeks. Few parents escape the complexities of home life with a tube.

Decannulation

This is the aim of all management, but is often not achieved easily or quickly. When the day arrives that the child can cry past the tracheostomy tube a plug may be inserted in the mouth of the tube for a trial period (under the closest observation!). If the natural laryngeal airway is adequate then the tube may be taken out. This is best done after laryngoscopy in theatre, because many have granulations in the trachea which can be removed. Once the tube is out the hole is covered with a finger, and if there is no stridor or dyspnoea an occlusive dressing is applied.[2] A pulse oximeter is very helpful. Reported difficulties with decannulation vary from very few[6] to 30%.[3] Excision of the fistulous tract and the upper margin of the tracheal stoma, with closure of the trachea and skin over an endotracheal tube, is recommended by Rogers[33] for difficult cases.

SURGICAL TREATMENT OF SUBGLOTTIC STENOSIS

The combination of growth and natural resolution make the effects of treatment difficult to assess.[11] Most patients with a tracheostomy for congenital subglottic stenosis were decannulated within 2–5 years without requiring any operative procedure on the larynx.

Steroids and serial dilatation

Some series have recommended this combination. Evans[15] advises that it is unhelpful when there is an abnormality of the cricoid cartilage, and Pashley[30] found it unsatisfactory in acquired stenosis.

Endoscopic resection

Retention cysts, fibrous webs and granulations have all been successfully treated endoscopically. The carbon dioxide laser is most helpful.[7,37]

Anterior cricoid split

The anterior wall of the cricoid cartilage is split in the midline to expose the endotracheal tube, which is then replaced with a larger one to act as a stent in the cricoid ring for 2 weeks.[12] This is probably best for treating mild stenosis of the soft tissue type. Should extubation fail after the 2 weeks both tracheostomy and reintubation are difficult because of the earlier wound and loose cartilage edge.

Laryngotracheal reconstruction

The larynx is split in the midline and a free graft of costal cartilage inserted anteriorly to widen the cricoid ring and

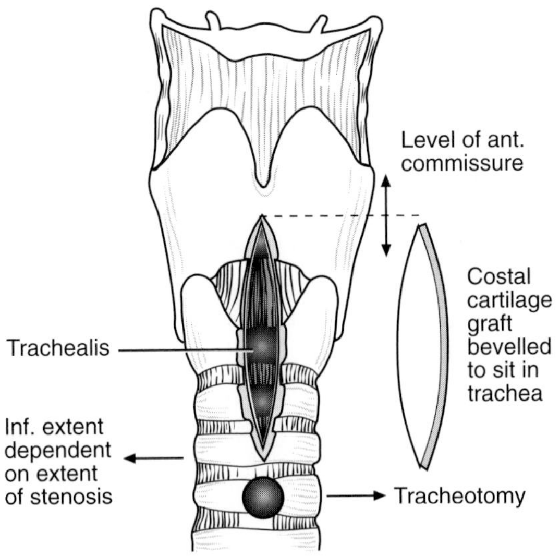

Fig. 29.109 Technique of laryngotracheoplasty.

upper trachea[9] (Fig. 29.109). If the arytenoids are bound together by scar tissue the posterior wall of the cricoid cartilage may be divided and a second cartilage graft inserted.[32] In a series of 37 children with severe subglottic stenosis from Colorado, 27% remained aphonic and dependent upon a tracheostomy despite radical surgery; the rest were successfully decannulated.[30]

Laryngotracheal resection

Although laryngotracheal reconstruction remains the operation of choice in most centres, Monnier et al[27] describe 26 cases treated by anastamosing the trachea to laryngeal cartilage after excising the stricture and cricoid ring; 96% of the patients were successfully decannulated in this way.

CONCLUSION

Congenital subglottic stenosis usually responds to tracheostomy and spontaneous growth. Acquired subglottic stenosis often requires laryngeal surgery. Fortunately, surgical procedures do not appear to suppress laryngeal growth.[10] The acquired condition is minimized by skill in the care of neonates requiring intubation. Bronchial injury from inappropriately deep suction is to be avoided.

REFERENCES

1. Benjamin B 1986 Posterior glottic pathology. International Journal of Paediatric Otorhinolaryngology 12: 23–31
2. Birrell J F, Cowan D L, Kerr A I G 1986 Intubation, tracheostomy and subglottic stenosis. In: Paediatric otolaryngology, 2nd edn. John Wright, Bristol, pp. 228–233
3. Black R J, Baldwin D L, Johns A N 1984 'Decannulation panic' in children: fact or fiction? Journal of Laryngology and Otology 98: 297–304
4. Brodsky L, Reidy M, Stanievich J F 1987 The effects of suctioning techniques on the distal tracheal mucosa in intubated low birth weight infants. International Journal of Paediatric Otorhinolaryngology 14: 1–14
5. Brown O E, Burns D K, Smith T H, Rutledge J C 1987 Bilateral posterior choanal atresia: a morphological and histological study, and computed tomographic correlation. International Journal of Paediatric Otorhinolaryngology 13: 125–142
6. Carter P, Benjamin B 1983 Ten year review of paediatric tracheostomy. Annals of Otology, Rhinology and Laryngology 92: 398–400
7. Carruth J A S, Morgan N J, Nielsen M S, Phillips J J, Wainwright A C 1986 The treatment of laryngeal stenosis using the CO_2 laser. Clinical Otolaryngology 11: 145–148
8. Corbally M T 1993 Laryngo-tracheo-oesophageal cleft. Archives of Disease in Childhood 68: 532–533
9. Cotton R T 1978 Management of subglottic stenosis in infancy and childhood: a review of a consecutive series of cases managed by surgical reconstruction. Annals of Otology, Rhinology and Laryngology 87: 649–657
10. Cotton R T, Evans J N G 1981 Laryngotracheal reconstruction in children. Five year follow-up. Annals of Otology, Rhinology and Laryngology 90: 516–520
11. Cotton R T, Myer C M 1984 Contemporary surgical management of laryngeal stenosis in children. American Journal of Otolaryngology 5: 360–368
12. Cotton R T, Seid A B 1980 Management of the extubation problem in the premature child: anterior cricoid split as an alternative to tracheostomy. Annals of Otology, Rhinology and Laryngology 89: 508–511
13. Desnos J, Andrieu-Grutancourt J, Dehesdin D, Dubin J 1980 Vascular strictures of the respiratory tract in children. International Journal of Paediatric Otorhinolaryngology 2: 269–285
14. Dinwiddie R 1988 A respiratory physician's view of acquired subglottic stenosis. Journal of Laryngology and Otology Suppl. 17: 31–34
15. Evans J N G 1987 Stenosis of the larynx. In: Keir A G (ed) Scott-Brown's otolaryngology, 5th edn, Vol 6. Butterworths, London, pp. 495–502
16. Freeland A P 1988 The laryngologist in the neonatal unit. In: Gray R F, Rutka J (eds) Recent advances in otolaryngology. Churchill Livingstone, Edinburgh, pp 109–124
17. Friedberg J, Forte V 1987 Acquired bronchial injury in neonates. International Journal of Paediatric Otolaryngology 14: 223–228
18. Glossop L P, Smith R J H, Evans J N G 1984 Posterior larnygeal cleft: an analysis of ten cases. International Journal of Paediatric Otorhinolaryngology 7: 133–143
19. Gray L, Denenny J C, Carvajal H, Jahrsdoefer R 1985 Fourier analysis of infantile stridor: preliminary data. International Journal of Paediatric Otorhinolaryngology 10: 191–199
20. Holinger P H, Kutnick S L, Schild J A, Holinger L D 1976 Subglottic stenosis in infants and children. Annals of Otology, Rhinology and Laryngology 85: 591–599
21. Inouye T 1983 Examination of child larynx by flexible fiberoptic laryngoscope. International Journal of Paediatric Otorhinolaryngology 5: 317–323
22. Kauten J R, Konrad H R, Wichterman K A 1984 Laryngotracheooesophageal cleft in a newborn. International Journal of Paediatric Otorhinolaryngology 8: 61–71
23. Kearns D B, Miller R H 1987 Tracheal agenesis. International Journal of Paediatric Otorhinolaryngology 13: 143–148
24. Laing I A, Cowan D L, Hume R 1987 Prevention of subglottic stenosis. Journal of Laryngology and Otology Suppl. 17: 11–13
25. Lazar R H, Younis R T 1995 Transnasal repair of choanal atresia. Archives of Otolaryngology – Head and Neck Surgery, 121: 517–520
26. Marshak G, Grundfast K M 1981 Subglottic stenosis. Pediatric Clinics of North America 28: 941–948
27. Monnier P, Savary M, Chapuis G 1995 Cricotracheal resection for pediatric subglottic stenosis: update of the Lausanne experience. Acta Oto-Rhino-Laryngologica Belgica 49: 373–82.
28. Narcy P, Contencin P, Bobin S, Manac'h Y 1985 Treatment of infantile subglottic haemangioma. A report of 49 cases. International Journal of Paediatric Otolaryngology 9: 157–164
29. Parkin J L, Stevens M H, Jung A L 1976 Acquired and congenital subglottic stenosis in the infant. Annals of Otology, Rhinology and Laryngology 85: 573–581

30. Pashley N R T 1982 Risk factors and the prediction of outcome in acquired subglottic stenosis in children. International Journal of Paediatric Otorhinolaryngology 4: 1–6
31. Quiney R E, Gould S J 1985 Subglottic stenosis: a clinicopathological study. Clinical Otolaryngology 10: 315–327
32. Rethi A 1956 An operation for cicatricial stenosis of the larynx. Journal of Laryngology and Otology 70: 283–293
33. Rogers J H 1987 Tracheostomy and decannulation. In: Keir A G (ed) Scott-Brown's otolaryngology, 5th edn., Vol 6. Butterworths, London, pp. 471–486
34. Schlesinger A E, Tucker G F Jr, Young S A 1985 Postintubation granuloma of the anterior subglottic larynx. International Journal of Paediatric Otorhinolaryngology 10: 279–248
35. Seid A B, Park S M, Kearns M J, Gugenheim S 1995 Laser division of the aryepiglottic folds for severe laryngomalacia. International Journal of Paediatric Otorhinolaryngology 10: 153–158
36. Solomons N B, Prescott C A J 1987 Laryngomalacia. A review and the surgical management for severe cases. International Journal of Paediatric Otorhinolaryngology 13: 31–39
37. Strong M S, Healy G B, Vaughan C W, Freid M P, Shapsay S 1979 Endoscopic management of laryngeal stenosis. Otolaryngologic Clinics of North America 12: 797–806
38. Toriumi D R, Miller D R, Holinger L D 1987 Acquired subglottic cysts in premature infants. International Journal of Paediatric Otorhinolaryngology 14: 151–160
39. van der Broek P, Brinkman W F B 1979 Congenital laryngeal defects. International Journal of Paediatric Otorhinolaryngology 1: 71–78

30

Cardiovascular disease

Nick Archer

INTRODUCTION

Cardiac problems in the newborn period can be primary or secondary, structural or functional, congenital or acquired. Whatever category of abnormality is concerned, a similar systematic approach to history, examination and investigation is required in all types to allow correct management. In many situations an understanding of fetal as well as of neonatal cardiovascular physiology is necessary. The approach of this chapter is essentially pathophysiological problem-oriented with information on particular diagnoses being considered under the most appropriate heading. Prior to addressing cardiac problems in the newborn a brief view of fetal and perinatal cardiovascular physiology will be given and the growing practice of fetal cardiac diagnosis and therapy will be considered. Those seeking information on embryology of the heart are referred to reviews by Clarke,[17] Mahony,[53] Pickoff.[67]

FETAL CIRCULATION

The basic differences between fetal and postnatal circulations are firstly the presence of a low-resistance high-flow placental circulation in the fetus and secondly the fact that less than 10% of total cardiac output enters the fetal pulmonary circulation at term and even less reaches the lungs in early gestation. Three vascular pathways exist in the fetus which close soon after birth in a healthy term infant. These are the ductus venosus, the foramen ovale and the ductus arteriosus. The first two allow oxygenated blood from the placenta to be channelled into the left atrium and thereby via the left ventricle and ascending aorta to reach the coronary and cerebral circulations. The DA has right-to-left flow because of high pulmonary vascular resistance. The DA is kept patent in utero by prostaglandins both circulating and locally produced and as gestation progresses it becomes increasingly sensitive to the constricting influence of oxygen. The role of prostaglandins in maintaining fetal duct patency is important when considering the administration of prostaglandin synthetase inhibitors to pregnant women for any reason such as to suppress premature labour or to treat polyhydramnios. In these circumstances fetal DA constriction which is usually reversible has been documented.[58] However, there are reports of neonatal PPHN in association with maternal prostaglandin synthetase inhibitor ingestion (p. 527).[55,92] This problem is probably related both to constriction of the DA and to changes in the pulmonary vessels induced by the drug. At birth, arterial oxygen tension rises and pulmonary vascular resistance begins to fall allowing an increase in pulmonary blood flow. Also in response to higher oxygen tension the DA starts to constrict; this process is functionally complete within 60 hours in 93% of term infants.[31] Increased lung blood flow causes increased pulmonary venous return to the left atrium where pressure rises and the foramen ovale is pushed shut, although it may permit left-to-right shunting, even into adult life. The ductus venosus closes as umbilical venous flow ceases but it can provide vascular access to the right heart for a few days.[7] Closure of all these structures may be delayed in pathological circumstances and may precipitate clinical deterioration in various structural cardiac conditions (Table 30.1). Continued patency of the DA and foramen ovale may contribute to clinical problems in some conditions (Table 30.2).

Table 30.1 Clinical problems associated with closure of foramen ovale, ductus venosus and ductus arteriosus after birth

Foramen ovale	Poorer mixing in TGA Systemic/pulmonary venous obstruction in right/left heart obstructions
Ductus venosus	Worsening pulmonary venous obstruction in infradiaphragmatic TAPVC
Ductus arteriosus	Marked deterioration in duct-dependent pulmonary or systemic circulations

Table 30.2 Clinical problems associated with failure of closure of foramen ovale, ductus venosus and ductus arteriosus after birth

Foramen ovale	Allows right-to-left shunting in PPHN and (probably less often) in respiratory causes of high right heart pressures
Ductus venosus	No definite problem identified
Ductus arteriosus	Associated with major respiratory and other problems in preterm infants Important left-to-right shunting only rarely seen in the newborn period in term infants with PDA

Table 30.3 Conditions with increased risk of fetal cardiac abnormalities; offer of fetal cardiac scan appropriate

- Autosomal dominant condition with cardiac implications in either parent
- Structural congenital heart disease in parent or previous sibling
- Structural heart disease in two or more family members
- Maternal disease with increased risk of fetal cardiac problem, e.g. diabetes mellitus, collagen vascular disease
- Maternal teratogen exposure, e.g.
  - infection: rubella
  - medication: anticonvulsants, lithium
  - alcohol
- Abnormal four-chamber screening scan
- Non-cardiac abnormalities in fetus
- Suspected syndrome in fetus
- Maternal prostaglandin synthetase inhibitor therapy
- Abnormal heart rate/rhythm in fetus
- Hydropic fetus

FETAL CARDIOLOGY

DIAGNOSIS

Fetal cardiac structure and rhythm can be determined by maternal abdominal ultrasound examination from 18 weeks' gestation;[3] transvaginal ultrasound may be accurate a few weeks earlier. Screening fetal cardiac anatomy with a four-chamber view at 18 weeks is part of general anomaly scanning in many regions; this will pick up under 50% of cases of structural heart lesions even in experienced hands.[84,93] Heart lesions picked up by a four-chamber screening scan are generally the more complex ones with the poorer outlook both prenatally and after delivery. Detailed evaluation of fetal cardiac anatomy by ultrasound is much more time-consuming and is usually reserved for individuals with an increased risk of having a fetus with a cardiac problem (Table 30.3). However, when detailed echocardiography was used on all pregnancies, Stümpflen and colleagues reported an 86% sensitivity and 100% specificity;[84] the conditions being missed were atrial septal defects and small ventricular septal defects. Other workers have pointed out the great difficulty in diagnosing coarctation and TAPVC in the fetus.[1] Fetal heart rhythm can be determined by M mode and Doppler studies.[2,83] There are ethical issues involved in fetal diagnosis which parents need to be aware of, and they need to be free to make their views known. This dimension must be catered for in any fetal cardiac scanning programme which should be carried out in the context of expertise in all aspects of fetal medicine.

TREATMENT

Accurate diagnosis of structural heart disease in a fetus allows information to be given to families. Benefit from fetal diagnosis or exclusion of structural heart disease is hard to quantify. Some pregnancies will be terminated and others associated with spontaneous fetal loss. In pregnancies progressing to viable delivery, a cardiac diagnosis may influence the place, time or mode of delivery. Many factors will influence these decisions including the presence of chromosome disorders or abnormalities in other body systems. The most important point with respect to heart disease is whether or not the lesion is likely to be duct dependent, thereby allowing prostaglandin to be used postnatally before symptoms develop. Fetal interventions such as aortic valvuloplasty are just being explored. There is some evidence that fetal diagnosis of severe duct-dependent congenital heart disease results in infants reaching a cardiac centre in better condition than those not diagnosed until after delivery.[16] Reassurance of normality or the chance to prepare for the arrival of an abnormal baby is valued by many parents.

Accurate diagnosis of fetal arrhythmias is essential to avoid unnecessary intervention and to allow appropriate treatment which can improve outlook for the fetus with a haemodynamically compromising dysrhythmia. Arrhythmias are further discussed on page 705.

Table 30.4 Congenital heart disease diagnosed by any means, presenting in the first year of life, Alberta, 1981–1984 inclusive (Source: Grabitz et al 1988)[38]

Lesion/group	Rate/1000 live births	% of total
Ventricular septal defect	1.905	34.4
Left heart obstruction	0.716	12.9
Right heart obstruction	0.600	10.8
Atrial septal defect	0.580	10.5
Transposition of the great arteries	0.280	5.1
Patent ductus arteriosus	0.251	4.5
Atrioventricular septal defect	0.242	4.4
Tetralogy of Fallot	0.203	3.7
Complex	0.193	3.5
Double outlet right ventricle	0.145	2.6
Total anomalous pulmonary venous drainage	0.087	1.6
Other	0.338	6.1
Total	5.541	100

Notes: (i) cases given a principal diagnosis and only counted once; (ii) excludes bicuspid aortic valve; (iii) patent ductus arteriosus only included if symptomatic after day 10; (iv) left heart obstruction includes coarctation, aortic stenosis, hypoplastic left heart, mitral stenosis or atresia; (v) right heart obstruction includes pulmonary stenosis or atresia, tricuspid atresia; (vi) complex includes absent pulmonary valve, transposition with atrioventricular septal defect and truncus arteriosus; (vii) other includes congenital complete heart block, heart muscle disease and symptomatic vascular rings.

INCIDENCE AND AETIOLOGY OF FETAL AND NEONATAL HEART DISEASE

Structural congenital heart disease occurs in approximately 8 per 1000 live births;[45] between 30 and 40% of these children will be symptomatic in early infancy and about two-thirds of them will have been diagnosed by the end of the first year of life. There are various studies on the prevalence of congenital heart disease. Diagnostic methods and criteria vary but Table 30.4 gives figures for those presenting in the first year of life at a time when echocardiography was starting to be widely used. Fetal echocardiography has shown that some severe cardiac lesions result in death in utero.[3] Acquired heart disease such as endocarditis and myocarditis may also present in the newborn period. Metabolic disorders which may involve heart muscle can produce symptoms in the newborn period. There are no reliable figures for the incidence of these problems nor for the incidence of fetal and neonatal arrhythmias. Aetiological factors and important associations of congenital heart disease are outlined in Table 30.5.

CLINICAL IMPLICATIONS OF ADAPTATION TO BIRTH

NORMAL ADAPTATION

There are haemodynamic consequences to normal adaptation which have adverse haemodynamic effects in certain cardiovascular conditions. Similarly, failure of normal changes to occur may also be disadvantageous under certain circumstances. These two situations will be considered under the four headings of the particular structures concerned.

Foramen ovale

If exit of blood from the left atrium through the mitral valve is impaired, the presence of a foramen ovale is important in allowing decompression of the left atrium as the flap valve of the foramen ovale is forced open by the abnormally high pressure in the left atrium. Failure of this mechanism by virtue of a small foramen ovale results in pulmonary venous hypertension and respiratory distress.

Table 30.5 Aetiological factors in congenital heart disease, with examples (not comprehensive) (See also: Neill.[63])

Category	Example	Cardiac lesions include
Chromosome abnormality	Down syndrome (trisomy 21)	AVSD, VSD, tetralogy of Fallot
	Edwards syndrome (trisomy 18)	VSD
	Patau syndrome (trisomy 13)	VSD
	Turner syndrome (XO)	Coarctation, AS, MS, PAPVC
	Catch 22 (22 q 11 del)	Truncus, IAA, tetralogy of Fallot, any
	Williams syndrome (7 q del)	Supravalvar AS, PABS
Non-specific genetic	Parent or sibling with CHD	Any
Teratogen exposure	Virus: rubella	Coarctation, PABS, VSD, PDA
	Drug:	
	Alcohol	VSD
	Phenytoin	ASD
	Lithium	Ebstein's anomaly
	Warfarin	VSD, tetralogy of Fallot
Syndromes	AD:	
	Noonan	PS, ASD, HCM
	Holt–Oram	ASD
	AR: TAR	ASD, tetralogy of Fallot
	Sporadic:	
	DiGeorge	(p. 1100)
	Williams	(p. 872)
	Cornelia de Lange	VSD
Maternal disease	Diabetes mellitus	VSD, HCM
	Collagen vascular diseases	CHB
Association with non-cardiac malformations	Oesophageal atresia	VSD, tetralogy of Fallot
	Diaphragmatic hernia	Any
	Exomphalos	Any
	Pierre Robin	VSD

This problem is an important part of the pathophysiology of mitral atresia or hypoplasia. A restrictive foramen ovale is also important in obstructive lesions in the right heart such as tricuspid atresia, pulmonary atresia with intact ventricular septum and critical pulmonary stenosis. In such circumstances right atrial enlargement and hydrops fetalis may occur in utero, but even if it does not, there may be postnatal problems from systemic venous engorgement and poor cardiac output. In the context of TGA a small foramen ovale is a cause of poor mixing of oxygenated and deoxygenated blood. In many of these conditions, particularly TGA, enlargement of the foramen ovale by balloon septostomy is an important part of the initial management. In some circumstances surgical septostomy or septectomy may be indicated as in mitral atresia. Failure of the foramen ovale to close has the same consequences as the presence of an ASD, indeed distinguishing between PFO and ASD in newborn infants can be difficult. The consequences are right-to-left shunting in the presence of structural or functional obstruction to right heart flow and left-to-right shunting otherwise. The balance between favourable and deleterious effects is different for different lesions. In general, left-to-right shunting at atrial level in early infancy is rarely a major haemodynamic disadvantage whereas right-to-left shunting will worsen systemic arterial desaturation, but this may be less of a disadvantage than very high venous pressures or poor left ventricular filling resulting from poor forward flow through the right heart.

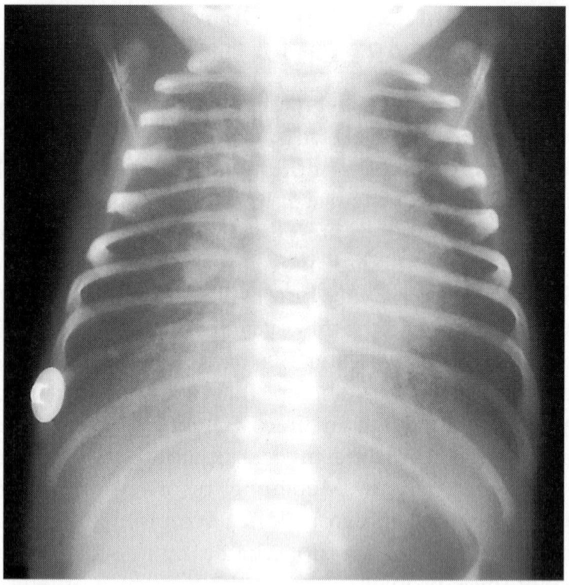

Fig. 30.1 CXR showing pulmonary venous engorgement and normal heart size in obstructed TAPVC.

Ductus venosus

Closure of the ductus venosus is of importance in that it removes the possibility of central venous access being obtained via the umbilical vein for monitoring, balloon septostomy or cardiac catheterization. It will also result in marked deterioration in cases of TAPVC to the portal vein as it will cause severe pulmonary venous obstruction with pulmonary oedema (Fig. 30.1). In this condition, closure of the ductus venosus may not occur until some days after birth. Delay in or failure of closure of the ductus venosus is probably rare and never of significance.

Ductus arteriosus

Closure of the DA will cause marked deterioration in duct-dependent pulmonary and duct-dependent systemic circulations; in the first instance worsening cyanosis will be caused and in the latter shock and heart failure result. Systemic arterial oxygenation in TGA will also deteriorate when the DA closes. These conditions are all discussed in more detail below (see Cyanosis and Collapse).

Pulmonary vascular resistance

Pulmonary blood flow increases rapidly at birth as pulmonary vascular resistance falls. This normal process will have adverse effects if an increase in pulmonary venous return is disadvantageous as discussed above in the context of restricted outflow from the left atrium or in the presence of pulmonary venous obstruction from any cause. Increased pulmonary blood flow secondary to lesions allowing left-to-right shunting will cause respiratory distress and heart failure as pulmonary vascular resistance falls. This usually is not a problem in the early newborn phase and often is not apparent until after the newborn period. A common exception to this statement is PDA in the preterm infant (see below). Any shunt lesion may become symptomatic at an earlier postnatal age in preterm infants than in term ones; this is attributed to less well developed pulmonary vascular musculature in the premature infant.[44] Delay in the normal fall in pulmonary vascular resistance may acutely result in a clinical problem (PPHN, p. 527) or it may become important in the pathophysiology of chronic lung disease and in the development of permanent pulmonary vascular changes in structural heart disease with unrestricted transmission of systemic pressures into the pulmonary circulation such as in large VSD and complete AVSD. PPHN may also be seen when there has been underdevelopment of the pulmonary vascular tree in utero, such as in diaphragmatic hernia, or if there has been in utero exposure to prostaglandin synthetase inhibitors as a result of maternal therapy with these drugs. Hypoxaemia in PPHN is due to right-to-left shunting which can be either within the lungs or extrapulmonary, in which case it can be at ductal level or intracardiac through the foramen ovale. Detailed consideration of PPHN is given on pages 527–537.

HISTORY AND EXAMINATION

These are basic in the evaluation of a newborn infant with suspected cardiac disease. History taking involves details of the current symptom as well as obtaining pregnancy, perinatal, family and social information. Much of this will be available in maternity records but clarification and expansion is often required when a particular clinical picture presents. Examination of the newborn is dealt with in Chapter 17; a number of points with specific reference to the cardiovascular system will be considered here.

DYSMORPHIC FEATURES AND NON-CARDIAC MALFORMATIONS

These must be carefully sought and described in detail in relation to all body systems. They are clearly important if a syndrome is to be diagnosed as well as in influencing and coordinating management decisions, in prognostication and in communicating fully with families. It may be relevant to investigate other systems on the basis of certain cardiac diagnoses, for example chromosome analysis or immune function testing. In some circumstances recognition of an abnormality in an infant will result in a diagnosis being made in a parent, for example Noonan syndrome. When certain non-cardiac structural abnormalities are recognized, a detailed cardiac evaluation is appropriate as in Down syndrome and many gastrointestinal abnormalities.[86]

PULSES

If femoral pulses cannot be felt easily because an infant is too active, a further attempt should be made when the baby is settled after a feed. Impalpable or weak femoral pulses in the presence of good volume upper limb pulses suggest coarctation of the aorta, in which case other signs may well be present and might include upper limb hypertension, systolic pressure difference of 20 mmHg or more between arms and legs, evidence of aortic valve abnormality (ejection click), a bruit between the scapulae and signs of heart failure. If all pulses are weak, then left ventricular outflow obstruction, hypovolaemia or left ventricular dysfunction should be considered. A preterm infant severely compromised by PDA may have very weak femoral pulses. An infant with interrupted aortic arch usually collapses in the first week of life; the diagnosis and the site of interruption can sometimes be deduced by comparing arm and neck pulses as they will be much stronger proximal to the interruption.

BLOOD PRESSURE

Blood pressure should be measured in both arms and in one leg in any newborn infant with cardiac symptoms and in an asymptomatic infant if other signs raise the possibility of coarctation. Blood pressure should also be measured in any unwell baby as well as in those with urinary tract abnormalities, those on steroids, in chronic lung disease and in the infants of drug-addicted mothers. It is essential that the infant is settled; results on crying or recently crying infants are misleading. Monitoring blood pressure is part of the management of severely ill babies; this should if possible be carried out invasively. Obtaining a definitive non-invasive blood pressure requires patience and attention to detail. The arterial pulse can be detected by palpation or with a Doppler probe. Both methods will only give a systolic value. Auscultation is very difficult and the flush method rarely used. Oscillometric monitors may be useful in sequential blood pressure monitoring of immobile babies but even then are subject to error at low pressures in extremely low-birthweight infants.[25] Cuff size is important and for the arm it should cover 75% of the distance from axilla to elbow or have a width which is 40–50% of the arm circumference.[62] The bladder should virtually encircle the arm. Leg blood pressure can be measured using the same cuff around the calf with detection of a dorsalis pedis or posterior tibial pulse. Normal blood pressure values are given in Appendix 4.

CYANOSIS

Peripheral cyanosis is very common in normal newborn infants. Central cyanosis can be mimicked by facial petechiae (traumatic cyanosis) and in markedly polycythaemic infants. Plethoric infants with a low normal oxygen saturation may have enough deoxygenated haemoglobin to give true central cyanosis. Pigmentation of the lips can also confuse the observer and it is important to look at the tongue to get the best possible assessment of saturation. Anaemia and desaturation make a baby look pale grey rather than really blue; methaemoglobinaemia gives babies a slate black or grey colour which is often mistaken for cyanosis. Cyanotic, often termed 'dusky', episodes are very common and are only occasionally a presenting feature for structural heart disease; persistent cyanosis is far more likely to be cardiac although it may vary in intensity. Cyanosis whilst crying is rarely pathological if colour and behaviour return to normal rapidly when the infant stops crying. Hypercyanotic episodes as seen in tetralogy of Fallot and related conditions are rare in the newborn period.

HEART FAILURE

The signs of heart failure in the newborn are listed in Table 30.6. These features can be masked or caused by respiratory disease and by circulatory collapse from any cause. Most causes of heart failure will be associated with other cardiovascular signs and with cardiomegaly on chest X-ray.

Table 30.6 Features of neonatal heart failure

- Poor feeding
- Excess or unexpected weight gain.
- Poor peripheral perfusion, clammy mottled skin, cold sweatiness
- Oedema – usually late but characteristic of fetal heart failure (hydrops) often with pericardial, pleural and peritoneal fluid
- Tachycardia (unless cause of failure is heart block)
- Hepatomegaly
- Respiratory distress, added sounds in chest
- Gallop rhythm
- Specific signs of causative lesion

HEART MURMUR

Heart murmurs in the newborn can be normal physiological findings and many serious cardiac conditions have unimpressive or even no murmurs. Other auscultatory and general cardiovascular signs are very important in assessing the significance of a murmur. The absence of any other features of cardiac disease as well as the presence of certain positive murmur characteristics are required to diagnose innocent heart murmurs. The typical normal heart murmur in newborn infants comes from the pulmonary artery branches (Table 30.7) and disappears before 6 months of age in term infants.

INVESTIGATIONS

History and examination often allow cardiac disease to be suspected or ruled out. They sometimes allow a definite diagnosis to be made. Investigations consist of those readily available in any neonatal nursery (chest X-ray, ECG, and hyperoxia test) and those only available at cardiac centres (cardiac catheterization and MRI). Echocardiography is being increasingly used outside cardiac centres and with suitable equipment and trained operators is very valuable in the care of the newborn, particularly to confirm or rule out a cardiac abnormality in those difficult cases where clinical assessment, ECG and chest X-ray have been inconclusive. It is not clear that ECG and chest X-ray have a large role in differentiating normal from abnormal murmurs in the newborn although they are widely used for such a purpose.

Table 30.8 Information obtainable from the electrocardiogram

- Rhythm
- Atrial:
  - position
  - enlargement
- Ventricular:
  - position
  - hypertrophy
  - strain/ischaemia

ELECTROCARDIOGRAM

The ECG provides useful information in a number of areas (Table 30.8) providing attention is paid to technical aspects of obtaining a good recording, which can be difficult in a neonatal nursery. Systematic reading of the ECG will optimize the information obtained and reference should be made to normal values for interpretation (see Appendix 3) and to a standard text for detailed consideration of ECGs.[65]

Heart rhythm

Abnormal heart rate can be confirmed on the ECG and heart rhythm usually can be ascertained. Sinus rhythm is characterized by normal P waves (frontal plane axis 0° to + 90°) preceding every QRS complex. Sinus rate varies between 70 and 180/min in healthy infants reaching as much as 220/min in sick babies. In these circumstances P waves can be hard to see but all leads should be examined and paper run at a faster speed (50 mm/s) if necessary. First degree heart block (prolonged PR interval) is rarely of importance in its own right in the newborn but may be a marker for structural heart disease such as ASD or Ebstein's anomaly. A short PR interval is a marker for an increased tendency to SVT although delta waves in the QRS complex may easily be overlooked in neonates. A short PR interval also accompanies some structural heart lesions (Ebstein's anomaly) and may be seen in glycogen storage disease. Partial AV dissociation (second degree heart block) and complete heart block are considered below as are SVT and VT.

Table 30.7 Features of innocent neonatal heart murmurs

Source/type	Characteristics	Comment
Pulmonary arteries	Base of heart, chest bilaterally	Gone by 6 months
Ductus arteriosus	No definite evidence that it can be heard whilst closing normally	
Tricuspid regurgitation (without structural heart disease)	Sounds like VSD	Often with perinatal stress and transient ST/T changes on ECG; resolves in days
Still's innocent murmur	Vibratory Mid-systolic Between LLSE and apex	Rarely heard in newborn period; lasts years

Abbreviations: LLSE – lower left sternal edge; ST/T – ST segment and T wave.

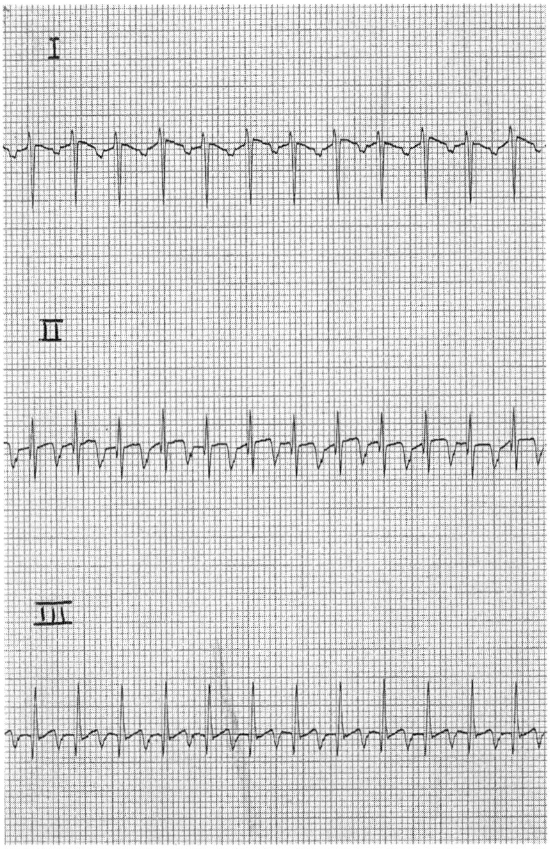

Fig. 30.2 ECG leads I, II and III showing inverted P wave in I. SVT at 190/min.

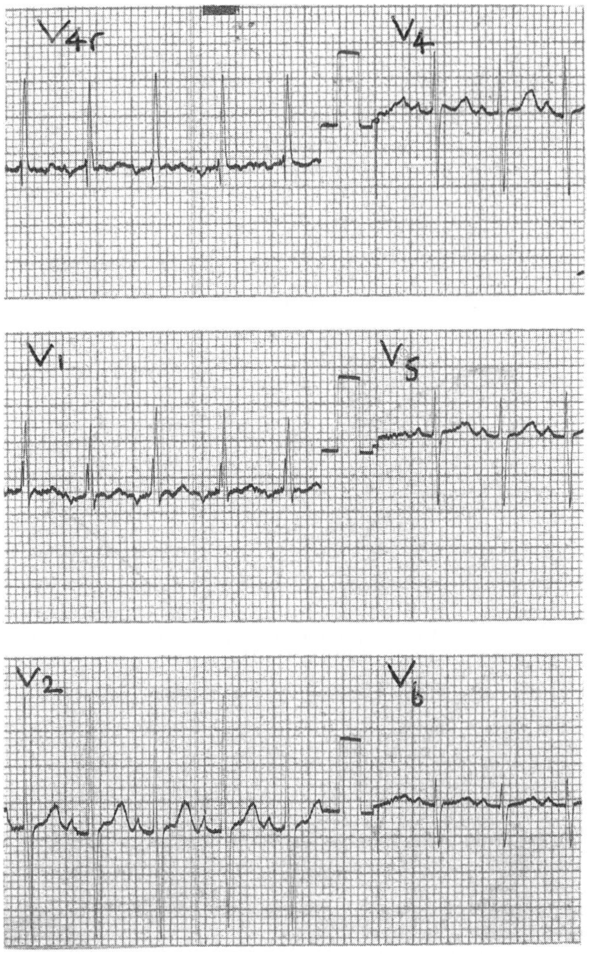

Fig. 30.3 ECG chest leads in 6-day-old infant. Neonatal R/S progression (normal) but upright T wave V_1 indicating RVH.

Information on the atria

Inverted P waves in lead 1 may be a sign of an incorrectly wired ECG (right arm/left arm reversed); this can be checked by looking at lead V_6. If I and V_6 look similar, the ECG is wired up correctly and negative P waves in I then suggest one of the following:

- not sinus rhythm (Fig. 30.2)
- heart in abnormal position
- heart in normal position but atria in abnormal spatial relationship to each other.

Right atrial enlargement is indicated by tall (> 2.5 mV) P waves and left atrial enlargement shown by broad P waves (> 3 mm) at standard paper speed (25 mm/s).

Information on the ventricles

Abnormal ventricular positions within the chest as in dextrocardia, or in relationship to each other as in congenitally corrected transposition, can be suspected from abnormalities in QRS progression across the chest leads. In dextrocardia, complexes do not evolve between V_1 and V_6 but simply get progressively smaller. Q waves in V_1 mean one of the following:

- abnormal intraventricular conduction (as in left bundle branch block or some cases of pre-excitation)
- severe right ventricular hypertrophy
- spatial relationship between right and left ventricles abnormal (as in congenitally corrected transposition).

RVH is suggested by one or more of:

- right axis deviation
- Q in V_1
- large RV_1 or SV_6 (see Appendix 3)
- upright T in V_1 after day 3 (Fig. 30.3).

It is important to note that conditions causing marked RVH in later infancy may cause no ECG abnormality in the immediate newborn period and only an upright T wave in V_1 in the later newborn period.

Left ventricular hypertrophy is suggested by one or more of:

- adult R/S progression V_1 to V_6 (dominant SV_1 dominant RV_6)
- large SV_1 or RV_6 (see Appendix 3).

Biventricular hypertrophy is indicated by a combination of these findings.

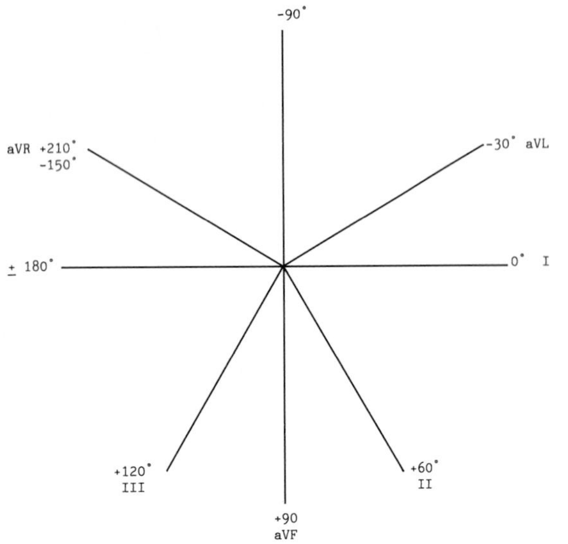

Fig. 30.4 Hexaxial reference system for calculating frontal plane axis of QRS complex (and of P and T waves if required).

Frontal axis of QRS complex can be estimated from the diagram showing polarity of ECG leads I, II, III, aVL, aVF and aVR. To obtain the frontal axis of a QRS complex:

1. Identify the lead in which R and S waves are most nearly of equal size.
2. Look at right angles (+ 90° and – 90°) to the lead identified in step 1.
3. One of the leads identified in step 2 will be predominantly positive; the other predominantly negative.
4. The predominantly positive lead identified by step 3 is approximately the QRS axis (depolarization towards a lead produces a positive deflection).
5. The approximate QRS axis obtained from step 4 can be made more accurate by estimating the equiphasic lead (step 1) more accurately by 'imagining' it between actual leads.

If all leads appear equiphasic, the QRS axis is described as indeterminate; this is rarely normal.

Ventricular strain or ischaemia is indicated by ST depression or T wave inversion in left chest leads (II, aVL, V_{5-6}) and may point to a primary cardiac muscle disorder or be secondary to a severe structural abnormality causing pressure or volume load on the heart. T wave changes are seen after perinatal stress and resolve in under a week. Pericarditis is rare in the newborn period but ST segment and T wave changes are seen.

QRS axis

The frontal QRS axis can be calculated as shown in Figure 30.4. An abnormal QRS axis may be an important diagnostic clue in a number of conditions including AVSD (Fig. 30.5) and tricuspid atresia (QRS usually −30°), in the former case it makes the ECG a valuable screening investigation in newborn infants with Down syndrome in whom clinical features of AVSD may be absent or very subtle.

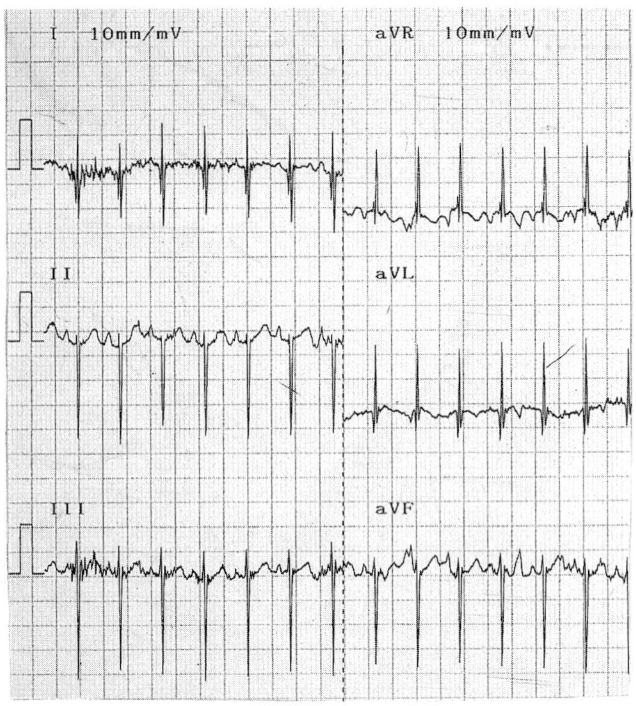

Fig. 30.5 ECG standard leads, superior QRS axis (– 90°), newborn with complete AVSD.

CHEST X-RAY

The plain CXR is widely used in the investigation of suspected cardiac disease. Features to look for in this context are listed in Table 30.9; examples are shown in Figures 30.6–30.9.

HYPEROXIA TEST

The hyperoxia test or nitrogen washout test is a way of standardizing and quantifying the effect of increasing inspired oxygen concentration in infants with suspected structural cyanotic congenital heart disease in whom the possibility of a respiratory cause of cyanosis exists. It was described before echocardiography imaging and Doppler assessment were available.[50] Babies with cyanotic heart disease in general show little increase in arterial oxygen tension in response to greater inspired oxygen. A rise of PaO_2 to a value below 20 kPa after 10 minutes in 85% or more inspired oxygen makes heart disease likely, whereas increase in PaO_2 above 20 kPa makes respiratory disease more likely. There are exceptions to this pattern in that desaturating cardiac disease with high lung blood flow (as in unobstructed TAPVC and double inlet ventricle for example) will pass, whereas infants with severe respiratory disease and with PPHN may fail. When it is essential to have an accurate measurement of arterial oxygen tension then an arterial blood sample must be obtained; further information of importance in the management of ill infants will also be available from a blood

Table 30.9 Features to assess on chest X-ray in infant with suspected cardiac disease

Feature	Comment
Quality of film	Adequate inspiration Normal penetration Centred on mid chest Not rotated
Abdominal situs Bronchial situs	Normal/inverted/ambiguous
Aortic arch side	Left or right
Heart	Side Direction of apex Size Contour
Lung vasculature	Plethora Oligaemia Pulmonary venous engorgement
Diaphragm	Distinct Side of apex should be more caudal
Lung fields	Any pathology
Musculoskeletal	Vertebral/rib abnormalities Fractures

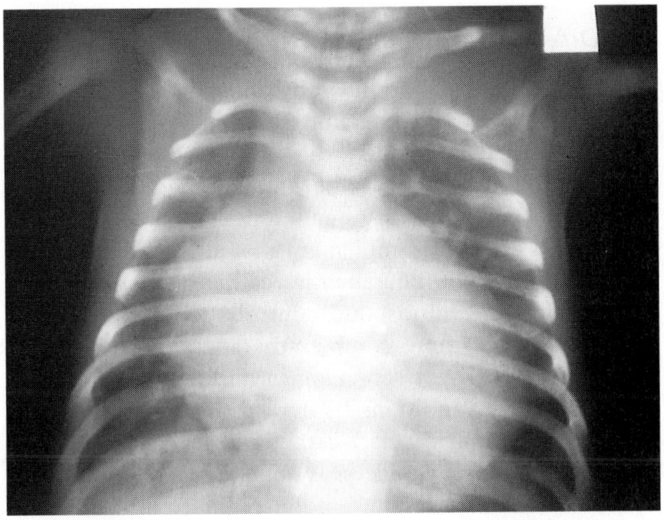

Fig. 30.6 CXR showing cardiomegaly and pulmonary plethora.

gas analysis. Transcutaneous oxygen tension monitors placed on the right upper chest (that is preductal) can be used instead of arterial sampling as a screening test in well infants. Oxygen pulse saturation monitors will not provide the same assurance of a pass as an infant will show 100% saturation at a PaO_2 value a long way below 20 kPa. A well infant who is clearly blue does not need a hyperoxia test; a sick infant on assisted ventilation in whom cardiac disease is suspected needs echocardiography irrespective of the hyperoxia test result, and, in any case, a look through the blood gas chart of such an infant is likely to serve the same purpose without a formal test. Babies for whom hyperoxia is potentially harmful (p. 909), even for a short period, should not be tested.

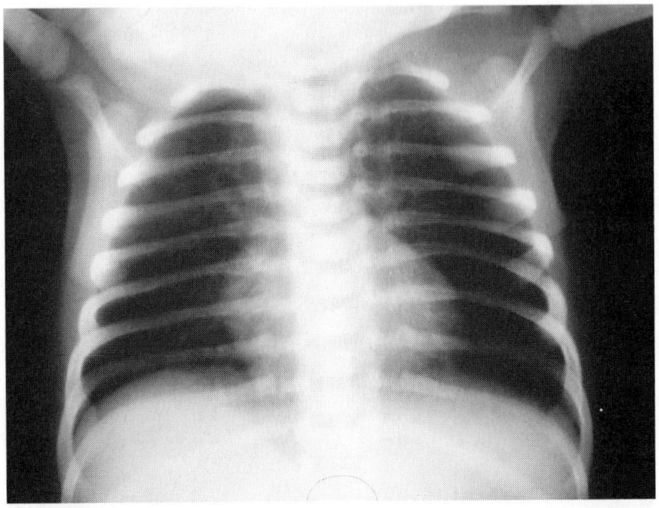

Fig. 30.7 CXR showing normal heart size and pulmonary oligaemia (tetralogy of Fallot).

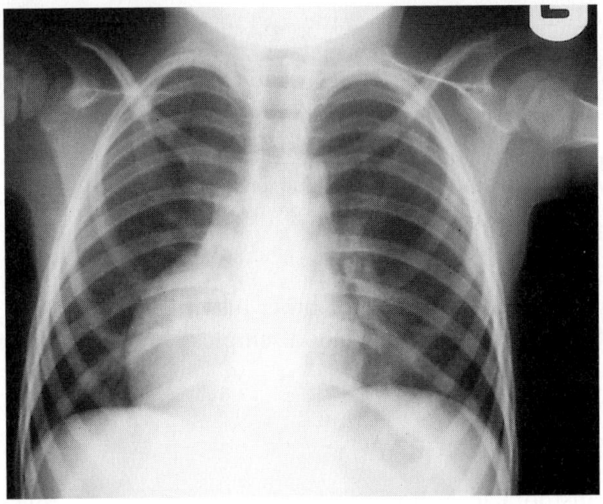

Fig. 30.8 CXR showing dextrocardia and apex to the right. Abdominal situs not seen (normal heart).

The role of the hyperoxia test has therefore changed since its description but it is still helpful in two additional circumstances.

1. When a well baby seems dusky and there is uncertainty as to whether a cyanotic cardiac condition is present. A failed transcutaneous or pulse oximeter hyperoxia test strongly points to cyanotic heart disease.
2. A well baby with signs of heart disease who looks pink may fail the hyperoxia test, thus alerting the physician to the presence of a more complex lesion.

It must be emphasized that the most accurate way to know the arterial oxygen tension is to perform an arterial blood gas sample; the use of non-invasive devices (transcutaneous oxygen tension monitors or pulse oximeters) will on occasion provide sufficient information when evaluating an infant for suspected cyanotic heart disease providing the limitations of these two techniques are

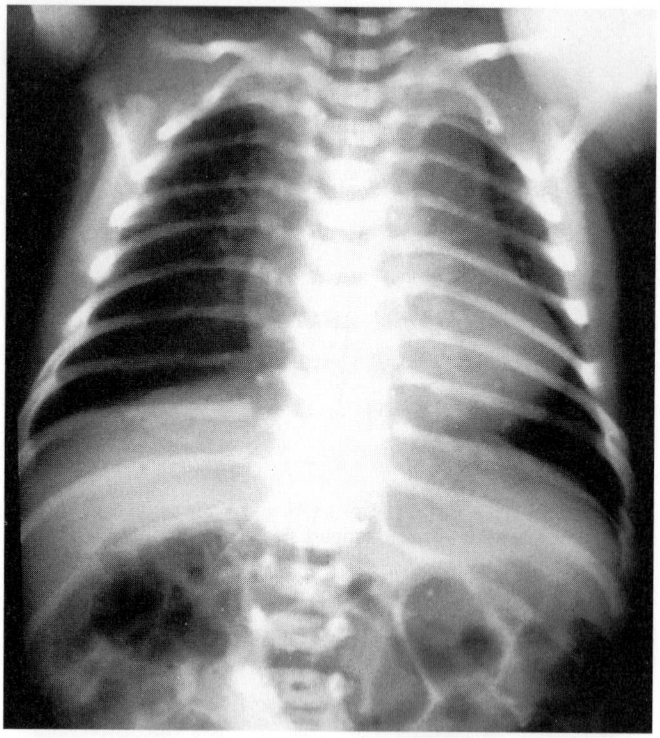

Fig. 30.9 CXR showing laevocardia, apex to the left, midline liver, stomach not clearly lateralized, pulmonary oligaemia (right isomerism, cardiac lesion with severe pulmonary outflow obstruction).

appreciated and providing other parameters measured or calculated from arterial blood samples are not needed for management.

ECHOCARDIOGRAPHY

Transthoracic echocardiography has a major role in diagnosis and management of neonatal heart disease. It has resulted in a dramatic reduction in the need for diagnostic cardiac catheterization and can be used to guide interventions such as balloon atrial septostomy. All ultrasound modalities have a role in evaluating the cardiovascular system (Table 30.10). Imaging gives anatomical detail. Doppler identifies or clarifies shunt lesions and regions of turbulent flow and allows quantification of stenosis by measuring blood velocity, which allows a pressure difference across a valve or between ventricles through a VSD to be calculated by the modified Bernouilli equation ($P = 4V^2$, where P = instantaneous peak systolic pressure gradient in mmHg, V = velocity distal to the site of obstruction in m/s). Detailed consideration of the ultrasound features of different conditions is outside the scope of this chapter but good reviews are available.[12,78] Standard echocardiographic windows and images of the heart are shown in Figure 30.10; examples of clinical scans are given in Figures 30.11–30.13; Transoesophageal echocardiography can be used on term newborn infants and has a role in postoperative assessment when precordial or subcostal images can be hard to obtain. The group of babies from whom transthoracic echocardiograms are most difficult to get are those with severe respiratory disease receiving assisted ventilation. Many of these infants are of low birthweight and too small to allow a TOE probe to be passed.

Table 30.10 Uses of different ultrasound modalities

Modality	Uses
2D imaging	Anatomical detail Chamber size, wall thickness Function
Doppler	Signals reflect direction and velocity of flow, turbulence and flow patterns
Colour flow	Rapid identification of site of abnormal pattern Detection of small shunt or regurgitant lesions
Pulsed wave	Sampling in a localized region Cannot measure high velocities
Continuous wave	Excellent for high velocities Not precisely localized
M mode	Dimensions and function

CARDIAC CATHETERIZATION

Cardiac catheterization may be diagnostic for haemodynamic or anatomical data or therapeutic. With present-day ultrasound capability, diagnostic catheterization is rarely required in the newborn infant and, when it is, there is usually only a small amount of information required in order to complement that already obtained by echocardiography. Therapeutic catheterization can be performed under ultrasound control such as for balloon septostomy[7] but more complex therapeutic interventions usually require X-ray screening in addition to or instead of ultrasound. Conditions treated in the newborn period by interventional cardiac catheterization are listed in Table 30.11. Vascular access is obtained via the umbilicus or percutaneously in the femoral region; cutdown techniques are rarely needed. Infants must have general and specific resuscitation before and during the procedure with particular reference to body temperature, blood glucose, circulating volume, acid–base balance and ventilation. If proper attention is paid to these things as well as ensuring adequate sedation or anaesthesia, complications are rare with vascular damage being the most common. Diminished leg arterial supply after femoral artery entry is usually reversible by heparin or streptokinase. Mortality in diagnostic catheterization in the newborn is less than 5%; for some interventions for serious conditions it is considerably more.[73]

MAGNETIC RESONANCE IMAGING

MRI provides excellent anatomical images but, in the newborn, echocardiography usually provides more than

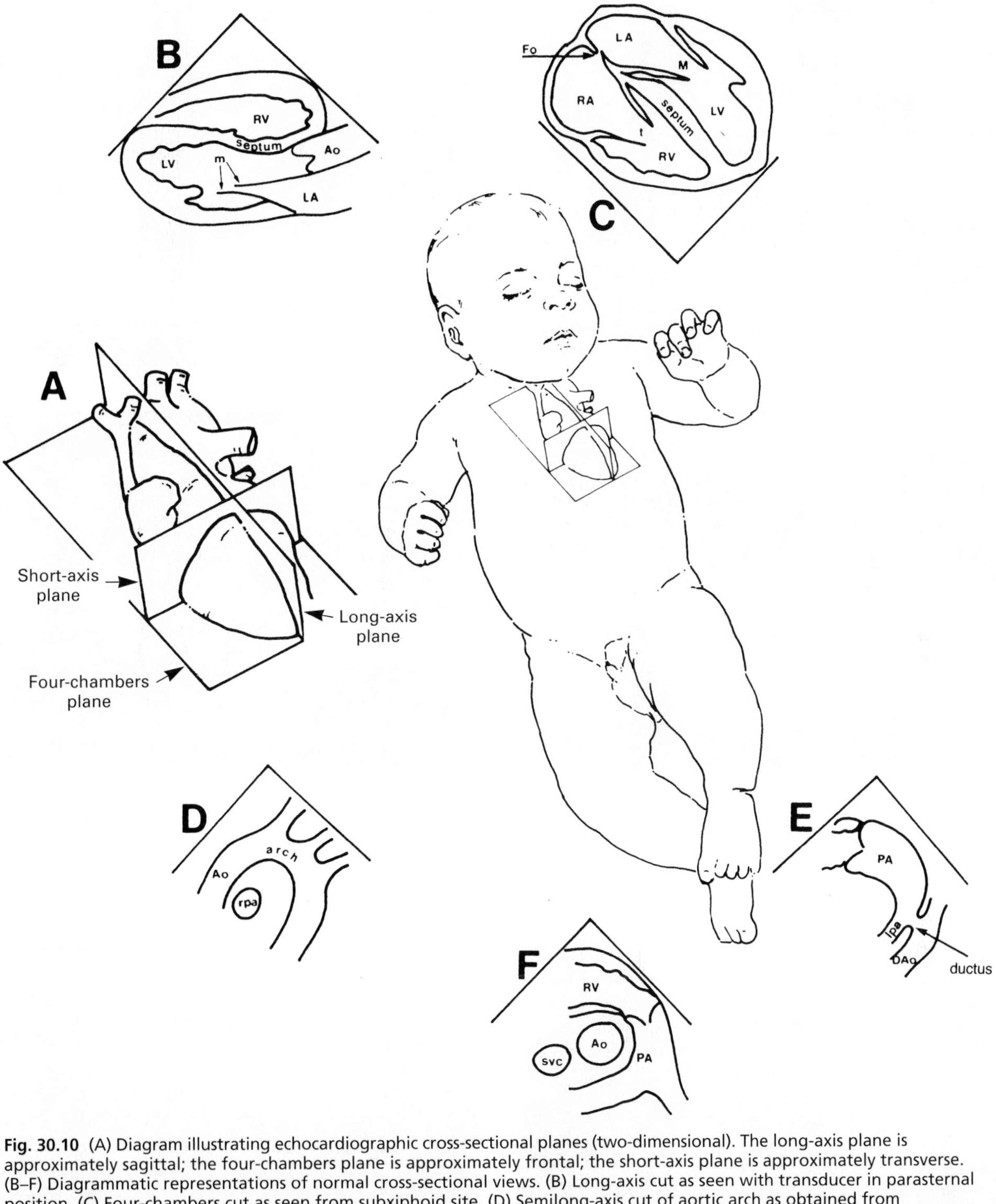

Fig. 30.10 (A) Diagram illustrating echocardiographic cross-sectional planes (two-dimensional). The long-axis plane is approximately sagittal; the four-chambers plane is approximately frontal; the short-axis plane is approximately transverse. (B–F) Diagrammatic representations of normal cross-sectional views. (B) Long-axis cut as seen with transducer in parasternal position. (C) Four-chambers cut as seen from subxiphoid site. (D) Semilong-axis cut of aortic arch as obtained from suprasternal view. (E) High long-axis cut (parasagittal) to show ductus arteriosus. (F) Short-axis cut through the great arteries just above the heart. Ao – aorta; DAo – descending aorta; Fo – foramen ovale; LA – left atrium; lpa – left pulmonary artery; LV – left ventricle; m – mitral valve leaflets; PA – pulmonary artery; RA – right atrium; rpa – right pulmonary artery; RV – right ventricle; svc – superior vena cava; t – tricuspid valve leaflets. Reproduced with permission from Wilkinson J L, Cooke R W I 1992 Cardiovascular disorders.

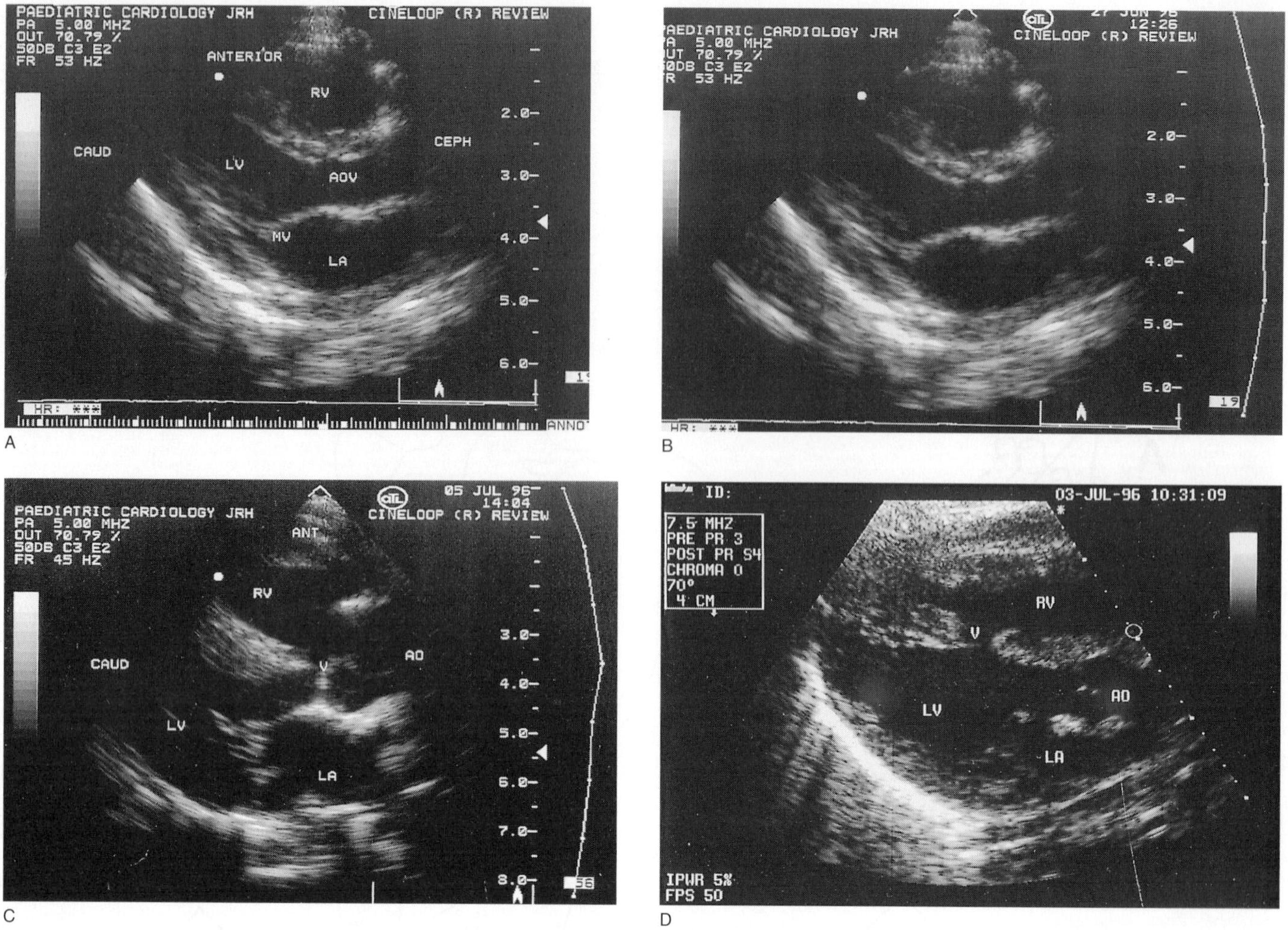

Fig. 30.11 Parasternal long-axis echocardiograms: (A) normal (systole) – annotated; (B) normal without annotation; (C) subaortic VSD (V) with aortic override; (D) midmuscular VSD (V). *Abbreviations:* ANT – anterior; AO – aorta; AOV – aortic valve; CAUD – caudal; CEPH – cephalad; LA – left atrium; LV – left ventricle; MV – mitral valve; RV – right ventricle.

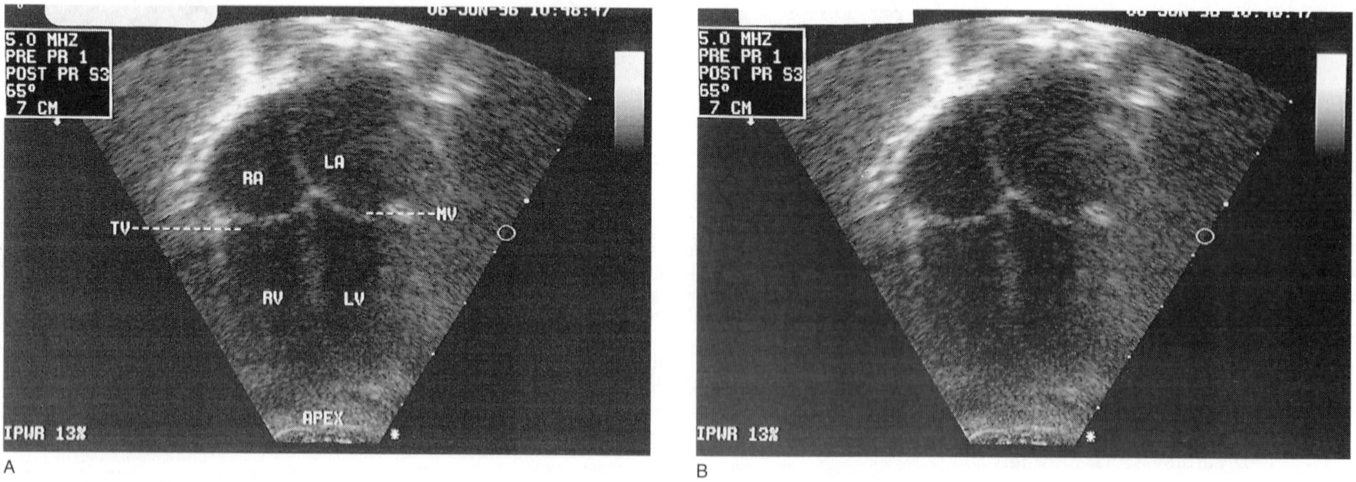

Fig. 30.12 Apical four-chamber echocardiograms: (A) normal (systole) – annotated; (B) normal without annotation.

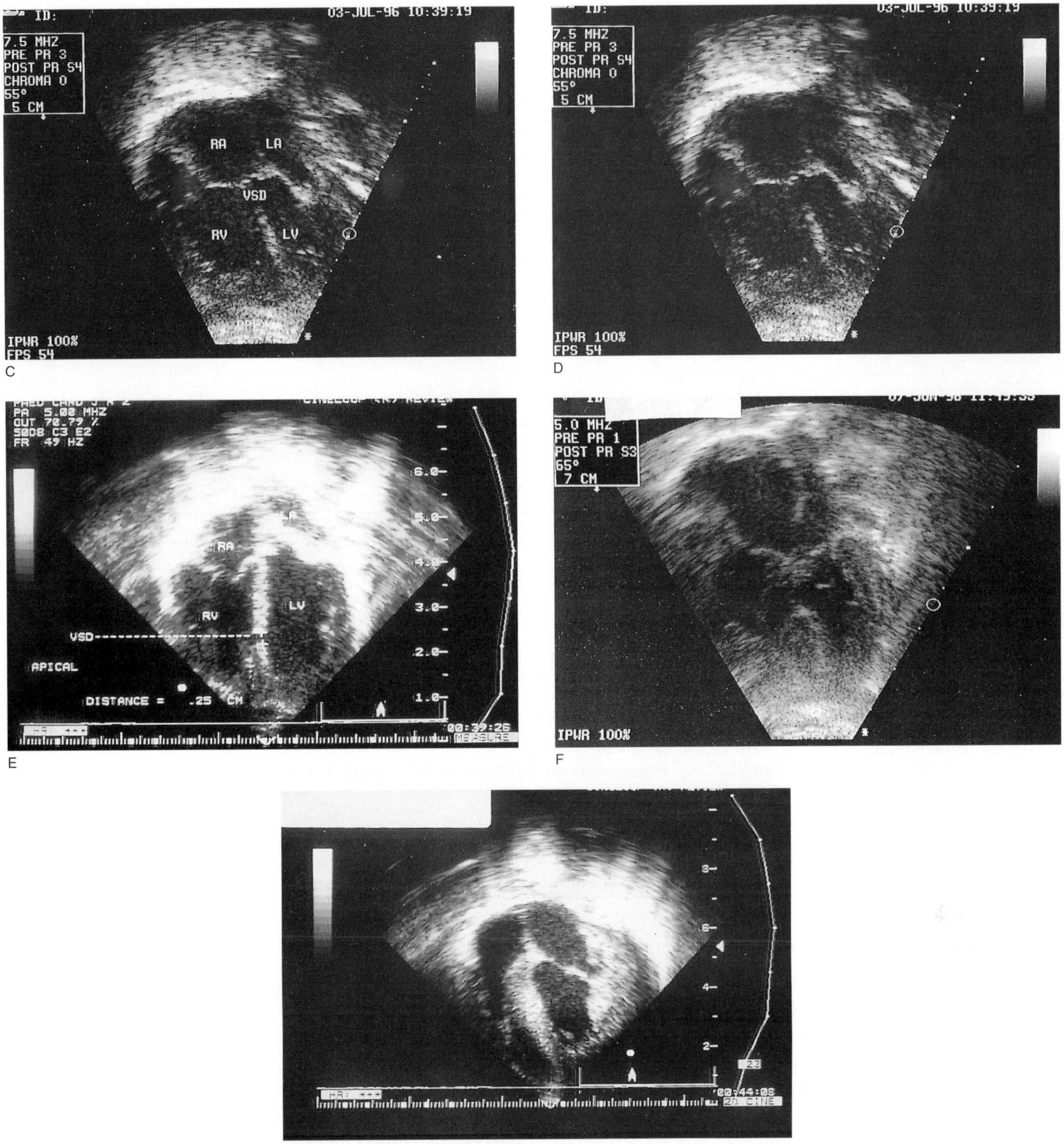

Fig. 30.12 (C) perimembranous VSD with annotation; (D) perimembranous VSD without annotation; (E) midmuscular VSD; (F) complete AVSD (systole) – common AV valve closed with adjacent large ASD and VSD; (G) massively thickened ventricular muscle, especially septum and LV (glycogen storage disease). *Abbreviations:* LA – left atrium; LV – left ventricle; MV – mitral valve; RA – right atrium; RV – right ventricle; TV – tricuspid valve.

adequate information. MRI is useful in older children in evaluating aortic arch and pulmonary arterial abnormalities. Whereas MRI involves no radiation hazard, it does require heavy sedation or general anaesthesia in an environment where detailed monitoring is rather more complicated to achieve and where instant access to the infant can be difficult.

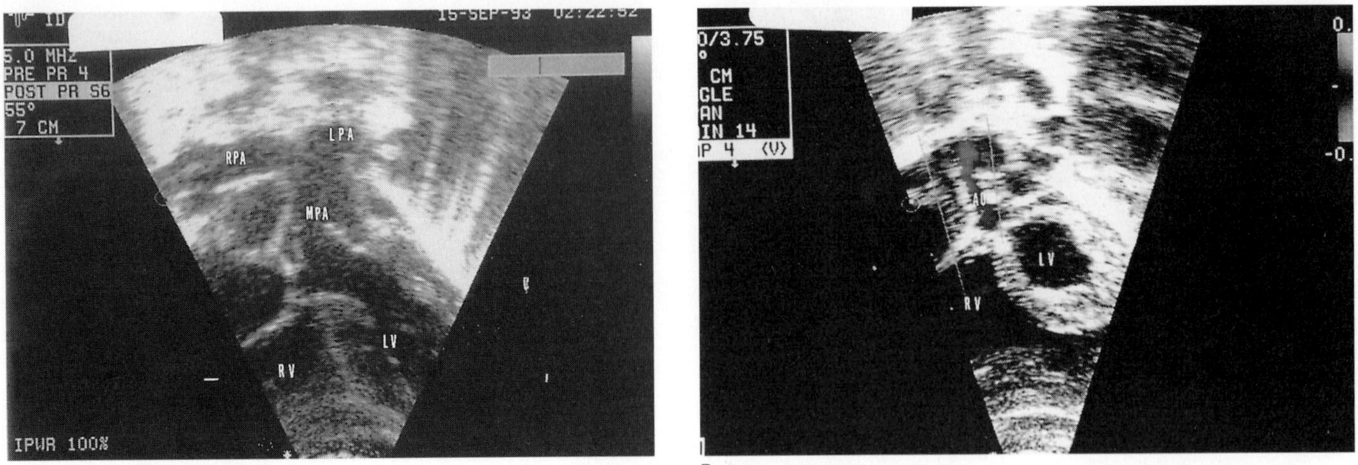

A B

Fig. 30.13 Subcostal echocardiograms. (A) Transposition. Main pulmonary artery (MPA) arising from LV divides into right and left pulmonary arteries (RPA, LPA). (B) Hypoplastic left heart. Tiny ascending aorta (AO) separated from thick-walled LV with small cavity by atretic aortic valve. Hugely dilated RV.

Table 30.11 Interventional cardiac catheterization in newborn infants

Technique	Comment
Balloon septostomy	First interventional catheter described For TGA and restrictive PFO in mitral obstruction or hypoplastic right heart
Balloon dilatation	
Pulmonary valve	Widely used as first choice
Aortic valve	An alternative to surgery, first choice in some centres
Coarctation	Lower success and higher complication rates than surgery
Infundibulum in Fallot's tetralogy	Used in a few centres in place of palliative shunt
Ductus arteriosus	Rarely, if prostaglandin fails
Laser techniques	
Pulmonary atresia without VSD	Being evaluated, surgical approaches more common
Stent techniques	
Ductus arteriosus	Being explored as part of initial palliation of hypoplastic left heart
Embolization techniques	
Cerebral AVM	Treatment of choice for neonates in heart failure

CONCLUSION

All newborn infants with cardiac problems should have ECG, chest X-ray and echocardiography. These provide immediate guidance as well as giving reference values to document future changes. The need for other investigations varies according to the diagnosis.

TREATMENT OF HEART DISEASE

General treatment principles, medication, interventional catheterization and surgery are all considered here with reference to other sections in the chapter as appropriate.

GENERAL PRINCIPLES

Good neonatal management before, during and after specific cardiac interventions is essential.

DUCTAL MANIPULATION

Establishing and maintaining an open DA is a crucial part of the resuscitation of infants with duct-dependent pulmonary or systemic circulations and usually greatly improves oxygenation in TGA. Prostaglandin E1 and prostaglandin E2 will both dilate the DA. Dosage regimes for both drugs are given in Table 30.12. Acute side-effects of prostaglandin include apnoea, jitteriness, convulsions, diarrhoea, flushing and fever. These are usually manageable without loss of therapeutic effect by stopping the infusion for a few minutes and restarting it at a lower dose. Long-term oral or nasogastric use[77] is sometimes of value, for example in a low birthweight infant with duct-dependent pulmonary circulation in whom somatic growth is considered desirable before surgical intervention. Whether this approach allows useful increase in the size of pulmonary arteries in term infants is unclear.[52]

Table 30.12 Prostaglandin dosage regimes

Drug and route	Dose	Comment
Prostaglandin E1 i.v.	0.005–0.1 µg/kg/min	Start at lowest dose, increase if necessary at 15-min intervals
Prostaglandin E2 i.v.	0.005–0.05 µg/kg/min	Side-effects increase with higher doses
Prostaglandin E2 oral/nasogastric	25–40 µg/kg/h	Start hourly at lower dose For long-term use can go stepwise to 4- to 6-hourly

Table 30.13 Heart failure management

Acute	Fluid restrict to approximately two-thirds maintenance Frusemide i.v. 1 mg/kg 6- to 12-hourly Optimize oxygenation, avoid hyperoxia Treat anaemia Consider dopamine or dobutamine if myocardial dysfunction (do not use in hypertrophic cardiomyopathy)
Chronic	Avoid fluid restriction if possible in order to maximize calorie intake Oral diuretic: frusemide 2–6 mg/kg/day (in two or three doses) and potassium-sparing diuretic or potassium supplement If heart muscle dysfunction, consider digoxin 4 µg/kg twice daily oral or ACE inhibitor (not in hypertrophic cardiomyopathy)

Important side-effects with gastric administration are rare. Bone periosteal reaction during chronic administration of prostaglandin is very uncommon with the doses currently recommended. When increasing the dose to allow for less frequent administration, it is advisable to observe the infant for apnoea. Manipulation of the DA in order to close it is considered on page 700.

HEART FAILURE

Management of heart failure is outlined in Table 30.13. In order to achieve as good a nutritional state as possible, it is desirable to minimize fluid restriction. In long-term management it is usually possible to regulate fluid status with diuretics and allow a good volume intake. Additives to increase the calorific value of milk are often needed and nasogastric feeding may be required. Loop diuretics may cause hyponatraemia; a reduction of dose with, if necessary, modest fluid restriction often brings this under control. Increasing sodium supplements in this context is to be avoided if possible, as this will also cause fluid retention. There is considerable experience of ACE inhibitor usage in infancy[60,75] but far less in newborn and, in particular, preterm newborn infants; this latter group appear to tolerate ACE inhibition poorly. If an ACE inhibitor is to be used, it is important not to have the patient dehydrated with diuretics before commencing the drug. Digoxin may be of value in chronic heart failure associated with poor muscle function but neither it nor ACE inhibitors should be used when dynamic left ventricular outflow obstruction is present.

PERSISTENT PULMONARY HYPERTENSION OF THE NEWBORN

Therapy is considered on pages 531–535.

ANTIARRHYTHMIC DRUGS

Arrhythmias and their management are considered on page 705. Doses of commonly used antiarrhythmic agents are given in Table 30.30.

INTERVENTIONAL CATHETERIZATION

This is considered on page 682 and in Table 30.11.

SURGERY

Cardiac surgery can be open as in intracardiac repairs or closed as in coarctation repair, clipping of the ductus arteriosus, Blalock–Taussig systemic-to-pulmonary anastomoses and pulmonary artery banding. Open cardiac surgery is generally performed through a median sternotomy using either hypothermic cardiac arrest or cardiopulmonary bypass or both. Closed operations are frequently performed through a posterolateral thoracotomy. There is an overall trend toward operations at a younger age and toward attempts at physiological, if not necessarily anatomical, corrections rather than palliation. Many conditions do not need surgery in the newborn period and a significant proportion of neonatal surgery is still palliative. Practice will vary from centre to centre but neonatal primary correction is the treatment of choice in simple TGA and in those cases of TAPVC that present in the newborn period. Operative mortalities are given in the discussion of particular conditions.

CARDIOVASCULAR PROBLEMS IN THE PRETERM INFANT

PATENT DUCTUS ARTERIOSUS

In the absence of RDS the DA closes in the same timescale after birth in preterm infants as it does in term ones, being closed in over 90% of infants by 60 hours of age.[31] Information on well, extremely preterm infants is obviously scarce. Closure of the DA in infants over 30 weeks' gestation with mild RDS takes place over a similar timescale with 90% being closed by the fourth day of life.[70] It therefore seems that failure of the DA to close in preterm infants is not primarily an abnormality of the DA but rather due to abnormal stimuli such as acidosis and continuing high circulating prostaglandin levels or due to the absence of normal stimuli such as an increase in oxygen tension. The DA is less sensitive to oxygen earlier in gestation but this does not appear to stop it closing in healthy preterm infants. Failure of the DA to close is associated with more severe RDS[23,47] and interventions to close the DA are associated with short-term improvements in respiratory status.[23,94]

Causative factors for PDA

Prematurity and RDS are the two major causative factors. Fetal exposure to indomethacin increases the likelihood of symptomatic PDA and is associated with a lower closure rate in response to postnatal indomethacin.[64]

Prevention of PDA

Antenatal steroid administration reduces the incidence and severity of RDS and one possible mechanism for this is steroid-induced reduction in ductal sensitivity to prostaglandin.[19,59] Postnatal management of RDS should include cautious fluid regimens as generous ones have been shown to be associated with higher incidence of sPDA (p. 512). Maintaining good oxygen delivery and avoiding acidosis make good theoretical sense. It is very attractive to close the DA actively in babies with RDS before sPDA becomes apparent; both surgery[15] and drug therapy[54] have been advocated. There are a number of difficulties with such an approach.

- Predicting which infants will develop sPDA is not particularly reliable.
- Surgery is an aggressive approach to use prophylactically as well as being logistically difficult for many neonatal intensive care units.
- Concerns about the safety of indomethacin, which is the most widely used DA-constricting drug, make it unclear that short-term benefits of prophylactic administration outweigh risks of the largely unknown long-term neurological sequelae.[33] However, there is considerable evidence that indomethacin reduces the occurrence of all grades of GMH/IVH and what long-term evidence there is suggests favourable rather than unfavourable long-term neurological consequences.[91] There is little evidence that prophylactic administration of indomethacin is associated with less short-term morbidity than use of the drug as soon as sPDA is detected,[18] although very early postnatal use of indomethacin has been advocated because of its effect in reducing intraventricular haemorrhage.[18] Ethamsylate used to prevent intraventricular haemorrhage has been associated with a reduced incidence of sPDA[5,9] but there is insufficient evidence to support its widespread use for DA prophylaxis.
- Prophylactic indomethacin has been reported to have a significant relapse rate[23] from a unit with an overall low incidence of sPDA.

Incidence, clinical features and diagnosis

Definitions of sPDA vary widely and quoted incidences therefore also show much variation but rates up to 50% or more in infants under 800 g have been reported;[85] rates diminish as birthweight and gestation increase. The picture of a baby with RDS, who is failing to improve or starts to deteriorate between 5 and 10 days of age, who has some or all of bounding pulses, an active precordium and a continuous murmur in the pulmonary area is easy to recognize (p. 512). Progressive cardiomegaly and worsening lung shadowing on X-ray may be seen but are rarely helpful. Less gross physical signs in the clinical context may still allow a diagnosis to be made even in the absence of a murmur.[6] Symptomatic PDA can occur well before 5 days of age, particularly in infants who have received exogenous surfactant;[24,69] indeed PDA may be important in the pathogenesis of pulmonary haemorrhage occurring after surfactant administration (p. 551). Apnoea in a non-ventilated baby is sometimes a manifestation of PDA, and necrotizing enterocolitis may be secondary to a widely patent duct. Echocardiography is more sensitive and specific than clinical signs[28] but is not always needed unless there is doubt about the diagnosis or other cardiac problems are suspected or surgery is intended. Echocardiographic features include volume overloading of the left heart, visualization of the ductus itself and Doppler evaluation of the pulmonary artery, the ductus and the descending aorta[28] (Fig. 30.14). Unless prophylactic drug therapy is intended, the significance of echocardiographic detection of PDA is evaluated in the light of the clinical picture.

Treatment of sPDA

The DA will close spontaneously in time in nearly all preterm infants without specific therapy but with considerable morbidity.[49] It is therefore appropriate to recommend early and aggressive treatment for sPDA in the preterm infant, although as discussed above prophylactic pharmacological treatment cannot yet be unreservedly advocated.[18,33] First-line treatment involves optimizing oxygen delivery by treating anaemia and achieving adequate arterial oxygen tension as well as employing fluid restriction and diuretics. Loop diuretics such as frusemide are the most commonly used although

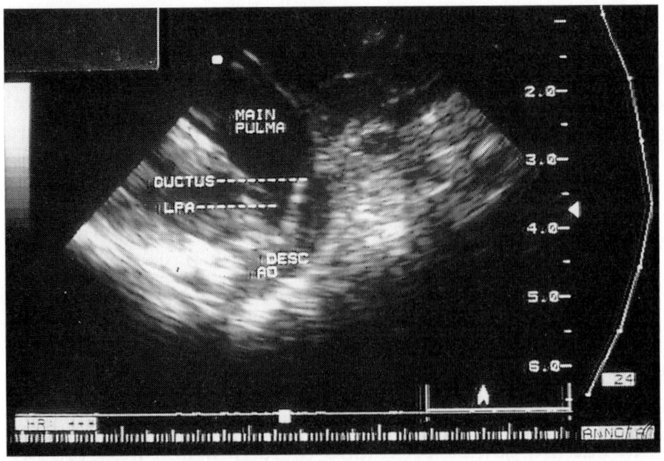

Fig. 30.14 High parasternal ultrasound scan showing PDA. *Abbreviations:* DESC AO – descending aorta; LPA – left pulmonary artery; MAIN PULMA – main pulmonary artery.

there are theoretical reasons as well as modest clinical evidence[40] to suggest that frusemide may promote ductal patency by its effect on renal prostaglandin synthesis. However, a short trial of fluid restriction and diuretic treatment is sometimes associated with clinical improvement, but if there is no improvement after 24 hours, ductal closure should be attempted by either indomethacin or surgery. Generally, indomethacin should be tried first unless a contraindication to its use exists. In a multicentre trial of babies under 1750 g birthweight,[35] 21% developed sPDA, and indomethacin closed the ductus within 48 hours of administration in 79% of the 135 infants who received it. Spontaneous closure occurred in only 28% of controls in the same timescale. One-third of responders relapsed but many of these did not require further intervention and many of those that did have further intervention responded to additional indomethacin administration. Overall, indomethacin had a 70% success rate which was not influenced by the application or not of prior fluid restriction and diuretic therapy. Many other studies have demonstrated similar results. Gestation under 28 weeks and postnatal age beyond 2 weeks are associated with lower success rates as is antenatal indomethacin exposure.[64]

Indomethacin is usually given intravenously in a dose of 0.2 mg/kg on three occasions with 8–12 h between each dose. If a response is seen but with later relapse, it is reasonable to give a further course of indomethacin. Indomethacin used in this way has a beneficial effect on ventilatory requirements and also allows improved nutrition. However, there is little clear evidence of long-term benefit in terms of survival, duration of hospital stay or improved neurodevelopmental outcome. Indomethacin interferes with platelet function and thrombocytopenia is a contraindication to its use, as are markedly elevated or rapidly rising blood urea or creatinine concentrations. As well as constricting the DA, indomethacin causes renal vasoconstriction resulting in oliguria, fluid retention, hyponatraemia and elevation of blood urea and creatinine concentrations. These effects are transitory and rarely serious if fluid restriction is applied during treatment; they may also be lessened by the use of dopamine during indomethacin treatment, although this has not been a consistent finding.[32] Peripheral vasoconstriction during indomethacin administration causes hypertension[27] and derangement of intestinal arterial haemodynamics.[21] The effect on gastrointestinal blood flow may be the explanation for gastrointestinal haemorrhage and perforation which are seen in less than 10% of recipients of indomethacin. Cranial Doppler ultrasound demonstrates significant falls in cerebral blood flow velocity after rapid intravenous administration of indomethacin[27] but not if the drug is given over 30 minutes.[20] However, near infrared spectroscopy shows marked and prolonged reduction in cerebral blood flow and volume, cerebral oxygen delivery and cerebral vascular responsiveness regardless of the speed of administration of the drug.[26] The evidence that indomethacin reduces cerebral blood flow is countered by clear evidence that it reduces the incidence of intraventricular haemorrhage[91] and that PDA has adverse effects on cerebral haemodynamics.[30,76] A 5-day course of indomethacin[42] has been shown to reduce relapse rate and a 6-day lower-dose (0.1 mg/kg/day) course[71] is associated with lower relapse rates and less biochemical disturbance. It is not known what cerebral haemodynamic disturbances accompany these longer courses of indomethacin. Ibuprofen has been shown to be effective at closing the ductus in a small group of extremely preterm infants but without disturbances of cerebral haemodynamics as demonstrated by near infrared spectroscopy.[66]

Surgery

Surgical occlusion of sPDA is indicated if a clear contraindication to indomethacin administration exists, or if the drug is ineffective. Relapse after a second short course of indomethacin or after a single 6-day course is also an indication for surgery. Surgery can be performed in the neonatal intensive care nursery with acceptable morbidity and low mortality.[22] If the above approaches are followed, most babies with sPDA should have had successful occlusion of it either pharmacologically or by surgery before 14 days of age, some even in the first week of life, and all well before they are 3 weeks old.

CHRONIC LUNG DISEASE

The pathogenesis of CLD is complex (Ch. 29, Part 3) and a contribution from PDA seems likely, although early intervention to close PDA has not been demonstrated to reduce the incidence of CLD. Other left-to-right shunt lesions may contribute to or be masked by chronic respiratory problems. CLD, particularly with sustained or recurrent hypoxaemia, results in elevation of pulmonary vascular resistance with consequent pulmonary hypertension, right heart enlargement and hypertrophy. Steroid administration may cause cardiac hypertrophy with or without systemic hypertension which may result in dynamic left ventricular outflow obstruction.[29] These changes are rarely of clinical significance and resolve with cessation of steroid therapy. Electrocardiographic and echocardiographic assessment of infants with CLD is appropriate to judge right ventricular hypertrophy and to get non-invasive (Doppler) evaluation of right heart pressures. Diuretics are of value in the condition as pulmonary oedema is a feature, and are also indicated if systemic venous engorgement occurs secondary to elevated right heart pressures. Reduced ventricular function or atrial dysrhythmias are late and very serious findings.

STRUCTURAL HEART DISEASE

Structural heart disease can be present in the preterm infant and may easily be overlooked because respiratory signs mask cardiac ones and chest X-rays can be hard to interpret. Any possibility of structural heart disease warrants echocardiographic evaluation if intervention for sPDA is contemplated, and such assessment is essential before surgery for PDA. Duct-dependent cardiac conditions can be particularly problematic in extremely preterm infants and long periods of intravenous or gastric prostaglandin administration may be required whilst growth to a size where corrective or palliative interventions are feasible occurs. Primary arrhythmias and acquired heart disease may occur in the preterm with morbidity and mortality being increased in the presence of severe RDS. Persistent pulmonary hypertension may complicate RDS (p. 489).

ENDOCARDITIS

Infective and non-infective thrombotic endocarditis occur in critically ill newborn infants with structurally normal hearts, particularly the preterm.[56,57] Clinical features are non-specific but recurrent or relapsing bacteraemia or the presence of multiple infected sites should raise suspicion of infective endocarditis. Splenomegaly and microscopic haematuria are often present but these have many other possible causes. Indwelling arterial or central venous cannulae are risk factors for thromboembolic phenomena and infection. Echocardiography is helpful in diagnosis by recognition of intracardiac vegetations. Treatment involves removal of infected or potentially infected lines and culture-guided antibiotic therapy which may require to be prolonged.

PERSISTENT PULMONARY HYPERTENSION

PPHN can occur in preterm or term infants and causes greater arterial desaturation than the underlying or associated disease would otherwise be expected to do. There are a number of possible pathogenetic associations with PPHN and the overall clinical picture will be influenced by the particular coexisting pathology. PPHN is dealt with in Chapter 29, Part 2.

STRUCTURAL HEART DISEASE IN THE NEWBORN

Heart disease in the newborn can be considered as presenting in one of four main ways, namely:

- cyanosis
- respiratory distress (heart failure)
- collapse
- asymptomatic.

Table 30.14 Conditions presenting with neonatal cyanosis

Category	Detail	Comment
Respiratory	Any respiratory disease	
Cardiac	Common mixing TAPVC DIV DOV Truncus arteriosus Right-to-left shunt Pulmonary atresia, IVS Pulmonary atresia, VSD Tricuspid atresia Tetralogy of Fallot Transposition	 Especially if obstructed Degree of cyanosis reflects severity of PS Heart failure common 20% cyanosed as newborn
Persistent pulmonary hypertension	See p. 527	
Haematological	Methaemoglobinaemia	Grey/black rather than blue, arterial oxygen tension normal

Table 30.15 Clinical features helpful in distinguishing respiratory from cardiac cyanosis. Note all categories have overlap between respiratory and cardiac causes

	Respiratory cyanosis	Cardiac cyanosis
History	Prematurity, meconium staining/ below cords, risk of infection (Table 29.13, pp. 498–499)	Family history of congenital heart disease
Respiration	Marked respiratory distress	Little or no respiratory distress unless shocked or metabolic acidosis
Cardiovascular examination	Normal	May have clear signs
Response to oxygen	Cyanosis likely to improve	Cyanosis unlikely to improve
Chest X-ray	Obvious respiratory pathology	No respiratory pathology, abnormal heart shadow or lung vasculature may be seen
ECG	Normal	May be normal, may be helpful
Blood gases	Hypercapnia	Hypo- or normocapnia

CYANOSIS

The causes of cyanosis are listed in Table 30.14. In practice it is often possible to distinguish respiratory and cardiac causes on clinical grounds; Table 30.15 gives details of helpful discriminating features. If cardiac disease is thought definite or likely, an approach to management is given in Table 30.16. Clinical features, ECG and chest X-ray often allow an approximate cardiac diagnosis to be made (Table 30.17). Echocardiography allows very precise diagnosis in the vast majority of cases. It is more important to stabilize an infant before transfer to a cardiac centre than to get a precise diagnosis by ultrasound. Differentiating cardiac disease from PPHN may require echocardiography and the two may coexist (Table 30.18). Basic clinical ECG and chest X-ray information on cyanotic conditions is given in Table 30.17; further details on each condition are given below.

Table 30.16 Management of newborn infant with suspected cyanotic congenital heart disease

1. General measures:
   - Maintain temperature
   - Avoid hypoglycaemia

If well proceed to 3

2. If ill:
   - Arterial blood gas
     - treat respiratory failure; ventilate if necessary
     - hypoxaemia alone not reason to ventilate
     - treat metabolic acidosis
     - consider hyperoxia test
   - Consider prostaglandin
3. Chest X-ray:
   - Diagnostic clues may be present
   - Aid in management
     - oligaemia: start prostaglandin
     - plethora: start prostaglandin if very hypoxaemic or metabolic acidosis
4. ECG: may point to specific diagnosis
5. Review:
   - Drugs
     - prostaglandin as above
     - alkali
     - diuretic if heart failure/pulmonary congestion
     - antibiotics if risk of serious infection
   - Need for hyperoxia test: it may help, see page 680
6. Echocardiography:
   - If infant requires transfer, stabilize first
   - Occasionally needed to confirm/rule out cardiac cause
   - Usually gives precise cardiac diagnosis

Transposition

Transposition of the great arteries represents approximately 5% of cases of structural congenital heart disease; it is rarely found in preterm infants and is rarely associated with extracardiac abnormalities or syndromes. It is commoner in males by a factor of 3. Associated cardiac conditions include ASD, VSD, PDA, valvar and subvalvar pulmonary stenosis and aortic coarctation. Clinical signs will be determined by the associated abnormalities and, in particular, the fewer and smaller the shunt lesions the more severe the cyanosis will be. Presentation is occasionally delayed beyond the first week of life but in those with no shunts is usually within a few hours of birth. Marked pulmonary outflow obstruction will result in worse cyanosis as well as a loud murmur with pulmonary oligaemia on chest X-ray, whereas in the absence of pulmonary stenosis, pulmonary plethora is the more usual finding. Cases with large shunt lesions will not require immediate intervention to improve oxygenation; those without large shunt lesions will usually improve oxygenation enough to avoid metabolic acidosis if the ductus arteriosus is opened with prostaglandin. In some cases enlargement of the foramen ovale by balloon septostomy will be necessary to obtain adequate entry of well-saturated blood into the right ventricle even if the ductus arteriosus has been reopened. Balloon septostomy can be done in the neonatal nursery under ultrasound control if cardiac catheterization and angiography are not needed for other reasons.[7] Balloon septostomy is likely to be needed if there is a poor response in oxygenation to prostaglandin administration or if early corrective surgery

Table 30.17 Clinical features of structural heart lesions presenting with cyanosis

Condition	Pulses	Respiratory distress	Precordium	Auscultation	ECG	CXR	Extracardiac abnormalities
Transposition	Normal	Mild	RV+	S2 single ± RVOT/LVOT systolic murmur	T↑V_1	RV+, lung fields normal or plethora Oligaemia if severe PS	Rare
Pulmonary atresia	Normal	Mild	Normal	S2 single ± TR	RA + LV + QRS 0° to 90°	Heart normal or large Oligaemia	Rare
Pulmonary atresia with VSD (+ MAPCAs)	Normal	Mild	Normal or RV+	S2 single ± continuous murmur (MAPCAs)	T↑V_1	Heart normal or large Small PA Right arch Oligaemia (plethora if many MAPCAs)	Common (GI, GU chromosomes)
Tetralogy of Fallot	Normal	None	RV+	S2 single RVOT systolic murmur	T↑V_1	Heart normal Small PA Oligaemia Right arch	Common (GI, GU chromosomes)
Tricuspid atresia	Normal	None	Normal	VSD or PS systolic murmur	RA + LAD (0° to −90°) LV+	Heart size normal RA+ Oligaemia	Rare
TAPVC (obstructed)	Normal or weak	Marked	RV+	S2 may be wide P2 loud No murmur	T↑V_1 RSRV_1	Heart normal if obstructed Pulmonary venous engorgement	Rare
Complex lesions	Normal, full or weak	Variable	Active	S2 often single Various murmurs	Abnormal P waves Abnormal QRS axis	Dextrocardia, situs inversus/ambiguus Oligaemia	Common including heterotaxy (p. 695)

Note: Any lesion may have ductal murmur in addition to signs listed.
Abbreviations:↑ – upright; ± – with or without; + – hypertrophied or enlarged.

Table 30.18 Features helpful in differentiating PPHN from cyanotic heart disease

	Persistent pulmonary hypertension	Cyanotic heart disease
History	Maternal prostaglandin synthetase inhibitor therapy	May have positive family history
Delivery	Fetal distress, birth asphyxia	Uneventful
Examination	Respiratory and/or neurological signs	May have clear cardiac signs
Chest X-ray	May have respiratory pathology	May have cardiac/pulmonary vascular signs. Often non-specific
ECG	May have RAH, ischaemic changes	May have clear abnormality
Hyperoxia test	Variable response, may pass, not if severe; fluctuating arterial oxygen tensions seen	Usually poor response
Upper/lower limb saturations	Lower limb often lower (if DA patent)	Occasionally marked discrepancy
Echocardiography	Usually can exclude heart abnormality but can be difficult	Usually diagnostic

Note: There can be marked overlap and both can coexist.

is not envisaged. Coexistent coarctation must be repaired and the arterial switch operation is performed in the newborn period unless there is marked fixed pulmonary outflow obstruction when the arterial switch operation is inappropriate. In these cases a systemic-to-pulmonary anastomosis will be needed and definitive surgery is deferred for some years. The arterial switch operation must be performed before left ventricular muscle has involuted in response to serving the lower-resistance pulmonary circulation; the timescale in which this happens is unclear but surgery under 3 weeks of age is within a safe margin. If there is a large VSD which does not reduce in size spontaneously, the timescale is not as pressing but there is no particular advantage in delaying surgery beyond 2 months. A baby with TGA who presents beyond the early newborn period needs careful echocardiography and sometimes catheterization to be sure that the left ventricular pressure remains high. If it is thought that the left ventricle is no longer capable of supporting the systemic circulation, a preliminary pulmonary artery banding is performed to prepare it. In these circumstances a systemic-to-pulmonary arterial anastomosis may also be needed to ameliorate profound cyanosis produced by the pulmonary artery band. Coronary artery anatomy is clearly important to the surgeon and can often be delineated by echocardiography, but even if it cannot, few centres now perform angiography to clarify it. Neonatal arterial switch operative mortality is < 10% for simple TGA. Repair of transposition by intra-atrial repair (Mustard or Senning operations) is uncommonly performed now because of long-term problems with arrhythmias and right ventricular failure.

Congenitally corrected transposition of the great arteries

This very rare abnormality (< 1% of structural heart lesions) involves not only ventriculoarterial discordance (as in TGA) but also atrioventricular discordance. Thus pulmonary venous blood passes from the left atrium through the tricuspid valve into the morphological right ventricle and then is ejected into the aorta. Desaturated systemic venous blood passes through the right atrium and morphological left ventricle into the pulmonary artery. There may be dextrocardia and sometimes situs inversus. If there are no associated defects, infants are pink and the condition is not suspected until long after the newborn period. Ventricular septal defects occur in 75–80% of patients and will often cause heart failure in infancy unless important pulmonary stenosis coexists, in which case cyanosis will occur, sometimes in the newborn period. Systemic atrioventricular valve regurgitation develops in about 30% of cases in later life and arrhythmias can develop at any age from fetal life onwards, including all degrees of atrioventricular block and SVT. Cyanosis or heart failure may be present; there is RVH and P2 is single. Murmurs depend on associated lesions. The ECG may have heart block of any degree or a pre-excitation pattern. There are Q waves in V_1 and none in V_{5-6}. Chest X-ray will be affected by associated lesions; it may show an abnormal heart position and often has a prominent left upper heart border due to the ascending aorta. Palliative surgery in the form of pulmonary artery banding or systemic-to-pulmonary anastomosis is indicated in symptomatic infants.

Pulmonary atresia

In all forms of this condition the pulmonary valve and sometimes the subvalvar ventricular outflow tract is completely blocked so there can be no forward flow from the right ventricle into the pulmonary artery. Valve morphology varies and may consist of two or three thin cusps which are fused or the valve cusps may be extremely thick, dysplastic and immobile. Whatever cusp morphology exists the valve ring itself is usually small in addition. Hearts with pulmonary atresia can be further subdivided as follows:

- with intact ventricular septum – pulmonary circulation always duct dependent (includes neonates with critical pulmonary valve stenosis)
- with ventricular septal defect – pulmonary circulation duct dependent or pulmonary blood supply from MAPCAs
- as part of complex cyanotic heart disease, for example as in asplenia with AVSD ± TGA.

Pulmonary atresia with intact ventricular septum

This condition always presents with severe cyanosis in the early newborn period, thereby making up 2.5% of symptomatic newborns with congenital heart disease but < 1% of all lesions. The main pulmonary artery and its branches are usually confluent and of reasonable size whereas the right ventricle and tricuspid valve are underdeveloped, sometimes severely so. The tricuspid valve is frequently malformed by displacement of its septal leaflet toward the apex (Ebstein's malformation). Anomalies of the coronary supply to the right ventricle are common and may affect outcome. There is total right-to-left shunting at atrial level. If the foramen ovale is or becomes restrictive, marked right atrial enlargement and systemic venous engorgement occur. Pulmonary blood flow is duct dependent and extreme cyanosis with metabolic acidosis develop as duct closure progresses. Clinical features are given in Table 30.17. Resuscitation includes prostaglandin and sometimes balloon atrial septostomy. Interventional catheterization is being explored as initial treatment[43] but most centres use a surgical approach, the exact sequence depending on echocardiographic assessment of right ventricular cavity and tricuspid valve sizes. In what way coronary abnormalities should affect management is unclear. Primary opening up of the right ventricle outflow tract is desirable if at all possible; systemic-to-pulmonary arterial anastomosis may be required in addition. These approaches give survival to school age in the region of 80%. If right ventricular hypoplasia is so severe that a biventricular circulation cannot ultimately be established, a systemic-to-pulmonary shunt is performed in the newborn period and the eventual aim is to achieve a Fontan-type circulation in which systemic veins are connected to the pulmonary arteries without passage of systemic venous blood through a ventricle. Critical pulmonary valve stenosis has many features in common with this situation except that there is forward flow through the pulmonary valve and the right heart is not markedly hypoplastic. Infants with critical pulmonary stenosis can be treated with either balloon dilatation or surgery with a good result even if further intervention in the form of pulmonary balloon dilatation is needed in later infancy.

Pulmonary atresia with VSD (Table 30.17)

These infants may have non-confluent and severely underdeveloped pulmonary arteries. Pulmonary blood supply may come entirely via the ductus arteriosus or it may come partly or entirely from other vessels arising from the aorta (MAPCAs) or head and neck branches. The degree of cyanosis and other physical signs will depend on the amount of flow into the pulmonary circulation. If MAPCAs are large or plentiful cyanosis is milder, continuous murmurs are heard all over the chest and heart failure may develop. This group of conditions has a significant association with extracardiac malformations, syndromes and chromosomal abnormalities. DiGeorge syndrome and 22q11 deletions must be remembered as they have important implications for management, with increased risk of symptomatic hypocalcaemia, immunodeficiency and, if transfused cellular blood products, of GVHD. If pulmonary blood flow is duct dependent, prostaglandin will be needed and early palliative surgery is indicated. If sources of lung blood supply are complex, detailed evaluation with angiography is required in early infancy in order to assess surgical options. Long-term outcome is variable but a survival of 80% or more is likely in those without complex sources of lung blood flow.

Pulmonary atresia as part of a complex lesion

These infants usually have duct-dependent pulmonary blood flow and their condition will be improved by prostaglandin. Obstruction to the systemic arterial outflow of the heart exceedingly rarely coexists, just as complex lesions with systemic outflow obstruction very rarely have significant pulmonary outflow obstruction. However, almost any other cardiac structural abnormality can coexist. Thus clinical features in addition to cyanosis vary, as do appropriate treatments. In the newborn period surgical interventions, if indicated at all, are likely to be only palliative. Extracardiac abnormalities are common and long-term outcome is often poor for both cardiac and non-cardiac reasons, particularly in those with dextro-isomerism (p. 696) in whom asplenia with a greatly increased risk of infection is usually present.

Tetralogy of Fallot (Table 30.17)

This constitutes 10% of all cases of structural heart disease but only 20% of cases of tetralogy of Fallot are cyanotic in the newborn period. Right ventricular outflow obstruction is always subvalvar (infundibular) but may be valvar and supravalvar in addition. Right ventricular outflow obstruction and a large VSD ensure right ventricular hypertrophy. The VSD is subaortic with the aorta arising in part from the right ventricle (overriding aorta); it is rarely restrictive and additional significant VSDs are occasionally found. Patent foramen ovale or ASD commonly coexist, rarely the pulmonary valve is absent (see below) and the condition can coexist with complete AVSD. The cases presenting with cyanosis as newborns may have pulmonary atresia or a very narrow but patent right ventricular outflow tract. Those with pulmonary atresia will be duct dependent. Tetralogy of Fallot without cyanosis in the newborn period is associated with a pulmonary outflow murmur although it is frequently not recognized as such. Cyanosis is progressive during the first year of life as subvalvar muscular right ventricular outflow tract obstruction increases. Hypercyanotic spells due to infundibular constriction are rare in the newborn period but are an indication for palliative or corrective surgery. Emergency management of spells includes:

- intermittent knee-chest position if feasible
- facial oxygen (although whilst the spell occurs it is unlikely to improve oxygenation)
- morphine (50–100 μg/kg s.c., i.m. or i.v.)
- phenylephrine 20 μg/kg i.v.
- propranolol 20 μg/kg slowly i.v., may be repeated once
- heavy sedation/anaesthesia and assisted ventilation.

It is rare to need to progress beyond morphine in this protocol. Intravenous drugs should only be used in a setting where ventilation and full cardiopulmonary resuscitation can be given. Spells are usually mild initially and get progressively more frequent, more severe and prolonged. Oral propranolol (1–2 mg/kg) three times daily usually prevents recurrent spells in the short and medium term whilst surgical strategies are decided. Cardiac catheterization is often carried out prior to corrective surgery for tetralogy of Fallot to assess coronary anatomy, to look for additional VSDs and to display pulmonary artery anatomy in detail. Cardiac catheterization is not required prior to the creation of a systemic-to-pulmonary anastomosis.

Tetralogy of Fallot with absent pulmonary valve

This rare variant of tetralogy (<5% of cases) has small dysplastic pulmonary valve leaflets resulting in marked pulmonary regurgitation, and dilatation, often massive, of the pulmonary arteries. The large pulmonary arteries compress the bronchi so that bronchomalacia develops in utero. Presentation in the newborn period is with airway obstruction causing pulmonary collapse or overinflation. Cyanosis is not usually marked in early infancy. Impressive systolic and diastolic murmurs from the right ventricular outflow tract with a single S2 in the context of airway obstruction strongly suggest the diagnosis. The dilated pulmonary arteries are seen on CXR; RVH is apparent on ECG. Severe bronchomalacia and pulmonary hypoplasia often cause death even if technically satisfactory cardiac surgical repair is achieved. Surgical mortality in those with severe pulmonary problems may be as high as 50%.

Tricuspid atresia (Table 30.17)

Tricuspid atresia represents about 2% of structural heart lesions. Associated abnormalities include VSD and TGA. Those without TGA may have pulmonary stenosis; those with TGA may have coarctation. Blood leaves the right atrium via the foramen ovale or an ASD. If the VSD is large or there is TGA, pulmonary blood flow will be high and cyanosis mild with the possibility of heart failure developing. A restrictive VSD and/or severe pulmonary stenosis will produce duct-dependent pulmonary circulation. Coarctation with TGA may result in collapse from duct-dependent systemic circulation. Clinical features are given in Table 30.17. Coarctation should be repaired at presentation. The long-term goal is a Fontan circulation, and either systemic-to-pulmonary anastomosis or pulmonary artery banding are usually required in infancy as palliation and, if the VSD is large, to ensure undamaged pulmonary vasculature. In the context of tricuspid atresia with TGA, an arterial switch operation may be performed. Although in this circumstance the switch is only palliative, it does ensure that the systemic ventricle is the morphologically left ventricle, an advantage for long-term ventricular function. Tricuspid atresia is the lesion with the best long-term outlook with a Fontan circulation, with an operative mortality in childhood of under 10% and a 15-year good-quality survival thereafter of 75%.

Total anomalous pulmonary venous connection (Table 30.17)

Entry of pulmonary veins into systemic venous pathways can be at one site or several (mixed TAPVC). Most commonly the pulmonary veins all enter a confluence behind, but separate from, the left atrium. The confluence then drains directly or indirectly into the right atrium. Drainage can be classified as in Figure 30.15. Obstruction to the pulmonary venous return can occur at a number of sites including the pulmonary vein orifices, on entry of the confluence to the systemic veins, on passage through the diaphragm and on passage through the liver after the ductus venosus closes in infradiaphragmatic TAPVC. Obstruction to the pulmonary veins will cause worse cyanosis, marked respiratory distress and less cardiomegaly than unobstructed TAPVC. There is always a PFO and often an ASD with entry of blood to the left heart only through these means; thus varying degrees of left ventricular underdevelopment are common. Coarctation and even severe hypoplasia of the left heart are occasionally present. Total anomalous pulmonary venous connection forms part of the complex abnormalities associated with heterotaxy states (left and right isomerism). These are considered in more detail. In

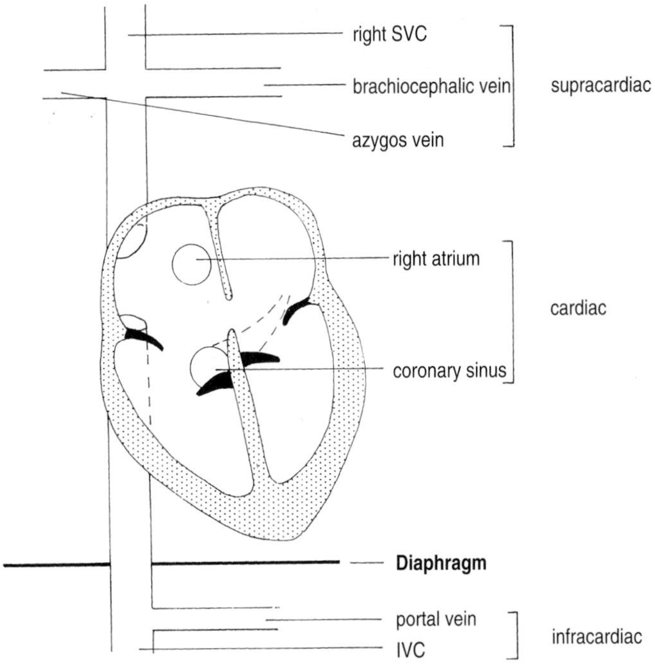

Fig. 30.15 Possible sites of total anomalous pulmonary venous connection; mixed connections can occur.

general, the more severe the pulmonary venous obstruction the earlier the infant is symptomatic. Infradiaphragmatic TAPVC to the portal vein is associated with marked cyanosis and respiratory distress which gets dramatically worse when the ductus venosus shuts. Infants with completely unobstructed TAPVC are sometimes not recognized until after the newborn period when recurrent or chronic chestiness and failure to thrive occur. As they sometimes present early and are very blue, infants with obstructed TAPVC often receive prostaglandin, sometimes with benefit to their general state. This improvement is presumably due either to opening of the ductus arteriosus and decompression of the right heart or to opening the ductus venosus and ameliorating pulmonary venous hypertension in TAPVC to the portal vein. Management is by corrective surgery with mortality below 10% and an excellent long-term outlook unless pulmonary vein stenosis is present.

Complex structural cyanotic congenital heart disease (Table 30.17)

These conditions often include more than one of the above abnormalities as well as shunt lesions and obstruction to either systemic or pulmonary arterial outflow tracts. Important pulmonary and systemic obstruction only very rarely coexist. Association with extracardiac abnormalities is common and in addition to specific system abnormalities the occurrence of heterotaxy states must be considered. Heterotaxy states, sometimes termed situs ambiguus, exist when abdominal, bronchial and atrial anatomy is neither the usual arrangement (situs solitus) nor a mirror image of the usual arrangement (situs inversus). The usual arrangement of viscera involves spleen and stomach being on the left-hand side and liver on the right, a morphologically left lung being on the left and a morphologically right lung (three-lobed) being on the right with a morphologically left atrium being to the left of the morphologically right atrium. Situs inversus is a mirror image of this arrangement and situs ambiguus exists when both lungs are of the same morphology (right or left) and both atria are of the same morphology (right or left), i.e. right or left isomerism. When these situations exist the liver tends to be midline, stomach position is variable and there is either asplenia (in right isomerism) or polysplenia (in left isomerism). Very rarely the situation is less clear cut and there are features of more than one arrangement of situs. Generally speaking, right isomerism is associated with severe cyanotic congenital heart disease including TAPVC, complete AVSD and pulmonary atresia or severe pulmonary stenosis. Often there will be transposition as well. The cardiac abnormalities associated with left isomerism are more variable in range and severity but abnormalities of the pulmonary venous drainage are common, although often only partially anomalous. Cardiac lesions with left isomerism are not always cyanotic. Clues to the presence of a complex abnormality include a midline liver and dextrocardia. Immediate management principles include deciding whether prostaglandin is indicated: the same criteria apply in these circumstances as in any other.

Conclusion

There are other structural lesions which may present with cyanosis in the newborn infant, such as truncus arteriosus and double inlet or double outlet ventricle, but frequently they are not diagnosed until beyond the newborn period. They are considered under respiratory distress.

RESPIRATORY DISTRESS

Cardiac conditions presenting with respiratory distress are listed in Table 30.19 and clinical details given in Tables 30.20 and 30.21. Some of these conditions may present with collapse and, in retrospect, a period of respiratory distress may have been present prior to collapse. Cardiac conditions causing respiratory distress usually do so through heart failure, the signs of which are given in Table 30.6. Cardiac disease will also cause respiratory distress if there is marked pulmonary venous engorgement or metabolic acidosis has developed; these two occurrences can be associated with cyanotic cardiac conditions. Some conditions characteristically cause both cyanosis and heart failure (Table 30.22). Signs of cardiac disease will be absent in respiratory causes of respiratory distress and a chest X-ray usually allows the distinction to be made with confidence; in addition cardiac causes of respiratory distress are likely to have signs related to the cardiac diagnosis.

Table 30.19 Cardiac conditions presenting with neonatal respiratory distress

Category	Comments
Heart muscle disease	
Ischaemia	With birth asphyxia
Myocarditis	Any cause
Cardiomyopathy	Hypertrophic or dilated
Arrhythmias	
Arteriovenous malformation	Cranial or other often with PPHN
Structural heart disease	
Week 1	
Hypoplastic left heart Interrupted arch Aortic atresia/critical stenosis Coarctation	May also present with collapse, see Tables 30.24 and 30.25
Week 2–3	
Truncus DOV, DIV, TAPVC TGA + VSD	May also present with cyanosis see Table 30.14
Week 3	
Left-to-right shunt lesions	Any
Time variable	
Tetralogy with absent pulmonary valve	Neonatal symptoms are due to airway obstruction

Abbreviations: DIV – double inlet ventricle; DOV – double outlet ventricle; TAPVC – total anomalous pulmonary venous connection; TGA – transposition of the great arteries; VSD – ventricular septal defect.

Arrhythmias (Table 30.20)

These are considered in detail on page 705.

Heart muscle disease (Table 30.20)

There is no information on the incidence of heart muscle disease in the newborn; many conditions associated with cardiomyopathy will not present in the newborn period or cardiac manifestations may not be apparent at that stage.

Myocardial ischaemia

Subclinical myocardial ischaemia in birth-asphyxiated and otherwise stressed infants is quite common.[48] Involvement severe enough to cause hypotension is less common although a transient murmur from tricuspid regurgitation in association with ST depression and T wave inversion in the left chest leads is a common finding. Specific therapy for heart failure is sometimes required; these infants usually have neurological and renal impairment in addition. Myocardial infarction in neonates may cause heart failure or sudden collapse; ECG changes include deep and wide Q waves, initial elevation of the ST segment followed by T wave inversion

Table 30.20 Clinical features of cardiovascular conditions not involving intracardiac structural abnormalities presenting with respiratory distress in the newborn

Condition	Pulses	Precordium	Auscultation	ECG	Extracardiac associations
Arrhythmia	Normal or weak	Normal	Gallop	Diagnostic	Rare
Heart muscle disease					
Myocarditis	Normal or weak	Normal	Gallop, MR murmur, rub	Small QRS ST↑, T↓	Common (hepatitis etc.)
Ischaemia	Normal or weak	Normal	Gallop, MR murmur, TR murmur	ST↑, T↓	Features of perinatal asphyxia
DCM	Normal or weak	Normal	Gallop, MR murmur	LV+, ST↓, T↓	Rare
EFE	Weak	Normal or active	Gallop, MR murmur	LV+, ST↓, T↓ V_{5-6}	Rare
HCM	Normal or jerky	Normal or active	Gallop, LVOT or RVOT systolic murmur	LV/RV+ ST↑ or ↓ T↓	Common (macrosomia, usually maternal diabetes)
AVM					
Cranial	Normal or weak femorals	Active	Gallop, MR murmur, cranial bruit	LV/RV+ ST↓, T↓	Neurological signs
Coronary	Full	Active	Gallop, continuous murmur	LV or RV+ ST↓, T↓	

Note: Cyanosis is not present in any condition unless PPHN occurs and all have cardiomegaly and pulmonary congestion on chest X-ray.

Table 30.21 Structural heart lesions presenting with respiratory distress (heart failure) after the first week of life

Condition	Pulses	Cyanosis	Precordium	Auscultation	ECG	Extracardiac associations
Truncus arteriosus	Normal or full	Mild	Active	S2 single, EC Systolic ± diastolic murmur	RV+ ± LV + ST↓, T↓ V_{5-6}	Common (DiGeorge)
TGA + VSD	Normal	Mild/moderate	RV+	S2 single ± VSD murmur	LV+ or RV+	Rare
TAPVC (unobstructed)	Normal or weak	Mild/moderate	RV+	S2 wide, P2 loud ± RVOT murmur	RV+ $RsRV_1$	Rare
DIV/DOV without PS	Normal	Mild	Active	P2 loud VSD murmur	Variable	Rare
PDA	Full	None	Active	Continuous murmur at base	LV+ ±RV+	Occasional
VSD	Normal	None	Active	P2 loud PSM LLSE	LV+ ± RV+	Occasional
Complete AVSD	Normal	None	Active	P2 loud VSD murmur LLSE MR murmur apex	RA+ RV+ Superior QRS axis	Very common (Down syndrome)
AP window	Normal or full	None	Active	P2 loud, continuous murmur at midsternal edge	LV+ RV+	Rare

some days later. Q waves persist indefinitely but ST segment changes resolve in a week or so and T waves return to normal over a much longer timescale. Enzyme studies can be difficult to interpret in the early newborn period as other tissues may be the source of the enzymes and cardiac-specific isoenzymes need to be measured. Myocardial infarction can occur as part of generalized perinatal asphyxia or secondary to thromboembolic events. Anomalous origin of the left coronary artery from the pulmonary artery is rarely symptomatic in early weeks of life as it is well tolerated whilst the pulmonary artery pressure remains high. It is a cause of pale sweating episodes (presumably angina), heart failure from dilated cardiomyopathy and myocardial infarction after the newborn period. Ischaemia secondary to birth asphyxia usually recovers fully without any apparent long-term sequelae even if intravenous inotrope support is required acutely.

Table 30.22 Structural cardiac conditions in which cyanosis and heart failure commonly coexist in the newborn

- Transposition
  - with coarctation
  - with large VSD
- Truncus arteriosus
- Tricuspid atresia
  - with large VSD
  - with TGA and coarctation
- Double inlet ventricle
- Total anomalous pulmonary venous connection
  - with obstructed pulmonary veins
- Hypoplastic left heart syndrome
- Arteriovenous malformation – usually intracerebral, often have PPHN

If significant pulmonary stenosis coexists heart failure is unlikely and cyanosis is more marked.

Myocarditis

Myocarditis is usually presumed rather than definitely proven to be viral in origin, although occasionally a virus is identified directly or by serology, often in the context of a generalized viraemic illness with hepatitis and meningoencephalitis. Heart failure and either tachy- or bradyarrhythmias can occur. Detection of a pericardial rub is rare in the newborn; pericardial effusion and even tamponade can occur. There is no specific therapy of benefit; heart failure should be treated in the usual way but digoxin used cautiously because of the risk of arrhythmias. Digoxin should not be used if tamponade is suspected as it will slow the heart rate and reduce cardiac output if venous return is already impaired. Symptomatic, large or increasing pericardial effusions should be drained. Usually this is possible percutaneously (p. 1382). Precise outcome figures are scarce but if death does not occur there may be complete recovery or the development of chronic dilated cardiomyopathy.

Dilated cardiomyopathy

This usually presents after the newborn period but fetal and neonatal presentation with heart failure do occur. Tachyarrhythmia must be excluded as a cause as must anomalous origin of the left coronary artery. Detailed investigations for infective and metabolic causes are appropriate[13] (Table 30.23) if perinatal asphyxia is not clearly responsible. If any of the screening investigations reveal possible aetiologies, enzyme studies on lymphocytes, fibroblasts or other tissue biopsies are indicated. If a metabolic cause is suspected from investigations or other clinical features such as skeletal myopathy, the question of blind treatment needs to be considered if the infant is critically ill. This may be appropriate if one of the carnitine deficiency states is suspected.[46] First degree relatives of infants with DCM should be evaluated clinically and by echocardiography as familial occurrence is recognized even when precise metabolic diagnoses are lacking.

Table 30.23 Blood and urine screening tests for hypertrophic and dilated cardiomyopathy in infants if no clinical diagnosis apparent. Abnormal findings need detailed investigation

- Blood for:
  - vacuolated lymphocytes
  - carnitine and acyl carnitine
  - lactate and pyruvate (fasting)
  - creatine kinase MM isoenzyme
  - thyroid function
  - autoimmune screen
  - amino acids
- Urine for:
  - amino and organic acids
  - glycosaminoglycans

Endocardial fibroelastosis

This can be primary in which case it has close clinical similarities to DCM with marked left ventricular hypertrophy on ECG. The endocardium is very echogenic on ultrasound. Information on prognosis is difficult to interpret as diagnostic criteria differ but complete recovery is described. EFE is often secondary to obstructive left heart lesions, in which case the clinical picture and prognosis are influenced by the nature and severity of the accompanying pathology.

Hypertrophic cardiomyopathy

This can be primary as a manifestation of an autosomal dominant genetic disease or in association with Noonan's syndrome, also autosomal dominant. Most commonly so far as symptomatic newborn infants are concerned HCM is secondary to hyperinsulinism, usually maternal diabetes mellitus (or at least maternal glucose intolerance during pregnancy which may not have been recognized as a diabetic state). Other rarer causes of hyperinsulinism can also cause neonatal cardiac hypertrophy. Infants receiving corticosteroids for chronic lung disease may develop reversible cardiac hypertrophy out of proportion to the degree of hypertension; they rarely show symptoms.[29] The majority of infants born to mothers with diabetes or gestational diabetes have no clinical effects from HCM. Some have a left ventricular outflow murmur and a few develop respiratory distress attributed more often to impaired left ventricular filling than to outflow obstruction. Hypertrophy can be global or localized and this is reflected in the ECG and echocardiographic findings. The infants of diabetic mothers also have an increased incidence of structural heart disease (5%), making detailed assessment including echocardiography important if there are any cardiac symptoms or signs in such infants. If maternal glucose intolerance cannot be confirmed, a search for metabolic causes of cardiac hypertrophy is indicated[11,41] (Table 30.23). Management of symptomatic cases should not usually include digoxin, inotropes or vasodilators as these all may exacerbate left ventricular outflow obstruction. Propranolol is occasionally indicated in severely symptomatic cases although hypoglycaemia needs to be carefully guarded against if it is used. Cardiac hypertrophy in association with maternal diabetes resolves over 6–12 months.[90]

Arteriovenous malformation (Table 30.20)

Arteriovenous fistulae may present in the newborn period with heart failure; there may be associated PPHN. Intracranial fistulae are the most common; intrahepatic fistulae are occasionally encountered and may coexist with intracranial shunts. As well as heart failure, signs include a bruit over the affected site. Management consists of medical support for the circulation and intervention to stop or at least reduce the shunt through the AVM. This involves catheter embolization for intracranial abnormalities which are most commonly vein of Galen aneurysms (p. 1309). The outcome is determined by the ability to achieve a marked reduction in or abolition of the arteriovenous shunt and by the severity of secondary hydrocephalus and cerebral ischaemic lesions.

Duct-dependent systemic circulation

This group of conditions comprises hypoplastic left heart syndrome, interrupted aortic arch, coarctation, aortic atresia and critical aortic stenosis and is discussed in detail under Collapse (p. 701).

Truncus arteriosus (Table 30.21)

This malformation constitutes <1% of congenital heart lesions; it is associated with DiGeorge syndrome in 30% of cases. A single artery arises from the heart giving rise to coronary and pulmonary circulations as well as to the aortic arch which is right sided in 30% of cases and interrupted in 5–10%, in which case the association with DiGeorge syndrome is very high. The VSD is usually large and the common arterial trunk overrides it; the truncal valve is abnormal and may be regurgitant or stenosed. Pulmonary arteries arise either laterally from the truncus, adjacent and posteriorly or from a short main pulmonary artery. Absence of one pulmonary artery occasionally occurs. Stenosis at the origin of a pulmonary artery if present is rarely severe; thus high pulmonary blood flow and pressure result in pulmonary vascular disease if the baby survives infancy without surgery. Clinical presentation is with tachypnoea or heart failure in the later newborn period. Severity of cyanosis varies but is usually only mild; other features are listed in Table 30.21. The severity and haemodynamic effect of the truncal valve abnormality influence the signs detected as does the pulmonary vascular resistance. Definitive diagnosis is by ultrasound, and providing both pulmonary arteries can be demonstrated further cardiac investigation is not normally required before surgery. Corrective surgery is favoured over palliation (pulmonary artery banding) and must be performed in infancy to avoid irreversible progressive pulmonary vascular disease. Chromosome 22q11 deletion and immune status should be investigated preoperatively. The long-term outlook is determined not only by the cardiac state but also by neurodevelopmental and immunological aspects of DiGeorge syndrome. Corrective surgery in early infancy has a mortality of 10–20% and further surgery in the form of replacement of the right ventricular to pulmonary artery graft will be required in later childhood. In addition, many cases will need truncal valve surgery at some stage although not usually at initial intervention; if valve replacement is required in early infancy surgical mortality can be up to 50%.

Transposition with ventriculoseptal defect (Table 30.21)

Transposition is discussed in detail in the section on cyanosis (p. 691). Clinical features of TGA + VSD are given in Table 30.21.

Total anomalous pulmonary venous connection (Table 30.21)

Unobstructed TAPVC presents with respiratory distress; it is discussed on page 695. Clinical features are given in Tables 30.17 and 30.21.

Double inlet and double outlet ventricle (Table 30.21)

These terms cover a wide spectrum of abnormalities. Double inlet ventricle is one type of univentricular AV connection when both atria empty into one ventricle; this is sometimes termed single ventricle. The other form of single ventricle is when one AV valve is atretic, that is tricuspid or mitral atresia (absent right or absent left AV connection respectively). A double inlet ventricle may receive atrial blood through one common or two separate AV valves. If there are two AV valves draining into one ventricle it is most usually the morphological left ventricle, double inlet left ventricle. Double outlet ventricle exists when both great arteries arise chiefly from the same ventricle. Double outlet right ventricle is the usual form; details of AV valve anatomy and great arterial arrangements vary greatly. Thus blood flow patterns and pathophysiology in DORV may resemble large VSD, TGA + VSD or tetralogy of Fallot depending on the associated abnormalities. Single ventricle arrangements and double outlet ventricle anatomy each constitute 1% of structural heart lesions. The clinical features in common between double inlet and double outlet ventricle are that heart failure is likely to develop as pulmonary vascular resistance falls unless there is important pulmonary stenosis in which case cyanosis will be the presenting feature. Coarctation may be present in cases without pulmonary stenosis.

Left-to-right shunt lesions (Table 30.21)

These conditions have a lot of features in common. Some lesions may be small and asymptomatic as is the case with many VSDs. Symptoms do not develop until pulmonary vascular resistance falls enough to permit excessive pulmonary blood flow; this may happen more quickly in preterm infants related to the relative paucity of muscularity in immature lung arterioles. In some circumstances when the defect is large, pulmonary vascular resistance may not fall sufficiently to result in excessive lung blood flow. These infants remain relatively well and pass into the phase of progressive vascular damage without heart failure occurring. Whether or not a period of heart failure occurs, the development of pulmonary vascular changes is universal and rapid in complete AVSD, but unusual and not until adult life in secundum type ASD. Other lesions lie between these extremes in both frequency and rapidity of progression to pulmonary vascular disease. Extracardiac factors may influence the risk and hasten the development of PVD. These include extreme prematurity, chronic lung disease, airway obstruction, life at high altitude and Down syndrome.

Patent ductus arteriosus

Prematurity and PDA are considered on pages 687–689. As an isolated lesion outside the context of respiratory distress syndrome and prematurity, PDA accounts for nearly 10% of congenital heart lesions. Clinical features are given in Table 30.21; diagnosis is often clinical and confirmed by echocardiography. Symptomatic PDA in term infants is an indication for surgical closure. If the infant is asymptomatic without evidence of pulmonary hypertension, intervention is often delayed until after infancy when occlusion by catheter-delivered coil or umbrella device, or by surgical clipping is performed. The size at which catheter closure can be performed is being reduced by the use of coils rather than umbrella devices. Surgery and transcatheter closure both have high success rates and excellent long-term prognosis. The factors influencing which method is chosen are many and are evolving.[39,72]

Atrial septal defect

Isolated ostium secundum ASDs very rarely if ever cause symptoms in newborn infants but are occasionally suspected on auscultation. Left-to-right shunting at atrial level is often found on echocardiography either as an isolated finding or in conjunction with physiological pulmonary artery branch stenosis, PDA or more complex lesions. It is not always clear whether the shunt is through an ASD or merely through a prolapsing PFO (p. 676). 85–90% of atrial shunts detected by ultrasound in the newborn period disappear and defects sized 3 mm or less always do.[68]

Ventricular septal defect

Ventricular septal defects without associated abnormalities account for at least 15% of structural heart lesions; up to 65% of them resolve spontaneously. They may be single or multiple and can occur in any part of the ventricular septum. The site is of importance with respect to associated lesions, likely natural history and surgical approaches. Symptoms may never occur and if heart failure does develop it frequently does not do so until after the newborn period; indeed there may be no murmur until several weeks of age. This is because there is little flow across a VSD whilst pulmonary vascular resistance is high. Diagnosis is usually clinical (Table 30.21) with echocardiographic confirmation and identification of precise location. Heart failure is treated as necessary (Table 30.13). Surgery is rarely needed in the newborn period unless there are associated lesions such as coarctation. Surgery is indicated for cases in which heart failure cannot be well enough controlled to permit satisfactory weight gain or if pulmonary artery pressure is over 50% of systemic; this can usually be assessed by Doppler echocardiography. Surgical repair of VSD has a low mortality (<3%) even in the newborn period. Palliative pulmonary artery banding is only considered when there are multiple VSDs or if surgery is indicated for another lesion such as coarctation. When VSD is part of a more complex lesion, strategies are different; in some circumstances a sizeable VSD is essential for satisfactory haemodynamics, for example in DILV with TGA.

Atrioventricular septal defect (Table 30.21)

The basic abnormality in this condition is in the AV septum which in a normal heart separates the left ventricle from the right atrium. A defect here will always be associated with an abnormality of the AV valves. There may be an intra-atrial defect (ostium primum ASD or partial AVSD), or additionally an intraventricular defect may also exist, in which case a complete AVSD is present and the AV valve has a single large orifice rather than two separate ones. In both forms there can be AV regurgitation including left ventricular to right atrial shunting. Partial AVSD constitutes <2% of congenital heart disease and complete AVSD accounts for 2% of congenital heart disease. Either lesion can be part of the complex cardiac abnormalities found in left isomerism (partial AVSD) or right isomerism (complete AVSD) as described above (p. 695). Partial AVSD is frequently undetected in the newborn period and may not cause heart failure in infancy although surgical correction is required in childhood to prevent right heart failure or PVD in adult life. Those presenting with heart failure in infancy often have left AV valve regurgitation as well as left-to-right shunting at atrial level and require valve repair as well as surgical closure of the shunt. 80% of cases of complete AVSD are associated with Down syndrome; in the region of 35% of infants with Down syndrome and congenital heart disease have complete AVSD. Occasionally tetralogy of Fallot coexists with AVSD as may PDA or coarctation. In some cases of complete AVSD one ventricle is much larger than the other; usually they are approximately equal sizes with volume overloading of the right ventricle. Clinical features of complete AVSD are given in Table 30.21. Heart failure may never develop and as PVD develops rapidly, particularly in Down syndrome, it is desirable to make the diagnosis in the newborn period. It is for this reason and because signs can be subtle, that at least an ECG is desirable by way of cardiac investigation in newborn infants with Down syndrome; if this is done, complete AVSD will not be overlooked as the QRS axis is superior ('north-west', + 180° to + 270°/– 90°). Diagnosis is by echocardiography; angiography is not usually needed. Survival without surgery is not always beyond infancy because of heart failure but in those alive at 1 year, survival may be expected into the late teens or early twenties. Corrective surgery for cases detected in infancy improves outlook with a surgical mortality of under 15%.

Aortopulmonary window (Table 30.21)

This rare abnormality involves a connection between the ascending aorta and the main pulmonary artery. It has haemodynamic and clinical features similar to large PDA and truncus arteriosus; it may coexist with PDA and with aortic arch interruption. (Table 30.21). It can be easily overlooked on echocardiography especially if a coexistent lesion is recognized. Surgical treatment at diagnosis is appropriate and has a high success rate.

Coronary arteriovenous fistula

This is another rare shunting lesion which presents with systolic and diastolic murmurs with or without bounding pulses and heart failure depending on the size of the shunt. The coronary fistula can be into any heart chamber or to the pulmonary artery. Ultrasound usually delineates the anatomy but angiography may be needed. Surgery or less commonly transcatheter occlusion is indicated for cases detected in the newborn period.

Conclusion

All the diseases and conditions discussed above may present in other ways such as asymptomatic murmurs and coincidental findings in investigations done for other reasons. In such circumstances management will need to be tailored in the light of the clinical picture and likely natural history.

Table 30.24 Cardiac conditions which may present with collapse

Arrhythmias – primary or secondary
Duct-dependent circulation
Transposition – without ASD, VSD, PDA
Pulmonary
Pulmonary atresia – without collaterals
Tricuspid atresia – with restrictive VSD
Systemic
Hypoplastic left heart
Aortic atresia
Critical aortic stenosis
Interrupted arch
Coarctation

Duct-dependent cardiac conditions often present with other signs (cyanosis or respiratory distress) before collapse occurs.

COLLAPSE

Conditions which commonly present with collapse are listed in Table 30.24. Differentiating cardiac from non-cardiac causes is usually not difficult although conditions with duct-dependent circulation can, when the duct closes, mimic septicaemia and primary metabolic disorders.

Arrhythmias

These are discussed in a separate section (p. 705). In the newborn period arrhythmias which cause sudden unexpected collapse with no signs and a normal ECG between episodes are very rare.

Duct-dependent pulmonary circulation and transposition

These infants will normally be recognized as cyanosed and are discussed under that heading (p. 691). Duct-dependent pulmonary circulation will result in extreme cyanosis and metabolic acidosis when ductal closure occurs, as will TGA if there is no mixing between systemic and pulmonary circulations via a VSD or a large ASD.

Duct-dependent systemic circulation (Table 30.25)

These lesions are listed in Table 30.24 with clinical features being given in Table 30.25. They are all likely to have at least mild respiratory distress and some physical signs prior to collapse but those features may have been unrecognized especially if early discharge home occurred. Resuscitation with prostaglandin (Table 30.12) will usually be carried out before definitive diagnosis by ultrasound has been performed; resuscitation must not be

Table 30.25 Structural heart lesions presenting with respiratory distress or collapse in the early newborn period. All may have cyanosis if PPHN or shocked; all have cardiomegaly with congested lung fields on chest X-ray

Condition	Pulses	Cyanosis	Precordium	Auscultation	ECG	Extracardiac associations
Hypoplastic left heart	Weak, femoral stronger if DA open	Mild	Active	Gallop	Small LV voltages	Uncommon
Aortic arch interruption	Strong proximal to lesion	None	Active	Gallop LVOT, systolic murmur	LV/RV+ T↓V_{5-6}	Common (DiGeorge)
Coarctation	Weak femoral	None	Active	Gallop, EC, LVOT, systolic murmur Murmur between scapulae	RA+ RV+ T↓V_{5-6}	Uncommon (Turner)
Critical aortic stenosis	Weak	None	Active	Gallop, EC, LVOT, systolic murmur	LV+ ST↓, T↓V_{5-6}	Uncommon

delayed awaiting echocardiography if the clinical picture is at all suggestive of the possibility of duct-dependent systemic circulation.

Hypoplastic left heart syndrome (Table 30.25)

This constitutes 1% of congenital heart disease but nearly 10% of symptomatic neonatal congenital heart disease in series dating from the era before fetal diagnosis. Extracardiac abnormalities are only occasionally encountered in liveborn infants with HLHS. The condition consists of a small left atrium, atresia of mitral and aortic valves and extreme hypoplasia of the left ventricle and aorta proximal to the ductus arteriosus. There is coarctation in 60–70% of cases. The right heart is dilated and hypertrophied with a large pulmonary artery. Head and coronary arterial flow is through retrograde filling of the transverse and ascending aorta via the ductus arteriosus. Clinical features are given in Table 30.25; before ductal closure occurs femoral pulses may be stronger than upper limb pulses. Death occurs rapidly after ductal closure and usually between 5 and 10 days after birth; occasional survival to a few months can occur. Until ultrasound was available for diagnosis and before prostaglandin therapy was discovered, HLHS made a major contribution to the high mortality of cardiac catheterization in the newborn period. The advent of prostaglandin and ultrasound and more recently still, fetal diagnosis has meant that most liveborn infants with HLHS can be stabilized whilst treatment options for this universally fatal condition are considered. The treatment options are:

- No active treatment.
- Heart transplantation. There are major problems with organ availability and, even if initially resuscitated and stabilized, infants may not be able to be kept in good condition long enough for a donor organ to become available. Long-term sequelae of transplantation need to be discussed with families before embarking on this pathway. Neonatal heart transplantation has up to 80% survival at 5 years.[8]
- Palliative measures in the form of surgery described by Norwood are subject to a number of variations.[82] This essentially consists of reconstruction of the systemic outflow of the heart using the native pulmonary artery with repair of coarctation if present. Pulmonary blood flow is established via a systemic-to-pulmonary anastomosis. The left atrium must be decompressed by balloon septostomy or surgical septectomy. The final goal is to establish a Fontan circulation with the right ventricle as the systemic ventricle, a far from ideal physiological situation. Norwood and a few others have been able to achieve this situation in 40% of those who commenced the process. Survival with this arrangement is approximately 50% 4 years after establishing a Fontan circulation. It is envisaged that organ availability for young children will be better than for neonates and so the Norwood approach can be considered palliative until heart transplant is possible. Most centres have been unable to match Norwood's results. Other palliative options being explored include stenting the ductus arteriosus at catheterization with surgical banding of the pulmonary artery branches[36] in the hope of achieving survival and satisfactory quality of life until transplant after fewer surgical interventions than the Norwood approach.

Aortic valve atresia

This lesion very occasionally occurs without hypoplasia of the remainder of the left heart. The ascending aorta is very small. Presentation and clinical features resemble HLHS but an attempt to establish a biventricular circulation may be successful.

Critical aortic stenosis (Table 30.25)

This lesion lies at the end of a spectrum of severity of aortic valve abnormalities, the mildest of which may cause no symptoms even in adult life. It is more common in males and the possibility of Turner syndrome must be considered in affected females. The aortic valve may have one, two or three cusps and there is often post-stenotic dilatation of the ascending aorta. Aortic stenosis of any degree may be associated with some AR, MS, VSD and coarctation. Symptomatic aortic stenosis at sub- or supravalvar levels is rare in the newborn but subvalvar AS may develop in treated or untreated valvar AS and in association with VSD and aortic coarctation or interruption. Symptomatic AR in neonates and infants is rare and is usually due to an aorticoventricular tunnel rather than a valvar abnormality. Progression of aortic stenosis and its unfavourable effect on the left ventricle in fetal life has been documented by ultrasound.[74] Death may occur in utero. The postnatal clinical picture (Table 30.25) may be of an asymptomatic murmur with heart failure developing in early infancy or of pulseless collapse when the ductus arteriosus shuts. Angiography is not required for diagnosis but cardiac catheterization may be performed for balloon dilatation although many centres prefer surgical valvotomy. Survival or not is determined by the state of the left ventricle which may either be dilated and have EFE or be severely hypertrophied with ischaemic changes on ECG. It is a matter of debate as to whether the most severe forms should be subject to Norwood-type surgery (see HLHS above). Fetal intervention has yet to establish a role. Surgery is successful in most symptomatic infants;[14] in some centres balloon dilatation is the treatment of choice[10] with a similarly low mortality. All infants requiring intervention in the newborn period will ultimately have further interventions either for residual or recurrent stenosis or for aortic regurgitation.

Aortic arch interruption (Table 30.25)

This abnormality is present in 1% of congenital heart lesions. The ductus arteriosus supplies the descending aorta distal to the site of interruption which is distal to the left subclavian artery in 30% (type A), between left carotid and left subclavian arteries in 45% (type B) and between innominate and left carotid in the remainder (type C). Approximately 50% of type A interruptions are associated with DiGeorge syndrome. Associated cardiac lesions always include VSD, often valvar or subvalvar aortic stenosis, sometimes mitral valve abnormalities and very occasionally truncus arteriosus or AP window. Clinical features are given in Table 30.25. Diagnosis can be strongly suspected clinically by careful attention to the pulses and is confirmed with clarification of associated lesions by ultrasound. Corrective surgery is usually performed through a median sternotomy with concurrent repair of intracardiac abnormalities with up to 90% survival. Left ventricular outflow obstruction may progress even after successful neonatal surgery and often requires surgery in infancy; further surgery to the repaired aortic arch may also be required.

Coarctation (Table 30.25)

This makes up 10% of congenital heart disease, being more common in males but having a strong association with Turner syndrome, 15% or more of whom have the condition. The position of the discrete narrowing of the aorta is distal to the left subclavian artery opposite the point of entry to the aorta of the ductus arteriosus. The exact position varies and may actually evolve in relation to ductal closure and postnatal growth. Terms such as pre-, juxta- and post-ductal are used to describe the site of coarctation and bear some relationship to the age of presentation and clinical picture. Not all cases of coarctation cause symptoms in the newborn period or infancy; some remain asymptomatic for years or occasionally decades. Other lesions in the left heart are very commonly associated, as are VSDs. Transposition and more complex cyanotic conditions may have accompanying coarctation. In the newborn with coarctation and PDA, there is systemic pressure in the right ventricle although, until the ductus arteriosus starts to close, shunting is predominantly left-to-right at ductal and atrial levels. Thus as heart failure starts to develop, the infant is pink with RVH on ECG. When the duct shuts, some constriction of the descending aorta probably occurs as well in those babies who then collapse. In others, duct closure is tolerated although heart failure and hypertension are apparent in the early weeks of life. Those infants who remain asymptomatic in the newborn period may develop heart failure in later infancy with LVH on ECG. After infancy and before middle age, coarctation presents with asymptomatic abnormalities of the pulses, with a murmur or with hypertension and its complications. The time and mode of presentation of infants with associated intracardiac lesions is influenced by the nature of the associated lesion. If the coexistent lesion presents early, great care must be taken not to overlook coarctation. Coarctation can be difficult to diagnose clinically (Table 30.25) in the newborn as pulses and upper/ lower limb blood pressures may be normal while the ductus is open, and if collapse occurs all pulses can be weak if left ventricular dysfunction is marked. Similarly, echocardiography imaging and Doppler assessment can sometimes be inconclusive whilst the ductus is wide open; even angiography and direct pressure measurements can be inconclusive. If there is doubt, careful observation and serial echocardiography over a period of a few days is required until the ductus arteriosus constricts and the characteristic features develop. Coarctation causing collapse is resuscitated with prostaglandin and heart failure is treated with diuretics. Inotrope support is needed in critically ill infants and renal function must be watched carefully as occasionally renal failure develops. Infants who collapse or who are in heart failure should undergo surgical repair when stabilized. Coarctation as part of a more complicated lesion must be repaired before or at the same time as the intracardiac abnormality. In some circumstances pulmonary artery banding is performed with coarctation repair if there is a cardiac lesion which will cause pulmonary plethora and which is not to be corrected in the newborn period, for example multiple muscular VSDs or DILV with VSD and TGA. There are disadvantages to pulmonary artery banding which mean it is desirable to avoid it if possible. Coarctation in the newborn period is commonly repaired by using the left subclavian artery (subclavian flap repair). This results in an absent brachial pulse in the left arm but very rarely leads to ischaemic problems. Some surgeons prefer excision of the coarctation and end-to-end repair in newborns. This is the technique after infancy. Mortality of coarctation repair without major intracardiac lesions is <5%. Asymptomatic infants or those with easily controlled heart failure can be operated on in later infancy with the intention of achieving a lower recurrence rate, which may be as high as 20% in those repaired in the newborn period.

Conclusion

Any of the causes of collapse considered above may present less dramatically, usually with evidence of heart failure which often precedes collapse. The precise diagnosis of which duct-dependent condition exists is not important at the resuscitation stage and if a collapsed infant could have structural heart disease as the cause, prostaglandin should be given. This is likely to be rapidly therapeutic as well as helpful in confirming a cardiac cause for the collapse. Absence of response to prostaglandin at doses at the top of the range (Table 30.12) makes duct-dependent systemic circulation unlikely but not impossible. Balloon dilatation of the ductus has been advocated in this unresponsive group of patients.[89] Risks of surgery are increased if renal or multiorgan failure are present.

CARDIAC CONDITIONS LIKELY TO PRESENT IN THE ASYMPTOMATIC NEWBORN (Table 30.26)

The commonest asymptomatic presentation of heart disease in the newborn period is the detection of a heart murmur which may be a feature of many of the conditions already discussed before symptoms develop.

Innocent heart murmurs

Detailed history and other features on physical examination are an important part of the evaluation of a heart murmur. The features of innocent murmurs in the newborn are given in Table 30.7. It is important to note that innocent murmurs have positive characteristics as well as being associated with no other clinical evidence of cardiovascular disease. It is unclear whether ECG and CXR help the experienced observer distinguish innocent from pathological murmurs but they are frequently used. A practical approach following the detection of a heart murmur is given below.

Table 30.26 Cardiac disease presenting in an asymptomatic newborn infant

Category	Detail	Comments
Fetal diagnosis	Any cardiac condition	Diagnosis known/ suspected before birth can be confirmed before infant becomes symptomatic
Murmur	Causes include: VSD Tricuspid regurgitation Aortic stenosis Pulmonary stenosis Patent ductus arteriosus Atrial septal defect AV septal defect Tetralogy of Fallot Innocent	See Table 30.7
Weak femoral pulses	Coarctation	Many non-cardiac causes of weak pulses
Rhythm or rate abnormality	Fast/slow/irregular	Some are normal variants See arrhythmia section

Some cardiac conditions are diagnosed when cardiac assessment is requested following a non-cardiac diagnosis being made (e.g. neonatal surgical conditions or certain syndromes).

Pathological asymptomatic heart murmurs

The likely causes for such murmurs detected in the newborn are given in Table 30.26. The conditions listed are considered elsewhere in the chapter. As a general rule obstructive lesions cause a murmur from birth although mild pulmonary stenosis, trivial aortic stenosis or simple bicuspid aortic valve are frequently not heard. Pulmonary and particularly aortic stenosis may progress in severity. Lesions associated with left-to-right shunts frequently cause no murmur in the immediate newborn period and may not be detected until a routine check at 6 or 8 weeks. If a pansystolic murmur suggesting VSD is heard in the newborn period, it may be due to tricuspid regurgitation which will resolve over a matter of a few weeks. A VSD detected immediately after birth is likely to be small. Tricuspid regurgitation and VSD can coexist.[51] If a structural abnormality is suspected as the cause of an asymptomatic murmur, an ECG and CXR should be performed. These investigations may have diagnostic features and are of some help in deciding the severity of the lesion and therefore the timescale in which cardiology review and echocardiography are indicated.

Practical approach to neonatal heart murmurs

When a heart murmur is detected in the early newborn period a number of options are open which will be influenced by local considerations, particularly availability of specialist cardiological services and echocardiography. The following are common approaches:

Table 30.27 Features in an infant with an asymptomatic murmur which suggest the possibility of a serious (duct-dependent) lesion

Feature	Comment
No weight loss after birth or excessive weight gain, especially if feeding poorly	May suggest incipient heart failure
Any suggestion of symptoms	If 'dusky', a transcutaneous hyperoxia test may help (p. 680)
Any doubt about quality of femoral pulses	Suggests coarctation
Right arm systolic blood pressure > 20 mmHg above leg pressure	
Murmur loudest between scapulae	Suggests coarctation, innocent pulmonary murmur well heard front and sides
Cardiomegaly on CXR	
Ventricular hypertrophy on ECG	

- If symptoms or other signs of cardiac disease exist, an ECG and CXR should be performed and cardiology referral made.
- If no symptoms or other signs are present but the murmur has features suggesting a structural lesion, an ECG and CXR should be performed and cardiology referral made.
- If no symptoms or other signs of cardiac disease are present and the murmur has features compatible with an innocent one (Table 30.7) or a VSD (harsh early-to-middle or pansystolic maximal at lower left sternal edge) and the baby is due for discharge, an ECG and CXR should be performed. If these are abnormal, cardiology referral is appropriate; if they are normal, follow-up can be arranged at 4–6 weeks. If for other reasons the baby is not yet due for discharge, no investigation need be performed but the baby should be listened to again prior to discharge. If the murmur has gone, no further action is required; if it persists, an ECG and CXR should be performed with cardiology referral taking place if there is an abnormality in these tests and clinic follow-up arranged at 4–6 weeks if the investigations are normal.

An infant with an asymptomatic murmur should not be allowed home until it is clear that no form of duct-dependent congenital heart disease is present; this is usually apparent on clinical grounds (Table 30.27). If there is any doubt, either a further period of observation in hospital is indicated or, preferably, echocardiography should be arranged.

ARRHYTHMIAS

Primary cardiac arrhythmias in the newborn requiring treatment are uncommon. Tachy- or bradyarrhythmias are much more likely to be secondary to extracardiac pathology which must be identified and treated.

Table 30.28 Approach to ECG interpretation of an arrhythmia

QRS complexes	Rate	Slow/normal/fast
	Rhythm	Regular/irregular If irregular: premature/delayed
	Configuration	Normal/abnormal
P waves	Seen/not seen	
	Rate	Slow/normal/fast
	Rhythm	Regular/irregular If irregular: premature/delayed
	Axis	Normal/abnormal
	Relationship to QRS complexes	None/constant/variable If constant: before/within/after If before, PR interval: Normal/long Fixed/changing

RECOGNITION OF ARRHYTHMIAS

Infants with an arrhythmia may be asymptomatic or present with heart failure or very rarely with collapse. Some will have been recognized in utero. An ECG will usually allow precise diagnosis although occasionally this will not be possible, either because the abnormal rhythm is intermittent or because the ECG is difficult to interpret. Sinus rhythm exists if each QRS complex is preceded by a P wave with an axis of 0° to + 90° and with a normal PR interval (90–120 ms). An approach to assessing the ECG in a possible arrhythmia involves answering the questions given in Table 30.28. Arrhythmias can be classified in a number of ways. They will now be considered under the headings supraventricular or ventricular.

SUPRAVENTRICULAR ARRHYTHMIAS

Supraventricular arrhythmias usually have narrow QRS complexes which resemble those seen when the patient is in sinus rhythm.

Sinus bradycardia

When asleep or when straining the interval between QRS complexes can lengthen transiently up to 1.5 s but sustained rates even during sleep below 80/min in term or 100/min in preterm infants are not normal. Sinus bradycardia is associated with normal P waves before every QRS complex; the QRS complexes are normal. Sinus bradycardia is seen most commonly in association with apnoeic episodes. It may also be a manifestation of hypoxaemia, raised intracranial pressure of any cause and hyperkalaemia. It is seen in association with stress from handling and interventions in critically ill infants. Drugs may cause sinus bradycardia, for example heavy sedation, digoxin and propranolol. Sustained sinus bradycardia or failure to increase heart rate when stressed in a relatively well infant may be a feature of hypothyroidism. Episodes of extreme symptomatic sinus bradycardia are a feature of reflex anoxic seizures, usually not recognized until after the newborn period when anticholinergic therapy aimed at preventing profound bradycardia is sometimes considered.

Sinus arrhythmia and sinus arrest

These result in variable slowing of the heart rate. Neither is common in the newborn infant. Sinus arrhythmia is an increase in the heart rate during inspiration and results in a regular irregularity of heart rate in time with the respiratory cycle. Sinus arrest or pauses result in an occasional abnormally long pause (> 1.6 s) between P waves, producing an irregular irregularity of the heart rate. These two variations of normal are of no significance of themselves. If they are very pronounced they can be a marker of sinoatrial dysfunction which may be associated with symptomatic bradycardia or tachycardia.

Atrial ectopics

These are due to premature depolarization of a site in an atrium earlier than the sinus node discharge so that either a premature QRS complex follows or, if the ectopic is so early as to occur whilst the ventricle is in its refractory period, there is no QRS complex (blocked atrial ectopics, Fig. 30.16). Intermediate between these two timings for the atrial ectopic, a QRS complex will be conducted aberrantly and be broad. If non-conducted atrial ectopics occur regularly alternating with normally conducted sinus impulses, there will be bradycardia in the region of 60–80/min. If ectopics are frequent or non-conducted but not alternating with sinus beats, the heart rate will be irregular (Fig. 30.16). Atrial ectopics are harmless but may cause confusion when detected in the fetus causing bradycardia with or without an irregular rhythm. They can be correctly diagnosed by fetal ultrasound[83] and thereby prevent unnecessary concern about fetal well-being being engendered. They are markers for an increased incidence of supraventricular tachycardia which may not necessarily be symptomatic.[79] Atrial ectopics resolve within 3 months in 90% of cases.

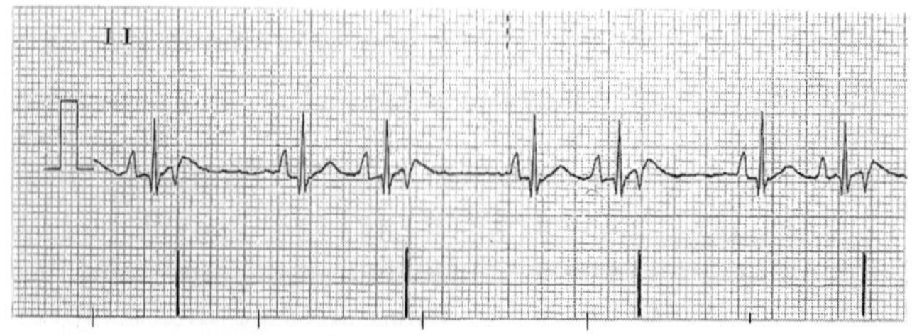

Fig. 30.16 ECG lead II, 25 mm/s. Blocked atrial ectopics on the upstroke of T wave of complexes 1, 3, 5 and 7.

Table 30.29 Simple classification of SVT

Site	Rhythm	Comment
Sinus node	Sinus tachycardia	Always secondary
Atrium	Atrial flutter	Rare
	Atrial fibrillation	Very rare
	Atrial tachycardia	Very rare
AV junction	AV re-entry tachycardia	Common
	AV nodal re-entry tachycardia	Rare
Below AV node	His bundle tachycardia	Very rare
	(junctional ectopic tachycardia)	Usually postoperative

Sinus tachycardia

Sinus tachycardia is a heart rate above 160/min in term and above 180/min in preterm infants. P waves have a normal axis and precede every QRS complex. Sinus tachycardia is always secondary, usually to a non-cardiac cause. Causes to be considered include fever, hypovolaemia, pain, respiratory failure, anaemia, fluid overload, drugs (in particular methylxanthines and inotropes) and septicaemia. Structural heart disease or heart muscle disease may cause sinus tachycardia. The cause should be identified and treated; therapy for sinus tachycardia itself is not indicated. In the newborn, sinus tachycardia can reach 230 beats/min so that at its higher rates it can be difficult to distinguish from the pathological types of supraventricular tachycardia.

Supraventricular tachycardia

A simple classification of SVT is given in Table 30.29.

Atrial flutter

This is a rare rhythm in the newborn; it may be diagnosed in utero. There is an association with myocarditis, myocardial ischaemia and structural heart disease although the heart is often normal in neonates with atrial flutter. Atrial rates usually exceed 300/min and ventricular rate and rhythm will vary with the degree and constancy of atrioventricular block. Consistent 2 : 1 AV block can make the rhythm hard to recognize as the characteristic flutter waves are hidden by QRS complexes but they may become apparent when the degree of block varies spontaneously or with adenosine administration. Fetal or neonatal heart failure often develops. The rhythm can be well tolerated for short periods but attempts to restore sinus rhythm or at least to control ventricular rate are appropriate to prevent deterioration in heart muscle function. Adenosine will not restore sinus rhythm but may transiently increase AV block allowing a diagnosis to be made if the rhythm has not been recognized prior to its use (Fig. 30.17). Shocked infants and those in severe heart failure warrant DC cardio-

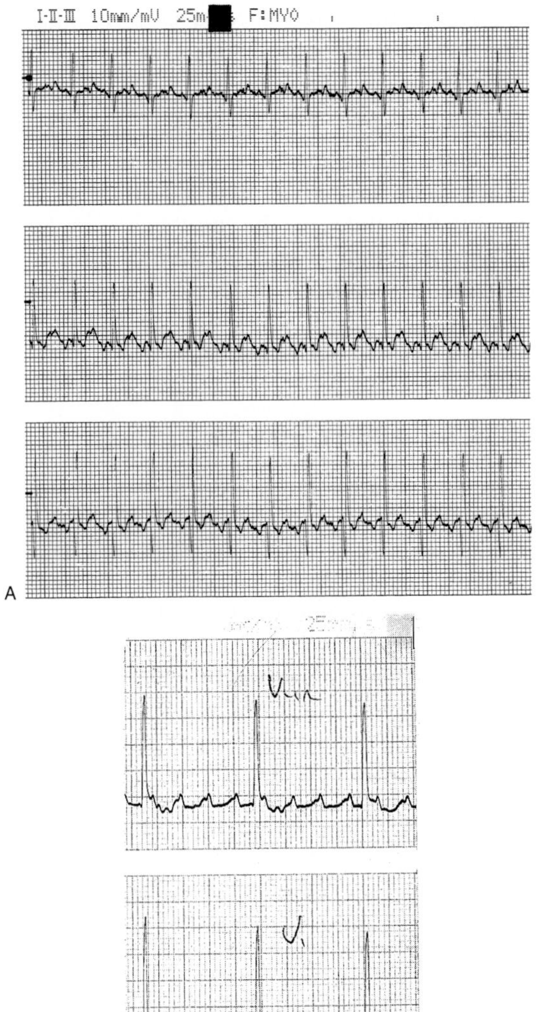

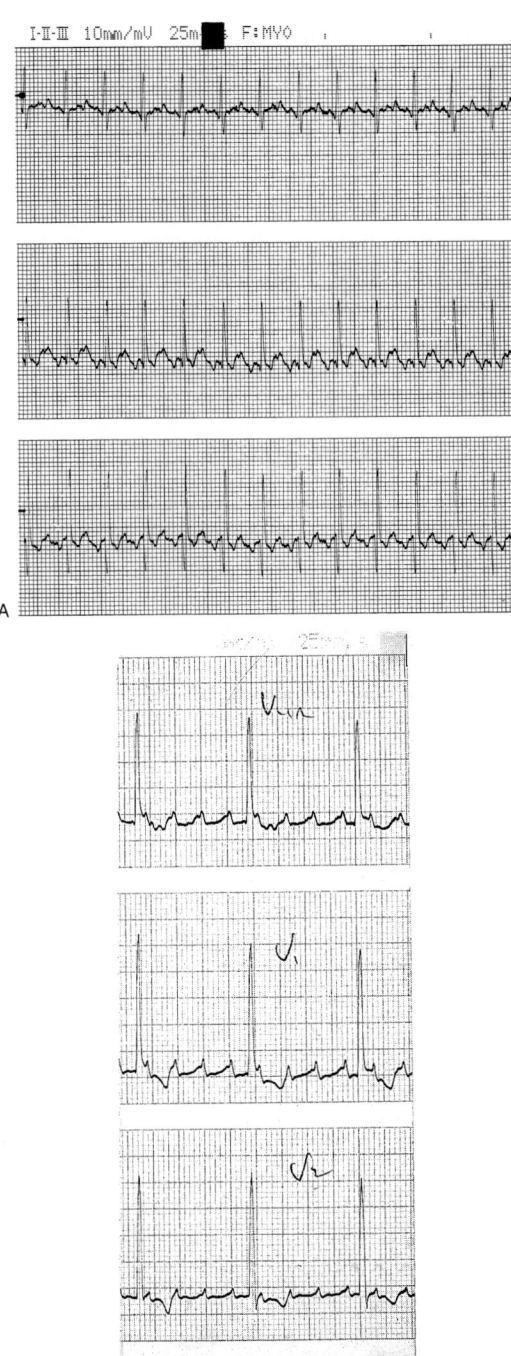

Fig. 30.17 (A) ECG leads I, II, III, 25 mm/s. Atrial flutter with 2 : 1 AV block. (B) ECG leads V_{4r}, V_1, V_2, 25 mm/s. Atrial flutter with 4 : 1 AV block. Flutter waves much easier to see than in A.

version or an attempt at oesophageal overpacing of the atria so as to establish sinus rhythm; neither of these therapies should be carried out without sedating the infant. Recurrence after cardioversion by either of these techniques may occur but is less likely in the newborn than in older children. Digoxin is used to slow ventricular rate and to help maintain sinus rhythm when achieved. Propranolol may be added to digoxin therapy to achieve further control of ventricular rate. If symptoms can be controlled and the heart is otherwise healthy spontaneous resolution can be hoped for. A minority of patients have an underlying pre-excitation ECG. The arrhythmia carries a mortality of 10–15% in the newborn, either from intractable heart failure or from progression to more malignant arrhythmias spontaneously or in response to electrical or pharmacological intervention.

Atrioventricular re-entry tachycardia

This is the commonest form of SVT in the newborn. The ECG in sinus rhythm may have a pre-excitation pattern (short PR interval and delta wave on QRS upstroke) allowing Wolfe–Parkinson–White syndrome to be diagnosed. Even if present, a pre-excitation pattern may be intermittent or disappear with age. The QRS complexes are narrow when SVT occurs, unless aberrant conduction occurs, which is very unusual in the newborn. P waves may be visible between QRS complexes but if they are they have an abnormal axis. QRS rates vary from 180–300/min (Fig. 30.2). Distinction from sinus tachycardia is occasionally difficult but the overall clinical picture, in conjunction with a careful examination of the ECG for features mentioned above, usually allows this. Infants can be asymptomatic or have episodes of pallor and breathlessness or be in heart failure. Any form of structural heart disease, myocardial tumours, myocarditis, electrolyte disturbances or indwelling right atrial lines should be considered as causes but the heart is usually normal. Myocardial dysfunction and mitral regurgitation develop secondary to the arrhythmia and can be expected to resolve once control is achieved. If the infant's condition allows, facial immersion in cold water until conversion or for a maximum of 10 s (Fig. 30.18) is the treatment of choice with an 85–90% success rate.[81] If this fails or is impracticable, application of ice to the face may be tried but has a lower success rate, and adenosine intravenously should be used. Adenosine also has an 85% success rate in restoring sinus rhythm and it may unmask atrial flutter if present. Contraindications to adenosine in the newborn are few. Dipyridamole will potentiate its effects. Side-effects include transient profound bradycardia. If these measures fail and the baby is collapsed, synchronized DC shock should be given. Digoxin should be given if heart failure is marked; propranolol may be used instead if heart failure is not severe or in addition if it is. If these measures fail but DC shock is not indicated, a further trial of cold water or adenosine should take place before progressing to amiodarone or a type I antiarrhythmic (disopyramide, flecainide, quinidine) all of which should be discussed with a cardiology centre. Verapamil is not recommended for intravenous administration in the newborn period or infancy because of the incidence of bradycardia and hypotension associated with its use. If the rhythm is well tolerated it is acceptable to give digoxin at least 6–12 hours to work even if loading doses

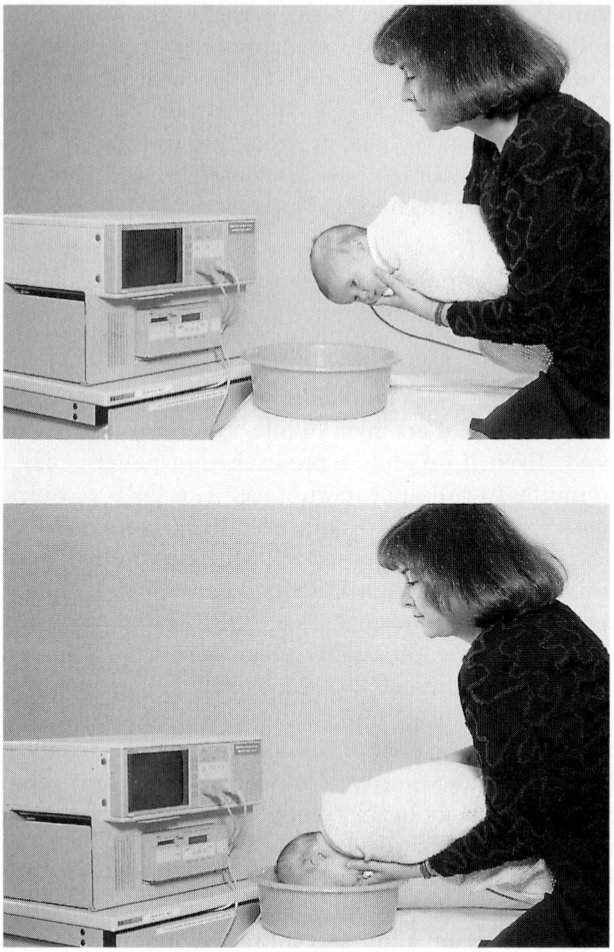

Fig. 30.18 Simulated facial immersion in cold water for treatment of SVT. Note ECG monitor interfaced to paper printer.

have been used. In summary, acute treatment of SVT is as follows (drug doses are in Table 30.30):

- DC cardioversion if collapsed (sedate unless unconscious).
- Facial immersion/ice bag.
- Intravenous adenosine if vagotonic manoeuvre fails.
- Intravenous propranolol if no heart failure and adenosine has failed.
- Start intravenous digitalization if heart failure or if two doses of propranolol fail
- Review need for cardioversion. Retry facial immersion and intravenous adenosine if DC cardioversion still not indicated.
- If baby stable without heart failure, continue digitalization regime and oral maintenance propranolol; infant may be watched for 6–12 hours. Further attempts at facial immersion and intravenous adenosine can be tried after 6–8 hours.
- If in heart failure, observation is not appropriate and amiodarone or a type 1 antiarrhythmic (disopyramide, flecainide, quinidine) should be considered in conjunction with discussion with cardiology service.
- When sinus rhythm established, decide on appropriate maintenance preventive treatment (see text).

Once sinus rhythm is restored, maintenance therapy with whatever agent(s) restored it is usually given for about 6 months. Drug doses are given in Table 30.30. Fetal SVT can be treated by administration of digoxin, quinidine or flecainide to the mother[4,37] in specialist centres. Administration of antiarrhythmics directly to the fetus is being explored. It is preferable to bring the arrhythmia under control before delivery but in extreme circumstances this will not be possible.

VENTRICULAR ARRHYTHMIAS

Ventricular arrhythmias have QRS-T complexes which are always different in configuration and polarity from those in sinus rhythm; the QRS complexes are usually but not necessarily broad. Broad complexes can be hard to recognize in the newborn as the upper limit of normal for QRS duration is only 70 ms. Associated and causative conditions for ventricular arrhythmias include any type of cardiomyopathy, myocarditis, intracardiac tumours, electrolyte disturbances, hypoxaemia and acidosis and only rarely structural congenital heart disease. Familial long QT syndromes[34] may be detected in the newborn if the family history is known or if ventricular arrhythmias occur.

Premature ventricular complexes

These are recognized by being abnormal premature QRS complexes without a preceding P wave. They are followed by a compensatory pause. Sometimes complexes with features of both the ventricular ectopic and the normal QRS complex are seen (fusion complexes). Ventricular ectopics have been found in up to 33% of healthy newborn infants.[80] They are rarely a sign of cardiac disease but conditions listed above must be considered. Occasional unifocal VEs with normal clinical examination and ECG require no action in the newborn period, merely review at 6–8 weeks. Very frequent VEs, the presence of a family history suggesting a long QT syndrome, cardiac physical signs or ECG abnormalities (particularly a long QT[87] or evidence for heart muscle disease) are an indication for echocardiography and 24h ECG monitoring (looking for ventricular tachycardia). Isolated VEs with a normal heart require no treatment and will resolve within 2 months; if they do not, echocardiography and 24h ECG monitoring should be performed or repeated.

Ventricular tachycardia

This is rare in the newborn and consists of a series of ventricular ectopics occurring sequentially with a rate of 150–250/min. Close examination reveals that there are

Table 30.30 Antiarrhythmic drug doses

Drug	Dose and route	Comment
Adenosine	0.05–0.25 mg/kg rapid i.v.	Start low and increase at 2-min intervals
Digoxin	10 μg/kg i.v. over 15 min, then 5 μg/kg i.v. after 6 h; repeat after a further 6 h After digitalization regime start maintenance at: 4 μg/kg/dose oral 12-hourly (give 60% of this if using i.v. route)	Acute loading doses. Ensure infant not hypokalaemic
Propranolol	0.05 mg/kg i.v. over 2 min. 1–2 mg/kg/dose oral 8-hourly	Acute, may repeat once. Avoid in severe heart failure Beware hypoglycaemia Never use after verapamil
Verapamil		Better avoided in newborns Never use after propranolol
Lignocaine	1 mg/kg i.v., then 1 mg/kg/h i.v.	
DC shock	SVT (synchronized) 0.5–1 joule/kg VT/VF 1–2 joule/kg	Sedation/anaesthesia required unless infant unconscious

Note: Other drugs used vary with local expertise. Advice should be sought.

minor irregularities in rate and that the P waves if recognized are either dissociated from the QRS complexes or conducted retrogradely. The rhythm may be paroxysmal or sustained; if paroxysmal, fusion beats may be seen. Neonates with VT may have underlying diseases as listed above but may have normal hearts. A well infant with no underlying disease may be asymptomatic; most cardiologists would still advocate preventive treatment in such cases initially. Severely collapsed infants should receive synchronized DC shock; less severely symptomatic infants should be treated with lignocaine intravenously by bolus and then infusion. Amiodarone should only be used after discussion with a cardiologist. Propranolol is the oral preventive of choice (Table 30.30). If the rhythm reflects underlying electrolyte disturbance this should be rapidly corrected.

Idioventricular rhythm

This has the morphology of VT but is slower (110–120/min), being around the same speed as sinus rhythm. It is rarely a sign of heart disease, is usually well tolerated and has a benign natural history.

Ventricular fibrillation

The QRS complexes are fast, bizarre and irregular. Full cardiopulmonary resuscitation should be instituted if the underlying pathology is unknown or considered remediable. Ventricular fibrillation is very rare in neonates and is usually terminal whatever the cause.

ATRIOVENTRICULAR CONDUCTION DISTURBANCES (HEART BLOCK)

There are three degrees of AV conduction block.

First degree heart block

This is present when the PR interval exceeds the upper limit of normal for age and heart rate, the maximum interval being 110 ms in the newborn. It is never symptomatic but may reflect underlying structural heart disease such as ASD, heart muscle disease or drug effect (e.g. digoxin). It can occur in families and may progress to more severe degrees of block.

Second degree heart block

This is present when not every P wave is followed by a QRS complex. There are two forms. Mobitz type I second degree AV block shows the Wenckebach phenomenon in which the PR interval progressively increases until after 3–6 cycles the P wave is not conducted; the sequence then commences again. This phenomenon may be seen in sleep or under anaesthesia at any age and does not necessarily reflect underlying heart disease. Mobitz type II block has a fixed normal or long PR interval with intermittent non-conduction of the P wave. Failure to conduct the P wave is often at regular intervals such as 2 : 1, 3 : 1 and so on. Mobitz type II block is much more likely to reflect underlying cardiac disease and frequently progresses to complete heart block.

Third degree heart block

This is also termed complete heart block. The P waves and QRS complexes in CHB are totally dissociated, with most commonly a normal atrial rate and responsiveness and a ventricular rate between 40 and 80/min (Fig. 30.19). Fetal and neonatal CHB may be associated with a variety of usually complex structural heart lesions, in

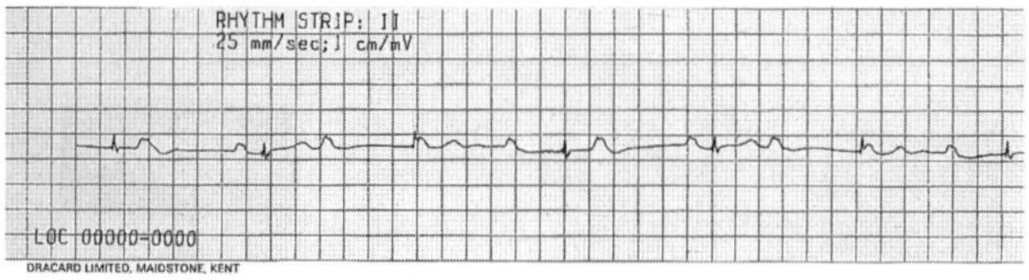

Fig. 30.19 ECG lead II, 25 mm/s. Complete heart block. Atrial rate 82 min (sleeping infant), ventricular rate 48 min.

which case heart failure is the norm and outlook is frequently poor. Another group of patients with congenital CHB have structurally normal hearts. A high proportion of these infants have His bundle fibrosis secondary to maternal antibodies, termed anti Ro or SS Ro antibodies. The mothers with these antibodies may have connective tissue disorders but more usually are well with serological markers for connective tissue disease, especially systemic lupus erythematosus. Many neonates with normal hearts and CHB are asymptomatic. Heart failure may occur pre- or postnatally; Stokes–Adams attacks are rare. A number of factors identify infants likely to have a poor outlook without intervention: these include structural heart disease, symptoms, resting heart rate below 55/min, little increase in heart rate in response to stress and broad QRS complexes. If necessary, specific emergency management should include inotropes and diuretics and if possible temporary pacing through the oesophagus or transvenously. Permanent pacemaker insertion is usually epicardial in newborn infants rather than endocardial. Complete heart block in the fetus is usually well tolerated; if hydrops starts to develop thought should be given to delivery. Evidence that the fetal heart rate can be significantly increased by drug administration to the mother is unclear; maternal steroid administration to prevent His bundle damage has been advocated but is not universally accepted. Fetal pacemaker insertion has yet to be successful.

HYPERTENSION

Measurement of neonatal blood pressure is discussed on page 677. Ill infants are likely to have direct invasive blood pressure measurements. Normal blood pressure increases with gestational and postnatal ages. Hypertension exists if blood pressure is found above the upper limit of normal in a calm infant. Normal values are given in Appendix 3. Causes of hypertension are given in Table 30.31. Hypertension is rarely symptomatic but may cause heart failure, irritability and other neurological signs.

Table 30.31 Causes of neonatal hypertension

System	Examples	Comment
Renal	Renal artery emboli/thrombosis	May be UAC related (p. 923) May be acutely symptomatic Often improves over 12 months
	Renal vein thrombosis	Hypertension may be delayed onset
	Dysplastic renal disease	
	Polycystic renal disease	
	Urinary tract obstruction	
	Renal infection	
	Renal failure	Any cause
Cardiovascular	Coarctation	
Endocrine	Congenital adrenal hyperplasia	
	Hyperaldosteronism	
	Hyperthyroidism	
	Phaeochromocytoma	
	Neuroblastoma	
Respiratory disease	Acute hypercapnia	Any cause
	Chronic lung disease	Often steroid induced
Neurological disease	Raised intracranial pressure	Any cause Treating BP alone will reduce cerebral perfusion pressure
	Convulsions	Probably mediated via intracranial pressure, convulsion may be subtle or masked by drugs
Drugs	Neonatal exposure	
	Corticosteroids	
	Methylxanthines	
	Phenylephrine	In eye drops
	Inotropes	Overdose
	Fetal exposure	
	Maternal cocaine	

Table 30.32 Drugs for treating systemic hypertension

Drug	Dose	Route	Comment
Vasodilators			
Phentolamine	0.1–0.5 μg/kg/min	i.v.	Alpha blocker
Captopril	0.1–1 mg/kg/dose	Oral	ACE inhibitor Acute or chronic Start low and increase Beware marked hypotension Watch renal function
Nifedipine	0.2 mg/kg/dose	Oral	Calcium channel blocker
	0.1–0.5 mg/kg/dose	Oral	Acute Chronic, 8-hourly
Hydrallazine	0.1–0.3 mg/kg/dose	i.v.	Acute, can repeat after 20–30 min
	0.2–0.5 mg/kg/dose	Oral	Chronic, 8-hourly
Diuretics			
Frusemide	1 mg/kg/dose	i.v.	Acute, 8-hourly
	1–2 mg/kg/dose	Oral	Chronic, 8- to 12-hourly
Chlorothiazide	25 mg/kg/dose	Oral	Chronic, 8- to 12-hourly
Beta blocker			
Propranolol	1–2 mg/kg/dose	Oral	Chronic, 8-hourly

Specific treatment is appropriate if there are symptoms; in their absence therapy should be aimed at the underlying disease and hypotensive therapy commenced only if there is severe hypertension or evidence of progressive left ventricular hypertrophy. Some drugs commonly used to treat neonatal hypertension are listed in Table 30.32. It is unusual for rapid reduction in blood pressure to be required in the newborn but intravenous alpha blockade with phentolamine, oral ACE inhibitor (captopril) or oral nifedipine will usually achieve this. Intravenous hydrallazine, nitroprusside or diazoxide are rarely used. The prognosis in hypertension is that of the underlying cause, providing malignant hypertension is avoided or treated rapidly and effectively.

CARDIAC TUMOURS

Symptomatic cardiac tumours are extremely rare in the newborn but asymptomatic ones are found more commonly since the widespread use of ultrasound scanning. So-called 'golf-ball' tumours, usually in the left ventricle, are a fetal echocardiographic finding; they have usually resolved by term and are of no functional significance. They may be a fetal marker for a syndrome if found in both ventricles. Cardiac tumours in the newborn may cause arrhythmias[61] or less commonly physical obstruction within the heart. Over 95% of intracardiac tumours in the newborn are benign and at least 75% of them are rhabdomyomata. Rhabdomyomata are often multiple and may resolve, which is a reason for being cautious about surgical intervention even if symptoms are present.[61] Multiple intracardiac tumours suggest the possibility of tuberous sclerosis (TS); 50% of individuals with TS will have cardiac tumours detected by echocardiography if looked for in infancy.[88] Pericardial tumours may present with pericardial effusion and tamponade in the newborn period.

REFERENCES

1. Allan L D 1995 Echocardiographic detection of congenital heart disease in the fetus: present and future. British Heart Journal 74: 103–106
2. Allan L D, Anderson R H, Sullivan I 1983 Evaluation of fetal arrhythmias by echocardiography. British Heart Journal 50: 240–245
3. Allan L D, Crawford D C, Anderson R H, Tynan M 1985 Spectrum of congenital heart disease detected echocardiographically in pre-natal life. British Heart Journal 54: 523–526
4. Allan L D, Chita S K, Sharland G K, Maxwell D, Priestley K 1991 Flecainide in the treatment of fetal tachycardias. British Heart Journal 65: 46–48
5. Amato M, Huppi P S, Markus D 1992 Prophylaxis of patent ductus arteriosus using ethamsylate in pre term infants treated with exogenous surfactant. Acta Paediatrica 81: 351–352
6. Archer L N J, Glass E J, Godman M J 1984 The silent ductus arteriosus in the idiopathic respiratory distress syndrome. Acta Paediatrica Scandinavica 73: 652–656
7. Ashfaq M, Houston A B, Gnanapragasam J P, Lilley S, Murtagh E P 1991 Balloon atrial septostomy under echocardiographic control: six years experience and evaluation of the practicability of cannulation via the umbilical vein. British Heart Journal 65: 148–151
8. Bailey L I, Gundry S R, Razzook A J 1993 Bless the babies: one hundred fifteen late survivors of heart transplantation during the first year of life. Journal of Thoracic and Cardiovascular Surgery 105: 805–815
9. Benson J W, Drayton M R, Hayward C et al 1986 Multicentre trial of ethamsylate for prevention of periventricular haemorrhage in very low birth weight infants. Lancet ii: 1297–1300
10. Bu'Lock F A, Joffe H S, Jordan S C, Martin R P 1993 Balloon dilatation (valvoplasty) as first line treatment for severe stenosis of the aortic valve in early infancy; medium term results and determinants of survival. British Heart Journal 70: 546–553
11. Burch M 1994 Hypertrophic cardiomyopathy. Archives of Disease in Childhood 71: 488–489
12. Burch M 1996 Oxford paediatric echo course video. Oxford Medical Illustration, Oxford OX3 9DU
13. Burch M, Runciman R 1996 Dilated cardiomyopathy. Archives of Disease in Childhood 74: 479–481
14. Burch M, Reddington A N, Carvallo J S et al 1990 Open valvotomy for critical aortic stenosis in infancy. British Heart Journal 63: 37–40
15. Cassady G, Crouse D T, Kirklin S W et al 1989 A randomised controlled trial of very early prophylactic ligation of the ductus arteriosus in babies who weighed 1000 g or less at birth. New England Journal of Medicine 320: 1511–1516
16. Chang A C, Huhta J C, Yoon G Y et al 1991 Diagnosis, transport and outcome in fetuses with left ventricular outflow obstruction. Journal of Thoracic and Cardiovascular Surgery 102: 841–848
17. Clark E B 1995 Morphogenesis, growth and biomechanics. In: Emmanouilides E C, Riemans-Schneider T A, Allen H A, Gutgesell H P (eds) Heart disease in infants children and adolescents, 5th edn. Williams & Wilkins, Baltimore, pp 1–15
18. Clyman R I 1996 Recommendations for the post natal use of indomethacin: an analysis of four separate treatment strategies. Journal of Pediatrics 128: 601–607
19. Clyman R I, Mauray F, Roman C, Rudolph A M, Heymann M A 1981 Glucocorticoids alter the sensitivity of the lamb ductus arteriosus to prostaglandin E2. Journal of Pediatrics 98: 126–128

20. Colditz P, Murphy D, Rolfe P, Wilkinson A R 1989 Effect of infusion rate of indomethacin on cerebrovascular responses in pre term neonates. Archives of Disease in Childhood 64: 8–12
21. Coombs R C, Morgan M E I, Durbin G M, Booth I W, McNeish A S 1990 Gut blood flow velocities in the newborn: effects of patent ductus arteriosus and parenteral indomethacin. Archives of Disease in Childhood 65: 1067–1071
22. Coster D D, Gorton M E, Grooters R K, Thieman K C, Schneider R F, Soltanzader H 1989 Surgical closure of the patent ductus arteriosus in the neonatal intensive care unit. Annals of Thoracic Surgery 48: 386–389
23. Cotton R B, Haywood J L, Fitzgerald G A 1991 Symptomatic patent ductus arteriosus following prophylactic indomethacin. Biology of the Neonate 60: 273–282
24. Couser R J, Ferrata B, Wright G B et al 1996 Prophylactic indomethacin therapy in the first twenty-four hours of life for the prevention of patent ductus arteriosus in pre term infants treated prophylactically with surfactant in the delivery room. Journal of Pediatrics 128: 631–637
25. Diprose G K, Evans D H, Archer L N J, Levene M I 1986 Dinamap fails to detect hypotension in very low birth weight infants. Archives of Disease in Childhood 61: 771–773
26. Edwards A D, Wyatt J S, Richardson C et al 1990 Effects of indomethacin on cerebral haemodynamics in very pre term infants. Lancet 335: 1491–1495
27. Evans D H, Levene M I, Archer L N J 1987 The effect of indomethacin on cerebral blood flow velocity in premature infants. Developmental Medicine and Child Neurology 29: 776–782
28. Evans N 1993 Diagnosis of patent ductus arteriosus in the pre term newborn. Archives of Disease in Childhood 68: 58–61
29. Evans N 1994 Cardiovascular effects of dexamethasone in the pre term infant. Archives of Disease in Childhood 70: F25–F30
30. Evans N, Kluckow M 1996 Early ductal shunting and intraventricular haemorrhage in ventilated pre term infants. Archives of Disease in Childhood 75: F183–F186
31. Evans N J, Archer L N J 1990 Postnatal circulatory adaptation in healthy term and pre term neonates. Archives of Disease in Childhood 65: 24–26
32. Fajardo C A, Whyte R K, Steele B T 1992 Effect of dopamine on failure of indomethacin to close the patent ductus arteriosus. Journal of Pediatrics 121: 771–775
33. Fowlie P W 1996 Prophylactic indomethacin: systematic review and meta-analysis. Archives of Disease in Childhood 74: F81–F87
34. Garson A 1990 Ventricular arrhythmias. In: Gillette P C, Garson A (eds) Pediatric arrhythmias: electrophysiology and pacing. W B Saunders Philadelphia, pp 427–500
35. Gersony W M, Peckham G J, Ellison R C, Miettinen O S, Nadas A S 1983 Effects of indomethacin in premature infants with patent ductus arteriosus: results of a national collaborative study. Journal of Pediatrics 102: 895–906
36. Gibbs J L, Wren C, Watterson K G, Hunter S, Hamilton J R L 1993 Stenting of the arterial duct combined with banding of the pulmonary arteries and atrial septectomy or septostomy: a new approach to palliation for the hypoplastic left heart syndrome. British Heart Journal 69: 551–555
37. Gow R, Hamilton R 1991 Diagnosis and therapy for fetal tachycardia and other fetal rhythm abnormalities. Current Opinion in Pediatrics 3: 838–843
38. Grabitz R G, Joffres M R, Collins-Nakai R L 1988 Congenital heart disease: incidence in the first year of life. American Journal of Epidemiology 128: 381–383
39. Gray D T, Fyler D C, Walker A M, Weinstein M C, Chalmers T C 1993 Clinical outcomes and costs of transcatheter as compared with surgical closure of patent ductus arteriosus. New England Journal of Medicine 329: 1517–1523
40. Green T P, Thompson T R, Johnson D E, Lock D E 1983 Furosemide promotes patent ductus arteriosus in premature infants with respiratory distress syndrome. New England Journal of Medicine 308: 743–748
41. Guenthard J, Wylie F, Fowler B, Baumgartner R 1995 Cardiomyopathy in respiratory chain disorders. Archives of Disease in Childhood 72: 223–226
42. Hammerman C, Aramburo M J 1990 Prolonged indomethacin therapy for the prevention of recurrences of patent ductus arteriosus. Journal of Pediatrics 117: 771–776
43. Hanley F L, Sade R M, Freedom R M, Blackstone E H, Kirklin J W 1993 Outcomes in critically ill neonates with pulmonary stenosis and intact ventricular septum: a multi institutional study. Journal of the American College of Cardiology 22: 183–192
44. Heymann M A 1995 Fetal and postnatal circulations, pulmonary circulation. In: Emmanouilides E C, Riemens-Schneider T A, Allen H D, Gutgesell H P (eds) Heart disease in infants children and adolescents, 5th edn. Williams & Wilkins, Baltimore, pp 41–47
45. Hoffman J I E, Christianson R 1978 Congenital heart disease in a cohort of 19,502 births with long-term follow up. American Journal of Cardiology 42: 641–647
46. Ino T, Sherwood G, Benson L N, Wilson G J, Freedom R M, Rowe R D 1988 Cardiac manifestations in disorders of fat and carnitine metabolism in infancy. Journal of the American College of Cardiology 11: 1301–1308
47. Jacob J, Gluck L, Di Sessa T et al 1980 The contribution of PDA in the neonate with severe RDS. Journal of Pediatrics 96: 79–87
48. Jedeikin R, Primhak R, Shennan A T, Swyer P R, Rowe R D 1983 Serial electrocardiographic changes in healthy and stressed neonates. Archives of Disease in Childhood 58: 605–611
49. Jones R W A, Pickering D 1977 Persistent ductus arteriosus complicating the respiratory distress syndrome. Archives of Disease in Childhood 52: 274–281
50. Jones R W A, Baumer J H, Joseph M C, Shinebourne E A 1976 Arterial oxygen tension and response to oxygen breathing in differential diagnosis of congenital heart disease in infancy. Archives of Disease in Childhood 51: 667–673
51. Kelly J R, Gunteroth W G 1988 Pansystolic murmur in the newborn, tricuspid regurgitation versus ventricular septal defect. Archives of Disease in Childhood 63: 1172–1174
52. Macmahon P, Gorham P R, Arnold R, Wilkinson J L, Hamilton D I 1983 Pulmonary artery growth during treatment with oral prostaglandin E2 in ductus dependent cyanotic congential heart disease. Archives of Disease in Childhood 58: 187–189
53. Mahony L 1995 Development of myocardial structure and function. In: Emmanouilides E C, Riemens-Schneider T A, Allen H, Gutgesell H P (eds) Heart disease in infants children and adolescents, 5th edn. Williams & Wilkins, Baltimore, pp 17–29
54. Mahony L, Carnero V, Brett C, Heymann M A, Clyman R I 1982 Prophylactic indomethacin therapy for patent ductus arteriosus in very low birth weight infants. New England Journal of Medicine 306: 506–510
55. Manchester D, Margolis H S, Sheldon R E 1976 Possible association between maternal indomethacin therapy and primary pulmonary hypertension in the newborn. American Journal of Obstetrics and Gynecology 126: 467–469
56. Mecrow I K, Ladusans E J 1994 Infective endocarditis in newborn infants with structurally normal hearts. Acta Paediatrica 83: 35–39
57. Millard D D, Shulman S T 1988 The changing spectrum of neonatal endocarditis. Clinics in Perinatology 15: 587–608
58. Moise K J, Huhta J C, Sharif D S et al 1988 Indomethacin in the treatment of premature labor. New England Journal of Medicine 319: 327–331
59. Momma K, Takao A 1989 Increased constriction of the ductus arteriosus with combined administration of indomethacin and betamethasone in fetal rats. Pediatric Research 25: 69–75
60. Montigny M, Biron P, Fournier A, Elie R, Davignon A, Fouron J-C 1989 Captopril in infants for congestive heart failure secondary to a large ventricular left to right shunt. American Journal of Cardiology 63: 631–633
61. Muhler E G, Kienas W, Turniski-Harder V, von Bernuth G 1994 Arrhythmias in infants and children with primary cardiac tumours. European Heart Journal 15: 915–921
62. National Institutes of Health 1987 Report of the second task force on blood pressure control in children. Pediatrics 79: 1–25
63. Neill C A 1990 Genetics and risks of congenital heart disease. In: Long W A (ed) Fetal and neonatal cardiology. W B Saunders, Philadelphia, pp 125–155
64. Norton M E, Merrill J, Cooper B A B, Kuller J A, Clyman R I 1993 Neonatal complications after the administration of indomethacin for pre term labor. New England Journal of Medicine 329: 1602–1607
65. Park M, Guntheroth W G 1992 How to read pediatric ECGs, 3rd edn. Year Book, Chicago
66. Patel J, Marks K A, Roberts I, Azzopardi O, Edwards A D 1995

Ibuprofen treatment for patent ductus arteriosus. Lancet 346: 255
67. Pickoff A S 1995 Development and function of the cardiac conduction system. In: Emmanouilides E C, Riemens-Schneider T A, Allen H D, Gutgesell H P (eds) Heart disease in infants children and adolescents, 5th edn. Williams & Wilkins, Baltimore, pp 29–41
68. Radzik D, Davignon A, van Doesburg N, Fournier A, Marchand T, Ducharme G 1993 Predictive factors for spontaneous closure of atrial septal defect diagnosed in the first 3 months of life. Journal of the American College of Cardiology 22: 851–853
69. Raju T N K, Langenberg P 1993 Pulmonary hemorrhage and exogenous surfactant therapy: a meta analysis. Journal of Pediatrics 123: 606–610
70. Reller M D, Colasurdo M A, Rice M C, McDouall R W 1990 The timing of spontaneous closure of the ductus arteriosus in infants with respiratory distress syndrome. American Journal of Cardiology 66: 75–78
71. Rennie J M, Cooke R W I 1991 Prolonged low dose indomethacin for persistent ductus arteriosus of prematurity. Archives of Disease in Childhood 66: 55–58
72. Report of the European Registry 1992 Transcatheter occlusion of persistent arterial duct. Lancet 340: 1062–1066
73. Salmon A P, Keeton B R, Sethia B 1993 Developments in interventional catheterisation and progress in surgery for congenital heart disease: achieving a balance. British Heart Journal 69: 479–480
74. Sharland G K, Chita S K, Fagg N L K et al 1991 Left ventricular dysfunction in the fetus: relation to aortic valve anomalies and endocardial fibroelastosis. British Heart Journal 66: 419–424
75. Shaw N J, Wilson N, Dickinson D F 1988 Captopril in heart failure secondary to a left to right shunt. Archives of Disease in Childhood 63: 360–363
76. Shortland D B, Gibson N A, Levene M I, Archer L N, Evans D H, Shaw D E 1990 Patent ductus arteriosus and cerebral circulation in preterm infants. Developmental Medicine and Child Neurology 32: 386–393
77. Silove E D, Roberts D G U, De Giovanni J V 1985 Evaluation of oral and low dose intravenous prostaglandin E2 in management of ductus dependent congenital heart disease. Archives of Disease in Childhood 60: 1025–1030
78. Silverman N H 1993 Pediatric echocardiography. Williams & Wilkins, Baltimore
79. Southall D P, Johnson A M, Shinebourne E A, Johnstone P G B, Vulliamy D G 1981 Frequency and outcome of disorders of cardiac rhythm and conduction in a population of newborn infants. Pediatrics 68: 58–66
80. Southall D P, Richard J, Mitchell P, Brown D J, Johnston P G B, Shinebourne E A 1980 Study of cardiac rhythm in healthy newborn infants. British Heart Journal 43: 14–20
81. Sreeram N, Wren C 1990 Supraventricular tachycardia in infants: response to initial treatment. Archives of Disease in Childhood 65: 127–129
82. Starnes V A, Griffin M L, Pitlick P T et al 1992 Current approach to hypoplastic left heart syndrome. Journal of Thoracic and Cardiovascular Surgery 104: 189–195
83. Steinfield L, Rappaport H L, Rossbach H C, Martinez E 1986 Diagnosis of fetal arrhythmias using echocardiographic and Doppler techniques. Journal of the American College of Cardiology 8: 1425–1433
84. Stümpflen I, Stümpflen A, Wimmer M, Bernaschek G 1996 Effect of detailed fetal echocardiography as part of routine pre natal ultrasonographic screening on detection of congenital heart disease. Lancet 348: 854–857
85. Trus T, Winthrop A L, Pyle S, Shah J, Langer J C, Lau G Y P 1993 Optimal management of patent ductus arteriosus in the neonate weighing less than 800 g. Journal of Pediatric Surgery 28: 1137–1139
86. Tulloh R M R, Tansey S P, Parashar K, De Giovanni J V, Wright J G C, Silove E D 1994 Echocardiographic screening in neonates undergoing surgery for selected gastrointestinal malformations. Archives of Disease in Childhood 70: F206–F208
87. Villain E, Levy M, Kachaner J, Garson A 1992 Prolonged QT interval in neonates: Benign, transient or prolonged risk of sudden death. American Heart Journal 124: 194–197
88. Wallace G, Smith H C, Watson G H, Rimmer S, D'Souza S W 1990 Tuberous sclerosis presenting with fetal and neonatal cardiac tumours. Archives of Disease in Childhood 65: 377–379
89. Walsh K P, Sreeram N, Franks R, Arnold R 1991 Balloon dilatation of the arterial duct in congenital heart disease. Lancet 339: 331–332
90. Way G L, Woolfe R R, Eshaghpour E, Bender R L, Jaffe R B, Ruttenberg H D 1979 The natural history of hypertrophic cardiomyopathy in infants of diabetic mothers. Journal of Pediatrics 95: 1020–1025
91. Wells J T, Ment L R 1995 Prevention of intraventricular hemorrhage in pre term infants. Early Human Development 42: 209–233
92. Wilkinson A R, Aynsley-Green A, Mitchell M D 1979 Persistent pulmonary hypertension and abnormal prostaglandin E levels in pre term infants after maternal treatment with naproxen. Archives of Disease in Childhood 54: 942–945
93. Wyllie J, Wren C, Hunter S 1994 Screening for fetal cardiac malformations. British Heart Journal 71(suppl): 20–27
94. Yeh T F, Luken J A, Thalji A, Raval D, Carr I, Pildes R S 1981 Intravenous indomethacin therapy in premature infants with persistent ductus arteriosus – a double-blind controlled study. Journal of Pediatrics 98: 137–145

31

Gastroenterology

Part 1

Neonatal jaundice

N. Kevin Ives

INTRODUCTION

Jaundice is the most common clinical sign in neonatal medicine, but only rarely is it the harbinger of disease or associated with neurotoxicity. Some two-thirds of entirely healthy term newborns,[70] and a greater proportion of preterms, develop jaundice in the first week of life. This usually reflects the immaturity of the liver's excretory pathway for bilirubin at a time of heightened production. The resultant jaundice is referred to as 'physiological'. Every jaundiced baby, however, demands assessment as to whether they possess features of 'pathological' jaundice, prompting further investigation and treatment. In the current era of early postnatal discharge from hospital,[8] the paediatrician's responsibility for detecting significant jaundice in the newborn is shared with midwives, health visitors and family practitioners. Neonatal jaundice is the most common reason for readmission of babies to hospital in the first week of life.[97]

Despite improved understanding of the mechanisms of bilirubin's neurotoxicity,[110] our ability to predict which babies are at greatest risk remains imprecise. Present-day treatment guidelines reflect this uncertainty by erring on the side of caution. A 'kinder, gentler approach' to the management of jaundice in healthy full-term newborns is evolving,[22,80] but it is wrong to consider such infants as being immune to kernicterus at any bilirubin level.[65]

BILIRUBIN BIOCHEMISTRY

Bilirubin is formed as a result of the two-stage catabolism of haem in the reticuloendothelial system (Fig. 31.1). The

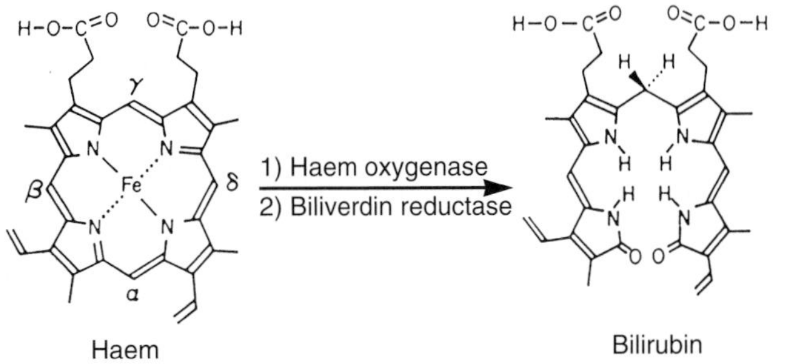

Fig. 31.1 Production of bilirubin from haem degradation. (Reproduced with permission from McDonagh and Lightner[72])

majority of haem arises from the turnover of haemoglobin released from naturally decommissioned or pathologically destroyed erythrocytes. Haem (ferroprotoporphyrin IX) has a porphyrin ring structure which is split open at its α-methene bridge by haem oxygenase. The intermediate pigment, biliverdin IXα, is water soluble, non-toxic, and serves as the excretory product of haem in amphibians, reptiles and birds. In mammals enzymatic reduction of biliverdin IXα by biliverdin reductase results in the production of bilirubin IXα.

Bilirubin IXα is the only toxic isomer of bilirubin. The small amounts of the IXβ and IXδ isomers produced are non-toxic. Our clinical concern regarding unconjugated hyperbilirubinaemia in the newborn thus arises from the preferential cleavage of the haem molecule at its α-methene bridge. Why mammalian species should expend energy producing and excreting a potentially neurotoxic haem byproduct is unclear. The need for products of fetal haem degradation to be able to cross the placenta is an important consideration.[32] Another explanation stems

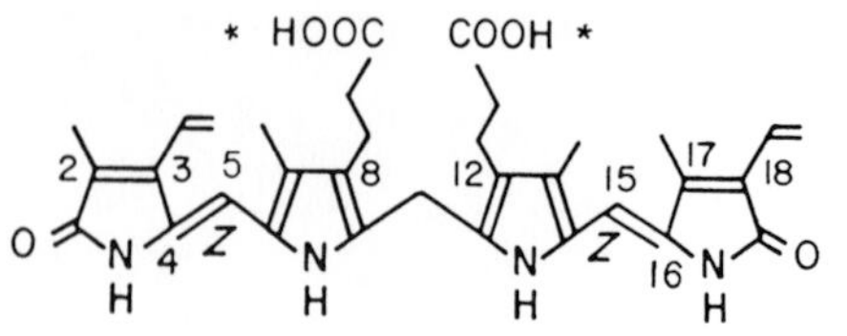

Fig. 31.2 Linear representation of bilirubin IXα with central propionic acid groups [**]. (Reproduced with permission from McDonagh and Lightner[72]) Z – see text.

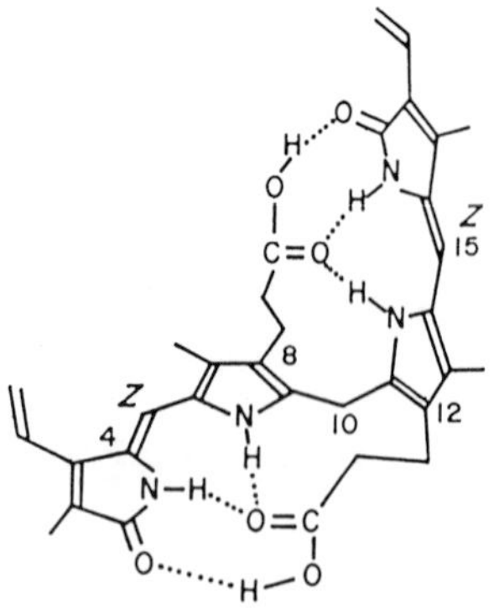

Fig. 31.3 Preferred conformation of bilirubin. (Reproduced with permission from McDonagh and Lightner[72])

from the discovery that bilirubin is a significant antioxidant, prompting the question: 'Is bilirubin good for you?'[71]

Diagrammatic representation of the bilirubin molecule conveys the impression of a tetrapyrrole aligned in a single plane (Fig. 31.2). The preferred conformation of the molecule is known to be partially folded at its mid-methylene bridge (Fig. 31.3).[7] This shape facilitates intramolecular hydrogen bonding, which saturates the hydrophilic polar groupings, rendering bilirubin virtually insoluble in water at physiological pH. The aqueous solubility of bilirubin dianion at a pH of 7.4 is as low as 7 nmol/l.[10] In this form bilirubin has lipophilic properties which enable it to cross cell membranes and biological boundaries, such as the placenta and blood–brain barrier.[41]

Within the physiological pH range bilirubin exists primarily as a dianion, with less than 1% taking on a proton to form the monoanion, and an even smaller fraction incorporating a futher proton to produce bilirubin acid. The propionic acid groups attached to the inner two pyrrole rings of the bilirubin molecule are the site of conjugation with glucuronic acid. The mono and diglucuronides of bilirubin so formed retain the more open, water-soluble conformation by reducing or preventing intramolecular hydrogen bonding. Polar groupings remain similarly exposed in the naturally occurring β and δ isomers of bilirubin, and in the major products of phototherapy, enabling them to be freely excreted in bile.[27]

BILIRUBIN METABOLISM AND EXCRETION

Most of the neonatal bilirubin pool originates from the breakdown of red cells, but up to a quarter comes from such sources as ineffective erythropoiesis, and from other haem-containing compounds such as myoglobin and cytochromes. This additional input to the bilirubin pool is known as 'shunt bilirubin'. Bilirubin is transported in the blood bound reversibly to serum albumin. Albumin has one high-affinity site which binds bilirubin in a molecular ratio of 1:1. Binding also occurs at lower-affinity sites, bringing the molar bilirubin–albumin ratio up to 3:1. Under normal circumstances the proportion of potentially toxic unbound, or free, bilirubin circulating in the jaundiced newborn is extremely low (<5 nmol/l). Changes in serum pH do not affect the binding of bilirubin to albumin, but a fall in pH will increase the concentration of bilirubin acid and promote binding of bilirubin to cell membranes and organelles.[9]

A carrier assists the transfer of bilrubin across the hepatocyte membrane, and specific binding proteins (e.g. ligandin or Y protein) are thought to increase net uptake by reducing the efflux of bilirubin from the hepatocyte.[16] Conjugation with glucuronic acid occurs in the smooth endoplasmic reticulum to form water-soluble mono- and diglucuronides of bilirubin. These reactions are catalysed by the microsomal enzyme hepatic uridine diphosphoglucuronosyl transferase.[6] Conjugated bilirubin (chiefly the monoglucuronide in the newborn) is actively transported out of the liver cell and into the biliary canaliculi as a component of bile.[16]

In adults, most of the conjugated bilirubin is converted by colonic flora to urobilinogen before elimination in the stool. In the newborn, however, a significant proportion is hydrolysed by small gut β-glucuronidase to yield glucuronic acid and unconjugated bilirubin. This bilirubin readily re-enters the circulating pool via the enterohepatic circulation.

BIOCHEMICAL BASIS OF PHOTOTHERAPY

Phototherapy detoxifies bilirubin and facilitates its excretion from the body via routes other than conjugation in the liver.[27,72] There are three photochemical reactions that can occur when bilirubin interacts with a photon of light energy. These are:

- photo-oxidation
- configurational isomerization
- structural isomerization.

Photo-oxidation, the first of these reactions to be discovered, involves disruption of the bilirubin molecule to form colourless polar fragments that are readily excreted in urine. Although this process reminds us of the need to avoid exposing serum samples to direct sunlight,[17] it is

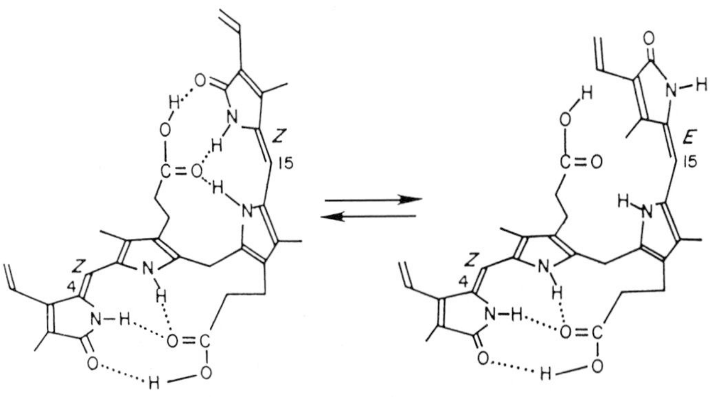

Fig. 31.4 Configurational photoisomerization of bilirubin. (Reproduced with permission from McDonagh and Lightner[72])

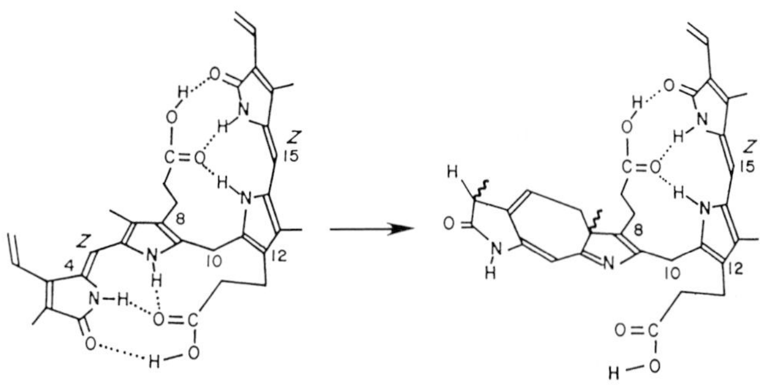

Fig. 31.5 Structural photoisomerization of bilirubin to form lumirubin. (Reproduced with permission from McDonagh and Lightner[72])

thought to play only a minor role in bilirubin excretion during phototherapy.

The bilirubin molecule remains intact in the other two reactions, undergoing either a configurational or a structural change. Configurational isomerization occurs by virtue of the double bonds between carbon atoms 4–5 and 15–16 of the molecule (Fig. 31.2). In the natural form the arrangement of these double bonds, and hence the alignment of the end pyrrole rings, is classified as bilirubin-4Z, 15Z (Z = *zusammen*, together). Photons of light striking the bilirubin molecule can temporarily disrupt the double bonds and initiate a 180° rotation of one or both end pyrrole rings to produce three isomeric forms, designated 4Z, 15E; 4E, 15Z; and 4E, 15E (E = *entgegen*, apart).

The formation of bilirubin-Z,E is favoured during phototherapy by the nature of the binding between bilirubin and albumin. While bound to albumin the configurational isomers remain stable for a number of hours. As shown in Figure 31.4, the conformation of bilirubin-Z,E maintains the exposure of polar groups at one end of the molecule, enabling it to be excreted unconjugated in bile. Once in bile a rapid reversal of the reaction occurs, such that unconjugated bilirubin-Z,Z enters the gut and is available for uptake via the enterohepatic circulation.

Configurational isomerization was originally thought to be the principal excretory mechanism of phototherapy. It is now realized that, although rapidly produced, these isomers are only slowly cleared in humans. The serum half-life of bilirubin-Z,E is about 15 hours, and after some 6–12 hours of phototherapy a steady state is achieved in which approximately 20% of the total serum bilirubin is in the form of the configurational isomer.[27] Importantly, this means that up to one-fifth of the circulating bilirubin is detoxified, despite not being in a form that is readily excreted.

The structural isomer, lumirubin, is currently considered to be the major excretory product of phototherapy.[27] Lumirubin is formed by 'cyclization' of one end of the bilirubin molecule, as shown in Figure 31.5. This structural change is irreversible and allows the more polar product to be excreted in bile and urine. Lumirubin's more efficient elimination is reflected in its half-life of less than 2 hours and steady-state concentration of 2–6% of the total serum bilirubin.[27] The production of lumirubin follows a dose–response relationship with the irradiance of phototherapy applied, and may be favoured by the use of light of a longer wavelength than that of conventional phototherapy[26] (see later, p. 727).

PHYSIOLOGICAL JAUNDICE

The fetus excretes unconjugated bilirubin via the placenta and maternal liver. In the absence of pathological fetal hyperbilirubinaemia or maternal liver disease, the mean bilirubin level in cord blood at birth is in the region of 20–35 μmol/l.[55,56] Postnatally most newborns exhibit a further elevation in serum bilirubin.[70] In healthy term infants the serum bilirubin peaks on the 3rd to 4th days of life, attaining clinically detectable levels (>80 μmol/l) in approximately two-thirds of the population.[70] Following this phase I peak, serum bilirubin levels fall rapidly for 2–3 days and then more gradually, reaching normal adult values between 1 and 2 weeks of age (phase II). Phase II may be prolonged in the breast-fed infant.[2] Physiological jaundice is the result of increased bilirubin production at a time when the mechanisms for liver uptake, transport and conjugation are immature. At higher serum bilirubin levels the carrier-mediated and saturable excretion of bilirubin into bile may also become rate limiting. The biphasic pattern of physiological jaundice results from a deficiency of UDPGT activity in the first phase[47] and low ligandin levels in the second.[33]

Premature infants exhibit a higher peak serum bilirubin level, occurring on days 5–6, and a longer second phase, persisting for 2–4 weeks. Even newborns bordering on prematurity are likely to exhibit heightened jaundice. This was demonstrated in a study population in which babies of 37 weeks' gestation were four times as likely to attain bilirubin levels greater than 220 μmol/l as those of 40 weeks' gestation.[30]

Table 31.1 Factors that exacerbate physiological jaundice in the newborn

Polycythaemia
Delayed cord clamping
Maternofetal transfusion
Recipient of twin–twin transfusion
Extravasated blood
Bruising (e.g. cephalhaematoma)
Birth trauma
Internal haemorrhage
Delayed passage of meconium
Swallowed blood
Hypocaloric feed intake
Dehydration
Breast-feeding
Prematurity

Bilirubin production during the first weeks of life is more than double that of the adult. Factors responsible for this excess bilirubin load in the newborn include the higher haematocrit,[89] increased red cell turnover, and a greater contribution from sources of haem other than senescent erythrocytes (shunt bilirubin). The lifespan of red cells is about 60–70 days in the healthy term infant, and as low as 30 days in the sick premature. A 10-fold higher level of β-glucuronidase in the small bowel brush border of the newborn reverses the conjugation process,[32] liberating more unconjugated bilirubin to enter the enterohepatic circulation. The high bilirubin content of meconium and the initial absence of gut bacteria are also thought to contribute. Other risk factors that heighten physiological jaudice are listed in Table 31.1.

Although the term 'physiological jaundice' is helpful in our understanding of the common pattern of newborn jaundice, it falsely conveys the impression of a totally benign condition. For this reason some clinicians prefer to place numerical limits on physiological jaundice. Serum bilirubin levels of more than two standard deviations above large population study means are chosen to denote pathological jaundice. Hence bilirubin values quoted as representing the upper limit of physiological jaundice are often in the region of 220 μmol/l for term and 250 μmol/l for premature infants. Higher levels should undoubtedly prompt consideration of pathological states contributing to a newborn's jaundice, but in the absence of a contributory disease process the term 'exaggerated physiological jaundice' may be more appropriate.[32] It must be remembered, however, that 'exaggerated physiological jaundice' may attain unconjugated bilirubin levels capable of transient[105] and occasionally permanent neurological damage.[65] It is a dangerous fallacy to assume that the otherwise healthy, non-haemolysing term infant is immune to bilirubin encephalopathy.

EPIDEMIOLOGY

Attempts to define physiological jaundice precisely are further confounded by a number of significant epidemiological determinants. Why certain Greek, Chinese and Japanese babies develop a marked idiopathic hyperbilirubinaemia (unrelated to their higher incidence of G-6PD deficiency) remains a mystery. Explanations are also sought as to why male infants have higher bilirubin levels than females[28,69] and caucasians higher than blacks.[28] Certain infants would appear to have a familial predisposition to hyperbilirubinaemia in the absence of any identifiable pathological cause. If one child in a family has exhibited marked physiological jaundice, subsequent siblings are statistically more likely to follow suit.[49] The prevalence of breast-feeding and the incidence of preterm birth will influence the pattern of jaundice within a population. Maternal smoking, probably through its negative correlation with breast-feeding, is associated with a lower incidence of neonatal jaundice.[69] The obstetric practices of oxytocin infusion and delivery by ventouse extraction have been associated with a mild increase in jaundice of the newborn. In the case of maternal diabetes, heightened jaundice may be the result of polycythaemia[5] or the higher incidence of preterm delivery. The higher concentration of β-glucuronidase in diabetic mothers' milk could also be contributory.[5]

JAUNDICE IN THE HEALTHY BREAST-FED INFANT

Breast-fed babies develop more marked and prolonged jaundice than those who are purely formula fed.[70] A review of the combined results from 12 studies involving more than 8000 newborns reveals that breast-fed babies are more than three times as likely to develop serum bilirubin levels greater than 205 μmol/l, and over six times as likely to exceed levels of 256 μmol/l as their formula-fed contempories.[92] The peak bilirubin level in the breast-fed baby may not occur until the 4th to 6th days of life.[3,52] Thus breast-fed babies are more likely to require extended hospitalization or readmission for investigation and treatment of early jaundice.

Up to one-third of breast-fed babies remain clinically jaundiced beyond 2 weeks of age,[2] and thus represent the majority of infants presenting at 2–3 weeks for a prolonged jaundice screen. The diagnosis of breast-milk jaundice can only reliably be made on exclusion of pathological causes. Once the diagnosis is confirmed, parents should be warned that resolution of jaundice in the breast-fed baby may take as long as 2–3 months. Although interruption of breast-feeds for 24 hours is frequently associated with a marked decline in serum bilirubin and lower rebound level on reintroduction, the practice cannot be justified clinically. Also to be discouraged is the vogue for supplementing breast-fed infants with water, regardless of their state of hydration. Newborns supplemented in this way have been shown to have significantly higher maximum serum bilirubin levels,[19] and may have their chances of successful breast-feeding jeopardized. The phenomenon of breast-milk jaundice also applies to babies born prematurely.[62]

Several hypotheses have been put forward to explain the association between breast-feeding and heightened jaundice. The subject has recently been reviewed,[35] and it would appear that the pathogenesis is likely to be multifactorial. Different mechanisms may account for what appears to be an early and a late phase of breast-milk associated jaundice, but our understanding is not greatly advanced by describing these as 'breast-feeding jaundice' and 'breast-milk jaundice' respectively.[3] Although the earlier phase may stem from a relative lack of milk and the second from factors within breast milk, the two undoubtedly overlap. Enhanced enterohepatic circulation of bilirubin in the breast-fed baby would appear to be a significant factor throughout. This may result from delayed passage of meconium, the presence of β-glucuronidase in breast milk, and decreased formation of urobilinogen, secondary to altered bacterial colonization of the gut. In addition, impaired bilirubin metabolism is thought to contribute as a result of decreased caloric intake, or inhibition of UDPGT by factors such as metal ions, steroids, nucleotides and free fatty acids in breast milk.[35]

One pattern of marked early exacerbation of jaundice in the breast-fed newborn has been more aptly referred to as 'lack-of-breast-milk jaundice'.[37] In this case infrequent and insufficient breast-feeds may predispose to severe jaundice through poor caloric intake, excessive weight loss and slow clearance of meconium. An early initial breast-feed and frequent subsequent feeds are advocated to lessen the peak bilirubin attained in the breast-fed infant.[31]

PATHOPHYSIOLOGY OF BILIRUBIN ENCEPHALOPATHY

KERNICTERUS

Kernicterus is the name given to the characteristic pattern of yellow staining of parts of the brain stem, hippocampus, cerebellum and certain brain-stem nuclei seen at autopsy in infants dying from acute bilirubin toxicity.[110] The clinical manifestations of bilirubin encephalopathy arise from the susceptibility to damage of the basal ganglia, brain-stem auditory pathways and oculomotor nuclei.[110] This anatomical preference for bilirubin deposition and vulnerability to toxicity has not been fully explained, but may be a consequence of increased blood flow and metabolic activity in these areas.[12] Regional variations in bilirubin detoxification and clearance may also play a part.

The blood–brain barrier is anatomically derived from tight junctions between the endothelial cells of cerebral blood vessels. This barrier remains permeable to lipid-soluble substances, but while intact excludes water-soluble substances and large molecules, such as proteins. Free bilirubin influxes and effluxes across the intact blood–brain barrier with a permeability in keeping with the behaviour of a lipid-soluble molecule.[41] Additional stripping of bilrubin from albumin during a single brain capillary transit (approximately 1 second) is limited by the kinetics of dissociation of bilirubin from albumin. Transport of bilirubin into the brain may be promoted by prolongation of the capillary transit time – as a result, for example, of increased venous pressure. Increases in blood flow to specific brain regions will also be expected to facilitate bilirubin deposition.

The exact mode of entry of bilirubin into the brain remains unclear. One recent hypothesis points to the detergent-like properties of the monovalent anion of bilirubin and its ability to align at the plasma-to-plasma membrane interface.[115] Once in this position it is proposed that the addition of a further proton will produce bilirubin acid capable of entering the lipid phase of the membrane. At the other side of the membrane a reversal of this process would enable bilirubin monoanion to enter the cytoplasm.

Disruption of the blood–brain barrier will allow an influx of albumin-bound as well as free bilirubin into the brain. In terms of toxicity, the significance of albumin-bound bilirubin within the brain is uncertain. Of note is the lack of correlation between bilirubin staining and histological evidence of neuronal injury observed in the brains of premature infants dying in the the so-called 'low bilirubin kernicterus' era.[107] In surviving infants, however, this pool of bound bilirubin could theoretically liberate further free bilirubin if coincident acidosis promoted bilirubin acid precipitation within brain tissue.

BILIRUBIN TOXICITY

Bilirubin's toxicity would appear to be that of a generalized cellular poison. Disruption of membrane function, lowering of action potentials, compromise of energy metabolism, and disturbance of neurotransmitter synthesis and neurotransmission, are some of the mechanisms implicated.[110] A progression of neuronal insult has been suggested,[13] with bilirubin first attaching reversibly to nerve terminals, lowering their membrane potential and reducing nerve conduction. With prolonged exposure, or in the presence of a combined insult, such as acidosis or hypoxia, bilirubin may enter nerve terminals and pass retrogradely towards the neuronal body, causing progressive and ultimately permanent intracellular damage en route. In this context axonal swelling has been observed prior to mitochondrial swelling, pyknosis, gliosis and bilirubin staining of affected neurons.[110]

Neuronal vulnerability to bilirubin would appear to be both gestational and postnatal age dependent, possibly reflecting the functional status of specific brain areas at the time of the metabolic insult. This may explain why VLBW infants do not exhibit the classic clinical signs of kernicterus. Attempts to reproduce bilirubin neurotoxicity experimentally have often required concentrations of bilirubin grossly in excess of those found in the brain of newborns who have suffered bilirubin encephalopathy. Studies point to the importance of coexisting risk factors, such as acidosis,[114] hypoxia,[43] hypercapnia[114] and blood–brain barrier disruption[42] as being prerequisites for bilirubin's toxicity. Hypercapnia should not be underestimated as a risk factor. Respiratory acidosis will increase cerebral blood flow, and at high levels can open the blood–brain barrier. In addition, the solubility of carbon dioxide enables it to rapidly influence brain intracellular pH, with obvious implications for bilirubin membrane binding and precipitation.

Toxicity is also known to be promoted by agents that interfere with the binding of bilirubin to serum albumin. The devastating effect of sulphisoxazole[100] in the 1960s serves as a reminder that all drugs entering use in neonatology should be assessed in terms of their potential to displace bilirubin from albumin.[86] Such testing has shown the antibiotics ceftriaxone, rifampicin and fusidic acid to be theoretically hazardous in this context. Also to be avoided in jaundiced infants are the diuretic chlorthiazide and large doses of radiographic contrast media. Free fatty acids, if they reach a molar ratio with albumin in excess of 4:1, interfere with bilirubin binding. Intravenous lipid preparations in themselves are not implicated but, following their administration, the resultant elevation in free fatty acids may attain such ratios in sick immature newborns. For this reason lipid infusions are commonly reduced or stopped during the peak phase of jaundice in sick preterm babies. A cautious approach to the use of any preparation that has been shown experimentally to displace bilirubin from albumin would appear wise. However, apart from sulphisoxazole, no other drug or biochemical agent has been implicated as a cause of clinical kernicterus in humans.

CLINICAL BILIRUBIN ENCEPHALOPATHY

The word kernicterus originated as a description of yellow nuclear staining of the brain, but has become synonymous with the acute and chronic neurological sequelae of what is more correctly called bilirubin encephalopathy. Most descriptions of 'classic kernicterus' arise from observations of markedly jaundiced infants with erythroblastosis fetalis before the advent of exchange transfusion. Three clinical phases have been identified.[14] The first few days are characterized by lethargy, hypotonia and poor sucking. Towards the end of the first week a second phase is heralded by hypertonia, which may include opisthotonus. At this stage the baby commonly exhibits a high-pitched cry and fever, and may have seizures. The third phase is entered as the hypertonia subsides to be replaced by hypotonia. Intervention during phase 1 with phototherapy and exchange transfusion may prevent long-term damage, but hypertonia during the second phase is a poor prognostic sign and is predictive of neurological sequelae.

The long-term features of bilirubin encephalopathy include extrapyramidal disturbances, auditory impairment, upward gaze palsies and dental enamel dysplasia. The resulting cerebral palsy typically has an element of athetosis, which can develop as early as 18 months or be delayed for several years. High-frequency sensorineural deafness frequently accompanies the cerebral palsy, but may evolve in isolation, as described in low-birthweight infants.[20] Mental retardation may result from bilirubin encephalopathy, but is not invariably seen.

IDENTIFYING THE NEWBORN AT RISK OF BILIRUBIN ENCEPHALOPATHY

Healthy term infants: total serum bilirubin concentration

Treatment thresholds for phototherapy and exchange transfusion have, until recently, reflected clinical experience gained with severe erythroblastosis fetalis more than 40 years ago. Early exponents of exchange transfusion determined that kernicterus was unlikely to occur in affected infants if serum bilirubin levels were kept below 20 mg/dl (342 μmol/l). Wherever this threshold for treatment has been adopted kernicterus resulting from newborn haemolytic disease has virtually been eradicated. However, those campaigning for 'a kinder, gentler approach'[80] to healthy, non-haemolysing term infants question the 'irrational fear of 20 mg/dl' ('vigintiphobia')[112] and its adoption as the exchange threshold for all infants, regardless of the cause of jaundice.

From clinical experience it would appear that the healthy, non-haemolysing full-term infant with a serum bilirubin level >340 μmol/l is at lower risk of developing bilirubin encephalopathy than an infant with haemolytic disease. In the one controlled trial[50] to address this question, 94 full-term infants with hyperbilirubinaemia not due to rhesus isoimmunization were randomized to receive exchange transfusion or no treatment when their serum bilirubin concentration reached 20 mg/dl (342 μmol/l). The lack of bilirubin encephalopathy in either group was falsely reassuring, as only seven infants had bilirubin levels in excess of 428 μmol/l (four in the treatment group), of whom in six the level was no greater than 465 μmol/l, with the one outlying value peaking at 539 μmol/l. The authors concluded that 425 μmol/l may be an appropriate threshold for exchange transfusion in healthy term infants.

A more recent study assessed 42 children who had experienced a serum bilirubin level of 340 μmol/l or greater as newborns.[25] When assessed more than 3 years later, only two had sequelae that may have been related to hyperbilirubinaemia. One child with rhesus disease and a peak serum bilirubin of 556 μmol/l had borderline abnormalities on psychological testing, but did not exhibit athetoid cerebral palsy or deafness. The other child with a peak serum bilirubin of 397 μmol/l had mild sensorineural hearing loss. The cause of her jaundice was ABO incompatibility, and she had also suffered birth asphyxia. Of the infants followed, 14 had been born at term with no pathological cause of jaundice identified. Their mean maximal serum bilirubin was only 365 μmol/l (standard deviation 29.8). The authors of this study have decided to maintain 340 μmol/l as the threshold for exchange in rhesus disease, but moved to thresholds of 420 μmol/l in cases of ABO incompatibility, G-6PD deficiency or sepsis, and 495 μmol/l in healthy term infants, while monitoring outcome prospectively.

What, then, is the evidence that an otherwise healthy, non-haemolysing baby can develop kernicterus at any bilirubin level? Maisels and Newman reviewed the files of 22 cases referred to them by lawyers throughout the United States, in which neonatal hyperbilirubinaemia was alleged to be responsible for brain damage in apparently healthy, non-isoimmunized full-term babies.[65] Six infants were identified, born at 37 or more weeks' gestation, who met the criteria that they manifested the classic signs of acute bilirubin encephalopathy, and had typical neurological sequelae. The babies had normal perinatal histories and appeared healthy at the time of discharge. They exhibited no clinical or laboratory evidence of haemolysis or infection, and were all breast-feeding. None of the infants were noted to be jaundiced within the first 24 hours after birth, and they all had the same blood group as their mothers. Their peak recorded bilirubin levels occurred between days 4 and 10 and ranged from 663 to 845 μmol/l. Anecdotal cases of this nature are difficult to place in clinical context because, as the authors point out, they represent 'numerators without denominators'.

As full-blown kernicterus is rare, the focus has shifted towards attempts to identify more subtle effects of bilirubin on intelligence, behaviour and hearing. Newman and Maisels carried out an extensive review of the existing literature before proposing their more relaxed approach to the healthy jaundiced term infant.[80] With respect to hearing, they could find no consistent association between sensorineural hearing loss and serum bilirubin levels in healthy term newborns. It should be noted, however, that the six studies reviewed reflect very little experience of bilirubin levels in excess of 440 μmol/l. On the question of bilirubin levels and IQ, Newman and Maisels suggest that 'statistical significance has been mistaken for clinical significance'. From the results of the Collaborative Perinatal Project, which studied the progress of babies born to a cohort of more than 53 000 American women who became pregnant between 1959 and 1965, they estimate that the statistically significant correlation between IQ and bilirubin represents a deficit in IQ of only one point per 85 μmol/l increase in serum bilirubin concentration.[80] The relevance of this correlation to the healthy term infant is further undermined by the fact that the study population included babies with haemolysis and prematures weighing more than 2.5 kg.

The more recent finding of an association between an IQ < 85 and serum bilirubin > 342 μmol/l in 17-year-old male Israeli army draftees[99] has met with similar controversy in its interpretation. These men had been born at term and were documented as having a negative Coombs' test. However, no association was seen in women draftees, and nor was any shown between serum bilirubin level and mean IQ, neurological abnormality or hearing loss.

Our clinical experience to date can be no more precise than to place the risk of bilirubin encephalopathy in healthy term newborns at a threshold of serum bilirubin somewhere between 400 and 650 μmol/l. Arbitrary action lines for phototherapy and exchange transfusion set within this range should err on the side of caution. Ideally, significant changes in management should be matched with prospective data collection on neurodevelopmental outcome and audiometry screening.[25] Major complications of jaundice in this group of infants are, however, extremely rare, and are perhaps more likely to surface through medical litigation than medical research.

Premature infants: total serum bilirubin concentration

Premature babies are generally considered to be more prone to bilirubin encephalopathy than their full-term counterparts. The greater risk to the preterm brain was overstated in the past by false interpretation of autopsy findings in the so-called 'low-bilirubin kernicterus era' (1965–1982). This was a time when all yellow staining of the basal ganglia merited the description kernicterus, regardless of histological confirmation. Agonal changes in blood–brain barrier permeability to albumin-bound as well as free bilirubin in infants dying from other causes have been implicated in this pattern of staining. Elevated serum bilirubin levels do appear to be a risk factor for hearing loss in premature babies. The high incidence of bilateral sensorineural deafness in a population of sick VLBW infants with serum bilirubin levels >240 μmol/l[20] was dramatically reduced when lower thresholds for intervention were adopted.[21] Deafness in this population was also shown to correlate with the mean duration of hyperbilirubinaemia.[20] It is now common clinical practice to adopt a sliding scale of lower threshold values of serum bilirubin for phototherapy and exchange transfusion in infants of lower gestational age.

There has been a recent call to relax the more aggressive treatment regimens applied to jaundiced preterm babies.[111] Those suggesting such changes base their argument on experience gained in a pre-intensive care era (1950–1965) with relatively more mature

(28–36-week gestation) infants, very few of whom were exposed to serum bilirubin levels in excess of 340 μmol/l. False reassurance is also gained from recent trials conducted against the backdrop of more interventionalist therapeutic regimens.

A study relating the neurodevelopmental outcome of preterm infants to their peak serum bilirubin levels (range 39–385 μmol/l) failed to demonstrate any causal relationship with cerebral palsy or early developmental delay.[36] However, only three of the 249 preterm infants assessed had serum bilirubin levels greater than 250 μmol/l. The large NICHHD phototherapy trial failed to demonstrate an association between maximal serum bilirubin level and neurodevelopmental outcome in term or preterm infants.[90] The strict criteria for exchange transfusion, however, had meant that serum bilirubin levels were kept relatively low. Nevertheless, four low-birthweight infants in the trial were found to have histopathological evidence of kernicterus at autopsy.[61]

Markers of bilirubin toxicity

The imprecise relationship between total serum bilirubin levels and adverse neurological outcome has encouraged research seeking to identify more accurate markers of bilirubin toxicity. Assessment of free bilirubin levels,[29] bilirubin binding capacity, brain-stem auditory evoked responses[29,109] and computer analysis of abnormality of the jaundiced infant's cry[109] have been proposed. Such markers may prove of value in research environments, but are not universally available, or indeed feasible, in the acute clinical situation.

More accessible is the bilirubin/albumin ratio, which acts as an indirect guide to the free bilirubin level.[1] The bilirubin/ albumin ratio, in conjunction with assessment of an individual baby's clinical risk factors, may help with the decision as to whether an exchange transfusion is indicated in borderline cases. On the basis of unbound bilirubin estimations an upper limit for an acceptable bilirubin/albumin ratio has been proposed as being 0.8 in the healthy term newborn.[1] This ratio would be achieved in a baby with a serum bilirubin of 485 μmol/l and an albumin concentration of 606 μmol/l (i.e. albumin 40 g/l × conversion factor of 15.15). In infants with lower serum albumin concentrations of 35 g/l (530 μmol/l), 30 g/l (454 μmol/l) and 25 g/l (379 μmol/l) the ratio of 0.8 would be attained at bilirubin concentrations of 424, 364 and 303 μmol/l, respectively. In a sick term infant an upper limit ratio of 0.72 has been suggested, and for the sick premature infant of < 1250 g one of 0.4 is advised. Clinicians using this ratio to assist decision making propose that the criteria for exchange transfusion for a given infant should be based on the bilirubin/albumin ratio and/or the total serum bilirubin, on the basis of whichever parameter is exceeded first (Table 31.2).[1] It is rightly cautioned that the bilirubin/albumin ratio could be falsely reassuring in the presence of agents competing with bilirubin for binding sites on albumin.

Table 31.2 Total bilirubin and bilirubin/albumin ratio as criteria for exchange transfusion*

	Birthweight (g)				
	<1250	1250–1499	1500–1999	2000–2499	≥2500
Standard risk	223	256	291	308	427–496
Or bilirubin/alb ratio	0.52	0.60	0.68	0.72	0.80
High risk[†]	171	223	256	291	308
Or bilirubin/alb ratio	0.40	0.52	0.60	0.68	0.72

Bilirubin and albumin measured in μmol/l
* Exchange transfusion at whichever comes first
[†]Risk factors: Apgar <3 at 5 minutes; PaO_2 < 40 mmHg ≥ 2 h; pH ≤ 7.15 ≥ 1 h; birthweight < 1000 g; haemolysis; clinical or central nervous system deterioration. (Converted to SI units and reproduced with permission from Ahlfors[1])

CLINICAL APPROACH TO THE DIAGNOSIS OF THE JAUNDICED INFANT

VISUAL INSPECTION

Clinical jaundice becomes apparent at serum bilirubin levels of 80–90 μmol/l, and is observed in the majority of newborns during the first week of life.[70] Significant jaundice of the skin can be missed in black infants, in whom examination of the sclerae and gums may be more informative. Visual assessment is also unreliable under artificial light, and is obviously meaningless once phototherapy has been commenced.

Newborns jaundiced within 24 hours of birth and all preterms with detectable jaundice, regardless of their postnatal age, should have their serum bilirubin determined. Clinical judgement should be exercised in assessing the need to investigate an otherwise healthy term infant, with no known risk factors, who develops jaundice from day 2 onwards. The cephalocaudal progression of dermal jaundice, which has long been observed,[57] has recently been validated by transcutaneous bilirubinometry.[54] The dermal zones of jaundice described by Kramer[57] can be used as a rough guide as to when to formally measure the serum bilirubin level in a term infant. From Kramer's observations, jaundice limited to the head and neck had an average value of 100 μmol/l, with a range of 70–130 μmol/l. If dermal jaundice had reached beyond the elbows and knees, but not as far as the hands and feet, an average value of 250 μmol/l was found (range 190–310 μmol/l). Dermal jaundice of the hands and feet calls for a formal serum bilirubin estimation, as a value >300 μmol/l is to be anticipated.

A recent hypothesis has been proposed to explain the cephalocaudal advance of jaundice based on the nature of the binding process of bilirubin with albumin.[54] After release from the reticuloendothelial system bilirubin enters a binding process with albumin. The initial association occurs very rapidly, but several seconds then elapse before a higher-affinity configuration of the bilirubin–albumin complex is established. The initial lower-affinity binding state is thought to facilitate bilirubin deposition proximally, whereas by the time the blood reaches the peripheries bilirubin is more tightly bound. Variations in skin blood flow and lipid content may also be factors.

NON-INVASIVE MEASUREMENTS OF BILIRUBIN

Two non-invasive techniques of serum bilirubin estimation are available and may be successfully used in selected populations to screen for significant hyperbilirubinaemia. Neither supplants laboratory measurement, but used optimally they should reduce the number of blood tests taken to monitor mild to moderate jaundice.

Icterometry

The Gosset Icterometer provides an estimation of the bilirubin level by visual comparison of yellow colour panels on an otherwise transparent perspex strip pressed against the skin of the baby's nose.[34] This simple method has been validated alongside transcutaneous bilirubinometry in term infants, and has recently been shown to be of value as a screening investigation in healthy premature infants.[75]

Transcutaneous bilirubinometry

The Minolta Air Shields Jaundice Meter is a handheld spectrophotometric device that emits and then analyses light reflected back from the skin. It provides a transcutaneous bilirubin index, expressed in arbitrary units, as a measure of the yellow pigment in the skin.[94] It is to be recommended that correlation curves for serum bilirubin are established for individual patient populations, because measurements are influenced by racial pigmentation, postnatal age and gestational age.[94] Future advances in the technology of transcutaneous bilirubin monitoring may improve its accuracy and encourage a wider clinical acceptance.

Transcutaneous bilirubinometry has a role in screening otherwise healthy term and near-term newborns, provided that a safe threshold is established beyond which invasive assessment is mandatory. A recent study cautions its use in the sick premature infant in view of unpredictable results.[53] Although relatively expensive, the jaundice meter should prove cost-effective in terms of a reduction in the invasive measurement of serum bilirubin of newborns,[103] both in hospital and at home. Access to a transcutaneous bilirubinometer by community midwives and health visitors may reduce the traffic in capillary tubes or babies to and from hospital.

Table 31.3 Clinical features that suggest a pathological cause of jaundice in the newborn

Jaundice appearing in the first 24 hours of life
Jaundice in a sick neonate
Total serum bilirubin level
> 250 μmol/l on day 2
> 300 μmol/l thereafter
Rapidly rising serum bilirubin > 100 μmol/24 h
Prolonged jaundice
> 14 days in term infants
> 21 days in preterm infants
Conjugated serum bilirubin > 25 μmol/l
Acholuric stools and dark urine

IDENTIFYING PATHOLOGICAL JAUNDICE

Every jaundiced newborn merits evaluation to identify underlying pathology and to assess the risk potential for bilirubin encephalopathy. Family, maternal and infant history should be reviewed and the baby examined. Appropriate early investigation aims to identify treatable disease states, such as isoimmunization, infection, hypothyroidism, biliary atresia and galactosaemia. Clinical features that suggest a pathological cause of jaundice and prompt further investigation are listed in Table 31.3. In cases where an exchange transfusion may be necessary blood should be sent for urgent grouping and cross-matching. A number of causes of unconjugated hyperbilirubinaemia are listed in Table 31.4.

Jaundice within the first 24 hours of life is likely to be the result of isoimmunization or other cause of marked haemolysis. Urgent investigation (Table 31.5) is essential. Maternal rhesus status and blood group should be sought. The infants of known rhesus-negative mothers must have cord or postnatal blood sent for grouping and Coombs' testing. The same approach to all infants born to blood group O mothers with the potential for the more frequently encountered ABO incompatibility has been suggested. Some institutions prefer to store cord blood on all newborns, and to retrieve individual samples for urgent testing if the baby subsequently develops significant early jaundice. Despite an ABO incompatibility set-up in 10–15% of pregnancies, the proportion that result in significant haemolysis is small. The finding of a positive direct Coombs' test is not predictive of the severity of jaundice, which in many cases does not become clinically significant. Cord bilirubin levels may be more useful in this context. Values > 68 μmol/l have been found to be predictive of hyperbilirubinaemia > 273 μmol/l at 12–36 hours in term infants with ABO incompatibility.[85] A direct Coombs' test is more likely to be positive on cord blood than from samples taken from the baby postnatally. Even so, a positive result should be interpreted with caution. Most importantly, documentation of ABO incompatibility should not prevent consideration of coexisting pathology.

Other blood group incompatibilities will usually be known from the maternal history. The Kell group incompatibilities can cause severe haemolytic disease of the

Table 31.4 Causes of unconjugated jaundice in the newborn

Haemolysis
Isoimmunization
Rhesus
ABO
Minor blood groups
Other
Spherocytosis*
G-6PD deficiency
Pyruvate kinase deficiency†
Sepsis§
Disseminated intravascular coagulation
α-thalassaemia
Polycythaemia
Small for dates
Twin–twin transfusion
Delayed cord clamping
Maternofetal transfusion
Infant of diabetic mother
Extravasated blood
Bruising, e.g. cephalhaematoma
Pulmonary haemorrhage
Cerebral haemorrhage
Intra-abdominal haemorrhage
Increased enterohepatic circulation
Pyloric stenosis
Bowel obstruction
Swallowed blood
Endocrine/metabolic
Hypothyroidism
Hypopituitarism§
Hypoadrenalism§
Glucuronosyl transferase deficiency
Galactosaemia§
Tyrosinosis§
Hypermethioninaemia§

§ conjugated jaundice often coexists
*and other red cell morphological abnormalities
† and other red cell enzyme defects

Table 31.5 Investigation of jaundice in the newborn

Early-onset jaundice
Blood group and DCT
Haematocrit and FBC
Blood film and reticulocyte count
Infection screen if indicated
Serology for congenital infections
Urine for CMV culture
Stool for virology
G-6PD screen
Red cell enzyme assays
Prolonged jaundice
Total and conjugated serum bilirubin
Thyroid function tests
Urine culture
Urine Clinitest for reducing substances
Liver function tests
α_1-antitrypsin assay and phenotype
Cystic fibrosis DNA screen
Immunoreactive trypsin
Plasma cortisol level
Serum amino acid screen

newborn, whereas complications of the Duffy, Kidd and MNS systems are usually less severe. A reticulocyte count of more than 6% after 3 days is suggestive of a haemolytic process, but it must be remembered that reticulocyte counts and blood films carry a low sensitivity and specificity for diagnosing haemolysis in the newborn.[79] The accuracy of an automated end-tidal carbon monoxide analyser as an early warning device for significant haemolysis is currently being assessed.[116] Carbon monoxide excretion serves as a useful marker, being produced in equimolar quantities with bilirubin during haem catabolism.[4,102]

The maternal record should be checked for documentation of syphilis and hepatitis serology, as well as any history suggesting congenital infection. Specific red cell morphological abnormalities, such as spherocytosis, or inborn errors of metabolism, such as galactosaemia or Crigler–Najjar syndrome types I and II, may be implicated from the family history. The jaundice associated with galactosaemia is likely to be predominantly unconjugated in the first week of life. Diagnostic pointers such as hepatomegaly, poor feeding and vomiting should prompt early screening for galactosaemia, with urinalysis for non-glucose reducing substances (Clinitest). This test is non-specific and may provide false negative and false positive results in the first few weeks of life.[78] Confirmation of the diagnosis of galactosaemia is made by assessment of erythrocyte galactose-1-phosphate uridyl transferase activity (p. 998).

The Crigler–Najjar syndromes characteristically present in the first few days of life, with a rapidly evolving, non-haemolytic unconjugated hyperbilirubinaemia. The type I disorder results from a complete absence of UDPGT within the hepatocyte, and is inherited in an autosomal recessive manner. Affected individuals frequently require exchange transfusions in the newborn period and subsequent nocturnal phototherapy in early childhood. Definitive treatment involves liver transplantation. Crigler–Najjar syndrome type II is a less severe condition in that there is defective, as opposed to absent, UDPGT activity. Inheritance is thought to be autosomal dominant with variable expression, and serum bilirubin levels can be adequately controlled with a UDPGT inducer such as phenobarbitone.

With parents of Mediterranean, Asian and African ethnicity the increased likelihood of G-6PD deficiency, especially in males, needs to be considered. Screening cord blood for evidence of G-6PD deficiency may be appropriate in populations with a high incidence of this condition. It should be remembered that G-6PD levels can be falsely elevated in the context of a high reticulocyte count. Marked jaundice may not present in affected babies until 3–5 days of age. The differing severity of jaundice probably reflects the variety of isoenzyme deficiencies involved. Recent studies suggest that the pronounced jaundice in neonates with G-6PD deficiency is largely the result of an associated partial defect in bilirubin conjugation.[44] This is in keeping with end-tidal carbon monoxide measurements that have failed to demonstrate appreciable early haemolysis in such infants.[95] After the newborn period an affected individual is at risk of haemolytic episodes triggered by a number of common drugs. Parents and family practitioners should be given a list of medications to be avoided (p. 826).

Details of gestational age and evidence of birth asphyxia and trauma may explain heightened or prolonged jaundice. The mode and success of feeding should be noted, and assessment made of the infant's state of hydration and weight trend since birth. Examination of the newborn should confirm gestational age and identify growth retardation. Polycythaemia, anaemia, hydrops, purpura and frank bruising should be looked for, along with signs of infection.

Serum unconjugated bilirubin levels in excess of 300 μmol/l in an otherwise healthy newborn may reflect exaggerated physiological jaundice, but this is a diagnosis of exclusion and the peak bilirubin will still need to be monitored. Unless there are diagnostic pointers to the more rarely encountered causes of neonatal jaundice, stepwise investigation should aim to identify the more common aetiologies first (Table 31.5). Early-onset jaundice demands prompt attention to identify possible causes of haemolysis. A low threshold for performing a full infection screen should be adopted. The set-up for a common blood group incompatibility should not delay consideration of coexisting infection. A full infection screen is not, however, an automatic requirement for cases of hyperbilirubinaemia in otherwise well newborns. No instance of bacterial septicaemia was identified from a study reporting the investigation of over 300 newborns readmitted with a mean peak serum bilirubin level of 316 μmol/l (range, 217–498 μmol/l).[68] However, failure of unconjugated hyperbilirubinaemia to respond to phototherapy should alert the clinician to the possibility of infection.[60] A raised component of conjugated bilirubin may also suggest infection.

PROLONGED JAUNDICE

Visibly detectable jaundice beyond 2 weeks of age in the term infant and 3 weeks in the preterm merits the description 'prolonged jaundice'. The majority of term infants presenting with prolonged jaundice exhibit an unconjugated hyperbilirubinaemia and will be breast-feeding. Provided there are no features in the history or on clinical examination that suggest a pathological cause (in particular, the urine and stool colour are normal), screening investigations can be safely performed between 2 and 3 weeks of age. At that stage the following first-phase tests are appropriate:

- Total and conjugated serum bilirubin;
- Full blood count, including reticulocytes;
- Examination of blood film;
- Thyroid function tests;
- Urinalysis for reducing sugars (Clinitest);
- Urine culture.

Further tests (Table 31.5 and Chapter 31 Part 2) will be indicated according to the outcome of this initial screen. Greater urgency and a more direct approach to investigations are necessary in cases where a specific pathology, such as biliary atresia, is suspected.

CONJUGATED JAUNDICE

Definitions of conjugated hyperbilirubinaemia vary. Serum conjugated bilirubin levels greater than 25 or 30 μmol/l are commonly adopted cut-offs; an alternative is to allow a value of up to 10% of the total serum bilirubin. Pale acholuric stools and dark bile-stained urine are the clinical markers of established conjugated jaundice, but neither may be present in the first weeks of many hepatic disease states, including biliary atresia. The absence of bilirubin in the urine on early testing may also be falsely reassuring because the renal threshold for conjugated bilirubin is reached at 40 μmol/l. Diagnosis of any associated clotting abnormality and its correction may be an urgent requirement in the infant with conjugated jaundice. Several of the conditions already mentioned present with a mixture of raised unconjugated and conjugated bilirubin. Notable among these are the intrauterine infections, bacterial sepsis, galactosaemia, aminoacidaemias and congenital hypopituitarism. Some of the causes of conjugated hyperbilirubinaemia are listed in Table 31.6, and the initial investigations are listed in Table 31.5. If an obstructive aetiology is suspected liver ultrasound and methylbromo-IDA scan will be indicated (p. 736). Visualization of the gall bladder on ultrasound does not rule out biliary atresia. The importance of making an early diagnosis of biliary atresia and its prompt referral to a centre specializing in the medical and surgical management of childhood

Table 31.6 Causes of conjugated jaundice in the newborn

Intrauterine infections
Toxoplasmosis
Rubella
Cytomegalovirus
Herpes simplex
Coxsackie and other viruses
Syphilis
Bacterial sepsis
Severe haemolysis, e.g. erythroblastosis
Prolonged parenteral nutrition
Biliary atresia
Intrahepatic biliary hypoplasia
α_1-antitrypsin deficiency
Cystic fibrosis
Cryptogenic hepatitis
Choledochal cyst
Spontaneous bile duct perforation
Inspissated bile plug syndrome
Galactosaemia
Tyrosinosis
Hypermethioninaemia

liver disorders cannot be overstated.[77] Conjugated hyperbilirubinaemia is further discussed in Part 2 of this chapter.

CLINICAL MANAGEMENT OF THE JAUNDICED INFANT

INVASIVE MEASUREMENT OF BILIRUBIN

No consistent differences in serum bilirubin have been demonstrated between simultaneously taken blood samples of capillary, venous or arterial origin. However, results do vary greatly according to the method of estimation. Laboratory measurement by the diazo reaction to determine the total and direct bilirubin is not a straightforward assay, and in past years the method has gained a reputation for being inaccurate. Interlaboratory variability in results from standard solutions are disconcerting.[93] One group has gone so far as to suggest that estimations of conjugated bilirubin would be more meaningful if quoted in bands of 25 μmol/l.[113] More recently the precision of the assay has been improved by the use of commercially produced reagents and automated methodology.

For practical purposes a bilirubinometer employing direct spectrometry is used in most neonatal units to provide rapid estimation of total serum bilirubin. It should be remembered that such instruments reflect the sum value of all species of bilirubin, conjugated and unconjugated, including photoisomers. Significant errors can arise from incorrect spectrometer use and poor maintenance. Failure by the operator to note that serum specimens are grossly lipaemic, or that the outside of the capillary tube or cuvette is dirty, will give misleading results. A daily check of instrument calibration by technical staff is to be recommended, and a varied quality control sample should be analysed amid a routine batch of clinical specimens on a weekly basis. Attention to quality control should provide early warning of machine drift, and will hopefully reassure clinicians that the bilirubinometer is accurate to within 30 or, ideally, 20 μmol/l. It is customary to confirm pre-exchange transfusion values of total serum bilirubin with a laboratory measurement, but transfusion should not be delayed if this service is not readily available. Equally, depending on the quality assessment of the laboratory, the result provided by the diazo reaction may or may not be more accurate than that from the bilirubinometer.

TREATMENT

The different modes of treatment of unconjugated jaundice are shown in Table 31.7. Scientific evidence supporting these various therapies, and trial data guiding us in their optimal use, is limited.[67] The two established approaches are phototherapy and exchange transfusion. A number of drug therapies have been shown to modify neonatal jaundice, but have yet to enter routine clinical practice. It is essential that any infant undergoing treatment for jaundice should be adequately investigated for the cause of hyperbilirubinaemia. Unconjugated hyperbilirubinaemia that is judged to be above treatment thresholds, but below those that prompt immediate exchange transfusion, is most commonly controlled using phototherapy. A lack of response to adequate phototherapy may imply significant underlying haemolysis, necessitating exchange transfusion.

Table 31.7 Unconjugated jaundice: modes of treatment

Phototherapy
Exchange transfusion
Pharmacological agents
Competitive inhibition of haem oxygenase, e.g. metalloporphyrins
Liver enzyme induction, e.g. phenobarbitone
Suppression of isoimmune haemolysis, e.g. intravenous immunoglobulin
Inhibition of the enterohepatic circulation, e.g. agar and cholestyramine

Phototherapy

Observation of the effect of sunlight on the serum bilirubin level of premature infants nursed outdoors prompted the first use of a 'cradle illumination machine' in 1958.[17] It took a decade for phototherapy to gain clinical acceptance throughout the world,[63] and a further 12 years before its mode of action started to be unravelled (see p. 716).[73] Phototherapy alone has not been shown to influence neurodevelopmental outcome or cognitive performance in recipients,[90,98] but it remains a convenient and safe means of lowering serum bilirubin. Most importantly, phototherapy reduces the need for the more hazardous alternative, namely exchange transfusion. The use of phototherapy has enabled countless isoimmunized infants to be less exposed to exchange transfusions or to avoid them entirely (p. 821). Likewise, optimal use of phototherapy in preterm physiological jaundice has made the need to resort to exchange transfusion in that context a rarity.

Phototherapy's ease of use has encouraged its overuse. Many newborns are 'placed under the lights' unnecessarily, or treated for too long. The vogue for 'prophylactic' phototherapy from birth in VLBW infants has been shown neither to reduce the peak nor to shorten the duration of their jaundice.[18] Phototherapy would only appear to be effective as bilirubin enters the skin at serum levels >80 μmol/l.[106] Similarly, a small study randomizing term infants with physiological jaundice to receive phototherapy at a threshold of either 250 or 320 μmol/l failed to demonstrate any significant difference in peak serum bilirubin levels between the two groups.[59]

The maximal effect of phototherapy is during the first 24–48 hours of its use. It has been suggested that the enterohepatic circulation of bilirubin-ZZ, reconstituted from configurational photoisomers in bile, causes this decay in response. Even without an impact on the serum bilirubin level, however, it can be argued that within a matter of hours of commencing phototherapy up to a fifth of the circulating bilirubin has been detoxified in the form of configurational photoisomers.[27]

Phototherapy has a benign reputation but it is not without side-effects. The most commonly encountered are:

- diarrhoea
- increased fluid loss via the skin
- temperature instability
- erythematous rashes
- tanning
- bronze baby syndrome.

The diarrhoea asssociated with phototherapy is thought to result from an irritant effect of photoisomers on the bowel. This and increased insensible water loss from the skin makes attention to fluid balance mandatory in any infant receiving phototherapy. A general prescription of additional fluid is often used in these circumstances, but individualized assessment of fluid requirements, especially in the premature or sicker infant, is to be advised. Close attention to thermoregulation is also important, with the risks of cooling from surface exposure and overheating from phototherapy lamps. Nursing care should include regular monitoring of the infant's temperature, documentation of stool frequency and urine output, and a daily assessment of weight. The eyes of an infant receiving lamp phototherapy should be shielded in view of the potential risk of retinal damage.[76] Shielding the gonads with a nappy has evolved as a precautionary practice.[101] In vitro evidence of light-induced DNA damage, particularly in the presence of bilirubin,[87] has not been mirrored by skin damage in clinical experience with newborns, or from long-duration phototherapy in children with Crigler–Najjar syndrome. The bronze baby syndrome results from an interaction between cholestatic jaundice and phototherapy.[82] The brown pigment produced (bilifuscin) stains the infant's skin and lingers for some time after phototherapy has been discontinued.

The recently developed fibreoptic systems for delivering phototherapy via a body pad or wrap have made its application more versatile. These devices are likely to gain greater acceptance in the context of healthy term infants nursed without eye pads and alongside their mothers. Trials have shown fibreoptic phototherapy to be as effective as conventional phototherapy in preterm infants,[15,104] but less so in term infants.[38,104] The fibreoptic pad devices can, however, be put to great advantage in combination with a conventional light unit to provide double phototherapy.[39]

Optimal use of phototherapy

The efficacy of phototherapy depends on the dose and wavelength of light used and the proportion of the infant's surface area to which it is applied. The dose administered is conventionally expressed in terms of spectral irradiance ($\mu W/cm^2/nm$). Before the mode of action of phototherapy was better understood it was thought that saturation of dose-response occurred within the blue light range at a spectral irradiance of 4 $\mu W/cm^2/nm$. This is true of the configurational isomer bilirubin-Z,E. However, it is now known that the production of the most important photoisomer, lumirubin, has a dose–response relationship that does not attain saturation until a spectral irradiance of 25–30 $\mu W/cm^2/nm$ is achieved.[27] Increasing the dose of phototherapy is most readily achieved by operating the light source at the minimum recommended safe distance from the infant. The fibreoptic Biliblanket at its highest setting delivers a spectral irradiance in the region of 35 $\mu W/cm^2/nm$ to an area of skin limited by the 10×20 cm pad size.

Early phototherapy lights were designed to emit blue light at a wavelength of around 450 nm, in keeping with the maximal absorbance of bilirubin. Pure blue light is poorly tolerated by staff and can mask cyanosis in a sick infant. Combinations of broad-spectrum white light and blue light have proved more acceptable. There are theoretical reasons why green light phototherapy would be the most efficient choice. Compared with blue light, green preferentially favours the formation of lumirubin, the main excretory photoisomer, and its longer wavelength enhances skin penetration.[26,27] Exponents of a new blue-green phototherapy lamp have reported such high 'phototherapeutic efficiency' that the majority of their preterm infants require only 1 day's duration of treatment.[23]

The efficiency of treatment can also be improved by using more than one phototherapy lamp, or by combining a conventional lamp with a fibreoptic system. Double phototherapy applied to a greater body surface area is more effective than single lights,[39] and should be adopted in cases of severe jaundice or while awaiting blood for an exchange transfusion. With less severe hyperbilirubinaemia it may be safe to use intermittent phototherapy. In such cases parents should be reassured that in taking their baby out of the lights for feeds and cuddles they are not jeopardizing therapy. The fact that it takes up to 3 hours for bilirubin to return to the skin following the removal of photoisomers has prompted intermittent phototherapy regimens based on 1 in 4 hours' exposure to lights. It should be recognized that claims that such regimens have been shown to be equally effective as continuous phototherapy are based on experience with moderate physiological jaundice.[58] Jaundice that has reached a level that is within 50 μmol/l of the exchange threshold should be treated with continuous phototherapy.

Pharmacological agents

Drug treatments designed to prevent or ameliorate unconjugated hyperbilirubinaemia are listed in Table 31.7. These agents act either by reducing bilirubin production or by hastening its clearance from the body. The use of synthetic metalloporphyrins to reduce bilirubin production through competitive inhibition of haem oxygenase has been an interesting development.[64] Haem does not accumulate as a result of these therapies because it can be excreted directly in the bile, as occurs in fetal life. The potential for metalloporphyrins to induce photosensitivity has led to a cautious approach to their use and to the development of less toxic variants, such as tin mesoporphyrin. Tin protoporphyrin has been used to modify the course of hyperbilirubinaemia in ABO isoimmunization.[46] Similarly, tin mesoporphyrin has been shown to supplant the need for phototherapy in term and near-term newborns with physiological jaundice,[45] and to significantly reduce phototherapy requirements in preterms.[108] The therapeutic potential of tin, zinc and chromium metalloporphyrins and their possible side-effects are discussed in a recent review.[116] These agents are likely to find a role in the preventative treatment of certain populations at high risk of significant pathological jaundice, or where conventional management with phototherapy and exchange transfusion is less readily available. Whether they are destined to revolutionize our management of most forms of neonatal jaundice will depend on their safety record.

Another preventative therapy that may be of benefit to newborns presenting with severe rhesus or ABO isoimmunization is early administration of high-dose intravenous γ-globulin. This treatment has been shown to inhibit haemolysis, and significantly reduce the need for exchange transfusion in rhesus incompatibility.[88] The requirement for exchange in rhesus disease can also be reduced by antenatal induction of fetal UDPGT, which is achieved by giving phenobarbitone to mothers carrying affected fetuses. Phenobarbitone is rarely used in this context, and its widespread use postnatally in unconjugated hyperbilirubinaemia is precluded by side-effects. Other inducers of UDPGT, lacking the sedative effects of phenobarbitone, are currently under investigation. Phenobarbitone does, however, currently have a role to play in moderating the level of jaundice in patients with Crigler–Najjar syndrome type II.

The use of agents such as agar and cholestyramine to bind gut bilirubin, and so prevent its reabsorption via the enterohepatic circulation, have met with disappointing results. Minimal benefit has been demonstrated in association with phototherapy, but in the case of cholestyramine these are outweighed by potential side-effects, including hyperchloraemic acidosis.

The administration of 1 g/kg of albumin prior to an exchange transfusion is not of proven benefit, but tends to be given in the context of a delay in obtaining blood and a bilirubin value well in excess of the exchange level. There are theoretical reasons why currently available solutions of albumin are poor binders of bilirubin,[1] and a suggestion that the heat-stabilizing agents present in such preparations may be displacers of bilirubin.[11] Albumin should be given to hydropic infants with caution and attention to CVP, to avoid precipitating heart failure.

Exchange transfusion

The practicalities of exchange transfusion are covered elsewhere (Chapter 51). The indications for exchange transfusion vary according to the underlying condition. In cases where there has been severe in-utero haemolysis, early exchange, irrespective of the bilirubin level, may be required to correct anaemia and to remove sensitized red cells. Previous guidelines based on cord blood values no longer apply, as most infants with severe erythroblastosis will have received in-utero transfusion. The timing of their last top-up and a Kleihauer estimation of the proportion of circulating fetal red cells are more likely to be predictive of the need for an early exchange. Many such infants respond to intensive phototherapy followed by a later top-up transfusion. If, despite double phototherapy, the serum bilirubin continues to rise by more than 10 μmol/l/h exchange transfusion is to be anticipated.

In addition to the low risk of bloodborne infection, exchange transfusion carries a significant risk of morbidity and mortality from vascular accidents, cardiac complications and biochemical or haematological disturbance.[48] This is especially the case in sick premature newborns. The mortality rate from the procedure is often quoted as being around 0.3%. It should be noted that this figure originates from a well conducted trial,[91] performed during an era when exchange transfusion was a more frequent event in neonatal medicine. Refinement in the antenatal management of haemolytic disease of the newborn, and the optimal use of phototherapy for other causes of hyperbilirubinaemia, has meant that exchange transfusions are now rarely necessary. With dwindling practical expertise there is a danger that the procedure will become more hazardous.

Exchange transfusion will remain necessary for infants who fail to respond to adequate phototherapy, or who present late with bilirubin levels in excess of a given exchange value. In the latter case the infant should be placed under double phototherapy, pending the availability of blood for the exchange. Attention should also be paid to correcting disturbances of hydration or acid–base balance, and to the treatment of any underlying infection. Symptoms and signs characteristic of acute bilirubin encephalopathy are an absolute indication for exchange transfusion.

GUIDELINES FOR THE USE OF PHOTOTHERAPY AND EXCHANGE TRANSFUSION

In contrast to the pre-exchange transfusion era of almost five decades ago, when up to half of infants with severe rhesus disease developed kernicterus, we now find that more than half the practising paediatricians in the UK are unlikely to have encountered the clinical sequelae of bilirubin toxicity.[22] Kernicterus has been virtually eradicated by the adoption of thresholds for exchange transfusion taken from early experience with severe erythroblastosis, and by the pre-emptive use of phototherapy to prevent, whenever possible, the exchange threshold being attained.

Two groups of term-born infants would appear to remain at greater risk from bilirubin toxicity, i.e. newborns with haemolysis, and those born with Crigler–Najjar syndrome. It is prudent to maintain our respect for a total bilirubin level of 20 mg/dl (342 μmol/l) as being the indication for exchange transfusion in these patient groups. Why such infants are more prone to bilirubin encephalopathy than healthy term newborns is not entirely clear. In the case of haemolysis, it has been proposed that red cell breakdown products may be capable of interfering with bilirubin–albumin binding. Haematin has the potential to compete with bilirubin for binding sites on albumin, but would not appear to reach sufficiently high concentrations to be clinically relevant.[51] Alternatively, albumin binding may be altered in sick newborns through mechanisms unrelated to haemolysis.

Formerly, no distinction was made between the thresholds for treatment of jaundiced term and preterm infants. Recognition that preterm newborns are at higher risk of bilirubin toxicity[20] has given rise to sliding scales prompting earlier intervention on the basis of birthweight or gestational age. Some clinicians prefer to apply a single treatment protocol to all preterm babies,[22] but it would appear logical to have a greater margin for error in the lower-gestation infant. Sick low-birthweight newborns are more likely to have been exposed to a number of specific risk factors, such as hypoxia, acidosis, hypercapnia, sepsis and hypoalbuminaemia, increasing their susceptibility to bilirubin toxicity. An example of a sliding scale of bilirubin values for intervention in preterm newborns is shown in Table 31.8. Phototherapy should be commenced in all preterm infants who become clinically jaundiced within the first 24 hours. Investigation of the cause of jaundice and assessment of the need for an early exchange transfusion are urgent considerations. From the second day onwards phototherapy and exchange transfusion should be considered if the serum bilirubin has reached the values shown in Table 31.8. On current evidence, calls to greatly relax such an approach to the jaundiced preterm population[111] should be resisted.[40]

The fact that healthy term infants would appear to tolerate higher levels of bilirubin than their haemolysing or sick contemporaries has prompted calls for a more relaxed approach to the management of their jaundice from days 2 or 3 onwards.[66,80,81] Over the past decade most paediatricians caring for healthy jaundiced newborns in the UK have been willing participants in a cautious relaxation of the threshold for phototherapy, from 250 μmol/l to 300–350 μmol/l, and for exchange transfusion from 340 μmol/l to 400–450 μmol/l.[22] This has reduced the number of infants receiving phototherapy and, by overcoming the previously universal 'vigintiphobia', has meant fewer babies being subjected to the perils of exchange transfusion.

How much further can this shift in practice be taken without placing such infants at greater risk of bilirubin toxicity? Newman and Maisels carried out an extensive review of the topic and proposed new treatment regimens for full-term infants, as summarized in Table 31.9.[80] The wide ranges of bilirubin values chosen were 'intended to encourage individualization of treatment, taking preferences and biases of the parent and pediatrician into account.' When such 'preference' or 'bias' dictates that an infant's serum bilirubin level may be allowed to reach 500 μmol/l, it should be acknowledged that the evidence supporting the safety of such practice is very sparse beyond bilirubin levels of 425 μmol/l.[80]

In the case of babies with proven or suspected haemolysis or who are otherwise sick, Newman and Maisels maintain a more conventional range for exchange transfusion at bilirubin levels between 300 and 400 μmol/l.[80] They suggest use of the lower end of this range for infants with severe haemolysis, or who are sick for other reasons, and values closer to 400 μmol/l for equivocal cases, such as breast-feeding babies with ABO incompatibility and positive Coombs' test but no anaemia.

Most treatment guidelines rely on total bilirubin level, but faced with the decision as to whether or not to perform an exchange transfusion, subtraction of a conjugated component of > 50 μmol/l would appear logical. Others recommend the more cautious approach of not subtracting the direct bilirubin concentration from the total until it reaches 50%.[66] Although conjugated bilirubin is nontoxic, there is some evidence to suggest that it may compete with unconjugated bilirubin for albumin-binding

Table 31.8 Guidelines for treatment of preterms babies with phototherapy and exchange transfusion

Gestational age	Serum bilirubin concentration (μmol/l) Phototherapy	Exchange transfusion	
		Sick*	Well
36 weeks	250	300	350
32 weeks	150	250	300
28 weeks	100	200	250
24 weeks	80	150	200

* Rhesus disease, perinatal asphyxia, hypoxia, acidosis, hypercapnia

Table 31.9 Newman and Maisels' treatment regimens for full-term infants[80]

Treatment	Total bilirubin level (μmol/l) Well baby, no haemolysis	Haemolysis likely, or sick
Phototherapy	300–375	225–300
Exchange transfusion	425–500	300–400

Table 31.10 Management of jaundice in the healthy term newborn: American Academy of Pediatrics Guidelines[83]

Age (h)	Total serum bilirubin level (μmol/l)			
	Consider phototherapy	Phototherapy	Exchange if intensive phototherapy fails*	Exchange and intensive phototherapy
25–48	≥170	≥260	≥340	≥430
49–72	≥260	≥310	≥430	≥510
> 72	≥290	≥340	≥430	≥510

* failure of intensive phototherapy to reduce serum bilirubin by 17 to 34 μmol/l within 4–6 hours
(Reproduced with permission from Pediatrics[83])

sites.[24] In this context, an anecdotal case has been reported in which a full-term infant developed clinical kernicterus when the total serum bilirubin level was 472 μmol/l with a direct-reacting component of 149 μmol/l.[66]

When considering an exchange transfusion in a baby receiving phototherapy, should allowance also be made for the fact that up to one-fifth of the circulating bilirubin pool may be in the form of non-toxic photoisomers? This practice could be hazardous, because the certainty of such an assumption depends on the duration and efficiency of phototherapy provided. The best practice is to agree on a set of guidelines for exchange transfusion in healthy and sick, term and preterm infants, and to stick by them. As thresholds for exchange transfusion are relaxed the margin for error is diminished, and excuses for not performing an exchange should be discouraged. Taking into account the serum albumin concentration may be a better arbiter in truly borderline cases, or indeed may prompt exchange at a threshold lower than that predicted by the total serum bilirubin alone[1] (see: Markers of bilirubin toxicity and Table 31.2.)

The so-called 'kinder, gentler approach' to the jaundiced term infant, proposed by Newman and Maisels,[80] has been tailored and incorporated in a 'practice parameter' issued by a subcommittee of the American Academy of Pediatrics (AAP), of which they were members.[83] The AAP recommendations for the management of hyperbilirubinaemia in the healthy term newborn are shown in Table 31.10. Predictably, these guidelines have been criticized, both for their laxity[84] and for their stringency.[96] Confidence in the use of such guidelines will evolve if prospective ascertainment of cases of clinical kernicterus and its sequelae is performed and remains reassuring. Controlled trials of this change in clinical management are an unlikely prospect. Extension of the current clinical practice of performing formal audiology tests on infants undergoing exchange transfusion for hyperbilirubinaemia to any term infant with a peak serum bilirubin in excess of 400 μmol/l may help in this respect.

A potential danger of this move to a more relaxed attitude to jaundice in the healthy term infant, particularly at a time when the majority of newborns are at home by 24–48 hours of age, may be that of delaying the diagnosis in cases of more sinister jaundice. Heightened awareness of aspects of the history and clinical examination that suggest a pathological cause for a newborn's jaundice will need to be maintained. Failure to do so may result in more infants being readmitted with bilirubin levels at or above exchange levels, with conditions such as ABO incompatibility and G-6PD deficiency.[74]

REFERENCES

1. Ahlfors C E 1994 Criteria for exchange transfusion in jaundiced newborns. Pediatrics 93: 488–494
2. Alonso E M, Whitington P F, Whitington S H, Rivard W A, Given G 1991 Enterohepatic circulation of non-conjugated bilirubin in rats fed with human milk. Journal of Pediatrics 118: 425–430
3. Auerbach K G, Gartner L M 1987 Breast feeding and human milk: their association with jaundice in the neonate. Clinics in Perinatology 14: 89–107
4. Bartoletti A L, Stevenson D K, Ostrander C R, Johnson J D 1979 Pulmonary excretion of carbon monoxide in the human infant as an index of bilirubin production. I. Effects of gestational age and postnatal age and some common neonatal abnormalities. Journal of Pediatrics 94: 952–955
5. Berk M A, Mimouni F, Miodovnik M, Herzberg V, Valuck J 1989 Macrosomia in infants of insulin-dependent diabetic mothers. Pediatrics 83: 1029–1034
6. Bock K W, Burchell B, Dutton G J et al 1983 UDP-glucuronosyl transferase activities: guidelines for the consistent interim terminology and assay conditions. Biochemical Pharmacology 32: 953–955
7. Bonnett R, Davies J E, Hursthouse M B 1976 Structure of bilirubin. Nature 262: 326–328
8. Britton J R, Britton H L, Beebe S A 1994 Early discharge of the term newborn: a continued dilemma. Pediatrics 94: 291–295
9. Brodersen R, Stern L 1990 Deposition of bilirubin acid in the central nervous system: a hypothesis for the development of kernicterus. Acta Paediatrica Scandinavica 79: 12–19
10. Brodersen R 1979 Bilirubin solubility and interaction with albumin and phospholipid. Journal of Biological Chemistry 254: 2364–2369
11. Brodersen R, Hansen P 1977 Bilirubin displacing effect of stabilizers added to injectable preparations of human serum albumin. Acta Paediatrica Scandinavica 66: 133–135
12. Burgess G H, Oh W, Bratlid D, Brubakk A-M, Cashore W J, Stonestreet B S 1985 The effects of brain blood flow on brain bilirubin deposition in newborn piglets. Pediatric Research 19: 691–696
13. Cashore W J 1990 The neurotoxicity of bilirubin. Clinics in Perinatology 17: 437–447
14. Connolly A M, Volpe J J 1990 Clinical features of bilirubin encephalopathy. Clinics in Perinatology 17: 371–379
15. Costello S A, Nyikal J, Yu V Y H, McCloud P 1995 BiliBlanket phototherapy system versus conventional phototherapy: a randomized controlled trial in preterm infants. Journal of Paediatrics and Child Health 31: 11–13
16. Crawford J M, Howswer S C, Gollan J L 1988 Formation, hepatic metabolism, and transport of bile pigments: a status report. Seminars in Liver Disease 8: 105–118
17. Cremer R J, Perryman P W, Richards D H 1958 Influence of light on the hyperbilirubinaemia of infants. Lancet i: 1094–1097
18. Curtis-Cohen M, Stahl G E, Costarino A T, Polin R A 1985 Randomised trial of prophylactic phototherapy in the infant with very low birth weight. Journal of Pediatrics 107: 121–124
19. De Carvalho M, Hall M, Harvey D 1981 Effects of water supplementation on physiological jaundice in breast-fed babies. Archives of Disease in Childhood 56: 568–569
20. DeVries L S, Lary S, Whitelaw A G et al 1987 Relationship of serum bilirubin levels and hearing impairment in newborn infants. Early Human Development 15: 269–277
21. DeVries L S, Lary S, Dubowitz L M S 1985 Relationship of serum bilirubin levels to ototoxicity and deafness in high-risk low birth-weight infants. Pediatrics 76: 351–354

22. Dodd K L 1993 Neonatal jaundice – a lighter touch. Archives of Disease in Childhood 68: 529–533
23. Donzelli G P, Agati G 1995 1-day phototherapy of neonatal jaundice with blue-green lamp. Lancet 346: 184–185
24. Ebbesen F 1982 Low reserve albumin for binding of bilirubin in neonates with deficiency of bilirubin excretion and bronze baby syndrome. Acta Paediatrica Scandinavica 71: 415–420
25. Eberhard B A, Drew J H 1994 Perhaps vigintiphobia should only apply to infants with rhesus erythroblastosis. Journal of Paediatrics and Child Health 30: 341–344
26. Ennever J R 1990 Blue light, green light, white light, more light: treatment of neonatal jaundice. Clinics in Perinatology 17: 467–481
27. Ennever J F 1992 Phototherapy for neonatal jaundice. In: Polin R A, Fox W W (eds.) Fetal and neonatal physiology. W B Saunders, Philadelphia, pp 1165–1173
28. Friedman L, Lewis P J, Clifton P, Bulpitt C J 1978 Factors influencing the incidence of neonatal jaundice. British Medical Journal i: 1235–1237
29. Funato M, Tamai H, Shimada S, Nakamura H 1994 Vigintiphobia, unbound bilirubin, and auditory brainstem responses. Pediatrics 93: 50–53
30. Gale R, Seidman D S, Dollberg S et al. 1990 Epidemiology of neonatal jaundice in the Jerusalem population. Journal of Pediatric Gastroenterology and Nutrition 10: 82–86
31. Gartner L M 1994 On the question of the relationship between breastfeeding and jaundice in the first 5 days of life. Seminars in Perinatology 18: 502–509
32. Gartner L M 1994 Neonatal jaundice. Pediatrics in Review 15: 422–432
33. Gartner L M, Lee K-S, Vaisman S, Lane D, Zarafu I 1977 Development of bilirubin transport and metabolism in the newborn rhesus monkey. Journal of Pediatrics 90: 513–531
34. Gosset I H 1960 A Perspex icterometer for neonates. Lancet 1: 87–89
35. Gourley G R 1992 Pathophysiology of breast milk jaundice. In: Polin R A, Fox W W (eds.) Fetal and neonatal physiology. W B Saunders, Philadelphia, pp 1173–1179
36. Graziani L J, Mitchell D G, Kornhauser M et al 1992 Neurodevelopment of preterm infants: neonatal neurosonographic and serum bilirubin studies. Pediatrics 89: 229–234
37. Hansen T W R 1995 Kernicterus in a full-term infant: the need for increased vigilance (letter). Pediatrics 95: 798–799
38. Holtrop P C, Madison K, Maisels M J 1992 A clinical trial of fibreoptic phototherapy vs conventional phototherapy. American Journal of Diseases of Children 146: 235–237
39. Holtrop P C, Ruedisueli K, Maisels M J 1992 Double vs single phototherapy in low birthweight infants. Pediatrics 90: 674–677
40. Ives N K 1992 Kernicterus in preterm infants: lest we forget (to turn on the lights). Pediatrics 90: 757–759
41. Ives N K, Gardiner R M 1990 Blood–brain barrier permeability to bilirubin in the rat: studies using intracarotid bolus injection and in situ brain perfusion techniques. Pediatric Research 27: 436–441
42. Ives N K, Bolas N M, Gardner R M 1989 The effects of bilirubin on brain energy metabolism during hyperosmolar opening of the blood–brain barrier: an in vivo study using 31P magnetic resonance spectroscopy. Pediatric Research 26: 356–361
43. Ives N K, Cox D W G, Gardner R M, Bachelard H S 1988 The effects of bilirubin on brain energy metabolism during normoxia and hypoxia: an in vitro study using 31P magnetic resonance spectroscopy. Pediatric Research 23: 569–573
44. Kaplan M, Rubaltelli F F, Hammerman C et al 1996 Conjugated bilirubin in neonates with glucose-6-phosphate dehydrogenase deficiency. Journal of Pediatrics 128: 695–697
45. Kappas A, Drummond G S, Henschke C, Valaes T 1995 Direct comparison of Sn-mesoporphyrin, an inhibitor of bilirubin production, and phototherapy in controlling hyperbilirubinemia in term and near-term newborns. Pediatrics 95: 468–474
46. Kappas A, Drummond G S, Manola T, Petmezaki S, Valaes T 1988 Sn-protoporphyrin use in the management of hyperbilirubinemia in term newborns with direct Coombs'-positive ABO incompatibility. Pediatrics 81: 485–497
47. Kawade N, Onishi S 1981 The prenatal and postnatal development of UDP-glucuronyl transferase activity toward bilirubin and the effect of premature birth on this activity in the human liver. Biochemical Journal 196: 257–260
48. Keenan W J, Novak K K, Sutherland J M, Bryla D A, Fetterly K L 1985 Morbidity and mortality associated with exchange transfusion. Pediatrics 75 (Suppl): 417–421
49. Khoury M J, Calle E E, Joesoef R M 1988 Recurrence risk of neonatal hyperbilirubinemia in siblings. American Journal of Diseases of Children 142: 1065–1069
50. Killander A, Michaelsson M, Muller-Eberhard U, Sjolin S 1963 Hyperbilirubinaemia in full term newborn infants: a follow-up study. Acta Paediatrica Scandinavica 52: 481–484
51. Kirk J J, Ritter D A, Kenny J D 1984 The effect of haematin on bilirubin binding in bilirubin-enriched neonatal cord serum. Biology of the Neonate 45: 53–57
52. Kivlahan C, James E J P 1984 The natural history of neonatal jaundice. Pediatrics 74: 364–370
53. Knudsen A, Ebbesen F 1996 Transcutaneous bilirubinometry in neonatal intensive care units. Archives of Disease in Childhood 75: F53–56
54. Knudsen A 1990 The cephalocaudal progression of jaundice in newborns in relation to the transfer of bilirubin from plasma to skin. Early Human Development 22: 23–28
55. Knudsen A 1989 Prediction of the development of neonatal jaundice by increased umbilical cord blood bilirubin. Acta Paediatrica Scandinavica 78: 217–221
56. Knudsen A, Lebech M 1989 Maternal bilirubin, cord bilirubin and placental function at delivery in the development of neonatal jaundice in mature newborns. Acta Obstetrica et Gynecologica Scandinavica 68: 719–724
57. Kramer L I 1969 Advancement of dermal icterus in the jaundiced newborn. American Journal of Diseases of Children 118: 454–458
58. Lau S P, Fung K P 1984 Serum bilirubin kinetics in intermittent phototherapy of physiological jaundice. Archives of Disease in Childhood 59: 892–894
59. Lewis H M, Campbell R H A, Hambleton G 1982 Abuse of phototherapy for physiological jaundice of newborn infants. Lancet ii: 408–410
60. Linder N, Yatsiv I, Tsur M et al 1988 Unexplained neonatal jaundice as an early diagnostic sign of septicemia in the newborn. Journal of Perinatology 8: 325–327
61. Lipsitz P J, Gartner L M, Bryla D A 1985 Neonatal and infant mortality in relation to phototherapy. Pediatrics 75(suppl): 423–426
62. Lucas A, Baker B A 1986 Breast milk jaundice in premature infants. Archives of Disease in Childhood 61: 1063–1067
63. Lucey J, Ferreiro M, Hewitt J 1968 Prevention of hyperbilirubinemia of prematurity by phototherapy. Pediatrics 41: 1047–1054
64. Lucey J F 1988 A new era in therapy for hyperbilirubinemia. Pediatrics 81: 579
65. Maisels M J, Newman T B 1995 Kernicterus occurs in otherwise healthy, breast-fed term newborns. Pediatrics 96: 730–733
66. Maisels M J 1994 Jaundice. In: Avery G B, Fletcher M A, MacDonald M G (eds). Neonatology: pathophysiology and management of the newborn, 4th edn. J B Lippincott, Philadelphia, pp 630–725
67. Maisels M J 1992 Neonatal jaundice. In: Sinclair J C, Bracken M B (eds) Effective care of the newborn infant. Oxford University Press, Oxford, pp 507–561
68. Maisels M J, Kring E 1992 Risk of sepsis in newborns with servere hyperbilirubinemia. Pediatrics 90: 741–743
69. Maisels M J, Gifford K L, Antle C E, Leib G R 1988 Jaundice in the healthy newborn infant: a new approach to an old problem. Pediatrics 81: 505–511
70. Maisels M J, Gifford K L 1986 Normal serum bilirubin levels in the newborn and the effect of breast feeding. Pediatrics 78: 837–843
71. McDonagh A F 1990 Is bilirubin good for you? Clinics in Perinatology 17: 359–369
72. McDonagh A F, Lightner D A 1985 'Like a shrivelled blood orange': bilirubin, jaundice and phototherapy. Pediatrics 75: 443–455
73. McDonagh A F, Palma L A, Lightner D A 1980 Blue light and bilirubin excretion. Science 208: 145–151
74. MacDonald M G 1995 Hidden risks: early discharge and bilirubin toxicity due to glucose-6-phosphate dehydrogenase deficiency. Pediatrics 96: 734–738
75. Merritt K A, Coulter D M 1994 Application of the Gosset icterometer to screen for clinically significant hyperbilirubinemia in premature infants. Journal of Perinatology 14: 58–65

76. Messner K H, Maisels M J, Leure-DuPree A E 1978 Phototoxicity to the newborn primate retina. Investigative Ophthalmology and Visual Sciences 17: 178–182
77. Mieli-Vergani G, Howard E R, Portmann B, Mowat A P 1989 Late referral for biliary atresia: missed opportunities for effective surgery. Lancet i: 421–423
78. Mowat A P 1994 Hepatitis and cholestasis in infancy: intrahepatic disorders. In: Liver disorders in childhood, 3rd edn. Butterworths, London, pp 43–78
79. Newman T B, Esterling M J 1994 Yield of reticulocyte counts and blood smears in term infants. Clinical Pediatrics 33: 71–76
80. Newman T B, Maisels M J 1992 Evaluation of jaundice in the term newborn: a kinder, gentler approach. Pediatrics 89: 809–818
81. Newman T B, Maisels M J 1990 Does hyperbilirubinemia damage the brain of healthy full-term infants? Clinics in Perinatology 17: 331–358
82. Onishi I, Itoh S, Isobe K et al 1982 Mechanism of development of the bronze baby syndrome in neonates treated with phototherapy. Pediatrics 69: 273–276
83. Provisional Committee for Quality Improvement and Subcommittee on Hyperbilirubinemia 1994 Practice parameter: management of hyperbilirubinemia in the healthy term newborn. Pediatrics 94: 558–565
84. Rabinovitz J J, Washburn E R 1995 Bilirubin guidelines are a setback! Pediatrics 95: 616–617
85. Risemberg H M, Mazzi E, MacDonald M G, Peralta M, Heldrich F 1977 Correlation of cord bilirubin levels with hyperbilirubinemia in ABO incompatibility. Archives of Disease in Childhood 52: 219–222
86. Robertson A, Carp W, Brodersen R 1991 Bilirubin displacing effect of drugs used in neonatology. Acta Paediatrica Scandinavica 80: 1119–1127
87. Rosenstein B S, Ducore J M 1984 Enhancement by bilirubin of DNA damage induced in human cells exposed to phototherapy light. Pediatric Research 18: 3–6
88. Rubo J, Albrecht K, Lasch P et al 1992 High dose intravenous immune globulin therapy for hyperbilirubinemia caused by Rh hemolytic disease. Journal of Pediatrics 121: 93–97
89. Saigal S, O'Neill A, Suraínder Y, Chua L-B, Usher R 1972 Placental transfusion and hyperbilirubinemia in the premature. Pediatrics 49: 406–419
90. Scheidt P C, Graubard B I, Nelson K B et al 1991 Intelligence at six years in relation to neonatal bilirubin level: follow-up of the National Institute of Child Health and Human Development Clinical Trial of Phototherapy. Pediatrics 87: 797–805
91. Scheidt P C, Bryla D A, Nelson K B, Hirtz D G, Hoffmann H J 1990 Phototherapy for neonatal hyperbilirubinemia: six year follow-up of the NICHD clinical trial. Pediatrics 85: 455–463
92. Schneider A P 1986 Breast milk jaundice in the newborn – a real entity. Journal of the American Medical Association 255: 3270–3274
93. Schreiner R L, Glick M R 1982 Interlaboratory bilirubin variability. Pediatrics 69: 277–281
94. Schumacher R E 1990 Non-invasive measurements of bilirubin in the newborn. Clinics in Perinatology 17: 417–435
95. Seidman D S, Shiloh M, Stevenson D K, Vreman H J, Paz I, Gale R 1995 Role of hemolysis in neonatal jaundice associated with glucose-6-phosphate dehydrogenase deficiency. Journal of Pediatrics 127: 804–806
96. Seidman D S, Stevenson D K 1995 The issues of hyperbilirubinemia. Pediatrics 96: 543–544
97. Seidman D S, Stevenson D K, Zivanit E, Gale G 1995 Hospital readmission due to neonatal hyperbilirubinemia. Pediatrics 96: 726–729
98. Seidman D S, Paz I, Stevenson D K, Laor A, Danon Y L, Gale R 1994 Effects of phototherapy for neonatal jaundice on cognitive performance. Journal of Perinatology 14: 23–28
99. Seidman D S, Paz I, Stevenson D K, Laor A, Danon Y L, Gale R 1991 Neonatal hyperbilirubinemia and physical and cognitive performance at age 17 years. Pediatrics 88: 828–833
100. Silverman W A, Andersen D H, Blanc W A et al 1956 A difference in mortality rate and incidence of kernicterus among premature infants allotted to two prophylactic antibacterial regimens. Pediatrics 18: 614–625
101. Speck W T, Rosenkranz P G, Behrman M, Rosenkranz H S 1981 The embryotoxic effect of phototherapy: separation of therapeutic and gametotoxic activities. Photochemistry and Photobiology 33: 121–122
102. Stevenson D K, Vreman H J 1994 Bilirubin production in healthy term infants as measured by carbon monoxide in breath. Clinical Chemistry 40: 1934–1939
103. Suckling R J, Laing I A, Kirk J M 1995 Transcutaneous bilirubinometry as a screening tool for neonatal jaundice. Scottish Medical Journal 40: 14–15
104. Tan K L 1994 Comparison of the efficacy of fiberoptic and conventional phototherapy for neonatal hyperbilirubinemia. Journal of Pediatrics 125: 607–612
105. Tan K L, Skurr B A, Yip Y Y 1992 Phototherapy and the brain-stem auditory evoked response in neonatal hyperbilirubinemia. Journal of Pediatrics 120: 306–308
106. Tan K L 1982 The pattern of bilirubin response to phototherapy for neonatal hyperbilirubinemia. Pediatric Research 16: 670–674
107. Turkel S B, Miller C A, Guttenberg M E, Moynes D R, Hodgman J E 1982 A clinical pathologic reappraisal of kernicterus. Pediatrics 69: 267–272
108. Valaes T, Petmezaki S, Henschke C, Drummond G S, Kappas A 1994 Contol of jaundice in preterm newborns by an inhibitor of bilirubin production: studies with tin mesoporphyrin. Pediatrics 93: 1–11
109. Vohr B R, Lester B, Rapisardi G et al 1989 Abnormal brain-stem function (brain-stem auditory evoked response) correlates with acoustic cry features in term infants with hyperbilirubinemia. Journal of Pediatrics 115: 303–308
110. Volpe J J 1995 Neurology of the newborn 3rd edn. W B Saunders, Philadelphia, pp 490–515
111. Watchko J F, Oski F A 1992 Kernicterus in preterm newborns: past, present, and future. Pediatrics 90: 707–715
112. Watchko J, Oski F 1983 Bilirubin 20 mg/dl = vigintiphobia. Pediatrics 71: 660–663
113. Watkinson L R, St John A, Penberthy L A 1982 Investigation into paediatric bilirubin analysis in Australia and New Zealand. Journal of Clinical Pathology 35: 52–58
114. Wennberg R P, Gospe S M Jr, Rhine W D, Seyal M, Saeed D, Sosa G 1993 Brainstem bilirubin toxicity in the newborn primate may be promoted and reversed by modulating pCO_2. Pediatric Research 34: 6–9
115. Wennberg R P 1991 Cellular basis of bilirubin toxicity. New York State Journal of Medicine 91: 493–496
116. Yao T C, Stevenson D K 1995 Advances in the diagnosis and treatment of neonatal hyperbilirubinemia. Clinics in Perinatology 22: 741–758

Part 2

Liver disease

Giorgina Mieli-Vergani Alex P. Mowat*

INTRODUCTION

Liver disease in infancy is rare but is a serious cause of morbidity and mortality. A better awareness of the causes of liver disease in this age group and their mode of presentation would lead to earlier diagnosis of treatable conditions, with considerable improvement in prognosis, and genetic counselling for those families with hereditary disorders.

Jaundice is usually the first sign of liver dysfunction, but its importance is often underestimated because of the frequent occurrence of physiological jaundice (Chapter 31, Part 1) in the neonatal period. A raised serum bilirubin with a conjugated component of 20–80%, and urine which contains bile pigment, is always pathological even if the total bilirubin is as low as 80 μmol/l (5 mg/dl). Awareness that jaundice could be due to liver disease should prompt health workers to check the colour of the urine and the stools to ascertain whether the jaundice is due to cholestasis. A baby's urine is usually pale yellow and often colourless. Dark yellow urine (unless during phototherapy) and stools which are not yellow or green in an infant of whatever age, should suggest liver disease and trigger appropriate investigations. A persistently unconjugated bilirubin, not explained by haemolysis or other neonatological problems, should suggest the possibility of liver-based inherited disorders of bilirubin metabolism.

HEPATITIS SYNDROME OF INFANCY

Hepatitis syndrome of infancy is characterized by clinical and laboratory features of liver dysfunction, of which the most distinct is conjugated hyperbilirubinaemia. Patients usually have inflammatory changes in the liver histology – hence the name hepatitis – but the cause is only rarely infective. In most cases the infant presents with conjugated jaundice, which follows physiological jaundice; the urine becomes dark and the stools pale. Less commonly, infants may present with complications of liver dysfunction such as a bleeding diathesis, hypoglycaemia or fluid retention. The bleeding diathesis is usually due to vitamin K deficiency associated with fat malabsorption, which may also cause failure to thrive. Unless parenteral vitamin K is given these infants may bleed catastrophically. Hepatomegaly is almost universal. Palpable splenomegaly occurs in 40–60% of cases.

Hepatitis syndrome of infancy most commonly is due to intrahepatic disease, for which there are many associated disorders. It may be due to lesions of the biliary system. All infants require urgent investigation to identify disorders for which there is specific treatment and to prevent complications of cholestasis. If the stools contain no yellow or green pigment, cholestasis is complete and biliary atresia must be suspected. It is essential to arrange urgent referral to a specialist centre with the experience and skills to confirm the diagnosis and provide corrective surgery as early as possible.[28,51]

PATHOLOGY

Four main pathological entities cause the syndrome:

1. Hepatocellular disease (hepatitis);
2. Inflammation and bile duct reduplication in the portal tracts, leading in some instances to paucity of interlobular bile ducts;
3. Disorders of the main intrahepatic bile ducts, leading to sclerosing cholangitis;
4. Disorders of the extrahepatic bile ducts, most commonly biliary atresia.

Hepatocellular disease may be associated with a wide range of infective, genetic, endocrine, vascular, toxic, familial or chromosomal disorders.[56] Most frequently there are no associated factors and the disorder is cryptogenic. Chronic liver disease rarely follows in cryptogenic, infective or endocrine disorders, but occurs in at least 50% of genetic or familial disorders. Pathological categories 2, 3 and 4 are invariably associated with chronic liver disease unless surgery is effective. Infants with a normal serum γ-glutamyl transpeptidase activity or cholesterol concentration in the presence of jaundice and abnormal biochemical tests of liver function,[48] and infants with sclerosing cholangitis,[2,5] have a particularly poor prognosis.

For all pathological entities, in the acute stages the intrahepatic pathology as revealed by liver biopsy is dominated by cholestasis, with varying degrees of giant cell transformation of hepatocytes and inflammatory cell infiltrate in the portal tracts. In metabolic disorders abnormal accumulation of metabolites may be found in hepatocytes or Kupffer cells. Portal tract widening with oedema, accumulation of fibrous tissue and bile duct proliferation is characteristic of disorders of the major bile ducts, the most common of which is biliary atresia. It may occur in genetic disorders such as α_1-antitrypsin deficiency and is a harbinger of chronic liver disease.

* Professor Mowat died in November 1995

Table 31.11 Clinical signs of diagnostic importance in conjugated hyperbilirubinaemia

Abnormal signs	Disorder
Skin lesions, purpura, choroidoretinitis, myocarditis	Generalized viral infection (p. 1156)
Cataract	Galactosaemia (p. 998) or intrauterine infection or hypoparathyroidism (p. 967)
Multiple congenital anomalies	Trisomy 21, 13 or 18
Cystic mass below the liver	Choledochal cyst
Ascites and bile-stained herniae	Spontaneous perforation of the bile ducts
Systolic murmur, abnormal facies, posterior embryotoxon	Arteriohepatic dysplasia (Alagille syndrome)
Cutaneous haemangiomata	Hepatic or biliary haemangioma
Situs inversus with or without polysplenia	Extrahepatic biliary atresia
Optic nerve hypoplasia and/or micropenis	Septo-optic dysplasia

CLINICAL FEATURES

The majority of infants with hepatitis syndrome present with conjugated hyperbilirubinaemia starting in the first 4 weeks of life, but may occasionally present as late as 4 months of age. The second most common presentation is spontaneous bleeding, usually secondary to vitamin K malabsorption, the jaundice being mild or ignored because it is considered physiological by parents and their medical advisers. Rarely patients present with features of hypoglycaemia or hypoalbuminaemia. Review of the perinatal case record and past medical history may reveal features suggesting intrauterine infection, exposure to toxins, drugs or intravenous nutrition, familial, genetic or metabolic disease or consanguinity.

Clinical examination is likely to show hepatomegaly and splenomegaly. Patients with intrahepatic disease may show failure to thrive, but patients with biliary atresia typically are well nourished and have no stigmata of chronic liver disease in the first 2 months of life. Rarely, there are clinical signs of diagnostic importance (Table 31.11). If the stools are white or grey there may be complete cholestasis and conditions such as biliary atresia enter into the differential diagnosis. Standard tests of liver function, such as serum bilirubin, alkaline phosphatase, aspartate transaminase, γ-glutamyl transpeptidase, albumin and prothrombin time, may be equally abnormal in each of the four main groups of disorders. Serum lipids and cholesterol are usually normal in the first 4 months of life but may increase thereafter, particularly in infants with bile duct hypoplasia. Serum α-fetoprotein values are high, particularly in tyrosinaemia and bile duct hypoplasia, in which values may exceed 5000 ng/ml.[47,56]

MANAGEMENT (Table 31.12)

The first priority on admission to hospital is to identify the causes and complications for which urgent treatment is required.[56] These are septicaemia, urinary tract infection, toxoplasmosis, syphilis, malaria, herpes simplex and the metabolic disorders galactosaemia and fructosaemia. The main complication is spontaneous haemorrhage due to vitamin K malabsorption. Such haemorrhage may well be intracranial. The initial investigations must therefore include blood cultures, urine culture, urinalysis for non-glucose reducing substances, full blood count and prothrombin time. Galactose and fructose must be excluded from the diet until it is shown that there is no metabolic abnormality primarily affecting their metabolism.[57,60] After these bloods have been taken, diagnostic investigations such as α_1-antitrypsin phenotyping and galactose-1-phosphate uridyl transferase activity in red cells can be carried out.

If septicaemia is suspected broad-spectrum antibiotic therapy is indicated. Even if septicaemia is confirmed there may still be serious underlying disease, such as galactosaemia, α_1-antitrypsin deficiency or biliary atresia. The finding of non-glucose reducing substances in the urine does not necessarily indicate galactosaemia, as they may occur in normal infants in the first 2 weeks of life

Table 31.12 Investigations in conjugated hyperbilirubinaemia

Immediate investigations in all cases
Bacterial culture of blood and urine
Urine microscopy and analysis for reducing substances
Prothrombin time
Full blood count and reticulocyte count
Blood sugar, creatinine and urea
Serum sodium, potassium, bicarbonate, calcium
Blood group and cross-match
Investigations when full laboratory service is available
Biochemical tests of liver function, including split bilirubin and γ-glutamyl transpeptidase
IgM/G to toxoplasma, listeria, cytomegalovirus, herpes virus, rubella, hepatitis A and C, HIV
Syphilis serology
Hepatitis B surface antigen
α_1-Antitrypsin phenotype or genotype
Red blood cell galactose-1-phosphate uridyl transferase
Sweat electrolytes and immunoreactive trypsin
Serum and urine amino acids
Urine succinyl acetone and organic acids
Direct Coombs' test (if appropriate)
T4, TSH, cortisol
Chest X-ray for cardiac lesions
Wrist X-ray for rickets
In the presence of ascites: tap for biochemical testing + culture
Ultrasound of liver to detect focal lesions and dilated bile ducts
Methylbromo-IDA scan following phenobarbitone (in selected cases)
Endoscopic retrograde cholangiopancreatography (in selected cases)
Tissue diagnosis
Percutaneous liver biopsy
Skin biopsy for fibroblast culture and enzyme analysis (in selected cases)
Bone marrow aspirate for Niemann–Pick C disease
Laparotomy, intraoperative cholangiography

Table 31.13 Surgically correctable disorders causing bile duct obstruction (see text)

Extrahepatic biliary atresia
Choledochal cyst
Spontaneous perforation of the bile ducts
Duodenal and low bile duct atresia
Gallstones
Haemangiomata
Extrinsic compression
Bile plugs in extrahepatic bile ducts

Table 31.14 Infections associated with conjugated hyperbilirubinaemia (see Ch. 43, Part 2)

Cytomegalovirus	Epstein–Barr virus
Rubella virus	Varicella-zoster virus
Hepatitis A	Psittacosis
Hepatitis B	Bacterial infections
Hepatitis C	Listeria
Non A–C hepatitis	*Treponema pallidum*
Herpes simplex virus	*Toxoplasma gondii*
Coxsackie A9, B	Malaria
Echovirus 9, 11, 14, 19	Tuberculosis
Adenovirus	Human immunodeficiency virus
Reo virus type III	

Table 31.15 Inherited metabolic disorders associated with hepatitis syndrome in infancy (see Ch. 38, Part 3)

Galactosaemia
Fructosaemia
Tyrosinaemia
α_1-Antitrypsin deficiency
Cystic fibrosis
Niemann–Pick type C
Gaucher's disease
Wolman's disease
Zellweger syndrome
Infantile polycystic disease (p. 1031)
Haemophagocytic lymphohistiocytosis
Neonatal iron storage disease (congenital haemochromatosis, p. 741)
Defects in synthesis of primary bile acids

and are common in all forms of liver damage.[56] Conversely, the absence of non-glucose reducing substances does not exclude galactosaemia, as very ill infants may feed poorly or vomit. If the prothrombin time is found to be prolonged, vitamin K 1 mg i.v. should be given and, if bleeding is still occurring, fresh-frozen plasma should be infused or exchange transfusion performed. The next priority is to identify those infants who require surgical correction of bile duct obstruction (Table 31.13). Ultrasound examination should be undertaken to exclude a choledochal cyst.

In all infants, infective (Table 31.14), metabolic (Table 31.15) and endocrine (Table 31.16) causes of liver damage affecting this age group must be excluded. With regard to infective conditions it must be remembered that cytomegalovirus, rubella and hepatitis B virus have been found to occur in all types of hepatobiliary disease.[56] Positivity for these viruses should not preclude investigation of other causes of liver damage. Galactosaemia, fructosaemia and tyrosinaemia must be investigated promptly because dietary intervention in the first two conditions and treatment with 2-(-2-nitro-4-trifluoromethyl-benzoyl)-,3-cyclohexanedione (NTBC)[42] in the last, need to be instituted urgently to avoid severe deterioration. α_1-Antitrypsin deficiency, cystic fibrosis and Niemann–Pick type C need also to be sought in all infants because these are relatively common genetic conditions for which antenatal diagnosis is possible. α_1-Antitrypsin deficiency must be excluded in all cases by determining the α_1-antitrypsin phenotype, rather than by means of the α_1-antitrypsin concentration, which can be within the normal range in the presence of hepatitis, as α_1-antitrypsin is an acute-phase reactant. This is perhaps the most important investigation in distinguishing severe hepatitis with complete cholestasis from extrahepatic biliary atresia, as the liver disease associated with α_1-antitrypsin deficiency (phenotype PiZZ, p. 740) has many clinical and pathological similarities with biliary atresia.[57,82] Investigation for rarer metabolic disease should be performed only if suggested by the family history or findings on percutaneous liver biopsy. The frequency with which infectious, genetic, pharmacological and toxic causes of hyperbilirubinaemia or structural biliary abnormalities can be identified depends not only on the prevalence of these in the community studied, but also on referral patterns and the sophistication of investigation facilities.[56]

In a study in southeast England of 54 infants who had conjugated hyperbilirubinaemia[22] of at least 2 weeks' duration, it was found that intrahepatic idiopathic disorders were approximately three times more common than biliary atresia and four times as frequent as disease associated with α_1-antitrypsin deficiency or the combined incidence of all other specific disorders. The relative frequency of the causes of conjugated hyperbilirubinaemia in infants referred to King's College Hospital, a tertiary referral centre, is shown in Table 31.17.

Table 31.16 Endocrine disorders associated with hepatitis syndrome in infancy (see Ch. 38, Part 1)

Hypopituitarism
Diabetes insipidus
Hypoadrenalism
Hypothyroidism
Hypoparathyroidism

IDENTIFYING BILE DUCT OBSTRUCTION

A most useful observation is the stool colour. Specimens of all stools passed are saved in the dark (e.g. in a black bag) and examined for yellow or green pigment; if absent, cholestasis is complete and biliary atresia must be excluded. Referral to a specialist centre with experience in the identification of this condition and a reputation for its successful surgical correction is essential.[45] A skilfully

Table 31.17 Relative frequency of causes of conjugated hyperbilirubinaemia in infants referred to the Paediatric Liver Service, King's College Hospital

Disorder	Referred cases
Biliary atresia	337
Idiopathic hepatitis	331
α_1-Antitrypsin deficiency	189
Alagille syndrome	41
Choledochal cyst	34
Spontaneous perforation of bile duct	6
Others	94

interpreted percutaneous liver biopsy performed under local anaesthesia using a Menghini technique is diagnostic in up to 90% of cases. If all portal tracts show increased oedema, fibrosis and bile duct reduplication, this strongly suggests major bile duct disease, of which the most common is biliary atresia. This appearance can be found also in such genetic disorders as α_1-antitrypsin deficiency (PiZZ), cystic fibrosis and endocrine disorders associated with septo-optic dysplasia. It occurs in some infants who will ultimately develop bile duct hypoplasia and in disorders of the intrahepatic bile ducts.[20,47] All of these disorders can cause complete cholestasis. It is essential that some of the material obtained is frozen at –70°C for subsequent biochemical analysis for inherited disorders (Table 31.15) if indicated by the liver histology or other investigations.

If there are doubts as to whether there is pigment in the stools, a helpful investigation is radionucleotide demonstration of bile duct patency. This is only useful if isotope is demonstrated in the gut, thereby excluding biliary atresia and avoiding an unnecessary and potentially dangerous laparotomy. No excretion in the gut does not equate with biliary atresia. A ^{99m}Tc-tagged imminodiacetic acid derivative, such as methylbromo-IDA, with good hepatic uptake and relatively poor renal uptake, must be used. Discrimination from intrahepatic cholestasis is enhanced if the infant is pretreated with phenobarbitone (5 mg/kg for at least 3 days). Repeated imaging up to 24 hours after intravenous injection may be required to demonstrate isotope in the gut. Equally effective discrimination may be achieved by computer analysis of distribution between the liver and heart within 10 minutes of intravenous injection.[25] Daily observation of the stool colour is essential even if patency of the bile ducts is demonstrated. If the stools remain acholic the liver biopsy should be repeated, and further radionucleotide studies may be necessary to identify the rare instances of late-onset biliary atresia.

The real difficulty arises if there is no excretion, the biopsy is not indicative of atresia and no genetic or endocrine disorder causing complete cholestasis has been identified. Unless filling of the intrahepatic ducts can be demonstrated by endoscopic retrograde cholangiography, such patients should have a laparotomy.[86] It is essential that this be undertaken by an experienced surgeon who can correctly assess the changes in the porta hepatis and, being confident of the diagnosis, proceed to portoenterostomy.[45] Final confirmation of the diagnosis comes from histological examination of the excised biliary remnants, by which time an irreversible operation has been performed! Even with intraoperative cholangiography extrahepatic ducts which are hypoplastic as a result of severe intrahepatic cholestasis may be considered atretic, leading to an unnecessary destructive operation.[48]

SURGICALLY CORRECTABLE DISORDERS

Biliary atresia

Biliary atresia is the most frequent surgically correctable liver disorder in infancy, affecting 1:14 000 liveborns. It is unique to infancy and is characterized by complete obstruction of the bile flow owing to obliteration or destruction of part or all of the extrahepatic biliary tree. Study of bile duct remnants removed at surgery, and from macroserial sectioning and reconstruction of surgical and necropsy liver specimens, indicates that biliary atresia arises from a sclerosing inflammatory process affecting previously formed bile ducts.[27,30] Recently, comparative anatomical studies have suggested that, in at least some cases, biliary atresia may be caused by failure of the intrauterine remodelling process at the hepatic hilum, with persistence of fetal bile ducts poorly supported by mesenchyme. As bile flow increases perinatally, bile leakage from these abnormal ducts may trigger an intense inflammatory reaction, with consequent obliteration of the biliary tree.[83] The extrahepatic ducts are primarily affected, whereas the intrahepatic bile ducts remain patent in early infancy but then also become affected, obliterated and eventually disappear. Cirrhosis with complications such as portal hypertension may appear at any time from 2 months of age, and death by 2 years of age is usual.

The cause of biliary atresia is unknown. Familial cases are extremely rare and, of 17 cases occurring in twins, in only two instances were both affected.[77] Up to 25% of infants have minor or major abnormalities outside the biliary system, with a particularly high frequency of abnormalities of the vasculature below the diaphragm. Polysplenia and splenic hypoplasia with or without situs inversus is another association. It has been suggested that children with these abnormalities may represent an aetiological subgroup, having, for example, a different HLA phenotype.[78] It has also been suggested that the precarious blood supply to the biliary tree may be further jeopardized with such abnormalities. An increased incidence of maternal diabetes mellitus has been associated with the splenic malformation syndrome.[19] Another suggested aetiological factor is a long common channel for the pancreatic and biliary ducts as they enter the duodenum, with the suggestion that pancreatic juice may enter the biliary system and initiate mucosal damage and subsequent inflammatory response. There have been many suggestions that perinatal infection may initiate biliary atresia, but all of the candidate viruses, e.g. Reo virus type III, infect atresia patients no more frequently than other infants.[54]

A specific problem in the diagnosis of biliary atresia is that, as mentioned above, in most cases it results from an obliterative disorder starting in formed extrahepatic ducts which eventually leads to their destruction.[27,30] Thus the extrahepatic bile ducts and intrahepatic bile ducts may be patent[38] in the first weeks of life, but become atretic later. Thus, in up to 30% of infants with atresia stools are pigmented in the first weeks after birth, before bile flow is completely obstructed.[12,18] All too frequently the infant's apparent well-being causes paediatricians and other health workers to dismiss consideration of this disorder in early infancy, when the chances of successful surgery are high.[28,51] The longer biliary atresia has been present the greater the likelihood that the intrahepatic bile ducts will have been obliterated and that portoenterostomy will be less likely to be successful. It is essential to refer infants with acholic stools to units with experience in the interpretation of the diagnostic investigations outlined above, and in the surgical and postoperative management of biliary atresia[31,33] (Table 31.18).

At laparotomy, the surgeon must first confirm that the bile ducts are absent or atretic. This is not a simple task, and narrow but patent bile ducts in infants with intrahepatic disease and complete cholestasis have been removed by experienced surgeons.[48] In 5–10% of infants the surgeon can identify a patent common bile duct containing bile and in continuity with intrahepatic bile ducts.[33] In these infants a biliary–intestinal anastomosis via a long Roux-en-Y loop may allow bile to drain satisfactorily. In the majority of patients, however, the proximal common hepatic duct is completely obliterated or absent up to where it enters the liver, and at the porta hepatis it is replaced by fibrous tissue. This tissue is transected flush with the liver and a Roux-en-Y loop of jejunum is anastomosed around the fibrous edges of the transected tissue, forming a hepaticoportoenterostomy (Kasai procedure). For surgery to be effective the intrahepatic bile ducts must be patent to the porta hepatitis. Modifications of the Kasai procedure undertaken to reduce the risks of cholangitis fail to do so and increase the risks of liver transplantation if this becomes subsequently necessary. Patients are started on phenobarbitone preoperatively at a dose of 45 mg/day to promote bile flow, and this is continued indefinitely, without dose modification with increasing weight, unless jaundice worsens or reappears, when the dose is increased to 60–90 mg/day. With an experienced surgeon good bile flow with normal serum bilirubin values can be achieved in more than 80% of children operated on by 60 days of age, but in only 20–30% with later surgery.[51,60] If bilirubin returns to normal, a 90% 15-year survival has been reported,[60,61] with a good quality of life into the fourth decade.[13,39] If the bilirubin is not reduced the rate of progression of cirrhosis is not slowed and survival beyond the second birthday is unusual. If bile drainage is partially effective death may be delayed to 6 or 7 years of age.

Table 31.18 Requirements to improve the management of biliary atresia

All infants jaundiced after 14 days of age should have urinalysis and total and direct serum bilirubin determination
If conjugated bilirubin is present the infant should be referred to a paediatrician for urgent investigation
If the stools have no yellow or green pigment the infant should be referred to a specialist centre to exclude or treat biliary atresia
'Well baby' clinics should be at 4 rather than 6 weeks of age to identify jaundice sufficiently early to increase the chances of successful treatment

An important postoperative complication is cholangitis. This is due to a wide range of microorganisms and occurs in over 50% of cases in the first 2 years after surgery. It is characterized by fever, recurrence or aggravation of jaundice, and frequently features of septicaemia. Blood culture, ascitic aspirate or liver biopsy to identify the organism responsible should precede intravenous antibiotic therapy, which is continued for 14 days. Often, however, the diagnosis of cholangitis is not obvious and unexplained fever may be the only symptom. Antibiotics are then started empirically, after taking a blood culture and assessing liver function tests and full blood count. If the fever responds to antibiotics, these are continued for 5 days. Should the fever recur after stopping antibiotics, a liver biopsy is performed for histological examination and culture. Amoxycillin and ceftazidime are currently our initial choice pending in-vitro sensitivities. Prophylactic antibiotics are of no proven value.

Portal hypertension is present in almost all cases at the time of initial surgery. Approximately 50% of all survivors aged 5 years, even those with normal bilirubin levels, have oesophageal varices, but only 10–15% have alimentary bleeding. For these, injection sclerotherapy is the treatment of choice. In approximately 10% of cases in whom the serum bilirubin returns to normal, intrahepatic cholangiopathy progresses and complications of biliary cirrhosis ultimately develop.[58] For these patients, and those for whom surgery has not been effective, liver transplantation should be considered.[64] With 2-year survival rates as high as 80%,[62] and 5-year survival rates ranging from 64 to 78%[36] liver transplantation is now a therapeutic option,[50,76] but it remains a formidable surgical procedure. The recipient is likely to have one or more life-threatening complications in the perioperative or postoperative period. Lifelong immunosuppressive therapy is required, with a high risk of opportunist and community-acquired infections demanding close medical and surgical supervision. Most of the survivors have a good quality of life and attend school, although the long-term medical and psychological effects of liver transplantation in childhood are as yet unknown. The supply of donors of suitable size (even if reduction hepatectomy is used) and blood group remains a major limiting factor in liver transplantation in childhood. Segmental graft transplant from living relatives has given survival rates of 90% in infants in whom Kasai portoenterostomy had been unsuccessful.[63] The results are better in children transplanted after the age of 1 year (or 10 kg) and if the procedure is done electively rather than as an emergency.[62] The precise indications and timing, and the optimum management of some of the intraoperative and postoperative problems, including the control of rejection, remain the subject of ongoing research and assessment. Although an important mode of management for end-stage liver disease, the role of liver transplantation in biliary atresia is secondary to that of portoenterostomy, except for infants in whom decompensated cirrhosis has developed because of delayed diagnosis.

Choledochal cysts

Choledochal cysts are dilatations of the biliary ducts which are usually associated with intermittent biliary obstruction. If uncorrected they lead to increasing biliary fibrosis and ultimately cirrhosis. In the newborn period the presentation is indistinguishable from neonatal hepatitis or biliary atresia. They may be diagnosed prenatally on routine ultrasound.[80] Cholangitis, rupture, pancreatitis and gallstones are important complications which can occur even in early infancy, and carcinoma of the cyst wall may be a long-term complication.

A cystic echo-free mass demonstrated in the biliary tree by ultrasound is strong evidence for this diagnosis. The intrahepatic bile ducts may be dilated. Diagnosis is confirmed by operative cholangiography. The treatment is surgical removal with biliary drainage via a Roux-en-Y loop.[34,84] With adequate surgery the long-term prognosis is good.[80]

Spontaneous perforation of the bile duct[36]

Spontaneous perforation of the bile duct at the junction of the cystic duct and common hepatic duct occurs when, for some unexplained reason, the common bile duct becomes blocked, usually at its distal end. Affected infants have mild jaundice, failure to gain weight and abdominal distension due to ascites, which classically causes the development of bile-stained herniae. The stools are white or cream in colour, the urine is dark. Abdominal paracentesis confirms the presence of bile-stained ascites.

If operative cholangiography shows free drainage of contrast into the duodenum the ruptured duct may be sutured, but more commonly it is necessary to establish cholecystojejunostomy drainage to a Roux-en-Y loop. With effective surgery the prognosis is excellent. Delay in instituting surgery may lead to severe malnutrition, peritonitis and septicaemia.

Miscellaneous conditions

The remaining surgical conditions listed in Table 31.13 are very rare, and are usually dealt with either by flushing out the obstruction with a percutaneous or operative cholangiogram or by a bypass procedure.

CONJUGATED HYPERBILIRUBINAEMIA ASSOCIATED WITH ERYTHROBLASTOSIS

No specific treatment is available. No long-term hepatic sequelae such as cirrhosis or portal hypertension have been recorded.

The condition must be distinguished from the inspissated bile plug syndrome, a very rare condition in which the distal bile duct is obstructed by debris which can be flushed into the duodenum at percutaneous or operative cholangiography. The diagnosis of this disorder is made by ultrasonography and liver biopsy.

PAUCITY OF INTERLOBULAR BILE DUCTS (INTRAHEPATIC BILIARY HYPOPLASIA)

This is a pathological diagnosis in which there is a decrease in the number of interlobular bile ducts seen in the portal tracts. It is found in many conditions causing hepatitis in infancy (Table 31.19). If it occurs with cardiovascular, skeletal and ocular anomalies it is called Alagille syndrome (syndromic paucity of the intrahepatic bile ducts; arteriohepatic dysplasia)[1] and is inherited in an autosomal dominant fashion with variable expression. The estimated incidence is 1:100 000 livebirths. It is caused by mutations in the human *Jagged 1* gene on chromosome 20p12.[71] There is long-standing cholestasis causing jaundice, pruritus, hypercholesterolaemia and xanthoma. The severity of the cholestasis varies. Mild cases may have pruritus only. The majority have jaundice

Table 31.19 Causes of paucity of interlobular bile ducts

Syndromic
Alagille syndrome or arteriohepatic dysplasia
Non-syndromic
Idiopathic
α_1-Antitrypsin deficiency
Biliary atresia after 6 months of age
Zellweger syndrome
Impaired cholic acid synthesis
Down syndrome
Intrauterine infection, e.g. rubella
Acquired
Graft-versus-host disease
Advanced chronic liver transplant rejection

from the neonatal period, which in severe cases may persist but in others clears in late childhood or early adult life. The long-term prognosis is uncertain, but some 15% may go on to develop cirrhosis[66] and 5–10% die from liver disease. In one series 25% died from cardiac involvement, classically a peripheral pulmonary stenosis, or infection.[1] Diagnosis is supported by the finding of the typical facies: deep-set eyes, mild hypertelorism, overhanging forehead, a straight nose which in profile is in the same plane as the forehead, a small pointed chin, posterior embryotoxon (a remnant of an embryonic membrane between iris and cornea, seen by slit lamp), and vertebral arch defects on spinal radiographs. A high serum cholesterol supports the diagnosis. The treatment is that of chronic cholestasis, with particular emphasis on adequacy of vitamin E replacement and the control of pruritus.[20]

LIVER DAMAGE ASSOCIATED WITH PARENTERAL NUTRITION

Prolonged intravenous nutrition, particularly in early infancy, causes cholestasis and hepatocellular damage, which may progress to cirrhosis and liver cancer if intravenous feeding continues with no oral intake. The aetiology is unknown.[26,49] Prevalence increases with the degree of prematurity, the duration of intravenous feeding and in the absence of any oral food intake. Cholestatic jaundice, defined as a direct-reacting bilirubin concentration of greater than 34 μmol/l, occurred in 8.6% of 267 infants receiving intravenous nutrition.[65] The incidence was inversely proportional to the gestation, being 13.7% in infants of less than 32 weeks, 5.3% in infants of 32–36 weeks and 1.4% in infants of greater than 36 weeks. In each gestational age group the duration of parenteral therapy in infants with cholestasis was significantly longer than in those who remained free from this complication. The infants with cholestasis also tended to be without oral feeding for longer – 23 days as opposed to 15 days. Sepsis, hypoxia, shock, blood transfusion, intra-abdominal surgery and potentially hepatotoxic drugs may aggravate the liver damage.

Pathologically there is a distinctly cholestatic hepatitis, with bile stasis within the hepatocytes and in the bile canaliculi, and bile in the Kupffer cells. These cells also contain marked accumulation of para-aminosalicylic acid-positive pigment. The hepatocytes are distended and may have increased numbers of nuclei. There is lobular disarray with distension of portal tracts by inflammatory cell infiltrate, bile duct proliferation and fibrous tissue. A fine panlobular sinusoidal or pericellular fibrosis may be noted in up to 50% of cases. Severe fibrosis, cirrhosis and hepatocellular carcinoma may develop if total intravenous feeding cannot be stopped. Acute acalculous cholecystitis, biliary sludge and cholelithiasis are complications. Follow-up biopsies 5–9 months after the height of the illness still show mild hepatocellular cholestasis, lobular disarray with ballooning of hepatocytes, and increased fibrosis.

The aetiology of the hepatobiliary complications of total parenteral nutrition is unknown.[70] Intravenous administration of amino acids, dextrose and protein hydrolysates can cause a rise in serum alkaline phosphatase concentrations above baseline levels during the first 3 weeks of administration. Intravenous amino acids, in addition, may cause hyperaminoacidaemia, metabolic acidosis or hyperammonaemia. Intravenous lipids cause a progressive rise in the concentration of lipoprotein X. How these abnormalities are associated with disturbances of intrahepatocyte metabolism is at present unknown. Other factors which have been postulated as possibly contributing to impaired hepatic function include a lack of essential nutrients, trace elements or an 'unbalanced' supply of amino acids. Other postulated causes include endotoxaemia, chronic hypoxia, toxins leached from central venous catheters and lack of intestinal stimulation of bile secretion because of lack of oral intake. Hypersensitivity reactions to drugs must also be considered.

The first clinical indication of hepatic involvement is usually the appearance of conjugated hyperbilirubinaemia. Hepatomegaly may be noted. Biochemical tests of liver function are abnormal. It is important to consider other causes of cholestasis in this age group before concluding that the disorder is due to intravenous nutrition. If intravenous nutrition can be withdrawn the jaundice settles within 4 weeks, although liver function tests may remain abnormal for 5 months and liver biopsy changes persist for up to a year.

There are no reported long-term follow-up studies. It is clearly important, therefore, to monitor closely liver function tests in infants who are receiving intravenous nutrition, particularly if they are premature. Intravenous nutrition should be curtailed as much as possible if conjugated hyperbilirubinaemia or other signs of hepatocellular injury appear in infancy. Tests of liver function should be carried out at least weekly during intravenous feeding. Treatment of the liver dysfunction associated with parenteral nutrition aims at improving bile flow with the use of ursodeoxycholic acid (15 mg/kg/day) or phenobarbitone (5 mg/kg/day). The most effective treatment, however, is the reintroduction of total or partial enteral nutrition, if tolerated.

LIVER DISEASE ASSOCIATED WITH α_1-ANTITRYPSIN DEFICIENCY

α_1-Antitrypsins are glycoproteins synthesized largely in the liver. In vitro they act as protease inhibitors. Over 90 different alleles, controlled by a single gene, may be isolated and are identified in alphabetical nomenclature as protease inhibitors (Pi). The predominant type is PiM. The alleles of α_1-antitrypsin are inherited in an autosomal codominant fashion, the most common being PiMM. Disease is associated with the PiZZ, Pinulnul or PiZnul variants. These are among the most common single gene defects, occurring in about 1:2000–1:7000 newborns of European origin.[69,73] The plasma deficiency of the glycoprotein is associated with a defect in secretion from the endoplasmic reticulum rather than a defect in the synthesis of the Z polypeptide.[11]

The clinical features associated with the deficiency state are very variable, with some having no overt disease, up to 20% developing liver disease of variable severity, and up to 60% developing emphysema. Cigarette smoking is closely associated with the development of emphysema, but the cause of the liver disease is unknown.[24,74] It is likely that a second genetic factor or environmental factors contribute to liver disease and its severity. Mechanisms of liver damage which have been suggested are defects in chemotaxis,[17] liver-specific autoimmune reactions,[54] possession of HLA DR3,[24] complement activation,[44] lack of breast-feeding and male sex,[42] accumulation of abnormal α_1-antitrypsin in the liver cells and the consequent increase in synthesis of heat-shock/stress proteins, particularly during episodes of pyrexia.[45]

Although over 50% of infants with the deficiency state have abnormal biochemical tests of liver function, and these remain abnormal in over 30% throughout the first 12 years of life, only 10–15% develop symptomatic liver disease.[81] In 90% this takes the form of a conjugated hyperbilirubinaemia with hepatosplenomegaly and disturbed biochemical tests of liver function presenting in the first 4 months of life. In 10% of these infants a serious bleeding diathesis due to vitamin K malabsorption is an important component of their illness, frequently leading to intracranial bleeding and permanent neurological abnormality;[57] 1–2% present in later childhood or adult life with cirrhosis with no history of prior jaundice in infancy.[25] Emphysema usually has its onset in early adult life.

The identification of liver disease associated with α_1-antitrypsin deficiency in the individual infant is important for diagnostic, prognostic and genetic reasons.[55] Such infants could be considered on clinical, biochemical and liver biopsy evidence to have extrahepatic biliary atresia and be subjected to the risks of unnecessary laparotomy. Infants with liver disease associated with α_1-antitrypsin deficiency have a significantly worse prognosis than those with hepatitis of unknown cause. In an epidemiological study in southeast England, seven cases of hepatitis in infants were associated with α_1-antitrypsin deficiency.[22] By 3 years of age four had died of cirrhosis, and cirrhosis was present in one of two reviewed at 10 years of age. In contrast only two of 28 with idiopathic hepatitis in this study died, and none at 10 years had cirrhosis. Our experience with 82 children with PiZ phenotype and liver disease was that approximately 25% died of cirrhosis by adolescence, a further 25% had histologically proven cirrhosis, 25% had persisting liver disease with possible cirrhosis, and 25% apparently recovered from liver disease showing no clinical or biochemical abnormality.[69]

In general the outcome of the liver disease is related to the severity and duration of the acute hepatitis in early infancy. In the individual patient the liver biopsy is the most helpful guide to prognosis. In those who die or have persistent hepatic abnormality there is a marked increase in portal tract oedema and fibrosis in the first 6 months of life. Unfortunately, there is no specific treatment for this form of liver disease.

Patients with cirrhosis associated with α_1-antitrypsin deficiency may have renal involvement with a variety of glomerulonephropathies.[79] Renal involvement may cause haematuria and/or proteinuria and contribute to hypoalbuminaemia. The development of renal complications adds to the difficulties after liver transplantation, particularly severe hypertension.

Reliable methods of genotyping from chorionic villus sampling at 8–10 weeks of gestation are available. Genetic counselling is difficult because of the varying severity of the clinical associations and difficulties in predicting the prognosis. From an analysis of our own and reported experience on the outcome of liver disease in 47 families with more than one PiZZ child, we conclude that if the firstborn has unresolved or fatal liver disease there is a 75% chance that a further PiZZ child in that family will have similar liver disease.[69] Such families should be carefully counselled and offered the option of prenatal diagnosis.

CRYPTOGENIC (IDIOPATHIC) HEPATITIS IN INFANCY

Despite an increasing number of specific disorders associated with hepatitis syndrome in infancy, in the majority the cause is cryptogenic. These children are frequently born after an abnormal pregnancy and are often of low birthweight. Frequently they come to medical attention for complications of prematurity or intrauterine growth retardation, and then subsequently develop evidence of liver disease. Although the liver disease may be severe, the mortality in such cases is usually less than 15% and long-term hepatic problems occur in less than 10%. The prognosis tends to be worse if exploratory laparotomy is carried out. Other indicators of poor prognosis are liver biopsy showing marked cholestasis with proliferation and/or damage of the intralobular bile ducts; cholangiography showing sclerosing cholangitis,[2,5] normal serum α-glutamyl transpeptidase in the presence of abnormality of other liver function tests indicating persistent liver disease,[46] family history of liver disease in childhood, or consanguinity.[21,22,32,59] In children with cholestatic liver disease and normal γ-glutamyl transpeptidase a genetic abnormality of bile salt formation must be excluded, as treatment with oral primary bile salts will reverse liver damage.[14,15]

NEONATAL HAEMOCHROMATOSIS

Neonatal haemochromatosis, or neonatal iron storage disorder, is a rare and often fatal disorder which causes either death in utero or acute liver failure in the neonatal period. The pathogenesis is uncertain. It has been observed in siblings and it has been suggested to have an autosomal recessive mode of inheritance.[16,40] However, we[37] and others[85] have observed it in neonates conceived by different fathers, suggesting a specific role for maternal factors, possibly mitochondrial[85] or related to pregnancy. Often the pregnancy is complicated by oligohydramnios and/or megaplacenta. Histologically, the condition is characterized by intense deposition of stainable iron in the liver, hepatocellular necrosis, and diffuse hepatic fibrosis with nodular regeneration. Other organs affected include the pancreas, heart, thyroid and salivary glands, with a characteristic sparing of the reticuloendothelial system. Although it has been reported that liver failure due to iron storage disease in the neonate may respond favourably to iron chelation (desferioxamine), prostaglandin E_1, and antioxidant (α-tocoferol, *n*-acetylcysteine and selenium),[75] our experience in five neonates with this condition treated with the antioxidant cocktail has been disappointing,[37] two dying and three requiring liver transplantation, which was successfully performed at the age of 5, 19 and 39 days. Liver transplant therefore remains the only real therapeutic option in the presence of liver failure.[8]

MANAGEMENT OF DISORDERS CAUSING HEPATITIS SYNDROME IN INFANCY

The essence of management is to define the site of the main pathological involvement and to identify any associated disorder, particularly those for which there is specific therapy. Infections must be treated with appropriate anti-infective agents.

Fructose and galactose are omitted from the diet until fructosaemia and galactosaemia have been excluded by specific tests. Fat-soluble vitamin deficiencies must be prevented by oral or parenteral supplements.[56] The exact vitamin requirements depend on the degree of malabsorption and metabolic demands. It is mandatory to monitor the prothrombin time (vitamin K), serum calcium, phosphate and wrist X-rays (vitamin D) and serum vitamin E and A concentrations to assess adequacy of supplementation. Vitamin K deficiency is an immediate risk.

If cholestasis persists for more than 3 months laboratory or radiological signs of vitamin D deficiency are likely to appear, with pathological evidence of vitamin E deficiency occurring after 5 months. Clinical evidence of vitamin A deficiency develops after some years, but biochemical evidence may be present earlier.[3] Oral supplements are given in doses of 3–5 times normal requirements if cholestasis is incomplete. In complete cholestasis doses of vitamin K 1 mg orally per day, vitamin D 30 000 units intramuscularly at 4-weekly intervals, and vitamin A 50 000 units intramuscularly at 4-weekly intervals will usually prevent laboratory evidence of deficiency. Vitamin E parenterally in a dose of 10 mg/kg at 2-weekly intervals is required to maintain the serum vitamin E level.[29] In infants with failure to thrive dietary supplements of carbohydrate polymers and medium-chain triglycerides (if defects of fat oxidation have been excluded) are required.

Cholestyramine with or without phenobarbitone, ursodeoxycholic acid or rifampicin may be required for pruritus. There is no medical treatment that influences the progression of idiopathic disorders.

INHERITED DISORDERS OF BILIRUBIN METABOLISM

GILBERT SYNDROME

A chronic, mild, variable unconjugated hyperbilirubinaemia with serum bilirubin levels around 32–85 μmol/l (2–5 mg/dl) and without significant haemolysis or abnormality of liver function is the characteristic feature of this condition. The pathogenesis is undetermined. Impaired hepatic uptake of bilirubin, deficient uridine diphosphate glucuronyl transferase activity and a mild excretory defect have been suggested. An abnormality of the promotor region of the UDPGT1 gene, inherited in an autosomal recessive fashion, has been demonstrated.[10,52] The frequency of the abnormal promotor among the normal population is 40%. Because clinically manifested Gilbert syndrome occurs in 5% of the population, other factors, such as an increased bilirubin production, must be present to bring this disease to expression. The diagnosis is rarely made with confidence before 10 years of age and is based on exclusion of other causes of unconjugated hyperbilirubinaemia. Whether the condition contributes to hyperbilirubinaemia in the newborn is difficult to ascertain.

CRIGLER–NAJJAR DISEASE

This disorder is characterized by elevated unconjugated hyperbilirubinaemia from birth. Crigler–Najjar disease type 1 results from a complete and type 2 from a partial deficiency of UDPGT. In Crigler–Najjar disease type 1 serum bilirubin values are in excess of 350 μmol/l and the bile contains only traces of bilirubin conjugates. Crigler–Najjar disease type 2 is less severe, with serum bilirubin values not exceeding 350 μmol/l. The bile of these patients contains bilirubin mono- and diglucoronides in low concentration. Genetically both diseases result from mutations of the UDPGT1 gene.[4,8,72] Crigler–Najjar type 1 is inherited in an autosomal recessive fashion, whereas type 2 is thought to be inherited in an autosomal dominant fashion with variable expression. Diagnosis is suspected on the basis of the clinical features and needs to be confirmed by measuring bilirubin conjugation in the bile collected at endoscopy, or by measuring UDPGTase activity in a percutaneous liver biopsy specimen. In Crigler–Najjar type 2 serum bilirubin levels decrease by at least 30% with phenobarbitone treatment. Patients with Crigler–Najjar type 1 are at risk throughout their life of developing neurological damage and kernicterus.[7] Most patients require exchange transfusion to control hyperbilirubinaemia in the newborn period, and thereafter require continuous phototherapy of sufficient intensity to keep the serum bilirubin below 340 μmol/l. This is most conveniently achieved by sleeping for up to 12–15 hours under a specially built phototherapy device incorporating as many as 32 phototherapy tubes.[87] Oral cholestyramine may reduce the phototherapy requirement by binding bilirubin in the gut. After 4 years of age phototherapy gradually becomes less effective and liver transplantation becomes necessary to prevent kernicterus.[67] Auxiliary liver transplant, where the left lateral segment of the recipient is removed and substituted with the donor's left lateral segment, has proved successful in correcting the enzymatic defect and minimizing the risks of transplantation.[6]

REFERENCES

1. Alagille D, Estrada A, Hadchouel M et al 1987 Syndromic paucity of interlobular bile ducts (Alagille's syndrome or arteriohepatic dysplasia): review of eighty cases. Journal of Pediatrics 110: 195–200
2. Amedee-Manesme O, Bernard O, Brunelle F et al 1987 Sclerosing cholangitis with neonatal onset. Journal of Pediatrics 111: 225–229
3. Amedee-Manesme O, Mourey M S, Couturier M, Alvarez F, Hanck A, Bernard O 1988 Short- and long-term vitamin A treatment in children with cholestasis. American Journal of Clinical Nutrition 47: 690–693
4. Aono S, Yamada Y, Keino H et al 1993 Identification of defect in the genes for bilirubin UDP-glucuronosyl-transferase in a patient with Crigler–Najjar syndrome type-II. Biochemical Biophysical Research Communications 197: 1239–1244
5. Baker A, Portmann B, Westaby D, Wilkinson M L, Karani J, Mowat A P 1993 Neonatal sclerosing cholangitis in two siblings: a category of progressive intrahepatic cholestasis. Journal of Pediatric Gastroenterology and Nutrition 17: 317–322
6. Baker A, Rela M, Muiesan P et al 1996 Auxiliary liver transplantation for metabolic diseases. Hepatology 24(suppl): 426A
7. Blaschke T F, Berk P D, Scharschmidt B F, Guyther J R, Vergalla J M, Waggoner J G 1974 Crigler–Najjar syndrome: an unusual course with development of neurologic damage at age eighteen. Pediatric Research 8: 573–590
8. Bonatti H, Muiesan P, Connelly S et al 1997 Hepatic transplantation in children under 3 months of age: a single centre's experience. Journal of Pediatric Surgery 32: 486–488
9. Bosma P J, Chowdhury H R, Goldhoorn B G et al 1992 Sequence of exons and the flanking regions of human bilirubin-UDP-glucuronosyltransferase gene complex and identification of a genetic mutation in a patient with Crigler–Najjar syndrome, type-I. Hepatology 15: 941–947
10. Bosma P J, Goldhoorn B, Bakker C et al 1994 Presence of an additional TA in the TATAA box of B-UGT1 correlates with Gilbert's syndrome. Hepatology 20:266A
11. Brantly M, Courtney M, Crystal R G 1988 Repair of the secretion defect in the Z form of alpha 1-antitrypsin by the addition of a second mutation. Science 242: 1700–1702
12. Brown W R, Sokol R J, Levin M J et al 1988 Lack of correlation between infection with reovirus 3 and extrahepatic biliary atresia or neonatal hepatitis. Journal of Pediatrics 113: 670–676
13. Chiba T, Ohi R, Nio M, Ibrahim M 1992 Late complications in long term survivors of biliary atresia. European Journal of Pediatric Surgery 2: 22–25
14. Clayton P T, Casteels M, Mieli-Vergani G, Lawson A M 1995 Familial giant cell hepatitis associated with greatly increased urinary excretion of bile alcohols; a new inborn error of bile acid synthesis? Pediatric Research 37: 424–431
15. Clayton P T, Leonard J V, Lawson et al 1987 Familial giant cell hepatitis associated with synthesis of 3,7-dihydroxy and 3,7, 12-trihydroxy-5-cholenoic acids. Journal of Clinical Investigation 79: 1031–1038
16. Collins J, Goldfischer S 1990 Perinatal hemochromatosis: one disease, several diseases or a spectrum? Hepatology 12: 176–177
17. Cox D W 1989 Alpha 1-antitrypsin deficiency. In: Scriver C R, Beautt M L, Hubbard R C, Curiel D T, States D J, Holmes M D (eds) The metabolic basis of inherited disease, 6th edn. McGraw-Hill, New York, pp 2409–2437
18. Daum F, Fisher S E (eds) 1983 Extrahepatic biliary atresia. Marcel Dekker, New York
19. Davenport M, Savage M, Mowat A P, Howard E R 1991 The biliary atresia–splenic malformation syndrome. Proceedings of the 5th International Sendai Symposium on Biliary Atresia. Professional Postgraduate Services, Japan, pp 11–14
20. Deprettere A, Portmann B, Mowat A P 1987 Syndromic paucity of the intrahepatic bile ducts: diagnostic difficulty; severe morbidity throughout childhood. Journal of Pediatric Gastroenterology and Nutrition 6: 865–871
21. Deutsch J, Smith A L, Danks D, Campbell P E 1985 Long-term prognosis for babies with neonatal liver disease. Archives of Disease in Childhood 60: 447–451
22. Dick M C, Mowat A P 1985 Hepatitis syndrome in infancy – an epidemiological study with 10-year follow-up. Archives of Disease in Childhood 60: 512–515
23. Doherty D G, Donaldson P T, Whitehouse D B et al 1990 HLA phenotypes and gene polymorphisms in juvenile liver disease associated with alpha 1-antitrypsin deficiency. Hepatology 12: 218–223
24. El Tumi M A, Clark M D, Barrett J J, Mowat A P 1987 A ten minute radiopharmaceutical test in suspected biliary atresia. Archives of Disease in Childhood 62: 180–184
25. Eriksson S, Carlson J, Velez R 1986 The risk of cirrhosis and primary liver cancer in alpha 1-antitrypsin deficiency. New England Journal of Medicine 314: 736–739
26. Farrell M K, Balistreri W F 1986 Parenteral nutrition and hepatobiliary dysfunction. Clinics in Perinatology 13: 197–212
27. Gautier M, Elliot N 1981 Extrahepatic biliary atresia: morphological study of 94 biliary remnants. Archives of Pathology and Laboratory Medicine 105: 397–402
28. Gautier M, Laurent J, Bernard O, Valayer J 1991 Improvement of results after Kasai operation. The need for early diagnosis and surgery. Proceedings of the 5th International Sendai Symposium on Biliary Atresia. Professional Postgraduate Services, Japan, pp 139–147
29. Guggenheim N A, Ringel S B, Silverman A, Grabert P E 1982 Progressive neuro-muscular disease in children with chronic cholestasis and vitamin E deficiency: diagnosis and treatment with alpha-tocopherol. Journal of Pediatrics 100: 51–58
30. Haas J E 1978 Bile duct and liver pathology in biliary atresia. World Journal of Surgery 2: 561–569
31. Hays D M, Kimura K 1980 Biliary atresia – the Japanese experience. Harvard University Press, Cambridge, MA
32. Henriksen N T, Drablos P A, Aagenaes O 1981 Cholestatic jaundice in infancy. The importance of familial and genetic factors in the aetiology and prognosis. Archives of Disease in Childhood 56: 622–627
33. Howard E R 1989 Biliary atresia. In: Schwartz C, Ellis H (eds) Maingot's abdominal operations, 9th edn. Appleton-Century-Crofts, Norwalk, CT, pp 1355–1364
34. Howard E R 1989 Choledochal cysts. In: Schwarz C, Ellis H (eds) Maingot's abdominal operations, 9th edn. Appleton-Century-Crofts, New York, p. 1366
35. Howard E R, Johnstone D I, Mowat A P 1976 Spontaneous perforation of the common bile duct in infants. Archives of Disease in Childhood 51: 883–886
36. Iwatsuki S, Starzl T E, Todo S et al 1988 Experience in 1000 liver transplants under cyclosporine-steroid therapy:

A survival report. Transplantation Proceedings 20S: 498–504
37. Kallas M B E, Baker A, Nash R, Mieli-Vergani G 1997 Chelation/antioxidant treatment is unsuccessful in neonatal hemochromatosis presenting with acute liver failure. Hepatology 26: 534A
38. Kasai M, Ohi R, Kiba T 1980 Intrahepatic bile ducts in biliary atresia. In: Kasai M, Shiraki K (eds) Cholestasis in infancy. Japan Medical Research Foundation, University of Tokyo Press, pp 181–188
39. Kasai M, Ohi R, Chiba T, Hayashi Y 1988 A patient with biliary atresia who died 28 years after hepatic portojejeunostomy. Journal of Pediatric Surgery 23: 431–434
40. Knisely A S 1992 Neonatal hemochromatosis. Advances in Pediatrics 39: 383–403
41. Labrune P, Odievre M, Alagille D 1989 Influence of sex and breastfeeding on liver disease in alpha 1-antitrypsin deficiency (letter). Hepatology 10: 122
42. Lindstedt S, Holme E, Lock E A et al 1992 Treatment of hereditary tyrosinaemia by inhibition of 4-hydroxyphenylpyruvate dioxygenase. Lancet 340: 813–817
43. Littleton E T, Bevis L, Hensen L J et al 1991 Alpha 1-antitrypsin deficiency, complement activation and chronic liver disease. Journal of Clinical Pathology 44: 855–858
44. Lomas D A, Evans D L, Finch J T, Carrell R W 1992 The mechanism of Z alpha$_1$-antitrypsin accumulation in the liver. Nature 357: 605–607
45. McClement J W, Howard E R, Mowat A P 1985 Results of surgical treatment of extrahepatic biliary atresia in the United Kingdom. British Medical Journal 290: 345–349
46. Maggiore G, Bernard O, Riely C A, Hadchouel M, Lemonnier A, Alagille D 1987 Normal serum gamma-glutamyl-transpeptidase activity identifies groups of infants with idiopathic cholestasis with poor prognosis. Journal of Pediatrics 111: 251–252
47. Manolaki A G, Larcher V F, Mowat A P, Barrett J J, Portmann B, Howard E R 1983 The pre-laparotomy diagnosis of biliary atresia. Archives of Disease in Childhood 58: 591–595
48. Markowitz J, Daum F, Kahn E I et al 1983 Arteriohepatic dysplasia. I. Pitfalls in diagnosis and management. Hepatology 3: 74–76
49. Merritt R J 1986 Cholestasis associated with total parenteral nutrition. Journal of Pediatric Gastroenterology and Nutrition 5: 9–22
50. Mieli-Vergani G, Mowat A P 1995 Disorders of infancy and childhood. In: Williams R, Portmann B, Tan KC (eds) The practice of liver transplantation. Churchill Livingstone, Edinburgh, pp 83–91
51. Mieli-Vergani G, Howard E R, Portmann B, Mowat A P 1989 Late referral for biliary atresia: missed opportunities for effective surgery. Lancet i: 421–423
52. Monaghan G, Ryan M, Seddon R, Hume R, Burchell B 1996 Genetic variation in bilirubin-UDP-glucuronosyltransferase gene promotor and Gilbert's syndrome. Lancet 347: 578–581
53. Mondelli M, Mieli-Vergani G, Eddleston ALWF, Williams R, Mowat A P 1984 Lymphocyte cytotoxicity to autologous hepatocytes in alpha 1-antitrypsin deficiency. Gut 25: 1044–1049
54. Morecki R, Glaser J 1989 Reovirus 3 and neonatal biliary disease: discussion of divergent results. Hepatology 10: 515–517
55. Mowat A P 1982 Familial inherited abnormalities: Hepatic disorders. Clinical Gastroenterology 11: 171–206
56. Mowat A P 1994 Hepatitis and cholestasis in infancy: intrahepatic disorders. In: Liver disorders in childhood, 3rd edn. Butterworths, London, pp 43–78
57. Mowat A P 1994 Alpha 1-antitripsin deficiency (PiZZ) and other glycoprotein storage diseases. In: Liver disorders in childhood, 3rd edn. Butterworths, London, pp 335–348
58. Nietgen G W, Vacanti J P, Perez-Atayade A 1992 Intrahepatic bile duct loss in biliary atresia despite portoenterostomy: a consequence of ongoing obstruction. Gastroenterology 102: 2126–2133
69. Odievre M, Hadchouel M, Landrieu C, Alagille D, Elliot N 1981 Long-term prognosis for infants with intrahepatic cholestasis and patent extrahepatic biliary tract. Archives of Disease in Childhood 56: 373–376
60. Ohi R, Nio M, Chiba T, Endo N, Goto M, Ibrahim M 1990 Long-term follow-up after surgery for patients with biliary atresia. Journal of Pediatric Surgery 25: 442–445
61. Ohkohchi N, Chiba T, Ohi R, Mori S 1989 Long-term follow-up of patients with cholangitis after successful Kasai operation in biliary atresia: selection of recipients for liver transplantation. Journal of Pediatric Gastroenterology and Nutrition 9: 416–420
62. Otte J B, Yandza T, De Ville De Goyet J, Tan K C, Salizzoni M, De Hemptinne B 1988 Pediatric liver transplantation: report on 52 patients with a 2-year survival of 86%. Journal of Pediatric Surgery 23: 250–253
63. Ozawa K, Uemoto S, Tanaka K et al 1992 An appraisal of pediatric liver transplantation from living relatives. Initial clinical experience in 20 pediatric liver transplantations from living relatives as donors. Annals of Surgery 216: 547–553
64. Paradis K J G, Freese D K, Sharp H L 1988 A pediatric perspective on liver transplantation. Pediatric Clinics of North America 35: 409–433
65. Pereira G R, Sherman M S, Digiacimo J 1981 Hyper-alimentation induced cholestasis. American Journal of Diseases of Children 135: 842–845
66. Perrault J 1981 Paucity of interlobular bile ducts. Digestive Disease and Science 26: 481–487
67. Pett S, Mowat A P 1987 Crigler–Najjar syndrome types I and II. Clinical experience – King's College Hospital 1972–1987. Phenobarbitone, phototherapy and liver transplantation Molecular Aspects of Medicine 9: 473–482
68. Povey S 1990 The genetics of alpha 1-antitrypsin deficiency in relation to neonatal liver disease. Molecular Biology and Medicine 7: 161–172
69. Psacharopoulos H T, Mowat A P, Cook P J L, Carile P A, Portman B, Rodeck C 1983 Outcome of liver disease associated with alpha 1-antitrypsin deficiency (PiZ); implications for genetic counselling and antenatal diagnosis. Archives of Disease in Childhood 58: 882–887
70. Quigley E M, Marsh M N, Shaffer J L, Markin R S 1993 Hepatobilary complications of total parenteral nutrition. Gastroenterology 104: 1583–1584
71. Rand E B 1998 The genetic basis of the Alagille syndrome. Journal of Pediatric Gastroenterology and Nutrition 26: 234–236
72. Ritter J K, Yeatman M T, Ferreira P, Owens I S 1992 Identification of a genetic alteration in the code for bilirubin UDP-glucoronosyltransferase in the UGT1 gene complex of a Crigler–Najjar type-I patient. Journal of Clinical Investigation 90: 150–155
73. Schroeder W T, Miller M T E, Woo S L C, Saunders G F 1985 Chromosomal localisation of the human alpha 1-antitrypsin gene (Pi) to 14q31–32. American Journal of Human Genetics 37: 868–872
74. Schwarzenberg S J, Sharp H L 1990 Pathogenesis of alpha 1-antitrypsin deficiency-associated liver disease. Journal of Pediatric Gastroenterology and Nutrition 10: 5–12
75. Shamieh I, Kibort P K, Suchy F J, Freese D K 1993 Antioxidant therapy for neonatal iron storage disease. Pediatric Research 33: 109A
76. Shaw B W, Wood R P, Kaufman S S et al 1988 Liver transplant therapy for children. Journal of Pediatric Gastroenterology and Nutrition 7: 157–166 and 797–815
77. Silveira T R, Salzano F M, Howard E R, Mowat A P 1991 Extrahepatic biliary atresia and twinning. Brazilian Journal of Medical and Biological Research 24: 67–71
78. Silveira T R, Salzano F M, Donaldson P T, Mieli-Vergani G, Howard E R, Mowat A P. Association between HLA and extrahepatic biliary atresia. Journal of Pediatric Gastroenterology and Nutrition 1993; 16: 114–117
79. Strife C F, Hug G, Chuck et al 1983 Membranoproliferative glomerulonephritis and alpha 1-antitrypsin deficiency in children. Pediatrics 71: 88–92
80. Stringer M D, Dhawan A, Davenport M, Mieli-Vergani G, Mowat A P, Howard E R 1995 Choledochal cysts: lessons from a 20 year experience. Archives of Disease in Childhood 73: 528–531
81. Sveger T 1988 The natural history of liver disease in alpha 1-antitrypsin deficient children. Acta Paediatrica Scandinavica 77: 847–851
82. Talbot I C, Mowat A P 1975 Liver disease in infancy: histological features and relationship of alpha 1-antitrypsin phenotype. Journal of Clinical Pathology 28: 559–563
83. Tan C E, Driver M, Howard E R, Moscoso G J 1994 Extrahepatic biliary atresia: a first trimester event? Clues from light microscopy and immunohistochemistry. Journal of Pediatric Surgery 29: 808–814
84. Tan K C, Howard E R 1988 Choledochal cyst: a fourteen year surgical experience with 36 patients. British Journal of Surgery 75: 892–895
85. Verloes A, Temple I K, Hubert A F et al 1996 Recurrence of neonatal haemochromatosis in half sibs born of unaffected mothers. Journal of Medical Genetics 33: 444–449
86. Wilkinson M L, Mieli-Vergani G, Ball C, Portmann B, Mowat A P 1991 Endoscopic retrograde cholangiopancreatography (ERCP) in infantile cholestasis. Archives of Disease in Childhood 66: 121–123
87. Yohannan M D, Perry M J, Littlewood J M 1983 Long-term phototherapy in Crigler–Najjar syndrome. Archives of Disease in Childhood 58: 460–462

Part 3

Gastrointestinal disorders

Simon J. Newell

STRUCTURE AND FUNCTION OF THE DEVELOPING GASTROINTESTINAL TRACT

BASIC EMBRYOLOGY

Embryological development is described in Chapter 9.

NEONATAL GASTROINTESTINAL FUNCTION

Digestion and absorption

This is dealt with in detail in Chapter 19, Part 1.

Motility

The ontogeny of motility lags behind digestive and absorptive function (Fig. 31.6). Disordered motor function presents clinically as 'poor tolerance of feeds'. Symptoms include vomiting, high gastric residual volume, bile staining of the gastric aspirate, abdominal distension and reduced stool frequency.

The oesophagus has two complementary functions: swallowing and the prevention of gastro-oesophageal reflux. Nutritive swallowing is seldom present in the infant of less than 34 weeks' postmenstrual age,[85] and 75% of healthy preterm infants require tube feeding until this postconceptional age.[96] The fetus, however, begins to swallow liquor at around 16 weeks' gestation. Initially small volumes are taken, and by term around 500 ml are swallowed each day, an important mechanism in the regulation of liquor volume, explaining the polyhydramnios seen in oesophageal atresia or in fetuses with neuromuscular conditions that reduce swallowing.[203]

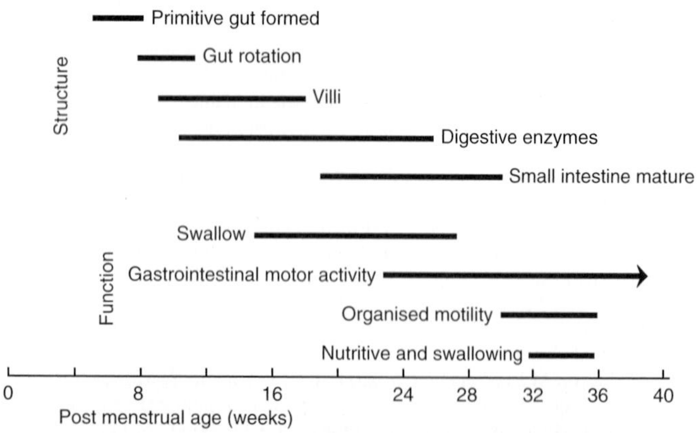

Fig. 31.6 Ontogenic timetable of gut structural and functional development. (Reproduced with permission from Newell[184])

Swallowed liquor may be important ontogenetically. Liquor contains small quantities of protein, carbohydrate and triglyceride, which may be luminal nutrients, and swallowed liquor may encourage the secretion of enteric hormones which have a trophic effect.[153] The observation that gut hypoplasia results from tying off the oesophagus in fetal rabbits even if saline is instilled into the distal gut, suggests a central role for the constituents of liquor. Epidermal growth factor originating from amniotic membrane is an important candidate for promoting fetal gut growth.[122,179]

In the term infant the full complex integrated mechanism of swallowing, with the movement of the bolus of milk into the stomach, protection of the airway, inhibition of respiration, and appropriate relaxation of oesophageal sphincter and gastric fundus, is achieved within a day or two of birth.[143] The mature manometric suck–swallow pattern is characterized by bursts of sucks at a rate of two per second, with associated oesophageal transit occurring on a few occasions during each burst of sucking.[85] In the preterm infant, using the same technique, uncoordinated motor activity is found,[85] with a pattern of motility similar to that seen in older children with reflux oesophagitis.[55]

Competent lower oesophageal sphincter activity is essential to prevent reflux. Pressure within the sphincter must exceed that in the fundus of the stomach.[182] The high pressure in the sphincter is partly a function of the diaphragm and the intra-abdominal segment of the oesophagus, although a muscular anatomical equivalent of the sphincter has now been recognized.[148] Early studies suggested the absence of an effective sphincter pressure in the first weeks of life, but newborn infants do not reflux continuously. More recent studies have demonstrated that term infants have LOS pressures equal to or greater than those seen in older children,[177] but in the preterm infant pressure is low, ranging from a mean of 4 mmHg before 29 weeks' gestation to 18 mmHg at term.[188] Control of the LOS is not well understood, but pressure is known to be reduced by the administration of caffeine[185] and is not greatly disrupted by nasogastric intubation.[2]

Gastric emptying can be observed in the fetus during the second trimester,[64] but may be slow in the preterm infant, presenting as failure to tolerate milk feeds.[35] Pressure in the fundus[188] and antrum[19] rises in the preterm infant with increasing postmenstrual age. Half emptying time for breast milk has been estimated as

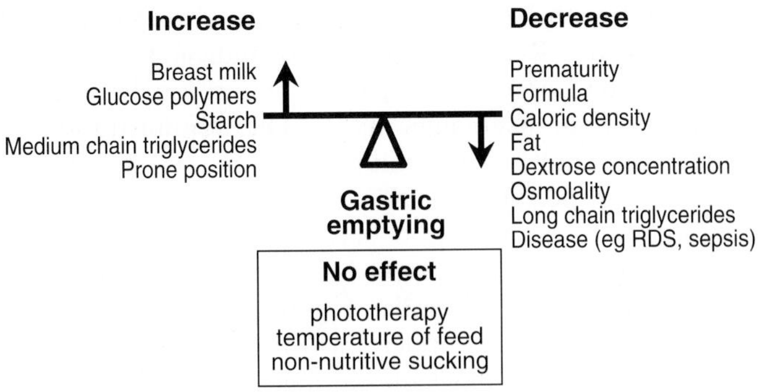

Fig. 31.7 Factors affecting gastric emptying. (Reproduced with permission from Newell[184])

20–40 minutes.[36,73,186] Emptying is faster with breast milk than formula.[73] A number of other factors affect gastric emptying (Fig. 31.7).[122] The addition of breast milk fortifier does not affect gastric emptying during the introduction of milk feeds.[166]

In the preterm infant propagative small intestinal motility is poorly organized, with short bursts of motor activity before 30 weeks' gestation, which subsequently become coordinated, coincident with the timing of nutritive sucking.[278] The coordination of gastric antral activity and duodenal and small intestinal motility occurs with increasing gestation.[19,35] Small intestinal motility and tolerance of feeds is enhanced by previous exposure to enteral nutrition.[17,20,113]

Total gut transit time in our recent study of minimal enteral feeding varied between 1 and 5 days. Passage of stool occurs within 24 hours of birth in 94–98% of healthy infants.[239] The passage of stools is slower in the preterm infant, and frequency is inversely related to gestation (Fig. 31.8).[42,223] Around half of infants under 28 weeks' gestation have not passed their first stool within the first 3 days.[267]

Barrier function

Mucosal protection is afforded by luminal, mucosal and systemic mechanisms (Table 31.20). Gastric acid, the first-line defence against the ingestion of potentially pathogenic bacteria, reduces gastric pH below 4 within hours of birth in all but the most immature infants, in whom this occurs within the first week.[123] The effect of enteral feeding may be to buffer feeds for considerable periods, particularly in the preterm infant.[226] The protective effect of gastric acid is implied by the observation that cimetidine, by reducing gastric acid secretion, may predispose towards NEC.[250]

Intact absorption of large molecules occurs across the neonatal gut. In the milk-fed infant β-lactoglobulin concentrations in the circulation in the preterm infant are 10–100 times higher than those seen in the term infant,[210] whereas absorption of α-lactalbumin diminishes

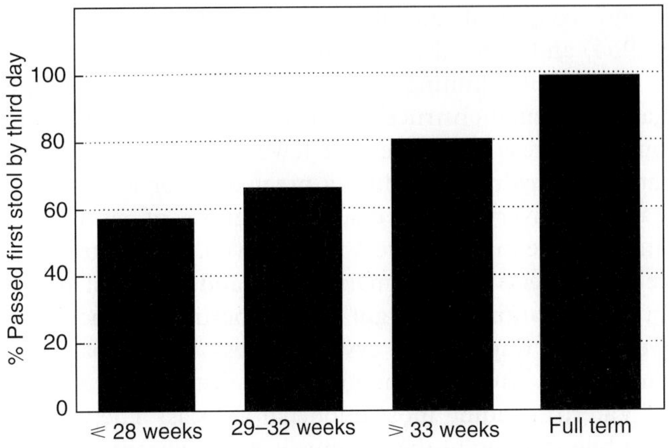

Fig. 31.8 Time of passage of first stool after birth.[42,223,267]

Table 31.20 The gastrointestinal barrier: factors which may protect against intestinal pathogens, toxins and antigens

Non-immune
Intraluminal
gastric acid
motility
pancreaticobiliary secretions
breast milk factors
lysozyme
lactoferrin
oligosaccharides
Mucosal
mucus, bicarbonate and glycocalyx
microvillous membrane
Immune
Secretory IgA
Cellular immunity (GALT and milk)
macrophages
lymphocytes
leukocytes
complement

over the first months of life. This process of gut closure may occur more rapidly if breast milk is given rather than cow's milk formula.[266] The biological and clinical significance of macromolecular absorption in the human is unclear.

SYMPTOMS AND SIGNS OF GASTROINTESTINAL DISEASE

VOMITING

Vomiting is a common symptom and assessment should take account of volume, frequency and content of the vomitus and associated symptoms. Effortless regurgitation may represent gastro-oesophageal reflux (see below). Vomiting is often a symptom of disease outside the gastrointestinal tract, notably infection (meningitis p. 1139, pyelonephritis p. 1148, hepatitis p. 1160), disease of the central nervous system (intracranial haemorrhage p. 1223, hydrocephalus p. 1305), metabolic disorders (galactosaemia

p. 997, congenital adrenal hyperplasia p. 973, thyrotoxicosis p. 964) and heart disease (cardiac failure p. 677).

Persistent vomiting may indicate obstruction. Upper gastrointestinal obstruction leads to vomiting shortly after birth, whereas incomplete or lower obstruction presents later. Polyhydramnios during pregnancy, or a 'mucousy' baby at delivery, should enable a diagnosis of oesophageal atresia to be made before a feed is given. Fetal ultrasound reliably detects diaphragmatic hernia and duodenal atresia, but malrotation, upper gut atresia, partial obstruction or web, and duplication cysts are less often diagnosed antenatally. Most obstruction occurs distal to the ampulla of Vater, including most duodenal atresias. The result is that bile staining of the vomitus is an important indicator of possible obstruction. Bile-stained vomiting indicates a surgical problem (p. 774) until proved otherwise. Herniae are an important site of obstruction at all ages (p. 790).

Vomiting later in the neonatal period is less specific. Functional obstruction occurs in NEC and ileus. Luminal obstruction may occur in meconium ileus (p. 799), meconium plug syndrome (p. 782) and, rarely, lactobezoar. In malrotation the initial symptoms may be intermittent. Hirschsprung's disease may not present with the typical features of abdominal distension and vomiting, and this diagnosis should always be considered if there is delayed passage of meconium (p. 783). Hypertrophic pyloric stenosis (p. 773) is a difficult diagnosis to make when symptoms begin.

UPPER GASTROINTESTINAL BLEEDING

The appearance of small amounts of fresh blood or 'coffee grounds' in vomitus is not rare. In most infants a cause is not found and the prognosis is good. Swallowed maternal blood may lead to haematemesis or melaena. If blood is fresh, Apt's test differentiates between adult and fetal haemoglobin. One part of vomitus or gastric aspirate is mixed with five parts of sterile water and centrifuged; 1 ml of 0.25% sodium hydroxide solution is added to 5 ml of the supernatant, which turns yellow-brown if adult haemoglobin is present but remains pink for a number of minutes if the sample contains fetal haemoglobin. The newborn may ingest maternal blood from a cracked nipple during breast-feeding.

Gastrointestinal bleeding may mark a bleeding diathesis. Classic haemorrhagic disease of the newborn (p. 798) still occurs if adequate vitamin K prophylaxis is not given.[205] Late HDN is more common in liver disease. Disseminated intravascular coagulation, often associated with severe sepsis, and inherited clotting disorders make assessment of coagulation status imperative if there is gastrointestinal bleeding.

Upper gastrointestinal ulceration occurs in the fetus,[12,271] the newborn after perinatal stress[59] and in infants receiving intensive care.[161] At endoscopy, an oesophagogastritis of unknown aetiology occurs in a proportion of infants presenting with haematemesis, frequent regurgitation, or poor growth.[59] Rarely, haematemesis indicates congenital varices, true peptic ulcer, gastric or intestinal volvulus, duplications or haemangioma.[257] The administration of dexamethasone[189] or tolazoline[31] may be associated with bleeding or perforation. We therefore routinely use a ranitidine infusion (0.06–0.12 mg/kg/h) to maintain gastric pH > 4 as prophylaxis in infants receiving dexamethasone.[121] A similar regimen is used for stress bleeding, and other upper gastrointestinal bleeding.[12] Routine use of H_2 blockade during intensive care is not recommended, and may predispose to NEC.[250]

RECTAL BLEEDING

Rapid intestinal transit may allow upper gastrointestinal bleeding to appear as fresh blood per rectum. A small amount of fresh rectal bleeding is commonly due to anorectal fissures, which may be evident on simple inspection by inserting a lubricated auriscope speculum into the anal canal. Rectal perforation is a rare complication of use of a rectal thermometer.[279] A wide variety of intestinal conditions may lead to rectal bleeding, including malrotation, volvulus, intussusception and Hirschsprung's disease (p. 775). Meckel's diverticulum, haemangiomata and bowel telangiectasia most commonly present after the neonatal period. In the preterm infant rectal bleeding may denote NEC (see below).

Colitis, with blood and mucus per rectum, may be secondary to dietary protein intolerance (see below).

DIARRHOEA

The immediate and universal consequence of diarrhoea is loss of water and electrolytes. Dehydration may be rapid because of low body mass and the relative importance of colonic water and electrolyte conservation. Infective causes are common, and a history of contact and stool culture is important (p. 1147). Loose, abnormal stools mark NEC (see below) or even Hirschsprung's disease. In persistent diarrhoea, rare disorders of mucosal function should be considered (see below). In some of these conditions, diarrhoea in utero may produce polyhydramnios and stool output may be enormous. Pancreatic malabsorption occurs in cystic fibrosis, Schwachmann syndrome and pancreatic hypoplasia, but does not usually present in the neonatal period (see below).

CONSTIPATION

Delayed passage of meconium may indicate obstruction or Hirschsprung's disease (p. 783). Meconium ileus, with thick, inspissated stools and abdominal distension, often associated with palpable faecal masses, is almost pathognomonic of cystic fibrosis (see below). In

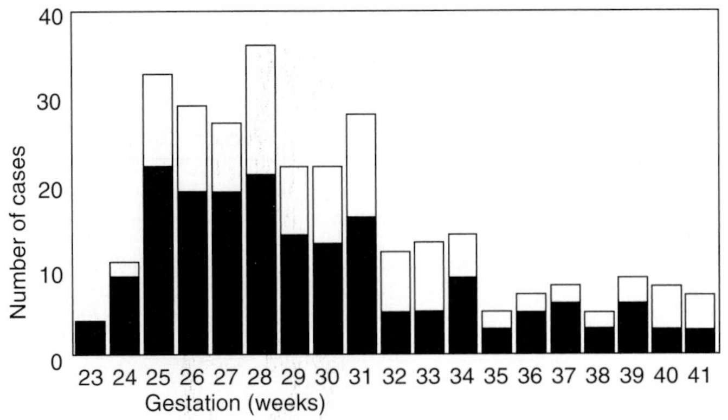

Fig. 31.9 Gestation at diagnosis of NEC: results of a survey in the UK over a period of 1 year. All cases are shown by the open bars. Cases confirmed at surgery, with gas in the portal tract, or free gas in the abdomen are shaded. (Reproduced with permission from Lucas A and Abbott R in collaboration with the Royal College of Paediatrics and Child Health Research Unit)

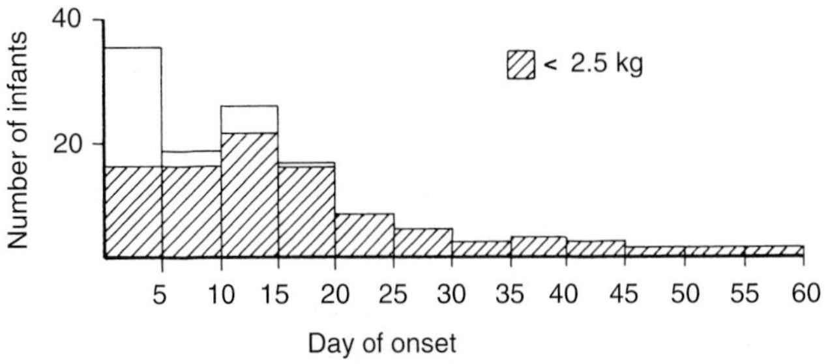

Fig. 31.10 Age of onset of NEC in 129 cases notified to the Communicable Diseases Surveillance Centre, July 1980 to June 1981. (Reproduced with permission from the Communicable Disease Surveillance Centre)[47]

meconium plug syndrome symptoms usually resolve after the first passage of meconium. Hypothyroidism, hypercalcaemia, diabetes insipidus and renal tubular acidosis may all present with constipation. Rare disorders of intestinal pseudo-obstruction often have a history going back to the neonatal period.[255]

In VLBW infants infrequent or delayed passage of meconium or stool may be associated with poor tolerance of feeds, particularly if preterm delivery has been preceded by poor intrauterine growth.[74] Suppositories may be helpful in inducing defecation. If infrequent passage of stools remains a problem, a small dose of lactulose may be justified.

Table 31.21 'Risk' factors incriminated in the aetiology of NEC

Prematurity
Intrauterine growth retardation
Abruptio placentae
Premature rupture of membranes
Perinatal asphyxia
Low Apgar score
Umbilical catheterization
Hypoxia and shock
Hypothermia
Patent ductus arteriosus
Non-human milk formula
Hypertonic feeds
Rapid introduction of enteral feeds
Fluid overload
Pathogenic bacteria
Polycythaemia
Thrombocytosis
Anaemia
Exchange transfusion
Cyanotic congenital heart disease

NECROTIZING ENTEROCOLITIS

EPIDEMIOLOGY

The incidence of NEC is between one and three cases per 1000 livebirths. NEC occurs in 2–5% of VLBW infants, and in 1–8% of NICU admissions.[13,131,135] Based on these figures, some 500–1500 cases could be expected each year in England and Wales. A survey was carried out by the British Paediatric Surveillance Unit, ending in 1994, and reported 300 new cases over 1 year, with an overall mortality of 22%.[27] As in previous studies, most infants were preterm with a median gestation of 29 weeks (Fig. 31.9). However, 12% of infants with NEC are born at term.[13,44,131] Onset of symptoms is most commonly in the second week (Fig. 31.10). There are no seasonal, sexual or geographic patterns with NEC. The NICHHD made the startling observation of a variation in prevalence from 4 to over 20% of VLBW infants between centres across North America.[248] It has been suggested that this variability in the incidence of NEC between neonatal centres suggests an iatrogenic component.[44]

NEC is a common end-point precipitated by a number of different circumstances (Table 31.21). Infants with NEC may be divided into three groups:[13] in the term infant, it is almost universally associated with risk factors for gut ischaemia, principally perinatal asphyxia. NEC may occur at term in Hirschsprung's disease.[13,60] Preterm infants under 30 weeks' gestation who develop NEC usually have no risk factors other than their prematurity. In contrast, preterm infants of 30–36 weeks' gestation have greater evidence of perinatal asphyxia than case controls, and a higher rate of intrauterine growth retardation.[13] When perinatal asphyxia is the main underlying factor NEC occurs in the first days of life. In most preterm infants, NEC develops in the second or third week after the introduction of enteral feeds (Fig. 31.10).[47,163]

PATHOLOGY

NEC may affect any part of the gastrointestinal tract. In infants who come to surgery or die the commonest sites of damage are the terminal ileum, caecum and ascending colon.[218] NEC is a transmural disease. The bowel appears purple and discoloured, and is often distended, with areas of serosal damage. Pneumatosis, the presence of submucosal and subserosal gas within the bowel wall, is the most characteristic appearance of the gut at laparotomy, histologically and radiographically. This gas is largely nitrogen and hydrogen and is produced by gas-forming bacteria.[71]

Histologically the earliest signs are a coagulative necrosis of the mucosa, with microthrombus formation, leading to patchy mucosal ulceration, oedema and haemorrhage.[102] Early in the disease the inflammatory cell infiltrate is small, suggesting that infection does not initiate the process, although later cellular infiltrate is considerable.

Cytokines have an important role in mediating intestinal inflammation and damage in NEC.[131] The relative importance of individual cytokines is difficult to determine. Their presence locally may represent a secondary or non-specific response to tissue insult, and any systemic response may not reflect local activity. Raised levels of interleukins 1, 3 and 6, TNFα, and platelet-activating factor may predict the severity of the disease[175] and the presence of sepsis.[91] Current evidence points to a central role for the lipid-derived proinflammatory cytokine PAF.[131] Administration of PAF results in histological NEC in rats exposed to hypoxia,[180] and pretreatment with PAF receptor antagonists reduces the incidence and severity of NEC induced by TNFα, lipopolysaccharide, hyperosmolar feeds and early exposure to non-pathogenic coliforms.[33,106] Human infants with NEC have high levels of PAF and reciprocally low levels of PAF-acetylhydrolase, an enzyme important in PAF degradation.[106,131] PAF levels increase after enteral feeds in infants developing subsequently proven NEC.[159] Glycosaminoglycans, important for maintaining mucosal integrity, are greatly reduced in NEC.[3]

AETIOLOGY

Numerous potential risk factors have been explored (Table 31.21). It is clear that none is in itself necessary or sufficient to produce NEC in the newborn infant. The major candidates are hypoxia, prematurity and poor mucosal integrity, the bacterial flora and the presence of a metabolic substrate – milk – in the intestinal lumen (Fig. 31.11). These subjects will be discussed individually and have been extensively reviewed.[44,100,131,133,135]

Gut hypoxia

The pathology of NEC, with vascular congestion, haemorrhage and ulceration, accords with the importance of hypoxia, and the cytokines involved in this condition may mediate their effects through reduction of local perfusion. The small intestine is served by the superior mesenteric artery, which divides into branches in the mesentery, forming arcades of arterioles supplying the submucosa and mucosa.

In the term infant, risk factors for gut hypoxia are almost invariably present when NEC occurs. NEC is well recognized after severe generalized hypoxia, maternal cocaine abuse and exchange transfusion.[13,274] Experimentally, in lambs, polycythaemia reduces oxygen delivery to the gut[67] and produces NEC.[144,280] In the infant a high PCV increases the risk of NEC, but may only do so when an exchange transfusion is performed.[275]

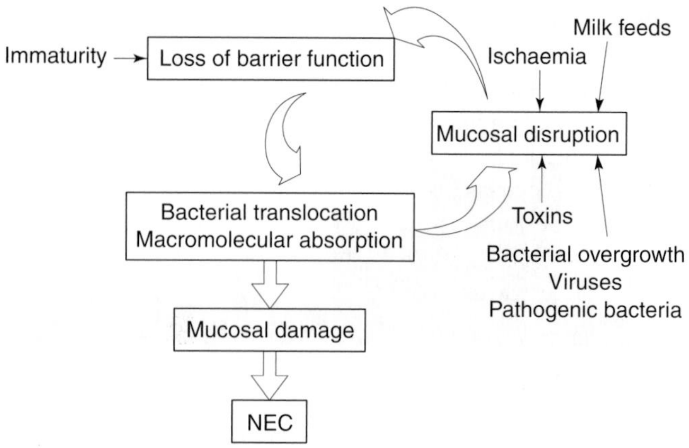

Fig. 31.11 Interaction of the main factors involved in the pathogenesis of NEC.

An adverse intrauterine environment leads to chronic fetal hypoxia and intrauterine growth restriction, and diversion of cardiac output away from the gut.[88] Small studies have shown that abnormal fetal Doppler studies do predispose to NEC.[88,162,168] A large multicentre European study showed increased perinatal mortality but no increase in NEC in infants with abnormal Doppler studies of fetal blood flow velocities.[119] In IUGR fetuses, oligohydramnios and fetal echogenic bowel predict feed intolerance.[74] Intrauterine growth restriction is an important risk factor for NEC in infants above 29 weeks' gestation, although this group are less likely to need surgery.[13,243]

The preterm infant is at particular risk of intestinal hypoxia during intensive care. In the animal model, bacterial colonization and excessive formula feeding do not precipitate NEC unless hypoxia is also present.[32] In the adult pig gut blood flow increases after feeds, whereas in the newborn oxygen extraction is increased but not blood flow, thereby predisposing to tissue hypoxia.[53] Patent ductus arteriosus, with left-to-right shunting and retrograde flow in the aorta during diastole, diminishes superior mesenteric artery blood flow.[127] PDA is more common in infants with NEC,[214] but its causative role has not been borne out in infants with congenital heart disease.[146] Indomethacin reduces gut perfusion and, if given to the mother for more than 2 days immediately before delivery, predisposes to NEC.[48,160]

Some of the earliest reports of NEC were in infants after exchange transfusion for rhesus haemolytic disease through a UVC.[195] Umbilical arterial cannulation has since been held to reduce gut blood supply and provoke embolization or thrombus formation, predisposing to NEC. However, the studies confirming this relationship were all published prior to 1980.[135] More recent prospective studies have shown no difference in the rate of NEC between high and low umbilical artery catheters,[43,124] or with early or late introduction of milk feeds.[56] The umbilical venous catheter, even if malpositioned and associated with other complications, appears not to predispose towards NEC.[204]

Mucosal integrity

Loss of mucosal integrity disrupts barrier function, allowing macromolecular absorption and bacterial translocation, and interferes with digestion. The preterm gut has an immature microvillous membrane with a relative deficiency of mucus and secretory IgA.[258] Prematurity results in increased permeability to small and large molecules.[15,265] Any further mucosal damage increases permeability to microorganisms and toxins.[109,264] Extreme prematurity, or the combination of prematurity and gut hypoperfusion, therefore results in invasion of bacteria, or the entry of toxins and the products of digestion into the mucosa. This process may initiate NEC.[44,109,142] Antenatal corticosteriod administration induces intestinal maturation, decreases permeability and protects against NEC.[10,109,110]

Microbial infection

NEC is not infectious. In sporadic disease the presence of bacteria is probably necessary for NEC to occur, but not sufficient without other risk factors. In epidemics of NEC there may be an infectious agent. During epidemics, a high frequency of gastrointestinal illness among intensive care staff and other infants on the neonatal unit has been recognized. A large number of infectious agents have been found in epidemics of NEC (Table 31.22).[44,212] Infection with *Clostridia*, which produce a potent toxin, occurs in epidemics.[89] *Clostridia* infection is less frequently seen in sporadic cases,[240] but is important in Hirschsprung's enterocolitis.[241] Infants with NEC during epidemics may fare better than infants with sporadic disease, although this may be related to heightened awareness and earlier detection of NEC on the neonatal unit.[44]

Table 31.22 Organisms associated with epidemics of NEC[44,212]

Klebsiella spp.
Non-pathogenic *Escherichia coli*
Enterotoxigenic *Escherichia coli*
Enterobacter spp.
Clostridium difficile
Clostridium butyricum
Clostridium perfringens
Salmonella spp.
Pseudomonas aeruginosa
Rotavirus
Coronavirus

Table 31.23 Organisms isolated from blood cultures in infants with NEC

	A	B	C	D	E
Coagulase-negative staphylococci	–	10	6	11	2
Staphylococcus aureus	1	4	–	2	2
Escherichia coli	24	3	8	3	3
Klebsiella	6	1	7	5	–
Enterobacter spp.	–	–	1	4	4
Proteus mirabilis	1	1	–	1	–
Clostridium spp.	1	5	2	–	–
Streptococcus faecalis	2	1	1	–	–
Pseudomonas aeruginosa	2	–	–	–	1
Candida albicans	1	–	–	–	–
Miscellaneous	4	2	–	5	–

Reference numbers: A[129]; B[47]; C[13]; D[169]; E[38]

In sporadic disease a large variety of microorganisms have been found, and no single organism is reliably associated with its pathogenesis (Table 31.23).[44,47,87,142] Positive blood cultures are found in 10–50% of cases, and correlate with isolates from stool or peritoneal fluid.[8,13,38,169] Overall, the microbiological picture is dominated by *Escherichia coli*, *Klebsiella*, *Enterobacter* and coagulase-negative staphylococci. In surgical patients, most of whom had gut perforation, peritoneal culture showed a wider variety of microorganisms in ELBW infants than in larger preterm infants. A predominance of *E. coli* was found in the latter.[214] Staphylococcal infection may be more important in infants who have not received milk.[169]

In the bacteriologically peculiar environment of the hospitalized preterm infant, unhindered proliferation of a small number of potentially pathogenic species may occur, promoting bacterial translocation and absorption of toxic products.[142] Gram-positive organisms in the stool of infants with NEC may interact with *E. coli* to increase the pathogenic properties of the latter.[196] Among *Klebsiellae* rapid carbohydrate fermenters are more pathogenic,[34,272] but this is not the case with some other bacteria.[87]

Enteral nutrition

The role of milk in NEC remains contentious. All studies have demonstrated that most infants with NEC have received milk.[13,29,129,214,218,234] In the BPSU survey, 90% of subjects had received enteral feeds prior to the onset of NEC.[27] In unfed infants with NEC symptoms present early, often following an asphyxial insult.[44] Intraluminal milk may simply promote bacterial proliferation or increase bacterial endotoxin production by Gram-negative bacteria.[29,240] Bacterial action upon unabsorbed nutrients results in gas formation[71] and the production of short-chain fatty acids, which can be toxic to the intestinal epithelium. Long-chain fats and undigested casein may contribute to inflammation and injury,[131] and the lipid in milk increases mucosal permeability.[54] In healthy infants who do not develop NEC milk induces a cellular and humoral inflammatory mucosal reaction, with an increase in circulating cytokines.[131,159]

Early studies showed reduced NEC when enteral feeds were delayed or replaced with parenteral nutrition.[75,81] Two other studies support the view that delayed oral feeding does not prevent NEC, but the later study was not randomized.[22,140] The evidence that aggressive enteral feeding with a rapid increase in feed volume is causative, is more compelling.[169] Hyperosmolar feeds produce mucosal damage,[61] and in one study NEC was seen in almost 90% of infants fed milk with twice the osmolality of breast milk.[21]

Breast milk protects against NEC:[30,155] infants given breast milk are 7–10 times less likely to suffer NEC, a benefit which is attenuated when breast milk is given with formula. Putative important factors in breast milk include immunoglobulins, lysozyme, complement, macrophages, growth factors and PAF-acetylhydrolase.[131,178] In the rat, maternal milk protects against NEC produced by hypoxia and heavy bacterial colonization.[7] In the same model the addition of milk macrophages to formula also offered a degree of protection.[201]

Immature patterns of motility and decreased digestive capacity predispose the preterm infant to NEC.[16,184] Trophic feeding – the use of minimal enteral feeds with parenteral nutrition – is of established value in improving gastrointestinal function, and may protect against NEC.[139]

CLINICAL FEATURES

Presentation may vary from insidious deterioration, with non-specific symptoms, lethargy, temperature instability and apnoeic episodes, to a rapidly progressive illness with shock, peritonitis and death. In the infant without gastrointestinal symptoms, early recognition of NEC requires a high index of suspicion. The infant's general condition is similar to that seen in sepsis, with pallor, skin mottling and jaundice. Bleeding may be due to DIC. Some infants have initial mild feed intolerance and then demonstrate the classic triad of abdominal distension, bloody mucousy stools and bile-stained vomit or aspirates.

The commonest abdominal sign is distension (Table 31.24). Careful assessment should be made for tenderness. Often distended loops are palpable and an intra-abdominal mass may represent localized perforation. Blue abdominal discoloration suggests disease progression, and occasionally the abdominal wall becomes indurated and red, a sign of underlying peritonitis. Proctoscopy with an auroscope may reveal friable haemorrhagic mucosa, but should be performed with care.[78] Equally important is a general assessment of cardiorespiratory function, blood pressure and perfusion.

Table 31.24 Presenting features of NEC (%)

	A	B	C
Abdominal distension	78	75	58
Lethargy	9	71	30
Visible blood in stool	28	70	68
Hypotonia	–	63	–
Vomiting/aspirates (± bile)	28	52	46
Abdominal tenderness	21	43	–
Apnoea	27	41	54
Bleeding diathesis	–	20	–
Abdominal wall oedema	–	19	–
Shock/sepsis	24	–	26

Reference numbers: A[129]; B[47]; D[280]

INVESTIGATION

Immediate investigations include haemoglobin, white cell and platelet counts, coagulation studies, urea, electrolytes and albumin and blood gas analysis. The platelet count initially rises, but falls with disease progression and DIC. Blood and fluid losses into the abdomen are often larger than appreciated, and abnormalities of perfusion, anaemia and electrolyte balance are common. Metabolic acidosis is usually a marker of shock. Carbon dioxide retention or hypoxia may represent respiratory failure due to apnoea or diaphragmatic splinting, and indicates the need for ventilatory support.

Abdominal radiography is mandatory. The bowel appearance varies from a gasless abdomen (Fig. 31.12) to

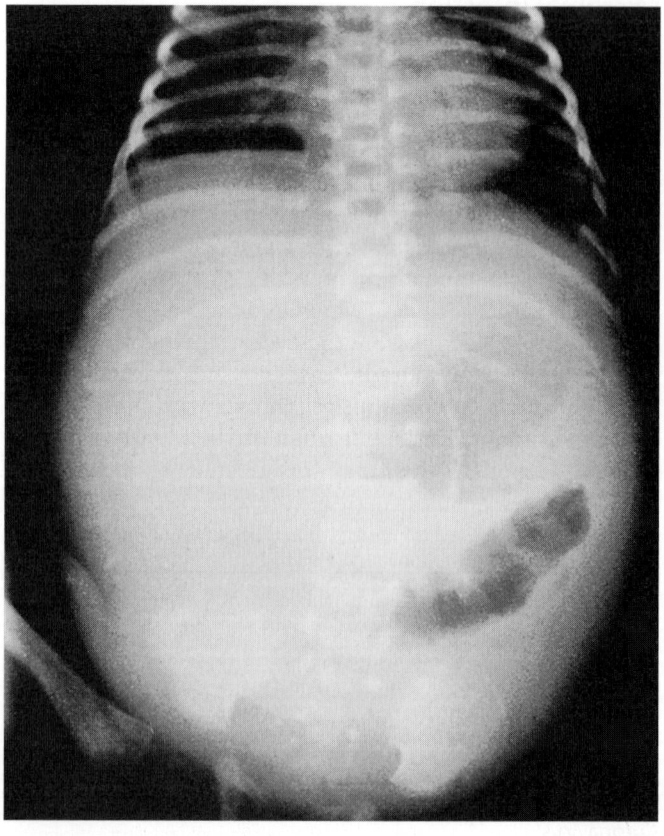

Fig. 31.12 Plain abdominal X-ray showing ascites in NEC.

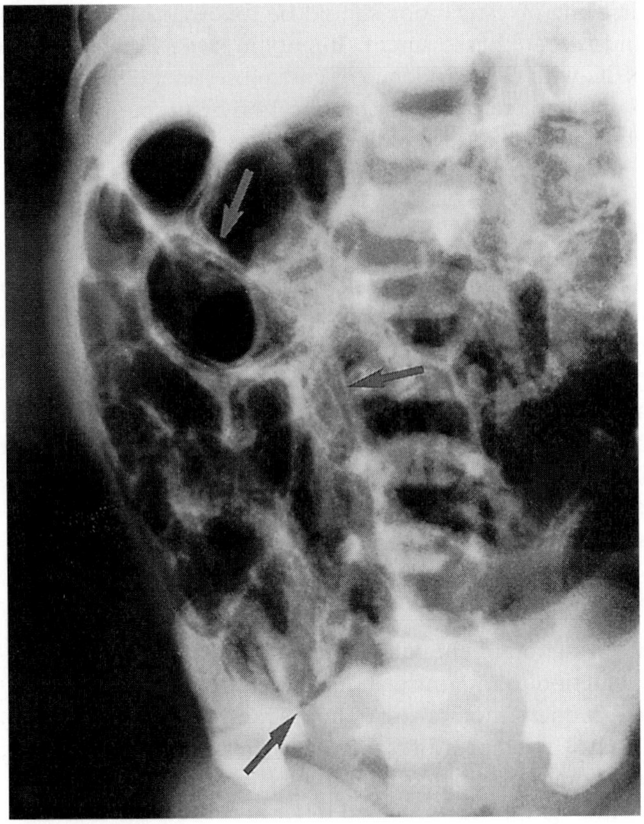

Fig. 31.13 Plain abdominal X-ray showing intraluminal gas (arrows) in NEC.

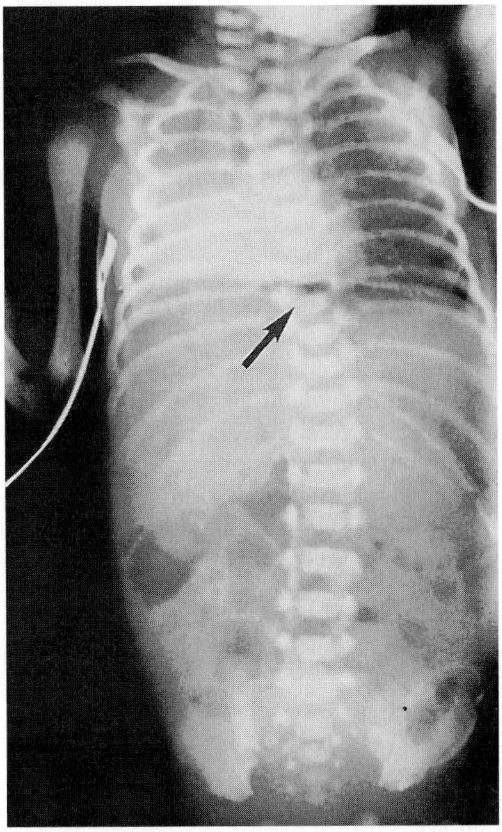

Fig. 31.14 Plain abdominal X-ray (antero-posterior, supine) in the presence of a perforation: free gas is seen under the diaphragm (arrowed).

dilated loops of thick-walled gut with fluid levels. The pathognomonic radiographic appearance is pneumatosis intestinalis due to bubbles of gas in the gut wall (Fig. 31.13). In severe disease gas collects within the portal venous system.[135,214]

Radiological detection of perforation is not easy (Figs 31.14, 31.15). Free air may be seen in only two-thirds of infants in whom perforation is present. A lateral horizontal beam shoot-through X-ray may allow easier detection of an anterior collection of gas, but on a supine film, free gas is best seen between the liver and the diaphragm.

Acute-phase proteins (CRP) are helpful in monitoring progress.[221] Stool contains reducing substances[23] and gut protein loss is increased with increased stool α_1-antitrypsin.[224] T-cryptantigen status, which can change in

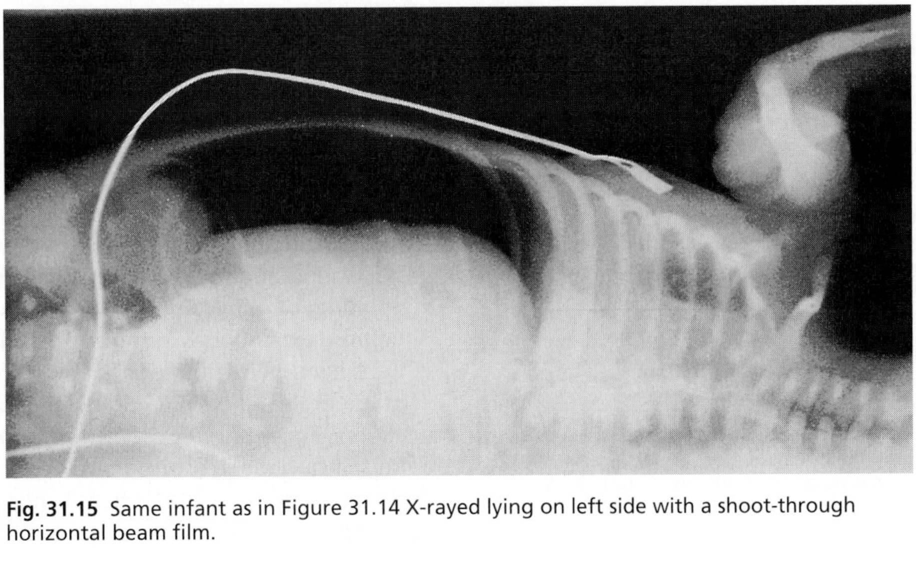

Fig. 31.15 Same infant as in Figure 31.14 X-rayed lying on left side with a shoot-through horizontal beam film.

severe colitis, should be determined as it predisposes to massive haemolysis with blood product administration.[190] Abdominal ultrasound may allow the detection of masses or ascites. Contrast studies are usually avoided during the acute phase of the disease, and should not be done outside a centre capable of providing immediate surgery.

DIFFERENTIAL DIAGNOSIS

In most cases recognition of NEC is not difficult, and once abdominal signs are present the diagnosis is clear. Other causes of gut ischaemia, including malrotation, volvulus and hernia, should be considered. Isolated rectal bleeding has a differential diagnosis, discussed above (p. 746). Abdominal distension with regurgitation of one or two feeds is common and, although NEC should be considered, it is reasonable simply to stop oral feeds for a few hours and observe the infant who has no other signs. 'NEC' may be the presenting feature of Hirschsprung's disease or cystic fibrosis.[241,277] Isolated perforation without evidence of NEC probably represents a different process, and occurs typically in the least mature infant in the ileum or duodenum.[163,249,270] Management of isolated perforation is similar to that of perforated NEC.

TREATMENT

The spectrum of clinical presentations makes it difficult and inappropriate to define a rigid regimen of management. Staging criteria may be helpful in tailoring treatment to the natural history of the disease[15,136,260] (Table 31.25). Stage 1 is suspected NEC, and requires full investigation to exclude other pathologies, notably infection. The initial management steps including cessation of enteral feeds, nasogastric suction, intravenous access, and first-line investigations should be followed by monitoring and repeated assessment. Infants in stage 2 have definite NEC with clear evidence of gastrointestinal disease. Stage 3 is characterized by complication with perforation or clinical signs of severe illness.[15]

Table 31.25 Clinical staging system for NEC[15]

Stage 1: Suspect
- History of perinatal stress
- Systemic signs of ill health: temperature instability, lethargy, apnoea
- Gastrointestinal manifestations: poor feeding, increased volume of gastric aspirate, vomiting, mild abdominal distension, faecal occult blood (no fissure)

Stage 2: Confirmed
- Any of features of stage 1 *plus*:
- Persistent occult, or gross gastrointestinal bleeding, marked abdominal distension
- Abdominal radiograph: intestinal distension, bowel wall oedema, unchanging bowel loops, pneumatosis intestinalis, portal vein gas

Stage 3: Advanced
- Any of features of stages 1 or 2 *plus*:
- Deterioration in vital signs, evidence of shock or severe sepsis, or marked gastrointestinal haemorrhage
- Abdominal radiograph shows any of features of stage 2 *plus* pneumoperitoneum

Medical

The overall aim of treatment is to rest the gut, control infection, restore metabolic equilibrium and maintain the infant in an optimal condition until the bowel heals. The preterm infant is particularly vulnerable to undernutrition and, with the suspension of enteral feeding, parenteral nutrition should be provided. Surgery is indicated if intestinal perforation occurs, if the infant's general condition deteriorates, or if intra-abdominal pathology persists beyond a few days.

The major components of medical management are as follows:

- Cessation of enteral feeding and regular nasogastric suction to minimize abdominal distension;
- Frequent monitoring of temperature, pulse, respiratory rate, blood pressure, fluid balance and abdominal girth;
- Plain abdominal radiography. If symptoms persist, radiographs are repeated 6–12-hourly on the first day of NEC, and while perforation remains likely;
- Peripheral venous access for antibiotics, blood and plasma;
- Blood cultures and septic screen; a lumbar puncture is not usually performed;
- Intravenous antibiotics: a triple antibiotic regimen is commonly used. Second-generation β-lactamase-resistant cephalosporins (e.g. cefuroxime) are not effective against Gram-negative organisms, notably enterobacter. In general, Gram-negative cover is best achieved with gentamicin or a third-generation cephalosporin (e.g. ceftazidime), although resistance to the latter is emerging. Gram-positive cover with amoxycillin or vancomycin is suitable. The broad-spectrum regimen should also include metronidazole. A regimen taking account of the dominant flora on a NICU is wise and may need revision in the light of bacterial cultures.[38]
- Volume replacement: fluid losses from the circulation into the gut or peritoneum can be easily underestimated. Immediate management of suspected NEC in an infant who appears unwell includes 15 ml/kg of 4.5% albumin solution or other suitable volume expander. Monitoring should include peripheral perfusion, peripheral–core temperature gradient, urine output and plasma bicarbonate or base excess. Aggressive circulatory support with volume and, if necessary, inotropes should be given to maintain peripheral and hence, hopefully, splanchnic perfusion;

- Regular blood gas analysis and early recourse to assisted ventilation if there is evidence of respiratory distress, failure or apnoeic episodes;
- Maintenance of normal urea, electrolytes, calcium and hydration by daily or twice-daily adjustments to rate and composition of i.v. fluids. Prompt treatment of intercurrent problems such as hypoglycaemia (p. 947), jaundice (p. 726) and DIC (p. 803);
- Transfuse to maintain haemoglobin. The platelet count may fall and transfusion may be necessary if the count is $<30 \times 10^9$/l;
- Removal of umbilical cannulae;
- Insertion of a percutaneous central venous line for total parenteral nutrition;
- Total parenteral nutrition (Chapter 20) is always necessary in definite NEC, for which enteral starvation for at least 7–10 days is needed. During the first 24–48 hours, and when an infant is very unwell, amino acid load is reduced and lipid infusion is avoided. In suspected NEC, if NEC is disproved feeds may be recommenced after 48–72 hours and TPN may not be necessary;
- Analgesics should be used liberally. Infants with NEC suffer pain and considerable stress.[4] An opiate infusion (e.g. morphine or alfentanyl) is recommended. Opiate-induced apnoea is not a problem in a neonatal unit where IPPV is available;
- Barrier nursing: in most units scrupulous handwashing and prevention of cross-infection is standard for all patients. True barrier nursing may be needed in the event of an outbreak of NEC.

The majority of infants managed medically recover steadily. Antibiotics, enteral starvation and TPN are usually given for at least 7 days from the time of recovery from the initial severe illness. Perforation most often occurs in the first 48 hours, but may become apparent at any time during the illness. By 7–14 days from diagnosis, most infants are free of signs of infection, have a soft abdomen, normal bowel sounds and a normal abdominal X-ray. Enteral feeding is restarted cautiously, using 0.5–1.0 ml/h for the first 24 hours and thereafter increasingly slowly. Expressed breast milk is the milk of choice; alternatively a preterm formula is used. Most infants who recover without the need for surgery will tolerate one of these milks (see surgical management for alternative feeds).

Surgical

Of infants with NEC 20–50% require surgery.[13,128,230] Unfortunately, aetiological risk factors are poor predictors of the need for operative treatment.[9]

Indications

The commonest indication for surgery is intestinal perforation, seen in 40–70% of infants who require surgery.[103,145,214] The commonest site of perforation is the terminal ileum, and multiple perforations are not unusual. Perforation may occur without visible gas on the plain abdominal radiograph. Abdominal air from pulmonary airleak is usually differentiated by its coincidence with pneumothorax (p. 525). Paracentesis showing at least 0.5 ml of brown-stained fluid, or the presence of bacteria on Gram stain, usually indicates perforation. Paracentesis, however, may be positive with extensive necrosis, and may be falsely reassuring. It is not widely used in the UK.[134,137,230]

Clinical deterioration despite intensive medical treatment is more difficult to define. Abdominal signs, including a fixed dilated loop of intestine on serial radiographs, abdominal wall erythema, or the development of an inflammatory mass, point to the need for surgery, as does general worsening in the infant's condition[134,230] or a failure of intra-abdominal signs to resolve.

Operation

At surgery bowel necrosis is most commonly ileocaecal, and in around a third is limited to the colon, but it may occur at any point in the gut.[145] Extensive gut necrosis may be inoperable and lethal.[214] The choice of operation depends upon the extent of necrosis, the extent of NEC in non-necrotic gut, and the general condition of the infant. Among the numerous surgical procedures described, four main options exist.[206]

The commonest procedure is laparotomy, resection of necrotic bowel, and creation of a proximal stoma and a distal mucous fistula.[103,206] This necessitates a second procedure to restore gut continuity. Large fluid, electrolyte and nutrient losses may occur through a small bowel stoma, especially when milk is reintroduced. This has led to earlier timing of the second procedure, which is often performed within 2 months of the initial surgery.[213,269] The possibility of stricture in the distal limb necessitates contrast study before the second operation and, if needed, the stricture can be successfully resected at the same time.[80] Postoperative complications include systemic, wound and intra-abdominal sepsis which, perhaps surprisingly, occur only in a small minority.[103] Stoma-related complications such as dehiscence are unusual, and less likely if good nutritional status can be achieved.[269]

Secondly, in the infant who is stable, with well-circumscribed disease, primary anastomosis may be performed at the time of initial gut resection. The anastomosis heals well, problems with losses from the stoma are avoided, and hospital stay may be reduced.[230] In the two-stage procedure strictures are nearly always in the distal loop of gut[220] and, following primary anastomosis, it is possible that the likelihood of late stricture is reduced.[181]

An alternative strategy is peritoneal drainage performed on the NICU under local anaesthesia. This comprises the insertion of one or two soft drains into the right lower quadrant, together with broad-spectrum antibiotic cover and nasogastric aspiration. Initially used in infants who were judged too unwell for surgery, it was noted that some infants thereby avoided surgery.[116] This technique has its proponents, but is now less frequently used and is usually reserved for small infants who are clinically unstable and deemed unsuitable for laparotomy.[70,176] If clinical deterioration occurs after drainage, laparotomy is indicated.

Finally, in a group with a generally poor prognosis[230] disease may be so extensive that resection cannot be performed or would entail extensive resection of the intestine. A proximal jejunostomy can be used to defunction distal bowel. A 'second-look' laparotomy is performed in the next few days, and necrotic gut resected.

Postoperative management

Nutritional support and intensive care is usually needed for 1–3 weeks. Enteral feeds are reintroduced slowly, using breast milk if available, as described above. If milk is not tolerated, a lactose-free formula containing hydrolysed protein and medium-chain triglycerides is used, and in some centres this is the feed of choice. If rapid gut transit and diarrhoea persist loperamide may be used, sometimes combined with a feed thickener. In the infant who is tolerating feeds but not gaining weight, salt and water depletion, malabsorption, and intestinal, systemic or urinary tract infection should be considered. Calories and protein may be added to breast milk using a commercial fortifier[166] (p. 340). Formula may be supplemented with a powdered carbohydrate/fat mixture in 2–5% solution, but this may provoke or exacerbate diarrhoea. Joint management with a paediatric dietitian is advised.

Late strictures caused by submucosal thickening and fibrosis[220] may have become more common.[141] In the infant who does not need surgery, strictures are less common and shorter.[141,145] Most are apparent within 6 weeks, and almost all within 4 months.[145,220] Overall strictures occur in 10–40%, and although some narrowing seen on contrast studies may resolve spontaneously, strictures that lead to symptoms of acute or subacute obstruction need surgery. Most are colonic, but strictures occur at the site of anastomosis and in the small bowel[117,145] (Fig. 31.16). Short bowel syndrome may require long-term management, especially if the ileocaecal valve has been resected (see below).

OUTCOME

In about 10% of cases, usually within a month of initial presentation, relapse occurs. Management is no different from that of the first attack. It is not clear if management of the first attack can alter risk of recurrence. The later complications of NEC are shown in Table 31.26.[130]

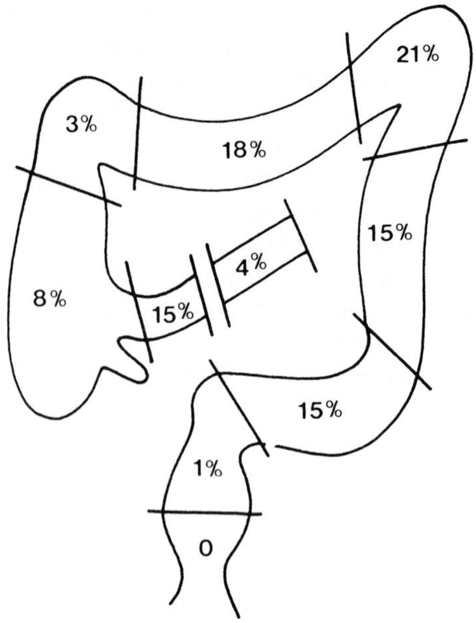

Fig. 31.16 Sites of intestinal stricture formation after NEC. (Reproduced with permission from Janik et al[117])

Table 31.26 Late complications of NEC

Recurrence
Intestinal stricture
Enterocyst
Short gut syndrome
Enterocolic fistula
Anastomotic leak
Cholestasis
Malabsorption
Atresias and aganglionosis
Salt and water depletion
Polyposis
Treatment complications

Mortality is higher in infants of less than 28 weeks' gestation and birthweight less than 1000 g. The presence of extensive disease, bacteraemia, DIC or persistent ascites is also a bad prognostic indicator.[103,129,145,167,214] Intestinal perforation and the need for surgery does not necessarily spell a higher mortality.[128] There has been an improvement in survival over the last two decades, with overall survival rates of 70–90%.[29,103,112,130,145,214]

The nutrition, growth and gastrointestinal function of survivors depend upon the site and extent of disease and resection: in the absence of short bowel syndrome (see below) prognosis is generally very good, although not infrequently short-term problems with rapid gut transit, diarrhoea and malabsorption are seen as gut adaptation occurs.[1,112,149,233] Specific nutritional deficiencies due to terminal ileal resection (particularly vitamin B_{12}) should not be forgotten.[46]

Long-term neurodevelopmental follow-up is needed in view of the high rate of disability in survivors of more severe NEC.[112] In a case control study a larger proportion of infants who had needed surgical treatment had neurodevelopmental problems, compared to gestation- and birthweight-matched infants without NEC, or those with NEC who needed only medical treatment.[243]

PREVENTION

In the term infant, measures that reduce perinatal asphyxia would reduce NEC.[13,44] Prompt resuscitation and restoration of normal circulation and acid–base status may be of further benefit. After significant birth asphyxia our practice includes the delayed, slow introduction of enteral feeds, which are avoided during any acute encephalopathy.

Antenatal steroids given to the mother at risk of preterm delivery reduces the risk of NEC.[10] This may be mediated through the amelioration of preterm lung disease, or by a direct effect upon gut maturation and mucosal integrity.[109] Maternal antibiotics in prolonged rupture of the membranes have no effect upon NEC.[68] Surfactant replacement therapy in respiratory distress syndrome makes NEC less likely.[50] General measures such as the maintenance of good tissue perfusion, blood pressure, hydration, and avoidance of hypotension, hypoxia and hypothermia are all likely to reduce NEC. Excessive fluids have been implicated in the pathogenesis of NEC.[14] In the preterm infant with hypotension resistant to volume expansion, inotropes improve gut perfusion.[94] Umbilical artery catheters should be removed if there is evidence of thrombosis, or reduced blood flow to the buttocks or lower limbs.

The timing, method and composition of enteral feeds in the face of immaturity of digestion, absorption, gut motility and barrier function has attracted most attention.[184] Breast milk should be given whenever possible, either alone or, if there are problems with adequate lactation, with formula.[155] Hyperosmolar feeds should be avoided, and care taken when adding electrolytes to milk.[21]

Although prolonged delay in enteral feeding for the prevention of NEC cannot be recommended,[140] rapid, incautious introduction and increase in enteral feeds in the face of poor feed tolerance is likely to lead to NEC.[16,169] In the UK more units are giving milk feeds during neonatal intensive care,[165] yet there is no apparent increase in NEC. The administration of small amounts of milk – minimal enteral feeding – is increasingly used, and leads to the promotion of gut development and possible avoidance of NEC.[139] Special care is needed with the introduction of milk in the infant with intrauterine growth retardation.[74,168]

Control of infection is essential in the management of epidemic NEC,[256] and is good practice in all cases. The prophylactic use of systemic antibiotics is not advised.[86,90] The administration of enteral aminoglycosides is not without risk, as absorption may occur, but it may reduce the risk of NEC.[256] Oral administration of immunoglobulins has been tried in a small number of centres.[69] Direct comparison of oral IgA–IgG and oral gentamicin suggests that the latter is more effective in a high-risk group.[77] Future possibilities include the addition of non-antibody immune factors such as lactoferrin to formula milk, the use of prostaglandins or their analogues, modification of cytokine activity, and treatment with growth factors.[44,109,256]

SHORT BOWEL SYNDROME

This follows the loss of a significant portion of the small intestine, and comprises malabsorption, diarrhoea and growth failure due to loss of mucosal surface area and rapid gastrointestinal transit. Loss of bowel may follow pre- or postnatal damage to the gut[49,66,149,235,261] (Table 31.27). The commonest cause is NEC in the preterm infant, which occurs at a time when, in fetal life, the small intestine is doubling in length,[247] leaving these infants at particular disadvantage. Among infants with NEC who require surgery and survive, 4–10% have SBS.[112,145]

Infants with less than 50% or 100 cm of small bowel are at high risk of SBS.[37,149] Parenteral nutrition is usually needed when less than 40 cm of small intestine remains, and is likely to be needed for longer if the ileocaecal valve is absent.[37,82,207,273]

The central tenet of management is nutritional support and the maintenance of fluid and electrolyte balance, allowing a period of gradual intestinal adaptation during which growth in the length and diameter of the remaining bowel, and mucosal hypertrophy, occurs.[37,149,281] In a group of infants with SBS, almost all had achieved 90% absorption of carbohydrate and fats by 3 months.[149] This remarkable process of adaptation has allowed infants with less than 10 cm of small bowel to achieve full enteral feeds.[235] Preservation of the ileum is important as it has a greater ability to adapt than the jejunum, a longer transit time and the unique ability to absorb vitamin B_{12} and bile acids.

Most infants require initial TPN (Chapter 20). If TPN is needed long term, home administration has allowed these children good quality of life.[208] Enteral feeds should be introduced cautiously. Most infants tolerate a feed containing protein hydrolysate, medium-chain triglycerides and glucose polymers but no lactose (e.g. Peptijunior (Cow & Gate), Pregestimil (Mead Johnson)).[45,235] Caloric content may be increased by the addition of starch, glucose polymers or fats, although the former may be better tolerated. In some infants a modular feed is

Table 31.27 Aetiology of short bowel

Prenatal	Postnatal
Vascular accidents	Necrotizing enterocolitis
Intestinal atresia	Midgut or segmental volvulus
Abdominal wall defects	Inflammatory bowel disease
Volvulus	Abdominal trauma
Meconium peritonitis	Vascular thrombosis

necessary to allow manipulation of individual nutrient components. Continuous feeds are usually tolerated well, although bolus feeds have the theoretical advantage of better promotion of gut development.[225,245] Enteral feeds are important for gut adaptation.[82] Specific nutrients may be used as primary therapy.[26,235] Pectin, a dietary fibre, is metabolized by colonic bacteria to short-chain fatty acids, which have important nutritional and trophic properties. In the animal model, pectin increases small intestinal length, weight and crypt depth.[132] Glutamine, an important gastrointestinal nutrient, has been shown to protect the gut from atrophy in enteral starvation, but has not proved to be beneficial in SBS.[254]

The diet must contain adequate calcium, magnesium, iron, fat and water-soluble vitamins and trace elements.[281] Vitamin B_{12} supplements may be necessary after terminal ileal resection.[46] SBS is often accompanied by initial hypergastrinaemia, which exacerbates symptoms. H_2-antagonists (ranitidine) or proton pump inhibitors may be required. Antimotility agents (loperamide) may be effective[217] but should be used with care.[268] Cholestyramine is indicated if there is evidence of bile acid diarrhoea after ileal resection.[45] Close attention to dietary detail, careful follow-up and monitoring are essential, and require multidisciplinary support.[235] Feeding and speech development should not be overlooked.

In a small proportion, who are dependent upon TPN and who have had at least a year to allow adaptation, surgery may be helpful. Procedures aim at slowing intestinal transit time or increasing the absorptive surface area by reconstruction of the ileocaecal valve, the interposition of colon or anti-peristaltic segments, recirculating loops or increasing intestinal length.[18,37,174,207,242] In children who cannot be maintained on TPN, small bowel transplantation may be considered.[120]

The prognosis for SBS is now a great deal better than it was 20 years ago, with survival rates exceeding 90%, even in those with less than 40 cm of small bowel.[82] Growth is often initially slow. Linear growth may be impaired in the first year, although most climb back into the normal weight range by their third year, albeit on the lower centiles.[49,66,149,273]

NEONATAL APPENDICITIS

Appendicitis in the neonate is very rare, representing only 0.1–0.2% of childhood appendicitis.[63] The commonest presentation is with perforation and diffuse peritonitis, with signs like those of NEC[164] (Table 31.28). NEC may be localized to the appendix.[11] Neonatal appendicitis has a high mortality. The combination of physical signs in the right iliac fossa, an abnormal gas pattern in that area on plain abdominal X-ray and red and white cells in the urine point strongly to the diagnosis.[222] Treatment is surgical, with intensive medical support and broad-spectrum antibiotic cover.

Table 31.28 Signs of intra-abdominal neonatal appendicitis in 55 infants[164]

Sign	% with finding
Abdominal distension	90
Vomiting	60
Refusal to feed	40
Temperature ≥ 38°C	40
Temperature 37–38°C	30
Temperature ≤ 37°C	30
Pain (crying, restlessness)	30
Lethargy	30
Erythema/oedema of right lower quadrant	20
Mass in right lower quadrant	20
Diarrhoea	20
Passage of bloody stools	20

INTRACTABLE DIARRHOEA

Severe diarrhoea which is persistent and protracted, beginning soon after birth, may be due to congenital abnormality of gastrointestinal function. All are rare and investigation and management require the support of a specialist centre. Intestinal mucosal biopsy is indicated, and fluid and electrolyte balance and support of nutrition are the central objectives of treatment.[152]

MICROVILLOUS INCLUSION DISEASE (CONGENITAL MICROVILLOUS ATROPHY)

This is an autosomal recessive disorder of the cytoskeleton of the apical region of the enterocyte, in which there is atrophy and involution of microvilli of the small and large bowel.[199] Massive diarrhoea is unresponsive to stopping feeds. To establish a diagnosis, mucosal biopsy is examined by electron microscopy. TPN is given, but the prognosis is very poor.[200] The future may lie in small intestinal transplantation.

CONGENITAL ELECTROLYTE TRANSPORT DEFECTS

Congenital chloride diarrhoea is autosomal recessive and caused by defective Cl^-/HCO_3^- transport in the ileum and colon.[101] Fetal diarrhoea produces polyhydramnios. Severe watery diarrhoea, which may be mistaken for urine in the nappy, abdominal distension, hypochloraemic alkalosis and rapid weight loss occur in the newborn period. Stool chloride is high. Congenital sodium diarrhoea, caused by defective sodium/ proton exchange, produces a similar picture but with high stool sodium losses.[24] Both conditions have been successfully managed with intravenous, and subsequently oral, mineral replacement.[62]

CONGENITAL LACTASE DEFICIENCY

Symptoms immediately follow the introduction of milk feeds, with acidic stools that contain lactose. Diagnosis is made by withdrawal of lactose-containing feeds and the demonstration of absent lactase activity on a jejunal mucosal biopsy.[219] It is very rare compared to secondary lactose intolerance.

CONGENITAL GLUCOSE/GALACTOSE MALABSORPTION

Watery acidic stools containing reducing substances, but possibly not lactose, are seen in the first days after birth. After rehydration a fructose-based formula is given, and the prognosis is good.[62,72]

AUTOIMMUNE ENTEROPATHY

Intractable diarrhoea, characteristically with a family history of autoimmune disease, may be due to an antienterocyte antibody and associated with a patchy enteropathy on biopsy.[173] A favourable response to cyclosporin has been reported.[216]

GASTRO-OESOPHAGEAL REFLUX

CLINICAL PRESENTATION

Gastro-oesophageal reflux leads to vomiting, oesophagitis, recurrent apnoea, pulmonary aspiration, exacerbation of bronchopulmonary dysplasia and failure to thrive.[95,104,161,172,185,197] Most episodes occur during transient relaxation of the lower oesophageal sphincter.[193] Reflux is more common in infancy than childhood.[252] The preterm infant is at high risk because of low resting LOS pressure (see above) and slow gastric emptying.[186,188] Reflux is often seen after repair of oesophageal atresia[41] (p. 772). Feeds, the supine position, nursing care, chest physiotherapy and xanthine administration increase reflux.[185,237,244,253] Reflux is reduced by small-volume tube feeds and during ventilation.[2,187,202,237]

Silent reflux, without the clinical clues of vomiting, should be suspected in infants with apnoea or respiratory problems resistant to the usual therapy, or with unexplained deterioration.[25,104,138,185] Diagnosis is best made by oesophageal pH studies. Contrast studies lack sensitivity but rule out anatomical abnormality. In some a trial of therapy is used.[58,185,238] Oesophagitis may lead to bleeding, and endoscopy is now feasible.[59,161]

TREATMENT

Changes in feed composition have little effect, although breast milk may be beneficial.[92,246] The prone, 30° head-up position reduces reflux, but can only be recommended during inpatient monitoring, and the left lateral position may be effective.[244,253] Feed thickening reduces regurgitation but is ineffective in older children with respiratory problems.[194,251] Cisapride, a prokinetic agent, is becoming the drug of choice in paediatric reflux.[183] It has been used in the newborn, and appears effective.[171] Cisapride should not be used with macrolide antibiotics (e.g. erythromycin) or the imidazole or triazole antifungal agents, because QT prolongation may occur.[147] Metoclopropamide should not be used. In oesophagitis, Infant Gaviscon (Reckitt & Colman) or ranitidine may be used. Infant Gaviscon contains approximately 1 mmol of sodium per dose. None of these agents is licensed in the UK for use in the newborn. Surgical fundoplication is rarely necessary in the neonatal period, except in severe reflux-related respiratory disorder.[104,125]

Treatment may lead to improved respiratory function[104] or resolution of apnoea.[185] Prognosis is good, and in most infants reflux resolves with maturation of the antireflux barrier. Infants with complicated reflux should be followed up. Persistent reflux is more common in those with neurodevelopmental problems.[58,227,231]

MILK PROTEIN INTOLERANCE

Antigens provoking milk protein intolerance include cow's milk whey proteins, β-lactoglobulin and α-lactalbumin, casein, other cow's milk proteins and soya proteins.[57] Immunogenic proteins may be absorbed and secreted in breast milk,[114] explaining uncommon reactions in exclusively breast-fed infants.[5] In the newborn gut, barrier function is poor (Table 31.20) and macromolecular absorption is high (p. 745). This is particularly the case in preterm infants, in whom atopic symptoms are common.[115,154] MPI may also occur after any gastrointestinal insult, and itself leads to immune-mediated mucosal disruption.[57,97,111]

Over 90% of cases of MPI present in the first months of life.[192] In a large prospective study of healthy term infants MPI was proven in 2.2%,[79] although over 50% with an atopic family history may develop MPI.[192] Infants with MPI often react to other antigens.

CLINICAL FEATURES

The commonest gastrointestinal symptoms are vomiting and diarrhoea. Other symptoms vary from mild to life-threatening (Table 31.29).[57,79,107,118,192] MPI enteropathy may result in weight loss, abdominal distension and

Table 31.29 Gastrointestinal manifestations of milk protein intolerance

Vomiting
Gastro-oesophageal reflux
Diarrhoea
Failure to thrive
Colic
Villous atrophy and malabsorption
Protein losing enteropathy
Occult blood loss
Colitis

steatorrhoea with patchy subtotal villous atrophy and crypt hyperplasia.[57,111] MPI is the commonest cause of colitis in the young infant, with rectal bleeding and loose stools containing mucus.[118] MPI may be accompanied by lactose intolerance. The non-gastrointestinal effects of MPI range from acute reactions, including urticaria and anaphylaxis, to chronic atopic disease (rhinorrhoea, eczema and asthma).[57]

Diagnosis rests upon remission of symptoms on an exclusion diet, and relapse on challenge. Intestinal biopsy, estimation of total IgE and specific antibodies (RAST), the skin-prick test and stool analysis may support the diagnosis. A hypoallergenic lactose-free milk substitute based upon hydrolysed whey (Peptijunior) or casein (Pregestimil, Nutramigen) is given. Infants with severe MPI, notably colitis, may be exquisitely sensitive to milk proteins, and may require an amino-acid formula or, if breast-fed, restriction of the maternal diet.[5,170] Management demands close dietetic supervision.[108,157] Challenge, to substantiate the diagnosis and to demonstrate resolution of MPI, should be in hospital and not usually in the neonatal period.[57] The vast majority of MPI resolves in the first 3 years.

PREVENTION

Prevention of MPI is contentious.[276] Non-exposure to cow's milk protein reduces the risk of atopic symptoms in preterm infants with an atopic family history.[154] Early breast-feeding may prevent atopic symptoms.[39,215,232] The infant at high risk is less likely to develop MPI if breast-fed during exclusion of cows' milk, egg and fish from the maternal diet, or if given a highly hydrolysed formula.[39,192]

CYSTIC FIBROSIS

Cystic fibrosis is an autosomal recessive condition affecting about 1 in 2500 livebirths in the UK.[65] The cystic fibrosis transmembrane conductance regulator acts as a channel for chloride ions leaving the cell. CF is caused by mutations of both CFTR alleles on the long arm of chromosome 7.[209] The commonest mutation is a single amino-acid substitution, ΔF508, but over 600 are known.[228] The carrier rate of CF mutations is about 1 in 25. All families of an infant with CF should be offered genetic counselling.

SCREENING

Neonatal screening (Table 31.30) uses the dried blood spot collected in the first week. Serum immune-reactive trypsin is elevated in almost all infants with CF in the neonatal period, but over 90% of infants with a single positive result do not have CF.[93,198,211] Combination of the IRT assay and examination of the same dried blood spot for commoner mutations reduces the false positive rate.[84,198] Recall of infants for a second IRT assay may generate parental anxiety, but increases sensitivity. Most authorities agree that neonatal screening is beneficial, and it has been shown to reduce early respiratory morbidity.[40,263]

Table 31.30 Neonatal presentations of cystic fibrosis

Antenatal mutation analysis
Fetal hyperechogenic bowel
Fetal gut dilatation
Fetal intra-abdominal calcification
Neonatal screening
Meconium peritonitis
Meconium ileus
Cholestasis
Respiratory infection
Exocrine pancreatic insufficiency
Failure to thrive

CLINICAL PRESENTATION

The mean birthweight in affected infants is below normal,[105] but most clinical presentation occurs in late infancy or childhood. 15–20% of affected infants present in the neonatal period with meconium ileus,[211] which is sometimes predictable from fetal ultrasound[51,236] (Table 31.30). Meconium ileus results in intestinal obstruction within 48 hours of birth. It is associated with pre- or postnatal perforation, volvulus, chemical or bacterial peritonitis, intestinal atresia and microcolon. Conservative management with intravenous fluids, antibiotics and water-soluble hyperosmolar contrast enema under fluoroscopic control, should only be attempted in a specialized centre, in collaboration with a paediatric surgeon (p. 779). Meconium ileus may be a difficult diagnosis in the preterm infant:[126] neonatal mortality is 10–20%, but in survivors outcome is similar to that seen in other children with CF.[52] CF should not be forgotten in infants with cholestasis[156] (Table 31.15, p. 735).

The sweat test with pilocarpine iontophoresis, essential to the diagnosis of CF, requires specialized expertise.[150,259] Sweat testing is possible in the neonatal period,[76] but we do not usually attempt it before 4–6 weeks post-term. A single test is not diagnostic. Mutation analysis is usually diagnostic, but even apparent homozygous ΔF508 status may be misleading.[262]

MANAGEMENT

The most important management step is referral to a specialized multidisciplinary team. In the infant with ventilator-dependent respiratory disease we have found dexamethasone helpful. Newborn infants with CF who do not have meconium ileus are usually asymptomatic. The philosophy behind their management is one of early intervention, and aggressive treatment of pathogens which

Table 31.31 Nutritional management of cystic fibrosis[83,158]

Energy	
Routine	100–130 cal/kg/day
Poor growth	150–200 cal/kg/day
Milk	
Routine	breast milk standard infant formula
Poor growth	supplement formula with: glucose polymer *or* fat emulsion (e.g. Calogen) and glucose polymer *or* mixed fat and carbohydrate (e.g. Duocal) to maximum total energy content of 100 cal/100 ml
Postoperative period or after meconium ileus	Peptijunior, Pregestimil
Pancreatic enzymes (acid-resistant microspheres)	
third to half capsule with feeds (e.g. Creon, Pancrease)	
mix enteric-coated granules with milk and give from a spoon before a feed	
Vitamins	
Vitamin A 4000 IU/day (e.g. Abidec 0.6 ml)	
Vitamin D 400 IU/day (e.g. Abidec 0.6 ml)	
Vitamin E 25–50 mg/day	
Vitamin K routine neonatal prophylaxis, repeat before surgery	
(Monitor vitamin status and adjust)	

colonize the respiratory tract soon after birth.[6] Chest physiotherapy should begin early. Prophylactic anti-staphylococcal antibiotics reduce pulmonary morbidity, hospital admission and the need for other antibiotics.[263] The increased energy requirements in CF may relate to respiratory morbidity, or be a primary effect of the gene defect.[83,191,229]

Breast-feeding should be encouraged.[83,99] Breast milk has lipolytic and anti-infective properties which may be of advantage. Alternatively, a standard infant formula is used. Sodium supplements (2 mmol/kg/day) may be necessary. Energy supplements need only be used if growth is suboptimal[158] (Table 31.31). A lactose-free hydrolysed protein feed containing medium-chain triglycerides (e.g. Peptijunior, Pregestimil) may be better tolerated after meconium ileus or surgery or in coexisting cow's milk protein intolerance.[98] Pancreatic function is abnormal before birth,[83] and malabsorption occurs in 60% of infants by 8 weeks of age, rising to over 90% at 1 year.[28] Pancreatic enzyme replacement therapy should be started as soon as there is clinical or laboratory evidence of steatorrhoea.[151]

REFERENCES

1. Abbasi S, Pereira G R, Johnson L, Stahl G E, Duara S, Watkins J B 1984. Long-term assessment of growth, nutritional status, and gastrointestinal function in survivors of necrotizing enterocolitis. Journal of Pediatrics 104: 550–554
2. Abe T, Hata Y, Sasaki F, Uchino J, Aoyama K, Nannbu H 1993 The effect of tube feeding on postprandial gastroesophageal reflux. Journal of Pediatric Surgery 28: 56–58
3. Ade-Ajayi N, Spitz L, Kiely E M, Drake D, Klein N 1996 Intestinal glycosaminoglycans in neonatal necrotizing enterocolitis. British Journal of Surgery 83: 415–418
4. Anand K J, Hickey P R 1987 Pain and its effects in the human neonate and fetus. New England Journal of Medicine 317: 1321–1329
5. Anveden Hertzberg L, Finkel Y, Sandstedt B, Karpe B 1996 Proctocolitis in exclusively breast-fed infants. European Journal of Pediatrics 155: 464–467
6. Armstrong D S, Grimwood K, Carzino R, Carlin J B, Olinsky A, Phelan P D 1995 Lower respiratory infection and inflammation in infants with newly diagnosed cystic fibrosis. British Medical Journal 310: 1571–1572
7. Barlow B, Santulli T V, Heird W C, Pitt J, Blanc W A, Schullinger J N 1974 An experimental study of acute necrotizing enterocolitis: the importance of breast milk. Journal of Pediatric Surgery 9: 587–595
8. Barnard J, Greene H, Cotton R 1983 Necrotizing enterocolitis. In: Kretchmer N, Minkowski A (eds) Nutritional adaptation of the gastrointestinal tract of the newborn. Raven Press, New York, pp 107–126
9. Barnard J A, Cotton R B, Lutin W 1985 Necrotizing entercolitis. Variables associated with the severity of disease. American Journal of Diseases of Children 139: 375–377
10. Bauer C R, Morrison J C, Poole W K et al 1984 A decreased incidence of necrotizing enterocolitis after prenatal glucocorticoid therapy. Pediatrics 73: 682–688
11. Bax N M A, Pearse R, Dommering M, Molenaar J C 1980 Perforation of the appendix in the neonatal period. Journal of Pediatric Surgery 15: 200–202
12. Bedu A, Faure C, Sibony O, Vuillard E, Mougenot J F, Aujard Y 1994 Prenatal gastrointestinal bleeding caused by esophagitis and gastritis. Journal of Pediatrics 125: 465–467
13. Beeby P J, Jeffrey H 1992 Risk factors for necrotising enterocolitis: the influence of gestational age. Archives of Disease in Childhood 67: 432–435
14. Bell E F, Warburton D, Stonestreet B S, Oh W 1980 The effect of fluid administration on the development of symptomatic patent ductus arteriosus and congestive heart failure in premature infants. New England Journal of Medicine 302: 598–603
15. Bell M J, Ternberg J L, Feigin R D et al 1978 Neonatal necrotizing enterocolitis: therapeutic decisions based upon clinical staging. Annals of Surgery 187: 1–7
16. Berseth C L 1994 Gut motility and the pathogenesis of necrotizing enterocolitis. Clinics in Perinatology 21: 263–270
17. Berseth C L, Nordyke C 1993 Enteral nutrients promote postnatal maturation of intestinal motor activity in preterm infants. American Journal of Physiology 264: G1046–1051
18. Bianchi A 1984 Intestinal lengthening: an experimental and clinical review. Journal of the Royal Society of Medicine 77: 35–41
19. Bisset W M, Watt J B, Rivers JPA, Milla P J 1988 Ontogeny of fasting small intestinal motor activity in the human infant. Gut 29: 483–488
20. Bisset W M, Watt J B, Rivers J P A, Milla P J 1989 Postprandial motor response of the small intestine to enteral feeds in preterm infants. Archives of Disease in Childhood 64: 1356–1361
21. Book L S, Herbst J J, Atherton S O, Jung A L 1975 Necrotizing enterocolitis in low birth weight infants fed an elemental formula. Journal of Pediatrics 87: 602–605
22. Book L S, Herbst J J, Jung A L 1976 Comparison of fast and slow feeding rate schedules to the development of necrotizing enterocolitis. Journal of Pediatrics 89: 463–466
23. Book L S, Herbst J J, Jung A L 1976 Carbohydrate malabsorption in necrotizing enterocolitis, Pediatrics 57: 201–205
24. Booth I W 1985 Defective jejunal brush border Na^+/H^+ exchange: a cause of congenital secretory diarrhoea. Lancet i: 1066–1069
25. Booth I W 1992 Silent gastro-oesophageal reflux: how much do we miss? Archives of Disease in Childhood 67: 1325–1327
26. Booth I W 1994 Enteral nutrition as primary therapy in short bowel syndrome. Gut 35: S69–S72
27. British Paediatric Surveillance Unit 1997 Annual Report. Royal College of Paediatrics and Child Health, London
28. Bronstein M N, Sokol R J, Abman S H et al 1992 Pancreatic insufficiency, growth, and nutrition in infants identified by newborn screening as having cystic fibrosis. Journal of Pediatrics 120: 533–540
29. Brown E G, Sweet A Y 1982 Neonatal necrotizing enterocolitis. Pediatric Clinics of North America 29: 1149–1170
30. Bunton G L, Durbin G M, McIntosh N 1977 Necrotising enterocolitis:

a controlled study of 3 years' experience in a neonatal intensive care unit. Archives of Disease in Childhood 52: 772–777
31. Butt W, Auldist A, McDougall P, Duncan A 1986 Duodenal ulceration: a complication of tolazoline therapy. Australian Paediatric Journal 22: 221–223
32. Caplan M S, Hedlund E, Adler L, Hsueh W 1994 Role of asphyxia and feeding in a neonatal rat model of necrotizing enterocolitis. Pediatric Pathology 14: 1017–1028
33. Caplan M S, Hedlund E, Adler L, Lickerman M, Hsueh W 1997 The platelet activating factor receptor antagonist WEB 2170 prevents neonatal necrotizing enterocolitis in rats. Journal of Pediatric Gastroenterology and Nutrition 24: 296–301
34. Carbonaro C A, Clark D A, Elseviers D 1988 A bacterial pathogenicity determinant associated with necrotizing enterocolitis. Microbiological Pathology 5: 427–436
35. Carlos M A, Babyn P S, Marcon M A, Moore A M 1997 Changes in gastric emptying in early postnatal life. Journal of Pediatrics 130: 931–937
36. Cavell B 1982 Reservoir and emptying function of the stomach of the premature infant. Acta Paediatrica Scandinavica Suppl 396: 60–61
37. Chaet M S, Farrell M K, Ziegler M M, Warner B W 1994 Intensive nutritional support and remedial surgical intervention for extreme short bowel syndrome. Journal of Pediatric Gastroenterology and Nutrition 19: 295–298
38. Chan K L, Saing H, Yung R W H, Yeung Y P, Tsol N S 1994 A study of pre-antibiotic bacteriology in 125 patients with necrotizing enterocolitis. Acta Paediatrica Suppl 396: 45–48
39. Chandra R K, Puri S, Hamed A 1989 Influence of maternal diet during lactation and use of formula feeds on development of atopic eczema in high risk infants. British Medical Journal 229: 228–230
40. Chatfield S L, Owen G, Ryley H C et al 1991 Neonatal screening for cystic fibrosis in Wales and the West Midlands: clinical assessment after five years of screening. Archives of Disease in Childhood 66: 29–33
41. Chetcuti P, Myers N A, Phelan P D, Beasley S W 1988 Adults who survived repair of congenital oesophageal atresia and tracheo-oesophageal fistula. British Medical Journal 297: 344–346
42. Clark D A. 1977 Times of first void and first stool in 500 newborns. Pediatrics 60: 457–459
43. Clark D A Barkemeyer B M, Miller M J S 1993 Perinatal hypoxic–ischemic risk factors and necrotizing enterocolitis. Pediatric Research 32: 207
44. Clark D A, Miller M J S 1996 What causes neonatal necrotising enterocolitis and how can it be prevented? In: Hansen T N, Mclntosh N (eds) Current topics in neonatology. W B Saunders, London, pp 160–176
45. Clark J H 1984 Management of short bowel syndrome in the high-risk infant. Clinics in Perinatology 11: 189–197
46. Collins J E, Rolles C J, Sutton H, Ackery D 1984 Vitamin B_{12} absorption after necrotizing enterocolitis. Archives of Disease in Childhood 59: 731–734
47. Communicable Disease Report 1982 Neonatal necrotising enterocolitis surveillance. In: Communicable disease report 82/05 Communicable Disease Surveillance Centre, London
48. Coombs R C, Morgan M E, Durbin G M, Booth I W, McNeish A S 1992 Abnormal gut blood flow velocities in neonates at risk of necrotising enterocolitis. Journal of Pediatric Gastroenterology and Nutrition 15: 13–18
49. Cooper A, Floyd T F, Ross A J, Bishop H C, Templeton J M, Ziegler M M 1984 Morbidity and mortality of short-bowel syndrome acquired in infancy: an update. Journal of Pediatric Surgery 19: 711–718
50. Corbet A, Gerdes J, Long W et al 1995 Double-blind, randomized trial of one versus three prophylactic doses of synthetic surfactant in 826 neonates weighing 700 to 1100 grams: effects on mortality rate. American Exosurf Neonatal Study Groups I and IIa. Journal of Pediatrics 126: 969–978
51. Corteville J E, Gray D L, Langer J C 1996 Bowel abnormalities in the fetus – correlation of prenatal ultrasonographic findings with outcome. American Journal of Obstetrics and Gynecology 175: 724–729
52. Coutts J A, Docherty J G, Carachi R, Evans T J 1997 Clinical course of patients with cystic fibrosis presenting with meconium ileus. British Journal of Surgery 84: 555
53. Crissinger K D 1994 Regulation of hemodynamics and oxygenation in developing intestine: insight into the pathogenesis of necrotizing enterocolitis. Acta Paediatrica Suppl 396: 8–10
54. Crissinger K D, Tso P 1992 The role of lipids in ischemia/reperfusion-induced changes in mucosal permeability in developing piglets. Gastroenterology 102: 1693–1699
55. Cucchiara S, Staiano A, Di Lorenzo C et al 1986 Esophageal motor abnormalities in children with gastroesophageal reflux and peptic esophagitis. Journal of Pediatrics 108: 907–910
56. Davey A M, Wagner C L, Cox C, Kendig J W 1994 Feeding premature infants while low umbilical artery catheters are in place: a prospective, randomized trial. Journal of Pediatrics 124: 795–799
57. David T J 1993 Cow's milk intolerance. In: Food and food additive intolerance in children. Blackwell, Oxford, pp 25–84
58. Davies AEM, Sandhu B K 1995 Diagnosis and treatment of gastro-oesophageal reflux. Archives of Disease in Childhood 73: 82–86
59. de Boissieu D, Dupont C, Barbet J P Bargaoui K, Badoual J 1994 Distinct features of upper gastrointestinal endoscopy in the newborn. Journal of Pediatric Gastroenterology and Nutrition 18: 334–338
60. de Gamarra E, Helardot P, Moriette G, Relier J P 1983 Necrotizing enterocolitis in full term newborns. Biology of the Neonate 44: 185–192
61. De Lemos R A, Rogers J H, McLaughlin W 1974 Experimental production of necrotizing enterocolitis in newborn goats. Pediatric Research 8: 380–387
62. Desjeux J 1996 Congenital transport defects. In: Walker W A, Durie P R, Hamilton J R, Walker-Smith J A, Watkins J B (eds) Pediatric gastrointestinal disease. B C Dekker: Philadephia, pp 792–816
63. Dessanti A, Porcu A, Scanu A, Dettori G 1995 Neonatal acute appendicitis in an inguinal hernia. Pediatric Surgery International 10: 561–562
64. Devane S P, Soothill P W, Candy D C A 1993 Temporal changes in gastric volume in human fetus in late pregnancy. Early Human Development 33: 109–116
65. Dodge J A, Goodall J, Geddes D et al 1988 Cystic fibrosis in the United Kingdom 1977–85: an improving picture. British Medical Journal 297: 1599–1602
66. Dorney S F, Ament M E, Berquist W E, Vargas J H, Hassall E 1985 Improved survival in very short small bowel of infancy with use of long-term parenteral nutrition. Journal of Pediatrics 107: 521–525
67. Edelstone D I, Holzman I R 1984 Regulation of perinatal intestinal oxygenation. Seminars in Perinatology 8: 226–233
68. Egarter C, Leitich H, Karas H et al 1996 Antibiotic treatment in preterm rupture of membranes and neonatal morbidity: a metanalysis. American Journal of Obstetrics and Gynecology 174: 589–597
69. Eibl M M, Wolf H M, Furnkranz H, Rosenkranz A 1988 Prevention of necrotizing enterocolitis in low birth weight infants by IgA-IgG feeding. New England Journal of Medicine 319: 1–7
70. Ein S H, Shandling B, Wesson D, Filler R M 1990 A 13 year experience with peritoneal drainage under local anesthesia for necrotizing enterocolitis. Journal of Pediatric Surgery 25: 1034–1037
71. Engel R R, Virnig N L, Hunt C E, Levitt M D 1973 Origin of mural gas in necrotizing enterocolitis. Pediatric Research 7: 292
72. Evans L, Grasset E, Heyman M, Dumontier A M, Beau J P, Desjeux J F 1985 Congenital selective malabsorption of glucose and galactose. Journal of Pediatric Gastroenterology and Nutrition 4: 878–886
73. Ewer A K, Durbin G M, Morgan M E, Booth I W 1994 Gastric emptying in preterm infants. Archives of Disease in Childhood 71: F24–F27
74. Ewer A K, McHugo J M, Chapman S, Newell S J 1993 Fetal echogenic gut: a marker of intrauterine gut ischaemia. Archives of Disease in Childhood 69: 510–513
75. Eyal E, Sagi E, Arad I, Avital A 1982 Necrotising enterocolitis in the very low birth weight infant: expressed breast milk compared with parenteral feeding. Archives of Disease in Childhood 57: 274–276
76. Farrell P M, Koscik R E 1996 Sweat chloride concentrations in infants homozygous or heterozygous for F508 cystic fibrosis. Pediatrics 97: 524–528
77. Fast C, Rosegger H 1994 Necrotizing enterocolitis prophylaxis: oral antibiotics and lyophilized enterobacteria vs oral immunoglobulins. Acta Paediatrica Suppl 396: 86–90
78. Fenton T R, Walker Smith J A, Harvey D R 1981 Proctoscopy in infancy with reference to its use in necrotising enterocolitis. Archives of Disease in Childhood 56: 121–124

79. Ford R P, Schluter P J, Taylor B J, Mitchell E A, Scragg R 1996 Allergy and the risk of sudden infant death syndrome. Members of the New Zealand Cot Death Study Group. Clinical and Experimental Allergy 26: 580–584
80. Gobet R, Sacher P, Schwobel M G 1994 Surgical procedures in colonic strictures after necrotizing enterocolitis. Acta Paediatrica Suppl 396: 77–79
81. Goldman H L 1980 Feeding and necrotizing enterocolitis. American Journal of Diseases of Children 134: 553–555
82. Goulet O J, Revillon Y, Jan D 1991 Neonatal short bowel syndrome. Journal of Pediatrics 119: 18–23
83. Green M R, Buchanan E, Weaver L T 1995 Nutritional management of the infant with cystic fibrosis. Archives of Disease in Childhood 72: 452–456
84. Gregg R G, Simantel A, Farrell P M et al 1997 Newborn screening for cystic fibrosis in Wisconsin: comparison of biochemical and molecular methods. Pediatrics 99: 819–824
85. Gryboski J D 1965 The swallowing mechanism of the neonate I: eosphageal and gastric motility. Pediatrics 35: 445–452
86. Grylack L J, Scanlon J W 1978 Oral gentamicin therapy in the prevention of neonatal enterocolitis: a controlled double blind trial. American Journal of Diseases of Children 132: 1192–1194
87. Gupta S, Morris J G, Panigrahi P, Nataro J P, Glass R I, Gewolb I H 1994 Epidemic necrotizing enterocolitis; lack of association with a specific infectious agent. Pediatric Infectious Disease Journal 13: 728–734
88. Hackett G A, Campbell S, Gamsu H, Cohen-Overbeek T, Pearce J M F 1987 Doppler studies in the growth retarded fetus and prdiction of neonatal necrotising enterocolitis haemorrhage, and neonatal morbidity. British Medical Journal 294: 13–16
89. Han V K M, Sayed H, Chance G W, Brabyn D G, Shaheed W A 1983 An outbreak of *Clostridium difficile* necrotizing enterocolitis: a case for oral vancomicin therapy. Pediatrics 71: 935–941
90. Hansen T N, Ritter D A, Speer M E, Kenny J D, Rudolph A J 1980 A randomized controlled study of oral gentamicin and the treatment of neonatal necrotizing enterocolitis. Journal of Pediatrics 97: 836–839
91. Harris M C, Costarino A T Jr, Sullivan J S et al 1994 Cytokine elevations in critically ill infants with sepsis and necrotizing enterocolitis. Journal of Pediatrics 124: 105–111
92. Heacock H J, Jeffery H E, Baker J L, Page M 1992 Influence of breast versus formula milk on physiological gastroesophageal reflux in healthy, newborn infants. Journal of Pediatric Gastroenterology and Nutrition 14: 41–46
93. Heeley A F, Heeley M E, King D N, Kuzemko J A, Walsh M P 1982 Screening for cystic fibrosis by dried blood spot trypsin assay. Archives of Disease in Childhood 57: 18–21
94. Hentschel R, Hensel D, Brune T, Rabe H, Jorch G 1995 Impact on blood pressure and intestinal perfusion of dobutamine or dopamine in hypotensive preterm infants. Biology of the Neonate 68: 318–324
95. Herbst J J, Minton S D, Book L S 1979 Gastroesophageal reflux causing respiratory distress and apnoea in newborn infants. Journal of Pediatrics 95: 763–768
96. Hey E N 1983 Special care nurseries: admitting to a policy. British Medical Journal 287: 1524–1527
97. Heyman M, Darmon N, Dupont C et al 1994 Mononuclear cells from infants allergic to cow's milk secrete tumor necrosis factor alpha, altering intestinal function. Gastroenterology 106: 1514–1523
98. Hill S M, Phillips A D, Mearns M, Walker Smith J A 1989 Cow's milk sensitive enteropathy in cystic fibrosis. Archives of Disease in Childhood 64: 1251–1255
99. Holliday K E, Allen J R, Waters D L, Gruca M A, Thompson S M, Gaskin K J 1991 Growth of human milk-fed and formula-fed infants with cystic fibrosis. Journal of Pediatrics 118: 77–79
100. Hollwarth M E 1994 Necrotizing enterocolitis: an editorial. Acta Paediatrica Suppl 396: 1
101. Holmberg C 1986 Congenital chloride diarrhoea. Clinics in Gastroenterology 15: 583–602
102. Hopkins G B, Gould V E, Stevenson J K, Oliver T K 1970 Necrotizing enterocolitis in premature infants: a clinical and pathologic evaluation of autopsy material. American Journal of Diseases of Children 120: 229–232
103. Horwitz J R, Lally K P, Cheu H W, Vazquez W D, Grosfield J L, Ziegler M M 1995 Complications after surgical intervention in necrotizing enterocolitis: a multicenter review. Journal of Pediatric Surgery 30: 994–999
104. Hrabovsky E E, Mullett M D 1986 Gastroesophageal reflux and the premature infant. Journal of Pediatric Surgery 21: 583–587
105. Hsia D Y 1959 Birth weight in cystic fibrosis of the pancreas. Annals of Human Genetics 23: 289–299
106. Hsueh W, Caplan M S, Sun X, Tan X, MacKendrick W, Gonzalez-Crussi F 1994 Platelet activating factor, tumour necrosis factor, hypoxia and necrotizing enterocolitis. Acta Paediatrica Supp 396: 11–17
107. Iacono G, Carroccio A, Cavataio F et al 1996 Gastroesophageal reflux and cow's milk allergy in infants: a prospective study. Journal of Allergy and Clinical Immunology 97: 822–827
108. Isolauri E 1995 The treatment of cow's milk allergy. European Journal of Clinical Nutrition 49: S49–S55
109. Israel E J 1994 Neonatal necrotizing enterocolitis, a disease of the immature intestinal mucosal barrier. Acta Paediatrica Suppl 396: 27–32
110. Israel E J, Schiffrin E J, Carter E A, Freiberg E, Walker W A 1990 Prevention of necrotizing enterocolitis in the rat with prenatal cortisone. Gastroenterology 99: 1333–1338
111. Iyngkaran N, Yadav M, Boey C G, Lam K L 1988 Severity and extent of upper small bowel mucosal damage in cow's milk protein-sensitive enteropathy. Journal of Pediatric Gastroenterology and Nutrition 7: 667–674
112. Jackman S, Brereton R J, Wright V M 1990 Results of surgical treatment of neonatal necrotising entercolitis. British Journal of Surgery 77: 146–148
113. Jadcherla S R, Berseth C L 1995 Acute and chronic intestinal motor activity responses to two infant formulas. Pediatrics 96: 331–335
114. Jakobsson I, Lindberg T, Benediktsson B, Hansson B G 1985 Dietary bovine betalactoglobulin is transferred to human milk. Acta Paediatrica Scandinavica 74: 342–345
115. Jakobsson I, Lindberg T, Lothe L, Axelsson I, Benediktsson B 1986 Human α-lactalbumin as a marker of macromolecular absorption. Gut 27: 1029–1034
116. Janik J S, Ein S H 1980 Peritoneal drainage under local anaesthesia for necrotizing enterocolitis. Journal of Pediatric Surgery 15: 565–568
117. Janik J S, Ein S H, Mancer K 1981 Intestinal stricture after necrotizing enterocolitis. Journal of Pediatric Surgery 16: 438–443
118. Jenkins H R, Pincott J R, Soothill J F, Milla P J, Harries J T 1984 Food allergy: the major cause of infantile colitis. Archives of Disease in Childhood 59: 326–329
119. Karsdrop V H M, Van-Vugt J M G, Van-Geijn H P et al 1994 Clinical significance of absent or reversed end diastolic velocity waveforms in umbilical artery. Lancet 344: 1664–1668
120. Kelly D A, Buckels J A C 1995 The future of small bowel transplantation. Archives of Disease in Childhood 72: 447–451
121. Kelly E J, Chatfield S L, Brownlee K G et al 1993 The effect of intravenous ranitidine on the intragastric pH of preterm infants receiving dexamethasone. Archives of Disease in Childhood 69: 37–39
122. Kelly E J, Newell S J 1994 Gastric ontogeny: clinical implications. Archives of Disease in Childhood 71: F136–F141
123. Kelly E J, Newell S J, Brownlee K G, Primrose J N, Dear P R 1993 Gastric acid secretion in preterm infants. Early Human Development 35: 215–220
124. Kempley S T, Bennett S, Loftus B G, Cooper D, Gamsu H R 1993 Randomised trial of umbilical arterial position: clinical outcome. Acta Paediatrica 83: 173–176
125. Kiely E M 1990 Surgery for gastro-oesophageal reflux. Archives of Disease in Childhood 65: 1291–1292
126. King A, Mueller R F, Heeley A F, Roberton N R C 1986 Diagnosis of cystic fibrosis in premature infants. Pediatric Research 20: 536–541
127. Kitterman J A 1975 Effects of intestinal ischemia. In: Moore T D (ed) Necrotizing enterocolitis in the newborn infant. 68th Ross conference on Pediatric Research. Ross Laboratories, Columbus, OH, pp 38–40
128. Kliegman R, Fanaroff A A 1981 Neonatal necrotizing enterocolitis: a nine year experience. II. Outcome assessment. American Journal of Diseases of Children 135: 608–611
129. Kliegman R M, Fanaroff A A 1981 Neonatal necrotizing enterocolitis: a nine year experience. I. Epidemiology and uncommon observations. American Journal of Diseases of Children 135: 603–607
130. Kliegman R M, Fanaroff A A 1984 Necrotizing enterocolitis. New England Journal of Medicine 310: 1093–1103
131. Kliegman R M, Walker W A, Yolken R H 1993 Necrotizing enterocolitis: research agenda for a disease of unknown etiology and pathogenesis. Pediatric Research 34: 701–708

132. Koruda M J, Rolandelli R H, Settle R G, Saul S H, Rombeau J L 1986 The effect of a pectin-supplemented elemental diet on intestinal adaptation to massive small intestinal resection. Journal of Parenteral and Enteral Nutrition 10: 343–350
133. Kosloske A M 1984 Pathogenesis and prevention of necrotizing enterocolitis: a hypothesis based on personal observation and a review of the literature. Pediatrics 74: 1086–1092
134. Kosloske A M 1994 Indications for operation in necrotizing enterocolitis revisited. Journal of Pediatric Surgery 29: 663–666
135. Kosloske A M 1994 Epidemiology of necrotizing enterocolitis. Acta Paediatrica Suppl 396: 2–7
136. Kosloske A M, Musemeche C A 1989 Necrotizing enterocolitis of the neonate. Clinics in Perinatology 16: 97–111
137. Kosloske A M, Papile L, Burstein J 1980 Indications for operation in acute nectrotizing enterocolitis of the neonate. Surgery 87: 502–508
138. Krishnamoorthy M, Mintz A, Liem T, Applebaum H 1994 Diagnosis and treatment of respiratory symptoms of initially unsuspected gastroesophageal reflux in infants. American Surgery 60: 783–785
139. La Gamma E F, Browne L E 1994 Feeding practices for infants weighing less than 1500 G at birth and the pathogenesis of necrotizing enterocolitis. Clinics in Perinatology 21: 271–306
140. La Gamma E F, Osterag S G, Birenbaum H 1985 Failure of delayed oral feedings to prevent necrotizing enterocolitis. Results of a study in very low birth weight neonates. American Journal of Diseases of Children 139: 385–389
141. Lamireau T, Llanas B, Chateil J F et al 1996 Fréquence accrue et difficultés diagnostiques des sténose intestinales après entérocolite ulceronécrosante. Archives de Pediatrie 3: 9–15
142. Lawrence G, Bates J, Gaul A 1982 Pathogenesis of neonatal necrotising enterocolitis. Lancet i: 137–139
143. Lebenthal E, Leung Y K 1988 Feeding the premature and compromised infant: gastrointestinal considerations. Pediatric Clinics of North America 35: 215–238
144. LeBlanc M H, D'Cruz C, Pate K 1984 necrotizing enterocolitis can be caused by polycythemic hyperviscosity in the newborn dog. Journal of Pediatrics 105: 804–809
145. Lemelle J L, Schmitt M, de Miscault G, Vert P, Hascoet J M 1994 Neonatal necrotizing enterocolitis: a retrospective and multicentric review of 331 cases. Acta Paediatrica Suppl 396: 70–73
146. Leung M P, Chau K, Hui P et al 1988 Necrotizing enterocolitis in neonates with symptomatic congenital heart disease. Journal of Pediatrics 12: 1044–1046
147. Lewin M B, Bryant R M, Fenrich A L, Grifka R G 1996 Cisapride-induced long Q T interval. Journal of Pediatrics 128: 279–281
148. Liebermann-Meffert D, Allgower M, Schmid P, Blum A L 1979 Muscular equivalent of the lower esophageal sphincter. Gastroenterology 76: 31–38
149. Liefaard G, Heineman E, Molenaar J C, Tibboel D 1995 Prospective evaluation of the absorptive capacity of the bowel after major and minor resections in the neonate. Journal of Pediatric Surgery 30: 388–391
150. Littlewood J M 1986 The sweat test. Archives of Disease in Childhood 61: 1041–1043
151. Littlewood J M 1996 Management of malabsorption in cystic fibrosis: Influence of recent developments on clinical practice. Postgraduate Medical Journal 72: S56–S62
152. Lo C W, Walker W A 1983 Chronic protracted diarrhoea of infancy: a nutritional disease. Pediatrics 72: 786–800
153. Lucas A, Bloom S R, Aynsley Green A 1980 Development of gut hormone response to feeding in neonates. Archives of Disease in Childhood 55: 678–682
154. Lucas A, Brooke O G, Morley R, Cole T J, Bamford M F 1990 Early diet of preterm infants and development of allergic or atopic disease: randomised prospective study. British Medical Journal 300: 837–840
155. Lucas A, Cole T J 1990 Breast milk and neonatal necrotising enterocolitis. Lancet 336: 1519–1523
156. Lykavieris P, Bernard O, Hadchouel M 1996 Neonatal cholestasis as the presenting feature in cystic fibrosis. Archives of Disease in Childhood 75: 67–70
157. Mabin D C, Sykes A E, David T J 1995 Nutritional content of few foods diet in atopic dermatitis. Archives of Disease in Childhood 73: 208–210
158. MacDonald A 1996 Nutritional management of cystic fibrosis. Archives of Disease in Childhood 74: 81–87
159. Mackendrick W, Hill N, Hsueh W, Caplan M S 1993 Increase in plasma platelet activating factor levels in enterally fed preterm infants. Biology of the Neonate 64: 89–95
160. Major C A, Lewis D F, Harding J A, Porto M A, Garite T J 1994 Tocolysis with indomethacin increases the incidence of necrotizing enterocolitis in the very low birth weight neonate. American Journal of Obstetrics and Gynecology 170: 102–106
161. Maki M, Ruuska T, Kuusela A 1993 High prevalence of asymptomatic esophageal and gastric lesions in preterm infants in intensive care. Critical Care Medicine 21: 1863–1867
162. Malcolm G, Ellwood D, Devonald K, Beilby R, Henderson-Smart D 1991 Absent or reversed end diastolic flow velocity in the umbilical artery and necrotising enterocolitis. Archives of Disease in Childhood 66: 805–807
163. Marchildon M B, Buck B E, Abdenour G 1982 Necrotizing enterocolitis in the unfed infant. Journal of Pediatric Surgery 17: 620–624
164. Marcy S M, Overturf G D 1996 Focal bacterial infections. In: Remington J S, Klein J O (eds) Infectious diseases of the fetus and newborn infant, 4th edn. W B Saunders, Philadelphia, pp 936–979
165. McClure R J, Chatrath M K, Newell S J 1996 Changing trends in feeding policies for ventilated preterm infants. Acta Paediatrica 85: 1123–1125
166. McClure R J, Newell S J 1996 Effect of fortifying breast milk on gastric emptying. Archives of Disease in Childhood 74: F60–F62
167. McCormack C J, Emmens R W, Putnam T C 1987 Evaluation of factors in high risk neonatal necrotizing enterocolitis. Journal of Pediatric Surgery 22: 488–491
168. McDonnell M, Serra Serra V, Gaffney G, Redman C W, Hope P L 1994 Neonatal outcome after pregnancy complicated by abnormal velocity waveforms in the umbilical artery. Archives of Disease in Childhood 70: F84–F89
169. McKeown R E, Marsh T D, Amarnath U, Garrison C Z, Addy C L, Thompson S J 1992 Role of delayed feeding and of feeding increments in necrotizing enterocolitis. Journal of Pediatrics 121: 764–770
170. McLeish C M, MacDonald A, Booth I W 1995 Comparison of an elemental with a hydrolysed whey formula in intolerance to cows' milk. Archives of Disease in Childhood 73: 211–215
171. Melis K, Janssens G 1990 Long-term use of cisapride Prepulsid in premature neonates. Acta Gastroenterologica Belgica 53: 372–375
172. Menon A P, Schefft G L, Thach B T 1985 Apnea associated with regurgitation in infants. Journal of Pediatrics 106: 625–629
173. Mirakian R, Richardson A, Milla P J et al 1986 Protracted diarrhoea of infancy: evidence in support of an autoimmune variant. British Medical Journal 293: 1132–1136
174. Mitchell A, Watkins R M, Collin J 1984 Surgical treatment of the short bowel syndrome. British Journal of Surgery 71: 329–333
175. Morecroft J A, Spitz L, Hamilton P A, Holmes S J K 1994 Plasma cytokine levels in necrotizing enterocolitis. Acta Paediatrica Suppl 396: 18–20
176. Morgan L J, Shochat S J, Hartman G E 1994 Peritoneal drainage as primary management of perforated NEC in the very low birth weight infant. Journal of Pediatric Surgery 29: 310–315
177. Moroz S P, Espinoza J, Cumming W A, Diamant N E 1976 Lower esophageal sphincter function in children with and without gastroesophageal reflux. Gastroenterology 71: 236–241
178. Moya F R, Eguchi H, Zhao B et al 1994 Platelet-activating factor acetylhydrolase in term and preterm human milk: a preliminary report. Journal of Pediatric Gastroenterology and Nutrition 19: 236–239
179. Mulvihill S J, Stone M M, Fonkalsrud E W, Debas H T 1986 Trophic effect of amniotic fluid on fetal gastrointestinal development. Journal of Surgical Research 40: 291–296
180. Musemeche C A, Baker J L, Feddersen R M 1995 A model of intestinal ischemia in the neonatal rat utilizing superior mesenteric artery occlusion and intraluminal platelet-activating factor. Journal of Surgical Research 58: 724–727
181. Musemeche C A, Kosloske A M, Ricketts R R 1987 Enterostomy in necrotizing enterocolitis: an analysis of techniques and timing of closure. Journal of Pediatric Surgery 22: 479–483
182. Newell S J 1988 Development of the lower oesophageal sphincter in the preterm infant. In: Milla P J (ed) Disorders of gastrointestinal motility in childhood. John Wiley & Sons, Chichester, pp 39–53
183. Newell S J 1990 Cisapride: its use in children. British Journal of Hospital Medicine 44: 408–409

184. Newell S J 1996 Gastrointestinal function and its ontogeny: how should we feed the preterm infant; In: Ryan S (ed) Seminars in neonatology. W B Saunders, London, pp 59–66
185. Newell S J, Booth I W, Morgan M E, Durbin G M, McNeish A S 1989 Gastro-oesophageal reflux in preterm infants. Archives of Disease in Childhood 64: 780–786
186. Newell S J, Chapman S, Booth I W 1993 Ultrasonic assessment of gastric emptying in the preterm infant. Archives of Disease in Childhood 69: 32–36
187. Newell S J, Morgan M E, Durbin G M, Booth I W, McNeish A S 1989 Does mechanical ventilation precipitate gastro-oesophageal reflux during enteral feeding? Archives of Disease in Childhood 64: 1352–1355
188. Newell S J, Sarkar P K, Durbin G M, Booth I W, McNeish A S 1986 Maturation of the lower oesophageal sphincter in the preterm baby. Gut 29: 167–172
189. Ng P C, Brownlee K G, Dear P R 1992 Gastroduodenal perforation in preterm babies treated with dexamethasone for bronchopulmonary dysplasia. Archives of Disease in Childhood 66: 1164–1166
190. Novak R W, Abbott A E, Klein R L 1993 T-cryptantigen determination affects mortality in necrotizing enterocolitis. Surgery Gynecology and Obstetrics 176: 368–370
191. O'Rawe A, Dodge J A, Redmond A O B, McIntosh J, Brock D J H 1990 Gene–energy interaction in cystic fibrosis. Lancet ii: 552–553
192. Oldaeus G, Anjou K, Bjorksten B, Moran J R, Kjellman N M 1997 Extensively and partially hydrolysed infant formulas for allergy prophylaxis. Archives of Disease in Childhood 77: 4–10
193. Omari T I, Miki K, Fraser R et al 1995 Esophageal body and lower esophageal sphincter function in healthy premature infants. Gastroenterology 109: 1757–1764
194. Orenstein S R, Shalaby T M, Putnam P E 1992 Thickened feedings as a cause of increased coughing when used as therapy for gastroesophageal reflux in infants. Journal of Pediatrics 121: 913–915
195. Orme R L, Eades S M 1968 Perforation of the bowel in the newborn as a complication of exchange transfusion. British Medical Journal iv: 349–351
196. Panigrahi P, Gupta S, Gewolb I H, Morris J G 1994 Occurrence of necrotizing enterocolitis may be dependent on patterns of bacterial adherence and intestinal colonisation: studies in Caco-2 tissue culture and weaning rabbit models. Pediatric Research 36: 115–121
197. Papaila J G, Wilmot D, Grosfeld J L, Rescorla F J, West K W, Vane D W 1989 Increased incidence of delayed gastric emptying in children with gastroesophageal reflux. A prospective evaluation. Archives of Surgery 124: 933–936
198. Phelan P D 1995 Neonatal screening for cystic fibrosis. Thorax 50: 705–706
199. Phillips A D, Jenkins P, Raafat F, Walker Smith J A 1985 Congenital microvillous atrophy: specific diagnostic features. Archives of Disease in Childhood 60: 135–140
200. Phillips A D, Schmitz J 1992 Familial microvillous atrophy: a clinicopathological review of 23 cases. Journal of Pediatric Gastroenterology and Nutrition 14: 380–396
201. Pitt J, Barlow B, Heird W C 1977 Protection against experimental necrotizing enterocolitis by maternal milk I: role of milk leukocytes. Pediatric Research 11: 906–909
202. Pradeaux L, Boggio V. Gouyon J B 1991 Gastro-oesophageal reflux in mechanically ventilated preterm infants. Archives of Disease in Childhood 66: 793–796
203. Pritchard J A 1966 Fetal swallowing and amniotic fluid volume. Obstetrics and Gynecology 28: 606–610
204. Raval N C, Gonzalez E, Bhat A M, Pearlman S A, Stefano J L 1995 Umbilical venous catheters: evaluation of radiographs to determine position and associated complications of malpositioned umbilical venous catheters. American Journal of Perinatology 12: 201–204
205. Rennie J M, Kelsall A W 1994 Vitamin K prophylaxis in the newborn – again. Archives of Disease in Childhood 70: 248–251
206. Rescorla F J 1995 Surgical management of pediatric necrotizing enterocolitis. Current Opinions in Pediatrics 7: 335–341
207. Ricketts R R 1994 Surgical treatment of necrotizing enterocolitis and the short bowel syndrome. Clinics in Perinatology 21: 365–387
208. Ricour C, Gorski A M, Goulet O J 1990 Home parenteral nutrition in children: 8 years of experience with 112 patients. Clinical Nutrition 9: 65–71
209. Riordan R J, Rommens J M, Kerem B et al 1989 Identification of the cystic fibrosis gene: cloning and characterization of complementary DNA. Science 245: 1066–1073
210. Roberton D M, Paganelli R, Dinwiddie R, Levinsky R J 1982 Milk antigen absorption in the preterm and term neonate. Archives of Disease in Childhood 57: 369–372
211. Roberts G, Stanfield M, Black A, Redmond A 1988 Screening for cystic fibrosis: a four year regional experience. Archives of Disease in Childhood 63: 1438–1443
212. Rotbart H A, Levin M J 1983 How contagious is necrotizing enterocolitis? Pediatric Infectious Disease Journal 2: 406–410
213. Rothstein F C, Halpin T C, Keigman R J, Izant R J 1982 Importance of early ileostomy closure to prevent chronic salt and water losses after necrotizing enterocolitis. Pediatrics 70: 249–253
214. Rowe M I, Reblock K K, Kurkchubasche A G, Healey P J 1994 Necrotizing enterocolitis in the extremely low birth weight infant. Journal of Pediatric Surgery 29: 987–990
215. Saarinen U M, Kajosaari M 1991 Breast feeding and health in the 1980s: prospective follow up study until 17 years old. Lancet 346: 1065–1069
216. Sanderson I R, Phillips A D, Spencer J, Walker Smith J A 1991 Response of autoimmune enteropathy to cyclosporin A therapy. Gut 32: 1421–1424
217. Sandhu B K, Tripp J H, Milla P J, Harries J T 1983 Loperamide in severe protracted diarrhoea. Archives of Disease in Childhood 58: 39–43
218. Santulli T V, Schullinger J N, Heird W C 1975 Acute necrotizing enterocolitis in infancy: a review of 64 cases. Pediatrics 55: 376–387
219. Savilathi E, Launiala K, Kuitunen P 1983 Congenital lactase deficiency: a clinical study of 16 patients. Archives of Disease in Childhood 58: 246–252
220. Schimpl G, Hollwarth M E, Fotter R, Becker H 1994 Late intestinal strictures following successful treatment of necrotizing enterocolitis. Acta Paediatrica Suppl 396: 80–83
221. Schober P H, Nassiri J 1994 Risk factors and severity indices in necrotizing enterocolitis. Acta Paediatrica Suppl 396: 49–52
222. Shaul W L 1981 Clues to the early diagnosis of neonatal appendicitis. Journal of Pediatrics 98: 473–476
223. Sherry S N, Kramer I 1955 The time of passage of the first stool and first urine by the newborn infant. Journal of Pediatrics 46: 158–159
224. Shulman R J, Buffone G, Wise L 1985 Enteric protein loss in necrotizing enterocolitis as measured by alpha1-antitrypsin excretion. Journal of Pediatrics 107: 287–290
225. Shulman R J, Redel C A, Stathos T H 1994 Bolus versus continuous feedings stimulate small intestinal growth and development in the newborn pig. Journal of Pediatric Gastroenterology and Nutrition 18: 350–354
226. Sondheimer J M, Clark D A, Gervaise E P 1985 Continuous gastric pH measurement in young and older healthy healthy preterm infants receiving formula and clear liquid feedings. Journal of Pediatric Gastroenterology and Nutrition 4: 352–355
227. Sondheimer J M, Morris B A 1979 Gastro-oesophageal reflux among severely retarded children. Journal of Pediatrics 94: 710–714
228. Southern K W 1997 DeltaF508 in cystic fibrosis: willing but not able. Archives of Disease in Childhood 76: 278–282
229. Spicher V, Roulet M, Schutz Y 1991 Assessment of total energy expenditure in free living patients with cystic fibrosis. Journal of Pediatrics 118: 865–872
230. Spitz L, Stringer M D 1993 Surgical management of neonatal necrotising enterocolitis. Archives of Disease in Childhood 69: 269–271
231. Staiano A, Cucchiara S, Del Giudice E, Andreotti M R, Minella R 1991 Disorders of oesophageal motility in children with psychomotor retardation and gastro-oesophageal reflux. European Journal of Pediatrics 150: 638–641
232. Standing Committee on Nutrition of the British Paediatric Association 1994 Is breast feeding beneficial in the UK? Archives of Disease in Childhood 71: 376–380
233. Stevenson D K, Kerner J A, Malachowski N, Sunshine P 1980 Late morbidity among survivors of necrotizing enterocolitis. Pediatrics 66: 925–927
234. Stoll B J 1994 Epidemiology of necrotizing enterocolitis. Clinics in Perinatology 21: 205–218
235. Stringer M D, Puntis J W L 1995 Short bowel syndrome. Archives of Disease in Childhood 73: 170–173

236. Stringer M D, Thornton J G, Mason G C 1996 Hyperechoic bowel. Archives of Disease in Childhood 74: F1–F2
237. Sutphen J L, Dillard V L 1988 Effect of feeding volume on early postcibal gastroesophageal reflux in infants. Journal of Pediatric Gastroenterology and Nutrition 7: 185–188
238. Tappin D M, King C, Paton J Y 1992 Lower oesophageal pH monitoring – a useful clinical tool. Archives of Disease in Childhood 67: 146–148
239. Tejavej A, Siripoonya P, Rusmemala L, Tinasulanan K, Auksukasate J 1984 The times of passage of the first urine and the first stool by Thai newborn infants. Journal of the Medical Association of Thailand 67: 86–88
240. Thomas D F M, Fernie D S, Bayston R, Spitz L 1984 Clostridial toxins in neonatal necrotising enterocolitis. Archives of Disease in Childhood 59: 270–272
241. Thomas D F M, Fernie D S, Malone M, Bayston R, Spitz L 1982 Association between *Clostridium difficile* and enterocolitis in Hirschprung's disease. Lancet i: 78–79
242. Thompson J S, Rikkers L F 1987 Surgical alternatives for the short bowel syndrome. American Journal of Gastroenterology 82: 97–106
243. Tobiansky R, Lui K, Roberts S, Veddovi M 1995 Neurodevelopmental outcome in very low birthweight infants with necrotizing enterocolitis requiring surgery. Journal of Paediatrics and Child Health 31: 233–236
244. Tobin J C, McCloud P, Cameron D J S 1997 Posture and gastro-oesophageal reflux: a case for left lateral positioning. Archives of Disease in Childhood 76: 254–258
245. Toce S S, Keenan W J, Homan S M 1987 Enteral feeding in very low birth weight infants: a comparison of two nasogastric methods. American Journal of Diseases of Children 141: 439–444
246. Tolia V, Lin C H, Kuhns L R 1992 Gastric emptying using three different formulas in infants with gastroesophageal reflux. Journal of Pediatric Gastroenterology and Nutrition 15: 297–301
247. Touloukian R J, Walker Smith J A 1983 Normal intestinal length in preterm infants. Journal of Pediatric Surgery 18: 720–723
248. Uauy R, Fanaroff A A, Korones S B, Phillips E A, Phillips J B, Wright L L 1991 Necrotizing enterocolitis in very low birth weight infants: biodemographic and clinical correlates. Journal of Pediatrics 119: 630–638
249. Uceda J E, Laos C A, Kolni H W, Klein A M 1995 Intestinal perforations in infants with a very low birth weight: a disease of increasing survival? Journal of Pediatric Surgery 30: 1314–1316
250. Udall J N 1990 Gastrointestinal host defence and necrotizing enterocolitis. Journal of Pediatrics 117: S33–S44
251. Vandenplas Y, Ashkenazi A, Belli D et al 1993 A proposition for the diagnosis and treatment of gastro-oesophageal reflux disease in children: a report from a working group on gastro-oesophageal reflux disease. Working Group of the European Society of Paediatric Gastro-enterology and Nutrition ESPGAN. European Journal of Pediatrics 152: 704–711
252. Vandenplas Y, Goyvaerts H, Helven R, Sacre L 1991 Gastroesophageal reflux, as measured by 24-hour pH monitoring, in 509 healthy infants screened for risk of sudden infant death syndrome. Pediatrics 88: 834–840
253. Vandenplas Y, Sacre Smits L 1985 Seventeen-hour continuous esophageal pH monitoring in the newborn: evaluation of the influence of position in asymptomatic and symptomatic babies. Journal of Pediatric Gastroenterology and Nutrition 4: 356–361
254. Vanderhoof J A 1996 Short bowel syndrome. Clinics in Perinatology 23: 377–386
255. Vargas J H, Sachs P, Ament M E 1988 Chronic intestinal pseudo-obstruction syndrome in pediatrics: results of a national survey of members of NASPGAN. Journal of Pediatric Gastroenterology and Nutrition 7: 323–332
256. Vasan U, Gotoff S P 1994 Prevention of neonatal necrotizing enterocolitis. Clinics in Perinatology 21: 425–435
257. Vinton N E 1994 Gastrointestinal bleeding in infancy and childhood. Gastroenterology Clinics of North America 23: 93–122
258. Walker W A 1985 Absorption of protein and protein fragments in the developing intestine: role in immunologic/allergic reactions. Pediatrics 75: 167–171
259. Wallis C 1997 Diagnosing cystic fibrosis: blood sweat and tears. Archives of Disease in Childhood 76: 85–88
260. Walsh M C, Kliegman R M 1986 Necrotizing enterocolitis: treatment based on staging criteria. Pediatric Clinics of North America 33: 179–201
261. Warner B W, Ziegler M M 1993 Management of short bowel syndrome in the pediatric population. Pediatric Clinics of North America 40: 1335–1350
262. Warren W S, Hamosh A, Egan M, Rosenstein B J 1997 False-positive results of genetic testing in cystic fibrosis. Journal of Pediatrics 130: 658–660
263. Weaver L T, Green M R, Nicholson K et al 1994 Prognosis in cystic fibrosis treated with continuous flucloxacillin from the neonatal period. Archives of Disease in Childhood 70: 84–89
264. Weaver L T, Laker M F, Nelson R 1984 Enhanced intestinal permeability in preterm babies with bloody stools. Archives of Disease in Childhood 59: 280–281
265. Weaver L T, Laker M F, Nelson R 1984 Intestinal permeability in the newborn. Archives of Disease in Childhood 59: 236–241
266. Weaver L T, Laker M F, Nelson R, Lucas A 1987 Milk feeding and changes in intestinal permeability and morphology in the newborn. Journal of Pediatric Gastroenterology and Nutrition 6: 351–358
267. Weaver L T, Lucas A 1990 Maturation of large bowel function in relation to gestational and postnatal age, feed volumes and composition in the newborn. Pediatric Reviews and Communications 4: 250
268. Weaver L T, Richmond S W J, Nelson R 1983 Loperamide toxicity in severe protracted diarrhoea. Archives of Disease in Childhood 58: 568
269. Weber T R, Tracy T F, Silen M L et al 1995 Enterostomy and its closure in newborns. Archives of Surgery 130: 534–537
270. Weinberg G, Kleinhaus S, Boley S J 1989 Idiopathic intestinal perforation in the newborn: an increasingly common entity. Journal of Pediatric Surgery 24: 1007–1008
271. Wen H H, Chen M H, Ho M M, Hwang K C 1992 Fetal gastric ulcer presenting with bloody amniotic fluid. Journal of Pediatric Gastroenterology and Nutrition 15: 455–457
272. Westra-Meijer C M M, Degener S E, Dzoljic-Danolivic G, Michel M F, Mettau J W 1983 Quantitative study of the aerobic and anaerobic faecal flora in neonatal necrotising enterocolitis. Archives of Disease in Childhood 58: 523–529
273. Wilmore D W 1972 Factors correlating with a successful outcome following extensive intestinal resection in newborn infants. Journal of Pediatrics 80: 88–95
274. Wilson R, del Portillo M, Schmidt E, Feldman R A, Kanto W P 1983 Risk factors for necrotizing enterocolitis in infants weighing more than 2000 grams at birth: a case control study. Pediatrics 71: 19–22
275. Wiswell T E, Cornish J D, Northam R S 1986 Neonatal polycythemia: frequency of clinical manifestations and other problems. Pediatrics 78: 26–28
276. Wolfe S P 1995 Prevention programmes – a dietetic minefield. European Journal of Clinical Nutrition 49: S92–S99
277. Wood C M, Spicer R D, Beddis I R, Puntis J W L 1995 Pancreatic exocrine failure in cystic fibrosis presenting as necrotising enterocolitis. Journal of Pediatric Gastroenterology and Nutrition 20: 104–106
278. Wozniak E R, Fenton T R, Milla P J 1983 The development of fasting small intestinal motility in the human neonate. In: Roman C (ed) Gastrointestinal motility. MTP Press, Lancaster, pp 265–270
279. Young D G 1965 Spontaneous rupture of the rectum. Proceedings of the Royal Society of Medicine 58: 615–616
280. Yu V Y, Joseph R, Bajuk B, Orgill A, Astbury J 1984 Necrotizing enterocolitis in very low birthweight infants: a four-year experience. Australian Paediatric Journal 20: 29–33
281. Ziegler M M 1986 Short bowel syndrome in infancy: etiology and management. Clinics in Perinatology 13: 163–173

Part 4

Congenital defects and surgical problems

Carl F. Davis Daniel G. Young

INTRODUCTION

Although each condition in this chapter is discussed in isolation, it must be remembered that many infants with one congenital anomaly may also have other structural defects. Establishing the diagnosis of one anomaly should make one more, rather than less, alert to the possibility of other anomalies. Some combinations are well recognized, such as the group that has attracted the title of VACTERL complex, i.e. an infant with vertebral, anorectal, cardiac, tracheo-oesophageal, renal and radial claw-hand anomalies. Other less common associations are not so well recognized.

The anomalies will be discussed in sequence from mouth to anus, rather than in order of their importance in regard to frequency of occurrence, morbidity or mortality from the defect. Sections will deal with mouth and nasopharynx, oesophagus and stomach, small bowel, large bowel and anorectal anomalies, followed by a discussion of abdominal wall defects and herniae.

MOUTH AND NASOPHARYNX

CLEFT LIP AND PALATE

For when born, my poor lip,
From the first there was a slip,
Which prevented me to talk,
Strangely seemed my Face at fault.

These lines, from Thomas Ragwaldson's *Psalm of Praise of the Still Deformed*, are part of his 50-verse description of the repair of his cleft lip in 1763, when he was 39 years old.[66] With continuing surgical experience the age at which repair of cleft lip or palate is carried out has progressively decreased, and discussion has arisen on the possibility and practicability of intrauterine repair of cleft lip, as intrauterine healing is associated with less scar formation than postnatal wound healing. However, although cleft lip in the fetus can be diagnosed by ultrasound, treatment is not normally commenced until after birth.[43]

CLEFT LIP

This defect may vary from a minor degree of cleft, in which the skin is intact and there is a hardly noticeable dimple on the vermilion border, to the severe degree of bilateral cleft. The more common varieties are the incomplete or complete unilateral forms of cleft (Figs 31.17, 31.18). Less frequently, severe bilateral cleft presents a much more unsightly appearance (Fig. 31.19) and is a much greater challenge to both surgeon and orthodontist. The prevalence of cleft lip is approximately 1 in 1000 births. Genetic factors play a part in the aetiology of this condition and it is not uncommon to find a positive family history. This can be of help in some instances in dealing with the immediate concerns and

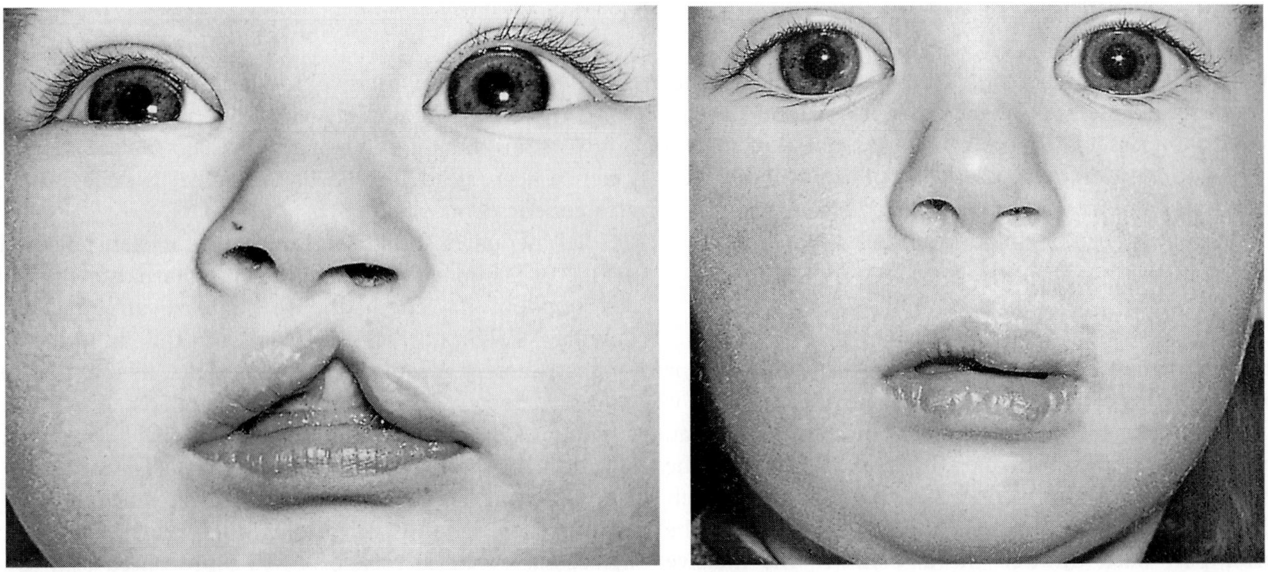

A B

Fig. 31.17 (A) Incomplete cleft lip showing mild nostril deformity. (B) Lip following repair. Slight excess of tissue on cleft side.

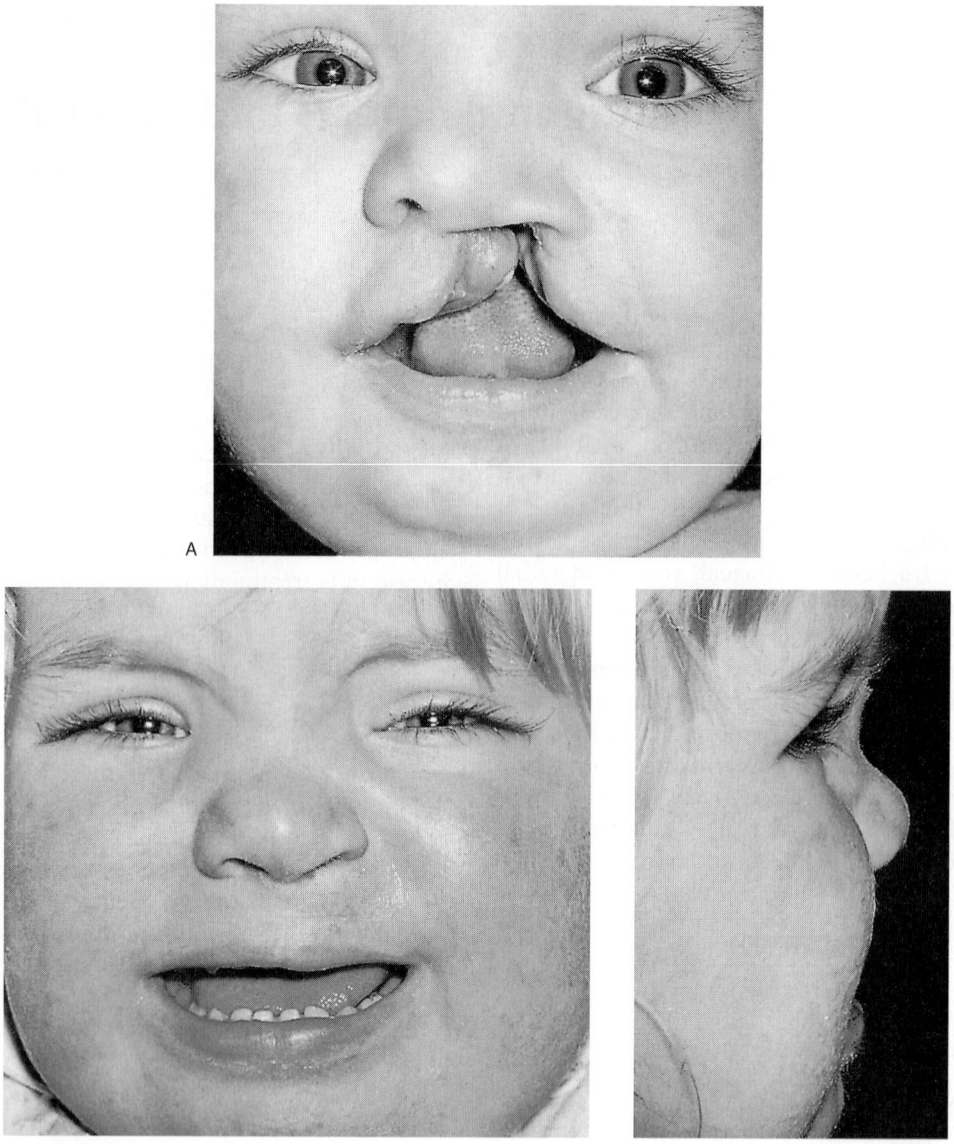

Fig. 31.18 (A) Complete unilateral cleft lip. (B) One year after repair.

apprehensions experienced by the parents. Having an affected first-degree relative increases the risk by a factor of about 40. Associated anomalies are not uncommon and need to be identified. Cleft lip with or without cleft palate is also one of the three most common anomalies found in infants born of epileptic mothers.[73]

CLEFT PALATE

Cleft palate may not be obvious at birth unless it is associated with a cleft lip. The prevalence of cleft palate is also approximately 1 in 1000 births, but with the overlap in infants who have both cleft lip and cleft palate the overall prevalence of both conditions is 1.5 in 1000. Cleft of the palate may be a primary cleft which affects the anterior part back through the alveolus to the incisive foramen, or a secondary cleft which extends forward from the uvula to the incisive foramen. The clefts may be incomplete, or complete cleft lip and palate. Genetic factors in the different types of cleft palate vary, and hence accurate definition of the defect is necessary prior to genetic counselling.

All neonates should be examined for cleft palate (Fig. 31.20) To do this it is necessary to visualize the palate throughout its length and to visualize an intact single uvula. Palpation of the roof of the mouth is an unsatisfactory means of detecting clefts, as only the more gross defects will be found. Cleft soft palate cannot be palpated by an examiner's finger in the baby's mouth. Submucous cleft of the palate is usually noted by the presence of a bifid uvula. This indicates a defect in the closure of the muscle forming the palate. Operation is necessary if nasal escape is to be prevented and speech development is to be normal.

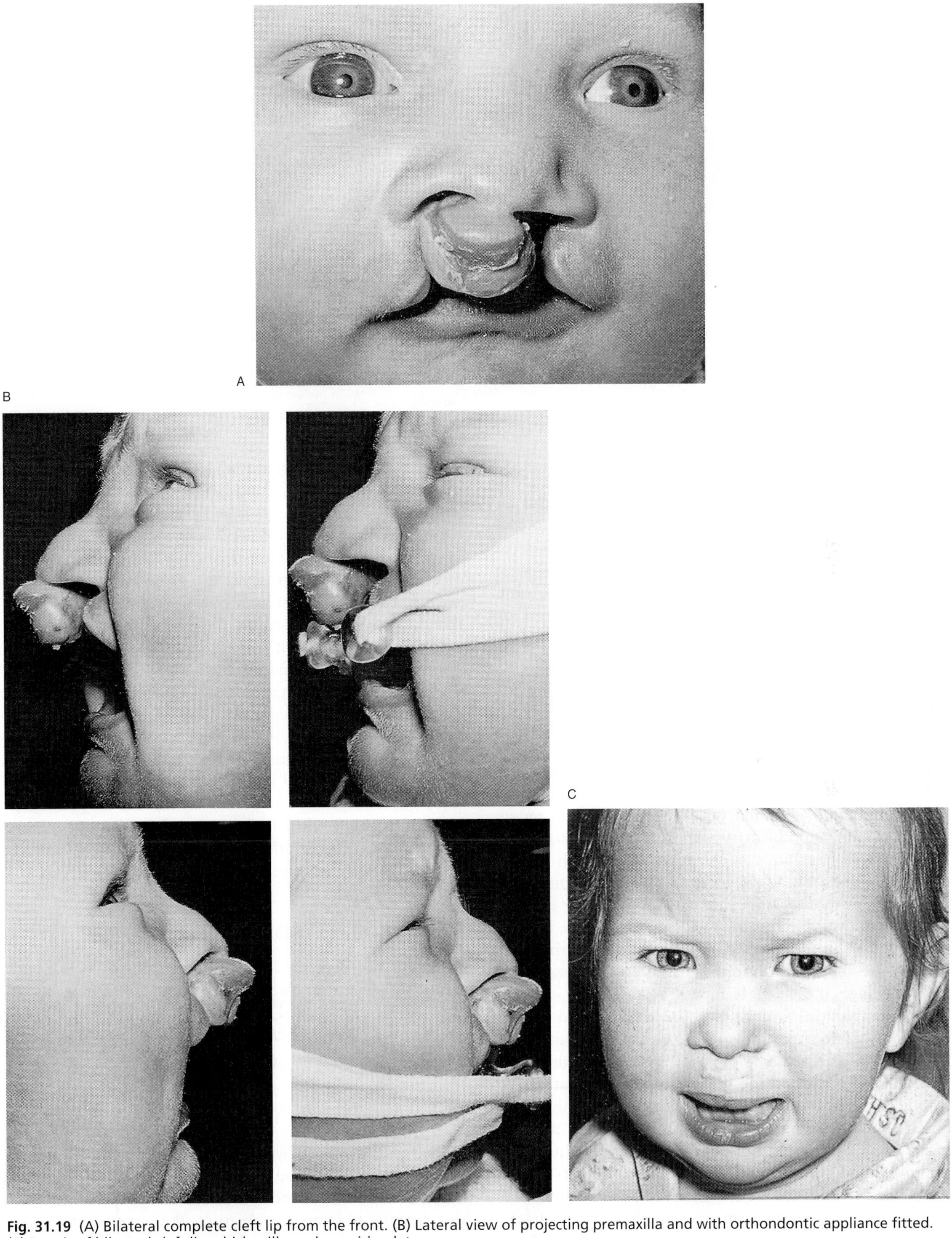

Fig. 31.19 (A) Bilateral complete cleft lip from the front. (B) Lateral view of projecting premaxilla and with orthondontic appliance fitted. (C) Repair of bilateral cleft lip which will require revision later.

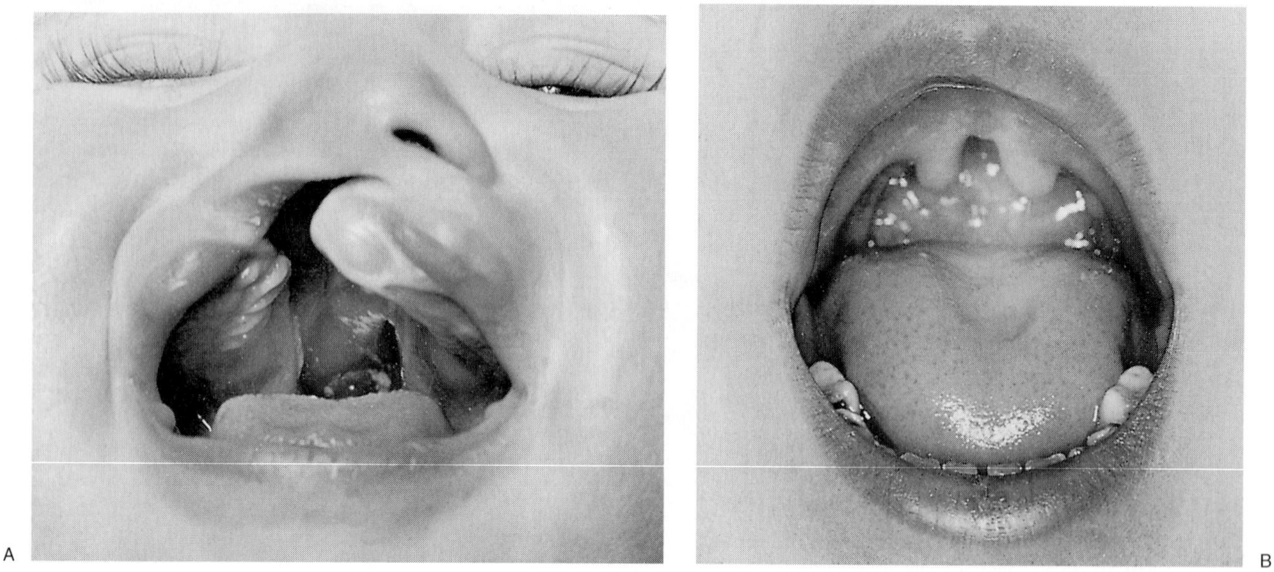

Fig. 31.20 (A) Complete cleft palate. (B) Bifid uvula which accompanies cleft of the soft palate.

Management

The unsightly nature of the cleft lip defect is an immediate shock. Some comfort can be given to the parents by the neonatal unit having photographs of previous patients with a similar condition and showing these together with photographs of the child some time after repair. Early consultation with the paediatric or plastic surgeon and orthodontist should be arranged. Most large referral units have a Cleft Team, drawing on all relevant specialities in a coordinated fashion. The Royal College of Surgeons of England has published a parents' guide to the treatment of cleft lip and palate. The Cleft Lip and Palate Association was formed between health-care professionals and parents to provide parental support and advice.

The timing of operation varies. Some prefer to repair the cleft soon after birth, within the first week of life. These procedures can now be done with a high degree of safety. The benefit of early correction is the early improvement in appearance, and wound healing may be better in the very young infant. Also, this earlier correction will lead to less secondary deformity from the continuing stresses of the abnormal tissue on the developing nasal cartilages if the cleft is allowed to persist.

The approach which has been practised more commonly is to delay operation on the cleft until the infant is over the neonatal period.[57,72] Here, repair of the lip is carried out when the infant is about 3 months old, by which time there has been considerable growth of the lip. If the infant has an associated cleft of the primary palate, oral orthopaedic treatment may be instituted to improve the alveolar malalignment. This is not usually necessary in those with cleft of the secondary palate. It entails regular attention from the orthodontic specialist to fit a series of prostheses contoured for the roof of the infant's mouth. The infant sucks on this plate. Through the repeated pressure, stimulation of growth and better alignment of the segments is achieved so that the ultimate repair of the lip does not need to bridge such a relatively broad gap. Treatment at this early time may also be directed towards decreasing the projection of the premaxillary segment to bring it backwards into line with the remaining structures forming the arch of the upper jaw.

The success of repair of cleft lip and palate has steadily improved, but some infants have deficiency of tissues to such an extent that later surgery is necessary to improve the end result. This may be a cosmetic procedure on the lip or nose, or one to improve function, such as a pharyngoplasty, eliminating the nasal escape of air. Where there is marked hypoplasia of the mid-third of the face, major surgical procedures may have to be performed in the teenage years to improve the cosmetic result. Continuing orthodontic supervision or treatment is necessary until the permanent dentition is settled.

PIERRE–ROBIN SYNDROME

Although the degree of upper airway obstruction is not quite so severe in the Pierre–Robin syndrome as in choanal atresia (p. 664), the condition is a major management problem that can too often lead to sudden infant death.

Pathophysiology

In the Pierre–Robin syndrome there is both a midline posterior cleft of the palate and hypoplasia of the mandible. This produces an unstable upper airway, with the tongue tending to obstruct the oropharynx. The obstruction is most severe when the infant lies on his back, and least of a problem when he is nursed prone. Frequent attacks of obstructive apnoea, which are particularly likely to occur when the infant is asleep, may lead to carbon dioxide retention, cor pulmonale and even mental retardation. The obstruction tends to become less severe as the infant gets older and the mandible grows. The incidence is approximately 1 in 20 000.

Diagnosis

Provided the doctor is aware of the condition, diagnosis is not a problem. The infant will be noticed to have intermittent obstructive apnoea, particularly when supine, and to have a poorly developed lower jaw and a midline cleft palate. Unless the palate is routinely visualized as part of the routine neonatal examination, this feature may be missed until the first feed, when milk then trickles from the nostrils.

Management

If the infant has severe obstructive apnoea from birth, insert an oral airway and fix it carefully in position. This will relieve the obstruction. Some infants can cope with minimal obstruction if nursed prone on a cradle with support to their forehead, allowing the tongue and mandible to fall forward, clearing the airway. It has now proved possible to rear these infants satisfactorily by using nasopharyngeal or nasal CPAP for the first weeks of life (p. 561). This is the treatment of choice, avoiding the need for tracheostomy, which was previously the only way of relieving the obstruction in those with severe defects and is still required in the rare severe case.[44] Feeding the infant is often a problem that can be helped by fitting a temporary plate, or using a feeding bottle with a soft flange that covers the defect. Some infants will need either spoon feeding or even nasogastric tube feeds for many weeks. Despite these provisions, sudden death can occur, either in hospital or while attempting to rear the infant at home.

Repair of the cleft palate is performed occasionally in the neonatal period by those advocating very early surgery. More commonly repair is delayed until the infant is about 1 year of age. Repair of the entire palate is then performed if possible. If not, the important feature is to repair the soft palate and the posterior aspect of the hard palate. The anterior part can be occluded by an obturator and the repair carried out later.

Long-term follow-up is essential, partly to provide the parents with support and to ensure that arrangements for palatal and mandibular surgery go smoothly, but also because children who have palatal problems are particularly prone to middle-ear infections.[9] They are also at increased risk of mental handicap.

OTHER CLEFTS

These are rare, but more gross defects of the upper lip or nose may occur.[77] They are usually accompanied by other anomalies, as in the infant shown in Figure 31.21 who had Fallot's tetralogy, oesophageal atresia and

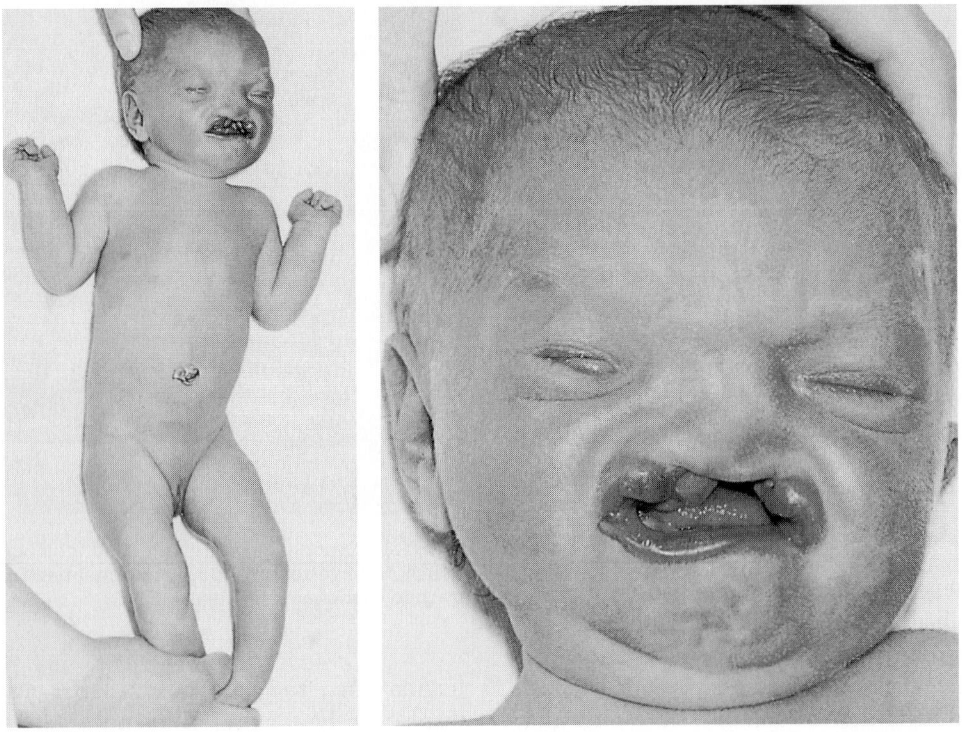

Fig. 31.21 More complex lip deformity showing single cleft opening to nose. Infant has multiple anomalies.

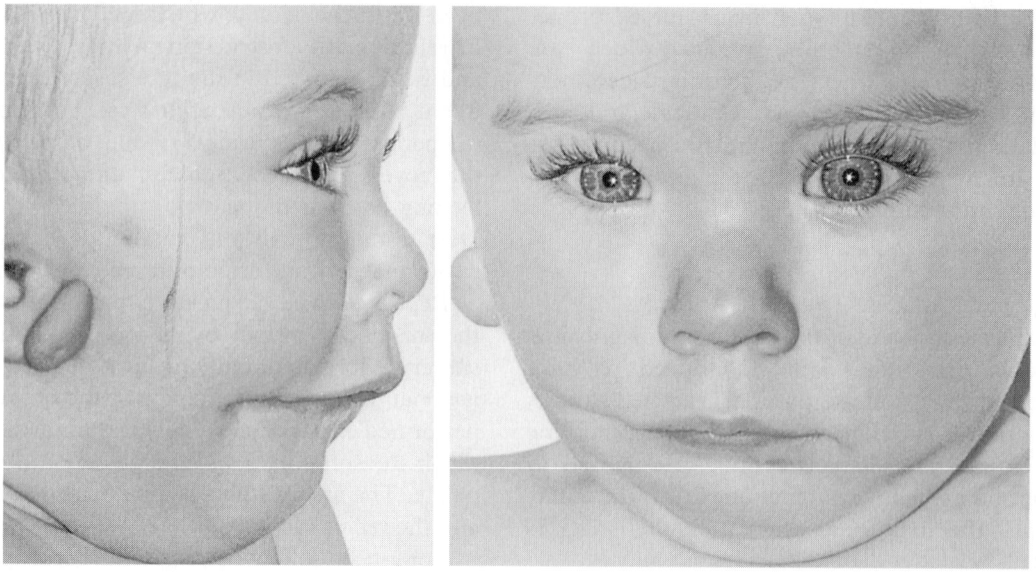

Fig. 31.22 Macrostoma with associated ear deformity.

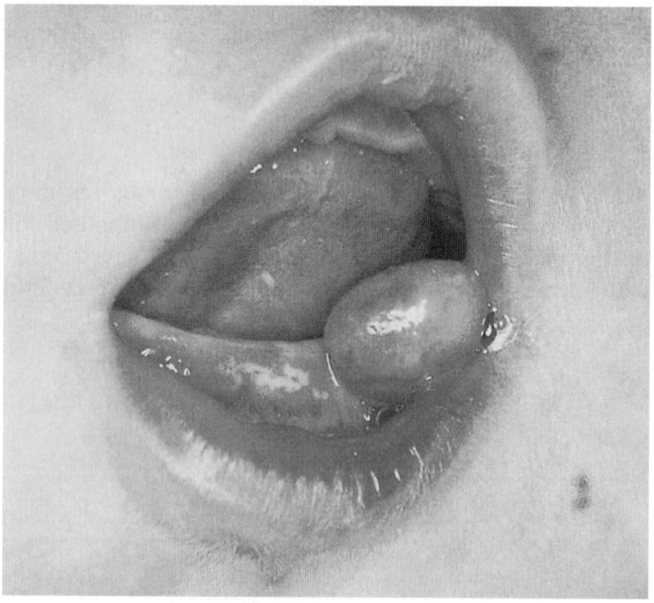

Fig. 31.23 Epulis arising from alveolar ridge.

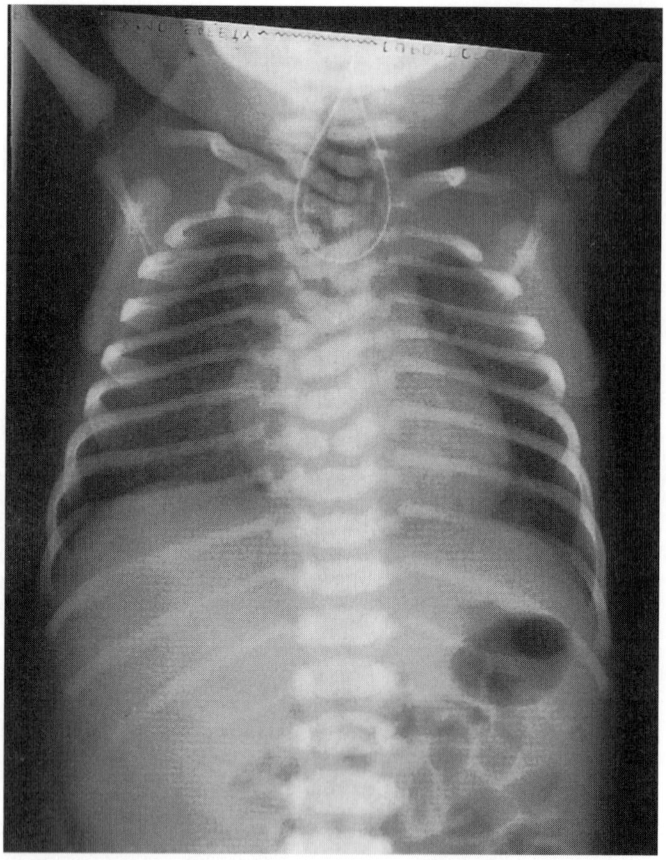

Fig. 31.24 Oesophageal atresia. Coiled feeding tube in proximal pouch. Note vertebral and rib abnormalities. Distal gas confirms a tracheo-oesophageal fistula.

tracheo-oesophageal fistula. Clefts or pits on the lower lip occur infrequently and require complete excision. Macrostoma (Fig. 31.22) is an infrequent anomaly which is amenable to surgical correction.[38]

MOUTH

Enlargement of the tongue may be due to hamartomatous malformation, such as haemangioma or lymphangioma, or to systemic disorders such as hypothyroidism (p. 961) or Weidemann–Beckwith syndrome (p. 945). These seldom require intervention in infancy. A ranula may occur in the floor of the mouth. This is usually the result of incomplete obstruction of the submandibular or sublingual duct, and can cause a large pearly-grey swelling, displacing the tongue. The ranula subsides spontaneously in many patients but if it persist or enlarges may require marsupialization. Retention mucus cysts on the lips, cheeks or mouth are simply excised. An epulis may arise from the alveolar ridge (Fig. 31.23) which may cause alarm. It is an hamartomatous lesion and treatment is simple excision.

OESOPHAGUS AND STOMACH

OESOPHAGEAL ATRESIA

Oesophageal atresia remains one of the major challenges in paediatric surgery, ever since the survival of two infants born in 1939 and treated by Leven[51] and Ladd.[50] Division of a tracheo-oesophageal fistula and primary anastomosis of oesophageal atresia was first successfully accomplished in 1941 by Haight.[42] In Britain, repair was first accomplished by Franklin in 1947.[31]

The prevalence of oesophageal atresia is 1 in 2500–3000 births. In 85% there is a blind proximal pouch and a fistula between the trachea and the distal oesophagus (Fig. 31.24). About 10% have oesophageal atresia without a fistula; here there is a long gap between oesophageal ends. Less commonly there is a tracheal fistula into the proximal oesophageal pouch, with or without a distal fistula.

Presentation

Antenatally polyhydramnios may alert the clinician to the possibility of the diagnosis, and on antenatal ultrasound screening the dilated proximal oesophageal pouch may be visualized. If a fistula is present there will be fluid in the stomach.

Postnatally there may be saliva or mucus dribbling from the infant's mouth and episodes of choking, cyanosis and coughing caused by overflow of secretions into the larynx and trachea. If fed, the infant will choke on swallowing and refuse further feeds. Attempted passage of a gastric tube will reveal a hold-up about 10 cm from the lips. The diagnosis is confirmed by passing a Franklin radio-opaque tube and obtaining anteroposterior and lateral X-rays of the chest and upper abdomen (Fig. 31.25) Air in the stomach indicates a fistula into the distal oesophagus. The presence of 13 pairs of ribs is not uncommon.

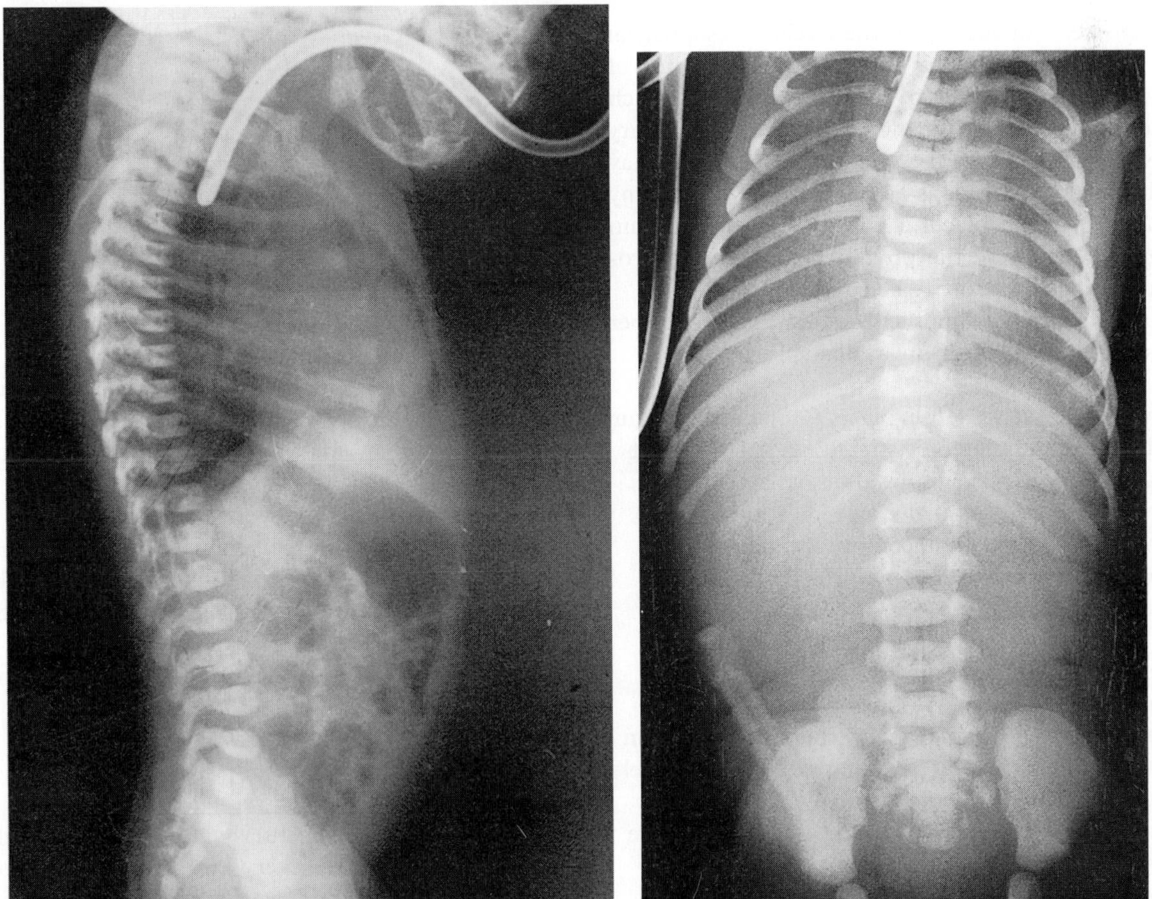

A B

Fig. 31.25 (A) Lateral X-ray with radio-opaque tube in proximal pouch confirming the diagnosis of oesophageal atresia. (B) Anteroposterior view of oesophageal atresia. A lack of gas in the abdomen indicates the lack of a distal tracheo-oesophageal fistula in this case.

Initial management is aimed at maintaining the airway free of secretions. The infant should be placed head-up, with a double-lumen (Replogle) tube (10 FG) in the proximal pouch on continuous effective suction to prevent aspiration of secretions. As these infants are prone to develop hypoglycaemia (p. 947) and hypocalcaemia (p. 966), appropriate intravenous fluids and electrolytes are given. Once stable, the infant should be transferred to a neonatal surgical unit for repair of the anomaly. Special care must be taken to identify associated anomalies (30–50%).[15,82] The VACTERL cluster (p. 883) is especially common, including cardiac, renal, vertebral, anorectal and limb anomalies. Intrinsic duodenal atresia is the commonest other gastrointestinal anomaly. More rarely, oesophageal atresia may be associated with the CHARGE (coloboma, heart defects, atresia of choanae, retarded growth, genital hypoplasia, ear anomalies) association.[49] Laryngotracheobronchial cleft anomalies must always be considered (p. 773).

The aim of surgery is to divide the fistula between the trachea and oesophagus and to unite the oesophageal ends by primary anastomosis.[65] This may not be possible if there is an excessive gap between the oesophageal ends, or if the physiological condition of the infant makes this approach unsafe.[64] In such cases the tracheo-oesophageal fistula is divided to protect the lungs from reflux of stomach secretions. In addition, either the proximal pouch can be left in place in the hope of delayed primary anastomosis, or the end of the proximal oesophagus may be brought out in the neck as a cervical oesophagostomy (Fig. 31.26). If left in place, it is necessary to maintain continuous aspiration of the proximal pouch. A gastrostomy allows enteral feeding to be commenced.

When a primary anastomosis is not feasible, a number of options for reconstruction are available:

- The proximal pouch is left in place. Growth may occur naturally or be stimulated by stretching.[46,80] Contrast studies of the proximal and distal oesophagus (the latter via the gastrostomy) give an indication of the likelihood of success. Thoracotomy and delayed oesophageal anastomosis are performed at about 3 months of age.
- A loop of colon or small bowel can be interposed between the proximal oesophagus and the distal oesophagus or stomach. This may be rotated on its vascular pedicle, as originally performed by Waterston in 1954.[2,34] Microvascular anastomosis of small bowel free graft has also been performed.
- A gastric tube, constructed from the greater curvature of the stomach, may be brought up through the left chest or retrosternally and anastomosed to the proximal oesophagus in the neck.[3,10]
- The stomach can be mobilized and a gastro-oesophageal anastomosis performed in the neck or mediastinum.[5,74]

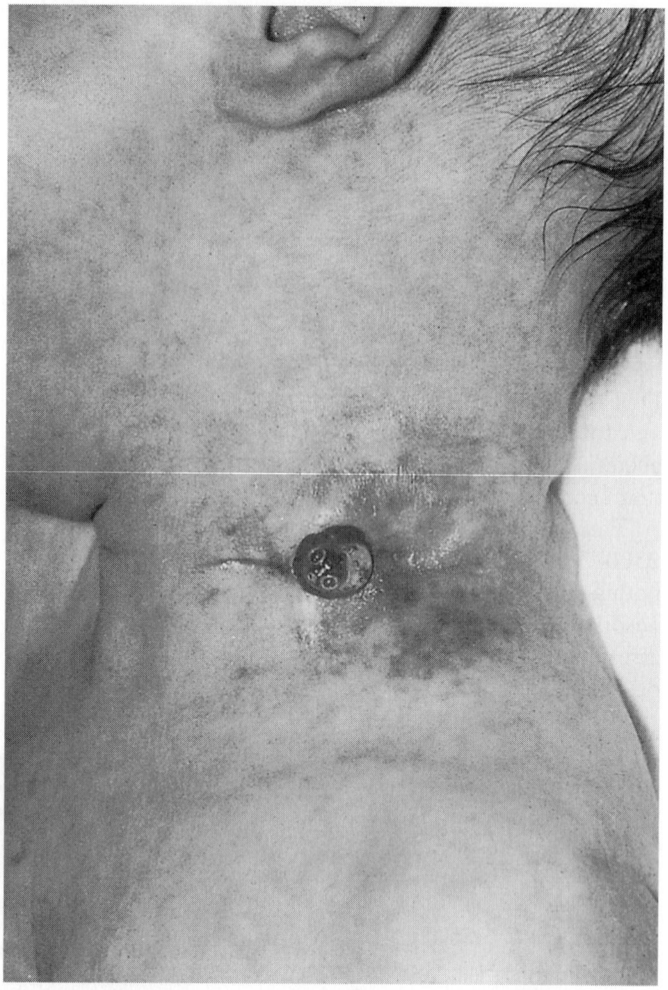

Fig. 31.26 Cervical oesophagostomy. This allows sham feeding.

The outlook for infants with oesophageal atresia is good. Mortality is dependent on the number and severity of associated major anomalies.[75] If birthweight is >1500 g with no other anomalies, survival rates approach 97%; weighing <1500 g in the presence of major cardiac anomalies reduces the overall survival rates to around 22%. Gastro-oesophageal reflux and oesophageal dismotility are common problems in children who have undergone repair of oesophageal atresia. Tracheomalacia may complicate recovery, and is exacerbated by the occurrence of an anastomotic stricture. Aortopexy is necessary in severe cases.[30]

TRACHEO-OESOPHAGEAL 'H' FISTULA

Tracheo-oesophageal fistula without oesophageal atresia occurs about once for every 20 infants with oesophageal atresia, but is not always obvious in the neonatal period.[19,58] Infants with larger tracheo-oesophageal fistulae present with problems earlier as a result of aspiration of material through the fistula into the trachea, causing respiratory problems. A small fistula may not cause clinical signs or symptoms for months or, on occasion, years. Infants with tracheo-oesophageal fistula in isolation do not have polyhdramnios in pregnancy and are of normal birthweight. Respiratory symptoms, particularly on feeding, are common. The commoner clinical signs are a right upper lobe pneumonia due to aspiration of material through the fistula, and gaseous distension of the abdominal contents due to air passing through the fistula into the oesophagus and down the alimentary tract. These infants, like those with oesophageal atresia, are more likely to have 13 pairs of ribs, and this can be a useful additional indicator.

The only simple test to help substantiate the diagnosis is to pass a tube into the upper oesophagus while placing the external end of this tube under water. If recurrent bubbles of air pass through the tube when the infant breathes or cries, a fistula is the likely explanation. The fistula may be visualized by tube oesophagogram. Here, contrast is instilled via a tube placed initially in the distal oesophagus and gradually withdrawn with the infant lying on the left side. Oesophagoscopy and bronchoscopy can also be used. Water-soluble methylene blue injected into the distal trachea will be seen to pass through the fistula into the oesophagus. Treatment is to divide the fistula. As it is always relatively high, it is best approached through a low neck incision rather than through a thoracotomy.

LARYNGOTRACHEO-OEOSOPHAGEAL CLEFT

This major anomaly, in which there is failure of complete separation of the trachea and oesophagus, can be associated with other oesophageal anomalies. Recognition of the disorder in infants presenting with respiratory problems in the neonatal period may not be easy on superficial inspection of the larynx at intubation. Difficulty in ventilating the infant may draw attention to the fact that all is not well. If there is doubt about the posterior aspect of the larynx, laryngoscopy will reveal whether it is cleft or intact. A minor sulcus posteriorly may be confused with a serious cleft. Treatment of the condition remains difficult and the longer-term problems are formidable.[32]

OESOPHAGEAL PERFORATION

Iatrogenic oesophageal perforation may occur unless care is taken when passing nasogastric or endotracheal tubes (p. 933). Non-ionic contrast can be used to show the site of perforation. Conservative management is usually successful, with surgery rarely required.

HYPERTROPHIC PYLORIC STENOSIS

This condition is uncommon in the neonatal period and more often presents just after, when an infant who has usually been progressing well develops projectile vomiting of gastric contents. The infant will often be dehydrated,

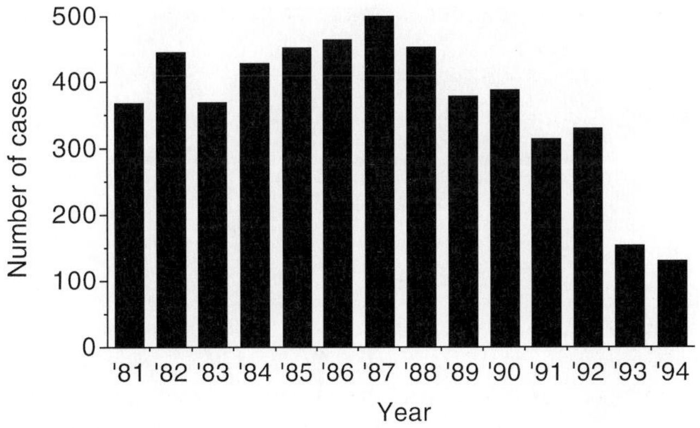

Fig. 31.27 Discharges from hospitals with diagnosis of hypertrophic pyloric stenosis in Scotland 1981–94.

typically has an anxious facies and feeds greedily. Of 130 cases seen in Glasgow during a 12-month period, 42% presented before 4 weeks when age was corrected for gestation, and 10% were born prematurely. The prevalence of hypertrophic pyloric stenosis varies, but has been reported as high as 8.8 in 1000 births.[47] More recently, the incidence has decreased (Fig. 31.27) There is a male to female ratio of 4:1. Breast-fed infants are less often affected, though not immune. Infants with nasojejunal tubes in situ for some time are at increased risk.[27,63] Infants who have had oesophageal atresia are also at increased risk.[36]

Electrolyte abnormalities are common, typified by hypochloraemic alkalosis. This may be severe and requires careful correction before surgery.

If hypertrophic pyloric stenosis is suspected, diagnosis is best made by feeling the hypertrophied pyloric muscle 'olive' when palpating the abdomen during a test feed, when the abdominal musculature is more relaxed. Gastric peristalsis is usually seen if looked for. If doubt remains ultrasound in experienced hands is very reliable (Fig. 31.28), and this has replaced barium meal examination.[59] Treatment of hypertrophic pyloric stenosis is by pyloro-

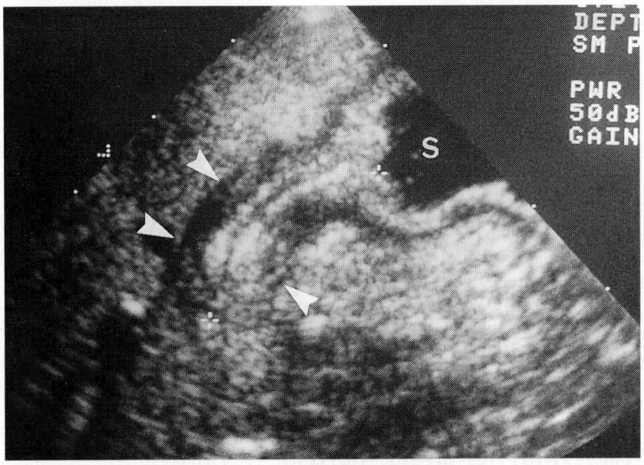

Fig. 31.28 Pyloric stenosis on ultrasound. The arrows outline the hypertrophied pyloric muscle. 'S' is the stomach.

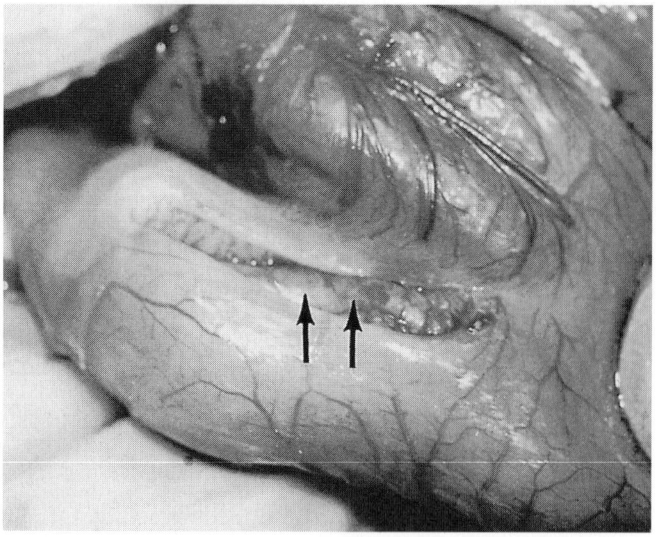

Fig. 31.29 Pyloromyotomy with mucosa projecting between the cut edges of the split hypertrophied muscle.

myotomy (Fig. 31.29). Feeding can be reintroduced within 12 hours of surgery.

PYLORIC ATRESIA

Atresia of the pyloric canal is a rare cause of neonatal intestinal obstruction. The association of this obstruction with severe aplasia of the skin and epidermolysis bullosa has been recorded.[25] Familial occurrence has also been recorded.[18]

DUPLICATIONS

Duplications of the upper alimentary tract are infrequent. They are usually cystic, and are referred to as para-oesophageal or paratracheal cysts. By pressure effects the cysts, particularly those situated in the lower neck at the thoracic inlet, may cause respiratory symptoms. When developing in the mediastinum the cysts have more room to expand and may not present in the neonatal period. They are usually lined by respiratory tract epithelium. Other oesophageal duplications may have gastric epithelium and may be seen as a posterior mediastinal shadow on X-ray (Fig. 31.30) These may cause ulceration and bleeding, and can even fistulate into the respiratory tract. There may be associated vertebral anomalies.

Duplication of the stomach is less common and presents with bleeding or vomiting.[45] Duodenal duplication is rare, and may present with vomiting or as an abdominal mass (Fig. 31.31).

Treatment is surgical, with excision of the duplication where possible. Subtotal excision may be all that is possible if the cyst and the bowel have a common wall.

DUODENUM AND SMALL BOWEL

Duodenal obstruction in the neonate may be divided into intrinsic and extrinsic causes.

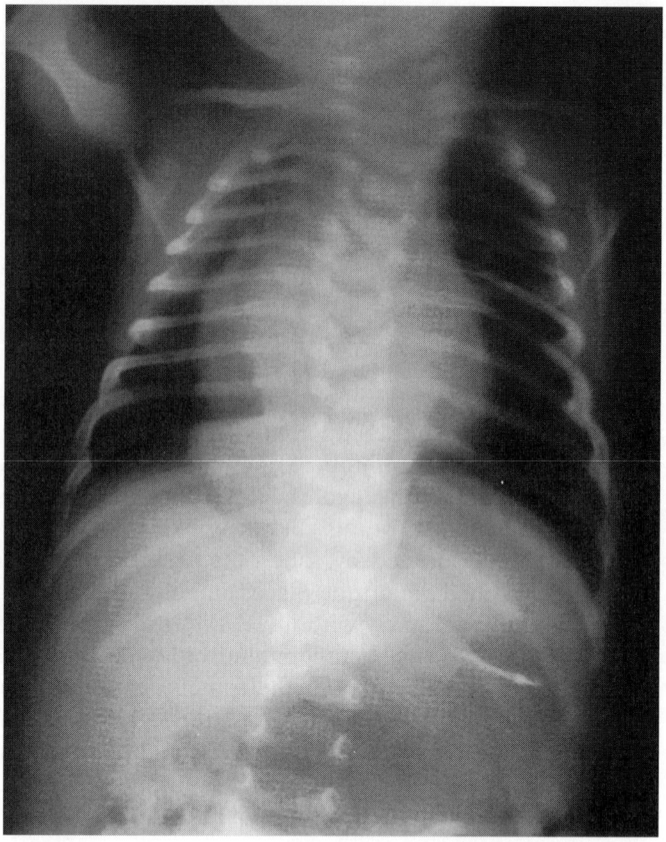

Fig. 31.30 Right-sided thoracic foregut duplication. Note associated vertebral abnormality.

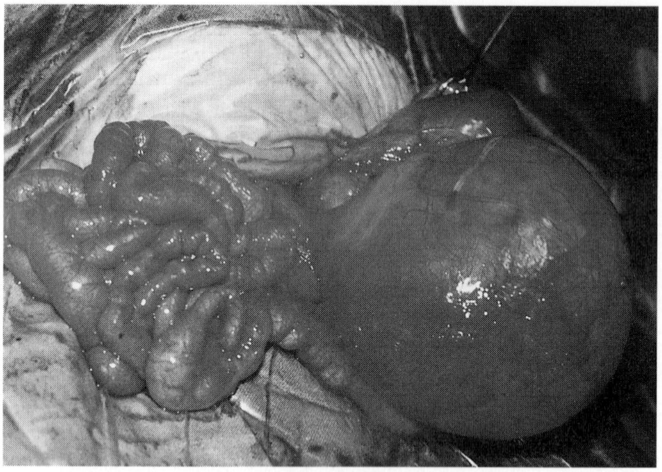

Fig. 31.31 Large duodenal duplication cyst at surgery. This could be seen to transilluminate preoperatively.

INTRINSIC DUODENAL OBSTRUCTION (DUODENAL ATRESIA)

Intrinsic obstruction of the duodenum may consist of atresia with a gap between duodenal ends (often with pancreas interposed), a duodenal membrane with continuity of duodenal wall, or duodenal stenosis causing bowel obstruction. The prevalence of intrinsic duodenal obstruction (atresia, membrane or severe stenosis) is 1 in

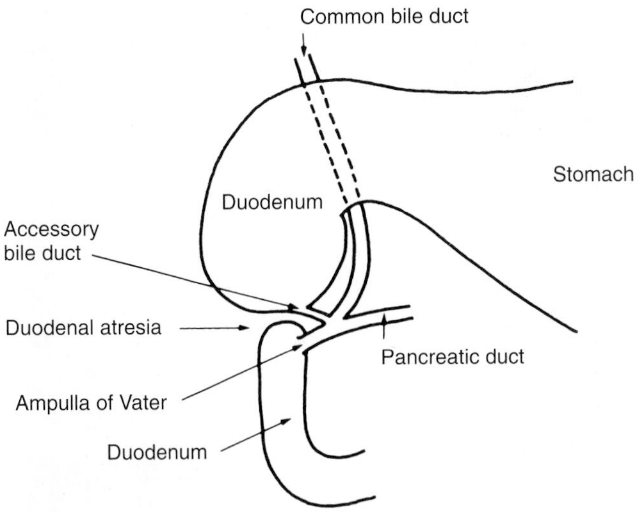

Fig. 31.32 Diagrammatic representation of the inverted Y termination of the common bile duct which may be present in infants with duodenal atresia.

6000 livebirths. Other major congenital anomalies are common. Down syndrome occurs in 30% of cases. There is no sex preponderance.

Whether the obstruction is due to failure of vacuolization of the duodenum or to a vascular mishap is not clear, but the atresia occurs usually in the region of the ampulla of Vater, a particularly active site embryologically. Anomalies of the distal bile duct have been found to provide the explanation why on rare occasions an infant may have bile-stained vomiting and pass normal-coloured meconium (Fig. 31.32).[4]

The frequent occurrence of polyhydramnios has resulted in intrinsic duodenal obstruction being often detected by antenatal ultrasound.[33] The characteristic 'double bubble' may be only intermittently seen because of fetal vomiting.

Postnatal presentation is with bile-stained vomiting within 24 hours of birth. In 10% the obstruction is proximal to the entrance of the bile duct into the duodenum and the vomitus will not contain bile. Examination will reveal a distended stomach with infrequent waves of gastric peristalsis passing from left to right across the upper abdomen. Passage of a gastric tube will reveal a large amount of bile-stained aspirate.

Plain X-ray of the abdomen will demonstrate the characteristic 'double bubble' sign of gas in the stomach, with a distended duodenum (Fig. 31.33). In most cases there is no distal gas, but a small volume of distal bowel gas may be present.

Management consists of early surgery. Only in cases where diagnosis has been delayed is correction of a resulting metabolic alkalosis necessary, and in such cases up to 72 hours of intravenous fluids may be necessary before surgery. At operation the duodenum proximal to the obstruction is anastomosed to the duodenum or jejunum distally. Great care must be taken not to damage the site of entrance of the bile duct(s) into the duodenum.

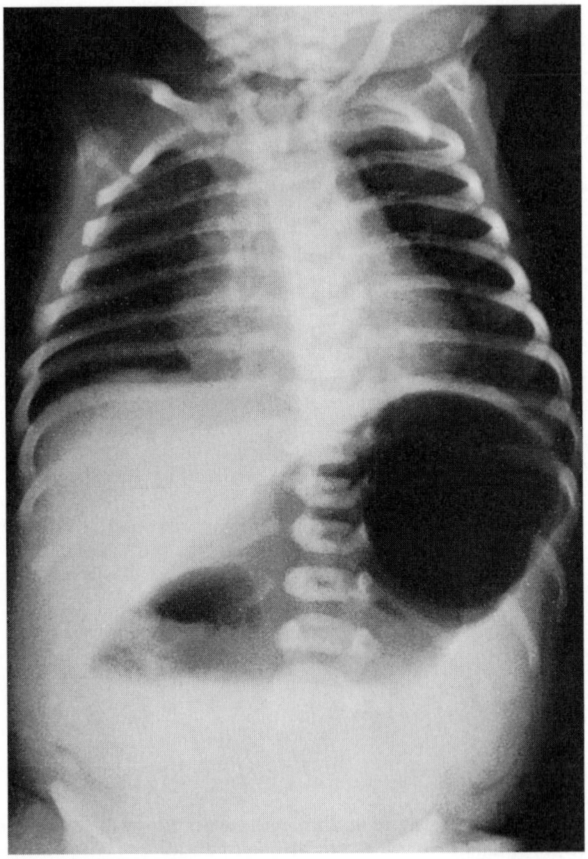

Fig. 31.33 Double bubble of duodenal atresia. The stomach is overlapping the duodenum with the second bubble being seen through the stomach.

Because of the gastric and duodenal dilatation there may be considerable delay in the return of normal peristalsis postoperatively. A gastrostomy tube is an alternative to a nasogastric tube for decompressing the stomach. Early feeding is preferred, supplemented as necessary by parenteral nutrition.

The outcome of intrinsic duodenal obstruction relates to associated anomalies, as the condition itself is amenable to surgical correction.

EXTRINSIC DUODENAL OBSTRUCTION (MALROTATION)

Unlike intrinsic duodenal obstruction, extrinsic duodenal obstruction is variable in the time of onset and may also be intermittent and incomplete. The usual cause is Ladd's bands running across the duodenum from a nonfixed caecum to the right subhepatic region. It is associated with incomplete rotation of the bowel. There is a male preponderance of 4:1.[79]

As obstruction may be intermittent and incomplete there may be difficulty in arriving at the diagnosis. This is especially dangerous as volvulus (see below) of the midgut may occur, with resultant catastrophic loss of bowel. Bile-stained vomiting is often the sole presenting sign.

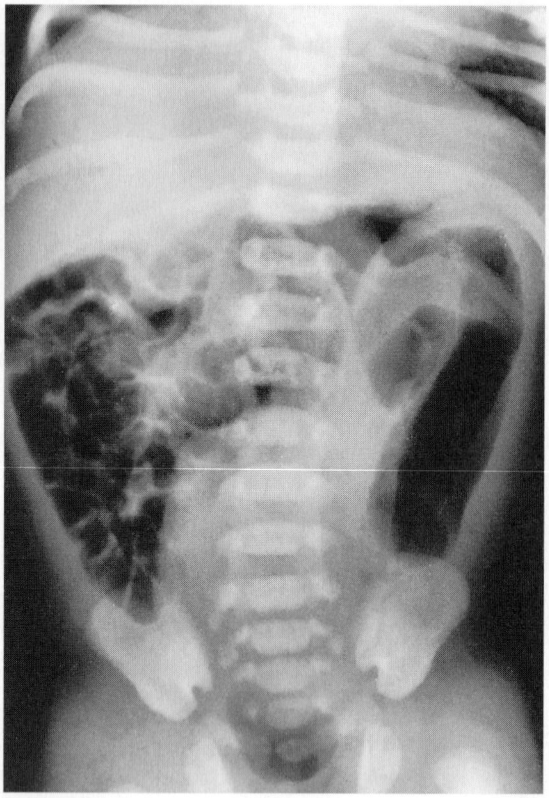

Fig. 31.34 Supine X-ray of abdomen showing non-rotation of the intestine. Small bowel on the right side of abdomen. Large bowel on the left side.

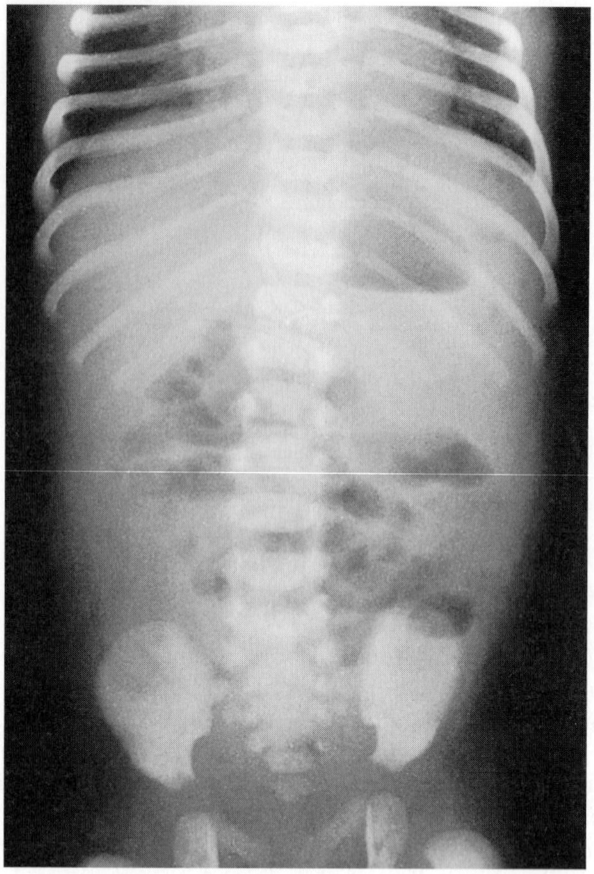

Fig. 31.35 Malrotation with fluid level in stomach and proximal small bowel lying in upper right abdomen. Large bowel not visualized as no gas is in it at time of X-ray.

Plain X-ray of the abdomen may show an alteration in the normal distribution of bowel gas, but there is no single characteristic picture. In some the diagnosis may be made as a result of small bowel being seen on the right, and obviously large bowel on the left of the abdomen (Figs 31.34, 31.35). Any infant presenting with bile-stained vomiting should have an upper gastro-intestinal series, which will show non-rotation of the duodenum (Figs 31.36, 31.37). Ultrasound may be of value, but should not be relied upon to exclude this diagnosis. A barium enema is not recommended, but may show incomplete rotation of the colon (Fig. 31.38).

Surgery is always warranted in symptomatic cases of malrotation, even if apparently incidentally diagnosed. This involves division of Ladd's bands, broadening the base of the small bowel mesentery, and placement of the small bowel to the right and the colon to the left. Appendicectomy should also be performed if the gut is viable. A rare though important association is situs inversus, polysplenia, a preduodenal portal vein and malrotation.

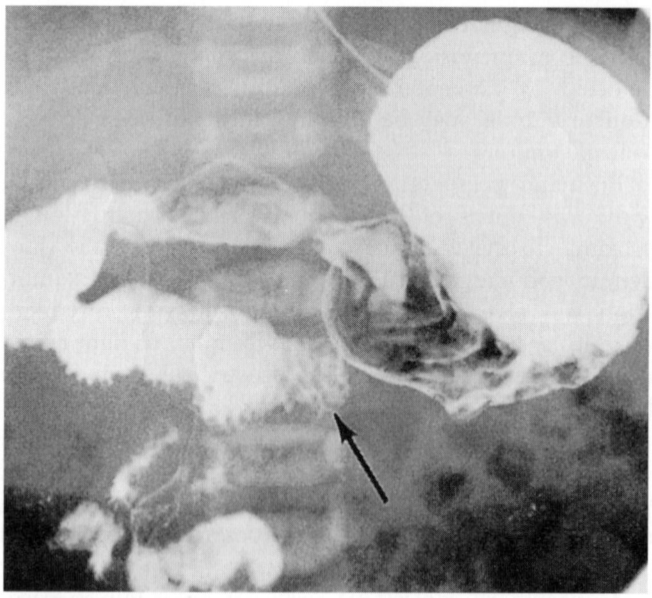

Fig. 31.36 Barium meal showing incomplete rotation of duodenum with the duodenojejunal flexure in front of the vertebrae rather than to the left side of the abdomen.

VOLVULUS

Volvulus of the midgut segment may occur in any infant who has incomplete rotation of the gut. Because of failure of normal fixation of the mesentery from the left upper to the right lower quadrant of the abdomen, the midgut loop, suspended on the superior mesenteric vessels, may

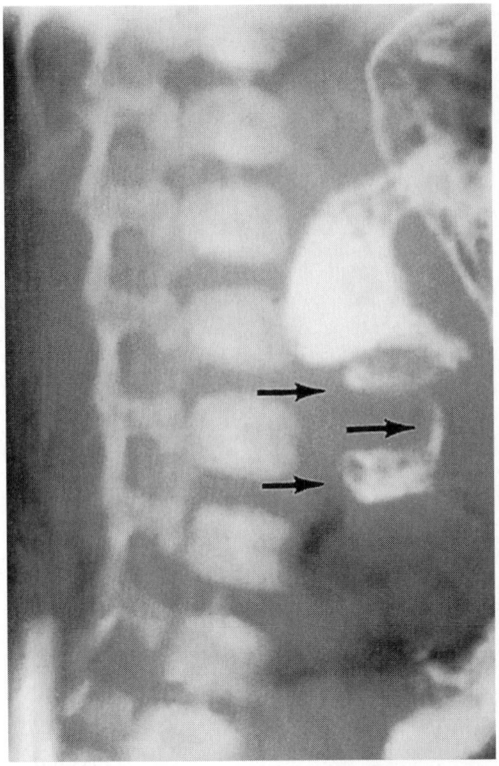

Fig. 31.37 Lateral X-ray showing barium passing down the duodenum and then being passed round a cork-screw segment of distal duodenum which is thus shaped due to volvulus having occurred but being completely obstructive.

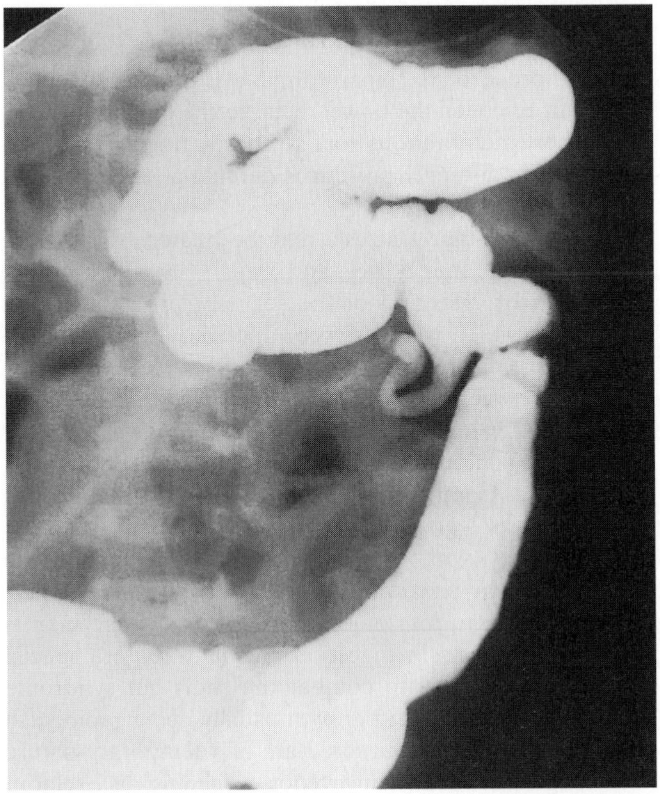

Fig. 31.38 Barium enema showing caecum and appendix in left upper quadrant in case of malrotation.

rotate, usually clockwise, causing volvulus and signs of extrinsic duodenal obstruction (Fig. 31.37). Volvulus may also be intermittent, twisting enough to cause obstruction and then untwisting, allowing relief of the obstruction. This feature contributes to delay in diagnosis. The importance of early diagnosis is that the superior mesenteric vessels are in the core of the mesentery of the twisting bowel and may become obstructed. Venous obstruction results in oozing of blood from the congested bowel into the lumen, with passage of blood per rectum in addition to bilious vomiting. Progression to arterial occlusion results in rapid onset of gangrene of the midgut segment. Although volvulus of the midgut loop is more common, volvulus of just a segment of small bowel may occur, giving rise to a similar clinical presentation.

The diagnosis of volvulus may be suspected prior to laparotomy, especially if blood is passed per rectum in addition to signs of extrinsic duodenal obstruction. Contrast studies will demonstrate the incomplete rotation and volvulus (Figs 31.36, 31.37). Peritonism, when present, is an ominous sign of ischaemic gut with incipient or actual perforation.

Urgent operation is necessary to undo the volvulus. This should not be delayed beyond rapid initial resuscitation. Chylous ascites may be seen at laparotomy. If the bowel is of dubious viability it should be replaced in the abdominal cavity and a second-look laparotomy performed 24 hours later, by which time considerable improvement may be seen. A prosthetic patch on the abdominal wound may help to reduce intra-abdominal pressure and provide optimum conditions for reperfusion of the damaged gut. Occasionally, volvulus of loops of small intestine may occur without an apparent precipitating cause. Such infants present with signs of obstruction and require urgent treatment.

JEJUNAL AND ILEAL ATRESIA

Atresia of the small bowel is usually a consequence of interference with the blood supply to the gut. This was shown initially experimentally by Louw.[52] The same causation probably accounts for most small bowel atresias in humans. Another intrauterine cause of atresia is volvulus of loops of small bowel with loss of blood supply to the involved bowel, necrosis and subsequent reabsorption of bowel, leaving a residual jejunal or ileal atresia. This is uncommon but may occur in the fetus with meconium ileus and cystic fibrosis.

Louw[53] suggested that jejunoileal atresia or stenosis be classified into four types, and Martin and Zerella[56] proposed the following classification:

- Type I: Single atresia consisting of a membrane or diaphragm with the bowel wall in continuity. The total bowel length is normal.
- Type II: Single atresia with discontinuity of the bowel

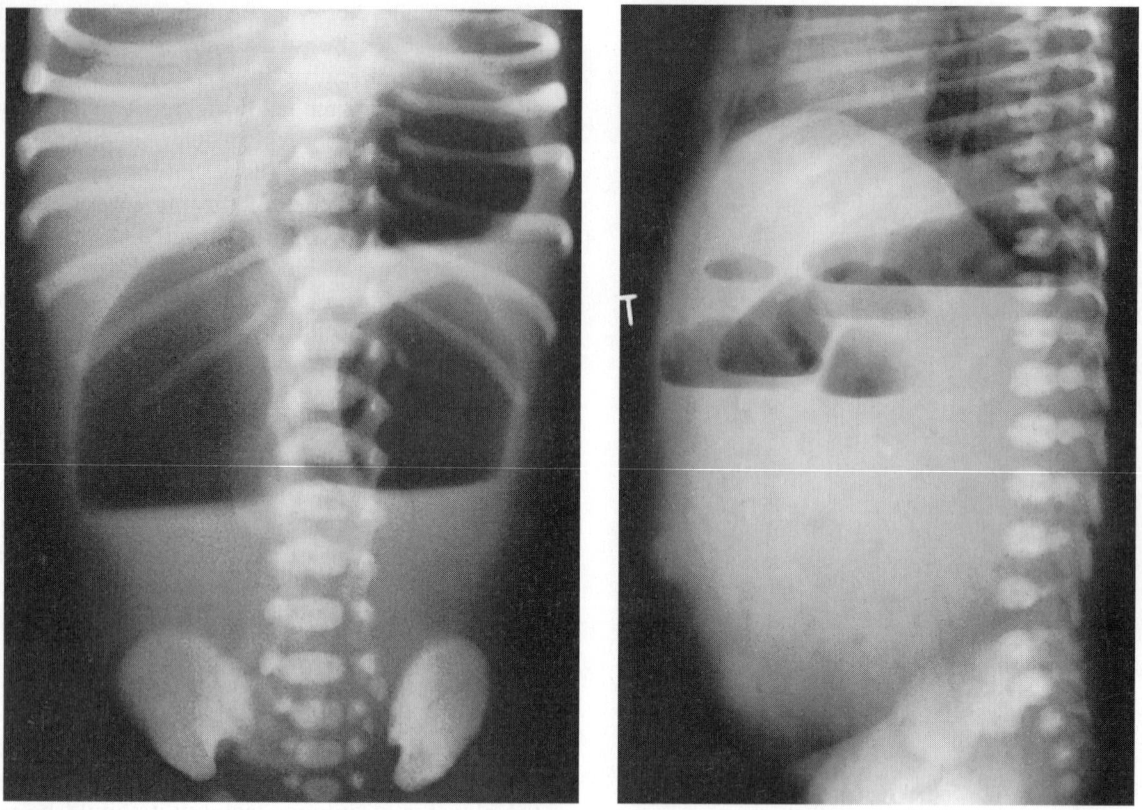

A B

Fig. 31.39 (A) Anteroposterior X-ray showing dilated bowel and fluid levels, indicating a proximal jejunal obstruction. (B) Lateral X-ray showing proximal loops of dilated bowel and fluid levels, indicating jejunal obstruction.

wall, but the blind ends may be connected by a fibrous band. The total bowel length is often significantly reduced.
- Type III: Multiple atresias.
- Type IV: The 'apple peel' deformity, in which atresia is accompanied by a deficiency of the dorsal mesentery and the total bowel length is reduced.

The significance of this classification is related to the management and complications that may follow, rather than to the initial presentation of infants with jejunal or ileal atresia.

Infants with small bowel stenosis may present later in infancy, but rarely the stenosis is so marked that they present in the neonatal period as a nearly complete obstruction.

Apart from having a lower birthweight than average, the infant with small bowel atresia may appear normal at birth. The higher the obstruction the earlier the vomiting occurs. Vomiting commences within 24–72 hours of birth and persists, the vomit becoming bile-stained. There is a failure to pass normal meconium. Increasing abdominal distension develops and is more marked with lower small bowel obstruction. X-ray of the abdomen shows the characteristic intestinal obstruction picture of dilated loops of bowel with fluid levels (Figs 31.39, 31.40).

Treatment is to rehydrate the infant if necessary and then to proceed to laparotomy. At laparotomy it is important to check the bowel distal to the obvious atresia, as further membranous or atretic segments may be present. The anomaly present is defined at this time and classified as type I–IV.[56]

Infants with type I atresia may be treated by a simple incision along the bowel and repair in a transverse fashion, or by resection of the segment proximal to the membrane, which is always very dilated, with end-to-end anastomosis of the gut. Owing to the discrepancy in diameter between the dilated proximal and narrow distal gut, the latter may be cut obliquely to give a better anastomosis in each of these so-called end-to-end anastomoses. Complications are infrequent and the long-term prognosis is good.

For infants with type II lesions resection of the terminal dilated proximal end with anastomosis is performed. Owing to loss of bowel prenatally, some infants will have problems in digestion and may require special feeds postoperatively to combat the short gut syndrome (p. 755). Adaptation and growth usually occur rapidly, so that the problems encountered are of a temporary nature and long-term total intravenous feeding is seldom necessary.

Less common are patients with type III and type IV

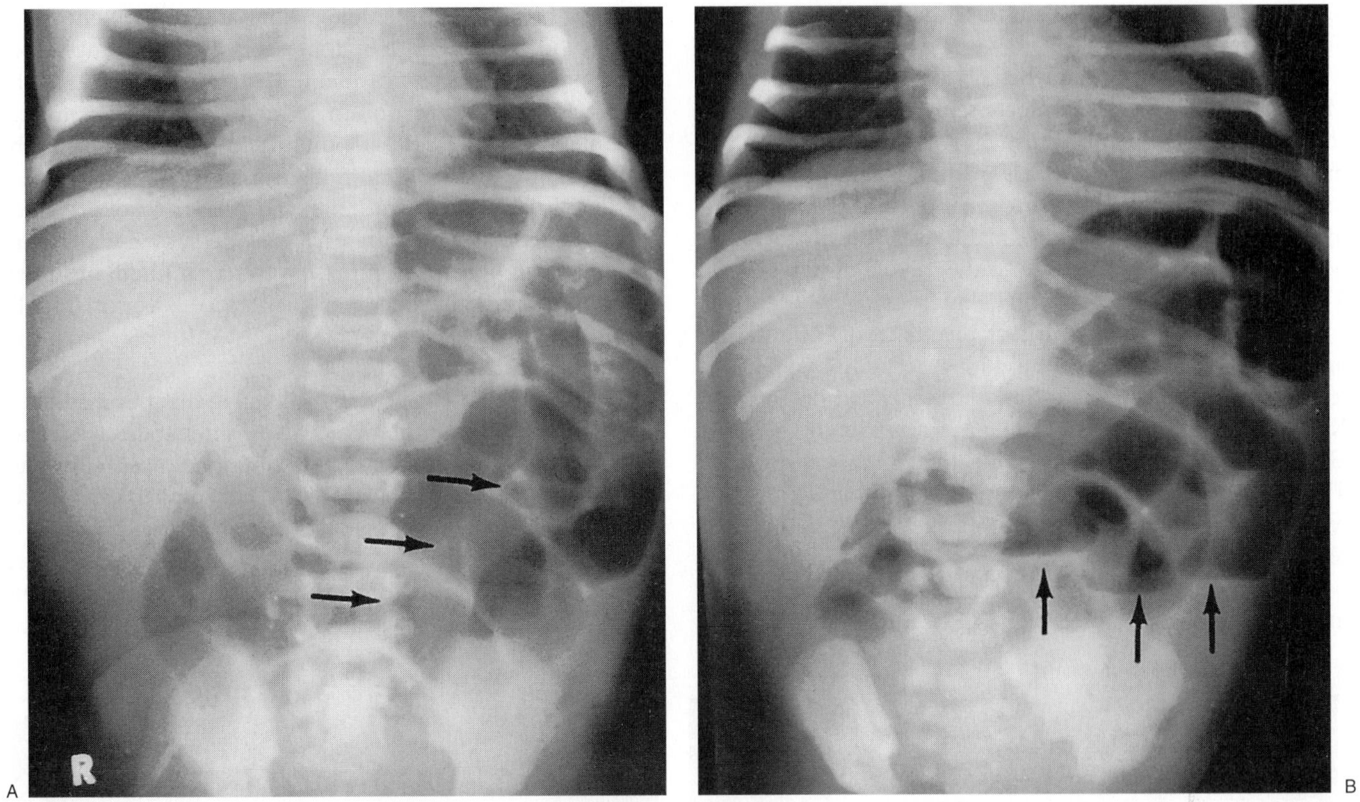

Fig. 31.40 (A) Supine X-ray showing ladder pattern of obstructed small bowel. (B) Erect film of same baby showing dilated bowel with fluid levels indicating ileal obstruction.

anomalies. The problems encountered following reconstruction of the alimentary canal in cases with multiple atresias (type III), which may necessitate more than one anastomosis to preserve the maximum length of the small bowel, are dependent on the length of bowel remaining and also on the function of that bowel. These infants appear to have had a more extensive insult to the bowel, including the mucosa, so that malfunction is more common. More prolonged intravenous feeding is necessary until adequate digestion and absorption is attained. Associated anomalies have been recognized with multiple atresias. The outlook is good.[37]

Type IV, the 'apple peel' deformity (Fig. 31.41), may present great problems for the surgeon.[22] Management depends on the viability of the distal bowel, with end-to-end anastomosis. Less commonly an end-to-side anastomosis is performed, bringing the distal end on to the abdominal wall as an 'ostomy' to allow inspection of the gut to ensure viability. Intravenous feeding is usually necessary for a time.

MECONIUM ILEUS

This is caused by hyperviscous meconium in the small bowel causing obstruction. Cystic fibrosis is almost invariably the underlying cause, though rare exceptions do occur.[69] Approximately 10% of infants with CF

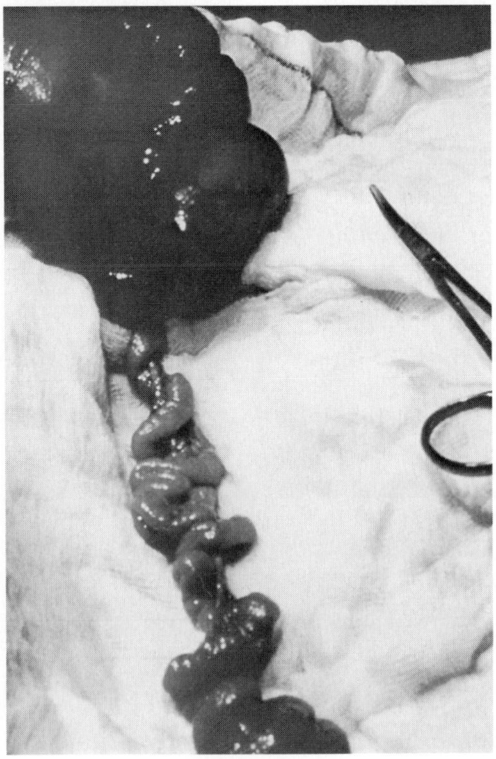

Fig. 31.41 'Apple peel' malformation of bowel in association with ileal atresia. Small bowel entwined around a narrow vascular pedicle.

present with meconium ileus or other related intestinal obstruction.

Meconium ileus may be uncomplicated or complicated. Uncomplicated meconium ileus presents with small bowel obstruction, usually at the mid-ileum. A progressive increase in the size of the meconium bolus in the small bowel results in secondary dilatation and hypertrophy of the more proximal bowel. The distal small bowel is narrow and packed with grey-coloured pellets. The colon is unused, becoming a microcolon.

Complicated meconium ileus results from intrauterine mishaps. The obstructed bowel may perforate, giving rise to meconium peritonitis (often with calcification seen on X-ray); the heavy dilated segment may undergo volvulus. Gangrene may supervene, with meconium peritonitis. The involved bowel may undergo resorption, with resulting ileal atresia of varying complexity or, if not, may result in a pseudocyst.

The clinical presentation of meconium ileus is with marked abdominal distension and, in some, palpable loops of bowel on abdominal examination. The abdominal distension is greater than that seen with uncomplicated ileal atresia and is probably a consequence of the stickiness of the meconium, which cannot be vomited. The ileum, distended with the viscid meconium, may be palpable as a mobile abdominal mass.

The infant does not pass meconium, though small plugs or pellets of pale material may be passed which may be mistaken for meconium by the untrained observer. Vomiting gradually becomes marked, the vomit initially being of gastric secretions and feeds, but later being bile stained.

A family history of CF will suggest the diagnosis. Meconium ileus can be detected by antenatal ultrasound, with a cluster of dense echoes in the lower abdomen caused by the viscid meconium. Biochemical analysis of amniotic fluid or DNA analysis can make the diagnosis of cystic fibrosis (p. 758).[14] Plain X-ray of the abdomen shows marked bowel distension with few, if any, fluid levels. The erect and supine films may be almost identical

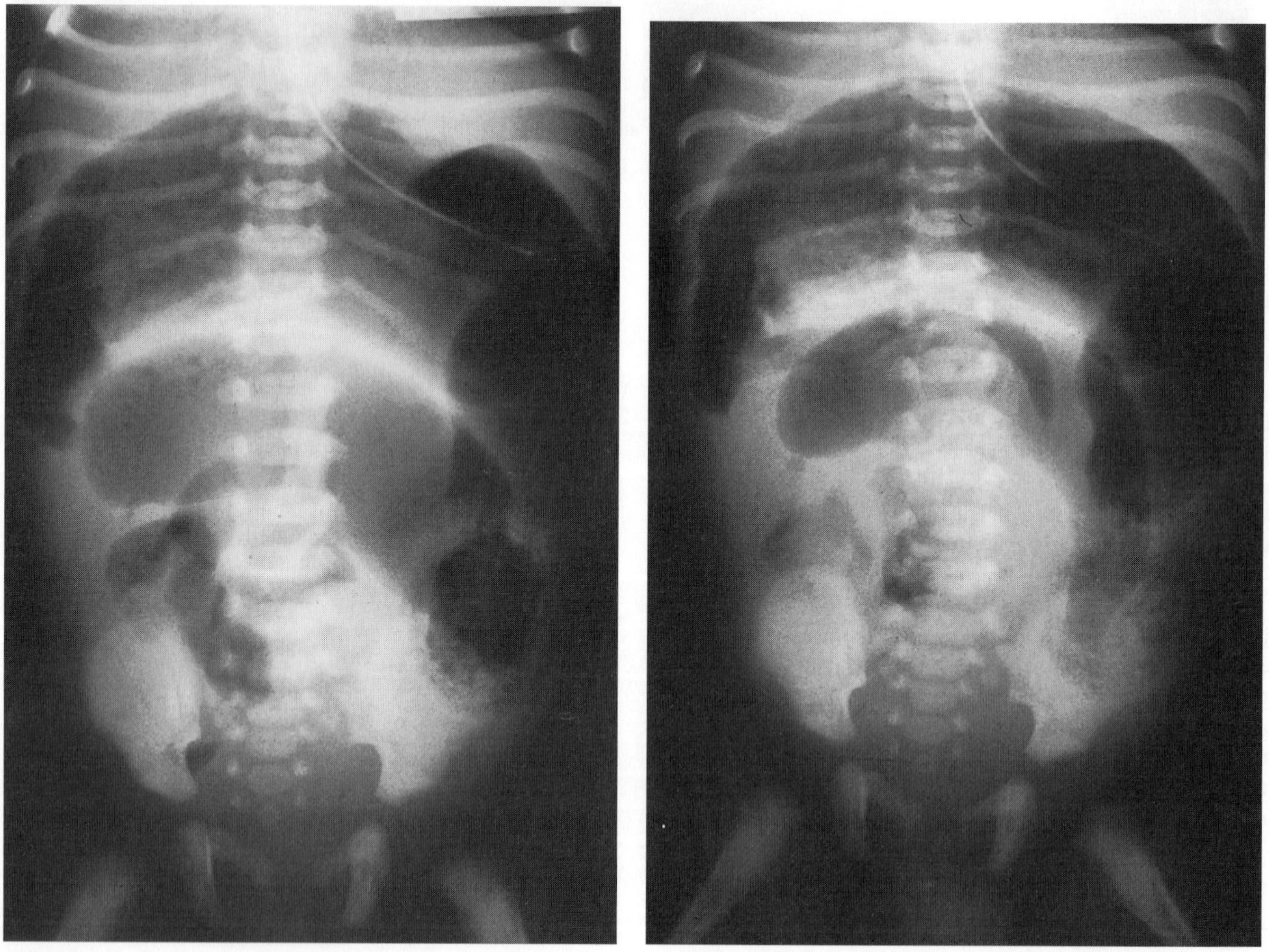

A B

Fig. 31.42 (A) Erect and (B) supine views of abdomen in same baby with meconium ileus. Note lack of fluid levels and similar appearances of both views because of heavy meconium-laden loops of intestine.

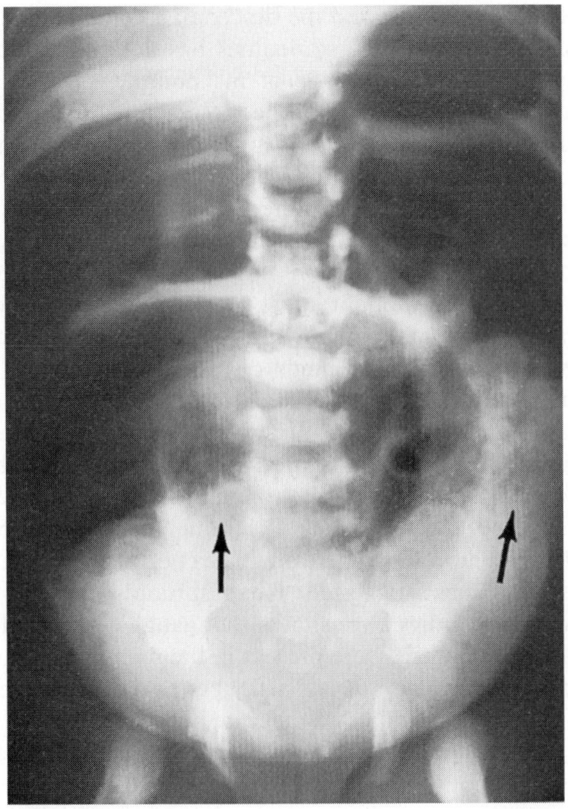

Fig. 31.43 Grossly dilated bowel and snowstorm appearance of mixture of air and viscid meconium in meconium ileus.

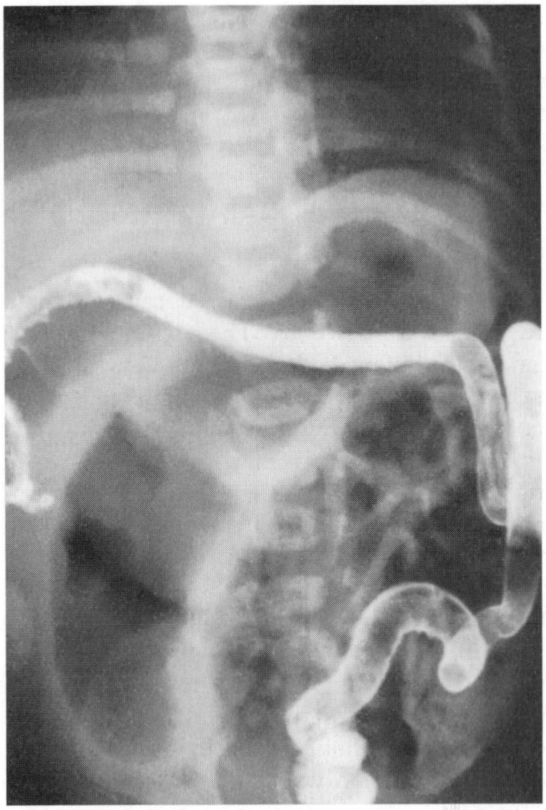

Fig. 31.44 Gastrografin enema showing microcolon and dilated loops of proximal small bowel in meconium ileus.

(Fig. 31.42). A 'snowstorm' appearance, caused by admixture of air and viscid meconium, may be seen in the abdomen (Fig. 31.43). In complicated cases intraperitoneal calcification may be visible. This is secondary to meconium peritonitis.

A dilute Gastrografin or an isotonic contrast enema may be therapeutic as well as diagnostic. The contrast solution is warmed to body temperature before use. The unused microcolon will be demonstrated (Fig. 31.44). Provided the contrast can be passed along the ileum into the distended bowel, the patency of the bowel is proven (Fig. 31.45). Once this is determined, a conservative line of management may be followed. Repeating the procedure at daily intervals for 4–5 days may be necessary before normal bowel movement is achieved.[8] With each enema the contrast has to be passed to a more proximal level or conservative management is discontinued. Care is essential, as hyperosmolar solutions are irritant and draw fluid into the lumen of the gut, making the meconium less tenacious. Adequate intravenous fluids are required to compensate for fluid lost in this fashion.

If the contrast enemas do not pass into dilated bowel, an ileal atresia may be present and operation required. Any suggestion that the meconium ileus is complicated precludes the use of enemas and warrants surgery. Even after apparently successful enemas, perforation of the distal small bowel or proximal colon has been recognized.

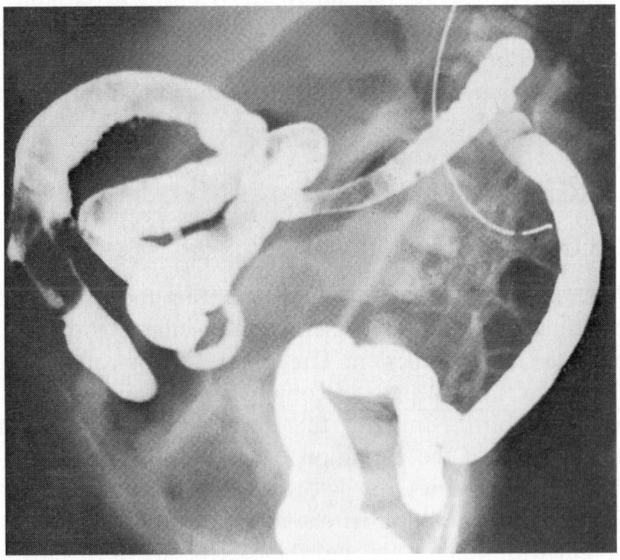

Fig. 31.45 Repeat Gastrografin enema 24 hours later filling the caecum and terminal ileum and outlining patency of the gut and plugging of meconium in the distal ileum confirming the diagnosis of meconium ileus.

The reason for this is unclear. Conservative management is successful in about 60% of cases, but perforation has occurred in almost 10%. Infants not responding to conservative management require surgery. A study of complicated meconium ileus from 1972 to 1990 showed a 1-year survival rate of 75%.[23] The occurrence of meconium ileus does not correlate with severity of subsequent pulmonary disease. A relatively good prognosis has been demonstrated for infants with CF who presented with meconium ileus.[17]

OTHER CAUSES OF NEONATAL INTESTINAL OBSTRUCTION

There are numerous other isolated causes of intestinal obstruction in the newborn. The presentation is similar to that of the infant with ileal atresia, with abdominal distension, vomiting and usually failure to pass normal meconium. Vitello-intestinal remnants with adhesion bands or internal hernia may occur. Giant Meckel's diverticulum, which may be mistaken on ultrasound examination for a duplication cyst, is another cause of neonatal obstruction which is amenable to resection and anastomosis.[20]

Duplications of the small bowel and Meckel's diverticulum may present either with obstruction or with haemorrhage from the bowel. The exact cause of the haemorrhage is not always clear, as the duplication may be encysted and, although lined by gastric mucosa, it is not in communication with the gut and therefore not a cause of peptic ulceration of the intact bowel. On other occasions the duplication may communicate with the bowel and peptic ulceration may be the cause of the passage of blood per rectum. With Meckel's diverticulum the usual cause of passage of blood is from peptic ulceration in the ileum adjacent to the Meckel's, or on occasion from within the diverticulum. Laparotomy with appropriate resection is the treatment.[45]

LARGE BOWEL

COLONIC ATRESIA

This is a rare form of atresia, accounting for only 5% of intestinal atresias. The presentation in infants is that of a low intestinal obstruction. The infant develops abdominal distension, fails to pass meconium and vomits within 72 hours of birth. Initially the vomit may be of clear material, but if the condition is not relieved bile-stained vomiting supervenes.

X-ray of the abdomen shows increasing dilatation of the gut with fluid levels, and the precise site of the atresia is usually determined at laparotomy. A contrast enema will demonstrate the level of the atresia. A two-stage procedure is often required, with initial relief of the obstruction by colostomy, followed later by closure of the colostomy.

MECONIUM PLUG OBSTRUCTION

Meconium plug obstruction frequently occurs in the low-birthweight infant in whom there has been no passage of material in utero beyond the descending colon or sigmoid colon. The infant also sometimes has additional factors likely to delay the passage of meconium, e.g. hypoxia, hypothermia, medication of the mother in labour or birth trauma, and presents a difficult diagnostic problem. A balance has to be drawn between subjecting the infant to what may prove to be unnecessary investigations and missing organic disease. The main differential is between meconium plug obstruction and Hirschsprung's disease. The latter was thought of as a disease of the above-average weight male infant, but the apparent increase in long-segment Hirschsprung's disease, which has no sex preponderance, and the recognition that Hirschsprung's disease can occur in low-birthweight infants have made diagnosis more difficult. Contrast enema studies done on these infants may be misinterpreted as showing evidence of Hirschsprung's disease. The same mistake has been made at laparotomy, where an apparent transition zone in the bowel has suggested Hirschsprung's disease but subsequent studies have shown that ganglion cells, which could be immature, were present in the rectum.

In preterm infants it is usually better to have patience and wait for the infant to defecate spontaneously. However, if abdominal distension is becoming marked, a large bowel washout with warm saline usually relieves the obstruction and produces a pale plug of meconium (Fig. 31.46). Alternatively, warmed Gastrografin may be instilled into the large bowel via a rectal tube and an X-ray film taken to demonstrate the meconium plug. Fluid and electrolyte balance has to be maintained by intravenous infusion during this procedure because of the hydroscopic effect of Gastrografin, although this has probably been overstressed in the past. This procedure provokes passage of the plug and, once the infant has started passing motions, further difficulty is unlikely to ensue, although he may continue with infrequent bowel actions. This is an indication for keeping the infant under close observation during his stay in the unit, and for careful follow-up after discharge.

In full-term infants, delay in passage of meconium beyond 48 hours merits active investigation along the lines outlined above, whereas for the preterm infant no investigation needs to be instigated during the first week of life, unless additional signs develop that indicate the need for exclusion of an alimentary tract abnormality.

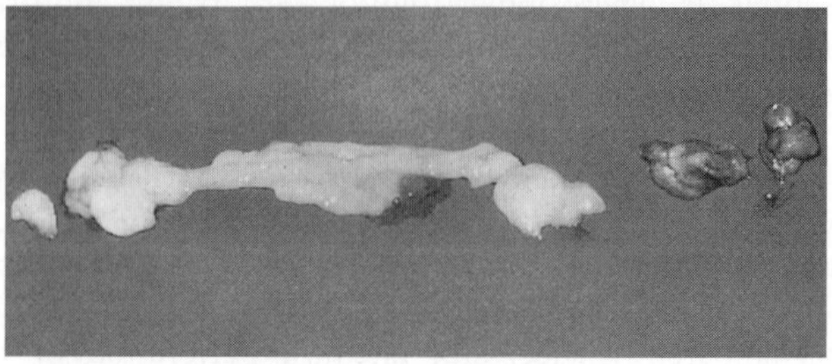

Fig. 31.46 Meconium plug.

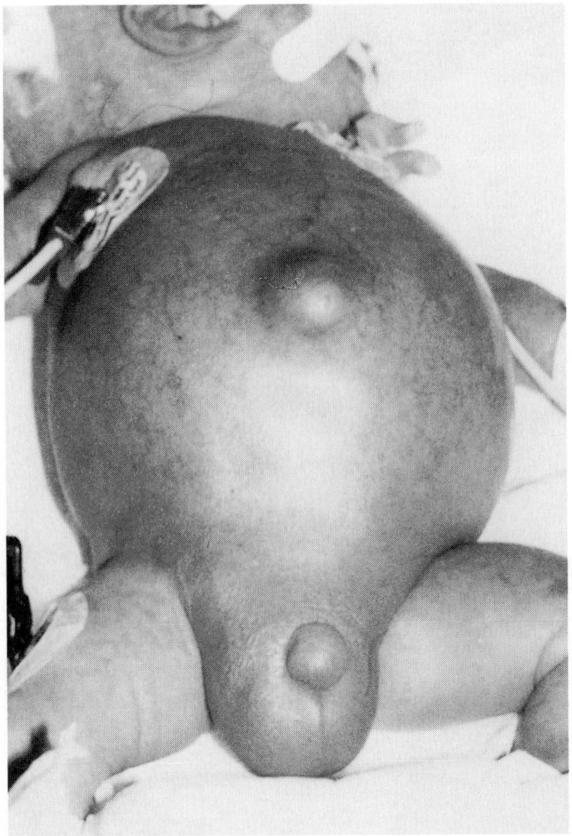

Fig. 31.47 Abdominal distension in a premature neonate with Hirschsprung's disease.

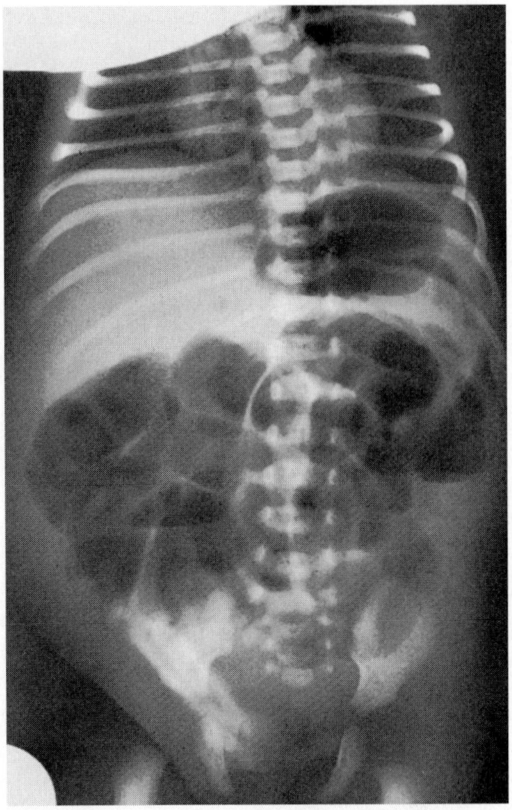

Fig. 31.48 Abdominal X-ray 30 hours after birth showing lack of gas in distal large bowel, suggesting Hirschsprung's disease.

DUPLICATION

Duplications of the colon or rectum occur less frequently than duplications of the foregut or midgut. They may also be associated with more complex anomalies than those with small bowel duplication, and the genitourinary tract may be involved.[45] Treatment must be tailored toward the specific anatomical anomaly present.

HIRSCHSPRUNG'S DISEASE

Although the clinical entity of Hirschsprung's disease was well recognized in the 19th century, the histopathological basis of the disease was only clarified by Bodian in 1949.[6] Congenital intestinal aganglionosis has been increasingly recognized, and current estimates are of a prevalence of 1 in 5000 births. A familial incidence of 8% has been reported, and in these cases associated anomalies may be more common.[26] Originally considered to be confined to high-birthweight infants, in recent years it has been increasingly recognized in low-birthweight infants. The multiple other problems of low-birthweight infants may distract attention from the colon, and as Hirschsprung's disease causes incomplete obstruction this makes the diagnosis all the more difficult. There is a male preponderance of 4:1, except in long segment disease, which has a ratio nearer 2:1.[67]

In utero, the neuroenteric ganglion cells migrate from the neural crest into the upper end of the alimentary tract and then migrate distally towards the most distal gut. In Hirschsprung's disease this migration is incomplete, resulting in aganglionosis of the distal rectum and extending proximally for a variable distance.

Hirschsprung's disease should be suspected in infants with delayed passage of meconium: 69% of newborns pass meconium within 2 hours and 94% within 24 hours of birth; 2–3% of otherwise healthy infants fail to pass meconium by 48 hours.[16] Infants who have not passed meconium by 24 hours should be suspected of having Hirschsprung's disease. Abdominal distension (Fig. 31.47) and vomiting occur. If failure to pass meconium persists then the vomit will become bile stained.

Plain X-ray of the abdomen will show a lack of gas in the distal large bowel (Fig. 31.48). It is important to include the pelvis on the film, and a lateral view is often helpful (Fig. 31.49). On occasion air may pass into the aganglionic distal bowel, showing the transition from dilated to non-dilated bowel. A contrast study with barium will usually clearly demonstrate the features of Hirschsprung's disease, and is diagnostic in experienced hands in 95% of cases (Fig. 31.50). It is of no value in

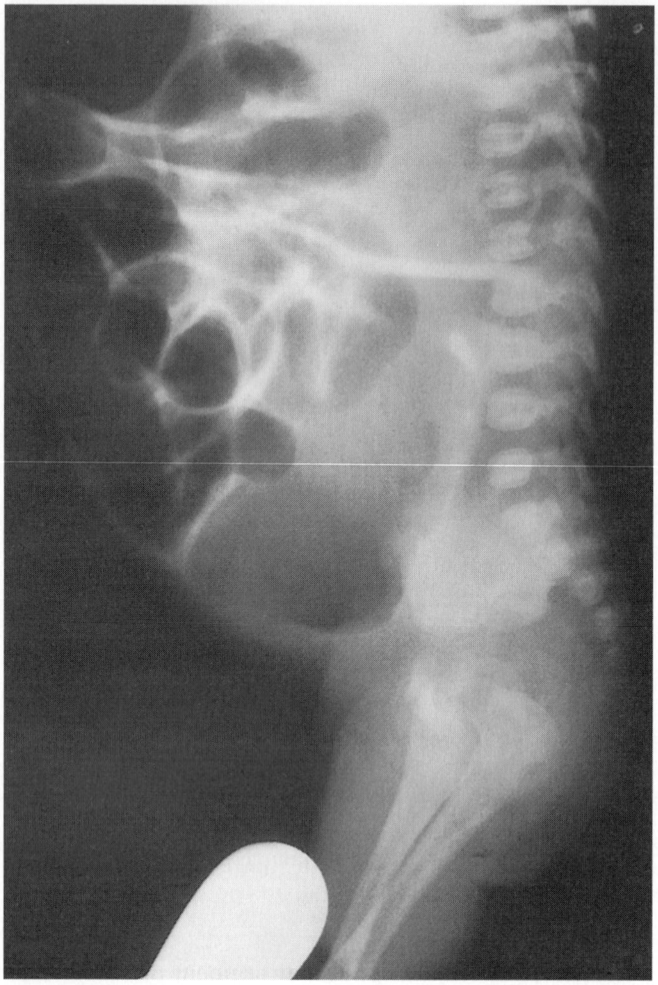

Fig. 31.49 Lateral X-ray of abdomen including pelvis showing grossly distended colon with lack of gas in pelvis suggesting Hirschsprung's disease.

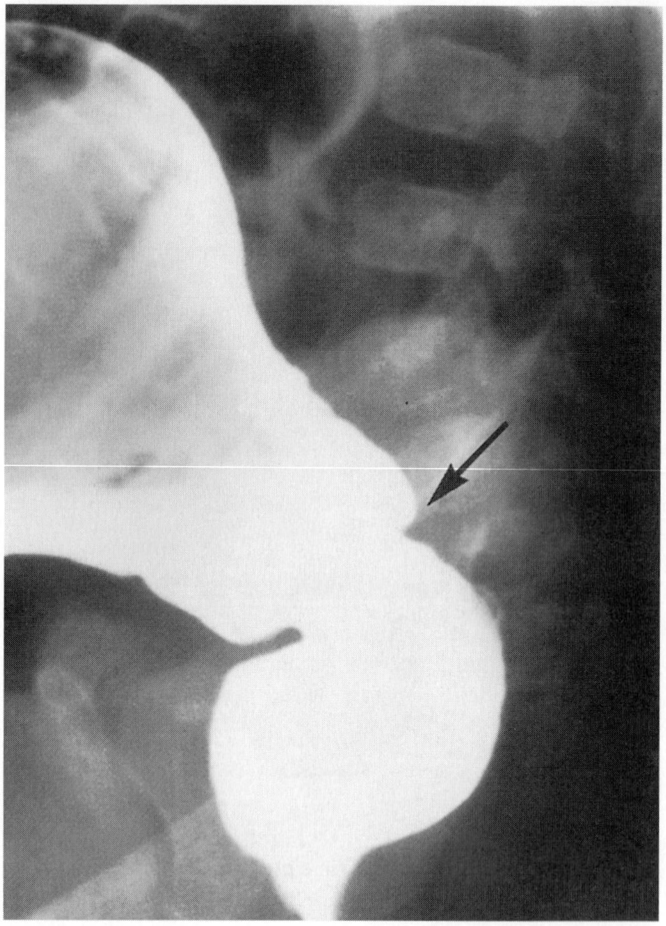

Fig. 31.50 Barium enema showing short segment Hirschsprung's disease. Note arrow at start of transition zone.

total colonic aganglionosis and in the very rare case of aganglionosis extending into the small bowel.

Definitive diagnosis is made on histological examination of a distal rectal biopsy. A suction biopsy of the rectum[12] 3 cm from the anus will allow examination of the submucous plexus to determine lack of nerve cells and the presence of abnormal nerve fibres.[6] Acetylcholinesterase staining techniques are preferred in some centres.[35] Manometric studies may be a useful aid to diagnosis in some cases.[1]

Diagnosis of Hirschsprung's disease can be dangerously delayed. Passage of meconium can be stimulated by digital rectal examination, the passage of a rectal thermometer or saline washouts. This may lead to a sense of false security, as the abdominal distension may be relieved and the infant may feed normally. This exposes him to the development of enterocolitis, with its high associated mortality. This can easily be misinterpreted as gastroenteritis, further delaying the correct diagnosis.

There has been an increasing move towards definitive surgery in the neonatal period, obviating the need for colostomy and staged surgery. Until surgery is undertaken, daily rectal washouts with warm saline keep the intestine decompressed. This is a time-consuming technique, requiring up to 2 litres of saline daily (Fig. 31.51), but it is well tolerated.

The aim of definitive surgery for Hirschsprung's disease is to resect the aganglionic bowel and to join the ganglionic colon (or the ileum in cases of total colonic aganglionosis) to the rectal stump. Surgeons have individual preferences as to the technique used.[7,24,55,71,76]

Results are dependent on the surgeon's technical ability with the particular procedure. In general the results of the various operative techniques are comparable, with 81% of children gaining good bowel control by 5 years after surgery.[70] Anal dilatation may be required following surgery. Most of the mortality associated with Hirschsprung's disease is related to the severe enterocolitis that can occur. This is particularly true in the neonatal period, but it may occur at any time, even after colostomy and after definitive surgery. *Clostridium difficile* has been linked to the aetiology of the enterocolitis,[78] but obstruction is probably the underlying common factor in most cases.

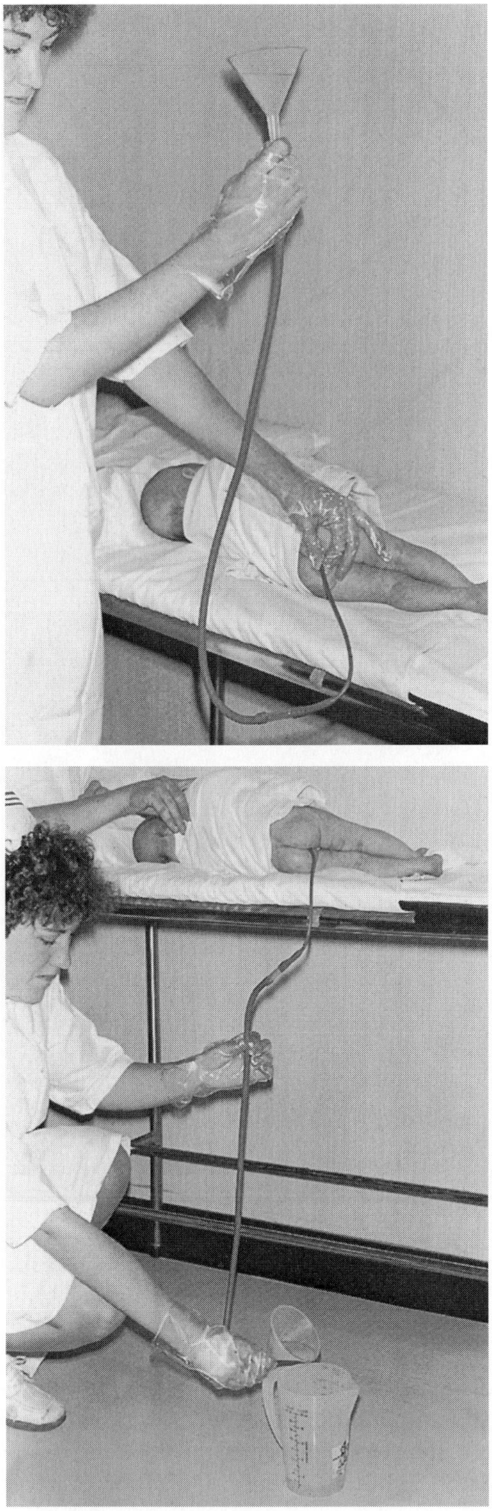

Fig. 31.51 Rectal washout in Hirschsprung's disease.

ANORECTAL MALFORMATIONS

The nomenclature in cases of anorectal anomalies is notoriously complicated, with many cases not fitting easily into any major category. In 1970, a workshop was convened in Melbourne, Australia, which developed a complicated classification system. This was subsequently modified in 1984 in Wingspread, Wisconsin, to a more simplified version of the male/female, high, intermediate and low (relating to the levator ani) 1970 classification. This 'Wingspread' classification is shown in Table 31.32.

Table 31.32 'Wingspread' classification of anorectal anomalies

Female	Male
High	
1. Anorectal agenesis	1. Anorectal agenesis
• with rectovaginal fistula	• with rectoprostatic urethral fistula
• without rectovaginal fistula	• without fistula
2. Rectal atresia	2. Rectal atresia
Intermediate	
1. Rectovestibular fistula	1. Rectobulbar urethral fistula
2. Rectovaginal fistula	2. Anal agenesis without fistula
3. Anal agenesis without fistula	
Low	
1. Anovestibular fistula	1. Anocutaneous fistula
2. Anocutaneous fistula	2. Anal stenosis
3. Anal stenosis	
Cloacal malformations	
Rare	Rare

A lateral X-ray of the pelvis taken at 24 hours after birth – a pronogram – with the infant lying prone and the pelvis elevated on a pillow, delineates the rectal pouch (Fig. 31.52). Ultrasound, in experienced hands, may also be of value in differentiating between high and low anomalies (Fig. 31.53).

In the male, if an orifice is found then the defect is low (except for rectal atresia). There may be an anocutaneous fistula (Fig. 31.54) or an anal stenosis. If an external orifice is found, except in the case of rectal atresia, a local anoplasty is normally sufficient and outlook for bowel control is good. If no orifice is found, then the defect is high or intermediate. In most cases there will be a fistula between the distal bowel and the urinary tract, usually

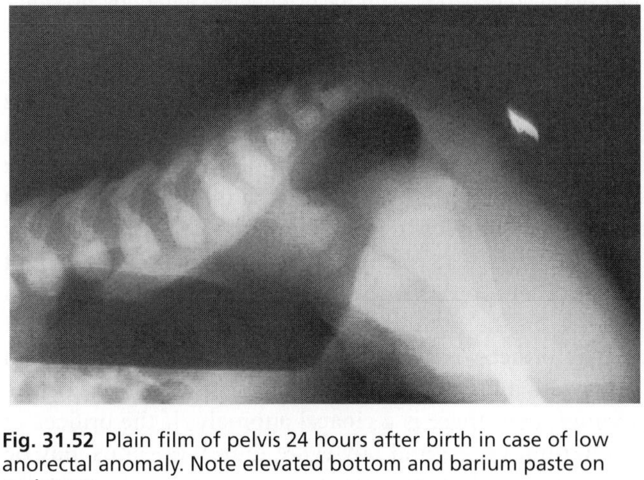

Fig. 31.52 Plain film of pelvis 24 hours after birth in case of low anorectal anomaly. Note elevated bottom and barium paste on perineum.

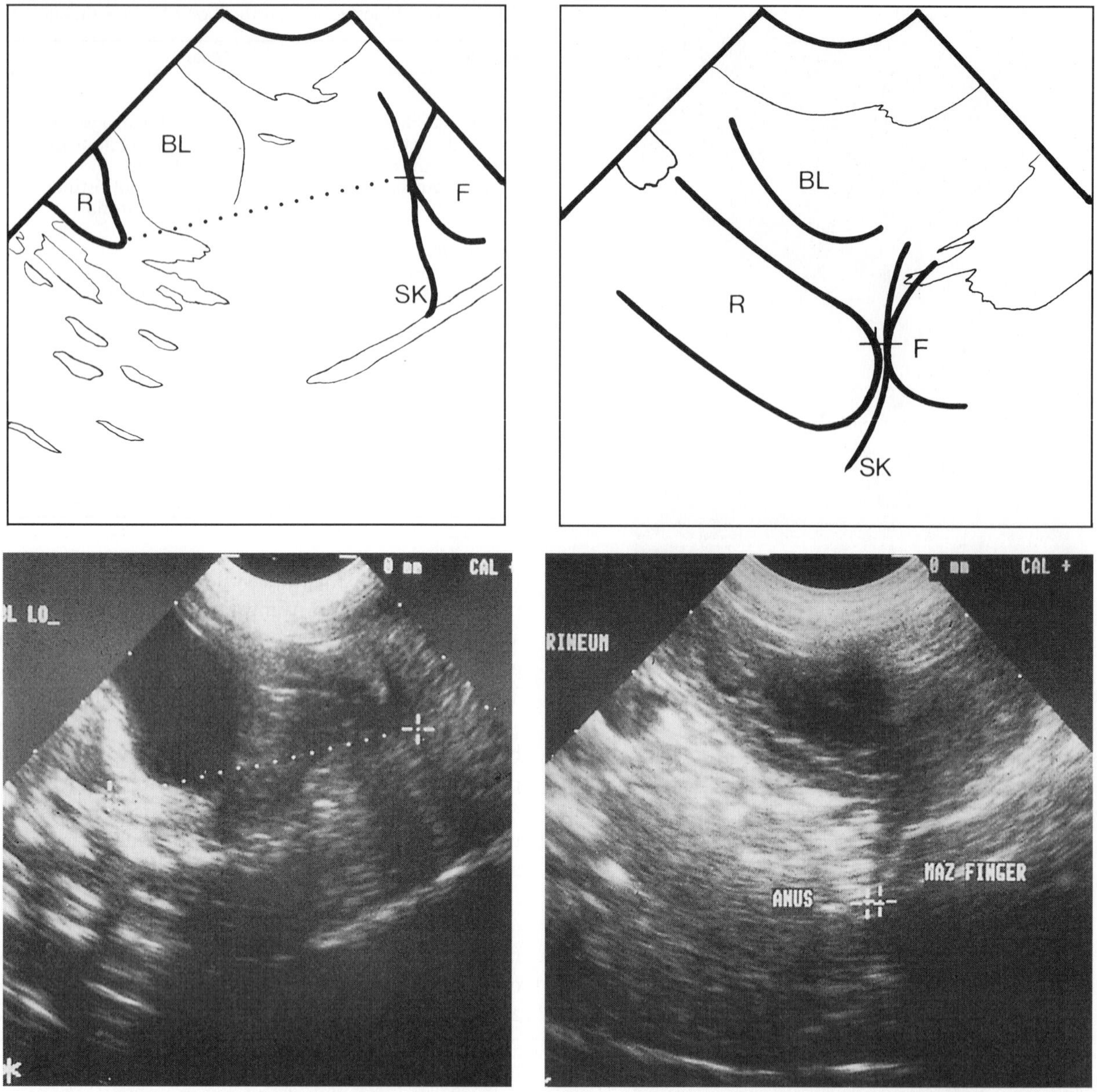

A B

Fig. 31.53 (A) Ultrasound of a high anorectal anomaly showing the distance from the outlined rectal pouch (R) to the perineal skin (SK) and the examining finger (F), with the bladder (BL) anteriorly. (B) Outline of the meconium-filled pouch seen in a low defect, with a very short gap between the bowel (R) and the perineal skin (SK) and the examining finger (F).

to the prostatic or bulbar urethra, and this may be recognized by meconium or bubbles in the urine. In these cases a colostomy will be required, with later definitive surgery to divide the fistula and bring the bowel through the 'muscle complex' to the perineum as a rectoplasty.[21]

In the female it is important to count the number of orifices that open to the surface, as the classification depends on the number of orifices found. If urethral and vaginal orifices are found then there is a rectovaginal fistula with a high or intermediate defect. If just one orifice is found, then there is a cloacal anomaly. If the orifices of the urethra, vagina and bowel are found, the anus may be normally sited but stenotic; the orifice may be anteriorly situated or may be at the vestibule, i.e. an anovestibular fistula. Treatment depends on the individual findings. For all high defects an initial colostomy is necessary, before later definitive surgery. Dilatation is necessary for anal stenosis and for some cases of anteriorly placed anus, but others may require anoplasty. Anovestibular fistula may be treated by anal transposition or dilatation. Non-communicating defects are rare in females.

Anal stenosis and rectal stenosis are not obvious on routine postnatal examination. If rectal examination is attempted, the tight band constricting the anal canal or distal rectum obstructs the examining finger. If not detected, diagnosis may be delayed until the patient is

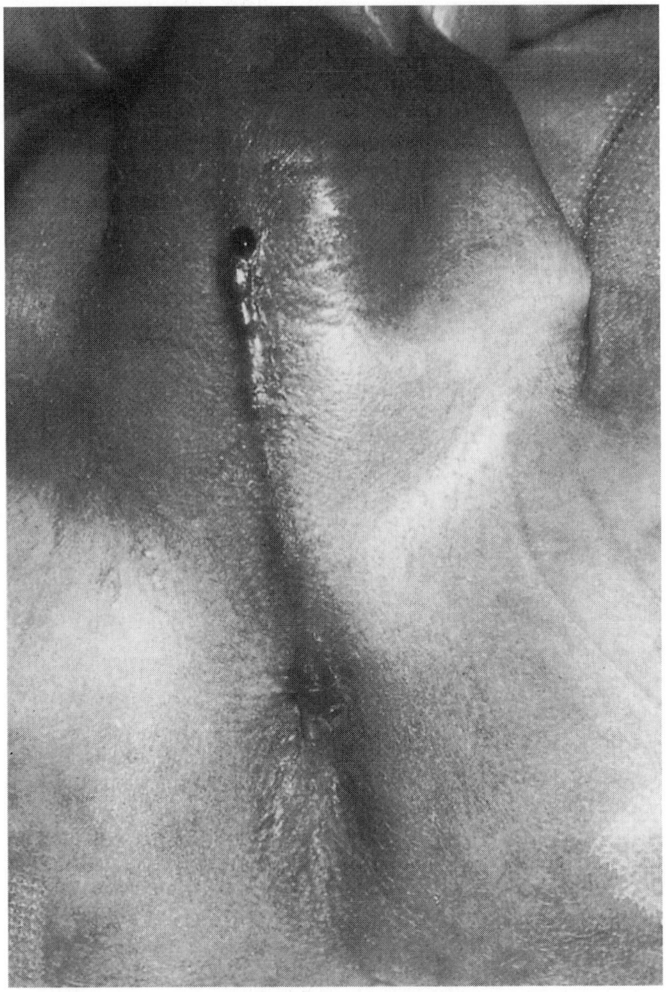

Fig. 31.54 Anorectal anomaly. Anocutaneous fistula with long subcutaneous track of meconium toward scrotum.

seen to pass toothpaste-like stool. When diagnosis is delayed, a secondary megarectum may develop with poor ability to attain satisfactory bowel habit.[48]

Associated conditions are common. The VACTERL complex (p. 765) is well recognized. Sacral anomalies have an important bearing on long-term bowel control. Urinary tract anomalies, in addition to the recognized fistula, are common.

Surgical repair of low anomalies is relatively straightforward and excellent long-term results can be expected. The posterior sagittal anorectoplasty (PSARP)[21] has been a breakthrough in the management of high and intermediate anorectal malformations, but with variable long-term continence figures reported.[60] In most cases, following early colostomy, the operation is performed at 9–15 months, followed by closure of the colostomy at 3 months postoperatively if the calibre of the anal orifice is satisfactory. It may be that the best results are obtained by early correction of the anomaly and early establishment of the neuroexcitatory pathways.

MICROCOLON–MEGACYSTIS SYNDROME

This rare entity remains a curiosity.[62] The viscera appear to be structurally normal but just do not function. This lack of propulsive activity persists despite the presence of apparently normal sympathetic and parasympathetic nerves. The infants have delay in the passage of meconium, which does not respond to any form of therapy.

DELAYED GUT FUNCTION

Two groups of infants suffer from disordered peristalsis in the newborn period. Preterm or very low-birthweight infants often have delay in establishing propulsive activity in the gut (p. 744). In preterm and full-term infants it may be due to hypoxia around delivery or intrapartum, hypothermia postnatally, hypothyroidism, or any severe illness such as RDS or sepsis. In the healthy preterm infant, once meconium has been passed, this can be followed by the gradual introduction of milk in small quantities and increasing this daily in strength and volume (pp. 395, 506). Stimulation of the bowel may be achieved by insertion of a glycerine suppository. In infants with other causes for the delayed peristalsis the primary cause must be corrected and patience exercised until normal activity is established. Intravenous feeding is necessary in the intervening period.

ANTERIOR ABDOMINAL WALL DEFECTS

The prevalence of abdominal wall defects is about 1 in 6000–8000 births. The male/female ratio is 1:1.

The anterior abdominal wall is formed by four separate embryological folds – cephalic, caudal, and right and left lateral – each of which has a splanchnic and a somatic aspect. Failure of the cephalic fold to close results in omphalocoele with a sternal/diaphragmatic defect, as seen in ectopia cordis, or the pentalogy of Cantrell.[13] Failure of the caudal fold to close results in omphalocoele with ectopia vesicae or the more complicated vesicointestinal fissure. Failure of the lateral folds to close results in omphalocoele. Gastroschisis has been considered to be the result of a failure of differentiation of mesoderm forming the muscles between the peritoneum and the skin, with secondary breakdown of this plate as can occur with the buccal plate. Many defects are, in practice, a spectrum of the above main types.

Subdivision of anterior abdominal wall defects is useful clinically and, although infants predominantly fall into one of two groups – exomphalos and gastroschisis – separation is not absolute. Exomphalos may be either with a small defect at the umbilicus, with gut prolapsing into the sac, i.e. the 'hernia into the cord', or the large exomphalos which has been called omphalocoele in the past. The terms exomphalos major, omphalocoele, exomphalos minor, hernia into the cord and gastroschisis

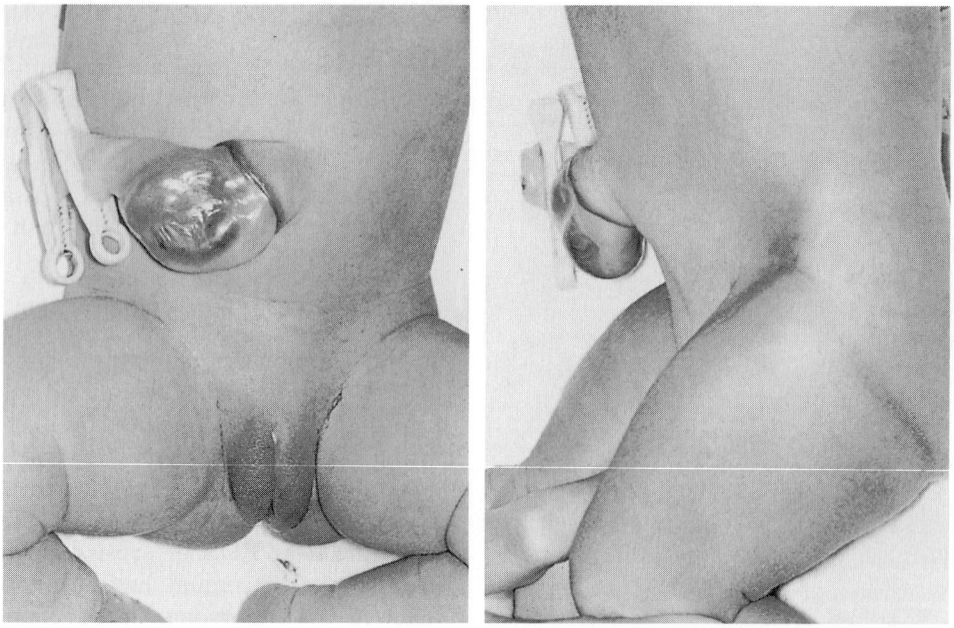

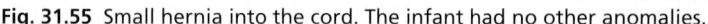

Fig. 31.55 Small hernia into the cord. The infant had no other anomalies.

have not always been used by authors with clear precision, as the anomalies are a spectrum of disorders rather than a single defect.

Intrauterine diagnosis of anterior abdominal wall defects has advanced in recent years, especially with the use of detailed antenatal ultrasound scanning and maternal serum α-fetoprotein estimates, the latter being raised in these conditions. The intestine has usually returned to the abdominal cavity by 12 weeks in the fetus, and large defects should be detected by 14–16 weeks; smaller defects may not be recognized until 18–20 weeks. It should be possible to differentiate omphalocoele from gastroschisis, and this is especially important in the case of omphalocoele. Amniocentesis or chorionic villous sampling should be done to rule out a chromosomal anomaly. Other major anomalies can be expected in over 50% of cases with large exomphalos.

HERNIA INTO THE CORD

Here the bowel has failed to return into the abdominal cavity, and in consequence there is incomplete rotation of the gut. The abdominal wall defect is less than 4 cm and there is minimal, if any, skin defect (Fig. 31.55). The incomplete rotation is rarely of any significance and is simply a consequence of persistence of the hernia into the cord. Infants with this condition are of lower birthweight than average but seldom have other major anomalies. They may have alimentary tract abnormalities, usually atresia or stenosis of the gut, probably secondary to a vascular accident because of the long course that vessels have to take to reach the herniated intestine. These occur in 25% of cases.

It is best to explore the defect, reduce the herniated bowel, inspect the gut to rule out atresia or stenosis, and formally repair the abdominal wall defect. The long-term outcome of these infants is good.

LARGE EXOMPHALOS

Prolapsing into the exomphalos sac there is liver as well as bowel (Fig. 31.56) and the liver lobulation is usually abnormal. Infants with this condition frequently have other major anomalies and hence, even though the

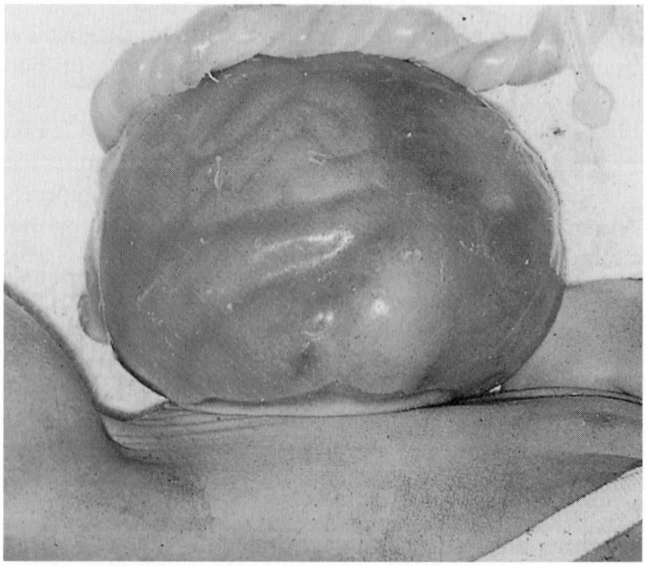

Fig. 31.56 Omphalocoele defect with bowel visible through sac in the lower part and abnormally lobulated liver in the sac in the upper part.

umbilical defect can be adequately treated, the infant may succumb from severe cardiac malformation or other anomaly. Chromosomal abnormalities are common.

Reduction of the prolapsed bowel and viscera into the relatively small abdominal cavity is problematic, and historically there has been a high associated mortality. Because of this, conservative methods were developed which consisted of treating the sac with desiccating agents or stimulants of epithelial growth. Mercurochrome was popular[39] but has been linked to mercury intoxication,[28] and enthusiasm has abated. Gross[40] favoured a two-stage repair, the initial step being to cover the intact sac with umbilical skin flaps and the second stage a late repair of the resulting ventral hernia. A major advance was the use of a silastic pouch (silo) sutured to the edge of the abdominal wall defect, with gradual reduction of the abdominal contents over a period of 7–10 days, followed by closure of the fascia and skin.[68] Most of the smaller exomphalos defects can be closed primarily. Large defects over 5 cm (exomphalos major), which account for about 20% of cases, almost invariably require the use of a silo. Outlook is dependent on the presence and severity of associated malformations, rarely being related to the defect or surgery per se.

GASTROSCHISIS

This condition was originally described in Glasgow in 1733.[11] Doubt was expressed as to the authenticity of the condition as recently as the late 1960s, when two patients were presented at the Royal Society of Medicine in London.[81] Currently, the differentiation between gastroschisis and exomphalos is well recognized.

Like infants with hernia into the cord, those with gastroschisis are of low birthweight and do not usually have other life-threatening anomalies. Associated intestinal abnormalities (e.g. atresia) have been noted in 22%.[41] The anterior abdominal wall defect is always to the right of the umbilicus and through this the midgut prolapses (Fig. 31.57). In some infants, not only will almost all the alimentary tract from stomach to sigmoid colon prolapse, but an ovary, fallopian tube or testis may also be present.

Infants with gastroschisis lose fluid and heat readily from the exposed gut after birth. They require more intravenous fluid than usual and great care must be taken in preventing hypothermia. Cellophane wrapping allows the bowel to be visualized and reduces heat and fluid loss. In utero transfer to a centre with paediatric surgical services is preferable to postnatal transfer.

There is a variable amount of thickening of the bowel wall. Most have adhesions between loops of bowel. In some infants there is dense matting of the gut (Fig. 31.58) with meconium staining of the bowel, but in others the bowel may remain quite pliable.

Reduction of the bowel and repair of the defect is relatively easy in those with pliable bowel and a small

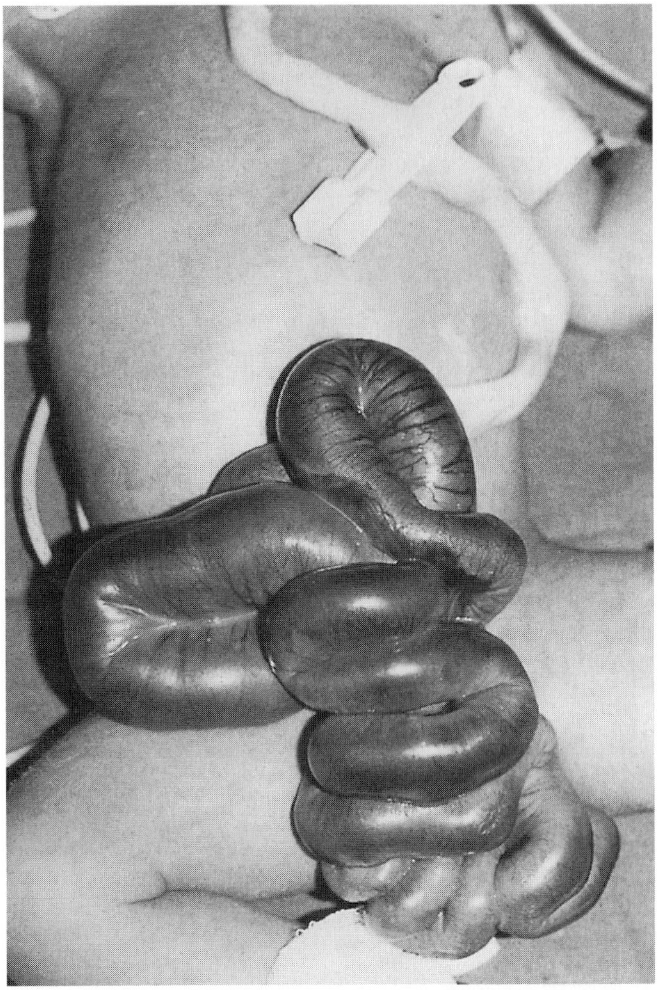

Fig. 31.57 Gastroschisis showing prolapsed intestine to the right of umbilical cord.

defect (about 85% of cases). Repair of a larger protrusion with matted bowel is complicated by an abdominal cavity too small to accommodate the bowel. In such a case, attaching a silastic silo at initial surgery which is reduced in size daily before final closure, is best (Figs 31.59, 31.60). These infants characteristically require prolonged parenteral nutrition while gut function slowly normalizes. Long-term survival figures are around 90% in most centres.[41]

CLOACAL EXTROPHY (VESICOINTESTINAL FISSURE)

This is an uncommon condition that affects the alimentary and urinary tracts. The gut may prolapse between parts of the ectopic bladder on either side, and many variations of this are encountered (Figs 31.61, 31.62). One problem with these infants is determining their sex because of the major genitourinary as well as the alimentary tract anomaly, and experienced assessment should be sought before informing parents of the sex of

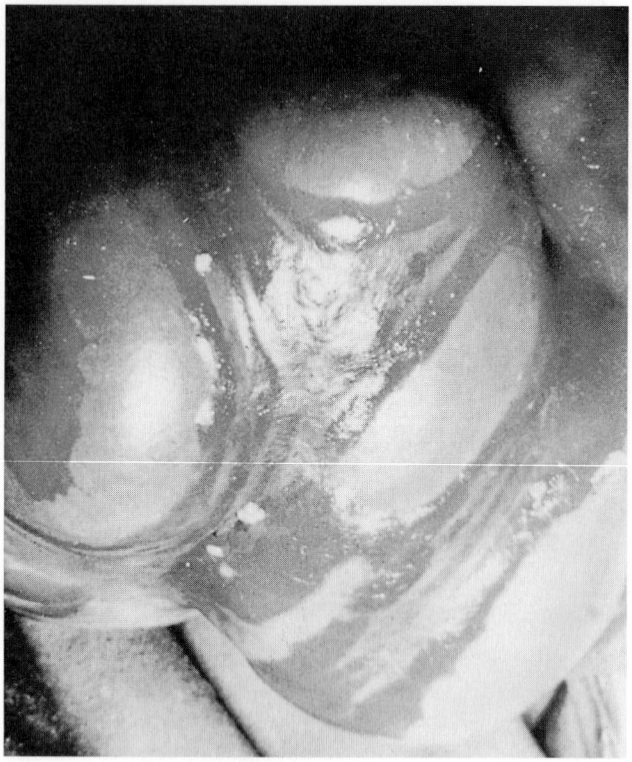

Fig. 31.58 Close-up of intensely matted gut in case of gastroschisis.

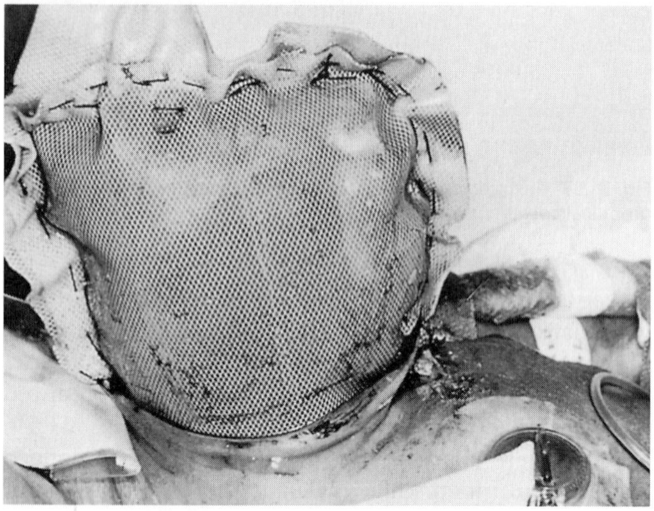

Fig. 31.59 Silastic pouch applied to the abdomen enclosing prolapsed gut in gastroschisis.

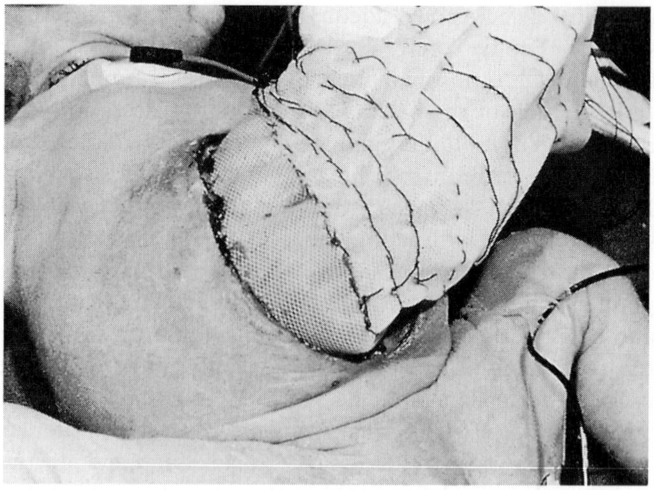

Fig. 31.60 Silastic pouch after 1 week with repeated tucks being taken to reduce the size of sac and move the gut intraperitoneally.

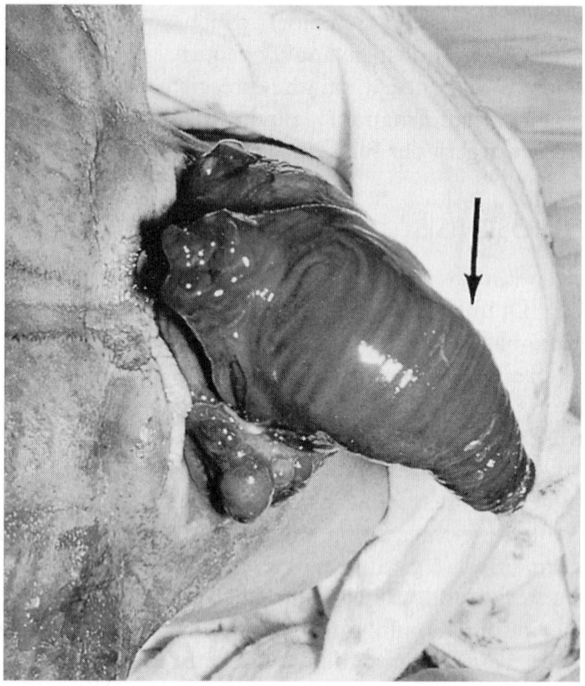

Fig. 31.61 Vesicointestinal fissure with prolapsing ileum (arrow).

the child if there is doubt. Associated with the abnormalities there often may be a short gut, colonic deficiency and an imperforate anus. Reconstruction is complicated and requires careful planning.[54]

PRUNE BELLY SYNDROME

The alternative name for this is the triad syndrome, with absent abdominal wall muscles, dilatation of the urinary tract and cryptorchidism. The title of prune belly is appropriate only in the immediate postnatal period, because beyond that the infant swallows air and distends the gut so that the abdomen becomes protuberant rather than flat. An integrated management approach is essential.[29]

HERNIAE

INGUINAL

Failure of obliteration of the processus vaginalis after testicular descent exposes the infant to the development of an inguinal hernia. The incidence of inguinal hernia is highest during the first years of life, peaking during the neonatal period. Boys are affected six times more

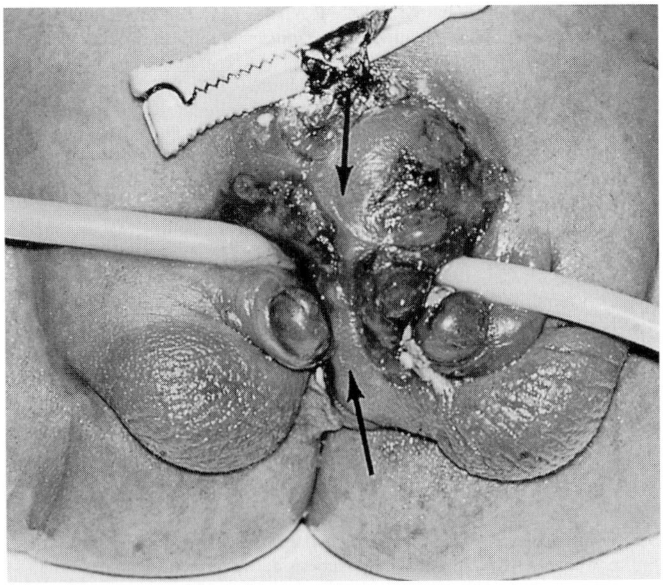

Fig. 31.62 Vesicointestinal fissure with bridge of skin across to perineum. Rubber tube passed through below the skin tag.

frequently than girls. There is a predominance of right-sided hernias in boys: 60% occur on the right, 30% on the left and 10% bilaterally.

Premature infants have an increased incidence of inguinal hernias, and this is proportional to the degree of prematurity. The risk of incarceration in this group is increased and strangulation can occur in the first few months, but rarely thereafter. Bilateral hernias are more common in premature infants (Fig. 31.63).

Premature infants should have their inguinal hernia repaired prior to discharge from hospital. This can be delayed as long as possible, provided the hernia is kept under inspection. Postoperative apnoea is less often seen in infants over 42 weeks' corrected gestation at the time of surgery. Many surgeons will explore both groins because of the high prevalence (about 50%) of a patent processus vaginalis on the contralateral side. Emergency surgery for incarcerated inguinal hernias can usually be avoided by gentle manual reduction of the hernia and early surgery. Epidural anaesthetics have facilitated surgery on premature infants with chronic lung disease, reducing the need for intubation and general anaesthesia.[61]

UMBILICAL

Umbilical hernias, though unsightly, rarely give rise to complications. As there is little risk and the majority will close if left alone, there is little place for surgery before 4 years of age at the earliest.

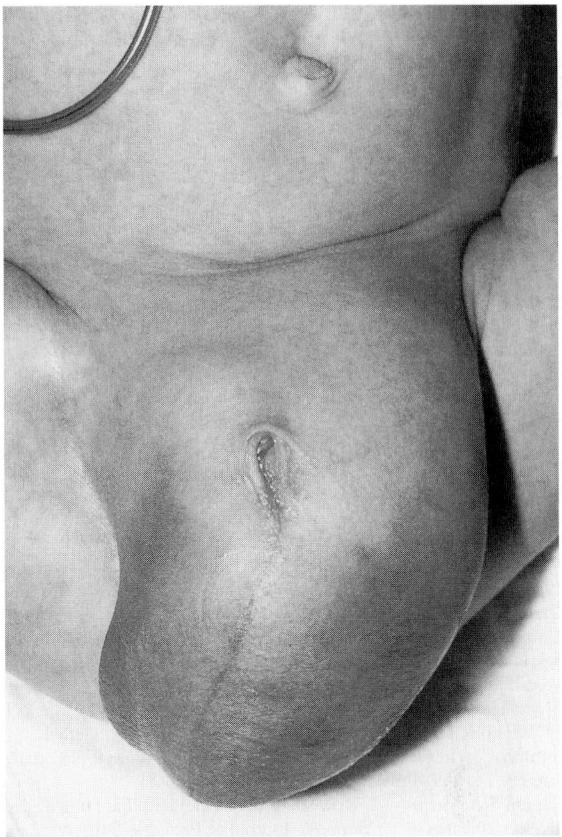

Fig. 31.63 Large bilateral inguinal herniae in a preterm neonate.

REFERENCES

1. Aaronson I, Nixon H H 1972 A clinical evaluation of anorectal pressure studies in the diagnosis of Hirschsprung's disease. Gut 13: 138–146
2. Ahmed A, Spitz L 1986 The outcome of colonic replacement of the esophagus in children. Journal of Pediatric Surgery 19: 37–54
3. Anderson K D, Randolph J G 1973 The gastric tube for esophageal replacement in children. Annals of Surgery 66: 333–342
4. Astley R 1969 Duodenal atresia with gas below the obstruction. British Journal of Radiology 42: 351–353
5. Atwell J D, Harrison G S 1980 Observation on the role of esophagogastrostomy in infancy and childhood with particular reference to the long term results and operative mortality. Journal of Pediatric Surgery 15: 303–309
6. Bodian M, Stephens F D, Ward B C H 1949 Hirschsprung's disease and idiopathic megalocolon. Lancet i: 6–11
7. Boley S J 1964 New modification of the surgical treatment of Hirschsprung's disease. Surgery 56: 1015–1017
8. Boyd A, Carachi R, Azmy A, Raine P A M, Young D G 1988 Gastrografin enema in meconium ileus: the persistent approach. Pediatric Surgery International 3: 139–140
9. Bull M J, Givan D C, Sadove A M, Bixler D, Hearn D 1990 Improved outcome in Pierre–Robin sequence: effect of multidisciplinary evaluation and management. Pediatrics 86: 293–301
10. Burrington J D, Stephens C A 1968 Esophageal replacement with gastric tube in infants and children. Journal of Pediatric Surgery 3: 246–252
11. Calder J 1733 In: Medical essays and observations relating to the practice of physics and surgery (abridged from Philosophical Discussions). Reviewed and published by J. Newberry, Edinburgh, vol. 1, pp 203–204
12. Campbell P E, Noblett H 1969 Experience with rectal suction biopsy in the diagnosis of Hirschsprung's disease. Journal of Pediatric Surgery 4: 410–414
13. Cantrell J R, Haller J A Jr, Ravitch M M 1958 A syndrome of congenital defects involving the abdominal wall, sternum, diaphragm, pericardium and heart. Surgery Gynecology and Obstetrics 197: 602–614
14. Carachi R, Whiteford M 1996 The role of cystic fibrosis genotyping in meconium ileus. Presented to the BAPS Congress, Jersey

15. Chittmittrapap S, Spitz L, Kiely E M, Brereton R I 1989 Oesophageal atresia and associated anomalies. Archives of Disease in Childhood 64: 364–368
16. Cockburn F, Drillien C M 1974 In: Neonatal medicine. Blackwell Scientific, Oxford, p 805
17. Coutts J, Docherty J G, Carachi R, Evans T J 1997 Clinical course of cystic fibrosis presenting with meconium ileus. British Journal of Surgery 84: 555
18. Cowton J A L, Beattie T J, Gibson A A M, Mackie R, Skerrow C J, Cockburn F 1982 Epidermolysis bullosa in association with aplasia cutis congenita and pyloric atresia. Acta Paediatrica Scandinavica 71: 155–160
19. Crabbe D C G, Kiely E M, Drake D P, Spitz L 1996 Management of the isolated congenital tracheo-oesophageal fistula. European Journal of Pediatric Surgery 6: 67–69
20. Craft A W, Watson A J, Scott J E S 1976 'Giant Meckel's diverticulum' causing intestinal obstruction in the newborn. Journal of Pediatric Surgery 11: 1037–1038
21. de Vries P A, Pena A 1982 Posterior sagittal anorectoplasty. Journal of Pediatric Surgery 17: 638–643
22. Dickson J A S 1970 Apple peel small bowel: an uncommon variant of duodenal and jejunal atresia. Journal of Pediatric Surgery 5: 595–600
23. Docherty J G, Zaki A, Coutts J A P, Evans T J, Carachi R 1992 Meconium ileus: a review 1972–1990. British Journal of Surgery 79: 571–573
24. Duhamel B 1956 Une nouvelle opération pour le mégacolon congénital. L'abaissement rectorectal et transanal du colon et son application possible au traîtment de quelques autres malformations. Presse Médicale 64: 2249–2250
25. El Shafie M, Stidham GI, Klippel C H, Katzman G H, Weinfield I J 1979 Pyloric atresia and epidermolysis bullosa lethalis: a lethal combination in two premature newborn siblings. Journal of Pediatric Surgery 14: 446–449
26. Engum S A, Petrites M, Rescorla F et al 1993 Familial Hirschsprung's disease: 20 cases in 12 kindreds. Journal of Pediatric Surgery 28: 1286–1290
27. Evans N J 1982 Pyloric stenosis in premature infants after transpyloric feeding. Lancet ii: 665
28. Fagan D G, Pritchard J S, Clarkson T W, Greenwood M R 1977 Organ mercury levels in infants with omphaloceles treated with organic mercurial antiseptic. Archives of Disease in Childhood 52: 962–964
29. Fallat M E, Skoog S J, Belman A B, Eng G, Randolph J G 1989 The prune belly syndrome: A comprehensive approach to management. Journal of Urology 142: 802–805
30. Filler R M, Messineo A, Vinograd I 1992 Severe tracheomalacia associated with esophageal atresia: results of surgical treatment. Journal of Pediatric Surgery 27: 1136–1141
31. Franklin R H 1948 Congenital atresia of the oesophagus. Annals of the Royal College of Surgeons of England 2: 69–72
32. Fuzesi K, Young D G 1976 Congenital laryngo-tracheo-esophageal cleft. Journal of Pediatric Surgery 11: 933–937
33. Gee H, Abdulla U 1978 Antenatal diagnosis of fetal duodenal atresia by ultrasonic scan. British Medical Journal ii: 1265
34. German J C, Waterston D J 1976 Colon interposition for the replacement of the esophagus in children. Journal of Pediatric Surgery 11: 227–233
35. Gibson A A M, Young D G 1975 Diagnosis of Hirschsprung's disease. Lancet ii: 1149
36. Glasson M J, Bandrevics V, Cohen D H 1973 Hypertrophic pyloric stenosis complicating esophageal atresia. Surgery 74: 530–535
37. Gobara O, Carachi R 1996 Multiple small bowel atresias. Presented to the Scottish Surgical Paediatric Society, Edinburgh
38. Gould G M, Pyle W L 1898 In: Anomalies and Curiosities of Medicine. W B Saunders, Philadelphia, p 253
39. Grob M 1963 Conservative treatment of exomphalos. Archives of Disease in Childhood 38: 148–150
40. Gross R E 1948 A new method for surgical treatment of large omphaloceles. Surgery 24: 277–292
41. Haddock G, Davis C F, Raine P A M 1996 Gastroschisis in the decade of prenatal diagnosis. European Journal of Pediatric Surgery 6: 18–22
42. Haight C, Towsley H 1943 Congenital atresia of the esophagus with tracheo-esophageal fistula. Report of successful ligation of the fistula and end to end anastomosis of the esophageal segments. Surgery Gynecology and Obstetrics 76: 672–688
43. Harrison M R, Globus M S, Filly R A 1981 Management of the fetus with a correctable congenital defect. Journal of the American Medical Association 246: 774–777
44. Heaf D P, Helms P J, Dinwiddie R, Matthew D J 1982 Nasopharyngeal airways in Pierre–Robin syndrome. Journal of Pediatrics 100: 698–703
45. Hocking M, Young D G 1981 Duplications of the alimentary tract. British Journal of Surgery 68: 92–96
46. Howard R, Myers N S 1965 Esophageal atresia: a technique for elongating the upper pouch. Surgery 58: 725–727
47. Kerr A M 1980 Unprecedented rise in incidence of infantile hypertrophic pyloric stenosis. British Medical Journal 281: 714–715
48. Kiely E M, Chopra R, Corkery J J 1979 Delayed diagnosis of congenital anal stenosis. Archives of Disease in Childhood 54: 68–79
49. Kutiyanawala M, Wyse RKH, Brereton R J et al 1992 CHARGE and esophageal atresia. Journal of Pediatric Surgery 27: 1136–1141
50. Ladd W E 1944 The surgical treatment of esophageal atresia and tracheo-esophageal fistulas. New England Journal of Medicine 230: 628–637
51. Leven N L 1941 Congenital atresia of the esophagus with tracheoesophageal fistula. Report of successful extrapleural ligation of fistulous communication and cervical esophagostomy. Journal of Thoracic and Cardiovascular Surgery 10: 648–657
52. Louw J H 1959 Congenital intestinal atresia and stenosis in the newborn. Observations of pathogenesis and treatment. Annals of the Royal College of Surgeons of England 25: 209–234
53. Louw J H 1966 Jejunoileal atresia and stenosis. Journal of Pediatric Surgery 1: 8–22
54. Lund D P, Hendren W H 1993 Cloacal extrophy: experience with 20 cases. Journal of Pediatric Surgery 28: 1360–1369
55. Martin L W, Altemier W A 1962 Clinical experience with a new operation (modified Duhamel procedure) for Hirschsprung's disease. Annals of Surgery 156: 678–681
56. Martin L W, Zerella J T 1976 Jejunoileal atresia: a proposed classification. Journal of Pediatric Surgery 11: 399–403
57. Muir I K 1974 Cleft lip and palate – management. British Medical Journal iii: 162–164
58. Myers N A, Egami K 1987 Congenital tracheo-oesophageal fistula. 'H' or 'N' type fistula. Pediatric Surgery International 2: 198–211
59. Neilson D, Hollman A S 1994 The ultrasonic diagnosis of infantile hypertrophic pyloric stenosis: technique and accuracy. Clinical Radiology 49: 246–247
60. Pena A 1988 Posterior sagittal anorectoplasty: results in the management of 332 cases of anorectal malformations. Pediatric Surgery International 3: 94–104
61. Peutrell J M, Hughes D G 1992 Epidural anaesthesia through caudal catheters for inguinal herniotomies in awake ex-premature babies. Anaesthesia 47: 128–131
62. Puri P, Lake B D, German-F, O'Donnel B, Nixon H H 1983 Megacystis–microcolon–intestinal hypoperistalsis syndrome. A visceral myopathy. Journal of Pediatric Surgery 18: 64–69
63. Raine P A M, Goel K, Young D G, Galea P, Maclaurin J C 1982 Pyloric stenosis and transpyloric feeding. Lancet ii: 821–822
64. Randolph J G, Newman K D, Anderson K D 1989 Current results of oesophageal atresia with tracheoesophageal fistula using physiologic status as a guide to therapy. Annals of Surgery 209: 526–531
65. Richter H M 1913 Congenital atresia of the oesophagus; an operation designed for its cure. Surgery Gynecology and Obstetrics 17: 397–402
66. Rintala A E 1976 How a patient experienced a cleft lip operation in 1763. Journal of Plastic Reconstructive Surgery 57: 158–162
67. Russell M B, Russell C A, Niebuhr E 1994 An epidemiological study of Hirschsprung's disease and additional anomalies. Acta Paediatrica 83: 68–71
68. Schuster S R 1967 A new method for the staged repair of large omphaloceles. Surgery Gynecology and Obstetrics 125: 837–850
69. Shigemoto H, Endo S, Isomoto T, Sano K, Taguchi K 1978 Neonatal meconium obstruction in the ileum without mucoviscidosis. Journal of Pediatric Surgery 13: 475–479
70. Sieber W K 1986 In: Welch K H, Randolph J G, Ravitch M M, O'Neill J A Jr, Rowe M I (eds) Pediatric surgery, 4th edn. Year Book Medical Publishers, Chicago, pp 995–1016
71. Soave F 1964 A new surgical technique for Hirschsprung's disease. Surgery 56: 1007–1014
72. Sommerland BC 1978 Cleft lip and palate management. British Journal of Hospital Medicine 19: 28–38

73. Speidel B D, Meadow S R 1972 Maternal epilepsy and abnormalities for the fetus and newborn. Lancet ii: 839–843
74. Spitz L 1992 Gastric transposition for esophageal substitution in children. Journal of Pediatric Surgery 27: 252–259
75. Spitz L, Kiely E M, Morecroft J A, Drake D P 1994 Esophageal atresia: at risk groups for the 1990s. Journal of Pediatric Surgery 29: 723–725
76. Swenson O, Bill A H 1948 Resection of rectum and rectosigmoid with preservation of sphincter for benign spastic lesions producing megacolon. Surgery 24: 212–220
77. Tessier P 1976 Anatomical classification of facial, cranio-facial and later-facial clefts. Journal of Maxillofacial Surgery 4: 69–92
78. Thomas D F M, Fernie D S, Malone M, Bayston R, Spitz L 1982 Association between *Clostridium difficile* and enterocolitis in Hirschsprung's disease. Lancet i: 78–79
79. Tryfonas G, Young D G 1975 Extrinsic duodenal obstruction. British Journal of Surgery 62: 125–129
80. Young D G 1967 Successful primary anastomosis in oesophageal atresia after reduction of a long gap between the blind ends by bouginage of the upper pouch. British Journal of Surgery 54: 321–324
81. Young D G 1967 Gastroschisis. Proceedings of the Royal Society of Medicine 60: 15–16
82. Young D G, Drainer I K 1972 Oesophageal atresia. British Journal of Hospital Medicine 7: 629–635

32

Haematology

Part 1

Coagulation disorders

Thomas L. Turner

INTRODUCTION

The coagulation system of the newborn is distinctly different in many respects from that of older children and adults, and changes physiologically with gestation.[5,6,7,8] It is remarkable, for example, how infrequently thrombotic episodes occur in babies, whereas in haemorrhagic disease of the newborn we see a disorder which is almost uniquely neonatal. Haemostatic defects are relatively common in LBW infants and those of short gestation. It has been demonstrated that 79% of 58 normally formed VLBW infants have some aberration of coagulation in the first day of life.[47] Surveys have shown the prevalence of thrombocytopenia (platelet count $<150 \times 10^9$/l) in a random population of infants admitted to a regional referral centre to be 22%, the majority recovering by day 10 following a nadir on day 6.[15] Term infants are more likely to have acquired bleeding problems, although bleeding due to temporary deficiency states also occurs. Inherited disorders are uncommon, but need to be considered in the differential diagnosis of bleeding at all gestations.

It is essential that a rational approach to coagulation problems in the newborn has its basis in a thorough knowledge of the physiological processes involved. Gestation-related variations occur and must be considered when interpreting laboratory results. Progressive changes in postnatal development of the human coagulation system in term infants have been demonstrated, reinforcing the need for adequate standards (Appendix 2). Differences in laboratory technique and sampling difficulties bedevilled earlier investigative work, but the impetus for standardization and improved techniques has come from the increasing realization that therapy can be of value. The availability of refined blood and coagulation products, with evidence of their safety, has increased their use in the newborn, in whom the majority of bleeding syndromes are likely to be temporary.

PHYSIOLOGY OF HAEMOSTASIS

There are three components of normal haemostasis: vascular factors, platelets and the coagulation system (procoagulants, fibrinolysis and procoagulant inhibitors).

VASCULAR

Moncada[36,37] discovered that the vessel wall synthesizes and releases a powerful inhibitor of platelet aggregation, prostacyclin. It was also shown by the same group that PGI_2 inhibits thrombus formation and may explain the lack of platelet adherence to healthy intact vascular endothelium. PGI_2 is also a very potent vasodilator, as well as having fibrinolysis-enhancing properties. Damage to the vascular lining reduces the available PGI_2. This, coupled with the exposure of collagen and myofibrils, results in platelet aggregation and the formation of the primary haemostatic plug. Furthermore, tissue factor III (tissue thromboplastin) and factor VII are produced in the vessel wall and play active roles in the coagulation cascade, along with high molecular weight kininogen and prekallikrein. Thromboxane A_2, a platelet-released prostaglandin, is responsible for vasoconstriction, allowing consolidation of the primary haemostatic plug. Nitric oxide is similar in action to PGI_2 and is a potent inhibitor of platelet activation and adhesion to damaged vessels. The vessel endothelial cells have other interesting capabilities, including fibrinolytic activity, being capable of releasing compounds such as tissue plasminogen activator, plasminogen activator inhibitor-1 and urokinase. Endothelial cells can also influence the protein-C and protein-S systems.

PLATELETS

Platelets are derived from megakaryocytes. They are of small volume (mean 7–9 fl) and play an extremely active role in haemostasis. There are no major disparities in either platelet count, shape or size between the adult and newborn, and the lifespan of platelets is probably very little different from that of the adult (around 7–10 days). Platelets have two granules: the α granules, which contain lysosomal enzymes, growth factors, coagulation proteins and adhesive proteins such as thrombospondin, and the high electron density granules containing calcium, serotonin, ATP and ADP. Cord platelets have similar properties to those of more mature platelets. Platelet membrane contains HLA and membrane-specific antigen (HPA1, HPA2, KOa, KOb etc.) as well as the vital arachidonic acid which is converted by cyclo-oxygenase to the cyclic endoperoxides PGG_2 and PGH_2. These in turn are rapidly converted to TXA_2, a potent platelet aggregator and vessel constrictor. The platelet also releases factors essential in the coagulation cascade; platelet factor 3 and platelet factor 4, a heparin-neutralizing substance. A delicate balance therefore exists between vessel wall and TXA_2. This balance is disturbed by vessel damage, with the subsequent formation of the primary haemostatic or platelet plug. This is caused by the adherence of platelets to the subendothelial layers and subsequent changes in shape and binding together of platelets. The adhesive properties of platelets may be less well developed than those in adults and platelet aggregation appears similarly less well developed. In vivo the bleeding time is the usual test for assessment of platelet function, and standardized tests have shown this to be shortened in the first week of life, probably owing to increased amounts of adhesive proteins, although this shortened bleeding time does not persist and indeed becomes prolonged after the first week of life. However, there are difficulties with the technique[4] and results require careful evaluation.

COAGULATION SYSTEM

The fact that blood remains fluid within intact blood vessels is remarkable in itself. The procoagulants lie in a state of readiness in their inactive forms, ready to produce thrombin from prothrombin if and when initiated by either the contact system (intrinsic system) or by exposure to TF. Tissue factor is the most important coagulation activation pathway in the newborn. All clotting factors (procoagulants) are high molecular weight proteins which in their inactive form (zymogens) do not cross the placenta. With the exception of factors III, VIII and possibly XIII they are manufactured by the liver, and inherited deficiencies of all except factors VIII and IX, which are sex-linked, share the autosomal recessive pattern of inheritance. The amino acid and nucleic acid frequencies, and the gene locus of almost all coagulation proteins, have now been established. Factor VIII molecule also provides the factor VIII-related antigen (von Willebrand factor) necessary for normal platelet adhesion.

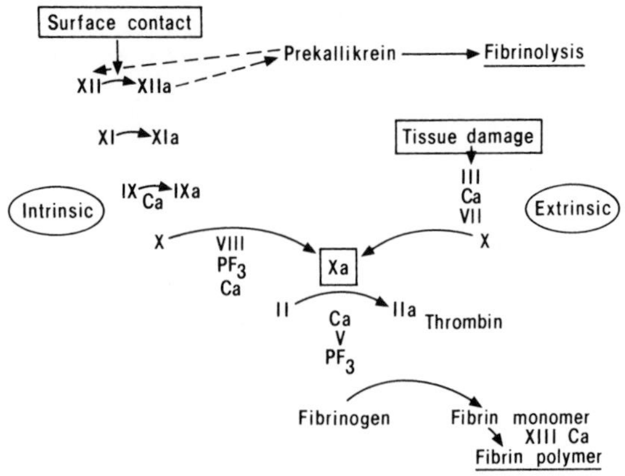

Fig. 32.1 Schematic representation of the coagulation cascade.

Following activation these zymogens behave as serine proteases, with very narrow substrate specificity. Fibrin is ultimately formed to produce the stable haemostatic clot. By a cascade process (Fig. 32.1) the intrinsic system factor XII, activated by vessel wall exposure (to collagen?), activates factor X by a series of steps. The extrinsic pathway operates more rapidly and, following release of tissue factors from vascular endothelium, factor X is again activated.

Factor Xa, factor V, PF3 and calcium convert prothrombin to the proteolytic enzyme thrombin, which is capable of converting fibrinogen (factor I) into fibrin monomer. Thrombin achieves its action by splitting off fibrinopeptides A and B from the fibrinogen molecule by division of arginyl-glycine bonds. This facilitates polymerization to insoluble fibrin strands by end-to-end and side-to-side combination. Once incorporated in the primary platelet plug, factor XIII activated by thrombin converts the loose strands of fibrin into a tough flexible polymer, which produces the stable haemostatic plug behind which vessel wall reconstitution begins.

FIBRINOLYSIS AND PROCOAGULANT INHIBITORS

Fibrinolysis and procoagulant inhibitors complete the normal balance between the hypercoagulable and the bleeding state. Fibrinolysis is responsible for the breakdown of fibrinogen and fibrin to FDPs. Early (high molecular weight) split products are likely to remain within the lysing fibrin clot, whereas the late (smaller) products appear in the serum and constitute the bulk of measurable FDPs. D-dimers are among the earliest degradation products found in the plasma, but their usefulness in assessing neonatal haemostasis has not been clarified,[26] as there appears to be a wide range of levels in apparently normal infants. In adults the range of normal concentrations is narrow, hence the value of measuring D-dimers in the early assessment of coagulopathy. Fibrinolysis can be activated by exogenous substances (e.g. streptokinase) or by labile endogenous activators. Plasminogen, the precursor of plasmin, the main enzyme in fibrinolysis, circulates in two forms. Tissue plasminogen activator is the most important; urokinase is another important plasminogen activator. The concentration of plasminogen is around half adult values, whereas the level of t-PA is higher than that found in adults, particularly in the hours following birth. It is likely that plasminogen has a fetal form, which is probably functionally less active. Although there is evidence that the fibrinolytic system is activated at birth, the reduced capacity to manufacture plasmin leads to a decreased fibrinolytic capacity. Following activation, plasminogen is converted to plasmin. This attacks fibrin and fibrinogen, producing FDPs, which themselves are powerful anticoagulants. Except in pathological situations, plasmin is rapidly inhibited by antiplasmins such as α_2-macroglobulin and α_1-antitrypsin. Antithrombin III also acts as an antiplasmin. Epsilon-aminocaproic acid and aprotinin (Trasylol) also act as antiplasmins and are used therapeutically and in FDP sample collection. Clearly, uncontrolled or inappropriate activation of fibrinolysis can rapidly produce defibrination.

Procoagulant inhibitors

Abilgaard et al[2] showed that ATIII is the most potent physiological inhibitor of procoagulant activity. Other direct inhibitors of thrombin include α_2M and heparin cofactor. ATIII is a single-chain polypeptide capable of inactivating serine proteases, particularly thrombin and factor Xa and, to a lesser extent, other activated factors. Low concentrations have been found at birth, and McDonald et al[31] showed the level to be half the adult value. These low levels which one imagines might lead to increased thrombosis are probably balanced by higher levels of α_2M, which may be twice adult levels. Heparin and heparin sulphate, released from endothelial cells, accelerate the inhibitory action of ATIII, whereas the prolonged intravenous use of heparin induces a reduction in ATIII levels. Other actions of heparin include interference with the activation of factors IX and X. $\alpha_1$antitrypsin and α_2M are also inhibitors, but less potent than ATIII itself; however, higher levels of α_2M persist throughout childhood, contributing to the reduced thrombotic risk. Deficiencies in either may result in thrombotic problems in the newborn.

Protein C[16] and protein S,[50] both of which are vitamin K dependent, are also important inhibitors which promptly inactivate activated factors V and VIII. Inherited deficiencies of protein C and protein S are rare in infancy, but can lead to a significant risk of thrombotic complications (p. 804). Resistance to activated protein C is the most common coagulation abnormality associated with venous thrombosis in adults, and has caused thrombotic complications in neonates.[29] This resistance arises from a guanidine to adenine substitution in the gene for factor V.[10] The resulting protein, factor V Leiden, is resistant to the usual inactivation effects of activated protein C, and the balance between the coagulation and anticoagulation systems is tipped to a procoagulable state (see p. 801 for more detail on the neonatal presentations of this condition).

SCREENING INVESTIGATIONS OF HAEMOSTASIS (Appendix 2)

Bleeding time

Using a standardized method the BT is normally less than 6 minutes and may be as short as 90 seconds. It reflects platelet function and number (see above). The clotting time is too insensitive for neonatal use. Studies of function (e.g. aggregation and adhesion) should not be considered as screening tests.

Platelet count

Platelet counting is now performed by an electronic particle counter (e.g. Coulter counter). The specimen must not contain microclots. A standard prepared blood film should also be examined.

Prothrombin time

Factors I, II, V, VII and X (extrinsic pathway) are measured by this assay, which is moderately heparin sensitive.

Partial thromboplastin time

When a phospholipid (cephalin) and kaolin (surface-activating agent) are added to plasma with calcium, the time taken to form the resultant clot gives a good index of intrinsic pathway integrity (factors I, II, V, VIII, IX, XII and prekallikrein). This assay is extremely heparin sensitive and may be used to guide heparin therapy.

Thrombotest

This rapid test assays the combined effects of the vitamin K-dependent factors (II, VII, IX, X).

Plasma fibrinogen concentration

Biological and immunological assays are available, but most depend on the ability of the patient's plasma to clot exogenous thrombin. FDPs interfere with the assay. Dysfibrinogenaemia can occur and cause difficulties in interpreting fibrinogen concentrations using biological methods.

Thrombin time

Fibrinogen concentration and function are assayed by this test, which is heparin and FDP sensitive. Any heparin effect can be neutralized by the addition of protamine sulphate.

Reptilase time

The venom of *Bothrops atrox* clots fibrinogen by cleavage of fibrinopeptide A, causing end-to-end polymerization of fibrin. This is unlike the A and B fibrinopeptide cleavage and full polymerization measured by the thrombin time. FDPs, but not heparin, affect the reptilase time. A prolonged PTT and TT in the presence of a normal reptilase time is probably due to heparin contamination; a prolonged PTT, TT and reptilase time in the newborn usually indicates DIC.

Fibrin degradation products

Several tests for FDP exist, including the latex agglutination test (Thrombo-Wellcotest). Specimens must be collected into fibrinolysis inhibitors (e.g. Aprotinin). D-Dimers, the D fragments of fibrinogen, may prove to be more sensitive markers of DIC (see above).

Blood film

In addition to screening platelet numbers, the presence of schistocytes (fragmented red cells) produced by mechanical damage or fibrin supports the diagnosis of active fibrinolysis.

Procoagulant assays

Specific assays of procoagulant activity are not performed routinely unless indicated by a family history or screening investigations.

METHODS OF INVESTIGATION

A well-documented history and family history are invaluable. Sample collection is difficult, as aspirated tissue factors rapidly convert a sample to a solid clot within the syringe. The following are sampling guidelines:

- Use a fresh needle, syringe and site for each venous sample.

Table 32.1 Volume of blood (ml) required to maintain constant 1:10 anticoagulant/blood ratio with 0.1 ml citrate anticoagulant

Packed cell volume (%)	30	35	40	45	50	55	60	65	70	75
Specimen volume (ml)	0.8	0.85	0.9	1.0	1.1	1.2	1.3	1.5	1.8	2.15

- Capillary collection methods are feasible if the foot is prewarmed to 42°C for 5 minutes.
- Catheter samples must be heparin free. First remove 3–4 ml of blood and return this after sample collection.
- Samples must be placed immediately into the appropriate anticoagulant or inhibitor. Table 32.1 gives appropriate anticoagulant volumes related to haematocrit.

The thrombotest can be performed on capillary samples, whereas a 3 ml venous sample will allow assessment of most other screening tests. Specialized laboratories are, however, progressively developing techniques to analyse smaller sample sizes.

NORMAL HAEMOSTATIC VALUES

Each laboratory should attempt to establish its own normal values for mature and preterm infants. For most factors other than V and VIII there is an appreciable gestational age variation (Appendix 2). This also affects the screening tests. Plasminogen and ATIII levels at term are both approximately half adult values. Preterm infants have 25% of adult values, increasing with gestational age.

SPECIFIC HAEMOSTATIC DEFECTS

COAGULATION FACTOR DEFICIENCIES

The vast majority of haemostatic defects in apparently healthy term infants are due to vitamin K1 deficiency or inherited specific coagulation factor disorders. In sick newborn infants secondary coagulation deficiencies, in particular DIC, are frequent. They are associated with hypoxia, infection, liver damage and rhesus isoimmunization.

Deficiency of vitamin K1-dependent factors

Haemorrhagic disease of the newborn – vitamin K deficiency bleeding

VKDB has been known since 1894, when Townsend[46] described a group of breast-fed infants who mostly developed gastrointestinal bleeding in the first week of life, with subsequently normal haemostasis in the survivors. Many authors have since confirmed these original observations and linked them with hypoprothrombinaemia,[12,41] the presence of breast-feeding,[45] reduction in the thrombotest and prolongation of the prothrombin time.[1]

It appeared from work in the 1960s and earlier that VKDB was a common disorder linked to breast-feeding, which could readily be prevented by giving vitamin K1 supplements either to the mother antenatally or to the infant after birth.

Vitamin K crosses the placenta poorly. Although the maternal plasma concentration may be 1–2 μg/l, cord plasma concentrations have been recorded as less than 0.05 μg/l. Mature human breast milk has been shown to have a mean vitamin K content of 2.1 μg/l (foremilk 1.4 μg/l, hindmilk 2.5 μg/l), whereas colostrum has a mean content of 2.3 μg/l. Formula milks are supplemented to 30 μg/l. The recommended daily intake of vitamin K is 1.0 μg/kg/day. Assays in formula-fed infants at 6 weeks have shown concentrations of 6.0 μg/l, whereas entirely breast-fed infants have concentrations of 0.13 μg/l at the same age. The bacterial flora of the gut, which provide an important source of vitamin K in older children and adults, do not contribute in the early neonatal period, accentuating the low supplies of vitamin K for breast-fed infants. As a result of these data, most infants, including those who were bottle-fed, were vitamin K1 supplemented and VKDB became very rare. It became clear, however, that factors other than breast-feeding were associated with VKDB. These included low maternal levels of vitamin K1, abnormal fat absorption and hepatic dysfunction in the neonate, and interfering compounds such as cephalosporins and high levels of vitamin E.

Vitamin K is available in three forms: phytomenandione (vitamin K1), its synthetic analogue menandiol sodium diphosphate, and menadione (vitamin K3) which does not possess a phytyl side-chain. Phytomenandione (Konakion) is the most widely used form. Vitamin K1 is essential to the hepatocyte for its role in conferring biological coagulant activity on factors II, VII, IX and X. This is achieved by carboxylation with carboglutamic acid. In the absence or lack of vitamin K1, partially carboxylated factors are produced and released from the hepatocytes (e.g. des-γ-carboxyprothrombins). These proteins induced by the absence of vitamin K (PIVKAs) have been detected in the blood of infants in the first 3 days of life. Shearer[43] showed by chromatography techniques that many term infants are indeed severely vitamin K1 deficient at birth, whereas hepatic vitamin K content is at least 20% of adult concentrations. The value to the infant of maternal prenatal vitamin K1, despite a low concentration gradient across the placenta, has also been demonstrated.

VKBD occurs in three forms in the newborn. Early haemorrhagic disease of the newborn presents within the first 48 hours of life. It is usually associated with maternal anticonvulsant therapy and the risk can be minimized by giving such mothers vitamin K1 during the latter weeks of pregnancy.

Classic VKDB occurs in breast-fed infants between the second and sixth days of life, and has an incidence of 1–1.6/1000 infants in the UK. Gastrointestinal tract bleeding is common and may be severe. To distinguish between swallowed maternal blood and neonatal gastrointestinal haemorrhage Apt's test was devised, but is frequently unhelpful. There may also be catastrophic bleeding into the central nervous system, but more often there is epistaxis, unexplained bruising, or oozing from the umbilicus or the Guthrie test site. Having confirmed the diagnosis (reduced thrombotest and/or prolonged prothrombin time), treat immediately with intravenous vitamin K1 (1 mg) and fresh-frozen plasma; vitamin K takes some hours to work. Consider blood transfusion. Rapid recovery of the clotting tests usually ensues.

Prophylaxis is the key to the prevention of this disorder. Vitamin K1 should be given to all babies at delivery. The intramuscular route gives the dual benefits of prevention of early, classic and late haemorrhagic disease (see later). The recommended standard intramuscular dose is 1 mg Konakion for term infants and 0.5 mg for infants less than 34 weeks' gestation. In response to concerns that the high plasma levels of vitamin K1 achieved following standard intramuscular use might be potentially carcinogenic (see below), the author and colleagues have used a lower intramuscular dose of 0.5 mg Konakion in term infants and 0.25 mg for infants of less than 34 weeks' gestation without a concomitant increase in VKDB. McNinch et al[32] have demonstrated the effectiveness of a similar oral dose in term infants, but the plasma concentrations reached, although reducing the risk of early and classic disease, will not prevent late haemorrhagic disease if only a single dose is used. It has been suggested that oral prophylaxis of the standard (intramuscular) vitamin K1 preparation (Konakion) given at birth and on days 3 and 7 and thereafter at monthly intervals, at least until the age of 3 months (in breast-fed babies), may reduce the development of late haemorrhagic disease; however, compliance with such a regimen is difficult.[17] Many other studies in children and adults have shown compliance rates for oral treatments to be as low as 50%. A new preparation of vitamin K1 (mixed micellar)[3] is better absorbed and produces higher plasma levels. Large studies on this compound are still awaited and the problems of compliance still exist, in addition to the increased costs that would accrue. The author has maintained his reliance on intramuscular vitamin K at birth, although where there is parental concern (see below) both forms of oral preparation have been used.

Late haemorrhagic disease of the newborn occurs between the ages of 8 days and 6 months. Bleeding is unfortunately often into the central nervous system, and frequently without warning. The most frequent association has been with prolonged breast-feeding without adequate vitamin K prophylaxis, although many infants have had gastrointestinal or hepatic disorders. Treatment is by prevention and, in the acute circumstance, with vitamin K1 intravenously, fresh-frozen plasma and/or blood transfusion. Neurological handicap is likely in those infants who have suffered substantial intracranial haemorrhage. It is a disorder which is largely preventable. It is important that infants who are on prolonged parenteral nutrition or who have persisting hepatic dysfunction have regular (usually intramuscular) vitamin K prophylaxis. It has been suggested that mothers who intend breastfeeding beyond 1 month should consider supplementing their diet with oral vitamin K1 (200 mg twice weekly), but few are likely to comply. Late VKDB has not been reported in infants given prophylactic intramuscular vitamin K1 at birth, unless they also had liver dysfunction.

Maternal anticonvulsant therapy

Infants of epileptic mothers who have taken therapeutic doses of phenytoin and phenobarbitone in pregnancy are more prone to develop VKDB. This is preventable by maternal supplementation or by routine administration of vitamin K1 at birth.

Vitamin K and cancer controversy

Golding and her co-workers in 1990[24] and 1992[23] reported a concerning association with childhood cancers and the neonatal administration of intramuscular, but not oral, vitamin K (odds ratio 2:1). This observation was set upon by the media, and as a consequence intramuscular vitamin K1 prophylaxis became extremely unfashionable in some centres because of parental concern. This is turn led to a recrudescence of haemorrhagic disease in some clinicians' practice. Fortunately it also led to increased work on oral preparations and encouraged the development of the newer forms of oral vitamin K. These observations by Golding have since failed to be borne out by subsequent studies of much larger populations in the USA[28] and Scandinavia.[22]

Experience in Denmark[39] found no difference in the incidence of childhood cancer over three time periods which spanned the introduction of vitamin K1. They concluded that intramuscular vitamin K prophylaxis could not be clearly associated with an increased cancer risk in childhood. However, there is undoubtedly, a need for vigilance and continuing awareness of associations between prophylactic vitamin K1 and longer-term effects. Negative results produced by von Kreis[48] in a fully designed case control study, and Ansell,[9] are encouraging.

Golding's observations, however, should not be dismissed entirely as there are associated in vitro observations of potential carcinogenicity by vitamin K in lymphocyte suspensions, with increased rates of sister chromatid exchanges which correlate with a compound's mutagenicity.[27] Other investigations failed to confirm this observation in the newborn, and at present there is no conclusive experimental evidence that vitamin K is a potential carcinogen in humans. It is important, however, that we continue to explore the possibility of effective and reliable methods of vitamin K prophylaxis by the oral route.

Maternal anticoagulant therapy

Oral anticoagulants taken in late pregnancy can increase the risk of fetal bleeding during delivery. It is recommended that oral anticoagulants should not be used during either the first or the third trimester to reduce the risks of malformation in the former (p. 192) and fetal and neonatal bleeding in the latter. However, provided the infant is given prophylactic vitamin K1 at birth, there is little risk of bleeding. The alternative is to use heparin throughout the entire pregnancy.

Nursing mothers transfer very significant amounts of coumarin derivatives in breast milk, but warfarin is safe because it is not transferred in breast milk. Heparin may also be continued while lactating with no risk to the baby.

Gastrointestinal and hepatic disorders, total parenteral nutrition

For a variety of reasons VLBW infants may be nourished for long periods by vitamin K1-poor parenteral nutrition. They should be given appropriate parenteral vitamin K1 supplementation weekly. Infants with malabsorptive disorders (e.g. cystic fibrosis, chronic diarrhoea) should also have vitamin K1 supplements. Infants with severe hepatic disease may be unable to synthesize vitamin K1-dependent factors, and in this circumstance vitamin K1 therapy is of limited value.

Inherited factor disorders

Fibrinogen

Afibrinogenaemia and hypofibrinogenaemia occur rarely, and usually present as haematoma, cord haemorrhage or bleeding after neonatal surgery. A family history can usually be established. Rare cases of dysfibrinogenaemia also occur where the fibrinogen has defective biological activity.

Treatment of bleeding fibrinogen deficiency states is best approached by the use of FFP 15 ml/kg or preferably cryoprecipitate (1 unit = 200 mg fibrinogen). Fibrinogen concentrate (2 g vial) is also available.

Prothrombin

Factor II deficiency is rare, usually presents as above and occurs even following vitamin K1 administration. Treatment, if necessary, involves replacement with FFP or with prothrombin complex concentrate, which contains 25 times the normal adult plasma concentration of factors II, VII, IX and X, and 10 units/ml heparin.

Factors V, VII and XI

Inherited deficiencies of these factors are extremely rare and respond to treatment with FFP (10–15 ml/kg), but factor concentrates are now available for factors V and VII.

Factor V Leiden

Activated protein C is a potent anticoagulant which is formed in the blood on the endothelium from an inactive precursor. During normal haemostasis APC limits clot formation by proteolytic inactivation of factors Va and VIIIa. To do this efficiently the enzyme needs a non-enzymatic cofactor, protein S. Recently it was found that the anticoagulant effect of APC was weak in the plasma of 21% of adult patients with thrombosis and in 50% of those with thrombosis with a positive family history or thrombosis in pregnancy.[18] The phenotype of APC resistance is associated with homozygosity or heterozygosity for the point mutation that produces factor V Leiden[10] (p. 804). This mutation is present in 2–5% of the population.[18] The locus of the gene is on chromosome 1. Healthy heterozygous individuals are at a 5–10-fold increased risk of thrombosis. Factor V Leiden is thus a much more common genetic risk factor than those previously recognized – protein C, protein S or anti-thrombin III deficiency – and has already been recognized as a risk factor for thrombotic disease in the neonate. Because the gene is quite common, individuals who are heterozygous for factor V Leiden and protein C deficiency are not rare. In a recent German series of 24 infants with porencephalic cysts 16 were found on careful investigation to have either heterozygous factor V Leiden, protein C deficiency, protein S deficiency, increased lipoprotein or a combination of two of these.[20]

Haemophilia A

Although it is unusual for the newborn infant with haemophilia to present with bleeding it can occur occasionally. I have seen the disorder in a male infant bleeding from a scalp pH electrode site. Local pressure may control bleeding, but factor VIII concentrates or cryoprecipitate may be necessary. Cryoprecipitate contains 110 units of factor VIII per donor unit (1 unit factor VIII per kilogram raises the plasma level by 2%). Increasingly prenatal diagnosis makes early postnatal confirmation possible.

Christmas disease

Neonatal factor IX deficiency is similar to haemophilia A. Specific factor IX is the treatment of choice; if it is unobtainable FFP provides sufficient quantities of factor IX.

Factor VIII-related antigen, von Willebrand's disease

Although this is not a true factor deficiency disorder, the autosomal dominant coagulation deficiency of factor VIII-related antigen is accompanied by consistently reduced levels of factor VIII. It produces a platelet function disorder, with bleeding and oozing from mucous membranes in the newborn. Diagnosis is confirmed by the failure of ristocetin to induce platelet aggregation, and the bleeding time is prolonged. Unlike haemophilia A, where the response to factor VIII replacement is short, in von Willebrand's disease it is prolonged.

Factor X

Deficiency of factor X is rare and prothrombin complex concentrate or FFP may be used in the bleeding state.

Factor XIII

Deficiency states often present with persistent umbilical stump oozing. There is an increased risk of intracranial haemorrhage, and replacement treatment is effective with monthly doses of FFP, cryoprecipitate or factor XIII concentrate. The diagnosis is established by observing overnight clot solubility in 5 M urea or monochloroacetic acid or by factor assay.

The management of all these deficiencies requires frequent assay to establish replacement frequency because of the variable in vivo half-life of these products. Careful genetic counselling is also indicated.

THROMBOCYTOPENIA

Isolated thrombocytopenia is uncommon in healthy infants, whereas a low platelet count in sick infants is the most common coagulation system defect, often with other coagulation disturbances. Thrombocytopenia can be confirmed when the platelet count is less than 100×10^9/l, although spontaneous bleeding seldom occurs if the count is above 40×10^9/l. The clinical features are purpura, especially in the flexures, pressure area bruising, e.g. skull or breech, and infrequently gastrointestinal haemorrhage. When more severe, haemorrhage elsewhere, especially in the brain and lung, can be catastrophic.

One per cent of term infants and between 15 and 22% of preterm infants will have some degree of thrombocytopenia at some time in the first 2 weeks of life.[15] Excessive platelet consumption, abnormally low production or a combination of both are the usual causes of thrombocytopenia. When due to either underlying cause the usual therapy involves platelet transfusion using compatible irradiated platelet concentrate if the platelet count falls below 20×10^9/l. Other forms of treatment have been suggested, but have not as yet been established as effective. These novel management modalities have been difficult because of the unusual physiology of platelet production. Whereas red and white cell progenitors can be stimulated to replicate by binary fission under the influence of erythropoietin and G-CSF, platelets multiply by a different system.

Instead of binary fission the precursor megakaryocyte undergoes endoreduplication. This leads to increasing maturity of the megakaryocyte, with a stepwise increase in the complement of chromosomes (up to 64 copies). This process is also called ‘endomitosis’. Bruno et al[13] have attempted to evaluate factors that might increase the numbers of megakaryocyte colony-forming units (CFU-Mks) and also increase endomitosis. They have demonstrated a role for a number of cytokines, including interleukins 3, 6 and 11. There is also a positive influence of G-CSF.

IMMUNE THROMBOCYTOPENIA

Neonatal alloimmune thrombocytopenia

This condition results from the transplacental passage of maternal specific IgG antiplatelet antibody from a platelet antigen-negative sensitized mother. This sensitization can occur at any time before or during pregnancy. Therefore, it can occur in all pregnancies and it is unusual for it to become progressively more severe. A moderately prolonged (3–4 weeks) thrombocytopenia is produced, which is often severe and symptomatic. Deaver[19] has shown that in 85% of cases the maternal antibody formed is to the HPA1 antigen present in 98% of the population. The remainder of the population are HPA2 antigen positive, i.e. HPA1 negative. Women who are HPA1 negative and tissue type DR52a make up the vast majority of affected mothers. If the thrombocytopenia is only mild (platelet count 40–100×10^9/l) careful observation alone is indicated, unless bleeding occurs. Where the platelet count is 10–40×10^9/l, some authors suggest corticosteroids. There is still controversy. No large control study of corticosteroid therapy has been reported and many, myself included, doubt its value. Against corticosteroid use is the observation that cerebral haemorrhage, probably the severest symptom, usually occurs prenatally and only occasionally intranatally or later. If corticosteroids have a role it may be in improving vessel wall integrity by reducing prostacyclin generation there.[11] Prednisolone 2 mg/kg/day orally is the usual recommended dose. Obviously intramuscular drugs should be avoided. Intravenous gammaglobulin has been used in affected infants with some success[21] when the platelet count reaches 20×10^9/l. In more severe cases (platelet count below 10×10^9/l), transfusion with random platelets will lead to a very short improvement in the platelet count. This, coupled with a normal maternal platelet count, should alert clinicians to the likelihood of NAITP. Exchange transfusion with fresh O-negative blood will reduce the concentration of antiplatelet antibody while washed maternal or HPA1-negative irradiated CMV-negative donor platelets (the most effective treatment) are sought.

When NAITP has occurred in a previous pregnancy antenatal management should be considered and may reduce the risk to the fetus[14,30,44] (p. 215). It is important to investigate the antigen status of other family members, especially women of childbearing age, to allow early recognition of affected women and hence discussion of appropriate antenatal management. Such a search may also identify a source of PLA1 antigen-negative platelet donors.

Autoimmune neonatal thrombocytopenia

Passive transfer of IgG platelet autoantibodies from mothers who have had ITP has been confirmed. Previous studies have indicated a high risk of thrombocytopenia in infants of mothers with ITP and, to a lesser extent, with SLE; 79% of infants developed thrombocytopenia if the maternal platelet count was less than 100×10^9/l, compared to 27% of infants whose maternal counts were greater. Although the perinatal mortality is low (less than 2%) morbidity is more significant: 4% of infants will be severely thrombocytopenic, 10% have platelet counts below 50×10^9/l, and a further 50% will show a fall during the first week of life. Mothers who have been splenectomized may still produce autoantibodies and have affected infants.

Severely affected infants with symptoms may respond to steroid therapy or intravenous IgG, which attempts to block the unbound platelet autoantibodies. Platelet transfusion is of no value.

HLA system-specific antileukocyte–platelet antibody is well documented but produces less severe thrombocytopenia. Here both maternal and infant plasma contain IgG antibody to platelet and leukocytes (often lymphocytes), although there is seldom evidence of leukopenia. The immediate management is as in NAITP. Investigation of the antigen status of other family members is also recommended. The antenatal management of such cases is described on page 216.

INFECTION

Infection-induced thrombocytopenia may be mediated by either megakaryocyte damage, endotoxin platelet damage, DIC or increased splenic removal. Congenital viral infections, particularly cytomegalovirus and rubella (p. 1168), can produce marked thrombocytopenia, which is usually considered to be secondary to both bone marrow damage and DIC. However, thrombocytopenia is much less frequent in congenital syphilis and toxoplasmosis. Bacterial infections frequently produce a dramatic fall in the platelet count, which may precede major clinical deterioration in Gram-negative septicaemia. The thrombocytopenia of bacterial infection is not always associated with DIC, but variably with neutropenia or neutrophilia.

DRUGS

Maternal drugs have frequently been implicated as a cause of neonatal thrombocytopenia, but tolbutamide is the only one with a substantial literature to support this association. It is now clear that thiazide diuretics[35] and salicylates affect function only, and there is a link between the use of Intralipid in parenteral nutrition and thrombocytopenia and platelet function.

BONE MARROW DEFECTS

Bone marrow replacement by acute neonatal leukaemia, histiocytosis-X and metastatic neuroblastoma can produce thrombocytopenia, and in Down syndrome[51] reduced or increased production lasting several weeks is frequently observed. The thrombocytopenia absent radii complex[25] with megakaryocyte absence is well described, and occasionally thrombocytopenia is seen in association with Fanconi's pancytopenia. Pure congenital amegakaryocytic thrombocytopenia akin to Diamond–Blackfan red cell aplasia has been described. In the sex-linked Wiskott–Aldrich syndrome thrombocytopenia has frequently been described.[52]

Following exchange transfusion, usually for rhesus isoimmunization, temporary thrombocytopenia may occur because of the washout effect of exchange, delayed marrow release and immune complexes (see later).

PLATELET FUNCTION DISORDERS

These are rare and seldom give rise to symptoms in the neonatal period.

HEREDITARY VARIETIES

Glanzmann's disease (thrombasthenia) is a rare autosomal recessive disorder producing chronic generalized purpura and prolonged bleeding. Platelet adhesion to collagen, release of ADP and PF4 in response to collagen, thrombin and ristocetin-induced aggregation are all normal. Studies suggest that there are deficiencies of membrane components, notably actomyosin and platelet membrane-specific glycoproteins.

Decreased ADP storage pool disease is also inherited in an autosomal recessive manner, with the clinical features of mild bruising or bleeding. The bleeding time is prolonged and there appears to be defective formation of the platelet granules that store ADP, ATP, serotonin and calcium.

Bernard–Soulier syndrome is a rare autosomal, incompletely recessive disorder of moderate clinical severity characterized by giant platelets, variable thrombocytopenia, prolonged bleeding time and decreased platelet adhesiveness. Platelet aggregation by ristocetin is abnormal and the platelets lack a critical receptor site for factor VIII-related antigen.

ACQUIRED VARIETIES

Drugs are the principal cause of this variety of platelet disorder in the neonatal period, although uraemia may also provoke platelet dysfunction. Aspirin, phenylbutazone, promethazine, indomethacin and carbenicillin have all been shown to produce platelet dysfunction, presumably by inhibiting cyclo-oxygenase, which converts arachidonic acid to prostaglandin endoperoxides, thus reducing TXA_2 and prolonging the bleeding time. The bulk of these disorders, both inherited and acquired, do not require active treatment but in an emergency would respond to platelet concentrate or platelet-rich plasma infusions.

DISSEMINATED INTRAVASCULAR COAGULATION (CONSUMPTION COAGULOPATHY, SECONDARY HAEMORRHAGIC DISEASE)

DIC has frequently been described, but often without sufficient delineation of the process. The definition used hereafter is a process characterized by widespread activation of the coagulation system with the formation of soluble or insoluble fibrin, and in which clotting factors and platelets are consumed with secondary activation of fibrinolysis.[40] There is, as a result, extensive intravascular thrombosis, with tissue damage and subsequent disturbance of function. The blood may be hyper- or hypocoagulable depending on the stage and degree of the process, the amount of FDP present and the infant's ability to replace the consumed coagulation factors and platelets. DIC may be generalized or localized, acute or chronic.

GENERALIZED DIC

Trigger factors are necessary to initiate the process of consumption, and these may act directly or indirectly to activate coagulation. In the direct variety, TF is released by hypoxia, acidosis or the placenta (e.g. chorioangioma, dead twin, abruption), with subsequent activation of the extrinsic pathway. Rivers et al[42] described tissue factor release by neonatal monocytes on exposure to Gram-negative endotoxins and the IgG anti-D erythrocyte immune complexes of rhesus isoimmunization. If the infant is able to restore consumed factors rapidly and the trigger is speedily removed (e.g. in acute asphyxia), the process may not progress to full-blown DIC. However, if hypoxia and/or acidosis persist in the presence of hepatic immaturity the scene is set for progressive, generalized DIC. Indirect activation of DIC occurs when the intrinsic pathway is stimulated by substances such as endotoxins, antigen–antibody complexes and cytokines, which may produce platelet membrane defects and widespread endothelial cell damage. Exposure of collagen and the release of platelet factors (PF3 and TXA_2) activate the intrinsic mechanism in the face of PGI_2 and plasminogen activator depletion. The low levels of ATIII and protein C accentuate the risk of DIC in the presence of continuing procoagulant activation.

CHRONIC DIC

This form of DIC is less frequently observed but may occur in moderate rhesus isoimmunization as described above, and in untreated polycythaemia, small for gestational age infants, twin-to-twin transfusion and Down syndrome.

LOCALIZED DIC

The outstanding example of this disorder is the Kasabach–Merritt syndrome (giant haemangioma) (p. 892), in which local consumption of platelets and coagulation factors may occur, with resultant generalized bleeding. Fortunately, regression, either induced by corticosteroids or spontaneous, terminates the consumption process. Occasionally in severe cases interferon-α_{2a} may be useful.

DIAGNOSIS

Clinical aids to the diagnosis of DIC include spontaneous bleeding from the gastrointestinal tract, haematuria and prolonged or renewed bleeding from heel stab and injection sites. The diagnosis of established DIC is confirmed by thrombocytopenia, often severe ($<50 \times 10^9$/l), in the presence of prolongation of the PT and PTT, and severely diminished plasma fibrinogen concentrations (<1 g/l), in the absence of heparin effect. Elevated FDPs (>80 mg/ml) D-dimers and schistocytes in the peripheral blood film are also found.

MANAGEMENT

In mild to moderate DIC expectant therapy is indicated unless there is persistence of the trigger factor or serious bleeding. Hypoxia, infection and acidaemia should be corrected, with careful attention to fluid balance and blood pressure control. Where trigger factors cannot readily be relieved and in severe DIC, controversy still exists over management. Exchange transfusion with fresh irradiated blood is indicated in rhesus disease, polycythaemia and sepsis-induced DIC, followed by platelet concentrate and appropriate coagulation factor replacement (e.g. FFP and cryoprecipitate) to return clotting studies to normal. There have been no extensive prospective studies on the treatment of DIC. If DIC persists I would encourage replacement therapy rather than exchange transfusion, despite the theoretical risks of accentuating the DIC process.

The major controversy surrounds the use of heparin, with which I have had little success, although in sepsis there may be successful arrest of DIC. Theoretically heparin may reduce ATIII, thus increasing the risk of thrombotic lesions, but others have used heparin successfully in the newborn in doses of 15 units/kg/h as a continuous infusion. Once fibrinogen concentration and platelet counts stabilize it would appear prudent to tail off heparin therapy. An alternative approach is the use of intravenous ATIII,[49] and this may prove to be a valuable addition to component replacement. In summary, the treatment of DIC principally depends on removal of the trigger, supportive therapy and, less frequently, exchange transfusion, replacement therapy and rarely heparinization, ATIII therapy and/or fibrinolytic agents.

THROMBOEMBOLISM

Major blood vessel thrombosis occurs infrequently (5/100 000 births)[38] and has usually been associated with the use of umbilical arterial or venous catheters (p. 919). Preterm infants are at the greatest risk. Arterial thrombosis may occur following umbilical arterial catheterization in any aortic branch vessel and lead to gut infarction, necrotizing enterocolitis, buttock infarction and aortic bifurcation thrombosis or embolus. Renal artery thrombosis can also develop, leading to neonatal hypertension.

The renal vein is probably the commonest site for venous thrombosis, but multiple sites are not uncommon. It occurs in infants of diabetic mothers, presumably related to the polycythaemia frequently found, but more commonly is associated with sepsis, asphyxia and DIC. If there is a family history of thrombosis the possibility of ATIII, protein S, and protein C deficiency should be explored. Factor V Leiden should be considered (p. 801). If clinically indicated, heparinization with (a) 100 units/kg 4-hourly or (b) 25–35 units/kg stat., followed by 10–15 units/kg/h by continuous infusion is suggested. Control of heparinization is difficult, but heparin plasma levels, if available, are of value (0.5–1.0 unit/ml). Alternatively, prolongation of the whole blood clotting time or prolongation of the PTT (to twice normal values) can be used as an indicator of successful heparinization. If ATIII deficiency is confirmed, ATIII concentrate

(0.6–0.8 units/kg) will satisfactorily raise ATIII levels.[33] Major vessel thrombosis or catheter-related thrombosis can also be treated by the use of fibrinolytic agents (e.g. tPA), and we have used such therapy in preterm infants with thrombus formation in the right heart from central line placement.

PROTEIN C DEFICIENCY

Complete deficiency of protein C is associated with massive thrombosis in the neonatal period. The syndrome is rare, but treatment can be lifesaving and recognition of the severe neonatal cases allows counselling for the heterozygous family members. Neonatal cases have skin bruises which rapidly spread and become necrotic (purpura fulminans); limbs have been lost. Central nervous system thromboses have been described, as with factor V Leiden (p. 801). In the acute phase the laboratory results are consistent with DIC, but in addition protein C levels are undetectable.[34] Emergency treatment is with fresh frozen plasma every 12 hours. In the long term oral anticoagulant therapy has been used, and one child had a successful liver transplant.

COAGULATION PROBLEMS IN PRETERM INFANTS

Preterm infants, particularly those of VLBW and under 32 weeks' gestation, appear particularly prone to haemostatic defects. This is partly due to their increased risk of sepsis and necrotizing enterocolitis, coupled with their proclivity for hypoxia, hypothermia and acidaemia. They also have gestation-related lower plasma procoagulant levels, probable vitamin K1 deficiency and low levels of ATIII. Hepatic immaturity provides a further handicap to haemostasis. DIC does occur, but less commonly than might be expected, especially if the diagnostic criteria above are adhered to. There is no evidence that coagulation defects are primarily responsible for the common bleeding disorders in preterm infants, pulmonary haemorrhage and GMH-IVH, although they may play a secondary role. Reduction in mortality from GMH-IVH, although not statistically significant, has been reported when attempts have been made to maintain normal haemostatic levels (p. 1262). It may well be that extension of intraventricular haemorrhages can be limited by maintenance of haemostasis. Other workers have demonstrated that ethamsylate, a capillary stabilizer, reduced the ultrasound detected incidence of GMH-IVH. Thus it may well be logical to combine its use with haemostatic correction in the prevention and limitation of GMH-IVH. Severe pulmonary haemorrhage has also responded to replacement therapy concomitant with full supportive measures (p. 554). The author recommends that all VLBW infants should have regular investigations of their haemostatic status at least daily during the first 3 days of life, and appropriate correction performed even if asymptomatic. In sick VLBW infants the need for such investigation and treatment is all the greater.

REFERENCES

1. Aballi A J, de Lamarens S 1962 Coagulation changes in the neonatal period and early infancy. Pediatric Clinics of North America 9: 785–817
2. Abilgaard U, Fagerol M K, Egeberg O 1970 Comparison of progressive antithrombin activity and the concentration of three thrombin inhibitors in human plasma. Scandinavian Journal of Clinical Laboratory Investigation 26: 349–354
3. Amedee-Manesme O, Lambert W E, Alagille D, de Leenheer A P 1992 Pharmacokinetics and safety of a new solution of vitamin K1 in children with cholestasis. Journal of Paediatric Gastroenterology and Nutrition 14: 160–165
4. Andrew M, Castle V, Mitchel L, Paes B 1989 Modified bleeding time in the infant. American Journal of Hematology, 30: 190–191
5. Andrew M, Paes B, Johnston M 1990 Development of the haemostatic system in the neonate and young infant. American Journal of Pediatric Hematology and Oncology 12: 95–104
6. Andrew M, Paes B, Milner R et al 1987 Development of the human coagulation system in the full-term infant. Blood 70: 165–172
7. Andrew M, Paes B, Milner R et al 1988 Development of the human coagulation system in the healthy premature infant. Blood 72: 1651–1657
8. Andrew M, Vegh P, Johnston M, Bowker J, Ofosu F, Mitchell L 1992 Maturation of the hemostatic system during childhood. Blood 80: 1998–2005
9. Ansell P, Bull D, Roman E 1996 Childhood leukaemia and intramuscular vitamin K: findings from a case-control study. British Medical Journal 313: 204–205
10. Bertina R M, Koeleman BBC, Koster T et al 1994 Mutation in blood coagulation factor V associated with resistance to activated protein C. Nature 369: 64–67
11. Blajchman M A, Senji A F, Hirsch J, Surya Y, Buchanan M, Mustard J F 1979 Shortening of the bleeding time in rabbits by hydrocortisone caused by inhibition of prostacyclin generation by the vessel wall. Journal of Clinical Investigation 63: 1026–1035
12. Brinkhous K M, Smith H P, Warner E D 1937 Plasma prothrombin levels in normal infancy and in haemorrhagic disease of the newborn. American Journal of Medical Sciences 193: 475–481
13. Bruno E, Cooper R J, Briddell R A, Hoffman R 1991 Further examination of the effects of recombinant cytokines on the proliferation of human megakaryocyte progenitor cells. Blood 77: 2339–2346
14. Bussel J B, Berkowitz R L, McFarland J G, Lynch L, Chitkara U 1988 Antenatal treatment of neonatal alloimmune thrombocytopenia. New England Journal of Medicine 319: 1374–1378
15. Castle V, Andrew M, Kelton J et al 1986 Frequency and mechanism of neonatal thrombocytopenia, Journal of Pediatrics 108: 749–755
16. Clouse L H, Comp P C 1986 The regulation of hemostasis: the protein C system. New England Journal of Medicine 314: 1298–1304
17. Croucher C, Azzopardi D 1994 Compliance with recommendations for giving vitamin K to newborn infants. British Medical Journal 308: 894–895
18. Dahlback B 1995 Factor V gene mutation causing inherited resistance to activated protein C as a basis for venous thromboembolism. Journal of Internal Medicine 237: 221–227
19. Deaver J E, Leppert P C, Zaroulis C 1986 Neonatal alloimmune thrombocytopenic purpura. American Journal of Perinatology 3: 127–131
20. Debus O, Koch HG, Kurlemann G, Vielhaber H, Weber P, Nowak-Gottl U 1998 Factor V Leiden and genetic defects of thrombophilia in neonatal porencephaly. Archives of Disease in Childhood 78: F121–124
21. Derycke M, Dreyfus M, Ropert J C, Tchernia G 1985 Intravenous immunoglobulin for neonatal iso-immune thrombocytopenia. Archives of Disease in Childhood 60: 667–669
22. Ekelund H, Finnstrom O, Gunnarskog J, Kallen B, Larsson Y 1993 Administration of vitamin K to newborn infants and childhood cancer. British Medical Journal 307: 89–91

23. Golding J, Greenwood R, Birmingham K, Mott M 1992 Childhood cancer, intramuscular vitamin K, and pethidine given during labour. British Medical Journal 305: 341–346
24. Golding J, Paterson M, Kinlen L J 1990 Factors associated with childhood cancer in a national cohort study. British Journal of Cancer 62: 304–308
25. Hall J G, Levin J, Kuhn J P, Ottenheimer E J, van Berkhum KAP, McKusick V A 1969 Thrombocytopenia with absent radius (TAR). Medicine 48: 411–439
26. Hudson I R B, Gibson B E S, Brownlie J, Holland B M, Turner T L, Webber R G 1990 Increased concentration of D-dimers in newborn infants. Archives of Disease in Childhood 65: 383–389
27. Israels L G, Friesen E, Jansen A H, Israels E D 1987 Vitamin K1 increases sister chromatid exchange in vitro in human leukocytes and in vivo in fetal sheep cells: a possible role for 'vitamin K deficiency' in the fetus. Pediatric Research 22: 405–408
28. Klebanoff M A, Read J S, Mills J L, Shiono P H 1993 The risk of childhood cancer after neonatal exposure to vitamin K. New England Journal of Medicine 329: 905–908
29. Kodish E, Potter C, Kirschbaum N E, Foster P A 1995 Activated protein C resistance in a neonate with venous thrombosis. Journal of Pediatrics 127: 645–648
30. Kroll H, Kiefel V, Giers G et al 1994 Maternal intravenous immunoglobulin treatment does not prevent intracranial haemorrhage in fetal alloimmune thrombocytopenia. Transfusion Medicine 4: 293–296
31. McDonald M M, Hathaway W E, Reeve E B, Leonard B D 1982 Biochemical and functional study of antithrombin III in newborn infants. Thrombosis and Haemostasis 47: 56–58
32. McNinch A W, Upton C, Samuels M et al 1985 Plasma concentrations after oral or intramuscular vitamin K in neonates. Archives of Disease in Childhood 60: 814–818
33. Mannucci P M, Boyer C, Wolf M, Tripodi A, Larrien M J 1982 Treatment of congenital antithrombin III deficiency with concentrates. British Journal of Haematology 50: 531–535
34. Marlar R A, Montgomery R R, Broekmans A W 1989 Diagnosis and treatment of homozygous protein C deficiency. Report of the Working Party on Homozygous Protein C deficiency. Journal of Pediatrics 114: 528–534
35. Merenstein G B, O'Loughlin E O, Plunket D C 1970 Effects of maternal thiazides on platelet function. Journal of Pediatrics 76: 766–777
36. Moncada S, Vane J R 1979 Arachidonic acid metabolites and the interactions between platelets and blood-vessel walls. New England Journal of Medicine 300: 1142–1147
37. Moncada S, Gryglewski R, Bunting S, Vane J R 1976 An enzyme isolated from arteries transforms prostaglandin endoperoxidases to an unstable substance that inhibits platelet aggregation. Nature 263: 663–665
38. Nowak-Gohl U, von Kries R, Gobel U, 1997 Neonatal symptomatic thromboembolism in Germany: two year survey. Archives of Disease in Childhood 76: F163–F167
39. Olsen J H, Hertz H, Blinkengorg K, Verder H 1992 Vitamin K regimens and incidence of childhood cancer in Denmark. British Medical Journal 308: 895–896
40. Preston F E 1982 Disseminated intravascular coagulation. British Journal of Hospital Medicine 28: 129–137
41. Quick A J, Grossman A M 1939 Prothrombin concentration in newborn. Proceedings of the Society for Exerimental Biology and Medicine 41: 227–228
42. Rivers R P A, Hathway W E, Weston W L 1975 The endotoxin induced coagulant activity of human monocytes. British Journal of Haematology 30: 311–313
43. Shearer M J, Barkham P, Rakin S, Stimmler L 1982 Plasma vitamin K_1 in mothers and their newborn babies. Lancet ii: 460–463
44. Sidiropoulos D, Herman U J, Morrell A, von Mutret G, Barandum S 1986 Transplacental passage of intravenous immunoglobulin in the last trimester of pregnancy. Journal of Pediatrics 109: 505–509
45. Sutherland J M, Glueck H I, Gleser G 1967 Hemorrhagic disease of the newborn. American Journal of Diseases of Children 113: 524–533
46. Townsend C W 1894 The haemorrhagic disease of the newborn. Archives of Paediatrics ii: 559–565
47. Turner T L, Prowse C V, Prescott R J, Cash J D 1981 A clinical trial on the early detection and correction of haemostatic defects in selected high risk neonates. British Journal of Haematology 47: 65–75
48. von Kries R, Gobel U, Hachmeister A, Kaletsch U, Michaelis J 1996 Vitamin K and childhood cancer: a population based case-control study in Lower Saxony, Germany. British Medical Journal 313: 199–203
49. von Kries R, Stannigel H, Gobe U 1985 Anticoagulant therapy by continuous heparin-antithrombin III infusion in newborns with disseminated intravascular coagulation. European Journal of Pediatrics 144: 191–194
50. Walker F J 1981 Regulation of inactivated protein C by protein S: the role of phospholipid in factor Va inactivation. Journal of Biological Chemistry 256: 1123–1131
51. Weinberger M M, Olenick A 1980 Congenital marrow dysfunction in Down's syndrome. Journal of Pediatrics 77: 273–279
52. Wolff J A 1967 Wiskott–Aldrich syndrome: clinical, immunologic and pathologic observations. Journal of Pediatrics 70: 273–279

Part 2

Anaemia in the newborn

Elizabeth A. Letsky

DEVELOPMENTAL HAEMOPOIESIS

ERYTHROPOIESIS

Erythropoiesis in the human embryo can be detected 2–3 weeks after conception. Blood islands form in the yolk sac, the peripheral cells of which differentiate to form the first blood vessels, the central cells becoming the primitive haemocytoblasts.[29,139]

Haemopoiesis in intrauterine life is conventionally divided into three periods: mesoblastic, hepatic and myeloid (Fig. 32.2). The earliest blood cells have megaloblastic features, are nucleated and contain the embryonic haemoglobins which are virtually confined to the mesoblastic period.

Normoblastic red cell production begins in the fetal liver by the fifth week. The liver is the major site of fetal erythropoiesis in the human, but blood production there decreases by 24 weeks and is virtually undetectable by birth.[57]

Marrow erythropoiesis can be detected by 9–11 weeks, and by 28 weeks this is the major blood-producing organ. Haemopoietic tissue in the bone marrow continues to increase until term, and for a short time after birth.[93]

During the second trimester haemopoietic tissue is also found in the connective tissue of the thymus, kidney and

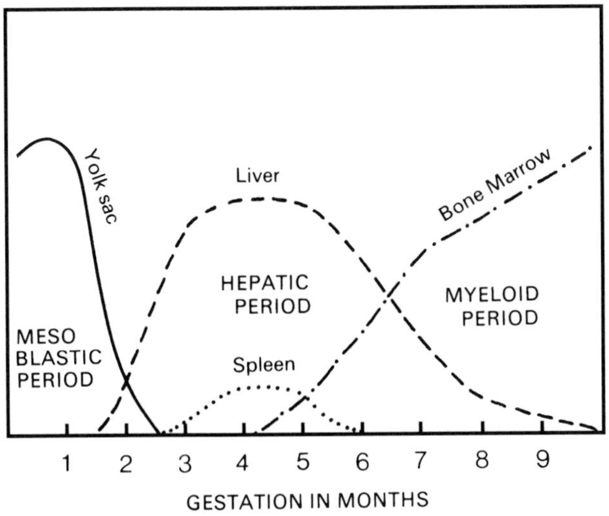

Fig. 32.2 Stages of haemopoiesis in the developing embryo and fetus.[141]

Table 32.2 Globin chain composition of human haemoglobins

Haemoglobin	Globin composition	Site of production	Stage of development
Gower 1	$\zeta_2\ \varepsilon_2$		Embryo
Gower 2	$\alpha_2\ \varepsilon_2$	Yolk sac	Embryo
Portland	$\zeta_2\ \gamma_2$		Embryo
Fetal	$\alpha_2\ \gamma_2$		Embryo
Fetal	$\alpha_2\ \gamma_2$	Liver	Fetus
Adult	$\alpha_2\ \beta_2$	Bone marrow	Fetus
HbA_2	$\alpha_2\ \delta_2$		Fetus
Fetal	$\alpha_2\ \gamma_2$		Adult
Adult	$\alpha_2\ \beta_2$	Bone marrow	Adult
HbA_2	$\alpha_2\ \delta_2$		Adult

spleen. The total contribution from these sites is negligible at birth.[56]

Control of erythropoiesis in the fetus is partially influenced by maternal factors, but is mainly controlled by fetal erythropoietin in the hepatic and myeloid phases.[199] Erythropoietin levels in the cord blood in non-anaemic premature infants are similar to normal adult levels, but rise with gestation and at term are greater than normal adult plasma levels.[83]

The main site of erythropoietin production in the human fetus is probably hepatic. In the sheep, the change-over from liver to kidney as the major site of erythropoietin synthesis occurs after birth. This change has not been demonstrated in the human, but neonates with renal agenesis are not anaemic.[199] More recent evidence suggests that the liver–kidney 'switch' during ontogeny is a genetically predetermined event, rather than a result of postnatal environmental factors.[68] The whole subject of developmental haematology is well covered in recent reviews.[29,84,139]

Physical characteristics and rate of production of red cells during development[29,84,139,179,184]

In the embryo the red blood cell count, the PCV and haemoglobin concentrations are very low compared to those found at term; the RBCs are very large (MCV approximately 200 fl), contain large amounts of haemoglobin (MCH 60 pg), and the majority are nucleated. As the fetus develops the circulating cells become smaller, contain less haemoglobin and there are fewer nucleated immature forms. The total haemoglobin concentration, PCV and RBC count increase, but the MCHC remains relatively constant (Appendix 1). Up to 10% of the total erythroid cells are nucleated at 10 weeks' gestation; the number decreases to about 1% at 20 weeks and continues to drop until term, when only 0.01% of the circulating red cells are nucleated. The reticulocyte count falls from around 40% at 10 weeks to 5–19% by 20 weeks, and to 3–7% at term.

Developmental changes in haemoglobins

There are three embryonic haemoglobins, Hb Gower 1 and 2 and Hb Portland. These disappear by 12 weeks' gestation, and it is thought that they are restricted to the primitive RBC in the yolk sac (Table 32.2). Fetal haemoglobin (HbF:$\alpha_2\gamma_2$) can be detected in embryos of 6–12 weeks' gestation[197] and is the major respiratory pigment throughout intrauterine life. From as early as 8–10 weeks of gestation it is possible to detect about 5–10% adult haemoglobin (HbA:$\alpha_2\beta_2$), which increases to 10% by 32 weeks. Between 32 and 36 weeks the production of HbA increases, coincident with a sharp decline in HbF production (Fig. 32.3). The decline of fetal haemoglobin in the perinatal period appears to be strictly regulated, and is not related to birth but to

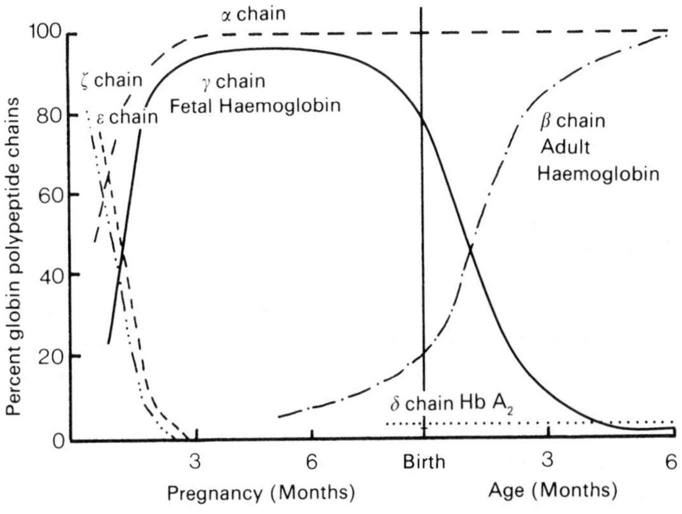

Fig. 32.3 Stages of haemopoiesis in the developing embryo and fetus.[141]

postconceptional age.[174] Studies have failed to produce a clear picture of the molecular basis of this changeover from fetal to adult haemoglobin in recent years.[174] HbA_2 ($\alpha_2\delta_2$), the minor adult haemoglobin, is detectable in the third trimester in small amounts, and reaches its adult level of about 2.5% by 6 months of age. The intracellular distribution of the haemoglobins has not been studied in detail, but HbA is present in most – probably all – red cells, although the amount varies from cell to cell.

Changes in red cell metabolism during development

The red cell is a dying cell from the moment it enters the circulation, and the activity of most of its enzymes decreases with age, so that the increased metabolic rate of fetal cells may be a reflection of younger cells in cord blood.[140] There are some unique metabolic characteristics which are not accounted for by cell age alone. These include the increased activity of phosphoglycerate kinase, enolase, glyceraldehyde-3 phosphate dehydrogenase, glucose phosphate isomerase, and decreased activity of phosphofructokinase on the Embden–Myerhof pathway. A relative deficiency of PFK may be responsible for the impairment of glycosis which is observed in the neonatal erythrocyte.[29,139] There is also widespread documented evidence that the newborn infants' erythrocytes are peculiarly sensitive to oxidant injury. It is possible that several factors are responsible for the susceptibility of neonatal cells to oxidant damage, including reduced levels of methaemoglobin reductase and catalase, reduced levels of membrane sulphydryl groups[176] and decreased levels of membrane antioxidants such as vitamin E (see below).

Red cell lifespan in premature and term neonates

The overall picture is that neonatal red cells have a shortened mean lifespan of between 45 and 70 days, compared to 120 days in the adult. There have been fewer studies on preterm newborns, but they all report an even shorter survival time.[29,139]

RBC membrane function and structure in the neonate

The majority of the cells are slightly more resistant to osmotic lysis and they are less filtrable.[80] The A and B blood group antigens, although detectable in early fetal life, are not fully expressed at birth and only reach adult strength by 2–4 years of age. The Lewis group antigens are very weakly expressed at birth. Cord blood reacts weakly with anti-I sera and strongly with anti-i. In the adult these reactions are reversed, and there is very little, if any, reaction with anti-i.[129]

Morphology of RBC in the term newborn

There are striking variations in size and shape, with some very large cells, moderate numbers of spherocytes, target cells, crenated cells, burr cells and fragments being seen. By approximately 8–9 weeks of life the red cells of the newborn are indistinguishable from those of the adult.

Morphology of RBC in premature infants

Preterm RBC show more marked anisocytosis and increased numbers of nucleated cells and bizarre fragments compared with term cells, and they persist in the circulation for a longer time.

LEUKOPOIESIS

The total white blood cell count at birth ranges from 9 to 36×10^9/l (9000–36 000/mm^3), with the mean between 15 and 20×10^9/l (15 000–20 000/mm^3). There is usually a rise in the total WBC count in the first few hours, and then a gradual fall to a mean of 12×10^9/l (12 000/mm^3) by the end of the first week (Appendix 1).

Granulopoiesis

There are very few circulating granulocytes in the first 20 weeks of gestation.[71,126,152] During the last trimester the numbers increase rapidly, and at term the total count is greater than in adults (Appendix 1). In the first 24 hours of life the neutrophil count rises in both term and premature infants. It remains relatively stable during the first few days and approximately 60% of the cells are granulocytes. Band-forms and myelocytes are commonly seen and occasional promyelocytes and even blast cells have been observed in healthy term infants, although these immature forms are more frequently observed in the premature neonate.[198] Between the fourth and seventh days the total count falls and the lymphocyte becomes the predominant cell, remaining so throughout early childhood.[161] Under stressed conditions neonatal neutrophils have a reduced phagocytic and bactericidal activity.[36,64] As well as infection p. 1124, which may often cause neutropenia rather than neutrophilia, conditions which increase the neutrophil count during the first week of life include maternal hypertension, intrapartum maternal pyrexia, haemolytic disease, intraventricular haemorrhage and birth asphyxia.[116]

Eosinophils

In the term infant the mean absolute eosinophil count is 0.267×10^9/l (267/mm^3, 2.2%) during the first 12 hours of life. This rises gradually and reaches a mean of 0.483×10^9/l (483/mm^3) by the end of the first month. Premature infants have very low counts at birth,[30] but this increases to 0.9–1.65 × 10^9/l (900–1650/mm^3) by the end of the first month. Sick premature babies have a marked eosinopenia.

Lymphopoiesis

Unlike granulocytes, circulating lymphocytes can be identified from the third fetal month and by 20 weeks there are 10 × 10^9/l (10 000/mm^3). Thereafter the count falls to approximately 3 × 10^9/l (3000/mm^3) at term.[152] The proportion of T and B lymphocytes in cord blood is similar to that found in adult blood.

Neonatal lymphocytes undergo a greater degree of spontaneous transformation into blasts and, up to 3 months of age, incorporate larger amounts of thymidine than adult lymphocytes. The lymphocytes of the newborn may be less active in effect or function than adult lymphocytes.[24]

Fetal development, leukopoiesis and neonatal white blood cell disorders are discussed by Engle et al, Cairo et al and Oski.[32,64,141]

THROMBOPOIESIS

Megakaryocytes can be seen in the yolk sac at 5 weeks' gestation, in the bone marrow from 12 weeks and in the liver until term. The platelet count from the 30th week of gestation is similar to the adult: 150–450 × 10^9/l.[1,70,126]

Recently a meg-CSF thrombopoietin-like protein has been purified and cloned which promotes proliferation and maturation of megakaryocytosis. The protein binds to and activates the C-mpl protein, one of the cytokine receptor superfamily. The isolated Mpl ligand shares homology with erythropoietin and stimulates both megakaryocytopoiesis and platelet production.[53]

PHYSIOLOGICAL ANAEMIA OF INFANCY

POSTNATAL CHANGES IN HAEMOGLOBIN IN TERM INFANTS

At birth up to a third of the blood volume of the conceptus is in the placenta. If the infant is held below the level of the placenta, one half of this volume is transferred to the neonate within a minute. If clamping the cord is delayed further an even larger transfusion will be achieved.

The cord blood haemoglobin concentration averages 16.8 g/dl in normal infants (Appendix 1), with a range of 14–20 g/dl. More extreme values (12–25 g/dl) are thought to depend on either large fetomaternal or maternal–fetal transfusion.[29,139] Male neonates may have a slightly higher haemoglobin than females, and firstborn infants are 0.5 g/dl higher than subsequent births.[109] The haemoglobin may rise by up to 6.0 g/dl in the first few hours after birth. The magnitude of this rise depends on the amount of the placental transfusion, as the infant responds to this by rapidly decreasing the plasma volume while the red cell mass remains unchanged. After this initial rise on day 1, the haemoglobin level returns to the cord blood value by 1 week (Appendix 1). There is no real decrease in haemoglobin concentration in the term infant until some time between the first and third weeks of life. Significant decreases in haemoglobin during the first week of life indicate either blood loss or haemolysis. A capillary haemoglobin of less than 14.5 g/dl[29,139] or a venous haemoglobin less than 13.0 g/dl[129] should be regarded as evidence of anaemia in the first 2 weeks of life in the term infant.

By 7–9 weeks, as a result of absent erythropoietin, the shortened RBC lifespan and the increasing blood volume, the haemoglobin level falls to 9.5–11.9 g/dl, irrespective of the size of the original placental transfusion. The PCV and RBC count also fall (Appendix 1).

In the first few days of life capillary samples have a haemoglobin concentration about 10% higher than simultaneously obtained venous samples, and the difference may be more marked in those infants with delayed clamping of the cord. The capillary–venous difference is thought to be due to the sluggish circulation in the peripheral vessels, with transudation of plasma.

At birth the reticulocyte count averages 5% (range 3–7%),[29,139] reflecting active erythropoiesis. This persists for the first 3 days and then drops abruptly to values of 1% or below by the seventh day of life. Persistent reticulocytosis suggests blood loss, hypoxia or a haemolytic process. About one nucleated RBC per 10 000 erythrocytes (0.01%) is present in the blood for the first 4 days of life. Despite the fact that it is common practice to express these as a percentage of the white cells, this is very inaccurate because of the variability of the white cell count. For what it is worth, in pre-electronic counter studies the term infant averaged 7.3 nucleated red cells per 100 leukocytes at birth (range 0–24).[4] All nucleated cells are included by electronic counters in the white blood cells, and then correction is made on examination of stained blood film. Absolute nucleated red cell counts range from 500/mm^3 in term infants, with higher counts in preterm infants. In those infants in which the numbers are even greater the most frequent causes are extreme prematurity, haemolytic disease of the newborn, maternal diabetes mellitus and intrauterine growth retardation. More recently the nucleated red cell count at birth has been used as a marker for fetal asphyxia and long-term neurological impairment. In one study the highest erythroblast counts were observed in pregnancies complicated by intrapartum fetal distress necessitating emergency caesarean section and directly related to the degree of fetal acidaemia.[178] Others have shown that increases in nucleated red cells identify the presence of fetal asphyxia, and that intrapartum injuries are associated with lower nucleated cell counts than those observed in pre-delivery fetal anoxia.[102,131,148]

Erythropoietin activity is very low immediately after birth.[83] This is interpreted as a physiological reaction to the greater availability of oxygen, and erythropoietin does not increase significantly in the serum until 8–12 weeks after birth. However, the erythroid activity in the bone marrow of term neonates starts to increase after 3–4 weeks, usually when the haemoglobin has fallen to about 10–11 g/dl. Erythroblasts in the bone marrow decline sharply during the first week, but hypoxic and anaemic infants do not show this fall[73] and continue to produce erythropoietin.[120]

ANAEMIA OF PREMATURITY

POSTNATAL HAEMOGLOBIN CHANGES IN PRETERM INFANTS

Although some investigators report that cord haemoglobin values rise steadily between 28 and 40 weeks' gestation, others have not confirmed this finding.[176] However, after birth the haemoglobin and RBC count fall more rapidly and earlier in preterm infants. The rapidity and magnitude of the fall is proportional to the immaturity of the infant. In those weighing 1.2–2.3 kg the haemoglobin falls to 9.6 ± 1.4 g/dl, whereas in those with birthweights less than 1.2 kg it falls to 7.8 ± 1.4 g/dl.[176] Babies with lower cord haemoglobin levels reach their nadir more rapidly than those born with higher levels, but the minimum haemoglobin reached is similar, indicating that the signal for marrow activity to return is probably the same for all premature babies.

Some infants tolerate very low levels of haemoglobin with none of the accepted signs of tissue anoxia, but others suffer considerable overt clinical difficulties, and the rapidity and extent of fall may be so great as to require blood transfusion. The aetiology of this anaemia is poorly understood, but in most babies it will have a multifactorial basis, resulting from a combination of iatrogenic blood sampling, varying oxygen availability and requirements, together with a variety of medical and surgical problems. As preterm infants have become viable extra utero at much earlier gestations over recent years, the anaemia of prematurity has become more complex.

AVAILABILITY OF OXYGEN AND SPECIAL PROBLEMS OF DEMAND AND SUPPLY

Tissue oxygen availability depends on arterial oxygen saturation, the concentration of haemoglobin and the position of the haemoglobin–oxygen dissociation curve. These are all different in VLBW infants, compared with term babies. Arterial oxygen saturation is frequently low because of diseases of the lung and apnoeic attacks. The concentration and type of haemoglobin are also different from those in a term baby.

The decline of fetal haemoglobin in the newborn period appears to be strictly regulated (see above). The switch from HbF to HbA synthesis occurs around 32 weeks' gestation;[174] it is not related to birth, but is based on postconceptional age. Thus the relative concentrations of HbF and HbA in cord blood depend on gestation. Babies at 32–34 weeks have a mean of 90% HbF; at term this is around 70–80%. HbF makes up <10% of haemoglobin at 3 months of age, and has fallen to the adult level of < 1% by 6 months to 1 year (Fig. 32.3).

The efficiency of oxygen delivery to the tissues is directly related to the interactions of haemoglobin with 2,3-DPG. High concentrations of 2,3-DPG push the oxygen dissociation curve to the right and facilitate oxygen delivery to the tissues. The reduction in the oxygen affinity of HbF by interaction with 2,3-DPG is only a fraction of that produced by the same concentration of 2,3-DPG with HbA. The effect of this reduced reaction of HbF with 2,3-DPG ensures that the oxygen affinity of fetal blood does not drop below that of the mother. This aids binding of oxygen from the maternal circulation in the placental villi. More than half of the oxygen bound in the placenta by the fetal blood can be released to fetal tissue, because the tissue oxygen levels in the fetus are much lower than those in the maternal tissues.

In the first few weeks of extrauterine life there is a progressive increase in the delivery of oxygen to the tissues. There is a gradual replacement of HbF by HbA, an increase in 2,3-DPG which shifts the oxygen dissociation curve to the right, and of course increased availability of oxygen. The net result of these changes is that although the haemoglobin level in the term infant falls from 17 to 11 g/dl in the first 12 weeks of life, the oxygen delivery to the tissues at 3 months is greater than that in the newborn infant.

However, the infant under 1000 g is unlikely to have reached 32 weeks postconception, and therefore the switch to predominant β-globin chain production has not even begun and it may be some weeks before significant amounts of HbA are produced.[7,151] This compromises the delivery of oxygen to the tissues by preventing the shift of the oxygen dissociation curve to the right.

ERYTHROPOIETIN

Maternal erythropoietin does not cross the placenta. Fetal erythropoiesis is endogenously controlled by fetally produced erythropoietin, which is structurally identical to the adult hormone.[92] High concentrations have been observed in the amniotic fluid and fetal blood[180] of pregnancies complicated by severe erythroblastosis fetalis. Elevated levels of erythropoietin have been demonstrated in the cord blood of babies who have undergone stressful

Table 32.3 Summary of clinical trials of erythropoietin in anaemia of prematurity

Ref. no.	Trial	No. of infants Epo	placebo	Mean GA (wks)	Age at start	Duration of Rx	Dose of r-HuEpo units/kg/wk	No. of transfusions Epo	Placebo	Oral Fe dose (mg/kg/day)
82	Halperin 1991	14	–	31	21–33 days	4 wks	75–300	3	–	2–5
12	Beck et al 1991	16	–	29	24–48 days	4 wks	10–200	4	–	3
168	Shannon et al 1991	10	10	27	10–35 days	6 wks	200	6	8	3
134	Obladen et al 1991	43	50	30	4 days	4 wks	70	30	34	2
135	Ohls and Christensen 1991	10	9	28	45+/–15 days	3 wks	700	0	5	2
169	Shannon et al 1992	4	4	28	8–28 days	6 wks	500–1000	1	3	3–6
34	Carnielli et al 1992	11	11	30	2 days	<8 wks	1200	NA	NA	3
173	Soubasi et al 1993 (C)	16	12	28	<7 days	6 wks	300	No difference		3
173	Soubasi et al 1993 (U)	9	7	30	<7 days	6 wks	300	3	6	3
11	Bechensteen et al 1993	14	15	30	21 days	4 wks	300	0	4	6–9
124	Messer et al 1993	31	20	30	10 days	6 wks	300–900	6	9	3–8
63	Emmerson et al 1993	15	8	30	8 days	5 wks	100–300	7	7	6
115	Maier et al 1994	121	120	29	3 days	6 wks	750	60	81	2
125	Meyer et al 1994	40	40	30	14–56 days (Mean 27 days)	6 wks	600	7	21	2–6
137	Ohls et al 1995	10	10	27	1 day	2 wks	200	2	14	2–6
167	Shannon et al 1995	77	80	27	23 days	6 wks	500	1.1*	1.6**	3–6

C = Complications
U = No complications
* 43% – No transfusion
** 31% – No transfusion

delivery or have suffered hypoxia in utero. However, the fetal response to hypoxia or anaemia is poor compared to that of the mature infant or adult. This reduced sensitivity to the stimulus of erythropoietin probably prevents accelerated erythropoiesis and hyperviscosity of the blood in the healthy fetus.[49]

Although term infants tend to respond appropriately to falls in haemoglobin concentration after birth by increases in erythropoietin production, the preterm infant retains its in-utero hyporesponsiveness to hypoxic stimuli, with an inappropriately impaired erythropoietic response.[175]

The least mature have the lowest levels of erythropoietin,[27] in spite of low haemoglobin concentration, high haemoglobin–oxygen affinity moving the oxyhaemoglobin dissociation curve to the left, with the potential for tissue hypoxia[87,88] and, often, lung disease causing hypoxaemia.

Shannon et al[170] have shown that progenitor cells committed to erythroid differentiation are present during the anaemia of prematurity and that the intrinsic responsiveness to erythropoietin in vitro is normal, leading to the conclusion that the anaemia of prematurity results from inadequate erythropoietin production. This may be due to a shift in the site of erythropoietin production.[49] In many mammalian species, including man, erythropoietin is produced in the liver in fetal life and there is a gradual shift to renal production of erythropoietin in the perinatal period. Erythropoietin produced in the fetal liver is much less sensitive to tissue hypoxia than that produced in the kidney, but this has not been confirmed in the human fetus. Human adult renal and hepatic erythropoietins have been shown to be structurally identical.[92]

Recombinant erythropoietin has been shown to stimulate erythroid proliferation in vitro.[171] The conclusion that the anaemia of prematurity results from inadequate erythropoietin production, and that there are circulating erythroid progenitors,[170] has led to the use of r-HuEpo as a therapeutic and prophylactic agent in the management of the anaemia of prematurity. However, this strategy has not had the strikingly successful outcome observed in those patients treated with r-HuEpo for the anaemia of chronic renal failure.

The mixed results obtained in a variety of reported pilot studies and, more recently, from randomized controlled trials, have been well reviewed.[177] The clinical use of r-HuEpo in the preterm infant is an important but confusing issue[11,12,34,63,82,115,124,125,134,135,137,167,168,169,173] (Table 32.3).

One of the earliest published pilot studies came from Halperin.[82] Treatment was not started until 21–33 days of life, and the dose given of 75–300 U r-HuEpo/kg/week was relatively small. All patients showed an increase in reticulocytes but an increase in haematocrit was variable and not universal, and in some infants a secondary decrease was observed. The effect of r-HuEpo was limited by a number of factors, the most important of which was iron deficiency, the serum iron and ferritin showing a rapid decrease after commencement of therapy.

In this study there was a tendency to early thrombocytosis and late neutropenia. The consensus retrospective opinion was that therapy was started too late and too little r-HuEpo was given.

The first randomized trial reported by Shannon et al[168] showed no improvement in haematocrit or need for transfusion due to the low dose of r-HuEpo and iron deficiency. In this group's second (1992) study[169] more r-HuEpo was given, with adequate iron supplements. The increased haematocrit and reticulocyte counts in the treated group led to a multicentre trial in the USA, which is not yet fully reported.

Many other small trials showed improvements in PCV and reticulocyte count, but no significant reduction in transfusion requirement.[11,34,63,124,135,173] The largest reported randomized trial to date[115] comes from the European multicentre Erythropoietin Study Group and involves 12 centres in six European countries. Of the 241 infants evaluated only 25% weighed less than 1000 g and 50% weighed more than 1250 g. The success rate, assessed by lack of need for transfusion and haematocrit never falling below 32%, was 4.1% in controls and 27.5% in the r-HuEpo group ($P = 0.008$). The results are broadly similar in the smaller randomized controlled trial by Meyer et al,[125] which also found significantly fewer transfused babies in the r-HuEpo-treated group (6 vs. 17 in the treatment vs. placebo groups). All of the babies in this study had a birthweight of less than 1500 g, the mean being 1059 and 1056 g in the r-HuEpo and placebo groups, respectively. The success of r-HuEpo in this study may be related to the small amount of blood taken for routine tests during the 6 weeks of the study – only 7.6 ± 1.7 ml in the treated cases and 8.1 ± 2.3 ml in the controls.

However, the effect of r-HuEpo may be overstated in studies with liberal indications for transfusion which will suppress erythropoiesis, and more babies under 1000 g need to be evaluated. The uncompleted US r-HuEpo Study group has published interim reports.[149,167] Of the 157 preterm infants entered from 11 centres, the mean gestational age was 27 weeks and the mean weight 924 g. The preliminary results show that r-HuEpo stimulates erythropoiesis and reduces the number and volume of transfusion. There was no difference in adverse effects. One control infant died of NEC. However, in appraising all of these studies we must bear in mind that there has been a fall in transfusion rate in recent years independent of the use of r-HuEpo.

Treatment with surfactant, modern ventilation, smaller blood losses for monitoring and conservative transfusion practices have all limited the need for r-HuEpo. It is clear from these reported trials that to achieve maximum efficiency enough erythropoietin has to be given, and it should probably be started during the first week to 10 days of life. In order to allow maximal response increased iron supplements must be administered. Benefits have not been clearly established for the infant under 1000 g who is sick.

Finally, one must address the cost of this therapy, which is very difficult to assess accurately. The cost of r-HuEpo has to be weighed against that of repeated transfusions. A comparison of the r-HuEpo-treated and control patients in the Zurich centre of the European trial assessed the cost of the r-HuEpo-treated as $1262 as opposed to $1203 in the control infants.

A small, recently reported controlled trial[137] from the US of the use of r-HuEpo in the first 2 weeks of life concluded that this resulted in fewer transfusions and was cost-effective. A similar analysis from the UK concluded that the reduction in transfusions was so small per baby that, overall, the use of r-HuEpo was not cost-effective.[196] In the UK the NHS cost of a 1000 U vial of r-HuEpo is £9. The current cost of an 'octopus' multisatellite unit of blood is £41.30.

Side-effects

- Neutropenia and sepsis. Although in vitro data suggest that erythropoietin suppresses granulopoiesis there was no evidence of significant neutropenia in the controlled trials. However, in the European multicentre trial there was an increased (non-significant) incidence of infection. The authors suggest that this may be due to depletion of iron stores, or the number of subcutaneous injections.
- Sudden infant death syndrome. Several cases have been reported in infants treated with r-HuEpo, but the controlled trials show no increased incidence associated with this therapy.
- Poor weight gain. This has been reported in some studies but not in others, and probably reflects the increased protein and calorie needs arising from the stimulation of erythropoiesis.[28]

Many questions remain to be answered.[42,66,104,136,166,175] At the time of writing the outcome of the US multicentre trial is still awaited. At best, this therapy will only be an adjunct to supportive therapy in the very low-birthweight infant and will not replace the need for red cell transfusion, although it may reduce it.[50]

IRON

Although iron transport to the fetus is unidirectional, with maternal–fetal serum ferritin ratios of 1:2–1:4, and there are adequate fetal iron stores even in cases of maternal iron deficiency, there is some evidence that there is a reduced red cell mass in the offspring of iron-deficient mothers and that iron stores, although high by adult standards, are reduced in these infants compared to those born to iron-replete mothers.[65] The fetus in utero normally recruits 75 mg iron per kilogram body weight, 75% of which is incorporated into RBC. Iron status at birth will therefore be related to birthweight and maturity and red cell mass.[5,51,88]

Iron deficiency is not likely to play a part in the early anaemia of prematurity unless there has been perinatal blood loss or repeated blood sampling for laboratory investigations.[113] The administration of medicinal iron will not prevent the initial fall in haemoglobin, but unless the premature infant is given iron supplements some time during the first 2–4 months of life, an anaemia, the so-called late anaemia of prematurity, inevitably develops as a result of iron deficiency.[176]

In general, infants with normal haemoglobin levels at birth will have depleted their iron stores and therefore limit the rate of haemoglobin synthesis by the time they have doubled their birthweight.[172] There is now a consensus of opinion that all premature infants, and particularly those weighing less than 1500 g at birth, require supplemental iron to prevent the development of late anaemia due to iron deficiency.[5,51]

Iron supplements in VLBW infants should be started on the 15th day of life in the following dosage regimen:[172]

2 mg/kg/24 h for infants from 1500 to 2500 g birthweight;
3 mg/kg/24 h for infants from 1000 to 1500 g birthweight;
4 mg/kg/24 h for those less than 1000 g birthweight.

Ideally these supplements should be continued for at least 12–15 months after birth,[138] although this is probably not necessary in bottle-fed babies if an infant formula with a high iron content (15 mg/l) is used.[81] If the infant is receiving adequate vitamin E in relation to polyunsaturated fat in the diet, the early introduction of supplemental iron causes no adverse effects.

It is important to give these supplements. The effects of maternal iron deficiency may have long-term effects on the fetus, neonate and developmental parameters in the first few years of life which have nothing to do with the Hb concentration and oxygen-carrying capacity of red cells. Animal experimentation has shown that early iron deficiency[189] irreversibly affects brain iron control and distribution, which results in neurotransmitter and behavioural alterations. Iron deficiency has been shown in the human infant to be associated with psychomotor delays in many studies.[90] Careful follow-up studies have shown that even after haematological correction the cognitive disadvantages persist at 5–6 years of age.[110] It is therefore very important to prevent iron deficiency during early development in the preterm infant, with appropriate maternal supplementation.[189]

COPPER

The diagnosis of copper deficiency anaemia is made by the demonstration of low serum copper (less than 40 μg/dl) or low caeruloplasmin values (less than 15 mg/dl), together with vacuolated erythroid precursors and maturation arrest in the granulocyte series. Anaemia and neutropenia due to nutritional copper deficiency will respond promptly to the administration of 400–600 μg of copper per day in a 1% copper sulphate solution.[138]

VITAMIN E

For a time it was fashionable to attribute any unexplained anaemia in the preterm infant to haemolysis associated with vitamin E deficiency. This was easy to substantiate, as all preterm babies are vitamin E deficient by adult standards and have a shortened red blood cell lifespan whether anaemic or not.

Haemolytic anaemia due to vitamin E deficiency in the newborn has now been shown to be an iatrogenic problem caused by inappropriate medication and excess PUFA in milks, as well as erroneous interpretation of findings.[202]

There are three variables in the diet of premature infants which increase haemolysis associated with lack of vitamin E:

- High PUFA
- Excess iron
- Low vitamin E content.

Correcting just one of the triad will prevent significant haemolysis or anaemia in the premature infant.[201]

Zipursky and colleagues[202] have shown that there is no haematological difference between infants supplemented with 25 i.u. oral vitamin E daily and a control group receiving no supplements, and it would appear that in standard neonatal care the hazard of vitamin E deficiency contributing to anaemia is negligible.

FOLIC ACID

Serum and red cell folate levels are higher in the newborn than in the normal adult regardless of birthweight or gestation, but fall quickly to levels which are often below the normal adult levels within several weeks of birth. This occurs more rapidly in the premature than in the term infant, as subnormal levels are reached within the first few weeks of life, whereas low levels do not develop in the term infant until after 6 months of age. Controlled studies have, however, failed to demonstrate any alteration in the early anaemia of prematurity by routine folate supplementation. The normal premature infant absorbs folic acid easily, and although there are no general recommendations for the prophylactic use of folic acid in the newborn,[176] a dietary provision of 20–50 μg/day will ensure sufficiency.

There is an increased risk of megaloblastic anaemia in the neonate of a folate-deficient mother, especially if delivery is preterm. The pathogenesis of development of such an anaemia is shown in Figure 32.4. The young infant's requirement for folate has been estimated at 20–50 μg/day (4–10 times the adult requirement on a weight basis). Serum and red cell folates are consistently higher in cord than in maternal blood, but the premature infant is in severe negative folate balance because of high growth rate and reduced intake. The usual fall in serum and red cell folate in the premature neonate, even in the absence of other complicating factors, may result in megaloblastic anaemia. This can be prevented by giving supplements of 50 μg/day.[85] In those infants whose dietary intake would be predictably poor, such as the very

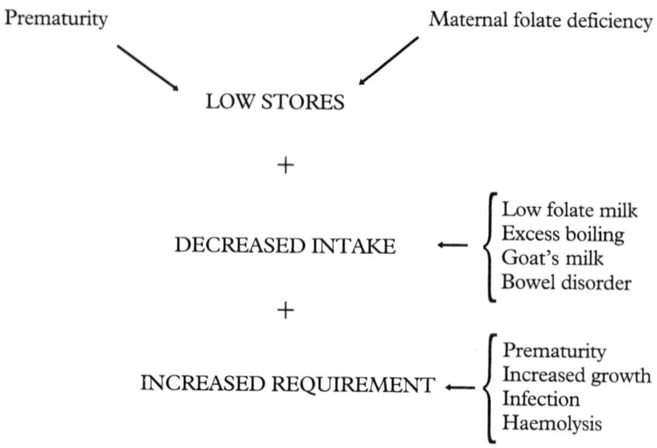

Fig. 32.4 The factors that contribute to the development of megaloblastic anaemia due to folate deficiency in infancy.

immature or those with chronic diarrhoea or recurrent infections, it would appear wise to give parenteral folic acid.

VITAMIN B_{12}

Serum B_{12} levels in all neonates are generally higher than in maternal serum. This is the result of active transfer of vitamin B_{12} across the placenta to the fetus at the expense of maintaining maternal vitamin B_{12} serum levels. This has little impact on the mother's reserves because adult stores are of the order of 3000 μg or more, and vitamin B_{12} stores in the newborn infant are about 50 μg.[156]

Because of these low reserves, and because of poor dietary intake of vitamin B_{12} during the period of rapid growth, most premature infants will have lower than normal adult levels by the fourth or fifth months of life. There is probably no significant relationship between deficiency of vitamin B_{12} and the early anaemia of prematurity. Sufficient B_{12} is present in breast milk and in all types of infant formula. Additional supplements are unnecessary even in premature infants.

PROTEIN

Protein synthesis and turnover are increased in preterm infants because of their very high metabolic rates. Adequate protein is necessary for healthy haemopoiesis, and therefore dietary intake of protein must be increased in these immature babies, particularly if they are being treated with rHuEpo.[28]

It has been shown[160] that human milk proteins promote general growth and erythropoiesis in very low-birthweight infants. The beneficial effect, particularly on erythropoiesis, promoting higher haemoglobin concentration in the early weeks of life, appears to be dependent on the human origin of this protein and an intake of 4 g/kg daily, which is double the usual intake.

PATHOLOGICAL ANAEMIA IN THE NEONATE

Anaemia in the neonate can result from haemorrhage, haemolysis, or failure of red cell production. Anaemia at birth is usually due to severe immune haemolysis or haemorrhage. Anaemia that becomes apparent after 24 hours is most often due to internal or external haemorrhage or non-immune haemolytic disorders. Infants with impaired red cell production do not usually develop anaemia until after 3 weeks.

Assessment of anaemia in the newborn infant has been well reviewed by Blanchette and Zipursky,[21] and more recently by Brugnara and Platt.[29] A practical approach is given in Figure 32.5.

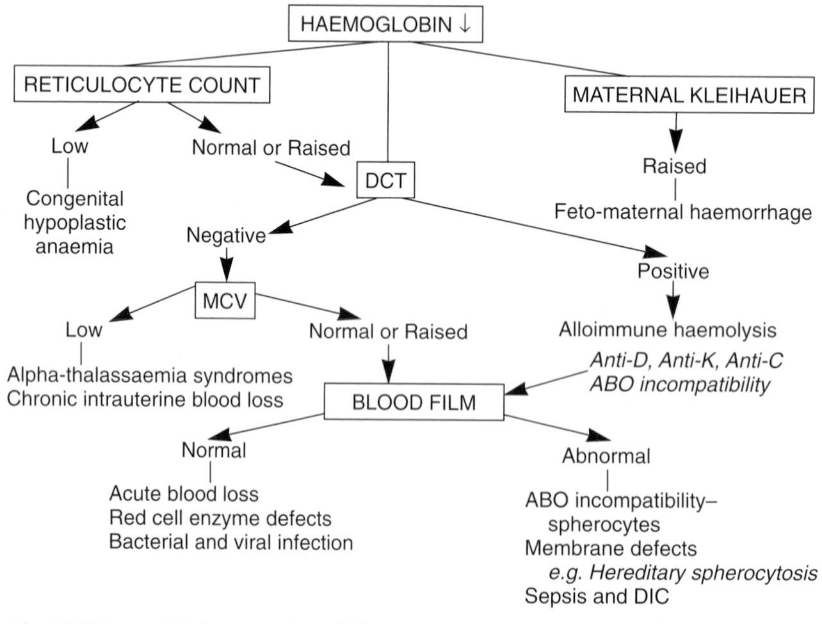

Fig. 32.5 A practical approach to differential diagnosis of anaemia in the neonate. MCV, mean corpuscular volume; DCT, direct Coombs' test.

Table 32.4 Conditions associated with anaemia in the newborn as a result of blood loss

Obstetric accidents	Rupture of normal umbilical cord Haematoma of cord or placenta Incision of placenta during caesarean section Placenta praevia Abruptio placentae
Malformations of placenta and cord	Rupture of anomalous vessels Rupture of abnormal umbilical cord Velamentous insertion Vasa praevia
Occult haemorrhage	Before birth or during delivery Fetomaternal spontaneous traumatic amniocentesis external cephalic version Fetoplacental Twin to twin
Internal haemorrhage	Intracranial Cephalhaematoma Retroperitoneal Ruptured liver Ruptured spleen Pulmonary
Iatrogenic blood loss	

ANAEMIA RESULTING FROM HAEMORRHAGE

The causes of anaemia due to blood loss in the early neonatal period can be divided broadly into three categories: haemorrhage due to obstetric accidents; occult blood loss and internal bleeding (Table 32.4).

Obstetric accidents

Umbilical vessels

Rupture of a normal umbilical cord may occur in an unattended precipitate delivery. The cord can also rupture in a normal delivery if there are vascular abnormalities such as an aneurysm, or if the cord is abnormally short or entangled around the fetus. Traction with forceps can result in rupture of the normal cord.[96]

Haematomas of the cord, although rare, may contain large volumes of blood, and a fetal mortality of over 47% has been reported associated with such blood loss.[91]

Velamentous insertion of the umbilical cord has been reported to occur in 1% of all pregnancies,[62] and is more common in twins where there is a low-lying placenta.

Only 1–2% rupture spontaneously or during labour.[29,112,139] The perinatal mortality rate, if the abnormal vessels do rupture, is high, many such infants being stillborn.[96]

Placenta

Massive fetal haemorrhage can be associated with accidental incision of the placenta at caesarean section, placenta praevia or abruptio placentae.

Lower-segment caesarean section with anterior placentae can result in direct placental injury.[132] Following caesarean section the placenta and membranes should always be examined for damage from the fetal side. Should such evidence be found, the infant's haemoglobin should be estimated at birth, and again 12–24 hours later because the initial haemoglobin may be normal. These estimations should also be carried out on all neonates born to mothers with unusual vaginal bleeding, placenta praevia or abruptio placentae. Placenta praevia is associated with anaemia in approximately 10% of the offspring,[133] and following abruptio placentae anaemia may well be present in surviving infants. Multilobed placentae may be associated with anomalous vessels crossing the internal os, termed vasa praevia. The infant is in double jeopardy with vasa praevia, as the vessels may well be compressed as well as lacerated during the second stage of labour. The perinatal death rate ranges from 58 to 80% in these cases, the majority of infants being stillborn.[96] In the minority born alive, death often occurs during the first 24 hours because of unrecognized severe anaemia.

Occult haemorrhage before and during delivery

Occult loss before birth may be due to fetomaternal haemorrhage, twin-to-twin transfusion or fetoplacental haemorrhage.

Fetomaternal haemorrhage

This is probably the commonest cause of unexpected/unanticipated anaemia in the newborn,[29,139] and is responsible for sensitizing the mother to fetal red cell antigens and the subsequent development of haemolytic disease of the newborn (see below).

Spontaneous fetomaternal bleeding is very common and usually occurs in the last trimester, with an increased rate during the first and second stages of labour. However, transplacental fetal bleeding has been identified as early as 4–8 weeks of gestation.[203] Occult fetomaternal haemorrhage may also be caused by the trauma incurred at amniocentesis, prenatal diagnostic fetal blood sampling, intrauterine transfusion and external cephalic version. Occasionally these blood losses are of such magnitude that they cause fetal anaemia, shock and, rarely, death. The degree of anaemia is variable. Very low haemoglobins in babies who may be hydropic and who survive are associated with chronic blood loss into the maternal circulation prior to delivery. If the haemorrhage is acute the baby may suffer hypovolaemic shock, but the haemoglobin may still be within the normal range at birth.

The way the fetal cells get into the maternal circulation is not understood. Erosions in the placental villi through which the cells could pass[99] and a correlation between occult placental haemorrhages and fetal red cells in the circulation[193] have been demonstrated.

It is possible to identify fetal blood in the maternal circulation by various techniques. The acid elution technique of Kleihauer-Betke is the most commonly used method, although for those fortunate enough to have the equipment, flow cytometry is increasingly being used. The Kleihauer test depends on the fact that in a blood film fetal red cells resist acid elution at low pH, whereas adult cells lose their haemoglobin more quickly, leaving, after appropriate staining, some deeply pigmented fetal cells in a sea of maternal ghost cells. It may be difficult to interpret this test if there is rapid removal of fetal red cells in the presence of ABO incompatibility, or if the mother has raised HbF levels. A rough quantitation of the volume of fetal blood lost can be made on the calculation that the fetal red cell count of 1% in the maternal circulation indicates a fetal haemorrhage of about 50 ml. Semiquantitative estimations are made by counting the number of fetal cells in the sample, comparing this with the number seen in standard reference films with known amounts of fetal blood diluted in adult blood. The invasion of the maternal circulation by a large amount of fetal blood may occasionally cause maternal transfusion reactions, which in one case has led to acute renal failure.[144]

Fetoplacental haemorrhage

In some instances the fetal blood may accumulate in the substance of the placenta[41] or retroplacentally.[95] During labour, approximately 20% of the infant's blood volume may be lost into the placenta if there is a tight nuchal cord.[37] Holding the infant above the uterus before clamping the cord at delivery results in loss of blood into the placenta, and this may account for the decreased blood volume in infants delivered by caesarean section.[98] In fetal lambs maternal hypotension immediately before delivery leads to neonatal hypovolaemia due to loss of blood into the placenta.[97]

Twin-to-twin transfusion[67]

In multiple pregnancy with dichorionic placentae vascular anastomoses are virtually unknown. A monochorial placenta occurs in 70% of monozygotic twins, and twin-to-twin vascular anastomoses occur in almost every instance. It has been estimated that significant twin-to-twin transfusion occurs in 15% of monochorial twins.[154] The twin transfusion syndrome can result in anaemia in the donor and polycythaemia in the recipient, and both have a significant morbidity and mortality. The condition is discussed in detail in Chapter 25.

Internal haemorrhage

Damage to organs during traumatic delivery is the usual cause of internal bleeding in the neonate. The common sites are subaponeurotic (subgaleal), subperiosteal (cephalhaematoma), cerebral and subarachnoid, and the liver, spleen, kidneys and lungs. Typical signs of bleeding occur 24–72 hours after birth, although problems can occur immediately.[29,111,139] Subgaleal haemorrhage can be much greater than subperiosteal haemorrhage because it is not confined by the periosteal attachments to the skull bones, and can spread over the whole calvarium, but both forms of bleeding into the scalp can result in severe anaemia and exsanguination.[8,157] These enclosed haemorrhages may cause severe jaundice.

Rupture of the liver probably occurs more often than is clinically recognized after traumatic delivery, with a prevalence of 1.2–9.6% in stillbirths and neonatal deaths.[26] If the haemorrhage remains confined by the liver capsule there may be abdominal swelling, decreased blood volume, anaemia and subsequent jaundice, but as the haematoma absorbs the baby recovers without complications. The capsule may rupture, usually 24–48 hours but occasionally up to 4 days, after delivery.[111]

Splenic rupture is unusual in the newborn infant, but can occur after a difficult delivery or during exchange transfusion, most commonly in association with the enlarged spleen of rhesus haemolytic disease.[150] Rarely the condition has been described in healthy full-term infants after an apparently normal delivery.[54]

Traumatic breech deliveries may cause haemorrhage into the kidneys, adrenals and retroperitoneal space. Adrenal haemorrhage, like splenic rupture, has also been described following the normal delivery of a large infant.

With any intra-abdominal haemorrhage there will be upper abdominal distension and shifting dullness, and straight X-rays or ultrasound of the abdomen may reveal free fluid. Paracentesis confirms the haemoperitoneum. The prognosis is poor, irrespective of which viscus is ruptured, but laparotomy and surgical repair are sometimes successful.[29,111,139] Bluish discoloration of the skin overlying a palpable flank mass suggests retroperitoneal haemorrhage; bleeding into the retroperitoneal space can also be caused by perforation or rupture of an umbilical artery by catheterization.[186]

Clinical features

The main differential diagnoses of pallor in the newborn and their clinical signs are listed in Table 32.5. Infants who have suffered chronic blood loss in utero vary in their clinical state at delivery, from a hydropic infant with severe anaemia requiring immediate resuscitation, to an asymptomatic, mildly anaemic thriving neonate who will require oral iron supplements only to raise the haemoglobin and replenish iron stores.

Acute haemorrhage before, during or after delivery is poorly tolerated by the neonate, and results in a pale, shocked, hypovolaemic infant whose haemoglobin, which may be normal initially, can fall rapidly within 6–8 hours.

Table 32.5 Pallor in the newborn – differential diagnosis. (Derived from Kirkman and Riley[96])

Acute blood loss	Asphyxia	Haemolytic disease
Blood pressure ↓	Response to oxygen	Hepatosplenomegaly
Tachycardia	Bradycardia	
Rapid shallow respiration	Recession	
Acyanotic	Cyanosis	Jaundice
	Moribund appearance	
		Positive Coombs' test
Drop in haemoglobin	Stable haemoglobin	Anaemia

Management

It is essential to have a planned programme of management on delivery of a pale, distressed infant. Kirkman and Riley[96] recommended a sensible routine which has been modified for optimum management today.

1. Maintain the airway and administer oxygen if necessary.
2. Insert an umbilical catheter and take blood for haemoglobin estimation, grouping, bilirubin, Coombs' test, cross-matching and blood gases.
3. Administer a plasma expander promptly to maintain blood volume. Albumin 4.5% is the product of choice until suitable red cell replacement is available.
4. If the arterial and venous pressure do not return to normal, repeat the procedure with a unit of group O-negative, CMV-negative packed red cells, which should be kept for emergency neonatal transfusion in the blood bank or delivery suite.
5. Search for the cause of haemorrhage:
   - careful examination of infant;
   - examine placenta and cord;
   - maternal blood Kleihauer test.

HAEMOLYTIC ANAEMIA

In adults the classic triad of anaemia, reticulocytosis and hyperbilirubinaemia is the basic laboratory feature of haemolytic anaemia. In the newborn, however, features of haemolysis are more variable and anaemia is rarely the presenting feature. Haemolytic jaundice in the newborn period can occur with only minimal changes in the haemoglobin level and without reticulocytosis, and has multiple aetiologies, which can be broadly grouped into three large categories: alloimmunization, congenital defects of the red cell, and acquired defects.

Acquired haemolytic anaemia can be due to drugs, toxins or infections, and may be secondary to disseminated intravascular coagulation (p. 803). The congenital defects of the red cell fall into three groups: membrane and morphological defects, enzyme abnormalities and abnormalities of haemoglobin.

In most parts of the world the commonest cause of haemolytic disease in the neonate is blood group incompatibility between the mother and the fetus.

Alloimmune anaemia in the fetus and neonate – haemolytic disease of the newborn

The anaemias that result from blood group incompatibility between mother and fetus are generally known as haemolytic disease of the newborn. Maternal IgG antibodies which cross the placenta are produced against paternally derived fetal blood group antigen, which the mother lacks. The most important type of HDN in terms of clinical severity and frequency in caucasian populations is that due to anti-D antibodies developing in a Rh-D-negative woman. Since the introduction of prophylaxis using maternally administered anti-D immunoglobulin the number of babies affected by severe HDN has fallen dramatically. The proportion of HDN due to antibodies other than anti-D has risen, but the severe cases with rare exceptions still result from anti-D antibodies. Access to the fetal circulation by ultrasound-guided needling of the umbilical vein has made direct investigation and in utero treatment a reality, but only if the fetus at risk is recognized and the mother referred to a specialist fetal care unit. The absolute reduction in numbers has led to a lack of experience in managing an affected pregnancy at any one individual centre. Paradoxically, optimum management of the sensitized woman has become more difficult to achieve in recent years because of the success of anti-D prophylaxis.

Rh blood group system

This is the most complex of the blood group systems. It is characterized by more than 30 known antigens and a much larger number of complex alleles. The Rh antigens are confined to the red-cell membrane. The system was first described by Landsteiner and Wiener in 1940.

The Wiener system proposed that the Rh phenotype is determined by a single genetic locus with many alleles. The Fisher–Race system, on the other hand, assumes that the inheritance of the Rh antigens is determined by three pairs of allelic genes, C-c, D-d and E-e, acting on three closely linked loci. Despite expansion over the years, the Fisher–Race system does not cover all the reactions that have been observed within the Rh system, but because the CDE/cde nomenclature is easy to use and enables practical visualization of how a given sample of cells will react with available antisera, the World Health Organization has recommended that the Fisher–Race system be adopted.

This classification follows the convention that the possession of a D gene and antigen is termed Rh-D positive, whereas the absence of a D gene and antigen is termed Rh-D negative.

DD homozygous	Rh-D positive
Dd heterozygous	Rh-D positive
dd	Rh-D negative

It follows that any Rh-D-positive offspring of a Rh-D negative mother has to be heterozygous *Dd* Rh-D positive, having received a D antigen from the father but not from the mother. It also follows that if the father is homozygous Rh-D positive then he can only have Rh-D-positive children, whereas if he is heterozygous (*Dd*) Rh-D positive, and his wife is Rh-D-negative, there is a 50:50 chance of his fathering a Rh-D-negative baby who will not be affected by maternal anti-D.

Approximately 15% of the caucasian population of the United Kingdom are Rh-D negative; the remaining 85% are Rh-D positive. Difficulties in determining the zygosity of a Rh-positive individual arose from the fact that there were no antisera that would identify the *d* antigen.

We now know that the Rh blood group system consists of three homologous but distinct transmembrane proteins. Two have immunologically distinct isoforms, Cc and Ee, but the principal protein D has no isoform d. The Rh locus on chromosome 1 consists of two homologous structural genes, Cc Ee and D. The Rh-D gene encodes the major antigen, RhD, in 'Rh-positive' individuals. In Rh-negative individuals the Rh-D gene is absent and there is no expression of D but normal Cc/Ee expression. This explains why an anti-d antibody has never been identified.

Preventing Rh-D immunization[106]

The development of successful prophylaxis programmes is an exciting and sometimes bizarre story which is eloquently recounted in a review article by Clarke, one of the pioneers in the field.[43] The observation that the incidence of haemolytic disease of the newborn in Rh-D-negative women who carried an ABO-incompatible fetus was less than expected[107] led to the hypothesis that ABO-incompatible matings may have a protective effect because the naturally occurring maternal anti-A or anti-B eliminated the fetal Rh-D-positive red cells from the maternal circulation and so blocked the production of Rh antibodies.[153] Clinical trials administering IgG anti-D, produced in male Rh-D-negative volunteers, to Rh-D-negative women in pregnancy were embarked upon in the 1960s. By 1967 collective experience from the United States, Germany and the United Kingdom clearly showed the protective effect of giving IgG anti-D intravenously to the mother within 48 hours of delivery of a Rh-positive ABO-compatible fetus compared to non-treated matched controls.

Without prophylaxis about one in six Rh-negative women who deliver a Rh-positive infant will develop anti-D antibodies resulting from fetomaternal haemorrhage occurring either during pregnancy or at delivery.[128] General recommendations for the administration of anti-D immunoglobulin to a non-sensitized Rh-D-negative woman in the UK should now include:

- post delivery if she gives birth to a Rh-D-positive infant;
- post-therapeutic abortion or identified spontaneous abortion;
- to cover antenatal procedures such as amniocentesis, CVS (chorionic villus sampling) or external cephalic version;
- if she threatens to abort or miscarry;
- antenatally at 28 and 34 weeks, particularly if she has no living children.

In Britain, however, the rate of Rh-D sensitization is still unacceptably high, at round 1.5%, i.e. more than 1000 Rh-negative women each year develop anti-D antibodies in association with delivery of a Rh-positive infant.

Until recently in the UK the standard dose at all centres was 500 iu (100 μg), which will suppress immunization from up to 5 ml Rh-positive red cells. It is known that 99% of women have a fetomaternal bleed of less than 4 ml at delivery. It is therefore the policy to give 100 μg anti-D postnatally and to perform tests to identify the few women who have a larger volume of fetal cells in their circulation and therefore require additional immunoglobulin.

A recent EC guideline which states that a larger standard dose of 1000–1500 iu may be given without a test to assess the size of the fetomaternal haemorrhage does not take account of the 0.3% of women (over 200 per year) who have a bleed into their circulation of greater than 15 ml, who would not be protected.

A significant cause of Britain's continuing relatively high sensitization rate is the failure to identify Rh-D-negative women at risk, and to give the standard postnatal dose postdelivery, but even with meticulous immunoprophylaxis postdelivery immunization occurs in about 1% of women owing to small fetomaternal haemorrhages that occur antenatally, particularly in the third trimester. Studies in Britain[183] and Canada[23] have shown that antenatal prophylaxis could reduce sensitization to less than 0.1%. Only a few obstetric units in the UK offer routine antenatal prophylaxis to Rh-negative women. This can no longer be justified by the shortage of anti-D immunoglobulin that existed when postnatal prophylaxis was first introduced, and we should now introduce routine antenatal prophylaxis at least for the first at-risk pregnancy.[158]

Development of synthetic anti-D human monoclonal antibody to Rh-D antigen. The in vitro production of human monoclonal antibodies has wide-ranging clinical potential. A monoclonal antibody directed against the Rh-D antigen can be a useful blood-typing reagent, but more importantly, if safe for human administration, could be used to prevent HDN, thus replacing the immune serum from immunized female and male volunteers used at present.

Monoclonal anti-D preparations are now widely used

in blood transfusion serology laboratories, but the development of the use of monoclonal anti-D antibodies to replace polyclonal antibodies in prophylaxis of HDN is as yet in its infancy.

An important problem to be overcome before these antibodies can be used for prophylaxis is how to ensure that the final preparation is free of viruses and DNA. Preliminary trials[89,103] have shown promising results and suggest that the use of therapeutic monoclonal anti-D will become a reality, but there are still many problems to overcome.[69]

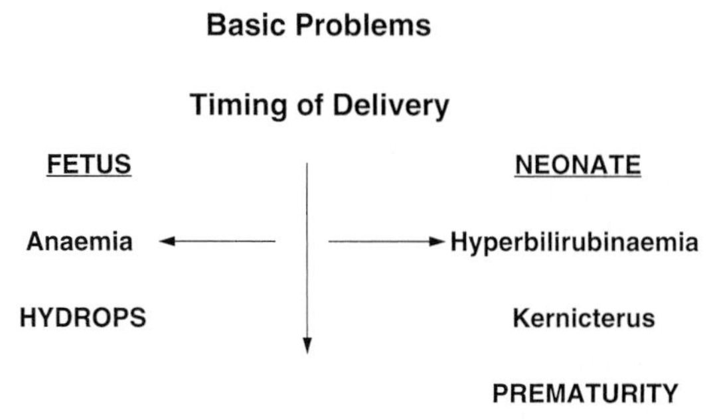

Fig. 32.6 Alloimmune haemolysis of the fetus and newborn.

Rh-D haemolytic disease of the newborn

The disease begins in intrauterine life and may result in death in utero. In liveborn infants the haemolytic process is maximal at the time of birth, and thereafter diminishes as the concentration of maternal antibody in the infant's circulation declines. During pregnancy the fetal and maternal circulations are separate. Red cells do not cross the placental barrier in large numbers in normal circumstances. Oxygen, nutrient and waste exchange takes place by diffusion across the intervillous space. IgG antibodies cross the placenta freely, carrying passive immunity for the fetus against infective agents to which the mother has had a healthy immune response. Following delivery of the infant, rupture of the placental villi and connective tissue at separation allows the escape of fetal blood cells into the maternal circulation prior to constriction of maternal vessels. Unless prevented, sensitization takes place in the majority of cases at this stage.

Antenatal management of Rh-D HDN

Antenatal screening. Routine serological testing of women is carried out to:

- identify pregnancies at risk of fetal and neonatal alloimmune disease (HDN);
- identify Rh-D-negative women who require antenatal anti-D prophylaxis;
- provide compatible blood swiftly in emergencies.[9]

All women who have no antibodies at 10–16 weeks at booking should be tested once again between 28 and 36 weeks' gestation. Some workers believe that Rh-D-negative women should have two tests, one at 28 weeks and one at 34–36 weeks, but sensitization late in pregnancy is unlikely to result in HDN requiring treatment.[194] If clinically significant antibodies are present at booking, e.g. anti-D, Kell and c, either alone or in combination, the partner's phenotype should be determined and the couple referred early to a specialist centre for assessment and further investigation, and treatment if indicated.

The Rh-D-negative pregnant woman with antibodies. If a woman has antibodies at booking, or if antibody is detected on subsequent testing, the pregnancy becomes high risk. Since the number of sensitized pregnancies has fallen dramatically, most peripheral centres will only see one or two women at risk per year. Although this is an advance in terms of public health, it means that very few groups now have expertise in monitoring progress, instituting therapy, prime-timing of delivery, and in the skilled procedures of intrauterine fetal transfusion.

It is essential that any woman at risk should, once identified, at least have her case drawn to the attention of one of the expert referral centres, so that collective experience may be applied and disasters in management avoided.

The changing incidence of HDN and the improvements in fetal and neonatal therapy have resulted in many review articles on the subject in recent years.[15,22,44,79,119,128,159,164,182,185,192]

The aim is to prevent hydrops in utero and to time delivery so that the infant has a maximal chance of survival (Fig. 32.6). Many babies delivered at 28 weeks' gestation survive, with no long-term handicap, and it is unusual for those of 32 weeks' gestation or more to present any more than routine problems for the average SCBU.

Monitoring severity of disease in the fetus. This is discussed in detail in Chapter 14.

Measures to suppress haemolytic disease in utero

Oral desensitization. Marked reduction of rhesus HDN has been reported following oral administration of Rh-D-positive red cell stroma in enteric-coated capsules.[19] The mechanism by which this interferes with maternal production of anti-D immunoglobulin and reduces the severity of Rh-D HDN is obscure. The results of the original study from France still await confirmation by other centres. Meanwhile, its use must be regarded as experimental.[20]

Intravascular immunoglobulin. In common with all immune-based diseases, the effect of high-dose IgG has been investigated. The possibility of modifying fetal red cell destruction by maternal (or fetal) high-dose IgG therapy is intriguing and deserves consideration. There are sporadic reports of apparent successful modification of disease using maternal Ig administration,[40,52,117] but these are not supported by the experience of other groups.[23]

Plasma exchange to reduce maternal antibody titre. Regular plasmapheresis two to three times weekly, from as early as 10 weeks' gestation, has been reported to reduce the severity of fetal haemolytic disease.[72] Although the anti-D levels may be reduced initially, they rise very rapidly when the plasma exchanges are discontinued. There are many practical problems. Results from various centres are conflicting. The reports from groups who believe plasmapheresis to be beneficial are not convincing because the outcomes are not compared with any suitable control group. Overall, the survival rate of infants is no better than from those centres who do not use plasmapheresis. The use of both i.v. IgG immunoglobulin and intensive plasma exchange at best only serves to delay the need for fetal blood sampling and intrauterine transfusion.[22]

Intrauterine transfusion

Death of the fetus from severe anaemia may be prevented by the introduction of compatible adult donor cells into the fetal circulation by the various methods described in Chapter 14.

Management of the baby after birth

Cord blood should be taken at delivery for ABO Rh-D grouping, direct antiglobulin (Coombs') test, serum bilirubin and haemoglobin. Babies who are born after a series of intrauterine transfusions often have a normal haemoglobin at delivery, negative direct Coombs' test and group as Rh-D negative because of successful replacement of fetal red cells by transfused donor blood combined with suppression of fetal marrow. These babies often require only phototherapy to control jaundice of prematurity and maybe a top-up transfusion to correct anaemia several weeks after delivery. The main problems are not haematological but those arising from immaturity, although many more fetuses are now kept in utero till 35–37 weeks' gestation. It should be appreciated that because HbA – with which the baby has been transfused – has a lower oxygen affinity than HbF, the haemoglobin concentration will drop to lower levels than usual in the neonatal period before erythropoietin production with reticulocytosis will be stimulated by hypoxia.[100,181] The infant may be thriving with the Hb between 6 and 7 g, and unnecessary top-up transfusions may be administered if these are undertaken because of Hb level alone.[127] Some workers have reported the successful use of erythropoietin to treat the late anaemia following intrauterine transfusions,[142,163] but the necessity for this treatment is questionable.

The management of the newborn following a series of intrauterine transfusions at a specialist centre usually involves delivery at the place of referral, and demands excellent communication between the fetal medicine unit concerned and the obstetrician, paediatrician and haematologist at the referring hospital. The predicted haematocrit/haemoglobin at delivery and the possible need for exchange or top-up transfusion should be assessed and communicated to those concerned from the degree of fetal marrow suppression and rate of fall of Hb. This is an area in which in the author's experience there is room for improvement.

Management of the infant who has not received intrauterine therapy. With current obstetric practice in the UK it is unlikely that a severely affected infant will be born requiring urgent treatment. Occasionally such infants who have not received intrauterine transfusions, or in whom delivery has been delayed inappropriately, will be born severely anaemic or even hydropic. They require urgent correction of the haemoglobin, together with routine resuscitation of a sick infant. The cord should be clamped immediately to reduce the volume of sensitized cells entering the neonatal circulation, and a top-up or partial exchange transfusion performed as soon as possible with partially packed red cells. Effective ventilation may be difficult in hydropic infants. If ascites is present rapid improvement may follow aspiration of fluid from the peritoneal cavity. Once the baby is in a stable state, double volume exchange transfusion should be performed in the usual way (see below).

The majority of infants who have been untreated in utero will be born in a stable condition. Although the haemoglobin may need correction, the main risk to the newborn is of hyperbilirubinaemia leading to kernicterus, if prompt measures are not taken to prevent this. Cord blood should be taken at delivery to determine direct Coombs' test, blood group, Hb and bilirubin.

Exchange transfusion for management and prevention of hyperbilirubinaemia. For sick infants exchange transfusion remains the mainstay of treatment. The indications for exchange transfusion vary with the age and condition of the infant and the level and rate of rise of bilirubin. A cord Hb of less than 10.0 g/dl and a bilirubin of greater than 70 μmol/l were taken as indications for exchange within 1 hour of birth, and still stand for the previously untreated neonate, but previous intrauterine transfusion together with improved phototherapy make guidelines for early exchange uncertain in the treated infant.[147]

Criteria for exchange transfusion. Clinical evidence of severe disease at delivery, such as pallor, petechiae or hepatosplenomegaly, are indications for immediate exchange transfusion without waiting for cord blood results. The baby who does not require immediate exchange should be monitored haematologically at regular 3–4-hour intervals, with particular reference to the bilirubin. A rapidly rising bilirubin is an indication for exchange. For all NICUs charts are available that indicate the levels of bilirubin at which exchange should be undertaken related to the birthweight and gestation, so that kernicterus will be prevented (see p. 719), but the clinician should always take into consideration the alternative therapies available and other relevant data before commencing exchange transfusion based on bilirubin levels or early rates of rise alone.

In addition to controlling existing hyperbilirubinaemia, exchange transfusion corrects anaemia and blood volume abnormalities. The first transfusion also washes out about one-third of the anti-D antibody in the neonatal circulation. A two-volume exchange (170 ml/kg) will remove 85–90% of the infant's circulating Rh-D-positive cells, which would otherwise contribute to the bilirubin pool, but only 25% of the infant's total bilirubin, because a large part of the total bilirubin is in the extravascular compartment. Maximum bilirubin reduction is achieved by a two-volume exchange. After the exchange transfusion serum levels may rapidly rebound to 70–80% of the pre-exchange values.

Whole blood in citrate phosphate dextrose is ideal for exchange transfusion in these circumstances. Although the final haematocrit may be in a lower range than the normal neonatal haematocrit, the adult haemoglobin transfused has a lower oxygen affinity. Added to this, the volume of one unit of whole blood is sufficient in the majority of cases for a double-volume (170 ml/kg) exchange, thus cutting down donor exposure. The blood should be as fresh as possible to minimize the metabolic changes due to storage, and always less than 5 days old. Group O Rh-D negative is the most suitable and should be cross-matched with the maternal serum. The standard HIV, HCV and hepatitis B tests should be performed and the unit should be CMV antibody negative. Although some authorities recommend routine irradiation, 'the likelihood of graft vs. host disease is so rare following exchange transfusion that providing the donor is not related to the affected infant non-irradiated blood may be used'.[22] The blood should be warmed, and exchange is best performed via the umbilical vein in 10 ml aliquots in the sick infant. A double-volume exchange will take a minimum of 2 hours. In the stable >37-week baby many exchanges have been performed using up to 20 ml aliquots.

The risks of exchange transfusion are many and have been reviewed.[76]

Complications and mortality. The overall mortality related to exchange transfusion depends on the premorbid condition of the infant and has been variably reported, but generally it is less than 1%.[45] Thrombocytopenia is a well-recognized complication of severe rhesus erythroblastosis fetalis, and usually corrects itself after 4–6 days. In some instances the thrombocytopenia appears to be the result of repeated exchange transfusions using platelet-poor blood. However, it may precede the exchange transfusion and, more recently, accompanying neutropenia has been described. The marked increase in erythropoiesis in fetuses with rhesus haemolytic disease can be accompanied by a down modulation of neutrophil and platelet production.[101] Regardless of the mechanism by which the neutropenia and thrombocytopenia are produced, these cytopenias are made worse by repeated exchange transfusions using neutrophil-poor and platelet-poor blood.

Other management

- Albumin administration. The binding of bilirubin to albumin is important in the prevention of bilirubin encephalopathy. There are no controlled trials to show that the administration of albumin reduces the number of exchange transfusions required, or the incidence of kernicterus, but before or during exchange transfusion it significantly increases the amount of bilirubin removed and increases the albumin-binding capacity of the infant's plasma after the transfusion. Albumin should not be added to blood used to exchange a severely anaemic or hydropic baby because the resulting increase in plasma colloid pressure may precipitate or augment heart failure.
- Jaundice. Techniques other than exchange transfusion to control hyperbilirubinaemia are described in Chapter 31, Part 1. In general babies with rhesus HDN should be nursed under phototherapy until it is clear that the bilirubin is stable or falling and further exchange transfusion will not be required.

Other causes of fetomaternal alloimmunization

In theory, any fetal red cell antigen may cause alloimmunization if the mother lacks that antigen. Thus any red cell antigen which the father possesses and the mother lacks, if inherited by the fetus, can cause maternal alloimmunization. A recent review documents the incidence of these antibodies in five series of patients.[75] In reality the three antibodies likely to cause significant anaemia in the fetus are anti-D, anti-c and anti-Kell, either alone or in combination with other antibodies.

Rh blood group c and E

Within the Rh blood group system the most immunogenic antigens after D are c and E.[129] These antibodies are found in women who are Rh-D positive and lack the c and E antigens, most usually those who have the genotype CDe/CDe (R_1R_1). The management of HDN caused by alloimmunization by antigens other than anti-D is the same as that for Rh-D HDN, and there is as yet no way of preventing these conditions. Some cases of HDN due to anti-c are as severe as anti-D HDN, and may end in hydrops if intrauterine transfusions are not given. If anti-c is found in the maternal serum this should be managed in much the same way as anti-D. Many transfusion centres now quantitate anti-c in the same way as anti-D. Guidance should be sought from individual centres regarding the significant levels at which invasive procedures are indicated antenatally.

Isolated anti-E antibodies are the ones most frequently found in antenatal serology. They are sometimes naturally occurring and very rarely cause any problems, either antenatally or post delivery. Occasionally a newborn may require phototherapy or, very unusually, exchange transfusion. However, if anti-c is found with anti-E, even in low concentration, the combination may result in very severe HDN, necessitating fetal intervention.

Kell blood group system

The Kell red cell blood group[129,155] occasionally causes severe problems. Ninety-two per cent of the British population are Kell negative (kk); the remaining 8% are Kell positive and the majority are heterozygous Kk. Only one in 500 individuals is found to be homozygous KK positive. The antibody anti-K is usually found in patients who have had multiple transfusions, either as a large number of donations to cover a single traumatic incident, or as recurrent supportive therapy over a long period. When anti-K is found in antenatal sera the majority of patients have a history of transfusion, but the partner's blood should be tested to determine his Kell status. There is no difficulty in finding blood for intrauterine or exchange transfusion as over 90% of the population are kk Kell negative. Kell haemolytic disease can be very severe and rapidly fatal in utero at a relatively early gestation.

For many years there have been reports suggesting that anti-K alloimmune disease behaves differently from Rh anti-D HDN. There may be severe anaemia, with low maternal anti-K concentrations. Anamnestic reactions (rising maternal antibody with a K-negative infant) are more frequent. Amniotic fluid bilirubin levels have been shown to be unhelpful or frankly misleading.[14,31,128] Clinical investigations suggest that the fetal anaemia results from erythroid suppression rather than haemolysis.[188,191] Moreover, recent in vitro work demonstrates that monoclonal anti-K inhibits K-positive red cell progenitors but has no effect on K-negative erythroid progenitors. A similar inhibition is seen with maternal sera containing anti-K, whereas there is no constant inhibition by anti-D of D-positive progenitors.[187] This has implications for the management of anti-K alloimmune anaemia. In all cases of paternal heterozygosity the K status of the fetus should be established early in pregnancy, preferably by DNA analysis of amniocytes[6] before potentially unnecessary, more hazardous, fetal blood sampling is embarked upon. The K-positive pregnancy should be followed by serial weekly ultrasound examination and early fetal blood sampling if in any doubt, as neither the maternal antibody quantitation nor the amniotic fluid bilirubin will give an indication of severity of anaemia.

Other blood groups

There are sporadic reports of unusually severe HDN due to other antibodies such as anti-Fya[47] and anti-M,[61] but these very rarely require intrauterine intervention.

All pregnant women have a group and antibody screen at booking, and this is repeated at 28–34 weeks' gestation. Specialist referral should occur early in pregnancy for all women with anti-D, anti-c or anti-K antibody.

Prevention of fetal alloimmune anaemia due to antibodies other than anti-D

The antibodies other than anti-D which are most frequently but much more rarely involved with severe fetal anaemia requiring intrauterine intervention are anti-c and anti-K, either alone or in combination with other antibodies, particularly c and E. It would not be cost-effective or practically feasible in terms of screening or preparing specific IgG antibody to have a prophylactic programme similar to the successful administration of anti-D immunoglobulin, but some measures can be taken to prevent maternal alloimmunization. In many centres, including our own, women in the reproductive years who require transfusion for any reason receive only K-negative pretyped units to prevent the development of anti-K antibodies. There is also a move afoot to transfuse all Rh-D-positive women with R_1R_1 (CDe/CDe) typed blood, to avoid the development of anti-c antibodies in those who lack the c antigen.

ABO blood group incompatibility

Even before the striking reduction in Rh-D HDN due to prophylaxis, the most frequent cause of HDN was the haemolysis due to ABO incompatibility. Although the incidence in the UK and the US has been found to be approximately 2% of all births, in only 1 in 3000 births does severe ABO HDN occur. Mild cases not requiring exchange transfusion are identified as 1 in 150 births. Less than 5% of affected newborns require phototherapy, and only in very rare cases is exchange transfusion required. There is a one in three chance that there will be ABO incompatibility, but the partner may be heterozygous in respect of the allele for the incompatible antigen, for example AO rather than AA (homozygous), so that the chance of ABO incompatibility between fetal red cells and maternal serum is one in five.

The vast majority of cases of HDN due to ABO incompatibility occur in group O mothers with A or B infants, because group O individuals make more avid antibody and are more likely to produce immune antibody; unlike rhesus disease, 40–50% of cases occur in firstborn infants and the disease does not become more severe with each subsequent pregnancy.

It is therefore surprising that ABO HDN is relatively

uncommon. There are several factors that explain this. A- and B-like substances are widespread in vegetable and animal life. The agglutinins, anti-A and -B, are often called naturally occurring antibodies, which is strictly a misnomer because they develop during the first few months of life, probably as a result of exposure to A- and B-like substances elaborated by Gram-negative bacteria that colonize the gut. Naturally occurring anti-A and anti-B are usually IgM immunoglobulins that will not cross the placenta. The maternal antibody can only cause HDN if it is one of the IgG type.

Group O women who have had ABO-incompatible pregnancies may develop IgG anti-A or -B (immune antibody). Also, group O individuals who have been vaccinated or immunized with preparations derived from hog stomach, or pneumococcal vaccine which contain an A substance, may develop immune lytic IgG anti-A antibody which can persist for some years (hog pepsin is used in the preparation of TAB and diphtheria toxoid). However, even if the group O mother has a high titre of lytic IgG anti-A or anti-B antibody, it is unlikely to cause problems for the ABO-incompatible fetus in utero because the A and B antigens, unlike Rh antigens, are present not only on the fetal red cells but also on cells of all other tissue and body fluids. Neutralization of maternal antibody by soluble fetal antigens, and by antigens carried on cells other than the red cells, will help to protect the incompatible fetal red cells.

Another factor which may help to protect the fetal red cells is that the A and B antigens, although detectable in the 5-week embryo, do not have the antigenic strength of adult red cells in the neonate, and therefore will not react fully with antibody that crosses the placenta.

There are distinct racial differences, and Asian and African babies, often group B, may suffer more severe ABO HDN than caucasian babies, usually group A, born to group O mothers. Apart from the occasional case with a history of other previously affected infants and/or lytic IgG in the maternal serum, screening of cord blood for ABO incompatibility is not usually performed. The diagnosis of ABO HDN is usually made in the work-up of a mature infant who develops jaundice in the first 24 hours of life. In fact, the diagnosis may be quite difficult to make because the direct antiglobulin (Coombs') test is not always strongly positive and there may be a very mild degree of anaemia, although such infants can develop a marked reticulocyte response and occasionally go on to develop jaundice of a severity which may lead to kernicterus. The danger is that with early discharge post delivery, the jaundice may develop at home. The confirmation of the diagnosis is made by finding IgG lytic antibody of the appropriate blood-group specificity in the maternal serum.[25] The blood film characteristically has large numbers of spherocytes. If exchange transfusion is undertaken in ABO HDN, group O red cells should be used. Ideally these should be washed and resuspended in AB plasma. However, the donors used for neonatal exchange transfusion do not have high-titre immune anti-A or anti-B, and the amount in CPD plasma of a whole blood donation will be negligible. One unit is usually sufficient for a double-volume exchange and this will cut down donor exposure.

Membrane defects

The membrane skeleton of the red cell consists of an extensive network of fibrous proteins that laminate the inner membrane surface and interact to form a self-supporting shell. Spectrin is the major skeletal component and accounts for 50–70% of the skeletal mass. Ankyrin, another skeletal protein, serves as the high-affinity binding site for the attachment of spectrin to the inner membrane surface.[13,74]

Hereditary spherocytosis

The basic membrane defect is expressed as a loss of surface area. Recent work has shown that all HS patients are spectrin-deficient and that the degree of deficiency correlates closely with the severity of the disease and the degree of spherocytosis assessed by the osmotic fragility.[13,74]

Hereditary spherocytosis is the most common of all red cell membrane defects. Inheritance is autosomal dominant in the majority (approximately 75%) and autosomal recessive in the remainder.[13,74] Its severity does not run true within families, probably because of other unrelated (not linked) factors, and a family history is absent in 25% of affected patients.[78] The observed decrease in spectrin may be secondary to reduced synthesis of spectrin or to loss of spectrin resulting from decreased ankyrin, the protein which anchors spectrin to the cytoskeleton of the red cell membrane.[48]

Spherocytes have an increased osmotic fragility in vitro which is exaggerated after 24 hours' incubation at 37°C. It is essential when measuring osmotic fragility in the newborn that each laboratory establishes its own normal values for control infant erythrocytes.[77]

Approximately 20% of patients present with haemolytic jaundice during the first week of life, but anaemia is mild and the haemoglobin rarely falls to less than 10.0 g/dl.

The finding of spherocytes in the blood film does not establish the diagnosis of hereditary spherocytosis, as there is a long list of conditions that injure the erythrocyte membrane, producing spherocytes. In the newborn period the cause is commonly ABO haemolytic disease of the newborn. The diagnosis of hereditary spherocytosis is made on the basis of family studies, an increased incubated red cell osmotic fragility, and by excluding other causes of spherocytosis – specialist laboratories can quantify spectrin in cells using molecular techniques.

Controlling jaundice by phototherapy and exchange transfusion is the most important aspect of therapy in the neonatal period. Once the diagnosis is made, the baby should be maintained on daily folic acid supplements to meet the requirements of the increased marrow turnover.

Hereditary elliptocytosis

Up to 15% of the cells in the circulation of normal individuals are elliptical. Those who have more than 25 and up to 75% are described as having hereditary elliptocytosis. Although approximately 0.04% of the population of the USA suffer from this condition, only 10% have active haemolysis at any time in their lives.[146] The usual mode of inheritance is autosomal dominant, although an autosomal recessive variant has been described.

Elliptocytosis probably results from several genetic determinants, one of which is linked to the Rh blood group locus. Homozygous hereditary elliptocytosis is associated with severe haemolytic anaemia in the neonatal period. Heterozygotes show much greater variation in clinical expression of the condition, ranging from no anaemia or evidence of haemolysis to relatively severe haemolysis with splenomegaly and jaundice. This clinical variability probably reflects underlying genetic heterogeneity.

Generally elliptocytosis is an incidental finding in the unrelated investigations of a haematologically healthy child. Occasionally the condition may present as neonatal jaundice with or without anaemia. The blood film in these cases usually contains a high proportion of poikilocytes and pyknocytes,[35] instead of a high proportion of elliptocytes.

Neonatal treatment is the control of jaundice by phototherapy, and occasionally exchange transfusion.

Hereditary pyropoikilocytosis

This very rare disease has only been reported in infants of African origin,[200] and presents in early infancy with severe haemolytic anaemia often requiring exchange transfusion, and later becoming transfusion dependent. There is extreme poikilocytosis, with budding red cells, burr cells, microfragments and other bizarre cells.[46] The unique diagnostic feature is the thermal sensitivity of the red cells.

Family studies of children with this condition reveal parents in whom one, both or neither exhibits elliptocytosis on examination of the blood film. Specialist laboratories demonstrate abnormalities in spectrin tetramer/dimer formation and specific amino acid substitutions on domains of the cytoskeleton required for tetramer stability.[118]

Hereditary stomatocytosis (hydrocytosis)

In this condition there is relative failure of the Na^+, K^+ pump, with passive cell wall permeability resulting in the influx of Na^+ and the loss of K^+, so that the cells swell as a result of the progressive gain of cations and water. The condition is characterized by variable numbers of stomatocytes in the circulating blood, but they are not unique to this disorder.[13,74] It may present in the neonatal period with severe jaundice requiring treatment.

Hereditary xerocytosis

This rare condition is characterized by an increased membrane permeability to potassium. The K^+ efflux exceeds the Na^+ influx and the cells become dehydrated. The inheritance is autosomal dominant. A stained blood film shows macrocytosis, target cells, shrunken spiculated cells and cells in which the haemoglobin seems to have collected in a puddle at one side.[13,74] Xerocytosis may present in the neonatal period with jaundice requiring treatment. It can be seen, therefore, that in any obscure congenital haemolytic anaemia an analysis of the cell content of sodium and potassium will be helpful.

Red cell enzyme abnormalities

Only two of these are of clinical significance, glucose-6-phosphate dehydrogenase deficiency and pyruvate kinase deficiency. The other very rare conditions are listed in Table 32.6. Detailed descriptions can be found in Luzzatto[114] and Mentzer.[123]

Glucose-6-phosphate dehydrogenase deficiency

This condition is the commonest enzymopathy, affecting 400 million people worldwide. It occurs (gene frequency 5–25%) in individuals originating from tropical Africa, the Middle East, some areas of the Mediterranean, tropical and subtropical Asia and Papua New Guinea.[16] As with thalassaemia and sickle cell trait, the carrier state is thought to give relative protection against malaria.[114] The gene for G6PD is located on the X chromosome, so that there are many more clinically affected males than females, but in contrast to several other X-linked conditions there are many populations in which the gene frequency is so high that homozygous females are not rare.[114] G6PD is genetically heterogeneous. More than 300 different mutants have been identified, and biochemical characterization shows that they all result from allelic mutations in the G6PD gene. Amino-acid analysis indicates that G6PD is similar to human haemoglobin in that the substitution of a single amino acid (among the 100–110 present) can result in profound deficiency in biological activity and clinical expression. In addition, structural variants without enzyme deficiency have been described. Recently the molecular basis of G6PD deficiency has been determined. Many different point mutations have been observed at gene level but no large deletions have

Table 32.6 Red cell glycolytic enzyme deficiencies

Enzyme pathway	Enzyme	Inheritance	Associated features
Embden–Myerhof pathway	Glucose phosphate isomerase	Autosomal recessive	Hydrops described. Haemolytic crisis precipitated by drugs or infection
	Phosphofructokinase	Autosomal recessive	Sometimes associated with myopathy
	Adolase	Unknown	One patient only described with mental retardation
	Triose phosphate isomerase	Autosomal recessive	Severe progressive neurological disorder. Susceptibility to bacterial infection
	Phosphoglycerate kinase	X-linked	Mental retardation and neurological disorders sometimes associated
	2,3-Diphosphoglycerate mutase	Unknown	Both haemolytic anaemia and polycythaemia described
	Pyruvate kinase (see text)	Autosomal recessive	Marked clinical variability. Many mutants described
Pentose phosphate pathway	Glucose-6-phosphate dehydrogenase (see text)	X-linked	Drug-induced and congenital haemolytic anaemia
	6-Phosphoglycerate dehydrogenase	Unknown	Clinical expression variable from no haemolysis to severe anaemia
	Glutathione peroxidase	Autosomal recessive	Possibly responsible for some drug-induced haemolytic anaemias
Glutathione metabolism	Glutathione synthetase	Autosomal recessive	Not always accompanied by haemolytic anaemia. May be associated with neurological defects and 5-oxoprolinuria
	γ-glutamyl-cysteine synthetase	Unknown	Profound depression of glutathione levels

been demonstrated to date. For a comprehensive review see Luzzatto.[114]

G6PD is a cytoplasmic enzyme present in all cells. It catalyses the first step in the hexose monophosphate pathway, producing NADPH, and is responsible for the generation and maintenance of GSH. This protects the cell membrane and metabolic pathways from the deleterious effects of oxidation. This is particularly true in red cells, which are exquisitely sensitive to oxidative damage and in which other NADPH-reducing enzymes are lacking.

The clinical expression of deficiency depends on which mutant is involved. The vast majority of individuals with G6PD deficiency are asymptomatic and go through life unaware of their deficiency. However, G6PD deficiency can cause the following syndromes:

- Drug-induced haemolysis (common);
- Infection-induced haemolysis (common);
- Favism;
- Neonatal jaundice;
- Chronic non-spherocytic haemolytic anaemia (rare);

of which only jaundice is common in the neonatal period.

G6PD deficiency and neonatal jaundice. G6PD deficiency is the commonest enzymopathy to cause neonatal jaundice with or without apparent haemolysis.

The earliest reports indicated that the incidence was maximal in Greece, Sardinia and the Far East, but it has emerged as a major problem in Africa in recent years.[143] As the incidence is higher among Africans in Africa than among black Africans in America,[18] and among Greeks in Greece than among those of Greek ancestry in Australia,[59] environmental or acquired factors are suggested to explain this wide variation,[143] rather than an additional genetic factor.

Jaundice is very rarely present at birth and the peak incidence of clinical onset is between days 2 and 3,[58] later than in Rh HDN and other blood group alloimmunization, and may persist for 2–3 weeks. The anaemia is seldom severe and there is always relatively more jaundice than anaemia;[121] no difference in the haematocrit values in the cord blood and on day 3 between jaundiced and non-jaundiced G6PD-deficient babies has been reported in one series. It has been suggested that in a majority of cases the jaundice may be of hepatic and not of haemolytic origin, but this view is still disputed.[114]

G6PD deficiency per se does not necessarily cause neonatal jaundice, and if it is found in association with neonatal jaundice it does not exonerate the paediatrician from looking for some oxidant stimulus, such as infection (common) or drugs (less common), including those taken by the mother. Fatal hydrops fetalis has been reported in one case of G6PD deficiency in a Chinese infant whose mother ate fava beans and ascorbic acid.[122]

The investigation for G6PD deficiency in the neonatal period should always involve enzyme assay of maternal as well as neonatal blood, because a high reticulocyte count in the baby's blood may well give near-normal levels of G6PD activity, especially in the milder varieties.

The management in the neonatal period is to control jaundice, and exchange transfusion can usually be avoided with early use of phototherapy. It has been suggested that phototherapy could increase haemolysis by leading to riboflavin deficiency and loss of antioxidant activity, but this has not been supported by several clinical studies, which have shown conclusively that phototherapy is effective. Other general measures would include avoiding oxidant drugs, and prompt treatment of coexistent hypoxia, sepsis and acidosis.

Table 32.7 Some of the therapeutic agents, chemicals and foodstuffs known to trigger haemolysis in G6PD-deficient subjects. These can also augment haemolysis in HbH disease (p. 828)

Antimalarials	*Sulfones*
Primaquine	Sulfoxone (Diazone)
Pamaquine	Thiazolsulfone (Promizole)
Mepacrine	Diaminodiphenyl sulphone (DDS)
Quinine	
Chloroquine	*Others*
	Dimercaprol (BAL)
Sulphonamides	Methylene blue
Sulphanilamide	Naphthalene (mothballs)
Sulphacetamide	Para-Aminosalicylic acid (PAS)
Sulphamethoxypyridazine (Lederkyn)	Phenylhydrazine
	Acetylphenylhydrazine
Sulphisoxazole (Gantrisin)	Probenecid (Benemid)
Sulphafurazole	Vitamin K (water-soluble analogues)
Nitrofurans	Chloramphenicol
Nitrofurantoin (Furadantin)	Quinidine
Furazolidone (Furazone)	Trinitrotoluene
Nitrofurazone (Furacin)	Mesantoin
	Broad beans
Antipyretics and analgesics	
Acetylsalicylic acid (aspirin)	
Acetanilide	
Acetophenetidin (phenacetin)	
Aminopyrine (Pyramidon)	
Antipyrine	

Parents of affected babies should be given a list of potentially dangerous oxidant drugs and toxins, some of which can be bought over the counter, e.g. aspirin and mothballs (Table 32.7). There is no need for folic acid maintenance as the chronic haemolysis is insignificant.

There are rare types of G6PD deficiency which cause chronic haemolysis in adults, requiring daily folate supplements, and which present in the neonatal period with severe jaundice uncontrolled by the above measures and requiring exchange transfusion.

Pyruvate kinase deficiency

This is an autosomal recessive disorder that occurs in all ethnic groups, although documented cases have come mainly from persons of north European stock. The frequency is of the order of hundreds of cases rather than the millions suffering from G6PD deficiency.[123]

The block in glycolysis at the lower end of the Embden–Myerhof pathway results in an accumulation of 2,3 diphosphoglycerate, a shift of the oxygen dissociation curve to the right and a reduction in oxygen affinity, which means that oxygen delivery to the tissues in the presence of PK deficiency may be normal or near normal, even with levels of haemoglobin between 6 and 8 g/dl. Clinically a child may thrive and require only the occasional transfusion when there is an extra stress on the bone marrow.

As a result, many cases of PK deficiency go undiagnosed for months or even years, but PK-deficient neonates may develop haemolytic jaundice and require phototherapy and exchange transfusion. The diagnosis is made by finding a low enzyme level in an anaemic but often thriving baby, and intermediate levels in the parents, who are not anaemic and who have no blood disorder. The neonatal blood film has no special characteristics to suggest PK deficiency.

Haemolysis due to haemoglobin disorders (haemoglobinopathies)

Haemoglobinopathies are divided into two broad groups, the haemoglobin variants (structural defects) and the thalassaemia syndromes (synthesis defects). The two most important haemoglobinopathies, numerically and clinically, are sickle cell disease and thalassaemia major (homozygous β-thalassaemia). Both are β-globin chain defects and therefore rarely cause problems before 3–6 months of age, when the β chain of adult haemoglobin (HbA:$\alpha_2\beta_2$) normally becomes predominant (Fig. 32.3, Table 32.2). However, a unique situation exists during the neonatal period because of the rapid evolutionary changes in respect of globin chain synthesis. γ-Chain defects may be seen at this time which spontaneously resolve as fetal haemoglobin ($\alpha_2\gamma_2$) disappears.

Haemoglobin variants

α-Chain structural defects are common to both adult and fetal haemoglobin and would be expected to have similar clinical manifestations in the neonate, older child and adult. Most α-chain mutants do not cause clinically significant disorders and are detected only as part of routine neonatal screening programmes. Haemoglobin Hasharon, an α-chain variant, is a mildly unstable haemoglobin which gives rise to a haemolytic anaemia in the newborn which resolves spontaneously during the first few months of life when adult haemoglobin appears, presumably because the defective α-chain is more stable with β chains than with the γ chains of fetal haemoglobin.[108]

γ-Chain structural defects will spontaneously resolve as fetal haemoglobin is replaced by adult haemoglobin in the first months of life. In general they are discovered in neonatal screening programmes and result in no haematological abnormality. An exception to this general rule is HbF Poole, an unstable γ-chain variant which persists as a Heinz body haemolytic anaemia during the first few weeks of life.[105]

As up to 30% of the haemoglobin at birth is haemoglobin A, β-chain variants can be a problem in the newborn period. Rarely homozygous sickle cell disease presents with jaundice, pallor, fever, respiratory distress and abdominal distension.[29,139] Massive sickling with severe jaundice has been described, occasionally with a fatal outcome. These episodes are triggered by anoxia and severe infection.

Any neonate with documented sickle cell disease who presents with symptoms or signs attributable to sickling is

	Normal	ALPHA-THAL+ TRAIT	ALPHA-THAL° TRAIT	HOMOZYGOUS ALPHA-THAL+	HbH DISEASE	Hb. BART'S HYDROPS
Alpha gene status	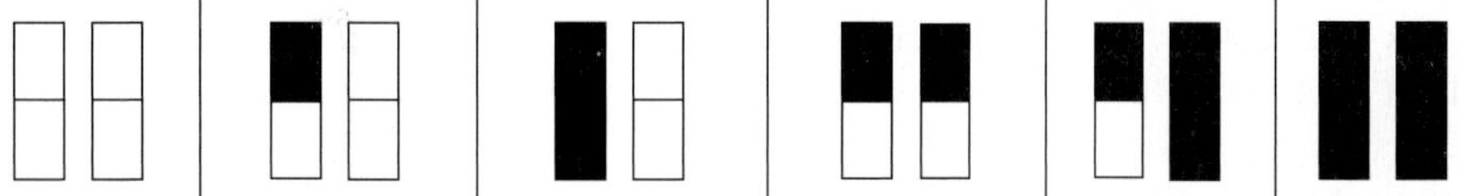					
Clinical presentation	Normal	Normal	Normal	Normal	Moderate haemolytic anaemia	Hydrops Fetalis
Haemoglobin pattern at birth	Normal	1–2% Hb. Bart's	5–10% Hb. Bart's	5–10% Hb. Bart's	25% Hb. Bart's <5% HbH	95% Hb. Bart's

Abnormal Gene

Fig. 32.7 The α-thalassaemias: classification based on genotype, clinical presentation and haemoglobin pattern at birth.

best treated with exchange transfusion. The infant with sickle cell syndrome can be identified early by a modification of conventional haemoglobin electrophoresis,[77] ideally using cord blood samples. This involves isoelectric focusing of Hb electrophoresis, which will separate HbF and HbA, which run together on conventional electrophoresis. Sickle cell trait will yield three distinct bands: HbF (major), HbA (minor) and HbS (minor). The haemolysate of the infant who has inherited HbSS sickle cell disease will exhibit two bands, HbF (major) and HbS (minor).

In some areas of the UK (including the northwest Thames region) routine screening of all babies is undertaken to identify haemoglobinopathies in those of multiethnic origin. Capillary samples are taken on days 7–10, at the same time as the Guthrie test. Alternatively, nearly all hospital laboratories will, on request, examine the blood of an infant at risk.

The β-chain variants or synthesis defects can only be diagnosed by appropriate modification of conventional tests to detect haemoglobinopathies in the adult. However, at term approximately 20% of the Hb present is HbA ($\alpha_2\beta_2$), and heterozygous and homozygous defects can be distinguished accurately as long as the laboratory is informed of the age and maturity of the infant.

Once the diagnosis is made parents should be warned of the signs of sickling infarcts and the conditions that precipitate them in the young infant, so that they can seek prompt medical treatment and advice early in any potential sickling crisis.

Thalassaemia syndromes

These are the most common inherited single-gene defects in the world.

α-Thalassaemia. α-Chains are common to fetal and adult haemoglobin and α-thalassaemia can therefore present at birth. α-Chain production is under the control of four genes, two on each of the homologous chromosomes 16. The majority of α-thalassaemia syndromes are due to gene deletion and their severity depends on how many of the α genes are affected (Fig. 32.7). α-Thalassaemia trait results from the deletion of one or two genes. The condition in which one gene is deleted (α^+-thalassaemia) results in no clinical manifestations and no obvious abnormality on initial blood screening. The diagnosis can only be made by analysis of globin chain synthesis and gene mapping. Homozygous α^+-thalassaemia (one gene missing on each chromosome) and α^0-thalassaemia (both genes missing on the same chromosome) will result in production of the typical thalassaemia red cell of small volume and reduced haemoglobin content. Under haematological stress such as pregnancy or infection a mild anaemia will develop.

Deletion of three of four α genes results in a haemolytic condition known as HbH disease. HbH is the name given to the haemoglobin formed by tetramers of the excess β chain – β4 – in the relative absence of α chains. If all four α genes are deleted the fetus can only make haemoglobin Bart's (tetramers of γ chain: γ4).

α-Thalassaemia syndromes are very common in oriental and Negro populations; however, the situation where both α genes have been deleted on one chromosome (α^0-thalassaemia trait) is very rare in Negroes, so that HbH disease, and particularly Hb Bart's hydrops (see below), are virtually limited to oriental populations. Many normal newborn infants in southeast Asia, Africa, the Mediterranean and the Middle East have elevated levels of haemoglobin Bart's detectable in cord blood that reflect the presence of an α-thalassaemia gene.

As β-chain production increases and γ-chain production wanes, haemoglobin Bart's disappears in the first few months of life.

Investigation of asymptomatic southeast Asian newborn infants has identified three different groups of haemoglobin Bart's values in cord blood: 1–2%, 5–10% and 25%. The first group have been interpreted as being carriers of α^+-thalassaemia, the second group as patients with α^0-thalassaemia or homozygous α^+-thalassaemia, and the third group are those with HbH disease. There is considerable overlap between the first two groups.[130] However, there is little doubt that an infant with 5% or more haemoglobin Bart's in his cord blood will, on average, have reduced haemoglobin concentrations and abnormal red cell indices later in life. In newborn Negro infants studies suggest a bimodal distribution of haemoglobin Bart's levels, with about 3% having levels in the 3–10% range.[86]

Of 345 Saudi Arabian neonates born in the eastern oasis 50% had elevated levels of haemoglobin Bart's, ranging from 1 to 16%.[145] The distribution of these levels forms a continuum.

Haemoglobin H disease. In the neonate with haemoglobin H disease there is anaemia and jaundice: electrophoresis demonstrates about 25% of haemoglobin Bart's (γ4) at birth, but as one α gene remains some haemoglobin F, A and A_2 is present as well as HbH and Hb Bart's. A full blood count with indices will reveal a low MCV and MCH, together with a reticulocytosis and abnormal HbH or Bart's inclusions. The infant becomes jaundiced, and the usual precautions to prevent kernicterus should be taken.

Subsequently transfusions are rarely needed, but folate supplements should be given. Typical HbH inclusions are seen in a film of an incubated reticulocyte preparation. It is not widely appreciated that because HbH is unstable these individuals are susceptible to increased haemolysis, induced by the same oxidant drugs and toxins that cause problems in G6PD-deficient patients (Table 32.7). In adult life they usually have moderate anaemia (Hb 8–9 g/dl), splenomegaly and a normal life expectancy.

Hb Bart's hydrops fetalis. This is the most severe type of α-thalassaemia (homozygous αO-thalassaemia), which is common in southeast Asia but rare in other parts of the world. Total suppression of α-chain synthesis, coupled with normal γ-chain production in the fetus, leads to the formation of Hb Bart's (γ_4), which has a high affinity for oxygen. This condition was first defined in a Chinese baby born at St Bartholomew's Hospital, London. Affected infants are either stillborn at about 34 weeks' gestation or, if liveborn, survive for about 1 hour. Usually of low birthweight, the infant is pale, very oedematous with ascites, and has gross hepatomegaly with variable splenomegaly. Severe anaemia is present (Hb <6 g/dl) and the blood film shows many nucleated red cells, anisopoikilocytosis, hypochromia, basophilic stippling and target cells. The reticulocyte count is high and serum bilirubin raised. Haemoglobin electrophoresis on starch gel shows Hb Bart's (90%) with small amounts of HbH (β4) and Hb Portland ($\varepsilon_2\gamma_2$) with an absence of HbA or HbF (Table 32.2).

This genetic disorder is transmitted in an autosomal recessive manner with a high risk of recurrence (1 in 4) for every pregnancy. Parents at risk can be identified early in pregnancy by confirming that they suffer from either αO-thalassaemia or HbH disease. Women carrying an α-thalassaemia hydrops have a high incidence of life-threatening hypertension and difficult vaginal delivery. The condition can be diagnosed by fetal amniotic cell or trophoblast DNA analysis, and termination of the non-viable child can be carried out before these complications become a problem.[190]

Rare cases of survival beyond the newborn period have been reported in fetuses detected and transfused in utero and supported by regular transfusions post delivery.[10,17]

γ-Thalassaemias. In the same way that γ-chain variants may cause transient effects in the newborn period, γ-thalassaemia can produce a mild to moderate anaemia in utero and at birth, with reduced levels of HbF. As there are multiple genes for γ-chain synthesis, the severity of the anaemia depends on the extent to which these genes are involved. The hypochromia and anaemia are transient because γ chains are replaced by β chains when adult haemoglobin synthesis replaces fetal haemoglobin during the first 3–6 months of life.

There have been several reports of infants with a combination of γ-and β-thalassaemia since it was first described in 1972 by Kan et al.[94] A term infant presented with a haemolytic anaemia, microcytosis, hypochromia and numerous nucleated red cells on the film. No Hb Bart's or HbH could be detected, but a synthesis deficiency of both γ and β chains could be demonstrated. The morphology of the blood film improved as the infant matured, and by 3 months of age this became identical with that of the father, who had β-thalassaemia trait.

β-Thalassaemia. One gene for β-globin chain production is inherited from each parent on chromosome 11. β-Thalassaemia occurs in heterozygous (minor) and homozygous (major) forms. β-Thalassaemia major represents a major public health problem in many countries of the world (e.g. in Cyprus the carrier rate is 1 in 7), with more than 100 000 affected babies born each year. Prenatal diagnosis by analysis of fetal blood samples or by DNA analysis of fetal cells obtained from amniotic fluid or, more usually nowadays, by transcervical or transabdominal chorion villus sampling, is available in many centres, but not always in areas where the disease is common. Successful prenatal diagnosis of thalassaemia and sickle cell anaemia has been reported using fetal cells harvested from maternal blood.[39]

In neonates with β-thalassaemia the haemoglobin will be in the normal range and the infant will thrive until 3–6 months of age, when β-chain production becomes predominant. In β-thalassaemia minor microcytosis will only become apparent later in the first 6 months of life. With β-thalassaemia major the first haematological sign is an increasing number of nucleated red cells in the blood film, together with the maintenance of high concentrations of HbF. Conditions such as intrauterine blood loss or alloimmune disease, which will lead to loss of fetal cells, may result in β-thalassaemia major presenting before 2–3 months of age. The diagnosis can only be made before this time by demonstrating a severe reduction in the synthesis of β-globin chains in the infant's blood, or by family DNA analysis of the β-globin gene locus.

Haemolytic anaemia due to acquired defects

Anaemia associated with infection

Both intrauterine and postnatally acquired infections are associated with anaemia and other haematological abnormalities in the neonatal period (Chapter 43, Part 2). Although these changes are sometimes produced by marrow suppression, severe neonatal infection is usually also accompanied by haemolysis and DIC (disseminated intravascular coagulation).

Haemolytic anaemia due to maternal autoimmune disease

The rare combination of AIHA and pregnancy carries great risk to both the woman and her fetus.[162] The degree of haemolysis in the fetus depends mainly on the amount and avidity of the transferred antibody for the fetal red cells. In one reported series of subjects with active maternal AIHA, four infants were stillborn, three had severe haemolytic disease postnatally, and the remaining 12 were normal.[38] Administration of prednisone, 2 mg/kg/24 h to the mother with active AIHA may reduce both maternal haemolysis and neonatal morbidity.[78] Fetal blood sampling will establish whether or not the fetus is affected (Chapter 14).

Although pregnancy may result in exacerbation of systemic lupus erythematosus, up to 50% of women with this condition are reported to improve during pregnancy, especially in the third trimester.[60] Haemolytic anaemia, leukopenia and thrombocytopenia have all been observed in infants of women with active disease,[165] presumably as a result of an IgG antibody involved in the disease crossing the placenta.

Management of the newborn in these conditions is directed primarily to the management of jaundice. Haemolytic anaemia in association with DIC is dealt with on page 804.

ANAEMIA IN THE NEONATE DUE TO IMPAIRED PRODUCTION OF RED CELLS

Congenital red cell aplasia (Diamond–Blackfan syndrome)

There have been well over 200 reports of this condition in the literature since it was first described in 1936.[2,3,55] The disorder has been called chronic congenital aregenerative anaemia, pure red cell aplasia, erythrogenesis imperfecta, congenital hypoplastic anaemia and chronic idiopathic erythroblastopenia. Evidence suggests the disorder is secondary to either a lack of erythroid stem cells or immune suppression of stem cell differentiation.[111] Inheritance appears to follow an autosomal recessive pattern. Of reported cases 25% present with neonatal pallor,[2] although the diagnosis may not be made until 6 years of age. It should be suspected in any newborn with anaemia and reticulocytopenia (<0.2%), together with normal platelets and leukocytes. The diagnosis is confirmed by examination of a bone marrow aspirate, which reveals a virtual absence of erythroid precursors. One-third of patients have physical abnormalities and the paediatrician may be alerted to the possibility by finding triphalangeal thumbs, characteristics of Turner syndrome or other musculoskeletal abnormalities. Once the diagnosis is established treatment with steroids should be started as soon as possible.

Congenital dyserythropoietic anaemia

There are a number of inherited disorders of erythropoiesis which result in anaemia, which is not due to aplasia but to ineffective erythropoiesis with morphological abnormalities of the erythroblasts. The various types of CDA are characterized by anaemia with an inappropriate low reticulocyte count and ineffective erythropoiesis.[3] There are multinuclear megaloblastoid cells with chromatin bridges and specific electron microscopy findings. In type II there is a positive acid lysis test of red cells with sera from normal individuals – so-called HEMPAS, hereditary erythroblastic multinuclearity with a positive acid serum test. Most cases present in the first decade of life or early teens, but there have been atypical cases which presented hydropic at birth[195] or in utero.[33] In the five hydropic infants reported in utero to date,[33] death occurred shortly after delivery or there was regular transfusion dependency in the survivors.

Anaemia as a result of impaired red cell production may also present in the newborn period or with hydrops in utero as a result of infection, particularly with parvovirus or with congenital leukaemia or osteopetrosis associated with ineffective erythropoiesis.

REFERENCES

1. Aballi, A J, Puapondh Y, Desposito F 1968 Platelet counts in thriving premature infants. Pediatrics 42: 685–689
2. Alter B P, Nathan D G 1979 Red cell aplasia in children. Archives of Disease in Childhood 54: 263–267
3. Alter B P, Young N S 1997 The bone marrow failure syndromes. In: Nathan D G, Orkin S H (eds) Nathan and Oski's hematology of infancy and childhood. WB Saunders, Philadelphia, pp 237–335
4. Anderson G W 1941 Studies on nucleated red cells in chorionic capillaries and cord blood of various ages of pregnancy. American Journal of Obstetrics and Gynecology 42: 1–14
5. Andrews N C, Bridges K R 1997 Disorders of iron metabolism and sideroblastic anemia. In: Nathan D G, Orkin S H (eds) Nathan and Oski's hematology of infancy and childhood. W B Saunders, Philadelphia, pp 440–462
6. Avent N D, Martin P G 1996 Kell typing by allele-specific PCR (ASP). British Journal of Haematology 93: 728–730
7. Bard H, Prosmanne J 1982 Postnatal fetal and adult hemoglobin synthesis in preterm infants whose birth weight was less than 1,000 grams. Journal of Clinical Investigation 70: 50–52
8. Barrow E, Peters R L 1968 Exsanguinating haemorrhage into the scalp in newborn infants. South African Medical Journal 42: 265
9. BCSH British Committee for Standards in Haematology Blood Transfusion Task Force 1996 Guidelines for blood grouping and red cell antibody testing during pregnancy. Transfusion Medicine 6: 71–74
10. Beaudry M A, Ferguson D J, Pearse K, Yanofsky R A, Rubin E M, Kan Y W 1986 Survival of a hydropic infant with homozygous alpha-thalassemia-1. Journal of Pediatrics 108: 713–716
11. Bechensteen A G, Haga P, Halvorsen S et al 1993 Erythropoietin, protein, and iron supplementation and the prevention of anaemia of prematurity. Archives of Disease in Childhood 69: 19–23
12. Beck D, Masserey E, Meyer M, Calame A 1991 Weekly intravenous administration of recombinant human erythropoietin in infants with the anaemia of prematurity. European Journal of Pediatrics 150: 767–772
13. Becker P S, Lux S E 1993 Disorders of the red cell membrane. In: Nathan D G, Oski F A (eds) Hematology of infancy and childhood. WB Saunders, Philadelphia, pp 529–633
14. Berkowitz R L, Beyta Y, Sadovsky E 1982 Death in utero due to Kell sensitisation without excessive elevation of the Δ OD 450 value in amniotic fluid. Obstetrics and Gynecology 60: 746–749
15. Berkowitz R L, Chitkara U, Goldberg J D, Wilkins I, Chervernak F A, Lynch L 1986 Intrauterine intravascular transfusion for severe red blood cell isoimmunization: ultra-sound guided percutaneous approach. American Journal of Obstetrics and Gynecology 155: 574–581
16. Beutler E 1971 Abnormalities of the hexose-monophosphate shunt. Seminars in Hematology 8: 311–347
17. Bianchi D W, Beyer E C, Stark A R, Saffan D, Sachs B P, Wolfe L 1986 Normal long-term survival with alpha-thalassemia. Journal of Pediatrics 108: 716–718
18. Bienzle U, Effiong C, Luzzatto L 1976 Erythrocyte glucose 6-phosphate dehydrogenase deficiency (G6PD type A-) and neonatal jaundice. Acta Paediatrica Scandinavica 65: 701–703
19. Bierme S J, Blanc M, Abbal M, Fournie A 1979 Oral Rh treatment for severely immunised mothers. Lancet i: 604–605
20. Bierme S J, Blanc M, Fournie A, Abbal M 1982 Desensitization by oral antigen. In: Frigoletto F D J, Figgis Jewett J, Konugres A A (eds) Rh hemolytic disease: new strategy for eradication. G K Hall, Boston, pp 249–266
21. Blanchette V S, Zipursky A 1984 Assessment of anaemia in newborn infants. Clinics in Perinatology 11: 489–510
22. Bowman J M 1996 Hemolytic disease of the newborn. Vox Sanguinis 70: 62–67
23. Bowman J M, Chown J M, Lewis M, Pollock J M 1978 Rh-isoimmunization during pregnancy: antenatal prophylaxis. Canadian Medical Association Journal 118: 623–627
24. Boxer L A 1978 Immunological function and leucocyte disorders in newborn infants. Clinics in Haematology 7: 123–146
25. Brouwers H A A, Overbeeke M A M, van Ertbruggen I et al 1988 What is the best predictor of the severity of ABO-haemolytic disease of the newborn? Lancet ii: 641–644
26. Brown J J M 1957 Hepatic haemorrhage in the newborn. Archives of Disease in Childhood 32: 480–483
27. Brown M S, Garcia J F, Phibbs R H, Dallman P R 1984 Decreased response of plasma immunoreactive erythropoietin to 'available oxygen' in anemia of prematurity. Journal of Pediatrics 105: 793–798
28. Brown M S, Shapiro H 1996 Effect of protein intake on erythropoiesis during erythropoietin treatment of anemia of prematurity. Journal of Pediatrics 128: 512–517
29. Brugnara C, Platt O S 1997 The neonatal erythrocyte and its disorders. In: Nathan D G, Orkin S H (eds) Nathan and Oski's hematology of infancy and childhood. W B Saunders, Philadelphia, pp 19–46
30. Burrell J M 1952 A comparative study of the circulating eosinophil levels in babies. Archives of Disease in Childhood 27: 337–340
31. Caine M E, Mueller-Heubach M D 1986 Kell sensitisation in pregnancy. American Journal of Obstetrics and Gynecology 154: 85–90
32. Cairo M S, Christensen R, Sender L S et al 1995 Results of a phase I/II trial of recombinant human granulocyte-macrophage colony-stimulating factor in very low birthweight neonates: significant induction of circulatory neutrophils, monocytes, platelets, and bone marrow neutrophils. Blood 86: 2509–2515
33. Cantu-Rajnoldi A, Zanella A, Conter U et al 1997 A severe transfusion dependent congenital dyserythropoietic anaemia presenting as hydrops fetalis. British Journal of Haematology 96: 530–533
34. Carnielli V, Montini G, Da Riol R, Dall'Amico R, Cantarutti F 1992 Effect of high doses of human recombinant erythropoietin on the need for blood transfusions in preterm infants. Journal of Pediatrics 121: 98–102
35. Carpentieri U, Gustavson L P, Haggard M E 1977 Pyknocytosis in a neonate: an unusual presentation of hereditary elliptocytosis. Clinical Pediatrics 16: 76–78
36. Carr R, Davies J M 1990 Abnormal FcRIII expression by neutrophils from very preterm neonates. Blood 76: 607–611
37. Cashore W J, Usher R H 1973 Hypovolemia resulting from a tight nuchal cord at birth (abstract). Pediatric Research 7: 399
38. Chaplin H, Cohen R, Bloomberg G, Kaplan H J, Moore J A, Dorner L 1973 Pregnancy and idiopathic auto-immune haemolytic anaemia. British Journal of Haematology 24: 219–239
39. Cheung M, Goldberg J D, Wai Kan Y 1996 Prenatal diagnosis of sickle cell anaemia and thalassaemia by analysis of fetal cells in maternal blood. Nature Genetics 14: 264–268
40. Chitkara U, Bussel J, Alvarez M, Lynch L, Meisel R L, Berkowitz R L 1990 High-dose intravenous gamma globulin: does it have a role in the treatment of severe erythroblastosis fetalis? Obstetrics and Gynecology 76: 703–708
41. Chown B 1955 The fetus can bleed. American Journal of Obstetrics and Gynecology 70: 1298–1308
42. Christensen R D, Hunter D D, Ohls R K 1994 Pilot study comparing recombinant erythropoietin alone with erythropoietin plus recombinant granulocyte-macrophage colony-stimulating factor for treatment of the anemia of prematurity. Journal of Perinatology 14: 110–113
43. Clarke C A 1989 Preventing rhesus babies: the Liverpool research and follow-up. Archives of Disease in Childhood 64: 1734–1740
44. Clarke C A, Whitfield A G W, Mollison P L 1987 Death from Rh haemolytic disease in England and Wales in 1984 and 1985. British Medical Journal 294: 1001
45. Cochran W D 1978 Increasing safety of exchange transfusion. Pediatric Research 12: 462
46. Coetzer T, Lawler J, Prchal J T, Palek J 1987 Molecular determinants of clinical expression of hereditary elliptocytosis and pyropoikilocytosis. Blood 70: 766–772
47. Cook S G, Baker J W, Weaver E W 1989 Intrauterine transfusion for anti-Duffy (Fy^a) haemolytic disease. Australian and New Zealand Journal of Obstetrics and Gynaecology 29: 263–264
48. Costa F F, Agre P, Watkins P C et al 1990 Linkage of dominant hereditary spherocytosis to the gene for the erythrocyte membrane-skeleton protein ankyrin. New England Journal of Medicine 323: 1046–1050
49. Dallman P R 1984 Erythropoietin and the anemia of prematurity. Journal of Pediatrics 105: 756–757
50. Dallman P R 1993 Anemia of prematurity: the prospects for avoiding

blood transfusions by treatment with recombinant human erythropoietin. Advances in Pediatrics 40: 385–403
51. Dallman P R, Yip R, Oski F A 1993 Iron deficiency and related nutritional anemias. In: Nathan D G, Oski F A (eds) Hematology of infancy and childhood. W B Saunders, Philadelphia, pp 413–450
52. de la Camara C, Arrieta R, Gonzalez A, Inglesias E, Omenaca F 1988 High-dose intravenous immunoglobulin as the sole prenatal treatment for severe Rh immunization. New England Journal of Medicine 318: 519–529
53. de Sauvage F J, Hass P E, Spencer S D et al 1994 Stimulation of megakaryocytopoiesis and thrombopoiesis by the c-Mpl ligand. Nature 369: 533–538
54. Delta B G, Eisenstein E M, Rothenberg A M 1968 Rupture of a normal spleen in the newborn: report of survival and review of the literature. Clinical Pediatrics 7: 373–376
55. Diamond L K, Wang W C, Alter B P 1976 Congenital hypoplastic anemia. Advances in Pediatrics 22: 349–378
56. Djaldetti M 1979 Hemopoietic events in human embryonic spleens at early gestational stages. Biology of the Neonate 36: 133–144
57. Djaldetti M, Ovadia J, Bessler O, Fishman P, Halbrecht I 1975 Ultrastructural study of the erythropoietic events in human embryonic livers. Biology of the Neonate 26: 367–374
58. Doxiadis S A, Valaes F 1964 The clinical picture of glucose-6-phosphate dehydrogenase deficiency in early childhood. Archives of Disease in Childhood 39: 545
59. Drew J H, Smith M B, Kitchen W H 1977 Glucose-6-phosphate dehydrogenase deficiency in immigrant Greek infants [letter]. Journal of Pediatrics 90: 659–660
60. Dubois E L 1966 Lupus erythematosus. McGraw-Hill, New York
61. Duguid J K, Bromilow I M, Entwistle G D, Wilkinson R 1995 Haemolytic disease of the newborn due to anti-M. Vox Sanguinis 68: 195–196
62. Earn A A 1951 Placental anomalies. Canadian Medical Association Journal 64: 113–120
63. Emmerson A J, Coles H J, Stern C M, Pearson T C 1993 Double blind trial of recombinant human erythropoietin in preterm infants. Archives of Disease in Childhood 68: 291–296
64. Engle W A, Schreiner R L, Baehner R L 1983 Neonatal white blood cell disorders. Seminars in Perinatology 7: 184–200
65. Fenton V, Cavill I, Fisher J 1977 Iron stores in pregnancy. British Journal of Haematology 37: 145–149
66. Fernandes C J, Hagan R, Frieberg A, Grauaug A, Kohan R 1994 Erythropoietin in very preterm infants. Journal of Paediatrics and Child Health 30: 356–359
67. Fisk N M 1995 The scientific basis of feto-fetal transfusion syndrome and its treatment. In: Ward R H, Whittle M (eds) Multiple pregnancy. RCOG Press, London, pp 235–250
68. Flake A W, Harrison M R, Adzick M S, Zanjani E D 1987 Erythropoietin production by the fetal liver in an adult environment. Blood 70: 542–545
69. Fletcher A, Thomson A 1995 The introduction of human monoclonal anti-D for therapeutic use. Transfusion Medicine Reviews 9: 314–326
70. Fogel B J, Arias D, Kung F 1968 Platelet counts in healthy premature infants. Journal of Pediatrics 73: 108–110
71. Forestier F, Daffos F, Galacteros F, Bardakjian J, Rainaut M, Beuzard Y 1986 Hematological values of 163 normal fetuses between 18 and 30 weeks of gestation. Pediatric Research 20: 342–346
72. Fraser I D, Bothamley J E, Bennett M O, Airth G R 1976 Intensive antenatal plasmapheresis in severe rhesus isoimmunisation. Lancet i: 6–8
73. Gairdner D, Marks J, Roscoe J D 1952 Blood formation in infancy. Part I. The normal bone marrow. Archives of Disease in Childhood 27: 128–133
74. Gallagher P G, Forget B G, Lux S E 1997 Disorders of the erythrocyte membrane. In: Nathan D G, Orkin S H (eds) Nathan and Oski's hematology of infancy and childhood. W B Saunders, Philadelphia, pp 544–664
75. Geifman-Holtzman O, Wojtowycz M, Kosmas E, Artal R 1997 Female alloimmunization with antibodies known to cause hemolytic disease. Obstetrics and Gynecology 89: 272–275
76. Gibson B E S 1991 Transfusion in the fetus and newborn. In: Hann I M, Gibson B E S, Letsky E A (eds) Fetal and neonatal haematology. Baillière Tindall, London, pp 189–217
77. Glader B E 1989 Recognition of anemia and red blood cell disorders during infancy. In: Alter B P (ed) Perinatal hematology. Methods in hematology 21. Churchill Livingstone, New York, pp 126–164
78. Glader B E, Platt O 1978 Haemolytic disorders of infancy. Perinatal haematology – Clinics in Haematology 7: 35–61
79. Grannum P A T, Copel J A 1988 Prevention of Rh isoimmunization and treatment of the compromised fetus. Seminars in Perinatology 12: 324–335
80. Gross G P, Hathaway W E 1972 Fetal erythrocyte deformability. Pediatric Research 6: 593–599
81. Hall R T, Wheeler R E, Benson J, Harris G, Rippetoe L 1993 Benefit from formula containing high iron content (15 mg/L) versus low (3 mg/L) during initial hospitalization to infants less than 1800 g birth weight. Pediatrics 92: 409–414
82. Halperin D S 1991 Use of recombinant erythropoietin in treatment of the anemia of prematurity. American Journal of Pediatric Hematology and Oncology 13: 351–363
83. Halvorsen S, Finne P H 1968 Erythropoietin production in the human fetus and newborn. Annals of the New York Academy of Sciences 149: 576–577
84. Hann I M 1991 Development of blood in the fetus. In: Hann I M, Gibson B E S, Letsky E A (eds) Fetal and neonatal haematology. Baillière Tindall, London, pp 1–28
85. Haworth C, Evans D I K 1981 Nutritional aspects of blood disorders in the newborn. Journal of Human Nutrition 35: 323–334
86. Higgs D R 1993 Alpha thalassaemia in haemoglobinopathies. In: Higgs D R, Weatherall D J (eds) Baillière's clinical haematology: The haemoglobinopathies. Baillière Tindall, London, pp 117–150
87. Holland B M, Jones J G, Wardrop C A F 1987 Lessons from the anemia of prematurity. Hematology/Oncology Clinics of North America 1: 355–366
88. Holland B M, Wardrop C A 1991 Oxygen transport in blood, haematinics and blood cell component therapy in the neonate. In: Rylance G, Aranda J, Harvey D (eds) Neonatal clinical pharmacology and therapeutics. Butterworths, Oxford, pp 211–223
89. Hughes-Jones N C 1988 Human monoclonal antibodies and haemolytic disease of the newborn. British Journal of Haematology 70: 263–265
90. Idjradinata P, Pollitt E 1993 Reversal of developmental delays in iron-deficient anaemic infants treated with iron. Lancet 341: 1–4
91. Irani P K 1964 Haematoma of the umbilical cord. British Medical Journal ii: 1436–1437
92. Jacobs K, Shoemaker C, Rudersdorf R et al 1985 Isolation and characterization of genomic and cDNA clones of human erythropoietin. Nature 313: 806–810
93. Kalpaktsoglou P K, Emery J L 1965 Human bone marrow during the last three months of intrauterine life. A histological study. Acta Haematologica 34: 228–238
94. Kan Y W, Forget B G, Nathan D G 1972 Gamma-beta thalassemia: a cause of hemolytic disease of the newborn. New England Journal of Medicine 286: 129–134
95. Kevy S 1962 Clinical pathologic conference. Journal of Pediatrics 60: 304–314
96. Kirkman H N, Riley H D 1959 Post-hemorrhagic anemia and shock in the newborn: a review. Pediatrics 24: 97–105
97. Kitterman J A, Schleuter M A 1974 Effects of intrauterine asphyxia on neonatal blood volume (abstract). Pediatric Research 8: 447
98. Kleinberg E, Phibbs R, Dong L 1973 Lack of placenta to infant transfusion with delayed cord clamping after Caesarean section delivery (abstract). Pediatric Research 7: 403
99. Kline P S 1948 Microscopic observations of the placental barrier in transplacental erythroblastosis fetalis in normal pregnancy. American Journal of Obstetrics and Gynecology 56: 226–237
100. Koenig J M, Ashton R D, DeVore G R, Christensen R D 1989 Late hyporegenerative anemia in Rh hemolytic disease. Journal of Pediatrics 115: 315–318
101. Koenig J M, Christensen R D 1989 Neutropenia and thrombocytopenia in infants with Rh hemolytic disease. Journal of Pediatrics 114: 625–631
102. Korst L M, Phelan J P, Ock Ahn M, Martin G I 1996 Nucleated red blood cells: an update on the marker for fetal asphyxia. American Journal of Obstetrics and Gynecology 175: 843–846
103. Kumpel B M, Goodrick M J, Pamphilon D H et al 1995 Human Rh D monoclonal antibodies (BRAD-3 and BRAD-5) cause accelerated clearance of Rh D+ red blood cells and suppression of Rh D immunization in Rh D– volunteers. Blood 86: 1701–1709

104. Lachance C, Chessex P, Fouron J C, Widness J A, Bard H 1994 Myocardial, erythropoietic, and metabolic adaptations to anemia of prematurity. Journal of Pediatrics 125: 278–282
105. Lee Potter J P, Deacon Smith R A, Simpkiss M J, Kamuzora H, Lehmann H 1975 A new cause of haemolytic anaemia in the newborn. A description of an unstable fetal haemoglobin: F Poole, alpha2-G-gamma2 130 tryptophan yields glycine. Journal of Clinical Pathology 28: 317–320
106. Letsky E A, De Silva M 1994 Preventing Rh immunisation. British Medical Journal 309: 213–214
107. Levine P 1943 Serological factors as possible causes in spontaneous abortions. Journal of Heredity 34: 71–80
108. Levine R L, Lincoln D R, Buchholz W M, Gribble J, Schwartz H C 1975 Hemoglobin Hasharon in a premature infant with hemolytic anemia. Pediatric Research 9: 7–11
109. Lind T, Gerrard J, Sheridan T S, Walker W 1977 Effect of maternal parity and infant sex upon the haematological values of cord blood. Acta Paediatrica Scandinavica 66: 333–337
110. Lozoff B, Jimenez E, Wolf A W 1991 Long-term developmental outcome of infants with iron deficiency. New England Journal of Medicine 325: 687–694
111. Lubin B, Vichinsky E 1979 Anemia in the newborn period. Pediatric Annals 8: 416–434
112. Lubin B H 1978 Neonatal anaemia secondary to blood loss. Clinics in Haematology 7: 19–34
113. Lundstrom U, Siimes M A, Dallman P R 1977 At what age does iron supplementation become necessary in low-birth-weight infants? Journal of Pediatrics 91: 878–883
114. Luzzatto L 1997 G6PD Deficiency and hemolytic anemia. In: Nathan D G, Orkin S H (eds) Nathan and Oski's hematology of infancy and childhood. W B Saunders, Philadelphia, pp 704–726
115. Maier R F, Obladen M, Scigalla P et al 1994 The effect of epoetin beta (recombinant human erythropoietin) on the need for transfusion in very-low-birth-weight infants. European Multicentre Erythropoietin Study Group. New England Journal of Medicine 330: 1173–1178
116. Manroe B L, Weinberg A G, Rosenfeld C R, Browne R 1979 The neonatal blood count in health and disease. I. Reference values for neutrophilic cells. Journal of Pediatrics 95: 89–98
117. Margulies M, Voto L S, Mathet E, Margulies M 1991 High-dose intravenous IgG for the treatment of severe rhesus alloimmunization. Vox Sanguinis 61: 181–189
118. Matsunaga A T, Lubin B H 1995 Hemolytic anemia in the newborn. Clinics in Perinatology 22: 803–828
119. McClure G 1992 Haemolytic disease of the newborn (erythroblastosis fetalis). In: Roberton N R C (ed) Textbook of neonatology, 2nd edn. Churchill Livingstone, Edinburgh, pp 725–732
120. Mclntosh S 1975 Erythropoietin excretion in the premature infant. Journal of Pediatrics 86: 202–206
121. Meloni T, Cutillo S, Testa U, Luzzatto L 1987 Neonatal jaundice and severity of glucose-6-phosphate dehydrogenase deficiency in Sardinian babies. Early Human Development 15: 317–322
122. Mentzer W C, Collier E 1975 Hydrops fetalis associated with erythrocyte G-6-PD deficiency and maternal ingestion of fava beans and ascorbic acid. Journal of Pediatrics 86: 565–567
123. Mentzer W C J 1997 Pyruvate kinase deficiency and disorders of glycolysis. In: Nathan D G, Orkin S H (eds) Nathan and Oski's hematology of infancy and childhood. W B Saunders, Philadelphia, pp 665–703
124. Messer J, Haddad J, Donato L, Astruc D, Matis J 1993 Early treatment of premature infants with recombinant human erythropoietin. Pediatrics 92: 519–523
125. Meyer M P, Meyer J H, Commerford A et al 1994 Recombinant human erythropoietin in the treatment of the anemia of prematurity: results of a double-blind, placebo-controlled study. Pediatrics 93: 918–923
126. Millar D S, Davis L R, Rodeck C H, Nicolaides K H, Mibashan R S 1985 Normal blood cell values in the early mid-trimester fetus. Prenatal Diagnosis 5: 367–373
127. Millard D D, Gidding S S, Socol M L et al 1990 Effects of intravascular, intrauterine transfusion on prenatal and postnatal hemolysis and erythropoiesis in severe fetal isoimmunization. Journal of Pediatrics 117: 447–454
128. Mollison P L, Engelfriet C P, Contreras M 1997 Haemolytic disease of the fetus and the newborn. In: Mollison P L, Engelfriet C P, Contreras M (eds) Blood transfusion in clinical medicine. Blackwell Science, Oxford, pp 390–424
129. Mollison P L, Engelfriet C P, Contreras M 1997 Blood transfusion in clinical medicine, 10th edn. Blackwell Science, Oxford
130. Na-Nakorn S P W 1970 Alpha-thalassaemia in Northern Thailand. American Journal of Human Genetics 22: 645–651
131. Naeye R L, Localio A R 1995 Determining the time before birth when ischemia and hypoxemia initiated cerebral palsy. Obstetrics and Gynecology 86: 713–719
132. Neligan G A, Russell J K 1954 Blood loss from the foetal circulation, a hazard of lower segment Caesarean section in cases of placenta previa. Journal of Obstetrics and Gynaecology of the British Empire 61: 206–212
133. Novak F 1953 Post-haemorrhagic shock in newborns during labour and after delivery. Acta Medica Jugoslavica 7: 280–292
134. Obladen M, Maier R, Segerer H et al 1991 Efficacy and safety of recombinant human erythropoietin to prevent the anaemias of prematurity. European Randomized Multicenter Trial. Contributions to Nephrology 88: 314–326
135. Ohls R K, Christensen R D 1991 Recombinant erythropoietin compared with erythrocyte transfusion in the treatment of anemia of prematurity. Journal of Pediatrics 119: 781–788
136. Ohls R K, Li Y, Trautman M S, Christensen R D 1994 Erythropoietin production by macrophages from preterm infants: implications regarding the cause of the anemia of prematurity. Pediatric Research 35: 169–170
137. Ohls R K, Osborne K A, Christensen R D 1995 Efficacy and cost analysis of treating very low birth weight infants with erythropoietin during their first two weeks of life: a randomized, placebo-controlled trial. Journal of Pediatrics 126: 421–426
138. Oski F A 1979 Nutritional anemias. Seminars in Perinatology 3: 381–395
139. Oski F A 1993 The erythrocyte and its disorders. In: Nathan D G, Oski F A (eds) Hematology of infancy and childhood. W B Saunders, Philadelphia, pp 18–43
140. Oski F A, Komazawa M 1975 Metabolism of the erythrocytes of the newborn infant. Seminars in Hematology 12: 209–221
141. Oski F A, Naiman J L (eds) 1982 Haematologic problems in the newborn, 3rd edn. W B Saunders, Philadelphia
142. Ovali F, Samanci N, Dagoglu T 1996 Management of late anemia in rhesus hemolytic disease: use of recombinant human erythropoietin (a pilot study). Pediatric Research 39: 831–834
143. Owa J A 1989 Relationship between exposure to icterogenic agents, glucose-6-phosphate dehydrogenase deficiency and neonatal jaundice in Nigeria. Acta Paediatrica Scandinavica 78: 848–852
144. Pasternack A, Furuhjelm V, Von Knoring J, Skrefvars B, Kuhlback B 1966 Acute renal failure after haemolysis probably due to foeto-maternal transfusion. Acta Medica Scandinavica 180: 13–15
145. Pembrey M E, Weatherall D J, Clegg J B, Bunch C, Perrine R P 1975 Haemoglobin Bart's in Saudi Arabia. British Journal of Haematology 29: 221–234
146. Penfold J B, Lipscomb J M 1943 Elliptocytosis in man, associated with hereditary telangiectasia. Quarterly Journal of Medicine 12: 157–167
147. Peterec S M 1995 Management of neonatal Rh disease. Clinics in Perinatology 22: 561–592
148. Phelan J P, Ock Ahn M, Korst L M, Martin G I 1995 Nucleated red blood cells: A marker for fetal asphyxia? American Journal of Obstetrics and Gynecology 173: 1380–1384
149. Phibbs R H, Keith J F I 1994 Recombinant human erythropoietin (r-HuEpo) stimulates erythropoiesis and reduces transfusions in preterm infants. Neonatology 155: 248A
150. Philipsborn H J J, Traisman H S, Greer D J 1955 Rupture of the spleen: a complication of erythroblastosis fetalis. New England Journal of Medicine 252: 158–162
151. Phillips H M, Holland B M, Jones J G, Abdel Moiz A L, Turner T L, Wardrop C A 1988 Definitive estimate of rate of hemoglobin switching: measurement of percent hemoglobin F in neonatal reticulocytes. Pediatric Research 23: 595–597
152. Playfair J H L, Wolfendale M R, Kay H E M 1963 The leucocytes of peripheral blood in the human fetus. British Journal of Haematology 9: 336–344
153. Race R R, Sanger R 1950 Blood groups in man. Blackwell Scientific, Oxford, pp 234–236

154. Rausen A R, Seki M, Strauss L 1965 Twin transfusion syndrome. Journal of Pediatrics 66: 613–628
155. Redman C M, Lee S 1995 The Kell blood group system. Transfusion Clinique et Biologique 2: 243–249
156. Roberts P D, James H, Petrie A, Morgan J O, Hoffbrand A V 1973 Vitamin B12 status in pregnancy among immigrants to Britain. British Medical Journal 3: 67–72
157. Robinson R J, Rossiter M A 1968 Massive subaponeurotic haemorrhage in babies of African origin. Archives of Disease in Childhood 43: 684–687
158. Robson S C, Lee D, Urbaniak S 1998 Anti-D immunoglobulin and RhD prophylaxis. British Journal of Obstetrics and Gynaecology 105: 129–134
159. Rodeck C H, Letsky E 1989 How the management of erythroblastosis fetalis has changed. British Journal of Obstetrics and Gynaecology 96: 759–763
160. Ronnholm K A, Siimes M A 1985 Haemoglobin concentration depends on protein intake in small preterm infants fed human milk. Archives of Disease in Childhood 60: 99–104
161. Rosse C, Kraemer M J, Dillon T L, McFarland R, Smith N J 1977 Bone marrow cell populations of normal infants; the predominance of lymphocytes. Journal of Laboratory and Clinical Medicine 89: 1225–1240
162. Sacks D A, Platt L D, Johnson C S 1981 Autoimmune hemolytic disease during pregnancy. American Journal of Obstetrics and Gynecology 140: 942–945
163. Scaradavou A, Inglis S, Peterson P, Dunne J, Chervenak F, Bussel J 1993 Suppression of erythropoiesis by intrauterine transfusions in hemolytic disease of the newborn: use of erythropoietin to treat the late anemia. Journal of Pediatrics 123: 279–284
164. Schumacher B, Moise K J J 1996 Fetal transfusion for red blood cell alloimmunization in pregnancy. Obstetrics and Gynecology 88: 137–150
165. Seip M 1960 Systemic lupus erythematosus in pregnancy with haemolytic anaemia, leucopenia, and thrombocytopenia in the mother and her newborn infant. Archives of Disease in Childhood 35: 364–366
166. Shannon K M 1990 Anemia of prematurity: progress and prospects. American Journal of Pediatric Hematology and Oncology 12: 14–20
167. Shannon K M, Keith J F, Mentzer W C, et al 1995 Recombinant human erythropoietin stimulates erythropoiesis and reduces erythrocyte transfusions in very low birth weight preterm infants. Pediatrics 95: 1–8
168. Shannon K M, Mentzer W C, Abels R I et al 1991 Recombinant human erythropoietin in the anemia of prematurity: results of a placebo-controlled pilot study. Journal of Pediatrics 118: 949–955
169. Shannon K M, Mentzer W C, Abels R I et al 1992 Enhancement of erythropoiesis by recombinant human erythropoietin in low birth weight infants: a pilot study. Journal of Pediatrics 120: 586–592
170. Shannon K M, Naylor G S, Torkildson J C et al 1987 Circulating erythroid progenitors in the anemia of prematurity. New England Journal of Medicine 317: 728–733
171. Sieff C A, Emerson S G, Mufson A, Gesner T G, Nathan D G 1986 Dependence of highly enriched human bone marrow progenitors on hemopoietic growth factors and their response to recombinant erythropoietin. Journal of Clinical Investigation 77: 74–81
172. Siimes M A 1981 A current perspective on the pathogenesis of iron deficiency in small children. European Journal of Pediatrics 137: 251–253
173. Soubasi V, Kremenopoulos G, Diamandi E, Tsantali C, Tsakiris D 1993 In which neonates does early recombinant human erythropoietin treatment prevent anemia of prematurity? Results of a randomized, controlled study. Pediatric Research 34: 675–679
174. Stamatoyannopoulos G, Nienhuis A W 1993 Haemoglobin switching. Part B, Cellular and molecular mechanisms. Alan R. Liss, New York
175. Stockman J A 1988 Erythropoietin: off again, on again. Journal of Pediatrics 112: 906–908
176. Stockman J A, Oski F A 1978 Physiological anaemia of infancy and the anaemia of prematurity. Clinics in Haematology 7: 3–18
177. Strauss R G 1995 Erythropoietin in the pathogenesis and treatment of neonatal anaemia. Transfusion 35: 68–73
178. Thilaganathan B, Athanasiou S, Ozmen S, Creighton S, Watson N R, Nicolaides K H 1994 Umbilical cord blood erythroblast count as an index of intrauterine hypoxia. Archives of Disease in Childhood 70: F192–F194
179. Thomas D E, Yoffey J M 1962 Human foetal haemopoiesis. I. The cellular composition of foetal blood. British Journal of Haematology 8: 290–295
180. Thomas R M, Canning C E, Cotes P M et al 1983 Erythropoietin and cord blood haemoglobin in the regulation of human fetal erythropoiesis. British Journal of Obstetrics and Gynaecology 90: 795–800
181. Thorp J A, O'Connor T, Callenbach J et al 1991 Hyporegenerative anemia associated with intrauterine transfusion in rhesus hemolytic disease. American Journal of Obstetrics and Gynecology 165: 79–81
182. Tovey L A D 1986 Haemolytic disease of the newborn – the changing scene. British Journal of Obstetrics and Gynaecology 93: 960–966
183. Tovey L A D, Townley A, Stevenson B J, Taverner J 1983 The Yorkshire antenatal anti-D immunoglobulin trial in primigravida. Lancet ii: 244–246
184. Turnbull E P N, Walker J 1955 Haemoglobin and red cells in the human foetus. Archives of Disease in Childhood 30: 102–110
185. Urbaniak S J 1985 Rh (D) haemolytic disease of the newborn: the changing scene. British Medical Journal 291: 4–6
186. Van Leeuwen G, Patney M 1969 Complications of umbilical vessel catheterisation: peritoneal perforation. Pediatrics 44: 1028–1030
187. Vaughan J I, Manning M, Warwick R M, Letsky E A, Murray N A, Roberts I A G 1998 Inhibition of erythroid progenitor cell growth by anti-Kell antibodies in fetal alloimmune anemia. New England Journal of Medicine 338: 798–803
188. Vaughan J I, Warwick R, Letsky E, Nicolini U, Rodeck C H, Fisk N M 1994 Erythropoietic suppression in fetal anemia because of Kell alloimmunization. American Journal of Obstetrics and Gynecology 171: 247–252
189. Walter T 1994 Effect of iron-deficiency anaemia on cognitive skills in infancy and childhood. Baillière's Clinical Haematology 7: 815–827
190. Weatherall D J 1991 Prenatal diagnosis of inherited blood disorders. In: Hann I, Gibson B, Letsky E A (eds) Fetal and neonatal haematology. Baillière Tindall, London, pp 285–314
191. Weiner C P, Widness J A 1996 Decreased fetal erythropoiesis and hemolysis in Kell hemolytic anemia. American Journal of Obstetrics and Gynecology 174: 547–551
192. Weiner C P, Williamson R A, Wenstrom K D, Sipes S L, Grant S S, Widness J A 1991 Management of fetal hemolytic disease by cordocentesis: I. Prediction of fetal anemia. American Journal of Obstetrics and Gynecology 165: 546–553
193. Wentworth P 1964 A placental lesion to account for foetal haemorrhage into the maternal circulation. Journal of Obstetrics and Gynaecology of the British Commonwealth 71: 379–387
194. Whittle M J 1996 Antenatal serology testing in pregnancy. British Journal of Obstetrics and Gynaecology 103: 195–196
195. Wickramasinghe S N, Illum N, Wimberley P D 1991 Congenital dyserythropoietic anaemia with novel intra-erythroblastic and intra-erythrocytic inclusions. British Journal of Haematology 79: 322–330
196. Williamson P, Griffiths G, Norfolk D, Levene M 1996 Blood transfusions and human recombinant erythropoietin in premature newborn infants. Archives of Disease in Childhood 75: F65–F68
197. Wood W G, Clegg J B, Weatherall D J 1977 Developmental biology of human hemoglobins., In: Brow E B (ed) Progress in hematology X. Grune & Stratton, New York, pp 43–90
198. Xanthou M 1970 Leucocyte blood picture in healthy full-term and premature babies during neonatal period. Archives of Disease in Childhood 45: 242–249
199. Zanjani E D, Poster J, Mann L I, Witsserman L R 1977 Regulation of erythropoiesis in the fetus. In: Fisher J W (ed) Kidney hormones. Vol. II, Erythropoietin. Academic Press, London, p 463
200. Zarkowsky H S, Mohandas N, Speaker C B, Shohet S B 1975 A congenital haemolytic anaemia with thermal sensitivity of the erythrocyte membrane. British Journal of Haematology 29: 537–543
201. Zipursky A 1984 Vitamin E deficiency anemia in newborn infants. Clinics in Perinatology 11: 393–402
202. Zipursky A, Brown E J, Watts J et al 1987 Oral vitamin E supplementation for the prevention of anemia in premature infants: a controlled trial. Pediatrics 79: 61–68
203. Zipursky A, Pollock J, Chown B, Israels L G 1963 Transplacental foetal haemorrhage after placental injury during delivery or amniocentesis. Lancet ii: 493–494

Part 3

Polycythaemia in the newborn

Elizabeth A. Letsky

INTRODUCTION

Polycythaemia in the neonatal period is a relatively common occurrence. Blood counts at birth or on the first day of life reveal many cases, only a fraction of whom develop overt clinical signs attributed to hyperviscosity.

Controversy centres on the need to screen all neonates within hours of birth[2] and whether or not prophylaxis of symptomless babies considered to be at risk has any effect on the incidence of late manifestations, such as cerebral defects affecting motor coordination and intellectual performance.

There is confusion among clinicians about which infants are likely to suffer effects in the neonatal period, and which, symptomatic or not, will have sequelae. The whole subject has been extensively reviewed over the years.[5,6,10,29,35,36,57]

DEFINITION

Polycythaemia and hyperviscosity are not synonymous terms. Three factors – the deformability of the red cells, the plasma viscosity and the haematocrit – determine the viscosity of the blood. Of these, the most important dependent variable affecting whole blood viscosity in the neonate is the haematocrit.[5,8] There is an almost linear relationship between viscosity and haematocrit below a haematocrit of 60–65%, but the relationship becomes exponential at higher haematocrits. Dunn[12] used a capillary haematocrit of 75% or greater to diagnose polycythaemia. A *central* venous haematocrit of 65% or more will, on in-vitro testing, prove to be hyperviscous; in contrast, hyperviscosity is never demonstrated, in vitro, in neonates with haematocrits below 60%. Blood with haematocrit values between 60 and 64% was shown to be hyperviscous on in-vitro examination in up to 23.0% of cases,[38] presumably because of the other variables that affect hyperviscosity. The red blood cells of the healthy neonate are less filtrable than those of normal adults. At low pH or in conditions of reduced oxygen tension the neonatal red cells become even less filtrable. Some babies have been shown to have hyperviscous blood on the basis of marked reduction in red cell filtrability.[16] Increases in osmolality and lipid concentrations will also result in increased whole blood viscosity.

INCIDENCE

The reported incidence of neonatal 'thick blood syndrome'[58] varies considerably depending on the criteria used for diagnosing the condition, which will be influenced by the age and maturity of the infant, the site of blood sampling and the method of analysis.[3,42,51] A central venous haematocrit of 65% or more is the generally accepted screening test today, but because the peripheral venous haematocrit is significantly higher than the central one, if a *peripheral* venous haematocrit of over 65% is used as a diagnostic screening test, the condition will be overdiagnosed. This may account for the fact that the majority of infants reported to have high haematocrits remain asymptomatic.[38] The incidence of polycythaemia from several prospective studies varies from 0.4% to 12%.[20,42,51] The overall incidence of hyperviscosity is not well established and reported prevalences vary from 4.0% to 0.4%.[3,38,51,62] A study of 494 healthy appropriate for gestational age newborns found that only 0.45% had venous haematocrits above 65%.[8]

TIMING OF HAEMATOCRIT DETERMINATION

The timing of the sampling for haematocrit estimation is obviously crucial to the diagnosis of 'at-risk' infants.[30,39,40] The haematocrit peaks at 2 hours and then decreases steadily, with significant changes occurring by 6 hours of age. The normal haematocrit of up to 70% for the term newborn at 2 hours of age is higher than that at birth or at 24 hours of age. Cord haematocrits of greater than 56% are associated with the development of polycythaemia, with a haematocrit of > 70% at 2 hours of age.[40,49,50]

METHOD OF HAEMATOCRIT DETERMINATION

Because viscosity determinations are unavailable to most physicians, venous haematocrit values are used to identify cases. However, if the haematocrit is determined by derivation of values obtained in an automatic electronic counter, the haematocrit is significantly lower than values obtained on the same sample by centrifugation. Inaccurate MCV estimation because of the poor deformability of the neonatal erythrocyte results in erroneous haematocrit calculations.[16] In one study the diagnosis of hyperviscosity would have been missed in 7 out of 10 infants if Coulter counter haematocrits of > 65% from venous blood had been used.[54] It is therefore strongly recommended that in infants with suspected hyperviscosity syndrome haematocrit values are measured by microcentrifugation.

Table 32.8 Neonatal polycythaemia

Active (increased intrauterine erythropoiesis)	**Passive (erythrocyte transfusion)**
Placental insufficiency	Maternal–fetal
Maternal smoking	Twin–twin
Maternal diabetes	Delayed cord clamping
Neonatal thyrotoxicosis	Unattended delivery
Congenital adrenal hyperplasia	
Chromosome abnormalities	

AETIOLOGY

The aetiology of hyperviscosity syndrome in the neonatal period is multifactorial, but the causes can be divided into two main groups, active and passive (Table 32.8, Fig. 32.8).

The active form occurs in those circumstances in which the fetus, in response to impaired placental function and/or intrauterine hypoxia[9,27,28,37,41,62] produces an increased number of red cells. The passive form develops when the fetus receives a transfusion. This may be maternal in origin, twin-to-twin, or result from delayed clamping of the cord (Table 32.8).

Maternal drugs such as propranolol have been incriminated,[13] but polycythaemia in the infant is probably due to the condition for which the mother is being treated. Hyperinsulinaemia in the fetus is associated with increased levels of erythropoietin.[59] Polycythaemia occurs frequently in the infants of mothers with both overt and gestational diabetes.[15,32,46,60] Down syndrome, trisomy 13 and trisomy 18 have all been associated with neonatal polycythaemia, thought to be the result of increased fetal erythropoietin activity. In Down syndrome a marked elevation of erythropoietin concentration has been reported. Other fetal conditions associated with polycythaemia include congenital hypothyroidism,[56] neonatal thyrotoxicosis and congenital adrenal hyperplasia.[36]

In normal term infants the most frequent cause of polycythaemia is delayed clamping of the cord. Infants with polycythaemia range in gestational age from 33 to 43 weeks. The condition is characteristically associated with the more mature infant, as the haematocrit rises with gestation. There is a higher incidence among term small-for-gestational-age infants and in postmature infants, compared to appropriate for gestational age term infants. Twin-to-twin transfusion is discussed in Chapter 25.

CLINICAL FINDINGS

The standard evaluation of newborn infants in most centres will not detect the majority of those who have polycythaemia and may therefore be at risk for hyperviscosity syndrome. When quiet these infants may not

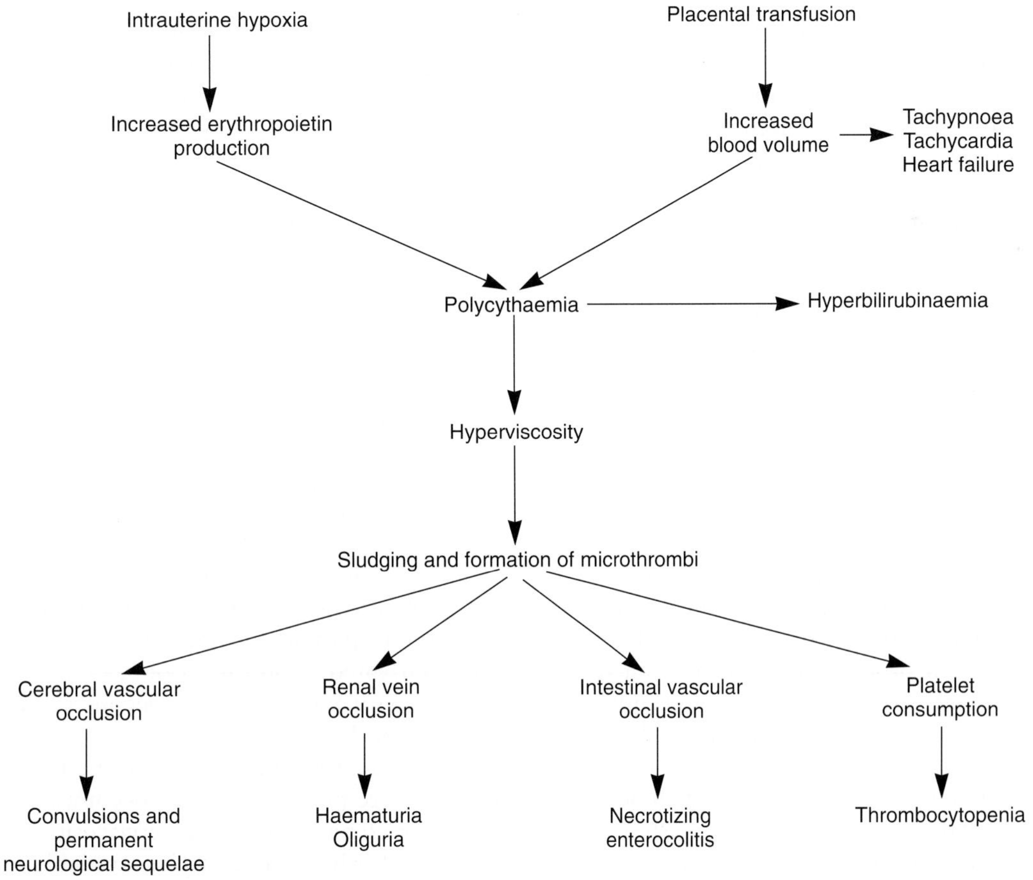

Fig. 32.8 Pathogenesis of polycythaemia and clinical manifestations of hyperviscosity in the newborn infant.

appear plethoric, and it is only when roused and active that they become very flushed or cyanosed. The signs usually become evident within the first 24 hours as the haematocrit rises as a result of a physiological decrease in plasma volume. The most consistent findings in newborns with established hyperviscosity are lethargy and hypotonia within 6 hours of birth, poor sucking, vomiting, difficulty in arousal, irritability when aroused, poor response to light, tremulousness and easy startlability. Some of these central nervous system signs and symptoms may be a result of the hypoglycaemia and hypocalcaemia[31] commonly associated with polycythaemia, rather than the direct result of a hyperviscosity itself. Observed complications include hyperbilirubinaemia with kernicterus due to breakdown of the increased red cell mass, heart failure, and problems due to vascular occlusion[44,45] (Fig. 32.8). Respiratory distress and cyanosis, together with congestive cardiac failure, may be severe enough to simulate cyanotic congenital heart disease. Thrombocytopenia is frequently observed, but it is not often associated with laboratory evidence of DIC and is thought to be due to local aggregation of platelets in the sluggish peripheral circulation.[22] In the full-blown syndrome thrombi in the peripheral circulation lead to tissue anoxia, with seizures,[1] priapism and testicular infarction,[21] renal vein thrombosis, renal failure,[19] gangrene,[45] distal bowel obstruction[25] and necrotizing enterocolitis.[17,63,64]

Follow-up studies do not differentiate the sequelae of polycythaemia per se from its antecedents. Late neurological sequelae described include running and laughing fits,[52] fine motor and speech abnormalities, spastic diplegia[7] and significant neurodevelopmental abnormalities. In addition, a prospective control study has shown significant lower achievement in terms of IQ scores, arithmetic and reading achievement at 7 years in 49 children with hyperviscosity in the neonatal period, compared with 40 controls.[11] However, most publications agree that in untreated neonatal polycythaemia with minor or no symptoms, significant late neurological manifestations are very rare.[4]

MANAGEMENT

Symptomatic infants with hyperviscosity require treatment in order to relieve the immediate clinical symptoms and perhaps to avoid late neurological sequelae. Dramatic improvement has been observed in patients with respiratory disturbance, cardiac failure, gastrointestinal and central nervous system signs and symptoms. The aim is to lower the haematocrit and thereby the viscosity. Partial exchange transfusion is performed, removing whole blood and replacing it with equal volumes of fresh (frozen) plasma or a plasma substitute to achieve a haematocrit of 55%, which is considered to be a 'safe' level.

An active area of controversy concerns the ideal replacement diluent fluid. Both HAS and FFP are widely used.[26] In addition, crystalloids have been favourably assessed in one Munich centre.[43] FFP has been advocated in infants with polycythaemia because they can develop sepsis associated with coagulopathy, and FFP provides not only coagulation factors but fibronectin, complement, opsonins and protease inhibitors, which enhance neutrophil function and may be deficient in these infants.

The argument against the use of FFP, which is after all the physiological diluent, is the very small risk in the UK of viral transmission[61] (p. 841). It is also argued that HAS has lower levels of fibrinogen than FFP, and will therefore be more effective in correcting hyperviscosity.[57]

The beneficial effect of partial exchange transfusion with human albumin has been reported.[23] There are no published randomized controlled trials of FFP vs. HAS in the management of polycythaemia/hyperviscosity syndromes in the neonate. Some units in the UK continue to use FFP from well characterized donors, which is our preferred diluent, but in the USA commercial plasma derivatives such as albumin are considered to be safer alternatives.

The formula used to calculate the volume to be exchanged is:

$$\text{Total blood volume} \times \frac{(\text{observed Hct} - \text{desired Hct})}{\text{observed Hct}}$$

assuming the neonatal blood volume to be 85 ml/kg.[29] Usually the volume exchanged is around 20 ml/kg. The exchange can be performed in 10 ml aliquots.

Although there is no doubt about the necessity or immediate efficacy of partial exchange transfusion in symptomatic infants, the problem of management arises in those who have been identified as having significant polycythaemia with or without hyperviscosity, and who are symptom free. These infants may be at risk particularly of late neurological sequelae. Do these patients receive 'prophylactic' exchange transfusion? Some paediatricians are in favour of universal screening and prompt treatment of any neonate with polycythaemia.[1,14] A beneficial effect on cerebral blood flow using partial plasma exchange transfusion has been demonstrated.[3,4,24] Improvements have also been documented in capillary perfusion[34,55] and cardiac function.[33] Others have been unable to demonstrate any significant benefit in babies with hyperviscosity but with no symptoms who have undergone partial exchange transfusion, compared with an untreated control group.[7,14,20,53] An increased incidence of necrotizing enterocolitis following exchange transfusion has been reported[6] but not confirmed.[18] It is felt by some that this fact should be taken into consideration before plasma exchange becomes an accepted treatment for all patients with hyperviscosity.[57]

Until further experience is available, the benefits of prophylactic exchange transfusion must remain speculative.[11] Because of the lack of evidence that plasma exchange benefits asymptomatic polycythaemic infants, the American Academy of Pediatrics[2] does not recommend routine screening of haematocrits in the term infant.[2]

SCREENING

There is no case for routine screening of all newborn infants for polycythaemia, but those at special risk of developing hyperviscosity, i.e. small and large for gestational age, infants of diabetic mothers, infants of mothers with pre-eclampsia and twins may have at least a blood count if they are admitted to the SCBU for the maternal or neonatal condition that put them at risk, or for clinical manifestations. It has been suggested that because of the changing haematocrit in the first few hours of life, significant results are not obtained until 8 hours post delivery.[48] If the capillary haematocrit is more than 65–70% a venous haematocrit should be performed. Those infants with a venous haematocrit of more than 65% established by microcentrifugation,[54] as well as a small proportion of those with venous haematocrits between 60 and 65%, will have hyperviscous blood. In laboratories with the facility, blood viscosity should be measured in these infants, who should be carefully examined for symptoms and signs of hyperviscosity. Symptoms are not usually present at birth but develop during the first 24 hours, when the concentration of red cells rises secondary to absorption of excess plasma. It is very unusual for symptoms to develop after the first 48 hours of life.[47] In addition, the blood sugar, calcium and bilirubin should be estimated. In this respect infants 3–4 days old may develop hyperbilirubinaemia because of transient polycythaemia but will no longer be polycythaemic at the time of identification.[38]

SUGGESTED PRACTICAL APPROACH

Healthy term infants appear to be at little risk of polycythaemia and hyperviscosity and need not be routinely screened.[2,8] In units where only the babies known to be at risk of significant polycythaemia are screened the paediatrician must remain constantly alert to early clinical signs of the condition. In those identified polycythaemic babies with mild or no symptoms of hyperviscosity, keeping the baby warm and well hydrated is probably all that is required to prevent sludging in the peripheral circulation.[22] All infants with significant symptoms should undergo partial exchange with fresh-frozen plasma or a substitute in order to bring the haematocrit down to a safe level of 55%.

REFERENCES

1. Allen J P, Chilcote R 1979 Transient erythrocytosis during the neonatal period: possible neurologic complications. Southern Medical Journal 72: 681–683
2. American Academy of Pediatrics Committee on Fetus and Newborn 1993 Routine evaluation of blood pressure, hematocrit, and glucose in newborns. Pediatrics 92: 474–476
3. Bada H S, Korones S B, Kolni H W et al 1986 Partial plasma exchange transfusion improves cerebral hemodynamics in symptomatic neonatal polycythemia. American Journal of the Medical Sciences 291: 157–163
4. Bada H S, Korones S B, Pourcyrous M et al 1992 Asymptomatic syndrome of polycythemic hyperviscosity: effect of partial plasma exchange transfusion. Journal of Pediatrics 120: 579–585
5. Black V D 1987 Neonatal hyperviscosity syndromes. Current Problems in Pediatrics 17: 73–130
6. Black V D, Lubchenco L O 1982 Neonatal polycythemia and hyperviscosity. Pediatric Clinics of North America 29: 1137–1148
7. Black V D, Lubchenco L O, Luckey D W et al 1982 Developmental and neurologic sequelae of neonatal hyperviscosity syndrome. Pediatrics 69: 426–431
8. Brooks G I, Backes C R 1981 Hyperviscosity secondary to polycythemia in the appropriate for gestational age neonate. Journal of the American Osteopathic Association 80: 415–418
9. Bureau M A, Shapcott D, Berthiaume Y et al 1983 Maternal cigarette smoking and fetal oxygen transport: a study of P50, 2,3-diphosphoglycerate, total hemoglobin, hematocrit, and type F hemoglobin in fetal blood. Pediatrics 72: 22–26
10. Danish E D 1986 Neonatal polycythemia. In: Brown EB (ed) Progress in hematology. Grune & Stratton, New York, pp 55–98
11. Delaney Black V, Camp B W, Lubchenco L O et al 1989 Neonatal hyperviscosity association with lower achievement and IQ scores at school age. Pediatrics 83: 662–667
12. Dunn P M 1970 Neonatal polycythaemia. Archives of Disease in Childhood 45: 273
13. Gladstone G R, Hordof A, Gersony W M 1975 Propranolol administration during pregnancy: effects on the fetus. Journal of Pediatrics 86: 962–964
14. Goldberg K, Wirth F H, Hathaway W E et al 1982 Neonatal hyperviscosity. II. Effect of partial plasma exchange transfusion. Pediatrics 69: 419–425
15. Green D W, Khoury J, Mimouni F 1992 Neonatal hematocrit and maternal glycemic control in insulin-dependent diabetes. Journal of Pediatrics 120: 302–305
16. Gross G P, Hathaway W E 1972 Fetal erythrocyte deformability. Pediatric Research 6: 593–599
17. Hakanson D O, Oh W 1977 Necrotizing enterocolitis and hyperviscosity in the newborn infant. Journal of Pediatrics 90: 458–461
18. Hein H A, Lathrop S S 1987 Partial exchange transfusion in term, polycythemic neonates: absence of association with severe gastrointestinal injury. Pediatrics 80: 75–78
19. Herson V C, Raye J R, Rowe J C, Philipps A F 1982 Acute renal failure associated with polycythemia in a neonate. Journal of Pediatrics 100: 137–139
20. Host A, Ulrich M 1982 Late prognosis in untreated neonatal polycythaemia with minor or no symptoms. Acta Paediatrica Scandinavica 71: 629–633
21. Jung A L, McGaughey H R, Matlak M E 1980 Neonatal testicular infarction and polycythemia. Journal of Urology 123: 781–782
22. Katz J, Rodriguez E, Mandani G, Branson H E 1982 Normal coagulation findings, thrombocytopenia, and peripheral hemoconcentration in neonatal polycythemia. Journal of Pediatrics 101: 99–102
23. Levy I, Merlob P, Ashkenazi S, Reisner S H 1990 Neonatal polycythemia: effect of partial dilutional exchange transfusion with human albumin on whole blood viscosity. European Journal of Pediatrics 149: 354–355
24. Maertzdorf W J, Tangelder G J, Slaaf D W, Blanco C E 1989 Effects of partial plasma exchange transfusion on cerebral blood flow velocity in polycythemic preterm, term and small for date newborn infants. European Journal of Pediatrics 148: 774–778
25. Malinowski B C, Kleinman L I 1979 Polycythemia in the newborn first observed as distal bowel obstruction. American Journal of Diseases of Children 133: 962–963
26. McClure G 1991 The use of plasma in the neonatal period [editorial]. Archives of Disease in Childhood 66: 373–374
27. Meberg A 1989 Hematologic syndrome of growth-retarded infants [letter; comment]. American Journal of Diseases in Childhood 143: 1260
28. Meberg A, Haga P, Sande H, Foss O P 1979 Smoking during pregnancy – hematological observations in the newborn. Acta Paediatrica Scandinavica 68: 731–734

29. Mentzer W C 1978 Polycythaemia and the hyperviscosity syndrome in newborn infants. Clinics in Haematology 7: 63–74
30. Merlob P 1989 Postnatal alteration in hematocrit and viscosity in normal infants and in those with polycythemia [letter]. Journal of Pediatrics 114: 169–170
31. Merlob, P, Amir J 1989 Pathogenesis of hypocalcemia in neonatal polycythemia. Medical Hypotheses 30: 49–50
32. Mimouni F, Miodovnik M, Siddiqi T A, Butler J B, Holroyde J, Tsang R C 1986 Neonatal polycythemia in infants of insulin-dependent diabetic mothers. Obstetrics and Gynecology 68: 370–372
33. Murphy D J Jr, Reller M D, Meyer R A, Kaplan S 1985 Effects of neonatal polycythemia and partial exchange transfusion on cardiac function: an echocardiographic study. Pediatrics 76: 909–913
34. Norman M, Fagrell B, Herin P 1992 Effects of neonatal polycythemia and hemodilution on capillary perfusion. Journal of Pediatrics 121: 103–108
35. Oh W 1986 Neonatal polycythemia and hyperviscosity. Pediatric Clinics of North America 33: 523–532
36. Oski F A 1982 Polycythemia and hyperviscosity in the neonatal period. In: Oski F A, Naiman J L (eds) Hematologic problems of the newborn. WB Saunders, Philadelphia, pp 87–96
37. Philip A G, Tito A M 1989 Increased nucleated red blood cell counts in small for gestational age infants with very low birth weight. American Journal of Diseases of Children 143: 164–169
38. Ramamurthy R S 1979 Neonatal polycythemia and hyperviscosity: state of the art. Perinatology–Neonatology 3: 38–40
39. Ramamurthy R S 1989 Postnatal alteration in hematocrit and viscosity in normal infants and in those with polycythemia. Journal of Pediatrics 114: 169–170
40. Ramamurthy R S, Berlanga M 1987 Postnatal alteration in hematocrit and viscosity in normal and polycythemic infants. Journal of Pediatrics 110: 929–934
41. Rawlings J S, Pettett G, Wiswell T E, Clapper J 1982 Estimated blood volumes in polycythemic neonates as a function of birth weight. Journal of Pediatrics 101: 594–599
42. Reisner S H, Mor N, Levy Y, Merlob P 1983 Incidence of neonatal polycythemia. Israel Journal of Medical Sciences 19: 848–849
43. Roithmaier A, Arlettaz R, Bauer K et al 1995 Randomized controlled trial of Ringer solution versus serum for partial exchange transfusion in neonatal polycythemia. European Journal of Pediatrics 154: 53–56
44. Schmidt B, Zipursky A 1984 Thrombotic disease in newborn infants. Clinics in Perinatology 11: 461–488
45. Scott F, Evans N 1995 Distal gangrene in a polycythemic recipient fetus in twin–twin transfusion. Obstetrics and Gynecology 86: 677–679
46. Shannon K, Davis J C, Kitzmiller J L, Fulcher S A, Koenig H M 1986 Erythropoiesis in infants of diabetic mothers. Pediatric Research 20: 161–165
47. Sheftel D N 1981 Neonatal polycythemia and the hyperviscosity syndrome. Wisconsin Medical Journal 80: 39–40
48. Shohat M, Merlob P, Reisner S H 1982 Neonatal polycythemia [letter]. Pediatrics 70: 155–156
49. Shohat M, Merlob P, Reisner S H 1984 Neonatal polycythemia: I. Early diagnosis and incidence relating to time of sampling. Pediatrics 73: 7–10
50. Shohat M, Reisner S H, Mimouni F, Merlob P 1984 Neonatal polycythemia: II. Definition related to time of sampling. Pediatrics 73: 11–13
51. Stevens K, Wirth F H 1980 Incidence of neonatal hyperviscosity at sea level. Journal of Pediatrics 97: 118–119
52. Sugimoto T, Matsumura T, Sakamoto Y, Taniuchi K 1979 Running and laughing fits as the sequelae of the neonatal hyperviscosity syndrome. Brain and Development 1: 323–326
53. Van Der Elst C, Molteno C D, Malan A F, de V Heese H 1980 The management of polycythaemia in the newborn infant. Early Human Development 4: 393–403
54. Villalta I A, Pramanik A K, Diaz Blanco J, Herbst J J 1989 Diagnostic errors in neonatal polycythemia based on method of hematocrit determination. Journal of Pediatrics 115: 460–462
55. Waffarn F, Tolle C D, Huxtable R F 1984 Effects of polycythemia and hyperviscosity on cutaneous blood flow and transcutaneous PO_2 and PCO_2 in the neonate. Pediatrics 74: 389–394
56. Weinblatt M E, Fort P, Kochen J, DiMayio M 1987 Polycythemia in hypothyroid infants. American Journal of Diseases of Children 141: 1121–1123
57. Werner E J 1995 Neonatal polycythemia and hyperviscosity. Clinics in Perinatology 22: 693–710
58. Wesenberg R L 1978 Neonatal 'thick blood' syndrome. Hospital Practice 13: 137–140
59. Widness J A, Susa J B, Garcia J F et al 1981 Increased erythropoiesis and elevated erythropoietin in infants born to diabetic mothers and in hyperinsulinemic rhesus fetuses. Journal of Clinical Investigation 67: 637–642
60. Widness J A, Teramo K A, Clemons G K et al 1990 Direct relationship of antepartum glucose control and fetal erythropoietin in human type 1 (insulin-dependent) diabetic pregnancy. Diabetologia 33: 378–383
61. Williamson L, Heptonstall J, Soldan K 1996 A SHOT in the arm for safer blood transfusion. British Medical Journal 313: 1221–1222
62. Wirth F H, Goldberg K E, Lubchenco L O 1979 Neonatal hyperviscosity: I. Incidence. Pediatrics 63: 833–836
63. Wiswell T E, Cornish J D 1986 Fresh frozen plasma partial exchange transfusion and necrotizing enterocolitis [letter]. Pediatrics 77: 786–787
64. Wiswell T E, Robertson C F, Jones T A, Tuttle D J 1988 Necrotizing enterocolitis in full-term infants. A case-control study. American Journal of Diseases of Children 142: 532–535

Part 4

Use of blood products

Elizabeth A. Letsky

INTRODUCTION

The indications for transfusion in the fetus and neonate, and the procedures undertaken by the blood bank to provide for these needs, have changed considerably over recent years. With the introduction of techniques that make the fetal circulation accessible (Chapter 14), intravascular transfusion of blood components has become a reality from as early as 18 weeks' gestation. Conversely, after birth there has been a dramatic reduction in the number of exchange transfusions required, in particular for haemolytic disease of the newborn. At the same time, the survival of very small preterm infants has resulted in the need for component therapy to manage the unique complications of this period.[22] (Fig. 32.9).

Newborn infants on special care baby units, whether term or preterm, are more likely to be transfused than any other patient in hospital. Transfusion in the preterm infant is needed to treat hypotension and replace blood

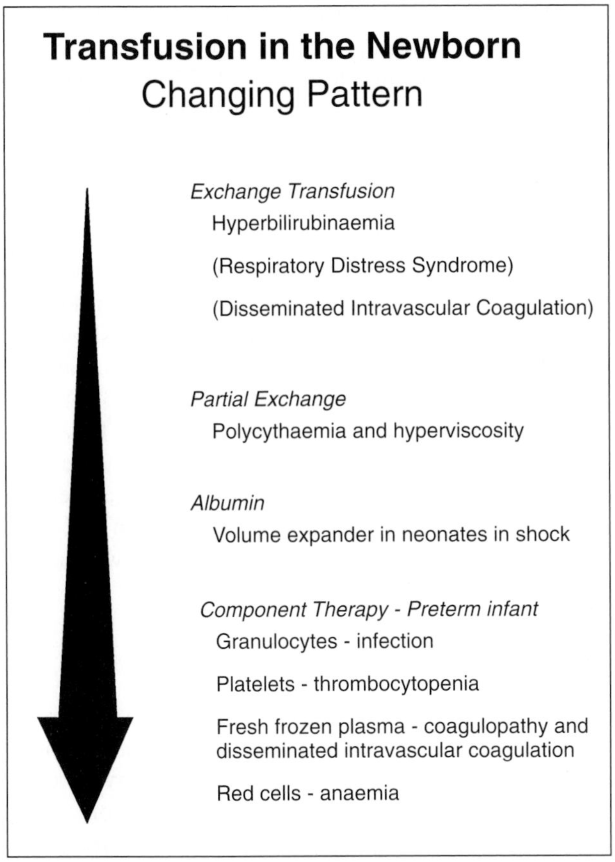

Transfusion in the Newborn
Changing Pattern
Exchange Transfusion
Hyperbilirubinaemia
(Respiratory Distress Syndrome)
(Disseminated Intravascular Coagulation)
Partial Exchange
Polycythaemia and hyperviscosity
Albumin
Volume expander in neonates in shock
Component Therapy - Preterm infant
Granulocytes - infection
Platelets - thrombocytopenia
Fresh frozen plasma - coagulopathy and disseminated intravascular coagulation
Red cells - anaemia

Fig. 32.9 Transfusion in the newborn – changing pattern.

loss from laboratory testing, FFP is given for coagulation problems and hypovolaemia, and platelets for symptomatic or hazardous thrombocytopenia. Transfusion of granulocytes to neutropenic infants with bacterial sepsis remains controversial and GCSF is still under investigation. All blood components for transfusion in the neonatal period make special demands on the regional service to provide small aliquots with minimal metabolic changes free from the risk of transmitting infection or the rare hazard of graft versus host disease. Guidelines for transfusion in these complex circumstances are not clear, and vary depending on local practice and the availability of suitable blood products and growth factors, rather than on controlled scientific investigations.[11,23,33]

RED CELL TRANSFUSION

The majority of transfusions are given to sick premature infants to treat hypotension and hypovolaemia, to replace blood withdrawn for laboratory testing, and because of their deficient erythropoietin response (see above). There is much to suggest[31] that the haemoglobin in such babies should be kept higher than 13 g/100 ml (PCV ≥ 40%).

Data are accumulating which suggest that morbidity, complications and costs can be reduced in the preterm infant by ensuring that the circulating red cell mass will meet the calculated physiological requirements. This can be achieved by optimum placentofetal transfusion at birth,[21] together with adequate single-donor blood transfusion when needed so as to reduce repeated small aliquot requirements. This whole question is well discussed in a recent review.[35]

It should be remembered that a blood transfusion is likely to be one of a series. The first will increase the concentration of HbA, shift the oxygen dissociation curve to the right, and lower the oxygen affinity of the circulating haemoglobin. This will then depress red cell production further and increase the delay before erythropoiesis is reactivated.

In older preterm infants with the anaemia of prematurity, the indications for transfusion are less clear-cut.

Ideally the indications should be based on assessing red cell mass or central venous oxygen tension,[16,20,30] but most nurseries do not have the facilities to measure these and until more precise guidelines are available the physician will continue to have to make clinical decisions based on the following:

1. For critically ill babies in intensive care:
   - All blood taken should be carefully recorded, and if 5–10% of the baby's blood volume is removed over a short space of time it should be replaced with packed red cells.
   - These babies may need to have their haemoglobin maintained in the range of 13–14 g/dl to ensure sufficient differential between arterial and venous oxygen tension, and an adequate blood pressure, cardiac output and tissue perfusion.[33]
2. For convalescent VLBW babies (p. 395) the haemoglobin should be measured on entry to the nursery and at regular (minimum weekly) intervals thereafter; the haemoglobin will drop 1 g/dl (on average) per week. Do not transfuse on level of haemoglobin alone. Although haemoglobin values of 7.0 g/dl or less require explanation, they may not need correction. Consider transfusion for late anaemia if:
   - weight gain is poor;
   - fatigue while feeding is noted;
   - tachypnoea and tachycardia are present.

Most transfusions are currently administered to those infants with birthweight less than 1.0 kg. For example, only 30% of infants weighing 1.0–1.3 kg at birth in an Iowa nursery (1993–4) were transfused, and this occurred without the use of recombinant r-HuEpo,[34] which may decrease the numbers of transfusions even further (pp. 810–812).[23] The results of a recent double-blind placebo-controlled study[32] of 158 infants under 1250 g at birth, of gestational age < 31 weeks, from 11 centres in the USA demonstrated quite clearly that the use of recombinant r-HuEpo reduces the number of red cell transfusions in very low-birthweight infants. A 1996 review of the published results of the use of r-HuEpo in the preterm neonate[38] shows that r-HuEpo has a role in reducing the need for transfusion in the anaemia of prematurity, but will not affect the need to replace blood loss due to massive iatrogenic blood-letting in the first weeks of life. The modest reduction in the number of red cell transfusions may be neither clinically useful nor cost-effective (p. 812).

COMPLICATIONS OF BLOOD TRANSFUSION

In principle all of the hazards associated with transfusion apply to the newborn, but there are, in addition, special complications and risks arising from the small size of the recipient, exposure to multiple donors[5] and increased vulnerability to transfusion-transmitted infection and metabolic disturbances due to the infant's immaturity.[33] There are also ill-defined risks arising from the immunological status of the VLBW infant, such as GVHD.[15]

METABOLIC PROBLEMS

On storage of blood in the anticoagulant CPD, the pH will fall in the first week from 7.0 to 6.8, and to 6.7 on 3 weeks' storage. The serum potassium level may reach 10 mmol/l by the end of the first week, but the 2,3-DPG levels are maintained during this time. The adult recipient can quickly adjust these adverse metabolic changes on storage of blood, but the immature neonate may find it a problem. Massive transfusions, as in exchange transfusions, can result in systemic acidosis followed by rebound alkalosis. Citrate binding results in hypocalcaemia, which is only occasionally symptomatic, and hypomagnesaemia. In addition, after exchange transfusion there is hyperglycaemia followed by rebound hypoglycaemia.

Another potential problem is the fact that the sodium content of CPD-stored blood is elevated. Because of these problems with CPD anticoagulation in the newborn, the use of heparin has been advocated. This has major disadvantages: blood taken into heparin has to be used within 12 hours of donation, tests for hepatitis and HIV have to be carried out on the donor before the blood is taken, and other components (e.g. FFP and platelets) cannot be obtained from heparinized fresh blood. Heparin is therefore no longer used in the UK.

More recently, whole blood taken into CPD has all the plasma removed for maximum production of components at the regional blood transfusion centre, and the red cells are resuspended in an additive solution containing sodium chloride, adenine, glucose and mannitol, known as SAG-M. The resulting red cell concentrate shelf-life is extended from 4 (28 days) to 5 weeks (35 days). When first introduced,[24] these preparations were thought to be unsuitable for neonates but they are now known to be safe for small 'top-up' transfusions. The metabolic disturbances are negligible and probably less than those observed with CPD red cell suspensions. They are, however, not suitable for exchange transfusion, when CPD blood should still be used.

The increased risks of multiple small RBC top-up transfusions can be reduced by prolonging the shelf-life of red cells to 35 days, and also by introducing multipacks with eight satellites (octopus) dedicated to one infant.[6,33]

A recent pilot study in a UK hospital has shown how this use of dedicated multipacks and prolongation of shelf-life reduced donor exposure from 4.9 ± 3.5 to 2.0 ± 0.9.[39] Similar results have been shown in the USA.[4] It is interesting that plasma potassium levels, the main metabolic complication feared in the past, were not significantly different following transfusion of blood stored for up to 35 days compared to blood with a shelf-life of 5 days or less.[39]

RED CELL INJURY

Haemolysis, caused by physical injury to the erythrocyte, is the usual cause of what appears to be a haemolytic transfusion reaction in the newborn. This may be caused by forcing red cells though a fine-bore needle or catheter, or by excessive heating in a blood warmer. Rarely a true immunohaemolytic transfusion reaction occurs; when this happens it is invariably the result of a clerical error.

ALLOIMMUNIZATION TO RED BLOOD CELL AND WHITE CELL ANTIGENS

Studies have shown that neonates do not readily form alloantibodies to either red cell or white cell antigens. Provided that there are no atypical antibodies demonstrable in maternal serum, and that the direct antiglobulin test (Coombs') on the infant's red cells is negative, a conventional first cross-match with maternal serum is unnecessary. Most regional transfusion centres provide group O Rh-D-negative units suitable for small top-up transfusions for all infants other than those with HDN. Recent guidelines[6] state that it is not necessary to continue donor red cell compatibility tests with the infant's serum for neonatal top-up transfusions because these do not result in the formation of red cell blood group antibodies. This results in a significant reduction in unnecessary blood-letting and laboratory workload.

As far as anti-HLA antibodies are concerned, a prospective study of 57 preterm infants has shown that some, but not all, have the ability to produce anti-HLA antibodies in response to multiple blood transfusions.[3] It has been recommended that a small-bore inline filter (Alpha-Micron-20) be used when administering transfusions.[39] The resulting leukocyte depletion will further reduce the risk of transmission of cell-associated viruses, e.g. HIV and CMV microaggregates which increase on storage will also be removed. This is of importance in preterm infants because the microaggregates are sequestered in the pulmonary vasculature. Many products for neonatal use, and all products for fetal use are now filtered before release from the transfusion centre.

TRANSMISSION OF INFECTION[18]

Viral hepatitis

Post-transfusion hepatitis is the most common and serious of all the problems associated with the transfusion of blood and blood products. In the preterm neonate the risk is increased for a chronic carrier state and for the development of cirrhosis and hepatic carcinoma, which may develop up to 17 years after infection with hepatitis C. The risk of hepatitis C-infectious donations entering the blood supply in England in 1996 for any reason has been calculated to be 1 in more than 200 000.[37] The risk is probably even less with the routine use of well characterized donors for neonatal and fetal transfusion.

CMV infection

Approximately 60% of all blood donors in the UK are CMV antibody positive. Unfortunately, this does not mean that their blood confers passive immunity, and transfusion-acquired CMV infection in premature newborns may be associated with significant morbidity and even mortality (p. 1162).

The infectivity of donor blood can be cut down by selecting CMV-negative donors, or by transfusing frozen or leukocyte-depleted red cells. It would appear that it is difficult to identify the potentially dangerous carrier of live virus within the 60% of donors who are antibody positive, therefore they must all be rejected if transfusion transmission is to be avoided. However, blood which has been stored at 4°C for 48 hours is much less likely to transmit CMV infection than fresh blood, even if there is live virus in the blood when collected from the donor. All blood for neonatal and intrauterine transfusion supplied by our and most other regional transfusion services in the UK is from documented CMV-negative donors.

Transmission of human immunodeficiency virus[10]

There are only two modes of transmission of HIV infection so far documented in the neonate:

- Parenteral contact with blood and blood products;
- Vertical transmission from an infected mother to her infant.

The first reported case of neonatally acquired AIDS came from California in 1982. A 20-month-old white boy, born preterm, who had received multiple top-up transfusions in the special care baby unit, developed hepatosplenomegaly, neutropenia, autoimmune haemolytic anaemia, thrombocytopenia, in vitro evidence of T-cell dysfunction, and opportunistic infection. One of the donors, although symptom free at the time, subsequently developed AIDS and died.[10]

There have been no cases of AIDS in the UK resulting from blood transfusion in the neonatal period, and the likelihood of a neonate acquiring AIDS from donor blood in the UK remains remote. The risk in 1987, estimated at less than 1 in 1 000 000 donations,[1] has now been even further reduced to 1 in more than 2 000 000 donations.[37] This is less than the risk of developing or dying from hepatitis, or being infected with CMV from the donor blood.

GRAFT VERSUS HOST DISEASE

GVHD has been described after transfusions of red cells, white cells, platelets, plasma exchange and intrauterine transfusion. In the neonate the clinical picture is one of skin rash, hepatitis and marrow aplasia. Lymphocyte engraftment in GVHD is directly related to the number of viable lymphocytes transfused.

It is possible to reduce the lymphocyte concentration in packed red cell transfusions by washing, filtration and freezing in glycerol, but GVHD can only be totally prevented by irradiation. However, potassium leakage from stored red cells postirradiation occurs, and there are no data to suggest that routine irradiation of blood for simple top-up transfusions to immunocompetent preterm infants is necessary.[2,25] There has been one report of fatal GVHD in an 855 g infant born at 25 weeks' gestation who received multiple small transfusions.[14] Evidence of donor engraftment was obtained by HLA and recombinant DNA analysis. The female infant was apparently genetically immunocompetent. GVHD is more likely to occur if first-degree relatives are used as donors, and this is a potent argument against using parental blood for transfusion. There are only two case reports in the UK of infants who developed GVHD following intrauterine transfusions for rhesus disease from a unit where repeated transfusions of non-irradiated maternal blood were given.[19] Guidelines recommend that all blood components for intrauterine transfusion should be irradiated. However, personal experience and that of others[7] has shown that, provided the transfused blood is from an unrelated donor and the fetus is immunocompetent (if immature), the risk of GVHD is negligible.

Although rare in normal preterm babies, it is obvious that the genetically immunocompromised fetus and neonate will be at increased risk from GVHD, and for these babies all blood products should be routinely irradiated before transfusion. GVHD has occasionally been reported following exchange transfusion in infants, particularly in those who have had prior intrauterine transfusions.[29,36] At the time of writing there are, however, no data to suggest that routine irradiation of all packed red cells before transfusion into very preterm infants is required.[36]

NECROTIZING ENTEROCOLITIS AND TRANSFUSION

Rare haemolytic transfusion reactions have been described in association with NEC and transfusion of blood products. Activation of the T antigen site of circulating red cells may occur as a result of bacteraemia in NEC, and it has been postulated that destruction of these autologous T-activated cells is brought about by naturally occurring anti-T present in all donor plasma. However, the haemolytic potential of anti-T is not firmly established,[27] and the issue is further complicated by the fact that intravascular haemolysis can be brought about by organisms such as *Clostridium perfringens*, sometimes associated with NEC, without involving anti-T in transfused plasma. The general consensus of those who have worked with neonates for 20 years or more on both sides of the Atlantic is that there is little objective evidence to justify withholding plasma products where indicated, or for routine screening for T-activation in infants suffering from NEC. If laboratory identification supports the diagnosis of T-activation in the rare infant with NEC who is haemolysing, transfusion of any product containing plasma should be avoided.[6] 'Top-up' red cell concentrates in SAG-M optimum additive solution will present no hazard in this situation, because virtually all the plasma has been removed.

PLATELET TRANSFUSION

Thrombocytopenia may result from sepsis or DIC and can be a complication of alloimmune and autoimmune processes resulting from fetal maternal interactions. Immune thrombocytopenias require specific therapy (p. 802).

Prophylactic transfusions are recommended at counts below 30×10^9/l, or in very sick infants even below 50×10^9/l.[36] A platelet concentrate from one donor is suspended in 50 ml plasma and contains more than enough platelets to correct the thrombocytopenia. The current recommendation from our regional transfusion centre is to raise the platelet count using the maximum tolerated volume of platelet suspension from a donor 50 ml aliquot. This will raise the platelet count as efficiently as a miniconcentrate. One point which seems to elude the stressed paediatric SHO on call is that platelets should *never* be stored in the refrigerator, so if they are on the unit awaiting administration they should be kept at room temperature. New developments will inevitably include the use of growth factors (meg-CSF),[12] but it will be some time before products are developed for safe routine administration in the nursery.

GRANULOCYTE TRANSFUSION

Although transfused donor granulocytes have been shown to be beneficial in the management of severe neonatal sepsis,[8] the technical problems of transfusing fresh preparations (the only effective mode of therapy) from the donor to the sick infant makes this form of treatment impractical in the majority of neonatal units in the UK. Recombinant cytokines and G-CSF have been shown to be effective in other situations where there is neutropenia or defects in neutrophil function, and trials of their use in the management of sepsis in the neonate are being reported.[9]

FRESH FROZEN PLASMA

The need for volume expansion occurs frequently in sick neonates. HAS and FFP are frequently used. FFP is not the component of choice for volume expansion in adults or children, but there is a case for using FFP in the immature neonate. Many of these sick babies are suffering from sepsis and may also have a coagulopathy. FFP contains opsonins and other factors which may improve neonatal neutrophil function,[13] as well as the procoagulants and the naturally occurring anticoagulants which become rapidly depleted in the course of coagulopathy.

The argument against the use of FFP is the small risk of viral transmission, which is absent with HAS. For those babies requiring repeated infusions, donor exposure is being reduced by some centres by preparing multipacks in much the same way as with packed red cells. There are measures currently being investigated that will inactivate virus without destroying the potential benefits of FFP. The addition of methylene blue is being used outside the UK, but may not be safe for administration to the sick neonate. Incubation of a plasma pool with organic solvent and detergent has an effective virus-killing effect without significant loss of coagulation factors, but each unit prepared involves multiple donations, with all the potential associated disadvantages. Meanwhile, plasma for administration to neonates should continue to be collected from long-standing safe, accredited donors. There is an obvious need for controlled studies of the benefits and hazards of FFP, HAS and other colloids.[26,40] There are several pilot studies in progress addressing the incidence of sepsis and GMH–IVH following volume expansion with FFP versus HAS.

One large trial of 776 babies of less than 32 weeks' gestation randomized to receive FFP, a gelatin-based plasma substitute, or maintenance infusion of glucose (controls) has been completed. No benefit was shown in any of the three groups at age 2 years in terms of neurological and developmental assessment.[28] Strategies for preventing GMH–IVH are controversial and vary with the geographical area in the UK, dependent on the areas in which trials are being carried out.[41] Meta-analysis has shown no consistent benefit for any preventive treatment.[17]

CONCLUSION

It is obvious from the above discussion that the indications for component transfusion in the neonatal period and the procedures undertaken by the blood bank to provide for those needs have changed considerably over recent years. For further practical clinical information the reader is referred to a valuable commentary[36] on the recent UK guidelines concerning transfusion of infants and neonates.[6]

REFERENCES

1. Acheson D 1987 Press release 1. Department of Health and Social Security 87/5, London
2. Anderson K C, Weinstein H J 1990 Transfusion associated graft versus host disease. New England Journal of Medicine 323: 315–321
3. Bedford Russell A R, Rivers R P A, Davey N 1993 The development of anti-HLA antibodies in multiply transfused preterm infants. Archives of Disease in Childhood 68: 49–51
4. Bell E F 1995 Reducing transfusion needs for preterm infants. European Society for Pediatric Research – Proceedings 81
5. Bifano E M, Curran C T R 1995 Minimizing donor blood expoure in the neonatal intensive care unit: current trends and future prospects. Clinics in Perinatology 22: 657–669
6. Blood Transfusion Task Force 1994 Working Party of the British Committee for Standards in Haematology (BCSH) British Society of Haematology. Guidelines for administration of blood products: transfusion of infants and neonates. Transfusion Medicine 4: 63–69
7. Bowman J M 1996 Hemolytic disease of the newborn. Vox Sanguinis 70: 62–67
8. Cairo M S 1987 Granulocyte transfusions in neonates with presumed sepsis. Pediatrics 80: 738–740
9. Cairo M S, Christensen R, Sender L S et al 1995 Results of a phase I/II trial of recombinant human granulocyte–macrophage colony-stimulating factor in very low birthweight neonates: significant induction of circulatory neutrophils, monocytes, platelets, and bone marrow neutrophils. Blood 86: 2509–2515
10. Connor M E, Minnefor A B, Okeske J M 1987 Human immunodeficiency virus infection in infants and children. In: Gottlieb E A (ed) Current topics in AIDS. Wiley, Chichester, pp 185–209
11. de Palma L, Luban N L C 1990 Blood component therapy in the perinatal period: guidelines and recommendations. Seminars in Perinatology 14: 403–415
12. de Sauvage F J, Hass P E, Spencer S D et al 1994 Stimulation of megakaryocytopoiesis and thrombopoiesis by the c-Mpl ligand. Nature 369: 533–538
13. Eisenfeld L, Krause P J, Herson V C et al 1992 Enhancement of neonatal neutrophil motility (chemotaxis) with adult fresh frozen plasma. American Journal of Perinatology 9: 5–8
14. Flidel O, Barak Y, Lifschitz Mercer B, Frumkin A, Mogilner B M 1992 Graft versus host disease in extremely low birth weight neonate [letter]. Pediatrics 89: 689–690
15. Funkhouser A W, Vogelsang G, Zehnbauer B et al 1991 Graft versus host disease after blood transfusions in a premature infant. Pediatrics 87: 247–250
16. Holland B M, Wardrop C A 1991 Oxygen transport in blood, haematinics and blood cell component therapy in the neonate. In: Rylance G, Aranda J, Harvey D (eds) Neonatal clinical pharmacology and therapeutics. Butterworths, Oxford, pp 211–223
17. Horbar J D 1992 Prevention of periventricular–intraventricular hemorrhage. In: Sinclair J C, Bracken M B (eds) Effective care of the newborn. Oxford University Press, Oxford, pp 562–583
18. Hurley R 1995 Infectious hazards associated with blood transfusion. Adverse Drug Reaction Toxicology Review 14: 157–174
19. Jan-Mohamed R, Hambley H, Gamsu H, Mufti G J 1993 Transfusion associated graft versus host disease – experience in a single centre. British Journal of Haematology 84: 10
20. Jones J G, Holland B M, Hudson I R, Wardrop C A 1990 Total circulating red cells versus haematocrit as the primary descriptor of oxygen transport by the blood. British Journal of Haematology 76: 288–294
21. Kinmond S, Aitchison T C, Holland B M, Jones J G, Turner T L, Wardrop C A 1993 Umbilical cord clamping and preterm infants: a randomised trial. British Medical Journal 306: 172–175
22. Letsky E A 1990 ABC of transfusion. Fetal and neonatal transfusion. British Medical Journal 300: 862–866 (New edition in press)
23. Luban N L 1994 Review of neonatal red cell transfusion practices. Blood Reviews 8: 148–153
24. Luban N L, Strauss R G, Hume H A 1991 Commentary on the safety of red cells preserved in extended-storage media for neonatal transfusions. Transfusion 31: 229–235
25. Luban N L C, Ness P M 1985 Irradiation of blood products: indications and guidelines. Transfusion 25: 301
26. McClure G 1991 The use of plasma in the neonatal period [editorial]. Archives of Disease in Childhood 66: 373–374
27. Mollison P L, Engelfriet C P, Contreras M 1997 Blood transfusion in clinical medicine, 10th edn. Blackwell Scientific, Oxford
28. Northern Neonatal Nursing Initiative Trial Group 1996. Randomised trial of prophylactic early fresh-frozen plasma or gelatin or glucose in preterm babies: outcome at 2 years. Lancet 348: 229–232
29. Parkman R, Mosier D, Umansky I, Cochran W, Carpenter C B, Rosen F S 1974 Graft-versus-host disease after intrauterine and exchange transfusions for hemolytic disease of the newborn. New England Journal of Medicine 290: 359–363
30. Phillips H M, Holland B M, Abdel Moiz A et al 1986 Determination of red-cell mass in assessment and management of anaemia in babies needing blood transfusion. Lancet i: 882–884
31. Roberton N R C 1987 Top up transfusions in neonates. Archives of Disease in Childhood 62: 984–986
32. Shannon K M, Keith J F, Mentzer W C et al 1995 Recombinant human erythropoietin stimulates erythropoiesis and reduces erythrocyte transfusions in very low birth weight preterm infants. Pediatrics 95: 1–8
33. Strauss R G 1991 Transfusion therapy in neonates. American Journal of Diseases of Children 145: 904–911
34. Strauss R G 1996 Neonatal anemia: pathophysiology and treatment. Vox Sanguinis 70: 57–61
35. Wardrop C A, Holland B M 1998 Blood transfusion for babies less than 1000 g. In: Harvey D, Cooke R W I, Levitt G A (eds) Baby under 1000 g. Wright, London
36. Warwick R, Modi N 1995 Guidelines for the administration of blood products. Archives of Disease in Childhood 72: 379–381
37. Williamson L, Heptonstall J, Soldan K 1996 A SHOT in the arm for safer blood transfusion. British Medical Journal 313: 1221–1222
38. Williamson P, Griffiths G, Norfolk D, Levene M 1996 Blood transfusions and human recombinant erythropoietin in premature newborn infants. Archives of Disease in Childhood 75: F65–F68
39. Wood A, Wilson N, Skacel P et al 1995 Reducing donor exposure in preterm infants requiring multiple blood transfusions. Archives of Disease in Childhood 72: F29–33
40. Wright I M, Levene M I, Arthur R, Martinez R 1995 Randomised trial of FFP and volume expansion in very low birthweight and sick preterm infants. Pediatric Research 38: 462 (abstract)
41. Wright I M R 1995 Prevention of intraventricular haemorrhage in preterm infants in Britain and Ireland [letter]. Archives of Disease in Childhood 72: F79

33

Non-immune hydrops fetalis

Philip C. Etches Nestor N. Demianczuk Nan B. Okun Radha Chari

INTRODUCTION

Hydrops fetalis is a term used to describe the fetus or neonate with generalized subcutaneous oedema, commonly associated with fluid collections within the pericardial, pleural, or peritoneal spaces. Fetal ultrasound allows for antenatal identification of hydrops with the potential for determining the underlying aetiology prior to birth, which may assist the obstetrician in the management of pregnancy and delivery, and forewarns the neonatologist regarding neonatal investigation and treatment. Associated antenatal ultrasound findings include polyhydramnios and placental oedema.[40] Confusion may occasionally occur with fetal adipose tissue, small (normal) amounts of pericardial or peritoneal fluid, or sometimes true transient fluid accumulation.[110,126]

CLASSIFICATION AND EPIDEMIOLOGY

There are two major categories of hydrops fetalis. Hydrops secondary to erythroblastosis fetalis from Rhesus isoimmunization or other maternal-fetal blood group incompatibilities is described as 'immune hydrops'. The second major group, 'non-immune hydrops', includes all other causes.

Historically, Rh isoimmunization was the leading cause of hydrops in the newborn. However, with the institution of passive maternal immunization.[31] and the development of fetal intrauterine transfusion over the last few decades, non-immune hydrops has become comparatively more prevalent. In 1992, Santolaya et al reported a series of 76 hydropic fetuses, 87% of which were non-immune.[120] Others have reported similar frequencies.[53,139] In addition, the use of antenatal ultrasound has facilitated the prenatal detection of fetal hydrops, resulting in an apparently increasing frequency of this disorder. The incidence of non-immune hydrops diagnosed antenatally appears greater than the neonatal incidence, which suggests that the affected pregnancies may not reach viability. The incidence of non-immune hydrops at delivery is reported to be 1 in 2000 to 1 in 3500.[53,70,88]

In utero diagnosis of non-immune fetal hydrops identifies a clinical entity, which has a myriad of underlying aetiologies and associations. This diagnosis also indicates that the fetus is significantly compromised and at imminent risk for serious morbidity or mortality. However, the risks and prognosis are dependent upon the actual aetiology of the hydrops and any antenatal or postnatal therapy that may be available. Consequently, the antenatal detection of non-immune fetal hydrops requires an expeditious and diligent search for the underlying cause, in order to direct appropriate pregnancy counselling and management. In addition, in a certain subset of patients, the underlying aetiology may be genetic in origin, and therefore may have a significant impact on subsequent pregnancies.

In general, unfortunately, the prognosis for non-immune hydrops remains poor, with a perinatal mortality rate approaching 80%.[26,70,140] Factors that contribute to this outcome are multiple, and include chromosomal anomalies, major malformations, pulmonary hypoplasia, and preterm delivery.[93]

PATHOPHYSIOLOGY

Interstitial fluid is produced at the level of the capillary, through the ultrafiltration of plasma. The normal transcapillary filtration rate is determined by the balance between the capillary and interstitial hydrostatic and colloid osmotic pressures, together with the permeability of the capillary membrane.[129] A disruption in the production, absorption, or distribution of this interstitial fluid can occur when there is a change in the capillary, plasma osmotic, or lymphatic pressures, or an alteration in the integrity of the capillary membrane.

Figure 33.1 summarizes the interrelationship between the more common, underlying aetiologies and the pathophysiological mechanisms that may lead to the

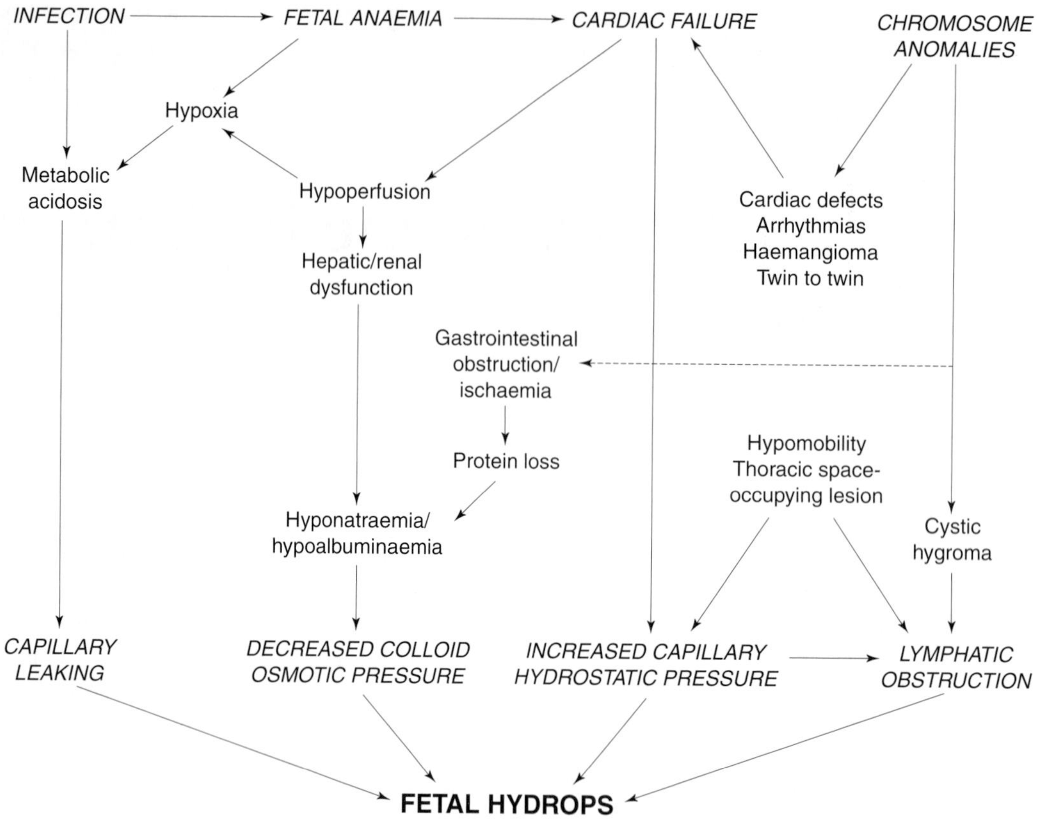

Fig. 33.1 Pathophysiological mechanisms whereby associated conditions may lead to fetal hydrops.

development of hydrops. Accumulation of interstitial fluid may lead to dysfunction of vital organs, including the heart, lungs, liver, or brain. As illustrated in the figure, a single aetiology may lead to hydrops through more than one pathophysiological mechanism.[7] Therefore, only by removing or correcting the underlying cause, may the abnormal accumulation of interstitial fluid be reversed. This principle is important when in utero shunting is being considered in order to drain body cavity fluid collections, for although one or two cavities may be decompressed, fluid accumulation in inaccessible vital areas of the fetus may still continue. Therefore, in generalized non-immune fetal hydrops, the treatment of specific symptoms may neither alter the overall course of the disease nor improve the prognosis.

DIAGNOSIS AND ANTENATAL MANAGEMENT

The presentation of non-immune hydrops includes a large-for-dates pregnancy, decreased fetal movement, a previous history of an hydropic fetus, or the incidental ultrasound diagnosis of hydrops. The condition is more common in twin pregnancies. Hydrops itself is not an adequate diagnosis, however, but a symptom of an underlying problem, so that referral to a tertiary centre is required for comprehensive investigation. A simple maternal blood type and routine antibody screen will rule out almost all immune causes of hydrops.

HISTORY AND PHYSICAL EXAMINATION

In our unit, we find it useful to perform a detailed ultrasound examination at the same time as obtaining the history, as one often guides the other and can make the entire process more efficient. Items to be considered include: consanguinity, Mediterranean or Asian ancestry, a family history of anaemia, antepartum haemorrhage, infection, polyhydramnios, and the 'mirror' syndrome in which the maternal status mimics that of the fetus with the development of peripheral oedema, pulmonary oedema, hypertension, proteinuria, and a hyperdynamic circulation.[100]

ULTRASOUND EXAMINATION

This includes the assessment of the severity, extent, and localization of the hydrops. There may be generalized anasarca, pleural effusions, pericardial effusions, ascites, or various combinations of these, with or without polyhydramnios, with different implications for management. In addition, an assessment of fetal well-being will guide immediate management plans in the viable fetus. At the same time as the quantity of movement is noted, so is the quality in terms of range of extension and flexion, and any postural abnormalities of the limbs suggesting particular chromosome anomalies or neuromuscular disorders.

The anatomic survey of the fetus must be very thorough. The estimated fetal weight is often falsely elevated by the hydropic state, so that the biparietal diameter and long bone length may more accurately reflect the small-for-gestational age fetus. A thorough fetal cardiac scan is indicated, as up to 26% of fetal hydrops cases are due to cardiac disease.[93] Occasionally, visualization of the heart is impeded by the pericardial or pleural effusion or another space-occupying lesion in the chest, so that some authors have found it helpful to drain pleural fluid, particularly when unilateral, to allow decompression of the heart and more complete visualization.[99,116] A search for cardiac dysrhythmia is also performed. Tachyarrhythmia may be intermittent and therefore not immediately evident, and prolonged monitoring is indicated to detect this relatively frequent cause of hydrops.[131]

The size and appearance of the liver and spleen should be evaluated, as these are helpful in suggesting congenital hepatitis and various inherited disorders of metabolism.[12,73,96]

A clinical geneticist should be involved in reviewing the ultrasound findings as he or she is often able to integrate seemingly unrelated findings and direct further investigations, including genetic testing, which may be more complicated than simple chromosome analysis.[130] For example, molecular genetic testing is now available for the diagnosis of myotonic dystrophy, which can present with fetal hydrops.[132]

The amount of amniotic fluid is quantified, either by the amniotic fluid index (wherein the deepest vertical pocket in each quadrant of the uterus is measured),[106] or by a single measurement of the deepest vertical pocket.[62] Initial quantitation is useful to follow effectiveness of therapy. The umbilical cord and placenta are scanned for evidence of masses that may relate to hydrops, particularly chorioangiomas.[123] A thickened placenta is more likely to be associated with fetal anaemia.[119]

INVESTIGATIONS

The maternal history and detailed ultrasound will in many cases determine the testing required. For those cases where the cause is not evident, reference to Table 33.1 may aid in determining appropriate investigation.

Some authors suggest maternal oral glucose tolerance testing for diabetes as part of the workup for fetal hydrops.[21] No association was found in the literature to substantiate or explain any association between these two.[88] There is an association between diabetes and polyhydramnios,[34] although the excessive fluid volume is not often severe, and may be a result of the increased size of the fetus with a resultant increased urine output.[49] Similarly, maternal workup for connective tissue disorder is often suggested. Again, no association can be found between this disease and hydrops, except by association of fetal bradycardia due to heart block, where the association with maternal autoantibody in systemic lupus erythematosus is well known.[87]

Other investigations are guided by the particular clinical situation. An aetiology can be found in up to 85% of hydrops if investigation is appropriate.[93] After the birth, the pathologist should be involved to examine placental and any other tissue which may be available.[79,93]

Maternal

Investigations to be considered are outlined in Table 33.2.

Fetal

Fetal investigation is outlined in Table 33.3.

For genetic testing, for either chromosomal defects or single gene disorders, fetal tissue is obtained by amniocentesis, chorionic villus sampling, or cordocentesis. The method chosen depends in part on the clinical urgency of the situation in that the results may take up to 3 weeks with amniocentesis or as little as 48 hours with CVS or cord blood sampling. With severe polyhydramnios, the only option may be amniocentesis, as both the umbilical cord and placenta may be inaccessible.

Fetal infection can be sought by maternal serology for toxoplasma, rubella, cytomegalovirus, herpes, and syphilis.[9] In addition, toxoplasma antigens may be found in fetal tissue, or the organism may be grown from culture of fetal tissues. Herpesvirus may be cultured from amniotic fluid,[54] and CMV may be grown from amniotic fluid or fetal urine or blood.[9] Parvovirus B19 may be demonstrated by specific IgM in maternal or fetal blood, or by the demonstration of DNA in fetal tissue.[44,135]

FETAL THERAPY: GENERAL CONSIDERATIONS

Only a limited number of causes of fetal hydrops, detailed below, are amenable to specific therapy. Hence, prior to viability, termination of pregnancy may be considered. If this occurs, careful examination of the fetus and products of conception by the pathologist is necessary to try to further elucidate aetiology and to allow appropriate counselling (Table 33.4).[79,93] If the fetus has achieved a greater gestational age compatible with a low mortality due to prematurity, and tests of fetal well-being are abnormal, then delivery following therapy with antenatal steroids (p. 491) should be strongly considered. Vaginal delivery may be difficult and traumatic, and therefore delivery by caesarean section is usually recommended. Clinicians should be prepared for maternal complications such as pre-eclampsia, anaemia, and postpartum haemorrhage.[52,64]

Table 33.1 Categorization of conditions associated with NIH, a frequency estimate as a percentage of cases of NIH, and possible pathophysiological mechanisms.[21,64,65,73,75,89,91,92,93,102,111,120,136,138] It must be emphasized that most, if not all, of these conditions may occur without NIH

FETAL: FOCAL ABNORMALITY		

Cardiac
Hypoplastic left heart
Subaortic stenosis
Pulmonary valve insufficiency
Ebstein's anomaly
Coarctation of the aorta
Hypoplastic right heart
Endocardial fibroelastosis
Rhythm abnormality
  Supraventricular tachycardia
  Atrial flutter
  Atrial fibrillation
  Heart block
Premature closure of the foramen ovale
Premature closure or restriction of ductus arteriosus
Intrapericardial teratoma
Rhabdomyoma
Myocarditis
Myocardial infarction
Idiopathic arterial calcification
Atrial septal defect
Ventricular septal defect
Truncus arteriosus
Tetralogy of Fallot
Transposition of the great vessels
	19–26%	Cardiac failure may be a cause of fetal hydrops due to chronic pressure load (valve abnormality), volume overload or severe anaemia. Both tachy- and bradyarrhythmias may lead to congestive heart failure. The observation of congenital heart block with bradycardia should suggest a possible diagnosis of autoimmune disease in the mother. Myocardial disease may cause hydrops by inadequate myocardial contraction and intracardiac tumours may interfere with cardiac function

Pulmonary Chylothorax Pulmonary lymphangiectasia Cystic adenomatoid malformation Extralobar pulmonary sequestration Mediastinal teratoma Hamartomatous malformation of lung Laryngeal atresia Mesenchymal malformation of lung Familial pulmonary lymphatic hypoplasia Diaphragmatic hernia	8–10%	Hydrops develops because of abnormal lymphatic drainage or obstructed venous return with increased intravascular pressure in the venous bed due to a space-occupying lesion within the thorax
Gastrointestinal Duodenal atresia Jejunoileal atresia Imperforate anus Volvulus Duodenal diverticulum	1%	Hydrops may develop because of decreased intravascular colloid osmotic pressure. Protein may be lost as a transudate into the bowel or there may be abnormalities of lymphatic drainage in the splanchnic bed
Hepatic Hepatic calcification Hepatic fibrosis Polycystic disease of the liver Cholestasis Cirrhosis with portal hypertension Congenital portal dysplasia Giant cell hepatitis	1%	There may be portal venous obstruction or hepatic dysfunction leading to hypoproteinaemia
Renal Congenital nephrosis (Finnish type) Renal dysplasia due to urethral obstruction Pelvic kidney Hypoplastic kidney Polycystic kidney Renal vein thrombosis	2–3%	The aetiology of hydrops in urinary tract anomalies could be fetal hypomobility due to oligohydramnios, decreased cardiac excursion because of urinary ascites, osmotic disturbances due to hypoalbuminaemia in nephrosis, and lymphatic vessel overload by urinary ascites

Table 33.1 Continued

Vascular Arteriovenous malformation Vena caval thrombosis Haemangioendothelioma Arterial calcification Vein of Galen aneurysm Fetal intracranial haemorrhage Fetal intracranial teratoma Sacrococcygeal teratoma Neuroblastoma Mesoblastic nephroma Hepatic adenoma	2–4%	Vascular malformations may lead to high-output cardiac failure or hypoxia due to haemorrhage. Hydrops occurring in fetuses with tumours may be due to circulatory obstruction or arteriovenous shunting resulting in high-output cardiac failure
FETAL: GENERALIZED ABNORMALITY		
Infectious causes Cytomegalovirus Coxsackie virus Syphilis Toxoplasmosis Parvovirus B19 Rubella Herpes simplex Chagas' disease Leptospirosis Respiratory syncytial virus Varicella	1–8%	Direct viral infection of the myocardium may lead to myocarditis and intrauterine congestive heart failure. Viraemia may also result in high-output congestive heart failure from severe anaemia by destruction of erythroid progenitor cells. Fetal infection can also cause alterations in organ blood flow and change microvascular hydrostatic pressures with escape of fluid through endothelial gaps and the basement membrane
Skeletal dysplasias Achondroplasia Achondrogenesis types I, IA, and II Osteogenesis imperfecta type II Lethal osteoporosis Asphyxiating thoracic dysplasia Thanatophoric dwarfism Isolated case reports of various other osteochondrodysplasias have been reported to be associated with hydrops	4%	The cause of hydrops in these cases is largely unknown. Hepatic enlargement with large vessel compression may occur secondary to proliferation of blood cell precursors to compensate for a small bone marrow volume. Thoracic abnormality secondary to various chondrodysplasias causes increased intrathoracic pressure leading to obstructed venous return
Metabolic disorders Gaucher's disease GM_1 gangliosidosis Mucopolysaccharidosis I and IVb Mucolipidosis types I and II Glucose phosphate isomerase deficiency Pyruvate kinase deficiency Carnitine deficiency Niemann–Pick diseases types A and C Sialic acid storage disorder Galactosialodosis	1%	Genetic metabolic diseases that cause hydrops may do so through myocardial involvement leading to congestive heart failure, or ascites secondary to hepatic sinusoidal infiltration resulting in disturbance of intrahepatic circulation. There may also be hypomobility secondary to muscle involvement. Erythrocyte enzymopathies can cause haemolytic anaemia with resultant hydrops
Chromosomal disorders Trisomy 21, 18, 13, 15, 16 45,XO (Turner syndrome) Partial duplication of chromosome 11, 15, 17, 18 Partial deletion of chromosome 13p Partial deletion of chromosome 18q Rearrangement of chromosome 22q 46, XX/XY mosaic Triploidy, tetraploidy	35%	There is no single clear pathogenesis for hydrops in chromosomally abnormal fetuses that have no cardiovascular abnormality or lymphatic drainage abnormality. In structurally normal fetuses, one theory for the hydrops involves fetal hypoxia from placental abnormalities
Fetal anaemia α-thalassaemia Fetal closed-space haemorrhage Haemolysis Maternal–fetal haemorrhage Twin-to-twin transfusion Acardiac twin	10–27%	Hydrops occurs due to severe anaemia and congestive heart failure. Usually there is extreme hepatic erythropoiesis in response to the anaemia, secondary portal hypertension, and hypoalbuminaemia/hypoproteinaemia

Table 33.1 Continued

Syndromes *Autosomal dominant* Opitz–Frias syndrome (G syndrome) Myotonic dystrophy Cornelia de Lange syndrome Noonan syndrome Yellow nail syndrome Tuberous sclerosis *Autosomal recessive* Orofaciodigital syndrome type II Polysplenia Pena–Shokeir syndrome Lethal multiple pterygium syndrome Neu–Laxova syndrome Idiopathic recurrent hydrops Isolated recurrent cystic hygroma Elejalde syndrome Hypophosphatasia Prune belly syndrome Klippel–Trenaunay–Weber syndrome Massive cystic hygroma Fanconi syndrome type III	8–9%	It is not known how hydrops develops in these various syndromes. In syndromes characterized by immobility, fetal hydrops may result from a lack of respiratory movement of the chest wall leading to a secondary rise in intrathoracic pressure. This in turn causes a rise in the systemic venous pressure, leading to oedema. In cases associated with cystic hygroma, the explanation is that of an embryonal malformation of the lymphatic ducts leading to a hypoplasia of the main lymphatic trunk with resulting fluid accumulation
Twinning Monozygotic twins with twin-to-twin transfusion syndrome (in recipient, donor, or both) Acardiac twins	4–8%	Hydrops in the recipient twin may be through reduced perfusion by hyperviscous blood. Hydrops in the donor is due to anaemia, cardiac failure, and hypoproteinaemia
PLACENTAL/UMBILICAL	2–6%	
Chorioangioma True knots of the cord Angiomyxoma of the umbilical cord Aneurysm of the umbilical artery Haemorrhagic endovasculitis of the placenta Chorionic vein thrombosis Placental and umbilical vein thrombosis Umbilical cord torsion		Chorioangioma acts as an arteriovenous shunt, bypassing normal placental tissue. The resultant physiological effects are increased pulse pressure, increased venous return to the heart, tachycardia, cardiac enlargement, and hypervolaemia
MATERNAL	<1%	
Maternal indomethacin use Lupus erythematosus		Hydrops may develop in these instances owing to premature closure or restriction of flow in the ductus arteriosus or because of fetal cardiac arrhythmia resulting in congestive heart failure

Table 33.2 Maternal investigation of fetal hydrops

Investigation	Underlying condition
Blood type, antibodies	Immune hydrops
Haemoglobin and peripheral smear	α-thalassaemia
Haemoglobin electrophoresis	
Serology	Infectious cause
Toxoplasma	
Rubella	
Cytomegalovirus	
Herpes	
Syphilis	
Parvovirus B19	
Kleihauer–Betke test	Fetomaternal haemorrhage
Lupus antibodies (fetal bradycardia)	Collagen vascular disease

Table 33.3 Fetal investigation of hydrops

Investigation	Underlying condition
Amniocentesis/CVS/PUBS	
Chromosomes	Fetal aneuploidy
Single gene disorders	
Haemoglobin, reticulocytes, film	Anaemia
Haemoglobin electrophoresis	α-thalassaemia
Blood type, antibodies	Immune cause
Protein, albumin	Hypoproteinaemia
Serology: toxoplasma, rubella, herpes, cytomegalovirus, parvovirus B19	Fetal infection
Culture	
Amniotic fluid	Viral infection
Fetal tissue	
Pleural fluid analysis	Chylothorax
Muscle biopsy	Muscular dystrophy

Table 33.4 Investigation of a stillbirth or neonatal death with hydrops fetalis

See investigations in Table 33.5
1. Detailed postmortem examination
2. Skin biopsy for fibroblast culture, karyotype
3. Liver biopsy for histopathology – freeze in liquid nitrogen
4. Tissue (liver, kidney, spleen) for B19 DNA
5. X-rays
6. Photograph

At gestations between previability and relative fetal maturity, the management is difficult and is individualized to the particular situation. Waiting runs the risk of stillbirth, although spontaneous resolution of hydrops has been described.[110,126] One study describes the measurement of the biventricular outer dimension in diastole as a useful prognostic tool.[20] Non-specific therapy using intra-abdominal injection of albumin or packed red cells has been employed by one group in Japan.[127] A team approach utilizing the input of the perinatologists, neonatologists, geneticist, surgeon, social worker, and most importantly the parents is necessary. The parents must be fully informed of the diagnosis as far as is known, prognosis, and possible risks and benefits of proposed management options.

SPECIFIC FETAL THERAPY

Fetal anaemia

In the case of Rhesus isoimmunization, fetal anaemia is known to produce a metabolic acidosis with elevation of plasma lactate.[128] Correction of anaemia by intravascular transfusion transiently makes this metabolic acidosis worse,[101] but the elevated umbilical venous pressure is rapidly corrected.[142]

α-thalassaemia (p. 827)

In the case of α-thalassaemia, the carrier state in pregnancy may present with pre-eclampsia, microcytic anaemia, and/or a large-for-dates pregnancy.[86] Although it is usually considered that the homozygous state is lethal for the fetus, occasional cases have been reported of prolonged postnatal survival when the infant is born alive.[11] Fetuses with Bart's haemoglobinopathy (p. 828) are known to be more hypoxic, acidotic, and hypercarbic than normal, which is explicable by the anaemia and the high oxygen affinity of Bart's haemoglobin.[66] Recently, a case has been described in which intrauterine intravascular exchange transfusions were utilized to maintain appropriate fetal growth, following which the baby survived and was being maintained postnatally with chronic blood transfusions.[23] However, this course of therapy should not be undertaken lightly, and the mainstay of management for this condition continues to be antenatal screening of susceptible populations, combined with prenatal diagnosis utilizing DNA hybridization techniques from fetal cells.[67,98]

Fetomaternal haemorrhage

Fetal anaemia may also occur secondary to severe fetomaternal haemorrhage, and there have been isolated case reports of successful treatment utilizing intrauterine transfusion.[19,134]

Fetal infection

Fetal toxoplasmosis

Untreated maternal toxoplasmosis infection results in a 20–50% rate of infection in the fetus, and approximately 10% of infected mothers will give birth to severely affected infants[25] (p. 1171). The risk to the fetus is increased with the presence of a high maternal antibody titre to toxoplasma.[124] Large studies from France have shown that antenatal diagnosis of fetal infection employing culture of fetal blood and amniotic fluid and testing of fetal blood for toxoplasma-specific IgM, combined with ultrasound examination, is reasonably sensitive (92%), and that maternal therapy with pyrimethamine and sulphonamides, or with spiramycin, alone or in combination, may be effective.[35,63] Prevention of infection by health education is extremely important.[72]

Parvovirus B19

In early pregnancy, parvovirus B19 may produce a disseminated fetal infection and embryopathy,[61,137] whereas later in gestation this virus is now well established as a cause of fetal hydrops by producing an aplastic crisis, leading to severe anaemia and high-output cardiac failure.[4,24] Additionally, there may be a direct cytopathic effect on myocardial cells.[61,97] Parvovirus B19 infection in pregnancy results in fetal death in 3–9% of cases,[32] although this may be an underestimate,[39] and it may be responsible for as many as 10% of non-malformed fetal deaths between 10 and 24 weeks' gestation.[144] Diagnosis is made by maternal seroconversion, positive IgM, and the detection of B19 DNA in fetal blood and amniotic fluid using the polymerase chain reaction.[44,135] B19 may account for approximately 10–15% of non-immune hydrops fetalis for which other causes are not apparent.[117,145] Although hydrops due to this virus may resolve spontaneously,[68,112] intrauterine transfusion to correct the anaemia has been shown to improve survival with apparently good long-term outcome,[44] although subsequent red cell aplasia following intrauterine parvovirus infection has been described.[16]

Syphilis

Syphilis was recognized as a cause of hydrops long before the description of Rhesus isoimmunization and must not be overlooked in view of the current resurgence of the disease (p. 1174). Appropriate diagnosis and maternal therapy with penicillin may allow the fetus to survive despite the presence of hydrops.[10]

Fetal arrhythmia

Tachyarrhythmia

Fetal tachyarrhythmia is thought to cause hydrops secondary to cardiac failure producing elevation in the umbilical venous pressure and a reduction in fetal lymph flow. Tachyarrhythmias are usually supraventricular in origin, and include paroxysmal supraventricular tachycardia, Wolff–Parkinson–White syndrome, atrial fibrillation, and atrial flutter. There are associated anatomical abnormalities in only 6 or 7% of cases.[114] The most commonly used therapy is maternal administration of digoxin,[3,143] which appears to achieve adequate levels in the fetus[121] unless there is severe hydrops.[146] Direct fetal therapy, by intravenous,[46] intramuscular,[57] or intraperitoneal[47] administration, has also been used. Other drugs employed include verapamil,[78] alone or in combination with digoxin;[104] quinidine;[55] propranolol;[114] amiodarone;[115] procainamide;[78] and flecainide.[80] Of these therapies, flecainide holds the most promise according to a recent series from the Netherlands of 49 fetuses with supraventricular tachycardia, 35 of which were treated transplacentally.[45] Digoxin restored sinus rhythm in 55% of nonhydropic, but only 8% of hydropic fetuses; whereas flecainide was effective in all nonhydropic fetuses where digoxin failed, and in 43% of hydropic fetuses, and was associated with reduced mortality. Another recent innovation is the direct intravenous injection into the fetus of adenosine, which terminates the supraventricular tachycardia, but is of short duration.[81] This approach, combined with long-acting therapy using digoxin and flecainide may be of most use.

Bradyarrhythmia

Fetal heart block is a less common cause of fetal hydrops, but is more difficult to treat antenatally. It may be associated with a structural congenital heart defect, in which case the prognosis is extremely poor.[48,125] In the presence of normal cardiac anatomy, hydrops fetalis is unusual, but has been reported in rare circumstances, e.g. congestive heart failure with sinus bradycardia and coronary artery embolus with myocardial infarction, premature delivery, and death.[77] The other well-known association of congenital heart block is with autoantibodies due to connective tissue disease,[22,58] in which case therapy with maternal steroids may be of help.[13,33] Other therapies that have been tried include maternal administration of sympathomimetic drugs,[122] intra-abdominal fetal administration of sympathomimetics,[95] and ventricular pacing.[37] If the fetus is near term, early delivery and pacing may be successful. Intrauterine pacing has been tried under ultrasound guidance, and although this was initially successful, the fetus died within 4 hours.[37] Some success with non-specific medical therapy (digoxin and diuretics) in the presence of complete heart block has also been reported.[59]

Fetal tumours

Sacrococcygeal teratoma

This tumour may be associated with arteriovenous shunting leading to high-output cardiac failure, hydrops fetalis, and death.[14,17] The fetal surgery group in San Francisco have reported their attempts at fetal surgery in one case; it resulted in reversal of the hydrops but the baby subsequently died.[84]

Intrathoracic space-occupying lesions

These include congenital cystic adenomatoid malformation of the lung, pulmonary sequestration, and congenital diaphragmatic hernia, which may produce pulmonary hypoplasia directly by compression or may reduce systemic venous return leading to hydrops.[17] Some of these lesions spontaneously resolve,[90] and although association with hydrops usually leads to fetal demise,[1,82] resolution of the hydrops occurs occasionally.[43] If this is not the case, palliative treatment by thoracocentesis[103] or shunting of cystic lesions[30,41] or pleural effusions[141] has been attempted, but these usually provide little long-term benefit. The San Francisco group has reported two cases of fetal surgery for cystic adenomatoid malformation, one of whom survived.[60]

Twin-to-twin transfusion

The twin transfusion syndrome occurs in multiple gestation when there are vascular anastomoses between monochorionic twins. It occurs extremely rarely in dichorionic twinning.[133] The syndrome can occur at any time during the pregnancy, but is most serious when it presents in the mid-second trimester, either as markedly discrepant growth, or a marked difference in fluid volumes between two amniotic sacs. The mortality with hydrops is extremely high, between 60 and 100%.[27,51,113] Hydrops can develop either in the twin who is the donor or in the recipient of excessive placental circulation. Management schemes have included maternal administration of digoxin[38] and indomethacin.[74] However, the current recommendation is repeated reduction amniocentesis. Although this may lead to complications such as abruption and preterm labour, several authors have shown success in improving survival with this method.[94,109]

Fetal fluid accumulation

Fetal pleural effusions may occur in conjunction with generalized hydrops, or may cause it by impeding venous return by shifting the mediastinum. The association of hydrops and pleural effusions carries a worse prognosis than isolated hydrops owing to the development of pulmonary hypoplasia. Some pleural effusions may resolve spontaneously,[56] occasionally after thoracocentesis.[2] If this does not occur, therapy consists of placement of a thoracoamniotic shunt under ultrasound guidance[15,17] (p. 221). This approach would usually be reserved for those cases in which congenital or chromosomal abnormalities have been excluded, and preliminary information suggests that it may be quite successful.[6] Similar approaches have been used to drain fetal ascites.[50]

NEONATAL MANAGEMENT OF HYDROPS FETALIS

Antenatal diagnosis allows transfer to a tertiary centre which allows for a planned delivery in a controlled setting, usually by caesarean section. This also permits the neonatal team to assemble all the equipment which may be required, and if necessary the appropriate surgical preparations to be made.

RESUSCITATION

Hydropic infants tolerate labour poorly, and are usually depressed at birth. Intubation is almost always required, which may be difficult because of oedema. Ventilation may require high pressures on account of pulmonary oedema and pulmonary hypoplasia secondary to pleural effusions and/or ascites. A prolonged initial breath at fairly high pressures (20–25 cmH_2O) for 1–4 s may help to establish a functional residual capacity, following which ventilation at rapid rates of 80–120 breaths/min is usually most effective.[107] Prophylactic surfactant may be given.

Preparations should be made for immediate thoracocentesis and/or paracentesis, which may be necessary in the course of initial resuscitation.

SUBSEQUENT MANAGEMENT

Umbilical arterial and venous catheterization will almost always be required, and these may be utilized to monitor arterial and central venous pressure. Although an intense vasoconstrictor response to asphyxia may produce elevated pressures, these babies are usually hypovolaemic.[108] Cautious correction of metabolic acidosis, volume replacement with blood or colloid depending on haematocrit, or exchange transfusion for severe anaemia is undertaken as indicated using central venous pressure as a guide. Fresh frozen plasma is usually preferable to albumin, both as a volume expander and also to raise plasma protein concentration and oncotic pressure, in view of the frequently associated DIC which will also benefit from platelets, cryoprecipitate, or exchange transfusion.[42,107]

Cardiovascular support with inotropic agents is often necessary to support blood pressure and maintain urine output. We use dopamine early,[76,118] but usually find adrenaline to be more effective.[8] Moderate fluid restriction (60–80 ml/kg per 24 h) and the use of diuretics such as frusemide (1 mg/kg/dose) help to promote a diuresis and the resolution of oedema. Haemoperfusion may be indicated, if the oedema is refractory.

Meticulous attention must be paid to biochemical measurements such as electrolytes, creatinine, liver function tests, and particularly glucose. Specific therapy for particular causative conditions as outlined in Table 33.1 may be necessary. Alternatively, if there are severe congenital abnormalities, discussion at this stage may take place with the parents regarding the withdrawal of active support. If this occurs, detailed pathological examination should be obtained with parental consent, as outlined in Table 33.4.

INVESTIGATION

Table 33.5 outlines tests which may be considered for the neonate with non-immune hydrops fetalis, guided by the nature of the case.

VENTILATION

The baby's respiratory status may improve rapidly after a few hours of ventilation at high pressure, but more

Table 33.5 Neonatal investigation of hydrops fetalis

Imaging	
X-rays	Chest, abdomen, skull, long bones
Ultrasound	Heart, abdomen, brain
Pleural/ascitic fluid	Cytology, karyotype
	Total protein, albumin, triglyceride
	Viral and bacterial culture
Urine	Urinalysis, protein
	Virus and bacterial culture
Blood	Blood count, platelets, reticulocytes, smear
	PT, PTT, fibrinogen, fibrin split products
	Blood group, direct Coombs' test
	Haemoglobin electrophoresis
	Electrolytes, creatinine, glucose
	Total protein, albumin, bilirubin
	Liver function tests
	Osmolality
	Serology for toxoplasma, rubella,
	cytomegalovirus, herpes,
	syphilis, parvovirus B19 (IgG and IgM)
	Karyotype
Electrocardiogram	

commonly there is ongoing respiratory insufficiency due to reaccumulation of pleural or peritoneal fluid, pulmonary oedema, HMD, PPHN or pulmonary hypoplasia. It is usually very difficult or impossible to determine the relative contribution of the last four of these factors. Effective pleural and/or peritoneal and/or pericardial drainage is essential. Pulmonary oedema may improve with diuretics and increased levels of PEEP, which will also be effective in HMD. Hopefully, antenatal steroids will have already been administered, and surfactant therapy will be indicated in most of these cases. High frequency ventilation may offer an advantage,[28,29] particularly when combined with surfactant therapy.[36,71] Inhaled NO has recently been shown to reduce death or the need for ECMO in near-term infants with respiratory failure,[18] and we have also found this therapy to be useful in preterm infants with 'pulmonary hypoplasia' from prolonged oligohydramnios.[105] However, no definitive trials of NO in preterm infants have been undertaken, and these results plus those of other newer therapies such as partial liquid ventilation are awaited.

EXTRACORPOREAL MEMBRANE OXYGENATION

If severe hypoxaemia persists, then it is probably due to pulmonary hypoplasia-associated pulmonary hypertension, which can be estimated echocardiographically. Both the degree of pulmonary hypoplasia and the reversibility of pulmonary hypertension are difficult to determine, but if the baby has at any time had a 'reasonable' PaO_2 (say 7 kPa), then it is possible that the situation may be salvageable. If the baby is at least 34 weeks' gestation, does not have any contraindications such as major malformations, chromosome anomalies, or intracranial bleeding, and meets the local ECMO criteria for severe refractory respiratory failure, then ECMO may permit lung rest and resolution of pulmonary hypertension. As of 30 January 1996, the ELSO Registry in the US records 29 cases of non-immune hydrops, with a mortality of 62% (T. N. DeLosh 1996, personal communication).

OUTCOME

Overall, the prognosis for non-immune hydrops is very poor with mortality rates ranging from 50–100%.[5,42] This poor prognosis is related to prematurity, associated lethal malformations, and the presence of pleural effusions producing pulmonary hypoplasia, which is the most consistent postmortem finding.[5,26,70] A recent series reports survival rates of around 15%, which is probably a realistic goal.[89] Iliff et al found that the three survivors from their series of 27 differed from the other 10 liveborn infants in that they were diagnosed antenatally, had no structural anomalies, and had normal concentrations of total plasma protein and albumin.[69] The major therapeutic hopes lie in identifying those fetuses who may be amenable to antenatal therapy, as outlined previously in this chapter.

The long-term outcome of survivors of non-immune hydrops fetalis is difficult to predict, and will clearly be related to any associated problems. In a recent pathological series of 38 cases, 23 were found to exhibit hypoxic ischaemic lesions, mostly in the white matter of the brain.[85] Similar findings were reported in the stillbirths and neonatal deaths described by Laneri et al.[83] Of the 10 survivors in this report, six were neurologically abnormal at the time of discharge. The neurodevelopmental outcome of these extremely sick babies is of great concern.

REFERENCES

1. Adzick N S, Harrison M R, Glick P L et al 1985 Fetal cystic adenomatoid malformation: prenatal diagnosis and natural history. Journal of Pediatric Surgery 20: 483–488
2. Aguirre O A, Finley B E, Ridgway L E III, Bennett T L, Cowles T A 1995 Resolution of unilateral fetal hydrothorax with associated non-immune hydrops after intrauterine thoracocentesis. Ultrasound in Obstetrics and Gynecology 5: 346–348
3. Allan L D, Crawford D C, Anderson R H, Tynan M 1984 Evaluation and treatment of fetal arrhythmias. Clinical Cardiology 7: 467–473
4. Anand A, Gray E S, Brown T, Clewley J P, Cohen B J 1987 Human parvovirus infection in pregnancy and hydrops fetalis. New England Journal of Medicine 316: 183–186
5. Andersen H M, Drew J H, Beischer N A, Hutchison A A, Fortune D W 1983 Non-immune hydrops fetalis: changing contribution to perinatal mortality. British Journal of Obstetrics and Gynaecology 90: 636–639
6. Ayida G A, Soothill P W, Rodeck C H 1995 Survival in non-immune hydrops fetalis without malformation or chromosomal abnormalities after invasive treatment. Fetal Diagnosis and Therapy 10: 101–105
7. Barnes S E, Bryan E M, Harris D A, Baum J D 1977 Oedema in the newborn. Molecular Aspects of Medicine 1: 187–282
8. Barrington K, Chan W 1993 The circulatory effects of epinephrine infusion in the anesthetized piglet. Pediatric Research 33: 190–194
9. Barron S D, Pass R F 1995 Infectious causes of hydrops fetalis. Seminars in Perinatology 19: 493–501
10. Barton J R, Thorpe E M Jr, Shaver D C, Hager W D, Sibai B M 1992 Nonimmune hydrops fetalis associated with maternal infection with syphilis. American Journal of Obstetrics and Gynecology 167: 56–58
11. Beaudry M A, Ferguson D J, Pearse K, Yanofsky R A, Rubin E M, Kan Y W 1986 Survival of a hydropic infant with homozygous α-thalassemia-1. Journal of Pediatrics 108: 713–716
12. Beck M, Braun S, Coerdt W, Merz E, Young E, Sewell A C 1992 Fetal presentation of Morquio disease type A. Prenatal Diagnosis 12: 1019–1029
13. Bierman F Z, Baxi L, Jaffe I, Driscoll J 1988 Fetal hydrops and congenital complete heart block: response to maternal steroid therapy. Journal of Pediatrics 112: 646–648
14. Bond S J, Harrison M Schmidt K G et al 1990 Death due to high-output cardiac failure. I. Fetal sacrococcygeal teratoma. Journal of Pediatric Surgery 25: 1287–1291
15. Booth P, Nicolaides K H, Greenough A, Gamsu H R 1987 Pleuro-amniotic shunting for fetal chylothorax. Early Human Development 15: 365–367
16. Brown K E, Green S W, de Mayolo J A et al 1994 Congenital anaemia after transplacental parvovirus infection. Lancet 343: 895–896
17. Bullard K M, Harrison M R 1995 Before the horse is out of the barn: fetal surgery for hydrops. Seminars in Perinatology 19: 462–473
18. Canadian Inhaled Nitric Oxide Study Group and the NICHD Neonatal Research Network 1996 The neonatal inhaled nitric oxide study (NINOS) in the term and near-term infant with hypoxic respiratory failure: a multicenter randomized trial. Presented at the Society for Pediatric Research Annual Meeting May 6–10, Washington, DC

19. Cardwell M S 1988 Successful treatment of hydrops fetalis caused by fetomaternal hemorrhage: a case report. American Journal of Obstetrics and Gynecology 158: 131–132
20. Carlson D E, Platt L D, Medearis A L, Horenstein J 1990 Prognostic indicators of the resolution of nonimmune hydrops fetalis and survival of the fetus. American Journal of Obstetrics and Gynecology 163: 1785–1787
21. Carlton D P, McGillivray B C, Schreiber M D 1989 Nonimmune hydrops fetalis: a multidisciplinary approach. Clinics in Perinatology 16: 839–851
22. Carpenter R J Jr, Strasburger J F, Garson A Jr, Smith R T, Deter R L, Engelhardt H T Jr 1986 Fetal ventricular pacing for hydrops secondary to complete atrioventricular block. Journal of the American College of Cardiology 8: 1434–1436
23. Carr S, Rubin L, Dixon D, Star J, Dailey J 1995 Intrauterine therapy for homozygous alpha-thalassemia. Obstetrics and Gynecology 85: 876–879
24. Carrington D, Whittle M J, Gibson A A M et al 1987 Maternal serum α-fetoprotein – a marker of fetal aplastic crisis during intrauterine human parvovirus infection. Lancet i: 433–435
25. Carter A O, Frank J W 1986 Congenital toxoplasmosis: epidemiologic features and control. Canadian Medical Association Journal 135: 618–623
26. Castillo R A, Devoe L D, Hadi H A, Martin S, Geist D 1986 Nonimmune hydrops fetalis: clinical experience and factors related to a poor outcome. American Journal of Obstetrics and Gynecology 155: 812–816
27. Chescheir N C, Seeds J W 1988 Polyhydramnios and oligohydramnios in twin gestations. Obstetrics and Gynecology 71: 882–884
28. Clark R H, Gerstmann D R, Null D M, deLemos R A 1992 Prospective randomized comparison of high-frequency oscillatory and conventional ventilation in respiratory distress syndrome. Pediatrics 89: 5–12
29. Clark R H, Yoder B A, Sell M S 1994 Prospective, randomized comparison of high-frequency oscillation and conventional ventilation in candidates for extracorporeal membrane oxygenation. Journal of Pediatrics 124: 447–454
30. Clark S L, Vitale D J, Minton S D, Stoddard R A, Sabey P L 1987 Successful fetal therapy for cystic adenomatoid malformation associated with second-trimester hydrops. American Journal of Obstetrics and Gynecology 157: 294–295
31. Clarke C A, Mollison P L 1989 Deaths from Rh haemolytic disease of the fetus and newborn, 1977–1987. Journal of the Royal College of Physicians of London 23: 181–184
32. Committee on Infectious Diseases 1990 Parvovirus, erythema infectiosum, and pregnancy. Pediatrics 85: 131–133
33. Copel J A, Buyon J P, Kleinman C S 1995 Successful in utero therapy for fetal heart block. American Journal of Obstetrics and Gynecology 173: 1384–1390
34. Cunningham F G, MacDonald P C, Gant N F, Leveno K J, Gilstrap L C 1993 Endocrine disorders. In: Williams' obstetrics, 19th edn. Appleton & Lange, pp 1201–1227
35. Daffos F, Forestier F, Capella-Pavlovsky M et al 1988 Prenatal management of 746 pregnancies at risk for congenital toxoplasmosis. New England Journal of Medicine 318: 271–275
36. Davis J M, Richter S E, Kendig J W, Notter R H 1992 High-frequency jet ventilation and surfactant treatment of newborns with severe respiratory failure. Pediatric Pulmonology 13: 108–112
37. Davison M B, Radford D J 1989 Fetal and neonatal congenital complete heart block. Medical Journal of Australia 150: 192–198
38. De Lia J, Emery M G, Sheafor S A, Jennison T A 1985 Twin transfusion syndrome: successful in utero treatment with digoxin. International Journal of Gynaecology and Obstetrics 23: 197–201
39. Dehner L P 1993 Parvovirus B19, hydrops fetalis, and fetal wastage. An etiologic sequence. American Journal of Clinical Pathology 96: 4–6
40. Driscoll S G 1966 Hydrops fetalis. New England Journal of Medicine 275: 1432–1434
41. Dumez Y, Mandelbrot L, Radunovic N et al 1993 Prenatal management of congenital cystic adenomatoid malformation of the lung. Journal of Pediatric Surgery 28: 36–41
42. Etches P C, Lemons J A 1979 Nonimmune hydrops fetalis: report of 22 cases including three siblings. Pediatrics 64: 326–332
43. Etches P C, Tierney A J, Demianczuk N 1994 Successful outcome in a case of cystic adenomatoid malformation of the lung complicated by fetal hydrops, using extracorporeal membrane oxygenation. Fetal Diagnosis and Therapy 9: 88–91
44. Fairley C K, Smoleniec J S, Caul O E, Miller E 1995 Observational study of the effect of intrauterine transfusions on outcome of fetal hydrops after parvovirus B19 infection. Lancet 346: 1335–1337
45. Frohnmulder I M, Stewart P A, Witsenburg M, Denhollander N S, Wladimiroff J W, Hess J 1995 The efficacy of flecainide versus digoxin in the management of fetal supraventricular tachycardia. Prenatal Diagnosis 15: 1297–1302
46. Gembruch U, Hansmann M, Bald R 1988 Direct intrauterine fetal treatment of fetal tachyarrhythmia with severe hydrops fetalis by antiarrhythmic drugs. Fetal Therapy 3: 210–215
47. Gembruch U, Hansmann M, Redel D A, Bald R 1988 Intrauterine therapy of fetal tachyarrhythmias: intraperitoneal administration of antiarrhythmic drugs to the fetus in fetal tachyarrhythmias with severe hydrops fetalis. Journal of Perinatal Medicine 16: 39–44
48. Gembruch U, Hansmann M, Redel D A, Bald R, Knopfle G 1989 Fetal complete heart block: antenatal diagnosis, significance and management. European Journal of Obstetrics and Gynecology and Reproductive Biology 31: 9–22
49. Girz B A, Divon M Y, Papajohn M, Merkatz I R 1990 Amniotic fluid volume in diabetic pregnancy. Presented at the Annual Meeting of the Society of Perinatal Obstetricians, Abstract 334
50. Goldberg J D, Mitty H, Dische M R, Berkowitz R L 1986 Prenatal shunting of fetal ascites in nonimmune hydrops fetalis. American Journal of Perinatology 3: 92–93
51. Gonsoulin W, Moise K J Jr, Kirshon B, Cotton D B, Wheeler J M, Carpenter R J Jr 1990 Outcome of twin-twin transfusion diagnosed before 28 weeks of gestation. Obstetrics and Gynecology 75: 214–216
52. Gough J D, Keeling J W, Castle B, Iliff P J 1986 The obstetric management of non-immunological hydrops. British Journal of Obstetrics and Gynaecology 93: 226–234
53. Graves G R, Baskett T F 1984 Nonimmune hydrops fetalis: antenatal diagnosis and management. American Journal of Obstetrics and Gynecology 148: 563–565
54. Greene D, Watson W J, Wirtz P S 1993 Non-immune hydrops with congenital herpes simplex infection. South Dakota Journal of Medicine 46: 219–220
55. Guntheroth W G, Cyr D R, Mack L A, Benedetti T, Lenke R R, Petty C N 1985 Hydrops from reciprocating atrioventricular tachycardia in a 27-week fetus requiring quinidine for conversion. Obstetrics and Gynecology 66: 29S–33S
56. Hagay Z, Reece A, Roberts A, Hobbins J C 1993 Isolated fetal pleural effusion: a prenatal management dilemma. Obstetrics and Gynecology 81: 147–152
57. Hallak M, Neerhof M G, Perry R, Nazir M, Huhta J C 1991 Fetal supraventricular tachycardia and hydrops fetalis: combined intensive, direct, and transplacental therapy. Obstetrics and Gynecology 78: 523–525
58. Hardy J D, Solomon S, Banwell G S, Beach R, Wright V, Howard F M 1979 Congenital complete heart block in the newborn associated with maternal systemic lupus erythematosus and other connective tissue disorders. Archives of Disease in Childhood 54: 7–13
59. Harris J P, Alexson C G, Manning J A, Thompson H O 1993 Medical therapy for the hydropic fetus with congenital complete atrioventricular block. American Journal of Perinatology 10: 217–219
60. Harrison M R, Adzick N S, Jennings R W et al 1990 Antenatal intervention for congenital cystic adenomatoid malformation. Lancet 336: 965–967
61. Hartwig N G, Vermeij-Keers C, Van Elsacker-Niele A M W, Fleuren G J 1989 Embryonic malformation in a case of intrauterine parvovirus B19 infection. Teratology 39: 295–302
62. Hill L M, Breckle R, Thomas M L, Fries J K 1987 Polyhydramnios: ultrasonically detected prevalence and neonatal outcome. Obstetrics and Gynecology 69: 21–25
63. Hohlfeld P, Daffos F, Thulliez P et al 1989 Fetal toxoplasmosis: outcome of pregnancy and infant follow-up after in utero treatment. Journal of Pediatrics 115: 765–769
64. Holzgreve W, Curry C J R, Golbus M S, Callen P W, Filly R, Smith J C 1984 Investigation of nonimmune hydrops fetalis. American Journal of Obstetrics and Gynecology 150: 805–812
65. Holzgreve W, Holzgreve B, Curry C J R 1985 Nonimmune hydrops fetalis: diagnosis and management. Seminars in Perinatology 9: 52–67
66. Hsieh F-J, Chang F-M, Ko T-M, Kuo P-L, Chang D-Y, Chen H-Y

1989 The antenatal blood gas and acid–base status of normal fetuses and hydropic fetuses with Bart's hemoglobinopathy. Obstetrics and Gynecology 74: 722–725
67. Hsieh F J, Ko T M, Chen H Y 1992 Hydrops fetalis caused by severe α-thalassaemia. Early Human Development 29: 233–236
68. Humphrey W, Magoon M, O'Shaughnessy R 1991 Severe nonimmune hydrops secondary to parvovirus B-19 infection: spontaneous reversal in utero and survival of a term infant. Obstetrics and Gynecology 78: 900–902
69. Iliff P J, Nicholls J M, Keeling J W, Gough J D 1983 Non-immunologic hydrops fetalis: a review of 27 cases. Archives of Disease in Childhood 58: 979–982
70. Im S S, Rizos N, Joutsi P, Shime J, Benzie R J 1984 Nonimmunologic hydrops fetalis. American Journal of Obstetrics and Gynecology 148: 566–569
71. Jackson J C, Truog W E, Standaert T A et al 1994 Reduction in lung injury after combined surfactant and high-frequency ventilation. American Journal of Respiratory and Critical Care Medicine 150: 534–539
72. Jeannel D, Costagliola D, Niel G, Hubert B, Danis M 1990 What is known about the prevention of congenital toxoplasmosis? Lancet 336: 359–361
73. Jones D C 1995 Nonimmune fetal hydrops: diagnosis and obstetrical management. Seminars in Perinatology 19: 447–461
74. Jones J M, Sbarra A J, Dilillo L, Cetrulo C L, D'Alton M E 1993 Indomethacin in severe twin to twin transfusion syndrome. American Journal of Perinatology 10: 24–26
75. Keeling J W, Gough D J, Iliff P 1983 The pathology of non-rhesus hydrops. Diagnostic Histopathology 6: 89–111
76. Klarr J M, Faix R G, Pryce C J E, Bhatt-Mehta V 1994 Randomized, blind trial of dopamine versus dobutamine for treatment of hypotension in preterm infants with respiratory distress syndrome. Journal of Pediatrics 125: 117–122
77. Kleinman C S, Donnerstein R L, Jaffe C C et al 1983 Fetal echocardiography. A tool for evaluation of in utero cardiac arrhythmias and monitoring of in utero therapy: analysis of 71 patients. American Journal of Cardiology 51: 237–243
78. Kleinman C S, Copel J A, Weinstein E M, Santulli T V Jr, Hobbins J C 1985 In utero diagnosis and treatment of fetal supraventricular tachycardia. Seminars in Perinatology 9: 113–129
79. Knisely A S 1995 The pathologist and the hydropic placenta, fetus, or infant. Seminars in Perinatology 19: 525–531
80. Kofinas A D, Simon N V, Sagel H et al 1991 Treatment of fetal supraventricular tachycardia with flecainide acetate after digoxin failure. American Journal of Obstetrics and Gynecology 165: 630–631
81. Kohl T, Tercanli S, Kececioglu D, Holzgreve W 1995 Direct fetal administration of adenosine for the termination of incessant supraventricular tachycardia. Obstetrics and Gynecology 85: 873–874
82. Kuller J A, Yankowitz J, Goldberg J D et al 1992 Outcome of antenatally diagnosed cystic adenomatoid malformations. American Journal of Obstetrics and Gynecology 167: 1038–1041
83. Laneri G G, Claassen D L, Scher M S 1994 Brain lesions of fetal onset in encephalopathic infants with nonimmune hydrops fetalis. Pediatric Neurology 11: 18–22
84. Langer J C, Harrison M, Schmidt K G et al 1989 Fetal hydrops and death from sacrococcygeal teratoma: rationale for fetal surgery. American Journal of Obstetrics and Gynecology 160: 1145–1150
85. Larroche J C, Aubry M C, Narcy F 1992 Intrauterine brain damage in nonimmune hydrops fetalis. Biology of the Neonate 61: 273–280
86. Liang S T, Wong V C, So W W, Ma H K, Chan V, Todd D 1985 Homozygous alpha-thalassaemia: clinical presentation, diagnosis, and management. A review of 46 cases. British Journal of Obstetrics and Gynaecology 92: 680–684
87. Litsey S E, Noonan J A, O'Connor W N, Cottrill C M, Mitchell B 1985 Maternal connective tissue disease and congenital heart block. Demonstration of immunoglobulin in cardiac tissue. New England Journal of Medicine 312: 98–100
88. Macafee C A J, Fortune D W, Beischer N A 1970 Non-immunological hydrops fetalis. Journal of Obstetrics and Gynaecology of the British Commonwealth 77: 226–237
89. McCoy M C, Katz V L, Gould N, Kuller J A 1995 Non-immune hydrops after 20 weeks' gestation: review of 10 years' experience with suggestions for management. Obstetrics and Gynecology 85: 578–582
90. MacGillivray T E, Harrison M R, Goldstein R B, Adzick N S 1993 Disappearing fetal lung lesions. Journal of Pediatric Surgery 28: 1321–1325
91. McGillvray B C, Hall J G 1987 Nonimmune hydrops fetalis. Pediatrics in Review 9: 197–202
92. Machin G A 1981 Differential diagnosis of hydrops fetalis. American Journal of Medical Genetics 9: 341–350
93. Machin G A 1989 Hydrops revisited: literature review of 1,414 cases published in the 1980s. American Journal of Medical Genetics 34: 366–390
94. Mahony B S, Petty C N, Nyberg D A, Luthy D A, Hickok D E, Hirsch J H 1990 The 'stuck twin' phenomenon: ultrasonographic findings, pregnancy outcome, and management with serial amniocentesis. American Journal of Obstetrics and Gynecology 163: 1513–1522
95. Martin T C, Arias F, Olander D S, Hoffman R J, Marbarger J P, Maurer M M 1988 Successful management of congenital atrioventricular block associated with hydrops fetalis. Journal of Pediatrics 112: 984–986
96. Meizner I, Levy A, Carmi R, Robinson C 1990 Niemann–Pick disease associated with nonimmune hydrops fetalis. American Journal of Obstetrics and Gynecology 163: 128–129
97. Morey A L, Keeling J W, Porter H J, Fleming K A 1992 Clinical and histopathological features of parvovirus B19 infection in the human fetus. British Journal of Obstetrics and Gynaecology 99: 566–574
98. Nakayama R, Yamada D, Steinmiller V, Hsia E, Hale R W 1986 Hydrops fetalis secondary to Bart hemoglobinopathy. Obstetrics and Gynecology 67: 176–180
99. Nicolaides K H, Azar G B 1990 Thoraco-amniotic shunting. Fetal Diagnosis and Therapy 5: 153–156
100. Nicolay K S, Gainey H L 1964 Pseudotoxemic state associated with severe Rh immunization. American Journal of Obstetrics and Gynecology 89: 41–45
101. Nicolini U, Santolaya J, Fisk N M et al 1988 Changes in fetal acid base status during intravascular transfusion. Archives of Disease in Childhood 63: 710–714
102. Norton M E 1994 Nonimmune hydrops fetalis. Seminars in Perinatology 18: 321–332
103. Nugent C E, Hayashi R H, Rubin J 1989 Prenatal treatment of type 1 congenital cystic adenomatoid malformation by intrauterine fetal thoracocentesis. Clinical Ultrasound 17: 675–677
104. Owen J, Colvin E V, Davis R O 1988 Fetal death after successful conversion of fetal supraventricular tachycardia with digoxin and verapamil. American Journal of Obstetrics and Gynecology 158: 1169–1170
105. Peliowski A, Finer N N, Etches P C, Tierney A J, Ryan C A 1995 Inhaled nitric oxide for premature infants after prolonged rupture of the membranes. Journal of Pediatrics 126: 450–453
106. Phelan J P, Smith C V, Broussard P, Small M 1987 Amniotic fluid volume assessment with the four quadrant technique at 36 to 42 weeks gestation. Journal of Reproductive Medicine 32: 540–542
107. Phibbs R H 1985–1986 Hydrops. In: Nelson N M (ed) Current therapy in neonatal–perinatal medicine. B C Decker, Toronto, pp 201–207
108. Phibbs R H, Johnson P, Kitterman J A, Gregory G A, Tooley W H, Schlueter M 1976 Cardiorespiratory status of erythroblastotic newborn infants. III. Intravascular pressure during the first hours of life. Pediatrics 58: 484–493
109. Pinette M G, Pan Y, Pinette S G, Stubblefield P G 1993 Treatment of twin–twin transfusion syndrome. Obstetrics and Gynecology 82: 841–846
110. Platt D, Collea J V, Joseph D M 1978 Transitory fetal ascites: an ultrasound diagnosis. American Journal of Obstetrics and Gynecology 132: 906–908
111. Poeschmann R P, Verheijen R H M, Van Dongen P W J 1991 Differential diagnosis and causes of nonimmunological hydrops fetalis: a review. Obstetrical and Gynecological Survey 46: 223–231
112. Pryde P G, Nugent C E, Pridjian G, Barr M Jr, Faix R G 1992 Spontaneous resolution of nonimmune hydrops fetalis secondary to human parvovirus B19 infection. Obstetrics and Gynecology 79: 859–861
113. Rausen A R, Seki M, Strauss L 1965 Twin transfusion syndrome. Journal of Pediatrics 66: 613–628
114. Reed K L 1989 Fetal arrhythmias: etiology, diagnosis, pathophysiology, and treatment. Seminars in Perinatology 13: 294–304
115. Rey E, Duperron L, Gauthier R, Lemay M, Grignon A, LeLorier J

1985 Transplacental treatment of tachycardia-induced fetal heart failure with verapamil and amiodarone: a case report. American Journal of Obstetrics and Gynecology 153: 311–312
116. Rodeck C H, Fisk N M, Fraser D I, Nicolini U 1988 Long-term in utero drainage of fetal hydrothorax. New England Journal of Medicine 319: 1135–1138
117. Rogers B B, Mark Y, Oyer C E 1993 Diagnosis and incidence of fetal parvovirus infection in an autopsy series: I. Histology. Pediatric Pathology 13: 371–379
118. Roze J C, Tohier C, Maingueneau C, Lefevre M, Mouzard A 1993 Response to dobutamine and dopamine in the hypotensive very preterm infant. Archives of Disease in Childhood 69: 59–63
119. Saltzman D H, Frigoletto F D, Harlow B L, Barss V A, Benacerraf B R 1989 Sonographic evaluation of hydrops fetalis. Obstetrics and Gynecology 74: 106–111
120. Santolaya J, Alley D, Jaffe R, Warsof S L 1992 Antenatal classification of hydrops fetalis. Obstetrics and Gynecology 79: 256–259
121. Schlebusch H, von Mende S, Grunn U, Gembruch U, Bald R, Hansmann M 1991 Determination of digoxin in the blood of pregnant women, fetuses and neonates before and during anti-arrhythmic therapy, using four immunochemical methods. European Journal of Clinical Chemistry and Biochemistry 29: 57–66
122. Schmidt K G, Ulmer H E, Silverman N H, Kleinman C S, Copel J A 1991 Perinatal outcome of fetal complete atrioventricular block: a multicenter experience. Journal of the American College of Cardiology 91: 1360–1366
123. Seifer D B, Ferguson J E, Behrens C M, Zemel S, Stevenson D K, Ross J C 1985 Nonimmune hydrops fetalis in association with hemangioma of the umbilical cord. Obstetrics and Gynecology 66: 283–286
124. Sever J L, Ellenberg J H, Ley A C et al 1988 Toxoplasmosis: maternal and pediatric findings in 23,000 pregnancies. Pediatrics 82: 181–192
125. Shenker L, Reed K L, Anderson C F, Marx G R, Sobonya R E, Graham A R 1987 Congenital heart block and cardiac anomalies in the absence of maternal connective tissue disease. American Journal of Obstetrics and Gynecology 157: 248–253
126. Sherer D M, Abramowicz J S, Eggers P C, Woods J R Jr 1992 Transient severe unilateral and subsequent bilateral primary fetal hydrothorax with spontaneous resolution at 34 weeks' gestation associated with normal neonatal outcome. American Journal of Obstetrics and Gynecology 166: 169–170
127. Shimokawa H, Hara K, Maeda H, Miyamoto S, Koyanagi T, Nakano H 1988 Intrauterine treatment of idiopathic hydrops fetalis. Journal of Perinatal Medicine 16: 133–138
128. Soothill P W, Nicolaides K H, Rodeck C H, Clewell W H, Lindridge J 1987 Relationship of fetal hemoglobin and oxygen content to lactate concentration in Rh isoimmunized pregnancies. Obstetrics and Gynecology 69: 268–271
129. Starling E H 1896 On the absorption of fluids from the connective tissue spaces. Journal of Physiology 19: 312–326
130. Steiner R D 1995 Hydrops fetalis: role of the geneticist. Seminars in Perinatology 19: 516–524
131. Stephenson T, Zuccollo J, Mohajer M 1994 Diagnosis and management of non-immune hydrops in the newborn. Archives of Disease in Childhood 70: F151–F154
132. Stratton R F, Patterson R H 1993 DNA confirmation of congenital myotonic dystrophy in non-immune hydrops fetalis. Prenatal Diagnosis 13: 1027–1030
133. Strong S J, Corney G 1967 The placenta in twin pregnancy. Pergamon Press, Oxford
134. Thorp J A, Cohen G R, Yeast J D et al 1992 Nonimmune hydrops caused by massive fetomaternal hemorrhage and treated by intravascular transfusion. American Journal of Perinatology 9: 22–24
135. Torok T J 1995 Human parvovirus B19. In: Remington J S, Klein J O (eds) Infectious diseases of the fetus and newborn infant, 4th edn. W B Saunders, Philadelphia, pp 668–702
136. Turkel B S 1982 Conditions associated with nonimmune hydrops fetalis. Clinics in Perinatology 9: 613–625
137. Van Elsacker-Niele A M W, Salimans M M M, Weiland H T, Vermey-Keers C H R, Anderson M J, Versteeg J 1989 Fetal pathology in human parvovirus B19 infection. British Journal of Obstetrics and Gynaecology 96: 768–775
138. Van Maldergem L, Jauniaux E, Fourneau C, Gillerot Y 1992 Genetic causes of hydrops fetalis. Pediatrics 89: 81–86
139. Warsof S L, Nicolaides K H, Rodeck C 1986 Immune and non-immune hydrops. Clinics in Obstetrics and Gynecology 29: 533–542
140. Watson J, Campbell S 1986 Antenatal evaluation and management in nonimmune hydrops fetalis. Obstetrics and Gynecology 67: 589–593
141. Weiner C, Varner M, Pringle K, Hein H, Williamson R, Smith W L 1986 Antenatal diagnosis and palliative treatment of nonimmune hydrops fetalis secondary to pulmonary extralobar sequestration. Obstetrics and Gynecology 68: 275–280
142. Weiner C P, Pelzer G D, Heilskov J, Wenstrom K D, Williamson R A 1989 The effect of intravascular transfusion on umbilical venous pressure in anemic fetuses with and without hydrops. American Journal of Obstetrics and Gynecology 161: 1498–1501
143. Wiggins J W, Bowes W, Clewell W et al 1986 Echocardiographic diagnosis and intravenous digoxin management of fetal tachyarrhythmias and congestive heart failure. American Journal of Diseases of Children 140: 202–206
144. Wright C, Hinchliffe S A, Taylor C 1996 Fetal pathology in intrauterine death due to parvovirus B19 infection. British Journal of Obstetrics and Gynaecology 103: 133–136
145. Yaegashi N, Okamura K, Yajima A, Murai C, Sugamura K 1994 The frequency of human parvovirus B19 infection in nonimmune hydrops fetalis. Journal of Perinatal Medicine 22: 159–163
146. Younis J S, Granat M 1987 Insufficient transplacental digoxin transfer in severe hydrops fetalis. American Journal of Obstetrics and Gynecology 157: 1268–1269

34

Malformation syndromes

Michael Baraitser   Robin M. Winter

SPECIFIC CHROMOSOMAL ABNORMALITIES

FREQUENCY OF CHROMOSOMAL ABNORMALITIES

At birth the frequency of sex chromosome abnormalities is about 3 per 1000, and of autosomal abnormalities about 4 per 1000. Of the latter group about 1.5 per 1000 represent autosomal trisomies (mainly Down syndrome), the remainder being translocations, mainly balanced. The frequency of chromosome abnormalities in miscarriages is much higher. Studies which include abortuses expelled up to the end of the second trimester show a frequency of 20–30%, whereas in those studies including only the early stages of pregnancy the figure is closer to 50%. A brief description of the more common chromosomal abnormalities recognizable at birth is given below. Fuller descriptions and photographs may be found in Jones.[92]

DOWN SYNDROME (Fig. 34.1)

The commonest autosomal anomaly is Down syndrome, or mongolism, which is present in about 1 in 600–700 livebirths. In the majority of cases there are 47 chromosomes, the extra chromosome being a small acrocentric, number 21.

This syndrome is usually due to non-disjunction during oogenesis in the mother. The incidence of Down syndrome due to non-disjunction shows a marked association with maternal age. The overall prevalence of Down syndrome in children born to 18-year-old mothers is about 1 in 2300, whereas at 40 it is 1 in 100, and at a maternal age of 46 it is about 1 in 45.

The clinical diagnosis of Down syndrome is seldom a problem to the neonatologist. Recognition is based on the upward slant of the eyes, prominent epicanthic folds, Brushfield spots in the iris, a flat nasal bridge, protruding tongue, short neck and flat occiput. In the limbs, short broad hands, short incurved little fingers, single transverse palmar creases and a sandal gap between the first and second toes are typical. Congenital heart disease occurs in about 40% of cases. Atrioventricular canal, atrial and ventricular septal defects are the commonest lesions.

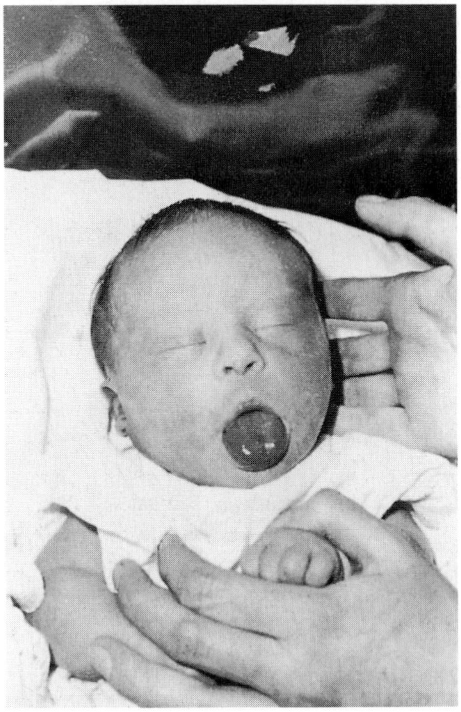

Fig. 34.1 Down syndrome (trisomy 21).

Although 95% of babies with Down syndrome are of the standard trisomic type, in about 2.5% there is mosaicism, with a population of normal cells being present, and in the remainder of cases a chromosome translocation involving chromosome 21 is involved. The translocations mostly involve a number 14 and 21 chromosome. Of these about three-quarters are de-novo events and one-quarter are inherited from a balanced translocation carrier parent. Very rarely, a parent carries a balanced Robertsonian translocation between two chromosomes 21. In this case all offspring will have Down syndrome.

Table 34.1 Recurrence risk figures in Down syndrome

	Risk
After one trisomic child (mother aged under 39 years)	1%
If mother aged over 39 years	Double maternal age risk
Mother is a 14/21 translocation carrier	10%
Father is a 14/21 translocation carrier	2%
One parent is a 21/21 translocation carrier	100%

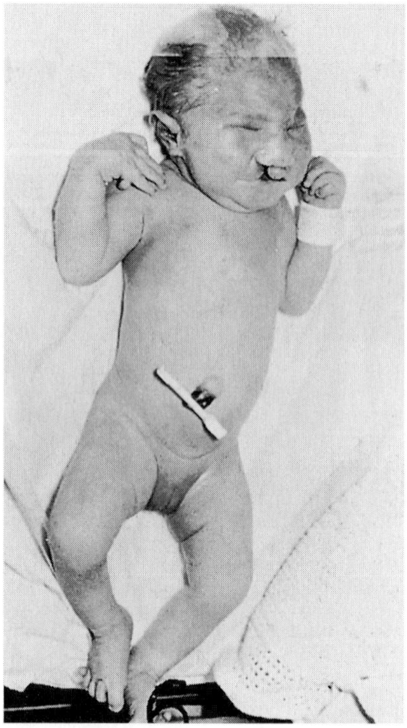

Fig. 34.2 Patau syndrome (trisomy 13).

Management

Almost all are agreed that the suspected diagnosis should be disclosed early on, provided the clinician is confident of the clinical diagnosis. Confirmation, by means of a chromosome analysis, should be available within a week. As well as advice about the management and prognosis of the infant, the parents will need counselling about risks to future children. This is best carried out some months after the birth, and should include full explanation of prenatal diagnosis (amniocentesis or chorion villus sampling) and the associated risk. A rough guide to the recurrence risk in Down syndrome is given in Table 34.1.

TRISOMY 13 (PATAU SYNDROME) (Fig. 34.2)

This aneuploidy has a frequency of 1 in 7000 live births. Survival after the first year of life is unusual, although survival until over the age of 5 years has been described. The head is small, triangular in shape (trigonocephaly), with a sloping forehead. The eyes are small and colobomata of the iris are common. Bilateral cleft lip and palate in the presence of the small head and jaw, in conjunction with the eye abnormalities, suggest the syndrome on inspection of the face alone. Congenital heart defects are present in more than 80% of cases, and in the limbs polydactyly (on the ulnar side) and the overlapping of fingers are frequent features, as are rocker-bottom feet. Urogenital abnormalities and malrotation of the gut frequently occur.

Most complete trisomy 13s are spontaneous events with a slight maternal age effect, but where the extra number 13 is in the form of an unbalanced translocation, an examination of the parental chromosomes is mandatory. Recurrence risks for another child with trisomy 13 are small; however, there is about a 1% risk of a numerical chromosome abnormality in future pregnancies. The most common problem would be Down syndrome. Under these circumstances most clinicians would offer an amniocentesis in subsequent pregnancies.

TRISOMY 18 (Figs 34.3, 34.4)

Trisomy 18 or Edward syndrome has a distinctive clinical picture. The incidence is about 1 in 5000. Those affected have a prominent occiput, a dolichocephalic (disproportionately long) head and a small chin. The ears are low-set and malformed (especially the auricles). The mouth opening is small, and ptosis and wide epicanthic folds are common. In the hands the second finger overlaps the third, and occasionally the fifth overlaps the fourth. Dermatoglyphic examination of the finger pads reveals a preponderance of low arches, and the distal crease on the fifth finger might be absent. Cryptorchidism is common and the majority of cases have congenital heart defects, especially an atrial septal defect or patent ductus arteriosus. Renal defects are also common. Mental retardation in survivors is severe, however: only 10% of babies survive the first year of life.

The association of trisomy 18 with increasing maternal age is not as obvious as in trisomy 21. However, the mean maternal age (32 years) is well above the population mean. Recurrence risks are similar to those for trisomy 13.

TRISOMY 8 (Fig. 34.5)

Most of these infants are mosaic for trisomy 8/normal cells. The most characteristic neonatal abnormality is the presence of deep grooves on the soles and palms. Mild camptodactyly and limitation of elbow extension might also be present. The face may not be very unusual, but there is a tendency for rather 'coarse' features, consisting of a broad nasal root, thick lips, prominent forehead and protuberant ears. Eventual development reveals mild to severe retardation.

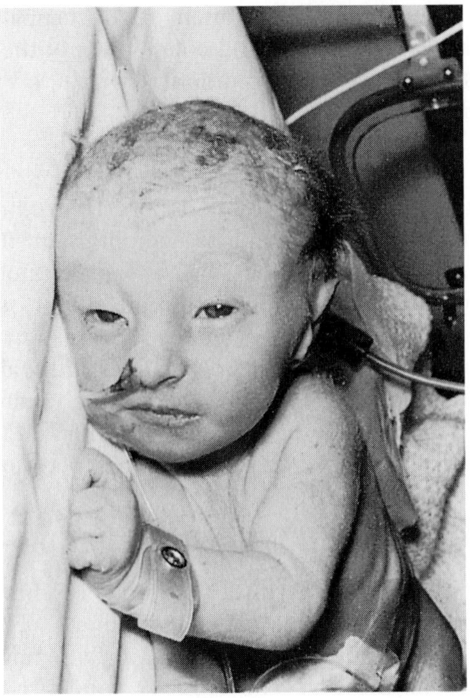

Fig. 34.3 Edward syndrome (trisomy 18).

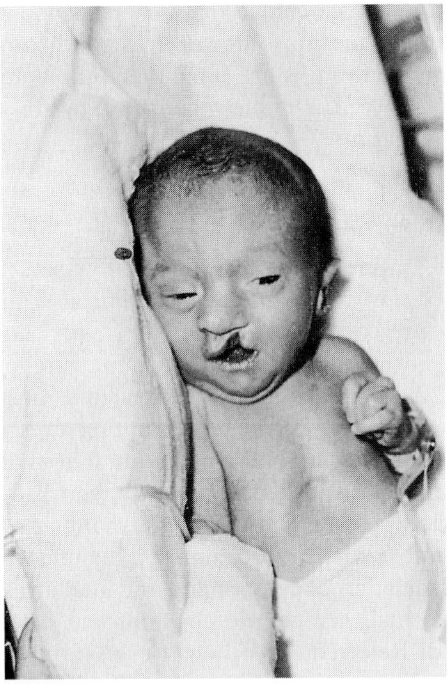

Fig. 34.4 Edward syndrome (trisomy 18).

DELETION OF THE SHORT ARM OF 4 (4p–) (WOLF–HIRSCHHORN SYNDROME) (Fig. 34.6)

Severe mental and growth retardation is invariably present. The head is small and midline scalp defects are common. Preauricular cutaneous pits and tags draw attention to the possible diagnosis, and colobomata of the iris, a fish mouth, cleft lip and palate and simple low-set

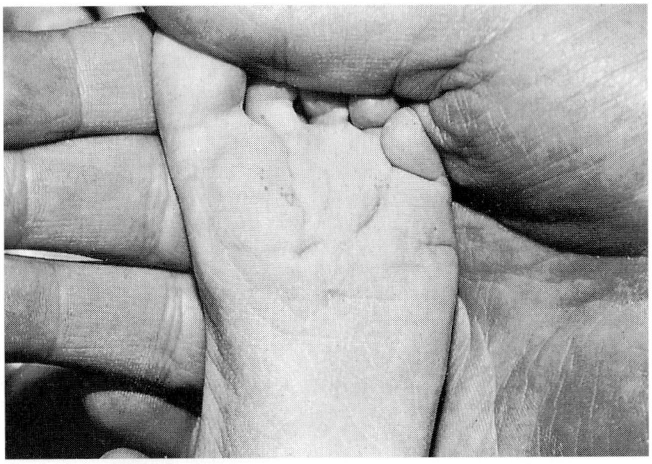

Fig. 34.5 Partial trisomy 8.

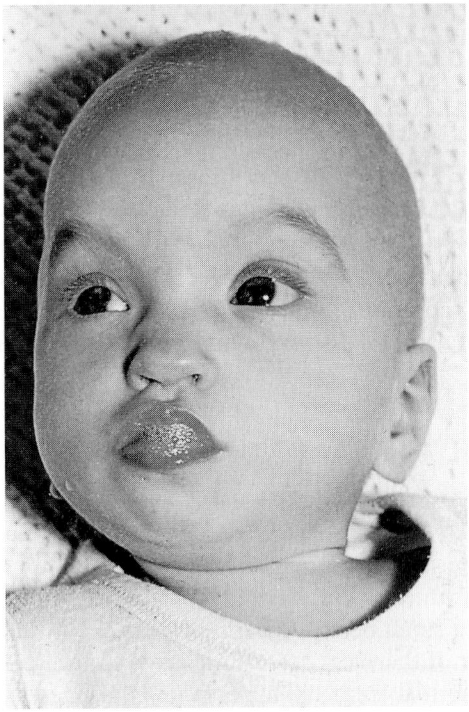

Fig. 34.6 Wolf–Hirschhorn syndrome (4p– syndrome).

ears are frequently found. The prominent glabella, lack of an angle between the forehead and the broad nasal bridge and hypertelorism give the face a 'Greek warrior helmet' appearance. Cardiac defects (atrial septal defects and ventricular septal defects) occur in one-third of cases. Grand mal epilepsy is common and half of those affected by the syndrome are dead before 6 months of age.

DELETION OF SHORT ARM OF 5 (5p–) (CRI DU CHAT SYNDROME) (Fig. 34.7)

Even in the absence of the typical neonatal cry (not invariably present), the cri du chat syndrome is in most instances recognizable because of the presence of a round

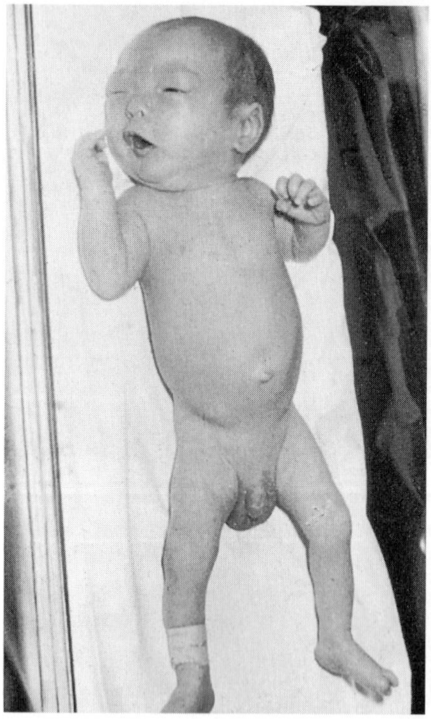

Fig. 34.7 Cri du chat syndrome (5p– syndrome).

face, small head, widely spaced eyes, prominent epicanthus, antimongoloid eye slant and low-set ears. Cleft lip and palate, cardiac and renal anomalies are sometimes present.

PARTIAL TRISOMY OF THE SHORT ARM OF 9

Trisomy 9p is now established as a definitive clinical entity. The facial appearance of this mental retardation syndrome is characterized by a large globulous nose, the effect of which is emphasized by deep-set, widely spaced eyes on a small head. Epicanthic folds, an antimongoloid obliquity of the eyes, downturned mouth, protruding ears with abnormal antihelix, hypoplastic phalanges, (especially the fifth finger middle phalanx) and extra skin folds in the neck are the other common features.

DELETION OF THE LONG ARM OF 11 (11q–)

The craniofacial abnormalities are sometimes distinctive. The occiput is flared and the forehead is keel-shaped. The eyes are downslanting and ptosis is sometimes present. The jaw is small, the ears low-set, the mouth is characteristically carp-shaped and the philtrum long. Congenital heart defects, especially a ventricular septal defect, are common. Multiple joint contractures may be present.

DELETION OF THE LONG ARM OF 13 (13q–)

There is usually a broad, prominent nasal bridge and glabella on a small and often trigonocephalic head. Epicanthic folds are wide and colobomata of the iris may be present. Ears are commonly large, low-set and malformed.

There is evidence to suggest that there is a difference in the clinical features when the distal or proximal segment is implicated in the deletion. Protruding upper incisor teeth are, for instance, common in the distal deletion, as is the frontal bossing, whereas retinoblastoma and mild mental retardation are more often found with proximal or interstitial deletions. Like most of the chromosomal syndromes, abnormalities are widespread. Absent or hypoplastic thumbs, congenital heart defect, cryptorchidism, hypospadias and webbing of the neck have all been described on more than one occasion.

DELETION OF THE LONG ARM OF 18 (18q–)

A deletion of the long arm of a number 18 chromosome can be diagnosed on clinical grounds. The most characteristic feature is the mild facial flattening, with a prominent jutting jaw. The eyes are widely spaced and nystagmus, epicanthus and pale optic discs are found. The ears are prominent with large antihelices and antitragi, but the external canal is narrow and deafness is common. The mouth is downturned and 'carp-like'. In the hands, the thumbs are proximally implanted and the fingers are tapered. Dimples over the extensor surfaces of joints are a feature.

TRISOMY 22

The head is small and the ears are low-set, malformed and angled forward. An unusual clinical feature is the frequent presence of preauricular skin tags which, although not unique to the syndrome, are pointers to trisomy 22. A beaked nose, anteverted nostrils, long philtrum, cleft palate and downslanting eyes occur frequently. The neck is short and redundant skin folds accentuate the short-necked appearance. Cardiac anomalies are found in 50% of cases. In the hands fingerized or broad thumbs are the more common manifestations.

The association of colobomata and anal atresia with an additional small acrocentric chromosome has long been recognized. Referred to as the cat eye syndrome (distinct from cat cry), most cases were described during the pre-banding era. It now appears that the syndrome represents a partial trisomy or tetrasomy of the long arm of 22.

MICRODELETION SYNDROMES

All neonates who look unusual or have one or more malformations need a G-banded chromosome analysis. There are, however, a small but significant number of conditions which, despite being chromosomal in origin, have changes (mostly small deletions) that cannot be detected in this way. Over the past few years new techniques have been developed to detect these submicroscopic deletions, the most commonly used being fluorescence in situ hybridization. The problem for the clinician is that a presumptive diagnosis needs to be made so that the laboratory can use the appropriate probes. The table below shows some of the more common conditions that may be diagnosed in this way.

Condition	Main features in neonate	Locus that needs attention
Williams	Supravalvular aortic stenosis Hypercalcaemia	7q11
Prader–Willi	Floppiness	15q11 (DNA studies should also be carried out)
Miller–Dieker	Lissencephaly	17p13
DiGeorge Shprintzen Velocardiofacial	Hypocalcaemia Interrupted aortic arch Cardiac lesion	22q11
Wolf–Hirschhorn	Specific facial dysmorphism (see Fig. 34.6)	4pter

SEX CHROMOSOME ABNORMALITIES

Of the common sex chromosome anomalies, fragile X (mental retardation), Klinefelter syndrome (47, XXY), 47,XXX females and 47,XYY males show few phenotypic abnormalities in the neonatal period and are rarely diagnosed at this time. In general all non-disjunction syndromes are maternal age-related, but not to the same extent as in Down syndrome.

TURNER SYNDROME (45,XO)

The prevalence of this disorder is 1 in 5000 births. The most striking features may be a webbed skin fold at the neck (pterygium colli), with a low, trident posterior hairline (Fig. 34.8). Lymphoedema of the dorsum of the hands and feet is common (Fig. 34.9). The chest may be broad with widespread nipples, and cardiac defects, especially coarctation of the aorta, occur in about 20% of cases. Minor abnormalities that might be noted at birth include small, convex, deep-set nails, pigmented naevi on the skin and an increased carrying angle at the elbow. Short stature is the rule, with a mean final height of 4 feet 7 inches. Streak gonads are usually present, with the consequence that normal menstruation does not occur and infertility is the rule. Replacement oestrogens are indicated at around the time of puberty. Outlook for final intelligence is good. Recurrence risks are small, probably less than those given for the autosomal trisomies.

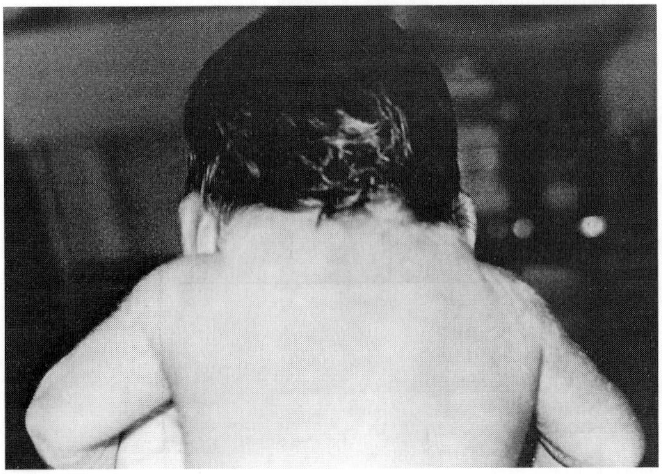

Fig. 34.8 Turner syndrome (45,XO).

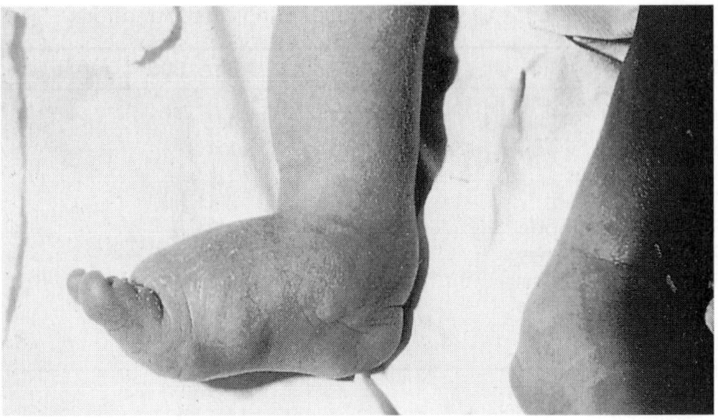

Fig. 34.9 Turner syndrome (45,XO).

HIGHER DEGREES OF SEX CHROMOSOME ANEUPLOIDY

With increasing numbers of sex chromosomes (e.g. 49,XXXXY; 48,XXXX, 49,XXXXX etc.) mental retardation becomes the rule. Pointers in the neonatal period include a tendency to mongoloid eye-slant, a short or webbed neck and joint abnormalities, especially radioulnar synostosis. There is an increased incidence of simple arched fingertip ridge patterns.

AN APPROACH TO THE CHROMOSOMALLY NORMAL MALFORMED NEONATE

GENERAL CONSIDERATIONS

One child in every 40 has a congenital malformation. Some of these are single, others are part of more complex dysmorphic syndromes. Single minor abnormalities are common (Table 34.2), but they also occur with an increased frequency in children with single or multiple major malformations. As pointed out by Marden et al,[115] multiple minor malformations occur alone in 0.8% of the population, whereas multiple minor malformations occur with single major malformations in 6.9% of affected infants. Multiple minor malformations occur in 56.2% of infants with multiple major malformations.

Table 34.2 Incidence of some common, minor malformations

Minor	Per 1000
Epicanthus	4.2
Small ears	1.4
Auricular sinus	1.2
Preauricular tags	2.3
Fifth finger clinodactyly	9.9
2/3 syndactyly, toes	1.6
Single palmar crease	
Unilateral	4%
Bilateral	1%

Syndrome recognition is an essential prerequisite for accurate genetic counselling, immediate management and prognosis. Syndrome identification in the neonate is based on an accurate evaluation of the dysmorphic features. For instance, hypertelorism (increased interpupillary distance) must be differentiated from telecanthus (increased distance between inner canthi).

Ideally this should be done with measurements and centile charts, and these do exist for certain modalities. Eventually photogrammetry might supersede clinical measurement, but at present a traditional clinical approach is used. Experience has shown that it is easier to make a syndrome diagnosis when a clearly delineated unusual feature or constellation of features is present. For example, cleft palate and polydactyly are more useful than those features that are common in normal neonates, such as inguinal hernia. Abnormal dysmorphic features might be thought of as 'handles', and there is a hierarchy

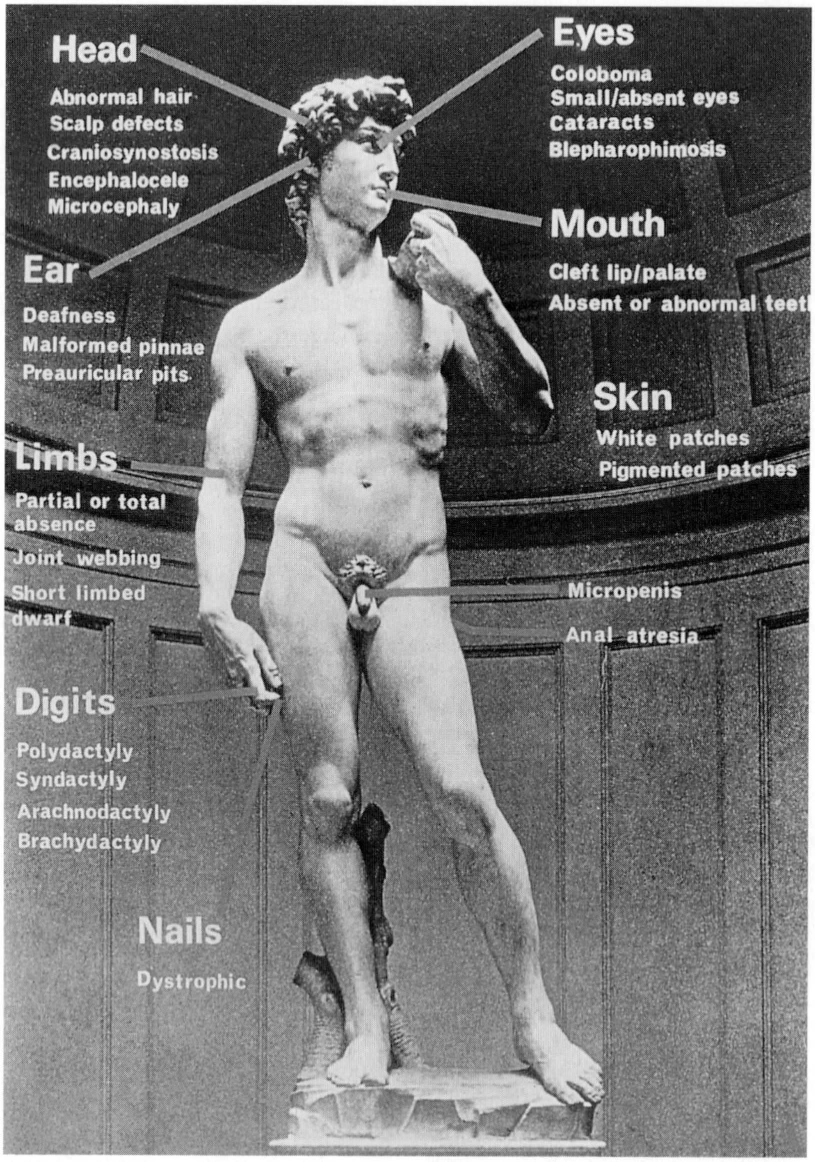

Fig. 34.10 An approach to the diagnosis of the dysmorphic child (see text).

of 'handles' in order of their usefulness for the syndromologist. Some malformations are minor and blend into normal variations; others are too frequent and therefore unhelpful. An approach to the diagnosis of the dysmorphic child will be discussed, using various 'handles' (Fig. 34.10).

DEVELOPMENTAL CONSIDERATIONS

In the assessment of the dysmorphic child it is necessary to decide whether there is (a) a malformation, (b) a deformation, or (c) a disruption. These can be defined as follows:[155]

a. A malformation results from an intrinsic abnormal developmental process. The developmental potential is abnormal (e.g. spina bifida).

b. A deformation results from mechanical alteration to a developing part after a period of normal development (e.g. talipes equinovarus caused by fetal constraint).

c. A disruption – after an initially normal development a breakdown of or an interference with organ development occurs, resulting in the destruction of that part (e.g. amniotic bands).

Having decided which of the three broad categories is appropriate, then, taking a malformation as an example, the designation to this category should be followed by the questions:

- Is it a single or multiple malformation?[92]
- If there are multiple malformations, are they part of a syndrome or a sequence?

If a single insult leads onto or initiates further defects then it is a *malformation sequence*. This implies that there is a cascade of secondary consequences. For example, renal agenesis causes oligohydramnios, which in turn gives rise to 'Potter's facies' and pulmonary hypoplasia. If the initial insult causes multiple defects but these are not the consequence of one another, then the term malformation syndrome might be appropriate. It should be noted that a syndrome is a pattern of malformations thought to be pathogenically related. If the multiple malformation complex under consideration is not thought to be a syndrome or sequence there could be a known association between the various components. An *association* is a non-random occurrence of multiple anomalies not known to be a sequence or a syndrome. It is a statistical concept. The importance of these distinctions is that deformations or disruptions are rarely genetically determined, whereas the malformation syndromes might be chromosomal, inherited in a Mendelian way.

Table 34.3 Important points in history taking

Questions	Relevance
Personal/family history	
(1) Elderly mother	? Chromosomal aneuploidy
(2) Elderly father	? New autosomal dominant mutation
(3) Maternal disease (e.g. diabetes)	Known associated fetal abnormalities (e.g. sacral agenesis with maternal diabetes)
(4) Poor social history	Possible alcohol/drug ingestion
(5) Racial origin of parents	Known genes of high frequency in certain racial group (e.g. Ellis van Creveld syndrome in the Amish)
(6) Parental consanguinity	Autosomal recessive disorders
(7) Other affected family members or multiple miscarriages/stillbirths	Single gene or chromosome disorders. Possible maternal uterine abnormalities
Pregnancy history	
(8) Maternal drug or alcohol ingestion	Teratogenic effects
(9) Exposure to radiation (especially therapeutic)	Possible mutagenic or teratogenic effects
(10) Early rupture of membranes	Possible fetal compression leading to deformation
(11) Oligohydramnios	Renal agenesis or outflow obstruction
(12) Polyhydramnios	Oesophageal atresia; neuromuscular disorders
(13) Poor fetal movements	Fetal compression, neuromuscular disorder
(14) Breech presentation	Neuromuscular disorder
(15) Early maternal infections	?Intra-uterine infection of the fetus

A CLINICAL APPROACH

History

Many important clues can be obtained by a careful history taken from the parents and detailed examination of the obstetric notes. A summary of important questions is given in Table 34.3.

Clinical examination

The malformed neonate with normal chromosomes might have a specific syndrome. Its recognition should be approached as follows:

Gestalt recognition

It might be that the individual malformation can easily be organized into a meaningful problem without consciously analysing the individual abnormalities. Recognition is

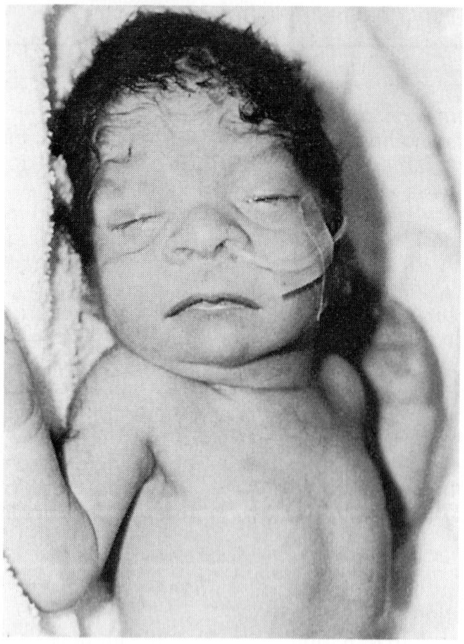

Fig. 34.11 De Lange syndrome.

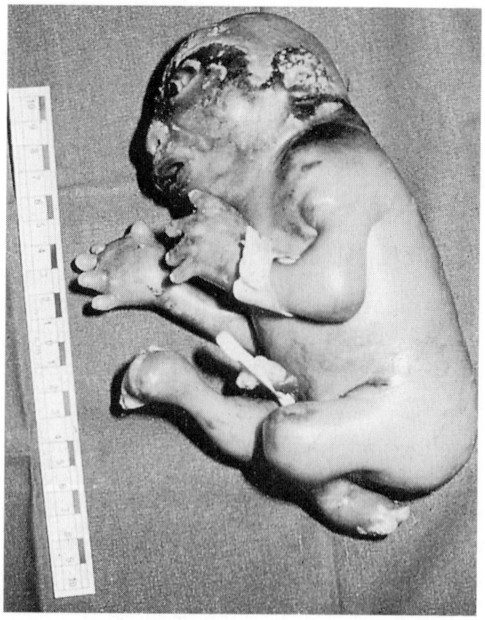

Fig. 34.12 Neu–Laxova syndrome.

immediate. For instance, diagnosis of the Cornelia de Lange syndrome (Fig. 34.11) is often possible from the examination of craniofacial features alone. Nevertheless, care should be taken not to overdiagnose syndromes on this basis, and a careful evaluation of other physical abnormalities which might help to confirm the initial diagnostic suspicion should be made.

Identification of suitable handles

Where immediate recognition is not possible it is necessary to identify one or more features (handles) which might lead the syndromologist to make a diagnosis. Useful handles are:

- well-defined but unusual physical signs, e.g. polydactyly. These should be carefully evaluated and described. For example, polydactyly can be of different degrees, associated with syndactyly, and can be on the radial side (preaxial) or ulnar side (postaxial);
- signs which are the subject of comprehensive reviews, e.g. anal atresia (see Pinsky[141]).

If one handle does not lead to a diagnosis then other combinations should be tried. Computer databases are now available which will furnish a manageable list of syndromes, with references for all possible combinations.[183] Lists of good handles are contained in Tables 34.4–34.41, which follow. The lists are not exhaustive but they attempt to cover most of the useful signs present in the neonate.

Abbreviations used in Tables 34.4–34.41

AD, autosomal dominant
AR, autosomal recessive
XLR, X-linked recessive
XLD, X-linked dominant.

Table 34.4 Microcephaly

Syndrome	Features present at birth	Features developing later	Inheritance	Location	Gene	References
Bloom	IUGR, malar hypoplasia	Facial telangiectasia, growth retardation, low IgA and IgM, lymphoreticular malignancy	AR	15q26	RecQ	51, 86
Coffin–Siris	see Nail abnormality (Table 34.33)					
de Lange (Fig. 34.11)	Synophrys, prominent philtrum, flared nostrils, thin upper lip, hirsutism, IUGR, limb defects, genital anomalies	Growth and mental retardation	Usually sporadic	3q26		88, 92
Dubowitz	IUGR, short palpebral fissures, ptosis, micrognathia, sparse hair	Short stature, mild mental retardation, eczema	AR			182
Fetal alcohol	IUGR, mid-face hypoplasia, short palpebral fissures, smooth philtrum, small finger nails, hirsutism	Mild to moderate mental retardation				
Fetal CMV	Hepatosplenomegaly, thrombocytopenia, jaundice, IUGR, intracranial calcification	Mental retardation				
Fetal rubella	IUGR, cataract, corneal opacity, chorioretinitis, microphthalmia, congenital heart disease, thrombocytopenia, jaundice, metaphyseal bone lesions	Deafness, mental retardation				
Johanson–Blizzard	see Aplastic alae nasi (Table 34.14)					
Lissencephaly	Wrinkled skin on forehead, seizures, hypotonia, cloudy cornea, jaundice	Early death	AR	17p13	LIS1	46, 48
Maternal phenylketonuria	IUGR, cardiac defects	Mental retardation				168
Meckel–Gruber	see Polydactyly (Table 34.27)					
Neu–Laxova (Fig. 34.12)	Hypoplastic nose, absent eyelids, micrognathia, multiple contractures, peripheral oedema, 'collodion' skin	Early death	AR			169
Roberts	see Radial defects (Table 34.34)					
Seckel	IUGR, prominent 'beaked' nose, low-set ears, dislocated elbow, hip	Mental retardation	AR			112, 167
Smith–Lemli–Opitz	Anteverted nostrils, ptosis, narrow frontal region, broad alveolar ridges, hypospadias, 2–3 syndactyly of toes	Mental retardation	AR	7q32.1	SLOS	92, 134
'True' microcephaly	Sloping forehead, large ears	Relatively good motor development. Mental retardation	AR			

Table 34.5 Macrocephaly (including hydrocephalus)

Syndrome	Features present at birth	Features developing later	Inheritance	Location	Gene	References
Achondroplasia	see Short limbs, moderate (Table 34.36)					
Albers–Schönberg	Osteopetrosis, pancytopenia		AR (severe type)	1p21-p13		92
Bannayan–Zonana	Capillary haemangiomas	Lipomas	AD	10q22-23	PTEN	119
Greig	see Polydactyly (Table 34.27)					
Hard [+ E]	Hydrocephalus, small encephalocele, retinal dysplasia, cataracts	Mental retardation	AR			47, 49
Neurofibromatosis	see Skin abnormalities (Table 34.41)		AD			
Robinow	see Hypertelorism (Table 34.12)					
Russell–Silver	Low birth weight		Sporadic	17		34, 135, 186
Sotos	Large birth weight, advanced bone age	Mild mental retardation	Possibly AD with reduced penetrance			
Sturge–Weber	see Skin abnormalities (Table 34.41)					
X-linked hydrocephaly	Adducted thumbs, aqueduct stenosis	Mental retardation	XLR	Xq28	L1CAM	60, 96

Table 34.6 Unusual-shaped skull

Syndrome	Features present at birth	Features developing later	Inheritance	Location	Gene	References
Apert (Figs 34.13, 34.14)	Craniostenosis, beaked nose, cleft palate, total syndactyly of hands and feet	Mild to moderate mental retardation	AD	10q25-26	FGFR2	92, 180
Baller–Gerold	see Radial defects (Table 34.34)					
Carpenter	see Polydactyly (Table 34.27)					
Crouzon	Craniostenosis, brachycephaly, prominent forehead, proptosis hypoplastic mid face	Normal intelligence	AD	10q25-26	FGFR2	92, 146
Fetal compression	see Multiple joint contractures/ dislocations (Table 34.37)					
Hypophosphatasia	see Very short limbs (Table 34.35)					
Pfeiffer	Brachycephaly, craniostenosis, broad thumb and hallux, 2–3 toe syndactyly	Normal intelligence	AD	8p11; 10q25-26	FGFR1/ FGFR2	92, 153
Saethre–Chotzen	Ptosis, asymmetric face, brachycephaly, prominent ear crus, mild syndactyly, clinodactyly	Usually, normal intelligence	AD	7p21	TWIST	84, 92, 145

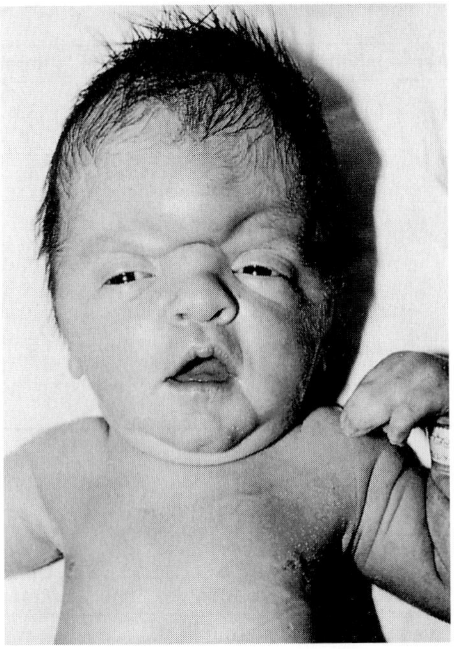

Fig. 34.13 Apert syndrome.

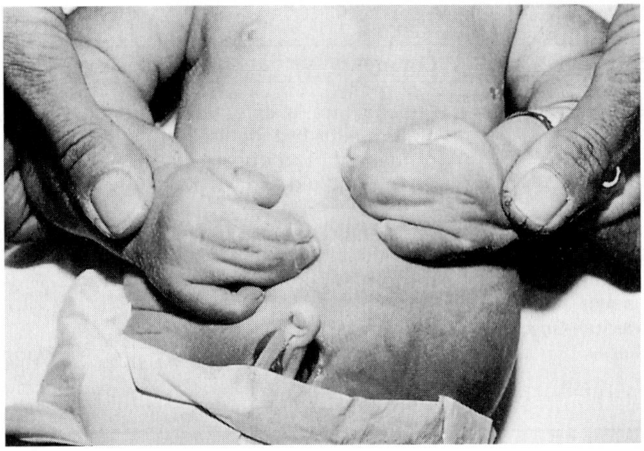

Fig. 34.14 Apert syndrome.

Table 34.7 Fontanelles – wide

Syndrome	Features present at birth	Features developing later	Inheritance	Location	Gene	References
Cleidocranial dysostosis	Prominent forehead, sloping shoulders, absent or hypoplastic clavicles	Widespaced, carious teeth, hypoplasia of distal phalanges	AD	6p21	$CBFA_1$	53, 92
Hallermann–Streiff	see Cataracts (Table 34.9)					
Hypophosphatasia	see Very short limbs (Table 34.35)			1p34-36	ALPL	
Hypothyroidism (p. 961)	Prolonged jaundice, constipation, umbilical hernia	Coarse facial features, large tongue, dry skin, sparse hair, developmental delay if untreated	Usually sporadic Some metabolic types AR			
Kenny	Hypocalcaemia. Thin medullary cavities of long bones on X-ray	Short stature, myopia	AD			92
Osteogenesis imperfecta congenita	see Very short limbs (Table 34.35)					
Pyknodysostosis	Beaked nose, small mandible, hypoplastic scapulae, short terminal phalanges, osteosclerosis	Fractures, short stature, crowded teeth	AR	1q21	Cathepsin K	11, 64
Fetal aminopterin	Small for dates, microcephaly, broad nasal bridge, upsweep of hair, low/dysplastic ears, synostosis	Occasional mental retardation				
Russell–Silver	see Macrocephaly (Table 34.5)					
Thanatophoric dysplasia	see Very short limbs (Table 34.35)					
Zellweger	see Cataracts (Table 34.9)					

Table 34.8 Coloboma

Syndrome	Features present at birth	Features developing later	Inheritance	Location	Gene	References
Charge association	Choanal atresia, external ear abnormality, hypogenitalism congenital heart disease	Short stature, deafness	Mostly sporadic			133
Cohen	Antimongoloid slant to eyes	Obesity, prominent teeth, thin fingers, mental retardation	AR	8q22-23		130, 164
Goltz	see Skin abnormalities (Table 34.41)					
Linear sebaceous naevus	see Skin abnormalities (Table 34.41)					
Meckel–Gruber	see Polydactyly (Table 34.27)					
Rieger	Aniridia, flat upper lip, prominent skin round umbilicus	Hypoplastic, widely spaced teeth	AD	4q25-27	RIEG	93, 157

Table 34.9 Cataract

Syndrome	Features present at birth	Features developing later	Inheritance	Location	Gene	References
Cerebro-oculo-facio-skeletal (COFS)	see Multiple joint contractures/dislocations (Table 34.37)					
Hallermann–Streiff	Brachycephaly, prominent forehead, sparse hair, micrognathia, pinched nose, neonatal teeth, skin atrophy over nose	Short stature, usually normal intelligence	Usually sporadic			28, 92
Incontinentia pigmenti	see Skin abnormalities (Table 34.41)					
Lowe	Glaucoma, amino-aciduria, renal tubular acidosis	Mental retardation	XLR	Xq25	OCRL	1, 104
Fetal rubella	see Microcephaly (Table 34.4)					
Neu–Laxova	see Microcephaly (Table 34.4)					
Rhizomelic chondrodysplasia punctata	see Short limbs – moderate (Table 34.36)					
Rothmund–Thomson	see Skin abnormalities (Table 34.41)					
Zellweger	Dolicocephaly, prominent forehead, stippled epiphyses, nystagmus, hypotonia, pipecolic aciduria	Mental retardation, early demise	AR	1p22-1p21; 7q11; 8q21.1	PXMP3/ PMP70	117, 120

Table 34.10 Dislocated lens

Syndrome	Features present at birth	Features developing later	Inheritance	Location	Gene	References
Homocystinuria	Arachnodactyly, pes cavus, pectus excavatum Homocystine in urine	Light, sparse hair, malar flush, arterial and venous thrombosis	AR	21q22	CBS	114
Marfan	see Arachnodactyly (Table 34.29)					
Sulphite oxidase deficiency	Sulphite and inorganic sulphate in the urine	Mental retardation, early demise	AR			110
Weill–Marchesani	Brachydactyly, spherical lens	Short stature	AR	15q21		185, 187

Table 34.11 Microphthalmia

Syndrome	Features present at birth	Features developing later	Inheritance	Location	Gene	References
Cerebro-oculo-facio-skeletal (COFS)	see Multiple joint contractures/ dislocations (Table 34.37)					
Cross	Hypopigmentation of skin, seizures	Mental retardation	AR			38
Cohen	see Coloboma (Table 34.8)					
Cryptophthalmos	Fused eyelids, syndactyly, genital anomalies, laryngeal stenosis, renal anomaly, cleft palate	Stillbirth common	AR			63, 65
Goltz	see Skin abnormalities (Table 34.41)					
Hallerman–Streiff	see Cataracts (Table 34.9)					
Incontinentia pigmenti	see Skin abnormalities (Table 34.41)					
Lenz	Prominent ears, genital abnormalities	Sloping shoulders, crowded teeth	XLR			9, 172
Neu–Laxova	See Microcephaly (Table 34.4)					
Meckel–Gruber	see Polydactyly (Table 34.27)					
Oculo-dento-digital	Pinched nose, syndactyly	Enamel hypoplasia of teeth, osteopetrosis	AD	6q22-6q24		66, 136

Table 34.12 Hypertelorism

Syndrome	Features present at birth	Features developing later	Inheritance	Location	Gene	References
Aarskog	Ptosis, 'shawl' scrotum	Short stature, mild mental retardation	XLR	Xp11	FGD1	12, 18, 143
Arteriohepatic dysplasia	Deepset eyes, mongoloid slant, pulmonary stenosis, liver disease		AD	20p11	Jagged 1	121, 123
Frontonasal dysplasia	Bifid nasal tip, anterior encephalocele, cleft palate		Sporadic			161
G/BBB	Hypospadias, swallowing difficulties (cleft larynx)	Mental retardation	AD	22q11; Xp22		62, 118
Greig	see Polydactyly (Table 34.27)					
Larsen	see Multiple contractures/ dislocations (Table 34.37)					
Noonan	see Short neck (Table 34.26)					
Otopalato-digital	see Cleft palate (Table 34.20)					
Robinow	Short limbs (mesomelia), prominent forehead, wide mouth, gingival hypertrophy, vertebral defects, micropenis/clitoris		AR and AD forms			92
Waardenburg	White forelock, heterochromia iris	Deafness	AD	I: 2q37 II: 3q12-3q14	PAX3 MITF	57, 92, 173

Table 34.13 Ptosis

Syndrome	Features present at birth	Features developing later	Inheritance	Location	Gene	References
Aarskog	see Hypertelorism (Table 34.12)		AD			
Blepharophimosis–ptosis–epicanthus inversus (BPES)	Short palpebral fissures, epicanthus inversus, dysplastic ears			3q22-23		132, 159
Dubowitz	see Microcephaly (Table 34.4)					
Fetal alcohol	see Microcephaly (Table 34.4)					
Moebius	Immobile face, limb defects, strabismus, syndactyly		Usually sporadic	13q12-13		6
Noonan	see Short neck (Table 34.26)					
Saethre–Chotzen	see Unusual-shaped skull (Table 34.6)					
Schwartz–Jampel	Small mouth/mandible, myotonia, flexion deformities, cataracts	Mild mental retardation, short stature	AR	1p34-1p36		10, 129
Smith–Lemli–Opitz	see Microcephaly (Table 34.4)					

Table 34.14 Aplastic alae nasi

Syndrome	Features present at birth	Features developing later	Inheritance	Location	Gene	References
Fetal warfarin	see Flat or depressed nasal bridge (Table 34.16)					
Freeman–Sheldon	see small mouth, (Table 34.18)					
Hallermann–Streiff	see Cataracts (Table 34.9)					
Johanson–Blizzard	Aplasia cutis of scalp, microcephaly, hypothyroidism, malabsorption, imperforate anus	Deafness, mental retardation, sparse hair	AR			85
Langer–Giedion	Microcephaly, bulbous nose, thin upper lip, prominent ears, cutis laxa	Sparse hair, cone-shaped epiphyses of phalanges	Possibly AD	8q24	TRPS1/ EXT1	82, 92
Oculodento-digital	see Microphthalmia (Table 34.11)					

Table 34.15 Beaked nose (i.e. convex outline)

Syndrome	Features present at birth	Features developing later	Inheritance	Location	Gene	References
Apert	see Unusual-shaped skull (Table 34.6)					
Crouzon	see Unusual-shaped skull (Table 34.6)					
Rubinstein–Taybi	Microcephaly, antimongoloid eye slant, ptosis, prominent nasal columella, hirsutism, broad thumbs	Mild microcephaly, mental retardation	Usually sporadic	16p13	CBP	92, 140
Seckel	see Microcephaly (Table 34.4)					

Table 34.16 Flat or depressed nasal bridge

Syndrome	Features present at birth	Features developing later	Inheritance	Location	Gene	References
Achondroplasia	see Short limbs – moderate (Table 34.36)					
Anhidrotic ectodermal dysplasia	Broad forehead, premaxillary hypoplasia, hyperthermia, poor sweating	Sparse, fine hair, dry skin hypodontia	Mostly XLR	Xq12-Xq13	EDA	92, 189
Blepharophimosis	see Ptosis (Table 34.13)					
Cleidocranial dysostosis	see Fontanelles – wide (Table 34.7)					
Fetal alcohol	see Microcephaly (Table 34.4)					
Fetal hydantoin	see Small or hypoplastic nails (Table 34.33)					
Fetal warfarin	Mid-face hypoplasia, stippled epiphyses on X-ray: short proximal segments of limbs	Mental retardation in some				
Larsen	see Multiple joint contractures/ dislocations (Table 34.37)					
Marshall–Stickler	Cleft palate, anteverted nostrils, flat mid-face, micrognathia	Epiphyseal dysplasia, cataract, joint stiffness, deafness	AD	12q13-12q14; 6p22-6p21	COL2A1/ COL11A27	7, 58
Williams (Fig. 34.15)	Blue eyes with stellate pattern to iris, thick lips, long philtrum, supravalvar aortic stenosis, hypercalcaemia	Mental retardation, mild, short stature	Mostly sporadic	7q11	Elastin (ELN)	39, 92

Table 34.17 Long philtrum

Syndrome	Features present at birth	Features developing later	Inheritance	References
de Lange	see Microcephaly (Table 34.4)			
Femoral hypoplasia, unusual facies	see Short limbs – moderate (Table 34.36)			
Langer–Giedion	see Aplastic alae nasi (Table 34.14)			
Robinow	see Hypertelorism (Table 34.12)			
Smith–Lemli–Opitz	see Microcephaly (Table 34.4)			
Williams	see Flat or depressed nasal bridge (Table 34.16)			

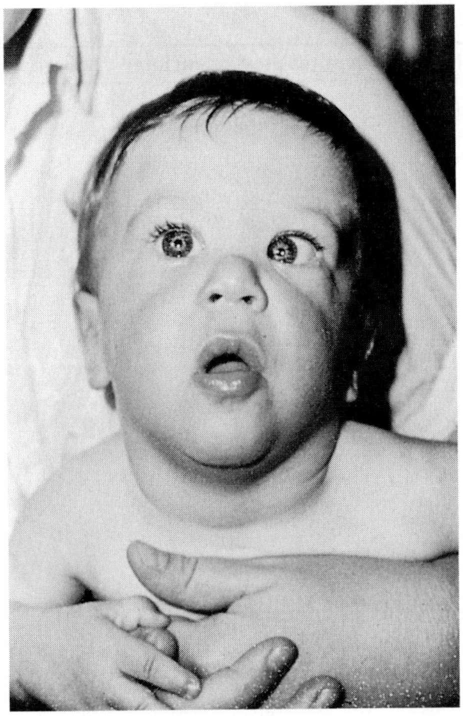

Fig. 34.15 Williams syndrome.

Table 34.18 Small mouth

Syndrome	Features present at birth	Features developing later	Inheritance	References
Freeman–Sheldon	Broad forehead, blepharophimosis, long philtrum, puckered lips, contractures with ulnar deviation of fingers, talipes	Short stature	AD	92
Marden–Walker	see Arachnodactyly (Table 34.29)			
Schwartz–Jampel	see Ptosis (Table 34.13)			

Table 34.19 Cleft lip

Syndrome	Features present at birth	Features developing later	Inheritance	Location	Gene	References
Amniotic bands	see Split hands/reduction defects (Table 34.31)					
Ectodermal dysplasia–ectrodactyly-clefting (EEC)	see Split hands/reduction defects (Table 34.31)					
Fetal hydantoin	see Small or hypoplastic nails (Table 34.33)					
Mohr	Broad nasal tip, midline cleft lip and palate, aberrant frenulae, cleft tongue with nodules, broad hallux, clinodactyly	Deafness, short stature	AR			116, 148
Orofacio-digital	see Syndactyly (Table 34.30)					
Popliteal web	Cleft lip and palate, web of skin at the knees		Mostly AD			61, 75
Rapp–Hodgkin	Dysplastic nails, pinched nose, cleft palate, hypospadias	Sparse hair	AD			17, 154
Roberts	see Radial defects (Table 34.34)					
Short rib polydactyly type 2	see Polydactyly (Table 34.27)					
Van der Woude	Lower lip 'pits', cleft palate		AD	1q32–1q41		92, 125

Table 34.20 Cleft palate

Syndrome	Features present at birth	Features developing later	Inheritance	Location	Gene	References
Apert	see Unusual-shaped skull (Table 34.6					
Camptomelic dysplasia	see Short limbs – moderate (Table 34.36)					
Cerebrocosto-mandibular	see Mandible – small (Table 34.24)					
Charge	see Coloboma (Table 34.8)					
Diastrophic dysplasia	see Very short limbs (Table 34.35)					
Fetal aminopterin	see Fontanelles – wide (Table 34.7)					
Fetal hydantoin	see Small or hypoplastic nails (Table 34.33)					
Femoral hypoplasia, unusual facies	see Short limbs – moderate (Table 34.36)					
Kniest	see Very short limbs (Table 34.35)					
Larsen	see Multiple joint contractures/ dislocations (Table 34.37)					
Marshall–Stickler	see Flat or depressed nasal bridge (Table 34.16)					
Mohr	see Cleft lip (Table 34.19)					
Otopalato-digital	Hypertelorism, flat mid-face, broad thumbs and tips to fingers	Prominent forehead and supraorbital ridges, short stature, deafness	XLR, some manifestations in females	Xq28		13, 138
Pierre–Robin sequence (p. 768)	Small mandible, glossoptosis	Mental retardation in a small proportion	Mostly sporadic			92
Popliteal web	see Cleft lip (Table 34.19)					
Spondyloepiphyseal dysplasia congenita	see Short limbs – moderate (Table 34.36)					
Van der Woude	see Cleft lip (Table 34.19)					

Table 34.21 Oral frenulae

Syndrome	Features present at birth	Features developing later	Inheritance	Location	Gene	References
C	see Polydactyly (Table 34.27)					
Ellis van Creveld	see Polydactyly (Table 34.27)					
Hypoglossia–hypodactyly	see Mandible – small (Table 34.24)					
Mohr	see Cleft lip (Table 34.19)					
Orofacio-digital	see Syndactyly (Table 34.30)					
Popliteal web	see Cleft lip (Table 34.19)					

Table 34.22 Tongue abnormalities

Syndrome	Features present at birth	Features developing later	Inheritance	Location	Gene	References
Beckwith (p. 945)	Large tongue, exomphalos, macrosomia, creases on ear lobe	Mental retardation in some, renal tumours in 5%	Mostly sporadic	11p15	CDKN1C	52, 80
GM_1 gangliosidosis	Large tongue, hypertrophied alveolar ridges, hepatomegaly, 'cloaking' of bones on X-ray	Hurleroid features	AR	3p21-3p14	GLB1	158
Hypothyroidism (p. 961)	Large tongue, large anterior fontanelles, prolonged jaundice	Cretinism if undetected and untreated	Mostly sporadic, some biochemical defects, AR			
Mohr	Cleft tongue, see Cleft lip (Table 34.19)					
Orofacio-digital syndrome	Tumours of the tongue, see also Syndactyly (Table 34.30)					

Table 34.23 Thick alveolar ridges

Syndrome	Features present at birth	Features developing later	Inheritance	Location	Gene	References
C	see Polydactyly (Table 34.27)					
GM_1-gangliosidosis	see Tongue abnormalities (Table 34.22)					
I-cell	Coarse facial features, 'stiff' skin, periosteal cloaking of long bones	Short stature, stiff joints, progressive coarsening of facial features, dysostosis multiplex	AR	4q21-4q23	GNPTA	106, 122
Robinow	see Hypertelorism (Table 34.12)					
Smith–Lemli–Opitz	see Microcephaly (Table 34.4)					

Table 34.24 Mandible – small

Syndrome	Features present at birth	Features developing later	Inheritance	Location	Gene	References
Bloom	see Microcephaly (Table 34.4)					
Cerebrocosto-mandibular	Cleft palate, defects of ribs, redundant skin	Mental retardation	AR			50, 105
Cerebro-oculo-facio-skeletal (COFS)	see Multiple joint contractures/dislocations (Table 34.37)					
de Lange	see Microcephaly (Table 34.4)					
Dubowitz	see Microcephaly (Table 34.4)					
Femoral hypoplasia, unusual facies	see Short limbs – moderate (Table 34.36)					
Goldenhar	see Ears – dysplastic (Table 34.25)					
Hallermann–Streiff	see Cataracts (Table 34.9)		Mostly sporadic			
Hypoglossia–hypodactyly	Small tongue, transverse limb defects					
Marshall–Stickler	see Flat or depressed nasal bridge (Table 34.16)					
Pierre–Robin sequence	see Cleft palate (Table 34.20)					

Table 34.25 Ears – dysplastic/small

Syndrome	Features present at birth	Features developing later	Inheritance	Location	Gene	References
Beal's contractural arachnodactyly	'Crumpled' ear, see Arachnodactyly (Table 34.29)					
Blepharophimosis	see Ptosis (Table 34.15)					
Branchio-oto and Branchio-otorenal dysplasia (BO and BOR)	Preauricular skin tags or pits. Renal abnormalities	Deafness in some	AD with variable penetrance	8q11		25, 31
Charge	see Coloboma (Table 34.8)					
Diastrophic dysplasia	Cystic ears – see Very short limbs (Table 34.35)					
Goldenhar	Preauricular skin tags, asymmetric facial hypoplasia, cervical vertebral defects, epibulbar dermoid		Usually sporadic			32, 92
Roberts	see Radial defects (Table 34.34)					
Townes	see Anal atresia (Table 34.39)					
Treacher Collins	Antimongoloid slant to eyes, lower lid coloboma, malar hypoplasia, micrognathia	Deafness, normal intelligence	AD	5q32	Treacle	45, 92
Wildervanck	see Short neck (Table 34.26)					

Table 34.26 Short neck (and/or webbing)

Syndrome	Features present at birth	Features developing later	Inheritance	Location	Gene	References
Goldenhar	see Ears – dysplastic (Table 34.25)					
Jarcho–Levin	Severe vertebral anomalies, broad forehead, short thorax, long fingers with camptodactyly	Early death from respiratory problems	AR			22, 95
Klippel–Feil	Fusion of cervical vertebrae, low hair line, webbed neck, torticollis	Kyphoscoliosis, deafness	Mostly sporadic	8q22-8q23		30
Multiple pterygium	see Multiple joint contractures/dislocations (Table 34.37)					
Noonan	Webbed neck, low hair line, antimongoloid eyeslant, ptosis, mild hypertelorism, pulmonary stenosis	Mild mental retardation	AD	12q22		91, 92
Wildervanck	Cervical vertebral abnormalities, Duane anomaly, cleft palate	Deafness, occasional mental retardation	Uncertain			179

Table 34.27 Polydactyly

Syndrome	Features present at birth	Features developing later	Inheritance	Location	Gene	References
C	Oral frenulae; trigonocephaly, loose skin, syndactyly	Mental retardation	AR			73, 152
Carpenter	Craniosynostosis, congenital heart defect, pre- and post-axial polydactyly	Mental retardation	AR			
Ellis van Creveld (Fig. 34.16)	Narrow thorax, congenital heart defect, oral frenulae, short limbs		AR	4p16		14, 142
Greig cephalo-polysyndactyly	Syndactyly, frontal bossing macrocephaly, hypertelorism		AD	7p13	GLI3	5, 69
Jeune	Narrow chest, short ribs, polydactyly	Renal dysfunction, cone-shaped epiphyses	AR	12p11-12p12		126
Kaufman–McKusick	see Anal atresia (Table 34.39)					
Laurence–Moon–Biedl		Obesity, retinitis pigmentosa, nephritis	AR	16q13, 3p11,15p,11q		92
Meckel–Gruber	Encephalocele, polycystic kidneys, early death	Severe mental retardation	AR	17q21-17q24		59, 151
Mohr	see Cleft lip (Table 34.19)					
Short-rib polydactyly	Very small thorax, short limbs; lethal		Three types All AR			92

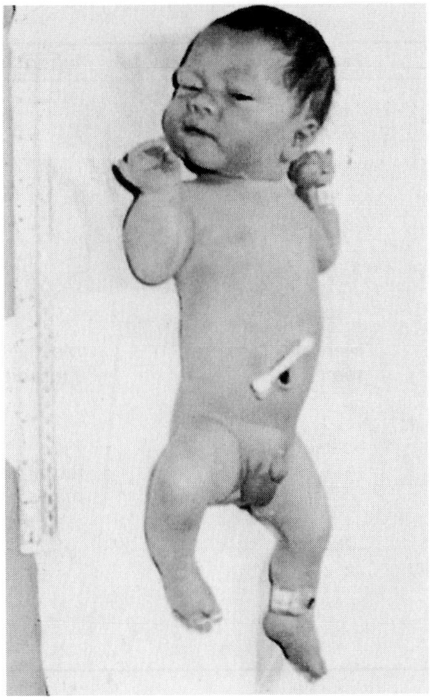

Fig. 34.16 Ellis van Creveld syndrome.

Table 34.28 Camptodactyly

Syndrome	Features present at birth	Features developing later	Inheritance	Location	Gene	References
Beal's contractural arachnodactyly	see Arachnodactyly (Table 34.29)					
Cerebro-oculo-facio-skeletal (COFS)	see Multiple joint contractures/dislocations (Table 34.37)					
Gordon	Talipes equinovarus, cleft palate		AD			87, 149
Marden–Walker	see Arachnodactyly (Table 34.29)					
Multiple pterygium	see Multiple joint contractures/ dislocations (Table 34.37)					

Table 34.29 Arachnodactyly

Syndrome	Features present at birth	Features developing later	Inheritance	Location	Gene	References
Beal's contractural arachnodactyly	Contracture of fingers and other joints. 'Crumpled' helix of ear	Kyphoscoliosis, contractures improve	AD	5q23-5q31	FBN2	75, 111
Frontometaphyseal dysplasia	Prominent forehead	Frontal bossing, joint limitation, deafness, optic atrophy, metaphyseal flaring	Possible AD			56, 67
Homocystinuria	see Dislocated lens (Table 34.10)					
Marden–Walker	Blepharophimosis, cleft palate, talipes equinovarus, congenital heart defect	Mental retardation	AR			89, 181
Marfan	Dislocated lens, high arched palate, pectus excavatum, aortic and mitral incompetence	Dissection of aorta	AD	15q21	FBN1	42, 92

Table 34.30 Syndactyly

Syndrome	Features present at birth	Features developing later	Inheritance	Location	Gene	References
Apert	see Unusual-shaped skull (Table 34.6)					
C	see Polydactyly (Table 34.27)					
Cryptophthalmos	see Microphthalmia (Table 34.11)					
Goltz	see Skin abnormalities (Table 34.41)					
Greig	see Polydactyly (Table 34.27)					
Incontinentia pigmenti	see Skin abnormalities (Table 34.41)					
Moebius	See Ptosis (Table 34.13)	Mental retardation in some	Mostly sporadic	13q12-13q13		6, 99
Mohr	see Cleft lip (Table 34.19)					
Neu–Laxova	see Microcephaly (Table 34.4)					
Orofacio-digital syndrome	Midline cleft lip, oral frenulae, cleft palate, cleft tongue, brachydactyly	Sparse hair	XLD, lethal in males	Xp22		8, 171
Pfeiffer	see Unusual-shaped skull (Table 34.6)					
Poland	Absence of pectoralis muscles unilaterally					41
Saethre–Chotzen	see Unusual-shaped skull (Table 34.6)					43

Table 34.31 Split hands/reduction defects

Syndrome	Features present at birth	Features developing later	Inheritance	Location	Gene	References
Amniotic bands	Facial clefts, ring constrictions (p. 1082)					
de Lange	see Microcephaly (Table 34.4)					
Ectodermal dysplasia–ectrodactyly-clefting (EEC)	Cleft lip and palate ectodermal dysplasia		AD	7q21		20, 100
Hypoglossia–hypodactyly	see Mandible – small (Table 34.24)					
Isolated cleft hand			AD			

Table 34.32 Abnormal thumbs

Syndrome	Features present at birth	Features developing later	Inheritance	Location	Gene	References
Aase	Triphalangeal thumbs, anaemia, leukopenia, VSD	Late closure of fontanelles, short stature	Possibly XLR			68, 124
de Lange	see Microcephaly (Table 34.4)					
Diastrophic dysplasia	'Hitchhiker' thumbs, see Very short limbs (Table 34.35)					
DOOR	see Small or hypoplastic nails (Table 34.33)					
Fanconi anaemia	Hypoplastic thumb, pigmented skin lesions, increased chromosome breakage, small penis	Pancytopenia lymphoreticular malignancies. Mental retardation in some.	AR	3p22-26; 9q22; 16q24.3	FA(A); FA(C)	144
Fibrodysplasia ossificans progressiva	Hypoplastic thumbs, great toes	Soft tissue calcification	AD			36, 37
Greig	Broad thumbs, see Polydactyly (Table 34.27)					
Holt–Oram	Hypoplastic thumbs and/or radius, ASD, VSD		AD variable expression	12q	TBX5	108, 127
Otopalato-digital	Broad thumbs, see Cleft palate (Table 34.20)					
Pfeiffer	Broad thumbs, see Unusual-shaped skull (Table 34.6)					
Rubinstein–Taybi	see Beaked nose (Table 34.15)					
Townes	Triphalangeal or hypoplastic thumbs, see Anal atresia (Table 34.39)					
Vater	Hypoplastic thumbs, see Vertebral anomalies (Table 34.40)					
X-linked hydrocephalus	Adducted thumbs, see Macrocephaly (Table 34.5)					

Table 34.33 Small or hypoplastic nails

Syndrome	Features present at birth	Features developing later	Inheritance	Location	Gene	References
Coffin–Siris	Sparse scalp hair, microcephaly, coarse facial features, thick lips	Mental retardation, body hirsutism	AR			23, 92, 107
DOOR (deaf, onycho-osteodystrophy osteolysis, retardation)	Triphalangeal thumb, small terminal phalanges	Mental retardation in some, deafness	AR			16, 137
Ellis van Creveld	see Polydactyly (Table 34.27)					
Fetal alcohol	see Microcephaly (Table 34.4)					
Fetal hydantoin	Hirsutism, cleft palate, mid-face hypoplasia	Short stature, mental retardation in some				
Goltz	see Skin abnormalities (Table 34.41)					
Nail patella	Talipes equinovarus and joint contractures, ileal spur on X-ray	Nephritis	AD	9q34		72, 92
Rapp–Hodgkin	see Cleft lip (Table 34.19)					

Table 34.34 Radial defects

Syndrome	Features present at birth	Features developing later	Inheritance	Location	Gene	References
Aase	See Abnormal thumbs (Table 34.32)		AR			
Baller–Gerold	Craniosynostosis		AR			33, 139
Fanconi anaemia	See Abnormal thumbs (Table 34.32)		AR			
Holt–Oram	Variable limb anomalies, see Abnormal thumbs (Table 34.32)		AD			
Juberg	Cleft lip and palate, microcephaly	Mental retardation	AR			94, 175
Roberts	Phocomelia, cleft lip and palate, mid-face haemangioma, hypertelorism, thin nares, malformed ears	Short stature, mental retardation	AR			3, 188
Thrombocytopenia, absent radius (TAR)	Thrombocytopenia		AR			74, 101
Vater	see Vertebral anomalies (Table 34.40)					

Table 34.35 Very short limbs

Syndrome	Features present at birth	Features developing later	Inheritance	Location	Gene	References
Achondrogenesis	Large head, underossification of skeleton	Lethal	Two types AR	5q31-5q34 (type 1B); 12q13 (type 2)	DTDST (type 1B); COL2A1 (type 2)	163
Diastrophic dysplasia	Adducted 'hitchhiker' thumbs, talipes equinovarus, cleft palate, respiratory difficulties	Kyphoscoliosis, cystic ear pinnae	AR	5q21-5q34	DTDST	79
Hypophosphatasia	Underossification of bones, low alkaline phosphatase, raised phosphoethanolamine in urine	Two forms, severe form lethal	AR in severe form	1p34-1p36	ALPL	71
Kniest	Broad chest, cleft palate, flat mid-face	Myopia and retinal detachment, kyphoscoliosis	Possibly AD	12q13-12q14	COL2A1	15
Osteogenesis imperfecta congenita (Fig. 34.17)	Blue sclerae, poor ossification of skull, multiple fractures, 'crumpled' bones on X-ray	Mostly lethal	AR in some	7q21-7q22; 17q21-17q22	COL1A1/ COL1A2	35
Short-rib polydactyly syndromes	see Polydactyly (Table 34.27)					
Thanatophoric dysplasia (Figs 34.18, 34.19)	Large head, small thorax	Lethal	Sporadic	4p16	FGFR3	165

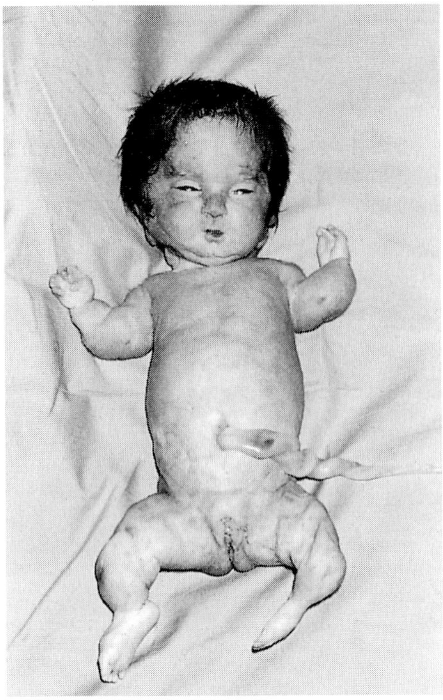

Fig. 34.17 Osteogenesis imperfecta congenita.

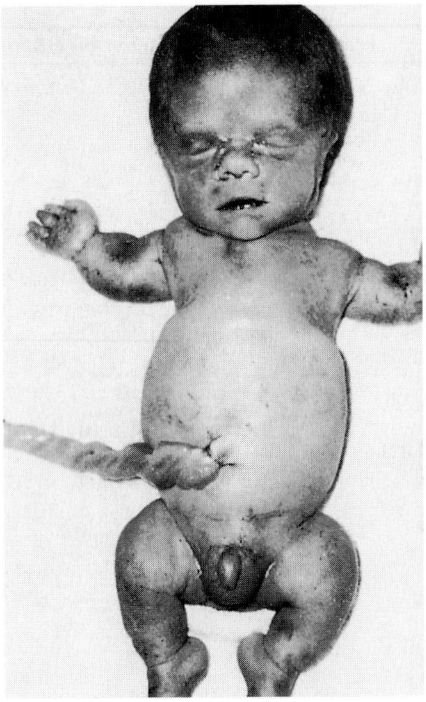

Fig. 34.18 Thanatophoric dysplasia.

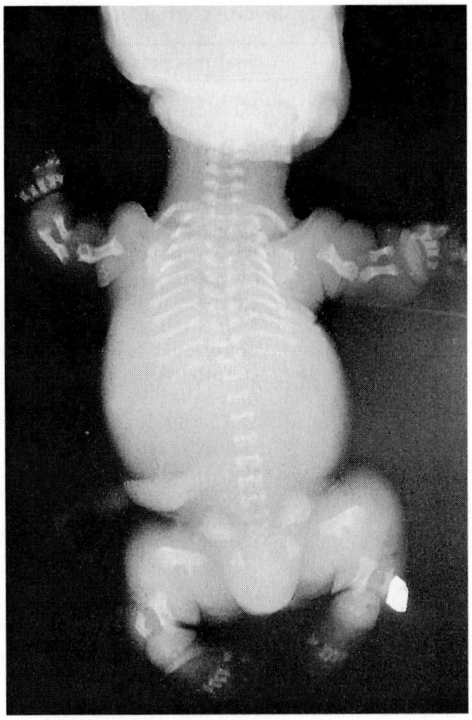

Fig. 34.19 Thanatophoric dysplasia.

Table 34.36 Short limbs – moderate

Syndrome	Features present at birth	Features developing later	Inheritance	Location	Gene	References
Achondroplasia	Large head, 'trident' hand, flat mid-face	Lumbar lordosis, short stature	AD	4p16	FGFR3	174
Camptomelic dysplasia	Bowing of long bones, hypoplastic scapulae, small thorax, sex reversal, cleft palate	Early demise, poor mental development	AR	17q24	SOX9	83, 113
Chondrodysplasia punctata epiphysealis (Conradi)	Flat mid-face, ichthyosis, stippled epiphyses, cataract	Short stature	AD, severe form is AR			76
Ellis van Creveld	see Polydactyly (Table 34.27)					
Femoral hypoplasia, unusual facies	Absent or hypoplastic femurs/ fibulae. Micrognathia/cleft palate, long philtrum, hypoplastic alae nasi		AD in some. Rule out maternal diabetes			
Hypochondroplasia	Short limbs	Characteristic X-ray appearance of spine, short femoral neck	AD	4p16	FGFR3	128
Leri–Weill	Madelung's deformity	Mild short stature	XLD	XpYp	SHOX	54, 109
Robinow	see Hypertelorism (Table 34.12)					
Spondyloepiphyseal dysplasia congenita	Cleft palate, flat mid-face, short trunk, delayed development of epiphyses	Progressive platyspondyly and scoliosis. Epiphyseal dysplasia, myopia and retinal detachment	AD	12q13	COL2A1	4, 78

Table 34.37 Multiple joint contractures/dislocations

Syndrome	Features present at birth	Features developing later	Inheritance	Location	Gene	References
Arthrogryposis	Multiple joint contractures	Many different causes, neuromuscular abnormalities should be excluded				97
Beal's contractural arachnodactyly	see Arachnodactyly (Table 34.29)					
C	see Polydactayly (Table 34.27)					
Cerebro-oculo-facio-skeletal (COFS)	Microcephaly, deep-set eyes, cataracts, rocker-bottom feet	Cachexia, mental retardation	AR			90, 184
Ehlers–Danlos	Dislocated joints, see Skin abnormalities (Table 34.41)					
Fetal compression	Unusual skull shape, micrognathia, cleft palate					
Gordon	See Camptodactyly (Table 34.28)					
Larsen	Flat mid-face, cleft palate		Mostly AD	3p14		103, 170
Marden–Walker	see Arachnodactyly (Table 34.29)					
Multiple pterygium	Folds of skin at elbow, neck, knees, groin, flat mid-face		AR			75, 106
Nail patella	see Small or hypoplastic nails (Table 34.33)					
Potter's sequence (Fig. 34.20)	Depressed nasal bridge, crumpled ears, talipes equinovarus, renal or urethral abnormalities leading to oligohydramnios	Lethal				
Schwartz–Jampel	see Ptosis (Table 34.13)					

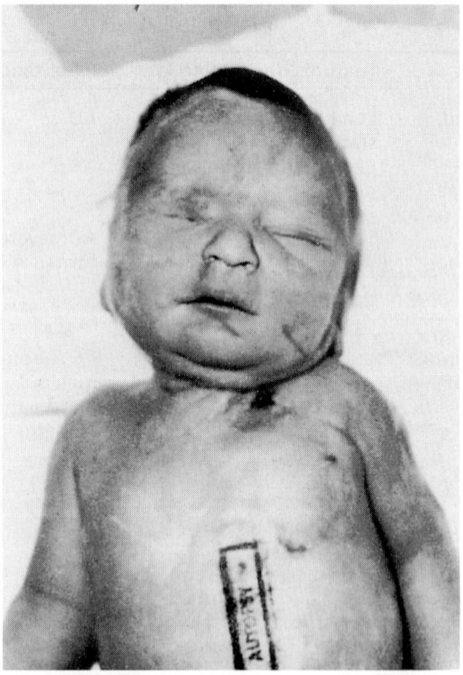

Fig. 34.20 Potter's sequence.

Table 34.38 Hypogenitalism (male)/hypospadias

Syndrome	Features present at birth	Features developing later	Inheritance	Location	Gene	References
Charge	see Coloboma (Table 34.8)					
de Lange	see Microcephaly (Table 34.4)					
G/BBB	see Hypertelorism (Table 34.12)					
Laurence–Moon–Biedl	see Polydactyly (Table 34.27)					
Meckel–Gruber	see Polydactyly (Table 34.27)					
Prader–Willi	Hypotonia; feeding difficulties	Obesity, almond-shaped eyes, small hands and feet	Mostly sporadic	15q11	SNRPN	21, 29
Robinow	see Hypertelorism (Table 34.12)					
Smith–Lemli–Opitz	see Microcephaly (Table 34.4)					

Table 34.39 Anal atresia (or abnormal placement)

Syndrome	Features present at birth	Features developing later	Inheritance	Location	Gene	References
Asymmetric crying facies	Asymmetric crying face, congenital heart defect		Mostly sporadic			
Cryptophthalmos	see Microphthalmia (Table 34.11)					
G/BBB	see Hypertelorism (Table 34.12)					
Johanson–Blizzard	see Aplastic alae nasi (Table 34.14)					
Kaufman–McKusick	Polydactyly, congenital heart defect, hydrometrocolpos		AR			27
Maternal diabetes	Congenital heart defects, sacral agenesis (rarely), limb defects					
Townes	Dysplastic ears, preauricular skin tags, abnormal thumbs		AD			131, 147
Vater	see Vertebral anomalies (Table 34.40)					

Table 34.40 Vertebral anomalies

Syndrome	Features present at birth	Features developing later	Inheritance	References
Costovertebral dysplasia	Rib defects		AD and AR forms	
Goldenhar	see Ears – dysplastic (Table 34.25)			
Jarcho–Levin	see Short neck (Table 34.26)			
Klippel–Feil	see Short neck (Table 34.26)			
Robinow	see Hypertelorism (Table 34.12)			
Spondyloepiphyseal dysplasia congenita	see Short limbs – moderate (Table 34.36)			
Vater association	Vertebral defects, anal atresia, tracheo-oesophageal fistula, renal and radial limb defects	Congenital heart disease	Mostly sporadic	
Wildervanck	see Short neck (Table 34.26)			

Table 34.41 Skin abnormalities

Syndrome	Features present at birth	Features developing later	Inheritance	Location	Gene	References
Conradi	Ichthyosis, see Short limbs – moderate (Table 34.36)					
Cutis laxa	Loose folds of skin	Bronchiectasis, premature aged appearance	AD and XLR forms			2
Ectodermal dysplasia–ectrodactyly-clefting	Ectodermal dysplasia, see Split hand (Table 34.31)					
Ehlers–Danlos	Hyperextensible skin, loose joints, blue sclerae	Abnormal scarring, vascular fragility, joint dislocation	At least 8 types, AD, AR or XLR	I: 9q34 II: 9q34 IV: 2q31 VI: 1p36 VII: 7q21-7q22/17q21-17q22	I: COL5A1 II: COL5A1 IV: COL3A1 VI: PLOD VII: COL1A1/COL1A2	19, 26, 81, 98
Fetal alcohol	Haemangiomas, see Microcephaly (Table 34.4)					
Goltz	Focal dermal hypoplasia with herniation of fat; telangiectasia, syndactyly, coloboma, microphthalmos	Abnormal teeth, alopecia, mental retardation	XLD –possibly lethal in the male	Xp22		70, 166
Hypomelanosis of Ito	Hypopigmented streaks of skin	Seizures, mental retardation in some				40, 150
I-cell	'Stiff' skin, see Thick alveolar ridges (Table 34.23)					
Incontinentia pigmenti	Bullous eruption of skin, cataracts	Whorls of skin pigmentation, microcephaly, seizures	XLD, lethal in males	Xp11 Xq28		24, 102
Klippel–Trenaunay–Weber	Cavernous or capillary haemangiomas, oedema, over-growth of limbs		Sporadic			178
Leopard	Multiple lentigenes, pulmonary stenosis, hypertelorism	Deafness, short stature	AD			
Leprechaunism	Hirsutism, loose skin, lack of subcutaneous tissue, enlarged penis/clitoris, hypoglycaemia	Growth deficiency; early demise	AR	19p13	INSR	44, 177
Limb reduction, ichthyosis	Unilateral ichthyosis with ipsilateral hypoplasia of limbs	Possible mental deficiency	Possibly AR			77, 92, 162
Linear sebaceous naevus	Raised, linear, pigmented, warty lesions, eye abnormalities	Seizures, mental retardation in some	Usually sporadic			
McCune–Albright (polyostotic fibrous dysplasia)	Café au lait patches with irregular borders	Fibrous dysplasia of bone, especially long bones, pelvis and skull	Sporadic	20q13	GNAS1	156
Rothmund–Thomson	Telangiectasia and atrophy giving 'marbled' appearance, cataract, hypoplastic thumbs	Short stature	AR			
Sturge–Weber	Facial capillary, haemangiomas, macrocephaly, intracerebral calcification	Seizures, mental retardation	Sporadic			
Von Recklinghausen neurofibromatosis	Café au lait patches, pseudarthroses	Neurofibromas of skin, peripheral nerves and central nervous system multiple possible complications, deafness	AD	17q11	NF1	176

REFERENCES

1. Abbassi V, Lowe C U, Calcagno P L 1968 Oculo-cerebro-renal syndrome: a review. American Journal of Diseases of Children 115: 145–168
2. Agha A, Sakati N O, Higginbottom M C et al 1978 Two forms of cutis laxa presenting in the newborn period. Acta Paediatrica Scandinavica 67: 775–780
3. Allingham-Hawkins D J, Tomkins D J 1991 Somatic cell hybridization of Roberts syndrome and normal lymphoblasts resulting in correction of both the cytogenetic and mutagen hypersensitivity cellular phenotypes. Somatic Cell and Molecular Genetics, 17: 455–462
4. Anderson I J, Goldberg R B, Marion R W et al 1990 Spondyloepiphyseal dysplasia congenita: genetic linkage to type II collagen (COL2A1). American Journal of Human Genetics 46: 896–901
5. Ausems M G E M, Ippel P F, Renardel de Lavalette P A W A 1994 Greig cephalopolysyndactyly syndrome in a large family: a comparison of the clinical signs with those described in the literature. Clinical Dysmorphology 3: 21–30
6. Baraitser M 1977 Genetics of the Moebius syndrome. Journal of Medical Genetics 14: 415–417
7. Baraitser M 1982 Marshall/Stickler syndrome. Journal of Medical Genetics 19: 139–140
8. Baraitser M 1986 The orofaciodigital (OFD) syndromes. Journal of Medical Genetics 23: 116–119
9. Baraitser M, Winter R M, Taylor D S I 1982 Lenz microphthalmia–a case report. Clinical Genetics 22: 99–101
10. Beighton P 1973 The Schwartz syndrome in Southern Africa. Clinical Genetics 4: 548–555
11. Bennani-Smires C, El Alamy N R, Bouchareb N 1984 Pyknodysostosis, typical and atypical features and report on seven cases. Journal of Radiology 65: 689–695
12. Berry C, Cree J, Mann T 1980 Aarskog's syndrome. Archives of Disease in Childhood 55: 706–710
13. Biancalana V, Le Marec B, Odent S et al 1991 Oto-palato-digital syndrome type I: further evidence for assignment of the locus to Xq28. Human Genetics 88: 228–230
14. Blackburn M G, Belliveau R E 1971 Ellis van Creveld syndrome. A report of previously undescribed anomalies in two siblings. American Journal of Diseases of Children 122: 267–270
15. Bogaert R, Wilkin D, Wilcox W R et al 1994 Expression, in cartilage, of a 7-amino-acid deletion in type II collagen from two unrelated individuals with Kniest dysplasia. American Journal of Human Genetics 55: 1128–1136
16. Bos C J M, Ippel P F, Beemer F A 1994 DOOR syndrome: additional case and literature review. Clinical Dysmorphology 3: 15–20
17. Breslau-Siderius E J, Lavrijsen A P M, Otten F W A et al 1991 The Rapp–Hodgkin syndrome. American Journal of Medical Genetics 38: 107–110
18. Brondum-Nielsen K 1988 Aarskog syndrome in a Danish family: an illustration of the need for dysmorphology in paediatrics. Clinical Genetics 33: 315–317
19. Burrows N P, Nicholls A C, Yates J R W et al 1996 The gene encoding collagen alpha 1(V) (COL5A1) is linked to mixed Ehlers–Danlos syndrome type I/II. Journal of Investigative Dermatology 106: 1273–1276
20. Buss P W, Hughes H E, Clarke A 1995 Twenty-four cases of the EEC syndrome: clinical presentation and management. Journal of Medical Genetics 32: 716–723
21. Butler M G, Meaney F J, Palmer C G 1986 Clinical and cytogenetic survey of 39 individuals with Prader Labhart Willi syndrome. American Journal of Medical Genetics 23: 793–809
22. Cantu J M, Urrusti J, Rosales G, Rojas A 1971 Evidence for autosomal recessive inheritance of costovertebral dysplasia. Clinical Genetics 2: 149–154
23. Carey J C, Hall B D 1978 The Coffin–Siris syndrome. American Journal of Diseases of Children 132: 667–671
24. Carney R G 1976 Incontinentia pigmenti: a world statistical analysis. Archives of Dermatology 112: 535–542
25. Chen A, Francis M, Ni L et al 1995 Phenotypic manifestations of branchio-otorenal syndrome. American Journal of Medical Genetics 58: 365–370
26. Chiodo A A, Hockey A, Cole W G 1992 A base substitution at the splice acceptor site of intron 5 of the COL1A2 gene activates a cryptic splice site within exon 6 and generates abnormal type I procollagen in a patient with Ehlers–Danlos syndrome type VII. Journal of Biological Chemistry 267: 6361–6369
27. Chitayat D, Hahm SYE, Marion R W et al 1987 Further delineation of the McKusick–Kaufman hydrometrocolpos–polydactyly syndrome. American Journal of Diseases of Children 141: 1133–1136
28. Christian C L, Lachman R S, Aylsworth AS et al 1991 Radiological findings in Hallermann–Streiff syndrome: report of five cases and a review of the literature. American Journal of Medical Genetics. 41: 508–514
29. Chu C E, Cooke A, Stephenson J B P et al 1994 Diagnosis in Prader–Willi syndrome. Archives of Disease in Childhood 71: 441–442
30. Clarke R A, Singh S, McKenzie H, Kearsley J H, Yip M-Y 1995 Familial Klippel–Feil syndrome and paracentric inversion inv(9)(q22.2q23.3). American Journal of Human Genetics 57: 1364–1370
31. Clarke-Fraser F, Ling D, Clogg D, Nogrady B 1978 Genetic aspects of the Bor syndrome – branchial fistulas, ear pits, hearing loss, and renal anomalies. American Journal of Medical Genetics 2: 241–252
32. Cohen M M Jr, Rollnick B R, Kaye C I 1989 Oculoauriculovertebral spectrum: an updated critique. Cleft Palate Journal 26: 276–286
33. Cohen MM Jr, Toriello H V 1996 Is there a Baller–Gerold syndrome? American Journal of Medical Genetics 61: 63–64
34. Cole T R P, Hughes H E 1994 Sotos syndrome: a study of the diagnostic criteria and natural history. Journal of Medical Genetics 31: 20–32
35. Cole W G, Dalgleish R 1995 Syndrome of the month. Perinatal lethal osteogenesis imperfecta. Journal of Medical Genetics 32: 284–289
36. Connor J M, Evans D A P 1982 Genetic aspects of fibrodysplasia ossificans progressiva. Journal of Medical Genetics 19: 35–39
37. Connor J M, Skirton H, Lunt P W 1993 A three generation family with fibrodysplasia ossificans progressiva. Journal of Medical Genetics 30: 687–689
38. Cross H E, McKusick V A, Breen W 1967 A new oculocerebral syndrome with hypopigmentation. Journal of Pediatrics 70: 398–406
39. Curran M E, Atkinson D L, Ewart A K et al 1993 The elastin gene is disrupted by a translocation associated with supravalvular aortic stenosis. Cell 73: 159–168
40. David T J 1981 Hypomelanosis of Ito: a neurocutaneous syndrome. Archives of Disease in Childhood 56: 798–800
41. David T J 1982 Familial Poland anomaly. Journal of Medical Genetics 19: 293–296
42. De Paepe A, Devereux R B, Dietz H C, Hennekam R C M, Pyeritz R E 1996 Revised diagnostic criteria for the Marfan syndrome. American Journal of Medical Genetics 62: 417–426
43. Der Kaloustian V M, Hoyme H E, Hogg H et al 1991 Possible common pathogenetic mechanisms for Poland sequence and Adams–Oliver syndrome. American Journal of Medical Genetics 38: 69–73
44. Der Kaloustian V M, Kronfol N M, Takla R, Habash A, Khazin A, Najjar S S 1971 Leprechaunism: a report of two new cases. American Journal of Diseases of Children 122: 442–445
45. Dixon MJ 1995 Syndrome of the month. Treacher–Collins syndrome. Journal of Medical Genetics 32: 806–808
46. Dobyns W B, Gilbert E F, Opitz J M 1985 Further comments on the lissencephaly syndromes. American Journal of Medical Genetics 22: 197–211
47. Dobyns W B, Kirkpatrick J B et al 1985 Syndromes with lissencephaly. II: Walker–Warburg and cerebro-oculomuscular syndromes and a new syndrome with type II lissencephaly. American Journal of Medical Genetics 157–195
48. Dobyns W B, Truwit C L 1995 Lissencephaly and other malformations of cortical development: 1995 update (Review). Neuropediatrics 26: 132–147
49. Donnai D, Farndon P A 1986 Walker–Warburg syndrome (Warburg syndrome). Hard ± E syndrome. Journal of Medical Genetics 23: 200–203
50. Drossou-Agakidou V, Andreou A, Soubassi-Griva V, Pandouraki M 1991 Cerebrocostomandibular syndrome in four sibs, two pairs of twins. Journal of Medical Genetics 28: 704–707
51. Ellis N A, German J 1996 Molecular genetics of Bloom's syndrome. Human Molecular Genetics 5: 1457–1463
52. Engstrom W, Lindham S, Schofield P 1988 Wiedemann-Beckwith syndrome. European Journal of Pediatrics 147: 450–457

53. Feldman G J, Robin N H, Brueton L A et al 1995 A gene for cleidocranial dysplasia maps to the short arm of chromosome 6. American Journal of Human Genetics 56: 938–943
54. Felman A H, Kirkpatrick J A 1970 Dyschondrosteosis: mesomelic dwarfism of Leri and Weill. American Journal of Diseases of Children 120: 329–331
55. Finegold DN, Armitage M M, Galiani M et al 1994 Preliminary localization of a gene for autosomal dominant hypoparathyroidism to chromosome 3q13. Pediatric Research 36: 414–417
56. Fitzsimmons J S, Fitzsimmons E M, Barrow M, Gilbert G B 1982 Fronto-metaphyseal dysplasia. Further delineation of the clinical syndrome. Clinical Genetics 22: 195–205
57. Foy C, Newton V, Wellesley D et al 1990 Assignment of the locus for Waardenburg syndrome type 1 to human chromosome 2q37 and possible homology to the splotch mouse. American Journal of Human Genetics 46: 1017–1023
58. Francomano C A, McIntosh I, Wilkin D J 1996 Bone dysplasias in man: molecular insights. Current Opinion in Genetic Development 6: 301–308
59. Fraser F C, Lytwyn A 1981 Spectrum of anomalies in the Meckel syndrome, 'or maybe there is a malformation syndrome with at least one constant anomaly'. American Journal of Medical Genetics 9: 67–73
60. Fried K 1972 X-linked mental retardation and/or hydrocephalus. Clinical Genetics 3: 258–263
61. Froster-Iskenius U G 1990 Syndrome of the month. Popliteal pterygium syndrome. Journal of Medical Genetics 27: 320–326
62. Funderburk S J, Stewart R 1978 The G and BBB syndromes: case presentations, genetics and nosology. American Journal of Medical Genetics 2: 131–144
63. Gattuso J, Patton M A, Baraitser M 1987 The clinical spectrum of the Fraser syndrome: report of the three new cases and review. Journal of Medical Genetics 24: 549–555
64. Gelb B D, Edelson J G, Desnick R J 1995 Linkage of pycnodysostosis to chromosome 1q21 by homozygosity mapping (Letter). Nature Genetics 10: 235–237
65. Ghose S, Sihota R, Dayal Y 1988 Symmetrical partial lateral 'cryptophthalmos': a new concept of its embryological pathogenesis. Ophthalmology Paediatrics and Genetics 1988; 9: 67–76
66. Gladwin A, Donnai D, Metcalfe K et al 1997 Localization of a gene for oculodentodigital syndrome to human chromosome 6q22–q24. Human Molecular Genetics 6: 123–127
67. Glass R B J, Rosenbaum K N 1995 Frontometaphyseal dysplasia: neonatal radiographic diagnosis. American Journal of Medical Genetics 57: 1–5
68. Gojic V, van't Veer-Korthof E T, Bosch L J et al 1994 Congenital hypoplastic anemia: another example of autosomal dominant transmission. American Journal of Medical Genetics 50: 87–89
69. Gollop T R, Fontes L R 1985 The Greig cephalopolysyndactyly syndrome: report of a family and review of the literature. American Journal of Medical Genetics 22: 59–68
70. Goltz R W, Henderson R R, Hitch J M, Ott J E 1970 Focal dermal hypoplasia syndrome: a review of the literature and report of two cases. Archives of Dermatology 101: 1–11
71. Greenberg C R, Evans J A, McKendry-Smith S et al 1990 Infantile hypophosphatasia: localization within chromosome region 1p36.1-34 and prenatal diagnosis using linked DNA markers. American Journal of Human Genetics 46: 286–292.
72. Guidera K J, Satter-White Y, Ogden J A et al 1991 Nail patella syndrome: a review of 44 orthopedic patients. Journal of Pediatric Orthopedics 11: 737–742
73. Haaf T, Hofmann R, Schmid M 1991 Opitz trigonocephaly syndrome. American Journal of Medical Genetics 40: 444–446
74. Hall J G 1987 Thrombocytopenia and absent radius (TAR) syndrome. Journal of Medical Genetics 24: 79–83
75. Hall J G, Reed S D, Rosenbaum K N, Gershanik J, Chen H, Wilson K M 1982 Limb pterygium syndromes: a review and report of eleven patients. American Journal of Medical Genetics 12: 377–409
76. Happle R 1979 X-linked dominant chondrodysplasia punctata: review of literature and report of a case. Human Genetics 53: 65–73
77. Happle R. Effendy I, Megahed M, Orlow S J, Kuster W 1994 CHILD syndrome in a boy. American Journal of Medical Genetics 62: 192–194
78. Harrod M J E, Friedman J M, Currarino G et al 1984 Genetic heterogeneity in spondyloepiphyseal dysplasia congenita. American Journal of Medical Genetics 18: 311–320
79. Hastbacka J, Sistonen P, Kaitila I et al 1991 A linkage map spanning the locus for diastrophic dysplasia (DTD). Genomics 11: 968–973
80. Hatada I, Morisaki H, Nakayama M et al 1996 An imprinted gene p57KIP2 is mutated in Beckwith–Wiedemann syndrome. Nature Genetics 14: 171–173
81. Hautala T, Byers M G, Eddy R L et al 1992 Cloning of human lysyl hydroxylase: complete cDNA-derived amino acid sequence and assignment of the gene (PLOD) to chromosome 1p36.3->p36.2. Genomics 13: 62–69
82. Hou J, Parrish J, Ludecke H J et al 1995 A 4-megabase YAC contig that spans the Langer–Giedion syndrome region on human chromosome 8q24.1: use in refining the location of the trichorhinophalangeal syndrome and multiple exostoses genes (TRPS1 and EXT1). Genomics 29: 87–97
83. Houston C S, Opitz J M, Spranger J W et al 1983 The Camptomelic syndrome: review: report of 17 cases and follow-up on the currently 17 year old boy first reported by Maroteaux in 1971. American Journal of Medical Genetics 15: 3–28
84. Howard T D, Paznekas W A, Green E D 1997 Mutations in TWIST, a basic helix-loop-helix transcription factor, in Saethre–Chotzen syndrome. Nature Genetics 15: 36–41
85. Hurst J A, Baraitser M 1989 Johanson-Blizzard syndrome. Journal of Medical Genetics 26: 45–48
86. Hustinix T W J, Ter Haar B G A, Scheres J M J C et al 1977 Bloom's syndrome in two Dutch families. Clinical Genetics 12: 85–96
87. Ioan D M, Belengeanu V, Maximilian C, Fryns J-P 1993 Distal arthrogryposis with autosomal dominant inheritance and reduced penetrance in females: the Gordon syndrome. Clinical Genetics 43: 300–302
88. Ireland M, English C, Cross I et al 1995 Partial trisomy 3q and the mild Cornelia de Lange syndrome phenotype (Letter). Journal of Medical Genetics 32: 837–838
89. Jaatoul N Y, Haddad N E, Khoury L A, Afifi A K, Bahuth N B, Deeb M E 1982 Brief clinical report and review: the Marden-Walker syndrome. American Journal of Medical Genetics 11: 259–271
90. Jaeken J, Klocker H. Schwaiger H et al 1989 Clinical and biochemical studies in three patients with severe early infantile Cockayne syndrome. Human Genetics 83: 339–346
91. Jamieson C R, van der Burgt I, Brady A F et al 1994 Mapping a gene for Noonan syndrome to the long arm of chromosome 12. Nature Genetics 8: 357–360
92. Jones K L 1988 Smith's recognizable patterns of human malformation, 4th Edn. W B Saunders, London, Philadelphia
93. Jorgenson R J, Levin L S, Cross H E, Yoder F, Kelly T E 1978 The Rieger syndrome. American Journal of Medical Genetics 2: 307–318
94. Juberg R C, Hayward J R 1969 A new familial syndrome of oral, cranial, and digital anomalies. Journal of Pediatrics 74: 755–762
95. Karnes P S, Day D, Berry S A, Pierpont M E M 1991 Jarcho–Levin syndrome: four new cases and classification of subtypes. American Journal of Medical Genetics 40: 264–270
96. Kenwrick S, Jouet M, Donnai D 1996 X linked hydrocephalus and MASA syndrome. Journal of Medical Genetics 33: 59–65
97. Kobayashi H, Baumbach L, Matise T C et al 1995 A gene for a severe lethal form of X-linked arthrogryposis (X-linked infantile spinal muscular atrophy) maps to human chromosome Xp11.3-q11.2. Human Molecular Genetics 4: 1213–1216
98. Kontusaari S, Tromp G, Kuivaniemi H et al 1992 Substitution of aspartate for glycine 1018 in type III procollagen (COL3A1) causes type IV Ehlers–Danlos syndrome: the mutated allele is present in most blood leukocytes of the asymptomatic and mosaic mother. American Journal of Human Genetics 51: 497–507
99. Kumar D 1990 Syndrome of the month. Moebius syndrome. Journal of Medical Genetics 27: 122–126
100. Kuster W, Majewski F, Meinecke P 1985 EEC syndrome without ectrodactyly? Report on 8 cases. Clinical Genetics 28: 130–135
101. Labrune P, Pons J C, Khalil M et al 1993 Antenatal thrombocytopenia in three patients with TAR (thrombocytopenia with absent radii) syndrome. Prenatal Diagnosis 13: 463–466
102. Landy S J, Donnai D 1993 Syndrome of the month. Incontinentia pigmenti (Bloch–Sulzberger syndrome). Journal of Medical Genetics 30: 53–59
103. Latta R J, Graham C B, Aase J, Scham A M, Smith D W 1971 Larsen's syndrome: a skeletal dysplasia with multiple joint dislocations and unusual facies. Journal of Pediatrics 78: 291–298

104. Leahey A-M, Charnas L R, Nussbaum R L 1993 Nonsense mutations in the OCRL-1 gene in patients with the oculocerebrorenal syndrome of Lowe. Human Molecular Genetics 2: 461–464
105. Leroy J G, Devos E A, Bulcke V L J, Robbe N S 1981 Cerebro-costomandibular syndrome with autosomal dominant inheritance. Journal of Pediatrics 99: 441–443
106. Leroy J G, Spranger J W, Feingold M, Opitz J M, Crocker A C 1971 I-cell disease: a clinical picture. Journal of Pediatrics 79: 360–365
107. Levy P, Baraitser M 1991 Syndrome of the month. Coffin–Siris syndrome. Journal of Medical Genetics 28: 338–341
108. Li Q Y, Newbury-Ecob R A, Terrett J A et al 1997 Holt–Oram syndrome is caused by mutations in TBX5, a member of the brachyury (T) gene family. Nature Genetics 15: 21–29
109. Lichtenstein J R, Sundaram M, Burdge R 1980 Sex-influenced expression of Madelung's deformity in a family with dyschondrosteosis. Journal of Medical Genetics 17: 41–43
110. McKusick V A 1978 Mendelian inheritance in man, 5th Edn. Johns Hopkins University Press, Baltimore, MD
111. MacNab A J, D'Orsogna L, Cole D E C et al 1991 Cardiac anomalies complicating congenital contractural arachnodactyly. Archives of Disease in Childhood 66: 1143–1146
112. Majewski F, Goecke T 1982 Studies of microcephalic primordial dwarfism. I: Approach to a delineation of the Seckel syndrome. American Journal of Medical Genetics 12: 7–21
113. Mansour S, Hall C M, Pembrey M E, Young I D 1995 A clinical and genetic study of camptomelic dysplasia. Journal of Medical Genetics 32: 415–420
114. Marble M, Geraghty M T, de Franchis R et al 1994 Characterization of a cystathionine beta-synthase allele with three mutations in cis in a patient with B6 nonresponsive homocystinuria. Human Molecular Genetics 3: 1883–1886
115. Marden P M, Smith D W, McDonald M J 1964 Congenital anomalies in the newborn infant, including minor variations. Journal of Pediatrics 64: 357–371
116. Martinot V L, Manouvrier S, Anastassov Y et al 1994 Orodigitofacial syndromes type I and II: clinical and surgical studies. Cleft Palate–Craniofacial Journal 31: 401–408
117. Masuno M, Kuroki Y, Shimozawa N et al 1994 Assignment of the human peroxisome assembly factor-1 gene (PXMP3) responsible for Zellweger syndrome to chromosome 8q21.1 by fluorescence in situ hybridization. Genomics 20: 141–142
118. McDonald-McGinn D M, Driscoll D A, Bason L et al 1995 Autosomal dominant 'Opitz' GBBB syndrome due to a 22q11.2 deletion. American Journal of Medical Genetics 59: 103–113
119. Miles J H, Zonana J, McFarlane J et al 1984 Macrocephaly with hamartomas: Bannayan–Zonana syndrome. American Journal of Medical Genetics 19: 225–234
120. Monnens L, Heymans H 1987 Peroxisomal disorders: clinical characterisation. Journal of Inherited Metabolic Disease 10 suppl.: 23–32
121. Moog U, Engelen J, Albrechts J, Hoorntje T, Hendrikse F, Schrander-Stumpel C 1996 Alagille syndrome in a family with duplication 20p11. Clinical Dysmorphology 5: 279–288
122. Mueller O T, Wasmuth J J, Murray J C, Lozzio C B, Lovrien E W, Shows T B 1987 Chromosomal assignment of *N*-acetylglucosaminyl phosphotransferase, the lysosomal hydrolase targeting enzyme deficient in mucolipidosis II and III (abstract). Cytogenetic Cell Genetics 46: 664
123. Mueller R F 1987 The Alagille syndrome (arteriohepatic dysplasia). Journal of Medical Genetics 64: 621–626
124. Muis N, Beemer F A, Van-Dijken P 1986 Aase syndrome. Case report and review of the literature. European Journal of Pediatrics 145: 153–157
125. Murray J C, Nishimura D Y, Buetow K H et al 1990 Linkage of an autosomal dominant clefting syndrome (Van der Woude) to loci on chromosome 1q. American Journal of Human Genetics 46: 486–491
126. Nagai T, Nishimura G, Kato R et al 1995 Del(12)(p11.21p12.2) associated with an asphyxiating thoracic dystrophy or chondroectodermal dysplasia-like syndrome. American Journal of Medical Genetics 55:16–18
127. Najjar H, Mardini M 1988 Variability of the Holt–Oram syndrome in Saudi individuals. American Journal of Medical Genetics 29: 851–856
128. Naski M C, Wang Q, Xu J, Ornitz D M 1996 Graded activation of fibroblast growth factor receptor 3 by mutations causing achondroplasia and thanatophoric dysplasia. Nature Genetics 13: 233–237
129. Nicole S, Ben Hamida C, Beighton P et al 1995 Localization of the Schwartz–Jampel syndrome (SJS) locus to chromosome 1p34-p36.1 by homozygosity mapping. Human Molecular Genetics 4: 1633–1636
130. North C, Patton M A, Baraitser M, Winter R M 1985 The clinical features of the Cohen syndrome: further case reports. Journal of Medical Genetics 22: 131–134
131. O'Callaghan M, Young I D 1990 Syndrome of the month. Townes–Brocks syndrome. Journal of Medical Genetics 27: 457–461
132. Oley C, Baraitser M 1988 Blepharophimosis, ptosis epicathus inversus syndrome (BPES syndrome). Journal of Medical Genetics 25: 47–51
133. Oley C A, Baraitser M, Grant D B 1988 A reappraisal of the Charge association. Journal of Medical Genetics 25: 147–157
134. Opitz J M, Penchaszadeh V B, Holt M C et al 1994 Smith–Lemli–Opitz (RSH) syndrome bibliography: 1964–1993. American Journal of Medical Genetics 50: 339–343
135. Patton M A 1988 Syndrome of the month: Russell–Silver syndrome. Journal of Medical Genetics 25: 557–560
136. Patton M A, Laurence K M 1985 Three new cases of oculodentodigital (ODD) syndrome. Development of the facial phenotype. Journal of Medical Genetics 22: 386–389
137. Patton M A, Krywawych S, Winter R M et al 1987 Door syndrome (deafness, onycho-osteodystrophy, and mental retardation), elevated plasma and urinary 2-oxoglutarate in three unrelated patients. American Journal of Medical Genetics 26: 207–215
138. Pazzaglia U E, Beluffi G 1986 Oto-palato-digital syndrome in four generations of large family. Clinical Genetics 30: 338–344
139. Pelias M Z, Superneau D W, Thurmon T F 1981. A sixth report (8th case) of craniosynostosis-radial aplasia (Baller-Gerold) syndrome. American Journal of Medical Genetics 10: 133–139
140. Petrij F, Peters D J M, Breuning M H et al 1995 Rubinstein–Taybi syndrome caused by mutations in the transcriptional co-activator CBP. Nature 76: 348–351
141. Pinsky L 1978 The syndromology of anorectal malformation (atresia, stenosis, ectopia). American Journal of Medical Genetics 1: 461–474
142. Polymeropoulos M H, Ide S E, Wright M et al 1996 The gene for the Ellis–van Creveld syndrome is located on chromosome 4p16. Genomics 35: 1–5
143. Porteous M E, Curtis A, Lindsay S et al 1992 The gene for Aarskog syndrome is located between DXS255 and DXS566 (Xp11.2–Xq13). Genomics 14: 298–301
144. Pronk J C, Gibson R A, Savoia A et al 1995 Localisation of the Fanconi anaemia complementation group A gene to chromosome 16q24.3 (Letter). Nature Genetics 11: 338–340
145. Reardon W, Winter R M 1994 Syndrome of the month. Saethre–Chotzen syndrome. Journal of Medical Genetics 31: 393–396
146. Reardon W, Winter R M, Rutland P et al 1994 Mutations in the fibroblast growth factor receptor 2 gene cause Crouzon syndrome. Nature Genetics 8: 98–103
147. Reid I S, Turner G 1976 Familial anal abnormality. Journal of Pediatrics 88: 992–994
148. Rimoin D L, Edgerton M T 1967 Genetic and clinical heterogeneity in the oral-facial-digital syndromes. Journal of Pediatrics 71: 94–102
149. Robinow M, Johnson G F 1981 The Gordon syndrome: autosomal dominant cleft palate, camptodactyly, and club feet. American Journal of Medical Genetics 9: 139–146
150. Ruiz-Maldonado R, Toussaint S, Tamayo L et al 1992 Hypomelanosis of Ito: diagnostic criteria and report of 41 cases. Pediatric Dermatology 9: 1–10
151. Salonen R 1984 The Meckel syndrome: clinicopathological findings in 67 patients. American Journal of Medical Genetics 18: 671–689
152. Sargent C, Burn J, Baraitser M et al 1985 Trigonocephaly and the Opitz C syndrome. Journal of Medical Genetics 22: 39–45
153. Schell U, Hehr A, Feldman G J et al 1995 Mutations in FGFR1 and FGFR2 cause familial and sporadic Pfeiffer syndrome. Human Molecular Genetics 4: 323–328
154. Schroeder H W, Sybert V P 1987 Rapp-Hodgkin ectodermal dysplasia. Journal of Pediatrics 110: 72–75
155. Spranger J, Benirschke K, Hall J G et al 1982 Errors of morphogenesis: concepts and terms. Journal of Pediatrics 100: 160–165
156. Schwindinger W F, Francomano C A, Levine M A 1992 Identification of a mutation in the gene encoding the alpha subunit of the stimulatory G protein of adenylyl cyclase in McCune–Albright syndrome. Proceedings of the National Academy of Sciences USA 1992 89: 5152–5156

157. Semina E V, Zabel B U, Carey J C et al 1996 Cloning and characterization of a novel bicoid-related homeobox transcription factor gene, RIEG, involved in Rieger syndrome. Nature Genetics 14: 392–399
158. Shows T B, Scrafford-Wolff L, Brown J A, Meisler M 1978 Assignment of a beta-galactosidase gene (beta-GAL-alpha) to chromosome 3 in man. Cytogenetic Cell Genetics 22: 219–222
159. Small K W, Stalvey M, Fisher L et al 1995 Blepharophimosis syndrome is linked to chromosome 3q. Human Molecular Genetics 4: 443–448
160. Spranger S, Spranger M, Meinck H-M, Tariverdian G 1995 Two sisters with Escobar syndrome. American Journal of Medical Genetics 57: 425–428
161. Stevens C A, Qumsiyeh M B 1995 Syndromal frontonasal dysostosis in a child with a complex translocation involving chromosomes 3, 7, and 11. American Journal of Medical Genetics 55: 494–497
162. Stosiek N, Ulmer R, von den Driesch P et al 1994 Chromosomal mosaicism in two patients with epidermal verrucous nervus. Demonstration of chromosomal breakpoint. Journal of the American Academy of Dermotology 30: 622–625
163. Superti-Furga A 1996 Achondrogenesis type 1B. Journal of Medical Genetics 33: 957–961
164. Tahvanainen E, Norio R, Karila E et al 1994 Cohen syndrome gene assigned to the long arm of chromosome 8 by linkage analysis. Nature Genetics 7: 201–204
165. Tavormina P L, Shiang R, Thompson L M et al 1995 Thanatophoric dysplasia (types I and II) caused by distinct mutations in fibroblast growth factor receptor 3. Nature Genetics 9: 321–328
166. Temple I K, MacDowall P, Baraitser M, Atherton D J 1990 Syndrome of the month. Focal dermal hypoplasia (Goltz syndrome). Journal of Medical Genetics 27: 180–187
167. Thompson E, Pembrey M E 1985 Seckel syndrome: an overdiagnosed syndrome. Journal of Medical Genetics 22: 192–201
168. Tolmie J L, Harvie A, Cockburn F 1992 The teratogenic effects of undiagnosed maternal hyperphenylalaninaemia: a case for prevention? British Journal of Obstetrics and Gynaecology 99: 347–348
169. Tolmie J L, Mortimer G, Doyle D et al 1987 The Neu-Laxova syndrome in female sibs: clinical and pathological features with prenatal diagnosis in the second sib. American Journal of Medical Genetics 27: 175–182
170. Topley J M, Varady E, Lestringant G G 1994 Larsen syndrome in siblings with consanguineous parents. Clinical Dysmorphology 3: 263–265
171. Toriello H V 1993 Review. Oral–facial–digital syndromes, 1992 Clinical Dysmorphology 2: 95–105
172. Traboulsi E I, Lenz W et al 1988 The Lenz microphthalmia syndrome. American Journal of Ophthalmology 105: 40–45
173. Van Camp G, Van Thienen M N, Handig I et al 1995 Chromosome 13q deletion with Waardenburg syndrome: further evidence for a gene involved in neural crest function on 13q. Journal of Medical Genetics 32: 531–536
174. Velinov M. Slaugenhaupt S A, Stoilov I et al 1994 The gene for achondroplasia maps to the telomeric region of chromosome 4p. Nature Genetics 6: 314–317
175. Verloes A, Le Merrer M, Davin J-C et al 1992 The orocraniodigital syndrome of Juberg and Hayward. Journal of Medical Genetics 29: 262–265
176. Wallace M R, Marchuk D A, Andersen L B et al 1990 Type 1 neurofibromatosis gene: identification of a large transcript disrupted in three NF1 patients. Science 249: 181–186
177. Wertheimer E, Lu S-P, Backeljauw P F et al 1993 Homozygous deletion of the human insulin receptor gene results in leprechaunism. Nature Genetics 5: 71–73
178. Whelan A J, Watson M S, Porter F D, Steiner R D 1995 Klippel–Trenaunay–Weber syndrome associated with 5:11 balanced translocation. American Journal of Medical Genetics 59: 492–494
179. Wildervanck L S, Hoksema P E, Penning L 1966 Radiological examination of the inner ear of deaf-mutes presenting the cervicooculo-acusticus syndrome. Acta Oto-Laryngologica 61: 445–453
180. Wilkie A O M, Slaney S F, Oldridge M et al 1995 Apert syndrome results from localized mutations of FGFR2 and is allelic with Crouzon syndrome. Nature Genetics 9: 165–172
181. Williams M S, Josephson K D, Wargowski D S 1993 Marden–Walker syndrome: a case report and a critical review of the literature. Clinical Dysmorphology 2: 211–219
182. Winter R M 1986 Dubowitz syndrome. Journal of Medical Genetics 23: 11–13
183. Winter R M, Baraitser M 1998 The London Dysmorphology Database; Oxford University Press, Oxford
184. Winter R M, Donnai D, Crawford M D'A 1981 Syndromes of microcephaly, microphthalmia, cataracts, and joint contractures. Journal of Medical Genetics 18: 129–133
185. Wirtz M K, Gorlin R J, Godfrey A et al 1996 Weill–Marchesani syndrome – possible linkage of the autosomal dominant form to 15q21.1 American Journal of Medical Genetics 65: 68–75
186. Wit J M, Beemer F A, Barth P G et al 1985 Cerebral gigantism (Sotos syndrome). Compiled data of 22 cases. Analysis of clinical features, growth and plasma somatomedin. European Journal of Paediatrics 144: 131–140
187. Young I D, Fielder A R, Casey T A 1986 The Weill-Marchesani syndrome in mother and son. Clinical Genetics 30: 475–480
188. Zergollern L, Hitrec V 1982 Four siblings with Robert's syndrome. Clinical Genetics 21: 1–6
189. Zonana J, Jones M, Browne D et al 1992 High-resolution mapping of the X-linked hypohidrotic ectodermal dysplasia (EDA) locus. American Journal of Human Genetics 51: 1036–1046

35

Neonatal dermatology

Neil P. J. Walker

INTRODUCTION

Anatomically the skin of the newborn is not very different from that of the adult. Nevertheless, the dermatological problems that commonly arise in the first month of life are special. This chapter will first highlight some of the ways in which neonatal skin is different, and will then consider some of the common disorders peculiar to infancy. Many of the several thousand named skin diseases can occur in early infancy. Some of those which are common, striking or important because of systemic implications will be briefly described.

Full details and bibliography for the diseases discussed in this chapter can be found in standard major dermatology textbooks[13,46] and in monographs and papers especially devoted to neonatal and paediatric dermatology.[21,23,32,33,49,53,60] The journal *Pediatric Dermatology* started in 1983.

THE NORMAL SKIN OF THE NEONATE

By the 28th week of gestation the infant's skin is well equipped with blood vessels, lymphatics, nerves and supporting structures. The appendages – hair follicles, sebaceous glands and sweat glands – have been present from the third or fourth month. The periderm has long since come and gone. However, although anatomically identifiable, not all these tissues are fully functional. For example, the various vascular plexuses characteristic of skin may not develop for some months after birth and depend on external stimuli for their proper development. Sweat glands do not begin to function until 2 or 3 days after birth and may take a year to two to function fully, even though no new glands are formed after fetal life.

Premature babies[27] have skin which is rather thin and has an often striking absence of subcutaneous fat. It may also be covered by fine lanugo hair which is normally shed in the last few weeks of gestation. Sweat gland functioning is delayed. Increased transepidermal water loss due to immaturity of the barrier function of the stratum corneum may be very significant compared with the full-term infant (p. 290).

Normal skin at birth is covered with vernix caseosa derived from sebaceous glands and from epidermal cell breakdown. This is shed over a few days and may have some antibacterial properties. Minor degrees of desquamation within the first week are physiological. For the first day or two the skin is red, partly attributable to the immaturity of the blood vessels and their controlling mechanism and partly to the increased blood viscosity and packed cell volume.[47] Sterile at birth, the skin normally starts to become colonized with the usual commensals within the first week. The neonatal skin has also been exposed to maternal stimuli, both physiological and pathological. Maternal hormones give rise to temporary sebaceous gland activity and even acne, as well as mammary changes (see also Transplacental diseases, p. 895).

GENERAL PRINCIPLES OF CARE[59]

A considerable folklore surrounds the routine care of neonatal skin. A physiological role for the vernix has traditionally been postulated and early removal associated with an increase in skin sepsis. It is customary for excess vernix to be wiped off, the scalp and face cleansed, and the baby not bathed formally for a few days. For bathing, detergents and foaming agents should be avoided. There is little scientific evidence on which to base a choice of agent. Aqueous cream is commonly used; it may be best to avoid preparations containing peanut oil (arachis oil) in case exposure to an allergen leads to sensitization.[30]

The residual umbilical cord will usually slough off within 10–14 days. The stump should be kept clean and dry. The regular use of talc may be the reason why granulomas are so common; the careful application of silver nitrate will usually aid their resolution.

When considering any form of topical therapy it must always be remembered that neonatal skin is less likely to develop allergic sensitization[11] and is more vulnerable to irritants. Even apparently straightforward skin preparation for procedures must be undertaken with care. Excess 70% isopropyl alcohol and iodine-containing preparations can cause chemical burns if a neonate is allowed to lie in them for any length of time (p. 931). The surface:volume ratio is much greater in infancy. This is important in relation to topical steroids and potential toxins like boric acid, mercury and hexachlorophane, which, especially when applied to damaged skin, may be absorbed in significant amounts. Topical steroids are potentiated by occlusion, and their use on the napkin area and flexures generally must be monitored carefully to avoid irreversible side-effects. Problems of insensible water loss, exacerbated by the lack of a stratum corneum in premature infants and which in severe neonatal skin disease may lead to renal failure, may be avoided by nursing in a humidified atmosphere and applying semi-permeable wound dressings. In other respects the general principles of therapy are the same as in adults.

VERY COMMON AND OFTEN TRIVIAL PROBLEMS SPECIAL TO THE NEONATE

ERYTHEMA NEONATORUM – TOXIC ERYTHEMA

This common disorder of infancy may occur in up to 50% of normal full-term babies, rather less in the premature. The aetiology is obscure.[6] Histology shows oedema and a mainly perivascular infiltrate in the dermis with a striking number of eosinophils. The eosinophils may also extend up into the epidermis to produce histologically and clinically evident eosinophilic abscesses. Blood eosinophilia is not uncommon. The eruption is rarely present at birth, commonly appearing within the first 3 days of life or up to 2 weeks. In mild forms there is a blotchy macular erythema, especially on the chest but often more widespread. The eruption is usually asymptomatic and unassociated with other problems. It regresses spontaneously in a few days and requires no treatment. It is seldom a problem to distinguish the disorder from impetigo and infected miliaria, but if raised papules or superimposed pustules appear then the correct diagnosis can be made by demonstrating the characteristic eosinophils in a smear from the lesion.

TRANSIENT NEONATAL PUSTULAR MELANOSIS

(Table 35.1)

This disorder was only described in 1976 but may well be quite common and in some ways resembles toxic erythema.[34,41] The eruption is present at birth and is more common in blacks. It starts with small superficial non-erythematous vesiculopustules, which rapidly progress to a collarette of scales, and finally a hyperpigmented macule which fades in a few weeks. The vesicles contain polymorphs rather than eosinophils. The cause is uncertain; the pustules are sterile and no treatment is required.

Table 35.1 Vesiculopapular diseases of neonates

Infectious	Non-infectious
Sepsis	Mastocytosis
Bullous impetigo	Incontinentia pigmenti
Staphylococcal scalded skin syndrome	Eosinophilic pustular folliculitis
	Epidermolysis bullosa
Neonatal herpes simplex	Erythema toxicum neonatorum
Neonatal varicella	Transient neonatal pustular melanosis
Congenital candidiasis	Miliaria
Syphilis	Acropustulosis infantum
Scabies	

HARLEQUIN CHANGE

This is a striking and common phenomenon of the neonatal period, especially in premature infants. The precise aetiology is unknown but it is attributed to vasomotor instability. It occurs within the first few days of life and may persist for a week or two. Particularly when the infant is lying on its side, there are episodes, lasting a few seconds or minutes, in which the upper half of the body becomes paler than the lower half, with a striking demarcation in the midline. The pattern may be reversed as the infant is turned onto its other side. This phenomenon is of no sinister significance and requires no treatment.

CUTIS MARMORATA/LIVEDO RETICULARIS

Potentially there is a network pattern in all normal skin due to the way the vessels are arranged. Cutis marmorata (marbled skin) is the name given to the minor physiological accentuation of this pattern. It is common in infancy and of no significance. It may be accentuated in various disorders, e.g. Down syndrome. Cutis marmorata telangiectatica congenita gives rise to more intense and often irregular mottling and sometimes thinning of the skin of, for example, one limb. It may be associated with other congenital defects.[44] It must be distinguished from genuine diffuse phlebectasia where the network discoloration is due to grossly dilated larger veins.

MILIA

Milia are tiny cysts which arise from the necks of either the pilosebaceous follicles or the sweat ducts. They are extremely common, and occur in almost half of normal neonates. They present as 1–2 mm yellowish-white spots, arising usually on normal skin. They are especially common on the nose and elsewhere on the face. There may be a few or many hundreds. They usually disappear spontaneously over a month or two. They should be distinguished from neonatally enlarged sebaceous glands.

COMMON SKIN DISEASES

A naevus is a circumscribed defect in the development of

predominantly one tissue, often with accompanying dysplasia of other tissues. There are no clear causative factors. They are commonly present at birth or become apparent within the neonatal period. They are often a source of great concern and an early specialist opinion should be sought. Naevi can be classified on the basis of the major tissue component.

EPITHELIAL NAEVI

Verrucous or warty naevus – naevus unius lateris

In these lesions there is an excessive development of the surface epidermis. They may be associated with mental retardation and ocular and other manifestations in the epidermal naevus syndrome.[54]

They may be present at birth as flesh-coloured or yellow-brown, linear, streaky and often warty lesions varying in size from 1 cm to half the body surface. They rarely disappear spontaneously and may thicken at puberty. Formal excision is the only sure way to eradicate the lesions but limited removal by diathermy, curette and cautery or laser vaporization may provide useful, if often temporary, cosmetic improvement.

Sebaceous naevus – naevus sebaceous of Jadassohn

These yellow-brown slightly raised plaques consist predominantly of sebaceous glands which histologically are entirely normal. They are usually present at birth as single lesions but may be multiple and extensive. Common sites are the sutural areas of the scalp. They may enlarge slowly through childhood or suddenly at puberty. They may be associated with convulsions, mental retardation, skeletal, ocular or other abnormalities.[37] Complex hamartomatous malformations may arise from them as may basal cell epitheliomas. Management is excision of the entire lesion although this may be delayed to early adulthood.

Naevus syringo-cystadenomatosus papilliferus

This defect of apocrine sweat duct development presents at birth or early childhood as 2–10 cm pink nodules, which may be discrete and scattered or grouped as a plaque with a warty often crusted surface. 50% occur on the scalp and may be associated with cicatricial alopecia. 10% turn malignant.

Comedo naevus

These consist of hair follicles containing horny plugs and may be very extensive. Some are present at birth.

CONNECTIVE TISSUE NAEVI

These are dysplasias of dermal connective tissue in which elastin or collagen fibres usually predominate, though clinically it may be difficult to define the major constituent. They may be single or multiple, small or of wide extent. They can be associated with other abnormalities, e.g. tuberous sclerosis.

MELANOCYTIC NAEVI

These are very common later in childhood. Less than 0.1% of all pigmented naevi are present at birth.[8] There is certainly a risk of malignant change occurring in the very large naevi. This has been assessed at as high as 42% in the giant lesions but is probably less than 10%.[18,25,52] The magnitude of the risk of malignant change in the smaller congenital pigmented naevi is uncertain, as also are opinions as to how these should be managed.[43] Formal surgical excision of the larger naevi can be a daunting procedure but is often considered appropriate. Of great interest recently has been the treatment of even large congenital naevi by such simple techniques as dermabrasion or curettage.[24] At first it was hoped that this could effect a virtual cure, but follow-up has indicated caution in accepting this claim and opinions are divided. If it is to be done it is best done in the first few months of life. Hence it is most important that congenital naevi should be assessed in the neonatal period by a plastic surgeon or a dermatologist. 'Q'-switched lasers can treat some of these naevi but their role is not clearly defined.

Mongolian blue spot

Blue/grey irregular macules up to 100 mm in diameter are present at birth in about 90% of Asians (hence the name) and Negroes, though only 5% of Caucasians. They are due to a deep dermal infiltrate of melanocytes and usually fade in infancy, though persistence throughout life has been reported. They are usually found over the lower back but can occur at other sites. They are entirely benign, unassociated with other pathology and require no treatment other than reassurance that they have nothing to do with Down syndrome or child abuse.

VASCULAR NAEVI

The clinical classification of these lesions can be difficult for though they can be broadly divided into two types many are obviously a combination.

Capillary malformation

This is a circumscribed defect of dermal capillaries which, if deep vessels are involved, is associated with connective tissue hypertrophy. As 'salmon patches' or 'stork marks' they occur in many neonates as pale pink lesions on the nape of the neck, forehead and eyelids and usually fade rapidly.

As 'port wine stains', a misnomer as many are initially no darker than a rosé, they present at birth and grow with the infant. Spontaneous improvement is rare. Usually the lesions become darker with age as the vessels become more ectatic. They are commonest on the face and trunk and may be associated with intracranial or spinal vascular anomalies (Sturge–Weber syndrome) or limb hypertrophy (Klippel–Trenaunay syndrome). Until recently, treatment has largely been unsatisfactory but the advent of lasers, particularly pulsed dye lasers, has meant that many of these lesions can be lightened very significantly.[55]

Capillary haemangioma ('strawberry marks')

These lesions are found in 10% of infants, being twice as common in girls. They may be superficial, subcutaneous or mixed and are probably due to isolated clusters of angiogenetic cells failing to establish normal communication with the circulation. 90% are manifest during the neonatal period, but very rarely at birth, appearing at any site. They usually increase rapidly in size over 3–9 months, the majority being 20–50 mm in diameter, before undergoing gradual, but usually complete, resolution. They can be very large. Haemorrhage may be alarming but is seldom serious. Ulceration may occur, especially in the napkin area. Thrombocytopenia may be caused by the very large strawberry marks (Kasabach–Merritt syndrome) and may demand active treatment, e.g. with systemic steroids or interferon.[12] On rare occasions the growth of a large lesion may both clinically and histologically resemble a malignant blood vessel neoplasm. Expectant treatment is best unless the site interferes with normal function or development, i.e. sucking or vision. If this is the case then reassurance, support and careful observation can be supplemented with steroids, either intralesional or systemic, interferon or pulsed dye laser treatment.[3] Surgical excision and radiotherapy may also be considered.

Diffuse haemangiomatosis with myriad small haemangiomas may or may not affect other organs so the prognosis is guarded.[20]

COMPLEX CONGENITAL ABNORMALITIES INVOLVING SKIN AND OTHER ORGANS

The skin may be involved in a wide range of complex congenital disorders which involve other organs as well as the skin. Most of these are rare. Details of some of them may be found elsewhere in this book (p. 34) or in standard dermatology texts.[46]

INFECTIONS

Cutaneous infections in the neonate can be a serious, life-threatening problem. Colonization of the skin by pathogenic organisms is an ever-present danger, especially in overcrowded nurseries. Great care in nursing and medical practice must be observed to reduce its incidence to a minimum and prevent cross-infection.

Bacteria

Bullous impetigo can be caused by *Staphylococcus aureus* or haemolytic streptococcus group A. The incidence is greatest in premature infants and the malnourished. Onset is usually within the first week with large bullae appearing which rapidly break down to leave a red, raw, moist surface.

Staphylococcal scalded skin syndrome (often associated with the names Ritter von Rittershain and Lyell) is produced by a toxin from a skin infection by *S. aureus* often of phage type 71, though other phage types have been implicated. There is a cleavage in the granular layer, with erythema, oedema and separation of large sheets of skin. Mortality for these conditions is high without treatment, which consists of general support and antistaphylococcal antibiotics, usually intravenously. The skin heals well.

Omphalitis. *Pseudomonas* can cause an omphalitis.

Listeriosis. In addition to systemic illness (p. 1149), the infant develops a generalized erythematous papular or petechial rash which may become pustular.

Congenital syphilis

This is rare. It is unusual for the skin lesions to appear within the first month.

Viruses

Congenital cytomegalovirus (p. 1170), and rubella infections (p. 1168) may present with jaundice and/or purpura.

Active genital herpes simplex in the mother is an indication for caesarean section within 4 hours of rupture of the membranes (but see p. 1158). Neonatal infection (p. 1156) can be overwhelming, though treatment with acyclovir may be successful.

Neonatal varicella is covered on page 1158.

The prevalence of HIV infection in children is increasing and the associated dermatological conditions, whilst morphologically usually the same as seen in immunocompetent children, tend to be severe and difficult to treat.

Candida

This dimorphic fungus is a frequent inhabitant of the genital and gastrointestinal tracts. Neonates frequently become colonized at birth or in early infancy.

All types of candidal infection are common after the use of antibiotics. There are three main clinical pictures.

1. In oral candidiasis early colonization is likely to be followed by the development of sharply defined patches of creamy, crumbly curd-like material on an erythematous base. There can be multiple lesions which extend to the pharynx and oesophagus. Therapy with oral nystatin is usually successful. If oral thrush is recurrent and/or resistant, immunodeficiency states including HIV infection should be considered.

2. Any opposing skin surfaces, areas subject to occlusion or close to an orifice may become colonized. Lesions present as extending patches of erythema with a fringed irregular edge, superficial pustules and satellite lesions.

3. As an extension of intertrigo, especially with an associated irritant dermatitis, *Candida* may colonize much of the napkin area, though at times the appearances are rather nondescript and the role of *Candida* dubious. Topical steroids modify the clinical picture and bacterial suppression with systemic or topical treatment may favour the yeast. Treatment with topical imidazoles or nystatin is usually adequate.

Scabies

Sarcoptes scabiei var. *hominis* is no respecter of age, and an eczema-like eruption, even in the first 4 weeks of life, which distresses the neonate should alert one to this possibility. The presence of symptoms in other members of the family is often a useful clue. The eruption in the neonate can be generalized, and burrows may be found on the palms and soles and should be distinguished from acropustulosis (see p. 896). The traditional treatment with gamma-benzene hexachloride is associated with a risk of systemic toxicity and should not be used.

The treatment of choice is crotamiton 10% cream or lotion.

INTERTRIGO

The term intertrigo describes the erythematous, sometimes exudative or even purulent, eruptions which occur in the folds of the skin. This is caused partly by microorganisms, commonly normal skin commensals, or sometimes by more pathogenic organisms (including staphylococci, streptococci and *Candida albicans*), with sweating, maceration and friction playing a considerable role. Minor degrees of intertrigo are sufficiently common as to be virtually physiological. Often no treatment other than elementary skin care is required. More severe episodes may require a topical antibiotic, occasionally with a weak topical steroid in addition. Miconazole/hydrocortisone cream is also useful. More severe examples of intertrigo merge into infantile seborrhoeic dermatitis.

INFANTILE ECZEMA AND DERMATITIS

Eczema in infancy is common, although somewhat less so in the neonatal period. The following types may be recognized:

Allergic contact dermatitis

This is very rare as a clinical problem at this age although neonates can be sensitized experimentally.

Irritant contact dermatitis

Because of the vulnerability of the infant skin, minor degrees of this are not uncommon. Diagnosis should seldom be in much doubt.

Atopic dermatitis

The aetiology of this disorder is complex.[57] IgE-mediated allergic reactions are only one facet, and often absent. In 70% of cases there is a family history of atopy. Atopic dermatitis in the neonatal period is quite uncommon and often atypical in that the infant is not capable of the scratching which so dominates the clinical picture in later childhood. In the early stages the characteristic flexural distribution of later childhood is not found. Some of the worst cases of atopic dermatitis, which may soon develop into the rare atopic erythroderma, may start soon after birth.

In the neonatal period treatment is unlikely to involve more than the use of simple emollients, like aqueous cream, or topical hydrocortisone. The role of diet is discussed on page 757.

Atopic dermatitis and other syndromes

Atopic dermatitis, or an eruption which may closely resembles it, may occur in various rare syndromes, e.g. Wiskott–Aldrich syndrome, phenylketonuria, Netherton syndrome. More bizarre patterns of eczema have been associated with rare abnormalities of biotin metabolism.[56]

Infantile seborrhoeic dermatitis (Fig. 35.1)

As with adult seborrhoeic dermatitis, the name is somewhat of a misnomer. There is no evidence to link the two types. The very existence of the neonatal disorder is disputed; however, until the aetiology is better understood it seems appropriate at present to retain it as a clinical entity. *Pityrosporum ovale* may play a role in the pathogenesis. The features which distinguish it from atopic dermatitis are lack of family history, early onset often in the first month of life, predominantly napkin, flexural and scalp distribution, and a distinctive morphology. The eruption usually consists of sheets of erythema, often with outlying islands and some scaling. About 20–40% of cases have clinical features overlapping with atopic dermatitis, which is not surprising as both are multifactorial diseases. Itching is seldom a problem and the general health is usually unimpaired. *Candida* can often be found,

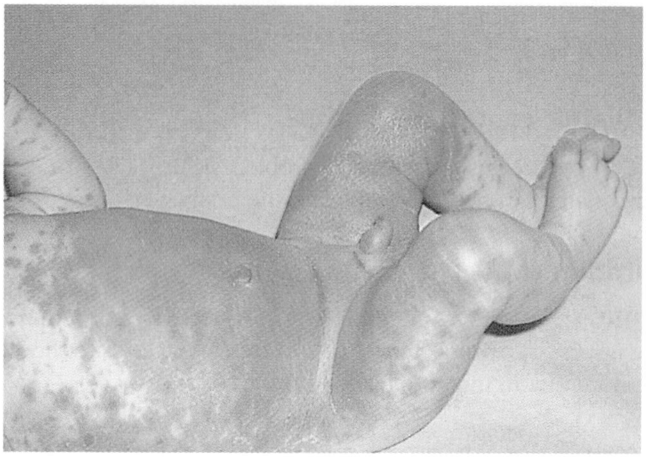

Fig. 35.1 Infantile seborrhoeic dermatitis.

although it may be difficult to decide whether it is a mere commensal or actively pathogenic. The prognosis is good and the eruption usually clears in a few weeks or months, except in that minority who change over into atopic dermatitis. Histiocytosis (p. 1059) may resemble seborrhoeic dermatitis. The adult form is unusual but may occur in association with HIV infection.

The treatment includes patience, exposure to fresh air, simple emollients like aqueous cream or emulsifying ointment, or a weak topical steroid like hydrocortisone cream. When the eruption is very inflammatory or more obviously exudative, a topical antibiotic can be added. If the clinical picture resembles candidiasis, with a peeling edge and outlying pustules, or if a swab grows *Candida*, topical nystatin or an imidazole can also be combined. There are proprietary preparations containing weak steroid/antibacterial and anticandida agents (e.g. Trimovate cream, Nystaform-HC cream and ointment).

Cradle cap

This is the lay name for the often greasy scaling which is so commonly found on the vertex of the scalp. It includes several different diagnoses. Often it is no more than a slight increase in normal physiological scaling. It can be part of the various types of ichthyosis. However, more commonly it is part, sometimes the only part, of infantile seborrhoeic dermatitis. In mild cases no treatment may be required, or the scales can be softened with oil left on for a few hours and then washed or combed off. More severe cases with inflammatory changes may be difficult to control or may respond to a weak steroid/antibiotic preparation.

Leiner's disease

This name is sometimes still applied to seborrhoeic dermatitis which has progressed to become a generalized erythroderma. As with any other erythroderma this can be a serious disease. There is associated diarrhoea, occasional vomiting and recurrent sepsis. There may be an association with breast-feeding. The disease tends to occur in sick infants or those with various immune defects – notably dysfunctional C5.[19] Treatment of the dermatitis demands skilled nursing but is otherwise as for seborrhoeic dermatitis.

Erythroderma

Erythroderma or exfoliative dermatitis is a universal inflammatory reaction of the skin, which becomes generally red, inflamed and often scaly. At any age it can be serious. In the neonate it is most often due to generalized atopic dermatitis, seborrhoeic dermatitis (Leiner's disease), psoriasis or ichthyosiform erythroderma. Treatment is that of the underlying disease. Particular care has to be taken with temperature control.

NAPKIN RASH

Napkin rashes have a multiplicity of causes, even for those who make some attempt at using the term in a rather more precise way than simply to describe any rash in the napkin area.

The traditional teaching is that napkin rash is due to the irritant effect of ammonia liberated by faecal organisms from urea in wet napkins. This is an oversimplification as ammonia alone will produce erythema only on previously damaged skin.[7] Other factors are also important including irritant faeces (freshly passed urine is not irritant), maceration, chafing, sweating, high humidity, bacterial and *Candida* colonization or even frank infection.[31,61] The harmful effects of plastic pants are often overemphasized. Napkin rashes are so common as to be normal at some stage. The clinical appearances are often those of erythema and oedema, perhaps with papules or even blisters, sometimes followed by scaling. These changes occur maximally on the convex surfaces of the thighs and buttocks. Sometimes, especially on the genitalia, there are quite discrete large eroded papules – the papuloerosive type.

Differential diagnosis of napkin eruptions must include especially intertrigo, seborrhoeic dermatitis, napkin psoriasis, contact dermatitis, perianal dermatitis, as well as less common disorders like congenital syphilis, acrodermatitis enteropathica, granuloma gluteale and juvenile pemphigoid.[46] Treatment is essentially removal of the various aetiological factors with careful attention to napkin technique. Fresh air can be very helpful. For prevention, any simple grease like Vaseline or other barrier cream is appropriate. For established cases a weak topical steroid and/or topical antibacterial preparation may be necessary for a short time. Where there is clinical indication, but not just on laboratory evidence, an anticandida preparation can be combined.

Perianal dermatitis

Minor erythema and more definite inflammatory changes occur very commonly in the first few days of life and regress without need of treatment. The aetiology is unknown.

Psoriasis/napkin psoriasis

Although psoriasis may affect 2% of the adult population, it is very rare in infancy, especially in the neonatal period. Very occasionally straightforward psoriasis may start in infancy with all the features of the adult disease. It may also be erythrodermic. Pustular psoriasis, with superadded sterile pustules, has also been recorded at this age. More commonly, an eruption with many features of infantile seborrhoeic dermatitis may gradually take on the appearances of psoriasis. Such eruptions usually clear in a few months but there may be a recurrence of more typical psoriasis later on. This type of napkin psoriasis can best be considered as an infantile seborrhoeic dermatitis, modified by the genetic background to develop psoriasis. Treatment is usually similar to that of seborrhoeic dermatitis.

TRAUMATIC LESIONS

A variety of traumatic lesions may be caused by or resemble the results of obstetric trauma. Amniocentesis may give rise to usually rather insignificant scars. Fetal electrodes may occasionally cause skin damage and herpes simplex type II infections may develop at that site. Blisters on the lips from sucking are a minor trauma that the infant inflicts upon himself. Similar blisters on the arms have been attributed to in utero sucking. Less immediately apparent are the diverse ways in which non-accidental injury may be manifest on the skin. Calcified nodules on the heels may follow multiple punctures to obtain blood (p. 930).

TRANSPLACENTAL DISEASE

Certain conditions which are associated with the presence of maternal circulating immunoglobulins may be manifest in the neonate, presumably because of the passage of IgG across the placenta. Idiopathic thrombocytopenic purpura (p. 802), systemic and discoid lupus erythematosus, pemphigus and bullous disorder of pregnancy (pemphigoid gestationis) are all reported.[36,42] Usually the neonatal disease is self-limiting but neonatal systemic lupus erythematosus, which may occur in infants of asymptomatic mothers, in whom nevertheless auto-antibodies can usually be demonstrated, is associated with congenital atrioventricular dissociation, cardiac fibrosis (p. 187), transient liver disease and thrombocytopenia. The skin disease is transient and does not scar.[29]

NEONATAL ACNE

A neonatal eruption similar to acne vulgaris with comedones, papules and pustules is presumed to be due to the effects of maternal androgens on the pilosebaceous unit. It is seen on the face, predominantly of boys, and resolves spontaneously within a few months. Resolution may be hastened by mild topical treatment with keratolytics, i.e. 0.5% salicylic acid in aqueous cream. If severe or prolonged, a virilizing syndrome should be suspected. There is no clear association with severe acne later in life.

PRENATAL DIAGNOSIS

The development of chorion biopsy, amniocentesis and fetoscopy has made it possible to obtain not only amniotic cells for culture but also fetal skin biopsies for histological examination. The enzyme defects in xeroderma pigmentosum can be found in amniotic cells. Recessive epidermolysis bullosa letalis (see below) and various ichthyoses have been diagnosed from skin biopsies. The list of disorders in which useful information may be found is increasing.[9,10]

ALPHABETIC GLOSSARY

Acrodermatitis enteropathica (Fig. 35.2)

The molecular basis of this rare autosomal recessive defect in the absorption of zinc is not yet fully characterized. It presents in infants under the age of 3 months but rarely under 1 month. The fully developed condition includes diarrhoea, failure to thrive, *Candida* infection, the characteristic rash and a low plasma zinc. The rash consists of sharp-edged areas of erythema, scaling and often pustulation around the mouth, ears, fingers and toes and anogenital region. This potentially fatal disease can now be completely reversed by oral zinc supplements

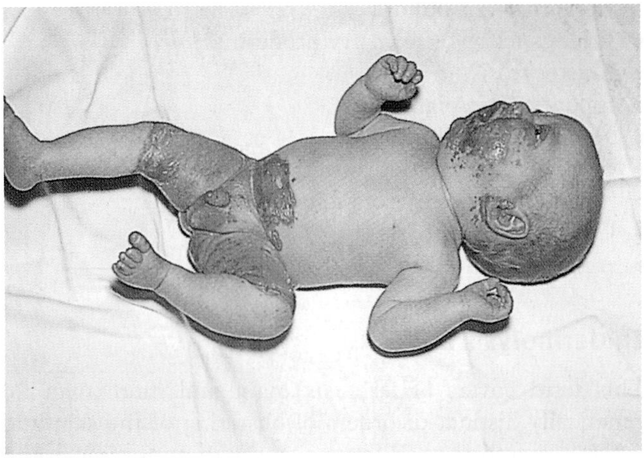

Fig. 35.2 Acrodermatitis enteropathica.

which usually need to be continued indefinitely. An exactly similar skin eruption can occur in parenterally fed premature babies and as a self-limiting form with transient zinc deficiency.[1,51]

Acropustulosis

This is an uncommon disease of unknown aetiology, characterized by crops of 2–4 mm papules which become vesiculopustules on the palms and soles but also on the dorsa of the hands and feet. It must be distinguished from scabies. It is often very itchy. Most cases have been in black infants from North America but it has been reported from England.[38] Severe cases may warrant the use of dapsone or of sulphapyridine.

Aplasia cutis[17]

A primary failure of differentiation in early embryonic life may lead to the absence, in circumscribed areas, of epidermis, dermis and subcutis. The severity varies from merely an absence of dermal appendages to full-thickness loss, which on the scalp can leave a defect down to dura. There may be a family history. The lesions are apparent at birth as raw, red, granulating wounds which might be considered to be the result of trauma, especially as 60% occur on the scalp. The area(s) heal slowly and care must be taken to avoid secondary infection. Plastic surgery may ultimately be required. Aplasia cutis may be associated with skeletal and other abnormalities.

Bullae

In the neonatal period bullae may be associated with a variety of congenital and acquired diseases. The possible diagnoses are listed below:

- Sucking
- Infection
  - staphylococcal
  - congenital syphilis
- Epidermolysis bullosa
- Bullous ichthyosiform erythroderma
- Mastocytosis
- Incontinentia pigmenti
- Neonatal pemphigus
- Pemphigoid gestationis (herpes gestationis)
- Acrodermatitis enteropathica
- Congenital porphyria
- Aplasia cutis.

Epidermolysis bullosa[14]

This term covers at least six main and more than 20 genetically distinct disorders of blistering of the skin and mucous membranes. Blisters occur with minor injury and in some cases spontaneously.

Autosomal dominant types usually present later in childhood or adolescence when areas of skin are subject to trauma. Depending on the level of cleavage the blisters heal with or without scarring. General physical development, including hair and nail growth, is usually normal.

Recessive dystrophic EB may present at birth and can be generalized or localized. Scarring is atrophic and large raw surfaces may pose real problems. The mucosae may be involved, which can complicate feeding, as can oesophageal and laryngeal involvement. Nails, hair and teeth may be affected, and pseudowebbing occurs later.

So-called recessive EB letalis (Herlitz type) may be so severe as to lead to early death. The abortion and stillbirth rate is high. The bullae, which are usually present at birth, are large and there is little tendency to heal. Nails are shed, teeth malformed and the mouth is usually involved. The long-term prognosis is, however, not so bad as the name implies.

Management

It is essential for treatment and future counselling that an accurate diagnosis is made. In the absence of a family history a clinical diagnosis may be inaccurate. Electron microscopic examination of skin biopsies is the best way to differentiate the various forms, although the use of immunofluorescence techniques to localize appropriate antigenic sites within the basement membrane zone may permit a rapid diagnosis. In all types of EB, infection of the raw surfaces is the major problem, compounded in some by scarring and contractures. Skilled nursing, preferably by those familiar with the disorder, is required. Protection is of paramount importance. The neonate should be nursed on silk sheets on foam padding, reducing the need for direct handling.[2,40] Eroded areas should be dressed with paraffin tulle and protected, as should pressure areas, with padding and bandages. If there is oral involvement, feeding may be eased by the use of large-hole teats. Antibiotics should be prescribed when indicated, and if the erosions are large plasma infusions may be necessary. There is controversy over the place of other systemic treatment. There are enthusiasts for the use of corticosteroids but the evidence is inconclusive and their use may contribute significantly to morbidity and mortality. Phenytoin may be of value in recessive dystrophic EB though toxicity is a problem.[4] The common view that early demise is normal for these infants probably reflects the outcome of an expectant policy. Active management, even of the most severe forms, is reflected in a marked improvement in prognosis. Antenatal diagnosis is now possible.

Ectodermal dysplasia[16]

This term covers a variety of syndromes and anomalies, of which some are still to be defined. The most important in the neonate is anhidrotic ectodermal dysplasia. Of reported cases, 90% are in males, suggesting an X-linked recessive inheritance, though some cases appear to be autosomal dominant. It is rare for the complete syndrome to be manifest in females. The clinical features are distinctive – prominent frontal ridges and chin, saddle nose, sunken cheeks, thick lips, large ears and sparse hair. The skin is smooth and dry owing to absent or reduced sweating and there is partial or complete anodontia. The main problem in neonates is hyperthermia due to defective sweating; they may present with fever for no apparent cause and placing them in an incubator will only aggravate the problem. Recognition can therefore be important for survival.

Eosinophilic pustular folliculitis[48]

This is a rare but distinct disorder that must be considered in the differential diagnosis of neonatal vesiculopustular diseases. It is characterized by crops of annular pustules of the scalp and recurring peripheral eosinophilia. It may simply be a persistent form of erythema neonatorum.

Erythema annulare

This has been reported in neonates, even as a familial trait.[5] It must be distinguished from annular pustular psoriasis and from lupus erythematosus.[35]

Granuloma gluteale infantum

This is a rare, characteristic, and often rather alarming eruption in the napkin area (Fig. 35.3). The aetiology is obscure but both *Candida* and topical steroids have been implicated. It usually settles with simple bland topical therapy.

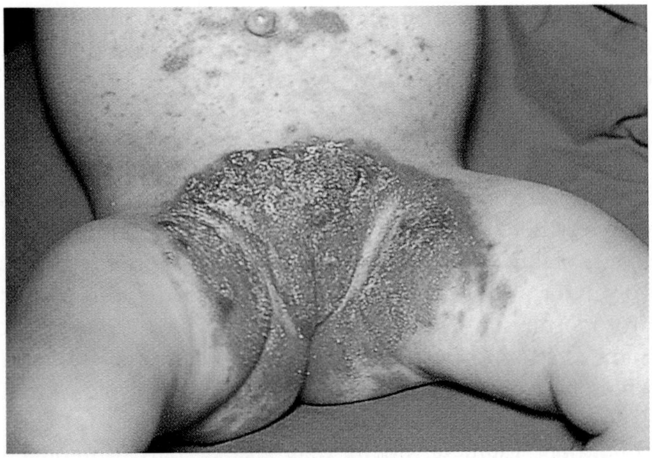

Fig. 35.3 Granuloma gluteale infantum.

Hair disorders[45]

The fetal lanugo hair is shed in utero at 7–8 months. It is rarely retained as long (20–100 mm) fine hair – hypertrichosis lanuginosa. Postnatally the neonate is generally covered in fine vellus hair with differentiation to medullated, long, coarse hairs apparent on the scalp. Fetal/neonatal hair growth cycles are initially in phase and there may be a transient alopecia as they all enter the telogen (resting) phase together; this synchronization is gradually lost.

Congenital alopecia may be either total or partial and present in association with many other anomalies.

Total alopecia is usually autosomal recessively inherited. There is often a normal scalp at birth, but over the first few months hair is lost which does not regrow. It may be confused with hidrotic ectodermal dysplasia. Diffuse hypotrichosis is a feature of many hereditary syndromes but is rarely apparent in the neonatal period.

Circumscribed alopecia is usually due to an epidermal naevus or aplasia cutis, and may occur in some cases of incontinentia pigmenti (see below).

Hypertrichosis may be a racial or familial feature of a normal child; it is seen in certain rare syndromes such as Cornelia de Lange (p. 867), and the mucopolysaccharidoses.

Localized patches of excess hair over the spine may be an important sign of spinal dysraphism.

Structural defects of hair may not be apparent in the neonate but the short kinky hair of Menkes syndrome (p. 1001) and the sparse frizzy coarse hair of hereditary trichodysplasia may be seen.

Ichthyoses[14]

This group of disorders, which is characterized by abnormal keratinization, with dryness and scaling, may provide diagnostic problems in the first weeks of life.

Ichthyosis vulgaris rarely presents within the first 3 months but occasionally can evolve from a collodion baby.

Sex-linked ichthyosis affects only males, though female carriers may exhibit certain features. Onset is within the first few weeks of life, with large pigmented scales on the anterior trunk and flexures. The palms and soles are spared. Slit-lamp examination of the cornea may show opacities. There is an association with steroid sulphatase deficiency.

Congenital non-bullous ichthyosiform erythroderma is an exceedingly rare autosomal recessive ichthyosis, often presenting at birth either as a collodion baby or as erythroderma with or without hyperkeratosis which gradually becomes more evident, especially in the flexures. The face is affected with ectropion, the scalp is very scaly, and the nails, palms and soles are usually affected. It may be difficult to differentiate from

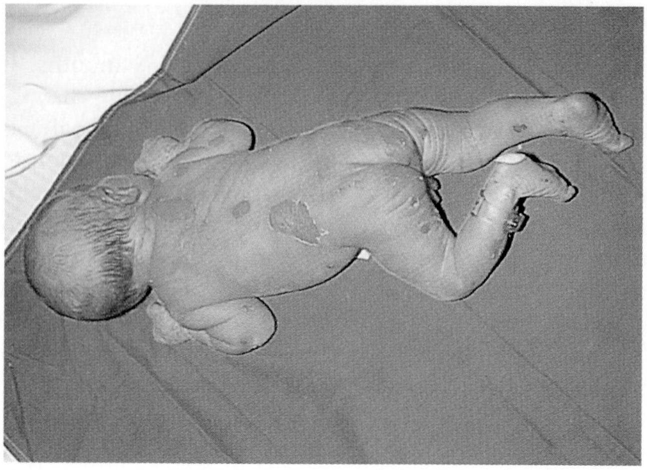

Fig. 35.4 Bullous icthyosiform erythroderma in a neonate, resembling epidermolysis bullosa.

erythrodermic psoriasis, severe infantile seborrhoeic dermatitis (Leiner's disease) or sometimes staphylococcal scalded skin syndrome.

In a rare but severe form the baby is born, often prematurely, covered in thick armour-like plates divided by deep red fissures – the harlequin fetus. Skin rigidity limits normal functions and the majority succumb rapidly. Oral retinoids may be able to improve this prognosis.[28]

Congenital bullous ichthyosiform erythroderma (Fig. 35.4) is an extremely rare autosomal dominant condition with variable penetrance for which antenatal diagnosis is possible. The baby may be normal at birth but within days widespread bullae and a generalized erythroderma develop. It must be differentiated from staphylococcal scalded skin syndrome and epidermolysis bullosa. The bullae become less frequent, eventually ceasing, and the erythroderma improves to leave hyperkeratosis, mainly over the anterior trunk and in the flexures.

Lamellar desquamation, often descriptively called 'collodion baby' (Fig. 35.5), may be a mild physiological event or very severe and a presenting feature of an ichthyosiform erythroderma. The bright red baby has a shiny translucent covering with immobile features. The covering dries and peels, in some cases only to reform. Treatment is initially supportive and after two or three episodes the underlying condition is usually apparent. If physiological, when it may be associated with placental insufficiency or post-maturity, the erythroderma is transient and normal skin evolves.

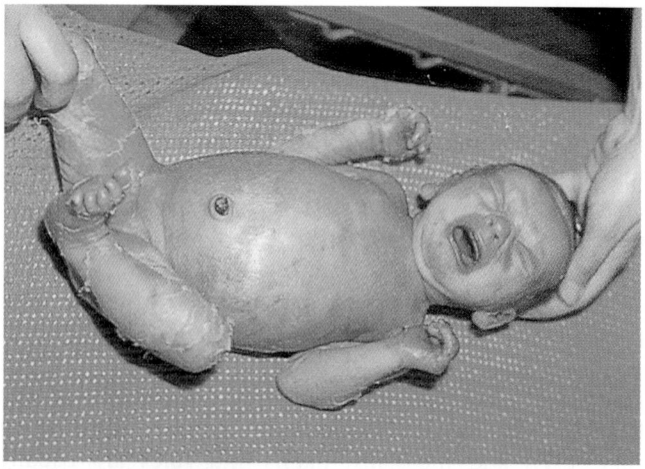

Fig. 35.5 Collodion baby.

Ichthyosis is also a feature of several important conditions including Conradi syndrome (p. 881), Netherton syndrome, Rud syndrome, Refsum syndrome and the Sjögren–Larsson syndrome.[46]

Treatment of ichthyosis

In mild forms, children with ichthyosis may be kept comfortable just by the regular use of emollients such as aqueous cream or Vaseline. Mild keratolytics, e.g. 1–2% salicylic acid in aqueous cream, may help, as may urea-containing preparations. In the severe forms, especially when bullous, careful nursing and medical care are required to avoid secondary infection and to compensate for losses of water, electrolytes and protein. There is some place for the use of oral retinoids but they are not without considerable problems.

Incontinentia pigmenti[15]

This is an infrequent syndrome, probably transmitted as an X-linked dominant; 95% of the reported cases are female. The disease progresses through four phases though the order and severity vary. The initial lesions, usually apparent within the first week, are clear tense bullae, often associated with erythematous nodules or plaques, which may be extensive. 50% of those affected have an eosinophilia at this stage. Hyperkeratotic, warty linear lesions appear between 2 and 6 weeks, notably on the backs of the hands and feet. Extensive pigmentation usually comes later, in a pattern which is often bizarre and streaky. Finally these areas may fade to be replaced by hypopigmented atrophic areas with no adnexae. In over 50% of reported cases there are associated dental, ocular or central nervous system defects.

Light sensitivity

This is rare in the neonatal period. It usually presents with erythema or photophobia, or less commonly with weals, plaques or blisters. It may be due to erythropoietic porphyria (Gunther's disease) or to erythropoietic protoporphyria. More importantly it may be the first manifestation of xeroderma pigmentosum (p. 901), in which case early diagnosis and advice about avoidance of exposure to ultraviolet light are imperative in early childhood. Light sensitivity may also be part of neonatal lupus erythematosus and of Hartnup disease.

The use of phototherapy in the neonatal period may make these disorders apparent at an early age. Such treatment may also produce the striking pigmentation of the bronze baby syndrome (p. 727).[39]

Lymphoedema, limb hypertrophy

Many cases of lymphoedema are due to congenitally defective lymphatics but are not manifest until later in childhood or even adult life. The term Milroy's disease should be restricted to those cases with a family history and abnormality apparent at birth. Lymphoedema may be part of the clinical picture of Turner syndrome (p. 863). Other causes of limb hypertrophy, e.g. neurofibromatosis, vascular malformation and epidermal naevus syndrome, must be considered in the differential diagnosis.

Lymphangiomas present in various ways: as circumscribed subcutaneous swellings; as widespread involvement of the subcutaneous tissues, for example of a whole limb; as superficial vesicles resembling frog-spawn; or as solitary large cystic spaces often around the neck – cystic hygroma. Surgical treatment is often far from straightforward.

Mastocytosis, urticaria pigmentosa (Fig. 35.6)

Mast cells appear in the skin and tissues towards the end of intrauterine life. They contain inflammatory mediators, release of which can lead to itching and flushing. Abnormal collections of mast cells may be confined to the skin or there may be systemic involvement.

Urticaria pigmentosa is occasionally seen at birth, but usually presents between 3 and 9 months of age as numerous generalized macular or nodular lesions which urticate when rubbed and occasionally spontaneously. Pigmentation may take 6 months to develop. The severity varies and it may present as a generalized bullous eruption; blisters are especially common with nodular lesions. Generalized flushing occurs and can be alarming.

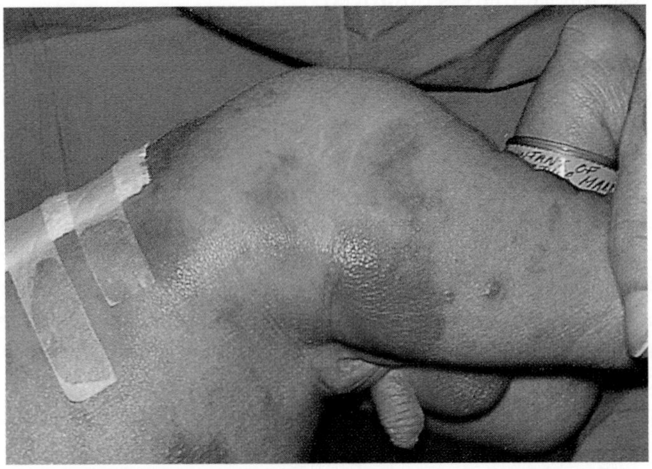

Fig. 35.6 Mastocytosis, an uncommon type presenting at birth with very vascular, infiltrated plaques and none of the pigmentation which is often present later.

Localized. 5–10% of patients with cutaneous mastocytosis have solitary or few lesions, usually presenting within the first weeks of life. Occasionally such areas are the start of widely disseminated disease.

Diffuse. This is very rare. The skin is thickened, yellow and diffusely infiltrated. Pigmentation may be absent. Large blisters occur spontaneously or following trauma.

Systemic. 10% of all cases have some systemic involvement particularly of the bones, liver, spleen, lymph nodes and gastrointestinal tract. The prognosis in these cases is variable, but often good.

The average duration of the skin lesions is 6 years. Treatment consists of general care. Antihistamines may relieve the flushing, as may oral cromoglycate. The wealing and flushing usually subside over a small number of years and the pigmentation may clear before puberty.

Miliaria

Miliaria, prickly heat or sweat rash is caused by obstruction of the sweat ducts. The visible changes develop following sweating when the sweat is unable to escape onto the surface. Bacterial colonization plays a role. The infant skin is particularly liable to this disorder, partly because of an uncharacterized immaturity of the sweat duct, and partly because the newborn infants are often occluded, overheated and their skin overhydrated.

The eruption consists of tiny vesicles (miliaria crystallina, sudamina) or more especially slightly deeper tiny erythematous papules (miliaria rubra), which develop around the sweat ducts. They can occur anywhere but especially on the chest or at sites of friction with clothing. Miliaria may arise on normal skin or quite commonly appears on skin damaged by some other eruption, e.g. a napkin rash or eczema. Secondary infection is not uncommon. The superficial miliaria crystallina is usually symptom-free. Miliaria rubra can cause distressing pricking or itching in the adult and distress in the neonate.

The main treatment is to reduce the necessity to sweat and also the humidity. In the tropics even a few hours a day in air conditioning can be helpful. Treatment of any preceding skin problems is important, but topical therapy is otherwise somewhat unsatisfactory.

Naevoxanthoendothelioma

This is a benign xanthomatous condition, largely confined to the skin, which appears within the first months of life and may be present at birth. Histology shows active xanthoma cells, giant cells and granuloma formation. Serum lipids are normal. The lesions, which vary from 1 mm to 2 cm in diameter and are often yellowish in colour, may occur anywhere but usually on the upper trunk and neck. They occur in crops and may be very numerous. They may grow a little before undergoing involution over several months to leave a hypopigmented atrophic macule. Rarely, systemic lesions occur but importantly the eye can be affected and blindness can ensue. In the majority no treatment is required. There is an association with neurofibromatosis.

Nail disorders

Isolated developmental anomalies of nails are rare but nail involvement is found with many diseases and is characteristic of some such as hidrotic ectodermal dysplasia. Anonychia may be isolated or associated with digital anomalies.

Pachyonychia congenita. Two syndromes of this name occur, both transmitted as an autosomal dominant. Both syndromes have grossly thickened nails which may be present at birth. There is associated palmoplantar keratoderma, which usually develops in the second or third year, and hyperhidrosis. There is either mucosal leukoplakia or multiple cysts.

Pigmentary changes

A wide range of disorders may produce increased or decreased pigmentation in the older child and adult but are seldom a problem in the neonate. The various types of albinism present at birth. Vitiligo appears later, but the otherwise somewhat similar patchy pigment loss of piebaldism is present at birth. The white forelock and other changes of the Waardenburg syndrome are present at birth. In a similar syndrome a white forelock may be a marker for the life-threatening neonatal intestinal obstruction of long-segment Hirschsprung's disease.[50]

The axillary freckling of von Recklinghausen's disease may be an early marker of the disease, as may the white 'ash-leaf' macules (named after the mountain ash) of tuberous sclerosis.

Purpura

Haematological causes of purpura are fully considered in Chapter 32, Part 1. In a dermatological chapter it is appropriate to mention the thrombocytopenia associated with giant haemangioma of the cavernous or strawberry naevus type (Kasabach–Merritt syndrome, p. 892).

The Wiskott–Aldrich syndrome consists of thrombocytopenia, eczema and poor resistance to infection. Any of the triad may precede the other manifestations and cause initial confusion.

The vascular types of purpura are very rare in the neonatal period. A rather characteristic type of purpura called the Cocarde type[26] may occur even in early infancy. Comparable in its pathology to Henoch–Schönlein purpura of older children, it may present with quite large purpuric or even erythematous macules or slightly raised lesions on the face or elsewhere and with a good prognosis.

Non-accidental injury must also be remembered as a cause of neonatal purpura.

Restrictive dermopathy

This is rare, autosomal recessive and characterized by universal tautness of the skin accompanied by generalized desquamation, joint contractures and facial hypoplasia. The outcome is fatal and prenatal diagnosis has not been possible.[22]

Subcutaneous fat disorders

There are three main disorders which involve the subcutaneous fat in the neonatal period and whose terminology is confusing. There is indeed some overlap in the aetiology, pathology and clinical features, and the aetiologies are not fully understood.

1. Neonatal cold injury, page 299.
2. Sclerema. This rare disorder, also known as either skin-bound induration or preagonal induration, may be confused in name with scleroderma and scleroedema, both of which are quite different. In sclerema there is firm, relatively non-pitting induration, clinically resembling fibrosis but more probably due to turgor of the fibrous trabeculae. The cut surface of the skin has been likened to bacon rind and is not obviously oedematous. There are no signs of inflammation or necrosis. This condition usually occurs in debilitated infants with other serious underlying problems, sometimes with cold as an added factor. The induration of the skin can occur over much of the body surface, often starting on the buttocks. The prognosis and treatment are those of the underlying disorder but the skin changes are reversible. The role of systemic steroids is unproven.
3. Subcutaneous fat necrosis of the newborn. This uncommon disease occurs in otherwise healthy infants within the first month or so of life. The aetiology is uncertain but obstetric trauma, exposure to cold, and maternal diabetes may contribute.

The fat shows patchy necrosis and infiltration with lymphocytes and epithelioid cells, giant cells and fat crystals. The disease presents with localized rather lobulated nodules or plaques of red or violaceous colour in the subcutaneous fat. The areas may be solitary or multiple. They may become fluctuant and may even discharge oily fluid, especially if inappropriately incised. The disorder regresses spontaneously over a few weeks and requires no treatment.

The fat deposits may calcify and they may be associated with hypercalcaemia. Poor feeding, failure to thrive and vomiting in children with these skin changes demands appropriate investigation.[58]

Other disorders of the subcutaneous fat which have very rarely been reported in the neonatal period include Farber's disseminated lipogranulomatosis, Weber–Christian disease (a localized inflammatory panniculitis with constitutional disturbance) and lipodystrophia centrifugalis abdominalis infantilis, which occurs mainly in Japanese.

Umbilicus

The cord usually separates in 1 week and has epithelialized within 15 days. During this period infection, omphalitis, can pose a real problem, especially if hygiene is poor. Staphylococci and streptococci are the common organisms but tetanus and pseudomonas may also cause problems. Clinically significant developmental anomalies are rare:

1. The omphalomesenteric duct connects the yolk sac to the digestive tract. There can be complete or partial failure of obliteration which usually occurs in the fourth to seventh week in utero. Complete patency presents as a faecal discharge with surrounding irritant dermatitis, whilst if partial the sinus intermittently discharges mucus.
2. The urachus is the intra-abdominal portion of the allantois from the umbilicus to the vertex of the bladder. The lower portion remains patent in about one-third of people. Persistence of the peripheral or intermediate portions may lead to symptoms. Complete patency presents with intermittent dribbling of urine (p. 276). The umbilicus may appear normal or there may be mucosal prolapse. There is a mild irritant dermatitis. Partial patency may be manifest as asymptomatic cysts or tender midline swellings which discharge via the umbilicus.

Urticaria

Urticaria is uncommon in neonates. Essentially it has the same multiplicity of causes as in the adult.

Xeroderma pigmentosum

This term covers an important group of hereditary disorders characterized by photosensitivity, freckling and the early development of cutaneous malignancies. Most cases are due to an inability to repair DNA damaged by ultraviolet radiation, and this defect can be diagnosed on cells obtained at amniocentesis. Early recognition of photosensitivity is important as the only currently effective treatment is protection from sunlight. Xeroderma pigmentosum may be associated with mental retardation, microcephaly, dwarfism and hypogonadism in the De Sanctis-Cacchione syndrome.

REFERENCES

1. Aggett P J, Atherton D J, More J, Davey J, Delves H T, Harries J H 1980 Symptomatic zinc deficiency in a breast-fed pre-term infant. Archives of Disease in Childhood 55: 547–550
2. Atherton D J 1990 Therapy and counselling in epidermolysis bullosa. In: Wojnarowska F, Briggaman R A (eds) Management of blistering diseases. Chapman & Hall, London, pp 173–188
3. Barlow R J, Walker N P J, Markey A C 1996 Treatment of proliferative haemangiomas with the 585 nm pulsed dye laser. British Journal of Dermatology 134: 700–704
4. Bauer E A, Cooper T W 1981 Therapeutic considerations in recessive dystrophic epidermolysis bullosa. Archives of Dermatology 117: 529–530
5. Beare J M, Froggatt P, Jones J H, Neill D W 1966 Familial annular erythema. An apparently dominant mutation. British Journal of Dermatology 78: 59–68
6. Berg F J, Solomon L M 1987 Erythema neonatorum toxicum. Archives of Disease in Childhood 62: 327–328
7. Berg R W, Buckingham K W, Stewart R L 1986 Etiologic factors in diaper dermatitis: The role of urine. Pediatric Dermatology 3: 102–106
8. Castilla E E, da Graca Dutra M, Orioli-Parreriras I M 1981 Epidemiology of congenital pigmented naevi. I. Incidence rates and relative frequencies. British Journal of Dermatology 104: 307–315
9. Dominey A M 1994 Recent advances in genodermatoses. Current Opinion in Dermatology 1: 127–132
10. Eady R A J 1992 Prenatal diagnosis. In: Rook A J et al (eds) Textbook of dermatology, 5th edn. Blackwell Scientific Publications, Oxford, pp 108–112
11. Epstein W L 1961 Contact-type delayed hypersensitivity in infants and children: induction of Rhus sensitivity. Pediatrics 27: 51–53
12. Ezekowitz A, Mulliken J, Folkman J 1991 Interferon alpha therapy of haemangiomas in newborns and infants. British Journal of Haematology 79 (suppl 1): 678
13. Fitzpatrick T B, Eisen A Z, Wolff K, Freedberg I M, Austen K F 1993 Dermatology in general medicine, 4th edn. McGraw-Hill, New York
14. Francis J S 1994 Genetic skin diseases. Current Opinion in Pediatrics 6: 447–453
15. Francis J S, Sybert V P 1995 Update on incontinentia pigmenti. Current Opinion in Dermatology 2: 55–60
16. Freire-Maia N, Pinheiro M 1985 Ectodermal dysplasias – a clinical and genetic study. Alan R Liss, New York
17. Frieden I J 1986 Aplasia cutis congenita. A clinical review and proposal for classification. Journal of the American Academy of Dermatology 14: 646–660
18. Gari L M, Rivers J K, Kopf A W 1988 Melanomas arising in large congenital nevocytic nevi; a prospective study. Pediatric Dermatology 5: 151–158
19. Glover M T, Atherton D J, Levinsky R J 1988 Syndrome of erythroderma, failure to thrive and diarrhoea in infancy, a manifestation of immunodeficiency. Pediatrics 81: 66–72
20. Golitz L E, Rudikoff J, O'Meara O P 1986 Diffuse neonatal haemangiomatosis. Pediatric Dermatology 4: 145–152
21. Gupta A K, Rasmussen J E 1988 What's new in pediatric dermatology. Journal of the American Academy of Dermatology 18: 239–259
22. Happle R, Stekhoven J H, Hamel B C *et al* 1992 Restrictive dermopathy in two brothers. Archives of Dermatology 128: 232–235
23. Harper J 1985 Handbook of paediatric dermatology. Butterworths, London
24. Johnson H A 1977 Permanent removal of pigmentation from giant hairy naevi by dermabrasion in early life. British Journal of Plastic Surgery 30: 321–323
25. Kopf A W, Bart R S, Hennessey P et al 1979 Congenital nevocytic nevi and malignant melanomas. Journal of the American Academy of Dermatology 1: 123–130
26. Lambert D, Laurent R, Bouilly D *et al* 1979 Oedeme aigu hémorragique du nourrisson. Donées immunologiques et ultrastructurales. Annales de Dermatologie et de Vénéréologie 106: 975–987
27. Lane A T 1987 Development and care of the premature infant's skin. Pediatric Dermatology 4: 1–5
28. Lawlor F, Peiris S 1985 Harlequin fetus successfully treated with etretinate. British Journal of Dermatology 112(5): 585–590

29. Lee L A 1993 Neonatal lupus erythematosus. Journal of Investigative Dermatology 100: 95–135
30. Lever L A 1996 Creams and ointments containing peanut oil may lead to sensitization. British Medical Journal 313: 299
31. Leyden J J, Kligman A M 1978 The role of micro-organisms in diaper dermatitis. Archives of Dermatology 115: 56–59
32. Maibach H I, Boisits E R 1982 Neonatal skin. Structure and function. Marcel Decker, New York
33. Mallory S B 1991 Neonatal skin disorders. Pediatric Clinics of North America 38: 745–761
34. Merlob P, Metzker A, Reisner S H 1982 Transient neonatal pustular melanosis. American Journal of Diseases of Children 136: 521–522
35. Miyagawa S, Kitamura W, Yoshioka J, Sakamoto K 1981 Placental transfer of anticytoplasmic antibodies in annular erythema of newborns. Archives of Dermatology 117: 569–572
36. Moncada B, Kettlesen S, Hernandez-Moctezuma J L, Ramirez F 1982 Neonatal pemphigus vulgaris: role of passively transferred pemphigus antibodies. British Journal of Dermatology 106: 465–468
37. Moskowitz R, Honig P J 1982 Nevus sebaceous in association with an intracranial mass. Journal of the American Academy of Dermatology 6: 1078–1080
38. Newton J A, Salisbury J, Marsden A, McGibbon D H 1986 Acropustulosis of infancy. British Journal of Dermatology 115: 735–739
39. Onishi S, Itoh S, Isobe K, Togari H, Kitoh H, Nishimura Y 1982 Mechanisms of development of bronze baby syndrome in neonates treated with phototherapy. Pediatrics 69: 273–276
40. Pessai A, Verdicchio J F, Caldwell D 1988 Epidermolysis bullosa. The pediatric dermatologic management and therapeutic update. In: Callen J P, Dahl M V, Golitz L E, Schacher L A, Stegman S J (eds) Advances in dermatology. Yearbook Medical Publishers, Chicago, vol 3, pp 99–119
41. Ramamurthy R S, Reveri M, Esterly N B, Fretzin D F, Pildes R S 1976 Transient neonatal pustular melanosis. Journal of Pediatrics 88: 831–835
42. Reunala T, Karvonen J, Tiilikainen A, Salo O P 1977 Herpes gestationis – a high titre of anti-HLS-B8 antibody in the mother and pemphigoid-like immunological findings in the mother and the child. British Journal of Dermatology 96: 563–568
43. Rhodes A R, Sober A J, Day C L et al 1982 The malignant potential of small congenital nevocellular nevi. An estimate of association based on histological study of 234 primary cutaneous melanomas. Journal of the American Academy of Dermatology 6: 230–241
44. Rogers M, Pyzer K G 1982 Cutis marmorata telangiectatica congenita. Archives of Dermatology 118: 895–899
45. Rook A, Dawber R 1991 Disease of the hair and scalp, 2nd edn. Blackwell Scientific Publications, Oxford
46. Rook A J, Wilkinson D S, Ebling F I G, Champion R H, Bunton J L 1998 Textbook of dermatology, 6th edn. Blackwell Scientific Publications, Oxford
47. Ryan T J 1992 Development of the cutaneous circulation. In: Polin R A, Fox W W (eds) Fetal and neonatal physiology. W B Saunders, Philadelphia, pp 555–565
48. Sahn E E 1994 Vesiculopustular diseases of neonates and infants. Current Opinion in Pediatrics 6: 442–446
49. Schachner L A, Hansen R C (eds) 1988 Pediatric dermatology. Churchill Livingstone, New York
50. Shah K N, Dalal S J, Desai M P, Sheth P N, Joshi N C, Ambani L M 1981 White forelock, pigmentary disorder of the irides and long segment Hirschsprung disease: possible variant of Waardenburg syndrome. Journal of Pediatrics 99: 432–435
51. Sharma N L, Sharma R C, Gupta N R, Sharma R P 1988 Self-limiting acrodermatitis enteropathica: a follow up study of three inter-related families. International Journal of Dermatology 27: 485–486
52. Solomon L M 1980 The management of congenital melanocytic nevi. Archives of Dermatology 116: 1017
53. Solomon L M, Esterly N B 1973 Neonatal dermatology. W B Saunders, Philadelphia
54. Solomon L M, Fretzin D F, Dewald R L 1968 The epidermal nevus syndrome. Archives of Dermatology 97: 273–285
55. Spicer M S, Goldberg D J 1996 Lasers in dermatology. Journal of the American Academy of Dermatology 34: 1–25
56. Tanaka K 1981 New light on biotin deficiency. New England Journal of Medicine 304: 839–840
57. Thestrup-Pedersen K 1996 The incidence and pathophysiology of atopic dermatitis. Journal of the European Academy of Dermatology and Venereology 7 (suppl 1): 53–57
58. Thomsen R J 1980 Subcutaneous fat necrosis of the newborn and idiopathic hypercalcaemia. Archives of Dermatology 116: 1155–1158
59. Vernon H J 1994 Advances in the care of neonatal skin. Current Opinion in Dermatology 1: 123–126
60. Wallach D 1979 Dermatologie neonatale. Vigot, Paris
61. Weston W L, Lane A T, Weston J A 1980 Diaper dermatitis: current concept. Pediatrics 66: 532–536

36

Neonatal ophthalmology

Anthony T. Moore

THE EYE AT BIRTH AND EARLY VISUAL DEVELOPMENT

At full term the eye is relatively well developed; the axial length is about 17 mm, compared with 24 mm for the average emmetropic adult eye,[119,122] and the ocular volume is about half that of the adult. Premature infants have smaller eyes and the axial length and volume are closely related to birthweight and postconceptional age. In contrast to other organs in the body, most of the increase from newborn to adult values occurs during the first 12–18 months of life. During this rapid infantile growth phase compensatory changes in the cornea and lens maintain the refraction of the eye close to emmetropia. Most newborn infants, however, are mildly hypermetropic, although premature infants tend to be myopic. There is also a high prevalence of astigmatism in infancy, but all types of refractive error tend to reduce with increasing age.[12,60,91] This process of emmetropization is dependent on visual feedback and may be disturbed in certain pathological conditions affecting vision, such as congenital retinal dystrophies,[126] in which high refractive errors are common.

The visual pathways are also immature at birth. Although the peripheral retina is relatively well developed, the macular region is very immature;[1,133] full development of the fovea may not be complete for 4 years after birth.[133] Similar maturational changes occur in the optic nerve[85] and posterior visual pathways[46] postnatally.

The immaturity of foveal cones and postreceptoral pathways is reflected in the poor acuity of neonates. Although such infants may show steady fixation, more sophisticated measurements of visual acuity using forced-choice preferential looking, opticokinetic nystagmus and neurophysiological techniques have shown an acuity of about 1 cycle per degree (20/600 Snellen equivalent) at birth. The acuity, however, develops rapidly over the next 6–9 months, although adult levels may not be reached until 3–5 years.[37] Other aspects of visual function, such as visual fields, binocularity and colour vision, show similar maturation during early infancy.

Table 36.1 Classification of amblyopia

Stimulus deprivation
Strabismic
Anisometropic
Meridional
Bilateral ametropic

ABNORMAL VISUAL DEVELOPMENT

Amblyopia

The infant visual system has a significant degree of plasticity in the first few years of life, and an abnormal visual experience of one or both eyes during this sensitive period for visual development may give rise to amblyopia, that is, visual loss without any evident organic cause. Clinical experience leads us to believe that the sensitive period in humans extends for as long as 7 years, although it is the first few months of life that are most important.

Amblyopia is the commonest cause of visual loss in childhood, and is classified according to its aetiology (Table 36.1). The most important and profound form of amblyopia seen in the neonatal period is due to stimulus deprivation, that is, the lack of a formed visual image on one or both foveae. If the underlying cause of the stimulus deprivation is not treated in early infancy, the visual results are poor despite apparent surgical success. For this reason complete unilateral ptosis, congenital cataracts and glaucoma should be detected and treated in early infancy if the best visual results are to be obtained.

Once any underlying ocular or lid pathology has been managed surgically, amblyopia is treated by correction of any refractive errors and patching of the preferred eye until vision is equal in the two eyes.

Delayed visual maturation

Illingworth[59] introduced the term delayed visual maturation to describe the condition of infants who appear to be blind or have severe visual impairment in early infancy but who subsequently improve and may attain normal vision. The infants may be otherwise normal or, more commonly, show neurological or developmental abnormalities.[41] In the latter case the visual abnormality is out of proportion to the other disabilities. A high proportion of infants with DVM are premature or small for dates, and it is likely that the visual abnormality is one manifestation of a wider neurological insult; it is only rarely that DVM occurs in otherwise completely normal infants.[7]

Affected infants show poor fixation and no following responses in the first few weeks of life and may develop transient nystagmus; pupil reactions and fundus examination are usually normal. The electroretinogram and pattern visually evoked potentials are normal compared to age matched controls.[77] Vision may improve dramatically within a few weeks, or take several months for full recovery.[41] The cause of this condition is unknown but may be related to cortical maturational delay.[58] It is in part a diagnosis of exclusion, and it is important to rule out other causes of apparent severe visual loss in an infant with a normal fundus examination such as a congenital retinal dystrophy, cortical blindness or ocular motor apraxia.[118] The diagnosis can only be made with certainty once vision has improved, but the finding of a normal ERG and pattern VEP responses in a child who appears to be functionally blind can strengthen confidence that recovery of vision is likely to occur within a few months.

COMMON EYE PROBLEMS IN THE NEONATE

Several transient ocular abnormalities may be found on routine examination of the neonate and are of no serious significance. Bruising of the face, including the lids, and subconjunctival and retinal haemorrhages are common after birth and resolve spontaneously. Transient ocular motor abnormalities are also common in the first few weeks of life, but any constant squint is abnormal.

Premature infants may show additional abnormalities which are related to their low gestational age and immaturity of ocular development. In infants of 28 weeks' gestation or less the lids are often fused, but are easily separated. Similarly, in early extrauterine life the lens is vascularized, and this vascularization (tunica vasculosa lentis) is frequently seen in premature infants and may be used to assess gestational age. The vessels gradually regress and regression is usually complete by 34 weeks.[52] Other transient abnormalities seen in premature infants include lens vacuoles,[82] mild corneal clouding, vitreous haze and persistence of the hyaloid artery.

Conjunctivitis is common in the neonate and is considered in detail on pages 1150–1151.

OCULOMOTOR ABNORMALITIES

STRABISMUS

The eyes of healthy neonates are frequently not aligned and intermittent squints are common in the first few weeks of life.[57,95] Transient VIth nerve palsies,[14,105] which may be related to birth trauma, and transient disorders of vertical gaze, may also be seen.[57] Any constant squint persisting after the age of 6 weeks is, however, abnormal and should be referred to an ophthalmologist. Strabismus may be the presenting sign of unilateral visual loss, for example in unilateral congenital cataract or retinoblastoma, hence the need for early referral.

Convergent strabismus (esotropia)

The commonest form of persistent strabismus in early infancy is congenital or infantile esotropia. In this disorder there is a large-angled convergent squint, which is often alternating. The infant may cross-fixate, that is, use the convergent eye to fixate objects to the opposite side, so it may be difficult to demonstrate full ocular movements with a target. Full abduction can, however, be demonstrated on rotation or by using the doll's head manoeuvre to elicit reflex eye movements. Other rare causes of esotropia in infancy include VIth nerve palsy, Duane's retraction syndrome or Moebius syndrome (p. 871), but in each case there is defective abduction of the affected eye.

Divergent strabismus (exotropia)

Many newborn infants have a transient divergent strabismus, but this usually recovers in the first 2 months of life.[95] Persistent exotropia is rare, and is usually seen in infants with severe neurological impairment.

Vertical strabismus

Vertical squints are only rarely evident in the neonatal period, except in the case of congenital IIIrd nerve palsy, when the marked ptosis is usually the presenting sign. Other causes, such as superior oblique palsy, Brown syndrome and double elevator palsy, usually present with an abnormal head posture in later infancy or childhood.[39]

NYSTAGMUS

Nystagmus is rarely evident at birth but usually presents in the first few weeks of life. It may be caused by severe bilateral visual loss, by central nervous system (usually cerebellar or brain stem) disease, or it may be idiopathic.[18,118] The most common cause is so-called congenital idiopathic motor nystagmus. Infants with this form usually have relatively good acuity and the horizontal nystagmus usually remains horizontal in all positions of gaze. The nystagmus may show variable amplitude and frequency in different positions of gaze, and older infants may adopt an abnormal head posture to use the position of gaze where nystagmus is least.

In infants with nystagmus it is important to rule out an anatomical abnormality of the eyes, such as aniridia, albinism or ocular colobomata, as a cause. Some of the inherited retinal dystrophies, for example Leber's amaurosis or achromatopsia, may have severe visual impairment, nystagmus and a normal eye examination, and optic nerve hypoplasia may be easily missed in an infant. It is therefore advisable to perform an ERG and VEPs in all infants who have nystagmus, poor vision and an apparently normal eye examination, to rule out these disorders. Infants with other neurological abnormalities or very atypical nystagmus may require CT or MRI scan to rule out a structural abnormality of the CNS.

OCULAR MOTOR APRAXIA

In this disorder there is an inability to generate horizontal fast (saccadic) eye movements; vertical saccades are normal.[50] Young infants with this disorder may be thought to have severe visual loss because of the lack of refixational eye movements. The diagnosis is made by demonstrating the absence of reflex fast-phase eye movements on rotating the infant. Older children with this disorder show an absence of horizontal saccades and the typical head thrusts, which are used to aid refixation. The disorder is usually benign and may improve with age, but may be associated with structural abnormalities of the CNS[115] or, rarely, be seen in association with brain-stem tumour.[81,121,134]

OTHER EYE MOVEMENT DISORDERS

Transient disorders of vertical gaze may be seen in healthy neonates but do not persist beyond a few weeks.[57] Vertical-gaze palsies may be seen in infantile hydrocephalus, when the lids may be retracted and the eyes deviated downwards (the 'setting sun sign'). This disorder, which is thought to be caused by pressure on the vertical gaze centre by an enlarged third ventricle, usually resolves after shunt surgery but may recur with shunt blockage.

Ocular flutter, in which there are intermittent rapid bursts of horizontal saccades or opsoclonus, in which both horizontal and vertical saccadic abnormalities occur, may be seen in infants with encephalitis or, rarely, as a remote effect of neuroblastoma. Often chaotic eye movements are seen, which may be associated with tremor of the arms or legs. The eye movements usually resolve spontaneously or will respond to adrenocorticotrophic hormone.

CONGENITAL ABNORMALITIES OF THE GLOBE

A failure of the development of the optic vesicle in early embryonic life may give rise to anophthalmos, microphthalmos or ocular colobomata. Other developmental disorders of the globe, such as aniridia, congenital glaucoma and congenital cataract, may also present in early infancy.

ANOPHTHALMOS AND MICROPHTHALMOS

In anophthalmos there is complete absence of the globe; the orbit is usually small and the palpebral fissure narrow, often with partial fusion of the eyelids. A CT or MRI scan of the orbit may be necessary to demonstrate that the globes are completely absent. Most cases are sporadic, although anophthalmos may be seen in chromosomal disorders, especially trisomy 13 (p. 860), and rarely may be inherited, when it is seen as the severe end of a spectrum of ocular malformation which includes microphthalmos and coloboma. Anophthalmos, like microphthalmos and coloboma, may be seen in association with a number of other congenital malformations.[129,130]

Microphthalmos, in which the globes are smaller than normal, is more common. Mild cases may have completely normal vision, but in severe microphthalmos the eye may be effectively blind. Many cases have associated ocular colobomata and, in some cases, there are associated orbital cysts which may cause proptosis or distend the lower lid. Most cases are sporadic, but autosomal dominant, autosomal recessive and X-linked inheritance have been described, as have a variety of associated malformations.[113,129,130]

OCULAR COLOBOMA

Failure of closure of the fetal fissure in early development gives rise to ocular coloboma, which may affect the iris, lens, retina, choroid and optic nerve. The tissue defect is usually seen in the 6 or 7 o'clock position inferiorly. There is a wide range of clinical expression. Vision may be normal in mild cases but is poor when there is severe optic nerve involvement or microphthalmia. The typical case shows absence of the iris inferiorly, so that the pupil is keyhole shaped. Chorioretinal defects are seen as linear or oval white areas in the inferior fundus.

Ocular colobomata are usually sporadic, but may be inherited as an autosomal dominant trait. They are also commonly seen in chromosomal abnormalities[131] and in a variety of other genetic syndromes, including the

CHARGE syndrome (p. 870), Aicardi syndrome, focal dermal hypoplasia and the Lenz microphthalmos syndrome (p. 871).[96,129,130]

CONGENITAL CATARACT

Congenital cataract is the commonest remediable cause of childhood blindness in the developed world, and the best visual results are achieved if surgery and optical correction are performed soon after birth, before stimulus-deprivation amblyopia becomes established. It is important, therefore, that infants with significant cataract are recognized during the routine neonatal examination performed by the paediatrician. This is best achieved using the direct ophthalmoscope to elicit the red reflex (p. 274) in all newborn infants. An absent or abnormal red reflex should prompt urgent referral to an ophthalmologist.

Congenital cataract may be an isolated finding or be associated with other systemic abnormalities. Many cases are genetic and most familial cataracts are inherited as an autosomal dominant trait, although X-linked and autosomal recessive inheritance have been reported. Many cases are sporadic, but some of these may represent new autosomal dominant mutations. Cataracts may form part of a more widespread genetic syndrome, as for example in Conradi syndrome (p. 881) or Hallermann–Streiff syndrome (p. 870), and metabolic causes include galactosaemia (p. 997), Lowe syndrome (p. 870) and neonatal hypoglycaemia (p. 941). Finally, many congenital cataracts are non-genetic, the commonest cause of which is the rubella syndrome (p. 1168).

All infants with congenital cataract should undergo further investigation to try to elucidate the cause. The ophthalmologist and paediatrician will be able to exclude many causes on clinical examination, and investigation should be tailored to the suspected diagnosis in each infant, rather than adopting a blanket series of screening investigations.

The management includes early surgery (lensectomy), correction of the resulting aphakic refractive error with contact lenses, and treatment of any associated amblyopia.[75] With advances in intraocular microsurgery and contact lens design, results are very good if surgery is performed early. The use of intraocular lenses in the management of neonates who have congenital cataract remains controversial: there is at present no evidence that the visual results are better than lensectomy and contact lens wear, and it is doubtful whether the increased risk of complications associated with intraocular lenses in such young infants can be justified.

CONGENITAL GLAUCOMA

Congenital glaucoma, although rare, is one of the commonest preventable causes of blindness in infancy.[36] The best results are achieved if the disorder is recognized and referred early. It is therefore important that paediatricians are aware of the common symptoms and signs. Congenital glaucoma presents at birth or in the first few months of life, with watering of the eyes and marked photophobia. The eyes are enlarged and the cornea hazy due to oedema; most cases are bilateral and occur in otherwise normal infants. Infantile glaucoma may, however, complicate other disorders such as the anterior segment cleavage syndrome, Sturge–Weber syndrome (p. 884), aniridia, neurofibromatosis (p. 884), congenital rubella syndrome (p. 1168), Lowe syndrome (p. 761) and the Rubenstein–Taybi syndrome. A form of secondary angle closure glaucoma may also complicate severe retinopathy of prematurity, retinal dysplasia and persistent hyperplastic primary vitreous (see below).

The management of this disorder is primarily surgical, and affected infants may need repeated examinations under anaesthesia to allow measurement of the intraocular pressure and assessment of optic disc cupping and growth of the eye. Once control of intraocular pressure is achieved and corneal clarity restored, management is concerned with treating the associated amblyopia, which is the major cause of visual morbidity in infants with this disorder.[27]

ANIRIDIA

Aniridia may be discovered in the neonatal examination or present in early infancy with nystagmus. Affected infants have poor vision and nystagmus due to foveal hypoplasia, and may develop corneal epithelial abnormalities and glaucoma; lens opacities are common. The iris may be completely absent or there may be a small peripheral rim of abnormal iris.

Aniridia is an autosomal dominant disorder caused by mutations of the *PAX6* gene on chromosome 11p.[35,65] *PAX6* is one of a family of developmental genes coding for transcription factors which regulate the expression of other genes during ocular development. Aniridia may be familial or sporadic. Infants with the sporadic form are at an increased risk of developing Wilms' tumour (p. 1056), as they are more likely to have large deletions which encompass both the *PAX6* and the adjacent Wilms' tumour locus. Chromosomal studies should be performed in infants with sporadic aniridia, as some show microscopic deletions of chromosome 11 (p. 1056).[107] In infants without microscopic deletions molecular genetic studies should be able to determine whether the mutation is confined to the *PAX6* gene or whether it involves the Wilms' tumour locus.

OTHER DEVELOPMENTAL ABNORMALITIES OF THE ANTERIOR SEGMENT

A number of other rare malformations of the anterior segment of the eye may be seen in the neonate.[38] In megalocornea the cornea is enlarged but otherwise normal. The normal intraocular pressure and absence of corneal oedema allow this disorder to be distinguished from congenital glaucoma. Bilateral corneal oedema without glaucoma is seen in a rare inherited ocular disorder, congenital hereditary endothelial dystrophy. The corneas are of normal size but have extensive stromal oedema due to impaired removal of fluid from the corneal stroma by the endothelium.

In Peters' anomaly there is a central corneal opacity with adhesions between the iris and posterior cornea; there may be associated glaucoma. Most cases are bilateral and are not associated with any systemic abnormalities. However, in Peters' plus syndrome the ocular abnormalities may be associated with a variety of systemic malformations, including cleft lip and palate, developmental delay and congenital heart disease. Some cases of Peters' anomaly are associated with mutations of the *PAX6* gene.

In sclerocornea there is peripheral corneal opacification and vascularization which, if extensive, may involve the central cornea. It is usually seen as an isolated ocular abnormality.

Rieger's anomaly is a developmental abnormality of the eye in which there is hypoplasia of the iris stroma, which may give rise to associated iris defects.[116] The pupil is often misshapen and eccentric, and there may be more than one pupil. Iridocorneal adhesions and peripheral corneal opacities are common. Glaucoma may complicate the disorder in infancy or childhood. Rieger's anomaly may be inherited as an autosomal dominant trait, but many cases have no family history. In Rieger's syndrome the ocular phenotype is accompanied by a number of systemic abnormalities, including facial and dental abnormalities, umbilical hernia and hypospadias. Rieger's syndrome is inherited as an autosomal dominant trait and exhibits very variable expression. Recently Semina et al[114] have identified mutations in a novel homoeobox gene in some patients with Rieger's syndrome.

ALBINISM

Infants with ocular or oculocutaneous albinism present in early infancy with coarse nystagmus and photophobia.[69] Affected infants may show very poor visual responses in early infancy which later improve – possibly an example of delayed visual maturation. Ocular examination shows nystagmus, iris translucency and a very blonde fundus owing to lack of pigment in the pigment epithelium. The fovea is hypoplastic. Infants with the purely ocular form are frequently misdiagnosed as having congenital idiopathic motor nystagmus, but the two conditions may be distinguished by performing slit-lamp examinations, which will demonstrate iris translucency in the former.[19] The distinction is of more than academic interest because of the different modes of inheritance of the two disorders. In infants where there is doubt about the diagnosis visual evoked potentials are useful, as a characteristic abnormality is seen in albinism.[110]

OPTIC NERVE ANOMALIES

Total absence of the optic nerve and retinal vessels (optic nerve aplasia) is rare and usually seen in congenitally abnormal eyes. Optic nerve hypoplasia, which is a non-progressive developmental abnormality in which the affected optic nerve is smaller than normal and has fewer axons, is, however, more common and is a significant cause of childhood visual loss.[61,86] There is a wide range of severity, and mild abnormalities are consistent with good visual acuity. Optic nerve hypoplasia is rarely diagnosed in the neonatal period unless it is severe and bilateral, when there is poor vision and nystagmus.

Optic nerve hypoplasia may be associated with midline brain abnormalities, especially absence of the septum pellucidum, and endocrine abnormalities, particularly growth hormone deficiency.[112] MRI scanning in infants with optic nerve hypoplasia may help predict those who will develop later endocrine problems.[17] Optic nerve hypoplasia may also occur in association with maternal intake of certain drugs, such as phenytoin,[56] LSD,[54], quinine,[84] alcohol[89] and crack cocaine,[48] and may be more common in infants born to diabetic mothers.[67]

LID AND ORBITAL DISORDERS

Lid and orbital disorders are uncommon in the neonatal period. Ptosis, the commonest abnormality, is usually due to a dystrophic levator muscle (congenital ptosis), although it may also be seen in congenital Horner syndrome or congenital IIIrd nerve palsy. Ptosis may also form part of a more widespread facial anomaly, such as in the blepharophimosis syndrome (p. 871). Lid surgery is usually deferred until age 4 or 5, although earlier intervention may become necessary if there is a significantly abnormal head posture or the risk of amblyopia. Other congenital lid abnormalities, such as coloboma, upper lid entropion and ectropion, are rare and usually need surgical correction in the neonatal period because of the risk of corneal exposure. Mild inturning of the lashes of the lower lid (epiblepharon) is relatively common, especially in oriental babies, and usually resolves spontaneously. Occasionally a minor plastic procedure is necessary to evert the lashes.

Ptosis may also develop secondary to a mass in the upper lid. Lymphangiomas and capillary haemangiomas may be present in the early neonatal period and, if large enough, may cause amblyopia by occlusion of the pupil or by inducing a high degree of astigmatism which blurs the retinal image. Haemangiomas may be treated with intralesional steroid injection or, if extensive, systemic steroids, which hasten regression. Lymphangiomas that threaten vision may need to be excised. Plexiform

Table 36.2 Proptosis in the neonate

Unilateral	Bilateral
Encephalocoele (p. 1300)	Craniofacial syndromes
Microphthalmos with cyst	Neuroblastoma
Haemangioma	
Lymphangioma	
Dermoid cyst	
Juvenile xanthogranuloma	
Teratoma (p. 1055)	
Optic nerve glioma	
Neurofibroma	
Rhabdomyosarcoma (p. 1058)	
Neuroblastoma (p. 1054)	

neuromas of the upper lid may cause similar problems in infants with neurofibromatosis type 1.

Proptosis in the neonatal period is rare, and is either due to the presence of shallow orbits associated with one of the craniofacial malformations, or is caused by tumour (Table 36.2). Most tumours are benign, although rarely malignant neoplasms such as neuroblastoma or rhabdomyosarcoma may present in early infancy.

Nasolacrimal duct obstruction is common in early infancy and may lead to a persistent watery sticky eye, and rarely to an acute dacryocystitis (p. 1151). In most cases the obstruction will clear spontaneously by 12 months of age. If symptoms persist after this time the duct may need to be probed to re-establish tear drainage.[132]

RETINAL DISORDERS

INFANTILE RETINAL DYSTROPHIES

Congenital retinal dystrophy (Leber's amaurosis)

Congenital retinal dystrophy is an unusual autosomal recessive disorder that presents in early infancy with poor vision and nystagmus. Fundus examination is usually normal, but the finding of abnormal pupil responses and an absent or subnormal ERG allows the correct diagnosis to be made.[92] Affected infants may be otherwise normal, but many are developmentally delayed or have other neurological abnormality. A similar retinal dystrophy may be seen in association with renal disease (juvenile nephronophthisis), so that infants with Leber's amaurosis should have renal function monitored throughout childhood.

It is now known that many different genetic disorders may give rise to a severe retinal dystrophy which presents in early infancy. Recently mutations of the retinal-specific guanylate cyclase gene[100] and *RPE65*, a gene coding for a retinal pigment epithelium-specific protein,[87] have been identified in some individuals with Leber's amaurosis; other causative genetic mutations remain to be disovered. An infantile retinal dystrophy indistinguishable from Leber's amaurosis may be seen, for example, in Joubert syndrome[68] and some of the peroxisomal disorders, Zellweger syndrome (pp. 1000, 1280), infantile adrenal leukodystrophy and infantile Refsum's disease (pp. 1000, 1280).

Achromatopsia and stationary night blindness may also present in infancy, with nystagmus and poor vision, but may be distinguished from Leber's amaurosis on ERG.[92]

RETINOBLASTOMA

Retinoblastoma is the commonest intraocular tumour of childhood, and many cases present in early infancy with an abnormal white reflex (leukocoria) in the pupil. This disorder is considered in detail on page 1058. Other causes of leukocoria in the neonate include retinal dysplasia, retinopathy of prematurity, congenital cataract, optic nerve coloboma and posterior hyperplastic primary vitreous.

RETINAL DYSPLASIA

Maldevelopment of the retina (retinal dysplasia) presents in the neonatal period with bilateral leukocoria caused by the disordered retina and vitreous forming a white mass behind the lens. Affected infants are blind or have severe visual loss, and there is unfortunately no effective treatment. It may be seen as an isolated anomaly or in association with various syndromes, such as Norrie disease,[16,127] incontinentia pigmenti (p. 898),[45,78] Warburg syndrome[128] and the osteoporosis–pseudoglioma–mental retardation syndrome.[93] Retinal dysplasia is also seen in chromosomal abnormalities, especially trisomy 13 (p. 860).

The gene for Norrie disease has recently been identified[15,21] and the identification of mutations in male infants with sporadic retinal dysplasia allows accurate genetic counselling.[16] Mutations of the Norrie gene have also been implicated in X-linked familial exudative vitreoretinopathy, a rare disorder in which male infants develop extensive bilateral retinal folds which run from the optic disc to the retinal periphery.[20] Rarely the dominant form of FEVR may present in infancy, with similar extensive bilateral retinal folds. This disorder shows a very wide range of expression, so it is important to perform a careful retinal examination of other family members. Gene carriers may be asymptomatic but show characteristic peripheral retinovascular abnormalities.[49] The appearance of the severe form of FEVR is similar to that of cicatricial retinopathy of prematurity, and the rare reports of ROP in full-term infants are probable examples of FEVR.

POSTERIOR HYPERPLASTIC PRIMARY VITREOUS

This disorder is a developmental abnormality of the eye in which the primary vitreous fails to regress. The majority of cases are unilateral and present at birth or in early infancy, with leukocoria. The affected eye is

Table 36.3 Classification of ROP. (Reproduced with permission from Committee for the Classification of ROP[28])

Stage 1	Demarcation line
Stage 2	Ridge
Stage 3	Ridge with extraretinal fibrovascular proliferation
Stage 4	Subtotal retinal detachment (a) extrafoveal (b) involving the fovea
Stage 5	Total retinal detachment

microphthalmic with a shallow anterior chamber and a dense white retrolental mass. There is often an associated lens opacity. Although surgical removal of the lens and abnormal retrolental tissue is possible, the visual results are generally poor.

RETINOPATHY OF PREMATURITY

Retinopathy of prematurity is a vasoproliferative retinopathy affecting premature infants. In its severe form it may lead to total retinal detachment and blindness. Although our understanding of the natural history and associated factors has improved since the original description by Terry,[124] the underlying disease mechanism is still ill-understood and the prevention of this serious disease remains a major challenge.

Classification

Retinal vascularization starts at about 16 weeks' gestation and proceeds from the optic disc towards the retinal periphery. The nasal retina is vascularized at about 32 weeks, and the temporal retina at term. Acute retinopathy of prematurity can be recognized in the preterm infant when specific morphological changes are seen in the immature peripheral retina at the junction between vascularized and non-vascularized retina. These acute changes usually regress spontaneously with or without cicatrization, but less commonly progress to retinal detachment. There is now an internationally agreed classification of acute ROP[28,29] which allows the severity, location and extent of the disease to be recorded. The disease is classified into five stages on the basis of findings on indirect ophthalmoscopy (Table 36.3). The various retinovascular and cicatricial retinal changes seen with regression are not included in the new classification, but may be recorded separately (Table 36.4).

In the normal premature infant the peripheral retina is incompletely vascularized and has a grey-white appearance. Stage 1 ROP is reached when there is a clear demarcation line between vascularized and non-vascularized retina (Fig. 36.1). As the disease advances the line is replaced by a ridge (Fig. 36.2), which projects anteriorly into the vitreous (stage 2), and in stage 3 fragile new vessels are seen projecting from the ridge forwards into the vitreous (Fig. 36.3). In stages 4 and 5 (Fig. 36.4(A),(B)) the retina is partially or completely detached. An eye is said to have 'plus' disease when there is marked dilatation and tortuosity of the posterior retinal vessels, vascular engorgement of the iris blood vessels, vitreous haze and pupillary rigidity.

The retina is divided into three zones, centred on the optic disc, with zone 1 posteriorly, zone 3 peripherally and zone 2 in between, so that the location of the disease can be defined (Fig. 36.5). The extent of disease is recorded as clock hours of retinal circumference affected:

Table 36.4 Regressed retinopathy of prematurity. (Reproduced with permission from Committee for the Classification of ROP[29])

Peripheral changes
Vascular
1. Failure to vascularize peripheral veins
2. Abnormal, non-dichotomous branching retinal veins
3. Vascular arcades with circumferential interconnection
4. Telangiectatic vessels

Retinal
1. Pigmentary changes
2. Vitreoretinal interface changes
3. Thin retina
4. Peripheral folds
5. Vitreous membranes with or without attachment to retina
6. Lattice-like degeneration
7. Retinal breaks
8. Traction/rhegmatogenous retinal detachment

Posterior changes
Vascular
1. Vascular tortuosity
2. Straightening of blood vessels in temporal arcade
3. Decrease in angle of insertion of major temporal arcade

Retinal
1. Pigmentary changes
2. Distortion and ectopia of macula
3. Stretching and folding of retina in macular region leading to periphery
4. Vitreoretinal interface changes
5. Vitreous membrane
6. Dragging of retina over disc
7. Traction/rhegmatogenous retinal detachment

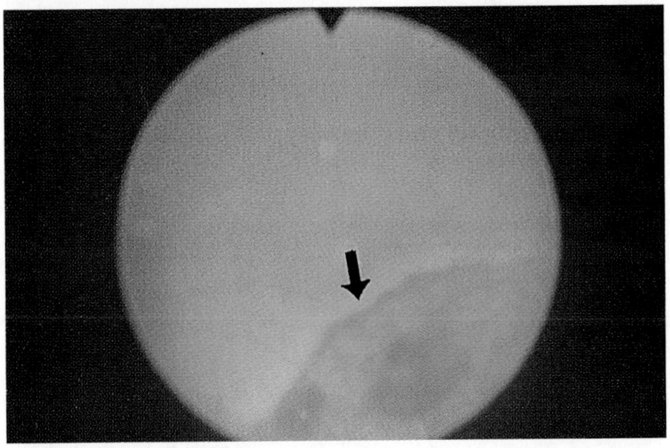

Fig. 36.1 Stage 1 ROP with peripheral demarcation line (arrow). Some retinal haemorrhages are evident posterior to the demarcation line.

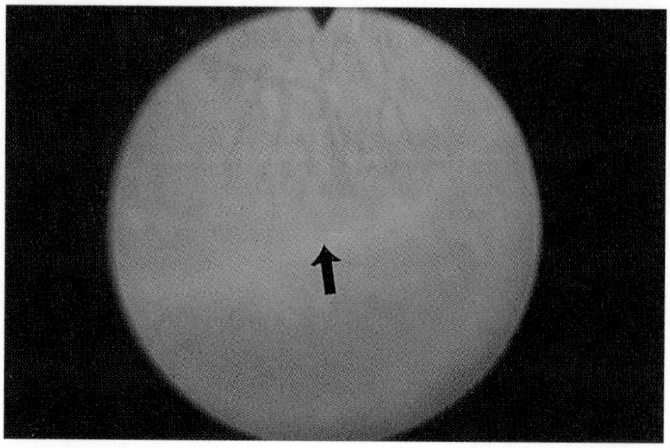

Fig. 36.2 Stage 2 ROP with ridge (out of focus) projecting forward into the vitreous (arrow).

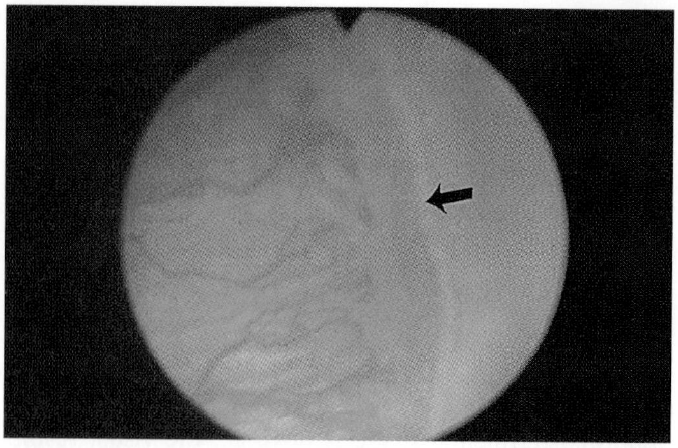

Fig. 36.3 Stage 3 ROP showing ridge with neovascular proliferation at posterior edge of the ridge (arrow).

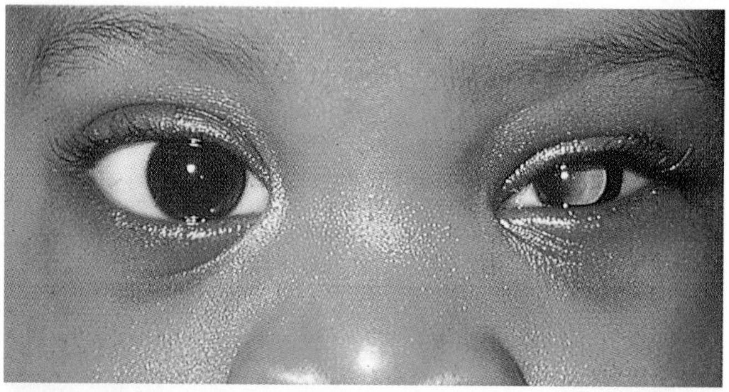

Fig. 36.4A Infant with leucocoria of the left eye.

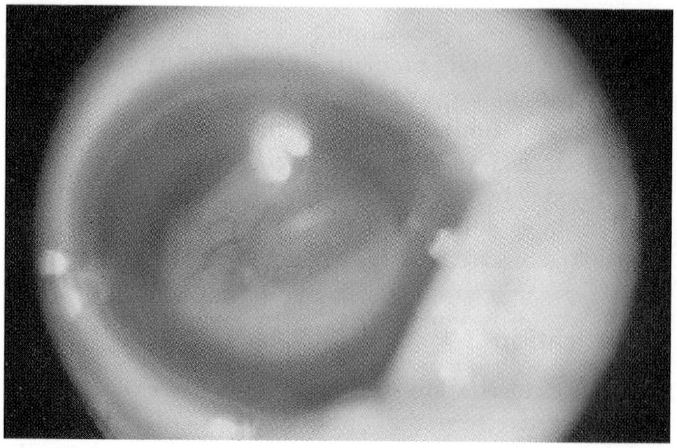

Fig. 36.4B Infant with leucocoria of the left eye due to a total retinal detachment.

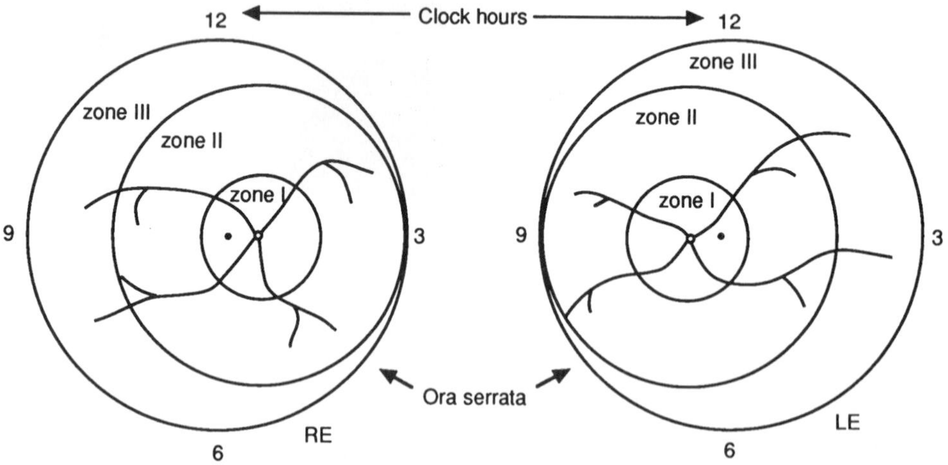

Fig. 36.5 Schematic representation of the retina of both eyes, showing the limits of each zone. The extent of disease may be described in clock hours as shown (the radius of zone 1 is twice the distance from the edge of the disc to the macula [shown as a black dot in the diagram]).

as the examiner looks at the eyes, the 3 o'clock position is on the right, i.e. the nasal side of the right eye and the temporal side of the left (Fig. 36.5).

Factors associated with the development of ROP

Although the original epidemic of ROP in the 1950s was clearly related to the introduction of oxygen into the premature nurseries, it is now evident that other factors apart from oxygen may play a role in its pathogenesis. A full discussion of these factors may be found in excellent reviews of the subject,[13,40,43,80] and they will be only briefly considered here.

Birthweight and gestational age

Most ROP is seen in very low-birthweight infants, and the incidence is inversely related to birthweight and gestational age.[44,71,94,106] About 70–80% of infants with birthweight less than 1000 g[44,94,106] show acute changes, whereas above 1500 g birthweight the frequency falls to less than 10%.[106] Furthermore, severe ROP (stages 3–5) is seen almost exclusively in infants of birthweight less than 1000 g. The increased risk of developing severe ROP in such infants is related not only to increased vulnerability of the very immature retinovascular system, but also to other factors associated with extreme prematurity or its treatment.

Oxygen administration

The early studies in the 1950s[70,79] demonstrated that preterm infants exposed to high levels of inspired oxygen developed significantly more acute and cicatricial ROP (Fig. 36.6) than infants with restricted oxygen. Subsequent reduction of oxygen usage in clinical practice led to a fall in the incidence of severe ROP, but was accompanied by increased neonatal mortality[10] and neurological morbidity.[83] It became necessary, therefore, to attempt to define a safe level of oxygen usage for clinical practice. A multicentre study[71] designed to assess the relationship between arterial oxygen and ROP failed to find any significant difference between PaO_2 values in infants with and without ROP. This trial suffered from a number of serious limitations, including the intermittent nature of the blood gas sampling, the fact that most babies had average PaO_2 values well within the danger zone, and that blood was sampled from the descending aorta which, in preterm infants, particularly those with a patent ductus, may not accurately reflect oxygen levels in the ophthalmic artery. More recently, a randomized controlled trial comparing continuous transcutaneous oxygen monitoring with standard neonatal care, although showing some benefit in larger infants (>1000 g), demonstrated no difference in the incidence or severity of ROP in infants of birthweight less than 1000 g.[44] This is disappointing, as it is in this latter group that ROP is most frequent and severe.

It is evident that careful control of oxygen administration will reduce the incidence of ROP,[70,79] but it has proved difficult to define a safe level of oxygen. The American Academy of Pediatrics[5] has recommended that arterial oxygen concentrations be kept in the region of 50–80 mmHg during neonatal care, and this view has gained general acceptance. Most neonatal units have well defined protocols for monitoring oxygen use in preterm infants, but despite this there is still a disappointingly high incidence of ROP.

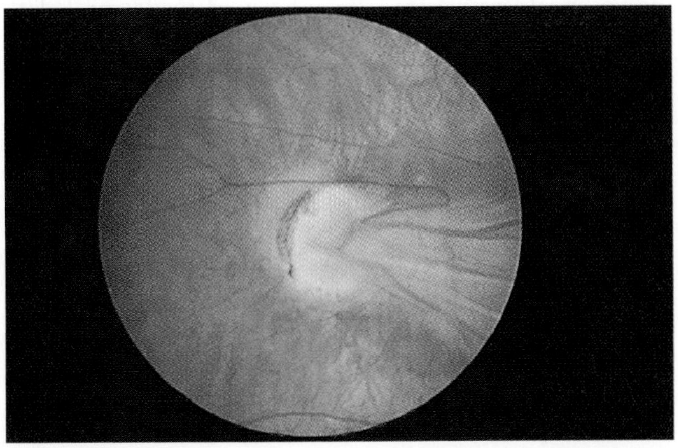

Fig. 36.6 Cicatricial ROP with dragging of the retinal vessels towards the retinal periphery.

The use of surfactant

Surfactant improves lung function in premature infants, and its use has led to a reduction in the duration of oxygen therapy which should, in theory, reduce the risk of developing ROP. However, surfactant use may result in greater fluctuations in arterial oxygen levels, which in animal models has been associated with more severe retinopathy.[98] Surfactant use is also associated with improved survival of infants at high risk of developing ROP. Studies to date on the effect of surfactant use on the incidence of ROP have given conflicting results.[11,66,99,123]

Exchange transfusions

Preterm infants requiring blood transfusion are given adult blood and run a theoretical risk of injury to the developing retinal vesels because of the higher tissue oxygen delivery of adult haemoglobin. Although several studies[25,117] have claimed to show an association between exchange transfusion and the incidence of ROP, it is still unclear whether exchange transfusion is an independent risk factor for the development of ROP or purely an indicator of the high-risk neonate.

Vitamin E

Kretzner and Hittner[73] suggested that vitamin E, a naturally occurring antioxidant, may play a role in preventing the retinal changes seen in preterm infants. In the developing retina, vascularization proceeds from the disc towards the periphery, and the developing vessels are preceded by migration of spindle cells, which are the precursors of the vascular endothelial cells. Preterm infants are relatively deficient in vitamin E, and the peripheral retina of preterm infants lacks interreceptor retinal-binding protein, a carrier protein for vitamin E.[62] It has been suggested[73] that spindle cells are normally protected from oxygen free radical damage by vitamin E, and that the relatively high levels of oxygen in the premature retina (compared with in utero) and the reduced levels of vitamin E result in spindle cell damage by free radicals. It follows from this hypothesis that supplementation with vitamin E may prevent the development of ROP. In an animal model vitamin E supplementation has been shown to reduce the severity of oxygen-induced retinopathy.[101]

Although there have been several trials of vitamin E supplementation in human preterm infants,[42,53,64,102] the protective effect of vitamin E has not been clearly demonstrated. Overall, high-dose vitamin E supplementation does not appear to reduce the incidence of ROP, although it may have an effect on the severity of disease. The possible side-effects of treatment, including sepsis,[63] necrotizing enterocolitis[63,64] and intraventricular[102] and retinal haemorrhage,[108] has meant that the risks of using high-dose vitamin E supplementation outweigh the possible benefits, and it is not in routine use.

Genetic factors

All very low-birthweight infants have a very immature retinal vasculature and most are exposed to oxygen and share common risk factors for the development of ROP. However, only a small minority develop severe disease leading to retinal detachment. The factors that underlie disease severity are ill understood, but it is apparent from variations in disease incidence and severity in different racial groups[47,111] that genetic factors may be important. The genetic basis for such disease susceptibility is poorly understood, but recently Shastry et al[119a] have identified missense mutations in the Norrie disease gene in some children with advanced ROP. This raises the possibility that polymorphisms or mutations in other genes involved in retinal vascular development (such as the vascular endothelial growth factor gene) may be important in determining disease severity. Research aimed at defining the genetic contribution to ROP is still at an early stage.

Other factors

Other factors that have been suggested to be associated with ROP include recurrent apnoea, hypercapnia, respiratory distress syndrome, blood viscosity and light levels in the premature nursery, but none has been confirmed.[13,80,88]

Pathogenesis of ROP

It is evident from clinical studies that the two major factors in determining the incidence and severity of ROP are the degree of retinal immaturity and the levels of arterial oxygen. The mechanism of oxygen toxicity has been studied in animal models, but these have limitations in that the experimental animals are not preterm, and oxygen exposure leads to vascular proliferation but not to retinal detachment. In the animal models of oxygen-induced retinopathy, both hyperoxia[9] and hypoxia[8] produce similar vasoproliferative changes. Furthermore, it appears that the degree of fluctuation in arterial oxygen levels may be important in determining the severity of retinopathy.[98] The effect of oxygen on the retinal vessels is to cause vasoconstriction, and on return to room air there is vasoproliferation similar to that seen in the acute stages of ROP. Recently it has been demonstrated that vascular endothelial growth factor is important in retinal vascular development and may act as a critical vascular survival factor in the developing retina.[4] Retinal endothelial cells have high-affinity VEGF receptors and respond to VEGF with increased cell growth.[2] Neonatal rats exposed to high oxygen show regression of retinal capillaries, and this is preceded by reduced production of VEGF by neighbouring neuroglial cells. Vessel regression occurs by apoptosis of endothelial cells, and intraocular injection of VEGF at the onset of hyperoxia prevents capillary loss.[4] A similar mechanism has been demonstrated in the neonatal murine[103] and feline retina.[120]

Hyperoxia appears to downregulate VEGF production by neuroglial cells and leads to capillary loss from apoptosis. The resulting retinal ischaemia and subsequent local hypoxia leads to upregulation of VEGF and subsequent vascular proliferation. This proposed mechanism has led to the suggestion that oxygen administration in the vasoproliferative stage may be used to downregulate VEGF and limit vascular proliferation.[103] It may be possible in future to limit neovascularization by suppressing VEGF production, preventing the activation of the VEGF receptor using specific VEGF inhibitors such as antisense oligonucleotides, or blocking the VEGF intracellular signal transduction cascade in the endothelial cell.[2,3]

Oxygen may have additional direct effects on retinal tissue through the formation of transient free radicals, to which the immature retina may be particularly vulnerable.[73] It has been suggested that natural antioxidants such as vitamin E and bilirubin may have a protective effect on the developing retinal vessels, but the evidence of a beneficial clinical effect is lacking. Similarly, there is no evidence that the administration of other synthetic antioxidants reduces the incidence or severity of ROP.[88]

The role of oxygen in the pathogenesis of ROP is complex. The animal studies suggest that the initiating event for vascular proliferation is retinal hypoxia, and that high arterial oxygen levels may cause local retinal hypoxia by vasoconstriction of the retinal arterioles. Vascular proliferation is maintained by upregulation of VEGF and other as yet unidentified factors, and it appears that the level of oxygen in the retina is the important factor in regulating such angiogenic factors and ultimately in determining the severity of ROP. Other factors such as the genetic background of the individual or other metabolic disturbances may influence the severity of the vascular proliferation once initiated. Neonatologists are able to measure arterial oxygen but not the degree of oxygenation of the retina. There is clearly a need both for further clinical and experimental studies to define the relationship between oxygen administration and ROP, and in the meantime neonatologists must strive to avoid episodes of hyperoxia or prolonged hypoxia. Advances in our understanding of the pathogenesis of ROP may lead to new treatment modalities aimed at preventing or suppressing the neovascular response in ROP.

Screening for ROP

It is important that all premature infants with a significant risk of developing ROP are examined by an ophthalmologist while on the special care baby unit. Palmer[97] suggested that the optimum time for a single screening examination for ROP is at 7–9 weeks, but it is evident from the data of Ng et al[94] that high-risk infants require more than one examination if significant retinopathy is not to be missed. The aim of screening is to identify infants with stage 3 threshold ROP at a stage when treatment may be effective. Screening can be confined to high-risk infants; this should include all infants less than 32 weeks' gestational age, and older infants whose birthweight is less than 1500 g. Ophthalmoscopic examinations need to start by 6 weeks postnatally and be continued until retinal vascularization has progressed to zone 3. Protocols for screening premature infants for ROP have been drawn up by working groups in the UK[6,109] and USA, and these documents are a useful resource when developing local screening protocols.

Practical aspects

Each unit should have a clear protocol. It is essential that all infants at risk of developing severe ROP are identified and screened at the appropriate time by an experienced ophthalmologist. When neonates are transferred between units it is important that there is good communication about screening examinations that have been performed, and the date at which the next examination is due.

The pupils should be dilated with cyclopentolate 0.5% and phenylephrine 2.5% repeated once, if necessary, 30 minutes before the examination. The use of a lid speculum, binocular indirect ophthalmoscopy and, in selected cases, a scleral depressor will allow a complete examination of the peripheral retina. The results may then be recorded on a standardized form using the international classification.

Infants with acute ROP should be reviewed every 1–2 weeks until regression occurs or the threshold for treatment has been reached. In most cases, complete regression occurs without cicatrization. The more severe and posterior the disease the more likely it is that significant cicatricial changes will develop. Visual loss will occur if there is retinal detachment or traction affecting the macula (Fig. 36.6). Infants with evidence of cicatricial disease should be followed up in the ophthalmology department during childhood because of the increased risk of high refractive errors, strabismus and amblyopia.[74]

Management

Cryotherapy of peripheral avascular retina has been shown to be effective in stage 3 in reducing the progression to blinding disease,[30,31,32] and it is suggested that the treatment protocol used in the trial be closely followed. The rationale for treatment is similar to that for photocoagulation in diabetic retinopathy and other vasoproliferative disorders. It is thought that the ischaemic peripheral retina produces an angiogenic factor which stimulates abnormal new vessel growth; ablation of the ischaemic retina is thought to reduce the level of the angiogenic factor and allows regression of new vessels. The recent development of laser delivery through the indirect ophthalmoscope has allowed the use of laser photocoagulation as an alternative to cryotherapy for the ablation of peripheral retina in ROP.[26] Laser therapy using either diode or argon lasers appears to be as effective as cryotherapy and has major advantages in treating zone 1 disease. Laser treatment may be associated with a lower incidence of myopia after treatment,[72] but there have been a number of reports of cataract developing after laser photocoagulation.[23,24] Further experience with laser therapy is needed before the relative effectiveness and complications of both treatment modalities can be compared.

The treatment of retinal detachment in advanced disease is controversial: although it has proved possible in some cases to reattach the retina with surgery, the visual results are generally poor.[22,51,90,104,125] It is hoped that with additional improvements in surgical technique and further experience of such procedures, the role of intraocular microsurgery in the management of stage 5 disease will become more clearly defined.

Prognosis

The prognosis for most infants who develop acute ROP is excellent. Most stage 1 and stage 2 disease regresses without cicatrization. Infants with stage 3 ROP that is confined to zone 3 also have a good prognosis.[33] Infants who develop stage 3 threshold disease (defined as stage 3 ROP in zone 1 or zone 2 involving five contiguous or eight cumulative clock hours with evidence of 'plus disease') have, without treatment, a 50% risk of progressing to total retinal detachment or severe retinal scarring. Prompt treatment once threshold disease has been reached halves the risk of developing such an outcome. About 20% of eyes with threshold disease will, however, progress to retinal detachment or severe cicatricial changes, even with optimum treatment. The prognosis with and without treatment is worse if the disease is in zone 1.[33] Longer-term follow-up of patients enrolled in this study[33] has shown that the anatomical results of treatment have remained constant, but the differences in functional outcome (as assessed by measurement of visual acuity) between treated and control eyes have narrowed.[32,34] It is likely that some of the difference between anatomical and functional outcome is related to coexisting ischaemic damage to the visual pathways, which may complicate extreme prematurity.[55] Furthermore, the results of Snellen visual acuity testing at $5\frac{1}{2}$ years show that in eyes which show regression fewer eyes in the treated group achieved normal visual acuity than controls, suggesting that although cryotherapy reduces the risk of blindness, there may be a cost in terms of visual acuity compared with those eyes that regress spontaneously.[34]

CORTICAL VISUAL IMPAIRMENT

Severe visual impairment in early infancy may be due to damage to the higher visual pathways. Affected infants have poor visual responses, with absence of normal fixation and following, but normal pupil reactions and usually a normal fundus examination or mild optic atrophy. Nystagmus is rarely present. Electrophysiological testing shows a normal electroretinogram but absent or abnormal visual evoked responses. CT or MRI may show abnormalities of the visual cortex or optic radiations, but in some cases there is no evidence of structural change. The visual prognosis appears best in those infants with a normal scan.[76] Most cases are associated with perinatal hypoxia or, in the case of preterm infants, PVL, but it is also seen in a variety of other disorders, such as meningitis, encephalitis and hydrocephalus.[76] It is rare that infants with damage to the visual cortex are totally blind and visual improvement may occur over a prolonged period, so parents should never be given a very pessimistic prognosis at diagnosis.

REFERENCES

1. Abramov I, Gordon J, Hendrickson A, Hainline L, Dobson V, La Bossiere E 1982 The retina of the newborn infant. Science 217: 265–267
2. Aiello L P 1996 Vascular endothelial growth factor and the eye. Past, present and future. Editorial. Archives of Ophthalmology 114: 1252–1254
3. Aiello L P 1997 Vascular endothelial growth factor 20th century mechanisms, 21st century therapies. Investigative Ophthalmology and Visual Science 38: 1647–1652
4. Alon T, Hemo I, Itin A et al 1995 Vascular endothelial growth factor acts as a survival factor for newly formed retinal vessels and has implications for retinopathy of prematurity. Nature Medicine 1: 1024–1028
5. American Academy of Pediatrics and American College of Obstetricians and Gynaecologists. 1988 Guidelines for perinatal care, 2nd edn, p 247
6. American Academy of Pediatrics, the American Association for Pediatric Ophthalmology and Strabismus and the American Academy of Ophthalmology 1997 Screening examination of premature infants for retinopathy of prematurity. Ophthalmology 104: 888–889
7. Anon 1984 Delayed visual maturation (editorial). Lancet i: 1158–1159
8. Ashton N, Henkind P 1965 Experimental occlusion of retinal arterioles. British Journal of Ophthalmology 49: 225–234
9. Ashton N, Ward B, Serpell G 1953 Role of oxygen in the genesis of retrolental fibroplasia. A preliminary report. British Journal of Ophthalmology 37: 513–520
10. Avery M E, Oppenheimer E H 1960 Recent increase in mortality from hyaline membrane disease. Journal of Pediatrics 57: 553–559
11. Axer-Siegel R, Snir M, Ma'ayan A et al 1996 Retinopathy of prematurity and surfactant treatment. Journal of Pediatric Ophthalmology and Strabismus 33: 171–174
12. Banks M 1990 Infant refraction and accommodation. International Ophthalmology Clinics 20: 205–232
13. Ben Sira I, Nissenkorn I, Kremer I 1988 Retinopathy of prematurity. Survey of Ophthalmology 33: 1–16
14. Benson P F 1962 Transient unilateral external rectus muscle palsy in newborn infants. British Medical Journal i: 1055
15. Berger W, van der Pol D, Warburg M et al 1992 Mutations in the candidate gene for Norrie disease. Human Molecular Genetics 1: 461–465
16. Black G, Redmond R M 1994 The molecular biology of Norrie disease. Eye 8: 491–496
17. Brodsky M C, Glazier C M 1993 Optic nerve hypoplasia. Clinical significance of associated central nervous system abnormalities on magnetic resonance imaging. Archives of Ophthalmology 111: 66–74
18. Casteels I, Harris C M, Shawkat F, Taylor D 1992 Nystagmus in infancy. British Journal of Ophthalmology 76: 434–437
19. Charles S J, Yates J R W, Grant J, Green J, Moore A T 1993 Clinical features of affected males in X-linked ocular albinism. British Journal of Ophthalmology 77: 222–227
20. Chen Z, Battinelli E M, Fielder A et al 1993 A mutation of the Norrie disease gene (NDP) associated with X-linked familial vitreoretinopathy. Nature Genetics 5: 180–183
21. Chen Z, Hendriks R W, Jobling A et al 1992 Isolation and characterisation of a candidate gene for Norrie disease. Nature Genetics 1: 203–208
22. Chong L P, Machemer R, de Juan R 1986 Vitrectomy for advanced stages of retinopathy of prematurity. American Journal of Ophthalmology 102: 710–716
23. Christiansen S P, Bradford J D 1995 Cataract in infants treated with argon laser photocoagulation for threshold retinopathy of prematurity. American Journal of Ophthalmology 119: 175–180
24. Christiansen S P, Bradford J D 1997 Cataract following diode laser photoablation for retinopathy of prematurity. Archives of Ophthalmology 115: 275–276
25. Clark C, Gibbs J A H, Maniello R et al 1981 Blood transfusions: a possible risk factor in retrolental fibroplasia. Acta Paediatrica Scandinavica 70: 535–539
26. Clark D J, Hero M 1994 Indirect diode laser treatment for stage 3 retinopathy of prematurity. Eye 8: 423–426
27. Clothier C M, Rice N S, Dobinson P, Wakefield R 1979 Amblyopia in congenital glaucoma. Transactions of the Ophthalmological Society of the United Kingdom 99: 427–431
28. Committee for the Classification of Retinopathy of Prematurity 1984 The international classification of retinopathy of prematurity. British Journal of Ophthalmology 68: 690–697
29. Committee for the Classification of Retinopathy of Prematurity 1987

II. The classification of retinal detachment. Archives of Ophthalmology 105: 906–912
30. Cryotherapy for Retinopathy of Prematurity Cooperative Group 1988 Multicentre trial of cryotherapy for retinopathy of prematurity (preliminary results). Archives of Ophthalmology 106: 471–479
31. Cryotherapy for Retinopathy of Prematurity Cooperative Group 1990 Multicentre trial of cryotherapy for retinopathy of prematurity. Three month outcome. Archives of Ophthalmology 108: 195–204
32. Cryotherapy for Retinopathy of Prematurity Cooperative Group 1993 Multicentre trial of cryotherapy for retinopathy of prematurity. $3\frac{1}{2}$ year outcome – structure and function. Archives of Ophthalmology 111: 339–344
33. Cryotherapy for Retinopathy of Prematurity Cooperative Group 1994 The natural outcome of premature birth and retinopathy. Status at one year. Archives of Ophthalmology 112: 903–912
34. Cryotherapy for Retinopathy of Prematurity Cooperative Group 1996 Multicentre trial of cryotherapy for retinopathy of prematurity. Snellen visual acuity and structural outcome at $5\frac{1}{2}$ years after randomisation. Archives of Ophthalmology 114: 417–424
35. Davis A. Cowell J K 1993 Mutations of the PAX6 gene in patients with hereditary aniridia. Human Molecular Genetics 2: 2093–2097
36. DeLuise V P, Anderson D R 1983 Primary infantile glaucoma (congenital glaucoma). Survey of Ophthalmology 28: 1–19
37. Dobson V, Teller D Y 1978 Visual acuity in human infants: a review and comparisons of behavioural and electrophysiological studies. Vision Research 18: 1469–1483
38. Elston J 1997 Developmental abnormalities of the anterior segment. In: Taylor DSI (ed) Paediatric ophthalmology, 2nd edn. Blackwell Scientific, Oxford, pp 252–265
39. Elston J 1997 Incomitant strabismus and cranial nerve palsies. In: Taylor D S I (ed) Paediatric ophthalmology, 2nd edn. Blackwell Scientific, Oxford, pp 937–968
40. Fielder A R 1997 Retinopathy of prematurity. Clinical Risk 3: 47–51
41. Fielder A R, Russell-Eggitt I R, Dodd K L, Mellor D H 1985 Delayed visual maturation. Transactions of the Ophthalmological Society of the United Kingdom 104: 653–661
42. Finer N N, Grant G, Schindler R F et al 1982 Effect of intramuscular vitamin E on frequency and severity of retrolental fibroplasia: a controlled trial. Lancet i: 1087–1091
43. Flynn J T 1987 Retinopathy of prematurity. Pediatric Clinics of North America 34: 1487–1516
44. Flynn J T, Bancalari E, Bawol R et al 1987 Retinopathy of prematurity. A randomised, prospective trial of transcutaneous oxygen monitoring. Ophthalmology 94: 630–638
45. Francois J 1984 Incontinentia pigmenti (Bloch Sulzberger syndrome) and retinal changes. British Journal of Ophthalmology 68: 19–25
46. Garey L J, De Courten C 1983 Structural development of the lateral geniculate body and visual cortex in monkey and man. Behavioural Brain Research 10: 3–13
47. Gilbert C, Rahi J, Eckstein M, O'Sullivan J, Foster A 1997 Retinopathy of prematurity in middle income countries. Lancet 350: 12–14
48. Good W V, Ferriero D M, Golabi M, Kobori J A 1992 Abnormalities of the visual system in infants exposed to cocaine. Ophthalmology 99: 341–346
49. Gow J, Oliver G L 1971 Familial exudative vitreoretinopathy: an expanded view. Archives of Ophthalmology 86: 150–155
50. Harris C M, Shawkat F, Russel-Eggitt I, Wilson J et al 1996 Intermittent horizontal saccade failure (ocular motor apraxia) in children. British Journal of Ophthalmology 80: 151–158
51. Hirose T, Katsumi O, Mehta M C, Schepens C L 1993 Vision in stage 5 retinopathy of prematurity after retinal reattachment by open sky vitrectomy. Archives of Ophthalmology 111: 345–349
52. Hittner H M, Hirsch N J, Rudolph A J et al 1977 Assessment of gestational age by examination of the anterior capsule of the lens. Journal of Pediatrics 91: 455–458
53. Hittner H M, Godio L B, Rudolph A J et al 1981 Retrolental fibroplasia: efficacy of vitamin E in double blind clinical study of preterm infants. New England Journal of Medicine 305: 1365–1371
54. Hoyt C S 1978 Optic disc anomalies and maternal ingestion of LSD. Journal of Pediatric Ophthalmology and Strabismus 15: 286–289
55. Hoyt C S 1993 Cryotherapy for retinopathy of prematurity. $3\frac{1}{2}$ year outcome for both structure and function (editorial). Archives of Ophthalmology 111: 319–320
56. Hoyt C S, Billson F A 1978 Maternal anticonvulsants and optic nerve hypoplasia. British Journal of Ophthalmology 62: 3–6
57. Hoyt C S, Mousel D K, Weber A A 1980 Transient supranuclear disturbances of gaze in healthy neonates. American Journal of Ophthalmology 89: 708–713
58. Hoyt C S, Jastrzebski G, Marg R 1983 Delayed visual maturation in infancy. British Journal of Ophthalmology 67: 127–130
59. Illingworth R S 1961 Delayed visual maturation. Archives of Disease in Childhood 36: 407–409
60. Ingram R M, Barr A 1979 Changes in refraction between the ages of 1 and $3\frac{1}{2}$ years. British Journal of Ophthalmology 63: 339–342
61. Jan J E, Robinson G C, Tinnis C et al 1977 Blindness due to optic nerve atrophy and hypoplasia in children. An epidemiological study (1944–1974). Developmental Medicine and Child Neurology 19: 353–363
62. Johnson A T, Kretzner F L, Hittner H M et al 1985 Development of the subretinal space in the preterm eye: ultrastructural and immunocytochemical studies. Journal of Comparative Neurology 232: 497–505
63. Johnson L, Baven F W, Abbasi S et al 1985 Relationship of prolonged pharmacologic serum levels of vitamin E to incidence of sepsis and necrotizing entercolitis in infants with birth weights 1500 grams or less. Pediatrics 75: 619–638
64. Johnson L, Quinn G E, Abbasi S et al 1988 Vitamin E and retinopathy of prematurity. Pediatrics 81: 329–331
65. Jordan T, Hanson I, Zaletayev D et al 1992 The human PAX6 gene is mutated in two patients with aniridia. Nature Genetics 1: 328–332
66. Kennedy J, Todd D A, Watts J, John E 1997 Retinopathy of prematurity in infants less than 29 weeks gestation: $3\frac{1}{2}$ years pre- and postsurfactant. Journal of Pediatric Ophthalmology and Strabismus. 34: 289–292
67. Kim R Y, Hoyt W F, Lessel S et al 1989 Superior segmental optic nerve hypoplasia: a sign of maternal diabetes. Archives of Ophthalmology 107: 1312–1315
68. King M D, Dudgeon J, Stephenson J B P 1984 Joubert's syndrome with retinal dysplasia; neonatal tachypnoea as the clue to a genetic brain-eye malformation. Archives of Disease in Childhood 59: 709–718
69. Kinnear P, Jay B, Witkop C J 1985 Albinism. Survey of Ophthalmology 30: 76–101
70. Kinsey V E, Twomey J T, Hamphill F M 1956 Retrolental fibroplasia and the use of oxygen. Archives of Ophthalmology 56: 481–529
71. Kinsey V E, Arnold H J, Kalina R E et al 1977 PaO_2 levels and retrolental fibroplasia: a report of the co-operative study. Pediatrics 60: 655–668
72. Knight-Nanan D M, O'Keefe M 1996 Refractive outcome in eyes with retinopathy of prematurity treated with cryotherapy or diode laser: 3 year follow up. British Journal of Ophthalmology 80: 998–1001
73. Kretzner F L, Hittner H M 1988 Retinopathy of prematurity: clinical implications of retinal development. Archives of Disease in Childhood 63: 1151–1167
74. Kushner B J 1982 Strabismus and amblyopia associated with regressed retinopathy of prematurity. Archives of Ophthalmology 100: 256–261
75. Lambert S L, Drack A V 1996 Infantile cataract. Survey of Ophthalmology 40: 427–458
76. Lambert S, Hoyt C S, Han J E, Barkovich J, Fiddmark O 1987 Visual recovery from hypoxic cortical blindness during childhood. Computed tomograhic and magnetic resonance imaging predictors. Archives of Ophthalmology 105: 1371–1377
77. Lambert S R, Kriss A, Taylor D 1989 Delayed visual maturation. A longitudinal clinical and electrophysiological assessment. Ophthalmology 96: 524–529
78. Landy S J, Donnai D 1993 Incontinentia pigmenti (Bloch–Sulzberger syndrome). Journal of Medical Genetics 30: 53–59
79. Lanman J T, Guy L P, Danus I 1954 Retrolental fibroplasia and oxygen therapy. Journal of American Medical Association 55: 223–226
80. Lucey J L, Dangman B 1984 A re-examination of the role of oxygen in retrolental fibroplasia. Pediatrics 73: 82–96
81. Lyle D J 1961 Discussion of ocular motor apraxia with a case presentation. Transactions of the American Ophthalmological Society 59: 274–285
82. McCormick A Q 1968 Transient cataracts in premature newborn infants – a new clinical entity. Canadian Journal of Ophthalmology 3: 202–205

83. McDonald A D 1963 Cerebral palsy in children of very low birth weight. Archives of Disease in Childhood 38: 579–588
84. McKinna A J 1966 Quinine-induced hypoplasia of the optic nerve. Canadian Journal of Ophthalmology 1: 261–265
85. Magoon E H, Robb R M 1981 Development of myelin in human optic nerve and tract. Archives of Ophthalmology 99: 655–659
86. Margalith D, Jan J E, McCormick A Q et al 1984 Clinical spectrum of optic nerve hypoplasia. Review of 51 patients. Developmental Medicine and Child Neurology 26: 311–322
87. Marlhens F, Bareil C, Griffoin J et al 1997 Mutations in RPE65 cause Leber's congenital amaurosis. Nature Genetics 17: 139–141
88. Marlow N 1997 Clinical care and the prevention of retinopathy of prematurity. Clinical Risk 3: 37–41
89. Miller M, Israel J, Cuttane J 1981 Fetal alcohol syndrome. Journal of Pediatric Ophthalmology and Strabismus 18: 6–15
90. Mintz-Hittner H A, O'Malley R E, Kretzer F L 1997 Long term form identification vision after early closed lensectomy–vitrectomy for stage 5 retinopathy of prematurity. Ophthalmology 104: 454–459
91. Mohindra I, Held R, Gwiazda J, Brill S 1978 Astigmatism in infants. Science 202: 329–330
92. Moore A T 1997 Inherited retinal dystrophies. In: Taylor DSI (ed) Paediatric ophthalmology, 2nd edn. Blackwell Scientific, Oxford, pp 557–598
93. Neuhauser G, Kaveggia E G, Opitz J M 1976 Autosomal recessive syndrome of pseudogliomatous blindness, osteoporosis and mild mental retardation. Clinical Genetics 9: 324–332
94. Ng Y K, Fielder A R, Shaw D E, Levene M I 1988 Epidemiology of retinopathy of prematurity. Lancet ii: 1235–1238
95. Nixon R B, Helveston E M, Miller K et al 1985 Incidence of strabismus in neonates. American Journal of Ophthalmology 100: 798–801
96. Pagon R A 1981 Ocular coloboma. Survey of Ophthalmology 25: 223–236
97. Palmer E A 1981 Optimal timing of examination for acute retrolental fibroplasia. Ophthalmology 88: 662–668
98. Penn J S, Henry M M, Wall P T, Tolman B L 1995 The range of PaO_2 variation determines the severity of oxygen induced retinopathy in newborn rats. Investigative Ophthalmology and Visual Science 36: 2063–2070
99. Pennefather P M, Tin W, Clarke M P et al 1996 Retinopathy of prematurity in a controlled trial of prophylactic surfactant treatment. British Journal of Ophthalmology 80: 420–424
100. Perrault I, Rozet J M, Calvas P et al 1996 Retinal specific guanylate cyclase gene mutations in Leber's congenital amaurosis. Nature Genetics 14: 461–464
101. Phelps D L, Rosenbaum A 1977 The role of tocopherol in oxygen induced retinopathy: kitten model. Pediatrics 59: 998–1005
102. Phelps D L, Rosenbaum A, Isenberg S J, Leake R D, Davey F J 1987 Tocopherol efficacy and safety for preventing retinopathy of prematurity: a randomised controlled double masked trial. Pediatrics 79: 489–500
103. Pierce E A, Foley E D, Smith L E 1996 Regulation of vascular endothelial growth factor by oxygen in a model of retinopathy of prematurity. Archives of Ophthalmology 114: 1219–1228
104. Quinn G E, Dobson V, Barr C C et al 1996 Visual acuity of eyes after vitrectomy for retinopathy of prematurity – follow up of 5 years. Ophthalmology 103: 595–600
105. Reisner S H, Perlman M, Ben Tovin N et al 1971 Transient lateral rectus muscle paresis in the newborn infant. Journal of Pediatrics 78: 461–465
106. Reisner S H, Amir I, Shohat M et al 1985 Retinopathy of prematurity: incidence and treatment. Archives of Disease in Childhood 60: 698–701
107. Riccardi V M, Sujansky E, Smith A E et al 1978 Chromosome imbalance in the aniridia, Wilms' tumour association: 11p interstitial deletion. Pediatrics 61: 604–610
108. Rosenbaum A, Phelps D, Isenberg S 1985 Retinal haemorrhage in retinopathy of prematurity associated with tocopherol treatment. Ophthalmology 92: 1012–1014
109. Royal College of Ophthalmologists and the British Association of Perinatal Medicine 1996 Retinopathy of prematurity: guidelines for screening and treatment. The report of a joint working party. Early Human Development 46: 239–258
110. Russell-Eggitt I, Kriss A, Taylor D S I 1990 Albinism in childhood: a flash VEP and ERG study. British Journal of Ophthalmology 74: 136–144
111. Saunders R A, Donahue M, Christmann L M et al 1997 Racial variation in retinopathy of prematurity. Archives of Ophthalmology 115: 604–608
112. Scarf B, Hoyt C S 1984 Optic nerve hypoplasia in children. Archives of Ophthalmology 102: 62–67
113. Schwartz J S, Lee D A, Isenberg S J 1989 Ocular size and shape. In: Isenberg S J (ed) The eye in infancy. Yearbook Medical Publishers, Chicago, pp 164–184
114. Semina E V, Reiter R, Leyesens N J et al 1996 Cloning and characterization of a novel bicoid-related homeobox transcription factor gene, RIEG, involved in Rieger syndrome. Nature Genetics 14: 392–399
115. Shawkat F S, Kingsley D, Kendall B et al 1995 Neuroradiological and eye movement correlates in children with intermittent saccade failure ('ocular motor apraxia'). Neuropaediatrics 26: 298–305
116. Shields M B, Buckley E. Klintworth G K, Thresher R 1985 Axenfield–Rieger syndrome. A spectrum of developmental disorders. Survey of Ophthalmology 29: 387–409
117. Shohat M, Reisner S H, Krikler R et al 1983 Retinopathy of prematurity: incidence and risk factors. Pediatrics 72: 159–163
118. Snead M, Moore A T 1996 The investigation of the apparently blind infant. In: Jay B, Kirkness C M (eds) Recent advances in ophthalmology. Churchill Livingstone, Edinburgh, pp 155–178
119. Sorsby A, Sheridan M L 1960 The eye at birth: measurements of the principal diameters in forty-eight cadavers. Journal of Anatomy 94: 192–197
119a. Shastry B S, Pendergast S D, Hartzer M K, Liu X, Trese M T 1997 Identification of missense mutations in the Norrie disease gene associated with advanced retinopathy of prematurity. Archives of Ophthalmology 115: 651–655
120. Stone J, Chan-Ling T Pe-er J et al 1996 Roles of vascular endothelial growth factor and astrocyte degeneration in the genesis of retinopathy of prematurity. Investigative Ophthalmology and Visual Science 37: 290–299
121. Summers C G, McDonald J T, Wirtschafter J D 1987 Oculomotor apraxia associated with intracranial lipoma. Journal of Pediatric Ophthalmology and Strabismus 24: 267–271
122. Swan K C, Wilkins J H 1984 Extraocular muscle surgery in early infancy – anatomical factors. Journal of Pediatric Ophthalmology and Strabismus 21: 44–49
123. Termote J U M, Schalij-Delfos N E, Wittebolpost D et al 1994 Surfactant replacement therapy: a new risk factor for developing retinopathy of prematurity. European Journal of Paediatrics 153: 113–116
124. Terry T L 1942 Extreme prematurity and fibroplastic overgrowth of persistent vascular sheath behind each crystalline lens. American Journal of Ophthalmology 25: 203–204
125. Trese M 1986 Visual results and prognostic factors for vision following surgery for stage V retinopathy of prematurity. Ophthalmology 93: 574–579
126. Wagner R S, Caputo A R, Nelson L, Zanoris D 1985 High hyperopia in Leber's congenital amaurosis. Archives of Ophthalmology 103: 1507–1509
127. Warburg M 1961 Norrie's disease: a new hereditary bilateral pseudotumour of the retina. Acta Ophthalmologica 39: 757–772
128. Warburg M 1971 The heterogeneity of microphthalmia in the mentally retarded. Birth Defects 7: 136–154
129. Warburg M 1991 An update on microphthalmos and coloboma: a brief survey of genetic disorders with microphthalmos and coloboma. Ophthalmic Paediatrics and Genetics 12: 57–63
130. Warburg M 1992 Update of sporadic microphthalmos and coloboma. Non-inherited anomalies. Ophthalmic Paediatrics and Genetics 13: 111–122
131. Warburg M, Freidrich U 1987 Coloboma and microphthalmos in chromosomal aberrations: chromosomal aberrations and neural crest cell developmental field. Ophthalmic Paediatrics and Genetics 8: 105–118
132. Young J D, MacEwan C J 1997 Managing congenital lacrimal obstruction in general practice. British Medical Journal 315: 293–296
133. Yuodelis C, Hendrickson A 1986 A qualitative and quantitative analysis of the human fovea during development. Vision Research 26: 847–855
134. Zaret C R, Myles M B, Eggers H M 1980 Congenital ocular motor apraxia and brain stem tumour. Archives of Ophthalmology 98: 328–330

37

Iatrogenic disorders

A. Jeffrey L. Brain N. R. C. Roberton Janet M. Rennie

Many conditions in the newborn have an iatrogenic component (Tables 37.1, 37.2): these are dealt with in other sections of this book and are well reviewed by Macpherson et al.[110] This chapter will concentrate on disorders which arise as complications of the procedures used during intensive care. We will deal with their prevention, recognition and, where relevant, their management.

UMBILICAL ARTERY CATHETERS

The technique of UAC insertion is described on page 1373 and its use in monitoring on page 363. The details of insertion, maintenance and removal of the catheter must be strictly adhered to, as this will minimize the likelihood of complications due to thrombosis or an embolism. In particular, we would emphasize:

- correct position of the catheter tip;
- use of appropriate heparinization;
- immediate removal when signs of vascular compromise occur.

Despite these precautions, however, the presence of a foreign body within the aorta will inevitably lead to thrombus formation in a small proportion of catheterized babies. Since our initial report[69] this has continued to be a relatively rare clinical phenomenon in our own experience, even though many neonatologists infuse most drugs through the UAC, including bicarbonate, antibiotics, inotropes and TPN. Whether the high incidence of intra-arterial thrombus formation reported in some series[129,196] arose because of infusion of high-osmolality solutions, inadequate heparinization[153] or some other unidentified problem remains unclear.

An impressive list of complications of UAC insertion has been assembled (Table 37.3).

Table 37.1 Neonatal disorders which may have an iatrogenic component

Condition	Damaging agent	Page nos
Retinopathy of prematurity	Oxygen	909–910
Necrotizing enterocolitis	Hypotension Enteral feeding, especially formula	748–750
Discrete intestinal perforation	Emboli from UAC, indomethacin	752
Airleaks, e.g. pneumothorax	High PIP, high MAP, inadequate humidity during IPPV	517, 521
Chronic lung disease	As for airleak Fluid overload Infection, oxygen	608, 610
GMH-IVH	Hypotension, hypoxia, hypercarbia, i.e. any asphyxial insult	1255–1257
PVL	Sepsis, hypotension, hypocarbia	1263–1264
Lung puncture	Treatment of pneumothorax	933
Gastric rupture	Mask/nasal IPPV	932
	Nasogastric tube erosion	933
Airway damage	ETT, oscillatory and jet ventilation	564, 569, 574
	Poor ET tube fixation	667–669
Obstructive jaundice	TPN	739
Complex metabolic upsets	TPN	354
Intestinal obstruction	High calorie density milks	746

Table 37.2 Drug-induced iatrogenic complications

Drug	Complication	Reference/page number
General	Incorrect dosage Incorrect drug Incorrect concentration	417–434
Specific		
Chloramphenicol	Grey baby syndrome	421–422
Sulphisoxazole	Kernicterus	720, 177
Tetracyclines	Stained teeth	91
Vitamin K analogues (menadione)	Jaundice	107
Vitamin E (Eferol)	Liver failure, haematuria	10
Tolazoline	Hypotension, haematuria, GI tract haemorrhage	203
Indomethacin	Fluid retention, GI tract haemorrhage, decreased cerebral blood flow velocity	4
Dexamethasone	GI tract haemorrhage & perforation, hypertension, sepsis, cardiomyopathy, glycosuria, adrenal suppression	163
Hexachlorophane	Vacuolative encephalopathy	176
Glycol in i.v. multivitamin preparation	Fits, GMH-IVH	109
Benzyl alcohol in i.v. saline	Acidaemia & collapse, kernicterus	79, 105
Heparin	GMH-IVH	101
Phenylephrine (mydriatic)	Hypertension	78
Transcutaneous		
Tribiotic (neomycin)	Deafness	126
Iodine-containing antiseptics	Transient hypothyroidism	184

Table 37.3 Complications of umbilical artery catheterization

Complication	Reference
Aortic thrombosis	198
Thromboses affecting	
legs/toes/buttocks	64
kidneys	117
gut	69
Urachal damage and urinary leak	46
Hypoglycaemia	197
Aortic aneurysm	49
Gluteal skin necrosis (gangrene)	114
Sciatic nerve damage	151
Hypertension	29, 142
Paraplegia	71
Haemorrhage	69
Fracture of catheter with embolism	179, 185

PROBLEMS DURING INSERTION

False passage

Although irritating to the operator, the rupture of the catheter either into a false passage within the arterial wall or right through the wall into the surrounding connective tissue is not only common but rarely causes any damage. It is usually obvious, as there is an increased resistance to passage of the catheter, and the attempt should therefore be abandoned.

Haematoma

In a small proportion of cases in which a false passage is created an asymptomatic haematoma may form, which is only recognized at autopsy. Occasionally the blood loss may be large, symptomatic and even fatal.[117,121] Such a lesion will present with signs of blood loss and should be identified on ultrasound. Treatment is initially transfusion and correction of any coagulation disorder, but occasionally surgery is required to ligate the bleeding site.[121]

Entry into the peritoneum

This occurs relatively easily if the operator is 'digging' to find a fresh piece of artery, either in a cord that has been cut flush with the abdominal wall or after initially creating a false passage. It may also occur if there is a very small omphalocoele in the base of the cord, in which case small intestine[181] or just the appendix may appear.[19] No harm is done in any of these situations; the hole should be closed with a suture, taking care that a loop of bowel is not included in the stitch.

Entry into the urachus

This is an unlucky complication.[46] Not only has the operator explored too far while probing for the umbilical artery, but he has done so in a baby with a large urachal remnant. If during the insertion of a UAC clear yellow fluid (urine) suddenly appears this suggests that part of the renal tract has been entered. Surgical help should be sought, but the fistula usually closes spontaneously if the bladder is kept empty via a urethral catheter.[84] In other cases the urinary leak may be intraperitoneal[46] and not recognized initially. Open surgery to repair the tear may then be required.

Catheterization of the wrong vessel

The angle at which the umbilical artery comes off the internal iliac artery makes it difficult for a catheter to do anything other than pass into the aorta. However, occasionally the tip passes into another branch of the internal iliac, including the superior and inferior gluteal arteries,[38] and this is probably the reason for some cases of damage to the pelvic bones and gluteal skin (superior gluteal artery) and the sciatic nerves (inferior gluteal arteries; see below) (Table 37.3). Malposition of the UAC in one of these vessels is one of the reasons for always confirming the position of the catheter tip by X-ray immediately after insertion. Should it be in one of these branches, Schreiber et al[168] have described a technique of passing another small (3.5 FG) UAC alongside the malpositioned one. This second catheter then enters the aorta and the original one can be removed.

Flow down these branches is also responsible for peripheral ischaemic change, which can be seen following 'blind' injection of high-toxicity drugs inadvertently into the umbilical artery in the umbilical cord during resuscitation at birth – usually in mistake for the umbilical vein[41] (pp. 257–258).

HAEMORRHAGE FROM THE UMBILICAL VESSELS

During insertion there may be brisk haemorrhage from the other umbilical artery or the vein. This can be prevented by having a ligature loosely around the stump before it is cut off for the procedure (p. 1374). After the catheter is inserted it must be tied in securely with a suture, which also prevents haemorrhage from the other cord vessels (p. 1374).

HAEMORRHAGE FROM THE CATHETER

This is an ever-present risk and is one of the commonest complications reported from the UAC.[69,188] It can and must be prevented by meticulous nursing observation of all connections to the catheter, and there must be a Luer lock between the catheter and the infusion line. These must never be hidden under bedding or clothing in an attempt to make the baby look 'nice' for the family, and the baby must never be laid prone on the catheter.

If haemorrhage of any type does occur the treatment is immediate transfusion, but the hypotension that accompanies large blood loss may already have done irreparable damage, particularly to the CNS of a preterm baby.

INFECTION FROM THE UAC

This has always been listed as one of the major hazards of UAC, and staphylococcal infection was relatively common in some early reports.[200] However, it has not been a major problem in our practice. We make a special effort to keep the umbilical stump sterile before insertion (p. 373). In addition, virtually all babies who require a UAC are suffering from a disorder for which antibiotics are indicated. If catheters are left in situ for a prolonged period of time, as is occasionally justified (p. 363), then it may be appropriate to discontinue antibiotics (p. 1137). In this situation the UAC, like any intravascular line, will predispose the baby to sepsis, in particular that caused by *Staphylococcus epidermidis* (p. 1133).[98,205]

Mycotic aneurysm

These usually occur at the site of the tip of an indwelling UAC and are most common with thoracic placement. Most occur in babies with coexisting staphylococcal septicaemia. Although true aneurysms do occur,[34,104] in many cases there is a false aneurysm, with the aorta communicating through its wall with a sac that does not contain the normal tissues of the aortic wall[49] or is composed of an organizing para-aortic haematoma.[154] In many reported cases, as well as the aneurysm there is associated thrombus of the aorta and its major branches.[54,104]

Rarely the aneurysm may rupture, with fatal results.[135] In some cases it has been an incidental finding at post-mortem,[104] but in others after treatment of the septicaemia with antibiotics and removal of the arterial catheter surgical repair has given good results.[54] Aneurysms have also presented as an incidental finding in babies over one year of age, and have then been successfully resected.[27,54]

AIR EMBOLI

If, as is usually the case, the UAC is maintained patent by a continuous infusion of heparinized saline, there is the ever-present risk of air being entrained in the line, creating systemic air embolism. However, because of the arterial pressure, leaks in the system are more likely to result in haemorrhage than in air being injected.

SEVERED CATHETER TIP

During removal a catheter may fracture or be cut across while the retaining suture is being freed and the umbilical stump cleaned. This can lead to brisk haemorrhage, the catheter tip being retained deep within the umbilical artery or even floating free and embolizing the arterial tree.[185] These problems should be avoided by careful technique when removing the catheter; if they do occur removal is best carried out with the techniques and expertise of cardiac catheterization.

PERIPHERAL ISCHAEMIA AND THROMBOSIS

This is the second most common complication after haemorrhage. Initially the features of peripheral ischaemia may be due simply to a large catheter occluding the aorta or iliac vessels, or to arterial spasm following infusion of (hypertonic) solutions or vasoconstricting drugs such as catecholamines. It is to prevent the latter problem that it is important to position the tip of the UAC well away from the major branches of the aorta (Fig. 21.1, p. 363),

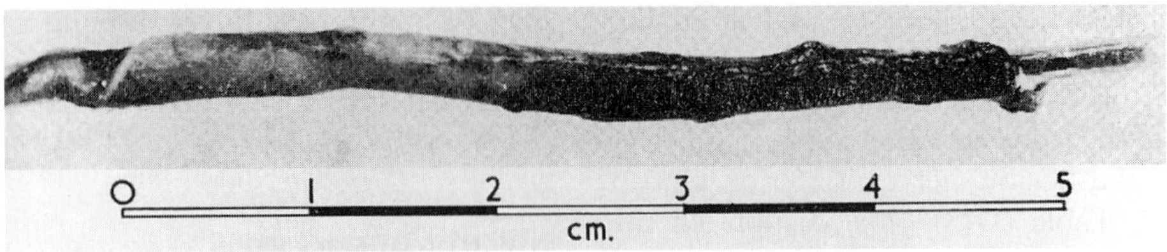

Fig. 37.1 Sheaths of thrombus surrounding a UAC found at postmortem. (From Gupta et al[69] with permission)

and if hypertonic drugs are being given they should be infused slowly so that they are instantaneously diluted in the rapidly flowing aortic blood.

The serious consequence is that thrombosis develops. The incidence of this complication varies widely in reported series, from as little as 1.5%[69] (where only clinically detected or autopsy-proven cases were reported) to as high as 95%, where aortography was used prior to removing the catheter.[129] Both the literature[64] and our own experience suggest that thombosis, if it is to occur, usually does so soon after the UAC is inserted and rarely thereafter. Another surprising feature of the reported studies on thrombosis is that normally grown term babies suffering from hypoxic–ischaemic encephalopathy seem to be significantly over-represented.[75,134,142,167,190,198]

Thrombus forms as a result of damage to the endothelial wall of the artery[31] and is likely to start by the hole in the catheter tip. Side-hole catheters, where the infusate impinges directly on to the endothelium of the artery, have been thought to create more problems than end-hole catheters, where the infusate is instantly diluted in the rapidly flowing arterial blood.[206] However, a recent report by Cohen et al[32] showed no increase in thrombotic complications in continuously recording side-hole catheters (Fig. 21.2, p. 364) compared with end-hole UACs.

Once thrombosis has formed it may propagate down the aorta alongside the catheter, down branches of the aorta such as the renal, mesenteric and lumbar arteries, and, once formed on the aortic wall, may propagate up the aorta, obstructing branches proximal to the tip of the catheter. Therefore, although it is standard teaching not to place the tip of the catheter opposite major branches of the aorta (Fig. 21.1, p. 363) this does not guarantee that thrombus will not form and propagate proximally or distally into these branches.

Thrombus may also disintegrate with embolization of any vessel which is peripheral to it. It is not clear how many episodes of peripheral ischaemia, such as NEC, haematuria or limb pallor, are due to emboli rather than to direct extension of the thrombus.

Clinical features

Many thrombi remain asymptomatic and are incidental findings on ultrasound scan or at postmortem (Fig. 37.1).[117,129,137] Thrombi can present in various ways. Rarely, there may be heart failure due to total aortic obstruction.[75] Much more common is evidence of ischaemia to a limb or organ (Table 37.4, Figs 37.2, 37.3, 37.4). These signs and symptoms may appear when the catheter is in situ, but may also occur just after its removal, presumably owing to dislodgement of thrombus on the aortic wall or to a sleeve of thrombus being left behind (Fig. 37.1). Occasionally signs develop several days after a UAC has been removed, presumably as a result of thrombus developing on the previously damaged intima.[2,95]

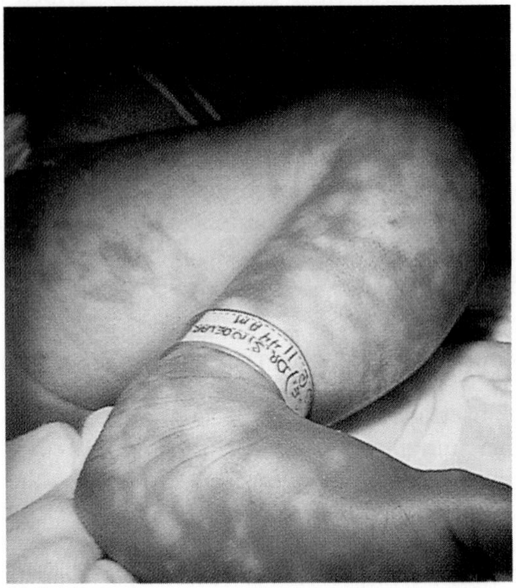

Fig. 37.2 Mottling of lower extremity in infant with umbilical artery catheter.

In babies with obstruction to the renal or iliac arteries the diagnosis is usually made promptly within minutes or hours of the obstruction, as the baby has haematuria, a reduced urinary output, or obvious poor peripheral perfusion, ischaemia and reduced pulses in the distribution of one artery (Figs 37.2, 37.3, 37.4, 37.6). However, with paraplegia the infant is often critically ill, hypotonic, and perhaps even paralysed on IPPV, and it is several days or even weeks before the paraplegia is recognized.

The role of UAC in the aetiology of NEC remains controversial, and most large epidemiological studies of this disorder do not show that the risk of NEC is greater

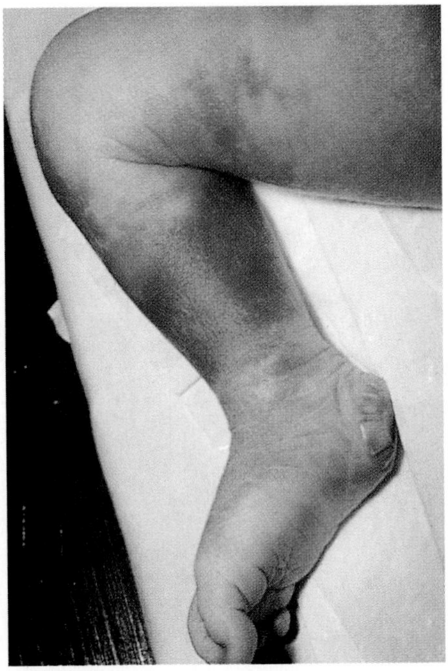

Fig. 37.3 Blanching and cyanosis in lower extremity in infant with umbilical artery catheter.

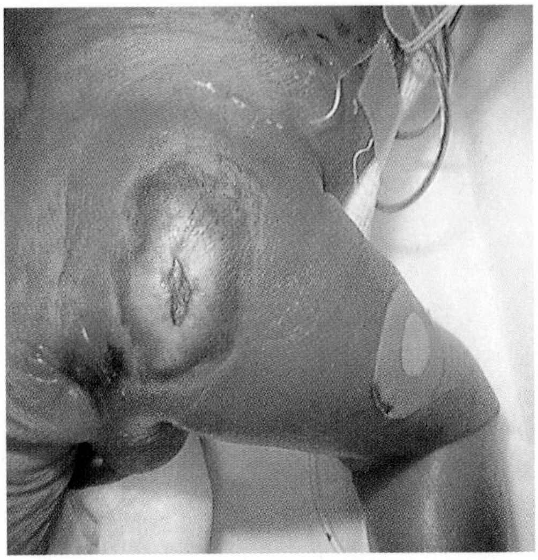

Fig. 37.4 Ischaemic injury in gluteal area.

in those babies who have UAC. However, in the separate entity of focal or discrete intestinal perforation emboli from a UAC are likely to be of importance.[133,162]

In addition to clinically obvious thrombotic or embolic lesions, autopsy studies have shown infarction secondary to UAC in the liver, adrenals, stomach, spleen and pancreas.[196]

Treatment

As soon as there is evidence of compromised circulation the catheter should be removed. In cases where there was simply obstruction of a blood vessel this, together with treatment to improve systemic pressure with volume expansion or inotropes, will usually result in prompt reversal of the ischaemia and no sequelae. In the typical cases occurring shortly after catheter insertion the ischaemic changes are usually due to arterial spasm, in addition to simple vessel obstruction. The application or infusion of vasodilators such as tolazoline or nitroglycerine[74,212] may be useful to reverse the peripheral ischaemia.

If there is clinical, radiological or ultrasound evidence of persistent ischaemia, thrombosis or arterial obstruction, careful assessment of the extent of the thrombus should be carried out by ultrasound or angiography. Renal involvement should be assessed with a DTPA or Hippuran scan.[29,198]

The treatment algorithm of Colburn et al[33] provides a good guide to subsequent treatment (Fig. 37.5). In most cases of aortic mural thrombosis conservative therapy is appropriate; the clot will clear, and this has been confirmed with ultrasound imaging.[2,171] However, if there are signs of persisting peripheral ischaemia or damage to other organs the baby should be heparinized and thrombolytic

Table 37.4 Clinical features of thrombotic or embolic obstruction secondary to umbilical artery catheterization

Artery	Clinical features	Reference
Renal	Haematuria	198
	Oliguria	142
	Renal failure	29
	Hypertension	
Superior/inferior mesenteric	Abdominal distension	
	Melaena	
	NEC	133
	Discrete intestinal perforation	
Common/external iliac	Leg pallor, ischaemia, gangrene	69, 124 Figs 37.2, 37.3
Internal iliac, superior and inferior gluteal	Buttock necrosis	114, Fig. 37.4
	Pelvic bone necrosis	38
	Sciatic nerve damage	151
Lumbar	Paraplegia	71, 95

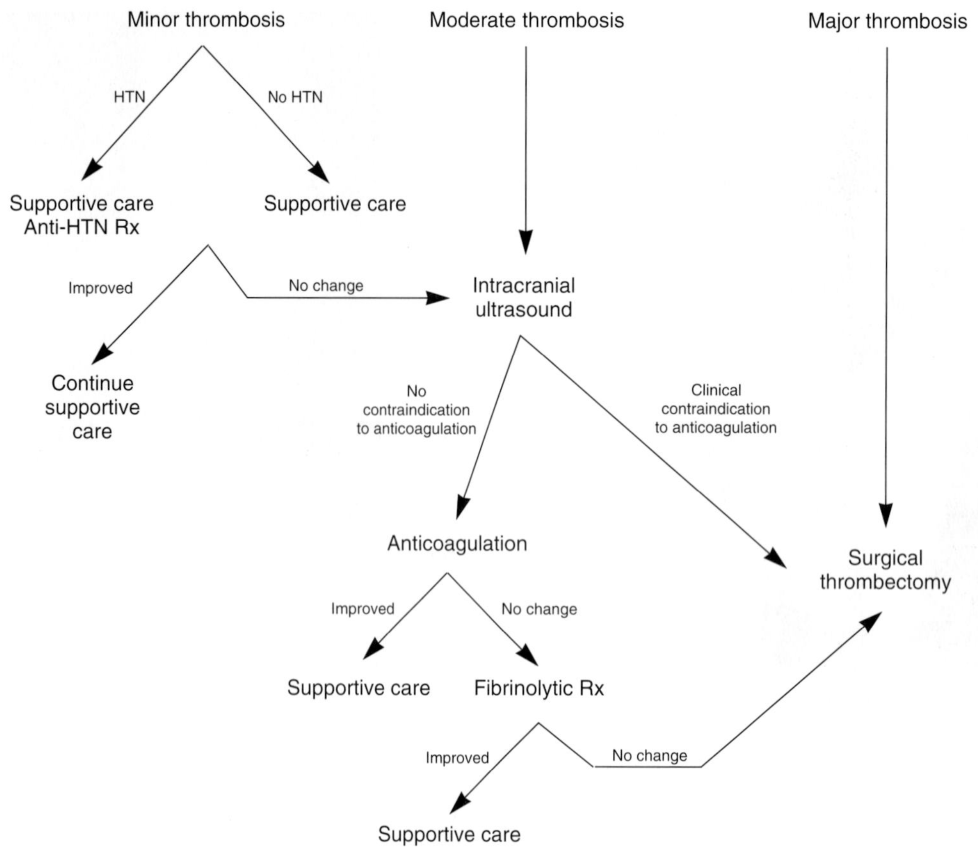

Fig. 37.5 Algorithm for management of neonatal aortic thrombosis. (From Colburn et al[33] with permission) (HTN = hypertension)

Table 37.5 Anticoagulants, thrombolytics in the neonate

Drug	i.v. bolus dose	i.v. maintenance dose	Reference
Heparin			
< 28 weeks' gestation	25 units/kg	15 units/kg/h	113
28–36 weeks' gestation	50 units/kg	20 units/kg/h	113
> 36 weeks' gestation	100 units/kg	25 units/kg/h	113
Streptokinase	1000 units/kg	1000 units/kg/h*	113
Urokinase	–	200 units/kg/h for 24 hours	7
Tissue plasminogen activator	0.5 mg/kg over 10 mins	0.5 mg/kg/h	2

*Monitor fibrinogen levels, stop treatment if less than 1 g/l

therapy commenced.[61] Heparinization may improve the outcome,[77,113,134] and should be given in the doses shown in Table 37.5. Rather more success has been reported with streptokinase or urokinase[113,158,190] (Table 37.5), although this is not always so.[52] More recently there have been reports of success with tissue plasminogen activator[2,88,134] (Table 37.5). Full intensive care should be continued as appropriate during attempts to dissolve the clot, in particular treating hypertension (see below) and renal failure.[29,112,142]

If these medical procedures do not result in a rapid improvement in perfusion, particularly to a leg, operation and thrombectomy or embolectomy can be extremely successful.[61,96,142]

Follow-up

The overall prognosis for aortic thrombosis and renal damage is surprisingly good, with the majority of babies surviving with hypertension that eventually resolves or is easily controlled.[29,112,198] However, some babies do develop renal failure and ultimately require transplants. Damage to the sciatic nerve is usually permanent, as is paraplegia. Where peripheral ischaemia occurs skin grafting may be required.

For limb ischaemia, if gangrene does not develop the prognosis is excellent. Leg growth is usually normal,[23] but one study reported that affected legs may be slightly wasted.[172] If gangrene does develop it may be very minor, involving the loss of just the pulp of one or two toes.[69]

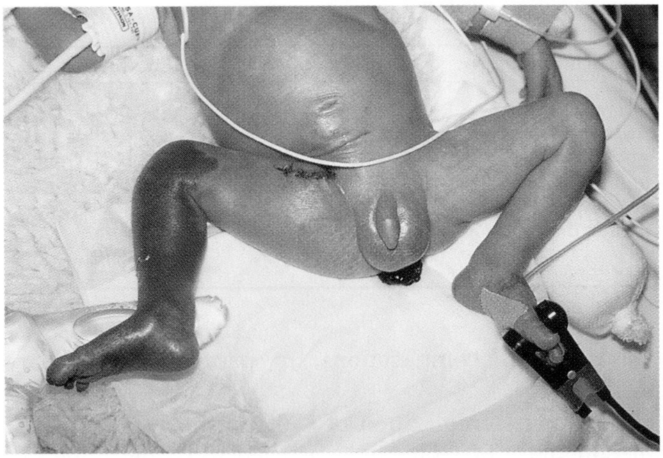

A

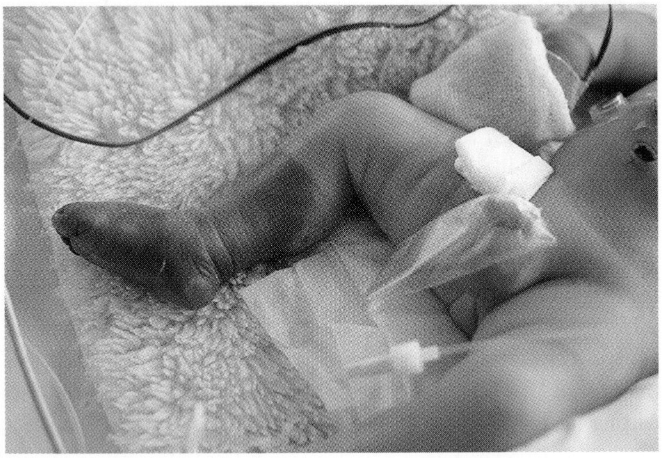

B

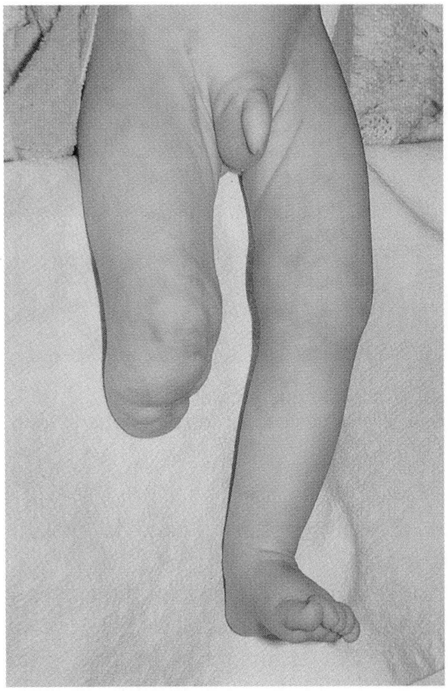

C

Fig. 37.6 (A) Acute ischaemia to the right leg following insertion of a femoral artery line. The level of injury appears to be above the knee. (B) Marked recovery with the line of demarcation below the knee. This resulted in below-knee amputation. (C) Immediately following the injury the artery had been explored, but this was unsuccessful in saving the limb.

Amputation for irreversibly ischaemic limbs

It is important to wait for a clean line of demarcation between viable and non-viable tissue. Only then can the level of amputation be determined. Too early surgery may result in a higher level of amputation, as there may be some proximal recovery (Fig. 37.6 A, B, C).

HYPERTENSION

This is a frequently reported complication of UAC, almost always in association with aortic thrombosis, which spreads to affect the renal arteries. At the time of the thrombosis the babies may have a high serum renin, and the cornerstone of early neonatal management is control of the hypertension with drugs[29,112] (p. 711). During long-term follow-up the hypertension resolves in many cases,[29,112,198] but not all.[142,149] If the hypertension is due to unilateral disease it may be cured by nephrectomy.[9,15]

HYPOGLYCAEMIA

If glucose is infused through a UAC whose tip is sited at the level of the coeliac axis the pancreas is exposed to a constant high concentration of glucose, and hyperinsulinaemia and hence hypoglycaemia results.[197] This complication should be prevented, and can be relieved by keeping the tip of the UAC away from the coeliac axis.

UMBILICAL VENOUS CATHETERS

These were widely used in the 1950s and 1960s when neonatology was in its infancy. One of the main indications for their use was exchange transfusion for rhesus haemolytic disease. Alarming complications were soon reported, which resulted in their use virtually disappearing from neonatal intensive care by the 1980s (Table 37.6). More recently, however, their use has again increased, particularly for making an attempt to measure central venous pressure (right atrial pressure) in critically ill babies on IPPV.

One of the problems with UVC is that there is no ideal site to place the tip. If it cannot be passed through the ductus venosus it becomes wedged within a branch of the hepatic venous tree, where infusions of hypertonic drugs cause liver necrosis[165,207] and vascular injury, leading to hepatic vein thrombosis[169] and, ultimately, portal hypertension with varices and splenomegaly.[99,139,193] The risk of thrombosis can be reduced by heparinization of the infusate using the usual concentration of 0.5–1 units/ml,

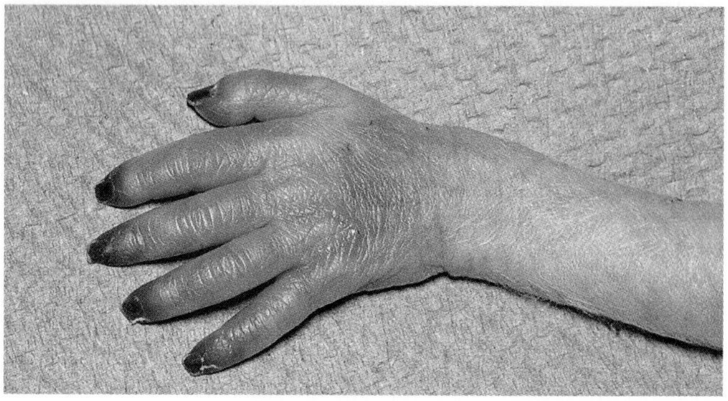

Fig. 37.7 Terminal digital ischaemia following accidental cannulation of the brachial artery while inserting a peripheral long line.

and if hepatic vein thrombosis does occur it can be relieved with streptokinase.[155]

If the UVC passes through into the inferior vena cava – probably the ideal position – there is still the risk of thrombosis, and the tip can easily pass the few extra millimetres that will take it into the right atrium. Indeed, getting into the right atrium is often the aim if CVP measurement is needed. Furthermore, many neonatologists feel that because of the risks of having the catheter tip wedged in the relatively stagnant hepatic venous blood flow, siting the tip in the right atrium is preferable, even for exchange transfusion. Once the catheter is placed anywhere above the diaphragm there is a major risk of air embolism,[90] as the catheter tip is then subject to the negative intrathoracic pressures of inspiration. For this reason, great care has to be taken not to leave the end off the catheter, as the risk of air being sucked in is greater than the risk of blood coming out, though this may also occur. Thrombi can form within the atria and these can become infected with candida.[80] An atrially sited catheter tip can provoke arrhythmias.[51]

Pushing the catheter in still further may cause it to cross the foramen ovale into the left atrium. This can cause various complications, in particular pulmonary haemorrhage.[20]

Table 37.6 Complications of umbilical venous catheterization

Complication	Reference
Air embolism	90
Cardiac arrhythmias	51
Sepsis	8, 193
Hepatic abscess	26, 210
Portal hypertension	83, 139
Hepatic infarction and necrosis	165
NEC	138, 195

The main complication of UVC in the 1960s was the introduction of infection, particularly that due to staphylococci,[8] which culminated in portal hypertension.[193] Liver abscess was also reported.[26,210] In part this was due to the catheterization taking place at several days of age (e.g. for exchange transfusion in rhesus HDN) through an umbilical stump that was necrotic and colonized with pathogenic organisms. Preventing this complication was one of the aims of improved methods of cord antisepsis in the neonatal period (p. 373).

Several reports in the late 1960s related the UVC used for exchange transfusion in rhesus HDN to NEC.[36,138] This may have been due to major pressure swings within the portal venous system during the infusion cycle of the exchange.[195] The plasticizers within the UVC were also implicated.[76]

PERIPHERAL ARTERIAL CANNULAE

Because of the risks of umbilical artery catheters, by the 1970s two alternatives were developed: first, intermittent sampling by puncture of the peripheral arteries, and then cannulation of these arteries. The former has only limited value, as not only is the artery irretrievably damaged by repeated punctures, even occasionally becoming aneurysmal,[136,156] but the handling associated with the

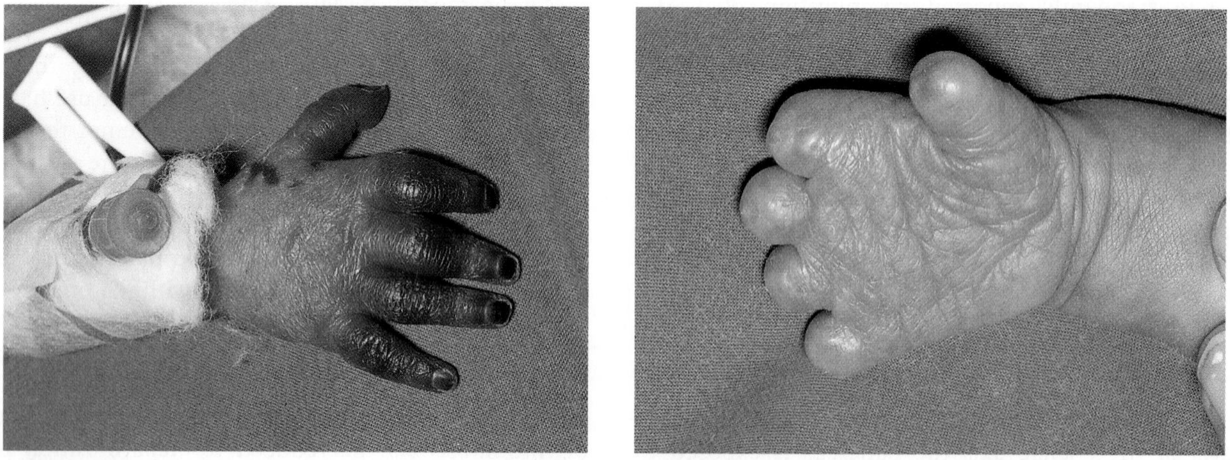

A B

Fig. 37.8 (A) Gangrenous fingers following radial artery catheterization. (B) Subsequent loss of fingers and thumb.

Table 37.7 Peripheral arterial cannulation in the neonate

Artery	Reference
Superficial temporal	150
Axillary	148
Brachial	157
Radial	143, 194
Ulnar	12, 202
Femoral	160
Posterior tibial	12, 187
Dorsalis pedis	202

procedure causes a fall in PaO_2 and the sample obtained does not therefore represent the stable status of the baby (p. 365). Furthermore, the spasm that follows an arterial stab may not resolve, and can be followed by peripheral ischaemia.[85]

Peripheral arterial cannulae have been placed in most accessible arteries (Table 37.7). As time has gone by it is clear that peripheral ischaemia is also a major complication at all these peripheral sites. In addition, the artery may go into spasm proximal to the site of cannulation and relatively extensive gangrene may result. The whole forearm can become ischaemic and need amputation following injury to the radial artery at the wrist.[85]

To minimize complications from peripheral arterial catheters the following rules should be adhered to:

- Catheters should only be used for sampling.
- Catheters should be perfused with 0.5 ml/h of heparinized saline.
- Catheters must be removed if there is more than extremely transient blanching of the periphery when the artery is flushed after sampling.

Over-vigorous flushing carries the theoretical hazard of dispersing emboli off the catheter tip into the systemic circulation,[106] and this may be responsible for some of the sequelae reported.

Peripheral arterial catheters must be clearly labelled to avoid the inadvertent injection of intravenous drugs, which can cause severe spasm, distal ischaemia and tissue loss. If this does occur administration of a vasodilator drug may be useful.[74,212]

SUPERFICIAL TEMPORAL ARTERY

This artery is no longer used since cannulation was found to cause ischaemic lesions of the underlying parietal lobe. Presumably spasm or emboli passed from the artery where it was cannulated alongside the ear down into the common carotid and then up the internal carotid into the middle cerebral artery.[28,178]

ARM ARTERIES

The axillary artery has recently been added to the list being cannulated,[148] and as yet no sequelae have been reported.

The brachial artery is an end artery and should not be cannulated, otherwise peripheral ischaemia is likely (Fig. 37.7). Furthermore, although it was one of the first arteries to be used for intermittent sampling,[157] even this use has decreased because the needling may damage the median nerve in the antecubital fossa,[141] or cause aneurysms.[156]

The radial and ulnar arteries are those usually chosen for cannulation. Whichever one is selected (usually the radial) it should only be cannulated after the other has been shown to be patent by manually compressing the artery to be cannulated and confirming that the hand remains pink and well perfused (Allen Test). It should be remembered that this is highly unlikely to be the case if one of the arteries has just been decannulated.[70] A wide variety of complications of radial artery catheterization have been reported in babies and adults,[183] of which by far and away the most important is peripheral ischaemia and gangrene (Fig. 37.8).[30] Other complications include ischaemic skin loss, carpal tunnel syndrome,[92] and fixed thumb adduction due to damage to the extensor muscles and tendons.[182] Although the artery remains occluded after decannulation for up to a month, recanalization is the norm.[70]

LEG ARTERIES

There is a general belief that the femoral artery should not be cannulated in neonates because it is an end artery and distal ischaemia is likely to lead to loss of the leg (Fig. 37.6 A, B, C). However, in our experience this is rare, and femoral arteries were cannulated extensively with minimal sequelae in the era of neonatal cardiac catheterization.[160] Posterior tibial artery cannulation[12,202] may be followed by peripheral ischaemia, with loss of toes or the foot.[1]

LONG LINES

CENTRALLY PLACED

Locating fine silastic or silicone catheters in a central site – the great veins or the right atrium – has been the standard way of administering TPN in many units[130] (Chapter 20). These catheters have been associated with five major groups of problems:

- Infections, including endocarditis, particularly with *Staph. epidermidis* (p. 1133) and fungi (p. 1163);
- Thrombosis;
- Ectopic placement with extravasation (Table 37.8);
- Retention;
- Air embolism.

The treatment of the first three is usually removal of the catheter. Thrombosis is relatively rare, occurring in less than 5% of catheterized neonates, and is more common

Table 37.8 Sites of extravascular infusions with TPN catheters

Site	Reference
Pericardial	86,191
Pleural, direct	86,170
Pleural, secondary to SVC obstruction	45
With permanent phrenic nerve injury	209
Intra-abdominal	132
Subdural	164, 215
Intrapulmonary	161 (Fig. 37.9)
Hydrocephalus secondary to vena caval obstruction	189
Lumbar vein/intrathecal	87

with the larger Broviac–Hickman type of catheter,[116,118] which take up more space in the blood vessel and are more rigid than fine silastic lines. Placement with the tip outside the right atrium leads to a high incidence of thrombosis, possibly due to intimal damage. Caution should be exercised when these lines are left in situ for long periods: the baby's growth will result in the tip leaving the right atrium, and thrombosis can follow. Thrombosis may occur in the great veins or, more characteristically, within the right atrium, where the thrombus can be seen bobbing about on a cardiac ultrasound image.[116,119] Such thrombi are frequently accompanied by a positive blood culture for *Staph. epidermidis* or candida, and may result in pulmonary or systemic embolization. They can resolve spontaneously,[119] but if infected should be treated with antibiotics, and thrombolytic therapy (Table 37.5) (urokinase, streptokinase, tissue plasminogen activator) should be considered.[3]

Where the tip lies in an inappropriate position (Table 37.8; Fig. 37.9) the situation must be handled accordingly. This usually includes aspiration of the extravasated material, plus appropriate treatment for the increasing respiratory failure (pleural fluid) or hypotension (pericardial fluid) that frequently coexists. One striking feature of this type of complication is that although a major vessel, or even the right atrium, is punctured for the extravasation to occur, haemorrhage is rare.

There are reports of the catheter becoming stuck by thrombus formation,[16,89] and we know of cases where the catheter has been severed and floated free, usually within the heart,[130] eventually becoming fixed to the endocardium. When tethered, catheters can be removed surgically.[16]

Catheters in the atria may provoke arrhythmias[39] and even cardiac arrest;[166] an air embolism has been reported in adults[145] and is a theoretical risk in neonates when infusion pumps are being used.

PERIPHERALLY PLACED

In many babies attempts to site a long line in the venae cavae or right atrium fail and the catheter tip lies, for example, in the subclavian or femoral veins. In this situation it is legitimate to leave lines in situ, in particular if achieving vascular access has proved difficult. The major complication is then venous obstruction in some cases complicated by thrombosis, with the limb becoming oedematous. The line should then be removed, and in our experience the oedema always resolves.

INTRAVENOUS DRIPS

The insertion of an i.v. infusion is probably the commonest procedure carried out on the neonate. Intravenous infusions have a high incidence of complications,

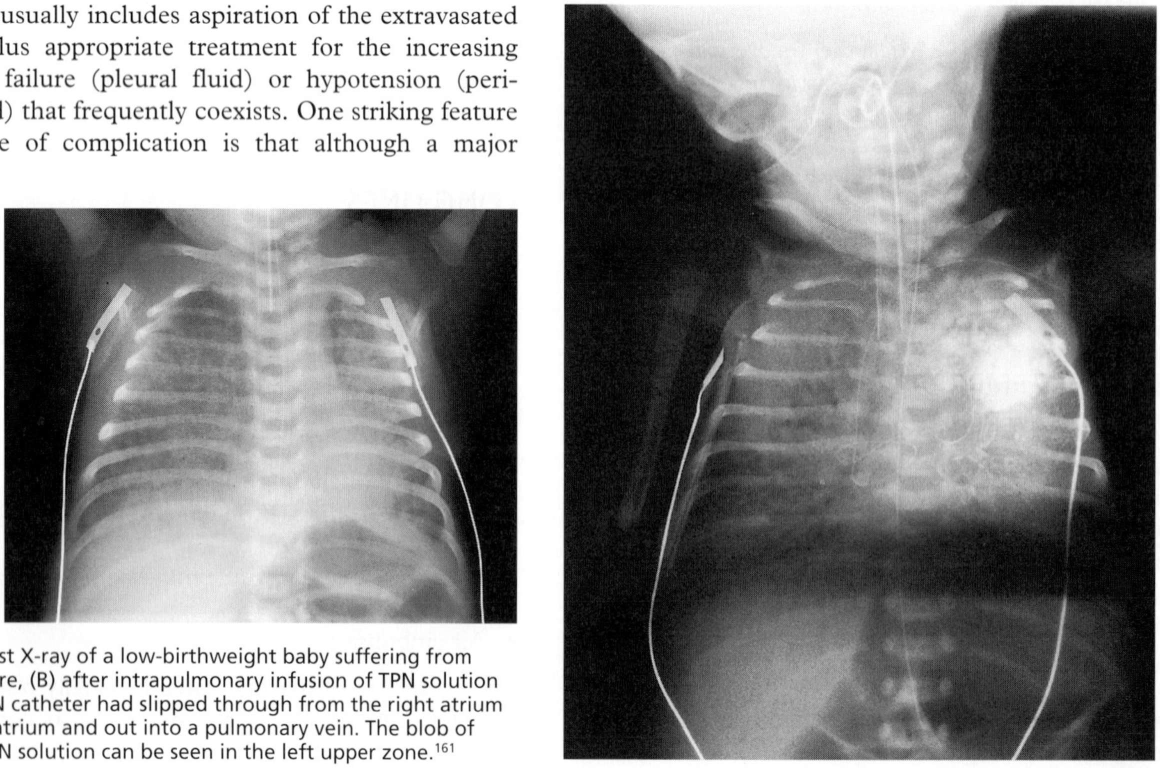
A B

Fig. 37.9 Chest X-ray of a low-birthweight baby suffering from CLD. (A) Before, (B) after intrapulmonary infusion of TPN solution when the TPN catheter had slipped through from the right atrium into the left atrium and out into a pulmonary vein. The blob of interstitial TPN solution can be seen in the left upper zone.[161]

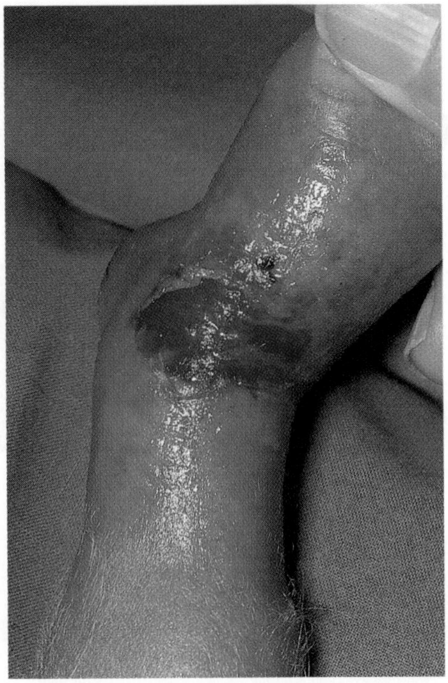

Fig. 37.10 Skin slough following infiltration of intravenous fluids.

of which the commonest is extravasation of the infusate into the subcutaneous tissues. Either the vessel leaks spontaneously, usually because the tip of the cannula ruptures the vessel wall, or it thromboses. Subcutaneous extravasation is therefore an unavoidable complication of neonatal care, and as hypertonic and irritant solutions such as drugs, TPN and base are frequently given, as are calcium salts which precipitate in the subcutaneous tissues, skin blistering and ischaemia are the commonest iatrogenic complications in neonatology. Other rarer complications of i.v. lines include infection,[192] local ischaemia and air emboli.[102]

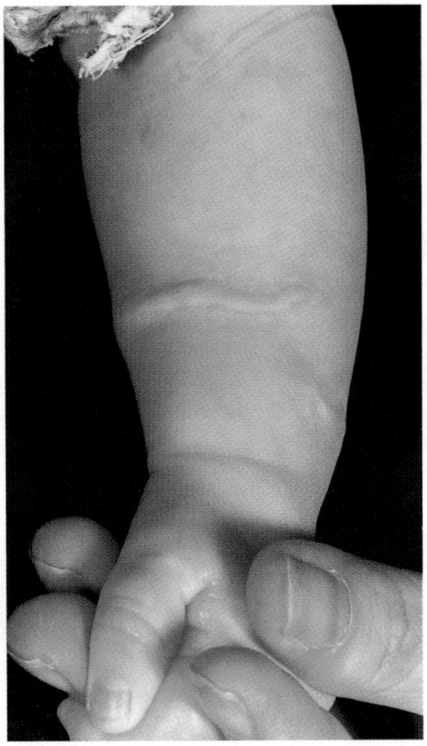

Fig. 37.12 Linear scar where an i.v. infusion had tissued proximal to a tightly occluded dressing.

SUBCUTANEOUS INFUSION

As many as 90% of i.v. infusions in the neonate result in the subcutaneous extravasation of the infusate.[58,122,146] Large areas of skin and subcutaneous tissue can be damaged (Fig. 37.10), with deformity from the subsequent scarring (Fig. 37.11 A, B). To minimize serious sequelae the i.v. cannulae should be immobilized in such a way that the infusion site is clearly visible and the vessel is not (partially) occluded by tightly binding the limb to a

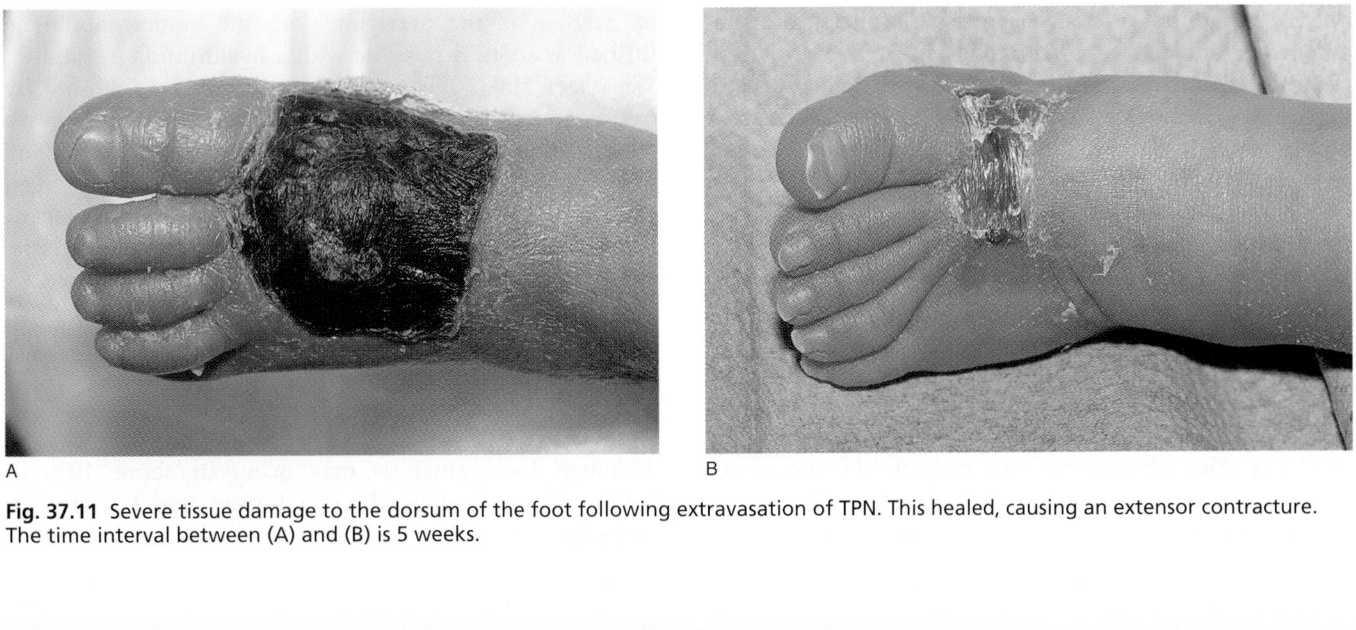

A B

Fig. 37.11 Severe tissue damage to the dorsum of the foot following extravasation of TPN. This healed, causing an extensor contracture. The time interval between (A) and (B) is 5 weeks.

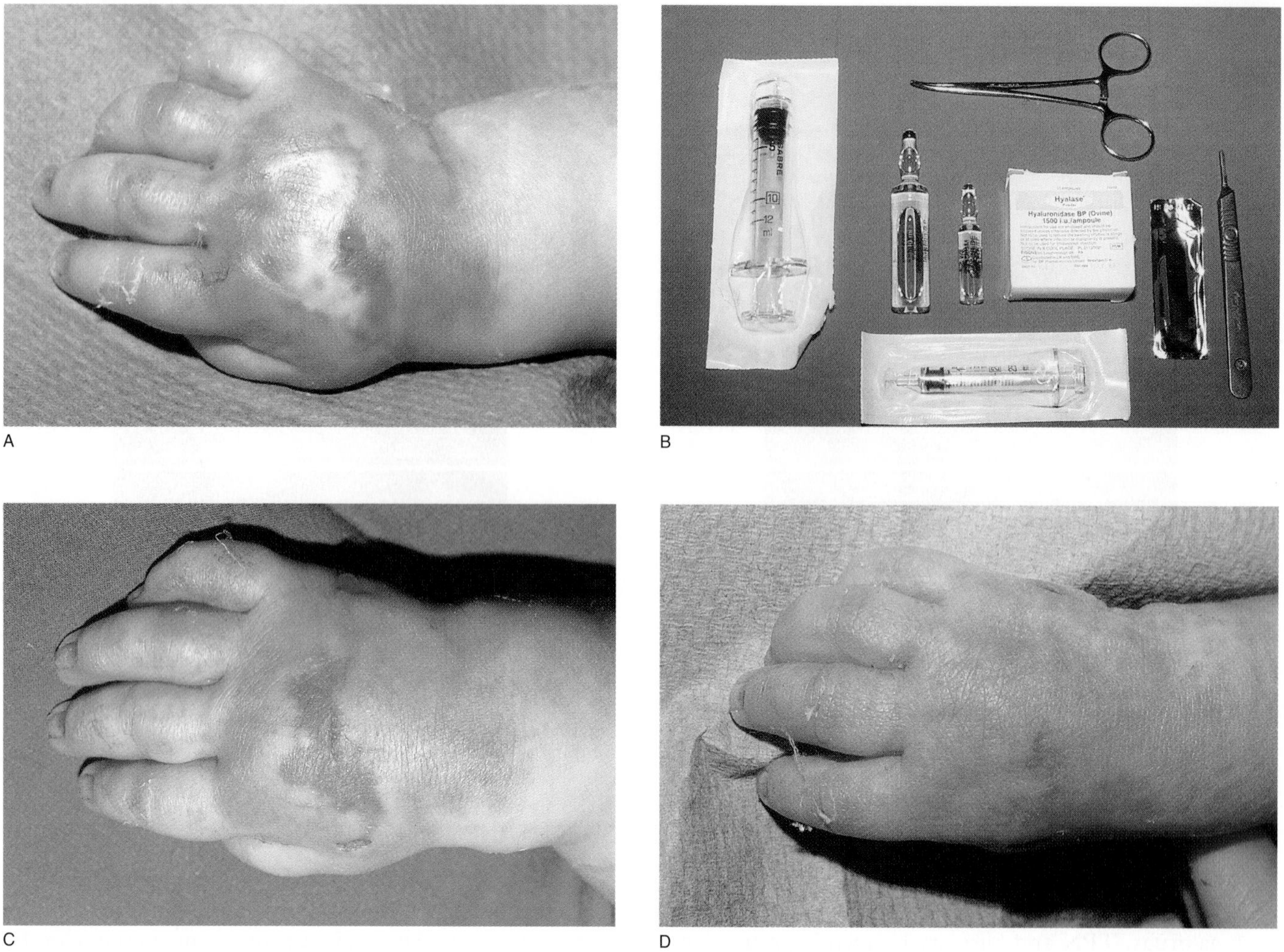

Fig. 37.13 (A) An acute TPN extravasation injury to the dorsum of the hand. (B) The simple kit needed to treat the problem by irrigation with hyaluronidase and saline. (C) Two small incisions made over the medial and lateral aspects of the dorsum of the hand using local anaesthesia. The tissue planes are opened with artery forceps. Hyaluronidase and saline are then introduced via one of the incisions irrigating the subcutaneous tissues on the back of the hand. The fluid exits from the incision on the other side. A marked improvement (C) can be seen immediately following this irrigation. (D) The result 24 hours after irrigation, with well vascularized skin and no sign of skin loss. Compare this with Figure 37.12

splint proximal to the infusion (Fig. 37.12). This may not only aggravate the tissue ischaemia by localizing the subcutaneous infusion to a 'tight blister' if the drip does extravasate, but the tightness may also damage adjacent nerves.[56] The site of an i.v. should always be checked hourly by the nursing staff for these complications.

In general the risk of extravasation is less with Teflon i.v. cannulae than with steel scalp vein needles,[14,146] and if 0.5 u/ml of heparin is added to the infusion.[122]

The risk of extravasation can also be reduced with the use of modern pressure-sensitive infusion devices, which will sound an alarm when the drip is obstructed or occluded. Once extravasation occurs the drip must be removed and the limb, if oedematous, should be elevated and kept dry. Why some babies develop necrosis of the overlying skin, whereas the vast majority do not, is not clear.

It is now recommended that if, when extravasation is recognized, there is impending or even established ischaemia or necrosis of the overlying skin, the tissues should be flushed as soon as possible with a hyaluronidase solution. We inject 500–1000 units of hyaluronidase followed by free irrigation using up to 500 ml normal saline to remove all irritant infusate (Fig. 37.13).[40] Our results in saving tissue have been very good when TPN has been extravasated, but not so good when the injurious agent has been a calcium compound. Once permanent tissue loss has occurred, plastic surgery will often be required.

OTHER COMPLICATIONS

Infection

Although local phlebitis may occur in about 10% of babies with a peripheral i.v. infusion, and bacteria, in particular *Staph. epidermidis*, may be grown using

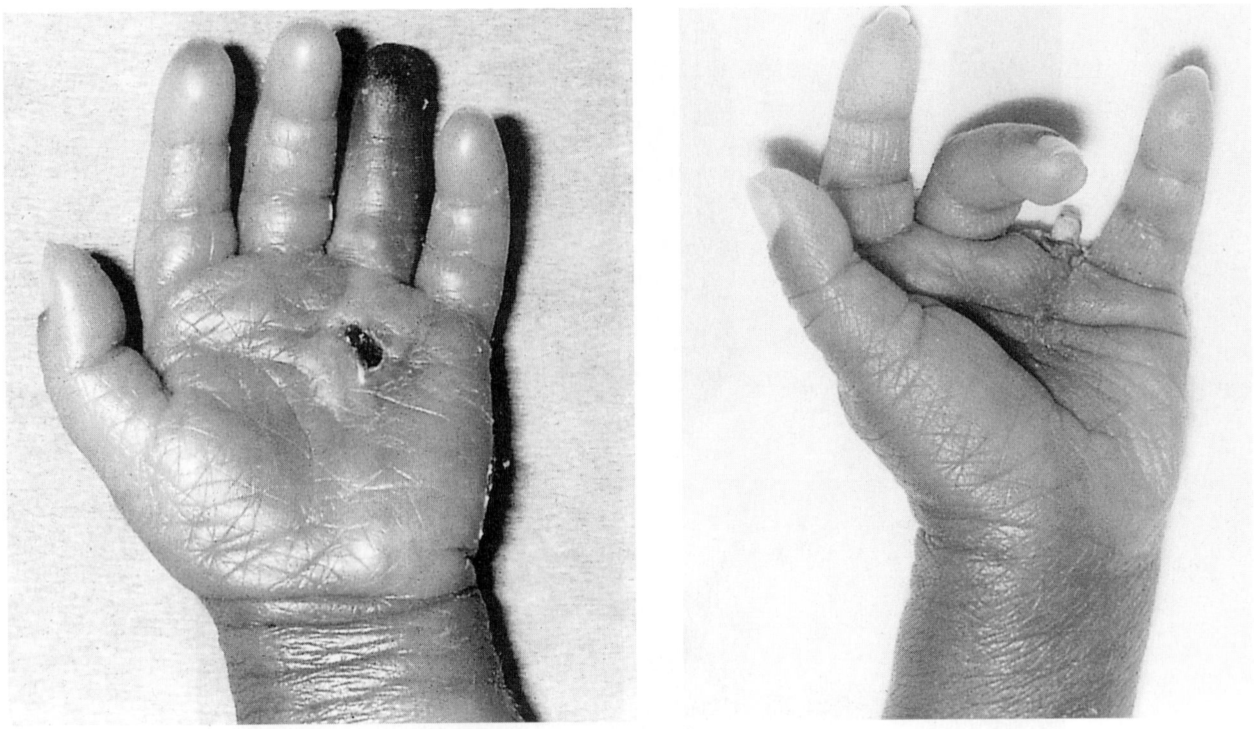

A B

Fig. 37.14 (A) Ischaemic change in a finger following subcutaneous infusion and deep infection at a drip site on the dorsum of the hand. (B) Subsequent tissue loss; the remnant of the proximal phalanx was easily removed with forceps.

sophisticated techniques from the site and the cannula at the time of removal, septicaemia from peripheral i.v. sites is rare.[58,192]

Ischaemic change

Subcutaneous i.v. infusion that compromises an arterial supply in the area can result in digital ischaemia[204] (Fig. 37.14). It may also damage adjacent nerves.[94]

Air embolism

Whenever a continuous infusion is being used there is a constant risk, as with long lines, of air being infused.[102] Nursing vigilance is essential for prevention. Small air emboli (the occasional bubble) are common and seem to be without effect, but if more than 5–10 ml of air are infused death or permanent CNS sequelae are likely.

LIMB INJURY

FRACTURES

Osteopenic VLBW babies have developed fractures in association with insertion of i.v. infusions[147] (Fig. 37.15), physiotherapy using a vibrating toothbrush[213] and when they trap their limbs over the edges of incubator trays.[42]

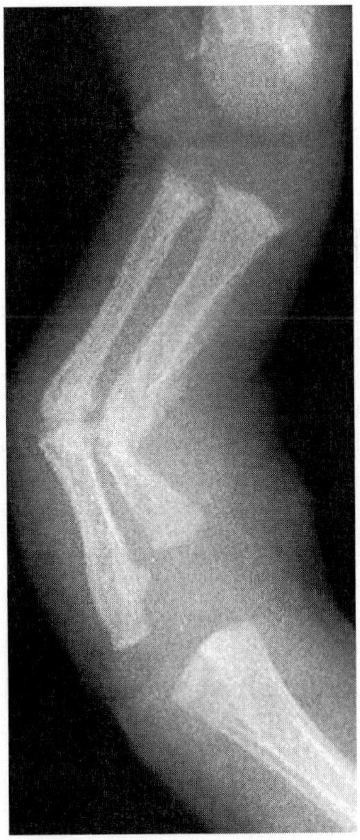

Fig. 37.15 X-ray showing fracture of the radius and ulna sustained during handling for intravenous line insertion in a baby with osteopenia of prematurity.

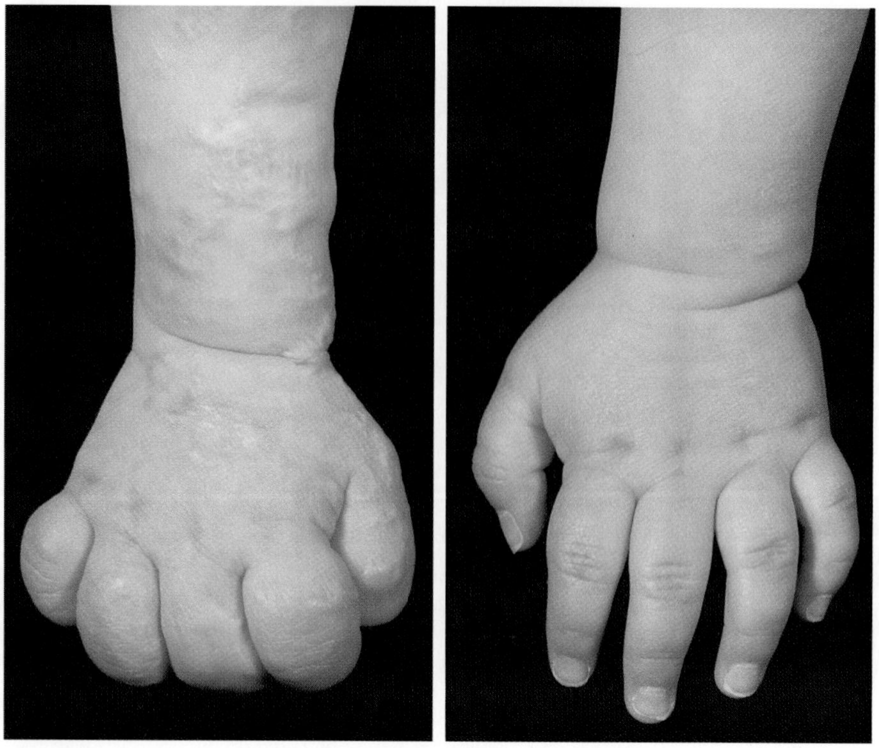

Fig. 37.16 Severe scarring and tissue distortion secondary to multiple venepunctures taken from the back of a low-birthweight baby's hand.

THREAD TOURNIQUET

Babies can get their fingers and toes caught in mittens or other pieces of thread, causing distal vascular obstruction with gangrene and some tissue loss.[13] Clothed extremities should be checked regularly to ensure that this does not occur.

BLOOD SAMPLING

The physical handling involved in taking arterial, venous or capillary blood can cause rapid deterioration in the unstable, ill preterm baby (p. 502). Preventing this is one of the many reasons for having indwelling arterial catheters, which allow frequent sampling without disturbing the baby. There are in addition some specific problems that result from blood sampling procedures.

BLOOD LOSS

Large quantities of blood may be removed from ill VLBW neonates, resulting in anaemia and hypotension: 'haemorrhage into the laboratory'. This is dealt with in Chapter 32, Part 4.

ARTERIAL SAMPLING

The hazards of intermittent arterial sampling are discussed above (p. 365).

VENOUS SAMPLING

Obtaining venous blood from VLBW neonates is not easy and the broken needle technique is frequently used (pp. 1372–1373), usually from a vein in the back of the hand. On follow-up such babies may show multiple tiny scars in this site[43] (Fig. 37.16).

Another problem that has received extensive media coverage recently is that after using the broken needle technique care must be taken to remove this hubless device from the incubator/ cot, otherwise it may work its way into the baby's subcutaneous tissues. We are aware of several instances in which this accident has occurred.

HEEL PRICKS

Incorrect technique (p. 1372)[21] can result in osteomyelitis/ osteochondritis of the os calcis,[103] and also the development of multiple painful calcific nodules at the site on the heel.[173]

INTRAMUSCULAR INJECTIONS

These have largely been abandoned in the neonate, other than for single-dose therapy such as vitamin K at birth or the use of paraldehyde (p. 1220), largely because the absorption of drugs is unpredictable and intravenous therapy is preferred.

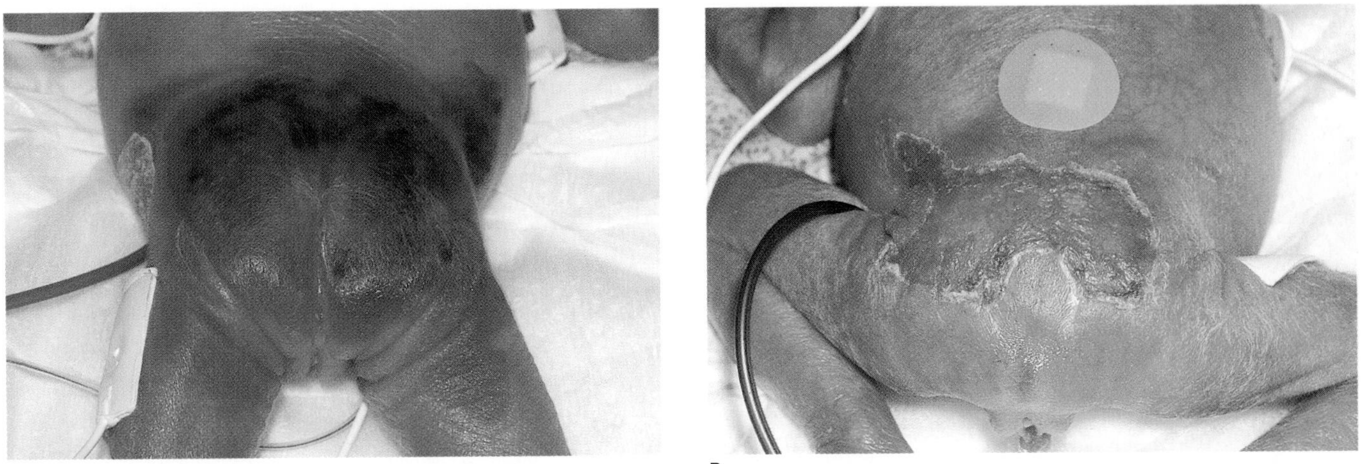

A B

Fig. 37.17 (A) Burn: black area and surrounding erythema on the buttocks of a 1200 g baby who had lain in a pool of antiseptic during umbilical artery catheterization. (B) Subsequent improvement in the lesion, with clean exposed tissue which healed with minimal scarring.

Injections into the legs and buttocks of preterm neonates with their low muscle mass has been associated with sciatic nerve damage[62] and fibrosis of the quadriceps (p. 1084),[131,174] with marked restriction of knee flexion and intramuscular calcification.[11]

SKIN DAMAGE

As well as skin damage from the conditions described above, babies' skin may be cut during caesarean section and scars result from the use of scalp clips.[5]

SCARS

Scarring from all surgical procedures in the newborn can be marked, because of the fragility of their skin, but can be minimized by special surgeons. Minor surgical procedures performed by physicians, such as cut-downs, can leave major scars. The site of a pneumothorax drain can also leave a large scar which may distort the underlying breast as a girl grows through puberty. It is imperative to avoid the nipple area. Damage to the tissue which will form the breast can result, giving rise to amazia.

ADHESIVE MATERIALS

Ordinary adhesive tape and the adhesive electrodes used in neonatal intensive care can damage neonatal skin. Often when plaster, urine bags and electrodes are removed, superficial layers of the preterm baby's skin detach as well. This must be painful, and will increase fluid loss and the baby's susceptibility to infection. Damage can be reduced by spraying the acrylic copolymer dressing Op-site, on to the skin,[55] but this has not been widely adopted in clinical practice.

CHEMICAL BURNS

The chemicals used in neonatal antiseptic solutions, in particular iodine and alcohol, can damage the preterm baby's skin. This is particularly likely to occur if the baby's back and buttocks are left on a nappy impregnated with these agents following, for example, their liberal application during umbilical catheterization (Fig. 37.17).[72,208]

THERMAL BURNS

Generalized burns have been described in infants with poor skin perfusion who have been placed under radiant heaters, or when the plastic backing of nappies on which they were lying became very hot.[57,180]

Localized burns are well recognized in certain situations. They occur with the use of TcPO_2 monitors, especially if they are heated to 44°C, the temperature at which they are most accurate.[25] The scarring that results may be deep and permanent.[65] The skin may also be damaged in the area around the burn by the adhesive disc used to fix the electrode to the skin. Both forms of damage can be minimized by spraying Op-site to the site before application.[55] Similar lesions, perhaps thermal in origin, perhaps due to pressure, have been recorded following pulse oximetry.[186,214] Burns have also been reported following the use of an incorrectly assembled transilluminator to identify the wrist arteries prior to cannulation.[108]

COMPLICATIONS OF IPPV

The complications of IPPV are severe and complicated (Table 37.1) and the majority are dealt with elsewhere in this book.

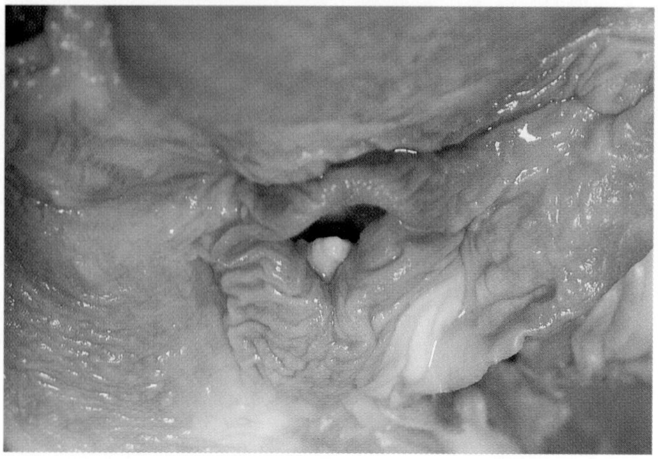

Fig. 37.18 Granuloma on interarytenoid fold in a baby of 30 weeks' gestation who had been on IPPV for 2 weeks.

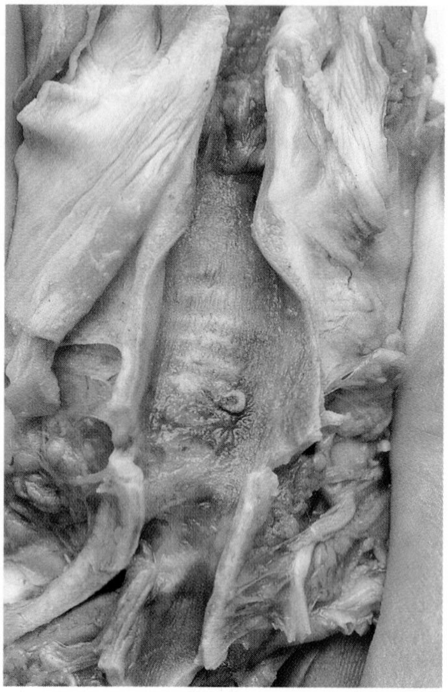

Fig. 37.19 Severe ulceration in distal trachea in a baby who had been on IPPV for several months.

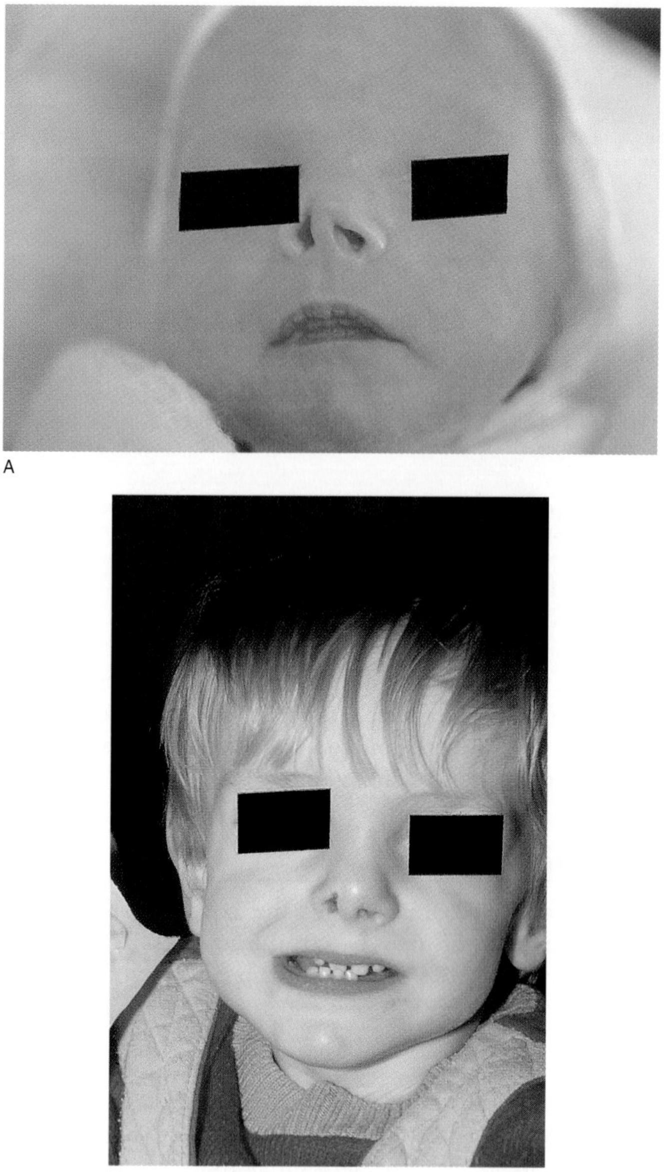

A

B

Fig. 37.20 (A) A notch in the nose caused by a nasoendotracheal tube during the neonatal period. (B) The same child more than 1 year later.

FACE MASK VENTILATION/CPAP

This is the least effective way of applying CPAP, and causes distortion and damage to the tissues of the face as well as intracerebellar haemorrhage if the strapping holding the mask on is too tight.[140] Another reported complication is corneal ulceration from the face mask.[35] Face mask and nasal prong ventilation may cause gastric perforation.[59]

LOCAL TRAUMA

The act of intubation causes widespread physiological responses of a stress type which can be very damaging, in particular increasing the risk of GMH-IVH. How to minimize this is discussed on pages 573–574.

A wide variety of local injuries can occur from acute and chronic trauma to the nose, mouth, pharynx, larynx (Fig. 37.18) and trachea (Fig. 37.19) following intubation (Table 37.9). Some of these are rare; others, like the palatal groove with oral ETT, may occur in 50% of neonates so treated,[53] although only a small proportion of these progress to perforation, causing iatrogenic cleft palate.[50] Nasal damage is more likely with endotracheal tubes (Fig. 37.20 A, B) than CPAP tubes, though it can still occur with double nasal CPAP prongs using the fluidic flip mechanism (Fig. 37.21). The longer the intubation and the smaller the baby the more severe and

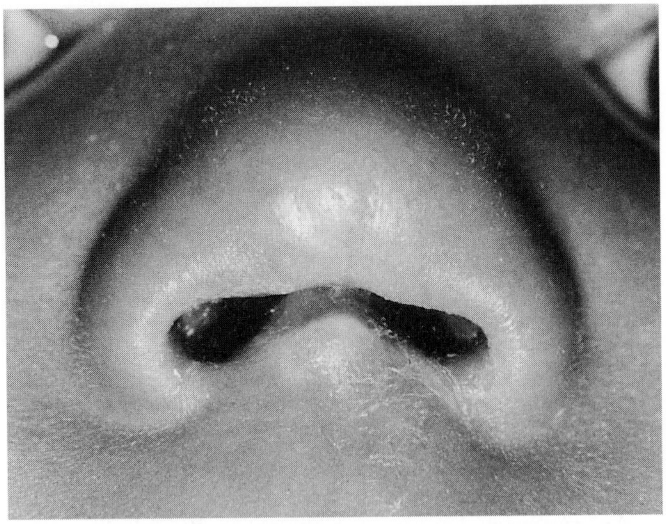

Fig. 37.21 Necrosis of the columella in a child aged 4 months from traumatic injury after CPAP had been given with a double-pronged nasal device in the early neonatal period. (From Robertson et al[159] with permission)

Table 37.9 Iatrogenic injury from intubation and in situ nasal or oral tubes

Injury	Reference
Local trauma to mouth, fauces with laryngoscope/ETT	
Nasal damage and stenosis	17, 67
Palatal grooves from oral ETT	53
Acquired cleft palate	50
Defective dentition*	127
Perforation of airway with ETT	110, 175

*This can be caused by pressure from the laryngoscope during intubation or from the indwelling oral ETT

marked destruction of the nasal margin that may occur, and there may be severe stenosis on healing.

It is perhaps noteworthy that most of these complications were reported in the early 1970s, and our own experience would suggest that they are now rarer, because of better nursing care, better immobilization of CPAP and IPPV tubes with the use of holding devices that do not cause tissue damage,[63] and probably owing to tubes being made to higher specifications from softer, more inert material.

AIRWAY DAMAGE

The most serious iatrogenic complications to the local airways and lungs following IPPV are those listed in Table 37.1. Other problems include metaplastic change in the laryngeal and tracheal mucosa,[60,82,211] which will eventually heal even with the ETT still in situ;[66] subglottic cysts,[37,48] which may occur in up to 7% of ex-intubated premature infants; tracheomegaly;[18] tracheobronchomalacia;[47] and bronchial stenosis,[128] though the latter is probably a complication of inappropriate and vigorous endotracheal tube suction.

The presence of the endotracheal tube compromises eustachian tube function, leading to otitis media.[44] Necrotizing tracheobronchitis[22] is an often fatal complication which is almost specific to HFJV (p. 569).

SUCTIONING

The frequency of ETT suctioning in the neonate should be tailored to the needs of the individual baby, but it is doubtful if it needs to be done more than 6-hourly in the standard baby with ventilator-dependent RDS (p. 573).

As well as the complex physiological deterioration that occurs during the act of suctioning, local trauma to the mucosa is common, as shown by the frequent presence of flecks of blood in the aspirate. In addition, granulomata may form at the carina or in the more peripheral airways[128] and the airways may be perforated by the suction catheter, resulting in pneumothorax, obviously with a big bronchopleural fistula.[68,201]

CHEST DRAINS

During insertion haemorrhage may occur if the vascular bundle in the intercostal groove below each rib is damaged. The area of the female breast should be avoided to prevent subsequent unsightly scarring (see above).

The lung may be transfixed by the pneumothorax drain in up to 25% of cases,[123] although this complication can be minimized by use of the appropriate insertion technique (p. 1381). The tip of the tube within the chest may damage the pericardium,[152] the thoracic duct[97] or one or both phrenic nerves.[6,115]

Suturing of the skin may not be necessary after removal of a chest drain. Following removal of the tube the tissue planes move over each other, occluding the hole. It is therefore important to pinch the skin around the tube as it is being removed, to prevent air entry. An airtight dressing can then be applied to minimize scarring. Lung damage could result from tissue being sucked into holes as the drain is removed, causing a pneumothorax.

GUT COMPLICATIONS

NASOGASTRIC TUBES

Bleeding gastric erosions and ulcers occur frequently in ill VLBW neonates,[111] and may be provoked/aggravated by indwelling nasogastric tubes. Coffee-ground aspirate is often noted by the nurses but frank haematemesis is rare. The tendency to haematemesis is aggravated by drugs, especially tolazoline, steroids and indomethacin (Table 37.2), and if overt haemorrhage does occur treatment with ranitidine is indicated (p. 746).

The gut may be perforated at any level by nasogastric or nasojejunal tubes, or by ETT, but most commonly this seems to occur in the pharynx and oesophagus.[81,93,100] It is

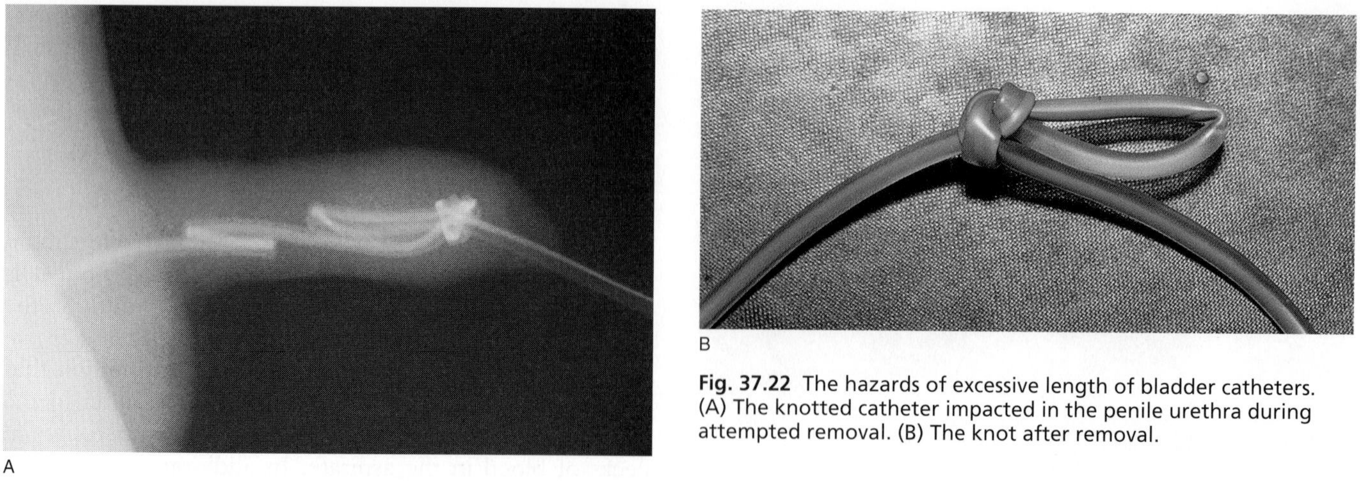

Fig. 37.22 The hazards of excessive length of bladder catheters. (A) The knotted catheter impacted in the penile urethra during attempted removal. (B) The knot after removal.

not justified to assume that this represents the use of excessive force: the viscus may have ruptured spontaneously through an area of congenital weakness, because of CPAP (p. 932) or from NEC (p. 747). These babies present with oesophageal obstruction if the leak is limited to the mediastinum, but if the leak reaches the pleural cavity respiratory distress results, as with any other pleural effusion. Treatment is conservative, with i.v. nutrition to bypass the lesion, draining of the pleural fluid and antibiotics.[81]

When the upper small intestine is perforated presentation is with clinical deterioration, and on abdominal X-ray the tube is seen to be incorrectly placed, together with a pneumoperitonium.[93,120] Many upper GI tract perforations occurred when PVC tubes were used for nasojejunal feeding as these tubes became hard and rigid after being in situ for some time[24,73] and transfixed the bowel wall. As a result silicone tubes are now used if nasojejunal feeding is required, though even these can perforate the bowel.[144] In one extraordinary case the lamina cribrosa of the ethmoid bone was perforated by a nasogastric tube; there were no sequelae after it was withdrawn.[199]

RECTAL PERFORATION

The risk of perforating a baby's rectum by inserting a thermometer or rectal probe is less than 1 in 2 million insertions. The data were reviewed by Morley et al.[125]

URINARY CATHETERS

Strict asepsis should be practised during catheterization. 'Catheter shock' with severe septicaemia may result from instrumentation of the urinary tract in the presence of infection. The administration of a broad-spectrum antibiotic before catheterization will reduce this risk.

Urethral stricture may result from traumatic catheterization. If the catheter does not pass into the bladder with ease, specialist advice should be sought.

An excessive length of catheter in the bladder may cause problems. Kinking of the catheter as the bladder empties, obstructing the lumen, leads to urine bypassing the catheter. The catheter may even tie itself into a knot, making removal very difficult (Fig. 37.22A, B).

REFERENCES

1. Abrahamson E L, Scott R C, Jurges E, Al-Jawad S, Madden N 1993 Catheterization of posterior tibial artery leading to limb amputation. Acta Paediatrica 82: 618–619
2. Ahluwalia J S, Kelshall A W R, Diederich S, Rennie J M 1994 Successful treatment of aortic thrombosis after umbilical catheterization with tissue plasminogen activator. Acta Paediatrica 83: 1215–1217
3. Alkalay A L, Mazereth R, Santuili T, Pomerance J J 1993 Central venous line thrombosis in premature infants. A case management and literature review. American Journal of Perinatology 10: 323–326
4. Archer N 1993 Patent ductus arteriosus in the newborn. Archives of Disease in Childhood 69: 529–532
5. Ashkenazi S, Metzker A, Merlob P, Ovadia J, Reisner S H 1985 Scalp changes after fetal monitoring. Archives of Disease in Childhood 60: 267–269
6. Ayra H, Williams J, Ponsford S N, Bissenden J G 1991 Neonatal diaphragmatic paralysis caused by chest drains. Archives of Disease in Childhood 66: 441–442
7. Bagnall H A, Gomperts E, Atkinson J B 1989 Continuous infusion of low dose urokinase in the treatment of central venous catheter thrombosis in infants and children. Pediatrics 83: 963–966
8. Balagatas R C, Bell C E, Edwards L D, Levin S 1971 Risk of local and systemic infections associated with umbilical vein catheterization: A prospective study in 86 newborn patients. Pediatrics 48: 359–367
9. Baldwin C E, Holder T M, Asheraft K W, Amoury R A 1981 Neonatal renovascular hypertension. A complication of aortic monitoring catheters. Journal of Pediatric Surgery 16: 820–821
10. Balistreri W F, Farrell M K, Bove K E 1986 Lessons from the E-ferol tragedy. Pediatrics 78: 503–506
11. Barak M, Herschkowitz S, Montag J 1986 Soft tissue calcification: a complication of the vitamin E injection. Pediatrics 77: 382–385
12. Barr P A, Sumners J, Wirtschafter D, Porter R C, Cassidy G 1977 Percutaneous peripheral arterial cannulation in the neonate. Pediatrics 59: 1058–1062
13. Barton D J, Sloan G M, Nichter L S, Reinisch J F 1988 Hair–thread tourniquet syndrome. Pediatrics 82: 925–928
14. Batton D G, Maisels M J, Appelbaum P 1982 Use of peripheral intravenous cannulas in premature infants. A controlled study. Pediatrics 70: 487–490
15. Bauer S B, Feldman S M, Gellis S S, Retik A B 1975 Neonatal hypertension: a complication of umbilical artery catheterization. New England Journal of Medicine 293: 1032–1033

16. Bautista A B, Ko S H, Sun S C 1995 Retention of percutaneous venous catheter in the newborn. A report of 3 cases. American Journal of Perinatology 12: 53–54
17. Baxter R J, Johnson J D, Guetsman B W, Hackel A 1975 Cosmetic nasal deformities complicating prolonged nasal tracheal intubation in critically ill newborn infants. Pediatrics 55: 884–886
18. Bhutani V K, Ritchie W G, Shaffer T G 1986 Acquired tracheomegaly in very preterm neonates. American Journal of Diseases of Children 140: 449–452
19. Biagtan J, Rosenfeld W, Salazar D, Velcek F 1980 Herniation of the appendix through the umbilical ring following umbilical artery catheterization. Journal of Pediatric Surgery 15: 672–673
20. Biorklund L J, Mahngren N, Lindroth M 1995 Pulmonary complications of umbilical venous catheters. Pediatric Radiology 25: 149–152
21. Blumenfeld T A, Turi G, Blanc W A 1979 Recommended site and depth of newborn heel stick punctures based on anatomical measurements and histopathology. Lancet i: 230–233
22. Boros S J, Mammel M C, Lewallen P K, Coleman J M, Gordon M J, Ophoven J 1986 Necrotizing tracheobronchitis: a complication of high-frequency ventilation. Journal of Pediatrics 109: 95–100
23. Boros S J, Nystrom J F, Thompson T R, Reynolds J W, Williams H J 1975 Leg growth following umbilical catheter associated thrombus formation: a 4 year follow-up. Journal of Pediatrics 87: 973–976
24. Boros S J, Reynolds J W 1974 Duodenal perforation: a complication of neonatal nasojejunal feeding. Journal of Pediatrics 85: 107–108
25. Boyle R J, Oh W 1980 Erythema following transcutaneous PO_2 monitoring. Pediatrics 65: 333–334
26. Brans Y W, Ceballos R, Cassady G 1974 Umbilical catheters and hepatic abscesses. Pediatrics 53: 264–266
27. Brill P W, Winchester P, Levin A R, Griffith A Y, Kazam E, Zirinsky K 1985 Aortic aneurysm secondary to umbilical artery catheterization. Journal of Pediatric Surgery 15: 199–201
28. Bull M J, Schreiner R L, Garg B P, Hutton N M, Lemons J A, Gresham E L 1980 Neurological complications following temporal artery catheterization. Journal of Pediatrics 96: 1071–1073
29. Caplan M S, Cohn R A, Langman C B, Conway J A, Shkolnik A, Brouillette R T 1989 Favourable outcome of neonatal aortic thrombosis and renovascular hypertension. Journal of Pediatrics 115: 291–295
30. Cartwright G W, Schreiner R L 1980 Major complication secondary to percutaneous radial artery catheterization in the neonate. Pediatrics 65: 139–141
31. Chidi C C, King D R, Boles E T 1983 An ultrastructural study of the intimal injury induced by an indwelling umbilical artery catheter. Journal of Pediatric Surgery 18: 109–115
32. Cohen R S, Ramachandran P, Kim E H, Glasscock G F 1995 Retrospective analysis of risks associated with an umbilical artery catheter system for continuous monitoring of arterial oxygen tension. Journal of Perinatology 15: 195–198
33. Colburn M D, Gelabert H A, Quinones–Baldrich W 1992 Neonatal aortic thrombosis. Surgery 111: 21–28
34. Colclough A B, Barson A J 1981 Infantile aortic aneurysm complicating umbilical arterial catheterization. Archives of Disease in Childhood 56: 795–797
35. Cole G F, Chaudhuri P R, Carroll L P 1982 Mask for continuous positive airways pressure: does it cause corneal abrasions? British Medical Journal 284: 19
36. Corkery J J, Dubowitz V, Lister J, Moosa A 1968 Colonic perforation after exchange transfusion. British Medical Journal iv: 345–349
37. Couriel J, Phelan P D 1981 Subglottic cysts: a complication of neonatal endotracheal intubation. Pediatrics 68: 103–105
38. Cumming W A, Burchfield D J 1994 Accidental catheterization of internal iliac branches: a serious complication of umbilical artery catheterization. Journal of Perinatology 14: 304–309
39. Daniels S R, Hannon D W, Meyer R A, Kaplan S 1984 Paroxysmal supraventricular tachycardia: a complication of jugular central venous catheters in neonates. American Journal of Diseases of Children 138: 474–475
40. Davies J, Gault D, Buchdahl R 1994 Preventing the scars of neonatal intensive care. Archives of Disease in Childhood 70: F50–51
41. de Curtis M, Mastropasqua S, Paludetto R, Orzalesi M 1985 Gangrene of the buttock: a devastating complication of the infusion of hyperosmolar solutions in the umbilical artery at birth. European Journal of Pediatrics 144: 261–262
42. Dellagrammaticas H D, Papageorgeou A 1994 Unfriendly incubators. Archives of Disease in Childhood 71: F 148
43. den Guden A L, Berger H M, Ruys J H 1986 Scarring of the hands after venepunctures in babies. European Journal of Pediatrics 145: 58–59
44. de Sa D J 1983 Mucosal metaplasia and chronic inflammation in the middle ear of infants receiving intensive care in the neonatal period. Archives of Disease in Childhood 58: 24–28
45. Dhande V, Kattwinkel J, Alford B 1983 Recurrent bilateral pleural effusions secondary to superior vena cava obstruction as a complication of central venous catheterization. Pediatrics 72: 109–113
46. Dmochowski R R, Crandell S S, Corrieri V N 1986 Bladder injury and uroascites from umbilical artery catheterization. Pediatrics 77: 421–422
47. Doull I J M, Mok Q, Tasker R C 1997 Tracheobronchomalacia in preterm infants with chronic lung disease. Archives of Disease in Childhood 76: F203–205
48. Downing G J, Hayen L K, Kilbride H W 1993 Acquired subglottic cysts in the low birthweight infant. American Journal of Diseases of Children 147: 971–974
49. Drucker D E M, Greenfield L J, Ehrich F, Salzberg A M 1986 Aorto-iliac aneurysms following umbilical artery catheterization. Journal of Pediatric Surgery 21: 725–730
50. Duke P M, Coulson J D, Santos J I, Johnson J D 1976 Cleft palate associated with prolonged orotracheal intubation in infancy. Journal of Pediatrics 89: 990–991
51. Egan E A, Eitzman D V 1971 Umbilical vessel catheterization. American Journal of Diseases of Children 121: 213–218
52. Emami A, Saldanha R, Knupp C, Kodroff M 1987 Failure of systemic thrombolytic and heparin therapy in the treatment of neonatal aortic thrombosis. Pediatrics 79: 773–777
53. Erenberg A, Nowak A J 1984 Palatal groove formation in neonates and infants with orotracheal tubes. American Journal of Diseases of Children 138: 974–975
54. Esper E, Krabill K A, St Cyr J A, Patton C, Foker J E 1993 Repair of multiple mycotic aneurysms in a newborn. Journal of Pediatric Surgery 28: 1553–1556
55. Evans N J, Rutter N 1986 Reduction of skin damage from transcutaneous oxygen electrodes using a spray-on dressing. Archives of Disease in Childhood 61: 881–884
56. Fischer A Q, Strasburger J 1982 Foot drop in the neonate secondary to use of foot boards. Journal of Pediatrics 101: 1003–1004
57. Fleischman A R 1977 Another potential hazard of radiant warmers (letter). Journal of Pediatrics 91: 984
58. Garland J S, Dunne W M, Havens P et al 1992 Peripheral intravenous catheter complications in critically ill children: a prospective study. Pediatrics 89: 1145–1150
59. Garland J S, Nelson D B, Rice T, Neu J 1985 Increased risk of gastrointestinal perforations in neonates mechanically ventilated with either face mask or nasal prongs. Pediatrics 76: 406–410
60. Gau G S, Ryder T A, Mobberley M A 1987 Iatrogenic epithelial change caused by endotracheal intubation of neonates. Early Human Development 15: 221–229
61. Gault D T 1992 Vascular compromise in newborn infants. Archives of Disease in Childhood 67: 463–467
62. Gilles F H, Matson D D 1970 Sciatic nerve injury following misplaced gluteal injection. Journal of Pediatrics 76: 247–254
63. Ginoza G, Cortez S, Modanlou H D 1989 Prevention of palatal groove formation in premature neonates requiring intubation. Journal of Pediatrics 115: 133–135
64. Goetzman B W, Stradalnik R C, Bogren H G, Blankenship W J, Ikeda R M, Thayer J 1975 Thrombotic complications of umbilical artery catheters. A clinical and radiographic study. Pediatrics 56: 374–379
65. Golden S M 1981 Skin craters: a complication of transcutaneous oxygen monitoring. Pediatrics 67: 514–516
66. Gould S J, Howard S 1985 The histopathology of the larynx in the neonate following endotracheal intubation. Journal of Pathology 146: 301–311
67. Gowdar K, Bull M J, Schreiner R L, Lemons J A, Gresham E L 1980 Nasal deformities in neonates. American Journal of Diseases of Children 134: 954–957
68. Grosfield J L, Lemons J L, Ballantine T V N, Schreiner R L 1980 Emergency thoracotomy for acquired bronchopleural fistula in the premature infant with respiratory distress. Journal of Pediatric Surgery 15: 416–421

69. Gupta J M, Roberton N R C, Wigglesworth J S 1968 Umbilical artery catheterization of the newborn. Archives of Disease in Childhood 43: 382–387
70. Hack W W M, Van der Lei J, Okken A 1990 Incidence and duration of total occlusion of the radial artery in newborn infants after catheter withdrawal. European Journal of Pediatrics 149: 275–277
71. Haldeman S, Fowler G W, Ashwal S, Schneider S 1983 Acute flaccid neonatal paraplegia: a case report. Neurology 33: 93–95
72. Harpin V, Rutter N 1982 Percutaneous alcohol absorption and skin necrosis in a preterm infant. Archives of Disease in Childhood 57: 477–479
73. Hayhurst E G, Wyman M 1975 Morbidity associated with prolonged use of polyvinyl feeding tubes. American Journal of Diseases of Children 129: 72–74
74. Heath R E 1986 Vasospasm in the neonate: response to tolazoline. Pediatrics 77: 405–408
75. Henry C G, Gutierrez F, Lee J T et al 1981 Aortic thrombosis presenting as congestive heart failure: an umbilical artery complication. Journal of Pediatrics 98: 820–822
76. Hillman L S, Goodwin S L, Sherman W R 1975 Identification and measurement of plasticizers in neonatal tissues after umbilical catheters and blood products. New England Journal of Medicine 292: 381–386
77. Horgan M J, Bartoletti A, Polansky S, Peters J C, Manning T J, Lamont B M 1987 Effect of heparin infusates in umbilical artery catheters on frequency of thrombotic complications. Journal of Pediatrics 111: 774–778
78. Isenberg S, Everett S 1984 Cardiovascular effects of mydriatics in low-birth-weight infants. Journal of Pediatrics 105: 111–112
79. Jardine D S, Rogers K 1989 Relationship of benzyl alcohol to kernicterus, intraventricular hemorrhage and mortality in preterm infants. Pediatrics 83: 153–160
80. Johnson D E, Base J L, Thompson T R et al 1981 Candida septicemia and right atrial mass secondary to umbilical vein catheterization. American Journal of Diseases of Children 135: 275–277
81. Johnson D E, Foker J, Munson D P, Nelson A, Athinarayanan P, Thompson T R 1982 Management of esophageal and pharyngeal perforation in the newborn infant. Pediatrics 70: 592–596
82. Joshi V V, Mandavia S G, Stern L, Wigglesworth F W 1972 Acute lesions induced by endotracheal intubation. American Journal of Diseases of Children 124: 646–649
83. Junker P, Egeblad M, Nielson O, Kamper J 1976 Umbilical vein catherization and portal hypertension. Acta Paediatrica Scandinavica 65: 499–504
84. Kaufman J M, Sharada P, Austin T L et al 1983 Neonatal bladder injury occurring after umbilical artery catheterization by cut down. Journal of the American Medical Association 250: 2968–2970
85. Keeling J W 1993 Fetal and neonatal pathology, 2nd edn. Springer-Verlag, London, p. 333
86. Keeney S E, Richardson C J 1995 Extravascular extravasation of fluid as a complication of central venous lines in the neonate. Journal of Perinatology 15: 284–288
87. Kelly M A, Finer N N, Dunbar L G 1984 Fatal neurological complication of parenteral feeding through a central vein catheter. American Journal of Diseases of Children 138: 352–353
88. Kennedy L A, Drummond W H, Knight M E, Millsaps M M, Wilhams J L 1990 Successful treatment of neonatal aortic thrombosis with tissue plasminogen activator. Journal of Pediatrics 116: 798–801
89. Khilnani P, Toce S, Reddy R 1990 Mechanical complications from very small percutaneous central venous silastic catheters. Critical Care Medicine 18: 1477–1478
90. Kitterman J A 1979 Fatal air embolism through an umbilical venous catheter. European Journal of Pediatrics 131: 71–73
91. Kline A H, Blattner R J, Lunin M 1964 Transplacental effect of tetracyclines on teeth. Journal of the American Medical Association 188: 178–182
92. Koenigsberger M R, Moessinger A C 1977 Iatrogenic carpal tunnel syndrome in the newborn infant. Journal of Pediatrics 91: 443–445
93. Krasna I H, Rosenfeld D, Benjamin B G, Klein G, Hiatt M, Hegyi T 1987 Esophageal perforation in the neonate: an emerging problem in the newborn nursery. Journal of Pediatric Surgery 22: 784–790
94. Kreusser K L, Volpe J J 1984 Peroneal palsy produced by intravenous fluid administration in a newborn. Developmental Medicine and Child Neurology 26: 522–524
95. Krishnamoorthy K S, Fernandex M D, Todres I D, DeLong G R 1976 Paraplegia associated with umbilical artery catheterization in the newborn. Pediatrics 58: 443–445
96. Krueger T C, Neblett W W, O'Neill J A, MacDonnell R C, Dean R H, Thiema G A 1985 Management of aortic thrombosis secondary to umbilical artery catheters in neonates. Journal of Pediatric Surgery 20: 328–332
97. Kumar S P, Belik J 1984 Chylothorax – a complication of tube placement in the neonate. Critical Care Medicine 12: 411–412
98. Landers S, Moise A A, Fraley J K, Smith E O'B, Baker C J 1991 Factors associated with umbilical catheter related sepsis in neonates. American Journal of Diseases of Children 145: 675–678
99. Larroche J C 1970 Umbilical catheterization: its complications. Biology of the Neonate 16: 101–116
100. Lee S B, Kahn J P 1976 Esophageal perforation in the neonate. American Journal of Diseases of Children 130: 325–329
101. Lesko S M, Mitchell A A, Epstein M F et al 1986 Heparin use as a risk factor for intraventricular hemorrhage in low birthweight infants. New England Journal of Medicine 314: 1156–1160
102. Levy I, Mosseri R, Garty B 1996 Peripheral intravenous infusion – another cause of air embolism. Acta Paediatrica 85: 385–386
103. Lilien L D, Harris V J, Ramamurthy R S, Pildes R D 1976 Neonatal osteomyelitis of the calcaneus: complication of heel puncture. Journal of Pediatrics 88: 478–480
104. Lobe T E, Richardson C J, Boulden T F, Swischuk L E, Hayden K E, Oldham K T 1992 Mycotic thromboaneurysm of the abdominal aorta in preterm infants: its natural history and its management. Journal of Pediatric Surgery 27: 1054–1060
105. Lovejoy F H 1982 Fatal benzyl alcohol poisoning in neonatal intensive care units. American Journal of Diseases of Children 136: 974–976
106. Lowenstein E, Little J W, Lo, H H 1971 Prevention of cerebral embolization from flushing radial artery cannulae. New England Journal of Medicine 285: 1414–1415
107. Lucey J F, Dolan R G 1959 Hyperbilirubinemia of newborn infants associated with the parenteral administration of a vitamin K analogue to the mothers. Pediatrics 23: 553–560
108. McArtor R D, Saunders B S 1979 Iatrogenic second degree burns caused by a transilluminator. Pediatrics 63: 422–424
109. MacDonald M G, Getson P R, Glasgow A M, Miller M K, Boeckx R L, Johnson E L 1987 Propylene glycol: increased incidence of seizures in low birthweight infants. Pediatrics 79: 622–625
110. MacPherson T A, Shen-Schwarz S, Valdes-Dapena M 1988 Prevention and reduction of iatrogenic disorders in the newborn. In: Guthrie R D (ed). Neonatal intensive care: Clinics in Critical Care Medicine No. 13. Churchill Livingstone, New York, p. 271–312
111. Maki M, Ruuska J, Kuusela A L, Karikoski-Leo R 1993 High prevalence of asymptomatic esophageal and gastric lesions in preterm infants in intensive care. Critical Care Medicine 21: 1863–1867
112. Malin S W, Baumgart S, Rosenberg H K, Foreman J 1985 Non-surgical management of obstructive aortic thrombosis complicated by renovascular hypertension in the neonate. Journal of Pediatrics 106: 630–634
113. Manco-Johnson M J 1990 Diagnosis and management of thromboses in the perinatal period. Seminars in Perinatology 14: 393–402
114. Mann N P 1980 Gluteal skin necrosis after umbilical artery catheterization. Archives of Disease in Childhood 55: 815–817
115. Marinelli P V, Ortiz A, Alden E R 1981 Acquired eventration of the diaphragm: a complication of chest tube placement in neonatal pneumothorax. Pediatrics 67: 552–554
116. Marsh D, Wilkerson S A, Cook L M, Pietsch J B 1988 Right atrial thrombus formation screening using two dimensional echocardiograms in neonates with central venous catheters. Pediatrics 81: 284–287
117. Marsh J L, King W, Barrett C, Fonkalsrud E W 1975 Serious complications after umbilical artery catheterization for neonatal monitoring. Archives of Surgery 110: 1203–1205
118. Mehta S, Connors A F, Danish E H, Grisoni E 1992 Incidence of thrombosis during central venous catheterization of newborns: a prospective study. Journal of Pediatric Surgery 27: 18–22
119. Mendoza G J B, Soto A, Brown E G, Dolgin S E, Steinfeld L, Sweet A W 1986 Intracardiac thrombi complicating central total parenteral nutrition: resolution without surgery or thrombolysis. Journal of Pediatrics 108: 610–613
120. Merton D F, Mumford L, Filstron H C, Brumley G W, Offman E L, Grossman H 1980 Radiological observations during transpyloric tube feeding in infants of low birthweight. Radiology 136: 67–75

121. Miller D, Kirkpatrick B V, Kodroff M, Ehrlich F E, Salzberg A M 1979 Pelvic exsanguination following umbilical artery catheterization in neonates. Journal of Pediatric Surgery 14: 264–269
122. Moclair A, Bates I 1995 The efficacy of heparin in maintaining peripheral infusions in neonates. European Journal of Pediatrics 154: 567–570
123. Moessinger A C, Driscoll J M, Wigger H J 1978 High incidence of lung perforation by chest tube in neonatal pneumothorax. Journal of Pediatrics 92: 635–637
124. Mokrohisky S T, Levine R L, Blumhagen J D, Wesenberg R L, Simmons M A 1978 Low positioning of umbilical artery catheters increases associated complications in newborn infants. New England Journal of Medicine 299: 561–564
125. Morley C J, Hewson P H, Thornton A J, Cole T J 1992 Axillary and rectal temperature measurements in children. Archives of Disease in Childhood 67: 122–125
126. Morrell P, Hey E, Mackee I W, Rutter N, Lewis M 1985 Deafness in preterm baby associated with topical antibiotic spray containing neomycin. Lancet i: 1167–1168
127. Moylan F M B, Seldin E B, Shannon D C, Todres I D 1980 Defective primary dentition in survivors of neonatal mechanical ventilation. Journal of Pediatrics 96: 106–108
128. Nagaraj H S, Shott R, Fellows R, Yacoub U 1980 Recurrent lobar atelectasis due to acquired bronchial stenosis in neonates. Journal of Pediatric Surgery 15: 411–415
129. Neal W A, Reynolds J W, Jarvis C W, Williams H J 1972 Umbilical artery catheterization: demonstration of arterial thrombosis by aortography. Pediatrics 50: 6–13
130. Neubauer A-P 1995 Percutaneous central i.v. access in the neonate: experience with 535 silastic catheters. Acta Paediatrica 84: 756–760
131. Norman M G, Temple A R, Murphy J V 1970 Infantile quadriceps femoris contracture resulting from intramuscular injections. New England Journal of Medicine 282: 964–966
132. Nour S, Puntis J W L, Stringer M D 1995 Intra-abdominal extravasation complicating parenteral nutrition in infants. Archives of Disease in Childhood 72: F207–208
133. Nowak C M, Waffarn F, Sills J H, Pousti T M, Warden M J, Cumingham M D 1994 Focal intestinal perforation in the extremely low birthweight infant. Journal of Perinatology 14: 450–453
134. Nowak-Gottl U, von Kries R, Gobel U 1997 Neonatal symptomatic thromboembolism in Germany: two year survey. Archives of Disease in Childhood 76: F163–167
135. O'Neill J A, Neblett W W, Born M L 1981 Management of major thromboembolic complications of umbilical artery catheters. Journal of Paediatric Surgery 16: 972–978
136. Ontell S J, Gauderer M W L 1985 Iatrogenic arteriovenous fistula after multiple arterial punctures. Pediatrics 76: 97–98
137. Oppenheimer D A, Carroll B A, Garth K E 1982 Ultrasonic detection of complications following umbilical artery catheterization in the neonate. Radiology 145: 667–672
138. Orme R. L'E, Eades S M 1968 Perforation of the bowel in the newborn as a complication of exchange transfusion. British Medical Journal iv: 349–351
139. Oski F A, Allen D M, Diamond L K 1963 Portal hypertension – a complication of umbilical vein catheterization. Pediatrics 31: 297–302
140. Pape K E, Armstrong D L, Fitzhardinge P M 1976 Central nervous system pathology associated with mask ventilation in the very low birthweight infant. A new etiology for intracerebellar hemorrhages. Pediatrics 58: 473–483
141. Pape K E, Armstrong D L, Fitzhardinge P M 1978 Peripheral median nerve damage secondary to brachial artery blood gas sampling. Journal of Pediatrics 93: 852–856
142. Payne R M, Martin T C, Bower R J, Canter C E 1989 Management and follow-up of arterial thrombosis in the neonatal period. Journal of Pediatrics 114: 853–858
143. Pearse R G 1978 Percutaneous catheterization of the radial artery in newborn babies using transillumination. Archives of Disease in Childhood 53: 549–554
144. Perez-Rodriguez J, Quero J, Frias E G, Omenaca F 1978 Duodenal perforation in a neonate by a tube of silicon rubber during transpyloric feeding. Journal of Pediatrics 92: 113–114
145. Peters J L, Armstrong R 1977 Air embolism as a complication of central venous catheterization. Annals of Surgery 187: 375–378
146. Phelps S J, Helms R A, 1987 Risk factors affecting infiltration of peripheral venous lines in infants. Journal of Pediatrics 111: 384–389
147. Phillips R R, Lee S H 1990 Fractures of long bones occurring in neonatal intensive therapy units. British Medical Journal 301: 225–226
148. Piotrowski A, Kawczynski P 1995 Cannulation of the axillary artery in critically ill newborn infants. European Journal of Pediatrics 154: 57–59
149. Plumer L B, Kaplan G W, Mendoza S A 1976 Hypertension in infants – a complication of umbilical arterial catheterization. Journal of Pediatrics 89: 802–805
150. Prian G W 1977 Complications and sequelae of temporal artery catheterization in the high risk newborn. Journal of Pediatric Surgery 12: 829–835
151. Purohit P M, Levkoff A H, de Vito P C 1978 Gluteal necrosis with foot drop. Complications associated with umbilical artery catheterization. American Journal of Diseases of Children 132: 897–899
152. Quak J M E, Szatmari A, van den Anker J N 1993 Cardiac tamponade in a preterm neonate secondary to a chest tube. Acta Paediatrica 82: 490–491
153. Rajani K, Goetzman B W, Wemberg R P, Tumer E, Abildgaard C 1979 Effect of heparinization of fluids infused through an umbilical artery catheter on catheter patency and frequency of complications. Pediatrics 63: 552–556
154. Rajs J, Finnstrom O, Wesstrom G 1976 Aortic aneursym developing after umbilical artery catheterization. Acta Paediatrica Scandinavica 65: 495–498
155. Rehan V K, Cronin C M G, Bowman J M 1994 Neonatal portal vein thrombosis successfully treated by regional streptokinase infusion. European Journal of Pediatrics 153: 456–459
156. Rey C, Marache P, Watel A, Francart C 1987 Iatrogenic false aneurysm of the brachial artery in an infant. European Journal of Pediatrics 146: 438–439
157. Reynolds E O R 1963 Arterial blood gas tensions in acute disease of lower respiratory tract in infancy. British Medical Journal i: 1192–1195
158. Richardson R, Applebaum H, Touran T et al 1988 Effective thrombolytic therapy of aortic thrombosis in the small premature infant. Journal of Pediatric Surgery 12: 1198–1200
159. Robertson N J, McCarthy L S, Hamilton P A, Moss A L H 1996 Nasal deformities resulting from flow driver continuous positive airway pressure. Archives of Disease in Childhood 75: F209–212
160. Rosenthal A, Anderson M, Thomson S J, Pappas A M, Fyler D C 1972 Superficial femoral artery catheterization. American Journal of Diseases of Children 124: 240–242
161. Rubin S P, Hewson P, Roberton N R C 1986 Pulmonary complications of total parenteral nutrition in a neonate. Journal of the Royal Society of Medicine 79: 545–547
162. Rubin S P, Roberton N R C 1991 Intestinal perforation without necrotizing enterocolitis in very low birthweight infants with umbilical arterial catheters. Pediatric Reviews and Communications 6: 51–54
163. Rush M G, Hazinski T A 1992 Current therapy of bronchopulmonary dysplasia. Clinics in Perinatology 19: 563–590
164. Rushforth A, Green M A, Levene M I, Puntis J W L 1991 Subdural fat effusion complicating parenteral nutrition. Archives of Disease in Childhood 66: 1350–1351
165. Sarrut S, Alain J, Alison F 1969 Les complications précoces de la perfusion par la veine ombilicale chez le prémature. Archives Français de Pédiatrie 26: 651–667
166. Sasidharan P, Bilhnan D, Heimler R, Nelin L 1996 Cardiac arrest in an extremely low birthweight infant: complication of percutaneous central venous catheter placement. Journal of Perinatology 16: 123–126
167. Schmidt B, Andrew M 1995 Neonatal thrombosis: report of a prospective Canadian and international registry. Pediatrics 96: 939–943
168. Schreiber M D, Perez C A, Kitterman J A 1984 A double-catheter technique for caudally misdirected umbilical artery catheters. Journal of Pediatrics 104: 768–769
169. Scott J M 1965 Iatrogenic lesions in babies following umbilical vein catheterization Archives of Disease in Childhood 40: 426–429
170. Seguin J H 1992 Right sided hydrothorax and central venous catheters in extremely low birthweight infants. American Journal of Perinatology 9: 154–158
171. Seibert J J, Lindley S G, Sutterfield S L, Seibert R W, Mollitt D L 1986 Umbilical artery clot in the neonate: spontaneous resolution. Journal of Pediatric Surgery 11: 973–974
172. Seibert J J, Northington F J, Miers J F, Taylor B J 1991 Aortic thrombosis after umbilical artery catheterization in neonates.

Prevalence of complications on long term follow-up. American Journal of Roentgenology 156: 567–569
173. Sell E J, Hansen R C, Struck-Pierce S 1980 Calcified nodules on the heel: a complication of neonatal intensive care. Journal of Pediatrics 96: 473–475
174. Sengupta S 1985 Pathogenesis of infantile quadriceps fibrosis and its correction by proximal release. Journal of Pediatric Orthopedics 5: 187–191
175. Serlin S P, Dally W J R 1975 Tracheal perforation in the neonate: a complication of endotracheal intubation. Journal of Pediatrics 86: 596–597
176. Shuman R M, Leech R W, Alvord E C 1974 Neurotoxicity of hexachlorophene in the human. 1. A clinical pathological study of 248 children. Pediatrics 54: 689–695
177. Silverman W A, Andersen D H, Blanc W A, Rozier D N 1956 A difference in mortality rate and incidence of kernicterus among premature infants alloted to two antibacterial regimes. Pediatrics 18: 614–625
178. Simmons M A, Levine R L, Lubehenko L O, Guggenheim M A 1978 Warning: serious sequelae of temporal artery catheterization. Journal of Pediatrics 92: 284
179. Sirnon-Fayard E E, Kroncke R S, Solarte D, Peverini R 1997 Non-surgical retrieval of embolised umbilical catheters in premature infants. Journal of Perinatology 17: 143–147
180. Simonsen K, Graem N, Rothman L P, Degn H 1995 Iatrogenic radiant heat burns in severely asphyxic newborn. Acta Paediatrica 84: 1438–1440
181. Simpson J S 1975 Misdiagnosis, complicating umbilical vessel catheterization. Clinical Pediatrics 14: 727–729
182. Skoglund R R, Giles E E 1986 The false cortical thumb. American Journal of Diseases of Children 140: 375–376
183. Slogoff S, Keats A S, Arlund C 1983 On the safety of radial artery cannulation. Anesthesiology 59: 42–47
184. Smerdely P, Boyages S C, Wu D et al 1989 Topical iodine-containing antiseptics and neonatal hypothyroidism in very low birthweight infants. Lancet ii: 661
185. Smith P L 1978 Umbilical catheter retrieval in the premature infant. Journal of Pediatrics 93: 499–502
186. Sobel D B 1992 Burning of a neonate due to a pulse oximeter: arterial saturation monitoring. Pediatrics 89: 154–155
187. Spahr R C, MacDonald H M, Holzrnan I R 1979 Catheterization of the posterior tibial artery in the neonate. American Journal of Diseases of Children 133: 945–946
188. Stavis R L, Krauss A N 1980 Complications of neonatal intensive care. Clinics in Perinatology 7: 107–124
189. Stewart D R, Johnson D G, Myers G G 1975 Hydrocephalus as a complication of jugular catheterization during total parenteral nutrition. Journal of Pediatric Surgery 10: 771–777
190. Strife J L, Ball W S, Towbin R, Keller M S, Dillon T 1988 Arterial occlusions of neonates. Use of fibrinolytic therapy. Radiology 166: 395–400
191. Sutcliffe A G 1995 Total parenteral nutrition tamponade. Journal of the Royal Society of Medicine 88: 173–174
192. Tager I B, Ginsberg M B, Ellis S E et al 1983 An epidemiological study of the risks associated with intravenous catheters. American Journal of Epidemiology 118: 839–851
193. Thompson E N, Sherlock S 1964 The aetiology of portal vein thrombosis with particular reference to the role of infection and exchange transfusion. Quarterly Journal of Medicine 33: 465–480
194. Todres L D, Rogers M C, Shannon D C, Moylan F C, Ryan J F 1975 Percutaneous catheterization of the radial artery in the critically ill neonate. Journal of Pediatrics 87: 273–275
195. Touloukian R J, Kadar A, Spencer R P 1973 The gastrointestinal complications of neonatal umbilical venous exchange transfusion. A clinical and experimental study. Pediatrics 51: 36–43
196. Tyson J E, de Sa D J, Moore S 1976 Thromboatheromatous complications of umbilical arterial catheterization in the newborn period: clinical pathological study. Archives of Disease in Childhood 51: 744–754
197. Urbach J, Kaplan M, Blondheim O, Hersch H J 1985 Neonatal hypoglycemia related to umbilical artery catheter malfunction. Journal of Pediatrics 106: 825–826
198. Vailas G N, Brouillette R T, Scott J P, Shkolnik A, Conway J, Wiringa K 1986 Neonatal aortic thrombosis: recent experience. Journal of Pediatrics 109: 101–108
199. van den Anker J N, Baerts W, Quak J M et al 1992 Iatrogenic perforation of the lamina cribrosa by nasogastric tube in an infant. Pediatric Radiology 22: 545–546
200. van Vliet P J K, Gupta J M 1973 Prophylactic antibiotics in umbilical catheterization in the newborn. Archives of Disease in Childhood 48: 296–300
201. Vaughan R S, Menke J A, Giacoia G P 1978 Pneumothorax: a complication of endotracheal tube suctioning. Journal of Pediatrics 92: 633–634
202. Wall P M, Kuhns L R 1977 Percutaneous arterial sampling using transillumination. Pediatrics 59: 1032–1035
203. Ward R M 1984 Pharmacology of tolazoline. Clinics in Perinatology 11: 703–713
204. Wehbe M A, Moore J H 1985 Digital ischemia following intravenous therapy. Pediatrics 76: 99–103
205. Wesstrom G, Finnstrom O 1979 Umbilical artery catheterization in newborns. II. Infections in relation to catheterization. Acta Paediatrica Scandinavica 68: 713–718
206. Wesstrom G, Finnstrom O, Stenport G 1979 Umbilical artery catheterization in newborns. 1. Thrombosis in relation to catheter type and position. Acta Paediatrica Scandinavica 68: 575–581
207. Wiedersberg H, Pawlowski P 1974 Anaemic necrosis of the liver after umbilical vein catheterization. Helvetica Paediatrica Acta 34: 53–62
208. Wilkinson A R, Baum J D, Keeling J W 1981 Superficial skin necrosis in babies prepared for umbilical arterial catheterization. Archives of Disease in Childhood 56: 237–238
209. Williams J H, Hunter J E, Kanto W P, Bhatia J 1995 Hemidiaphragmatic paralysis as a complication of central venous catheterization in a neonate. Journal of Perinatology 15: 386–388
210. Williams J W, Rittenberry A, Dillard R, Allen R G 1973 Liver abscess in newborn: complication of umbilical vein catheterization. American Journal of Diseases of Children 125: 111–113
211. Wiswell T E, Turner B S, Bley J A, Fritz D L, Hunt R E 1989 Determinants of tracheobronchial histologic alterations during conventional mechanical ventilation. Pediatrics 84: 304–311
212. Wong A F, McCulloch L M, Sola A 1992 Treatment of peripheral tissue ischemia with topical nitroglycerine ointment in neonates. Journal of Pediatrics 121: 980–983
213. Wood B P 1987 Infant ribs: generalized periosteal reaction resulting from vibrator chest physiotherapy. Radiology 162: 811–812
214. Wright I M R, Puntis J W L 1993 A case of skin necrosis related to a pulse oximeter probe. British Journal of Intensive Care 3: 394–398
215. Young S, MacMahon P, Kovar I Z 1989 Subdural intravenous fat collection – an unusual complication of central intravenous feeding in the neonate. Journal of Parenteral and Enteral Nutrition 13: 661–662

38

Metabolic disease

Part 1

Disorders of blood glucose homoeostasis in the neonate

J. M. Hawdon A. Aynsley-Green

INTRODUCTION

Neonatal hypoglycaemia has been recognized for many years,[38,130,143] although with time there have been wide swings of opinion regarding the definition of the condition, its clinical significance and its optimal management. For example, in the era when routine postnatal management involved the withholding of feeds from healthy infants for up to 24 hours, and even longer in sick or small babies, many were found to have low blood glucose concentrations, and this became accepted as a normal finding.[42,43] However, to others it was apparent that some of these babies had clinical signs of hypoglycaemia, and the risk of reduced glucose availability to the brain was acknowledged even for babies with no signs. Neligan[113] summarized the level of anxiety: 'Certainly the risk of such complications forms a cogent incentive to all concerned to make the diagnosis as early as possible in every case'.

Such anxieties were later reawakened by the publication of papers by Koh et al[90] and Lucas et al[101] which suggested that there were significant neurological sequelae of hypoglycaemia. This resulted in a swing towards the treatment of large numbers of infants with intravenous glucose, which involved separation from their mothers and placed at risk the establishment of breast-feeding. Subsequent research has demonstrated that many infants may be protected from the neurological effects of hypoglycaemia by virtue of the availability of alternative cerebral fuels, so that this management may be overly intensive if applied to all babies.[74] Therefore, it is important to identify those infants most at risk of neurological sequelae and determine the most effective and least invasive regimens for their prevention. To date, no controlled studies have addressed either of these issues.

Hyperglycaemia was recognized as a neonatal complication over a century ago,[89] but until recent times was a rare phenomenon. However, it is now commonly seen in the increasing numbers of extremely low-birthweight infants who are cared for in our neonatal units. As such, there is still some uncertainty as to its clinical significance and optimal management.

To manage these disorders of blood glucose homoeostasis it is essential to understand the metabolism of the fetus and neonate and the changes that occur at birth in the healthy infant. This chapter will summarize the current knowledge of the disorders of blood glucose homoeostasis, and aims to provide a practical and pragmatic approach to the management of babies with hypoglycaemia and hyperglycaemia.

GLUCOSE HOMOEOSTASIS IN THE HEALTHY FETUS AND NEONATE

FETAL METABOLISM

During pregnancy the human fetus receives from its mother, via the placental circulation, a supply of substrates necessary for growth, for the deposition of fuel stores which are essential after birth (see below), and for energy to meet the basal metabolic rate and requirements for growth. Glucose is transported across the placenta by facilitated diffusion, but during maternal starvation or placental insufficiency the fetus is capable of endogenous glucose production.[76] Glucose metabolism accounts for

65% of fetal energy production, with lactate probably accounting for most of the remainder.[27,76] Glucose is not the only fuel utilized by the fetal brain. Studies of perfused human fetal brain have demonstrated that uptake of ketone bodies, the products of β oxidation of fatty acids, is greater than that of glucose and it is likely that the fate of ketone bodies is both incorporation into brain lipids and for use as a cerebral energy source.[2] Lactate may also be metabolized.

The fetus is usually capable of regulating its glucose concentrations independently of maternal hormones. This capacity is seen in some cases of placental insufficiency (see above), when gluconeogenesis is activated, and in the fetus of the diabetic mother (Chapter 24), who responds to the high placental transfer of glucose by secreting high concentrations of insulin. However, the healthy fetus differs from adults in that there is a blunted insulin response to high glucose concentrations, and that insulin secretion is more sensitive to amino acids than glucose.[110,114] In fact, it appears that insulin has a greater role in fetal growth than in fetal metabolic control. Similarly, the fetus is less sensitive than the neonate to the glucose-mobilizing actions of glucagon, although sensitivity increases with gestational age.[145]

Under extreme circumstances fetal blood glucose control fails. For example, in some cases of placental insufficiency leading to intrauterine growth retardation fetal hypoglycaemia may occur.[69,141] If prolonged periods of postnatal hypoglycaemia cause long-term neurological damage, it is possible that such profound and prolonged fetal hypoglycaemia may have the same effect and may explain some of the handicap following intrauterine growth retardation, even when there have been no postnatal complications.

METABOLIC CHANGES AT BIRTH

These changes are essential to preserve fuel supplies for vital organ function when the continuous flow of nutrients from the placenta is abruptly discontinued. As oxygen supply also temporarily fails, anaerobic metabolism must occur and this requires higher substrate availability than aerobic metabolism. In addition, the newborn infant must adapt to the change in major energy source, from glucose from the placenta to fat from adipose tissue stores and in milk feeds, and to the fast-feed cycle. After birth, plasma insulin levels fall and there are rapid surges of catecholamine and pancreatic glucagon release.[31,64] These endocrine changes switch on the essential enzymes for glycogenolysis (the release of glucose stored as glycogen in liver, cardiac muscle and brain), for gluconeogenesis (glucose production from 3-carbon precursor molecules by the liver), lipolysis (release of fatty acids from adipose tissue stores), and ketogenesis (the β oxidation of fatty acids by the liver). Although glucose is the major metabolic fuel for most organs in the immediate postnatal period, there is evidence that lactate may be the preferred cerebral fuel over glucose and ketone bodies at this time.[106]

NEONATAL METABOLISM

The metabolic processes of fetal life and at birth are repeated on a smaller scale during the milk-fed infant's fast-feed cycles. Immediately after a feed there is availability of metabolic fuels, namely fatty acids and, to a lesser extent, sugars from milk. Some tissues, for example the kidney, are obligate glucose users, but others burn fatty fuels and the respiratory quotient falls after birth, reflecting the fact that fat oxidation accounts for about 75% of oxygen consumption. Of the organs that utilize alternative fuels to glucose, the brain is the most important in that it takes up and oxidizes ketone bodies at higher rates than seen in adults, and the neonatal brain uses ketone bodies more efficiently than glucose.[53]

Any excess glucose available after a feed is stored as glycogen in the liver or converted to fat for deposition in adipose tissue, along with fatty acids absorbed after milk feeds.

Between feeds, blood glucose levels start to fall and glycogenolysis and gluconeogenesis are again activated to ensure availability for organs which are obligate users (Fig. 38.1). Glycogenolysis is an exhaustible source of glucose whose capacity varies according to fetal growth and maturity,[135] and after approximately 2 hours gluconeogenesis must become the major glucose-providing process. Stable isotope turnover studies have shown that

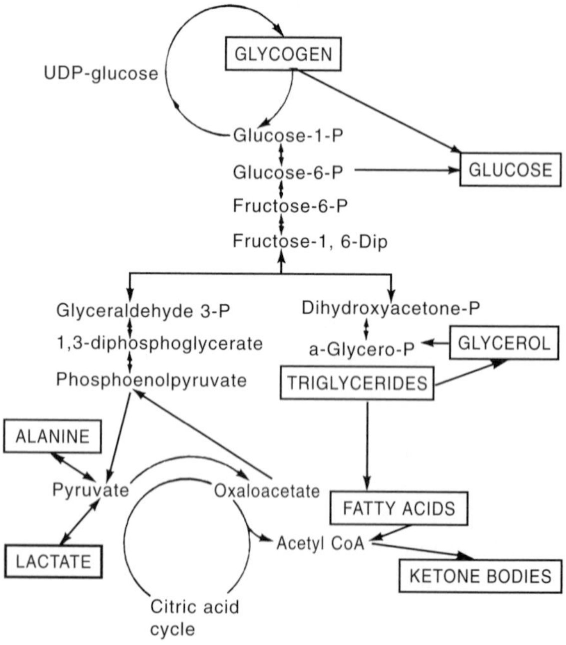

Fig. 38.1 Metabolic pathways involved in gluconeogenesis (pathways below glucose-6-P) and in glycogen synthesis (above glucose-6-P) and glycogenolysis. Galactose enters the pathways above glucose-6-P.

neonatal glucose production rates are 4–6 mg/kg/min.[29,32] Between feeds, lipolysis and ketogenesis provide alternative fuels to glucose for organs such as the brain, which are not obligate glucose utilizers.[69] The process of ketogenesis also provides energy and cofactors which are utilized in gluconeogenesis, again highlighting the importance of fatty fuels.

The control of neonatal metabolism is dependent first on the synthesis of key enzymes, such as hepatic phosphorylase for glycogenolysis, PEPCK for gluconeogenesis, and carnitine acyltransferases for ketogenesis, and secondly, on the induction of enzyme activity by hormonal changes. Glucagon is the major neonatal glucoregulatory hormone.[144] Its concentration increases when blood glucose levels fall, and it induces activity of the enzymes of glycogenolysis, gluconeogenesis and ketogenesis in the liver. The glucoregulatory role of insulin in the neonate is less clear and may well differ from that in the adult (see below). In most neonates insulin does not appear to have a major influence on normal blood glucose homoeostasis, but in some extreme cases (see below) high insulin concentrations may result in hypoglycaemia. Finally, it is unlikely that other hormones, such as the catecholamines, cortisol, thyroid hormones and growth hormone, are important regulators in the fast-feed cycle of the healthy neonate, but rare cases of hypopituitarism or cortisol deficiency (see below) may present with neonatal hypoglycaemia, which suggests that minimum basal levels are needed to maintain normoglycaemia.

Finally, the change from fetal to neonatal metabolism must take into account the important role of gastrointestinal adaptation. It is possible that the introduction of enteral feeding triggers the secretion of gastrointestinal regulatory peptides and hormones, which in turn induce the features of gut adaptation, namely gut growth, mucosal differentiation, induction of motor activity and the development of digestion and absorption.[19,100]

DIFFERENCES BETWEEN NEONATAL AND ADULT METABOLISM

It is apparent that neonates do not follow the same metabolic 'rules' as adults. Milk-fed neonates utilize ketone bodies to the extent seen in adults only after a prolonged fast, and thus have the mechanisms to support this. Other fuels such as lactate may also be used, in addition to glucose and ketone bodies. Insulin plays a lesser role in glucoregulation in the neonate than in the adult, in that its release in response to glucose is blunted and delayed when compared to the adult, and that there may be end-organ insensitivities to its action.[84] In fact, healthy neonates have insulin–glucose relationships that differ markedly from those of older subjects.[70,75] Therefore, when interpreting studies of impaired neonatal glucoregulation it is essential to have reference data from healthy infants, rather than comparing the neonatal concentrations and interrelationships of fuels and hormones with those of adults. Also, it is impossible to consider glucose alone, and the availability of alternative fuels must be established.

HYPOGLYCAEMIA

CLINICAL SIGNIFICANCE

The controversy regarding the clinical significance of neonatal hypoglycaemia mirrors that surrounding its definition.[45] Blood glucose levels fall immediately after birth but rise after a few hours either spontaneously or in response to feeding, in almost all healthy full-term infants.[69,119,146] This brief period of 'hypoglycaemia' cannot be considered of clinical significance, and indeed if it were so would lead to the admission of large numbers of infants to neonatal units for treatment. No studies of human neonates have addressed the duration of hypoglycaemia which is harmful, but a recent study of neonatal monkeys demonstrated that a duration of 6 hours was not associated with subsequent abnormalities, whereas 10 hours of severe hypoglycaemia were associated with 'motivational and adaptability' problems 8 months later.[128] In the light of the paucity of human neonatal data and the variability between babies with regard to exacerbating factors and protective mechanisms, it is impossible to state the duration of hypoglycaemia that is harmful to human neonates, but we suspect that prolonged periods (at least 12–24 hours) in the 'at-risk' groups of human neonates may lead to neurological sequelae, and that brief self-limiting episodes are of no neurological significance if not accompanied by clinical signs or coexisting clinical complications.

Acute neurophysiological changes at low blood glucose levels have been demonstrated in human neonates and those of other species.[90,156] However, the long-term significance of these acute changes is not clear. There is no doubt that a number of infants have fits or a reduced level of consciousness when blood glucose levels are low, and some authors have described adverse long-term outcomes when neurological signs have been present.[62,131] Profound hypoglycaemia, usually the result of serious inborn errors of metabolism, may even result in 'cot death' or apparent life-threatening events. Other clinical signs have often been associated with hypoglycaemia, namely tremor, irritability, 'jitteriness', apnoea, hypotonia, abnormal cry, tachypnoea, pallor and feeding difficulties. However, these are more likely to be the result of coexisting clinical complications such as perinatal asphyxia or the cause of hypoglycaemia (e.g. poor feeding) than the specific effects of hypoglycaemia.

No study has clearly demonstrated the independent contribution of hypoglycaemia (with or without signs) to neurodevelopmental outcome because all studies to date are of neonates who had other adverse clinical factors.[45]

However, it is possible that severe prolonged hypoglycaemia may have long-term as well as acute neurological effects, especially if there are coexisting adverse perinatal events such as asphyxia.

Although there is a paucity of information regarding the histopathological changes associated with neonatal hypoglycaemia, and the reports of past studies are conflicting, the current view is that hypoglycaemia must be both profound and prolonged before structural changes are seen in the brain.[9,16,25,63,142] Animal studies have shown that structural changes, when present, are in a distribution characteristic of dendritic loss secondary to a neurotoxic agent,[16] and authors have postulated that neuroexcitatory transmitters such as glutamate accumulate during hypoglycaemia and that their action on neuronal NMDA receptors causes depolarization and cell damage.[22]

For infants with multisystem problems (for example the preterm or asphyxiated infant) all *potential* causes of neurological damage should be prevented and treated as far as possible, and in practice the management of hypoglycaemia is often the easiest of clinical issues.

Finally, the impact of hypoglycaemia and its treatment on the mother and baby must be considered. The early neonatal period is an emotionally sensitive time, and the diagnosis of hypoglycaemia may create or add to anxiety for the parents. Treatment of the infant with intravenous glucose usually involves separation of the baby and mother, and may be perceived as invasive or painful. The implications for the establishment of breast-feeding must also not be forgotten.[54,65] Therefore, emphasis should be on the early prevention of hypoglycaemia and strategies of management that do not involve the separation of mother and baby.

PREVALENCE OF NEONATAL HYPOGLYCAEMIA

Because clinical practices have changed to such an extent since the risks of hypoglycaemia were first identified, and because of the controversy surrounding definition, it is difficult to comment on the prevalence of hypoglycaemia in the at-risk groups. For example, using the definition proposed by Cornblath,[42,43] prevalences in term infants ranged from 5% to 7.9% for term infants and 3.2% to 15% in preterm infants.[42,56,69,78] Using the more recently suggested level for blood glucose concentrations (2.6 mmol/l), Lucas et al[101] reported a prevalence of 67%, whereas a more recent study of clinically stable, AGA, term and preterm neonates reported prevalences of 10% and 4%, respectively.[69] The lower incidence reported in preterm infants in the most recent study[69] may reflect the trend away from clinicians' accepting the previous definitions of hypoglycaemia and thus aiming to maintain higher blood glucose levels in preterm infants. The prevalence of low blood glucose concentrations in the healthy, AGA term population is unlikely to be of clinical concern in the light of the protective ketone body response, but early monitoring and the prevention of hypoglycaemia in at-risk groups should take place in order to minimize its occurrence in such groups.

DEFINITION AND DIAGNOSIS

Definition

Much controversy and confusion has surrounded the definition of hypoglycaemia.[42,45,91] For example, Koh et al[91] demonstrated that the definition varied widely not only among standard paediatric textbooks but also among neonatologists, with values given ranging from below 1 mmol/l to below 4 mmol/l. The ideal definition of hypoglycaemia should include the blood glucose concentration considered to be the minimum safe level, the length of time beyond which the low blood glucose level is considered to be harmful, the presence of clinical signs, the group of infants studied, the consideration of alternative fuel availability, the conditions of sampling and the assay methods. Most of these criteria have never been adequately addressed by previous studies or publications.

Previous widely used definitions were based on cross-sectional samples from newborn babies, with the assumption that those with the lowest blood glucose levels were abnormal.[42,43] This led to definitions of hypoglycaemia as follows: term infants less than 48 hours old – blood glucose level less than 1.7 mmol/l; term infants more than 48 hours old – less than 2.2 mmol/l; preterm infants less than 1.1 mmol/l. However, these definitions were proposed at a time when, unlike the present, infants were starved for considerable periods after birth, and small and preterm infants received less milk than healthy term infants. Therefore, it is not surprising that so many infants on the first postnatal day had low blood glucose levels. The trend towards early feeding of infants has been associated with a more rapid increase in blood glucose concentration after the immediate postnatal fall[19,146] (Fig. 38.2). Fortunately, the long-standing belief that the brains of preterm infants were more able to withstand low blood glucose levels than those of term infants is now less widely accepted.[44,91,159]

More recently, this statistical definition of hypoglycaemia has been challenged and a 'functional' definition has been proposed, which is 'at what level of blood glucose is the body's function, particularly that of the brain, compromised?' It is not possible to define hypoglycaemia from the blood glucose level at which symptoms occur, because, unlike adults and older children, babies cannot complain of symptoms and by the time blood glucose levels have fallen so low that clinical signs of cerebral dysfunction occur in neonates there is a risk that brain damage may have been sustained. There is no doubt that any low blood glucose concentration of any duration which causes clinical signs, such as fits or coma, is *too low*, regardless of its numerical value, and must be treated. In

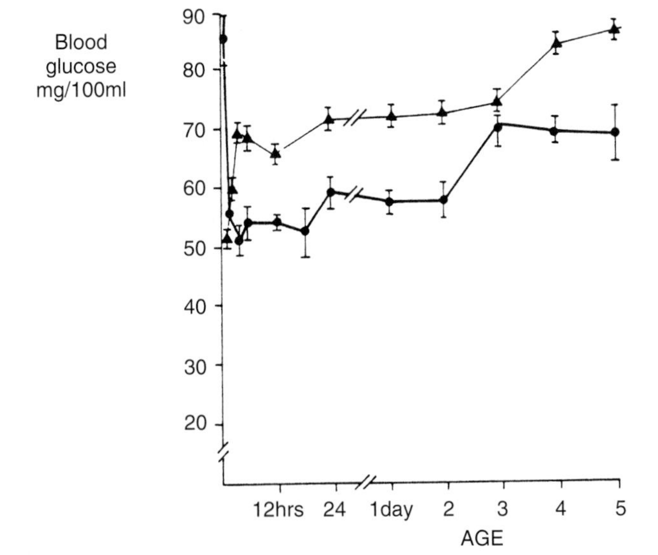

Fig. 38.2 Blood glucose levels (mean ± SE) in full-term infants showing the changing pattern of development during the first postnatal days in 1965, compared with 1986 (•, Cornblath & Reisner[42]; ▲, Srinivasan et al[146]). To convert mg/100 ml into mmol/l divide by 18.

fact, the rapid clinical resolution of the signs after the intravenous administration of glucose confirms the diagnosis of cerebral dysfunction secondary to hypoglycaemia.

Only two studies have addressed the 'safe level' for blood glucose concentrations in neonates without apparent clinical signs.[90,101] In a neurodevelopmental follow-up study of very low-birthweight preterm infants, Lucas et al[101] found that neonatal blood glucose concentrations below 2.6 mmol/l on at least 3 days were associated with a poor neurodevelopmental outcome. The neurophysiological study of Koh et al[90] demonstrated that in a group of subjects which included five neonates of varying birthweights and gestations, no baby with a blood glucose level above 2.6 mmol/l had abnormal sensory evoked brain-stem potentials. No differences were found in the blood glucose threshold for abnormal SEPs between subjects who had symptoms of hypoglycaemia and those who were asymptomatic. Thus both studies suggested that blood glucose levels less than 2.6 mmol/l are associated with abnormal acute and prolonged neurological function, and that levels above this could be considered safe. However, the subjects of the studies were not representative of all neonates, and there have been no prospective studies of the effects of neonatal hypoglycaemia in individual 'at-risk' groups which satisfactorily control for the effects of other neonatal complications.

No study has yet addressed the duration of hypoglycaemia or of acute neurological dysfunction which is harmful to the human neonate, but a study of rhesus monkeys has shown that a duration of neonatal hypoglycaemia (blood glucose less than 1.5 mmol/l) of 6.5 hours had no demonstrable long-term effects, whereas 10 hours of hypoglycaemia was associated with 'motivational and adaptability problems' but no motor or cognitive deficit on testing at 8 months of age.[128]

Another factor not previously addressed is that babies vary in their ability to mount protective metabolic responses when blood glucose levels are low. Indeed, there is evidence that glucose utilization by the neonatal brain is less than in subsequent months, and the role of alternative fuels must be considered.[87] For example, it has recently become apparent that neonates differ in terms of their ability to produce ketone bodies in response to hypoglycaemia. Low blood glucose concentrations (less than 2.6 mmol/l) are commonly found during the first 3 postnatal days in healthy AGA term neonates, particularly those who are breast-fed. However, these infants have high ketone body levels when blood glucose concentrations are low, and it is likely that this protects them from neurological sequelae, although this has yet to be proved in the human neonate.[69,153] Therefore, it is inappropriate to consider low blood glucose levels in such infants as a pathological diagnosis. However, other groups, such as those who are preterm, IUGR, asphyxiated or hyperinsulinaemic have impaired ketogenesis; in these babies circulating blood glucose concentrations acquire greater clinical significance and hypoglycaemia, if present, must be diagnosed and treated effectively.[66,67,69,71,74] The presence of additional neonatal complications which may add to neurological risks, such as asphyxia, acidosis, hyperbilirubinaemia and polycythaemia, must also be considered when deciding what level of blood glucose is acceptable.

In the light of the above discussion, it is difficult to identify a single 'cut-off' value for the definition of hypoglycaemia. However, we suggest that a blood glucose concentration below 2.6 mmol/l (as measured by accurate laboratory assay) for a prolonged period of at least 4–6 hours should be avoided in infants who are at risk of neurological sequelae by virtue of their inability to mobilize ketone bodies at low blood glucose levels (Table 38.1). It would be prudent to apply this most rigorously to infants with coexisting clinical complications. Regardless of the blood glucose concentration, neurological signs at low blood glucose levels should prompt investigations to establish a firm diagnosis of hypoglycaemia and the institution of urgent treatment.

Table 38.1 Mechanisms of hypoglycaemia

Increased glucose utilization
Hyperinsulinism
Inadequate glucose supply
Reduced availability of gluconeogenic precursors
Inactivity of enzymes of glycogenolysis and gluconeogenesis
Glucoregulatory hormone imbalance

Diagnosis

The accurate measurement of blood glucose levels is essential in the diagnosis of hypoglycaemia. It is well known that glucose reagent strips, commonly used in neonatal and maternity units, are insufficiently reliable for the diagnosis.[74,88,105,124] Therefore, if these strips are used for neonatal screening *all* low values should be confirmed by accurate measurement. These samples should be assayed promptly as blood glucose levels diminish with time, even in fluoridated tubes.[85] Accurate determination may be conveniently performed using a blood glucose analyser sited in a neonatal unit laboratory. Usually whole blood samples are taken, and it may be of relevance that plasma glucose samples are 13–18% higher than in whole blood. In terms of safety, accurate blood glucose measurements in whole blood samples will not underestimate the severity of hypoglycaemia, except in polycythaemia.

In addition to diagnosing hypoglycaemia, the underlying cause must be determined. This is usually self-evident from the obstetric history or clinical examination, but if this is not the case and the hypoglycaemia is profound or persistent despite treatment, further investigations must be performed to identify rare but serious inborn errors of metabolism or hormone deficiencies (Table 38.2). As these tests are most informative when carried out at the time of hypoglycaemia, it is important to take the necessary blood samples during such episodes and process and store them if necessary out of laboratory working hours. Each unit should devise an appropriate protocol for this in liaison with local and regional specialized laboratories.

MECHANISMS AND AT-RISK GROUPS

Hypoglycaemia may be secondary to increased utilization of glucose, to inadequate endogenous or exogenous supply of glucose, or to a combination of the two (Table 38.1).

Increased glucose utilization

The most common cause of excessive utilization of glucose is neonatal hyperinsulinism. Hyperinsulinism should be confirmed by the use of a highly specific insulin assay for plasma insulin concentrations and its interpretation with reference to normal neonatal insulin–glucose relationships[70,74,75] (Fig. 38.3). Clinical features are that glucose requirements to maintain normoglycaemia are high, in excess of the 4–6 mg/kg/min usually required by neonates, and the infant may be macrosomic (Fig. 38.4). Investigation of suspected hyperinsulinism will demonstrate low fatty acid and ketone body concentrations during hypoglycaemia, but this feature is not specific to hyperinsulinism as some infants who are *not* hyperinsulinaemic, such as those who are preterm or IUGR or, more rarely, those with congenital hypopituitarism, also fail to mount lipolytic and ketogenic responses.

Table 38.2 Infants who are at risk for the neurological sequelae of hypoglycaemia

At-risk group	Mechanisms	Management
Preterm (≤36 weeks)	Low substrate stores Immature hormone and enzyme responses Fluid/energy restriction Feeding difficulties	Early, frequent and adequate feeds i.v. glucose (if necessary)
Intrauterine growth retardation (b.wt <3rd percentile or clinically wasted)	Low substrate stores Immature hormone and enzyme responses Feeding difficulties	Early, frequent and adequate feeds i.v. glucose (if necessary) i.m./i.v. glucagon
Infant of diabetic mother (poor antenatal control) Beckwith–Wiedemann syndrome Rhesus haemolytic disease	Hyperinsulinism	Early, frequent and adequate feeds i.v. glucose (if necessary) Diazoxide Somatostatin
Islet-cell dysregulation syndrome Islet-cell adenoma	Hyperinsulinism	Pancreatectomy/resection adenoma
Perinatal asphyxia (requiring admission to NNU)	Low substrate stores 'Exhausted' stress response Hyperinsulinism Fluid/energy restriction Feeding difficulties	Adequate energy provision
Maternal β-blocker administration	Suppressed catecholamine response	Early, frequent and adequate feeds i.v. glucose (if necessary)
Septicaemia	Inhibition of counterregulatory enzymes Fluid/energy restriction Feeding difficulties	Adequate energy provision
Inborn errors of metabolism	Defects of enzymes of glycogenolysis, gluconeogenesis or fatty acid β oxidation	Investigate Adequate energy provision

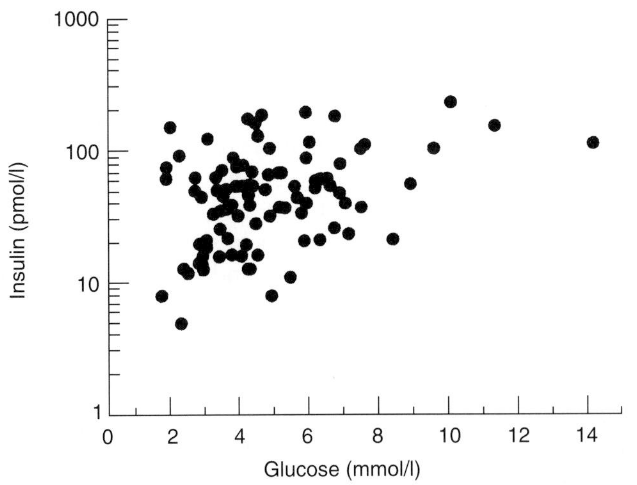

Fig. 38.3 Insulin–glucose relationship in preterm neonates, insulin concentrations measured using a highly specific immunoradiometric assay. (Reproduced with permission from Hawdon et al[75])

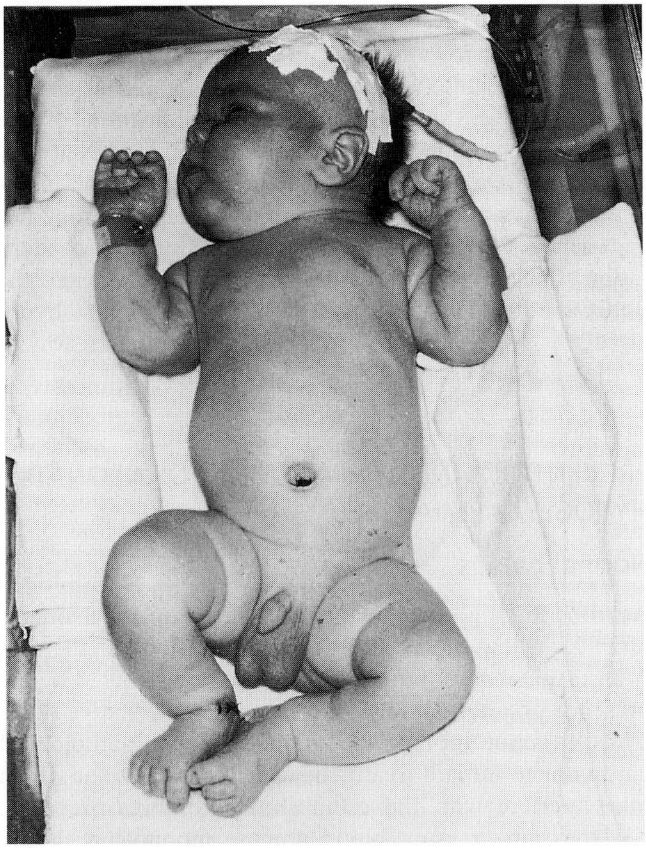

Fig. 38.4 Newborn infant with pancreatic islet cell dysregulation syndrome (nesidioblastosis) showing increased adiposity and resemblance to an infant of a diabetic mother.

Self-limiting hyperinsulinism

Hyperinsulinism may be a temporary phenomenon when the fetus has been rendered hyperglycaemic by poorly controlled maternal diabetes (Chapter 24), antenatal administration of thiazide diuretics or the administration of glucose to the mothers in labour, and in infants shortly after abrupt discontinuation of intravenous glucose infusions, after bolus doses of glucose, or if glucose has been infused through an umbilical arterial catheter whose tip is close to the coeliac axis.[99,120,126,132] Rhesus haemolytic disease and perinatal asphyxia have also been associated with transient fetal and neonatal hyperinsulinism, although the aetiological link is not known.[39,66,112] It has been suggested that hyperinsulinism contributes to hypoglycaemia after intrauterine growth retardation, but this is difficult to understand in the context of the wasting seen in this condition, and more recently normal insulin–glucose relationships (using neonatal reference data) have been demonstrated in IUGR neonates.[40,70–72]

Beckwith–Wiedemann syndrome

This condition, described independently by Beckwith[28] and Wiedemann,[160] is characterized by exomphalos, macroglossia, visceromegaly, earlobe abnormalities and an increased later incidence of malignancies. Hyperinsulinism is a common but not invariable feature causing high glucose requirements in the early neonatal period, and which usually resolves some time after birth. It is likely that the previously reported long-term developmental difficulties were related to undiagnosed and untreated hypoglycaemia, and it is anticipated that awareness of the condition and prevention of hypoglycaemia should result in improved outcome.

Islet-cell dysregulation syndrome

This is a rare condition, associated with macrosomia and extreme hyperinsulinism, which may be self-limiting in the neonatal period but more often is persistent, is associated with neurological signs of hypoglycaemia, and requires urgent treatment.[24] Many descriptive terms, such as 'nesidioblastosis' or 'persistent hyperinsulinaemic hypoglycaemia of infancy', have been applied to the histological appearance of the pancreas in this condition, and histochemical studies suggest that they are all related variants of inappropriate pancreatic development during fetal life.[18,121] More recently, the fundamental abnormality has been identified to be in the K^+ATP channel in the β-cell membrane. Molecular genetic analysis has shown a variety of mutations in the sulphonylurea receptor, which is functionally an integral part of the K^+ATP channel.[96,108] Recognition of the condition and early prevention and treatment of hypoglycaemia should reduce the incidence of permanent neurological damage which has been previously reported.[83,140]

Islet-cell adenoma

This is a very rare cause of permanent hyperinsulinism which is difficult to diagnose in the neonate using imaging techniques, and intraoperative ultrasound may be required to localize the tumour.[20,139] The tumour is benign and hyperinsulinaemic hypoglycaemia resolves after resection.

'Leucine-sensitive hypoglycaemia'

This was previously described as a distinct entity, but it is more likely that hypoglycaemia in response to leucine administration represents underlying hyperinsulinism and should be investigated and treated as such.[167]

Inadequate supply of glucose

Hypoglycaemia is most often the result of reduced delivery of glucose into the blood. In the enterally fed infant all the circulating glucose is provided either by the absorption and conversion of sugars or by glycogenolysis and gluconeogenesis, and in some babies there may be a contribution from intravenous glucose infusion. Thus, if the infant fails to switch on glycogenolysis or gluconeogenesis in response to falling blood glucose levels, or clinicians prescribe insufficient intravenous glucose, hypoglycaemia may occur. Three possible mechanisms may cause the failure of glucose production.

- Reduced availability of gluconeogenic precursors. First, glycogenolysis and gluconeogenesis may be limited by reduced availability of glycogen, gluconeogenic precursors or the energy provided by fatty acid oxidation. This may occur after preterm delivery, intrauterine growth retardation, placental insufficiency, perinatal asphyxia or fetal alcohol syndrome, or as a consequence of inadequate substrate intake after birth.[115,116,134,137]
- Inactivity of enzymes of glycogenolysis and gluconeogenesis. Secondly, there may be a failure of synthesis and activation of the key enzymes described above. This may be the result of a specific inherited metabolic disorder, in which case hypoglycaemia is recurrent or persistent, or there may be generalized immaturity of enzymes, as in preterm and IUGR infants, so that the infant is resistant to the effects of the counter-regulatory hormones, glucagon and the catecholamines. Finally, the activities of key enzymes may be suppressed, for example by inflammatory mediators in neonatal infection. Defective gluconeogenesis may also be the cause of hypoglycaemia complicating some cases of congenital heart disease and the now rare syndrome of neonatal cold injury.[77,104]
- Glucoregulatory hormone imbalance. Thirdly, there may be glucoregulatory hormone imbalances, so that enzymes are not activated and there is insufficient glucose production. As well as leading to increased glucose utilization, hyperinsulinism (see above) results in the suppression of glycogenolysis and gluconeogenesis. Insulin also inhibits lipolysis, so that fatty acids are not available for ketone body generation. Failure of release of the counter-regulatory hormones that stimulate the metabolic changes after birth may contribute to neonatal hypoglycaemia. Some preterm and IUGR infants do not have the glucagon surge described above, and maternal β-blocker medication in pregnancy is an additional risk factor.[31,115] Finally, there may be rare permanent causes for insufficiency of these hormones, for example low cortisol and growth hormone levels in septo-optic dysplasia and congenital hypopituitarism, and low glucocorticosteroid levels in adrenocortical deficiencies.[46,58,98]

Mechanisms of hypoglycaemia vary among groups of infants, and some may have more than one aetiological mechanism (Table 38.2). This is most applicable to neonates who have been subject to intrauterine growth retardation, which results in many reasons for failure of glycogenolysis and gluconeogenesis after birth. In addition, a failure of the ketogenic response to hypoglycaemia compromises total fuel availability, and animal studies have demonstrated that this does indeed reduce the availability of alternative fuels for cerebral metabolism.[51,67,71] It is important to note that not all IUGR infants will be 'small for gestational age' (Chapter 10), and clinical examination is important for the identification of the 'wasted' neonate. Conversely, not all small for gestational age infants will have been subject to placental insufficiency: they may be constitutionally small and may not experience the postnatal problems in metabolic adaptation. The early identification of at-risk neonates and the understanding of underlying mechanisms of hypoglycaemia are important for the diagnosis and treatment of the disorder.

PREVENTION AND MANAGEMENT OF NEONATAL HYPOGLYCAEMIA (Table 38.3)

Normal babies

As described above, healthy full-term AGA neonates often have low blood glucose concentrations in the first 2–3 postnatal days, but are thought to be protected by the presence of ketone bodies and lactate as alternative fuels. Thus, it is not appropriate to label this as a pathological entity nor to initiate treatment which is invasive or which may interfere with the establishment of breast-feeding. For the same reason, blood glucose monitoring should not be performed in healthy breast-fed babies whose birthweight is appropriate for gestational age. Because of the healthy infant's ability to counter-regulate, delayed establishment of successful breast-feeding is equally likely to present with excessive weight loss (in excess of 10% birthweight), dehydration and jaundice as with clinically significant hypoglycaemia. Therefore, breast-feeding advice and intervention should not be based on blood glucose levels. This does not preclude careful examination and observation of all newborn babies by midwives

Table 38.3 Prevention and management of hypoglycaemia

1. Identify at-risk infants (See Table 38.2)	
2. Early energy provision (within 1 hour of birth): *If enteral feeding planned*: Breast-feed Formula supplement of at least 12 ml/kg Minimum between feed interval of 3 hours	 *If enteral feeding contraindicated*: i.v. 10% glucose infusion of at least 3 ml/kg/h
3. Blood glucose monitoring: Before second feed, then frequency according to progress (at least 4–6 hourly in first 24 hours) Accurate method or confirm low (<2.6 mmol/l) reagent stick measurements with accurate method Discontinue when more than 2 readings >2.5 mmol/l Recommence if energy intake falls, e.g. vomiting	
4. Maintain energy provision: Minimum between feed interval of 3 hours: increase interval if BG >3 mmol/l *Mother plans to breast-feed*: Breast feeds offered before each formula feed Formula supplements by gavage, cup or bottle start at 100 ml/kg/day half volume if preceding BG >3 mmol/l then discontinue supplements when BG >3 mmol/l Continue milk feeds if tolerated even if i.v. therapy commenced *IV therapy*: Make gradual reductions, e.g. by 1–2 ml/h if blood glucose >2.5 mmol/l Resite drips promptly	 *Mother plans to bottle feed*: Start at 100 ml/kg/day Demand feed when BG >3 mmol/l
5. If blood glucose low (e.g. <2.6 mmol/l) on at least two occasions, but no clinical signs: *If enterally fed*: Increase feed volume and frequency Commence i.v. glucose if BG still low despite above If BG persistently low despite above, trial of glucagon i.m./i.v. 100 μg/kg	 *If i.v. 10% glucose already running*: Increase infusion rate Increase glucose concentration if volume restriction necessary
6. If clinical signs (fits, reduced level consciousness): Take sample for accurate BG but don't wait for result i.v. 10% glucose bolus of 3 ml/kg, repeated if signs do not resolve Followed immediately by i.v. glucose infusion of at least 3 ml/kg/h, adjust according to signs and BG If problems siting i.v. and diagnosis is hyperinsulinism, give glucagon i.m./i.v. 100 μg/kg Collect and freeze next urine sample	
7. If hypoglycaemia severe or persistent: Investigate as in Table 38.4	
8. Summary: Milk feeds: to maximum volume tolerated i.v. glucose: minimum necessary to maintain blood glucose >2.5 mmol/l	

and doctors to be alert to the possibility of dehydration and significant hypoglycaemia resulting from minimal milk intake after the third postnatal day if there is a failure of successful lactation, or to rare disorders, such as inborn errors of metabolism, which present with the neurological signs of hypoglycaemia and for which specific investigations should be performed (Table 38.4).

At-risk babies (Table 38.2)

For practical purposes, the following discussion focuses only on the infants who are at risk of the neurological sequelae of hypoglycaemia (Table 38.2). Early prevention of hypoglycaemia is optimal for these infants, so the first step in management must be to identify them. Although this is easy in some cases (such as the preterm baby), for others clinical observations are important (for example to identify the wasted appearance of the growth-retarded neonate who may not necessarily have a low birthweight).

These at-risk infants should have regular pre-feed blood glucose monitoring (at least 4–6-hourly initially). In addition, it is imperative that any infant with neurological signs, even if not in an at-risk group, should have urgent, accurate blood glucose measurement. The monitoring schedule for at-risk infants will vary according to local protocols, but we suggest that monitoring should be commenced before the first feed and that pre-feed monitoring be continued until the infant has had at least two satisfactory measurements. Monitoring should be recommenced if the infant's clinical condition worsens or energy intake decreases. If monitoring is by reagent strip, low levels must be confirmed by accurate measurement (see above).

The importance of early milk feeding has been appreciated for many years.[138] Both breast and formula milks provide important gluconeogenic precursors and fatty acids for β oxidation, and have a higher joule/ml content than 10% dextrose. In addition, enteral milk

Table 38.4 Samples for the investigation of severe or persistent hypoglycaemia. NB: Each condition is a rare cause of neonatal hypoglycaemia

Sample	Assay	Diagnosis
Blood	Glucose*	Confirm diagnosis
Blood	pH* Lactate*	Lactic acidosis in: glucose-6-phosphatase deficiency fructose-1,6-diphosphatase deficiency pyruvate carboxylase deficiency phosphoenolpyruvate carboxykinase deficiency Acidosis in disorders of amino acid metabolism
Blood	Intermediary metabolites	Disorders of gluconeogenesis
Blood	Ketone bodies	Disorders of fatty acid β oxidation (NB: low ketone body levels in preterm, IUGR and hyperinsulinaemic infants)
Plasma	Fatty acids	Disorders of fatty acid β oxidation
Plasma	Insulin+	Hyperinsulinism
Plasma	Glucagon Catecholamines Corticosteroids Growth hormone	Isolated hormone deficiency or in association with others, e.g. septo-optic dysplasia
Plasma/urine	Amino acid profile	Disorders of amino acid metabolism
Urine	Organic acids	Disorders of fatty acid β oxidation
Fibroblasts/leukocytes	Enzyme activities	Selected inborn errors of metabolism

* Analysers available for use in neonatal unit laboratory
\+ Use specific assay and neonatal reference data[70,75]

Total volume / % of Gluc. = G of Glucose
100 ml of 20% Dext. : 20g glucose = 20 × 1000 = 20000/24 = 833/60 = 13.8/wt. × 1000/24/60 = mg/kg/min

feeding stimulates the secretion of gut hormones, which may facilitate postnatal metabolic adaptation.[100] Therefore, all infants who are expected to tolerate enteral feeds should be fed with milk as soon as possible after birth, and at frequent intervals thereafter. Babies who are capable of sucking should be offered the breast at each feed (if this is the mother's wish), and feeds should be supplemented with formula milk by bottle, cup or gavage. For infants who are expected to tolerate enteral feeds, daily milk intakes of at least 100 ml/kg should be aimed for from birth. The need for formula supplementation will vary between babies, will diminish with the successful establishment of breast-feeding, and will be guided by regular pre-feed blood glucose monitoring.

When full enteral feeding is not anticipated, for example in the very preterm or sick infant, an intravenous glucose infusion should be commenced as soon as possible after birth. Usually 10% dextrose at 3 ml/kg/h (5 mg glucose/kg/min) is sufficient to prevent hypoglycaemia, but in some cases (such as hyperinsulinism) more is required. If the amount of glucose administered is limited by fluid restriction, more concentrated dextrose solutions may be required and central venous lines should be used, because these solutions are sclerotic to peripheral veins and cause tissue damage if they leak.

If hypoglycaemia develops in the milk-fed infant despite the above measures, it may be possible to increase further the volumes and/or frequencies of feeds. If this is not possible, or if the hypoglycaemia is resistant to this strategy, intravenous glucose will be required. If the infant is tolerating milk feeds these should be neither stopped nor reduced. The initial rate of 10% glucose infusion should be 3 ml/kg/h (5 mg/kg/min; Table 38.5), but adjusted according to frequent accurate blood glucose measurements. If the need for fluid restriction limits the amount of glucose that may be given more concentrated solutions may need to be infused (Table 38.5). If hypoglycaemia persists despite intravenous glucose, it is important to check the infusion site and the infusion apparatus to confirm glucose delivery. Leaking drips should be promptly resited. Boluses of concentrated glucose solution should be avoided because of the risk of rebound hypoglycaemia and cerebral oedema,[133] and if boluses are required (for example if there are neurological signs of hypoglycaemia) they should be of 10% dextrose

Table 38.5 Chart for conversion of rate of glucose infusion from ml/kg/24 h to mg/kg/min depending on strength of dextrose solution

Rate of infusion		Strength dextrose solution mg/kg/min 4%	10%	15%	20%
ml/kg/24h	ml/kg/h	mg/kg/min			
60	2.5	1.7	4.2	6.2	8.4
72	3.0	2.0	5.0	7.5	10.0
80	3.3	2.2	5.6	8.3	11.2
100	4.2	2.8	6.9	10.4	13.8
120	5.0	3.3	8.3	12.5	16.6
150	6.3	4.2	10.4	15.6	20.8
180	7.5	5.0	12.5	18.7	25.0
200	8.3	5.6	13.9	20.8	27.8

(3–5 ml/kg), given slowly, and always followed by an infusion. All reductions in infusion rate should be gradual. In cases of hyperinsulinism, intramuscular glucagon will have a temporary glycaemic effect if there is delay in siting an intravenous infusion (see below).

Specific treatments

Hyperinsulinism

This condition is usually self-limiting, but if the delivery of adequate amounts of intravenous glucose becomes a practical difficulty it is possible to administer diazoxide, which suppresses pancreatic insulin release. It may be given enterally (on a named-patient basis, Allen and Hanbury) or intravenously, starting with a dose of 5–10 mg/kg/day in three doses, and the effect is optimal if a daily dose of chlorthiazide (10 mg/kg) is given to potentiate the hyperglycaemic effect and prevent the fluid-retentive effect of diazoxide. Somatostatin analogue (Sandostatin, Sandoz Pharmaceuticals) administered subcutaneously at a dose of 1 μg/kg 4-hourly also suppresses insulin release.[82] However, tolerance may develop and there is concern about possible effects on the secretion of other hormones, and for this latter reason glucagon is often administered simultaneously.[18,68] In rare cases of islet-cell dysregulation syndrome subtotal pancreatectomy is required, and for this referral, should be made to regional neonatal surgical centres. Glucagon (200 μg/kg), i.v. or i.m., has a temporary glycaemic effect via its glycogenolytic action and may be a useful holding measure, for example when resiting glucose infusions.

Intrauterine growth retardation

Of more interest is the potential role of glucagon when hypoglycaemia is secondary to intrauterine growth retardation. It appears that its mechanism of action when given in pharmacological doses (30–200 μg/kg) is to mimic the postnatal glucagon surge and the 'switching on' of the enzymes of gluconeogenesis.[73,107] Thus it is a useful adjunct to intravenous glucose therapy and, after further evaluation, may prove an alternative treatment to intravenous glucose.

Adrenocortical insufficiency

Although parenteral hydrocortisone has been used for many years for the treatment of hypoglycaemia of various aetiologies, its place is solely as a replacement therapy for cortisol deficiency.

Inborn errors of metabolism

The management of the rare inborn errors of metabolism varies according to diagnosis and is beyond the scope of this chapter. In general, the aim is to provide adequate calories to prevent hypoglycaemia and catabolism.

NEONATAL HYPOGLYCAEMIA IN DEVELOPING COUNTRIES

In developing countries growth retardation, hypothermia, practices of late feeding and maternal nutritional factors are risk factors for hypoglycaemia.[163,164] However, there are few published data regarding the prevalence of hypoglycaemia in any developing country, and comparison of data with those from the developed world is hampered by differing definitions, populations, labour room practices, timing and technical methods. A study in Nepal using glucose test strips demonstrated that 38% of newborns during the first 3 days experienced a blood glucose of less than 2.6 mmol/l, compared to 18% of newborns of the same age in Newcastle upon Tyne, UK.[10,69] It is not known whether babies born in such circumstances are at risk of hypoketonaemia during hypoglycaemia, but if there is a high prevalence of intrauterine growth retardation the vulnerability of these infants to the potential sequelae of hypoglycaemia should be considered.

Therefore, it may not be appropriate to apply the guidelines described so far in this chapter to babies born in developing countries, and specific measures may be required to minimize the risk of neonatal hypoglycaemia. For example, the Baby Friendly Hospital initiative developed by UNICEF since 1992 has enjoyed considerable success in changing the culture of maternity hospitals, so that early breast-feeding is promoted, assisted by changes in facilities and procedures to ensure continual contact between mothers and their babies.[61] In addition, health education before and after childbirth, early suckling and promotion of breast-feeding, swaddling, early breast-feeding or skin-to-skin contact should reduce the risk of hypothermia and hypoglycaemia.[154]

Neonatal mortality accounts for 50–60% of all infant deaths in developing countries.[15] It is possible that neonatal hypoglycaemia, arising as a consequence of fetal malnutrition, birth asphyxia, postnatal hypothermia or infection, could be responsible for some of the hitherto unexplained neonatal deaths.

SUMMARY

The prevention and management of hypoglycaemia depends upon the administration of sufficient energy via either enteral or parenteral routes. In fact, many cases of hypoglycaemia are iatrogenic as a result of a failure to recognize poor milk intake in at-risk infants, or to prescribe sufficient glucose to fluid-restricted babies. Correcting these deficiencies is usually sufficient and only rarely are additional treatments required.

Neonatal hypoglycaemia is a common but usually preventable condition. Its prompt recognition, prevention and management are important to reduce the as yet unquantified but worrying risk of neurological sequelae.

HYPERGLYCAEMIA

Neonatal hyperglycaemia has been recognized for over a century,[89] and during this time it has become apparent that it represents several distinct clinical entities. As with hypoglycaemia, much uncertainty exists regarding definition, clinical significance and treatment.

NEONATAL DIABETES MELLITUS

Classic diabetes mellitus has been described as first presenting in the neonatal period, and is the subject of a recent British Paediatric Surveillance Unit study whose results yield exciting data regarding the genetics of the condition.[151,152] The condition is rare (1:500 000).[136] Early reports suggested that the condition was usually transient, characteristically occurring in small for gestational age infants in the first 6 postnatal weeks and presenting with very high blood glucose levels, low plasma insulin concentrations, dehydration, fever and failure to thrive despite adequate feeding.[79,80,118] The mean duration of insulin therapy, if required, was 69 days for the transient form, and it was thought that very few infants developed permanent diabetes in later life.[43,57] However, a more recent review of reported cases of neonatal diabetes mellitus, confirming its occurrence in predominantly small for gestational age infants, demonstrated that 46% developed permanent diabetes in the neonatal period, 23% developed permanent diabetes in childhood or adolescence, and in 31% diabetes resolved in the neonatal period. In this review, 10 cases had coexisting clinical conditions and six families had more than one affected individual (including two pairs of twins).[136,158]

SELF-LIMITING NEONATAL HYPERGLYCAEMIA

Neonatal hyperglycaemia is most often a transient disorder which resolves spontaneously and has few features in common with classic diabetes mellitus. The prevalence of transient hyperglycaemia appears to be increasing in parallel with the increased survival of extremely low-birthweight infants and the early use of parenteral nutrition solutions and corticosteroid therapy in these babies.[55,95] The following sections refer to the most common condition, transient hyperglycaemia in small or sick infants.

Clinical significance

It is of the utmost importance to remember that neonatal hyperglycaemia may be a sign of a serious underlying disorder, such as infection. However, it is still not known whether the high glucose concentrations themselves place the infant at further risk. Unlike adults with insulin deficiency, hyperglycaemic neonates do not develop ketosis or metabolic acidosis.[59] There is a risk that glycosuria and osmotic diuresis may cause fluid and electrolyte imbalance with dehydration, and such disturbances are themselves common in the groups of infants who develop hyperglycaemia, but studies of large numbers of infants have reported that osmotic diuresis is not an invariable consequence of neonatal hyperglycaemia.[47,122,148] There is also concern that changes in blood osmolality and fluid shifts may result in cerebral damage. However, cerebral pathology and adverse neurodevelopmental outcome have never been demonstrated to occur as the direct result of hyperglycaemia, and it is thought that blood glucose levels above 20 mmol/l are required to exert significant osmolar effects.[13,52,111]

As described above, neonatal hyperglycaemia is clinically significant in that it may herald a serious underlying disorder. Once such disorders have been ruled out and treated, there is no evidence that self-limiting hyperglycaemia secondary to immaturity of glucoregulation or excessive glucose intakes and not associated with osmotic diuresis, has adverse effects at blood glucose levels below 20 mmol/l.

Prevalence

Without a clear definition of hyperglycaemia it is difficult to comment on its frequency. Studies of prevalence vary according to their subjects, with hyperglycaemia found most frequently in very low-birthweight and preterm infants.[36,166] Small for gestational age infants who are preterm are more at risk for developing hyperglycaemia than hypoglycaemia when receiving standard intravenous infusions.[37] Reported prevalences vary from 29% to 86% in very low-birthweight neonates.[52,97]

Definition and diagnosis

There is no established definition of neonatal hyperglycaemia, but blood glucose levels above 7 mmol/l are usually considered to be high. However, the upper 'safe' limit of blood glucose concentration in the neonate is entirely unknown (see below) and, as with hypoglycaemia, there is likely to be great variation among practising neonatologists in terms of the diagnosis and management of hyperglycaemia.

The use of glucose reagent strips is more useful in the diagnosis of hyperglycaemia than for hypoglycaemia because the strips are more reliable at high blood glucose levels, and inaccuracies of 0.5–1.0 mmol/l are of less clinical relevance in the context of hyperglycaemia. However, clinicians should be urged to confirm the diagnosis with a laboratory measurement. It may also be useful to monitor urine for glycosuria, but it should be remembered that neonates, particularly those who are preterm, have a low renal threshold for glucose and fractional excretion of glucose varies widely, so that glycosuria may be present even in normoglycaemia.[161]

Mechanisms and at-risk groups

The mechanisms underlying neonatal hyperglycaemia vary and, as with hypoglycaemia, are best understood with reference to the expected metabolic changes at birth. In contrast to hypoglycaemia resulting from a low glucose production rate or a high glucose uptake rate, hyperglycaemia may be the result of a high glucose production or infusion rate or a low glucose uptake rate.

Neonatal hyperglycaemia is usually secondary to a high glucose appearance rate and it is often seen when glucose infusion rates are high.[72,97,111] To maintain control, the infant must be able to adapt to the exogenous administration of glucose (for example by intravenous infusion) by suppressing glucose production by the liver. The ability to glucoregulate in this way has been demonstrated in normoglycaemic neonates.[86,92] However, there is evidence from clinical and animal studies that some neonates do not suppress glucose production in response to glucose infusion and/or increased blood glucose levels.[23,34,48–50,72,155]

The inability to suppress gluconeogenesis may in turn be the result of disordered glucoregulatory hormone control. Although the glucoregulatory role of insulin in the neonate is unclear and may vary between infants, it has been suggested that hyperglycaemia results from decreased insulin secretion in immature subjects.[109,166] This is analogous to the adult insulin-dependent diabetic. Animal studies have also shown that after chronic hyperglycaemia the fetal pancreas cannot mount an insulin response to a further glucose surge.[35] This may be analogous to the condition in preterm babies receiving constant high-rate glucose infusions, whose pancreatic response to hyperglycaemia may be 'exhausted'.

Alternatively, circulating insulin concentrations may be appropriate for the blood glucose concentration, but hyperglycaemia may result from end-organ insensitivity to insulin. This is analogous to 'maturity-onset diabetes', which is characterized by insulin resistance. Neonatal insulin resistance has been demonstrated by the persistence of hyperglycaemia in the presence of raised insulin concentrations, the poor hypoglycaemic response to large exogenous doses of insulin, and the high insulin concentrations needed to suppress gluconeogenesis.[60,81,93,122,150] Insulin resistance may be secondary to immaturity or downregulation of peripheral receptors, to the effect of high fatty acid levels resulting from infusion of fat emulsion, or to the peripheral actions of counter-regulatory hormones.[165]

A recent study has shown that some hyperglycaemic preterm infants have inappropriately low plasma insulin concentrations and high plasma catecholamine levels, whereas others have apparently appropriate insulin concentrations and may have insulin resistance (Fig. 38.5) (Hawdon et al, unpublished data). The former group were those who had other clinical complications such as infection, and the latter were either very preterm or preterm and small for gestational age.

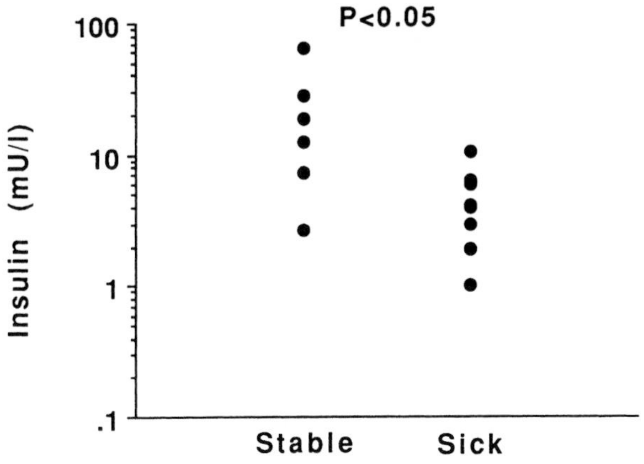

Fig. 38.5 Plasma insulin concentrations in preterm infants who were clinically stable or who had clinical complications such as infection or necrotizing enterocolitis (sick infants).

The excess secretion of counter-regulatory hormones, which themselves stimulate glycogenolysis and gluconeogenesis, may in addition block the secretion of insulin and inhibit its peripheral action, thereby contributing to insulin resistance.[34,41] This is the mechanism of hyperglycaemia secondary to exogenous corticosteroids, often administered in large doses to neonates with lung disease.[123,127] It has even been suggested that antenatal corticosteroid administration contributes to the failure to suppress postnatal gluconeogenesis.[155] Aminophylline, used for the prevention of apnoea of prematurity, mimics the action of catecholamines and induces glycogenolysis.[162] To date, growth hormone has not been implicated in the aetiology of neonatal hyperglycaemia.[166]

These hormonal disturbances may be the consequence of underlying clinical stresses such as infection, respiratory distress, pain or surgery.[5,6,33,94,97,147,149,166] Studies by Anand et al[3–8] demonstrated that with minimal anaesthesia for major surgical procedures in term and preterm neonates, high glucagon and catecholamine levels and inhibition of insulin secretion led to a number of metabolic abnormalities, including hyperglycaemia and hyperlactataemia. This response was in proportion to the severity of surgical stress and could be prevented by the addition of opioid analgesia or halothane to anaesthetic regimens. In some conditions associated with severe clinical stress, such as perinatal asphyxia, hyperglycaemia may occur as the result of high counter-regulatory hormone concentrations but hyperglycaemia is more often seen, probably because the latter represents the situation found after the stress response is exhausted.

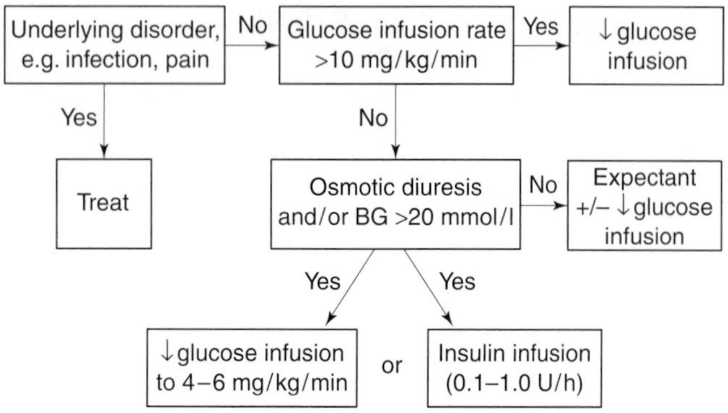

Fig. 38.6 Steps in the management of neonatal hyperglycaemia.

Despite the frequency with which hyperglycaemia is now observed, the aetiology and optimal management of this metabolic disorder have not been established. Clinical, animal and laboratory studies suggest that glucose production is not suppressed in the face of hyperglycaemia, but there are conflicting data regarding the role of defective glucoregulatory hormone responses.

Prevention and management (Fig. 38.6)

As neonatal hyperglycaemia is usually self-limiting and not associated with adverse sequelae, many clinicians choose not to treat raised blood glucose concentrations aggressively. However, the first step in management, especially in a baby who has previously been normoglycaemic, must be to seek and treat serious underlying disorders. The second step is to prevent the occurrence of high blood glucose concentrations secondary to high glucose infusion rates by instituting careful management of intravenous fluid prescriptions. Clinicians may increase fluid infusion rates to counter renal and extrarenal losses in the immature neonate. It is often forgotten that increasing the rate of administration of a glucose solution will result in a proportionate increase in glucose administration. For example, 200 ml/kg/day of 10% dextrose provides 14 mg/kg/min glucose, which is well in excess of the neonate's requirements. Thus it is not surprising that hyperglycaemia occurs and the extra glucose given is 'wasted'. Therefore, glucose infusion rates should be calculated and, if they are found to be excessive (for example above 4–6 mg/kg/min), more dilute solutions should be used.

Hyperglycaemia may still occur in some neonates who are clinically stable and who are not receiving excessive glucose intakes. These infants are usually of extremely low birthweight and less than 1 week old. Often they have received early parenteral nutrition and thus fairly high rates of glucose infusion in combination with amino acids. At the same time they may have high counter-regulatory hormone levels, rendering them 'catabolic' with or without peripheral insulin resistance, so that they cannot utilize the infused substrates. The condition is usually self-limiting and may be prevented by the more gradual introduction of parenteral nutrition solutions in those at risk.

There are three strategies for management of hyperglycaemia when it occurs in these circumstances. First, moderate hyperglycaemia may be 'tolerated' if it does not appear to be causing osmotic diuresis. Our experience is that the condition resolves within a few days even if no action is taken. Secondly, the rate of glucose infusion may be carefully reduced to the rate at which blood glucose levels become normal, and then gradually increased as tolerated. This carries the possible disadvantage of reducing the infant's energy intake, but it is likely that immature infants are unable to effectively utilize all the glucose offered, especially if at a rate in excess of 5 mg/kg/min.[155] Thirdly, insulin may be administered in order to lower the blood glucose concentration without reducing the glucose infusion rate. Controlled studies of insulin administration to adult intensive care patients on intravenous nutrition have demonstrated that although there is a short-term improvement in nitrogen balance, there is no advantage in terms of either weight gain or body composition, and that a number of patients become hypoglycaemic.[102,125] Although there are a number of reports of this practice in the neonatal literature, there is no consistency regarding the clinical situations in which insulin has been given, only short-term outcome measures have been reported, and there are few prospective controlled trials. For example, Ostertag et al[117] and Vaucher et al[157] reported that the administration of insulin (20–400 mU/h, and 2–86 mU/kg/h) was associated with the ability to tolerate increased glucose infusion rates. Binder et al[30] found that the babies who received insulin (53 mU/g glucose infused) had blood glucose concentrations, glucose and energy intakes and daily weight gain similar to those of other babies of <1000 g who did not receive insulin. However, as these studies were neither controlled nor randomized, and in the absence of long-term outcome measures, it is impossible to conclude that insulin therapy conferred a clinical advantage. All of these studies reported hypoglycaemia in some infants even after the discontinuation of insulin infusion.

One controlled trial of hyperglycaemic preterm neonates demonstrated that insulin administration(40–1000 mU/h) allowed glucose infusion rates of 20 mg/kg/min, compared to 13 mg/kg/min in infants who did not receive insulin (both are higher rates of glucose infusion than would be used in current clinical practice). There was more rapid early weight gain in the treated group, but this may have been related to higher rates of fluid infusion. Infected infants had extremely high insulin requirements and high circulating insulin concentrations, suggesting significant insulin resistance.[41]

There is marked variation between and within studies regarding the doses of insulin required, and some authors have raised the possibility of the development of tolerance in some babies, so that hyperglycaemia recurs despite large increases in insulin dosage.[30,41,60,117] This is surprising in the face of the clinical observation that without insulin treatment neonatal hyperglycaemia is usually a transient and self-limiting condition, and it may be that insulin administration in some way hinders spontaneous recovery.

Recent studies have suggested that intrauterine nutritional and endocrine status may influence adult metabolism and susceptibility to disease.[26] The long-term clinical significance of early high energy intakes in association with large doses of exogenous insulin in the preterm neonate, and of possible up- or downregulation of insulin receptors, has not yet been considered.

Finally, the introduction of enteral feeding with small volumes of milk as soon as the infant's gastrointestinal tract will tolerate this may hasten the control of blood glucose homoeostasis by inducing surges of gut hormones which may promote insulin secretion (the enteroinsular axis).[19]

The pathogenesis of neonatal hyperglycaemia and the mechanism of action of exogenous insulin administration are not clearly understood. Therefore, the increasing practice of prescribing insulin to neonates without understanding its mode of action is of concern. It is not known whether insulin administration promotes linear growth in neonates, or merely converts glucose into fat. A prospective randomized controlled trial of insulin therapy in preterm neonates who become glucose intolerant would assess the impact of insulin therapy on glucose tolerance, metabolism and growth in the short and long term. Until such a study is performed it is impossible to judge whether insulin therapy does confer clinical advantage over expectant management of a condition which is usually self-limiting.

SUMMARY

In this chapter an approach to the controversy surrounding the definition, diagnosis and management of babies with neonatal hypoglycaemia has been presented. Much more information is needed before the same aspects of the present pragmatic approach, based on the safest possible practice, can be established on a more secure scientific basis. The following summarizes the key questions that still need to be addressed.

First, the long-term effects of moderate and/or asymptomatic hypoglycaemia must be established. For example, we do not know whether the preterm infant's brain is more or less vulnerable to hypoglycaemia than that of the term infant, what duration of hypoglycaemia results in permanent disability, and whether the effects of hypoglycaemia are exacerbated by concurrent complications such as hyperbilirubinaemia. We do not know whether the differences that we have demonstrated between preterm and term infants in metabolic adaptation persist beyond the first postnatal week, and whether there are implications for the preterm infant in terms of persistent impairment of metabolic responses.

Secondly, more information must be gathered relating to other factors regulating glucose availability to the brain, namely cerebral blood flow, the ontogeny of glucose transporter proteins, and the role of the astrocyte in neuronal metabolic support.

Finally, as we realize the inadequacy of glucose reagent sticks for the diagnosis and monitoring of hypoglycaemia, improved accurate near-patient systems should be developed for the measurement of blood glucose concentrations, and the ability to measure blood ketone body concentrations in these circumstances would markedly enhance management.

In 1954, McQuarrie[103] urged the physician caring for children to be constantly aware of the risk of hypoglycaemia. This exhortation is still relevant in the 1990s, but much still needs to be learned and there are many challenging areas of research for the clinical investigator.

Acknowledgement

The authors wish to thank Dr A. M. de L. Costello for his contribution to the section on neonatal hypoglycaemia in developing countries.

REFERENCES

1. Adam P A J, Kind K, Schwartz R 1968 Model for the investigation of intractable hypoglycemia: insulin glucose interrelationships during steady state infusions. Pediatrics 41: 91–105
2. Adam P A J, Raiha N, Rahiala E C, Kekomahl M 1975 Oxidation of glucose and β hydroxybutyrate by the early human fetal brain. Acta Paediatrica Scandinavica 64: 17–24
3. Anand K J S, Aynsley-Green A 1988 Measuring the severity of surgical stress in newborn infants. Journal of Pediatric Surgery 23: 297–305
4. Anand K J S, Hickey P R 1987 Pain and its effects on the human neonate and fetus. New England Journal of Medicine 317: 1321–1329
5. Anand K J S, Brown M J, Causon R C, Christofides N D, Bloom S R, Aynsley-Green A 1985 Can the human neonate mount an endocrine and metabolic response to surgery? Journal of Pediatric Surgery 20: 41–48
6. Anand K J S, Sippell W G, Aynsley-Green A 1985 Metabolic and endocrine effects of surgical ligation of patent ductus arteriosus in the human neonate: are there implications for further improvement of postoperative outcome? In: Falkner R, Kretchner N, Rossi E (eds) Modern problems in paediatrics, Karger, Basle, pp 145–157
7. Anand K J S, Sippel W G, Aynsley-Green A 1987 Randomised trial of fentanyl anaesthesia in preterm neonates undergoing surgery. Effects on the stress response. Lancet i: 243–248
8. Anand K J S, Sipell W G, Schofield N, Aynsley-Green A 1988 Does halothane anaesthesia decrease the metabolic and endocrine stress response of newborn infants undergoing surgery? British Medical Journal 296: 668–672
9. Anderson J M, Milner R D G, Strich S J 1967 Effects of neonatal hypoglycaemia on the nervous system: a pathological study. Journal of Neurology, Neurosurgery and Psychiatry 30: 295–310
10. Anderson S, Shakya K N, Shrestha L N, Costello A M de L 1993 Hypoglycaemia: a common problem among uncomplicated newborn infants in Nepal. Journal of Tropical Pediatrics 39: 273–277
11. Anwar M, Vannucci R C 1988 Autoradiographic determination of

regional cerebral blood flow during hypoglycemia in newborn dogs. Pediatric Research 24: 41–45
12. Aranda J V, Dupont C 1976 Metabolic effect of theophylline in the premature neonate (letter). Journal of Pediatrics 89: 833
13. Arant B S, Gorsh W M 1978 Effects of acute hyperglycemia on the central nervous system of neonatal puppies. Pediatric Research 12: 549
14. Ashton J K, Aynsley-Green A 1978 Somatomedin in an infant with Beckwith's syndrome. Early Human Development 14: 357–362
15. Ashworth A, Waterlow J C 1982 Infant mortality in developing countries. Archives of Disease in Childhood 57: 882–884
16. Auer R N, Siesjo B K 1993 Hypoglycaemia: brain neurochemistry and neuropathology. In: Baillières Clinical Endocrinology and Metabolism 7: 611–625
17. Avery G B, Fletcher A B, Kaplan M, Brudno S 1985 Controlled trial of dexamethasone in respirator-dependent infants with bronchopulmonary dysplasia. Pediatrics 75: 106–111
18. Aynsley-Green A 1981 Nesidioblastosis of the pancreas in infancy. In: Randle P J, Steiner D F, Whelan W J (eds) Carbohydrate metabolism and its disorders. Academic Press, London, pp 181–204
19. Aynsley-Green A 1988 Metabolic and endocrine interrelationships in the human fetus and neonate: an overview of the control of the adaptation to postnatal nutrition In: Lindblad B A (ed) Perinatal nutrition. Academic Press, New York, pp 162–191
20. Aynsley Green A 1988. The adaptation of the human neonate to extrauterine nutrition: a pre-requisite for postnatal growth In: Cockburn F (ed) Fetal and neonatal growth. Wiley, Chichester, New York, pp 153–183
21. Aynsley-Green A 1988 The management of islet cell dysregulation syndromes in infancy and childhood. Zeitschrift für Kinderchirurgie 43: 267–272
22. Aynsley-Green A 1996 Glucose, the brain and the paediatric endocrinologist. Hormone Research 46: 8–25
23. Baarsma R, Chapman T E, Van Asselt W A, Berger R, Okken A 1990 Glucose kinetics in preterm and term small for gestational age newborn infants. In: Chapman T E, Berger R, Reijngold D J, Okken A (eds) Stable isotopes in paediatric nutritional and metabolic research. Intercept Press, Andover
24. Baker L, Stanley C A 1977 Hyperinsulinism in infancy: a pathophysiologic approach to diagnosis and treatment. In: Chiumello G, Laron Z (eds) Recent progress in pediatric endocrinology. Academic Press, London, pp 89–100
25. Banker B Q 1967 The neuropathological effects of anoxia and hypoglycaemia in the newborn. Developmental Medicine and Child Neurology 9: 544–550
26. Barker D J P 1992 Fetal and infant origins of adult disease. British Medical Journal, London
27. Battaglia F C, Hay W W 1984 Energy and substrate requirements for fetal and placental growth and metabolism. In: Beard R W, Nathanielsz P W (eds) Fetal physiology and medicine. Marcel Dekker, New York, pp 601–628
28. Beckwith J B 1963 Extreme cytomegaly of the adrenal fetal cortex, omphalocele, hyperplasia of kidneys and pancreas and Leydig cell hyperplasia. Another syndrome? Proceedings of the Western Society for Pediatric Research, November 1963, Los Angeles
29. Bier D M, Leake R D, Haymond M W et al 1977 Measurement of 'true' glucose production rates in infancy and childhood with 6, 6-dideuteroglucose. Diabetes 26: 1016–1023
30. Binder N D, Raschko R K, Benda G I, Reynolds J W 1989 Insulin infusion with parenteral nutrition in extremely low birthweight infants with hyperglycemia. Journal of Pediatrics 114: 273–280
31. Bloom S R, Johnston D J 1972 Failure of glucagon release in infants of diabetic mothers. British Medical Journal iv: 453–454
32. Bougneres P F 1987 Stable isotope tracers and the determination of fuel fluxes in newborn infants. Biology of the Neonate 52 (suppl. 1): 87–96
33. Bryan M H, Wei P, Hamilton J R, Chance G W, Swyer P R 1973 Supplemental intravenous alimentation in low birthweight infants. Journal of Pediatrics 82: 940–944
34. Burstein R L, Papile C A, Greenberg R E 1980 Mechanisms of hyperglycemia in small premature infants. Pediatric Research 14: 568
35. Carver T D, Anderson S M, Aldoretta P A, Esler A L, Hay W W 1995 Glucose suppression of insulin secretion in chronically hyperglycemic fetal sheep. Pediatric Research 38: 754–762
36. Chaivorarat O, Dweck H S 1976 Effect of prolonged continuous glucose infusion in preterm neonates. Pediatric Research 10: 406
37. Chance G W, Bower B D 1966 Hypoglycaemia and temporary hyperglycaemia in infants of low birth weight for maturity. Archives of Disease in Childhood 41: 279–285
38. Cobliner S 1911 Blutzuckeruntersuchungen bei Säuglingen. Zeitschrift für Kinderheilkunde 1: 207–216
39. Collins J E, Leonard J V 1984 Hyperinsulinism in asphyxiated and small for dates infants with hypoglycaemia. Lancet ii: 311–313
40. Collins J E, Leonard J V, Teale D et al 1990 Hyperinsulinaemic hypoglycaemia in small for dates babies. Archives of Disease in Childhood 65: 1118–1120
41. Collins J W Jr, Hoppe M, Brown K, Edidin D V, Padbury J, Ogata E S 1991 A controlled trial of insulin infusion and parenteral nutrition in extremely low birthweight infants with glucose intolerance. Journal of Pediatrics 118: 921–927
42. Cornblath M, Reisner S H 1965 Blood glucose in the neonate, clinical significance. New England Journal of Medicine 272: 378–381
43. Cornblath M, Schwartz R 1976 Disorders of carbohydrate metabolism in infancy, 2nd edn. W B Saunders, Philadelphia
44. Cornblath M, Schwartz R 1993 Hypoglycemia in the neonate. Journal of Pediatric Endocrinology 6: 113–129
45. Cornblath M, Schwartz R, Aynsley-Green A, Lloyd J K 1990 Hypoglycemia in infancy: the need for a rational definition. A Ciba Foundation discussion meeting. Pediatrics 85: 834–837
46. Costello J M, Gluckman P D 1988 Neonatal hypopituitarism: a neurological perspective. Developmental Medicine and Child Neurology 30: 190–199
47. Cowett R M, Schwartz R 1979 The role of hepatic control of glucose homeostasis in the aetiology of neonatal hypo and hyperglycemia. Seminars in Perinatology 3: 327
48. Cowett R M, Oh W, Schwartz R 1983 Persistent glucose production during glucose infusion in the neonate. Journal of Clinical Investigation 71: 467–475
49. Cowett R M, Andersen G E, Maguire C A, Oh W 1988 Ontogeny of glucose homeostasis in low birth weight infants. Journal of Pediatrics 112: 462–465
50. Cowett R M, Susa J B, Oh W, Schwartz R 1978 Endogenous glucose production during constant glucose infusion in the newborn lamb. Pediatric Research 12: 853–857
51. Dahlquist G 1976 Cerebral utilization of glucose, ketone bodies and oxygen in starving infant rats and the effect of intrauterine growth retardation. Acta Paediatrica Scandinavica 98: 237–247
52. Dweck H S, Cassady G 1974 Glucose tolerance in infants of very low birthweight. I. Incidence of hyperglycemia in infants of birthweights 1100 grams or less. Pediatrics 53: 189–195
53. Edmond J, Auestad N, Robbins R A, Bergstrom J D 1985 Ketone body metabolism in the neonate: development and effect of diet. Federal Proceedings 44: 2359–2364
54. Elander G, Lindberg T 1984 Short mother–infant separation during first week of life influences the duration of breast feeding. Acta Paediatrica Scandinavica 73: 237–240
55. Fiser R H Jr, Williams P R, Fisher D A, Delameter P V, Sperling M A, Oh W 1975 The effect of oral alanine on blood glucose and glucagon in the newborn infant. Pediatrics 56: 78–81
56. Fluge G 1974 Clinical aspects of neonatal hypoglycaemia. Acta Paediatrica Scandinavica 63: 826–832
57. Francois R, Hermier M, Jurlot B 1975 Occurrence of diabetes in infants less than one year old. In: Laron Z (ed) Diabetes in juveniles. Karger, Basle, pp 60–66
58. Gemelli M, De Luca F, Barberio G 1979 Hypoglycaemia and congenital adrenal hyperplasia. Acta Paediatrica Scandinavica 68: 285–286
59. Gentz J C H, Cornblath M 1969 Transient diabetes of the newborn. Advances in Pediatrics 16: 345–363
60. Goldman S L, Hirata T 1980 Attenuated response to insulin in very low birthweight infants. Pediatric Research 14: 50–53
61. Grant J 1995 UNICEF State of the World's Children. Oxford University Press, Oxford
62. Griffiths A D 1968 Association of hypoglycaemia with symptoms in the newborn. Archives of Disease in Childhood 43: 688–694
63. Griffiths A D, Lawrence K M 1974 The effects of hypoxia and hypoglycaemia on the brain of the newborn human infant. Developmental Medicine and Child Neurology 16: 308–319

64. Hägnevik K, Faxelius G, Irestedt L, Lagercrantz H, Lundell B, Persson B 1984 Catecholamine surge and metabolic adaptation in the newborn after vaginal delivery and caesarean section. Acta Paediatrica Scandinavica 73: 602–609
65. Hawdon J M 1993 Neonatal hypoglycaemia: the consequences of admission to the special care nursery. Maternal and Child Health Feb: 48–51
66. Hawdon J M, Ward Platt M P 1992 Metabolic and hormonal interrelationships in perinatal asphyxia. Biology of the Neonate 62: 300
67. Hawdon J M, Ward Platt M P 1993 Metabolic adaptation in small for gestational age infants. Archives of Disease in Childhood 68: 262–268
68. Hawdon J M, Ward Platt M P, Lamb W H, Aynsley-Green A 1990 Tolerance to Sandostatin in neonatal hyperinsulinaemic hypoglycaemia. Archives of Disease in Childhood 65: 341–343
69. Hawdon J M, Ward Platt M P, Aynsley-Green A 1992 Patterns of metabolic adaptation for preterm and term infants in the first neonatal week. Archives of Disease in Childhood 67: 357–365
70. Hawdon J M, Aynsley-Green A, Alberti K G M M, Ward Platt M P 1993 The role of pancreatic insulin secretion in neonatal glucoregulation. I Healthy term and preterm infants. Archives of Disease in Childhood 68: 274–279
71. Hawdon J M, Weddell A, Aynsley-Green A, Ward Platt M P 1993 Hormonal and metabolic response to hypoglycaemia in small for gestational age infants. Archives of Disease in Childhood 68: 269–273
72. Hawdon J M, Aynsley-Green A, Bartlett K, Ward Platt M P 1993 The role of pancreatic insulin secretion in neonatal glucoregulation. II Infants with disordered blood glucose homeostasis. Archives of Disease in Childhood 68: 280–285
73. Hawdon J M, Aynsley-Green A, Ward Platt M P 1993 Neonatal blood glucose concentrations: Metabolic effects of intravenous glucagon and intragastric medium chain triglyceride. Archives of Disease in Childhood 68: 255–261
74. Hawdon J M, Ward Platt M P, Aynsley-Green A 1994 Controversy. Prevention and management of neonatal hypoglycaemia. Archives of Disease in Childhood 70: 60–65
75. Hawdon J M, Hubbard M, Hales C N, Clark P 1995 Use of a specific immunoradiometric assay to determine preterm neonatal insulin-glucose relations. Archives of Disease in Childhood 73: F166–F169
76. Hay W W Jr, Sparks J W 1985 Placental, fetal and neonatal carbohydrate metabolism. Clinical Obstetrics and Gynecology 28: 473–485
77. Haymond M W, Strauss A W, Arnold K J, Bier D M 1979 Glucose homeostasis in children with severe cyanotic congenital heart disease. Journal of Pediatrics 95: 220–227
78. Heck L J, Erenberg A 1987 Serum glucose levels in term neonates during the first 48 hours of life. Journal of Paediatrics 110: 119–122
79. Hoffman W H, Knoury C, Byrd H A 1980 Prevalence of permanent congenital diabetes mellitus. Diabetologia 19: 487–488
80. Hutchinson J H, Keay A J, Kerr M N 1962 Congenital temporary diabetes mellitus. British Medical Journal ii: 436–440
81. Issad T, Pastor-Anglada M, Coupe C, Ferre P, Girard J 1990 Glucose metabolism and insulin sensitivity during suckling period in rats. In: Cuezva J M, Paseaud-Leone A M, Patel M S (eds) Endocrine development of the fetus and neonate. Plenum Press, New York, pp 61–66
82. Jackson J A, Hahn H B, Oltorf C E, O'Dorisio T M, Vinik A L 1987 Long-term management of refractory neonatal hypoglycemia with long-acting somatostatin analog. Journal of Pediatrics 111: 548–551
83. Jacobs D G, Haka-Ikse K, Wesson D E, Filler R M, Sherwood G 1986 Growth and development in patients operated on for islet cell dysplasia. Journal of Pediatric Surgery 21: 1184–1189
84. Johnston V, Frazzini V, Davidheiser S, Przybylski R J, Kleigman R M 1991 Insulin receptor number and binding affinity in newborn dogs. Pediatric Research 29: 611–614
85. Joosten K J, Schellehens A P, Waellens J J, Wulffraat N M 1991 Erroneous diagnosis 'neonatal hypoglycaemia' due to incorrect preservation of blood samples. Nederlands Tijdschrift Geneeskunde 135: 1691–1694
86. Kalhan S C, Oliver A, King K C, Lucero C 1986 Role of glucose in the regulation of endogenous glucose production in the human newborn. Pediatric Research 20: 49–52
87. Kinnala A, Suhonen-Polvi H, Aarimaa T et al 1996 Cerebral metabolic rate for glucose during the first six months of life: an FDG positron emission tomography study. Archives of Disease in Childhood 74: F153–F157
88. Kirkham P, Watkins A 1995 Comparison of two reflectance photometers in the assessment of neonatal hypoglycaemia. Archives of Disease in Childhood 73: F170–F173
89. Kitselle J F 1852 Kinderh Leipsic XVIII 313
90. Koh T H H G, Eyre J A, Aynsley-Green A 1988 Neural dysfunction during hypoglycaemia. Archives of Disease in Childhood 63: 1353–1358
91. Koh T H H G, Eyre J A, Aynsley-Green A 1988 Neonatal hypoglycaemia – the controversy regarding definition. Archives of Disease in Childhood 63: 1386–1389
92. Lafeber H N, Sulkers E J, Chapman T E, Sauer P J J 1990 Glucose production and oxidation in preterm infants during total parenteral nutrition. Pediatric Research 28: 153–157
93. Le Dune MA 1971 Insulin studies in temporary neonatal hyperglycaemia. Archives of Disease in Childhood 46: 392–394
94. Lilien L D, Rosenfield R C, Pildes R S 1979 Hyperglycemia in small stressed neonates. Journal of Pediatrics 94: 454–459
95. Lindblad B S, Settegren G, Feychting H 1977 Total parenteral nutrition in infants. Blood levels of glucose, lactate, pyruvate, free fatty acids, glycerol, D β hydroxybutyrate, triglycerides, free amino acids and insulin. Acta Paediatrica Scandinavica 66: 409–419
96. Lindley K J, Dunne M J, Kane C et al 1996 Ionic control of β cell function in nesidioblastosis. A possible role for calcium channel blockade. Archives of Disease in Childhood 74: 373–378
97. Louik C, Mitchell A A, Epstein M F, Shapiro S 1985 Risk factors for neonatal hyperglycemia associated with 10% dextrose infusion. American Journal of Diseases of Children 139: 783–786
98. Lovinger R D, Kaplan S L, Grumback M M 1975 Congenital hypopituitarism associated with neonatal hypoglycemia and microphallus. Journal of Pediatrics 87: 1171–1181
99. Lucas A, Adrian T E, Aynsley-Green A, Bloom S R 1980 Iatrogenic hyperinsulinism at birth. Lancet i: 144–145
100. Lucas A, Aynsley-Green A, Bloom S R 1981 Gut hormones and the first meals. Clinical Science 60: 349–353
101. Lucas A, Morley R, Cole T F 1988 Adverse neurodevelopmental outcome of moderate neonatal hypoglycaemia. British Medical Journal 297: 1304–1308
102. MacFie J, Yule A G, Hill G L 1981 Effect of added insulin on body composition of gastroenterologic patients receiving intravenous nutrition – a controlled clinical trial. Gastroenterology 81: 285–289
103. McQuarrie I 1954 Idiopathic spontaneously occurring hypoglycemia in infants. American Journal of Diseases of Children 87: 399–428
104. Mann T P, Elliot R I K 1957 Neonatal cold injury due to accidental exposure to cold. Lancet i: 229–231
105. Medical Devices Agency 1996 Extra-laboratory use of blood glucose meters and test strips: contraindications, training and advice to the users. Safety Notice MDA SN 9616
106. Medina J M, Fernandez E, Bolaros J P, Vicario C, Arizmendi L 1990 Fuel supply to the brain during the early postnatal period. In: Cueza J M, Pasaud-Leone A M, Patel M S (eds) Endocrine development of the fetus and neonate. Plenum Press, New York, pp. 175–194
107. Mehta A, Wootton R, Cheng K N, Penfold P, Halliday D, Stacey T E 1987 Effect of diazoxide or glucagon on hepatic glucose production rate during extreme neonatal hypoglycaemia. Archives of Disease in Childhood 62: 924–930
108. Milner R D G 1996 Nesidioblastosis unravelled. Archives of Disease in Childhood 74: 369–372
109. Milner R D G, Ferguson A W, Naidu S H 1971 Aetiology of transient neonatal diabetes. Archives of Disease in Childhood 46: 724–726
110. Milner R D G, Fekete M, Assan R 1972 Glucagon, insulin and growth hormone response to exchange transfusion in premature and term infants. Archives of Disease in Childhood 17: 186–189
111. Miranda L, Dweck H S 1977 Perinatal glucose homeostasis: the unique character of hyperglycemia and hypoglycemia in infants of very low birthweight. Clinics in Perinatology 4: 351–365
112. Molsted-Pedersen L, Trautner H, Jorgensen K R 1973 Plasma insulin and K values during intravenous glucose tolerance test in newborn infants with erythroblastosis fetalis. Acta Paediatrica Scandinavica 62: 11–16
113. Neligan G 1965 Idiopathic hypoglycaemia in the newborn. In: Gairdner D ed. Recent advances in paediatrics III. Churchill, London

114. Obershain S S, Adam P A J, King K C et al 1970 Human fetal response to sustained maternal hyperglycemia. New England Journal of Medicine 283: 566–572
115. Ogata E S 1986 Carbohydrate metabolism in the fetus and neonate and altered neonatal glucoregulation. Pediatric Clinics of North America 33: 25–45
116. Ogata E S, Paul R I, Finley S L 1987 Limited maternal fuel availability due to hyperinsulinemia retards fetal growth and development in the rat. Pediatric Research 22: 432–437
117. Ostertag S G, Jovanovic L, Lewis B, Auld P A M 1986 Insulin pump therapy in the very low birthweight infant. Pediatrics 78: 625–630
118. Pagliara A S, Karl I E, Kipnis D B 1973 Transient neonatal diabetes: delayed maturation of the pancreatic beta cell. Journal of Pediatrics 82: 97–101
119. Persson B, Gentz J 1966 The pattern of blood lipids, glycerol and ketone bodies during the neonatal period, infancy and childhood. Acta Paediatrica Scandinavica 55: 353–362
120. Philipson E H, Kalhan S C, Rika M M, Pimental R 1987 Effects of maternal glucose infusion on fetal acid–base status in human pregnancy. American Journal of Obstetrics and Gynecology 157: 866–873
121. Polak J M, Bloom S R 1980 Decrease of somatostatin content in persistent neonatal hyperinsulinaemic hypoglycaemia In: Andreani D, Lefebvre P J, Marks V (eds) Current views on hypoglycaemia and glucagon. Academic Press, London, pp 367–378
122. Pollack A, Cowett R M, Schwartz R, Oh M D 1978 Glucose disposal in low birthweight infants during steady state hyperglycemia: effects of exogenous insulin administration. Pediatrics 61: 546–549
123. Pomerance J, Puri A R 1980 Treatment of neonatal bronchopulmonary dysplasia with steroids. Pediatric Research 14: 649A
124. Reynolds G J, Davies S 1993 A clinical audit of cotside blood glucose measurement in the detection of neonatal hypoglycaemia. Journal of Paediatrics and Child Health 29: 289–291
125. Ross R J M, Miell J P, Buchanan C R 1991 Avoiding autocannibalism. British Medical Journal 303: 1147–1148
126. Rutter N, Spencer A, Mann N, Smith M 1980 Glucose during labour. Lancet ii: 155
127. Sanders R J, Cox C, Phelps D C, Sinkin R A 1994 Two doses of early intravenous dexamethasone for the prevention of bronchopulmonary dysplasia in babies with respiratory distress syndrome. Pediatric Research 36: 122–128
128. Schrier A M, Wilhelm P B, Church R M et al 1990 Neonatal hypoglycaemia in the Rhesus monkey: effect on development and behaviour. Infant Behaviour and Development 13: 189–297
129. Schwartz R 1991 Neonatal hypoglycaemia. Back to basics in diagnosis and treatment. Diabetes 40 (suppl 2): 71–73
130. Sedgwick J P, Ziegler M R 1920 The nitrogenous and sugar content of the blood of the newborn. American Journal of Diseases of Children 19: 429–432
131. Senior B 1973 Current concepts. Neonatal hypoglycemia. New England Journal of Medicine 289: 790–793
132. Senior B, Slone D, Shapiro S 1976 Benzothiazides and neonatal hypoglycaemia. Lancet ii: 377
133. Shah A, Stanhope R, Matthew D 1992 Hazards of pharmacological tests of growth hormone secretion in childhood. British Medical Journal 304: 173–174
134. Shelley H J, Basset J M 1975 Control of carbohydrate metabolism in the fetus and newborn. British Medical Bulletin 31: 37–43
135. Shelley H J, Neligan G S 1966 Neonatal hypoglycaemia. British Medical Bulletin 22: 34–39
136. Shield J P H, Gardner R J, Wadsworth E J K et al 1996 Transient neonatal diabetes: a study of its aetiopathology and genetic basis. Archives of Disease in Childhood 76(1): F39–42
137. Singh S P, Pullen G L, Snyder A K 1988 Effects of ethanol on fetal fuels and brain growth in rats. Journal of Laboratory and Clinical Medicine 112: 704–710
138. Smallpiece V, Davies P A 1964 Immediate feeding of premature infants with undiluted breast milk. Lancet ii: 1349–1356
139. Soltész G, Aynsley-Green A 1984 Hyperinsulinism in infancy and childhood In: Prader A (ed) Advances in internal medicine and paediatrics, Vol. 51. Springer, Berlin, pp 151–202
140. Soltész G, Jenkins P A, Anysley-Green A 1984 Hyperinsulinaemic hypoglycaemia in infancy and childhood: a practical approach to diagnosis and medical treatment based on experience of 18 cases. Acta Paediatrica Academiae Scientiarum Hungaricae 25: 319–322
141. Soothill P W, Nicolaides K H, Campbell S 1987 Prenatal asphyxia, hyperlacticaemia, hypoglycaemia and erythroblastosis in growth retarded fetuses. British Medical Journal 294: 1051–1053
142. Spar J A, Levine J D, Orrison W W Jr 1994 Neonatal hypoglycemia: CT and MR findings. American Journal of Neuroradiology 15: 1477–1478
143. Spence J C 1921 Some observations on sugar tolerance, with special reference to variations found at different ages. Quarterly Journal of Medicine 14: 314–326
144. Sperling M A, Grajwer L A, Leake R, Fisher D A 1976 Role of glucagon in perinatal glucose homeostasis. Metabolism 25 (suppl 1): 1385–1386
145. Sperling M A, Ganguli S, Leslie N, Landt K 1984 Fetal–perinatal catecholamine secretion: role in perinatal glucose homeostasis. American Journal of Physiology 247: E69–74
146. Srinivasan G, Pildes R S, Cattamanchi G, Voora S, Lilien L D 1986 Plasma glucose values in normal neonates: a new look. Journal of Pediatrics Surgery 21: 114–117
147. Srinivasan G, Jain R, Pildes R S, Kannon C R 1986 Glucose homeostasis during anaesthesia and surgery in infants. Journal of Pediatric Surgery 21: 718–721
148. Stonestreet B S, Rubin L, Pollack A, Cowett R M, Oh W 1980 Renal function of low birthweight infants with hyperglycemia and glucosuria produced by glucose infusion. Pediatrics 66: 561–567
149. Stubbe P, Wolf H 1971 The effect of stress on growth hormone, glucose and glycerol levels in newborn infants. Hormone Metabolism Research 3: 175–179
150. Susa J B, Cowett R M, Oh W 1979 Suppression of gluconeogenesis and endogenous glucose production by exogenous insulin administration in the newborn lamb. Pediatric Research 13: 594–599
151. Temple I K, James R S, Crolla J A et al 1995 An imprinted gene(s) for diabetes. Nature Genetics 9: 110–112
152. Temple I K, Gardner R J, Robinson D O et al 1996 Further evidence for an imprinted gene for neonatal diabetes localised to chromosome 6q22-q23. Human Molecular Genetics 5(8): 1117–1121
153. Thurston J H, Hawhart R E, Schiro J A 1986 β-hydroxybutyrate reverses insulin-induced hypoglycaemic coma in suckling–weanling mice despite low blood and brain glucose levels. Metabolism and Brain Research 1: 63–82
154. Van den Bosch C A, Bullough C H W 1990 The effect of suckling on term neonates' core body temperature. Annals of Tropical Paediatrics 10: 347–353
155. Van Goudoever J B, Sulkers E J, Chapman T E 1993 Glucose kinetics and glucoregulatory hormone levels in ventilated preterm infants on the first day of life. Pediatric Research 33: 583–589
156. Vannucci R C, Nardis E E, Vannucci J S, Campbell P A 1981 Cerebral carbohydrate and energy metabolism during hypoglycemia in newborn dogs. American Journal of Physiology 240: R192–199
157. Vaucher Y E, Watson P D, Morrow G 1982 Continuous insulin infusion in hyperglycemic, very low birthweight infants. Journal of Pediatric Gastrology and Nutrition 1: 211–217
158. Von Muhlendahl K E, Herkenhoff H 1995 Long term outcome of neonatal diabetes. New England Journal of Medicine 333: 704–708
159. Wariyar U, Ward Platt M P 1993 Neonatal hypoglycaemia: changing attitudes in the Northern Region. Health Trends 25: 150–152
160. Wiedemann H R 1964 Complexe malformatif familial avec hernie umbilicale et macroglossie. Un 'syndrome nouveau'? Journal de Génétique Humaine 13: 223–232
161. Wilkins B H 1992 Renal function in sick very low birthweight infants: 4: Glucose excretion. Archives of Disease in Childhood 67: 1162–1165
162. Wilkinson A R, Fok T-F, Au-Yeung H 1984 High incidence of clinical problems in the newborn possibly attributable to theophylline therapy (abstract). Pediatric Research 18: 89
163. World Bank 1995 World Development Report. Oxford University Press, Oxford
164. World Health Organisation 1991 Child health and development: health of the newborn. Report of the Director General of the World Health Organisation EB89/26: 15–17
165. Yunis K A, Oh W, Kalhan S, Cowett R M 1989 Mechanisms of glucose perturbation following intravenous fat infusion in the low birthweight infant. Pediatric Research 25: 299A
166. Zarif M, Pildes R S, Vidyasagar D 1976 Insulin and growth hormone responses in neonatal hyperglycemia. Diabetes 25: 428–433
167. Zuppinger K A 1975 Hypoglycaemia in childhood. Monographs in paediatrics 4. S Karger, Basle

Part 2

Endocrine disorders

Nick D. Barnes Tim D. Cheetham

The endocrine functions of mother, placenta and fetus are closely interwoven, and at birth the transition to independent life is associated with many changes in hormone release and handling. Knowledge of these changes and their impact on circulating hormone concentrations is important when investigating endocrine disease in the newborn. Although obvious physical signs, such as ambiguous genitalia, may occasionally indicate underlying endocrine pathology, more often, in conditions such as hypothyroidism or cortisol deficiency, the signs are subtle and a low threshold for the suspicion of endocrine disease is necessary. Endocrine problems in the newborn may be serious, even life-threatening, but are nearly always treatable, and so it is important that they are identified as soon as possible.

In this chapter space permits only a brief and largely practical discussion of the clinical aspects of the endocrine disorders that may present in the newborn. Advances in the field of molecular biology are now clarifying the cellular basis of many endocrine disorders. For fuller discussions of the clinical and molecular aspects of endocrine disease the reader is referred to standard works on paediatric or general endocrinology, such as Sperling,[165] Brook[13] or Wilson and Foster.[188]

HYPOTHALAMUS AND ANTERIOR PITUITARY

NORMAL FUNCTION

The hypothalamus and anterior pituitary form a neuroendocrine unit, mediating between the central nervous system and the peripheral tissues. The hypothalamic nerve fibres liberate humoral substances into the capillaries of the primary plexus in the median eminence, to be carried by the portal vessels to excite or inhibit the secretion of the cells of the anterior pituitary. Four hypothalamic releasing hormones, CRH, TRH, GnRH and GHRH, and two inhibitory hormones, somatostatin and dopamine, are well recognized. These modulate the secretion into the circulation of the pituitary trophic hormones ACTH, TSH, FSH, LH, GH and prolactin. With the exception of prolactin, these in turn elicit the secretion of further hormones from their target organs.

HYPOTHALAMIC AND ANTERIOR PITUITARY DISEASE

The disorders that may present in the newborn period are shown in Table 38.6. A high index of clinical suspicion and a competent endocrine laboratory are essential for diagnosis and management.

Table 38.6 Hypothalamic and anterior pituitary disease in the newborn

With associated congenital abnormality
Anencephaly, holoprosencephaly
Septo-optic dysplasia and related disorders
Cleft lip and palate
Congenital rubella syndrome
Hall–Pallister syndrome
Abnormal sella turcica

Without associated abnormality
Hypothalamic
- hypothalamic dysplasia, sporadic or genetic
- isolated hypothalamic hormone deficiency, sporadic or genetic
  - GHRH
  - TRH
  - CRH
  - GnRH
- multiple hypothalamic hormone deficiency, sporadic or genetic

Pituitary
- pituitary dysplasia, sporadic or genetic
- isolated pituitary hormone deficiency, sporadic or genetic
  - GH
  - TSH
  - ACTH
  - FSH
  - LH
- multiple pituitary hormone deficiency, sporadic or genetic including *Pit-1* deficiency

Midline developmental defects may be associated with anterior pituitary dysplasia. In anencephaly some anterior pituitary tissue is always present, although it may be hypoplastic and outside a malformed sella.[172] Holoprosencephaly is associated with various anomalies, including aplasia of the olfactory bulbs and tracts, facial dysplasia and pituitary defects. Congenital hypopituitarism may occur with trans-sphenoidal encephalocele and mid-facial anomalies.[37]

These are gross neuroanatomical abnormalities, but pituitary insufficiency of variable degree may also accompany less serious defects. It has been described in 4% of children with cleft lip and palate.[146] Hypothalamic–pituitary insufficiency may also occur in association with hypoplasia of the optic nerves: in fully expressed septo-optic dysplasia there is agenesis of the septum pellucidum and hypoplasia of the optic tracts and infundibulum; such infants are blind and have small optic discs, but partial forms of this syndrome occur.[166]

Absence of the pituitary has been reported in newborn infants with hypothalamic hamartoblastoma, imperforate anus, postaxial polydactyly and other congenital defects,[57] and partial pituitary deficiency of early onset has also been described in congenital rubella syndrome.[133] Familial hypopituitarism with diabetes insipidus but no other apparent CNS or midline abnormality has also been reported.[192] Birth trauma was thought to be the cause of many cases of 'idiopathic' hypopituitarism; there is a high incidence of breech and forceps delivery in some series,[24] and Rona and Tanner[142] calculated that a male firstborn delivered by the breech has an 11-fold increased risk of growth hormone deficiency. The fetus with isolated anterior pituitary aplasia[77] and most with hypothalamic hypopituitarism[171] still present in the cephalic position and an underlying brain malformation that is associated with altered movement in utero may be the common link between hypopituitarism and breech delivery.[33]

Gene defects resulting in isolated deficiencies of GH, TSH, ACTH or gonadotrophins[191] and the abnormal regulation of pituitary hormone release may cause hypopituitarism. *Pit-1* is a transcription factor involved in the regulation of GH, TSH and prolactin production, and *Pit-1* deficiency can present with hypopituitarism in the neonatal period.[34,128,129] The diagnosis should be considered if there is a family history of hypopituitarism, and where ACTH and gonadotrophin release are preserved.

Diagnosis

Clinical recognition of hypopituitarism in the newborn is difficult. Growth hormone deficiency leads to relatively subtle changes in body form, with a reduction in length of about 1 SD but a normal birthweight.[46] Micropenis is an important sign in the male with gonadotrophin deficiency,[149] but the first indicator of an underlying endocrinopathy is often hypoglycaemia[89] (p. 944). This can occasionally reflect isolated growth hormone deficiency (GH is an insulin antagonist), but it is seldom a prominent symptom in this disorder and severe early hypoglycaemia suggests adrenocortical insufficiency or panhypopituitarism, which must always be excluded in unexplained hypoglycaemia. Prolonged neonatal jaundice with a conjugated hyperbilirubinaemia has been described in association with congenital hypopituitarism[61] and is linked closely to cortisol deficiency. Symptomatic hypothyroidism is not usually a feature of hypopituitarism, reflecting the less profound effect on thyroid hormone production when the thyroid gland is intact although understimulated.

Biochemical confirmation of hypopituitarism requires measurement of pituitary hormones in the resting state and after stimulation, either with non-specific stimuli, such as hypoglycaemia, or with specific hypothalamic releasing hormones, TRH for TSH and prolactin, GnRH for LH and FSH, CRH for ACTH and GHRH for growth hormone. With the releasing hormones, an absent response typically indicates hypopituitarism and a partial and/or delayed response hypothalamic insufficiency. In practice such tests are only seldom needed and should probably be done in specialist units. GH levels are often elevated in the first days of life, and a single value can provide valuable information. A low or unrecordable GH concentration at the time of a documented hypoglycaemic episode suggests hypothalamopituitary disease. Non-specific stimulation of GH release with glucagon may also be used in the older infant. It should be remembered that drugs, such as dopamine, that are used in neonatal intensive care may interfere with endocrine investigations.[32]

Treatment

Hypopituitarism is treated by replacing either the missing pituitary hormones or the products of their target organs. For adrenal replacement hydrocortisone in a dose around 10–12 mg/m²/24 h (in two or three divided doses) is suitable. Although the cortisol production rate in the newborn is 6.6–8.8 mg/m²/24 h[99] absorption and bioavailability vary considerably and this needs to be taken into consideration. For thyroid replacement thyroxine in a single dose of 100 μg/m²/24 h, approximately 10 μg/kg/24 h in the newborn, is suitable initially (p. 962). Growth hormone replacement is not necessary to sustain growth in the first year of life, but it may be needed to control the hypoglycaemia of hypopituitarism if this proves intractable.

RESISTANCE TO THE ACTIONS OF ANTERIOR PITUITARY HORMONES

Endocrine disorders in which hormone action is impaired or absent due to abnormalities of the receptor or abnormal postreceptor events are now well recognized. The phenotypic features of these rare conditions may suggest hypopituitarism, but the levels of pituitary hormones are usually normal or elevated. The best-described example is probably insensitivity to GH (Laron syndrome), which can present with hypoglycaemia and micropenis in the newborn period. Resistance to TSH, ACTH and gonadotrophins[87,167,181] presenting with neonatal hypothyroidism, hypoadrenalism or micropenis, respectively, is also recognized.[191]

POSTERIOR PITUITARY[126]

NORMAL FUNCTION

From the end of the first trimester oxytocin and vasopressin (AVP/ADH) are elaborated from prohormones in the hypothalamic supraoptic and paraventricular nuclei and conveyed along the neurons of the neurohypophyseal tract in conjunction with specific carrier proteins, the neurophysins, to the posterior pituitary, where they are stored and released under neural control.

Oxytocin causes uterine contraction and milk ejection, but neonatal disease due to deficiency or excess is not recognized.

Vasopressin alters the permeability of the renal collecting tubules for water and urea, varying free water loss by up to 25 times. Secretion is controlled by the osmoreceptors of the hypothalamus, the stretch receptors of the left atrium and the baroreceptors in the carotid sinus; it is increased by hyperosmolality, hypovolaemia and the upright position, and decreased by hypo-osmolality, hypervolaemia and the recumbent position.

DIABETES INSPIDUS[126]

In the absence of vasopressin, urine volume and tonicity are changed only minimally in the distal tubule and collecting ducts; urine volume can reach nearly 10% of the glomerular filtrate, with an osmolality of 100 mmol/kgH_2O or less. Permanent severe pituitary diabetes insipidus occurs only with destruction of the supraoptic nucleus or high stalk section, more distal lesions usually causing only transient partial malfunction.[38] Congenital brain malformations such as septo-optic dysplasia may cause posterior as well as anterior pituitary dysfunction.[93]

Diabetes inspidus is increasingly recognized in the newborn. The causes are shown in Table 38.7.

Clinically the condition is characterized by excessive fluid output and intake. Congenital diabetes inspidus may be heralded by polyhydramnios. Diagnosis is difficult in the newborn because a high urine output is easily overlooked and persistent crying and weight loss are likely to be ascribed to a cause other than water loss. The low osmolar load of breast-feeding tends to reduce the symptoms. Infants may therefore present late, with non-specific symptoms such as anorexia, vomiting, poor weight gain, constipation or delayed development.

The diagnosis is confirmed by failure to concentrate the urine in spite of plasma hypertonicity, and reversal by administration of vasopressin or an analogue. Polyuria due to hypercalcaemia or potassium deficiency must be excluded, and allowance made for the lesser concentrating power of the neonatal kidney. Assays for plasma and urine vasopressin are available.[137] The principal differential diagnoses are nephrogenic diabetes insipidus, which is an inherited renal tubular anomaly (p. 1033), or a water-losing nephropathy (p. 1032).

Table 38.7 Causes of vasopressin-deficient diabetes insipidus

Primary
Familial
isolated-X-linked recessive
autosomal dominant
with other congenital anomalies such as septo-optic dysplasia
Laurence–Moon–Biedl syndrome
Wolfram (DIDMOAD) syndrome
Idiopathic sporadic
Secondary
Trauma, asphyxia
Intraventricular haemorrhage
Disseminated intravascular coagulation
Inflammation e.g. meningitis and CMV infection
Maternal drug therapy, e.g. lithium

Treatment

Treatment is by replacement of vasopressin or use of an analogue, of which the most effective available is desmopressin (DDAVP). This compound is more potent than the native molecule and has a five times longer half-life.[140] The standard solution (100 µg/ml) may be diluted with 0.9% NaCl solution to create a more manageable volume (for example 10 µg/ml – discuss with the hospital pharmacy) and can be instilled into the nose using a 1 ml syringe or with a graduated rhinyl catheter. A suitable starting dose in the newborn is 1.0 µg daily in one or two doses. The dose can be altered as necessary for adequate antidiuretic effect, since the absorption and therapeutic effects are variable in degree and duration. It is extremely important to be aware of the danger of water overload, which will develop in the presence of too much medication or excessive fluid administration, and osmolality should be checked regularly, particularly in the initial phase while the dose is being adjusted. It is safer in both the short and the long term for an infant with diabetes insipidus (and an intact sense of thirst) to be allowed to compensate for a relatively low dose of DDAVP by feeding or drinking more. Parents should be actively involved in management from an early stage and encouraged to gauge both fluid input and output. An oral preparation, Desmotabs, is now available, but experience of its use in the newborn period is limited.

EXCESS VASOPRESSIN SECRETION (SYNDROME OF INAPPROPRIATE ADH SECRETION)

This is described on pages 1024–1025.

THYROID

Disorders of thyroid development and/or function are relatively common, affecting approximately one newborn infant in 3000. Delay in diagnosis and treatment may have disastrous consequences. Improved methods for the measurement of thyroid axis hormones and the information gained from population screening for congenital hypothyroidism have greatly increased the understanding of neonatal thyroid disorders.

NORMAL FUNCTION

Thyroid hormones have a profound effect on the rate of cellular oxidation in most tissues except the central

Table 38.8 Developmental disorders of thyroid function

	Disorders	
	Permanent	**Transient**
Embryogenesis (0–12 weeks' gestation)		
Thyroid gland development		
anatomical	Aplasia, hypoplasia, ectopia	
biochemical	Dyshormonogenesis	
Pituitary development		
anatomical	Aplasia, hypoplasia	
biochemical	TSH deficiency	
Hypothalamic maturation (5–35 weeks' gestation)		
Hypothalamic development		
anatomical	Dysplasia	
biochemical	TRH deficiency	
Functional maturation of the thyroid axis (20 weeks' gestation to 4 weeks postnatal)		
Feedback control of TRH and TSH secretion		Hypothyroxinaemia
TSH control of thyroid function		Hyperthyrotrophinaemia
Thyroid gland metabolism		Hypothyroidism due to antithyroid drugs, iodine excess or deficiency
Peripheral thyroxine metabolism		Low T3 syndrome (non-thyroidal illness)
Protein binding of serum thyroid hormones	Binding protein abnormalities	
Tissue responsiveness	Thyroid hormone resistance	

nervous system. The key circulating thyroid hormone is free T3. TSH, modulated by TRH, stimulates the synthesis and release of T4 and T3 from the thyroid into the plasma, where they circulate, strongly bound to proteins. The greater part of the circulating T3, however, is derived from peripheral monodeiodination of the outer ring of T4, which therefore acts as a reservoir or prohormone for the more active T3. An alternative monodeiodination affects the inner ring of T4 and produces reverse T3, a totally inactive compound. This remarkably economical mechanism permits a balance between production of the most and least active thyroid hormones.

It is now recognized that maternal T4, but not TSH or T3, crosses the placenta in physiologically significant amounts, which explains the relatively normal phenotype in hypothyroid infants at birth.[17,34] Maternal and endogenous T4 is converted preferentially to reverse T3 by the fetus. Thyroid development can be considered in three partially overlapping phases, during each of which errors may occur. These are summarized in Table 38.8.

After birth there is an acute discharge of TSH, provoked by cooling, which reaches a peak at 30 minutes then falls to basal levels within the first 3 days. This evokes an appropriate release of thyroid hormones. In addition, within 4–6 hours of delivery there is a three to sixfold increase in T3, owing to enhanced peripheral conversion from T4. There is a further increase in total T3 and free T3 levels for about 36 hours, which coincides with the postnatal peak in T4 (Fig. 38.7). Preterm infants delivered before this maturational process is complete show similar but lesser changes in TSH and iodothyronine concentrations. T4 levels remain below those of full-term infants through the first few weeks of

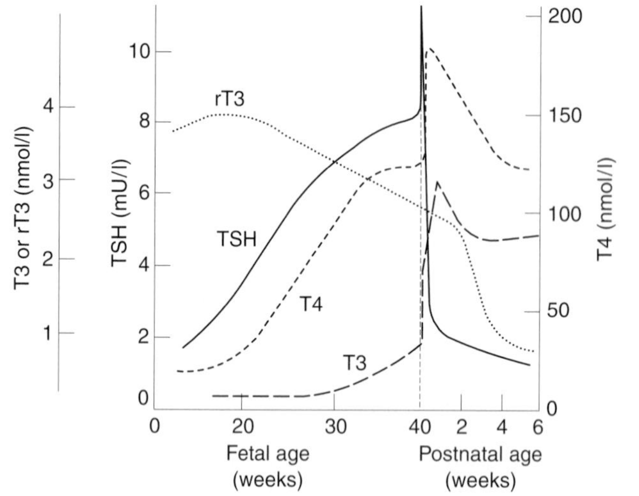

Fig. 38.7 The trend in fetal and neonatal plasma TSH/T4/T3 and rT3 levels. (Adapted from Fisher[41])

life,[44] and T3 levels climb gradually to normal postnatal levels.

NEONATAL SCREENING[54,55]

When radioimmunoassays were developed for measurement first of T4, and soon thereafter TSH, in very small samples of serum or whole blood spotted on to filter paper, screening was rapidly adopted in many countries. Most programmes used a single blood sample taken between the fifth and ninth days of life, by which age relative stability has returned to the thyroid axis after the abrupt postnatal perturbation. T4 screening alone proved inadequate because of the overlap between normal and hypothyroid values. The alternatives were therefore either to add a TSH assay in all cases or for the lower range of T4 values, or to use TSH as the primary test and accept that the rare cases of secondary hypothyroidism would be missed. Programmes based on both systems were successful and both retain advocates, but most have now adopted the primary TSH approach.[48] There remain pitfalls in this, as in all forms of screening.[113] Guidelines for neonatal screening programmes have been published.[5,54]

The returns from screening proved even greater than had been expected: in both America and Europe the frequency of congenital hypothyroidism was approximately 1 in 3500, almost double that suggested by retrospective surveys.[39,112] Isotope scanning showed that many infants had hypoplastic and/or ectopic thyroid tissue, and without screening would probably not have presented until later in childhood. Hypothyroidism had very seldom been suspected clinically by the time it was biochemically confirmed, and treatment could be started by 1–4 weeks of age.

HYPOTHYROIDISM

Thyroid dysgenesis

Embyrological defects causing thyroid dysgenesis are the most common causes of congenital primary hypothyroidism, and range from an ectopic and/or hypoplastic gland to thyroid agenesis. Some thyroid tissue is demonstrable in approximately two-thirds of affected infants, and there is a spectrum of severity of hypothyroidism. The frequency is around 1 in 3500, and although it is usually viewed as a sporadic condition of unknown cause there is increasing evidence that gene mutations of, for example, the TSH receptor may account for some cases of dysgenesis.[8] Thyroid dysgenesis is twice as common in females as in males and only minor racial and seasonal differences in incidence have been reported. Familial cases are very rare, but there is an association with Down syndrome.

Thyroid hormone replacement abolishes the physical manifestations of hypothyroidism but, as first reported by Smith et al in 1957,[159] the intellectual and neurological prognosis is poor unless treatment is started within the first few weeks of life. Because the early manifestations are non-specific and development of the typical features usually occurs only slowly (Table 38.9), even in the most medically advanced countries no more than half the affected infants could be diagnosed clinically by the age of 3 months, which is dangerously late for treatment to start.[4] The problem therefore was to identify affected infants promptly, and the need for screening was apparent.

Table 38.9 Clinical features of congenital hypothyroidism

May be present at birth
Postmaturity, large size
Large posterior fontanelle, delayed bone age
Umbilical hernia
Goitre
Early signs (first 4 weeks)
Placid, 'good', sleepy
Poor feeding
Constipation, abdominal distension
Respiratory problems
Mottling, hypothermia, peripheral cyanosis
Oedema
Prolonged 'physiological' jaundice
Late signs
Cretinous appearance
Large tongue
Hoarse cry
Dry skin, hair
Slow responses
Retarded development
Growth failure, infantile proportions

Diagnosis

It remains essential to exclude hypothyroidism in any infant in whom there is clinical suspicion because, first, errors inevitably occur in all screening programmes; secondly, mild hypothyroidism may escape detection by all screening methods; and thirdly, early acquired hypothyroidism does occasionally occur. The major clinical features are summarized in Table 38.9. Infants with low thyroxine values (less than 30 nmol/l) are more likely to have clinical signs such as feeding difficulties, lethargy, prolonged jaundice, umbilical hernia and macroglossia.[50] Such infants are more likely to have an aplastic rather than a hypoplastic or ectopic gland. A gestation over 40 weeks, induction of labour and a birthweight above 3500 g are all more common among infants with hypothyroidism. The diagnosis is made by finding a low serum T4 and high TSH. The T3 level is variable and is preserved in the normal range for longer. A TRH stimulation test is rarely indicated, but an exaggerated and prolonged TSH response is observed if TSH levels are mildly elevated because of a compromised thyroid gland.[135] Imaging can give further information about the nature, and hence the prognosis, of the underlying defect. In thyroid dysgenesis an isotope scan (technetium or ^{123}I) will reveal an absent, small or ectopic gland. This condition has a very low risk of recurrence in further children. If the gland is anatomically normal and the uptake is high, the hypothyroidism is probably due to dyshormonogenesis and inherited as an autosomal recessive condition. Scanning should be undertaken before or within a few days of starting thyroxine replacement treatment, when the TSH levels are still high. Ultrasound examination of the neck can be used as a means of identifying the size and site of the gland, but is an operator-dependent technique. A plain radiograph of the knee to assess epiphyseal maturity is often taken and may reflect the degree of fetal hypothyroidism, but is of limited clinical value.

Treatment[51]

Thyroxine is used for replacement and there is no advantage in giving tri-iodothyronine. It is a matter of some urgency to start treatment, and when the diagnosis is virtually certain it may be preferable to collect further specimens and start treatment without waiting for the results. If these do fail to confirm the diagnosis, reassessment can be undertaken sooner rather than later.

In hypothyroidism of postnatal onset the thyroid axis can be used to assess the correct dose of thyroxine in an individual patient, which can be defined as the smallest dose that suppresses the serum TSH into the normal range. In congenital hypothyroidism this is generally true, but in some infants the set-point of the thyroid axis may be abnormal and excessively large doses of thyroxine may be needed to suppress the TSH. Replacement is usually satisfactory if the serum total T4 and free T4 are in the upper part of the quoted laboratory normal range for age, and this should be checked on four or five occasions during the first year of life. There is some evidence to suggest that the initial dose of thyroxine may affect subsequent IQ, with higher doses related to higher IQ scores later in childhood, but this has not been a consistent observation.[50,144] Severe overdosage may cause accelerated bone maturation and even craniostenosis, but the danger of impaired neurological development from underdosage is greater. An appropriate starting dose of thyroxine in the newborn is 10–15 μg/kg/24 h given as a single daily dose.[5,36] It is satisfactory to start all full-term infants on 37.5–50 μg daily, and this brings the TSH into the normal range quickly. Tablets of 25 μg are available, and because of the long half-life of thyroxine the dose can be adjusted more accurately by giving a higher or lower dose on alternate days, such as 25 μg one day and 50 μg the next. Because thyroxine acts as a prohormone there is probably little to be gained by more exact weight-related dosage, and thyroxine suspensions can be unreliable.

Follow-up and prognosis

It is vital that parents understand the importance of this most unimpressive-looking medication. Growth, clinical progress and thyroid function should be checked after 6–8 weeks on treatment, and then at 2–3-monthly intervals through the first year and regularly thereafter. Persistently high TSH levels in spite of T4 levels at the upper end of the normal range may be observed in the first weeks of treatment, but an increase in dose should be considered if the TSH levels remain elevated beyond the first few weeks. The commonest reason for raised TSH levels at this, as at other, ages is probably lack of compliance.

Table 38.10 Reassessment protocol in congenital hypothyroidism

After 2 years of age
replace T4 with T3 20 μg daily for 4 weeks
stop all therapy for 10 days
check thyroid function (and isotope scan if needed)
resume previous T4 dose immediately
reassess when results available

If needed, definitive reassessment of thyroid status can be undertaken after the age of 2 years, when brief cessation of treatment will have no adverse effect. The interruption of treatment can be reduced if the maintenance preparation is changed from T4 to T3 beforehand to take advantage of the shorter half-life. A suitable protocol is shown in Table 38.10. In addition to the serological thyroid function tests, this opportunity can be taken to obtain or repeat an isotope thyroid scan.

Congenital hypothyroidism is associated with impaired motor development, a lower IQ and impaired hearing and language problems.[30,145] These features are related to the severity of hypothyroidism at birth. In one study T4 levels below 42 nmol/l in the neonatal period were associated with a 10-point deficit in IQ at school entry.[170] Individuals with T4 values above 42 nmol/l were no different from controls, indicating a threshold effect, and neither the average thyroxine dose nor thyroxine concentration during treatment in the first year affected IQ. Thus it seems that the degree of pre- and perinatal hypothyroidism has implications for central nervous system function in the long term.

Dyshormonogenesis[136]

Recessively inherited biochemical defects of iodothyronine synthesis are the second most common cause of permanent congenital hypothyroidism, with a frequency in Europe and North America of approximately 1 in 30–50 000, accounting for some 10–15% of patients identified by screening. The sex incidence is equal. A goitre may be present at birth but, unless large, may be difficult to detect and may not develop until later in life. The degree of clinical hypothyroidism is also variable but tends to be mild. Biochemically such infants, like those with thyroid dysplasia, show low T4 and high TSH concentrations. The T3 is often within the normal range and sometimes, in ‘compensated’ hypothyroidism, the T4 is also within the normal range. An isotope scan usually shows normal thyroid anatomy and increased or normal uptake, except in the rare disorder of iodine trapping. In Pendred syndrome of goitre and congenital deafness there is usually excessive discharge of iodide from the thyroid gland after administration of perchlorate (the perchlorate discharge test), due to an abnormality of organification of iodide into thyroglobulin. Compensated primary hypothyroidism with normal isotope imaging due to abnormalities of the TSH receptor has now been

Table 38.11 Inherited metabolic defects causing hypothyroidism

TSH resistance including TSH receptor defects
Iodine transport defect
Organification (peroxidase) defect
with deafness (Pendred syndrome)
without deafness
Defective iodotyrosine coupling
Defective iodotyrosine deiodinase activity
Aberrant thyroglobulin synthesis
Defective thyroid hormone secretion
Thyroid hormone resistance
at pituitary and peripheral tissues

described.[167] Delineation of the precise biochemical defect in these disorders does not alter the need for life-long replacement, but can be important when counselling families about the likelihood of recurrence. The chemical defects that have been defined are shown in Table 38.11.

Secondary (pituitary/hypothalamic) congenital hypothyroidism

These conditions are rare, causing hypothyroidism in approximately 1 in 60–100 000 infants. TSH deficiency is indicated by low bound and free T4 and T3 levels and a low TSH which is unresponsive to TRH stimulation. In hypothalamic hypothyroidism the iodothyronine values are similar but the TSH may be slightly raised, which can be misleading, and typically shows a delayed or sometimes normal response to TRH.

Abnormalities of binding proteins

The major carrier protein of the thyroid hormones is thyroxine-binding globulin. Deficiency of TBG is usually inherited as an X-linked dominant trait and has a frequency of approximately 1 in 10 000, with a male/female ratio of 9:1.[39] Affected patients are euthyroid. Total T4 and T3 levels are low, but the free fractions are normal and the resting and stimulated TSH values are also normal. TBG measurement is needed for definitive diagnosis.

TRANSIENT DISORDERS OF THYROID FUNCTION

Transient hypothyroxinaemia

All premature infants have some degree of hypothyroxinaemia, as cord serum T4 values increase with gestational age. Low values persist in the first 1–2 weeks in association with low free T4 and normal TSH levels. T4 values increase gradually from approximately 2 weeks onwards. This was thought to be of little consequence in the short term,[22] but recent evidence has suggested a relationship between thyroxine concentrations in preterm and low-birthweight infants and subsequent neurodevelopmental outcome.[29,97,138] Although these studies have attempted to consider potential confounding variables it is possible that in some infants thyroxine levels are simply a marker of fetal wellbeing. A low thyroxine concentration may therefore be an adaptation to illness in preterm infants, as in adults.[40] The impact of thyroxine administration on the short- and longer-term outcome following preterm delivery has also to be established. Improvements in survival have been reported in some studies[154] but not others,[22] and early neurodevelopmental outcome does not appear to be affected by treatment in those infants born between 27 and 30 weeks' gestation.[174,175] The effects of thyroxine administration may depend on the gestation and age of the infant treated, with protective mechanisms ensuring an adequate supply of tri-iodothyronine in all but the most preterm.

Transient hyperthyrotropinaemia

In this disorder T4 and T3 concentrations are normal but TSH is raised, returning to normal within the first few months of life. Treatment is not necessary but is safe if the diagnosis is in doubt. The cause may be delayed maturation of thyroid responsiveness to TSH, intra-uterine exposure to antithyroid drugs, and iodine deficiency or excess.[79] Artefactual hyperthyrotropinaemia in both mother and infant may also occur in the presence of antibodies that interfere with the TSH assay.

Transient hypothyroidism

Transient hypothyroidism (in contrast to infants with transient hypothyroxinaemia, TSH levels are raised, in addition to low iodothyronine levels) has been observed with variable frequency in different populations, probably in relation to iodine availability.[28] Premature babies are most frequently affected. A high incidence has also been described in infants exposed to routine use of topical iodinated antiseptic agents:[79,158] these are readily absorbed and should be avoided or carefully removed following initial application. Transient hypothyroidism may be due to the transplacental passage of thyrotropin receptor-blocking antibodies in approximately 2% of cases of congenital hypothyroidism.[16] Hypothyroidism develops in the first weeks of life and persists for a variable time, usually 2 or 3 months. Thyroxine replacement is needed to cover the period of hypothyroidism. Unless transient hypothyroidism is suspected, the precise diagnosis may not be made until reassessment is undertaken at a later stage. In some infants early acquired neonatal hypothyroidism has been observed, sometimes due to iodine exposure, to which the premature infant is especially susceptible, or to another exogenous environmental goitrogen. A brief reduction in thyroxine levels, with an associated rise in TSH lasting a few days, has been observed in neonates born to mothers who received antithyroid drugs in pregnancy.[21]

The 'low T3 syndrome' (non-thyroidal illness)

This term is used to describe thyroid function tests characterized by low serum T3 concentrations, normal or raised reverse T3, variable T4 and normal TSH. Fetal T3 levels are low throughout gestation because of enhanced conversion of T4 to reverse T3, and this picture is frequently observed in preterm infants. As in older patients, T3 levels may be further reduced by intercurrent illness and poor nutrition in infants of all gestational ages. Recent evidence has suggested a possible link between T3 levels below 0.3 nmol/l and lower intelligence in later life.[90] Thyroxine administration to infants of less than 30 weeks' gestation does not increase T3 levels.[174]

HYPERTHYROIDISM

Neonatal thyrotoxicosis

Neonatal thyrotoxicosis is a relatively rare but serious condition, usually caused by the transplacental passage of thyroid-stimulating immunoglobulins (TSI; a general term for antibodies mimicking TSH actions) from the serum of a mother with active, inactive or treated Graves' disease.[95,168] It may also occur when the mother has autoimmune thyroid disease other than Graves'.[14,65] The disease is usually transient, resolving within the timespan predictable from the half-life of the stimulating immunoglobulins. Neonatal hyperthyroidism is underrecognized but it can often be predicted and treated prenatally, and this may prove life-saving to the infant.

TSI may be demonstrated in the sera of nearly all patients with Graves' disease, and these antibodies cross the placenta freely. Thyrotoxicosis in the fetus may lead to preterm labour, low birthweight, stillbirth and neonatal death. Only about 1 in 70–100 infants of mothers with Graves' disease becomes overtly thyrotoxic, and the risk is related to the concentration of TSI in the maternal serum.[107,157,196] Thyrotropin-binding inhibitory immunoglobulins may be be present as well as TSI, and the clinical and biochemical picture will reflect the impact of the high thyroid hormone levels on hypothalamopituitary function as well as the prevailing immunoglobulin concentrations; thus an infant who is initially hyperthyroid can subsequently become hypothyroid.[59]

Although neonatal thyrotoxicosis is usually due to the transplacental passage of TSI, in some infants such antibodies are not present and the hyperthyroidism persists.[67] These children suffer more complications and long-term morbidity, in particular growth failure in spite of early accelerated skeletal maturity, behaviour problems, and even mental retardation. It is likely that most of the reported cases are due to constitutively active mutations of the TSH receptor.[80]

Clinical features (Table 38.12)

Table 38.12 Clinical features of neonatal hyperthyroidism

Thyroid	Goitre
Central nervous system	Irritability, restlessness, 'jitteriness'
Eyes	Stare, lid retraction, oedema, proptosis
Cardiovascular system	Tachycardia, cardiac failure, arrhythmia
Gastrointestinal tract	Excess appetite, weight loss, emaciation, diarrhoea
Other	Sweating, flushing, acrocyanosis, hepatosplenomegaly, lymphadenopathy, thymic enlargement, thrombocytopenia, bruising, petechiae, hyperviscosity, advanced skeletal maturation, craniosynostosis, microcephaly

The signs of thyrotoxicosis in the fetus include tachycardia and intrauterine growth retardation. Infants with perinatal thyrotoxicosis may show signs of hyperthyroidism immediately after birth, but symptoms may be delayed as long as 4–6 weeks.[157,195] This may be due to the effect of maternal antithyroid drugs or to the relative effects of both blocking and stimulating antibodies. Most infants have a palpable goitre, and although eye signs, especially proptosis and lid retraction, may be present at birth they are often mild or absent throughout the course of the disease. Very rarely a mother with euthyroid ophthalmic Graves' disease may produce an infant with eye involvement but no evidence of thyrotoxicosis. Signs of central nervous system stimulation, such as irritability, restlessness and 'jitteriness', usually predominate and there is tachycardia and occasionally arrhythmia, which may progress rapidly to severe and intractable heart failure. Other signs of hypermetabolism include an excessive appetite with weight loss or inadequate weight gain, diarrhoea, sweating and flushing. Less predictable clinical features include hepatosplenomegaly, jaundice and accelerated bone maturation, which can cause premature closure of the skull sutures, with craniosynostosis and occasionally microcephaly.[197] Mortality rates of 16–25% have been reported,[157,197] and the long-term outcome is uncertain.

Management

Hyperthyroid mothers should be treated with the antithyroid thiourea derivatives carbimazole or propylthiouracil.[143] The use of radioactive iodine is absolutely contraindicated during pregnancy, and surgery may precipitate preterm delivery. The antithyroid drugs cross the placenta, and the lowest dose that controls the hyperthyroidism should be used. This is often lower in pregnancy than the dose normally required in adults. The 'block and replace' regimen, using higher doses of antithyroid drugs in combination with replacement thyroxine, should be avoided. If maternal antithyroid treatment causes goitre formation and bradycardia in the fetus, it is possible to give thyroxine by intramniotic injection. There may be biochemical evidence of transient hypothyroidism in clinically euthyroid infants of mothers treated with antithyroid drugs.[21] If fetal tachycardia suggests hyperthyroidism, treatment should be adjusted to maintain the fetal heart rate below 160 beats per minute and careful assessment of fetal growth is necessary. Cordocentesis may be used to confirm the diagnosis.

Severe hyperthyroidism carries a high mortality in the newborn. The key to successful management is first, anticipation and prevention, then control of thyroid status until the disease runs its self-limited course. If the fetus was believed to be hyperthyroid and the mother received a thionamide during pregnancy, the wisest course will usually be to continue the same preparation in suitable neonatal dosage, propylthiouracil 10 mg/kg/24 h or carbimazole 1.0 mg/kg/24 h in divided doses by mouth every 6–8 hours. Regular assessment of thyroid function is necessary. As at other ages, it may be difficult to maintain a stable euthyroid state on treatment, and so it is sometimes easier and safer to give a generous dose of an antithyroid and simultaneously a replacement dose of thyroxine. Infants who are clinically euthyroid and subsequently show signs of hyperthyroidism will also need to be treated. Antithyroid medication should be continued for several weeks and then cautiously withdrawn. It is essential to maintain close observation until treatment has been successfully stopped and the infant is well, because fatal acute recurrent thyrotoxicosis has occurred at this stage. If an infant is thought to be at particular risk of hyperthyroidism, if a sibling was symptomatic or if there is a high titre of maternal antibodies, for example, then close clinical and biochemical surveillance should be continued for the first weeks of life. Treatment with an antithyroid preparation should be started promptly if necessary.

If acute thyrotoxicosis does occur, in addition to a thionamide, propranolol 2.0 mg/kg/24 h in divided doses by mouth 6–8-hourly can be used to control the peripheral stimulatory effects of thyroid hormones and/or potassium iodide, as aqueous iodine (Lugol's) solution (iodine 5%, potassium iodide 10%, in water), one drop 8-hourly, to prevent synthesis and release of thyroid hormones from the gland. Treatment may be needed for heart failure, infection or other complications. Radiographic iodine-containing agents have also been used in the treatment of neonatal Graves' disease, partly because of the relatively rapid response.[76] Neonatal hyperthyroidism due to the transplacental passage of antibody usually resolves by the time the infant is 4–6 months of age.

DISORDERS OF CALCIUM METABOLISM[84,85]

NORMAL PHYSIOLOGY

Calcium has a central role in many physiological processes, including transmission across membranes, activation and inhibition of enzymes, intracellular regulation of metabolic sequences, the secretion and action of hormones, blood coagulation, muscle contraction and nerve transmission. In addition, calcium gives structural stability to the skeleton, which contains approximately 99% of total body calcium. Most of this large calcium pool is metabolically inactive and can be mobilized only slowly, but a small available fraction is under close regulation.

Calcium is present in serum in three fractions, protein bound (30–50% of the total), diffusible non-ionized calcium, chiefly in complexes with phosphate and citrate (5–15%), and ionized (40–60%). The ionized fraction is metabolically active and available for regulation. Of the protein-bound calcium approximately 80% is attached to albumin and 20% to globulin, but this varies with the concentration of albumin and the pH. A rough 'correction' of the serum calcium concentration can be made by adding or subtracting 0.1 mmol/l for each 4 g/l of albumin above or below the mean serum albumin for age. Hydrogen ions compete with calcium for binding sites, so that a decrease in pH causes a release of calcium from albumin and an immediate increase in ionized calcium, then, once homoeostasis is restored, a decreased total serum calcium; the opposite effect occurs with alkalosis.

There is active transport of calcium and phosphate by the placenta to the fetus, particularly in the last trimester. Fetal serum calcium increases from around 1.38 mmol/l in mid-pregnancy to 2.75 mmol/l at term. Serum total and ionized calcium concentration are high in cord blood but decrease rapidly in the first hours after birth, remaining relatively low for the first 2–4 days[94] before rising and remaining fairly constant until adult life.

There are three major influences on calcium metabolism: the parathyroids, vitamin D and calcitonin.

The parathyroids

Parathyroid hormone has 84 amino acid residues, of which the amino-terminal 34 have full biological activity. The primary stimulus to PTH synthesis and secretion is a low serum calcium level, but the secretion of PTH is reduced by a low magnesium concentration. When PTH is released it is rapidly degraded into a number of fragments, the more active of which include the amino-terminal sequence and have a half-life of only a few minutes. Some inactive fragments remain in the circulation much longer. The primary action of PTH is on the osteoclasts and promotes the release of calcium from bone. In the kidney it increases the excretion of phosphate (and sodium, potassium and bicarbonate) and decreases that of calcium (and magnesium and hydrogen ion). These are the primary actions that regulate calcium levels acutely, but PTH also increases the formation of 1,25-dihydroxyvitamin D, and so indirectly increases calcium absorption from the gut in the longer term.

Vitamin D

This term describes a number of compounds related to cholesterol, the two naturally occurring forms being ergocalciferol (D2), which is derived from plants, and cholecalciferol (D3), which is derived from the effect of irradiation on precursors in the skin and is absorbed from animal sources in the diet. In the blood vitamin D and its metabolites are transported by vitamin D-binding protein, an α_2-globulin. Vitamin D is then hydroxylated, primarily by the liver, to 25-hydroxyvitamin D, which is the major circulating vitamin D metabolite. This undergoes 1-hydroxylation in the kidney to 1,25-dihydroxyvitamin D, the metabolically active form, or to 1,24,25-trihydroxyvitamin D or 24,25-dihydroxyvitamin D (see below). 1-hydroxylation is stimulated and 24-hydroxylation inhibited by hypocalcaemia, hypophosphataemia and PTH.

The net effect of vitamin D is to increase serum levels of calcium and phosphate by increasing their absorption from the gut, increasing mobilization of calcium and phosphate from bone in the presence of PTH and decreasing renal excretion of calcium and phosphate. The facilitation of bone mineralization by vitamin D is probably due to its impact on circulating calcium and phosphate levels. Fetal 1,25-dihydroxyvitamin D is probably the major stimulus to placental transfer of calcium.

The physiological significance of 1,24,25-trihydroxyvitamin D and 24,25-dihydroxyvitamin D is uncertain, although the latter may also be involved in the maintainance of bone mineralization and in the inhibition of PTH release.

Calcitonin

This 32 amino acid peptide hormone is secreted by the parafollicular C cells of the thyroid in response to hypercalcaemia. It lowers serum calcium by inhibiting bone resorption, increasing urinary calcium and phosphate loss, and probably by decreasing intestinal calcium absorption. Although it can produce hypocalcaemia in humans, neither removal of the thyroid gland nor massive hypersecretion in medullary thyroid carcinoma affects the serum calcium, and its chief physiological significance may be in promoting prenatal skeletal development and preserving maternal skeletal integrity during pregnancy.

RECEPTORS AND CALCIUM HOMEOSTASIS

Defects of vitamin D, PTH and calcium receptors and other abnormalities which cause altered signal transduction may cause hypo- and hypercalcaemia. The vitamin D receptor is one of a family of nuclear receptors,[62] whereas the PTH receptor is one of a group of G protein-coupled receptors.[15] Cellular resistance to the actions of vitamin D or PTH may result in hypocalcaemia; these disorders are described below. The extracellular calcium-ion sensing receptor is also 'G-protein coupled', and responds to alterations in the concentration of calcium ion, thereby regulating parathyroid hormone release and renal tubular calcium reabsorption.[124] This receptor is also involved in the regulation of calcitonin release. Gene mutations that result in impaired or enhanced receptor activity can alter the 'set-point' and lead to hypo- or hypercalcaemia. Autosomal dominant familial benign hypocalciuric hypercalcaemia (impaired receptor function) and hypocalcaemia with hypercalciuria (enhanced receptor function) may present in the neonatal period. Babies who are homozygous for mutations that usually lead to the 'benign' phenotype can have acute, life-threatening illness. These rare but important causes of neonatal hyper- and hypocalcaemia are also described below.

HYPOCALCAEMIA

Hypocalcaemia may be defined as a total serum calcium below 1.75 mmol/l and/or ionized calcium below 0.625 mmol/l. In infants, clinical features may include irritability, tremors, twitching and seizures, but some infants may in contrast be lethargic, feed poorly and vomit. The Chvostek and Trousseau signs are not reliable in the newborn. The QT interval of the ECG is increased and sudden cardiac death can occur.

Causes

The causes of hypocalcaemia are shown in Table 38.13.

Treatment

Severe symptoms of hypocalcaemia, such as seizures, may be treated with 10% calcium gluconate (9.4% calcium

Table 38.13 The causes of neonatal hypocalcaemia

Neonatal hypocalcaemia
early (preterm, asphyxia, infants of diabetic mothers)
late (inappropriate feeds)
Secondary to hypomagnesaemia
Hypoparathyroidism
X-linked
dominant
recessive
Microdeletions of chromosome 22 (including DiGeorge syndrome)
Pseudohypoparathyroidism (seldom presents in the newborn)
Maternal hypercalcaemia
Calcium sensing receptor defects (activating – hypocalcaemic hypercalciuria)
Vitamin D-dependent rickets (types I and II)
Alkalosis, bicarbonate therapy, citrate in blood transfusion
Malabsorption
Maternal vitamin D deficiency
Hypoalbuminaemia

by weight) 2 ml/kg by slow intravenous injection. If necessary this may be followed by continuous infusion of diluted 10% calcium gluconate, 5–8 ml/kg/24 h, with careful monitoring of cardiac rate and rhythm and serum calcium concentration. Oral calcium supplements and/or a vitamin D analogue may be needed for long-term management, but this will depend on the cause of the hypocalcaemia and will be discussed under the appropriate diagnoses.

Early hypocalcaemia

Symptomatic hypocalcaemia occurs more commonly in preterm babies, infants of diabetic mothers and those who suffer birth asphyxia or other perinatal stress, but not in small for gestational age infants. Although the mechanisms leading to low calcium levels in preterm infants are not well defined, the levels of PTH are not low.[141] A degree of PTH resistance may be present, and a sudden interruption in calcium supply at a time of high demand may also account for the fall in calcium levels. Calcitonin secretion is high in the neonatal period, and although it then falls rapidly during early infancy this may be another factor in the development of early neonatal hypocalcaemia.[9,27] A low milk intake, or blood transfusions which cause non-ionizable salt formation, can excacerbate hypocalcaemia still further. Many infants with early neonatal hypocalcaemia, especially those with diabetic mothers, also have low serum magnesium levels which, like the hypocalcaemia, usually improve spontaneously.

Late hypocalcaemia due to inappropriate feeds

This clinical picture is now much less common than it was when unmodified cow's milk formulas were widely used. It usually presented with multifocal fits in normal term infants on the fifth to seventh days of life. It was due to the high phosphate and relatively low calcium content of cow's milk (p. 327). Increased absorption of phosphate caused hyperphosphataemia, which in turn depressed the serum calcium. The treatment needed was to control the fits and change the feed to breast milk or a modified low-phosphate formula. Even with more modern formulas calcium levels may be reduced when compared to breast-fed infants.[162]

Hypomagnesaemia

Hypomagnesaemia may cause hypocalcaemia both by inhibiting the secretion of PTH and by reducing responsiveness to its actions. As many as 80% of infants with hypocalcaemic fits may be hypomagnesaemic, and hypocalcaemia may prove difficult to correct until the hypomagnesaemia has itself been corrected. This is most easily done by giving intramuscular magnesium sulphate in 50% solution 0.2 ml/kg every 4–8 hours. The serum magnesium should therefore be measured in all infants with persistent hypocalcaemia.

Hypoparathyroidism

Hypoparathyroidism is a rare cause of hypocalcaemia in the newborn period. Other biochemical findings include hyperphosphataemia, hypomagnesaemia and a normal or low alkaline phosphatase. The diagnosis is confirmed by the finding of low or absent immunoreactive PTH levels. This condition may be familial, with X-linked recessive, autosomal dominant and recessive patterns of inheritance described. Hypoparathyroidism, thymic aplasia, congenital abnormalities of the heart and great vessels and other dysmorphic features may result from deletions within chromosome 22q11. The DiGeorge syndrome links thymic hypoplasia with hypocalcaemia and forms part of this constellation of abnormalities, which collectively has been termed CATCH 22 (*C*ardiac defects, *A*bnormal facies, *T*hymic hypoplasia, *C*left palate, *H*ypocalcaemia).[186] The presence of hypocalcaemia with congenital abnormalities should prompt detailed genetic analysis,[88] but it should be remembered that calcium levels may return to normal spontaneously.

Hypoparathyroidism has been reported in association with a ring chromosome 16 or 18 and with production of a biologically inactive PTH. Prolonged transient hypoparathyroidism lasting up to 1 year has also been described. Autoimmune hypoparathyroidism, the most common cause in older children, probably does not occur in the newborn.

In the past high doses of vitamin D_2 were used for treatment, but the potent water-soluble analogues are preferable. A suitable dose in the newborn is α-calcidol (1α-hydroxycholecalciferol) or calcidol (1,25-dihydroxycholecalciferol) 0.03–0.08 μg/kg/24 h up to a maximum of 1–2 μg. The maintenance dose needed varies not only between patients but also in the same patient at different times; frequent measurement of the serum calcium is therefore necessary, with dose adjustments to keep the level within the normal range. Supplementary oral calcium is not essential but may help to stabilize the serum calcium.

Pseudohypoparathyroidism

The term pseudohypoparathyroidism is used to describe several related disorders characterized by peripheral unresponsiveness to the action of PTH as a result of receptor and/or postreceptor defects. The characteristic biochemical findings are hypocalcaemia with hyperphosphataemia, raised levels of PTH and an absent or impaired response to exogenous PTH. In some patients there are characteristic morphological abnormalities, including obesity, short stature and short fourth and/or fifth metacarpal and metatarsal bones, collectively known as Albright's hereditary osteodystrophy. Mild to moderate mental retardation is often present, and abnormal signal transduction may affect the activity of other hormones, such as TSH and gonadotrophins, thereby causing hypothyroidism and hypogonadism. These conditions are usually inherited as an autosomal dominant trait. Treatment of hypocalcaemia in this disorder usually requires calcium supplements and a vitamin D analogue.

Although PTH transduction defects do not usually present in the newborn period a transient form of parathyroid resistance, resolving by 6 months, has been described.[102]

Maternal hypercalcaemia

In the presence of maternal hypercalcaemia the fetus is exposed to chronic hypercalcaemia from excessive trans-placental passage of calcium. Parathyroid suppression may result in hypocalcaemia after birth,[169] but this generally resolves spontaneously. Maternal calcium levels should be checked whenever there is unexplained hypo-calcaemia in the newborn.

Hypocalcaemic hypercalciuria

Hypocalcaemia with hypercalciuria due to activating mutations of the calcium-sensing receptor may present in childhood with seizures. This rare condition should be suspected when hypocalcaemia is associated with PTH levels that are within the normal range, in contrast to infants with hypoparathyroidism.[125] It is important to be aware of this condition because vitamin D administration may lead to nephrocalcinosis.

Vitamin D-dependent rickets[62]

VDDR type I is due to defective renal hydroxylation of vitamin D, whereas in VDDR type II there is cellular resistance to hormone action. This may be due to mutations in the steroid-binding domain or the DNA-binding domain of the vitamin D receptor. Levels of 1,25-dihydroxyvitamin D are reduced in type I VDDR but elevated in type II. These rare, autosomal recessive conditions can present with rickets in infancy.

Vitamin D-deficient rickets

Hypocalcaemia and rickets may occur in association with maternal and infant vitamin D deficiency.[1] Although some racial groups are more susceptible to hypocalcaemia and rickets than others, this remains a worldwide problem.[7,163] The vitamin D status of an infant will reflect the mother's diet and her exposure to sunlight, as well as postnatal factors such as the type of feed. Most commercial milk preparations contain enough vitamin D to prevent rickets, but supplementation is advisable in breast-fed babies. A dose of 400 IU of vitamin D per day is appropriate in most infants.

Other causes

Hypocalcaemia may occur in alkalosis, with citrate administration in blood transfusion and in hypo-albuminaemic states. It may also arise in infants with renal failure who have hyperphosphataemia.

HYPERCALCAEMIA

This is generally defined as a serum calcium above 2.75 mmol/l. Clinical manifestations include hypotonia, weakness and irritability, poor feeding, weight loss, constipation, vomiting, polydipsia and polyuria. Nephro-calcinosis with hypertension can occur. Severe hyper-calcaemia is therefore dangerous and must be corrected rapidly.

Causes

The causes of hypercalcaemia are shown in Table 38.14.

Treatment

The primary cause must be corrected if possible. Generous hydration and frusemide diuresis promote urinary calcium loss. Glucocorticoids (e.g. hydrocortisone 1 mg/kg 6-hourly) reduce intestinal calcium absorption but the effect is slow, taking some days. Calcitonin (10 U/kg i.v.) may be useful and has its maximum effect in 1 hour; infusions may be repeated 4-hourly. The hormone is antigenic and so the synthetic derivative salcatonin should be used in the longer term.

Williams syndrome (pp. 872–873)

This rare but serious condition is characterized by intermittent hypercalcaemia, a characteristic 'elfin' or 'pekinese' facial appearance, moderate mental retardation and vascular stenoses, most commonly supravalvular

Table 38.14 The causes of hypercalcaemia

Williams syndrome
Phosphate depletion in low birthweight
Calcium sensing receptor defects (inactivating)
benign familial hypercalcaemia with hypocalciuria
neonatal severe hyperparathyroidism
Hyperparathyroidism
Excess vitamin D
Subcutaneous fat necrosis
Adrenal insufficiency
Hypophosphatasia
Malignancy
Vitamin A intoxication

aortic stenosis. There is early failure to thrive, with severe anorexia, vomiting and constipation, hypotonia, polyuria and polydipsia. The hypercalcaemia and consequent symptoms tend to resolve spontaneously, but the other features persist. Radiologically there is sclerosis of the skull base, spine and long bones, and there may be metastatic calcification. Most children with Williams syndrome, and particularly those in whom there are cardiovascular manifestations, have deletions of the elastin gene on chromosome 7.[116] The condition is usually sporadic, although familial, autosomal dominant inheritance has also been observed.[104] In the hypercalcaemic phase treatment is with a diet lacking vitamin D and as low as possible in calcium. Glucocorticoids may help to reduce the serum calcium in the early stages of treatment, but control of the serum calcium seems unfortunately to have no effect on the progression of the other features of the disease.

Hypercalcaemia due to phosphate depletion

Severe hypercalcaemia may occur in low-birthweight preterm infants with hypophosphataemia due to a low phosphate intake from breast milk or parenteral feeding (p. 1003). The hypercalcaemia responds to phosphate repletion.[91,100]

Benign familial hypocalciuric hypercalcaemia and neonatal severe hyperparathyroidism[124]

These conditions are associated with mutations in the extracellular calcium-ion sensing receptor which lead to loss of function. The set-point at which PTH is released is therefore altered. Benign familial hypercalcaemia is inherited as an autosomal dominant trait, whereas the severe neonatal form is associated with both heterozygous and homozyous mutations of the calcium-sensing receptor genes.[123,131] Factors influencing the phenotype in this disorder may therefore include the number of mutant genes and the extent to which the calcium receptor is compromised.[60,132] The neonatal form can lead to hypotonia, respiratory distress and failure to thrive, in association with hypercalcaemia and elevated PTH levels. There is skeletal undermineralization, with rib fractures and subperiosteal erosions. The treatment of severe cases, usually homozygous for receptor mutations, may entail urgent parathyroidectomy, but some neonatal cases appear to run a milder, self-limiting course.[185] Earlier reports of primary hyperparathyroidism in neonatal life probably included children with calcium receptor abnormalities.

Hyperparathyroidism

Hyperparathyroidism may occur in association with two dominantly inherited syndromes of multiple endocrine adenomatosis, type 1 with pituitary and pancreatic adenomas (and sometimes Zollinger–Ellison syndrome), and type 2 with medullary carcinoma of the thyroid, phaeochromocytoma and sometimes mucosal neuromata. The risk to an infant may therefore be anticipated, although the clinical manifestations occur later.

Secondary hyperparathyroidism may be due to untreated maternal hypoparathyroidism, which causes fetal hypocalcaemia and parathyroid hyperplasia; this condition is self-limiting but the hypercalcaemia may need treatment with steroids, calcitonin or diuretics. Other causes include rickets and renal osteodystrophy (p. 1031).

Hypercalcaemia in association with excess vitamin D

Infantile hypercalcaemia was common in the UK for some years when there was liberal vitamin D supplementation of foods. It generally presented with symptoms of hypercalcaemia in the early months of life, but was mild and self-limiting (Lightwood syndrome). The incidence fell when the use of vitamin D supplements was reduced, and it is thought to have affected infants with unusual sensitivity to vitamin D, when the cumulative daily dose could reach 2000–4000 IU or more. Hypercalcaemia due to excessive vitamin D intake has been reported in association with prolonged administration of preterm formula.[111]

Subcutaneous fat necrosis

Hypercalcaemia may occur in association with extensive neonatal subcutaneous fat necrosis (p. 900), which is seen especially after traumatic delivery of large infants. This may be due to unregulated production of 1,25-dihydroxyvitamin D by the affected adipose tissue.[83]

Others

Vitamin A excess, adrenal failure, hypophosphatasia and malignancy are rare causes of hypercalcaemia in early life. Constitutively activating PTH receptor mutations have recently been reported in association with hypercalcaemia and short-limbed dwarfism.[153]

ADRENAL

NORMAL DEVELOPMENT AND FUNCTION[68]

The adrenal gland has two embryologically and functionally distinct components. The medulla is formed from neural crest cells which enter the gland at about the seventh week of gestation and secrete catecholamines. Disorders of function are not recognized in the newborn.

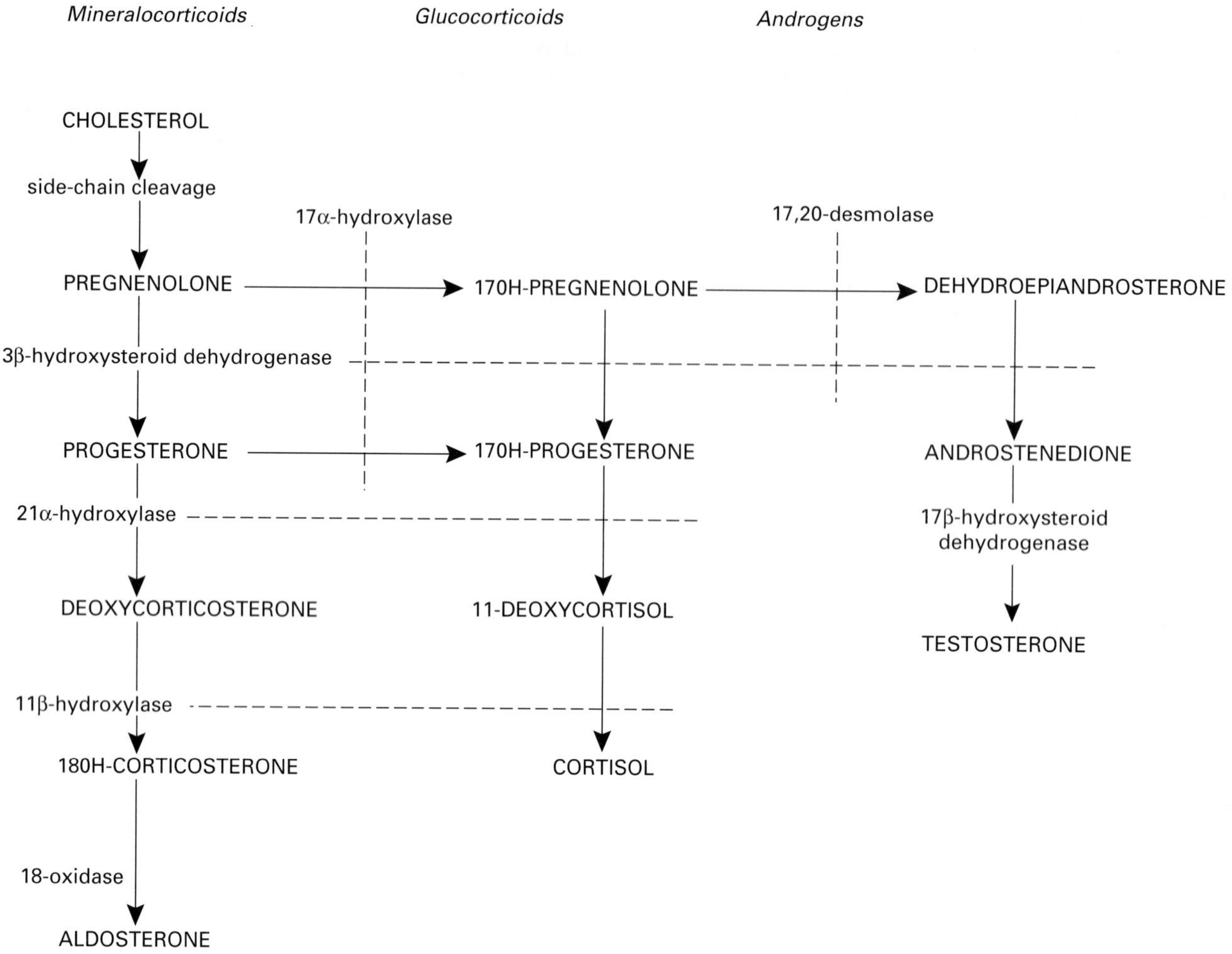

Fig. 38.8 Adrenal steroid biosynthesis.

The cortex is derived from mesodermal cells near the cephalic part of the mesonephros. It shares common primordial cells with the gonads, which also secrete steroids and may express similar enzyme deficiencies in inborn errors. The fetal adrenal is remarkably hyperplastic, 10–20 times larger than the adult gland relative to body weight. At birth both glands together weigh 7–9 g. They are largely composed of the histologically distinct fetal cortex, which comprises 80% of the gland at birth and then involutes rapidly, reducing to half its size by 2 weeks and disappearing by 6 months.

The enzyme activities of the fetal adrenal and the placenta are complementary; thus the placenta lacks the enzymatic activity necessary to generate adrenal androgens from the precursors, pregnenolone and progesterone (17α-hydroxylase and 17,20-desmolase; Fig. 38.8), whereas the fetal adrenal lacks the enzymatic activity to produce oestrogen from androgens, until the later stages of gestation. The adrenal androgens (primarily dehydroepiandrosterone and its sulphate) are therefore converted to oestrogen by the placenta, which expresses the necessary enzyme activity, including sulphatase and aromatase. Hence the fetal adrenal provides the precursors necessary for placental oestrogen production, and steroid production by the fetoplacental unit promotes maturation of organs such as the lungs. A case of placental aromatase deficiency has now been described which causes virilization of the mother and female infants during pregnancy.[156]

The adrenal cortex secretes three major groups of steroid hormones: glucocorticoids, mineralocorticoids and androgens. The chief biosynthetic pathways are shown in Figure 38.8. The gland has three histologically distinct zones. The outer zone, the zona glomerulosa, contains the enzymes for aldosterone biosynthesis but little 17α-hydroxylase, so it produces little cortisol or androgen. Aldosterone release is primarily controlled by the renin–angiotensin system and by the plasma concentrations of sodium and potassium, with ACTH playing a minor role. The two inner zones, fasciculata and reticularis, secrete cortisol and androgens respectively, but no aldosterone. ACTH is the primary regulator of cortisol and androgen synthesis and secretion. The normal circadian pattern of cortisol release is usually established by 3 months of age, but has been identified as early as 2 weeks post-delivery.[150]

Table 38.15 The causes of adrenocortical insufficiency

Primary
Panadrenocortical insufficiency
Congenital adrenal hypoplasia
sporadic
X-linked
autosomal recessive
Side-chain cleavage (cholesterol desmolase)
Adrenal necrosis or haemorrhage
Acute infection (Waterhouse–Friderichsen syndrome)
Lysosomal acid lipase deficiency (Wolman syndrome)
Maternal Cushing or steroid therapy
Selective adrenocortical insufficiency
Glucocorticoid
isolated glucocorticoid deficiency
glucocorticoid receptor resistance
congenital adrenal hyperplasia
• 21α-hydroxylase deficiency, non salt-losing
• 11β-hydroxylase deficiency
• 17α-hydroxylase deficiency
iatrogenic, post glucocorticoid therapy
Mineralocorticoid
hypoaldosteronism
• corticosterone methyl oxidase deficiency I
• corticosterone methyl oxidase deficiency II
aldosterone unresponsiveness (pseudohypoaldosteronism)
Gluco- and mineralocorticoid
congenital adrenal hyperplasia
• 21α-hydroxylase deficiency, salt-losing
• 3β-hydroxysteroid dehydrogenase deficiency
• congenital lipoid adrenal hyperplasia
Secondary
See under anterior pituitary problems (Table 38.6)

ADRENOCORTICAL INSUFFICIENCY[42]

A classification of the causes of adrenocortical insufficiency in the newborn is shown in Table 38.15.

Congenital adrenal hypoplasia

Primary adrenocortical insufficiency due to congenital hypoplasia or atrophy of the glands has been estimated to have a frequency of 1 in 12 500 births. The condition may be X-linked, sporadic or familial. The X-linked recessive form has been linked to mutations of the gene encoding a nuclear hormone receptor, DAX-1,[108] which resides in the region Xp21. The DAX-1 gene product is expressed in the adrenal and testis, and also has a role in the normal production of gonadotrophins by the hypothalamopituitary axis. Other genes in the vicinity of DAX-1 include loci for glycerol kinase and dystrophin. This form of adrenal hypoplasia may be associated with cryptorchidism, hypogonadotrophic hypogonadism, glycerol kinase deficiency and Duchenne muscular dystrophy.

The clinical presentation reflects the degree of glucocorticoid and mineralocorticoid deficiency. Severely affected infants may become hypoglycaemic within the first few days of life, which may manifest as fits or apnoeic spells. Later presentation may be with poor feeding, vomiting, dehydration, failure to thrive and sometimes fever. A misdiagnosis of upper intestinal obstruction has sometimes been made. Hyperpigmentation is rare until the third week of life, and cortisol deficiency may also present as prolonged jaundice.

The early biochemical findings include hypoglycaemia, hyponatraemia, hyperkalaemia and a metabolic acidosis. ACTH and renin levels are raised but cortisol and aldosterone reduced. Reduced ACTH levels and normal electrolytes suggest secondary adrenal insufficiency. Adrenal stimulation tests with tetracosactrin show an absent or greatly reduced response.

The diagnosis may be suspected antenatally if maternal oestriol values are very low, but adrenal hypoplasia cannot thus be differentiated from the more common – and also X-linked – placental sulphatase deficiency.

In the past most affected patients died, but some, presumably less severely affected, presented later in life. With prompt recognition and treatment the prognosis now should be good.

Adrenal haemorrhage

The large hyperaemic fetal gland is vulnerable to vascular damage. Birth trauma presumably accounts for most adrenal haemorrhage seen at autopsy in the newborn: 0.05% of 3657 infants were affected in the series of Snelling and Erb,[161] although haemorrhage has also been detected antenatally. Bilateral haemorrhage has also been described in neonatal tuberculosis or syphilis. The incidence is increased in preterm infants and after prolonged or complicated labour. The bleeding may be sufficient to form a palpable mass, which may be mistaken for a tumour, especially if unilateral, or may rupture into the peritoneum and cause intestinal obstruction or a scrotal haematoma. There may also be signs of acute blood loss or, at a later stage, anaemia and jaundice. If both glands are infarcted the baby can present acutely ill with hypoglycaemia, shock and Addisonian features.

The diagnosis is difficult unless a mass is palpable, but ultrasound is useful to confirm suspected haemorrhage.[103] Adrenal calcification has been observed as early as the fifth day, but usually occurs much later. The presentation of adrenal insufficiency may be delayed but the regenerative capacity of the adrenal is great, and most adrenal haemorrhage is not associated with significantly impaired function.

Maternal hyperadrenocorticism, steroid therapy and fetal adrenal function

Adrenocortical insufficiency in the newborn may arise following maternal Cushing syndrome or steroid therapy.[11,81] The potential for adrenal suppression must be considered in any infant exposed to glucocorticoid in pregnancy. Long-term dexamethasone administration during pregnancy to treat prenatally diagnosed fetal congenital adrenal hyperplasia usually leads to side-effects in the mother, but has not been associated with overt abnormalities in the babies.[120] These infants will have abnormal adrenal function and are routinely treated with glucocorticoid after delivery.

Adrenal (Addisonian) crisis

Crisis may supervene in all forms of adrenal insufficiency except those that only affect androgen production. It is often precipitated by acute illness, surgery, trauma or other insults. Hypoglycaemia can occur independently of salt and water loss. The onset is usually rapid, with vomiting, diarrhoea, vascular collapse, prostration and coma. Hypoglycaemia, hyponatraemia, hyperkalaemia and metabolic acidosis are present.

Treatment consists of i.v. glucose, fluid and electrolyte replacement, steroid replacement, and treatment of any underlying disease. A bolus of i.v. glucose (0.5–1.0 g/kg over several minutes) and a rapid infusion of albumin or normal saline (20 ml/kg initially) may first be needed, then, if the response is satisfactory, rehydration can be continued with i.v. normal saline with added glucose. Intravenous hydrocortisone hemisuccinate 12.5–50 mg should be given stat, then 4-hourly by bolus or continuous infusion until the baby's condition is stable, when the dose can be reduced. Hydrocortisone may also be administered intramuscularly if venous access is difficult. The mineralocorticoid effect of hydrocortisone is adequate at these doses but can be supplemented by fludrocortisone 25–50 μg 12-hourly by mouth. The serum potassium generally falls rapidly, but if the level is dangerously high, the ECG is abnormal and cardiac arrhythmia threatens, it may be necessary to give 10% calcium gluconate 2 ml/kg by slow i.v. injection, salbutamol and/or glucose and insulin, to achieve immediate control of the hyperkalaemia (p. 1024).

Waterhouse–Friderichsen syndrome

Acute adrenal insufficiency from adrenal haemorrhage and infarction complicating septicaemic illness with DIC is a rare event in the newborn, but can cause circulatory collapse and death. There is no evidence in favour of the prophylactic use of high-dose steroids in septicaemic shock.

Adrenoleukodystrophy[105] (pp. 1000, 1280)

Isolated glucocorticoid deficiency

There are at least two autosomal recessive causes of glucocorticoid deficiency characterized by high circulating ACTH levels: familial glucocorticoid deficiency and triple A syndrome.[3,106] Familial glucocorticoid deficiency presents with signs of cortisol deficiency in infancy, or later in childhood, when hyperpigmentation may provide a diagnostic clue. Some, but not all, cases are due to abnormalities of the ACTH receptor.[180,181] The triple A syndrome is the association of glucocorticoid deficiency with achalasia of the cardia and deficient tear production. Glucocorticoid deficiency, achalasia and more extensive neurological dysfunction, including mild dementia, has also been described.[49]

Glucocorticoid receptor resistance

This is a rare autosomal dominant cause of hypercortisolism where there is defective cortisol binding to the glucocorticoid receptor. Affected individuals do not have signs of glucocorticoid excess and presentation is usually in childhood[92] or adult life, with signs of androgen excess or hypertension.

Mineralocorticoid deficiency and pseudohypoaldosteronism

Severe isolated renal salt wasting is seen in the recessively inherited defects of aldosterone biosynthesis due to corticosterone methyl oxidase deficiency.[176] These respond to treatment with fludrocortisone. They are closely mimicked by the condition of pseudohypoaldosteronism, in which there is resistance to endogenous and exogenous mineralocorticoids.[127,152] Treatment requires generous salt supplements; spontaneous improvement occurs with age and, combined with the ability to choose a salty diet, usually allows these to be stopped later in childhood. This condition may be associated with polyhydramnios.[52]

Neonatal adrenal function and glucocorticoid therapy

Neonates who are oxygen or ventilator dependent may be treated with an exogenous glucocorticoid such as dexamethasone to assist weaning. The doses used in this situation are large, often starting at 500 μg/kg/day. Suppression of the HPA axis has been demonstrated both during and after dexamethasone treatment in these infants.[75,139,187] The degree of HPA suppression will depend on the dose of glucocorticoid used and the duration of therapy. If an infant has received glucocorticoid for more than 1 week it is wise to reduce the dose gradually and/or change to an alternate-day regimen prior to stopping treatment, bearing in mind that 50 μg of dexamethasone will probably suppress the adrenal gland completely.[63] It should also be remembered that an infant who has recently stopped glucocorticoid treatment may require steroid cover in association with subsequent illness or surgery.[115]

The reliability and interpretation of tests of the HPA are the subject of considerable debate, but a synacthen stimulation test with measurement of baseline levels may be of value if there is concern about adrenal function. Conventional doses of synacthen (for example 36 μg/kg or 250 μg/1.73 m^2) represent a pharmacological rather than a physiological stimulus, and a normal response does not exclude a degree of adrenal suppression.[118] The cortisol response to low-dose synacthen stimulation (0.5 μg/1.73 m^2) or to CRH may be a more sensitive means of assessing the integrity of the adrenal axis.[25,58,114,179] A two to three fold rise in baseline cortisol, or an increment of 2–300 nmol/l, would be expected 30 or 60 minutes after synacthen 36 μg/kg. Random plasma cortisol concentrations may be difficult to interpret, but adrenal suppression or insufficiency should be suspected if baseline cortisol values are below 140 nmol/l in stressed preterm infants[73] or when the response to synacthen stimulation is below 400 nmol/l.

During glucocorticoid treatment side-effects such as a rise in blood pressure, hyperglycaemia and glycosuria are seen. Steroids also make the infant catabolic, impair growth, and their long-term sequelae when used at this stage of development are unknown.

ADRENOCORTICAL HYPERFUNCTION[43]

Except in congenital adrenal hyperplasia, adrenocortical hyperfunction is extremely rare in the newborn.

Congenital adrenal hyperplasia[70]

CAH is a generic term used to describe a series of autosomal recessive disorders affecting adrenal steroidogenesis. It is the commonest adrenal problem in the newborn period and the leading cause of ambiguous genitalia. More than 95% of cases are due to 21α-hydroxylase deficiency, of which there are several allelic forms. Boys are underrepresented in most series, and some presumably die undiagnosed from salt depletion and its complications. The prevalence in the UK is approximately 1 in 10 000, and worldwide approximately 1 in 14 000.[119] Population screening in an Italian region revealed a frequency of 1 in 8600.[19]

Pathogenesis

A simplified schematic representation of adrenal steroid biosynthesis is shown in Figure 38.8 and with this background many of the consequences of a given enzyme defect can be determined. These are summarized in Table 38.16.

21α-Hydroxylase deficiency

This condition classically presents as 'salt-losing', 'simple virilizing' or 'late-onset' forms. The majority of affected individuals presenting in early life have salt loss, but some produce enough mineralocorticoid to maintain sodium homoeostasis; these children secrete sufficient aldosterone while on appropriate glucocorticoid replacement, despite impaired enzyme activity. The genetics of 21-hydroxylase deficiency have been extensively studied. There are two 21-hydroxylase genes, one of which is inactive (*CYP21A*) and one active (*CYP21B*). They are both located on chromosome 6, interspersed between the genes encoding the C4 component of complement and in close proximity to the HLA complex (Fig. 38.9). Most affected individuals will be compound heterozygotes for a relatively small number of gene defects; the *CYP21B* locus (normally the active gene sequence) is affected by a gene conversion whereby part or all of this gene is converted to the inactive gene sequence of *CYP21A*. Alternatively, there may be a gene deletion extending from a point within the *CYP21A* gene to a corresponding part of the *CYP21B* gene. Most patients with salt loss have gene deletions or conversions that severely impair enzyme activity, whereas the 'late-onset' form is an allelic variant

Table 38.16 Major clinical and biochemical features of enzymatic blocks in adrenocortical steroid biosynthesis

Enzyme defect	Clinical features/Sexual development		
	Male	Female	Salt status
21α-Hydroxylase			
simple virilizing	N	Virilized	N
salt losing	N	Virilized	Loss
11β-Hydroxylase	N	Virilized	Retention (usually)
3β-Hydroxysteroid	Inadequate virilization	N or mild virilization	Loss
17α-Hydroxylase	Female or inadequate virilization	N	Retention
Cholesterol desmolase	Female	N	Severe loss

N, normal

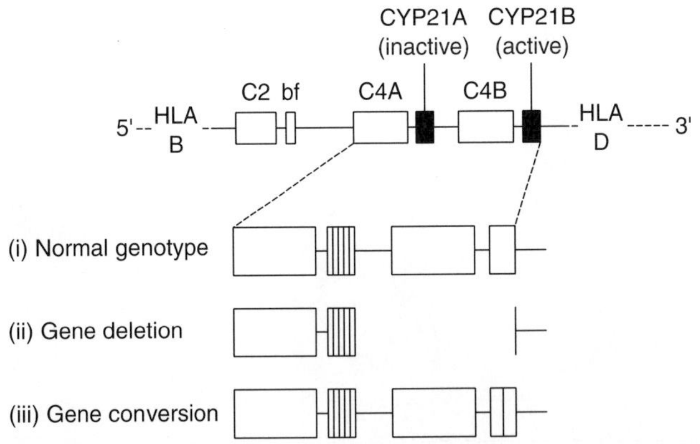

Fig. 38.9 Schematic diagram illustrating the proximity of the inactive (21A) and active (21B) 21α-hydroxylase genes to the HLA loci on chromosome 6. (i) The vertical lines in the 21A gene represent some of the mutations that lead to gene inactivity and that may be incorporated into the normally active 21B locus. (ii) The genotype of an affected infant will usually include 21B gene deletions and/or (iii) gene conversions, leading to impaired 21α-hydroxylase activity. C2, C4A, C4B genes coding for complement components. HLA B, HLA D genes for HLA antigens.

with higher enzyme levels that are sufficient to maintain health and a normal phenotype in the newborn period.

Clinical presentation

In the simple virilizing form the clinical features are due to overproduction of androgens, lack of cortisol and excess secretion of ACTH. In the fetus the low levels of circulating cortisol result in activation of the feedback pathway and, through secretion of CRH and ACTH, stimulation and eventually hyperplasia of the adrenal cortex and overproduction of androgen.

In male babies there may be some increase in pigmentation, especially of the scrotum, but there is no gross anatomical abnormality. If the condition is not treated continued postnatal overproduction of androgen causes rapid growth and virilization, but these do not generally become obvious until around the second year of life.

In females the prenatal androgen overproduction causes virilization, which can vary profoundly in appearance. The clitoris is enlarged and the labioscrotal folds undergo anterior migration and fusion. In the least virilized infants there may be only slight clitoral enlargement, but most commonly the clitoris becomes almost as large as a normal neonatal penis, with a considerable degree of chordee. The labioscrotal fusion leaves only a small common anterior perineal opening at the base of the phallus (Fig. 38.10). In very severely virilized female infants there may be complete fusion of the labioscrotal folds and the urethra may migrate along the phallus. If the urethral meatus reaches the tip of the glans the genital appearance much resembles a cryptorchid male, and is often misdiagnosed as such.

The cortisol deficiency can cause hypoglycaemia, but this occurs only infrequently, probably because the enzymatic block is incomplete.

In salt-losing CAH there is an enzymatic block at the 21α-hydroxylase step in the aldosterone as well as in the cortisol pathway. Inadequate production of aldosterone leads to renal salt loss. Affected neonates develop serious illness from sodium depletion, with a median age at presentation of around 12 days.[35] The early symptoms are vomiting, anorexia and sometimes diarrhoea which, if untreated, may develop into full Addisonian crisis (p. 972). The mineralocorticoid deficiency causes hyponatraemia, hyperkalaemia and acidosis. This characteristic picture should indicate the diagnosis if it has not been suspected previously. Conditions that may be confused with salt-wasting CAH include urinary tract infection and pyloric stenosis.

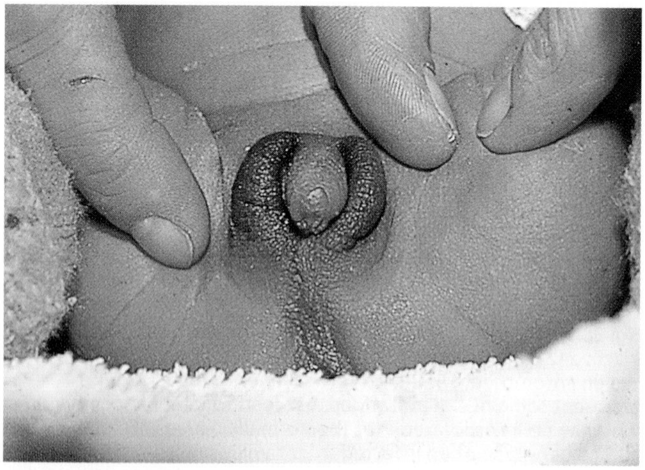

Fig. 38.10 Genitalia of a female infant with 21α-hydroxylase deficiency.

Diagnosis

Failure to make a prompt diagnosis may be disastrous. When the genitalia are ambiguous it is urgent to establish the genetic sex of the infant by examination of the karyotype. In 21α-hydroxylase deficiency there is gross elevation of the plasma 17-hydroxyprogesterone concentration. Assays for this steroid are now widely available. In the immediate newborn period there is assay interference from maternal and placental steroids, but the test is generally diagnostic after 24 hours. However, seriously ill preterm infants may show moderate elevation of plasma 17-OHP in the absence of adrenal hyperplasia.[109] The plasma ACTH level is raised in all states of cortisol deficiency, so this is a non-specific test and it is also a difficult and less widely available assay. 11β-hydroxylase deficiency is often misdiagnosed as simple virilizing 21α-hydroxylase deficiency, so it is desirable to assay plasma 11-deoxycortisol as well as 17-OHP. It is also wise to collect a sample of urine at presentation to be used for analysis of the urinary steroid profile by gas chromatography if the diagnosis proves to be more complex.

Prenatal diagnosis and treatment

There is now strong evidence that the prenatal administration of glucocorticoids to the mother of a female fetus with 21α-hydroxlase deficiency can reduce the degree of fetal virilization and hence the need for postnatal surgery.[98,101]

Before the pregnancy the potential benefits and risks of prenatal treatment must be explained to the parents. Some will decline treatment, especially if a previous affected child was only mildly virilized. Unfortunately, in some families the phenotype may vary, so it is not possible to state that subsequent children will not be more severely affected.[189]

In a pregnancy at risk the mother can be given dexamethasone in a dose of 20 μg/kg/day in 2–3 divided doses as soon as the pregnancy is confirmed. Dexamethasone crosses the placenta well and suppresses fetal ACTH secretion, and so the excess androgen production is curtailed. The treatment needs to be started as early as possible, and certainly before 8 weeks' gestation. It is then necessary to establish the sex of the fetus and whether or not it is affected. As the treatment is needed only for female fetuses with homozygous or compound heterozygote 21α-hydroxylase deficiency it can then be stopped in the seven out of eight pregnancies where the fetus is either male or an unaffected female.

The prenatal diagnosis of 21α-hydroxylase deficiency was first made by finding raised 17-OHP levels in amniotic fluid. More recently the likelihood of a pregnancy being affected has been established by HLA typing of the parents, index case and fetus, or by linkage analysis using markers in the region of the 21-OH gene. These techniques depend on the proximity of the locus for the 21α-hydroxylase gene to the HLA antigens on chromosome 6 or other 'adjacent' genes. In the last few years it has become possible to use specific DNA probes or allele-specific PCR to screen for one of the relatively few number of mutations in family members, and then in the fetus using tissue obtained by chorionic villus sampling at 10–12 weeks.[147,164,190]

Treatment of the mother with a potent steroid throughout pregnancy clearly carries some risk, and excessive weight gain, glucose intolerance, a rise in blood pressure, gastrointestinal upset and Cushingoid features have been recorded. No adverse effects on the fetus have been observed to date, but careful follow-up studies will be needed.

Population screening

Measurement of 17-OHP in dried capillary blood samples (like those collected for screening for phenylketonuria and hypothyroidism) (p. 380) is possible and screening has been implemented in some countries, notably New Zealand[26] and some States in the USA. There are currently no plans to include CAH in the UK national neonatal screening programme.

Treatment[20]

This entails replacing glucocorticoid and, if necessary, mineralocorticoid as well. The majority of affected girls will also require surgical correction of the virilization.

A baby presenting in Addisonian crisis should be treated as detailed above. Thereafter the need to suppress ACTH, and hence androgen levels, means that an initial dose of hydrocortisone of 15–25 mg/m^2/24 h is usually appropriate. This should be trebled to cover significant acute illness and *must* be given parenterally if the oral dose is vomited. An average dose for a full-term newborn infant, surface area 0.2 m^2, will therefore be around 2.5 mg b.d. or 2mg/2mg/1mg if a t.d.s. regimen is used. Liquid preparations tend to be unstable, but 2.5 mg tablets are available. Fludrocortisone can be given in an initial dose of 25–50 μg b.d. and then adjusted according to the salt balance, blood pressure and renin levels; divisible 100 μg tablets are available. Salt supplements may also be needed initially, and can be added to the milk: 2–4 g of additional sodium chloride daily will ensure adequate intake until the diet contains more salt and the child can select salty foods.

The long-term management consists of giving, first, enough glucocorticoid to maintain suppression of the excess androgen production but not enough to cause iatrogenic Cushing syndrome and growth retardation, and secondly, enough mineralocorticoid to ensure normal salt balance without excessive salt retention and hypertension. The key to the assessment of treatment in early life is close clinical observation with careful measurement of growth, electrolytes and blood pressure, supplemented with plasma steroid measurements. A profile of plasma 17-OHP (which can be estimated on finger-prick samples) probably gives the best simple estimate of biochemical control. Levels should be suppressed, but there should still be evidence of diurnal variation.[130]

Virilized girls require surgical reduction of the phallus and exposure of the vagina. This entails difficult surgery, and early assessment by an experienced paediatric urologist is needed. The operation can be done in a single stage but may need two stages if there is severe virilization. Clitoral reduction is best done when the girl has reached a reasonable size but before sexual identity has developed. Most surgeons favour the age range 6–18 months. Increased steroid cover is, of course, needed for surgery.

11β-Hydroxylase deficiency[183]

This is the second most common cause of congenital adrenal hyperplasia, but accounts for less than 5% of cases in the UK. There is a relatively high incidence in the Middle East. Affected females are virilized but males are normal at birth. Plasma 11-deoxycortisol, deoxycorticosterone and their metabolites are increased (there is also some increase of 17-OHP), and although the increased intermediate compounds in the aldosterone pathway usually prevent salt loss and may cause hypertension in later life, salt-wasting has been reported in infancy[64] and the potential for confusion with 21-hydroxylase deficiency is apparent.[66]

3β-Hydroxysteroid dehydrogenase deficiency

(see p. 978)

Congenital lipoid adrenal hyperplasia

(see p. 977)

17α-Hydroxylase deficiency and 17,20-desmolase deficiency (p. 978)

A single protein is responsible for these two separate enzyme activities. When this is deficient there are varying degrees of cortisol deficiency with excessive mineralocorticoid production, driven primarily by ACTH feedback, sometimes causing hypertension and hypokalaemic alkalosis in infancy. The glucocorticoid activity of the excess mineralocorticoid may in part compensate for a lack of cortisol. In later life affected females develop no secondary sexual characteristics and are amenorrhoeic, and males show absent or inadequate virilization.[151] This defect should be considered in the differential diagnosis of androgen insensitivity in genetic males and primary hypogonadism in females.

DISORDERS OF SEXUAL DEVELOPMENT[148]

NORMAL SEXUAL DIFFERENTIATION

The physical basis of the sex of an individual is the product of the genotype, the gonads, the internal sexual organs, the external sexual organs and the secondary sexual characteristics developed at puberty. In the disorders of sexual development there is abnormal or discordant development of one or more of these factors. Later in life discordance can also occur between physical sex, gender identity and psychosexual orientation.

The primary event in sexual determination is the fertilization of an ovum by either an X- or a Y-bearing spermatozoon. Normally this initiates a cascade of events which culminates in female or male development. A 46XX genotype determines that the undifferentiated bipotential gonads develop into ovaries by the 12th week of fetal life under the influence of genes on both the long and the short arms of the X chromosome, and probably also one or more autosomes. Subsequent female development, as first shown in the classic studies of Jost,[74] is a relatively passive process and proceeds normally in a castrated fetus irrespective of the genetic sex. There is persistence and development of the Mullerian ducts, which form the fallopian tubes, uterus and upper vagina, and the external genitalia take female form.

In contrast, male development is an active process, a 46XY genotype inducing testicular differentiation through the action of the testis-determining factor on the Y chromosome, which is now referred to as SRY (sex-determining region of the Y chromosome). SRY is a sequence of 14 kilobases adjacent to the pseudo-autosomal region of the short arm of the Y chromosome, and encodes a DNA-binding regulatory protein. Other genes 'downstream' of this initial event are also important in testicular development, but remain to be elucidated in detail. The presence of testes thus indicates the presence of a Y chromosome except in the rare occurrence of XX males, in whom there has usually been a translocation of the SRY onto the paternal X chromosome, and XX true hermaphrodites. Male sex is also associated with the presence of the histocompatibility Y (H-Y) antigen, a cell-surface protein found in the males of all mammalian species which has a role in spermatogenesis. In the presence of these factors, the indifferent gonads transform into testes by the fifth to sixth weeks of intrauterine life and then play an active role in development by secreting two hormones, testosterone and anti-Mullerian hormone.

Testosterone is secreted from the Leydig cells, initially under the stimulus of placental chorionic gonadotrophin (which explains why gonadotrophin deficiency is usually associated with micropenis and/or cryptorchidism, and not with ambiguous genitalia), and by a local effect stimulates development of the Wolffian ducts into epididymis, vas deferens and seminal vesicles. It also reaches androgen-sensitive peripheral cells via the circulation, where it binds to the androgen receptor in the cell cytoplasm and nucleus. Testosterone is also converted to the potent androgen dihydrotesterone in peripheral tissues by the enzyme 5α-reductase. In the fetus testosterone and DHT induce virilization of the urogenital sinus and the external genitalia. This process is complete by 13 weeks of embryonic life. The normal pattern of hCG, gonadotrophin and androgen release in the male fetus is shown in Figure 38.11.

The fetal testes also produce AMH, a high molecular weight glycoprotein secreted by the Sertoli cells, which causes local regression of the Mullerian ducts.

ABNORMAL SEXUAL DEVELOPMENT

In the neonatal period the most common presentation of disorders of sexual development is with ambiguity or abnormality of the genitalia in the female, or hypospadias

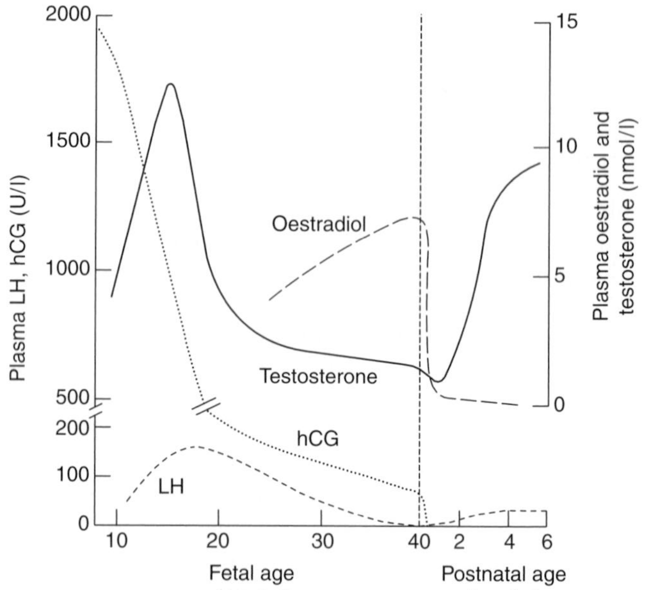

Fig. 38.11 The trend in fetal and neonatal plasma hCG, LH, testosterone and oestradiol concentrations in the male. (Adapted from Fisher[41])

in the male. The abnormalities can vary from a minor degree of labial fusion in the female or hypospadias in the male to gross virilization in a genetic female or lack of development in a genetic male, such that the 'wrong' sex is assigned without question.

The major disorders of sexual development can be classified by gonadal development into three groups:

- Male pseudohermaphroditism (an incompletely virilized male), in which there is an XY karyotype and testes, but inadequate or abnormal virilization;
- Female pseudohermaphroditism (a virilized female), in which there is an XX karyotype and ovaries but inappropriate virilization;
- Disorders of gonadal development, which include most of the disorders of the sex chromosomes and also true hermaphroditism, in which both testicular and ovarian tissue is present.

The sexual organs may also be involved in a wide variety of dysmorphic syndromes, which are not currently known to be related to specific disorders of sexual development but may sometimes closely mimic them.

MALE PSEUDOHERMAPHRODITISM (INCOMPLETE VIRILIZATION IN A GENETIC MALE)

This condition arises when a genotypically normal male with well-differentiated testes fails to virilize normally. The phenotype can vary from that of a normal female through all degrees of ambiguity to normal male external genitalia. These conditions can arise for one of three reasons:

- Impaired production or action of AMH;
- Inadequate production of testosterone from the fetal Leydig cells;
- Inadequate peripheral androgenic effect of testosterone due to end-organ resistance.

A classification of male pseudohermaphroditism is shown in Table 38.17.

Table 38.17 Causes of male pseudohermaphroditism

AMH deficiency
Testosterone deficiency
Deficiency of
congenital lipoid adrenal hyperplasia
3β-hydroxysteroid dehydrogenase
17α-hydroxylase
17,20-desmolase
17β-hydroxysteroid dehydrogenase
Leydig cell hypoplasia including luteinizing hormone receptor defects
Gonadotrophin deficiency
Impaired peripheral androgen responsiveness
5α-reductase deficiency
Androgen insensitivity
partial
complete
Dysmorphic syndromes
Drash syndrome
Other
Idiopathic

AMH deficiency

In the persistent Mullerian duct syndrome the uterus and fallopian tubes fail to regress during development. Affected infants usually present when undergoing surgery for cryptorchidism or inguinal hernia repair, when the Mullerian structures are identified.

A number of mutations of the AMH gene have now been described in this syndrome, and in some patients the problem appears to be end-organ resistance.[12,71]

Testosterone deficiency

The biosynthesis of testosterone can be affected at each stage by a recessively inherited disorder, resulting in a variable degree of inadequate testosterone production and fetal virilization, and often also inadequate virilization at puberty. In the metabolic blocks that affect the earlier stages of the biosynthetic pathways, steroid synthesis in the adrenal cortex as well as the testis is affected. These produce the most severe degrees of deficiency in virilization and may also be associated with cortisol deficiency; affected infants are therefore at risk from hypoglycaemia.

Luteinizing hormone receptor defects

It is now recognized that impaired androgen production by the testis may be due to end-organ insensitivity arising from molecular defects in the LH receptor.[82,87] The gonad is unable to respond normally to hCG in early pregnancy and then to LH in later gestation. Affected individuals may be described as having Leydig cell hypoplasia because of the associated histological findings.

Congenital lipoid adrenal hyperplasia

Congenital lipoid adrenal hyperplasia (lipoid CAH) was formerly referred to as side chain cleavage or cholesterol desmolase deficiency. Most cases of lipoid CAH are now known to be due to mutations in the steroidogenic regulatory protein (StAR) which promotes cholesterol transport into the mitochondria.[10] Impaired StAR activity leads to deficient synthesis of all steroid products including aldosterone, cortisol and androgen. The genitalia are therefore female in appearance and there is severe salt loss and hypoglycaemia. At postmortem the adrenals are enlarged and full of accumulated cholesterol. Survival is possible with prompt recognition and appropriate treatment.[78]

3β-Hydroxysteroid dehydrogenase deficiency (Fig. 38.8)

In this condition the variable degree of impaired enzyme activity can cause considerable phenotypic heterogeneity. Affected males are usually poorly virilized and may have perineal hypospadias. Females are either normal in appearance or are virilized, probably because of increased ACTH-stimulated production of the weak androgen dehydroepiandrosterone, which can be converted peripherally to more potent androgens such as testosterone. Some, but not all, affected children develop salt wasting or signs of glucocorticoid deficiency.[96,121]

17α-Hydroxylase deficiency and 17,20-desmolase deficiency (Fig. 38.8)

A single protein is responsible for these two separate enzyme activities. Affected males are inadequately virilized, whereas females are phenotypically normal in early life.[193]

17β-Hydroxysteroid dehydrogenase deficiency (Fig. 38.8)

This enzyme is responsible for the last step in testosterone production. At birth affected males are poorly virilized, and many have been reared as females before being investigated at puberty, when marked virilization occurs.[178] Presentation in infancy with herniae and palpable gonads has also been reported.[53]

Impaired peripheral androgen metabolism or responsiveness

5α-Reductase deficiency[134]

Genetic males with 5α-reductase deficiency have external genitalia that are largely female in appearance. The defect was described in families living in an isolated community in the Dominican Republic, where affected individuals were raised as females but at puberty there was virilization of the genitalia and body habitus and the development of male psychosexual orientation; most then converted to the male role.[72] The condition has now been recognized in many countries. Clinically there is normal fetal development of Wolffian structures, which are testosterone dependent, but poor development of the external genitalia, which require dihydrotestosterone. Biochemically the key finding is a high testosterone/dihydrotesterone ratio in serum and analogous changes on urinary steroid analysis.[117]

Partial androgen insensitivity

In this X-linked recessive condition the genital abnormality arising from the insensitivity to androgen varies widely, ranging from a near-normal female appearance to normal male virilization with azoospermia. This is an important cause of perineal hypospadias.[6] Many affected children have inherited defects of the androgen receptor (which maps to the long arm of the X-chromosome). The genetics of this disorder have been studied in detail.[122]

Complete androgen insensitivity

Complete androgen insensitivity, also inherited as an X-linked recessive condition, is seldom diagnosed in the neonatal period unless there is a positive family history or gonads are palpable in the groin, because affected infants are otherwise indistinguishable from normal females.[122] Mullerian regression occurs normally under the influence of AMH but the Wolffian ducts fail to differentiate. At puberty there is breast development but no virilization.[31] Plasma testosterone and LH levels are typically elevated.

FEMALE PSEUDOHERMAPHRODITISM (VIRILIZATION IN GENETIC FEMALES)

These conditions are characterized by a normal female karyotype, normal ovaries and normal female internal genitalia but virilized external genitalia. Exposure of a female fetus to excess androgen can occur in three ways. The first is relatively common whereas the second and third mechanisms are well recognized but extremely rare:

- Increased endogenous adrenal androgen production in congenital adrenal hyperplasia;
- Impaired conversion of androgens to oestrogen by the placenta in aromatase deficiency;
- Increased transplacental exposure to androgen, of either maternal or exogenous origin.

The causes are shown in Table 38.18.

Congenital adrenal hyperplasia

The three virilizing forms are discussed above (p. 973).

Aromatase deficiency

Normal conversion of fetal and maternal androgens to oestrogen by placental aromatase enzyme activity was

Table 38.18 Causes of female pseudohermaphroditism

Virilizing congenital adrenal hyperplasia
Deficiency of
21α-hydroxylase
11β-hydroxylase
3β-hydroxysteroid dehydrogenase
Aromatase deficiency
Maternal androgen excess
Endogenous
Exogenous
Dysmorphic syndromes

thought to be essential for survival of the conceptus, but recently there have been reports of aromatase gene mutations leading to impaired placental enzyme activity and subsequent maternal and fetal virilization.[23,156] It therefore appears that a pregnancy can be viable despite a marked reduction in oestrogen production, but that the associated rise in androgens in aromatase deficiency may lead to female pseudohermaphroditism.

Excess maternal androgens

Fetal virilization may rarely occur in response to excess maternal androgen production from an adrenal or ovarian tumour. The degree of virilization will depend on the timing and degree of androgen overproduction.[177]

Iatrogenic fetal virilization

Fetal virilization was formerly observed in female infants of mothers treated with androgens or androgenic progestins during pregnancy; these were given in an attempt to prevent recurrent spontaneous abortion,[184] but such treatment is now rarely used.

DISORDERS OF GONADAL DEVELOPMENT

These disorders (Table 38.19) are diverse but have in common a defect in the genetic programming of gonadal development. Diagnosis in the newborn period usually depends on recognizing an abnormality of the external genitalia, which is often but not always present. There is the potential for both Mullerian and Wolffian duct development in one individual and variable potential for germ cell development, neoplasia and endocrine function.

True hermaphroditism

This diagnosis rests on the histological demonstration of ovarian and testicular tissue in a single individual, either in separate gonads or, more commonly, in ovotestes. There is nearly always some genital ambiguity and the internal sexual organs are variable. In one large series 13% of individuals were mosaic 46XX/46XY, and 58% were XX.[173] Many affected children have been raised as males in the past,[18] but gender assignment should usually be female as there is good potential for sexual function and even fertility, and a high risk of tumour formation in dysgenetic testicular tissue.[56]

Table 38.19 Disorders of gonadal development

True hermaphroditism
XX male
Klinefelter syndrome
Mixed gonadal dysgenesis
Turner syndrome
Pure gonadal dysgenesis
Anorchia

XX males

Individuals with this rare condition (1 in 20 000) have testes despite an XX karyotype. The genitalia are usually male, although there may be ambiguity which can lead to presentation in infancy. Y-specific DNA sequences, sometimes including the *SRY* gene, can be identified in 80–90% of cases.[182]

Klinefelter syndrome

This remarkably common condition (around 1 in 1000 live male births) is associated with a 47XXY karyotype. It is not usually diagnosed until later childhood, puberty or adult life, but hypospadias, small testes and extension of the scrotal skin on to the shaft of a small penis may indicate its presence earlier.[86,155]

Mixed gonadal dysgenesis

Children with this condition have genetic mosaicism, including cell lines with and without Y-chromosome material. The phenotype is extremely varied, ranging from apparently normal male to apparently normal female, but is typified by a child with a testis with Wolffian structures on one side, a streak gonad with Mullerian structures on the other and a 45X/46XY karyotype. The genital appearance is variable but usually female, with some clitoral enlargement and labial fusion.[194] Stigmata of Turner syndrome are present in more than 50% of affected children. There is a high risk of gonadoblastoma, which may present at birth and occurs in approximately 75% of cases by 26 years.[194] Female sex assignment is usually appropriate. Virilization at puberty is inadequate and the gonads should be removed because of the risk of malignancy. However, studies on prenatal diagnosis have shed new light on the condition, since of cases diagnosed by prenatal screening more than 80% show an apparently male phenotype, and it is clear that there has been major ascertainment bias in identifying affected individuals.[69]

Turner syndrome (p. 863)

A clinical diagnosis may be made in the newborn period because of the characteristic lymphoedema of the hands and feet, or suspected because of the presence of other associated abnormalities such as aortic coarctation. This permits early counselling and detection of problems such as growth failure and lack of pubertal development.

Pure gonadal dysgenesis

Affected infants are phenotypic females (usually with an XX karyotype, but they may also be XY) with normal external genitalia and bilateral streak gonads. This condition usually presents in adolescence with primary amenorrhoea, rather than in the neonatal period. It has now been shown that some individuals with hypergonadotrophic ovarian dysgenesis have abnormalities of the FSH receptor.[2] Male gonadal development and spermatogenesis do not seem to be dependent on normal FSH receptor/signal transduction to the same extent.

Anorchia

The effect of anorchia depends on the stage of development at which it occurs. Involution early in fetal life results in phenotypically normal or slightly virilized female genitalia with neither Wolffian nor Mullerian internal structures.[47] Later involution may cause the 'micropenis with rudimentary testes' syndrome,[110] and, still later, results in absent testes in an otherwise normal male.[45] It has been suggested that testicular torsion in utero or in the perinatal period may be responsible for some cases.[160]

THE CLINICAL APPROACH TO PROBLEMS OF INTERSEX

Every mother asks first of her newborn child, 'Is it a boy or a girl?' and 'Is it all right?' There is inevitable distress when these questions cannot be answered immediately; problems of sexual differentiation are often particularly worrying. Full discussion at all stages with both parents is therefore especially important. The initial discussions should emphasize that:

- abnormalities of sexual development are intrinsically no more threatening than anomalies in any other system, and are usually, but not always, confined to the genital tract;
- the cause can be determined, the appropriate sex of rearing assigned and treatment planned with little delay in nearly all cases;
- the prognosis for life and health, and also for sexual function, is good, but that for fertility must be guarded.

An early anxiety of the parents will be what to tell grandparents, siblings, friends and colleagues. It may be possible to delay announcing the birth, or alternatively to announce only that the baby has a problem requiring treatment and that the parents would prefer not to discuss progress for a few days. The birth should not be registered until the sex of rearing is decided. Choice of a name suitable for either sex is probably unwise.

Deciding the appropriate sex of rearing only occasionally presents real difficulty. Whatever the genetic status and the anatomy of the internal sexual organs, successful integration in either sexual role depends on the configuration and function of the external genitalia, against the background of the prevailing social and religious attitudes. It is impossible, even with the most expert modern reconstructive surgery, to create an adequate erectile penis from inadequate tissue. In the past plastic surgeons and urologists sometimes took an optimistic view of what it might be possible to achieve with a small phallus, but the end results, often after multiple distressing operations, were very disappointing.

The prospects for development at puberty and for fertility must also be considered, but these are secondary.

There may be strong ethnic, social or religious pressures influencing the family's choice, and these must obviously be respected.

Psychological adjustment to the sex of rearing seldom causes problems as long as this is chosen early and accepted by those handling the child. Experience with 5α-reductase deficiency and other conditions has shown that greater flexibility in sexual role is possible than was previously believed. Nonetheless, the aim must be to select the sex of rearing as early in infancy as possible, and also to complete any genital surgery necessary to produce cosmetically acceptable external genitalia as early as is practicable, certainly before school age and preferably before 2 years, by which age gender identity is established.

The clinical management of the baby is directed to clarifying the aspects of gender detailed above. The essential steps can be summarized as follows:

1. Review the family history and the pre- and perinatal course for clues, such as maternal 'aunts' with amenorrhoea and infertility, or maternal exposure to drugs in pregnancy.
2. Examine the infant for pigmentation, palpable gonads or other relevant features.
3. Be prepared to keep the mother and baby in hospital for 10 days or longer in order to check regularly for hypoglycaemia, salt loss or other metabolic problems, to complete initial investigation, if possible to decide on the sex of rearing, and to help the parents with understanding and acceptance of the problem.
4. Obtain a karyotype as quickly as possible (the buccal smear is inadequate and especially unreliable in the first few days, as it is often negative in XX females).
5. Start appropriate biochemical investigation as soon as possible; this must be tailored according to the clinical and genetic findings, but initially should include plasma 17-OHP, 11-deoxycortisol and androgens (testosterone, dihydrotestosterone, androstenedione and dehydroepiandrosterone). Always remember to save a specimen of blood for future analysis.
6. Start appropriate anatomical investigation. Ultrasound scanning is non-invasive and of some value, but the most useful radiological investigation is a 'genitogram', in which radio-opaque dye is injected into the genital orifice. Good definition of the internal organs can generally be obtained (Fig. 38.12).

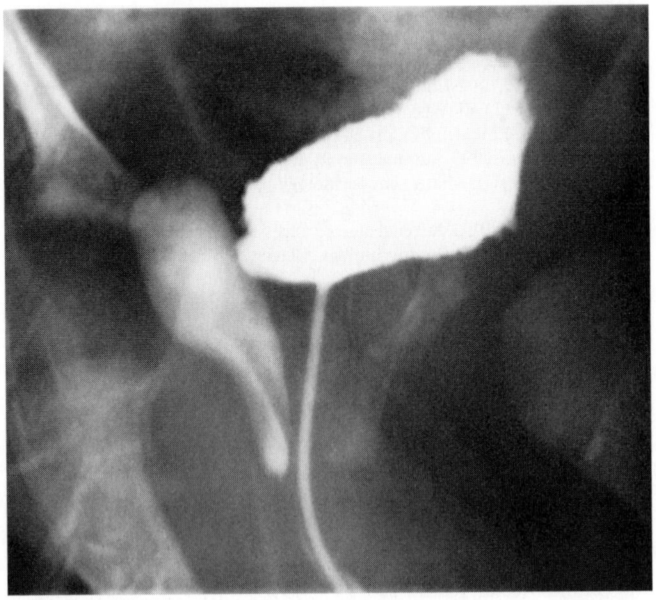

Fig. 38.12 The 'genitogram' of an infant with XY karyotype and ambiguous genitalia. Note the clearly defined blind-ending but adequately sized 'vaginal' cavity posterior to the urethra. This infant proved to have partial androgen unresponsiveness and was reared in the female sex.

The most common outcome will be the finding that the baby has an XX genotype, a high plasma 17-OHP and a normal or low plasma 11-deoxycortisol and cortisol, indicating congenital adrenal hyperplasia with a 21α-hydroxylase block. The presence or absence of salt wasting is then determined from the weight chart and serial plasma and urinary electrolytes, possibly supplemented by plasma renin and aldosterone measurements. 11β-Hydroxylase deficiency may be misdiagnosed as simple virilizing 21α-hydroxylase deficiency if the plasma 11-deoxycortisol is not estimated.

Girls with these defects have normal female internal genitalia and are potentially fertile, so there is no question that, whatever the degree of virilization, they must be reared in the female sex.

If the karyotype proves to be XY, investigation is more complex. Exact definition of the defect will depend on demonstration of a block in androgen synthesis, which may require an hCG stimulation test, or an abnormality of androgen receptor function. Such complex investigation may take time, but the choice of sex of rearing will depend on the external genitalia. If the phallus is very small, which is judged by feeling the corpora, not merely by assessing the amount of shaft and preputial skin, which may be misleading in the presence of normal or high androgen levels, the prospects for further phallic growth are poor and the female sex will probably be appropriate. If there is remaining doubt a course of depot testosterone, 25 mg i.m. monthly for 3 months, can be given, good phallic growth confirming the potential for virilization at puberty.

The genitogram will often reveal a 'vaginal' cavity, and if this is of reasonable size the prospect of female rearing is made more acceptable. Even in the absence of such a cavity, however, it is possible surgically to construct a functional vagina later in life. In the disorders of gonadal development there is such diversity and discordance between the genetic and anatomical findings that in addition to an investigation pathway as outlined above, it may be necessary to undertake laparotomy and gonadal biopsy.

REFERENCES

1. Ahmed I, Atiq M, Iqbal J, Khurshid M, Whittaker P 1995 Vitamin D deficiency rickets in breast-fed infants presenting with hypocalcaemic seizures. Acta Paediatrica 84: 941–942
2. Aittomäki K, Lucena J L D, Pakarinen P et al 1995 Mutation in the follicle-stimulating hormone receptor gene causes hereditary hypergonadotropic ovarian failure. Cell 82: 959–968
3. Allgrove J, Clayden G S, Grant D B, McCauley J C 1978 Familial glucocorticoid deficiency with achalasia of the cardia and deficient tear production. Lancet 1: 1284–1286
4. Alm J, Larsson A, Zetterstom I R 1978 Congenital hypothyroidism in Sweden. Incidence and age at diagnosis. Acta Paediatrica Scandinavica 67: 1–3
5. American Academy of Pediatrics A A P Section on Endocrinology and Committee on Genetics, and American Thyroid Association Committee on Public Health 1993 Newborn screening for congenital hypothyroidism: recommended guidelines. Pediatrics 91: 1203–1209
6. Batch J A, Evans B A J, Hughes I A, Patterson M N 1993 Mutations of the androgen receptor gene identified in perineal hypospadias. Journal of Medical Genetics 30: 198–201
7. Belton N R 1986 Rickets – not only the 'English disease'. Acta Paediatrica (Suppl) 323: 68–75
8. Biebermann H, Schöneberg T, Krude H, Schultz G, Gudermann T, Grüters A 1997 Mutations of the human thyrotropin receptor gene causing thyroid hypoplasia and persistent congenital hypothyroidism. Journal of Clinical Endocrinology and Metabolism 82: 3471–3480
9. Body J J, Chanoine J P, Dumon J C, Delange F 1993 Circulating calcitonin levels in healthy children and subjects with congenital hypothyroidism from birth to adolescence. Journal of Clinical Endocrinology and Metabolism 77: 565–567
10. Bose HS, Sugawara T, Strauss III J F, Miller W 1996. The pathophysiology and genetics of congenital lipoid adrenal hyperplasia. New England Journal of Medicine 335: 1870–1878
11. Bradley B S, Kumar S P, Mehta P N, Ezhuthachan S G 1994 Neonatal cushingoid syndrome resulting from serial courses of antenatal betamethasone. Obstetrics and Gynecology 83: 869–872
12. Brook C D G, Wagner H, Zachmann M 1973 Familial occurrence of persistent Mullerian structures in otherwise normal males. British Medical Journal i: 771–773
13. Brook C D G 1995 Clinical paediatric endocrinology. Blackwell Scientific, Oxford
14. Brookfield D S K, McCandless A E, Smith C S 1976 Thyrotoxicosis in a neonate of a mother with no history of thyroid disease. Archives of Disease in Childhood 55: 894–895
15. Brown E M, Segre G V, Goldring S R 1996 Serpentine receptors for parathyroid hormone, calcitonin and extracellular calcium ions. In: Sheppard M C, Franklyn J A (eds) Baillière's clinical endocrinology and metabolism. Baillière Tindall, London, pp 123–161
16. Brown R S, Bellisario R L, Botero D et al 1996 Incidence of transient congenital hypothyroidism due to maternal thyrotropin receptor-blocking antibodies in over one million babies. Journal of Clinical Endocrinology and Metabolism 81: 1147–1151
17. Burrow G N, Fisher D A, Larsen P R 1994 Maternal and fetal thyroid function. New England Journal of Medicine 331: 1072–1078
18. Butler L J, Snodgrass G J A I, France N E 1969 True hermaphroditism or gonadal intersexuality. Archives of Disease in Childhood 44: 666–680

19. Cacciari E, Balsamo A, Cassio A et al 1983 Neonatal screening for congenital adrenal hyperplasia. Archives of Disease in Childhood 58: 803–806
20. Cheetham T D, Hughes I A 1996 Optimizing the management of congenital adrenal hyperplasia. In: Kelnar C J H (ed) Baillière's clinical paediatrics. Baillière Tindall, London, pp 277–293
21. Cheron R G, Kaplan M M, Larsen P R, Selenkow H A, Crigler J F 1981 Neonatal thyroid function after propylthiouracil therapy for maternal Graves' disease. New England Journal of Medicine 304: 525–528
22. Chowdhry P, Scanlon J W, Auerbach R, Abbassi V 1984 Results of controlled double blind study of thyroid replacement in very low birth weight premature infants with hypothyroxinaemia. Pediatrics 73: 301–305
23. Conte F A, Grumbach M M, Ito Y, Fisher C R, Simpson E R 1994 A syndrome of female pseudohermaphrodism, hypergonadotropic hypogonadism, and multicystic ovaries associated with missense mutations in the gene encoding aromatase (P450arom). Journal of Clinical Endocrinology and Metabolism 78: 1287–1292
24. Craft W H, Underwood L E, Van Wyk J J 1980 High incidence of perinatal insult in children with idiopathic hypopituitarism. Journal of Pediatrics 96: 397–402
25. Crowley S, Hindmarsh P C, Honour J W, Brook C G D 1983 Reproducibility of the cortisol responses to stimulation with a low dose of ACTH(1–24): the effect of basal cortisol levels and comparison of low-dose with high-dose secretory dynamics. Journal of Endocrinology 136: 167–172
26. Cutfield W S, Webster D 1995 Newborn screening for congenital adrenal hyperplasia in New Zealand. Journal of Pediatrics 126: 118–121
27. David L, Salle B, Putet G, Grafmeyer D 1981 Serum immunoreactive calcitonin in low birth weight infants. Description of early changes in serum calcium, phosphorus, magnesium, parathyroid hormone and gastrin levels. Pediatric Research 15: 803–808
28. Delange F, Henderson P, Bourdoux P et al 1986 Regional variations of iodine nutrition and thyroid function during the neonatal period in Europe. Biology of the Neonate 49: 322–330
29. Den Ouden A L, Kok J H, Verkerk P H, Brand R, Verloove-Vanhorick S P 1996 The relation between neonatal thyroxine levels and neurodevelopmental outcome at age 5 and 9 years in a national cohort of very preterm and/or very low birth weight infants. Pediatric Research 39: 142–145
30. Derksen-lubsen Verkerk P H 1996 Neuropsychologic development in early treated congenital hypothyroidism: analysis of literature data. Pediatric Research 39: 561–566
31. Dewhurst C J 1971 The XY female. American Journal of Obstetrics and Gynecology 109: 675–688
32. De Zegher F, Van den Berghe G, Devlieger H, Eggermont E, Veldhuis J D 1993 Dopamine inhibits growth hormone and prolactin secretion in the human newborn. Pediatric Research 34: 642–645
33. De Zegher F, Kaplan S L, Grumbach M M, Van den Berghe G, Francois I, Vanhole C 1995 The foetal pituitary, postmaturity and breech presentation. Acta Paediatrica 83: 1100–1102
34. De Zegher F, Pernasetti F, Vanhole C, Devlieger H, Van den Berghe G, Martial J A 1995 The prenatal role of thyroid hormone evidenced by fetomaternal Pit-1 deficiency. Journal of Clinical Endocrinology and Metabolism 80: 3127–3130
35. Donaldson M D C, Thomas P H, Love J G, Murray G D, McNinch A W, Savage D C L 1994 Presentation, acute illness, and learning difficulties in salt-wasting 21-hydroxylase deficiency. Archives of Disease in Childhood 70: 214–218
36. Dubuis J-M, Glorieux J, Richer F, Deal C L, Dussault J H, van Vliet G 1996 Outcome of severe congenital hypothyroidism: closing the developmental gap with early high dose levothyroxine treatment. Journal of Clinical Endocrinology and Metabolism 81: 222–227
37. Ellyin F, Khatir A H, Singh S P 1980 Hypothalamic-pituitary function in patients with trans-sphenoidal encephalocele and mid-facial anomalies. Journal of Clinical Endocrinology and Metabolism 51: 854–856
38. Fenton L J, Kleinman L I 1974 Transient diabetes insipidus in a newborn infant. Journal of Pediatrics 85: 79–81
39. Fisher D A, Dussault J H, Foley T P Jr et al 1979 Screening for congenital hypothyroidism: results of screening one million North American infants. Journal of Pediatrics 94: 700–705
40. Fisher D A 1990 Euthyroid low thyroxine (T4) and triiodothyronine (T3) states in prematures and sick neonates. Pediatric Clinics of North America 37: 1297–1312
41. Fisher D A 1992 Endocrinology and fetal development. In: Wilson J D, Foster D W (eds) Williams textbook of endocrinology. W B Saunders, Philadelphia, pp 1049–1077
42. Forest M G 1995 Adrenal steroid deficiency states In: Brook C G D (ed) Clinical paediatric endocrinology. Blackwell Scientific, Oxford, pp 453–498
43. Forest M G 1995 Adrenal steroid excess. In: Brook C G D (ed) Clinical paediatric endocrinology. Blackwell Scientific, Oxford, pp 499–535
44. Frank J E, Faix J E, Hermos R J et al 1996 Thyroid function in very low birth weight infants: effects on neonatal hypothyroid screening. Journal of Pediatrics 128: 548–554
45. Glenn, J F, McPherson H T 1971 Anorchism: definition of a clinical entity. Journal of Urology 105: 265–270
46. Gluckman P D, Gunn A J, Wray A et al 1992 Congenital idiopathic growth hormone deficiency is associated with prenatal and early postnatal growth failure. Journal of Pediatrics 121: 920–923
47. Grant D B, Dillon M J 1975 Micropenis associated with testicular agenesis. Archives of Disease in Childhood 50: 247–249
48. Grant D B, Smith I 1988 Survey of neonatal screening for primary hypothyroidism in England, Wales and Northern Ireland 1982–1984. British Medical Journal 296: 1355–1358
49. Grant D B, Dunger D B, Smith I, Hyland K 1992 Familial glucocorticoid deficiency with achalasia of the cardia associated with mixed neuropathy, long-tract degeneration and mild dementia. European Journal of Pediatrics 151: 85–89
50. Grant D B, Smith I, Fuggle P W, Tokar S, Chapple J 1992 Congenital hypothyroidism detected by neonatal screening: relationship between biochemical severity and early clinical features. Archives of Disease in Childhood 67: 87–90
51. Grant D B 1995 Congenital hypothyroidism: optimal management in the light of 15 years' experience of screening. Archives of Disease in Childhood 72: 85–89
52. Greenberg D, Abramson O, Phillip M 1995 Fetal pseudohypoaldosteronism: another cause of hydramnios. Acta Paediatrica 84: 582–584
53. Gregory J W, Aynsley-Green A, Evans B A, Hughes I A, Werder E A, Zachmann M 1993 Deficiency of 17-ketoreductase presenting before puberty. Hormone Research. 40: 145–148
54. Grüters A, Delange F, Giovannelli G et al 1993 Guidelines for neonatal screening programs for congenital hypothyroidism. European Journal of Pediatrics 152: 974–975
55. Grüters A 1996 Screening for congenital hypothyroidism: effectiveness and clinical outcome. In: Kelnar C J H (ed) Baillière's clinical paediatrics. Baillière Tindall, London, pp 259–276
56. Hadjiathanasiou C G, Brauner R, Lortat-Jacob S et al 1994 True hermaphroditism: genetic variants and clinical management. Journal of Pediatrics 125: 738–744
57. Hall J G, Pallister P D, Clarren S K et al 1980 Congenital hypothalamic harmartoblastoma, hypopituitarism, imperforate anus, and postaxial polydactyly – a new syndrome? Part 1: Clinical, causal and pathogenic considerations. American Journal of Medical Genetics 7: 47–74
58. Hanna C E, Keith L D, Colasurdo M A et al 1993 Hypothalamic pituitary adrenal function in the extremely low birth weight infant. Journal of Clinical Endocrinology and Metabolism 76: 384–387
59. Hashimoto H, Maruyama H, Koshida R, Okuda N, Sato T 1995 Central hypothyroidism resulting from pituitary suppression and peripheral thyrotoxicosis in a premature infant born to a mother with Graves' disease. Journal of Pediatrics 127: 809–811
60. Heath H, Odelberg S, Jackson C E et al 1996 Clustered inactivating mutations and benign polymorphisms of the calcium receptor gene in familial benign hypocalciuric hypercalcemia suggest receptor functional domains. Journal of Clinical Endocrinology and Metabolism 81: 1312–1317
61. Herman S P, Baggenstoss A M, Cloutier M D 1975 Liver dysfunction and histologic abnormalities in neonatal hypopituitarism. Journal of Pediatrics 87: 892–895
62. Hewison M and O'Riordan J L H 1994 Vitamin D resistance. In: Sheppard M C, Stewart M C (eds) Baillière's clinical endocrinology and metabolism. Baillière Tindall, London, pp 305–315

63. Hindmarsh P C, Brook C G D 1985 Single dose dexamethasone suppression test in children: dose relationship to body size. Clinical Endocrinology 23: 67–70
64. Hochberg Z, Benderly A, Zadik Z 1984 Salt loss in congenital adrenal hyperplasia due to 11-beta-hydroxylase deficiency. Archives of Disease in Childhood 59: 1092–1094
65. Hoffman W H, Sahasrananan P, Ferandos S S, Burek C L, Rose N R 1982 Transient thyrotoxicosis in an infant delivered to a longacting thyroid stimulator (LATS) and LATS protector negative, thyroid stimulating antibody positive woman with Hashimoto's thyroiditis. Journal of Clinical Endocrinology and Metabolism 54: 354–356
66. Holcombe J H, Keenan B S, Nichols B L, Kirkland R T, Clayton G W 1980 Neonatal salt loss in the hypertensive form of congenital adrenal hyperplasia. Pediatrics 65: 777–781
67. Hollingsworth D R, Mabry C, 1976 Congenital Graves' disease. American Journal of Diseases of Children 130: 148–155
68. Honour J W 1995 The adrenal cortex. In: Brook C G D (ed) Clinical paediatric endocrinology. Blackwell Scientific, Oxford, pp 434–452
69. Hsu L Y F 1989 Prenatal diagnosis of 45X/46XY mosaicism – a review and update. Prenatal Diagnosis 9: 31–48
70. Huma Z, Crawford C, New M I 1995 Congenital adrenal hyperplasia In: Brook C G D (ed) Clinical paediatric endocrinology. Blackwell Scientific, Oxford, pp 536–557
71. Imbeaud S, Carre-Eusebe D, Rey R, Belville C, Josso N, Picard J Y 1994 Molecular genetics of the persistent mullerian duct syndrome: a study of 19 families. Human Molecular Genetics 3: 125–131
72. Imperato-McGinley J, Peterson R E, Gautier T, Sturla E 1979 Androgens and the evolution of male gender identify among pseudohermaphrodites with 5α-reductase deficiency. New England Journal of Medicine 300: 1233–1237
73. Jett P L, Samuels M H, McDaniel P A et al 1997 Variability of plasma cortisol levels in extremely low birthweight infants. Journal of Clinical Endocrinology and Metabolism 82: 2921–2925
74. Jost A 1953 Problems of fetal endocrinology: the gonadal and hypophyseal hormones. Recent Progress in Hormone Research 8: 379–413
75. Kari M A, Raivio K O, Stenman U-H, Voutilainen R 1996 Serum cortisol, dehydroepiandrosterone sulfate, and steroid-binding globulins in preterm neonates: effect of gestational age and dexamethasone therapy. Pediatric Research 40: 319–324
76. Karpman B A, Rapoport B, Filetti S, Fisher D A 1987 Treatment of neonatal hyperthyroidism due to Graves disease with sodium ipodate. Journal of Clinical Endocrinology and Metabolism 64: 119–123
77. Kato F, Kikudhi K, Miyamoto S, Ohie T, Yamaguchi S 1995 Congenital hypopituitarism with hypoplasia of the anterior pituitary gland. Acta Paediatrica 84: 1201–1203
78. Kirkland R T, Kirkland J L, Johnson C M, Horning M G, Librk L, Clayton G W 1973 Congenital lipoid adrenal hyperplasia in an 8 year old phenotypic female. Journal of Clinical Endocrinology and Metabolism 36: 488–496
79. Köhler B, Schnabel D, Biebermann H, Grüters A 1996 Transient congenital hypothyroidism and hyperthyrotropinemia: normal thyroid function and physical development at the ages of 6–14 years. Journal of Clinical Endocrinology and Metabolism 81: 1563–1567
80. Kopp P, van Sande J, Parma J et al 1995 Brief report: Congenital hyperthyroidism caused by a mutation in the thyrotropin-receptor gene. New England Journal of Medicine 332: 183–185
81. Kreines K, DeVaux W D 1971 Neonatal adrenal insufficiency associated with maternal Cushing's syndrome. Pediatrics 47: 516–519
82. Kremer H, Kraaij R, Toledo S P A et al 1995 Male pseudohermaphroditism due to a homozygous missense mutation of the luteinizing hormone receptor gene. Nature Genetics 9: 160–164
83. Kruse K, Irle U, Uhlig R 1993 Elevated 1,25-dihydroxyvitamin D serum concentrations in infants with subcutaneous fat necrosis. Journal of Pediatrics 122: 460–463
84. Kruse K 1995 Endocrine control of calcium and bone metabolism. In: Brook C G D (ed) Clinical paediatric endocrinology. Blackwell Scientific, Oxford, pp 713–734
85. Kruse K 1995 Disorders of calcium and bone metabolism. In: Brook C G D (ed) Clinical paediatric endocrinology. Blackwell Scientific, Oxford, pp 735–778
86. Laron Z, Hochman H 1971 Small testes in prepubertal boys with Klinefelter's syndrome. Journal of Clinical Endocrinology and Metabolism 32: 671–672
87. Latronico A C, Anasti J, Arnhold I J P et al 1996 Testicular and ovarian resistance to luteinizing hormone caused by inactivating mutations of luteinizing hormone receptor gene. New England Journal of Medicine 334: 507–512
88. Levy-Mozziconacci A, Wernert F, Scambler P et al 1994 Clinical and molecular study of DiGeorge sequence. European Journal of Pediatrics 153: 813–820
89. Lovinger R D, Kaplan S L, Grumbach M M 1975 Congenital hypopituitarism associated with neonatal hypoglycaemia and microphallus. Four cases secondary to hypothalamic hormone deficiencies. Journal of Pediatrics 87: 1171–1181
90. Lucas A, Morley R, Fewtrell M S 1996 Low triiodothyronine concentration in preterm infants and subsequent intelligence quotient (IQ) at 8 year follow up. British Medical Journal 312: 1132–1133
91. Lyon A J, McIntosh N, Wheeler K, Brooke O G 1984 Hypercalcaemia in extremely low birthweight infants. Archives of Disease in Childhood 59: 1141–1144
92. Malchoff C D, Javier E C, Malchoff D M et al 1990 Primary cortisol resistance presenting as isosexual precocity. Journal of Clinical Endocrinology and Metabolism 70: 503–507
93. Masera N, Grant D B, Stanhope R, Preece M A 1994 Diabetes insipidus with impaired osmotic regulation in septo-optic dysplasia and agenesis of the corpus callosum. Archives of Disease in Childhood 70: 51–53
94. Mayne P D, Kovar I Z 1991 Calcium and phosphorus metabolism in the premature infant. Annals of Clinical Biochemistry 28: 131–142
95. McKenzie J M, Zakarija M 1978 Pathogenesis of neonatal Graves' disease. Journal of Endocrinological Investigation 1: 183–189
96. Mébarki F, Sanchez R, Rhéaumes E et al 1995 Non salt-losing male pseudohermaphroditism due to the novel homozygous N100S mutation in the type II 3β-hydroxysteroid dehydrogenase gene. Journal of Clinical Endocrinology and Metabolism 80: 2127–2134
97. Meijer W J, Verloove-Vanhorick S P, Brand R, van den Brande J L 1992 Transient hypothyroxinaemia associated with developmental delay in very preterm infants. Archives of Disease in Childhood 67: 944–947
98. Mercado A B, Wilson R C, Cheng K C, Wei J-Q, New M I 1995 Prenatal treatment and diagnosis of congenital adrenal hyperplasia owing to steroid 21-hydroxylase deficiency. Journal of Clinical Endocrinology and Metabolism 80: 2014–2020
99. Metzger D L, Wright N M, Veldhuis J D, Rogol A D, Kerrigan J R 1993 Characterization of pulsatile secretion and clearance of plasma cortisol in premature and term neonates using deconvolution analysis. Journal of Clinical Endocrinology and Metabolism 77: 458–463
100. Miller R R, Menke J A, Menster M I 1984 Hypercalcaemia associated with phosphate depletion in the neonate. Journal of Pediatrics 105: 814–817
101. Miller W L 1994 Genetics, diagnosis, and management of 21-hydroxylase deficiency. Journal of Clinical Endocrinology and Metabolism 78: 241–246
102. Minagawa M, Yasuda T, Kobayashi Y, Niimi H 1995: Transient pseudohypoparathyroidism of the neonate. European Journal of Endocrinology 133: 151–155
103. Mittelstaedt C A, Volberg F M, Merten D F, Brill P W 1979 The sonographic diagnosis of neonatal adrenal hemorrhage. Radiology 131: 453–457
104. Morris C A, Thomas I T, Greenberg F 1993 Williams syndrome: autosomal dominant inheritance. American Journal of Medical Genetics 47: 478–481
105. Moser H W, Moser A E, Singh I, O'Neill B P 1984 Adrenoleukodystrophy: survey of 303 cases: biochemistry, diagnosis and therapy. Annals of Neurology 16: 628–641
106. Moshang T, Rosenfield R L, Bongiovanni A M 1973 Familial glucocorticoid insufficiency. Journal of Pediatrics 82: 821–826
107. Munro D S, Dirmikis S M, Humphries H, Smith T, Broadhead G D 1978 The role of thyroid stimulating antibodies of Graves' disease in neonatal thyrotoxicosis. British Journal of Obstetrics and Gynaecology 85: 837–843
108. Muscatelli F, Storm T M, Walker A P et al 1994 Mutations in the *Dax-1* gene give rise to both X-linked adrenal hypoplasia congenita and hypogonadotropic hypogonadism. Nature 372: 672–676
109. Murphy J F, Joyce B G, Dyas J, Hughes I A 1983 Plasma 17-hydroxyprogesterone concentration in ill newborn infants. Archives of Disease in Childhood 58: 532–534

110. Najjar S S, Takla R J, Nasser V H 1974 The syndrome of rudimentary testes: occurrence in five siblings. Journal of Pediatrics 84: 119–122
111. Nako Y, Fukushima N, Tomomasa T, Nagashima K 1993 Hypervitaminosis D after prolonged feeding with a premature formula. Pediatrics 92: 862–864
112. Newborn Committee of the European Thyroid Association 1979 Neonatal screening for congenital hypothyroidism in Europe. Acta Endocrinologica 90 (suppl. 223): 5–29
113. New England Congenital Hypothyroidism Collaborative 1982 Pitfalls in screening for neonatal hypothyroidism. Pediatrics 70: 16–20
114 Ng P C, Wong G W K, Lam C W K et al 1997 The pituitary–adrenal responses to exogenous human corticotropin-releasing hormone in preterm, very low birth weight infants. Journal of Clinical Endocrinology and Metabolism 82: 797–799
115. Ng P C, Wong G W K, Lam C W K et al 1997 Pituitary–adrenal suppression and recovery in preterm very low birthweight infants after dexamethasone treatment for bronchopulmonary dysplasia. Journal of Clinical Endocrinology and Metabolism 82: 797–799
116. Nickerson E, Greenberg F, Keating M T, McCaskill C, Shaffer L G 1995 Deletions of the elastin gene at 7qII.23 occur in ~90% of patients with Williams' syndrome. American Journal of Medical Genetics 56: 1156–1161
117. Odame I, Donaldson M D C, Wallace A M, Cochran W, Smith P J 1992 Early diagnosis and management of 5α-reductase deficiency. Archives of Disease in Childhood 67: 720–723
118. Oelkers W 1996 Dose–response aspects in the clinical assessment of the hypothalamopituitary–adrenal axis, and the low-dose adrenocorticotropin test. European Journal of Endocrinology 135: 27–33
119. Pang S, Wallace M A, Hofman L et al 1988 Worldwide experience in newborn screening for classical congenital adrenal hyperplasia due to 21-hydroxylase deficiency. Pediatrics 81: 866–874
120. Pang S, Clark A T, Freeman L C et al 1992 Maternal side effects of prenatal dexamethasone therapy for fetal congenital adrenal hyperplasia. Journal of Clinical Endocrinology and Metabolism 75: 249–253
121. Parks G A, Bermudez J A, Anast C S, Bongiovanni A M, New M I 1971 Pubertal boy with 3β-hydroxysteroid dehydrogenase defect. Journal of Clinical Endocrinology and Metabolism 33: 269–278
122. Patterson M N, McPhaul M J, Hughes I A 1994 Androgen insensitivity syndrome. In: Sheppard M C, Stewart P M (eds) Clinical endocrinology and metabolism. Volume 8, No 2, Baillière Tindall, London, pp 379–404
123. Pearce S H S, Trump D, Wooding C et al 1995 Calcium-sensing receptor mutations in familial benign hypercalcaemia and neonatal hyperparathyroidism. Journal of Clinical Investigation 96: 2683–2692
124. Pearce S H S, Brown E M 1996 The genetic basis of endocrine disease. Disorders of calcium ion sensing. Journal of Clinical Endocrinology and Metabolism 81: 2030–2035
125. Pearce S H S, Williamson C, Kifor O et al 1996 A familial syndrome of hypocalcaemia with hypercalciuria due to mutations in the calcium-sensing receptor. New England Journal of Medicine 335: 1115–1122
126. Perheentupa J. 1995 The neurohypophysis and water regulation. In: Brook C G D (ed) Clinical paediatric endocrinology. Blackwell Scientific, Oxford, pp 580–615
127. Peter M, Sippell W G 1996 Congenital hypoaldosteronism: the Visser–Cost syndrome revisited. Pediatric Research 39: 554–560
128. Pfäffle R W, DiMattia G E, Parks J S et al 1992 Mutation of the POU-specific domain of Pit-1 and hypopituitarism without pituitary hypoplasia. Science 257: 1118–1121
129. Pfäffle R, Kim C, Otten B et al 1996 Pit-1: clinical aspects. Hormone Research 45(supplement): 25–28
130. Pincus D R, Kelnar C J H, Wallace A M 1993 17-hydroxyprogesterone rhythms and growth velocity in congenital adrenal hyperplasia. Journal of Paediatrics and Child Health 29: 302–304
131. Pollak M R, Brown E M, Wu Chou Y-H et al 1993 Mutations in the human Ca^{2+}-sensing receptor gene cause familial hypocalciuric hypercalcemia and neonatal severe hyperparathyroidism. Cell 75: 1297–1303
132. Pollak M R, Wu Chou Y-H, Marx S J et al 1994 Familial hypocalciuric hypercalcemia and neonatal severe hyperparathyroidism. Effects of mutant gene dosage on phenotype. Journal of Clinical Investigation 93: 1108–1112
133. Preece M A, Kearney P J, Marshall W C 1977 Growth hormone deficiency in congenital rubella. Lancet ii: 842–844
134. Randall V A 1994 Role of 5α-reductase in health and disease. In: Sheppard M C, Stewart P M (eds) Clinical endocrinology and metabolism. Volume 8, No 2. Baillière Tindall, London, pp 405–431
135. Rapaport R, Sills I, Patel U et al 1993 Thyrotropin-releasing hormone stimulation tests in infants. Journal of Clinical Endocrinology and Metabolism 77: 889–894
136. Reed Larsen P, Ingbar S H 1992 The thyroid gland. In: Wilson J D, Foster D W (eds) Williams textbook of endocrinology. W B Saunders, Philadelphia, pp 458–459
137. Rees L, Forsling M L, Brook C G D 1980 Vasopressin levels in the newborn. Clinical Endocrinology 12: 357–363
138. Reuss M L, Paneth N, Pinto-Martin J A, Lorenz J M, Susser M 1996 The relation of transient hypothyroxinemia in preterm infants to neurologic development at two years of age. New England Journal of Medicine 334: 821–827
139. Rizvi Z B, Aniol H S, Myers T F, Zeller W P, Fisher S G, Anderson C L 1992 Effects of dexamethasone on the hypothalamic–pituitary–adrenal axis in preterm infants. Journal of Pediatrics 120: 961–965
140. Robinson A G 1976 DDAVP in the treatment of central diabetes insipidus. New England Journal of Medicine 294: 507–511
141. Romagnoli C, Zecca E, Tortorolo G, Diodato A, Fazzini G, Sorcini-Carta M 1987 Plasma thyrocalcitonin and parathyroid hormone concentrations in early neonatal hypocalcaemia. Archives of Disease in Childhood 62: 580–584
142. Rona R J, Tanner J M 1977 Aetiology of idiopathic growth hormone deficiency in England and Wales. Archives of Disease in Childhood 52: 197–208
143. Roti E, Minelli R, Salvi M 1996 Management of hyperthyoidism and hypothyroidism in the pregnant woman. Journal of Clinical Endocrinology and Metabolism 781: 1679–1682
144. Rovet J F, Ehrlich R M 1995 Long-term effects of L-thyroxine therapy for congenital hypothyroidism. Journal of Pediatrics 126: 380–386
145. Rovet J, Walker W, Bliss B, Buchanan L, Ehrich R 1996 Long-term sequelae of hearing impairment in congenital hypothyroidism. Journal of Pediatrics 128: 776–783
146. Rudman D, Davis T, Priest J H et al 1978 Prevalence of growth hormone deficiency in children with cleft lip and palate. Journal of Pediatrics 93: 378–382
147. Rumsby G, Honour J W, Rodeck C 1993 Prenatal diagnosis of congenital adrenal hyperplasia by direct detection of mutations in the steroid 21-hydroxylase gene. Clinical Endocrinology 38: 421–425
148. Saenger P 1995 Physiology of sexual determination and differentiation 1995 Congenital adrenal hyperplasia. In: Brook C G D (ed) Clinical paediatric endocrinology. Blackwell Scientific, Oxford, pp 41–52
149. Salisbury D M, Leonard J V, Dezateux C A, Savage M O 1984 Micropenis: an important early sign of congenital hypopituitarism. British Medical Journal 288: 621–622
150. Santiago L B, Jorge S M, Moreira A C 1996 Longitudinal evaluation of the development of salivary cortisol circadian rhythm in infancy. Clinical Endocrinology 44: 157–161
151. Savage M O, Chaussain J L, Evain D, Roger M, Canlorbe P, Job J C 1978 Endocrine studies in male pseudohermaphroditism in childhood and adolescence. Clinical Endocrinology 8: 219–231
152. Savage M O, Jefferson I G, Dillon M J, Milla P J, Honour J W, Grant D B 1982 Pseudohypoaldosteronism: severe salt wasting in infancy caused by generalized mineralocorticoid unresponsiveness. Journal of Pediatrics 101: 239–242
153. Schipani E, Langman C B, Parfitt A M et al 1996 Constitutively activated receptors for parathyroid hormone and parathyroid hormone-related peptide in Jansen's metaphyseal chondrodysplasia. New England Journal of Medicine 335: 708–714
154. Schonberger W, Grimm W, Emmrich P, Gempp W 1981 Reduction of mortality rate in premature infants by substitution of thyroid hormones. European Journal of Pediatrics 135: 245–253
155. Schwartz I D, Root A W 1991 The Klinefelter syndrome of testicular dysgenesis. Endocrinology and Metabolism Clinics of North America 20: 153–163

156. Shozu M, Akasofu K, Harada T, Kubota Y 1991 A new cause of female pseudohermaphroditism: placental aromatase deficiency. Journal of Clinical Endocrinology and Metabolism 72: 560–566
157. Skuza K A, Sills I N, Stene M, Rapaport R 1996 Prediction of neonatal hyperthyroidism in infants born to mothers with Graves disease. Journal of Pediatrics 128: 264–267
158. Smerdely P, Lim A, Boyages S C et al 1989 Topical iodine-containing antiseptics and neonatal hypothyroidism in very-low-birthweight infants. Lancet ii: 661–664
159. Smith D W, Blizzard R M, Wilkins L 1957 The mental prognosis in hypothyroidism of infancy and childhood. A review of 128 cases. Pediatrics 19: 1011–1022
160. Smith N M, Byard R W, Bourne A J 1991 Testicular regression syndrome – a pathological study of 77 cases. Histopathology 19: 269–272
161. Snelling C E, Erb E H 1955 Hemorrhage and subsequent calcification of the adrenal. Journal of Pediatrics 6: 22–41
162. Specker B L, Tsang R C, Ho M S, Landi T M, Gratton T L 1991 Low serum calcium and high parathyroid hormone levels in neonates fed 'humanized' cow's milk-based formula. American Journal of Diseases in Childhood 145: 941–945
163. Specker B L, Ho M L, Oestreich A et al 1992 Prospective study of vitamin D supplementation and rickets in China. Journal of Pediatrics 120: 733–739
164. Speiser P W, White P C, Dupont J, Zhu D, Mercado A B, New M I 1994 Prenatal diagnosis of congenital adrenal hyperplasia due to 21-hydroxylase deficiency by allele-specific hybridization and Southern blot. Human Genetics 93: 424–428
165. Sperling M (ed) 1996 Pediatric endocrinology. W B Saunders, Philadelphia
166. Stanhope R, Preece M A, Brook C G D 1984 Hypoplastic optic nerves and pituitary dysfunction. Archives of Disease in Childhood 59: 111–114
167. Sunthornthepvarakul T, Gottschalk M E, Hayashi Y, Refetoff S 1995 Resistance to thyrotropin caused by mutations in the thyrotropin-receptor gene. New England Journal of Medicine 332: 155–160
168. Teng C S, Tong T C, Hutchinson J H, Yeung R T T 1980 Thyroid stimulating immunoglobulins in neonatal Graves' disease. Archives of Disease in Childhood 55: 894–895
169. Thomas B R, Bennett J D 1995 Symptomatic hypocalcemia and hypoparathyroidism in two infants of mothers with hyperparathyroidism and familial benign hypercalcemia. Journal of Perinatology 15: 23–26
170. Tillotson S L, Fuggle P W, Smith I, Ades A E, Grant D B 1994 Relation between biochemical severity and intelligence in early treated congenital hypothyroidism: a threshold effect. British Medical Journal 309: 440–445
171. Triulzi F, Scotti G, di Natale B et al 1994 Evidence of congenital midline brain anomaly in pituitary dwarfs: a magnetic resonance imaging study in 101 patients. Pediatrics 93: 409–416
172. Tuchmann-Duplessis H 1959 A study of endocrine glands in anencephalics. Biology of the Neonate 1: 8–32
173. van Niekerk W A 1981 True hermaphroditism. In: The intersex child. Paediatric and adolescent endocrinology Vol. 8. Karger, Basle, pp 80–99
174. Van Wassenaer A G, Kok J H, Endert E, Vulsma T, de Vijlder J J 1993 Thyroxine administration to infants of less than 30 weeks' gestational age does not increase plasma triiodothyronine concentrations. Acta Endocrinologica (Copenhagen) 129: 139–146
175. Van Wassenaer A G, Kok J H, de Vijlder J J M et al 1997 Effects of thyroxine supplementation on neurologic development in infants born at less than 30 weeks' gestation. New England Journal of Medicine 336: 21–26
176. Veldhuis J D, Kulin H E, Santen R J 1980 Inborn error in the terminal steps of aldosterone biosynthesis. Corticosterone methyl oxidase type II deficiency in a North American pedigree. New England Journal of Medicine 303: 117–121
177. Verhoeven A T M, Mostblum J L, Van Lousden H A I M 1973 Virilisation in pregnancy coexisting with an ovarian mucinous cystadenoma: a case report and review of virilising ovarian tumours in pregnancy. Obstetric and Gynecological Survey 28: 597–622
178. Virdis R, Saenger P, Senior B 1978 Endocrine studies in a pubertal male pseudohermaphrodite with 17-ketosteroid reductase deficiency. Acta Endocrinologica 87: 212–224
179. Watterberg K L, Scott S M 1995 Evidence of early adrenal insufficiency in babies who develop bronchopulmonary dysplasia. Pediatrics 95: 120–125
180. Weber A, Clark A J 1994 Mutations of the ACTH receptor gene are only one cause of familial glucocorticoid deficiency. Human Molecular Genetics 3: 585–588
181. Weber A, Toppari J, Harvey R D et al 1995 Adrenocorticotropin receptor gene mutations in familial glucocorticoid deficiency: relationships with clinical features in four families. Journal of Clinical Endocrinology and Metabolism 80: 65–71
182. Weil D, Wang I, Dietrich A, Poustka A, Weissenbach J, Petit C 1994 Highly homologous loci on the X and Y chromosomes are hot-spots for ectopic recombinations leading to XX maleness. Nature Genetics 7: 414–419
183. White P C, Curnow K M, Pascoe L 1994 Disorders of steroid 11β-hydroxylase isoenzymes. Endocrine Reviews 15: 421–438
184. Wilkins L M 1960 Masculinisation of the female fetus due to the use of orally given progestagens. Journal of the American Medical Association 172: 1028–1032
185. Wilkinson H, James J 1993 Self limiting neonatal primary hyperparathyroidism associated with familial hypocalciuric hypercalcaemia. Archives of Disease in Childhood 69: 319–321
186. Wilson D I, Burn J, Scrambler P, Goodship J 1993 DiGeorge syndrome: part of CATCH 22. Journal of Medical Genetics 30: 852–856
187. Wilson D M, Baldwin R B Ariagno R L 1988 A randomized, placebo-controlled trial of effects of dexamethasone on hypothalamic–pituitary–adrenal axis in preterm infants. Journal of Pediatrics 120: 961–965
188. Wilson J D, Foster D W (eds) 1992 Williams textbook of endocrinology. W B Saunders, Philadelphia
189. Wilson R C, Mercado A B, Cheng K C, New M I 1995 Steroid 21-hydroxylase deficiency: genotype may not predict phenotype. Journal of Clinical Endocrinology and Metabolism 80: 2322–2329
190. Wilson R C, Wei J-Q, Cheng K C, Mercado, A B, New M I 1995 Rapid deoxyribonucleic acid analysis by allele-specific polymerase chain reaction for detection of mutations in the steroid 21-hydroxylase gene. Journal of Clinical Endocrinology and Metabolism 80: 1635–1640
191. Woods K A, Weber A, Clark A J L 1995 The molecular pathology of of pituitary hormone deficiency. In: Thakker (ed) Baillière's clinical endocrinology and metabolism. Baillière Tindall, London, pp 453–487
192. Yagi H, Nagashima K, Miyake H et al 1994 Familial congenital hypopituitarism with central diabetes insipidus. Journal of Clinical Endocrinology and Metabolism 78: 884–889
193. Zachmann M 1996 Prismatic cases: 17,20-desmolase (17,20-lyase) deficiency. Journal of Clinical Endocrinology and Metabolism 81: 457–459
194. Zah W, Kalderon A E, Tucci J R 1975 Mixed gonadal dysgenesis. Acta Endocrinologica 197 suppl.: 1–39
195. Zakarija M, McKenzie J M 1983 Immunoglobulin G inhibitor of thyroid-stimulating antibody is a cause of delay in the onset of neonatal Graves' disease. Journal of Clinical Investigation 72: 1352–1356
196. Zakarija M, McKenzie J M, Hoffman W H 1986 Prediction and therapy of intrauterine and late onset neonatal hyperthyroidism. Journal of Clinical Endocrinology and Metabolism 62: 368–371
197. Zimmerman D, Gan-Gaisano M 1990 Hyperthyroidism in children and adolescents. Pediatric Clinics of North America 37: 1273–1295

Part 3

Inborn errors of metabolism in the neonate

J. E. Wraith

INTRODUCTION

All paediatricians have been presented with a desperately sick neonate for whom no diagnosis is readily available. It is in this group of patients that an IEM is near the top of the differential diagnostic list. It is important to keep IEMs in mind as a possible cause of symptoms in the neonatal period, and to accept that it is worth investigating 10 babies to diagnose one. Most neonatologists find it easy to maintain this attitude towards bacterial infection, but difficult to sustain the same approach to IEMs. It is very important that a diagnosis of an IEM is established promptly as many disorders are now amenable to effective treatment, but also because of the genetic implications for the families concerned. Even in disorders where treatment is unsatisfactory prenatal diagnosis in subsequent pregnancies may allow parents to avoid the recurrence of a serious disease.

In most cases an IEM will be diagnosed during the newborn period because of severe clinical symptoms (Table 38.20), and the bulk of this chapter will concentrate upon the recognition of IEMs in babies who become ill without any prior warning. In some families the neonatologist or preferably the obstetrician will be alerted to the risk of a particular IEM which has been present in a previous sibling (or other family member in the case of X-linked disorders). In some families less specific but equally important clues may exist, such as previous unexplained neonatal deaths, particularly if there is a history of parental consanguinity. It is important always to take a very careful family history and examine the obstetric notes carefully.

Table 38.20 Clues to the presence of an IEM

Antenatal
Consanguinity
Previous neonatal death
Recurrent non-immune hydrops fetalis
Sibs with known IEMs
Clinical
Unexplained clinical deterioration in an infant who was well at birth
Persistent vomiting with no anatomical cause
Persistent hiccups
Major organ failure, e.g. heart or liver
Cardiomyopathy
Dysmorphism or multiple congenital anomalies
Unusual odours
Cataracts
Encephalopathy/coma and/or seizures
Biochemical
Unexplained metabolic acidaemia
Ketosis
Unexpected hypoglycaemia
Hyperammonaemia
Haematological
Neutropenia and thrombocytopenia
Postmortem
Fatty liver and/or heart

The importance of being prewarned about the possibility of an IEM cannot be overemphasized. Most disorders are much easier to treat before the onset of symptoms, and the prognosis for a good neurological outcome is often directly related to the age at which effective treatment commences. This is particularly true for disorders associated with neonatal encephalopathy, such as maple syrup urine disease, organic acidaemias or urea cycle defects. *Remember: the outcome is directly related to the speed of diagnosis.*

IEMs can present in other ways, for instance as a result of mass screening of newborn babies, giving the clinician the opportunity of starting treatment before damage is done. Unfortunately, this approach is not really practicable for most of the disorders that cause neonatal illness.

Although the primary concern of this chapter is with those IEMs that cause symptoms in the newborn period, it is important to recognize that a number of disorders which normally present in older infants are capable of producing profound abnormalities in the neonate. The neonatologist needs to be alert to the possibility of encountering these conditions for the first time, or even of encountering a new IEM not previously described.

Finally, it is important to remember that infants with IEMs can be severely dysmorphic, and investigation of this latter group of patients can never be considered complete until one has considered the possibility of an IEM in the infant, or indeed in the mother.

Details of the long-term management of individual IEMs and the laboratory methods used for detection and follow-up are beyond the scope of this chapter. This information is available in the major reference work on IEMs.[20]

THE ORGANIZATION OF CLINICAL AND LABORATORY SERVICES

A large number of IEMs present in the newborn period. A wide range of techniques are required for diagnosis,

Table 38.21 Investigations for diagnosis of an IEM

First-line investigations (available in all units providing neonatal care)
Full blood count
Urea and electrolytes
Blood gas and acid–base analysis
Blood ammonia
Urine-reducing substances
Urine ketones (dipstick)
Second-line investigations (available in each region)
Urine amino acids
Urine organic acids
Plasma amino acids
Blood and CSF lactate and/or pyruvate
Plasma carnitine
Urine orotic acid
Beutler test (for galactosaemia)
Specialized investigations (available on a supraregional basis)
Specific enzyme assays on blood or skin fibroblasts, e.g. lysosomal enzyme studies etc.
DNA mutation analysis
Special metabolite studies, e.g. very long-chain fatty acids, bile acid analysis etc.

and the level of clinical and biochemical experience required for their effective treatment is substantial. Ideally, clinical and laboratory services for IEMs should be integrated, as prompt clinical interpretation of abnormal results is required if treatment is to proceed smoothly. Neonatologists must initiate appropriate investigations (Table 38.21), but they must recognize that rapid and correct diagnosis and treatment of these conditions is a highly specialized skill. A high index of suspicion of an IEM is a reason for referral to a paediatrician expert in the management of metabolic diseases, and not just a reason for sending blood and urine samples to a laboratory.

Some of the investigations performed in the laboratory are relatively simple and can be applied to every patient in whom there is the slightest suspicion of an IEM. Other tests are very complex and should be used only in carefully defined situations. Errors or delays in the use of the right tests or the best forms of therapy can prove very damaging – even fatal – to the affected neonate, especially those with a disorder of intermediary metabolism such as an organic acid defect or a urea cycle disorder. Close collaboration between clinician and laboratory is essential. Each health region within the UK should have the facilities to screen for the commoner IEMs, as well as a clinician specializing in the clinical management of affected patients. Laboratory services for subacute and chronic disorders can be centralized for much larger populations and areas, giving rise to National Reference Laboratories for these groups of IEMs.

Before sending samples always:

- phone laboratory to indicate urgency;
- give all details of drugs, diet and previous blood transfusions;
- arrange suitable transport for samples;
- discuss which tests are indicated with the metabolic consultant;
- freeze and save all urine passed by the infant.

PATHOGENESIS OF IEMs

The majority of disorders are autosomal recessive, but a few are X-linked recessive, e.g. ornithine carbamyl transferase deficiency. Deficiency of the E1 α-subunit of pyruvate dehydrogenase is X-linked dominant, with almost all cases, both male and female, due to new mutations.[5] In the X-linked recessive disorders one occasionally sees partial manifestation in heterozygous females, e.g. OCT deficiency. The defective genotype is present from conception and in most cases the enzyme controlled by the gene in question is active during fetal life. Nonetheless, most IEMs have no effect on the health and development of the fetus, because placental perfusion can correct the disturbance in systemic metabolite levels caused by the enzyme defect. Consequently, most babies with IEMs are of normal birthweight and are in good general condition at birth.

This statement applies to those IEMs in which systemic accumulation of a toxic metabolite (or deficiency of an essential metabolite) damages cells of organs such as the brain. Hyperammonaemia can be taken as a classic example of this. Defective conversion of ammonia to urea in the liver leads to elevated levels of circulating ammonia and intoxicating effects on the brain. A readily dialysed compound such as ammonia is removed very effectively by the placenta before birth, and accumulation commences only after delivery.

There are some exceptions to this concept of 'placental protection'. Defects in cellular energy production (e.g. mitochondrial disorders) may have severe effects prenatally, including defects in embryonic development presenting as physical malformations at birth, or destructive processes later in fetal life (e.g. patchy brain destruction). In lysosomal storage disorders intracellular accumulation of the substrate of the defective enzyme can be demonstrated early in fetal life, even though the serious symptoms may not develop until some years after birth.

In some IEMs the primary defect is in cerebral metabolism (e.g. glycine encephalopathy, p. 995) and the abnormalities observed in blood and urine merely represent overflow from the brain. Placental perfusion may have a very small effect on this disease in utero, but not enough to prevent affected infants from being born with hypotonia, lethargy, seizures and often established structural brain damage.

Finally, symptoms of some IEMs develop after birth because of the substrate of the defective enzyme becomes available in large amounts only after the baby begins to feed, as in galactosaemia and hereditary fructose intolerance.

CLINICAL PRESENTATION OF IEMs

The affected child is likely to be normal at birth. The signs and symptoms produced by IEMs are non-specific and most are shared by many other more common neonatal disorders, especially serious generalized infections. The high frequency of bacterial infections in the newborn period makes it easy to forget the possibility of an IEM. To complicate the matter further, septicaemia is a frequent secondary event in some IEMs, e.g. galactosaemia.

A metabolic cause is particularly likely in babies who develop symptoms one or several days after birth, having been entirely normal for an initial period. Dramatic improvements during a period of intravenous fluid administration, followed by relapse when put back on milk feeding, is another strongly suggestive feature.

Although the range of possible symptoms is very wide indeed, there are two particularly frequent patterns of illness. The first begins with vomiting, acidosis and circulatory disturbance, followed by depressed consciousness and convulsions, and is particularly suggestive of one of the organic acidaemias. The second is dominated by neurological features, with lethargy, refusal to feed, drowsiness, unconsciousness and apnoea. Hypotonia may be a prominent feature. Primary defects of the urea cycle and glycine encephalopathy present in this way.

There are a few more specific symptoms of IEMs. Abnormal body odour is noted in some organic acidaemias, e.g. the smell of maple syrup in maple syrup urine disease, and of sweaty feet in isovaleric acidaemia or glutaric aciduria type II. *Most babies who have an unusual or powerful odour do not have an IEM, but there are exceptions.*

Jaundice and a haemorrhagic tendency occur in those diseases that damage the liver (galactosaemia and acute hereditary tyrosinaemia), but may also be seen as a very late sign in other IEMs, such as urea cycle defects. *The presence of cataracts in an infant with liver disease should lead to urgent investigation to exclude galactosaemia.*

Although convulsions may occur in many different IEMs, the pattern of convulsions in pyridoxine dependency is particularly characteristic and the onset is usually very early.[16] This classic pattern does not occur in every instance, and patients have been described whose convulsions began later than the first 24 hours or were of a very minor type, and some in whom there were considerable periods of freedom from convulsion without specific administration of pyridoxine.[2,8] Formal exclusion of this condition is desirable in all babies with persistent convulsions, regardless of the pattern of onset and progression and regardless of the existence of other apparent aetiological factors (e.g. birth asphyxia).

Hypoglycaemia is a very common finding in the newborn period and is only occasionally due to an IEM. However, this possibility must be borne in mind when hypoglycaemia occurs in atypical circumstances or recurs (p. 944). To have the best chance of making a diagnosis in a hypoglycaemic infant collect the samples whilst the sugar is low.

Some patients with IEMs present with prominent cardiac disease. Cardiac failure, particularly with an accompanying hypertrophic cardiomyopathy and hypotonia, is suggestive of a mitochondrial respiratory chain disorder or a defect in long-chain fatty acid oxidation. The multisystem carbohydrate deficient glycoprotein disorder (CDG type I) may also present soon after birth, with pericardial effusion. In addition, affected patients fail to thrive and have a variable dysmorphic appearance, which often includes abnormal fat distribution ('fat pads'), large ears and inverted nipples.[10]

Dysmorphic features can also be produced by other metabolic disturbances in the embryo. The resulting infants have physical malformations at birth, including abnormal facies and cardiac, cerebral, renal and skeletal defects. The conditions responsible are those that affect mitochondrial energy production directly (glutaric aciduria type II, pyruvate dehydrogenase deficiency) or indirectly (3-hydroxy isobutyryl CoA deoxylase deficiency). *Always remember IEMs as a possible cause of multiple congenital anomalies.*

Hypothermia may suggest hypothyroidism or, less often, Menkes disease. The majority of infants with this X-linked recessive disorder have temperature instability which can be noted in the newborn period, although most are not diagnosed until other features of the disease appear in later infancy.

Microcephaly, hydranencephaly and porencephaly with severe neurological deficits are other important presenting features seen in some peroxisomal defects and in pyruvate dehyrogenase deficiency ('cerebral' lactic acidosis, seen generally in females). Rapidly progressive cerebral degeneration starting in the newborn period is seen in both molybdenum cofactor deficiency and isolated sulphite oxidase deficiency. Severe peripheral arteriospasm with marked pallor may occur in primary lactic acidosis. This causes a particularly difficult differential because poor perfusion may cause secondary lactic acidosis.

A summary of some of the commoner presentations is given in Table 38.22. It should be recognized that this is not an exhaustive list and that some symptoms, such as poor feeding, lethargy and failure to thrive, are almost universal in infants with IEMs. Those who find alogorithms useful are guided to the chapter by Saudubray and Charpentier in Scriver et al.[20]

INVESTIGATION OF A BABY WHO MAY HAVE AN IEM

GENERAL APPROACH

The approach to diagnosis varies with the severity and nature of the symptoms. In some babies one can make a very good guess at the diagnosis clinically and choose the test or tests most likely to give the answer (e.g. a baby hypotonic at birth who becomes more depressed within the first 24 hours and who develops seizures with a 'burst-suppression' pattern on EEG is very likely to have glycine encephalopathy). However, it is more usual to need to perform a group of tests to reach a diagnosis, as many different IEMs may cause very similar symptoms.

It is important to discuss investigations with the laboratory and also to give some indication of urgency. Many non-urgent samples for amino acid and organic acid analysis are received by metabolic laboratories, and it is often difficult from the clinical information (if any is provided!) on the sample cards to obtain any idea of the urgency of the situation. In addition, appropriate transportation to the laboratory must be arranged if an urgent analysis is requested. Full details of drugs and feeding history should be provided so that proper interpretation of results can be made. If an infant has received a blood transfusion prior to metabolic screening this should be made known to the laboratory, as this will interfere with the commonly used screening test to exclude galactosaemia.

Some general tests are easily performed and should be used in all infants in whom there is even a slight possibility of an IEM (Table 38.22). These will include 'routine' tests of electrolyte analysis, bilirubin, acid–base balance, blood glucose and calcium, as well as haematological assessment. Plasma ammonia should be measured in all infants with neurological depression. A simple bedside test for ketones can be very useful. Neonates do not produce ketones readily and a heavy ketonuria in an infant with unexplained illness, especially if associated with metabolic acidosis, should be followed by urgent organic acid analysis. Urine testing for reducing substances should not be relied upon to make or refute a diagnosis of possible galactosaemia. Infants presenting with vomiting and acute liver disease, often with a secondary coagulopathy, must be screened urgently for galactosaemia using a specific screening test on blood. Ketosis is very unusual in the newborn period – regard its presence with great suspicion.

In patients with acidosis, calculation of the anion gap – the sum of the serum concentrations of sodium and potassium minus the sum of the serum concentrations of chloride and bicarbonate – can be helpful. Patients with an increased anion gap, and especially those with a value greater than 25 mmol/l (normal range 12–16 mmol/l), are likely to have a specific organic acidaemia. Patients with a normal anion gap and acidosis are most likely to have renal tubular acidosis or intestinal bicarbonate loss.[7] Never ignore a raised anion gap: if it is associated with ketosis an organic acidaemia is very likely.

SPECIFIC TESTS: 'THE METABOLIC SCREEN'

Occasionally experts are asked to give advice after an infant's death, and although it is possible to perform

Table 38.22 Signs and symptoms suggestive of an IEM

Sign or symptom	Disorder	Test(s)
Hydrops fetalis	Lysosomal storage disease	Urine MPS, WCEs
Coma/ encephalopathy	Organic acidaemias	UOAs
	Maple syrup urine disease	U/PAAs
	Urea cycle disorders	NH_4, orotic acid, U/PAAs
	Non-ketotic hyperglycinaemia	CSF/P glycine ratio
	Mitochondrial disease	P/CSF lactate
Coma + hypoglycaemia	GSD I	Enzyme assay
	Organic acidaemias	UOAs
	Fructose 1,6-bisphosphatase	Enzyme assay
	Fat oxidation defects	UOAs
	Hyperinsulinism	Insulin, c-peptide
	Other endocrine causes	GH, cortisol
Odours	Maple syrup urine disease	U/PAAs
	Isovaleric acidaemia	UOAs
	Glutaric aciduria type II	UOAs
Cataracts	Galactosaemia	Beutler test
Seizures	Pyridoxine dependency	Pyridoxine i.v.
	Non-ketotic hyperglycinaemia	CSF/P glycine ratio
Liver disease	Galactosaemia	Beutler test
	Tyrosinaemia	UOAs, P/UAAs
	α_1-antitrypsin deficiency	α_1-AT level
	Niemann–Pick type C	Cholesterol esterification
	Fat oxidation defects	UOAs
	Mitochondrial disease	P/CSF lactate
Severe diarrhoea	Congenital chloride diarrhoea	Blood and stool chloride
	Glucose/galactose malabsorption	Faecal sugars
	CDG syndrome	Plasma transferrins
Cardiomyopathy	Fat oxidation defects	UOAs
	Primary carnitine deficiency	Plasma carnitine, acylcarnitine
	Mitochondrial disease	P/CSF lactate
Severe hypotonia	Zellweger syndrome	VLCFAs, DHAP-AT
	Mitochondrial disease	P/CSF lactate
Dysmorphism	Peroxisomal disorders	VLCFAs, DHAP-AT
	Glutaric aciduria II	UOAs
	PDH deficiency	P/CSF lactate
	CDG syndrome	plasma transferrin
	Smith–Lemli–Opitz	plasma 7-dehydrocholesterol

MPS, mucopolysaccharides
WCEs, white cell enzymes
UOAs, urine organic acids
UAAs, urine amino acids
PAAs, plasma amino acids
GH, growth hormone
VLCFAs, very long-chain fatty acids
DHAP-AT, dihydroacetone phosphate acyl-transferase
P/CSF, plasma/CSF ratio
GSD, glycogen storage disease
PDH, pyruvate dehydrogenase
CDG, carbohydrate deficient glycoprotein disorder

some investigations post mortem, early suspicion and collection of the appropriate tissues and samples from a living child permit a more comprehensive screen for metabolic disease.

Although techniques will vary, most metabolic laboratories will require a sample of blood (1–2 ml in a heparinized tube) and urine (5–10 ml in a sterile container with no preservatives) for a metabolic screen. It is now essential that these basic samples are supplemented by a sample of blood (3–5 ml in an EDTA bottle) for subsequent DNA extraction and storage. This is particularly important in infants suspected of having the commonest fatty acid oxidation defect, MCAD deficiency, where analysis for the common genetic mutation is often the quickest way of establishing the diagnosis.[9]

It is good practice to save and freeze all urine passed by the infant for future analysis and to save a heparinized sample of blood from all infants who require an exchange transfusion (in case galactosaemia screening is thought to be necessary).

In the laboratory, amino acid concentrations can be estimated in blood and urine by one-dimensional paper chromatography. Abnormal results are then characterized quantitatively. Gas–liquid chromatography with mass spectrometry should be used for urinary organic acid analysis. In infants who are hyperammonaemic, amino acid analysis should be performed, and the urinary orotic acid level is determined by high-performance liquid chromatography. Occasionally more specialized investigations will be required, e.g. plasma carnitine or amino and organic acid analysis of CSF. If this is the case it is best to discuss the clinical problem with the laboratory to ensure that the appropriate samples are collected.

Infants with lactic acidosis present a difficult problem. It is often impossible to distinguish those with a primary defect in pyruvate metabolism from those with lactic acidosis secondary to hypoxia, cardiac disease, infection or convulsions. It is necessary to treat possible underlying causes aggressively while attempting to separate the two groups. Venous obstruction by tourniquet, crying or breath-holding may raise venous lactate and pyruvate levels as much as two- or threefold. Arterial samples are generally required, preferably from an arterial line which has been in place for some time. A persistent elevation of blood lactate greater than 2 mmol/l in an infant who was not asphyxiated and who was not hypoxic or suffering from other organ failure at the time of collection should lead to further mitochondrial investigations, especially if the clinical presentation is suggestive, e.g. prominent neuromuscular symptoms.

Urinary lactate (measured on the standard organic acid procedure) can be helpful. In those patients with secondary lactic acidosis the urinary lactate falls (although this may take 2–3 days) as the underlying disorder improves, but infants with a primary defect in pyruvate metabolism presenting in the newborn period are generally unresponsive to treatment. Often the child dies before a clear distinction can be made, and one has to rely upon formal assay of the enzymes known to cause lactic acidosis. This is an unsatisfactory approach, as many patients with strong evidence of a primary defect have no biochemical abnormality detectable on enzyme testing. Lactic acidosis is a heterogeneous group of disorders, and it is likely that many defects have not been fully defined or are tissue specific, e.g. limited to muscle or the central nervous system. Infants with primary disorders of pyruvate metabolism are very difficult to diagnose; the lactic acidosis is usually persistent and severe (>6 mmol/l).

In many cases these investigations will provide a definitive diagnosis or a high suspicion of a known IEM, and appropriate treatment can be commenced. The complete characterization of the particular condition involves more specific studies, such as enzyme assays, studies of in-vitro cofactor requirements, DNA mutation analysis and often further family studies. Most of the biochemical work-up can often be performed on cultured skin fibroblasts or transformed lymphoid lines.

MANAGEMENT WHILE AWAITING RESULTS

The severity of symptoms dictates the management. Very mild symptoms may occasion no change in management while awaiting results. It may be prudent to cease milk-containing feeds if symptoms are more than very mild, as protein catabolism is generally the source of the toxic metabolites. Glucose can be given orally or intravenously, but care must be taken to avoid inducing intestinal sugar intolerance by too large an oral glucose load.

In more severe cases intravenous fluids will certainly be needed, and bicarbonate may be necessary to correct acidosis. Other additives should be dictated by laboratory results, the aim being to achieve glucose and electrolyte homoeostasis. Dextrose 10% (with appropriate additives) should generally be used to try and inhibit catabolism, except when a primary lactic acidosis is possible, as some forms will be aggravated by a carbohydrate load.

If the patient is extremely ill, or is deteriorating rapidly, then very aggressive therapy may be warranted even before a diagnosis has been made.

MANAGEMENT OF BABIES WITH SEVERE ACUTE IEMs

There can be no doubt that the greatest impact on the prognosis for infants with severe acute IEMs has been the improvement in neonatal intensive care that has occurred over the last decade or so. In particular, improvements in mechanical ventilation techniques, the use of central access and the ability to dialyse very small infants have been critical, but if treatment is to be successful great emphasis must be placed on precision and attention to detail.

Appropriate intravenous fluids must be given, but care must be taken to avoid overhydration in the presence of impaired renal function.

Acid–base imbalance must be corrected promptly and adequately. This may require very large doses of sodium bicarbonate in some of the organic acidaemias (e.g. 20–30 mmol/kg/day), and this will lead to hypernatraemia of a degree sufficient to necessitate peritoneal dialysis, especially in the presence of impaired renal function. Correction of acidosis may unmask hypokalaemia, which must be corrected quickly. It is always important to check the electrolyte levels frequently (e.g. 6-hourly) during correction of acidosis and liaise closely with the metabolic team and nephrologists who will be involved in the acute management of these patients.

Good tissue perfusion is essential if secondary lactic acidosis is to be avoided. Oxygen therapy may be needed as well as blood transfusion to correct anaemia (which may occur as an iatrogenic problem). The most common reason for poor tissue oxygenation is hypoventilation due to cerebral depression, and most babies with severe IEMs will require mechanical ventilation. Direct toxic effects of accumulating metabolites (e.g. ammonia) upon the brain may cause cerebral oedema, and this can be easily aggravated by hypercapnia due to inadequate ventilation. Ventilatory support should therefore be used early in order to treat carbon dioxide retention long before measurable hypoxia develops, and should be continued until the baby is breathing vigorously. If an IEM causes coma (as in hyperammonaemia) one usually has to wait at least 48 hours after metabolic correction before clinical recovery occurs to a degree sufficient to cease ventilator support. Hypoglycaemia or hypocalcaemia may require correction initially or during the recovery phase.

Nutrition in the acute phase requires careful attention as most IEMs are aggravated by tissue catabolism, which is very difficult to reverse during the first 24 hours of severe illness. Intravenous glucose (with appropriate electrolyte additives) should be used initially and, when acid–base balance has been restored and tissue perfusion and oxygenation improved, one should attempt to encourage the development of an anabolic state. This may mean infusing 20% dextrose via a central venous catheter, the amount given being increased until a mild hyperglycaemia is induced (e.g. blood glucose 7–12 mmol/l). Small doses of insulin (0.05 U/kg/h as an infusion) may be used to help initiate anabolism, but this must be used with caution as some infants are exquisitely sensitive and become hypoglycaemic very rapidly. If tolerated, intravenous lipid emulsions can be used as a source of calories and in some units growth hormone is also being used as an anabolic agent.[14]

Oxygenation, good tissue perfusion, the correction of acidosis and anabolism are the cornerstones of supportive therapy.

Once the infant's catabolic state has been stabilized – often apparent as an increase in the amount of glucose tolerated, and accompanied by a diuresis (as well as improvement in general condition) – one should introduce protein into the diet fairly quickly. This should start at 0.5 g protein per kilogram body weight for the first 24 hours; this can then be increased (if tolerated) by 0.25–0.5 g/kg/day on successive days up to a maximum of around 1.5 g/kg/day. In addition one should supply 120 kcal/kg, and this combination of protein and energy should be sufficient to promote and sustain anabolism. In some infants, especially those with urea cycle defects, protein may need to be maintained at slightly lower levels (1.2 g/kg/day), but in all cases sufficient must be given to allow the infant to grow and gain weight. Usually the infant has recovered sufficiently to tolerate the protein as a formula given by nasogastric tube, but if not parenteral feeding regimens can also be used.

Peritoneal dialysis, haemodialysis and haemofiltration are important in the management of these patients. *Exchange transfusion is not a useful adjunct to therapy*, except in exceptional circumstances when access to dialysis is not immediately available. Often one will have to start one or other of these treatments while awaiting biochemical results, especially if the baby has a history strongly suggestive of an IEM and is unconscious or deteriorating rapidly despite supportive treatment. Peritoneal dialysis is effective in infants with organic acid defects or hyperammonaemia due to a urea cycle defect, and it can be used with safety in infants in whom vascular access proves difficult, although haemodialysis or haemofiltration remains the method of choice. Dialysis or haemofiltration will generally be required for 5–7 days, and one should continue with therapy until the baby is established on enough protein to maintain anabolism.

A number of metabolic disorders are known to have vitamin-responsive forms, and it has become traditional to administer a combination of vitamins in pharmacological dosages to sick infants while awaiting results. It is difficult to justify this blind approach to therapy, as the ready availability of metabolic investigations in most regions should allow for diagnosis to proceed rapidly. This can be followed by the use of the appropriate vitamin cofactor (in a dose approximately 100 times the daily requirement) once diagnosis has been confirmed. *'Blunderbuss' vitamin therapy is never indicated.*

LONG-TERM MANAGEMENT AFTER THE ACUTE PHASE HAS PASSED

The first problem is to achieve a form of treatment which can be continued in the long term and which is compatible with normal growth and development. This can be very difficult when the mainstay of treatment is protein restriction, as the amount of protein tolerated may be insufficient for growth.

The next step is to obtain some information about the margin of latitude available in the treatment of a particular patient. A patient who tolerates very little protein (e.g. <1.5 g/kg/day) will demonstrate metabolic imbalance very rapidly during the course of intercurrent infections, and will be at great risk if the parents or local paediatricians are not familiar with the child's illness. *An emergency regimen giving clear, written instructions on how to deal with infections*, particularly those associated with anorexia, diarrhoea or vomiting, should be discussed with the parents before the baby is discharged from hospital. A copy should also be made available for the GP and referring paediatrician. We instruct the parents to be cautious and to bring the child early to hospital for assessment, particularly during the first two or three episodes of intercurrent illness. This allows the metabolic team as well as the parents to get some idea of how the individual child responds to different stresses. With experience the parents become experts in judging how to respond to these intercurrent episodes. One must guard against undue complacency on the part of parents or of doctors in hospital emergency departments as well as in the community, who are not experienced with these conditions.

MANAGEMENT WHEN NO DIAGNOSIS CAN BE MADE

As all metabolic disorders have genetic implications for the family every effort must made be to keep the infant alive so that investigations can be completed. Even if the initial metabolic screen is normal, biochemical correction by dialysis or haemofiltration is still indicated in infants with hyperammonaemia, as severe *transient* hyperammonaemia is well recognized. These infants, often premature, may have very high plasma ammonia levels, but with aggressive treatment have a good prognosis and no long-term metabolic disturbance.

FURTHER MANAGEMENT WHEN DEATH IS INEVITABLE

If a baby cannot be kept alive it is still important to think very carefully about the possibility of an underlying metabolic disorder. An autopsy is essential, and this must be performed quickly if metabolic studies are to be interpretable.[18] In this situation it is always best to discuss the infant's poor prognosis fully and frankly with the parents and obtain permission for the autopsy or biopsies before the infant's demise. Tissues should be prepared for electron microscopy and portions of the relevant organs (usually liver, muscle and brain) snap-frozen in liquid nitrogen. Parallel samples should be taken for histology and histochemistry, and it is best to work in close liaison with the pathologist and metabolic specialist to ensure that the correct specimens are collected. It is important not to forget the appropriate viral and bacterial cultures. A careful examination for structural abnormalities of the brain, heart and other organs is also necessary, and it is therefore vital for the pathologist to be involved in the urgent autopsy irrespective of the time of day or night.

SPECIAL MANAGEMENT WHEN AN IEM CAN BE ANTICIPATED

Sometimes one knows in advance that a baby may be born with a particular IEM. This may be true when a sibling has the condition, or when the mother is a proven or suspected carrier of the gene for an X-linked IEM. The optimal treatment can be planned in advance and one can decide whether to treat the baby as affected from the time of delivery (or before), or to investigate promptly and treat only after a diagnosis has been established. The choice will vary from one disease to another.

In other circumstances the birth of a child who may have an IEM is anticipated without any precise information about what IEM may be present, e.g. when one or two children in a family have died in circumstances that suggest an IEM, but without adequate investigation or without achieving a diagnosis. In families like this consideration should be given to transfer to the metabolic unit soon after delivery.[6] All the investigations listed above should be done immediately and repeated again after the infant has started protein-containing feeds, if the initial set are negative.

By using this approach it is hoped to achieve a diagnosis before symptoms develop, and to initiate appropriate therapy. If symptoms develop without any diagnostic biochemical findings the prognosis is very poor.

POTENTIAL HAZARDS OF AGGRESSIVE TREATMENT

Some paediatricians are concerned that an aggressive approach to management may keep alive a grossly brain-damaged infant, but in practice this is not a significant problem. If improvement does not occur within a few days and the prospects of near-normal cerebral function appear remote, one can merely refrain from employing extraordinary measures in the next acute episode of deterioration which will inevitably occur. This approach does carry the risk of producing a survivor with a mild to moderate degree of brain damage, but this is true in all acute neonatal illnesses and in all IEMs that can affect the brain.

DETECTION OF IEMs BY MASS SCREENING

Screening for hypothyroidism is considered on page 960. Phenylketonuria is the only IEM which has received universal acceptance for mass newborn screening. It is worth reflecting on the characteristics of PKU, as it illustrates an almost ideal situation for mass screening and serves as a yardstick against which mass screening for other IEMs in the newborn period can be measured.

Babies with PKU are born in good health, protected by the intrauterine environment. They begin to be affected by their metabolic disorder after birth, but these effects are gradual and probably take several weeks before leading to severe, irreversible change. The outcome of treatment is excellent if it is initiated within the first 2–3 weeks of life, but is not good if treatment is delayed until symptoms are apparent. In addition, there are a number of cheap and simple laboratory methods available, using microsamples of blood, which are very reliable in detecting the disorder. Finally, PKU occurs with a frequency (1:10–15 000 in the UK) sufficient to justify detection by screening.

Tests suitable for mass screening have been developed for a large number of IEMs but none of these has achieved universal acceptance.[1] Presymptomatic identification of the conditions that cause acute illness in the newborn period would obviously be an advantage, but in practice this cannot be achieved, although this may change with the introduction of tandem-mass spectrometry techniques.[24] The sample used for PKU screening is collected between the fifth and 11th days of life by the visiting nurse (midwife or health visitor) in most regions of the UK, depending on the method used for analysis. This is too late for conditions that cause severe symptoms within the first week of life. Even if an additional earlier sample were collected (before discharge from the maternity hospital) it would not really be possible to organize a system that could handle the large number of samples concerned and get results back within the 24-hour period that might be available. Umbilical cord blood is unsuitable for the vast majority of disorders, as metabolite levels are too close to normal in the cord blood to be diagnostic in most diseases.

False negative results for PKU may occur if samples are taken too early or if the infant has not been established on a good protein intake.[23] Premature or sick babies may be receiving intravenous fluids at the time of the test. A false positive result may be obtained from a sick neonate on TPN. The elevation of phenylalanine will be accompanied by increases in the level of other amino acids, and in practice is not a diagnostic problem. Details of feeds should be recorded on the screening card and a further test performed when the infant has been established on a normal protein intake for 48–72 hours.

The PKU screening test identifies all babies with elevated levels of blood phenylalanine, but not all will have 'classic' PKU. Some will have mild hyperphenylalaninaemia (blood phe <500 µmol/l) and will not require dietary therapy, but all should be seen in the metabolic unit for assessment. Infants with defects in the synthesis or recycling of the tetrahydrobiopterin cofactor for phenylalnine hydroxylase activity (Fig. 38.13) need to be distinguished from those with 'classic' PKU, as the low phenylalanine diet has to be supplemented with neurotransmitter therapy in these patients. Specific enzyme assays for cofactor defects, combined with urine pterin analysis and/or tetrabiopterin loading tests, are necessary in all patients found to have raised phenylalanine on neonatal screening. It is important to remember that blood phenylalanine may only be marginally elevated in infants with cofactor disorders.

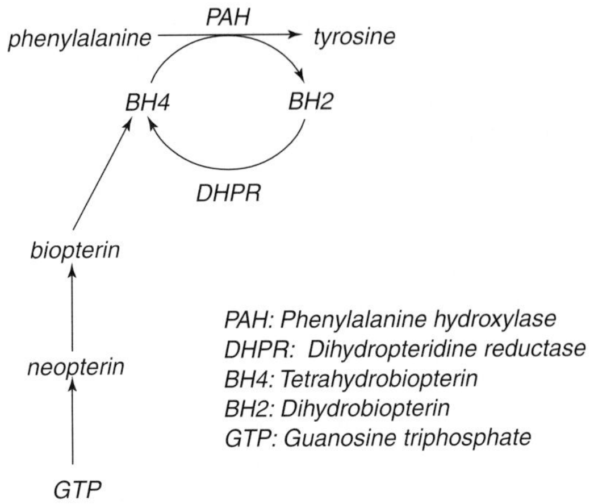

Fig. 38.13 Metabolic pathways for hyperphenylalaninaemia which in the classic form is due to lack of PAH. Rarer variants are due to defects in the tetrahydrobiopterin cofactor system.

Each metabolic unit will have its own approach to the management of PKU. We recommend dietary treatment for all infants with a blood phe >400 µmol/l. The treatment of PKU (like other metabolic disorders) should be carried out only by those with substantial experience, and details of management are beyond the scope of this chapter. In principle most of the infant's amino acid requirements are provided in synthetic form, and natural proteins are used in portions sufficient to supply the phenylalanine required for growth, leaving no excess to be broken down to tyrosine.

Galactosaemia has a prevalence of about 1:60 000 births, severe consequences if left untreated and an effective form of treatment for the early complications. Communities that do employ one of the several screening tests available for galactosaemia pick up about 60–70% of cases before serious symptoms have developed. The remainder have already presented with acute neonatal illness before the screening test sample has come back from the laboratory. Nonetheless, the result may still hasten diagnosis in these very sick infants. We regard the liberal use of the screening assay in symptomatic babies as preferable to mass screening. There is little evidence to suggest that diagnosis at or soon after birth gives a better long-term outlook than diagnosis by rapid screening of the symptomatic neonate.

A few communities (e.g. some American States, Ireland and Japan) regard the cost of screening for maple syrup urine disease as acceptable. However, the prevalence is very low (about 1:250 000 births) and some patients are already very ill before the test is performed. The outcome, however, is only good in those patients diagnosed in the first few days of life, before the onset of encephalopathy. If screening is to be successful in this disorder it needs to be performed in the first 2 or 3 days of life and the result available by 5–7 days. This is not possible with the current practice of neonatal screening in the UK.

Screening for tyrosinaemia may be justified in those few parts of the world (see below) where the condition is frequent, but it is certainly not justified elsewhere. Some methods of newborn screening for PKU (e.g. those using chromatography of plasma) will detect pyridoxine-unresponsive homocystinuria because of the raised levels of methionine associated with this disorder. Early diagnosis and treatment with a low-methionine diet is very successful in preventing complications of this disease, but its frequency (1:100 000 in the UK) does not justify specific screening for it.

Screening for biotinidase deficiency has been introduced in some centres following claims of high sensitivity and specificity for the test procedure and the high frequency of the disease.[28] However, wider experience has cast some doubt on all these characteristics.[1]

The increasing use of molecular analysis for the diagnosis of IEMs could lead to an expansion in the range of conditions for which accurate screening could be provided. MCAD deficiency is one disorder that has gained some support for screening (for discussion see Naylor[17]). However, we must not lose sight of the other criteria outlined above and, most important of all, screening should still be limited to those disorders that are treatable.

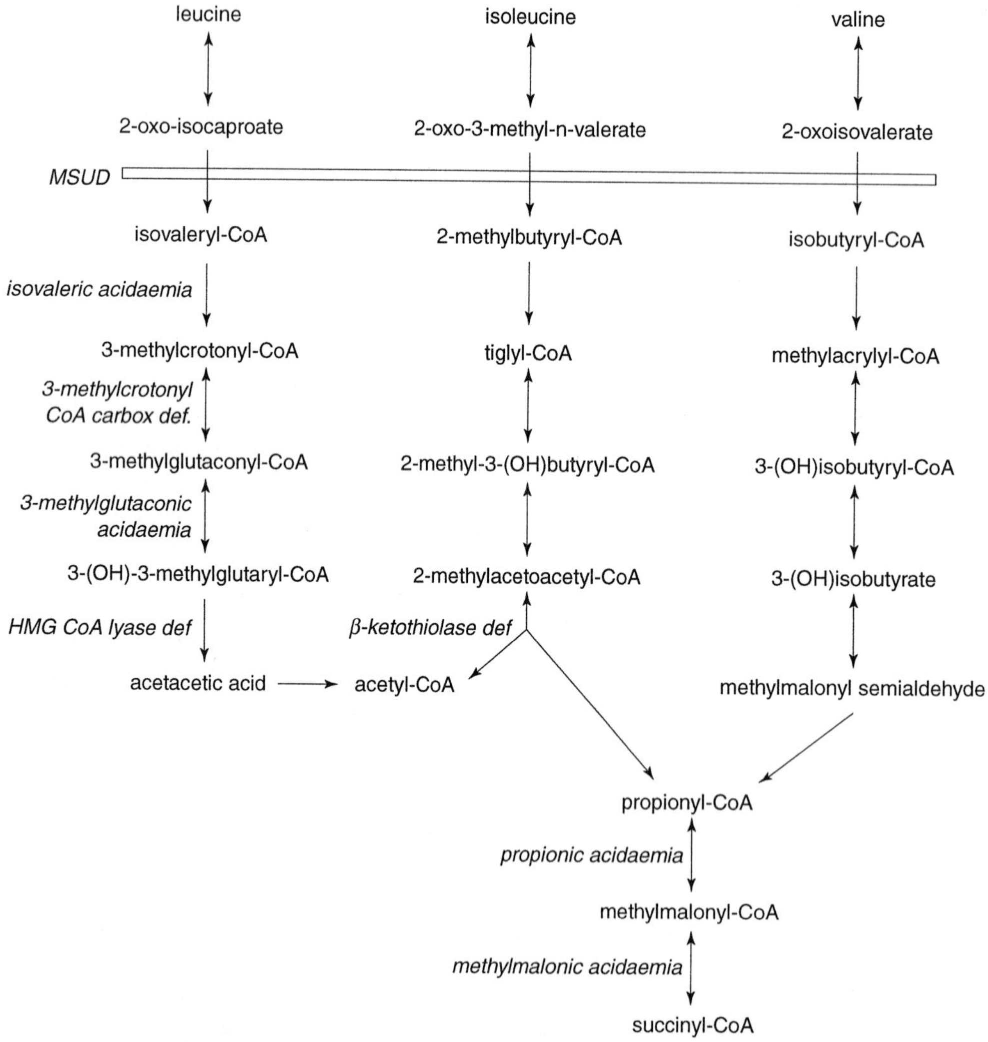

Fig. 38.14 Metabolic pathways in several important IEMs presenting in the neonatal period. The disorders (italics) are placed next to the metabolic step for which the enzyme (see text) is lacking.

CONSIDERATION OF SPECIFIC IEMs

AMINO ACID DISORDERS (Fig. 38.14)

Maple syrup urine disease

- Incidence: 1:250 000 (approx) – ethnic and regional variation
- Inheritance: autosomal recessive
- Enzyme deficiency: branched chain α-keto acid dehydrogenase (BCKAD)
- Mutation data: multienzyme complex consisting of E1α (chromosome 19q13.1-q13.2), E1β (6p21-p22), E2 (1p31) and E3 (7q31-q32) subunits
- Diagnosis: urine amino and organic acids. Confirm diagnosis on skin fibroblasts
- Initial treatment: dialysis
- Long-term treatment: diet low in branched-chain amino acids
- Prenatal diagnosis: direct enzyme assay on uncultured CVB cells.

This rare disorder usually presents towards the end of the first week of life, with vomiting and an encephalopathy characterized by drowsiness, seizures and dystonia. A maple syrup odour is often detectable and affected infants have severe ketoacidosis and are often hypoglycaemic.

Elevated levels of the branched-chain amino acids (leucine, isoleucine and valine) in blood and urine and of the corresponding 2-ketoacids in urine are characteristic. Deficiency of the branched-chain 2-ketoacid dehydrogenase complex can be demonstrated in cultured skin fibroblasts. The prognosis is directly related to the age at diagnosis,[12] and is guarded even in the most skilled hands as dietary treatment is difficult. Very rarely the disorder occurs as a thiamine-responsive variant.

Acute hereditary tyrosinaemia (tyrosinaemia type I)

- Incidence: <1:100 000 but marked ethnic and regional variation
- Inheritance: autosomal recessive
- Enzyme deficiency: fumarylacetoacetate hydrolase
- Mutation data: 15q23-q25 – several mutations identified
- Diagnosis: urine organic acids (succinyl acetone)
- Initial treatment: NTBC (see text)
- Long-term treatment: NTBC and low-tyrosine diet
- Prenatal diagnosis: succinyl acetone in amniotic fluid, FAH activity in CVB mutation analysis of DNA from CVB where mutations in family have been characterized.

The acute neonatal form of this disorder presents with progressive liver disease (occasionally acute hepatic necrosis) and renal tubular dysfunction. A diffuse hyperplasia of the pancreatic islet cells is seen in florid cases, and the subsequent hypoglycaemia can be resistant to treatment. Plasma tyrosine and methionine levels are raised, phosphate and potassium levels are low and there is usually a gross generalized aminoaciduria, glycosuria and phosphaturia. The diagnosis is established by demonstrating increased urinary succinyl acetone excretion on urinary organic acid analysis. The enzyme fumarylacetoacetase is deficient when assayed in lymphocytes or fibroblasts.

The prognosis for affected infants has been revolutionized by the introduction of treatment with 2-(2-nitro-4-trifluoromethylbenzoyl)-1,3-cyclohexanedione (NTBC). This chemical inhibits the enzyme 4-hydroxyphenylpyruvate dioxygenase and prevents the formation of maleylacetoacetate and fumarylacetoacetate, thus averting the risk of liver damage and normalizing porphyrin synthesis in affected patients.[13]

Although there is a panethnic incidence the disorder is particularly common in a French-Canadian isolate in Quebec, as well as in certain areas of Scandinavia.

Non-ketotic hyperglycinaemia (glycine encephalopathy)

- Incidence: 1:250 000 (USA) but marked ethnic and regional variation
- Inheritance: autosomal recessive
- Enzyme deficency: glycine cleavage enzyme
- Mutation data: multienzyme complex, P-protein (9p13), T-protein and U-protein
- Mutations in gene encoding P-protein described
- Diagnosis: ratio of CSF to blood glycine level (normal – 0.01–0.04, NKH – 0.09–0.25)
- Initial treatment: no effective therapy
- Prenatal diagnosis: enzyme assay on uncultured CVB cells.

This usually presents in the neonatal period, with drowsiness and lethargy, hypotonia and hypoventilation. Seizures are prominent and are often myoclonic in nature. The EEG often shows a 'burst-suppression' pattern. Hiccupping and opisthotonus are common features. These may be present at birth and some mothers have reported reduced fetal movements in utero. In these latter cases intracranial anomalies have been reported and the disorder is one cause of agenesis of the corpus callosum.

Plasma glycine levels are very variable in affected patients, and can be normal. Large amounts of glycine are usually excreted in the urine, but the glycine elevation is much more marked in the CSF, reflecting the primary disturbance of neuronal glycine metabolism. Organic acids are not increased in the urine as they are in the various forms of ketotic hyperglycinaemia.

The effects of the disease are caused by the excitatory effects of glycine at the cortical NMDA receptor. Treatment that modifies the systemic levels of glycine have little effect on the disease, and specific inhibitors of glycine at the NMDA receptor, such as strychnine or tryptophan,[15] may lead to an improvement in seizure control and hypotonia but do not usually affect the prognosis, which is very gloomy, death usually occurring in early childhood.

The basic defect is in the multicomplex glycine cleavage enzyme, and diagnosis can be confirmed on transformed lymphocytes or liver biopsy, but *not* cultured skin fibroblasts.[11]

UREA CYCLE DISORDERS (Table 38.23)

- Diagnosis: blood ammonia, urine orotic acid, blood and urine amino acids for all
- Initial treatment: Dialysis, sodium benzoate, sodium phenylbutyrate, sodium phenylacetate, arginine (not arginase deficency)
- Long-term treatment: low-protein diet, essential amino acids, sodium benzoate, sodium phenylbutyrate.

The predominant clinical features of all of these conditions are similar and are a result of the accumulation of ammonia. Presentation in the neonatal period is usually with episodes of vomiting and drowsiness, proceeding to unconsciousness and seizures. The absence of acidosis is an important point.

Once hyperammonaemia has been established by measurement of the blood ammonia level, the diagnosis of a primary urea cycle defect can usually be made after measuring plasma and urine amino acids and by screening the urine for organic acids and orotic acid. Hyperammonaemia secondary to an organic acidaemia will be excluded by a normal urinary organic acid profile and the absence of ketosis and metabolic acidosis.

In CPS deficiency and OTC deficiency, plasma ammonia levels are grossly elevated (2–3000 μmol/l), but plasma amino acid levels are usually normal apart from elevation of glutamate. The two conditions can be differentiated by measuring urinary orotic acid, which is grossly elevated in OTC deficiency but not in CPS deficiency. Citrullinaemia, argininosuccinic aciduria and arginase deficiency all show characteristic elevations of the respective amino acids in plasma and urine.

Table 38.23 Urea cycle disorders

	CPS	OTC	ASAS	ASAL	ARG
Incidence	1:100 000	1:100 000	1:100 000	1:100 000	1:100 000
Inheritance	AR	XLR	AR	AR	AR
Enzyme deficiency	CPS	OTC	ASAS	ASAL	ARG
Mutations	2p	Xp21.1	9q34	7cen-p21	6q23
Prenatal	Fetal liver or DNA	Fetal liver or DNA	Enz-CVB	Enz-CVB	Fetal blood or DNA

CPS, carbamyl phosphate synthetase
OTC, ornithine transcarbamylase
ASAS, argininosuccinic acid synthetase (citrullinaemia)
ASAL, argininosuccinic acid lyase (argininosuccinic aciduria)
ARG, arginase (argininaemia)

Definitive diagnosis is obtained by measuring the individual enzymes in a liver biopsy (all defects), cultured skin fibroblasts (citrullinaemia, argininosuccinic aciduria and arginase deficiency) or erythrocytes (argininosuccinic aciduria).

Treatment of urea cycle disorders includes arginine (which becomes an essential amino acid in all but arginase deficiency) supplementation (2 ml/kg of 10% arginine HCL) and the use of alternative pathways to excrete nitrogen waste. Amino acid nitrogen may be excreted as hippuric acid if sodium benzoate (250–500 mg/kg/day) is administered, or as phenylglutamine after phenylacetate (250–500 mg/kg/day) administration. These methods have made a great difference to the outcome of this group of patients.[3,4] Essential amino acid supplements can also be used to provide some of the nitrogen requirement.

It is important to remember that OTC deficiency is one of the X-linked IEMs. Female heterozygotes can be symptomatic in the newborn period and are often protein intolerant later in life. Carrier testing is possible by performing an allopurinol-loading test.[21] The OTC gene has been identified and a number of mutations characterized. Direct mutation analysis is playing an increasing role in both carrier detection and prenatal diagnosis in this disorder.

Transient neonatal hyperammonaemia

Plasma ammonia levels of over 1500 μmol/l have been described in a small number of comatose newborn infants who have recovered completely after very aggressive treatment with no biochemical evidence of a specific enzyme defect in the urea cycle. These babies have subsequently tolerated a normal protein intake without any symptoms. The biochemical basis of the condition is unknown, but as it mainly occurs in preterm infants immaturity of enzyme systems has been postulated.

ORGANIC ACID DISORDERS (Fig. 38.13)

Propionic acidaemia

- Incidence: 1:50–100 000 (NW England)
- Inheritance: autosomal recessive
- Enzyme deficiency: propionyl-CoA carboxylase
- Mutation data: α-subunit (13q32), β-subunit (3q13.3-q22) – mutations identified in β-subunit gene
- Diagnosis: urine organic acids, confirm on cultured skin fibroblasts
- Initial treatment: dialysis, bicarbonate, sodium benzoate, carnitine
- Long-term treatment: liver transplantation or low protein diet, bicarbonate, sodium benzoate, carnitine
- Prenatal diagnosis: enzyme assay, CVB.

In its acute form this disorder presents early in the newborn period, with severe metabolic acidosis, poor feeding, vomiting and drowsiness which rapidly proceeds to coma. Hyperammonaemia and hypoglycaemia are often present. The blood ammonia may be elevated to levels similar to those seen in primary urea cycle defects.

In less severe forms the features are poor feeding, failure to thrive and recurrent vomiting. Ketoacidosis and hyperglycinaemia are the main biochemical features, and some patients are neutropenic.

The urine contains large amounts of a wide variety of organic acids, including 3-hydroxypropionate, methylcitrate and tiglylglycine, as well as some unusual ketone bodies. Diagnosis is confirmed by assay of propionyl-CoA carboxylase in white blood cells or cultured skin fibroblasts.

Long-term treatment relies upon protein restriction, alkali therapy, sodium benzoate and carnitine replacement. Because of the poor prognosis for neurological outcome in most patients on conventional therapy, liver transplantation may offer a better prognosis.

Methylmalonic acidaemia

- Incidence: 1:20 000 (overall)
- Inheritance: all types are autosomal recessive
- Enzyme deficiency: (1) methylmalonyl-CoA mutase (MUT) mut°-(vitamin B_{12}-unresponsive MMA) (2) methylmalonyl-CoA mutase (MUT) mut^{-} (reduced affinity for cofactor adenosylcobalamin – vitamin B_{12} responsive MMA) (3) various defects in cobalamin metabolism (some associated with homocystinuria), known as cbl A, B, C, D and F mutations
- Mutation data: MUT 6p12-p21.2 – a number of mutations characterized
- Diagnosis: urine organic acids and confirmatory studies on skin fibroblasts
- Initial treatment: dialysis, sodium bicarbonate, vitamin B_{12}, carnitine
- Long-term treatment: liver transplantation or low-protein diet, bicarbonate, carnitine in vitamin B_{12}-unresponsive forms, vitamin B_{12} 1000 mg three times per week in vitamin B_{12}-responsive forms
- Prenatal diagnosis: enzyme assay or metabolic studies on cultured cells from CVB.

The clinical features of this disorder are very similar to those of propionic acidaemia. However, it can be distinguished by the excretion of methylmalonic acid and by specific enzyme assay. Methylmalonic acidaemia can be subdivided into a number of different categories, depending on whether the defect is in the methylmalonyl-CoA mutase enzyme or in one of the steps in the formation of its cofactor adenosylcobalamin. They all present with vomiting, acidosis and neurological symptoms and they can be differentiated only by careful enzyme studies in cultured cells to distinguish defects of different steps in adenosylcobalamin synthesis as well as responsiveness to vitamin B_{12} therapy. The degree of response to vitamin B_{12} varies depending on the step in cofactor synthesis that is affected.

Hyperammonaemia can occur in any of the more severe forms of methylmalonic acidaemia, as in propionic acidaemia, although it is usually not so severe. Methylmalonic acidaemia plus homocystinuria may be seen in defects in the early steps of cobalamin cofactor biosynthesis. Long-term therapy is relatively simple and very effective in the vitamin B_{12}-responsive cases, but difficult in the remainder, in whom stringent protein restriction is required. Intercurrent infective illnesses frequently cause exacerbations of acidosis requiring intravenous therapy. Late complications such as progressive renal damage or acute infarction of the basal ganglia may occur, and liver transplantation may be a better long-term therapy.

Isovaleric acidaemia

- Incidence: 1:100–200 000
- Inheritance: autosomal recessive
- Enzyme deficiency: isovaleryl-CoA dehydrogenase
- Mutation data: 15q14-q15, several mutations identified
- Diagnosis: urine organic acids, confirmatory studies on skin fibroblasts
- Initial treatment: dialysis, carnitine, glycine supplementation
- Long-term treatment: low-protein diet, carnitine, glycine
- Prenatal diagnosis: enzyme assay on cultured cells from CVB.

This disorder, caused by a deficiency of the enzyme isovaleryl-CoA dehydrogenase, may present in the newborn period with vomiting and severe ketoacidosis. Affected infants are often neutropenic and thrombocytopenic during the acute episode, and the urine has a characteristic 'sweaty feet' odour owing to the excretion of isovaleric acid. Treatment with protein restriction, carnitine and glycine supplementation generally results in normal development in those infants who survive the newborn period unscathed.

DEFECTS IN CARBOHYDRATE METABOLISM

Galactosaemia

- Incidence: 1:40–60 000 (UK)
- Inheritance: autosomal recessive
- Enzyme deficiency: galactose-1-phosphate uridyl transferase
- Mutation data: 9p13, several mutations identified, including a common Q188R mutation

- Diagnosis: Beutler test (screening), formal enzyme assay in blood
- Initial treatment: galactose-free diet
- Long-term treatment: galactose-free diet.

Infants with 'classical' galactosaemia due to deficiency of the enzyme galactose-1-phosphate uridyl transferase present towards the end of the first week of life with vomiting, failure to thrive and jaundice. Neurological symptoms are common and 30–40% develop a superadded septicaemia, usually due to *Escherichia coli* infection, which often starts as a urinary tract infection. This may be diagnosed and treated without recognizing the underlying metabolic disease, especially as milk feeds are stopped during the treatment of this acute illness. Recurrence of symptoms when milk is reintroduced may alert the neonatologist to the principal diagnosis. Hepatomegaly is always present and the clinical course is dominated by the progressive liver damage. Cataracts may appear even in the first week, and there may be early evidence of renal damage, with proteinuria and aminoaciduria.

The diagnosis may be suspected by the urinary excretion of galactose and is readily confirmed by measurement of erythrocyte galactose-1-phosphate uridyl transferase. If the infant has had a prior blood transfusion, enzyme analysis is unreliable and diagnosis is achieved by measuring galactose-1-phosphate levels in blood.

Long-term treatment is with a milk-free diet. Cataracts regress and the liver heals, but the intellectual outcome remains poor, with most affected adults having IQ scores of 60–80. There is often a specific speech delay, and a cerebellar syndrome with ataxia becomes prominent in some affected adults. Ovarian failure occurs in at least 80% of affected female patients and is not related to delays in postnatal treatment. An effect on fetal ovarian development has been postulated.

Fructose-1,6-bisphosphatase deficiency

- Incidence: 1:150–200 000
- Inheritance: autosomal recessive
- Enzyme deficiency: fructose-1,6-bisphosphatase
- Mutation data: 9q22.2-q22.3, a number of mutations identified
- Diagnosis: clinical, urine organic acids, enzyme assay on WBC
- Initial treatment: correct acidosis and hypoglycaemia
- Long-term treatment: avoid fasting
- Prenatal diagnosis: enzyme not expressed in CVB or amniocytes.

This disorder may present in the newborn period with severe lactic acidosis. Affected infants hyperventilate, are often hypoglycaemic and can deteriorate rapidly with apnoea and death. Later episodes in survivors are often triggered by intercurrent fasting or infections. Gluconeogenesis is severely impaired and hypoglycaemia is prominent, with the accumulation of gluconeogenic precursors such as lactate, amino acids and ketones. Unlike hereditary fructose intolerance, patients do not vomit after the ingestion of fructose and an aversion to sweets does not develop. The diagnosis can be established on white blood cell enzyme assay. A fructose tolerance test is not necessary.

Glycogen storage disease type I

- Incidence: GSD Ia – 1:100 000, GSD Ib – 1:200 000, GSD Ic and Id – very rare
- Inheritance: autosomal recessive
- Enzyme deficiency: GSD Ia – glucose-6-phosphatase, GSD Ib – glucose-6-phosphate translocase
- Mutation data: GSD Ia (chromosome 11), a number of mutations identified, GSD Ib – unknown
- Diagnosis: clinical, enzyme assay on fresh and frozen liver biopsy samples
- Initial treatment: correction of hypoglycaemia
- Long-term treatment: maintenance of normoglycaemia, corn starch, continuous overnight feeds
- Prenatal diagnosis: possible if mutation known in family (GSD Ia), enzymes not expressed in CVB or amniocytes.

All variants of GSD type I (a, b, c and d) can present in the newborn period with profound hypoglycaemia. In addition there is lactic acidosis, hyperuricaemia and hyperlipidaemia. Hepatomegaly is usually obvious, but the very soft liver in GSD I may be difficult to define by palpation. The diagnosis is established by enzyme assay (glucose 6-phosphatase) performed on a liver biopsy sample. Treatment is aimed at maintaining normoglycaemia with frequent daytime feeds and continuous nocturnal intragastric infusion of glucose.

Primary disorders of pyruvate metabolism

Pyruvate dehydrogenase deficiency

- Incidence: 1:200 000
- Inheritance: multienzyme complex, commonest deficiency E1α-subunit – X-linked dominant
- Enzyme deficiency: pyruvate dehydrogenase
- Mutation data: Xp22.1-22.2 – a number of mutations described
- Diagnosis: lactic acidosis, urine organic acids, confirmatory studies on skin fibroblasts
- Initial treatment: none effective, correction of acidosis
- Long-term treatment: none effective.

All the primary disorders of pyruvate metabolism are associated with lactic acidosis and all have similar clinical features, with profound peripheral circulatory disturbance and severe neurological abnormalities. Pyruvate dehydrogenase deficiency deserves special mention. This multienzyme complex is a major metabolic control point in the aerobic oxidation of carbohydrates and some gluconeogenic amino acids. The action of PDH is controlled by a specific kinase (inactivation) and phosphorylase (activation), which are tightly regulated in response to metabolite concentrations within the mitochondrion. The enzyme complex itself comprises three main enzymes, E1 or pyruvate decarboxylase (with α and β subunits), E2 or lipoyl transacetylase, and E3, a dihydrolipoyl-dehydrogenase. Defects in all three main components have been described, and early presentation is generally with severe acidosis or with profound neurological deficit in a baby with minimal or no acidosis (often with structural brain lesions, 'cerebral lactic acidosis'). Milder cases may present later with intermittent ataxia or acidosis. Deficiency of the E1α-subunit (the subunit which is subject to most of the acute metabolic controls over enzyme activity) is the most frequent defect. The gene for this subunit is on the short arm of the X chromosome.[5] Both hemizygous males and heterozygous females are affected, nearly all cases being the result of new mutations. The patients with the 'cerebral' form are females with severe enzyme lesions which destroy patches of the brain in which the mutant gene is active. Males predominate among those with early severe acidosis, and usually have an incomplete enzyme deficiency.

Patients with E3 deficiency may excrete large amounts of 2-ketoglutarate and branched-chain 2-ketoacids in addition to lactate, as this component appears to be common to all 2-ketoacid dehydrogenase complexes.

Patients with these defects deteriorate when given a high glucose intake, and prompt recognition is therefore important. It is very difficult to give the high-lipid high-protein low-carbohydrate regimes which in theory would be best for these patients. Occasional patients have been described who respond to large doses of thiamine, but there is no way of differentiating these patients clinically or biochemically from those with unresponsive forms.[26]

Lactic acidosis presents a very complex set of problems. The first difficulty arises in diagnosis in an acutely ill newborn infant. Primary lactic acidosis can cause the very effects (vasoconstriction, convulsions, severe acidosis) that can cause secondary lactic acidosis when present for other reasons. The matter is further complicated by the existence of some disorders leading to lactic acidosis which require treatment with carbohydrate supplementation (e.g. fructose 1,6-bisphosphatase deficiency and some other gluconeogenic defects), and others which are made worse by this regimen (e.g. pyruvate dehydrogenase deficiency and some other mitochondrial disorders). The presence of structural CNS defects makes the latter group more likely, but often one has to gamble. As the gluconeogenic defects generally have the better prognosis it is usually preferable to err on the side of carbohydrate supplementation in practice, especially as the profound hypoglycaemia which can occur in these disorders can cause severe brain damage.

In all forms of severe lactic acidosis muscle paralysis and ventilatory support have a specific role in reducing muscle lactate production and, as with other IEMs that can affect the brain, ventilatory support should be considered early, especially in infants with significant (pH <7.1) or persistent metabolic acidosis.

FATTY ACID OXIDATION DEFECTS

A number of defects in fatty acid oxidation have been identified. Some prevent uptake of fatty acids into the mitochondria and others affect specific steps in the β-oxidation within the mitochondria. These enzymes have specificity based on the length of fatty acid carbon chain. All can present in the newborn period and can commonly present with life-threatening or fatal illness. Deficiency of MCAD is the most frequently recognized. Diagnosis in this disorder has been considerably simplified by the finding of a common genetic mutation which accounts for nearly 90% of mutant chromosomes in the caucasian population. This disorder usually presents with hypoketotic hypoglycaemia between the ages of 3 and 18 months, although neonatal presentation is now well recognized.[27]

MCAD

- Incidence: 1:40 000
- Inheritance: autosomal recessive
- Enzyme deficiency: medium-chain fatty acyl-CoA dehydrogenase deficiency
- Mutation data: 1p31 – common A985G mutation in 90% caucasian MCAD patients
- Diagnosis: urine organic acids, DNA analysis
- Initial treatment: correct hypoglycaemia
- Long-term treatment: avoid fasting
- Prenatal diagnosis: possible on DNA analysis of CVB, but rarely asked for.

One other serious presentation of this group of disorders is with hypertrophic cardiomyopathy, which can cause heart failure or cardiorespiratory arrest in the newborn period. This occurs in multiple acyl-CoA dehydrogenase deficiency (glutaric aciduria type II), long-chain fatty acyl-CoA dehydrogenase deficiency, 3-hydroxyacyl-CoA dehydrogenase deficiency and the primary disorders of carnitine metabolism.[22]

Diagnosis of defects in fatty acid metabolism relies on a combination of biochemical abnormalities, which may include evidence of liver disease (raised transaminases, hyperammonaemia) and muscle disease (raised CPK). Urinary organic acid profiles may reveal a characteristic pattern of abnormalities, and the blood and urine carnitine status may be abnormal. Specific enzyme assays on cultured skin fibroblasts are a difficult and specialized investigation and are not readily available. Decreased rates of catabolism of radiolabelled fatty acid substrates can be used to demonstrate a defect somewhere in the β-oxidation pathway, and can be helpful when interpreted with the clinical presentation and supporting biochemical abnormalities.

DISORDERS OF SUBCELLULAR ORGANELLES

Mitochondrial disease

- Incidence: incidence of mitochondrial disorders as a group is unknown, but they are being increasingly recognized
- Inheritance: can be recessive, dominant, X-linked or maternal
- Enzyme deficiencies: components of the respiratory transport chain
- Mutation data: many point mutations in mitochondrial DNA (mtDNA) identified
- Diagnosis: combination of clinical features, enzyme activities, muscle biopsy histology and mtDNA analysis
- Initial treatment: none effective, correct acidosis, supplement with thiamine, riboflavin, coenzyme Q10 and ubiquinone
- Long-term treatment: continue supplements in patients that survive neonatal period
- Prenatal diagnosis: depends on specific defect, not readily available.

Mitochondria are unique among cytoplasmic organelles as they contain their own genetic material. The mitochondrial genome is a circular DNA molecule of approximately 16 500 base pairs which encodes some (but not all) of the polypeptides of the respiratory transport chain and some other components of mitochondrial transcription and translation (22 transfer RNAs and 2 ribosomal RNAs). There are multiple copies of mtDNA in each mitochondrion and many mitochondria in each cell, so that each cell contains several thousand mtDNA molecules. The phenotype and rate of progression of mitochondrial disorders appears to be determined by the proportion and segregation of abnormal mtDNA molecules at cell division, combined with a 'threshold effect' in various tissues depending on energy requirements and functional reserve. Brain and muscle appear to be most sensitive to mitochondrial dysfunction.

The other major characteristic of mtDNA is that it is transmitted between generations only by the mother, probably because at fertilization only the head of the sperm enters the egg and the mitochondria in the rest of the sperm are lost. Maternal inheritance patterns are seen in those disorders where there is a primary mtDNA mutation responsible for the disease.

Clinical features are extremely variable and the diagnosis should be suspected in infants where there is multiple organ involvement. Lactic acidosis is usual and there may be abnormalities on routine haematological and biochemical analyses, depending on the main target organs affected. Specific biochemical investigation will include assay of respiratory transport chain activity on muscle biopsy material. Histological changes in muscle tissue can be important, and the characteristic pathological finding in patients with many forms of mitochondrial disease is the 'ragged red fibre' on staining with Gomori trichrome.

In a number of mitochondrial disorders underlying or associated genetic changes have been defined in mtDNA. These include large structural rearrangements (deletions and duplications) and point mutations. When present, these are a highly specific and sensitive addition to the biochemical investigations.

Peroxisomal disorders (Table 38.24)

These disorders present in the neonatal period and are all disorders of peroxisomal biogenesis or peroxisomal protein transportation. Not all defects have been fully categorized and there are a number of different complementation groups described. Single peroxisomal enzyme defects have been described and some can present neonatally.[19]

- Prenatal diagnosis: direct enzyme assay on CVB, VLCFAs on cultured CVB or amniocytes.

There are over 15 different peroxisomal disorders, caused by an impairment of one or more peroxisomal functions. The more profound and complex disorders of peroxisomal biogenesis or of multiple peroxisomal enzyme deficiency present in the newborn period with severe neurological abnormalities plus various other features, including abnormal facies and body build, cataracts, punctate epiphyseal calcification, liver fibrosis, renal cysts and adrenal or hepatic failure. Increased levels of very long-chain fatty acids (VLCFA C26+) in plasma and/or deficiency of dihydroacetone phosphate acyl transferase (DHAP-AT) are useful biochemical markers.

Table 38.24 Peroxisomal disorders

	Zellweger	RCDP	NALD/ INF.REF.
Incidence	1:50 000	1:100 000	V. rare
Inheritance	AR	AR	AR
Enzyme deficiency	Membrane protein	Import protein	Membrane protein
Mutation data	8q21.1	?	?
Diagnosis	VLCFA/ DHAP-AT	As Zellweger	As Zellweger
Initial treatment	None	None	None
Long-term treatment	None	None	None

RCDP, rhizomelic chondrodysplasia punctata; NALD; neonatal adrenoleukodystrophy; INF.REF., infantile Refsum's disease

The absence of peroxisomes on liver histology is typical of Zellweger syndrome. There is no effective treatment, but prenatal diagnosis is possible.

Lysosomal disorders

The lysosomal disorders are conditions in which a defective lysosomal enzyme leads to the accumulation of specific substrates within the cell which eventually interfere with normal cellular function. The disorders are progressive and usually present in childhood or later, but some can produce dramatic neonatal presentation, usually in such cases with hydrops fetalis as a prominent feature. Diagnosis is established by enzyme assay on white blood cells or cultured skin fibroblasts.

MISCELLANEOUS DISORDERS

Carbohydrate-deficient glycoprotein syndromes

- Incidence: 1:40 000 (CDG type I)
- Inheritance: autosomal recessive
- Enzyme defect: abnormality in oligosaccharide processing on to glycoproteins
- Mutation data: CDG type I – 16p13.3-p13.2
- Diagnosis: isoelectric focusing of plasma transferrin
- Initial treatment: supportive
- Long-term treatment: supportive, hormone replacement when deficient
- Prenatal diagnosis: not yet available.

This newly described group of metabolic disorders is characterized by a deficiency in the carbohydrate moiety of secretory glycoproteins, including a characteristic change in transferrin, which can be used as a diagnostic test. A number of variants have been described, including a type which can produce severe neonatal disease.[10]

During the first 24 hours of life many CDG infants feed poorly and are often floppy and hypothermic. Birthweight is usually normal, but a variable dysmorphism is often present, including abnormalities of the skin (*peau d'orange*) or subcutaneous tissue (fat pads). A number of serious complications can develop, including pericardial effusion and liver dysfunction. Failure to thrive and psychomotor delay are usual.

Menkes disease

- Incidence: 1:200 000
- Inheritance: X-linked recessive
- Enzyme defect: ATPase copper transport protein
- Mutation data: Xq13, a number of mutations have been identified
- Diagnosis: clinical, copper and ceruloplasmin, copper kinetic studies on cultured skin fibroblasts
- Initial treatment: none effective
- Long-term treatment: supportive
- Prenatal diagnosis: copper studies on cultured CVB cells, DNA analysis when mutation known in family.

Most babies with this X-linked recessive disease have difficulty in maintaining body temperature in the neonatal period, but few are diagnosed at this stage. Most are diagnosed at 2–4 months because of poor development, seizures and abnormal 'steely' hair. Low plasma levels of copper confirm the diagnosis.

The basic defect is in copper transport across the intestinal mucosa and in body cells. Parenteral copper therapy improves copper enzyme levels, but has little effect on development. Treatment after symptomatic diagnosis can only prolong existence with severe brain damage.

Smith–Lemli–Opitz syndrome

- Incidence: 1:20 000
- Inheritance: autosomal recessive
- Enzyme defect: 7-dehydrocholesterol-δ-7-reductase
- Mutation data: 7q32.1
- Diagnosis: clinical, 7-dehydrocholesterol in plasma
- Initial treatment: high-cholesterol diet, bile acid supplementation – no firm evidence of efficacy
- Long-term treatment: as above
- Prenatal diagnosis: 7-dehydrocholesterol level in amniotic fluid.

This recessive disorder had been recognized as a 'dysmorphic syndrome' for many years prior to the identification of the defect in cholesterol metabolism responsible for the clinical phenotype. Affected patients have characteristic craniofacial features, cleft palate, hypospadias, postaxial polydactyly and toe syndactyly. A number of biochemical abnormalities were known to be associated with the syndrome, including a very low plasma cholesterol level. Further investigation led to the finding of grossly elevated 7-dehydrocholesterol levels in the plasma of affected children, and this is now the basis of the biochemical confirmation of this disorder. This compound is the immediate precursor in the cholesterol biosynthetic pathway. A deficiency of the enzyme 3β-hydroxysteroid-δ-7-reductase has been proposed as the primary genetic lesion in affected infants. Treatment with bile acid supplementation and a high cholesterol diet has been attempted in a number of patients, but it is too early to say whether this will be of benefit.[25]

REFERENCES

1. Bamforth F J 1994 Laboratory screening for genetic disorders and birth defects. Clinical Biochemistry 27: 333–342
2. Bankier A, Turner M, Hopkins I J 1983 Pyridoxine-dependent seizures – a wider clinical spectrum. Archives of Diseases in Childhood 58: 415–418
3. Batshaw M L, Brusilow S, Waber L et al 1982 Treatment of inborn errors of urea synthesis. Activation of alternative pathways of waste nitrogen synthesis and excretion. New England Journal of Medicine 306: 1387–1392

4. Batshaw M L, Brusilow S W, Danney M et al 1984 Treatment of episodic hyperammonemia in children with inborn errors of urea synthesis. New England Journal of Medicine 310: 1630–1634
5. Brown R M, Dahl H-H M, Brown G K 1989 X-chromosome localization of the functional gene for the E1α subunit of the human pyruvate dehydrogenase complex. Genomics 4: 174–181
6. Danks D M 1974 Management of newborn babies in whom serious metabolic disease is anticipated. Archives of Disease in Childhood 49: 576–578
7. Gabow P A, Kaeburg W D, Fennessey P V et al 1980 Diagnostic importance of an increased anion gap. New England Journal of Medicine 330: 854–858
8. Goutieres F, Aicardi J 1985 Atypical presentation of pyridoxine-dependent seizures: a treatable cause of intractable epilepsy in infants. Neurology 17: 117–120
9. Gregerson N, Blakemore A I F, Winter V et al 1991 Specific diagnosis of medium-chain acyl-CoA dehydrogenase (MCAD) deficiency in dried blood spots by a polymerase chain reaction (PCR) assay detecting a point mutation (G985) in the MCAD gene. Clinica Chimica Acta 203: 23–34
10. Hagberg B A, Blennow G, Kristiansson B et al 1993 Carbohydrate-deficient glycoprotein syndromes: peculiar group of new disorders. Pediatric Neurology 9: 255–262
11. Hayasaka K, Tada K, Fueki N, Nakamura Y, Nyhan W L, Schmidt K et al 1987 Non-ketotic hyperglycinemia: analysis of glycine cleavage system in typical and atypical cases. Journal of Pediatrics 110: 873–877
12. Kaplan P, Mazur A, Field M et al 1991 Intellectual outcome in children with maple syrup urine disease. Journal of Pediatrics 119: 46–50
13. Lindstedt S, Holme E, Lock E A et al 1992 Treatment of hereditary tyrosinaemia type I by inhibition of 4-hydroxyphenylpyruvate dioxygenase. Lancet 340: 813–817
14. Marsden D, Barshop B A, Capistrano-Estrada S et al 1994 Anabolic effect of human growth hormone: management of inherited disorders of catabolic pathways. Biochemical Medicine, Metabolism and Biology 52: 145–154
15. Matsuo S, Inoue F, Takeuchi Y et al 1995 Efficacy of tryptophan for the treatment of nonketotic hyperglycinemia: a new therapeutic approach for modulating the *N*-methyl-D-aspartate receptor. Pediatrics 95: 142–146
16. Minns R 1980 Vitamin B6 deficiency and dependency. Developmental Medicine and Child Neurology 22: 795–799
17. Naylor E W 1995 Biochemical versus molecular newborn screening. Screening 4: 41–45
18. Perry T L 1981 Autopsy investigation of disorders of amino acid metabolism. In: Barson A J (ed) Laboratory investigation of fetal disease. Wright, Bristol, Ch 19, pp 429–451
19. Roels F, de Bie S, Schutgens R B H, Besley G T N 1995 Diagnosis of human peroxisomal disorders. Journal of Inherited Metabolic Disease 18: Suppl. 1.
20. Scriver C R, Beaudet A L, Sly W S, Valle D (eds) 1995 The metabolic and molecular bases of inherited disease, 7th edn. McGraw-Hill, New York.
21. Sebesta I, Fairbanks L D, Davies P M et al 1994 The allopurinol loading test for identification of carriers for ornithine carbamoyl transferase deficiency: studies in a healthy control population and females at risk. Clinica Chimica Acta 224: 45–54
22. Servidei S, Bertini E, DiMauro S 1994 Hereditary metabolic cardiomyopathies. Advances in Pediatrics 41: 1–32
23. Starfield B, Holtzman N A 1975 A comparison of effectiveness of screening for phenylketonuria in the United States, United Kingdom and Ireland. New England Journal of Medicine 293: 118–121
24. Sweetman L 1996 Newborn screening by tandem mass spectrometry (MS-MS). Clinical Chemistry 42: 345–346
25. Tint G S, Irons M, Elias E et al 1994 Defective cholesterol biosynthesis associated with the Smith–Lemli–Opitz syndrome. New England Journal of Medicine 330: 107–113
26. Wick H, Schweizer K, Baumgartner R 1977 Thiamine dependency in a patient with congenital lactic acidaemia due to pyruvate dehydrogenase deficiency. Agents Actions 7: 405–410
27. Wilcken B, Carpenter K H, Hammond J 1993 Neonatal symptoms in medium chain acyl coenzyme A dehydrogenase deficency. Archives of Disease in Childhood 69: 292–294
28. Weissbecker K A 1985 Clinical findings in four children with biotinidase deficiency detected through a statewide neonatal screening programe. New England Journal of Medicine 313: 16–19

Part 4

Metabolic bone disease

N. J. Bishop

INTRODUCTION

The majority of neonatal metabolic bone disease is seen in preterm infants, in whom it is due largely to substrate deficiency. For these infants, factors such as the administration of steroids, diuretics and the effects of immobilization also merit consideration.

Diagnostic criteria vary considerably between centres, leading to estimates of incidence that vary from 32 to 92%.[9,29,38]

DIAGNOSING METABOLIC BONE DISEASE IN PRETERM INFANTS

Bone disease in preterm infants is characterized by a sequence of events which begins with biochemical evidence of disturbed mineral metabolism,[1,10,11,28,36,39,48,56] continues with reduced bone mineralization[13,26,31,58,59,62] (as assessed by absorptiometric techniques), and results in abnormal bone remodelling[22] and reduced linear growth velocity.[36] In extreme forms, fractures of ribs and the distal ends of long bones[34] and craniotabes have been reported.[22,38] In the longer term height may be reduced,[36] there is a trend towards earlier presentation with fracture (excluding non-accidental injury cases),[17] and bone mineral accretion in later childhood may also be influenced.[7]

AETIOLOGY

DISTURBED MINERAL METABOLISM

Calcium and phosphate

Whole blood ionized calcium falls within 18–24 hours of

delivery. This is a physiological rather than a pathological event, reflecting continued calcium accretion into bone in the face of reduced exogenous calcium input, and a postnatal surge in calcitonin production of unknown aetiology.[45] Ionized calcium may remain low in asphyxiated infants beyond 48 hours of age, indicating impaired transmembrane pumping. The initial manifestation of disturbed mineral metabolism is hypophosphataemia.[11,48] Plasma phosphate falls below 1.0 mmol/l at between 7 and 14 days of age, and is accompanied by hypophosphaturia, with tubular reabsorption of phosphorus typically greater than 90%.[1,56] Where persistent phosphate wasting is observed, investigations for renal tubular problems should be undertaken.

In phosphate-depleted infants both hypercalcaemia (plasma calcium >2.7 mmol/l) and hypercalciuria are frequently observed,[10,39] reflecting increased plasma 1,25-$(OH)_2D_3$ activity.

Phosphate depletion can be monitored by serial urinary calcium/phosphate ratios.[55] This test can be performed on a single untimed sample and should be less than 1 by age 3 weeks if the infant is phosphate replete (calcium and phosphate both measured in mmol/l).

In our prospective studies of 857 preterm infants fed different diets, we could not demonstrate a relationship between linear growth at 18 months post-term age and neonatal plasma phosphate[36] after adjusting for the effects of diet and plasma alkaline phosphatase activity. Ryan et al[47] found a weak negative correlation with forearm bone mineral content.

Plasma alkaline phosphatase activity

Bone alkaline phosphatase activity is widely thought to reflect the rate of new bone formation. Most reports of raised plasma alkaline phosphatase activity have given total values, rather than specific bone isoenzyme measurements. Other alkaline phosphatases can be raised around delivery and may confound interpretation (Clarke P, personal communication).

Plasma alkaline phosphatase activity typically rises over the first 3 weeks of postnatal life to levels two to threefold greater than the maximum of the adult normal range (typically <130 IU/l). Activity increases further (from age 5–6 weeks) in infants who receive diets low in mineral substrate compared to those who receive diets with increased mineral content.[28,36] In the short term, plasma alkaline phosphatase activity greater than five times the maximum of the adult normal range is associated with progressive slowing of linear growth velocity.[36]

Vitamin D and its metabolites

Where routine supplementation of doorstep milk and cereals is practised, cord blood levels of 25-OH D_3 are typically >20 ng/ml, indicating vitamin D sufficiency at all gestations. Maternal supplementation with vitamin D results in higher cord blood levels of 25-OH vitamin D, but not 1,25-$(OH)_2$ vitamin D.[18] Where maternal vitamin D intake during pregnancy has been poor, or where there is pre-existing maternal vitamin D deficiency, neonatal vitamin D stores may be low, and supplemental vitamin D of more than the normal 400 IU/day may be required. A number of studies have identified low/borderline plasma 25-OH vitamin D and elevated 1,25-$(OH)_2$ vitamin D levels in the plasma of preterm infants fed unsupplemented human milk,[27,51] suggesting an increased requirement for vitamin D during rapid bone turnover in phosphate-depleted infants. Many studies indicate that vitamin D supplementation does improve calcium absorption and retention, although the magnitude of this improvement is variable, possibly reflecting mineral as well as vitamin D status. There are no data indicating improved long-term outcome for infants receiving higher doses of vitamin D. There is no good evidence suggesting frank vitamin D deficiency in the majority of infants.

Osteocalcin (bone GLA protein)

Plasma osteocalcin is widely regarded as a measure of new bone formation. Cord blood osteocalcin increases between 22 and 27 weeks,[54] decreasing thereafter. This rise parallels the rate of mineral accretion calculated from the data of Ziegler.[4,67]

Plasma osteocalcin values correlated with plasma alkaline phosphatase activity, but not with plasma 25-OH vitamin D concentrations in a prospective study of VLBW infants fed human milk.[43] Higher levels of plasma osteocalcin were demonstrated in term infants who received human milk,[41] suggesting increased new bone formation in the face of dietary mineral restriction.

REDUCED OR STATIC BONE MINERALIZATION

The estimation of bone mineral content in enterally fed term and premature infants has been reported from many centres.[13,26,31,58,59,62] The studies undertaken, irrespective of the technique used, show that mineral accretion in the majority of sick infants lags behind that which would be expected had the infant remained in utero. Healthy preterm infants who received cow's milk-based diets supplemented with large amounts of calcium and phosphorus showed improved mineral accretion, which approached the in utero accretion rate.[13,26,62] There have as yet been no reports of reduced mineral accretion during the period of initial hospitalization being predictive of later outcome in terms of growth, fracture risk or later mineral accretion.

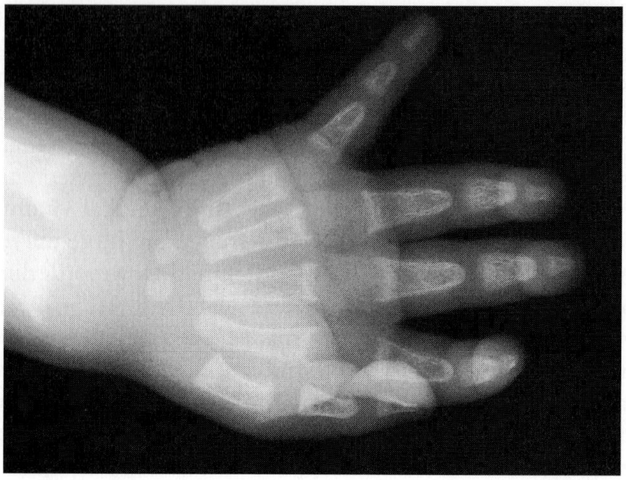

Fig. 38.15 X-ray of an ex-preterm infant showing rachitic changes.

Most studies have utilized techniques that measure principally cortical bone in a limb (e.g. distal forearm) by the attenuation of weak X-ray beams by techniques such as single photon absorptiometry. Such instruments have been superseded by new machines capable of measuring total body bone mineral, and also estimating total body water and fat mass. However, these new instruments (usually called dual-energy X-ray absorptiometers, DXA) are very large and often located several hundred metres from the NICU, severely limiting their usefulness. Some studies have been undertaken in preterm infants,[50] but the technique is not as yet in widespread use.

ABNORMAL BONE REMODELLING (Fig. 38.15)

Radiological abnormalities (rachitic changes, fractures) are occasionally seen at birth in very growth-retarded infants, presumably secondary to inadequate transplacental substrate supply. The majority of infants developing radiological abnormalities weigh less than 1000 g at birth, receive diets grossly deficient in mineral substrate, or both. Such diets include intravenous solutions formulated with inorganic mineral salts and unsupplemented breast milk.

A useful scoring system based on single-view radiographs of the wrist or ankle at postnatal ages 5 and 10 weeks was described by Koo in 1982.[33] Lyon[38] found that over 70% of infants weighing less than 1000 g had evidence of abnormal remodelling using this system. In older reports, epiphyseal cupping, splaying and fraying and craniotabes were observed in as many as 50% of infants of less than 33 weeks' gestation. Fractures of the ribs and long bones were also widely reported.[22,61,63] Perhaps the most comprehensive description is that of Eek et al in 1957,[22] which includes numerous plates showing the radiological changes that occur with increasing postnatal age.

EFFECTS OF DRUGS AND IMMOBILIZATION

Steroids reduce bone turnover, but also reduce linear growth. Despite the association of steroid use with osteoporosis in adults, there has been no convincing demonstration of a similar effect in preterm infants. There are, however, suggestions that steroid administration may lead to permanent stunting in some infants, and the appearance of the steroid-treated infant with BPD is certainly suggestive of Cushing syndrome and/or growth hormone deficiency. Frusemide causes hypercalciuria, but again no convincing effect on growth or mineral accretion has been demonstrated.

Immobilization leads to disuse osteoporosis in older children and adults. Moyer-Mileur et al[42] showed a substantial gain in forearm BMC in infants undergoing up to 10 minutes of passive exercise per day over a 4-week period compared to matched controls.

BONE OUTCOMES – GROWTH, RISK OF FRACTURES AND MINERAL ACCRETION

GROWTH

Raised plasma alkaline phosphatase activity (>5 times maximum normal adult range) during the period of hospitalization was associated with reduced stature at 18 months post-term age.[36] Other groups have reported similar findings.[35]

FRACTURES

In a retrospective analysis over a 7-year period we were unable to demonstrate any difference in fracture incidence between children born at term or preterm,[17] although there was a trend towards presentation with fracture at less than 2 years of age for infants born at less than 33 weeks' gestation. Others have reported an increased fracture incidence in preterm infants with rachitic changes.[34]

BONE MINERAL ACCRETION

Debate continues over the natural history of bone mineral accretion in preterm infants after discharge from hospital. Some suggest a period of rapid 'catch-up', usually by 8–16 weeks post-term age,[15,43,44] such that appendicular bone mineral content estimated for preterm infants is similar to that of term infants, but not all reports support these findings.[5,12] Increasing the mineral content of the post-discharge diet is associated with improved bone mineral accretion rates.[5,12] Many infants show a continuing deficit in radial bone mineral content up to age 1 year.[34,52] Beyond this time there appears to be a gradual catch-up,[53] and then from the age of 2 years continued mineral accretion to levels higher than those seen in children born at term.[46]

Diet may have an effect on bone mineral accretion in later childhood. We measured forearm BMC by SPA in 54 children who had received either donated pasteurized breast milk or preterm formula as a supplement to their own mother's milk.[3,7] The larger the proportion of human milk in the diet, the greater the later bone mineral content. The use of standard deviation scores adjusting for body size[6,19] showed that, compared to children of similar body size born at term, the children born prematurely who had received mostly human milk (maternal, donated or both) had significantly higher than expected bone mineral content.[7]

These follow-up studies together suggest that infants disconnected prematurely from placental growth-regulating activity tend to have greater than expected BMC in later childhood. There is also a clear effect of early dietary mineral intake on later BMC.

TREATMENT: PREVENTION IS BETTER THAN CURE

The objective of treatment should be first, the prevention of abnormal bone-remodelling activity during the period of hospitalization, and secondly the optimization of growth potential. It is clear that inadequate mineral supply, particularly of phosphate, is the principal aetiological factor, and therapeutic strategies are suggested with this in mind. As with all facets of neonatology, the smallest, sickest infants are at the greatest risk and pose the greatest challenge in terms of nutrient delivery.

Organic phosphate solutions (sodium glycerophosphate, glucose-1-phosphate) are now available for parenteral administration and, in combination with inorganic calcium solutions, could provide mineral substrate before intravenous feeding is started. The substantially improved cosolubility of these compounds with calcium salts means that the theoretical in-utero accretion rate of each could be maintained postnatally for any parenterally nourished infant.[16]

All enterally fed preterm infants should receive 2 mmol/kg/day of phosphate. Phosphate retention is of the order of 90–95%. For the infant receiving human milk, with a typical phosphate content of 0.5 mmol/100 ml, this means a total daily supplement when on full feeds of 1 mmol/kg/day of phosphate. For infants receiving preterm formula, further supplements should not be necessary. Term formula is not an acceptable diet for preterm infants.[37] The practice in most NICUs is to start oral phosphate supplements when the oral intake is 2 ml/hour. Once phosphate supplementation is adequate, a relative deficiency of calcium may become evident.[55] Such a deficiency is evidenced by radiological osteopenia and high plasma alkaline phosphatase activity in the face of normal plasma phosphate (i.e. >1.8 mmol/l). Calcium supplementation is then warranted. If both calcium and phosphate are being added to human milk, the phosphate should be added first and allowed to stand for at least 5 minutes, followed by the calcium; coprecipitation is thereby kept to a minimum. There is no place for the use of active metabolites of vitamin D, other than in the treatment of rare inherited disorders (see below).

At present, we support the recommendation that all infants should receive 400 IU/day vitamin D. It is not at all clear that supplements beyond this amount are associated with improved long-term outcome, except in situations where vitamin D deficiency can be shown.

Passive physical exercise substantially improves weight gain and bone mineral accretion in these infants, and should be considered a routine part of care.

INHERITED METABOLIC BONE DISEASE

RACHITIC DISORDERS

The three principal inherited types of rickets rarely present in the neonatal period, but clinical suspicion may indicate investigation where there is a relevant family history. Hypophosphatasia, although not generally classified as a form of rickets, is characterized by excessive osteoid accumulation and so is included here.

Familial (X-linked) hypophosphataemic rickets

Classic familial hypophosphataemic rickets is an X-linked dominant condition characterized by renal phosphate wasting and a defective osteoblastic response to vitamin D metabolites.[20,21] There are a few reported cases with autosomal recessive inheritance. Typical biochemical changes include hypophosphataemia, elevated plasma alkaline phosphatase activity and hyperphosphaturia. Treatment with oral phosphate and calcitriol is not usually tolerated until the age of 6 months. Although mutations in a specific region of the X chromosome have now been characterized,[30] it is unclear how the protein product of the affected gene (PEX) influences vitamin D and phosphate metabolism.

A variant form has been described ('hereditary hypophosphataemic rickets') in which affected infants show muscle weakness, hypercalciuria and elevated plasma calcitriol, in addition to hypophosphataemia.[25]

Hypocalcaemic vitamin D-resistant rickets

This rare autosomal recessive disorder arises because of a non-functioning vitamin D receptor. Neonatal presentation is unusual. Clinical signs are persistent hypocalcaemia, elevated plasma 1,25-(OH)2D3 and rachitic changes on X-ray, and alopecia.[40] Treatment is difficult. Some cases have responded to regular intravenous infusions of calcium[64] followed by large oral doses;[49] patients with alopecia respond less well.

Pseudo-vitamin D deficiency rickets

This autosomal recessive disorder results from defective activity of the 25-hydroxyvitamin D1α hydroxylase enzyme. The clinical picture is of a rachitic, apathetic infant, typically 4–6 months old, with hypocalcaemia who fails to thrive and may have fits.[2] The condition responds completely to treatment with calcitriol.[24]

Hypophosphatasia (p. 880)

Hypophosphatasia is an autosomal recessive disorder characterized by the congenital absence of bone/liver/kidney-specific alkaline phosphatase in all tissues and serum.[65] Other biochemical abnormalities include urinary excretion of inorganic pyrophosphate and phospho-ethanolamine. Chorionic villus sampling has been successfully applied in affected families.[8] Cases presenting early are characterized by severely defective osteogenesis and defective mineralization. There are case reports of successful treatment with frequent fresh plasma infusions,[66] but at least 50% of affected infants die.

DISORDERS OF OSTEOGENESIS

A problem with osteogenesis may be suggested antenatally by ultrasound demonstration of shortened limbs after 20 weeks' gestation.

Osteogenesis imperfecta

The diagnosis of osteogenesis imperfecta remains difficult because of the extreme variability in phenotype[57] and the lack of a definitive biochemical test for the disorder. Genetic studies looking for the individual mutations typical in types III and IV can be lengthy and tedious when using fibroblast cultures, although screening using heteroduplex analysis on cell extracts may give results after as little as 2 weeks (Roughley P, personal communication). Fractures at birth may occur in any type of OI, most frequently in children with types II–IV. OI type I (characterized by a 50% deficit in type I collagen production, autosomal dominant (AD) inheritance) rarely causes problems in the neonatal period. Types II–IV result from mutations in the collagen gene that affect the protein's ability to form the normal triple helices.

Type II is uniformly lethal. It is important to make the diagnosis, however, since parental germline mutations effectively create an AD inheritance, engendering a significant risk of a second affected child.[14]

Multiple early fractures leading to limb shortening are characteristic of OI III; affected infants typically have blue sclerae. In contrast to infants with OI II, there are few rib fractures and hence no thoracic dysplasia. Differentiating types III and IV is really only possible postneonatally, although children with OI IV usually have white rather than blue sclerae. Lax skin and ligaments are seen in all types. Postneonatally, the principal differential diagnosis is non-accidental injury; in such cases the debate can often only be resolved by the passage of time or the use of invasive techniques such as skin or bone biopsy.

Thanatophoric dwarfism

Both type I (cloverleaf skull, curved femora, marked platyspondyly) and type II (cloverleaf skull, short, straight long bones, mild platyspondyly) thanatophoric dwarfism result from mutations in fibroblast growth factor receptor 3 gene.[60] Mutations in other parts of the same gene are responsible for achondroplasia and hypochondroplasia.

OSTEOPETROSIS

The clinical features of 'marble bones' and immunodeficiency in the autosomal recessive form arise from defective osteoclastic (bone-resorbing) activity and reduced leukocyte superoxide production. Pancytopenia is common, and retinal degeneration reported from age 2 months.[23] Treatment with interferon-γ_{1b} is usually effective;[32] it is not yet clear whether this treatment obviates the need for later bone marrow transplantation.

REFERENCES

1. Atkinson S A, Ingeborg C, Radde M D, Anderson G H 1983 Macromineral balances in premature infants fed their own mothers' milk or formula. Journal of Pediatrics 102: 99–106
2. Balsan S 1991 Hereditary pseudo-deficiency rickets or vitamin D-dependency type I. In: Glorieux F H (ed.) Rickets. Vevey/Raven Press Ltd, New York, pp 155–165
3. Bishop N J 1993 Bone mineralisation in preterm infants: effect of early diet. MD Thesis, University of Manchester
4. Bishop N J 1994 Bone growth and mineralisation in infants born preterm. Growth Matters International 15: 10–12
5. Bishop N J, King F J, Lucas A 1993 Increased bone mineral content of preterm infants fed with a nutrient enriched formula after discharge from hospital. Archives of Disease in Childhood 68: 573–578
6. Bishop N J, DePriester J A, Cole T J, Lucas A 1992 Reference values for radial bone width and mineral content in healthy children aged 4 to 10 years. Acta Pediatrica 81: 463–468
7. Bishop N J, Dahlenburg S L, Fewtrell M S, Morley R, Lucas A 1996 Early diet of preterm infants and bone mineralisation at age 5 years. Acta Paediatrica 85: 230–236
8. Brock D J, Barron L 1991 First-trimester prenatal diagnosis of hypophosphatasia: experience with 16 cases. Prenatal Diagnosis 11: 387–391
9. Callenbach J, Sheenhan M B, Abramson S J, Hall R T 1981 Etiologic factors in rickets of very low-birth-weight infants. Journal of Pediatrics 98: 800–805
10. Carey D E, Hopfer S M 1987 Hypophosphataemic rickets with hypercalciuria and microglobulinuria. Journal of Pediatrics 111: 860–863
11. Carey D E, Goetz C A, Horak E, Rowe J C 1985 Phosphorus wasting during phosphorus supplementation of human milk feedings in preterm infants. Journal of Pediatrics 107: 790–794
12. Chan G M 1993 Growth and bone mineral status of discharged very low birth weight infants fed different formulas or human milk. Journal of Pediatrics 123: 439–443
13. Chan G M, Mileur L, Hansen J W 1988 Calcium and phosphorus

requirements in bone mineralization of preterm infants. Journal of Pediatrics 113: 225–229
14. Cole G C 1994 Osteogenesis imperfecta as a consequence of naturally occurring and induced mutations of type I collagen. In: Heersche J N M, Kanis J A (eds) Bone and mineral research. Elsevier, Amsterdam, pp 167–204
15. Congden P J, Horsman A, Ryan S W, Truscott J G, Durward H 1990 Spontaneous resolution of bone mineral depletion in preterm infants. Archives of Disease in Childhood 65: 1038–1042
16. Costello I, Powell C, Williams A F 1995 Sodium glycerophosphate in the treatment of neonatal hypophosphataemia. Archives of Disease in Childhood 73: F44–45
17. Dahlenburg S L, Bishop N J, Lucas A 1989 Are preterm infants at risk for subsequent fractures? Archives of Disease in Childhood 64: 1384–1385
18. Delvin E E, Salle B L, Glorieux F H, Adelaine P, David L S 1986 Vitamin D supplementation during pregnancy: effect on neonatal calcium homeostasis. Journal of Pediatrics 109: 328–334
19. DePriester J A, Cole T J, Bishop N J 1991 Bone growth and mineralisation in children aged 4 to 10 years. Bone Mineral 12: 57–65
20. Ecarot B, Caverzasio J, Desbarats M, Bonjour J-P, Glorieux F H 1994 Phosphate transport by osteoblasts from X-linked hypophosphataemic mice. American Journal of Physiology 266: E33–E38
21. Ecarot B, Glorieux F H, Desbarats M, Travers R, Labelle L 1992 Defective bone formation by hyp mouse bone cells transplanted into normal mice: evidence in favor of an intrinsic osteoblast defect. Journal of Bone and Mineral Research 7: 215–220
22. Eek S, Gabrielson L H, Halvorsen S 1957 Prematurity and rickets. Pediatrics 20: 63–77
23. Gerritsen E J, Vossen J M, van Loo I H et al 1994 Autosomal recessive osteopetrosis: variability of findings at diagnosis and during the natural course. Pediatrics 93: 247–253
24. Glorieux F H 1990 Calcitriol treatment in vitamin D-dependent and vitamin D-resistant rickets. Metabolism 39(Suppl 1): 10–20
25. Glorieux F H 1991 Rickets, the continuing challenge. New England Journal of Medicine 325: 1875–1877
26. Greer F R, McCormick A 1988 Improved bone mineralization and growth in premature infants fed fortified own mother's milk. Journal of Pediatrics 112: 961–969 [published erratum appears in 113(6): 1118]
27. Greer F R, Steichen J J, Tsang R C 1982 Calcium and phosphate supplements in breast milk-related rickets. American Journal of Diseases of Children 136: 581–583
28. Gross S J 1983 Growth and biochemical response of preterm infants fed human milk or modified formula. New England Journal of Medicine 308: 237–241
29. Hillman L S, Hoff N, Salmons S, Martin L, McAlister W, Haddad J 1985 Mineral homeostasis in very premature infants: serial evaluation of serum 25-hydroxyvitamin D, serum minerals, and bone mineralization. Journal of Pediatrics 106: 970–980
30. Hyp Consortium 1995 A gene (PEX) with homologies to endopeptidases is mutated in patients with X-linked hypophosphatemic rickets. Nature Genetics 11: 130–136
31. James J R, Congdon P J, Truscott J, Horsman A, Arthur R 1986 Osteopenia of prematurity. Archives of Disease in Childhood 61: 871–876
32. Key L L, Rodriguez R M, Willi S M et al 1995 Long-term treatment of osteopetrosis with recombinant interferon gamma. New England Journal of Medicine 332: 1594–1599
33. Koo W W K, Gupta J M, Nayanar V V, Wilkinson M, Posen S 1982 Skeletal changes in preterm infants. Archives of Disease in Childhood 57: 447–452
34. Koo W W, Sherman R, Succop P et al 1988 Sequential bone mineral content in small preterm infants with and without fractures and rickets. Journal of Bone and Mineral Research 3: 193–197
35. Kovar I, Mayne P, Barltrop D 1982 Plasma alkaline phosphatase activity: a screening test for rickets in preterm infants. Lancet i: 308–310
36. Lucas A, Brooke O G, Baker B A, Bishop N, Morley R 1989 High plasma alkaline phosphatase activity and growth in preterm neonates. Archives of Disease in Childhood 64: 902–909
37. Lucas A, Morley R, Cole T J et al 1990 Early diet in preterm infants and developmental status at 18 months. Lancet 335: 1477–1481
38. Lyon A J, McIntosh N, Wheeler K, Williams J E 1987 Radiological rickets in extremely low birthweight infants. Pediatric Radiology 17: 56–58
39. Lyon A J, McIntosh N, Wheeler K, Brooke O G 1984 Hypercalcaemia in extremely low birthweight infants. Archives of Disease in Childhood 59: 1141–1144
40. Marx S J 1991 1,25-dihydroxyvitamin D_3 receptors and resistance: implications in rickets, osteomalacia, and other conditions. In: Glorieux F H (ed) Rickets. Vevey/Raven Press Ltd, New York, pp 167–184
41. Michaelson K F, Johansen J S, Samuelson G, Price P A, Christiansen C 1992 Serum bone gamma-carboxyglutamic acid protein in a longitudinal study of infants: lower values in formula-fed infants. Pediatric Research 31: 401–405
42. Moyer-Mileur L, Luetkemeier M, Boomer L, Chan G M 1995 Effect of physical activity on bone mineralisation in preterm infants. Journal of Pediatrics 127: 620–625
43. Pettifor J M, Rajah R, Venter A et al 1989 Bone mineralization and mineral homeostasis in very low-birth-weight infants fed either human milk or fortified human milk. Journal of Pediatric Gastroenterology and Nutrition 8: 217–224
44. Pittard W B III, Geddes K M, Sutherland S E, Miller M C, Hollis B W 1990 Longitudinal changes in the bone mineral content of term and premature infants. American Journal of Diseases of Children 144: 36–40
45. Romagnolli C, Zecca E, Tortorolo G, Diodato A, Fazzini G, Sorcini-Carta M 1987 Plasma thyrocalcitonin and parathyroid hormone concentrations in early neonatal hypocalcaemia. Archives of Disease in Childhood 62: 580–584
46. Rubinacci A, Sirtori P, Moro G, Galli L, Minoli I, Tessari L 1993 Is there an impact of birth weight and early life nutrition on bone mineral content in preterm born infants and children? Acta Paediatrica 82: 711–713
47. Ryan S W, Truscott J, Simpson M, James J 1993 Phosphate, alkaline phosphatase and bone mineralisation in preterm neonates. Acta Paediatrica 82: 518–521
48. Sagy M, Birenbaum E, Balin A, Orda S, Barzilay Z, Brish M 1980 Phosphate-depletion syndrome in a premature infant fed human milk. Journal of Pediatrics 96: 683–685
49. Sakati N, Woodhouse N J Y, Niles N, Harfi H, de Grange D A, Marx S 1986 Hereditary resistance to 1,25-dihydroxyvitamin D: clinical and radiological improvement during high-dose oral calcium therapy. Hormone Research 24: 280–287
50. Salle B L, Glorieux F H 1993 Assessment of bone mineral content in infants: the new age. Acta Paediatrica 82: 709–710
51. Salle B L, Glorieux F H, Delvin E E 1988 Perinatal vitamin D metabolism. Biology of the Neonate 54: 181–187
52. Salle B L, Braillon P, Glorieux F H, Brunet J, Cavero E, Meunier P J 1992 Bone mineral content (BMC) of the lumbar spine in preterm infants: a longitudinal study during the first year of life. Pediatric Research 31: 294A
53. Schanler R J, Burns P A, Abrams S A, Garza C 1992 Bone mineralisation outcomes in human milk-fed preterm infants. Pediatric Research 31: 583–586
54. Seki K, Furuya K, Makimura N, Mitsui C, Hirata J, Nagata I 1994 Cord blood levels of calcium-regulating hormones and osteocalcin in premature infants. Journal of Perinatal Medicine 22: 189–194
55. Senterre J 1991 Osteopenia versus rickets in premature infants. In: Glorieux F H (ed) Rickets. Vevey/Raven Press Ltd, New York, pp 145–154
56. Senterre J, Salle B 1982 Calcium and phosphorus economy of the preterm infant and its interaction with vitamin D and its metabolites. Acta Pediatrica Scandinavica Suppl 296: 85–92
57. Sillence D D, Senn A, Danks D M 1979 Genetic heterogeneity in osteogenesis imperfecta. Journal of Medical Genetics 16: 101–116
58. Steichen J J, Asch P A, Tsang R C 1988 Bone mineral content measurement in small infants by single-photon absorptiometry: current methodologic issues. Journal of Pediatrics 113: 181–187
59. Steichen J J, Gratton T L, Tsang R C 1980 Osteopenia of prematurity: the cause and possible treatment. Journal of Pediatrics 96: 528–534
60. Tavormina P L, Shiang R, Thompson L M et al 1995 Thanatophoric dysplasia (types I and II) caused by distinct mutations in fibroblast growth factor receptor 3. Nature Genetics 9: 321–328
61. Tulloch A L 1974 Rickets in the premature. Medical Journal of Australia i: 137–140
62. Venkataraman P S, Blick K E 1988 Effect of mineral supplementation of human milk on bone mineral content and trace element metabolism. Journal of Pediatrics 113: 220–224
63. Von Sydow G 1946 A study of the development of rickets in premature infants. Acta Paediatrica 33(Suppl. 2)

64. Weisman Y, Bab I, Gazit D, Spirer Z, Jaffe M, Hochberg Z 1987 Long-term intracaval calcium infusion therapy in end-organ resistance to 1,25-dihydroxyvitamin D. American Journal of Medicine 83: 984–990
65. Whyte M P, McAlister W H, Patton L S et al 1984 Enzyme replacement for infantile hypophosphatasia attempted by infusions of alkaline-phosphatase-rich Paget plasma: results in three additional patients. Journal of Pediatrics 105: 926–933
66. Whyte M P, Magill H L, Fallon M D, Herrod H G 1986 Infantile hypophosphatasia: normalisation of circulating alkaline phosphatase activity followed by skeletal remineralisation. Journal of Pediatrics 108: 82–88
67. Ziegler E E, O'Donnell A M, Nelson S E 1976 Body composition of the reference fetus. Growth 40: 329–341

39

Disorders of the kidneys and urinary tract

Part 1

Renal function, fluid and electrolyte balance and neonatal renal disease

Neena Modi

PHYSIOLOGY

INTRODUCTION

Problems with fluid balance are not uncommon in newborn infants, who differ from other age groups in several important respects. Neonatal physiology is not static, as developmental changes continue and are particularly rapid in very immature infants. The immediate postnatal period is a time during which the transition from the fluid, intrauterine environment to the gaseous, postnatal environment must be successfully made, and postnatal adaptation of extrarenal systems may also affect fluid balance. Finally, the added influences of underlying pathology, acute illness and medication may be superimposed. This chapter will discuss the regulation of fluid balance and its management in the newborn from the perspective of the clinician.

DEVELOPMENTAL PHYSIOLOGY

Renal growth and blood supply

The first definitive nephrons arise during the fifth week of gestation and become functional by around 8 weeks. Nephrons are formed in a centrifugal manner, and at 22 weeks' gestation are all juxtamedullary.[128] These are the earliest nephrons to mature, are associated with the longest loops of Henle and have the greatest role in sodium conservation. The development of new glomeruli occurs only slowly in the last trimester, and is complete by 34–36 weeks' postconceptional age, by which time each kidney contains the full complement of one million nephrons.[104] Renal growth thereafter depends on an increase in the size and number of cells of the existing nephrons. Birth does not accelerate nephrogenesis.[127]

The renal blood supply arises from the aorta between T12 and L2, a relationship that remains constant between 24 and 44 weeks.[125] As the renal artery divides into segmental end-arteries, the renal tissue in their area of distribution is very vulnerable to ischaemia. Umbilical arterial catheters should therefore be positioned to end either above or below this region (p. 363). Division gives rise, in turn, to interlobar, arcuate and interlobular arteries, from the last of which afferent arterioles lead to glomeruli. The venous drainage, unlike the arterial system, has anastomoses at several levels. The fetal kidneys receive approximately 3% of the combined cardiac output, and after birth this rises to between 20 and 30%. During development there is a centrifugal redistribution of blood flow, in keeping with the pattern of glomerular and tubular growth. After birth, a fall in renal vascular resistance also increases renal blood flow.

An anatomical glomerulotubular imbalance exists, in that the glomeruli are relatively larger than the tubules, with a glomerular surface area/proximal tubular volume ratio about 10 times that seen in adults,[53] but glomerular and tubular functions develop in parallel. Kidney length increases from a mean of 27 mm at 24 weeks' gestation, to 37 mm at 32 weeks and 44 mm at term.[71]

The last decade has seen major advances in our understanding of the molecular basis of nephrogenesis. It is now known that many of the transcription factors, growth factors and oncogenes involved in the regulation of gene expression in the embryo are expressed during nephrogenesis.[10] This is discussed further in the section on congenital kidney disorders (p. 1031).

Glomerular filtration

Glomerular filtration is the process by which water and solutes pass across the glomerular membrane. Glomerular filtrate is identical in composition to plasma, except that it contains no fat and very little protein. Glomerular filtration is dependent on renal perfusion pressure and renal blood flow. It is difficult to assess in the newborn, requiring the measurement in plasma and urine of a substance that is freely filtered at the glomerulus and neither secreted nor reabsorbed by the renal tubules. Insulin clearance remains the 'gold standard', but in the newborn requires either a constant infusion over 24 hours or a single injection combined with urine collection and repeated blood sampling over 5 hours.[34] In practice, endogenous creatinine clearance is an acceptable alternative as it agrees closely with inulin clearance, if interference from non-creatinine chromogens in plasma is removed,[39] as is the case with modern automated creatinine analysers utilizing reaction rate analysis.

The interpretation of measurements of GFR has been an area of considerable confusion in the past, partly because of different methods of expression.[37] Although in adults GFR is expressed per unit surface area, it has long been argued that weight is the best standard in the newborn, as weight, rather than surface area, most closely reflects the size of the extracellular compartment, which is the fluid pool affected by the kidney.[103] During adult life the ratio of surface area to weight changes little. In contrast, it falls by a third between 27 weeks' gestation and term (Fig. 39.1). Table 39.1 shows how different methods of expression of GFR can give very different impressions of the relationship between GFR in a 1 kg baby with a surface area of approximately 0.1 m^2 and an adult weighing 70 kg, with a surface area of 1.7 m^2. The important point is that in both the GFR is appropriate to metabolic need.

The pattern of maturation of glomerular filtration has also been described in conflicting ways, but when differences in expression are eliminated, GFR can be shown to rise logarithmically with increasing postconceptional age and to be independent of postnatal age and birthweight[35] (Fig. 39.2).

In clinical practice the serum creatinine concentration is the most widely used index of glomerular filtration rate, and this is discussed further below. Urea is a very poor marker, as it is influenced by many non-renal factors.[39] In older children the accuracy of estimating glomerular filtration rate from serum creatinine concentration can be improved by factoring for body length, but in neonates

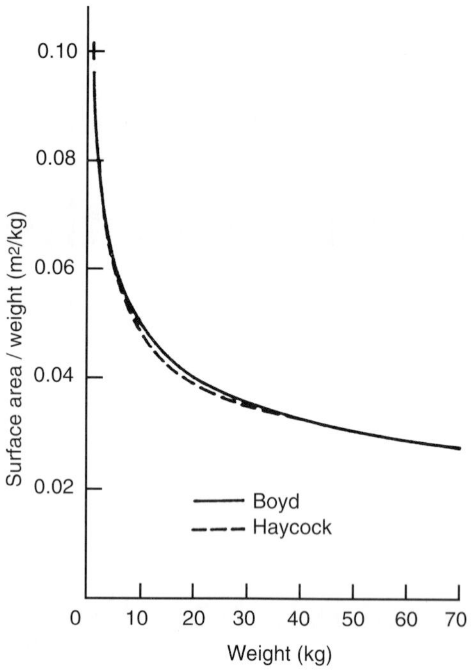

Fig. 39.1 Relation between surface area to weight ratio and body weight, calculated from the data of Boyd[23] and Haycock et al[77]. (Reproduced with permission from Coulthard and Hey[37])

Table 39.1 The effect of different methods of expression of GFR

	Adult	Preterm neonate
Weight (kg)	70	1
Surface area (m^2)	1.7	0.1
GFR expressed as		
ml/min	140	0.5
ml/min/m^2	80	5
ml/min/kg	2	0.5

this is unhelpful because, as discussed above, glomerular filtration does not vary with surface area.

Tubular function

Regulation of sodium balance

Neonates, especially if preterm, have a relatively limited capacity both to excrete and to conserve sodium. Limited sodium excretion is primarily responsible for most of the difficulties in the management of sodium balance in the first days after birth. In contrast, poor retention predominantly leads to difficulties after the first week.

The first step in sodium reabsorption occurs in the proximal tubule (Fig. 39.3). Here, the absorption of sodium and water is isotonic and regulated by hydrostatic and osmotic forces. The descending limb of the loop of Henle is impermeable to sodium. In the thick ascending limb chloride is actively transported in conjunction with other ions, followed by sodium. Finally, sodium is reabsorbed in the distal tubule and to a small extent (around 3%) in the collecting ducts. Distal tubular

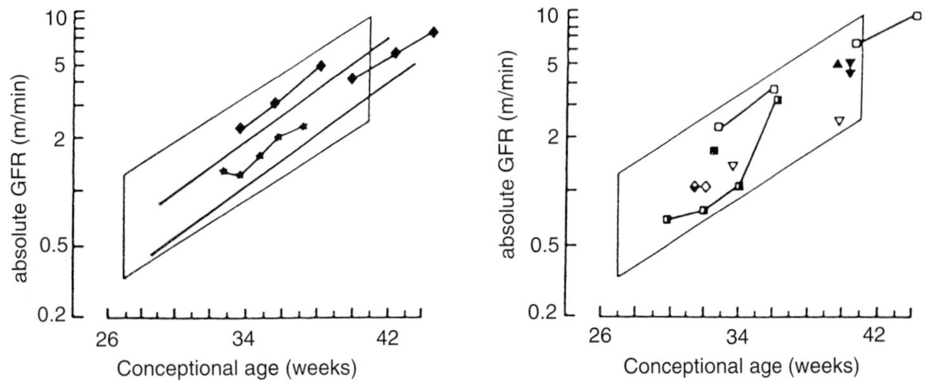

Fig. 39.2 Effect of postconceptional age on absolute GFR (taken from the data of Coulthard 1985[35]). The boxes represent the confidence limits for the data from that study and the other lines and symbols the results from 12 other studies. (Reproduced with permission from Coulthard[36])

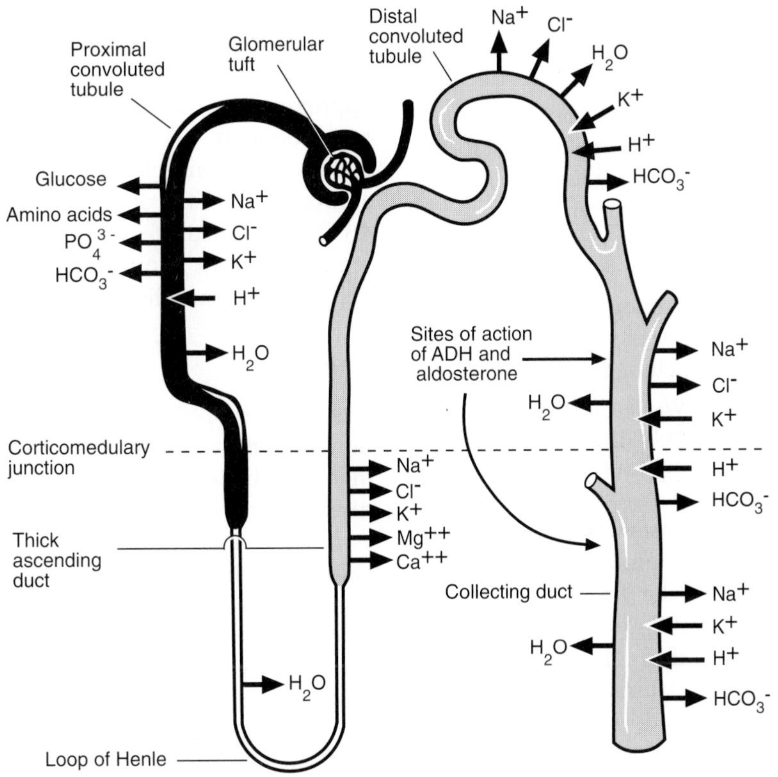

Fig. 39.3 Excretion of water and electrolytes. Water is reabsorbed in the proximal tubule together with glucose, amino acids, phosphate, sodium and bicarbonate, and from the distal nephron under the influence of ADH and the hypertonic medulla. In the distal tubule sodium is reabsorbed under the influence of aldosterone with associated excretion of potassium and hydrogen ions. (Reproduced with permission from Cumming and Swainson[42])

sodium reabsorption, exchanging sodium for potassium, is regulated via the renin–angiotensin–aldosterone system.

The sodium retention that characterizes growth is due to the influence of very high RAAS activity.[154] The renal salt wasting seen in preterm babies below 32 weeks' gestation is due both to impaired reabsorption at the proximal tubule, resulting in a higher distal sodium delivery, and to limited aldosterone responsiveness at the distal tubule.[160] Intestinal absorption is also limited.[3] Conversely, acute sodium loading in neonates results in only a blunted fall in RAAS activity and limited natriuretic response.[45] The limited capacity to excrete a sodium load cannot be attributed to a low GFR, because filtration, in even the most immature neonate, greatly exceeds the amount that is ultimately retained. Homeostasis is dependent on the regulation of tubular reabsorption, a process which also undergoes developmental maturation.

$Na^+K^+ATPase$ is the enzyme responsible for active sodium transport in all eukaryotic cells. There are many forms of $Na^+K^+ATPase$, each encoded by specific groups of $Na^+K^+ATPase$ genes. In renal tubular cells $Na^+K^+ATPase$, present on the basolateral membrane, creates an electrochemical gradient which is the energy source for the cotransport, involving specific transporter proteins, of Na^+ and glucose and Na^+ and amino acids and the countertransport of Na^+ and H^+ across the luminal membrane. The long-term regulation of sodium balance is brought about by changes in the abundance of sodium transporters. During ontogenesis there are tissue-specific patterns of increase in activity, accompanied by an increase in $Na^+K^+ATPase$ mRNA.[121] Glucocorticoid treatment, as used to promote lung maturation, increases the abundance of $Na^+K^+ATPase$ in both lungs and kidney, as well as enhancing the maturation of renal tubular transport (see below).

The postnatal enhancement in sodium conservation is brought about by increasing responsiveness of the distal tubule to aldosterone[2,159] and by an increase in the abundance of $Na^+K^+ATPase$ and transporter proteins.[76,80] The ability to excrete a sodium load also matures during development. An increase or decrease in the activity of renal $Na^+K^+ATPase$ is the final common pathway for the short-term regulation of natriuresis.[7] Downregulatory factors, which cause natriuresis, include ANP, dopamine and diuretics. Noradrenaline is an upregulatory factor, which results in sodium retention. The peptide regulatory factors bind to cell membrane receptors and exert their effects via a cascade of intracellular messengers. There is increasing evidence that these intracellular signalling systems are also subject to developmental maturation, with a resulting enhancement in the fine-tuning of the regulation of sodium balance.[47,57,88,109,155] Clinical observations offer some substantiation of these in vitro studies. Atrial natriuretic peptide stimulates membrane-bound guanylate cyclase, which leads to an increase in the intracellular second messenger, cGMP, generated from endogenous GTP. Cyclic GMP interacts with specific protein kinases, which in turn catalyse the phosphorylation of several protein substrates, and finally leads to a biological effect such as inhibition of sodium reabsorption. In a study of preterm babies[109] the ratio of urinary cGMP to ANP was found to increase exponentially in the first 3 days after birth, and then to reach a plateau. The ratio of sodium excretion to cGMP continued to increase over the 10 days of the study. This suggests a postnatal maturation in the ANP/cGMP/sodium excretion cascade and thus an increasing postnatal ability to excrete sodium.

These observations offer some insight into the cellular processes underlying the developmental regulation of sodium balance, and some explanation of why the end-organ responses to factors that govern sodium retention and excretion are blunted early in development, but undergo rapid maturation. They open a window onto future possibilities for therapeutic enhancement of tissue maturation.

Potassium

A major proportion of filtered potassium is actively reabsorbed in the proximal tubule and in the ascending limb of the loop of Henle. In the distal nephron aldosterone stimulates the active transport of potassium from the peritubular fluid into the cells, from where a potential gradient favours the diffusion of potassium from cells to lumen. Unrecognized negative potassium balance may be relatively common in neonates receiving intensive care. It is all too easy to mask a falling serum potassium if blood samples are slightly haemolysed. Engle and Arant[48] found that newborns with respiratory distress syndrome had a mean cumulative negative potassium balance of approximately 4 mmol/kg by day 4. This represents approximately 10% of the estimated total body potassium content of 46 mmol/kg. Preterm neonates should receive a potassium intake of 2 mmol/kg/day, commencing within 48 hours of birth if urine output is satisfactory and there are no concerns about renal function. Hyperkalaemia and hypokalaemia are discussed below.

Chloride

Chloride is predominantly an extracellular anion. The normal serum level is 90–110 mmol/l. Urinary losses are increased by loop diuretics, and infants with chronic lung disease on prolonged treatment with diuretics are especially vulnerable to hypochloraemia. A serum chloride below 90 mmol/l has been associated with a poorer outcome.[123] Hyperchloraemia may occur with some parenteral nutrition formulations and should be considered in the investigation of metabolic acidosis. Partly replacing chloride with acetate in parenteral nutrition has been shown to reduce hyperchloraemic metabolic acidosis.[124]

Renal water handling

As nutrition can only be provided to babies in liquid form, a high fluid intake is mandatory and the baby must have a high urine flow in order to maintain water balance. A high urine flow rate is achieved by a much greater fractional excretion of glomerular filtrate (Fe_{H_2O}). Reabsorption at the proximal tubule is isotonic, and in newborn babies decreased hydrostatic and osmotic forces across the peritubular space result in decreased proximal tubular reabsorption of filtered water. A greater proportion of water is therefore delivered distally, compared to older subjects. In the distal nephron water reabsorption is regulated by ADH (antidiuretic hormone, also known as arginine vasopressin, AVP). In the presence of ADH the collecting duct becomes permeable to water, which moves passively across the tubular membrane in response to the high concentration of the medullary interstitium. Fetal animals and preterm babies are sensitive to ADH.[49] Although preterm babies are able to achieve similar minimal urine osmolalities to adults, with values of 50 mmol/kg or less,[38,180] the maximum urine osmolality is about 600–800 mmol/kg, compared to twice this in older subjects. This difference is due both to shorter loops of Henle and to reduced tonicity of the medullary interstitium, as urea concentrations are low because of the highly anabolic state of the rapidly growing infant. Higher urine concentrations can, however, be produced under conditions of severe dehydration stress.

The peak urine flow of mature infants given a water load is the same as that of adults, when expressed per unit body water.[102] Coulthard and Hey[38] have also challenged the view that newborns have a limited capacity for water excretion. They showed that healthy preterm babies are able to adjust water excretion appropriately from the second day after birth, when their daily intakes were varied between 95 and 200 ml/kg, sodium intake remaining constant. The Fe_{H_2O} increased from a mean of 7.4% to 13.1% of the filtered volume with the higher intake. A similarly high Fe_{H_2O} in adults would result in a daily urine volume of over 20 l. It is of note that there was no concomitant increase in the loss of sodium in the urine, an observation that refutes the widely held view that babies are unable to sustain a high urine flow without an inevitable increase in the loss of sodium.

Given a diluting and concentrating capacity that extends from 50 to 600 mOsmol/kg and a renal solute load of approximately 10–15 mOsmol/kg,[180] the maximum and minimum urine flow rates that preterm infants can achieve are 300 and 25 ml/kg/24 h, respectively. The latter value, which represents the minimum urine flow rate beyond which solute retention would result, approximates to 1 ml/kg/h and is the justification for the use of this figure as a clinical indication of renal failure. The former volume is greater than the amount available from glomerular filtration in many preterm babies, so that diluting ability is unlikely to limit water excretion. For example, a baby below 30 weeks' gestation with a GFR of around 0.8 ml/kg/min[35,110] would have a maximum volume of about 230 ml/kg/day available for excretion, given that about 20% of the filtrate would be delivered distally. Certainly most preterm babies are able to achieve a urine flow rate of around 7 ml/kg/h, and Leake et al[95] showed that babies between 28 and 34 weeks' gestation could increase urine flow rate to a mean of 12 ml/kg/h during acute increases in infusion rates to 250 ml/kg/day. In the absence of evidence of renal impairment there is therefore no justification for 'running babies dry', a practice which increases the risks of hypernatraemia and reduces nutritional intake.

Renal regulation of acid–base balance

In order of speed of response, the regulation of acid–base status involves body buffers, respiratory function and renal function. In the proximal tubular cells carbon dioxide, derived from cellular metabolism or diffusion from the tubular lumen, combines with water to form carbonic acid. This dissociates to H^+ and HCO_3^-. The H^+ is actively pumped into the tubular lumen and combines with filtered bicarbonate to form carbonic acid, which dissociates to water and CO_2. The CO_2 then diffuses back into the tubular cell to repeat the cycle. The net effect is that for each hydrogen ion excreted one bicarbonate ion is retained, so that bicarbonate reserves are continuously regenerated.

$$CO_2 + H_2O \longleftrightarrow H_2CO_3 \longleftrightarrow H^+ + HCO_3^-$$

In mature subjects bicarbonate is regenerated by this process to maintain a plasma concentration of about 25 mmol/l, but preterm babies have a lower threshold.[25] Hydrogen ions are excreted all along the nephron and combine with other bases, chiefly phosphate and ammonia, in the tubular fluid, when bicarbonate reabsorption is complete. In health, renal excretion is the only route for acid loss. Acid gain may arise from respiratory or metabolic disorders.

Acidosis. Acidosis may be respiratory, metabolic or mixed. In respiratory failure carbon dioxide retention shifts the equation above to the right, with an increase in carbonic acid. Renal compensation is accomplished over a period of several days, by an increase in hydrogen ion excretion and bicarbonate regeneration. Blood gas analysis will reveal a compensated respiratory acidosis, with a high PCO_2, a raised bicarbonate and a normal pH (Fig. 39.4).

A metabolic acidosis is due to an increase in acid or a decrease in base. The most common cause for metabolic acidosis in neonatal intensive care is tissue hypoxia, leading to lactic acidosis. Metabolic acidosis also occurs with sepsis, renal failure, amino acid intolerance during parenteral nutrition, and in inborn errors of metabolism. In an otherwise normal subject a fall in pH will stimulate hyperventilation, shift the carbonic acid equation to the left, and increase CO_2 elimination. The features of a compensated metabolic acidosis are a low bicarbonate, low PCO_2 and normal pH.

Infants with both respiratory disease and a metabolic acidosis will show a mixed picture, with a high PCO_2, low bicarbonate and low pH.

Renal tubular acidosis is discussed below.

Alkalosis. A metabolic alkalosis is caused by a gain of base, as in the injudicious use of sodium bicarbonate, or loss of acid. Gastric acid loss may occur in high intestinal obstruction. In the distal tubule and collecting duct sodium is reabsorbed in exchange for either potassium or hydrogen ions, under the influence of aldosterone. If intracellular H^+ is low potassium is preferentially lost, and

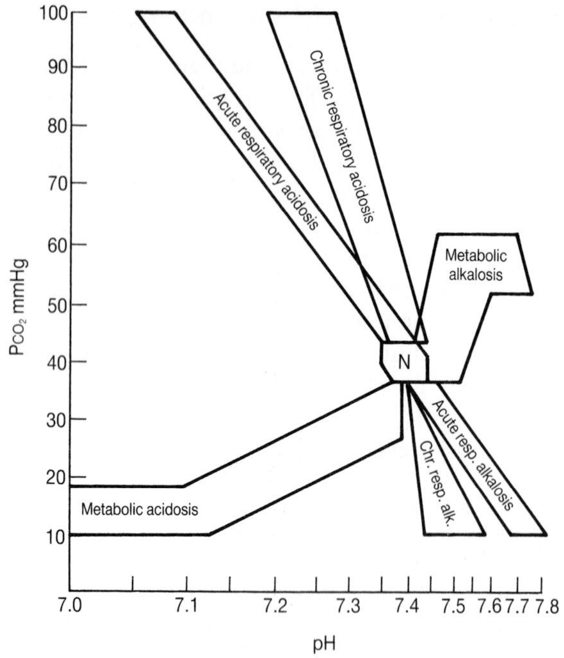

Fig. 39.4 Interpretation of changes in acid–base balance (simplified from Golberger[59]).

Table 39.2 Causes of metabolic alkalosis

Gastric loss	Vomiting, pyloric stenosis, high intestinal obstruction, continuous gastric suction
Excessive bicarbonate administration	
Hypokalaemia	Diuretic therapy, inadequate intake
Hypochloraemia	Diuretic therapy, diarrhoea
Adrenal hypersecretion	
Bartter syndrome	

vice versa. This explains the association between alkalosis and hypokalaemia. Causes of metabolic alkalosis are shown in Table 39.2. A respiratory alkalosis results from hyperventilation. The commonest cause in the neonatal unit is iatrogenic, during assisted ventilation. Hyperventilation may also be seen in neurologically damaged infants and in rare conditions such as Leigh's disease and Joubert's disease.

EXTRARENAL POSTNATAL ADAPTATION AND FLUID BALANCE

Insensible water loss

Insensible water loss occurs through the respiratory tract, in stool and across the skin. Stool water loss is small and usually less than 5 ml/kg/24 h in the first days after birth, but there may be increased losses from the respiratory tract with a rapid respiratory rate and if inspired gases are not adequately humidified. The upper respiratory tract both warms and humidifies inspired gases, and full saturation (44 mg/l) is achieved by the mid-trachea. For the spontaneously breathing infant a rise in ambient humidity, within either a head box or an incubator, will result in a substantial reduction in respiratory water loss. If the upper respiratory tract is bypassed with an endotracheal tube, or if the infant is breathing through nasal prongs, respiratory water loss must be reduced through adequate humidification of inspired gases. Care must therefore be taken when selecting humidifiers for use with neonatal ventilators, ensuring that this level of saturation is achieved within the operating temperature range.

Transepidermal water loss may be considerable in preterm babies and reflects both skin immaturity and the large suface area to weight ratio. During the first days after birth the skin is as (and occasionally more) important a determinant of postnatal water balance in extremely preterm babies as renal function. Sodium is not lost through the skin because babies born below 36 weeks' gestation do not sweat, although this develops within the first 2 weeks after birth.[73]

The stratum corneum of the skin consists of overlapping dead epidermal cells that have been filled with keratin, a fibrous protein, and this layer is the barrier to water loss. Although keratinization begins at around 18 weeks' gestation, the fetal epidermis is still very thin at 26 weeks and the stratum corneum barely visible. During the last trimester the epidermis and stratum corneum thicken and keratinization becomes more marked.[50] Transepidermal loss falls exponentially with increasing gestational and postnatal age (Fig. 39.5)[67,68,69,143] as skin maturation, unlike the maturation of renal function, is accelerated by birth. After 32 weeks' gestation water loss through the skin is low (around 12 ml/kg/day).[140] Trans-

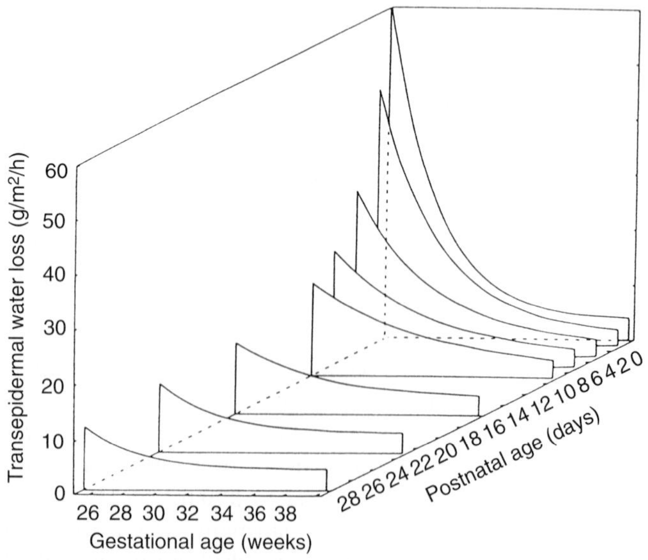

Fig. 39.5 Transepidermal water loss in relation to gestational age at birth at different postnatal ages in appropriate for gestational age infants. (Reproduced with permission from Sedin et al[143])

Table 39.3 Factors influencing insensible water loss

Increased loss	Lower gestational age	
	Lower postnatal age	
	Denuded/broken skin	
	Increased skin temperature	
	Activity	
	Increased environmental temperature	
	Radiant heat sources	Radiant warmers Phototherapy units
	Draughts	
	Crying	
	Tachypnoea	
Decreased loss	Clothing	
	High ambient humidity	
	High humidity microenvironment	Body box Plastic blanket
	Good skin care	
	Humidification of inspired gases	
	Topical agents	

epidermal loss is also influenced by ambient humidity, skin integrity, environmental and skin temperature, air speed and radiant heat sources, including phototherapy (Table 39.3). Radiant heat sources can increase transepidermal water loss by a factor of up to 0.5–2.[140]

In immature babies the highest transepidermal losses occur during the first days after birth (Table 39.4). Babies below 28 weeks' gestation, nursed naked under radiant warmers, are most vulnerable and in this group, without adequate measures to decrease losses, water lost through the skin may exceed urine volume.

Each millilitre of water that evaporates from the skin is accompanied by the loss of 560 calories of heat, and so it is also difficult to keep a baby with a high transepidermal water loss warm. A high ambient humidity reduces transepidermal water loss, and this effect is most marked in the most immature infants (Fig. 39.6). A decrease in ambient humidity from 60% to 20% will increase water lost through the skin by 100% in infants below 26 weeks' gestation.[67] Takahashi et al[162] showed that insensible water loss in infants weighing less than 1000 g is reduced to less than 40 ml/kg/day if ambient humidity is above 90%. Humidification is easier with an incubator, but a high-humidity microenvironment may be maintained immediately around the baby nursed under a radiant warmer, by using bubblewrap or other plastic sheeting and a humidified body box. The aim should be for a relative humidity of over 60%. Draughts should be eliminated. Stripping of the stratum corneum and deeper abrasions of the skin can be reduced by using non-abrasive tape such as micropore, neonatal electrodes and skin protectants, prior to affixing urine bags and transcutaneous oxygen electrodes.[27,51] Although a water-impermeable barrier, such as soft paraffin, applied to the skin, has been suggested, it is messy and impractical and has not entered into routine use. An adequate provision of fluid is also necessary, using a system which allows the glucose delivery rate to be altered independently of fluid volume, in order to avoid hyperglycaemia.[6]

The extent to which transepidermal water loss is

Table 39.4 Transepidermal water loss (ml/kg/24 h) at an ambient humidity of 50% (mean ± SD)[69]

		Postnatal age (days)					
Gestational age (weeks)	*n*	**0–1**	**3**	**7**	**14**	**21**	**28**
25–27	9	129 ± 39	71 ± 9	43 ± 9	32 ± 10	28 ± 10	24 ± 10
28–30	13	42 ± 13	32 ± 9	24 ± 7	18 ± 6	15 ± 6	15 ± 6
31–36	22	12 ± 5	12 ± 4	12 ± 4	9 ± 3	8 ± 2	7 ± 1
37–41	24	7 ± 2	6 ± 1	6 ±1	6 ±1	6 ± 0	7 ± 1

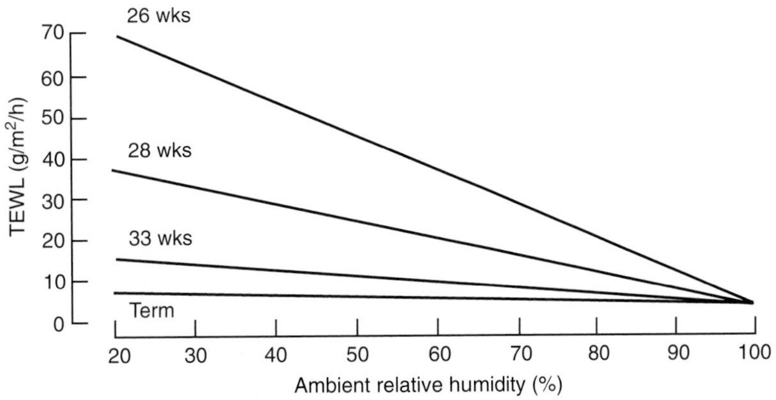

Fig. 39.6 The effect of ambient relative humidity on transepidermal water loss (based on the data of Hammarlund and Sedin[67]). (Reproduced with permission from Rutter[140])

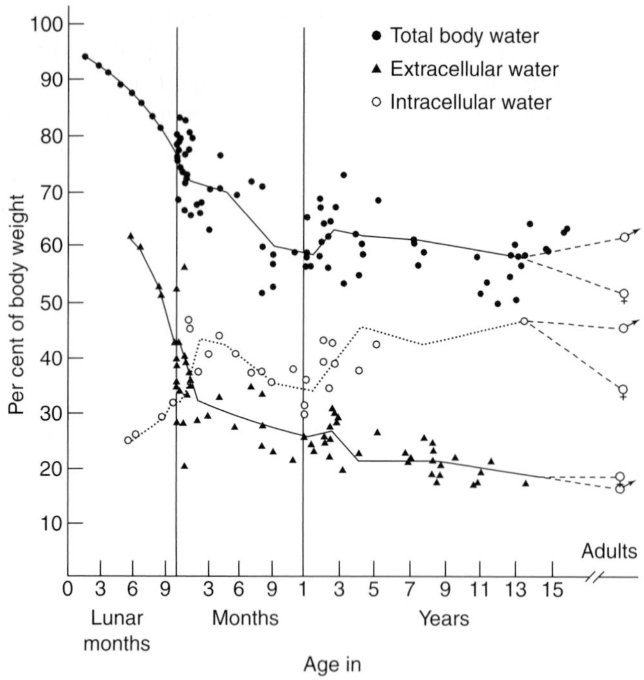

Fig. 39.7 Body water compartments as percentages of body weight from early fetal life to adult life. (Reproduced with permission from Friis-Hansen[55])

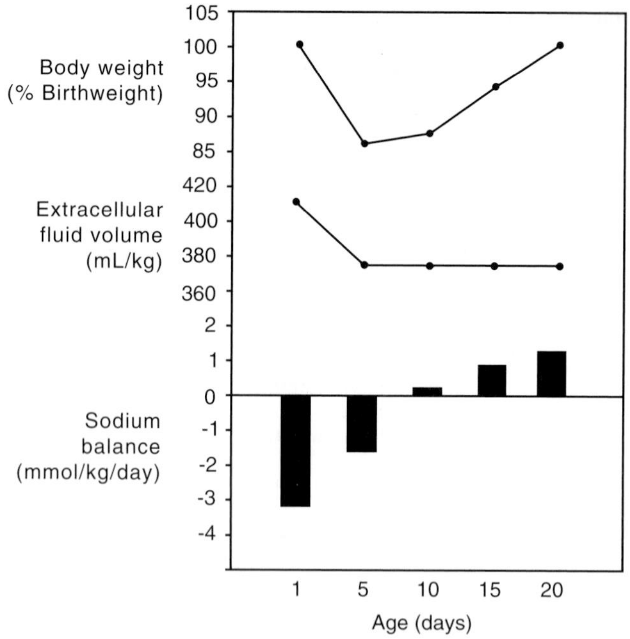

Fig. 39.8 Postnatal changes in body weight, extracellular volume and sodium balance. (Reproduced with permission from Shaffer and Weismann[147])

reduced, hypernatraemic dehydration and hyperglycaemia avoided and temperature stability maintained, may be regarded as an index of the overall quality of nursing and medical care.

Postnatal alterations in body water distribution

The size of the extracellular compartment decreases steadily throughout life, from around 65% of body weight at 26 weeks' gestation, to 40% at term and 20% by the age of 10 years[56] (Fig. 39.7). Superimposed on this gradual reduction with time there is a more abrupt contraction of the extracellular compartment, which occurs shortly after birth[14,15,79,145,146,151] owing to loss of interstitial fluid. This accounts, at least in part, for early postnatal weight loss. The onset of extracellular fluid loss appears to be closely interrelated with cardiopulmonary adaptation. In healthy babies loss of extracellular fluid occurs rapidly, but in babies with RDS this may be delayed.[115] Several studies now suggest that it is triggered by a surge in ANP release brought about by increased atrial stretch as pulmonary vascular resistance falls.[21,92,138,166] The intravascular compartment may also be acutely expanded during birth, because of reabsorption of lung liquid and a variable placental transfusion. As the timing of the diuresis/natriuresis is a consequence of the fall in pulmonary vascular pressure, it is not surprising that attempts to improve the course of RDS with the use of frusemide have shown no consistent benefit.[8]

A corollary of isotonic loss of extracellular fluid is that net water and sodium balance in the first days after birth is negative (Fig. 39.8). Negative sodium balance during this period is physiological, which is borne out by the observation that in newborn babies an early increase in the intake of sodium leads to an increase in sodium excretion.[94,131,146] However, all preterm babies have a limited, though variable, capacity to excrete a sodium load, so that, despite increasing excretion in response to an increase in intake, sodium retention readily occurs.[21,33] If the intake of water is limited hypernatraemia results, as shown in a study by Shaffer and Meade[146] of babies between 25 and 31 weeks' gestation in the first 10 days after birth. Babies were randomized to receive a sodium intake of 3 mmol/kg/day or 1 mmol/kg/day. Of the former group 50% became hypernatraemic, compared to 20% in the latter group. In this study the intake of water was restricted to 75 ml/kg/day on the first day, increasing by 10 ml/kg/day until day 5.

If a more liberal intake of water is allowed, in conjunction with the intake of sodium, extracellular tonicity is maintained by expansion of the extracellular compartment. This will be shown by weight gain at a time when weight loss is to be expected. In the majority of babies this cumulative positive balance is subsequently lost; in other words, the normal postnatal change in body water distribution occurs, but is delayed.[21] The well recognized diuresis that accompanies improving respiratory function in babies with RDS is in a fact a natriuresis,[115] and is an example of delayed postnatal adaptation.

CLINICAL IMPLICATIONS OF POSTNATAL AND DEVELOPMENTAL CHANGES

The first days after birth

The management of sodium balance during the period of postnatal adaptation is governed by principles that differ from those that govern management afterwards. The baby with RDS may be usefully regarded as a model of delayed postnatal maturation. In contrast, in the healthy preterm baby postnatal cardiopulmonary adaptation occurs over the same rapid timescale as in a full-term baby. Early fluid management during the period of postnatal adaptation should permit an isotonic contraction of the extracellular compartment and negative sodium and water balance.

As discussed above, babies with respiratory distress have a delayed postnatal diuresis and, if fluid balance is improperly managed, may gain weight in the first days after birth, when weight loss should be occurring. If the serum sodium concentration is normal, isotonic expansion of the extracellular compartment has occurred and sodium balance in these babies is positive, at a time when it should be negative.[21] This unsatisfactory situation will be missed unless changes in weight are being carefully monitored and the significance of inappropriate weight gain appreciated. Extracellular water overload increases the risks and severity of respiratory illness in the newborn[117,134,149,150] and weight gain in the first days after birth, in babies with RDS, appears to be associated with an increased risk of developing CLD.[167]

Costarino et al[33] confirmed some of these observations in a blind trial comparing sodium restriction in the first 5 days after birth with sodium supplementation of 3–4 mmol/kg/day from birth. Water was prescribed independently. Unfortunately, extracellular volume was not measured in this study, nor were the babies weighed. However, sodium balance was positive in the sodium-supplemented group on the first day after birth, and this group had a significantly higher incidence of CLD.

In most newborn babies the early administration of sodium will simply lead to an increase in excretion until the loss of extracellular fluid has occurred.[94,131,146] However, the limited capacity for sodium excretion still leaves the extremely preterm infant with RDS at risk of early sodium overload. Although the increasing use of antenatal glucocorticoids, which also induce maturation of sodium excretion, has resulted in a decrease in the number of affected infants, the immediate or early administration of 'maintenance' sodium is unnecessary and possibly harmful. Sodium will, in any case, almost inevitably be administered inadvertently, occasionally in large amounts, as flush fluids, with drugs and as colloid (Table 39.5). Routine sodium supplements should therefore be avoided until the physiological postnatal diuresis/natriuresis.[21,112,115] If this point is indeterminate, supplementation should be deferred until weight loss of the order of 5–7% of birthweight has occurred.[15,151,164] This figure is an approximation, as hydration at birth is variable[163] and birthweight does not correlate closely with extracellular water volume.[145] Early postnatal weight loss reflects both the loss of body water and the loss or gain of body solids. As nutritional support for sick preterm babies improves it is likely that overall weight loss will be diminished, although body water will still be lost to the same extent. This was shown in a study comparing healthy preterm babies with a group with RDS, during the first week after birth. Both groups lost an identical amount of body water, i.e. 10% of the total body water content at birth. However, the healthy babies lost a maximum of 5.9% of birthweight, in contrast to 8.6% in the RDS group. This was because although both groups gained in body solids during the period of weight loss, the healthy babies, who received a higher energy intake, gained solids to a significantly greater extent[164] (Fig. 39.9).

An adequate quantity of water should be provided, sufficient to allow the excretion of a relatively small initial renal solute load[179] and to maintain tonicity in the face of initially high, but rapidly falling, transepidermal losses (see above). The principal determinant of water requirements in the first days after birth in very immature babies is the magnitude of insensible water loss. Reducing this to a minimum should be regarded as a primary goal of nursing and medical care. Although negative water

Table 39.5 Sodium content of intravenous fluids and drugs

Fluid/drug	Proprietary name	Sodium content
Sodium chloride 30%		5 mmol/ml
Sodium chloride 0.9%		0.15 mmol/ml
Sodium chloride 0.45%		0.075 mmol/ml
Sodium bicarbonate 8.4%		1.0 mmol/ml
Sodium bicarbonate 4.2%		0.5 mmol/ml
Plasma substitutes		
gelatins	Gelofusine	0.15 mmol/ml
	Haemaccel	0.145 mmol/ml
fresh frozen plasma		0.145 mmol/ml
human albumin solution (4.5%)		0.140 mmol/ml
Amino acid solutions	Vaminolact	0 mmol/ml
	Vamin 9 glucose	0.05 mmol/ml
Antibiotics		
benzylpenicillin	Crystapen	1.68 mmol/600 mg
flucloxacillin	Floxapen	2.26 mmol/1000 mg
amoxycillin	Amoxil	3.3 mmol/1000 mg
ampicillin	Penbritin	0.73 mmol/250 mg
co-amoxiclav	Augmentin	1.6 mmol/600 mg
gentamicin/amikacin	Cidomycin/Amikin	< 0.5 mmol/500 mg
piperacillin	Pipril	1.94 mmol/1000 mg
cefotaxime	Claforan	2.09 mmol/1000 mg
ceftazidime	Fortum	2.3 mmol/1000 mg
vancomycin	Vancocin	0
Antifungals		
fluconazole	Diflucan	15 mmol/200 mg
Normal immunoglobulin	Sandoglobulin	4.95 mmol/1000 mg

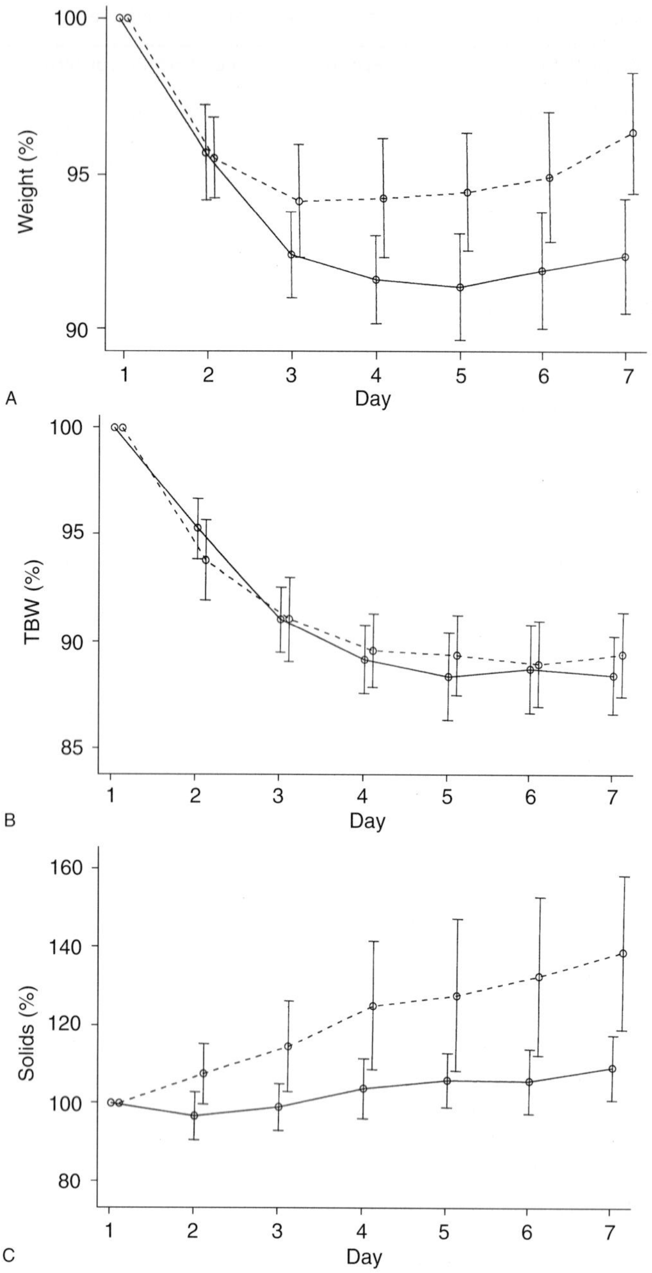

Fig. 39.9 Weight (A), total body water (B) and body solids (C) during the first week of life in healthy preterm babies (dotted line) and babies with respiratory distress syndrome (solid line). Values (mean ± 95% CI) are expressed as a percentage of the value at birth. (Reproduced with permission from Tang et al[164])

balance is the physiological norm during this period, the provision of sodium-free fluid does not routinely have to be restricted in order to achieve this. As already discussed, diluting capacity will not limit water excretion. In addition, although babies who are hypoxaemic and hypovolaemic are likely to have reduced glomerular filtration, this is not the case for well-supported infants with stable clinical parameters.[114] It is erroneous to assume that all babies with respiratory distress syndrome have an impaired glomerular filtration rate. Similarly, observations of the effects of positive airway pressure made in newborn animals with normal lungs should not be extrapolated to babies with non-compliant lungs. In the former, but not the latter, high inflation pressures will be transmitted to the intrathoracic contents, affecting venous return and altering intrarenal blood flow[118] and glomerular filtration.[54]

Nevertheless, neonatal paediatricians have long been concerned about 'excessive' fluid intake. Associations have been described between high fluid intakes and increased risk of symptomatic PDA,[19,156] NEC[18] and CLD.[26,33,167] In the former condition an expanded intravascular compartment might exacerbate left–right shunting and in the latter two interstitial oedema has been implicated in pathogenesis. In addition, an increased quantity of lung water will increase the amount of ventilatory support required and potentiate pulmonary barotrauma. Regrettably, sodium intake was not controlled in these studies, so that increased 'fluid' meant an increased intake of both sodium and water. The evidence suggests that it is the early intake of sodium and the resulting expansion of the extracellular compartment, and not the 'excessive' intake of water, that is responsible for the increase in morbidity. In the study referred to above,[164] comparing healthy preterm babies with a group with RDS, although the latter received the same volume of fluid as the healthy babies, both groups had lost an identical amount of body water by the end of the first week. In addition, there was no relationship between the volume of fluid administered and total body water lost.

The infant with RDS

For a baby requiring intensive care, such as one with RDS, a reasonable intravenous volume at which to start is with an allowance for urinary water of 30–60 ml/kg/day plus estimated insensible water loss[113] (Table 39.6). Glucose delivery may commence at 7 mg/kg/min. A didactic recommendation is inappropriate, given variations in nursing practice, humidity and clinical condition. With an understanding of the principles involved it is a straightforward matter to decide a starting prescription. First, make a judgement of likely insensible water loss, taking into account sources of radiant heat, ambient humidity, humidification of inspired gases, respiratory rate, gestational and postnatal age. For example, the insensible water loss in an infant below 1000 g birthweight during the first week after birth will be of the order of 40 ml/kg/day in ambient incubator humidity exceeding 90%,[162] but around 120 ml/kg/day under a radiant warmer in 50% humidity. The initial volume necessary might therefore be anything from 70 to 180 ml/kg/day. As neither transepidermal water loss, the integrity of renal function nor the timing of the postnatal natriuresis/diuresis can be predicted precisely, the adequacy of the estimate must be repeatedly assessed. At

Table 39.6 Estimated starting intravenous intake, at an ambient humidity of 50%

Gestational age (weeks)	Birthweight (kg)	Approximate[143] transepidermal water loss (ml/kg/24 h)	Allowance for urine output (ml/kg/24 h)	Estimated intake range (ml/kg/24 h)	Suggested starting volume† (ml/kg/24 h)
< 27	< 1.0	120	30–60	150–180	150*,§
27–30	1.0–1.5	40	30–60	70–100	90
31–36	1.5–2.5	15	30–60	45–75	60
> 36	> 2.5	10	30–60	40–70	60

* The most immature infants are particularly vulnerable to renal impairment and impaired water excretion, therefore a cautious approach, commencing at the lower end of the estimated intake requirement, is recommended.
§ If a higher humidity is achieved requirements will be correspondingly reduced.
† Once sustained weight loss of at least 5% is achieved, proceed to the intravenous volume necessary to provide total parenteral nutrition (usually 150 ml/kg/day), without stepwise increments.

6–8 hours, measure the serum sodium and potassium. At 24 hours, measure serum creatinine, sodium and potassium and weigh the baby. This should be repeated at least daily. Urine output should be assessed continuously.

It is important to ensure that blood glucose levels remain stable. The use of a single solution containing a fixed concentration of glucose will obviously increase the chances of hypoglycaemia or hyperglycaemia if the volume of fluid administered cannot be altered independently. The use of 5% and 50% glucose solutions delivered through a Y connection allows both the glucose delivery rate and the volume infused to be readily altered independently.[6] The 5% solution may also contain amino acids. For example, a 10% solution will provide a glucose delivery rate of 4.86 mg/kg/min at 70 ml/kg/24 h, and 9.7 mg/kg/min at 140 ml/kg/24 h. A constant glucose delivery rate of, for example, 7 mg/kg/min, could be achieved by the infusion of 5% glucose at 2.3 ml/h and 50% glucose at 0.3 ml/h (for a total of 70 ml/kg/24 h) or 5% glucose at 5.5 ml/h and 50% glucose at 0.3 ml/h (for 140 ml/kg/24 h). If the blood glucose rises, the glucose delivery rate may be reduced to 5 mg/kg/min by altering the proportion of 5% and 50% glucose to 2.6 ml/h and 0.3 ml/h, or 5.8 ml/h and 0 ml/h, with no change in the total volume infused.

Satisfactory management is marked by a urine flow rate of at least 0.5–1 ml/kg/h on the first day, rising to 2–3 ml/kg/h thereafter, daily weight loss of the order of 1–2%, a falling serum creatinine and serum electrolyte concentrations within the normal range (Table 39.7). If the serum sodium rises, increase the intake volume; if it falls, it should be decreased. The aims of fluid management in preterm infants with RDS are outlined in Table 39.8.

Chronic lung disease, heart failure, indomethacin treatment in PDA, NEC, birth asphyxia and post-operative management are other common conditions in neonatal intensive care where careful management of fluid balance is necessary. The principles underlying management are outlined in Table 39.9. Reference is also made in specific chapters.

Table 39.7 Monitoring fluid balance

Weight	Daily or twice daily	Steady initial loss of 1–2% daily. Weight gain should commence by 7–10 days
Urine output	Continuously, review 8-hourly	Should exceed 0.5 ml/kg/h on day 1 in extremely preterm infants, thereafter > 2–3 ml/kg/h in all infants; <1 ml/kg/h requires investigation of renal impairment
Serum sodium	Daily or twice daily	132–144 mmol/l; if high increase fluid intake; if low, decrease
potassium	Daily or twice daily	3.8–5.7 mmol/l; spurious elevation due to haemolysis common
creatinine	Daily	Exponential fall after birth

Table 39.8 Aims of fluid balance management in preterm babies with respiratory distress syndrome

• Reduce insensible water loss to a minimum	Incubator care; high humidity delivered to microenvironment using bubblewrap, plastic blanket or body box; skin care; draught elimination
• Facilitate early postnatal loss of extracellular interstitial fluid	Reduce the early intake of sodium to a minimum
• Maintain glucose homeostasis	Use a volume-independent, variable glucose delivery system
• Optimize nutritional support	Early provision of parenteral and minimal enteral nutrition
• Maintain renal perfusion	Monitor blood pressure, core–peripheral temperature gap, capillary refill time, urine output, cardiac output and central venous pressure; colloid and inotrope support as necessary

The phase of growth

Fluid volume

Once the phase of immediate postnatal adaptation is over, growth becomes of paramount importance. The total intravenous volume required may be given, without stepwise increments[38,114] once postnatal weight loss has been achieved, since, as discussed above, healthy preterm

Table 39.9 Common clinical problems in fluid balance management

Respiratory distress syndrome	Starting volume dependent on insensible water loss. Delay sodium supplementation until after postnatal diuresis/natriuresis and steady weight loss of at least 5%
Patent ductus arteriosus	Medical treatment of heart failure with fluid restriction and diuretics. Indomethacin toxicity exacerbated by dehydration
Indomethacin	Reduce fluid intake by 30% at start of treatment
Severe, full-term, birth asphyxia	Anticipate renal failure. Restrict salt-free intake to 20–30 ml/kg/day initially. Central vascular access required to maintain blood glucose
Chronic lung disease	Avoid prolonged periods of fluid restriction as poor nutrition will worsen prognosis. If diuretics are necessary beware chronic sodium depletion, which will further compromise growth
Necrotizing enterocolitis	Third-space fluid losses may be considerable. Monitoring weight unhelpful. Maintain intravascular volume assiduously
Postoperative	Reduce salt-poor fluid by 30%. Unrecognized hypovolaemia common and may contribute to postoperative hyponatraemia if inadequate replacement with saline or colloid

babies are capable of excreting large volumes of water. Enteral feeds may be commenced concurrently.

Sodium

Sodium is a permissive factor for growth, and a deficiency inhibits DNA synthesis in the most immature cells.[122] Chronic limitation of intake is associated not only with extracellular volume contraction and poor weight gain, but also with poor skeletal and tissue growth[28,74,76,170] and adverse neurodevelopmental outcome.[74] Human milk will provide a daily sodium intake of about 1 mmol/kg body weight, which is sufficient for normal growth if retained. The full-term baby is able to retain this virtually completely, by both renal tubular and intestinal reabsorption. However, extremely immature babies require a sodium intake of at least 4 mmol/kg/day, or more if on treatment with xanthines or other diuretics, in order to ensure the retention of 1 mmol/kg/day.[76] In babies below 36 weeks' gestation commence full sodium supplementation at 4 mmol/kg/day, once 5% weight loss has been achieved.

If preterm babies are fed unsupplemented or unfortified breast milk, chronic sodium depletion will be revealed in the first instance by poor weight gain. Sodium supplementation should continue until around 32–34 weeks' postconceptional age, by which time maturation of sodium conservation should have occurred.[4,136] It is not known whether supplementation beyond this time is harmful, for example in terms of chronic sodium retention and the development of hypertension.

DISORDERS OF FLUID AND ELECTROLYTE BALANCE

Disorders of renal function and fluid balance may commence antenatally, as a consequence of an abnormal pregnancy and possibly its treatment, or because of a malformation of the renal tract. Antenatal ultrasound screening is now widely used and will draw attention to oligohydramnios and polyhydramnios, an obstructed or distended renal tract, fetal hydrops, twin-to-twin transfusion syndrome and renal agenesis, hypoplasia or dysplasia.

The family history and history of maternal medication during pregnancy should be obtained. Angiotensin-converting enzyme inhibitors, when used in pregnancy, may cause irreversible renal failure in the newborn.[108] Indomethacin, a common tocolytic agent, results in a reduction in fetal urine flow (see below), and it is this action which has led to its use for the symptomatic treatment of polyhydramnios. Prolonged maternal exposure to indomethacin and other non-steroidal anti-inflammatory agents may cause neonatal renal failure and persistent pulmonary hypertension. Self-medication with these agents is a particular hazard during pregnancy.[17,84]

Difficulty in resuscitation at birth may first lead to suspicion of a renal disorder, as pulmonary hypoplasia may have resulted from severe fetal oliguria and oligohydramnios. At the extreme end of the spectrum, Potter syndrome comprises pulmonary hypoplasia and bilateral renal agenesis (pp. 641, 882). Findings on examination of the newborn baby which suggest a need for further investigation of the renal tract are an abdominal mass, a two-vessel cord, and ear or genital anomalies. Common postnatal presentations are oliguria or anuria, disordered electrolyte balance, excessive or inadequate weight gain, failure to observe the normal postnatal decline in plasma creatinine, haematuria and metabolic acidosis.

MONITORING RENAL FUNCTION

Fluid balance should be monitored meticulously in sick newborn babies requiring intensive care. All too often, a failure to detect a problem in its early stages leads to a potentially reversible situation becoming irreversible. Good monitoring is the responsibility of both medical and nursing staff. The serum sodium, potassium and creatinine should be assessed regularly, urine output carefully measured and the baby weighed at least daily (Table 39.7). As levels at birth reflect maternal values, a baseline measure of serum creatinine, sodium and potassium, obtained as soon as possible after birth, is necessary in order to be able to interpret subsequent

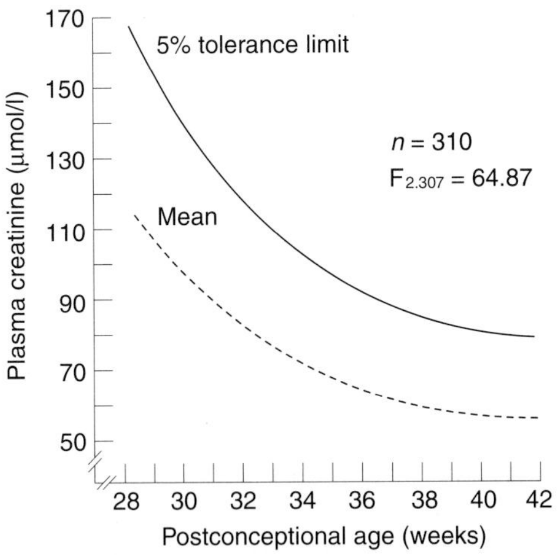

Fig. 39.10 Normal ranges for plasma creatinine by postconceptional age. (Reproduced with permission from Trompeter et al[165])

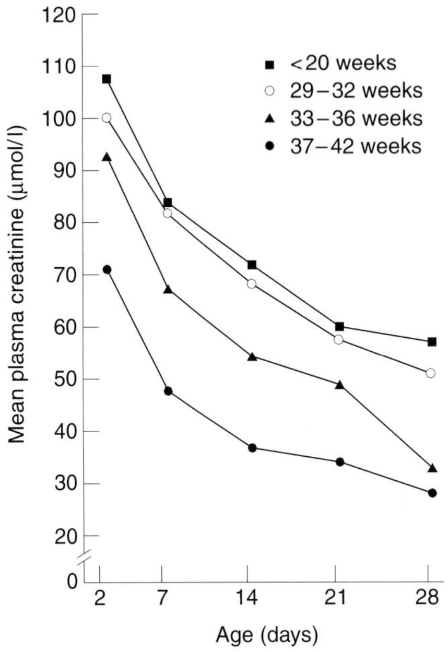

Fig. 39.11 Relationship between plasma creatinine and postnatal age in different gestational age groups. (Reproduced with permission from Rudd et al[139])

levels. Nursing charts should be designed so that hourly intake and output volumes can be clearly recorded.

Serum creatinine

Creatinine is derived from the turnover of phosphocreatine in muscle, and is excreted in the urine. At steady state, creatinine excretion is an indirect measure of muscle mass. In everyday clinical practice the serum creatinine is used as an index of GFR. The serum creatinine at birth is influenced by the maternal level. Subsequently, the level changes at a rate based on the balance between creatinine production rate, dependent on muscle mass,[116] and clearance rate which, as discussed above, is dependent on GFR, which in turn varies with postconceptional age (Fig. 39.10). The wide range of values seen for serum creatinine against postnatal age is due predominantly to the large variation that exists in weight for postconceptional age.

In the first weeks after birth plasma creatinine falls, initially exponentially as the maternally derived creatinine load is excreted, then more gradually.[139] A single measure of plasma creatinine provides no more than a crude estimate of renal function, and observing the change over days is more helpful. A useful clinical pointer to renal insufficiency is a failure to see the expected postnatal decline in plasma creatinine. The change in serum creatinine should therefore be considered, rather than the absolute level. Initially high, the neonatal serum creatinine level falls during the first week (Fig. 39.11). A sustained rise, or failure to fall, in serum creatinine is indicative of a fall in glomerular filtration rate. The blood urea is of little value in the newborn as it is influenced by numerous non-renal factors. For example, an elevated blood urea may be caused by blood in the gastrointestinal tract, or be due to catabolism during treatment with dexamethasone, despite normal renal function.

Urinary indices

The fraction of filtered sodium excreted (Fe_{Na}) and urinary sodium concentration rise transiently during the postnatal natriuresis and then fall with postnatal age. Values for the former, in babies between 25 and 34 weeks' gestation, in the first week after birth, often exceed 5%. The median urinary sodium concentration is around 80 mmol/l. The fractional sodium excretion is often used in the evaluation of the oliguric infant and is discussed on page 1028. 'Spot' urinary sodium concentrations bear no relationship to daily sodium balance and are of little use in determining the cause of hyponatraemia.

Well preterm infants are able to achieve a minimum urine osmolality of around 50 mOsmol/kg, and infants with RDS around 90 mOsmol/kg.[110] Maximum osmolality is of the order of 600–800 mOsmol/kg, though higher values exceeding 1000 mOsmol/kg are occasionally seen. A urine osmolality that lies between 200 and 400 mOsmol/kg usually suggests that fluid intake is satisfactory. However, as immature babies in the first days after birth may have even more limited concentrating abilities, they may become dehydrated while continuing to pass urine of low osmolality. Specific gravity is often measured in place of osmolality as it can easily be done on the ward. The presence of glucose or protein (both often found in samples from sick preterm babies) will, however, falsely elevate the specific gravity. In addition, the relationship between specific gravity, as measured with a refractometer, and osmolality differs between the newborn and older children, so that in the newborn an osmolality of 400 is indicative of a specific gravity

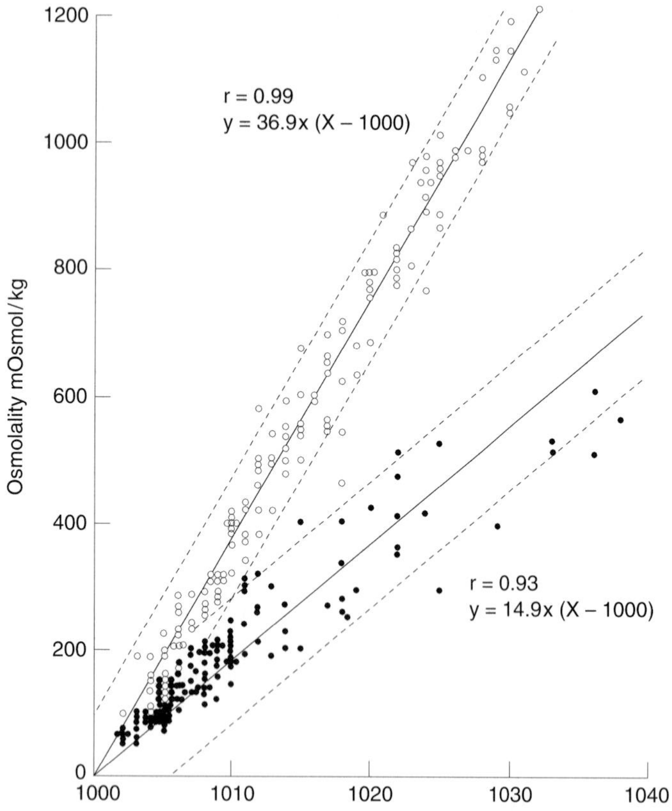

Fig. 39.12 Relationship between specific gravity and urinary osmolality in newborn infants (•) and older children (o). Dotted lines show 95% prediction limits for individual observations. (Reproduced with permission from Benitez et al[20])

between 1020 and 1030 (Fig. 39.12).[20] Reagent strip test measurement of urinary specific gravity is unsatisfactory.[61]

Dipstick urinalysis may be used as a screening test for proteinuria, haematuria and glycosuria. Bilirubin causes dark yellow to brown discoloration and suggests a conjugated hyperbilirubinaemia. Dark brown or red urine usually suggests haematuria, but may be caused by bile pigments, haemoglobin, rifampicin, porphyrins or urates. Urine microscopy is necessary to detect red blood cells, leukocytes and casts. Red blood cell casts imply renal parenchymal pathology. Haematuria may occur in renovascular disease, cortical and tubular necrosis, neoplasia, obstructive uropathy, coagulopathy, nephritis and infection. A clean-catch or suprapubic aspirate of urine should contain fewer than five white blood cells.[99] Leukocyturia is most often caused by infection, but pyrexia or any inflammatory process may also be responsible. Newborns excrete small amounts of protein (Table 39.10). The heaviest proteinuria is seen in congenital nephrotic syndrome.

Urine flow rate

Urine can be collected into adhesive bags, easily in boys but with more difficulty in girls. Self-adhesive urine bags in a wide variety of different sizes and designs are now commercially available. In order to protect the skin and prevent breakdown it is important to prepare the skin first and to use a suitable medical adhesive if necessary. Repeated application, because of poor adhesion, rapidly leads to excoriation of the delicate skin around the groin. Many urine bags are designed for once-only use and cannot be emptied though an integral port. If so, ensure that urine can be aspirated without having to remove the bag, by inserting a soft feeding tube into the bag before application. Collection into weighed nappies or cotton-wool balls is widely practised, but can be misleading, as evaporation, leading to volume loss and increased osmolality, may be appreciable.[172] Occasionally catheterization, using a soft feeding tube, may be necessary.

Table 39.10 Protein excretion in the newborn[44]

Gestational age (weeks)	Number of subjects	Protein excretion (mg/m²/24 h)	
		Mean	Range
< 28	5	21	4.8–31
30	12	50	0–226
32	15	56	0–125
34	15	60	0–314
36	17	30	0–110
40	26	31	0–146

It is generally held that a urine output less than 1 ml/kg/h is suggestive of impaired renal function. This is because in the presence of a renal solute load of 15 mOsmol/kg/day and an approximate maximum urinary concentration of 600–800 mOsmol/kg water, solute retention would occur if urine flow rate were less than 1 ml/kg/h. Extremely immature infants have considerably smaller solute loads on the first day after birth, and in these infants it may be more appropriate to regard a urine flow rate of less than 0.5 ml/kg/h on day 1 and 1 ml/kg/h thereafter, as abnormal. It has been estimated that the most immature preterm infants might achieve a maximum urine flow rate of around 7 ml/kg/h.[38] As neonates do not empty their bladders completely on voiding, and as 7% fail to void during the first 24 hours after birth, external urine collections of short duration may be inaccurate.

Alterations in body weight

The importance of accurate daily weighing as part of the assessment of fluid balance in babies requiring intensive care cannot be overemphasized. Isotonic expansion of the extracellular compartment can, and frequently does, occur in the preterm neonate. This will be missed if changes in body weight are not considered in conjunction with serum electrolytes. Poor growth in the face of an adequate energy intake may reflect chronic sodium depletion, and this may occur with a normal or low normal serum sodium concentration. Electronic scales, accurate to at least 5 g, are required. The net weight should be documented, taking into account the weights of attachments, as these may vary substantially from day to day for babies in intensive care.

HYPERNATRAEMIA AND HYPONATRAEMIA

A low serum sodium at birth suggests that the mother has received a large volume of salt-poor intravenous fluid during labour, resulting in an excess transfer of water to the baby. Labour ward policies should avoid the use of fixed-concentration solutions for intrapartum drug administration, as under these circumstances an increase in dose will result in increasing infusion volumes. Neonatal hyponatraemia has also been described following maternal diuretic and laxative abuse.

Changes in serum sodium concentration reflect both sodium and water balance. In the first few days after birth, prior to the postnatal diuresis/natriuresis and in the absence of substantial sodium intake, hyponatraemia is almost invariably dilutional, due to excessive water retention and not to sodium depletion. Early hypernatraemia in extremely preterm babies is usually due to excessive transepidermal water loss, possibly compounded by excessive sodium administration. The key to the sound management of hyponatraemia or hypernatraemia developing after birth is first to assess changes in weight carefully. Hyponatraemia with weight loss or inadequate weight gain suggests sodium depletion. Hyponatraemia with inappropriate weight gain suggests primary water excess (Table 39.11). Hypernatraemia with weight loss suggests dehydration, and hypernatraemia with weight gain, salt and water overload.

Chronic sodium loss will first be accompanied by extracellular volume contraction, poor weight gain and a normal serum sodium concentration. Hyponatraemia will only ensue as a late sign. Donor breast milk contains variable but inadequate quantities of sodium. Breast milk from mothers delivering preterm contains larger amounts, but this is not sustained and even in babies receiving this type of EBM, sodium supplementation is necessary by the third to fourth weeks. Many babies receive xanthines to treat apnoea of prematurity. These are weak diuretics, but chronic use will predispose to sodium depletion. Potent agents such as frusemide may cause large sodium losses. An acute fall in serum sodium usually reflects impaired water excretion, but may occur following a single dose of frusemide or with sudden gastrointestinal loss, as in necrotizing enterocolitis. Sodium loss may occur from the gastrointestinal tract as a visible external loss, as in vomiting or as ileostomy or colostomy losses, or as sequestered loss, as with an ileus or obstruction. In the latter case there will be no weight loss. Renal tubular loss of sodium may arise in acute pyelonephritis and following relief of obstructive uropathy. Endocrine causes of hyponatraemia are discussed in Chapter 38, Part 2. The diagnostic approach in suspected inappropriate ADH secretion is discussed below.

It is a reasonable assumption that hyponatraemia and hypernatraemia contribute to neurological morbidity in sick newborn babies, though quantification of the effect, particularly in preterm babies, is difficult. Brain cell volume is affected by acute changes in extracellular tonicity. The regulation of cell volume following cell swelling or shrinkage in response to changes in extracellular tonicity, is brought about by the accumulation or loss of inorganic ions and organic solutes. Compensatory changes in electrolyte content occur rapidly, so that during acute exposure to hypertonicity there is a rapid movement of electrolytes into the cell, in favour of water retention. Adaptation to chronic hyperosmolar states occurs by increasing the concentration of intracellular

Table 39.11 Causes of hyponatraemia in neonates

Primary water excess	
Excess intake	
to mother	Large intrapartum infusion of sodium-free fluid
to baby	Excessive intravenous intake
Impaired excretion	
intrinsic renal failure	
indomethacin	
syndrome of inappropriate ADH secretion	
adrenocortical failure	
Primary sodium depletion	
Insufficient intake	
Maternal laxative or diuretic abuse	
Use of non-sodium supplemented breast milk for preterm babies	
Excessive loss	
Renal	
Diuretics including xanthines	
Tubular dysfunction	
Pyelonephritis	
Nephrotoxic agents	
Obstructive uropathies	
Endocrine	
Salt-losing forms of congenital adrenal hyperplasia	
Hypoaldosteronism	
Gastrointestinal	
External	
Vomiting	
Ileostomy/colostomy loss	
Sequestered	
Ileus	
Obstruction	
Necrotizing enterocolitis	
Central nervous system	
Following repeated drainage of CSF in post haemorrhagic hydrocephalus	
Cerebral salt wasting	
Mixed	
Water excess and sodium depletion	
sodium and water depletion treated with continued infusion of sodium-free fluid	
Chronic lung disease treated with long-term diuretic therapy	
Water excess disproportionate to whole body sodium excess	
Effective central hypovolaemia	
Congestive cardiac failure	
Liver failure	
Nephrotic syndrome	

organic osmolytes.[158] Loss of organic osmolytes occurs more slowly than movement of electrolytes. Thus, if chronic hyperosmolality is corrected rapidly the influx of water into the cell continues, resulting in cell swelling and cerebral oedema. Cell swelling can lead to occlusion of blood flow, hypoxia and the release of cytotoxic neuro-excitatory amino acids. Conversely, an acute fall in serum sodium concentration will first lead to the movement of water into cells and the development of intracellular oedema and brain swelling. Over a period of time the concentration of intracellular osmolytes decreases, so as to favour the movement of water out of the cell. If extracellular hypotonicity is then corrected rapidly, the continued movement of water out of the cell will result in brain shrinkage.

Although the timescale over which the human brain adapts to alterations in tonicity by increasing or decreasing intracellular organic osmolytes is not clearly established, a chronic imbalance in tonicity should be corrected slowly over at least 48–72 hours. The management of acute imbalance may be quicker. In the extremely preterm baby hypernatraemic dehydration due to excessive insensible water loss may be managed by increasing the volume of infused dextrose/water. This does not imply the use of a salt-free infusate, as these babies will be receiving sodium from drugs, flush fluids and possibly colloid. Hypotonicity due to water overload should be treated by water restriction.

SERUM POTASSIUM

Potassium is the principal intracellular cation. It is important for the maintenance of intracellular fluid volume. Total body potassium is approximately 46 mmol/kg, a value that is similar in both babies and adults. A high potassium level may be reported if there has been difficulty in obtaining the blood sample or a delay in processing it, as potassium is released from damaged cells. True hyperkalaemia occurs in the context of extensive tissue damage, such as following extensive bruising, shock and ischaemia, and in renal failure. Management is discussed below and outlined in Table 39.12.

The causes of hypokalaemia are shown in Table 39.13. Hypokalaemia may arise through gastrointestinal or urinary loss. Most gastrointestinal disorders are also associated with sodium loss and the resulting increase in circulating aldosterone exacerbates potassium loss. Hypokalaemia is usually accompanied by a metabolic alkalosis.

Table 39.12 Treatment of hyperkalaemia

Serum potassium > 6.5 mmol/l
- Commence calcium resonium rectally, 150 mg/kg/dose, every 6 hours
- Rectal plug of calcium resonium can be removed by irrigation with 1–2 ml sodium chloride 0.9%
- Monitor ECG

Serum potassium > 8 mmol/l or ECG abnormalites (peaked T wave, widened QRS complex)
- Calcium gluconate 10%, 0.5 ml/kg diluted 10-fold with glucose 5%, i.v. bolus at a maximum rate of 0.1 ml/min
- Sodium bicarbonate 4.2%, 4 ml/kg (2 mmol/kg) i.v. over 5 minutes. Check base deficit immediately
- Glucose and insulin: add 25 units neutral insulin to 500 ml glucose 10% to produce 1 unit insulin to 2 g glucose. Infuse at 0.05–0.1 units/kg/h (1–2 ml/kg/h). Monitor blood glucose closely
- Salbutamol, i.v. infusion over 20 minutes, 4 μg/kg/dose

Table 39.13 Causes of potassium depletion

- Inadequate intake
- Gastrointestinal loss
  - Aspiration of gastrointestinal content
  - Vomiting
  - Pyloric stenosis
  - Ileus
  - Ileostomy loss
  - Diarrhoea
- Renal loss
  - *With metabolic alkalosis*
  - Excessive base administration
  - Frusemide and other loop diuretics
  - Congenital chloride diarrhoea
  - Hyperaldosteronism
  - Bartter syndrome
  - Cushing syndrome
  - *With metabolic acidosis*
  - Renal tubular acidosis
  - Diuresis during recovery from acute renal failure

APPROPRIATE AND INAPPROPRIATE ADH SECRETION

The release of the ADH is stimulated by a rise in osmolality and also by baroreceptors located in the heart and great vessels. ADH has two principal actions: it increases the permeability of the renal collecting ducts and thereby the reabsorption of water, and it is a potent vasoconstrictor, contributing to the maintenance of blood pressure. The ADH-dependent increase in water permeability is brought about by the insertion of water channels in the apical membranes of cells of the collecting ducts.[43] The pressor effect of ADH appears to be one of the mediators through which central arterial blood pressure is maintained, and both hypovolaemia and hypotension will result in a rise in circulating ADH.[46]

Under experimental conditions a rise in ADH occurs when intravascular volume falls by about 10%.[46] Little is known of the setting of baroreceptor responses in the human preterm newborn, though Rees et al[130] described a doubling of urinary arginine vasopressin after blood loss of the order of 10% in a 26-week, 800 g infant.

It has been suggested that the syndrome of inappropriate ADH secretion (SIADH) occurs frequently in the newborn.[130] Raised ADH levels and hyponatraemia are common in acutely ill infants. However, the maintenance of central blood pressure overrides the defence of tonicity. This was clearly demonstrated in experiments on human volunteers, in whom progressive salt depletion was induced by a salt-free diet and vigorous sweating.[101] The intake of water was unrestricted. Whole body sodium depletion was initially accompanied by isotonic contraction of the extracellular compartment and rapid weight loss. With increasing depletion baroreceptor-induced water reabsorption slowed down the rate of weight loss, but at the cost of a fall in plasma osmolality. In such a situation the release of ADH is not inappropriate for volume status. Evidence suggests that this effect underlies the impaired water excretion seen in ill infants. Gerigk et al,[58] in a large prospective study, found that although plasma osmolality was lower in acutely ill infants and children than in a control group, both ADH and PRA were raised, i.e. that there was also activation of the renin–angiotensin–aldosterone system. The best reduction in ADH and PRA levels was achieved by the intravenous infusion of isotonic saline, compared to hypotonic saline and oral fluids. This suggests that the elevated levels were due to baroreceptor stimulation, i.e. that ADH was appropriately elevated for volume status.

The recognition of an inadequate intravascular volume is often difficult. In the study by Gerigk et al,[58] described above, only a third of infants and children had overt signs of dehydration. Newborn babies are at particular risk of intravascular volume depletion.[169] Immediate cord clamping has been shown to result in a 50% lower blood volume than late clamping,[98] and this may be compounded by frequent blood sampling. Blood pressure measurements cannot be relied upon to detect hypovolaemia. The normal range for blood pressure in the newborn is wide, and blood pressure correlates poorly with blood volume.[11,13] Careful attention should be paid to assessment of the circulation, using central venous pressure monitoring,[152] capillary-refill time, core–peripheral temperature difference and Doppler echocardiographic assessment of cardiac output.[126] The core–peripheral temperature difference correlates with circulating AVP.[94]

Postoperatively a low serum sodium is usually a result of unrecognized intravascular volume depletion and continuing provision of salt-poor fluid, with ADH-driven water retention. The appropriate management of postoperative fluid balance includes relative restriction of salt-poor fluid and the liberal use of salt-containing fluid.[82] It is unclear whether normal saline or colloid, as either albumin or plasma, is the more appropriate fluid for volume support in neonates.[153] Once water retention and hyponatraemia have occurred, water restriction is necessary to correct the hyponatraemia safely.

True inappropriate ADH secretion is probably rare in the newborn.[75] The diagnosis should only be made in accordance with the classic criteria of Bartter and Schwartz, when hyponatraemia exists with normovolaemia, normal blood pressure normal renal and cardiac function and evidence of continuing sodium excretion.[12] The urine will not be maximally dilute. In the newborn, SIADH has been described in acute brain injury and central nervous system infection, and following maternal substance abuse.[173]

In pathological circumstances, such as heart failure and liver failure, hypotension accompanies a raised extracellular fluid volume and there is whole body sodium excess, despite hyponatraemia. Abnormal myocardial function, whether arising from ischaemia, metabolic acidosis, immaturity or another cause, is increasingly recognized during neonatal intensive care and may contribute to impaired water excretion. Hyponatraemia is also commonly observed in infants with CLD, often with clinical signs suggestive of an expanded extracellular compartment. Whole body sodium may be depleted by chronic diuretic therapy, but levels of ADH are raised and free water clearance reduced.[78] It is possible that abnormal transmural pressure gradients lead to effective central hypotension, increased ADH release and impaired water excretion. During acute episodes associated with air trapping, pulmonary hypovolaemia and decreased left atrial filling will lead to a similar situation.[129] However, the aetiology of disordered salt and water balance in CLD is inadequately understood. Pulmonary hypertension, initially reversible, is an almost invariable accompaniment of CLD and fluid retention may be attributable to cor pulmonale, though cardiac performance may be impaired by other factors such as chronic dexamethasone therapy.[24,70]

PHARMACOLOGICAL INFLUENCES ON FLUID BALANCE

INDOMETHACIN

Indomethacin is a prostaglandin synthetase inhibitor which is commonly used to facilitate the closure of a symptomatic patent ductus arteriosus. It is also administered antenatally as a tocolytic, and to reduce liquor volume in polyhydramnios. In older subjects it is known to reduce sodium excretion and urine flow by enhancing tubular reabsorption, but in addition to this there have been anxieties that it may lower GFR in preterm infants. This difference may reflect the dependence of these subjects on renal prostaglandins to maintain an adequate renal blood flow in the face of high RAAS activity; a parallel can be seen in a study in dogs, where indomethacin was shown to induce a fall in GFR only when RAAS activity was increased by sodium depletion.[120] Conversely, there is also evidence to suggest that inhibition of prostaglandin synthesis has no effect on renal blood flow.[9] Walker and colleagues,[168] studying the chronically catheterized fetal sheep, describe the amelioration of the oliguric response to indomethacin in the presence of an ADH V_2-receptor antagonist. They speculate that indomethacin stimulates circulating ADH levels, resulting in oliguria.

A temporary reduction of sodium and water excretion is described in all reports of babies given indomethacin for duct closure. In the early days of its use, salt and water retention and dilutional hyponatraemia were a common occurrence. The simultaneous administration of 1 mg/kg of frusemide has been shown to eliminate the renal side-effects of 0.3 mg/kg indomethacin without reducing its efficacy in duct closure.[175] In a randomized controlled trial, similar claims for concurrent dopamine therapy were found to be unsubstantiated.[52] If indomethacin is to be used in a dose of 0.2 mg/kg, 12-hourly, it is appropriate to restrict sodium and water intake by approximately 30% and monitor fluid balance carefully (Table 39.9). Smaller doses, of 0.1 mg/kg 24-hourly, as suggested by Rennie and Cooke,[132] are less likely to result in adverse renal effects. Other agents, such as ibuprofen, are currently being evaluated as alternatives to indomethacin, although oligohydramnios and neonatal renal failure have been described after maternal exposure to ibuprofen.[17,84] It is possible that the development of selective cyclo-oxygenase inhibitors may allow more precise therapeutic targeting.

STEROIDS

The synthetic glucocorticoids dexamethasone and betamethasone are widely used in perinatal medicine, antenatally to promote fetal lung maturation, and postnatally in the management of chronic lung disease. These drugs have a number of potent actions on several organ systems. They are gene transducers as well as having direct effects at the level of the cell membrane. They increase β_2-receptor density, antioxidant levels and the density of Na^+K^+ATPase, and also affect a variety of cytokines and growth factors, enhance surfactant production, increase clearance of lung liquid and suppress inducible nitric oxide synthase. Glucocorticoids are also catabolic agents. A temporary inhibition in growth is well documented during therapy, and this often results in a rise in blood urea.

The abundance of Na^+K^+ATPase is regulated by glucocorticoids[29] in an age-dependent manner.[30] In rats, betamethasone will increase Na^+K^+ATPase mRNA in the kidney during infancy, but not during fetal life, nor in adults. In contrast, lung tissue Na^+K^+ATPase is maximally induced by glucocorticoids during the perinatal period. The inference is that glucocorticoids interact with other transcriptional factors, expressed in an age-dependent fashion, to activate the genes for Na^+K^+ATPase, so that different tissues have different periods of sensitivity to glucocorticoid regulation. Glucocorticoids not only enhance renal tubular regulation of sodium balance, potentiate ANP stimulation of cGMP production[72] and enhance the maturation of renal acidification,[16] but also induce both Na^+K^+ATPase and Na^+ channels in lung epithelial cells, thus facilitating the clearance of lung liquid.[119] In addition to the well known effects on the lungs, antenatal exposure to dexamethasone accelerates the maturation of renal function in human preterm newborns.[5]

Paradoxically, glucocorticoids frequently appear to trigger a diuresis when used in the fluid-retaining baby with chronic lung disease.[63,142]

INOTROPIC AGENTS

Dopamine and dobutamine are now frequently used in neonatal intensive care, to support blood pressure and cardiac output, and also for their purported renal effects at low dose. In addition to cardiovascular effects that influence renal function, dopamine also has direct renal actions, inhibiting renal Na^+K^+ATPase and Na^+/H^+ exchanger activity and attenuating the actions of aldosterone and AVP.[144] The cellular signalling system that transduces the signal from activated dopamine receptor to inhibit renal Na^+K^+ATPase, undergoes developmental regulation.[57]

Three randomized clinical studies[64,89,137] comparing the efficacy of dopamine and dobutamine all showed that dopamine is more effective at raising and maintaining blood pressure than dobutamine. However, in only one of these studies was left ventricular output measured as well, and this showed that dopamine did not increase cardiac output, in contrast to dobutamine, which produced a mean increase in left ventricular output of 21%.[137] Seri et al[144] showed that dopamine at a dose of 2 µg/kg/min induced maximal diuresis and natriuresis in sick preterm neonates if systemic blood pressure was within the normal range. An increase to 4 µg/kg/min resulted in a further increase in blood pressure, but no change in urine output and sodium excretion. As dopamine raises blood pressure though its vasconstrictor actions, renal perfusion may in fact be impaired at higher doses.

RENAL DISEASE IN THE NEONATE

ACUTE RENAL FAILURE

Causes and incidence

Both chronic renal renal disease and acute renal failure occur in the newborn. The former, including fetal renal failure with oligoanuria of antenatal onset, is discussed below.

During the initiating phase of acute renal failure renal perfusion is decreased. Stimulation of the juxtaglomerular apparatus activates the RAAS, which further decreases renal blood flow and perpetuates a vicious cycle of further renal ischaemia. Varying degrees of glomerular and tubular injury are present during the established phase.

Acute renal failure is defined as a sudden and severe reduction in GFR. This will result in a rise in serum creatinine, and eventually in further metabolic distur-

Table 39.14 Causes of renal failure in the newborn

Prerenal	Intrinsic	Obstructive
Systemic hypovolaemia	*Congenital abnormalities*	*Congenital malformations*
Dehydration	Congenital dysplasias	Ureterocoele
Haemorrhage	Renal agenesis	Posterior urethral valves
Septic shock	Polycystic kidney disease	Vesicoureteric reflux
Systemic vasodilators	Glomerulosclerosis	Megacystis–megaureter
Necrotizing enterocolitis	Denys–Drash syndrome	PUJ obstruction
Operative fluid loss	*Maternal drugs*	Prune belly syndrome
Renal hypoperfusion	ACE inhibitors	*Extrinsic compression*
Cardiac failure	Cyclo-oxygenase inhibitors	Sacrococcygeal tumour
Respiratory failure	*Acute tubular necrosis*	Haematocolpos
Asphyxia	*Acute cortical necrosis*	*Intrinsic obstruction*
Indomethacin	*Haemoglobinuria*	Fungal ball
	Myoglobinuria	*Neurogenic bladder*
	Renal vascular thrombosis	Asphyxia
	Disseminated intravascular coagulation	Spina bifida
	Pyelonephritis	
	Nephrotoxins	

bance. The serum creatinine in newborns is very variable and an absolute cut-off value is not helpful in making a diagnosis of acute renal failure. It is more useful to suspect renal impairment if the serum creatinine rises or fails to show the normal postnatal fall.

Prerenal, renal and postrenal failure all occur in the newborn period (Table 39.14). Although non-oliguric renal failure has been described,[65] the usual form is oliguric. Renal failure should also be suspected in any neonate in whom urine flow rate falls abruptly or falls below 1 ml/kg/h.

Acute renal failure reportedly occurs in approximately 6–8% of neonates requiring intensive care, and has a mortality of around 50%,[85] although these figures will vary with both place and time, reflecting differences in diagnostic criteria, case-mix and the quality of supportive care. Renal failure was formerly most often seen in the context of severe respiratory disease, but with improvements in the management of this condition perinatal asphyxia, sepsis, NEC and major surgery have emerged as the four most common predisposing causes.

Other clinical settings in which acute renal failure may occur include intrapartum blood loss, as in acute fetomaternal or fetofetal haemorrhage. This may not be immediately obvious, unlike serious neonatal haemorrhage. Dehydration, through failure to replace high insensible water losses, occurs readily. Fluid may be lost acutely into the gastrointestinal tract, as in acute obstruction and NEC. Myocardial compromise, following asphyxia, in heart failure, in hypoplastic left heart syndrome or following cardiac surgery, will lead initially to decreased renal perfusion. Drug therapy may lead to catastrophic hypotension. Tolazoline, an α-agonist, is occasionally employed for its pulmonary vasodilator actions (p. 534). It is also a systemic vasodilator, and systemic hypotension, which may lead to renal failure, is a serious side-effect of therapy. Tolazoline acts rapidly and should not be used in hypotensive states. Blood pressure should be monitored continuously during the initial test dose of 1–2 mg/kg and colloid be available for immediate use. Acute falls in blood pressure have also been described following the use of fentanyl and the ACE inhibitors. Through different modes of action, antenatal exposure to ACE inhibitors and non-steroidal anti-inflammatory agents, including indomethacin, may lead to renal impairment in the newborn. Extracorporeal membrane oxygenation is associated with a transient impairment in renal function and marked fluid retention.[135]

Hydration and the adequacy of the circulation require careful and continuous assessment in neonatal intensive care. Failure to monitor urine output accurately, will delay recognition and increase the risk of prerenal impairment progressing to intrinsic renal failure. It is important to exclude congenital abnormalities of the kidneys, such as dysplasia and infantile-type polycystic disease, and to diagnose renal venous thrombosis or treatable obstructive lesions such as posterior urethral values. Acute retention of urine also occurs, particularly in full-term asphyxiated babies.

The spectrum of renal damage following hypoxic–ischaemic injury extends from mild tubular dysfunction to acute tubular necrosis or irreversible cortical necrosis. Myoglobinuria following rhabdomyolysis and haemoglobinuria due to intravascular haemolysis may also affect renal function.[91] The management of the severely asphyxiated infant should include anticipation of the possibility of renal failure (p. 1243). Careful monitoring of urine output should commence immediately on admission. Initial fluid intake in severely asphyxiated full-term babies should be restricted to 20–30 ml/kg/day until the situation is clear (Table 39.9). This is considerably more than the transepidermal insensible loss of full-term babies, which is around 12 ml/kg/day, and will not result in dehydration. Hypoglycaemia may be a problem at low infusion volumes, and hypertonic dextrose may be necessary, infused centrally. The circulation should be carefully supported. Colloid infusion will inevitably result in the concomitant infusion of sodium, and as sodium will probably also be administered with medications, routine supplementation should be avoided. Urinary retention may require catheterization.

Investigation and management of oligo/anuria

If the urine flow rate falls abruptly in a previously stable infant, or drops below 1 ml/kg/h in the first few days after birth, immediate investigation is mandatory. An obstructed renal tract can be easily identified using ultrasound. The intravenous urogram produces poor images in normal preterm babies and has no role in the assessment of acute renal impairment. Prerenal failure may result from either hypovolaemia or renal hypoperfusion. Hypovolaemic prerenal failure must be considered a matter of urgency, as it is reversible but will rapidly lead to established renal failure if untreated.

It has been suggested that the best indicator to distinguish prerenal from established renal failure in the oliguric neonate is the fractional excretion of sodium (Fe_{Na}). This is readily calculated from the sodium and creatinine concentrations of serum (S) and a spot urine (U) sample:

$$Fe_{Na}\ \% = (U/S)\ \text{sodium} \times (S/U)\ \text{creatinine} \times 100$$

If tubular function is intact and sodium reabsorption continues, the infant is in oliguric prerenal failure and the Fe_{Na} will be less than 3%. Once tubular necrosis has occurred the Fe_{Na} is usually above 10%. Prerenal oliguria demands urgent attention to renal perfusion, whereas a high Fe_{Na} suggests established renal failure and the equally urgent need for restriction of fluid intake. Unfortunately, the fractional sodium excretion, and other indices such as the renal failure index (U sodium × S/U creatinine), have poor sensitivity and specificity.[111] In extremely immature infants values for Fe_{Na} in prerenal and renal failure overlap. The urinary sodium concentration cannot be interpreted clearly if frusemide has already been used, nor is delaying further action until urinary sodium and creatinine estimations have been obtained acceptable.

The clinical context should be carefully evaluated. Poor perfusion results from several causes. Features include a low or low normal blood pressure, capillary refill time exceeding 3 seconds, and core–peripheral temperature gap of greater than 2°C. Dehydration will additionally result in weight loss, decreased skin turgor and hypernatraemia. An increase in maintenance volumes is mandatory, and should be preceded by a rehydration volume of 20 ml/kg over 1–2 hours.

If there are signs of extracellular volume overload, with weight gain or weight retention, or the infant appears frankly oedematous, a fluid challenge may well worsen the situation, and inotropic support of cardiac output with dobutamine 10–20 μg/kg/min, together with low-dose dopamine 2 μg/kg/min to improve renal perfusion, is recommended.

If the clinical assessment is equivocal, a cautious fluid challenge is an appropriate approach. Ensure that the intravascular compartment is adequately filled by administering a volume of 10–20 ml/kg, followed by frusemide. It is not known whether colloid or normal saline is the more suitable fluid.[153] A note of caution should be sounded as regards the critically ill neonate with severe respiratory failure. Impaired renal perfusion may be unresponsive to volume replacement, and indeed the risk of exacerbating respiratory function through the injudicious use of large intravenous volumes is substantial. A urine low rate of 0.5 ml/kg/h is acceptable on the first day after birth in such infants. Attention should be directed towards improving renal perfusion through optimal respiratory and cardiovascular support.

Frusemide increases the flow of tubular fluid but also stimulates prostaglandin release and reduces renal metabolic requirements by inhibiting the sodium pump. Although doses of 1–3 mg/kg have been recommended a higher dose of 4–5 mg/kg is probably more appropriate, as frusemide exerts its effects on the loop of Henle only after glomerular filtration, and high plasma levels are necessary when the GFR is low.[114] However, because the half-life of frusemide clearance is almost 24 hours in healthy preterm infants that are not in renal failure,[31] clearance will almost certainly be several days in babies remaining in renal failure, and there is no rationale for repeating the dose; this would only lead to accumulation and the risks of ototoxicity, interstitial nephritis and possibly persistence of ductal patency.

If a volume challenge does not produce a prompt diuresis the baby needs to be managed as one in established renal failure, and intake volume reduced immediately to no more than insensible water loss plus urine output.

ESTABLISHED RENAL FAILURE

The prime imperative in the management of the infant who is in established renal failure or has failed to respond to volume repletion is to avoid fluid overload and electrolyte imbalance. Meticulous monitoring of physiological variables and 'aggressive' supportive therapy is mandatory while establishing a prognosis.

The baby should be weighed 12-hourly. Intake volumes and losses should be carefully recorded. The adequacy of the circulation should be monitored, including regular assessment of capillary refill time, core–peripheral temperature gap, invasive blood pressure monitoring and, if possible, cardiac output and central venous pressure. Low-dose dopamine has been advocated in the management of established acute renal failure, though there is no evidence that it improves outcome. The renal actions of dopamine are described above. Dobutamine is currently the drug of choice if cardiac output is to be augmented. If the central venous pressure is below 4 cmH_2O colloid support is necessary.[152] Although albumin may be used, fresh frozen plasma may be more appropriate, as disseminated intravascular coagulation often accompanies acute renal failure.

Extremely careful attention should be paid to reduce the total intake of crystalloid to no more than insensible losses plus urine output and gastrointestinal losses, as water overload very readily occurs, making a bad situation considerably worse. Full-term infants will have an insensible water loss of less than 20 ml/kg/day, and effective fluid restriction will require central vascular access for the infusion of hypertonic glucose solution and for drug delivery. Sodium intake should similarly be limited to the replacement of losses, bearing in mind the occasional need for base in the form of sodium bicarbonate, and that substantial inadvertent sodium administration is very common (Table 39.5). In practical terms, therefore, no sodium should be prescribed and every effort should be made to minimize inadvertent administration. Weight gain with hyponatraemia in renal failure is due to water excess and suggests that fluid restriction has not been aggressive enough. Calcium may be added to the infusion fluid in a dose of 0.5–1.0 mmol/kg/24 h.

The cautious infusion of sodium bicarbonate may be necessary, but intractable metabolic acidosis is a poor prognostic sign. A reportedly high serum potassium in the newborn is most often due to a haemolysed blood sample. If in doubt, it should be repeated. Commence treatment for hyperkalaemia with rectal calcium resonium when the serum potassium exceeds 6.5 mmol/l. ECG abnormalities (peaked T waves, widened QRS complexes) are rarely seen in the newborn until the serum potassium exceeds 8 mmol/l. Emergency treatment is then necessary while preparing for dialysis. Calcium gluconate, sodium bicarbonate, and either dextrose and insulin or salbutamol may be employed (Table 39.12).

Hypertension in acute renal failure is usually secondary to volume overload, although activation of the renin–angiotensin–aldosterone system may be responsible as, for example, in renal artery occlusion. Treatment is rarely necessary, though it is clearly merited if the hypertension is severe or symptomatic. Hydrallazine is an effective first drug (100–500 μg/kg/dose 4-hourly i.v. or 250–700 μg/kg/dose 8-hourly orally). Propranolol (500 μg/kg/dose 8-hourly orally) may be used if tachycardia is a side-effect of hydrallazine therapy.

Current experimental approaches are directed at intervention during the therapeutic window that is believed to exist after hypoxic–ischaemic insult, before cell death ensues. Animal models of hypoxic–ischaemic renal injury have demonstrated that renal tubular damage progresses for several hours after renal blood flow has been restored. The infusion of ATP-$MgCl_2$ during this period has been shown, using nuclear magnetic resonance spectroscopy, to result in accelerated recovery of renal ATP.[157] Similar effects have been demonstrated with thyroxine.[161]

At present, the management of acute renal failure rests on aggressive support. If the insult that precipitated renal failure is no longer operative, meticulous medical management, optimizing renal perfusion and avoiding fluid overload, will allow even an anuric baby to remain in stable electrolyte and water balance for several days. To help determine the prognosis in an anuric baby, radionuclide scans such as ^{99}Tc-DTPA may be used to assess whether the kidneys are still perfused, but false negatives may occur[31] and an unequivocal distinction between bilateral cortical necrosis and tubular necrosis in the acute stages is difficult. Acute renal failure in the newborn usually occurs together with other major problems. If the overall prognosis is believed to be good, dialysis should be considered if medical management is no longer able to contain acidosis, severe electrolyte imbalance, hypoglycaemia and fluid overload. A rising serum creatinine is not, on its own, an indication for dialysis. Although haemodialysis and haemofiltration have been described in extremely preterm newborns,[40] peritoneal dialysis remains the only readily available approach.

Peritoneal dialysis

For most neonatal intensive care units, peritoneal dialysis is the only practicable technique for very small babies. In theory, the large peritoneal surface area to body ratio in preterm babies would be advantageous, and fortunately the technique is relatively simple. It has also been successfully reported after abdominal surgery,[107] although this is usually considered a contraindication. Rigid peritoneal dialysis catheters are unsuitable for extremely small babies as the side holes extend too far and they may damage the bowel. Various soft catheters are available or, alternatively, chest drain tubes with side holes may be used. They are inserted percutaneously, over a trocar or using the Seldinger technique[41,93,96,177] and lie curled up in the peritoneal space. Peripheral intravenous catheters are unsuitable as they almost invariably fail to drain adequately owing to the lack of side holes.

The technique for peritoneal dialysis is as follows: systemic analgesia (morphine 50–100 μg/kg, i.v.) is administered and local anaesthetic (0.5 ml 1% lignocaine) infiltrated into the skin and subcutaneous tissues. Although a midline insertion, below the umbilicus, is sometimes advocated, this will interfere will the fixation of a urine bag and insertion just lateral to the rectus sheath and just below the level of the umbilicus is the preferred approach, particularly in very small babies. A peripheral intravenous cannula is then inserted into the peritoneal cavity and a prefill instilled, of 20 ml/kg dialysis fluid, warmed to body temperature, in order to reduce the risk of bowel perforation. If this volume is tolerated well, a further 10–20 ml/kg may be instilled. The cannula is then removed and the dialysis catheter introduced and connected to the administration and drainage sets. Integrated sealed dialysis systems are available commercially and are to be preferred, as the risk of infection is reduced with the smaller number of connections. However, an adequate system can be put together with individual components if necessary (Fig. 39.13). These comprise the bag of dialysis fluid, a graduated burette to accurately measure inflow, a

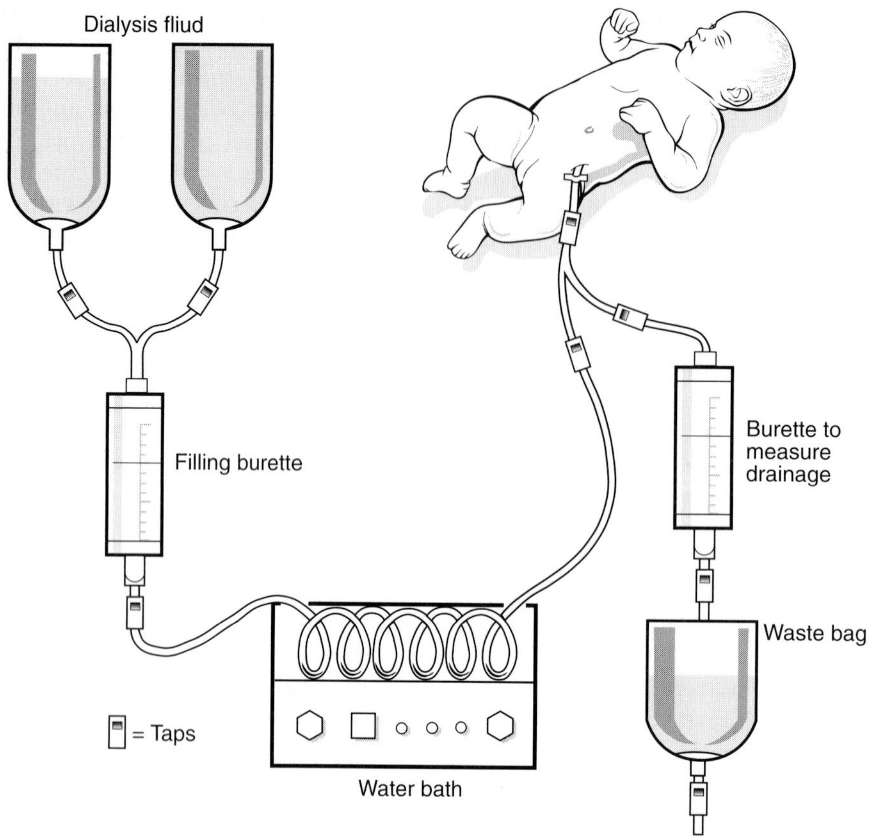

Fig. 39.13 Diagram of peritoneal dialysis circuit.

fluid warmer and a gravity drain outflow via a graduated burette, to accurately measure the volume of fluid drained. In practice the two most troublesome problems are the high incidence of leakage around the insertion site and catheter obstruction by omentum. The skin incision should therefore be kept as small as possible, as large a prefill used as is tolerated, and as long as possible a length of catheter with side holes inserted. A drop of collodion may be placed around the exit site. The catheter should be secured reliably, then connected to the system and the outflow opened.

Volumes of 15–20 ml/kg, instilled by gravity flow, are used initially, increasing to 40 ml/kg provided this does not cause respiratory difficulty. Commence with a cycle without a dwell period, in order to test for adequacy of drainage. Open the outflow port and begin gravity drainage. Once the effluent is no longer bloodstained, begin half-hourly or hourly cycles, lengthening further as dictated by the biochemical response. A typical dialysis prescription might be a 10-minute infusion time, 35-minute dwell and 15-minute drain time. Poor drainage may be addressed by flushing and repositioning the catheter.

Though there were initial concerns that very immature, unwell infants would be unable to adequately metabolize the lactate present in commercially available dialysis fluids this has proved unusual. Intravenous calcium supplements are usually necessary. Hyperglycaemia may result from glucose absorbed from the dialysis fluid. This should be managed by reducing the intravenous glucose delivery rate in the first instance, though an insulin infusion may be required. Hypertonic dialysis fluids should not be used in very immature babies as the sudden fluid shift may cause acute circulatory collapse. It is best to commence with an isotonic 1.36% solution and increase the concentration cautiously if necessary. Heparin (1 unit/ml) may be added to the dialysis fluid, particularly if the effluent is bloodstained, to prevent clots forming in the catheter holes. If an aminoglycoside is indicated this may be added to the dialysis fluid at the appropriate concentration to be achieved in the plasma (10 mg/l for gentamicin) and one loading dose given parenterally if it has not already been started. The dose of systemically administered penicillins should be halved during dialysis, and other renally excreted drugs individually adjusted. Once the serum potassium has fallen below 3.5 mmol/l, add potassium chloride 4 mmol/l to the dialysis fluid. Bacterial and fungal peritonitis are a major hazard of peritoneal dialysis at all ages. The risks can be minimized by using a complete neonatal administration set rather than making one up from separate components, and by obsessive nursing care. Clinical signs suggesting peritonitis include cloudy fluid, abdominal tenderness and pyrexia. Microscopy and culture of the effluent fluid should be carried out daily and antibiotics added to the dialysis fluid at the earliest suspicion of an infection. Infection may also occur at the catheter exit site.

The mortality in neonates requiring dialysis for acute renal failure is reported to be around 50% or higher, and is dependent on overall condition.[22]

Haemofiltration

The term filtration refers to the removal of plasma water across a membrane, in contrast to dialysis, which is the removal of plasma solutes by diffusion down a concentration gradient across a semipermeable membrane. Ultrafiltration requires a net pressure gradient between hydraulic and hydrostatic pressure, which favour filtration, and oncotic pressure, which opposes it. Dialysis fluid may be set up to flow countercurrent to blood flow, and so provide combined dialysis and filtration. Ultrafilters and dialysers suitable for use in tiny babies, with very small blood priming volumes, are now available commercially. If reliable arterial access is available, as with an umbilical catheter, and systolic blood pressure exceeds 45 mmHg, the baby's heart may be used to provide the pressure for filtration. If only venous access is available, or systemic blood pressure inadequate, a blood pump is necessary. This may consist of manual, syringe-driven pumping. These methods are technically highly demanding.[40,97,176,181] Though feasible, the overall reported prognosis for babies undergoing the procedure remains poor.[41] Very careful consideration should be given to the child's and the family's best interests, because renal failure so often occurs in a setting of multisystem impairment and poor ultimate outcome.

CHRONIC RENAL DISEASE

This term is used to denote impaired renal function arising as a consequence of a congenital abnormality of the kidneys or renal tract, which may be a developmental malformation or arise as an inherited disorder. The terminology of congenital and inherited kidney disease can be confusing, and this is probably a reflection of the fact that the abnormalities in embryogenesis that underlie these conditions are poorly understood. The molecular basis of nephrogenesis is now beginning to be unravelled[174] In situ hybridization, cell culture and transgenic animals are being used to identify and understand the role of the many transcription factors, oncogenes and growth factors expressed during normal and aberrant nephrogenesis. Genes that have a direct role in nephrogenesis are beginning to be identified. The Wilms' tumour suppressor gene *WT-1* is specifically involved in kidney development. Mutations may lead to Wilms' tumour, ambiguous genitalia and nephropathy, which may progress to renal failure.[100] There are now mouse models for both the autosomal recessive and dominant forms of polycystic kidney disease. The next decade will undoubtedly see better understanding of gene product regulation of renal differentiation.

In a multicystic kidney there is no continuity between glomeruli and calyces, and the kidney is non-functioning. The term dysplastic refers to disorganized renal architecture; there may be cysts present and ectopic tissue, such as cartilage and muscle. A polycystic kidney contains many cysts, but there is continuity of the lumen of the nephron with the urinary tract. In renal agenesis there is unilateral or bilateral absence of the kidney. Renal agenesis and the multicystic dysplastic kidney are discussed in Part 2 of this chapter.

The presentation of chronic renal disease may be antenatally, in the immediate newborn period, or later in life. As the placenta performs a renal role, even lethal kidney malformations may not result in biochemical disturbance for several days. Renal abnormalities are often associated with other conditions and are a feature of many dysmorphic syndromes. Renal cysts occur in Meckel, Jeune and Goldston syndromes. The antenatal onset of renal failure leads to the oligohydramnios sequence, in which there is uterine compression of the fetus due to decreased amniotic fluid. The infant has a Potter facies, limb contractures and pulmonary hypoplasia (pp. 641, 882).

Children with chronic renal disease may have a multiplicity of associated and related problems and their care and that of their families clearly requires a multidisciplinary approach. Management is frequently difficult. The underlying aetiology and the renal and extrarenal prognosis need to be determined. A decision to embark on treatment should not be undertaken lightly and parents need to be made fully cognisant of all the implications. Growth compromise, repeated hospitalization, a period of dialysis, possibly prolonged, leading to renal transplantation, and a heavy emotional cost for both the child and the family, are all factors to be taken into account.

POLYCYSTIC KIDNEY DISEASE

Polycystic kidney disease occurs in both AR and AD forms. Autosomal recessive polycystic kidney disease is a rare disorder with a reported prevalence ranging from 1:6000 to 1:55 000 livebirths. It arises from a mutation on chromosome 6. The condition often causes renal failure in infancy, and presentation may be with the oligohydramnios sequence. In the neonate, renal involvement is more prominent than hepatic. Kaplan et al[83] reported the long-term survival of 55 paediatric cases of ARPKD: 42% presented under the age of 1 month, with hepatomegaly, palpable kidneys, renal failure and respiratory failure. Diagnosis is based on the family history, liver biopsy and imaging. The presence of hepatic fibrosis with biliary dysgenesis strongly suggests ARPKD.[32]

Autosomal dominant polycystic kidney disease accounts for 5–10% of end-stage renal failure worldwide, and is one of the most common dominantly inherited conditions, with an estimated incidence of 1 in 1000. Clinical expression is variable but it should be regarded as a systemic disorder, with cysts affecting mainly the kidneys and liver, and other organs to a lesser extent. It is also associated with aneurysms of the cerebral and coronary arteries. It usually presents in adult life, but approximately 2% present with severe manifestations in childhood. Prenatal onset has also been reported.[178] The most common form, ADPKD-1, accounts for 85% of cases and is caused by a mutation on the short arm of chromosome 16, with the gene for ADPKD-2 on chromosome 4 and the location of ADPKD-3 as yet unknown.[62] The diagnosis may follow investigation of a known at-risk subject. Clinical presentation in an index case is commonly with haematuria, enlarged kidneys and hypertension. A rapid decline in renal function is not inevitable, but early treatment of hypertension is important.[171] Genetic counselling is integral to the management of the family.

In the absence of a definite family history, the differentiation of ARPKD from ADPKD in a neonate with large kidneys can be difficult. Clinicians should also be aware of the wide number of syndromes in children in which polycystic kidneys are a feature, such as tuberous sclerosis and von Hippel–Lindau disorder. Neither ultrasound nor intravenous pyelography will always differentiate between ARPKD and ADPKD, and an infant may manifest the disease before a parent. Hepatic and renal imaging of both parents should be carried out, as the presence of cysts will confirm a diagnosis of ADPKD. Prediction of ADPKD by DNA restriction-length polymorphisms is a promising development.

GLOMERULAR DISEASE

Glomerulonephritis and nephrotic syndrome are both rare in the newborn. Glomerulonephritis has principally been described in association with congenital syphilis, toxoplasmosis and cytomegalovirus. Presentation is with the features of the primary disease and haematuria or proteinuria. The features of congenital nephrotic syndrome are oedema, proteinuria, decreased plasma albumin and elevated plasma cholesterol. Other causes of oedema, such as cardiac failure, capillary leak syndrome and renal failure, are much more common. Nephrotic syndrome in the newborn may be inherited, as in the Finnish type, and the Galloway–Mowat and other rare syndromes, or occur with congenital syphilis and hepatitis B (Table 39.15). Congenital syphilis is treatable, and therefore this diagnosis should not be missed. Congenital nephrotic syndrome of the Finnish type is the best-known, followed by idiopathic nephrosis with the histopathological features of minimal change disease, diffuse mesangial proliferation and focal segmental glomerulosclerosis.[66]

Table 39.15 Causes of infantile nephrotic syndrome

Primary
Finnish type
Denys–Drash syndrome
Galloway–Mowat syndrome
Diffuse mesangial sclerosis
Minimal change disease
Focal segmental glomerulosclerosis
Secondary
Congenital syphilis
Toxoplasmosis
Cytomegalovirus
Hepatitis B
Mercury poisoning

Congenital nephrotic syndrome of the Finnish type is an autosomal recessive condition, with the locus on the long arm of chromosome 19.[87] The onset of proteinuria may be in utero. Maternal serum and amniotic fluid α-fetoprotein levels are elevated. The placenta is large, weighing more than 25% of the infant's birthweight in contrast to the normal 18%. The prevalence of the condition is 1.2 per 10 000 births in Finland. It has also been described in other racial groups. Oedema develops in half of affected infants in the first week after birth, and in all cases invariably within 3 months.[81] Renal histological evaluation shows dilatation of the proximal tubules, glomerular hypercellularity and mesangial accentuation. The condition is unresponsive to corticosteroids and immunosuppresive drugs. The clinical course is marked by growth failure and recurrent, severe bacterial infections, but although glomerular filtration rate declines with disease progression, renal failure is not an inevitable consequence. Management is largely supportive, optimizing nutrition, symptomatic treatment of oedema with diuretics and salt restriction, and aggressive treatment of infections. Genetic counselling is of paramount importance. If renal failure supervenes, bilateral nephrectomy and renal transplantation is an option, with a still poor but improving prognosis.[106]

INHERITED RENAL TUBULAR DISORDERS

The renal tubular disorders are a diverse group of conditions representing abnormalities of renal ion transport. Disordered renal tubular function may present antenatally, with polyhydramnios, or after birth with vomiting, failure to thrive and lethargy. Prenatal diagnosis, utilizing chorion villus sampling or amniocentesis, is possible for certain conditions, but usually relies on the diagnosis having first been made in a proband.

Bartter syndrome

The different forms of this disorder have yet to be fully

unravelled. The typical neonatal form frequently presents with polyhydramnios and preterm delivery, followed by volume depletion and hypokalaemic alkalosis in the newborn. There is marked hypercalciuria, with a urinary calcium to creatinine ratio exceeding 0.4, but no hypomagnesaemia. This form of the disorder has been shown to be linked to mutations in the Na-K-2Cl cotransporter gene *NKCC2*.[148] There is marked stimulation of renal and systemic prostaglandin E_2 production. The condition responds to treatment with indomethacin, a prostaglandin synthetase inhibitor, and adequate sodium and potassium replacement.[105]

Nephrogenic diabetes insipidus

This condition, arising from insensitivity of the distal nephron to ADH, may present with polyhydramnios. After birth the baby will excrete large quantities of hypotonic urine, become dehydrated and fail to thrive. The serum sodium, chloride and creatinine will be elevated and there is no response to exogenous ADH. In most patients with inherited nephrogenic diabetes insipidus the condition is X-linked. The mutation has been localized to Xq28 and prenatal diagnosis is possible. Treatment consists of indomethacin with hydrochlorothiazide, or hydrochlorothiazide with amiloride.[90]

Renal tubular acidosis

Although a metabolic acidosis is a common finding among the neonatal intensive care population, primary renal tubular acidosis is uncommon. Renal tubular acidosis should be suspected when a metabolic acidosis is accompanied by hyperchloraemia and a normal plasma anion gap. This implies loss of bicarbonate from either the gastrointestinal tract, as in chronic diarrhoea, or the kidneys. Together, bicarbonate and chloride account for most of the anions in plasma, with less than 16 mmol/l from proteins and inorganic and organic salts. The sum of the measured cations (Na^+ and K^+) is always slightly more than the measured anions (HCO_3^- and Cl^-) i.e. $[Na^+ + K^+] - [Cl^- + HCO_3^-] = 8–16$ mmol/l. A large anion gap in the newborn suggests the presence of other acids, as in the organic and inorganic acidaemias.

Before considering a diagnosis of renal tubular acidosis, ensure that hyperchloraemia is not a result of excessive chloride administration in, for example, parenteral nutrition formulations. The defect in renal tubular acidosis may be permanent, but the entity presenting in the newborn is more often transient.

In proximal renal tubular acidosis, bicarbonate reabsorption in the proximal tubule is impaired. Distal acidification by H^+ secretion is intact and the urine pH is therefore low. In the renal Fanconi syndrome, a generalized proximal tubular dysfunction results in proximal renal tubular acidosis as well as urinary loss of phosphate, glucose, amino acids, and low molecular weight proteins. Cystinosis is the most frequent cause of inherited Fanconi syndrome in infants.

A diagnosis of distal renal tubular acidosis may be made, if stool bicarbonate loss is excluded, if the urinary pH is above 6. Regardless of the site of the defect, treatment, consists of alkali in the form of oral bicarbonate or citrate. A dose of around 1–2 mmol/kg/day is usually sufficient for distal and 2–5 mmol/kg/day in proximal renal tubular acidosis.[60]

RENAL VASCULAR DISEASE

Renal arterial thrombosis

A report from a prospective registry involving 22 Canadian and 42 neonatal centres in North America, Europe and Australia, over a 42-month period, concluded that neonatal thrombosis is now fairly rare[141] and, with the exception of renal venous thrombosis, is almost always associated with indwelling catheters. Twenty-one cases of renal venous thrombosis were registered from 29 centres. Of the 33 reported arterial thromboses, 28 affected the aorta, iliac or femoral vessels and only five involved either the renal or pulmonary arteries. However, many episodes of catheter occlusion are clinically silent and renal involvement may present late, with impaired renal function and hypertension (p. 920). In the acute phase heparin or thrombolytic therapy should be considered, as discussed on page 922. Ultrasound and Doppler flow may be used to aid the diagnosis and assess the response to therapy. Renal size will initially be normal, but a radionuclide scan will show reduced uptake. Later scans may show renal atrophy. Plasma renin activity will be raised. Hypertension may be severe enough to warrant treatment, but limited follow-up information suggests that it will often resolve.[1]

Renal venous thrombosis

This is more common than renal arterial occlusion in the newborn. It is usually preceded by venous stasis and decreased renal perfusion, and is therefore associated with asphyxia, dehydration, hypotension, cyanotic congenital heart disease, polycythaemia and hyperosmolality states, and is seen in infants of diabetic mothers. Thrombosis begins in the arcuate and intralobular veins and is accompanied by parenchymal hypoxia, cellular disruption and haemorrhage. The commonest presenting feature is of a mass in the flank, followed by gross haematuria, microscopic haematuria, renal impairment and thrombocytopenia. Ultrasonography will reveal renal enlargement and possibly visible thrombus in the renal vein and inferior vena cava. The management of renal venous thrombosis is based on supportive therapy, treatment of the underlying condition and correction of polycythaemia and dehydration. Nephrectomy is no longer considered to be indicated and experience with thrombectomy is unsatisfactory. In the absence of evidence of ongoing intravascular coagulation the role of heparin is unclear, as extensive thrombosis is presumably present by the time of diagnosis. Fibrinolytic therapy may be a more effective approach, although experience is scanty. Survival rates after renal venous thrombosis range between 45 and 86%, with deaths caused by the underlying illness. The spectrum renal of impairment after recovery ranges from normal function to renal atrophy, hypertension and chronic renal failure.[86,133]

REFERENCES

1. Adelman R 1987 Long term follow up of neonatal renovascular hypertension. Pediatric Nephrology 1: 35–41
2. Al-Dahhan J, Haycock G B, Chantler C, Stimmler L 1983 Sodium homeostasis in term and preterm neonates. I. Renal aspects. Archives of Disease in Childhood 58: 335–343
3. Al-Dahhan J, Haycock G B, Chantler C, Stimmler L 1983 Sodium homeostasis in term and preterm neonates. II. Gastrointestinal aspects. Archives of Disease in Childhood 58: 343–345
4. Al-Dahhan J, Haycock G B, Nichol B, Chantler C, Stimmler L 1984 Sodium homeostasis in term and preterm neonates. III. Effect of salt supplementation. Archives of Disease in Childhood 59: 945–950
5. Al-Dahhan J, Stimmler L, Chantler C, Haycock G B 1987 The effect of antenatal dexamethasone administration on glomerular filtration rate and renal sodium excretion in premature infants. Pediatric Nephrology 1: 131–135
6. Al-Rubeyi B, Murray N, Modi N 1994 A variable dextrose delivery system for use in neonatal intensive care. Archives of Disease in Childhood 70: F79
7. Aperia A, Holtback U, Syren M L, Svensson L B, Fryckstedt J, Greengard P 1994 Activation/deactivation of renal Na^+, K^+-ATPase: a final common pathway for regulation of natriuresis FASEB Journal 8: 436–439
8. Aranda J V, Chemtob S, Laudignon N, Sasyniuk B I 1986 Furosemide and vitamin E: two problem drugs in neonatology. Pediatric Clinics of North America 33: 583–602
9. Arnold-Aldea S A, Auslender R A, Parer J T 1991 The effect of the inhibition of prostaglandin synthesis on renal blood flow in fetal sheep. American Journal of Obstetrics and Gynecology 165: 185–190
10. Bard J B L, Woolf A S 1992 Nephrogenesis and the development of kidney disease. Nephrology Dialysis Transplantation 7: 563–572
11. Barr P A, Bailey P E, Sumners J, Cassady G 1977 Relation between arterial blood pressure and blood volume and effect of infused albumin in sick preterm infants. Pediatrics 60: 282–289
12. Bartter F C, Schwartz W B 1967 The syndrome of inappropriate secretion of antidiuretic hormone. American Journal of Medicine 42: 790–806
13. Bauer K, Linderkamp O, Versmold H T 1993 Systolic blood pressure and blood volume in preterm infants. Archives of Disease in Childhood 69: 521–522
14. Bauer K, Versmold H 1989 Postnatal weight loss in preterm neonates less than 1500 g is isotonic dehydration of the extracellular volume. Acta Paediatrica Scandinavica Suppl 360: 37–42
15. Bauer K, Bovermann G, Roithmaier A, Gotz M, Proiss A, Versmold H 1991 Body composition, nutrition and fluid balance during the first two weeks of life in preterm neonates weighing less than 1500 g. Journal of Pediatrics 118: 615–620
16. Baum M, Quigley R 1993 Glucocorticoids stimulate rabbit proximal convoluted tubule acidification. Journal of Clinical Investigation 91: 110–114
17. Bavoux F 1992 Toxicité foetale des anti-inflammatoires non stéroidiens. Presse Médicale 21: 1909–1912
18. Bell E F, Warburton D, Stonestreet B, Oh W 1979 High volume fluid intake predisposes premature infants to necrotising enterocolitis. Lancet ii: 90
19. Bell E F, Warburton D, Stonestreet B, Oh W 1980 Effect of fluid administration on the development of symptomatic patent ductus arteriosus and congestive heart failure in premature infants. New England Journal of Medicine 302: 598–604
20. Benitez O A, Benitez M, Stijnen T, Boot W, Berger H M 1986 Inaccuracy in neonatal measurement of urine concentration with a refractometer. Journal of Pediatrics 108: 613–616
21. Bétrémieux P, Modi N, Hartnoll G, Midgley J 1995 Longitudinal changes in extracellular fluid volume, sodium excretion and atrial natriuretic peptide, in preterm neonates with hyaline membrane disease. Early Human Development 41: 221–222
22. Blowey D L, Mcfarland K, Alon U, McGraw-Houchens M, Hellerstein S, Warady B A 1993 Peritoneal dialysis in the neonatal period: outcome data. Journal of Perinatology 13: 59–64
23. Boyd E 1935 The growth of the surface area of the human body. Institute of Child Welfare Monograph Series No. 10 University of Minnesota Press.
24. Brand P L, van Lingen R A, Brus F, Talsma M D, Elzenga N J 1993 Hypertrophic obstructive cardiomyopathy as a side effect of dexamethasone treatment for bronchopulmonary dysplasia. Acta Paediatrica 82: 614–617
25. Brewer E D 1998 Urinary acidification. In Polin R A, Fox W W (eds) Fetal and neonatal physiology, 2nd edn. WB Saunders, Philadelphia, pp 1657–1660
26. Brown E R, Stark A, Sosneko I, Lawson E E, Avery M E 1978 Bronchopulmonary dysplasia: possible relationship to pulmonary oedema. Journal of Pediatrics 92: 982–984
27. Cartlidge P H T, Rutter N 1987 Karaya gum ECG electrodes for the preterm infant. Archives of Disease in Childhood 62: 1281–1282
28. Chance G W, Radde I C, Willis D M, Roy R N, Park E, Ackerman J 1977 Postnatal growth of infants of <1.3 kg birth weight; effects of metabolic acidosis, of caloric intake and of calcium, sodium and phosphate supplementation. Journal of Pediatrics 91: 787–793
29. Celsi G, Nishi A, Akusjärvi G, Aperia A 1991 Abundance of Na^+, K^+-ATPase mRNA is regulated by glucocorticoid hormones in infant rat kidneys. American Journal of Physiology 260: F192–F197
30. Celsi G, Wang Z M, Akusjarvi G, Aperia A 1993 Sensitive periods for glucocorticoid regulation of Na^+, K^+-ATPase mRNA in the developing lung and kidney. Pediatric Research 33: 5–9
31. Chevalier R L, Campbell F, Brenbridge A N A G 1984 Prognostic factors in neonatal acute renal failure. Pediatrics 74: 265–272
32. Cole B R, Conley S B, Stapleton F B 1987 Polycystic kidney disease in the first year of life. Journal of Pediatrics 111: 693–699
33. Costarino A T, Gruskay J A, Corcoran L, Pollin R A, Baumgart S 1992 Sodium restriction versus daily maintenance replacement in very low birth weight premature neonates: a randomised, blind therapeutic trial. Journal of Pediatrics 120: 99–106
34. Coulthard M G 1983 Comparison of methods of measuring renal function in preterm babies using inulin. Journal of Pediatrics 102: 923–930
35. Coulthard M G 1985 Maturation of glomerular filtration in preterm and mature babies. Early Human Development 11: 281–292
36. Coulthard M G 1989 Renal function. In: Harvey D R, Cooke R W I, Levitt G A (eds) The baby under 1000 g. Butterworths, London; p 214
37. Coulthard M G, Hey E N 1984 Weight as the best standard for glomerular filtration in the newborn. Archives of Disease in Childhood 59: 373–375
38. Coulthard M G, Hey E N 1985 Effect of varying water intake on renal function in healthy preterm babies. Archives of Disease in Childhood 60: 614–620
39. Coulthard M G, Hey E N, Ruddock V 1985 Creatinine and urea clearances compared to inulin clearance in preterm and mature babies. Early Human Development 11: 11–19
40. Coulthard M G, Sharp J 1995 Haemodialysis and ultrafiltration in babies weighing under 1000 g. Archives of Disease in Childhood 73: F162–F165
41. Coulthard M G, Vernon B 1995 Managing acute renal failure in very low birth weight babies. Archives of Disease in Childhood 73: F187–F192
42. Cumming A D, Swainson C P 1995 Disturbances in water, electrolyte and acid–base balance. In: Edwards C R W, Bouchier I A D, Haslett C, Chilvers E R (eds) Davidson's principles and practice of medicine. Churchill Livingstone, Edinburgh, p 587
43. Deen P M, Verdijk M A, Knoers N V et al 1994 Requirement of

human renal water channel aquaporin-2 for vasopressin dependent concentration of urine. Science 264: 92–95
44. De Luna M B, Hallet W H 1967 Urinary protein excretion in healthy infants, children and adults. Proceedings of the American Society of Nephrology 16: 16
45. Drukker A, Goldsmith D I, Spitzer A, Edelmann C M, Blaufox M D 1980 The renin angiotensin system in newborn dogs: developmental patterns and response to acute saline loading. Pediatric Research 14: 304–307
46. Dunn F L, Brennan T J, Neelson A E, Robertson G L 1976 The role of blood osmolality and volume in regulating vasopressin secretion by the rat. Journal of Clinical Investigation 52: 3212–3219
47. Ekblad H, Aperia A, Larsson S H 1992 Intracellular pH regulation in cultured renal proximal tubule cells in different stages of maturation. American Journal of Physiology 263: F716–F721
48. Engle W D, Arant B S 1984 Urinary potassium excretion in the critically ill neonate. Pediatrics 74: 259–264
49. Ervin M G 1988 Perinatal fluid and electrolyte regulation: role of arginine vasopressin. Seminars in Perinatology 12: 134–142
50. Evans N J, Rutter N 1986 Development of the epidermis in the newborn. Biology of the Neonate 49: 74–80
51. Evans N J, Rutter N 1986 Reduction of skin damage from transcutaneous oxygen electrodes using a spray-on dressing. Archives of Disease in Childhood 61: 881–884
52. Fajardo C A, Whyte R K, Steele B T 1992 Effect of dopamine on failure of indomethacin to close the patent ductus arteriosus. Journal of Pediatrics 121: 771–775
53. Fetterman G F, Shuplock N A, Philipp F G, Gregg H S 1965 The growth and maturation of human glomeruli and proximal convolutions from term to adulthood. Studies by microdissection. Pediatrics 35: 601–619
54. Fewell J E, Norton J B 1980 Continuous positive airway pressure impairs renal function in newborn goats. Pediatric Research 14: 1132–1134
55. Friis Hansen B 1961 Body water compartments in children: changes during growth and related changes in body composition. Pediatrics 28: 169–181
56. Friis Hansen B 1983 Water distribution in the fetus and newborn infant. Acta Paediatrica Scandinavica Suppl 305: 7–11
57. Fukuda Y, Bertorelli A, Aperia A 1991 Ontogeny of the regulation of Na^+, K^+-ATPase activity in the renal proximal tubular cell. Pediatric Research 30: 131–134
58. Gerigk M, Gnehm Hp E, Rascher W 1996 Arginine vasopressin and renin in acutely ill children: implications for fluid therapy. Acta Pædiatrica 85: 550–553
59. Golberger E 1986 A primer of water, electrolyte and acid–base disorders, 7th edn. Lea & Febinger, Philadelphia, p 55
60. Goldstein M B, Bear R, Richardson R M A, Marsden P A, Halperin M L 1986 The urine anion gap: a clinically useful index of ammonium excretion. American Journal of Medical Science 292: 198–202
61. Gouyon J B, Houchan N 1993 Assessment of urine specific gravity by reagent strip test in newborn infants. Pediatric Nephrology 7: 77–78
62. Grantham J J 1995 Polycystic kidney disease – there goes the neighbourhood. New England Journal of Medicine 333: 56–57
63. Greenough A, Chan V, Emery E F, Gamsu H R 1993 Respiratory status and diuresis following treatment with dexamethasone. Early Human Development 32: 87–91
64. Greenough A, Emery E F 1993 Randomised trial comparing dopamine and dobutamine in preterm infants. European Journal of Pediatrics 152: 925–927
65. Grylack L, Medani C, Hultzen C et al 1982 Nonoliguric acute renal failure in the newborn: a prospective evaluation of diagnostic indices. American Journal of Diseases of Children 136: 518–520
66. Habib R 1993 Nephrotic syndrome in the first year of life. Pediatric Nephrology 7: 347–353
67. Hammarlund K, Sedin G 1979 Transepidermal loss in newborn infants III. Relation to gestational age. Acta Paediatrica Scandinavica 68: 795–801
68. Hammarlund K, Sedin G, Stromberg B 1982 Transepidermal water loss in newborn infants VII. Relation to postnatal age in very preterm and full term appropriate for gestational age infants. Acta Paediatrica Scandinavica 71: 369–374
69. Hammarlund K, Sedin G, Stromberg B 1983 Transepidermal water loss in the newborn VIII. Relation to gestational age and postnatal age in appropriate and small for gestational age infants. Acta Paediatrica Scandinavica 72: 721–728
70. Haney I, Lachance C, van Doesburg N H, Fouron J C 1995 Reversible steroid induced hypertrophic cardiomyopathy with left ventricular outflow tract obstruction in two newborns. American Journal of Perinatology 12: 271–274
71. Hansmann M, Hackelöer B J, Staudach A 1985 Ultrasound diagnosis. In: Obstetrics and gynaecology. Springer-Verlag, Berlin, p 470
72. Hayamizu S, Kanda K, Ohmori S, Murata Y, Seo H 1994 Glucocorticoids potentiate the action of atrial natriuretic polypeptide in adrenalectomized rats. Endocrinology 135: 2459–2464
73. Harpin V A, Rutter N 1982 Sweating in preterm babies. Journal of Pediatrics 100: 614–619
74. Haycock G B 1993 The influence of sodium on growth in infancy Pediatric Nephrology 7: 871–875
75. Haycock G B 1995 The syndrome of inappropriate secretion of antidiuretic hormone. Pediatric Nephrology 9: 375–381
76. Haycock G B, Aperia A 1991 Salt and the newborn kidney. Pediatric Nephrology 5: 65–70
77. Haycock G B, Schwartz G J, Wisotsky D H 1978 Geometric method for measuring body surface area: a height–weight formula validated in infants, children and adults. Journal of Pediatrics 93: 62–66
78. Hazinski T A, Blalock W A, Engelhardt B 1988 Control of water balance in infants with bronchopulmonary dysplasia: role of endogenous vasopressin. Pediatric Research 23: 86–88
79. Heimler R, Doumas B T, Jendrzejczak B M, Nemeth P B, Hoffman R G, Nelin L D 1993 Relationship between nutrition, weight change and fluid compartments in preterm infants during the first week of life. Journal of Pediatrics 122: 110–114
80. Herin P, Aperia A 1994 Neonatal kidney, fluids and electrolytes. Current Opinion in Pediatrics 6: 154–157
81. Hoyer J R, Anderson C E 1981 Congenital nephrotic syndrome. Clinics in Perinatology 8: 333–356
82. Judd B A, Haycock G B, Dalton N, Chantler C 1987 Hyponatraemia in premature babies and following surgery in older children. Acta Paediatrica Scandinavica 76: 385–393
83. Kaplan B S, Fay J, Shah V, Dillon M J, Barratt T M 1989 Autosomal recessive polycystic kidney disease Pediatric Nephrology 3: 43–49
84. Kaplan B S, Restaino I, Raval D S, Gottlieb R P, Bernstein 1994 Renal failure in the neonate associated with in utero exposure to non-steroidal anti-inflammatory agents. Pediatric Nephrology 8: 700–704
85. Karlowicz M G, Adelman R D 1992 Acute renal failure in the neonate. Clinics in Perinatology 19: 139–158
86. Keidan I, Lotan D, Gazit G, Boichis H, Reichman B, Linder N 1994 Early neonatal renal venous thrombosis: long term outcome. Acta Paediatrica 83: 1225–1227
87. Kestila M, Manniko M, Holmberg C et al 1994 Congenital nephrotic syndrome of the Finnish type maps to the long arm of chromosome 19. American Journal of Human Genetics 54: 757–764
88. Kinoshita S, Jose P A, Felder R A 1989 Ontogeny of the dopamine 1 receptor in rat renal proximal convoluted tubule. Pediatric Research 25: 68A
89. Klarr J M, Faix R G, Pryce C J, Bhatt-Mehta V 1994 Randomised blind trial of dopamine versus dobutamine for treatment of hypotension in preterm infants with respiratory distress syndrome. Journal of Pediatrics 125: 117–122
90. Knoers N, Monnens L A H 1992 Nephrogenic diabetes insipidus; clinical symptoms, pathogenesis, genetics and treatment. Pediatric Nephrology 6: 476–482
91. Kojima T, Kobayashi T, Matsuzaki S, Iwase S, Kobayashi Y 1985 Effects of perinatal asphyxia and myoglobinuria on development of acute neonatal renal failure. Archives of Disease in Childhood 60: 908–912
92. Kojima T, Hirata Y, Fukuda Y, Iwase S, Koboyashi Y 1987 Plasma atrial natriuretic peptide and spontaneous diuresis in sick neonates. Archives of Disease in Childhood 62: 667–670
93. Lambert H, Morris K P, Sharp J, Coulthard M G 1990 Access for peritoneal dialysis in neonates and infants. Archives of Disease in Childhood 65: 914–915
94. Lambert H J, Coulthard M G, Palmer J M, Baylis P H, Matthews J N S 1990 Control of sodium and water balance in the preterm neonate. Pediatric Nephrology 4: C53
95. Leake R D, Zakauddin S, Trygstad C W, Fu P, Oh W 1976 The effect

of large volume intravenous fluid infusion on neonatal renal function. Journal of Pediatrics 89: 968–972
96. Lewis M A, Houston I B, Postlethwaite R J 1990 Access for peritoneal dialysis in neonates and infants. Archives of Disease in Childhood 65: 44–47
97. Lieberman K V, Nardi L, Bosch J P 1985 Treatment of acute renal failure in an infant using continuous arteriovenous hemofiltration. Journal of Pediatrics 106: 646–649
98. Linderkamp O, Nelle M, Kraus M, Zilow E P 1992 The effects of early and late cord clamping on blood viscosity and other haemorheological parameters in full term neonates. Acta Paediatrica 81: 745–750
99. Littlewood J M 1971 White cells and bacteria in voided urine of healthy newborns. Archives of Disease in Childhood 56: 167–172
100. Maalouf E, Ferguson J, van Heyningen V, Modi N 1998 Denys–Drash syndrome presenting in a newborn with end-stage renal failure of antenatal origin. Pediatric Nephrology (in press)
101. McCance R A 1936 Experimental sodium chloride defiency in man. Proceedings of the Royal Society of London (Biology) 119: 245–268
102. McCance R A, Naylor N J B, Widdowson E M 1954 The response of infants to a large dose of water. Archives of Disease in Childhood 29: 104–109
103. McCance R A, Widdowson E M 1952 The correct physiological basis on which to compare infant and adult renal function. Lancet ii: 860–862
104. MacDonald M S, Emery J L 1959 The late intrauterine and postnatal development of human renal glomeruli. Journal of Anatomy 93: 331–340
105. Mackie F E, Hodson E M, Roy L P, Knight J F 1996 Neonatal Bartter syndrome – use of indomethacin in the newborn period and prevention of growth failure. Pediatric Nephrology 10: 756–758
106. Mahan J D, Hoyer J R, Vernier R L 1988 Nephrotic syndrome in the first year of life. In: Cameron J S, Glassock R J (eds) The nephrotic syndrome. Marcel Dekker, New York, pp 401–422
107. Mattoo T K, Ahmad G S 1994 Peritoneal dialysis in neonates after major abdominal surgery. American Journal of Nephrology 14: 6–8
108. Mehta N, Modi N 1989 ACE inhibitors in pregnancy. Lancet ii: 96
109. Midgley J P, Modi N, Littleton P, Carter N, Royston P, Smith A 1992 Atrial natriuretic peptide, cyclic guanosine monophosphate and sodium excretion during postnatal adaptation in male infants below 34 weeks gestation with severe respiratory distress syndrome. Early Human Development 28: 145–154
110. Modi N 1988 Development of renal function. British Medical Bulletin 44: 935–956
111. Modi N 1989 Treatment of renal failure in neonates. Archives of Disease in Childhood 64: 630
112. Modi N 1993 Sodium intake and preterm babies. Archives of Disease in Childhood 69: 87–91
113. Modi N 1997 Management of postnatal disorders of fluid balance. In: Brace R (ed) Fetus and neonate volume IV – Body fluids and kidney. Cambridge University Press, Cambridge
114. Modi N, Coulthard M. Renal function. In: Harvey D R, Cooke R W I, Levitt G A (eds) The baby under 1000 g, 2nd edn. Butterworth-Heinemann, Oxford (in press)
115. Modi N, Hutton J L 1990 The influence of postnatal respiratory adaptation on sodium handling in preterm neonates. Early Human Development 21: 11–20
116. Modi N, Hutton J L 1990 Urinary creatinine excretion and estimation of muscle mass in infants of 25–34 weeks gestation. Acta Paediatrica Scandinavica 79: 1156–1162
117. Mohan P, Rojas J, Davidson K K et al 1984 Pulmonary air leak associated with neonatal hyponatraemia in premature infants. Journal of Pediatrics 105: 153–157
118. Moore E S, Galvez M B, Paton J B, Fisher D E, Behrman R E 1974 Effects of positive pressure ventilation on intrarenal blood flow in infant primates. Pediatric Research 8: 792–796
119. O'Brodovich H, Canessa C, Ueda J, Rafii B, Rossier B C, Edelson J 1993 Expression of the epithelial Na^+ channel in the developing rat lung. American Journal of Physiology 265: C491–C496
120. Oliver J A, Pinto J, Sciacca R R, Cannon P J 1980 Increased renal secretion of norepinephrine and prostaglandin E_2 during sodium depletion in the dog. Journal of Clinical Investigation 66: 748–756
121. Orlowski J, Lingrel J B 1988 Tissue-specific and developmental regulation of rat Na, K-ATPase catalytic α isoform and β subunit mRNAs. Journal of Biological Chemistry 263: 10436–10442
122. Ostlund E V, Eklof A C, Aperia A 1993 Salt deficient diet and early weaning inhibit DNA synthesis in immature rat proximal tubular cells. Pediatric Nephrology 7: 41–44
123. Perlman J M, Moore V, Siegel M J, Dawson J 1986 Is chloride depletion an important contributing cause of death in infants with BPD? Pediatrics 77: 212–216
124. Peters O, Ryan S, Matthew, Cheng K, Lunn J 1997 Randomised controlled trial of acetate in preterm neonates receiving parenteral nutrition. Archives of Disease in Childhood 77: F12–15
125. Phelps D L, Lachman R S, Leake R D, Oh W 1972 The radiological localisation of the major aortic tributaries in the newborn infant. Journal of Pediatrics 81: 336–339
126. Pladys P, Bétrémieux P, Lefrancois C, Schleich J M, Gourmelon N, Le Marec B 1994 Apport de l'échocardiographie Doppler dans l'évaluation des effets de l'expansion volémique chez le nouveau-né. Archives of Pediatrics 1: 470–476
127. Potter E L, Thierstein S T 1943 Glomerular development in the kidney as an index of fetal maturity. Journal of Pediatrics 22: 695–706
128. Potter E L 1965 Development of the human glomerulus. Archives of Pathology 80: 241–255
129. Rao M, Eid N, Herrod L, Parekh A, Steiner P 1986 Antidiuretic response in children with bronchopulmonary dysplasia during episodes of acute respiratory distress. American Journal of Diseases of Children 140: 825–828
130. Rees L, Brook C D G, Shaw J C L, Forsling M L 1984 Hyponatraemia in the first week of life in preterm infants. I. Arginine vasopressin secretion. Archives of Disease in Childhood 59: 414–422
131. Rees L, Shaw J C L, Brook C D G, Forsling M L 1984 Hyponatraemia in the first week of life. II Sodium and water balance. Archives of Disease in Childhood 59: 423–429
132. Rennie J, Cooke R W I 1991 Prolonged low dose indomethacin for persistent ductus arteriosus of prematurity. Archives of Disease in Childhood 66: 55–58
133. Ricci M A, Lloyd D A 1990 Renal venous thrombosis in infants and children. Archives of Surgery 125: 1195–1199
134. Rojas J, Mohan P, Davidson K K 1984 Increased extracellular water volume associated with hyponatraemia at birth in premature infants. Journal of Pediatrics 105: 158–161
135. Roy B J, Cornish J D, Clark R H 1995 Venovenous extracorporeal membrane oxygenation affects renal function. Pediatrics 95: 573–578
136. Roy R N, Chance G W, Radde I C, Hill D E, Willis D M, Sheepers J 1976 Late hyponatraemia in very low birthweight infants (< 1.3 kg). Pediatric Research 10: 526–531
137. Rozé J C, Tohier C, Maingueneau C, Lefèvre M, Mouzard A 1993 Response to dobutamine and dopamine in the hypotensive, very preterm infant. Archives of Disease in Childhood 69: 59–63
138. Rozycki J H, Baumgart S 1991 Atrial natriuretic factor and postnatal diuresis in respiratory distress syndrome. Archives of Disease in Childhood 66: 43–47
139. Rudd P T, Hughes E A, Placzek M M, Hodes D T 1983 Reference ranges for plasma creatinine during the first month of life. Archives of Disease in Childhood 58: 212–215
140. Rutter N 1989 The hazards of an immature skin. In: Harvey D R, Cooke R W I, Levitt G A (eds) The baby under 1000 g. Butterworths, London, pp 94–105
141. Schmidt B, Andrew M 1995 Neonatal thrombosis: report of a prospective Canadian and international registry. Pediatrics 96: 939–943
142. Schrod L, Frauendienst-Egger G, Forgber I, von Stockhausen H B 1991 Dexamethason in der Behandlung der bronchopulmonalen Dysplasie. Pneumologie 45: 892–896
143. Sedin G, Hammarlund K, Nilsson G E, Strömberg B, Oberg P 1985 Measurements of transepidermal water loss in newborn infants. Clinics in Perinatology 12: 79–99
144. Seri I, Rudas G, Bors Z, Kanyicska B, Tulassay T 1993 Effects of low dose dopamine infusion on cardiovascular and renal functions, cerebral blood flow and plasma catecholamine levels in sick, preterm neonates. Pediatric Research 34: 742–749
145. Shaffer S G, Bradt S K, Hall R T 1986 Postnatal changes in total body water and extracellular volume in the preterm infant with respiratory distress syndrome. Journal of Pediatrics 109: 509–514
146. Shaffer S G, Meade V M 1989 Sodium balance and extracellular volume regulation in very low birth weight infants. Journal of Pediatrics 115: 285–290

147. Shaffer S G, Weismann D N 1992 Fluid requirements in the preterm infant. Clinics in Perinatology 19: 233–250
148. Simon D B, Karet F E, Hamdan J M, Di Pietro A, Sanjad S A, Lifton R P 1996 Bartter's syndrome, hypokalaemic alkalosis with hypercalciuria, is caused by mutations in the Na-K-2Cl cotransporter NKCC2. Nature Genetics 13: 183–188
149. Singhi S C, Chookang E 1984 Maternal fluid overload during labour, tranplacental hyponatraemia and risk of transient neonatal tachypnoea in term infants. Archives of Disease in Childhood 59: 1155–1158
150. Singhi S C, Chookang E, Hall J S, Kalghatgi S 1985 Iatrogenic neonatal and maternal hyponatraemia following oxytocin and aqueous glucose infusion during labour. British Journal of Obstetrics and Gynaecology 92: 356–363
151. Singhi S C, Sood V, Bhakoo N K, Ganguly N K, Kaur A 1995 Composition of postnatal weight loss and subsequent weight gain in preterm infants. Indian Journal of Medical Research 101: 157–162
152. Skinner J R, Milligan D W A, Hunter S, Hey E 1992 Central venous pressure in the ventilated neonate. Archives of Disease in Childhood 67: 374–377
153. So K W, Fok T F, Ng P C, Wong W W, Cheung K L 1997 Randomised controlled trial of colloid or crystalloid in hypotensive preterm infants. Archives of Disease in Childhood 76: F43–46
154. Spitzer A 1982 The role of the kidney in sodium homeostasis during maturation. Kidney International 21: 539–545
155. Sposi N M, Bottero L, Cossu G, Russo G, Testa U, Peschle C 1989 Expression of protein kinase C genes during ontogenic development of the central nervous system. Molecular and Cellular Biology 9: 2284–2288
156. Stevenson J G 1977 Fluid administration in the association of patent ductus arteriosus complicating respiratory distress syndrome. Journal of Pediatrics 90: 257–261
157. Stromski M E, Cooper K, Thulin G et al 1986 Postischaemic ATP-$MgCl_2$ provides precursors for resynthesis of cellular ATP in rats. American Journal of Physiology 250: F834–F837
158. Strange K 1993 Maintenance of cell volume in the central nervous system. Pediatric Nephrology 7: 689–697
159. Sulyok E, Nemeth M, Tenyi I et al 1979 Postnatal development of renin–angiotensin–aldosterone system, RAAS, in relation to electrolyte balance in premature infants. Pediatric Research 13: 817–820
160. Sulyok E, Varga F, Gyory E, Jobst K, Csaba I F 1979 Postnatal development of renal sodium handling in premature infants. Journal of Pediatrics 95: 787–792
161. Sutter P M, Thulin G, Skromski M et al 1988 Beneficial effect of thyroxine in the treatment of ischemic acute renal failure. Pediatric Nephrology 2: 1–7
162. Takahashi N, Hoshi J, Nishida H 1994 Water balance, electrolytes and acid–base balance in extremely premature infants. Acta Paediatrica Japonica 36: 250–252
163. Tang W, Modi N, Clark P 1994 Dilution kinetics of $H_2{}^{18}O$ for the measurement of total body water in preterm babies in the first week after birth. Archives of Disease in Childhood 69: 28–31
164. Tang W, Ridout D, Modi N 1997 Influence of respiratory distress syndrome on body composition after preterm birth. Archives of Disease in Childhood 77: F28–31
165. Trompeter R S, Al-Dahhan J, Haycock G B, Chik G, Chantler C 1983 Normal values for plasma creatinine concentration related to maturity in normal term and preterm infants. International Journal of Pediatric Nephrology 4: 145–148
166. Tulassay T, Seri I, Rascher W 1987 Atrial natriuretic peptide and extracellular volume control after birth. Acta Paediatrica Scandinavica 76: 444–446
167. Van Marter L J, Leviton A, Allred E N, Pagano M, Kuban K C 1990 Hydration during the first days of life and the risk of bronchopulmonary dysplasia in low birth weight infants. Journal of Pediatrics 116: 942–949
168. Walker M P R, Moore T R, Brace R A 1994 Indomethacin and arginine vasopressin interaction in the fetal kidney: a mechanism of oliguria. American Journal of Obstetrics and Gynecology 171: 1234–1241
169. Wardrop C A, Holland B M 1995 The roles and vital importance of placental blood to the newborn infant. Journal of Perinatal Medicine 23: 139–143
170. Wassner S J 1991 The effect of sodium repletion on growth and protein turnover in sodium depleted rats. Pediatric Nephrology 5: 501–504
171. Watson M L 1996 Clinical developments in polycystic kidney disease. Nephrology Dialysis Transplantation 11: 764–766
172. Williams P R, Kanarek K S 1982 Urine evaporative loss and effects on specific gravity and osmolality. Journal of Pediatrics 100: 626–628
173. Winrow A P, Kovar I Z, Jani B R, Gatzoulis M 1992 Early hyponatraemia and neonatal drug withdrawal. Acta Paediatrica 81: 847–848
174. Woolf A S, Winyard P J D 1995 Unravelling the pathogenesis of cystic kidney diseases. Archives of Disease in Childhood 72: 103–105
175. Yeh T F, Wilks A, Singh J, Betkerur M, Lilien L, Pildes R S 1982 Furosemide prevents the renal side effects of indomethacin therapy in premature infants with patent ductus arteriosus. Journal of Pediatrics 101: 433–437
176. Yorgin P D, Krensky A M, Tune B M 1990 Continuous venovenous hemofiltration. Pediatric Nephrology 4: 640–642
177. Zaramella P, Andreeta B, Zanon G et al 1994 Continuous peritoneal dialysis in newborns. Peritoneal Dialysis International 14: 22–25
178. Zerres K, Weiss H, Bulla M, Roth B 1982 Prenatal diagnosis of an early manifestation of autosomal dominant adult type polycystic kidney disease. Lancet ii: 988
179. Ziegler E, Fomon S J 1971 Fluid intake, renal solute load and water balance in infancy. Journal of Pediatrics 78: 561–568
180. Ziegler M D, Ryu J E 1976 Renal solute load and diet in growing premature infants. Journal of Pediatrics 89: 609–611
181. Zobel G, Kuttnig M, Ring E 1990 Continuous arteriovenous hemodialysis in critically ill infants. Child Nephrology and Urology 10: 196–198

Part 2

Urology in the neonatal period

Pierre Mouriquand   Duncan Wilcox

URINARY TRACT ANOMALIES

ABNORMAL FORMATION, MIGRATION AND FUSION OF THE KIDNEY

The absence of a kidney on ultrasound can be due to a congenital deficiency (unilateral or bilateral), involution of a multicystic dysplastic kidney or, alternatively, it could represent an ectopically placed kidney which has yet to be identified.

Renal agenesis

Renal agenesis can be unilateral or bilateral and probably results from a failure of the ureteral bud to induce development in the kidney. This may be due to a defect either in the ureteral bud or in the developing kidney.[46]

The incidence of unilateral agenesis is between 1:1000 and 1:1500.[54] Increasingly unilateral agenesis is diagnosed on antenatal ultrasound; previously it was picked up on postnatal ultrasound or on intravenous urography.

Ectopic kidney needs to be excluded by performing a renal isotope nuclear scan (DMSA), which visualizes all functioning renal tissue.

Associated urogenital anomalies are common. The ipsilateral ureter is absent or partially atretic in all cases, as confirmed by cystoscopy. The contralateral kidney is either malrotated or ectopic in 15% of cases, and has associated vesicoureteric reflux in 37%.[61]

The incidence of bilateral renal agenesis (Potter syndrome) is 1:4000 births. Bilateral renal agenesis is more common in males and within the same family, suggesting a genetic component.[55] Diagnosis is usually made antenatally by ultrasonography, which reveals oligohydramnios and absence of the kidneys. False positive diagnoses have been reported.[56] The ureters are usually absent or partially developed. Testicular absence has been found in approximately 10% of cases, but the vas deferens is often present, suggesting that renal agenesis is not due to a failure of the Wolffian duct to develop.[5] Potter syndrome is, of course, fatal. The main differential diagnosis is bilateral involuted multicystic dysplastic kidneys.

Multicystic dysplastic kidney

Multicystic dysplastic kidney is increasingly being diagnosed during pregnancy. It is more commonly unilateral, although bilateral cases have been reported. Associated contralateral problems are frequently encountered. Postnatally, diagnosis is confirmed with an ultrasound showing multiple cysts which have completely replaced the kidney (Fig. 39.14). Nuclear renograms show that the multicystic dysplastic kidney is non-functioning. Anomalies in the contralateral kidney are seen in 25% of patients: these include pyeloureteric junction anomalies and vesicoureteric reflux; Consequently, most centres advocate a micturating cystourethrogram and prophylactic antibiotics.

Recently the management of these patients has changed to a non-operative approach. Serial ultrasounds show that these kidneys frequently involute. The size of the kidney at initial presentation appears to predict involution, with few multicystic dysplastic kidneys greater than 6 cm disappearing spontaneously. If the kidney is not decreasing in size many centres offer nephrectomy, as there have been reports of hypertension and malignant change associated with multicystic dysplastic kidneys.[30]

Ectopic kidneys

Ectopic kidneys are caused by an abnormality in renal ascent and/or renal fusion. If an ectopic kidney is suspected then an ultrasound and DMSA scan should be performed for diagnostic reasons, and a micturating cystourethrogram to exclude reflux. Ectopic kidneys can be divided into simple, horseshoe and crossed renal ectopia.

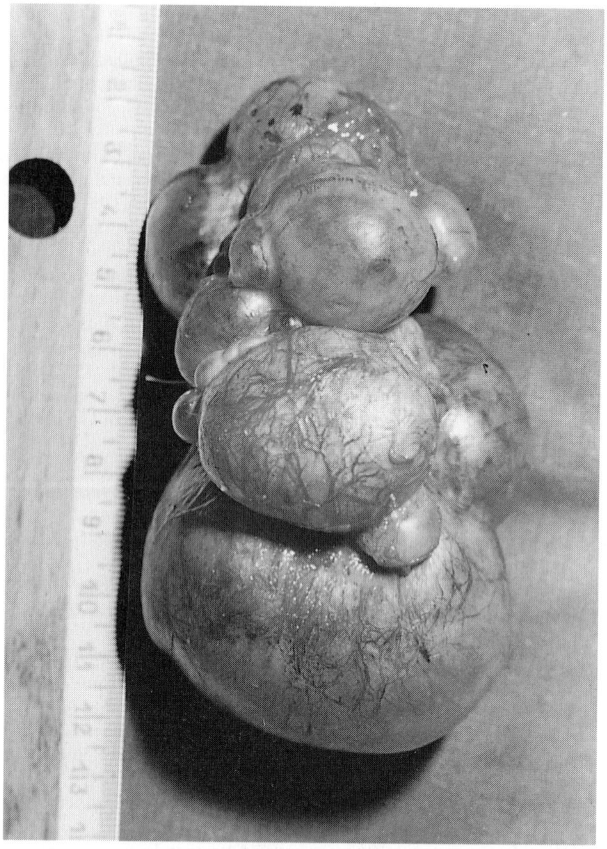

Fig. 39.14 Postmortem specimen showing a multicystic dysplastic kidney.

Simple

The most common location for a simple ectopic kidney is pelvic, which occurs in 60% of cases. It is usually unilateral, with a slight predilection for the left side, but is found bilaterally in 10% of cases.[54] In addition to its abnormal location, a pelvic kidney is frequently small and irregular in shape. The remaining ectopic kidneys lie between the pelvis and the normal position. Very rarely the kidney can be found within the thorax.

Ectopic kidneys are often associated with genital and contralateral urinary abnormalities, such as absence of the vagina,[34] retrocaval ureter, bicornuate uterus, supernumerary kidney[23] and contralateral ectopic ureter.[11] The ectopic kidney can be a component of more complex syndromes, such as the Mayer–Rokitansky–Küster–Hauser syndrome,[8] Fanconi anaemia[20] or conjoined twins.[62]

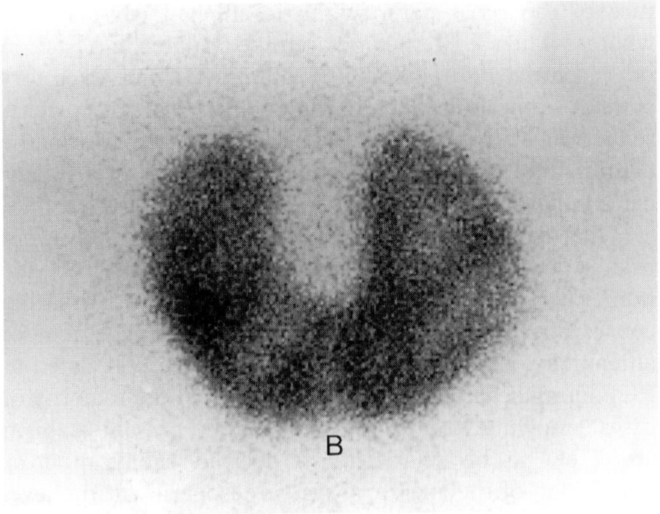

Fig. 39.15 MAG 3 renogram showing a horseshoe kidney; the bridge of renal tissue connecting the right and left kidneys can be seen (B).

Horseshoe kidney

The incidence of horseshoe kidney varies between 1:400 and 1:1800[13] autopsies, and is more common in males. In 95% of cases the lower poles of the two kidneys are joined by a bridge of renal tissue, which can be normal, dysplastic or fibrous (Fig. 39.15). In about 40% of cases the isthmus lies at the level of L4, just beneath the origin of the inferior mesenteric artery. In 20% the isthmus is in the pelvis; in the rest it lies at the level of the lower poles of normally placed kidneys.[34] A small number of horseshoe kidneys have fusion at their upper poles. The ureters arch anteriorly to pass over the isthmus,[12] which may explain the relatively high incidence of pyeloureteric anomalies (20%) associated with horseshoe kidneys. Associated abnormalities are common: these can involve the central nervous system, gastrointestinal tract, and the skeletal and cardiovascular systems.

Crossed renal ectopia

There are four varieties of crossed renal ectopia:

- with renal fusion (85%);
- without fusion (< 10%);
- solitary;
- bilateral.

There is a slight male predominance and crossing from left to right occurs more frequently than right to left. The fusion, when it exists, is usually between the upper pole of the crossed kidney and the lower pole of the normally positioned kidney (unilateral fused type) (Fig. 39.16). Associated anomalies are commonly found with renal ectopia. In addition renal ectopia may also be a component of more complex syndromes, such as the VACTERL syndrome[27] and agenesis of the corpus callosum.[24]

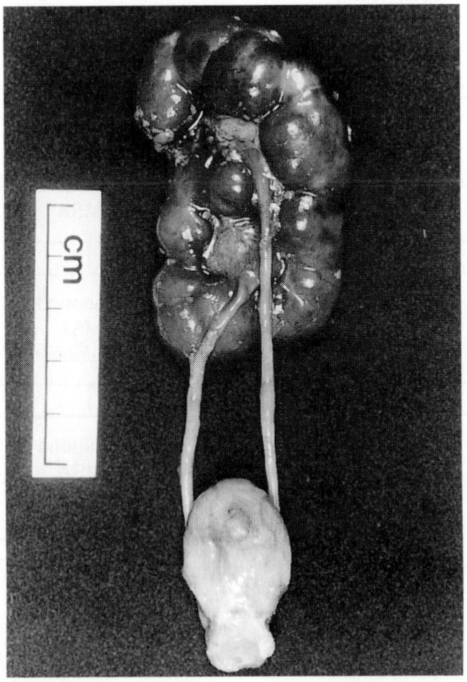

A

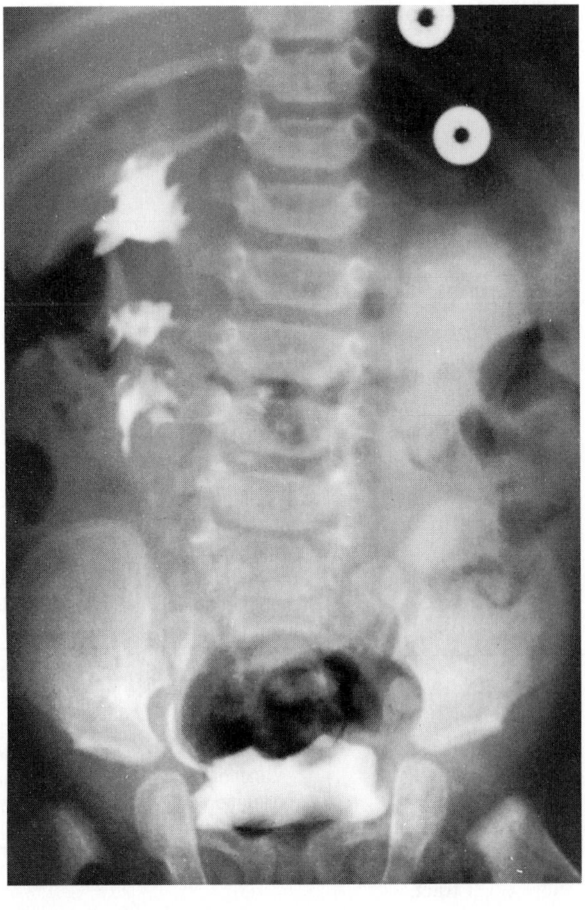

B

Fig. 39.16 (A) Postmortem specimen showing a crossed fused ectopia. (B) Intravenous urogram showing a crossed fused ectopia, with both collecting systems visualized on the right side.

URINARY TRACT DILATATION

Urinary tract dilatation is increasingly being detected by antenatal ultrasound, with 1:800 pregnancies having an antenatally diagnosed uropathy.[58] Despite improvements in technique, some children with an abnormal urinary tract still avoid detection and present during childhood with signs and symptoms of a urinary tract infection. Urinary tract dilatation can occur either as a result of an impairment of urine flow, or from urine back-flow caused by vesicoureteric reflux.

Urine flow impairment

Urine flow impairment can occur at any level in the urinary tract, and may affect one or both sides. The common causes are pyeloureteric junction anomaly, vesicoureteric junction anomaly, ureteroceles and posterior urethral valves. These sites are where two embryological components join to form the renal tract. Regardless of the underlying pathology, during pregnancy UFI leads to a similar pattern of anatomical and functional pathophysiology.

Dilatation of the pelvis and calyces is the first anatomical response to UFI and may lead to histological damage of the renal parenchyma and changes in renal function. Histological damage is related to the degree, the level of UFI and its duration. Renal atrophy is the ultimate response to UFI related to the onset of a unique form of programmed cell death (apoptosis).[26]

When UFI is significant early in pregnancy the structure of the renal parenchyma is affected (dysplasia),[25] whereas when UFI becomes significant later in gestation or is partial, it generates dilatation of the excretory system[9,33] without affecting the parenchymal structure. A reduction of the ipsilateral GFR and an increase in the contralateral GFR are the ultimate responses to a significant unilateral UFI.

The natural history of UFI located in the upper urinary tract is now better understood owing to the numerous randomized clinical studies[10,44,51] comparing conservative management with surgical management of antenatally diagnosed dilated upper tracts. UFI related to PUJ anomalies improves spontaneously in the majority of cases, implying that most cases of UFI present at birth are likely to be related to a delayed canalization or maturation of the excretory system, especially at the level of the PUJ. However, the degree of dilatation at birth does not consistently predict outcome and mild dilatation of the pelvis can occasionally deteriorate, suggesting that long-term deterioration of antenatally diagnosed UFI is always a possibility.[22,32,49] Conversely, severely dilated upper tracts may improve with time, confirming that the anatomical assessment is of poor prognostic value. Likewise, functional studies may improve or deteriorate with time regardless of the initial assessment. This shows that the management of UFI can only be decided upon after a period of regular assessment. A simple approach to the management of these complex problems is given in Figure 39.17.

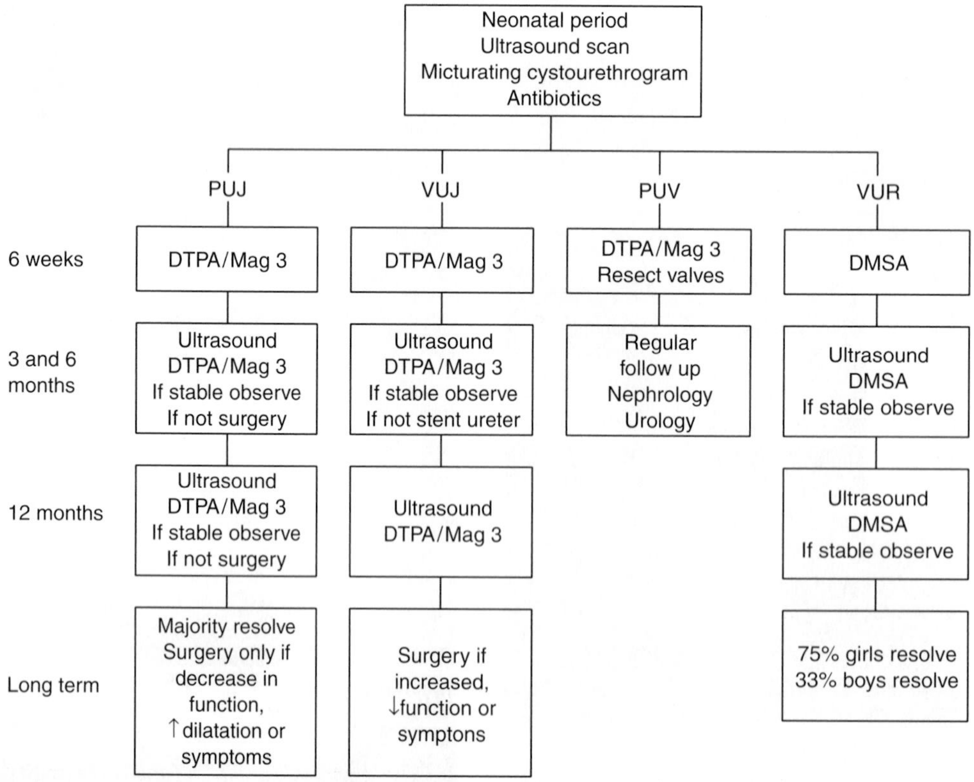

Fig. 39.17 Postnatal assessment of patients with an antenatally diagnosed dilatation of the urinary tract.

Pyeloureteric junction anomalies

Fetal uropathies occur in 1 in 800 pregnancies[4,60] and PUJ anomalies are the most common.[63,65] There are three types of PUJ anomaly: extraluminal, luminal and intraluminal. Extraluminal anomalies are mainly caused by aberrant vessels, although kinks, bands, adhesions and arteriovenous malformation have also been described[15] which span the PUJ and reduce the urine flow intermittently. In these cases the dilatation of the pelvis and symptoms are often intermittent. Luminal anomalies are the most common and are due to an abnormal distribution of the muscular and collagen fibres at the level of the PUJ. Intraluminal anomalies are rare and mainly described as valve-like processes and benign fibroepithelial polyps.[43] Association between extraluminal and luminal anomalies is common, hence the difficulty in establishing the exact cause of UFI.

The diagnosis of unilateral or bilateral PUJ anomaly can be suspected antenatally when an ultrasound scan of the fetus shows a dilated renal pelvis. However, antenatal pelvic dilatation may also reflect:

- transient physiological dilatation of the urinary tract due to the slow canalization and slow maturation of the excretory system;[1,28,57]
- pathological transitory dilatation of the urinary tract due to transient fetal UFI;
- permanent pathological UFI due to another urological malformation (ureterovesical anomaly; vesicourethral anomaly; vesicoureteric reflux).

Therefore, the exact cause of UFI can only be established formally after birth.

Significant pathology may be suspected after 18 weeks' gestation if the pelvis is dilated, associated with changes in the parenchymal appearance[48] or with a reduction in the amount of amniotic fluid when the anomaly is bilateral. In that case, oligohydramnios is usually detected during the second half of pregnancy.

Although many PUJ anomalies are diagnosed antenatally, they may continue to cause problems in childhood. Recurrent urinary tract infections are a common symptom in infants with PUJ anomalies. Abdominal mass was one of the principal symptoms of PUJ anomaly in babies before the ultrasound era.[21] Loin pain reflects the intermittent distension of the renal pelvis. Haematuria and hypertension are rare symptoms of PUJ anomalies.

However the diagnosis of a PUJ anomaly is suspected, complementary investigations are required. Ultrasound demonstrates and measures the pelvic and calyceal dilatation. If the degree of pelvic dilatation is greater than 5 mm then it should be investigated further as outlined in Figure 39.17. Pelvic dilatation, detected during the neonatal period is considered minimal between 5 and 12 mm (anteroposterior diameter), between 12 and 20 mm as moderate and over 20 mm as severe (Fig. 39.18). Ultrasound demonstrates important negative signs, such as the absence of dilatation of the ureters (which, when it exists, is more in favour of vesicoureteric junction anomalies, megaureter or reflux) or the absence of a thick-walled bladder (which would favour a lower urinary tract anomaly, posterior urethral valve or bladder dysfunction). Ultrasound can also show the echogenicity of the kidney itself and the possible association of the PUJ anomaly with other urological anomalies, such as a duplex system, a horse shoe kidney or a ureterocoele.

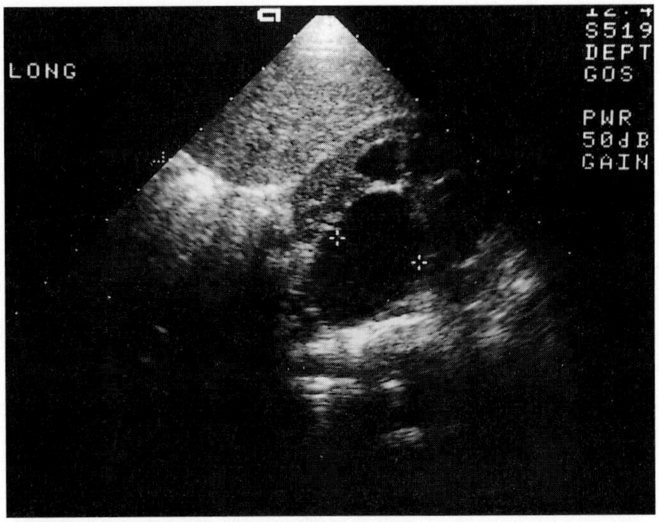

Fig. 39.18 Ultrasound scan showing a pyeloureteric junction anomaly. The markers indicate the lateral margins of the dilated renal pelvis.

Ultrasound is the investigation of choice, but IVU is still used in some centres. In the case of PUJ anomaly this shows three main signs:

- a delayed excretion of contrast;
- distended pelvis and calyces;
- a delayed passage of contrast medium through the PUJ (> 20 minutes).

These signs are mainly anatomical and poorly reflect the function of the kidney itself.

In neonates with pelvic dilatation of more than 5 mm it is important to exclude vesicoureteric reflux. This is assessed using an MCUG: this can be performed during the neonatal period, but requires antibiotic cover. Increasingly ultrasound is being used to try and minimize the number of MCUGs done: however, a large study looking at the success of ultrasound in excluding reflux concluded that postnatal ultrasound correlated poorly with the presence and degree of reflux in children with antenatally diagnosed hydronephrosis.[64] It is therefore important to perform an MCUG on all children with antenatally diagnosed hydronephrosis (greater than 5 mm).

Isotope studies examine several parameters:

- The perfusion of the kidney (during the first 15 seconds after the i.v. injection);

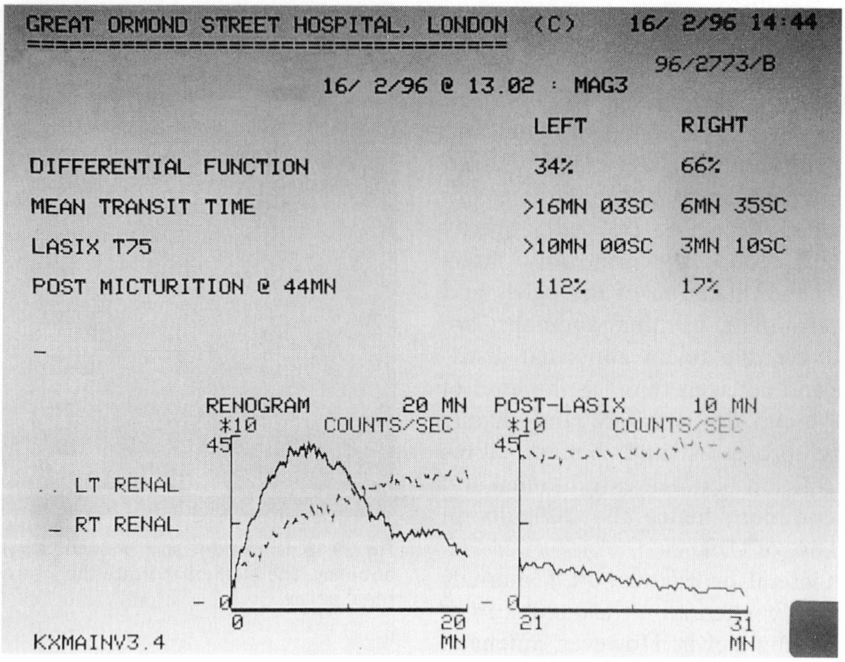

Fig. 39.19 MAG 3 renogram showing a left unilateral pyeloureteric junction anomaly. The dotted line represents the radioactivity in the left kidney, the plain line represents the radioactivity in the right kidney. The right kidney takes up the radioactive marker promptly and then within 20 minutes, as shown by the down-sloping line, has excreted the marker. This is a normal curve. The left kidney has poor uptake indicating reduced function, confirmed by the differential function of 34%, and by 30 minutes the radioactivity remains high showing impaired urinary excretion.

- The relative function of each kidney, which reflects the glomerular function (during the first 30 seconds);
- The parenchymal transit time of the isotope;
- The washout or clearance of the isotope from the upper tract, which reflects the drainage;
- Finally, reascent of the radioactivity in the renal areas may be an indirect sign of vesicoureteric reflux (Fig. 39.19).

The drainage curves are dependent on the degree of hydration of the child as well as the function of the lower urinary tract. If they are normal and if the relative function of the ipsilateral kidney is not too low (>30%), there is no UFI. If they are abnormal this suggests that there is a drainage problem, but not necessarily at the PUJ level.

There are essentially two types of renal scan assessing function or structure (Chapter 47). ^{99m}Technetium-DTPA and Mag 3 are both isotopes excreted by glomerular filtration and tubular secretion;[69] both therefore evaluate the relative function and the drainage capability of the kidneys. ^{99m}Technetium-DMSA specifically localizes in the proximal convoluted tubule and gives an image of the renal mass structure.[29] The isotopes are poorly taken up into the newborn kidney and only after 4–6 weeks has the kidney matured enough to give accurate reproducible results.

It is essential to define whether the PUJ anomaly is an isolated condition or is associated with other anomalies. Associated urological anomalies include ureteric hypoplasia,[2] vesicoureteric reflux,[36,50] partial or complete ureteric duplication[39,45] and horseshoe kidney. PUJ anomalies also can be associated with anorectal anomalies, congenital heart disease and VATER syndrome.[22]

There are four possible therapeutic approaches to PUJ anomalies:

- Conservative management;
- Temporary diversion of pelvic urine (percutaneous nephrostomy);
- Surgical treatment of the anomaly;
- Fetal surgery diversion; this is still in the experimental stage and will not be discussed further.

Conservative management of PUJ anomalies is justified in most cases during the first year of life. Three conditions are required to follow a unilateral PUJ anomaly conservatively:

- The child must be asymptomatic;
- The pelvic dilatation should either be stable on repeated ultrasound scans or should decrease;
- The relative function on repeated isotopic studies should either be stable or should improve.

Antibiotic prophylactic cover is recommended, although no studies have to date proved that it prevents urinary tract infections. This conservative approach, initially proposed by Ransley et al,[51] is now followed by many centres.

Temporary diversion of the pelvic urine is indicated in infants with severe unilateral pelvic dilatation and poor relative function. The question is, should this kidney be repaired or removed? To answer the question it is necessary to place a percutaneous nephrostomy for 3 or 4 weeks, followed by reassessment of the relative function. Either the function has improved and a pyeloplasty can be performed, or the function remains poor and a nephrectomy should be discussed.

Surgical treatment of the PUJ anomaly is advocated by most urologists, in four main circumstances:

- Symptomatic PUJ anomaly;
- Declining function in the dilated kidney;
- Increasing pelvic dilatation;
- Bilateral moderate to severe dilatation of the pelvis.

When surgery is performed the most common operation is a dismembered pyeloplasty (Anderson–Hynes technique).

Vesicoureteric junction anomaly

Many classifications of megaureter have been reported[41] but practically there are two categories:

- Megaureters related to an abnormal vesicoureteric junction (obstructed vesicoureteric junction, primary megaureter or vesicoureteric reflux);
- Megaureters secondary to a dysfunctioning or obstructed lower urinary tract.

A megaureter may be due to a structural anomaly of the distal segment of the ureter caused by collagen deposition, cellular hypoplasia, muscular disarray or some other as yet undefined injury or deficiency at the microscopic level. Regardless of the primary pathology, a loss of functional continuity results. Most studies have documented hyperplasia and hypertrophy of smooth muscle cells within the walls of the dilated proximal ureter. These presumably represent the ureter's compensatory response to distal UFI.

Anatomical studies include ultrasound scan of the urinary tract (Fig. 39.20), intravenous urography and an MCUG. All three may show the degree and extent of urinary tract dilatation; the MCUG may also show the presence of vesicoureteric reflux. Distal anatomical obstruction of the ureter and vesicoureteric reflux may occur together. Functional studies (diuresis renography) are useful to assess the degree of functional UFI; however, it is sometimes difficult to distinguish a PUJ from a VUJ anomaly, as they can occur together. In these difficult cases a contrast antegrade pyelogram may be the only way to differentiate the two conditions.

Spontaneous improvement of ureteric dilatation is a

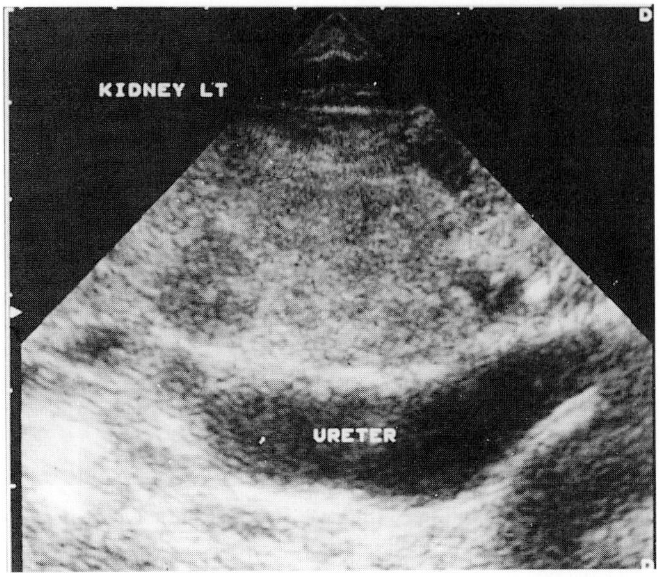

Fig. 39.20 Ultrasound scan showing a dilated megaureter which has a tortuous route.

frequent event in megaureters related to a faulty vesicoureteric junction. Resolution of UFI is common and conservative management of megaureters is recommended when renal function and dilatation of the upper tract remain stable (or improve), and when the child remains asymptomatic.[53] Antibiotic prophylaxis is recommended, especially in refluxing megaureters. Regular isotope assessments are required to follow these children.

When the conservative approach fails, i.e. when infections recur in spite of an adequate antibiotic prophylactic cover, or when renal function decreases on repeated isotope studies or when dilatation of the urinary tract increases, ureteric reimplantation is usually recommended, except where renal function is poor (<15%), when nephroureterectomy is indicated. The aim of the operation is to excise the distal obstructive segment of the ureter and reimplant the ureter with an antireflux mechanism.

Ureterocoeles

Ureterocoeles are a cystic dilatation of the intravesical portion of the ureter. They occur in approximately 1:500 people. In children they are almost always associated with a duplex kidney and occur in the ureter draining the upper pole.

Ureterocoeles occur more frequently in girls and in the white population. Ureterocoeles have been classified in many ways, but a simple classification is to divide them into those arising from a single or duplex kidney, and then further into intravesical and extravesical types.

Ureterocoeles can cause UFI either to a single system or, more commonly in children, to the upper pole of a duplex system. Urine flow impairment during gestation

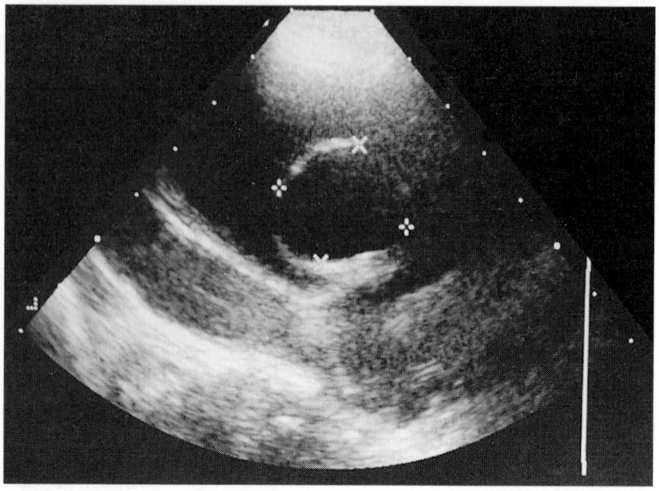

Fig. 39.21 Ultrasound scan. The cystic structure outlined by the markers is a ureterocoele situated within the bladder.

results in upper tract dilatation, which is increasingly being detected on antenatal ultrasound scans. Postnatally ureterocoeles can present in a variety of ways, including:

- urinary tract infection, which can be secondary to stasis due to the ureterocoele or due to reflux in the lower pole of either the ipsilateral or contralateral kidney;
- bladder outlet obstruction if the ureterocoele encroaches into the bladder neck;
- occasionally in girls the ureterocoele prolapses through the bladder neck and can be seen at the urethral orifice; the differential diagnosis is a urethral prolapse.

Investigations include:

- ultrasound, which can visualize both the ureterocoele within the bladder and the duplex kidney (Fig. 39.21);
- IVU, which is excellent at identifying duplex kidneys and can identify ureterocoeles within the bladder, either as a filling defect or as a 'cobra head' deformity (this occurs only if the upper pole is functioning) (Fig. 39.22);
- it is essential to perform an MCUG, so that vesicoureteric reflux into both the ipsilateral and contralateral ureters can be excluded (Fig. 39.23);
- finally, an isotope scan should be performed to assess the function of both moieties of the duplex kidney.

There is considerable controversy over the management of ureterocoeles, which varies from simple endoscopic puncture of the ureterocoele to upper pole heminephrectomy and bladder reconstruction. Increasingly a more conservative approach is being adopted. In patients who present in the neonatal period the first procedure is endoscopic puncture: this was the only procedure required in 73%, and resulted in drainage and preservation of the upper pole in over 90% of patients.[10] In this and other studies ureteric reflux was created in 20–40% of patients, and further surgery including upper pole nephrectomy plus or minus bladder reconstruction was required in 20–80%.[10,17]

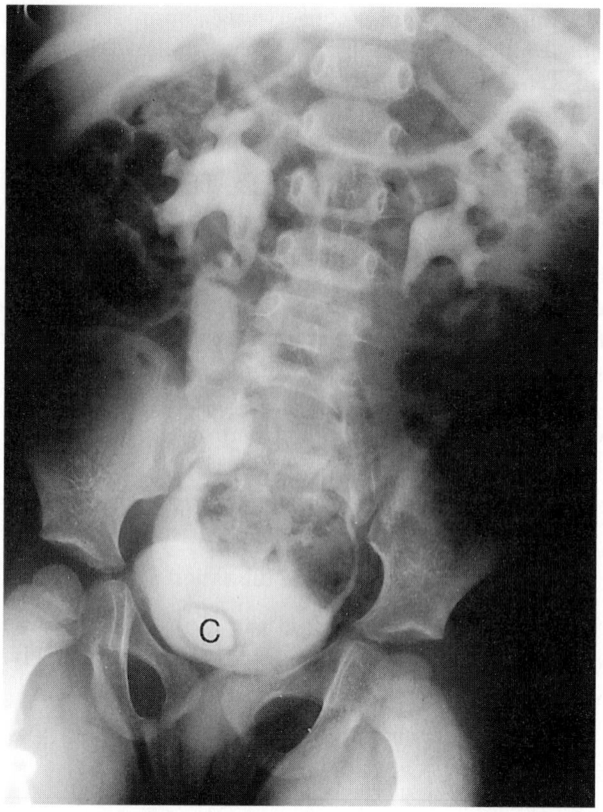

Fig. 39.22 Intravenous urogram showing a dilated right collecting system, with dilated renal pelvis and ureter. In the bladder there is a 'cobra head deformity' (C): this represents a ureterocoele and the halo effect is caused by the wall of the ureterocoele. The upper tract dilatation is therefore secondary to the ureterocoele.

Posterior urethral valves

A posterior urethral valve is a congenital membrane obstructing or partially obstructing the posterior urethra. Rarely described in females,[7] it is the most common cause of lower urinary obstruction in males. The incidence is between 1:4000 and 1:25 000.[6,40]

The anatomical effects of PUV on the urinary tract are mainly dilatation and elongation of the posterior urethra, thickening of the bladder neck, which can be wide open or very narrow, and thickening of the detrusor,[68] which is often trabeculated. In addition to the anatomical problems bladder dysfunction is frequently seen in association with PUV. Variable urodynamic bladder profiles have been reported, although it is sometimes difficult to know whether these are related to the congenital disorder or its treatment. Vesicoureteric reflux is often noticed, with a marked dilatation of the upper tract and poor renal function. The thick bladder wall can cause a secondary UFI at the level of the vesicoureteric junction and at the bladder outlet. Some associated lesions of the urinary

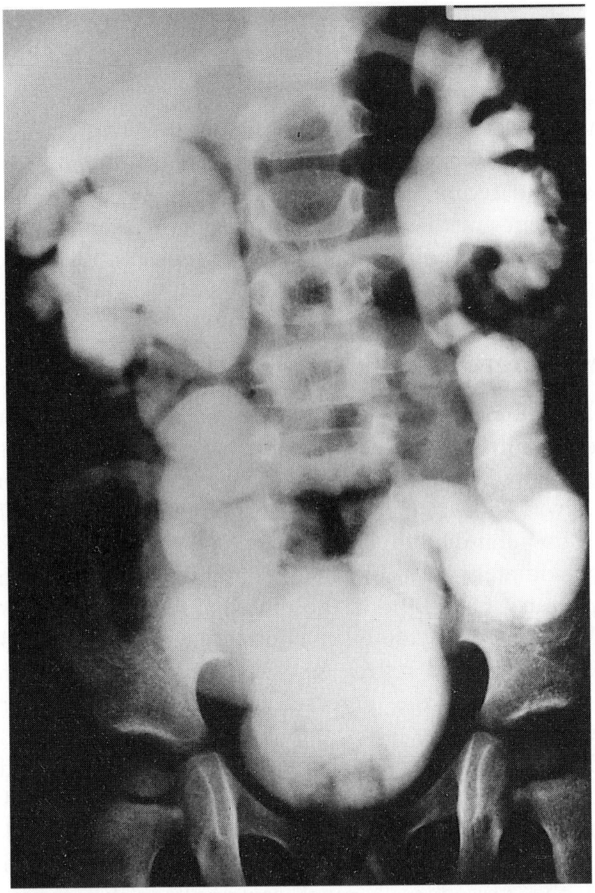

Fig. 39.23 Micturating cystogram showing bilateral vesicoureteric reflux. There is gross bilateral dilatation of the ureters and marked clubbing of the calyces and renal pelvis.

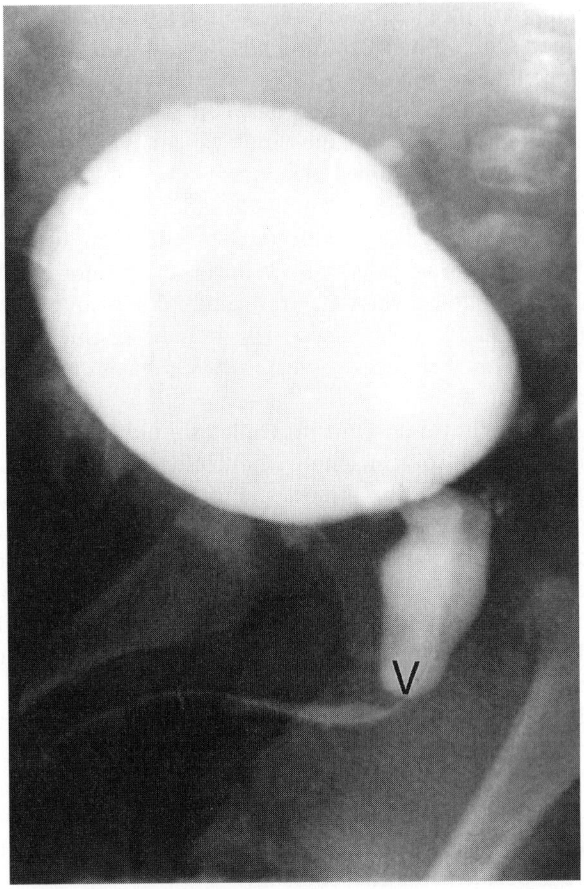

Fig. 39.24 Micturating cystogram showing a posterior urethral valve. Below the bladder is the dilated posterior urethra, from which runs a fine line of contrast. The posterior urethral valves are situated at the transition between the dilated posterior urethra and the thin urethra (V).

tract, such as vesicoureteric reflux (22–70% of patients),[40] bladder diverticula and urine extravasation (with or without ascites) can provide a pressure pop-off mechanism which minimizes the renal consequences of PUV.

Renal dysplasia is frequently associated with PUV;[35] this often leads to chronic renal failure and, owing to the failure of the renal tubules to concentrate urine, large quantities of urine are passed. Hyperdiuresis may then become a significant factor in urinary incontinence associated with PUV.[19]

PUV should be suspected in a fetus with a thick-walled bladder and bilateral dilatation of the upper urinary tract, whether or not associated with renal dysplasia and oligohydramnios. Oligohydramnios is usually noticed during the second part of pregnancy, when most of the amniotic fluid is fetal urine. Despite modern ultrasonic equipment, only 16–55% of patients with PUV are detected before 24 weeks' gestation.[18] Children with antenatal diagnosis of PUV seem to have a worse renal prognosis than those with later diagnosis, and earlier diagnosis and treatment do not improve the clinical prognosis.[52]

Children who are not diagnosed antenatally usually present in the following ways. In the newborn there are symptoms of severe metabolic disorders related to renal failure, respiratory failure (spontaneous pneumothorax or pneumomediastinum) and urinary tract infection.[59] Palpation of the kidney(s) and the bladder is usually easy.

In infants and young children urinary symptoms are more common (dysuria, haematuria, urinary tract infection, septicaemia), sometimes accompanied by rectal prolapse. Renal failure may be present. In the older child, urinary incontinence, urgency and dysuria are sometimes seen.

Ultrasound scan of the urinary tract is the first-line investigation. This shows the dilatation of the upper urinary tract, the possible abnormal echogenicity of the renal parenchyma, the thick bladder wall associated or not with bladder diverticula, and the dilated posterior urethra. Perineal ultrasound is increasingly able to detect urethral anomalies. An MCUG is still the gold standard investigation to detect PUV (Fig. 39.24). Insertion of a transurethral catheter can damage the anatomy of the valve, and some paediatric urologists prefer to perform an MCUG via a suprapubic catheter. Isotope studies are essential to assess the renal consequences of PUV.[31,66]

Antenatal treatment is rarely indicated but may be justified when oligohydramnios is deteriorating in a fetus with bilateral dilatation of the upper urinary tract. Insertion of a double-J stent between the fetal bladder or the dilated kidneys and the amniotic cavity, under ultrasound guidance, allows decompression of the urinary tract, possible preservation of development of the fetal kidney, and possible maturation of the fetal lungs by restoration of an adequate volume of amniotic fluid. These antenatal diversions are usually done quite late in pregnancy and, once again, the benefit of such interventions in children with PUV has not been demonstrated.

After birth, three main principles should be respected: it is essential to resuscitate the child when necessary, adequately drain the bladder and destroy the valves. Resuscitation implies hydration, electrolyte replacement and antibiotics, and should be done in a neonatal intensive care unit. Urine drainage can usually be achieved either by inserting a transurethral or a suprapubic catheter. Occasionally a surgical vesicostomy is required to drain the bladder.

If the child is severely ill and infected, drainage of the upper tract may be the best option (ureterostomy or, preferably, percutaneous nephrostomy). Destruction of the valve is performed when resuscitation is achieved, usually a few days after birth. Surgical destruction of the valve is performed endoscopically.

Renal failure is a common complication of PUV and is seen in 40–50% of cases at the time of diagnosis. The type of primary surgical treatment does not seem to influence the progression of renal failure or body growth in children with PUV. Regardless of the surgical or medical treatment, which can greatly influence mortality, renal failure develops in almost 50% of children with PUV.[52] Four factors have been identified as being associated with poor long-term outcome: presentation before the age of 1 year, bilateral vesicoureteric reflux, proteinuria, and daytime incontinence at the age of 5.

Incontinence is reported to be between 14 and 38%[14,38] after treatment of PUV. The incontinence tends to improve at puberty, presumably as a result of further prostatic development. The association of bad outcome with incontinence may point to continuing bladder dysfunction as a major determinant of long-term outcome for renal function.

However, hyperdiuresis due to chronic renal failure may also contribute to the association of urinary incontinence and poor prognosis in PUV.[19]

Prune-belly syndrome

Prune-belly syndrome is an extremely rare condition in which the infant has three characteristic features:

- Congenital absence or hypoplasia of the abdominal musculature;
- A massively dilated urinary tract from both kidneys to the prostatic urethra;
- Bilateral cryptorchidism.

The incidence of this condition appears to be decreasing, probably associated with an increase in antenatal diagnosis and termination of the pregnancy. Because of the infrequency with which this condition is seen, management needs to be individualized. Prognosis is usually poor and dependent on the renal situation.[42]

Vesicoureteric reflux

Vesicoureteric reflux occurs when urine flows from the bladder into the ureters. Previously reflux was diagnosed in patients being investigated for urinary tract infections; however, with improvements in antenatal scanning reflux can be identified during pregnancy, and accounts for approximately 10% of all antenatally diagnosed hydronephrosis.[3] Over 90% of those with antenatally diagnosed reflux are boys; this is in contrast to those with postnatally diagnosed reflux, who are mainly girls, and may be explained by the increased voiding pressure required in male fetuses.[3]

Investigation of an antenatally diagnosed hydronephrosis has already been outlined, but when reflux has been identified (Fig. 39.23), it is important to proceed to a DMSA isotope scan so that individual renal function and the presence of renal scarring can be assessed. Approximately 60% of kidneys with reflux, within the first 4 weeks of life, have an abnormal renogram; in the majority this was before a urinary tract infection had occurred. These data suggest that abnormalities in renal development occur with reflux during intrauterine life.[3]

Treatment of reflux is initially non-operative. All patients should be placed on prophylactic antibiotics in an attempt to avoid infection. Although this is current dogma there is little evidence to prove that prophylactic antibiotics prevent infection, and it is possible that long-term antibiotics can alter the bowel flora from relatively harmless organisms to more virulent strains. Despite this, long-term antibiotics are still recommended. Some authors suggest that circumcision can reduce the number of urinary tract infections, but this has not been proved by a controlled trial despite being supported by considerable anecdotal evidence.[67] When these methods fail to prevent recurrent urinary tract infections, or when there is a significant decrease in renal function associated with scarring, then reimplantation of the ureter is required to surgically correct the reflux.

GENITOURINARY TRACT ANOMALIES

EPISPADIAS AND BLADDER EXSTROPHY

Epispadias, bladder exstrophy and cloacal exstrophy represent a spectrum of congenital malformations in

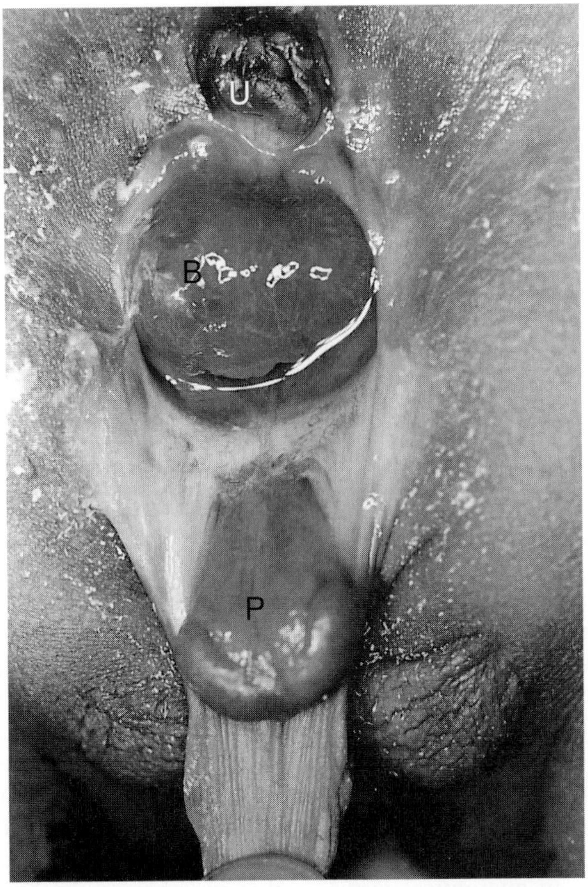

Fig. 39.25 A child with bladder exstrophy. The umbilicus is at the top of the photograph (U); below this is the bladder plate (B) with an open bladder neck and an epispadic penis (P).

which there is an abnormal development of the cloacal membrane and consequently incomplete midline fusion of the cloacal structures.

Epispadias is the mildest form: it is rare, with an incidence of 1 in 100 000, and can occur in both sexes, although it is more common in boys. In epispadias the bladder is covered and the urethra opens on to the dorsal surface of the penis; in addition the penis is often short and wide, with marked dorsal chordee. In girls the urethra is patulous and the clitoris has not fused in the midline. Treatment consists of reconstructing the genitalia; however, as the bladder neck and sphincter are often involved, further treatment to ensure urinary continence is often required.

Bladder exstrophy occurs in 1 in 30 000 livebirths. In this anomaly the bladder opens on to the abdominal wall, there is marked separation of the pubic bones and epispadias of the genitalia (Fig. 39.25). Like epispadias, this is more common in boys. Treatment requires closure of the bladder and pubic ring within the first few days of life, then a staged approach to correct the epispadias and reconstruct the bladder neck. These patients will require lifelong follow-up, but despite the many problems

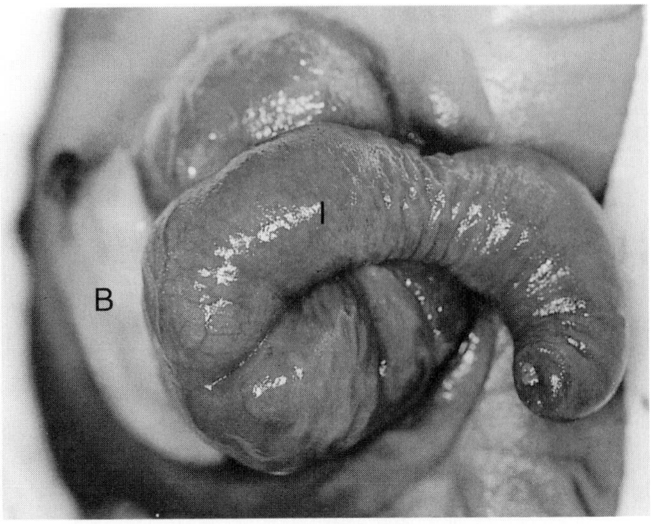

Fig. 39.26 Child with cloacal exstrophy. Prolapsed ileum (I) is seen coming from the exstrophied caecum; on the left side is an exstrophied hemibladder (B).

the majority are socially continent and sexually active. Cloacal exstrophy is the most severe and fortunately the rarest form of the exstrophy complex. It has an incidence of 1 in 250 000 and, unlike bladder exstrophy, is more common in girls.[16] In cloacal exstrophy the bowel, usually at the ileocaecal valve, opens in the midline with two hemibladders lateral to it (Fig. 39.26). There is also epispadias of the genitalia and pubic bone separation.[37] Until 1960 this was uniformly fatal, but since 1980 the survival rate has been over 90% (see also pp. 789, 1081).[37]

HYPOSPADIAS

Hypospadias occurs in 1 in 300 male births. This congenital abnormality consists of three features: an abnormally placed urethral meatus, which can be found anywhere from the glans to the penoscrotal junction; chordee of the penis, which forces the penis to point towards the scrotum when erect; and a foreskin which, instead of being wrapped around the penis, is present only on the dorsal side (Fig. 39.27).[47] The underlying pathology is not fully understood, but it is probably caused by an incomplete virilization of the penis. The important consideration when examining a child with hypospadias is to be certain that this is not an overvirilized female or an XY/XO mosaic. This can usually be assessed by palpation of the testes: if there are two the karyotype is XY; however, if there is only one palpable a karyotype of XY/XO must be considered. If no testes are palpable then an overvirilized female must be excluded. If there is any doubt the child should be investigated as a case of ambiguous genitalia (p. 976). In the majority the hypospadias is an isolated problem and requires surgical reconstruction between 1 and 2 years of age.

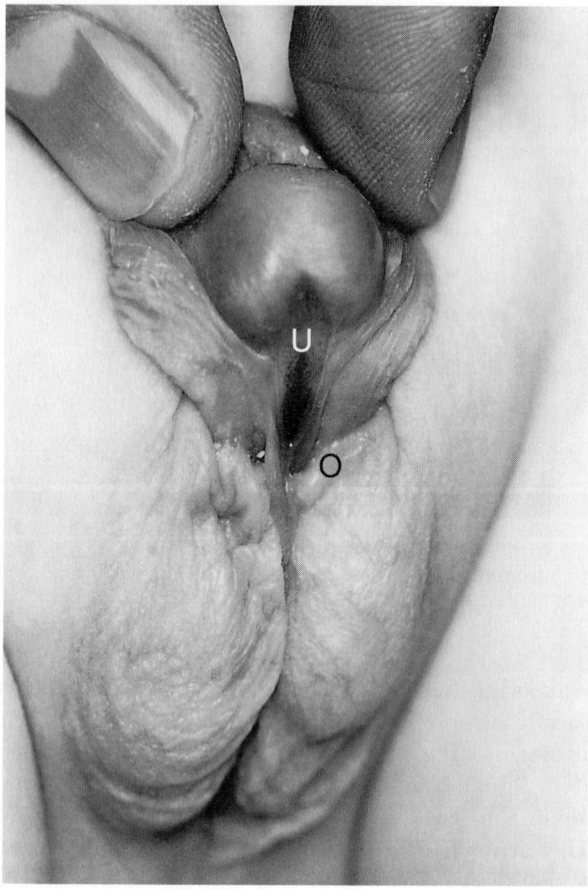

Fig. 39.27 Boy with hypospadias. This shows the urethral plate (U) with the urethral opening (O) on the scrotum and the hooded foreskin all behind the penis.

UNDESCENDED TESTICLE

At birth, in term boys, both testicles have usually descended. The incidence of undescended testicles at term is 1:50 to 1:100, but as the testicles descend from the fifth to the seventh months of gestation premature boys have an increased risk of undescended testicles. The left testicle descends first, therefore a right undescended testicle is slightly more common. Undescended testicles can be of two types: true undescended testicles (20%), which lie along the original line of descent but which have not reached the scrotum, and ectopic testicles, which have deviated from the normal line of descent, the most common place being in the superficial pouch above the external inguinal ring.

Once the diagnosis of undescended testicle is made it is important to keep the child under review, because occasionally a previously undescended testicle can complete descent, and also there is a high association between undescended testicle and a hernia sac. If a hernia occurs it is necessary both to repair the hernia and to perform an orchidopexy soon in order to prevent a strangulated hernia. In most cases of undescended testicle a definitive operation to bring the testicle down into the scrotum is performed between 1 and 2 years of age.

The rationale for performing an orchidopexy includes the following:

- There is a sixfold increase in the rate of testicular cancer; although this may not decrease when the testicle is placed in the scrotum it improves surveillance.
- The testicle out of the scrotum is kept at a higher temperature, which reduces sperm production.
- Cosmetically it is important to have two testicles in the scrotum, and this is the most common reason for parents to seek advice about their son's undescended testicle.

HYDROCOELES

Congenital hydrocoele results from an incomplete obliteration of the patent processus vaginalis. Normally the processus vaginalis, which accompanies the descending testicle into the scrotum, has been obliterated by the seventh month of pregnancy. If the processus remains patent around the testicle and there is a small lumen connecting it to the peritoneal cavity, fluid can enter and stay in the processus vaginalis, forming a hydrocoele. The only difference between a hydrocoele and hernia, therefore, in anatomical terms, is that in a hernia the lumen allows the bowel to enter the processus.

Hydrocoeles usually present with a scrotal swelling. The features which differentiate it from a hernia are that hydrocoeles transilluminate, and that it is possible to get above a hydrocoele, whereas a hernia extends into the peritoneal cavity. It is vital that a hernia is excluded in the diagnosis as the two conditions have very different treatments.

Most hydrocoeles can be left, as the vast majority spontaneously resolve by 2 years of age. Surgical ligation of the processus vaginalis is carried out if the hydrocoele remains, becomes symptomatic (very rare), or cannot be differentiated from a hernia.

NEONATAL TESTICULAR TORSION

Neonatal or intrauterine torsion of the testicle usually presents as a swollen testicle. The scrotum is often red, oedematous, and may be tender on examination. Often a black testicle can be identified within the scrotum. Occasionally the initial event is not identified and the torted testicle is only noticed when a fibrotic atrophied testicle is seen during exploration for an undescended testicle. The treatment is often early surgical exploration. However, in the neonatal period the testicle is always necrotic and it is now more common practice to treat the boy with analgesia and antibiotics alone.

PHIMOSIS

At birth the prepuce and the glans of the penis are firmly adherent, gradually separating over the first 5 years. During this time retraction of the foreskin is not possible; this is the so-called physiological phimosis. It is therefore unusual to require circumcision during the neonatal period. The indications for circumcision are for religious reasons and recurrent balanitis; other indications are considerably less definite. Pathological phimosis does occur but, as mentioned above, is rare before 5 years of age, and even then can usually be successfully treated with gentle parental retraction of the foreskin. Many factors have been put forward in defence of circumcision, including a decreased incidence of penile and cervical cancer and a reduction in the incidence of urinary tract infections. However, once religion, social class and social activity are taken into consideration many of these factors lose their significance. The one definite contraindication for circumcision is in boys with hypospadias, where the prepuce may be required to reconstruct the urethra; even for religious reasons parents can be reassured that once the hypospadias repair has been performed their child will be circumcised.

REFERENCES

1. Alcaraz A, Vinaixa F, Tejedo-Mateu A et al 1991 Obstruction and recanalization of the ureter during embryonic development. Journal of Urology 145: 410–416
2. Allen T D, Husmann D A 1989 Ureteropelvic junction obstruction associated with ureteral hypoplasia. Journal of Urology 142: 353–355
3. Anderson P A, Rickwood A M K 1991 Features of primary vesicoureteric reflux detected by prenatal sonography. British Journal of Urology 67: 267–271
4. Arthur R J, Irving H C, Thomas D F M 1989 Bilateral fetal uropathy; what is the outlook? British Medical Journal 298: 1419–1420
5. Ashley D J B, Mostofi F K 1960 Renal agenesis and dysgenesis. Journal of Urology 83: 211–230
6. Atwell J D 1983 Posterior urethral valves in the British Isles: a multicenter BAPS review. Journal of Pediatric Surgery 18: 70–74
7. Bakker N J 1958 Valves in the female urethra. Urology International Basel 6: 187–190
8. Barakat A Y, Seikaly M G, Der Kaloustian V M 1986 Urogenital abnormalities in genetic disease; Journal of Urology 136: 778–785
9. Beck A D 1971 The effect of intra-uterine urinary obstruction upon the development of the fetal kidney. Journal of Urology 105: 784–789
10. Blyth B, Snyder H M, Duckett J W 1993 Antenatal diagnosis and subsequent management of hydronephrosis. Journal of Urology 149: 693–698
11. Borer J G, Corgan F J, Krantz R, Gordon D H, Maiman M, Glassberg K I 1993 Unilateral single vaginal ectopic ureter with ipsilateral hypoplastic pelvic kidney and bicornuate uterus. Journal of Urology 149: 1124–1127
12. Boullier J, Chehval M J, Purcell M H 1992 Removal of a multicystic half of a horseshoe kidney: significance of preoperative evaluation in identifying abnormal surgical anatomy. Journal of Pediatric Surgery 27: 1244–1246
13. Campbell M F 1970 Anomalies of the kidney. In: Campbell M F, Harrison J H (eds) Urology, 3rd edn, vol 2. W B Saunders, Philadelphia, p 1416
14. Cass A S, Stephens F D 1974 Posterior urethral valves: diagnosis and management. Journal of Urology 112: 519–525
15. Chung B H, Chung K H, Lee J H, Kim J H, Choi J Y 1992 Hydronephrosis secondary to congenital pelvic arteriovenous malformation: a case report. Journal of Urology 148: 1877–1879
16. Diamond D A 1990 Cloacal exstrophy: associated anomalies. Dialogues in Pediatric Urology 13: 6–8
17. Di Benedetto V, Meyrat B J, Sorrentino G, Monfort G 1995 Management of duplex ureteroceles detected by prenatal ultrasound. Pediatric Surgery International 10: 485–487
18. Dinneen M D, Dhillon H K, Word H C, Duffy P G, Ransley P G 1993 Antenatal diagnosis of PUV. British Journal of Urology 72: 364–369
19. Dinneen M D, Duffy P G, Barratt T M, Ransley P G 1994 Persistent polyuria after valve ablation. British Journal of Urology 75: 236–240
20. Evans D G, Rees H C, Spreadborough A et al 1994 Radial ray defects, renal ectopia, duodenal atresia and hydrocephalus: the extended spectrum for Fanconi anæmia. Clinical Dysmorphology 3: 200–206
21. Flashner S C, Lower R K 1992 Ureteropelvic junction. In: Kelalis P P, King L R, Belman A B (eds) Clinical pediatric urology, 3rd edn. W B Saunders, Philadelphia, pp 693–725
22. Flashner S C, Mesrobian H G J, Flatt J A, Wilkinson R H, King L R 1993 Nonobstructive dilatation of upper urinary tract may later convert to obstruction. Urology 42: 569–573
23. Flyer M A, Haller J O, Feld M, Kantor A 1994 Ectopic supernumerary kidney: another cause of a pelvic mass. Abdominal Imaging 19: 374–375
24. Franco I, Kogan S, Fisher J et al 1993 Genitourinary malformations associated with agenesis of the corpus callosum. Journal of Urology 149: 1119–1121
25. Glick P L, Harrison M R, Noall R A, Villa R L 1983 Correction of congenital hydronephrosis in utero III. Early mid-trimester ureteral obstruction produces renal dysplasia. Journal of Pediatric Surgery 18: 681–687
26. Gobe G C, Axelsen R A 1987 Genesis of renal tubular atrophy in experimental hydronephrosis in the rat. Role of apoptosis. Laboratory Investigation 56: 273–281
27. Golomb J, Ehrlich R M 1989 Bilateral ureteral triplication with crossed ectopic fused kidneys associated with the VACTERL syndrome. Journal of Urology 141: 1398–1399
28. Gonzales J 1984 Relation structure et fonction dans le développement de l'appareil urinaire du fetus. Journal d'Urologie (Paris) 91: 108–117
29. Gordon I 1987 Indications for ^{99m}technetium dimercapto-succinic acid scan in children. Journal of Urology 137: 464–467
30. Gough D C S, Postlethwaite R J, Lewis M A, Bruce J 1995 Multicystic renal dysplasia diagnosed in the antenatal period: a note of caution. British Journal of Urology 76: 244–248
31. Groshar D, Embdon O M, Sazbon A, Koritny E S, Frenkel A 1988 Radionuclide assessment of bladder outlet obstruction: a noninvasive (1-step) method for measurement of voiding time, urinary flow rates and residual urine. Journal of Urology 139: 266–269
32. Hanna H K 1991 The case for early operation. Dialogues in Pediatric Urology 14(2)
33. Harrison M R, Nakayama D K, Noall R, DeLorimier A A 1982 Correction of congenital hydronephrosis in utero; decompression reverses the effects of obstruction on the fetal lung and urinary tract. Journal of Pediatric Surgery 17: 965–974
34. Hendren W H, Donahoe P K 1986 Renal fusions and ectopia. In. Welch K J, Randolph J G, Ravitch M M, O'Neill J A Jr, Rowe M I (eds) Pediatric surgery, 4th edn. Year Book Medical Publishers, Chicago, pp 1134–1145
35. Henneberry M O, Stephens F D 1980 Renal hypoplasia and dysplasia in infants with posterior urethral valves. Journal of Urology 123: 912–915
36. Hollowell J G, Altman H G, Snyder H M, Duckett J W 1989 Coexisting ureteropelvic junction obstruction and vesicoureteral reflux: diagnostic and therapeutic implications. Journal of Urology 142: 490–493
37. Hurwitz R S, Mansoni G A M, Ransley P G, Stephens F D 1988 Cloacal exstrophy: a report of 34 cases. Journal of Urology 138: 1065–1068
38. Johnson J H, Kulatilake A E 1971 The sequelae of posterior urethral valves: British Journal of Urology 43: 743–748
39. Joseph D B, Bauer S B, Colodny A H, Mandell J, Lebowitz R L, Retik A B 1989 Lower pole ureteropelvic junction obstruction and incomplete renal duplication. Journal of Urology 141: 896–899
40. Kaplan G W, Scherz H L 1992 Infravesical obstruction in clinical pediatric urology, 3rd edn. WB Saunders, Philadelphia, pp 821–864
41. Kass E J 1992 Megaureter. In: Kelalis P P, King L R, Belman A B (eds) Clinical pediatric urology. WB Saunders, Philadelphia, p782
42. Keating M A, Duckett J W 1993 Prune belly syndrome. In: Ashcraft K W, Holder T M (eds) Pediatric surgery. W B Saunders, Philadelphia, pp 721–739

43. Macksood M J, Roth D R, Chang C H, Perlmutter A D 1985 Benign fibroepithelial polyps as a cause of intermittent ureteropelvic junction obstruction in a child: a case report and review of the literature. Journal of Urology 134: 951–952
44. Madden N P, Thomas D F M, Gordon A C, Arthur R J, Irving H C, Smith S E W 1991 Antenatally detected pelviureteric junction obstruction. Is non-operation safe? British Journal of Urology 68: 305–310
45. Mesrobian H G J 1986 Ureteropelvic junction obstruction of the upper pole moiety in complete ureteral duplication. Journal of Urology 136: 452–453
46. Mesrobian H G J, Sulik K K 1992 Characterization of the upper urinary tract anatomy in the Danforth spontaneous murine mutation. Journal of Urology 148: 752–755
47. Mouriquand P D E, Mollard P 1995 Hypospadias repair: the paediatric urologist's point of view. European Urology Update Series. 4: 106–111
48. Nicolini U, Fisk N M, Rodeck C H, Beacham J 1992 Fetal urine biochemistry: an index of renal maturation and dysfunction. British Journal of Obstetrics and Gynæcology 99: 46–50
49. Noe H N, Magill H L 1987 Progression of mild ureteropelvic junction obstruction in infancy. Urology 30: 348–351
50. Paltiel H J, Lebowitz R L 1989 Neonatal hydronephrosis due to primary vesico-ureteric reflux: trends in diagnosis and treatment. Radiology 170: 787–789
51. Ransley P G, Dhillon H K, Gordon I, Duffy P G, Dillon M J, Barratt T M 1990 The postnatal management of hydronephrosis diagnosed by prenatal ultrasound. Journal of Urology 144: 584–587
52. Reinberg Y, De Castano I, Gonzales R 1992 Prognosis for patients with prenatally diagnosed posterior urethral valves. Journal of Urology 148: 125–126
53. Rickwood A M K, Jee L D, Williams M P L, Anderson A P 1992 Natural history of obstructed and pseudo-obstructed megaureters detected by prenatal ultrasonography. British Journal of Urology 70: 322–325
54. Ritchey M 1992 Anomalies of the kidney. In: Kelalis P P, King L R, Belman A B (eds) Clinical pediatric urology, 3rd edn. WB Saunders, Philadelphia, pp 500–529
55. Rizza J M, Downing S E 1971 Bilateral renal agenesis in two female siblings. American Journal of Diseases of Children 121: 60–63
56. Romero R, Cullen M, Grannum P 1985 Antenatal diagnosis of renal anomalies with ultrasound: III. Bilateral renal agenesis, American Journal of Obstetrics and Gynecology 151: 38–43
57. Ruano-Gil D, Coca-Payeras A, Tejedo-Mateu A 1975 Obstruction and normal recanalization of the ureter in the human embryo: its relation to congenital ureteric obstruction. European Urology 1: 287–293
58. Scott J E S, Renwick M 1988 Antenatal diagnosis of congenital abnormalities in the urinary tract. Results from the northern region fetal abnormality survey. British Journal of Urology 62: 295–300
59. Sheldon C A 1995 In: Male external genitalia. Rowe M I, O'Neill J A, Grosfeld J L, Fonkalsrud E W, Coran AG (eds) Essentials of pediatric surgery. Mosby, St. Louis, pp 775–776
60. Smith D, Egginton J A, Brookfield D S K 1987 Detection of abnormality of fetal urinary tract as a predictor of urinary tract disease. British Medical Journal 294: 27–28
61. Song J T, Ritchey M L, Zerin M, Bloom D A 1995 Incidence of vesicoureteral reflux in children with renal agenesis. Journal of Urology 153: 1249–1251
62. Spitz L, Stringer M D, Kiely E M, Ransley P G, Smith P 1994 Separation of brachio-thoraco-ischiopagus bipus conjoined twins. Journal of Pediatric Surgery 29: 477–481
63. Thomas D F, Irving H C, Arthur R J 1985 Prenatal diagnosis: how useful is it? British Journal of Urology 57: 784–787
64. Tibballs J M, De Bruyn R 1996 Primary vesicoureteric reflux – how useful is postnatal ultrasound? Archives of Disease in Childhood 75: 444–447
65. Turnock R R, Shawis R 1984 Management of fetal urinary tract anomalies detected by prenatal ultrasonography. Archives of Disease in Childhood 59: 962–965
66. Van Der Vis Melsen M J E, Baert R J M, Rajnherc J R, Groen J M, Bemelmans L M M J, De Nef J J E M 1989 Scintigraphic assessment of lower urinary tract function in children with and without outflow tract obstruction. British Journal of Urology 64: 263–269
67. Wiswell T E, Smith F R, Bass J W 1985 Decreased incidence of urinary tract infections in circumcised male patients. Pediatrics 75: 901–903
68. Workman S J, Kogan B A 1990 Fetal bladder histology in posterior urethral valves and the prune belly syndrome. Journal of Urology 144: 337–339
69. Young D W 1991 The use of nuclear renography and assessment of hydronephrosis. Dialogues in Pediatric Urology 14(2)

40

Malignancy in the neonate

Valerie A. Broadbent

Neonatal cancer is rare, a surprising fact in view of the rapid cell division and growth occurring throughout fetal life. Our understanding of the factors affecting cell growth has recently undergone rapid expansion.[20,56] Central regulation of normal cell growth is by proto-oncogenes. Once such a gene is altered by mutation it becomes an oncogene, giving rise to excessive cell growth or inappropriate cell proliferation. Recently a new class of oncogenes has been discovered which act in normal cells to suppress proliferation, and have been termed anti-oncogenes or tumour-suppressor genes. If a tumour-suppressor gene is inactivated the normal constraint to growth is removed and target cells are allowed to proliferate in an uncontrolled way.

Knudson's[34] 'two-hit' theory of carcinogenesis, which he subsequently expanded,[35] has been verified by this recent knowledge of the genetic factors that control cell growth. The 'hits' could be a wide variety of agents – viral, chemical, radiation[6] – and cause mutation of a proto-oncogene or inactivation or loss of a tumour-suppressor gene. This first 'hit' would allow all cells in the body, including the germ cells, to carry the defect, which could thus be passed on to the next generation. The second 'hit' would be in the somatic cells of a target organ, in which the proto-oncogene would become an oncogene, or the loss of a homologous tumour-suppressor gene would allow uncontrolled cellular growth. The time during which the second 'hit' could occur is probably confined to the period when the cells of the target organ are undergoing mitotic activity, but ceases when they are fully mature. For example, retinoblasts differentiate to become photoreceptor cells (cones) by the age of 3 years, and this may explain why retinoblastoma is not found in older children or adults.

Oncogenes exert their effect on cells through a variety of mechanisms. These include control of cellular growth factors or their receptors, or by modifying the signals sent from growth receptors to the nucleus of the cell. This may result in an effect on DNA repair, programmed cell death (apoptosis) or the cells' ability to metabolize toxins. For instance, the *p53* gene,[21] which is found on chromosome 17, encodes a nuclear phosphoprotein which acts as a transcription factor in programmed cell death. Mutant *p53*, found in a wide variety of cancers, prevents this apoptosis and the cell becomes immortal.

INCIDENCE

A reliable incidence figure is difficult to ascertain as many large series are from single centres rather than population based, or are cancer registry figures and may not include benign neoplasms. A recent population based study from the West Midlands Health Authority region incorporated data from cases of both benign and malignant neoplasms over a 30-year period in children from birth to 3 months of age,[44] and found an incidence rate of 7.2 per 100 000 live births. This is a much higher incidence than the United Kingdom Children's Cancer Study Group's (UKCCSG) figure of 2.27 per 100 000 live births (Table 40.1)[50] or the 3.64 per 100 000 livebirths reported in the United States Third National Cancer Survey.[1]

In Parkes' series[44] over half the cases were diagnosed at birth or within the first month of life, similar to the

Table 40.1 Neonatal cancer in Great Britain in children born during 1985–92

	Male		Female		Total	
	n	Rate	*n*	Rate	*n*	Rate
Neuroblastoma	25	0.81	19	0.65	44	0.73
Acute leukaemia	16	0.52	11	0.38	27	0.45
Soft tissue sarcoma	7	0.23	13	0.44	20	0.33
Malignant germ cell (extracranial)	4	0.13	7	0.24	11	0.18
Intracranial germ cell	1	0.03	5	0.17	6	0.10
Other CNS	7	0.23	6	0.21	13	0.22
Retinoblastoma	5	0.16	3	0.10	8	0.13
Wilms' tumour	1	0.03	2	0.07	3	0.05
Hepatoblastoma	2	0.07	1	0.03	3	0.05
Malignant melanoma	0	–	1	0.03	1	0.02
Total	68	2.21	68	2.32	136	2.27

Rates are incidence per 100 000 live births.

Toronto series reported by Campbell,[10] in which 42/102 (38%) presented on the first day of life and 50% by the end of the first week, and the Philadelphia series[22] where 30% were diagnosed at birth and 50% by the end of the first week.

In all series, including a large series from Los Angeles,[30] solid tumours, predominantly teratomas, neuroblastomas and sarcomas, are most common, followed by brain tumours and leukaemias.

SURVIVAL

Malignant tumours in the neonatal period can cause death during birth, when their size or position may cause obstructed labour. They can rupture at birth, causing exsanguination, or they can obstruct vital organs such as airways. Metastatic disease may be overwhelming.

Although it is widely thought that neonatal malignancy behaves in a more benign fashion than its counterpart in older children, there was only a 45% 2-year actuarial survival in the Philadelphia series,[22] which is similar to a 47% 5-year survival in Parkes'[44] group. Sixty-five per cent of the neonates in Isaacs' group[30] died, compared to 41% in the Toronto series.[10] Of the 34 neonates presenting at St Judes Research Hospital between 1962 and 1988, 23 (68%) were alive and free of disease 2 months to 24 years after diagnosis.[14] All these series have been collected over several decades, during which time the overall survival in older children with malignancy has increased steadily[51] and therapeutic practice has changed.

NEUROBLASTOMA

This is the commonest neonatal malignancy, accounting for 30–50% of all cases. It originates from neural crest cells that normally give rise to the adrenal medulla and the sympathetic ganglia. Neural crest cells are also located in nearly all viscera and in the skin. Tumours can arise at any site where there is neural crest tissue. Host-dependent mechanisms may be important in controlling proliferation of these cells, as the frequency of neuroblastoma-in-situ in the adrenal medulla in autopsies of infants dying of other causes may be as high as 1 : 40,[25] and spontaneous regression of widespread disease (stage 4s) is well documented in very young infants (see below).

CLINICAL FEATURES

Sixty per cent of tumours arise within the abdomen or pelvis, giving rise to an abdominal swelling and palpable mass. Thoracic neuroblastomas develop in the posterior mediastinum, causing respiratory obstruction or obstruction of the superior vena cava. A unilateral Horner syndrome may be a sign of disease in this area. Anaemia from extensive bone marrow involvement is common, and bluish subcutaneous nodules are found in 30% of cases presenting in the neonatal period. Spinal cord compression giving rise to paraplegia, or abnormal neurological signs in the lower limbs due to intravertebral extension of a tumour arising in the sympathetic chain, constitutes a medical emergency. Rarely, neonatal neuroblastomas may metastasize to the placenta[52,54] and the circulating catecholamines produced give rise to symptoms of hypertension, palpitations and agitation in the mother.

STAGING

As with most tumours, the clinical stage at presentation is a useful predictor of ultimate survival and must be established in order to institute appropriate therapy. The system proposed by Evans et al[18] has been replaced by the Forbeck criteria:[9]

Stage 1 Tumour confined to organ or structure of origin. Complete gross excision; sampled ipsi- and contralateral lymph nodes microscopically negative;

Stage 2a Unilateral tumour with incomplete gross excision. Sampled nodes as in stage I;

Stage 2b Unilateral tumour with complete or incomplete gross excision; positive ipsilateral nodes; sampled contralateral nodes negative;

Stage 3 Tumour infiltrating across midline with or without regional lymph node involvement, or unilateral tumour with contralateral regional node involvement, or midline tumour with bilateral regional node involvement;

Stage 4 Remote disease involving skeleton, organs, soft tissues or distant lymph node groups;

Stage 4s Cases in those under 1 year old which would otherwise be stage 1 or 2, but who have remote disease involving soft tissues only (liver, skin, bone marrow) without bony metastases.

Of the 31 neonates in Parkes'[44] series, 10 were low stage (1 or 2), five had stage 3, seven had stage 4 and 9 stage 4s. Of the 14 neonates presenting with this condition in Isaacs'[30] series nine had stage 4s disease, two stage 4, two stage 2 and one stage 1.

INVESTIGATIONS

The diagnosis of neuroblastoma can be made without biopsy of the lesion if the following features are positive:

- Raised urinary vanillylmandelic acid (VMA) or other urinary catecholamines;
- Compatible radiological evidence, i.e. calcification on plain X-ray and/or a mass on CT or ultrasound in a compatible site;
- Positive bone marrow aspiration showing typical morphology of clumps of tumour cells arranged in rosettes, which stain with monoclonal antibody to neuroblastoma.

Table 40.2 Prognostic factors in neuroblastoma

	Prognosis		
Factors	**Good**	**Intermediate**	**Poor**
Age (years)	< 1	1–2	> 2
Stage (INSS)	1; 2a; 4s	2b; some 3	some 3; 4
Primary site	Mediastinal	Pelvic, cervical	Retroperitoneal
Histology	Ganglioneuro-blastoma	Differentiated neuroblastoma	Undifferentiated neuroblastoma
Ferritin levels	Normal	–	Abnormal (raised)
NSE levels (ng/ml)	< 20	20–100	> 100
No. of n-*myc* copies	2	3–10	> 10
Ploidy	Hyperdiploid		Diploid
Chromosome 1	Normal		Abnormal

INSS, International Neuroblastoma Staging System[9]
NSE, Neuron-specific enolase.

However, needle biopsy under CT or ultrasound scanning will not only confirm diagnosis but may give additional useful prognostic information, such as ploidy and chromosome analysis, as well as number of copies of the n-*myc* oncogene in the tumour cells (Table 40.2). Staging of disease is not complete without a bone scan. ^{131}I-labelled meta-iodobenzylguanidine (MIBG) is taken up by neurosecretory granules and gives a positive scan of both primary and metastatic disease in 90% of patients.

TREATMENT

Total surgical excision is the treatment of choice for stage 1 and 2 cases, and is usually curative.[33] Chemotherapy is not usually indicated in these stages. A wide variety of chemotherapeutic agents will cause regression of disease in stage 3 and 4 patients. A combination of vincristine (Oncovin), cisplatinum/carboplatin, etoposide and cyclophosphamide (OPEC/OJEC) is most effective. Spinal cord compression constitutes a medical emergency, and immediate treatment with dexamethasone and chemotherapy is the treatment of choice. Surgery is usually too mutilating for initial therapy but may have a place to remove residual disease.

STAGE 4s DISEASE (Fig. 40.1)

The most important group to recognize are patients with stage 4s disease. Spontaneous regression is the rule for these patients.[45] No active treatment is indicated, but close observation with regular clinical monitoring of disease regression, together with urinary VMA estimation

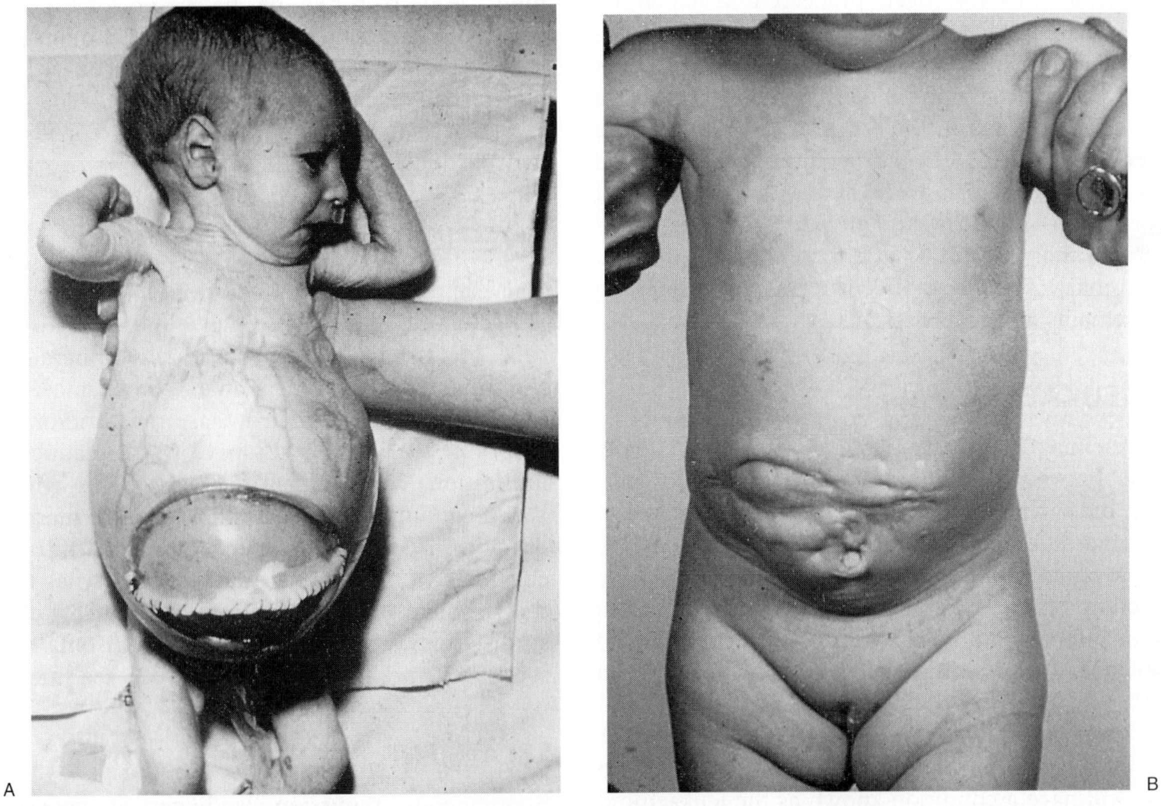

Fig. 40.1 (A) Stage 4s neuroblastoma presenting in the neonatal period as extreme hepatomegaly causing profound respiratory and nutritional embarrassment. A silastic pouch was constructed into which the liver was allowed to expand with relief of symptoms. (Courtesy of Dr A. Mowat.) (B) Reconstruction of the abdominal wall 20 months later after spontaneous regression of tumour.

and appropriate radiological confirmation, is essential. Hypertension due to catecholamine release may require treatment. A grossly enlarging liver causing life-threatening episodes of respiratory embarrassment and failure to thrive may require urgent surgical relief, or shrinkage by irradiation or chemotherapy. Late relapses may occur outside the neonatal period and careful continued surveillance is necessary.

PROGNOSIS

All stages of neuroblastoma have a much better prognosis than the corresponding stage occurring in older children. The prognosis for stage 1 and 2 disease is excellent, with 100% survival. Deaths in stage 4s disease are more likely to occur from respiratory and nutritional distress due to gross hepatomegaly than from the disease per se. Prognosis is excellent once spontaneous regression occurs. Even with extensive disease (stages 3 and 4), children under 1 year fare better than their older counterparts.

SCREENING

Over 90% of patients with neuroblastoma have raised urinary vanillylmandelic and homovanillic acid levels. The remaining 10% are non-secreting. A screening test based on the detection of a raised urinary concentration of these metabolites has been pioneered in Japan by Sawada.[49] This is performed at 6 months of age and has been reported to improve survival rates,[42] but these results have not been confirmed by subsequent large studies in Quebec[53] and in the north of England.[3] In the former series 41 673 3-week-old neonates were screened and four neuroblastomas were detected, only one of which was stage 4, and in the latter 20 829 babies were screened at 6 months and only two were found to have neuroblastoma. The cost-effectiveness of screening therefore remains controversial.

ACUTE LEUKAEMIA

Acute leukaemia during the neonatal period is equally distributed between lymphoid and myeloid subtypes, whereas in older children there is a 7:1 preponderance of the lymphoid subtype. Rearrangements of the MLL (major leukaemia locus) gene on chromosome 11q23 are the most common genetic abnormalities, and are found in 70–80% of infant acute lymphoblastic leukaemia (ALL) and 60% of those with acute myeloid leukaemia (AML).[46]

In a quarter of cases there is an associated trisomy 21 (Down syndrome). A number of infants with Down syndrome will have a condition known as the leukaemoid reaction, or transient myeloproliferative disorder. This is clinically indistinguishable from true leukaemia and the cellular characteristics of the marrow and peripheral blast cells are the same as in true leukaemic blast cells. The two conditions may be distinguished by karyotypic analysis of bone marrow cells, which show only Down trisomy 21 in the majority of cultured cells in TMD, whereas with progression to frank leukaemia they are more likely to show extra chromosome abnormalities. For instance, in the series reported by Hayashi[27] two out of 15 patients with TMD later developed acute leukaemia; one had a normal male Down syndrome karyotype (47, XY+21) during the period of TMD, but developed a 48, XY+8+21 karyotype when he developed acute leukaemia. The other patient was a mosaic (46, XY/47, XY+21) during TMD but again developed a 48, XY+8+21 karyotype in his leukaemia cells. Although a proportion of children with TMD go on to develop acute leukaemia, in the majority the signs and symptoms spontaneously regress over a 1–6-month period, after which time the infant is haematologically normal. Serial analysis of bone marrow chromosomes will indicate whether a transition to acute leukaemia has occurred.

CLINICAL FEATURES

Hepatosplenomegaly may be present at birth, with widespread petechiae and ecchymoses. Plaques of skin infiltration commonly occur in the neonate, and respiratory distress may be due to leukaemic infiltration of the lungs. Bone pain may be the reason for the opisthotonic position adopted by these babies, and a bulging fontanelle may suggest meningeal involvement or an intracranial haemorrhage due to thrombocytopenia.

Congenital leukaemia has been reported to cause hydrops (p. 846) and stillbirth.[24]

INVESTIGATIONS

The haemoglobin may be normal in the neonate and the WBC count high or normal with a neutropenia. Blast cells are usually present in the peripheral blood and thrombocytopenia is invariable. The diagnosis is made by examining a bone marrow aspirate and/or a trephine biopsy of the marrow. Biopsy of skin plaques will reveal infiltration with immature blast cells. Morphological classification of these and those in the marrow may be difficult on routine staining, but the introduction of enzyme and monoclonal marker studies has helped solve this problem. Peripheral blood and marrow chromosome studies may reveal an associated trisomy 21, Turner syndrome, mosaic trisomy 9 or 11q23 rearrangement.

TREATMENT

Spontaneous remission is likely in cases of TMD associated with Down syndrome, and in such patients supportive treatment is all that is indicated, giving blood and platelet transfusions together with antibiotics if infection supervenes, in the expectation that spontaneous remission will occur. Leukaemia occurring in the neonatal period is almost always fatal, especially if the MLL gene is present, and in no other malignancy of this period are the ethics of treatment more questionable. Neonates tend to have the features associated with the worst prognosis of acute leukaemia, that is, a high presenting WBC, undifferentiated or myelogenous cell types with chromosomal abnormalities, and central nervous system involvement.[38] Intensive chemotherapy is poorly tolerated. However, if treatment is the chosen option it should be according to the current relevant MRC protocol.

In Pui's[46] review of the current literature, the reported event-free survival (EFS) in ALL in infancy (up to 1 year) was around 30–50%, but Chessel's report of the MRC UK trials[11] showed a significantly worse survival for those children under 26 weeks of age at diagnosis (5-year EFS 40% over 26 weeks versus 10% under 26 weeks ($P = 0.00005$)). In Parkes' series[44] only 1/21 was alive at 5 years, and this was a patient with Down syndrome who was thought to have megakaryoblastic leukaemia at age 19 days, was not treated and had a normal marrow at 3 months, and was therefore probably a case of TMD. Only 7/21 were treated with chemotherapy.

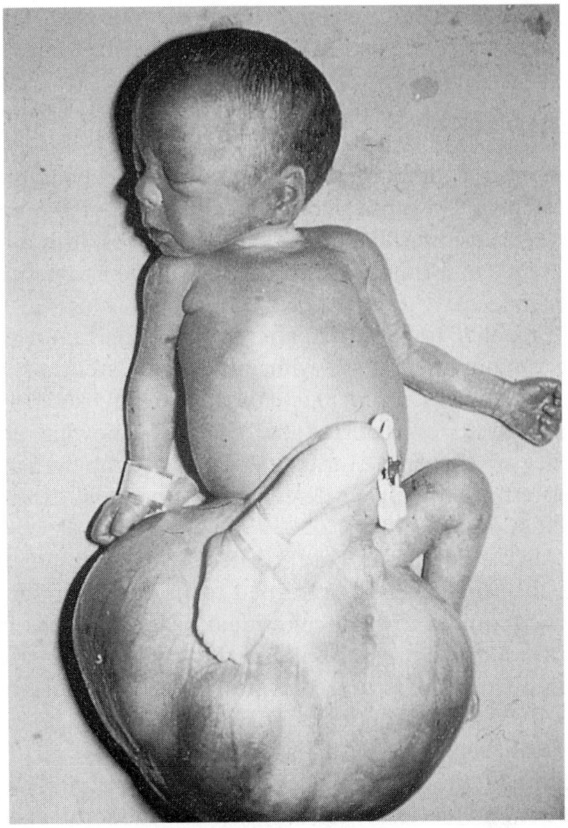

Fig. 40.2 Sacrococcygeal teratoma. (Courtesy of Dr J. Berry.)

TERATOMAS

Teratomas are tumours derived from all three embryonic germ cell layers – ectoderm, mesoderm and endoderm. They are predominantly found in the midline or in the gonads. In the neonate the commonest site of presentation is in the sacrococcygeal region, and there is a 4:1 female to male preponderance. Tumours in this region may be postsacral (external), presacral (internal) or dumb-bell-shaped (both external and internal portions). Only 10% of neonatal teratomas are malignant, the greatest risk being in those that are presacral;[43] 45% arise in the sacral area, 20% in the ovary, 20% in the testis, and approximately 10% intracranially. The cervical region and the mediastinum account for 5%.[15]

CLINICAL FEATURES

The most common presentation in the newborn is a readily recognizable tumour lying postanally between the buttocks. The tumour varies in size, from one which appears as a slight elevation or discoloration over the coccyx to one which equals the size of the baby (Fig. 40.2) and causes difficulty during delivery. There is usually very little presacral extension in these tumours, but a few will have intra-abdominal extension which can be palpated abdominally as a mass arising in the pelvis. Presacral tumours may not be as rare in this age group as supposed, as they may be unsuspected and only become apparent in the older child when they are recognized as having a greater chance of being malignant. Tumours of the head, neck and mediastinum may be extensive and cause difficulty in delivery and airways obstruction.

INVESTIGATIONS

A lateral X-ray of the abdomen may show anterior displacement of the rectum and possible calcification within the tumour. A chest X-ray (posteroanterior and lateral views) is important to rule out pulmonary metastases. A CT scan of the abdomen and pelvis with bowel contrast may determine whether primary surgery is feasible. The serum level of AFP should be measured. A high level is found in the normal newborn (mean 50 000 U/ml), with a gradual fall to adult levels (less than 10 U/ml) over the first year of life.[5] This protein is produced by cells derived embryologically from either fetal yolk sac or liver, and the level is grossly elevated (often to several million U/ml) in malignant teratoma, where the yolk sac tissue is the malignant element, but is normal in benign tumours. Serial readings are therefore important to plot the rate of fall and compare it with that expected based on the half-life of AFP (5 days). Failure to fall at the expected rate after surgery, or a subsequent rise, would indicate residual malignant yolk sac elements or the development of metastases. Malignant teratomas sometimes secrete β-HCG, which can then also be used as a tumour marker.

In 10% of cases malignant elements (usually teratocarcinoma) may be present, but the markers are negative.

TREATMENT

Ninety per cent of neonatal teratomas are benign and treatment is by surgical removal. Removal of the entire coccyx is essential. Failure to do this will result in a local recurrence in 30% of cases,[16] despite the benign nature of the lesion.

Functional impairment after surgery, particularly for large tumours and those with intrapelvic extension, may be commoner than previously thought, with 11/27 (41%) of a large series reported by Malone[40] showing either bladder or bowel dysfunction or lower limb weakness. Long-term follow-up to detect these functional deficits is therefore mandatory.

Malignant tumours are treated with chemotherapy until the AFP level has returned to normal, but surgery may be required to remove residual disease. Deaths from benign teratoma are confined to the group where size or location causes obstructed labour. Fortunately, diagnosis by antenatal ultrasound scanning may allow a planned caesarean section for delivery, but the baby may still succumb if the tumour is in a site causing vital organ obstruction (cervical lesions). With modern chemotherapy, using platinum-based drug regimens, the very small number of neonates with malignant teratoma have an excellent chance of cure.

BRAIN TUMOURS

Brain tumours are rarely diagnosed in neonatal life unless they are growing rapidly. Gordon[23] reported 21 cases under the age of 2 years presenting to a single institution over a 15-year interval, of whom three were under the age of 6 months at presentation. Wakai[55] reported two cases and extensively researched the literature, recording a 14% survival in 171 patients in whom postoperative courses were described.

CLINICAL FEATURES

Signs of raised intracranial pressure with vomiting, an increased head circumference with separation of the sutures, and a bulging fontanelle can occur in the neonate with a rapidly expanding tumour. However, most will be too small to cause symptoms during this period of life and only become apparent when the child is a few months old.

INVESTIGATIONS

Ultrasound and CT scanning have revolutionized the diagnosis of lesions within the brain. MRI may be the investigation of choice for tumours arising in the posterior fossa and brain stem.

TREATMENT

Treatment of brain tumours has traditionally been by surgery and radiotherapy. Immature brains are extremely susceptible to damage by irradiation, and the chances of avoiding intellectual as well as physical handicap after central nervous system irradiation in the newborn are slight. Therefore, treatment should aim at reducing raised pressure by decompression using a shunt device, together with surgical removal of the tumour if feasible. The value of chemotherapy is currently being assessed.

KIDNEY TUMOURS (MESOBLASTIC NEPHROMA), NEPHROBLASTOMA (WILMS' TUMOUR)

The commonest type of renal tumour in neonates is the mesoblastic nephroma.[7] This is a leiomyomatous hamartoma composed of spindle-shaped mesenchymal cells in which there are entrapped tubules and glomeruli. The appearances of a rubbery grey-yellow whorled tumour (not unlike a uterine fibroid) on macroscopic cut section are diagnostic. These tumours are usually benign and are cured surgically, but there are more aggressively behaving variants[31] which may recur locally or metastasize.

True Wilms' tumour, derived from mesenchymal blastema, which may differentiate into glomerular, tubular or stromal structures, is rare in the neonatal period. These histological variants are termed favourable and are associated with a good prognosis. The anaplastic Wilms', the bone-metastasizing renal tumour first described by Marsden et al in 1978[41] (the clear cell sarcoma of American literature), and the malignant rhabdoid tumour of the kidney, are treated as unfavourable-histology Wilms' tumours. Malignant rhabdoid tumour is occasionally associated with an intracranial tumour, which is usually of neuroepithelial origin. Two of the seven infants with this variant reported in Bonnin et al's series[8] presented in the neonatal period.

The condition of nephroblastomatosis – the abnormal persistence of metanephric blastema beyond 36 weeks' gestation[28] – is thought by some to be a precursor of Wilms' tumour, being present in 20–40% of kidneys containing a Wilms' tumour. This relationship may be analogous to that seen between neuroblastoma and neuroblastoma-in-situ; the subject has been extensively reviewed by Beckwith et al.[2] An interesting feature of Wilms' tumour is its association with a wide variety of congenital abnormalities, of which the most common are hemihypertrophy, aniridia, the WAGR syndrome (Wilms', aniridia, genitourinary tract abnormalities, mental retardation) and Beckwith–Wiedemann syndrome (p. 945), associated with loss of the tumour-suppressor gene *WT1* at 11p13.[47] Denys–Drash syndrome (ambiguous genitalia, Wilms' and nephritis) is thought to involve the *WT2* gene at the 11p15 locus.

CLINICAL FEATURES

Most renal tumours in neonates are found as an abdominal mass on routine examination. Haematuria is rare. Hydrocephalus due to associated cerebral tumour, a presentation unique to neonates, has been recorded.[8] There may be features associated with the syndromes described above.

INVESTIGATIONS

Abdominal ultrasound and CT scan with intravenous contrast are now the investigations of choice for location of abdominal masses. A chest X-ray (both posteroanterior and lateral views) should always be taken to look for lung metastases and, if clear, a chest CT performed to confirm the absence of disease. Hypercalcaemia may occur in association with both Wilms' tumour and mesoblastic nephroma, possibly owing to secretion of parathormone in the former and excessive PGE_2 in the latter.[12] Treatment of this phenomenon is surgical resection of the tumour, but it may respond to steroids if surgery has to be delayed for any reason.

STAGING

Staging of the tumour is important in order to institute appropriate therapy.

Stage I Tumour confined to kidney and totally resected;
Stage II Tumour extending beyond kidney but completely resected;
Presurgical biopsy or local tumour spillage at operation;
Hilar lymph node involvement;
Stage III Residual tumour confined to abdomen;
Positive lymph nodes other than hilar;
Gross tumour spillage;
Stage IV Haematogenous spread (lungs, liver);
Stage V Bilateral tumours.

TREATMENT

The common neonatal tumour, the mesoblastic nephroma, is usually curable by surgery alone; the rare ones with vascular invasion or other aggressive features, or those that spill at operation, may recur or metastasize. However, the role of chemotherapy in these cases is controversial.

For Wilms' tumours, histology (favourable or unfavourable – see above), as well as staging and initial operability, is taken into account in the current national UKCCSG treatment protocol. In favourable-histology tumours abdominal irradiation has been omitted from stage I and II treatment regimens. Vincristine is given weekly for 10 weeks in all stages, with the addition of actinomycin alone 3-weekly in stage II but with adriamycin in addition in stages III and IV. Abdominal irradiation is added in stage III disease, together with pulmonary irradiation in stage IV disease in older children. Unfavourable-histology tumours are treated with more intensive chemotherapy using the same agents.

PROGNOSIS

The prognosis of neonates with mesoblastic nephroma is excellent, as most can be completely surgically resected. There was a 98% survival in 51 children reported from the USA National Wilms' Tumour Study by Howell et al.[29] The prognosis for neonates with true Wilms' probably does not differ from that in older children, and is dependent on stage. It is a highly curable tumour, with an 87% 5-year survival rate in patients registered in the UKCCSG Wilms' 2 study between 1986 and 1991. Most neonates presenting with Wilms' have stage I or II disease, although all stages are represented, and survival is likely to be even greater in this group, who may require only surgery for cure.

SCREENING

From the known incidence of Wilms' tumour (1 in 10 000 births), and the known incidence of aniridia (1 in 50 000), Beckwith syndrome (1 in 17 000) and hemihypertrophy (1 in 53 000), it can be calculated that the chance of Wilms' tumour in the three conditions is approximately 5% in aniridia, 2% in Beckwith's and between 5 and 10% in hemihypertrophy. Abdominal ultrasound screening of patients with these syndromes has been advocated, but the value of screening in this highly curable condition was not known. Craft et al[13] have recently looked at the role of screening and found no difference in stage distribution or outcome in any of the three groups, whether they were unscreened, screen positive or screen negative. In future, with more precise delineation of the loci involved in the syndromes and more sensitive tests for minor deletions, it will be possible to use karyotypic analysis to predict those with deletions which are more likely to develop the full picture. In the meantime, routine screening is not now advocated in the UK. Teaching parents to palpate the abdomen and giving them quick and easy access to investigation if symptoms or signs develop is the preferred action.

SARCOMAS

Malignant soft-tissue tumours arising from mesenchyme comprise about 10% of neonatal tumours. Of the 170 neonatal malignancies in Parkes'[44] series 17 were of this nature, but the majority of mesenchymal tumours in the newborn are benign. The commonest benign lesion is congenital fibromatosis, which may be solitary or multi-

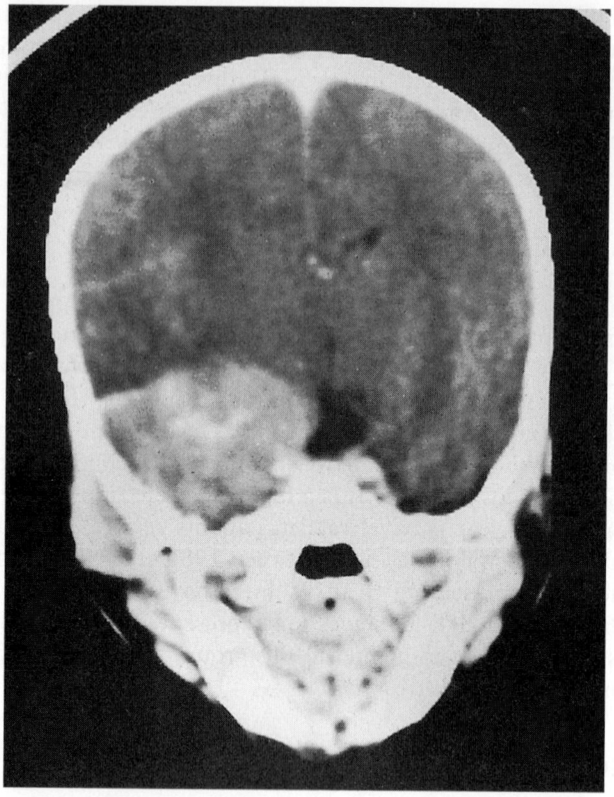

Fig. 40.3 Extensive facial rhabdomyosarcoma with intracranial extension. (Courtesy of Dr J. Pritchard.)

focal, and predominates in the head, neck and extremities. The histological distinction between this entity and fibrosarcoma is difficult, but neonatal fibrosarcoma may behave much more like fibromatosis than in older children or adults, and may spontaneously remit.[39] In Isaacs'[30] series fibrosarcomas tended to be much larger lesions than fibromata, and histologically showed an increased cellularity and mitotic rate, with nuclear atypia. True sarcomas (rhabdomyosarcomas) may present at birth at any site, but tend to arise in the head and neck area. They are often extensive (Fig. 40.3). Of the 357 patients with soft tissue sarcoma entered into the German study reported by Koscielniak et al,[36] six cases were diagnosed in the first month of life.

CLINICAL FEATURES

Soft-tissue tumours are easily recognizable as a mass. Sixty per cent will arise in the head and neck region (Fig. 40.3) or involve the extremities. Occasionally a mass is so large that it causes difficulty in delivery, or may rupture, causing exsanguination.

INVESTIGATIONS

The extent of lesions can be imaged with CT or MRI. Diagnosis is made by biopsy, and it is important to obtain fresh or frozen tissue for electron microscopy, monoclonal marker studies and tumour chromosomes.

TREATMENT

Wide surgical excision of malignant lesions is the treatment of choice. If this is impossible without gross disfiguration (amputation of a limb, for example), a trial of chemotherapy to shrink the tumour may be indicated. In the German series reported by Koscielniak,[36] 20–50% of the recommended chemotherapy doses for older children were used. Radiation therapy, which is a useful treatment modality in this tumour in older patients, is not indicated in neonates because of its damaging effects on the growth and function of immature tissues.

PROGNOSIS

Prognosis is good in those patients in whom primary resection is possible. Local recurrence of fibromatosis and fibrosarcoma is likely if surgical margins are not clear of disease, although all four neonates with fibrosarcoma treated with chemotherapy in the German series[36] after inadequate resection are long-term survivors. The prognosis of extensive rhabdomyosarcomatous lesions and those with metastases is very poor. Those arising in the head and neck may cause death from respiratory obstruction.

RETINOBLASTOMA

Retinoblastoma accounts for 3% of childhood tumours and is familial in 40% of cases. The incidence in the neonatal period will depend on the local screening policy of those with a family history. In the Toronto series[10] 11.5% were diagnosed as neonates. Of the 17 infants, 13 had bilateral disease. Four cases were diagnosed on elective screening. In the British series reported by Parkes[44] 14 cases were identified, 11 bilateral and three unilateral. Seven patients had a family history. Six patients died, all of a second malignancy and all having had bilateral disease. The retinoblastoma gene was identified by Friend et al[19] on chromosome 13q14, and is either partially or totally deleted in retinoblastoma and osteosarcoma. In the familial disease both copies of the retinoblastoma (*Rb*) gene are missing from all cells, but in the sporadic cases there is one intact copy and one defective copy. If the intact copy is lost through somatic mutation at the target organ (retinoblast), a tumour results. It may be possible to predict the occurrence of these tumours by fetal chromosome analysis in the future, especially in familial cases.

CLINICAL FEATURES

Those tumours not detected by elective screening are

most likely to present with leukocoria (the typical white reflex seen through the pupil), heterochromia of the iris and strabismus.

INVESTIGATION

Staging is by ophthalmoscopic examination under anaesthetic, together with CT or MRI scanning.

Stage I Confined to retina;
Stage II Retinal detachment;
Stage III Optic nerve involved but not beyond cut end;
Stage IV Optic nerve involved beyond cut end;
Stage V Extraocular spread.

TREATMENT

Enucleation is the treatment of choice for tumours greater than stage II, although if they are bilateral conservative management (radiotherapy, cryotherapy or light coagulation) is usually attempted for the less severely affected eye.

PROGNOSIS

The overall 3-year survival in Sanders et al's series[48] was 88%, with older patients having a worse prognosis. Long-term follow-up is essential, as there is an 8% chance of developing a second tumour,[17] many of which will be osteosarcomas, the locus for which is closely linked to that of the retinoblastoma gene.

HEPATOBLASTOMA

Hepatoblastomas occasionally occur in the very young and may be associated with hemihypertrophy or Beckwith–Wiedemann syndrome (p. 945). Hepatomegaly may cause respiratory embarrassment or gastrointestinal symptoms. Surgical removal is the treatment of choice for stage I disease, but large tumours may be rendered operable by chemotherapy using adriamycin and cisplatinum.

LANGERHANS' CELL HISTIOCYTOSIS, FORMERLY HISTIOCYTOSIS X

This is a rare 'reactive' disease in which cells having the characteristics of epidermal Langerhans' cells are found in the dermal skin layer or in other organs, where they cause tissue damage by producing excessive interleukins and PGE_2.[32] It is included in this chapter as it is usually treated by oncologists, although it is no longer thought to be a malignant disease.

Neonatal presentation is usually with a skin rash, which may resemble either healing chickenpox with widely scattered purple papules involving all areas of the body, including palms and soles, and described by Hashimoto and Pritzger as congenital self-healing histiocytosis,[26] or seborrhoeic dermatitis involving the groins, axillary folds, 'necklace area' and scalp. The latter form is usually associated with involvement of other organs, commonly lung, liver and bone marrow. Diagnosis is made on skin biopsy and the extent of organ involvement determined by investigations, which should include full blood count and differential, liver function tests, including clotting studies, skeletal survey and chest X-ray.

Table 40.3 Tumours associated with specific malformations, syndromes and chromosomal abnormalities. (Reproduced with permission from Berry[4])

Inherited syndrome	Childhood cancer
Phakomatoses and hamartoses	
Neurofibromatosis (p. 884)	Brain tumours, sacromas, leukaemia
Tuberous sclerosis	Brain tumours
Basal cell naevus syndrome	Medulloblastoma, basal cell carcinoma
Turcot syndrome	Medulloblastoma
Multiple mucosal neuroma syndrome	Medullary thyroid carcinoma, phaeochromocytoma
Metabolic disorders	
Glycogenosis type I	Hepatocellular carcinoma
Hereditary tyrosinaemia (p. 995)	Hepatocellular carcinoma
Alpha-1-antitrypsin deficiency (p. 739)	Hepatocellular carcinoma
Chromosome breakage and repair defects	
Bloom syndrome (p. 867)	Leukaemia, gastrointestinal tumours
Ataxia telangiectasia	Leukaemia, lymphoma
Fanconi's anaemia	Leukaemia, hepatoma
Xeroderma pigmentosum (p. 901)	Skin cancers, melanoma
Immune deficiency disorders	
Wiscott–Aldrich syndrome (p. 803)	Leukaemia, lymphoma (often in the central nervous system)
Sex-linked lymphoproliferative syndrome	B-cell lymphoma
Severe combined immunodeficiency (p. 934)	Leukaemia, lymphoma
Bruton's agammaglobulinaemia	Leukaemia, lymphoma
Chromosomal anomaly	
Down syndrome (trisomy 21) (p. 859)	Acute leukaemia
Turner syndrome (45XO) (p. 863)	Neurogenic tumours
13q-syndrome (p. 862)	Retinoblastoma
11p-syndrome (p. 862)	Nephroblastoma
Monosomy 7	Preleukaemia and non-lymphoblastic leukaemia
XY gonadal dysgenesis (p. 979)	Gonadoblastoma
Trisomy 18 (p. 860)	Nephroblastoma
Klinefelter syndrome (p. 863)	Leukaemia, teratoma, breast carcinoma
Congenital anomaly	
Hemihypertrophy and Beckwith syndrome (p. 945)	Nephroblastoma, adrenal cortical carcinoma, hepatoblastoma
Sporadic aniridia	Wilms' tumour
Poland syndrome (p. 878)	Leukaemia
Hirschsprung's disease (p. 783)	Neuroblastoma

Congenital self-healing histiocytosis heals spontaneously over 4–8 weeks, whereas systemic chemotherapy[37] is usually indicated in the multisystem variety.

TUMOURS ASSOCIATED WITH SPECIFIC MALFORMATIONS, SYNDROMES AND CHROMOSOMAL ABNORMALITIES

Specific malformations, syndromes and chromosomal abnormalities (Table 40.3) are recognizable in the neonatal period, although the tumours associated with them usually appear much later in life. However, early detection of a tumour may be possible if a patient known to be susceptible is regularly screened.

ANTENATAL ULTRASOUND DETECTION OF SOLID TUMOURS

With the advent of routine antenatal screening, solid tumours are being diagnosed more frequently in the fetus. This understandably causes both parents and obstetrician grave concern. As a general rule, early diagnosis and premature induction of labour does not confer a prognostic benefit in these circumstances. The preferred option is to allow the pregnancy to continue to term, so that, if treatment is indicated, it is better tolerated. However, the growth of these lesions should be monitored so that elective caesarean section can be planned at term if there is a risk of obstructed labour.

REFERENCES

1. Bader J L, Miller R W 1979 US cancer incidence and mortality in the first year of life. American Journal of Diseases of Children 133: 157–159
2. Beckwith J B, Kiviat N B, Bonadio J F 1990 Nephrogenic rests, nephroblastomatosis and the pathogenesis of Wilms' tumour. Pediatric Pathology 10: 1–36
3. Bell S, Parker L, Craft A et al 1994 False positive results in neuroblastoma screening. Medical and Pediatric Oncology 24: 271–273
4. Berry P J 1987 In: Keeling J W (ed) Congenital tumours in foetal and neonatal pathology. Springer Verlag, London, pp 229–247
5. Blair J I, Carachi R, Gupta R et al 1987 Plasma α fetoprotein reference ranges in infancy: effect of prematurity. Archives of Disease in Childhood 62: 362–369
6. Bolande R P 1994 Pre-natal carcinogenesis: an appraisal. Cancer 74: 1674–1679
7. Bolande R P, Brough A J, Izant Jr R J 1967 Congenital mesoblastic nephroma of infancy Pediatrics 40: 272–278
8. Bonnin R P, Brough A J, Palmer N F, Beckwith J B 1984 The association of embryonal tumours originating in the kidney and in the brain. A report of seven cases. Cancer 54: 2137–2146
9. Brodeur G M, Pritchard J, Berthold F et al 1993 Revision of the international criteria for neuroblastoma diagnosis, staging and response to treatment. Journal of Clinical Oncology 11: 1466–1477
10. Campbell A N, Chan H S, O'Brien A et al 1987 Malignant tumours in the neonate. Archives of Disease in Childhood 62: 19–23
11. Chessels J M, Eden O B, Bailey CC et al 1994 Acute lymphoblastic leukaemia in infancy: experience in the MRC UKALL trials. Report from the Medical Research Council working party on childhood leukaemia. Leukaemia 8: 1275–1279
12. Coppes M 1993 Serum biologic markers and paraneoplastic syndromes in Wilms' tumour. Medical and Pediatric Oncology 21: 213–221
13. Craft A W, Parker L, Stiller C, Cole M 1995 Screening for Wilms' tumour in patients with aniridia, Beckwith syndrome or hemihypertrophy. Medical and Pediatric Oncology 24: 231–234
14. Crom D B, Williams J A, Green AA et al 1989 Malignancy in the neonate. Medical and Pediatric Oncology 17: 101–104
15. Dehner L P 1983 Gonadal and extragonadal germ cell neoplasia of childhood. Human Pathology 14: 493–511
16. Donellan W A, Swenson O 1968 Benign and malignant sacrococcygeal teratomas. Surgery 64: 834–846
17. Draper G J, Saunders B M, Kingston J E 1986 Retinoblastoma and second primary tumours. British Journal of Cancer 53: 661–671
18. Evans A E, D'Angio G J, Randolph J 1971 A proposed staging for children with neuroblastoma. Cancer 27: 374–378
19. Friend S H, Bernards R, Rogelj et al 1986 A human DNA segment with properties of the gene that predisposes to retinoblastoma and osteosarcoma. Nature 329: 642–645
20. Friend S H, Thaddeus P D, Weinberg R A 1998 Oncogenes and tumour suppressing genes. New England Journal of Medicine 318: 618–622
21. Fung C Y, Fisher D E 1995 p53: From molecular mechanisms to prognosis in cancer. Journal of Clinical Oncology 13: 808–811
22. Gale G B, D'Angio G J, Uri A et al 1982 Cancer in neonates: the experience at the Children's Hospital of Philadelphia. Pediatrics 70: 409–413
23. Gordon G S, Wallace S J, Neal J W 1995 Intracranial tumours during the first two years of life: presenting features. Archives of Disease in Childhood 73: 345–347
24. Gray E S, Balch N J, Kohler H et al 1986 Congenital leukaemia: an unusual cause of stillbirth. Archives of Disease in Childhood 61: 1001–1006
25. Guin G H, Gilbert E F, Jones B 1969 Incidence of neuroblastoma in infants dying of other causes. American Journal of Clinical Pathology 51: 127–136
26. Hashimoto K, Pritzker M G 1973 Electron microscopic study of reticulohistiocytoma: an unusual case of congenital, self-healing reticulohistiocytosis. Archives of Dermatology 107: 263–270
27. Hayashi Y, Eguchi M, Sugita K et al 1988 Cytogenetic findings and clinical features in acute leukaemia and myeloproliferative disorder in Down's syndrome. Blood 72: 15–23
28. Hou L T, Holman R L 1961 Bilateral nephroblastomatosis in a premature infant. Journal of Pathology and Bacteriology 82: 249–255
29. Howell C G, Otherson H B, Kiviat N E et al 1982 Therapy and outcome in 51 children with mesoblastic nephroma: a report of the National Wilms' Tumour Study. Journal of Pediatric Surgery 17: 826–831
30. Isaacs H 1985 Perinatal (congenital and neonatal) neoplasms: a report of 110 cases. Pediatric Pathology 3: 165–216
31. Joshi V J, Kasznica J, Walters T R 1986 Atypical mesoblastic nephroma: pathologic characterisation of a potentially aggressive variant of conventional congenital mesoblastic nephroma. Archives of Pathology and Laboratory Medicine 110: 100–106
32. Kannourakis G, Abbas A 1994 The role of cytokines in the pathogenesis of Langerhans' cell histiocytosis. British Journal of Cancer 70 (suppl xxiii): s37–s40
33. Keily E M 1994 The surgical challenge of neuroblastoma. Journal of Pediatric Surgery 29: 128–133
34. Knudson Jr A G 1971 Mutation and cancer: a statistical study of retinoblastoma. Proceedings of the National Academy of Science USA 68: 820–823
35. Knudson Jr A G 1985 Hereditary cancer, oncogenes and antioncogenes. Cancer Research 45: 1437–1443
36. Koscielniak E, Harms D, Schmidt D et al 1989 Soft tissue sarcomas in infants younger than 1 year of age: a report of the German soft tissue sarcoma study group (CWS-81). Medical and Pediatric Oncology 17: 105–110
37. Ladisch S, Gadner H 1994 Treatment of Langerhans' cell histiocytosis – evolution and current approaches. British Journal of Cancer 70 (suppl xxiii): s41–s46
38. Leiper A D, Chessels J 1986 Acute lymphoblastic leukaemia under 2 years. Archives of Disease in Childhood 61: 1007–1012
39. Madden N P, Spicer R D, Allibone E B, Lewis I J 1992 Spontaneous regression of fibrosarcoma. British Journal of Cancer 66 (suppl xviii): s72–s75
40. Malone P S, Spitz L, Keily E M et al 1990 The functional sequelae of sacrococcygeal teratoma. Journal of Pediatric Surgery 25: 679–680

41. Marsden H B, Lawler W, Kumar P M 1978 Bone metastasising renal tumour of childhood. Cancer 42: 1922–1928
42. Nishi M, Miyake H, Takeda T et al 1987 Effects of mass screening of neuroblastoma in Sapporo city. Cancer 60: 433–436
43. Noseworthy J, Lack E E, Kosakewich HPW et al 1981 Sacrococcygeal germ cell tumours of childhood: an updated experience with 118 patients. Journal of Pediatric Surgery 16: 358–364
44. Parkes S E, Muir K R, Southern L et al 1994 Neonatal tumours: a thirty year population based study. Medical and Pediatric Oncology 22: 309–317
45. Pritchard J, Hickman J A 1994 Why does stage 4s neuroblastoma regress spontaneously? Lancet 344: 869–870
46. Pui G H, Kane J R, Crist W M 1995 The biology and treatment of infant leukaemias. Leukaemia 9: 762–769
47. Riccardi V M, Hittner HM Franke U et al 1980 The aniridia–Wilms' tumour association: the critical role of chromosome band 11p13. Cancer Genetics and Cytogenetics 2: 131–137
48. Sanders B M, Draper G J, Kingston J E 1986 Retinoblastoma in Great Britain 1969–80: incidence, treatment and survival. British Journal of Ophthalmology 72: 576–583
49. Sawada T, Hirayama M, Nakata T et al 1984 Mass screening in infants in Japan. Lancet ii: 271–273
50. Stiller C A 1995 Childhood Cancer Research Group, Oxford. Personal communication
51. Stiller C A, Birch K J 1990 Trends in survival for childhood cancer in Britain diagnosed 1971–1985. British Journal of Cancer 62: 806–815
52. Strauss L, Driscoll G 1964 Congenital neuroblastoma involving the placenta. Pediatrics 34: 23–31
53. Tuchman M, Lemieux B, Auray BC et al 1990 Screening for neuroblastoma at 3 weeks of age; methods and preliminary results from the Quebec Neuroblastoma Screening project. Pediatrics 86: 765–773
54. Voute Jr P A, Wadman S K, van Putten W J 1970 Congenital neuroblastoma: symptoms of the mother during pregnancy. Clinical Pediatrics 9: 206–208
55. Wakai S, Toshimoto A, Masakatsu N 1984 Congenital brain tumours. Surgical Neurology 21: 597–609
56. Weinberg R A 1988 Finding the anti-oncogene. Scientific American 259: 34–41

41

Orthopaedic problems in the newborn

Robert N. Hensinger Eric T. Jones

INTRODUCTION

Historically, orthopaedic participation in the care of the newborn infant has been limited. In the neonatal intensive care unit musculoskeletal deformities are less serious than the demanding and life-threatening paediatric problems, and their treatment was deferred until the infant was discharged from the nursery or until the child was 'big enough' to undergo orthopaedic management. Unfortunately, for many children this led to an increase in the deformity, and the problems associated with treatment became significantly more extensive. We have found that orthopaedic problems in the newborn can be reduced in size by early recognition and treatment.[33]

THE IMPORTANCE OF GROWTH

The effect of growth on the musculoskeletal system may be positive or negative. Growth can produce deformity, as in cerebral palsy, in which the spastic and unbalanced muscle forces gradually deform the bones and joints that were normal at birth (Figs 41.1, 41.2). However, the rapid growth in the neonate enables the orthopaedist to utilize growth to direct the development of the affected part along a more normal tract.

NORMAL ORTHOPAEDIC DEVELOPMENT

There is presumptive evidence, but scant experimental documentation, of a temporary ligamentous laxity in the neonate secondary to maternal hormones such as relaxin and oestrogen. This short period of hyperelasticity coupled with rapid growth can facilitate the correction of deformities such as metatarsus adductus, clubfoot or dislocation of the hip. If the deforming forces are appropriately managed, the adaptive pathological changes can be rapidly reversed; if treatment is delayed the problem becomes more complex and the treatment required more extensive.

SPINE

The axial skeleton changes shape with growth. The neonate has a relatively large head and long spine, with

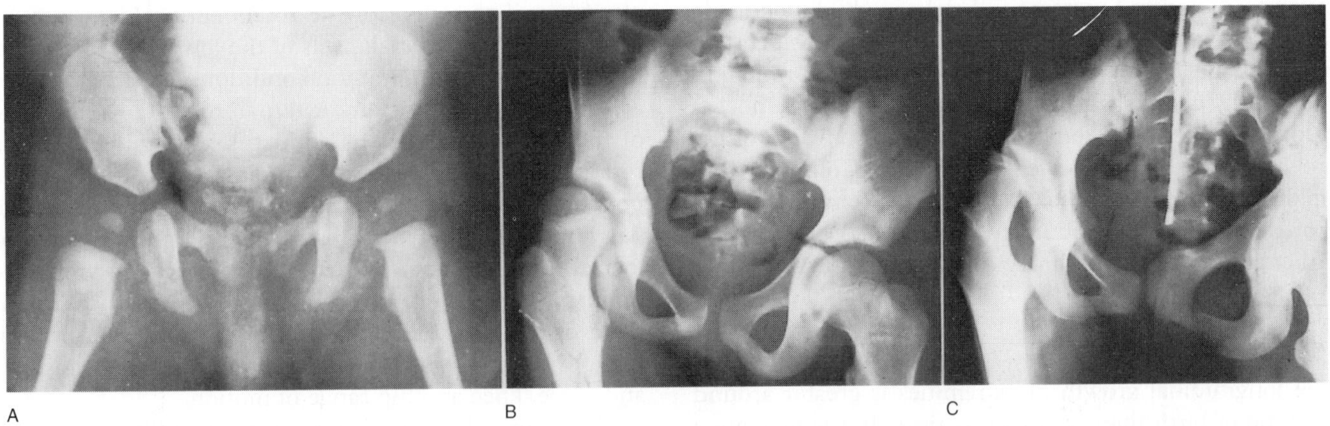

Fig. 41.1 Serial X-rays of the hips of a girl with right-sided spastic hemiplegia secondary to cerebral palsy. (A) Normal radiographic appearance of the hips at 8 months of age. (B) and (C) Progression to a dislocated hip at age 13 years, with no treatment of the spastic adductors of the right hip. The bones and joints are normal at birth. With growth, the abnormal spastic muscles, if untreated, will cause the proximal femur to develop extreme valgus, acetabular dysplasia and subsequently a dislocated hip.

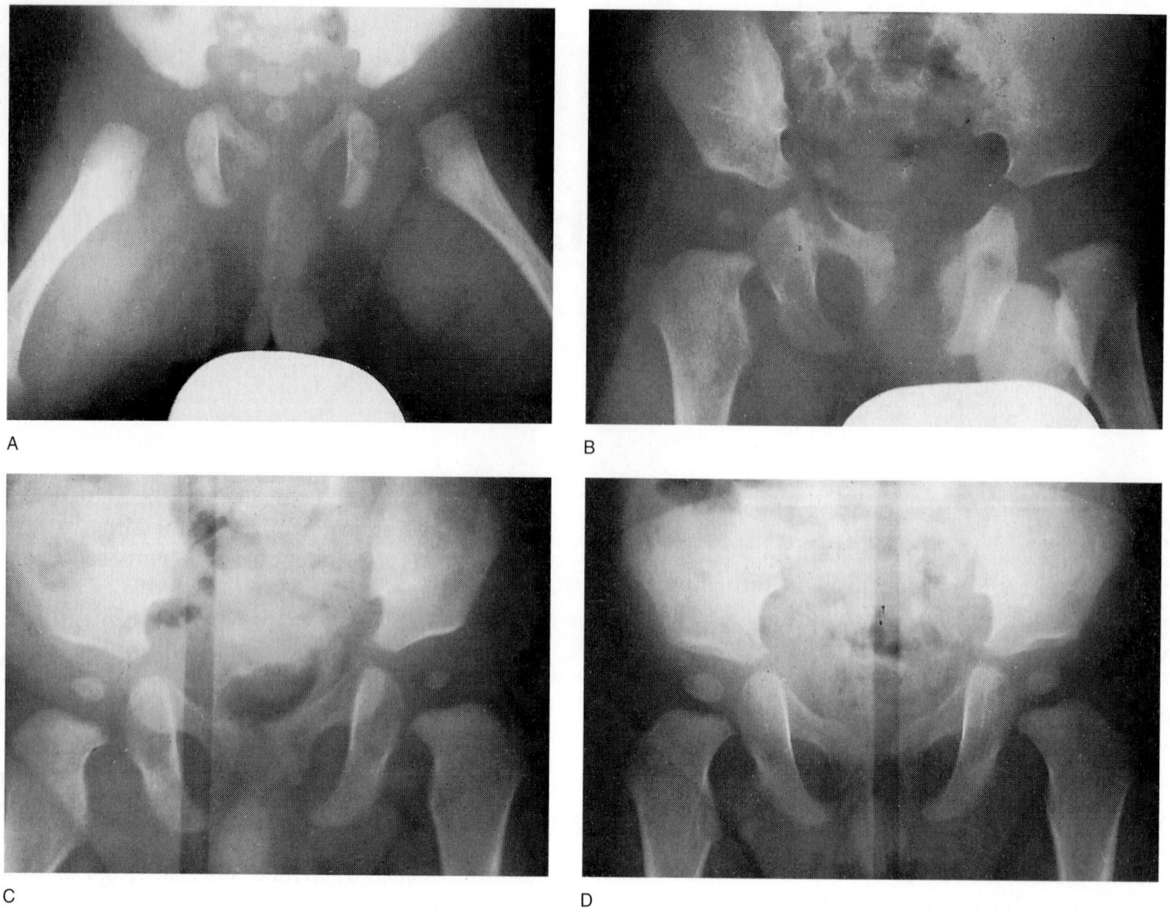

Fig. 41.2 Successive X-rays of a newborn with bilateral dislocated hips. (A) Treatment within the first week of life with a Pavlik harness. The right hip was clinically reducible and the left hip reduced quickly in the harness. Films at 3 months (B), 6 months (C) and 1 year (D) demonstrate growth to a near-normal appearance by walking age.

proportionately shorter limbs than the adult; the entire spine is concave anteriorly. In the first 3 months of life, with the acquisition of head control, a cervical lordosis appears. Similarly, lumbar lordosis begins with sitting. By the age of 1 year, 50% of the total growth of the spine has occurred[85] and the axial skeleton does not contribute as much to the overall increase in height in childhood as do the lower extremities. This is an important consideration in the management of a congenital spine deformity. In the young child short-segment spinal fusion is not as stunting to the ultimate height as premature fusion of the growth plates of the lower extremities. Conversely, in children with congenital scoliosis/kyphosis, continued spinal growth may not contribute to longitudinal growth, but rather to growth in a pathological direction (curvature).

LIMBS

The longitudinal growth of extremities is greater around the time of birth than at any other time. In the neonate a growth plate injury or infection can cause a significant limb length and/or angular discrepancy. As the extremities grow longitudinally they also change rotationally and angularly, and there are important physiological variations in normal growth during the first 2 years of life. Most of the lower extremity rotational ‘problems’ seen in the newborn and infant represent either side of the normal bell-shaped curve, so it is important to understand the normal physiological variations at each stage of growth and development. The source of the rotational problem may be at one level or at several levels of the lower extremities. In the infant the most common conditions causing variation are medial tibial torsion, external rotatory contracture of the hip and metatarsus adductus. All children with a rotational variation should be examined to rule out the possibility of a pathological condition such as cerebral palsy, myelodysplasia, diastematomyelia or a subtle neurological problem, particularly if they have asymmetric findings or a history of progressive deformity. Examination of the non-walking child should include inspection for foot deformity, tibial or femoral rotation or bowing, and ankle, knee and hip range of motion.

The natural history of most of these conditions favours improvement with time. Most respond to simple conservative treatment, such as stretching and night splints; rarely, a patient may require surgical intervention.

FEMORAL ANTEVERSION[23]

Internal femoral torsion is an abnormal relationship of the knee to the head and neck of the femur. The newborn has physiological femoral anteversion of approximately 40°, i.e. when the knee points straight ahead the femoral head is pointing slightly anteriorly, and not directly at the pelvis. This usually decreases quite rapidly during the first 2 years of life, and 15° of anteversion is normal in the older child and adult.

EXTERNAL ROTATORY CONTRACTURE[72]

Many children in the first few months have marked external rotation of the entire leg. Examination in the supine or prone position will demonstrate excessive external rotation and markedly diminished internal rotation of the lower extremity at the hip. This condition is due to an abduction/external rotation contracture of the soft tissues around the hip secondary to intrauterine position. Spontaneous correction normally occurs once the child has been walking for a few months.[72] The parent can be instructed in exercises to stretch the posterior hip capsule by internally rotating the lower extremities. This can be done with each nappy change. Radiographic examination of the hips may be wise in some of these children to rule out developmental displacement of the hip.

MEDIAL TIBIAL TORSION

In this condition the tibia is rotated medially on its long axis, causing the foot to point inward (Fig. 41.3). The majority of neonates have this positioning of their tibiae, probably related to intrauterine posture.

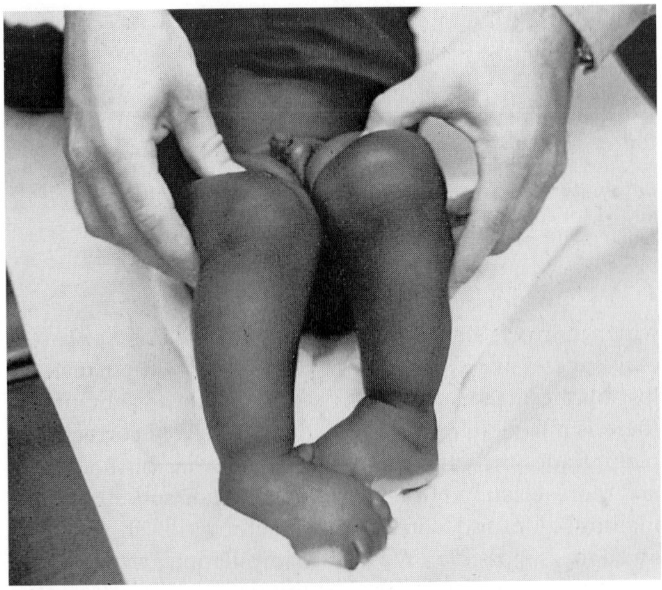

Fig. 41.3 A 6-month-old with persistent internal tibial torsion. Tibial torsion is best examined with the femur placed in neutral rotation, the thighs directly in front of the hip joint and the heels against a flat surface.

Most examiners use the relationship of the medial to the lateral malleolus to determine the transmalleolar axis and its relationship to the long axis of the tibia or a specific protuberance of the tibia, such as the anterior tibial tubercle. The transmalleolar axis is usually rotated externally, approximately 5° in the neonate, increasing with growth to an average of 22° in the adult.[71] The greatest increase occurs in the first $1\frac{1}{2}$ years of life.[72] A lateral bowing of the tibia – a common finding in children under 18 months of age – can accentuate the appearance of internal tibial torsion.

PHYSIOLOGICAL BOW LEGS

Mild bowing of the lower extremities (apex laterally) is a normal finding in the neonate and young child under 18 months of age. Generally the bowing (approximately 15°) is confined to the tibia (genu varum), but occasionally it can be noted in the distal femur as well. It is often accompanied by internal tibial torsion and is usually symmetrical. This should correct spontaneously at 18–24 months of age.[66] Pathological conditions that lead to bowing are uncommon in the neonate; however, in the infant rickets, Blount's disease and metaphyseal dysplasia can cause bowing, but this can usually be distinguished radiographically from physiological bowing. Blount's disease or pathological tibia vara should be suspected in children in whom the physiological bowing does not regress by 18–24 months of age.

NEWBORN FOOT PROBLEMS

METATARSUS ADDUCTUS[10]

Turning in of the forepart of the foot, or metatarsus adductus (Fig. 41.4), is a frequent finding in the newborn

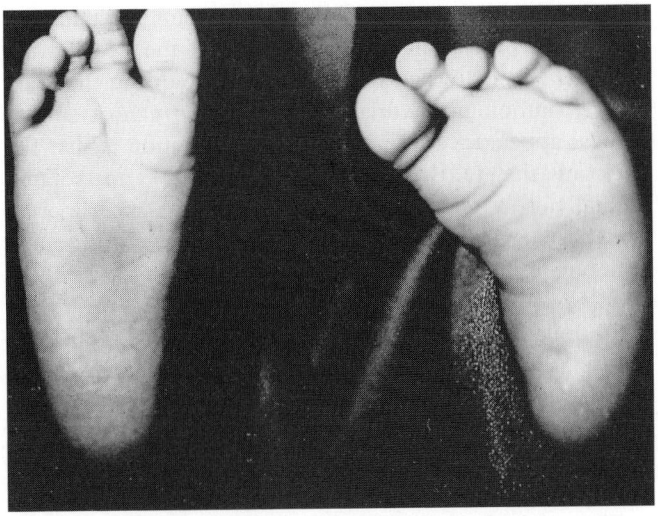

Fig. 41.4 Infant with unilateral metatarsus adductus, demonstrating a convex lateral border of the left foot with the curve beginning at the base of the fifth metatarsal.

and may be related in part to intrauterine positioning. Many children with metatarsus adductus also have an associated medial tibial torsion. Diagnosis is made by inspecting the sole of the foot and can be easily documented by a footprint. The lateral border of the normal foot is straight, but in metatarsus adductus that border of the forefoot is convex, with the curve beginning at the base of the fifth metarsal.[10] Up to 90% may spontaneously improve without specific treatment.[65] Unfortunately, guidelines for determining those that will improve and those that will persist are not yet available. Children with rigid metatarsus adductus, or flexible (easily passively correctable) metatarsus adductus who still supinate and medially rotate (adduct) the forefoot on dorsiflexion by 2–3 months of age are probably best treated by serial casts[10] or corrective shoes. Five to 10% of children with metatarsus adductus also have developmental displacement of the hip, and should therefore be examined appropriately.[40]

CLUBFOOT (CONGENITAL TALIPES EQUINOVARUS)

This is a common problem in the newborn. The prevalence is about 1 per 1000 livebirths, with a male/female ratio of about 2:1. There seems to be a multifactorial inheritance pattern,[89] and the aetiology is still the subject of debate.

Anatomically the entire foot is inverted and supinated, and the forefoot adducted (Fig. 41.5(A)). The heel is rotated inward (varus) and in equinus with the calcaneus inverted beneath the talus. The talus is in equinus as well as the os calcis. The navicular is medial to the head of the talus, and often the talus is prominent in the dorsolateral aspect of the foot, stretching the skin over that area. Whether these changes are due to alterations in the soft tissues with dislocation of the foot about the talus, or arise because of congenital distortion of the neck of the talus, has been studied in great detail. No doubt there are several pathological variations which can give a similar clinical appearance, but a popular explanation is that the neck of the talus is congenitally short and rotated medially in a plantar direction. However, experimental evidence suggests that intrauterine problems of positioning and oligohydramnios also play a significant role in the aetiology.

In unilateral cases the calf is noticeably smaller and the foot is shorter on the affected side. There may be a prominent crease in the arch of the foot, which is believed to indicate a more severe, rigid deformity which will be less responsive to conservative management and more likely to need surgical correction.

The goal of treatment is both clinical and roentgenographic correction. Because the deformity varies in the newborn, from a very rigid and resistant foot to one which corrects easily with simple passive manipulation, early aggressive treatment is indicated.[33] Much can be lost by the slightest delay. The best results are obtained if there is a flexible foot which can be passively corrected to plantigrade in the first few hours following birth. Infants are more elastic at this time, and soft tissue stretching, manipulation and correction of deformities should start as soon as possible. We use manipulation accompanied by tape to maintain the position[33,50] (Fig. 41.5(B)). When the foot is corrected or the child discharged from the neonatal nursery the foot is placed in a cast. Casts are changed at 1–2-week intervals until the foot is large

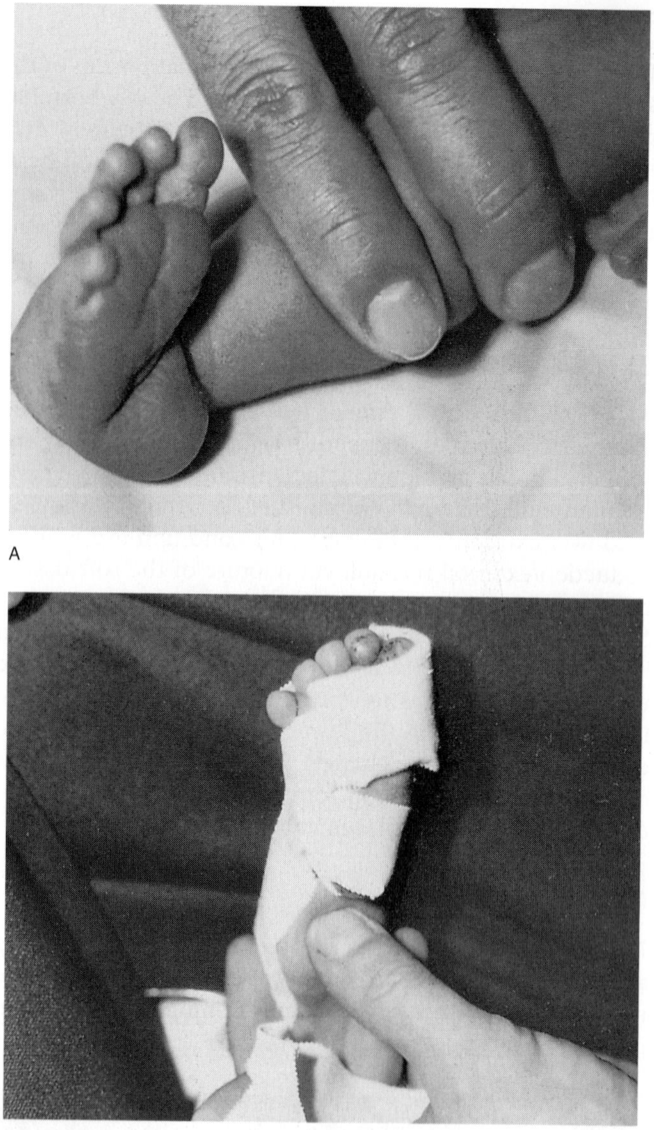

A

B

Fig. 41.5 (A) Typical clinical appearance of the newborn with a unilateral clubfoot (congenital talipes equinovarus). The entire foot is inverted and supinated; the forefoot is adducted. The heel is rotated inward and is in equinus. (B) After passive correction of the deformity the foot is held in a corrected position with tapes. This allows for continued regular stretching and further correction while maintaining the foot position.

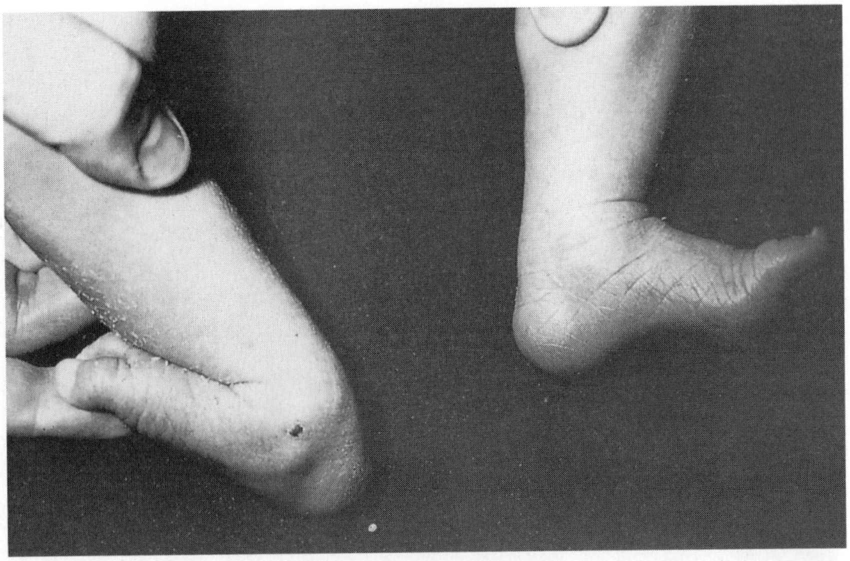

A

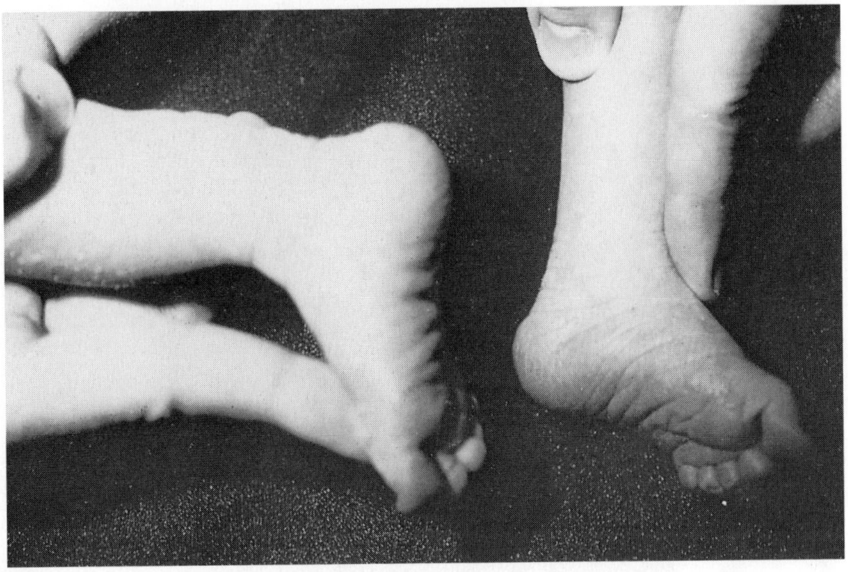

B

Fig. 41.6 Calcaneovalgus (flexible flat foot), a common postnatal finding that may be related to intrauterine moulding. (A) The foot and ankle seem to be unusually lax and dorsiflex nearly to the tibia. (B) Plantar flexion is restricted and the heel remains in a valgus position. Spontaneous resolution is the rule, and the condition seldom requires treatment.

enough to be controlled in a shoe, or until it is clear that since stretching and serial casts are not improving the foot operative management will be required. Non-operative management can be expected to achieve a satisfactory result in more than two-thirds of children.[61]

PES VALGUS

Infantile calcanceovalgus

This is a common neonatal finding (Fig. 41.6). The foot and ankle seem unusually lax and dorsiflex nearly to the tibia. Plantar flexion is restricted, and the heel is in a valgus position. It may be partly related to – or at least occurs frequently with – external rotatory contracture of the hips. The condition may be related to intrauterine moulding, as it is more common in the firstborn child. The vast majority correct spontaneously. Treatment, when required, consists of stretching exercises, which are usually sufficient, but tape or plaster may be necessary in more rigid deformities. Calcaneovalgus may be confused with congenital vertical talus or 'rocker bottom' foot (see below). If there is doubt, a lateral X-ray of the foot will be helpful.

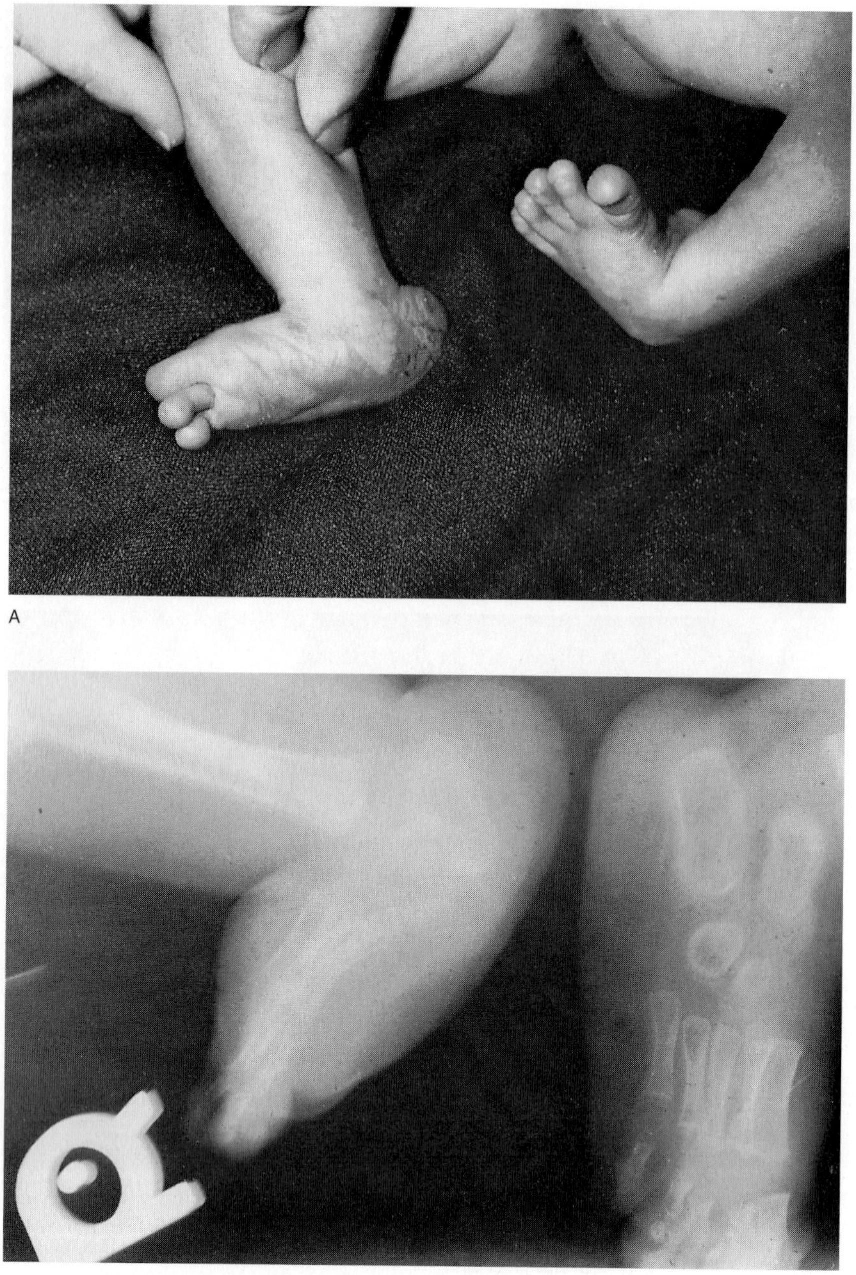

Fig. 41.7 (A) Clinical appearance of a newborn with a vertical talus (congenital 'rocker-bottom' foot). This is a rigid deformity, and when viewed from the side the plantar surface of the foot appears curved with the apex at the midtarsal joint. (B) X-ray appearance of the deformity. Note the equinus position of the hindfoot, as seen in the foot on the right (large R on X-ray), versus the normal appearance on the left. The heel cord is contracted, the talonavicular joint subluxed and the forefoot is dorsiflexed at the midtarsal joint.

Vertical talus ('rocker-bottom' foot)

This is an uncommon condition in which the child is born with a very rigid flat foot (congenital pes planus). When viewed from the side the plantar surface of the foot appears curved, with the apex at the midtarsal joint (Fig. 41.7). The deformity includes an equinus position of the hindfoot owing to a contracted heelcord and talonavicular subluxation, with the talus being vertical in the foot and palpable on the plantar surface. The anterior tibial tendon and extensors of the toes are shortened, as well as the peroneal tendons, which are often subluxed anterior to the lateral malleolus, causing the forefoot to be abducted and dorsiflexed at the midtarsal joint.

In the neonate the deformity is very rigid, and may be associated with arthrogryposis, Turner and Edward syndromes (pp. 860, 863) and other congenital anomalies, particularly those that involve the central nervous system, such as myelodysplasia (p. 1302), sacral agenesis (p. 1080) and diastematomyelia. Eighty-five per cent of children with congenital vertical talus can be expected to have a neurological abnormality. Early treatment is necessary and successful. Long-term follow-up indicates that the untreated foot is stiff and rigid, and leads to considerable difficulty even in the young child.

DEVELOPMENTAL DYSPLASIA OF THE HIP

The term 'developmental dysplasia of the hip' has been proposed to replace the possibly misleading term 'congenital dislocation of the hip', which has been used for the last 70 years.[44] The latter rigidly indicates a prenatally established malformation of the hip which is present at birth. The term developmental dysplasia of the hip is broader and indicates a more dynamic disorder, and would include children with displacement of the hip regardless of the time or aetiology. It is well established that hips can become displaced in the antenatal, neonatal or postnatal periods, that the hips are sometimes stable and sometimes unstable, and that the aetiology is multifactorial, including the broad category of idiopathic displacement of the hip. However, dysplastic, teratogenic, paralytic and post-traumatic displacements of the hips may also occur, and traditionally have been referred to as congenital dislocation of the hip. The term developmental dysplasia of the hip more accurately describes the problems that occur in infants, as it is well known that hips can displace postnatally, even as late as walking age. During the neonatal period most children with hip displacement have idiopathic, recently displaced hips, which aptly fit the description of 'congenital dislocation'.

DDH occurring in the perinatal period has a prevalence of approximately 10 per 1000 livebirths.[14,38] The incidence may be higher if children are examined in the immediate newborn period.[7] Some of these hips are 'dislocatable' and stabilize in the first few days. Females outnumber males 6:1.[67] Early recognition and treatment have met with spectacular success, with approximately 96% of affected children developing radiologically and functionally normal hips.[25,63] The longer the dislocation remains undiscovered and untreated, the greater are the problems in returning the femoral head to its normal position within the acetabulum and the poorer the chances of obtaining a satisfactory result. In the newborn the diagnosis of dislocation is best made by clinical examination using Ortolani and Barlow tests. Those experienced in the examination can include these tests, which take only a few seconds, in the routine neonatal examination. Routine screening for DDH should be an integral part of neonatal and follow-up examinations during infancy. The hip at risk is a new term that has been introduced to highlight those children who are more susceptible to DDH. The clinical profile of the hip at risk includes children who are firstborn, breech, have a positive family history and other problems due to intrauterine moulding, such as torticollis and metatarsus adductus. It is currently recommended that children with this profile have a hip examination at each 'well baby' visit until 1 year of age, and that a single anteroposterior X-ray of the pelvis and hips be taken at 3 months of age.

AETIOLOGY

There is no single cause of DDH. Rather, the aetiology is multifactorial with both mechanical and physiological factors on the part of the mother and infant, and occasionally postnatal and environmental factors combining to produce hip instability and subsequently dislocation. The typical congenital dislocation occurs just prior to or following delivery in an otherwise normal infant. The mechanical factors that predispose to the typical dislocation occur primarily in the last trimester of pregnancy. All have the effect of restricting the space available for the fetus in the uterus. It is believed that the pelvis of the fetus becomes trapped in the maternal pelvis. The fetus is then unable to kick and change positions, which prevents the normal flexion of the hip and knee or limb folding. Sixty per cent of children with DDH are firstborns, suggesting that the tight unstretched maternal abdominal and uterine musculature restricts fetal movement.[32,33,58]

Breech presentation also plays a significant role in the aetiology of DDH: 30–50% of children with DDH are delivered in this presentation.[67] If, in addition, the knees are extended (frank breech), the increased tension in the hamstrings further contributes to hip instability.

The left hip is more frequently involved (55%) in DDH than the right. It is believed that a fetus in the breech position tends to lie most often with the right shoulder anterior and with the left thigh against the maternal sacrum.[67] Thus the fetal pelvis is held securely in the maternal pelvis, with the thigh trapped tightly against the maternal sacrum, forcing the hip into a posture of flexion and adduction. In this position the femoral head is covered more by the joint capsule than by the bony acetabulum. The right hip only is dislocated in 20% of patients and both hips in 25%.[58] The incidence of DDH is increased in children who have other deformities caused by intrauterine moulding, such as congenital muscular torticollis,[39] metatarsus adductus and talipes calcaneovalgus.

The physiological factors in the development of DDH are maternal oestrogens and those hormones that affect pelvic relaxation just prior to delivery. Their pharmacological effect is not limited to the maternal pelvis, but may also lead to temporary laxity of the pelvic joints and hip capsule in the newborn.

Postnatal environmental factors contribute to the

development of hip instability and dislocation. In the first months after delivery the normal physiological position of the hip is that of flexion and abduction. In societies where infants are customarily wrapped to a cradle board or swaddled to maintain the legs in extension, the incidence of congenital hip dislocation is 10 times greater than normal.[67]

PATHOMECHANICS

The mechanism of a typical congenital dislocation is probably quite simple. Near the time of birth the cramped interuterine position in the presence of maternal hormones results in a stretched elastic joint capsule. Following delivery the femoral head is loose within the joint and free 'to fall out' of the acetabulum. If the dislocation is recognized in the newborn period the femoral head can easily be returned to its normal position (reduced). At this early stage the shape of the joint and soft tissue structures is very close to normal. Thus for a stable hip to develop it is only necessary to maintain a normal relationship between the femoral head and the acetabulum for a few weeks while the joint capsule returns to its normal configuration. In this case the hip has the potential for an excellent long-term result. However, if the dislocation is allowed to persist, the soft tissue and bone adjacent to the joint gradually undergo adaptive changes, the dislocation becomes more difficult to reduce and the chance of obtaining a successful long-term result diminishes significantly.

RECOGNITION AND DIAGNOSIS

Examination of the newborn and infant

(Fig. 41.8)

The most reliable clinical method of diagnosing DDH in the newborn period is with the examinations described by Ortolani[59] and Barlow.[6] The Ortolani examination is a test of hip reduction: when the infant with a dislocated hip is examined the femoral head returns to the acetabulum with the Ortolani manoeuvre. This finding is known as a 'positive Ortolani'. The Ortolani test is initiated with the hips and knees in 90° of flexion (Fig. 41.8) and the hips are examined one at a time. The examiner grasps the baby's thighs with the middle finger over the greater trochanter and the thumb around the distal medial femur. This allows for steady gentle traction on the thigh, with simultaneous abduction to pull the hip anteriorly from its dislocated position to 'clunk' into the acetabulum. This examination takes only a few seconds and should be part of all newborn and follow-up examinations, and is also important in assessing the progress of treatments; this lesion is called a type 1 dislocated hip.

The Barlow portion of the examination is the reverse. When the infant is examined the femoral head is located within the acetabulum. However, if the hip is flexed and the thigh brought into an adducted position the femoral head falls 'or can be gently pushed' posteriorly out of the acetabulum, demonstrating an unstable hip joint which is dislocatable. This is a type 2 dislocated hip. A type 3 dislocated hip is in fact just unstable or subluxable on the Barlow test. The femoral head is loose in the acetabulum but cannot be completely dislocated.

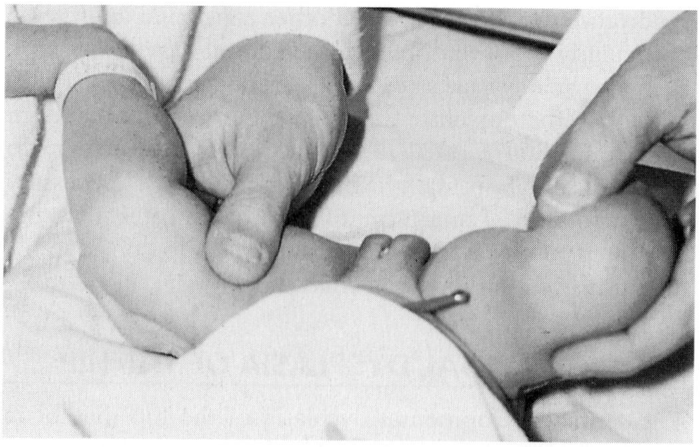

Fig. 41.8 Examination of a quiet comfortable child for dislocated hips should require but a few seconds in a routine examination. If the child's hip is dislocated, gentle traction with abduction of the hips in 90–100° of flexion should produce a 'clunk' characteristic of a 'positive Ortolani', as the dislocation is reduced and the femoral head goes back into the acetabulum.

These are not forceful examinations and the infant must be relaxed and content. Cooperation by the patient and patience on the part of the examiner significantly affect the accuracy of the examination. A kicking, crying child can prevent a satisfactory examination by tightening the adductors and hamstrings, leading to a false result.

As the child grows the clinical findings of an untreated dislocated hip become more obvious (Fig. 41.9). The surrounding soft tissue and bone gradually adapt to the

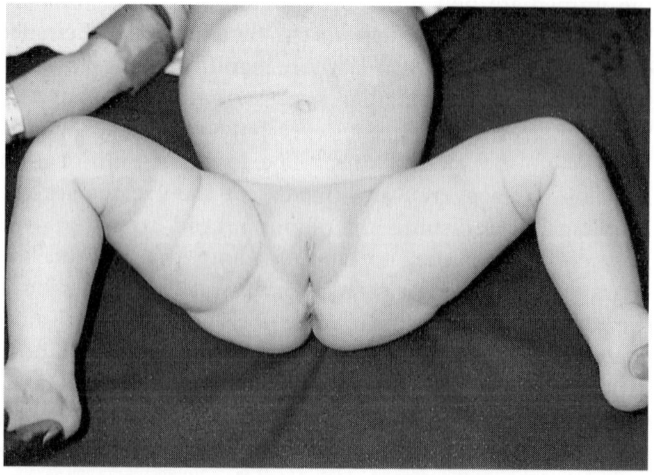

Fig. 41.9 In the older child with a dislocated hip there is limitation of abduction, shortening of the thigh and extra skin folds (on the left of the picture).

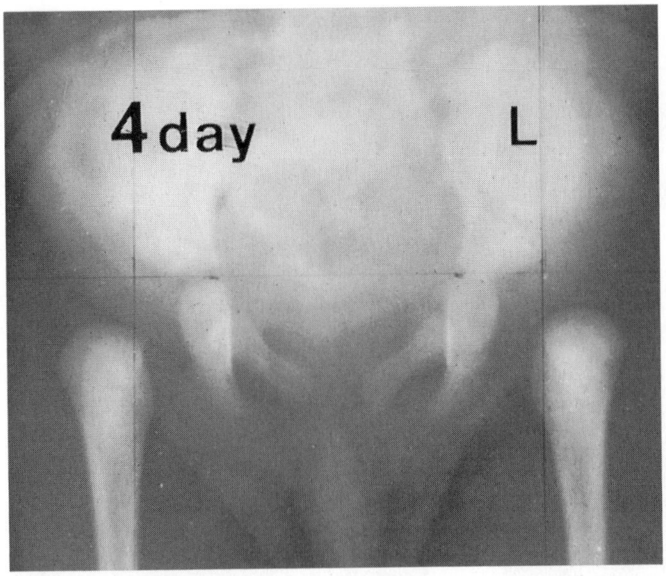

Fig. 41.10 A radiograph at 4 days of age of a dislocated left hip. The hip is being held in the dislocated position. A normal-appearing X-ray in this age group does not exclude the presence of a dislocation.

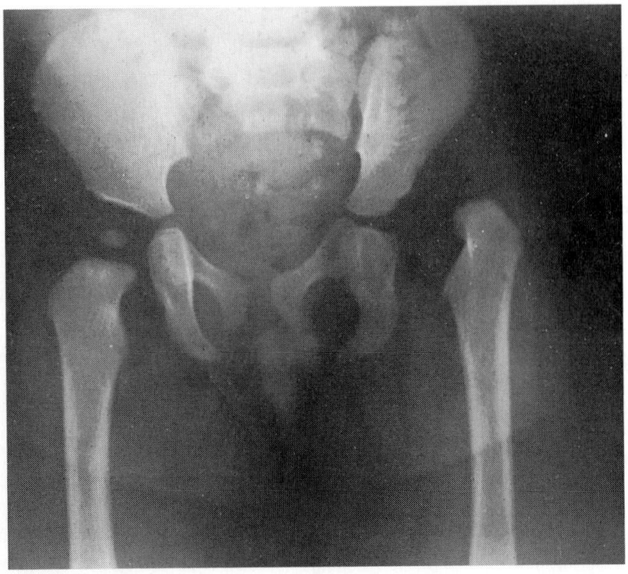

Fig. 41.11 A radiograph of a 2-year-old child with a unilateral dislocation of the left hip. The typical X-ray findings of proximal lateral migration of the neck of the femur, dysplasia of the acetabulum and development of false acetabulum are seen. With growth both the clinical and X-ray deformities become more obvious.

abnormal position of the femoral head. With time it becomes more difficult to reduce the femoral head into the acetabulum and the Ortolani test becomes negative. In other words, the femoral head becomes trapped outside the acetabulum. All muscle groups about the hip become shortened and contracted. Adductor tightness, which is reflected in limited thigh abduction, is most apparent. As the thigh is shortened the skin and subcutaneous tissues bunch up and extra skin folds can be observed; with the patient supine and the knees flexed, the knees will not be at the same level (Allis', Galeazzi's sign). The femur can be freely moved up and down, which is described as 'pistoning' or 'telescoping'.

RADIOLOGICAL FINDINGS

Radiological examination of the newborn to detect a typical congenital dislocation is not reliable.[15] The X-rays may not reveal the dislocation even if the hip is clinically held in a dislocated position (Fig. 41.10). The usual bony landmarks are not visible, as much of the infant's pelvis is cartilaginous and consequently radiolucent. In addition, the dislocation is so recent that many of the pathological changes characteristically associated with DDH have not had sufficient time to develop, and therefore are not apparent on the X-rays. Thus, a normal hip X-ray does not rule out the presence of a dislocation.

The earliest age at which one can reliably recognize the radiological changes of a typical dislocated hip on a single X-ray is approximately 6 weeks. As the child grows, the adaptive changes of the hip joint and femur become evident on routine anteroposterior views of the pelvis and hips. The characteristic findings (Fig. 41.11) include proximal lateral migration of the femoral neck adjacent to the ilium, a shallow incompletely developed acetabulum, and delayed ossification of the femoral ossific nucleus.

Rarely (1%) will advanced radiological changes be found in the newborn. This type of dislocation is referred to as a teratological dislocation and is usually associated with conditions such as arthrogryposis, chromosomal abnormalities and severe congenital anomalies, such as sacral agenesis and myelodysplasia.

ULTRASONOGRAPHY

Ultrasonography has proved to be an excellent non-invasive and non-irradiating technique to diagnose developmental displacement of the hip.[28,29] In the infant a great deal of the hip joint is cartilaginous, and so the relationship of the femoral head to the acetabulum can be examined soon after birth, which is a significant improvement over the use of X-rays in the newborn[13] (Fig. 41.12(A–C)). As investigators have become more familiar with the procedure, reliable and reproducible standards have been obtained to determine acetabular dysplasia and hip displacement.[56] However, sonography can be too sensitive to minor degrees of instability or immaturity of the hip, which can lead to unnecessary treatment and result in a significant increase in costs and the potential for problems for the child and the family.[35] The dynamic ultrasound examination coordinated with a careful clinical examination may help to reduce the incident of false positives.[30] As experience is gained, these normal variations in hip maturation should be better understood. Ossification of the femoral head prevents

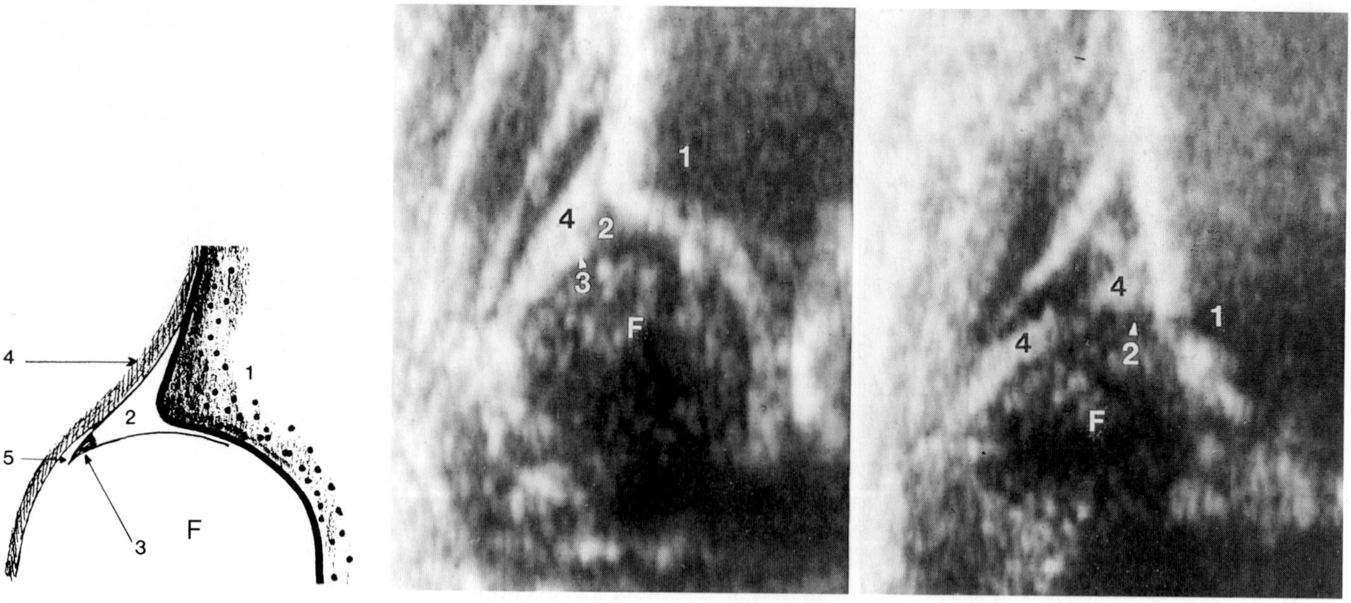

Fig. 41.12 (A) Drawing of the acetabular rim area (right hip): 1, osseous rim; 2, cartilaginous rim; 3, fibrocartilaginous limbus; 4, joint capsule; 5, recess between the limbus and periosteum; F, femoral head. (Reproduced with permission from Graf.[28]) (B) Ultrasound scan of a normal right hip in a 1-month-old child with the same structures identified. (C) Ultrasound scan of a dislocated right hip in a 1-month-old child with same structures identified.

satisfactory visualization of the acetabulum, and as a consequence this technique is not as useful as X-rays in children over 6 months of age. Sonography is helpful to follow the progress of treatment, particularly with the Pavlik harness, to demonstrate that the hip is stable and the acetabulum is remodelling. Ultrasound is helpful for assessing fluid accumulation in the joint and can assist in identifying a septic dislocation secondary to pyarthrosis.

TREATMENT AND FOLLOW-UP

Selection of one treatment device over another is determined by the age of the patient, the ease of reduction and, importantly, the potential for redislocation. The majority of children found to have hip instability (type 3 DDH) at birth will spontaneously recover in the first few weeks of life.[6] A simple positioning device (such as triple nappies or a Frejka pillow) to maintain the hip flexed and abducted during this period may be sufficient. However, the child must be observed closely, and if the hip continues to be unstable more definitive management will be required. In the newborn with marked instability (positive Ortolani type 1 DDH) or a dislocatable hip (type 2 DDH) it is best to resort directly to a secure restraint (such as a Pavlik harness, Fig. 41.13), anticipating that the reduction will have to be maintained for a few weeks before the joint structures return to normal. Many restraints have been described that maintain the hip reduced in the infant. Nearly all can achieve a successful end result provided the device is properly applied and maintains the femoral head reduced in a comfortable and physiologically safe position of flexion–abduction. Conversely, any restraint, if improperly applied or adjusted, can cause problems such as redislocation or avascular necrosis of the femoral head.

The duration of the treatment is directly related to the age at which it is initiated. The earlier the dislocation is discovered, the less pathological change there is to reverse and the shorter the period needed to achieve clinical stability and a radiologically normal hip joint. The long-term consequences of developmental dysplasia of the hip are not fully understood. Seventeen per cent of those who have a clinical and radiographically perfect treatment result at age 3 can develop acetabular dysplasia in a 12-year average follow-up.[82] It is therefore essential that all children treated for DDH be followed until maturity with X-rays every 2–3 years.

CONGENITAL DISLOCATION OR SUBLUXATION OF THE KNEE

Congenital dislocation of the knee is an uncommon neonatal problem but a true orthopaedic emergency. Immediate management can result in a satisfactory solution for a high percentage of patients.[57,73] The knee may be simply hyperextended (recurvatum), or in the severe form there may be complete dislocation with the proximal tibia anterior and lateral to the femur.[17] The dislocation is bilateral in the majority, but may not be equal in severity (Fig. 41.14). There is a mild hereditary or familial tendency.[57] Many have associated congenital abnormalities such as torticollis or dislocation of the elbow,

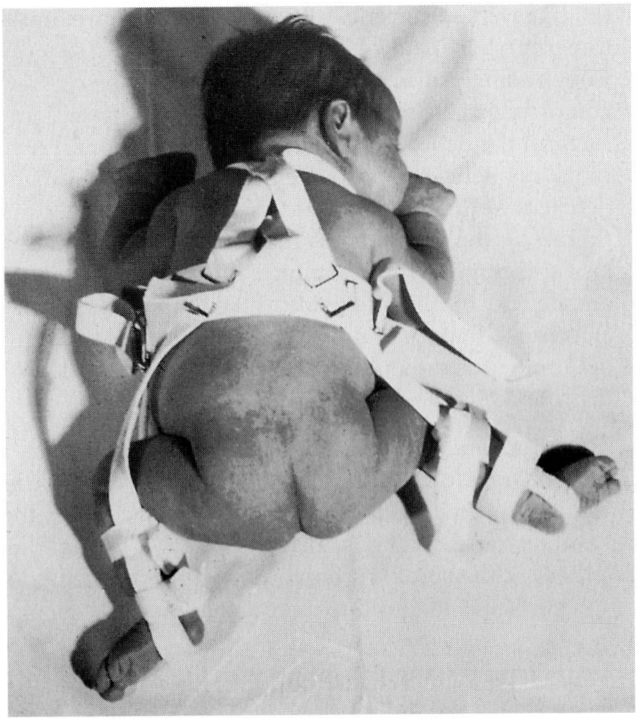

Fig. 41.13 Pavlik harness. This restraint maintains the lower extremities in the proper position by the use of shoulder harness, foot cuffs and straps with Velcro closures. The harness is applied loosely, the hips are reduced with the Ortolani manoeuvre, flexion is maintained at 90°. The posterior strap is adjusted to maintain the thigh in the safe zone of Ramsey.[63] Adjustment of the posterior strap is critical, and it should not be clinched down tightly. It is meant to serve as a checkrein to prevent the thigh from adducting to the point where the femoral head will redislocate.

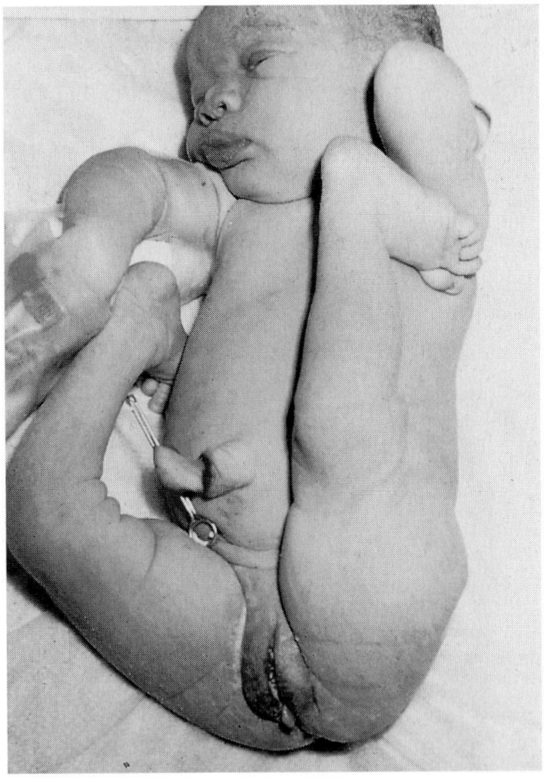

Fig. 41.14 Newborn with bilateral dislocation of the knees and hips. The infant has been placed in the intrauterine position, with the feet tucked in the axillae. The right knee is frankly dislocated, the left knee is subluxed.

and in 50% the ipsilateral hip is dislocated.[73] Hyperextension or dislocation of the knee is a frequent finding in children with arthrogryposis and myelodysplasia.[17,55] In these conditions the aetiology is related to muscle imbalance, usually contracture of the quadriceps with weak or absent hamstrings. In an otherwise normal child the aetiology is believed to be due to intrauterine position (frank breech), with locking of the feet beneath the mandible or in the axilla.[73]

Clinically the knee appears hyperextended, and in the severe type the joint may be further extended until the leg touches the chest (Fig. 41.14). The medial hamstrings may be displaced forward, anterior to the axis of the knee, and function as extensors. The patella may be displaced laterally. The condyles of the femur are prominent posteriorly, but the circulation below the knee is usually intact. Few neonates with this problem have been examined pathologically; consequently, little is known about the posterior capsule or the cruciate ligaments. In the older child these structures are stretched, hypoplastic and occasionally absent, but these changes may be secondary to persistent dislocation. Fibrosis of the vastus lateralis or vastus intermedius has been described, but usually in children with arthrogryposis, myelodysplasia or postinjection fibrosis.

X-ray evaluation will confirm the severe genu recurvatum with the tibia and femur malaligned. Deformity of the epiphyses of the distal femur and proximal tibia is not seen in the neonate, but is found in the untreated child and represents modelling changes secondary to the malalignment.

Treatment for both dislocation and subluxation should be immediate, with passive stretching, bringing the knee gradually into flexion within a few hours of birth[73] (Fig. 41.15). Usually the knee can be manipulated and held by a cast, a splint or taping. The splint should be changed daily and the joint gently stretched and put through the full range of passive movements, until approximately 90° flexion is obtained. X-rays should be obtained to document a satisfactory reduction, as clinically one can easily be misled that the flexed knee is anatomically reduced. The earlier the joint is reduced prior to the development of a fixed contracture, the better the long-term result[17,73] and the fewer adaptive and modelling changes that will have to be reversed.

ANOMALIES OF THE EXTREMITIES

These highly visible problems attract a great deal of attention in the newborn period. Many will not require immediate treatment, but counselling for the parents is

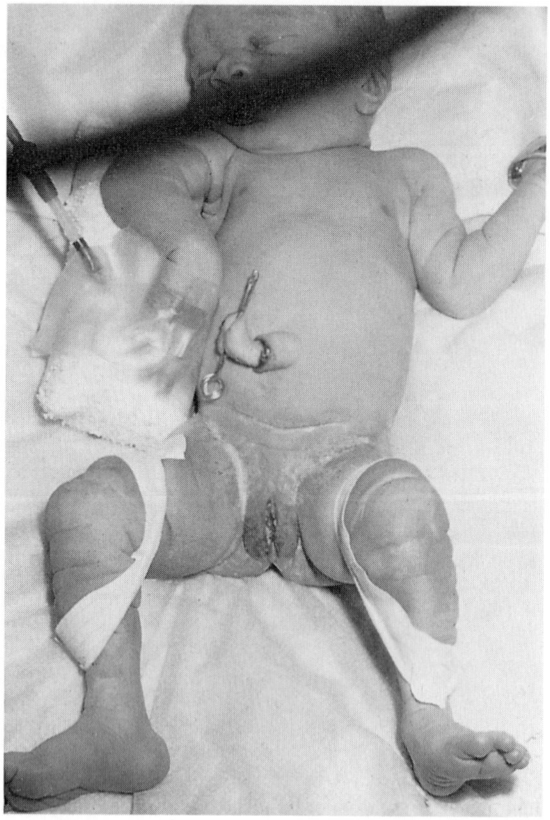

Fig. 41.15 The same child as pictured in Fig. 41.14. Treatment for dislocation of the knees should be immediate with passive stretching and gradual flexion of the knee in the nursery. If this is done within a few hours of birth, as was done with this infant, the knees can usually be brought into a flexed attitude, and the position maintained by a cast, splint or, in this case, taping. The child gradually obtained full range of knee motion and at 2 weeks was transferred to a Pavlik harness to maintain the dislocated hips reduced.

important at this time. Discussion here will be limited to the common anomalies. Others are listed in Table 41.1, with appropriate references.

Several classifications have been proposed for congenital limb malformations. In more recent times, the classification as proposed by Swanson[74] has gained widespread acceptance. There are seven categories:

I Failure of formation of parts (arrest of development);
II Failure of differentiation (separation of parts);
III Duplication;
IV Overgrowth (gigantism);
V Undergrowth (hypoplasia);
VI Congenital constriction band syndrome;
VII Generalized skeletal abnormalities.

Failure of formation (category I) has been further divided into:

1. Terminal – no normal parts distal to the amputation. This is believed to represent a complete arrest of formation of the limb anlage, the most common being the transverse deficiencies at the level of the proximal forearm (short below-elbow amputation).
2. Longitudinal – arrested or defective formation, complete or partial, of an individual bone. In the forearm the deficit can be radial, central or ulnar. A radial ray deficiency (radial club hand) may be a slight deficiency of the thenar muscles, a short floating thumb, or the entire radius may be absent; a central loss is exemplified by the typical lobster-claw hand, and deficits on the ulnar side of the limb by the ulnar club hand. Failure of differentiation includes such deformities as radioulnar synostosis, syndactyly of digits and elbow synostosis.

The problem common to all classification systems is that the X-rays obtained when the child is very young, particularly neonates, do not demonstrate the bones that are not yet ossified. Thus, diagnosis in the young child should be considered tentative and subject to revision until he or she is followed to a more mature age.

DEFORMITIES OF THE UPPER EXTREMITY

About 1 in every 600 newborns will have a congenital anomality of the hand or forearm, with almost the same frequency in males and females. Congenital deficiencies of the upper extremities occur twice as often as in the lower extremities, and bilateral involvement occurs in approximately 30%.[33] With the exception of radial and ulnar club hand, congenital upper extremity problems do not require immediate treatment in the neonate.

Sprengel's deformity (congenital elevation of the scapula)

The scapula is elevated and hypoplastic. The affected side of the neck is fuller and shorter, with a decrease in the cervicoscapular line and the appearance of torticollis. Abduction of the affected shoulder is limited because of a decrease in the scapulocostal motion. Scapulohumeral joint motion is usually normal. There is no right or left preponderance, and one-third are bilateral. Associated congenital scoliosis and/or diastematomyelia is common, and one-third have renal anomalies. No treatment is necessary in the neonatal period. Approximately a third of the children will have sufficient deformity to warrant surgical intervention in early childhood.

Congenital amputation

The terminal short below-elbow amputation is the most common. Frequently there are small skin tags, probably remnants of unformed digits.

Initial limb fitting is simple and is generally done when the child is ready to sit (6 months) and reach out for toys, but before he is ready to crawl. The prostheses used in the young child are simple, non-articulated devices

Table 41.1 Extremity anomalies

Condition	Characteristic	Associated conditions	Treatment required in the newborn	Reference
Shoulder				
Congenital pseudarthrosis of the clavicle	Painless swelling, predominantly right sided	—	—	48
Congenital absence of the pectoralis musculature (Poland syndrome p. 878)	Absent anterior axillary fold	Absent breast and nipple	—	33
Cleidocranial dysostosis	Absence of part or all of the clavicles	Short stature and soft skull	—	24, 33, 60
Elbow				
Congenital fusion of the elbow	Absent elbow motion	—	—	33, 54
Congenital radioulnar synostoses	Absent forearm rotation	—	—	
Congenital dislocation of the radial head	Decreased elbow flexion or extension	Arthrogryposis, De Lange and Russell–Silver syndrome	—	33
Forearm				
Congenital absence of the radius	Radial club hand (see text)	VATER	+	27, 33
Congenital absence of the ulna	Shortened, ulnarly-bowed forearm	—	+	33
Lobster claw hand	Central cleft in hand	—	—	33
Hand				
Syndactyly	Webbing of the fingers	—	+	33
Acrosyndactyly	Skin web distally	Annular bands	—	33
Macrodactyly	Enlarged digit	—	—	33
Polydactyly	Extra digit	—	+	33
Symphalangism	Stiffness of the proximal interphalangeal joint	—	—	33
Hip and thigh				
Congenital short femur	Shortened thigh	—	—	33
Proximal focal femoral deficiency	Severe shortening of the thigh (Fig. 41.16)	Associated fibular and tibial anomalies (40–60%)	—	3, 33
Calf				
Congenital absence of the fibula (paraxial fibular hemimelia)	Short calf with valgus foot (Fig. 41.17)	Femoral shortening	+	33, 78, 84
Congenital absence of the tibia (paraxial tibial hemimelia)	Shortened calf with varus foot often familial (Fig. 41.18)	Absence of medial rays	+	33, 41
Congenital posterior bow of the tibia	Bowed tibia (Fig. 41.19)	—	—	11, 33, 36
Anterior bow of the tibia (the high risk tibia)	Bowed tibia (Fig. 41.20)	Neurofibromatosis	+	33, 47, 64

which encourage the child to use the extremities away from the body. The use of a sample plastic paddle in a child 6–12 months old is sufficient. Later a padded hook is added, but the child can rarely learn to use a shoulder cable and harness for pinch before 18–24 months.

Congenital absence of the radius (radial club hand)

This may be a partial or, more commonly (50%), a complete longitudinal deficiency. The ulna is usually shortened and curved, the concavity directed toward the radial side, and the hand tends to deviate radially as well. If the deformity remains untreated the hand deviation will increase with growth, and may form an angle of 80% or more with the forearm. The thumb, if present, is usually hypoplastic (80%) and the first metacarpal is absent. The elbow is often limited in extension. The radial nerve is usually absent and the sensory supply is from a normal median and ulnar nerve. A very high percentage (77%) can be expected to have significant abnormalities of other organ systems, particularly those with bilateral involvement. Radial aplasia is a major component of the VATER association (p. 883), which is an acronym to indicate a constellation of congenital anomalies that are frequently associated: Vertebral defects, Anal atresia, Tracheo-oesophageal fistula (with or without oesophageal atresia)

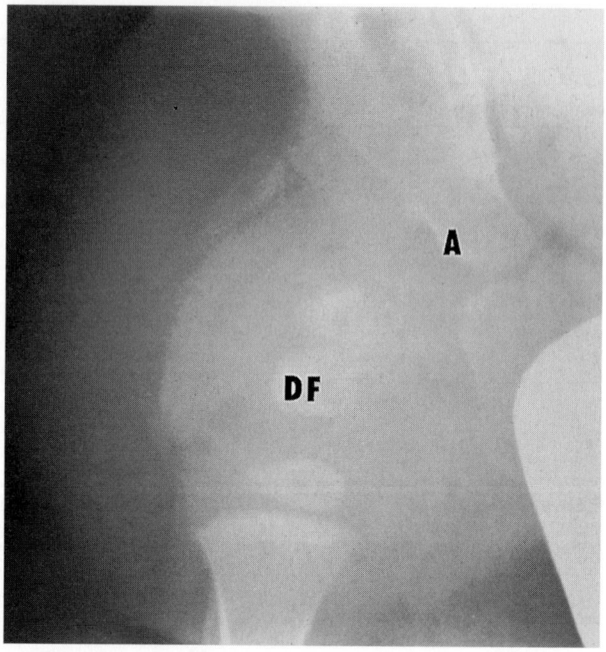

Fig. 41.16 Severe proximal femoral focal deficiency: complete absence of the femur with only the most distal portion present (DF). The acetabulum (A) is poorly developed (dysplastic) suggesting the absence of the femoral head. There may be flexion, abduction and external rotation deformity of the entire thigh. In severe deformity surgical ablation of the foot may be necessary with the fitting of an above-knee prosthesis.

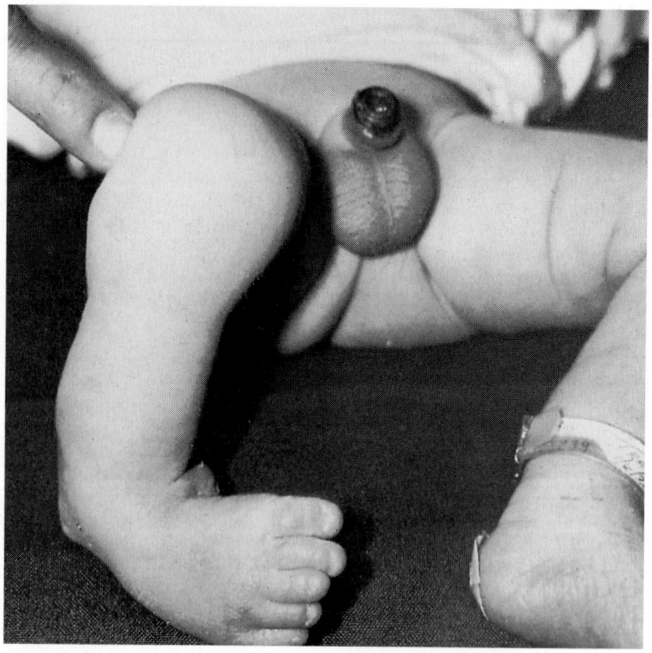

Fig. 41.18 Congenital absence of the tibia. Clinical appearance of a 5-day-old child with absence of the tibia. Note the varus deformity of the foot and the subluxation of the knee. The knee joint is usually unstable. This is a rare anomaly which results in a severe shortening, often associated with flexion contracture of the knee, and absence of one or more medial rays of the foot.

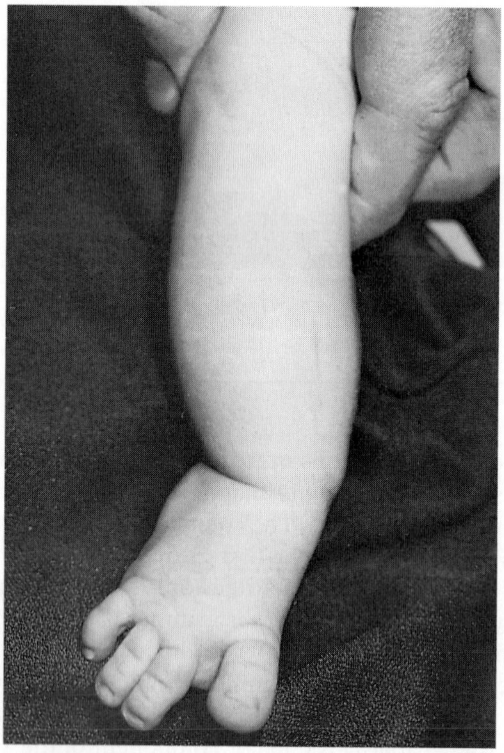

Fig. 41.17 Congenital absence of the fibula. Clinical appearance of the short extremity with valgus attitude of the foot, absence of the lateral ray. The majority of children will have a severe limb length discrepancy, the average being greater than 12 cm at maturity, and a foot deformity which cannot be corrected.

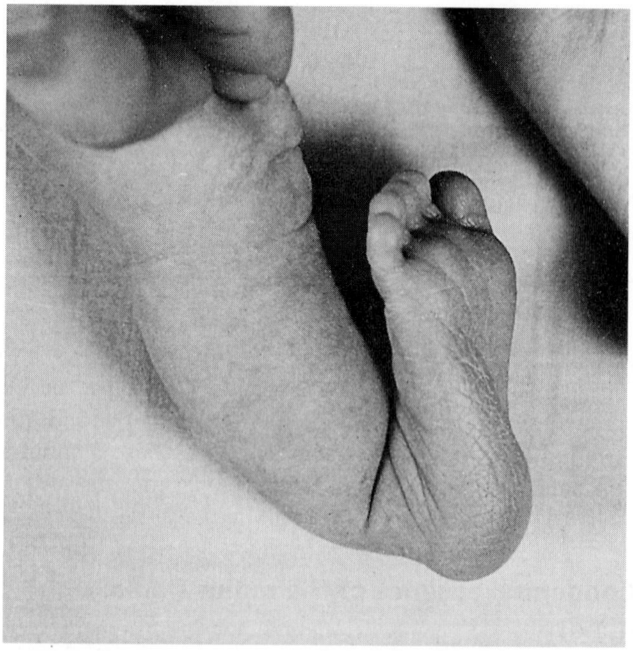

Fig. 41.19 Congenital posterior bow of the tibia. The apex of the bow is directed posteromedially at the junction of the lower and middle thirds of the tibia. The foot is of calcaneovalgus type and can be dorsiflexed to the shin.

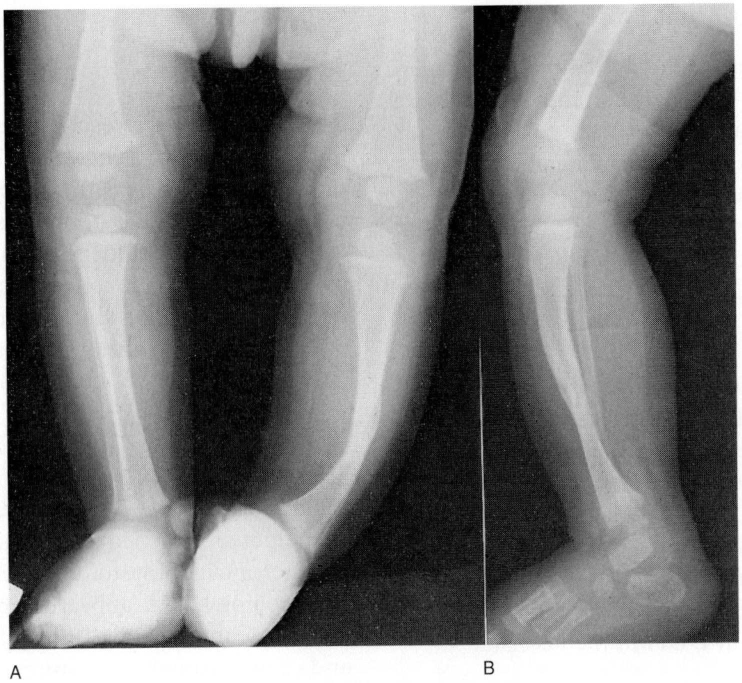

Fig. 41.20 Anterior bow with cyst. (A) Anteroposterior roentgenographic view demonstrating a bowed tibia with a cyst at the junction of the middle and distal thirds. (B) Lateral view. The medullary canal is present but narrowed, with sclerotic changes. A large percentage of these will fracture before 1 or 2 years of age. This child's tibia fractured with minimal trauma shortly after these X-rays were obtained.

and Radial limb dysplasia.[8] The child with radial defects should be carefully evaluated for these other anomalies.

Treatment should begin immediately following birth and is similar to the management of a club foot, with every effort being made to align the radially deviated hand and wrist over the ulna and increase elbow flexion.

Hand and finger deformities

Lobster-claw hand

Congenital cleft of the hand is usually inherited as an autosomal dominant, is frequently bilateral, and may occur in the feet as well. Usually the central ray, the middle or ring finger and their metacarpals are absent; occasionally the index and/or thumb may be absent.

Syndactyly

Webbing of the fingers is the most common congenital anomaly of the hand. Syndactyly may occur as a developmental defect due to arrested fetal development at 7–8 weeks, or as a dominantly inherited deformity. There is a variety of combinations of skin bridges, from very slight, hardly perceptible, to complete involvement extending to the tips of the fingers as an Apert syndrome (pp. 868–869). Syndactyly may be associated with other anomalies, such as Poland syndrome (p. 878), constriction bands, polydactyly, and most often with syndactyly of the feet. If the syndactyly includes a bony fusion or causes distortion of growth such as rotation or an angulation problem, this may worsen unless the fingers are separated early.

Acrosyndactyly

The fingers are fused distal to the skin webs, with a small open slit proximal to the web at the base of the involved digits. The fingers appear as though they have been tied together with a narrow string, and this is usually seen with congenital constriction bands (see Annular bands, p. 1082).

Polydactyly

Duplication anomalies of the fingers are often hereditary and the most common hand anomaly in blacks, and may be accompanied by supernumerary toes. The extra digit may be a simple skin tag or a normally functioning sixth digit. An obviously atrophic floppy remnant should be removed, usually prior to discharge from the nursery. We recommend that this be done surgically, and discourage the older method of ligating it with a suture, as this leaves an unsightly skin tag. If you are unsure about this recommendation, ask the parents. They will often demonstrate a long-term follow-up.

DEFORMITIES OF THE LOWER EXTREMITY

Defects in the femur range from a slight difference in length and an otherwise normal extremity to severe defects such as complete absence of the proximal femur and absent distal parts, usually the fibula and lateral rays of the foot (see Fig. 41.16). Partial absence or severe loss of the femur is usually referred to as proximal focal femoral deficiency. The aetiology is unknown.

Proximal focal femoral deficiency

This is a term used to describe more severe forms of femoral shortening, usually accompanied by a lack of development of part of the proximal femur (Fig. 41.16). Classifications have been developed to aid in prognosis and treatment, but in the neonate exact classification is usually not possible.[33]

The shortening of the thigh is readily apparent at birth and X-rays confirm the diagnosis, although the milder defects may be confused with DDH in the neonate.

Anterior bow of the tibia (the 'high-risk' tibia)

(Fig. 41.20)

Rathgeb et al[64] have classified anterior bow of the tibia into three types: (1) simple anterior bow, (2) anterior bow with cyst at the apex, and (3) pseudarthrosis of the tibia. Although there will be some overlap in radiological appearance, in general the classification represents the progressive increase in the risk of fracture for the infant, which is greatest with pseudarthrosis.

Anterolateral bowing of the tibia with a narrow, sclerotic intramedullary canal or cystic change is an urgent problem and treatment should begin immediately, as fracture and pseudarthrosis usually follow in the weeks following delivery. Unfortunately many patients sustain fracture while awaiting bracing or surgery. A custom-made plastic orthosis should be used to protect the extremity until the child is ready for a standard orthosis or surgery.

Congenital lower extremity amputation

Lower extremity terminal (complete) amputations are often associated with amputation in the other three extremities. In the lower extremity, a prosthesis is fitted when the child is interested in standing. A prosthesis may be fitted earlier in a child with complete amelia so the lower extremities can be utilized for sitting balance.

Failure of formation of parts can be due to either genetic or environmental factors or a combination of both. Most of the transverse amputations may be due to environmental factors such as anoxia, radiation and chemicals. Absent tibia is often familial, and children with this deformity should have a genetic consultation.

SPINE

Torticollis

Torticollis, or wry neck, is a common clinical sign found in a wide variety of childhood illnesses. When torticollis is recognized at or near the time of birth the usual cause is congenital muscular torticollis. However, X-rays of the cervical spine should be obtained to exclude other less common congenital conditions, such as fixed or bony torticollis due to Klippel–Feil syndrome (pp. 876, 1079) and/or injuries and anomalies of the atlantoaxial articulation.[33]

Congenital muscular torticollis

This is usually discovered in the first 4–8 weeks of life. In the infant's neck a non-tender, soft, mobile 'tumour' can be palpated attached to, or located within, the body of the sternocleidomastoid muscle. By 4–6 months of age the swelling has disappeared and the only clinical findings are the contracture of the sternocleidomastoid muscle and the torticollis posture: head tilted towards the involved side and the chin rotated towards the opposite shoulder (Fig. 41.21).

The birth records of these children demonstrate a preponderance of breech or difficult forceps deliveries or primiparous births. A common misconception is that the neck is contused during delivery and the resultant haematoma leads to fibrosis and contracture. However, experimental work suggests that the fibrosis within the muscle is due to oedema and muscle necrosis following

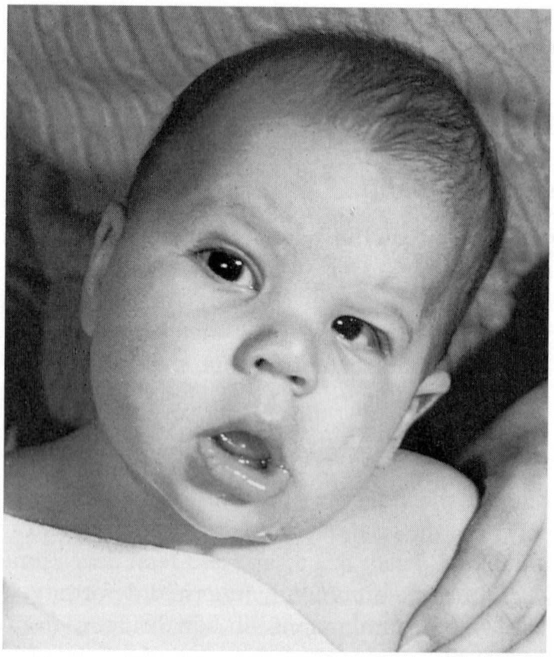

Fig. 41.21 A 6-month-old infant with congenital muscular torticollis. Note the rotation of the skull, asymmetry and flattening of the face and depression adjacent to the left eye on the side of the contracted sternocleidomastoid.

venous occlusion during delivery, from pressure on the neck in the birth canal.[12] Congenital muscular torticollis may represent the sequel of an intrauterine compartment syndrome. Recent MRI evidence suggests that the soft tissue findings in the muscle body of the sternocleidomastoid are similar to those found in compartment syndromes due to ischaemia. Similarly, anatomical studies of the muscle sheath suggest that a compartment syndrome is possible.[19]

The clinical deformity is probably related to the ratio of muscle fibrosis to the remaining viable functional muscle after the initial insult. If sufficient normal muscle is present, it will stretch with growth and the child will not develop the torticollis posture, whereas a severely fibrotic area has little elastic potential. Further support for an intrauterine aetiology comes from two additional factors: three out of four children have lesions on the right side,[46] and up to 20% have DDH.[39]

Sandifer syndrome

Children with torticollis may present in the first several months of life with symptoms of hiatal hernia and gastro-oesophageal reflux. Often, Sandifer syndrome[43] may be associated with violent posturing, body stiffening and apnoea due to reflux and aspiration. In mild forms of this condition torticollis may be the only evident finding. An accurate diagnosis of Sandifer syndrome allows the appropriate therapy for the gastro-oesophageal reflux, which when treated results in disappearance of the torticollis. Usually the diagnosis can be made by upper gastrointestinal studies, although occasionally oesophageal pH monitoring may also be necessary. In children with Sandifer syndrome it is proposed that the associated torticollis may be the result of extreme sensitivity of the oesophagus to the reflux of gastric acid.[83]

Klippel–Feil syndrome

The term Klippel–Feil syndrome describes all individuals with congenital fusion of the cervical vertebrae, whether it be two segments (congenital block vertebrae) or the entire cervical spine. Congenital cervical fusion is the result of failure of the normal segmentation of the cervical somites during the third to eighth weeks of fetal life. The aetiology is as yet undetermined. However, the embryological abnormality is not limited to the cervical spine.

Clinical description

The classic description of the syndrome is a triad: low posterior hairline, short neck and limitation of head and neck motion. Fixed bony deformities frequently prevent proper positioning for radiographs. Overlapping shadows from the mandible, occiput or foramen magnum may obscure the upper cervical vertebrae. Scoliosis and/or kyphosis is the most frequent anomaly found in association with this syndrome.

Children with Klippel–Feil syndrome, even those with minor cervical fusions, may be at risk of having other less apparent but serious defects.[34] One-third may have a significant urinary tract anomaly; hearing loss is common and, less frequently, Klippel–Feil syndrome may be associated with congenital heart disease. There are no symptoms directly attributed to the fused cervical vertebrae. The associated malformations are the major threat to these infants.

Congenital scoliosis

Congenital scoliosis seldom poses a serious problem for the neonate; however, early recognition of a vertebral anomaly is important, as if not controlled they can quickly lead to significant deformities, both cosmetic and life-threatening.[87] In the neonate there may be no visible curvature to suggest a vertebral anomaly. There are, however, other clinical and X-ray findings which should alert the examiner to the possibility of an undetected vertebral anomaly, such as cutaneous abnormalities in the region of the back, dermal sinuses, hairy patches, dimples and haemangiomata, and anomalies of the cervical spine, including bony torticollis, Klippel–Feil anomaly and Sprengel's deformity.[34] Children with congenital problems of the lower extremities, foot deformities and particularly asymmetrical findings such as atrophy and hemihypertrophy, should be suspected of having an underlying vertebral deformity, diastematomyelia, myelodysplasia or sacral agenesis. Children with congenital scoliosis have a 20% frequency of kidney and bladder malformations, and a 15% frequency of heart defects. Urological evaluation should be routine for all children who have vertebral anomalies.[49] It has been found that ultrasonography offers a non-invasive way to screen adequately for the anomalies associated with Klippel–Feil syndrome.[21] Careful follow-up is essential for all cases, and progression requires surgery at any age.[86]

Congenital kyphosis

Congenital kyphosis is often more progressive than congenital scoliosis, leading to severe deformity early in life. The most common site of kyphosis is at the thoracolumbar junction, between T10 and L2. Congenital kyphosis is caused by the same embryological mechanism as congenital scoliosis:

- Failure of formation, with complete or partial absence of the anterior portion of the vertebral body;[33]
- Failure of segmentation, with anterior fusion of vertebral bodies.

Progressive and severe deformity occurs because of one or more of the following mechanisms:

- Absence of growth anteriorly;
- Mechanical collapse;
- Anterior tethering;
- Continued growth of the posterior elements.

Steady progression can be expected as the child grows, particularly when sitting, and this is accentuated with standing and walking.[88] Initially the deformity is painless. Later, neurological problems and even complete paraplegia can result if the kyphosis is allowed to progress.[88] Compression of the spinal cord or cauda equina has been reported in 25% of the published cases.[76]

Posterior surgical stabilization prior to severe deformity may be required as early as 3–6 months of age, particularly in infants with an absent vertebral body.

Diastematomyelia

Diastematomyelia is an uncommon congenital disturbance of the vertebral architecture, in which the neural elements, the spinal cord or the intraspinal nerve roots, are split into two columns by a midline mass in the spinal canal, fixed anteriorly to the vertebral body. The mass may be an osseous or cartilaginous spicule or a fibrous septum, partially or completely dividing the neural canal. Diastematomyelia may be localized at one vertebral level or extend over several segments, and is commonly found in the lumbar region. It is presumed that the clinical consequences are due to the 'tethering' effect of the diastematomyelia on the normal ascent of the spinal cord. It may act as a 'checkrein' to upward migration of the neural elements, and possibly cause progressive neurological deficit in the lower extremities. It should be emphasized that the greatest change occurs in the last 6 months of intrauterine skeletal growth. Differential growth during childhood is slower, with more time for adaptive changes in the spinal cord and nerve roots.

The majority of patients have a cutaneous abnormality in the midline of the back, which serves as an important clue to the diagnosis. This may be a patch of hair, a discrete dimple, a subcutaneous fatty tumor, pigmented naevi or a haemangioma.[33] Association with a dermal sinus is rare but important, and must be carefully searched for as it may represent a portal of entry of bacteria into the spinal canal. The orifice may be quite discrete and innocuous in its appearance, yet lead to abscess formation and meningitis or a frank neurocutaneous fistula. Similarly, incidental discovery of such a defect should raise suspicion of a diastematomyelia.

Lumbosacral agenesis

The degree of disability with this malformation is dependent on the level of the vertebral lesion. Those with a partial sacral or coccygeal agenesis may be asymptomatic. In contrast, the patient with lumbar or complete sacral agenesis is severely deformed.

The aetiology of this malformation has not been completely delineated. Clinically a large percentage of children afflicted with this condition are offspring of diabetic mothers or have a strong family history of diabetes, and Duraiswami[22] induced rumplessness in developing chicks by injecting insulin into the egg.

If there is complete absence of the sacrum the posture of the lower extremities has been likened to a 'sitting Buddha', with flexion–abduction contractures of the hips, knees flexed at 60° with popliteal webbing, and the feet tucked under the buttocks in equinovarus. Inspection of the back reveals a bony prominence, which is the last vertebral segment, and often excessive mobility between it and the pelvis. The buttocks are narrowed and compressed, with dimpling 4–6 cm lateral to the gluteal cleft. The anus is patulous and horizontal. When the patient sits unsupported, the pelvis rolls up under the thorax. Flexion– extension may occur at the junction of the spine and pelvis rather than the hips. Walking is not possible.

The neurological deficit is one of the most unusual features of this condition. Motor paralysis is profound, with no voluntary, involuntary or reflex activity, and anatomically corresponds within one level to what might be expected from the vertebral loss. In contrast, the sensory disturbance does not parallel the motor or vertebral lesion. Even the most severely involved patients have sensation to the knees and spotty hypaesthesia distally. Trophic ulceration of the feet is quite uncommon, suggesting at least protective sensation. Unfortunately, bladder incontinence is a consistent feature in even the relatively minor hemisacral defect, but the mechanism is not the same in each patient. There are no clinical or radiological findings that provide a reliable guide to identifying the variable patterns of urinary function. Perineal sensation is preserved in almost all patients.

With the low-level lesions the foot and leg deformities are similar to those found in the patient with a resistant club foot. It is not unusual for these children to be misdiagnosed for several years, or until the problems of toilet training call attention to the sacral anomalies.

Scoliosis, hemivertebrae, spina bifida and meningocoele are commonly associated spinal anomalies. Visceral anomalies have been reported in about 35% of patients, and are usually confined to the anogenital region. Imperforate anus is the most common, but urinary tract problems occur, with bladder dysfunction, hydronephrosis, vesicoureteric reflux and diverticula, fused or absent kidneys, exstrophy and hyposadias.

Treatment

If the sacropelvic ring is intact the patient will generally have a stable spinopelvic junction and should learn to walk with minimal or no brace support. Deformities of the feet and legs, particularly severe resistant club foot, require early and vigorous correction. Surgical release may be necessary if conservative measures fail. An important part of the management of these children is the treatment of their urinary abnormalities.

EXSTROPHY OF THE BLADDER

Bladder exstrophy is an uncommon anomaly which includes failure of anterior closure of the bladder, with the mucosal surface remaining exposed on the abdomen. It represents a very challenging reconstructive problem for the urological surgeon. Orthopaedically, the pubic bones are widely separated and the two halves of the pelvis, along with the acetabulae and the femoral heads, are externally rotated. If orthopaedically untreated, the gait is broad-based, especially in the young child. This skeletal anomaly usually causes little long-term orthopaedic disability. However, it is often necessary to osteotomize the ilium to facilitate soft tissue repair of the exstrophy.[51] This allows the two halves of the pelvis to be manipulated into a more normal relationship anteriorly and reduces the tension on the repair of the abdominal wall and bladder. The exact site of the osteotomy and its postoperative fixation has not been resolved.[69]

FRACTURES IN NEONATES

LONG BONES

Fractures usually occur at the time of delivery and are either epiphyseal separations, particularly of the humerus or femur, or midshaft fractures of long bones. Studies suggest that fractures are uncommon, occurring in less than 1% of newborn infants.[52] The vast majority are clavicular, and are often only recognized when callus is palpable. Similarly, many epiphyseal separations are only slightly displaced and thus may be undetected for long periods. Traumatic fracture separation of the upper femoral epiphysis often presents as a pseudodislocation of the hip. This fracture may not be recognized until after the development of the inflammatory phase of healing, and if previously untreated may be mistaken for an infection.[77] In contrast, midshaft fractures of the long bones are generally recognized immediately, often by the obstetrician at the precise moment they occur.

As might be expected, injury to a bone or joint occurs more often with complicated obstetrical procedures, big babies or breech deliveries, and is rare in routine deliveries.[52] Injury is more common with firstborns, but with the exception of the clavicular injuries the mother seldom has a narrow pelvis and relatively few (14%) of the children are premature.

Clinically the child has a tender, swollen extremity, often noted the day following delivery. The fractured extremity hangs limply and the child avoids voluntary movement of the limb (pseudoparalysis). Swelling may be extensive, the soft tissues are tense, the skin erythematous, and the child may have a low-grade fever. The clinical and radiographic appearances are similar to a bone or joint infection, and the two problems are often confused, particularly in the child with an epiphyseal separation. An ultrasound or arthrogram of the joint can be helpful in differentiating the two conditions. Fractures in the newborn respond to simple splinting and heal quickly: problems can occur with overtreatment. Fractures of the humerus are easily treated with a long-sleeved shirt, pinning the sleeve to the chest.[33] Femur fractures usually require a spica cast for 2–3 weeks. Clavicular fractures require no treatment.

CERVICAL SPINE INJURIES IN THE NEONATE

Cervical injury would appear to be uncommon, or at least not commonly recognized, and occurs at two levels, at the C1–2 articulation and at C6–7 or C7–T1. However, there is seldom X-ray evidence of a bony injury. The vertebral elements of a neonatal spine are more elastic than the spinal cord itself.

The newborn spine can stretch 5 cm without bony disruption, but the spinal cord only stretches by 6–8 mm.[81] Stretching can therefore cause a complete transection of the spinal cord without X-ray evidence of bony disruption. Consequently, if a dislocation or fracture of the cervical vertebrae is discovered, it suggests a severe transection-type injury to the spinal cord. C1–2 injuries are more common following cephalic delivery and are believed to be due to excessive rotational forces, whereas C6–T1 injury more often follows breech delivery with excessive traction (Fig. 41.22).

Following a spinal cord injury the infant has a period of 'spinal shock' – hyporeflexia, hypotonia and hypoventilation. There may be an Erb's palsy and paralysis of the diaphragm. Later, if the external muscles of respiration remain paralysed, the child will develop a bell-shaped chest. If an early myelogram is performed it usually demonstrates a subarachnoid block due to haemorrhage; however, laminectomy and decompression of the cord have not been helpful. Later, localized cord atrophy may be identified. Recently, magnetic resonance imaging has provided an excellent means of diagnosing and defining a suspected cervical spinal cord injury, with a relatively low risk.[45] If a fracture occurs it is usually through the epiphyseal plate of the vertebral body, and simple positioning in extension usually achieves anatomical reduction of the bony elements and rapid healing of the fracture. Most survivors have some degree of paraparesis or quadriparesis.

The 'flying fetus' (also called the 'star-gazing fetus' or 'fetal opisthotonus') is frequently associated with cervical spinal cord injury. The distinguishing feature is intrauterine hyperextension of the fetal cervical spine, which may be so marked that the occiput is at the level of the 11th thoracic vertebra. Approximately 70 cases have been

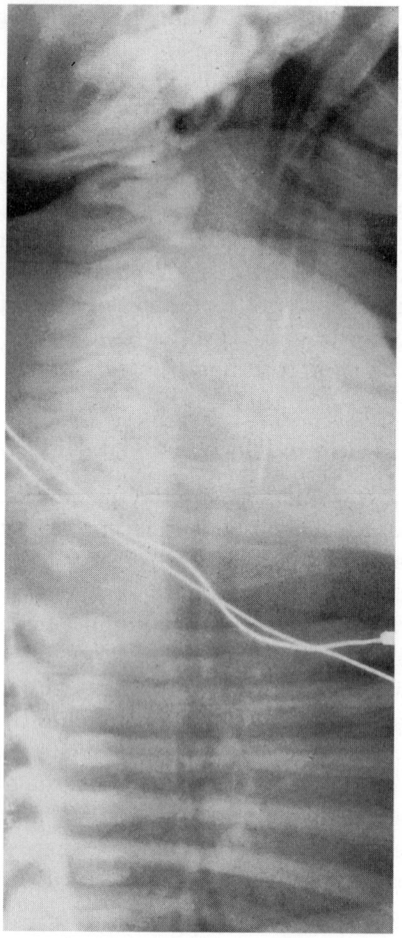

Fig. 41.22 This newborn sustained an upper thoracic spinal cord disruption during a difficult breech delivery. Upper cervical injuries are more often found following cephalic delivery.

reported[1,9] and current estimates are that 25% of fetuses with these features, delivered vaginally, will have a significant cord injury.[1] However, spinal cord injury has been reported in a case delivered by caesarean section.[53] The hyperextension posture may persist for 1–2 months after delivery.

OCCULT CERVICAL INJURIES

Autopsy studies of newborns dying within the first week of life suggest that the incidence of spinal injury is more common than clinically appreciated. Routine autopsies of neonatal deaths indicate only a 1% prevalence of spinal cord damage, whereas autopsies done specifically to search for this problem suggest a much higher prevalence, with haemorrhage in joint capsules, torn ligaments and dura and extensive bruising or bleeding in the spinal cord and nerves. Complete destruction of the cord is uncommon.[42,80,91]

This evidence suggests a significant incidence of occult cervical trauma in survivors, with clinical findings at birth ranging from mild respiratory depression to complete areflexia and hypotonia, and normal spine X-rays. Allen,[4] who reviewed 31 children initially classified as having infantile spinal muscular atrophy (Werdnig–Hoffmann disease) or amyotonia congenita, reported that 58% had a clinically non-progressive, non-familial neurological disorder which could have been due to spinal cord trauma at the time of birth.

GANGRENE OF THE NEWBORN

About 50% of children with this uncommon condition present in the first day of life. There are a variety of causes,[33] and knowledge of the exact sequence of events that precede the development of gangrene is helpful in determining the aetiology and treatment. In approximately two-thirds of cases a single major vessel in the extremity appears to have been involved.

It is important to distinguish gangrene of the newborn from necrotizing fasciitis (p. 1152) of the newborn, a much more virulent condition with rapidly developing sepsis and tissue destruction. The latter is associated with a high mortality rate and demands an entirely different course of treatment from gangrene, including prompt and vigorous supportive measures and surgical debridement. If the obstructed artery is of sufficient size and the problem recognized quickly, then embolectomy or thrombectomy may be considered, and has been successful. Otherwise the initial treatment is supportive, with adequate hydration, maintaining an aseptic environment for the extremity, preventing infection (or controlling it if it occurs) and surgical drainage if an abscess develops. As a general rule it is better to let the area demarcate rather than attempt early surgical debridement. Usually this results in a considerably smaller loss of tissue than first anticipated (p. 923).

CONGENITAL ANNULAR BANDS

Congenital annular constricting bands of the extremities are rare but regularly accompanied by other orthopaedic anomalies, including congenital amputation (Fig. 41.23), distal syndactyly and club foot. Torpin and Faulkner[79] reported on the dissection of 14 placentae and documented the origin of the amniotic bands in these patients.

Although the amnion may rupture with the loss of amniotic fluid, the chorion remains intact. The amnion may form bands that are free-floating and may encircle extremities, the umbilical cord or even the neck. The band may extend through the fascia and as far as bone. Depending on the depth of the band, there may be oedema and enlargement of the distal portion. Syndactyly of the fingers is common, and it appears as if the fingers have been tied together at their tips with an open space between them proximal to the distal syndactyly (acrosyndactyly). Club foot occurs in approximately 50% of these children and may be bilateral.[16] Autoamputation

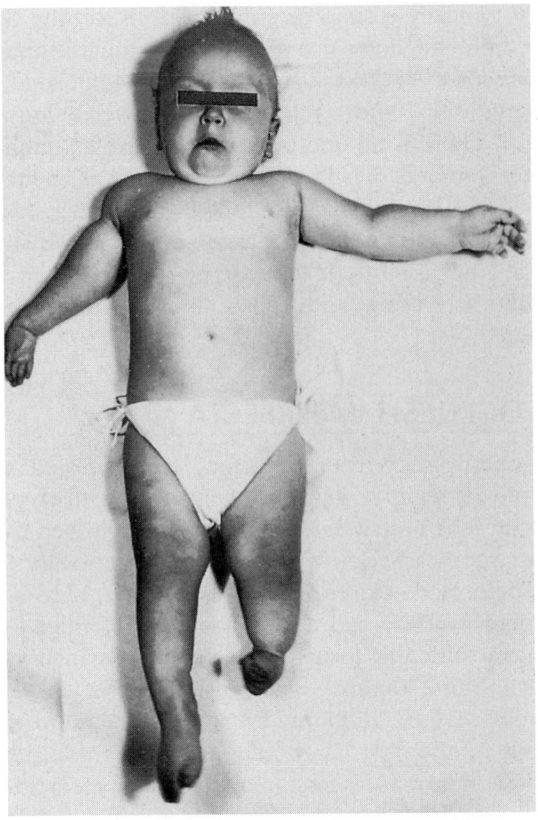

Fig. 41.23 Infant with multiple congenital annular bands. Clinical appearance of the bands in the mid-portion of the right arm and distal portions of both lower extremities.

of fingers and toes is common, but it can be an entire arm or leg. It is not unusual to have bilateral loss.

Shallow grooves seldom require either immediate or late treatment. Early release may be required in the infant who has a lymphatic obstruction or neurovascular complication distal to a deep band; attempted release is preferable even in small digits, rather than allowing the part to go on to amputation. Excision must be performed down to and including the fascia, and to normal skin on either side. Surgical correction of distal syndactyly is indicated in early childhood to improve the function of the digits and to prevent further deformity with growth. Treatment of club foot should be begun immediately after birth.

ARTHROGRYPOSIS

Arthrogryposis multiplex congenita (multiple congenital curved joints) is a syndrome that probably encompasses several different conditions.

This disorder is non-progressive and the aetiology is unclear, but it may be caused by any of a number of conditions that restrict fetal joint motion and lead to stiff, contracted extremities, such as oligohydramnios. One form may be due to an intrauterine infection, probably viral, causing failure of development or deterioration of the anterior horn cells, with resultant loss of muscle tone and mobility, leading by the time of birth to chronically immobile stiff joints with muscle fibrosis and atrophy. There may be a primary myogenic type of arthrogryposis which is autosomally inherited as a non-progressive form of congenital muscular dystrophy.[90] Arthrogryposis has been associated with other conditions such as tuberous sclerosis, neurofibromatosis (p. 884), myelodysplasia (p. 1302) and sacral agenesis (p. 1080). The differential diagnosis includes Larsen syndrome (p. 882), congenital contractual arachnodactyly (p. 882), Marfan syndrome (p. 877) and trisomy 18 (p. 860).

Children with arthrogryposis may be born in the breech position secondary to the intrauterine contractures. The antenatal history may reveal a relatively inactive fetus. They may also have fractures of the thin spindly bones, especially in the leg.

Examination of the newborn is striking, in that there are multiple rigid deformities that are usually bilateral but always symmetrical. The characteristic posture is adduction and internal rotation of the upper extremities, and stiff 'diamond-shaped' lower extremities (Fig. 41.24).

The condition may, however, be limited to the upper extremities, the lower extremities, or occur in all four. The extremities are rather featureless as there are few

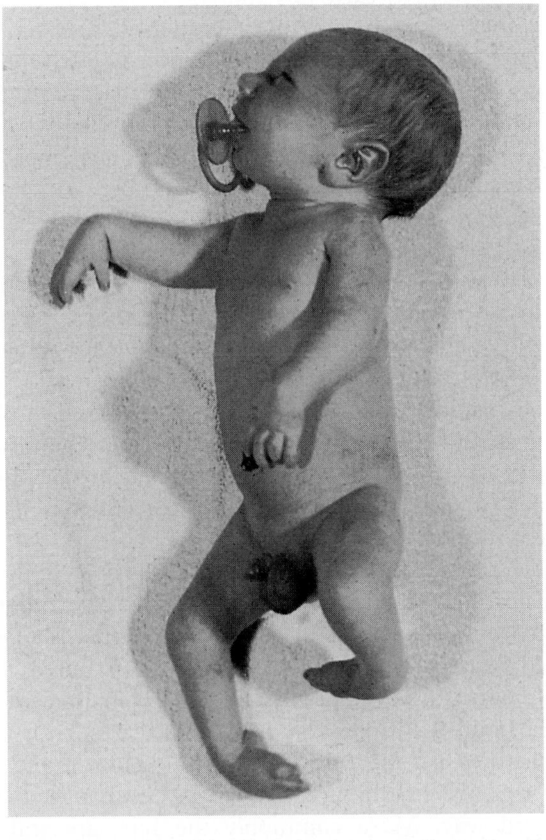

Fig. 41.24 A 5-day-old child with arthrogryposis, illustrating the diamond-shaped extremities and equinovarus deformity of the feet. The flexion deformity of the wrists and absent skin creases (featureless joints) are evident.

joint skin creases, and there may be soft-tissue webbing on the flexion side of the immobile joints. The skin is thin and smooth and the subcutaneous tissue is scanty. There is striking muscle atrophy proximal and distal to the stiff joints, especially in the lower extremities, and the joints may appear enlarged. Radiographically there is an increase in the angle of the proximal carpal row that is opposite to the decrease in the carpal angle described for Turner syndrome.[62] Otherwise, the radiographic findings are not diagnostic and serve only to confirm the clinical condition. Similarly, there are no diagnostic laboratory studies.

These children have normal sensation and potential for normal intelligence, and good general health. The majority (85%) will be able to walk and be independent with bowel and bladder control.[33]

TREATMENT

In the newborn period the management is directed towards both the deformity and the muscle weakness. Early correction is encouraged via vigorous physical therapy and stretching casts. Care should be taken to avoid undue force, as the bones are thin and fracture easily.

The elbows may be fixed in either flexion or extension. If fixed in flexion, early physiotherapy and splinting may be all that is required. More commonly, however, they are fixed in extension and, in addition to early physiotherapy and splinting, may require muscle transfers in later childhood to provide elbow flexion. The wrist and hand are usually severely involved, but most are surprisingly functional in later life.

The foot is commonly involved, usually in a rigid equinovarus deformity, but congenital vertical talus ('rocker bottom' foot) is not uncommon. Treatment should be initiated as early in the newborn period as possible, including early vigorous adhesive strapping and regular stretching exercises.

The majority will require surgical treatment and the family should be aware that in severe cases the feet will need to be braced or otherwise splinted throughout the growing years, to maintain satisfactory alignment and prevent recurrence.

The knees are usually stiff in extension or hyperextension and, rarely, in flexion.[20] Early physiotherapy, assisted by splints, casts or adhesive strapping, should be started, but surgical treatment may be required if the knee motion fails to improve with conservative treatment.

The hip deformities are of two types, soft-tissue contractures and dislocations. Dislocated hips in the child who is only mildly involved may be managed in a standard way. More commonly the hips are stiff and dislocated, with advanced adaptive changes (teratologic) similar to those found in the older child with DDH. In this situation the dislocation is best left untreated, as surgery typically results in stiff hips.[20] Recently, Staheli has recommended the use of a medial adductor approach for reduction of the dislocated hips associated with arthrogryposis, and reported improved long-term results.[75] There is no question that the stable relationship between femoral head and acetabulum is better for ambulation, but this must be balanced against the potential for stiffness and limitation of motion. If surgical reduction is performed, it must be accomplished when the child is young and the soft tissues are not yet contracted.

OSTEOGENESIS IMPERFECTA (p. 1006)

Osteogenesis imperfecta congenita is manifested at the time of birth and may be confused with types of dwarfism. The individuals appear as short-limbed dwarfs, with a large head relative to the trunk, secondary to the short deformed extremities. Most have blue sclera, prominent eyeballs and a depressed nasal bridge. There are several different forms of this disease, which vary in severity. Some infants with osteogenesis imperfecta congenita may be stillborn, or not survive more than a few days or months. They may die from the trauma of birth, secondary to intracranial haemorrhage and fracture. Osteogenesis imperfecta is not a difficult diagnosis to make in the newborn period, as it is one of the few disorders that manifests itself at birth with multiple fractures and generalized osteoporosis. The orthopaedic management of those infants who survive is splinting the extremities for pain relief and to prevent deformity and contracture, and yet maintaining as much motion as possible to prevent further osteoporosis.[33]

IDIOPATHIC FIBROSIS OF MUSCLE

This is a problem which may be identified in infancy, but only rarely in the neonate. The presentation is usually the progressive and insidious development of contractures of the deltoid, triceps, gluteal and quadriceps muscles. This is believed to represent fibrosis secondary to intramuscular injection (p. 930), as nearly all the children have a history of neonatal illness and many a history of injection into the muscle involved. The most frequently involved muscles are in areas where an intramuscular injection might be expected to have been administered. Pathologically the fibrosis is similar to that associated with sternocleidomastoid contracture in congenital muscular torticollis. To date, treatment has been distal (tendinous) surgical release later in childhood.

CONGENITAL HEMIHYPERTROPHY

Asymmetry of the extremities – hemihypertrophy or hemiatrophy – is an occasional neonatal finding. Depending on the degree of involvement the problem may not be recognized for several months, particularly idiopathic congenital hypertrophy, as the extremities are normal in every respect except for a subtle difference in length and girth. However, all cases should have a thorough investigation to seek an underlying cause such as neurofibromatosis (p. 884), Wilms' tumour (p. 1057), haemangiomata and lymphangiomata. Pathological thinness – hemiatrophy – is less common and usually associated with a neurological problem, such as diastematomyelia or sacral agenesis (see above). Some children may have partial enlargement of, for example, just the foot or below the knee, whereas others have complete hemihypertrophy, with the entire lower extremity, abdomen, chest, upper extremity and face involved. The skin may be thicker on one side, there may be different amounts of hair, teeth may appear at different ages, the pupils may vary in size, as well as hypertrophy of all supporting structures, bones, blood vessels and nerves. In congenital hemihypertrophy the percentage of difference can be expected to remain constant with growth.

KLIPPEL–TRENAUNAY SYNDROME

Klippel–Trenaunay syndrome is a combination of varicose veins, soft tissue and bony hypertrophy, together with cutaneous haemangiomata of the extremities. It is unilateral in more than 90% of cases and is more common in the lower extremity. There is almost invariably overgrowth of the extremity secondary to increased blood supply. Thus the degree of asymmetry will increase during growth. Arteriovenous fistulae are multiple and not localized to any portion of the extremity, which is typically warm with many dilated superficial veins and cutaneous haemangiomata. Cardiac enlargement due to high-output cardiac failure may occur in infancy.

CONGENITAL MULTIPLE AND GENERALIZED FIBROMATOSIS

Congenital multiple fibromatosis is a rare condition recognized in the perinatal period in which benign fibrous tumours involve, to a varying degree, the subcutaneous tissues, muscle, viscera and bones. These histological benign lesions grow for varying periods of time after birth. If the viscera are involved to a great extent – congenital generalized fibromatosis – the result is death within the first 4 months of life in 80%. If there is no visceral involvement the lesions stabilize or regress by 3–4 months of age and the child seems to have a normal life expectancy. When bone is involved there are multiple well-circumscribed lytic lesions with sclerotic borders similar to histiocytosis disease. Neurofibromatosis and metastatic neuroblastoma should be considered in the differential diagnosis. Pathological fractures through the areas of involved bone have been treated similarly to traumatic fractures, with good results.

NERVE INJURIES

BRACHIAL PLEXUS INJURY IN THE NEWBORN

These injuries are due to traction on the brachial plexus during delivery. The usual mechanism is distraction of the upper extremity away from the head and neck and stretching the nerve roots as they exit from the cervical spine. The delivery is often prolonged or traumatic and the infant large.[2]

During a cephalic presentation, following delivery of the head, shoulder dystocia may develop, resulting in inadvertent traction injury to the brachial plexus. The majority of brachial plexus injuries arise in this way. In a breech presentation the problem is more likely to be due to cephalopelvic disproportion, with traction on the infant's trunk in an attempt to deliver the head. Improvements in obstetric care have reduced the prevalence of brachial plexus injury this century from 1.56 to 0.38 per 1000 livebirths, but there has been no significant change in the last decade.[5] The injuries are divided into three types:

- Erb's palsy: the C5–6 lesion with denervation of the deltoid, supraspinatus, biceps and brachioradialis;
- Klumpke: C8–T1 lesion, denervation of the intrinsics of the hand, flexors of the wrist and fingers and sympathetics (Horner's syndrome), typically associated with hyperabduction of the shoulder and arm;
- Erb–Duchenne–Klumpke, or a combined lesion involving the entire arm. Paralysis of the diaphragm may be expected in those injuries that are high enough to involve the C4 nerve root.

The infant holds the arm loosely at the side of the thorax; the entire arm is internally rotated at the shoulder, with extension at the elbow, pronation of the forearm and flexion at the wrist ('headwaiter's tip' position) (Fig. 41.25). The Moro reflex is diminished on the involved side. If the lesion is the T1 (Klumpke) type the wrist and finger flexors are involved, with a claw-hand deformity. Swelling may be found in the region of the shoulder and supraclavicular fossa. The clavicle may be fractured. Initially there will be a full passive range of motion, but no active motion will be detected in the denervated areas.

The differential diagnosis includes fracture of the clavicle or proximal humerus, which usually results in limitation of passive motion due to pain and crepitance. The appearance of the upper extremity is similar in infants with arthrogryposis, but in the latter the passive motion of the joints will be limited and both upper and lower extremities are usually involved. Erb's palsy may be confused with an injury to the cervical spine, and the two may coexist.

The primary goal is to avoid contractures of the involved joints by preserving a full range of passive motion.[5,31] The importance of maintaining normal joint

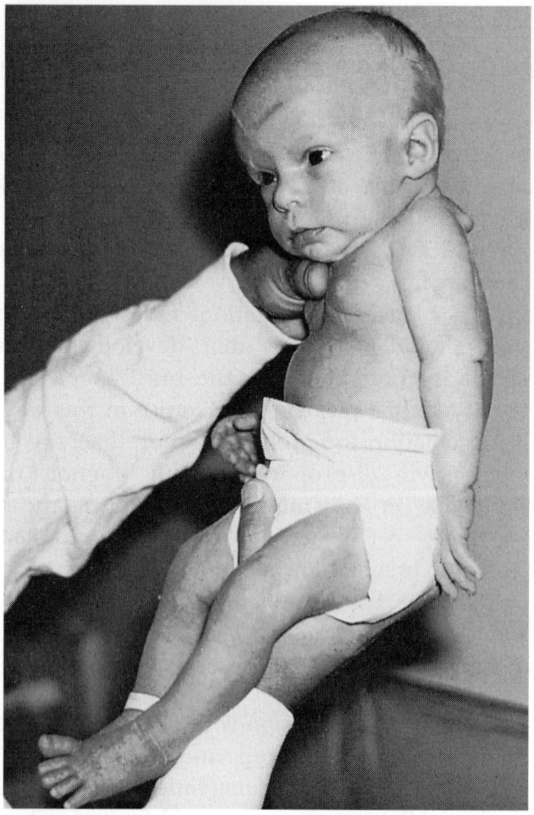

Fig. 41.25 A newborn baby showing a left-sided Erb's palsy with the left arm hanging at his side with the hand in the headwaiter's tip position.

motion must be emphasized to the parent: if there is neurological recovery the reinnervated musculature will require supple joints, and if there is no recovery prevention of contractures will allow a greater latitude in the choice of reconstructive procedures.

The majority of neurological recovery is within the first 6 months, commonly within the first month, but may extend to 18 months.[2,5] Less than 20% obtain full neurological return,[2] although in most the functional outcome is good. Reconstructive procedures can be considered prior to school age, when the child can cooperate with an accurate assessment of the remaining functional muscles.[37]

SCIATIC NERVE INJURIES (p. 921)

Sciatic nerve injury occurs in two ways:

- Direct injection of medication intramuscularly near the nerve: this complication is less frequent because of changes in injection techniques;[18,26]
- Indirectly by parenteral administration of agents through the umbilical vessels, particularly the umbilical artery.[68]

In direct injury there is an immediate loss of motor and sensory function of the nerve, with both local and referred pain.[26] The child is unable actively to dorsiflex (foot drop) and evert the foot,[68] and has anaesthesia of the foot and lateral aspect of the leg. The area of injection is locally tender and a firm mass (granuloma) may be palpable in the buttock. Recovery may occur in 6 weeks to 18 months (in some cases as long as 3 years), but only one-third recover completely.[26]

Indirect injury is the result of material injected into the umbilical artery shortly after birth (p. 258). This can then pass down the internal iliac (usually the left) and enter the inferior gluteal or superior gluteal artery and cause thrombosis. The baby is usually debilitated and hypotensive at the time of the injury, which increases the risk of vascular thrombosis. There may be a firm, non-mobile mass in the left upper buttock consisting of fat necrosis and early calcification. Circulatory changes may be evident, with purple, mottled discoloration over the affected parts, and induration, ulceration and sloughing of the skin. In some cases thrombosis of the common iliac artery, with loss of the inferior mesenteric vessels causing gangrene and perforation of the sigmoid colon, may occur.[68] Nerve involvement has varied from mild paresis to complete flaccidity. Recovery is good if paralysis is initially incomplete, or if improvement occurs within a few days, but such improvement is rare.[70]

REFERENCES

1. Abroms I F, Fresnan M J, Zuckerman J E, Fischer E G, Strand R 1973 Cervical cord injuries secondary to hyperextension of the head in breech presentations. Obstetrics and Gynecology 41: 369–378
2. Adler J B, Patterson R L 1967 Erb's palsy: long-term results of treatment in 88 cases. Journal of Bone and Joint Surgery 49A: 1052–1064
3. Aitken G T 1969 Proximal femoral focal deficiency – definition, classification and management. In: Aitken G T (ed) Proximal femoral focal deficiency: a congenital anomaly. Symposium held in Washington, June 13, 1968. National Academy of Sciences, Washington, pp 1–22
4. Allen J P 1970 Birth injury to the spinal cord. Northwest Medicine 69: 323–326
5. Aston Jr J W 1977 Brachial plexus birth palsy. Orthopaedics 2: 594–601
6. Barlow T G 1962 Early diagnosis and treatment of congenital dislocation of the hip. Journal of Bone and Joint Surgery 44B: 292–301
7. Barlow T G 1966 Congenital dislocation of the hip in the newborn. Proceedings of the Royal Society of Medicine 59: 1103–1108
8. Beals R K, Rolfe B 1989 Current concepts review: VATER association. Journal of Bone Joint Surgery 71A: 948–950
9. Bhagwanani S G, Price H V, Laurence K M, Cinz B 1973 Risks and prevention of cervical cord injury in the management of breech presentation with hyperextension of the fetal head. American Journal of Obstetrics and Gynecology 115: 459–1161
10. Bleck E E 1983 Metatarsus adductus: classification and relationship to outcomes of treatment. Journal of Pediatric Orthopedics 3: 2–9
11. Bray C B, Follows J W 1975 Congenital posterior angulation of tibia and fibula. Southern Medical Journal 68: 292–296
12. Brooks B 1922 Pathological changes in muscle as a result of disturbances of circulation. Archives of Surgery 5: 188–216
13. Clarke N M P: 1986 Sonographic clarification of the·problems of neonatal hip instability. Journal of Pediatric Orthopedics 6: 527–532
14. Coleman S S 1956 Diagnosis of congenital dysplasia of the hip in the newborn infant. Journal of the American Medical Association 162: 548–554
15. Coleman S S 1965 Treatment of congenital dislocation of the hip in the infant. Journal of Bone and Joint Surgery 47A: 590–601
16. Cowell H R, Hensinger R N 1976 The relationship of club foot to

congenital annular bands. In: Batemann J E (ed) Foot science. W B Saunders, Philadelphia, pp 41–46
17. Curtis B H, Fisher, R L 1969 Congenital hyperextension with anterior subluxation of the knee. Journal of Bone and Joint Surgery 51A: 255–269
18. Curtiss P H Jr 1960 Sciatic palsy in premature infants. Journal of the American Medical Association 17: 1586–1588
19. Davids J R, Wenger D R, Mubarak S J 1993 Congenital muscular torticollis: sequela of intrauterine or perinatal compartment syndrome. Journal of Pediatric Orthopedics 13: 141–147
20. Drachman D C 1971 The syndrome of arthrogryposis multiplex congenita. Birth Defects: Original Article Series 7: 90–97
21. Drvaric D M, Ruderman R J, Conrad R W et al 1987 Congenital scoliosis and urinary tract abnormalities: are intravenous pyelograms necessary? Journal of Pediatric Orthopedics 7: 441
22. Duraiswami P K 1952 Experimental causation of congenital skeletal defects and its significance in orthopaedic surgery. Journal of Bone and Joint Surgery 34B: 646–698
23. Fabry J, MacEwen, G D, Shands A R Jr 1973 Torsion of the femur. The follow-up study in normal and abnormal conditions. Journal of Bone and Joint Surgery 55A: 1726–1738
24. Fairbanks T A H 1949 Cranio-cleido-dysostosis. Journal of Bone and Joint Surgery 31B: 608–617
25. Fredensborg N 1976 The results of early treatment of typical congenital dislocation of the hip in Malmo. Journal of Bone and Joint Surgery 58B: 272–278
26. Gilles F H, French J H 1969 Postinjection sciatic nerve palsies in infants and children. Journal of Pediatrics 68: 195–204
27. Goldberg M J, Meyn M 1976 The radial club hand. Orthopedic Clinics of North America 7: 341–353
28. Graf R 1983 New possibilities of the diagnosis of congenital hip joint dislocation by ultrasonography. Journal of Pediatric Orthopaedics 3: 354–359
29. Graf R 1984 Fundamentals of sonographic diagnosis of infant hip dysplasia. Journal of Pediatric Orthopedics 4: 735–740.
30. Harcke H T, Grissom L E 1990 Performing dynamic sonography of the infant hip. American Journal of Radiology 155: 837–844
31. Hensinger R N 1977 Orthopedic problems to the shoulder and neck. Pediatric Clinics of North America 4: 889–902
32. Hensinger R N 1979 Congenital dislocation of the hip. CIBA Clinical Symposium Vol. 31 No. 1
33. Hensinger R N, Jones E T 1981 Neonatal Orthopedics. Grune & Stratton, New York
34. Hensinger R N, Lang J R, MacEwen G D 1974 The Klippel–Feil syndrome: a constellation of related anomalies. Journal of Bone and Joint Surgery 56A: 1246–1253
35. Hernandez R J U, Cornell R G, Hensinger R N 1994 Ultrasound diagnosis of neonatal congenital dislocation of the hip. A decision analysis assessment. Journal of Bone and Joint Surgery 76: 539–543
36. Heyman C H, Herndon C H, Heiple K G 1959 Congenital posterior angulation of the tibia with talipes calcaneus. Journal of Bone and Joint Surgery 41A: 476–488
37. Hoffer M M, Wichenden R, Roper B 1978 Brachial plexus birth palsies. Results of tendon transfers to the rotator cuff. Journal of Bone and Joint Surgery 60A: 691–695
38. Howorth B 1977 Development of present knowledge of congenital displacement of the hip. Clinical Orthopaedics 125: 68–87
39. Hummer C D Jr, MacEwen G D 1972 The coexistence of torticollis in congenital dysplasia of the hip. Journal of Bone and Joint Surgery 54A: 1255–1256
40. Jacobs J E 1960 Metatarsus varus and hip dysplasia. Clinical Orthopaedics 16: 203–212
41. Jayakumar S S, Eilert R E 1979 Fibular transfer for congenital absence of the tibia. Clinical Orthopaedics 139: 97–101
42. Jones L 1970 Birth trauma in the cervical spine. Archives of Disease in Childhood 45: 147–154
43. Kinsbourne M, Oxen D M 1964 Hiatus hernia with contortions of the neck. Lancet i: 1058–1061
44. Klisic P G 1989 Congenital dislocation of the hip – a misleading term. Journal of Bone and Joint Surgery 71B: 136
45. Lanska M J, Roessmann U, Wiznitzer M: 1990 Magnetic resonance imaging in cervical cord birth injury. Pediatrics 85: 760–764
46. Ling C M, Low Y S 1972 Sternomastoid tumor in muscular torticollis. Clinical Orthopaedics 86: 144–150
47. Lloyd-Roberts G C, Shaw N E 1969 The prevention of pseudarthrosis in congenital kyphosis of the tibia. Journal of Bone and Joint Surgery 51B: 100–105
48. Lloyd-Roberts G D, Apley A G, Owen R 1975 Reflections upon the aetiology of congenital pseudarthrosis of the clavicle with a note on cranio-cleido-dysostosis. Journal of Bone and Joint Surgery 57B: 24–29
49. MacEwen G D, Hardy J H 1972 Evaluation of kidney anomalies in congenital scoliosis. Journal of Bone and Joint Surgery 54A: 1451–1454
50. McGillicuddy D M, Jones E T, Hensinger R N 1980 The early treatment of talipes equinovarus with adhesive taping. Orthopedics 3: 33–37
51. McKenna P H, Khoury A E, McLorie G A, Churchill B M, Babyn P B, Wedge J H 1994 Iliac osteotomy: a model to compare the options in bladder and cloacal exstrophy reconstruction. Journal of Urology 151: 182–187
52. Madsen E T 1955 Fractures of extremities in the newborn. Acta Obstetrica et Gynaecologica Scandinavica 34: 41–75
53. Maekawa K, Masaki T, Kokubun Y 1976 Fetal spinal-cord injury secondary to hyperextension of the neck: no effect of caesarean section. Developmental Medicine and Child Neurology 18: 229–238
54. Mnaymneh W A 1978 Congenital radiohumeral synostosis. Clinical Orthopaedics and Related Research 131: 183–184
55. Nason S S, Jackman K V, McKay D W 1978 Congenital subluxation of the knee – an anatomic dissection. Orthopedics 1: 49–51
56. Nichols G W Schwentker E P, Boal D K 1986 Correlation of anatomy and ultrasonographic images in the infant hip: an experimental cadaver study. Journal of Pediatric Orthopedics 6: 410–415
57. Niebauer J J, King D E 1960 Congenital dislocation of the knee. Journal of Bone and Joint Surgery 42A: 207–225
58. Ogden J A, Moss H L 1978 Pathological anatomy of congenital hip disease. In: Weill U H (ed) Progress in orthopaedic surgery. Vol. 2: Acetabular dysplasia. In: Skeletal Dysplasias in Childhood. Springer-Verlag, Berlin, pp 1–45
59. Ortolani M 1937 Umsegno poco noto e sua importanza per la diagnosis precore di prelussazione congenita dell'onca. Pediatria (Napoli) 45: 129–136
60. Outland T, Sherk H 1961 Cleidocranial dysostosis; the hereditary aspects. Clinical Orthopaedics and Related Research 20: 241–244
61. Ponseti I V, Smoley E M 1963 Congenital club foot: the results of treatment. Journal of Bone and Joint Surgery 45A: 261–275
62. Poznanski A K, La Rowe P C 1970 The radiographic manifestations of the arthrogryposis syndrome. Radiology 95: 353–358
63. Ramsey P L, Lasser S, MacEwen G D 1976 Congenital dislocation of the hip. Journal of Bone and Joint Surgery 58A: 1000–1004
64. Rathgeb J M, Ramsey P L, Cowell H R 1974 Congenital kyphoscoliosis of the tibia. Clinical Orthopaedics 103: 178–190
65. Rushforth G F 1978 The natural history of the hooked forefoot. Journal of Bone and Joint Surgery 60B: 530–532
66. Salenius P, Vankka E 1975 The development of the tibial-femoral angle in children. Journal of Bone and Joint Surgery 57A: 259–261
67. Salter R B 1968 Etiology, pathogenesis and possible prevention of congenital dislocation of the hip. Canadian Medical Association Journal 98: 933–945
68. San Agusting M, Nitowsky H M, Borden J N 1962 Neonatal sciatic palsy after umbilical vessel injection. Journal of Pediatrics 60: 408–413
69. Schmidt A H, Keenen T L, Tank E S, Bird C B, Beals R K 1993 Pelvic osteotomy for bladder exstrophy. Journal of Pediatric Orthopedics 13: 214–219
70. Shaw N E 1960 Neonatal sciatic palsy from injection into the umbilical cord. Journal of Bone and Joint Surgery 42B: 736–741
71. Staheli L T, Engle G M 1972 Tibial torsion. A method of assessment in a study of normal children. Clinical Orthopaedics 86: 183–186
72. Staheli L T, Corbett M, Weiss C, King C H 1985 Lower extremity rotational problems in children. Journal of Bone and Joint Surgery 67A: 39–47
73. Stern M B 1968 Congenital dislocation of the knee. Clinical Orthopaedics 61: 261–268
74. Swanson A B 1976: A classification for congenital limb malformations. Journal of Hand Surgery 1: 8–22
75. Szoke G, Staheli L T, Jaffe K, Hall J G 1996 Medial-approach open reduction of hip dislocation in amyoplasia-type arthrogryposis. Journal of Pediatric Orthopedics 16: 127–130
76. Tachdjian M O 1972 Pediatric orthopaedics. W B Saunders, Philadelphia, Ch. 6

77. Theodorou S D, Mitsou M N I, Mitsou A 1982 Obstetrical fractures: separation of the upper femoral epiphysis. Acta Orthopaedica Scandinavica 53: 239–243
78. Thompson T C, Straub L R, Arnold W D 1957 Congenital absence of the fibula. Journal of Bone and Joint Surgery 39A: 1229–1237
79. Torpin R, Faulkner A 1966 Intrauterine amputation with the missing member found in the fetal membranes. Journal of the American Medical Association 198: 185–187
80. Towbin A 1964 Spinal cord and brain stem injury at birth. Archives of Radiology 77: 620–623
81. Towbin A 1969 Latent spinal cord and brain stem injury in newborn infants. Developmental Medicine and Child Neurology 11: 54–68
82. Tucci J J, Kumar S J, Guille J T, Rubbo E R 1991 Late acetabular dysplasia following early successful Pavlik harness treatment of congenital dislocation of the hip. Journal of Pediatric Orthopedics 11: 502–505
83. Werlin S L, D'Souza B D, Hogan W J, Dodds W J, Arndorfer R C 1980 Sandifer syndrome: an unappreciated clinical entity. Developmental Medicine and Child Neurology 22: 374–378
84. Westin W, Sakai D N, Wood W L 1976 Congenital longitudinal deficiency of the fibula. Follow-up of treatment by Syme amputation. Journal of Bone and Joint Surgery 58A: 492–496
85. Winter R B 1977 Scoliosis and spinal growth. Orthopaedic Review 6: 17–20
86. Winter R B 1981 Convex anterior and posterior hemiarthrodesis and hemiepiphyseodesis in young children with progressive congenital scoliosis. Journal of Pediatric Orthopedics 1: 361–366
87. Winter R B, Moe J H, Eilers V E 1968 Congenital scoliosis – a study of 234 patients treated and untreated. Journal of Bone and Joint Surgery 50A: 1–11
88. Winter R B, Moe J H, Wang J F 1973 Congenital kyphosis. Its natural history and treatment as observed in a study of 130 patients. Journal of Bone and Joint Surgery 55A: 223–256
89. Wynne-Davies R 1964 Family studies and the cause of congenital club foot. Talipes equino varus, talipes calcano valgus, and metatarsus varus. Journal of Bone and Joint Surgery 46B: 445–463
90. Wynne-Davies R 1978 Heritable disorders in orthopedics. Orthopedic Clinics in North America 9: 1–14
91. Yates, P O 1959 Birth trauma to the vertebral arteries. Archives of Disease in Childhood 34: 436–441

42

Neonatal gynaecology

D. K. Edmonds

Gynaecological problems in neonatal life are unusual and rare. Many conditions which are thought to be pathological are commonly physiological or anatomical variants, but these variants cause considerable anxiety amongst parents. A knowledge of the physiology and anatomy of the development of the genital tract during fetal life is therefore important, so that an explanation of these variations can be offered to parents in a reassuring manner.

THE PHYSIOLOGY OF THE FETAL HYPOTHALAMO-PITUITARY AXIS

The early fetal brain undergoes rapid development and by 5 weeks of gestation gonadotrophin-releasing hormone can be detected in whole brain extract.[25] GnRH can be localized to the hypothalamus by 8–13 weeks' gestation[2,11] and the hypothalamic GnRH content of female fetuses reaches a maximum at between 22 and 25 weeks' gestation and thereafter declines.[21] This is almost certainly in response to negative feedback of circulating oestradiol.

Luteinizing hormones and follicle-stimulating hormone (FSH) can be identified within the pituitary gland by 9–11 weeks' gestation[6,9] and the portal circulation linking the hypothalamus with the pituitary is known to be intact by 12 weeks' gestation.[23] In response to GnRH release, FSH and LH reach their maximum between 16 and 24 weeks.[22] Subsequently FSH levels decline, almost certainly owing to active secretion of inhibin from the granulosa cells in the ovary. During the latter part of fetal life, gonadotrophin levels are reduced and remain at low levels until birth.[22] Both inhibin and circulating oestradiol exhibit this negative feedback mechanism.

Following birth, the contribution of placental oestradiol to the fetal circulation is withdrawn, the fetal hypothalamo-pituitary axis becomes activated and both GnRH and gonadotrophin levels rise immediately.[24] FSH levels and LH levels remain elevated for several months after birth, but subsequent central suppression of GnRH leads to decline in gonadotrophin levels by around 6 months of age. The central suppression of the pulse generator in the arcuate nucleus of the hypothalamus may be brought about by several modulators, including noradrenaline, dopamine, central opiates, neuropeptide Y, glutamate or aspartate.[5,8,12,20] The cell receptors on the GnRH-secreting neurons are controlled by a gene encoding for transforming growth factor alpha,[14] and this gene may well itself be controlled by the secretion of leptin,[15] a hormone produced by adipose tissue; decreasing the body mass index towards later infancy and increasing body mass at puberty may be intimately involved in the activation of the gene.

Thus, throughout fetal and early neonatal life, the hypothalamo-pituitary ovarian uterine axis is fully developed and active, and capable of responding to all of the appropriate integrated mechanisms. It is only the genetic downregulation of central receptors that suppresses activity after birth.

NEONATAL BREAST DEVELOPMENT

Breast development occurs during fetal life and is well described as proceeding in female infants during neonatal life for several months after birth. It is occasionally associated with secretions similar to lactation. Two studies suggest that after birth circulating levels of oestriol, which would be maternally derived, decline rapidly and yet breast development continues for several months after birth.[1,16] Elevated levels of oestradiol and prolactin in the neonate are directly related to breast size, particularly the relationship to prolactin. Therefore it would seem that the infant's own gonadal secretions are responsible for the control of the breast. Histological studies further support this theory.[17] Breast development in early neonatal life therefore is a normal physiological process and ceases at 3–6 months of age; the breast bud may thereafter regress.

Supernumerary nipples are a common finding; they extend along the nipple line on either side of the chest wall, down the abdomen and may occur in the labia. Bilateral ectopic breast tissue has been described in the vulva.[13]

VULVAL PROBLEMS

Labial cysts in the newborn are rare, and occur in about 6 per 1000 female infants. These congenital cysts require no treatment whatsoever, and conservative management leads to complete resolution within 2–3 months of life. No surgical approach should be taken in these circumstances.[18]

Occasionally, inguinal masses may be detected in female infants in the differential diagnosis of ambiguous genitalia. Ultrasound of these masses can be extremely useful, and will differentiate ovarian tissue when present in the hernia sac and also aid in differentiating the presence of ovary and testis. Early diagnosis in these cases of the presence of an ovary herniating into the labia may be extremely important, as correction of this anatomical defect may reduce the risk of infarction and subsequent loss of the ovary.

PROBLEMS OF THE HYMEN

The hymen at birth is usually annular or fimbriated and commonly associated with external ridges. Hymenal tags are extremely common at birth,[19] and are often misdiagnosed as 'prolapse'. The hymen changes its characteristics during the first 3 years of life and becomes crescentic by age 3 years in the vast majority, with the external ridges disappearing.[3] Problems in neonatal life which are associated with peripheral oedema often lead to oedema of the hymen which may protrude beyond the vulval entrance and again be mistaken for a prolapse.

Failure of the hymen to perforate during embryological life may lead to retention of vaginal secretions which cannot escape and the vagina distends proximal to the hymen. Although these membranes are often referred to as imperforate hymen, it is likely that this is not strictly correct and that these membranes are transverse vaginal septae, resulting from failure of fusion of the urogenital sinus and the downgrowth of the vaginal plate from the müllerian structures. When a large quantity of fluid collects, there may be difficulty in emptying the bladder, as the distended vagina fills the pelvis and the child may be very fretful and clearly in discomfort. The physical signs are of a lower abdominal cystic swelling and a bulging membrane at the introitus (Fig. 42.1). Diagnosis is extremely important, as misdiagnoses abound in which laparotomy has been performed, and even hysterectomy, and this is absolutely unnecessary. The most common misdiagnoses are to believe that this is either a swelling which is an ovarian cyst or, occasionally, a full bladder with a urethral prolapse. Ultrasound imaging is extremely important to identify the anatomy involved. It is simple to demonstrate the uterus sitting above a distended vagina when the diagnosis is hydrocolpos. Treatment is simple in most cases: the intact membrane is incised and the retained fluid released. Redundant portions of the membrane may be excised and the procedure completed. If the obstruction is more extensive owing to a wide transverse septum, great care is needed to avoid damage to the bladder and rectum, but an end-to-end anastomosis can be achieved to result in a normal vagina. One can only presume that these cases of hydrocolpos are exceptional, as most cases of transverse vaginal septum are not diagnosed until puberty.[7]

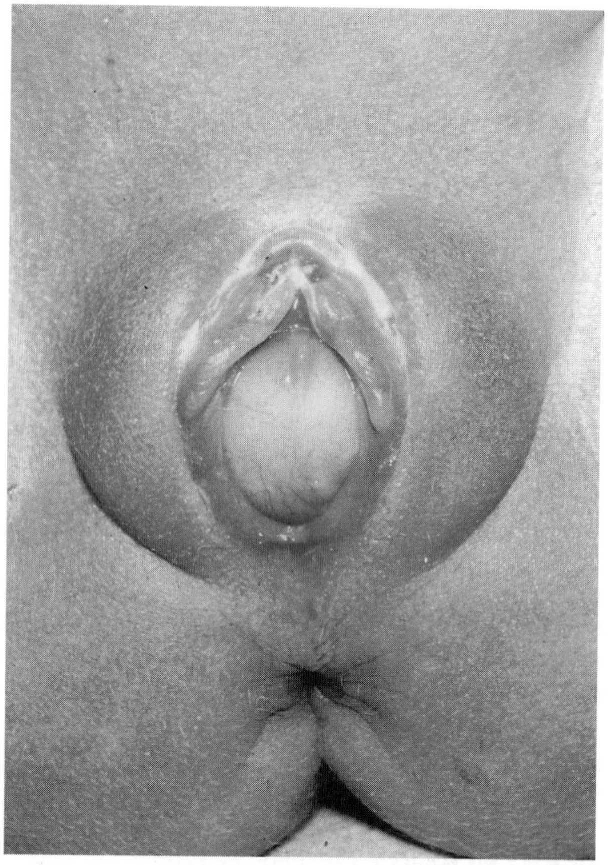

Fig. 42.1 Bulging membrane at the introitus in a case of transverse vaginal septum presenting in a newborn.

MENSTRUAL PROBLEMS

Bleeding from the genital tract in the newborn period is well described. A study from Huber in 1976[10] showed that vaginal bleeding occurs in 25% of newborn girls, although it is only macroscopically visible in 3.3%. Vaginal bleeding in the first week of life is extremely common. Persistent vaginal bleeding beyond the first year of life demands further investigation. The development of rhabdomyosarcoma, whilst extraordinarily rare in immediate neonatal life, may present as bleeding at 2–3 months of age. Most of the genital lesions associated with rhabdomyosarcoma of the perineum, vulva and vagina occur in early childhood.

UTERINE PROLAPSE

Prolapse in the neonatal period is extremely rare, but may present with the cervix protruding through the vagina. A number of cases have been described and, although the etiology of the problem remains obscure, some cases are associated with neurological abnormalities, e.g. spina bifida. Treatment is conservative and involves digital replacement of the prolapse into the vagina. This may have to be repeated on a number of occasions but eventually, by 3 months of age at the latest, all of these prolapses have resolved. Occasionally pessaries may be required if the prolapse remains persistent. No data exist to suggest whether or not these female infants develop prolapse problems in a later stage of their life, but it is likely that this will be the case as the occurrence of prolapse in these circumstances may be associated with poor collagen development in the supporting tissue of the genital tract.

URETHRAL PROLAPSE

Urethral prolapse in the neonatal period is extremely rare, but may present with vaginal bleeding. The urethral mucosa prolapses through the meatus and forms a sensitive vulval mass that bleeds on touch. The passage of urine may be unimpaired when the lesion is small, and in these circumstances the use of oestrogen cream may be beneficial. However, occasionally urinary retention may be present, or the prolapse may recur following repeated oestrogen treatments and recurrence may require surgical excision if the lesion is large. This tends to be only rarely necessary and is usually only employed when urinary retention is present.

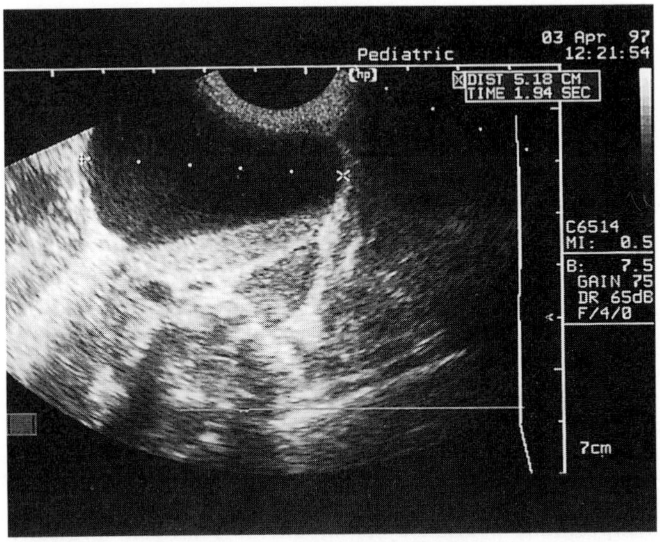

Fig. 42.2 Pelvic ultrasound scan showing an ovarian cyst 5 cm in diameter in a newborn girl.

OVARIAN CYSTS

Ultrasound of the fetus during pregnancy is now sophisticated enough to diagnose ovarian cysts in mid-pregnancy, and these may be detected as early as 16–18 weeks' gestation. The vast majority of these cysts are

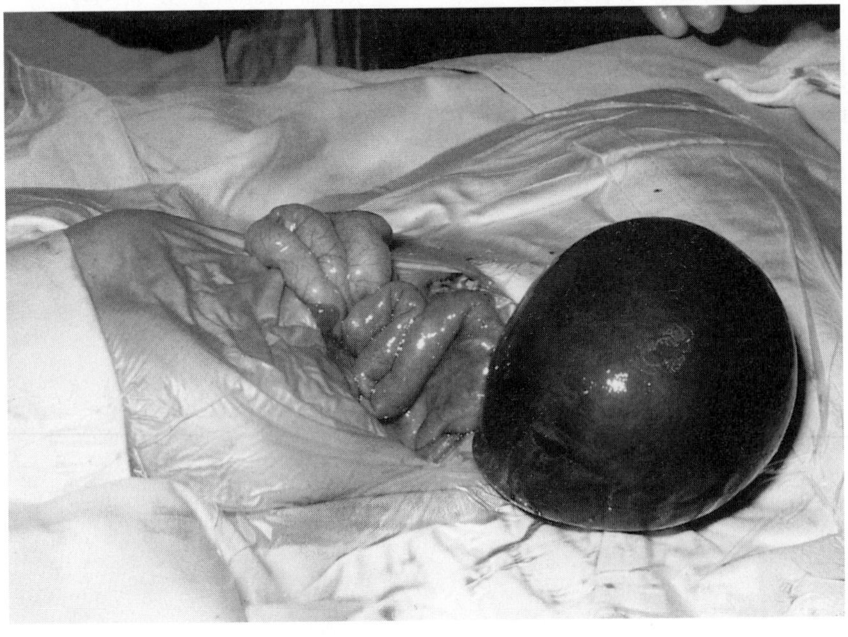

Fig. 42.3 Torted ovarian cyst at laparotomy in a young girl.

functional, benign follicular cysts and do not interfere with the course of pregnancy or birth. If these cysts are less than 5 cm as diagnosed during the postnatal period, then they may be managed conservatively with serial ultrasound and the vast majority will resolve spontaneously.[4] This may take as long as 6 months to a year and this relates to stimulation of the ovary by elevated FSH levels which persist during this time. Cysts that are larger than 5 cm in diameter (Fig. 42.2) but do not contain any solid elements may be managed by percutaneous aspiration under local anaesthesia. Should this be performed, cytology should always be carried out for confirmation of a benign lesion. All cysts of 4 cm or more have the risk of torsion, and therefore care must be taken in their management and also in the advice that is given to parents. All complex cystic masses or symptomatic ovarian cysts should be removed surgically (Fig. 42.3) and histology performed to ensure that the cyst is benign. Antenatal torsion of a cyst has been described in a pregnancy that resulted in premature birth, although the clinical course of the neonate was uneventful.

REFERENCES

1. Anbazhagan R, Bartek J, Monaghan P, Gusterson B A 1991 Growth and development of human infant breast. American Journal of Anatomy 192: 407–17
2. Aubert M L, Grumbach M M, Kaplan S L 1977 The autogenesis of human fetal hormones. Journal of Clinical Endocrinology and Metabolism 44: 1130–1141
3. Berenson A B 1995 A longitudinal study of hymenal morphology in the first three years of life. Pediatrics 95: 490–495
4. Brandt M L, Luks F I, Filiatrault D, Garel L, DesJardins J G, Youssef S 1991 Surgical indications in antenatally diagnosed ovarian cysts. Journal of Pediatric Surgery 26: 276–281
5. Brann D W 1995 Glutamate: a major excitatory transmitter in neuroendocrine regulation. Neuroendocrinology 61: 213–225
6. Currie R W, Fairman C, Thliveris J A 1981 An immunocytochemical and routine electron microscopic study of LH & FSH cells in the human fetal pituitary. American Journal of Anatomy 161: 281–297
7. Edmonds D K 1988 Practical Paediatric and Adolescent Gynaecology. Butterworths, London, pp 86–95
8. Gore A C, Mitshushima D, Terasawa E 1993 A possible role for neuropeptide Y in the control of the onset of puberty in female rhesus monkeys. Neuroendocrinology 58: 23–24
9. Hagen C, McNeilly A S 1977 The gonadotrophins and their sub units in fetal pituitary glands and circulation. Journal of Steroid Biochemistry 8: 537–544
10. Huber A 1976 Häufigkeit der physiologischen vaginalen neugeboren Blutung. Zentralblatt fur Gynäkologie 98: 1017–1020
11. Kaplan S L, Grumback M M, Aubert M L 1976 The autogenesis of pituitary hormones and hypothalamic factors in the human fetus. Recent Progress in Hormone Research 32: 161–243
12. Lee P A 1988 The neuroendocrinology of puberty. Seminars in Reproductive Medicine 6: 13–20
13. Levin N, Diener R L 1968 Bilateral ectopic breast of the vulva. Obstetrics and Gynaecology 32: 274–276
14. Ma Y J, Costa H E, Ojeda S R 1994 Developmental expression of the genes encoding transforming growth factor alpha and its receptor in the hypothalamus of the female rhesus macaque. Neuroendocrinology 60: 346–359
15. MacDougald O A, Hwang C S, Fan H, Lane M D 1995 Regulated expression of the obese gene product, leptin, in white adipose tissue. Proceedings of the National Academy of Science 92: 9034–9037
16. McKiernan J F, Hull D 1981 Prolactin maternal oestrogens and breast development in the newborn. Archives of Disease in Childhood 56: 770–774
17. McKiernan J F, Coyne J, Cahalane S 1988 Histology of breast development in early life. Archives of Disease in Childhood 63: 136–139
18. Merlob P, Bahari C, Liban E, Reisner S H 1978 Cysts of the female external genitalia in the newborn infant. American Journal of Obstetrics and Gynaecology 132: 607–610
19. Mor N, Merlob P, Reisner S H 1983 Tags and bands of the female external genitalia in the newborn infant. Clinics Pediatrics Philadelphia 22: 122–124
20. Prasad B, Conover C D, Barker D K, Rabii J, Advis J P 1993 Feed restriction in prepubertal lambs: effect on puberty, LHRH, neuropeptide Y, and beta-endorphin release from the postero-lateral median eminence. Neuroendocrinology 57: 1171–1181
21. Sider-Khodr T M 1978 Studies in human fetal endocrinology. LHR factor content of the hypothalamus. American Journal of Obstetrics and Gynecology 130: 795–800
22. Takagi S, Yoshida T, Tsubata K et al 1977 Sex differences in fetal gonadotrophins and androgens. Journal of Steroid Biochemistry 8: 609–620
23. Thliveris J A, Currie R W 1980 Observations of the hypothalamo-hypophysial portal vasculature in the developing human fetus. American Journal of Anatomy 157: 441–444
24. Winter J S D 1975 Pituitary-gonadal relating in infancy. Journal of Endocrinology and Metabolism 42: 545
25. Winters A J, Eskay R L, Porter J C 1974 Concentration and distribution of TRH and LRH in human fetal brain. Journal of Endocrinology and Metabolism 39: 960–963

43

Neonatal infection

Part 1

Neonatal immunology

Colin M. Stern

INTRODUCTION

Perinatal infection is uncommon in healthy, term, breast-fed infants nursed by their mothers in a clean environment. Conversely, babies born early and cared for away from their mothers in, for example, neonatal units, run a significantly greater risk of infection, especially by bacteria. This increased risk is considerably heightened by coexisting neonatal illness and less than meticulous standards of hygiene. Many authorities ascribe this high infection risk to the immaturity of the immune system at birth and, tacitly or explicitly, consider the newborn infant immunodeficient.

It would be more accurate to say that the term newborn infant has an immune system which, at birth, is appropriate for his or her needs. Most, but not all, failures of the neonatal immune system to respond adequately to pathogenic attack are the consequence of antigenic naiveté. The earlier a preterm infant is born, the less maternal immunoglobulin is transferred via the placenta. In vitro deficiencies of neonatal cellular immune function have been demonstrated, although these have not been supported by demonstrations of immune response impairment in vivo.

The invasion of tissues by microorganisms elicits, first, an early innate host response, which is capable of reacting against a wide variety of organisms and limits the spread of infection. More slowly, the adaptive response to the infection gathers strength and eventually supersedes the early innate reaction, in both specificity and potency. The adaptive immune response is an immune reaction which selects immunoreactive molecules and cells with increasing specificity and avidity for antigens. The innate immune response, which is non-specific with respect to antigens is, in general, less effective in the newborn infant than the adaptive response, compared with older children.

It has become possible to enhance or inhibit the activity of specific elements of the immune response and of inflammation. Early examples of such therapies are the use of interferons and of G-CSF. The neonatologist needs to be in a position to consider the effect of modulating interactions between ligands and their receptors. Table 43.1 describes briefly the nature of some important cytokines, and Table 43.2 lists some of the more important CD markers.

In the last 5 years there has been an explosive increase of information about the molecular signals, the receptors, lectins and sequences of actions that permit the regulation of an effective immune response. It is of vital importance for the neonatologist to understand these events, because significant immune modulation is on the brink of providing useful therapy for the infected newborn infant. Those who seek detailed information on the development of the immune system and its constituents are referred to two excellent textbooks.[49,101]

THE MATERNOFETAL IMMUNOLOGICAL RELATIONSHIP

The embryo and the fetus grow and differentiate in close physiological contact with the mother.[45] It has become clear that this relationship has important effects upon the development of the fetal immune system, modifying the fetal response to infection and, rarely, generating specific fetal diseases.

Table 43.1 Cytokines with important functions in the immune response. Some future clinical interventions in diseases caused by immune dysfunction may act by modulating the action of specific cytokines. The most likely candidates are described here (R = receptor)

Cytokine	Cytokine family	CD binding molecule	Action
IL2 (T-cell growth factor)	Haematopoietin	CD25 (α); CD 122 (β)	T-lymphocyte proliferation
IL4	Haematopoietin	CD124, γc	B-lymphocyte activation, IgE switch
IL5	Haematopoietin	CD125, γc	Eosinophil growth & differentiation
IL6	Haematopoietin	CD26, CD_w130	T- & B-lymphocyte growth & differentiation, acute phase protein production
IL9	Haematopoietin	IL-9R, γc	Mast cell stimulation
IL13	Haematopoietin	IL-13R, γc	B-lymphocyte growth & differentiation, macrophage stimulation
G-CSF	Haematopoietin	G-CSFR	Stimulates neutrophil development
IFN-α	Interferons	CD118	Viral inhibition, MHC Class I synthesis
IFN-β	Interferons	CD118	Viral inhibition, MHC Class I synthesis
IFN-γ	Interferons	CD119	Macrophage activation and MHC synthesis
CD80	Immunoglobulin superfamily	CD28, CTLA-4	T-lymphocyte stimulator
B70	Immunoglobulin superfamily	CD28, CTLA-4	T-lymphocyte stimulator
TNF-α	TNF family	CD120a & b, p55 & p75	Activates endothelial cells, promotes inflammation
TNF-β	TNF family	CD120a & b, p55 & p75	Cytotoxic, activates endothelial cells
CD40 ligand	TNF family	CD40	Activates B-lymphocytes, Ig class switch
Fas ligand	TNF family	CD95 (Fas)	Lymphocyte proliferation
CD27 ligand	TNF family	CD27	T-lymphocyte proliferation
CD30 ligand	TNF family	CD30	T- & B-lymphocyte proliferation
4-1BBL	TNF family	4-1BB	T- & B-lymphocyte proliferation
IL-8	Chemokine family	CD_w128	Neutrophil chemotactic factor
MCP-1	Chemokine family	Unknown	Monocyte chemotactic factor
TGF-β	Not assigned	Unknown	Inhibitor of inflammation
IL1α	Not assigned	CD_w121a	Fever, T-lymphocyte & macrophage stimulation
IL1β	Not assigned	CD_w121a	Fever, T-lymphocyte & macrophage stimulation
IL10	Not assigned	Unknown	Macrophage function inhibitor
IL12	Not assigned	Unknown	NK-cell activator, TH_1-cell inducer
MIF	Not assigned	Unknown	Inhibits macrophage migration

Table 43.2 The more important clusters of differentiation. Some future clinical interventions in diseases caused by immune dysfunction may act by modulating the action of specific clusters of differentiation. The most likely candidates are described here

CD number	Cytokine family	Cells on which found	Function
CD1a,b,c	Immunoglobulin superfamily	Cortical thymocytes, Langerhans' cells, dendritic cells, B cell, intestinal epithelium	MHC class II-like May present antigen to γ/δ cells
CD2	Immunoglobulin superfamily	T cells, thymocytes, NK cells	Binds CD58 Can activate T cells
CD3	Immunoglobulin superfamily	Thymocytes, T cells	Needed for surface expression of T-cell receptor, and signal transduction
CD4	Immunoglobulin superfamily	Thymocyte subsets, TH_1 & TH_2 cells, monocytes, macrophages	MHC class II coreceptor Binding site for HIV-1 & HIV-2
CD8	Immunoglobulin superfamily	Thymocytes, cytotoxic T cells	MHC class I coreceptor
CD11a	None	Lymphocytes, granulocytes, monocytes and macrophages	α^L subunit of LFA_1 (integrin)
CD11b	None	Myeloid & NK cells	α^M subunit of integrin CR3, binds CD54, and iC3b
CD11c	None	Myeloid cells	α^X subunit of integrin CR4, binds fibrinogen
CD16	Immunoglobulin superfamily	Neutrophils, NK cells, macrophages	Part of low-affinity Fc receptor; mediates phagocytosis & ADCC
CD18	None	Leukocytes	Integrin β_2 subunit, binds CD11a, b, c
CD19	Immunoglobulin superfamily	B cells	
CD21	Complement control protein superfamily	Mature B cells, dendritic cells	C3d & EB virus receptor. B-cell coreceptor with CD19 & CD81
CD23	C-type lectin	Mature B cells, activated macrophages, eosinophils, dendritic cells, platelets	Low-affinity IgE receptor. CD19:CD21:CD81 receptor ligand

Table 43.2 (*Contd*)

CD number	Cytokine family	Cells on which found	Function
CD25	Complement control protein superfamily	Activated T cells, B cells & monocytes	IL-2 receptor α chain, links to CD122 & IL-2Rγ chain
CD28	Immunoglobulin superfamily	T-cell subsets; activated B cells	Receptor for costimulatory signal for activation of naive T cells, binds CD80 & B7.2
CD34	None	Haemopoietic precursors and capillary endothelial cells	Ligand for CD62L (L-selectin)
CD35	Complement control protein superfamily	B cells, dendritic cells, red cells, monocytes, eosinophils & neutrophils	Binds C3b & C4b to mediate phagocytosis. Complement receptor 1
CD40	NGF receptor superfamily	B cells, monocytes, dendritic cells	Receptor for costimulatory signal for B cells, binds CD40 ligand (CD40L)
CD40-L	TNF family	Activated CD4 + T cells	Ligand for CD40
CD45	None	Leukocytes	Amplifier for T- & B-cell antigen receptor signalling. Phosphotyrosine phosphatase; many isoforms (other CD45s)
CD54	Immunoglobulin superfamily	Haemopoietic & other cells	Intercellular adhesion molecule (ICAM-1). Binds LFA-1 & Mac-1. Rhinovirus receptor
CD55	Complement control protein superfamily	Haemopoietic & other cells	Binds C3b; breaks down C3/C5 convertase
CD59	Ly-6 superfamily	Haemopoietic & other cells	Binds C8/C9, blocks assembly of membrane attack complex
CD62E	C-type lectin. EGF & CCP superfamily	Endothelium	Adhesion molecule mediating rolling adherence of leukocytes to endothelium
CD62L	C-type lectin. EGF & CCP superfamily	T cells, NK cells, B cells and monocytes	Adhesion molecule mediating rolling adherence of leukocytes to endothelium
CD62P	C-type lectin. EGF & CCP superfamily	Platelets, megakaryocytes and endothelium	Adhesion molecule mediating rolling adherence of leukocytes to endothelium
CD74	None	B cells, macrophages, MHC class II + cells, monocytes	Invariate chain associated with MHC class II
CD79α,β	Immunoglobulin superfamily	B cells	Needed for cell–cell interactions & signal transduction. Like CD3
CD80	Immunoglobulin superfamily	B-cell subset	Costimulator: ligand for CD28
CD81	Membrane proteins spanning tetra	Lymphocytes	B-cell coreceptor when linked to CD19 & CD21
CD95	NGF receptor superfamily	Many cell lines	Binds Fas ligand: induces apoptosis
CD102	Immunoglobulin superfamily	Lymphocytes, monocytes & vascular endothelial cells	Binds CD11a (LFA-1) & CD18, *not* CD11b (Mac-1)
CD106	Immunoglobulin superfamily	Endothelial cells	Adhesion molecule (ligand) for VLA-4
CD117	Immunoglobulin superfamily (tyrosine kinase)	Haemopoietic precursor cells	Stem cell factor receptor
CD119	None	Macrophages, monocytes, B cells & endothelium	Interferon-γ receptor
CD120a	NGF receptor superfamily	Many cell types, highest on epithelial cells	TNF receptor for TNF-α & TNF-β
CD122	None	NK cells, resting T-cell subsets, some B cells	IL-2 receptor β-chain
CD124	Cytokine & type III fibronectin superfamilies	Mature T & B cells; haemopoietic precursor cells	IL-4 receptor
CD128	Rhodopsin superfamily	Neutrophils, basophils and a T-cell subset	IL-8 receptor

TH_1 cells are 'inflammatory' T lymphocytes; TH_2 cells are 'helper' T lymphocytes

Pregnant women are exposed to a variety of paternal and fetal antigens, including transplantation antigens, both by direct contact with the placenta and its membranes and by the transportation of fetal cells into their circulation.[53] There is clear evidence for the expression of fetal transplantation antigens on placental cells.[25] These antigens, although inevitably derived from one or other parent, are not expressed by them in postnatal life.[58]

Mothers make both cell-mediated and antibody responses against fetal antigens.[21,33] These responses are not normally damaging, although some, such as against the rhesus D antigen, cause neonatal disease.[57] Some claim that maternal antifetal responses are not regular events, but a majority maintain that not only is this not the case, but that these immune responses help to maintain a normal gestation.[8,108,122]

The effects of maternal isoimmunization against blood group antigens such as Rh, ABO and Kell, or against platelet or white cell antigens, are well-known (pp. 802, 817). Other maternally derived antibodies which may have fetal effects include those directed against the acetylcholine receptor, which may cause neonatal myasthenia gravis

(p. 1291) or against thyroid components which lead to neonatal thyrotoxicosis (p. 964).[92] An antibody known as anti-Ro (SS-A), produced by some women suffering from SLE, may cause miscarriage, fetal heart block and transient neonatal skin lesions, thrombocytopenia and heart block.[93]

There are many of these autoantibodies, which are capable of binding to fetal antigens.[86] Why do only a few bring about neonatal illness? The explanation centres on the nature of those fetal antigens expressed in the centre of the placental villus. Transferred maternal immunoglobulin passes through this region, which is called the 'placental sink'.[35,121] Maternal antibody directed against a fetal antigen expressed here binds to it and never reaches the baby. Some antigens expressed by highly differentiated cells, such as thyroid and erythrocyte, or at special sites like the neuromuscular junction, are not found in the placental villus and consequently antibodies to them reach the fetus, causing disease.

Two conditions which can lead to fetal loss may share an immune-related aetiology. Pre-eclampsia is associated with maternal HLA antigen homozygosity, and it has been suggested that this may impair the maternal immune response to the fetus so as to generate the disease.[80] This hypothesis remains unconfirmed, but there are several reports of linkage to HLA-DR4 in a manner which suggests the effect of an autosomal recessive gene shared by both the mother and her fetus.[17,55] Recurrent spontaneous fetal loss, however, is associated both with parental HLA antigen sharing[105] and with a deficient maternal antipaternal cytotoxic reaction.[69] Immunotherapy, using a variety of paternal white cell preparations, has been shown to improve the chances of carrying a fetus to term.

It seems that a minority of mothers in whom endocrinological, chromosomal, anatomical and other known disorders have been excluded may lose their babies because they are unable to mount an appropriate immune response.[102]

TRANSFER OF IMMUNOGLOBULIN FROM MOTHER TO FETUS

Mammalian mothers transfer immunoglobulin to their offspring transplacentally and/or in colostrum.[97] In humans, all maternal immunoglobulin transfer to the fetus occurs across the placenta by a selective process known as transcytosis.[35] This begins at about 14 weeks' gestation and, by term, the levels of IgG in cord serum are usually higher than those found in maternal blood. The bulk of transferred immunoglobulin belongs to the subclasses IgG_1 and IgG_3. The relative lack of IgG_2 makes rapid responses to the capsular polysaccharides of some organisms, such as the group B streptococcus, poor.[15] No IgM, IgA, IgD or IgE is transported and, if these immunoglobulins are found in cord blood, they have been synthesized by the fetus.[26]

IgG transfer is mediated by a receptor, FcγRN, which is expressed upon the surface of syncytiotrophoblast. FcγRN has close structural homology with class I MHC molecules, but has an occluded peptide-binding groove. Consequently, it binds in a different way to IgG. Two molecules of FcγRN link to one IgG molecule and transport it across the placenta. The process starts slowly at about 12 weeks' gestation, accelerating first at around 22 weeks' gestation and transporting large quantities of IgG after 30 weeks' gestation. At 28 weeks' gestation, cord IgG levels are about 0.04 g/l. By term, they reach 1.8 g/l, a 45-fold increase.[26]

THE IMMUNE SYSTEM IN THE TERM INFANT

IMMUNODEFICIENT OR IMMUNOEFFECTIVE?

Deficiencies in immunological reactivity have been described in term babies, especially of phagocytic function. Poor motility of polymorphonuclear leukocytes, possibly as a result of infection, has been shown in the human newborn. Reductions in chemotactic and phagocytic activity have been demonstrated[98] and the efficiency both of the oxidative burst and of bacterial killing has been found to be less than the responses of adult leukocytes.[43] However, limitations on opsonizing capacity create conditions under which bacteria are ingested in a greater state of activity and may damage cells more readily.[47] Reductions in T-lymphocyte killing and NK-cell activity[6] are typical of responses seen in gnotobiotic animals.

Some studies have described limitations of the size of the granulocyte progenitor pool in bone marrow and shown that there is a reduction in the neutrophil storage pool, leading to a rapid depletion of circulating neutrophils during episodes of neonatal sepsis.[15] These observations should be placed in context. It is known that estimations of stem cell pool size are inaccurate because, first, the most pluripotent of these cells adhere to the inner cortical surface of the bone marrow and are not effectively removed by aspiration, and secondly the movement of neutrophils through the circulating pool requires kinetic measurement, observations inadequately made by simple counts.[56] Neonatal bone marrow stem cells, and peripheral blood cells, respond to factors such as GM-CSF and, more recently used, G-CSF, 10 times more efficiently than adult cells.[68,76] As babies are able to generate these factors in significant amounts and to induce measurable responses, this may not be a significant deficiency in vivo. CD molecules (Table 43.2) interact with soluble cytokines (Table 43.1), such as complement components, interleukins, B-cell growth factors and interferons, which are produced in low but adequate quantities in term babies.[23,100,106] When sepsis is overwhelming, the newborn baby's defences lack the resilience that derives from years of activation to a wide variety of antigens. However, when a healthy baby is nursed in a natural maternal environment, his immune system has been ideally established to initiate appropriate and adequate responses.

The low level of IgM antibody present at birth increases susceptibility to infection by Gram-negative bacteria and, coupled with low C3b production, accounts in part for the predominance of such infections in the newborn. In addition, relatively smaller amounts of IgG_2 are transferred, which reduces the ability to bind capsular polysaccharide antigen.

POSTNATAL CHANGES IN IMMUNE REACTIVITY

There are a series of non-specific mechanisms, including the alternative pathway of complement activation and some monokines and macrophage functions, which do not require the induction of antigen-specific responses. These immune reactions, often called *non-adaptive immune responses*, are of vital importance in immune defence during early neonatal life.

The skin is the first barrier against infection[65] and uses three different systems of defence. The first is a mechanical defence, depending upon the cornification of the skin and the adherence, through their tight junctions, of neighbouring epithelial cells. The movement of air over the skin helps to prevent pathogens from gaining a foothold. The second is a chemical defence, consisting of a variety of enzymes, such as lysozyme; a group of antibacterial peptides called defensins; and fatty acids.

Thirdly, the alternative pathway of complement activation can be activated immediately upon contact with the surfaces of many microorganisms. Bacteria do not express CR1, MCP or DAF on their cell membranes: proteins which protect against the activation of the alternative pathway. Penetration of the gastric mucosa is limited by the low environmental pH. Bronchial mucosa is protected by the continuous production and removal of mucus. In addition, skin colonization by normal flora is protective, and if these benign surface organisms are removed there is a greater risk of infection by pathogenic bacteria.

Neutrophils are attracted to local sites of infection and inflammation by an array of cytokines that are released in this initial phase of the infection. These phagocytose and kill bacteria, even in the absence of antibody, but are aided by the binding of the lipopolysaccharide-binding protein in plasma and by the activation of the alternative pathway of complement activation.[85] They represent a critical component of the infant's protection against infection: congenital deficiency of neutrophils results in early, catastrophic infection by bacteria and fungi. Macrophages possess receptors which can bind directly to certain bacterial cell membrane components, leading to their engulfment and killing.

Three families of cytokines play important roles during early innate responses to infection: two of these are *monokine* groups (i.e. produced by monocytes), the third consists of *interferons*. IL1, IL6 and TNFα are endogenous pyrogens, because they raise body temperature in infection. Interferons α and β can be produced by many different cells early during virus infections. They have two main effects: the inhibition of viral replication within cells and the inhibition of the translation of viral RNA. IFNα and IFNβ also stimulate the surface expression of MHC Class I molecules, thus increasing the cell's susceptibility to attack by passing CD8-positive cytotoxic T cells. In addition, IFNα and IFNβ activate natural killer cells, which can kill virus-infected cells early.[106]

Although absolute levels of serum immunoglobulins fall over the first 3 months of life, there is expansion of the plasma volume and a dilutional effect upon serum protein levels.[97] However, the total quantity of immunoglobulin in the infant remains constant as the fall in serum level is matched by endogenous immunoglobulin production. Serum levels begin to rise again after 3 months of age. The amount of transferred maternal immunoglobulin with specificity for any given pathogen is low and, although too small to have much effect in limiting infection, is very potent in the early and rapid triggering of the baby's primary immune response. At birth, most immunoglobulin is in plasma and as the baby responds to antigenic stimuli, mostly from dietary antigens, there is a progressive rise in intracellular immunoglobulin, which first matches and then outstrips the catabolism of maternal immunoglobulin.

The nature of IgG produced by the infant differs from that in the adult. Although the synthesis of IgG_1 and IgG_4 occurs fairly early and rapidly, normal circulating amounts of IgG_3 are not achieved until the age of 10 years, nor of IgG_2 until 12 years. Their ability to generate adequate antibody responses to polysaccharide antigens are not achieved until about 2 years.[81]

Notwithstanding bacterial colonization, dietary antigen challenge is the most important way in which the newborn baby's immune system becomes primed and activated.[115] These challenges include not only milk components but also ingested bacteria and viruses, which in normal circumstances derive from the mother.[12,64] Most research on atopic dermatitis emphasizes the importance of IgE in mediating the allergic reaction.[63] However, the relationship between breast-feeding and infantile eczema sheds light on the manner in which maternal macrophages modify the immune response of their babies.[51] Some authorities recommend breast-feeding on the grounds that cow's milk allergy will be less likely.[50]

Recent studies have shown that infantile eczema is more common in breast-fed infants whose mothers are atopic.[64] Furthermore, antigen avoidance by these allergic mothers while breast-feeding reduces the incidence of eczema to that of the breast-fed babies of non-atopic parents.[14,114] Unsurprisingly, atopic mothers who bottle-feed their babies increase the risk of infantile eczema very considerably. On the other hand, breast-feeding by non-atopic mothers is associated with less infantile eczema than artificial feeding.[27]

These observations have been held to indicate that the small amount of antigen present in breast milk is capable of inducing an allergic response in the offspring.[13] From an immunological point of view this might seem more likely to induce antigen unresponsiveness. Breast milk contains a large number of macrophages, which are important in protecting the newborn infant from bowel infection.[48,61] However, it seems certain that, in atopic mothers with cow's milk protein sensitivity, some of these cells bear on their surfaces small quantities of processed cow's milk antigen, which can cooperate with neonatal lymphocytes and prime infants to cow's milk proteins (see below).[22,36,51,61]

It is not known whether any maternally derived mechanism for accelerating the immune response, possibly mediated through the enhanced upregulation of T-lymphocyte antigen receptors, exists for T lymphocytes. However, the peripheral blood of the newborn infant contains significant numbers of NK cells. Some serious virus infections, such as croup and bronchiolitis, occur in babies in the post-neonatal period, but their damaging effects tend to be limited to the respiratory tract.

Serious systemic virus infections in the first year of life are relatively infrequent and are limited not only by transferred maternal immunoglobulin, but by the presence of these cells, which have the capacity to kill virus-infected cells in a non-antigen specific fashion.[79] Thus, virus infections may be life-threatening as a consequence of local invasion, for example respiratory syncytial virus on bronchi, especially when damaged by CLD. Enhanced systemic antiviral defence in the infant declines in the second year of life.

Thus, the healthy newborn baby at term is adequately prepared to deal with the wide variety of antigenic challenges that lie in wait, as the essential components of the immune system develop early in fetal life.[99] However, the principal difference between the immune system of these neonates and that of older children and adults is its antigenic innocence.

Bacterial and fungal colonization of the skin and respiratory tract of the newborn is rapid.[7] When the baby is nursed with the mother, organisms are derived from her and, by the protection mechanisms already described, neonatal immune responses to these antigens rapidly follow.

PASSIVELY ACQUIRED IMMUNOGLOBULIN AND THE PRIMARY IMMUNE RESPONSE

It is generally assumed that transferred maternal immunoglobulin protects the newborn child by acting purely as passive antibody, binding to antigens commonly found in the maternofetal environment.

The kinetics of the primary immune response in the healthy adult are normally quite slow. Ten days elapse, during which time a peak of IgM production is reached and after which IgG antibody is generated in significant quantity. Similarly, cytotoxic T lymphocytes begin to be produced after 4 days and are maximally effective by 10 days. Meanwhile, NK cells limit virus spread.[79] A subsequent exposure to antigen induces a secondary immune response, in which accelerated IgG production peaks at 4–5 days. In the term newborn infant the presence of high levels of maternal antibody allows the primary immune response to develop much faster.[71]

When experimental animals are immunized, the presence of passive antibody accelerates the rate and increases the potency of the primary immune response, improving antigen presentation by accessory cells and amplifying the central phase of the immune response.[71] One might imagine that such a mechanism would be of significant benefit to the antigenically naive infant.[110] The acquisition of maternal immunoglobulin would thus help the newborn infant to accelerate primary immune responses, and induces a paradigm of antigenic experience. Antibodies with specificities capable of binding antigens previously encountered by the mother and present in the maternal environment act as passive opsonins; they are also capable of reducing the requirement for T-lymphocyte help.[116] This phenomenon depends upon the formation of a complex between antigen and antibody in such a way that they behave like a T-independent antigen, shortening the time required for antigen to be presented on the surface of the accessory cell.[71]

It is probable that this mechanism allows the healthy, term, newborn infant to generate primary immune responses in which significant quantities of high-affinity IgG are produced over a timespan closer to that after the typical secondary antigen challenge.

The best evidence to support this effect of maternal immunoglobulin transfer upon neonatal defence rests upon an analysis of the effect of infused immunoglobulin on endogenous antibody production.[15] It seems likely that the presence in the bowel of large amounts of maternal IgA allows a similar reaction in GALT. It is significant that there are many IgA antibody specificities in breast milk directed against dietary antigens, reflecting a lymphocyte recirculation pattern common to GALT and to breast parenchyma, for the same population of primed, stimulated B lymphocytes derived originally from the bowel.[61] There is an obvious beneficial effect to the breast-fed baby, initiating an early neonatal immune response to dietary antigens.

THE IMMUNE SYSTEM IN THE PRETERM INFANT

Survival in infants of less than 23 weeks' gestation, or weighing less than 500 g, is uncommon.[18,89,103] By this gestational age the fetus possesses T and B lymphocytes, macrophages, monocytes, polymorphonuclear cells and the capacity to synthesize all the immune factors that are currently known,[2,37,111,120] lacking only adequate amounts of transferred maternal immunoglobulin. The ability of neonatal T and B lymphocytes to generate cytokines is less than that of adults, but they are capable of generating appropriate adaptive immune responses.[62,119]

Some viruses are able to infect the fetus. These include CMV, rubella, some parvoviruses and HIV. The placenta is not very susceptible to virus infection, because its microvillous surface is shed continually into the maternal circulation. For a virus to reach the fetus, it requires to be transported within a cell traversing the placenta. Some maternal lymphocyte subpopulations do just this, and those viruses found to infect the fetus are known to have intralymphocytic phases.

When a fetus is infected by a virus the immune response is muted. The reasons for this difference are complex. Viral access to the fetus, within a transplacentally migrating maternal cell, is via the placental vein, through the liver and avoiding the lungs. Consequently, peripheral fetal organs are exposed to the virus. Viral replication is rapid in a manner that inactivates those T lymphocytes that express the appropriate specificities. However, the rapid spread of virus is limited by a highly efficient NK-like population of T cells. This response inhibits the fetus from eliminating the virus, although significant amounts of antibody are produced and may be found eventually in cord blood. Postnatally, virus may continue to replicate for a prolonged period and may be detected in urine. The reasons for this persistence lie most probably in the inactivation of antigen-reactive T lymphocytes, causing antigen unresponsiveness.[70] Eventually, this blockade is overcome and the virus may not be eliminated until many months after birth.

Postnatally, the preterm baby is frequently the victim of bacterial infection. Thompson[107] collected blood and culture specimens from 82 consecutive babies weighing less than 1500 g at birth. Samples were collected prospectively, at least twice weekly for the whole of each baby's stay in the neonatal unit. Laboratory measurements were correlated with a computer model of neonatal clinical risk factors. He showed that there were 927 suspected episodes of neonatal infection in these babies, of which half proved to have been genuine by standard criteria. Others have shown a similar incidence of infection in this group. However, the inadequacy of these babies' response to infection is directly related to their very low levels of maternal immunoglobulin, and is supported by the poor reaction both to dietary antigen and to natural bacterial colonization.

An important limitation on the ability of preterm babies to restrict invasion by microorganisms is the tenuous nature of their skin compared with term infants (see Maibach and Boisits[65] for an excellent review). The alternative pathway of complement activation is functional in preterm infants, even at the earliest gestations. However, levels of complement components are low, even at term, and the earlier the gestation the lower the concentrations. Rapidly progressive infections exhaust the complement system quickly. Cornification is poor and there are few cell layers to be penetrated. Fatty acid production is low and, after 2 weeks, gastric acid production falls steeply. The ability to produce local enzymes and defensins is not known. This is reflected by a high transepidermal water loss, which is directly related to gestational age and which falls in step with cornification.

On the other hand, although a direct skin breach may encourage local infection, the most important local cell of the immune system, the Langerhans' cell, is present by 18 weeks' gestation and, as antigen contacts grow, so the collections of plasma cells around Langerhans' cells increase. Integumental fragility is, therefore, one basis of increased risk of local infection in preterm babies, coupled with antigenic inexperience.

The cells of the GALT are present by 18 weeks' gestation and permit antigen processing in the bowel wall in as efficient a manner as in the term infant.[12,75] Consequently, milk feeding, even in extremely premature babies, is quite safe from an immunological point of view, and indeed may have much to commend it as it exposes babies to a wide range of antigens, safely, as early as possible.[10]

The preterm infant receives smaller amounts of maternal immunoglobulin than the term infant: the earlier the gestational age, the lower the quantity transferred. Babies who are born early and have low immunoglobulin levels take several months to achieve adequate circulating concentrations.[26,91] The serological response of these babies to routine immunization is less than that of term infants, although there is no evidence that there is a consequential increase in infection risk. Babies who have been given passive immunoglobulin in the neonatal period respond to immunization by generating higher antibody titres.[16,109]

Although there is conflict concerning the protection that passive immunoglobulin donation confers against infection in the preterm baby,[31,52,60] some published data reveal that there is a marked increase in circulating concentrations not only of IgG, the only immunoglobulin present in the commercial preparation used, but also of IgA and IgM in the serum of treated VLBW babies compared with controls.[39] The probable immunological basis of this effect is discussed above.

A recent meta-analysis of a series of papers on the effects of passive immunoglobulin donation to low birthweight infants suggested that no reduction in the rate of infection was demonstrable.[60] However, the majority of these studies were carried out in neonatal units with low rates of infection.[96] Furthermore, there have been no observations on subsequent morbidity and mortality after discharge from the neonatal unit, nor of the responses to routine immunization. More recent evidence supports the effectiveness of passive immunoglobulin donation to preterm infants.[52] Consequently, the value of passive immunoglobulin infusion to the preterm infant is, as yet, contentious and it is likely to be at least as valuable to the preterm neonate as G-CSF,[59,84] as phagocytosis is far more efficient when bacteria have been liberally opsonized.

NEONATAL IMMUNODEFICIENCY DISEASES

Congenital immunodeficiency diseases rarely present in the neonatal period, unless they affect granulocytes, and should be considered when there is a family history of immunodeficiency disease or recurrent infection, when there are abnormalities of the aortic arch, when hypocalcaemia is refractory to treatment or when the umbilical cord is slow to separate. The absence of lymph nodes, spleen, thymus or tonsils may alert the neonatologist to the possibility.

Newborn babies who develop pleomorphic or evanescent but recurrent skin rashes may have GVHD, to which T-lymphocyte deficiency states predispose. The common skin rash, erythema toxicum, is histologically similar to the rash of GVHD and may be a neonatal reaction to the infusion of maternal white cells during labour.[95]

Defects of phagocytosis and bacterial killing, involving polymorphonuclear cells and macrophages and dependent upon efficient opsonization, have the earliest effects. Commonly, they present in the first 3 months of life. Conversely, defects of lymphocyte function are rarely detected as a consequence of neonatal infection.[40] When the di George syndrome is diagnosed in the first month it usually follows the identification of a typical congenital cardiovascular anomaly, and not infection. However, recently it has become clear that deletions at 22q11 are relatively common and that the di George syndrome, consequent upon a 22q11.2 deletion, represents only one of these.[117]

Reticular dysgenesis, a condition in which all the white cells are deficient, is one of a few conditions involving a lymphocyte defect which may present neonatally with indolent infection.

Table 43.3 shows the various clinical symptoms that lead one to suspect the presence of an immunodeficiency state. Classically, the presence of persistent oral or perianal thrush, intractable diarrhoea and failure to thrive, suppurative otitis media and pleomorphic skin rashes are signs of immunodeficiency, but they are rarely seen in the first month of life.[11,87] The absence of those immunocompetent cells required for an adequate immune response is likely to allow tissue necrosis at the site of an infection, rather than suppuration: there may be no pus cells to congregate.

Table 43.3 Clinical clues to the possibility of neonatal immunodeficiency

Prenatal	
Family history of:	
Immunodeficiency disease	
Recurrent serious infections	
Autoimmune disease	
Unexplained infant death	
Glucose-6-phosphatase deficiency	
Short stature	
Isoimmunization	
Passive immunoglobulin given to mother	
Specific infection in pregnancy (e.g. cytomegalovirus)	
Maternal drug therapy (e.g. quinine, chlorpromazine)	
Clinical signs and symptoms	*Possible syndrome*
Non-specific dermatitis Persistent pneumonia Chronic otitis media Persistent diarrhoea Poor growth/failure to thrive Chronic moniliasis Very large or very small lymph nodes	Non-specific
Typical facies Persistent hypocalcaemic tetany Congenital heart disease Absent thymus on X-ray	Thymic aplasia (di George)
Absent eyebrows and thin friable hair	Cartilage–hair hypoplasia
Hepatosplenomegaly	Possible graft-versus-host disease
Seborrhoeic dermatitis and bleeding due to thrombocytopenia	Possible C5 deficiency Wiskott–Aldrich syndrome
Absent spleen on ultrasound	Asplenia
Delayed separation of the umbilical cord	Possible C3D receptor deficiency

PRIMARY IMMUNODEFICIENCIES PRESENTING IN THE NEONATE

Primary B-cell immunodeficiency

B-cell deficiencies rarely present in the neonatal period because the immune response, including the alternative pathway of complement activation in the presence of transferred maternal immunoglobulin, offers some protection from infection. The classic disease is the X-linked variety, which is most commonly caused by an abnormal gene at Xq22 which causes defective synthesis of tyrosine kinase. Other atypical forms have been reported.[19]

di George syndrome

This condition is the consequence of a deletion at 22q11.2 and leads to maldevelopment of the third and fourth pharyngeal pouches in early embryonic life.[117] Absence or hypoplasia of the parathyroid glands leads to neonatal hypocalcaemic tetany, which is resistant to treatment. Abnormalities of the aortic arch, commonly right-sided or double, sometimes together with complex congenital heart disease, cause neonatal symptoms and signs. Absence of the thymus prevents normal differentiation of T lymphocytes and is followed by postneonatal infection. Consequently, this is a deficiency primarily affecting T lymphocytes. These children also have a characteristic facies, with a small chin, down-slanting palpebral fissures, simple protuberant ears and a broad forehead.

The prognosis for children with thymic aplasia is that of their congenital heart disease. Calcium metabolism eventually self-regulates. In time, T lymphocytes mature in alternative bone marrow nurseries. Early treatment with bone marrow transplantation is successful but unnecessary, and aggressive treatment of infections is rewarded by the emergence of a competent immune system.[87] Table 43.4 outlines the various primary immunodeficiencies affecting the newborn child.

Severe combined immunodeficiency

Babies with severe combined immunodeficiency rarely present in the neonatal period. Maternal immunoglobulin, normal accessory cells, macrophages and granulocytes protect affected babies from infection. However, when infants with these syndromes are born preterm and denied adequate levels of maternal immunoglobulin, they may present with intractable infections, particularly with viruses or fungi. Furthermore, the clinical features of this condition are similar to those of AIDS, when it presents in early infancy.[28,112]

Mainly T-lymphocytes affected

This group includes Nezelof syndrome, purine nucleotide phosphorylase deficiency, defective T-cell-C3D receptor and SCID with normal immunoglobulin levels.[44,72]

Table 43.4 Description of primary immunodeficiencies, including those affecting the newly born. Deficiencies of phagocyte function tend to present in the youngest babies and in those affecting T-lymphocyte function next. B-lymphocyte abnormalities present later, which underlines the limited protection provided by maternal immunoglobulin

Immunodeficiency	Chromosomal site	Functional deficiency	Presents at term	Presents preterm	Presents in infancy
Mainly B cells affected					
Transient hypogammaglobulinaemia of infancy	–	None	Yes	Yes	Yes
X-linked agammaglobulinaemia (classical)	Xq22: Tyrosine kinase mutation	Antibody	No	No	Yes
X-linked agammaglobulinaemia: atypical type 1	Xq22: SH2 domain	Antibody	No	No	Yes
X-linked agammaglobulinaemia: atypical type 2	Xq22: N-terminal domain	Antibody	No	No	Yes
X-linked lymphoproliferative hypogammaglobulinaemia	Xq24–26	Anti-EBV NA antibody, T-cell defect?	No	No	Rarely
Common variable hypogammaglobulinaemia	6p21.3?	Antibody	No	No	Sometimes
Selective IgA deficiency	6p21.3?	IgA antibody	No	No	No
IgG Sub-class deficiencies	Unknown	Antibody	No	No	Rarely
Immunoglobulin heavy chain deletion	14q32.3	Antibody	No	No	Rarely
κ-chain deficiency	2p11	Antibody	No	No	Rarely
Mainly T cells affected					
di George syndrome	22q11.2	T cells; some antibody	Yes	Yes	Yes
X-linked immunodeficiency with hyper-IgM	Xq26	IgG and IgA	No	No	Rarely
Defective T-cell receptor-C3D immunodeficiency	11	T cells and anti-polysaccharide antibodies	No	No	Sometimes
Defective cytokine production	Unknown	IL2 IL4, IL5 & others	No	Not known	Yes
CD8 lymphopenia	2q12	T cells, some antibodies	No	Not known	Yes
Both T and B cells affected					
Combined (Nezelof) immunodeficiency (purine nucleotide phosphorylase deficiency)	14q13.1	CD3+ T-cell depletion	Yes	Yes	Yes
Cartilage–hair hypoplasia	(AR)	T-cell depletion (G1-phase block)	Yes	Yes	Yes
Severe combined immunodeficiency	Various (see below)	–	–	–	–
Autosomal recessive severe combined deficiency	(AR)	T & B cells depleted	Yes	Yes	Yes
Adenosine deaminase deficiency	20q13-ter	T & B cells depleted	Yes	Yes	Yes
X-linked severe combined immunodeficiency	Xq13	T & B cells depleted	Yes	Yes	Yes
Reticular dysgenesis	Unknown	No stem cells	Yes	Yes	Yes
Defective HLA expression: class I	6 ? site	No HLA class I expression	Yes	Yes	Yes

Table 43.4 (*contd*)

Immunodeficiency	Chromosomal site	Functional deficiency	Presents at term	Presents preterm	Presents in infancy
Defective HLA expression: class II	6 ? site	No HLA class II expression	Yes	Yes	Yes
Defective HLA expression: class I & II	6 ? site	No HLA class I *or* II expression	Yes	Yes	Yes
Omenn syndrome	(AR)	Very low immunoglobulins; impaired IFN-γ secretion	Yes	Yes	Yes
Wiskott–Aldrich syndrome	Xp11.22-23	No isohaemagglutinins; low response to polysaccharide antigens	Sometimes	Unknown	Yes
Ataxia telangiectasia	11q22.3	WASP protein	No	No	Rarely
Hyper-IgE syndrome	(AD?)	TH_1/TH_2 cell imbalance?	No	No	Rarely
Phagocytes affected					
'Septic' neutropenia	–	Reduced neutrophils	Yes	Yes	Yes
Neutropenia secondary to material hypertension	–	Reduced neutrophils	Yes	Yes	Yes
Chronic benign neutropenia	–	None	No	No	Rarely
Autoimmune neutropenia	–	Reduced neutrophils	Yes	No	Yes
Genetic infantile agranulocytosis (Kostmann's disease)	(AR)	Neutropenia secondary to low GM-CSF	Yes	Yes	Yes
Cyclic neutropenia	Unknown	Neutropenia with reduced phagocytosis	No	No	Rarely
Chediak–Higashi syndrome	(AR)	Abnormal neutrophil fluidity	Yes	Unknown	Yes
Myeloperoxidase deficiency	17-q.22-23	Reduced production of myeloperoxidase	No	No	No
Specific granule deficiency	Unknown	Absence of neutrophil alkaline phosphatase	No	No	No
X-linked chronic granulomatous disease type 1	X-p21	Reduced neutrophil NADPH oxidase	Yes	Yes	Yes
X-linked chronic granulomatous disease type 2	X-p21	Reduced neutrophil NADPH oxidase	Yes	Yes	Yes
Autosomal chronic granulomatous disease type 1	Unknown	Reduced neutrophil NADPH oxidase	Yes	Yes	Yes
Autosomal chronic granulomatous disease type 2	Unknown	Reduced neutrophil NADPH oxidase	Yes	Yes	Yes
Neutropenia in type 1b glycogen storage disease	(AR)	Reduced neutrophil production of glucose-6-phosphatase	Yes	Unknown	Yes
Schwachmann–Diamond syndrome	(AR)	Chemotactic defect	No	No	No
Barth syndrome	X-q2.8	Neutrophil dysfunction	Yes	Unknown	Yes
(Cartilage–hair hypoplasia)	(AR)	T-cell depletion (G1-phase block)	Yes	Yes	Yes
Dyskeratosis congenita	X-linked	Low neutrophils	Yes	Unknown	Yes
Onchotrichodysplasia and neutropenia	(AR)	Neutropenia: low GM-CSF?	Yes	Yes	Yes
Adhesion molecule deficiencies					
Type 1 leukocyte adhesion deficiency	Unknown	Absence of CD11a,b,c	Yes	Yes	Yes
Type 2 leukocyte adhesion deficiency	Unknown	Sialyl Lewis-X absence	Yes	Yes	Yes
Cell motility & chemotactic disorders					
Neonatal neutrophil hypomobility	Unknown	Slow chemotactic receptor expression	Yes	Yes	Yes
Neutrophil actin dysfunction	Unknown	Reductin actin contractility	Unknown	Unknown	Unknown
Hypophosphataemia	–	Low neutrophil alkaline phosphatase	No	No	Later
Kartagenar syndrome	–	Myofibrillar dysfunction	No	No	Later
Chromosome 7 abnormalities	7 ? site	Unknown	Unknown	Unknown	Unknown
Acrodermatitis enteropathica (zinc deficiency)	(AR)	Reduced intracellular bacterial killing	No	No	Yes
Increased microtubule assembly	Unknown	Myofibrillar dysfunction	Unknown	Unknown	Unknown

WASP, Wiskott–Aldrich serum protein

PNP deficiency is the consequence of a single-gene defect at 14q13.1, and the consequent defect in purine metabolism underlies the immunodeficiency. Affected children have very low levels of plasma and urinary uric acid. Two-thirds of patients have a wide variety of neurological abnormalities, from developmental delay through ataxia to severe spastic quadriparesis. They have also a tendency to develop autoimmune disease: up to 60% may have autoimmune haemolytic anaemia, idiopathic thrombocytopenia or systemic lupus erythematosus. Enzyme replacement therapy has not been effective, although bone marrow transplantation has been. Significant numbers of children diagnosed as having Nezelof syndrome have been found to be deficient in PNP, but there may be other causes of this form of SCID.[67]

T and B lymphocytes affected

This group includes adenosine deaminase deficiency (see below), the 'bare lymphocyte' syndrome (defective cell-surface HLA expression), autosomal recessive SCID, X-linked SCID due to the absence of IL2-γ chain, Omenn syndrome and reticular dysgenesis.[32,101]

ADA deficiency is the result of a single-gene defect on the short arm of chromosome 20.[94] X-linked SCID is due to a deletion at Xq13 which leads to a failure to synthesize the γ chain of IL2, a component of several critically important cytokine receptors. Omenn syndrome children lack the ability to synthesize interferon-γ and respond to it when given passively.

Babies with severe combined immunodeficiency may present in the neonatal period in a variety of ways. Some develop recurrent pleomorphic skin rashes, hair loss and increasingly severe erythroderma. This presentation may be similar to that seen in Letterer–Siwe disease. The presence of dramatic lymphadenopathy and hepatosplenomegaly should suggest the possibility of GVHD or chronic virus or fungal infections, as does intractable infection with *Candida albicans*, not only systemically but also superficially in multiple sites. A common syndrome in this group is chronic diarrhoea and failure to thrive, a consequence of the inability to generate an appropriate immune response to dietary antigens and to bacteria colonizing the bowel.

With dysmorphic features

Two varieties of SCID present with typical dysmorphisms: SCID with short limbed dwarfism, and SCID with cartilage–hair hypoplasia.

SCID with short-limbed dwarfism is a consequence of ADA deficiency: ADA is required for the normal development of the skeleton and these babies have chondro-osseous dysplasia, mostly seen at the costochondral junctions, the iliac apophyses and the vertebrae. There is a variety of point mutations and deletions from 20q13 to the N-terminus. The lack of adenosine deaminase leads to intracellular accumulation of adenosine and its metabolites, which causes lymphocyte apoptosis by inhibiting S-adenosylhomocysteine hydrolase. SAH inhibits intracellular methylation. The condition responds both to passive bovine ADA donation and to bone marrow transplantation.

SCID with cartilage–hair hypoplasia falls into the SCID with low lymphocytes group, but no particular genetic site has been ascribed to it as yet, although it is inherited as an autosomal recessive. It was initially described amongst the Pennsylvanian Amish, but cases have been described in other races. Children have hyperelastic skin and hypermobile joints, thin fine hair and sclerotic, cystic and eroded areas in the bony metaphyses. Survival is variable, the oldest surviving patients being in their 70s. Some children show poor antibody responses. Some are Nezelof-like, and about one-third have mixed T- and B-cell SCID.

Phagocyte deficiency

Infantile genetic agranulocytosis (Kostman's disease) and familial severe neutropenia are two rare disorders affecting granulocytes which may present neonatally. The former is due to an inability to synthesise G-CSF, but the abnormal gene has not yet been identified. Chediak–Higashi syndrome also presents in the newborn. The failure of phagocytic function found in these children probably resides in abnormal cell membrane fluidity and fusion, and causes the appearance of very large intracellular granules. Apart from the appropriate use of antibiotics, good effects have been seen with acyclovir, and bone marrow transplantation can help.[4,46]

The lazy leukocyte syndrome and Schwachmann syndrome do not usually present in the newborn period, nor do Job syndrome, chronic granulomatous disease or myeloperoxidase deficiency.[83]

Types I and II leukocyte adhesion deficiency present in the newborn. These depend upon the presence of a variety of mutations and deletions at 22q21.3, the site on chromosome 22 where the common β-subunit of LFA-I, MAC-I and p150.95 is encoded. The lack of these adhesion molecules reduces the effective margination of neutrophils to areas of infection, and so such children suffer from a variety of bacterial and fungal infections.[4,85]

Abnormalities of granulocyte chemotaxis and mobility have been described.[24] G6PD deficiency is associated with an increase in neonatal infections, probably as a consequence of hypofunction of the oxidative burst in bacterial killing.

When a newborn infant presents with recurrent bacterial infection, and when these infections seem more severe and intractable than one might expect for that infant's gestation and other clinical problems, an abnormality of granulocyte function should be considered.

DEFICIENCIES OF COMPLEMENT COMPONENTS AND RECEPTORS

Classical Pathway
C1q/C1r/C1s→C4→C2→C3→C5/C6/C7→C8/C9
Alternative Pathway
Factor B→Factor D→C3→C5/C6/C7→C8/C9

Deficiency of the early complement components, C1, C4, C2 and C3, may be associated with neonatal bacterial infection, but presentation and diagnosis at this age are uncommon.[54] Leiner's disease is the consequence of C5 dysfunction and presents with staphylococcal skin sepsis in the neonatal period, peeling skin and failure to thrive.

Deficiency of the CR3/CFA1/p150,95 membrane glycoprotein (a complement receptor) presents neonatally with delayed separation of the umbilical cord and recurrent bacterial infections.[88]

SECONDARY IMMUNODEFICIENCIES PRESENTING IN THE NEONATE

There remains a group of immunodeficiencies, some poorly defined, in which the condition is temporary or acquired.[41,101]

Transient and other immunodeficiencies

Some babies present with recurrent bacterial infections but have only marginal abnormalities of their immune systems. They may be found to have opsonic defects with respect to specific microorganisms, but a few are found to have a low-grade neutropenia, which returns to normal after some months. Immunodeficiency has been ascribed to drug therapy or to the presence of co-existing disorders, such as neonatal leukaemia, DIC or the loss of immunoglobulin and immunocompetent cells through damaged skin or enteropathy. When congenital virus infection is detected, an associated failure to demonstrate a normal immune response to the infecting organism has been designated an immunodeficiency disease. Abnormal immune responses in babies with Down syndrome have acquired the same cachet.[101]

Congenital aplastic anaemia is a special case, in that when the condition affects more than erythrocyte precursors a primary immunodeficiency is present. When only the red cells are affected, however, the consequent anaemia is associated with an increased rate of infection. Maintenance of an adequate haemoglobin level is sufficient treatment. Deficiency of folate or vitamin B_{12} leads to an increased infection rate, by a process analogous to the increase in the number of bacterial infections seen in babies with G6PD.[77]

HIV attacks the CD4-positive lymphocyte and slowly eliminates this lymphocyte subpopulation.[20,73] As these cells decline in number, so microorganisms are better able to infect the human host, especially opportunistic organisms of low pathogenicity.[9] There have been reports that suggest significant symptomatic benefit from treating HIV-infected babies with frequent doses of intravenous immunoglobulin, about 0.4 g/kg/month.[38]

INVESTIGATIONS

The most useful precept is to *think* that recurrent infection may indicate an underlying immunodeficiency disease. The next step is to have a helpful set of preliminary investigations, and the most important end-point is to know when further tests are not necessary. Table 43.5 describes a two-stage approach to the infant who may be immunodeficient. If the investigations

Table 43.5 Tests of immune function in the newborn infant

Stage I
Full blood count
White cell morphology, ideally by an experienced haematologist
HLA and CD cell surface markers on lymphocyte subsets
Serum C-reactive protein level
Serum immunoglobulins, with isotypes and subclasses
Serological response to (routine) tetanus immunization
Cultures of infected surfaces, blood, urine, stool, cerebrospinal fluid; for bacteria, fungi and viruses
Chest X-ray
Stage II
Clinical
Delayed hypersensitivity to streptokinase/streptodornase
Dinitrochlorobenzene sensitivity induction
Rebuck skin window, with observation of migratory responses
Lymph node biopsy, before and after local immunization
Humoral responses
B-cell subsets by CD markers
Specific antibody responses to *Salmonella* (IgM to O antigen, IgG to H antigen)
T- and B-cell coculture in vitro for specific antibody production
Immunoglobulin genetic typing (e.g. for Gm and Inv subgroups)
Cellular responses
Antibody responses to diphtheria and tetanus toxoids (for TH_1 cell function)
Thymic hormone levels
Mitogenic responses to phytohaemagglutinin, concanavalin A and human T-lymphocyte antigen
Mixed lymphocyte reactivity
T-cell responses in coculture with semiallogeneic T cells (e.g. from parent)
Phagocytic function
Nitroblue tetrazolium test
Bacterial and fungal phagocytosis and killing
Polymorphonuclear leukocyte mobility and chemotaxis
Glucose-6-phosphatase levels
Cytokine production
Specific measurement of cytokine production by selected cell subsets
Genetic studies
DNA analysis for specific nucleotide deletion, missense or translational defects

described in stage I are normal, no further investigations are required. Stage II is a more comprehensive study of the neonatal immune system and is most appropriately carried out in specialist centres, where the normal range of responses and values can be more reliably interpreted.[101]

TREATMENT OF THE IMMUNODEFICIENT NEONATE

MODE OF CARE

Babies with immunodeficiency disease should be cared for in the same manner as any low-birthweight newborn infant at risk from infection or suffering from severe sepsis. When a particular pathogen infects such a baby, dedicating specific nursing staff to their care may prevent the organism from spreading. Babies with serious immunodeficiency disease may require isolation in a positive air pressure room.

SUPPORTIVE TREATMENT

Infections of immunodeficient babies often have paradoxical effects. There may be no pus, because there are no pus cells; changes in temperature may not occur because mediators such as interleukin-1 are not generated; and there may be no lymphadenopathy, because lymphocytes are few. On the other hand, supportive treatment of these infected babies is more complex than for immunocompetent babies, because they are less able to limit the toxic effects of pathogens.

The choice of the appropriate antibiotic regimen should, ideally, wait upon the identification of the infecting organism. In practice, the antibiotic policy for the treatment of suspected infection used by most neonatal intensive care units – a penicillin together with an aminoglycoside – is adequate. However, many would advocate the use of a tertiary cephalosporin, such as ceftriaxone, although there is no evidence that this is more effective. The risk of fungal infection, with *Candida albicans* for example, is higher in this group and chronic virus infection is more likely to occur.

Nutrition

Babies with SCID or reticular dysgenesis may suffer from intractable diarrhoea and fail to thrive.[11,87] Nutrition must be adequate and digestible, as progressive catabolism may restrict their chances of successful bone marrow transplantation. Oral feeds with predigested milk, Pregestimil or Neocate may provide adequate sustenance. Carefully devised parenteral feeding regimens for the newborn have improved survival for the VLBW baby and are very useful in sustaining the immunodeficient infant. However, meticulous insertion and maintenance of the long intravenous lines necessary for this treatment is critically important to prevent septicaemia or fungaemia.

Transfusion

Blood transfusion is often needed by infected babies, but when there is immunodeficiency there is a risk of engraftment by immunocompetent donor cells and subsequent GVHD.[41] For this reason, transfusion using irradiated donor blood is recommended. There is evidence of long-term engraftment of donor cells in immunocompetent infants, for example following neonatal transfusion with large volumes of blood for rhesus D isoimmunization.[3,34,113] There is no evidence that engraftment in these otherwise healthy babies is clinically important. However, when immunodeficiency is a possibility it is prudent to irradiate any transfusion of blood cells, including platelet packs.

Immunization

Babies with immunodeficiency diseases may be peculiarly susceptible to persistent infection and illness following immunization with live attenuated virus vaccines. However, they will be even more at risk of severe morbidity from infection by 'wild' virus, so it is important to consider protecting them by immunization with appropriate immunogens. For example, children who have intact cellular immune responses may be able to tolerate live virus vaccines, or alternatively may be immunized safely with killed virus forms of the vaccine, such as that available to protect against poliomyelitis. It is best to define the immunodeficiency present in each child from a functional viewpoint and to choose an immunization protocol that is appropriate to their clinical risks.

Immune factors

A range of soluble products derived from various cells of the immune system have been employed in attempts to boost the immune response in a variety of clinical situations. These include transfer factor, IFN-γ, IL1 and IL2.[66,112] More recently, G-CSF has been used.[42,84] Recent studies of the effects of passive immunoglobulin donation demonstrate its value in clinical situations where there is a high risk of infection.[1] Now that some immunodeficiencies have been found to depend upon the absence of particular molecules, such as variants of SCID with deficiencies of IL2 or receptor abnormalities, these therapies can be employed in a much more disease-specific fashion.[59]

Interferons may be valuable in congenital infections with viruses such as Coxsackie, by promoting the differentiation of NK precursors and by protecting uninfected cells.[76] New factors with special functions are being reported and may have potential roles in the treatment of neonatal infection.

Bone marrow transplantation

The general aim of BMT in immunodeficiency is to replace a 'missing' subset of immunosignificant cells. However, BMT is also used as a vehicle for the transfer of genes, to replace missing or defective allotypes which have been identified as the bases of a wide range of metabolic diseases.

Organ transplantation in the newborn is technically more difficult, because of constraints imposed both by size and by the need for subsequent growth. However, BMT requires less manual dexterity than that of the heart, but the greater ease with which immunological unresponsiveness develops has permitted early heart transplantation. Where feasible, BMT should be deferred until the second year of life. In spite of this stricture, there are case reports and some small series of BMT as therapy for congenital immunodeficiency disease and haemoglobinopathies, as well as combined BMT plus homologous thymic transplantation for some athymic children.[82,104]

Initial identification of the immunodeficient baby's HLA haplotypes is essential. This can be performed by cDNA hybridization on nuclear material prepared from a frozen specimen of whole peripheral blood, so there is no need for a sample containing a significant number of circulating cells of the immune system bearing these antigens on their surfaces.[118] The development of the polymerase chain reaction has allowed us to produce very large numbers of copies of single genes from individuals.

Clearly, the more HLA genes are shared both by bone marrow donor and recipient, the more likely is BMT to be effective. However, parent-to-child BMT carries a high risk of GVHD, as the baby possesses an HLA haplotype from the other parent.[5] Sibling grafts from a brother or sister whose HLA type matches or closely matches that of the patient are the most effective.

However, the chances of a matching sibling are small, and this has led to the establishment of bone marrow donor registers, as the odds against finding an HLA match from many unrelated volunteers are high. Unfortunately, BMT using unrelated matched donors is far less successful than using siblings, but this has not prevented continuing attempts because of the lack of therapeutic alternatives.

The management of BMT is complex and a matter for the specialist. Babies suitable for treatment should be transferred to a recognized centre after establishing, first, whether the child has an appropriate condition for BMT and, secondly, whether there is an HLA-matched donor. An increasing armamentarium of supportive treatment, such as antilymphocyte serum, interferons, prednisolone and cyclosporin A, which are capable of interfering with cell communication in a variety of ways, has increased the success of BMT and made it available to younger patients. The commoner complications, such as cytomegalovirus infection and other chronic lung infections, can be more effectively treated and sometimes their incidence reduced by pre-BMT immunization.

Graft-versus-host disease

When a bone marrow transplant is carried out, haemopoietic stem cells seed the host's marrow. The mature cells of the immune system that they produce must share at least some of the cell surface molecular markers of the MHC with the host, in order to recognize and cooperate with host cells. When there are MHC differences between them, grafted lymphocytes may attack host cells, causing GVHD.[78]

Maternal cells cross routinely from mother to fetus. This normal situation does the fetus no harm as the fetal immune system eliminates these cells, while mothers tolerate a balanced state of chimerism with respect to fetal lymphocytes that cross into their circulation. The immunodeficient fetus, however, is unable to limit the action of maternal lymphocytes and may develop GVHD. The characteristic features of GVHD are a maculopapular skin rash, cholestatic hepatitis, and enteritis with diarrhoea. The characteristic papules are identical with the rash of erythema toxicum, both clinically and histologically. It seems likely that erythema toxicum is an expression of a *forme fruste* of GVHD in an immunologically competent baby. As loose stools are common and cholestatic jaundice not infrequent in the newly born, it is not easy to investigate this possibility.[74]

Babies with severe combined immunodeficiency may present with erythroderma, hair and eyebrow loss, diarrhoea and jaundice as a consequence of maternal antifetal GVHD. The progression of GVHD can lead to chronic multisystem autoimmune disease, including a lupus-like syndrome and biliary cirrhosis.

The risk of inducing a secondary GVHD in babies with congenital immunodeficiency disease by blood transfusion is serious. Consequently, it is vital to maintain a high index of suspicion and to use only irradiated matched genotyped blood for transfusion when congenital immunodeficiency is thought to be a possibility.[29,30]

Gene therapy

Genes are being manufactured and presented as artificial transposons (genes which are capable of transfecting the DNA of one individual to the DNA of another), but attempts to pass them into the DNA of living human cells and make them susceptible to appropriate biological activation are proving much more difficult. The identification of deleterious genes made before conception, by the extension of longitudinal family studies and analysis in chorionic villus samples, is offering tantalizing opportunities for therapy which cannot yet be realized. Fetuses with immunodeficiency diseases will eventually be treatable with the appropriate artificial transposon, as will any identified genetic disorder in which survival past embryogenesis is possible. Whether this approach will be preferable to the elimination of abnormal fetuses by termination of pregnancy is a complex ethical issue.[90]

REFERENCES

1. Acunas B A, Peakman M, Liossis G et al 1994 Effect of fresh frozen plasma and gammaglobulin on humoral immunity in neonatal sepsis. Archives of Disease in Childhood 70: F182–F187
2. Adinolfi M 1988 New and old aspects of the ontogeny of immune responses. In: Stern C M M (ed) Immunology of pregnancy and its disorders. Kluwer, Dordrecht, pp 33–60
3. Almeida J M de, Rosado L 1972 Rh blood group of grandmother and incidence of erythroblastosis. Archives of Disease in Childhood 47: 609–612
4. Anderson D C 1989 Neonatal neutrophil dysfunction. American Journal of Pediatric Hematology and Oncology 11: 224–231
5. Atkinson K 1990 Chronic graft-versus-host disease. Bone Marrow Transplantation 5: 69–84
6. Baker D A, Milch P O, Salvatore W, Luft J 1987 Enhancement of maternal and neonatal natural killer cell activity with interleukin 2. American Journal of Obstetrics and Gynecology 157: 780–781
7. Bayley J E, Kleigman R M, Boxerbaum B, Fanaroff A A 1986. Fungal colonisation in very low birthweight babies. Pediatrics 78: 225–232
8. Beer A E 1988 Immunotherapy in reproductive disorders. In: Stern C M M (ed) Immunology of pregnancy and its disorders. Kluwer, Dordrecht, pp 165–196
9. Bernstein I J, Kreiger B Z, Novck B et al 1985 Bacterial infections in the acquired immunodeficiency syndrome of children. Pediatric Infectious Disease Journal 4: 472–475
10. Björkstein B 1986 Immune response to ingested antigens in relation to feeding pattern in childhood. Annals of Allergy 57: 143–146
11. Buckley R H 1994 Breakthroughs in the understanding and therapy of pediatric immunodeficiency. Pediatric Clinics of North America 41: 665–708
12. Cadranel S, Zeglache S, Jonckheer T et al 1987 Factors affecting antibody response of newborns to repeated administration of the rotavirus vaccine RIT 4237. Journal of Pediatric Gastroenterology 6: 525–528
13. Cavagni G, Paganelli R, Caffarelli C et al 1988 Passage of food antigen into circulation of breastfed infants with atopic dermatitis. Annals of Allergy 61: 361–365
14. Chandra R K, Puri S, Suraiya C, Cheema P S 1986 Influence of maternal food antigen avoidance during pregnancy and lactation on incidence of atopic eczema in infants. Clinical Allergy 16: 563–567
15. Christenson K L, Christenson P 1988 IgG subclasses and neonatal infections with group B streptococcus. Monographs in Allergy 88: 138–147
16. Conway S, James J, Balfour A, Smithells R 1993 Immunization of the preterm infant. Journal of Infection 27: 143–150
17. Cooper D W, Hill J A, Chesley L C, Bryant C I 1988 Genetic control of susceptibility to eclampsia and miscarriage. British Journal of Obstetrics and Gynaecology 13: 496–499
18. Costeloe K, for the EPICure Study Steering Group 1997 Survival and morbidity of infants born at the extremes of life. Proceedings of the First Annual Meeting of the Royal College of Paediatrics and Child Health, pp 31, P5
19. Cunningham-Rundles C 1989 Clinical and immunologic analyses of 103 children with common variable immunodeficiency. Journal of Clinical Immunology 9: 22–34
20. Cunningham-Rundles S, Chen C, Bussel J B et al 1993 Human immune development: implications for congenital HIV infection (review). Annals of the New York Academy of Sciences 693: 20–34
21. Davies M, Browne L M 1985 Anti-trophoblast antibody responses during normal human pregnancy. Journal of Reproductive Immunology 7: 285–297
22. de Martino M, Rossi M E, Novembre E, Vierucci A 1988 Occurrence and subclass distribution of IgG antibodies to dietary antigens in children with atopic dermatitis and in their mothers. Annals of Allergy 61: 253–258
23. Dinarello C A 1996 Biology of interleukin 1 in disease. Blood 57: 2095–2147
24. Downey G P 1994 Mechanisms of leukocyte mobility and chemotaxis. Current Opinion in Immunology 6: 113–124
25. Ellis S A, Sargent I L, Redman C W G, MacMichael A J 1986 Evidence for a novel HLA antigen found on human extravillous trophoblast and a chorioncarcinoma cell line. Immunology 6: 167–174
26. Evans H E, Akpata S O, Glass L 1971 Serum immunoglobulin levels in premature and full term infants. American Journal of Clinical Pathology 56: 416–421
27. Falth-Magnussen K, Kjellman N I, Magnussen I L E 1988 Antibodies IgG, IgA and IgM to food antigens during the first eighteen months of life in relation to feeding and development of atopic disease. Journal of Allergy and Clinical Immunology 81: 743–749
28. Fauci A S 1993 Multifactorial nature of human immunodeficiency virus disease: implications for therapy. Science 262: 1011–1018
29. Filipovitch A H, Shapiro R S, Ramsay N K C et al 1992 Unrelated donor bone marrow transplantation for correction of lethal congenital immunodeficiencies. Blood 80: 270–276
30. Fischer A, Landais P, Friedrich W et al 1994 Bone marrow transplantation (BMT) in Europe for primary immunodeficiencies other than severe combined immunodeficiency: a report from the European Group for BMT and the European Group for Immunodeficiency. Blood 83: 1149–53
31. Fischer G W 1988 Therapeutic uses of intravenous gammaglobulin for pediatric infections. Pediatric Clinics of North America 35: 97–126
32. Geha R S, Reinherz E 1983 Identification of T- and B-lymphocytes in uncomplicated severe combined immunodeficiency by HLA typing of sub-populations of T-cells separated by the fluorescence-activated cell sorter, and of EB-virus-derived clones. Journal of Immunology 130: 2493–2496
33. Genetet N, Genetet B, Amice V, Fauchet R 1985 Allogeneic responses in vivo induced by feto-maternal allo-immunization. American Journal of Reproductive Immunology 2: 90–96
34. Gill T J III 1977 Chimerism in humans. Transplantation Proceedings IX: 1423–1428
35. Gitlin D, Kumate J, Urrusti J, Morales C 1964 The selectivity of the human placenta in the transfer of plasma proteins from mother to fetus. Journal of Clinical Investigation 43: 1938–1951
36. Goodman A S, Ham-Pong A J, Goldblum R M 1985 Host defences: development and maternal contributions. Advances in Pediatrics 32: 71–100
37. Griffiths-Chu S, Patterson J A K, Berger C L, Edelson R C, Chu A L 1984 Characterisation of immature T-cell sub-populations in neonatal blood. Blood 64: 296–300
38. Hague R A, Yap P L, Mok J Y O et al 1989 Intravenous immunoglobulin in HIV infection: evidence for efficacy of treatment. Archives of Disease in Childhood 64: 1146–1150
39. Haque K N, Zaidi M H, Haque S K, Bahakim H, El-Hazmi M, El-Swailam M 1986 Intravenous immunoglobulin for prevention of sepsis in pre-term and low birthweight infants. Pediatric Infectious Disease Journal 5: 622–625
40. Hayward A R 1976 Immunodeficiency. In: Turk J (ed) Current topics in immunology, 6, 125–147
41. Hayward A R 1983 Development of immunity mechanisms. In: Soothill J F, Hayward A R, Wood C B S (eds) Paediatric immunology. Blackwell, Edinburgh, pp 48–55
42. Hibi S, Yoshihara T, Nakajima F, Misu H, Mabuci O, Imashuku S 1994 Effect of recombinant human granulocyte-colony stimulating factor (rhG-CSF) on immune system in pediatric patients with aplastic anaemia. American Journal of Pediatric Hematology and Oncology 11: 19–23
43. Hill H R 1987 Biochemical, structural and functional abnormalities of polymorphonuclear leukocytes in the neonate. Paediatric Research 22: 375–382
44. Hirschhorn R 1990 Adenosine deaminase deficiency. Immunodeficiency Reviews 2: 175–198
45. Hunt J S 1992 Biology of pregnancy. Current Opinion in Immunology 4: 1–244
46. Hutchinson R, Boxer L A 1990 Disorders of granulocyte and monocyte

production. In: Benz E J, Cohen H J, Furie B (eds) Hematology: basic principles and practice. Churchill Livingstone, New York. pp 193–204
47. Isberg R R 1991 Discrimination between intracellular uptake and surface adhesion of bacterial pathogens. Science 252: 934–938
48. Jain L, Viyasagar D, Xanthou M, Ghai V, Shimada S, Bueno M 1976 In vivo distribution of human milk leukocytes after ingestion by newborn baboons. Archives of Disease in Childhood 64: 930–933
49. Janeway C A, Travers P 1996 Immunobiology: the immune system in health and disease, 2nd edn. Current Biology, London
50. Jakubovsky J, Brozman M, Hereeny K et al 1988 Morphological changes in the proximal jejunum and in the skin of children with atopic eczema are of a similar nature. Bratislavske Lakarske Listy 89: 483–494
51. Jelliffe D B, Jelliffe E F 1985 Breast-feeding and immunity: adaptable defense in depth. Journal of Tropical Paediatrics 31: 66–67
52. Jensen H B, Powrie B H 1997 Meta-analysis of the effectiveness of intravenous immunoglobulin for the prevention and treatment of neonatal sepsis. Pediatrics, 99: e2: 246
53. Johnson P M 1984 Immunobiology of human trophoblast. In: Crichton D B (ed) Immunological aspects of reproduction in mammals. Butterworths, London, pp 56–71
54. Johnson R B Jr 1995 Disorders of the complement system. In: Stiehm E R (ed) Immunological disorders in infants and children, 4th edn. W B Saunders, Philadelphia, pp 125–146
55. Kilpatrick D C, Liston W A, Gibson F, Livingstone J 1989 Susceptibility to pre-eclampsia within families is associated with HLA-DR4. Lancet ii: 369–375
56. Kind C 1986 What does neutropenia tell about the existence of sepsis in the newborn? Helvetica Paediatrica Acta 41: 277–289
57. Kochenour N K, Scott J R 1985 Rhesus iso-immunization in pregnancy. In: Scott J R, Roten S (eds), Immunology in obstetrics and gynaecology. Appleton-Century-Crofts, Norwalk, pp 853–872
58. Kovats S, Main E L, Librach C, Stubblebine M, Fischer S J, DeMars R 1990 A class I antigen, HLA-G, expressed in human trophoblast. Science 248: 220–223
59. Kruskal B A, Ezekowitz A B 1994 Cytokines in the treatment of primary immunodeficiency. Biotherapy 7: 249–259
60. Lacey J B, Ohlsson A 1995 Administration of intravenous immunoglobulins for prophylaxis or treatment of infection in pre-term infants: meta-analyses. Archives of Disease in Childhood 72: F151–155
61. Lascelles A K, Gurnor B W, Coombs R R A 1969 Some properties of human colostral cells. Australian Journal of Experimental Biology and Medical Science 47: 349–360
62. Lawton A R 1994 Immunization of the neonate (review). International Journal of Technology Assessment in Health Care 10: 154–160
63. Leung D Y, Schneerberger E E, Siraganian R P, Geha R S, Bhan A K 1987 The presence of IgE on macrophages and dendritic reticulum cells infiltrating into the lesion of atopic dermatitis. Clinical Immunology and Immunopathology 42: 328–337
64. Leventhal J M, Shapiro E D, Aten C B, Berg A T, Egerton S A 1986 Does breastfeeding protect against infections in infants less than three months of age? Pediatrics 78: 896–903
65. Maibach H A, Boitsis E R 1982 Neonatal skin: structure and function. Marcel Dekker, New York
66. Male D, Champion B, Cooke A 1987 Lymphokines. In: Male D, Champion B, Cooke A (eds) Advanced immunology. Mosby, London pp 11.1–11.8
67. Markert M L 1991 Purine nucleotide phosphorylase deficiency. Immunodeficiency Reviews 3: 45–62
68. Metcalfe D 1986 The molecular biology and functions of the granulocyte–macrophage colony stimulating factor. Blood 67: 257–271
69. Mowbray J F, Gibbings C, Liddell H, Reginald P, Underwood J L, Beard R W 1985 Controlled trial of treatment of recurrent spontaneous abortion by immunization with paternal cells. Lancet i: 941–943
70. Müller G (ed) 1993 Peripheral T-cell immunological tolerance. Immunological Reviews 133: 1–240
71. Müller G, Coutinho A 1975 Factors influencing activation of B-cells in immunity. Annals of the New York Academy of Science 249: 68–88
72. Noguchi M, Yi H, Rosenblatt H M et al 1993 Interleukin-2 receptor gamma-chain mutation results in X-linked severe combined immunodeficiency. Cell 73: 147–157
73. Nadal D, Hunziker U A, Schupbach J et al 1989 Immunological evaluation in the early diagnosis of prenatal or perinatal HIV infection. Archives of Disease in Childhood 64: 662–669
74. Nash R A, Pepe M S, Storb R et al 1992 Acute graft-versus-host disease: analysis of risk factors after allogeneic marrow transplantation and prophylaxis with cyclosporin and methotrexate. Blood 80: 1838–1844
75. Ogura H 1987 Serum antibodies to *Escherichia coli* in breastfed infants. Acta Medica Okayama 41: 161–163
76. Paulnock D M 1992 Macrophage activation by T-cells. Current Opinion in Immunology 4: 344–349
77. Pletsityi K D 1993 Vitamins and immunity. Vaprosy Pitaniia 3: 4–9
78. Quinones R R 1993 Haematopoietic engraftment and graft failure after bone marrow transplantation. American Journal of Pediatric Hematology and Oncology 15: 3–18
79. Raulet D H, Held W 1995 Natural killer cell receptors: the offs and ons of NK cell recognition. Cell 82: 697–700
80. Redman C W G 1985 Immunological aspects of eclampsia and pre-eclampsia. In: Hearn J P (ed) Immunological aspects of reproduction and fertility control. MTP Press, Lancaster pp 83–103
81. Reth M 1992 Antigen receptors on B lymphocytes. Annual Review of Immunology 10: 97–118
82. Robertson K A 1993 Pediatric bone marrow transplantation. Current Opinion in Pediatrics 5: 103–121
83. Ricevuti G, Mazzone A 1987 Clinical aspects of neutrophil locomotor disorders. Biomedicine and Pharmacotherapy 41: 355–367
84. Rodwell, Gray P H, Taylor K M, Manchester R 1996 Granulocyte colony stimulating factor treatment for auto-immune neonatal neutropenia. Archives of Disease in Childhood 75: F57–58
85. Rosales C, Brown E J 1993 Neutrophil receptors and modulation of the immune response. In: Abramson J S, Wheeler J G (eds) The natural immune system. IRL Press, New York, pp 24–62
86. Rose N R, MacKay I R 1992 The immune response in autoimmunity and autoimmune disease. In: Rose N R, MacKay I R (eds) The autoimmune diseases II. Academic Press, Orlando, pp 1–26
87. Rosen F S 1986 Defects in cell-mediated immunology. Clinical Immunology and Immunopathology 41: 1–7
88. Ross G D 1987 Abnormalities of membrane complement receptors associated with disease. Recent Advances in Clinical Immunology 4: 61–78
89. Saigal S, Rosenbaum P, Stotskopf B, Sinclair J C 1984 Outcome in infants 501–1000 g birthweight delivered to residents of the McMaster health region. Journal of Pediatrics 105: 969–976
90. Salvetti A, Heard J M, Danos O 1995 Gene therapy for lysozymal storage disorders. British Medical Bulletin 51: 106–122
91. Sasidharan P 1988 Postnatal IgG levels in very-low-birthweight babies: preliminary observations. Clinical Pediatrics 27: 271–274
92. Scott J R 1985 Immunologic diseases in pregnancy. In: Scott J R, Rote N S (eds) Immunology in obstetrics and gynaecology. Appleton-Century-Crofts, Norwalk, pp 165–196
93. Scott J S, Maddison P J, Taylor P V, Escher E, Scott O, Skinner R P 1983 Connective tissue, antibodies to ribonucleoprotein and congenital heart block. New England Journal of Medicine 309: 209–212
94. Schuurman R K B, Mansink E J B M, Schot J O L 1987 Molecular biology and genetics of the immune system and immunodeficiency disease. Advances in Clinical Immunology 4: 201–220
95. Schwartz R A, Janniger C K 1996 Erythema toxicum neonatorum. Cutis 58: 153–155
96. Sideropoulos D, Boehme U, von Muralte G et al 1981 Immunoglobulin supplementation in the management of neonatal sepsis. Schweizerische Medizinische Wochenschrift 111: 1649–1653
97. Solomon J B 1971 Fetal and neonatal immunology. In: Neuberger A, Tatum E L (eds) Frontiers of biology. North Holland, Amsterdam, pp 96–138
98. Speer C P, Johnson R B 1984 Phagocyte function. In: Pearay W (ed) Neonatal infections: nutritional and immunologic interactions. Raven Press, New York:
99. Splawski J B, Jelinek D F, Lipsky P E 1991 Delineation of the functional capacity of human neonatal lymphocytes. Journal of Clinical Investigation 87: 545–553
100. Splawski J B, Lipsky P E 1991 Cytokine regulation of immunoglobulin secretion by neonatal B-cells. Journal of Clinical Investigation 88: 967–977
101. Stiehm E R (ed) 1995 Immunological disorders in infants and children, 4th edn. W B Saunders, Philadelphia
102. Stern C M M 1988 Genetics of reproduction. In: Stern C M M (ed) Immunology of pregnancy and its disorders. Kluwer, Dordrecht, pp 197–214

103. Stewart A 1985 Follow-up bei kinder mit sehr niedrigem Geburtsgewicht (VLBW). In: Kleiniches Management 'Kleinen' Frühgebornen (<1500 g), Georg Thieme Verlag, Stuttgart, pp 9–17
104. Storb R, Thomas E D 1988 Transplantation of bone marrow. In: Samfer S, Talmage D W, Frank M, Austen K F, Claman H N (eds) Immunological disease, 4th edn. Marcel Dekker, New York, pp 467–495
105. Thomas M L, Harger J H, Wagener D K, Rabin D S, Gill T J III 1985 HLA sharing and spontaneous abortion in humans. American Journal of Obstetrics and Gynecology 151: 1053–1057
106. Thompson A (ed) 1994 The cytokine handbook, 2nd edn. Academic Press, San Diego
107. Thompson A R 1992 The incidence of infection in very low birthweight neonates: correlation with endotoxinaemia. MD thesis, University of Cambridge, Cambridge
108. Toivanen P, Uksila J, Leino A, Lassila O, Hirunen T, Ruuskanen O 1983 Development of mitogen-responsive T-cells and natural killer cells in the human fetus. Immunological Reviews 57: 89–105
109. Topsis J, Kandace S, Weinstein J, Wilets I, 1994 Tolerance of initial diphtheria–tetanus–pertussis immunization in preterm infants. Journal of Perinatology 16: 98–102
110. Tsuji T, Nibu R, Iwai K et al 1994 Effective induction of immunoglobulin production in neonatal naive B-cells by memory CD4+ T cell subset expressing homing receptor L-selectin. Journal of Immunology 152: 4417–4424
111. Tucci A, Mouzaki A, James H, Bennefoy J Y, Zubler R H 1991 Are cord blood B cells functionally mature? Clinical and Experimental Immunology 84: 389–394
112. Voss S D, Hong R, Sondel P M 1994 Severe combined immunodeficiency, interleukin-2 (IL-2) and the IL-2 receptor: experiments of nature continue to point the way. Blood 84: 626–632
113. Walkanowska J, Conte F A, Grumbach M M 1969 Practical and theoretical implications of fetal–maternal lymphocyte transfer. Lancet i: 1119–1120
114. Walker W A 1986 Allergen absorption in the intestine: implications for food allergy in children. Journal of Allergy and Clinical Immunology 78: 1003–1009
115. Walker W A 1987 Pathophysiology of intestinal uptake and absorption of antigens in food allergy. Annals of Allergy 59: 7–16
116. Watson W, Oen K, Ramdahin R, Harman C 1991 Immunoglobulin and cytokine production by neonatal lymphocytes. Clinical and Experimental Immunology 83: 169–174
117. Webber S A, Hatchwell E, Barber J C et al 1996 Incidence of microdeletions of chromosome 22q11 as a cause of selected malformations of the ventricular outflow tracts and aortic arch. Journal of Pediatrics 129: 26–32
118. Weiss E H, Kuon W, Dorner C, Lang M, Reithmüller G 1985 Ontogeny, sequence and expression of the HLA-B27 gene: a molecular approach to analyse HLA and disease associations. Immunology 170: 367–380
119. Wilson C B 1986 Immunological basis for increased susceptibility of the neonate to infection. Journal of Pediatrics 108: 1–12
120. Wilson C B, Lewis D B, English B K 1991 T-cell development in the fetus and neonate. Advances in Experimental Medicine and Biology 310: 17–27
121. Wood G W, Bjerrum K, Johnson B 1982 Detection of IgG bound within the human placenta. Placenta 2: 355–370
122. Wosler L B, Lawton R 1985 Ontogeny of B-cells and humoral immune function. Clinical Immunology and Allergy 5: 235–252

Part 2

Infection in the newborn

Peter Dear

Infection, as either prime pathology or a complication of other illness, is a major cause of neonatal mortality and morbidity throughout the world. The incidence of culture-confirmed neonatal sepsis in the USA is in the region of 0.7%.[832] Most infections occur in babies admitted to neonatal units, and a comprehensive study of systemic bacterial and fungal infections in neonatal units in Australia produced incidence figures of 0.22% for early-onset and 0.44% for late-onset sepsis.[535] The mortality rate for early-onset sepsis was 15% and for late-onset sepsis 9%. In a recent prospective study of bloodstream infections in three North American neonatal units 11.2% of all babies had culture-proven sepsis.[79] Among infants requiring neonatal intensive care the incidence of infection is twice as high, with a mortality rate of about 16%,[400] although interestingly, in a recent review of the rate of infection among 5000 babies treated with extracorporeal membrane oxygenation, a rate of infection of only 3.5% was documented.[266] Among very low birthweight infants undergoing prolonged intensive care the rate of culture-proven sepsis may be as high as 30%, with a mortality rate of 30%.[832] In the developing world neonatal sepsis is a greater problem. A recent study from Malaysia reported rates of neonatal sepsis of 5–10%, with case fatality rates of between 23 and 52%. Septicaemia accounted for between 11 and 30% of all neonatal deaths.[127] In Ghana the mortality rate for culture-proven neonatal sepsis is 37%.[36]

The impact of infection can be reduced, as international comparisons show, but even in the most technologically advanced countries the contribution of sepsis to neonatal mortality and morbidity remains unacceptably high. The combination of a susceptible host, non-specific clinical presentation and an ever-changing population of pathogens makes for a great challenge. This chapter presents a systematic review of the pathogenesis, prevention, diagnosis and treatment of neonatal infection.

THE PATHOGENESIS OF NEONATAL INFECTION

The fetus normally encounters no microorganisms during development, and the newborn infant becomes harmlessly colonized by bacteria acquired from the birth canal and the environment. This happy state of affairs is evidence of the integrity of the barrier to infection provided by the placenta and membranes, the low pathogenicity of most colonizing organisms and the relative competence of the baby's defence mechanisms. It is usually when one or other of these factors is altered that fetal or neonatal infection occurs. These ideas provide a useful conceptual framework within which to discuss specific infections in detail.

EXPOSURE TO MICROORGANISMS

Transplacental

Certain infective agents have an inherent ability to penetrate the placental barrier, often damaging the placenta in the process, e.g. rubella virus (p. 1168). The effects on the fetus are often devastating.

Ascending

Ascent of vaginal organisms into the uterine cavity prior to rupture of the membranes is rare but well recognized.[90] Once the membranes rupture the risk increases progressively with time.

Intrapartum

Vaginal delivery inevitably results in contamination and the beginning of colonization of the skin and the gut. The pattern of organisms and the heaviness of colonization are usually closely similar between mother and baby[687] (Fig. 43.1). Vaginal flora vary considerably from woman to woman,[687] and many cases of early-onset neonatal sepsis result from the vaginal carriage of opportunistic pathogens. Another potential source of intrapartum bacterial contamination is from the water used for 'water births'.[489]

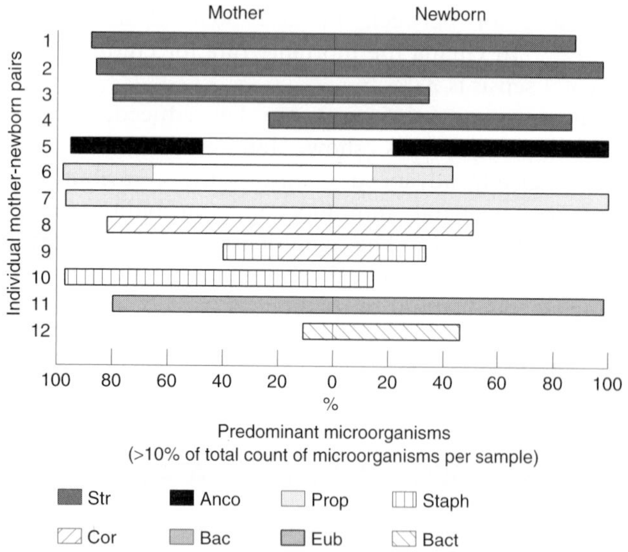

Fig. 43.1 Relationship between maternal and infant colonizing flora. The figure shows the predominant species of microorganism grown from the baby's ear and the maternal vagina in 12 mother–infant pairs. (From Mandar and Mikelsaar[687] with permission) *Str, streptococci; Anco, anaerobic cocci; Prop, propionibacteria; Staph, staphylococci; Cor, corynebacteria; Bac, bacilli; Eub, eubacteria; Bact, bacteroides.*

Postnatal

In addition to the organisms acquired during birth, all babies are subject to further microbiological contamination from the environment. People are the main source of such contamination.

COLONIZATION

Bacterial colonization is the inevitable lot of all creatures and it generally brings advantages. Competitive inhibition of potential pathogens is an important benefit, and as an example it can be shown that pharyngeal colonization of the newborn with *Streptococcus viridans* reduces the risk of serious bacterial illness.[343]

Colonization of normal infants

The nature of colonizing organisms is determined by the pattern of flora in the birth canal and in the environment. Babies born at home are colonized by organisms derived primarily from the mother.[575] These organisms, and those acquired from other family members, tend to be community-derived antibiotic-sensitive organisms of limited pathogenicity, although even women choosing home delivery may harbour serious potential pathogens such as GBS. On the postnatal ward the baby will acquire organisms from the ward environment, other babies and the clinical staff. The chance of encountering pathogens and their variety is considerably greater here than in the home environment.

The predominant intestinal organisms acquired by normal babies are enterobacteria (including *Escherichia coli*, *Klebsiella* sp. and *Citrobacter* sp., *Bacteroides* sp., enterococci, staphylococci, *Lactobacillus* sp. and *Bifidobacteria* sp. Breast-feeding reduces the intensity of colonization by the Enterobacteriaceae[13] and *Bifidobacteria* sp. tend to predominate in breast-fed infants.[64,65,1137]

Colonization of the upper respiratory tract occurs rapidly, and 90% of infants have positive pharyngeal cultures by the third day. Coagulase-negative staphylococci are commonest, followed by *Str. viridans* and *Staphylococcus aureus*.[343] Exclusive breast-feeding does not influence the pattern of nasopharyngeal colonization compared with exclusive formula feeding.[562]

Skin colonization is very rapid, with the number of bacteria increasing 100-fold during the first week. Coagulase-negative staphylococci predominate, but *Staph. aureus* may be found in 65% of infants.[1001] A host of other organisms can be found, including yeasts and a range of saprophytic bacteria. The umbilicus, perineum and axillae are most heavily colonized.

Colonization of infants on a neonatal unit

These babies are at greatest risk of becoming colonized by pathogens, which often show resistance to antibiotics.[655] The pattern of bowel colonization is very different among sick preterm infants. CONS and antibiotic-resistant Gram-negative organisms predominate.[312,313] Such organisms make a significant contribution to late-onset sepsis in these infants, and bacterial translocation through the gut wall is a likely mechanism in some cases.[1056] The results of an attempt to replace this faecal reservoir of potential pathogens with virtually harmless *Lactobacillus* sp. have been reported.[718] Bowel colonization with *Lactobacilli* was achieved, but unfortunately the reservoir of potential nosocomial pathogens was not significantly reduced and no clinical benefit was found.

Skin colonization on the NICU is mainly by CONS, which can be isolated from over 90% of all positive cultures.[577] *Staphylococcus epidermidis* accounts for 80% and *Staphylococcus haemolyticus* for almost all of the remainder.[112] These organisms show increasing resistance to antibiotics as the babies grow older[577] (Fig. 43.2). Interestingly, the skin of the preterm infant is much less heavily colonized than that of the adult, supports fewer species of bacteria and tends to have a transient rather than a stable resident population of organisms. Molecular biological techniques such as DNA fingerprinting, plasmid analysis and multilocus enzyme electrophoresis are increasingly being used to investigate the epidemiology of colonization and infection with these and many other organisms.[112,650,812,822,1025,1126]

BALANCE BETWEEN COLONIZATION AND INFECTION

Most babies become colonized without becoming infected, but in others various host factors or the pathogenicity of the organisms result in tissue invasion and sepsis. It is useful to consider host and organism factors separately.

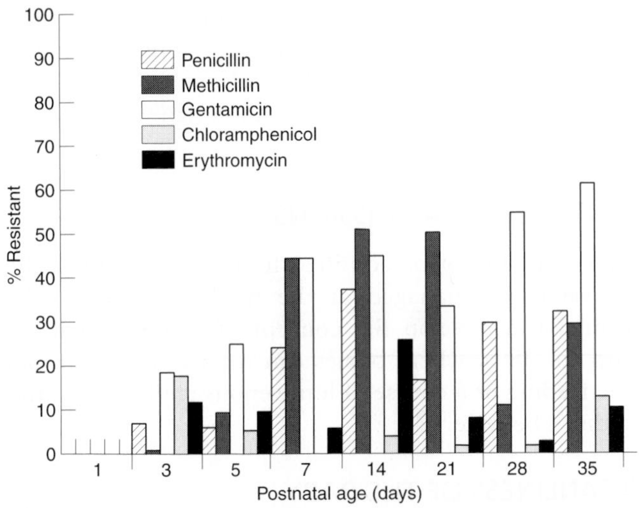

Fig. 43.2 Changes in percentage of cutaneous staphylococcus resistant to antibiotics with postnatal age. Measurements taken in all neonates at all sites. (From Keyworth et al[577] with permission)

Features of the host

Portals of entry

Intact skin and mucous membranes present a formidable barrier to microorganisms. Abrasions and cuts, mucosal injury, cannulae, catheters and endotracheal tubes all open the way for bacterial invasion. Among inmates of a NICU the risk of bacterial infection plummets as soon as intubation and vascular access are no longer required.[379]

Host immunity

Babies are less able than older children or adults to combat infection, an ability which is further compromised by prematurity. Particularly poor is the local inflammatory response, so that infecting organisms easily enter the circulation. Accordingly, a much higher proportion of infections in babies have a septicaemic component than is the case with older children or adults.

Antibiotic exposure

Antibiotics are used freely in neonatology and increasingly so in obstetrics. The resulting obliteration of colonizing flora predisposes to superinfection with pathogens, such as yeasts, and antibiotic resistance becomes common.[243,655,662,719,968]

Prematurity

Premature babies have poorer immunity (p. 1098), less effective cutaneous and mucosal barriers, more portals of entry secondary to invasive procedures, and greater exposure to potential pathogens from their environment. There is a clear inverse relationship between birthweight and risk of sepsis.[269,571]

Features of the microorganisms

Pathogenicity

The following are notoriously pathogenic to babies: GBS, *Staph. aureus*, CONS, *Listeria monocytogenes*, *Haemophilus influenzae*, *E. coli*, *Pseudomonas aeruginosa*, *Klebsiella* sp., *Serratia marcescens*, *Candida albicans* and herpes simplex.

Dose

The heavier the colonization the greater the risk of invasion and sepsis.[1001] Efforts to reduce the level of colonization by measures such as umbilical cord care, mouth care and bathing are important, even though complete eradication of the organisms is usually impossible.

Competition

Competition between bacteria is a controlling influence on the level of colonization and risk of infection, for example the inhibition of yeasts by bacteria and the competitive inhibition of Gram-negative organisms by *Lactobacillus bifidus* in the gut of the breast-fed infant.

PREVENTION OF INFECTION

If the newborn infant has little contact with anyone other than his mother and is breast-fed from the outset, the risk of significant nosocomial infection is negligible. When babies are retained in a hospital environment with multiple carers the risk is increased substantially. At the extreme end of the spectrum of risk is the tiny immature baby who spends weeks on a neonatal intensive care unit, constantly invaded by tubes, needles and catheters and cared for by a multiplicity of staff, who are also caring for a large number of other similarly disadvantaged infants. Then, nosocomial infection is virtually inevitable and the emphasis is on early detection and treatment as much as on prevention. The principles of control of cross-infection in hospital are well established, and in the account that follows those principles will be related mainly to the case of a baby on a neonatal unit.

ENVIRONMENT

There are several important factors in the environment that can contribute, either by creating circumstances in which cross-infection is more likely to occur or by creating environmental reservoirs of potential pathogens.

Unit design

To minimize cross-infection adequate space should be allowed around the cots. The Department of Health[248] recommends that the minimum space allocated to each incubator in a six-cot intensive care nursery should be 3 m^2 (100 sq feet). The ventilation to the rooms should deliver a maximum of 2.7 m^3/s,[248] though in general there is no need to have special ventilation systems. Enough sinks must be provided so that hand-washing protocols are easy to implement. There should be sufficient single rooms equipped for intensive care, so that sick babies can be isolated if necessary. The floors, walls and all flat surfaces should be cleaned regularly,[48] and ideally the unit should be sufficiently spacious for rooms to be vacated for cleaning on a regular rotational basis.

Equipment

Any medical equipment that comes into close contact with the baby is a potential source of infection, except for the moment when it is first removed from its sterile wrapping. Each baby in a normal nursery should have his own thermometer, and in the NICU he should have his own suction unit and stethoscope. If the equipment has to be shared it should either be wiped clean between patients (for example ultrasound transducers) or disposable devices should be used to connect the equipment to each patient (for example blood pressure cuffs). Equipment that comes into contact with potentially infective body fluids should be disposable. Three-way taps on intravenous or arterial lines should be changed every 24–48 hours and a meticulous regimen should be established for changing the drips and three-way taps connected to central lines used for total parenteral nutrition.

Humidified incubators are an infection hazard because Gram-negative bacilli, particularly *Pseudomonas* sp., thrive in the wet and humid environment.[481] Modern incubators are efficient when run dry, and many units only use humidification when they are having difficulty maintaining the temperature of particularly small babies. If incubator humidification is used the humidifier should be drained daily and refilled with sterile distilled water. It should be swabbed regularly to look for Gram-negative colonization. Incubators should be cleaned between babies, using conventional detergents, and they should be allowed to dry thoroughly before being reused. Routine fumigation of incubators is unnecessary and it is not necessary to change a baby's incubator on a routine basis.

Ventilators pose an infection risk as many parts of the circuit are inaccessible to sterilization. Most ventilator circuits are now disposable, but the expense involved in changing them frequently is prohibitive. Changing them weekly seems a reasonable compromise between reducing infection risk and expense. As soon as the ventilator comes out of use it is important to thoroughly clean the humidifier and all removable, cleanable items. The system should be allowed to dry thoroughly before being reused.

CONTROLLING ADMISSIONS

Babies should not be admitted to a neonatal unit if they can safely be managed at the mother's bedside. Any hospital can develop the concept of a transitional care ward (p. 389), where babies can receive incubator care, tube feeding or a course of intravenous antibiotics at their mother's bedside.[239]

CLEANLINESS OF THE BABY

Bacterial colonization of the newborn is inevitable, but as the risk of invasive infection increases with the level of colonization,[1001] and as heavily colonized sites may cross-infect other sites on the same baby,[283] attempts to control the level of colonization are warranted. Babies should be kept socially clean by the use of soap and water, but in the management of outbreaks of *Staph. aureus* infection a limited period of use of an antibacterial agent for bathing babies is justified. An example of the effectiveness of such a regimen is the recently reported eradication of an outbreak of MRSA in a neonatal nursery brought about by bathing babies using a preparation containing 0.3% triclosan (Bacti-Stat).[1140]

CORD CARE

The cord stump is generally the most heavily colonized area of the baby's surface, and invasive infection, particularly with *Staph. aureus*, can be reduced by cord care regimens aimed at preventing heavy colonization. At intervals cord care regimens are abandoned because of doubts about efficacy or concerns about toxicity or the induction of antibiotic resistance. Such changes in practice have invariably been followed by an increase in the incidence of staphylococcal infection.[23,51] This is well illustrated in Figure 43.3. Many cord-care preparations have been advocated, although the published literature prevents firm conclusions being drawn about what is best. A common approach in the UK is to clean the cord stump with alcohol swabs and to apply chlorhexidine powder[51] or to use antibiotic sprays (p. 373). Hexachlorophane powder is also effective,[23] as is triple dye.[453] In the developing world improved attention to the care of the umbilical cord can make a major impact on serious neonatal morbidity and on neonatal mortality.[377]

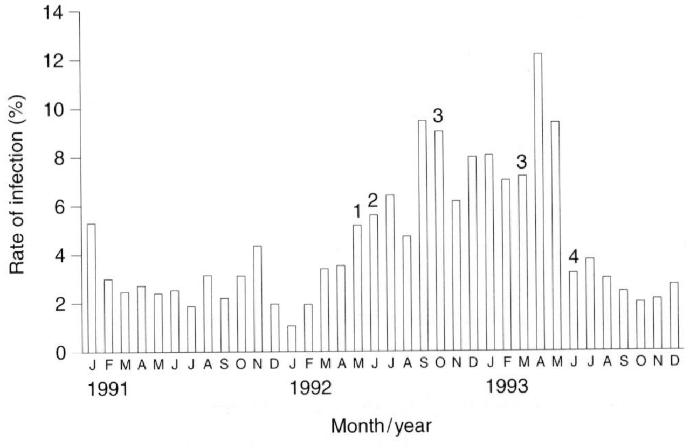

Fig. 43.3 Incidence of staphylococcal cord infection over time in relation to changes in cord care regimen. (From Allen et al[23] with permission)

INVASIVE PROCEDURES

All invasive procedures can introduce colonizing bacteria into the circulation. Areas of heavy colonization, such as the groins, should be low down on the list of desirable sites for vascular access. The skin should be cleaned thoroughly, with either an iodine- or an alcohol-containing solution, which should be allowed to dry before the procedure is undertaken. A recent study[682] shows that more effective decontamination is obtained with a 30-second period of cleaning than with the conventional 5–10 second wipe. There is convincing evidence that catheter-related sepsis is more likely if the line is used frequently,[380,749] and every effort should be made to avoid doing so by the use of peripheral cannulae for blood transfusions and drug administration.

OTHER BABIES, STAFF AND VISITORS

The greatest threat to an individual baby comes from bacteria colonizing the skin, pharynx and gastrointestinal tract of other babies, visitors and staff, although the risk of acquiring infection from healthy visitors is trivial in relation to the social benefits of a reasonably open visiting policy (p. 378), as several studies have shown.[138,468,601] However, it should not be thought that visitors pose a zero risk, and epidemics of RSV and rotavirus may be introduced by visiting siblings. Visitors must be shown how to wash their hands properly and must not touch babies other than their own.

HANDWASHING

The hands of the medical and nursing staff are the main potential route of cross-infection and, of all the measures for preventing nosocomial infection, hand-washing is by far the most important. Hands should be washed before touching any baby and again immediately afterwards. Sleeves should be rolled up to the elbow and watches and jewellery removed. The highest bacterial kill rates are obtained with solutions or soaps containing iodine or alcohol. An effective approach is to use betadine- or chlorhexidine-containing solutions to thoroughly wash the hands and forearms occasionally during a stint of duty on the neonatal intensive care unit, and then to simply rinse the hands in an alcohol-containing solution prior to and after touching each baby. Unfortunately, compliance with good hand-washing practice is often poor. In a study conducted in a North American unit, good hand-washing practice was carried out by the medical staff on only 37.5% of occasions prior to handling babies, and the nursing staff were only slightly better at 53.9%. Wrist ornaments were removed prior to hand-washing on only 75% of occasions.[871] In another study hand-washing was found to follow patient contact on only 29% of occasions, and the average duration of a hand-wash was

14.5 seconds.[613] Staff who only occasionally visit the neonatal unit, such as radiographers or physiotherapists, may have less opportunity to be educated in good hand-washing habits.

GOWNS, MASKS, CAPS AND SHOES

Routine use of gowns, masks, caps and shoes by staff or visitors is unnecessary on either the NICU[14,207] or the postnatal wards.[116]

STRESS AND OVERWORK

Overcrowding and understaffing are associated with an increased incidence of nosocomial infection.[453]

INFECTIOUS DISEASE IN STAFF AND PARENTS

Medical and nursing staff with significant intercurrent infections should ideally stay away from work. Parents and siblings should take similar precautions, and be kept away from newborn babies. Staff with conditions such as gastroenteritis or skin infection should stay off duty, or stay away from babies. Infected parents, if they cover infected lesions and take appropriate precautions (masks, hand-washing), can usually be allowed access to their baby (pp. 374, 1115). Herpes simplex is a problem (p. 1156) and staff with herpetic lesions should stay off duty. Herpetic lesions in parents should be treated with topical acyclovir and covered. Hand-washing must be meticulous.

For serious infections in the mother and father, the routines outlined in Table 43.6 should be followed. Siblings and more distant family relations should be kept away from the baby.

ANTIBIOTIC USE

Antibiotic use affects the pattern of nosocomial infection by influencing the colonizing flora and by predisposing to antibiotic resistance.[563] In a recent study of antibiotic use in a North American NICU[350] 75% of all infants, and 92% of VLBW babies, received antibiotics within 48 hours of birth. Five cross-sectional studies in the nursery showed point-prevalence rates of antibiotic use to be between 27% and 43% of the whole NICU population. These figures are almost certainly representative of most NICUs. It is difficult to know how, with the limitations of present investigational methods, the rate of initiating courses of antibiotics can safely be reduced, but there is a good deal that can be done in terms of stopping antibiotics sooner and rationalizing the treatment once the infecting organisms have been identified (p. 1137).

Prophylactic antibiotic therapy is almost always undesirable, as although it may protect the individual from infections by sensitive organisms, it predisposes to infection by resistant organisms and adds to the total amount of antibiotics prescribed, which over time encourages the emergence of resistant strains. Two randomized controlled trials[560,993] have recently demonstrated a convincing reduction in the incidence of CONS sepsis in infants who received parenteral nutrition fluids containing vancomycin. However, this practice will increase the risk of the emergence of strains of CONS and enterococci resistant to vancomycin, and that would be a very serious problem. The practice of adding antibiotics to infusion fluids as prophylaxis is mistaken.

HUMAN MILK

Human milk confers significant protection against infection, particularly in the developing world[44,447,740] but also in affluent populations.[251] Apart from protection against necrotizing enterocolitis the evidence for human milk protection against systemic sepsis in preterm babies is less good, but there is a dearth of good literature on the subject. Many units in the UK have abandoned milk banking since HIV came on the scene, but all presumably do (and certainly should) encourage the use of the baby's own mother's milk. Safe practice in running a breast milk bank is described on page 344. It is important to be aware, though, that human milk can be a vehicle for transmission of bacterial infection,[113] and to culture milk when such an occurrence is suspected. Routine culture of milk is unnecessary.

MICROBIOLOGICAL SURVEILLANCE

The NICU and the microbiology department should collaborate in a continuous microbiological surveillance programme, so that the pattern of infecting organisms and their antibiotic sensitivity is known at all times. It is very helpful to have a microbiologist on the NICU ward round on a regular basis to discuss prevention measures and antibiotic policy.

CONTROL OF OUTBREAKS OF INFECTION

When an outbreak of bacterial infection occurs within an NICU or on the postnatal wards the following steps should be taken. How far down the list it is necessary to go will depend on many factors, and should be decided in discussion with a microbiologist and the control of infection officer. It will also depend on the available human resources.

1. Isolate the infected babies together, so far as is practical. They may need to be transferred to a satellite unit. Clean and disinfect vacated rooms before readmitting to them.
2. Increase attention to measures designed to minimize cross-infection, especially hand-washing. The use of gowns by staff is also important, with a separate gown for each baby.[677] The use of gloves seems to have been useful in curtailing some outbreaks.[1060]

Table 43.6 Effect of perinatal maternal infections

Illness in mother	Access to normal baby	Treatment
Varicella	Access restricted until lesions crusted: mother gowned, masked and gloved	Give 250 mg of zoster immune globulin i.m. to infant if maternal disease <7 days predelivery; consider prophylaxis with acyclovir (p. 1158)
Zoster	Access	None: baby immune because of trans-placental maternal IgG
Measles	Access	Give 250 mg of human normal immuno-globulin i.m. to infant (hyperimmune if available)
Mumps	Access	Nil
Rubella	Access	No problem to neonate but keep mother away from antenatal patients
Herpes simplex (labial)	Access, but mother to wear face mask and treat lesion with acyclovir	None for baby
Herpes simplex (genital overt)	Access but meticulous hand washing and gloves	Acyclovir orally to mother
Infectious hepatitis A (current)	Access	Give 250 mg of human normal immuno-globulin i.m. to baby
Recent acute hepatitis B or hepatitis B carrier	Access	Give 200 units of anti-hepatitis B immuno-globulin stat.; immunize baby with HBV vaccine stat. with booster at 1–6 months (p. 1162)
HIV-positive (with or without AIDS)	Access	Nil. Breast-feeding probably contraindicated
TB open	Access	INAH to infant. BCG at 6 months if infant Mantoux negative: or give INAH-resistant BCG at once (p. 1153)
TB closed, on treatment or in the past	Access	BCG to infant
Brucella (active)	Access	Avoid breast-feeding[182a]
Syphilis active	Access, meticulous hand washing, gloves for 24 hours	Penicillin to infant and mother (pp. 1175–1176)
Gonorrhoea	Access	Treat mother and consort. Eye prophylaxis (p. 1150)
Malaria (active)	Access	Test infant's blood for parasites, especially if mother has falciparum malaria or if the infant develops symptoms. Treat congenital infection with chloroquine
Acute enteric infections (cholera, typhoid)	Nil during acute phase: mother too ill	Nil. Encourage breast-feeding if possible: immunize infant
Leprosy	Access	Continue maternal treatment
Other tropical diseases (i.e. trypanosomiasis, schistomiasis, filariasis)	Access	Nil but consult local tropical disease hospital if infant symptomatic
Chlamydia	Access	Nil
Cytomegalovirus	Access	Nil
Acute respiratory infection (RSV, flu)	Access with masking and hand washing	Nil
Gastroenteritis	Access with meticulous hand washing	Nil
Streptococcal illness or carriage	Access, mask for group A streptococcal respiratory infection, hand washing for all	Nil
Skin infection (boils, impetigo)	Access. Meticulous hand washing. Antibiotic ointment to maternal lesions	Nil
Glandular fever	Access	Nil

INAH = Isonicotinic acid hydrazide

3. Cohort the staff so that those caring for infected or colonized babies do not also care for non-colonized ones.
4. Culture all infants on the unit to identify asymptomatic carriers, and isolate them together if possible. Clean and disinfect vacated rooms before readmitting to them.
5. Change skin and cord care regimens, e.g. in a *Staph. aureus* outbreak.[1140]
6. Culture equipment such as incubators, ventilators, and blood gas analysers,[415] and use settle plates to study the environment.
7. Where relevant, obtain surface cultures from all the unit staff to look for possible reservoirs and modes of transmission of infection.
8. Consider the use of prophylactic antibiotics for a short period, e.g. in an outbreak of streptococcal infection.
9. Restrict admissions or close the NICU until contacts are discharged or are known not to be carriers. This is a last resort and should only be done after discussion with the control of infection team. Very rarely it will be necessary to close the maternity unit.

GENERAL CONSIDERATIONS REGARDING CLINICAL PRESENTATION, INVESTIGATION AND MANAGEMENT OF NEONATAL SEPSIS

Neonatal infections can be caused by an extraordinary variety of microorganisms and can present many specific features. There are, though, many common principles relating to presentation, investigation and management which can usefully be considered before moving on to classify and deal with specific conditions.

CLINICAL PRESENTATION AND ASSESSMENT OF THE INFANT

Early recognition, diagnosis and treatment of serious infection in the neonate is essential because of the extreme rapidity with which the risk of permanent morbidity or mortality can develop. Progression from mild symptoms to death can occur in less than 24 hours.[548] Most neonatal bacterial infections have an early bacteraemic phase preceding the development of a full-blown septicaemia or the localization of infection in organs and tissues. During this phase the clinical signs are subtle, but this is when treatment must be started if there is to be intact survival. These factors dominate the clinician's approach to infants with apparently minor symptoms, and lead to an apparent, but totally justified, tendency to over investigate and over treat. It is undoubtedly better to be proved wrong and to withdraw treatment after 48 hours from a well infant whose cultures are negative than to procrastinate for even a few hours with fatal consequences.

History

Ask about maternal, perinatal and neonatal events that put the baby at increased risk of infection.[989] If there is a possibility of congenital infection take a detailed pregnancy history, enquiring about apparently trivial episodes of pyrexia or skin rash, as well as contact with known cases of infectious disease. Take the intrapartum history: was the mother unwell or febrile; did she have a tender uterus or a vaginal discharge; when did the membranes rupture (pp. 165, 1130); were there any potentially infectious lesions on her cervix or vulva? If the mother has overt intrapartum infection, 15.2% of preterm babies and 4.1% of term babies will develop infection.[994] Maternal urinary tract infection is an important risk factor for neonatal sepsis.[434,947] Are there factors predisposing to nosocomial infection, such as a history of possible contact with an infected person or environment? Has there been contact between the mother or other family members and patients with infectious disease? Do any of the staff have infections? What organisms are around the NICU at the time, and is there any evidence of an epidemic of infectious disease? Are there portals of entry for infection, such as a long line? Other factors which predispose to neonatal sepsis include iron overload[71] and G6PD deficiency.[4] If the baby presents with pyrexia, is this environmental in origin? If the baby is ventilated, have the requirements increased? Has jaundice or a bleeding tendency developed? Is there abdominal distension or blood in the stools?

Signs of neonatal sepsis

In the early stages signs are subtle and often noted first by the nurses or the mother. Such concerns must always be taken seriously and should not be overridden by the findings of a single clinical examination, especially when risk factors for sepsis are present.

Early signs

- *'Going off'*. This is difficult to define, yet is often the earliest and most important sign. The mother or an experienced nurse thinks the baby is just not 'right'. He is slightly floppy, pale or mottled (cutis marmorata). He may be slightly irritable or unresponsive. He loses interest in feeding or sucks poorly.
- *Temperature change*. After excluding the effect of an abnormal environmental temperature (p. 300) and pyrexia in the first 1–2 hours of age in a baby of a pyrexial mother,[1071] a temperature below 36°C or above 37.8°C sustained for more than an hour must be regarded as probably due to infection until proved otherwise.[301,1071]
- *Jaundice*. Jaundice is far too common among newborn babies to have a useful positive predictive value for infection. However, infection enters into the differential list of causes of jaundice and should be considered if there is no other obvious explanation. Jaundice during sepsis is due to the effect of bacterial endotoxin on the liver, plus an increase in haemolysis.[902,975]
- *Apnoea*. In the preterm baby apnoeic attacks are an early and significant sign of all types of infection.
- *Tachypnoea/recession*. Mild respiratory distress, as evidenced by a raised respiratory rate (sustained above 60 breaths per minute) and slight recession are among the first non-specific sign of sepsis.
- *Cardiovascular signs*. A tachycardia > 160/min is often present early in sepsis.[416] In cases of myocarditis or endocarditis (pp. 698, 1146) cardiovascular signs will be more marked. Poor cutaneous circulation is common and is indicated by mottling and delayed capillary filling after the skin has been blanched by gentle pressure. The colour should normally return within 3 seconds.
- *Gastrointestinal*. The baby may vomit, have mild diarrhoea, or may develop an ileus with associated abdominal distension.

- *Irritability*. Infection may cause pain and may make the baby restless or whimper. Persistent moaning respiration is an ominous early sign.
- *Poor weight gain*. This may be a marker of chronic low-grade infection, such as a urinary tract infection or an infected central line or shunt.
- *Skin*. Petechiae may be present (p. 1124) or there may be paronychia, septic spots or omphalitis.

Late signs of infection

The more obvious signs only appear with advanced infection, and if they occur it usually means that the subtle signs have been present for some time beforehand.

- *Respiratory*. Cyanosis, grunting and dyspnoea are the classic signs of neonatal lung disease (p. 495). If present within the first 4–6 hours of life pneumonia is a possibility, but many other diagnoses are possible (Table 29.13). Beginning beyond 6–12 hours of age, these signs mean pneumonia until proved otherwise (pp. 497, 1142–1143).
- *Abdominal*. Signs of intestinal obstruction may be due to generalized sepsis as well as NEC (p. 747) and structural malformations of the gastrointestinal tract (Chapter 31, Part 4). Bilious vomiting and abdominal distension are non-specific signs of obstruction, but flank lividity, abdominal redness and induration and periumbilical staining are late features of intraperitoneal sepsis.
- *Central nervous system*. A high-pitched cry, neck retraction, bulging fontanelle and convulsions are late features of neonatal meningitis, which has probably progressed to a cerebritis and cortical thrombophlebitis with a poor prognosis. In no other neonatal infection is it more important to consider the diagnosis as early as possible on the basis of the non-specific features.
- *Haemorrhagic diathesis*. DIC with petechiae and bleeding from puncture sites, the gut or the renal tract is a late sign of sepsis. Thrombocytopenia without evidence of DIC is also common with severe infection, especially fungal (p. 1164).
- *Sclerema* (p. 900). This is a non-specific feature of any serious neonatal illness. It may be seen in babies who have been septic for days, but is rarely found at presentation.
- *Pseudoparalysis*. The failure to move one limb, sometimes combined with the baby crying when moved, may be the only clue to septic arthritis or osteomyelitis.

Physical examination

Have the baby completely naked and look for:

- lesions of the skin or subcutaneous tissues;
- signs of respiratory distress, such as tachypnoea or expiratory grunting;
- signs of dehydration, suggesting fluid loss from vomiting or diarrhoea, or that the pyrexia is due to dehydration (p. 384);
- a red or discharging umbilicus or periumbilical flare.

In the formal examination the following procedures should always be carried out:

- Examine the chest – is there tracheal shift, decreased air entry or added sounds?
- Check the heart rate and note the pulse volume – are there murmurs or a triple rhythm, suggesting myocarditis or endocarditis?
- Look for hepatosplenomegaly, which may accompany generalized septicaemia as well as hepatitis.
- Carefully palpate the kidneys – with pyelonephritis a baby may have loin tenderness. Enlarged kidneys are a non-specific finding in early septicaemia.
- Is the abdomen tender, suggesting peritonitis? Is there redness or induration of the abdominal skin? Are there any underlying masses? Is peristalsis visible, and are bowel sounds present?
- Check the fontanelle tension, measure the head circumference and check the spinal column and skull for pits or other skin defects, which might be the entry site for meningeal infections.
- Try to get an overall picture of the baby's neurological state. Is he obtunded or in coma?
- Can oesteomyelitis and septic arthritis be excluded by the presence of full and painless limb movements?
- Do not forget otitis media (p. 1151).
- Measure the blood pressure – always.

INVESTIGATION OF NEONATAL SEPSIS

Principles of investigation and the value of tests

If the history and examination suggest infection, either investigation alone or else investigation followed immediately by treatment is indicated. The decision to treat will be determined mainly by the clinical assessment, but since septic infants deteriorate so rapidly the threshold for a pre-emptive strike with antibiotics, pending further evaluation, should be low: that is, the clinical test(s) used to make a decision about prescribing antibiotics for newborn infants are adjusted towards a high sensitivity, and the well-trained paediatrician will give antibiotics to a considerable number of non-infected infants.[384] To improve on this diagnostic accuracy various tests have been developed and evaluated. Unfortunately, most evaluations have assessed the likelihood of a positive test in babies who have infection, and a negative test in babies shown not to have infection. This approach gives values for the sensitivity and specificity of the test (Appendix 14). The question that the doctor wants the answer to, however, is 'what is the likelihood of this baby being infected, given the results of the test(s)?' This question refers to the predictive value of the test(s) when used in a population of babies suspected of having infection. A recent study from Switzerland illustrates this point.[97] In a population of 195 sick infants suspected to be septicaemic during the first 3 days of life, the sensitivity and specificity of an elevated CRP were found to be 75% and 86% respectively, and for a reduced white cell count 67% and 90%. However, the positive predictive value of a raised CRP was only 32% and of leukopenia 37%. I am not aware of a formal study to compare the predictive value of any laboratory test with the predictive value of a clinical opinion, and the value of such a study would in any case be limited by the impossibility of standardizing clinical opinion.

Given the limited predictive power of existing tests, and the fact that few of them can produce results rapidly enough, decisions about antibiotic prescribing for unwell babies should continue to be made on clinical grounds. However, positive test results suggestive of infection may be sufficient reason to begin therapy even when the level of clinical suspicion is not high, for example a low WBC count (say, $<5 \times 10^9$/l) in a slightly grunty term baby. The only test results that are more or less immediately available and sufficiently sensitive to endorse a decision to go ahead with antibiotic therapy are CSF and urine microscopy, bacterial antigen tests, buffy coat microscopy and, possibly, the chest X-ray. The rest of the tests subserve one or both of the following functions:

- To provide retrospective evidence for or against the clinical diagnosis of infection;
- To establish the nature and antimicrobial sensitivity of the infecting organism.

The possible investigations are listed in Table 43.7.

Any baby who is suspected of being infected should have all of the routine tests performed immediately on presentation. The rest of the tests in Table 43.7 can be selected according to the circumstances. All are discussed below.

Table 43.7 Investigation of neonatal sepsis

Routine septic screen
Full blood count, including film
Blood culture
Swab from any site of inflammation
Throat and ear swab (in the case of suspected early-onset infection)
Urine microscopy and culture
Chest X-ray
C-reactive protein
Additional routine tests, indicated by the clinical situation/availability
Lumbar puncture
Culture and Gram stain of gastric aspirate
Culture and Gram stain of a maternal high vaginal swab
Culture of endotracheal tube tip or tracheal aspirate
Culture of chest drain tip
Culture of removed vascular catheter
Quantitative blood cultures or multiple site blood cultures
Organism-specific serial IgG concentrations
Organism-specific IgM concentration
Buffy coat microscopy
Non-routine or novel tests
Latex agglutination tests
Serum interleukin and TNFα
Immunoelectrophoresis
Acridine orange leukocyte cytospin test
NBT

Microbiological investigation

Blood culture

This is the definitive test, as the vast majority of neonatal infections are associated with bacteraemia. Continuous monitoring methods usually allow a positive blood culture to be reported within 12–24 hours, and virtually all cultures that are going to be positive have grown by 48 hours whatever the culture method.[704,912] Possible exceptions are *Listeria monocytogenes*, *Haemophilus influenzae* and yeasts, which may all take longer to grow. There are several pitfalls in collecting blood for culture and interpreting the findings.

Collecting blood for culture. Ideally, blood for culture should be taken from a peripheral vein after thoroughly cleaning the overlying skin with an antiseptic solution and allowing it to dry. Chlorhexidine with alcohol or an iodine-containing solution should be used. A better result can be obtained if the skin is cleansed for 30 seconds rather than the usual 5–10 seconds.[682] With good technique, skin contamination of blood cultures taken from peripheral veins can be reduced to an acceptable level. In a study of 677 paired cultures from blood and skin access sites, only 9 of 58 positive blood cultures grew the same organism that was grown from the skin.[463] With modern laboratory techniques 0.5 ml of blood may be sufficient for a successful culture,[573] but increasing the volume to 1 or 2 ml definitely increases the chance of a positive culture.[533,946]

Cultures from long lines and umbilical artery catheters also give acceptable results.[849,1022] Allowing the blood to drip directly into the culture bottle through a needle from which the hub has been removed, and capillary sampling, can be adapted to give acceptable results if vascular access is a major problem,[593] but contamination is more likely using these methods.

Interpreting blood culture results. The problem lies in distinguishing septicaemia from skin contamination. A pure growth appearing within 24–48 hours is virtually always significant, but mixed organisms, bizarre organisms or growth that does not appear until after 72 hours of incubation should raise suspicion. However, in the case of the VLBW infant it is unwise to ignore bizarre organisms (Table 43.8), or polymicrobial infection.[126,546]

CONS present the greatest difficulty because they colonize the skin of all babies and yet are the commonest pathogen among NICU inmates. Multiple-site blood

Table 43.8 Organisms reported to cause neonatal sepsis (not specifically referred to in the main text). Most of these organisms cause a septicaemic type of illness and only focal features are referred to here

Organism	Focal and other features	References
Gram-positive cocci		
Group A streptococcus	Meningitis Fasciitis	Coulter et al 1984 Lancet ii:356 Nutman et al 1979 Arch. Dis. Child. 54:637
Group C streptococcus (*Streptococcus equisimilis*)	Meningitis	Hervas et al 1985 Ped. Inf. Dis. J. 4:694
Group D streptococcus		
1. α-haemolytic (viridans) (*Strep. sanguis, mitis*)	Meningitis	Freedman and Baltimore 1990 J. Perinatol. 10:272 Heath et al 1980 Am. J. Obs. Gyn. 138:343 Haftar et al 1983 J. Clin. Microb. 18:101 Spigelblatt et al 1984 Ped. Inf. Dis. J. 4:56
2. *Strep. bovis*	Meningitis	Alexander & Giacoia 1978 J. Pediatr. 93:489 Fikar & Levy 1979 Am. J. Dis. Child 133:1149
3. *Strep. faecalis*	Meningitis Abscess	Dobson and Baker 1990 Ped. Inf. Dis. J. 9:165 Jeffery et al 1977 Arch. Dis. Child. 52:683 Luginbuhl et al 1987 Ped. Inf. Dis. J. 6:1022
α-haemolytic streptococcus (non-group D)	Meningitis	Broughton et al 1981 J. Pediatr. 99:450
Group F streptococcus		Well & Keeney 1980 Pediatrics 66:820
Group G streptococcus		Brans 1975 Pediatrics 55:745 Dyson & Reld 1981 J. Pediatr. 99:944
Strep. Mulleri (usually group F, can be C, A, G)		Cox et al 1987 J. Clin. Pathol 40:190
Streptococcus pneumoniae	Meningitis	Alzahawi et al 1988 Br. J. Obs. Gyn. 95:1198 Geelen et al 1990 J. Perinat. Med. 18: 125 Jacobs et al 1990 Scand. J. Infect. Dis. 22:493 Kaplan et al 1993 Am. J. Perinatol. 10:1 Robinson 1990 Rev. Inf. Dis. 12:799 Westh et al 1990 Rev. Inf. Dis. 12:416 Wright et al 1990 J. Infect. 20:59
Leuconostoc	Meningitis	Friedland et al 1990 J. Clin. Microbiol. 28:2125
Peptostreptococcus (anaerobic)		Chow et al 1974 Pediatrics 54:736 Noel et al 1988 Ped. Inf. Dis. J. 7:858
Gram-positive bacilli		
Bacillus fragilis	Osteomyelitis	Brock 1980 Clin. Pediat. 19:639
Bacillus licheniformis	Meningitis	Thompson et al 1990 Pediat. Rev. Comm. 4:147
Bacillus cereus	Meningitis Pneumonia	Feder et al 1988 Pediatrics 82:909 Jevon et al 1993 Ped. Inf. Dis. J. 12:251
Bifidobacterium		Noel et al 1988 Ped. Inf. Dis. J. 7:858
Clostridium perfringens (Welchii)	Congenital infection Meningitis NEC	Gallaher and Marks 1991 Am. J. Perinatol. 8:370 Orzel et al 1983 Ped. Inf. Dis J. 2:457 Long et al 1985 Ped. Inf. Dis J. 4:752 Noel et al 1988 Ped. Inf. Dis J. 7:858
Lactobacillus	Meningitis	Broughton et al 1983 Ped. Inf. Dis. J. 2:382
Gram-negative cocci		
Moraxella catarrhalis	Meningitis Pneumonia Cellulitis	Daoud et al 1996 Ann. Trop. Paediatr. 16:199 Ohlsson & Bailey 1985 Scand. J. Inf. Dis. 17:225 Leighton et al 1982 Ped. Inf. Dis. J. 1:339
Neisseria gonorrhoea	Ventriculitis Ophthalmia Vaginitis	Bland et al 1983 Am. J. Obs. Gyn. 147:1781 Desenclos et al 1992 Sex. Transm. Dis. 19:105 Stark & Glade 1979 J. Pediatr 94:298
Neisseria meningitidis	Intrauterine infection Abscess Meningitis	Bhutta et al 1991 Ped. Inf. Dis. J. 10:868 Chugh et al. 1988 Ped. Inf. Dis. J. 7:136 Embree et al 1987 Ped. Inf. Dis. J. 6:299

Table 43.8 (*contd*)

Organism	Focal and other features	References
Gram-negative bacilli		
Acinetobacter sp	Meningitis	Ibrahim 1995 West. Afr. J. Med. 14:59 Horrevorts et al 1995 J. Clin. Microb. 33:1567 Morgan & Hart 1982 Arch. Dis. Child. 57:557 Stone & Das 1985 J. Hosp. Inf. 6:42 Vesikari et al 1985 Arch. Dis. Child. 60:542
Achromobacter xylosoxidans	Meningitis	Hearn and Gander 1991 Am. J. Clin. Pathol. 96:211 Namuyak et al 1985 J. Clin. Microb. 22:470
Alkaligenes xylosoxidans	Meningitis	Boukadida et al 1993 Ped. Inf. Dis. J. 12:696 Kishan et al 1987 Ind. J. Ped. 54:789 Praczek & Whitelaw 1983 Arch. Dis. Child. 58:728
Bacteroides fragilis	Meningitis – metronidazole may be useful	Chow et al 1974 Pediatrics 54:736 Ketter & Monif 1988 Obs & Gynecol 71:463 Webber & Tuohy 1988 Ped. Inf. Dis. J. 7:886 Noel et al 1988 Ped. Inf. Dis. J. 7:858
Brucella	Enterocolitis	Lubani et al 1988 Eur. J. Pediatr. 147:520 Labrune et al 1990 Acta. Paed. Scand. 79:707
Campylobacter jejuni	Meningitis Gastroenteritis	Youngs et al 1985 Arch. Dis. Child. 60:480 Goosens et al 1986 Lancet ii: 146 Forbes & Scheifele 1987 Ped. Inf. Dis. J. 6:494
Capnocytophaga		Feldman et al 1985 Ped. Inf. Dis. J. 4:415
Citrobacter (freundii, diversus)	Meningitis – abscesses common	Rae et al 1991 Drug Intell. Clin. Pharm. 25:27 Kline et al 1988 J. Pediatr. 113:430 Goering et al 1992 Ped. Inf. Dis. J. 11:99 Saraswathi et al 1995 Ind Pediatr. 32:359
Corynebacterium amycolatum		Berner et al 1997 J. Clin. Microb. 35:1011
Edwardsiella tarda	Meningitis	Vohra et al 1988 Ped. Inf. Dis. J. 7:814
Eikenella		Sporken et al 1985 Acta Obs. Gynecol. Scand. 64:683
Enterobacter cloacae	Meningitis	Acolet et al 1994 J. Hosp. Infect. 28:273 Bannon et al 1988 Arch. Dis. Child. 64:1388 Lacey and Want 1995 J. Infect. 30:223 Modi et al 1987 Arch. Dis. Child. 62:148 Verweij et al 1995 Infect. Control. Hosp. Epidemiol. 16:25
	NEC	Millar et al 1992 Arch. Dis. Child. 67:53
E. sakazakii	Meningitis	Muytjens et al 1983 J. Clin. Microb. 18:115 Willis & Robinson 1988 Ped. Inf. Dis. J. 7:196
Flavobacterium meningosepticum	Meningitis – consider rifampicin	Thong et al 1981 J. Clin. Pathol. 34:429 Linder et al 1984 Arch. Dis. Child. 59:582 Tam et al 1989 Ped. Inf. Dis. J. 8:252
Fusobacterium	NEC	Noel et al 1988 Ped. Inf. Dis. J. 7:858
Haemophilus influenzae	Pneumonia and meningitis	al Mofada 1994 J. Infect. 29:283 Bale & Watkins 1978 J. Pediatr. 92:233 Berg et al 1981 Scand. J. Inf. Dis. 13:299 Barton et al 1982 Am. J. Dis. Child. 136:463 Kinney et al 1993 Ped. Inf. Dis. J. 12:739 Lilien et al 1978 Pediatrics 62:299 Meis et al 1991 Scand. J. Infect. Dis. 23:649 Mendoza and Roberts 1991 J. Perinatol. 11:126 Wong and Ng 1991 J. Paediatr. Child Health. 27:113 Webster et al 1995 Aust. N. Z. J. Obst. Gynecol. 35:102 Milne et al 1988 Arch. Dis. Child. 63:83
	Osteomyelitis	Williams et al 1994 J. Infect. 29:203
H. parainfluenzae	Meningitis	Nakamura et al 1984 Am. J. Clin. Pathol. 81:388
Helicobacter cinaedi	Meningitis	Orlicek et al 1993 J. Clin. Microb. 31:569
Klebsiella oxytoca		Tullus et al 1992 Acta Pathol. Microb. Imm. Scand. 100:1008
Klebsiella pneumoniae	UTI	Reish et al 1993 J. Hosp. Inf. 25:287 Coovadia et al 1992 J. Hosp. Infect. 22:197
	Meningitis	Cherubin et al 1982 Rev. Inf. Dis. 4, S:453 McCracken et al 1980 Lancet i:187 Morgan et al 1984 J. Hosp. Inf. 5:377

Table 43.8 *(contd)*

Organism	Focal and other features	References
Mycobacterium cheloni		Speert et al 1980 J. Pediatr. 96:681
Pasteurella multocida	Meningitis – from animals	Thompson et al 1984 Ped. Inf. Dis. J. 3:559
Pasteurella pestis (plague)	Skin	White et al 1984 Am. J. Dis. Child. 135:418
Pleisomonas shigelloides	Meningitis	Waeker et al 1988 Ped. Inf. Dis. J. 7:877 Billiet et al 1989 J. Inf. 19:267
Proteus mirabilis	Meningitis – abscesses common	Smith & Mellor 1980 Arch. Dis. Child. 55:308 Velvis et al 1986 Ped. Inf. Dis. J. 5:591
Pseudomonas aeruginosa	Meningitis	Eisele et al 1990 Ear Nose Throat J. 69:119 Gupta et al 1993 J. Trop. Pediatr. 39:32 Jeffrey et al 1977 Arch. Dis. Child. 52:683 Leigh et al 1995 Ped. Inf. Dis. J. 14:367 Turkel et al 1986 Ped. Pathol. 6:131 Ruderman et al 1983 Clin. Pediatr. 22:630
	Noma neonatorum	Juster Reicher et al 1993 Am. J. Perinatol. 10:409
Pseudomonas pseudomallei	Meningitis	Lumbiganon et al 1988 Ped. Inf. Dis. J. 7:634
Salmonella eimsbuettel	Gastroenteritis	McAlister et al 1986 Lancet i: 1262
Salmonella typhi	Gastroenteritis Typhoid fever	Chin et al 1986 Arch. Dis. Child. 61:1228 Reed and Klugman 1994 Ped. Inf. Dis. J. 13:774
Salmonella oranienburg	Gastroenteritis	Mehta et al 1987 Ind. J. Med. Res. 75:482
Salmonella sp. *(heidelberg, typhimurium dublin, enteriditis, urbana, poona)*	Meningitis	McCracken et al 1980 Lancet i: 787 Davis 1981 Am. J. Dis. Child. 135:1096 Gogate & Deodhar 1984 Ind. J. Pediat. 51:549
	Gastroenteritis	Kumar et al 1995 Indian Pediatr. 32:881 Mahajan et al 1995 J. Commun. Dis. 27:10 Umasankar et al 1996 J. Hosp. Inf. 34:117 Sirinavin et al 1991 J. Hosp. Inf. 18:231 Stone et al 1993 Am. J. Inf. Control. 21:270
Serratia marcescens	Meningitis	Lewis et al 1983 Brit. Med. J. 287:1701 Smith et al 1984 Lancet i: 151
Shigella sonnei	Late-onset gastroenteritis	Ruderman et al 1986 Ped. Inf. Dis. J. 6:379
Shigella flexneri	Gastroenteritis and bowel perforation	Starke & Baker 1985 Ped. Inf. Dis. J. 4:405
Vibrio cholera		Coovadia et al 1982 S. Afr. Med. J. 64:405
Yersinia enterocolitica	Gastroenteritis	Paisley and Laver 1992 Ped. Inf. Dis. J. 11:331
Leptospira sp.		
Leptospirosis		Shaked et al 1993 Clin. Infect. Dis. 17:241
Legionella		
Legionella pneumophila	Pneumonia	Luck et al 1994 Eur. J. Clin. Microb. Inf. Dis. 13:565 Holmberg et al 1993 Pediatrics. 92:450 Greene et al 1990 J. Perinatol. 10:183
Viruses		
Adenovirus	Systemic infection	Abzug and Levin 1991 Pediatrics 87:890 Piedra et al 1992 Ped. Inf. Dis. J. 11:460 Montone et al 1995 Diagn. Cytopathol. 12:341 Chiou et al 1994 Ped. Inf. Dis. J. 13:664
Coronavirus	Pneumonia	Sizun et al 1995 Acta Paediatr. 84:617
Enteroviruses	Systemic infection Respiratory illness	Abzug et al 1993 Ped. Inf. Dis. J. 12:820 Pruekprasert et al 1995 J. Assoc. Acad. Minor. Phys. 6:134
Rhinovirus	In BPD	Chidekel et al 1997 Ped. Inf. Dis. J. 16:43
Parasites		
Blastocystis hominis	Diarrhoea	Galatowicz et al 1993 Ped. Inf. Dis. J. 12:345
Giardia lamblia	Gastroenteritis	Morrow et al 1992 J. Pediatr. 121:363

cultures may improve the distinction between genuine septicaemia and skin contamination.[1114] However, a recent study of multiple-site cultures, using plasmid typing and antibiotyping, has shown an incidence of unrelated strains of CONS from different sites of greater than 50%,[579] suggesting a high frequency of contamination. There is no easy answer to the problem of contamination in the case of CONS, and clinical assessment combined with the results of tests such as the blood count and CRP is often the only way to make a judgement about the likelihood of infection.

In septicaemia secondary to a long line, semi-quantitative cultures on blood drawn from the line may be valuable in establishing the site of infection.[872] The magnitude of the bacteraemia may also correlate with outcome, at least in the case of *Staph. aureus*.[954]

If conventional bacterial cultures are negative in a baby who has signs suggestive of septicaemia it is important to exclude viral and fungal infection by sending appropriate samples after consultation with the clinical microbiologist.

Surface swabs

Swabbing sites of inflammation is important, but routine swabbing of sites such as the umbilicus, groin, ear, nose, throat, pharynx and rectum is much less so. Surface swabs are informative about colonization, but all babies are soon colonized. Numerous studies have shown that the results of surface cultures are of limited value in diagnosis[553,861,1144] and can probably be abandoned without detriment.[257] A recent study of the value of surveillance of pharyngeal colonization in the detection of bacterial illness found concordance between pharyngeal isolates and blood-culture isolates in only 11% of cases.[343] Occasional studies, however, have concluded differently, such as the demonstration that nasal culture has a high negative predictive value (99%) and a low false-negative rate (7%) in identifying babies with early-onset sepsis.[456] On balance, it seems reasonable to limit routine surface culture to a throat and ear swab in the investigation of suspected early-onset sepsis.

Gastric aspirate

This can be viewed as a sample of amniotic fluid, plus or minus some swallowed secretions from the birth canal. About one-third of gastric aspirates show bacteria on Gram stain (often potential pathogens, such as the Enterobacteriaceae, GBS and enterococci) and a similar proportion contain some polymorphs.[132] The great majority of these babies do not become septic, and the results of gastric aspirate microbiology cannot be considered an argument for antibiotic therapy. If a baby is thought to be infected on clinical grounds, however, it is important to choose antibiotic therapy that will cover any organisms seen in the gastric aspirate.

Maternal HVS

When babies present with signs of infection within the first 24–48 hours of birth the source is likely to be the maternal vagina, and an HVS may well grow the responsible organism. Like the gastric aspirate and surface swabs, however, the HVS tells about possible exposure to pathogens and not about infection, and the results are available too late to influence initial decision-making about therapy. They may help, though, to decide about the need to continue with therapy and on the choice of therapeutic agent.

Urine

There are two practical ways to obtain urine from babies for the purpose of diagnosing infection. One is to use a urine collection bag and the other is to perform an SPA (p. 1379). SPA overcomes the problem of contamination, and pus cells or organisms in a technically satisfactory SPA indicate urinary infection. To avoid delay and uncertainty it may be worth performing an SPA in the initial assessment of the sick baby who is thought to be septicaemic.

As part of the routine septic screen it is usual to begin with a urine specimen collected in a bag applied to the perineum. The perineum should be cleaned carefully before the bag is applied and the bag removed as soon as the urine is passed. It is not satisfactory to cover a urine bag with a nappy and remove it at the next nappy change! Urine should be microscoped as soon after voiding as possible. If bacteria and white cells are seen this strongly suggests UTI. Because of the long-term implications of a diagnosis of UTI (p. 1148) the result of urinalysis must be interpreted with great care. The main value of bag urines is that if they are clear they exclude UTI. Positive bag urines should always be viewed with suspicion unless there are many white cells (>150/mm^3) and a pure growth of at least 10^8 organisms per litre of urine (10^5/ml). A mixed growth, or an organism other than *E. coli*, obtained from a bag urine should always be confirmed by performing an SPA.

It is also possible to screen for UTI in babies by means of dipsticks. These measure the concentrations of leukocyte esterase, nitrites and protein by a colour change which can be read using a photometer. One study has shown a negative predictive value for UTI of 99.4% in a cohort of newborn babies and infants.[629] Sticks have not yet been evaluated in the neonatal intensive care setting.

Tracheal secretions and endotracheal tube-tip culture

Undoubtedly, microorganisms recovered from the upper airway may be those causing septicaemia and lower respiratory tract infection, and this has been shown in the case of CONS, using ribotyping techniques,[109] and also with *Candida* sp.[911] The results of cultures of respiratory secretions should therefore be used to inform the choice of antimicrobial agents for suspected pulmonary infection. However, it is naive to base the diagnosis of pulmonary infection solely on the results of culture of respiratory secretions, as illustrated by a recent study comparing tracheal aspirate cultures from babies showing signs of respiratory deterioration with cultures from babies who were stable. No significant difference was found in the rate of positive cultures for bacteria, viruses, chlamydia or ureaplasmas. Cultures were positive in about one-third of the babies in each group.[1030] Other studies, however, have reported that culturing respiratory secretions has clinical value,[484,616,971] and it has been suggested that using a bronchial brush technique may give better results.[889]

Vascular lines and thoracentesis tubes

The tips of umbilical cannulae, central lines and thoracentesis tubes should be sent for culture when removed. Central lines can be cultured using the 'Macki roll' technique, in which the line is rolled across the culture plate and a subsequent colony count performed. This can help to distinguish genuine line infection from skin contamination during removal of the line.

Lumbar puncture

Neonatal bacterial meningitis carries such a high morbidity and mortality (p. 1139), especially if diagnosis and treatment are delayed, that an LP should be performed as part of the infectious disease work-up of most ill babies before antibiotics are started. Exemptions can be made for babies with pulmonary infection complicating long-term IPPV (pp. 615, 1145), babies with overt localized infection such as NEC or osteomyelitis, and babies who would not be able to tolerate the procedure.[461,1087] However, these are rare and specific exemptions. As the LP is being used as a screening procedure a large number of negative CSF results can be expected. In a recent survey 99.05% of all CSF results were normal,[521] although it must be said that the threshold for performing an LP was extremely low, with 42% of all babies admitted to the neonatal unit concerned having their CSF examined. In keeping with this finding, the positive predictive value was low, at 46%. Whether or not babies presenting with respiratory distress syndrome soon after birth should be added to the exemption list is debatable. Most clinicians probably do not routinely LP preterm babies with respiratory distress syndrome before starting antibiotics, and there is literature to support this stance.[497] However, there is a slight risk of missing or delaying the diagnosis of meningitis in preterm infants if the LP is omitted from the early sepsis screening.[1113] In general the LP is more likely to produce a positive result in late-onset than in early-onset sepsis.[959]

Lumbar puncture should be performed with strict sterile precautions (p. 1113). It is best performed with the baby sitting upright,[401,1087] but if the baby is on its side it is important to avoid excessive flexion of the trunk as this may cause respiratory embarrassment or apnoea.[461] If it is essential to examine the CSF in an unstable baby, it may be safer to intubate and ventilate before proceeding.

CSF analysis. Although high WBC counts in CSF have sometimes been reported in babies without meningitis, a polymorphonuclear leukocyte count higher than $20/mm^3$ should be regarded with suspicion, and counts above $30/mm^3$ are strongly indicative of meningitis. When bloodstained CSF is obtained, the ratio of red cells to white cells should be calculated. In uninfected CSF this is usually >500:1.

Microscopy of the CSF is crucial and may, with caution, be used to direct the choice of initial antimicrobial therapy, although broad-spectrum antibiotics should be used until the results of the cultures are known. The isolation of *Candida* sp. from the CSF of infants in the absence of other CSF abnormality usually suggests contamination.[37]

The upper normal limit of CSF protein is 1.5–2.0 g/l in the term and 3.7 g/l in the preterm baby.[893] The levels are usually raised in meningitis. CSF glucose levels should be related to a simultaneous measurement of blood glucose. The CSF glucose should be 50% or more of the blood glucose level, and a low level (<1.0 mmol/l or a value less than 30% of the blood glucose) suggests bacterial meningitis.

The CSF should be tested for the presence of group B streptococcal or *E. coli* K1 antigen, which gives accurate and prompt diagnostic information.[868]

A new development in the diagnosis of meningitis in neonates and infants is the measurement of cytokines such as IL-6 and TNFα in the CSF. A recent study found IL-6 to be present in the CSF of each of 20 infants with bacterial meningitis and absent in all 20 infants without bacterial meningitis. In cases of aseptic meningitis IL-6 was found in about half, but at only about 10% of the concentration found in bacterial meningitis. TNFα was found to be a less sensitive indicator of bacterial meningitis.[272] More research is needed to define the predictive value of tests for neonatal meningitis based on cytokine measurements. Another investigation that has been performed on neonatal CSF in an attempt to improve on the diagnostic accuracy has been the measurement of β_2-microglobulin by enzyme immunoassay.[371] A cut-off concentration of 2.25 mg/l was found to provide an accurate distinction between babies with and without CNS infection.

Radiology

All babies with suspected sepsis should have a chest X-ray. An abdominal X-ray and ultrasound are indicated if there are abdominal signs or suspicion of urinary tract infection. X-rays are not a good way to detect bone or joint infection in the early stages (p. 1147).

Haematological investigation

White blood cell count. Abnormal white cell indices are useful adjuncts to clinical opinion but do not have sufficient predictive value to be allowed to override a decision to treat suspected infection. A repeat full blood count taken about 24 hours after the onset of the illness is a better predictor of infection than the one performed as part of the initial septic screen.[423] Interpreting blood films requires considerable skill and familiarity with the appearances of neonatal white cells.

Total white cell count is the least useful index because the normal range is so wide (Appendix 1), varies with gestation and postnatal age, can be confused by machines including nucleated RBC in the count, and can be 30–40% lower in blood obtained from a central catheter than in a capillary sample.[1031] Furthermore, many non-infective catastrophes such as periventricular haemorrhage, convulsions and asphyxia can raise the total WBC count.

The neutrophil count is of more value. There are well-documented normal ranges in term and preterm infants at various postnatal ages[428,689] (Appendix 1). Manroe's reference range for the total neutrophil count in the VLBW infant has recently been extended.[742] Within the first 48 hours of life, neutropenia ($<2.0–2.5 \times 10^9$/l) suggests bacterial infection,[143] and at this cut-off value the sensitivity is around 20%.[446] Thereafter, both neutropenia and neutrophilia ($>7.5–8.0 \times 10^9$/l) have useful predictive power, although in neither case is the specificity or sensitivity greater than about 80%.[97]

The appearance of the circulating neutrophils changes in infection, so that more immature forms are seen in the peripheral blood. These are commonly known as band forms. The absolute value for band forms is not of much use because it tends to rise late in infection, and in the most severely affected infants band cell production is limited as the marrow becomes exhausted. A slightly more useful indicator of infection is the ratio of immature to total neutrophils (I/T ratio). The maximum normal value is 0.16 during the first 24 hours, 0.14 by 48 hours and 0.13 by 60 hours, where it remains until 5 days of age. Thereafter, the maximum normal I/T ratio is 0.12 until the end of the first month.[689] Several,[385,833,895] but by no means all, studies[451,585] have found that an I/T ratio >0.2 is a useful marker of infection and that a ratio <0.2 makes infection unlikely. Using a higher I/T ratio of 0.3 or 0.4 has been reported to marginally increase the positive predictive value of the tests.[451] An abnormal I/T ratio in the presence of a low absolute neutrophil count is more strongly suggestive of infection.

Another feature suggesting infection is the presence of toxic granulation in the neutrophils. Manroe et al[689] found this in only 11% of normal infants, compared to 63% of infants with confirmed sepsis.

It has been recommended that in neutropenic infected babies the WBC storage pool should be assessed by marrow puncture. However, as the test is invasive, the neutropenia is usually transient[306] and treatment by granulocyte transfusions is still experimental,[59,171] there seems little purpose in doing this.

The lymphocyte count. Babies who have lymphoctye counts persistently below 2.8×10^9/l should be investigated for severe combined immunodeficiency.[452]

Acridine orange test. Direct staining of micro-organisms within white blood cells using the acridine orange technique is a useful way of diagnosing septicaemia and fungaemia.[183,585,587] In a study comparing CRP, acridine orange and nitroblue tetrazolium in the diagnosis of central venous catheter sepsis, acridine orange was shown to be most accurate (87% sensitivity and 94% specificity).[920] Microscopy of a buffy-coat smear stained with methylene blue is also a useful test with a high rate of concordance with blood culture results.[870]

Platelet count. In 50% of babies with bacterial infection the platelet count will fall below 100×10^9/l, but this usually occurs after the baby is obviously septic. In a recent study, the sensitivity and specificity of thrombocytopenia for the diagnosis of septicaemia were reported as 65% and 47%, respectively.[97]

Viral infections, both congenital (e.g. rubella, CMV and herpes) and acquired (e.g. enterovirus, CMV, herpes) may cause a profound thrombocytopenia (p. 1168).

Acute-phase proteins

C-reactive protein. This globulin is produced by the liver during any generalized inflammatory process, probably as a result of stimulation by IL-1[786] and IL-6 (see below). Systemic bacterial and fungal infections produce a sharp rise in the blood CRP concentration of newborn infants, but there is a delay of about 10–12 hours between the onset of infection and the CRP increase,[695,1013] which limits the usefulness of the CRP in the initial evaluation of the septic infant. Viral infections often do not cause a rise in the CRP.[847]

CRP is a more accurate predictor of infection than the WBC indices,[97,446] especially if serial measurements are made[848] and a receiver operator characteristic curve is constructed to establish the best cut-off value. In a recent study of the value of the CRP in predicting culture-proven sepsis in a cohort of infants below 30 weeks' gestation[1072] the following results were obtained. On day 1 of the illness: sensitivity 62.7%, specificity 87.7%, negative predictive value 92.2%; on day 2 of the illness (combining the results with those of day 1): sensitivity 90.2%, specificity 80.6%, negative predictive value 97.7%. In another recent study[569] the negative predictive value for proven sepsis in term and preterm infants was found to be 99.0% and 97.8% respectively, although the sensitivity and specificity were 61.5% and 75%. These results indicate that culture-proven sepsis is most unlikely if the CRP does not rise within 24–48 hours of the onset of the illness, and the combination of a normal CRP and negative cultures at 48 hours is a generally safe basis for stopping antibiotic therapy which was started on clinical suspicion.[294]

Serial measurements of CRP are useful in monitoring the progress of infection. Persistently elevated CRP during antibiotic therapy for presumed bacterial infection should suggest the possibility of fungal infection, resistant organisms or the development of a complication such as bacterial endocarditis or abscess formation. A raised CRP is often seen in association with meconium aspiration, even when there is no evidence of bacterial infection.

Other acute-phase proteins. Orosomucoid (α_1-acid glycoprotein), haptoglobin, α_1-antitrypsin and α_1-antichymotrypsin have all been used in assessing neonatal infection, but add little if anything to what is learnt from studying CRP.[833,938,1013] The same applies to fibronectin assays,[258,385] although it is worth pointing out that many septic preterm infants develop significantly low plasma fibronectin concentrations, which may impair their ability to combat infection.[279,290]

IL-6 and TNFα

Because IL-6 plays a critical role in inducing CRP synthesis it should provide an earlier indicator of infection than CRP. A recent study measuring serial IL-6 and CRP plasma concentrations prospectively in a cohort of infants admitted to a neonatal unit found that on admission IL-6 was more sensitive than CRP in diagnosing sepsis – 73% vs 58%.[157] Increased concentrations of IL-6, in association with raised serum CRP, have also been reported in the bronchoalveolar lavage fluid of babies born after prolonged rupture of the membranes.[432]

TNFα has not yet been studied extensively as a mediator of inflammation in the newborn or as a possible diagnostic test. However, raised TNFα concentrations have been found in the lung lavage fluid of babies with pneumonia[158] and elevated plasma concentrations have been found in infants with culture-proven sepsis.[798] A comparison between IL-6 and TNFα concentrations in septic infants has suggested that IL-6 is the more reliable indicator of bacterial sepsis.[485]

Granulocyte elastase concentration

Elevation of the amniotic fluid granulocyte elastase concentration has recently been shown to have a useful predictive value for neonatal sepsis and merits further evaluation as an early screening test.[696]

Serum procalcitonin

Elevated serum concentrations of procalcitonin have recently been shown to predict neonatal sepsis with considerable accuracy, but further studies are needed.[382,735]

Serum granulocyte colony-stimulating factor

Using a cut-off value of 120 pg/ml, the serum G-CSF concentration has been shown to have a sensitivity of 95%, a specificity of 73%, a positive predictive value of 40% and a negative predictive value of 99% in the diagnosis of culture-proven neonatal sepsis.[574]

Immunological studies

Antigen detection tests. Counterimmunoelectrophoresis has been used to detect the presence of bacterial antigens in blood, urine or CSF, but it is little used in neonatal practice. However, rapid screening for GBS using latex particle agglutination is in quite widespread use, for detecting both maternal and neonatal colonization.[365,421,466,868] In screening neonates it has been suggested that it may be best to concentrate the urine before testing.[80] However, a recent evaluation of the test on concentrated urine in screening for GBS within the first 24 hours of life found a sensitivity of 90%, a specificity of 70%, a positive predictive value of 12% and negative predictive value of 99%.[1112] These results suggest that the main value of the test may be in providing reassurance of the absence of GBS.

Antibody detection tests. These are of more value in viral infections, when a fourfold or greater rise in antibody titre in samples drawn 2 weeks apart is diagnostic. If there is suspicion of congenital infection, organism-specific IgM should be sought (p. 1169), although this is not reliable for HIV (p. 1177).

Genetic techniques

It is now possible to amplify highly conserved DNA sequences from a variety of Gram-positive and Gram-negative organisms, as well as many viruses, using PCR, while avoiding the simultaneous amplification of associated human DNA.[654] This method has the potential to be automated and to provide rapid diagnosis of bacteraemia. Other DNA amplification techniques are also becoming available.

TREATMENT OF NEONATAL SEPSIS

In this section the general principles of treatment of the septicaemic infant will be outlined. The overriding consideration is prompt and effective treatment, as infants with systemic sepsis deteriorate very rapidly because of poor host defences, and morbidity and mortality rates are high.

ANTIBIOTICS

The choice and administration of antibiotics for early-onset sepsis are discussed on page 1129 and for late-onset sepsis on pages 1136–1137. Other comments on antibiotics are linked to the discussion of focal infections.

ADJUNCTIVE THERAPIES

Although antibiotics are the mainstay of treatment of neonatal bacterial infection, experience with immunodeficient patients shows that antibiotics alone are often unsuccessful in defeating bacteria if not supplemented by host defences. Because all neonates are to an extent immunodeficient, and preterm infants especially so, various attempts have been made to employ adjunctive therapies to improve host defences.

Immunoglobulin therapy

The prophylactic use of immunoglobulins is discussed on page 1137. The therapeutic use of immunoglobulin infusions in clinically suspected sepsis has been less well studied. There is evidence of improved humoral immunity in babies after immunoglobulin infusion,[9] of enhanced opsonophagocytosis of CONS by neonatal blood after the addition of immunoglobulin,[218] and of enhanced production of TNFα by cord blood monocytes following incubation with IgG,[234] but there is as yet inconclusive evidence of efficacy in reducing morbidity or mortality (see pp. 1137–1138 for further comment).

Fresh frozen plasma

Fresh frozen plasma is commonly used as part of the treatment of the septic infant in an attempt to enhance humoral immunity.[1011] Adult FFP enhances neonatal neutrophil chemotaxis in vitro.[295] However, when FFP was infused into infants no effect on the serum concentrations of components of humoral immunity was found.[9] There are also concerns about the safety of FFP[160] (p. 842). Unless evidence of the efficacy of FFP in treating neonatal sepsis is forthcoming from randomized controlled trials, there is little justification for its use in septic infants other than in treating associated DIC (p. 804).

Exchange transfusion

Exchange transfusion provides humoral factors and removes some noxious products of septicaemia, such as bacterial toxins, fibrin degradation products and cytokines. Some studies have suggested that exchange transfusion with fresh whole blood is beneficial in neonatal sepsis,[1049] but well-designed, prospective randomized controlled trials are conspicuous by their absence. However, the improvement in some septicaemic babies after exchange with fresh blood is occasionally dramatic, and the technique should not necessarily be abandoned.

Granulocyte transfusion

Granulocytes obtained from donor blood, or by plasmapheresis, have been given to septic babies, in particular when their illness has been complicated by neutropenia and granulocyte storage pool depletion, as judged by bone marrow aspiration (p. 1124). Several efficacy studies are published but are too flawed in their design to allow clear conclusions to be reached.[174,197,617] The most recently published randomized trial has suggested a possible benefit,[176] but overall the literature is not convincing.

Granulocyte colony stimulating factor and granulocyte macrophage colony stimulating factor

G-CSF and GM-CSF are important in inducing granulocyte production and activation in the newborn during sepsis.[388,922] and may be a useful marker of infection.[574] The mononuclear cells of the newborn are less able to produce G-CSF than those from adults,[175] and this may be part of the explanation for the granulocytopenia that often accompanies severe neonatal sepsis. In newborn rats the administration of recombinant G-CSF induces granulocyte production and improves survival from GBS sepsis.[173] In human newborns several trials of recombinant G-CSF in suspected sepsis have shown an increase in neutrophil counts and enhanced functional activity, as judged by C3bi expression.[82,172,394,906] There are no published studies of the influence of G-CSF on outcome in neonatal sepsis, although there is a single case report of probable benefit in a neutropenic 654 g infant with recurrent GBS sepsis.[891] In infants suffering from alloimmune neutropenia or congenital agranulocytosis G-CSF and GM-CSF can be very effective.[894]

Other innovations

Pentoxifylline

Pentoxifylline is an immunomodulating agent which can augment impaired neutrophil function in newborn infants. It has a wide range of effects, including altering neutrophil deformability and increasing NBT reduction and H_2O_2 production.[603] Its use in septic infants has not been evaluated.

Antilipid A monoclonal antibodies

Lipid A is responsible for the toxic effects of lipopolysaccharide in Gram-negative shock, and antilipid A monoclonal antibody decreases mortality in infected newborn rats.[410] Interestingly from a perinatal point of view, the antilipid antibody was administered to the pregnant female rat and passed transplacentally.

Supportive therapy

The septicaemic baby often requires full neonatal intensive care, as described in Chapter 21 and Chapter 29, Part 2. There are, though, one or two specific points that require special attention.

Arterial and venous lines

The preferred course of action is to remove any central lines that have been in place for more than 24 hours and to replace them with peripheral lines until the sepsis has been dealt with. This option may prove impossible to implement in tiny babies with difficult vascular access, in whom, despite the hazards, leaving the lines in place for both infusion and sampling in the early stages of the illness may be totally justified.

Bleeding diathesis

Thrombocytopenia and DIC are both common complications of neonatal septicaemia. Their management is discussed in detail on pages 804 and 842.

Nutrition

Septicaemic babies are usually catabolic but rarely tolerate enteral feeds because of a paralytic ileus, NEC or gastroenteritis. Intravenous feeding, particularly fat, is poorly tolerated during septicaemia. For this reason, dextrose and electrolytes alone should be used for the first 24–48 hours of infection. More complete parenteral or enteral nutrition should be established as soon as there is improvement in the baby's condition.

CLASSIFICATION OF NEONATAL INFECTIONS

Classification is useful in so far as it facilitates consideration of common principles of causation, presentation or treatment. The following is the most helpful to the practice of neonatal medicine.

- **Early-onset sepsis.** Definitions range from 24 hours to 7 days, but here the term means infection presenting within the first 48 hours of life and commonly caused by microorganisms acquired from the mother before or during birth. Other terms used for this pattern of infection are 'vertically transmitted' (meaning from mother to infant) and 'perinatally acquired'.
- **Late-onset sepsis.** This term means infection presenting after 48 hours of age and generally caused by microorganisms acquired from the environment rather than from the mother. The other terms used for this pattern of infection are 'nosocomial' and 'horizontally transmitted'. Nosocomial means literally 'of, or related to, a hospital'. In this sense many vertically transmitted infections are nosocomial, but it is more useful in studying epidemiology to separate infections acquired from the mother during birth from those acquired after birth.
- **Transplacental infection.** This is self-explanatory and is the usual term for infections such as congenital rubella, toxoplasmosis and CMV. It is also appropriate for many cases of HIV infection and hepatitis, and some cases of herpes simplex infection.

EARLY-ONSET NEONATAL SEPSIS

Early-onset sepsis is usually a fulminating septicaemic illness, often complicated by meningitis or pneumonia. It is caused by pathogens acquired from the mother prior to, or during, birth. Important predisposing factors are prolonged rupture of the membranes, maternal urinary tract infection, prematurity, and bad luck in the form of a particularly pathogenic microorganism. It has also recently been reported that a significant proportion of the babies of mothers with severe pre-eclampsia are neutropenic and more than usually vulnerable to early-onset sepsis.[169,264,360,741] Although prematurity is an important risk factor, the mean birthweight of babies suffering from early-onset sepsis is significantly higher than that of babies suffering from late-onset sepsis. In two recent studies the mean birthweight of babies with early-onset sepsis was 2472 g and 2213 g and for babies with late-onset sepsis 1960 g and 1711 g respectively.[269,535]

The incidence of early-onset sepsis (as defined here) is around two to three cases per 1000 livebirths.[535] The incidence of early-onset sepsis may be falling in developed countries, especially among low birthweight infants, possibly owing to antibiotic prophylaxis for group B streptococcal infection[832] (p. 1130).

Most early-onset sepsis is caused by *Streptococcus agalactiae*, commonly known as GBS.[400,535,599,832] Other important organisms are *E. coli*, streptococci other than GBS, *H. influenzae*, *L. monocytogenes*, Gram-negative anaerobes,[149] fungi and *Chlamydia trachomatis*. The pattern of presentation is similar with most of the causative organisms, and early-onset sepsis with GBS will serve as the model for all.

EARLY-ONSET SEPSIS DUE TO THE GROUP B STREPTOCOCCUS

Epidemiology

There are seven identifiable subtypes of GBS, based on capsular polysaccharide antigens: Ia, Ib, II, III, IV, V, VI, and one non-typable group. All are implicated in early-onset disease, but most neonatal infections are caused by types I, II and III. In addition to the polysaccharide antigens there are surface-exposed protein antigens which may also contribute to the pathogenicity of particular strains,[203] although tissue invasiveness seems unrelated to known surface antigens.[1054]

Recent publications have reported the incidence of early-onset GBS sepsis in different countries as follows. In the USA, 1.8 per 1000 livebirths;[140] in Canada, 1.75 per 1000;[205] in Australia, 1.3 per 1000;[535] in Spain, 1.2 per 1000.[500] In the UK, the most recently reported incidences have been in the range 0.3–1 per 1000,[548,701,880] but these data are quite old. From time to time major outbreaks are reported during which the incidence may be as high as 14 per 1000 livebirths.[10]

The two major factors influencing the prevalence of GBS sepsis are vaginal carriage rates among pregnant women and the effectiveness of strategies to prevent contamination of the baby at birth. During the last 5 years, vaginal and rectal carriage rates have been variously reported as 18.5%,[391] 12%,[549] 16.3%,[863] 23%[38] and 7.1%.[500] The lowest rates are reported from European centres, and this is mirrored in the lower reported incidence of early-onset GBS sepsis in Europe, certainly compared with the USA.

Clinical picture

Most cases of GBS sepsis develop within the first 4–6 hours (Fig. 43.4) and almost 90% of cases present within 24 hours of birth.[375,1130] GBS sepsis may masquerade as severe birth asphyxia[653,820] or present immediately after resuscitation with respiratory failure, cyanosis and shock. More often, the baby presents with the early signs of sepsis (pp. 1116–1117), and this is when the condition **must be suspected**. Without prompt recognition and treatment the baby's condition rapidly worsens and he requires intubation and IPPV for apnoea and severe hypoxaemia, often demonstrating the cardiorespiratory features of PPHN (p. 527). Hypotension, metabolic acidaemia, tachycardia and poor peripheral perfusion develop in severe cases, and then the prognosis is poor.[168]

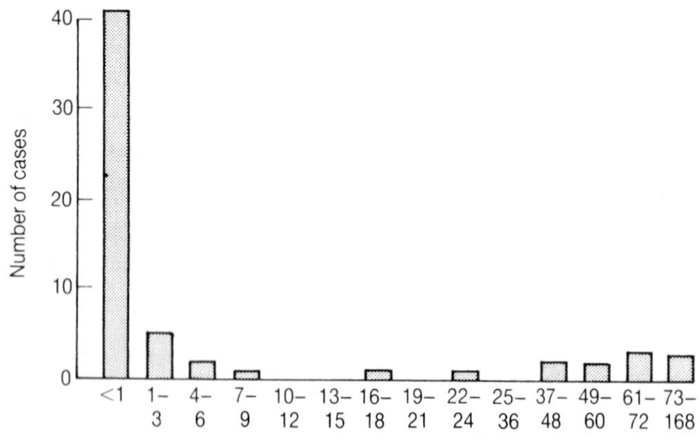

Fig. 43.4 Distribution of 61 cases of early-onset GBS infection. (Reproduced with permission from Boyer and Gotoff[141])

Pathophysiology

The hypotension, hypoxaemia and lung injury that characterize early-onset GBS sepsis in the newborn are very reminiscent of the septic shock syndrome caused by the endotoxin of Gram-negative organisms. Gram-negative endotoxin exerts its effects mainly by stimulating the release of cytokines, such as TNFα, IL-1[1055] and IL-6 from antigen-presenting cells, including macrophages and monocytes. TNFα causes progressive hypotension, decreased cardiac output, hypoxaemia and lung injury when infused directly into animals. TNFα can be detected in the serum and urine of babies with GBS sepsis (but not from healthy controls), and in the laboratory, heat-killed washed GBS can induce the production of TNFα from monocytes and macrophages[1110] (Fig. 43.5). Interestingly, mixed mononuclear cells from neonates produced significantly more TNFα in response to GBS than did cells from adults[1110] (Fig. 43.6). The cellular component of GBS responsible for TNFα release

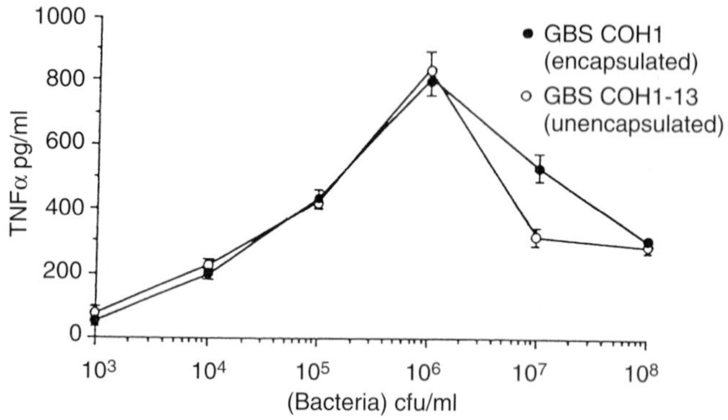

Fig. 43.5 Production of TNFα by monocytes and macrophages in response to encapsulated (COH1) and unencapsulated (COH1-13) type III GBS. (From Williams et al[1110] with permission)

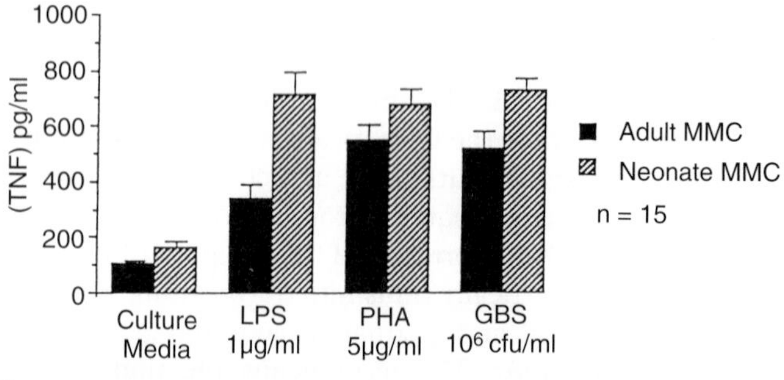

Fig. 43.6 Comparison of TNFα production by mixed mononuclear cells from adults and newborn infants in response to stimulation by GBS, phytohaemagglutinin (PHA) and *E. coli* endotoxin (LPS = lipopolysaccharide). (From Williams et al[1110] with permission)

is not yet identified, but seems not to be the polysaccharide surface antigen. These observations could shed fresh light on the pathophysiology of GBS sepsis and may lead to novel immunological therapies, such as antibodies directed against TNFα.

Another feature of the GBS is its ability to invade pulmonary endothelial cells,[311] especially the cells of the microvasculature, and lead to the release of the eicosanoids, such as prostacyclin and PGE_2.[392] In animals, injection of heat-killed GBS causes dose-dependent increases in pulmonary arterial pressure and pulmonary and systemic vascular resistance, and decreases in cardiac output and heart rate. The quantitative response of the pulmonary vascular resistance is strain dependent, with serotype Ib having a greater effect than serotype III.[219] Infection with different strains might go some way towards explaining different severities of illness.

Host defences against GBS include polymorphonuclear leukocytes, complement and type-specific antibodies directed against the polysaccharide and protein antigens. A baby is most susceptible to GBS when his mother, despite having GBS in her vagina, has little or no circulating anti-GBS IgG.[54,1068] This is particularly likely if the baby is born prematurely.[30] A concentration of IgG-specific antibody of >2 μg/ml in the serum of newborns seems protective.[397] Neonatal white cells find it difficult to kill the organism[1012] and, if antibody is present, GBS antigen causes neutrophil aggregation in the lung, with the consequent release of a multiplicity of cytokines which further contribute to tissue injury.[663]

Postmortem findings

There are no specific features although many infants have alveolar hyaline membranes, as well as pneumonia.[2,814] In the preterm infant surfactant-deficient HMD may coexist,[543] but in term babies the hyaline membranes are a non-specific change caused by GBS toxicity.[900] The presence of hyaline membranes may in the past, in the absence of adequate bacteriological investigation, have resulted in many deaths due to GBS or other similar infections being attributed to surfactant-deficient RDS.

Investigation

On no account should the treatment of suspected early-onset sepsis be delayed pending the results of tests. The objective of performing tests is to provide retrospective confirmation of the diagnosis, to identify the responsible organism and to look for complications.

Microbiological

The blood culture will almost invariably be positive if the mother has not been treated with antibiotics. GBS is easy to culture and will usually grow from most surface swabs and from the gastric aspirate (which often contains numerous Gram-positive cocci), although there is little benefit in investigating these sites in addition to blood. Meningitis is unusual in infants presenting in the first hours of life, but an LP should be performed in infants presenting with signs of early-onset sepsis[1113] (p. 1123). GBS antigen can be identified by latex particle agglutination tests on the infant's serum and concentrated urine[365,868] (p. 1125). However, in a recent multicentre study evaluating the latex particle agglutination test in the urine of babies with culture-proven GBS sepsis, only 53.5% of infected babies had a positive test.[80]

The organism is invariably present in the mother's high vaginal swab, and new techniques may enable rapid detection of the organism in this site when the mother is admitted in labour.[1006] The specificity of these tests appears to be good, but their sensitivity is relatively poor.[421]

Haematological

Neutropenia and the presence of primitive cells in the peripheral blood are common[143,688] and neutropenia $< 1.5 \times 10^9$/l is an ominous sign.[814] However, the sensitivity, specificity and predictive values of haematological values in the diagnosis of early-onset sepsis are poor.[423,451] Anaemia and thrombocytopenia may develop in survivors. Acute-phase reactants such as the C-reactive protein are generally highly elevated in GBS sepsis, but there may be a delay of 12 hours or so between the onset of signs and the rise in CRP.[831]

Radiological

The chest X-ray may be virtually normal or show widespread homogeneous opacity in those with coexisting RDS,[638] and is rarely helpful in differential diagnosis. Pleural effusions may occur.[814]

Treatment

Intravenous antibiotics, at the high end of the recommended dose range, must be started immediately the diagnosis is suspected. A combination of ampicillin and gentamicin is a good choice for blind treatment of early-onset sepsis in the newborn because of synergism between these antibiotics against GBS,[56,1019] and because it is necessary to cover other organisms responsible for the syndrome (p. 1131). A cephalosporin alone is unsatisfactory initial therapy for early-onset sepsis, as it will not treat *L. monocytogenes* or enterococci. Once the diagnosis of GBS sepsis is confirmed therapy can be simplified to intravenous benzylpenicillin alone, continued for 10 days. GBS is very sensitive to penicillin, with most isolates having a minimal inhibitory concentration of less than 0.06 μg/ml.

Exchange transfusions using blood from a donor with anti-GBS antibodies have been considered helpful.[59,457,972] Infusions of immunoglobulins have been advocated and are used by some clinicians as supplementary therapy. The published evidence relating to the benefits of immunoglobulin infusions in the treatment of early-onset neonatal sepsis is fairly persuasive, but is based mainly on small studies which are not amenable to meta-analysis because of significant differences in study design and evaluation criteria.[478,1090] These trials have been reviewed recently.[476] Part of the problem may be the highly variable immunological activity of standard immunoglobulin preparations.[397] Specially prepared GBS-hyperimmune globulin will produce higher antibody titres, and such a product has been effective in experimental animals.[1085] However, because immunoglobulin infusions may increase the risk of white cells aggregating in the lungs, they should be used with caution.[1084]

Recent studies of GBS disease in experimental animals have shown a halving of mortality rate with the use of recombinant human GM-CSF as adjunctive therapy.[398]

Outcome

In the late 1970s early-onset GBS sepsis had a mortality rate of around 50%,[53] rising to 100% for babies <1.50 kg.[862] The results have improved since then, and the overall mortality rate for early-onset disease is now reported to be 15% or less.[535,1130] For mature babies, and those with late-onset disease, the mortality should now be <10%.[141,535,1130] Low-birthweight babies still do less well, with a mortality rate of 27%.[1088]

Preventing GBS sepsis

Maternal prophylaxis

Approximately 1% of babies born vaginally to mothers who carry GBS at the time of birth become infected. Important predisposing factors are evidence of chorioamnionitis, such as maternal pyrexia; prolonged labour; prolonged rupture of the membranes; frequent pelvic examinations in labour; and low birthweight.[10,204,375,391,676] One or more of these predisposing factors is present in 82% of cases of early-onset neonatal GBS sepsis.[375]

The main approach to preventing vertical transmission is intrapartum antibiotic prophylaxis, given to women who have been shown to carry GBS on screening during pregnancy and/or who have obstetric risk factors.[99,834] Many individual studies have reported significant benefits of this policy in terms of reducing neonatal colonization and infection,[376,549,863,1042] although this finding has not been universal.[43] A meta-analysis of all published randomized controlled trials up to 1994 concluded that although there was convincing evidence of a reduction in neonatal colonization with GBS, there was no demonstrated significant reduction in the incidence of serious maternal or neonatal outcome.[789] Also of concern is the observation that the use of antibiotics to prevent neonatal GBS infection can be associated with serious neonatal infection with resistant Enterobacteriaceae.[662]

On the balance of the existing evidence it seems advisable to use maternal antibiotic prophylaxis in an attempt to prevent neonatal infection, and the American Academy of Pediatrics has recently recommended two possible approaches.[27] One is to screen all pregnant women for GBS at 35–37 weeks' gestation and to give intrapartum penicillin or ampicillin to all who screen positive, regardless of other risk factors. The second approach is not to screen, but to give intrapartum antibiotics to all women with a risk factor. Risk factors include a previous baby with GBS disease, GBS bacteriuria during pregnancy, preterm labour, ruptured membranes for more than 18 hours prior to delivery, and intrapartum fever.

A promising new approach is the possibility of immunizing pregnant women to induce transplacental transmission of anti-GBS IgG.[567] Another approach to reducing vertical transmission of GBS is the use of vaginal chlorhexidine disinfection during labour. One randomized double-blind placebo-controlled study of this method[162] has shown benefit in terms of a significant reduction in the number of babies admitted to the NNU within 48 hours of delivery, while another[908] has shown no benefit.

Management of premature rupture of the membranes and preterm, premature rupture of the membranes[408,714]

Once the amnion ruptures the amniotic cavity and the fetus become accessible to microorganisms present in the vagina. The likelihood of such ascending infection increases with time. When the membranes rupture prior to the onset of labour (known simply as 'premature rupture of the membranes') the interval between membrane rupture and the birth of the baby may be prolonged. When the membranes rupture at less than 37 weeks' gestation (known as 'preterm, premature rupture of the membranes') an even greater interval between membrane rupture and birth often occurs.

The evidence concerning the risk of neonatal sepsis following premature rupture of the membranes at term is conflicting. Some studies suggest relatively little increased risk,[641] whereas others show a high risk and a high mortality.[17] Meconium staining of the liquor increases the risk of intra-amniotic infection.[1096] A randomized controlled trial of the management of PROM at term has recently been concluded and shows no benefit in terms of neonatal sepsis of induction of labour over expectant management for up to 4 days.[471] The overall rate of neonatal sepsis in this study was around 2–3%.

There is no doubt that PPROM carries a significant risk of sepsis,[46,136,502,633,641,1062] although when membrane rupture occurs before 28 weeks of gestation pulmonary hypoplasia is probably the greater threat to survival.[672] The risk of neonatal sepsis following PPROM has been reported to be about 3.5 times that without PPROM.[633] The risk can be reduced by prompt delivery following membrane rupture, but this has to be balanced against the risk of premature birth. There have been no satisfactory randomized trials comparing different delivery strategies following PPROM.

Several meta-analyses of published randomized controlled trials of prophylactic antibiotics in preterm labour, with or without ruptured membranes, suggest little benefit.[291,292,713] There have been several randomized controlled trials of antibiotic prophylaxis following PPROM,[314,669] but no convincing evidence of a reduction in the incidence of neonatal sepsis. As might be expected, prophylactic antibiotics following PPROM have induced neonatal sepsis with resistant organisms.[662] There is, though, reasonable evidence of a prolongation of the duration of pregnancy as a result of antibiotic therapy for PPROM.[408]

Neonatal prophylaxis

Whether or not to give prophylactic antibiotics to asymptomatic babies considered to be at risk of GBS sepsis is a controversial issue. Some studies have shown that giving prophylactic penicillin to all babies,[788,974] or just those <2.00 kg,[645] will cause a significant reduction in the incidence of GBS sepsis, but others have failed to demonstrate this benefit.[862] Giving prophylactic penicillin to all babies hardly seems to be justified, but giving penicillin to asymptomatic babies of women who have grown GBS from vaginal swabs, but have not themselves received appropriate antibiotics, is a common practice which seems reasonable.

Recurrent GBS infection

Some unfortunate infants experience more than one distinct episode of GBS sepsis, although the risk of this is no more than about 1%. In a recently reported series of nine cases the mean age at the second infection was 42 days;[422] six cases had septicaemia without a focus of infection and three had meningitis. In more than half of the cases the organism causing the first and subsequent infection was shown by means of restriction enzyme digestion and pulsed-field gel electrophoresis to be the same. Whether these cases represent a relapse of the initial infection or a reinfection is unclear.

Table 43.9 Conditions caused by GBS. (Reproduced with permission from Baker and Edwards)[53]

Early-onset septicaemia
Asymptomatic bacteraemia
Meningitis
Pneumonia
Empyema
Peritonitis
Suprarenal abscess
Arthritis
Osteomyelitis
Brain abscess
Subdural empyema
Cerebritis
Endocarditis
Pericarditis
Myocarditis
Ethmoiditis
Otitis media
Conjunctivitis
Endophthalmitis
Breast abscess
Cellulitis
Fasciitis
Impetigo
Purpura fulminans
Omphalitis
Dactylitis
Superficial abscess
Urinary infection

OTHER ORGANISMS CAUSING EARLY-ONSET NEONATAL SEPSIS

Many other organisms besides GBS can cause acute early-onset sepsis with a pattern of illness very similar to that described above (Table 43.8). These organisms can also cause late-onset septicaemia, as well as many of the specific infections listed in Table 43.9. It is because of this common presentation with such a diversity of pathogens that antibiotic therapy must be broad spectrum until the results of culture allow refinement. A few specific causes of early-onset sepsis warrant further discussion.

Haemophilus influenzae

H. influenzae, especially the non-capsulate non-serotypable strains, has an affinity for the female genital tract and is responsible for almost 10% of early-onset sepsis,[712] third only in importance to GBS and *E. coli*.[921] The incidence of neonatal *H. influenzae* infection was recently reported to be 4.6 per 100 000 births in the Oxford region.[331] The same obstetric risk factors operate as for GBS, and a recent study of early-onset *H. influenzae* sepsis reported preterm labour in 92%, PROM >12 hours in 63%, maternal fever in 64%, chorioamnionitis in 43% and vaginal discharge in 44%.[584] Most infants present immediately after birth with respiratory distress due to pneumonia. Meningitis and conjunctivitis are relatively common. The reported mortality is in the region of 50%.[1116] Most *H. influenzae* causing early-onset sepsis in newborn infants in the UK are currently sensitive to ampicillin, and this is one of the reasons why ampicillin is preferable to benzylpenicillin as part of the blind initial treatment. However, ampicillin resistance is progressively emerging and cefotaxime should be added when there is good reason to suspect *H. influenzae* sepsis.

Listeria monocytogenes (see also p. 1149)

Early-onset neonatal sepsis with *L. monocytogenes* is becoming commoner and the reported incidence from Denmark in 1986 was 25.3 cases per 100 000 livebirths.[361] The mortality rate recently reported from a UK centre is about 15%.[555] Most vertically transmitted listeria infections present at, or within 24 hours of, birth as septicaemia, pneumonia or meningitis. Diarrhoea and an erythematous skin rash may occur. It is very important to realize that listeria is not effectively treated by third-generation cephalosporins, and high dose ampicillin is the drug of choice.

Coagulase-negative staphylococci

Although a common cause of late-onset sepsis, CONS are also occasionally implicated in early-onset sepsis in preterm babies, and may cause pulmonary haemorrhage.[1008]

LATE-ONSET SEPSIS

Most neonatal infections which begin more than 48 hours after birth are caused by organisms acquired from the postnatal environment, rather than transplacentally or from the birth canal. The spectrum of late-onset sepsis ranges from minor skin infection to life-threatening septicaemia. In a recent prospective epidemiological study carried out in Australian neonatal units (using the 48 hour cut-off, as adopted here), the incidence of late-onset systemic sepsis was 4.4 per 1000 livebirths, compared to 2.2 per 1000 for early-onset sepsis.[535] The mortality rate from late-onset sepsis was 9% as opposed to 15% for early-onset sepsis, and numerous studies have reported a much higher mortality rate from early-onset than from late-onset sepsis. The vast majority of episodes of serious late-onset sepsis occur in preterm infants on the NICU, and life-threatening late-onset infections in term babies are rare. Rates of nosocomial infection on an NICU have been variously reported to have an incidence density as high as 22 infections per 1000 patient days[269] and as low as 4.8 infections per 1000 patient days.[341]

The commonest organisms causing late-onset systemic sepsis are CONS, Gram-negative bacilli (such as *Klebsiella* sp., *E. coli*, *Serratia marcescens* and *Pseudomonas* sp.), *Staph. aureus* and various *Candida* sp. (Fig. 43.7 and Table 43.10). Numerous other species of microorganism are involved from time to time (see Table 43.8), most of

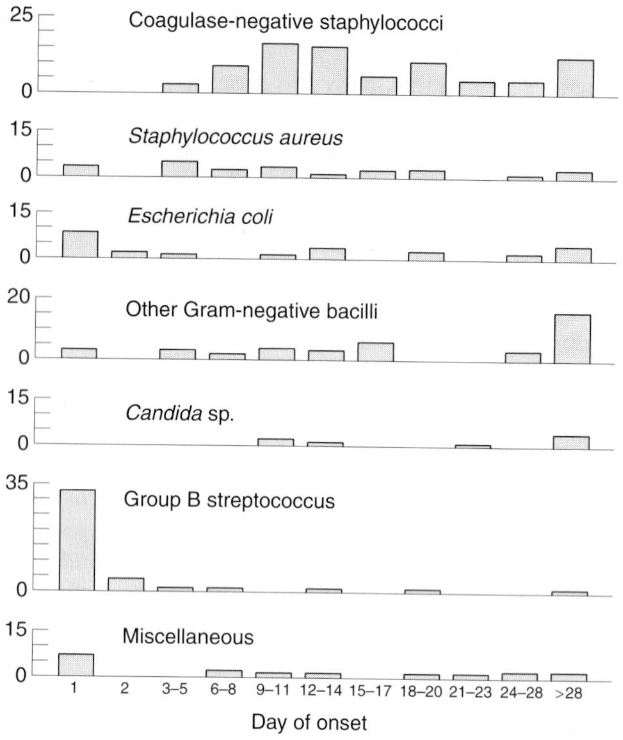

Fig. 43.7 Pattern of organisms causing neonatal sepsis. Organisms isolated from 234 babies with 241 episodes of sepsis in relation to postnatal age. (From Isaacs et al[535] with permission)

Table 43.10 Distribution of pathogens associated with episodes of late-onset sepsis treated with antibiotics for 5 or more days. (From Stoll et al[1009] with permission)

Organism	No.	%
Gram-positive organisms		
Staphylococcus – coagulase-negative	1288	55
Staphylococcus aureus	209	9
Enterococcus/group D streptococcus	111	5
Group B streptococcus	53	2
Other	52	2
Gram-negative organisms		
Enterobacter	102	4
Escherichia coli	101	4
Klebsiella	85	4
Pseudomonas	53	2
Other	82	4
Fungi		
Candida albicans	111	5
Candida parapsilosis	57	2
Other	51	2
Total	2355	100

which are normally commensals. Most minor superficial infections are caused by *Staph. aureus* and Gram-negative bacilli.

EPIDEMIOLOGY OF NOSOCOMIAL SPREAD OF INFECTION

The important reservoirs of microorganisms involved in late-onset sepsis are people, including the subject's own skin and gastrointestinal tract, other babies, hospital staff and visitors. Rarely, the source is the physical environment. Occasionally a specific contaminated source is discovered, for example mineral oil spreading *Listeria* sp.[955] or parenteral nutrition solutions containing *Acinetobacter* sp.[767] Modern methods of identifying specific strains of bacteria are proving useful in understanding the ecology of nosocomial pathogens, a step which is essential if the increasing rates of nosocomial infection and antibiotic resistance on the NICU are to be controlled.[334,441,571,812]

Predisposing factors to nosocomial infection

Any baby may acquire an infection from another person or from an environmental source, but certain babies and certain circumstances greatly increase this risk. Some of the more general predisposing factors relating to cross-infection were discussed in the section relating to preventative measures (p. 1112), but there are two crucial factors over which there is little control.

Prematurity and low birthweight and the use of medical devices

There is a strong relationship between prematurity and low birthweight and the risk of late-onset sepsis, especially that caused by CONS.[79,418,534,535,578,948,1007] In recent studies of NICU inmates, rates of nosomial infection among babies weighing less than 1000 g have been reported as 44.4% and 22.6%, and among those weighing more than 2000 g as 10.1% and 0.6%.[269,534] This undoubtedly has something to do with the inherent susceptibility of such babies to infection,[169] but is also strongly influenced by factors in the NICU environment, such as the adverse microbiological ecology and the use of medical devices. Many studies have demonstrated a strong positive correlation between rate of nosocomial infection and the use – and duration of use – of ventilators, lines for central vascular access, intravenous fat emulsions and implanted shunts for hydrocephalus.[84,170,362,373,374,379,380,845] The importance of exposure to these risk factors has been illustrated by the finding of a positive association between the rate of nosocomial infection and the overall average duration of stay on the NICU,[379] (Fig. 43.8), as well as the individual duration of stay on the NICU.[418] These findings show the importance of correcting for average duration of admission when making interhospital comparisons of nosocomial infection rates.

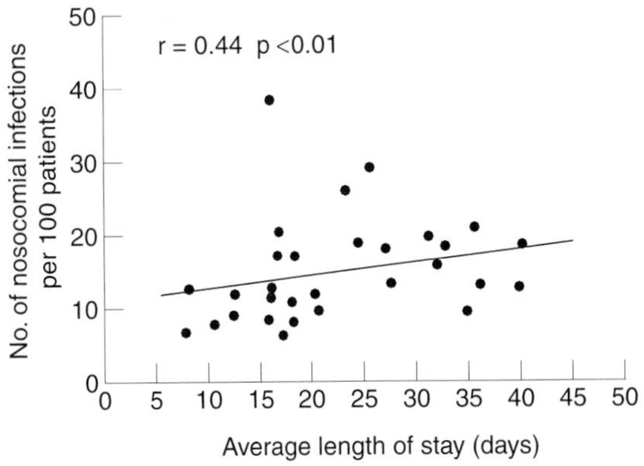

Fig. 43.8 Overall nosocomial infection rates in the NICUs plotted against average length of stay. (From Gaynes et al[379] with permission)

bacilli.[535,578] In developing countries the organisms causing late-onset sepsis are quite different. In rural India most cases are due to *Salmonella typhimurium* and *Pseudomonas* sp.,[875] whereas in Jordan, Gram-negative organisms predominate.[939] However, as countries implement modern neonatal medicine practices CONS seem inevitably to emerge as the most important pathogens.[477]

Epidemiology

The CONS constitute a ubiquitous group of organisms found in abundance on human skin. They can be found on the skin of some premature infants from as early as 6 hours of age, and increase rapidly to colonize all infants during the first week of life[577] (Fig. 43.9). The most heavily colonized sites are the umbilicus and the nose.[112] CONS are found in the stools of 90% of preterm infants.[945] There are more than 20 species of CONS, but 60–80% of the isolates from babies are *Staph. epidermidis*, with *Staph. haemolyticus* making up most of the remainder and *Staph. warnerii* and *Staph. capitis* a long way behind.[112,577,763] Strains of CONS isolated from preterm infants exhibit low rates of susceptibility to penicillins and aminoglycosides.[763]

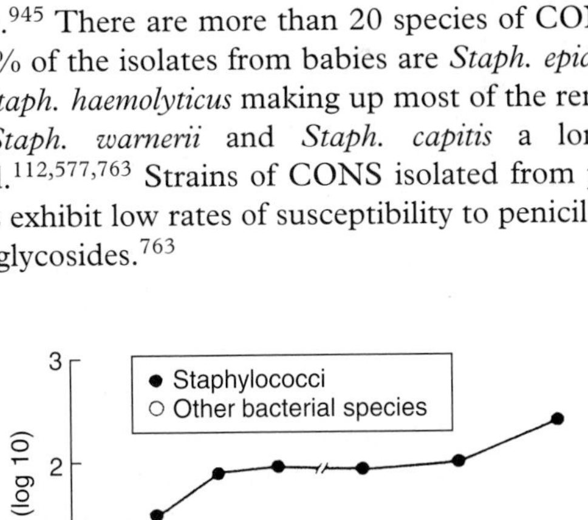

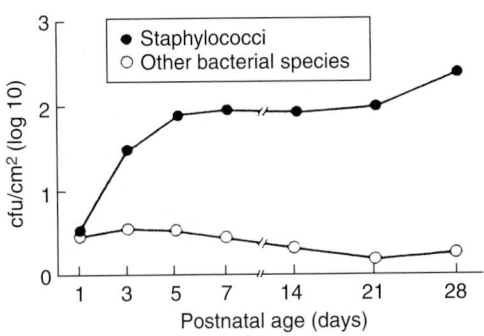

Fig. 43.9 Quantitative changes in cutaneous microflora with postnatal age. Measurements are logarithmically transformed and taken at eight sites in nine neonates. (From Keyworth et al[577] with permission)

SPECIFIC EXAMPLES OF NOSOCOMIAL INFECTION

Coagulase-negative staphylococci

CONS currently account for the majority of late-onset sepsis in developed countries, followed by Gram-negative

Infected infants are typically long-stay NICU patients on ventilators and with central venous access. Preterm infants seem particularly vulnerable to attack by CONS, and their deficiency of complement-mediated opsonic activity against *Staph. epidermidis* may be an important factor in this.[218] Infection is commonly with slime-producing strains.[442,458,524,949] Slime is a viscous extra-cellular polysaccharide substance which facilitates adherence to smooth surfaces, such as the plastic or silicone used for vascular lines, shunts and endotracheal tubes.[195,828] Slime also inhibits neutrophil chemotaxis and phagocytosis and suppresses blastogenesis.[417,552] There is also some evidence that the slime can inhibit the action of glycopeptide antibiotics such as vancomycin.[335]

Clinical features

The clinical presentation of CONS sepsis is very variable. Ordinarily there is septicaemia without focal complication, although the longer the septicaemia persists the more likely is the infection to localize. Occasionally the baby is acutely ill and shows all the signs of fulminant sepsis described previously (p. 1128), but more often the onset is subtle,[810,949] even in those with endocarditis.[776,777] Transient apnoeic attacks, tachypnoea, mottled skin, abdominal distension, loose stools, the occasional vomit, a few spikes of fever up to 37.6 or 38°C and the need for increased ventilatory support are typical. The importance of intravascular catheters and shunts in CONS infection is such as to warrant a detailed discussion.

Catheter-related infections. The diagnosis of catheter-related sepsis can be established by one of the following criteria:

- A positive catheter-tip culture yielding the same organism as is grown from a peripheral blood sample;
- Differential quantitative blood cultures with significantly greater colony counts from the catheter specimens than from peripheral blood cultures (pp. 1118–1119);
- Clinical and culture-proven sepsis which is resistant to antibiotic therapy but which resolves when the catheter is removed.

More often the diagnosis is assumed when CONS, or another common skin commensal, grows in blood cultures from a baby who has a central line in place.

The emphasis is on central lines, which have a higher rate of bacterial colonization than peripheral lines,[759] albeit that peripheral lines can sometimes act as portals of entry for CONS septicaemia.[374] Catheter-related sepsis rates among newborn infants have been variously reported as 10.3 per 1000 catheter days,[931] 10 per 1000 catheter days[522] and 3.7 per 1000 catheter days.[589] Most catheter-related infections occurring within a few days of insertion are probably caused by CONS migrating along the catheter from the skin around the insertion site. Infections of later onset, especially beyond 30 days, are probably due to colonization of the catheter hub, followed by intraluminal migration into the bloodstream.[932] In a recent study of newborn infants with presumed catheter-related sepsis, 30% were found to have positive cultures for CONS from the entry site and 30% from the catheter hub.[1025] Interestingly, molecular techniques showed that the isolates from blood and catheter hub were from identical clones in every case, but this was not so with the entry-site cultures, suggesting that the hub was the more likely source of infection. Further support for this is provided by a prospective study of catheter-hub contamination, in which 54% of episodes of catheter-related sepsis were preceded by, or associated with, contamination of the hub.[931]

There is a positive relationship between the length of time that a catheter is in place and the risk of infection.[170,180,188,374,380] Another important predisposing factor is the frequency with which the catheter is used for procedures such as giving drugs or blood transfusions.[380,749]

Catheter infections generally present with the low-grade clinical features outlined above, but occasionally may be complicated by blood vessel perforation,[68] central venous thrombosis,[919] bacterial endocarditis[876] even when the heart is structurally normal,[705] and intestinal perforation.[715] The clinical presentation of vessel perforation is usually fairly dramatic, with peritonitis, respiratory distress or cardiac tamponade, depending on the location of the perforation. Endocarditis due to CONS is usually less dramatic, presenting as a persistent septicaemia despite appropriate antibiotics and catheter removal. Diagnosis is by echocardiography (p. 1148). The prognosis for endocarditis due to CONS is much better than for endocarditis due to Gram-negative organisms.

Shunt infections. The shunt infection rate for children under 6 months of age was recently reported as 15.7%, with 67% of these due to CONS.[845] High skin bacterial density prior to surgery and the presence of CONS with high adherence properties (a marker of pathogenicity) were found to be important risk factors.

Investigation

The problem of interpreting the results of blood cultures has already been discussed in some detail (pp. 1118–1119). In babies with shunts, as well as performing the blood culture, which is positive in almost all those with ventriculoatrial shunts but only in 25% of those with ventriculoperitoneal shunts, the shunt reservoir or tubing should also be aspirated and the CSF sent for culture. The LP may be negative in the presence of shunt infection.[373]

Haematological changes are fairly common and include a rise in WBC and a fall in platelet count and haemoglobin concentration. The mean platelet volume often increases during CONS septicaemia, and this may be a useful adjunct to conventional tests.[783] The high specificity of the acridine orange leucocyte cytospin test for excluding line infection[920] (p. 1124) bears another mention here. Depression of the plasma fibronectin concentration has a usefully high specificity of 94% in suspected late-onset sepsis among VLBW babies.[290] Serial measurements of the CRP are useful in monitoring the response to therapy,[811] and a failure of the CRP to fall as expected should lead to the consideration of line colonization or a complication such as endocarditis.

Therapy is discussed below in the section on antibiotics for nosocomial infection.

Staphylococcus aureus

Staph. aureus is inherently far more pathogenic than CONS, and epidemiological evidence suggests that some strains are more virulent than others. During the 1950s' heyday of perinatal *Staph. aureus* infection phage type 80/81 showed itself to be particularly virulent.[339] This is partly explained by extracellular factors, especially the α-haemolysin, epidermolytic-toxin, enterotoxin, coagulase and leukocidin, and partly by surface components such as teichoic acid[24] which confers mucosal-binding properties. *Staph. aureus* was once the scourge of the newborn,[407,494] but nowadays (in the developed world at least) it is a much rarer cause of systemic neonatal infection than either GBS, CONS or the Gram-negative bacilli. *Staph. aureus* remains, however, the commonest cause of infection in bones and joints,[93,255,539] skin and umbilical cord, and a common cause of eye infection. Systemic infections with *Staph. aureus* carry high morbidity and mortality rates. In the developing world *Staph. aureus* is a common cause of neonatal sepsis and in Nigeria[18] it is the commonest pathogen causing neonatal meningitis (interestingly, GBS was not encountered in this series, which is a common finding in developing countries). In Pakistan *Staph. aureus* accounts for 15% of nosocomial infections, second only to *Salmonella typhi* and group A β-haemolytic streptococci (*Streptococcus pyogenes*).[111]

Epidemiology

Staph. aureus colonizes the skin and upper gastrointestinal tract of many infants,[343] although is nowhere near as ubiquitous as CONS. In a recent study of *Staph. aureus* colonization of the umbilicus, rates of 68% and 65% were found at 48 hours and 8/9 days respectively.[1001] In that study the rate of infection with *Staph. aureus* was 12% and there was a significant positive relationship between the level of colonization and the risk of infection. *Staph. aureus* gains a foothold very easily, and quantitative studies have shown that fewer than 10 bacteria can initiate colonization of the umbilicus in up to 50% of newborn infants. As with CONS, molecular methods are valuable in studying the epidemiology of outbreaks of *Staph. aureus*.[674,822,1126]

Clinical features

Septicaemia with *Staph. aureus* is anything but subtle, and very urgent action is required if death or serious morbidity is to be avoided. There is a clear association between the severity of bacteraemia as judged by semiquantitative blood cultures and the mortality rate.[954] Pustular or impetiginous skin lesions are common and provide a clue to the offending organism. Rapid seeding of organs occurs, especially to bones, joints and lungs. *Staph. aureus* is a relatively rare cause of meningitis and an even rarer cause of UTI.

Blood and other cultures are usually positive within 24 hours, and neutropenia and thrombocytopenia are common. Interpretation of a positive blood culture with *Staph. aureus* is less problematic than with CONS. The CRP usually soars and concentrations above 100 mg/l are often encountered within 12–24 hours of the onset of illness.

Therapy is discussed below in the section on antibiotics for nosocomial infection.

Gram-negative bacilli

These are a diverse group of organisms of widely differing genera. Most of those causing neonatal sepsis belong to the Enterobacteriaceae family, a large and heterogeneous group of Gram-negative rods whose natural habitat is the intestinal tract of humans and animals. Most of the species causing neonatal sepsis are part of the normal bowel flora, and only incidentally cause disease when they reach tissues outside the gut lumen. The most important Gram-negative bacilli causing neonatal sepsis in developed countries are *E. coli*, *Klebsiella pneumoniae*, *Pseudomonas aeruginosa*, *Serratia marcescens*, *Citrobacter diversus*, *Proteus mirabilis* and *Enterobacter cloacae*. In the developing world these same organisms are prominent,[110] but in addition more overtly pathogenic members of the Enterobacteriaceae, such as the Salmonellae and Shigellae, are important causes of neonatal sepsis.[875] A recent study comparing intestinal organisms between babies born in Sweden and in Pakistan showed that the babies in Pakistan were more rapidly colonized by the Enterobacteriaceae, and that a much wider spectrum of organisms was present.[13] The Swedish babies harboured either *E. coli* or *Klebsiella* sp., but the Pakistani babies often harboured *E. coli*, *Klebsiella* sp., *Proteus* sp., *Enterobacter* sp. and *Citrobacter* sp. simultaneously.

Epidemiology

Gram-negative bacilli currently account for 20–30% of cases of late-onset sepsis.[400] Figure 43.7 shows the distribution of cases of sepsis due to Gram-negative bacilli in relation to postnatal age and other causes of sepsis.[535] In developing countries, Gram-negative organisms are more prominent and in a recent study from Northern Jordan, *Klebsiella* sp. accounted for 64% of cases of culture-proven neonatal sepsis.[939] However, the Jordanian babies were totally spared infection by the GBS. In Kuala Lumpur, *Klebsiella* sp. are again the commonest cause of neonatal sepsis.[127] As with other organisms, molecular methods are proving useful in understanding the epidemiology of nosocomial infection.[114]

Clinical features

Systemic sepsis due to Gram-negative bacilli is usually fulminant and the mortality and morbidity are high, especially among very low-birthweight infants. A mortality rate of 50% was recently reported from the USA among a group of VLBW infants with *Ps. aeruginosa* septicaemia,[628] and from India a mortality rate of 23% for all babies with *Pseudomonas* sepsis.[448] In the United Arab Emirates the mortality rates from *Ps. aeruginosa* and *Klebsiella* sp. sepsis have been reported as 71% and 59% respectively.[599]

Therapy is discussed below in the section on antibiotics for nosocomial infection.

Enterococci

These are mostly non-β-haemolytic. They are normal bowel organisms which only cause disease when they get out of their proper place. The organism causing most disease in babies is *Enterococcus faecalis*, with *Enterococcus faecium* a poor second.[198] Enterococci are a notorious cause of nosocomial infection in both adult and neonatal intensive care units. In the NICU enterococci are an important cause of serious late-onset sepsis among VLBW infants.[256] Molecular methods are useful in establishing whether epidemic increases in enterococcal sepsis are due to the dissemination of a clonal strain or to multiple strains,[198] and this can be useful in planning antibiotic therapy for suspected cases. Enterococci are notoriously antibiotic resistant, especially *E. faecium*. This resistance is partly intrinsic, but extrachromosomal resistance transferred by plasmid genes is also very important. Septicaemia with antibiotic-resistant enterococci carries a mortality rate of 75%.

Therapy is discussed below in the section on antibiotics for nosocomial infection.

ANTIBIOTIC THERAPY FOR LATE-ONSET BACTERIAL INFECTION

There should be a low threshold for starting antibiotic therapy pending the results of clinical observation, cultures and other tests. Antibiotics should be given intravenously in appropriate doses and at appropriate intervals for the age and gestation of the baby. The difficulty lies in the choice of antibiotics, given the wide range of potential pathogens and the propensity of some of the common bacteria responsible for late-onset infection to possess, or acquire, antibiotic resistance. The initial choice is guided by three considerations:

- Knowledge of the species of bacteria most likely to cause infection on the particular unit. This local knowledge is best acquired by the formal collection of data by the department of microbiology in the hospital.
- Knowledge of the antibiotic resistance patterns of the bacteria most likely to be responsible for the infection, from the information obtained from the point above. These vary from unit to unit and within a particular unit over time, mainly as a result of antibiotic use.[243]
- Knowledge of the patient's previous antibiotic therapy. This is important because previous antibiotic exposure predisposes to infection with multiply resistant organisms. It is wise to choose different antibiotics from those used in a recently completed course.

Initial therapy

Unless there are local reasons to think otherwise, initial antibiotic therapy should be aimed at CONS and Gram-negative bacilli. If the locally endemic strains of CONS are sensitive to flucloxacillin, this should be the first choice. Commonly, though, CONS are flucloxacillin resistant and vancomycin should be used instead, given as a loading dose of 15 mg/kg body weight, followed by 20–30 mg/kg/day maintenance, with the dose interval adjusted according to the baby's gestation and postnatal age (Chapter 52).[661,1077] Careful monitoring of serum drug concentration is required as the pharmacokinetics are very variable.[42]

The choice of an antibiotic for Gram-negative bacilli rests between an aminoglycoside and a third-generation cephalosporin, such as ceftazidime, and should be based on local knowledge of antibiotic resistance, the site of infection and the toxicity of particular combinations. For example, suspicion of Gram-negative meningitis might lead to cefotaxime being preferred over gentamicin (p. 1140), and concerns about impaired renal function might lead to vancomycin and a cephalosporin being preferred over vancomycin and gentamicin. If *Pseudomonas* sp. are suspected, ceftazidime should be used in preference to cefotaxime.

Although a combination of vancomycin and either a third-generation cephalosporin or an aminoglycoside will cover the majority of late-onset infections on the neonatal unit, neither combination is a panacea and a definitive choice can only be made when, and if, the organism responsible for the infection is identified and its antibiotic susceptibility established. Several newer antibiotics are finding a useful role in difficult cases. Aztreonam is valuable in the treatment of Gram-negative sepsis[719,980,1015,1045] in the newborn, as is imipenem.[1014]

Definitive antibiotic therapy

Once the infecting organism is identified, therapy is rationalized to maximize efficacy and to minimize the risk of inducing resistance. The following are suitable antibiotic choices for the common neonatal nosocomial pathogens.

CONS. Vancomycin is the current drug of choice. The strains of CONS responsible for sepsis among babies on an NICU are commonly insensitive to penicillin, flucloxacillin and gentamicin. Routine susceptibility testing sometimes indicates that a CONS resistant to methicillin is sensitive to cephalosporins, but cross-resistance is common and all CONS that are resistant to penicillinase-resistant penicillins should be considered resistant to cephalosporins.[494] Persistent infection with CONS despite vancomycin therapy has been treated successfully with a combination of vancomycin and rifampicin.[1024]

For shunt infections routine i.v. antibiotics should be given, and the CSF examined every other day to check that the infection is clearing. If not, it may be necessary to give intraventricular antibiotics, including vancomycin, either by direct infusion into the shunt or by inserting an Ommaya/Rickham reservoir.[357] In general, however, the best results are obtained by removing the shunt and giving 10–14 days of antibiotics. The shunt can then be reinserted once the infection has cleared.[74,373,1135]

Staph. aureus. An antistaphylococcal penicillin, such as flucloxacillin, should be used in preference to vancomycin if the organism is sensitive.

Methicillin-resistant Staph. aureus. Vancomycin is currently the drug of choice. Persistent infection with MRSA despite vancomycin therapy has been treated successfully with a combination of vancomycin and rifampicin.[1024]

Escherichia coli. An aminoglycoside or a third-generation cephalosporin, depending on sensitivity pattern, should be used.

Klebsiella. An aminoglycoside or a third-generation cephalosporin, depending on sensitivity pattern, should be used.

Enterobacter, *Citrobacter*, *Serratia* and *Pseudomonas*. An aminoglycoside and a third-generation cephalosporin in combination should be used. Ceftazidime should be used if *Pseudomonas* is suspected.

Enterococci. Ampicillin or vancomycin plus an aminoglycoside should be used.

Combination therapy is recommended partly to exploit synergistic antibiotic combinations and partly to prevent the emergence of antibiotic resistance.

Administering antibiotic therapy

Antibiotics should be given intravenously, with careful attention to the recommended dosage, frequency, and the procedure for intravenous administration. If there is impaired renal or hepatic function the antibiotic regimen will require modification if a safe course is to be steered between efficacy and toxicity. When gentamicin or vancomycin is used serum concentrations should be monitored.

Duration of therapy

The duration of a course of antibiotic therapy will depend on whether or not infection is confirmed, the nature of the infecting organism and the location of infection. Little research exists to inform practice, but some guidelines can be given, as follows.

- If the clinical signs that led to treatment remit rapidly, and if after 48 hours there has been no rise in the CRP, no significant change in the WBC profile and the blood culture is negative, antibiotics can be stopped with minimal risk. A recent report has suggested that it may even be safe to stop antibiotics after 24 hours, by the application of a decision rule.[315] However, if the level of clinical suspicion at the time of starting treatment was high, then even in the absence of supportive or confirmatory tests 5 days of treatment is easy to justify.
- In most cases where bacterial infection is confirmed by culture, or where there is strong clinical suspicion, supported by a CRP rise or a suggestive change in the WBC profile, but there is minimal or absent evidence of focal infection and a good clinical response to therapy, 7–10 days of appropriate antibiotic therapy is adequate. The duration of antibiotic therapy required to eradicate CONS infection is mainly determined by whether or not it is possible to remove indwelling vascular catheters or other foreign bodies. Systemic infection with *Staph. aureus* should be treated for 3 weeks.
- In the case of focal infections much depends on the location and the pathogen, and advice on these will be given in the sections that follow.

PROPHYLACTIC USE OF IMMUNOGLOBULIN

Preterm infants have lower serum IgG concentrations than their term counterparts and show a progressive fall in IgG concentration for many weeks after birth. Unsupplemented, about 15% of VLBW babies will develop IgG concentrations of less than 200 mg/dl by about 12 weeks of age.[213] There is evidence that VLBW babies who develop hospital-acquired infection have significantly lower serum IgG concentrations than those who do not.[615] It was found that if the serum IgG was less than 350 mg/dl during the first week, or less than 230 mg/dl in the second week, the risk of sepsis was five times greater than among babies with higher levels.

It is possible to maintain IgG concentrations in these infants by giving regular infusions of immunoglobulin.

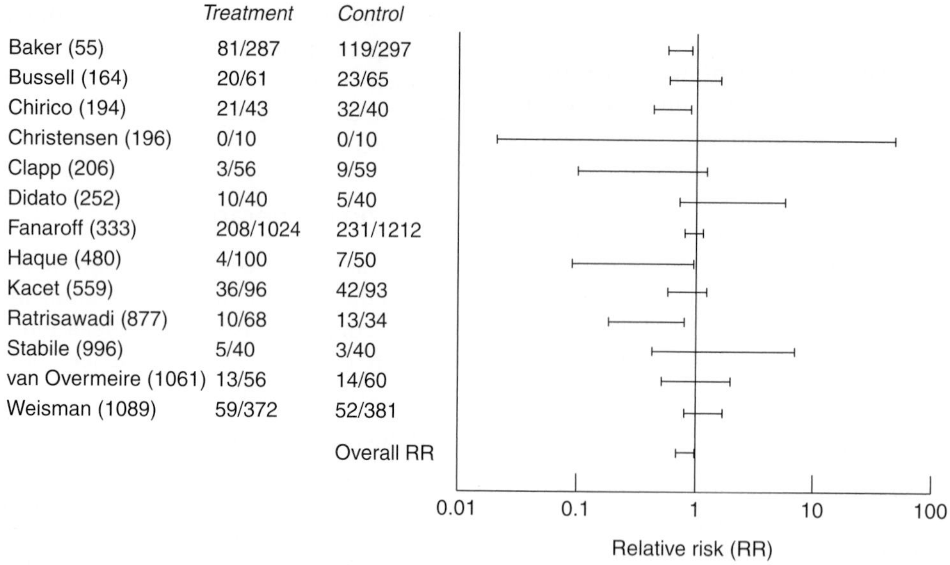
Treatment
Control
Baker (55) 81/287 119/297
Bussell (164) 20/61 23/65
Chirico (194) 21/43 32/40
Christensen (196) 0/10 0/10
Clapp (206) 3/56 9/59
Didato (252) 10/40 5/40
Fanaroff (333) 208/1024 231/1212
Haque (480) 4/100 7/50
Kacet (559) 36/96 42/93
Ratrisawadi (877) 10/68 13/34
Stabile (996) 5/40 3/40
van Overmeire (1061) 13/56 14/60
Weisman (1089) 59/372 52/381
Overall RR
0.01
0.1
1
10
100
Relative risk (RR)

Fig. 43.10 A meta-analysis of the effects of prophylactic immunoglobulin on the incidence of *infection* among preterm infants. Infection defined as clinical signs in conjunction with positive cultures from normally sterile body fluids. Overall RR = 0.81 (95%CI = 0.67–0.97). If only studies given a high scientific rating by the reviewers(55,164,196,206,252,333,1089) are included, the RR rises to 0.90 (95% CI = 0.72–1.11). (From Lacy and Ohlsson[608] with permission)

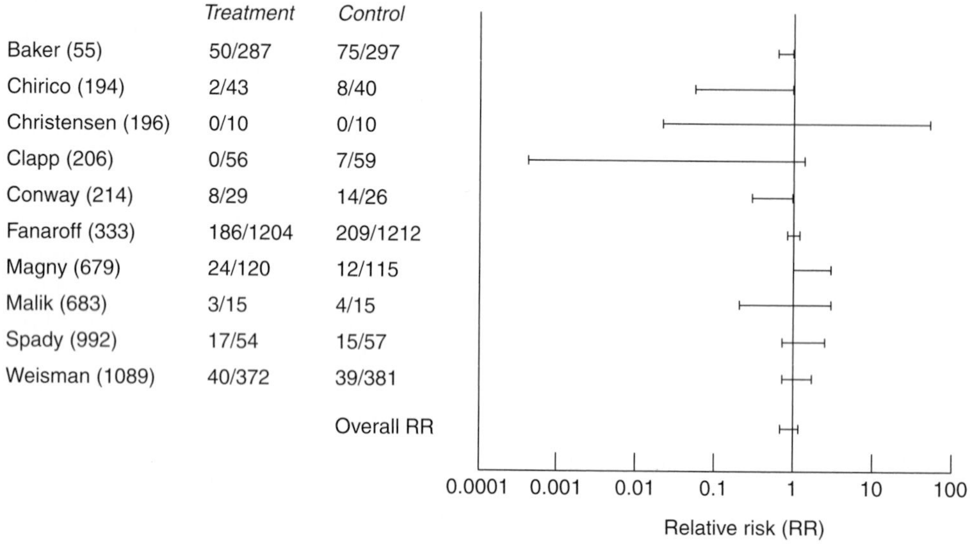

Fig. 43.11 A meta-analysis of the effects of prophylactic immunoglobulin on the incidence of *septicaemia* among preterm infants. Septicaemia defined as clinical signs in conjunction with positive blood culture. Overall RR = 0.87 (95% CI = 0.66–1.13). If only studies given a high scientific rating by the reviewers(55,196,206,333,679,1089) are included the RR rises to 0.94 (95%CI = 0.69–1.28). (From Lacy and Ohlsson[608] with permission)

The question, though, is does this reduce the incidence or severity of infection? Numerous studies have looked into this.[55,164,194,196,206,214,252,333,478,479,480,559,679,683,877,992,996,1061,1089,1090] These trials have recently been the subject of an independent (but not uncontroversial[475]) meta-analysis[608] and the main findings are shown in Figures 43.10 and 43.11. One problem is the variation in antibody activity between different batches of immunoglobulin.[25,345,1086] This may be improved by the development of immunoglobulin preparations with enhanced specific activity (p. 1130). On balance it seems reasonable to advocate immunoglobulin prophylaxis in the developing world, where infection plays such a large role in determining neonatal mortality and morbidity, but to regard the benefits as probably marginal in UK practice.

FOCAL BACTERIAL INFECTIONS IN THE NEWBORN

MENINGITIS

The incidence of neonatal meningitis in the technologically developed world is falling according to some surveys,[970] but not according to others.[87,1020] The current incidence is in the region of 0.25–0.5 cases per 1000 births.[354,520,535,1113] In the developing world it is more like 2 per 1000.[18] Meningitis complicates 20% of cases of early-onset and 10% of cases of late-onset sepsis.[535] The risk increases with decreasing gestational age and, as a group, preterm infants carry two or three times the risk that term infants do, and account for an even greater majority of the late-onset cases.[520]

Organisms

In the UK, GBS (mostly type III) and *E. coli* are responsible for just over 60% of all cases of neonatal bacterial meningitis, with *L. monocytogenes* a poor third at about 7%[1020] (Table 43.11) (Fig. 43.12). GBS is commoner in the early-onset cases and *E. coli* and other Gram-negative organisms in the late-onset ones.[520] About 80% of *E. coli* causing neonatal meningitis carry the K1 capsular antigen,[745] and many show reduced interaction with host neutrophils[790] and aerobactin production.[1041] In addition to the organisms mentioned, neonatal meningitis, like other forms of neonatal sepsis, can be caused by a host of bacteria (Table 43.8). The three organisms traditionally associated with meningitis in the older child, *H. influenzae*, *Streptococcus pneumoniae* and *Neisseria meningitidis*, are usually only found in the late neonatal period or in the second month of life.[308,354]

Table 43.11 Laboratory reports of bacterial meningitis: England and Wales, 1975–91 (bacteria identified in cerebrospinal fluid and blood); figures are total (%). (From de Louvois[244])

Organisms or group	Neonates	All other ages
Group B streptococcus	633 (34.3)	368 (1.4)
Escherichia coli	526 (28.5)	523 (2.0)
Listeria monocytogenes	125 (6.8)	448 (1.7)
Streptococcus pneumoniae	98 (5.3)	5 025 (19.5)
Other streptococci (excluding *S. pneumoniae*)	59 (3.2)	538 (2.1)
Neisseria meningitidis	50 (2.7)	8 870 (34.4)
Proteus sp.	44 (2.4)	84 (0.3)
Staphylococcus aureus	43 (2.3)	612 (2.4)
Klebsiella sp.	42 (2.3)	159 (0.6)
Haemophilus influenzae	42 (2.3)	7 200 (27.9)
Pseudomonas sp.	39 (2.1)	170 (0.7)
Enterobacter sp.	28 (1.5)	65 (0.3)
Staphylococcus epidermidis/albus	28 (1.5)	586 (2.3)
Citrobacter sp.	21 (1.1)	12 (<0.1)
Salmonella sp.	18 (0.9)	55 (0.2)
Serratia sp.	15 (0.8)	23 (0.9)
Coagulase negative staphylococci	14 (0.8)	124 (0.5)
Mycobacteria	0	433 (1.7)
Other*	21	462 (1.8)
Total	1846 (100)	25 757 (100)

*Includes *Acinetobacter* sp. (4), *Bacteroides* sp. (3), *Clostridium* sp. (3), coliforms (3), *Pasteurella* sp. (3), achromobacter/alcaligenes (2), *Haemophilus parainfluenzae* (1), *Corynebacterium* sp. (1), *Flavobacterium* sp. (1).

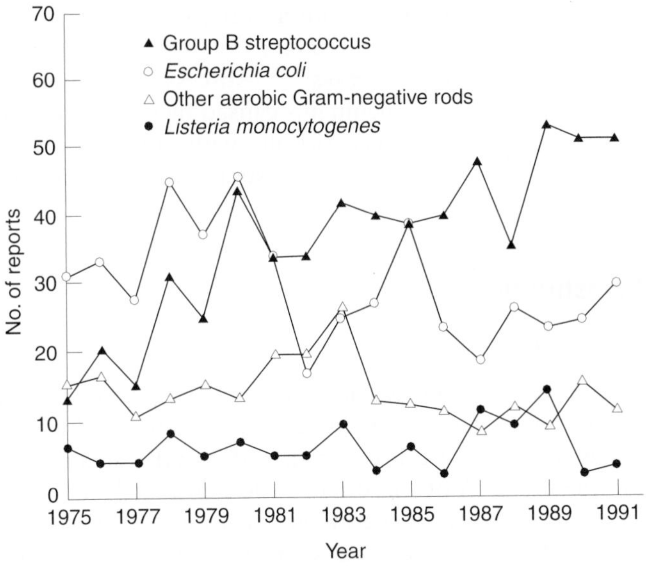

Fig 43.12 Secular trends of neonatal bacterial meningitis: laboratory reports from England and Wales 1975–91. (From Synnott et al[1020] with permission)

Clinical features

Neonatal meningitis must be diagnosed on the basis of the 'softer' signs of early neonatal infection (p. 1116), as by the time that signs such as a bulging fontanelle, high-pitched cry, altered consciousness or seizures occur the disease has advanced to the stage at which permanent neurological sequelae are likely. In VLBW infants recurrent apnoea, abdominal distension, hyponatraemia and loss of glucose homoeostasis are common.[826]

During clinical examination the head circumference should be measured and the skull and axial skeleton scrutinized for skin defects or pits that might have provided a portal of entry for infection.

Pathology

Inflammation, oedema and arachnoiditis are widespread in most cases of neonatal meningitis, as are vasculitis and superficial cortical thrombophlebitis, which cause superficial ischaemic damage to the brain. A useful rat model for neonatal meningitis has been developed.[583] Ventriculitis occurs in 70–90% of cases of neonatal meningitis,[100,395] but is less common with GBS than with Gram-negative organisms. Severe encephalopathic changes often occur,[100] probably as a result of direct penetration of the infection into the brain,[89] and may result in widespread cerebral atrophy. The choroid plexus may be damaged, permanently compromising CSF production, and exudate may obstruct intraventricular foramina and arachnoid granulations, leading to hydrocephalus in around one-third of cases.[520] Abscess formation is commonly seen with meningitis caused by *Citrobacter* and *Proteus* sp.,[590,885] and occasionally with other coliforms. Abscess formation begins with a suppurative ventriculitis and progresses to periventricular abscess formation.[990]

Investigation

CSF analysis

The criteria for diagnosing meningitis are given on page 1123. Gram-negative meningitis generally produces a higher CSF white cell count than does GBS meningitis, in which the WBC is often <100/mm^3.[521,940] In most cases bacteria can be identified when the CSF is stained by the Gram or acridine orange method, and if no bacteria are seen the possibility of a viral pathogen such as herpes simplex should also be considered. Occasionally, in the early stages of fulminating infection, organisms may be seen without a significant pleocytosis. If no organisms are seen on Gram stain, latex agglutination testing on the CSF will identify GBS infection with a high degree of specificity.[466,868] Measurement of CSF β_2-microglobulin concentration provides a valuable distinction between babies with CNS infection and those without, at a cut-off level of 2.25 mg/l.[371]

Lumbar punctures should be performed daily, or at least every other day, from the time of diagnosis until it is clear that the meningitis is improving. Failure of the lumbar CSF to improve is an indication for further investigation by ventricular puncture or ultrasound. Once the CSF is clearing LPs can be discontinued, as long as the infant's condition continues to improve. However, an LP should be checked weekly and before therapy is stopped. The last CSF may not show complete clearing of cells, but the sugar and protein values should be within the normal range, no organisms should be seen, and the culture must, of course, be negative.

Blood culture

Blood culture is commonly positive because neonatal meningitis is usually secondary to a septicaemia. However, negative blood cultures may be found in around 15% of cases of neonatal meningitis with positive CSF culture.[520,1067] The likelihood of a negative blood culture in meningitis is lowest in early-onset sepsis,[497,520] and this is when an LP may most safely be deferred if the baby is too ill to tolerate handling.[521]

Other tests

Cerebral ultrasonography will identify the cause of a rising OFC. It can also be used to detect ventriculitis,[506] and to monitor the response to therapy. Parenchymal changes or ventriculomegaly identify babies at high risk of sequelae.[469] If there is doubt about ultrasound findings a CT or MRI scan is justified. In VLBW infants progressive ventriculomegaly and the development of thalamic echodensities are quite common late findings, and suggest the need for serial brain ultrasound scanning.[826]

The EEG may be a useful guide to prognosis in neonatal meningitis and, when considered along with the presence or absence of seizures and alterations in conscious level, can predict outcome accurately in 93% of cases.[189]

Daily head circumference measurements are the simplest way of detecting the increasing cranial volume that occurs with cerebral oedema, hydrocephalus or subdural effusion (although this third complication is rare in neonatal meningitis).

Treatment

Antibiotics

Initial therapy. The safest initial blind treatment for suspected early-onset meningitis is still probably a combination of ampicillin and an aminoglycoside. This will effectively begin to treat meningitis caused by GBS, *L. monocytogenes*, enterococci, *H. influenzae* and many Gram-negative organisms. The alternative choice is a third-generation cephalosporin, such as cefotaxime or ceftriaxone, plus ampicillin. A combination of a third-generation cephalosporin and an aminoglycoside is sometimes used, but this will not effectively treat *L. monocytogenes* or enterococci. For late-onset cases the blind choice is more difficult, but the combination of a third-generation cephalosporin and an aminoglycoside probably offers the best chance of immediately effective therapy. Table 43.12 shows how the pattern of initial antibiotic prescribing in the UK and the USA has changed during recent years.[244,586,1120] The routine use of chloramphenicol is no longer justified.

When the Gram stain indicates the likely type of organism, prescribing is less speculative. For Gram-positive cocci, Gram-negative cocci or Gram-positive bacilli, ampicillin and an aminoglycoside should be used, and for Gram-negative bacilli a combination of cefotaxime or ceftriaxone and an aminoglycoside. When the sensitivity pattern suggests that vancomycin is indicated it is worth knowing that there is effective CSF penetration of vancomycin in preterm infants below about 32 weeks' gestation.[882]

Definitive therapy. GBS should be treated with benzylpenicillin, plus or minus gentamicin, with which there is some synergy. *L. monocytogenes* and enterococci are treated with ampicillin and gentamicin.[256] Gram-negative bacilli vary so much in their sensitivity patterns that definitive therapy can only be decided after the microbiology department has carried out sensitivity

Table 43.12 Neonatal meningitis. Antibiotic prescribing in America and the UK. (From de Louvois[244])

	Neonates (%)				Infants (%)			
	USA 1987[a]	USA 1989[b]	USA 1992[c]	UK 1992[d]	USA 1987[a]	USA 1989[b]	USA 1992[c]	UK 1992[d]
Aminoglycoside + Amp/Pen	59	60	39	16	12	11	1	8
Chloramphenicol + Amp/Pen	0	0	0	8	9	5	0	21
Cefotaxime + Amp/Pen	33	33	58	45	52	68	78	53
Ceftriaxone + Amp	7	2	1	0	15	11	13	0
Ceftazidime + Amp/Pen	0	0	0	13	0	0	0	10
Ceftazidime or cefotaxime + aminoglycoside	0	0	0	11	0	0	0	9

[a]Word & Klein[1120]
[b]Word & Klein[1121]
[c]Klass & Klein[586]
[d]de Louvois, unpublished data.
Amp, Ampicillin; Pen, penicillin.

testing. This is especially so in the case of nosocomial infections among the inmates of an NICU, who may acquire some very unusual and resistant pathogens. Combination therapy with cefotaxime or ceftriaxone and an aminoglycoside will be the most common choice. Aztreonam is emerging as a useful treatment for Gram-negative infections, including meningitis.[1015] Antibiotic therapy for neonatal meningitis should be continued intravenously for at least 21 days.

Adjunctive treatment

Neonatal meningitis is such a potentially damaging condition, even with prompt and appropriate antibiotic therapy, that there is a need for additional interventions. In experimental animals dexamethasone has been shown to prevent the brain injury associated with GBS meningitis almost completely.[583] There is no systematic study of steroid therapy in neonatal meningitis, and until such work is undertaken it is difficult to recommend steroids as part of routine treatment. It is likely that interventions aimed at the cytokines mediating inflammation and injury will eventually become routine. In experimental animals the use of chemical agents to inhibit the binding of excitatory amino acids to neuronal receptors has been shown to lessen brain injury.[627]

Intraventricular antibiotic therapy

Ventriculitis is common in neonatal meningitis, especially when caused by Gram-negative bacilli. Before the introduction of the third-generation cephalosporins, ventriculitis with persistently positive CSF cultures was relatively common. The explanation for this is probably the poor CSF penetration of the aminoglycoside antibiotics which have so commonly been used to treat neonatal meningitis – with peak CSF concentrations often approximating to the minimal inhibitory concentration. Third-generation cephalosporins, such as cefotaxime and ceftriaxone, have very good CSF penetration and their introduction has led to a great reduction in the number of cases where ventriculitis has persisted. In a recently reported large study of neonatal meningitis in the UK no baby required treatment with intraventricular antibiotics.[520] In the very unusual case of persistent ventriculitis despite adequate doses of appropriate antibiotics, recourse may still be made to CSF drainage procedures and direct instillation of antibiotics into the ventricles. However, controlled trials of both intrathecal[657] and intraventricular[658] aminoglycoside administration have failed to show significant benefit over systemic therapy.

Viral meningitis (p. 1156)

Mycoplasma meningitis (p. 1152)

Fungal meningitis (p. 1163)

Neurological complications

Cerebral abscess

This mainly occurs when meningitis is caused by *Citrobacter* or *Proteus* sp.,[590,885] but may occasionally complicate meningitis caused by many other organisms, including *E. coli*, *Staph. aureus*, *Mycoplasma hominis*[344] and GBS.[52] Abscesses may present with signs of increased intracranial pressure in a baby who is responding poorly to treatment, but in some cases produce no obvious change in the clinical state.[995] Ultrasound or CT establishes the diagnosis. Multiple or small abscesses can be treated with high-dose intravenous antibiotics. If only one or two abscess cavities are present, or if abscesses fail to resolve with antibiotics, the cavities should be aspirated and an appropriate antibiotic instilled. Systemic antibiotic therapy should be maintained for at least 4 weeks.

Hydrocephalus

This may occur during the second week of the illness while the infant still has ventriculitis, or may present with increased head growth and CNS signs at almost any stage after bacteriological cure of the meningitis. If infection is still present an intraventricular reservoir should be inserted and intraventricular and systemic antibiotics continued. External ventricular drainage is an alternative. In most cases a permanent CSF shunt will be required after the infection is controlled.

Deafness

Bacterial meningitis is the single most important cause of acquired sensorineural hearing loss in childhood, and neonates are especially vulnerable.[353] All survivors of neonatal meningitis should routinely undergo audiological screening soon after recovery, and audiological follow-up.

Prognosis

Mortality

The mortality rate varies with the nature of the organism and the maturity of the patient, and there is limited value in quoting overall mortality rates for neonatal meningitis. For what it is worth, the overall mortality rate seems to have fallen during the last five decades, from around 60% in the 1950s and 1960s[649] to around 30% more recently.[656,745] There is some evidence to suggest that mortality rates may have reached a plateau, and Volpe[1069,1070] showed no significant change over a 6-year period in the outlook for neonates with meningitis (Table 43.13) as far as either death or severe sequelae are concerned.

In some reports the mortality rate associated with Gram-negative meningitis is up to three times that seen with meningitis caused by Gram-positive organisms.[358] Meningitis due to Gram-negative enteric organisms still carries a mortality rate of around 25–30%, with lower rates reported for GBS and lower rates still for other Gram-positive organisms.[244] In a recent British study the mortality rate for neonatal *E. coli* meningitis was 25%.[245]

Mortality is higher in preterm infants. Mulder et al[746] found a mortality in *E. coli* meningitis of 66% in babies of <31 weeks' gestation, 30% at 32–34 weeks, reducing to 19% in babies >35 weeks.

Table 43.13 Outcome of neonatal meningitis. (Data from Volpe[1069,1070])

Organism	Dead (%)		Severe sequelae (%)*		Mild sequelae (%)*		Normal (%)*	
	1981	1987	1981	1987	1981	1987	1981	1987
GBS	15	21	11	21	11	29	64	50
Coliform (70% *E. coli*)	32	19	6	11	19	38	43	51

*Among survivors.

Permanent CNS damage

In most series adverse neurological sequelae occur in 30–50% of survivors[656] (Table 43.13). It is commonly believed that babies with GBS meningitis do better than those with Gram-negative bacillary disease, with up to 70% of survivors being normal.[191] However, some studies have found that only 50% of GBS meningitis survivors are intact.[289] The prognosis is worse in preterm babies. All forms of cerebral palsy, mental subnormality, epilepsy and cortical blindness may occur singly or in combination. In the most recently reported follow-up study 38% of survivors were normal, 38% had mild disabilities and 24% moderate to severe disabilities.[358]

PNEUMONIA

Neonatal pneumonia may be an isolated focal infection but is commonly part of a more widespread infective illness.[542] Definition and ascertainment of cause is generally more difficult with pneumonia than with other focal infections. This is partly because non-infective pulmonary pathology is so common in babies, and often impossible to distinguish radiologically, and partly because the isolation of bacteria from respiratory secretions is not synonymous with pneumonia in the same way that bacteria in the CSF are synonymous with meningitis. These uncertainties should be borne in mind when assessing the reported incidence of neonatal pneumonia. Using a rigorous approach to diagnosis, in a prospective study the incidence of neonatal pneumonia in an Oxford hospital was reported to be 3.7 per 1000 livebirths.[1082] This was among a population of almost 20 000 babies born in a tertiary referral centre and included all cases of pneumonia occurring before discharge. This probably represents the best available estimate of the current incidence of neonatal bacterial pneumonia.

There are several ways to classify neonatal pneumonia, but from a problem-orientated point of view classification according to age of onset is most useful:

- Congenital or intrauterine pneumonia;
- Pneumonia presenting within the first 48 hours of life and commonly due to pathogens acquired from the birth canal;
- Pneumonia occurring after 48 hours and usually acquired nosocomially.

Congenital or intrauterine pneumonia

This is rare and mainly occurs secondary to ascending infection and chorioamnionitis following PROM. The mortality rate is high and many affected infants appear asphyxiated at birth. Much of what is known about the pathogenesis has come from postmortem histology, and this presents some paradoxes. Bacteria are by no means always to be seen and many of the histological changes usually associated with pneumonia are absent in congenital cases, particularly evidence of a pleural reaction and of infiltration and destruction of bronchopulmonary tissue.[238] This has led to the suggestion that many cases of so-called congenital pneumonia are predominantly cases of asphyxia. There is very little up-to-date literature to be found on the subject.

Early-onset pneumonia

The reported incidence of early-onset pneumonia is 1.79 per 1000 livebirths.[1082] GBS accounts for 70% of cases, but *H. influenzae*,[584,921] *S. pneumoniae*,[544,566,1125] *L. monocytogenes*[509] and Gram-negative enteric bacilli contribute. Rarely, yeasts may be involved.[769] The same predisposing factors operate as for early-onset septicaemia (p. 1127), and bronchoalveolar lavage fluid from ventilated babies, born following prolonged rupture of the membranes, contains increased numbers of WBCs and a high concentration of IL-6.[432] Numerous viruses may also cause early-onset pneumonia, e.g. adenovirus[6,192,736,836] and CMV.[958]

Clinical features

In term infants early-onset pneumonia is comparatively easy to suspect, but in preterm infants distinction from HMD is difficult and sometimes impossible (p. 497). Typically, in term infants signs of respiratory distress accompanied by signs of systemic sepsis develop within a few hours of birth and progress rapidly. Pulmonary hypertension with hypoxaemia secondary to right-to-left shunting is a common complication, and in the case of GBS infection may be triggered by damage to the lung endothelium and the release of vasoconstrictor substances[392] (p. 529).

Investigation

Blood culture is usually positive, and culture of nasopharyngeal aspirates grows the same organism as the blood culture in a high proportion.[1082] If intubation is necessary, tracheal secretions should be obtained for microscopy and culture. Unfortunately, positive cultures from respiratory secretions do not prove pneumonia, but in rationalizing the choice of antibiotics it is important to know what is grown. Cultures from other sites are less helpful. The radiological changes are quite variable and usually not of themselves diagnostic. They include nodular or coarse infiltrates, a diffuse picture with air bronchograms rather like HMD, perihilar streaking and well-defined areas of consolidation.

To make the diagnosis of pneumonia there should be evidence of an inflammatory process, such as a rise in the CRP or an abnormal WBC, convincing chest X-ray appearances, clinical findings and a positive blood culture. In many cases the evidence is less compelling. Babies with pneumonia have higher concentrations of IL-1 and TNFα in tracheal aspirates than babies with uncomplicated RDS,[158] and tests based on recovered cytokines hold promise as discriminators in the future.

Differential diagnosis

The principal differential diagnosis in the preterm infant is HMD and, as pneumonia can damage surfactant production and function, the two conditions may coexist[624] (p. 497). Bacterial pneumonia should be suspected when there are features such as hypotension, poor tissue perfusion, metabolic acidosis and leucopenia. However, as it is impossible to exclude early pneumonia in preterm infants with apparent RDS, many neonatologists prescribe antibiotics for 48 hours until cultures are negative and the CRP has been seen not to rise.

If a previously well baby becomes dyspnoeic after 6 hours of age, pneumonia is the most likely diagnosis (see Table 29.13). Pulmonary oedema in infants with heart disease, and the very rare infant who presents late with a pneumothorax or an intrathoracic malformation, can usually be differentiated easily by a clinical examination, chest X-ray and, if necessary, an echocardiograph. Care must also be taken to exclude other causes of tachypnoea, in particular that secondary to metabolic acidaemia.

Treatment

Antibiotics. All babies showing signs of respiratory distress which does not have a clear non-infective cause must be treated with antibiotics, pending the results of further observation, cultures, CRP and other appropriate investigations. If the cultures are negative, the CRP does not rise and the baby makes a rapid recovery (as is often the case), treatment can be stopped. The safest 'blind' choice of antibiotic for presumed neonatal pneumonia is a combination of ampicillin and an aminoglycoside. A third-generation cephalosporin is an alternative if there is little likelihood of the pneumonia being due to *L. monocytogenes* or enterococci, and it does offer the benefit of reliable cover against *H. influenzae*, increasing numbers of which are now resistant to ampicillin. Antibiotic therapy for proven pneumonia should continue for 10 days, unless the pathogen is *Staph. aureus*, in which case at least 3 weeks should be employed.

Outcome

With modern neonatal intensive care early-onset pneumonia in otherwise normal term babies carries a low mortality rate, but among preterm babies the mortality rate approaches 50%, especially when the chest X-ray shows widespread atelectasis.[1082] In infants with staphylococcal or coliform pneumonia pneumatocoeles may develop,[605] as, rarely, may lung abscess (p. 1146) and empyema.[449] Abscesses and pneumatocoeles should be treated conservatively in the first place using long-term i.v. antibiotics for the abscess. Empyema requires insertion of a thoracentesis tube for closed chest drainage, and intravenous antibiotics for several weeks.

Late-onset pneumonia

Pneumonia developing more than 48 hours after birth is commonest among preterm babies who are receiving IPPV. In the Oxford study referred to earlier, 92% of babies with late-onset pneumonia were preterm and 87% were on IPPV at the time of onset.[1082] The mean postnatal age at onset was 35 days. The reported incidence of pneumonia in intubated babies varies from 10 to 35%. Halliday et al[462] reported an incidence of pneumonia of 35% among intubated babies with RDS. Using more stringent immunological criteria, Giacoia et al[389] diagnosed pneumonia in 24% of intubated babies, but in the Oxford study, using strict radiological and laboratory criteria, only 10% of intubated babies had late-onset pneumonia.

Organisms and pathogenesis

The organisms implicated in late-onset pneumonia are in many respects similar to those already described as causing late-onset septicaemia (p. 1132), except that Gram-negative bacilli are clear winners over CONS (Tables 43.14, 43.15). In long-stay patients with CLD unusual organisms, including fungi, mycoplasma and chlamydia, as well as viruses such as RSV and CMV, must be considered.[177] Other unusual causes of nosocomial neonatal pneumonia are reported from time to time, e.g. *Legionella pneumophila*,[424,516,651] coronavirus[979] and rhinovirus.[190]

Pneumonia in ventilated babies can occur secondary to septicaemia or secondary to colonization of the endotracheal tube. In contrast to early-onset cases, blood cultures are negative in most instances of late-onset pneumonia.

Clinical features

In an infant with primary lung disease already on IPPV, infection presents with deteriorating lung function (p. 615) plus non-specific signs of infection (p. 1116). An increase in endotracheal tube aspirate suggests infection, but can be confused with the bronchorrhoea seen in CLD. Localized and generalized crepitations may be heard.

Investigation

A method of surveillance for possible pneumonia in ventilated babies must be found, as it is a potentially serious cause of deterioration and additional lung injury.

Table 43.14 Bacterial isolates from seven babies with pneumonia of late onset (presenting after 48 hours of age). (From Webber et al[1082])

Case No	From blood culture	From culture from nasopharynx or endotracheal tube
1	*Pseudomonas aeruginosa* *Achromobacter xylosoxidans*	No growth
2*	*P. aeruginosa, Streptococcus faecalis*	No growth
3	*S. epidermidis*	*S. aureus*
4	*S. epidermidis*	Coliform sp. *S. faecalis*
5	*P. aeruginosa*	*P. aeruginosa*
6	*S. epidermidis*	*P. aeruginosa* Coliform sp.
7	*S. epidermidis*	Coliform sp.

*Baby subsequently diagnosed as having cystic fibrosis and died.

Table 43.15 Bacterial isolates from nasopharyngeal or endotracheal secretions of 32 babies during 34 probable episodes of pneumonia of late onset. (From Webber et al[1082] with permission)

Gram negative bacilli:	30
Coliform sp.	15
P. aeruginosa	12
Escherichia coli	2
Proteus mirabilis	1
S. aureus	5
S. epidermidis	2
Group B streptococcus	1
H. influenzae	1
No organism identified	4

Our approach is to perform routine, twice-weekly CRP estimations on all ventilated babies, and to undertake a chest X-ray, blood cultures and culture of respiratory secretions in any baby whose ventilatory requirement increases significantly or who develops a raised CRP. Interpretation of the results of tracheal secretion culture is discussed on pages 588 and 1145. In older babies, viral cultures and immunofluorescence studies for chlamydia (p. 1145) and RSV (p. 1145) are indicated.

Treatment

The choice of initial antibiotic therapy for neonatal pneumonia is difficult because the list of potential pathogens is long and because it is more or less essential to cover CONS. Unless local knowledge suggests otherwise, a third-generation cephalosporin plus vancomycin is a good choice. Therapy should subsequently be modified to cover organisms grown from the blood or tracheal secretions, along the lines suggested for specific bacteria (p. 1137 et seq).

If the baby is already on antibiotics when deterioration from presumed pneumonia occurs, it is usually advisable to change the drugs and to broaden the spectrum of cover, often to include an antibiotic effective against *Pseudomonas* sp. In babies on IPPV for several weeks, in whom *Chlamydia* sp., *Mycoplasma* sp., *Bordetella pertussis* or even *Pneumocystis carinii* are possible pathogens, antibiotics such as erythromycin and septrin should be considered.

Pneumonia in the baby with CLD (p. 615)

In babies with long-term respiratory disease pneumonia should always be at the top of the list of differential diagnosis if the lung disease deteriorates. Some of these babies are several months old and, in addition to the usual pathogens, the respiratory viral infections characteristic of that age group are common.[836] There is a suggestion from the literature that respiratory tract colonization with Gram-negative organisms is associated with more severe CLD.[216] Babies with CLD who acquire added pulmonary infection often become extremely ill, and frequently require IPPV. Antibiotics should always be given. Viral respiratory infections in babies with CLD lead to a worsening of chronic respiratory morbidity, with signs of increased airway resistance compared to those who avoid viral infection.[1139]

SOME SPECIFIC NEONATAL LUNG INFECTIONS

Ureaplasma urealyticum

Ureaplasma urealyticum is a common vaginal commensal. It may be implicated in some cases of chorioamnionitis and premature delivery,[280,934] along with *Mycoplasma hominis*.[1051] There is growing speculation that these organisms may cause acute neonatal pneumonia[793] and have a role in the pathogenesis of CLD (pp. 609, 1152).[182,280,370] Unfortunately, ureaplasma require a special culture medium and may take several weeks to grow. Recently, however, a detection method for ureaplasma antibody has been described which should be useful in both clinical and research contexts.[865] Erythromycin is the antibiotic of choice for both ureaplasma and mycoplasma infections in the newborn.[1074]

Respiratory syncytial virus

RSV infections are comparatively rare on the neonatal unit, but small epidemics occur from time to time and the effects on individual babies can be devastating, especially among those with severe chronic lung disease.[437,454,707,760,1047,1053] Such babies may rapidly develop almost complete airway obstruction and become impossible to ventilate. Recurrent bradycardia is a common presenting feature,[352] and the clinical course is occasionally complicated by atrial tachycardia.[40,262] RSV infection must always be considered when a baby with CLD experiences a deterioration in lung function, even if the typical physical signs of a bronchiolitis are absent.[437] RSV is easily diagnosed by immunofluorescence on respiratory secretions. Stringent measures to limit cross-infection are required if a case of RSV infection occurs on an NICU.[677] Babies with CLD also remain very vulnerable to RSV infection for many months after discharge from the NICU.[976] Early institution of treatment with ribavirin is recommended;[501] although there is little evidence of efficacy in this group of patients, it seems a reasonable therapy to try in such a potentially serious condition.[26] Extracorporeal membrane oxygenation should be considered early in deteriorating cases. Prevention of RSV infection in vulnerable preterm infants using RSV hyperimmune globulin has been tried and recent reports are quite encouraging, showing a significant reduction in the incidence of RSV infection compared to controls.[435,436,438,708] Another approach to prevention is immunization of pregnant women, on the grounds that the babies of mothers with high levels of neutralizing RSV antibody seem protected.[307] This has not been put to trial as yet.

Other respiratory viruses

VLBW babies who remain on the NICU for many months may contract the usual viral respiratory infections of early childhood from their visitors and from nursing and medical staff. Symptoms are usually of a mild URTI accompanied by a low-grade pyrexia.[220,597,707,1053] More severe viral pneumonia, other than that caused by RSV, may also occur at any time in the neonatal period, and adenoviruses and coronaviruses are often responsible.[698,836,979]

Pertussis

Severe pertussis can occur in the late neonatal period, presenting with paroxysmal cough, vomiting, apnoea and choking spells. Whooping is rare. Prolonged ventilatory support is often required.[467] Diagnosis is by culture of nasopharyngeal swabs or, in the case of babies who have started antibiotic therapy, by PCR.[287] Treatment is with erythromycin and sedation. In recent reports the baby has acquired the infection from his unimmunized mother, who developed the disease perinatally.[85, 199]

Chlamydia

Chlamydia trachomatis and *Chlamydia pneumoniae* can cause severe early-onset disease similar to that seen with GBS.[45,692] Even birth by caesarean section with intact membranes does not preclude the possibility of vertical transmission,[88] and the organism can cross the intact membranes, causing fetal pneumonic stillbirth.[1029] Chlamydial infection during pregnancy should be treated with either ampicillin or erythromycin in order to prevent perinatal transmission.[933] Chlamydial pneumonia in term infants is characteristically a disease in those over 4 weeks of age,[486] but it can occur in the first week of life.[927] The diagnosis is made by culture or immunofluorescence techniques in the presence of a suggestive clinical picture, which includes an afebrile pneumonia with tachypnoea and rales, diffuse chest X-ray changes, an eosinophilia and previous neonatal conjunctivitis.[887] Like other neonatal lung diseases, chlamydial pneumonia can cause long-term pulmonary damage.[1091] Treatment is with erythromycin.

Lung abscess

This is a rare occurrence in the newborn, presenting usually with dyspnoea and an area of opacification on chest X-ray. It usually follows previous pneumonia and is usually caused by Gram-negative organisms, but can be caused by *Staph. aureus*. It should be treated initially with broad-spectrum antibiotics. If the lesion does not resolve, bronchoscopy or surgery may be indicated.[967,973]

CARDIAC INFECTION

Endocarditis

Endocarditis is being recognized with increasing frequency in VLBW babies[720] with structurally normal hearts. Virtually all of these babies have had central lines lying in the right atrium or right ventricle.[777,782] The organisms responsible for most cases are CONS, but enterococci, *Staph. aureus* and *Candida* sp. are well recognized causal agents.[705,824,876] Endocarditis in this group of infants usually presents with no more than persistent signs of sepsis and positive blood cultures despite appropriate antibiotic therapy, although in a few cases there are changing murmurs, heart failure, persisting haematuria or thrombocytopenia. A baby who presents any of these features and who has, or has recently had, an intracardiac central line should have an echocardiogram performed. The demonstration of intracardiac vegetations, which are present in most patients,[785] confirms the diagnosis.

Treatment and outcome

Remove the central line and check that the appropriate antibiotics are being given for the organism grown from the blood, at the correct dose and dose interval. If the signs of sepsis remit within a few days, and blood cultures become negative, antibiotic therapy should be continued for 10–14 days.[867] The prognosis for catheter-related endocarditis due to CONS is better than might be thought, with recovery rates of more than 60% recently reported from small series.[705,876] Endocarditis due to *Candida albicans* carries a poor prognosis. Rarely, vegetations persist or severe valve damage occurs, and then surgery may be indicated.

Pericarditis

This is extremely rare, and usually develops as a complication of pre-existing sepsis or an abscess near the mediastinum. Implicated organisms include *Staph. aureus*, *E. coli*, *H. influenzae*, *Klebsiella* sp., *Pseudomonas* sp. and *Candida* sp.[340,1127] The chest X-ray shows an increase in the size of the cardiac silhouette, but signs of tamponade are unusual. ECG changes are present, and the diagnosis can be confirmed by echocardiography and pericardial tap. The treatment is surgical drainage and long-term antibiotics.

Myocarditis (p. 698)

BONE AND JOINT INFECTION

Septic arthritis and osteomyelitis are rare in the newborn, although their incidence does seem to vary quite a lot. Only four cases have occurred at St James's University Hospital in Leeds during the last 15 years (in over 75 000 births), whereas a recent report from an Australian tertiary centre describes an incidence of 9.6 cases per 1000 NICU admissions.[538] Osteomyelitis and septic arthritis are mainly caused by *Staph. aureus*,[255,539] but GBS is important[1130] and several other organisms may be involved, including *H. influenzae*,[1111,1116] *U. urealyticum*,[399] *Candida* sp.[403,1093] and *Neisseria gonorrhoea*.[531] Osteomyelitis and septic arthritis often coexist, and are often indistinguishable clinically. There are two reasons for this. The infected metaphysis of the bone often lies within the capsule of the joint, and when the thin metaphyseal cortex collapses infection enters the joint. In addition, blood vessels frequently pass through the thin epiphyseal plate of neonatal long bones, transmitting metaphyseal infection to the joint capsule.[787]

Osteomyelitis/septic arthritis takes two forms. One is seen in acutely ill babies with complex problems, and often with indwelling cannulae, in whom multiple bone involvement may occur.[539] The other form is a more subtle presentation and usually only one site is affected.[732] GBS is quite often responsible for this latter form.[288] The sites most commonly affected are the pelvis, hip, knee and humerus,[95,592,732] but any site may be involved. Skull osteomyelitis may occur following infection of a cephalhaematoma[622,730] or a scalp puncture for fetal pH monitoring.[620,670] Vertebral disease occasionally develops,[296] and calcaneal disease may follow heel puncture.[637] Isolated arthritis is rarely reported, but the organisms isolated are similar to those reported for osteomyelitis,[840] except for the preponderance of coliform arthritis of the hip when this complicates femoral venepuncture.[511]

Clinical features

These disorders usually present in one of three ways:

- With pseudoparalysis of the affected limb due to pain. The affected area may be warm and swollen;

- Following investigation of the baby with non-specific signs of sepsis;
- Incidentally on X-ray in a baby with multisystem disease.

Investigation and diagnosis

The affected bone or joint must be X-rayed as a baseline, although no changes are usually seen for 10–14 days, when bone rarefaction, lytic lesions, periosteal elevation and periosteal new bone formation are seen.[732,1092] Isotope scans are also useful in identifying 'hot spots' in joints or bones. Magnetic resonance imaging can be very valuable, especially to look at the spine and pelvis.[703] Aspiration of the affected joint or bone should usually be attempted, not only to achieve prompt bacteriological diagnosis by Gram stain and culture, but because decompression is an important part of therapy.

Treatment

Vancomycin and a third-generation cephalosporin is a reasonable starting point until the results of blood cultures are available. Thereafter, the appropriate antibiotic(s) (p. 1137) should be given intravenously for at least 4–6 weeks. When pus is obtained at aspiration, orthopaedic advice should always be sought about surgical drainage of the bone or joint.

Prognosis

Mortality relates almost entirely to multisytem disease, but there is a high morbidity rate. Following staphylococcal and Gram-negative infections permanent damage to the epiphyseal plate or the metaphysis is common. This may cause permanent arthritis, long-term growth problems or deformity, particularly in those with an acute onset or multiple sites of involvement, in whom up to 50% may have significant long-term orthopaedic problems.[95,592,732,830] Long-term clinical and radiological follow-up is essential, especially as impaired growth may not become evident for several years.[830] The prognosis for complete recovery from GBS infections is somewhat better.[711]

GASTROENTERITIS

Neonatal gastroenteritis in Britain is commonly sporadic and usually mild. Infection may be acquired from the mother during birth, or subsequently by cross-infection or from contaminated feeds. Many nursery outbreaks are initiated by an asymptomatic infant who sheds the virus or bacterium. For some viral pathogens, such as rotavirus, nursery outbreaks often coincide with seasonal peaks of the disease in the community.[1002] Breast-feeding is strongly protective, in the developing world at least.[648,1136]

Organisms

Most neonatal gastroenteritis is due to rotavirus,[73,240,923] which may also be endemic in some nurseries without there being any evidence of it causing symptoms other than a mild increase in stool frequency.[200,433] *E. coli*, *Salmonella* sp. and *Shigella* sp. all may cause neonatal gastroenteritis.[444,1046] Neonatal campylobacter gastroenteritis has been described, often contracted from the baby's mother,[29] as have infections with adenovirus, echovirus, coxsackie virus and astrovirus.[444]

Symptoms and signs

Diarrhoea, rather than vomiting, is usually the predominant feature in neonatal gastroenteritis, and copious watery stools may be passed. Bloody stools are rare, except in infection with *Salmonella*, *Shigella* or *Campylobacter* sp. Signs of dehydration soon appear and shock may develop, especially in preterm babies, who may rapidly lose more than 10% of their body weight. The infant is often pale and listless, with a distended abdomen and a metabolic acidosis.

Differential diagnosis and investigation

Healthy breast-fed babies may pass up to 10 loosish yellow stools per day, but are thriving and otherwise completely asymptomatic. Frequent loose green stools are often seen in infants receiving phototherapy (p. 727) and do not require further investigation. Severe diarrhoea can occasionally be caused by the inherited abnormalities of sugar absorption (p. 756), congenital chloride diarrhoea (p. 756) or cystic fibrosis (p. 758). If these conditions are excluded, copious diarrhoea is almost always due to gastroenteritis. Stool culture is essential and, if appropriate, stools should also be examined by electron microscopy for virus particles.

Treatment

If the symptoms are mild and dehydration minimal, it may be worth persisting with breast- or formula feeding, giving small frequent feeds. If the major problem is vomiting, this can usually be controlled with a glucose–electrolyte solution (e.g. Pedialyte, Dioralyte).[493] In more severe cases oral feeds should be stopped for 48 hours and intravenous fluids started. Infusions of sodium bicarbonate may need to be given to acidaemic preterm babies. After 48 hours oral glucose–electrolyte solutions are usually well tolerated, and the baby can promptly restart milk feeds in the next 24–48 hours. There is no need to regrade the feeds from quarter to half to full strength.[39] If diarrhoea returns, lactose intolerance (pp. 756–757) or milk intolerance should be considered and, if present, the baby should be started on an appropriate lactose-free hydrolysed milk such as Pregestimil.

Antibiotics should not be given routinely. However, if an epidemic of bacterial gastroenteritis develops, oral non-absorbable antibiotics such as neomycin or colomycin may be indicated.[659] If *Salmonella* sp., *Shigella* sp. or campylobacter are grown, and particularly if the infant has systemic symptoms or is premature, parenteral antibiotics should be given using co-trimoxazole or a third-generation cephalosporin for *Salmonella*, ampicillin or co-trimoxazole for *Shigella*, and erythromycin or gentamicin for campylobacter. Antidiarrhoeal agents should not be used in the neonatal period.

Isolation

Term babies who develop mild symptoms on a postnatal ward can be isolated with their mothers. Sporadic cases on a neonatal unit should be isolated within the unit or, if appropriate facilities exist, transferred to the paediatric infectious disease unit. The management of epidemics is outlined on pages 1114–1115.

URINARY TRACT INFECTION

The true incidence of urinary tract infection in the newborn is difficult to establish because the methods of urine collection employed in epidemiological surveys are all likely to lead to overdiagnosis, because of contamination. In term infants the reported incidence is in the range 0.1–3%, and among low-birthweight infants at least three times as high and possibly as much as 10 times as high.[1,98,268,286,411,644,680,1097,1115] If the higher quoted figures are true, most neonatal UTIs remain undiagnosed. There is a two- to threefold higher incidence in males at any gestation. Infants of cocaine users seem to be unusually susceptible to UTI.[411] UTI in the newborn is believed to occur mainly as a result of bloodstream spread of organisms to the kidney during a septicaemia, although no doubt the reverse situation can also apply. Breast-feeding offers a significant degree of protection.[838]

Organisms

The commonest pathogen by far is *E. coli*, and responsible strains are associated with P-fimbria, a limited number of serotypes, resistance to the bactericidal effects of serum, adhesion to epithelial cells and the production of haemolysins.[540,1018] In addition, many Gram-negative enteric bacteria and some Gram-positive cocci, including CONS, *Staph. aureus* and enterococci, can cause neonatal UTI. In VLBW babies, and the occasional mature baby with urinary tract obstruction, *C. albicans* is a well-recognized cause of UTI[835] and, in the case of the VLBW baby, this is usually one component of a multisystem infection (p. 1164).

Symptoms and signs

Neonatal UTI may present acutely with all the signs of septicaemia (pp. 1116–1117), or insidiously with poor feeding, listlessness, poor weight gain and low-grade fever. Some infections only come to light if urinalysis is done as part of the routine investigation of a baby with, say, persisting jaundice, unexplained anaemia or poor weight gain. On examination, signs particularly relevant to the diagnosis of UTI include distress during renal palpation, renal enlargement due to hydronephrosis or some other congenital abnormality, and an enlarged bladder, suggesting outflow tract obstruction. The external genitalia must be examined to exclude stenoses or fistulae, and the blood pressure should be checked.

Investigation

If the UTI is part of a septicaemic illness there will commonly be a positive blood culture in addition to a positive urine culture. The technique of urine collection and the diagnostic criteria for UTI are given on page 1122, and should be adhered to. All babies with a proven UTI must have their serum biochemistry checked.

Further investigation is essential, as between 35 and 50% will have an underlying abnormality, which in about two-thirds will be vesicoureteric reflux.[1,643,901] A renal ultrasound scan will demonstrate the presence, position and size of the kidneys, the size and thickness of the bladder and dilatation of the collecting systems. Ultrasound may also show echogenic fungal material in the renal pelvis or ureter in around a third of cases of proven UTI due to *C. albicans*.[835] Ultrasound alone, however, cannot be relied upon to show scars or exclude vesicoureteric reflux,[982,983] and all children under the age of 1 year being investigated following proven UTI should have an MCUG and a DMSA scan in addition to ultrasound.[915] The MCUG will exclude bladder neck obstruction and urethral valves, but its most important role is to exclude vesicoureteric reflux. The DMSA can show scarring, which is probably commoner after renal infection than was once thought to be the case.[545] The intravenous urogram has fallen out of fashion but may be necessary on occasion to fully delineate an abnormality and plan further treatment. In children over 1 year of age the diagnostic work-up is different.[402]

Treatment

If the baby presents with a systemic illness the usual antibiotic combinations for either early or late-onset sepsis should be used, and the treatment refined when the results of cultures are available. If UTI is confirmed, antibiotics should be continued for 10–14 days. Resolution of infection should be confirmed with further urine cultures. Once the infection has been treated, prophylaxis with low-dose trimethoprim, given in a single dose at night, should continue until radiological investigations have excluded underlying abnormalities. If the investigations are normal prophylaxis can be discontinued, but the infant should be followed with urinalyses every 3 months for at least a year. If there is evidence of reflux, antibiotic prophylaxis should be continued. UTI due to *C. albicans* has traditionally been treated with amphotericin alone or in combination with one of the newer antimycotic drugs. A recent report has suggested that good results can also be obtained with a combination of fluconazole and flucytosine.[510]

LISTERIOSIS

L. monocytogenes is a short Gram-positive rod which can be found both inside and outside cells. The most important reservoir for transmission to humans is probably food, especially dairy products, contaminated by infected farm animals.[348,381] Almost half of all documented infections occur in pregnant women,[555] and the currently reported incidence of fetomaternal listeriosis in Denmark is 25 cases per 100 000 livebirths.[361] Women infected with HIV are considerably more susceptible to *L. monocytogenes* than the general population.[323] Newborn infants are particularly susceptible for a variety of immunological reasons, including defects in macrophage response[541] and low opsonic activity.[134] Three main types of fetal and neonatal infection are found.[614]

Transplacental infection

L. monocytogenes causes a non-specific influenzal or gastroenteritic illness in the pregnant woman, during which the organism may infect the fetus, either by haematogenous spread across the placenta or via infection of the amniotic fluid. First- or second-trimester infection may cause fetal death or miscarriage, and recurrent abortion due to listeria has been recorded in humans.[420] Later in pregnancy infection may precipitate preterm labour,[137,381] with fetal distress and meconium staining of the liquor.[630] Because meconium staining of the liquor is rare at gestations below 34 weeks, its presence should raise the suspicion of listeria. Liveborn babies are often extremely ill at birth. They may have a severe pneumonia, and hepatomegaly and meningitis may already be present.[630,1026] Blood and stool cultures are invariably positive. Characteristically, small (2–3 mm) pinkish-grey cutaneous granulomas are present and, at autopsy, similar small granulomatous lesions are widespread in the lung, liver, CNS and many other tissues and organs.

Early-onset infection, acquired intrapartum

Most cases of neonatal listeriosis are sporadic, but epidemics are described.[81,630,1026] At least two-thirds of infants who acquire listeria infection intrapartum are preterm, and almost all become ill within 24 hours of birth.[664] Most have disseminated infection, with pneumonia, meningitis, thrombocytopenia, anaemia and sometimes conjunctivitis. Small cutaneous granulomas may be found in some babies.

Late-onset infection, usually meningitis, probably due to nosocomial infection

Nosocomial spread of listeria is well documented.[336,665,762,821,890] Late-onset listeria infection is usually in the form of a meningitis (p. 1139) with or without concomitant septicaemia or colitis.[614] The median age of onset is about 2 weeks.

Investigation

The routine investigations of early-onset sepsis and meningitis reveal the diagnosis. However, listeria can pose problems for the microbiologist, as its uptake of the Gram stain can be variable and it may be slow-growing.

Therapy

The most effective antibiotic therapy is ampicillin plus gentamicin, and in units where listeria is a common pathogen there is much to be said for using this combination as the routine for early-onset sepsis. Listeria is resistant to all third-generation cephalosporins. Intrathecal treatment is not required for listerial meningitis. ECMO has recently been used successfully in the treatment of severe early-onset listeriosis.[509]

Outcome

The mortality for neonatal listeriosis is in the range 5–15%.[361,555] The prognosis for listerial meningitis is better than that for other neonatal bacterial meningitis.

SUPERFICIAL INFECTIONS

Umbilical cord infections

Divitalized tissue provides a good culture medium and the thrombosed cord vessels are a potential portal of entry into the circulation. In the days before effective prophylactic measures were introduced, staphylococcal infection of the cord and surrounding tissues, often leading to systemic infection, was commonplace. In the developing world neonatal tetanus occurs mainly as a result of contamination of the umbilical cord stump by *Clostridium tetani*.[330,930]

Despite good cord care, minor umbilical infection still occurs in 2% of preterm and 0.5% of term neonates.[673] Although *Staph. aureus* is still the most important pathogen, Gram-negative enteric bacilli, especially *E. coli* and *Klebsiella* sp., are relatively common.[694] In most cases the clinical features are limited to periumbilical erythema, often with a small amount of discharge,[223] but in other cases there is a spreading cellulitis of the abdominal wall, or even fasciitis.[694]

Investigation and treatment

Swab any exudate and take a blood culture. Usually local treatment with an antiseptic such as chlorhexidine powder will suffice, but if there is evidence of invasion of the surrounding tissues or of systemic upset, a broad-spectrum antibiotic combination, effective against *Staph. aureus* and Gram-negative bacilli, should be given intravenously. A combination of vancomycin or flucloxacillin and a third-generation cephalosporin, or flucloxacillin and gentamicin, would be suitable initial treatment.

Skin infections

Staphylococcal

The commonest presentation is with a few flaccid intraepidermal bullae which are filled with a yellowish opalescent fluid, but occasionally larger bullae may be present, in which case the condition merges into bullous impetigo (p. 892). Paronychia may also occur. The infant is usually well, with little or no local inflammation and no regional lymphadenitis. After taking swabs from the lesions, treatment should be with oral flucloxacillin. If there is any suggestion of a systemic illness, staphylococcal septicaemia should be suspected, appropriate investigations carried out and parenteral antibiotics started.

Candida (thrush) (see pp. 892–893)

Conjunctivitis

Up-to-date and useful epidemiological information on neonatal conjunctivitis is hard to come by. A recent study in Norway found an overall incidence of neonatal conjunctivitis of approximately 19%, of which 7% were classed as severe.[232] The incidence of conjunctivitis was approximately 15% among infants not receiving silver nitrate prophylaxis, and approximately 20% among those who did.

Organisms

Infective conjunctivitis can be caused by a wide variety of pathogens and the pattern varies considerably between reported series. In the UK, the top five would normally include *Staph. aureus*, *C. trachomatis*, *H. influenzae*, *S. pneumoniae* and '*Streptococcus viridans*'. *N. gonorrhoeae* is rare in the UK at the present time. In all ill children with conjunctival discharge, in addition to the organisms mentioned, always consider herpes simplex (p. 1156), *L. monocytogenes* and *N. meningitidis*.

General considerations

Conjunctivitis can develop at any stage in the neonatal period. Late-onset and recurrent conjunctivitis is much more common if there is a blocked lacrimal duct with epiphora (p. 908). The spectrum of severity ranges from mild crusting on the eyelids, through purulent discharge, conjunctival injection and eyelid oedema, to invasion of the eye and retro-orbital structures.

In infants with mild conjunctivitis no treatment other than regular cleaning/bathing of the lids with a sterile saline swab 4–6-hourly for 2–3 days is required. However, if cultures are positive, discharge persists for more than 48 hours, or there is conjunctival or lid oedema, topical antibiotics should be started. Chloramphenicol, neomycin or gentamicin eye drops are common choices, administered 6-hourly. Because an important part of the therapy is irrigation, drops are preferable to ointment. Both eyes should be treated, even though infection is only apparent in one. In infants with epiphora, after instilling the antibiotics the lacrimal duct should be gently massaged towards the eye in an attempt to unblock it. Rarely, probing the lacrimal duct under anaesthesia may be necessary later in infancy (p. 908).

Gonococcal ophthalmia

This usually presents within 24 hours of delivery with a profuse, bilateral, purulent conjunctival discharge, but can present less dramatically at any time in the first month.[952] Significant systemic upset is unusual, but because of the speed with which the infection can damage the cornea it is important that the diagnosis is made and treatment started immediately. A swab must be sent to the laboratory promptly for Gram stain and culture in an enriched medium. If Gram-negative intracellular diplococci are seen on microscopy, this confirms the diagnosis and treatment must be started immediately pending culture. Penicillin is given intravenously for 7 days, together with penicillin or chloramphenicol eye drops, which should be instilled hourly for 24 hours, and 4-hourly thereafter for the next 6 days. The third-generation cephalosporins should be used for penicillin-resistant strains.[609] The infected baby must be isolated with his mother from all other babies, and the mother and her contacts should be treated.

Chlamydial ophthalmia

This is now among the commonest causes of neonatal conjunctivitis, and some babies infected as neonates will develop chlamydial pneumonia later in infancy, which is often severe enough to require hospital admission. In Western Europe chlamydial pneumonia is probably quite rare, and a recent study in Germany reported that only 1% of infants with pneumonia had evidence of chlamydia.[547] However, in areas of the world where chlamydial genital infection is much more common, 50% of all pneumonia in early infancy may be due to this organism.[887,1032]

The risk of vertical transmission of *C. trachomatis* has been variously reported. In some studies 50% of babies delivered to mothers with genital chlamydia become infected, although only half of these are symptomatic with conjunctivitis or pneumonia.[88,887,943,986] However, a study in the UK reported that only 25% of infants of infected mothers were infected, with only 14% being symptomatic, and of those who did become symptomatic only one-quarter developed pneumonia.[854]

Chlamydial conjunctivitis usually presents between 5 and 12 days' postnatal age. It may be unilateral initially, but often becomes bilateral. Rarely it can cause adhesions between the bulbar and tarsal conjunctiva, with some persisting pannus,[937,1081] but it almost never causes permanent visual impairment.[887] Conventional cultures are negative and treatment with standard topical antibiotics is rarely successful: in many cases chlamydia is first suspected for these very reasons. Several tests are available for the identification of chlamydia from eye swabs, including enzyme immunoassay and immunofluorescence techniques,[274,464,887] the immune dot-blot test[117] and tissue culture. It is not clear from the literature which is best, and no doubt others, including the use of PCR, will soon be available in routine laboratories.

Chlamydial eye infection should be treated with tetracycline eye drops or ointment and oral erythromycin for 2 weeks. This should also prevent the baby developing chlamydial pneumonia in infancy.[491,886]

Attempts have been made to prevent both the neonatal conjunctivitis and pneumonia in infancy by some form of early neonatal prophylaxis. Silver nitrate eye drops and tetracycline or erythromycin eye ointment applied at delivery have all been used, with varying degrees of success.[246,465] It has recently been shown that a 2.5% ophthalmic solution of povidone–iodine is a more effective form of prophylaxis than either silver nitrate or erythromycin.[538] If maternal infection is detected antenatally, treatment with erythromycin for 1 week considerably reduces the risk of neonatal infection.[22,668,744,944,986] Alternatively, the mother can be treated with ampicillin.[22] The risk of perinatal transmission is reduced by caesarean section,[88] but few would consider this an indication for the operation.

Pseudomonal ophthalmia

Although a relatively rare cause of neonatal ophthalmia, *Ps. aeruginosa* has a remarkable ability to invade ocular tissue and to cause severe damage.[646] Most cases occur in preterm infants, usually as a result of cross-infection from an environmental source. Many of these infants develop septicaemia as well as ophthalmia. If pseudomonal ophthalmia is suspected, or if the organism is grown from an eye swab, parenteral therapy with a suitable antibiotic, such as gentamicin or ceftazidime, should be begun at once, in addition to locally applied gentamicin drops or ointment. Subconjunctival gentamicin should be considered if there is evidence of corneal inflammation.

Dacrocystitis

This presents within the first week as a reddish-purple swelling over the course of the lacrimal duct and sac on the medial and inferior margin of the eye. Local pressure often results in a squirt of purulent material from the lacrimal punctum. The usual cause is *Staph. aureus*. Treatment is with systemic and topical antibiotics, usually in drops rather than ointment. Sequelae are rare.

OTITIS MEDIA

This diagnosis is often ignored in the neonatal period, probably because of the great difficulty in visualizing the oblique, downward-facing immobile tympanic membrane through the hairy, narrow neonatal external auditory meatus. However, otitis media has been reported to occur in two-thirds of infants ventilated through a nasotracheal tube, which compromises normal function at the lower end of the Eustachian tube,[101] and infection may still be present at autopsy.[250] However, in those who survive the infection resolves.[414] Otitis media is virtually universal in infants with cleft palate,[412] in whom there is reflux of milk and secretions into the Eustachian tube. Finally, otitis media may occur in a previously healthy baby[123] and in long-stay patients on an NICU who develop signs of an upper respiratory tract infection.

Among the inmates of an NICU, the organisms responsible are often *E. coli* and *Staph. aureus*, but *H. influenzae* and *S. pneumoniae* may be grown from previously asymptomatic babies who present later in the neonatal period. In many cases fluid obtained by tympanocentesis is sterile.[163]

Treatment of otitis media in the ill low-birthweight baby on IPPV should be with the usual broad-spectrum antibiotic combination. In older infants with upper respiratory tract infection and/or cleft palate, oral treatment with an antibiotic active against *S. pneumoniae* and *H. influenzae*, such as amoxicillin or trimethoprim, is usually adequate.

OTHER NEONATAL BACTERIAL INFECTIONS

Localized abscesses

These may develop anywhere, but are most common at the site of heel pricks, intravenous infusions, or where the skin has been abraded by electrode adhesive or some other piece of monitoring equipment. There is localized swelling, redness and tenderness. The infection may spread to more important local tissues, such as bone, causing an osteomyelitis or, rarely, septicaemia may develop. If a fluctuant area develops, incision or aspiration under local anaesthesia, using a wide-bore needle, is helpful. Broad-spectrum antibiotic cover should be given intravenously, but if the baby is well this can be changed to an appropriate oral antibiotic once the culture and sensitivities are available. Treatment should usually be given for 7–10 days.

Breast abscess

Breast enlargement and redness in babies of either sex is not unusual and represents a transient hormonal stimulus, rather than infection. However, if tenderness and erythema are present with fluctuation, pyrexia or a purulent discharge from the nipple (not to be confused with neonatal breast milk/lactorrhoea, p. 275), then treatment with systemic antibiotics should be given.

Liver abscess

Postmortem examinations indicate that multiple microabscesses in the liver may occur in both preterm and term babies as a complication of generalized sepsis, vascular cannulae or abdominal surgery. In life there are few clues to their presence, although they may be associated with hepatomegaly and abnormal liver enzymes. Solitary liver abscesses have occasionally been reported in the newborn, mostly in preterm infants who have had umbilical vein catheterization, but all of the references are quite old.[145,960] Most cases are caused by *Staph. aureus*. Ultrasound examination of the liver will discover an abscess quite reliably.[693] True bacterial hepatitis is very rare, but is a well documented feature of congenital listeriosis. *C. albicans* can cause multiple liver abscesses in babies with immunodeficiency states.

Therapy for multiple microabscesses is that for septicaemia. Solitary abscesses may require drainage in addition, either percutaneously under ultrasound guidance[917] or by open operation.

Sialadenitis

Both the parotid and submandibular glands may become infected, with the latter more often involved in premature babies.[66,619] Presentation is with a red indurated area over the gland, with pus draining from either Stensen's or Wharton's duct. *Staph. aureus* is the usual pathogen. Treatment is with intravenous antibiotics, which should always include flucloxacillin.

Necrotizing fasciitis

Bacterial infection of the subcutaneous tissues and fascia is rare in neonates. It can arise from any site, including the umbilicus.[694] It presents as a rapidly progressive fluctuant subcutaneous swelling, for which the appropriate treatment is wide surgical debridement and appropriate broad-spectrum antibiotic cover.[390]

MYCOPLASMA AND UREAPLASMA INFECTIONS[652]

If present in the mother's birth canal, these organisms may colonize as many as 50% of babies,[254,934,936] but their importance in causing infectious disease is incompletely understood.

The probable role of *U. urealyticum* in neonatal pneumonia and CLD has been discussed (p. 1145). There is also little doubt that both *U. urealyticum* and *M. hominis* may occasionally cause focal infection[925] or septicaemia in ill low-birthweight babies (Table 43.16). Some epidemiological studies, however, have found little evidence to suggest that babies colonized by either *U. urealyticum* or *M. hominis* are disadvantaged compared to those who are not.[490] Improved methods of detecting these organisms, such as PCR, should help to define their role further.[121]

Treatment

The most effective antibiotic against both mycoplasmas and ureaplasmas is erythromycin, and this should be given intravenously.[1075]

Table 43.16 Neonatal infections caused by *ureaplasmas and mycoplasmas*

Organism	Infection	Reference
Mycoplasma hominis	Surgical wound infection	Brooker et al 1994 Ped. Inf. Dis. J. 13:751
	Abscess	Sacker et al 1970 Pediatrics 46:303–4
	Sialadenitis	Powell et al 1979 Pediatrics 63:789–99
	Meningitis	Hjelm et al 1980 Acta. Paed. Scand 69:415
		Waites et al 1988 Lancet i:17
		McDonald & Moore 1988 Ped. Inf. Dis. J. 7:795
	Septicaemia	Unsworth et al 1985 J. Inf. 10:163
	Pericarditis	Miller et al 1982 Am. J. Dis. Child. 136:271
Ureaplasma sp.	Meningitis	Waites et al 1988 Lancet I:17
		Garland & Murton 1987 Ped. Inf. Dis. J. 6:868.

TUBERCULOSIS

Tuberculosis is prevalent in almost all tropical developing countries and constitutes a special risk during pregnancy and lactation to mothers and babies. In the UK, perinatal tuberculosis is currently extremely rare. Transplacental infection usually occurs when the pregnant woman has clinical tuberculosis or a recent primary infection. In the former, but not in the latter, miliary lesions are present in the placenta. There is an absence of cellular response in the baby, and the primary focus and lymph nodes are caseous, with abundant tubercle bacilli. The peripheries of the lesions contain few lymphocytes and no giant cells.

Criteria for the diagnosis of congenital tuberculosis were first laid down by Beitzke,[86] and are rigorous enough for all time. There must be proof that the lesion is tuberculous, and in this regard a primary complex in the liver is almost certainly of intrauterine origin. If the liver primary complex is absent, the infection should be obvious in the fetus or in the neonate at birth or during the first week. Neonatal tuberculosis is the result either of intrauterine infection or of inhalation of tubercle bacilli during or soon after birth, through intimate contact with an adult with active pulmonary tuberculosis.

Clinical picture

The onset of symptoms is usually within the first month of life. The primary focus is often in the liver, and congenitally infected infants may present with hepatomegaly and jaundice caused by obstruction of bile drainage by enlarged lymph nodes at the porta hepatis.[351] Sometimes a primary complex is found in the lung as a result of dissemination through the ductus venosus. The infant may then present with pneumonia, anaemia and hepatosplenomegaly, with radiological evidence of widespread pulmonary infection involving both lungs and mediastinal and hilar lymph nodes. There is usually no liver lesion in this clinical syndrome, the source of infection probably being the amniotic fluid or the maternal genital tract.[405] Examination of the gastric aspirate for acid-fast bacilli is the best diagnostic test. The infected neonate is not sensitive to tuberculin. Occasionally localized infection is reported, such as otitis.[766]

Management

Results are best when infected mothers have been detected by antenatal screening and antituberculous treatment instituted during pregnancy.[495] The management of an infant of a mother with the disease poses special problems. Isolation of the baby from the infected mother is usually not feasible and is in any case undesirable, because it would signal the end of breast-feeding and expose the infant to all the hazards of artificial feeding. Breast-feeding seems to be safe for the infant of a mother taking antituberculous drugs.[988] The policy advocated here for asymptomatic infants of tuberculous mothers has been proved effective, and is as follows:

- Maintain breast-feeding (except where this is precluded by the gravity of the maternal illness).
- Treat the mother for tuberculosis.
- Give the infant prophylactic isoniazid in a single dose of 10 mg/kg daily, this to continue until the mother is confirmed to be sputum negative by repeated sputum examination.
- Carry out BCG immunization in the infant using isoniazid-resistant BCG.

Treatment of proven neonatal infection is not well researched because of the relative rarity of the condition, although regimens that are effective in treating adults and children should be effective.[28] One recommended regime is isoniazid (20 mg/kg/day) plus rifampicin(20 mg/kg/day) and pyrazinamide (30 mg/kg/day) for 2 months, followed by 4 months of isoniazid and rifampicin. An alternative is a 9-month course of isoniazid and rifampicin. If isoniazid resistance is suspected, usually on the basis of the likely geographical source of the infection, at least one additional drug should be used until sensitivities are known. Streptomycin (20 mg/kg/day i.m.), ethambutol (20 mg/kg/day) or pyrazinamide (30 mg/kg/day) are suitable choices. Steroids have no place in treatment because of the lack of a host reaction. The infant with congenital tuberculosis should be vaccinated with isoniazid-resistant BCG to encourage active immunity. Breast-feeding should be encouraged, and if the mother is infected she must also be treated with antituberculous drugs.

NEONATAL TETANUS

Tetanus is an important cause of neonatal death (up to 60 per 1000 livebirths) worldwide because of local conditions and customs, rather than climate. Neonatal tetanus still accounts for between 25 and 65% of all neonatal deaths in some countries.[310,1122] In rural India the walls of the village houses are made of a mixture of earth and cowdung, and the ash of cowdung fires is used to dress the umbilical stump. Neonatal tetanus is known as the '8-day disease' in the Punjab, because so many babies die of tetanus on the eighth day of life.[409] Infection of the umbilical stump caused by septic management of the cord and harmful cultural practices are the main reasons for the high frequency of neonatal tetanus in rural communities in the tropics.

The organism

Clostridium tetani is a Gram-positive rod and a strict anaerobe. It is present in animal faeces, though usually absent from human faeces. Spores of *Cl. tetani* are highly resistant to heat, chemicals and antibiotics, but can be destroyed if autoclaved. They can survive for many years in dry dust or earth. During germination and growth in anaerobic conditions the organism produces two toxins, tetanospasmin and tetanolysin. Tetanospasmin is a potent exotoxin with high affinity for nervous tissue. It is produced by the vegetative form of *Cl. tetani* in conditions of reduced oxygen. Within the central nervous system the toxin is bound to gangliosides, where it suppresses inhibitory influences on motor neurons and interneurons, directly enhancing excitatory synaptic action. Its action is similar to that of strychnine, inducing hypertonicity, spasms and seizures. The toxin also produces overactivity of the sympathetic nervous system, resulting in tachycardia, arrhythmias, labile hypertension, peripheral vasoconstriction, sweating, hypercarbia and increased urinary excretion of catecholamines. The site of absorption of tetanus toxin is at the peripheral motor and autonomic nerve endings. Toxin ascends the nerve fibres and crosses the synaptic cleft into the presynaptic endings of adjacent inhibitory spinal interneurons, where it is bound. Antitoxin inhibits tetanospasmin only before it is fixed on to the presynaptic terminal.

Clinical features

The incubation period of neonatal tetanus varies from 3 to 14 days or more,[930] the severity of the disease being greater with a shorter incubation period. Both muscle rigidity and spasms are typical of tetanus. Muscle rigidity persists throughout the illness and principally involves the masseters, the abdominal muscles and the erectors of the spine. Muscle spasm is intermittent, at intervals that vary with the severity of the disease.

Trismus, caused by spasm of the masseter muscles, a few days after birth is the presenting symptom in more than half of patients with neonatal tetanus. This is followed by stiffness of the neck muscles and difficulty in swallowing. The infant is irritable, restless and unable to feed. Spasm of the facial muscles produces risus sardonicus. Tonic contractions of the lumbar and abdominal musculature occur next, and result in opisthotonus. This is accompanied by flexion and adduction of the arms and clenching of the fists. Spasms which initially last a few seconds become more prolonged, and may persist for minutes as the disease progresses. The patient is conscious and crying because of intense pain from muscle spasms that become more powerful, and which are easily precipitated by any tactile, visual or auditory stimulus. Fever is a feature, probably because of overactivity of the muscles. Spasms of laryngeal and respiratory muscles may lead to obstruction, asphyxia and cyanosis. The natural history of tetanus is one of increasing severity during the first 7 days, followed by a plateau in the second week and gradual abatement over the next 2–6 weeks. Tetanus is often fatal in the neonate, with mortality as high as 60–90%.[310,470,929] Bronchopneumonia, aspiration pneumonia and atelectasis are common complications.[929] When assisted ventilation and intensive care are available the death rate can be substantially reduced.[330,580,930]

Management

The use of meagre resources to treat a serious infection with high mortality which can be eliminated by preventive measures raises some awkward ethical and administrative problems. The improved survival of patients with neonatal tetanus in centres where assisted ventilation, curarization, intravenous nutrition and new spasmolytic drugs have been applied raises questions about the reasons for the disparity in medical services which, on the one hand, are insufficiently developed to prevent this dreadful disease but which on the other hand can employ expensive modern technology to treat it.

There is currently no agreed standard regimen of management of neonatal tetanus. Efficacy of treatment will be influenced by factors of prognostic significance, such as incubation period, interval between the first symptom and the first spasm (onset interval), frequency and duration of spasms, fever and respiratory complications. The aims of treatment are to neutralize existing toxin before it enters the nervous system, to reduce further production of toxin, to control the neuromuscular and autonomic features and to sustain the patient until the effects of toxin resolve.

General management includes skilful nursing care to prevent aspiration pneumonia and atelectasis, and the reduction to a minimum of stimuli that can precipitate a convulsion. Patients are best cared for in open wards, where they are in easy view and within access of nurses and resuscitation equipment, rather than being confined to a darkened quiet place with no attention from medical staff. Provision must be made to accommodate mothers to ensure a supply of breast milk, and they should be encouraged to participate in the observation and care of the patient.

The infant has to be fed by nasogastric tube as he is unable to suck. Transpyloric feeding is preferred as it reduces the danger of aspiration of gastric contents. Breast milk should be given and supplemented by an intravenous infusion through which drugs can be administered.

Penicillin 60 mg (100 000 units) kg/day is given for 5 days to eliminate *Cl. tetani.* Concomitant infections should be treated with appropriate broad-spectrum antibiotics.

Tetanus antitoxin can only neutralize unbound circulating toxin and has no effect on toxin fixed in nerve cells. Although the central nervous system is often affected by toxin before symptoms appear, patients given antitoxin have usually fared better than those not given antitoxin. Specific antitetanus human immunoglobulin is the preparation of choice. A single dose of 3000–5000 units given by intramuscular injection is recommended. Equine antitetanus serum remains the most widely used tetanus antitoxin. It should be used as early as possible in the course of the disease, as either a single intramuscular injection of 5000 units or 750–1500 units daily for three doses. Massive doses of ATS have no significant advantage over smaller doses. There may be benefit in giving 1500 units of ATS intrathecally early in the disease. There is a significantly lower death rate in babies given intrathecal therapy (45%) compared to controls (82%) given intramuscular ATS. Infants who receive intrathecal ATS also have fewer complications than controls.[734] There is no convincing evidence that periumbilical infiltration of ATS has a significant effect on the outcome of neonatal tetanus.

Paraldehyde for immediate control of spasms, followed by phenobarbitone and chlorpromazine or diazepam for continued sedation, is effective in the control of spasms. The mortality from neonatal tetanus has been strikingly reduced by the use of muscle relaxants and intermittent positive-pressure ventilation, and this approach should be used wherever the facilities to apply it exist.

The following regimen of sedation is recommended for general use in tetanus neonatorum, where intensive care is not available.

1. Immediate control of spasms: Paraldehyde 0.3 ml/kg i.m. and/or:
   Diazepam 1–2 mg/kg i.m. or i.v.
   Diazepam should be administered slowly to avoid respiratory arrest.
2. Continued sedation (via nasogastric or nasotranspyloric tube):
   Phenobarbitone 5 mg/kg 6-hourly
   Chlorpromazine 2 mg/kg 6-hourly
   Diazepam 1–2 mg/kg 6-hourly.

Failure to control spasms on this regimen in the early phase of treatment calls for intermittent injections of paraldehyde or diazepam. The value of corticosteroids in the management of neonatal tetanus remains unproven.

Prevention

Tetanus in the newborn can be prevented by aseptic management of the umbilical cord at birth. The persistence of neonatal tetanus in many developing countries reflects the lack of rudimentary obstetric services for large sections of the population.[330] Education of traditional birth attendants in hygienic handling of the umbilical cord at birth has resulted in a sharp decline in the prevalence of neonatal tetanus. This provides a model which should be adopted with this disease in developing countries.

Active immunization of pregnant women with tetanus toxoid prevents the disease, but unfortunately those in greatest need of protection are not likely to attend antenatal clinics. At least two doses of tetanus toxoid, 0.5 ml each separated by 2 months, affords satisfactory immunity.[953]

Passive immunization of neonates at risk is the most frequently employed preventive measure in paediatric practice. The administration of 750 units of antitetanus serum to infants born in high-risk circumstances will provide protection.

Tetanus control and elimination

The Eighth International Conference on Tetanus in 1987 recognized that tetanus kills about 800 000 infants each year in developing countries. Recommendations for the control and elimination of neonatal tetanus arising from the meeting included: immunizing all women of child-bearing age with five doses of tetanus toxoid; assuring hygienic delivery and umbilical cord care through training and supervision of birth attendants; and investigating tetanus cases to determine what action could have prevented them.[1124]

LEPROSY

Babies of mothers with leprosy

Babies of mothers with leprosy are of lower than average birthweight.[709] Intrauterine growth retardation has been observed in babies of mothers with lepromatous leprosy as early as the 16th week of pregnancy. IgA antibodies to *M. leprae* have been found in 30% of cord sera of babies of mothers with active lepromatous leprosy. Specific IgA and IgM anti-*M. leprae* antibody production occurs during the first 6 months of life of these babies infected in utero. The prevalence of leprosy in children under 2 years of age whose mothers have active lepromatous leprosy is 5%. Diagnosis in these children has been made with positive skin tests to *M. leprae*, together with a marked increase in serum IgA and IgM anti-*M. leprae* antibody activity.

Management

The pregnant mother should receive multidrug therapy of dapsone 2 mg/kg daily, clofazimine 1 mg/kg daily and rifampicin 10 mg/kg monthly. Clofazimine will turn her milk pink, so mothers should be reassured that the colour change does not affect the quality of their milk. Folate supplements should be given. Women with leprosy should be encouraged to breast-feed their babies while they are receiving effective treatment. Heavy breast milk infection only occurs in advanced leprosy involving the nipple and milk ducts.

Newborn babies of mothers who were not treated during pregnancy should be treated with clofazimine 1 mg/kg daily, which may be also be given to babies of treated women if indicated. Unlike dapsone, clofazimine will not induce haemolysis in children with G6PD deficiency.

PERINATAL VIRAL INFECTIONS

Several viral agents can cause serious neonatal illness with high mortality and morbidity rates. Most of these infections are acquired by vertical transmission, but some are the result of cross-infection postnatally.

HERPESVIRUSES

Herpes simplex virus

Herpes simplex is a large virus containing double-stranded DNA, which encodes for some 70 polypeptides. It exists in two antigenically distinct forms, HSV-1, the cause of orolabial, ophthalmic and encephalitic herpes in older children and adults, and HSV-2, which until recently caused 80–85% of genital herpes and the majority of neonatal infections. The remaining 15–20% of cases of genital herpes, and up to 30% of neonatal infections, were due to HSV type 1.[1106] Lately, genital infection with HSV-1 has become commoner in the UK (probably as a result of the fear of HIV leading to more oral sex) and the most recent incidence report has HSV-1 and HSV-2 accounting for equal proportions of neonatal infection.[1034]

The incidence of neonatal herpes in the UK is around 1 case per 50 000 births,[459,1034] but 100-fold higher incidences are reported from North America.[598,963,1104] Neonatal herpes is often fatal and neurological handicap is common in survivors. The preterm infant is most susceptible.[1101]

Modes of transmission

Transplacental infection. Transplacental transmission of HSV is rare and usually associated with primary maternal infection with HSV-2. This route accounts for around 5% of all cases of neonatal herpes,[527] and some 70 cases have been reported in the literature.[1103] The infection may ascend through intact membranes.[529,823] The congenitally infected baby is usually profoundly damaged, with microcephaly or hydranencephaly, chorioretinitis and skin lesions, but occasionally may just have mild eye involvement.[527] No treatment is available for these babies.

Vertical transmission. Neonatal HSV occurs as a result of maternal genital herpes in about 85% of cases,[671] although most of the mothers are either asymptomatic at the time of birth or have no history of genital herpes.[686,1132] Rarely, the virus may reach the fetus in utero following prolonged rupture of the membranes, in which case the baby may be born with skin and eye lesions. This form of infection is rare and carries a relatively good prognosis with effective antiviral treatment.[1103] Usually infection is acquired during passage down the birth canal. If the mother has an active primary infection at the time of vaginal delivery the risk of neonatal infection is about 50%,[152] but if she has a secondary recurrence of genital herpes, lower concentrations of virus are shed and the risk is reduced to around 3%.[151,855]

Nosocomial infection. HSV can be acquired from other neonatal cases, or from orolabial or cutaneous herpes in staff or family.[265,636,1058,1059] Although this form of transmission is allegedly rare, the fact that the incidence of type I neonatal HSV is roughly double that of type I genital herpetic infections[1103] (see above) suggests that non-genital sources of neonatal infection may be more common than previously thought.[525]

Table 43.17 Change in type of neonatal herpes virus infection at the time of diagnosis (percentage). (Reproduced with permission from Whitley et al[1106])

Period	Superficial	Meningoencephalitis	Disseminated
1973–80 (95 patients)	17.89	31.58	50.53
1981–87 (196 patients)	43.37	33.67	22.96

Clinical features

Neonatal HSV infection occurs in three distinct forms, albeit with a degree of overlap[299,686] (Table 43.17).

Localized to skin, mouth and eyes. Superficial infection ordinarily occurs during the second week of life and is a more common presentation if the mother has recurrent rather than primary infection.[684] The baby may develop a vesicular skin rash, keratoconjunctivitis or, rarely, intraoral vesicles. The disease can be localized to just one of these sites or may affect any combination of them. The skin vesicles are usually 1–2 mm in diameter, but may be much larger. They can be multiple or occur in clusters.

Babies who present with superficial infection generally do not develop disseminated disease, but a surprisingly high proportion (maybe up to 30%) show subsequent neurodevelopmental abnormalities.[1103] Conversely, infants who present with disseminated disease may later develop cutaneous and eye lesions.

CNS disease. About one-third of babies with HSV infection present with isolated meningoencephalitis and symptoms similar to those seen in neonatal bacterial meningitis. The usual age of onset is around 10–14 days of age.[756] Many subsequently develop cutaneous or ocular herpes. This form of the disease may result either from haematogenous spread or from neural spread, with retrograde axonal transmission of the virus to the CNS.[429,1103]

Disseminated disease. This most severe form of neonatal herpes presents during the first week of life,[684] and is probably a viraemia with secondary seeding of the CNS.[1103] About half of the cases will have only systemic disease and/or pneumonia,[31] but the rest will have co-existing meningoencephalitis;[536] 20% have no cutaneous manifestations, making diagnosis difficult.[1079]

Infants with disseminated disease present like any critically ill septic baby (pp. 1116–1117). They have respiratory distress as a result of pneumonitis, and usually require IPPV. They are often hypotensive, peripherally vasoconstricted, and have renal failure. Severe hepatitis[91,425] may occur with or without hepatosplenomegaly. DIC, causing petechiae and generalized bleeding, is common.[536] Hypotonia, seizures and coma are common whether or not meningoencephalitis is present.

Diagnosis

Cutaneous vesicles, ocular or oral lesions strongly suggest herpes. Other vesicular lesions, such as staphylococcal skin infection or varicella, are usually easily differentiated by the history and their clinical appearance (pp. 892, 896, 1158).[928]

The most rapid and useful diagnostic test that is widely available is immunofluorescence performed on vesicle fluid. Viral culture should also be undertaken on vesicle fluid, conjunctival scrapings, nasopharyngeal swab and, where obtained, CSF. Cultures may show cytopathic changes within a few days. The virus may also grow from blood.[406] Serology is much less useful because of the difficulty in distinguishing between passively acquired maternal antibody and endogenously produced antibody. DNA amplification tests are also available.

In the absence of a maternal history of genital disease or of suspicious skin, eye or mouth lesions, disseminated HSV infection will only be diagnosed if viral cultures are a routine part of the investigation of all septic babies, with or without meningitis, from whom no bacterial pathogen is grown after 24–48 hours. Neonatal viral meningitis is usually a mild illness, so that if the CSF findings suggest it (p. 1159) but the baby is seriously ill, herpes is the most likely diagnosis. In some cases of herpetic meningoencephalitis, however, the CSF contains more than 1000 WBC/mm^3, many of them polymorphs, together with many red cells, a markedly raised protein and a low glucose.[537,717] Differentiating these cases from bacterial meningitis depends on cultures.

If herpes is suspected an EEG should be performed, as it may show characteristic temporoparietal high-voltage low-frequency activity. A CT scan should be performed to look for the characteristic necrosis and haemorrhage in the temporal lobes. These may only appear late in the disease, although MRI changes may occur earlier.[594] Visceral calcification has been reported with disseminated disease.[499]

If there is even a suspicion that systemic illness in a baby is due to herpes, treatment should be begun (see below) until a definite diagnosis is established. Nevertheless, some fulminating cases only come to light at postmortem, when widespread herpetic microabscesses are found, or the virus is grown or detected by PCR.[771]

Treatment

Treatment is with either acyclovir or adenine arabinoside. Although a recent prospective controlled trial showed no differences between the two agents in the treatment of neonatal herpes,[1105] controlled trials comparing acyclovir with adenine arabinoside in adults with meningoencephalitis have previously shown a distinct benefit from acyclovir.[981] Alarmingly, acyclovir-resistant neonatal HSV infection has recently been reported.[780] In experimental animals a combination of anti-HSV antibody and acyclovir is far superior to acyclovir alone in reducing mortality,[146] but there is no such study in newborn infants as yet.

Acyclovir is given intravenously, 8-hourly, in a total daily dose of 30 mg/kg. As recurrences have occurred after a 10-day course[231] this should be continued intravenously for at least 14 days. Topical acyclovir should be applied to eye and skin lesions.

Prognosis

The outcome of neonatal herpes before effective antiviral therapy was available was poor (Table 43.18).[757] More recently the results have improved, partly because more cases are diagnosed early and have only localized disease (Table 43.17).[1106] The mortality rate for disseminated disease is now between 35 and 60%,[1100,1102,1104] and for disease isolated to the CNS between 10 and 15%.[1104] HSV-2 carries a much higher mortality rate than HSV-1[684,1099]

In terms of morbidity the picture remains poor, with major adverse sequelae in some 85% of survivors of disseminated disease and in some 50–75% of survivors of meningoencephalitis.[537] HSV-2 infection has a worse

Table 43.18 Outcome of neonates with herpes infections. (Reproduced with permission from Nahmias et al[757])

	No. of cases	Dead (%)	Alive but handicapped (%)	Alive and normal (%)
Disseminated herpes without CNS involvement	157	91	2	7
Disseminated herpes with CNS involvement	154	73	15	12
Localized CNS disease	116	41	42	17
Other localized disease	76	7	24	70

prognosis than HSV-1,[685] and in one study only 25% of babies with HSV-2 infection were normal on follow-up compared to 100% of those with HSV-1.[217] An abnormal EEG in the neonatal period is a poor prognostic sign.[685]

Recurrent infection

Despite apparent complete resolution of the initial infection there is a high incidence of recurrence in the following 6–12 months, owing to a defective immunological response to the virus.[595] In one series, relapses occurred in all congenital cases and 12 out of 25 neonatal cases.[1016] Kohl[595] reports that most treated neonates will develop cutaneous recurrences in the first year of life. Encephalitic relapses may also occur,[1016] and Gutman et al[450] have reported progressive neurological deterioration during the first year of life in a group of infants with neonatal encephalitis. The virus is, however, still sensitive to and may respond to further courses of antiviral drugs.[869]

Prevention

The risk of transplacental infection is low,[152] only around 0.3% of women excreting the virus intrapartum.[151,856] The risk of neonatal infection is extremely small in babies born to the asymptomatic HSV excreter,[151,855] yet 60–80% of cases of neonatal herpes occur in babies whose mothers have neither a history of genital herpes nor any evidence of intrapartum infection.[796] These facts suggest that there is little point in routinely screening for HSV during pregnancy,[550,635] and that there is no need to deliver asymptomatic women with a history of herpes by caesarean section. The risk of neonatal herpes infection following vaginal delivery when the mother has overt primary genital herpes, however, is around 50%, and can be reduced to less than 20% if delivery is by caesarean section within 24 hours of membrane rupture. An apparently successful alternative approach is to treat women who have a primary herpes infection in pregnancy with acyclovir from 36 weeks' gestation until delivery.[961] Arguably, the best strategy for the prevention of neonatal herpes, without greatly increasing the number of caesarean sections, is physical examination of the mother at the time of labour, with caesarean section for those who have lesions.[635]

Postnatally the baby of the mother with covert genital herpes requires no treatment. Following vaginal delivery in the presence of overt genital herpes, the baby should stay with its mother and should be treated with intravenous acyclovir, although this is not always effective.[338] If the mother has orolabial or cutaneous herpes the baby should stay with her (p. 1115, Table 43.6) but her lesions should be covered, treated with topical acyclovir, and her hand-washing technique should be meticulous. Other family members or staff with open herpes should stay away.

VARICELLA ZOSTER VIRUS

This is a member of the herpesvirus family. It causes varicella (chickenpox) as an acute primary infection, but when reactivated from its dormant site in the dorsal root ganglia it causes the cutaneous eruption known as zoster (shingles). Primary infection can occur in the fetus and newborn, sometimes with devastating effect. Reactivation of the virus to cause zoster is rare in the newborn period. Primary VZV infections can be classified as congenital, perinatal or postnatal. Congenital varicella is discussed on page 1173.

Perinatally acquired varicella

If a mother develops varicella during the 3 weeks prior to delivery there is a 25% chance of her baby developing the illness.[751] Some babies may be born with the rash,[472,723] in which case the prognosis is good, as it is if the baby develops a rash within 4 days of birth. The usual interval between the onset of the rash in the mother and the onset of rash in the fetus or infant is between 9 and 15 days.[758] The timing of birth in relation to the maternal infection is critical to outcome. Babies born 5 or more days after the mother develops the rash receive some transplacental immunity, have an excellent prognosis, and all reported cases have survived. Babies born less than 5 days after the mother develops the rash develop the disease some 5–10 days after delivery and experience a high mortality (Table 43.19).

Postnatally acquired varicella

Varicella acquired later in the neonatal period is usually a benign disease, although occasional fatalities occur.[916]

Clinical features of neonatal varicella

The disease in the newborn can range from a few vesicles in a relatively well baby to severe disseminated infection complicated by pneumonitis. When pneumonitis occurs the mortality is high.

Treatment

Babies born to mothers who develop varicella between 7 days antenatally and 14 days postnatally should receive

Table 43.19 Outcome of neonates with varicella. (Reproduced with permission from Hanshaw & Dudgeon[473])

	Total	Survived	Died (%)
Maternal varicella > 5 days from delivery, neonatal varicella 0–4 days	27	27	0
Maternal varicella < 4 days from delivery, neonatal varicella 5–10 days	23	16	7 (30%)

a dose of ZIG, 100 mg, as soon after delivery as possible, or as soon as possible after the mother becomes symptomatic.[723] This will reduce the severity of the disease in the baby but will usually not prevent it.[472,723] Miller et al[723] reported that 78 of 125 such babies developed varicella – 15 severely – but none died. This is a much better prognosis than suggested by Table 43.19. However, there are reports of neonatal deaths[514] in the high-risk group born within 7 days of the maternal presentation, despite the use of ZIG. For this group, therefore, in addition to giving ZIG, consider giving acyclovir 60 mg/kg/day, 8-hourly, if vesicles appear. Babies born to mothers with perinatal varicella should be isolated from other babies from birth.

If a baby is exposed to varicella postnatally, whether or not treatment is required depends on its immune status. All exposed infants should have their immune status checked using the varicella zoster ELISA test in order to avoid unnecessary treatment with a blood product.[768] If the baby is seronegative ZIG should be administered, especially if it is less than 32 weeks' gestation or in some other high-risk category. If the baby has antibody there is no need to give ZIG, unless it is more than 2 months old and still in an NICU.[364,809]

Zoster infection

Zoster has been reported in the neonate,[147] but the accuracy of the diagnosis must be questioned in the absence of confirmation by culture.[153] In babies who have congenital varicella (p. 1173), zoster may appear shortly after the first month of life[505] and may also occur in early infancy in babies who develop perinatal varicella.[723] Maternal zoster does not usually affect the baby,[304,723] although there are occasional reports of fetal damage.[505]

HUMAN HERPES VIRUS TYPE 6

Human herpes virus type 6 may be transmitted perinatally but does not cause serious neonatal disease.[455,618]

ENTEROVIRUSES

These are small spherical viruses containing a single strand of RNA. There are traditionally three main subgroups, namely polioviruses, echoviruses and coxsackieviruses, but newly classified enteroviruses are now being numbered outside this classification, e.g. enterovirus 72 is hepatitis A virus.

Most neonatal enterovirus infections are mild and occur after the first week, often coinciding with epidemics in the community.[551] Poliovirus infections are rare in developed countries, and becoming rarer in developing countries, but both echoviruses and coxsackieviruses regularly cause serious neonatal infection.[7] Enterovirus infection in the newborn can be acquired by both vertical and horizontal transmission. Infection due to vertical transmission tends to be more severe[536,537] and earlier in onset.[7] Horizontal spread is mainly via the faecal–oral route, but respiratory secretions may also be infectious.

Echovirus

Many neonatal echovirus infections are asymptomatic,[551] but some antigenic types, e.g. 6, 7, 11, 12 and 14, can cause serious disease. Echovirus 11 has been responsible for the most severe cases.[728,754] Echovirus infection tends to follow one of three patterns.

Mild malaise

This is the commonest pattern. There is fever, malaise and mild gastrointestinal upset lasting for 3 or 4 days, and a full recovery is made.[536] These cases are most often diagnosed during epidemiological surveys of outbreaks of serious disease. Investigation, apart from isolating the virus, is usually negative except for a few atypical mononuclear white cells on the differential WBC. Recently it has become possible to detect enteroviruses in the serum and urine of infected babies using PCR.[8,942]

Viral meningitis

This is usually mild, and seizures and other major neurological signs are rare.[602] CSF analysis will show features typical of viral meningitis with up to 100–200 WBC/mm^3, mainly lymphocytes, and comparatively normal protein and sugar concentrations. No organisms are seen on Gram stain. The virus will grow from the CSF, and also usually from a throat swab and the stools. Atypical mononuclear cells may be seen on the blood film. Recovery is the rule, although evidence of focal encephalitis is increasingly recognized using modern imaging techniques.[907]

Severe viraemic illness

This is commonly caused by serotypes 6, 7 and 11, and is often acquired vertically. It is a serious infection, usually associated with hepatitis and often with meningoencephalitis, pneumonitis, myocarditis, gastroenteritis and disseminated intravascular coagulation.[139,729,857] There is rapid deterioration, with acidaemia, jaundice, apnoea, internal and external haemorrhage and profound hypotension resistant to volume expansion and inotropic drugs. Renal failure often develops and the condition commonly progresses to death within 48 hours.[537] The autopsy findings are very characteristic, with massive hepatic necrosis and haemorrhagic necrosis of adrenals, renal tubules and myocardium.[103]

Coxsackievirus

Coxsackievirus infections can be acquired by both vertical

and horizontal transmission, but unlike the echovirus the mode of transmission has little effect on the severity of illness. Most neonatal infections are due to type B. The spectrum ranges from a mild febrile illness, with or without diarrhoea, to meningoencephalitis,[492,729] myocarditis (p. 698) and a severe viraemic illness similar to that seen with the echoviruses.[1117] The non-specific illnesses may progress to the more severe illnesses over several days and sometimes a biphasic illness is seen, with apparent recovery in between a mild illness and a fatal myocarditis.[270] Coxsackievirus infections are often accompanied by a rash, which is sometimes petechial.

Coxsackievirus B myocarditis may present gradually with tachycardia, breathlessness and poor feeding, or acutely with circulatory collapse. There is invariably cardiomegaly, often a murmur, and the ECG shows ST-segment depression and sometimes a supraventricular tachycardia. Viral RNA can be demonstrated in the myocardium using PCR.[507] This illness carries a high mortality rate and is often associated with signs of encephalitis or hepatitis.[565]

Meningoencephalitis usually occurs in small epidemics, and outbreaks due to many group A and B serotypes have been reported. The CSF shows a typical picture of viral meningitis and the virus can be grown from a throat swab, stools or CSF. The infant is rarely severely ill and usually recovers completely within 7–10 days. Neurological sequelae are extremely unusual.

It has recently been suggested that the children of women whose serum contained IgM to coxsackievirus B at delivery are at significantly increased risk of childhood-onset diabetes.[226]

Poliomyelitis

Neonatal polio typically presents with fever, listlessness, poor feeding, diarrhoea and flaccid paralysis of one or more limbs. There is often a CSF pleocytosis, and virus can usually be grown from the stools and CSF. Neonatal polio may occur following contact with an older patient known to have polio, or following birth to a mother who herself develops polio around the time of delivery.

Treatment of enterovirus infections

There is no specific antiviral agent. Injections of pooled IVIG have been advocated to reduce the severity of illness as well as prevent transmission of an epidemic within an NICU,[755,1050] although some studies have shown little benefit once the infection is established.[537] More recently, it has been suggested that higher doses of IVIG, or IVIG selected for its high titres of antibody to virulent enterovirus serotypes, may be beneficial.[5] Clinical trials are needed. Successful treatment of fulminant neonatal echovirus 11 infection by means of orthotopic liver transplantation has been recorded.[201]

MEASLES

Measles in pregnancy is even rarer than varicella. There is a substantial complication rate among pregnant women with measles, with high hospitalization rates and pneumonia in around a quarter of cases.[285] The measles virus is probably not teratogenic, but measles in pregnancy may lead to high rates of fetal loss and prematurity, mostly occurring within 2 weeks of the appearance of the rash.[285] If the mother has measles around the time of delivery the baby may be infected transplacentally and either be born with the rash or develop it within the first 10 days of life. Perinatal measles is often a mild illness, but may be severe and complicated by a fatal pneumonitis. The older literature reports a high mortality rate but it is doubtful if this still applies in an era of broad-spectrum antibiotics and neonatal intensive care.[387] The effect of hyperimmune antimeasles globulin in this situation has not been adequately evaluated, but it could be beneficial.[379a] There is a putative link between perinatal measles and the subsequent occurrence of Crohn's disease.[297]

MUMPS

There is an unresolved controversy over whether congenital mumps infection can cause endocardial fibroelastosis in the neonate. Apart from this, prenatal mumps infection is apparently benign. Neonatal mumps seems to be extremely rare and is a mild disease.[556]

RUBELLA

With a high level of maternal immunity in the community (p. 1168) and a 3-week incubation period, primary rubella is highly unlikely to occur in the neonate, and when it does it is usually mild.

NEONATAL HEPATITIS

Neonatal hepatitis can be due to congenital, perinatal or postnatal infections. The main congenital causes are rubella (p. 1169), CMV (p. 1170), herpes simplex (p. 1156), toxoplasmosis (p. 1172) and syphilis (p. 1174). Perinatal infections, following intrapartum contact with infected maternal blood or secretions, include herpes simplex (p. 1157), CMV (p. 1162), enteroviruses[7] (p. 1159), varicella (p. 1158), adenovirus,[6] hepatitis A, B and C and non-A, B or C hepatitis (see below). CMV is the only common postnatal cause of viral hepatitis.

Clinical presentation

Infants with congenital infective hepatitis are usually jaundiced within 24 hours of birth. Of the perinatally acquired causes of hepatitis, only herpes simplex is likely to present within the first week of the neonatal period.[796] Hepatitis A, B and C usually present towards, or beyond, the end of the neonatal period, because of their long incubation times. Acquired CMV usually comes from blood transfusion (pp. 841, 1162) and often presents in the postneonatal period in VLBW survivors who have had to stay in a neonatal unit for many weeks (p. 1162).

Babies with hepatitis are jaundiced and unwell. They usually have hepatosplenomegaly and often have dark urine and pale stools. A considerable proportion of the total bilirubin is conjugated and the liver enzymes are elevated. The commonest differential diagnosis is from conditions such as the inspissated bile syndrome following haemolytic jaundice, TPN-related cholestasis (p. 739) and α_1-antitrypsin deficiency. The more complex metabolic possibilities and whether or not the infant has biliary atresia are outlined on page 733.

Hepatitis A

Transplacental hepatitis A infection has not been reported, and perinatal infection, even if the mother has active hepatitis at delivery, is extremely unusual.[1033] Epidemics of hepatitis A in neonatal units have been reported, some associated with transfusion from an infected donor[588,625,775,905] and others with postnatal transmission from mother to baby.[1080] No treatment for hepatitis A is available, but it is prudent to give 0.5–1.0 ml of pooled immunoglobulin to all infants delivered to women who have active hepatitis A within 2 weeks of delivery.

Hepatitis B

Epidemiology and vertical transmission

The majority of the 300 million asymptomatic carriers of hepatitis B virus live in developing countries.[1123] Two-fifths of children with persistent infection who survive to adulthood die as a result of chronic liver disease and carcinoma. The prevalence of hepatitis B surface antigen, HBsAg, the marker for the carrier state of hepatitis B virus in apparently healthy adults, varies from 0.1% in parts of Europe and North America to between 15 and 20% in parts of West Africa and East Asia. In Africa the majority of carriers are infected during childhood, whereas in Asia perinatal infection is the most important route of transmission of the virus from carrier mothers to their newborn infants.[727] Transplacental passage of hepatitis B virus is uncommon.[792] Perinatal infection is probably a result of the leak of infected maternal blood into the infant's circulation during labour, or its ingestion at birth.

The risk of infection is high for babies born to carrier mothers in countries with high carrier rates, e.g. Taiwan, where the perinatal transmission rate is about 40%.[1005] Ethnic group susceptibility to infection is significant. Chinese HBsAg carrier mothers transmit infection more frequently to their infants than carriers among Africans, Asians or Caucasians in the UK.[249,1119] The presence of HBeAg in mother's blood greatly increases the risk of infection in the baby.[386,844,1119] This 'e' antigen is associated with a defective immune response to hepatitis B virus, which permits continued replication of virus in liver cells.[1043] The expression of 'e' antigen, HBeAg, appears to be genetically determined. More Chinese women carriers (40%) of hepatitis B virus are HBeAg-positive than are African carrier mothers (15%). Of children born to Chinese carrier mothers between 40 and 70% become carriers; to African mothers about 30%; to Indian mothers 6–8%; and to European mothers almost none. Perinatal transmission of hepatitis B virus among Arab women is low.

Clinical picture

The majority of infected infants do not develop neonatal jaundice and remain asymptomatic. HBsAg appears in their blood between 6 weeks and 4 months after birth,[249,1119] and usually persists. Most of these infants become chronic carriers of hepatitis B virus. A small number of infants with hepatitis B develop a fulminant illness and die with massive liver necrosis. The reasons for this are not understood. Although the clinical course for infected infants is usually mild, the long-term prognosis is blighted by their increased risk of chronic liver disease and primary hepatic carcinoma in adulthood. Convincing evidence of an association between HBsAg and hepatoma has emerged from a prospective study of 22 707 Chinese men in Taiwan, 15% of whom were HBsAg positive. Forty of the 41 cases of hepatocellular carcinoma detected in the 5-year study had HBsAg in their blood.[76]

Management and prevention

Once the carrier state has developed it cannot be terminated by any therapeutic agent currently available. Prevention is therefore extremely important, and regimens based on a combination of active and passive immunization are most effective.

For active immunization, two types of vaccine are currently available. The plasma vaccine is prepared from plasma of carriers of hepatitis B. Non-infectious subunits of the HBsAg are separated, purified and inactivated by three processes, each of which inactivates all known viruses, including HIV. The plasma-derived vaccine is effective for at least 5 years in subjects who produce an initial high antibody titre, and in a recent study from China at least 9 years of protective immunity was found.[253] The recombinant vaccine is produced by yeast, into which a plasmid containing the gene for the HBsAg has been inserted. It is adsorbed onto an aluminium hydroxide adjuvant. Currently there are two available preparations in the UK, Energix B (SmithKline Beecham) and H-B-VaxII (Pasteur Mérieux MSD). The recombinant vaccine is cheaper than the plasma-derived vaccine and has the advantage of not requiring a supply of plasma from hepatitis B carriers, but it is not yet known for how long it maintains effective antibody levels.

Active immunization of all susceptible infants in areas where there is a high carrier rate is highly desirable, although not yet economically feasible. However, the genetically engineered vaccine could provide the 300 million or so doses required by the year 2000 to prevent the spread of hepatitis B worldwide.

Passive immunization is with specific hepatitis B immunoglobulin given soon after birth. This therapy alone, if given repeatedly, will prevent persistent carriage in most exposed infants by modifying the infection. A 75% protection rate was reported from Taiwan in a controlled trial of hepatitis B immunoglobulin given at birth and repeated twice at intervals of 3 months.[77]

A combination of active and passive immunization is the preferred protection regimen and is very effective.[33,247,774,962] It is even possible to provide this combined regimen on the basis of the results of intrapartum screening.[827] In Britain, where an estimated 400 non-Caucasian babies are at risk of becoming persistent carriers of hepatitis B virus each year after exposure at birth, a national programme of hepatitis B immunoglobulin administration to at-risk babies was introduced in 1982. Since 1985, infants also receive a course of vaccination from birth.[842] Studies have shown that 90% of fully immunized infants have high levels of protective antibody at 1 year. Reactions have been reported after 11% of vaccine doses and 8% of specific immunoglobulin doses, but none of these reactions was considered to be severe.

In the UK at present the following scheme of passive–active immunization is recommended for the babies of women who are HBsAg positive or who have had acute hepatitis during pregnancy. All infants should receive the vaccine at birth or as soon as possible after birth, irrespective of the maternal HBe antigen or antibody status.[78,702] In addition, hepatitis B immunoglobulin (200 IU) should be given intramuscularly within 24 hours, or at the latest within 48 hours, of delivery to all infants of HBsAg-positive women, other than those who possess anti-HBe antibody. Further doses of vaccine are given at 1 and 6 months of age.

Breast-feeding should not be discouraged because transmission of the virus through breast milk or by ingestion of blood from excoriated nipples is negligible compared to the infant's exposure to contaminated maternal blood at delivery.[75] Furthermore, the dangers of not breast-feeding in developing countries outweigh the very small chance of the baby becoming infected exclusively by the breast milk of the carrier mother. If given hepatitis B vaccine at birth these babies will not even be exposed to this small risk of infection from breast milk.

Hepatitis C

Hepatitis C can undoubtedly be transmitted vertically,[640,791,1028,1094,1095] especially when the mother is coinfected with HIV.[346,799,1141] Breast-feeding, however, seems relatively safe.[639] This infection can also be acquired from transfusion, but in the UK all blood and blood products are now screened for hepatitis C. The incubation period is long and cases are unlikely to present within the neonatal period.

Hepatitis non-A, B or C

Other hepatitis viruses are uncommon in the UK, but vertical transmission of hepatitis E causing serious neonatal hepatitis is well documented in developing countries.[581]

CYTOMEGALOVIRUS

Serious illness, including hepatitis and pneumonia, is described in babies given CMV-positive blood during exchange transfusion,[94,1131] and following multiple top-up transfusions in VLBW babies.[12,1133] The pneumonitis can cause marked deterioration in lung function, especially among those with CLD.[941] Acquiring CMV may also predispose the VLBW baby to other serious infections.[606] It is important to use only CMV-negative donors for transfusion of VLBW babies, even those of seropositive mothers,[241] or to treat donor blood to remove the lymphocytes which are the vectors of CMV (p. 841).[733]

Babies may also acquire CMV from staff or infected babies, or from the mother's cervix or expressed breast milk.[278,888] Neonatal CMV is more likely to occur in babies of CMV-seronegative mothers, but also occurs in babies born to seropositive mothers after the titre of maternal antibody has declined postnatally.[242,1134]

Treatment is supportive. The use of high-titre CMV immunoglobulin and drugs such as ganciclovir, which have met with limited success in older immunosuppressed patients, has not been evaluated in neonates. VLBW babies who acquire CMV perinatally may have an increased incidence of handicap on follow-up, though more data are required.[806]

FUNGAL INFECTIONS

Newborn infants are susceptible to invasive fungal infection because of their relative immunodeficiency. Particular factors are the 'naive' state of neonatal T cells,

Table 43.20 Reported fungal infections in the neonate

Organism	Symptoms	Treatment and comment	References
Alcaligenes xylosoxidans	Meningitis		Boukadida et al 1993 Ped. Inf. Dis. J. 12:696
Aspergillus fumigatus	Sepsis	None diagnosed in life. All fatal	Schwartz et al 1988 Ped. Inf. Dis. J. 7:349
Blastomycosis	Presented as SIDS	Presumed transplacental infection	Watts et al 1983 Ped. Inf. Dis. J. 2:308
Candida parapsilosis	NICU outbreak of septicaemia		Welbel et al 1996 Ped. Inf. Dis. J. 15:998
Coccidioides	Pneumonia	Present in maternal cervical swab. Proved fatal	Bernstein et al 1981 J. Pediatr 99:752
Curvularia lunata	Wound infection	Surgical excision	Yau et al 1994 Clin. Infect. Dis. 19:735
Hansenula anomala	Sepsis, meningitis	Amphotericin and flucytosine Epidemic ceased with oral nystatin and betadine to venepuncture sites	Murphy et al 1986 Lancet i:291
Malassezia furfur	Facial pustules confused with neonatal acne or miliaria	Ketoconazole cream Remove lines and stop i.v. fat	Rapelanoro et al 1996 Arch. Dermatol. 132:190 Powell et al 1984 J. Pediatr. 105:987 Aschner et al 1987 Pediatrics 80:535
Malassezia pachydermatis	Sepsis: common skin commensal	Amphotericin. Remove lines stop i.v. fat. Outlook good	Nickelsen et al 1988 J. Inf. Dis. 157:1163 Larocco et al 1988 Ped. Inf. Dis. J. 7:398
Rhizopus	Disseminated infection in a preterm infant	Surgery and amphotericin, but proved fatal	Craig et al 1994 Pediatr. Dermatol. 11:346
	Skin abscess	Amphotericin. Resolved	Ng & Dear 1989 Arch. Dis. Child. 64:862
Torulopsis glabrata	Systemic infection in 2 preterm infants	Amphotericin. Successful outcome	Reich et al 1997 South. Med. J. 90:246
Trichophyton rubrum	Systemic infection		Singal et al 1996 Pediatr. Dermatol. 13:488
Trichosporon beigelii	Cysto-peritoneal shunt infection	Shunt removal and antifungal agents	Ashpole et al 1991 Br. J. Neurosurg. 5:515
	Outbreak of systemic infection in a NICU	Resistant to amphotericin	Fisher et al 1993 Ped. Inf. Dis. J. 12:149 Giacoia 1992 South. Med. J. 85:1247 Rowen et al 1995 Pediatrics 95:682
	Systemic illness		del Palacio et al 1990 Ped. Inf. Dis. J. 9:520
Zygomyosis	Disseminated or necrotizing cellulitis	Severe forms fatal	Grim et al 1984 Ped. Inf. Dis. J. 3:61 White et al 1986 Pediatrics 78:100

mainly CD45RA type, and reduced T-cell cytotoxicity.[483] Invasive candidiasis has been reported in as high a proportion as 4.5% of VLBW infants.[329]

C. albicans accounts for about 75% of neonatal fungal infections, with *C. parapsilosis* and *C. tropicalis* accounting for most of the rest. Several other species of fungi have been known to cause neonatal infection from time to time (Table 43.20).

CANDIDA ALBICANS

Cutaneous candidiasis is described on pages 892–893.

Congenital candidiasis

Vaginal candidiasis is common in pregnancy and ascending fetal infection occasionally occurs, especially if an intrauterine contraceptive device is left in situ or a cervical suture is inserted.[1107] It is associated with preterm labour.[1063] The infection spreads over the external and internal body surface rather than invading the bloodstream, and congenitally infected babies characteristically have skin and mucosal involvement and often a pneumonia.[526,769] *Candida* sp. can be cultured from gastric aspirates, superficial lesions and the lung, but rarely from the blood or CSF.[165] Treatment is with amphotericin and flucytosine (see below) but, as with postnatally acquired systemic candidiasis, the mortality is high.[647] *C. albicans* amnionitis has been successfully treated by amnioinfusion with amphotericin.[966]

Acquired systemic candidiasis[765]

This is an increasing problem in VLBW survivors of neonatal intensive care, affecting some 2–3%.[165,710] The majority have been colonized by *C. albicans* from birth,[61] although around 15% acquire the organism nosocomially. As risk factors, such as the presence of central lines,[932] ventriculoperitoneal shunts,[193] tracheal tubes[911] and extensive antibiotic use accumulate, the probability of invasive infection grows.[60,329,1083] The use of intravenous hydrocortisone for the treatment of hypotension soon after birth may predispose to systemic candidiasis.[135]

Disseminated candidiasis presents like bacterial sepsis,[60,327,985] and the spectrum of illness includes pneumonia, septicaemia with or without endocarditis, septic arthritis, osteomyelitis, endophthalmitis, intraperitoneal infection, liver abscesses, meningitis and renal tract infection. Preceding mucocutaneous candidiasis is common[329] and skin lesions are almost universal. Baley and Silverman[63] described mucocutaneous candidiasis in about half their cases of systemic disease, and the other half had a characteristic bright, erythematous, macular patchy dermatitis, usually on the trunk, often presenting within the first 72 hours. Localized cutaneous abscesses may also occur.[498]

Neonatal sepsis caused by other *Candida* species, such as *C. parapsilosis*[300,985] and *C. lusitaniae*,[935] presents a clinical picture indistinguishable from that caused by *C. albicans*.[328] Recently there have been reports of invasive fungal dermatitis, occurring during the first week or so of life in very immature infants[910] and, as larger numbers of such babies are now surviving, this is something to watch out for.

Investigation

It is harder to diagnose fungal infection than bacterial infection because positive blood cultures are less common. Even when the organisms are in the blood it takes several days longer for cultures to become positive than is the case with most bacteria. In one study, the average time between the onset of symptoms and the initiation of antifungal therapy was 11 days.[60] When there is no typical mucocutaneous rash or some other clue to suggest fungal infection, the diagnosis is usually made during the routine investigation of an infant with suspected sepsis. In addition to culturing blood, urine and CSF where indicated, endotracheal tube aspirate and tubes removed from the baby, including chest drains and intravascular cannulae, can be examined microscopically for budding yeasts or fungal hyphae. A useful additional test is to examine a buffy-coat smear for the characteristic intracellular inclusions.[183] Thrombocytopenia is common[281] and should raise the level of suspicion. Serological tests to demonstrate the presence of both candida antigen and antibody have been developed, but have not as yet shown sufficient sensitivity or specificity to be of much use. Acute-phase proteins are usually very elevated in systemic candida infection.

In all cases of suspected or proven candidiasis the following investigations should be undertaken. The renal tract should be examined with ultrasound to look for evidence of fungal and cellular debris, which may cause obstruction.[50] If there is, or has recently been, a central line in situ, echocardiography should be performed to look for evidence of fungal endocarditis.[705] The CSF should be examined[37] and ophthalmological examination should be performed to look for endophthalmitis. In the case of NICU outbreaks of candida infection, DNA fingerprinting may help to understand the mechanism of spread.[108]

Prevention

Limiting exposure to broad-spectrum antibiotics is important, and is in any case sound practice. The early introduction of enteral feeding allows risk factors such as central lines and intravenous fat emulsions to be dispensed with. Attempts to prevent systemic candida infection by oral prophylaxis with antifungals have generally not been successful,[969,1073] although one report suggests some benefit in controlling an outbreak of infection.[228]

Treatment

Immediately the diagnosis has been made, or even when there is a high level of suspicion in a sick infant, treatment with intravenous amphotericin B should be started. Because of the toxicity of amphotericin, it is preferable to use the liposomal form of the drug, ambisone.[236,607] This should be started at a dose of 0.5 mg/kg/day, given as a single infusion over 6 hours, and increased to 1 mg/kg/day after 3 or 4 days.[403] Flucytosine acts synergistically with amphotericin,[841] and many authorities advocate their combined use in the initial treatment of fungal infection in the newborn. The dose of flucytosine is 100 mg/kg/day, given as a single infusion.[62] Flucytosine may depress the marrow and damage the liver, so that plasma levels should be monitored and weekly blood counts checked. Miconazole has been used successfully,[1039] but there are limited data on the newer agents, such as ketoconazole, fluconazole or itraconazole. Fluconazole has good urinary tract penetration, including tubular excretion, and is recommended for treatment of renal candidiasis[510] and for fungal infection resistant to conventional treatment.[337] Intrathecal treatment is not usually required for candidal meningitis, as amphotericin has good CSF penetration.[62] Central vascular catheters should be removed if systemic candidiasis is diagnosed or strongly suspected.[926,932] Fungal material in the renal tract, demonstrated by ultrasound, usually disappears with medical treatment, although surgery is sometimes required.[49,510]

Malsezzia species seem to be lipid dependent, and only occur if Intralipid is being given. Although amphotericin has been used in such patients, most cases resolve if the catheter is withdrawn and intravenous fat discontinued.

Prognosis

The reported mortality rate associated with systemic candidiasis in the newborn period ranges from 18%[647] to 50%.[60,327] A significant proportion of cases are first diagnosed at postmortem. The prognosis for candidal meningitis is very bleak.[156]

Other neonatal fungal infections

Data on other fungi which have become opportunistic

pathogens in ill VLBW babies are summarized in Table 43.20.

PARASITIC INFECTIONS

PNEUMOCYSTIS CARINII

Cases of *Pneumocystis carinii* pneumonia were common, mainly in premature babies, in postwar Europe.[368] They usually presented just outside the neonatal period with progressive dyspnoea and increasing oxygen requirements, and with symptomatic treatment the mortality rate was around 50%. *Pneumocystis carinii* infection in the developed world now occurs almost exclusively among babies with an underlying immunodeficiency state,[518] often in combination with CMV infection. Prenatal or perinatal transmission of HIV infection has not been reported to cause *Pneumocystis carinii* infection in the neonate (pp. 1176–1177). The presentation is usually insidious, with progressive respiratory distress and a diffusely hazy chest X-ray. The diagnosis requires a high level of clinical suspicion and acumen, and may be confirmed by direct microscopy of bronchial lavage material, although lung biopsy is much more likely to be successful. A PCR-based test is now a possibility.[978] Treatment is with high-dose co-trimoxazole or, if this is not successful, with pentamidine (4 mg/kg/day).

TRICHOMONAS VAGINALIS

This protozoon has occasionally been reported to cause vaginitis and urinary tract infections in the neonate.[20,124,229] Case reports suggest that rarely it might cause pneumonia.[504,675] If the organism is found on direct microscopy of a tracheal aspirate, or is isolated from any other infected site, treatment with metronidazole should be started.

MALARIA

Pregnancy is associated with an increased susceptibility to malaria and with more severe infection. Primigravidae in Africa[666] and Papua New Guinea[144] have a peak prevalence of parasitaemia between 9 and 16 weeks of pregnancy. Parasitaemia and parasite density are higher in primigravidae than in multigravidae, and both decline progressively with parity. Involvement of the placental tissue is common, but fetal infection is relatively uncommon in endemic areas where there are high rates of maternal immunity. The risk of fetal infection increases with both the density of maternal parasitaemia and the severity of involvement of the placenta.[879] Simultaneous maternal HIV infection also increases the risk of fetal infection.[1003]

Specific malaria antibody responses are not depressed during pregnancy. In the Gambia, the highest titres of specific malaria antibody were recorded in parasitized pregnant women.[666] Alterations of cell-mediated immune responses have been found, and these probably influence susceptibility to *Plasmodium falciparum* infection in pregnancy. The spleen plays a major role in the control of parasitaemia, with splenomegaly occurring in early pregnancy but regressing in the third trimester.[144]

Pathology

Malaria commonly involves the placenta, where microscopic examination shows large intervillous accumulations of parasitized erythrocytes together with monocytes containing ingested pigment. The trophoblastic basement membrane shows irregular thickening, with protrusion of syncytiotrophoblast into the basement membrane.[369] The resulting placental dysfunction leads to intrauterine growth retardation[293] and, in a recent study from Zambia, the mean birthweight of infants from infected mothers was 469 g lower than that of controls.[612] In a study from Sierra Leone the reduction in birthweight was reported as 265 g.[738] Neither of these studies found an increase in the rate of premature birth, but other studies have.[881,1004] For some unexplained reason heavy infections of the placenta with *P. falciparum* are more likely to occur in immune mothers, particularly primiparae.[369,667,881]

Congenital malaria

In endemic areas it is difficult to distinguish congenital malaria from malaria acquired soon after birth, because the lifecycle of the protozoon means that symptoms from congenital malaria may be delayed for weeks or even months. However, a recent study in Nigeria estimated that 75% of neonatal malaria was of congenital origin.[530] Infection may occur with *P. falciparum*, *P. vivax* and *P. malariae*, and there is no evidence that one of these organisms is more likely to cause a congenital infection than any of the others. Congenital malaria is much more likely to occur when the mother has a clinical attack of malaria during pregnancy than when she has a chronic subclinical infection. This is mainly due to protection from maternally derived IgG antibody, which may protect the fetus even when there is major placental invasion.

Malarial parasites find it harder to thrive in erythrocytes containing fetal haemoglobin.[808] This may explain the high gene frequencies of the thalassaemias and sickle cell anaemias in malaria-endemic areas.

The prevalence of malaria in pregnancy has recently been reported as 63% in Zambia in the rainy season[612] and 21% in Zaire,[779] despite some use of prophylaxis (see below) in both countries. The overall incidence of fetal parasitaemia in Zambia was 29%, and in Zaire 9%. A recent study in southwestern Nigeria reported a 23.7% prevalence of parasitaemia among newborn infants.[19]

Congenital malaria usually presents between 10 and 26 days of age, with the same symptoms as the acquired disease, namely fever, jaundice, severe anaemia and massive splenomegaly. Non-specific findings include poor feeding and failure to thrive, loose stools and diarrhoea. In the tropics, many infants with congenital malaria also suffer from other infections such as septicaemia and pneumonia.

An exclusive breast-milk diet has been shown to suppress malarial infection in infants and experimental animals by depriving the parasite of para-aminobenzoic acid, which is required for its growth in the erythrocyte.[604]

Treatment

Chloroquine is the drug of choice in the treatment of congenital malaria, particularly in regions of stable malaria. An initial dose of 10 mg/kg is followed by a similar dose 6 hours later. A further two doses of 5 mg/kg are given at 24 and 48 hours. The preferred route of administration is by mouth, as parenteral administration of chloroquine may be complicated by hypotension.

Quinine is preferred for treatment in regions of chloroquine-resistant *P. falciparum* malaria, such as in Papua New Guinea, East Africa, some areas of Central and West Africa, and in most regions of unstable (epidemic) malaria. Quinine, which binds plasmodial DNA, is administered in a dose of 10 mg/kg every 8 hours for 7 days by mouth, or by intravenous infusion in 30 ml of 5% dextrose over 8 hours. Cardiac arrythmias (prolonged QT interval and T-wave flattening), hypotension and hypoglycaemia may follow rapid intravenous infusion.

Chloroquine will eliminate sensitive strains of *P. falciparum*, *vivax*, *malariae* and *ovale*, but it will not prevent relapses of *P. vivax* and *P. ovale* infection. To ensure eradication of the exoerythrocytic forms of *P. vivax* and *P. ovale* a 14-day course of primaquine 0.5 mg/kg/day is given following the chloroquine. Primaquine should not be administered to infants with G6PD deficiency because of the danger of haemolysis.

Babies who require blood transfusions or exchange transfusion in malaria-endemic areas might be at risk of transfusion-acquired malaria. It is recommended that these infants receive a curative course of chloroquine following their transfusion. In areas now known to have chloroquine-resistant malaria, the treatment described above should be prescribed.

Antimalarial protection for pregnant women

It is prudent to protect all pregnant women in the tropics from malaria. A recent study from Malawi has estimated that such prevention could reduce the incidence of preventable low birthweight by more than 30%.[1004] In areas with no evidence of chloroquine resistance in *P. falciparum* parasites, proguanil 200 mg daily or chloroquine 300 mg weekly gives adequate protection. Folic acid supplement is advisable with proguanil. Where chloroquine resistance is commonplace (southeast Asia, India, Latin America, East and Central Africa), a combination of daily proguanil and weekly chloroquine is recommended. In parts of southeast Asia and Papua New Guinea, where chloroquine resistance is common and the combination of proguanil and chloroquine apparently ineffective, the current WHO recommendation for prophylaxis is chloroquine 300 mg and dapsone-pyrimethamine (Maloprim) one tablet weekly. However, agranulocytosis has been reported with maloprim in Europeans on malarial chemoprophylaxis,[366] and maloprim resistance has developed in strains of *P. falciparum* in Thailand. Fansidar (pyrimethamine with sulphadoxine) has been used successfully to protect against *P. falciparum* in Malawi.[956] Newer antimalarials such as mefloquine and halofantrine have been reserved for treatment, but in spite of restricted use some strains of *P. falciparum* in Thailand have become resistant to mefloquine. Visitors who leave a malarious country must remember to continue chemoprophylaxis for at least 4 weeks. Adequate protection against biting mosquitoes is recommended in addition to chemoprophylaxis. Sleeping under a mosquito net impregnated with permethrin 0.2 g/m^2 protects against mosquito bites even when there are holes in the net.

Malaria vaccine development

Naturally acquired immunity to malaria develops slowly and is incomplete. Evidence of this is the high (20–25%) parasitaemia rate in adults living in areas of high malarial endemicity. However, in spite of more than 15 years of research into malarial vaccines, no effective product has emerged. The development of an effective vaccine to prevent malaria will not be easy, even with the application of genetic engineering techniques.[202]

TRYPANOSOMIASIS

Trypanosomes are protozoa and produce two distinct diseases in man. African sleeping sickness is caused by *Trypanosoma (brucei) gambiense* and *T. (brucei) rhodesiense* and is transmitted by *Glossina* (tsetse) flies. Chagas' disease, found in Latin America, is caused by *Trypanosoma cruzi* and transmitted by large Triatomidae bugs.

African trypanosomiasis

Trypanosomiasis during pregnancy often leads to abortion, hydramnios and preterm delivery.[167] Congenital African trypanosomiasis has been reported with both

T. gambiense and *T. rhodesiense*, although most cases involve *T. gambiense*.[161,237,794] Fever and anaemia, with trypanosomes in the blood and/or cerebrospinal fluid of the infant in the first weeks of life, is the usual presentation of congenital infection. In congenital infection in endemic areas, trypanosomes are found in the CSF by the end of the first week even before they are detected in the blood. Increased rouleau formation in the blood should raise the suspicion of trypanosomiasis. IgM is usually high in the blood and low in the CSF during the neonatal period in infected infants. Lymphadenopathy is not a feature of the congenital disease, although it is characteristic of infection acquired after birth.

Management

Treatment is hazardous because highly toxic drugs such as suramin, an organic urea, and melarsoprol, an arsenical compound, have to be used. Irrespective of species, congenital trypanosomiasis is treated initially with three injections of suramin (5 mg, 10 mg and 20 mg/kg) given on alternate days. This is followed by intravenous melarsoprol 3.6% solution in three courses of 3 days each: 0.1 ml (0.36 mg) given on 3 consecutive days, 0.2 ml (0.72 mg) on 3 consecutive days, and finally 0.4 ml (1.44 mg) on 3 consecutive days.

Congenital Chagas' disease

Chagas' disease is a major public health problem in South and Central America, where more than 65 million people living in rural areas are exposed to infection by *Trypanosoma cruzi*. The frequency of congenital Chagas' disease is higher than suggested by the number of cases reported. Studies in Chile, Argentina and Brazil have shown that between 0.5 and 2% of low-birthweight infants have congenital Chagas' disease.[119]

Trypanosoma cruzi enters the fetal circulation through the placental trophoblast in acute, latent or chronic maternal disease. In most cases of transplacental infection the mother is asymptomatic.[519] The diseased placenta is large, and in cases in which the fetus is hydropic it is indistinguishable from the placentitis of syphilis or toxoplasmosis. Abortions occur when the placenta is massively diseased.[118] Congenital Chagas' disease has been observed to recur in subsequent pregnancies.

Most newborn infants with Chagas' disease are of low birthweight and may be either preterm or small for dates. Clinical manifestations of congenital infection may be obvious at birth or occur after a few months. Anaemia, jaundice, oedema, petechiae, hepatosplenomegaly, tremor and convulsions are common features. Anaemia may be so severe as to require blood transfusion. Dysphagia, with inflammatory infiltration of the oesophagus and absence of nerve cells of the myenteric plexus, interferes with feeding and has been described in a few cases. Prognosis of congenital infection depends upon the intensity of parasitaemia. Several organs, including the heart, oesophagus, brain, skin and skeletal muscle, show pathological changes, with inflammation, giant cells (a distinctive feature) and granulomas. Parasites have been found either in the muscle fibres or in the reticuloendothelial system. Long-term follow-up has shown a high frequency of neurological sequelae, such as mental retardation or behavioural and learning disabilities.

Diagnosis

Diagnosis of congenital Chagas' disease in the newborn is made on the presence of *Trypanosoma cruzi* amastigotes in the blood using a fresh thin blood smear or a thick drop preparation. An indirect immunofluorescence reaction detects IgM of fetal origin specific for *T. cruzi*.[997] High levels of fetal IgM and IgA have been observed on the first and 15th days after birth. A direct agglutination test using sera treated with 2-mercaptoethanol has also been introduced as a simple method of diagnosing congenital Chagas' disease.[1021] Recently ELISA has been used with success.

Management

No satisfactory treatment for Chagas' disease is currently available. Symptomatic treatment for heart failure may give temporary relief, but the prognosis remains gloomy because *T. cruzi* invades many organs and there is no satisfactory drug to eradicate it. Nifurtimox, a nitrofuran derivative, has been used in the acute phase of the disease with the elimination of parasitaemia and remission of clinical symptoms, but it is very toxic. Infants with congenital Chagas' disease may be treated with nifurtimox, 25 mg/kg daily for at least 3 months, together with phenobarbitone 5 mg/kg daily to prevent neurological side-effects of treatment and irritability.

AMOEBIASIS

Entamoeba histolytica, a unicellular protozoal parasite, has a global distribution and frequently causes intestinal disease in warm climates in communities with poor sanitation. Pregnant women may transmit the parasite to their newborn infants through faecal contamination at birth. The infant will usually present with bloody diarrhoea within a few days of birth. Amoebic proctocolitis and liver abscess have been reported.[47]

Metronidazole 50 mg/kg daily in three divided doses for 5–7 days is the treatment of choice for amoebiasis.

STRONGYLOIDES

A syndrome of respiratory distress, generalized pitting oedema and abdominal distension with ascites has been described in young infants from the age of 2 weeks in

Table 43.21 Rubella-associated defects following maternal rubella (without laboratory confirmation) by time of infection. (Reproduced with permission from Munroe et al[750])

Gestational week	1–2	3–4	5–6	7–8	9–10	11–12	13–14	15–16	17–18	19–20	>20	Total	
Number of cases	**4**	**27**	**30**	**60**	**44**	**45**	**40**	**20**	**15**	**8**	**23**	**316**	**%**
Heart defects	–	15	13	22	6	4	2	1	1	1	1	66	21
CNS defects	3	12	13	15	11	8	5	4	2	1	3	77	24
Eye defects	2	18	20	26	15	5	6	3	1	–	1	97	31
Deafness	2	21	22	48	38	35	31	16	9	5	6	233	74
No defects	–	1	1	5	2	9	6	3	5	3	16	51	16

the Gulf Province of Papua New Guinea.[1066] Other prominent features of this syndrome include severe hypoproteinaemia with low serum albumin and heavy infestation of the stool with a *Strongyloides* species similar to *S. fulleborni*.

Management of this unusual illness consists of plasma infusion and thiabendazole 50 mg/kg daily in two divided doses for 3 days. The infection responds readily to thiabendazole.

CONGENITAL INFECTIONS

CONGENITAL RUBELLA

The incidence of congenital rubella is now less than 2 cases per 100 000 births in countries with high rates of immunization, and a recent report from Western Australia reported an incidence of less than 2 cases per 10 000 births.[211] In Britain, 20–30 cases per annum were being notified to the congenital rubella surveillance programme in the mid-1980s.[987] This had approximately halved by the mid-1990s;[724] a majority of the mothers of affected babies were from the immigrant population.

Pathogenesis

The embryo or fetus becomes infected with rubella virus transplacentally during maternal viraemia. The placenta often sustains cellular and tissue damage in the process, and this may result in abortion, stillbirth or impaired fetal nutrition and oxygenation. In the embryo the virus can cause widespread tissue injury and, despite evoking a vigorous antibody response, persists in the tissues until delivery and for some time thereafter. The timing of maternal infection has a major influence on outcome. When it occurs in the first 12–16 weeks of pregnancy, even within days of conception,[305] there is virtually always embryonal or fetal infection. By the end of the second trimester only a third of infected women transfer infection to their fetus.[722] The risk of rubella-induced congenital abnormality also falls with advancing gestation. Malformations occur in 90% of infected infants whose mothers are infected in the first 2 months of pregnancy, but in only 50% of those infected in the third month and 20% of those infected in the fourth and fifth months.[305,721,817] Congenital rubella is rare after 20 weeks of gestation because of maturation of fetal immune mechanisms. The type of defect caused by congenital infection at different stages of pregnancy is shown in Table 43.21.

Secondary infection with rubella in pregnancy

The risk of reinfection with rubella after the natural illness is around 5%, but after immunization may be as high as 50%, as judged by serology.[517] The risk of fetal damage from reinfection is less than 5%.[159,802] There are, though, well-documented instances of fetal damage following secondary rubella infection in pregnancy.[107,235,572,804]

Clinical features[309] (Fig. 43.13)

The extended rubella syndrome presents as a sick baby with jaundice, petechiae and hepatosplenomegaly. On detailed examination eye and bone abnormalities may be found and a murmur heard. About one-third of affected babies are below the third centile for birthweight. A long-term follow-up of cases from the 1963–1965 epidemic reported ocular disease in 78%, sensorineural hearing loss in 66%, psychomotor retardation in 62%, cardiac abnormalities in 58% and mental retardation in 42%.[396]

Eye defects

Cataracts may be detected at birth and may affect the whole of the lens or be central. Glaucoma also occurs, and requires urgent treatment (p. 906). Microphthalmia is common. A fine pigmentary retinopathy (pepper-and-salt retinopathy) may be seen.

Deafness

This is usually sensorineural and bilateral. It is caused by inflammatory changes within the cochlea or the organ of Corti and, as its incidence increases throughout childhood, damage to these tissues is progressive. All babies suspected of congenital rubella should have auditory evoked responses checked as soon after delivery as possible.[1108]

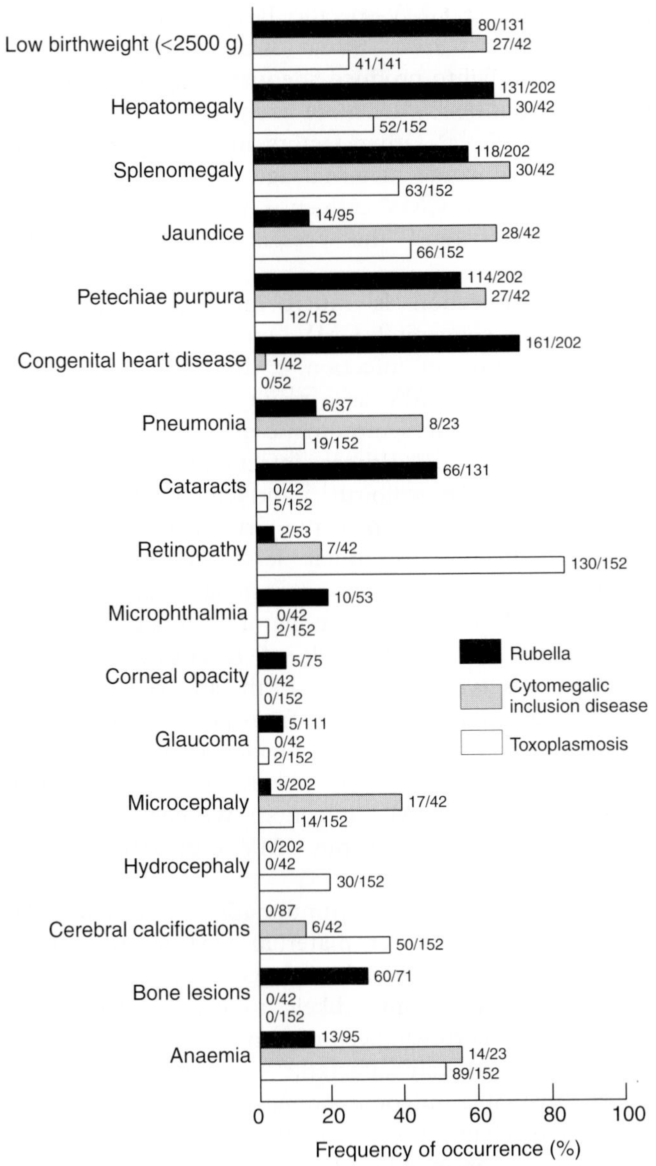

Fig. 43.13 Manifestations of symptomatic congenital rubella, CMV and toxoplasmosis. (Reproduced with permission from Overall and Glasgow[797])

Central nervous system

Microcephaly, delayed motor development, various types of cerebral palsy and mental retardation, which in some cases can be profound, are common in isolation or in combination.

Cardiovascular

Virus damage to the endothelium of large blood vessels results in a high incidence of patent ductus arteriosus and peripheral pulmonary artery stenosis.

Bone

In rubella osteitis there are irregular translucencies and an irregular trabecular pattern in the long bones. The radiological appearance is of a 'celery-stick'.

Liver

Hepatitis causing prolonged jaundice is common in the extended rubella syndrome (p. 1160).

Thrombocytopenia

This is found in most neonatal cases of rubella, though it is rarely found in cases presenting later in life.

Affected infants may present outside the neonatal period with neurological and eye defects, deafness and congenital heart disease. In infants presenting later with these conditions it may not be possible to establish the diagnosis of congenital rubella by antibody studies, but culturing the virus from, for example, the lens at a cataract operation strongly suggests prenatal infection. Infants presenting in the neonatal period, and those with a delayed presentation, may in later life develop a rubelliform rash, interstitial pneumonitis, hypogammaglobulinaemia, reduced cellular immunity, thyroid autoantibodies, thymic hypoplasia and diabetes mellitus.

Diagnosis

Congenital rubella is differentiated from the other organisms in Figure 43.13 by culturing the virus from a throat swab or urine, and by demonstrating rubella-specific IgM in plasma. There is no value in screening otherwise normal SFD babies for congenital rubella.[681] Whenever the diagnosis is established in Britain, the baby must be notified to the Congenital Rubella Surveillance Programme.

Treatment

No specific treatment is available. Some babies with the extended rubella syndrome are quite ill and need intensive care. Platelet transfusion is often required, as are phototherapy or exchange transfusion. Cataracts and glaucoma must be treated early, and hearing aids fitted if there is any evidence of deafness.

The infants are highly infectious during the first few months of life and are a hazard to female members of the nursing and medical staff. Appropriate precautions should be taken, the most important of which is to ensure that these personnel are rubella immune.

Prevention

In Britain in 1988, the immunization policy was changed from one in which only schoolgirls were given monovalent rubella vaccine, to one of giving children of both sexes the rubella vaccine as part of the MMR vaccine at 18 months of age. Such a policy has virtually eliminated rubella in the USA. However, because of the risk to the fetus from secondary infection, pregnant women should avoid people with rubella. Immunization during pregnancy is also best avoided, although there is no convincing evidence that it is teratogenic.[851]

Any woman who has a rubella contact or who develops a febrile, exanthematous illness in the first few months of pregnancy should have rubella serology checked as soon as possible, and again 2–3 weeks later. If both rubella IgM and IgG are present in the first sample, recent infection is very likely and termination of pregnancy should be offered. If there is a rising titre between the two samples the same applies. If the IgG level shows no rise and the IgM level is low, the diagnosis of recent infection remains in doubt and decision-making should reflect this uncertainty. Rubella RNA may be detected by PCR on tissue obtained by chorionic villus sampling early in the second trimester if further confirmation of fetal infection is required,[1027] although there is still limited experience with this technique.[1052] The measurement of IgM in fetal cord blood has been described.[528]

CONGENITAL CYTOMEGALOVIRUS

Epidemiology and incidence

CMV is the commonest cause of congenital infection, affecting 1–2% of infants worldwide,[1000] and probably the commonest cause of infection-related congenital abnormality.[57] The annual cost of treating the complications of congenital CMV in the USA has recently been put at $2 billion.[230] There are large international differences in incidence, and the estimated frequency in the UK is 0.3–0.4%.[853] In the UK, just over half of all women presenting at antenatal clinics are seropositive for CMV.[1035]

Transmission

Unlike rubella and toxoplasmosis, congenital acquisition of CMV occurs as a consequence of both recurrent and primary infection. The risk of transplacental transmission during reactivated infection is only around 2% (as opposed to as high as 25% during primary infection), but the high incidence of CMV seropositivity among pregnant women worldwide means that transplacental transmission during reactivated infection accounts for a high proportion of all congenitally acquired CMV infection. It has been estimated that 30–50% of congenital infections are due to reactivation of maternal virus,[853,999] and there are well-documented cases of women having two affected infants.[302,772,958]

Of pregnant women who develop a primary infection 10–25% will transmit the virus to the fetus, as assessed by the presence of CMV-specific IgM in cord blood, or positive cultures from throat swab or urine.[342,852,998] Women who fail to produce adequate amounts of CMV-neutralizing antibody are more likely to transmit the virus transplacentally.[128] Other factors increasing the risk of transmission include maternal age less than 20 years, a weak response to CMV antigen in the lymphocyte transformation test, and the presence of CMV in the urine.[342,355]

Primary infection is much more likely to cause symptomatic congenital CMV and long-term sequelae than reactivation of infection.[356] In one study of 125 infants acquiring CMV as a result of primary maternal infection, 18% were symptomatic at birth and 25% had long-term sequelae.[356] Primary infection may also increase the risk of abortion, stillbirth[430] and fetal hydrops.[324]

Congenital acquisition of the virus during reactivated maternal infection is much less likely to lead to problems.[591,998] although occasional fatalities are reported.[846] In one study[356] none of 64 infants acquiring congenital CMV as a result of reactivated maternal infection was symptomatic at birth, and only 8% developed later sequelae. Women from poor socioeconomic backgrounds who have a high incidence of seropositivity to CMV[187] are, therefore, less likely to have babies with serious congenital CMV infection. Women with AIDS may be more likely to transmit CMV to the fetus during a reactivation of infection.[958]

The observation that symptomatic congenital CMV is associated with lower maternal IgM levels at term than asymptomatic infection suggests that early congenital infection is more likely to cause symptomatic disease.[130,148] Surprisingly, only one member of a twin pair may be severely affected,[277] and there is even a report of variable outcome among infected quads.[951] An emerging mechanism of congenital CMV infection is that seen in the offspring of liver transplant patients.[610]

Clinical signs

Over 90% of infants with congenital CMV (culture and IgM positive) are asymptomatic in the neonatal period, though of slightly reduced birthweight.[96,853] In the minority who are symptomatic, severe multisystem disease may be present which is clinically similar to congenital rubella or toxoplasmosis (Fig. 43.13). CMV hepatitis can lead to intrahepatic and extrahepatic bile duct destruction[487,561] as well as haemochromatosis.[576] CMV infection of the fetal brain causes microcephaly, with calcification in periventricular areas where the infection has caused brain necrosis. These lesions are clearly seen on ultrasound scanning.[166] The pattern of CNS damage probably varies with the timing of injury, so that lissencephaly is a feature of early injury, and polymicrogyria of slightly later injury. When the gyral pattern is normal the injury has probably occurred in the third trimester of pregnancy.[69]

Hydrocephalus has been reported.[359,1044] Eye involvement, with chorioretinitis, cataract and blindness, occurs in 10–20% of cases presenting in the neonatal period. Pneumonitis may develop in the first few months after birth, even in infants who were initially asymptomatic.[853]

Diagnosis

Fetal infection can be confirmed by cordocentesis in the mid-second trimester.[706] In the absence of screening most cases of congenital CMV will go unrecognized. Screening on saliva has been reported.[58] If the baby develops the severe form of the disease with jaundice and purpura, the diagnosis is confirmed by culturing CMV from a throat swab or urine, and by demonstrating CMV-specific IgM in the infant's serum. CMV DNA can also be detected in the urine,[227,426,784,977] CSF[233,1037] and serum[761] by means of PCR. There is no need to screen asymptomatic SFD babies for congenital CMV.[681]

Treatment

CMV-infected infants excrete the virus for months or years, and should be segregated from potentially pregnant female members of staff. Whether there is a place for using anti-CMV chemotherapy in the neonatal period remains uncertain,[1138] although there are some encouraging case reports on the use of ganciclovir.[367] One recent report showed benefit from a regimen of ganciclovir 7.5 mg/kg twice daily for 2 weeks followed by 10 mg/kg three times weekly for 3 months.[773]

Prognosis

Most infants with congenital CMV who are asymptomatic in the neonatal period develop normally and have a normal IQ,[816] and this includes the majority of cases caused by reactivation of maternal infection. About 10% of asymptomatic infants become deaf later in life, and constitute a major group of children with congenital deafness.[356,503,819,853] A small percentage may have other neurological defects,[474] but this seems to be very rare except in those who are deaf.[15,210]

The mortality from symptomatic neonatal CMV infection is between 10%[131] and 30%,[554] although much higher if the baby is premature.[825] Of those without signs of CNS involvement in the neonatal period 30% will have neurological sequelae. If there is evidence of neurological involvement, including evidence of chorioretinitis, some 75% will have permanent neurological disability.[873] Intracerebral calcification shown by CT imaging is associated with a bad neurological outcome.[129]

Prevention

There is no successful CMV vaccine but there is a need to develop one,[11,431,1138] as reactivation of CMV in immune women rarely causes sequelae in the baby (see above). If primary CMV infection is suspected in pregnancy, prenatal diagnosis may be attempted by examination of amniotic fluid, fetal blood or chorionic tissue for specific IgM and the presence of the virus, by culture or PCR.[260,261,439,770] As yet, though, the diagnostic accuracy of available tests is relatively poor in early pregnancy.[261,770]

CONGENITAL TOXOPLASMOSIS

Toxoplasmosis is caused by the intracellular coccidian protozoan parasite *Toxoplasma gondii*. The definitive host, in which the organism completes its sexual cycle, is the cat. Toxoplasma organisms exist in three forms: the oocyst, which is excreted by the million in cat faeces; the tachyzoite, which is the active form and can migrate in tissues; and the cyst, which is a dormant form.

Incidence

In North America, Scandinavia and the UK the number of women developing toxoplasmosis during pregnancy is in the range 1–6 per 1000.[16,558,626,884,965] If only 5–10% of the babies of infected women develop symptomatic disease (see below) the incidence of significant congenital infection would be about 1:10 000, which was the incidence reported in Britain by Hall.[460] The risk is probably increased in infants of HIV-positive mothers, who are themselves at risk from toxoplasmosis.[726]

Pathogenesis

Humans become infected either by direct contamination from infected cats or their excreta, or as a result of toxoplasma entering the human food chain through the intermediate host of the domestic farm animal. If meat is not adequately cooked toxoplasma cysts are not destroyed and the organism is liberated during digestion. Contaminated vegetables used in salads are another important source. The world's largest reported outbreak of toxoplasmosis was in Canada in 1995, as a result of water contamination.[748]

Infected adults may remain asymptomatic or develop an influenza or glandular fever type of illness. Infection can reach the fetus at any stage of gestation, but whereas the risk of transplacental infection is greatest during the third trimester, first- and second-trimester infection is more likely to damage the fetus (Table 43.22). Fetal infection occurs only during primary maternal infection. During primary infection in pregnancy the overall risk of fetal infection is about 25%.[1076] However, the proportion of pregnant women who are seropositive for toxoplasmosis varies widely between populations, and is the major influence on the incidence of the congenital form

Table 43.22 Incidence of congenital toxoplasmosis by gestational age at maternal infection. (Reproduced with permission from Remington and Desmonts[884])

	Trimester of infection		
	1	2	3
Total women infected	126	246	128
SB or NND	6	5	0
Congenital toxoplasmosis			
Severe	7	6	0
Mild	1	13	8
Subclinical	3	49	68
No congenital infection	109 (86%)	173 (71%)	52 (41%)

Severe = overt clinical disease in neonatal period or subsequently;
mild = no clinical sequelae except chorioretinitis, IQ normal;
subclinical = serological evidence of infection only.
These data may underestimate the incidence since about two-thirds of these women were treated during pregnancy.

of the disease. In the UK about 30% of women are seropositive, and congenital infection occurs in fewer than 1 per 1000 infants. Of those fetuses infected, approximately 25% have subclinical disease affecting only the eyes, and only 5–10% develop widespread infection.[225,512,883]

Clinical features

The classic tetrad of congenital toxoplasmosis is hydrocephalus, epilepsy, cerebral calcification and chorioretinitis.[215] Congenital toxoplasmosis may also involve the reticuloendothelial system, liver, lungs and muscles, including the myocardium (Fig. 43.13). CNS infection causes extensive cortical and periventricular necrosis. This necrotic tissue may become calcified, and can then be seen as diffuse intrahemispheric calcification on ultrasound. Periventricular damage around the aqueduct of the midbrain may obstruct CSF flow and lead to congenital hydrocephalus. Patchy myelitis with ascending paralysis has been reported.[21]

About a third of congenitally infected infants, i.e. around 5–10% of all babies born to mothers infected during pregnancy (Table 43.22), have neonatal symptoms and about 25% of these die as a result. These babies are often small for dates and can present with the classic tetrad. Hydrocephalus may obstruct delivery or be noted at birth. Eye abnormalities may occur, including microphthalmia and cataract. Congenital toxoplasmosis can also present with the typical congenital infection syndrome of jaundice, hepatosplenomegaly and petechiae (Fig. 43.13).

Diagnosis

Diagnosis is by antibody assay although, for reasons that are not fully understood, tests for toxoplasma-specific IgM are often initially negative. If there is doubt about the serological diagnosis a repeat test can be performed 4 weeks later. Other approaches to distinguishing between active and passive antibody include measurement of IgG avidity[515] and measurement of specific IgE[1118] and specific IgA.[106,440,837] CSF analysis may show a lymphocytosis, raised protein and tachizoites in centrifuged CSF. Positive serological tests for toxoplasmosis on CSF confirm the diagnosis. The pattern of intracerebral calcification is very specific for toxoplasmosis, and is different from the periventricular calcification seen with congenital CMV.

Treatment

Unlike rubella and CMV, toxoplasmosis is a potentially treatable condition. If infection is diagnosed in pregnancy the woman should be treated with spiramycin to reduce the risk of fetal infection. The diagnosis of fetal infection can be established by PCR for toxoplasma DNA in amniotic fluid[513] at 20 weeks' gestation. If the diagnosis is confirmed at that stage termination of the pregnancy should be considered, although if antiparasitic therapy is given and serial fetal ultrasound scans are normal this may not be necessary.[102,697] Fetal infection occurring after the first trimester can be treated with pyrimethamine and sulphadiazine, but these drugs are contraindicated in the first trimester.

Whether or not there are clinical signs, the congenitally infected baby should be given spiramycin (100 mg/kg/day) for 4–6 weeks, alternating with 3 weeks of pyrimethamine (1 mg/kg/day) plus sulphadiazine (50 mg/kg/day). The drugs in this regimen are synergistic against toxoplasma[482] and should be continued for 1 year. Several novel and less toxic drugs are under evaluation.[383]

Prognosis

For seropositive infants with no intracranial calcification and, at most, chorioretinitis in the neonatal period (subclinical and mild cases in Table 43.22), the long-term prognosis is good, although new areas of chorioretinitis may appear in untreated patients until early adult life.[596] For those with neurological features or systemic disease the outlook without treatment is bleak. About a quarter die and most of the survivors are handicapped. With treatment as outlined above the outlook may be improved,[899] but there has been no controlled trial.

Prevention

Antenatal diagnosis can be achieved by regular serological testing of pregnant women. If this is combined with PCR to confirm fetal infection in mothers who seroconvert, antenatal treatment of the mother can be given or the pregnancy can be terminated (see above). In these ways,

Daffos et al[225] suggest that symptomatic congenital toxoplasmosis can be eliminated. Whether or not antenatal screening is justifiable in the UK is debatable,[496,818] but it is not currently recommended. The other purpose of screening would be to educate those at risk about avoidance measures. Women who have high-avidity specific IgG during the first trimester are most unlikely to have a primary infection and their fetuses are at low risk.[611]

Screening of newborn infants has been evaluated in both New England and Denmark, and there is no doubt that it can identify infected babies without overt clinical signs.[284,443,621] Infected infants were treated and appeared to have a better long-term outcome than expected, but there were no untreated controls, for obvious reasons.

CONGENITAL VARICELLA

Ninety-five per cent of women of childbearing age in the UK have had varicella in childhood and are immune. Varicella in pregnancy is therefore rare,[363,505] and prospective studies have shown it to be no more severe than at other times of life.[393] The incidence of varicella in pregnancy is around 5 cases per 10 000,[964] and among those who develop varicella in early pregnancy the risk of fetal damage is around 2%.[304,557,805,807,850,866]

VZV is teratogenic and infection during early pregnancy can cause chromosomal aberrations as well as a host of congenital structural defects, affecting the brain, eye, skeleton, gastrointestinal tract and renal tract.[557,678] Vocal cord paralysis has been reported.[874] A particular feature of congenital varicella is cutaneous scarring in a dermatomal distribution, which probably represents reactivation of the virus to cause zoster. Limb defects may be associated with severe cutaneous scarring.

Prevention

Pregnant women who are exposed to varicella, but are uncertain of their immune status, should have their antibody levels checked. Most will be found to be immune. Infection after 20 weeks of gestation will not cause congenital varicella (see above). With modern techniques of fetal imaging and blood sampling it is now possible to assess the fetus for congenital infection in time to terminate the pregnancy if indicated.

CONGENITAL EPSTEIN–BARR VIRUS INFECTION

Maternal infection with the EB virus is uncommon, as most women of childbearing age are immune.[347] Whether or not maternal EB infection can cause fetal malformations is still unclear, but rare cases have been described with low birthweight, abnormal facies, eye defects and congenital heart disease.[363]

CONGENITAL HERPES (see p. 1156)

CONGENITAL PARVOVIRUS B19 INFECTION

Human parvovirus B19 is best known as the cause of erythema infectiosum (fifth disease) in children. The virus has a predilection for rapidly dividing cells, including erythrocyte precursors, and can cause a haemolytic anaemia in the fetus,[1078] as well as haemolytic crises in the haemoglobinopathies. The incidence of parvovirus infection in pregnancy is in the range 0.3–3.7%.[378,413] In about 25–30% of these cases there is serological evidence of fetal infection[413,445] and in 1–2% of these the infection results in abortion, stillbirth or hydrops.[859,892] Between 10 and 25% of cases of non-immune hydrops are thought to be related to parvovirus.[737,1129] In a significant proportion of cases the hydrops resolves as the infection subsides,[858,1036] but in the remainder the prognosis seems to be very poor, with many infants dying. In some survivors the anaemia persists into childhood,[150] but in others lasts only for a few weeks.[1040] In the light of the significant spontaneous remission rate the benefits of prenatal diagnosis and fetal transfusion at cordocentesis are difficult to evaluate,[803,829] although some new data are encouraging.[326] Newer diagnostic techniques using PCR or ELISA may allow the prenatal diagnosis of parvovirus infection.[600,1128] It has recently been suggested that fetal parvovirus B19 infection can cause congenital structural abnormalities, by disrupting cell lines other than those involved in erythropoesis,[568] but more data are required to evaluate this possibility. Parvovirus can cause myocarditis,[991] cardiomyopathy,[72] and liver disease,[1098] and possible neonatal meningitis due to parvovirus has been reported.[1017]

CONGENITAL INFECTIONS IN THE DEVELOPING WORLD

The intrauterine infections described in industrialized countries also occur in developing countries. Congenital rubella probably occurs more frequently in the absence of routine immunization, but congenital CMV infection is relatively uncommon because most women of childbearing age in the developing world possess antibodies to CMV.[1023] *Toxoplasma gondii* infects the fetus in the pregnant mother who eats inadequately cooked infected meat. Syphilis and tuberculosis are rife in many cities in the developing world. Malaria is endemic throughout the tropics, hepatitis B virus infection is a major public health problem in southeast Asia, and trypanosomiasis is endemic in tropical Africa. Congenital infections caused by these agents are encountered, but in the cases of tuberculosis, malaria and trypanosomiasis congenital infections occur much less frequently than might be anticipated from the prevalence of these diseases in the population at large. As a cause of congenital abnormality

Table 43.23 Incidences of congenital infection among 1688 Malaysian infants with congenital abnormalities. (From Balasubramaniam et al[57])

Type of infection	Proportion of children affected (%)
CMV	11.4
Syphilis	4.0
Rubella	3.7
Toxoplasmosis	1.0

the intrauterine infections are important,[57] as shown by Table 43.23.

The clinical manifestations of congenital rubella, CMV, herpes simplex and toxoplasmosis in the tropics show no essential differences from those described in industrial countries, and will not be further considered in this section.

SYPHILIS

The classic sequence of events in untreated syphilis in a woman of childbearing age is one or more abortions followed by stillbirth[795] or the livebirth of an affected infant. Fetal infection occurs in 40–50% of women with primary syphilis. Reactive syphilis serology is a significant risk factor for perinatal mortality in developing countries,[125,660] where the prevalence of seropositivity among pregnant women may be as high as 10%.[427] In the USA the annual case rate for syphilis among women has been in the range 5–8 per 100 000 population during the past decade,[184] although there are wide regional variations and evidence of increasing prevalence in some large cities.[757a]

Clinical manifestations of congenital syphilis

Many infants appear normal at birth and only develop signs of the disease weeks, months or, occasionally, years later. Early manifestations of congenital syphilis resemble the lesions of secondary syphilis in adults, and later manifestations correspond more to tertiary syphilis.[322] Prematurity and low birthweight are commonly associated.[115,259]

Early-onset congenital syphilis is a serious life-threatening disease, often presenting with general constitutional disturbance such as anaemia, oedema, jaundice, failure to thrive and pyrexia, in the absence of the more typical mucocutaneous lesions and other local signs of the disease. Conversely the infant may initially show quite florid mucocutaneous lesions in the absence of significant constitutional disturbance.[92] Hepatomegaly is usual and splenomegaly and lymphadenopathy are common.

Skin eruptions are common but vary considerably both in character and in distribution.[928] Usually the rash is maculopapular, but circinate lesions occur and are among the most characteristic eruptions encountered. Involvement of the skin of the palms and the soles is usual and provides one of the typical localizing features of the rash of congenital syphilis. The palms and soles may become red, mottled and swollen, with superficial desquamation. A characteristic early sign is rhinitis, and ulceration of the nasal mucosa produces a profuse mucopurulent discharge which may be bloodstained and frequently causes excoriation around the nose and on the upper lip. Destruction of the nasal cartilage and bone will in time produce the flattened nasal bridge and 'saddle-nose' of congenital syphilis. Lesions at the mucocutaneous junctions of the mouth, nose, anus and vulva are common and produce moist fissuring and bleeding. Healing of deep fissures around the mouth leads to radiating scars called rhagades, one of the typical stigmata of congenital syphilis. Flat raised plaques with moist surfaces, called condylomata, may occur around the anus and female genitalia. Osteochondritis is a frequent and typical manifestation of the disease and may present as dactylitis, fracture or pseudoparalysis. Radiological examination of the bones is a most useful adjunct to the clinical diagnosis of congenital syphilis.[632] Radiological changes are usually multiple and widespread, and most easily evident around the wrists, elbows and knees (Fig. 43.14). Osteochondritis is manifest by widening and alteration in the

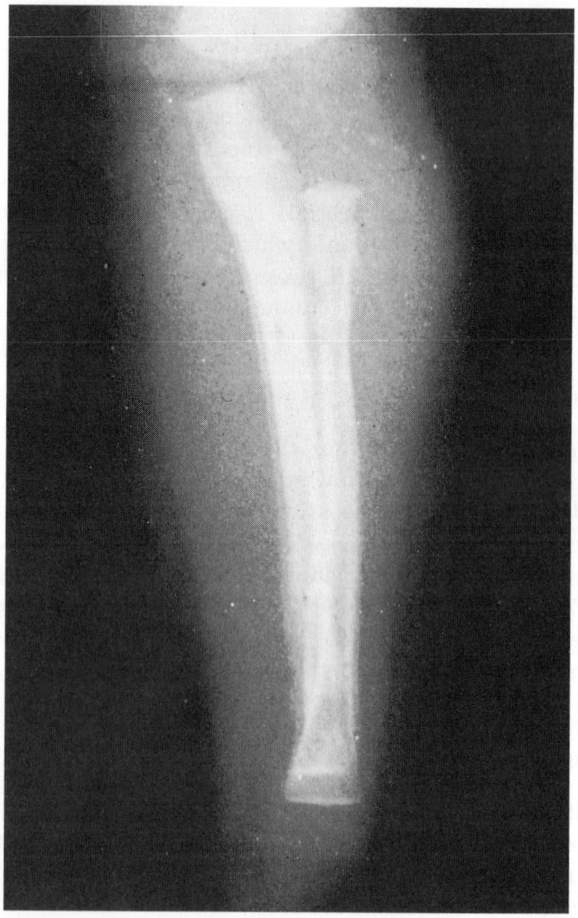

Fig. 43.14 Widespread periostitis of the radius and ulna in an infant with congenital syphilis.

density of the epiphyseal line and by irregular destructive lesions in the epiphyseal end of the metaphyses. Periostitis can be widespread in the bones of the limbs and may also involve the skull. The radiological signs of congenital syphilis may not be very evident in the immediate neonatal period, but become more obvious during the early months of life. They may show spontaneous regression after the sixth month.

Signs of meningitis may occur with congenital syphilis, as may evidence of hydrocephalus. Even when there is no clinical evidence of central nervous system involvement the CSF may be abnormal, although probably not often enough to justify routine lumbar puncture in asymptomatic at-risk infants.[83] The classic changes in the CSF are a moderate increase in cells, mainly lymphocytes, an increased protein, normal sugar levels and positive serological tests for syphilis.

Investigation and diagnosis

The diagnosis of congenital syphilis relies on awareness of the condition and a high index of clinical suspicion. Syphilis has a justifiable reputation as a great imitator, and this is certainly true of the congenital form of the disease. Diagnosis is based on the following approaches:

- Making the diagnosis of syphilis in the mother;
- Observing suspicious or diagnostic clinical features in the infant;
- Observing characteristic radiological features;
- Demonstrating spirochaetes in samples from suspicious lesions;
- Serological testing.

Making the diagnosis in the mother

All pregnant women in the UK undergo routine serological testing for syphilis at booking. In the tropics there might also be a case for screening by colposcopy.[631] False-positive results may occur in women previously infected with yaws (*Treponema pertenue*). Women who are seropositive for syphilis are twice as likely to be HIV-positive than those who are seronegative.[582]

Demonstrating spirochaetes in samples from suspicious lesions

Spirochaetes can sometimes be demonstrated in the placenta or umbilical cord, or in material aspirated from bullae or papules. In a recent study spirochaetes were identified in 89% of cords from babies born to mothers with untreated syphilis, using a combination of silver stains and immunofluorescence.[957]

Serological testing

Despite continuing improvements, serological tests for syphilis still lack sufficent diagnostic precision to give a confident answer to the question: Is this possibly infected but asymptomatic infant infected or not? Serological tests for syphilis are traditionally of two kinds, those aimed at detecting non-treponemal antibodies, such as those to cardiolipin (VDRL test), and those aimed at detecting antitreponemal antibodies (FTA and TPHA tests). Serological testing for syphilis in the newborn is problematic because IgG antibody is transferred across the placenta. In non-infected babies the VDRL test usually reverts to negative within 6 months, and the TPHA and FTA-ABS tests, based on IgG, within 1 year.[186] Persistence of positive tests beyond these times is usually considered diagnostic. Basing the tests on IgM antibodies is preferable because IgM does not cross the intact placenta.[634] Using modern tests based on detection of antitreponemal IgM (such as FTA-ABS IgM, IgM capture ELISA for *T. pallidum* and IgM immunoblotting), sensitivities between 70 and 83% and specificities between 97 and 100% have been reported.[950,1010] At the present time, however, an approach to diagnosis which combines epidemiological, clinical and serological information is advisable.

Treatment

An algorithm to guide the investigation and treatment of the baby at risk of congenital syphilis has been produced by the Centres for Disease Control in the USA. This is illustrated in Figure 43.15. Penicillin is the drug of choice in treatment, preferably aqueous penicillin G (benzylpenicillin) 50 000 units/kg (i.e. 30 mg/kg) intravenously, twice daily for 10 days. In circumstances where follow-up is unlikely or doubtful, and meningeal involvement has been excluded, long-acting benzathine penicillin 100 000 units/kg may be given in a single intramuscular dose, although published evidence on the efficacy of this approach is lacking.

HIV INFECTION AND AIDS[419]

The prevalence of HIV-positive women in the population varies enormously between communities. In the USA, HIV is now the commonest congenital infection and the seventh leading cause of death in the paediatric age group.[896] As of September 1996, a total of 7472 cases of AIDS in children had been reported in the USA, and the number of children infected annually (the vast majority in the perinatal period) was estimated to be between 1000 and 2000.[185] In urban centres in sub-Saharan Africa the prevalence in antenatal populations may be as high as 30%. Among European populations the prevalence of HIV positivity in antenatal populations is in the range 0.0002–0.26%.[532]

In the UK the prevalence of HIV positivity in the childbearing population remains relatively low, but is

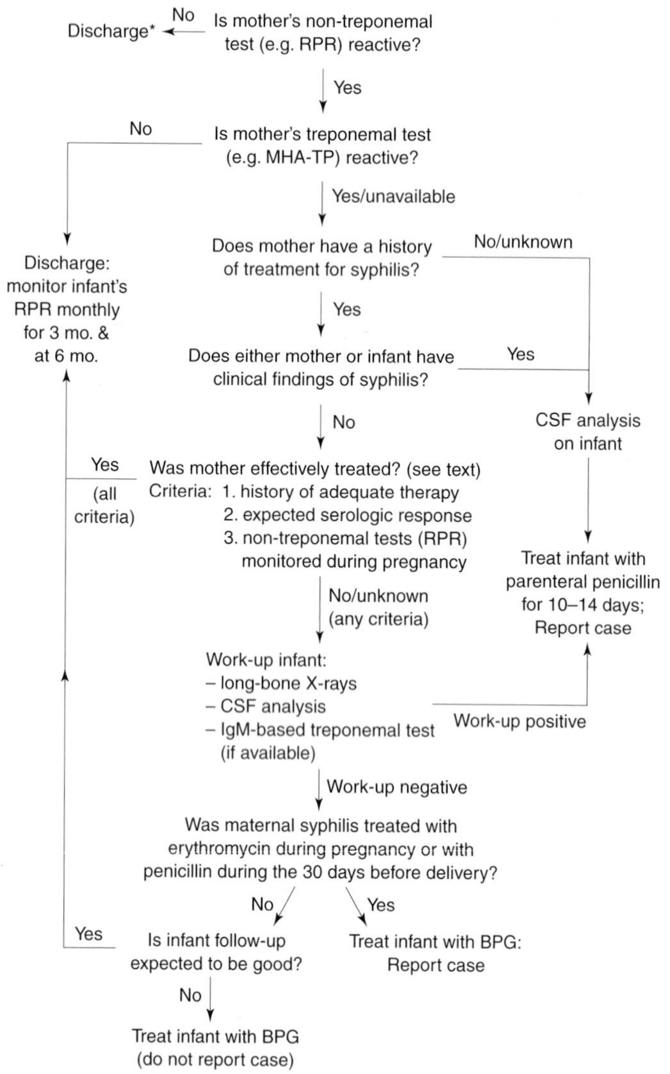

Fig. 43.15 Algorithm to aid the management of an infant at risk of congenital syphilis. The RPR non-treponemal test is equivalent to the VDRL test. Effective treatment of the mother is penicillin therapy, appropriate for the stage of syphilis in the mother, started at least 30 days before delivery. Reporting criteria are for the USA. BPG, benzathine penicillin. (From Zenker and Berman[1142] with permission)

rising. In the previous edition of this book it was reported that by January 1991 the Communicable Diseases Surveillance Centre had had only 21 notifications of congenital AIDS. The recently published British Paediatric Surveillance Unit 11th Annual Report,[914] however, records that by January 1997 a total of 1132 children had been born to HIV-infected women in the UK, of whom 420 had confirmed infection and 239 had developed AIDS. The report also states that there has been a substantial increase in the number of children in London requiring care because of HIV infection. In Yorkshire, between January 1990 and December 1996, the unlinked anonymous antenatal survey found 30 HIV-positive women out of a total of 249 623 women screened, a prevalence of 0.01%.

Transmission

Mother to infant

The exact mechanisms of vertical transmission of HIV remain unclear,[739] but recent evidence suggests that approximately one-third of vertically transmitted infections occur transplacentally and the other two-thirds during delivery.[154,275,909] An important mechanism of transmission may be materno-fetal transfusion during placental separation.[271]

The transmission rate varies between populations, from as high as 40% in parts of Africa[508,924] to as low as 13% in parts of Europe.[320,815] The risk of transmission is heightened if the mother is severely immunodeficient, as evidenced by a low CD4 lymphocyte count and the presence of immune complex-dissociated p24 antigenaemia, which may in turn be reflections of a high maternal viral load.[3,142,903] Preterm birth is associated with a higher transmission rate,[3] and in the European Collaborative Study[320] babies of less than 34 weeks' gestation were three times more likely to be infected than mature babies. How much of this effect is directly due to HIV status and how much to confounding factors, such as intravenous drug abuse, is unclear.[316] Membrane rupture more than 4 hours before delivery is associated with an increased rate of mother–infant transmission.[725]

Breast-feeding is an established mechanism for vertical transmission of HIV, increasing the risk by some 14% overall.[276] In women infected with HIV during lactation the risk of mother–infant transmission may be almost 30%.[801]

Blood transfusion

Hopefully this method of transmission has been virtually eliminated. The estimated risk in the USA is 1 in 153 000 transfusions[222] and in the UK 1 in 1 million.[34]

Nosocomial spread

Casual household transmission of HIV has been documented on very few occasions[878] and spread within a family is rare.[263,564] The risk of a non-breast-feeding HIV-positive mother infecting her baby during the activities of normal care must be extremely slight.[747]

Prevention of vertical transmission

In Europe 82% of cases of AIDS in childhood are the result of vertical transmission,[178] and so the prevention of AIDS in children now depends crucially on preventing perinatal transmission. There are many possible approaches to this, including health education, prevention of pregnancy and a combination of antenatal screening and termination of pregnancy. Once pregnancy in an HIV-positive woman has occurred, and is to continue, there is still the possibility of successful intervention. The antiretroviral drug zidovudine has recently been shown to reduce the risk of perinatal transmission from 25.5% (in the placebo group) to 8.3% (in the treated group).[212] In the treatment group, zidovudine was given during late pregnancy, during labour and to the baby for 6 weeks after birth. The women enrolled in the trial were all in an early stage of HIV infection and would not normally have been receiving antiviral therapy, and there is a danger in extrapolating the result of this study to other patient groups.[897,1048] However, there is a suggestion that this policy (implemented in the USA in 1994), combined with a policy of routine counselling and voluntary screening (implemented in the USA in 1995), may have resulted in a decline in the rate of perinatally acquired HIV infection.[185,1109] The cost-effectiveness of such a policy requires careful evaluation, and although there might be cost savings in developed countries, where the HIV prevalence rate among pregnant women is 5% or so,[699] the choice may be driven by different considerations in parts of the world where health-care resources are very limited.[690] The role of caesarean section in reducing perinatal transmission is still not completely clear,[1065] although evidence for benefit is mounting.[316,319]

Identifying the congenitally infected baby

Very occasionally an HIV-infected baby presents with features such as hepatosplenomegaly, lymphadenopathy or thrombocytopenia, but as a rule they are indistinguishable from normal babies on clinical grounds. Earlier reports of an associated dysmorphic syndrome have not been substantiated.[303,316,321,864]

Because maternal IgG to HIV crosses the placenta, all babies born to HIV-positive women are initially seropositive. Most non-infected children become seronegative by about 9 months of age, although some may remain so for up to twice as long.[32,318,731] A small number of at-risk but seronegative infants have evidence of infection on clinical or virological grounds.[133] Because of the prolonged persistence of maternal antibody, an infant can only be declared free from HIV if there are no stigmata of disease and he or she is free of antigen and antibody after 18 months of age.[317,332] Conversely, if antibody persists beyond this age it strongly suggests that the child is infected. Neonatal screening has been argued for in certain populations, and the pros and cons of this have been discussed.[273]

Currently, the best approach to the definitive diagnosis of neonatal HIV infection is by means of PCR for HIV proviral DNA,[716] and criteria have been proposed for the definition of prenatal versus intrapartum transmission of HIV based on the results of this and serology.[813] Feasibility studies have shown the potential for screening newborn populations using the 'Guthrie card'[208,224] (p. 380).

Cross-infection

HIV is not a highly contagious disease,[263,691,898] unless there is direct contact with the patient's body fluids. The number of hospital staff infected by contact with HIV-positive patients worldwide is in the region of 90–100 cases, and the estimated risk of acquiring infection from a single cutaneous exposure is 0.3% (95% CI 0.18–0.46%).[282] The labour ward, though, is one of the most bloody places in the hospital, and until all pregnant women are screened (and the pros and cons of this are much debated) labour ward staff are only likely to know the HIV status of women who have voluntarily agreed to testing, or who have already developed AIDS. For untested women in labour, a somewhat pejorative assessment of the risk can be made on the basis of their lifestyle and social circumstances, although a recent study has cast significant doubt on the validity of this approach.[488] In all situations, however, much greater care needs to be taken now than formerly, by all personnel, in dealing with blood or fomites potentially contaminated by HIV.[642] In the labour ward this includes the following:

- Avoid mouth-held mucus extractors.
- Do not give direct mouth-to-mouth resuscitation.
- Wear gloves during resuscitation and other risky procedures.
- Wear basic protective clothing (aprons, face masks, overshoes).
- Clean all equipment carefully after use, in particular the laryngoscope and suction apparatus.
- Postexposure prophylaxis with an antiretroviral drug is now a consideration, although precise guidelines are not yet available.[282]

For the baby of the known HIV-positive mother more stringent precautions should be instituted, including the use of full protective clothing.[642,913] Measures to reduce the risk of contaminating the baby with its mother's blood are also probably worth undertaking, such as avoiding airway suction where possible and avoiding crushing the umbilical cord with a clamp in the presence of maternal blood.[1064]

Breast-feeding and breast milk banking

The advice from both the American Academy of Pediatrics[209] and the Department of Health[35] is that HIV-positive mothers should not breast-feed. It is difficult to quibble with this advice in a western context. In the developing world breast-feeding should not be discouraged,[120,523,623,1057] as the decrease in mortality it affords outweighs the risk of acquiring HIV infection in this way. However, beyond about 6 months of age this risk/benefit balance may reverse,[298,753] and there is a significant late-postnatal rate of acquisition of HIV by babies of infected mothers of around 4%.[104]

Table 43.24 Congenital infections

Organism/disease	Symptoms	Treatment	Reference
Babesia microti	Fever, haemolytic anaemia	Clindamycin	Esernio Jenssen et al 1987 J. Padiatr. 110:570
Borrelia burgdorferi (Lyme disease)	Early neonatal death following birth asphyxia	Penicillin	Weber et al 1988 Ped. Inf. Dis. J. 7:286
Respiratory papillomatosis	Presents with loss of voice or airways obstruction post extubation Condylomata not always present in the mother	Laser coagulation if severe	Sedlacek et al 1989 Am. J. Obs. Gyn. 161:55 Chipps et al 1990 Ped. Pulmonol. 9:125

Immunization

Infants of HIV-positive mothers should be immunized at the normal times using DPT vaccine and substituting the Salk killed-polio vaccine for the Sabin oral polio vaccine. MMR should also be given, as the severity of these illnesses, especially measles, is increased in infants with AIDS. For measles immunization to be maximally effective in HIV-infected children it should be given between 6 and 12 months of age.[918] BCG can safely be given in the neonatal period to babies from at-risk groups, but should not be given beyond the neonatal period for fear of disseminated infection if immunodeficiency has developed.[105,781] Hepatitis B vaccination is relatively unsuccessful in babies who subsequently progress to AIDS, and failure to seroconvert may be a marker for a poor prognosis.[1143] Similarly, a single dose of polyvalent polysaccharide pneumococcal vaccine does not seem to confer lasting immunity in children with perinatally acquired HIV infection.[41]

Prognosis

A few babies with undoubted HIV infection seem to recover completely and become seronegative.[155,764,800,904] For the rest the prognosis is grim. In a recent large outcome study involving 2148 perinatally HIV-infected children, there was a 50% chance of developing AIDS, and a 25% chance of dying, by 5 years of age. The mean time from birth to developing AIDS was 4.8 years and the mean survival time was 9.4 years.[70] In a recent report from Australia the median duration of survival was 8 years.[179] The prognosis is worse in those born with hepatosplenomegaly or adenopathy, in those with a low proportion of CD4+ cells at birth, and in those who are culture or PCR positive.[700,839] HIV-infected infants also exhibit impaired physical growth and development relative to controls.[743,843] Respiratory infection and cor pulmonale are common findings even in the first year of life.[67] Early treatment, especially of *Pneumocystis carinii* pneumonia, may improve the outlook,[752] and in a recent study 65% were still alive at 5 years.[122] In general, those who present early or are born prematurely[3,404] do less well. The rapidity of virus growth in culture at 3 months of age has recently been shown to have considerable predictive value for outcome at 1 year.[372] Coinfection with CMV is associated with a more rapid disease progression.[267]

CONGENITAL HTLV I/II INFECTION

These viruses, the cause of T-cell lymphoma and adult T-cell leukaemia, are carried by a large number of women from Japan and the Caribbean. In Britain up to 5% of women in London of Afro-Caribbean descent are antibody positive.[221]

Although congenital infection with this virus is thought not to occur, some 40% of babies of infected women become infected, probably by breast milk.[778] Seropositive women should therefore be counselled not to breast-feed their babies, with the intention of significantly reducing the incidence of lymphatic malignancy in their babies 50 years later.[1038]

HUMAN PAPILLOMAVIRUS

Perinatal transmission of human papillomavirus and the persistence of viral DNA in infants is well described.[181,349,570,860,984] The risk of vertical transmission is in the region of 70%. Infected infants may present with minor hyperplastic growths of the oral mucosa or, rarely, with laryngeal papillomatosis. The human papillomavirus is associated with anogenital carcinoma in adults, although the potential seriousness of perinatal transmission has yet to be established.

OTHER CONGENITAL INFECTIONS

Various other organisms have been shown to cause congenital infection by direct transplacental or intrapartum spread. Some of these are listed in Table 43.24.

REFERENCES

1. Abbot G D 1972 Neonatal bacteriuria: a prospective study of 1460 infants. British Medical Journal i: 267–269
2. Ablow R C, Driscoll S G, Effmann E L et al 1976 A comparison of early onset group B streptococcal infection and the respiratory distress

syndrome of the newborn. New England Journal of Medicine 294: 65–70
3. Abrams E J, Matheson P B, Thomas P A et al 1995 Neonatal predictors of infection status and early death among 332 infants at risk of HIV-1 infection monitored prospectively from birth. New York City Perinatal HIV Transmission Collaborative Study Group. Pediatrics 96: 451–458
4. Abu-Osba Y K, Mallouh A A, Hann R W 1989 Incidence and causes of sepsis in glucose-6-phosphate dehydrogenase deficient newborn infants. Journal of Pediatrics 114: 748–752
5. Abzug M J, Keyserling H L, Lee M L, Levin M J, Rotbart H A 1995 Neonatal enterovirus infection: virology, serology, and effects of intravenous immune globulin. Clinical Infectious Diseases 20: 1201–1206
6. Abzug M J, Levin M J 1991 Neonatal adenovirus infection: four patients and review of the literature. Pediatrics 87: 890–896
7. Abzug M J, Levin M J, Rotbart H A 1993 Profile of enterovirus disease in the first two weeks of life. Pediatric Infectious Disease Journal 12: 820–824
8. Abzug M J, Loeffelholz M, Rotbart H A 1995 Diagnosis of neonatal enterovirus infection by polymerase chain reaction. Journal of Pediatrics 126: 447–450
9. Acunas B A, Peakman M, Liossis G et al 1994 Effect of fresh frozen plasma and gammaglobulin on humoral immunity in neonatal sepsis. Archives of Disease in Childhood 70: F182–F187
10. Adams W G, Kinney J S, Schuchat A et al 1993 Outbreak of early onset group B streptococcal sepsis. Pediatric Infectious Disease Journal 12: 565–570
11. Adler S P 1995 Immunoprophylaxis against cytomegalovirus disease. Scandinavian Journal of Infectious Diseases Suppl 99: 105–109
12. Adler S P, Chandrika T, Lawrence L, Baggett J 1983 Cytomegalovirus infection in neonates acquired by blood transfusions. Pediatric Infectious Disease Journal 2: 114–118
13. Adlerberth I, Carlsson B, de Man P et al 1991 Intestinal colonization with Enterobacteriaceae in Pakistani and Swedish hospital-delivered infants. Acta Paediatrica Scandinavica 80: 602–610
14. Agbayani M, Rosenfield W, Evans H, Salazar D, Jhaveri R, Braun J 1981 Evaluation of modified gowning procedures in a neonatal intensive care unit. American Journal of Diseases of Children 135: 650–652
15. Ahlfors K, Ivarsson S-A, Harris S et al 1984 Congenital cytomegalovirus infection and disease in Sweden and the relative importance of primary and secondary maternal infections. Scandinavian Journal of Infectious Diseases 16: 129–137
16. Ahlfors K, Börjeson M, Huldt G, Forsberg E 1989 Incidence of toxoplasmosis in pregnant women in the city of Malmo, Sweden. Scandinavian Journal of Infectious Diseases 21: 315–321
17. Airede A I 1992 Prolonged rupture of membranes and neonatal outcome in a developing country. Annals of Tropical Paediatrics 12: 283–288
18. Airede A I 1993 Neonatal bacterial meningitis in the middle belt of Nigeria. Developmental Medicine and Child Neurology 35: 424–430
19. Akindele J A, Sowunmi A, Abohweyere A E 1993 Congenital malaria in a hyperendemic area: a preliminary study. Annals of Tropical Paediatrics 13: 273–276
20. Al-Salihi F, Curran J P, Wang J-S 1974 Neonatal trichomonas vaginalis. Pediatrics 53: 196–200
21. Al Shahwan S, Rossi M L, al Thagafi M A 1996 Ascending paralysis due to myelitis in a newborn with congenital toxoplasmosis. Journal of Neurological Science 139: 156–159
22. Alary M, Joly J R, Moutquin J M et al 1994 Randomised comparison of amoxycillin and erythromycin in treatment of genital chlamydial infection in pregnancy. Lancet 344: 1461–1465
23. Allen K D, Ridgway E J, Parsons L A 1994 Hexachlorophane powder and neonatal staphylococcal infection. Journal of Hospital Infection 27: 29–33
24. Aly R, Shinefield H R, Litz C 1980 Teichoic acid in the binding of *Staphylococcus aureus* to nasal epithelial cells. Journal of Infectious Diseases 141: 463–467
25. Amato M, Huppi P, Imbach P, Llauto A, Burgi W 1995 Immunoglobulin subclass concentration in preterm infants treated prophylactically with different intravenous immunoglobins. American Journal of Perinatology 12: 306–309
26. American Academy of Pediatrics Committee on Infectious Diseases 1996 Reassessment of the indications for ribavarin therapy in respiratory syncytial virus infections. Pediatrics 97: 137–140
27. American Academy of Pediatrics Committee on Infectious Diseases and Committee on Fetus and Newborn 1997 Revised guidelines for prevention of early-onset group B streptococcal (GBS) infection. Pediatrics 99: 489–496
28. American Thoracic Society and the Centres for Disease Control 1986 Treatment of tuberculosis and tuberculous infection in adults and children. American Review of Respiratory Disease 134: 355–363
29. Anders B J, Lauer B A, Paisley J W 1981 Campylobacter gastroenteritis in neonates. American Journal of Diseases of Children 135: 900–902
30. Anderson D C, Hughes B J, Edwards M S, Buffone G J, Baker C J 1983 Impaired chemotaxigenesis by type III group B streptococci in neonatal sera: relationship to diminished concentration of specific anticapsular antibody and abnormalities of serum complement. Pediatric Research 17: 496–502
31. Anderson R D 1987 Herpes simplex virus infections of the neonatal respiratory tract. American Journal of Diseases of Children 141: 274–276
32. Andiman W A, Simpson J, Olson B 1990 Rate of transmission of human immunodeficiency virus type-1 from mother to child and short-term outcome of neonatal infection. American Journal of Diseases of Children 144: 758–766
33. Andre F E, Zuckerman A J 1994 Review: protective efficacy of hepatitis B vaccines in neonates. Journal of Medical Virology 44: 144–151
34. Anon 1987 Blood transfusion and AIDS. British Medical Journal 294: 192
35. Anon 1988 HIV infection, breast-feeding and human milk banking. Lancet ii: 143–144
36. Anyebuno M, Newman M 1995 Common causes of neonatal bacteraemia in Accra, Ghana. East African Medical Journal 72: 805–808
37. Arisoy E S, Arisoy A E, Dunne W M J 1994 Clinical significance of fungi isolated from cerebrospinal fluid in children. Pediatric Infectious Disease Journal 13: 128–133
38. Armer T, Clark P, Duff P, Saravanos K 1993 Rapid intrapartum detection of group B streptococcal colonization with an enzyme immunoassay. American Journal of Obstetrics and Gynecology 168: 39–43
39. Armitstead J, Kelly D, Walker-Smith J 1989 Evaluation of infant feeding in acute gastroenteritis. Journal of Pediatric Gastroenterology and Nutrition 8: 240–244
40. Armstrong D S, Menahem S 1993 Cardiac arrhythmias as a manifestation of acquired heart disease in association with paediatric respiratory syncitial virus infection. Journal of Paediatrics and Child Health 29: 309–311
41. Arpadi S M, Back S, O'Brien J et al 1994 Antibodies to pneumococcal capsular polysaccharides in children with human immunodeficiency virus infection given polyvalent pneumococcal vaccine. Journal of Pediatrics 125: 77–79
42. Asbury W H, Darsey E H, Rose W B, Murphy J E, Buffington D E, Capers C C 1993 Vancomycin pharmacokinetics in neonates and infants: a retrospective evaluation. Annals of Pharmacotherapy 27: 490–496
43. Ascher D P, Becker J A, Yoder B A et al 1993 Failure of intrapartum antibiotics to prevent culture-proved neonatal group B streptococcal sepsis. Journal of Perinatology 13: 212–216
44. Ashraf R N, Jalil F, Zaman S et al 1991 Breast feeding and protection against neonatal sepsis in a high risk population. Archives of Disease in Childhood 66: 488–490
45. Attenburrow A A, Barker C M 1985 Chlamydial pneumonia in the low birthweight neonate. Archives of Disease in Childhood 60: 1169–1172
46. Averbuch B, Mazor M, Shoham Vardi I et al 1995 Intra-uterine infection in women with preterm premature rupture of membranes: maternal and neonatal characteristics. European Journal of Obstetrics Gynecology and Reproductive Biology 62: 25–29
47. Axton J H M 1972 Amoebic protocolitis and liver abscess in a neonate. South African Medical Journal 46: 258–259
48. Ayliffe G A J, Coates D, Hoffman P N 1984 Chemical disinfection in hospitals. Public Health Laboratory Service, London
49. Babut J M, Coeurdacier P, Bawab F, Treguier C, Fremond B 1995

Urinary fungal bezoars in children–report of two cases. European Journal of Pediatric Surgery 5: 248–252
50. Baetz-Greenwalt B, Debaz B, Kumar M L 1988 Bladder fungus-ball: a reversible cause of neonatal obstructive uropathy. Pediatrics 81: 826–829
51. Bain J 1994 Midwifery: umbilical cord care in pre-term babies. Nursing Standard 8: 32–36
52. Baker C J, Edwards M S 1983 In: Remington J S, Klein J O (eds) Infectious diseases of the fetus and newborn infant. W B Saunders, Philadelphia, pp 820–881
53. Baker C J, Edwards M S 1990 Group B streptococcal infections. In: Remmington J S, Klein J O (eds) Infectious diseases of the fetus and newborn infant. W B Saunders, Philadelphia, 3rd edn, pp 742–811
54. Baker C J, Kasper D L 1976 Correlation of maternal antibody deficiency with susceptibility to neonatal group B streptococcal infection. New England Journal of Medicine 294: 753–756
55. Baker C J, Melish M E, Hall R T, Casto D T, Vasan U, Givner L B 1992 Intravenous immune globulin for the prevention of nosocomial infection in low birthweight neonates. New England Journal of Medicine 327: 213–219
56. Baker C N, Thornsberry C, Facklam R R 1981 Synergism killing kinetics and antimicrobial susceptibility of group A and B streptococci. Antimicrobial Agents and Chemotherapy 19: 716–725
57. Balasubramaniam V, Sinniah M, Tan D S, Redzwan G, Lo'man S G 1994 The role of cytomegalovirus (CMV) infection in congenital diseases in Malaysia. Medical Journal of Malaysia 49: 113–116
58. Balcarek K B, Warren W, Smith R J, Lyon M D, Pass R F 1993 Neonatal screening for congenital cytomegalovirus infection by detection of virus in saliva. Journal of Infectious Diseases 167: 1433–1436
59. Baley J E 1988 Neonatal sepsis: the potential for immunotherapy. Clinics in Perinatology 15: 755–771
60. Baley J E, Kliegman R M, Fanaroff A A 1984 Disseminated fungal infection in very low birthweight infants. Clinical manifestations and epidemiology. Pediatrics 73: 144–152
61. Baley J E, Kliegman R M, Boxerbaum B, Fanaroff A A 1986 Fungal colonization in the very low birthweight infant. Pediatrics 78: 225–232
62. Baley J E, Meyers C, Kliegman R M, Jacobs M R, Blumer J L 1990 Pharmacokinetic outcome of treatment and toxic effects of amphotericin B and 5 fluorocytosine in neonates. Journal of Pediatrics 116: 791–797
63. Baley J E, Silverman R A 1988 Systemic candidiasis: cutaneous manifestations in low birthweight infants. Pediatrics 82: 211–215
64. Balmer S E, Wharton B A 1989 Diet and fecal flora in the newborn: breast milk and infant formula. Archives of Disease in Childhood 64: 1672–1677
65. Balmer S E, Scott P H, Wharton B A 1989 Diet and fecal flora in the newborn: casein and whey proteins. Archives of Disease in Childhood 64: 1678–1684
66. Banks W W, Handler S D, Glade G B, Turner H D 1980 Neonatal submandibular sialadenitis. American Journal of Otolaryngology 1: 261–263
67. Bannerman C, Chitsike I 1995 Cor pulmonale in children with human immunodeficiency virus infection. Annals of Tropical Paediatrics 15: 129–134
68. Bansal V, Strauss A, Gyepes M, Kanchanapoom V 1993 Central line perforation associated with *Staphylococcus epidermidis* infection. Journal of Pediatric Surgery 28: 894–897
69. Barkovich A J, Lindan C E 1994 Congenital cytomegalovirus infection of the brain: imaging analysis and embryologic considerations. American Journal of Neuroradiology 15: 703–715
70. Barnhart H X, Caldwell M B, Thomas P et al 1996 Natural history of human immunodeficiency virus disease in perinatally infected children: an analysis from the Pediatric Spectrum of Disease Project. Pediatrics 97: 710–716
71. Barry DMJ, Reeve A W 1977 Increased incidence of Gram negative neonatal sepsis with intramuscular iron administration. Pediatrics 60: 908–912
72. Barton L L, Lax D, Shehab Z M, Keith J C 1997 Congenital cardiomyopathy associated with human parvovirus B19 infection. American Heart Journal 133: 131–133
73. Bates P R, Bailey A S, Wood D J 1993 Comparative epidemiology of rotavirus, subgenus F (types 40 and 41) adenovirus, and astrovirus in children. Journal of Medical Virology 39: 224–230
74. Bayston R 1985 Hydrocephalus shunt infections and their treatment. Journal of Antimicrobial Chemotherapy 15: 259–261
75. Beasley R P, Stevens C E, Shaio I-S, Meng H-C 1975 Evidence against breast feeding as a mechanism for vertical transmission of hepatitis B. Lancet ii: 740–741
76. Beasley R P, Lin C-C, Hwang L-Y, Chien C-S 1981 Hepatocellular carcinoma and hepatitis B virus; a prospective study of 22707 men in Taiwan. Lancet ii: 1129–1132
77. Beasley R P, Hwang L-Y, Lin C-C, Stevens C E, Wang K Y, Sim T S, Hsieh F J, Szmuness W 1981 Hepatitis B immunoglobulin (HBIG) efficacy in the interruption of perinatal transmission of hepatitis B carrier state. Lancet ii: 388–393
78. Beasley R P, Hwang L-Y, Lee G C-Y, Lan C-C, Roan C-H, Huang F-Y, Chen C-L 1983 Prevention of perinatally transmitted hepatitis B virus infections with hepatitis B immune globulin and hepatitis B vaccine. Lancet ii: 1099–1102
79. Beck Sague C M, Azimi P, Fonseca S N et al 1994 Bloodstream infections in neonatal intensive care unit patients: results of a multicenter study. Pediatric Infectious Disease Journal 13: 1110–1116
80. Becker J A, Ascher D P, Mendiola J et al 1993 False-negative urine latex particle agglutination testing in neonates with group B streptococcal bacteremia. A function of improper test implementation? Clinical Pediatrics (Philadelphia) 32: 467–471
81. Becroft D M O, Farmer K, Seddon R J et al 1971 Epidemic listeriosis in the newborn. British Medical Journal iii: 747–751
82. Bedford Russell A R, Graham Davies E, Ball S E, Gordon-Smith E 1995 Granulocyte colony stimulating factor treatment for neonatal neutropenia. Archives of Disease in Childhood 72: 53–54
83. Beeram M R, Chopde N, Dawood Y, Siriboe S, Abedin M 1996 Lumbar puncture in the evaluation of possible asymptomatic congenital syphilis in neonates. Journal of Pediatrics 128: 125–129
84. Beganovic N, Verloove-Vanhorick S P, Brand R, Ruys J H 1988 Total parenteral nutrition and sepsis. Archives of Disease in Childhood 63: 66–67
85. Beiter A, Lewis K, Pineda E F, Cherry J D 1993 Unrecognized maternal peripartum pertussis with subsequent fatal neonatal pertussis. Obstetrics and Gynecology 82: 691–693
86. Beitzke H 1935 Uber die angeborne tuberculose infektion Ergebnisse der Gesamten. Tuberkulose-Forschung 7: 1–30
87. Bell A H, Brown D, Halliday H L, McClure G, Reid M McC 1989 Meningitis in the newborn – a 14 year review. Archives of Disease in Childhood 64: 873–874
88. Bell T A, Stamm W E, Kuo C C, Wang S P, Holmes K K, Grayston J T 1994 Risk of perinatal transmission of *Chlamydia trachomatis* by mode of delivery. Journal of Infection 29: 165–169
89. Bell W E, McGuinness G A 1982 Suppurative central nervous system infections in the neonate. Seminars in Perinatology 6: 1–24
90. Ben David Y, Hallak M, Evans M I, Abramovici H 1995 Amnionitis and premature delivery with intact amniotic membranes involving *Staphylococcus aureus*. A case report. Journal of Reproductive Medicine 40: 485–486
91. Benador N, Mannhardt N, Schranz D et al 1990 Three cases of neonatal herpes simplex virus infection presenting as fulminant hepatitis. European Journal of Pediatrics 149: 555–559
92. Bennett M L, Lynn A W, Klein L E, Balkowiec K S 1997 Congenital syphilis: subtle presentation of fulminant disease. Journal of the American Academy of Dermatology 36: 351–354
93. Bennett O M, Namnyak S S 1992 Acute septic arthritis of the hip joint in infancy and childhood. Clinical Orthopedics 123–132
94. Benson J W T, Bodden S J, Tobin J O H 1979 Cytomegalovirus and blood transfusion in neonates. Archives of Disease in Childhood 54: 538–541
95. Bergdahl S, Ekengren K, Eriksson M 1985 Neonatal hematogenous osteomyelitis: risk factors for long term sequelae. Journal of Pediatric Orthopedics 5: 564–568
96. Berge P, Stagno S, Federer W et al 1990 Impact of asymptomatic congenital cytomegalovirus infection on size at birth and gestational duration. Pediatric Infectious Disease Journal 9: 170–175
97. Berger C, Uehlinger J, Ghelfi D, Blau N, Fanconi S 1995 Comparison of C-reactive protein and white blood cell count with differential in neonates at risk for septicaemia. European Journal of Pediatrics 154: 138–144
98. Bergström T, Larson H, Lincoln K, Winberg J 1972 Studies on

urinary tract infections in infancy and early childhood. Journal of Pediatrics 80: 858–866
99. Beri R, Lourwood D L 1997 Chemoprophylaxis for group B streptococcus transmission in neonates. Annals of Pharmacotherapy 31: 110–112
100. Berman P H, Banker B Q 1966 Neonatal meningitis: a clinical and pathological study of 29 cases. Pediatrics 38: 6–24
101. Berman S A, Balkany T J, Simmons M A 1978 Otitis media in the neonatal intensive care unit. Pediatrics 62: 198–201
102. Berrebi A, Kobuch W E, Bessieres M H et al 1994 Termination of pregnancy for maternal toxoplasmosis. Lancet 344: 36–39
103. Berry P J, Nagington J 1982 Fatal infection with echovirus 11. Archives of Disease in Childhood 57: 222–229
104. Bertolli J, St Louis M E, Simonds R J et al 1996 Estimating the timing of mother-to-child transmission of human immunodeficiency virus in a breast feeding population in Kinshasa, Zaire. Journal of Infectious Diseases 174: 722–726
105. Besnard M, Sauvion S, Offredo C 1993 Bacillus Calmette–Guerin infection after vaccination of human immunodeficiency virus-infected children. Pediatric Infectious Disease Journal 12: 993–997
106. Bessieres M H, Roques C, Berrebi A, Barre V, Cazaux M, Seguela J P 1992 IgA antibody response during acquired and congenital toxoplasmosis. Journal of Clinical Pathology 45: 605–608
107. Best J M, Banatvala J E, Morgan-Capner P, Miller E 1989 Fetal infection after maternal reinfection with rubella: criteria for defining reinfection. British Medical Journal 299: 773–775
108. Betremieux P, Chevrier S, Quindos G, Sullivan D, Polonelli L, Guiguen C 1994 Use of DNA fingerprinting and biotyping methods to study a *Candida albicans* outbreak in a neonatal intensive care unit. Pediatric Infectious Disease Journal 13: 899–905
109. Betremieux P, Donnio P Y, Pladys P 1995 Use of ribotyping to investigate tracheal colonisation by *Staphylococcus epidermidis* as a source of bacteremia in ventilated newborns. European Journal of Clinical Microbiology and Infectious Diseases 14: 342–346
110. Bhutta Z A 1996 Enterobacter sepsis in the newborn – a growing problem in Karachi. Journal of Hospital Infection 34: 211–216
111. Bhutta Z A, Naqvi S H, Muzaffar T, Farooqui B J 1991 Neonatal sepsis in Pakistan. Presentation and pathogens. Acta Paediatrica Scandinavica 80: 596–601
112. Bialkowska Hobrzanska H, Jaskot D, Hammerberg O 1993 Molecular characterization of the coagulase-negative staphylococcal surface flora of premature neonates. Journal of General Microbiology 139: 2939–2944
113. Bingen E, Denamur E, Lambert Zechovsky N et al 1992 Analysis of DNA restriction fragment length polymorphism extends the evidence for breast milk transmission in *Streptococcus agalactiae* late-onset neonatal infection. Journal of Infectious Diseases 165: 569–573
114. Bingen E H, Mariani Kurkdjian P, Lambert Zechovsky N Y et al 1992 Ribotyping provides efficient differentiation of nosocomial *Serratia marcescens* isolates in a pediatric hospital. Journal of Clinical Microbiology 30: 2088–2091
115. Bique Osman N, Folgosa E, Gonzalez C, Bergstrom S 1995 Low birth weight and genital infections. An incident case-reference study. Gynecologic and Obstetric Investigation 40: 183–189
116. Birenbaum H J, Glorioso L, Rosenberger C, Arshad C, Edwards K 1990 Gowning on a post-partum ward fails to decrease colonisation in the newborn infant. American Journal of Diseases of Children 144: 1031–1033
117. Bishop P N, Tullo A B, Killough R, Richmond S J 1991 An immune dot-blot test for the diagnosis of ocular infection with *Chlamydia trachomatis*. Eye 5: 305–308
118. Bittencourt A L 1969 The congenital transmission of Chagas disease as a cause of abortion. Gazette Medicina Bahia 69: 118–122
119. Bittencourt A L 1976 Congenital Chagas disease. American Journal of Diseases of Children 130: 97–103
120. Black R F 1996 Transmission of HIV-1 in the breast-feeding process. Journal of the American Diet Association 96: 267–274
121. Blanchard A, Hentschel J, Duffy L, Baldus K, Cassell G H 1993 Detection of *Ureaplasma urealyticum* by polymerase chain reaction in the urogenital tract of adults, in amniotic fluid, and in the respiratory tract of newborns. Clinical Infectious Diseases 17 Suppl 1: S148–153
122. Blanche S, Tardieu M, Duliege A-M et al 1990 Longitudinal study of 94 symptomatic infants with perinatally acquired immunodeficiency virus infection. American Journal of Diseases of Children 144: 1210–1215
123. Bland R D 1972 Otitis media in the first 6 weeks of life: diagnosis, bacteriology and management. Pediatrics 49: 187–197
124. Blattner R J 1967 Trichomonas vaginalis infection in a newborn infant. Journal of Pediatrics 71: 608–610
125. Bloland P, Slutsker L, Steketee R W, Wirima J J, Heymann D L, Breman J G 1996 Rates and risk factors for mortality during the first two years of life in rural Malawi. American Journal of Tropical Medicine and Hygiene 55: 82–86
126. Bonadio W A 1988 Polymicrobial bacteremia in children. American Journal of Diseases of Children 142: 1158–1160
127. Boo N Y, Chor C Y 1994 Six year trend of neonatal septicemia in a large Malaysian maternity hospital. Journal of Pediatrics and Child Health 30: 23–27
128. Boppana S B, Britt W J 1995 Antiviral antibody responses and intrauterine transmission after primary maternal cytomegalovirus infection. Journal of Infectious Diseases 171: 1115–1121
129. Boppana S B, Fowler K B, Vaid Y et al 1997 Neuroradiographic findings in the newborn period and long-term outcome in children with symptomatic congenital cytomegalovirus infection. Pediatrics 99: 409–414
130. Boppana S B, Pass R F, Britt W J 1993 Virus-specific antibody responses in mothers and their newborn infants with asymptomatic congenital cytomegalovirus infections. Journal of Infectious Diseases 167: 72–77
131. Boppana S B, Pass R F, Britt W J, Stagno S, Alford C A 1992 Symptomatic congenital cytomegalovirus infection: neonatal morbidity and mortality. Pediatric Infectious Disease Journal 11: 93–99
132. Borderon E, Desroches A, Tescher M, Bondeux D, Chillou C, Borderon J C 1994 Value of examination of the gastric aspirate for the diagnosis of neonatal infection. Biology of the Neonate 65: 353–366
133. Borkowsky W, Paul D, Bebenroth D 1987 Human immunodeficiency virus in infants negative for anti-HIV by enzyme-linked immunoassay. Lancet i: 1168–1171
134. Bortolussi R, Issekutz T B, Faulkner A 1986 Opsonization of *Listeria monocytogenes* type 4b by human adult and newborn sera. Infection and Immunity 52: 493–495
135. Botas C M, Kurlat I, Young S M, Sola A 1995 Disseminated candidal infections and intravenous hydrocortisone in preterm infants. Pediatrics 95: 883–887
136. Botet F, Cararach V, Sentis J 1994 Premature rupture of membranes in early pregnancy. Neonatal prognosis. Journal of Perinatal Medicine 22: 45–52
137. Boucher M, Yonekura M L 1986 Perinatal listeriosis (early onset): correlation of antenatal manifestations and neonatal outcome. Obstetrics and Gynecology 68: 593–597
138. Boxall J, Orme R L, Cruickshank J G 1982 Shared care and infection in a special care baby unit. Nursing Times 78: 1848–1850
139. Boyd M T, Jordan S W, Davis L E 1987 Fatal pneumonitis from congenital Echo 6 infection. Pediatric Infectious Disease Journal 6: 1138–1139
140. Boyer K M 1995 Neonatal group B streptococcal infections. Current Opinion in Pediatrics 7: 13–18
141. Boyer K M, Gotoff S P 1988 Antimicrobial prophylaxis of neonatal group B streptococcal sepsis. Clinics in Perinatology 15: 831–850
142. Boyer P J, Dillon M, Navaie M et al 1994 Factors predictive of maternal–fetal transmission of HIV-1. Preliminary analysis of zidovudine given during pregnancy and/or delivery. Journal of the American Medical Association 271: 1925–1930
143. Boyle R J, Chandler B D, Stonestreet B S, Oh W 1978 Early identification of sepsis in infants with RDS. Pediatrics 62: 744–750
144. Brabin B J, Brabin L R, Sapau J, Alpers M P, van der Kaay H J 1988 A longitudinal study of splenomegaly in pregnancy in a malaria endemic area in Papua New Guinea. Transactions of the Royal Society of Tropical Medicine 82: 677–682
145. Brans Y W, Ceballos R, Cassady G 1974 Umbilical catheters and hepatic abscesses. Pediatrics 53: 264–267
146. Bravo F J, Bourne N, Harrison C J et al 1996 Effect of antibody alone and combined with acyclovir on neonatal herpes simplex virus infection in guinea pigs. Journal of Infectious Diseases 173: 1–6
147. Brazin S A, Simkovich J W, Johnson W 1979 Herpes zoster during pregnancy. Obstetrics and Gynecology 53: 175–181
148. Britt W J, Vugler L G 1990 Antiviral antibody responses to mothers and their newborn infants with clinical and subclinical cytomegalovirus infection. Journal of Infectious Diseases 161: 214–219

149. Brook I 1995 Bacteroides infections in children. Journal of Medical Microbiology 43: 92–98
150. Brown K E, Green S W, Antunez de Mayolo J et al 1994 Congenital anaemia after transplacental B19 parvovirus infection. Lancet 343: 895–896
151. Brown Z A, Benedetti J, Ashley R et al 1991 Neonatal herpes simplex virus infection in relation to asymptomatic maternal infection at the time of labor. New England Journal of Medicine 324: 1247–1252
152. Brown Z A, Vontver L A, Benedetti J 1987 Effects on infants of a first episode of genital herpes during pregnancy. New England Journal of Medicine 317: 1246–1251
153. Brunell P A 1983 Fetal and neonatal varicella zoster infection. Seminars in Perinatology 7: 47–56
154. Bryson Y J, Lazuriaga K, Wara D W 1993 Proposed definition for in utero versus intrapartum transmission of HIV-1. New England Journal of Medicine 327: 1246–1247
155. Bryson Y J, Pang S, Wei M S 1995 Clearance of HIV infection in a perinatally infected infant. New England Journal of Medicine 332: 833–838
156. Buchs S 1985 Candida meningitis. A growing threat to premature and fullterm infants. Pediatric Infectious Disease Journal 4: 122–123
157. Buck C, Bundschu J, Gallati H, Bartmann P, Pohlandt F 1994 Interleukin-6: a sensitive parameter for the early diagnosis of neonatal bacterial infection. Pediatrics 93: 54–58
158. Buck C, Gallati H, Pohlandt F, Bartmann P 1994 Increased levels of tumor necrosis factor alpha (TNF-alpha) and interleukin 1 beta (IL-1 beta) in tracheal aspirates of newborns with pneumonia. Infection 22: 238–241
159. Burgess M A 1992 Rubella reinfection – what risk to the fetus? Medical Journal of Australia 156: 824–825
160. Burgner D 1994 Fresh frozen plasma and neonatal sepsis. Archives of Disease in Childhood 71: F233
161. Burke J, Bengoni K, Diantete N L 1974 Un cas de trypanosomiase africaine (*T. gambianse*) congenitale. Annales de la Société Belge de Médecine Tropicale (Bruxelles) 54: 1–4
162. Burman L G, Christensen P, Christensen K et al 1992 Prevention of excess neonatal morbidity associated with group B streptococci by vaginal chlorhexidine disinfection during labour. The Swedish Chlorhexidine Study Group. Lancet 340: 65–69
163. Burton D M, Seid A B, Kearns D B, Pransky S M 1993 Neonatal otitis media. An update. Archives of Otolaryngology Head and Neck Surgery 119: 672–675
164. Bussel J R 1990 Intravenous gammaglobulin in the prophylaxis of late sepsis in very-low-birthweight infants: preliminary results of a randomised, double-blind, placebo-controlled trial. Review of Infectious Disease 12S: 457–462
165. Butler K M, Baker C J 1988 Candida: an increasingly important pathogen in the nursery. Pediatric Clinics of North America 35: 543–563
166. Butt W, Mackay R J, de Crespigny L C, Murton L J, Roy R N 1984 Intracranial lesions of congenital cytomegalovirus infection detected by ultrasound scanning. Pediatrics 73: 611–614
167. Buyst H 1973 Pregnancy complications in Rhodesian sleeping sickness. East African Medical Journal 50: 19–21
168. Cabal L A, Siassi B, Cristofani C, Cabal C, Hodgman J E 1990 Cardiovascular changes in infants with β haemolytic streptococcus sepsis. Critical Care Medicine 18: 715–718
169. Cadnapaphornchai M, Faix R G 1992 Increased nosocomial infection in neutropenic low birth weight (2000 grams or less) infants of hypertensive mothers. Journal of Pediatrics 121: 956–961
170. Cairns P A, Wilson D C, McClure B G, Halliday H L, McReid M 1995 Percutaneous central venous catheter use in the very low birth weight neonate. European Journal of Pediatrics 154: 145–147
171. Cairo M S 1990 The use of granulocyte transfusion in neonatal sepsis. Transfusion Medical Review 4: 14–22
172. Cairo M S, Christensen R, Sender L S et al 1995 Results of a phase I/II trial of recombinant human granulocyte–macrophage colony-stimulating factor in very low birthweight neonates: significant induction of circulatory neutrophils, monocytes, platelets, and bone marrow neutrophils. Blood 86: 2509–2515
173. Cairo M S, Plunkett J M, Mauss D, van de Ven C 1990 Seven-day administration of recombinant human granulocyte colony-stimulating factor to newborn rats: modulation of neonatal neutrophilia, myelopoiesis, and group B streptococcus sepsis. Blood 76: 1788–1794
174. Cairo M S, Rucker R, Bennetts G A 1984 Improved survival of newborns receiving leukocyte transfusions for sepsis. Pediatrics 74: 887–892
175. Cairo M S, Suen Y, Knoppel E et al 1992 Decreased G-CSF and IL-3 production and gene expression from mononuclear cells of newborn infants. Pediatric Research 31: 574–578
176. Cairo M S, Worcester C C, Rucker R W et al 1992 Randomized trial of granulocyte transfusions versus intravenous immune globulin therapy for neonatal neutropenia and sepsis. Journal of Pediatrics 120: 281–285
177. Campbell J R 1996 Neonatal pneumonia. Seminars in Respiratory Infection 11: 155–162
178. Canosa C A 1994 Epidemiology of HIV infection in children in Europe. Acta Paediatrica Suppl 400: 8–14
179. Carlin J B, Langdon P, Hurley S F et al 1996 Health care and its costs for children with perinatally acquired HIV infection. Journal of Paediatrics and Child Health 32: 42–47
180. Casado Flores J, Valdivielso Serna A, Perez Jurado L et al 1991 Subclavian vein catheterization in critically ill children: analysis of 322 cannulations. Intensive Care Medicine 17: 350–354
181. Cason J, Kaye J N, Jewers R J et al 1995 Perinatal infection and persistence of human papillomavirus types 16 and 18 in infants. Journal of Medical Virology 47: 209–218
182. Cassell G H, Waites K B, Watson H L, Crouse D T, Harasawa R 1993 *Ureaplasma urealyticum* intrauterine infection: role in prematurity and disease in newborns. Clinical Microbiology Review 6: 69–87
182a. Cataldo F, Scotto E, De Gregoriio T 1983 Brucellosis in a five month old infant infected by mother. Acta Mediterranea Patologica Infettia et Tropica 62: 302–304
183. Cattermole HEJ, Rivers RPA 1987 Neonatal candida septicaemia, diagnosis on buffy smear. Archives of Disease in Childhood 62: 302–304
184. Centres for Disease Control and Prevention 1993 Special focus: surveillance for sexually transmitted diseases. Morbidity and Mortality Weekly Report 42: SS3
185. Centres for Disease Control and Prevention 1996 AIDS among children – United States, 1996. Morbidity and Mortality Weekly Report 45: 1005–1010
186. Chang S N, Chung K Y, Lee M G, Lee J B 1995 Seroreversion of the serological tests for syphilis in the newborns born to treated syphilitic mothers. Genitourinary Medicine 71: 68–70
187. Chandler S H, Alexander E R, Holmes K K 1985 Epidemiology of cytomegaloviral infections in a heterogeneous population of pregnant women. Journal of Infectious Diseases 152: 249–255
188. Chathas M K, Paton J B, Fisher D E 1990 Percutaneous central venous catheterization. Three years' experience in a neonatal intensive care unit. American Journal of Diseases of Children 144: 1246–1250
189. Chequer R S, Tharp B R, Dreimane D, Hahn J S, Clancy R R, Coen R W 1992 Prognostic value of EEG in neonatal meningitis: retrospective study of 29 infants. Pediatric Neurology 8: 417–422
190. Chidekel A S, Rosen C L, Bazzy A R 1997 Rhinovirus infection associated with serious lower respiratory illness in patients with bronchopulmonary dysplasia. Pediatric Infectious Disease Journal 16: 43–47
191. Chin K C, Fitzhardinge P M 1985 Sequelae of early onset group B hemolytic streptococcal neonatal meningitis. Journal of Pediatrics 106: 819–822
192. Chiou C C, Soong W J, Hwang B, Wu K G, Lee B H, Wang H C 1994 Congenital adenoviral infection. Pediatric Infectious Disease Journal 13: 664–665
193. Chiou C C, Wong T T, Lin H H et al 1994 Fungal infection of ventriculoperitoneal shunts in children. Clinical Infectious Diseases 19: 1049–1053
194. Chirico G, Rondini G, Plebani A, Chiara A, Massa M, Ugazio A G 1987 Intravenous gammaglobulin therapy for prophylaxis of infection in high risk neonates. Journal of Pediatrics 110: 437–442
195. Christensen G D, Simpson W A, Bisno A L 1982 Adherence of slime-producing strains of *Staphylococcus epidermidis* to smooth surfaces. Infection and Immunity 37: 318–322
196. Christensen R D, Hardman T, Thornton J, Hill H R 1989 A randomised, double-blind, placebo-controlled investigation of the safety of intravenous immune globulin administration to preterm neonates. Journal of Perinatology 9: 126–130

197. Christensen R D, Rothstein G, Anstall H B 1982 Granulocyte transfusions in neonates with bacterial infection, neutropenia and depletion of mature marrow neutrophils. Pediatrics 70: 1–6
198. Christie C, Hammond J, Reising S, Evans Patterson J 1994 Clinical and molecular epidemiology of enterococcal bacteremia in a pediatric teaching hospital. Journal of Pediatrics 125: 392–399
199. Christie CDC, Baltimore R S 1989 Pertussis in neonates. American Journal of Diseases of Children 143: 1199–1202
200. Chrystie I L, Totterdell B M, Banatvala J E 1978 Asymptomatic endemic rotavirus infections in the newborn. Lancet i: 1176–1178
201. Chuang E, Maller E S, Hoffman M A, Hodinka R L, Altschuler S M 1993 Successful treatment of fulminant echovirus 11 infection in a neonate by orthotopic liver transplantation. Journal of Pediatric Gastroenterology and Nutrition 17: 211–214
202. Chulay J D 1989 Development of sporozoite vaccines for malaria. Transactions of the Royal Society of Tropical Medicine and Hygiene 83 (suppl.) (Malaria and Babesiosis): 61–66
203. Chun C S, Brady L J, Boyle M D, Dillon H C, Ayoub E M 1991 Group B Streptococcal C protein-associated antigens: association with neonatal sepsis. Journal of Infectious Diseases 163: 786–791
204. Churgay C A, Smith M A, Blok B 1994 Maternal fever during labor – what does it mean? Journal of the American Board of Family Practice 7: 14–24
205. Cimolai N, Roscoe D L 1995 Contemporary context for early-onset group B streptococcal sepsis of the newborn. American Journal of Perinatology 12: 46–49
206. Clapp D W, Kliegman R M, Baley J E et al 1989 Use of intravenously administered immune globulin to prevent nosocomial sepsis in low birthweight infants: report of a pilot study. Journal of Pediatrics 115: 973–978
207. Cloney D L, Donowitz L G 1986 Overgown use for infection control in nurseries and neonatal intensive care units. American Journal of Diseases of Children 140: 680–883
208. Comeau A M, Hsu H W, Schwerzler M et al 1993 Identifying human immunodeficiency virus infection at birth: application of polymerase chain reaction to Guthrie cards. Journal of Pediatrics 123: 252–258
209. Committee on Pediatric AIDS 1995 Human milk, breastfeeding and transmission of human immunodeficiency virus in the United States. Pediatrics 96: 977–979
210. Conboy T J, Pass R F, Stagno S et al 1986 Intellectual development in school aged children with asymptomatic congenital cytomegalovirus infection. Pediatrics 77: 801–806
211. Condon R J, Bower C 1993 Rubella vaccination and congenital rubella syndrome in Western Australia. Medical Journal of Australia 158: 379–382
212. Connor E M, Sperling R S, Gelber R 1994 Reduction of maternal–infant transmission of human immunodeficiency virus type 1 with zidovudine treatment. New England Journal of Medicine 331: 1173–1180
213. Conway S P, Dear P R F, Smith I 1985 Immunoglobulin profile of the preterm baby. Archives of Disease in Childhood 60: 208–212
214. Conway S P, Ng P C, Howell D, Macdain B, Gooi H C 1990 Prophylactic immunoglobulin in preterm infants: a controlled trial. Vox Sanguinis 59: 6–11
215. Cook G C 1990 *Toxoplasma gondii* infection. A potential danger to the unborn fetus and AIDS sufferer. Quarterly Journal of Medicine 74: 3–19
216. Cordero L, Ayers L W, Davis K 1997 Neonatal airway colonization with Gram-negative bacilli: association with severity of bronchopulmonary dysplasia. Pediatric Infectious Disease Journal 16: 18–23
217. Corey L, Whitley R J, Stone E F, Mohan K 1988 Difference between herpes simplex type I and type II neonatal encephalitis in neurological outcome. Lancet i: 1–4
218. Correa A G, Baker C J, Schutze G E, Edwards M S 1994 Immunoglobulin G enhances C3 degradation of coagulase-negative staphylococci. Infection and Immunity 62: 2362–2366
219. Covert R F, Schreiber M D 1993 Three different strains of heat-killed group B beta-hemolytic streptococcus cause different pulmonary and systemic hemodynamic responses in conscious neonatal lambs. Pediatric Research 33: 373–379
220. Crain E F, Gershel J C 1988 Which febrile infants younger than 2 weeks of age are likely to have sepsis? Pediatric Infectious Disease Journal 7: 561–564
221. Cruickshank J K, Richardson J H, Morgan O St C et al 1990 Screening for prolonged incubation of HTLV I infection in British and Jamaican relatives of British patients with tropical spastic paraperesis. British Medical Journal 300: 300–304
222. Cumming P D, Wallace E L, Schorr J B, Dodd R Y 1989 Exposure of patients to human immunodeficiency virus through the transfusion of blood components that test antibody negative. New England Journal of Medicine 321: 941–946
223. Cushing A H 1985 Omphalitis: a review. Pediatric Infectious Disease Journal 4: 282–285
224. Dadswell J V, Dowding B, Fletcher M, Pinney G J, Sellwood J, Williams D L 1992 A pilot study of dried blood spot testing for HIV antibody in neonates. Communicable Disease Reports, CDR Reviews 1992; 2: R126–7
225. Daffos F, Forestier F, Capella-Pavlovsky M et al 1988 Prenatal management of 746 pregnancies at risk from congenital toxoplasmosis. New England Journal of Medicine 318: 271–275
226. Dahlquist G, Frisk G, Ivarsson S A, Svanberg L, Forsgren M, Diderholm H 1995 Indications that maternal coxsackie B virus infection during pregnancy is a risk factor for childhood-onset IDDM. Diabetologia 38: 1371–1373
227. Daiminger A, Schalasta G, Betzl D, Enders G 1994 Detection of human cytomegalovirus in urine samples by cell culture, early antigen assay and polymerase chain reaction. Infection 22: 24–28
228. Damjanovic V, Connolly C M, van Saene H K et al 1993 Selective decontamination with nystatin for control of a Candida outbreak in a neonatal intensive care unit. Journal of Hospital Infection 24: 245–259
229. Danesh I S, Stephen J M, Gorbach J 1995 Neonatal *Trichomonas vaginalis* infection. Journal of Emergency Medicine 13: 51–54
230. Daniel Y, Gull I, Peyser M R, Lessing J B 1995 Congenital cytomegalovirus infection. European Journal of Obstetrics Gynecology and Reproductive Biology 63: 7–16
231. Dankner W M, Spector S A 1986 Recurrent herpes simplex in a neonate. Pediatric Infectious Disease Journal 5: 582–586
232. Dannevig L, Straume B, Melby K 1992 Ophthalmia neonatorum in northern Norway. I: Epidemiology and risk factors. Acta Ophthalmologica (Copenhagen) 70: 14–18
233. Darin N, Bergstrom T, Fast A, Kyllerman M 1994 Clinical, serological and PCR evidence of cytomegalovirus infection in the central nervous system in infancy and childhood. Neuropediatrics 25: 316–322
234. Darville T, Tabor D, Simpson K, Jacobs R F 1994 Intravenous immunoglobulin modulates human mononuclear phagocyte tumor necrosis factor-alpha production in vitro. Pediatric Research 35: 397–403
235. Das B D, Lakhani P, Kurtz J B et al 1990 Congenital rubella after previous maternal immunity. Archives of Disease in Childhood 65: 545–546
236. da Silva L P, Amaral J M, Ferreia N C 1993 Which is the most appropriate dosage of liposomal amphotericin B for the treatment of fungal infections in infants of very low birthweight? Pediatrics 91: 1217–1218
237. Daveloose P 1972 Un cas de trypanosomiase africaine congenitale. Annales de la Société Belge Médecine Tropicale (Bruxelles) 52: 63
238. Davies P A, Aherne W 1962 Congenital pneumonia. Archives of Disease in Childhood 37: 598–602
239. Dear P R F, McLain B I 1987 Establishment of an intermediate care ward for babies and mothers. Archives of Disease in Childhood 62: 597–601
240. Dearlove J, Latham P, Dearlove B, Pearl K, Thomson A, Lewis I G 1983 Clinical range of neonatal rotavirus gastroenteritis. British Medical Journal 286: 1473–1475
241. de Cates C R, Gray J, Roberton N R C, Walker J 1994 Acquisition of cytomegalovirus infection by premature neonates. Journal of Infection 28: 25–30
242. deCates C R, Roberton N R C, Walker J R 1988 Fatal acquired cytomegalovirus in a neonate with maternal antibodies. Journal of Infection 17: 235–240
243. de Champs C, Franchineau P, Gourgand J M, Loriette Y, Gaulme J, Sirot J 1994 Clinical and bacteriological survey after change in aminoglycoside treatment to control an epidemic of *Enterobacter cloacae*. Journal of Hospital Infection 28: 219–229
244. de Louvois J 1994 Acute bacterial meningitis in the newborn. Journal of Antimicrobial Chemotherapy 34 Suppl A: 61–73

245. de Louvois J, Blackbourn N, Hurley R, Harvey D 1991 Infantile meningitis in England and Wales. Archives of Disease in Childhood 66: 603–607
246. de Toledo A R, Chandler J W 1992 Conjunctivitis of the newborn. Infectious Diseases Clinics of North America 6: 807–813
247. Delage G, Remy Prince S, Montplaisir S 1993 Combined active–passive immunization against the hepatitis B virus: five-year follow-up of children born to hepatitis B surface antigen-positive mothers. Pediatric Infectious Disease Journal 12: 126–130
248. Department of Health 1989 Health building note No. 21. Maternity Department. HMSO, London
249. Derso A, Boxall E H, Tarlow M J, Flewett T H 1978 Transmission of HBsAg from mother to infant in four ethnic groups. British Medical Journal i: 949–952
250. deSa D J 1983 Mucosal metaplasia and chronic inflammation in the middle ear of infants receiving intensive care in the neonatal period. Archives of Disease in Childhood 58: 24–28
251. Dewey K G, Heinig M J, Nommsen Rivers L A 1995 Differences in morbidity between breast-fed and formula-fed infants. Journal of Pediatrics 126: 696–702
252. Didato M A, Gioeli R, Prisolisi A 1988 The use of intravenous gamma-globulin for prevention of sepsis in preterm infants. Helvetica Paediatrica Acta 43: 283–294
253. Ding L, Zhang M, Wang Y, Zhou S, Kong W, Smego R A J 1993 A 9-year follow-up study of the immunogenicity and long-term efficacy of plasma-derived hepatitis B vaccine in high-risk Chinese neonates. Clinical Infectious Diseases 17: 475–479
254. Dinsmoor M J, Ramamurthy R S, Gibbs R S 1989 Transmission of genital mycoplasmas from mother to neonate in women with prolonged membrane rupture. Pediatric Infectious Disease Journal 8: 483–487
255. Dirschl D R 1994 Acute pyogenic osteomyelitis in children. Orthopedic Review 23: 305–312
256. Dobson S R, Baker C J 1990 Enterococcal sepsis in neonates: features by age at onset and occurrence of focal infection. Pediatrics 85: 165–171
257. Dobson S R, Isaacs D, Wilkinson A R, Hope P L 1992 Reduced use of surface cultures for suspected neonatal sepsis and surveillance. Archives of Disease in Childhood 67: 44–47
258. Domula M, Bykowska K, Wegrzynowicz A, Lopaciuk S, Weissbach G, Kopec M 1985 Plasma fibronectin concentrations in healthy and septic infants. European Journal of Pediatrics 144: 49–52
259. Donders G G, Desmyter J, De Wet D H, Van Assche F A 1993 The association of gonorrhoea and syphilis with premature birth and low birthweight. Genitourinaty Medicine 69: 98–101
260. Dong Z W, Yan C, Yi W, Cui Y Q 1994 Detection of congenital cytomegalovirus infection by using chorionic villi of the early pregnancy and polymerase chain reaction. International Journal of Gynaecology and Obstetrics 44: 229–231
261. Donner C, Liesnard C, Brancart F, Rodesch F 1994 Accuracy of amniotic fluid testing before 21 weeks' gestation in prenatal diagnosis of congenital cytomegalovirus infection. Prenatal Diagnosis 14: 1055–1059
262. Donnerstein R L, Berg R A, Shehab Z, Ovadia M 1994 Complex atrial tachycardias and respiratory syncytial virus infections in infants. Journal of Pediatrics 125: 23–28
263. Donowitz L G 1989 Practical infection control for human immunodeficiency virus infection in children. Pediatric Infectious Disease Journal 8: 133–135
264. Doron M W, Makhlouf R A, Katz V L, Lawson E E, Stiles A D 1994 Increased incidence of sepsis at birth in neutropenic infants of mothers with preeclampsia. Journal of Pediatrics 125: 452–458
265. Douglas J, Schmidt O, Corey L 1983 Acquisition of neonatal HSV I infection from a paternal source contact. Journal of Pediatrics 103: 908–910
266. Douglass B H, Keenan A L, Purohit D M 1996 Bacterial and fungal infection in neonates undergoing venoarterial extracorporeal membrane oxygenation: an analysis of the registry data of the extracorporeal life support organization. Artificial Organs 20: 202–208
267. Doyle M, Atkins J T, Rivera Matos I R 1996 Congenital cytomegalovirus infection in infants infected with human immunodeficiency virus type 1. Pediatric Infectious Disease Journal 15: 1102–1106
268. Drew J H, Acton C M 1976 Radiological findings in newborn infants with urinary tract infection. Archives of Disease in Childhood 51: 628–631
269. Drews M B, Ludwig A C, Leititis J U, Daschner F D 1995 Low birth weight and nosocomial infection of neonates in a neonatal intensive care unit. Journal of Hospital Infection 30: 65–72
270. Druyts Voets E, Van Renterghem L, Gerniers S 1993 Coxsackie B virus epidemiology and neonatal infection in Belgium. Journal of Infection 27: 311–316
271. Duliege A M, Amos C I, Felton S 1995 Birth order, delivery route and concordance in the transmission of HIV type 1 from mothers to twins. Pediatrics 126: 625–632
272. Dulkerian S, Kilpatrick L, Costarino A T J et al 1995 Cytokine elevations in infants with bacterial and aseptic meningitis. Journal of Pediatrics 126: 872–876
273. Dumois A O 1995 The case against mandatory newborn screening for HIV antibodies. Journal of Community Health 20: 143–159
274. Dumornay W, Roblin P M, Gelling M, Hammerschlag M R, Worku M 1992 Comparison of a chemiluminometric immunoassay with culture for diagnosis of chlamydial infections in infants. Journal of Clinical Microbiology 30: 1867–1869
275. Dunn D T, Brandt C D, Krivine A et al 1995 The sensitivity of HIV-1 DNA polymerase chain reaction in the neonatal period and the relative contributions of intra-uterine and intra-partum transmission. AIDS 9: F7–11
276. Dunn D T, Newell M L, Ades A E, Peckham C 1992 Risk of human immunodeficiency virus type 1 transmission through breastfeeding. Lancet 340: 585–588
277. Duvekot J- J, Theewes B A M, Wesdorp J M, Roumen F J M E, Boukaert P X J M 1990 Congenital cytomegalovirus infection in a twin pregnancy: a case report. European Journal of Pediatrics 149: 261–262
278. Dworsky M, Yow M, Stagno S, Pass R F, Alford C 1983 Cytomegalovirus in breast milk and transmission in infancy. Pediatrics 72: 295–299
279. Dyke M P, Forsyth K D 1993 Decreased plasma fibronectin concentrations in preterm infants with septicaemia. Archives of Disease in Childhood 68: 557–560
280. Dyke M P, Grauaug A, Kohan R, Ott K, Andrews R 1993 *Ureaplasma urealyticum* in a neonatal intensive care population. Journal of Paediatrics and Child Health 29: 295–297
281. Dyke M P, Ott K 1993 Severe thrombocytopenia in extremely low birthweight infants with systemic candidiasis. Journal of Paediatrics and Child Health 29: 298–301
282. Easterbrook P, Ippolito G 1997 Prophylaxis after occupational exposure to HIV. British Medical Journal 315: 557–558
283. Eastick K, Leeming J P, Bennett D, Millar M R 1996 Reservoirs of coagulase negative staphylococci in preterm infants. Archives of Disease in Childhood 74: F99–104
284. Eaton R B, Petersen E, Seppanen H, Tuuminen T 1996 Multicenter evaluation of a fluorometric enzyme immunocapture assay to detect toxoplasma-specific immunoglobulin M in dried blood filter paper specimens from newborns. Journal of Clinical Microbiology 34: 3147–3150
285. Eberhart-Phillips J E, Frederick P D, Baron R C, Mascola L 1993 Measles in pregnancy: a descriptive study of 58 cases. Obstetrics and Gynecology 82: 797–801
286. Edelman C M, Ogwo J E, Fine B P 1973 The prevalence of bacteriuria in full-term and premature newborn infants. Journal of Pediatrics 82: 125–129
287. Edelman K, Nikkari S, Ruuskanen O, He Q, Viljanen M, Mertsola J 1996 Detection of *Bordetella pertussis* by polymerase chain reaction and culture in the nasopharynx of erythromycin-treated infants with pertussis. Pediatric Infectious Disease Journal 15: 54–57
288. Edwards M S, Baker C J, Wagner M L, Taber L H, Barrett F F 1978 An etiologic shift in infantile osteomyelitis: the emergence of Group B streptococcus. Journal of Pediatrics 93: 578–583
289. Edwards M S, Rench M A, Haffar A A M, Murphy M A, Desmond M M, Baker C J 1985 Long term sequelae of group B streptococcal meningitis in infancy. Journal of Pediatrics 106: 717–722
290. Edwards M S, Rench M A, Hall M A, Baker C J 1993 Fibronectin levels in premature infants with late-onset sepsis. Journal of Perinatology 13: 8–13
291. Egarter C, Leitich H, Husslein P, Kaider A, Schemper M 1996 Adjunctive antibiotic treatment in preterm labor and neonatal

morbidity: a meta-analysis. Obstetrics and Gynecology 88: 303–309
292. Egarter C, Leitich H, Karas H et al 1996 Antibiotic treatment in preterm premature rupture of membranes and neonatal morbidity: a metaanalysis. American Journal of Obstetrics and Gynecology 174: 589–597
293. Egwunyenga O A, Ajayi J A, Popova Duhlinska D D, Nmorsi O P 1996 Malaria infection of the cord and birthweights in Nigerians. Central African Journal of Medicine 42: 265–268
294. Ehl S, Gering B, Bartmann P, Hogel J, Pohlandt F 1997 C-reactive protein is a useful marker for guiding duration of antibiotic therapy in suspected neonatal bacterial infection. Pediatrics 99: 216–221
295. Eisenfeld L, Krause P J, Herson V C, Block C, Schick J B, Maderazo E 1992 Enhancement of neonatal neutrophil motility (chemotaxis) with adult fresh frozen plasma. American Journal of Perinatology 9: 5–8
296. Eismont F J, Bohlman H H, Soni P L, Goldberg V M, Freehafer A 1982 Vertebral osteomyelitis in infants. Journal of Bone and Joint Surgery 64B: 32–35
297. Ekbom A, Wakefield A J, Zack M, Adami H O 1994 Perinatal measles and subsequent Crohn's disease. Lancet 344: 1161–1162
298. Ekpini E R, Wiktor S Z, Satten G A et al 1997 Late postnatal mother to child transmission of HIV-1 in Abidjan, Côte d'Ivoire. Lancet 349: 1054–1059
299. Elder D E, Minutillo C, Pemberton P J 1995 Neonatal herpes simplex infection: keys to early diagnosis. Journal of Paediatrics and Child Health 31: 307–311
300. el Mohandes A E, Johnson Robbins L, Keiser J F, Simmens S J, Aure M V 1994 Incidence of *Candida parapsilosis* colonization in an intensive care nursery population and its association with invasive fungal disease. Pediatric Infectious Disease Journal 13: 520–524
301. El Radhi A S, Jawad M H, Mansor N, Ibrahim M, Jamil I I 1983 Infection in neonatal hypothermia. Archives of Disease in Childhood 58: 143–145
302. Embil J A, Ozere R L, Haldane E V 1970 Congenital cytomegalovirus infection in two siblings from consecutive pregnancies. Journal of Pediatrics 77: 417–421
303. Embree J E, Braddick M, Datta P, Muriithi J, Hoff C, Kreiss J K 1989 Lack of correlation of maternal immunodeficiency virus infection with neonatal malformations. Pediatric Infectious Disease Journal 8: 700–704
304. Enders G, Miller E, Cradock Watson J, Bolley I, Ridehalgh M 1994 Consequences of varicella and herpes zoster in pregnancy: prospective study of 1739 cases. Lancet 343: 1548–1551
305. Enders G, Nickerl-Pacher U, Miller E, Cradock-Watson J E 1988 Outcome of confirmed periconceptional maternal rubella. Lancet i: 1445–1447
306. Engle W A, McGuire W A, Schreiner R L, Yu P-L 1988 Neutrophil storage pool depletion in neonates with sepsis and neutropenia. Journal of Pediatrics 113: 747–749
307. Englund J A 1994 Passive protection against respiratory syncytial virus disease in infants: the role of maternal antibody. Pediatric Infectious Disease Journal 13: 449–453
308. Enzenauer R W, Bass J W 1983 Initial antibiotic treatment of purulent meningitis in infants 1–2 months of age. American Journal of Diseases of Children 137: 1055–1056
309. Epps R E, Pittelkow M R, Su W P 1995 TORCH syndrome. Seminars in Dermatology 14: 179–186
310. Eregie C O, Ofovwe G 1995 Factors associated with neonatal tetanus mortality in northern Nigeria. East Africa Medical Journal 72: 507–509
311. Eriksen N L, Blanco J D 1993 Group B streptococcal infection in pregnancy. Seminars in Perinatology 17: 432–442
312. Eriksson M, Bennett R, Nord C E, Zetterstrom R 1986 Fecal bacterial microflora of newborn infants during intensive care management and treatment with five antibiotic regimes. Pediatric Infectious Disease Journal 5: 533–539
313. Eriksson M, Melen B, Myrback K-E, Winbladh B, Zetterstrom R 1982 Bacterial colonization of newborn infants in a neonatal intensive care unit. Acta Paediatrica Scandinavica 71: 779–783
314. Ernest J M, Givner L B 1994 A prospective, randomized, placebo-controlled trial of penicillin in preterm premature rupture of membranes. American Journal of Obstetrics and Gynecology 170: 516–521
315. Escobar G J, Zukin T, Usatin M S et al 1994 Early discontinuation of antibiotic treatment in newborns admitted to rule out sepsis: a decision rule. Pediatric Infectious Disease Journal 13: 860–866
316. European Centre for the Epidemiological Monitoring of AIDS 1994 AIDS surveillance in Europe. Quarterly Report No 44: 41–53
317. European Collaborative Study 1988 Mother to child transmission of HIV infection. Lancet ii: 1039–1043
318. European Collaborative Study 1991 Children born to women with HIV-1 infection: natural history and risk of transmission. Lancet 337: 253–260
319. European Collaborative Study 1994 Caesarean section and risk of vertical transmission of HIV-1 infection. Lancet 343: 1464–1467
320. European Collaborative Study 1992 Risk factors for mother-to-child transmission of HIV-1. Lancet 339: 1007–1012
321. European Collaborative Study 1994 Perinatal findings in children born to HIV-infected mothers. British Journal of Obstetrics and Gynaecology 101: 136–141
322. Evans H E, Frenkel L D 1994 Congenital syphilis. Clinics in Perinatology 21: 149–162
323. Ewert D P, Lieb L, Hayes P S, Reeves M W, Mascola L 1995 *Listeria monocytogenes* infection and serotype distribution among HIV-infected persons in Los Angeles County, 1985–1992. Journal of Acquired Immune Deficiency Syndrome and Human Retrovirology 8: 461–465
324. Fadel H E, Ruedrich D A 1988 Intrauterine resolution of non-immune hydrops associated with cytomegalovirus infection. Obstetrics and Gynecology 71: 1003–1005
325. Faer M J, Taybi H 1977 Mycotic aortic aneurysm in premature infants. Radiology 125: 177–180
326. Fairley C K, Smoleniec J S, Caul O E, Miller E 1995 Observational study of effect of intrauterine transfusions on outcome of fetal hydrops after parvovirus B19 infection. Lancet 346: 1335–1337
327. Faix R G 1984 Systemic candida infections in infants in intensive care nurseries. Journal of Pediatrics 105: 616–622
328. Faix R G 1992 Invasive neonatal candidiasis: comparison of albicans and parapsilosis infection. Pediatric Infectious Disease Journal 11: 88–93
329. Faix R G, Kovarik S M, Shaw T R, Johnson R V 1989 Mucocutaneous and invasive candidiasis among very low birthweight infants in intensive care nurseries: a prospective study. Pediatrics 83: 101–107
330. Fajemilehin B R 1995 Neonatal tetanus among rural-born Nigerian infants. Maternal and Child Nursing Journal 23: 39–43
331. Falla T J, Dobson S R, Crook D W et al 1993 Population-based study of non-typable *Haemophilus influenzae* invasive disease in children and neonates. Lancet 341: 851–854
332. Falloon J, Eddy J, Wiener L, Pizzo P A 1989 Human immunodeficiency virus infection in children. Journal of Pediatrics 114: 1–30
333. Fanaroff A, Korones S B, Wright L L, Wright E C, Poland R L, Bauer C B 1994 A controlled trial of intravenous immune globulin to reduce nosocomial infections in very-low-birthweight infants. New England Journal of Medicine 330: 1107–1113
334. Fang F C, McClelland M, Guiney D G et al 1993 Value of molecular epidemiologic analysis in a nosocomial methicillin-resistant *Staphylococcus aureus* outbreak. Journal of the American Medical Association 270: 1323–1328
335. Farber B F, Kaplan M H, Clogston A G 1990 *Staphylococcus epidermidis* extracted slime inhibits the antimicrobial action of glycopeptide antibiotics. Journal of Infectious Diseases 161: 37–41
336. Farber J M, Peterkin P I, Carter A O, Varughese P V, Ashton F E, Ewan E P 1991 Neonatal listeriosis due to cross-infection confirmed by isoenzyme typing and DNA fingerprinting. Journal of Infectious Diseases 163: 927–928
337. Fasano C, O'Keeffe J, Gibbs D 1994 Fluconazole treatment of neonates and infants with severe fungal infections not treatable with conventional agents. European Journal of Clinical Microbiology and Infectious Diseases 13: 351–354
338. Feder H M 1988 Disseminated herpes simplex infection in a neonate during prophylaxis with vidarabine. Journal of the American Medical Association 259: 1054–1055
339. Fekety F R, Buchbinder L, Shaffer E L 1958 Control of an outbreak of staphylococcal infections among mothers and infants in a suburban hospital. American Journal of Public Health 48: 298–303
340. Feldman W E 1979 Bacterial etiology and mortality of purulent

pericarditis in pediatric patients. Review of 162 cases. American Journal of Diseases of Children 133: 641–647
341. Ferguson J K, Gill A 1996 Risk-stratified nosocomial infection surveillance in a neonatal intensive care unit: report on 24 months of surveillance. Journal of Paediatrics and Child Health 32: 525–531
342. Fernando S, Pearce J M, Booth J C 1993 Lymphocyte responses and virus excretion as risk factors for intrauterine infection with cytomegalovirus. Journal of Medical Virology 41: 108–113
343. Finelli L, Livengood J R, Saiman L 1994 Surveillance of pharyngeal colonization: detection and control of serious bacterial illness in low birth weight infants. Pediatric Infectious Disease Journal 13: 854–859
344. Fischer E G, McLennan J E, Suzuki Y 1981 Cerebral abcess in children. American Journal of Diseases of Children 135: 746–749
345. Fischer G W 1994 Use of intravenous immune globulin in newborn infants. Clinical and Experimental Immunology 97 Suppl 1: 73–77
346. Fischler B, Lindh G, Lindgren S et al 1996 Vertical transmission of hepatitis C virus infection. Scandinavian Journal of Infectious Diseases 28: 353–356
347. Fleisher G, Bolognese R 1984 Epstein–Barr virus infections in pregnancy: a prospective study. Journal of Pediatrics 104: 374–379
348. Fleming D W, Cochi S L, MacDonald K L 1985 Pasteurised milk as a vehicle of infection in an outbreak of listeriosis. New England Journal of Medicine 312: 404–407
349. Fletcher J L J 1991 Perinatal transmission of human papillomavirus. American Family Physician 43: 143–148
350. Fonseca S N, Ehrenkranz R A, Baltimore R S 1994 Epidemiology of antibiotic use in a neonatal intensive care unit. Infection Control and Hospital Epidemiology 15: 156–162
351. Foo A L, Tan K K, Chay O M 1993 Congenital tuberculosis. Tubercular Lung Disease 74: 59–61
352. Forster J, Schumacher R F 1995 The clinical picture presented by premature neonates infected with the respiratory syncytial virus. European Journal of Pediatrics 154: 901–905
353. Fortnum H, Davis A 1993 Hearing impairment in children after bacterial meningitis: incidence and resource implications. British Journal of Audiology 27: 43–52
354. Fortnum H M, Davis A C 1993 Epidemiology of bacterial meningitis. Archives of Disease in Childhood 68: 763–767
355. Fowler K B, Stagno S, Pass R F 1993. Maternal age and congenital cytomegalovirus infection: screening of two diverse newborn populations, 1980–1990. Journal of Infectious Diseases 168: 552–556
356. Fowler K B, Stagno S, Pass R F, Britt W J, Boll T J, Alford C A 1992 The outcome of congenital cytomegalovirus infection in relation to maternal antibody status. New England Journal of Medicine 326: 663–667
357. Frame P T, McLaurin R L 1984 Treatment of CSF shunt infections with intrashunt plus oral antibiotic therapy. Journal of Neurosurgery 60: 354–360
358. Franco S M, Cornelius V E, Andrews B F 1992 Long-term outcome of neonatal meningitis. American Journal of Diseases of Children 146: 567–571
359. Fraser S H, O'Keefe R J, Scurry J P, Watkins A M, Drew J H, Chow C W 1994 Hydrocephalus ex vacuo and clasp thumb deformity due to congenital cytomegalovirus infection. Journal of Paediatrics and Child Health 30: 450–452
360. Fraser S H, Tudehope D I 1996 Neonatal neutropenia and thrombocytopenia following maternal hypertension. Journal of Paediatrics and Child Health 32: 31–34
361. Frederiksen B, Samuelsson S 1992 Feto-maternal listeriosis in Denmark 1981–1988. Journal of Infection 24: 277–287
362. Freeman J, Goldman D A, Smith N E, Sidebotton D G, Epstein M F, Platt R 1990 Association of intravenous lipid emulsion and coagulase negative staphylococcal bacteremia in neonatal intensive care units. New England Journal of Medicine 323: 301–308
363. Freij B J, Sever J L 1988 Herpes virus infections in pregnancy. Clinics in Perinatology 15: 203–231
364. Friedman C A, Temple D M, Robbins K K, Rawson J E, Wilson J P, Feldman S 1994 Outbreak and control of varicella in a neonatal intensive care unit. Pediatric Infectious Disease Journal 13: 152–154
365. Friedman C A, Wender D F, Rawson J E 1984 Rapid diagnosis of Group B streptococcal infection utilizing a commercially available latex agglutination assay. Pediatrics 73: 27–30
366. Friman G, Nystrom-Rosander C, Jonsell G, Bjorkman A, Ledas G, Svendsrup B 1983 Agranulocytosis associated with malaria prophylaxis with Maloprim. British Medical Journal 286: 1244–1245
367. Fukuda S, Miyachi M, Sugimoto S, Goshima A, Futamura M, Morishima T 1995 A female infant successfully treated by ganciclovir for congenital cytomegalovirus infection. Acta Paediatria Japonica 37: 206–210
368. Gajdusek D C 1957 *Pneumocytis carinii* – etiologic agent of interstitial plasma cell pneumonia of perinatal and young infants. Pediatrics 19: 543–565
369. Galbraith R M, Fox H, Hsi B, Galbraith G M P, Bray R S, Faulk W P 1980 The human materno-fetal relationship in malaria II. Histological, ultrastructural and immunopathological studies of the placenta. Transactions of the Royal Society of Tropical Medicine and Hygiene 74: 61–72
370. Gannon H 1993 Ureaplasma urealyticum and its role in neonatal lung disease. Neonatal Network 12: 13–18
371. Garcia Alix A, Martin Ancel A, Ramos M T et al 1995 Cerebrospinal fluid beta 2-microglobulin in neonates with central nervous system infections. European Journal of Pediatrics 154: 309–313
372. Garcia Rodriguez M C, Bates I, de Jose I et al 1995 Prognostic value of immunological data, in vitro antibody production, and virus culture in vertical infection with HIV-1. Archives of Disease in Childhood 72: 498–501
373. Gardner P, Leipzig T, Phillips P 1985 Infections of central nervous system shunts. Medical Clinics of North America 69: 297–314
374. Garland J S, Dunne W M J, Havens P et al 1992 Peripheral intravenous catheter complications in critically ill children: a prospective study. Pediatrics 89: 1145–1150
375. Garland S M 1991 Early onset neonatal group B streptococcus (GBS) infection: associated obstetric risk factors. Australia and New Zealand Journal of Obstetrics and Gynaecology 31: 117–118
376. Garland S M, Kelly N 1995 Early-onset neonatal group B streptococcal sepsis: economics of various prevention strategies. Medical Journal of Australia 162: 413–417
377. Garner P, Lai D, Baea M, Edwards K, Heywood P 1994 Avoiding neonatal death: an intervention study of umbilical cord care. Journal of Tropical Paediatrics 40: 24–28
378. Gay N J, Hesketh L M, Cohen B J et al 1994 Age specific antibody prevalence to parvovirus B19: how many women are infected in pregnancy? Communicable Disease Reports. CDR Reviews 4: 104–107
379. Gaynes R P, Martone W J, Culver D H et al 1991 Comparison of rates of nosocomial infections in neonatal intensive care units in the United States. National Nosocomial Infections Surveillance System. American Journal of Medicine 91: 192S–196S
379a. Gazala E, Karplus M, Liberman J R, Sarov I 1985 The effect of maternal measles on the fetus. Pediatric Infectious Disease Journal 4: 203–204
380. Gellert G A, Ewert D P, Bendana N et al 1993 A cluster of coagulase-negative staphylococcal bacteremias associated with peripheral vascular catheter colonization in a neonatal intensive care unit. American Journal of Infection Control 21: 16–20
381. Gellin B G, Broome C V 1989 Listeriosis. Journal of the American Medical Association 261: 1313–1320
382. Gendrel D, Assicot M, Raymond J et al 1996 Procalcitonin as a marker for the early diagnosis of neonatal infection. Journal of Pediatrics 128: 570–573
383. Georgiev V S 1994 Management of toxoplasmosis. Drugs 48: 179–188
384. Gerdes J S 1991 Clinicopathologic approach to the diagnosis of neonatal sepsis. Clinics in Perinatology 18: 361–381
385. Gerdes J S, Polin R A 1987 Sepsis screens in neonates with evaluation of plasma fibronectin. Pediatric Infectious Disease Journal 6: 443–446
386. Gerety R J, Schweitzer I L 1977 Viral hepatitis type B during pregnancy, the neonatal period, and infancy. Journal of Pediatrics 84: 661–665
387. Gershon A A 1990 Chickenpox, measles and mumps. In: Remington JS, Klein JO (eds) Infectious disease of the fetus and newborn infant, 3rd Edn WB Saunders, Philadelphia, pp 395–445
388. Gessler P, Kirchmann N, Kientsch Engel R, Haas N, Lasch P, Kachel W 1993 Serum concentrations of granulocyte colony-stimulating factor in healthy term and preterm neonates and in those with various diseases including bacterial infections. Blood 82: 3177–3182
389. Giacoia G P, Neter E, Ogra P 1981 Respiratory infections in infants on mechanical ventilators. The immune response as a diagnostic aid. Journal of Pediatrics 98: 691–695
390. Gibboney W, Lemons J A 1986 Necrotizing fasciitis of the scalp in neonates. American Journal of Perinatology 3: 58–60

391. Gibbs R S, McDuffie R S J, McNabb F, Fryer G E, Miyoshi T, Merenstein G 1994 Neonatal group B streptococcal sepsis during 2 years of a universal screening program. Obstetrics and Gynecology 84: 496–500
392. Gibson R L, Soderland C, Henderson W R J, Chi E Y, Rubens C E 1995 Group B streptococci (GBS) injure lung endothelium in vitro: GBS invasion and GBS-induced eicosanoid production is greater with microvascular than with pulmonary artery cells. Infection and Immunity 63: 271–279
393. Gilbert G L 1993 Chickenpox during pregnancy. British Medical Journal 306: 1079–1080
394. Gillan E R, Christensen R D, Suen Y, Ellis R, van de Ven C, Cairo M S 1994 A randomized, placebo-controlled trial of recombinant human granulocyte colony-stimulating factor administration in newborn infants with presumed sepsis: significant induction of peripheral and bone marrow neutrophilia. Blood 84: 1427–1433
395. Gilles F H, Jammes J L, Berenberg W 1977 Neonatal meningitis. The ventricle as a bacterial reservoir. Archives of Neurology 34: 560–562
396. Givens K T, Lee D A, Jones T, Ilstrup D M 1993 Congenital rubella syndrome: ophthalmic manifestations and associated systemic disorders. British Journal of Ophthalmology 77: 358–363
397. Givner L B 1990 Human immunoglobulins for intravenous use: comparison of available preparations for group B streptococcal antibody levels, opsonic activity, and efficacy in animal models. Pediatrics 86: 955–962
398. Givner L B, Nagaraj S K 1993 Hyperimmune human IgG or recombinant human granulocyte–macrophage colony-stimulating factor as adjunctive therapy for group B streptococcal sepsis in newborn rats. Journal of Pediatrics 122: 774–779
399. Gjuric G, Prislin Muskic M, Nikolic E, Zurga B 1994 Ureaplasma urealyticum osteomyelitis in a very low birth weight infant. Journal of Perinatal Medicine 22: 79–81
400. Gladstone I M, Ehrenkranz R A, Edberg S C, Baltimore R S 1990 A ten-year review of neonatal sepsis and comparison with the previous fifty-year experience. Pediatric Infectious Disease Journal 9: 819–825
401. Gleason W A, Martin R J, Anderson J V, Carlo W A, Sanniti K J Fanaroff A A 1983 Optimal position for spinal tap in preterm infants. Pediatrics 71: 31–35
402. Gleeson F V, Gordon I 1991 Imaging in urinary tract infection. Archives of Disease in Childhood 66: 1282–1283
403. Glick C, Graves G R, Feldman S 1993 Neonatal fungemia and amphotericin B. Southern Medical Journal 86: 1368–1371
404. Goedert J J, Mendez H, Drummond J E et al 1989 Mother to infant transmission of human immunodeficiency virus type I. Association with prematurity or low anti-gp 120. Lancet ii: 1351–1354
405. Gogus S, Umer H, Akcoren Z, Sanal O, Osmanlioglu G, Cimbis M 1993 Neonatal tuberculosis. Pediatric Pathology 13: 299–304
406. Golden S E 1988 Neonatal herpes simplex viremia. Pediatric Infectious Disease Journal 7: 425–426
407. Goldmann D A, Durbin W A, Freeman J 1981 Nosocomial infections in a neonatal intensive care unit. Journal of Infectious Diseases 144: 449–459
408. Gomez R, Ghezzi F, Romero R, Muñoz H, Tolosa J E, Rojas I 1995 Premature labour and intra-amniotic infection. Clinics in Perinatology 22: 281–342
409. Gordon J E, Singh S, Wyon J B 1961 Tetanus in villages of the Punjab: an epidemiological study. Journal of the Indian Medical Association 37: 157–161
410. Goto M, Zeller W P, Hurley R M, Jong J S, Lee C H 1991 Prophylaxis and treatment of newborn endotoxic shock with anti-lipid A monoclonal antibodies. Circulatory Shock 35: 60–64
411. Gottbrath Flaherty E K, Agrawal R, Thaker V, Patel D, Ghai K 1995 Urinary tract infections in cocaine-exposed infants. Journal of Perinatology 15: 203–207
412. Grant H R, Quiney R E, Mercer D M, Lodge S 1988 Cleft palate and glue ear. Archives of Disease in Childhood 63: 176–179
413. Gratacos E, Torres P J, Vidal J et al 1995 The incidence of human parvovirus B19 infection during pregnancy and its impact on perinatal outcome. Journal of Infectious Diseases 171: 1360–1363
414. Gravel J S, McCarton C M, Ruben R J 1988 Otitis media in neonatal intensive care unit graduates. A one year prospective study. Pediatrics 82: 44–49
415. Gravel Tropper D, Sample M L, Oxley C, Toye B, Woods D E, Garber G E 1996 Three-year outbreak of pseudobacteremia with *Burkholderia cepacia* traced to a contaminated blood gas analyzer. Infection Control and Hospital Epidemiology 17: 737–740
416. Graves G G, Rhodes P G 1984 Tachycardia as a sign of early onset neonatal sepsis. Pediatric Infectious Disease Journal 3: 404–406
417. Gray E S, Peters G, Verstegen M 1984 Effect of extracellular slime substance from *Staphylococcus epidermidis* on the human cellular immune response. Lancet i: 365–367
418. Gray J E, Richardson D K, McCormick M C, Goldmann D A 1995 Coagulase-negative staphylococcal bacteremia among very low birth weight infants: relation to admission illness severity, resource use, and outcome. Pediatrics 95: 225–230
419. Gray J 1997 HIV in the neonate. Journal of Hospital Infection 37: 181–198
420. Gray M L 1960 Genital listeriosis as a cause of repeated abortion. Lancet ii: 296–297
421. Green M, Dashefsky B, Wald E R, Laifer S, Harger J, Guthrie R 1993 Comparison of two antigen assays for rapid intrapartum detection of vaginal group B streptococcal colonization. Journal of Clinical Microbiology 31: 78–82
422. Green P A, Singh K V, Murray B E, Baker C J 1994 Recurrent group B streptococcal infections in infants: clinical and microbiologic aspects. Journal of Pediatrics 125: 931–938
423. Greenberg D N, Yoder B A 1990 Changes in the differential white blood cell count in screening for group B streptococcal sepsis. Pediatric Infectious Disease Journal 9: 886–889
424. Greene K A, Rhine W D, Starnes V A, Ariagno R L 1990 Fatal postoperative *Legionella* pneumonia in a newborn. Journal of Perinatology 10: 183–184
425. Greenes D S, Rowitch D, Thorne G M, Perez Atayde A, Lee F S, Goldmann D 1995 Neonatal herpes simplex virus infection presenting as fulminant liver failure. Pediatric Infectious Disease Journal 14: 242–244
426. Greenfield C, Sinickas V, Harrison L C 1991 Detection of cytomegalovirus by the polymerase chain reaction. A simple, rapid and sensitive non-radioactive method. Medical Journal of Australia 154: 383–385
427. Greenwood A M, D'Allesandro U, Siay F, Greenwood B M 1992 Treponemal infection and outcome of pregnancy in a rural area of The Gambia, West Africa. Infectious Diseases 166: 842–846
428. Gregory J, Hey P 1972 Blood neutrophil response to bacterial infection in the first month of life. Archives of Disease in Childhood 47: 747–753
429. Gressens P, Langston C, Martin J R 1994 In situ PCR localization of herpes simplex virus DNA sequences in disseminated neonatal herpes encephalitis. Journal of Neuropathology and Experimental Neurology 53: 469–482
430. Griffiths P D, Baboonian C 1984 A prospective study of primary cytomegalovirus infection during pregnancy: final report. British Journal of Obstetrics and Gynaecology 91: 307–315
431. Griffiths P D, Baboonian C, Rutter D, Peckham C 1991 Congenital and maternal cytomegalovirus infections in a London population. British Journal of Obstetrics and Gynaecology 98: 135–140
432. Grigg J M, Barber A, Silverman M 1992 Increased levels of bronchoalveolar lavage fluid interleukin-6 in preterm ventilated infants after prolonged rupture of membranes. American Review of Respiratory Disease 145: 782–786
433. Grillner L, Broberger U, Chrystie I, Ransjö U 1985 Rotavirus infections in newborns: an epidemiological and clinical study. Scandinavian Journal of Infectious Diseases 17: 349–355
434. Grio R, Porpiglia M, Vetro E et al 1994 Asymptomatic bacteriuria in pregnancy: maternal and fetal complications. Panminerva Medicine 36: 198–200
435. Groothuis J R 1994 Role of antibody and the use of respiratory syncytial virus immunoglobulin in the prevention of respiratory syncytial virus disease in preterm infants with and without bronchopulmonary dysplasia. Pediatric Infectious Disease Journal 13: 454–457
436. Groothuis J R 1994 Role of antibody and use of respiratory syncytial virus (RSV) immune globulin to prevent severe RSV disease in high-risk children. Journal of Pediatrics 124: S28–32
437. Groothuis J R, Gutierrez K M, Lauer B A 1988 Respiratory syncytial virus infection in children with bronchopulmonary dysplasia. Pediatrics 82: 199–203
438. Groothuis J R, Simoes E A, Hemming V G 1995 Respiratory syncytial virus (RSV) infection in preterm infants and the protective effects of

RSV immune globulin (RSVIG). Respiratory Syncytial Virus Immune Globulin Study Group. Pediatrics 95: 463–467
439. Grose C, Meehan T, Weiner C P 1992 Prenatal diagnosis of congenital cytomegalovirus infection by virus isolation after amniocentesis. Pediatric Infectious Disease Journal 11: 605–607
440. Gross U, Roos T, Appoldt D, Heesemann J 1992 Improved serological diagnosis of *Toxoplasma gondii* infection by detection of immunoglobulin A (IgA) and IgM antibodies against P30 by using the immunoblot technique. Journal of Clinical Microbiology 30: 1436–1441
441. Grundmann H, Kropec A, Hartung D, Berner R, Daschner F 1993 *Pseudomonas aeruginosa* in a neonatal intensive care unit: reservoirs and ecology of the nosocomial pathogen. Journal of Infectious Diseases 168: 943–947
442. Gruskay J A, Nachamkin I, Baumgart S 1986 Predicting the pathogenicity of coagulase negative staphylococci in the neonate: slime production, antibiotic resistance and predominance of *S. epidermidis* species. Pediatric Research 20: 397A
443. Guerina N G, Hsu H W, Meissner H C et al 1994 Neonatal serologic screening and early treatment for congenital *Toxoplasma gondii* infection. The New England Regional Toxoplasma Working Group. New England Journal of Medicine 330: 1858–1863
444. Guerrant R L, Cleary T G, Pickering L K 1990 Microorganisms responsible for neonatal diarrhoea. In: Remington J S, Klein J O (eds) Infectious diseases of the fetus and newborn infant, 3rd edn W B Saunders, Philadelphia, pp 901–980
445. Guidozzi F, Ballot D, Rothberg A D 1994 Human B19 parvovirus infection in an obstetric population. A prospective study determining fetal outcome. Journal of Reproductive Medicine 39: 36–38
446. Guillois B, Donnou M D, Sizun J, Bendaoud B, Youinou P 1994 Comparative study of four tests of bacterial infection in the neonate. Total neutrophil count, CRP, fibrinogen and C3d. Biology of the Neonate 66: 175–181
447. Gunnlaugsson G, da Silva M C, Smedman L 1995 Does age at the start of breast feeding influence infantile diarrhoea morbidity? A case-control study in periurban Guinea-Bissau. Acta Paediatrica 84: 398–401
448. Gupta A K, Shashi S, Mohan M, Lamba I M, Gupta R 1993 Epidemiology of *Pseudomonas aeruginosa* infections in a neonatal intensive care unit. Journal of Tropical Pediatrics 39: 32–36
449. Gustavson EE 1986 *Escherichia coli* empyema in the newborn. American Journal of Diseases of Children 140: 408–411
450. Gutman L T, Wilfert C M, Eppes S 1986 Herpes simplex virus encephalitis in children: analysis of cerebrospinal fluid and progressive neurodevelopmental deterioration. Journal of Infectious Diseases 154: 415–421
451. Hachey W E, Wiswell T E 1992 Limitations in the usefulness of urine latex particle agglutination tests and hematologic measurements in diagnosing neonatal sepsis during the first week of life. Journal of Perinatology 12: 240–245
452. Hague R A, Rassam S, Morgan G, Cant A J 1994 Early diagnosis of severe combined immunodeficiency syndrome. Archives of Disease in Childhood 70: 260–263
453. Haley R W, Cushion N B, Tenover F C et al 1995 Eradication of endemic methicillin-resistant *Staphylococcus aureus* infections from a neonatal intensive care unit. Journal of Infectious Diseases 171: 614–624
454. Hall C B, Kopelman A E, Douglas R G, Geiman J M, Meagher M P 1979 Neonatal respiratory syncytial virus infection. New England Journal of Medicine 300: 393–396
455. Hall C B, Long C E, Schnabel K C et al 1994 Human herpesvirus-6 infection in children. A prospective study of complications and reactivation. New England Journal of Medicine 331: 432–438
456. Hall R T, Kurth C G 1995 Value of negative nose and ear cultures in identifying high-risk infants without early-onset group B streptococcal sepsis. Journal of Perinatology 15: 356–358
457. Hall R T, Shigeoka A O, Hill H R 1983 Serum opsonic activity and peripheral neutrophil counts before and after exchange transfusion in infants with early onset Group B streptococcal septicemia. Pediatric Infectious Disease Journal 2: 356–358
458. Hall R T, Hall S L, Barnes W G, Izuegbu U J, Rogolsky M, Zorbas I 1987 Characteristics of coagulase negative staphylococci from infants with bacteremia. Pediatric Infectious Disease Journal 6: 377–383
459. Hall S, Glickman B 1991 The British Paediatric Surveillance Unit. New England Journal of Medicine 323: 344–346
460. Hall S M 1983 Congenital toxoplasmosis in England, Wales and Northern Ireland: some epidemiological problems. British Medical Journal 287: 453–455
461. Halliday H L 1989 When to do a lumbar puncture in a neonate. Archives of Disease in Childhood 64: 313–316
462. Halliday H L, McClure G, Reid M Mc C, Lappin T R J, Meban C, Thomas P S 1984 Controlled trial of artifical surfactant to prevent respiratory distress syndrome. Lancet i: 476–478
463. Hammerberg O, Bialkowska Hobrzanska H, Gregson D, Potters H, Gopal J, Reid D 1992 Comparison of blood cultures with corresponding venipuncture site cultures of specimens from hospitalised premature neonates. Journal of Pediatrics 120: 120–124
464. Hammerschlag M R, Herrmann J E, Cox P, Worku M, Laux R, Howard L V 1985 Enzyme immunoassay for diagnosis of neonatal chlamydial conjunctivitis. Journal of Pediatrics 107: 741–743
465. Hammerschlag M R, Cummings C, Roblin P M, Williams T H, Delke I 1989 Efficacy of neonatal ocular prophylaxis for the prevention of chlamydial and gonococcal conjunctivitis. New England Journal of Medicine 320: 769–772
466. Hamoudi A C, Marcon M J, Cannon H J, McClead R E 1983 Comparison of three major antigen detection methods for the diagnosis of Group B streptococcal sepsis in neonates. Pediatric Infectious Disease Journal 2: 432–435
467. Hampl S D, Olson L C 1995 Pertussis in the young infant. Seminars in Respiratory Infection 10: 58–62
468. Hamrick W B, Reilly L 1992 A comparison of infection rates in a newborn intensive care unit before and after adoption of open visitation. Neonatal Network 11: 15–18
469. Han B K, Babcock D S, McAdams L 1985 Bacterial meningitis in infants – sonographic findings. Radiology 154: 645–650
470. Handalage D C M A, Wickramasinghe S Y D C 1976 Neonatal tetanus – some observations from Sri Lanka. Journal of Tropical Paediatrics and Environment Child Health 22: 167–171
471. Hannah M E, Ohlsson A, Farine D et al 1996 Induction of labor compared with expectant management for prelabor rupture of the membranes at term. TERMPROM Study Group. New England Journal of Medicine 334: 1005–1010
472. Hanngren K, Grandien M, Granstrom G 1985 Effect of zoster immunoglobulin for varicella prophylaxis in a newborn. Scandinavian Journal of Infectious Diseases 17: 343–347
473. Hanshaw J B, Dudgeon J A 1978 Viral disease of the fetus and newborn. W B Saunders, Philadelphia p 198
474. Hanshaw J B, Scheiner A P, Moxley A W, Gaev L, Abel V, Scheiner B 1976 School failure and deafness after 'silent' congenital cytomegalovirus infection. New England Journal of Medicine 295: 468–470
475. Haque K N 1995 Pitfalls in meta-analysis. Archives of Disease in Childhood 73: 196–199
476. Haque K N 1997 Should intravenous immunoglobulins be used in the treatment of neonatal sepsis? British Journal of Intensive Care 7: 12–17
477. Haque K N, Chagia A H, Shaheed M M 1990 Half a decade of neonatal sepsis, Riyadh, Saudi Arabia. Journal of Tropical Pediatrics 36: 20–23
478. Haque K N, Remo C, Bahakim H 1995 Comparison of two types of intravenous immunoglobulins in the treatment of neonatal sepsis. Clinical and Experimental Immunology 101: 328–333
479. Haque K N, Zaidi N H, Bahakim H 1988 IgM enriched intravenous immunoglobulin therapy in neonatal sepsis. American Journal of Diseases of Children 142: 1293–1296
480. Haque K N, Zaidi M H, Haque S K et al 1986 Intravenous immunoglobulin for prevention of sepsis in preterm and low birthweight infants. Pediatric Infectious Disease Journal 5: 622–625
481. Harpin V A, Rutter N 1985 Humidification of incubators. Archives of Disease in Childhood 60: 219–224
482. Harris C, Salgo M P, Tanowitz H B, Witner M 1988 In vitro assessment of antimicrobial agents against toxoplasma gondii. Journal of Infectious Diseases 157: 14–22
483. Harris D T, Schumacher M J, Locascio J 1992 Phenotypic and functional immaturity of human umbilical cord blood T lymphocytes. Proceedings of the National Academy of Sciences USA 89: 10006–10010
484. Harris H, Wirtschafter D, Cassady G 1976 Endotracheal intubation and its relationship to bacterial colonization and systemic infection in newborn infants. Pediatrics 58: 816–825

485. Harris M C, Costarino A T J, Sullivan J S et al 1994 Cytokine elevations in critically ill infants with sepsis and necrotizing enterocolitis. Journal of Pediatrics 124: 105–111
486. Harrison H R, English M G, Lee C K, Alexander E R 1978 *Chlamydia trachomatis* infant pneumonitis. New England Journal of Medicine 298: 702–708
487. Hart M H, Kaufman S S, Vanderhoof J A et al 1991 Neonatal hepatitis and extrahepatic biliary atresia associated with cytomegalovirus infection in twins. American Journal of Diseases of Children 145: 302–305
488. Hawken J, Chard T, Costeloe K, Jeffries D J, Hudson C N 1995 Risk factors for HIV infection overlooked in routine antenatal care. Journal of the Royal Society of Medicine 88: 634–636
489. Hawkins S 1995 Water vs conventional births: infection rates compared. Nursing Times 91: 38–40
490. Heggie A D, Jacobs M R, Butler V T, Baley J E, Boxerbaum B 1994 Frequency and significance of isolation of *Ureaplasma urealyticum* and *Mycoplasma hominis* from cerebrospinal fluid and tracheal aspirate specimens from low birth weight infants. Journal of Pediatrics 124: 956–961
491. Heggie A D, Jaffee A C, Stuart L A, Thombre P S, Sorensen R U 1985 Topical sulphacetamide vs oral erythromycin for neonatal chlamydial conjunctivitis. American Journal of Diseases of Children 139: 564–566
492. Helin I, Widell A, Borulf S, Walder M, Ulmsten U 1987 Outbreak of coxsackie virus A-14 meningitis among newborns in a maternity hospital ward. Acta Paediatrica Scandinavica 76: 234–238
493. Helmy N, Abdalla S, El Essaily M, Nasser S, Hirschhorn N 1988 Oral rehydration therapy for low birthweight neonates suffering from diarrhoea in the intensive care unit. Journal of Pediatric Gastroenterology and Nutrition 7: 417–423
494. Hemming V G, Overall J C, Britt M R 1976 Nosocomial infections in a newborn intensive care unit. New England Journal of Medicine 294: 1310–1316
495. Henderson C E 1995 Management of tuberculosis in pregnancy. Journal of the Association for Academic Minority Physicians 6: 38–42
496. Henderson J B, Beattie C, Hale E G, Wright T 1984 The evaluation of new services: possibilities for preventing congenital toxoplasmosis. International Journal of Epidemiology 13: 65–72
497. Hendricks Munoz K D, Shapiro D L 1990 The role of the lumbar puncture in the admission sepsis evaluation of the premature infant. Journal of Perinatology 10: 60–64
498. Hensey O J, Hart C A, Cooke R W I 1984 Candida albicans skin abscesses. Archives of Disease in Childhood 59: 479–480
499. Herman T E, Siegel M J 1994 Special imaging casebook. Congenital disseminated herpes simplex infection with visceral calcifications. Journal of Perinatology 14: 80–82
500. Hervas J A, Gonzalez L, Gil J, Paoletti L C, Madoff L C, Benedi V J 1993 Neonatal group B streptococcal infection in Mallorca, Spain. Clinical Infectious Diseases 16: 714–718
501. Herzog K D, Long S S, McGuigan M, Fisher M C, Deforest A 1990 Impact of treatment guidelines on use of Ribavirin. American Journal of Diseases of Children 134: 1001–1004
502. Hibbard J U, Hibbard M C, Ismail M, Arendt E 1993 Pregnancy outcome after expectant management of premature rupture of the membranes in the second trimester. Journal of Reproductive Medicine 38: 945–951
503. Hicks T, Fowler K, Richardson M, Dahle A, Adams L, Pass R 1993 Congenital cytomegalovirus infection and neonatal auditory screening. Journal of Pediatrics 123: 779–782
504. Hiemstra I, Van Bel F, Berger H M 1984 Can trichomonas vaginalis cause pneumonia in newborn babies? British Medical Journal 289: 355–356
505. Higa K, Dan K, Manabe H 1987 Varicella zoster virus infection during pregnancy. Hypothesis concerning the mechanisms of congenital malformations. Obstetrics and Gynecology 69: 214–222
506. Hill A, Shackelford G D, Volpe J J 1981 Ventriculitis with neonatal bacterial meningitis: identification with real time ultrasound. Journal of Pediatrics 99: 133–136
507. Hilton D A, Variend S, Pringle J H 1993 Demonstration of Coxsackie virus RNA in formalin-fixed tissue sections from childhood myocarditis cases by in situ hybridization and the polymerase chain reaction. Journal of Pathology 170: 45–51
508. Hira S K, Kamanga J, Bhat G J et al 1989 Perinatal transmission of HIV I in Zambia. British Medical Journal 289: 1250–1252
509. Hirschl R B, Butler M, Coburn C E, Bartlett R H, Baumgart S 1994 *Listeria monocytogenes* and severe newborn respiratory failure supported with extracorporeal membrane oxygenation. Archives of Pediatrics and Adolescent Medicine 148: 513–517
510. Hitchcock R J, Pallett A, Hall M A, Malone P S 1995 Urinary tract candidiasis in neonates and infants. British Journal of Urology 76: 252–256
511. Ho N K, Low Y P, See H F 1989 Septic arthritis in the newborn. A 17 years clinical experience. Singapore Medical Journal. 30: 356–358
512. Hohlfeld P, Daffos F, Thulliez P et al 1989 Fetal toxoplasmosis: outcome of pregnancy and infant follow-up after in-utero treatment. Journal of Pediatrics 115: 765–769
513. Hohlfeld P, Daffos F, Costa J M, Thulliez P, Forestier F, Vidaud M 1994 Prenatal diagnosis of congenital toxoplasmosis with a polymerase-chain-reaction test on amniotic fluid. New England Journal of Medicine 331: 695–699
514. Holland P, Isaacs D, Moxon E R 1986 Fatal neonatal varicella infections. Lancet ii: 1156
515. Holliman R E, Raymond R, Renton N, Johnson J D 1994 The diagnosis of toxoplasmosis using IgG avidity. Epidemiology and Infection 112: 399–408
516. Holmberg R E J, Pavia A T, Montgomery D, Clark J M, Eggert L D 1993 Nosocomial *Legionella* pneumonia in the neonate. Pediatrics 92: 450–453
517. Horstmann D M, Schluederberg A, Emmons J E, Evans B K, Randolph M F, Andiman W A 1985 Persistence of vaccine-induced immune response to rubella: comparison with natural infection. Review of Infectious Diseases 7(Suppl): 80–85
518. Hostoffer R W, Litman A, Smith P G, Jacobs H S, Tosi M F 1993 *Pneumocystis carinii* pneumonia in a term newborn infant with a transiently depressed T lymphocyte count, primarily of cells carrying the CD4 antigen. Journal of Pediatrics 122: 792–794
519. Howard J E, Rubio M 1968 Entermedad de Chagas congenital: I. Estudio clinico y epidemiologico de 30 casos. Boletin Chileno de Parasitologia 23: 107–112
520. Hristeva L, Booy R, Bowler I, Wilkinson A R 1993 Prospective surveillance of neonatal meningitis. Archives of Disease in Childhood 69: 14–18
521. Hristeva L, Bowler I, Booy R, King A T, Wilkinson A R 1993 Value of cerebrospinal fluid examination in the diagnosis of meningitis in the newborn. Archives of Disease in Childhood 69: 514–517
522. Hruszkewycz V, Holtrop P C, Batton D G, Morden R S, Gibson P, Band J D 1991 Complications associated with central venous catheters inserted in critically ill neonates. Infection Control and Hospital Epidemiology 12: 544–548
523. Hu D J, Heyward W L, Byers R H J et al 1992 HIV infection and breast-feeding: policy implications through a decision analysis model. AIDS 6: 1505–1513
524. Huebner J, Pier G B, Maslow J N et al 1994 Endemic nosocomial transmission of *Staphylococcus epidermidis* bacteremia isolates in a neonatal intensive care unit over 10 years. Journal of Infectious Diseases 169: 526–531
525. Hufert F T, Diebold T, Ermisch B, Von Laer D, Meyer Konig U, Neumann Haefelin D 1995 Liver failure due to disseminated HSV-1 infection in a newborn twin. Scandinavian Journal of Infectious Diseases 27: 627–629
526. Hung F C, Huang C B, Huang S C, Liu S T 1994 Congenital cutaneous candidiasis – report of two cases. Chang Keng I Hsueh 17: 63–67
527. Hutto C, Arvin A, Jacobs R et al 1987 Intrauterine herpes simplex virus infection. Journal of Pediatrics 110: 97–101
528. Hwa H L, Shyu M K, Lee C N, Wu C C, Kao C L, Hsieh F J 1994 Prenatal diagnosis of congenital rubella infection from maternal rubella in Taiwan. Obstetrics and Gynecology 84: 415–419
529. Hyde S R, Giacoia G P 1993 Congenital herpes infection: placental and umbilical cord findings. Obstetrics and Gynecology 81: 852–855
530. Ibhanesebhor S E 1995 Clinical characteristics of neonatal malaria. Journal of Tropical Pediatrics 41: 330–333
531. Ingram D L 1994 *Neisseria gonorrhoeae* in children. Pediatric Annals 23: 341–345
532. Ippolito G, Stegagno M, Girardi E et al 1996 Temporal and geographical trends of anti-HIV-1 antibodies screening among

newborns in Italy, 1990–1993. Italian Collaborative Study Group for HIV Prevalence in Newborns. Journal of Acquired Immune Deficiency Syndrome and Human Retrovirology 12: 63–68
533. Isaacman D J, Karasic R B, Reynolds E A, Kost S I 1996 Effect of number of blood cultures and volume of blood on detection of bacteremia in children. Journal of Pediatrics 128: 190–195
534. Isaacs D, Barfield C, Clothier T et al 1996 Late-onset infections of infants in neonatal units. Journal of Paediatrics and Child Health 32: 158–161
535. Isaacs D, Barfield C P, Grimwood K, McPhee A J, Minutillo C, Tudehope D I 1995 Systemic bacterial and fungal infections in infants in Australian neonatal units. Australian Study Group for Neonatal Infections. Medical Journal of Australia 162: 198–201
536. Isaacs D, Dobson S R M, Wilkinson A R, Hope P L, Eglin R, Moxon E R 1989 Conservative management of an Echovirus 11 outbreak in a neonatal unit. Lancet ii: 543–545
537. Isaacs D, Moxon E R 1991 Neonatal infections. Butterworth Heinemann, Oxford, pp 149–166
538. Isenberg S J, Apt L, Wood M 1995 A controlled trial of povidone–iodine as prophylaxis against ophthalmia neonatorum. New England Journal of Medicine 332: 562–566
539. Ish Horowicz M R, McIntyre P, Nade S 1992 Bone and joint infections caused by multiply resistant *Staphylococcus aureus* in a neonatal intensive care unit. Pediatric Infectious Disease Journal 11: 82–87
540. Israele V, Darabi A, McCracken G H 1987 The role of bacterial virulence factors and Tamm–Horsfall protein in the pathogenesis of *Escherichia coli* urinary tract infection in infants. American Journal of Diseases of Children 141: 1230–1234
541. Issekutz T B, Evans J, Bortolussi R 1984 The immune response of human neonates to *Listeria monocytogenes* infection. Clinical Investigative Medicine 7: 263–266
542. Itoh K, Aihara H, Takada S et al 1990 Clinicopathological differences between early-onset and late-onset sepsis and pneumonia in very low birth weight infants. Pediatric Pathology 10: 757–768
543. Jacob J, Edwards D, Gluck L 1980 Early onset sepsis and pneumonia observed as respiratory distress syndrome. American Journal of Diseases of Children 134: 766–768
544. Jacobs J, Garmyn K, Verhaegen J, Devlieger H, Eggermont E 1990 Neonatal sepsis due to *Streptococcus pneumoniae*. Scandinavian Journal of Infectious Diseases 22: 493–497
545. Jakobsson B, Berg U, Svensson L 1994 Renal scarring after acute pyelonephritis. Archives of Disease in Childhood 70: 111–115
546. Jarvis W R, Highsmith A K, Allen J R, Haley R W 1983 Polymicrobial bacteremia associated with lipid emulsions in a neonatal intensive care unit. Pediatric Infectious Disease Journal 2: 203–208
547. Jantos C A, Wienpahl B, Schiefer H G, Wagner F, Hegemann J H 1995 Infection with *Chlamydia pneumoniae* in infants and children with acute lower respiratory tract disease. Pediatric Infectious Disease Journal 14: 117–122
548. Jeffery H, Mitchison R, Wigglesworth J S, Davies P A 1977 Early neonatal bacteraemia. Archives of Disease in Childhood 52: 683–686
549. Jeffery H E, McIntosh E D 1994 Antepartum screening and non-selective intrapartum chemoprophylaxis for group B streptococcus. Australia and New Zealand Journal of Obstetrics and Gynaecology 34: 14–19
550. Jeffries D J 1991 Intra-uterine and neonatal herpes simplex virus infection. Scandinavian Journal of Infectious Diseases: Suppl 80: 21–26
551. Jenista J A, Powell K P, Menegus M A 1984 Epidemiology of neonatal enteroviral infection. Journal of Pediatrics 104: 685–690
552. Johnson G M, Lee D A, Regelmann W E 1986 Interference with granulocyte function by *Staphylococcus epidermidis* slime. Infection and Immunity 54: 13–16
553. Jolley A E 1993 The value of surveillance cultures on neonatal intensive care units. Journal of Hospital Infection 25: 153–159
554. Jones C A, Isaacs D 1995 Predicting the outcome of symptomatic congenital cytomegalovirus infection. Journal of Paediatrics and Child Health 31: 70–71
555. Jones E M, McCulloch S Y, Reeves D S, MacGowan A P 1994 A 10 year survey of the epidemiology and clinical aspects of listeriosis in a provincial English city. Journal of Infection 29: 91–103
556. Jones J F, Ray C G, Fulginiti V A 1980 Perinatal mumps infection. Journal of Pediatrics 96: 912–914
557. Jones K L, Johnson K A, Chambers C D 1994 Offspring of women infected with varicella during pregnancy: a prospective study. Teratology 49: 29–32
558. Joynson D H M, Payne R 1988 Screening for toxoplasma in pregnancy. Lancet ii: 795–796
559. Kacet N, Gremillet C, Zaoui C, Pierrat V, Racoussot S, Dubos J P 1991 Prevention of late-onset infections in preterm infants with intravenous gamma-globulin: a randomized clinical trial. European Journal of Pediatrics 150: 604
560. Kacica M A, Horgan M J, Ochoa L, Sandler R, Lepow M L, Venezia R A 1994 Prevention of gram-positive sepsis in neonates weighing less than 1500 grams. Journal of Pediatrics 125: 253–258
561. Kage M, Kosai K, Kojiro M, Nakamura Y, Fukuda S 1993 Infantile cholestasis due to cytomegalovirus infection of the liver. A possible cause of paucity of interlobular bile ducts. Archives of Pathology and Laboratory Medicine 117: 942–944
562. Kaleida P H, Nativio D G, Chao H P, Cowden S N 1993 Prevalence of bacterial respiratory pathogens in the nasopharynx in breast-fed versus formula-fed infants. Journal of Clinical Microbiology 31: 2674–2678
563. Kalenic S, Francetic I, Polak J, Zele Starcevic L, Bencic Z 1993 Impact of ampicillin and cefuroxime on bacterial colonization and infection in patients on a neonatal intensive care unit. Journal of Hospital Infection 23: 35–41
564. Kaplan J E, Oleske J M, Getchell J P et al 1985 Evidence against transmission of human T lymphotropic virus/lymphadenopathy-associated virus (HTLV III/LAV) in families of children with acquired immunodeficiency syndrome. Pediatric Infectious Disease Journal 4: 468–471
565. Kaplan M, Klein S W, McPhee J 1983 Group B coxsackievirus infections in infants younger than 3 months of age: a serious childhood illness. Review of Infectious Diseases 5: 1019–1032
566. Kaplan M, Rudensky B, Beck A 1993 Perinatal infections with *Streptococcus pneumoniae*. American Journal of Perinatology 10: 1–4
567. Kasper D L 1995 Designer vaccines to prevent infections due to group B streptococcus. Proceedings of the Association of American Physicians 107: 369–373
568. Katz V L, McCoy M C, Kuller J A, Hansen W F 1996 An association between fetal parvovirus B19 infection and fetal anomalies: a report of two cases. American Journal of Perinatology 13: 43–45
569. Kawamura M, Nishida H 1995 The usefulness of serial C-reactive protein measurement in managing neonatal infection. Acta Paediatrica 84: 10–13
570. Kaye J N, Starkey W G, Kell B et al 1996 Human papillomavirus type 16 in infants: use of DNA sequence analyses to determine the source of infection. Journal of General Virology 77: 1139–1143
571. Kazembe P, Simor A E, Swarney A E et al 1993 A study of the epidemiology of an endemic strain of *Staphylococcus haemolyticus* (TOR-35) in a neonatal intensive care unit. Scandinavian Journal of Infectious Diseases 25: 507–513
572. Keith C G 1991 Congenital rubella infection from reinfection of previously immunised mothers. Australia and New Zealand Journal of Ophthalmology 19: 291–293
573. Kennaugh J K, Gregory W W, Powell K R, Hendley J O 1984 The effect of dilution during culture on detection of low concentrations of bacteria in blood. Pediatric Infectious Disease Journal 3: 317–322
574. Kennon C, Overturf G, Bessman S, Sierra E, Smith K J, Brann B 1996 Granulocyte colony stimulating factor as a marker for bacterial infection in neonates. Journal of Pediatrics 128: 765–769
575. Kerr M M, Hutchison J H, McVicar J, Givan J, McAllister T A 1976 The natural history of bacterial colonization of the newborn in a maternity hospital. Scottish Medical Journal 21: 111–117
576. Kershisnik M M, Knisley A S, Sun C C, Andrews J M, Wittwer C T 1992 Cytomegalovirus infection, fetal liver disease and neonatal hemochromatosis. Human Pathology 23: 1075–1080
577. Keyworth N, Millar M R, Holland K T 1992 Development of cutaneous microflora in premature neonates. Archives of Disease in Childhood 67: 797–801
578. Khadilkar V, Tudehope D, Fraser S 1995 A prospective study of nosocomial infection in a neonatal intensive care unit. Journal of Paediatrics and Child Health 31: 387–391
579. Khatib R, Riederer K M, Clark J A, Khatib S, Briski L E, Wilson F M 1995 Coagulase-negative staphylococci in multiple blood cultures: strain relatedness and determinants of same-strain bacteremia. Journal of Clinical Microbiology 33: 816–820
580. Khoo B H, Lee E L, Lam K L 1978 Neonatal tetanus treated with

high dose diazepam. Archives of Disease in Childhood 53: 737–739
581. Khuroo M S, Kamili S, Jameel S 1995 Vertical transmission of hepatitis E virus. Lancet 345: 1025–1026
582. Kidan K G, Fantahun M, Azeze B 1995 Seroprevalence of human immunodeficiency virus infection and its association with syphilis seropositivity among antenatal clinic attenders at Debretabor Rural Hospital, Ethiopia. East African Medical Journal 72: 579–583
583. Kim Y S, Sheldon R A, Elliott B R, Liu Q, Ferriero D M, Tauber M G 1995 Brain injury in experimental neonatal meningitis due to group B streptococci. Journal of Neuropathology and Experimental Neurology 54: 531–539
584. Kinney J S, Johnson K, Papasian C, Hall R T, Kurth C G, Jackson M A 1993 Early onset *Hemophilus influenzae* sepsis in the newborn infant. Pediatric Infectious Disease Journal 12: 739–743
585. Kite P, Millar M R, Gorham P, Congdon P 1988 Comparison of five tests used in the diagnosis of neonatal bacteraemia. Archives of Disease in Childhood 63: 639–643
586. Klass P E, Klein J O 1992 Therapy of bacterial sepsis, meningitis and otitis media in infants and children: 1992 poll of directors of programs in pediatric infectious diseases. Pediatric Infectious Disease Journal 11: 702–705
587. Kleiman M B, Reynolds J K, Schreiner R L, Smith J W, Allen S D 1984 Rapid diagnosis of neonatal bacteremia with acridine orange-stained buffy coat smears. Journal of Pediatrics 105: 419–421
588. Klein B S, Michaels J A, Rytel M W, Berg K G, Davis J P 1984 Nosocomial hepatitis A. Journal of the American Medical Association 252: 2716–2721
589. Klein J F, Shahrivar F 1992 Use of percutaneous silastic central venous catheters in neonates and the management of infectious complications. American Journal of Perinatology 9: 261–264
590. Kline M W 1988 Citrobacter meningitis and brain abscess in infancy: epidemiology, pathogenesis and treatment. Journal of Pediatrics 113: 430–434
591. Knox G E 1983 Cytomegalovirus: patient counselling. Seminars in Perinatology 7: 43–46
592. Knudsen C J M, Hoffman E B 1990 Neonatal osteomyelitis. Journal of Bone and Joint Surgery 72B: 846–851
593. Knudson R P, Alden E R 1980 Neonatal heelstick blood culture. Pediatrics 65: 505–507
594. Kohl S 1988 Herpes simplex virus encephalitis in children. Pediatric Clinics of North America 35: 465–483
595. Kohl S 1989 The neonatal human's immune response to herpes simplex virus infection: a critical review. Pediatric Infectious Disease Journal 8: 67–74
596. Koppe J G, Loewer-Sieger D H, de Roever-Bonnet H 1986 Results of a 20 year follow-up of congenital toxoplasmosis. Lancet i: 254–256
597. Korones S B 1988 Uncommon virus infections of the mother, fetus and newborn – influenza, mumps and measles. Clinics in Perinatology 15: 259–272
598. Koskiniemi M, Happonen J-M, Järvenpää A-I, Pettay O, Vaheri A 1989 Neonatal herpes simplex virus infection: a report of 43 patients. Pediatric Infectious Disease Journal 8: 30–35
599. Koutouby A, Habibullah J 1995 Neonatal sepsis in Dubai, United Arab Emirates. Journal of Tropical Pediatrics 41: 177–180
600. Kovacs B W, Carlson D E, Shahbahrami B, Platt L D 1992 Prenatal diagnosis of human parvovirus B19 in nonimmune hydrops fetalis by polymerase chain reaction. American Journal of Obstetrics and Gynecology 167: 461–466
601. Kowba M D, Schwirian P M 1985 Direct sibling contact and bacterial colonisation of newborns. Journal of Obstetric, Gynecologic and Neonatal Nursing 14: 412–417
602. Krajden S, Middleton P J 1983 Enterovirus infections in the neonate. Clinical Pediatrics 22: 87–92
603. Krause P J, Maderazo E G, Contrino J et al 1991 Modulation of neonatal neutrophil function by pentoxifylline. Pediatric Research 29: 123–127
604. Kretschmar W 1966 bie Bedeutung der p- Aminobenzoeasäure für den Krankheitsverlauf und die Immunität bei der Malaria im Tier und im Menschen (Plasmodium falciparum) I, II, III. Zeitschrift für Tropenmedizin und Parasitologie 17: 301, 369, 375
605. Kuhn J P, Lee S B 1973 Pneumatoceles associated with *Escherichia coli* pneumonias in the newborn. Pediatrics 51: 1008–1011
606. Kumar M L, Jenson H B, Dahms B B 1985 Fatal staphylococcal epidermidis infections in very low birthweight infants with cytomegalovirus infections. Pediatrics 76: 110–112
607. Lackner H, Schwinger W, Urban C 1992 Liposomal amphotericin B for treatment of disseminated fungal infections in two infants of very low birthweight. Pediatrics 89: 1259–1261
608. Lacy J B, Ohlsson A 1995 Administration of intravenous immunoglobulins for prophylaxis or treatment of infection in preterm infants: meta-analyses. Archives of Disease in Childhood 72: F151–155
609. Laga M, Naamara W, Brunham R C et al 1986 Single dose therapy of gonococcal ophthalmia neonatorum with ceftriaxone. New England Journal of Medicine 315: 1382–1385
610. Laifer S A, Ehrlich G D, Huff D S, Balsan M J, Scantlebury V P 1995 Congenital cytomegalovirus infectious in offspring of liver transplant recipients. Clinical Infectious Diseases 20: 52–55
611. Lappalainen M, Koskiniemi M, Hiilesmaa V et al 1995 Outcome of children after maternal primary *Toxoplasma* infection during pregnancy with emphasis on avidity of specific IgG. Pediatric Infectious Disease Journal 14: 354–361
612. Larkin G L, Thuma P E 1991 Congenital malaria in a hyperendemic area. American Journal of Tropical Medicine and Hygiene 45: 587–592
613. Larson E L, McGinley K J, Foglia A et al 1992 Handwashing practices and resistance and density of bacterial hand flora on two pediatric units in Lima, Peru. American Journal of Infection Control 20: 65–72
614. Larsson S, Cronberg S, Winbald S 1979 Listeriosis during pregnancy and the neonatal period in Sweden 1958–1974. Acta Paediatrica Scandinavica 68: 485–493
615. Lassiter H A, Tanner J E, Cost K M, Steger S, Vogel R L 1991 Diminished IgG, but not complement C3 or C4 or factor B, precedes nosocomial bacterial sepsis in very low birth weight neonates. Pediatric Infectious Disease Journal 10: 663–668
616. Lau Y L, Hey E N 1991 Sensitivity and specificity of daily tracheal aspirate cultures in predicting organisms causing bacteremia in ventilated neonates. Pediatric Infectious Disease Journal 10: 290–294
617. Laurenti F, Ferro R, Isacchi G 1981 Polymorphonuclear transfusion for the treatment of sepsis in the newborn infant. Journal of Pediatrics 98: 118–123
618. Leach C T, Newton E R, McParlin S, Jenson H B 1994 Human herpesvirus 6 infection of the female genital tract. Journal of Infectious Diseases 169: 1281–1283
619. Leake D, Leake R D 1970 Neonatal suppurative parotitis. Pediatrics 46: 203–207
620. Leatherman J, Parchman M L, Lawler F H 1992 Infection of fetal scalp electrode monitoring sites. American Family Physician 45: 579–582
621. Lebech M, Petersen E 1995 Detection by enzyme immunosorbent assay of *Toxoplasma gondii* IgG antibodies in dried blood spots on PKU-filter paper from newborns. Scandinavian Journal of Infectious Diseases 27: 259–263
622. LeBlanc C M, Allen U D, Ventureyra E 1995 Cephalhematomas revisited. When should a diagnostic tap be performed? Clinical Pediatrics (Philadelphia) 34: 86–89
623. Lederman S A 1992 Estimating infant mortality from human immunodeficiency virus and other causes in breast-feeding and bottle-feeding populations. Pediatrics 89: 290–296
624. Lee D R, Moore G W, Hutchins G M 1991 Lattice theory analysis of the relationship of hyaline membrane disease and fetal pneumonia in 96 perinatal autopsies. Pediatric Pathology 11: 223–233
625. Lee K K, Vargo L R, Le C T, Fernando L 1992 Transfusion-acquired hepatitis A outbreak from fresh frozen plasma in a neonatal intensive care unit. Pediatric Infectious Disease Journal 11: 122–123
626. Lee R V 1988 Parasites and pregnancy: the problems of malaria and toxoplasmosis. Clinics in Perinatology 15: 351–363
627. Leib S L, Kim Y S, Ferriero D M, Tuber M G 1996 Neuroprotective effect of excitatory amino acid antagonist kynurenic acid in experimental bacterial meningitis. Journal of Infectious Diseases 173: 166–171
628. Leigh L, Stoll B J, Rahman M, McGowan J J 1995 *Pseudomonas aeruginosa* infection in very low birth weight infants: a case-control study. Pediatric Infectious Disease Journal 14: 367–371
629. Lejeune B, Baron R, Guillois B, Mayeux D 1991 Evaluation of a screening test for detecting urinary tract infection in newborns and infants. Journal of Clinical Pathology 44: 1029–1030
630. Lennon D, Lewis B, Mantell C et al 1984 Epidemic perinatal listeriosis. Pediatric Infectious Disease Journal 3: 30–34

631. Leroy V, De Clercq A, Ladner J, Bogaerts J, Van de Perre P, Dabis F 1995 Should screening of genital infections be part of antenatal care in areas of high HIV prevalence? A prospective cohort study from Kigali, Rwanda, 1992–1993. The Pregnancy and HIV (EGE) Group. Genitourinary Medicine 71: 207–211
632. Levin T L, Schulman M, Zieba P, Goldman H S 1994 Absence of lower extremity ossification centers in term infants with congenital syphilis. Journal of Perinatology 14: 106–109
633. Levine C D 1991 Premature rupture of the membranes and sepsis in preterm neonates. Nursing Research 40: 36–41
634. Lewis L L 1992 Congenital syphilis. Serologic diagnosis in the young infant. Infectious Disease Clinics of North America 6: 31–39
635. Libman M D, Dascal A, Kramer M S, Mendelson J 1991 Strategies for the prevention of neonatal infection with herpes simplex virus: a decision analysis. Review of Infectious Diseases 13: 1093–1104
636. Light T J 1979 Postnatal acquisition of herpes simplex virus by the newborn infant: a review of the literature. Pediatrics 63: 480–482
637. Lilien L D, Harris V J, Ramamurthy R S, Pildes R S 1976 Neonatal osteomyelitis of the calcaneus: complication of heel puncture. Journal of Pediatrics 88: 478–480
638. Lilien L D, Harris V J, Pildes R S 1977 Significance of radiographic findings in early onset Group B streptococcal infection. Pediatrics 60: 360–363
639. Lin H H, Kao J H, Hsu H Y et al 1995 Absence of infection in breast-fed infants born to hepatitis C virus-infected mothers. Journal of Pediatrics 126: 589–591
640. Lin H H, Kao J H, Hsu H Y et al 1994 Possible role of high-titer maternal viremia in perinatal transmission of hepatitis C virus. Journal of Infectious Diseases 169: 638–641
641. Linder N, Ohel G, Gazit G, Keidar D, Tamir I, Reichman B 1995 Neonatal sepsis after prolonged premature rupture of membranes. Journal of Perinatology 15: 36–38
642. Lissauer T 1989 Impact of AIDS on neonatal care. Archives of Disease in Childhood 64: 4–7
643. Littlewood J M 1972 66 infants with urinary tract infection in the first month of life. Archives of Disease in Childhood 47: 218–226
644. Littlewood J M, Kite P, Kite B 1969 Incidence of neonatal urinary tract infection. Archives of Disease in Childhood 44: 617–621
645. Lloyd D J, Belgaumkar T K, Scott K C, Wort A J, Aterman K, Krause V W 1979 Prevention of Group B beta-haemolytic streptococcal septicaemia in low birth-weight neonates by penicillin administered within 2 hours of birth. Lancet i: 713–715
646. Lohrer R, Belohradsky B H 1987 Bacterial endophthalmitis in neonates. European Journal of Pediatrics 146: 354–359
647. Loke H L, Verber I, Szymonowicz W, Yu V Y H 1988 Systemic candidiasis and pneumonia in preterm infants. Australian Pediatric Journal 24: 138–142
648. Lopez Alarcon M, Villalpando S, Fajardo A 1997 Breast-feeding lowers the frequency and duration of acute respiratory infection and diarrhea in infants under six months of age. Journal of Nutrition 127: 436–443
649. Lorber J 1974 Neonatal bacterial meningitis. Medicine (Baltimore) 27: 1579–1582
650. Low D E, Schmidt B K, Kirpalani H M et al 1992 An endemic strain of *Staphylococcus hemolyticus* colonizing and causing bacteremia in neonatal intensive care unit patients. Pediatrics 89: 696–700
651. Luck P C, Dinger E, Helbig J H et al 1994 Analysis of *Legionella pneumophila* strains associated with nosocomial pneumonia in a neonatal intensive care unit. European Journal of Clinical Microbiology and Infectious Diseases 13: 565–571
652. Lyon A J 1996 Genital mycoplasmas and infection in the neonate. In: Hansen T N, McIntosh N (eds) Current topics in neonatology. W B Saunders, Philadelphia, pp 1–20
653. Maberry M C, Ramin S M, Gilstrap L C, Leveno K L, Dax J S 1990 Intrapartum asphyxia in pregnancies complicated by intra-amniotic infection. Obstetrics and Gynecology 76: 351–354
654. McCabe K M, Khan G, Zhang Y H, Mason E O, McCabe E R 1995 Amplification of bacterial DNA using highly conserved sequences: automated analysis and potential for molecular triage of sepsis. Pediatrics 95: 165–169
655. McCarthy A E, Victor G, Ramotar K, Toye B 1994 Risk factors for acquiring ampicillin-resistant enterococci and clinical outcomes at a Canadian tertiary-care hospital. Journal of Clinical Microbiology 32: 2671–2676
656. McCracken G H 1984 Management of bacterial meningitis; current status and future prospects. American Journal of Medicine 76: 215–223
657. McCracken G H, Mize S G 1976 A controlled study of intrathecal antibiotic therapy in Gram negative enteric meningitis of infancy. Journal of Pediatrics 89: 66–72
658. McCracken G H, Mize S G, Threkeld N 1980 Intraventricular gentamicin therapy for gram-negative bacillary meningitis in infancy. Lancet i: 787–791
659. McCracken G H, Nelson J D 1983 Antimicrobial therapy for newborns 2nd Edn. Grune & Stratton, New York
660. McDermott J, Steketee R, Wirima J 1996 Perinatal mortality in rural Malawi. Bulletin of the World Health Organization 74: 165–171
661. McDougal A, Ling E W, Levine M 1995 Vancomycin pharmacokinetics and dosing in premature neonates. The Drug Monitor 17: 319–326
662. McDuffie R S J, McGregor J A, Gibbs R S 1993 Adverse perinatal outcome and resistant Enterobacteriaceae after antibiotic usage for premature rupture of the membranes and group B streptococcus carriage. Obstetrics and Gynecology 82: 487–489
663. McFall T L, Zimmerman G A, Augustine N H, Hill H R 1987 Effect of group B streptococcal type-specific antigen on polymorphonuclear leucocyte function and polymorphonuclear leucocyte endothelial cell interaction. Pediatric Research 21: 517–523
664. MacGowan A P, Cartlidge P H, MacLeod F, McLaughlin J, Maternal listeriosis in pregnancy without fetal or neonatal infection. Journal of Infection 22: 53–57
665. MacGowan A P, O'Donaghue K, Nicholls S, McLauchlin J, Bennett P M, Reeves D S 1993 Typing of *Listeria* spp. by random amplified polymorphic DNA (RAPD) analysis. Journal of Medical Microbiology 38: 322–327
666. McGregor I A 1984 Epidemiology, malaria and pregnancy. American Journal of Tropical Medicine and Hygiene 33: 517–525
667. McGregor I A, Wilson M E, Billewicz W Z 1983 Malaria infection of the placenta in the Gambia, West Africa; its incidence and relationship to stillbirth, birthweight and placental weight. Transactions of the Royal Society of Tropical Medicine and Hygiene 77: 232–244
668. McGregor J A, French J L 1991 *Chlamydia trachomatis* infection during pregnancy. American Journal of Obstetrics and Gynecology 164: 1782–1789
669. McGregor J A, French J I, Seo K 1991 Antimicrobial therapy in preterm premature rupture of membranes: results of a prospective, double-blind, placebo-controlled trial of erythromycin. American Journal of Obstetrics and Gynecology 165: 632–640
670. McGregor J A, McFarren T 1989 Neonatal cranial osteomyelitis: a complication of fetal monitoring. Obstetrics and Gynecology 73: 490–492
671. McIntosh D, Isaacs D 1992 Herpes simplex virus infection in pregnancy. Archives of Disease in Childhood 67: 1137–1138
672. McIntosh N, Harrison A 1994 Prolonged premature rupture of membranes in the preterm infant: a 7 year study. European Journal of Obstetrics Gynecology and Reproductive Biology 57: 1–6
673. McKenna H, Johnson D 1977 Bacteria in neonatal omphalitis Pathology 9: 111–113
674. Mackenzie A, Johnson W, Heyes B, Norrish B, Jamieson F 1995 A prolonged outbreak of exfoliative toxin A-producing *Staphylococcus aureus* in a newborn nursery. Diagnostic Microbiology and Infectious Disease 21: 69–75
675. McLaren L C, Davis L E, Healy G R, James C G 1983 Isolation of *Trichomonas vaginalis* from the respiratory tract of infants with respiratory disease. Pediatrics 71: 888–890
676. McLaren R A, Chauhan S P, Gross T L 1996 Intrapartum factors in early-onset group B streptococcal sepsis in term neonates: a case-control study. American Journal of Obstetrics and Gynecology 174: 1934–1937
677. Madge P, Paton J Y, McColl J H, Mackie P L 1992 Prospective controlled study of four infection-control procedures to prevent nosocomial infection with respiratory syncytial virus. Lancet 340: 1079–1083
678. Magliocco A M, Demetrick D J, Sarnat H B, Hwang W S 1992 Varicella embryopathy. Archives of Pathology and Laboratory Medicine 116: 181–186
679. Magny J F, Bremard Oury C, Brault D, Menguy C, Voyer M, Landais P 1991 Intravenous immunoglobulin therapy for prevention

of infection in high-risk premature infants: report of a multi-centre, double-blind study. Pediatrics 88: 437–443
680. Maherzi M, Guignard J P, Torrado A 1978 Urinary tract infection in high-risk newborn infants. Pediatrics 62: 521–524
681. Mahon B E, Yamada E G, Newman T B 1994 Problems with serum IgM as a screening test for congenital infection. Clinical Pediatrics (Philadelphia) 33: 142–146
682. Malathi I, Millar M R, Leeming J P, Hedges A, Marlow N 1993 Skin disinfection in preterm infants. Archives of Disease in Childhood 69: 312–316
683. Malik S, Giacoia G P, West K, Miller G 1990 Intravenous immunoglobulin to prevent infections in infants with bronchopulmonary dysplasia. Pediatric Research 27: 273A
684. Malm G, Berg U, Forsgren M 1995 Neonatal herpes simplex: clinical findings and outcome in relation to type of maternal infection. Acta Paediatrica 84: 256–260
685. Malm G, Forsgren M, el Azazi M, Persson A 1991 A follow-up study of children with neonatal herpes simplex virus infections with particular regard to late nervous disturbances. Acta Paediatrica Scandinavica 80: 226–234
686. Malouf D J, Oates R K 1995 Herpes simplex virus infections in the neonate. Journal of Paediatrics and Child Health 31: 332–335
687. Mandar R, Mikelsaar M 1996 Transmission of mother's microflora to the newborn at birth. Biology of the Neonate 69: 30–35
688. Manroe B L, Rosenfield C R, Weinberg A G, Browne R 1977 The differential leucocyte count in the assessment and outcome of early onset Group B streptococcal disease. Journal of Pediatrics 91: 632–637
689. Manroe B L, Weinberg A G, Rosenfield C R, Browne R 1979 The neonatal blood count in health and disease. I. Reference values for neutrophilic cells. Journal of Pediatrics 95: 89–98
690. Mansergh G, Haddix A C, Steketee R W et al 1996 Cost-effectiveness of short-course zidovudine to prevent perinatal HIV type 1 infection in a sub-Saharan African developing country setting. Journal of the American Medical Association 276: 139–145
691. Marcus R and the CDC Co-operative Needlestick Surveillance Group 1988 Surveillance of health care workers exposed to blood from patients infected with human immunodeficiency virus. New England Journal of Medicine 319: 1118–1193
692. Mårdh P A, Johansson B J H, Svenningsen N 1984 Intrauterine lung infection with *Chlamydia trachomatis* in a premature infant. Acta Paediatrica Scandinavica 73: 569–572
693. Martin D J 1985 Neonatal disorders diagnosed with ultrasound. Clinics in Perinatology 12: 219–231
694. Mason W H, Andrews R, Ross L A, Wright H T 1989 Omphalitis in the newborn infant. Pediatric Infectious Disease Journal 8: 521–525
695. Mathers N J, Pohlandt F 1987 Diagnostic audit of C reactive protein in neonatal infection. European Journal of Pediatrics 146: 147–151
696. Matsuda Y, Maruyama H, Kuraya K 1995 Relationship between granulocyte elastase levels and perinatal infections. Gynecologic and Obstetric Investigation 39: 162–166
697. Matsui D 1994 Prevention, diagnosis, and treatment of fetal toxoplasmosis. Clinics in Perinatology 21: 675–689
698. Matsuoka T, Naito T, Kubota Y et al 1990 Disseminated adenovirus (Type 19) infection in a neonate. Acta Paediatrica Scandinavica 79: 568–571
699. Mauskopf J A, Paul J E, Wichman D S, White A D, Tilson H H 1996 Economic impact of treatment of HIV-positive pregnant women and their newborns with zidovudine. Implications for HIV screening. Journal of the American Medical Association 276: 132–138
700. Mayaux M J, Burgard M, Teglas J P 1996 Neonatal characteristics in rapidly progressive perinatally acquired HIV-1 disease. Journal of the American Medical Association 275: 606–610
701. Mayon White D, Holm S E, Christensen P (eds) 1982 Basic concepts of streptococci and streptococcal diseases. Reedbooks Ltd, Chertsey
702. Mazel J A, Schalm S W, de Gast B C, Nuijten A S M, Heijtink R A, Botman M J 1984 Passive-active immunisation of neonates of HBsAg positive carrier mothers: preliminary observations. British Medical Journal 288: 513–515
703. Mazur J M, Ross G, Cummings J, Hahn G A J, McCluskey W P 1995 Usefulness of magnetic resonance imaging for the diagnosis of acute musculoskeletal infections in children. Journal of Pediatric Orthopedics 15: 144–147
704. Meadow W L, Schwartz I K 1986 Time course of detection of positive blood cultures in childhood. Pediatric Infectious Disease Journal 5: 333–336
705. Mecrow I K, Ladusans E J 1994 Infective endocarditis in newborn infants with structurally normal hearts. Acta Paediatrica 83: 35–39
706. Meisel R L, Alvarez M, Lynch L, Chitkara U, Emanuel D J, Berkowitz RL 1990 Fetal cytomegalovirus infection: a case report. American Journal of Obstetrics and Gynecology 162: 663–664
707. Meissner H C, Murray S A, Kiernan M A, Snydman D R, McIntosh K 1984 A simultaneous outbreak of respiratory syncytial virus and parainfluenza virus type 3 in the newborn nursery. Journal of Pediatrics 104: 680–684
708. Meissner H C, Welliver R C, Chartrand S A, Fulton D R, Rodriguez W J, Groothuis J R 1996 Prevention of respiratory syncytial virus infection in high risk infants: consensus opinion on the role of immunoprophylaxis with respiratory syncytial virus hyperimmune globulin. Pediatric Infectious Disease Journal 15: 1059–1068
709. Melsom R, Harboe M, Duncan M E 1982 IgA, IgM and IgG anti-*M leprae* antibodies in babies of leprosy mothers during the first 2 years of life. Clinical and Experimental Immunology 49: 532–540
710. Melville C, Kempley S, Graham J, Berry C L 1996 Early onset systemic *Candida* infection in extremely preterm neonates. European Journal of Pediatrics 155: 904–906
711. Memon I A, Jacobs N M, Yeh T F, Lilien L D 1979 Group B streptococcal osteomyelitis and septic arthritis. Its occurrence in infants less than 2 months old. American Journal of Diseases of Children 133: 921–923
712. Mendoza J C, Roberts J L 1991 Early-onset *Hemophilus influenzae* sepsis in the neonate. Journal of Perinatology 11: 126–129
713. Mercer B M, Arheart K L 1995 Antimicrobial therapy in expectant management of preterm premature rupture of the membranes. Lancet 346: 1271–1279
714. Merenstein G B, Weisman L E 1996 Premature rupture of the membranes: neonatal consequences. Seminars in Perinatology 20: 375–380
715. Meyer C L, Payne N R, Roback S A 1991 Spontaneous, isolated intestinal perforations in neonates with birth weight less than 1,000 g not associated with necrotizing enterocolitis. Journal of Pediatric Surgery 26: 714–717
716. Midani S, Rathore M H 1997 Polymerase chain reaction testing for early detection of HIV infection in children. Southern Medical Journal 90: 294–295
717. Mikati M A, Krishnamoorthy K S 1985 Hypoglycorrhachia in neonatal herpes simplex virus meningoencephalitis. Journal of Pediatrics 107: 746–748
718. Millar M R, Bacon C, Smith S L, Walker V, Hall M A 1993 Enteral feeding of premature infants with *Lactobacillus* GG. Archives of Disease in Childhood 69: 483–487
719. Millar M R, MacKay P, Levene M, Langdale V, Martin C 1992 Enterobacteriaceae and neonatal necrotising enterocolitis. Archives of Disease in Childhood. 67: 53–56
720. Millard D D, Shulman S T 1988 The changing spectrum of neonatal endocarditis. Clinics in Perinatology 15: 587–608
721. Miller E 1991 Rubella in the United Kingdom. Epidemiology and Infection 107: 31–42
722. Miller E, Craddock-Watson J E, Pollock T M 1982 Consequences of confirmed maternal rubella at successive states of pregnancy. Lancet ii: 781–784
723. Miller E, Craddock-Watson J E, Ridehalgh M K S 1989 Outcome in newborn babies given anti-varicella-zoster immunoglobulin after perinatal maternal infection with varicella-zoster virus. Lancet ii: 371–373
724. Miller E, Tookey P, Morgan Capner P et al 1994 Rubella surveillance to June 1994: third joint report from the PHLS and the National Congenital Rubella Surveillance Programme. Communicable Disease Report CDR Review 4: R146–152
725. Minkoff H, Burns D N, Landesman S et al 1995 The relationship of the duration of ruptured membranes to vertical transmission of human immunodeficiency virus. American Journal of Obstetrics and Gynecology 173: 585–589
726. Mitchell C S, Erlich S S, Mastrucci M T, Hutton S C, Parks W P, Scott G B 1990 Congenital toxoplasmosis occurring in infants perinatally infected with human immunodeficiency virus 1. Pediatric Infectious Disease Journal 9: 512–518
727. Mittal S K, Rao S, Rastogi A, Aggarwal V, Kumari S 1996 Hepatitis B

– potential of perinatal transmission in India. Tropical Gastroenterology 17: 190–192
728. Modlin J F 1986 Perinatal echovirus infection: insights from a literature review of 61 cases of serious infection and 16 outbreaks in nurseries. Reviews of Infectious Diseases 8: 918–926
729. Modlin J F 1988 Perinatal echovirus and group B Coxsackie virus infections. Clinics in Perinatology 15: 233–246
730. Mohon R T, Mehalic R F, Grimes C K, Philip A G S 1986 Infected cephalhematoma and neonatal osteomyelitis of the skull. Pediatric Infectious Disease Journal 5: 253–256
731. Mok J 1991 HIV infection in children: millions will suffer. British Medical Journal 302: 921–922
732. Mok P M, Reilly R J, Ash J M 1982 Osteomyelitis in the neonate. Radiology 145: 677–682
733. Mollison P L, Engelfriet C P, Contreras M 1987 Blood transfusion in clinical medicine, 8th Edn. Blackwell Scientific Publications, Oxford, p 795
734. Mongi P S, Mbise R L, Msengi A E, Amsi O M D 1987 Tetanus neonatorum – experience with intrathecal serotherapy at Mumimbili Medical Centre, Dar es Salaam, Tanzania. Annals of Tropical Paediatrics 7: 27–31
735. Monneret G, Labaune J M, Isaac C, Bienvenu F, Putet G, Bienvenu J 1997 Procalcitonin and C-reactive protein levels in neonatal infections. Acta Paediatrica 86: 209–212
736. Montone K T, Furth E E, Pietra G G, Gupta P K 1995 Neonatal adenovirus infection: a case report with in situ hybridization confirmation of ascending intrauterine infection. Diagnostic Cytopathology 12: 341–344
737. Morey A L, Porter H J, Keeling J W, Fleming K A 1992 Non-isotopic in-situ hybridisation and immunophenotyping of infected cells in the investigation of human fetal parvovirus infection. Journal of Clinical Pathology 45: 673–678
738. Morgan H G 1994 Placental malaria and low birthweight neonates in urban Sierra Leone. Annals of Tropical Medicine and Parasitology 88: 575–580
739. Morrison J, Alp N J 1997 Vertical transmission of human immunodeficiency virus. Quarterly Journal of Medicine 90: 5–12
740. Morrow A L, Reves R R, West M S, Guerrero M L, Ruiz Palacios G M, Pickering L K 1992 Protection against infection with *Giardia lamblia* by breast-feeding in a cohort of Mexican infants. Journal of Pediatrics 121: 363–370
741. Mouzinho A, Rosenfeld C R, Sanchez P J, Risser R 1992 Effect of maternal hypertension on neonatal neutropenia and risk of nosocomial infection. Pediatrics 90: 430–435
742. Mouzinho A, Rosenfeld C R, Sanchez P J, Risser R 1994 Revised reference ranges for circulating neutrophils in very-low-birth-weight neonates. Pediatrics 94: 76–82
743. Moye J, Rich K C, Kalish L A et al 1996 Natural history of somatic growth in infants born to women infected by human immunodeficiency virus. Women and Infants Transmission Study Group. Journal of Pediatrics 128: 58–69
744. Much D H, Yeh S Y 1991 Prevalence of *Chlamydia trachomatis* infection in pregnant patients. Public Health Report 106: 490–493
745. Mulder C J J, Zanen H C 1984 A study of 280 cases of neonatal meningitis in the Netherlands. Journal of Infection 9: 177–184
746. Mulder C J J, van Alphen L, Zanen H C 1984 Neonatal meningitis caused by *Escherichia coli* in the Netherlands. Journal of Infectious Diseases 150: 935–940
747. Mulder D W, Nunn A, Kamali A et al 1996 Post-natal incidence of HIV-1 infection among children in a rural Ugandan population: no evidence of transmission other than mother to child. Tropical Medicine and International Health 1: 81–85
748. Mullens A 1996 'I think we have a problem in Victoria': MDs respond quickly to toxoplasmosis outbreak in BC. Canadian Medical Association Journal 154: 1721–1724
749. Mulloy R H, Jadavji T, Russell M L 1991 Tunneled central venous catheter sepsis: risk factors in a pediatric hospital. Journal of Parenteral and Enteral Nutrition 15: 460–463
750. Munro N D, Sheppard S, Smithells R W, Holzel H, Jones G 1987 Temporal relations between maternal rubella and congenital defects. Lancet ii: 201–204
751. Myers J D 1974 Congenital varicella in term infants: risk reconsidered. Journal of Infectious Diseases 129: 215–216
752. Nadal D, Hunziker U A, Schupbach J et al 1989 Immunological evaluation in the early diagnosis in prenatal or perinatal HIV infection. Archives of Disease in Childhood 64: 662–669
753. Nagelkerke N J, Moses S, Embree J E et al 1995 The duration of breastfeeding by HIV-infected mothers in developing countries: balancing benefits and risks. Journal of Acquired Immune Deficiency Syndrome and Human Retrovirology 8: 176–181
754. Nagington J, Wreghitt T G, Gandy G M, Roberton N R C, Berry P J 1978 Fatal Echovirus 11 infections in outbreak in special care baby unit. Lancet ii: 725–728
755. Nagington J, Gandy G M, Walker J, Gray J J 1983 Use of normal immunoglobulin in an Echo 11 outbreak in a special care baby unit. Lancet ii: 443–446
756. Nahmias A, Whitley R, Vistine A M 1982 Herpes simplex virus encephalitis: laboratory evaluations and their diagnostic significance. Journal of Infectious Diseases 145: 829–836
757. Nahmias A J, Keyserling H L, Kerrick G M 1983 Herpes simplex. In Remington J S, Klein J O (eds) Infectious diseases of the fetus and newborn infant, 2nd Edn. Saunders, Philadelphia, pp 636–678
757a. Nakashima A K, Rolfs R T, Flock M L, Greenspan J R 1996 Epidemiology of syphilis in the United States. Sexually Transmitted Diseases 23: 16–23
758. Nankervis G A, Gold E, Kaplan A S (eds) 1973 The herpesviruses. Academic Press, New York, pp 327–333
759. Narendran V, Gupta G, Todd D A, John E 1996 Bacterial colonization of indwelling vascular catheters in newborn infants. Journal of Paediatrics and Child Health 32: 391–396
760. Neligan G A, Steiner H, Gardner P S, McQuillin J 1970 Respiratory syncytial virus infection of the newborn. British Medical Journal iii: 146–147
761. Nelson C T, Istas A S, Wilkerson M K, Demmler G J 1995 PCR detection of cytomegalovirus DNA in serum as a diagnostic test for congenital cytomegalovirus infection. Journal of Clinical Microbiology 33: 3317–3318
762. Nelson K E, Warren D, Tomasi A M, Raju T N, Vidyasagar D 1985 Transmission of neonatal listeriosis in a delivery room. American Journal of Diseases of Children 139: 903–905
763. Neumeister B, Kastner S, Conrad S, Klotz G, Bartmann P 1995 Characterization of coagulase-negative staphylococci causing nosocomial infections in preterm infants. European Journal of Clinical Microbiology and Infectious Diseases 14: 856–863
764. Newell M L, Dunn D T, De Maria A 1996 Detection of virus in vertically exposed HIV antibody negative children. Lancet 347: 213–215
765. Ng P C 1994 Systemic fungal infections in neonates. Archives of Disease in Childhood 71: F130–135
766. Ng P C, Hiu J, Fok T F, Nelson E A, Cheung K L, Wong W 1995 Isolated congenital tuberculosis otitis in a preterm infant. Acta Paediatrica 84: 955–956
767. Ng P C, Herrington R A, Beane C A, Ghonheim A T M, Dear P R F 1989 An outbreak of acinetobacter septicaemia in a neonatal intensive care unit. Journal of Hospital Infection 14: 363–368
768. Ng P C, Lyon D J, Wong M Y et al 1996 Varicella exposure in a neonatal intensive care unit: emergency management and control measures. Journal of Hospital Infection 32: 229–236
769. Ng P C, Siu Y K, Lewindon P J, Wong W, Cheung K L, Dawkins R 1994 Congenital *Candida* pneumonia in a preterm infant. Journal of Paediatrics and Child Health 30: 552–554
770. Nicolini U, Kustermann A, Tassis B et al 1994 Prenatal diagnosis of congenital human cytomegalovirus infection. Prenatal Diagnosis 14: 903–906
771. Nicoll J A, Love S, Burton P A, Berry P J 1994 Autopsy findings in two cases of neonatal herpes simplex virus infection: detection of virus by immunohistochemistry, in situ hybridization and the polymerase chain reaction. Histopathology 24: 257–264
772. Nigro G, Clerico A, Mondaini C 1993 Symptomatic congenital cytomegalovirus infection in two consecutive sisters. Archives of Disease in Childhood 69: 527–528
773. Nigro G, Scholz H, Bartmann U 1994 Ganciclovir therapy for symptomatic congenital cytomegalovirus infection in infants: a two-regimen experience. Journal of Pediatrics 124: 318–322
774. Niu M T, Targonski P V, Stoll B J, Albert G P, Margolis H S 1992 Prevention of perinatal transmission of the hepatitis B virus. Outcome of infants in a community prevention program. American Journal of Diseases of Childhood 146: 793–796

775. Noble R C, Kane M A, Reeves S A, Roeckel I 1984 Post transfusion hepatitis A in a neonatal intensive care unit. Journal of the American Medical Association 252: 2711–2715
776. Noel G J, Edelson P J 1984 *Staphylococcus epidermidis* bacteremia in neonates: further observations and the occurrence of focal infection. Pediatrics 74: 832–837
777. Noel G J, O'Loughlin J E, Edelson P J 1988 Neonatal *Staphylococcus epidermidis* right sided endocarditis: description of 5 catheterized infants. Pediatrics 82: 234–239
778. Nyambi P N, Ville Y, Louwagie J et al 1996 Mother-to-child transmission of human T-cell lymphotropic virus types I and II (HTLV-I/II) in Gabon: a prospective follow-up of 4 years. Journal of Acquired Immune Deficiency Syndrome and Human Retrovirology 12: 187–192
779. Nyirjesy P, Kavasya T, Axelrod P, Fischer P R 1993 Malaria during pregnancy: neonatal morbidity and mortality and the efficacy of chloroquine chemoprophylaxis. Clinical Infectious Diseases 16: 127–132
780. Nyquist A C, Rotbart H A, Cotton M et al 1994 Acyclovir-resistant neonatal herpes simplex virus infection of the larynx. Journal of Pediatrics 124: 967–971
781. O'Brien K L, Ruff A J, Louis M A et al 1995 Bacillus Calmette–Guérin complications in children born to HIV-1 infected women with a review of the literature. Pediatrics 95: 414–417
782. O'Callaghan C, McDougall P 1988 Infective endocarditis in neonates. Archives of Disease in Childhood 63: 53–57
783. O'Connor T A, Ringer K M, Gaddis M L 1993 Mean platelet volume during coagulase-negative staphylococcal sepsis in neonates. American Journal of Clinical Pathology 99: 69–71
784. Oda K, Oki S, Tsumura N, Nakao M, Motohiro T, Kato H 1995 Detection of cytomegalovirus DNA in urine from newborns in NICU using a polymerase chain reaction. Kurume Medical Journal 42: 39–44
785. Oelberg D G, Fisher D G, Gross D M, Denson S E, Adcock E W 1983 Endocarditis in high risk neonates. Pediatrics 71: 392–397
786. O'Garra A 1989 Interleukins and the immune system. Lancet ii: 943–946
787. Ogden J A, Lister G 1975 The pathology of neonatal osteomyelitis. Pediatrics 55: 474–478
788. Ohlsson A, Myhr T L 1994 Intrapartum penicillin prophylaxis of early-onset streptococcal infection. Canadian Medical Association Journal 150: 1197–1198
789. Ohlsson A, Myhr T L 1994 Intrapartum chemoprophylaxis of perinatal group B streptococcal infections: a critical review of randomized controlled trials. American Journal of Obstetrics and Gynecology 170: 910–917
790. Ohman L, Tullus K, Katouli M, Burman L G, Stendahl O 1995 Correlation between susceptibility of infants to infections and interaction with neutrophils of *Escherichia coli* strains causing neonatal and infantile septicemia. Journal of Infectious Diseases 171: 128–133
791. Ohto H, Terazawa S, Sasaki N et al 1994 Transmission of hepatitis C virus from mothers to infants. The Vertical Transmission of hepatitis C Virus Collaborative Study Group. New England Journal of Medicine 330: 744–750
792. Okada K, Yamada T, Miyakawa A Y, Mayumi M 1975 Hepatitis B surface antigen in the serum of infants after delivery from asymptomatic carrier mothers. Journal of Pediatrics 87: 360–363
793. Ollikainen J, Hiekkaniemi H, Korppi M, Sarkkinen H, Heinonen K 1993 *Ureaplasma urealyticum* infection associated with acute respiratory insufficiency and death in premature infants. Journal of Pediatrics 122: 756–760
794. Olowe S A 1975 A case of congenital trypanosomiasis in Lagos. Transactions of the Royal Society of Tropical Medicine and Hygiene 69: 57–59
795. Osman N B, Folgosa E, Gonzales C, Bergstrom S 1995 Genital infections in the aetiology of late fetal death: an incident case-referent study. Journal of Tropical Pediatrics 41: 258–266
796. Overall J C J 1994 Herpes simplex virus infection of the fetus and newborn. Pediatric Annals 23: 131–136
797. Overall J C, Glasgow L A 1970 Virus infections of the fetus and newborn infant. Journal of Pediatrics 77: 315–333
798. Ozdemir A, Oygur N, Gultekin M, Coskun M, Yegin O 1994 Neonatal tumor necrosis factor, interleukin-1 alpha, interleukin-1 beta, and interleukin-6 response to infection. American Journal of Perinatology 11: 282–285
799. Paccagnini S, Principi N, Massironi E et al 1998 Perinatal transmission and manifestation of hepatitis C virus infection in a high risk population. Pediatric Infectious Disease Journal 14: 195–199
800. Palasanthiran P, Ziegler J B, Dwyer D E 1994 Early detection of human immunodeficiency virus infection in Australian infants at risk of infection and factors affecting transmission. Pediatric Infectious Disease Journal 13: 1083–1090
801. Palasanthiran P, Ziegler J B, Stewart G J et al 1993 Breast-feeding during primary maternal human immunodeficiency virus infection and risk of transmission from mother to infant. Journal of Infectious Diseases 167: 441–444
802. Paludetto R, van den Heuvel J, Stagni A, Grappone L, Mansi G 1994 Rubella embryopathy after maternal reinfection. Biology of the Neonate 65: 340–341
803. Panero C, Azzi A, Carbone C, Pezzati M, Mainardi G, di Lollo S 1994 Fetoneonatal hydrops from human parvovirus B19. Case report. Journal of Perinatal Medicine 22: 257–264
804. Partridge J W, Flewett T H, Whitehead J E M 1981 Congenital rubella infecting an infant whose mother had rubella antibodies before conception. British Medical Journal 282: 187–189
805. Paryani S G, Arvin A M 1986 Intrauterine infection with varicella-zoster-virus after maternal varicella. New England Journal of Medicine 314: 1542–1546
806. Paryani S G, Yeager A S, Hosford-Dunn H et al 1985 Sequelae of acquired cytomegalovirus infection in premature and sick term infants: Journal of Pediatrics 107: 451–456
807. Pastuszak A L, Levy M, Schick B et al 1994 Outcome after maternal varicella infection in the first 20 weeks of pregnancy. New England Journal of Medicine 330: 901–905
808. Pasvol G, Weatherall D J, Wilson R J M, Smith D H, Gilles H M 1976 Fetal haemoglobin and malaria. Lancet i: 1269–1272
809. Patou G, Midgeley P, Meurisse E V, Feldman R G 1990 Immunoglobulin prophylaxis for infants exposed to varicella in the neonatal unit. Journal of Infection 20: 207–213
810. Patrick C C 1990 Coagulase negative staphylococci; pathogens with increasing clinical significance. Journal of Pediatrics 116: 497–507
811. Patrick C C, Kaplan S L, Baker C J, Parisi J T, Mason E O 1989 Persistent bacteremia due to coagulase negative staphylococci in low birthweight neonates. Pediatrics 84: 977–985
812. Patrick C H, John J F, Levkoff A H, Atkins L M 1992 Relatedness of strains of methicillin-resistant coagulase-negative staphylococcus colonizing hospital personnel and producing bacteremias in a neonatal intensive care unit. Pediatric Infectious Disease Journal 11: 935–940
813. Paul M O, Tetali S, Lesser M L et al 1996 Laboratory diagnosis of infection status in infants perinatally exposed to human immunodeficiency virus type 1. Journal of Infectious Diseases 173: 68–76
814. Payne N R, Burke B A, Day D L, Christenson P D, Thompson T R, Ferrieri P 1988 Correlation of clinical and pathological findings in early onset neonatal Group B streptococcal infection with disease severity and prediction of outcome. Pediatric Infectious Disease Journal 7: 836–847
815. Paz I, Seidman D S, Mashiach S, Stevenson D K 1994 Maternal transmission of human immunodeficiency virus. Obstetric and Gynecologic Survey 49: 577–584
816. Pearl K N, Preece P M, Ades A, Peckham C S 1986 Neurodevelopmental assessment after congenital cytomegalovirus infection. Archives of Disease in Childhood 62: 323–326
817. Peckham C 1972 Clinical and laboratory study of children exposed in utero to maternal rubella. Archives of Disease in Childhood 47: 571–577
818. Peckham C, Logan S 1993 Screening for toxoplasmosis during pregnancy. Archives of Disease in Childhood 68: 3–5
819. Peckham C S, Stark O, Dudgeon J A, Martin J A M, Hawkins G 1987 Congenital cytomegalovirus infection: a cause of sensorineural hearing loss. Archives of Disease in Childhood 62: 1233–1237
820. Peevy K J, Chalhub E G 1983 Occult group B streptococcal infection: an important cause of intrauterine asphyxia. American Journal of Obstetrics and Gynecology 146: 989–990
821. Pejaver R K, Watson A H, Mucklow E S 1993 Neonatal cross-infection with *Listeria monocytogenes*. Journal of Infection 26: 301–303
822. Pekkala D H, Low D E, Wyper P A et al 1992 The utility of restriction endonuclease analysis and phage typing in the epidemiologic investigation of a *Staphylococcus aureus* outbreak in a

neonatal nursery. Diagnostic Microbiology and Infectious Disease 15: 307–311

823. Peng J, Krause P J, Kresch M 1996 Neonatal herpes simplex virus infection after cesarean section with intact amniotic membranes. Journal of Perinatology 16: 397–399
824. Perez Benavides F, Park J M, Myers M K, Graham S C, Shehata B M 1993 Sudden death in neonate with staphylococcal endocarditis. Journal of Perinatology 13: 285–287
825. Perlman J M, Argyle C 1992 Lethal cytomegalovirus infection in preterm infants: clinical, radiological, and neuropathological findings. Annals of Neurology 31: 64–68
826. Perlman J M, Rollins N, Sanchez P J 1992 Late-onset meningitis in sick, very-low-birthweight infants. Clinical and sonographic observations. American Journal of Diseases of Children 146: 1297–1301
827. Petermann S, Ernest J M 1995 Intrapartum hepatitis B screening. American Journal of Obstetrics and Gynecology 173: 369–373
828. Peters G, Loscci R, Pulverer G 1982 Adherence and growth of coagulase-negative staphylococci on surfaces of intravenous catheters. Journal of Infectious Diseases 146: 479–482
829. Peters M T, Nicoliades K H 1990 Cordocentesis for the diagnosis and treatment of fetal parvovirus infection. Obstetrics and Gynecology 75: 501–504
830. Peters W, Irving J, Letts M 1992 Long-term effects of neonatal bone and joint infection on adjacent growth plates. Journal of Pediatric Orthopedics 12: 806–810
831. Philip A G S 1985 Response of C reactive protein in neonatal group B streptococcal infection. Pediatric Infectious Disease Journal 4: 145–148
832. Philip A G S 1994 The changing face of neonatal infection: experience at a regional medical center. Pediatric Infectious Disease Journal 13: 1098–1102
833. Philip A G S, Hewitt J R 1980 Early diagnosis of neonatal sepsis. Pediatrics 65: 1036–1041
834. Philipson E H, Herson V C 1996 Intrapartum chemoprophylaxis for group B streptococcus infection to prevent neonatal disease: who should be treated? American Journal of Perinatology 13: 487–490
835. Phillips J R, Karlowicz M G 1997 Prevalence of *Candida* species in hospital-acquired urinary tract infections in a neonatal intensive care unit. Pediatric Infectious Disease Journal 16: 190–194
836. Piedra P A, Kasel J A, Norton H J et al 1992 Description of an adenovirus type 8 outbreak in hospitalized neonates born prematurely. Pediatric Infectious Disease Journal 11: 460–465
837. Pinon J M, Chemla C, Villena I et al 1996 Early neonatal diagnosis of congenital toxoplasmosis: value of comparative enzyme-linked immunofiltration assay, immunological profiles and anti-*Toxoplasma gondii* immunoglobulin M (IgM) or IgA immunocapture and implications for postnatal therapeutic strategies. Journal of Clinical Microbiology 34: 579–583
838. Pisacane A, Graziano L, Mazzarella G, Scarpellino B, Zona G 1992 Breast-feeding and urinary tract infection. Journal of Pediatrics 120: 87–89
839. Pitt J, Brambilla D, Reichelderfer P 1997 Maternal immunologic and virologic risk factors for infant human immunodeficiency virus type 1 infection: findings from the Women and Infants Transmission Study. Journal of Infectious Diseases 175: 567–575
840. Pittard W B, Thullen J D, Fanaroff A A 1976 Neonatal septic arthritis. Journal of Pediatrics 88: 621–624
841. Polak A 1988 Combination therapy with antifungal drugs. Mykoses 31 (suppl. 2): 45–53
842. Polakoff S, Vandervelde E M 1988 Immunisation of neonates at high risk of hepatitis B in England and Wales: a national surveillance. British Medical Journal 297: 249–253
843. Pollack H, Kuchuk A, Cowan L et al 1996 Neurodevelopment, growth and viral load in HIV-infected infants. Brain Behaviour and Immunity 10: 298–312
844. Pongpipat D, Suvatte V, Assateerawatts A 1980 Vertical transmission of the hepatitis B surface antigen in Thailand. South-East Asian Journal of Tropical Medicine and Public Health 11: 582–587
845. Pople I K, Bayston R, Hayward R D 1992 Infection of cerebrospinal fluid shunts in infants: a study of etiological factors. Journal of Neurosurgery 77: 29–36
846. Portolani M, Cermelli C, Sabbatini A M et al 1995 A fatal case of congenital cytomegalic inclusion disease following recurrent maternal infection. New Microbiology 18: 427–428
847. Pourcyrous M, Bada H S, Korones S B, Barrett F F, Jennings W, Lockey T 1991 Acute phase reactants in neonatal bacterial infection. Journal of Perinatology 11: 319–325
848. Pourcyrous M, Bada H S, Korones S B, Baselski V, Wong S P 1993 Significance of serial C-reactive protein responses in neonatal infection and other disorders. Pediatrics 92: 431–435
849. Pourcyrous M, Korones S B, Bada H S, Patterson T, Baselski V 1988 Indwelling umbilical artery catheter: a preferred sampling site for blood culture. Pediatrics 81: 821–824
850. Preblud S, Cochi S, Orenstein W 1986 Varicella-zoster infection in pregnancy. New England Journal of Medicine 315: 1415–1421
851. Preblud S R, Williams N M 1985 Fetal risk associated with rubella vaccine: implications for vaccination of susceptible women. Obstetrics and Gynecology 66: 121–123
852. Preece P M, Blount J M, Glover J, Fletcher G M, Peckham C S, Griffiths P D 1983 The consequences of primary CMV infection in pregnancy. Archives of Disease in Childhood 58: 970–975
853. Preece P M, Pearl K N, Peckham C S 1984 Congenital cytomegalovirus infection. Archives of Disease in Childhood 59: 1120–1126
854. Preece P M, Anderson J M, Thompson R G 1989 *Chlamydia trachomatis* infection in infants: a prospective study. Archives of Disease in Childhood 64: 525–529
855. Prober C G, Sullender W M, Yasukawa L L, Au D S, Yeager A S, Arvin A M 1987 Low risk of herpes simplex virus infections in neonates exposed to the virus at the time of vaginal delivery to mothers with recurrent genital herpes simplex virus infections. New England Journal of Medicine 316: 240–244
856. Prober C G, Hensleigh P A, Boucher F D, Yasukawa L L, Au D S, Arvin A M 1988 Use of routine viral cultures at delivery to identify neonates exposed to herpes simplex virus. New England Journal of Medicine 318: 887–891
857. Pruekprasert P, Stout C, Patamasucon P 1995 Neonatal enterovirus infection. Journal of the Association for Academic Minority Physicians 6: 134–138
858. Pryde P G, Nugent C E, Pridjian G, Barr M J, Faix R G 1992 Spontaneous resolution of nonimmune hydrops fetalis secondary to human parvovirus B19 infection. Obstetrics and Gynecology 79: 859–861
859. Public Health Laboratory Service 1990 Prospective study of human parvovirus (B19) infection in pregnancy. British Medical Journal 300: 1166–1170
860. Puranen M, Yliskoski M, Saarikoski S, Syrjanen K, Syrjanen S 1996 Vertical transmission of human papillomavirus from infected mothers to their newborn babies and persistence of the virus in childhood. American Journal of Obstetrics and Gynecology 174: 694–699
861. Puri J, Revathi G, Faridi M M, Talwar V, Kumar A, Parkash B 1995 Role of body surface cultures in prediction of sepsis in a neonatal intensive care unit. Annals of Tropical Paediatrics 15: 307–311
862. Pyati S P, Pildes R S, Ramamurthy R S, Jacobs N 1981 Decreasing mortality in neonates with early onset Group B streptococcal infection. Reality or artefact? Journal of Pediatrics 98: 625–628
863. Pylipow M, Gaddis M, Kinney J S 1994 Selective intrapartum prophylaxis for group B streptococcus colonization: management and outcome of newborns. Pediatrics 93: 631–635
864. Qazi Q H, Sheikh T M, Fikrig S, Menikoff H 1988 Lack of evidence for craniofacial dysmorphism in perinatal human immunodeficiency virus infection. Journal of Pediatrics 112: 7–11
865. Quinn P A, Li HC, Th'ng C, Dunn M, Butany J 1993 Serological response to *Ureaplasma urealyticum* in the neonate. Clinical Infectious Diseases 17 Suppl 1: S136–143
866. Qureshi F, Jacques S M 1996 Maternal varicella during pregnancy: correlation of maternal history and fetal outcome with placental histopathology. Human Pathology 27: 191–195
867. Raad I I, Sabbagh M F 1992 Optimal duration of therapy for catheter-related *Staphylococcus aureus* bacteremia: a study of 55 cases and review. Clinical Infectious Diseases 14: 75–82
868. Rabalais G P, Bronfin D R, Daum R S 1987 Evaluation of commercially available latex agglutination test for rapid diagnosis of group B streptococcal infection. Pediatric Infectious Disease Journal 6: 177–181
869. Rabalais G P, Nusinoff-Lehrman S, Arvin A M, Levin N J 1989 Antiviral susceptibilities of herpes simplex virus isolates from infants with recurrent mucocutaneous lesions after neonatal infection. Pediatric Infectious Disease Journal 8: 221–224

870. Rabasa A I, Okolo A A 1996 Early diagnosis of septicaemia in infants with respiratory distress in the tropics. Tropical Doctor 26: 62–64
871. Raju T N, Kobler C 1991 Improving handwashing habits in the newborn nurseries. American Journal of Medical Science 302: 355–358
872. Ramanathan R, Durand M 1987 Blood cultures in neonates with percutaneous central venous catheters. Archives of Disease in Childhood 62: 621–623
873. Ramsay M E B, Miller E, Peckham C S 1991 Outcome of confirmed symptomatic congenital cytomegalovirus infection. Archives of Disease in Childhood 66: 1068–1069
874. Randel R C, Kearns D B, Nespeca M P, Scher C A, Sawyer M H 1996 Vocal cord paralysis as a presentation of intrauterine infection with varicella-zoster virus. Pediatrics 97: 127–128
875. Rao P S, Baliga M, Shivananda P G 1993 Bacteriology of neonatal septicaemia in a rural referral hospital in south India. Journal of Tropical Pediatrics 39: 230–233
876. Rastogi A, Luken J A, Pildes R S, Chrystof D, LaBranche F 1993 Endocarditis in neonatal intensive care unit. Pediatric Cardiology 14: 183–186
877. Ratrisawadi V, Srisuwanporn T, Paupondh Y 1991 Intravenous immunoglobulin prophylaxis for infection in very low birthweight infants. Journal of the Medical Association of Thailand 74: 14–18
878. Razel M 1997 Evidence for casual household transmission of HIV: review and analysis. Harefuah 132: 156–162
879. Redd S C, Wirima J J, Steketee R W, Breman J G, Heymann D L 1996 Transplacental transmission of *Plasmodium falciparum* in rural Malawi. American Journal of Tropical Medicine and Hygiene 55: 57–60
880. Reid T M S 1975 Emergence of group B streptococci in obstetric and neonatal infections. British Medical Journal ii: 533–536
881. Reinhardt M C 1978 A survey of mothers and their newborns in Abidjan (Ivory Coast). Helvetica Paediatrica Acta 41 (suppl.): 1–32
882. Reiter P D, Doron M W 1996 Vancomycin cerebrospinal fluid concentrations after intravenous administration in premature infants. Journal of Perinatology 16: 331–335
883. Remington J S, Desmonts G 1983 Toxoplasmosis. In: Remington J S, Klein J O (eds) Infectious diseases of the fetus and newborn infant. 2nd Edn. W B Saunders, Philadelphia, pp 143–263
884. Remington J S, Desmonts G 1990 Toxoplasmosis. In: Remington J S, Klein J O (eds) Infectious diseases of the fetus and newborn infant. 3rd Edn. W B Saunders, Philadelphia, pp 89–195
885. Renier D, Flandin C, Hirsch E, Hirsch J F 1988 Brain abscess in neonates. Journal of Neurosurgery 69: 877–882
886. Rettig P J 1986 Chlamydial infection in pediatrics: diagnostic and therapeutic considerations. Pediatric Infectious Disease Journal 5: 158–161
887. Rettig P J 1988 Perinatal infections with *Chlamydia trachomatis*. Clinics in Perinatology 15: 321–350
888. Reynolds D W, Stagno S, Hosty T S, Tiller M, Alford C A 1973 Maternal cytomegalovirus excretion and perinatal infection. New England Journal of Medicine 289: 1–5
889. Rigal E, Roze J C, Villers D et al 1990 Prospective evaluation of the protected specimen brush for the diagnosis of pulmonary infections in ventilated newborns. Pediatric Pulmonology 8: 268–272
890. Roberts R J, Quoraishi A H, Evans M R 1994 Neonatal listeriosis in twins due to cross-infection in theatre recovery room. Lancet 344: 1572
891. Roberts R L, Szelc C M, Scates S M et al 1991 Neutropenia in an extremely premature infant treated with recombinant human granulocyte colony-stimulating factor. American Journal of Diseases of Children 145: 808–812
892. Rodis J F, Hovick T J, Quinn D L, Rosengren S S, Tattersall P 1988 Human parvovirus infection in pregnancy. Obstetrics and Gynecology 72: 733–738
893. Rodriguez A F, Kaplan S L, Masen E O 1990 Cerebrospinal fluid values in the very low birthweight infant. Journal of Pediatrics 116: 971–974
894. Rodwell R L, Gray P H, Taylor K M, Minchinton R 1996 Granulocyte colony stimulating factor treatment for alloimmune neonatal neutropenia. Archives of Disease in Childhood 75: 57–58
895. Rodwell R L, Leslie A L, Tudehope D I 1988 Early diagnosis of neonatal sepsis using a hematologic scoring system. Journal of Pediatrics 112: 761–767
896. Rogers M F, Caldwell M B, Gwinn M L, Simonds R J 1994 Epidemiology of paediatric human immunodeficiency virus infection in the United States. Acta Paediatrica Suppl 400: 5–7
897. Rogers M F, Mofenson L M, Moseley R R 1995 Reducing the risk of perinatal HIV transmission through zidovudine therapy: treatment recommendations and implications. Journal of American Medical Women's Association 50: 78–82, 93
898. Rogers M F, White C R, Sanders R et al 1990 Lack of transmission of human immunodeficiency virus from infected children to their household contacts. Pediatrics 85: 210–214
899. Roizen N, Swisher C N, Stein M A et al 1995 Neurologic and developmental outcome in treated congenital toxoplasmosis. Pediatrics 95: 11–20
900. Rojas J, Stahlman M 1984 The effect of Group B streptococcus and other organisms on the pulmonary vasculature. Clinics in Perinatology 11: 591–599
901. Rolleston G L, Maling T M J, Hodson C J 1974 Intrarenal reflux and the scarred kidney. Archives of Disease in Childhood 49: 531–539
902. Rooney J C, Hill D J, Danks D M 1971 Jaundice associated with bacterial infection in the newborn. American Journal of Diseases of Children 122: 39–41
903. Roques P, Marce D, Courpotin C 1993 Correlation between HIV provirus burden and in-utero transmission. AIDS 7 (Supplement 2) 39–43
904. Roques P A, Gras G, Parnat-Methieu F 1995 Clearance of HIV infection in 12 perinatally infected children: virological and immunological data. AIDS 9: 19–26
905. Rosenblum L S, Villarino M E, Nainan O V et al 1991 Hepatitis A outbreak in a neonatal intensive care unit: risk factors for transmission and evidence of prolonged viral excretion among preterm infants. Journal of Infectious Diseases 164: 476–482
906. Rosenthal J, Healey T, Ellis R, Gillan E, Cairo M S 1996 A two-year follow-up of neonates with presumed sepsis treated with recombinant human granulocyte colony-stimulating factor during the first week of life. Journal of Pediatrics 128: 135–137
907. Rotbart H A 1995 Enteroviral infections of the central nervous system. Clinical Infectious Diseases 20: 971–981
908. Rouse D J, Hauth J C, Andrews W W, Mills B B, Maher J E 1997 Chlorhexidine vaginal irrigation for the prevention of peripartal infection: a placebo-controlled randomized clinical trial. American Journal of Obstetrics and Gynecology 176: 617–622
909. Rouzioux C, Costagliola D, Burgard M 1993 Timing of mother-to-child transmission depends on maternal status. AIDS 7(Suppl 2): 49–52
910. Rowen J L, Atkins J T, Levy M L, Baer S C, Baker C J 1995 Invasive fungal dermatitis in the < or = 1000-gram neonate. Pediatrics 95: 682–687
911. Rowen J L, Rench M A, Kozinetz C A, Adams J M J, Baker C J 1994 Endotracheal colonization with *Candida* enhances risk of systemic candidiasis in very low birth weight neonates. Journal of Pediatrics 124: 789–794
912. Rowley A H, Wald E R 1986 Incubation period necessary to detect bacteremia in neonates. Pediatric Infectious Disease Journal 5: 590–591
913. Royal College of Obstetricians and Gynaecologists 1987 Report of the RCOG sub-committee on problems associated with AIDS in relation to obstetrics and gynaecology. RCOG, London
914. Royal College of Paediatrics and Child Health 1997 British Paediatric Surveillance Unit 1997. 11th Annual Surveillance Report
915. Royal College of Physicians 1991 Guidelines for the management of acute urinary tract infection in childhood Journal of the Royal College of Physicians, London 25: 36–42
916. Rubin L, Leggiadro R, Elie M T, Lipsitz P 1986 Disseminated varicella in a neonate: implications for immunoprophylaxis of neonates postnatally exposed to varicella. Pediatric Infectious Disease Journal 5: 100–102
917. Rubinstein Z, Heyman Z, Morag B 1983 Ultrasound and computed tomography in the diagnosis and drainage of abscesses and other fluid collections. Israel Journal of Medical Science 19: 1050–1060
918. Rudy B J, Rutstein R M, Pinto-Martin J 1994 Responses to measles immunization in children infected with human immunodeficiency virus. Journal of Pediatrics 125: 72–74
919. Rupar D G, Herzog K D, Fisher M C 1990 Prolonged bacteremia with catheter-related central venous thrombosis. American Journal of Diseases of Children 144: 879–882

920. Rushforth J A, Hoy C M, Kite P, Puntis J W 1993 Rapid diagnosis of central venous catheter sepsis. Lancet 342: 402–403
921. Rusin P, Adam R D, Peterson E A, Ryan K J, Sinclair N A, Weinstein L 1991 *Hemophilus influenzae*: an important cause of maternal and neonatal infections. Obstetrics and Gynecology 77: 92–96
922. Russell A R, Davies E G, McGuigan S, Scopes G J, Daly S, Gordon Smith E C 1994 Plasma granulocyte-colony stimulating factor concentrations (G-CSF) in the early neonatal period. British Journal of Haematology 86: 642–644
923. Ruuska T and Veskari T 1991 A prospective study of acute diarrhoea in Finnish children from birth to $2^1/_2$ years of age. Acta Paediatrica Scandinavica 80: 500–4
924. Ryder R W, Nsa W, Hassig S E, Behets F, Rayfield M, Ekungola B 1989 Perinatal transmission of the human immunodeficiency virus type I to infants of seropositive women in Zaire. New England Journal of Medicine 320: 1637–1642
925. Sacker I, Brunell P A 1970 Abscess in newborn infants caused by mycoplasma. Pediatrics 46: 303–304
926. Sadiq H F, Devaskar S, Keenan W J, Weber T R 1987 Broviac catheterisation in low birthweight infants: incidence and treatment of associated complications. Critical Care Medicine 15: 47–50
927. Sagy M, Barzilay Z, Yahav J, Ginsberg R, Sumpolinsky D 1980 Severe neonatal chlamydial pneumonitis. American Journal of Diseases of Children 134: 89–90
928. Sahn E E 1994 Vesiculopustular diseases of neonates and infants. Current Opinion in Pediatrics 6: 442–446
929. Salimpour R 1977 Cause of death in tetanus neonatorum – study of 233 cases with 54 necropsies. Archives of Disease in Childhood 52: 587–589
930. Saltigeral Simental P, Macias Parra M, Mejia Valdez J, Sosa Vazquez M, Castilla Serna L, Gonzalez Saldana N 1993 Neonatal tetanus experience at the National Institute of Pediatrics in Mexico City. Pediatric Infectious Disease Journal 12: 722–725
931. Salzman M B, Isenberg H D, Shapiro J F, Lipsitz P J, Rubin L G 1993 A prospective study of the catheter hub as the portal of entry for microorganisms causing catheter-related sepsis in neonates. Journal of Infectious Diseases 167: 487–490
932. Salzman M B, Rubin L G 1995 Intravenous catheter-related infections. Advances in Pediatric Infectious Disease 10: 337–368
933. Samson L, MacDonald N E 1995 Management of infants born to mothers who have *Chlamydia* infection. Pediatric Infectious Disease Journal 14: 407–408
934. Sanchez P J 1993 Perinatal transmission of *Ureaplasma urealyticum*: current concepts based on review of the literature. Clinical Infectious Diseases 17 Suppl 1: S107–111
935. Sanchez P J, Cooper B H 1987 Candida lusitaniae sepsis and meningitis in a neonate. Pediatric Infectious Disease Journal 6: 758–759
936. Sanchez P J, Regan J A 1987 Vertical transmission of *Ureaplasma urealyticum* in full term infants. Pediatric Infectious Disease Journal 6: 825–828
937. Sandström I 1987 Ophthalmia neonatorum with special reference to *Chlamydia trachomatis*. Acta Paediatrica Scandinavica suppl. 330
938. Sann L, Bienvenu F, Bienvenu J, Bourgeois J, Bethenod M 1984 Evolution of serum pre-albumin, C-reactive protein and orosomucoid in neonates with bacterial infection. Journal of Pediatrics 105: 977–981
939. Saoud A S, Abuekteish F, Obeidat A, el Nassir Z, al Rimawi H 1995 The changing face of neonatal septicaemia. Annals of Tropical Paediatrics 15: 93–96
940. Sarff L D, Platt L H, McCracken G H 1976 Cerebrospinal fluid evaluation in neonates: comparison of high risk infants with and without meningitis. Journal of Pediatrics 88: 473–477
941. Sawyer M H, Edwards D K, Spector S A 1987 Cytomegalovirus infection and bronchopulmonary dysplasia in premature infants. American Journal of Diseases of Children 141: 303–305
942. Sawyer M H, Holland D, Aintablian N, Connor J D, Keyser E F, Waecker N J J 1994 Diagnosis of enteroviral central nervous system infection by polymerase chain reaction during a large community outbreak. Pediatric Infectious Disease Journal 13: 177–182
943. Schachter J, Grossman M, Sweet R L, Holt J, Jordan C, Bishop E 1986 Prospective study of perinatal transmission of *Chlamydia trachomatis*. Journal of the American Medical Association 255: 3374–3377
944. Schachter J, Sweet R L, Grossman M, Landers D, Robbie M, Bishop E 1986 Experience with the routine use of erythomycin for chlamydial infections in pregnancy. New England Journal of Medicine 314: 276–279
945. Scheifele D W, Bjornson G L, Dyer R A 1987 Delta-like toxin produced by coagulase-negative staphylococci is associated with neonatal necrotising enterocolitis. Infection and Immunity 55: 2268–2271
946. Schelonka R L, Chai M K, Yoder B A, Hensley D, Brockett R M, Ascher D P 1996 Volume of blood required to detect common neonatal pathogens. Journal of Pediatrics 129: 275–278
947. Schieve L A, Handler A, Hershow R, Persky V, Davis F 1994 Urinary tract infection during pregnancy: its association with maternal morbidity and perinatal outcome. American Journal of Public Health 84: 405–410
948. Schiff D E, Stonestreet B S 1993 Central venous catheters in low birth weight infants: incidence of related complications. Journal of Perinatology 13: 153–158
949. Schmidt B K, Kirpalani H M, Corey M, Low D E, Philip A G S, Ford-Jones E 1987 Coagulase negative staphylococci as true pathogens in newborn infants: a cohort study. Pediatric Infectious Disease Journal 6: 1022–1026
950. Schmitz J L, Gertis K S, Mauney C, Stamm L V, Folds J D 1994 Laboratory diagnosis of congenital syphilis by immunoglobulin M (IgM) and IgA immunoblotting. Clinical and Diagnostic Laboratory Immunology 1: 32–37
951. Schneeberger P M, Groenendaal F, De Vries L S, van Loon A M, Vroom T M 1994 Variable outcome of a congenital cytomegalovirus infection in a quadruplet after primary infection of the mother during pregnancy. Acta Paediatrica 83: 986–989
952. Schofield C B S, Shanks R A 1971 Gonococcal ophthalmia neonatorum despite treatment with antibacterial eyedrops. British Medical Journal i: 257–259
953. Schofield F D, Tucket V M, Westbrook G R 1961 Neonatal tetanus in New Guinea. Effect of active immunization in pregnancy. British Medical Journal ii: 785–789
954. Schonheyder H C, Gottschau A, Friland A, Rosdahl V T 1995 Mortality rate and magnitude of *Staphylococcus aureus* bacteremia as assessed by a semiquantitative blood culture system. Scandinavian Journal of Infectious Diseases 27: 19–21
955. Schuchat A, Lizano C, Broome C V, Swaminathan B, Kim C, Winn K 1991 Outbreak of neonatal listeriosis associated with mineral oil. Pediatric Infectious Disease Journal 10: 183–189
956. Schultz L J, Steketee R W, Macheso A, Kazembe P, Chitsulo L, Wirima J J 1994 The efficacy of antimalarial regimens containing sulfadoxine-pyrimethamine and/or chloroquine in preventing peripheral and placental *Plasmodium falciparum* infection among pregnant women in Malawi. American Journal of Tropical Medicine Hygiene 51: 515–522
957. Schwartz D A, Larsen S A, Beck Sague C, Fears M, Rice R J 1995 Pathology of the umbilical cord in congenital syphilis: analysis of 25 specimens using histochemistry and immunofluorescent antibody to *Treponema pallidum*. Human Pathology 26: 784–791
958. Schwebke K, Henry K, Balfour H H J, Olson D, Crane R T, Jordan M C 1995 Congenital cytomegalovirus infection as a result of nonprimary cytomegalovirus disease in a mother with acquired immunodeficiency syndrome. Journal of Pediatrics 126: 293–295
959. Schwersenski J, McIntyre L, Bauer C R 1991 Lumbar puncture frequency and cerebrospinal fluid analysis in the neonate. American Journal of Diseases of Children 145: 54–58
960. Scott J 1965 Iatrogenic lesions in babies following umbilical vein catheterisation. Archives of Disease in Childhood 40: 426–428
961. Scott L L, Sanchez P J, Jackson G L, Zeray F, Wendel G D Jr 1996 Acyclovir suppression to prevent cesarean delivery after first-episode genital herpes. Obstetrics and Gynecology 87: 69–73
962. Sehgal A, Sehgal R, Gupta I, Bhakoo O N, Ganguly N K 1992 Use of hepatitis B vaccine alone or in combination with hepatitis B immunoglobulin for immunoprophylaxis of perinatal hepatitis B infection. Journal of Tropical Pediatrics 38: 247–251
963. Selin L K, Hammond G W, Aoki F Y 1988 Neonatal herpes simplex virus infection in Manitoba 1980–86 and implications for preventive strategies. Pediatric Infectious Disease Journal 7: 733–734
964. Sever J A, White L R 1969 Intrauterine viral infections. Annual Review of Medicine 19: 471–486

965. Sever J L, Ellenberg J, Ley A C et al 1988 Toxoplasmosis: maternal and pediatric findings in 23,000 pregnancies. Pediatrics 82: 181–192
966. Shalev E, Battino S, Romano S, Blondhaim O, Ben Ami M 1994 Intraamniotic infection with *Candida albicans* successfully treated with transcervical amnioinfusion of amphotericin. American Journal of Obstetrics and Gynecology 170: 1271–1272
967. Shamir R, Horvev G, Merlob P, Nutman J 1990 *Citrobacter diversus* lung abscess in a preterm infant. Pediatric Infectious Disease Journal 9: 221–222
968. Shamseldin el Shafie S, Smith W, Donnelly G 1995 An outbreak of gentamicin-resistant *Klebsiella pneumoniae* in a neonatal ward. Central European Journal of Public Health 3: 129–131
969. Sharp A M, Odds F C, Evans E G 1992 *Candida* strains from neonates in a special care baby unit. Archives of Disease in Childhood 67: 48–52
970. Shattuck K E, Chonmaitree T 1992 The changing spectrum of neonatal meningitis over a fifteen-year period. Clinical Pediatrics (Philadelphia) 31: 130–136
971. Sherman M P, Chance K H, Goetzman B W 1984 Gram stains of tracheal secretions predict neonatal bacteremia. American Journal of Diseases of Children 138: 848–850
972. Shigeoka A O, Hall R T, Hill H R 1978 Blood transfusion in group B streptococcal sepsis. Lancet i: 636–638
973. Siegel J D, McCracken G H 1979 Neonatal lung abscess. American Journal of Diseases of Children 133: 947–949
974. Siegel J D, McCracken G H, Threlkeld N, Milvenan B, Rosenfield C R 1981 Single dose penicillin prophylaxis against neonatal group B streptococcal infections. New England Journal of Medicine 303: 769–776
975. Sikuler E, Guetta V, Keynan A, Neumann L, Schlaeffer F 1989 Abnormalities of bilirubin and liver enzyme levels in adult patients with bacteremia. Archives of Internal Medicine 149: 2246–2248
976. Simoes E A, King S J, Lehr M V, Groothuis J R 1993 Preterm twins and triplets. A high-risk group for severe respiratory syncytial virus infection. American Journal of Diseases of Children 147: 303–306
977. Siritantikorn S, Nantharukchaikul S, Chavalidthamrong P, Sutthent R, Wasi C, Thongcharoen P 1994 Detection of human cytomegalovirus in urine of infants by polymerase chain reaction. Journal of the Medical Association of Thailand 77: 414–420
978. Sison A V 1992 Maternal and fetal infections. Current Opinion in Obstetrics and Gynecology 4: 48–54
979. Sizun J, Soupre D, Legrand M C et al 1995 Neonatal nosocomial respiratory infection with coronavirus: a prospective study in a neonatal intensive care unit. Acta Paediatrica 84: 617–620
980. Sklavunu Tsurutsoglu S, Gatzola Karaveli M, Hatziioannidis K, Tsurutsoglu G 1991 Efficacy of aztreonam in the treatment of neonatal sepsis. Review of Infectious Diseases 13 Suppl 7: S591–593
981. Skölderberg B, Forsgren M, Alestig K et al 1984 Acyclovir versus vidarabine in herpes simplex encephalitis. Lancet ii: 707–711
982. Smellie J M, Rigden S P A 1995 Pitfalls in the investigation of children with urinary tract infection. Archives of Disease in Childhood 72: 251–258
983. Smellie J M, Rigden S P A, Prescod N P 1995 Urinary tract infection: a comparison of four methods of investigation. Archives of Disease in Childhood 72: 247–250
984. Smith E M, Johnson S R, Cripe T et al 1995 Perinatal transmission and maternal risks of human papillomavirus infection. Cancer Detection and Prevention 19: 196–205
985. Smith H, Congdon P 1985 Neonatal systemic candidiasis. Archives of Disease in Childhood 60: 365–369
986. Smith J R, Taylor Robinson D 1993 Infection due to *Chlamydia trachomatis* in pregnancy and the newborn. Baillières Clinical Obstetrics and Gynaecology 7: 237–255
987. Smithells R W, Sheppard S, Holzel H, Dickson A 1985 National congenital rubella surveillance programme. British Medical Journal 291: 40–41
988. Snider D E, Powell K E 1984 Should women taking antituberculous drugs breastfeed? Archives of Internal Medicine 144: 589–590
989. Soman M, Green B, Daling J 1985 Risk factors for early neonatal sepsis. American Journal of Epidemiology 121: 712–719
990. Soriano A L, Russell R G, Johnson D, Lagos R, Sechter I, Morris J G J 1991 Pathophysiology of *Citrobacter diversus* neonatal meningitis: comparative studies in an infant mouse model. Infection and Immunity 59: 1352–1358
991. Soulie J C 1995 Cardiac involvement in fetal parvovirus B19 infection. Pathologie Biologie (Paris) 43: 416–419
992. Spady D W, Pabst H F, Byrnes P 1994 Intravenous immunoglobulin (IVIG) shortens the stay for low birthweight infants. Pediatric Research 35: 304A
993. Spafford P S, Sinkin R A, Cox C, Reubens L, Powell K R 1994 Prevention of central venous catheter-related coagulase-negative staphylococcal sepsis in neonates. Journal of Pediatrics 125: 259–263
994. Sperling R S, Newton E, Gibbs R S 1988 Intra-amniotic infection in low-birth-weight infants. Journal of Infectious Diseases 157: 113–117
995. Spirer Z, Jurgenson U, Lazewnick R, Reider-Grossvasser I 1982 Complete recovery from an apparent brain abscess treated without neurosurgery: the importance of early CT scanning. Clinical Pediatrics 21: 106–109
996. Stabile A, Sopo M, Romanelli V, Pastore R, Pesaresi M A 1988 Intravenous immunoglobulin for prophylaxis of neonatal sepsis in premature infants. Archives of Disease in Childhood 63: 441–443
997. Stagno S, Hurtado R 1971 Enfermedad de Chagas congenita: Studio immunologico y diagnostico mediante immuno fluorescencia con anti IgM. Boletin Chileno de Parasitologia 26: 20–27
998. Stagno S, Whitley R J 1985 Herpes virus infections in pregnancy. I. Cytomegalovirus and Epstein-Barr virus infections. New England Journal of Medicine 313: 1270–1274
999. Stagno S, Pass R F, Dworsky M C et al 1982 Congenital cytomegalovirus infection. The relative importance of primary and recurrent maternal infection. New England Journal of Medicine 306: 945–949
1000. Stagno S, Pass R E, Dworsky M C, Alford C A 1983 Congenital and perinatal cytomegalovirus infections. Seminars in Perinatology 7: 31–42
1001. Stark V, Harrisson S P 1992 *Staphylococcus aureus* colonization of the newborn in a Darlington hospital. Journal of Hospital Infection 21: 205–211
1002. Steele A D, Sears J F 1996 Characterisation of rotaviruses recovered from neonates with symptomatic infection. South African Medical Journal 86: 1546–1549
1003. Steketee R W, Wirima J J, Bloland P B et al 1996 Impairment of a pregnant woman's acquired ability to limit *Plasmodium falciparum* by infection with human immunodeficiency virus type-1. American Journal of Tropical Medicine and Hygiene 55: 42–49
1004. Steketee R W, Wirima J J, Hightower A W, Slutsker L, Heymann D L, Breman J G 1996 The effect of malaria and malaria prevention in pregnancy on offspring birthweight, prematurity, and intrauterine growth retardation in rural Malawi. American Journal of Tropical Medicine and Hygiene 55: 33–41
1005. Stevens C E, Beasley R P, Tsui J, Lee W-C 1975 Vertical transmission of hepatitis B antigen in Taiwan. New England Journal of Medicine 292: 771–774
1006. Stiller R J, Blair D O, Clark P, Tinghitella T 1989 Rapid detection of vaginal colonization with Group B streptococci by means of latex agglutination. American Journal of Obstetrics and Gynecology 160: 566–568
1007. Stoll B, Gordon T, Korones S B et al 1996 Late-onset sepsis in very low birthweight neonates: a report from the National Institute of Child Health and Human Development Neonatal Research Network. Journal of Pediatrics 129: 63–71
1008. Stoll B J, Fanaroff A 1995 Early-onset coagulase-negative staphylococcal sepsis in preterm neonate. National Institute of Child Health and Human Development (NICHD) Neonatal Research Network. Lancet 345: 1236–1237
1009. Stoll B J, Gordon T, Korones S B et al 1996 Early-onset sepsis in very low birthweight neonates: a report from the National Institute of Child Health and Human Development Neonatal Research Network. Journal of Pediatrics 129: 72–80
1010. Stoll B J, Lee F K, Larsen S et al 1993 Clinical and serologic evaluation of neonates for congenital syphilis: a continuing diagnostic dilemma. Journal of Infectious Diseases 167: 1093–1099
1011. Strauss R G, Levy G J, Sotelo-Avila C 1993 National survey of neonatal transfusion practices: II. Blood component therapy. Pediatrics 91: 530–536
1012. Stroobant J, Harris M C, Cody C S, Polin R A, Douglas S D 1984 Diminished bactericidal capacity for group B streptococcus in neutrophils from stressed and healthy neonates. Pediatric Research 18: 634–637

1013. Stuart J, Whicher J-T 1988 Tests for detecting and monitoring the acute phase response. Archives of Disease in Childhood 63: 115–117
1014. Stuart R L, Turnidge J, Grayson M L 1995 Safety of imipenem in neonates. Pediatric Infectious Disease Journal 14: 804–805
1015. Stutman H R 1991 Clinical experience with aztreonam for treatment of infections in children. Review of Infectious Diseases 13 Suppl 7: S582–585
1016. Sullender W M, Miller J L, Yasukawa L L et al 1987 Humoral and cell mediated immunity in neonates with herpes simplex virus infection. Journal of Infectious Diseases 155: 28–37
1017. Suzuki N, Terada S, Inoue M 1995 Neonatal meningitis with human parvovirus B19 infection. Archives of Disease in Childhood 73: F196–197
1018. Svanborg C, Hausson S, Jodal U 1988 Host-parasite interaction in the urinary tract. Journal of Infectious Diseases 157: 421–425
1019. Swingle H M, Bucciarelli R L, Ayoub E M 1985 Synergy between penicillin and low concentrations of gentamicin in the killing of group B streptococci. Journal of Infectious Diseases 152: 515–520
1020. Synnott M B, Morse D L, Hall S M 1994 Neonatal meningitis in England and Wales: a review of routine national data. Archives of Disease in Childhood 71: 75–80
1021. Szarfman A, Otatti L, Schmunis A, Vilches A M 1973 A simple method for the detection of human congenital Chagas disease. Journal of Parasitology 59: 723
1022. Tafuro P, Colbourn D, Gurevich I et al 1986 Comparison of blood cultures obtained simultaneously by venepuncture and from vascular lines. Journal of Hospital Infection 7: 283–288
1023. Tan D S K, Stern H 1981 A serological study of cytomegalovirus and herpes simplex virus infections in Peninsular Malaysia. Bulletin of the World Health Organization 59: 909–912
1024. Tan T Q, Mason E O J, Ou C N, Kaplan S L 1993 Use of intravenous rifampin in neonates with persistent staphylococcal bacteremia. Antimicrobial Agents and Chemotherapy 37: 2401–2406
1025. Tan T Q, Musser J M, Shulman R J, Mason E O J, Mahoney D H J, Kaplan S L 1994 Molecular epidemiology of coagulase-negative staphylococcus blood isolates from neonates with persistent bacteremia and children with central venous catheter infections. Journal of Infectious Diseases 169: 1393–1397
1026. Teberg A-J, Yonekura M L, Salminen C, Pavlova Z 1987 Clinical manifestations of epidemic neonatal listeriosis. Pediatric Infectious Disease Journal 6: 817–830
1027. Terry G M, Ho-Terry L, Warren R C, Rodeck C H, Cohen A, Rees K P 1986 First trimester perinatal diagnosis of congenital rubella: a laboratory investigation. British Medical Journal 292: 930–933
1028. Thaler M M, Park C K, Landers D V et al 1991 Vertical transmission of hepatitis C virus. Lancet 338: 17–18
1029. Thorp J M, Katz V L, Fowler L J, Kurtzman J T, Bowes W A 1989 Fetal death from chlamydial infection across intact amniotic membranes. American Journal of Obstetrics and Gynecology 161: 1245–1246
1030. Thureen P J, Moreland S, Rodden D J, Merenstein G B, Levin M, Rosenberg A A 1993 Failure of tracheal aspirate cultures to define the cause of respiratory deteriorations in neonates. Pediatric Infectious Disease Journal 12: 560–564
1031. Thurlbeck S M, McIntosh N 1987 Preterm blood counts vary with sampling site. Archives of Disease in Childhood 62: 74–75
1032. Tipple M A, Beem M O, Saxon E M 1979 Clinical characteristics of the afebrile pneumonia associated with *Chlamydia trachomatis* infection in infants less than 6 months of age. Pediatrics 63: 192–197
1033. Tong M J, Thursby M, Rakela J 1981 Studies on the maternal–infant transmission of the viruses which cause acute hepatitis. Gastroenterology 80: 999–1004
1034. Tookey P, Peckham C S 1996 Neonatal herpes simplex virus infection in the British Isles. Paediatric and Perinatal Epidemiology 10: 432–442
1035. Tookey P A, Ades A E, Peckham C S 1992 Cytomegalovirus prevalence in pregnant women: the influence of parity. Archives of Disease in Childhood 67: 779–783
1036. Torok T J, Wang Q Y, Gary G W, Yang C F, Finch T M, Anderson L J 1992 Prenatal diagnosis of intrauterine infection with parvovirus B19 by the polymerase chain reaction technique. Clinical Infectious Diseases 14: 149–155
1037. Troendle Atkins J, Demmler G J, Williamson W D, McDonald J M, Istas A S, Buffone G J 1994 Polymerase chain reaction to detect cytomegalovirus DNA in the cerebrospinal fluid of neonates with congenital infection. Journal of Infectious Diseases 169: 1334–1337
1038. Tsuji Y, Doi H, Yamabe T, Ishimaru T, Miyamoto T, Aino S 1990 Prevention of mother-child transmission of human T lymphotropic virus type I. Pediatrics 86: 11–17
1039. Tuck S 1980 Neonatal systemic candidiasis treated with miconazole. Archives of Disease in Childhood 55: 703–706
1040. Tugal O, Pallant B, Shebarek N, Jayabose S 1994 Transient erythroblastopenia of the newborn caused by human parvovirus. American Journal of Pediatric Hematology and Oncology 16: 352–355
1041. Tullus K, Brauner A, Fryklund B et al 1992 Host factors versus virulence-associated bacterial characteristics in neonatal and infantile bacteraemia and meningitis caused by *Escherichia coli*. Journal of Medical Microbiology 36: 203–208
1042. Tuppurainen N, Hallman M 1989 Prevention of neonatal group B streptococcal disease: intrapartum detection and chemoprophylaxis of heavily colonised parturients. Obstetrics and Gynecology 73: 583–587
1043. Turner G, Green H T, Blundell V D 1978 e-antigen: a link between immune response and infectivity in hepatitis B? Journal of Hygiene 81: 405–414
1044. Twickler D M, Perlman J, Maberry M C 1993 Congenital cytomegalovirus infection presenting as cerebral ventriculomegaly on antenatal sonography. American Journal of Perinatology 10: 404–406
1045. Umana M A, Odio C M, Castro E, Salas J L, McCracken G H J 1996 Evaluation of aztreonam and ampicillin vs. amikacin and ampicillin for treatment of neonatal bacterial infections. Pediatric Infectious Disease Journal 9: 175–180
1046. Umasankar S, Mridha E U, Hannan M M, Fry C M, Azadian B S 1996 An outbreak of *Salmonella enteritidis* in a maternity and neonatal intensive care unit. Journal of Hospital Infection 34: 117–122
1047. Unger A, Tapia L, Minnich L L, Ray C G 1982 Atypical neonatal respiratory syncytial virus infection. Journal of Pediatrics 100: 762–764
1048. US Public Health Service Task Force on the use of zidovudine to reduce perinatal transmission of human immunodeficiency virus. 1994 Morbidity and Mortality Weekly Report 43: 1–20
1049. Vain N E, Mazlumian J R, Swarner W 1980 Role of exchange transfusion in the treatment of severe septicemia. Pediatrics 66: 693–698
1050. Valduss D, Murray D L, Karna P, Lapour K, Dyke J 1993 Use of intravenous immunoglobulin in twin neonates with disseminated coxsackie B1 infection. Clinical Pediatrics (Philadelphia) 32: 561–563
1051. Valencia G B, Banzon F, Cummings M, McCormack W M, Glass L, Hammerschlag M R 1993 *Mycoplasma hominis* and *Ureaplasma urealyticum in* neonates with suspected infection. Pediatric Infectious Disease Journal 12: 571–573
1052. Valente P, Sever J L 1994 In utero diagnosis of congenital infections by direct fetal sampling. Israel Journal of Medical Science 30: 414–420
1053. Valenti W M, Clarke T A, Hall C B, Menegus M A, Shapiro D L 1982 Concurrent outbreaks of rhinovirus and respiratory syncytial virus in an intensive care nursery: epidemiology and associated risk factors. Journal of Pediatrics 100: 722–726
1054. Valentin Weigand P, Chhatwal G S 1995 Correlation of epithelial cell invasiveness of group B streptococci with clinical source of isolation. Microbial Pathogenesis 19: 83–91
1055. Vallette J D Jr, Goldberg R N, Suguihara C et al 1995 Effect of an interleukin-1 receptor antagonist on the hemodynamic manifestations of group B streptococcal sepsis. Pediatric Research 38: 704–708
1056. Van Camp J M, Tomaselli V, Coran A G 1994 Bacterial translocation in the neonate. Current Opinion in Pediatrics 6: 327–333
1057. Van de Perre P 1995 Postnatal transmission of human immunodeficiency virus type 1: the breast-feeding dilemma. American Journal of Obstetrics and Gynecology 173: 483–487
1058. Van der Wiel H, Weiland H T, van Doornum G J J, van der Straaten P J, Berger H M 1985 Disseminated neonatal herpes simplex virus infection acquired from the father. European Journal of Pediatrics 144: 56–57
1059. Van Dyke R B, Spector S A 1984 Transmission of herpes simplex virus type I to a newborn infant during endotracheal suctioning for meconium aspiration. Pediatric Infectious Disease Journal 3: 153–156
1060. van Ogtrop M L, van Zoeren-Grobben D, Verbakel-Salomans E M A, van Boven C P A 1997 *Serratia marcescens* infections in neonatal

departments: description of an outbreak and review of the literature. Journal of Hospital Infection 36: 95–103
1061. Van Overmeire B, Bleyart S, Van Reempts P, Van Assche F A 1993 The use of intravenously administered immunoglobulins in the prevention of severe infections in very low birthweight neonates. Biology of the Neonate 64: 110–115
1062. Van Reempts P, Kegelaers B, Van Dam K, Van Overmeire B 1993 Neonatal outcome after very prolonged and premature rupture of membranes. American Journal of Perinatology 10: 288–291
1063. Van Winter J T, Ney J A, Ogburn P L J, Johnson R V 1994 Preterm labor and congenital candidiasis. A case report. Journal of Reproductive Medicine 39: 987–990
1064. Verkuyl D A A 1995 Practising obstetrics and gynaecology in areas with a high prevalence of HIV infection. Lancet 346: 293–296
1065. Villari P, Spino C, Chalmers T C, Lau J, Sacks H S 1993 Cesarean section to reduce perinatal transmission of human immunodeficiency virus. A metaanalysis. Online Journal of Current Clinical Trials Doc No 74: 5107
1066. Vince J D, Ashford R W, Gratten M J, Bana-Koiri J 1979 Strongyloides species infestation in young infants of Papua New Guinea: association with generalized oedema. Papua New Guinea Medical Journal 22: 120–127
1067. Visser V E, Hall R T 1980 Lumbar puncture in the evaluation of suspected neonatal sepsis. Journal of Pediatrics 96: 1063–1067
1068. Vogel L C, Boyer K M, Gadzala C A, Gotoff S P 1980 Prevalence of type specific Group B streptococcal antibody in pregnant women. Journal of Pediatrics 96: 1047–1051
1069. Volpe J J 1981 Neurology of the newborn. W B Saunders, Philadelphia, Ch. 19
1070. Volpe J J 1987 Neurology of the newborn, 2nd edn. W B Saunders, Philadelphia, Ch. 20
1071. Voora S, Srinivasan G, Lilien L D, Yeh T F, Pildes R S 1982 Fever in full term newborns in the first 4 days of life. Pediatrics 69: 40–44
1072. Wagle S, Grauaug A, Kohan R, Evans S F 1994 C-reactive protein as a diagnostic tool of sepsis in very immature babies. Journal of Paediatrics and Child Health 30: 40–44
1073. Wainer S, Cooper P A, Funk E, Bental R Y, Sandler D A, Patel J 1992 Prophylactic miconazole oral gel for the prevention of neonatal fungal rectal colonization and systemic infection. Pediatric Infectious Disease Journal 11: 713–716
1074. Waites K B, Crouse D T, Cassell G H 1993 Therapeutic considerations for *Ureaplasma urealyticum* infections in neonates. Clinical Infectious Diseases 17 Suppl 1: S208–214
1075. Waites K B, Sims P J, Crouse D T et al 1994 Serum concentrations of erythromycin after intravenous infusion in preterm neonates treated for *Ureaplasma urealyticum* infection. Pediatric Infectious Disease Journal 13: 287–293
1076. Walpole I R, Hodgen N, Bower C 1991 Congenital toxoplasmosis: a large survey in Western Australia. Medical Journal of Australia 154: 720–724
1077. Wandstrat T L, Phleps S J 1994 Vancomycin dosing in neonatal patients: the controversy continues. Neonatal Network 13: 33–39
1078. Ware R 1989 Human parvovirus infection. Journal of Pediatrics 114: 343–348
1079. Wareham J, Harris H, Whitman I 1995 Herpes simplex type II infection in monozygotic twins. American Journal of Perinatology 12: 75–77
1080. Watson J C, Fleming D W, Borella A J, Olcott E S, Conrad R E, Baron R C 1993 Vertical transmission of hepatitis A resulting in an outbreak in a neonatal intensive care unit. Journal of Infectious Diseases 167: 567–571
1081. Watson P G, Gairdner D 1968 TRIC agent as a cause of neonatal eye sepsis. British Medical Journal ii: 527–528
1082. Webber S, Wilkinson A R, Lindsell D, Hope P L, Dobson S R M, Isaacs D 1990. Neonatal pneumonia. Archives of Disease in Childhood 65: 207–211
1083. Weese-Mayer D E, Fonriest D W, Brouilette R T, Shulman S T 1987 Risk factors associated with candidemia in the neonatal intensive care unit: a case controlled study. Pediatric Infectious Disease Journal 6: 190–196
1084. Weisman L E, Lorenzetti P M 1989 High intravenous doses of human immune globulin suppress neonatal Group B streptococcal immunity in rats. Journal of Pediatrics 115: 445–450
1085. Weisman L E, Anthony B F, Hemming V G, Fischer G W 1993 Comparison of group B streptococcal hyperimmune globulin and standard intravenously administered immune globulin in neonates. Journal of Pediatrics 122: 929–937
1086. Weisman L E, Cruess D F, Fischer G W 1993 Standard versus hyperimmune intravenous immunoglobulin in preventing or treating neonatal bacterial infections. Clinics in Perinatology 20: 211–224
1087. Weisman L E, Merenstein G B, Steenbarger J R 1983 The effect of lumbar puncture position on sick neonates. American Journal of Diseases of Children 137: 1077–1079
1088. Weisman L E, Stoll B J, Cruess D F 1992 Early-onset group B streptococcal disease; a current assessment. Journal of Pediatrics 121: 428–433
1089. Weisman L E, Stoll B J, Kueser T J, Rubio T T, Frank C G, Heiman H S 1994 Intravenous immune globulin prophylaxis of late-onset infection in premature neonates. Journal of Pediatrics 125: 922–930
1090. Weisman L E, Stoll B J, Kueser T J et al 1992 Intravenous immune globulin therapy for early-onset sepsis in premature neonates. Journal of Pediatrics 121: 434–443
1091. Weiss S G, Newcomb R W, Beem M O 1986 Pulmonary assessment of children after chlamydial pneumonia of infancy. Journal of Pediatrics 108: 659–664
1092. Weissberg E D, Smith A L, Smith D H 1974 Clinical features of neonatal osteomyelitis. Pediatrics 53: 505–510
1093. Weisse M E, Person D A, Berkenbaugh J T J 1993 Treatment of *Candida* arthritis with flucytosine and amphotericin. Journal of Perinatology 13: 402–404
1094. Wejstal R, Norkrans G 1989 Chronic non A- non B hepatitis in pregnancy: outcome and possible transmission to the offspring. Scandinavian Journal of Infectious Diseases 21: 485–490
1095. Wejstal R, Widell A, Mansson A S, Hermodsson S, Norkrans G 1992 Mother-to-infant transmission of hepatitis C virus. Annals of Internal Medicine 117: 887–890
1096. Wen T S, Eriksen N L, Blanco J D, Graham J M, Oshiro B T, Prieto J A 1993 Association of clinical intra-amniotic infection and meconium. American Journal of Perinatology 10: 438–440
1097. Wettergren B, Jodal U, Jonasson G 1985 Epidemiology of bacteruria during the first year of life. Acta Paediatrica Scandinavian 74: 925–930
1098. White F V, Jordan J, Dickman P S, Knisley A S 1995 Fetal parvovirus B19 infection and liver disease of antenatal onset in an infant with Ebstein's anomaly. Pediatric Pathology and Laboratory Medicine 15: 121–129
1099. Whitley R, Arvin A, Prober C et al 1991b Predictors of morbidity and mortality in neonates with herpes simplex virus infections. The National Institute of Allergy and Infectious Diseases Collaborative Antiviral Study Group. New England Journal of Medicine 324: 450–454
1100. Whitley R, Hutto C 1985 Neonatal herpes simplex virus infections. Paediatrics in Review 7: 119–126
1101. Whitley R, Corey L, Arvin A et al 1988 Changing presentation of neonatal herpes simplex encephalitis. Journal of Infectious Diseases 158: 109–112
1102. Whitley R, Nahmias A, Seng-Jaw Song 1980 Vidarabine therapy of neonatal herpes simplex viral infection. New England Journal of Medicine 266: 495–501
1103. Whitley R J 1988 Neonatal herpes simplex virus infections. Clinics in Perinatology 15: 903–960
1104. Whitley R J 1993 Neonatal herpes simplex virus infections. Journal of Medical Virology Suppl 1: 13–21
1105. Whitley R J, Arvin A, Prober C et al 1991 A controlled trial comparing vidarabine with acyclovir in neonatal herpes simplex virus infection. New England Journal of Medicine 324: 444–449
1106. Whitley R J, Corey L, Arvin A et al 1988 Changing presentation of herpes simplex virus infection in neonates. Journal of Infectious Diseases 158: 109–116
1107. Whyte R K, Hussan Z, DeSa D J 1982 Antenatal infection with candida species. Archives of Disease in Childhood 57: 528–535
1108. Wild N J, Sheppard S, Smithells R W, Holzel H, Jones G 1989 Onset and severity of hearing loss due to congenital rubella infection. Archives of Disease in Childhood 64: 1280–1283
1109. Wilfert C M 1996 Prevention of perinatal transmission of human immunodeficiency virus: a progress report 2 years after completion of AIDS Clinical Trials Group trial 076. Clinical Infectious Diseases 23: 438–441
1110. Williams P A, Bohnsack J F, Augustine N H, Drummond W K, Rubens C E, Hill H R 1993 Production of tumor necrosis factor by

human cells in vitro and in vivo, induced by group B streptococci. Journal of Pediatrics 123: 292–300

1111. Williams R, Kirkbride V, Corcoran G D 1994 Neonatal osteomyelitis in Down's syndrome due to non-encapsulated *Haemophilus influenzae*. Journal of Infection 29: 203–205

1112. Williamson M, Fraser S H, Tilse M 1995 Failure of the urinary group B streptococcal antigen test as a screen for neonatal sepsis. Archives of Disease in Childhood 73: 109–111

1113. Wiswell T E, Baumgart S, Gannon C M, Spitzer A R 1995 No lumbar puncture in the evaluation for early neonatal sepsis: will meningitis be missed? Pediatrics 95: 803–806

1114. Wiswell T E, Hachey W E 1991 Multiple site blood cultures in the initial evaluation for neonatal sepsis during the first week of life. Pediatric Infectious Disease Journal 10: 365–369

1115. Wiswell T E, Roscelli J D 1986 Corroborative evidence for the decreased incidence of urinary tract infections in circumcised male infants. Pediatrics 78: 96–99

1116. Wong S N, Ng T L 1991 *Haemophilus influenzae* septicaemia in the neonate: report of two cases and review of the English literature. Journal of Paediatrics and Child Health 27: 113–115

1117. Wong S N, Tam A Y C, Ng T H G, Ng N T, Tong C Y, Tang T S 1989 Fatal coxsackie B1 virus infection in neonates. Pediatric Infectious Disease Journal 8: 638–641

1118. Wong S Y, Hajdu M P, Ramirez R, Thulliez P, McLeod R, Remington J S 1993 Role of specific immunoglobulin E in diagnosis of acute toxoplasma infection and toxoplasmosis. Journal of Clinical Microbiology 31: 2952–2959

1119. Woo D, Cummins M, Davies P A, Harvey D R, Hurley R, Waterson A P 1979 Vertical transmission of hepatitis B surface antigen in carrier mothers in two west London hospitals. Archives of Disease in Childhood 54: 670–675

1120. Word B M, Klein J O 1988 Current therapy of bacterial sepsis and meningitis in infants and children: a poll of directors of programs in pediatric infectious diseases. Pediatric Infectious Disease Journal 7: 267–270

1121. Word B M, Klein J O 1989 Therapy of bacterial sepsis and meningitis in infants and children: 1989 poll of directors of programs in pediatric infectious diseases. Pediatric Infectious Disease Journal 8: 635–637

1122. World Health Organization 1982 Expanded programme on immunization: prevention of neonatal tetanus. Weekly Epidemiological Records 57: 137–142

1123. World Health Organization 1988 Progress in the control of viral hepatitis: memorandum from a WHO meeting. Bulletin of the World Health Organization 66: 443–455

1124. World Health Organization 1988 Expanded Programme on Immunization: neonatal tetanus elimination. EPI Global Advisory Group Meeting. EPI/GAG/88/WP.9

1125. Wright E D, Lortan J E, Perinpanayagam R M 1990 Early-onset neonatal pneumococcal sepsis in siblings. Journal of Infection 20: 59–63

1126. Wu S, Shen L 1993 Plasmid analysis and phage typing in the study of staphylococcal colonization and disease in newborn infants. Chinese Medical Science Journal 8: 157–161

1127. Wynn R J 1979 Neonatal *E. coli* pericarditis. Journal of Perinatal Medicine 7: 23–24

1128. Yaegashi N, Okamura K, Tsunoda A, Nakamura M, Sugamura K, Yajima A 1995 A study by means of a new assay of the relationship between an outbreak of erythema infectiosum and non-immune hydrops fetalis caused by human parvovirus B19. Journal of Infection 31: 195–200

1129. Yaegashi N, Okamura K, Yajima A, Murai C, Sugamura K 1994 The frequency of human parvovirus B19 infection in non-immune hydrops fetalis by polymerase chain reaction. Journal of Perinatal Medicine 22: 159–163

1130. Yagupsky P, Menegus M A, Powell K R 1991 The changing spectrum of group B streptococcal disease in infants: an eleven-year experience in a tertiary care hospital. Pediatric Infectious Disease Journal 10: 801–808

1131. Yeager A S 1974 Transfusion acquired cytomegalovirus infection in newborn infants. American Journal of Diseases of Children 128: 478–483

1132. Yeager A S, Arvin A M. Reasons for the absence of a history of recurrent genital infections in mothers of neonates infected with herpes simplex virus. Pediatrics 73: 188–193

1133. Yeager A S, Grumet F C, Hafleigh E B, Arvin A M, Bradley J S, Prober C G 1981 Prevention of transfusion acquired cytomegalovirus infections in newborn infants. Journal of Pediatrics 98: 281–287

1134. Yeager A S, Palumbo P E, Malachowski N, Ariagno R L, Stevenson D K 1983 Sequelae of maternally derived cytomegalovirus infections in premature infants. Journal of Pediatrics 102: 918–922

1135. Yogev R 1985 Cerebrospinal fluid shunt infections: a personal view. Pediatric Infectious Disease Journal 4: 113–118

1136. Yoon P W, Black R E, Moulton L H, Becker S 1996 Effect of not breastfeeding on the risk of diarrheal and respiratory mortality in children under 2 years of age in Metro Cebu, The Philippines. American Journal of Epidemiology 143: 1142–1148

1137. Yoshioka H, Iseki K-I, Fujita K 1983 Development and differences of intestinal flora in the neonatal period in breast-fed and bottle-fed infants. Pediatrics 72: 317–321

1138. Yow M D 1989 Congenital cytomegalovirus; a *now* problem. Journal of Infectious Diseases 159: 163–167

1139. Yuksel B, Greenough A 1994 Viral infections acquired during neonatal intensive care and lung function of preterm infants at follow-up. Acta Paediatrica 83: 117–118

1140. Zafar A B, Butler R C, Reese D J, Gaydos L A, Mennonna P A 1995 Use of 0.3% triclosan (Bacti-Stat) to eradicate an outbreak of methicillin-resistant *Staphylococcus aureus* in a neonatal nursery. American Journal of Infection Control 23: 200–208

1141. Zanetti A R, Tanzi E, Paccagnini S et al 1995 Mother-to-infant transmission of hepatitis C virus. Lombardy Study Group on Vertical HCV Transmission. Lancet 345: 289–291

1142. Zenker P N, Berman S M 1991 Congenital syphilis: trends and recommendations for evaluation and management. Pediatric Infectious Disease Journal 10: 516–522

1143. Zuccotti G V, Riva E, Flumine P et al 1994 Hepatitis B vaccination in infants of mothers infected with human immunodeficiency virus. Journal of Pediatrics 125: 70–72

1144. Zuerlein T J, Butler J C, Yeager T D 1990 Superficial cultures in neonatal sepsis evaluations. Impact on antibiotic decision making. Clinical Pediatrics (Philadelphia) 29: 445–447

44

Neurological problems in the newborn

Part 1

Assessment of the neonatal nervous system

Janet M. Rennie

INTRODUCTION

Suspicion of neurological illness in the neonatal period is always important. As in any organ system disease, diagnosis and prognosis must be based on the findings of a full examination together with the results of appropriate investigation. Neonatal neurological assessment includes repeated careful examination, which of necessity is dominated by examination of the baby's state of alertness and the motor system. Neurological examination of an infant receiving intensive care is difficult, but is not impossible, and can be supplemented by a wide range of diagnostic tests. Cranial ultrasound scanning is now commonplace in neonatal units, and specific atlases can help interpret the findings.[16,35] More experience has been gained with MRI scanning of the neonatal brain.[4,14] Normal ranges exist for somatosensory, auditory and visual evoked potentials, and recording the EEG can prove helpful. The information in this chapter can be supplemented by further reading from more detailed texts.[2,49] For advice on general examination of the newborn see Chapter 17.

BEHAVIOURAL STATES

The initial assessment of the infant's nervous system should involve evaluation of behavioural state, a sensitive indicator of neural integrity. Behavioural states can be described on the basis of four features (Table 44.1).[34]

BEHAVIOURAL STATES OF THE NEONATE 36 WEEKS OR OLDER[7,29,34]

Term babies spend about 50 minutes of each hour asleep, about 50% of the time in quiet sleep (state 1). Babies usually cycle between states, and failure to do so is abnormal; examples of conditions which cause this are drug withdrawal and hypoxic– ischaemic encephalopathy.

Table 44.1 Features of neonatal behavioural states[34]

	Eyes open	Respiration regular	Gross movements	Vocalization
State 1	−1	+1	−1	−1
State 2	−1	−1	0	−1
State 3	+1	+1	−1	−1
State 4	+1	−1	+1	−1
State 5	0	−1	+1	+1

+1 = present; −1 = absent; 0 = present or absent

State 1 (deep or quiet sleep)

A state 1 epoch begins when breathing becomes regular in an infant who keeps his eyes closed (Table 44.1). Sighs or short apnoeic spells may occur, but respiration rapidly becomes regular again. Marked irregularities are always transient and associated with brief gross motor activity. There are no eye movements under the closed eyelids. The infant is generally still and not moving. Spontaneous clonus may occur in the extremities or the jaw. Rhythmical mouthing movements appear for seconds to a maximum of a few minutes; each burst usually lasts 10–20 seconds. Although gross motor movements are rare, startles do occur.

State 2 (light or rapid eye movement sleep)

Onset of a state 2 epoch after an awake state is determined at the moment the infant closes his eyes.

Respirations are now irregular; furthermore, if an antigravity posture was present while awake, this will disappear either gradually or stepwise after each body movement during the onset of sleep. The transition from state 1 into state 2 is frequently marked with a startle, gross movements, or at least with a sigh. Apnoeic spells may occur, frequently heralded by gross movements. Under the closed eyelids slow eye movements can be observed immediately after the onset of state 2, and after 1–4 minutes the typical rapid eye movements appear. Small twitches are common in state 2 and are visible in the face, hands and feet. Grimaces, smiles and rhythmical mouthing are observable at times. Gross movements of one limb or of the whole body and head are the most characteristic transitory events in state 2. Although startles may occur, they are less stereotyped than in state 1. The many movements result in frequently changing posture.

State 3 (awake; drowsy)

In state 3 the infant lies still and keeps his eyes open, although they may be heavy lidded. Although there may be moments of staring, most of the time the infant seems to scan the environment with rapid eye movements. A stable posture and regular respiration are usual. State 3 epochs can be very brief, lasting only a few minutes. Babies have a dazed look in this half-awake state. The longest such periods occur after a feed.

State 4 (alert)

The infant has his eyes open and moves his arms, legs and head. In the prone position the head lifts and some motion occurs; in the supine position, limb movements are frequently less patterned. Periods with large and small movements alternate; respiration is more irregular, especially at the time of large movements. Posture changes frequently.

State 5 (crying)

The infant is crying. Cry is a communication signal, and it is clear that mothers and nurses can often discriminate between cries of discomfort, hunger and pain. Brazelton and Nugent[7] classify crying as state 6, and insert another state between 4 and 6, that of awake and fussing.

Consolability/cuddliness

During an examination, or while in state 5, infants cry but are consolable. Brazelton and Nugent[7] stress that normal infants are 'cuddly' and will mould into the crook of an arm or nestle in the examiner's neck. Persistent high-pitched crying is abnormal, as is the stiff 'uncuddly' tone of a baby with encephalopathy.

BEHAVIOURAL STATE OF THE NEONATE YOUNGER THAN 36 WEEKS

Babies born before 36 weeks' gestation spend a great deal of time asleep, but their sleep states cannot be classified so easily as quiet and active sleep. Prechtl et al,[32] on the basis of a longitudinal study of very low-risk preterm infants, came to the following conclusion: 'Cycles of rest and activity, regular and irregular breathing, and epochs with and without eye movements may alternate independently and may accidentally overlap, but often do not coincide at all before 35–37 weeks'.

ABNORMAL STATES, ABNORMAL STATE CYCLING, AND COMA

Nearly every disorder that affects the central nervous system disturbs the level of alertness at some time.[49] A baby older than 36 weeks who cannot be classified into one of the five behavioural states is sick or under the influence of medication. Infants are usually arousable, that is, they will awaken to the sound of a bell or a bright light. Failure to do so means that they are stuporose or comatose. Both in utero[33] and after birth stereotyped movements are an indicator of disease, and a rich variety of movement is an indicator of health.

In conclusion, in healthy newborns, both full term and preterm, cycles of activity should be present: after 36 weeks these are recognized as distinct behavioural state cycles as described above; before 36 weeks they consist of more or less independently occurring cycles of activity and quiescence, of regular and irregular breathing, and of periods with and without rapid eye movements. Recognition of these cycles can be helped by looking at the ECG, respiratory pattern and $TcPO_2$, especially when complemented by good behavioural observations by the nursing staff. Attention to assessment of behavioural state and behavioural state cycling may be the single most sensitive way to assess the integrity of the neonatal central nervous system, and should be the starting point for examination of the nervous system.

SYSTEMATIC EXAMINATION: 1. POSTURE, SPONTANEOUS MOVEMENT AND TONE

Normal muscle offers a resistance to stretch which is felt by the examiner as tone. Passive flexor tone appears between 28 and 34 weeks and matures from the feet and legs upwards.[1] This is clear from the posture adopted by term babies, who lie with their limbs flexed and adducted, unlike preterm infants, who adopt an extended posture. Asymmetrical tone does not always indicate asymmetrical pathology in the newborn period. A pattern of mixed change in tone, with hypertonia in the limbs and hypotonia in the trunk, is abnormal, as is arching of the trunk at any age. When the whole body is arched the term 'opisthotonos' is used. Tone can alter considerably in relation to feeds and sleep state, and repeated examinations are required to confirm physical signs.

A term newborn makes smooth, varied, spontaneous and symmetrical limb movements which stop when the infant's attention is diverted.[31] Finger movements are elegant and varied, involving the thumb, which can be abducted away from the palm by term.[15] A persistently adducted thumb (cortical thumb) is abnormal, and brain-damaged infants often have fisted hands and a paucity of fine finger movements.

FACIAL EXPRESSION

Spontanteous facial movements are frequently seen in the normal newborn, although bilateral facial paralysis (as in

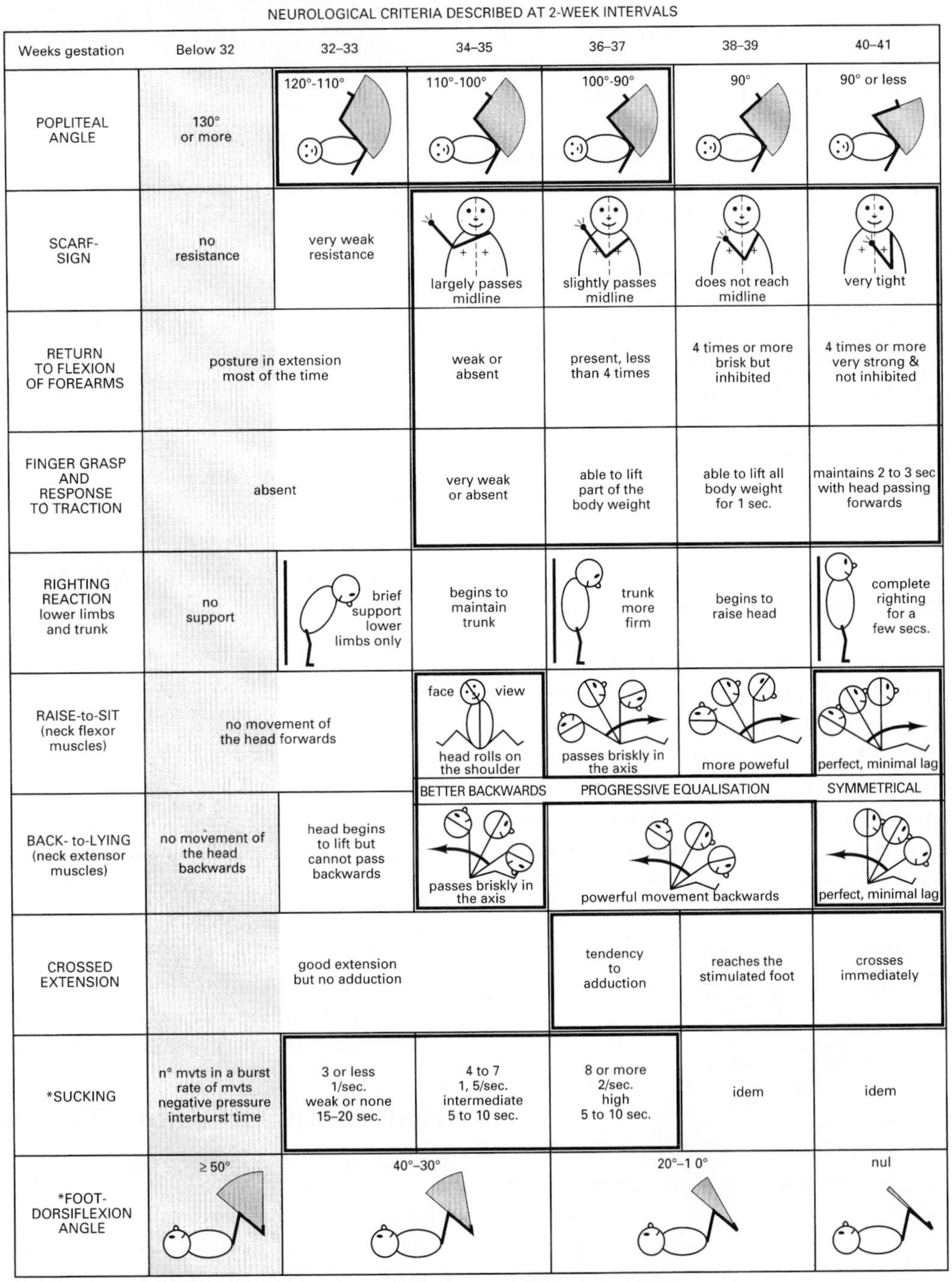
NEUROLOGICAL CRITERIA DESCRIBED AT 2-WEEK INTERVALS
Weeks gestation
Below 32
32–33
34–35
36–37
38–39
40–41
POPLITEAL ANGLE
130° or more
120°-110°
110°-100°
100°-90°
90°
90° or less
SCARF-SIGN
no resistance
very weak resistance
largely passes midline
slightly passes midline
does not reach midline
very tight
RETURN TO FLEXION OF FOREARMS
posture in extension most of the time
weak or absent
present, less than 4 times
4 times or more brisk but inhibited
4 times or more very strong & not inhibited
FINGER GRASP AND RESPONSE TO TRACTION
absent
very weak or absent
able to lift part of the body weight
able to lift all body weight for 1 sec.
maintains 2 to 3 sec with head passing forwards
RIGHTING REACTION lower limbs and trunk
no support
brief support lower limbs only
begins to maintain trunk
trunk more firm
begins to raise head
complete righting for a few secs.
RAISE-to-SIT (neck flexor muscles)
no movement of the head forwards
face view
head rolls on the shoulder
passes briskly in the axis
more poweful
perfect, minimal lag
BETTER BACKWARDS
PROGRESSIVE EQUALISATION
SYMMETRICAL
BACK- to-LYING (neck extensor muscles)
no movement of the head backwards
head begins to lift but cannot pass backwards
passes briskly in the axis
powerful movement backwards
perfect, minimal lag
CROSSED EXTENSION
good extension but no adduction
tendency to adduction
reaches the stimulated foot
crosses immediately
*SUCKING
n° mvts in a burst rate of mvts negative pressure interburst time
3 or less 1/sec. weak or none 15–20 sec.
4 to 7 1, 5/sec. intermediate 5 to 10 sec.
8 or more 2/sec. high 5 to 10 sec.
idem
idem
*FOOT-DORSIFLEXION ANGLE
≥ 50°
40°–30°
20°–1 0°
nul

Fig. 44.1 Aspects of the neurological examination of the preterm and term newborn, documented at 2-weekly intervals, to show changes in tone. Boxes highlight periods of rapid maturation, the most discriminative period for this item. * identifies items which are non-discriminatory during ex utero life. Shaded area, below 32 weeks, indicates period unable to be evaluated by this system. (Reproduced with permission from Amiel-Tison[1])

Moebius syndrome) is much more difficult to diagnose than the more common unilateral facial palsy. Normal facial expression in an otherwise hypotonic and flaccid infant suggests a spinal cord problem. Babies of just a few days old will often imitate facial gestures, for example putting out their tongues.

LIMB TONE AND POWER

Before passive movements are used to assess tone it may be possible to observe spontaneous movements of the limbs against gravity. Failure to move part or the whole of a limb may be due to pain or paralysis. Limb tone in newborns is influenced by the tonic neck reflex, which means it is important to have the head in the midline before beginning to elicit passive movements. These involve gentle flexion of the upper and lower limbs, then rapid extension and observation of recoil. A summary is contained within the protocol suggested by Dubowitz and Dubowitz.[10] This examination system, like that of Amiel-Tison[1] (Fig. 44.1), involves assessing the angles created by bending and manipulating the limbs and trunk (Fig. 44.2). These include the popliteal angle, the foot dorsiflexion angle and the scarf sign. A reduced popliteal angle and clusters of abnormal signs are sensitive indicators of later outcome.[11]

Jitteriness

The normal term newborn is in a state of hypertonicity, with brisk reflexes tending to clonus. This 'transient spasticity' gradually relaxes over the first 8–10 months in a caudocephalad direction. The high tone can lead to the clinical sign of jittering. Jittering is a high-frequency generalized symmetrical tremor of the limbs which is stilled by flexion or by inducing the infant to suck on a finger. It is common in the first 2 or 3 days in term babies, but if it is excessive or persistent deserves investigation (see Seizures, p. 1215). Repetitive chewing

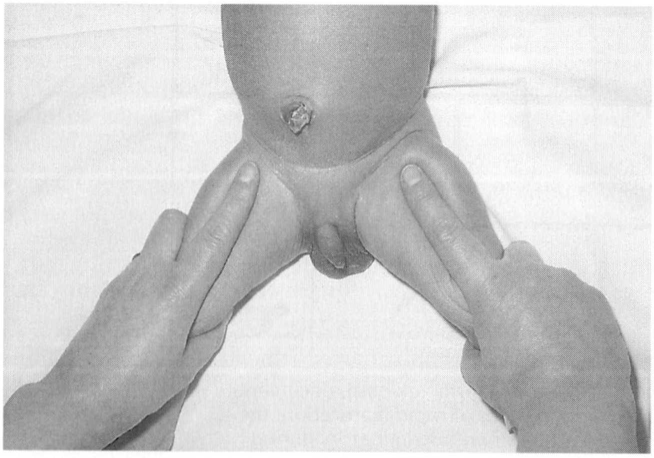

Fig. 44.2 Assessment of the adductor angle of the legs.

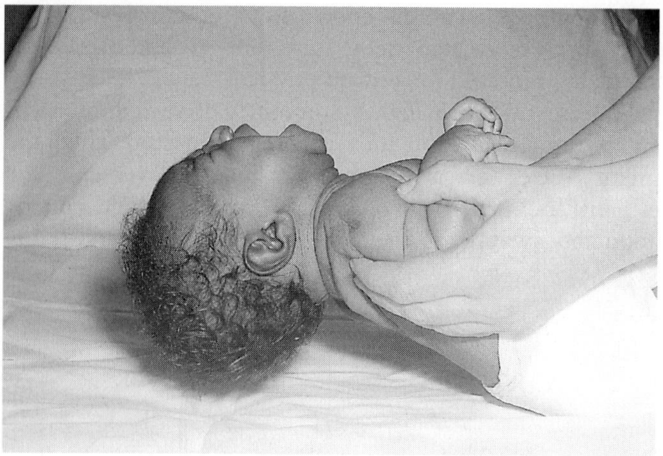

Fig. 44.3 Pull-to-sit manoeuvre: this full-term baby is attempting to raise his head.

movements or tongue thrusting are not part of jitteriness and imply seizures. Jitteriness is stimulus sensitive, whereas seizures are not. In seizure the movement has a fast and a slow component, whereas in jittering the tremor is symmetrical. Jittering is never accompanied by physiological changes due to the activation of the autonomic nervous system, such as tachycardia, hypertension or apnoea.

TRUNK AND NECK TONE AND POWER

Normal term infants have sufficient power in their neck muscles to lift their heads slightly when prone or supine. Preterm babies can manage to turn their heads from side to side, but have much less power, with complete head lag when pulled to sit. In order to judge tone in the neck and trunk, babies should be pulled to sit by holding them at the shoulders (Fig. 44.3). The pull-to-sit manoeuvre elicits an attempt to raise the head in a normal term newborn (Fig. 44.3). If the head is unsupported it will gradually fall forwards or backwards; normal term infants will be able to raise their heads to the vertical again from either direction (Fig. 44.4). Truncal tone can be assessed by placing the infant on his side, with one hand on the back and the other manipulating the legs. It is normally easier to flex the infant's trunk than to extend it.

SYSTEMATIC EXAMINATION 2: REFLEXES

TENDON AND BABINSKI REFLEXES

Eliciting tendon reflexes is of less value in the newborn period than later in childhood. Knee and biceps jerks can usually be obtained. Reflexes at term are very brisk because of the high tone, and a few beats of clonus at the ankle are usual. Very brisk reflexes and clonus are not reliable indicators of an upper motor neuron lesion until about 6 months of age.[3] A crossed adductor response to

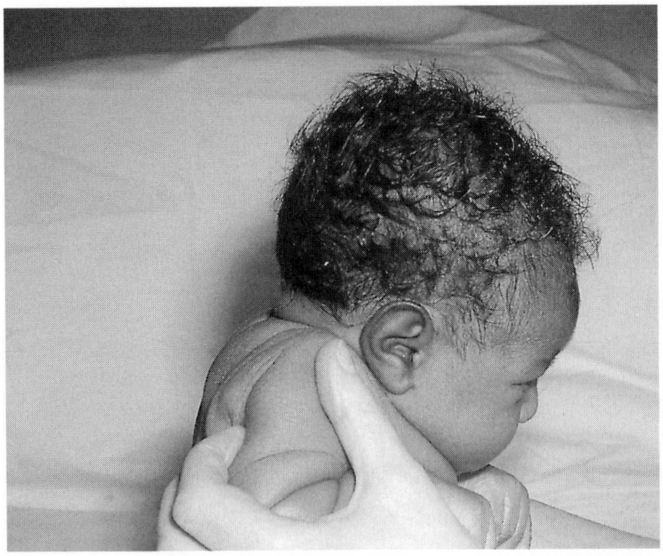

Fig. 44.4 After being pulled to sit the baby has raised his head to the vertical position, having let it fall forward.

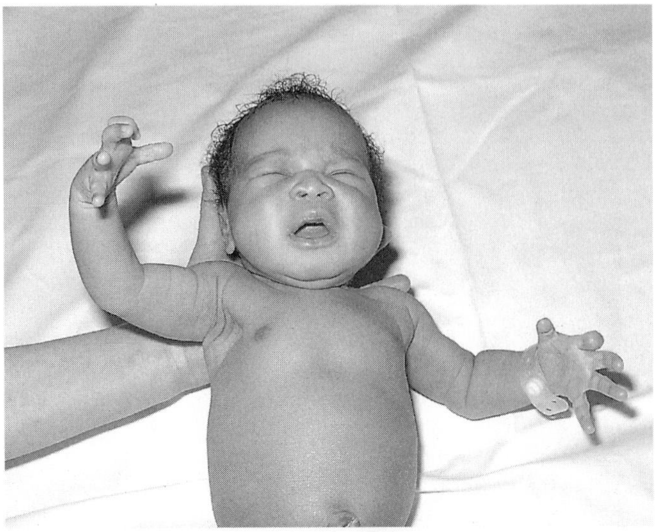

Fig. 44.5 The abduction phase of the Moro response: the baby's head has been allowed to fall back slightly, but is then supported by the examiner's hand.

the knee jerk (see below for description of this reflex) is also usual in the first months of life, whereas the sign is abnormal later on. The plantar reflex of Babinski is always extensor in babies, and is best omitted as the stimulus is painful and often results in a withdrawal response.

PRIMARY NEONATAL REFLEXES

Although these responses are undoubtedly fascinating to doctors and parents alike, it is necessary to have a working knowledge of only a few. Primitive reflexes normally habituate after repeated performance. Persistence of the primitive reflexes can considerably inhibit normal movement in children with cerebral palsy.

Moro

This reflex is usually elicited by allowing the previously supported head of a baby to fall backwards slightly, whereupon the baby extends and adducts both upper limbs, opening the hands (Fig. 44.5). Babies of greater than 33 weeks' gestation subsequently adduct their arms. The Moro response is present from 28 weeks of gestation and usually disappears by 4 months. Persistence beyond 6 months is always abnormal.

Asymmetric tonic neck reflex

Starting with the infant supine and the head in the midline, the head is slowly turned to one side. This results in increased extensor tone in the arm on the side to which the head is turned, and increased flexor tone in the arm on the opposite side (fencing posture). The reflex appears by 35 weeks' gestation, is very prominent by about 1 month of age and disappears by about 7 months.

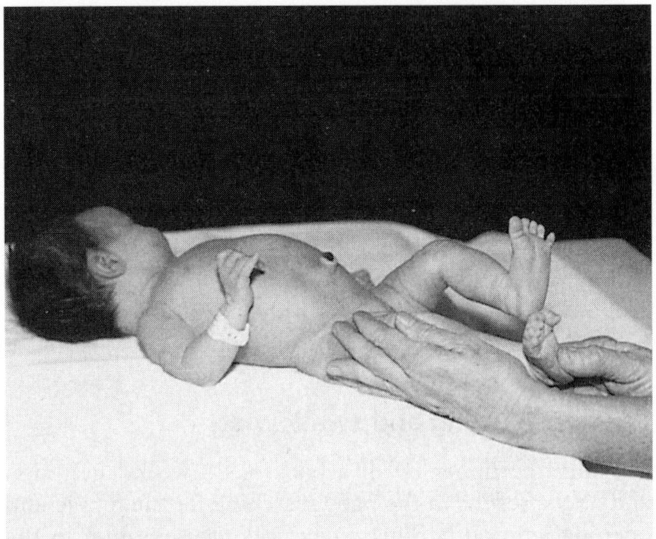

Fig. 44.6 The crossed extension reflex. Stimulating one foot has led to withdrawal and then extension of the other leg, fanning of the toes, and finally adduction. (Reproduced with permission from Amiel-Tison[1])

Crossed extension (adduction) reflex (Fig. 44.6)

One leg is held in extension and the sole of the foot is rubbed. The other leg first withdraws and then extends, with fanning of the toes. The third and final component of the fully developed reflex brings the other foot towards the side that was stimulated. Eliciting the knee jerk often produces this reflex in the neonatal period, which should not persist after 8 months of age.

Placing and stepping

By stimulating the dorsum of the foot, usually by bringing it into contact with the edge of the couch, a mature baby

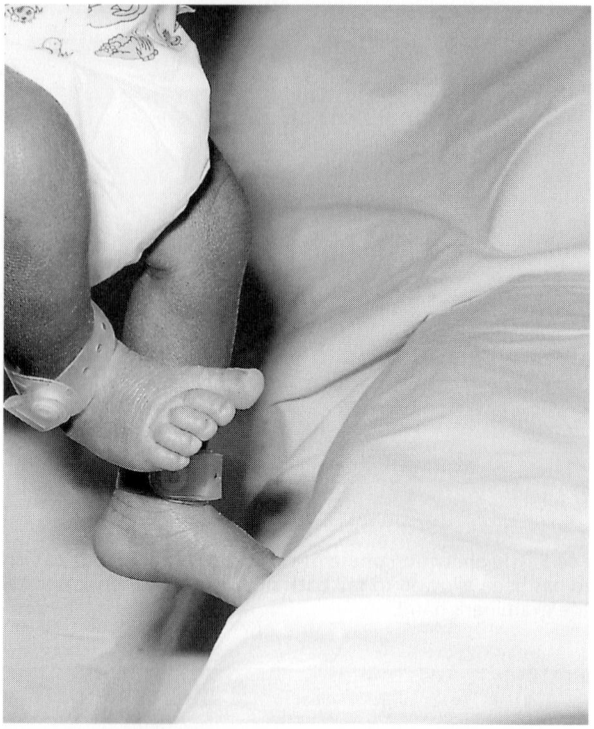

Fig. 44.7 The stepping reflex, elicited by bringing the dorsum of the baby's foot into contact with the couch.

can be induced to 'step' over the edge (Fig. 44.7). The baby's toes fan out and he lifts his foot up and then places it on the surface. Babies will extend their legs on to a flat surface and 'support' their weight when held under the arms. With the feet in contact with a solid surface and the body tilted forwards the baby will 'walk'.

Rooting, sucking and swallowing

Stroking the upper lip of a baby of 28 weeks' gestation and above results in the baby searching for the nipple and opening its mouth. This reflex tests the sensation in the distribution of the Vth cranial nerve and the motor pathways of cranial nerves V, VII, XII (Fig. 44.8). Swallowing also involves cranial nerves IX and X. The sensory input for the sucking reflex comes from the hard palate, not the tongue or cheek. Sucking begins during the 11th week of intrauterine life. Coordination between sucking and swallowing exists from 28 weeks' gestation, but the strength to sustain it and to synchronize the process with breathing is only adequate after 32–34 weeks' gestation. Sucking gradually builds up from bursts of three sucks at a time to eight or more, with a reduction in the interburst interval. If sucking is absent test the gag reflex by gently stroking the soft palate with a cotton bud.

Palmar and plantar grasp

The palmar reflex results from stroking the palmar surface of the hand, eliciting a grasp that is often strong

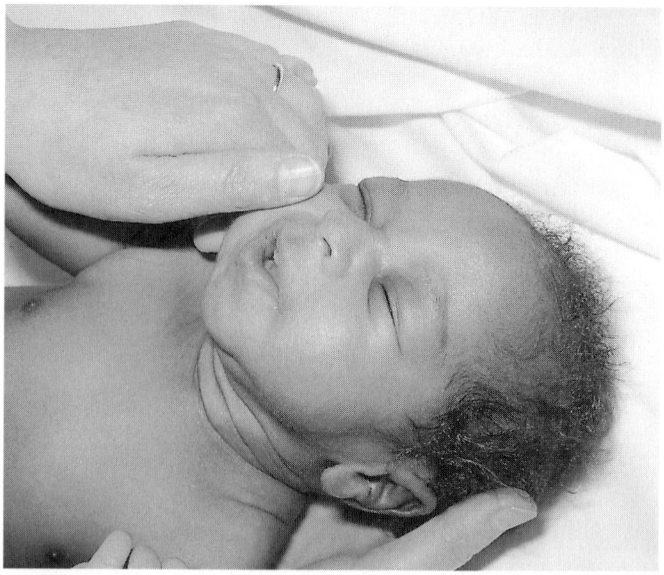

Fig. 44.8 The rooting reflex.

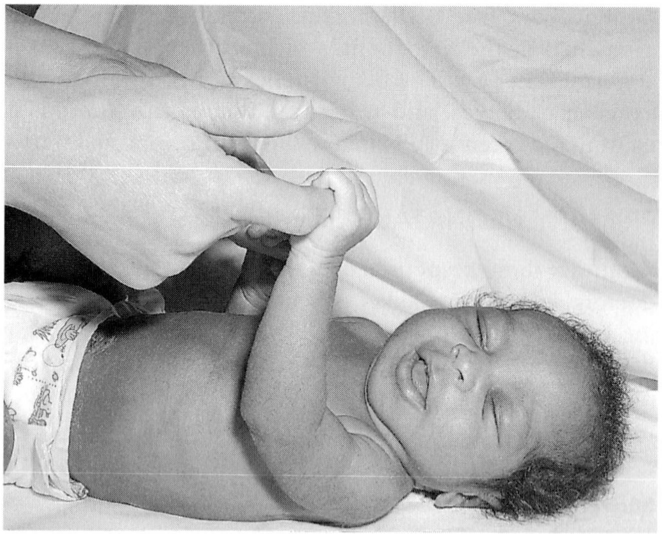

Fig. 44.9 The grasp reflex.

enough to lift the baby from the crib (Fig. 44.9). It is present from 26 weeks' gestation and persists for up to 4 months. Stroking the ball of the foot results in curling of the toes in a similar manner to the palmar response.

Pupillary reflex

The pupils respond to light only after 30 weeks' gestation, and the response was present in all infants after 35 weeks.[37] The size of the pupil gradually decreases after the development of the light reflex. The amplitude of the response – that is, the difference in size of the pupil before and after the light exposure – increases up to term. A small pupil on the side of an Erb's palsy suggests Horner syndrome due to the involvement of C8 and T1 nerve roots. A large pupil can indicate a congenital or acquired IIIrd nerve palsy.

NEONATAL NEUROLOGICAL ALARM SIGNALS

Certain neonatal neurological signs are generally recognized as potential indicators of serious disease. These 'alarm signs' are derived from the work of many authors:[2,8,22,30,40,45]

- Persistent irritability
- Difficulty in feeding
- Persistent deviation of head and/or eyes
- Persistent asymmetry in posture and movements
- Opisthotonus
- Apathy and immobility
- Floppiness
- Hyperexcitability, jitteriness
- Convulsions
- Abnormal cry
- The combination of setting-sun sign, vomiting, wide sutures and/or abnormal increase in skull circumference
- The occurrence and, especially, the recurrence of respiratory difficulties and apnoea
- The loss of variability in respiration, heart rate and transcutaneous oxygen tension.

Respiratory difficulties and apnoea can be signs of neurological dysfunction, although apnoea of prematurity is the commonest cause on a modern neonatal unit. In one large study, recurrent apnoea (i.e. three or more episodes of apnoea of longer than 20 seconds' duration) occurred in 1% of 25 154 infants evaluated between 1974 and 1979.[19] Of the affected infants, apnoea commenced in the first 2 days of life in 77% and was unlikely to commence after 7 days.[19] The gestational age at birth had a major impact with respect to the postnatal age when the last apnoea was detected (Fig. 44.10).

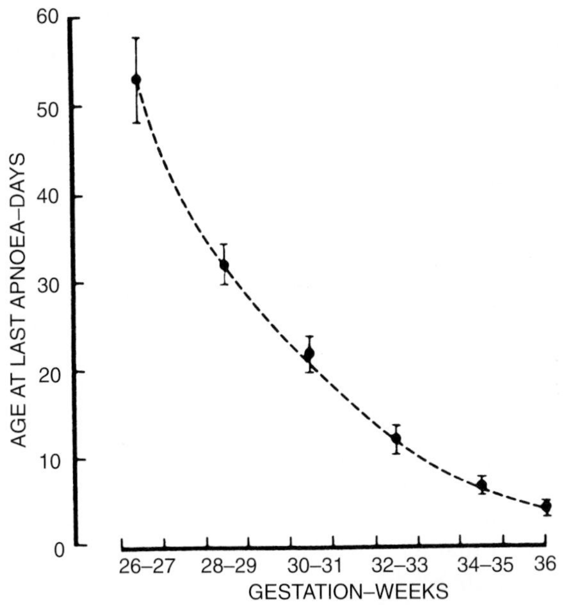

Fig. 44.10 Mean and standard deviation of the postnatal age when last apnoea was detected versus gestational age at birth in 24 145 infants. (Reproduced with permission from Ellison et al[19])

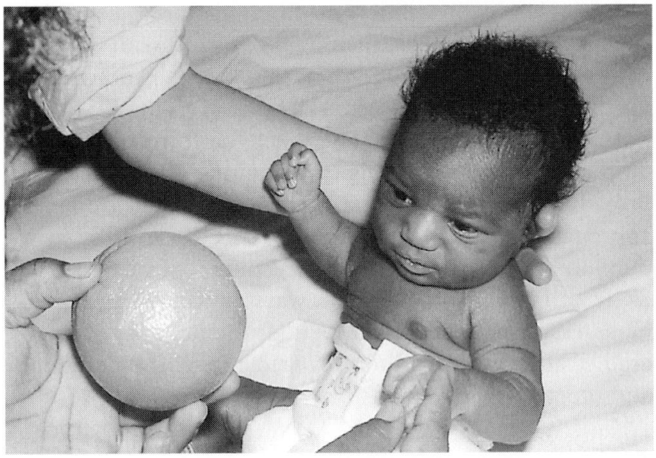

Fig. 44.11 Fixing and tracking an orange at term.

SPECIAL SENSES

EXAMINATION OF VISION, VISUAL EVOKED POTENTIALS

The 26-week gestation preterm infant blinks in response to light; by 32 weeks there is eye closure; by 34 weeks a baby is able to track a bright object briefly. By 37 weeks a baby will turn to soft light, and can track reliably (Fig. 44.11). Optokinetic nystagmus is present when a term baby looks at a striped rotating drum, or a striped tape is moved in front of his eyes. Changing the width of the stripes or forced-choice preferential looking at striped grids can be used to test visual acuity, which is equivalent to 20/150 vision at term.

The interpretation of deficient neonatal visual responses, however, is much more difficult. Dubowitz and Dubowitz[10] stress the importance of the loss of previously good visual performance as a disturbing sign.

Babies' eyes are usually in alignment, although a slight horizontal divergence is normal until 6 weeks of age, particularly in preterm babies. Vertical or skew deviation is always abnormal and has been seen in association with GMH-IVH.[49] For more information on abnormal and delayed visual development, and squint, see Chapter 36.

Visual evoked potentials are produced within the occipital cortex as a result of repeatedly applying an appropriate visual stimulus so that the minute electrical response to it, which will be identical each time, can be extracted from the random background electrical noise (EEG) by computerized averaging. Strobosocopic or flashing red lights are used which can penetrate closed eyelids. The electrical response 'matures' with advancing gestation, and can be detected from 25 weeks. VEPs have been found to be of value in predicting outcome after birth asphyxia,[43] and are a sensitive test for the integrity of the visual pathway. Absent VEPs predicted cortical blindness in preterm infants with extensive cystic leukomalacia.[9]

AUDITORY TESTING IN THE NEONATAL PERIOD

The fetus responds to sound from 19 weeks of gestation.[20] Infants from 28 weeks of gestation respond to noise by turning their heads, arousing from sleep or increasing their body movements. Bilateral sensorineural deafness occurs in about 1.5 per 1000 children (Chapter 7). Young children who are fitted with hearing aids early have an excellent chance of developing normal speech, but the current average age when hearing aids are given to children is often almost 2 years.[36] This has led to the suggestion that all newborns, and certainly those at high risk of deafness because of a positive family history, neonatal illness, cleft palate or low birthweight, should be screened for hearing loss.[24,41] The latter approach will identify 40% of the hearing-impaired children for the work of screening about 10% of the whole population. Hearing loss will still occur from acquired conditions such as glue ear or after meningitis. A successful universal neonatal screening programme has been established in north London,[51] and is being developed in the US, but is not supported by all.[5] The poor performance of the current distraction testing programme at 9 months is providing a stimulus for discussion regarding a different approach to hearing screening in the UK, and the introduction of universal neonatal screening looks increasingly likely.[17] There are three main ways in which hearing can be assessed in the neonatal period: the auditory response cradle, automated auditory evoked brainstem potentials, and otoacoustic emissions.

Auditory response cradle

This involves placing the infant in a special crib which monitors body movement, respiration and head turning via a pressure-sensitive mattress. The infant is exposed to sounds with a threshold of 90 dB. Of 6000 children 1.7% failed this test in one west London hospital; 20% of these were subsequently confirmed to have significant hearing loss.[48] Seven children who passed the test in the neonatal period were subsequently found to be deaf: five had a progressive hereditary condition or definite postnatal factors. The test also had a high false positive rate in a group of babies tested in Nottingham, and has not been widely adopted.[25] The US equivalent, the Crib-O-Gram, has not proved a success either.

Brain-stem auditory evoked potential

These indicate electrical events generated in the brain-stem auditory pathway in response to sound (usually a click) presented at the ear. The electrical signals are recorded with EEG electrodes on the scalp. The results of many click stimulations are summed by a computer, which uses coherent averaging to eliminate the background noise generated by the local EEG signal. The mature pattern consists of seven waves, but these are poorly developed with increased latency and require a larger stimulus in order to elicit them in babies, in whom the response is present from 24 weeks. Prolongation of brain-stem auditory evoked potentials has been described with hyperbilirubinaemia and gentamicin toxicity. Automated brain-stem response equipment eliminates the need for extensive operator training, and is the most widely used method of hearing screening. Ex-preterm infants are tested as near to term as possible in order to reduce the false positive failure rate to a minimum.

Otoacoustic emissions

Otoacoustic emissions were discovered in 1978. They are low-amplitude sound waves produced by the inner ear, and occur spontaneously as well as in response to a click stimulus. The automated method depends on the fact that a click stimulus, when presented to an intact hearing ear, evokes an otoacoustic emission which can be detected by a probe lying in the ear canal. Programmable software for measuring otoacoustic emissions has been developed (POEMS) and the system evaluated as a screening method in high-risk newborn babies in Sheffield and Southampton.[24,42] POEMS was quicker to administer than the automated evoked brain-stem response method (no scalp electrodes), but there were more false positive results.

IMAGING

For advice on the best imaging modality to choose when investigating the central nervous system see Chapter 47.

EXAMINATION OF CEREBROSPINAL FLUID, INTRACRANIAL PRESSURE

Lumbar puncture is often done in babies because the signs of meningitis are subtle. For practical advice on how to perform the procedure see Chapter 51. In the neonatal period cerebrospinal fluid may be xanthochromic because of jaundice or old GMH-IVH. The cell count is higher than later in childhood. In preterm neonates the red and white cell counts can each be up to 30/mm^3 (Appendix 11). In term infants after the first week of life more than 10 cells of each type per cubic millimetre is abnormal. A white cell count of more than 30/mm^3 with neutrophils more than 66% of the total, is suspicious, although in cases of meningitis the white cell count is usually more than 100/mm^3. Seizures do not influence the results. Red cell counts of more than 1000/mm^3 make the interpretation of cerebrospinal fluid results impossible: applying correction factors using the ratio of white cells to red cells has been shown to be inaccurate.[28,39] The only course of action is to repeat the lumbar puncture after 12 hours.

Measured accurately with pressure transducers at lumbar puncture, the intracranial pressure was 0–5.5 mmHg[23] in one study and 2 mmHg in another.[26] The upper limit of normal pressure is thus 7 cmH_2O.

ELECTROENCEPHALOGRAPHY

Conventional multichannel EEG recordings can be difficult to obtain in newborn infants. The montage of electrodes is hard to apply and maintain, and many babies requiring investigation are in intensive care units, which are electrically noisy. Short recordings are of less value than prolonged ones, as the EEG shows wide variability and changes not only with sleep state but also

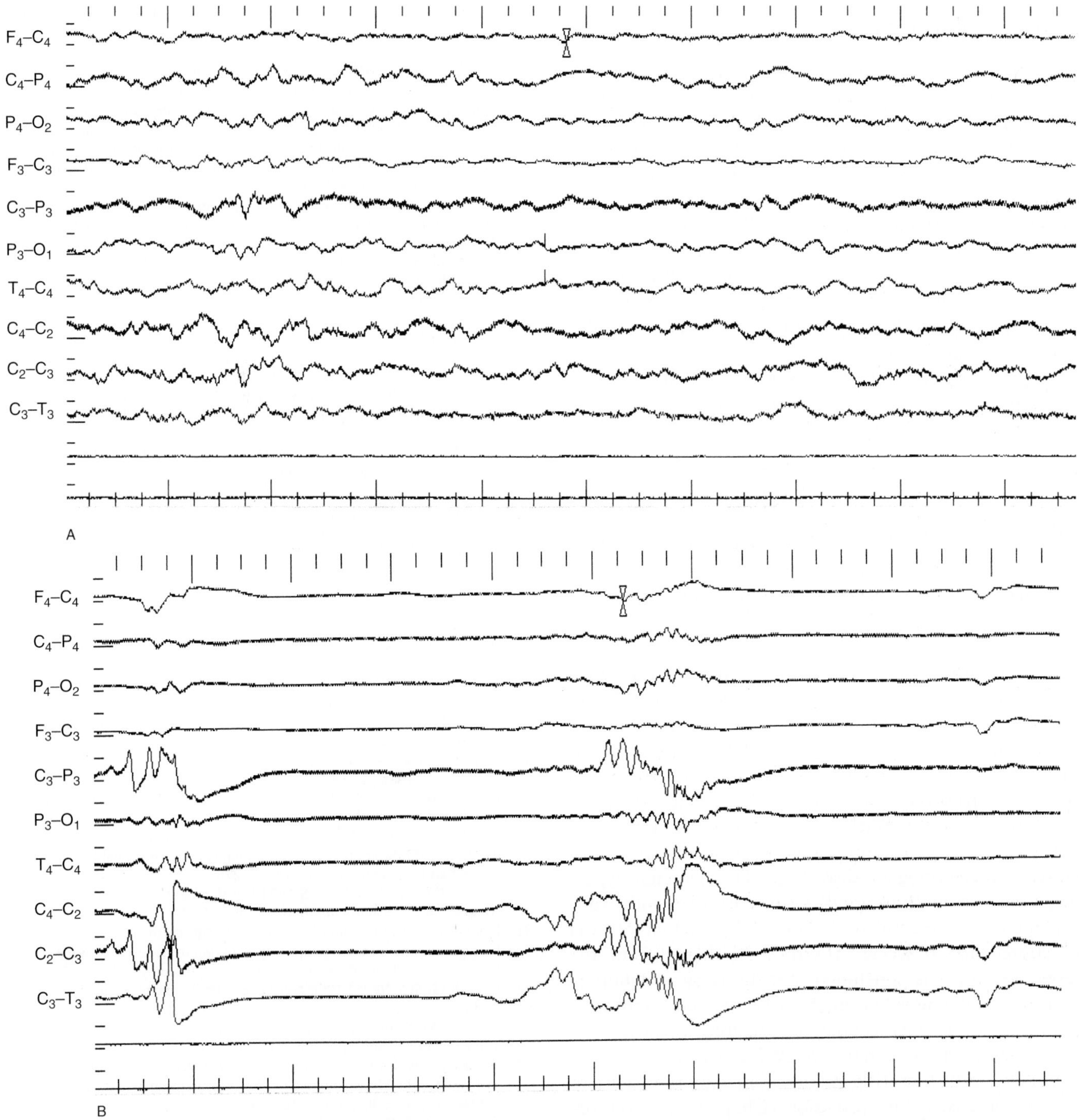

Fig. 44.12 (A) 12-lead EEG recorded from a normal full-term infant. Recorded using a modified 10–20 system of electrode placement normal continuous pattern at term. (B) 12-lead EEG recorded from a normal preterm infant of 25 weeks' gestation. Discontinuous pattern.

with the length of the preceding sleep epoch.[13,38] Continuous monitoring is possible with either a cerebral function monitor, which displays the amplitude of one or two channels of processed EEG, or the Oxford Medilog system, which records up to eight channels of EEG on to audio tape, requiring later analysis. Unless a dedicated laptop computer is connected to the system the Oxford Medilog does not allow for cotside display. Video-EEG telemetry is becoming more established on neonatal units.[6]

MATURATION OF EEG

The EEG of very preterm babies is markedly discontinuous (Fig. 44.12),[13] and consists of long periods of quiescence, interspersed with bursts of high-voltage mixed frequency activity termed 'trace discontinu'. Delta brushes are a specific feature of the preterm EEG, maximal at 32 weeks. They are delta waves with fast frequency superimposed on top. With increasing gestation the interburst intervals decrease and the record becomes more continuous. High-voltage slow activity intermixed with periods of voltage attenuation can be seen during quiet sleep in mature babies, and is called 'trace alternant'. Abnormal background EEG activity, such as severe amplitude depression or burst suppression, correlates well with later adverse outcome in both preterm and asphyxiated term babies.[12,18,21,50]

NEUROLOGICAL EXAMINATION BEFORE DISCHARGE, AND FOLLOW-UP

When assessing the predictive value of the neurological examination before discharge a distinction should be made between studies of low-risk and of high-risk newborns. In low-risk full-term infants there is a low but significant correlation between the neonatal neurological evaluation and follow-up evaluations to school age.[44,47] In high-risk preterm infants Touwen[46] found a much higher correlation between the neonatal and follow-up examinations during infancy. The neonatal hemisyndrome and hypertonia syndrome have distinct prognostic value, but hypotonia does not. With asphyxia, however, hypotonia which evolves to hypertonia correlates significantly with subsequent neurological disorders.[8] The neonatal hyperexcitability syndrome appears to correlate with subsequent developmental difficulties only when it persists for more than 6 weeks. If, upon discharge from the neonatal unit, it is concluded that the baby is definitely neurologically abnormal, on the basis of such established abnormalities as microcephaly or seizures, a nearly 100-fold increased risk of cerebral palsy does exist.[27]

Follow-up of high-risk infants is an important part of neonatal intensive care provision (Chapter 7). Monitoring of head growth and neurodevelopment over the first months can give early warning of neurodevelopmental problems. A failure to achieve a normal pattern of head growth is an ominous sign.

REFERENCES

1. Amiel-Tison C 1995 Clinical assessment of the infant nervous system. In: Levene, M I, Lilford R J (eds) Fetal and neonatal neurology and neurosurgery, 2nd edn. Churchill Livingstone, Edinburgh, pp 83–104
2. Amiel-Tison C, Grenier A 1986 Neurological assessment in the first year of life. Oxford University Press, New York
3. Amiel-Tison C, Stewart A 1994 Apparently normal survivors: neuromotor and cognitive function as they grow older. In: Amiel-Tison C, Stewart A. (eds) The newborn infant: one brain for life. INSERM, Paris, pp 227–237
4. Ball W S 1997 Pediatric neuroradiology. Lippincott-Raven, Philadelphia
5. Bess F H, Paradise J L 1994 Universal screening for infant hearing: not simple, not risk-free and presently not justified. Pediatrics 93: 330–334
6. Boylan G B, Pressler R, Rennie J M, Binnie C B. Electroclinical, electrographic and clinical seizures in the newborn infant. (In press)
7. Brazelton T B, Nugent J K 1995 Neonatal behavioural assessment scales. MacKeith Press, London
8. Brown J K, Purvis R J, Forfar J O, Cockburn F 1974 Neurological aspects of perinatal asphyxia. Developmental Medicine and Child Neurology 16: 567–580
9. de Vries L S, Connell J, Dubowitz L M S, Oozeer R C, Dubowitz V, Pennock J M 1987 Neurological, electrophysiological and MRI abnormalities in infants with extensive cystic leukomalacia. Neuropediatrics 18: 61–66
10. Dubowitz L M S, Dubowitz V 1981 The neurological assessment of the preterm and full term newborn infant. MacKeith Press, London
11. Dubowitz L M S, Dubowitz V, Palmer P G, Miller G, Fawer C-L, Levene M I. 1984 Correlation of neurological assessment in the preterm newborn infant with outcome at age 1 year. Journal of Pediatrics 105: 452–456
12. Eken P, Toet M C, Groenendaal F, de Vries L S 1995 Predictive value of early neuroimaging, pulsed Doppler and neurophysiology in full term infants with hypoxic ischaemic encephalopathy. Archives of Disease in Childhood 73: f75–f81
13. Eyre J A, Nanei S, Wilkinson A R 1988 Quantification of change in normal neonatal EEGs with gestation. Developmental Medicine and Child Neurology 30: 599–607
14. Faerber E N 1995 CNS Magnetic resonance imaging in infants and children. MacKeith Press, London
15. Ferrari F, Cioni G, Prechtl H F R 1990 Qualitative changes of general movement in preterm infants with brain lesions. Early Human Development 23: 193–231
16. Govaert P, de Vries L S 1997 An atlas of neonatal brain sonography. MacKeith Press, London
17. Haggard M P 1990 Hearing screening in children – state of the art(s). Archives of Disease in Childhood 65: 1193–1198
18. Hellstrom-Westas L, Rosen I, Svenningsen N W 1995 Predictive value of early continuous amplitude integrated EEG recordings on outcome after severe birth asphyxia in full term infants. Archives of Disease in Childhood 72: F34–F38
19. Henderson-Smart D J 1981 The effect of gestational age on the incidence and duration of recurrent apnoea in newborn babies. Australian Paediatric Journal 17: 273–276
20. Hepper P G, Shahidullah B S 1994 Development of fetal hearing. Archives of Disease in Childhood 71: F81–F87
21. Holmes G, Rowe J, Schmidt R, Testa M, Zimmerman A 1982 Prognostic value of the electroencephalogram in neonatal seizures. Electroencephalography and Clinical Neurophysiology 53: 60–72
22. Joppich G, Schulte F J 1968 Neurologie des Neugeborenen. Springer, Berlin
23. Kaiser A M, Whitelaw A G L 1986 Normal cerebrospinal fluid pressure in the newborn. Neuropediatrics 17: 100–102
24. Kennedy C R, Kimm L, Caferelli Dees D et al 1991 Otoacoustic emissions and auditory brainstem responses in the newborn. Archives of Disease in Childhood 66: 1124–1129
25. McCormick B, Curnock D A, Spavins F 1984 Auditory screening of special care neonates using the auditory response cradle. Archives of Disease in Childhood 59: 1168–1172

26. Minns R A 1984 Intracranial pressure monitoring. Archives of Disease in Childhood 59: 486–488
27. Nelson K B, Ellenberg J H 1979 Neonatal signs as predictors of cerebral palsy. Pediatrics 64: 225–232
28. Novak R W 1984 Lack of validity of standard corrections for white blood cell counts of blood-contaminated cerebrospinal fluid in infants. American Journal of Clinical Pathology 82: 95–97
29. Prechtl H F R 1974 The behavioural states of the newborn infant. Brain Research 76: 185–212
30. Prechtl H F R 1980 The optimality concept. Early Human Development 4: 201–206
31. Prechtl H F R 1990 Qualitative changes of spontaneous movements in fetus and preterm infant as a marker of neurological dysfunction. Early Human Development 23: 151–158
32. Prechtl H F R, Fargel V W, Weinaman H M, Bakker H H 1979 Postures, motility and respiration of low risk preterm infants. Developmental Medicine and Child Neurology 21: 3–7
33. Prechtl H F R, Nolte R 1984 Motor behaviour of preterm infants. In: Precht H F R (ed) Continuity of neural functions from prenatal to postnatal life. MacKeith Press, London
34. Prechtl H F R, O'Brien M J 1982 Behavioural states of the full term newborn. In: Stratton P (ed) Pschychobiology of the human newborn. John Wiley, New York, pp 53–73
35. Rennie J M 1997 Neonatal cranial ultrasound. Cambridge University Press, Cambridge
36. Robertson C, Aldrige S, Jarman F, Saunders K, Poulakis Z, Oberklaid F 1995 Late diagnosis of congenital sensorineural hearing impairment: why are detector methods failing? Archives of Disease in Childhood 72: 11–15
37. Robinson J, Fielder A R 1990 Pupillary diameter and reaction to light in preterm infants. Archives of Disease in Childhood 65: 35–38
38. Roffwarg H P, Muzio J N, Dement, W C 1966 Ontogenetic development of human sleep dream cycles. Science 152: 604–619
39. Rubenstein J S, Yogev R 1985 What represents pleocytosis in blood contaminated ('traumatic tap') cerebrospinal fluid in children? Journal of Pediatrics 107: 249–252
40. Saint-Anne Dargassies S 1977 Neurological development in the full term and premature neonate. Elsevier, Amsterdam
41. Stapells D R, Kurtzberg D 1998 Evoked potential assessment of auditory system integrity in infants. Clinics in Perinatology 18: 497–518
42. Stevens J C, Webb H D, Hutchinson J, Connell J, Smith M F, Buffin J T 1989 Click evoked otoacoustic emissions compared with brain stem electrical response. Archives of Disease in Childhood 64: 1105–1111
43. Taylor M J, Murphy W J, Whyte H E 1992 Prognostic reliability of somatosensory and visual evoked potentials in asphyxiated term newborns. Developmental Medicine and Child Neurology 34: 507–515
44. Touwen B C L 1972 The relationship between neonatal and follow up findings. In: Saling E, Schulte F J (eds) Perinatale Medizin. Thieme Verlag, Stuttgart, pp 303–306
45. Touwen B C L 1976 Neurological development in infancy. Heinemann, London
46. Touwen B C L 1978 Early detection of developmental neurological disorders. In: Jonxis J H P (eds) Growth and development of the full term and premature neonate. The Jonxis lectures. Excerpta Medica, Amsterdam, pp 244-261
47. Touwen B C L, Lok-Mejjer T Y, Huisjes H J, Olinga A A 1982 The recovery rate of neurologically deviant newborns. Archives of Disease in Childhood 67: 911–919
48. Tucker S M, Battacharya J 1992 Screening of hearing impairment in the newborn using the auditory response cradle. Archives of Disease in Childhood 67: 911–919
49. Volpe J J 1995 The neurological examination: normal and abnormal features. In: Neonatal neurology, 3rd edn. W B Saunders, Philadelphia, pp 95–124
50. Watanabe K, Miyazaki S, Hara K, Hakamanda A 1980 Behavioral state cycles, background EEGs and prognosis of newborn with perinatal hypoxia. Electroencephalography and Clinical Neurophysiology 49: 618–625
51. Watkin P M 1996 Neonatal otoacoustic emission screening and the identification of deafness. Archives of Disease in Childhood 74: F16–F25

Part 2

Seizures in the newborn

Janet M. Rennie

INTRODUCTION

The immature central nervous system is particularly susceptible to seizures, which are more common in newborn babies than at any other time of life. The vulnerability of the neonatal brain to seizures is thought to be due to a combination of enhanced excitability, with an abundance of NMDA binding sites, and low levels of the inhibitory neurotransmitter GABA.[56] All those who care for the newborn therefore need a working knowledge of the likely causes and a management plan for this important emergency. Prompt diagnosis, investigation and treatment are vital, as delayed recognition of a treatable cause can have a significant impact on the child's subsequent neurological outcome. In neonates seizures are associated with conditions such as GMH-IVH, cerebral infarction (stroke), hypoglycaemia, infection, cerebral malformations and HIE. Seizures represent the brain's final common response to insult. The initial injury may be brief, but membrane damage releases excitotoxic substances such as glutamate, which trigger further epileptic activity. If convulsions are not controlled the electrical activity can continue to circulate, a phenomenon known as kindling. Prolonged fits cause progressive cerebral hypoxia, cerebral oedema, lactic acidosis and further excitotoxicity. Permanent brain damage is associated with neonatal seizures; magnetic resonance imaging of the brain showed markedly reduced myelination in childhood in several cases.[51] A single bout of seizures permanently inhibited DNA synthesis in the neonatal rat brain.[77,78] These animal data suggest that abnormal elecrical activity may be damaging per se, although evidence that it is the seizures rather than the underlying cause that damages the brain is more difficult to find in human neonates.

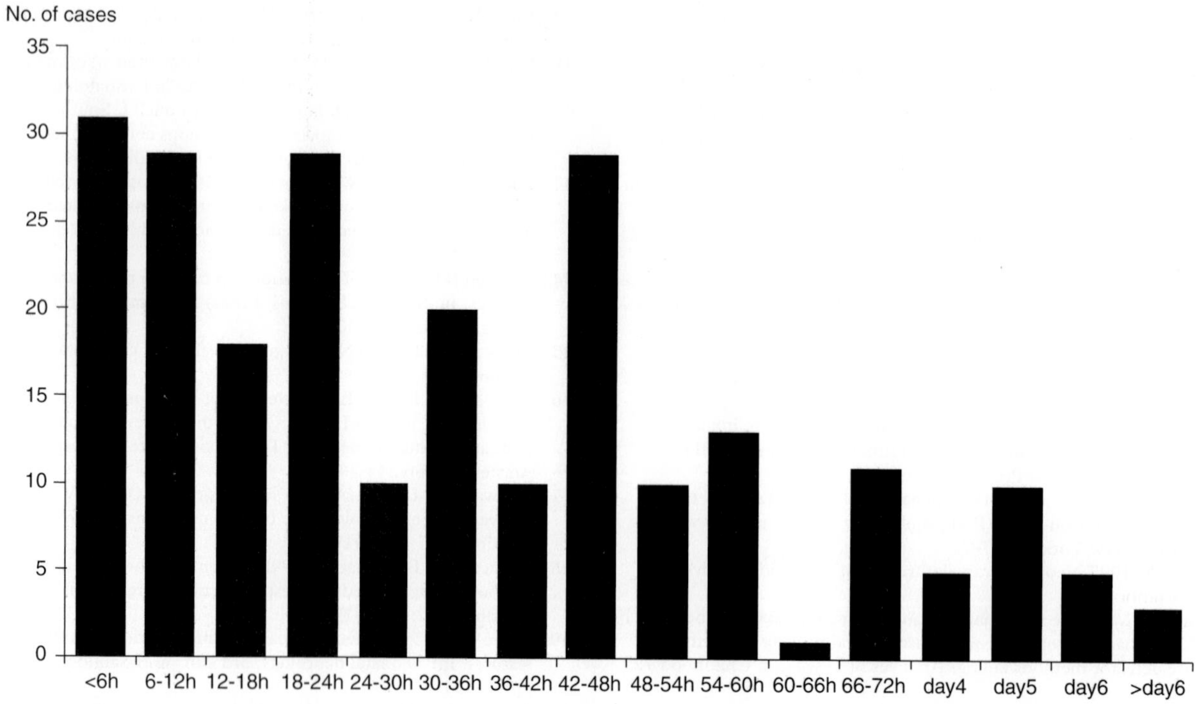

Fig. 44.13 Time of onset of seizures in 277 neonatal cases: data from the National Collaborative Perinatal Project.[36] Note the scale on the *x* axis starts as 6-hourly periods, and is then grouped by days.

INCIDENCE

Seizures occur in 6–13% of very low-birthweight infants, and in 1–2 per 1000 of infants born at term.[14,44,45,48,80] Older series did not usually discriminate between term and preterm infants, and reported higher incidence figures. Many term cases were due to late-onset hypocalcaemia. Brown et al[6] reported an incidence of 14 per 1000 and Keen and Lee[39] 12:1000 infants. The incidence of early (<48 hours) seizures in term infants has been proposed as an indicator of the quality of perinatal care because the most common cause in this group is hypoxic–ischaemic encephalopathy.[16] The incidence of early seizures varies, being 0.87 per 1000 in Dublin between 1980 and 1984,[14] 1.3 per 1000 in Cardiff during 1970–79[54] and 2.8 per 1000 in Fayette County, Kentucky, in 1985–89.[44] The incidence of early seizures at term seems likely to become a core item in a minimum dataset requested from UK maternity units, but there are many problems in definition which will become apparent to the reader. Subtle seizures are the most common type, particularly in premature infants, being present in 75% of the cases described by Sher et al.[65]

TIME OF ONSET

Seizures apparent in the delivery room are rare, and from personal experience and case reports these are often due to a severe prolonged hypoxic–ischaemic insult and are associated with a poor outlook. Pyridoxine-dependent seizures can begin very early. Most neonatal seizures start between 12 and 48 hours after birth. Late-onset seizures suggest meningitis, benign familial seizures or hypocalcaemia. Figure 44.13 shows the time of onset recorded in 277 neonatal cases.[36]

DIAGNOSIS AND CLASSIFICATION

A seizure is a paroxysmal alteration in neurological function, either behavioural, motor or autonomic.[75] Four main types are recognized (Table 44.2), and within each type the seizures can be unifocal, multifocal or generalized. In the newborn there is the additional problem of electroclinical dissociation (see below).

Table 44.2 Types of seizure in the newborn. (Adapted from Volpe[75])

Type	Clinical manifestation
Subtle	Eye signs: eyelid fluttering, eye deviation, fixed open stare, blinking; apnoea, cycling, boxing, stepping, swimming movements of limbs, mouthing, chewing, lip smacking, smiling. EEG changes most likely with ocular manifestations
Tonic	Stiffening. Decerebrate posturing. EEG variable
Clonic	Repetitive jerking, distinct from jittering. Can be unifocal or multifocal. Usually EEG change.
Myoclonic	Rare, sleep myoclonus is benign. EEG often normal, although background EEG can be abnormal

SUBTLE

The clinical manifestations of seizures in infants can be extremely subtle. They can be divided into orofacial manifestations including eye deviation, eyelid blinking, sucking, chewing and lip smacking, and limb movements (often described as swimming, boxing or cycling). In addition, apnoeic episodes can be due to seizures and this diagnosis should be considered if there is slow response to bag and mask ventilation, particularly in a preterm neonate with an intracranial lesion. Another clue may be associated movements such as eyelid or mouth opening, and a bradycardia which starts soon after the collapse.

TONIC

Sustained posturing of the limbs or trunk, or deviation of the head or eyes, are the usual manifestations of tonic seizures in the newborn. This type of seizure is usually associated with a characteristic EEG signature of high-frequency sharp waves.

CLONIC

Clonic seizures usually involve one limb or one side of the face or body jerking rhythmically at a frequency of 1–4 times per second. This type of seizure is associated with a characteristic EEG discharge consisting of runs of focal sharp wave complexes which spread ipsilaterally from the hemisphere in which they originate. Clonic seizures in the neonate can have more than one focus or migrate in a non-Jacksonian fashion: for example, jerking of one leg can be followed by similar movements in the opposite hand. Clonic seizures are often a clue to an underlying focal lesion such as a cortical infarction, but they can have a metabolic cause. Infants are not usually unconscious during clonic seizures.

MYOCLONIC

Myoclonic jerks tend to occur in the flexor muscle groups. Generalized myoclonic seizures resemble salaam spasms and are the type most likely to be unassociated with EEG change. Any type of myoclonic seizure (focal, multifocal or generalized) can occur in benign neonatal sleep myoclonus.[13]

JITTERINESS (p. 1206)

Jitteriness is an extremely common phenomenon among normal newborns, being observed in 44% of a sample of 936 babies.[58] It is more common in infants born to mothers who use marijuana. Jittering is a symmetrical tremor, without the fast and slow component of a clonic or myoclonic seizure, and occurs at a faster rate of 5–6 times per second. It does not involve the face (unlike subtle seizures), is markedly stimulus sensitive, and ceases when the limb is held. The autonomic nervous system changes of a seizure, such as tachycardia or hypertension, are never seen in jittering.

HYPEREKPLEXIA

Hyperekplexia is a rare autosomal dominant disorder characterized by hypertonia, especially in infancy, and an exaggerated startle response.[72] The startles can look like myoclonic jerks, and the high tone, hyper-reflexia and jitteriness can lead to an erroneous diagnosis of seizure.[27] Hyperekplexia is probably the same condition previously known as hereditary stiff-baby syndrome.[49] Treatment with clonazepam or diazepam results in marked improvement. The disorder is caused by mutations in the α-subunit of the inhibitory glycine receptor,[69] and very low cerebrospinal fluid GABA levels (11 nmol/l) were found in one case.[17] This finding may not be specific, as newborns have low cerebrospinal fluid GABA levels of 20–100 nmol/l. Low levels have also been found in pyridoxine-dependent seizures.[43]

PHYSIOLOGICAL CHANGES DURING SEIZURES

Blood glucose remains normal or rises during seizure, but brain glucose falls markedly. This implies that brain transport mechanisms are unable to keep up with the increased demand. The demand for oxygen is also increased, and cerebral blood flow rises to try to meet the need for oxygen and glucose. That metabolic demand outstrips supply in the newborn is supported by magnetic resonance spectroscopic data showing a shift in spectra from the high-energy phosphate compounds towards inorganic phosphate.[82] Glucose pretreatment is effective in reducing the high mortality of status epilepticus in rats, a benefit which is not seen with ketone body supplementation, although the neonatal brain is known be able to utilize alternative fuels. Lactate accumulates during seizure, and the arterial pH falls. Systemic blood pressure increases in seizures with marked pathological activity.

EEG DIAGNOSIS OF SEIZURES

NORMAL NEONATAL EEG

The EEG of the preterm newborn is characterized by a degree of discontinuity which would be abnormal at term.[9] The interburst interval falls from 15 seconds at 28 weeks to 5 seconds at term (Fig. 44.14). Ellison et al[19] characterized the neonatal EEG mainly on the basis of the interburst interval, categorizing the EEG of infants <30 weeks as abnormal if the interval was >60 seconds, and using a figure of 30 seconds at term. There is a trend towards increasing frequency (from 0.5–1 Hz to 1–2 Hz) and reducing amplitude with increasing gestational age. Delta brushes (p. 1212) are high-frequency components which appear superimposed on the baseline amplitude change, and these are common between 30 and 36 weeks' gestation. The EEG is symmetrical in healthy infants.

ELECTROGRAPHIC SEIZURES

Electrographic seizures are brief in the newborn, usually lasting about 2 minutes in term infants, with about 8 minutes between seizures in most cases. Clancy and Ledigo[8] used an arbitrary cut-off of 10 seconds as a minimum duration, and this definition was also adopted by Scher et al.[66] Others have used 5 seconds.[67] Very short bursts of abnormal electrical activity have also been termed BIRDS – brief intermittent rhythmic discharges. Electrograpic seizures characteristically consist of monophasic repetitive discharges or spike and wave activity (Fig. 44.14). An electrographic seizure should have a clear onset and conclusion, but these can be difficult to identify. Electrographic seizures may or may not be accompanied by stereotyped movements (see below).

ELECTROCLINICAL DISSOCIATION

There is asynchrony between the clinical and the electrical diagnosis of neonatal seizures: in only one-third of cases studied with video surveillance were the clinical and electrical manifestations simultaneous.[40,81] Subtle stereotyped behaviour may or may not be associated with characteristic EEG changes, and continuous electrical monitoring detects many clinically silent seizures.[10,20,32] One explanation is that the motor manifestations arise because of discharges from the brain stem and spinal cord which are 'released' because of lack of inhibition from higher centres. An alternative explanation is that scalp electrodes are incapable of recording from every part of the brain; depth electrodes reveal an otherwise unsuspected electrical focus in 10% of adult patients. Of the orofacial manifestations only tonic horizontal deviation of the eyes was consistently associated with EEG paroxysms in one video EEG study.[55] The neurological effects of clinically silent (electrographic) seizures are not known, nor is it certain that treatment of clinically manifest seizures to electrical silence is required. This is an important question because phenobarbitone treatment

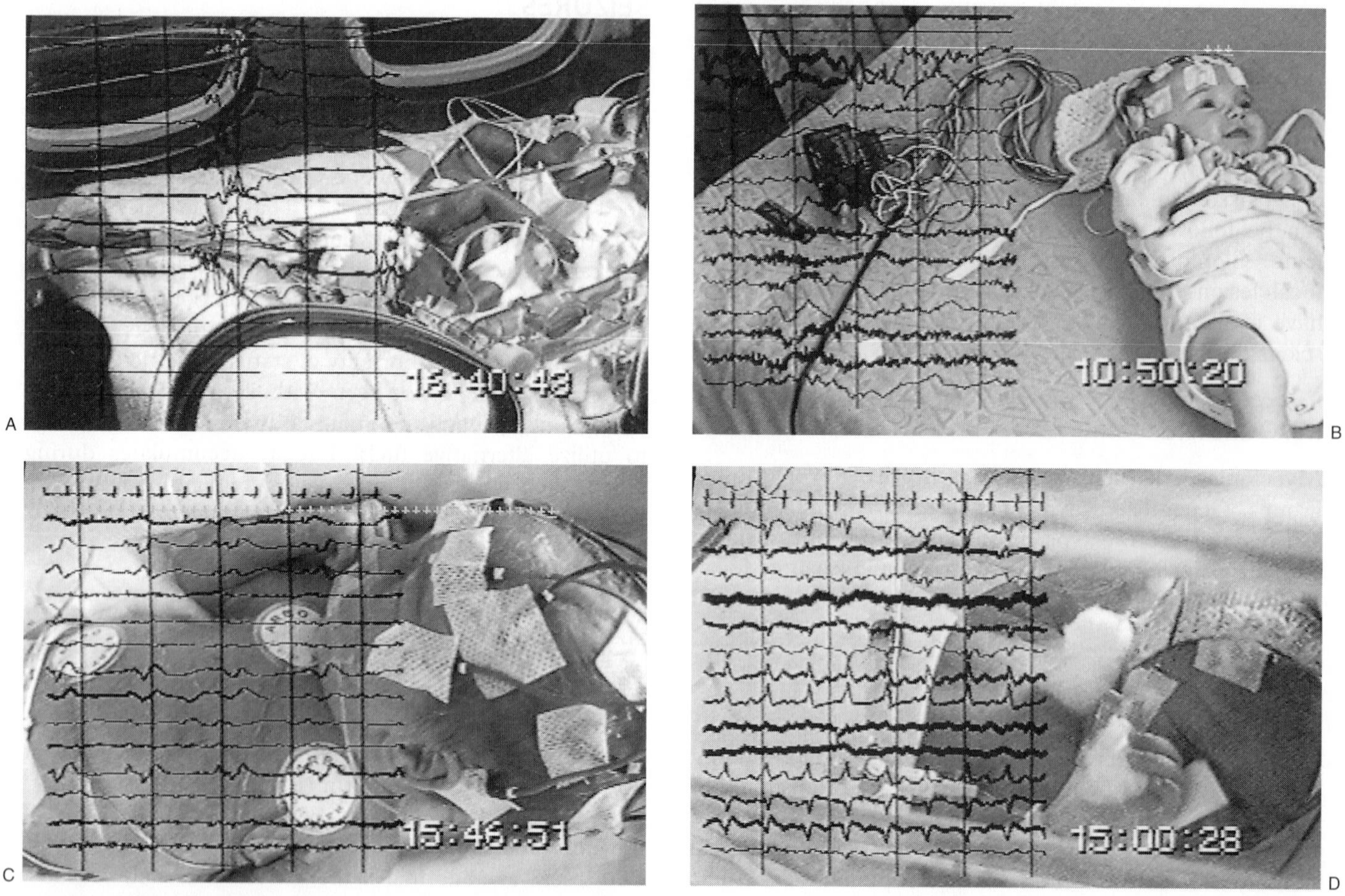

Fig. 44.14 EEG recordings showing normal preterm activity (A), normal term activity (B) and seizures in both preterm (C) and term (D) infants. EEG montage same as that shown in Figure 44.12. Top two channels show respiration and ECG.

frequently abolishes the clinical manifestations while the electrical paroxysms continue.

Our video EEG studies have shown that all cases seen so far with 'clinical only' seizures had normal background EEG and normal neuroimaging.[7] The motor manifestations did not involve orofacial movements. These preliminary findings require confirmation, but imply that EEG is mandatory before starting treatment in cases with tonic-clonic or myoclonic seizures involving the limbs only. Current clinical practice is to commence anticonvulsant treatment without obtaining an EEG in the newborn; this may be acceptable if orofacial twitching is seen. There is as yet no information regarding any clinical benefits of treating to electrical quiescence, and in the current state of knowledge it is acceptable practice to treat only the clinically apparent seizures. Treating to electrical quiescence is in any case virtually impossible with the currently available anticonvulsants considered suitable for the newborn.

AETIOLOGY

Causes of neonatal seizures in current order of importance are shown in Table 44.3. Data in column 1 are from Levene and Trounce,[47] column 2 from Goldberg et al,[25] column 3 from Andre et al,[1] column 4 from Bergman et al,[4] column 5 from Estan and Hope[19a] and column 6 from Lien et al.[48]

Table 44.3 Causes of neonatal seizure. Blank spaces indicate no reports of infants with these conditions in the series.

	1	2	3	4	5*	6+
Number of cases			**71**	**131**	**100**	**40**
Hypoxic–ischaemic encephalopathy	53%	16%	49%	30%	49%	37%
Intracranial haemorrhage	17%		14%		7%	12%
Cerebral infarction (stroke)					12%	17%
Meningitis	8%	3%	2%	7%	5%	5%
Maternal drug withdrawal			4%			
Hypoglycaemia	3%	2%	0.1%	5%	3%	
Hypocalcaemia, hypomagnasaemia				22%		
Rapidly changing serum sodium						
Congenitally abnormal brain		8%		4%	3%	17%
Fifth-day fits		52%				
Benign familial neonatal seizures						
Pyridoxine-dependent seizures						
Hypertension			1.4%			
Kernicterus					1%	
Inborn errors of metabolism					3%	

*this series included >31 week gestation infants only
+this series was limited to cases presenting in the first 48 hours of life.

HYPOXIC–ISCHAEMIC ENCEPHALOPATHY

This is the most common cause of neonatal seizures at term, contributing over half the cases to most series. The characteristic time of onset is within 24 hours of birth, and seizures often begin in the first 12 hours (Fig. 44.13). For more information on management and prognosis of this condition, see pages 1231–1248.

INTRACRANIAL HAEMORRHAGE

Germinal matrix or intraventricular haemorrhage is the most frequent cause of seizures in preterm infants (p. 1252 et seq.). The incidence of clinically recognized convulsions in the Cambridge very low-birthweight population between 1985 and 1992 was 9%, and 58/72 cases (80%) had periventricular haemorrhage (personal observations). Scher found that 45% of fitting preterm infants had GMH-IVH.[65]

FOCAL CEREBRAL INFARCTION

Preterm infants with GMH-IVH often have an associated IPL caused by haemorrhagic venous infarction, which acts as a focus for seizure (Chapter 44, Part 5). Seizures in term infants with normal Apgar scores are likely to be due to focal lesions, most commonly middle cerebral artery infarction[19a] (p. 1228). These may require MRI for identification.[53] Focal infarcts may be caused by polycythaemia (Chapter 32, Part 3), protein C or S deficiency (Chapter 32, Part 1), maternal lupus (Chapter 32, Part 1), Factor V Leiden (p. 32, Part 1) or emboli from the placenta.

MENINGITIS

Intracranial infections, both bacterial (p. 1139 et seq.), non-bacterial and congenital, cause neonatal seizures usually after the first week of life. Lumbar puncture is mandatory in babies with seizures.

DRUG WITHDRAWAL (Chapter 28)

Maternal methadone addiction is more likely to be associated with neonatal withdrawal seizures than is heroin.[35] Withdrawal seizures can occur for the first time at any age up to 3 weeks, with a median time of onset of 10 days, and can persist for several months. EEG abnormalities are present in 50% of cocaine-exposed neonates, persist for up to 1 year, and are associated with an adverse neurodevelopmental outcome. Tremors have been noted in children who received prolonged infusions of narcotics for analgesia.[21]

METABOLIC CAUSES

Hypoglycaemia (p. 939)

Hypoglycaemia can be the sole cause of neonatal seizures and other neurological symptoms such as apnoea, lethargy and jitteriness. Often hypoglycaemia complicates hypoxic–ischaemic encephalopathy or infection, and hypoglycaemia is also common in infants who are small for gestational age. The adverse outcome, associated with the underlying cause, makes it difficult to determine the prognosis of uncomplicated hypoglycaemia. There is no doubt that severe prolonged hypoglycaemia can cause brain damage,[41] but there is less certainty regarding brief episodes of treated hypoglycaemia even if symptomatic.[12] Howarth[37] summarized the literature in an editorial comment and concluded that the outcome of symptomatic hypoglycaemia was poor, with a quarter to a half of the survivors brain damaged. However, the distribution and mechanism of injury in hypoglycaemic brain damage differs from ischaemic damage. MRI in five cases of neisidioblastosis showed damage to the parietal and occipital lobes.[3a] This pattern of damage does not reflect the pattern of cerebral glucose uptake in neonates. The vulnerability of the immature rat brain to hypoxic–ischaemic injury is enhanced by hypoglycaemia.[73] The cerebral protection afforded by glucose after hypoxic injury suggests that a low intracellular glucose is involved in the mechanism of damage.[31] Volpe has suggested that hypoglycaemia or hypoxia which alone would not cause brain injury might do so when acting in concert. He is persuaded that 'there are good data to suggest additive and potentiating effects of hypoglycaemia' in hypoxia.[76] Persistent moderate hypoglycaemia in the preterm newborn may be associated with a worse neurodevelopmental outcome.[50]

Hypocalcaemia (p. 966)

Half the babies in the series of Brown et al[6] were hypocalcaemic (total serum calcium less than 1.75 mmol/l). Rose and Lombroso found an incidence of 20% in Harvard between 1958 and 1963.[63] High incidences of late (days 4–7) hypocalcaemic seizures were reported prior to the introduction of low-phosphate milks: in the late 1960s infants were consuming doorstep cow's milk or a high-phosphate formula. Hypocalcaemic seizures occasionally occur secondary to maternal hypercalcaemia (prolonged intrauterine exposure to high levels) or maternal vitamin D deficiency, and the neonatal diagnosis should prompt estimation of the maternal serum calcium. Hypomagnesaemia frequently accompanies hypocalcaemia and may require correction before the seizures will respond. Hypocalcaemia is common in ill VLBW babies and in babies with HIE, and is not causally related to the seizures in these cases.

Hyponatraemia

A very high, very low or rapidly changing serum sodium occurring in conditions such as the syndrome of inappropriate ADH secretion (p. 1024), Bartter syndrome or severe dehydration can cause seizures.

CONGENITAL MALFORMATIONS OF THE BRAIN

Disorders of neuronal migration such as lissencephaly or schizencephaly can present with neonatal seizures. Diagnosis has been facilitated with the advent of magnetic resonance imaging, but is sometimes possible with ultrasound (pp. 1308–1309).

INBORN ERRORS OF METABOLISM

Pyridoxine-dependent seizures

The first case of an infant with intractable seizures controlled by pyridoxine was reported by Hunt et al in 1954.[38] Such seizures can begin during intrauterine life and are very resistant to treatment, stopping usually within minutes of parenteral pyridoxine (50 mg) and returning within days of withdrawal. This therapeutic trial can cause hypotonia requiring ventilatory support, and should be carried out in an intensive care unit.[42] The seizure type is non-specific, but generalized tonic–clonic seizures were the most common in a series of 76 cases.[30] Atypical cases who respond more slowly and who have late-onset seizures requiring unusually high doses of pyridoxine have been described.[3,30] Very large amounts of pyridoxine may need to be given for 2 weeks before this rare disorder can be excluded beyond doubt. The underlying defect is thought to be defective binding of the pyridoxal phosphate coenzyme with glutamic acid decarboxylase (GAD), the rate-limiting enzyme in GABA synthesis.[28] Low levels of GABA in cerebrospinal fluid have been reported in this condition.[43] The condition is autosomal recessive and the gene for GAD resides on chromosome 2, although so far no specific mutation has been found. Supplementation of the diet with pyridoxine (vitamin B_6) 20–100 mg b.i.d. is required for life. Unfortunately many of these children are retarded despite early diagnosis and treatment.

Glycine encephalopathy (p. 995)

Non-ketotic hyperglycinaemia is a rare inborn error of metabolism in which large amounts of glycine accumulate, causing intractable seizures (p. 995). Hiccups can be troublesome. Levels of glycine in blood, urine and cerebrospinal fluid are very high. In one case dextromethorphan monotherapy (35 mg/kg/day) was associated with cessation of seizures and normalization of the EEG,[68] but this regimen was not successful in another infant.[83]

BENIGN FAMILIAL NEONATAL CONVULSIONS

This fascinating autosomal dominant condition was first recognized in 1964.[62] The seizures are dramatic and clonic, 80% beginning on the second or third day of life and ceasing at the age of 6 months. Genetic markers have shown a mutation on chromosome 20.[46] It is interesting that the gene for autosomal dominant nocturnal frontal lobe epilepsy maps to the same gene (20q13.2).[60] In contrast to pyridoxine-dependent seizures these fits can be controlled by conventional medication and the prognosis for development is excellent.

BENIGN NEONATAL SLEEP MYOCLONUS

In this condition the myoclonic jerks only occur during sleep, when the EEG is normal. The myoclonus is present in all sleep states, although its frequency is state dependent and greatest during quiet sleep. The movements disappear by 6 months of age. No treatment is required and parents should be reassured that the jerks will cease eventually.

FIFTH-DAY FITS

This benign self-limiting condition reached epidemic proportions in some Australian maternity units in the late 1970s.[25,61] Reports also came from France, but only two cases have been seen in Nancy since 1985 and the diagnosis has not been made in Sydney since 1989.[2,57] The seizures began between days 3 and 5 and lasted for up to 2 weeks. The cause remains a mystery, although low cerebrospinal fluid zinc was found in a few cases.[24]

HYPERTENSION

Rapid lowering of the blood pressure with captopril was accompanied by a seizure in one case,[59] and Andre et al[1] reported two cases of hypertensive seizure. With the increasing incidence of hypertension due to steroid treatment in chronic lung disease (p. 617) this may become more of a problem in coming years.

INVESTIGATION

Essential laboratory investigations include:

- blood glucose
- serum calcium, ionized if possible
- serum magnesium
- arterial pH
- serum sodium
- serum urea and creatinine
- lumbar puncture
- blood culture
- cranial ultrasound scan.

If the cause is not revealed second-line investigations include specimens for virology and a congenital infection screen, CT or magnetic resonance imaging, samples such as hair or urine to look for maternal 'street' drugs, urinary and blood amino acid estimation, chromosomal analysis, blood ammonia and measurement of urinary organic acids. Consideration should be given to a trial of pyridoxine in resistant cases. The value of an EEG examination has already been discussed and an EEG should be obtained if at all possible, and certainly in difficult cases.

TREATMENT

INDICATIONS

The special problems of electroclinical dissociation and the short duration of neonatal seizures make it difficult to be sure when to start and stop anticonvulsant treatment. There are good theoretical reasons for suppressing seizure activity completely, but so far there is no clinical evidence that the generally poor outcome can be improved with anticonvulsant treatment to electrical quiescence. In part this may be because the available treatments are ineffective in supressing abnormal electrical activity.[11,29] Alternatively, the prognosis may be so completely determined by the underlying condition that treatment cannot influence the outcome. Given the current state of knowledge, most neonatologists would treat if there were more than three brief seizures in an hour, or the baby had a single seizure lasting more than 3 minutes. Current clinical practice is to treat to clinical, rather than electrical, silence (see p. 1217).

GENERAL GUIDELINES

Treatment is best started intravenously as absorption is erratic from intramuscular or enteral administration, and the neonate has little muscle mass. Facilities to site and maintain intravenous lines and to institute artificial ventilation are necessary before treating seizures, as most of the available drugs depress respiration and ventilation can become inadequate owing to frequent convulsions. The high total body water of the neonate means there is a large volume of distribution, hence the relatively large loading doses suggested in Table 44.4. Many of the drugs are protein bound and can interact with other drugs and bilirubin. Elimination half-lives are calculated from blood levels and take no account of the volume of distribution; the drug can take much longer to be eliminated from the body (e.g. diazepam). Probably the best advice is to use phenobarbitone in an adequate dose with an early blood level, and to follow with intravenous phenytoin, then midazolam or rectal paraldehyde. Thiopentone coma did not improve the outcome in a controlled clinical trial.[26] There is little clinical experience with valproate in babies, but in resistant cases I would currently consider sodium valproate, dexamethasone[5] or lamotrigine. There is very little experience with lignocaine.[33]

Table 44.4 Anticonvulsant drug use in the newborn

Drug	Initial dose	Route	Maintenance dose	Route	Half-life	Mode of excretion	Note	Therapeutic level
Phenobarbitone	15–30 mg/kg	i.v.	4–5 mg/kg/24 h	oral	100–200 h	hepatic P_{450} cytochrome oxidase	slow oral absorption: liver enzyme inducer	20–40 mg/l 90–180\ micromol/l
Phenytoin	20 mg/kg in 2 doses	i.v. slowly	5 mg/kg/24 h in 2 doses	i.v./ oral	20 h (75 prems)	liver glucuronidation	vitamin K antagonist	10–20 mg/l 40–80 mmol/l
Paraldehyde	0.2 ml/kg i.m. *or* 0.3 ml/kg p.r. (0.6 ml/kg of mixture)	deep i.m. rectal	for rectal use dilute 1:1 with arachis oil, give no more than t.d.s.		10 h	mainly liver, some lungs	protect from light and plastic	
Diazepam	0.2 mg/kg	i.v.	0.2 mg/kg repeat no more than 3 times	i.v.	20–60 h	liver glucuronidation	very long half-life: infusions not recommended	
Clonazepam	100 microg/kg	i.v.	4 microg/kg/h	i.v.	30 h	liver glucuronidation	excessive oral secretions	30–100 microg/l
Carbamazepine	5 mg/kg	oral	5–15 mg/kg/12 hourly	oral	3–15 h	liver	maintenance only	4–12 microg/l (17–50 microg/l)
Valproate	20 mg/kg	i.v.	10 mg/kg/12 hourly	oral	26–47 h	hepatic	GABA modifier increased ammonia	40–50 mg/l 275–350 micromol/l
Lignocaine	2 mg/kg	i.v.	2 mg/kg/h maximum 6 mg/kg/h	i.v.	200 min	liver and kidney	toxic metabolites accumulate in 24 hours	2.4–6 mg/l in adults? levels of little value in infants
Midazolam	200 microg/kg	i.v.	30–60 microg/kg/h	i.v.	12 h	liver glucuronidation	possible withdrawal syndrome	
Lamotrigine	–	–	0.2 mg/kg	oral			no i.v. preparation yet available	

PHENOBARBITONE

Give a large loading dose: it is reasonable to give 30 mg/kg if the patient is already ventilated, otherwise use 15 mg/kg initially. Gilman et al[23] achieved seizure control with phenobarbitone alone in 77% of cases using a rapid sequential method in which they gave 15–20 mg/kg initially then further doses of 5–10 mg/kg every 30 minutes, up to a maximum of 40 mg/kg to achieve a serum level of over 40 mg/l (20–40 mg/l = 90–180 μmol/l). The half-life is very long and there have been concerns about toxic effects on the developing brain. Nevertheless, the drug has other actions, reducing cerebral metabolic rate and acting as a free radical scavenger, which make it a good choice as a first-line anticonvulsant. EEG response to phenobarbitone treatment is variable, as the drug undoubtedly produces electroclinical dissociation.

PHENYTOIN

There is some suggestion that more rapid control of seizures can be achieved with this agent, although its usefulness is limited by the myocardial depressant effect in some babies. Long-term treatment is not suggested because of the side-effects and unpredictable metabolism.

PARALDEHYDE

Rectal administration of paraldehyde has been used for many years with safety and the drug is a useful second-line anticonvulsant. There is some experience with intravenous infusions, which can be inconvenient as the drug must be light protected. Concern has been raised regarding pulmonary oedema and hepatic necrosis. Intramuscular administration often leads to sterile abscess formation and should be abandoned.

CLONAZEPAM

Clonazepam is sometimes used as an infusion in intractable neonatal seizures, although the half-life is such that intermittent dosing is probably just as good. Midazolam has a shorter half-life and may be a better current choice.

SODIUM VALPROATE

Concern about the hepatotoxic effects, hyperammonaemia and hyperglycinaemia limits the use of this drug in the newborn. Valproate proved effective in six intractable cases of neonatal seizure.[22] The oral solution is absorbed from the rectum.[70]

DURATION OF TREATMENT

Concern about the effects of anticonvulsant treatment on the developing brain means that many neonatologists would only discharge a baby on maintenance phenobarbitone if the neurological examination was abnormal, discontinuing treatment before discharge in those who were neurologically normal. Only two of 55 Swedish infants discharged without medication relapsed.[34] Some would perform an EEG at a month and continue anticonvulsants only if this was abnormal. Only 3% of US neonatologists discontinued treatment prior to discharge.[52] As many as 56% of infants developed subsequent epilepsy in one series,[45] although 20–30% is probably a more realistic figure.[4,65] For infants who are discharged on anticonvulsants consider discontinuation of treatment if the baby is seizure free at 9 months.

MAINTENANCE ANTICONVULSANTS

Phenobarbitone in a dose of 5 mg/kg/day is the usual maintenance anticonvulsant chosen for the newborn. There is very little experience with alternative maintenance therapy at the present time and combinations are best avoided. Phenytoin is not a good choice for long-term therapy. Resistant cases should be treated with a combination of phenobarbitone and carbamazepine.

PROGNOSIS

This is mainly related to the cause of the seizures (Table 44.5). Following hypoxic–ischaemic encephalopathy at term 25% of those who develop grade II Sarnat and Sarnat encepalopathy (p. 1239) will suffer sequelae. The combination of a 5-minute Apgar score < 5, fits and signs of encephalopathy was a poor one, with 33% dead and 55% with handicap.[18] Of 70 cases of clinical seizure in very low-birthweight infants followed in Cambridge 43 (59%) died, 16 (22%) had a major handicap and 11 (15%) were normal at 18 months (personal observations). These data are remarkably similar to those of Watkins et al[80] (n = 65), Van Zeben et al[74] (n = 72) and Scher et al (n = 62)[65], although as many as 90% of the preterm infants in some series died.[4] The prognosis after hypocalcaemic seizure and in familial neonatal seizure is excellent. Symptomatic hypoglycaemia and meningitis have a 50% chance of sequelae in the survivors.[4,63] A normal background interictal EEG at term is a good prognostic factor, with fewer than 10% of such infants experiencing sequelae.[79] Electroclinically dissociated seizures are not benign: 50% of babies with electrically silent seizures were dead or handicapped at follow-up[4] and 40% of those with electical seizures alone were doing badly at a year.[64] The value of a normal neurological examination at discharge in providing early reassurance should not be underestimated: 11 of 14 infants with seizures who were normal at 4 years were assessed as normal at this stage.[15] However, this apparently normal group of Oxford children then had problems with spelling and memory in adolescence.[71]

Table 44.5 Outcome of neonatal seizures by cause (%)

	Dead	Handicap	Normal	Reference
HIE grade II, III	50	25	25	74, 80
Preterm	58	23	18	64, 74, 80
Meningitis	20	40	40	
Malformations	60	40		63
Late onset Hypocalcaemia			100	63
Hypoglycaemia		50	50	4, 41, 63

REFERENCES

1. Andre M, Matisse N, Vert P, Debruille Ch 1988 Neonatal seizures – recent aspects. Neuropediatrics 19: 201–207
2. Andre M, Selton D 1993 Convulsions in the fifth day of life. A critical study. Archives of French Pediatrics 50: 197–200
3. Bankier A, Turner M, Hopkins I J 1983 Pyridoxine dependent seizures: a wider clinical spectrum. Archives of Disease in Childhood 58: 415–418

3a. Barkovich A J, Al Ali F, Rowley H A, Bass N 1998 Imaging patterns of neonatal hypoglycaemia. American Journal of Neuroradiology 19: 523–528

4. Bergman I, Painter M J, Hirsch R P, Crumine P K, David R 1983 Outcome in neonates with convulsions treated in ICU. Annals of Neurology 14: 642–647
5. Boor R, Schmitt-Mechelke T, Stopfkuchen H, Reitter B 1993 Dexamethasone in refractory seizures of premature infants. Acta Paediatrica Scandinavica 82: 100–101
6. Brown J K, Cockburn F, Forfar J O 1972 Clinical and chemical correlates in convulsions of the newborn. Lancet i: 135
7. Boylan G, Pressler R M, Rennie J M, Binnie C 1997 Electroclinical, electrographic and clinical seizures in the newborn infant (in press)
8. Clancy R R, Ledigo A 1987 The exact ictal and interictal duration of electroencephalographic neonatal seizures. Epilepsia 28: 537–541
9. Connell J, Oozeer R C, Dubowitz V 1987 Continuous 4 channel EEG monitoring: a guide to interpretation, with normal values, in preterm infants. Neuropediatrics 18: 138–145
10. Connell J, Oozeer R C, de Vries L S, Dubowitz L M S, Dubowitz V 1989 Continuous EEG monitoring of neonatal seizures: diagnostic and prognostic considerations. Archives of Disease in Childhood 64: 452–458
11. Connell J, Oozeer R, de Vries L S, Dubowitz L M S, Dubowitz V 1989 Clinical and EEG response to anticonvulsants in seizures. Archives of Disease in Childhood 64: 459–464
12. Cornblath M, Schwartz R 1991 In: Disorders of carbohydrate metabolism in infancy. Blackwell Scientific, Oxford, pp 96–97
13. Coulter D L, Allen R J 1982 Benign neonatal sleep myoclonus. Archives of Neurology 39: 191–192
14. Curtis P D, Matthews T G, Clarke T A et al 1988 Neonatal seizures: the Dublin Collaborative Study. Archives of Disease in Childhood 63: 1065–1067
15. Dennis J 1978 Neonatal convulsions: aetiology, late neonatal status and long term outcome. Developmental Medicine and Child Neurology 20: 143–158
16. Dennis J, Chalmers I 1982 Very early neonatal seizure rate: a possible indicator of the quality of perinatal care. British Journal of Obstetrics and Gynaecology 89: 418–426
17. Dubowitz L M, Bouza H, Hird M F, Jaeken J 1992 Low cerebrospinal fluid concentration of free gamma-aminobutyric acid in startle disease. Lancet 340: 430–431
18. Ellenberg J H, Nelson K B 1988 Cluster of perinatal events identifying infants at high risk of death or disability Journal of Pediatrics 113: 546–552

19. Ellison P, Franklin S, Brown P, Jones M G 1989 The evolution of a simplified method for interpretation of EEG in the preterm neonate. Acta Paediatrica Scandinavica 78: 210–216
19a. Estan J, Hope P L 1997 Unilateral cerebral infarction in full term infants. Archives of Diseases in Childhood 76: F88–F93
20. Eyre J A, Oozeer R C, Wilkinson A R 1983 Diagnosis of neonatal seizures by continuous recording. Archives of Disease in Childhood 58: 785–790
21. French J P, Nocera M 1994 Drug withdrawal symptoms in children after continuous infusions of fentanyl. Journal of Pediatric Nursing 9: 107–113
22. Gal P, Oles K S, Gilman J T, Weaver R 1988 Valproic acid efficacy, toxicity, and pharmacokinetics in neonates with intractable seizures. Neurology 38: 467–471
23. Gilman J T, Gal P, Duchowny M S, Weaver R L, Ransom J L 1989 Rapid sequential phenobarbital treatment of neonatal seizures. Pediatrics 83: 674–678
24. Goldberg H J 1982 Fifth day fits – an acute zinc deficiency syndrome? Archives of Disease in Childhood 57: 633–635
25. Goldberg H J 1983 Neonatal convulsions: a ten year review. Archives of Disease in Childhood 58: 976–978
26. Goldberg P N, Moscoso P, Bauer C R 1986 Use of barbiturate therapy in severe perinatal asphyxia. Journal of Pediatrics 109: 851–856
27. Gordon N 1993 Startle disease or hyperekplexia. Developmental Medicine and Child Neurology 35: 1015–1024
28. Gospe S M, Olin K L, Keen C L 1994 Reduced GABA synthesis in pyridoxine dependent seizures. Lancet 343: 1133–1134
29. Hakeen V F, Wallace S J 1990 EEG monitoring of therapy for neonatal seizures. Developmental Medicine and Child Neurology 32: 858–864
30. Haenggeli C A, Girardin E, Paunier L 1991 Pyridoxine-dependent seizures, clinical and therapeutic aspects. European Journal of Pediatrics 150: 452–455
31. Hattori H, Wasterlain C G 1990 Posthypoxic glucose supplementation reduces hypoxic–ischemic brain damage in the neonatal rat. Annals of Neurology 28: 122–128
32. Hellstrom-Westas L, Rosen I, Svenningsen N W 1985 Silent seizures in sick infants in early life. Acta Paediatrica Scandinavica 74: 741–748
33. Hellstrom-Westas L, Westergren U, Rosen I, Svenningsen N W 1988 Lidocaine for treatment of severe seizures in newborn infants. Acta Paediatrica Scandinavica 77: 79–84
34. Hellstrom-Westas L, Blennow G, Lindroth M, Rosen I, Svenningsen N W 1995 Low risk of seizure recurrence after early withdrawal of anticonvulsants in the neonatal period. Archives of Disease in Childhood 72: F97–F101
35. Herzlinger R A, Kandall S R, Vaughan H G 1977 Neonatal seizures associated with drug withdrawal. Journal of Pediatrics 91: 638–641
36. Holden K R, Mellits D, Freeman J M 1982 Neonatal seizures I: correlation of prenatal and perinatal events with outcomes. Pediatrics 70: 165–176
37. Howarth J C 1974 Neonatal hypoglycaemia: how much does it damage the brain? Pediatrics 54: 3–4
38. Hunt A D, Stokes J, McCrory W W, Stroud H H 1954 Pyridoxine dependency: report of a case of intractable convulsions in an infant controlled by pyridoxine. Pediatrics 13: 140–145
39. Keen J H, Lee D 1973 Sequelae of neonatal convulsions. Archives of Disease in Childhood 48: 542–548
40. Kellaway P Mizrahi E M 1990 Clinical, electroencephalographic, therapeutic and pathophysiologic studies of neonatal seizures. In: Wasterlain C G, Vert P (eds) Neonatal seizures. Raven Press, New York, pp 1–13
41. Koivisto M, Blanco-Sequeiros M, Krause U 1972 Neonatal symptomatic and asymptomatic hypoglycaemia: a follow up study of 151 children. Developmental Medicine and Child Neurology 14: 603–614
42. Kroll J S 1985 Pyridoxine for neonatal seizures: an unexpected danger. Developmental Medicine and Child Neurology 27: 377–379
43. Kurlemann G, Ziegler R, Gruenberg M, Bomelburg T, Ullrich K, Palm D G 1992 Disturbance of GABA metabolism in pyridoxine dependent seizures. Neuropediatrics 23: 257–259
44. Lanska M J, Lanska R J, Baumann R J, Kryscio R J 1995 A population based study of neonatal seizures in Fayette County, Kentucky. Neurology 45: 724–732
45. Legido A, Clancy R R, Berman P H 1991 Neurologic outcome after electroencephalographically proven neonatal seizures. Pediatrics 88: 583–596
46. Leppert M, Anderson V E, Quattlebaum T et al 1989 Benign familial neonatal convulsions linked to genetic markers on chromosome 20. Nature 337: 647–648
47. Levene M I, Trounce J Q 1986 Causes of neonatal convulsions. Archives of Disease in Childhood 61: 78–79
48. Lien J M, Towers C V, Quilligan E J, de Veciana M, Toohey J S, Morgan M A 1995 Term early-onset neonatal seizures: obstetric characteristics, etiologic classifications, and perinatal care. Obstetrics and Gynecology 85: 163–169
49. Lingham S, Wilson J, Hart E W 1981 Hereditary stiff-baby syndrome. American Journal of Diseases of Children 135: 909–911
50. Lucas A, Morley R, Cole T J 1988 Adverse neurodevelopmental outcome of moderate hypoglycaemia. British Medical Journal 297: 1304–1308
51. Martin E, Boesch C, Zuerrer M et al 1990 MR imaging of brain maturation in normal and developmentally handicapped children. Journal of Computer Assisted Tomography 14: 685–692
52. Massingale T W, Buttross S 1993 Survey of treatment practices for neonatal seizures. Journal of Perinatology 13: 107–110
53. Mercuri E, Cowan F, Rutherford M, Acolet D, Pennock J, Dubowitz L S 1995 Ischaemic and haemorrhagic brain lesions in newborn infants with seizures and normal Apgar scores. Archives of Disease in Childhood 73: F67–F74
54. Minchom P, Niswander K, Chalmers I et al 1987 Antecedents and outcome of very early neonatal seizures in infants born at or after term. British Journal of Obstetrics & Gynaecology 49: 431–439
55. Mizrahi E M, Kellaway P 1987 Characterization and classification of neonatal seizures Neurology 37: 1837–1844
56. Moshe S L 1993 Seizures in the developing brain. Neurology 43 (Suppl 5): S3–S7
57. North K N, Storey G N, Henderson-Smart D J 1989 Fifth day fits in the newborn. Australian Paediatric Journal 25: 284–287
58. Parker S, Zuckerman B, Bauchner H, Frank D, Vinci R, Cabral H 1990 Jitteriness in full term neonates: prevalence and correlates. Pediatrics 85: 17–23
59. Perlman J M, Volpe J J 1989 Neurologic complications of captopril treatment of neonatal hypertension. Pediatrics 83: 47–52
60. Phillips H A, Scheffer I E, Berkovic S F, Hollway G E, Sutherland G R, Mulley J C 1995 Localisation of a gene for autosomal dominant nocturnal frontal lobe epilepsy to chromosome 20q 13.2. Nature Genetics 10: 117–118
61. Pryor D S, Don N, Macourt D C 1981 Fifth day fits: a syndrome of neonatal convulsions. Archives of Disease in Childhood 56: 753–758
62. Rett A, Teubel R 1964 Neugeborenen Krampfe im Rohmen einer epileptisch belasten familie. Wiener Klinische Wochenschrift 76: 609–613
63. Rose A L, Lombroso C T 1970 Neonatal seizures. Pediatrics 45: 404–425
64. Scher M S, Painter M J, Bergman I, Barmada M A, Brunberg J 1989 EEG diagnoses of neonatal seizures: clinical correlates and outcome. Pediatric Neurology 5: 17–24
65. Scher M S, Aso K, Beggarly M E, Hamid M Y, Steppe D A, Painter M J 1993 Electrographic seizures in preterm and full term neonates: clinical correlates, associated brain lesions and risk for neurologic sequelae. Pediatrics 91: 128–134
66. Scher M S, Hamid M Y, Steppe D A, Beggarly M E, Painter M J 1993 Ictal and interictal electrographic seizure durations in preterm and term neonates. Epilepsia 34: 284–288
67. Shewman D A 1990 What is a neonatal seizure? Problems in definition and quantification for investigative and clinical purposes. Journal of Clinical Neurophysiology 7: 315–368
68. Schmitt B, Steinmann B, Gitzelmann R, Thun-Hohenstein L, Mascher H, Dumermuth G 1993 Nonketotic hyperglycinaemia: clinical and electrical effects of dextromethorphan, an antagonist of the NMDA receptor. Neurology 43: 421–424
69. Shiang R, Ryan S G, Fielder T J et al 1995 Mutational analysis of familial and sporadic hyperekplexia. Annals of Neurology 38: 85–91
70. Steinberg S A, Shalev R S, Amr N 1986 Valproic acid in neonatal status convulsivus. Brain Development 8: 278–280
71. Temple C M, Dennis J, Carney R, Sharich J 1995 Neonatal seizures: long term outcome and cognitive development among 'normal' survivors. Developmental Medicine and Child Neurology 37: 108–118
72. Tohier C, Roze J C, David A, Veccierini M F, Renaud P, Mouzard A 1991 Hyperekplexia or stiff baby syndrome. Archives of Disease in Childhood 66: 460–461

73. Vannucci R C, Vannucci S J 1978 Cerebral carbohydrate metabolism during hypoglycemia and anoxia in newborn rats. Annals of Neurology 4: 73–79
74. Van Zeben D M, Veerlove-Vanhorick S P, den Ouden L, Brand R, Ruhy J H 1990 Neonatal seizures in very preterm and low birthweight infants: mortality and handicaps at two years in a nationwide cohort. Neuropediatrics 21: 62–65
75. Volpe J J 1989 Neonatal seizures: current concepts and revised classification. Pediatrics 84: 422–428
76. Volpe J J 1995 Neurology of the newborn, 3rd edn. WB Saunders, Philadelphia, p 478
77. Wasterlain C G 1976 Effects of neonatal status epilepticus on rat brain development. Neurology 26: 975–986
78. Wasterlain C G, Plum F 1973 Vulnerability of developing rat brain to electroconvulsive seizures. Archives of Neurology 29: 38–42
79. Watanabe K 1980 Behavioural state cycles, background EEGs and prognosis of newborns with perinatal hypoxia. EEG and Clinical Neurophysiology 49: 618–625
80. Watkins A, Szymonowicz W, Jin X, Yu V Y H 1988 Significance of seizures in very low birthweight infants. Developmental Medicine and Child Neurology 30: 162–169
81. Weiner S P, Painter M J, Geva D, Guthrie R D, Scher M S 1991 Neonatal seizures: electroclinical dissociation. Pediatric Neurology 7: 363–368
82. Younkin D P, Delivoria-Papdopoulos M, Maris J, Donlon E, Clancy R, Chance B 1986 Cerebral metabolic effects of neonatal seizures measured with in vivo P-31 NMR spectroscopy. Annals of Neurology 20: 513–519
83. Zammarchi E, Donati M A, Ciani F, Pasquini E, Pela I, Fiorini P 1994 Failure of early dextromethorphan and sodium benzoate therapy in an infant with nonketotic hyperglycinaemia. Neuropediatrics 25: 274–276

Part 3

Intracranial haemorrhage at term

Malcolm I. Levene

INTRODUCTION

Bleeding into the brain and related structures is a very common neonatal event and is most frequently recognized in premature infants. Intracranial haemorrhage involving the term baby occurs less commonly than in the preterm, and the affected sites and pathogenesis of the bleeding are far more heterogeneous. The pattern of intracranial haemorrhage in the term baby has changed over the last 40 years. Subdural haemorrhage was a common cause of death following traumatic delivery, but its incidence has fallen with improved obstetric management. In recent years subdural haemorrhage has again become more frequently recognized, mainly owing to improved imaging techniques, which allows identification of smaller (and sometimes asymptomatic) lesions.

Intracranial haemorrhage in the term infant may occur at many sites (Fig. 44.15). In addition, it is important to consider other forms of intracranial pathology which predispose to bleeding or haemorrhagic infarction and which may be mistaken for primary haemorrhage. In particular, infarction of a cerebral artery and venous sinus thrombosis are two important causes that need to be considered.

Intracranial haemorrhage detected by imaging studies in apparently healthy term infants is relatively common. Studies have reported an overall incidence of 3.1–5.5%.[20] A study of 1000 unselected low-risk apparently healthy

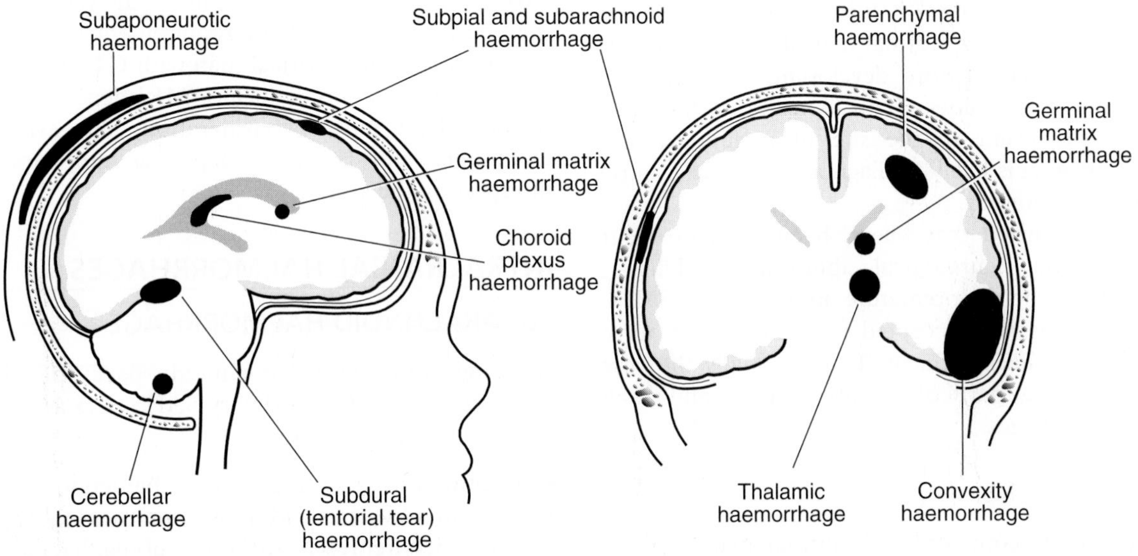

Fig. 44.15 Sites of intracranial haemorrhage.

asymptomatic term babies showed that intracranial haemorrhage was present in 3.5%, and all were periventricular in origin.[20] Before discussing in detail the various sites of intracranial bleeding in mature infants, this chapter will initially review the presentation and investigation of intracranial haemorrhage in this group of infants.

PRESENTATION

Intracranial haemorrhage in the term neonate usually presents with neurological symptoms and signs, but these are often non-specific in that they do not point to a focal site of cerebral pathology. Signs may be very general and not point directly to the brain as the source of the problem, and in some cases clues to the cause of the haemorrhage may be obtained by general examination.

NEUROLOGICAL SIGNS

The major neurological feature of intracranial pathology is seizures. Seizures occur commonly and are a feature of many different forms of brain pathology (p. 1217), but in the mature brain overt seizures occur as a result of intracranial haemorrhage more frequently than in the premature infant.

A complicating factor in evaluating the significance of abnormal neurological signs is that they may be present as the result of underlying pathology, which is the cause of the haemorrhage rather than the effect. Severe intrapartum asphyxia is an example of this sequence: the baby may develop seizures and other abnormal signs from shortly after birth and the development of intracranial haemorrhage may not be considered because the abnormal signs are thought to be due to the more obvious pathology. Imaging must be carried out in all term babies with abnormal neurology. Ultrasound is a useful first-line investigation but is not as sensitive as MRI, which should be considered if the cranial ultrasound scan is normal.

A common clinical course is for a baby to be born in good condition and show normal neurological behaviour for a number of days before developing an acute and major encephalopathic illness. This focuses the clinician's attention to the brain as the site of pathology, and appropriate imaging is likely to diagnose the precise cause if haemorrhage is present.

It is well recognized that 'silent' haemorrhages occur with little or no neurological abnormality. This is particularly common in premature infants with GMH-IVH, but it is now well accepted to occur also in term infants with brain haemorrhage. This is usually the case with minor bleeding, particularly subarachnoid and small subdural haemorrhages.

NON-SPECIFIC SIGNS

Fever is relatively common with intracranial haemorrhage. Meningitis must always be considered in a baby with fever and abnormal neurology, and lumbar puncture may reveal leucocytes and low CSF glucose levels, together with bloodstained CSF. This is a common finding following GMH-IVH and may make the distinction between meningitis and intraventricular haemorrhage very difficult.

ASSOCIATED SIGNS

Intracranial bleeding can occur as the result of a coagulopathy, and petechial or purpuric skin lesions may be widespread. Thrombocytopenia (pp. 801–802) or a congenital clotting factor abnormality (p. 801) must be considered as the cause. Multiple cutaneous haemangiomata may rarely be associated with rupture of an intracranial haemangioma. A neurologically abnormal infant with extensive bruises also suggests the possibility of intracranial birth trauma, and this should be considered.

INVESTIGATIONS

Imaging is the most important method for confirming or excluding the diagnosis of intracranial haemorrhage.

Ultrasound is widely used in neonatal intensive care units for brain imaging and is valuable in term neonates as a screening technique when intracranial haemorrhage is suspected. However, its limitations must be recognized. It is very poor at diagnosing subarachnoid and/or subdural haemorrhages unless they are large. In addition, ultrasound may miss important associated pathology which predisposes to haemorrhage, such as cerebral artery infarction and venous sinus thrombosis.

I recommend that all infants in whom intracranial haemorrhage is clinically suspected should have either CT or MR imaging. MRI is probably the most versatile and sensitive imaging modality currently available. Pathology not detected on CT scan may be recognized on MRI, but the process of acquiring the data for the scan may be prolonged and the requirement for the infant to remain still is more critical than with CT. The decision as to whether to undertake CT or MRI depends on the type of pathology under consideration, the availability of techniques and the local expertise and experience in interpreting the scans.

INTRACRANIAL HAEMORRHAGES

SUBARACHNOID HAEMORRHAGE

Bleeding into the subarachnoid space may be either primary or secondary. Primary SAH arises as the result of two separate mechanisms:

- Rupture of veins bridging the subarachnoid space;
- Rupture of vessels within the leptomeningeal plexus, which may represent ruptured subpial haemorrhage with consequent SAH.

Secondary SAH occurs as the result of haemorrhage from another site, usually intraventricular, draining into the subarachnoid space. SAH may also occur overlying an area of arterial infarction.

SAH is a very common finding at autopsy and does not necessarily indicate the presence of underlying brain injury. Many of these small lesions may actually represent subpial haemorrhages,[14] which are most commonly seen over the temporal or parietal lobes.[9,11] Larger lesions appear as a reddish-yellow layer of jelly-like consistency over the surface of the brain.[6] Large SAH is particularly likely in babies with coagulopathy.[5,14] Traumatic delivery has been reported to cause SAH in surviving infants.[45]

Diagnosis

Convulsions are the most common sign associated with SAH in the term infant and are usually present within the first 24 hours of life. Characteristically the baby is said to be neurologically normal between seizures, but the larger the SAH, the more neurologically abnormal the baby is likely to be.

Diagnosis is made by CT or MRI. Ultrasound is an unreliable method for diagnosing this condition. A small SAH is most likely to appear on CT scan as an area of increased attenuation within the posterior interhemispheric fissure. It may be impossible to distinguish a large convexity SAH from subdural haemorrhage.

The prognosis for primary SAH is good unless there is massive convexity bleeding.

CONVEXITY HAEMORRHAGE

In this condition a large collection of clotted subarachnoid blood causes a convex space-occupying lesion, usually over the temporal or occipital region.[34] The convexity haemorrhage commonly causes compression of cortical and subcortical structures, with localized venous infarction adjacent to the lesion. Histologically it may be difficult to identify the origin of the bleeding, which in some cases has been reported to be subpial in origin.[11]

Convexity haemorrhage is particularly associated with neonatal coagulopathy (see below), and Larroche[23] has reported its association with exchange transfusion. The lesion is usually well seen with ultrasound imaging (Fig. 44.16).

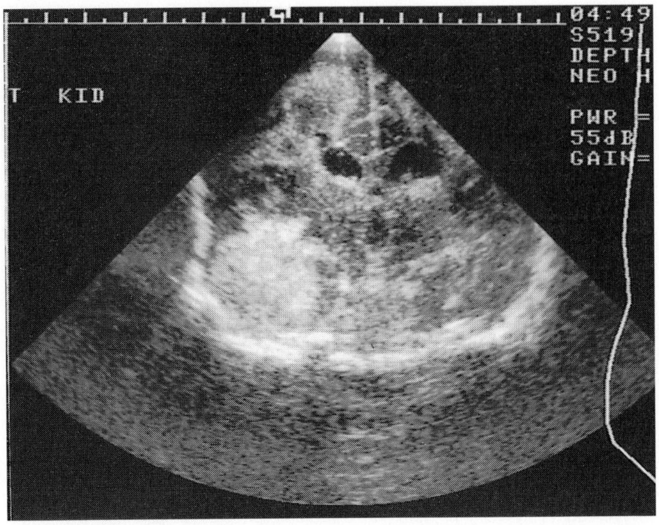

Fig. 44.16 Convexity haemorrhage. Ultrasound scan showing echodense haemorrhage in right temporal area.

The prognosis for a large convexity haemorrhage is poor and is dependent on the degree of infarction of normal brain immediately adjacent to the lesion.

SUBDURAL HAEMORRHAGE

Massive subdural haemorrhage causing death is now a rare occurrence, but with the increased availability of modern imaging techniques a second type of less severe SDH is recognized more frequently in surviving infants.

Subdural haemorrhage arises as the result of three different mechanisms:

- Rupture of bridging veins;
- Tearing of the dural membranes owing to distorting forces;
- Laceration of the dura from skull displacement (osteodiastasis); this latter variant is commonly associated with associated cerebellar haemorrhage (see below).

The cause of subdural haemorrhage is basically trauma to the head. This may be direct, which is now rare, or as a result of abnormal forces associated with instrumental delivery, particularly vacuum extraction.

The dura is a thick membrane which compartmentalizes the brain. Folds of dura form the sagitally lying falx, which separates the two cerebral hemispheres. The posterior dural reflection forms the axially lying tentorium, which separates the cerebellum from the cerebral hemispheres. The venous sinuses lie within the folds of the dura and a tear to the dural membrane is likely to be associated with rupture of a venous sinus, causing extensive intradural and subdural haemorrhage. Bridging veins run from the dural membranes to the superior sagittal sinus, and these may rupture also resulting in subdural haemorrhage.

SDH may be supratentorial or lie within the posterior fossa. In the latter case blood may be visible either between the superior surface of the cerebellum and the tentorium or between the convexity of the cerebellar hemisphere and the occipital bone.[39] This type of SDH is often associated with severe HIE and a tear of the tentorium. The lesion is difficult to treat and has a very poor prognosis. On the other hand, vault SDH presents later, can be treated, and can have a good outcome. Intracerebellar haemorrhage is commonly seen in association with neonatal SDH.

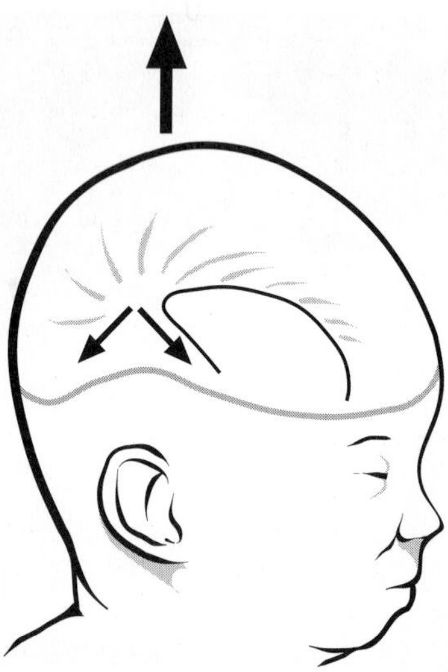

Fig. 44.17 Forces on the tentorium (small arrows) as the result of traction on the vertex, as occurs in vacuum extraction delivery (large arrow).

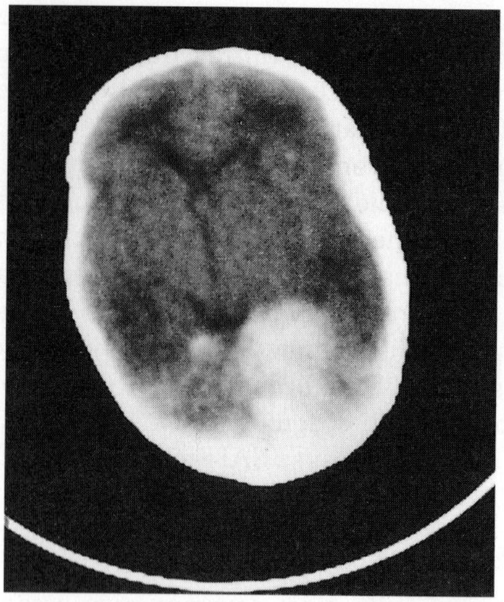

Fig. 44.18 CT scan of subdural haemorrhage associated with tentorial tear.

Aetiology

Trauma is the underlying cause of SDH in almost all cases. Fetal SDH has been described as the result of direct trauma to the maternal abdomen at term.[24] The commonest cause of SDH is maldistribution of compressive forces on the head during delivery. If the head is distorted excessive stress is applied to the tentorium and falx, causing a tear to the free edge of the tentorium (Fig. 44.17) with associated rupture of the vein of Galen or straight sinus. This is likely to occur as the result of prolonged labour, uncontrolled delivery of the fetal head where the compressive forces rapidly change, or to traction from forceps or vacuum extraction. SDH is increasingly being recognized as a complication of vacuum extraction.[3,19] Elongation of the head by traction causes a particular strain on the apex of the tentorium, with rupture of bridging veins or venous sinuses. In one study 10 unselected asymptomatic infants delivered by vacuum extraction showed evidence of intracranial bleeding, of which intradural or subdural haemorrhage was most common, although no baby appears to have sustained adverse neurodevelopmental outcome as a result.[1]

Subdural haemorrhage is well recognized to occur in infants with severe HIE. Rebleeding up to 4 days after the first bleed has been described following primary non-fatal SDH.[6] The delayed bleed may occur as the result of restoration of blood pressure or as a result of falling intracranial pressure in the few days after the original bleed.[44]

Diagnosis

Govaert et al[15] reviewed 78 cases of subdural haemorrhage diagnosed during life. A recognizable symptom complex has been described, including tense fontanelle, hypotonia, lethargy with reduced primitive reflexes and facial palsy. Symptoms related to posterior fossa injury include apnoea, irregular sighing respiration, fixed bradycardia, opisthotonos and skew deviation of the eyes. Seizures may not occur in subtentorial bleeding.

Imaging

Subdural haemorrhage most commonly occurs in the posterior fossa and is recognized on CT or MRI scanning (Fig. 44.18). Autopsy studies have shown that a small intradural haemorrhage may be missed on CT.[27]

Management

There is little consensus as to the indications for craniotomy and drainage of the clot. Review of reported cases suggests that there is some benefit to surgery,[15] but this may represent case selection for surgery in that only those thought to have the best prognosis were operated on. Hydrocephalus may occur as a secondary event, but spontaneous resolution of CSF blockage is well recognized.

Complications

SDH can cause acute obstruction to the fourth ventricle, with impairment of CSF flow and brain-stem compression. This may require urgent intervention. Infarction of the middle or posterior cerebral artery is now a recognized complication following supratentorial subdural haemorrhage.[16] This occurs as the result of supratentorial subdural clot, leading to uncal herniation with occlusion of the ipsilateral posterior and middle cerebral artery. A convexity subdural or subarachnoid haemorrhage may cause obstruction to more peripheral branches of the middle cerebral artery.

GERMINAL MATRIX AND INTRAVENTRICULAR HAEMORRHAGE

GMH-IVH is a generic term which does not indicate the origin of the bleeding. In term babies there are three major sites of origin:

- Germinal matrix
- Choroid plexus
- Extension of an intraparenchymal haemorrhage.

In premature infants the germinal matrix is the most likely origin of GMH-IVH, and this becomes progressively less common as the baby matures (Chapter 44, Part 5). Germinal matrix haemorrhage is well recognized to occur at term,[29,38] and is reported to occur in 2% of asymptomatic, unselected and apparently normal term infants.[20] Others have reported an incidence for symptomatic IVH of 0.036%.[22]

Haemorrhage from the choroid plexus is the commonest cause of large GMH-IVH in term infants, and was reported to occur in 1.1% of unselected healthy term infants.[20] Choroid plexus haemorrhage is discussed in detail below.

Rupture of an intraparenchymal haemorrhage (see below) into the ventricle is a relatively uncommon cause of GMH-IVH. These babies are usually symptomatic, with major signs of neurological disturbances. GMH-IVH has been reported in conjunction with deep venous thrombosis.[32] Massive GMH-IVH occurring prenatally in mature fetuses is well described[25] and may be associated with fetal or maternal coagulopathy.

GMH-IVH has also been reported to occur as the result of abdominal compression in a term infant[43] and following gentle aspiration of CSF from a ventricular reservoir in babies with hydrocephalus.[30] GMH-IVH is seen in infants who have survived ECMO treatment.[4,40]

Diagnosis

Small GMH-IVH may be asymptomatic. Larger haemorrhages present with severe neurological abnormalities, including convulsions, signs of raised intracranial pressure, and feeding difficulties. Hyperpyrexia has been reported as a frequent finding.[22,32] Diagnosis is suspected on the basis of abnormal neurological signs. Lumbar puncture reveals frankly bloodstained CSF with an excess of seven red blood cells per cubic millimetre.

Prognosis

Jocelyn and Casiro[22] report the outcome of 15 term infants with symptomatic GMH-IVH. One died, and of the survivors followed up for a mean age of 35 months 36% had severe handicaps. They reported a correlation between severity of GMH-IVH and adverse outcome, but others have reported much better outcome even in babies with extensive GMH-IVH.[38] Posthaemorrhagic hydrocephalus is an important complication of GMH-IVH at term. The incidence of hydrocephalus requiring shunt placement is 35%.[22,38]

CHOROID PLEXUS HAEMORRHAGE

Haemorrhage from the veins of the choroid plexus is well described as a cause of intraventricular haemorrhage occurring in term neonates. The most frequent site of bleeding is into the posterior tufts at the level of the glomus. Choroid plexus haemorrhage was diagnosed by ultrasound in 1.1% of asymptomatic, non-selected term infants.[20]

Diagnosis is made by detection of thrombus adherent to the choroid plexus (Fig. 44.19). In infants with clot filling the major part of a lateral ventricle it may not be possible to determine the origin of the bleed. The presence of intraventricular haemorrhage with no pathology in the germinal matrix is strongly suggestive of the choroid plexus as its site of origin. Clinical presentation is as for any cause of GMH-IVH.

INTRAPARENCHYMAL LESIONS

Intraparenchymal lesions (IPL) in the term infant represent a heterogenous group of conditions. For a discussion of IPLs in preterm infants see page 1258.

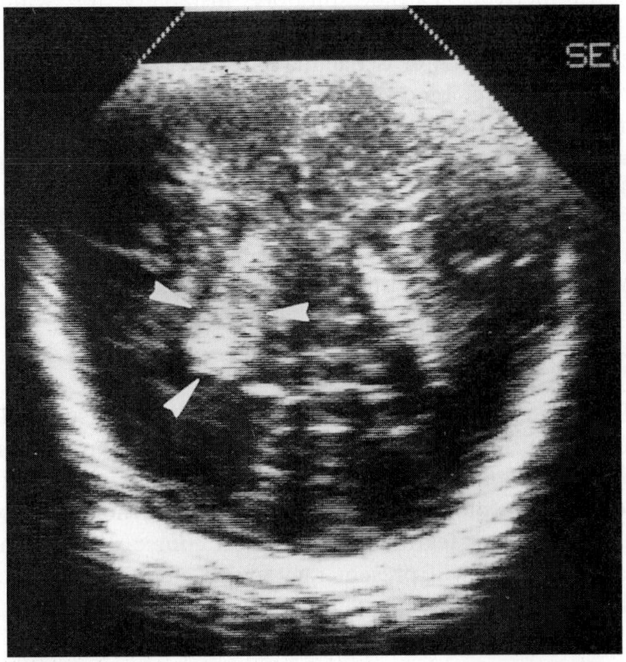

Fig. 44.19 Choroid plexus haemorrhage. Ultrasound scan showing echogenic clot adherent to one choroid plexus. (Reproduced with permission from Spastics International Medical Publications)

Table 44.6 Causes of intraparenchymal lesions at term

Coagulopathy
Trauma
Arterial infarction
Sinus thrombosis
Hypoxia–ischaemia
Extracorporeal membrane oxygenation therapy
Arteriovenous malformation
Aneurysm
Tumour
Protein C deficiency
Protein S deficiency
Factor V Leiden

Aetiology

Table 44.6 lists the causes of IPLs. In some cases there is bleeding into an area of existing infarction, which may be either arterial or venous. Arterial infarcts are recognized by their distribution on CT or MRI scans. An unrecognized sinus thrombosis is an important cause of parenchymal haemorrhage. The haemorrhage may be multifocal, which is suggestive of intrapartum asphyxia, an underlying coagulopathy or, rarely, a multiple embolic cause.

Coagulopathy due to clotting factor abnormality, α_1-antitrypsin deficiency or vitamin K deficiency is one of the most common causes of intraparenchymal haemorrhage at term. Birth trauma has been implicated as the cause for supratentorial intraparenchymal haemorrhage[45] and intrapartum asphyxia causes haemorrhage within both grey and white matter,[8] although this may represent bleeding into a previously infarcted area. IPL is a well recognized complication of ECMO. This may be due to the underlying cardiorespiratory instability for which ECMO was given, anticoagulation necessary during the course of ECMO, or ischaemia induced by impairment of carotid artery blood flow. All forms of intracranial haemorrhage are common in babies requiring ECMO, and intraparenchymal haemorrhage has been reported in 3–18%.[4,18,40]

Arterial aneurysm[28] and arteriovenous malformation[42] are rare causes of IPL at term. Sinus thrombosis has also been reported in conjunction with IPL.[2]

Diagnosis

There is often a history of symptoms occurring suddenly at 1–5 days of age in an infant who had previously been apparently normal. At presentation the baby is usually severely neurologically abnormal, but convulsions are not always a major feature of the clinical course. Focal signs rarely occur but if present may give a clue to the site of the lesion.

Investigations

The diagnosis may be suspected on ultrasound examination, but CT or MRI is much more reliable in accurately defining the position and possible aetiology of the lesion. If an aneurysm or venous thrombosis is suspected to be the underlying cause magnetic resonance angiography is the investigation of choice; carotid or vertebral angiograms should be avoided if at all possible. Repeated imaging in the weeks after the acute insult usually shows resolution of the lesion to a porencephalic cavity in the majority of cases.

Prognosis

This depends on the underlying cause of the lesion. It is reported that approximately one-third of infants die, one-third are handicapped and one-third are subsequently neurologically normal.

CEREBELLAR HAEMORRHAGE

Bleeding into the posterior fossa is a well recognized complication of breech delivery in a term infant. Haemorrhage may be due to subdural rupture, with bleeding from the venous sinus or from haemorrhage within the cerebellum. It is not uncommon for both types of bleeding to occur together. Although not all causes of cerebellar haemorrhages in term infants are related to trauma, this accounts for the majority of cases.

Cerebellar haemorrhage occurs as the result of:

- germinal matrix bleeding from the roof of the fourth ventricle;
- trauma to the cerebellum, of which occipital osteodiastasis with breech delivery is the most common cause.

As well as the cerebellar germinal matrix adjacent to the fourth ventricle, there is an area of poorly formed vascular tissue just below the pial layer of the cerebellum. These vessels are easily damaged, with ensuing haemorrhage into the cerebellar cortex. This appears to occur in both premature and term infants, but is not usually severe.

More severe bleeding into the cerebellum occurs as the result of trauma, usually sustained during breech delivery (Fig. 44.20). Overextension of the neck during delivery causes separation of the squamous and lateral portions of the occipital bone, with direct trauma to the cerebellum.[46] This is termed occipital osteodiastasis and is commonly associated with subdural tears.

A tight-fitting band around the head to maintain the position of a face mask has also been implicated in occipital diastasis with cerebellar infarction or haemorrhage.[33]

Diagnosis

Seizures are a less frequent presenting sign associated with cerebellar haemorrhage. The baby is usually lethargic, has

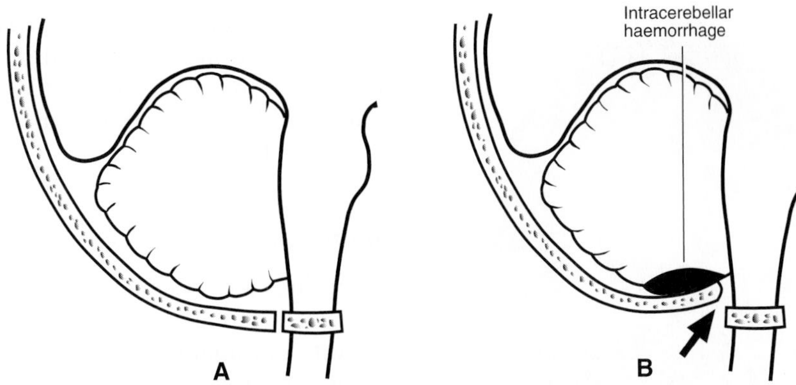

Fig. 44.20 Occipital diastasis. (A) Normal. (B) Diastasis with the occipital bone subluxing into the cerebellum.

episodes of apnoea or irregular ventilation, and bradycardia. He does not suck well and may show signs of raised intracranial pressure. Nystagmus and facial nerve palsy may be seen on examination.

Management

The role of craniotomy and evacuation of the clot is not certain (see Management of subdural haemorrhage). Successful conservative management of cerebellar haematomas has been described.[10]

Prognosis

There is little known about the long-term outcome.

THALAMIC HAEMORRHAGE

This is now a well recognized form of haemorrhage in the term baby.[7,37,41] Extension into the thalamus from GMH-IVH in the premature infant is a different condition (pp. 1253–1254). It is almost always unilateral and must be distinguished from bilaterally bright basal ganglia, which are seen in severely asphyxiated infants (Chapter 44, Part 4). These babies are severely neurologically abnormal from birth, whereas primary thalamic haemorrhage arises de novo in an otherwise normal infant.

The cause of thalamic haemorrhage is unknown in most cases, but rarely haemorrhagic infarction, meningitis, coagulation disorders and sinus thrombosis have been associated factors.

Diagnosis

The baby is usually normal at birth and causes no concern until the development of dramatic and severe neurological abnormality 2–14 days later. This not uncommonly occurs after discharge from hospital. A particular feature of the neurological presentation is dramatic ocular signs, with sunsetting and eye deviation downward and outwards to the side of the thalamic lesion.[41] The abnormal eye posture is due to close proximity of the haemorrhage of the lesion to the frontomesencephalic pathway of the optic tract.

The lesion is easily recognized on ultrasound imaging as well as CT and MRI. Evidence of associated venous thrombosis has been reported on CT[37] and MRI.[13] A vascular malformation causing the haemorrhage is very rare, and if MRI does not suggest such a lesion further invasive procedures are not warranted.

Prognosis

Initial reports of outcome were optimistic but this has not been borne out on longer-term follow-up. Roland et al[37] reported that less than 29% of term babies with primary thalamic haemorrhage were normal at follow-up. Cerebral palsy is a common sequel, but is often not severe. Cognitive deficit is common and this may be severe.

SUBAPONEUROTIC (SUBGALEAL) HAEMORRHAGE

Bleeding into the loose connective tissue below the aponeurotic membrane is referred to as subaponeurotic or subgaleal haemorrhage. It is not an intracranial form of bleeding, but may be life-threatening and deserves consideration here. A considerable volume of blood may be extravasated into this potential space before the extent of the bleeding has been realized, leading to hypovolaemia and possibly death.

The overall incidence of subaponeurotic haemorrhage is approximately 1:1250 deliveries,[31] but is particularly common following vacuum extraction, with an incidence of 1:150.[31] It may be due to vitamin K deficiency and appears to be more common in babies of Afro-Caribbean descent.

Diagnosis

A history of fetal distress is noted in half of cases, and the infant may show abnormal neurological signs secondary

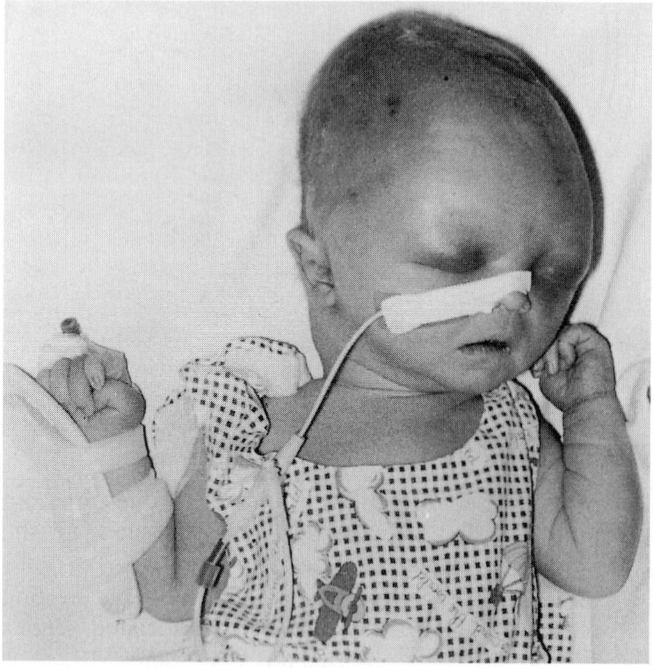

Fig. 44.21 Massive scalp enlargement caused by subaponeurotic haemorrhage.

to shock. This may make the distinction between fetal distress or bleeding as the primary cause of the encephalopathy a difficult clinical problem. A large volume of blood may extravasate into the subaponeurotic space before signs of haemorrhage are obvious. The first indication of abnormality may be anaemia, a rapid drop in haematocrit, or shock. The head size increases rapidly and may become enormous owing to the accumulation of blood (Fig. 44.21). The soft tissue swelling crosses suture lines. Each centimetre enlargement has been said to correspond to a blood loss of 40 ml.

Management

Rapid diagnosis and blood replacement is the key to management, which may need to be directed towards supporting organs such as the kidneys and brain if shock has occurred.

Prognosis

Mortality from subaponeurotic haemorrhage is reported to be 17–25%.[17,31,35]

CEREBRAL SINUS AND VENOUS THROMBOSIS

Thrombosis of the cerebral veins or sinuses is rarely diagnosed in life, but probably occurs more frequently than initially thought. It may occur in association with intracranial haemorrhage or be mistaken for haemorrhage on imaging of the brain.

Thrombosis of the cerebral veins may occur spontaneously, but has been found in association with sepsis, trauma to the skull and underlying structures, dehydration with reduction in venous flow, and congenital protein C deficiency.

Diagnosis

There are no specific neurological signs that suggest neonatal cerebral venous thrombosis, but it should be suspected in infants with dehydration or those with pre-existing neurological disease if exacerbation of neurological features occurs. General signs include features of intracranial hypertension, convulsions, hypertonia and opisthotonus. Unexplained lethargy has been reported to be a consistent feature.[36]

Cerebral ultrasound and colour flow Doppler do not appear to offer diagnostic benefit. CT and MRI are the only methods for diagnosing this condition in life. On CT the diagnosis is suspected by increased density of the vein of Galen and straight sinus or a high-density thrombus in a cerebral cortical vein. CT enhancement and MRI may reveal specific abnormalities.[26]

Management

Only two case reports exist on the management of sinus thrombosis with urokinase.[12,21] The role of thrombolysis in this condition is uncertain, but may be appropriate in symptomatic cases.

REFERENCES

1. Avrahami E, Frishman E, Minz M 1993 CT demonstration of intracranial haemorrhage in term newborn following vacuum extractor delivery. Neuroradiology 35: 107–108
2. Bergman I, Bauer R E, Barmada M A et al 1985 Intracerebral hemorrhage in the full-term neonatal infant. Pediatrics 75: 488–496
3. Castillo M, Fordham L A 1995 M R of neurologically symptomatic newborns after vacuum extraction delivery. American Journal of Neuroradiology 16: 816–818
4. Cilley R E, Zwischernberger J B, Andrews A F, Bowerman R A, Roloff D W, Bartlett R H 1986 Intracranial hemorrhage during extracorporeal membrane oxygenation in neonates. Pediatrics 78: 699–704
5. Chaou W-T, Chou M-L, Eitzman D V 1984 Intracranial hemorrhage and vitamin K deficiency in early infancy. Journal of Pediatrics 105: 880–884
6. Craig W S 1938 Intracranial haemorrhage in the new-born. Archives of Disease in Childhood 13: 89–124
7. De Vries L S, Smet M, Goemans N, Wilms G, Devlieger H, Casaer P 1992 Unilateral thalamic haemorrhage in the pre-term and full-term newborn. Neuropediatrics 23: 153–156
8. Eken P, Jansen G H, Groenendaal F, Rademaker K J, de Vries L S 1994 Intracranial lesions in the fullterm infant with hypoxic ischaemic encephalopathy: ultrasound and autopsy correlation. Neuropediatrics 25: 301–307
9. Fenichel G M, Webster D L, Wong W K T 1984 Intracranial hemorrhage in the term newborn. Archives of Neurology 41: 30–34
10. Fishman M A, Percy A K, Cheek W R, Speer M E 1981 Successful conservative management of cerebellar hematomas in term neonates. Journal of Pediatrics 98: 466–468

11. Friede R L 1972 Subpial hemorrhage in infants. Journal of Neuropathology and Experimental Neurology 31: 548–556
12. Gebara B M, Goetting M G, Wang A-M 1995 Dural sinus thrombosis complicating subclavian vein catheterization: treatment with local thrombolysis. Pediatrics 95: 138–140
13. Govaert P, Acten E, Vanhaesebrouck P, de Praeter C, van Damme J 1992 Deep cerebral venous thrombosis in thalamo-ventricular hemorrhage of the term newborn. Pediatric Radiology 22: 123–127
14. Govaert P, Bridger J, Wigglesworth J 1995 Nature of the brain lesion in fetal allo-immune thrombocytopenia. Developmental Medicine and Child Neurology 37: 485–495
15. Govaert P, Calliauw L, Vanhaesebrouck P, Martens F, Barrilari A 1990 On the management of neonatal tentorial damage. Eight case reports and a review of the literature. Acta Neurochirurgica 106: 52–64
16. Govaert P, Vanhaesebrouck P, de Praeter C 1992 Traumatic neonatal intracranial bleeding and stroke. Archives of Disease in Childhood 67: 840–845
17. Govaert P, Vanhaesebrouck P, De Praeter C, Moens K, Leroy J 1992 Vacuum extraction, bone injury and neonatal subgaleal bleeding. European Journal of Pediatrics 151: 532–535
18. Grayck E N, Meliones N J, Kern F H, Hansell D R, Ungerleider R M, Greeley W J 1995 Elevated serum lactate correlates with intracranial hemorrhage in neonates treated with extracorporeal life support. Pediatrics 96: 914–917
19. Hanigan W C, Morgan A M, Stahlberg L K, Hiller J L 1990 Tentorial hemorrhage associated with vacuum extraction. Pediatrics 85: 534–539
20. Heibel M, Heber R, Bechinger D, Kornhuber H H 1993 Early diagnosis of perinatal cerebral lesions in apparently normal fullterm newborns by ultrasound of the brain. Neuroradiology 35: 8591
21. Higashida R T, Helmer E, Helbach V V 1989 Direct thrombolytic therapy for superior sagittal sinus thrombosis. American Journal of Neuroradiology 10: 54–56
22. Jocelyn L J, Casiro O G 1992 Neurodevelopmental outcome of term infants with intraventricular hemorrhage. American Journal of Diseases of Children 146: 194–197
23. Larroche J-C 1977 Developmental pathology in the neonate. Excepta Medica, Amsterdam
24. Larroche J-C 1986 Fetal encephalopathies of circulatory origin. Biolology of the Neonate 50: 61–74
25. Laroche J-C 1995 Fetal cerebral pathology of circulatory origin. In: Levene M I, Lilford R J, Bennett M J, Punt J (eds) Fetal and neonatal neurology and neurosurgery, 2nd edn. Churchill Livingstone, Edinburgh, pp 321–331
26. Levene M I, de Vries L S 1995 Neonatal intracranial haemorrhage. In: Levene M I, Lilford R J, Bennett M J, Punt J (eds) Fetal and neonatal neurology and neurosurgery, 2nd edn. Churchill Livingstone, Edinburgh, pp 335–359
27. Ludwig B, Brand M, Brockerhoff P 1980 Postpartum C T examination of the heads of full term infants. Neuroradiology 20: 145–154
28. McLellan N J, Prasad R, Punt J 1986 Spontaneous subhyaloid and retinal haemorrhages in an infant. Archives of Disease in Childhood 61: 1130–1132
29. Mitchell W, Tuama L 1980 Cerebral intraventricular hemorrhages in infants: a widening age spectrum. Pediatrics 65: 35–39
30. Moghal N E, Quinn M W, Levene M I, Puntis J W L 1992 Intraventricular haemorrhage after aspiration of ventricular reservoirs. Archives of Disease in Childhood 67: 448–449
31. Ng P C, Siu Y K, Lewindon P J 1995 Subaponeurotic haemorrhage in the 1990s: a 3-year surveillance. Acta Paediatrica 84: 1065–1069
32. Palma P A, Miner M E, Morriss F H, Adcock E W, Denson S E 1979 Intraventricular hemorrhage in the neonate born at term. American Journal of Diseases of Children 133: 941–944
33. Pape K E, Armstrong D L, Fitzhardinge P M 1976 Central nervous system pathology associated with mask ventilation in the very low birthweight infant: a new etiology for intracerebellar hemorrhage. Pediatrics 58: 473–483
34. Pape K E, Wigglesworth J S 1979 Haemorrhage, ischaemia and the perinatal brain. Clinics in Developmental Medicine 69/70, London
35. Plauche W C 1980 Subgaleal haematoma. A complication of instrumental delivery. Journal of the American Medical Association 244: 1597–1598
36. Rivkin M J, Anderson M L, Kaye E M 1992 Neonatal idiopathic cerebral venous thrombosis: an unrecognized cause of transient seizures or lethargy. Annals of Neurology 32: 51–56
37. Roland E H, Flodmark O F, Hill A 1990 Thalamic hemorrhage with intraventricular hemorrhage in the full-term newborn. Pediatrics 85: 737–742
38. Scher M S, Wright F S, Lockman L A, Thompson T R 1982 Intraventricular hemorrhage in the full-term neonate. Archives of Neurology 39: 769–772
39. Scotti G, Flodmark O, Harwood-Nash D C, Humphries R P 1981 Posterior fossa hemorrhages in the newborn. Journal of Computer Assisted Tomography 5: 68–72
40. Taylor G A, Fitz C R, Glass P, Short B L 1989 C T of cerebrovascular injury after neonatal extracorporeal membrane oxygenation: implications for neurodevelopmental outcome. American Journal of Roentgenology 153: 121–126
41. Trounce J Q, Dodd K L, Fawer C-L, Fielder A R, Punt J, Levene M I 1985 Primary thalamic haemorrhage in the newborn: a new clinical entity. Lancet i: 190–192
42. Wakai S, Andoh Y, Nagai M, Teramoto C, Tanaka G 1990 Choroid plexus arteriovenous malformation in a full-term neonate. Journal of Neurosurgery 72: 127–129
43. Wehberg K, Vincent M, Garrison B, Dilustro J F, Frank L M 1992 Intraventricular hemorrhage in the full-term neonate associated with abdominal compression. Pediatrics 89: 327–329
44. Welch K 1980 The intracranial pressure in infants. Journal of Neurosurgery 52: 693–699
45. Welch K, Strand R 1986 Traumatic parturitional intracranial haemorrhage. Developmental Medicine and Child Neurology 28: 156–164
46. Wigglesworth J S, Husemeyer R P 1977 Intracranial birth trauma in vaginal breech delivery: the continued importance of injury to the occipital bone. British Journal of Obstetrics and Gynaecology 84: 684–691

Part 4

Hypoxic–ischaemic injury

David J. Evans Malcolm I. Levene

INTRODUCTION

INCIDENCE

Throughout the world intrapartum hypoxic–ischaemic insults remain an important cause of perinatally acquired brain injury in full-term infants. The incidence varies depending upon the clinical definition used. Table 44.7 gives incidence figures from studies in term infants using neonatal encephalopathy as a main diagnostic criterion. The risk of death or severe neurological impairment following hypoxia–ischaemia is 0.5–1.0 per 1000 live births in this era of perinatal care, representing approxi-

Table 44.7 Incidence of neonatal encephalopathy and death or severe neurological impairment following intrapartum hypoxia–ischaemia

Place	Year	Total births	Criteria	Incidence per 1000 live births		Reference
				Intrapartum hypoxia–ischaemia	Death and/or severe neurological disability	
Edinburgh, Scotland	1969–73	14 020	Encephalopathy	6.7	2.3	16
Edmonton, Canada	1974–78	20 155	Sarnat HIE	4.7	0.9	35
Leicester, England	1980–84	20 975	Levene HIE	6.0	1.1	66
Gothenburg, Sweden	1985–91	42 203	Apgar < 7 at 5 min + HIE	1.8	0.5	130

mately 750 infants per year in the United Kingdom alone.

In developing countries intrapartum hypoxic–ischaemic injury appears to be more common, although studies in such countries often include preterm as well as full-term infants. Countries reporting incidences include Kuwait[3] (9.4 per 1000), Malaysia[15] (18.7 per 1000), Nigeria[2] (26.5 per 1000), India[118] (New Delhi 59 per 1000) and Tanzania[58] (229 per 1000). Neonatal mortality in the first 24 hours following hypoxic–ischaemic injury in normal-birthweight infants was 18 per 1000 live births in the Tanzanian study.[58] Follow-up programmes are not well developed in these countries and the numbers of survivors with severe neurological impairment are unknown, but it is likely that hypoxic–ischaemic injury produces a huge burden of worldwide disability.

Having established that hypoxia–ischaemia is an important cause of death and disability, it is disappointing to note that the management of these infants is still largely empirical and virtually no treatment regimen has been the subject of a randomized controlled trial.

TERM VERSUS PRETERM

It is unclear to what extent preterm infants can manifest similar clinical features following hypoxic–ischaemic injury compared to term infants. The immature central nervous system may respond differently to such insults, although clinical features of hypoxic–ischaemic encephalopathy have been described in an infant of 31 weeks' gestation.[91] Preterm infants are also at risk from additional insults outside the intrapartum period. Antenatal insults, including infection, may be more common than previously thought, and could be responsible for the onset of preterm labour. Postnatal problems such as respiratory illness, GMH-IVH and leukomalacia may cause further injury that lead to neurological morbidity. These additional insults can mask the significance of intrapartum hypoxia–ischaemia and can confound the study of preterm hypoxia–ischaemia. Therefore, the majority of information discussed in this chapter will refer to hypoxic–ischaemic injury in the term infant, occurring most commonly as the result of an intrapartum insult.

PATHOPHYSOLOGY OF HYPOXIA–ISCHAEMIA

Asphyxia is etymologically derived from the Greek word meaning 'pulseless', but the term birth asphyxia has become widely used to describe a presumed intrapartum hypoxic–ischaemic insult. The preferred term is hypoxia–ischaemia, which descibes a pathophysiological process at tissue level comprising hypoxaemia with ischaemia and resultant hypercarbia and acidosis. Hypoxia–ischaemia produces a heterogeneous clinical 'syndrome', the nature of which is determined by the aetiology of the insult and the fetal response to that insult.

AETIOLOGY OF HYPOXIC–ISCHAEMIC INSULTS

As the intrauterine pressure exceeds 30 mmHg during contractions in active labour, the perfusion of the intervillous space is impaired, transiently interrupting placental gas exchange. This can be accommodated by the healthy fetoplacental unit, provided the contractions are of less than 60 seconds' duration, with sufficient respite (2.3 minutes) in between.[95]

Several additional stresses may occur; some represent acute hypoxic–ischaemic insults, others chronic or acute-on-chronic insults:

- Interruption of the umbilical circulation (e.g. cord compression or cord prolapse);
- Altered placental gas exchange (e.g. abruption, placental insufficiency);
- Reduced maternal placental perfusion (e.g. maternal hypotension or hypertension);
- Impaired maternal oxygenation;
- Failure to establish adequate cardiopulmonary circulation after birth.

FETAL RESPONSES TO HYPOXIA–ISCHAEMIA

The healthy fetus is able to use a variety of adaptive responses in order to help it overcome the hypoxic–ischaemic insult. These include:

- Reduction in body movements, breathing movements and REM sleep, thus reducing energy consumption and oxygen demand;[100]
- Increased oxygen extraction from the blood. The maternofetal circulation represents a high-output oxygen supply such that almost twice the amount of oxygen can be extracted by fetal haemoglobin before cardiac output needs to increase.[14] Erythropoietin concentrations are increased, stimulating fetal erythrocyte production;[108]
- Redistribution of blood supply to the central nervous system, myocardium and adrenals at the expense of the kidneys, gastrointestinal tract, liver and muscle;[23]
- Within the brain, preferential oxygenation is maintained by diverting blood flow to the brain stem, midbrain and cerebellum;[101]
- Sympathetic response. The high catecholamine levels seen during hypoxia–ischaemia increase peripheral vascular resistance and myocardial contractility in order to maintain perfusion, despite the fetal bradycardic response. The sympathetic stimulus also accelerates anaerobic glycolysis, with mobilization of liver glycogen stores, thus maintaining the CNS and myocardial energy substrate;
- The immature CNS can more readily utilize the lactate, pyruvate and ketones generated by anaerobic glycolysis as an alternative to glucose.[150] Infants with hyperinsulinaemia (e.g. those born to mothers with diabetes) are less able to generate these alternative energy sources and are therefore at greater risk from hypoxic–ischaemic injury.

MECHANISMS OF BRAIN INJURY

Although brain injury begins during the initial insult (primary neuronal injury), it continues despite resuscitation. The term secondary neuronal injury is used to describe damage that occurs during recovery from the initial insult and is the consequence of numerous processes set in motion by the hypoxic–ischaemic insult. Many of these individual processes have been characterized by observations in animal models and are summarized in Figure 44.22. It has proved difficult to determine the relative importance of individual mechanisms as they are intricately interrelated and may not necessarily occur to the same degree or in the same sequence, depending upon the nature of the insult.

Primary neuronal injury

During the insult, intracellular energy depletion occurs. In the cells most affected, complete energy exhaustion leads to membrane pump failure. Water then enters the cells, resulting in cytotoxic cerebral oedema and primary neuronal death.[54] It is the fate of the surviving cells following resuscitation that has been the subject of much research. These surviving neurons appear vulnerable to further injury because of postischaemic cerebrovascular dysfunction and excessive movement of calcium into the cell.

Postischaemic cerebrovascular dysfunction

During hypoxia–ischaemia cerebral blood flow is severely reduced. Immediately following resuscitation elevated levels have been documented, probably due to the 'washout' of lactic acid and other products of acute hypoxia–ischaemia.[55] This may be followed by a further period of marked reduction in cerebral blood flow, referred to as the no reflow phenomenon,[5] documented using near-infrared spectroscopy in asphyxiated infants.[133] Other studies have reported persisting high cerebral blood flow after hypoxia–ischaemia, characterized by a reduced vascular reactivity to changes in arterial PCO_2. This is thought to represent loss of cerebrovascular autoregulation and is associated with severe brain injury.[98] It is likely that following a severe hypoxic–ischaemic insult there is an early stage of impaired cerebral blood flow which gives way to vasoparalysis with increased blood flow. Several mechanisms may play a role in the development of such cerebrovascular dysfunction.

Neutrophils

Hypoxic–ischaemic injury to the vascular endothelium results in activation of neutrophils, which then cause further injury to the endothelium, obstruct the microvasculature and infiltrate the CNS parenchyma. Neutropenic animals show less disturbance in cerebral blood flow and improved cortical evoked responses following induced cerebral ischaemia.[31]

Platelet-activating factor and eicosanoids

During ischaemic injury platelet-activating factor is synthesized from the action of phospholipase A_2 upon lipid membranes. PAF activates neutrophils, promotes platelet aggregation, increases vascular permeability resulting in vasogenic cerebral oedema, and stimulates the release of vasoactive eicosanoids (thromboxanes, prostaglandins and leukotrienes).[152]

Free radicals

Reperfusion following hypoxia–ischaemia leads to the formation of free radicals from free fatty acid and prostaglandin metabolism. In addition, the degradation of

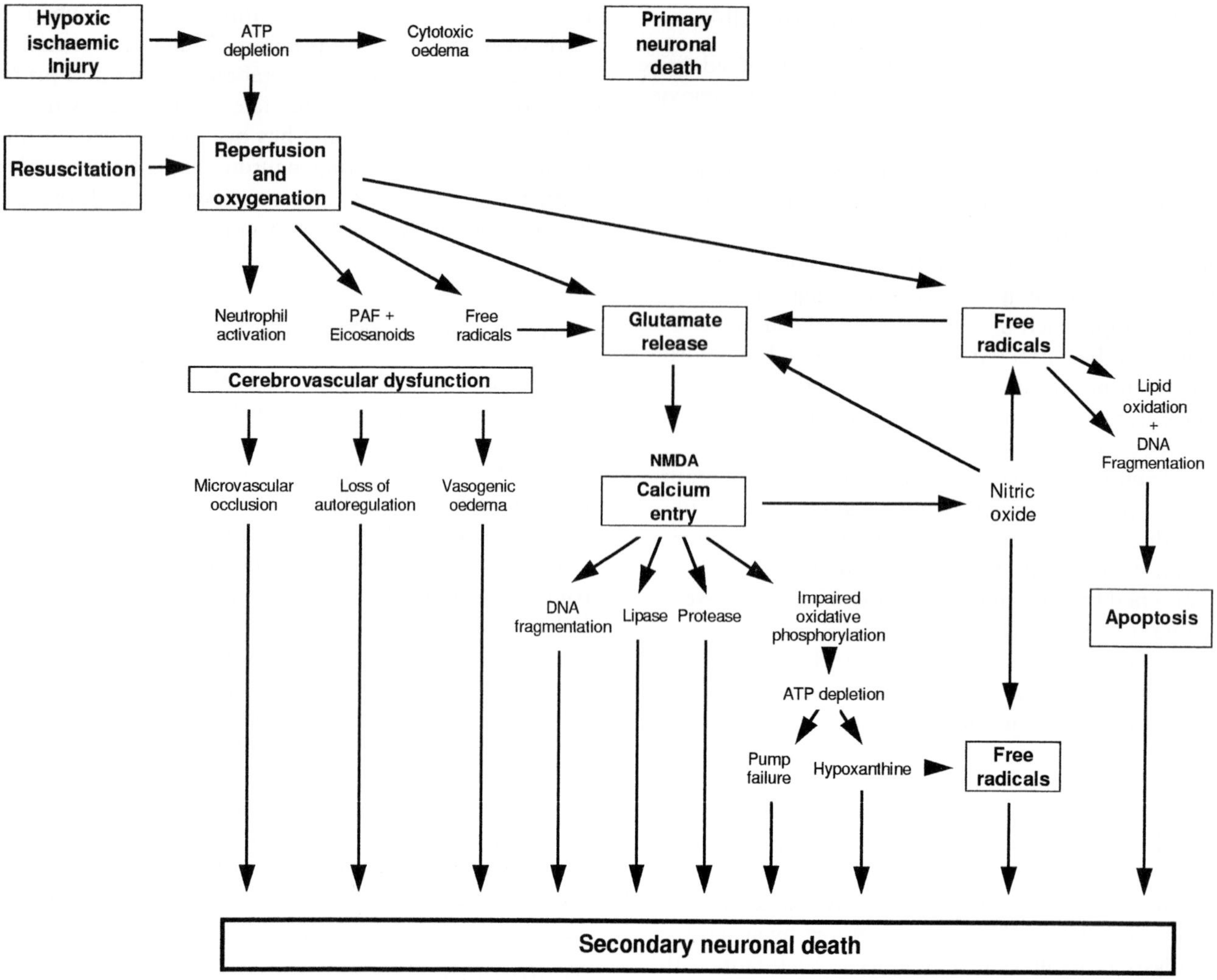

Fig. 44.22 Simplified schematic representation of the mechanisms involved in secondary neuronal injury following hypoxia–ischaemia.

ATP to hypoxanthine during ischaemia results in free radical formation as the hypoxanthine is converted to xanthine and uric acid by xanthine oxidase.[77] Free radicals act directly on the vasculature to increase the permeability of the blood–brain barrier,[22] and also indirectly by activation of neutrophils and stimulation of PAF production. These abnormalities in cerebrovascular autoregulation may compromise the ability of surviving neurons to recover and may contribute to secondary neuronal injury.

Secondary neuronal injury and apoptosis

The death of neurons in the postasphyxial period may be initiated by necrosis as the direct result of the hypoxic–ischaemic insult, or occur as the result of apoptosis. Apoptosis is the now well accepted concept of programmed cell death due to failure of a complicated and incompletely understood intercellular signalling process. Secondary neuronal death probably occurs as a combination of these two interrelated processes.

In the asphyxiated newborn piglet model, the intracellular phosphocreatinine to inorganic phosphate ratio (PCr/Pi) can be determined by ^{31}P magnetic resonance spectroscopy. The PCr/Pi ratio represents the phosphorylated energy status within the neuron and shows a biphasic pattern following hypoxic–ischaemia. The initial precipitate fall is largely reversed by resuscitation, but is followed by a delayed fall as the remaining neurons succumb to secondary neuronal death.[71]

Calcium entry into the neuron appears to be a key stage in the commencement of a cascade of processes leading to cell death. It uncouples oxidative phosphorylation, which results in futile ATP consumption. It also activates the enzymes responsible for DNA fragmentation and free radical formation.[117]

A stimulus for calcium entry involves excessive release from neurons of glutamate, a fast excitatory neurotransmitter. Glutamate acts upon the *N*-methyl-D-aspartate (NMDA) receptor, a postsynaptic ion channel, permitting calcium influx. Activation of the NMDA receptor leads to the production of nitric oxide (NO) by neuronal nitric oxide synthetase (NOS). NO can diffuse through membranes and act as a retrograde messenger, further stimulating glutamate release.[61] It can also react with molecular oxygen to form superoxide, peroxide and peroxynitrite free radicals. These free radicals cause DNA damage and membrane lipid oxidation, and are potent inducers of apoptosis.[19]

NO is also produced by vascular endothelial NOS. In contrast to its neuronal effects, NO may have beneficial effects on the vasculature, including vasodilatation, inhibition of neutrophil activation and inhibition of platelet aggregation.[56]

Neuronal repair

During the 72 hours following the hypoxic–ischaemic insult there is an induction of trophic factors, particularly in the developing CNS. Of those characterized, insulin-like growth factor 1 (IGF-1) is produced by astrocytes in the area of damage and is highly neurotrophic. These trophic factors may act to rescue neurons from secondary cell death by an unknown mechanism.[40]

An understanding of the processes involved in secondary neuronal death becomes important when developing treatments that can protect the brain from further injury following resuscitation.

PATHOLOGY

There is no single distinct or uniform pathological appearance of the brain following hypoxia–ischaemia. Cell death will occur when the metabolic demand fails to be met by substrate delivery via the blood. The pattern of injury depends upon the severity of asphyxial insult (total versus partial), its timing and duration (acute versus chronic), the developmental maturity of the brain and regional variations in vulnerability (due to local vascular factors, distribution of NMDA receptors etc.).

OBSERVED PATTERNS OF INJURY FOLLOWING HYPOXIA–ISCHAEMIA

Cerebral oedema

Within 24–48 hours gross swelling of the cerebral tissue may occur, with marked flattening and widening of the gyri plus obliteration of the sulci, seen on imaging or at postmortem. It arises through two mechanisms: *cytotoxic*, when membrane pump failure leads to *intracellular* fluid accumulation, and *vasogenic*, when the impaired blood–brain barrier permits capillary leak and *interstitial* fluid accumulation.

Selective neuronal necrosis

This is the most commonly observed pathology following hypoxia–ischaemia in term infants, affecting neurons in a scattered fashion and often widely distributed throughout the grey matter. The cerebral cortex layers III and IV and the hippocampus appear particularly vulnerable.[120] This may reflect differing metabolic rates of the various cortical structures.[60] Light-microscopy changes are apparent 24–36 hours following the insult, with cytoplasmic eosinophilia and nuclear fragmentation. Overt necrosis follows within a few days.

Basal ganglia and brain stem

In animal models this pattern of injury is seen following acute total asphyxia rather than chronic partial asphyxia.[84] Basal ganglia injury is thought to be responsible for the dyskinetic type of cerebral palsy seen in survivors of hypoxia–ischaemia, and abnormal signal intensity in the basal ganglia is a common MRI finding.[110] Within the first weeks abnormal capillary proliferation and microcalcification can be seen on histology.[115] Abnormalities detected at this stage by ultrasound or CT are thought to represent these pathological processes (Fig. 44.23).[137] If the infant survives for several months, an abnormal myelination pattern occurs which is detectable on MRI scan. This is responsible for the marble-like appearance of the basal ganglia seen at postmortem, known as status marmoratus.

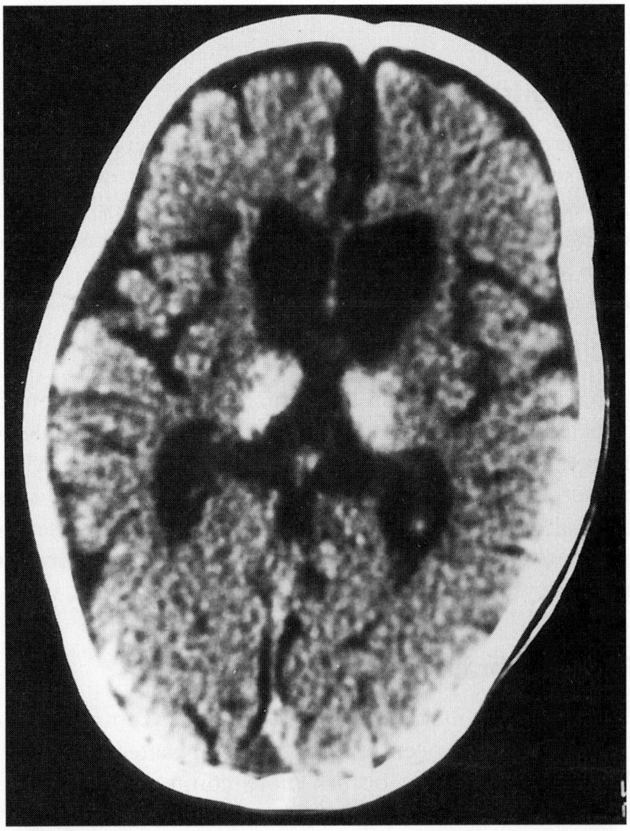

Fig. 44.23 CT brain of asphyxiated neonate aged 18 months. Note the bilateral bright thalami and generalized cortical atrophy.

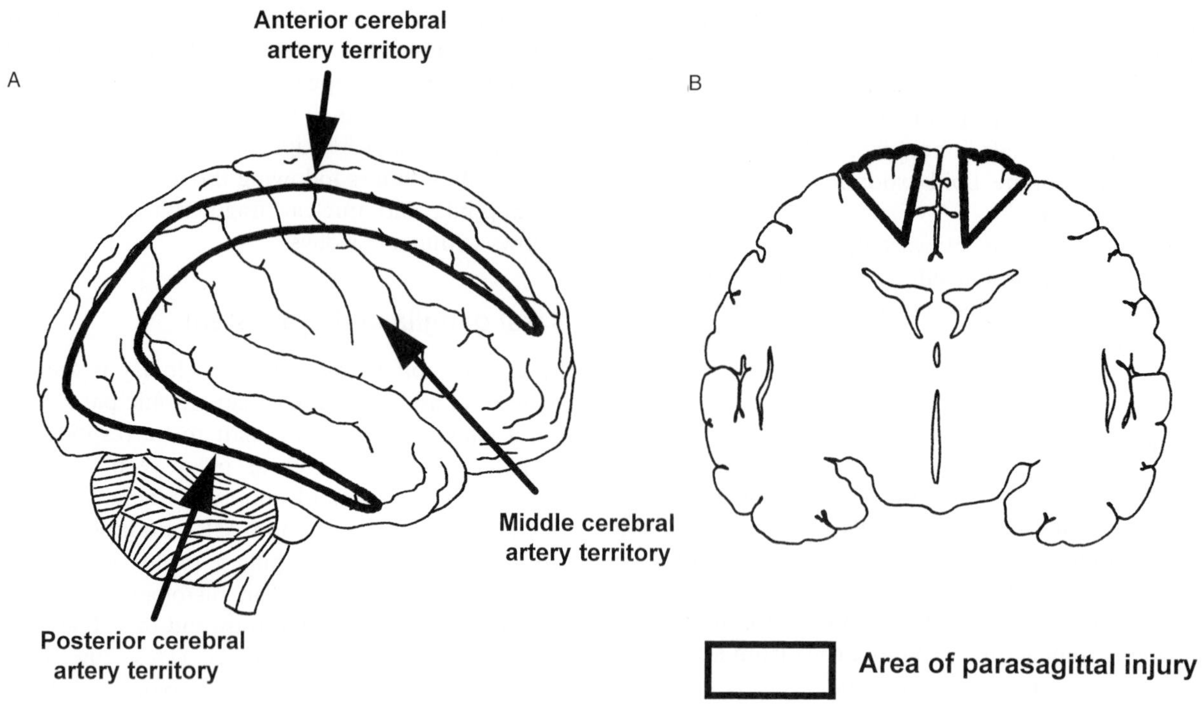

Fig. 44.24 Parasagittal injury. (A) Lateral view of the cerebral cortex. (B) Coronal section.

Haemorrhage and haemorrhagic infarction affecting the thalami following hypoxia–ischaemia are also well recognized phenomena.

Parasagittal injury

This is an ischaemic injury affecting the cerebral cortex and subcortical white matter in vascular watersheds between the anterior, middle and posterior cerebral arteries, giving rise to a parasagittal distribution, and is often symmetrical (Fig. 44.24).[139]

White matter injury

Ischaemic insults in preterm infants produce periventricular leukomalacia. Periventricular glia are vulnerable to ischaemia in preterm infants. When ischaemic white matter injury occurs at term, it usually results in subcortical leukomalacia. The survivors of the most severe insults usually show a mixed pattern of injury, referred to as multicystic leukoencephalopathy (Fig. 44.25).

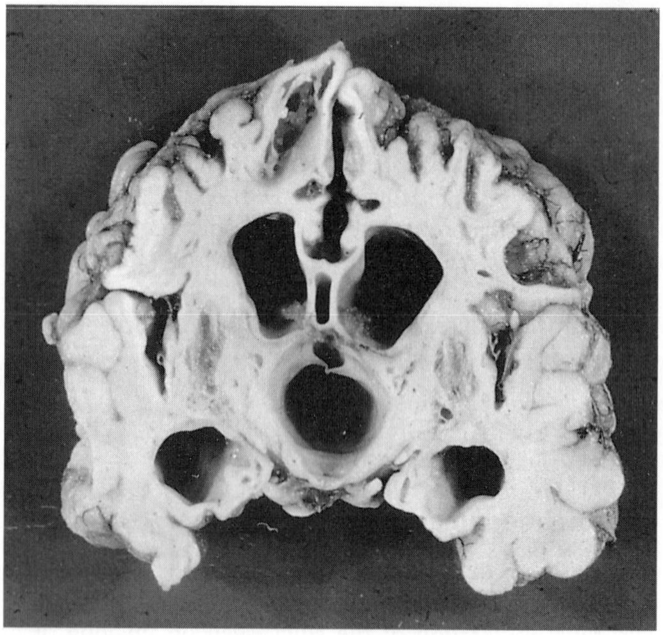

Fig. 44.25 Multicystic leukoencephalopathy. Coronal section of a pathological specimen with areas of cystic degeneration throughout the periventricular white matter, subcortical white matter and basal ganglia. Also note the generalized cortical atrophy with ventricular enlargement.

Focal cerebral infarction

Infarction of a major cerebral artery, most commonly the middle, has also been reported in asphyxiated infants.[141] Although this lesion occurs more commonly in infants with no evidence of intrapartum asphyxia (67%),[138] hypoxia–ischaemia does represent the largest identifiable cause of such infarction.

CLINICAL DEFINITION: 'THE ASPHYXIA SYNDROME'

Despite the increasing knowledge of the pathophysiology of perinatal asphyxia, there is little agreement over its

Table 44.8 Evidence for intrapartum hypoxic–ischaemic injury causing cerebral palsy

Evidence for intrapartum asphyxia	Fetal distress Fetal acidosis Depressed Apgar scores Delayed onset of respiration Hypoxic–ischaemic encephalopathy Multiorgan involvement
Exclusion of alternative causes of neonatal encephalopathy (Table 44.9)	
Supporting evidence	Normal fetal brain growth until birth, followed by failure of normal brain growth Pattern of MRI abnormality suggestive of intrapartum hypoxia–ischaemia
Pattern of disability	Spastic quadriplegia Dyskinetic cerebral palsy

Table 44.9 Aetiology of early neonatal encephalopathy

Hypoxia–ischaemia	
Infection	Neonatal meningitis
Drug-related	Maternal anaesthesia/analgesia Maternal drug abuse Neonatal sedatives/anticonvulsants
CNS malformations	
Intracranial haemorrhage	
Metabolic	Hypoglycaemia Hyponatraemia/hypocalcaemia Bilirubin encephalopathy Amino acidaemias (e.g. non-ketotic hyperglycinaemia) Organic acidaemias Pyridoxine dependency Lactate acidaemias Urea cycle disorders

clinical definition. This is reflected in the multitude of differing definitions used in studies of incidence, treatment and outcome. There are many clinical and biochemical features that are used as possible markers but, as with the definition of many other syndromes, no single feature alone should be taken as defining perinatal asphyxia. One problem in evaluating the relative importance of such features (or a combination of features) has been the lack of a 'gold standard' by which to weight their value. We cannot yet clinically define the nature, timing or severity of the asphyxial insult, and in many cases the observed outcome may not necessarily be a consequence of that insult. To diagnose 'asphyxia syndrome' it is necessary to ascertain positive features (Table 44.8), together with excluding alternative conditions which may mimic some of these features (Table 44.9).

FETAL DISTRESS

The fetus is well adapted to cope with the physiological stress normally imposed by labour. The aim of intrapartum monitoring is to detect fetal 'distress', rather than 'stress', which is normal. If fetal distress is detected it cannot be assumed that the insult has occurred during labour. A fetus that has sustained an hypoxic–ischaemic insult before labour may not be able to mount the normal physiological coping responses during labour. Therefore, evidence of 'fetal distress' may in some cases be a marker of compromise prior to the onset of labour.

Intrapartum fetal monitoring

Electronic fetal monitoring

In the 1970s electronic fetal monitoring (EFM) was introduced and it was assumed that more precise information about fetal heart rates would lead to improved outcomes.[147] Fetal blood sampling (FBS) can be used as an adjunct to EFM: the pH and/or blood gases of fetal scalp capillary blood are measured intermittently at appropriate intervals, often in response to equivocal EFM recordings. However, meta-analyses of randomized controlled trials comparing EFM +/– FBS versus intermittent auscultation do not show a reduction in intrapartum deaths or cerebral palsy, despite an increase in caesarean section rates.[86,126] However, the randomized controlled trials published to date, comparing EFM +/– FBS versus intermittent auscultation, did not have sufficient statistical power to demonstrate a reduction in the incidence of perinatal death or subsequent neurological impairment secondary to hypoxia–ischaemia.

The only benefit in neonatal outcome seen after electronic fetal monitoring was a reduction in the incidence of early neonatal seizures. The prevalence of cerebral palsy in the two randomized controlled trials with follow-up data was not significantly altered by EFM + FBS.[42,73] One meta-analysis reported a reduction in perinatal mortality due to fetal hypoxia.[136] However, this study did not show a reduction in overall perinatal mortality rate and, as there is no specific marker for hypoxic death, it is difficult to reliably ascertain the mortality due to fetal hypoxia.[8] In conclusion, it appears that a normal heart rate pattern may be reassuring (negative predictive value of adverse outcome >96% in most studies) but an abnormal pattern is poorly predictive of fetal compromise. It appears that abnormal fetal heart rate patterns are unreliable markers of intrapartum antecedents of neurological damage, leading to obstetric intervention without proven benefit. It remains to be seen whether better markers can be developed from future work on the newer techniques of intrapartum monitoring.

Fetal ECG analysis

During myocardial ischaemia anaerobic glycolysis changes the ion gradients across the myocardial cell membranes,

Table 44.10 The outcome associated with latest* very low Apgar score (0–3)[88]

	<2501 g				>2500 g			
Time (min)	Number liveborn	Death by 1 year (%)	Number known to 7 years	Cerebral palsy (%)	Number liveborn	Death by 1 year (%)	Number known to 7 years	Cerebral palsy (%)
1	428	25.5	257	1.9	1729	3.1	1330	0.7
5	163	55.2	56	7.1	286	7.7	217	0.9
10	67	67.2	15	6.7	66	18.2	43	4.7
15	51	84.3	8	0.0	23	47.8	11	9.1
20	139	95.7	7	0.0	39	59.0	14	57.1

*Counts at each time include only those children with very low Apgar scores at that time and no later very low Apgar score.

resulting in a raised ST segment and a raised T/QRS ratio.[105] When tested in a randomized controlled trial, this technique enabled a reduction in operative intervention without worsening outcome.[145]

Systolic time intervals

Fetal ECG analysis in combination with Doppler analysis of the cardiac cycle has been used to assess myocardial function. The pre-ejection period (an electromechanical interval from initial deflection of the QRS complex to aortic valve opening) and the ventricular ejection time (duration of aortic valve opening) are thought to be sensitive indicators of myocardial contractility, and have been used to detect deteriorating function during asphyxia.[68]

Fetal pulse oximetry

Continuous fetal oxygen saturation monitoring is possible and corresponds to results from fetal blood analysis.[74] However, signal quality is limited and the technique has not been tested in large-scale clinical practice.

Near-infrared spectroscopy (NIRS)

Light of near-infrared wavelengths can penetrate brain tissue for distances up to 8 cm. It is possible to obtain continuous quantification of changes in cerebral haemoglobin oxygen saturation and total cerebral haemoglobin concentration (representing cerebral blood volume) by analysis of the absorption spectra. During labour, an optical probe is inserted through the dilated cervix and on to the fetal head. A study of 41 fetuses during labour demonstrated good correlation between the mean cerebral oxygen saturation shortly before delivery and the umbilical arterial acid–base status immediately after birth.[4] This technique has not been applied in a large series or trial.

Passage of meconium

This occurs in 10–20% of all term deliveries but it is often taken as a marker of fetal distress. However, only 0.4% of term infants with meconium-stained liquor during labour subsequently developed cerebral palsy.[89] Richey et al found no correlation between the passage of meconium and markers of acute asphyxia (umbilical arterial pH, lactate and hypoxanthine).[102]

CONDITION AT BIRTH

Apgar scores

A method of assessing an infant's condition at birth was first described by Virginia Apgar.[6] Originally scored at 1 minute of life by summation of five scored signs (p. 242), this was later extended to 5-minute intervals. A hypoxic–ischaemic insult can cause depression of the Apgar score, but this is not invariable unless the insult occurs immediately prior to birth. Many non-asphyxial factors can cause depression, for example prematurity, maternal analgesia or anaesthetic. Nevertheless, prolonged depression of the Apgar score is related to death or major neurological disability.[88] (Table 44.10). It is notable that almost 75% of children with cerebral palsy had Apgar scores of 7–10 at 5 minutes of life.

Acidosis

Metabolic acidosis is an index of anaerobic metabolism and is widely used as retrospective evidence of tissue hypoxia and 'fetal distress'. However, umbilical arterial acidaemia at delivery, considered on its own, is not associated with a poor outcome:[28,109] it is associated with a poor outcome only when in combination with abnormal fetal heart rate patterns, depressed Apgar scores and significant neonatal encephalopathy.[151] Severe fetal acidosis occurs in the moribund fetus, but may also occur in the fetus who has compensated by preserving function in vital organs. Thus there is only a very loose association between fetal acidosis and severe fetal distress.

CLINICAL FEATURES AFTER BIRTH

Hypoxic–ischaemic encephalopathy (HIE)

Very young infants recovering from a near-miss sudden infant death syndrome (SIDS) often show a predictable

Table 44.11 A clinical grading system for hypoxic–ischaemic encephalopathy[66]

Grade I (mild)	Grade II (moderate)	Grade III (severe)
Irritability 'hyperalert'	Lethargy	Comatose
Mild hypotonia	Marked abnormalities in tone	Severe hypotonia
Poor sucking	Requires tube feeds	Failure to maintain spontaneous respiration
No seizures	Seizures	Prolonged seizures

progression of neurological symptoms.[25] Initially there is a period of near normality, followed by the onset of seizures and a gradual deterioration in their conscious level. Similar behaviour is seen in severely asphyxiated term infants. Sarnat and Sarnat introduced a grading system to describe the neurological abnormality,[113] which was modified by Levene et al (Table 44.11).[66]

Mild (grade I) encephalopathy

This stage is characterized by apparent hyperalertness, staring (decreased frequency of blinking), normal or decreased spontaneous motor activity and a lower threshold for all stimuli, including the easily elicited Moro reflex.

Moderate (grade II) encephalopathy

Seizures occur commonly. There is lethargy, hypotonia with reduced spontaneous movements, a higher threshold for primitive reflexes, and mainly parasympathetic responses. A consistent feature is differential tone between the upper and lower limbs, with the arms being relatively hypotonic compared to the legs.

Severe (grade III) encephalopathy

These neonates are comatose, with hypotonia and no spontaneous movements. Primitive reflexes and the suck reflex are often absent. Seizures may be frequent and prolonged, although in the most severe cases there may be no seizure activity and an isoelectric EEG.

It is important to consider alternative causes for a neonatal encephalopathy (Table 44.9). Meningitis is the most common treatable condition that can produce encephalopathic features, and may coexist with hypoxia–ischaemia.

In a meta-analysis of studies examining the outcome of neonates with different HIE grades, it appears that stage I (mild HIE) does not confer an increased risk of death or disability. Table 44.12 shows the risks of death and neurological abnormalities in survivors associated with

Table 44.12 Risk of death or severe handicap in remaining survivors associated with grade of hypoxic–ischaemic encephalopathy[96]

HIE grade	Risk of death or severe handicap in survivors		
	Percentage	Likelihood ratio	(95% CI)
Mild (I)	1.6	0.05	0.02–0.15
Moderate (II)	24	0.94	0.71–1.23
Severe (III)	78	10.71	6.71–17.1

HIE grade from this analysis.[96] A significant reduction in IQ at 8 years has been reported in children who had suffered from grade II HIE, but who were neurologically normal, compared to children with grade I HIE.[104]

In a comparison of depression of Apgar scores with HIE grading in predicting outcome, an Apgar score of 5 or less at 10 minutes was found to be a more specific predictor of death or major neurological sequelae than HIE grades II and III (95% versus 78%), although it was less sensitive (57% versus 96%).[67]

Multiorgan dysfunction

During hypoxia–ischaemia blood flow is redistributed in order to preserve circulation to the most vital organs, namely the brain, heart and adrenals. This is at the expense of the kidneys, liver and gastrointestinal tract, which are therefore vulnerable to hypoxic–ischaemic damage. Such damage to these and other organs serves as a further marker of hypoxia–ischaemia (Table 44.13).

INVESTIGATIONS

Many advances have been made in imaging techniques, enabling a greater understanding of the pathophysiology of perinatal asphyxia and allowing a more accurate

Table 44.13 Multiorgan dysfunction following hypoxia–ischaemia

Renal	Acute renal failure Myoglobinuria Haematuria
Gastrointestinal	Abnormal motility and feed intolerance Necrotizing enterocolitis
Cardiovascular	Reduced ventricular function Myocardial ischaemia (ECG) Papilliary muscle necrosis
Pulmonary	Meconium aspiration Persistent pulmonary hypertension Apnoea
Haematological	Disseminated intravascular coagulation
Metabolic	Hyponatraemia/inappropriate ADH Hypoglycaemia Hypocalcaemia Elevated liver enzymes Elevated ammonia Metabolic acidosis

prognosis. This is particularly important because accurate early detection is required in assessing the efficacy of potential neuroprotective therapies. However, some of the newer imaging techniques have not been fully evaluated because accurate neurodevelopmental follow-up is still awaited.

CRANIAL ULTRASOUND

Ultrasound has proved most useful in the detection of GMH-IVH and ischaemic lesions in preterm infants, and it can also be of use in asphyxiated term infants. Initially, cerebral oedema can be recognized by a generalized increase in echodensity, a loss of anatomical landmarks, indistinct sulci and compression of the ventricles. 'Slit-like' ventricles are seen normally in the first 24 hours in term infants, and are only abnormal if persisting for more than 36 hours. Later ultrasound scan findings associated with a poor neurodevelopmental outcome include bilateral, uniformly echogenic thalami, which represents severe basal ganglia hypoxic–ischaemic injury;[24] diffuse parenchymal echodensities (thought to represent neuronal necrosis); multifocal cystic changes; periventricular echodensities; and ventriculomegaly with cortical atrophy.[116] One of the major limitations of ultrasound in asphyxia has been its inability to assess peripheral cortical damage, but with the recent use of higher-resolution probes (10 mHz) increased cortical echogenicity associated with hypoxic–ischaemic damage can be detected.[32]

Cerebral blood flow velocities

Using pulsed-wave duplex Doppler with real-time spectral analysis of the back-scattered Doppler signal from a major cerebral artery (often the anterior), the cerebral blood flow velocities in that vessel can be determined. A relative increase in the end-diastolic blood flow velocity compared to the peak systolic blood flow velocity (Pourcelot's resistivity index <0.55) is associated with a poor outcome in asphyxiated infants.[7] It was later demonstrated that if the anterior cerebral artery blood flow velocity rose to above three standard deviations from the normal mean, this was also associated with an adverse outcome (positive predictive value 94%).[64] This increased velocity lacked the normal variation with changing PCO_2 and was thought to represent vasoparalysis of the cerebral vasculature. The cerebral blood flow velocities can take 24 hours to become abnormal following hypoxia–ischaemia, and have been found to be of little prognostic value if performed at 6 hours.[33]

CEREBRAL BLOOD FLOW

In studies of infants with hypoxic–ischaemic encephalopathy using near-infrared spectroscopy, the cerebral blood volume was found to be increased, the normal response to changing CO_2 tension was markedly attenuated, and cerebral autoregulation to changing arterial pressure was also impaired.[149] Studies using the xenon clearance method for measuring cerebral blood flow have found that high flow and loss of autoregulation to changes in PCO_2 are associated with a poor prognosis following hypoxia–ischaemia.[98]

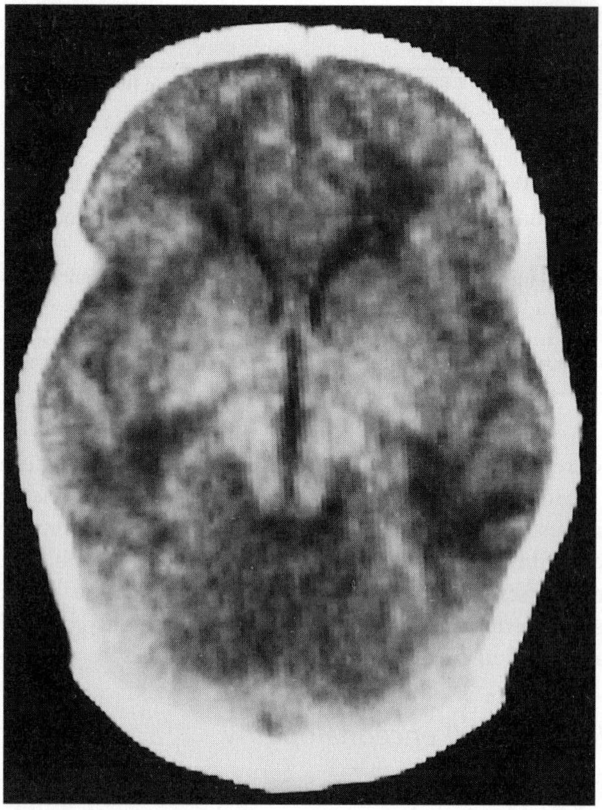

Fig. 44.26 CT brain of asphyxiated neonate aged 10 days. There is a generalized reduction in cortical density surrounding the more prominent basal ganglia.

COMPUTED TOMOGRAPHY

In a study of 43 asphyxiated term infants cerebral CT scans were performed in the first 2 weeks and the appearances classified as normal or decreased density (subdivided into patchy, diffuse or global).[1] Diffuse or global decreased density (Fig. 44.26) indicates a poor prognosis (sensitivity 93%, specificity 80%). Other studies have shown little correlation unless the scans are performed after the first week.[69]

MAGNETIC RESONANCE IMAGING

MRI has had an enormous impact on neuroimaging because of its higher sensitivity and specificity for maturational changes, such as visualization of myelination, and its better anatomical resolution, particularly the basal ganglia and the peripheral cortex. Late MRI findings associated with a poor neurodevelopmental outcome are delayed myelination, which is a marker of neuronal destruction, and other abnormalities, including cortical atrophy with thinning of the corpus callosum, persisting abnormal signal intensity in the basal ganglia, ventricular dilatation and extensive white matter changes (Fig. 44.27).[20,112] Patchy white matter changes, most obvious posteriorly, have recently been demonstrated in late MRI scans of asphyxiated infants who presented with mild HIE and were apparently normal at 1 year.[112] It will be interesting to discover whether these children have any minor neurological dysfunction at school age. There has been increasing interest in the early MRI changes. Initially there is evidence of brain swelling, which clears during the first week revealing abnormal signal intensity in the cortex, white matter, basal ganglia and the posterior limb of the internal capsule (Fig. 44.28). These changes are associated with severe hypoxic–ischaemic injury and adverse neurodevelopmental outcome.[59,111,112] In the second week further loss of white matter and subcortical breakdown occurs, with injury to the basal ganglia becoming more obvious.[9] Basal ganglia enhancement with MRI contrast within the first 10 days may indicate a particularly poor prognosis.[146]

In a comparison with ultrasound, early MRI was found to be superior at diagnosing cerebral arterial infarcts, cortical atrophy and basal ganglia lesions, although ultrasound proved more able to detect periventricular haemorrhage. With MRI the risk of adverse outcome appeared to be related to the severity of basal ganglia and thalamic injury seen.[110]

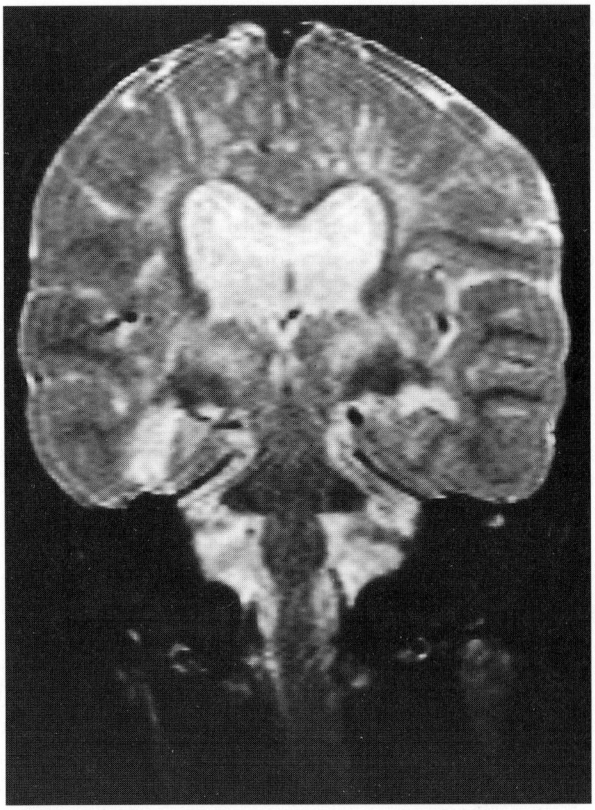

Fig. 44.27 MRI brain (T2-weighted coronal image) performed 2 years following an hypoxic–ischaemic insult. There is extensive abnormal high signal intensity in the periventricular white matter plus ventricular enlargement.

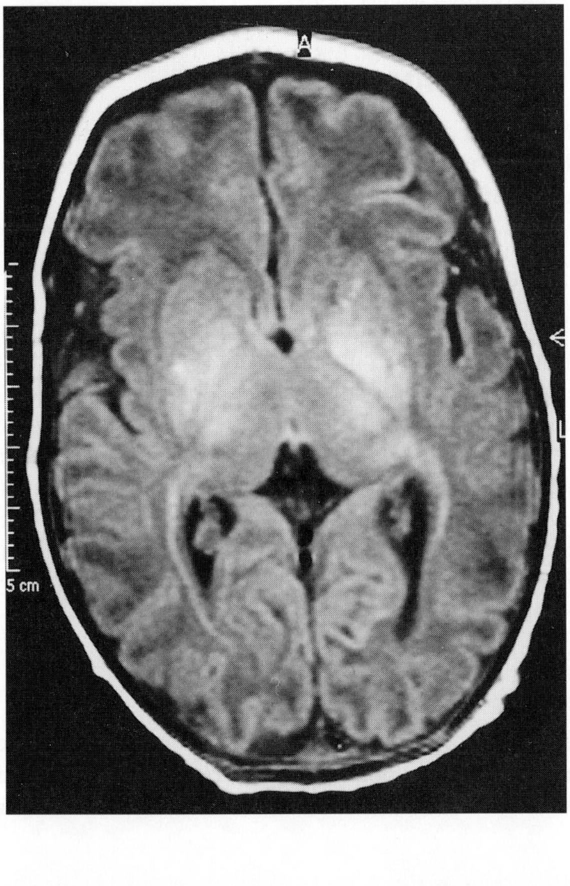

A

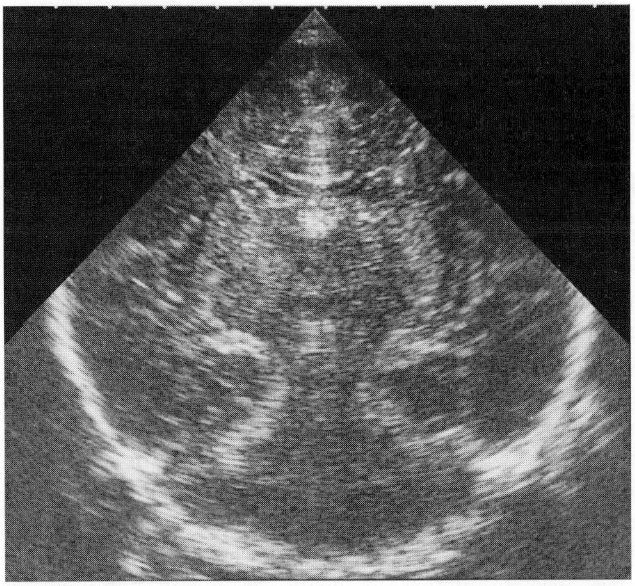

B

Fig. 44.28 (A) MRI brain (T1-weighted axial section) performed 8 days following hypoxia–ischaemia, with abnormal high signal in the basal ganglia, prominence of the cortical ribbon in the left frontal lobe and areas of abnormal low signal intensity in the subcortical areas (particularly frontal lobes). (B) Cranial ultrasound of the same patient (7.5 MHz, coronal section) showing bilateral echogenic basal ganglia but failing to detect any cortical abnormalities.

Magnetic resonance spectoscopy

Phosphocreatinine (PCr) and inorganic phosphate (Pi) can be measured from the ^{31}P magnetic resonance spectra. The PCr/Pi ratio represents the phosphorylated energy status within the brain, and a low PCr/Pi ratio in asphyxiated neonates is associated with later neurodevelopmental impairment,[82] with a sensitivity of 88% and specificity of 83%. Proton MRS detects a rise in lactate and a fall in *N*-acetyl-aspartate (Naa) following hypoxic–ischaemic injury. A low Naa/creatinine or Naa/choline ratio has been shown to be associated with a poor prognosis.[44,94] It appears that information from the proton resonance spectra can be gained before changes in the ^{31}P spectra occur, i.e. before cellular energy levels have been depleted.

ELECTROPHYSIOLOGY

Electroencephalography

Studies of neonatal EEGs in term infants with evidence of perinatal asphyxia have shown that background activity is an important prognostic indicator.[124] Continuous computer EEG analysis, allowing quantification and grading of the background activity, demonstrates that the more discontinuous the background, the poorer the associated outcome.[144] However, there are many practical difficulties in obtaining extended EEG monitoring, thereby limiting its use. Cerebral function monitors record amplitude-integrated EEG on a compressed timescale, providing a continuous trend of cerebral activity using just three electrodes. Hellstrom-Westas et al applied this technique in the first 6 hours and predicted the outcome correctly in 92% of infants.[50]

Evoked potentials

Persistently absent auditory brain-stem evoked responses (ABRs) and visual evoked potentials (VEPs) are predictive of sensorineural deafness and visual impairment, respectively.[83,123] Somatosensory evoked potentials (SEPs) are technically the most difficult to perform but are useful in predicting neurological outcome because of the close proximity of sensory and motor axons within the deep periventricular white matter. In a study of term infants following hypoxic–ischaemic insult, a normal median nerve SEP within the first 24 hours accurately predicted normal outcome (sensitivity 94%), whereas an absent response was predictive of death or major handicap (specificity 59%).[30]

MARKERS OF TISSUE INJURY

A number of biochemical markers have been proposed as indicators of hypoxic–ischaemic injury and as possible predictors of outcome. These include plasma lactate, CSF lactate dehydrogenase (LDH) and hydroxybutyrate dehydrogenase (HBDH),[26] plasma hypoxanthine, vasopressin and erythropoietin.[108] Many of the studies are in mixed preterm and term populations and the precise sensitivity and specificity of each assay requires further study. Of particular recent interest is the brain-specific isoenzyme of creatine kinase (CK-BB). In an analysis of three reports measuring CK-BB in term infants following hypoxic–ischaemia, those who died or were subsequently handicapped had a higher weighted mean CK-BB level in the first 6 hours than those without subsequent neurological impairment.[96] CSF CK-BB may be a more specific marker for adverse outcome.[29] Other CSF markers of recent interest include neuron-specific enolase,[39] glial fibrillary acidic protein (GFAP)[13] and excitatory amino acids.[46]

MANAGEMENT FOLLOWING HYPOXIA–ISCHAEMIA

NEONATAL RESUSCITATION

- It is important to establish adequate oxygenation and restore circulation by rapid and effective resuscitation.
- There is evidence that air is as effective as 100% oxygen in resuscitation,[99] and may cause less potentially harmful cerebral vasoconstriction.[72]
- If effective resuscitation fails to establish spontaneous cardiac output by 10 minutes, or respiratory activity by 20–30 minutes, the outlook for preterm and term infants alike is very poor.

SYSTEMIC MANAGEMENT

The cornerstone of management following hypoxia–ischaemia is still supportive care and the careful maintenance of systemic homeostasis.

Respiratory support

Following resuscitation, respiratory support may be required for those patients with severe encephalopathy, co-existing lung disease (e.g. meconium aspiration syndrome, ARDS) or frequent and prolonged convulsions. Hypoxia should be avoided. Hyperoxia may promote oxygen free radical formation and may also be detrimental. Spontaneously breathing infants should be electively ventilated if their PCO_2 rises above 7 kPa (53 mmHg). The relationship between PCO_2, cerebral blood flow and cerebral oedema is discussed later.

Cardiovascular support

Continuous intra-arterial monitoring and the prompt treatment of hypotension is recommended because systemic blood pressure needs to be adequate to maintain cerebral perfusion. Hypotension following hypoxia–ischaemia is common, owing to myocardial compromise rather than hypovolaemia. Therefore, caution must be used when using colloid infusions in order not to further impair cardiac function. If there is not a rapid response to 10 ml/kg of colloid, or the central venous pressure is elevated, the early use of inotropes is recommended. Dopamine at doses of 7 microg/kg/min and above reduces cerebral blood flow through α-mediated vasoconstriction in beagle dogs.[140] Therefore, dobutamine (which lacks α effect), in combination with dopamine at a low dose (2–5 microg/kg/min), should be used. Although echocardiography may demonstrate poor myocardial contractility, it may not reliably exclude hypovolaemia.

Fluid and electrolyte therapy

Fluid restriction is commonly practised as a method of limiting cerebral oedema, although there is little evidence that fluid intake contributes to cerebral oedema. However, renal impairment and inappropriate antidiuretic hormone (ADH) are common sequelae of hypoxic–ischaemia, and therefore water overload can occur. The infant should be given only the volume of fluid necessary for adequate hydration, and a reasonable starting point is restricting to 20% less than the normal maintenance rate for the first 48 hours. Regular assessment of hydration, serum electrolytes, urine output and specific gravity or osmolality is required, aiming to maintain the serum osmolality in the region of 290 mmol/l and the urine specific gravity at 1010.

Infection

Early neonatal meningitis may have a similar presentation to hypoxic ischaemic encephalopathy, and if there is any doubt a lumbar puncture must be performed. The routine use of antibiotics, without clinical indication, is not recommended.

Haemostasis

Disseminated intravascular coagulation (DIC) can occur, and therefore tests of clotting function must be performed following hypoxia–ischaemia. Treatment is with additional vitamin K, plasma or clotting factors and platelet transfusions, in sufficient quantity to restore clotting function.

Nutrition

Asphyxiated infants are at risk of developing necrotizing enterocolitis, and also of aspiration if there is pharyngeal incoordination. A transient intolerence to enteral feeds is common because of the reduced small intestinal motility.[11] Enteral feeds should be introduced cautiously and it may take some time for the infant to breast-feed or feed from a bottle. In some cases the infant may be discharged with tube feeds continuing at home.

TRADITIONAL BRAIN-ORIENTED MANAGEMENT

Much of the clinical management following hypoxia–ischaemia is largely empirical and has not been the subject of large randomized controlled clinical trials. When assessing the effectiveness of a particular treatment, problems arise because extrapolation from animal studies is difficult and comparison between clinical studies may not be possible if different definitions of hypoxia–ischaemia are used. Testing treatments in clinical trials with meaningful numbers of infants is, however, logistically difficult given the relatively low incidence of hypoxia–ischaemia for any individual centre. Table 44.14 summarizes a pragmatic approach to the management of an asphyxiated term infant.

Cerebral oedema and intracranial hypertension

If cerebral oedema leads to reduced cerebral perfusion and cerebrovascular dysfunction, it is argued that treatment directed at reducing the oedema may be protective against further compromise. It is questionable whether cerebral oedema has a significant role in the development of further cerebral injury. Where intracranial pressure (ICP) has been measured with a subarachnoid catheter, raised ICP was found in 14 out of 23 asphyxiated infants and in only five cases could the raised ICP be medically controlled. Treatment of intracranial hypertension appears to have little influence on final outcome.[63]

Hyperventilation

Hypocapnia due to hyperventilation leads to an increase in cerebrovascular resistance, which reduces cerebral perfusion and may potentially compound an ischaemic insult. Hyperventilation appears to increase the risk of ischaemic lesions in preterm infants.[37] If vasoparalysis occurs following hypoxia–ischaemia,[98] the relationship between PCO_2 and cerebrovascular resistance no longer holds. This vasoparalysis may result in increased perfusion to damaged areas at the expense of the less damaged areas with intact autoregulation (a 'reverse steal' effect). Mildly elevated PCO_2 levels have been found to be more neuroprotective than normal PCO_2 levels (both associated with less severe brain damage than hypocapnia) in the 7-day postnatal rat model.[134] Therefore, hyperventilation cannot be recommended.

Steroids

These are only of benefit in treating cerebral oedema associated with cerebral mass lesions. Studies in adults following stroke, head trauma or hypoxic events have failed to show any benefit, and there are no data from

Table 44.14 Suggested standard treatment of a term infant following intrapartum hypoxia–ischaemia

Respiratory	*Indications for ventilation* Frequent apnoea, $PCO_2 > 7$ kPa, hypoventilation secondary to anticonvulsants, meconium aspiration syndrome/pulmonary hypertension
	Maintain PCO_2 4.0–6.5 kPa
Blood pressure	Maintain mean arterial pressure > 40 mmHg in term infants
	Cautious use of volume expansion (10 ml/kg colloid)
	Use dopamine (2–5 microg/kg/min) and dobutamine (5–15 microg/kg/min) if no response within 30 minutes
Fluids and electrolytes	Restrict to 20% less than maintenance for first 48 hours (anticipating SIADH or renal failure)
	Monitor fluid balance, infant's weight, serum electrolytes and osmolality, urine specific gravity and urinanalysis
	Aim for neutral fluid balance (i.e. replacement of losses)
	Mannitol (1 g/kg) can be used if clinical signs of raised intracranial pressure (renally excreted)
	Treat hypocalcaemia if Ca < 1.7 mmol
Seizures	Treat if frequent (> 3 per hour), prolonged (3 or more minutes), or interfering with respiration or ventilation.
Glucose	Treat hypoglycaemia (< 2.6 mmol) and hyperglycaemia (> 8.0 mmol)
Infection	Blood cultures, consider lumbar puncture Antibiotics if clinically indicated
Haematology	Check clotting, give parenteral vitamin K Treat DIC with plasma, clotting factors, platelet transfusions, as necessary
Nutrition	Observe for NEC and aspiration of gastric contents Caution and patience with enteral feeds
Temperature	If pyrexial (> 37.0°C), lower enviromental temperature, use antipyretics Maintain environmental temperature in thermoneutral range
No indications for	Hyperventilation Corticosteroids Prophylactic anticonvulsants

perinatal animal models of hypoxia–ischaemia demonstrating that steroids improve outcome. In a case series of seven asphyxiated neonates, dexamethasone treatment reduced ICP but was accompanied by a fall in systemic blood pressure and no improvement in cerebral perfusion pressure.[62] Therefore, there is no evidence supporting the use of steroids following hypoxia–ischaemia.

Osmotic agents

Mannitol has been used in a number of uncontrolled case series. In a heterogeneous group of 225 asphyxiated infants 1 g/kg of mannitol was given either early (before 2 hours) or late following hypoxic–ischaemia in a non-randomized fashion; the early treatment group had a better outcome.[75] In a small study, four infants with raised ICP (measured by subarachnoid catheter) were given 1 g/kg mannitol over 20 minutes. This produced a transient fall in ICP and an improvement in cerebral perfusion pressure for around 4 hours.[62] Mannitol is also a free radical scavenger and has been shown to reduce brain injury following hypoxia–ischaemia, when given with another free radical scavenger and magnesium, in the rat model.[128] Although there is no good evidence for a beneficial effect, in practice mannitol can be used when there are clinical signs of raised intracranial pressure (e.g. bulging anterior fontanelle), provided renal function is adequate for its excretion.

Anticonvulsants (see also Chapter 44, Part 2)

Seizure control

HIE is the most common cause of neonatal seizures at term. Seizures can substantially increase CNS metabolic demand, cause the release of excitatory neurotransmitters such as glutamate, lead to fluctuations in systemic arterial pressure, and may cause hypoxia and hypercapnia. A variety of anticonvulsants have been employed to control seizures, and most experience relates to the use of barbiturates. In addition to their anticonvulsant activity, they are known to decrease CNS metabolic rate in high dose, reduce calcium entry postischaemia, and are free radical scavengers. However, long-term use leads to inhibition in brain growth and development in animal models.

There is no good evidence that post hypoxic–ischaemic convulsions cause further injury in the perinatal brain, and there are few data to suggest that all seizures should be abolished. Our practice is to treat seizures when frequent (more than three per hour) or prolonged (3 or more minutes), particularly if they are interfering with respiration or ventilation. Initially a 20 mg/kg loading dose of phenobarbitone is used (a further 10 mg/kg loading may be given), followed by a maintenance dose of 3 mg/kg every 12 hours. Clonazepam may be added as a second line: 100–200 microg/kg loading followed by an infusion at 10–30 microg/kg/h. If necessary, further treatment with phenytoin (20 mg/kg), given as a loading dose only, may also be effective in stopping frequent seizures. The anticonvulsants can be discontinued once seizure control has been attained and the infant is neurologically normal. In the majority of cases anticonvulsants can be stopped prior to discharge.

Prophylaxis

Administration of barbiturates following hypoxia–ischaemia for neuroprotection has been attempted. The only prospective randomized controlled trial reported used thiopentone following hypoxia–ischaemia, but failed to show any significant differences in outcome.[41] There were only 17 treated and 15 control infants; 14 of the 17 treated required inotropic support for hypotension, compared to only seven of the controls. Thus, there are no clinical studies to date that support the prophylactic use of barbiturates in term infants with HIE.

Glucose

Hypoglycaemia

Animals rendered hypoglycaemic by insulin administration have a greatly reduced capacity to survive hypoxia–ischaemia.[135] However, 7-day postnatal rats which have been rendered hypoglycaemic through fasting prior to induced hypoxia–ischaemia show a reduction in brain damage compared to insulin-treated or normoglycaemic controls.[150] This neuroprotective effect may be due to the increased capacity of the immature brain to utilize lactate, pyruvate and ketones as an alternative energy source to glucose. The immature blood–brain barrier is more able to transport ketones, and the enzymes involved in ketone metabolism are induced rapidly after birth, in contrast to glycolytic enzymes. However, there is no evidence that depriving infants of glucose after hypoxia–ischaemia is neuroprotective, and the administration of ketones has not been tested. Best clinical practice is to maintain normoglycaemia.

Hyperglycaemia

Can further neuronal injury be prevented by the administration of additional glucose (i.e. hyperglycaemia) in an attempt to maintain ATP levels by glycolysis? In mature animals hyperglycaemia prior to the insult accentuates hypoxic–ischaemic injury.[85] The excessive accumulation of lactate appears responsible for this detrimental effect, possibly by causing endothelial damage. The converse occurs in the immature CNS: 7-day postnatal rats rendered hyperglycaemic prior to induced hypoxia–ischaemia survived twice as long as normoglycaemic counterparts.[142] The immature CNS has a lower capacity for glucose uptake and lactate production, and is more able to utilize lactate as an energy substrate, thereby preventing harmful lactate accumulation. These differences in carbohydrate metabolism may account for the apparent paradox seen when comparing studies of hypoxic–ischaemic damage following hyperglycaemia in both adults and neonates. The evidence that inducing hyperglycaemia in immature animals following hypoxia–ischaemia is beneficial remains controversial, with conflicting results in the 7-day postnatal rat model.[49,114]

At present there is insufficient evidence to justify any other course of clinical management than the maintenance of normoglycaemia following hypoxia–ischaemia.

NEW NEUROPROTECTIVE APPROACHES

Many neuroprotective approaches designed to be administered after hypoxic–ischaemic insult and calculated to protect the central nervous system from secondary neuronal injury are emerging from animal models, but are yet to be applied clinically. It seems unlikely that a single agent will confer complete neuroprotection, and therefore a combination of such agents may eventually be required.

Prevention of cerebrovascular dysfunction

Non-steroidal anti-inflammatory drugs improve post-ischaemic recovery in dogs,[43] and aspirin improves recovery following stroke in adults.[34] By inhibiting cyclooxygenase they attenuate postischaemic cerebral hypoperfusion and inhibit platelet aggregation. A variety of PAF antagonists have been used successfully to reduce ischaemic injury in animal models,[152] although there are no studies in immature animals.

Prevention of free radical injury

Allopurinol

This is a xanthine oxidase inhibitor. When given in high dosage (135 mg/kg) 15 minutes after hypoxic–ischaemic injury in 7-day old rats it has been shown to reduce brain injury.[93] It appears to be effective at higher doses than simple enzyme inhibition; other effects include inhibition of neutrophil lysosomal enzyme release and scavenging of hydroxyl free radicals. When used to prevent free radical mediated injury in preterm infants it was found to be ineffective, although a relatively low oral dose was used (20 mg/kg).[107]

Elimination of free iron

Free iron is able to transfer electrons and catalyse free radical-forming reactions. A hydroxyethyl starch conjugate of the iron chelating agent desferrioxamine has been used, as desferrioxamine alone causes cardiogenic shock in humans. This conjugate has been shown to reduce lipid peroxidation and neurological injury post-hypoxia–ischaemia in a rat model.[106]

Nitric oxide synthetase (NOS) inhibitors

The NOS inhibitor nitro-L-arginine is effective in limiting postarterial occlusion injury in a rat model.[17,48,131]

Free radical scavengers

Once formed, free radicals can be scavenged by drugs such as vitamin C and E, mannitol,[128] barbiturates and polyethylene glycol-linked endogenous scavengers such as superoxide dismutase.[21]

Prevention of calcium entry

Calcium channel blockers are neuroprotective in animals[127] but their negative inotropic effect in asphyxiated infants has prevented their clinical use.[65] Excessive release of glutamate following hypoxia–ischaemia acts upon the NMDA receptor and results in excessive calcium influx. The release of glutamate could theoretically be inhibited by such agents as baclofen, but this has not been attempted. Attention has therefore focused on NMDA receptor antagonists.

MK-801

This is an NMDA antagonist which, when given systemically to rats after stereotactic NMDA injection into the cerebral hemispheres, protects against hippocampal neuronal necrosis. When MK-801 was given immediately after the insult 90% protection was seen;[78] this fell to 75% if administration was delayed until 120 minutes after the insult.[79] Unfortunately, MK-801 is toxic and is unlikely to find clinical application.

Magnesium

This has been found to block the NMDA ion channel under resting conditions, occupying a binding site within the ion channel.[92] This block is voltage dependent and is overcome during the axonal depolarization that occurs with hypoxia–ischaemia.[53] If the extracellular magnesium concentrations are raised, this blockade can be restored.[51] The systemic administration of magnesium after a simulated hypoxic–ischaemic insult limits neurological damage in several animal models, including rat,[80,81,148] piglet[52] and mouse.[76] Magnesium has also been effective when used in combination with oxygen free radical scavengers, L-methionine and mannitol,[128] and has the advantage of being less toxic than MK-801. It has been used in obstetric practice for over 60 years, and readily crosses the placenta without apparent harm to the fetus or neonate. Indeed, from epidemiological studies, the use of antenatal maternal magnesium therapy is associated with a lower incidence of periventricular–intraventricular haemorrhage (PV-IVH)[97] and cerebral palsy in the preterm population.[90] The efficacy of magnesium given postnatally or antenatally in providing neuroprotection has not been established in controlled clinical trials.

Hypothermia

Hypothermia is thought to reduce the cerebral metabolic rate, limit the damage from free radicals,[57] and to reduce the release of excitatory amino acids and peroxidation of lipids.[18] Animal models suggest that hypothermia may be neuroprotective and have renewed interest in its potential role following hypoxia–ischaemia. In one animal model newborn piglets were subjected to hypoxia–ischaemia until their PCr/Pi ratio, measured by ^{31}P MRS, had fallen to almost zero before resuscitation was commenced. Mild hypothermia following resuscitation (35°C for 12 hours) prevented the secondary energy failure seen in normothermic animals.[129] A reduction in post-hypoxic– ischaemic neuronal loss was also observed in infant rats subjected to mild hypothermia, although maintenance of the hypothermia was required for 72 hours following the insult.[119] Despite these encouraging animal models, there are no data from controlled clinical trials to recommend using hypothermia in human infants at present.

Other neuroprotective agents

Gangliosides, which are polar sugar-containing lipids and major constituents of neuronal membranes, are neuroprotective in fetal sheep.[125] They are thought to maintain membrane integrity, bind calmodulin and inhibit NO synthetase.[27] Other agents shown to be neuroprotective in animal models include trophic factors such as IGF-1[40] and Felbamate, which blocks the glycine site of the NMDA receptor.[143]

OUTCOME

INTERPRETING CLINICAL STUDIES

The risk of death or major neurological sequelae following hypoxic–ischaemic insult is one of the foremost concerns of parents and clinicians alike. Many of the studies described in this chapter examine the outcome associated with a particular predictive factor. Table 44.15 gives the relative efficacy of methods for predicting outcome following severe hypoxic–ischaemic injury. However, comparison between studies is difficult because of potential confounding variables:

- Variation in the clinical definition of asphyxia;
- Gestational age: factors associated with an adverse outcome identified by studies on a preterm population may not be applicable to the term infant;
- Variation in the technique and timing of investigations, and definition of an abnormal result;
- Variation in outcome variable assessed (e.g. mortality, cognitive, motor, neurological, behavioural) and definition of severe disability;
- Age of assessment: early assessment allows for better inference as to the relationship between a perinatal event and later outcome. Later follow-up enables a more detailed assessment of higher-order cognitive functioning, but is more likely to be confounded by environmental influences.

WITHDRAWAL OF VENTILATORY SUPPORT

Following severe hypoxia–ischaemia many neonatologists consider that discontinuation of artificial ventilation is

Table 44.15 Prognostic abilities of various techniques following hypoxia–ischaemia

Test	Result	Time assessed	Number in study	Sensitivity (%)	Specificity (%)	Predictive value of positive result for adverse outcome (%)	Predictive value of negative result for good outcome (%)	Prevalence of adverse outcome in study (%)	Ref
Apgar score	5 or less	10 minutes	122	57	95	72	90	19	67
Encephalopathy	Sarnat grade III		200	50	100	100	84	28	103
	Sarnat grades II + III		200	100	52	43	100	28	103
Doppler ultrasound	PRI < 0.55	24 hours	43	100	81	67	100	29	7
CT	Diffuse/global Decreased density	7–14 days	43	93	80	90	86	65	1
MRI	Diffuse hyperintensity of cerebral hemispheres *or* Basal ganglia changes (moderate–severe)	2–14 days	43	100	92	70	100	16	59
MRS	PCr/Pi below normal	1–5 days	32	88	83	64	95	25	82
	Naa/choline < 0.80	1–20 days	21	90	73	75	89	48	44
Amplitude integrated EEG (cerebral function monitor)	Burst suppression, low voltage or flat	1–6 hours	47	95	89	86	96	40	50
Standard EEG	Burst suppression, low voltage or flat	1–4 days	44	84	88	84	88	41	50
Median nerve SSEP	Absent or delayed	24 hours	40	94	59	65	93	45	30

Sensitivity: Proportion of infants with an adverse outcome correctly predicted by the investigation
Specificity: Proportion of infants with a normal outcome correctly predicted by the investigation
Predictive values: Positive: Proportion of infants with positive or abnormal result that have an adverse outcome
Negative: Proportion of infants with negative or normal result that are normal on follow-up
Adverse outcome: Death or major neurological impairment

justified if the prognosis is poor. Early accurate information about prognosis is required in this situation. Unfortunately, the maximal degree of HIE may not be determined for a few days. The best early predictors of poor outcome are sustained low-voltage states and discontinuous activity on EEG, appearing by 6 hours, and abnormal Doppler cerebral blood flow velocities, appearing by 24 hours. Our personal practice is to perform these tests, and if the results of these investigations are unequivocally abnormal on two separate occasions after the first 24 hours, to explain the results and the poor prognosis to the parents. We offer to consider withdrawal of ventilatory support. If the parents choose this option care continues but is redirected towards supporting the parents and ensuring the infant does not suffer distress. The parents are warned that the baby may not die if artificial ventilation is withdrawn.

FOLLOW-UP

Term infants with mild HIE are unlikely to have any subsequent neurodevelopmental problems and their parents should be strongly reassured. Severe HIE is clearly associated with a poor outcome. Unfortunately, the majority of infants admitted to a neonatal unit following hypoxia–ischaemia show signs of moderate HIE, making it difficult for the clinician to counsel the parents. A cluster of abnormal perinatal signs, including fetal heart rate pattern, acid–base status, depressed Apgar scores and multiorgan dysfunction, with such an encephalopathy, is associated with later impairment.[151] Encouraging clinical features are the early establishment of breast or bottle feeds and the absence of neurological abnormalities on discharge. Many of the widely available investigations have good negative predictive powers but are poor at predicting subsequent impairment. It remains to be seen whether newer techniques, such as MRI, will become useful when more available.

The infant will need to be followed up until at least 12 months of age; 2 years or more if preterm. The classic disability suffered by survivors of hypoxia–ischaemia is cerebral palsy, in particular spastic quadriplegia and dyskinetic cerebral palsy. There may be associated intellectual impairment, blindness or epilepsy. Mental retardation alone is not a recognized sequel.

MEDICOLEGAL IMPLICATIONS (Chapter 50)

In the 19th century, work by Little[70] suggested that the major cause of cerebral palsy and mental retardation was intrapartum 'brain damage', later translated into terms such as 'birth asphyxia' or 'hypoxic–ischaemic injury'. This resulted in undue emphasis being placed on the causative role of intrapartum events in cerebral palsy by the medical profession, lawyers and lay people. However, the incidence of cerebral palsy is largely unchanged despite increasing obstetric intervention.[45,122] In a case note analysis of the 183 cases of spastic cerebral palsy from the Western Australia Cerebral Palsy Register 1975–1980, 14.1% were judged to have suffered perinatal asphyxia. However, only 8.2% of cerebral palsy was judged to have been *caused* by asphyxia, as there were many cases of perinatal asphyxia in the control population without cerebral palsy.[12] Similar figures have been derived from other epidemiological studies.[87] MRI studies also suggest that the majority of cerebral palsy is due to prenatal brain injury.[132] Intrapartum asphyxia may be the first presentation of cerebral palsy if this prenatal insult impairs the ability of the fetus to cope with the physiological stress of labour.[47] Gaffney et al[38] found that there had been a suboptimal clinical response to fetal distress (judged by case note review) in only 6.8% of children with cerebral palsy born to residents in the Oxford Region 1984–1987.[38] Lawyers and expert witnesses need to be aware that only a small proportion of cerebral palsy can be prevented by improvements in intrapartum care.[36,121]

TERMINOLOGY

In this increasingly litigious world medical note-keeping following the birth of an infant in poor condition needs to be accurate and non-judgemental. Terms such as 'birth asphyxia' may be valid, but only if there is evidence to support the diagnosis (which should be documented). However, depressed Apgar scores alone do not make the diagnosis and the infant should be described as being born in 'poor condition' or with 'low Apgar scores', not 'asphyxiated'. Likewise, neonatal encephalopathy may not be asphyxial in origin, and therefore the term 'hypoxic–ischaemic encephalopathy' should be avoided until specific evidence for its origin becomes available.[10]

EVIDENCE FOR MEDICOLEGAL CASES

When giving evidence in medicolegal cases the neonatal paediatrician will be required to consider whether the adverse outcome (e.g. cerebral palsy) resulted from intrapartum hypoxia–ischaemia. Table 44.8 gives the information required from the case notes for the paediatrician to be confident of causation. The obstetrician will need to consider liability when commenting upon the obstetric management. In order for a court to make a decision in such cases, three separate issues need to be addressed in light of the evidence presented by the paediatrician and obstetrician:

1. Was the adverse outcome a consequence of intrapartum hypoxia–ischaemia?
2. Was negligence demonstrated by the medical team responsible for management of the patient in labour?
3. Would a reasonable alternative management have resulted in a more favourable outcome?

REFERENCES

1. Adsett D B, Fitz C R, Hill A 1985 Hypoxic–ischaemic cerebral injury in the term newborn: correlation of CT findings with neurological outcome. Developmental Medicine and Child Neurology 27: 155–160
2. Airede A I 1991 Birth asphyxia and hypoxic–ischaemic encephalopathy: incidence and severity. Annals of Tropical Paediatrics 11: 331–335
3. Al-Alfry A, Carroll J E, Devarajan L V, Moussa M A 1990 Term infant asphyxia in Kuwait. Annals of Tropical Paediatrics 10: 355–361
4. Aldrich C J, D'Antona D, Wyatt J S, Spencer J A, Peebles D M, Reynolds E O R 1994 Fetal cerebral oxygenation measured by near-infrared spectroscopy shortly before birth and acid–base status at birth. Obstetrics and Gynecology 84: 861–865
5. Ames A, Wright R L, Kowada M 1968 Cerebral insult: II. The no reflow phenomenon. American Journal of Pathology 52: 437–453
6. Apgar V 1953 A proposal for a new method of evaluation of the newborn infant. Anesthesia and Analgesia 32: 260–267
7. Archer L N J, Levene M I, Evans D H 1986 Cerebral artery Doppler ultrasonography for prediction of outcome after perinatal asphyxia. Lancet ii: 1116–1118
8. Bader T J, Morgan M A 1995 Intrapartum electronic fetal heart rate monitoring versus intermittent auscultation: a meta-analysis (letter). Obstetrics and Gynecology 85: 643
9. Barkovitch A J, Westmark K, Partridge C, Sola A, Ferriero D M 1995 Perinatal asphyxia: M R findings in the first 10 days. American Journal of Neuroradiology 16: 427–438
10. Bax M, Nelson K B 1993 Birth asphyxia: a statement. World Federation of Neurology Group. Developmental Medicine and Child Neurology 35: 1022–1024
11. Berseth C L, McCoy H H 1992 Birth asphyxia alters neonatal intestinal motility in term neonates. Pediatrics 90: 669–673
12. Blair E, Stanley F J 1988 Intrapartum asphyxia: a rare cause of cerebral palsy. Journal of Pediatrics 112: 515–519
13. Blennow M, Hagberg H, Rosengren L 1995 Glial fibrillary acidic protein in the cerebrospinal fluid: a possible indicator of prognosis in full-term asphyxiated newborn infants? Pediatric Research 37: 260–264
14. Bocking A D, White S E, Homan J, Richardson B S 1992 Oxygen consumption is maintained in fetal sheep during prolonged hypoxaemia and hypercapnia in sheep. Journal of Developmental Physiology 17: 169–174
15. Boo N Y, Lye M S 1991 Factors associated with clinically significant perinatal asphyxia in the Malaysian neonates: a case-control study. Journal of Tropical Pediatrics 38: 284–289
16. Brown J K, Purvis R J, Forfar J O, Cockburn F 1974 Neurological aspects of perinatal asphyxia. Developmental Medicine and Child Neurology 16: 567–580
17. Buisson A, Plotkine M, Boulu R G 1992 The neuroprotective effect of a nitric oxide inhibitor in a rat model of focal cerebral ischaemia. British Journal of Pharmacology 106: 766–767
18. Busto R, Globus M Y T, Dietrich W D, Martinez E, Valdes I, Ginsberg M D 1989 Effect of mild hypothermia on ischemia-induced release of neurotransmitters and free fatty acids. Stroke 20: 904–910
19. Buttke T M, Sandstrom P A 1994 Oxidative stress as a mediator of apoptosis. Immunology Today 15: 7–10
20. Byrne P, Welch R, Johnson M A, Darrah J, Piper M 1990 Serial magnetic resonance imaging in neonatal hypoxic–ischaemic encephalopathy. Journal of Pediatrics 117: 694–700
21. Cerchiari E L, Hoel T M, Safar P, Sclabassi R J 1987 Protective effect of combined superoxide dismutase and desferrioxamine on recovery of cerebral blood flow and function after cardiac arrest in dogs. Stroke 18: 869–878
22. Chan P H, Schmidley J W, Fishman R A, Longar S M 1984 Brain injury, edema and vascular permeability changes induced by oxygen-derived free radicals. Neurology 34: 315–320
23. Cohn H E, Sachs E J, Heyman M A, Rudolph A M 1974 Cardiovascular responses to hypoxemia and acidaemia in fetal lambs. American Journal of Obstetrics and Gynecology 120: 817–824
24. Connolly B, Kelehan P, O'Brien N et al 1994 The echogenic thalamus in hypoxic–ischaemic encephalopathy. Pediatric Radiology 24: 268–271
25. Constantinou J E C, Gillis J, Ouvrier R A, Rahilly P M 1989 Hypoxic–ischaemic encephalopathy after near miss sudden infant death syndrome. Archives of Disease in Childhood 64: 703–708
26. Dalens B, Viallard J-L, Raynauld E-J, Dastuge B 1981 CSF levels of

lactate and hydroxybutyrate dehydrogenase as indicators of neurological sequelae after neonatal brain damage. Developmental Medicine and Child Neurology 23: 228–233
27. Dawson T M, Hung K, Dawson V L, Steiner J P, Snyder S H 1995 Neuroprotective effects of gangliosides may involve inhibition of nitric oxide synthetase. Annals of Neurology 37: 115–118
28. Dennis J, Johnson A, Mutch L, Yudkin P, Johnson P 1989 Acid–base status at birth and neurodevelopmental outcome at four and one-half years. American Journal of Obstetrics and Gynecology 161: 213–220
29. De Praeter C, Vanhaesebrouck P, Govaert P, Delanghe J, Leroy J 1991 Creatine kinase concentrations in the cerebrospinal fluid of newborns: relationship to short-term outcome. Pediatrics 88: 1204–1210
30. De Vries L S 1993 Somatosensory evoked potential in term neonates with postasphyxial encephalopathy. Clinics in Perinatology 20: 463–482
31. Dukta A J, Kochanek P M, Hallenbeck J M 1989 Influence of granulocytopenia on canine cerebral ischaemia induced by air embolism. Stroke 20: 390–395
32. Eken P, Jansen G H, Groenendaal F, Rademaker K J, de Vries L S 1994 Intracranial lesions in the fullterm infant with hypoxic–ischaemic encephalopathy: ultrasound and autopsy correlation. Neuropediatrics 25: 301–307
33. Eken P, Toet M C, Groenendaal F, de Vries L S 1995 Predictive value of early neuroimaging, pulsed Doppler and neurophysiology in full term infants with hypoxic-ischaemic encephalopathy. Archives of Disease in Childhood 73: F75–F80
34. Fields W S, Lemak N A, Frankowski R F, Hardy R J 1977 Controlled trial of aspirin in cerebral ischaemia. Stroke 8: 301–315
35. Finer N N, Robertson C M, Richards R T, Pinnell L E, Peters K L 1981 Hypoxic–ischemic encephalopathy in term neonates: perinatal factors and outcome. Journal of Pediatrics 98: 112–117
36. Freeman J M, Nelson K B 1988 Intrapartum asphyxia and cerebral palsy. Pediatrics 82: 240–249
37. Fujimoto S, Togari H, Yamaguchi N, Mizutani F, Suzuki S, Sobajima H 1994 Hypocarbia and cystic periventricular leukomalacia in premature infants. Archives of Disease in Childhood 71: F107–F110
38. Gaffney G, Sellers S, Flavell V, Squier M, Johnson A 1994 Case-controlled study of intrapartum care, cerebral palsy, and perinatal death. British Medical Journal 308: 743–750
39. Garcia-Alix A, Cabanas F, Pellicer A, Hernanz A, Stiris T, Quero J 1994 Neuron-specific enolase and myelin basic protein: relationship of cerebrospinal fluid concentrations to the neurologic condition of asphyxiated full-term infants. Pediatrics 93: 234–240
40. Gluckman P, Klempt N, Guan J et al 1992 A role for IGF-1 in the rescue of CNS neurons following hypoxic–ischemic injury. Biochemical and Biophysical Research Communications 182: 593–599
41. Goldberg R, Moscoso P, Bauer C 1986 Use of barbiturate therapy in severe perinatal asphyxia: a randomised controlled trial. Journal of Pediatrics 109: 851–856
42. Grant A, O'Brien N, Joy M, Hennessy E, MacDonald D 1989 Cerebral palsy among children born during the Dublin randomised trial of intrapartum monitoring. Lancet ii: 1233–1236
43. Grice S C, Chappel E T, Prough D S, Whitley J M, Su M, Watkins W D 1987 Ibuprofen improves cerebral blood flow after global ischaemia in dogs. Stroke 18: 787–791
44. Groenendaal F, Veenhoven R H, van der Grond J, Jansen G H, Witkamp T D, de Vries L S 1994 Cerebral lactate and *N*-acetyl-aspartate/choline ratios in asphyxiated full-term neonates demonstrated in vivo using proton magnetic resonance spectroscopy. Pediatric Research 35: 148–151
45. Hagberg B, Hagberg G, Olow I 1993 The changing panorama of cerebral palsy in Sweden VI. Prevalence and origin during the birth year period 1983–1986. Acta Paediatrica 82: 387–393
46. Hagberg H, Thornberg E, Blennow M et al 1993 Excitatory amino acids in the cerebrospinal fluid of asphyxiated infants: relationship to hypoxic–ischemic encephalopathy. Acta Paediatrica 82: 925–929
47. Hall D M 1994 Intrapartum events and cerebral palsy. British Journal of Obstetrics and Gynaecology 101: 745–747
48. Hamada Y, Hayakawa T, Hattori H, Mikawa H 1994 Inhibitor of nitric oxide synthesis reduces hypoxic–ischemic brain damage in the neonatal rat. Pediatric Research 35: 10–14
49. Hattori H, Wasterlain C G 1990 Posthypoxic glucose supplement reduces hypoxic–ischemic brain damage in the neonatal rat. Annals of Neurology 28: 122–128
50. Hellstrom-Westas L, Rosen I, Svenningsen N W 1995 Predictive value of early continuous amplitude integrated EEG recordings on outcome after severe birth asphyxia in full term infants. Archives of Disease in Childhood 72: F34–F38
51. Henneberry R C, Novelli A, Cox JA, Lysko P G 1989 Neurotoxicity at the *N*-methyl-D-aspartate receptor in energy-compromised neurons. An hypothesis for cell death in aging and disease. Annals of the New York Academy of Science 568: 225–233
52. Hoffman D J, Marro P J, McGowan J E, Mishra O P, Delivoria-Papadopoulos M 1994 Protective effect of $MgSO_4$ infusion on NMDA receptor binding characteristics during cerebral cortical hypoxia in the newborn piglet. Brain Research 644: 144–149
53. Hori N, Carpenter D O 1994 Transient ischaemia causes a reduction of Mg^{2+} blockade of NMDA receptors. Neuroscience Letters 173: 75–78
54. Hossman K A 1983 Neuronal survival and revival during and after cerebral ischaemia. American Journal of Emergency Medicine 1: 191–197
55. Hossman K A, Kleihues P 1973 Reversibility of ischaemic brain damage. Archives of Neurology 29: 375–385
56. Huang Z, Huang P L, Panahian N, Dalkara T, Fishman M C, Moskowitz M A 1994 Effects of cerebral ischaemia in mice deficient in neuronal nitric oxide synthetase. Science 265: 1883–1885
57. Karibe H, Chen S F, Zarow G J et al 1994 Mild intraischemic hypothermia suppresses consumption of endogenous antioxidants after temporary focal ischemia in rats. Brain Research 649: 12–18
58. Kinoti S N 1993 Asphyxia of the newborn in east, central and southern Africa. East African Medical Journal 70: 422–433
59. Kuenzle C, Baenziger O, Martin E et al 1994 Prognostic value of early MR imaging in term infants with severe perinatal asphyxia. Neuropediatrics 25: 191–200
60. Laroche J-C 1984 Perinatal brain damage. In: Adams J H, Corsellis J A N, Duchen L W (eds) Greenfield's neuropathology. Edward Arnold, London
61. Lawrence A J, Jarrott B 1993 Nitric oxide increases interstitial excitatory amino acid release in the rat dorsomedial medulla oblongata. Neuroscience Letters 151: 126–129
62. Levene M I, Evans D H 1985 Medical management of raised intracranial pressure after severe birth asphyxia. Archives of Disease in Childhood 60: 12–16
63. Levene M I, Evans D H, Forde A, Archer L N 1987 Value of intracranial pressure monitoring of asphyxiated newborn infants. Developmental Medicine and Child Neurology 29: 311–319
64. Levene M I, Fenton A C, Evans D H, Archer L N J, Shortland D B, Gibson N A 1989 Severe birth asphyxia and abnormal cerebral blood flow velocity. Developmental Medicine and Child Neurology 31: 427–434
65. Levene M I, Gibson N A, Fenton A C, Papathoma E, Barnett D 1990 The use of a calcium-channel blocker, nicardipine, for severely asphyxiated newborn infants. Developmental Medicine and Child Neurology 32: 567–574
66. Levene M I, Kornberg J, Williams T H C 1985 The incidence and severity of post-asphyxial encephalopathy in full-term infants. Early Human Development 11: 21–26
67. Levene M I, Sands C, Grindulis H, Moore J R 1986 Comparison of two methods of predicting outcome in perinatal asphyxia. Lancet i: 67–69
68. Lewinsky R M 1994 Cardiac systolic time intervals and other parameters of myocardial contractility as indices of fetal acid–base status. Baillières Clinical Obstetrics and Gynecology 8: 663–681
69. Lipp-Zwahlen A E, Deonna T, Chrzanowski R, Micheli J L, Calame A 1985 Temporal evolution of hypoxic–ischaemic brain lesions in the asphyxiated full-term newborn assessed by computerized tomography. Neuroradiology 27: 138–144
70. Little W J 1862 On the influence of abnormal parturition, difficult labours, premature birth, and asphyxia neonatorum, on the mental and physical condition of the child, especially in relation to deformities. Transactions of the Obstetrical Society of London 3: 293–344
71. Loreck A, Takei Y, Cady E B et al 1994 Delayed ('secondary') cerebral energy failure after acute hypoxia–ischaemia in the newborn piglet: continuous 48-hour studies by phosphorus magnetic resonance spectroscopy. Pediatric Research 36: 699–706
72. Lundstrom K E, Pryds O, Greisen G 1995 Oxygen at birth and prolonged cerebral vasoconstriction in preterm infants. Archives of Disease in Childhood 73: F81–F86

73. Luthy D A, Shy K K, van Belle G et al 1987. A randomised trial of electronic fetal monitoring in preterm labour. Obstetrics and Gynecology 69: 687–695
74. Luttkus A, Fengler T W, Friedmann W, Dudenhausen J W 1995 Continuous monitoring of fetal oxygen saturation by pulse oximetry. Obstetrics and Gynaecology 85: 183–186
75. Marchal C, Costagliola P, Leveau P, Dulucq P, Steckler R, Rouquier F 1974 Traitement de la souffrance cérébrale néonatale d'origine anoxique par le mannitol. Revue de Pediatrie 9: 581–589
76. Marret S, Gressens P, Gadisseux J-F, Evrard P 1995 Prevention by magnesium of excitotoxic neuronal death in the developing brain: an animal model for clinical intervention studies. Developmental Medicine and Child Neurology 37: 473–484
77. McCord J M 1985 Oxygen-derived free radicals in postischemic tissue injury. New England Journal of Medicine 312: 159–163
78. McDonald J W, Roeser N F, Silverstein F S, Johnston M V 1989 Quantitive assessment of neuroprotection against NMDA-induced brain injury. Experimental Neurology 106: 289–296
79. McDonald J W, Silverstein F S, Cardona D, Hudson C, Chen R, Johnson M V 1990 Systemic administration of MK-801 protects against *N*-methyl-D-aspartate- and quisqualate-mediated neurotoxicity in perinatal rats. Neuroscience 36: 589–599
80. McDonald J W, Silverstein F S, Johnston M V. 1990. Magnesium reduces *N*-methyl-D-aspartate (NMDA)-mediated brain injury in perinatal rats. Neuroscience Letters 109: 234–238
81. McIntosh T K, Vink R, Yamakami I, Faden A I 1989 Magnesium protects against neurological deficit after brain injury. Brain Research 482: 252–260
82. Moorcraft J, Bolas N M, Ives N K et al 1991 Global and depth resolved phosphorus magnetic resonance spectroscopy to predict outcome after birth asphyxia. Archives of Disease in Childhood 66: 1119–1123
83. Muttitt S C, Taylor M J, Kobyashi J S, MacMillan L, Whyte H E 1991 Serial evoked visual potentials and outcome in full term birth asphyxia. Pediatric Neurology 7: 86–90
84. Myers R E 1972 Two patterns of perinatal brain damage and their conditions of occurrence. American Journal of Obstetrics and Gynecology 112: 246–276
85. Myers R E, Yamaguchi S 1977 Nervous effects of cardiac arrest in monkeys. Preservation of vision. Archives of Neurology 34: 65–74
86. Neilson J P 1994 EFM + scalp sampling vs intermittent auscultation in labour: In: Enkin M W, Keirse M J N C, Renfew M J, Neilson J P (eds) Pregnancy Database of Systematic Reviews': Review No. 03297, 4 May 1994. Published through 'Cochrane Updates on Disk', Oxford: Update Software, 1994, Disk Issue 1
87. Nelson K B 1988 What proportion of cerebral palsy is related to birth asphyxia? Journal of Pediatrics 112: 572–573
88. Nelson K B, Ellenberg J H 1981 Apgar scores as predictors of chronic neurologic disability. Pediatrics 68: 36–44
89. Nelson K B, Ellenberg J H 1984 Obstetric complications as risk factors for cerebral or seizure disorder. Journal of the American Medical Association 251: 1843–1848
90. Nelson K B, Grether J K 1995 Can magnesium sulfate reduce the risk of cerebral palsy in very low birthweight infants? Pediatrics 95: 263–269
91. Niijima S, Levene M I 1989. Post-asphyxial encephalopathy in a preterm infant. Developmental Medicine and Child Neurology 31: 391–397
92. Nowak L, Bregestovski P, Ascher P, Herbet A, Prochiantz A 1984 Magnesium gates glutamate-activated channels in mouse central neurones. Nature 307: 462–465
93. Palmer C, Towfighi J, Roberts R L, Heitjan D F 1993 Allopurinol administered after inducing hypoxic–ischemia reduces brain injury in 7 day old rats. Pediatric Research 33: 405–411
94. Peden C J, Rutherford M A, Sargentoni J, Cox I J, Bryant D J, Dubowitz L M S 1993. Proton spectroscopy of the neonatal brain following hypoxic-ischaemic injury. Developmental Medicine and Child Neurology 35: 502–510
95. Peebles D M, Spencer J A, Edwards A D et al 1994 Relation between frequency of uterine contractions and human fetal cerebral oxygen saturation studied during labour by near infrared spectroscopy. British Journal of Obstetrics and Gynaecology 101: 44–48
96. Peliowski A, Finer N N 1992 Birth asphyxia in the term infant. In: Sinclair J C, Bracken M B (eds) Effective care of the newborn infant. Oxford University Press, Oxford, pp 249–279
97. Perlman J, Fernandez C, Gee J, Leveno K, Risser R 1995 Magnesium sulphate (Mg) administered to mothers with pregnancy-induced hypertension (PIH) is associated with a reduction in periventricular–intraventricular hemorrhage (PV-IVH). Pediatric Research 37: 231A
98. Pryds O, Greisen G, Lou H, Friis-Hansen B 1990 Vasoparalysis associated with brain damage in asphyxiated term infants. Journal of Pediatrics 117: 119–125
99. Ramji S, Ahuja S, Thirupuram S, Rootwelt T, Rooth G, Saugstad O D 1993 Resuscitation of asphyxic newborn infants with room air or 100% oxygen. Pediatric Research 34: 809–812
100. Richardson B S, Carmichael L, Homan J, Patrick J E 1992 Electrocortical activity and breathing movements in fetal sheep with prolonged and graded hypoxemia. American Journal of Obstetrics and Gynecology 167: 553–558
101. Richardson B S, Rurak D, Patrick J E, Homan J 1989 Cerebral oxidative metabolism during sustained hypoxaemia in fetal sheep. Journal of Developmental Physiology 11: 37–43
102. Richey S D, Ramin S M, Bawdon R E et al 1995 Markers of acute and chronic asphyxia in infants with meconium-stained amniotic fluid. American Journal of Obstetrics and Gynecology 172: 1212–1215
103. Robertson C, Finer N 1985 Term infants with hypoxic–ischemic encephalopathy: outcome at 3.5 years. Developmental Medicine and Child Neurology 27: 473–484
104. Robertson C M T, Finer N N, Grace M G A 1989 School performance of survivors of neonatal encephalopathy associated with birth asphyxia at term. Journal of Pediatrics 114: 753–760
105. Rosén K G 1986 Alterations in the fetal electrocardiogram as a sign of fetal asphyxia – experimental data with a clinical implimentation. Journal of Perinatology 14: 355–364
106. Rosenthal R E, Chanderbhan R, Marshall G, Fiskum G 1992 Prevention of post-ischemic brain lipid conjugated diene production and neurological injury by hdroxyethyl starch-conjugated desferrioxamine. Free Radical Biolology and Medicine 12: 29–33
107. Russell G A B, Cooke R W I 1995 Randomised controlled trial of allopurinol prohylaxis in very preterm infants. Archives of Disease in Childhood 73: F27–F31
108. Ruth V, Autti-Ramo I, Granstrom M-L, Korkman M, Raivio K O 1988 Prediction of perinatal brain damage by cord plasma vasopressin, erythropoietin, and hypoxanthine values. Journal of Pediatrics 113: 800–815
109. Ruth V J, Raivio K O 1988 Perinatal brain damage: predictive value of metabolic acidosis and the Apgar score. British Medical Journal 297: 24–27
110. Rutherford M A, Pennock J M, Dubowitz L M S 1994 Cranial ultrasound and magnetic resonance imaging in hypoxic–ischaemic encephalopathy: a comparison with outcome. Developmental Medicine and Child Neurology 36: 813–825
111. Rutherford M A, Pennock J M, Schwieso J E, Cowan F M, Dubowitz L M 1995 Hypoxic ischaemic encephalopathy: early magnetic resonance imaging findings and their evolution. Neuropediatrics 26: 183–191
112. Rutherford M, Pennock J, Schwieso J, Cowan F, Dubowitz L 1996 Hypoxic–ischaemic encephalopathy: early and late magnetic resonance imaging findings in relation to outcome. Archives of Disease in Childhood 75: F145–F151
113. Sarnat H B, Sarnat M S 1976 Neonatal encephalopathy following fetal distress. Archives of Neurology 33: 696–705
114. Sheldon R A, Partridge J C, Ferriero D M 1992 Postischemic hyperglycemia is not protective to the neonatal rat brain. Pediatric Research 32: 489–493
115. Shewmon D A, Fine M, Masdeu J C, Palacios E 1981 Postischemic hypervascularity of infancy: a stage in the evolution of ischemic brain damage with characteristic CT scan. Annals of Neurology 9: 358–365
116. Siegel M J, Shackelford G D, Perlman G M, Fulling K H 1984 Hypoxic–ischaemic encephalopathy in term infants: diagnosis and prognosis evaluated by ultrasound. Radiology 152: 395–399
117. Siesjo B K 1992 Pathophysiology and treatment of focal cerebral

ischaemia. Part II: Mechanisms of damage and treatment. Journal of Neurosurgery 77: 337–354
118. Singh M, Deorari A K, Khajuria R C, Paul V K 1991 A four year study on neonatal morbidity in a New Delhi hospital. Indian Journal of Medical Research 94: 186–192
119. Sirimanne E S, Blumberg R M, Bossano D et al 1996 The effect of prolonged modification of cerebral temperature on outcome after hypoxic–ischemic brain injury in the infant rat. Pediatric Research 39: 591–597
120. Smith M L, Auer R N, Siesjo B K 1984 The density and distribution of ischemic brain injury in the rat following 2–10 min of forebrain ischemia. Acta Neuropathologica 64: 319–332
121. Stanley F 1994 Cerebral palsy. The courts catch up with the sad realities. Medical Journal of Australia 161: 236
122. Stanley F J 1994 Cerebral palsy trends. Implications for perinatal care. Acta Obstetrica et Gynecologica Scandinavia 73: 5–9
123. Stockard J E, Stockard J J, Kleinberg F, Westmoreland B F 1983 Prognostic value of brainstem auditory evoked potentials in neonates. Archives of Neurology 40: 360–365
124. Takeuchi T, Watanabe K 1988 The EEG evolution and neurological prognosis of perinatal hypoxia in neonates. Brain Development 11: 115–120
125. Tan W K, Williams C E, Mallard G E, Gluckman P D 1994 Monosialoganglioside GM1 treatment after a hypoxic–ischemic episode reduces the vulnerability of the fetal sheep brain to subsequent injuries. American Journal of Obstetrics and Gynecology 170: 663–669
126. Thacker S B, Stroup D F, Peterson H B 1995 Efficacy and safety of intrapartum electronic fetal monitoring: an update. Obstetrics and Gynecology 86: 613–620
127. Thiringer K, Hrbek A, Karlsson K, Rosen K-G, Kjellmer I 1987 Postasphyxial cerebral survival in newborn sheep after treatment with oxygen free radical scavengers and a calcium antagonist. Pediatric Research 22: 62–66
128. Thordstein M, Bagenholm R, Thiringer K, Kjellmer I 1993 Scavengers of free oxygen radicals in combination with magnesium ameliorate perinatal hypoxic–ischaemic brain damage in the rat. Pediatric Research 34: 23–26
129. Thoresen M, Penrice J, Lorek A et al 1995 Mild hypothermia after severe transient hypoxia–ischemia ameliorates delayed energy failure in the newborn piglet. Pediatric Research 37: 667–670
130. Thornberg E, Thiringer K, Odeback A, Milson I 1995 Birth asphyxia: incidence, clinical course and outcome in a Swedish population. Acta Paediatrica 84: 927–932
131. Trifiletti R R 1992 Neuroprotective effects of NG-nitro-L-arginine in focal stroke in the 7-day old rat. European Journal of Pharmacology 218: 197–198
132. Truwit C L, Barkovich A J, Koch T K, Ferriero D M 1992 Cerebral palsy: MR findings in 40 patients. American Journal of Neuroradiology 13: 67–78
133. van Bel F, Dorrepaal C A, Benders M J, Zeeuwe P E, van deBor M, Berger H M 1993 Changes in cerebral haemodynamics and oxygenation in the first 24 hours after birth asphyxia. Pediatrics 92: 365–372
134. Vannucci R C, Towfighi J, Heitjan D F, Brucklacher R M 1995 Carbon dioxide protects the perinatal brain from hypoxic–ischemic damage: an experimental study in the immature rat. Pediatrics 95: 868–874
135. Vannucci R C, Vannucci S J 1978 Cerebral carbohydrate metabolism during hypoglycaemia and anoxia in newborn rats. Annals of Neurology 4: 73–79
136. Vintzileos A M, Nochimson D J, Guzman E R, Knuppel R A, Lake M, Schifrin B S 1995 Intrapartum electronic fetal heart rate monitoring versus intermittent auscultation: A meta-analysis. Obstetrics and Gynecology 85: 149–155
137. Voit T, Lemburg P, Neuen E, Lumenta C, Stork W 1987 Damage of thalamus and basal ganglia in asphyxiated full-term neonates. Neuropediatrics 18: 176
138. Volpe J J 1995 Hypoxic–ischemic encephalopathy: neuropathology and pathogenesis. In: Volpe J J. Neurology of the newborn, 3rd edn. Saunders, Philadelphia, pp 279–313
139. Volpe J J, Herscovitch P, Perlman J M, Kreusser K L, Raiche M E 1985 Positron emission tomography in the asphyxiated term newborn: parasagittal impairment of cerebral blood flow. Annals of Neurology 17: 287–296
140. von Essen C, Zervas N T, Brown D R, Koltun W A, Pickren K S 1980 Local cerebral blood flow in the dog during intravenous infusion of dopamine. Surgical Neurology 13: 181–188
141. Voorhies T M, Ehrlich M E, Frayer W, Lee B, Vannucci R C 1983 Occlusive vascular disease in perinatal cerebral hypoxia–ischaemia. American Journal of Perinatology 1: 1–5
142. Voorhies T M, Rawlinson D, Vannucci R C 1988 Glucose and perinatal hypoxic–ischemic brain damage in the rat. Annals of Neurology 24: 638–646
143. Wasterlain C G, Adams L M, Schwartz P H, Hattori H, Sofia R D, Wichmann J K 1993 Posthypoxic treatment with felbamate is neuroprotective in a rat model of hypoxia–ischaemia. Neurology 43: 2303–2310
144. Wertheim D, Mercuri E, Faundez J C, Rutherford M, Acolet D, Dubowitz L 1994 Prognostic value of continuous electroencephalographic recording in full term infants with hypoxic ischaemic encephalopathy. Archives of Disease in Childhood 71: F97–F102
145. Westgate J, Harris M, Curnow J S H, Greene K R 1993 Plymouth randomised trial of cardiotocogram only versus ST waveform plus cardiotocogram for intrapartum monitoring in 2400 cases. American Journal of Obstetrics and Gynecology 169: 1151–1160
146. Westmark K D, Barkovitch A J, Sola A, Ferriero D, Partridge J C 1995. Patterns and implications of MR contrast enhancement in perinatal asphyxia: a preliminary report. American Journal of Neuroradiology 16: 685–692
147. Wheble A M, Gillmer M D G, Spencer J A D, Sykes G S 1989 Changes in fetal monitoring practice in the UK: 1977–1984. British Journal of Obstetrics and Gynaecology 96: 1140–1147
148. Wolf G, Keilhoff G, Fischer S, Hass P 1990 Subcutaneously applied magnesium protects reliably against quinolinate-induced *N*-methyl-D-aspartate (NMDA)-mediated neurodegeneration and convulsions in rats: are there therapeutical implications? Neuroscience Letters 117: 207–211
149. Wyatt J S, Edwards A D, Azzopardi D et al Cerebral haemodynamics during failure of oxidative phosphorylation following birth asphyxia. Pediatric Research 26: 511A
150. Yager J Y, Heitjan D F, Towfighi J, Vannucci R C 1991 Effect of insulin induced and fasting hypoglycaemia on perinatal hypoxic–ischemic brain damage. Pediatric Research 31: 138–142
151. Yudkin P L, Johnson A, Clover L M, Murphy K W 1994 Clustering of perinatal markers of birth asphyxia and outcome at age five years. British Journal of Obstetrics and Gynaecology 101: 774–781
152. Yue T L, Feuerstein G Z 1994 Platelet activating factor. A putative neuromodulator and mediator in the pathophysiology of brain injury. Critical Reviews in Neurobiology 8: 11–24

Part 5

Preterm brain injury

Linda S. de Vries Janet M. Rennie

PRETERM CEREBRAL HAEMORRHAGE

TERMINOLOGY

Since the decline in subdural haemorrhage secondary to birth trauma, bleeding into the brain of preterm infants has become the most common type of neonatal intracranial haemorrhage. Diagnosis in life using cranial ultrasound imaging has been possible since 1978. Cohort screening with this technique has given new knowledge about the incidence, timing and evolution of neonatal cerebral lesions. In the past the term 'periventricular haemorrhage', was widely used in the generic sense to embrace germinal matrix haemorrhage, intraventricular haemorrhage and haemorrhage into the brain parenchyma. In our view this term should be abandoned: it is now realized that neither are all parenchymal lesions haemorrhagic, nor are they all periventricular. The Papile classification,[116] which was based on CT scan appearances, is also outmoded. The Papile classification was designed to grade a single CT 'snapshot' taken during the first week of life. In this system grade I described a haemorrhage confined to the subependymal region, grade II was used for bleeding into the ventricular cavity but not distending it, grade III for an intraventricular bleed with ventricular enlargement, and grade IV for any parenchymal lesion. There are several disadvantages to this system, including the fact that grade IV 'lumps' all parenchymal lesions together, whereas modern neuroimaging can distinguish many different types.

A more specific descriptive system is clearly required, and the new system needs to be able to classify both early and late ultrasound appearances. A system of classification must be applicable to the early appearances, because some infants will die before the evolving lesion can be studied. However, the evolution of a parenchymal lesion often provides the best clue as to which type of lesion it is. 'Germinal matrix haemorrhage–intraventricular haemorrhage' (GMH-IVH) is the most appropriate generic term for the common form of intracranial haemorrhage seen in preterm infants which does not involve the brain parenchyma. Parenchymal lesions are not all periventricular in location or haemorrhagic in origin, so that a better all-embracing term for these is intraparenchymal lesion (IPL).

A classification system must acknowledge the limitations of ultrasound, because this is the main method of neuroimaging in the neonatal period. Ultrasound cannot reliably distinguish between infarction and haemorrhage, so we prefer not to use the term haemorrhagic periventricular infarction (HPI) (p. 89). Direct extension into the parenchyma from pressure of blood in the ventricle is now considered unlikely; some take the view that all parenchymal lesions are originally ischaemic in origin, any bleeding being a secondary complication. However, most agree that a unilateral parenchymal lesion accompanying GMH-IVH is most often caused by the presence of the GMH, leading to impaired venous drainage and venous infarction, at the same time accepting that ischaemic white matter damage can be associated with haemorrhage in severe cases. Intraparenchymal lesions seen early in life using ultrasound should be carefully described as to size, echogenicity and location. A permanent image should be made, together with a written description, which can be invaluable if the image degrades or is lost. The progress of the parenchymal lesion should be followed. When first seen with ultrasound most parenchymal lesions are echoreflectant, or 'bright'. Over the next weeks some resolve, many evolve into multiple small cysts, and others evolve into single large cysts. Using ultrasound it is not possible to make a certain pathological diagnosis, so the terms 'grade IV intraventricular haemorrhage' and 'parenchymal extension of intraventricular haemorrhage' should be abandoned. As yet there is no universal agreement on how to classify GMH-IVH or intraparenchymal lesions. A classification system suitable for describing early and late ultrasound appearances and based on that suggested by Volpe[182] and de Vries[31] is given in Table 44.16. An attempt has been made to give equivalents (Table 44.16C) so that alternative classification systems, for example that used in Chapter 7, can be interpreted.

GERMINAL MATRIX HAEMORRHAGE–INTRAVENTRICULAR HAEMORRHAGE (GMH-IVH)

Incidence

The first studies, using CT and ultrasound, were performed between 1978 and 1983 and showed an incidence of all forms of intracranial haemorrhage (encompassing GMH-IVH and IPL) to be 40–50% in infants with a birthweight of less than 1500 g.[13,33] In the 1990s many groups have noted a decline in the incidence of GMH-IVH and IPL together, to about 20% of very low-birthweight infants,[6,125,159] but this has not been confirmed by others.[22] The incidence and severity of

Table 44.16 Classification of ultrasound appearances of neonatal intracranial lesions

A Description of neonatal intracranial lesions seen early in life with ultrasound

Description	Generic term
Germinal matrix haemorrhage	GMH-IVH
Intraventricular haemorrhage without ventricular dilatation	GMH-IVH
Intraventricular haemorrhage with acute ventricular dilatation (measure the ventricle)	GMH-IVH and ventriculomegaly
Intraparenchymal lesion: describe size, location, degree of echogenicity (see B) and permanently record the image	IPL

B Description of neonatal intraparenchymal lesions using ultrasound

Classification	Description
Flare or echodensity	Periventricular echodense area. Loss of the normal pattern of alternating echoreflectant and echopoor lines. Record size, side and position. Monitor duration of abnormal ultrasound appearance for at least a month and describe duration in days
Frontoparietal cystic PVL	Localized small frontoparietal cysts; lesions not involving the occipital cortex
Parieto-occipital cystic PVL	Multiple cysts in the parieto-occipital white matter
Subcortical cystic PVL	Multiple subcortical cysts in the deep white matter (multicystic leukoencephalomalacia, MCLE)
Porencephalic cyst	Single large cavity adjoining a ventricle and in communication with it

C Table of ultrasound descriptions with equivalent terms and pictorial examples

Description of ultrasound appearances, equivalent terms	Nomenclature used in this chapter	Examples of ultrasound appearances Early	Mid	Late
Germinal matrix haemorrhage which forms a subependymal cyst; Subependymal haemorrhage; Uncomplicated periventricular haemorrhage; Grade I PVH. **NB** not equivalent to subependymal pseudocyst which forms in a different place[55,134]	Uncomplicated GMH-IVH	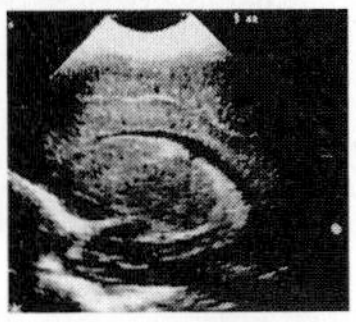	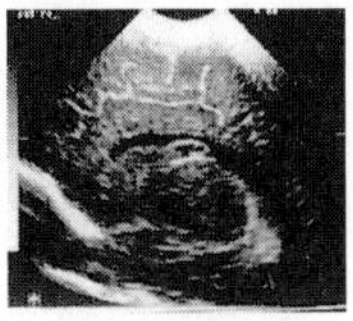	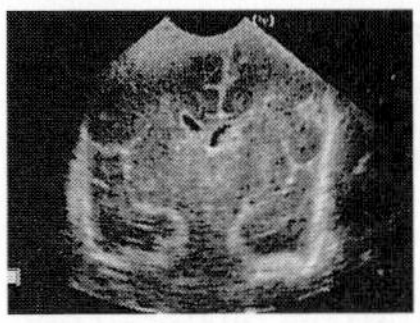
Intraventricular haemorrhage which resolves without ventricular enlargement IVH; Intraventricular haemorrhage, grade II PVH Uncomplicated periventricular haemorrhage	Uncomplicated GMH-IVH	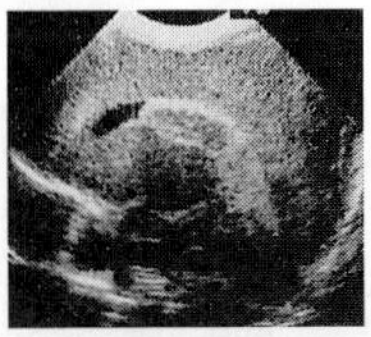	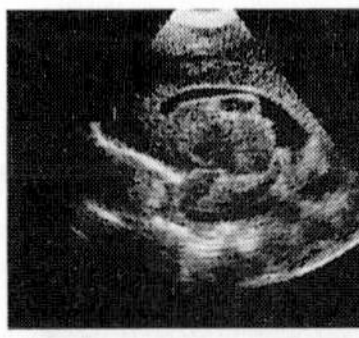	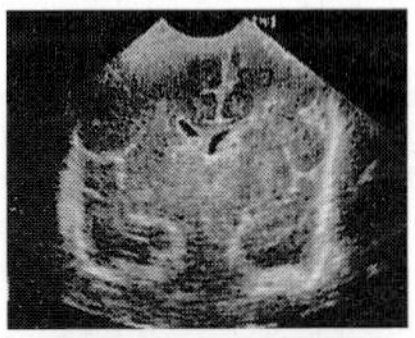
Intraventricular haemorrhage which at some stage is associated with enlarged ventricles (>97th centile of Levene[80b]) which does not progress to hydrocephalus Ventricular dilatation, grade III PVH	Complicated GMH-IVH; GMH-IVH with non-progressive ventriculomegaly	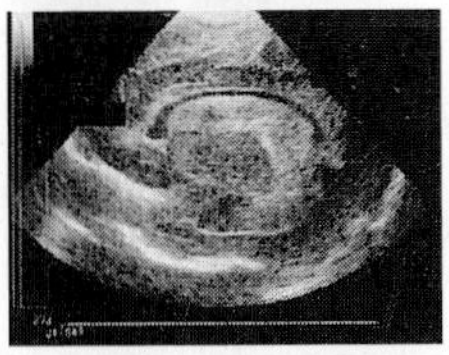	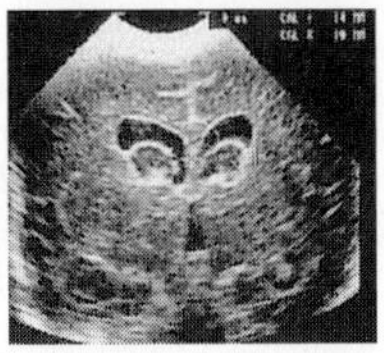	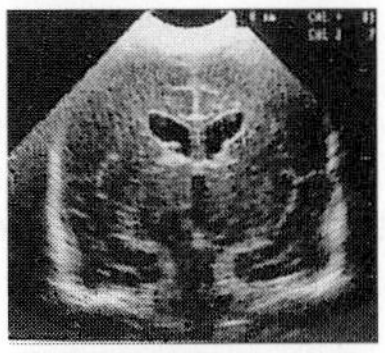
Intraventricular haemorrhage associated with enlarged ventricles and which progresses to hydrocephalus with symptomatic raised intracranial pressure or excessive head growth; Posthaemorrhagic hydrocephalus	Complicated GMH-IVH; GMH-IVH with progressive hydrocephalus; Posthaemorrhagic hydrocephalus	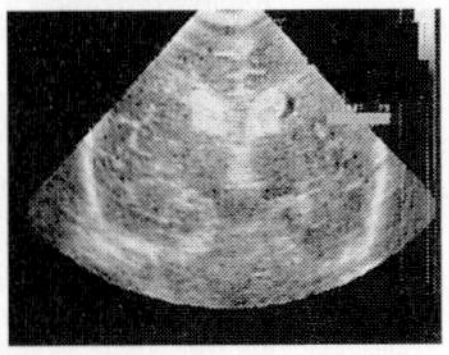	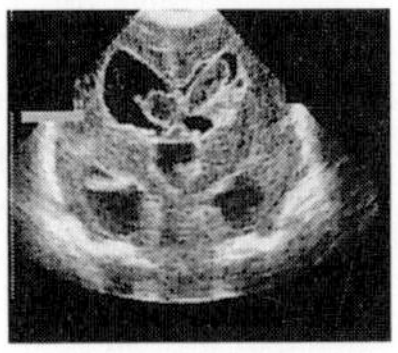	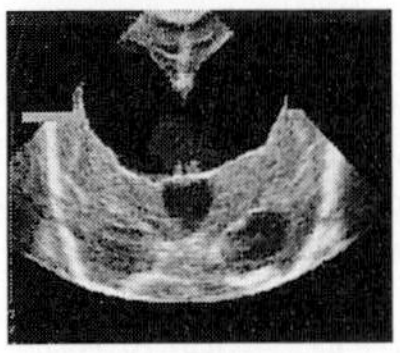

Table 44.16C (Cont'd)

Description of ultrasound appearances, equivalent terms	Nomenclature used in this chapter	Examples of ultrasound appearances		
		Early	Mid	Late
Enlarged ventricles (usually with irregular margins) without preceding GMH-IVH Ventriculomegaly; cerebral atrophy	Enlarged ventricles without GMH-IVH; Non-haemorrhagic ventriculomegaly; Cerebral atrophy	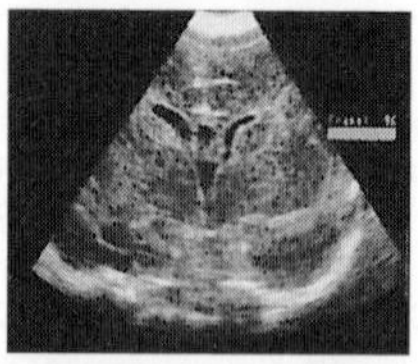		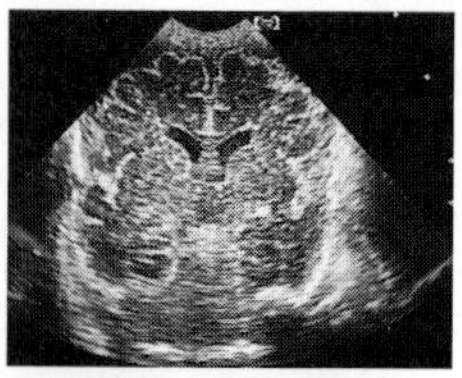
IPL (usually globular and unilateral, and usually associated with GMH-IVH) evolving to a single large porencephalic cyst Haemorrhagic periventricular infarction associated with PVH; Grade IV PVH	Globular IPL with or without GMH-IVH evolving into porencephalic cyst	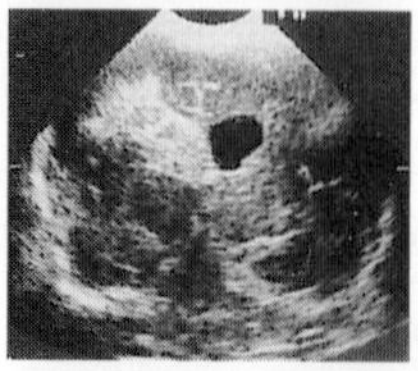	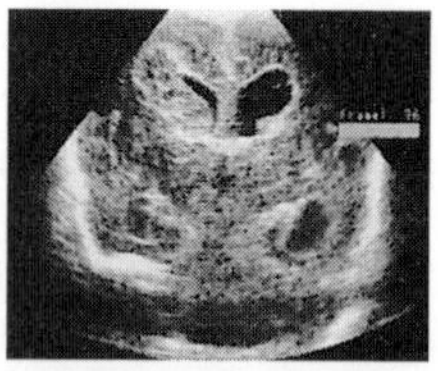	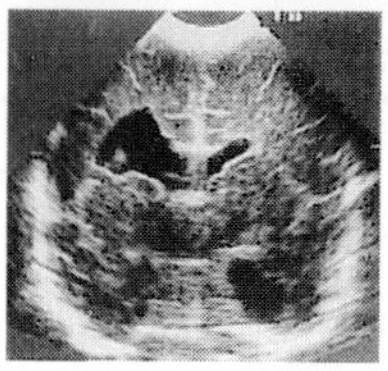
IPL, usually unilateral, fan-shaped and associated with GMH-IVH but partially separate from the ventricle, evolving into multiple cysts	Fan-shaped IPL Evolving into multiple cysts – describe anatomical location	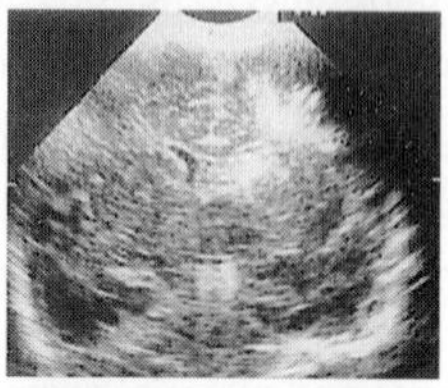	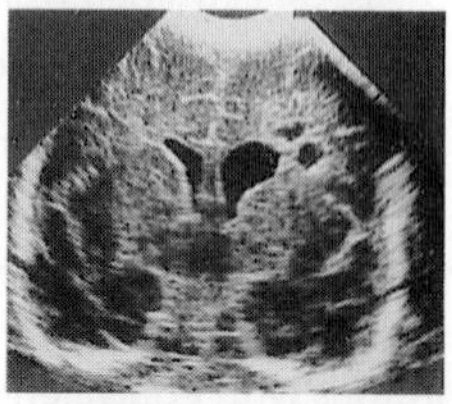	
IPL (usually bilateral) persisting for at least 48 hours without cystic evolution. Can be associated with GMH-IVH, usually not. Transient flare; Periventricular flare	IPL persisting for 48 hours; transient flare	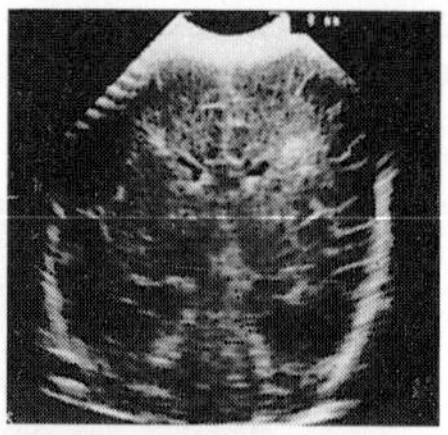	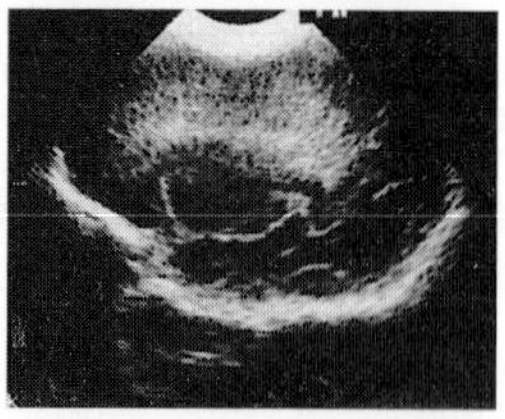	
IPL (usually bilateral) persisting for at least 7 days without cystic evolution. Can be associated with GMH-IVH, usually not; Persistent flare; Mild PVL; grade I PVL[28]	IPL persisting for 7 days; prolonged flare	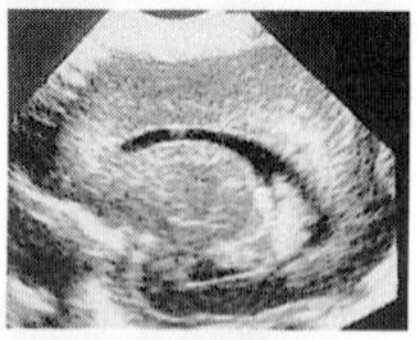	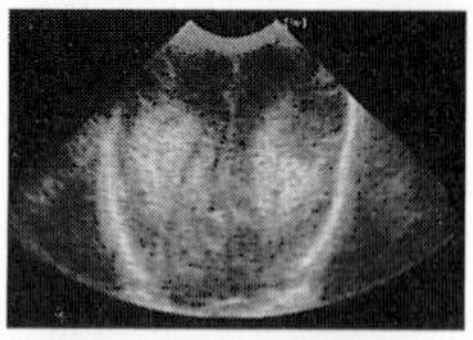	
IPL persisting for 7 days and evolving into localized small frontoparietal cysts; lesions not involving the occipital cortex Cystic PVL; grade II PVL[28]	IPL persisting for 7 days and evolving into localized small frontoparietal cysts; Frontoparietal cystic PVL	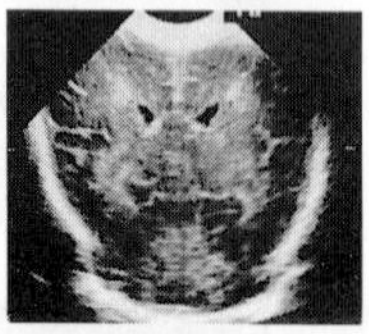	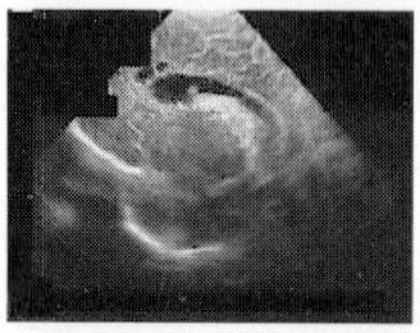	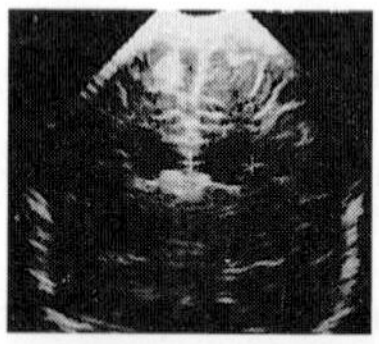
IPL persisting for days and evolving into multiple cysts in the parieto-occipital white matter; Cystic PVL; grade III PVL[28]	IPL persisting for days and evolving into multiple cysts in the parieto-occipital white matter; Parieto-occipital cystic PVL	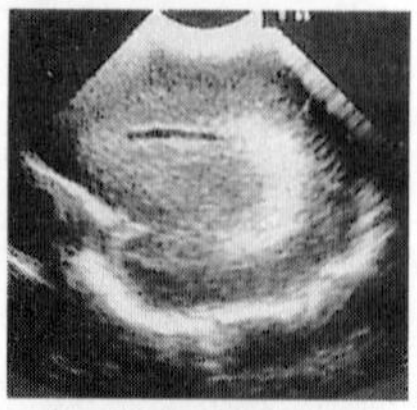	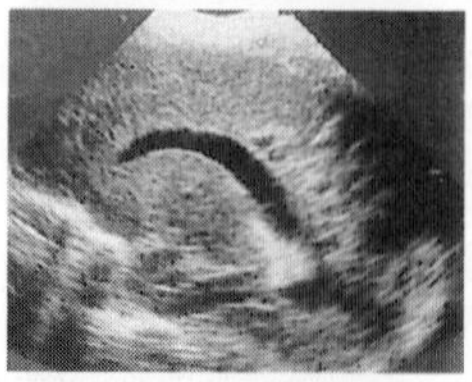	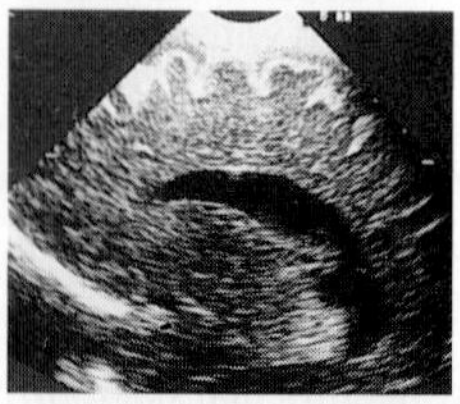
IPL persisting for days and evolving into multiple subcortical cysts in the deep white matter; Cystic PVL; grade IV PVL[28]	IPL persisting and evolving into multicystic leukoencephalomalacia (MCLE); Subcortical cystic PVL	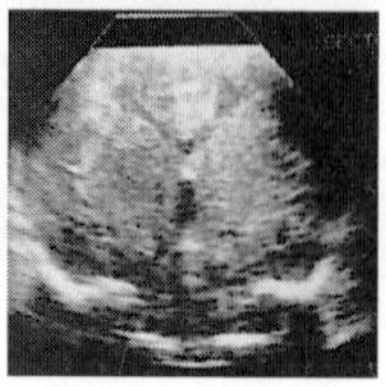	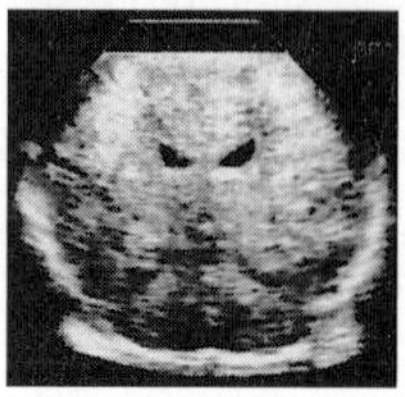	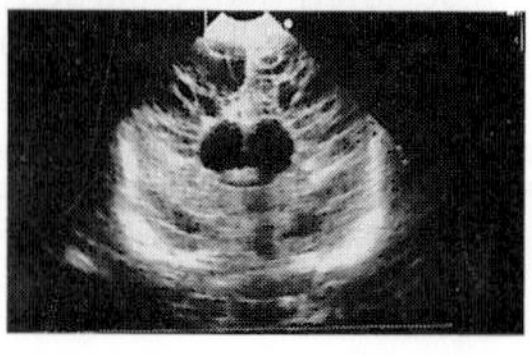

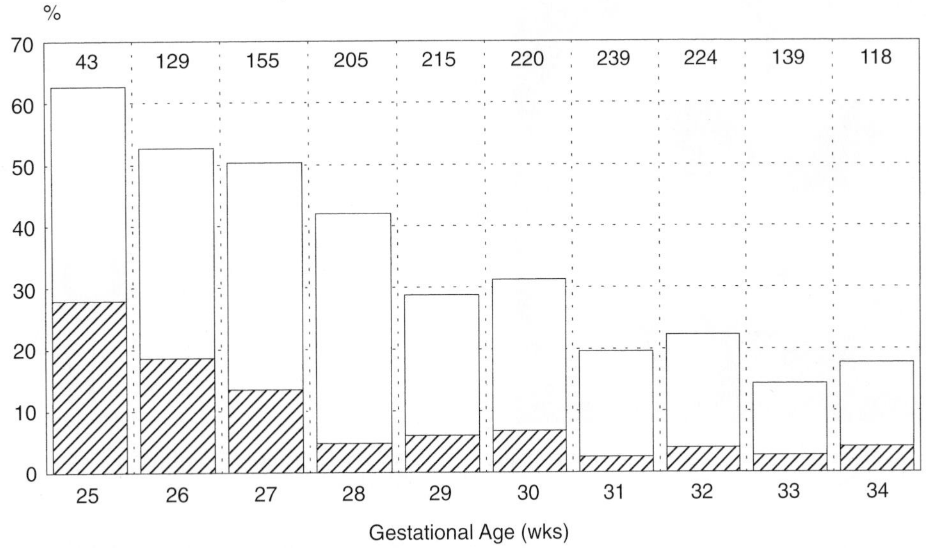

Fig. 44.29 Incidence of GMH-IVH in premature infants in relation to gestational age. The number at the top of each column refers to the number of infants in each group. The unfilled bars represent cases of uncomplicated GMH-IVH; the cross-hatched bars represent complicated GMH-IVH and/or IPL.

GMH-IVH is tightly related to gestational age (Fig. 44.29). A quarter of the cases are bilateral.[180]

Timing

Although GMH-IVH can occasionally occur antenatally, the majority of preterm infants develop the lesion after birth. Before the era of neuroimaging, timing was assessed using radioactively labelled red cells and by looking at the proportion of mature red cells in the clot at autopsy,[168] and suggested an onset of haemorrhage within the first 48 hours of life. Sequential ultrasound studies enabled accurate timing of the onset after birth.[50] These studies showed that the majority of lesions occurred within 72 hours, almost half during the first 24 hours.[33,94,96,169] In 10–20% of cases extension occurs over the next 24–48 hours[83,145] (Fig. 44.30). According to others[85,97] 20–25% of the lesions develop within the first 12 hours of life, and GMH-IVH has been reported to occur very soon after birth in the least mature infants.[121,123] Only about 10% of GMH-IVH occurs beyond the end of the first week, in contrast to periventricular leukomalacia, where late onset is not uncommon.[27,139,145]

Pathogenesis

Anatomy and pathology of the preterm brain

Ruckensteiner and Zollner[137] were the first to point out that GMH-IVH developed following haemorrhage in the subependymal germinal matrix, a structure which is most prominent between 24 and 34 weeks of gestation and which has almost completely regressed by term. Germinal matrix tissue is abundant over the head of the caudate nucleus, and can also be found in the periventricular zone. Recently magnetic resonance imaging has confirmed just how extensive this tissue is in preterm infants.

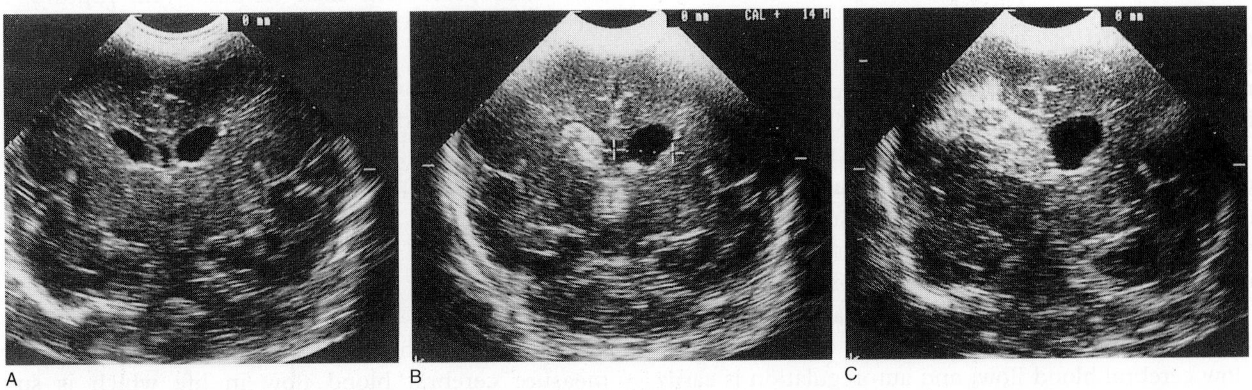

Fig. 44.30 Coronal view at 3, 12 and 36 hours. (A) Mild ventricular dilatation. (B) Right-sided IVH. (C) Parenchymal involvement.

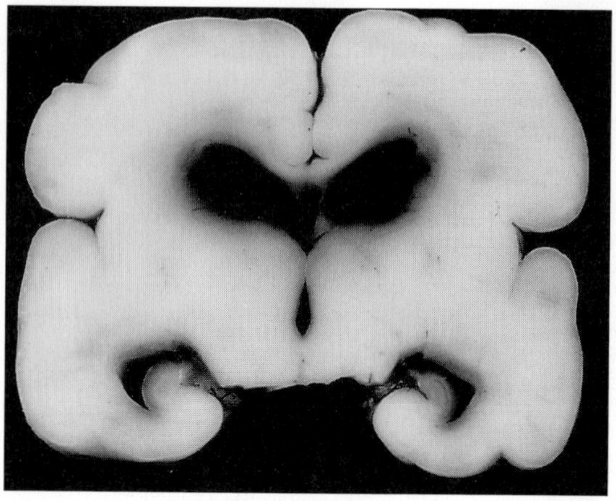

Fig. 44.31 Germinal matrix–intraventricular haemorrhage in an infant with a gestational age of 26 weeks. Coronal section of brain.

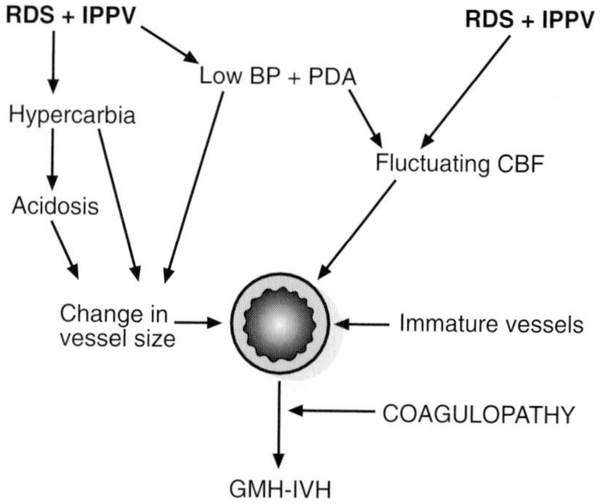

Fig. 44.32 Interaction of factors involved in the genesis of GMH-IVH.

The germinal matrix contains neuroblasts and glioblasts, which undergo mitotic activity before the cells migrate to other parts of the cerebrum. Bleeding into the caudo-thalamic part of the germinal matrix was predominant in the large autopsy series from New Jersey, but more than a third of cases also had bleeding into the temporal or occipital germinal matrix outer zones.[113] Choroid plexus bleeding was also common.

The germinal matrix receives its main blood supply from a branch of the anterior cerebral artery known as Heubner's artery. The rest is derived from the anterior choroidal artery and the terminal branches of the lateral striate arteries.[63] Venous drainage of the deep white matter occurs through a fan-shaped leash of short and long medullary veins, through which blood flows into the germinal matrix and subsequently into the terminal vein, which lies below the germinal matrix.[161] The anatomical distribution of parenchymal lesions associated with GMH-IVH suggested venous infarction due to obstruction of this vein.[54] The blood can fill part of or the entire ventricular system (Fig. 44.31), spreading through the foramen of Monro, the third ventricle, the aqueduct of Sylvius, the fourth ventricle and the foramina of Luschka and Magendie, to eventually collect around the brain stem in the posterior fossa.

Cerebral blood flow and vascular factors

Prematurity and the presence of respiratory distress syndrome are the main risk factors for GMH-IVH. The best unifying hypothesis (Fig. 44.32) is that GMH-IVH occurs as a result of a combination of vulnerable immature anatomy, haemodynamic instability and the propensity to bleeding which is intrinsic to the newborn.[114] The neonatal platelet has a storage pool defect and the substances released by the neonatal endothelium tend to be vasodilators. The newborn of most species have low cerebral blood flow, and autoregulation is easily disturbed by insults such as hypoxia or acidosis, which are more likely to be present if there is respiratory disease. Impaired autoregulation renders the cerebral circulation 'pressure passive' and hence unprotected from any wide swings or changes in blood pressure. All these factors combine to increase the risk of intracranial haemorrhage. Changes in cerebral blood flow have been documented with pneumothorax, handling and endotracheal suction,[66,119,189] all of which have been implicated in the genesis of GMH-IVH. Carbon dioxide retention, artificial ventilation, hypoxia, hypoglycaemia, anaemia and seizures also alter cerebral blood flow.[66,88,130] Various prenatal and postnatal factors have been found to be associated with GMH-IVH in preterm infants (Table 44.17).[67,100,157,183,184]

The precise nature and origin of GMH-IVH remains uncertain. Although some groups have suggested that the capillaries in the germinal matrix do not rupture easily, others have suggested that they can, owing to the fact that the vessels are immature in structure with little evidence of basement membrane protein, and are relatively large in diameter.[61] Early neuropathologists considered subependymal bleeding to be entirely venous in origin. This theory was rebutted by the work of Hambleton and Wigglesworth[63] and Pape and Wigglesworth,[114] who suggested from their injection studies that capillary bleeding was more prominent than terminal vein rupture. Most recently there has been a return to the concept that most IPLs are due to venous infarction,[54,161] or to a reperfusion injury following an ischaemic insult.[180] Ultrasound cannot reliably distinguish between haemorrhage and infarction in the early stages,[109,139] hence the classification system proposed in Table 44.16A.

Cerebral blood flow measurements in the newborn

There is no method that can accurately and repeatedly measure cerebral blood flow in life which is suitable for repeated use in sick preterm infants, so the

Table 44.17 Factors associated with an increased risk of GMH-IVH in preterm infants

Factor	Reference
Prenatal	
Failure to give antenatal steroids (pp. 165, 491)	5, 24, 39,135,149
Maternal aspirin therapy	138
Maternal smoking	5, 155
Reason for prematurity other than pre-eclamptic toxaemia	78
Male sex	135
Breech vaginal delivery (some studies)	97
Very preterm delivery	most studies
At delivery	
Birth depression; asphyxia	97, 135
Birth trauma; bruising	157
Postnatal	
Respiratory distress syndrome, particularly if complicated by	
pneumothorax	67, 157, 183
hypercarbia	157, 183
acidosis	5
hypoxia	5
Hypotension, low right ventricular output	4, 39, 100, 138, 184
Fluctuating cerebral blood flow	118, 171
Bruising and associated hyperkalaemia	151
Coagulation disturbance (prematurity/bruising/sepsis)	94, 163
Tolazoline therapy	163
Patent ductus arteriosus (low BP, cerebral steal)	39

pressure-passive circulation/ischaemia theories remain hypotheses.[179] Using radioactive Xenon, Lou et al[90] showed a direct linear relationship between blood pressure and cerebral blood flow in a small number of infants. A fluctuating cerebral blood flow, mirroring changes in arterial blood pressure, was demonstrated using Doppler ultrasound and this pattern was associated with an increased risk of GMH-IVH.[118] Muscle paralysis stabilized the fluctuating blood flow pattern and was followed by a reduction in GMH-IVH.[120] The importance of the fluctuating pattern was subsequently confirmed by some,[4,171] but not by others.[101] The origin of the fluctuating pattern is almost certainly the infant fighting the ventilator, and may be exaggerated in hypovolaemia.[58,129,131] Administration of surfactant has also been noted to cause a transient increase in cerebral blood flow by some,[65,170] but not by others.[23] The benefits of surfactant therapy in ameliorating the severity of respiratory distress syndrome, hence reducing hypoxia, hypotension and hypercarbia, clearly outweigh these theoretical risks, and surfactant therapy has generally been associated with fewer cases of GMH-IVH[70,89] (p. 494).

Hypotension and cerebral ischaemia

Hypotension is a common complication of severe respiratory distress syndrome, and in the presence of a pressure-passive cerebral circulation may lead to hypoxia–ischaemia of the germinal matrix and parenchyma. The brain may be damaged in the ischaemic phase or during subsequent reperfusion. Several groups have shown that arterial hypotension precedes the development of both GMH-IVH and IPL.[100,184] It has been suggested that the protective effect of antenatal steroids is due to a reduction in the need for blood pressure support, or by direct stabilization of the capillary endothelium.[102] Early administration of gelofusin or fresh frozen plasma did not prevent either GMH-IVH or later handicap,[108] perhaps because hypotension can be due to either cardiac dysfunction or hypovolaemia.[53] A reduction in GMH-IVH has been seen during an era of closer attention to blood pressure, gentle handling, synchronous ventilation and less severe respiratory distress syndrome due to antenatal steroid and postnatal surfactant therapy, rather than to any specific drug used as prophylaxis.[75,125,186]

Diagnosis

Clinical

Volpe[179] describes three clinical syndromes, the first being *catastrophic deterioration*. A sudden deterioration is noted in the baby's clinical state; examples include an increase in oxygen or ventilatory requirement, a fall in blood pressure and/or peripheral mottling, pallor, feed intolerance, and acidosis. This change in condition is non-specific, but if accompanied by a drop in haematocrit, the occurrence of clinical seizures and a full fontanelle, is very suggestive of GMH-IVH. The *saltatory syndrome* is more common and gradual in onset, presenting with a change in spontaneous general movements. The quality of the infant's movements may change from fluid and elegant to a paucity of cramped or stylized movements; there may be subtle seizures, with eye deviation or lip-smacking (p. 1215). The third and most frequent presentation is *asymptomatic*: 25–50% of infants with GMH-IVH have no obvious clinical signs. Dubowitz et al[35] were also able to recognize three phases on careful neurological assessment. With the current ready availability of ultrasound in most neonatal units around the world, any abnormal central nervous system signs or symptoms or a sudden unexplained deterioration in the general condition of a preterm neonate are indications for cranial imaging.

Ultrasound diagnosis

Cranial ultrasound is a reliable, portable and cheap non-invasive technique with which to diagnose GMH-IVH and IPL and to study their evolution over time. Good correlations with autopsy findings have been reported.[15,115,166] Most neonatal units routinely screen all VLBW admissions, partly as a form of audit and partly in order to provide an early warning of problems and to inform counselling

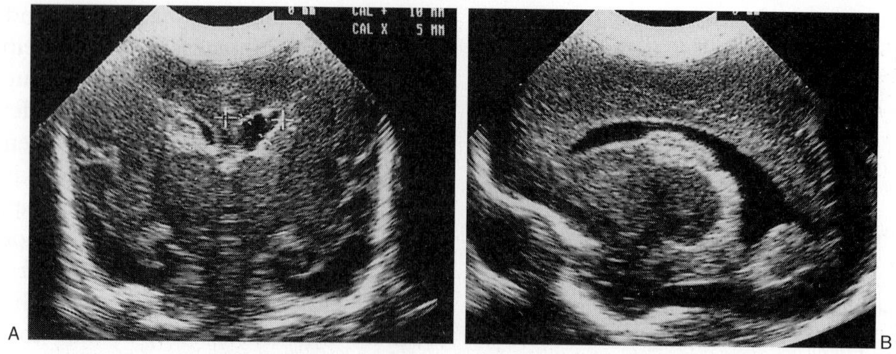

Fig. 44.33 (A) Coronal and (B) parasagittal views showing a small GMH. Also note a small clot on the floor of the occipital horn.

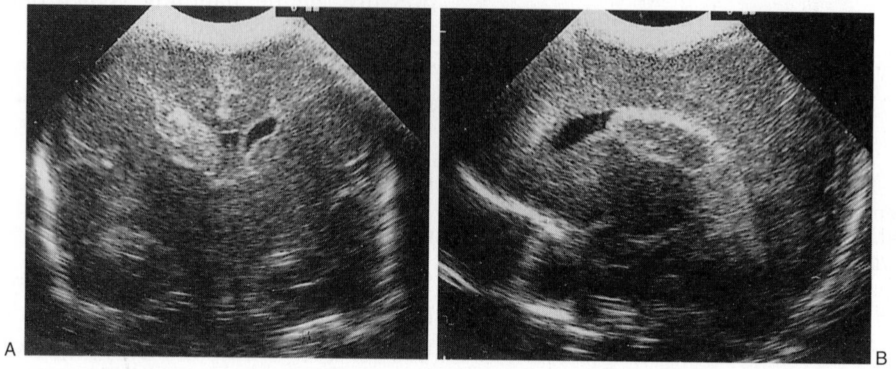

Fig. 44.34 (A) Coronal and (B) parasagittal views, showing an IVH, with a clot filling more than 50% of the right ventricle.

about prognosis. The ideal protocol would include an admission scan, together with daily scans for the first week, reducing to twice weekly or weekly thereafter. Frequent scans enable accurate timing of the onset of lesions and monitoring of their evolution to assist in the final classification (Table 44.16C). The records can be very helpful for audit and for medicolegal purposes, as lesions may have been evident before a given clinical event. If the available manpower or equipment allows for only a single scan then the optimal time is at the end of the first week, but repeated imaging is required to detect all lesions reliably. For more information on normal cranial ultrasound appearances see Chapter 47. Several atlases exist.[55,113,134]

A germinal matrix haemorrhage can be recognized as an echogenic area between the caudate nucleus and the ventricle, which evolves over a 2–4-week period into a cystic lesion which will eventually disappear (Fig. 44.33). An intraventricular bleed can be recognized as an echogenic structure within the normally echolucent ventricle (Fig. 44.34). When the amount of blood in the lateral ventricle is small, it is often difficult to make a distinction between a GMH and a GMH associated with a small IVH. A large IVH is easy to recognize and distends the ventricle in the acute stage (Fig. 44.34). Infants with GMH-IVH sufficiently large to form a cast of the entire ventricle are almost certain to develop posthaemorrhagic ventricular dilatation (see next section). A very large GMH-IVH which balloons the ventricle can be confused with an IPL.[113]

Unilateral IPL associated with GMH-IVH is usually due to venous infarction.[54] This type of lesion is classically triangular or fan-shaped, with the apex at the outer border of the lateral ventricle (Fig. 44.35). In some cases the lesion is globular, with the apex of the triangle at the midline and a smooth outer border (Fig. 44.35C, D) This globular type of lesion (usually unilateral) evolves over 2–3 weeks into a porencephalic cyst (Fig. 44.36), whereas those IPLs which are clearly separate from the ventricle at the start often form multiple small cysts[133] (Fig. 44.37). Porencephalic cysts do not disappear with time like those of PVL.

Complications

Posthaemorrhagic ventricular dilatation (PHVD)

About 30% of infants with GMH-IVH go on to develop ventricular dilatation;[81] the more severe the GMH-IVH the higher the risk of developing PHVD. This condition is considered to be due to an obliterative arachnoiditis.[79] In this condition the arachnoid villi, situated over the vault of the brain, are damaged and cease to reabsorb cerebrospinal fluid, causing a communicating form of hydrocephalus. Less commonly there is blockage of the aqueduct of Sylvius, leading to a non-communicating

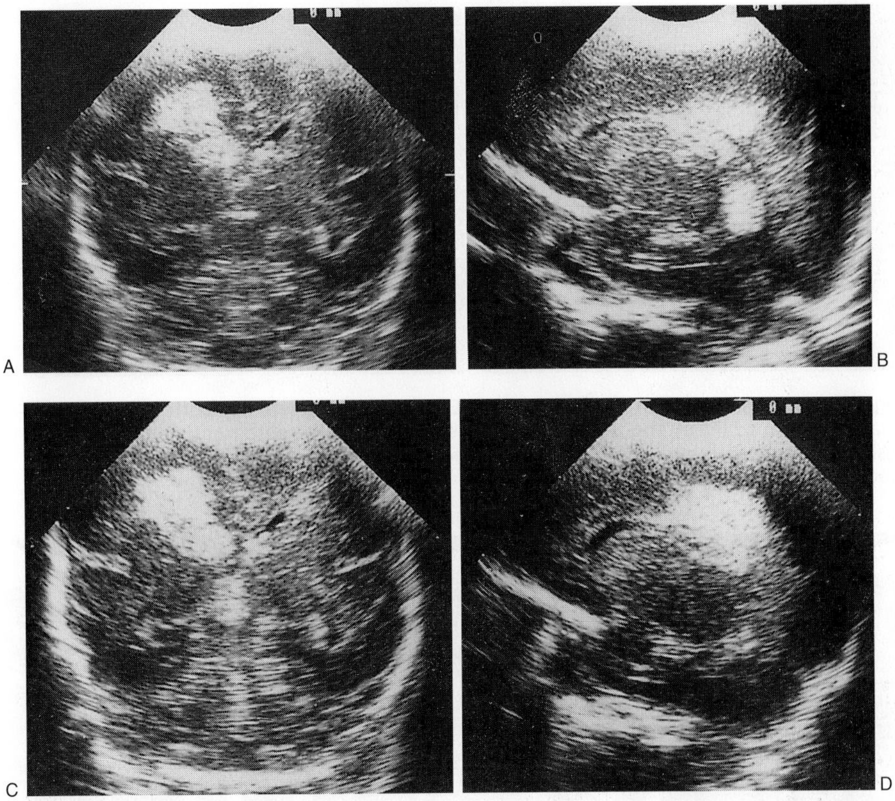

Fig. 44.35 Coronal and parasagittal views at 3 and 24 hours of age. On the first scan (A, B) the parenchymal involvement is smaller and still separate from the lateral ventricle. On the second scan (C, D) the lesion looks more globular and appears to be in communication with the lateral ventricle.

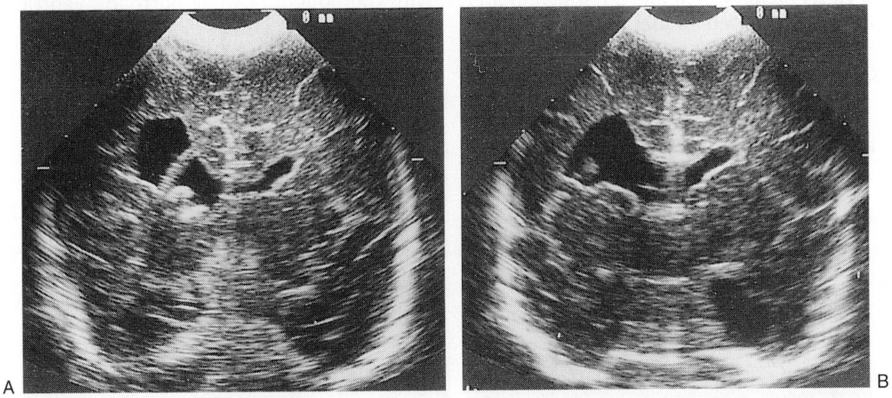

Fig. 44.36 Cranial ultrasound at 4 weeks of age, same infant as in Fig. 43.30, showing the development of a porencephalic cyst, which is partially separate and partially in communication with the lateral ventricle.

form of hydrocephalus. The former usually develops between 10 and 20 days following the onset of the GMH-IVH. Ventricular dilatation seen using cranial ultrasound precedes the development of clinical symptoms by days or even weeks. The clinical signs are a full fontanelle, diastasis of the sutures and an increase in head size. Sunsetting of the eyes is a late sign. PHVD is transient in about half of the infants and is persistent or rapidly progressive in the remaining cases (Fig. 44.38). Once it has been recognized that the ventricles are enlarged the baseline size should be measured using ultrasound. The most widely adopted measurement system is that of Levene.[80a,81] This 'ventricular index' is the distance between the midline and the lateral border of the ventricle measured in a coronal view in the plane of the third ventricle (Figs 44.38(B), 44.39). The measurement made from the scan image can then be compared to the chart of normal ranges (Fig. 44.40). There are many

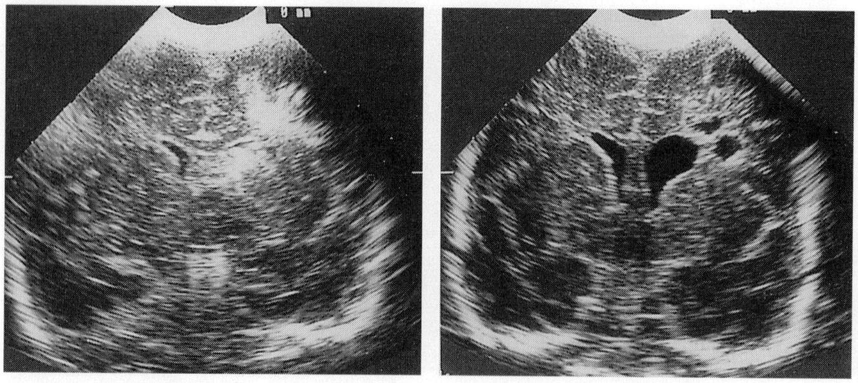

A B

Fig. 44.37 Coronal views on day 3, showing a GMH-IVH on the left side with a triangular shaped IPL on the same side, which over time evolves into multiple cystic lesions associated with mild ventricular dilatation on the affected side. (With permission from Rademaker et al[133])

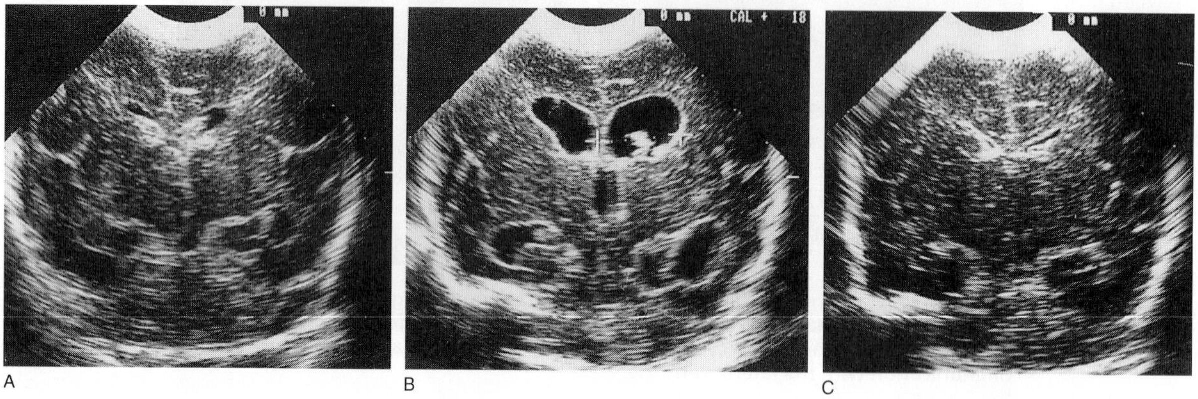

A B C

Fig. 44.38 Coronal views on days 2, 14 and 35, showing an IVH with subsequent posthaemorrhagic ventricular dilatation, which resolved following repeated lumbar punctures.

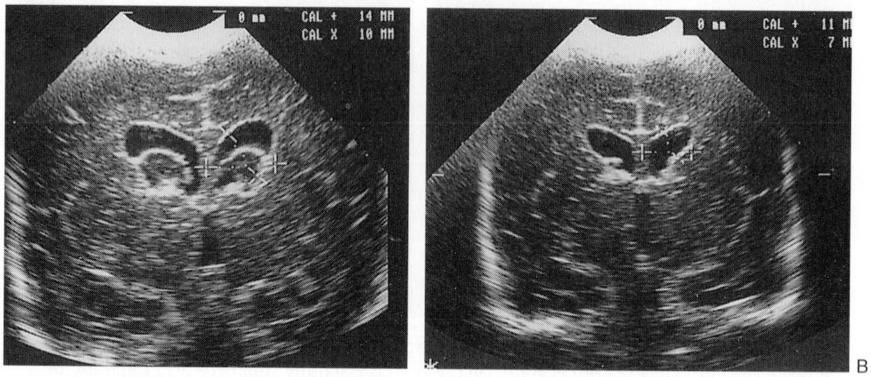

A B

Fig. 44.39 Coronal views showing posthaemorrhagic ventricular dilatation before and after repeated punctures from a reservoir. Both the width and the diagonal size are measured.

other reported measurement systems, including area and volume estimation, but this simple linear index has proved repeatable and robust and has a well established normal range. Another common measurement is the depth of the frontal horn taken just in front of the thalamic notch, a height of >3 mm being used to define ventriculomegaly and one of >5 mm to suggest hydrocephalus[55] (Chapter 7).

The key to the management of PHVD is to distinguish between cases that will require surgical treatment for progressive hydrocephalus (i.e. those with raised intracranial pressure) from those in whom the dilatation is due to cerebral atrophy (low pressure), who will not require surgery. Accurate measurement of pressure is a vital part of this assessment; the size of the ventricles cannot indicate the pressure. Progressive hydrocephalus is very

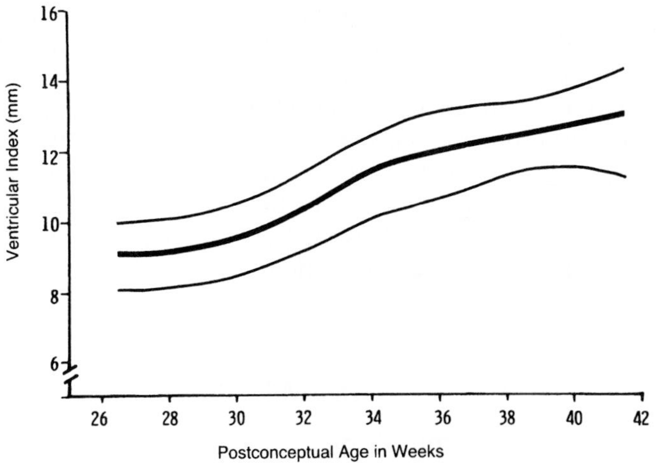

Fig. 44.40 Normal range for the ventricular index. (Reproduced with permission from Levene[80a])

likely if the cerebrospinal fluid pressure, measured via the lumbar route in communicating hydrocephalus or via the ventricle in non-communicating cases, is more than 1.6 kPa (12 mmHg or 15.6 cm of cerebrospinal fluid).[74,173] The upper limit of normal cerebrospinal fluid pressure for newborns is 0.7 kPa (5.25 mmHg or 6.8 cm cerebrospinal fluid).[74] Late progression has been described[122] and serial monitoring of head circumference is required for up to a year, with further ultrasound examinations if there is any concern about the pattern of head growth.

In the early stages PHVD should be monitored with serial ultrasound scans and head circumference measurements at least thrice weekly. Raised cerebrospinal fluid pressure can cause symptoms, including visual disturbance, seizure, feed intolerance and apnoea. In the long term pressure-induced destruction of neuronal tissue causes motor handicap and mental retardation. Short-term adverse effects on the nervous system have been confirmed using somatosensory and visual evoked potentials,[30,37] Doppler estimates of cerebral blood flow velocity[143] and near-infrared spectroscopy.[16] Cerebrospinal fluid hypoxanthine levels were also found to be raised in infants with PHVD.[7]

Despite these findings there is no evidence that early drainage of cerebrospinal fluid alters the natural history of outcome of PHVD, which is that about half of the infants will develop progressive hydrocephalus.[173,174] Once the diagnosis of ventriculomegaly has been made a single lumbar puncture is indicated in order to measure the cerebrospinal fluid pressure, assess whether there is communication between the lumbar and ventricular cerebrospinal fluid, and to exclude a low-grade meningitis as a cause for the ventriculomegaly. If the pressure is low at lumbar puncture but the hydrocephalus is rapidly progressive the cause is likely to be non-communicating hydrocephalus, and ventricular drainage through an external drain or via a surgically inserted subcutaneous reservoir should be considered. Repeated ventricular taps are not recommended as they can result in multiple needle tracks through the brain, and the need for a shunt will not be prevented by this treatment.[173,174] Acetazolamide cannot be recommended.[150] Preliminary results of a European randomized trial of diuretic therapy with acetazolamide in PHVD have shown no benefit from this combination treatment either; indeed, the treated group did worse. Isosorbide is sometimes advocated,[142] and is better tolerated than acetazolamide by sick preterm infants. A few infants have been treated with intraventricular fibrinolytic therapy, which remains experimental.[188]

There is no absolute consensus regarding the point at which drainage is indicated. Some would argue that the following indications, derived from the collaborative ventriculomegaly trials, let the situation deteriorate too far and that earlier treatment leads to better results. However, there can be no doubt that absolute indications for cerebrospinal fluid drainage include:

- symptoms such as apnoea, seizure, irritability or vomiting (visual deterioration in older infants), associated with an intracranial pressure of more than 10 cm cerebrospinal fluid;
- head circumference crossing two centile lines, or enlarging at twice the normal rate for more than 2 weeks.

Clues that the ventriculomegaly is likely to become progressive and that the child may need surgical drainage are a cerebrospinal fluid pressure greater than 1.6 kPa at any stage (12 mmHg; 15.6 cm cerebrospinal fluid), and a rapid progression of the ventricular index measurement. This knowledge may allow early transfer of an infant to a centre with a paediatric neurosurgeon before symptoms develop. Once it is established that treatment is required the timing of the insertion of a suitable ventriculo-peritoneal shunt can be discussed. Many neurosurgeons will insert such devices straight away even in very small infants, but some advocate temporary external drainage or drainage via a surgically implanted subcutaneous reservoir, in order to allow the infant to gain weight. Temporary external drainage systems are prone to infection in this immunocompromised group and are less preferable to an indwelling device if shunt surgery has to be delayed. Some neurosurgeons regard a high cerebrospinal fluid protein level of more than 1.5 or 2 g/l as a contraindication for permanent shunt insertion, and use repeated intermittent drainage until the protein level has reduced.[52,187]

Prevention of GMH-IVH

A reduction in the incidence of GMH-IVH has been reported in many large neonatal units without any specific pharmacological prophylaxis. The importance of good general care, with attention to careful control of blood pressure, temperature and blood gases, gentle handling, gentle ventilation and the appropriate use of antenatal steroids and postnatal surfactant, cannot be overemphasized.[181] With the low incidence of parenchymal lesions seen in most neonatal units nowadays the use of prophylaxis against GMH-IVH, which will benefit only a few infants while exposing many to potentially serious side-effects, is not recommended. The most promising specific prophylactic drug, excluding prenatal dexamethasone, is indomethacin.[48,98] Unfortunately, the long-term outcome study[99] showed that no protection against neurodevelopmental handicap was gained from the early reduction in GMH-IVH. The following section is a brief review of the history of drug prophylaxis against GMH-IVH.

Antenatal administration of several drugs has been advocated. Antenatal phenobarbitone was shown to be protective in some but not all studies.[71,103,146,148,164] Maternal vitamin K administration was noted to be associated with a significant reduction in the risk of preterm infants developing GMH-IVH.[104,128] Marked benefit has been achieved with the use of antenatal steroids in both the short and the long term.[24,51,86,135,149] The effect may be due to the amelioration of the severity of respiratory distress syndrome, capillary stabilization, closure of the ductus or a positive inotropic effect.

Phenobarbitone has also been given postnatally and was shown to be effective.[34] Subsequent studies did not confirm the protective effect of phenobarbitone and a detrimental effect was noted in one study.[77] Perlman et al[120] found a significant reduction in GMH-IVH following muscle paralysis. Other drugs, such as ethamsylate and vitamin E, are considered to have a stabilizing effect on the fragile vessels in the germinal matrix. Ethamsylate looked promising at first,[11] but a recent multicentre study was unable to show a protective effect.[162] The data for vitamin E are controversial.[18,46,154]

Prognosis: neurodevelopmental outcome

Uncomplicated GMH-IVH has a good prognosis. The risk of handicap in VLBW survivors with uncomplicated GMH-IVH or normal cranial ultrasound scans at discharge is 4%.[91,156,178] PHVD carries a high risk of adverse neurodevelopmental outcome – about 50% – and this increases to 75% if a shunt procedure is required.[44,111,117,147,173,174] Only 11 of 112 infants enrolled in the multicentre ventriculomegaly trial were normal at follow-up, underlining the poor prognosis for this group.[174] Prognosis after diagnosis of parenchymal involvement has become more difficult since the realization that not all these lesions are haemorrhagic,[62] and this will be discussed in the next section. Many older studies did not clearly distinguish between parenchymal involvement, ventriculomegaly and progressive hydrocephalus.[17] What is clear is that there is the occasional child with a large porencephalic cyst who is entirely normal. This is also true for a child with a few isolated cysts of periventricular leukomalacia isolated to the anterior frontoparietal region. However, the mortality in series reporting the outcome of large IPL is high: 59% in one study,[62] with 86% of the survivors suffering hemiplegia or spastic quadriplegia. Bilateral parieto-occipital cystic periventricular leukomalacia has an even more dismal prognosis (see next section).

PERIVENTRICULAR LEUKOMALACIA (PVL)

History and terminology

Damage to the deep white matter in the centrum semiovale is the main reason for spastic diplegia, the most common adverse neurodevelopmental sequel of prematurity. The characteristic pattern of late white matter loss, particularly marked in the posterior trigone, is best demonstrated with MRI. Ultrasound remains important in the early evaluation of PVL, despite its limitations. Myelination is actively proceeding in infants and damage to the myelin-producing cells (oligodendroglia) leads to lipid accumulation, necrotic foci and cellular reaction. White matter damage in babies was observed by pathologists as early as 1867, when Virchow first described abnormal areas in the periventricular zone.[177] The term periventricular leukomalacia (PVL) was coined in 1962 by Banker and Larroche, who described changes in histology in 51 infants.[3] The term PVL was chosen as white (leukos) spots and softening (malacia) were seen in the periventricular white matter. Most of the infants in the study of Banker and Larroche were born at more than 28 weeks' gestation (74% were preterm) and were several weeks old at the time of death. Anoxic events were recorded in all the cases; jaundice, sepsis and surgery were also mentioned as possible risk factors.

More recently Paneth et al[112] reported on autopsy findings in 22 very preterm infants who died after 5 days. Although 15 of them had white matter necrosis, only three had the classic changes of PVL. Further observations were made by the same authors in their excellent monograph.[113] Twenty-five infants with white matter damage were autopsied. Only one had 'classic' PVL, but the pathological changes of PVL were associated with GMH-IVH in 20 babies. Thirteen had been noted to have an increase in echogenicity in the periventricular white matter on ultrasound, and nine had ventriculomegaly, apparently without GMH-IVH. We should be aware of these very important pathological studies when we are tempted to use the term PVL to describe a bright area in the brain parenchyma in a 26-week gestation infant on the first day of life. Classifying the ultrasound appearance as an IPL at this stage, as suggested by us, avoids a number of assumptions.

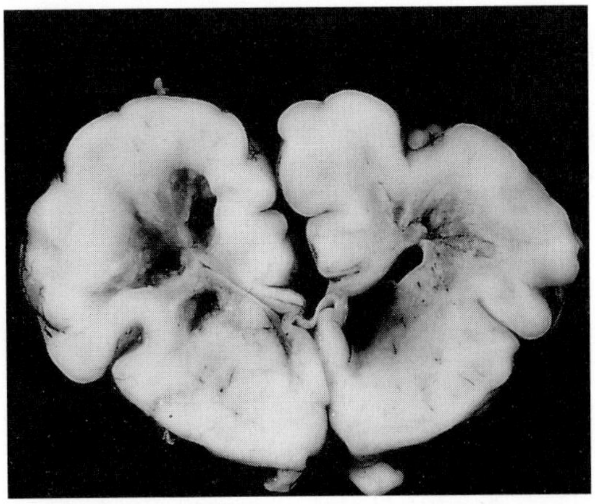

Fig 44.41 Germinal matrix haemorrhage on the left and bilateral extensive cystic leukomalacia.

Pathology and vascular factors

Pathological changes include coagulation necrosis at 3–6 hours, followed by microglial activation at 6–8 hours. Several days later there is astrocytic degeneration and karyorrhexis, with macrophage infiltration. Precisely when the earliest changes can be seen with ultrasound is not known; certainly a 'flare' can be seen 24–48 hours after a hypoxic–ischaemic insult in many cases. Less severe injury may never be detectable with ultrasound, although some develop late ventriculomegaly, and in others earlier imaging may show changes. Microcavities appear in the brain between 8 and 12 days, with macroscopic cavities by 2 weeks, and these can be imaged with ultrasound. The pathological hallmark of PVL is coagulation necrosis. Liquefaction of the centre of the necrotic area can occur after 10–20 days and these small cavities are usually not in communication with the lateral ventricle when imaged with ultrasound (Fig. 44.41). The abnormalities reflect a response to tissue injury which is specific to highly metabolically active white matter undergoing rapid myelination. PVL has long been thought to be vascular in origin and due to hypoperfusion of the boundary zones between ventriculofugal and ventriculopetal arteries.[2,3,160] The major arteries of the brain encircle the cerebrum and send off penetrating branches oriented towards the lateral ventricles. The discovery of a further radially arranged set of vessels travelling out from the ventricles (ventriculofugal) was thought to create a 'boundary zone' or 'watershed' susceptible to a reduction in blood supply. More recently, the existence of ventriculofugal and ventriculopetal arteries has been questioned.[76,93,107] This work used high-power stereomicroscopic instruments and the results suggested that ventriculofugal and ventriculopetal arteries are in fact transcerebral venous channels. These recent studies, suggesting that there is no ventriculofugal circulation and that the vessels previously thought to be arteries are in fact veins, have dealt a blow to the ischaemia theory. However, no better alternative explanation has been offered and the pathological findings clearly suggest hypoxia–ischaemia.

Incidence and timing

It is difficult to get a good idea about the incidence of PVL, as different research groups have used different classification systems in different cohorts. Often only infants with extensive cystic lesions are included, and sometimes globular unilateral IPL, usually due to haemorrhage into an area of venous infarction, is lumped together with cases of bilateral cystic PVL. Most large studies report an incidence of 3–10% for bilateral cystic leukomalacia.[28,40,165] When non-cystic PVL (bilateral IPL which does not progress to cystic change ('flare') is included an incidence of 26% has been found,[165] which is comparable to our own experience (Fig. 44.42).

The time of onset of PVL is much more variable than that of GMH-IVH. Occasionally the injury is of antenatal onset, for example following the death of a co-twin, chorioamnionitis, prolonged rupture of membranes or antepartum haemorrhage.[9,60,80,105,106,124,158] In these situations fully developed cysts can be seen on the first image made shortly after birth. The time taken for an IPL of the 'flare' category (Table 44.16B) to develop into cystic PVL is usually 2 weeks. Sometimes the initial IPL develops several weeks after birth following an acute clinical deterioration such as septicaemia or necrotizing enterocolitis.[27,139]

Pathogenesis

The pathogenesis of PVL is multifactorial and less well understood than that of GMH-IVH. Hypoxic–ischaemic or toxic injury to the metabolically active oligodendroglia is thought to be important.[110] These cells appear to be particularly vulnerable: it was recently shown in a culture model that glutamate is highly toxic to differentiating oligodendroglia.[110] Several groups have found an association between bacterial infection and white matter injury.[8,25a,84,105,124,153,175] Leviton[87] has suggested that there may be release of tumour necrosis factor (TNF) in response to endotoxins, producing hypotension, disseminated intravascular coagulation and the production of platelet-activating factor. TNF promotes destruction of oligodendrocytes and the proliferation of astrocytes.

As with GMH-IVH, changes in blood pressure are more likely to matter if there is a pressure-passive cerebral circulation, because autoregulation is lost. Studies using continuous blood pressure measurements have so far been unable to identify hypotension as an independent risk factor.[167,184] Cerebral 'steal' occurs when there is a large PDA. When this occurs there is an abnormal reversal of cerebral blood flow in diastole, rather than the normal situation of continuous forward flow, and this

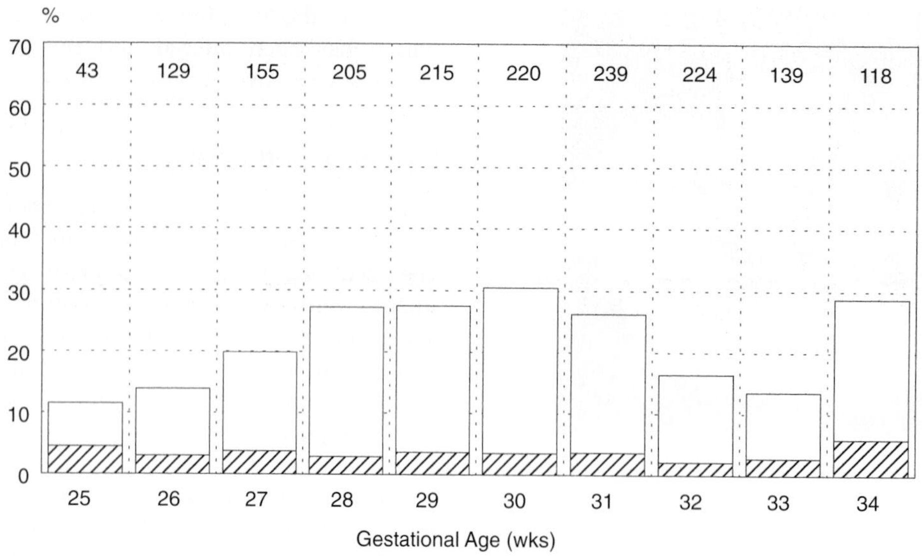

Fig. 44.42 Incidence of PVL in premature infants in relation to gestational age. The number at the top of each column refers to the number of infants in each group. The unfilled bars represent cases of 'flare' or mild PVL; the cross-hatched bars represent cases of cystic PVL.

flow pattern has been linked to PVL.[152] Severe hypocarbia, which causes a decrease in cerebral blood flow, has been identified as an independent risk factor for periventricular leukomalacia.[14,49,57,59,72,190] Both cerebral blood flow and cerebral oxygen delivery were found to be significantly reduced in infants who went on to develop PVL.[132]

The pathogenesis of bilateral IPL which evolves into cystic PVL appears to be very different from a globular unilateral IPL which evolves into a porencephalic cyst. Bilateral cystic PVL occurs with or without GMH-IVH, the age of onset is much more variable, and the lesion much less tightly linked to gestational age. More subtle white matter damage also occurs in the neonatal period and gives rise later to loss of white matter, but goes undetected with ultrasound. These cases form the 'ultrasound-negative' group of ex-preterm children who develop cerebral palsy with an apparently normal neonatal cranial ultrasound scan, who are shown to have loss of myelin volume on MRI in later childhood.

Diagnosis and evolution

Clinical diagnosis

Compared with large GMH-IVH the clinical signs occurring in infants who develop cystic PVL are less obvious and may easily go unnoticed. In the acute phase hypotonia and some degree of lethargy can be observed. Six to 10 weeks later a characteristic clinical picture emerges.[36] The infants become very irritable and are hard to pacify. They are hypertonic and show increased flexion of the arms and extension of the legs. Frequent tremors and startles can be noted and the Moro reaction is usually abnormal. General movement studies have reported these infants to have a 'cramped synchronized' movement pattern.[19] In spite of the cortical visual impairment that is often noted in later infancy in this group, visual tracking still appears normal at this stage.[38]

Electrographic diagnosis

Positive Rolandic sharp waves on the EEG are an abnormal finding. These transient sharp waves are specifically associated with periventricular leukomalacia in preterm infants and may assist in distinguishing those with a poor prognosis.[92] EEG has also proved a useful additional tool in the hands of other groups.[5a,21]

Ultrasound diagnosis

Since 1983 many groups have shown that cystic PVL can be diagnosed using cranial ultrasound scans.[12,68,82] The angle of insonation should be wide enough to visualize the periventricular white matter and the resolution of the transducer should be high (7.5 MHz) in order to detect small cystic lesions.[31] Serial ultrasound scans, at least weekly until discharge, are essential for case ascertainment. Correlation with autopsy findings has shown that ultrasound is less sensitive for the detection of periventricular leukomalacia than for GMH-IVH.[28,40,166] The sensitivity was very high in infants who died with cystic lesions diagnosed using ultrasound.[109] However, there have been many missed diagnoses in infants with noncavitating PVL. Small areas of diffuse gliosis have often been seen at autopsy which had gone unnoticed with cranial ultrasound.[69,112] In the series described by Paneth et al[113] most of the cases with haemorrhagic PVL were

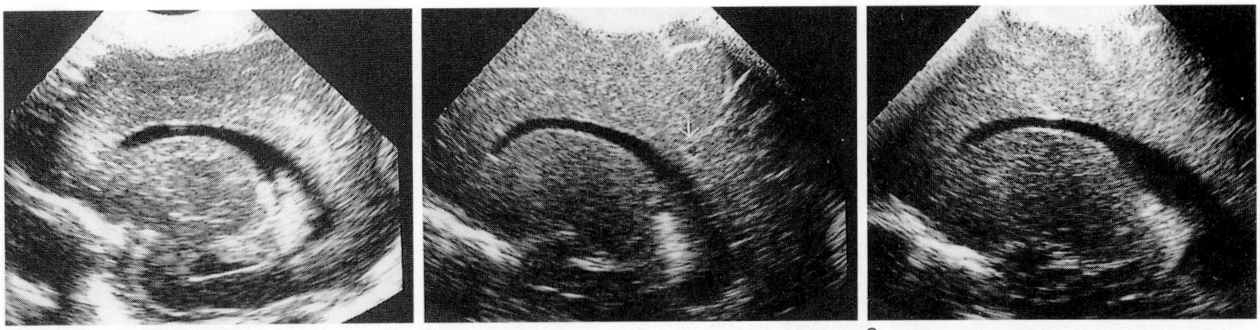

A B C

Fig 44.43 Parasagittal views taken on days 2, 16 and 45, showing increased echogenicity in the periventricular white matter, posterior to the occipital horn, evolving into small cystic lesions (arrow) and subsequently into dilatation of the occipital horn of the lateral ventricle.

correctly diagnosed with ultrasound, but those with focal non-haemorrhagic PVL were frequently missed.

Eventually the cystic lesions disappear and ventricular dilatation is often seen. The ventricular cavity typically has a scalloped inner wall and/or a square, straight-edged appearance of the trigone when imaged with MR, even years later. These findings can appear without preceding cysts or flare, probably because the damage to the oligodendroglia is too subtle to be detected with ultrasound. A glial scar can be left. There is no generally accepted classification system for PVL. Table 44.16B gives a suggested classification.[31] Others[25] have suggested a subclassification of 'flare' into those of brief duration (1–6 days), intermediate (7–13 days) and prolonged (14 days or more).

Diagnosis of periventricular flare. The main difficulty with ultrasound diagnosis of early PVL occurs with the requirement for a distinction between a genuinely echogenic patch and the normal peritrigonal 'blush' which is often seen in the brain of the very preterm infant. Ultrasound interpretation is prone to artefact because of poor transducer–skin contact and excessive gain settings, and requires experience for accurate recognition. Interpretation is still subjective. Any abnormality of white matter will increase echogenicity, so that the ultrasound findings are not specific. A truly abnormal echogenic area is as bright as the choroid plexus, and the abnormality can be confirmed in more than one scan plane on more than one occasion. The genuinely abnormal area of confluent high-intensity echoes completely obliterates the normal pattern of finely interlaced echogenic and echopoor lines that fan out from the periventricular zone. These gracile lines, which can normally be seen in the periventricular region, are thought to represent interfaces between the neural and vascular bundles. This abnormal ultrasound appearance, when present for more than 48 hours, is classified as a transient flare, and when present for more than 7 days as a persistent flare (Table 44.16B, C). A flare can coexist with GMH-IVH; if the echogenic area is globular and unilateral it may represent a parenchymal venous infarction, as already discussed.

Areas of increased echogenicity (IPL) are usually seen 24–48 hours after the insult, whether it be a venous infarction with the globular type of IPL or the fan shaped 'flare' that usually precedes bilateral cystic PVL. Bilateral flare can resolve within days. If areas of increased echodensity persist beyond day 7, but do not become cystic, they can be considered to represent mild leukomalacia. Mild ventricular dilatation with widening of the interhemispheric fissure is often seen with ultrasound studies later in infancy in these cases, suggesting cerebral atrophy. Gliosis has indeed been found in a few cases who died after neonatal cranial ultrasound appearances of flare evolved into mild ventriculomegaly.[28,40,95,166] In other cases the echobright area evolves into localized small cysts a few millimetres in diameter over 2–3 weeks (Fig. 44.43). These are often located in the frontoparietal periventricular white matter. In a minority of the infants extensive cystic lesions develop, which are often especially prominent in the parieto-occipital periventricular white matter (Fig. 44.44). The cysts do not communicate with the lateral ventricle. They collapse after several weeks and are no longer visible with cranial ultrasound once the child is 2–3 months old. At this stage irregular ventricular dilatation can be noted owing to atrophy of the periventricular white matter (Fig. 44.44C). Magnetic resonance imaging (MRI) performed in the second year of life confirms the irregular dilatation of the lateral ventricle and can also show white matter loss, particularly marked in the trigone, with extensive gliosis in the areas where the cysts were initially seen.[32,47]

Prevention

In contrast to GMH-IVH, where many intervention studies have been performed both before and after delivery, hardly any data are available with regard to the prevention of PVL. Prevention of systemic hypotension is considered to be important. Normal blood pressure data continue to accrue, but an arterial pressure of 30 mmHg is generally considered to represent a threshold suitable for most preterm infants.[64,176,184]

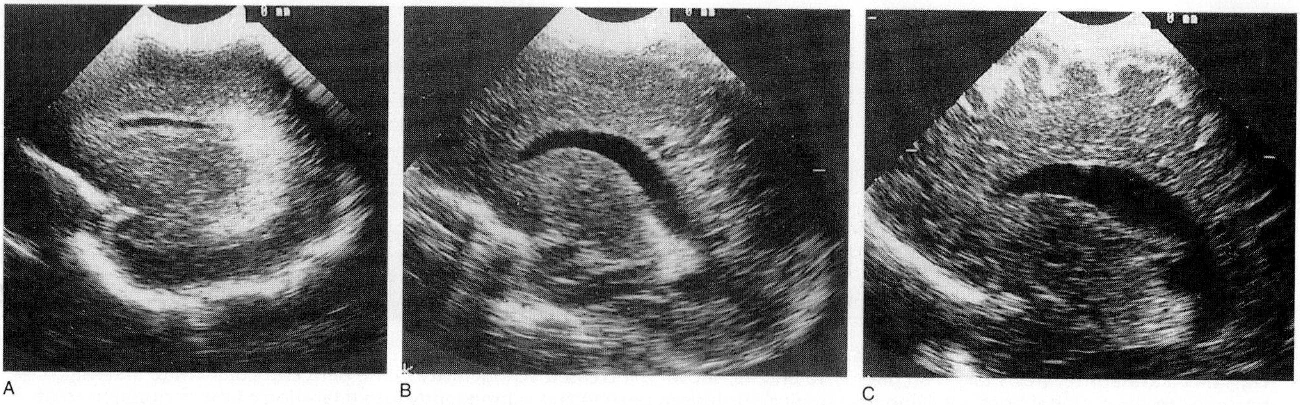

A B C

Fig 44.44 Parasagittal views on days 2 and 16 and at 3 months, showing evolution from increased echogenicity into extensive cysts and finally dilatation ex vacuo. (With permission from de Vries et al[32])

Adjusting ventilator settings in order to avoid severe hypocarbia can also be recommended on the basis of both animal studies as well as risk factor data in humans.[14,43,57,59,72,172,172a,190,191] This may be especially important in infants ventilated with high-frequency oscillation.[191]

High hypoxanthine levels were present at birth in infants who went on to develop PVL, suggesting that free radical damage might be important.[140] One randomized double-blind study used allopurinol, an inhibitor of xanthine oxidase, but no protective effect could be shown.[141] Another retrospective case control study showed that infants who were exposed to magnesium sulphate in utero were less likely to develop cystic PVL.[45] A prospective study is needed to support these findings.

Prognosis: neurodevelopmental outcome

There is no doubt that cystic periventricular leukomalacia is the most powerful predictor of cerebral palsy (usually spastic diplegia) among the neonatal cranial ultrasound lesions so far described.[12,185] In many cohort follow-up studies almost all the cases of cerebral palsy had bilateral parieto-occipital leukomalacia in the neonatal period.[10,43,56,126,127,136,192] Earlier studies, reporting an association between ventricular dilatation and adverse outcome,[17,156] probably included some undiagnosed cases of periventricular leukomalacia due to poor resolution of the older ultrasound scanners. Single cysts and cysts confined to the frontal region appear to have a better outcome than multiple bilateral parieto-occipital cysts, where the outlook is universally dismal.[17,39,49] Cerebral visual impairment is another important sequel and attempts should be made to recognize this early in infancy, for example using visual acuity cards.[20,38,144] Bilateral occipital cystic white matter damage carries a significantly higher risk of developing a major handicap than a large unilateral parenchymal haemorrhage.[26] As leukomalacia is almost always bilateral there is little scope for compensation by the contralateral hemisphere.

Although transient densities were not taken very seriously to start with, they are now generally considered to be a mild form of leukomalacia, provided they persist for at least 7–14 days. Both short- and long-term follow-up studies have shown an adverse effect on neurodevelopmental outcome, with a risk of developing spastic diplegia of 5–10%.[1,29,41,95] In the early follow-up studies almost half of infants surviving with persistent echodensity without cystic change were found to have transient abnormalities in tone. When these children were assessed again at the age of 6 years and compared with preterm infants with normal ultrasound scans, no difference was found in cognitive abilities. However, the results of standardized motor assessment showed that performance decreased significantly if there had been prolonged periventricular echodensity.[73] Other groups have also noted abnormal neuromotor signs as well as lower cognitive abilities.[42]

CONCLUSION

The use of cranial ultrasound imaging over almost 20 years has allowed documentation of a changing pattern of brain injury in preterm infants. In particular, the realization that not all parenchymal lesions are of uniform aetiology has been an important finding. In view of the fact that the prognosis for bilateral occipital cystic white matter damage is so poor, the challenge for the next decade is to increase our understanding of this condition. Neonatology would achieve much if a reduction in incidence of similar magnitude to that which has been accomplished in GMH-IVH could be obtained.

REFERENCES

1. Appleton R E, Lee R E J, Hey E N 1990 Neurodevelopmental outcome of transient neonatal intracerebral echodensities. Archives of Disease in Childhood 65: 27–29
2. Armstrong D, Norman M G 1974 Periventricular leukomalacia in neonates: complications and sequelae. Archives of Disease in Childhood 49: 367–375

3. Banker B Q, Larroche J-C 1962 Periventricular leukomalacia in infancy: a form of neonatal anoxic encephalopathy. Archives of Neurology 7: 386–410
4. Bada H S, Korones S B, Perry E H et al 1990 Mean arterial blood pressure changes in premature infants and those at risk for intraventricular hemorrhage. Journal of Pediatrics 117: 607–614
5. Bada H S, Korones S B, Perry E H et al 1990 Frequent handling in the neonatal intensive care unit and intraventricular hemorrhage. Journal of Pediatrics 117: 126–131
5a. Bagioni E, Bartelena L, Biver P, Pieri R, Cioni G 1996 Electroencephalographic dysmaturity in preterm infants: a prognostic tool in the early postnatal period. Neuropediatrics 27: 311–316
6. Batton D G, Holtrop P, Dewitte D, Pryce C, Roberts C 1994 Current gestational age-related incidence of major intraventricular hemorrhage. Journal of Pediatrics 125: 623–625
7. Bejar R, Saugstad O D, James H, Gluck L 1983 Increased hypoxanthine concentrations in cerebrospinal fluid of infants with hydrocephalus. Journal of Pediatrics 103: 44–48
8. Bejar R, Wozniak P, Allard M et al 1988 Antenatal origin of neurologic damage in newborn infants. I. Preterm infants. American Journal of Obstetrics and Gynecology 159: 357–363
9. Bejar R, Vigliocco G, Gramajo H et al 1990 Antenatal origin of neurologic damage in newborn infants. II. Multiple gestations. American Journal of Obstetrics and Gynecology 162: 1230–1236
10. Bennett F C, Silver G, Leung E J, Mack L A 1990 Periventricular echodensities detected by cranial ultrasonography: usefulness in predicting neurodevelopmental outcome in low-birth weight, preterm infants. Pediatrics 85: 400–404
11. Benson J W T, Drayton M R, Haywood C et al 1986 Multicentre trial of ethamsylate for prevention of periventricular haemorrhage in very low birth weight infants. Lancet ii: 1297–1300
12. Bozynski M E, Nelson M N, Matalon T A S et al 1985 Cavitary periventricular leukomalacia: incidence and short term outcome in infants weighing <1200 grams at birth. Developmental Medicine and Child Neurology 27: 572–577
13. Burstein J, Papile L, Burstein R 1979 Intraventricular hemorrhage in premature newborns: a prospective study with CT. American Journal of Radiology 132: 631–635
14. Calvert S A, Hoskins E M, Fong K W, Forsyth S C 1987 Etiological factors associated with the development of periventricular leukomalacia. Acta Paediatrica Scandinavica 76: 254–259
15. Carson S C, Hetzberg B S, Bowie J D, Burger P C 1990 Value of sonography in the diagnosis of intracranial hemorrhage and periventricular leukomalacia: a postmortem study of 35 cases. American Journal of Neuroradiology 11: 677–683
16. Casaer P, von Siebenthal K, van der Vlugt A, Lagae L, Devlieger H 1992 Cytochrome aa3 and intracranial pressure in newborn infants: a near infrared spectroscopy study (letter) Neuropediatrics 23:111
17. Catto-Smith A G, Yu V Y H, Bajuk B, Orgill A A, Astbury J 1985 Effect of neonatal periventricular haemorrhage on neurodevelopmental outcome. Archives of Disease in Childhood 60: 8–11
18. Chiswick M L, Johnson M, Woodhall C et al 1983 Protective effect of vitamin E (dl-alpha-tocopherol) against intraventricular haemorrhage in premature babies. British Medical Journal 287: 81–84
19. Cioni G, Prechtl H F R 1990 Preterm and early post-term motor behaviour in low-risk premature infants. Early Human Development 23: 159–191
20. Cioni G, Fazzi B, Ipata A E, Canapicchi R, van Hof-van Duin J 1996 Correlation between cerebral visual impairment and MR imaging in children with neonatal encephalopathy. Developmental Medicine and Child Neurology 38: 120–132
21. Connell J A, Oozeer R C, Regev R, de Vries L S, Dubowitz L M S, Dubowitz V 1987 Continuous 4 channel monitoring in the evaluation of echodense ultrasound lesions. Archives of Disease in Childhood 62: 1019–1024
22. Cooke R W I 1991 Trends in preterm survival and incidence of cerebral haemorrhage 1980–89. Archives of Disease in Childhood 56: 425–431
23. Cowan F, Whitelaw A, Wertheim D, Silverman M 1991 Cerebral blood flow velocity after rapid administration of surfactant. Archives of Disease in Childhood 66: 1105–1109
24. Crowley P 1997 Corticosteroids prior to preterm delivery. In: Neilson J P et al (eds) Pregnancy and childbirth module of the Cochrane Collaboration Database of Systematic Reviews. The Cochrane Collaboration Issue 3, Update Software, Oxford
25. Damman O, Leviton A 1997 Duration of transient hyperechoic images of white matter in very low birthweight infants: a proposed classification. Developmental Medicine and Child Neurology 39: 2–5
25a. Damman O, Leviton A 1997 Maternal intrauterine infection, cytokines, and brain damage in the preterm newborn. Pediatric Research 42: 1–8
26. de Vries L S, Dubowitz L M S, Dubowitz V et al 1985 Predictive value of cranial ultrasound: a reappraisal. Lancet ii: 137–140
27. de Vries L S, Regev R, Dubowitz L M S 1986 Late onset cystic leukomalacia. Archives of Disease in Childhood 61: 298–299
28. de Vries L S, Wigglesworth J S, Regev R, Dubowitz L M S 1988 Evolution of periventricular leukomalacia during the neonatal period and infancy: correlation of imaging and postmortem findings. Early Human Development 17: 205–219
29. de Vries L S, Regev R, Pennock J M, Wigglesworth J S, Dubowitz L M S 1988 Ultrasound evolution and later outcome of infants with periventricular densities. Early Human Development 16: 225–233
30. de Vries L S, Pierrat V, Minami T, Casaer P 1990 Short latency cortical somatosensory evoked potentials in infants with hydrocephalus. Neuropediatrics 21: 136–139
31. de Vries L S, Eken P, Dubowitz L M S 1992 The spectrum of leukomalacia using cranial ultrasound. Behavioural Brain Research 49: 1–6
32. de Vries L S, Eken P, Groenendaal F, van Haastert I C, Meiners L C 1993 Correlation between the degree of periventricular leukomalacia diagnosed using cranial ultrasound and MRI later in infancy in children with cerebral palsy. Neuropediatrics 24: 263–268
33. Dolfin T, Skidmore M B, Fong K W, Hoskins E M, Shannon A T 1983 Incidence, severity and timing of subependymal and intraventricular hemorrhages in preterm infants born in a perinatal unit as detected by serial real-time ultrasound. Pediatrics 71: 541–546
34. Donn S M, Roloff D W, Goldstein G W 1981 Prevention of intraventricular haemorrhage in preterm infants with phenobarbital. Lancet ii: 215
35. Dubowitz L M S, Levene M I, Morante A, Palmer P, Dubowitz V 1981 Neurological signs in neonatal intraventricular hemorrhage: correlation with real-time ultrasound. Journal of Pediatrics 99: 127–133
36. Dubowitz L M S 1987 Clinical assessment of the infants nervous system. In: Levene M I, Bennett M J, Punt J (eds) Fetal and neonatal neurology and neurosurgery, 1st edn. Churchill Livingstone, Edinburgh, pp 51–58
37. Ehle A, Sklar F 1979 Visual evoked potentials in infants with hydrocephalus. Neurology 29: 1541–1544
38. Eken P, van Nieuwenhuizen O, van der Graaf Y, Schalij-Delfos N E, de Vries L S 1994 Relation between neonatal cranial ultrasound abnormalities and cerebral visual impairment in infancy. Developmental Medicine and Child Neurology 36: 3–15
39. Evans N, Kluckow M 1996 Early ductal shunting and intraventricular haemorrhage in ventilated preterm infants. Archives of Disease in Childhood 75: F183–F190
40. Fawer C-L, Calame A, Perentes E, Anderegg A 1985 Periventricular leukomalacia: a correlation study between real-time ultrasound and autopsy findings. Neuroradiology 27: 292–300
41. Fawer C-L, Diebold P, Calame A 1987 Periventricular leukomalacia and neurodevelopmental outcome in preterm infants. Archives of Disease in Childhood 62: 30–36
42. Fawer C-L, Calame A 1991 Significance of ultrasound appearances in the neurological development and cognitive abilities of preterm infants at 5 years. European Journal of Pediatrics 150: 515–520
43. Fazzi E, Orcesi S, Caffi L et al 1994 Neurodevelopmental outcome at 5–7 years in preterm infants with periventricular leukomalacia. Neuropediatrics 25: 134–139
44. Fernell E, Hagberg G, Hagberg B 1993 Infantile hydrocephalus in preterm, low-birth-weight infants: a nationwide Swedish cohort study 1979–1988. Acta Paediatrica 82: 45–48
45. FineSmith R B, Roche K, Yellin P B et al 1997 Effect of magnesium sulfate on the development of cystic periventricular leukomalacia. American Journal of Perinatology 14: 303–307
46. Fish W H, Cohen M, Franzek D, Williams J M, Lemons J A 1990 Effects of intramuscular vitamin E on mortality and intracranial hemorrhage in neonates of 1000 grams or less. Pediatrics 85: 578–584

47. Flodmark O, Lupton B, Li D et al 1989 MR imaging of periventricular leukomalacia in childhood. American Journal of Neuroradiology 10: 111–118
48. Fowlie 1996 Prophylactic indomethacin: systematic review and meta-analysis. Archives of Disease in Childhood 74: F81–F87
49. Fujimoto S, Togari H, Yamaguchi N, Mizutani F, Suzuki S, Sobajima H 1994 Hypocarbia and cystic periventricular leukomalacia in preterm infants. Archives of Disease in Childhood 71: F107–F110
50. Funato M, Tamai H, Noma K et al 1992 Clinical events in association with timing of intraventricular hemorrhage in preterm infants. Journal of Pediatrics 121: 614–619
51. Garland J S, Buck S, Leviton A 1995 Effect of maternal glucocorticoid exposure on risk of severe intraventricular hemorrhage in surfactant-treated preterm infants. Journal of Pediatrics 126: 272–279
52. Gaskill S J, Marlin A E, Rivera S 1988 The subcutaneous ventricular reservoir: an effective treatment for posthaemorrhagic hydrocephalus. Child's Nervous System 4: 291–295
53. Gill A B, Weindling A M 1993 Randomised controlled trial of plasma protein fraction versus dopamine in hypotensive very low birthweight infants. Archives of Disease in Childhood 64: 678–686
54. Gould S J, Howard S, Hope P L, Reynolds E O R 1987 Periventricular intraparenchymal cerebral haemorrhage in preterm infants: the role of venous infarction. Journal of Pathology 151: 197–202
55. Govaert P, de Vries L S 1997 An atlas of neonatal brain sonography. Clinics in Developmental Medicine No 141–142. MacKeith Press, London
56. Graham M, Levene M I, Trounce J Q, Rutter N 1987 Prediction of cerebral palsy in very low birth weight infants: prospective ultrasound study. Lancet ii: 593–596
57. Graziani L, Spitzer A R, Mitchell D G et al 1992 Mechanical ventilation in preterm infants: neurosonographic and developmental studies. Pediatrics 90: 515–522
58. Greenough A, Wood S, Morley C J, Davis J A 1984 Pancuronium prevents pneumothoraces in ventilated premature babies who actively expire against positive pressure inflation. Lancet i: 1–3
59. Greisen G, Munck H, Lou H 1987 Severe hypocarbia in preterm infants and neurodevelopmental deficit. Acta Paediatrica Scandinavica 76: 401–404
60. Grether J K, Nelson K B, Emery E S, Cummins S K 1996 Prenatal and perinatal factors and cerebral palsy in very low birth weight infants. Journal of Pediatrics 128: 407–414
61. Grunnet M R L 1989 Morphometry of blood vessels in the cortex and germinal plate of premature neonates. Paediatric Neurology 5: 12–16
62. Guzzetta F, Shackelford G D, Volpe S, Perlman J M, Volpe J J 1986 Periventricular intraparenchymal echodensities in the premature newborn: critical determinant of neurologic outcome. Pediatrics 78: 995–1006
63. Hambleton G, Wigglesworth J S 1976 Origin of intraventricular haemorrhage in the preterm infant. Archives of Disease in Childhood 51: 651–659
64. Hegyi T, Carbone M T, Anwar M et al 1994 Blood pressure ranges in premature infants I. The first hours of life. Journal of Pediatrics 124: 627–633
65. Hellström-Westas L, Bell A H, Skov L, Greisen G, Svenningsen N W 1992 Cerebroelectrical depression following surfactant treatment in preterm neonates. Pediatrics 89: 643–647
66. Hill A, Volpe J J 1981 Seizures, hypoxic–ischemic brain injury and intraventricular hemorrhage in the newborn. Annals of Neurology 10: 109–121
67. Hill A, Perlman J M, Volpe J J 1982 Relationship of pneumothorax to occurrence of intraventricular hemorrhage in the premature newborn. Pediatrics 69: 144–149
68. Hill A, Melson G L, Clark H B, Volpe J J 1982 Haemorrhagic leukomalacia: diagnosis by real-time ultrasound and correlation with autopsy findings. Pediatrics 69: 282–284
69. Hope P L, Gould S J, Howard S, Hamilton P A, Costello A M de L, Reynolds E O R 1988 Ultrasound diagnosis of pathologically verified lesions in the brains of very preterm infants. Developmental Medicine and Child Neurology 30: 457–471
70. Horbar J D, Soll R F, Schachinger H et al 1990 A European multicenter randomized controlled trial of single dose surfactant therapy for idiopathic respiratory distress syndrome. European Journal of Pediatrics 149: 416–423
71. Horbar J D 1992 Prevention of periventricular–intraventricular haemorrhage. In: Sinclair J C, Bracken M B (eds) Effective care of the newborn infant. Oxford University Press, Oxford, pp 562–589
72. Ikonen R S, Kuusinen E J, Janas M O, Koivikko M J, Sorto A E 1988 Possible etiological factors in extensive periventricular leukomalacia of preterm infants. Acta Paediatrica Scandinavica 77: 489–495
73. Jongmans M, Henderson S, de Vries L S, Dubowitz L M S 1993 Duration of periventricular densities in preterm infants and neurological outcome at six years of age. Archives of Disease in Childhood 69: 9–13
74. Kaiser A, Whitelaw A 1986 Cerebrospinal fluid pressure during posthaemorrhagic ventricular dilatation in newborn. Archives of Disease in Childhood 60: 920–924
75. Kollee L A, Verloove-Vanhorick P P, Verwey R A, Brand R, Ruys J H 1988 Maternal and neonatal transport: results of a national collaborative survey of preterm and very low birth weight infants in the Netherlands. Obstetrics and Gynecology 72: 729–732
76. Kuban K C K, Gilles F H 1985 Human telencephalic angiogenesis. Annals of neurology 17: 539–548
77. Kuban K C K, Leviton A, Krishnamoorthy K S et al 1986 Neonatal intracranial hemorrhage and phenobarbital. Pediatrics 77: 443–450
78. Kuban K C K, Leviton A, Pagano M, Fenton T, Strassfeld R, Wolff M 1992 Maternal toxemia is associated with reduced incidence of germinal matrix hemorrhage in premature babies. Journal of Child Neurology 7: 70–76
79. Larroche J C 1972 Posthaemorrhagic hydrocephalus in infancy. Biologia Neonatorum 20: 287–299
80. Larroche J C 1986 Fetal encephalopathies of circulatory origin. Biology of the Neonate 50: 61–74
80a. Levene M I 1981 Measurement of the growth of the lateral ventricles in preterm infants with real-time ultrasound. Archives of Disease in Childhood 56: 900–904
81. Levene M I, Starte D R 1981 A longitudinal study of posthaemorrhagic ventricular dilatation in the newborn. Archives of Disease in Childhood 56: 905–910
82. Levene M I, Wigglesworth J S, Dubowitz V 1983 Hemorrhagic periventricular leukomalacia in the neonate: a real-time ultrasound study. Pediatrics 71: 794–797
83. Levene M I, de Vries L S 1984 Extension of neonatal intraventricular haemorrhage. Archives of Disease in Childhood 59: 631–636
84. Leviton A, Gilles F H 1984 Acquired perinatal leukoencephalopathy. Annals of Neurology 16: 1–8
85. Leviton A, Pagano M, Kuban K C K, Krishnamoorthy K S, Sullivan K F, Alfred E N 1991 The epidemiology of germinal matrix haemorrhage during the first half day of life. Developmental Medicine and Child Neurology 33: 138–145
86. Leviton A, Kuban K C, Pagano M, Allred E N, Marter L V 1993 Antenatal corticosteroids appear to reduce the risk of postnatal germinal matrix hemorrhage in intubated low birth weight newborns. Pediatrics 91: 1083–1088
87. Leviton A 1993 Preterm birth and cerebral palsy: is tumor necrosis factor the missing link? Developmental Medicine and Child Neurology 35: 553–558
88. Lipp-Zwahlen A E, Miller A, Tuchschmid P, Duc G 1989 Oxygen affinity of haemoglobin modulates cerebral blood flow in premature infants. A study with the non-invasive xenon-133 method. Acta Paediatrica Scandinavica. Supplement 360: 26–32
89. Long W, Corbet A, Cotton R et al 1991 The American exosurf neonatal study group, and the Canadian exosurf neonatal study group. A controlled trial of synthetic surfactant in infants weighing 1250 g or less with respiratory distress syndrome. New England Journal of Medicine 325: 1696–1703
90. Lou H C, Lassen N A, Friis-Hansen B 1979 Impaired autoregulation of cerebral blood flow in the distressed newborn infant. Journal of Pediatrics 94: 118–121
91. Lowe J, Papile L A 1990 Neurodevelopmental performance of very low birth weight infants with mild periventricular, intraventricular hemorrhage. American Journal of Diseases of Children 144: 1242–1245
92. Marret S, Parain D, Jeannot E, Eurin D, Fessard C 1992 Positive rolandic sharp waves in the EEG of the premature newborn: a five year prospective study. Archives of Disease in Childhood 67: 948–951
93. Mayer P L, Kier E L 1991 The controversy of the periventricular white matter circulation: a review of the anatomic literature. American Journal of Neuroradiology 12: 223–228

94. McDonald M M, Rumack C M, Johnson M L 1984 Timing and antecedents of intracranial hemorrhage in the newborn. Pediatrics 74: 32–36
95. McMenamin J B, Shackelford D G, Volpe J J 1984 Outcome of neonatal intraventricular hemorrhage with periventricular echodense lesions. Annals of Neurology 15: 285–290
96. Ment L R, Duncan C C, Ehrenkrantz R A 1984 Intraventricular hemorrhage of the preterm neonate: timing and cerebral blood flow changes. Journal of Pediatrics 104: 419–425
97. Ment L R, Oh W, Philip A G S et al 1992 Risk factors for early intraventricular hemorrhage in low birth weight infants. Journal of Pediatrics 121: 776–783
98. Ment L R, Oh W, Ehrenkranz R A et al 1994 Low-dose indomethacin and prevention of intraventricular hemorrhage: a multicenter randomized trial. Pediatrics 93: 543–550
99. Ment L R, Vohr B, Oh W et al 1996 Neurodevelopmental outcome at 36 months corrected age of preterm infants in the multicenter indomethacin trial. Pediatrics 98: 714–718
100. Miall-Allen V, de Vries L S, Whitelaw A G L 1987 Mean arterial pressure and neonatal cerebral lesions. Archives of Disease in Childhood 62: 1068–1069
101. Miall-Allen V, de Vries L S, Dubowitz L M S, Whitelaw A G L 1989 Blood pressure fluctuation and intraventricular hemorrhage in the preterm infant of less than 31 weeks gestation. Pediatrics 83: 657–661
102. Moise A A, Wearden M E, Kozinetz C A, Gest A L, Welty S E, Hansen T E 1995 Antenatal steroids are associated with less need for blood pressure support in extremely premature infants. Pediatrics 95: 845–850
103. Morales W J, Koerten J 1986 Prevention of intraventricular hemorrhage in very low birth weight infants by maternally administered phenobarbital. Obstetrics and Gynecology 68: 295
104. Morales W J, Angel J L, O'Brien W F, Knuppel R A, Marsalisi F 1988 The use of antenatal vitamin K in the prevention of early neonatal intraventricular hemorrhage. American Journal of Obstetrics and Gynecology 159: 774–779
105. Murphy D J, Sellers S, MacKenzie I Z, Yudkin P L, Johnson A M 1995 Case control study of antenatal and intrapartum risk factors for cerebral palsy in very preterm singleton babies. Lancet 346: 1449–1454
106. Nelson K B, Ellenberg J H 1985 Antecedents of cerebral palsy; I univariate analysis of risk factors. New England Journal of Medicine 315: 81–86
107. Nelson M D, Gonzalez-Gomez I, Gilles F H 1991 The search for human telencephalic ventriculofugal arteries. American Journal of Neuroradiology 12: 215–222
108. Northern Neonatal Nursing Initiative Trial Group 1996 Randomised trial of prophylactic early fresh frozen plasma or gelatin or glucose in preterm babies: outcome at 2 years. Lancet 348: 229–232
109. Nwaesei C G, Pape K E, Martin D J, Becker L E, Fitz C R 1984 Periventricular infarction diagnosed by ultrasound: a postmortem correlation. Journal of Pediatrics 105: 106–110
110. Oka A, Belliveau M J, Rosenberg P A, Volpe J J 1993 Vulnerability of oligodendroglia to glutamate: pharmacology, mechanisms and prevention. Journal of Neuroscience 13: 1441–1453
111. Palmer P, Dubowitz L M S, Levene M I, Dubowitz V 1982 Developmental and neurological progress of preterm infants with intraventricular haemorrhage and ventricular dilatation. Archives of Disease in Childhood 57: 748–752
112. Paneth N, Rudelli R, Monte W et al 1990 White matter necrosis in very low birth weight infants: neuropathologic and ultrasonographic findings in infants surviving six days or longer. Journal of Pediatrics 116: 975–984
113. Paneth N, Rudelli R, Kazam E, Monte W 1994 Brain damage in the preterm infant. Clinics in Developmental Medicine No 131. MacKeith Press, London
114. Pape K E, Wigglesworth J S 1979 Haemorrhage, ischaemia and the perinatal brain. Clinics in Developmental Medicine no 69/70. SIMP/Heinemann, London, pp 133–148
115. Pape K E, Bennett-Button S, Szymonowicz W, Martin D J, Fitz C R, Becker L 1983 Diagnostic accuracy of neonatal brain imaging: a postmortem correlation of computed tomography and ultrasound scans. Journal of Pediatrics 102: 275–280
116. Papile L A, Burstein J, Burstein R, Koffler H 1978 Incidence and evolution of subependymal and intraventricular hemorrhage: a study of infants with birth weights less than 1500 gm. Journal of Pediatrics 92: 529–534
117. Pellicer A, Cabanas F, Garcia-Alix A, Rodriguez J P, Quero J 1993 Natural history of ventricular dilatation in preterm infants: prognostic significance. Paediatric Neurology 9: 108–114
118. Perlman J M, McMenamin J B, Volpe J J 1983 Fluctuating cerebral blood flow velocity in respiratory distress syndrome: relation to the development of intraventricular hemorrhage. New England Journal of Medicine 309: 204–209
119. Perlman J M, Volpe J J 1983 Suctioning in the preterm infant: effect on cerebral blood flow velocity, intracranial pressure and arterial blood pressure. Pediatrics 72: 329–334
120. Perlman J M, Goodman S, Kreusser K L, Volpe J J 1985 Reduction in intraventricular hemorrhage by elimination of fluctuating cerebral blood flow velocity in preterm infants with respiratory distress syndrome. New England Journal of Medicine 312: 1353–1357
121. Perlman J M, Volpe J J 1986 Intraventricular hemorrhage in extremely small premature infants. American Journal of Diseases of Children 140: 1122–1124
122. Perlman J M, Lynch B, Volpe J J 1990 Late development after arrest and resolution of neonatal posthaemorrhagic hydrocephalus. Developmental Medicine and Child Neurology 32: 725–742
123. Perlman J M, Rollins N, Burns D, Risser R 1993 Relationship between periventricular intraparenchymal echodensities and germinal matrix-intraventricular hemorrhage in the very low birth weight neonate. Pediatrics 91: 474–480
124. Perlman J M, Risser R, Broyles R S 1996 Bilateral cystic periventricular leukomalacia in the premature infant: associated risk factors. Pediatrics 97: 822–827
125. Philip A G S, Allan W C, Tito A M, Wheeler L R 1989 Intraventricular hemorrhage in preterm infants: declining incidence in the 1980s. Pediatrics 84: 797–801
126. Pidcock F S, Graziani L J, Stanley C, Mitchell D G, Merton D 1990 Neurosonographic features of periventricular echodensities associated with cerebral palsy in preterm infants. Journal of Pediatrics 116: 417–422.
127. Pinto-Martin J A, Riolo S, Cnaan A, Holzman C, Susser M W, Paneth N 1995 Cranial ultrasound prediction of disabling and nondisabling cerebral palsy at age two in a low birth weight population. Pediatrics 95: 249–254
128. Pomerance J J, Teal J G, Gogolok J F et al 1987 Maternally administered antenatal vitamin K1: effect on neonatal prothrombin activity, partial thromboplastin time, and intraventricular hemorrhage. Obstetrics and Gynecology 70: 235–241
129. Pryds O, Greisen G, Lou H, Friis-Hansen B 1989 Heterogeneity of cerebral vasoreactivity in preterm infants supported by mechanical ventilation. Journal of Pediatrics 115: 638–645
130. Pryds O, Christensen N J, Friis-Hansen H B 1990 Increased cerebral blood flow and plasma epinephrine in hypoglycemic, preterm neonates. Pediatrics 85: 172–176
131. Pryds O 1991 Control of cerebral circulation in the high-risk neonate. Annals of Neurology 30: 321–329
132. Pryds O 1994 Low neonatal cerebral oxygen delivery is associated with brain injury in preterm infants. Acta Paediatrica 93: 1233–1236
133. Rademaker K J, Groenendaal F, Jansen G H, Eken P, de Vries L S 1994 Unilateral haemorrhagic parenchymal lesions in the preterm infant: shape, site and prognosis. Acta Paediatrica 83: 602–608
134. Rennie J M 1997 Neonatal cerebral ultrasound. Cambridge University Press, Cambridge
135. Rennie J M, Wheater M, Cole T J 1996 Antenatal steroid administration is associated with an improved chance of intact survival in preterm infants. European Journal of Pediatrics 155: 576–579
136. Rogers B, Msall M, Owens T et al 1994 Cystic periventricular leukomalacia and type of cerebral palsy in preterm infants. Journal of Pediatrics 125: S1–8
137. Ruckensteiner E, Zollner F 1929 Uber die Blutungen im Gebiete der vena terminalis bei Neugeborenen. Frankfurt Zeitschrift für Pathologie 37: 568–578
138. Rumak C M, Guggenheim M A, Rumak B H, Peterson R G, Johnson M L, Braithwaite W R 1981 Neonatal intraventricular hemorrhage and maternal use of aspirin. Obstetrics and Gynecology 58: 52S–55S
139. Rushton D I, Preston P R, Durbin G M 1985 Structure and evolution of echodense lesions in the neonatal brain. Archives of Disease in Childhood 60: 798–808

140. Russell G A B, Jeffers G, Cooke R W I 1992 Plasma hypoxanthine: a marker for hypoxic–ischaemic induced periventricular leukomalacia. Archives of Disease in Childhood 67: 388–392
141. Russell G A B, Cooke R W I 1995 Randomised controlled trial of allopurinol prophylaxis in very preterm infants. Archives of Disease in Childhood 73: F27–F31
142. Salfield A W, Lorber J, Lonton T 1981 Isosorbide in the management of infantile hydrocephalus. Archives of Disease in Childhood 56: 806
143. Saliba E, Santini J J, Arbeille Ph et al 1985 Mesure non invasive du flux sanguin cérébral chez le nourisson hydrocéphale. Archives Francaise Pédiatrie 42: 97–102
144. Scher M S, Dobson V, Carpenter N A, Guthrie R D 1989 Visual and neurological outcome of infants with periventricular leukomalacia. Developmental Medicine and Child Neurology 31: 353–365
145. Shankaran S, Slovis T L, Bedard M P, Poland R L 1982 Sonographic classification of intracranial hemorrhage in the premature newborn infant. Journal of Pediatrics 100: 469–475
146. Shankaran S, Cepeda E E, Ilagan N et al 1986 Antenatal phenobarbital for the prevention of neonatal intracerebral hemorrhage. American Journal of Obstetrics and Gynecology 154: 53–57
147. Shankaran S, Koepke T, Woldt E et al 1989 Outcome after posthemorrhagic ventriculomegaly in comparison with mild hemorrhage without ventriculomegaly. Journal of Pediatrics 114: 109–114
148. Shankaran S, Papile L-A, Wright L L et al 1997 The effect of antenatal phenobarbital therapy on neonatal intracranial haemorrhage. New England Journal of Medicine 337: 466–471
149. Shankaran S, Bauer C R, Bain R, Wright L L, Zachary J 1995 Relationship between antenatal steroid administration and grades III and IV intracranial hemorrhage in low birthweight infants. American Journal of Obstetrics and Gynecology 173: 305–312
150. Shinnar S, Gammon K, Bergman E W, Epstein M, Freedom J M 1985 Management of hydrocephalus in infancy: use of acetazolamide and furosemide to avoid cerebrospinal fluid shunts. Journal of Pediatrics 107: 31–36
151. Shortland D B, Trounce J Q, Levene M I 1987 Hyperkalaemic cardiac arrythmias and cerebral lesions in high risk infants. Archives of Disease in Childhood 62: 1139–1143
152. Shortland D B, Gibson N A, Levene M I, Archer L N J, Evans D H, Shaw D E 1990 Patent ductus arteriosus and cerebral circulation in preterm infants. Developmental Medicine and Child Neurology 32: 386–393
153. Sims M E, Beckwitt Turkel S, Halterman G, Paul R H 1985 Brain injury and intrauterine death. American Journal of Obstetrics and Gynecology 151: 721–723
154. Speer M E, Blifield C, Rudolph A J, Chadda P, Holbein M E, Hittner A J, 1984 Intraventricular hemorrhage and vitamin E in the very low birth weight infant: evidence for efficacy of early intramuscular vitamin E administration. Pediatrics 74: 1107–1112
155. Spinillo A, Ometto A, Bottino R, Piazzi G, Iasci A, Rondini G 1995 Antenatal risk factors for germinal matrix hemorrhage and intraventricular hemorrhage in preterm infants. European Journal of Obstetrics Gynecology and Reproductive Biology 60: 13–19
156. Stewart A L, Thorburn R J, Hope P L, Goldsmith M, Lipscomb A P, Reynolds E O R 1983 Ultrasound appearance of the brain in very preterm infants and neurodevelopmental outcome at 18 months of age. Archives of Disease in Childhood 58: 598–604
157. Szymonowicz W, Yu V Y H, Wilson F E 1984 Antecedents of periventricular haemorrhage in infants weighing 1250 gram or less at birth. Archives of Disease in Childhood 59: 13–17
158. Szymonowicz W, Preston H, Yu V Y H 1986 The surviving monozygotic twin. Archives of Disease in Childhood 61: 454–458
159. Szymonowicz W, Yu V Y H, Bajuk B, Astbury J 1986 Neurodevelopmental outcome of periventricular haemorrhage and leukomalacia in infants 1250 g or less at birth. Early Human Development 14: 1–7
160. Takashima J, Tanaka K 1978 Development of cerebral architecture and its relationship to periventricular leukomalacia. Archives of Neurology 35: 11–16
161. Takashima S, Takashi M, Ando Y 1986 Pathogenesis of periventricular white matter haemorrhage in preterm infants. Brain Development 8: 25–30
162. The EC Ethamsylate Trial Group 1994 The EC randomised controlled trial of prophylactic ethamsylate for very preterm neonates: early mortality and morbidity. Archives of Disease in Childhood 70: F201–F205
163. Thorburn R J, Lipscomb A P, Stewart A L, Reynolds E O R, Hope P L 1982 Timing and antecedents of periventricular haemorrhage and of cerebral atrophy in very preterm infants. Early Human Development 7: 221–238
164. Thorp J A, Parriott J, Ferrette-Smith D, Meyer B A, Cohen G R, Johnson J 1994 Antepartum vitamin K and phenobarbital for preventing intraventricular hemorrhage in the premature newborn: a randomised double-blind, placebo-controlled trial. Obstetrics and Gynecology 83: 70–76
165. Trounce J Q, Rutter N, Levene M I 1986 Periventricular leukomalacia and intraventricular haemorrhage in the preterm neonate. Archives of Disease in Childhood 61: 1196–1202
166. Trounce J Q, Fagan D, Levene M I 1986 Intraventricular haemorrhage and periventricular leukomalacia: ultrasound and autopsy correlation. Archives of Disease in Childhood 61: 1203–1207
167. Trounce J Q, Shaw O E, Levene M I, Rutter N 1988 Clinical risk factors and periventricular leukomalacia. Archives of Disease in Childhood 63: 17–22
168. Tsiantos A, Victorin L, Relier P et al 1974 Intracranial hemorrhage in the prematurely born infant. Timing of clots and evaluation of clinical signs and symptoms. Journal of Pediatrics 85: 854–859
169. van de Bor M, Verloove-Vanhorick S P, Brand R, Keirse M J N C, Ruys J H 1987 Incidence and prediction of periventricular–intraventricular hemorrhage in very preterm infants. Journal of Perinatal Medicine 15: 333–339
170. van de Bor M, Ma E J, Walther F J 1991 Cerebral blood flow velocity after surfactant installation in preterm infants Journal of Pediatrics 118: 285–287
171. van Bel F, van de Bor M, Stijnen T, Baan J, Ruys J H 1987 Aetiological role of cerebral blood-flow alterations in development and extension of peri-intraventricular haemorrhage. Developmental Medicine and Child Neurology 29: 601–614
172. Vanucci R C, Towfighi J, Heitjan D F, Brucklacher R M 1995 Carbon dioxide protects the perinatal brain from hypoxic–ischemic damage: an experimental study in the immature rat. Pediatrics 95: 868–874
172a. Vannuci R C, Brucklacher R M, Vannuci S J 1997 Effect of carbon dioxide on cerebral metabolism during hypoxia–ischaemia in the immature rat. Pediatric Research 42: 24–29
173. Ventriculomegaly Trial Group 1990 Randomised trial of early tapping in neonatal posthaemorrhagic ventricular dilatation. Archives of Disease in Childhood 65: 3–10
174. Ventriculomegaly Trial Group 1994 Randomised trial of early tapping in neonatal posthaemorrhagic ventricular dilatation: results at 30 months. Archives of Disease in Childhood 70: F129–F136
175. Verma U, Tejani N, Klein S et al 1997 Obstetric antecedents of intraventricular hemorrhage and periventricular leukomalacia in the very low birthweight infant. American Journal of Obstetrics and Gynaecology 176: 275–281
176. Versmold H T, Kitterman J A, Phibbs R H, Gregory G A, Tooley W H 1981 Aortic blood pressure during the first 12 h of life in infants with birthweight 610 to 4222 grams. Pediatrics 67: 607–613
177. Virchow R 1867 Zur pathologischen Anatomie des Gehirns I: congenitale encephalitis und myelitis. Virchows Archiv 38: 129–142
178. Vohr B R, Garcia-Coll C, Flanagan P, Oh W 1992 Effects of intraventricular hemorrhage and socioeconomic status on perceptual, cognitive, and neurologic status of low birth weight infants at 5 years of age. Journal of Pediatrics 121: 280–285
179. Volpe J J 1977 Neonatal intracranial hemorrhage: pathophysiology, neuropathology and clinical features. Clinics in Perinatology 4: 77–102
180. Volpe J J 1989 Intraventricular hemorrhage in the premature infant–current concepts. Part I. Annals of Neurology 25: 3–11
181. Volpe J J 1990 Brain injury in the premature infant: is it preventable? Pediatric Research 27: 28–33
182. Volpe J J 1995 Neonatal Neurology, 3rd edn. Saunders, Philadelphia, pp 403-463
183. Wallin L A, Rosenfeld C R, Laptook A R et al 1990 Neonatal intracranial haemorrhage: II. Risk factor analysis in an inborn population. Early Human Development 23: 129–137
184. Watkins A M C, West C R, Cooke R W I 1989 Blood pressure and cerebral haemorrhage and ischaemia in very low birthweight infants. Early Human Development 19: 103–110

185. Weindling A M, Rochefort M J, Calvert S A, Fok T F, Wilkinson A 1985 Development of cerebral palsy after sonographic detection of periventricular cysts in the newborn. Developmental Medicine and Child Neurology 27: 800–806
186. Wells J T, Ment L R 1995 Prevention of intraventricular haemorrhage in preterm infants. Early Human Development 42: 209–233
187. Weninger M, Salzer H R, Pollak A et al 1992 External ventricular drainage for treatment of rapidly progressive posthemorrhagic hydrocephalus. Neurosurgery 31: 52–58
188. Whitelaw A, Rivers R P, Creighton L, Gaffney P 1992 Low dose intraventricular fibrinolytic treatment to prevent posthaemorrhagic hydrocephalus. Archives of Disease in Childhood 67: 12–14
189. Wimberley P D, Lou H C, Pedersen H 1982 Hypertensive peaks in the pathogenesis of intraventricular haemorrhage in the newborn: abolition by phenobarbitone sedation. Acta Paediatrica Scandinavica 71: 537–542
190. Wiswell T E, Graziani L J, Kornhauser M S et al 1996 Effects of hypocarbia on the development of cystic periventricular leukomalacia in premature infants treated with high frequency jet ventilation. Pediatrics 98: 918–924
191. Wiswell T E, Graziani L J, Kornhauser M S et al 1996 High frequency jet ventilation in the early management of respiratory distress syndrome is associated with a greater risk for adverse outcomes. Pediatrics 98: 1035–1043
192. Zorzi C, Angonese I, Zaramella P et al 1988 Periventricular intraparenchymal cystic lesions: critical determinant of neurodevelopmental outcome in preterm infants. Helvetica Paediatrica Acta 43: 195–202

Part 6

Hereditary and degenerative central nervous system disease

Alan Hill

INTRODUCTION

Most hereditary disorders with central nervous system involvement which result in clinical manifestations during the newborn period relate either to chromosomal abnormalities and genetic syndromes or to inborn errors of metabolism. These conditions are discussed more appropriately elsewhere (see Chapter 34 Inherited genetic disease and Chapter 38 Metabolic disease). However, there are several rare hereditary degenerative disorders that affect principally the central nervous system in the newborn, which are not categorized easily according to the above classifications but which nevertheless may have important prognostic, genetic and therapeutic implications. These rare hereditary disorders may be classified according to whether they affect predominantly grey matter, white matter or a combination of both.[64] Clearly, there is considerable overlap in the clinical features and neuropathology between these major categories.

DISORDERS PRIMARILY AFFECTING GREY MATTER

The clinical presentation of disorders with primary grey matter involvement usually includes prominent seizures or myoclonus, regression or lack of cognitive development, retinal disease and epileptiform abnormalities on electroencephalography. Some of these disorders have associated visceral storage, e.g. GM-1 gangliosidosis, Sandhoff variant of GM-2 gangliosidosis, Niemann–Pick disease (types A and C), infantile Gaucher disease, Farber disease and infantile sialic acid storage disease. Clinically such visceral storage may be recognized by hepatosplenomegaly, often associated with coarse facies and long bone abnormalities.

All of these disorders are inherited in an autosomal recessive manner, except Menkes' disease, which is X-linked. Prenatal diagnosis is available in all instances. The major hereditary degenerative disorders affecting grey matter are summarized in Table 44.18.

TAY–SACHS DISEASE (INFANTILE GM-2 GANGLIOSIDOSIS)

This autosomal recessive disorder, which occurs most commonly in infants of Ashkenazi Jewish ancestry, is caused by a deficiency of the enzyme hexosaminidase A. In the Sandhoff variant there is a deficiency of both isozymes of hexosaminidase (A and B). This disorder appears to have considerable genetic heterogeneity.

Clinical features

Symptoms begin insidiously during the first months of life, with listlessness, hypotonia, irritability and hyperacusis following initially normal growth and development. Affected infants develop marked sensitivity to sound and other sensory stimuli, which characteristically elicit massive startle responses which do not habituate. Careful fundoscopy reveals the classic cherry-red spot in the macular region which results from ganglioside storage in retinal ganglion cells surrounding the normally red fovea. This abnormality is invariably present when neurological symptoms develop, and has been identified as early as 2 days of age.[19] There is usually rapid deterioration of neurological status, with intractable seizures (especially myoclonic), complete blindness with preserved pupillary light reflexes, loss of all voluntary movement, spasticity and opisthotonus, and progressive macrocephaly after

Table 44.18 Hereditary degenerative diseases primarily affecting grey matter

Disease	Enzyme defect	Sotroge material (in brain)	Visceromegaly	Major clinical features
Tay–Sachs disease (GM-2 gangliosidosis)	(a) Hexosaminidase A (b) Hexosaminidase A & B (Sandhoff variant) (c) Activator deficiency	GM-2 ganglioside Sandhoff variant: globoside in viscera	– Sandhoff variant: +	Hyperacusis, cherry-red macula, seizures, blindness, Sandhoff variant: hepatosplenomegaly
Infantile neuronal ceroid-lipofucsinosis (Santavuori disease)	Unknown	Ceroid-lipofuscin	–	Severe seizures, microcephaly later vegetative state
Alper disease	? Mitochondrial dysfunction	Possibly elevated lactate/pyruvate levels in CSF or blood	–	Seizures, myoclonus, developmental arrest and regression, late hepatic dysfunction
Menkes' disease (kinky hair disease)	Copper-containing enzymes	Copper	–	Hypothermia, seizures, developmental repression, colourless 'steely' hair
GM-1 gangliosidosis	β-galactosidase	GM-1 ganglioside	+	Coarse facies, cherry red macula, bony abnormalities
Niemann–Pick disease (types A and C)	Type A: sphingomyelinase Type C: defective esterification of cholesterol	Sphingomyelin non-esterified cholesterol	+	Failure to thrive, seizures, peripheral neuropathy
Infantile Gaucher disease (type 2)	Glucocerebrosidase	Glucocerebroside, glucosphingosine	+	Skin abnormalities, hydrops, laryngeal spasm, fractures, spasticity
Farber disease	Ceramidase	Ceramide	±	Joint swelling, hyperaesthesia, hoarse cry, vomiting, recurrent infections
Infantile sialic acid storage disease and sialidosis	Abnormal sialic acid transport, sialidase	Oligosaccharides (sialic acid)	+	Hydrops, dysostosis, corneal opacification

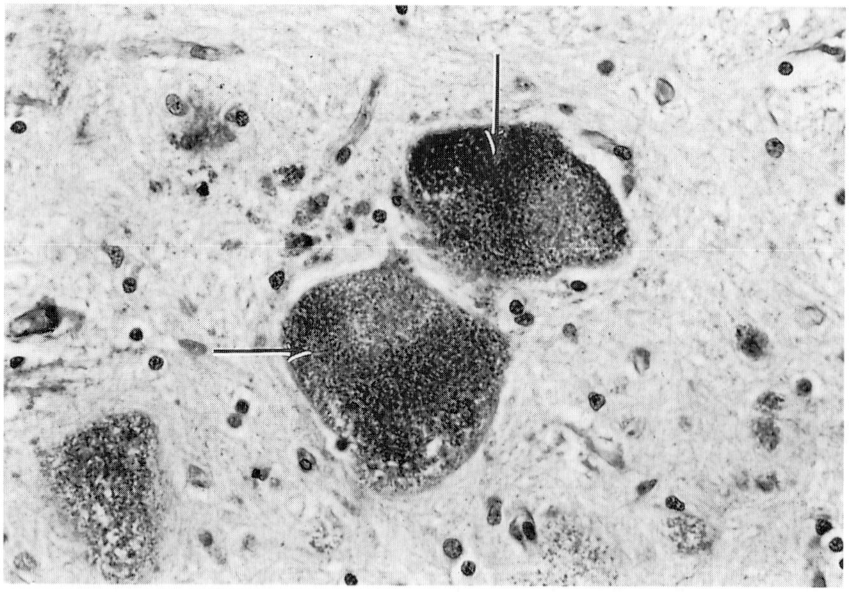

Fig. 44.45 Tay–Sachs disease. Photomicrograph of motor neurons of anterior horn of spinal cord. Note dark-coloured storage material which is PAS positive within cytoplasm (arrows). (×280)

12 months of age. There is no effective treatment and death usually occurs before 4 years of age. In the Sandhoff variant there is also progressive hepatosplenomegaly and cardiac involvement.

Diagnosis

Diagnosis as well as detection of carrier/heterozygote status is achieved by serum hexosaminidase assay or by identification of the enzyme defect in leukocytes or

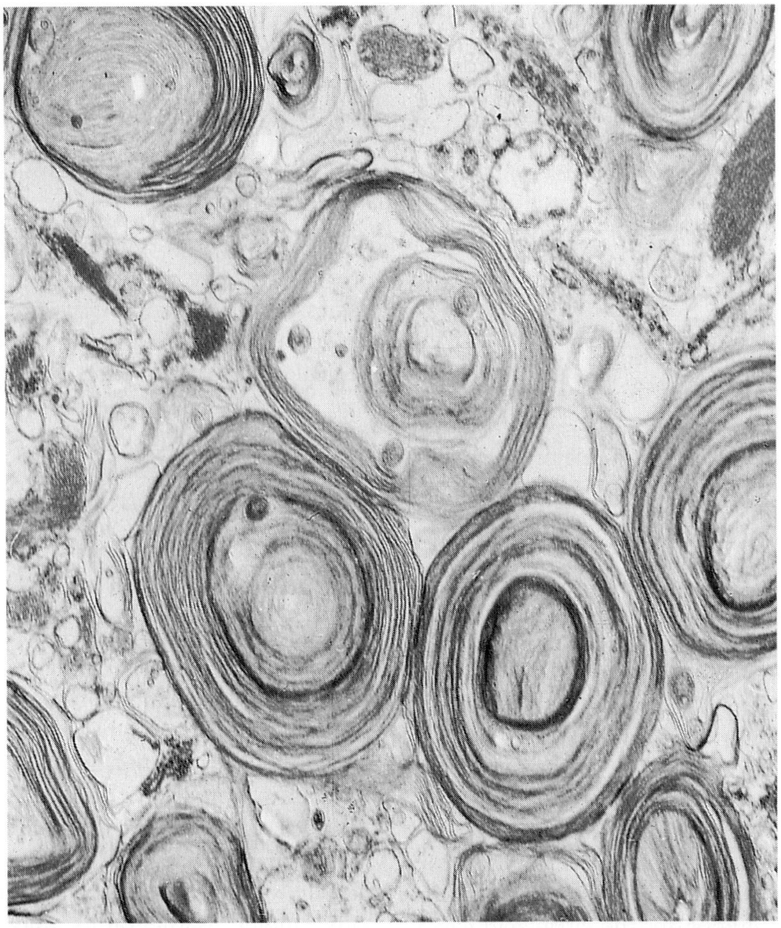

Fig. 44.46 Tay–Sachs disease. Electron micrograph of membranous cytoplasmic bodies. (×7360)

cultured fibroblasts. The serum hexosaminidase assay has been automated and mass screening programmes have been established to establish carrier states in high-risk populations.[30]

In affected infants routine cerebrospinal fluid studies are normal. Serum glutamic-oxaloacetic transaminase and lactic dehydrogenase levels may be elevated. Neuroimaging demonstrates low density and occasionally increased volume of thalami, basal ganglia and white matter on CT scans, as well as increased signal in these regions on T2-weighted MRI. The EEG may demonstrate a hypsarrhythmic pattern or multifocal spike activity. Electroretinography is usually normal.

Prenatal diagnosis and detection of carriers is possible by enzymatic assay of cultured amniotic fluid cells or chorionic villus sampling.[20]

Pathology

Depending on the time of death in relation to the stage of progression of the disease, the brain may be either increased or decreased in total weight and volume. Histological examination and electron microscopy reveal decreased numbers of neurons, which are distorted and swollen. The neurons are filled with membranous cytoplasmic inclusions which contain GM-2 ganglioside and displace the cell nuclei peripherally. (Figs 44.45, 44.46) There is astrocytic proliferation with fusiform swelling of axons (termed 'torpedoes'). The liver, spleen, anterior horn cells and serum also contain increased amounts of GM-2 ganglioside. The ganglioside content of other viscera is normal.

EARLY INFANTILE NEURONAL CEROID LIPOFUSCINOSIS (SANTAVUORI DISEASE)

The early infantile form of neuronal ceroid lipofuscinosis has been linked to the short arm of chromosome 1.[29] The precise biochemical abnormality is unknown.

Clinical features

Although symptoms begin most commonly between 9 and 18 months of age, rare cases have presented during the neonatal period, with severe seizures and microcephaly followed by rapid progression to a vegetative state with severe spasticity and death during the first weeks of life.[69] There is no retinal cherry-red spot, although pigmentary retinal degeneration may occur.[5]

Diagnosis

Diagnosis is based on identification of the autofluorescent lipopigments (ceroid and lipofuscin) in lymphocytes, skin or rectal mucosa.

The MRI scan demonstrates severe progressive cerebral atrophy.[13] Other characteristic abnormalities include the early loss of electroretinographic and visual evoked responses and subsequent development of an isoelectric EEG.[24,47]

Prenatal diagnosis may be made by electron microscopy of chorionic villus sampling or by DNA analysis.[28,46]

Pathology

The affected brain is small, with cortical atrophy due to diffuse severe neuronal loss. Microscopic examination demonstrates mild neuronal distension by accumulation of granular, PAS and Sudan black-positive, autofluorescent ceroid–lipofuscin in neurons, glia and macrophages.

ALPER DISEASE

This progressive degenerative disease of the grey matter may be a mitochondrial disorder possibly related to disturbances in pyruvate metabolism, the citric acid cycle or abnormalities of complex 1 of the electron transport chain.[60]

Clinical features

Affected infants are hypotonic and demonstrate seizures and stimulus-sensitive myoclonus and vomiting during the first weeks of life. Clinical liver dysfunction usually becomes evident after 9 months of age, but may be suspected early on the basis of elevated serum transaminase levels. Most infants die before the age of 3.

Diagnosis

There is no specific diagnostic investigation.

Pathology

Affected infants have major cortical neuronal loss and gliosis, often associated with capillary proliferation, which is most evident in deep cortical layers and striate (occipital) cortex.

MENKES' DISEASE

This X-linked disorder results from impaired transport of copper across cellular compartments such that body copper is unavailable for synthesis of copper-containing enzymes, e.g. caeruloplasmin, superoxide dismutase, cytochrome oxidase, and especially lysyl oxidase (causing failure in elastin and collagen cross-linking).

Clinical features

Symptoms appear during the newborn period and include hypothermia, hyperbilirubinaemia and poor feeding. The facies are described as 'cherubic', with a depressed nasal bridge and fine, colourless hair. There is rapid neurological deterioration with marked hypotonia and seizures and development of the characteristic, friable, kinky hair. There may be hydronephrosis and bladder diverticulum and long bone changes, including metaphyseal spurring and diaphyseal periosteal reaction.

Diagnosis

Diagnosis is confirmed by serial serum copper and caeruloplasmin levels, which are normally low in the newborn period and subsequently fail to rise to adult levels during the first month of life. Alternatively, serum levels may be normal initially but decrease rather than increase normally during subsequent weeks. Cultured fibroblasts or lymphocytes demonstrate increased levels of copper. Copper levels are low in the liver and brain, but elevated in other tissues, e.g. intestine, muscle, spleen and kidney. Radiographs may demonstrate long bone changes. CT and MRI invariably demonstrate cerebral atrophy and encephalomalacia, asymptomatic subdural haematomas and tortuosity of the intracranial vessels. Electroencephalography demonstrates multifocal epileptiform discharges or hypsarrhythmia. Visual evoked responses are absent or diminished in amplitude.

Prenatal diagnosis may be made on the basis of increased copper content of chorionic villi during the first trimester or cultured amniotic fluid cells during the second trimester.[59]

Pathology

Cerebral abnormalities result from vascular lesions or copper deficiency and include cortical neuronal loss, gliosis and severe axonal degeneration in the white matter and cerebellum. Electron microscopy may demonstrate increased numbers of abnormal mitochondria.

GM-1 GANGLIOSIDOSIS (PSEUDO-HURLER SYNDROME) TYPE I

In generalized GM-1 gangliosidosis there is deficiency of the enzyme β-galactosidase, which results in the accumulation of GM-1 ganglioside in cerebral grey matter, liver and spleen.

Clinical features

Severe type 1 GM-1 gangliosidosis may present during the newborn period with hypotonia, abnormalities of sucking and swallowing and delayed development. Affected infants have characteristic coarse facies, with hirsutism, frontal bossing, low-set ears and hypertrophy of the gums and tongue. Non-pitting generalized oedema may be striking and ascites may occur in the newborn period.[1] Ocular abnormalities include a retinal cherry-red spot in approximately 50% of cases, corneal clouding or optic atrophy.[51] Abnormalities of skeletal and cardiac muscle may occur.[11] Seizures and hepatosplenomegaly occur most commonly after 6 months of age, and death usually occurs during the second year.

Diagnosis

The diagnosis may be suspected in infants who have clinical and radiological bone changes similar to those observed in Hurler syndrome, with normal excretion of mucopolysaccharides. Diagnosis may be confirmed by demonstration of reduced activity of β-galactosidase in leukocytes, cultured fibroblasts or conjunctival biopsy. Cholera toxin B and its antibody may be used to demonstrate accumulation of ganglioside in the cerebral cortex and peripheral nerves.[27]

Prenatal diagnosis may be made by enzyme analysis of either cultured amniocytes or cell-free amniotic fluid.[36]

Pathology

The monosialoganglioside (GM-1) normally comprises approximately 20% of brain tissue gangliosides. In generalized type 1 GM-1 gangliosidosis the quantity of stored GM-1 increases dramatically to 80–90% of total grey matter gangliosides. Although the concentration of GM-1 is highest in the cerebral cortex, it is also deposited in peripheral nerves, liver and spleen.[27] A unique feature of type 1 GM-1 gangliosidosis is the deposition of a mucopolysaccharide which resembles keratin sulphate, especially in the liver and other organs.[43,54] The basis for storage of the mucopolysaccharide material is unknown.

INFANTILE NIEMANN–PICK DISEASE

Two varieties of lysosomal storage disease (types A and C) may have an acute infantile presentation. These autosomal recessive lysosomal storage disorders result in accumulation of sphingomyelin in the reticuloendothelial system. In type A Niemann–Pick disease there is deficiency of the lysosomal (acid) sphingomyelinase enzyme secondary to a gene mutation on the short arm of chromosome 11.[34] This results in a marked accumulation of sphingomyelin and non-esterified cholesterol, as well as glucosyl ceramide and glycerol-phospholipid in viscera. In type C Niemann–Pick disease there is relatively normal sphingomyelinase activity but defective esterification of cholesterol, which leads to lysosomal storage of non-esterified cholesterol and sphingomyelin.[8]

Clinical features

Early clinical features include feeding difficulties and failure to thrive during the first weeks of life. Persistent neonatal jaundice and massive hepatosplenomegaly are common symptoms during the newborn period. Neurological deterioration often becomes apparent by 6 months of age, and is characterized by deterioration of motor function (hypotonia, areflexia) related to slowed nerve conductions and general 'apathy'. Macular degeneration and the presence of a retinal cherry-red spot are observed in approximately 25–50% of cases. As the disease progresses there is further deterioration in both motor and intellectual function, resulting ultimately in rigidity and obtundation. Seizures, especially myoclonic seizures, occur frequently but are less common early in the disease than in Tay–Sachs disease. There is variable progression, but death occurs usually before 5 years of age.[8,52]

Diagnosis

Niemann–Pick disease type A may be confirmed by deficiency of sphingomyelinase activity in leukocytes and skin fibroblasts to less than 10% of normal. In Niemann–Pick disease type C, sea-blue histiocytes and foam cells are seen in the bone marrow.[62] More specific diagnosis may be possible by measurement of increased amounts of unesterified cholesterol in fibroblasts. Nerve conduction studies may be slowed and peripheral nerve biopsy may demonstrate inclusion bodies in Schwann cells.[21]

Prenatal diagnosis of type A disease may be made by demonstration of decreased sphingomyelinase activity in cultured amniotic fibroblasts.[61]

Pathology

Large lipid-laden cells are found in the reticuloendothelial systems, e.g. spleen, bone marrow, liver, lymph nodes and lungs. In the brain there are ballooned ganglion cells and foam cells, especially in the cerebellum, brain stem and spinal cord, as well as lipid storage in perivascular cerebral tissues, choroid plexus and meninges.

INFANTILE GAUCHER'S DISEASE (TYPE 2)

The enzyme defect in this autosomal recessive disease involves lysosomal glucocerebrosidase, which results in storage of cerebrosides in the reticuloendothelial system. The defective gene is located on the long arm of chromosome 1, but there appears to be no direct correlation between an individual's genotype and phenotype. The disease types tend to be similar in siblings.[9] In the infantile disease there may be focal increase in glucocerebroside in the brain as well as accumulation of glucosphingosine.

Clinical features

A rapidly progressive neonatal variety presents with congenital ichthyosis or collodion skin, hepatosplenomegaly and hydrops fetalis.[49] Neurological abnormalities which may be seen during the newborn period include hyperextension of the head, spasticity and strabismus, followed by profound irritability and psychomotor retardation. Laryngeal spasm and seizures may occur. Bones become rarefied and fractures are common. Death occurs usually before 2 years of age.

Diagnosis

A definitive diagnosis is achieved by demonstration of diminished β-glucosidase in leukocytes, skin fibroblasts or liver. Serum acid phosphatase is elevated and characteristic modified macrophages (Gaucher cells) are present in spleen and bone marrow. Heterozygotes may be recognized by reduced enzyme activity in leukocytes.

Prenatal diagnosis is possible by demonstration of the enzyme defect or restriction fragment polymorphism in cultured amniotic fluid cells or chorionic villus sampling.

There is a possibility for therapy of affected infants by bone marrow transplantation or retrovirus-mediated gene transfer.[6]

Pathology

Gaucher cells, which are pathognomonic of this disease, are found in liver, bone marrow, spleen, lymph nodes and other organs. Their cytoplasm has a unique architecture, with a wrinkled or pleated appearance. Electron microscopic studies demonstrate large, membrane-enclosed sacs containing tubular structures. Examination of the nervous system reveals neuronophagia, decreased numbers of neurons, especially in the cerebral cortex, brain stem and cerebellar nuclei. In infantile Gaucher's disease there is no apparent neuronal storage.

FARBER DISEASE (LIPOGRANULOMATOSIS)

This extremely rare lysosomal storage disease has absent ceramidase activity in the brain, kidneys and skin fibroblasts, with a marked increase in ceramide in affected tissues. There is also increase in gangliosides in subcutaneous nodules.

Clinical features

Onset is in early infancy and the initial signs include periarticular swelling of the hands and feet associated with hyperaesthesia and a hoarse cry. Later, flexion contractures of the joints develop and subcutaneous nodules are found on the dorsum of the hands and feet. Dyspnoea may occur as a result of infiltration of the lungs. There are ongoing problems with vomiting, diarrhoea, recurrent infections and failure to thrive. Neurological features include hypotonia, weakness, muscle atrophy and hyporeflexia due to anterior horn cell and peripheral nerve involvement. Hepatosplenomegaly occurs in 50% of cases. Death from pulmonary disease occurs before 2 years of age.[40]

Diagnosis

Diagnosis is made on the basis of the characteristic clinical features described above, and the typical histological features of the subcutaneous nodules. Routine laboratory investigations are usually normal except for elevation of cerebrospinal fluid protein. The defective enzyme, ceramidase, can be measured in cultured skin fibroblasts and prenatal diagnosis is made by analysis of cultured amniotic fluid cells.

Pathology

The yellowish firm subcutaneous nodules contain granulomas with fibrous tissue and numerous histiocytes, which often have foamy cytoplasm. There is extra fibrous tissue in the larynx (which accounts for the hoarseness). The perialveolar and peribronchial regions contain histiocytes and there may be pulmonary fibrosis. Neuronal storage and cell loss occurs, especially in anterior horn cells.

INFANTILE SIALIC ACID STORAGE DISEASE AND SIALIDOSIS

Sialic acid is an oligosaccharide component of glycoproteins. Problems may relate to disorders of sialic acid transport (sialuria or sialic acid storage disease)[16] or relate to a defect in the lysosomal enzyme (sialidase) that degrades oligosaccharides (sialidosis).[58]

Clinical features

Both sialuria and sialidosis may present during the neonatal period, with generalized oedema (hydrops), hepatosplenomegaly with ascites, coarse dysmorphic facies, dysostosis of long bones and corneal opacification. Infants with sialuria also have thin, white hair. Subsequently they have severe anaemia, failure to thrive and developmental regression.

Diagnosis

In sialuria (infantile sialic acid storage disease) there is increased free sialic acid in plasma and urine and normal

Table 44.19 Hereditary degenerative diseases affecting primarily white matter

Disease	Clinical features	Diagnosis	Antenatal diagnosis	Inheritance	Pathology
Krabbe's leukodystrophy	Irritability, stiffening, feeding difficulties, peripheral neuropathy Death before age 2 years	Galactosyl Ceramidase I High CSF protein	+	Autosomal recessive	Paucity of myelin in CNS Globoid cells in white matter Segmental demyelination in peripheral nervous system
Pelizaeus–Merzbacher disease	Nystagmus, head lag, microcephaly, stridor	Clinical features DNA analysis	–	X-linked	Cerebral and cerebellar atrophy Patchy demyelination
Canavan's disease	Excessive head growth, lethargy, irritability, hypotonia, sucking and swallowing problems	Clinical features Neuroimaging Increased *N*-acetylaspartic acid in urine	–	Autosomal recessive	Paucity of myelin, spongy appearance Swelling of astrocytes of cerebral and cerebellar cortex Abnormal mitochondria
Alexander's disease	Excessive head growth Spasticity Seizures	Clinical features Neuroimaging Pathology	–	Usually sporadic	Soft white matter Loss of myelin Rosenthal fibres in cerebral cortex and white matter
Metachromatic leukodystrophy	Rare in neonatal period	Arylsulphatase A	+	Autosomal recessive	Metachromatic lipids in CNS and in Schwann cells

activity of α-neuraminidase activity in fibroblasts. Sialidosis is diagnosed by deficiency of α-neuraminidase activity in fibroblasts.

Similarly, prenatal diagnosis of infantile sialic acid storage disease is made by demonstration of increased free sialic acid levels in cultured amniotic fluid cells. Sialidosis is diagnosed prenatally by decreased α-neuraminidase activity.

Pathology

In sialidosis the brain has membrane-bound vacuoles in the cerebral cortex and Purkinje cells and 'zebra bodies' in spinal cord neurons, with storage of sialic acid-containing oligosaccharides.

DISORDERS AFFECTING PRIMARILY WHITE MATTER

The major hereditary-degenerative disorders affecting principally the white matter are summarized in Table 44.19.

KRABBE LEUKODYSTROPHY (GLOBOID CELL LEUKODYSTROPHY, GALACTOCEREBROSIDE LIPIDOSIS)

In this autosomal recessive disorder the basic defect is deficiency of galactosylceramidase 1 (galactocerebroside β-galactosidase) in leukocytes, brain liver, spleen and cultured skin fibroblasts, which breaks down galactosyl sphingosine (psychosine) which is toxic to oligodendroglial cells. With the destruction of oligodendroglia and accumulation of galactosylsphingosine there is arrest of myelin formation.[55]

Clinical features

The various modes of presentation at different ages have been reviewed.[55] Approximately 25% of cases present before 3 months of age, and onset in the newborn period has been reported.[23] It is associated with hyperirritability, increased muscle tone, hypersensitivity to stimulation, unexplained recurrent fever and poor feeding. There is no hepatosplenomegaly but the head circumference often increases disproportionately. There is progressive deterioration, resulting in death before 1 year of age in 70% of cases.[55] Peripheral neuropathy, which may be suspected on the basis of depressed tendon reflexes and markedly increased levels of cerebrospinal fluid protein, may be an early feature of Krabbe's disease and can be confirmed by nerve conduction studies.[35]

Clarke et al[12] reported a case of Krabbe's disease which presented with irritability and 'twitchiness' from birth. By 2 weeks of age there were feeding difficulties, drowsiness, respiratory distress with tachypnoea and seizures. Chest radiographs demonstrated evidence of diffuse inflammatory lung disease. There was progressive neurological deterioration, followed by death at 15 weeks of age. At autopsy the lungs were firm with a fine granular appearance in cut sections. Galactocerebroside β-galactosidase activity was absent in leukocytes.

Diagnosis

Identification of affected children and carriers is achieved by absence or greatly reduced β-galactosidase galactosylceramidase in the serum, leukocytes or skin fibroblasts, and prenatal diagnosis is possible using this enzyme assay on amniotic fluid cells or chorionic villus sampling.[56] Motor nerve conduction velocities are often slow, with evidence of denervation on electromyography. Computed tomography demonstrates increased density in the thalami and posterior limb of the internal capsule, as well as non-specific changes in white matter[3] which may be better defined by increased signal on T2-weighted MRI images, especially in the parietal lobes.[14]

Pathology

The principal neuropathological findings are paucity of myelin within the CNS (Fig. 44.47) and segmental demyelination in peripheral nerves, which results in moderate cortical atrophy. Vast numbers of globoid cells are observed in white matter, but also in lungs, spleen and lymph nodes. Electron microscopy of these cells reveals intracellular and extracellular crystalline inclusions (Fig. 44.48).

PELIZAEUS–MERZBACHER DISEASE

Pelizaeus–Merzbacher disease is considered to be a sudanophilic leukodystrophy. The inheritance pattern may be X-linked recessive, involving a gene on the long arm of

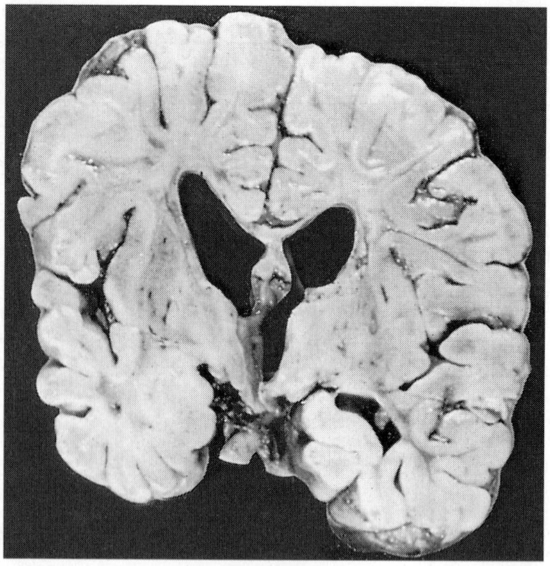

Fig. 44.47 Krabbe's disease. Note widespread atrophy and demyelination of white matter and previous secondary ventricular enlargement.

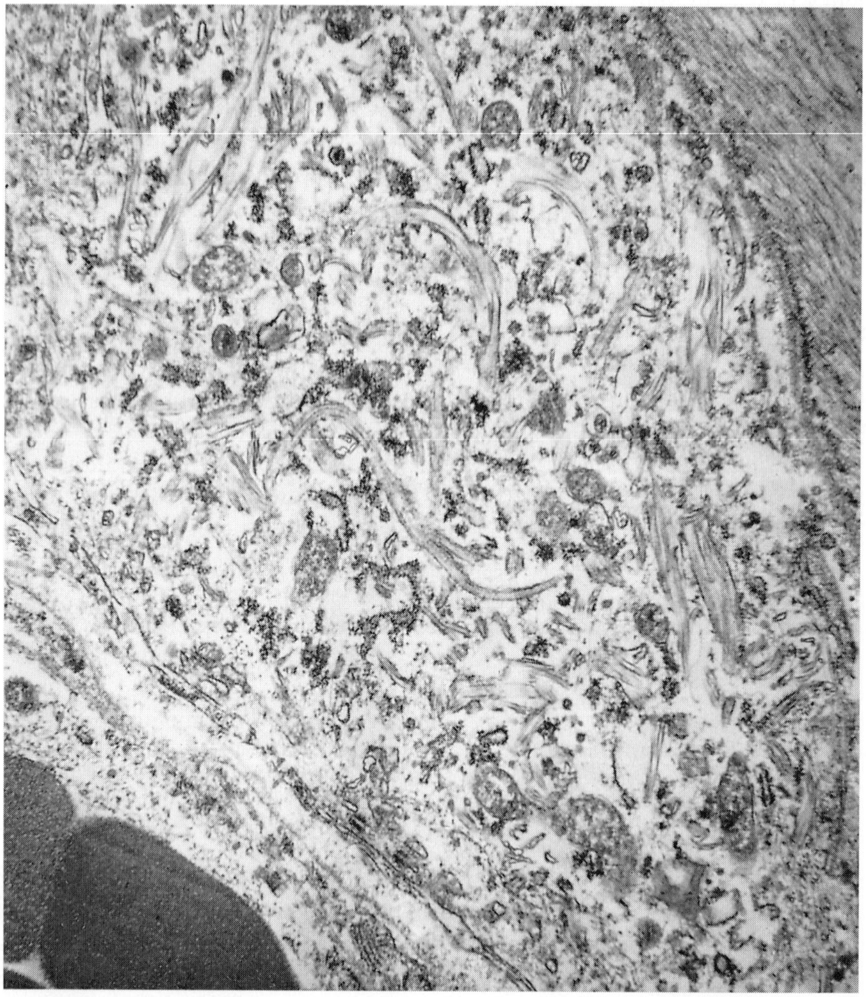

Fig. 44.48 Krabbe's disease. Electron micrograph of globoid cell. Red blood cells are seen in vascular lumen in left upper corner. Note spicules of storage material within cytoplasm.

the X-chromosome (Xq21.2-Xq22), which encodes proteolipid protein and DM20, two structural proteins of myelin.[44] Alternatively, the inheritance pattern may be autosomal recessive. The molecular deficit of this variety is unknown.

Clinical features

Several clinical variants with early onset have been described. The connatal type (type II disease) begins in the neonatal period and is associated with rapid deterioration and death in infancy or childhood. Initial features include nystagmus and trembling, roving eye movements, tremor, poor head control often associated with stridor, dysarthria and optic atrophy. Seizures occur in 75% of cases. Microcephaly, poor somatic growth, choreoathetosis and spasticity develop subsequently.[7,22,48] Type III disease may also have early onset followed by slower progression and death later in the first decade of life.

Diagnosis

Diagnosis may be suspected on the basis of the distinctive clinical features, but may be difficult to prove by biochemical or neuroimaging techniques. MRI may show a marked decrease in quantity and increased signal in white matter on T2-weighted images.[50] The CSF is normal. Visual evoked potentials are usually abnormal.

More recently, restriction enzyme DNA analysis with appropriate probes may permit definitive diagnosis as well as prenatal diagnosis.[10]

Pathology

There is cerebral and cerebellar atrophy. A distinctive feature is patchy demyelination with sudanophilic degradation products deposited in the centrum semiovale, cerebellum and brain stem. Small islands of myelin may be preserved.[67]

CANAVAN DISEASE (SPONGY DEGENERATION OF THE CEREBRAL WHITE MATTER)

This autosomal recessive disease is characterized by decreased activity of *N*-acetylaspartoacylase enzyme and increased levels of *N*-acetylaspartic acid in the brain.

Clinical features

Symptoms may become evident during the first weeks of life and include marked hypotonia, decreased visual responses, nystagmus and failure to achieve developmental milestones. Initial hypotonia progresses to spasticity, decorticate posture, seizures and occasional choreoathetosis. A significant feature is the disproportionate enlargement of the head, which is noted usually before 3–6 months of age. Visual impairment and optic atrophy occur between 12 and 18 months. Paroxysmal episodes of sweating, hyperthermia, vomiting and hypotension (autonomic dysfunction) may occur before death, which is usually before 5 years of age.[2,17]

Diagnosis

The diagnosis is confirmed by demonstration of increased excretion of *N*-acetylaspartic acid in the urine and decreased activity of *N*-acetylaspartacylase activity in cultured fibroblasts.[37] An increased ratio of *N*-acetylaspartic acid to creatinine and choline in the brain has been documented in vivo by magnetic resonance spectroscopy.[4] Visual evoked responses are abnormal early, before blindness develops. Cranial ultrasonography or CT may demonstrate cystic changes in white matter, whereas on MRI there is high signal in cerebral white matter on T2-weighted images.[31]

Elevated levels of *N*-acetylaspartic acid have been documented in the urine of a mother with an affected 4-month-old fetus,[15] which may permit prenatal diagnosis.

Pathology

The major pathological abnormalities are oedema, axonal swelling and cystic degeneration of the white matter. There is increased water content and decreased lipids in the white matter.[2] Axonal degeneration with clumping of peripheral nerves occurs.

ALEXANDER DISEASE

The majority of cases of Alexander disease are sporadic. The basic metabolic defect is not known, but there are characteristic neuropathological changes of deposition of crystalline protein and eosinophilic material in fibrillary astrocytes (Rosenthal fibres).[42]

Clinical features

An inappropriate increase in head size (either with or without hydrocephalus) may become evident during the first weeks of life. There is variable psychomotor deterioration, with seizures and spasticity. Death usually occurs before 3 years of age.[45]

Diagnosis

Diagnosis may be suspected on the basis of clinical features and neuroimaging. Computed tomography demonstrates decreased attenuation in cerebral white matter, which may be most marked in the frontal regions.[25] Definitive diagnosis depends on microscopic examination of the brain. There is no identifiable enzymatic or biochemical derangement of storage material.

Pathology

Brain weight is usually increased. The white matter is soft and there is marked loss of myelin. There are large numbers of Rosenthal fibres in the cerebral cortex and in white matter. These structures arise from degeneration of fibrillary astrocytes.

METACHROMATIC LEUKODYSTROPHY

This autosomal recessive disorder is occasionally evident during the newborn period. There is deficiency of the cerebroside sulfatase enzyme (arylsulfatase A), with accumulation of a sulfatide, i.e. metachromatic material that is a constituent of myelin. The gene coding for arylsulfatase A is located on the long arm of chromosome 22.

Clinical features

The age at onset is extremely variable. Early abnormalities include hypotonia, psychomotor regression with spasticity, and death between 3 and 6 years of age.[32]

Diagnosis

Diagnosis is confirmed by reduction in urinary or leukocyte arylsulfatase A activity in urine or leukocytes. Other features include elevated CSF protein levels, slowed motor nerve conduction velocities and abnormal brain-stem auditory evoked potentials. The electroretinogram is normal.

Cultured amniotic fluid cells or chorionic villus sampling permit prenatal diagnosis.

Pathology

There is decreased myelin in central and peripheral neurons, with accumulation of metachromatic material (sulfatide) in macrophages, glial and Schwann cells.

DISORDERS AFFECTING BOTH GREY AND WHITE MATTER

PEROXISOMAL DISORDERS

Several inherited and progressive metabolic disorders of genetic and phenotypic heterogeneity have been identified as disorders of peroxisome metabolism. Peroxisomes are subcellular organelles that contain numerous enzymes involved in anabolic and catabolic reactions, especially bile acid biosynthesis, gluconeogenesis, oxidation of very long-chain fatty acids, and purine catabolism. Human peroxisomal disorders are classified according to whether there are absent or reduced numbers of peroxisomes (group 1), normal numbers of peroxisomes with abnormal activity of a single enzyme (group 2), or multiple peroxisomal enzyme abnormalities (group 3).[39] The two peroxisomal disorders that present most commonly during the newborn period are neonatal adrenoleukodystrophy (ALD) and Zellweger's cerebrohepatorenal syndrome. Both conditions have an autosomal recessive inheritance pattern and are associated with reduced numbers of peroxisomes and abnormal activities of multiple peroxisomal enzymes (group 1). Affected infants are unable to synthesize phospholipids or oxidize very long-chain fatty acids or phytanic acid.

Clinical features

Because of the ubiquitous distribution of peroxisomes, clinical abnormalities may be identified in almost every organ and tissue of affected children. Table 44.20 compares the major clinical features of peroxisomal disorders that may present in the newborn. The dysmorphic

Table 44.20 Clinical features of major peroxisomal disorders

Abnormalities	Zellweger syndrome	Neonatal adrenoleukodystrophy	Infantile Refsum's disease	Hyperpipecolic acidaemia	Pseudo-Zellweger
Neurological					
Seizures	++	+	+	+	++
Severe hypotonia	++	+	+	+	++
Hyporeflexia	++	+	+	+	++
Impaired hearing	++	++	++	++	++
Craniofacial dysmorphism	++	++	+	++	++
Ocular					
Cataracts	++	±	–	–	++
Abnormal retina	++	++	++	++	++
Optic atrophy	++	++	±	++	++
Other organs					
Liver	++	++	±	+	++
Renal	++ (cysts)	–	–	–	±
Adrenal	±	++	–	–	++

++ = always present; + = present; ± = variably present; – = absent.
In the 'other organs' section of the table, the + signs indicate the degree of infiltration of the organ, which may or may not be enlarged.

craniofacial features of Zellweger syndrome are more marked than those of neonatal adrenoleukodystrophy. The disturbances of neuronal migration (heterotopias) which have been identified in cerebral and cerebellar cortex may account for the profound hypotonia, delayed development and neonatal seizures. After the first year of life significant demyelination, similar to that observed in X-linked ALD of older children, may cause additional neurological regression. There is usually macrocephaly, visual and auditory impairment and deterioration of neurological status, with death occurring at approximately 3 years of age.

Although many of the clinical features of neonatal ALD may be considered a milder variant of Zellweger syndrome, with fewer dysmorphic features, absence of renal cortical cysts, or calcific stippling of patellae, hips and epiphyses and longer survival, the two conditions are definitely distinct. Thus, the biochemical abnormalities and cerebral migration abnormalities are more severe in Zellweger syndrome, whereas the adrenal atrophy of neonatal ALD is absent in Zellweger syndrome. The clinical features of infantile Refsum syndrome resemble neonatal ALD and Zellweger syndrome. However, affected individuals may survive beyond the first decade.[65] It has not been determined whether hyperpipecolic acidaemia, which is an extremely rare disorder, is distinct from Zellweger syndrome.

Disorders with normal numbers of peroxisomes but deficient activity of several peroxisomal enzymes include two conditions that may present early. Pseudo-Zellweger syndrome (β-ketothiolase deficiency) is a term coined by Goldfischer et al to describe a patient who had features of classical Zellweger syndrome both clinically and biochemically, but who had abundant peroxisomes.[18] Furthermore, the rhizomelic form of chondrodysplasia punctata is an autosomal recessive disorder characterized by punctate epiphyseal and extraepiphyseal calcifications, psychomotor retardation, short limbs and cataracts, which results in death during the first year of life. Peroxisomes are abundant in this disorder but multiple enzymes are deficient.[26]

Diagnosis

Peroxisomal disorders can be diagnosed prenatally or postnatally by demonstrating increased very long-chain fatty acids in plasma, cultured skin fibroblasts or amniocytes. In addition to the characteristic clinical features of dysmorphism, retinopathy, calcific stippling of epiphyses and renal cysts, cultured skin fibroblasts may confirm a reduction in peroxisome number. Infantile Refsum's disease may demonstrate decreased numbers of liver peroxisomes as well as varying degrees of elevation of phytanic acid levels in blood and tissues. Aminocytes or chorionic villus samples permit prenatal diagnosis of affected fetuses.[39,65]

Pathology

Pathological investigations have revealed abnormalities in numerous organ systems, particularly the CNS. The CNS abnormalities include neuronal migration defects as well as degenerative features, e.g. cortical neuronal loss, gliosis, globoid cells, storage of fat in astrocytes, glycogen in cortical neurons and lamellar membrane and lipid inclusions. The liver is often enlarged, with severe fibrosis and micronodular cirrhosis. Electron microscopy may confirm absent or reduced numbers of peroxisomes and distorted mitochondria.[65]

MITOCHONDRIAL DISORDERS

Leigh's disease is an autosomal recessive disorder which results from a number of errors in energy metabolism and may involve the pyruvate dehydrogenase complex, cytochrome C oxidase (complex IV), NADH-CoQ reductase (complex I) or complex V.[53]

Clinical features

Onset is within the first year of life in 60% of cases, and most frequently in the first few months. Early features include loss of motor abilities and brain-stem dysfunction. Abnormalities of sucking and swallowing, together with vomiting, result in poor nutrition. There may be respiratory dysfunction, with unexplained hyperventilation which may last hours to days. Abnormalities of cranial nerve function present as gaze palsies, ptosis or mydriasis. Nystagmus, dysphagia, facial weakness, choreoathetosis and blindness may occur. Deterioration in neurological function often coincides with intercurrent infection. Most children with early-onset disease die within the first year of life, although transient spontaneous remissions have been described.

Diagnosis

Increases in blood lactate and pyruvate, or pyruvate/lactate ratio, are often found. Elevations of lactate level are even more consistent. Fibroblast or other tissue cultures have demonstrated various abnormalities in energy metabolism, as outlined previously. Computed tomography of the brain may demonstrate a characteristic appearance, with symmetrical areas of low attenuation in the putamen of the basal ganglia (Fig. 44.49). T2-weighted MRI images demonstrate increased signal in the putamen, often associated with abnormalities in periventricular white matter, midbrain and lower brain stem.[38] Nuclear magnetic resonance spectroscopy has shown elevated lactate levels in involved regions of the brain.[33] Position emission tomography has demonstrated decreased glucose utilization in the caudate and putamen in a child with cytochrome C oxidase deficiency.[68]

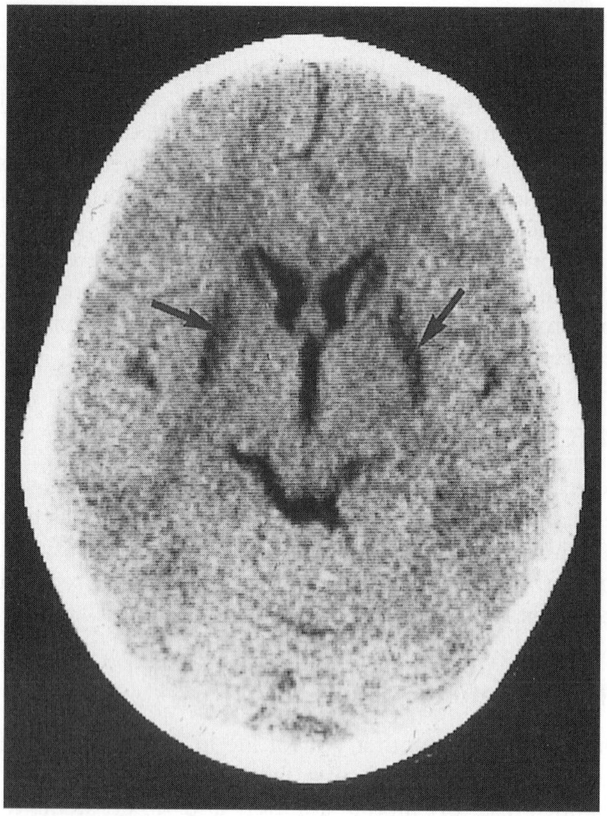

Fig. 44.49 Leigh's disease. CT scan of head. Note bilateral decreased tissue attenuation in basal ganglia (arrows).

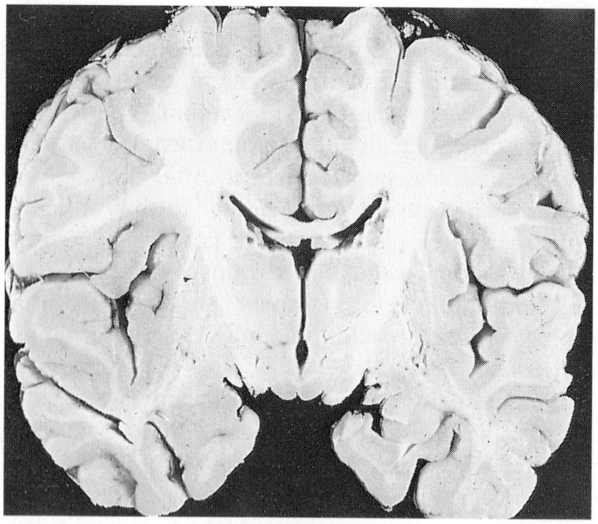

Fig. 44.50 Leigh's disease. Coronal section at level of mamillary bodies. Note spongy atrophy of basal ganglia and normal mamillary bodies.

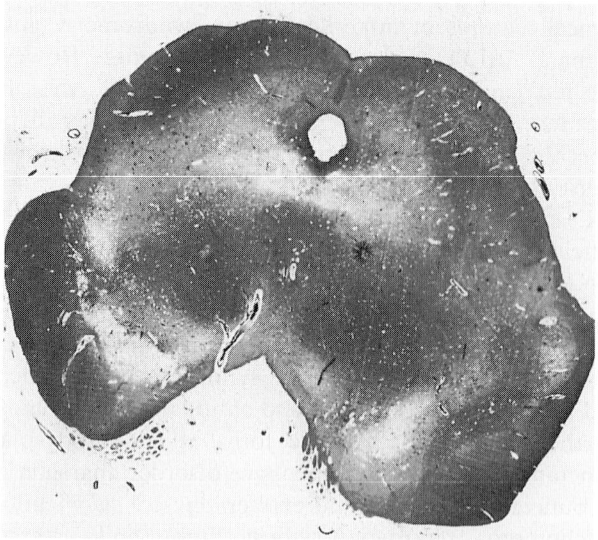

Fig 44.51 Leigh's disease. Histological section of midbrain. Note spongy atrophy in the light areas in periaqueductal grey matter and in substantia nigra.

Pathology

Focal necrosis with vascular proliferation occurs in a symmetrical pattern in the dorsal brain stem, thalamus, basal ganglia, optic nerves, cerebellum and spinal cord. Sparing of the mamillary bodies is a characteristic feature. Spongy atrophy of the basal ganglia, the periaqueductal grey matter and the substantia nigra occurs (Figs 44.50, 44.51). Electronmicroscopy of affected neurons may demonstrate abnormal mitochondria.

CYTOSKELETAL DISORDERS

Infantile neuroaxonal dystrophy is a disorder of neurofilaments, which are a major cytoskeletal component of both grey and white matter. It involves a molecular defect in the gene for α-*N*-acetylgalactosaminidase.[66]

Clinical features

The onset of this disorder is usually later in the first year of life, although several cases with neonatal abnormalities have been reported. Abnormalities may include disturbances of muscle tone, abnormal eye movements and pupillary reaction and poor sucking. Later, infants develop seizures and spasticity, and death usually occurs within the first 2 years.[41,63]

Diagnosis

Diagnosis is made by demonstration of axonal spheroids on nerve biopsy. There may be calcification of basal ganglia and thalami on CT scan by 1 month of age.[57] The T2-weighted MRI scans show cerebellar atrophy and hyperintensity of the cerebellar cortex.[57]

Pathology

Axonal spheroids are characteristic findings in central and peripheral axons. Changes are most marked in the dorsal horns and columns of the spinal cord, brain stem and cerebellum. Cerebral white matter is decreased in quantity.

REFERENCES

1. Abu-Dalu K I, Tamary H, Livni N, Rivkind A I, Yatziv S 1982 G M_1 gangliosidosis presenting as neonatal ascites. Journal of Pediatrics 100: 940–943
2. Adachi M, Schneck L, Cara J, Volk B W 1973 Spongy degeneration of the central nervous system (van Bogaert and Bertrand type; Canavan's disease). A review. Human Pathology 4: 331–347
3. Baram T Z, Goldman A N, Percy A K 1986 Krabbe disease: specific MRI and CT findings. Neurology 36: 111–115
4. Barker P B, Bryan R N, Kumar A J, Naidu S 1992 Proton NMR spectroscopy of Canavan's disease. Neuropediatrics 23: 263–267
5. Bateman J B, Philippart M 1986 Ocular features of the Hagberg–Santavuori syndrome. American Journal of Ophthalmology, 102: 262–271
6. Bentler E, Grabowski 1995 Gaucher disease. In: Scriver C R, Beaudet A L, Sly W S et al (eds) The metabolic basis of inherited disease, 7th edn. McGraw-Hill, New York, pp. 2641–2670
7. Boulloche J, Aicardi J 1986 Pelizaeus–Merzbacher disease: clinical and nosological study. Journal of Child Neurology 1: 233–239
8. Brady R O, Filling-Katz M R, Barton N W, Pentchev P G 1989 Niemann–Pick disease types C and D. Neurologic Clinics 7: 75–88
9. Brady R O, O'Neill R R, Barton N W 1993 Glucosylceramide lipidosis: Gaucher disease. In: Rosenberg RN et al (eds) The molecular and genetic basis of neurological disease. Butterworth-Heinemann, Boston, pp. 467–484
10. Bridge P J, MacLeod P M, Lillicrap D P 1991 Carrier detection and prenatal diagnosis of Pelizaeus–Merzbacher disease using a combination of anonymous DNA polymorphisms and the proteolipid protein (PLP) gene cDNA. American Journal of Medical Genetics 38: 616–621
11. Charrow J, Hvizd M G 1986 Cardiomyopathy and skeletal myopathy in an unusual variant of GM_1 gangliosidosis. Journal of Pediatrics 108: 729–732
12. Clarke J T R, Ozere R L, Krause V W 1981 Early infantile variant of Krabbe globoid cell leucodystrophy with lung involvement. Archives of Disease in Childhood 56: 640–642
13. Confort-Gouny S, Chabrol B, Vion-Dury J, Mancini J, Cozzone P J 1993 MRI and localized proton MRS in early infantile form of neuronal ceroid-lipofuscinosis. Pediatric Neurology 9: 57–60
14. Demaerel P, Wilms G, Verdru P, Carlton H, Baert A L 1990 MR findings in globoid leukodystrophy. Neuroradiology; 32: 520–522
15. Elpeleg ON 1992 *N*-acetylaspartic aciduria in young age. Neuropediatrics 23: 112
16. Gahl W A, Schneider J A, Avla P P 1995 Lysosomal transport disorders: cystonosis and sialic acid storage disorders. In: Scriver C R, Beaudet A L, Sly W S et al (eds) The metabolic basis of inherited disease, 7th edn. McGraw-Hill, New York, pp. 3763–3799
17. Gascon G G, Ozand P T, Mahdi A et al 1990 Infantile CNS spongy degeneration – 14 cases: clinical update. Neurology 40: 1876–1882
18. Goldfischer S, Collins J, Rapin I et al 1986 Pseudo-Zellweger syndrome deficiencies in several peroxisomal oxidative activities. Journal of Pediatrics 108: 25–32
19. Gravol R A, Clarke J T R, Koback M M et al 1995 The GM_2 gangliosidoses. In: Scriver C R, Beaudet A L, Sly W S et al (eds) The metabolic and molecular basis of inherited disease, 7th edn. McGraw-Hill, New York, pp. 2839–2882
20. Grebner E, Wenger D A 1987 Use of 4-methylumbelliferyl-6-sulpho-2-acetamido-2-deoxy-beta-d-glucopyranoside for prenatal diagnosis of Tay–Sachs disease using chorionic villi. Prenatal Diagnosis 7: 419–423
21. Gumbinas M, Larsen M, Liu HM 1975 Peripheral neuropathy in classic Niemann–Pick disease: ultrastructure of nerves and skeletal muscles. Neurology 25: 107–113
22. Haenggeli C A, Engel E, Pizzolato G P 1989 Connatal Pelizaeus–Merzbacher disease. Developmental Medicine and Child Neurology 31: 803–807
23. Hagberg B 1984 Krabbe's disease: clinical presentation of neurological variants. Neuropediatrics 15: 11–15
24. Harden A, Pampliglione G, Picton-Robinson N 1973 Electroretinogram and visual evoked responses in a form of 'neuronal lipidosis' with diagnostic EEG features. Journal of Neurology, Neurosurgery and Psychiatry 36: 61–67
25. Hess D C, Asma Q F, Yaghmai F, Figueroa R, Akamatsu Y 1990 Comparative neuroimaging with pathologic correlates in Alexander's disease. Journal of Child Neurology 5: 248–252
26. Heymans H S A, Oorthuys J W E, Nelck G et al 1986 Peroxisomal abnormalities in chondrodysplasia punctata. Journal of Inherited Metabolic Diseases 9 (suppl 2): 329–331
27. Iwamasa T, Ohshita T, Nashiro K, Iwananga M 1987 Demonstration of GM_1 ganglioside in nervous system in generalized GM_1 gangliosidosis using choleral toxin B subunit. Acta Neuropathologica 73: 357–360
28. Jarvela I, Rapola J, Peltonen L et al 1991 DNA-based prenatal diagnosis of the infantile form of neuronal ceroid lipofuscinosis (INCL, CLNI). Prenatal Diagnosis 11: 323–328
29. Jarvela I, Santavuori P, Puhakka L, Haltia M, Peltonen L 1992 Linkage map of the chromosomal region surrounding the infantile neuronal ceroid lipofuscinosis on 1p. American Journal of Medical Genetic 42: 546–548
30. Kaback M, Lim-Steele J, Dabholkar D, Brown D, Levy N, Zeiger K 1993 Tay–Sachs disease – carrier screening, prenatal diagnosis and the molecular era. An international perspective, 1970–1993. The International TSD Data Collection Network. Journal of the American Medical Association 270: 2307–2315
31. Kendall B E 1992 Disorders of lysosomes, peroxisomes and mitochondria. American Journal of Neuroradiology 13: 621–653
32. Kolodny E H, Fluharty A L 1995 Metachromatic leukodystrophy and multiple sulfatase deficiency: sulfatide lipidosis. In: Scriver C R, Beaudet A L, Sly W S et al (eds) The metabolic basis of inherited disease, 7th edn. McGraw-Hill, New York, pp. 2693–2740
33. Krageloh-Mann I, Grodd W, Schoning M, Marquard K, Nagele T, Ruitenbeek W 1993 Proton spectroscopy in 5 patients with Leigh's disease and mitochondrial enzyme deficiency. Developmental Medicine and Child Neurology 35: 769–776
34. Levran O, Desnick R J, Schuchman E H 1991 Niemann–Pick disease. A frequent missense mutation in the acid sphingomyelinase gene of Ashkenazi Jewish type A and B patients. Proceedings of the National Academy of Sciences 88: 3748–3752
35. Lieberman J S, Oshtory M, Taylor R G, Dreyfus P M 1980 Perinatal neuropathy as an early manifestation of Krabbe's disease. Archives of Neurology 37: 446–447
36. Lowden J A, Cutz E, Conen P, Rudd N, Doran T A 1973 Prenatal diagnosis of GM_1-gangliosidosis. New England Journal of Medicine 288: 225–228
37. Matalon R, Kaul R, Michals K 1993 Canavan disease: biochemical and molecular studies. Journal of Inherited Metabolic Disease 16: 744–752
38. Medina L, Chi T L, DeVivo D C, Hilal S K 1990 MR findings in patients with subacute necrotizing encephalomyelopathy (Leigh syndrome): correlation with biochemical defect. American Journal of Neuroradiology 11: 379–384
39. Moser H W 1993 Peroxisomal disorders. In: Rosenberg R N et al (eds) The molecular and genetic basis of neurological disease. Butterworth-Heineman, Boston, pp. 351–387
40. Moser H W 1995 Ceramidase deficiency: Farber lipogranulomatosis. In: Scriver C R, Beaudet A L, Sly W S et al (eds) The metabolic basis of inherited disease, 7th edn. McGraw-Hill, New York, pp. 2589–2600
41. Nagashima K, Suzuki S, Ichikawa E et al 1985 Infantile neuroaxonal dystrophy: perinatal onset with symptoms of diencephalic syndrome. Neurology 35: 735–738
42. Neal J W, Cave E M, Singhrao S K, Cole G, Wallace S J 1992 Alexander's disease in infancy and childhood – a report of 2 cases. Acta Neuropathologica 84: 322–327
43. O'Brien J S 1969 Generalized gangliosidosis. Journal of Pediatrics 75: 167–186
44. Otterbach B, Stoffel W, Ramaekers V 1993 A novel mutation in the proteolipid protein gene leading to Pelizaeus–Merzbacher disease. Biological Chemistry Hoppe–Seyler 374: 75–83
45. Pridmore C L, Baraitser M, Harding B, Boyd S G, Kendall B, Brett E M 1993 Alexander's disease: clues to diagnosis. Journal of Child Neurology 8: 134–144
46. Rapola J, Salonen R, Ammala P, Santavuori P 1990 Prenatal diagnosis of the infantile type of neuronal ceroid lipofuscinosis by electron microscopic investigation of human chorionic villi. Prenatal Diagnosis 10: 553–559
47. Santavuori P, Haltia M, Rapola J 1974 Infantile type of so-called neuronal ceroid-lipofuscinosis. Developmental Medicine and Child Neurology 16: 644–653
48. Scheffer I E, Baraitser M, Wilson J, Harding B, Kendall B, Brett E M 1991 Pelizaeus–Merzbacher disease: classical or connatal? Neuropediatrics 22: 71–78
49. Sidransky E, Sherer D, Ginns E I 1992 Gaucher disease in the neonate:

a distinct Gaucher phenotype is analogous to a mouse model created by targeted disruption of the glucocerebrosidase gene. Pediatric Research 32: 494–498
50. Silverstein A M, Hirsch D K, Trobe J D, Gebarski S S 1990 MR imaging of the brain in five members of a family with Pelizaeus–Merzbacher disease. American Journal of Neuroradiology 11: 495–499
51. Sorcinelli R, Sitzia A, Loi M 1987 Cherry-red spot, optic atrophy and corneal clouding in a patient suffering from GM_1 gangliosidosis type 1. Metabolic Pediatric Systemic Ophthalmology 10: 62–63
52. Spence M W, Callahan J W 1989 Sphingomyelin-cholesterol lipidoses: the Niemann–Pick group of disease. In: Scriver C R et al (eds) The metabolic basis of inherited disease, 6th edn. McGraw-Hill, New York, pp. 1655–1676
53. Sperl W, Ruitenbeek W, Sengers R C et al 1992 Combined deficiencies of the pyruvate dehydrogenase complex and enzymes of the respiratory chain in mitochondrial myopathies. European Journal of Pediatrics 151: 192–195
54. Suzuki K 1968 GM_1-gangliosidosis. Chemical pathology of visceral organs. Science 159: 1471–1472
55. Suzuki K, Suzuki Y 1989 Galactosylceramide lipidosis: globoid cell leukodystrophy (Krabbe's disease). In: Scriver C R, Beaudet A L, Sly W S et al (eds) The metabolic basis of inherited disease, 6th edn. McGraw-Hill, New York, pp. 1699–1720
56. Swaiman K 1989 Lysosomal disorders. In: Pediatric neurology: principles and practice, 2nd edn. Mosby, St. Louis, pp. 1017–1066
57. Tanabe Y, Lai M, Ishii M et al 1993 The use of magnetic resonance imaging in diagnosing infantile neuroaxonal dystrophy. Neurology 43: 110–113
58. Thomas G H, Beaudet A L 1995 Disorders of glycoprotein degradation: mannosidosis, fucosidosis, sialidosis and aspartylglycosaminuria. In: Scriver C R, Beaudet A L, Sly W S et al (eds) The metabolic basis of inherited disease, 7th edn. McGraw-Hill, New York, pp. 3763–3799
59. Tonnesen T, Horn N 1989 Prenatal and postnatal diagnosis of Menkes' disease, an inherited disorder of copper metabolism. Journal of Inherited Metabolic Diseases 12 (Suppl.1): 207–214
60. Tulinius M H, Holme E, Kristiansson B, Larsson N G, Oldfors A 1991 Mitochondrial encephalomyopathies in childhood II. Clinical manifestations and syndromes. Journal of Pediatrics 119: 251–259
61. Vanier M T, Rousson R, Garcia I, Baiilourd G et al 1985 Biochemical studies in Niemann–Pick disease. III In vitro and in vivo assays of sphingomyelin degradation in cultured skin fibroblasts and amniotic fluid cells for diagnosis of various forms of the disease. Clinical Genetics 27: 20–32
62. Vanier M T, Wenger D A, Comly M E, Rousson R, Brady R O, Pentchev P G 1988 Niemann–Pick disease group C: clinical variability and diagnosis based on defective cholesterol esterification. A collaborative study on 70 patients. Clinical Genetics 33: 331–348
63. Venkatesh S, Coulter D L, Kemper T D 1994 Neuroaxonal dystrophy at birth with hypertonicity and basal ganglia mineralization. Journal of Child Neurology 8: 74–76
64. Volpe J J 1995 Degenerative diseases of the newborn. In: Volpe J J (ed.) Neurology of the newborn, 3rd edn. W B Saunders, Philadelphia, pp. 565–582
65. Wanders R J A, Heymans H S A, Schutgens R B H et al 1988 Peroxisomal disorders in neurology. Journal of Neurological Science 88: 1–39
66. Wang A M, Schindler D, Desnick R J 1990 Schindler disease. The molecular lesion in the alpha-*N*-acetylgalactosaminidase gene that causes infantile neuroaxonal dystrophy. Journal of Clinical Investigation 86: 1752–1756
67. Watanabe I, Patel V, Goebel H H et al 1973 Early lesion of Pelizaeus–Merzbacher disease: electron microscopic and biochemical study. Journal of Neuropathology Experimental and Neurology 32: 313–333
68. Yanai K, Iinuma K, Matsuzawa T et al 1987 Cerebral glucose utilization in pediatric neurological disorders determined by positron emission tomography. European Journal of Nuclear Medicine 13: 292–296
69. Yoshiokawa H, Yamada K, Sakuragawa N 1992 MRI in the early stage of Tay–Sachs disease. Neuroradiology 34: 394–395

Part 7

Muscle disease in the newborn

Elke H. Roland

INTRODUCTION

Neuromuscular disease implies dysfunction of the motor system at some level between the motor cortex and muscle. In the newborn infant neuromuscular disease may present a difficult diagnostic challenge. Management of these disorders is often associated with serious ethical and genetic implications. Although this chapter focuses principally on disorders of muscle, other diseases of the lower motor neuron, which must be considered in the differential diagnosis, e.g. anterior horn cell disease, peripheral neuropathy and disorders of the neuromuscular junction, will be reviewed briefly.

DIAGNOSIS OF NEUROMUSCULAR DISORDERS

Accurate diagnosis of neuromuscular disease in the newborn depends on a detailed history and physical examination performed in conjunction with appropriate laboratory investigations. Table 44.21 lists the major clinical features that may assist in the differentiation

Table 44.21 Classification of hypotonia

Clinical features	Central origin	Neuromuscular origin
Encephalopathy (altered consciousness, seizures)	Present	Usually absent
Dysmorphic features	Other organ involvement	Micrognathia, undescended testes
Tendon reflexes	Normal or brisk	Normal or decreased
Recoil strength of limbs	Strong	Weak
Improvement of tone over time	Yes	Variable
Other motor abnormalities		
Fasciculations, facial diplegia, ptosis	Rare	May be present
Orthopaedic problems		
Dislocated hips, arthrogryposis	Variable	Present

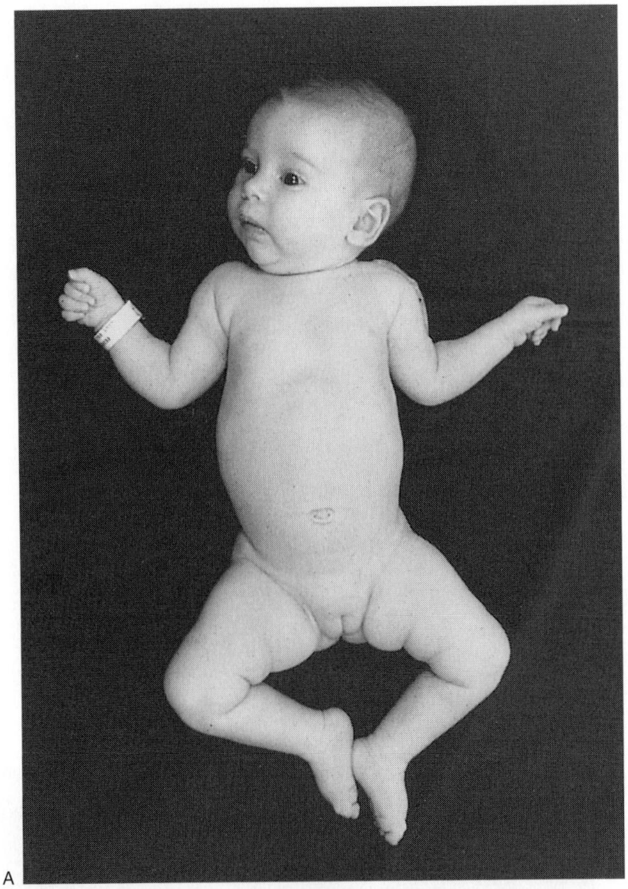

A

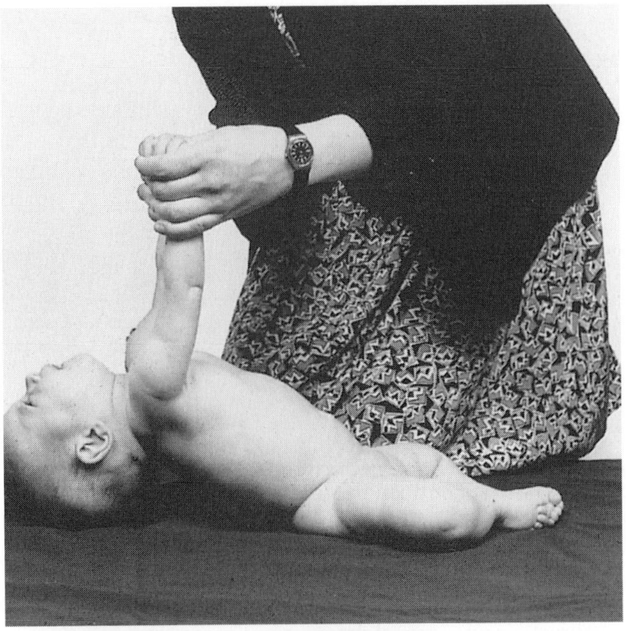

B

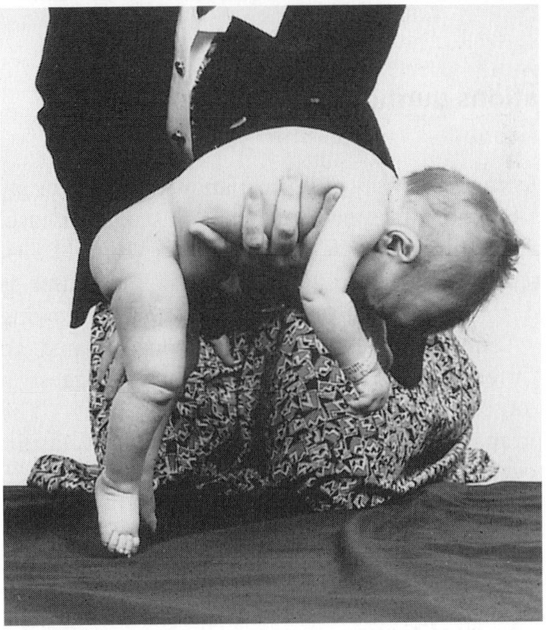

C

Fig. 44.52 (A) Hypotonic infant with spinal muscular atrophy. Abnormal resting posture with fully abducted legs (frog-leg position). (B) Abnormal traction response in hypotonic newborn. The head falls backwards as the body is pulled forward and there is no resistance in the limbs. (C) Abnormal horizontal suspension in hypotonic newborn. The head, body and limbs hang limply.

between hypotonia which is central in origin and that associated with primary neuromuscular disease. In general, disorders of the lower motor neuron should be considered whenever a newborn presents with hypotonia and/or weakness in association with a normal level of consciousness (Fig. 44.52). However, this approach may be too simplistic because many traditional muscle disorders, such as congenital muscular dystrophy, may have significant central nervous system involvement or should be considered as multisystem disorders, e.g. mitochondrial cytopathies, myotonic dystrophy. Furthermore, it must be emphasized that infants with neuromuscular disorders may sustain secondary hypoxic–ischaemic cerebral insult related to weakness of respiratory muscles or pulmonary hypoplasia. For example, in one series of 17 newborns with muscle disease nine had low Apgar scores suggestive of a possible hypoxic–ischaemic insult.[9] In such instances hypotonia and weakness may be attributed erroneously to hypoxic–ischaemic encephalopathy alone and the underlying neuromuscular disease may be overlooked, unless a high index of suspicion is maintained.[81]

HISTORY

Family history

Because the majority of neuromuscular disorders are inherited, a detailed family history is of paramount importance. In fact, in certain inherited neuromuscular diseases, e.g. Duchenne/Becker muscular dystrophy, affected infants are asymptomatic during the first year of life and a positive family history may provide the only clue that leads to investigation, e.g. measurement of serum creatine phosphokinase, and early diagnosis prior to the emergence of clinical signs.[5,14] Whenever the possibility of neuromuscular disease is suspected in a newborn, specific inquiries should be made about consanguinity, previous childhood deaths, delayed motor

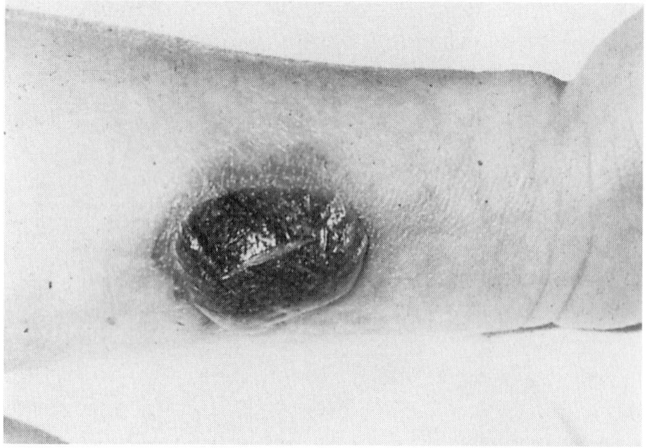

Fig. 44.53 Area of pressure necrosis related to decreased fetal movement noted at birth on the forearm of a newborn with congenital myotonic dystrophy. (The baby had a corresponding area of pressure necrosis on the scalp, where the arm rested against the head during pregnancy.)

milestones and wheelchair requirements in family members.

Complications during pregnancy, labour and delivery

Certain complications of pregnancy are strongly suggestive of antenatal onset of neuromuscular disease. These include diminished fetal movements (Fig. 44.53), breech presentation and polyhydramnios. The latter is considered to be related to impaired fetal swallowing activity.[81] Abnormal progression of labour, related to abnormal uterine muscle contraction, may suggest a diagnosis of congenital myotonic dystrophy.[30,37,65] The risk of intrapartum hypoxic–ischaemic cerebral insult, related to respiratory muscle weakness, has been discussed previously (see above).

PHYSICAL EXAMINATION

Motor abnormalities

Whenever neuromuscular disease is suspected, specific attention must be directed towards assessing muscle tone, bulk and power, as well as the presence of diminished tendon reflexes and primitive reflexes. Careful examination for evidence of myotonia, fatiguing of muscle, fasciculations, facial diplegia and ptosis may support the notion that hypotonia is probably of neuromuscular origin.

Neurological examination of the parents is an integral part of the evaluation of the newborn with suspected neuromuscular disease. For example, the presence of myotonia in the mother may confirm the diagnosis of congenital myotonic dystrophy in the newborn. Similarly, evidence of fatiguing of muscles in the mother raises the possibility of transient neonatal myasthenia gravis.

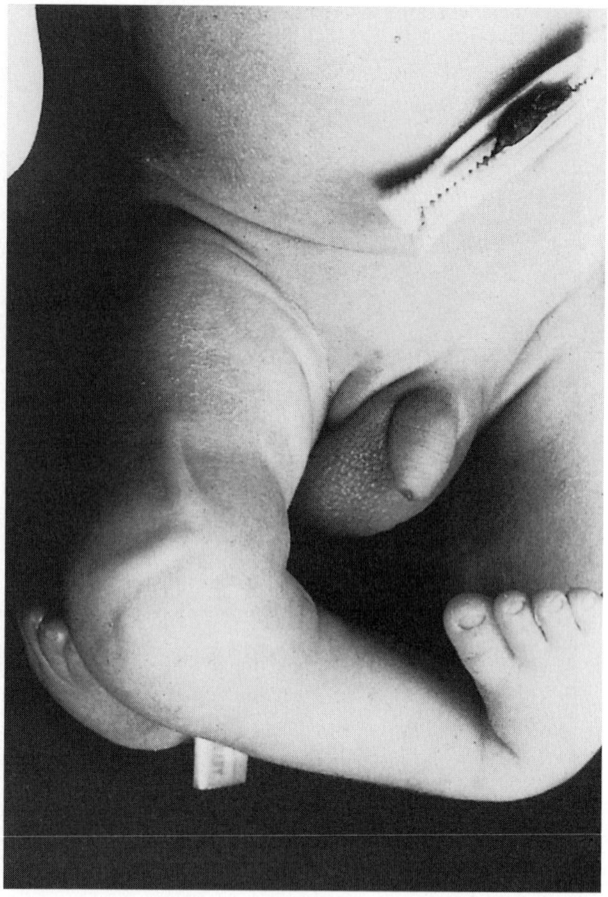

Fig. 44.54 Arthrogryposis multiplex congenita. Flexion contractures of hips, knees and ankles.

Congenital abnormalities

Minor congenital abnormalities, e.g. micrognathia, indistinct palmar creases, undescended tests in males, high-arched palate and a prominent, box-like forehead, have been described in the context of neuromuscular disease. In contrast, major congenital anomalies of other organ systems are often associated with hypotonia of central origin. Orthopaedic abnormalities which may be indicative of neuromuscular disease include congenital foot deformities, dislocation of the hips and scoliosis.

Arthrogryposis multiplex congenita

A fixed position and limitation of range of movement at multiple joints may occur with abnormalities originating at all levels of the motor system. In neuromuscular disease the joint contractures are often more severe distally, e.g. talipes equinovarus and flexion deformities of the wrists (Fig. 44.54).[1] Atrophic muscles may create a fusiform appearance of the joints. Occasionally, intrauterine mechanical restrictions associated with oligohydramnios or amniotic bands may produce arthrogryposis.[27,29]

LABORATORY INVESTIGATIONS

Serum creatine phosphokinase

Elevated levels of this enzyme may indicate significant skeletal or cardiac muscle necrosis. Unfortunately, increased CK levels may occur also in the context of acute hypoxic–ischaemic cerebral injury and acidosis.[61] In such instances it is useful to assay CK isoenzyme levels, to distinguish between skeletal, cardiac muscle or brain involvement. Moreover, up to 10-fold elevations of CK have been reported in normal newborns up to 1 week following vaginal delivery (related presumably to muscle trauma).[3,14,75] Thus, in instances where there are no other factors suggestive of neuromuscular disease it is recommended that the CK level be measured on several occasions after 2 or 3 weeks of age, before embarking on more extensive investigations.

Aspartate aminotransferase (AST)

This enzyme may be mildly elevated in liver and skeletal muscle disease. Persistent elevation may indicate a neuromuscular disorder with hepatic involvement, e.g. Pompe's disease.

Chest X-ray

Thin ribs on chest X-ray, presumably related to diminished fetal respiratory movements, are a useful clue to antenatal onset of neuromuscular disease (Fig. 44.55).[53] Thin ribs have been reported in a variety of neuromuscular disorders, including spinal muscular atrophy, congenital myotonic dystrophy and other severe congenital myopathies. An enlarged cardiac silhouette, related to cardiomyopathy, may suggest metabolic myopathy, e.g. mitochondrial myopathy, Pompe's disease.

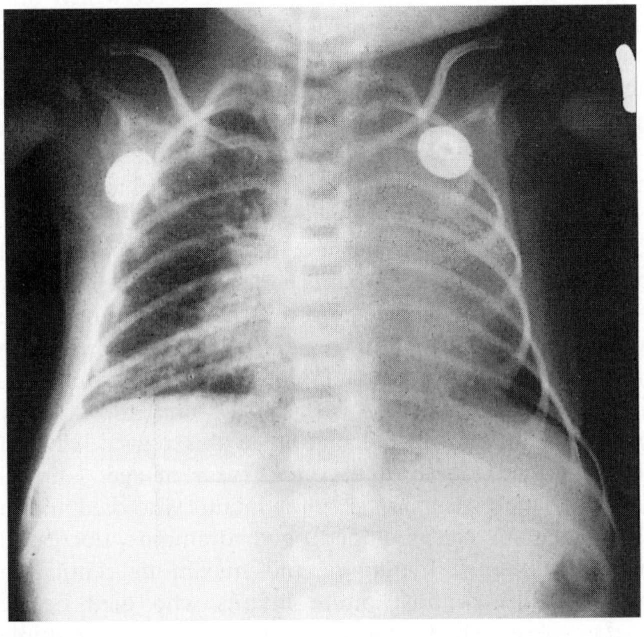

Fig. 44.55 Chest radiograph of a newborn with congenital myotonic dystrophy. Note thin ribs of normal length and mineralization.

Nerve conduction velocity/electromyography

It has been reported that the level of involvement of the motor system may be established by electrical studies in approximately 80% of hypotonic infants before 3 months of age.[54] However, both the technical performance and interpretation of EMG data are difficult in the newborn.[11,41,42]

Nerve conduction velocities, especially motor nerve conduction velocity measured in ulnar and peroneal nerves, have been shown to be a consistent and reliable determinant of gestational age after 32 weeks. This may be particularly useful in small-for-dates infants.[2] Nerve conduction velocities are lower in the newborn than in older individuals.[26,42] Characteristically, nerve conduction velocities are diminished in peripheral neuropathy, especially in the demyelinating varieties (i.e. motor nerve conduction often less than 5 m/s or unrecordable).

EMG, which assesses the intrinsic electrical activity of muscle, may be abnormal as a result of dysfunction at various levels of the motor system. Thus, in resting muscle there may be fasciculations in anterior horn cell disease, or fibrillations in both anterior horn cell and peripheral nerve diseases. Increased amplitude and duration of motor unit responses is observed in anterior horn cell disease, whereas there is decreased amplitude of motor responses in peripheral neuropathy and muscle disorders. Myotonic discharges, i.e. spontaneous bursts of potentials with gradual waning, which occur in older individuals with myotonic dystrophy, are rarely elicited in the newborn, although they have been observed during the first week of life.[81] A decremental response of motor unit amplitude to repetitive nerve stimulation may be obtained in newborns with myasthenia gravis.[31,80]

Imaging of muscle

Derangements of muscle architecture by infiltration of adipose or connective tissue may be visualized as increased muscle echogenicity on high-resolution real-time ultrasonography.[32] Image variation, related to interobserver variability, has been minimized by computerization of this technique.[21] Ultrasonography may have particular value for selection of the optimal site for needle muscle biopsy.[32,33]

Recently, both computed tomography[6] and magnetic resonance imaging[45,82] have had application in the investigation of muscle disease. However, to date there is minimal experience with these imaging techniques in the newborn.

Muscle biopsy

This procedure is technically feasible using either open surgical or needle techniques.[15,18,34,67,68] Most biopsies are taken from the quadriceps (vastus lateralis), except in cases with selective involvement of muscles. Problems may arise with histological interpretation of the biopsy during the newborn period, related principally to the presence of non-specific abnormalities which are observed during the early stages of progressive muscular dystrophies.[77] The potential benefit of repeated muscle biopsies has been reported previously.[9,59] Thus, it has been proposed that muscle biopsy be postponed until several months of age, especially in view of the absence of effective treatment for most myopathies in this age group.[77] However, in some instances, particularly if there is severe respiratory muscle involvement, early biopsy may provide a definitive diagnosis and more accurate prognosis, which assists further management decisions. Electron microscopy and immunocytochemistry have significantly improved the diagnostic capabilities of muscle biopsy (e.g. desmin and vimentin staining for myotubular myopathy,[69] dystrophin for Duchenne/Becker dystrophy, and merosin for congenital muscular dystrophy.[8]

Sural nerve biopsy

This procedure, which may be useful for diagnosis of peripheral neuropathy, is performed only rarely in the newborn.

Cerebrospinal fluid examination

Increased protein concentration in CSF may be detected in peripheral nerve disease and in degenerative diseases of the central nervous system which have an associated neuropathy, e.g. Krabbe's disease.

Neuroimaging (cranial ultrasonography, computed tomography, magnetic resonance imaging)

Cerebral abnormalities, which may be demonstrated by imaging techniques, have been reported in several neuro-degenerative conditions as well as in primary muscular dystrophies. Thus, diminished cerebral white matter is a feature of Krabbe's leukodystrophy.[81] Dilatation of cerebral ventricles, possibly related to cerebral dysgenesis or periventricular leukomalacia, has been reported in congenital myotonic dystrophy.[23,58,76] In several variants of congenital muscular dystrophy there is prominent cerebral involvement, including cerebral dysgenesis and decreased cerebral white matter.[10,16,17,57,78]

Molecular genetic techniques (Chapter 11)

It is difficult to overstate the significance of molecular genetics, which is revolutionizing the diagnosis and classification of neuromuscular disease. The identification of numerous gene locations, characterization of gene abnormalities and their protein products will permit accurate diagnosis and prenatal testing in affected individuals, reduce the necessity for invasive investigations and provide a rational basis for intervention. Clearly, clinical assessment will continue to direct costly genetic investigations.

Miscellaneous biochemical investigations

Rhabdomyolysis without myoglobinuria has been described as a presentation of X-linked recessive muscular dystrophy in a newborn who was shown subsequently to have a gene deletion at the Duchenne/Becker locus.[4] Furthermore, rhabdomyolysis and myoglobinuria have been documented in asphyxiated infants, presumably as a consequence of extensive ischaemic muscle injury.[43] There are other investigations which have limited application for diagnosis of specific neuromuscular conditions, e.g. serum lactate level in mitochondrial cytopathies. Because of the specific nature of these investigations, they will be described in greater detail in relevant sections later in this chapter.

MANAGEMENT OF NEONATAL NEUROMUSCULAR DISEASE

The management of a newborn with neuromuscular disease involves principally supportive care, which may include mechanical ventilation and/or oxygen therapy, nasogastric feeding and physiotherapy to minimize joint contractures. Specific therapies exist for some conditions, e.g. pyridostigmine for myasthenia gravis (see below).

Major ethical dilemmas may arise over the duration of mechanical ventilatory support, which is considered reasonable in infants with severe neuromuscular disease. Unfortunately, few scientific guidelines exist. It is not clear whether the use of mechanical ventilation simply prolongs survival or also improves the quality of life in affected individuals. Our review of 17 newborns with muscle disease, who were admitted to British Columbia's Children's Hospital between 1983 and 1990, may provide some useful information in this regard. Five of the 17 infants survived beyond 1 year of age. Clinical features which were similar in the infants who died and in those who survived included polyhydramnios, decreased fetal movements, hypotonia and maximum ventilation pressures. In contrast, more infants who died before 1 year of age had arthrogryposis (9/12) and multiple congenital anomalies unexplained by fetal inactivity (3/12). Infants who died were of lower gestational age (mean 30 weeks, range 29–39 weeks) than those who survived (mean 36.8 weeks, range 35–40 weeks). Six of the 12 infants who died had pulmonary complications of prematurity, including pulmonary hypoplasia, pneumothorax, respiratory distress syndrome and bronchopulmonary dysplasia. The duration of mechanical ventilation was longer in infants who died (mean 44 days, range 3–120 days) than in infants who survived (two infants required oxygen therapy only; in the remainder the mean duration of ventilation was 15 days, range 10–21 days).[9]

In another reported series of seven patients with congenital neuromuscular disease who received long-term mechanical ventilation before 2 years of age, the mortality rate was high (57%). Long-term survival did not appear to correlate with the primary diagnosis, but rather with the development of the electrocardiographic changes of cor pulmonale. It is speculated that cardiopulmonary deterioration may relate to prolonged, constant mechanical ventilation.[38]

BASIC ANATOMY AND MATURATION OF MUSCLE

The understanding of congenital myopathies requires a basic understanding of the histology and development of muscle. Human muscle tissue is comprised of two histologically distinct fibre types, type I, which are involved in slow, sustained motor activity and which contain predominantly oxidative enzymes, and type II, which contain glycolytic enzymes and which control rapid bursts of activity. There is a recognized maturational process of muscle development during gestation, with predominance of type II fibres prior to 25 weeks' gestation and differentiation of type I and type II after 20 weeks of gestation. Subsequently there is increasing formation of type I fibres, until at term there are approximately equal numbers of type I and type II, which are arranged in a 'chequerboard' pattern.[67,68] Motor end plates develop after 14 weeks' gestation.

MUSCLE ABNORMALITIES ASSOCIATED WITH DISTURBANCES OF THE CENTRAL NERVOUS SYSTEM

Experimental animal data suggest that developmental abnormalities of the central and peripheral nervous systems may result in aberrations of muscle development.[40] Thus, denervation of the soleus muscle in rats during the myotubular stage of development is associated with persistence of immature myoblasts and failure of differentiation of fibre types.[19] In the human newborn several abnormalities of skeletal muscle have been documented in infants with cerebral abnormalities, especially malformations of the cerebellum and brain stem.[44] These include failure of fibre type differentiation, type I or type II fibre predominance, or type I fibre disproportion. These observations raise the possibility that such abnormalities of muscle may account, in part, for the hypotonia which is often observed in children with cerebral malformations.[70] Furthermore, it is possible that abnormalities of motor innervation may produce the type I fibre predominance which is recognized as a non-specific feature in several congenital myopathies, including congenital fibre type disproportion, nemaline rod disease and central core disease.[40,68] However, because of the paucity of neuropathological data the effect of lesions of the upper motor neuron on muscle development in the human newborn must be considered to be speculative.

In contrast, primary diseases of the lower motor neuron, e.g. anterior horn cell disease and peripheral neuropathy, are associated with recognizable secondary changes of denervation in muscle.

ANTERIOR HORN CELL DISEASE

Diseases of the anterior horn cell, particularly type I spinal muscular atrophy (Werdnig–Hoffman disease), account for approximately 35% of all newborn cases of severe generalized hypotonia of neuromuscular origin.[7] Less common disorders of the anterior horn cell which may present in the newborn include type II glycogen storage disease (Pompe's disease),[15] neurogenic arthrogryposis multiplex congenita[1] and neonatal poliomyelitis.[15] The clinical features of the major types of anterior horn cell disease which may present in the newborn are summarized in Table 44.22.

Neuropathology

The primary pathological processes in Werdnig–Hoffmann disease involve progressive severe degeneration and depletion of anterior horn cells in the spinal cord and the motor nuclei of the cranial nerves, especially cranial nerves V, VII, IX, XI and XII.[81] Muscle biopsy demonstrates severe denervation, with grouped atrophy of muscle fibres and marked hypertrophy of type I fibres[15,81] (Fig. 44.56).

The genetic defect has been identified on chromosome 5q11.2–13.3, which has led to the development of molecular diagnostic tests and prenatal testing with chorionic villus sampling.[48,49]

Clinical features

Prenatal onset of anterior horn cell disease may be indicated by decreased fetal movements and severe respiratory distress at birth. Nevertheless, despite reports of decreased fetal movements, joint contractures are uncommon. Characteristically affected infants appear very alert, with a characteristic posture of abducted limbs

Table 44.22 Clinical features of common anterior horn cell diseases in the newborn

	Werdnig–Hoffmann disease	Neurogenic arthrogryposis multiplex	Type II glycogen storage disease (Pompe's disease)	Neonatal poliomyelitis (other enteroviruses)
Onset	In utero to several weeks of age	In utero	Several weeks of age	Birth to several weeks
Pattern of weakness	Generalized, proximal > distal	Generalized or localized	Generalized, muscles enlarged	Asymmetric
Joint contractures	Rare	Multiple, severe	Rare	Rapid postnatal progression
Cranial nerve dysfunction	Bulbar dysfunction, tongue atrophy, fasciculations	None	Bulbar dysfunction Enlarged tongue with fasciculations	Variable
Tendon reflexes	Absent	Absent	Variable	Asymmetric
Other organs affected	None	None	Cardiac, liver, brain	Brain (encephalitis)
Clinical course	Variable, relates to complications	Static	Rapid deterioration	Rapid deterioration
Pathogenesis/inheritance pattern	Autosomal recessive, chromosome 5q11.2–13.3	Sporadic ± spinal cord dysgenesis	Acid maltase deficiency, glycogen deposition in tissues Autosomal recessive	Prenatal or postnatal infection Polio or enterovirus

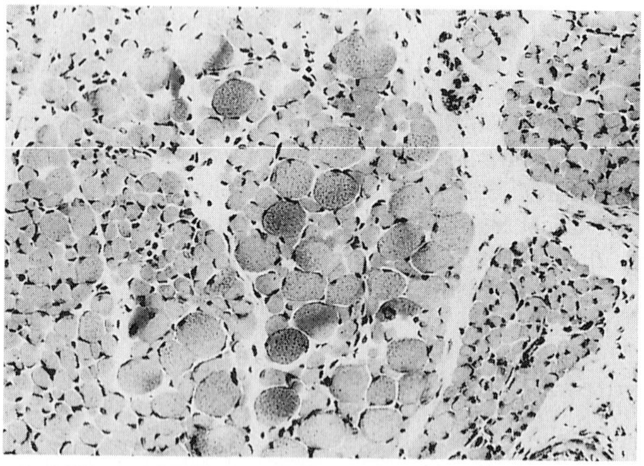

Fig. 44.56 Werdnig–Hoffmann disease. The muscle biopsy demonstrates neurogenic atrophy at 4 months of age. Note groups of small, atrophic fibres interspersed with hypertrophied type I fibres (H&E × 50).

(frog-leg position) and paradoxical diaphragmatic respiratory movements (Fig. 44.52). Involvement of the motor nuclei of cranial nerves may result in bulbar dysfunction, with impaired sucking and swallowing, atrophy and fasciculations of the tongue. Sphincter and sensory functions are normal.

Recent observations suggest that Werdnig–Hoffmann disease may not be a true degenerative condition, and more prolonged survival is possible. Muscle strength appears to remain relatively static and survival and deterioration relate more directly to frequency of aspiration from impaired swallowing, respiratory infections, prolonged immobility and hospitalizations.[39,60]

In addition to the evidence of denervation on muscle biopsy, EMG demonstrates spontaneous fasciculations and fibrillations and increased amplitude of evoked motor unit potentials. The serum CK level is usually normal in the infantile variety of spinal muscular atrophy.

Table 44.23 Peripheral nerve disorders in the newborn

Neuronal–axonal disease ± Werdnig–Hoffmann disease
Hypomyelinative neuropathy
Giant axonal neuropathy
Metabolic neuropathies: mitochondrial (Leigh's disease), lysosomal (Krabbe's leukodystrophy)
Sensory neuropathies: congenital sensory neuropathy, ± anhidrosis and mental retardation, familial dysautonomia (Riley–Day syndrome)
? Acute postinfectious polyneuropathy

DISORDERS OF PERIPHERAL NERVE

Disorders of peripheral nerve (Table 44.23) present rarely in the newborn period.[81] Clinical features include generalized weakness and hypotonia, with more marked weakness and atrophy of distal limb musculature and absent tendon reflexes. Feeding difficulties are common. There is variable involvement of the respiratory muscles, cranial nerves and joint contractures. Clinical or electrophysiological evidence of sensory deficits may be difficult to demonstrate reliably, but they are a valuable diagnostic clue. The clinical course is variable and may be non-progressive,[81] or even reversible.[24]

Investigations

Measurement of nerve conduction velocity is the principal investigation. Muscle biopsy may demonstrate denervation and sural nerve biopsy may demonstrate

Table 44.24 Disorders of neuromuscular transmission

Autoimmune
Neonatal transient myasthenia gravis
Genetic defects of neuromuscular junction
Familial infantile myasthenia gravis (autosomal recessive): postsynaptic defect in acetylcholine synthesis, packaging or release
End-plate actylcholinesterase deficiency (autosomal or X-linked recessive)
High-conductance fast channel syndrome
Congenital myasthenia: end-plate acetylcholine receptor deficiency (autosomal recessive)
Toxic–metabolic
Infantile botulism
Drug-induced, e.g. hypermagnesaemia, aminoglycosides

dysmyelination, i.e. hypomyelination or onion bulb formation related to repeated demyelination and remyelination. Other useful investigations include measurement of CSF protein concentration, which may be increased in demyelinating neuropathy. Serum and CSF lactate levels may be elevated in infants with Leigh's disease.

DISORDERS OF THE NEUROMUSCULAR JUNCTION

Disorders of neuromuscular transmission, which present clinically as fluctuating muscle weakness or fatiguing, may be difficult to recognize in the newborn. Other major clinical features of these disorders include variable ptosis, ophthalmoplegia, impaired sucking and swallowing, hypoventilation, facial diplegia and autonomic disturbances, e.g. impaired pupillary response to light or urinary retention. Early diagnosis is critical because these conditions often respond to treatment and timely intervention may prevent serious complications, e.g. respiratory failure. The major disorders of neuromuscular transmission which present during the neonatal period are summarized in Table 44.24.

MYASTHENIA GRAVIS

Transient neonatal myasthenia gravis

This condition develops in approximately 20% of infants of mothers with myasthenia gravis. The risk increases to 75% for an infant whose mother has had a previously affected child. There is no direct correlation between the severity or duration of maternal disease and the severity of symptoms in the newborn. In fact, severe neonatal disease may occur despite maternal remission.[50,52]

The syndrome results from circulating maternal anti-acetylcholine receptor antibodies compromising the infant's acetylcholine receptors. Thus, there is a direct correlation between the degree of elevation of the maternal antibody titre and the severity of symptoms in affected infants. However, asymptomatic infants may have similarly elevated titres.[50] It appears that symptomatic infants may synthesize acetylcholine receptor antibodies in addition to passive transfer of maternal antibody, and the half-life of this antibody is increased four- to eightfold in affected newborns. It may be critical that affected infants appear to have the same human leukocyte antigen (HLA) associated with myasthenia that is exhibited by their mothers.[55]

Clinical abnormalities usually become evident within hours after birth, but may be delayed for several days. In addition to generalized hypotonia and weakness there is dysphagia, weak sucking, ptosis and respiratory inadequacy. The Moro reflex is often diminished. In contrast to older patients, ptosis and ophthalmoplegia occur in only approximately 15% of cases. Symptoms usually last between 1 and 4 weeks, but may persist for months. Rarely, there may be evidence of intrauterine onset of weakness, including arthrogryposis, polyhydramnios and pulmonary hypoplasia.

When the mother's disease is not established the diagnosis may require evaluation of the infant's clinical response to anticholinesterase medication by observing changes in crying, sucking or swallowing, respiration or strength of limb movement. A test dose of edrophonium (0.15 mg/kg) administered intramuscularly or subcutaneously, or 0.1 mg/kg administered intravenously, should produce improvement within 3–5 minutes which lasts 10–15 minutes. Alternatively, neostigmine methylsulfate 0.15 mg/kg administered intramuscularly or subcutaneously will produce maximum response within 15–30 minutes. This has the major advantage that the beneficial effect is more prolonged, lasting 1–3 hours.

Management of transient myasthenia gravis involves both supportive therapy and anticholinesterase therapy with neostigmine (0.05 mg/kg), administered intramuscularly or subcutaneously approximately 20 minutes prior to feeding. Exchange transfusion has been reported to be a helpful adjunct in some cases.

Familial infantile myasthenia

This rare autosomal recessive disorder is often indistinguishable clinically from neonatal transient myasthenia gravis, but treated infants generally improve gradually although there may be episodic recurrences in association with respiratory infections. Prolonged anticholinesterase treatment and close surveillance is recommended for the risk of sudden recurrence.

Congenital myasthenia: abnormal neuromuscular junction

Several anatomical defects of the neuromuscular junction, e.g. congenital end-plate anticholinesterase deficiency and end-plate acetylcholine receptor deficiencies, have been reported.[81] Affected infants have prominent ptosis and ophthalmoplegia, with less severe feeding problems and minimal hypotonia and weakness. The clinical course is often benign. The response to anticholinesterase drugs is variable.[20]

TOXIC–METABOLIC DISTURBANCES

Impaired presynaptic release of acetylcholine by toxins may lead to disturbed neuromuscular transmission. Hypermagnesaemia, following treatment of maternal eclampsia with magnesium sulphate, may result in rapidly progressive flaccid weakness, bulbar dysfunction, apnoea and autonomic dysfunction, e.g. pupillary dilation and urinary retention.[47] Aminoglycoside antibodies may produce similar adverse effects, which may be compounded in infants with myasthenia gravis or botulism.[83] In many instances the rapid deterioration of the infant may be misdiagnosed as sepsis, which in turn may lead to further antibiotic therapy and aggravation of the weakness.

INFANTILE BOTULISM

This condition occurs most commonly between 6 weeks and 6 months of life as a result of intestinal absorption of toxin produced by ingested *Clostridium botulinum* organisms. It has been reported as early as 9 days of age. Honey has been often implicated as the offending food containing the botulinum spores. Affected infants usually present with constipation, in addition to ophthalmoplegia, bulbar dysfunction, generalized weakness, hypotonia and areflexia. The diagnosis may be suspected by culture of *Clostridium* organisms in stools, in addition to an incremental response to repetitive nerve stimulation on EMG. Supportive treatment is of paramount importance because eventual full recovery can be anticipated if secondary complications are avoided.

MUSCLE DISORDERS

Generalized muscle diseases which are clinically symptomatic during the newborn period may be classified as

- muscular dystrophies, which usually have non-specific histological features of muscle necrosis, regeneration and fibrosis;
- 'non-progressive' congenital myopathies, which are often characterized by distinctive histological abnormalities.

Myopathies are diseases that involve primarily striated muscle. The term 'muscular dystrophy' is applied to genetically determined myopathies which are characterized clinically by worsening weakness and pathologically by progressive muscle degeneration. The recent discovery of many gene mutations and the associated abnormalities in protein products may eventually result in reclassification of the muscular dystrophies according to their specific abnormalities at a cellular level.

MUSCULAR DYSTROPHIES WITH NON-SPECIFIC HISTOLOGY

Congenital myotonic dystrophy

Although myotonic dystrophy is generally considered to have an autosomal dominant inheritance pattern, the neonatal variety of the disease is inherited almost exclusively from the mother. The earlier the onset and more severe the disease in the mother, the greater the risk of congenital myotonic dystrophy in the newborn. The early onset of problems in utero, e.g. polyhydramnios and prematurity, is associated with more severe neonatal disease. Clinical or electromyographic myotonia, which is characteristic of this disease in older individuals, cannot usually be elicited in affected newborns. Affected infants commonly present with generalized hypotonia, proximal weakness, impaired sucking and swallowing, facial diplegia, ptosis, arthrogryposis and respiratory impairment (Fig. 44.57). Less severely affected newborns with hypotonia and facial weakness may remain undetected during the newborn period.

Congenital myotonic dystrophy is a multisystem disorder with cognitive impairment and evidence of dysmaturity of other organs. Neuroimaging may demonstrate dilatation of the cerebral ventricles, related to cerebral dysgenesis or periventricular leukomalacia.[23,58,76]

Until recently the diagnosis was based most frequently on a positive family history and clinical or electromyographic evidence of myotonia in the mother. At the present time, diagnosis is based on molecular genetic studies in the mother or affected newborn which demonstrate an increase in trinucleotide repeats (CTG) in an unstable DNA region of the myotonic dystrophy gene at chromosome 19q13.3.[51,73] The serum CK and EMG are often normal in affected newborns. Muscle

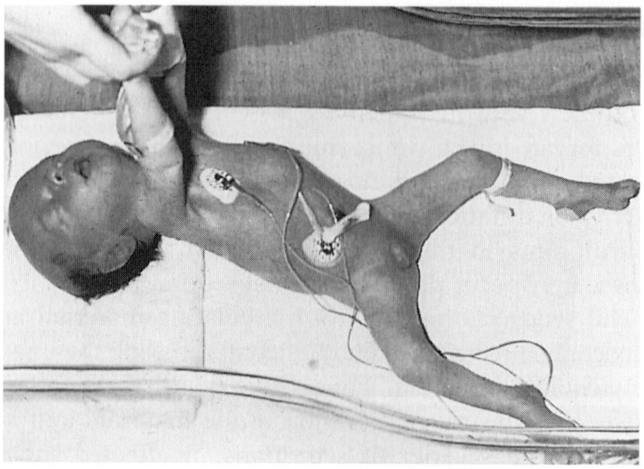

Fig. 44.57 Premature infant with congenital myotonic dystrophy. Note facial diplegia and frog-leg position.

biopsy may reveal changes distinct from the adult form of the disorder, i.e. maturational arrest with predominance of type II fibres and poorly differentiated small fibres with large internal nuclei, reminiscent of fetal myotubes, which are usually seen at approximately 20 weeks' gestation.[66]

The clinical course is variable and relates to the severity of the disease. The mortality rate is high (approximately 50%). Survivors are usually able to suck and swallow adequately by 12 weeks of age. Thereafter, muscle weakness is often static or slowly progressive and there is associated moderate intellectual impairment, which may also show progressive deterioration.[15,81]

Congenital muscular dystrophy

The congenital muscular dystrophies are a group of disorders that present with muscle weakness at birth and have a dystrophic pattern on muscle biopsy. They usually have autosomal recessive inheritance. Congenital muscular dystrophy may be classified according to whether there is myopathy alone or a combination of central nervous system and skeletal muscle involvement.

In the newborn infant CMD usually presents with generalized hypotonia, disproportionate weakness of the neck flexors and some degree of facial diplegia, with normal extraocular muscle function. Difficulties with swallowing and breathing lead to respiratory failure in approximately one-third of cases. Significant contractures and scoliosis are often present at birth, or develop rapidly postnatally. In infants without central nervous system involvement the muscle weakness is often static, and affected individuals may have functional improvement and attain ambulation despite greatly reduced muscle bulk ('stick-man dystrophy').

In contrast, several variants of CMD have prominent central nervous system involvement, including cerebral dysgenesis with migration abnormalities,[22,25] decreased cerebral white matter[17] and ocular abnormalities (muscle–eye–brain disease, Santavuori, variant) and Walker–Warburg syndrome.[13,62,63] Central nervous system involvement may be suspected clinically if there is evidence of seizures, glaucoma, optic nerve abnormalities or cataracts. The clinical course of patients who have central nervous system involvement is often progressive, with reduced survival.[46]

Investigations include normal or moderate elevations of CK levels, a myopathic pattern on EMG and a dystrophic process on muscle biopsy, which should not be used as an index of prognosis or severity of the disease. Occasionally muscle histopathology may demonstrate a significant inflammatory process.[56] Delayed or diminished cerebral white matter or cerebral dysgenesis may be documented by CT or MRI. Western blot and immunocytochemical assessment of the muscle biopsy reveals normal dystrophin but a deficiency of merosin (laminin M or α_2), a protein attached to the dystrophin-associated glycoproteins on the outside of the muscle membrane, in the biopsies of cases with cerebral white matter abnormalities.[8,57,71] Furthermore, merosin-negative cases appear to link to chromosome 6, the locus for the merosin gene,[35] which strengthens the impression that merosin may have a major role in the pathogenesis of CMD.

CONGENITAL MYOPATHIES WITH DISTINCT HISTOLOGY

There are numerous congenital myopathies, which may be classified according to their distinct histological appearance on muscle biopsy (Table 44.25). With the exception of nemaline myopathy and X-linked myotubular myopathy, which may be associated with

Table 44.25 Congenital myopathies with distinct muscle histology

Myopathy	Inheritance pattern	Histological features	Major clinical features
Central core disease	Autosomal dominant	Single or multiple central cores of closely packed, degenerating myofibrils in type I fibres; absent oxidative enzymes in cores	Kyphoscoliosis Pes cavus Dislocated hips
Nemaline (rod body) myopathy	Autosominal dominant (incomplete penetrance)	Multiple, small rod-like protein particles in continuity with Z-band on electron microscopy	Dysmorphic features, facial weakness, may develop fulminant respiratory failure
Myotubular myopathy	Autosomal dominant or recessive, X-linked, sporadic	Internal nuclei, central area of increased oxidative enzymes and decreased ATPase activity; resemble fetal myotubes	Fulminant respiratory failure (X-linked), Facial diplegia, Ptosis Ophthalmoplegia Central nervous system abnormalities
Congenital variable fibre type disproportion		Increased number of type I fibres (>55%) Size of type I fibres < type II	Proximal weakness Dysmorphic features Normal reflexes Contractures Kyphoscoliosis

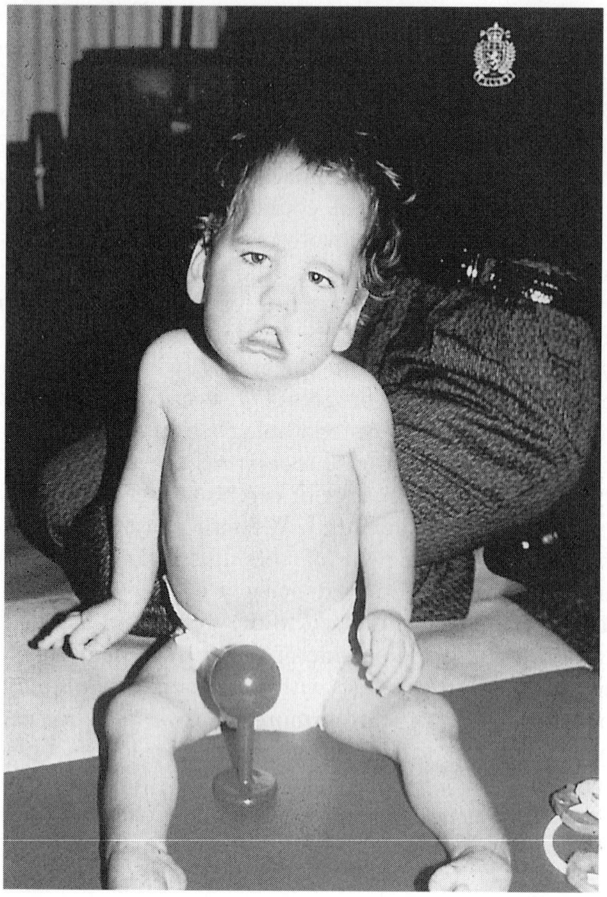

Fig. 44.58 Child with myotubular myopathy. Note facial diplegia and foot deformities.

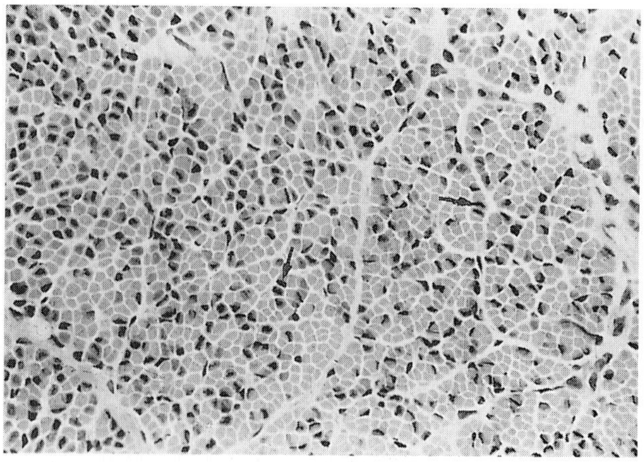

Fig. 44.59 Muscle biopsy of myotubular myopathy. Note central nuclei and myotubes in type I fibres (arrows).

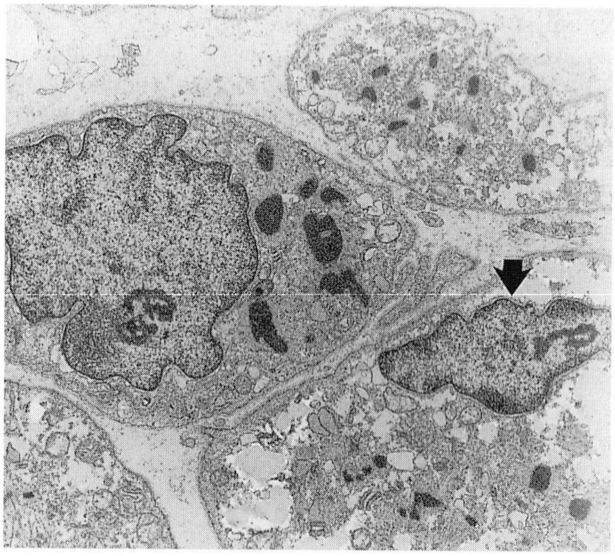

Fig. 44.60 Nemaline myopathy. Note nemaline rods in subsarcolemmal location (arrow).

fulminant respiratory failure in early infancy, these conditions present with relatively mild static hypotonia and weakness, which is often worse proximally.[15,81] Facial weakness occurs commonly (Fig. 44.58). Diagnosis is based on the specific histological or electron microscopic abnormalities on muscle biopsy. For example, Figure 44.59 illustrates the typical histological appearance of myotubular myopathy and Figure 44.60 demonstrates the electron microscopic features of nemaline myopathy. Serum CK and EMG, which may be normal, are not usually helpful in diagnosis.

Isolated case reports of numerous other myopathies with distinctive histological features on muscle biopsy have been reported. These include such conditions as reducing body myopathy, tubular aggregate myopathy, fingerprint body myopathy, multicore myopathy, sarcotubular myopathy and spheroid body myopathy.[15] Further delineation of the specificity, clinical features and pathogenesis of these rare congenital myopathies may be expected.[64]

METABOLIC MYOPATHIES

With the availability of electron microscopy, muscle enzyme assays and magnetic resonance spectroscopy there has been increasing recognition of metabolic myopathies characterized by primary functional derangements of energy metabolism in muscle. Normal muscle activity depends on the metabolic pathways within the mitochondria, including the Krebs cycle and oxidative phosphorylation, glycogen and lipid metabolism and β-oxidation of long-chain fatty acids which enter the inner mitochondrial space in the presence of carnitine and carnitine palmityl transferase. Clearly, a comprehensive discussion of the biochemical aspects of these complex disorders is beyond the scope of this chapter, and is presented elsewhere.[15,36]

Mitochondrial myopathies

Mitochondrial myopathies are multisystem disorders which have variable presentation, with features of growth failure and exacerbation of muscle fatigue and weakness associated with exercise or infection. In addition to myopathic features, central nervous system involvement frequently occurs. Symptoms may include microcephaly, mental retardation, myoclonic seizures, ataxia and stroke-like episodes. In view of this great variability in clinical presentation a high index of suspicion must be maintained for mitochondrial disorders whenever there is evidence of fluctuating neurological abnormalities.

Laboratory investigations may reveal lactic acidosis, with normal or mild elevations of CK level. The EMG is often normal. Histopathology on muscle biopsy may demonstrate excessive red-staining material on modified Gomori trichrome stain ('ragged red fibres'), and electron microscopy may demonstrate increased numbers of mitochondria with abnormal configuration. More recently it has become possible to document disturbed mitochondrial function (enzyme levels) as well as relevant gene deletions. A rational classification of these disorders, based on genetic, biochemical and clinical features, is gradually emerging.[12]

Several infants with severe myopathy related to deficiency of cytochrome C oxidase (complex IV of the mitochondrial respiratory chain) have been reported. Clinical features include severe generalized weakness, areflexia, severe lactic acidosis and respiratory failure, which results in death during early infancy.[12] There is often facial weakness and weak sucking, although eye movements are normal. There may be associated hepatic, renal and cardiac dysfunction. Infants usually have progressive deterioration, with death in the first year.

A remarkably benign and reversible variant of cytochrome C oxidase deficiency also occurs. In these infants the symptoms, which may be severe initially, improve gradually after several months, and the child may be normal by 2–4 years. Thus it is recommended that life support be continued in affected infants long enough to distinguish between the benign and malignant varieties of cytochrome C oxidase deficiency. Benign disease is suggested by increasing muscle strength, declining blood lactate and increasing cytochrome C oxidase activity in repeated biopsies. It is also possible to distinguish between these two varieties by immunohistochemistry with antibodies directed against different subunits of cytochrome C oxidase.[12,79]

Carnitine deficiency

The absence of this cofactor, which is required for the transport of long-chain fatty acids into mitochondria for β-oxidation, may result in clinical abnormalities during early infancy, including hypotonia, mild proximal muscle weakness, failure to thrive, encephalopathy, hypoketotic hypoglycaemia and cardiomyopathy. Muscle histology demonstrates lipid-containing vacuoles. Carnitine levels in serum and muscle are low. Treatment consists of long-term administration of oral carnitine.[28,72]

Carnitine palmityl transferase deficiency

Although this disorder presents in later childhood, an infantile variety with severe hypoglycaemia and absent liver carnitine palmityl transferase activity has been described.[74]

Disorders of glycogen and lipid metabolism

Rarely, disorders of glycogen and lipid metabolism may present with moderate or severe muscle weakness in the newborn. Additional features include joint contractures, liver dysfunction and hypoglycaemia. Diagnosis depends on identification of glycogen or lipid-containing vacuoles in muscle biopsy.[81,36]

REFERENCES

1. Banker B Q 1986 Arthrogryposis multiplex congenita: spectrum of pathologic changes. Human Pathology 17: 656–672
2. Blom S, Finnstrom O 1971 Studies on maturity in newborn infants v. motor conduction velocity. Neuropediatrics 3: 129–139
3. Bodensteiner J, Zellweger H 1971 Creatine phosphokinase in normal neonates and young infants. Journal of Laboratory and Clinical Medicine 77: 853–858
4. Brenningstall G N, Grover W D, Barbera S, Marks H G 1988 Neonatal rhabdomyolysis as a presentation of muscular dystrophy. Neurology 38: 1271–1272
5. Brooke M H 1986 A clinician's view of neuromuscular diseases. Williams & Wilkins, Baltimore, p. 127
6. Calo M, Crisi G, Martinelli C, Colombo A, Schoenhuber R, Gibertoni M 1986 CT and the diagnosis of myopathies. Neuroradiology 28: 53–57
7. Carroll J E 1983 The floppy infant. Neurology Neurosurgical Update Series 4:1
8. Connolly A M, Pestronk A, Planer G J, Yue J, Mehta S, Choksma R 1996 Congenital muscular dystrophy syndromes distinguished by alkaline and acid phosphatase, merosin and dystrophin staining. Neurology 46: 810–814
9. Connolly M B, Roland E H, Hill A 1992 Clinical features for prediction of survival in neonatal muscle disease. Pediatric Neurology 8: 285–288
10. Cook J D, Gascon G G, Haider A et al 1992 Congenital muscular dystrophy with abnormal radiographic myelin pattern. Journal of Child Neurology 7 (Suppl): 551–563
11. David W S, Jones H R 1994 Electromyography and biopsy correlation with suggested protocol for evaluation of the floppy infant. Muscle and Nerve 17: 424–430
12. DiMauro S 1993 Mitochondrial encephalomyopathies. In: Rosenberg R N, Prusiner S B, DiMauro S et al. (eds) The molecular and genetic basis of neurological disease. Butterworth-Heinemann, Boston, pp 665–694
13. Dobyns W B, Pagon R A, Armstrong D et al 1989 Diagnostic criteria for Walker–Warburg syndrome. American Journal of Medical Genetics 32: 195–210
14. Drummond L M 1979 Creatine phosphokinase levels in the newborn and their use in screening for Duchenne muscular dystrophy. Archives of Disease in Childhood 54: 362–366
15. Dubowitz V 1995 Muscle disorders in childhood, 2nd ed. Saunders, London
16. Dubowitz V 1994 Workshop report: 22nd ENMC-sponsored workshop on congenital muscular dystrophy. Neuromuscular Disorders 4: 72–81
17. Echenne B, Arthuis M, Billard C et al 1986 Congenital muscular dystrophy and CT scan anomalies. Report of a collaborative study of the Société de Neurologie Infantile. Journal of Neurological Sciences 75: 7–22
18. Edwards R H T, Round J M, Jones D A 1983 Needle biopsy of skeletal muscle: a review of 10 years' experience. Muscle and Nerve 6: 676–683
19. Engel W K, Karpati G 1968 Impaired skeletal muscle maturation following neonatal neurectomy. Developmental Biology 17: 713–723

20. Engel A G 1988 Congenital myasthenic syndromes. Journal of Child Neurology 3: 233–246
21. Fischer A Q, Carpenter D W, Hartlage P L, Carroll J E, Stephens S 1988 Muscle imaging in neuromuscular disease using computerized real-time sonography. Muscle and Nerve 11: 270–275
22. Fukuyama Y, Osawa M, Suzuki H 1981 Congenital progressive muscular dystrophy of the Fukuyama type – clinical, genetic and pathological considerations. Brain Development 3: 1–29
23. Garcia-Alix A, Cabanas F, Morales C et al 1991 Cerebral abnormalities in congenital myotonic dystrophy. Pediatric Neurology 7: 28–32
24. Ghamdi M, Armstrong D L, Miller G 1997 Congenital hypomyelinating neuropathy: a reversible case. Pediatric Neurology 16: 71–73
25. Goebel H H, Fidzianski A, Lenard H G et al 1983 A morphological study of non-Japanese congenital muscular dystrophy associated with cerebral lesions. Brain Development 5: 292–301
26. Goeschen K, Pluta M, Rothe J, Saling E 1983 Measurement of motor nerve conduction velocity: precise method of estimating maturity in the newborn. British Journal of Obstetrics and Gynaecology 90: 61–68
27. Hageman G, Willemse J, Van Ketch B A et al 1987 The pathogenesis of fetal hypokinesia. Neuropediatrics 18: 22–33
28. Hale D E, Bennett M J 1992 Fatty acid oxidation disorders: a new class of metabolic disease. Journal of Pediatrics 121: 1–11
29. Hall J G 1985 Genetic aspects of arthrogryposis. Clinical Orthopedics 194: 44–53
30. Harper P S 1989 Myotonic dystrophy, 2nd edn. Saunders, London
31. Hays R M, Michaud L J 1988 Neonatal myasthenia gravis: specific advantages of repetitive stimulation over edrophonium testing. Pediatric Neurology 4: 245–247
32. Heckmatt J Z, Dubowitz V 1987 Ultrasound imaging and directed needle biopsy in the diagnosis of selective involvement in neuromuscular disease. Journal of Child Neurology 2: 205–213
33. Heckmatt J Z, Pier N, Dubowitz V 1988 Real-time ultrasound imaging of muscles. Muscle and Nerve 11: 56–65
34. Heckmatt J Z, Moosa A, Hutson C, Maunder-Sewry C A, Dubowitz V 1984 Diagnostic needle muscle biopsy: a practical and reliable alternative to open biopsy. Archives of Disease in Childhood 59: 528–532
35. Hillaire D, Leclerc A, Faure S et al 1994 Localization of merosin-negative congenital muscular dystrophy to chromosome 6q2 by homozygosity mapping. Human Molecular Genetics 3: 1657–1661
36. Hilton-Jones D, Squier M, Taylor D, Matthews P 1995 Metabolic myopathies. W B Saunders, London
37. Jaffe R, Mock M, Abramowicz J, Ben-aderet N 1986 Myotonic dystrophy and pregnancy: a review. Obstetrics and Gynecology 41: 272–278
38. Iannaccone S T, Guilfoile T 1988 Longterm mechanical ventilation in infants with neuromuscular disease. Journal of Child Neurology 2: 30–32
39. Iannaccone S T, Brown R H, Samaha F J et al 1993 Prospective study of spinal muscular atrophy before age 6 years. Pediatric Neurology 9: 187–193
40. Jacob P, Sarnat H B 1989 Influences of the brain on normal and abnormal muscle development. In: Hill A, Volpe J J (eds) Fetal neurology. Raven Press, New York, p. 269
41. Jones H R 1990 EMG evaluation of the floppy infant. Differential diagnosis and technical aspects. Muscle and Nerve 13: 338–347
42. Jones H R 1993 Pediatric electromyography. In: Brown W F, Bolton C F (eds) Clinical electromyography. Butterworth-Heinemann, Boston
43. Kasik J W, Leuschen M P, Bolan D L, Nelson R N 1985 Rhabdomyolysis and myoglobinemia in neonates. Pediatrics 76: 255–258
44. Kyriakides T, Silberstein J M, Jongpiputvanichi et al 1993 The clinical significance of type 1 fiber predominance. Muscle and Nerve 16: 418–423
45. Lamminen A E 1990 Magnetic resonance imaging of primary skeletal muscle diseases: patterns of distribution and severity of involvement. British Journal of Radiology 63: 946–950
46. Leyton Q U Y, Gabreals F J M, Renier W O, Terlaak H J, Sengers R C A, Mullaart R A 1989 Congenital muscular dystrophy. Journal of Pediatrics 115: 214–222
47. Lipsitz P J 1971 The clinical and biochemical effects of excess magnesium in the newborn. Pediatrics 47: 501–509
48. MacKenzie A, Roy N, Besner A et al 1993a Genetic linkage analysis of Canadian spinal muscular atrophy kindreds using flanking microsatellite 5q13 polymorphisms. Human Genetics 90: 501–504
49. Mackenzie A, Besner A, Roy N 1993b Rapid diagnosis of infantile spinal muscular atrophy by direct amplification of amniocyte and GVS DNA. Journal of Medical Genetics 30: 162–164
50. Morel E, Eymard B, Garabedian V et al 1988 Neonatal myasthenia gravis: a new clinical and immunologic appraisal in 30 cases. Neurology 38: 138–142
51. Mulley J C, Staples A, Donnolly A et al 1993 Explanation for exclusive maternal origin for congenital form of myotonic dystrophy. Lancet 341: 236–237
52. Namba T, Brown S B, Grobd 1970 Neonatal myasthenia gravis: report of two cases and review of the literature. Pediatrics 45: 488–504
53. Osborne J P, Murphy E G, Hill A 1983 Thin ribs on chest X-ray: a useful sign in the differential diagnosis of the floppy newborn. Developmental Medicine and Child Neurology 25: 343–345
54. Packer R J, Brown M J, Bermann P H 1982 The diagnostic value of electromyography in infantile hypotonia. American Journal of Diseases of Children 54: 331–338
55. Papazian O 1992 Transient neonatal myasthenia gravis. Journal of Child Neurology 7: 135–141
56. Pegoraro E, Mancias P, Swerdlow S H et al 1996 Congenital muscular dystrophy with primary laminin alpha 2 (merosin) deficiency presenting as inflammatory myopathy. Annals of Neurology 40: 782–791
57. Philpot J, Topaloglu H, Pennock J, Dubowitz V 1995 Familial concordance of brain magnetic resonance imaging changes in congenital muscular dystrophy. Neuromuscular Disorders 5: 227–231
58. Regev R, de Vries L S, Heckmatt J Z et al 1987 Cerebral ventricular dilation in congenital myotonic dystrophy. Journal of Pediatrics 111: 372–376
59. Ricoy J, Cabello 1981 Dysmaturative myopathy. Evolution of the morphological picture in three cases. Acta Neuropathology Supplement VII: 313–316
60. Russman B S, Iannacone S T, Buncher C R et al 1992 Spinal muscular atrophy: new thoughts on the pathogenesis and classification scheme. Journal of Child Neurology 7: 347–353
61. Ruth V J 1989 Prognostic value of creatine kinase-BB-isoenzyme in high risk newborn infants. Archives of Diseases in Childhood 64: 563–568
62. Santavuori P, Somer H, Sainio K et al 1989 Muscle–eye–brain disease (MEB). Brain and Development 11: 147–153
63. Santavuori P, Pihko H, Sainio K et al 1990 Muscle–eye–brain disease and Walker–Warburg syndrome. American Journal of Medical Genetics 36: 371–374
64. Sarnat H B 1994 New insights into the pathogenesis of congenital myopathies. Journal of Child Neurology 9: 193–201
65. Sarnat H B, O'Connor T, Byrne P A 1976 Clinical effects of myotonic dystrophy on pregnancy and the neonate. Archives of Neurology 33: 459–465
66. Sarnat H B, Silbert S W 1976 Maturational arrest of fetal muscle in neonatal myotonic dystrophy. Archives of Neurology 33: 466–474
67. Sarnat H B 1978 Diagnostic value of the muscle biopsy in the neonatal period. American Journal of Diseases of Children 132: 782–785
68. Sarnat H B 1983 Muscle pathology and histochemistry. American Society of Clinical Pathologists Press, Chicago
69. Sarnat H B 1990 Myotubular myopathy: arrest of morphogenesis of myofibers associated with persistence of fetal vimentin and desmin. Canadian Journal of Neurological Sciences 17: 109–123
70. Sarnat H B 1986 Cerebral dysgeneses and their influence on fetal muscle development. Brain Development 8: 495–499
71. Sewry C, Philpot D, Mahony D, Wilson L A, Mutoni F, Dubowitz V 1995 Expression of laminin subunits in congenital muscular dystrophy. Neuromuscular Disorders 5: 307–316
72. Shapira Y, Glick B, Harel S et al 1993 Infantile idiopathic myopathic carnitine deficiency: treatment with L-carnitine. Pediatric Neurology 9: 35–38
73. Shelbourne P, Davies J, Buxton J et al 1993 Direct diagnosis of myotonic dystrophy with a disease-specific DNA marker. New England Journal of Medicine 328: 471–475
74. Smith S 1989 Congenital and metabolic myopathies. In: Swaiman K F (ed) Pediatric neurology: principles and practice, Vol II. C V Mosby, St. Louis, pp. 1165–1170
75. Sutton T M, O'Brien J F, Kleinberg F et al 1981 Serum levels of creatine phosphokinase and its isoenzymes in normal and stressed neonates. Mayo Clinic Proceedings 56: 150–154

76. Tanabe Y, Iai M, Tamai K et al 1992 Neuroradiological findings in children with congenital myotonic dystrophy. Acta Paediatrica 81: 613–617
77. Thompson C E 1985 Pitfalls in muscle biopsies of hypotonic children. Developmental Medicine and Child Neurology 27: 675–685
78. Topaloglu H, Yalaz K, Renda Y et al 1991 Occidental type cerebromuscular dystrophy: a report of eleven cases. Journal of Neurology, Neurosurgery and Psychiatry 54: 226–229
79. Tritschler H J, Bonilla E, Lombes A et al 1991 Differential diagnosis of fatal and benign cytochrome C oxidase-deficient myopathies of infancy. Neurology 41: 300–305
80. Vial C, Charles N, Chouplannaz G et al 1991 Myasthenia gravis in childhood and infancy. Usefulness of electrophysiologic studies. Archives of Neurology 48: 847–849
81. Volpe J J 1995 Neurology of the Newborn, 3rd edn. Saunders, Philadelphia, pp 606–608
82. Wallgren-Pettersson C, Kivisaari L, Jaskelainen J et al 1990 Ultrasonography, CT and MRI of muscles in congenital nemaline myopathy. Pediatric Neurology 6: 20–28
83. Wright E A, McQuillen M P 1971 Antibiotic-induced neuromuscular blockade. Annals of the New York Academy of Sciences 183: 716–719

Part 8

Central nervous system malformations

Janet M. Rennie

EPIDEMIOLOGICAL ASPECTS

INCIDENCE AT BIRTH

Congenital malformations of the CNS, consisting principally of spina bifida, anencephalus and hydrocephalus, form a large but progressively diminishing proportion of all major congential malformations (Table 44.26, Figs 44.61, 44.62). Since the last edition of this book there has been a sustained reduction in the prevalence of NTD at birth, due only in part to antenatal diagnosis and termination of pregnancy. At the same time there has been an increase in the diagnosis during life of cerebral malformations such as lissencephaly using magnetic resonance imaging. Antenatal diagnosis has created new dilemmas, particularly for parents whose fetus has a condition for which the prognosis is uncertain, such as mild unilateral ventriculomegaly, isolated agenesis of the corpus callosum, hemimegalencephaly or a middle cranial fossa arachnoid cyst. In addition a great deal of parental anxiety is engendered by the antenatal finding of a minor CNS malformation, such as a choroid plexus cyst or an enlarged cisterna magna. This evolution in clinical practice has required a change of emphasis from the second edition, to which the reader is referred for an excellent and detailed account of neural tube defects.

In 1974 almost 5000 babies were conceived with CNS defects of all types in England and Wales. By 1993 this figure had reduced to just over 1000, and among livebirths CNS defects had reduced tenfold. During the same period other malformations increased from 158.8 to 190.8 per 10 000 deliveries.[55,56] Anencephalic births fell from 13.1 to 0.2 per 10 000 between 1974 and 1993; spina bifida from 18.3 to 1.2 and hydrocephalus from 4.8 to 1.0 per 10 000.

The causes of this decline are only partly known, but in 1974 only 34 abortions were carried out because of fetal CNS defects compared to about 500 per annum in the last decade. The increased number of terminations does not entirely account for the decline in CNS defects at birth. Figure 44.61 shows the impact of terminations of pregnancy for fetal malformations on perinatal mortality in the Northern region of the UK between 1982 and

Table 44.26 The number of babies (live and stillborn) with CNS defects born in England and Wales, together with the number of abortions carried out for CNS defects (Source: Office of National Statistics 1993)

Year	Terminations of pregnancy	Anencephalus births	Spina bifida births	Congenital hydrocephalus	Other CNS malformation births	Total CNS malformation births	Total CNS malformations
1974	34	849	1185	313	105	2452	4938
1976	81	644	880	267	124	1915	3911
1979	285	455	845	227	110	1637	3559
1983	511	114	422	194	187	917	2345
1987	529	31	202	117	161	511	1551
1990	452	26	120	92	122	360	1172
1993	536	14	81	71	88	255	1045

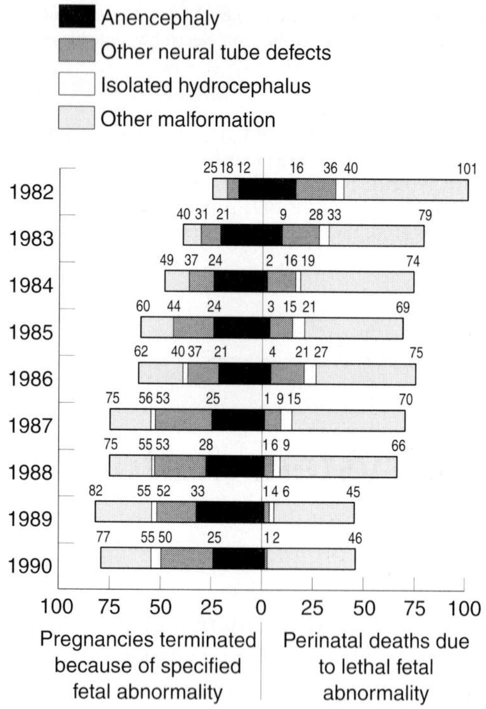

Fig. 44.61 Neural tube defects, congenital hydrocephalus and other lethal fetal abnormalities in the Northern region 1982–1990, their increasing antenatal recognition and the impact of this on perinatal mortality. (From Northern Regional Survey Steering Group,[54] with permission)

1990.[54] Figure 44.62 shows the decline in CNS births recorded by the Office of National Statistics, with the annual termination rate for CNS malformations also shown. Unfortunately, the national statistics are probably an underestimate; the South East Thames congenital malformation register alone recorded over 200 cases of anencephaly and spina bifida as liveborn or terminations between April 1992 and April 1995, and the Northern region recorded about 50 cases per year with the same diagnosis (Fig. 44.61).

Regional variations

There are large variations in the incidence of CNS defects in different parts of the world[26,74] and at different periods. In the British Isles the highest incidence is in Ireland, followed by Wales. In England the highest incidence was in the northwest and the lowest in the southeast, but these differences have been almost eliminated by antenatal diagnosis and terminations of pregnancies.

Sex incidence

In anencephalus and in encephalocoele the sex ratio of females to males is 7:3, and in spina bifida it is 55:45, but

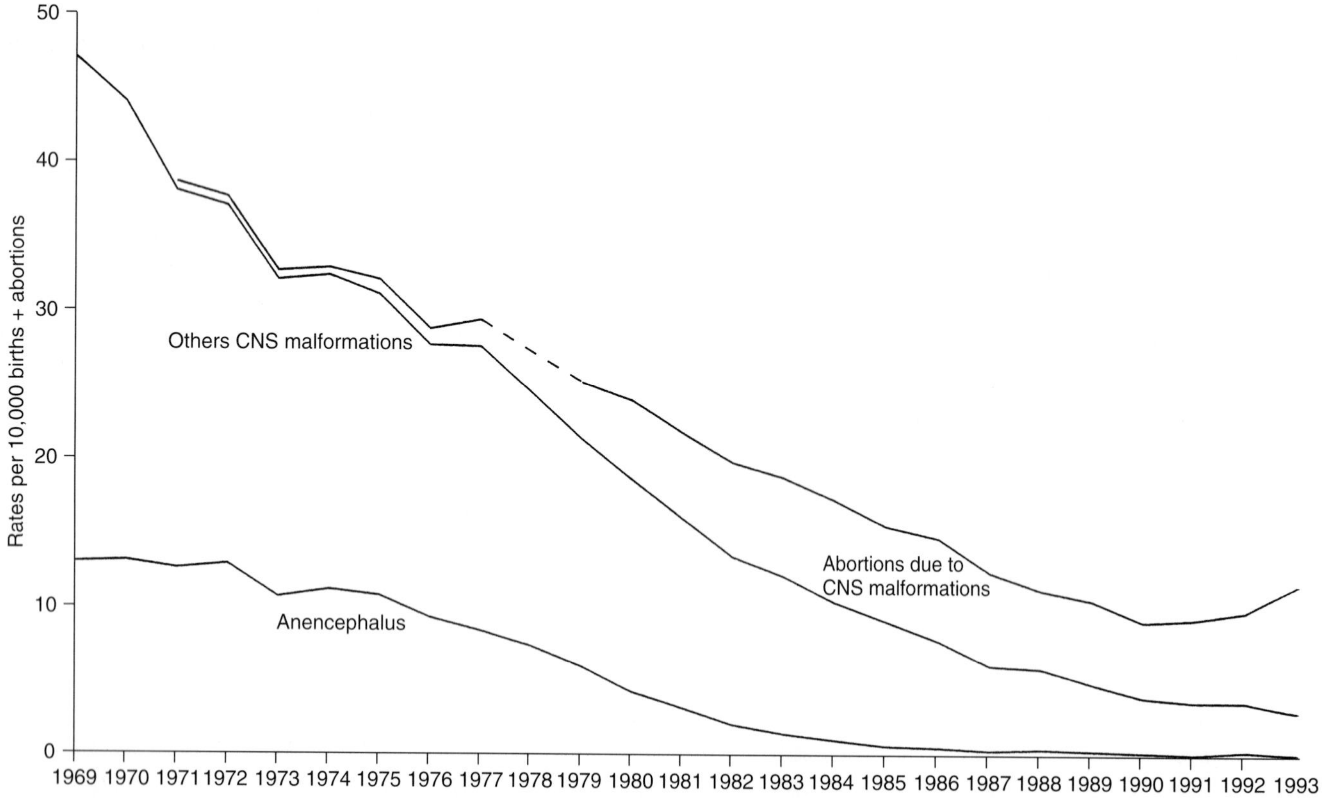

Fig 44.62 The annual incidence of CNS malformations among liveborn infants in England and Wales, together with the reported terminations of pregnancy for CNS malformations. (Source: National Statistics Office 1993)

in congenital hydrocephalus it is 4:6. An explanation of these differences might provide one possible clue to the causation of CNS defects.

Twins

Both twins are rarely affected by NTD. Both affected twins may have different malformations. Analysis of a series of 887 pairs (which was in part personal and in part collected from the world literature), in which at least one twin had either anencephalus or spina bifida, showed that the concordance rate was 4.9%. In twin pairs with spina bifida alone the concordance in like-sexed twins was 9% and in unlike-sexed twins it was 1%. In monozygous twins the concordance was 12% of pairs.[47]

Family history and recurrence risks of spina bifida, anencephalus and congenital hydrocephalus

The risk of recurrence to siblings following the birth of a fetus or baby with a NTD is around 5%[14,15,42] and may be related to the incidence in the area at a given time. For example, in the British Isles the highest recurrence rate recorded was 8.8% in the high-incidence area of Belfast, relating to births in the 1960s,[52] and the lowest 3.4% in the southeast of England during the 1970s.[67] The recurrence risk is approximately 10% if the mother has already had two or more affected babies.[17,42,69] The risk to children of a parent who had spina bifida is of the same order as to siblings after a single affected case.[16] The risk to more distant relations is far less. There is a considerably increased risk of CNS malformations in the siblings of a baby with congenital hydrocephalus unassociated with spina bifida. In Sheffield 187 patients with congenital hydrocephalus had 338 siblings: 3.8% had CNS defects, five (1.5%) hydrocephalus and eight (2.3%) spina bifida or anencephalus, so at least a part of the 'congenital hydrocephalus' group is of similar or identical aetiology to spina bifida and anencephalus.[44,45] In Belfast in a smaller group the recurrence rate of 1.9% for congenital hydrocephalus was 26 times higher than in the local population.[1] Cohen et al[21] collected data from various parts of the world to show that following the birth of a baby with isolated hydrocephalus the risk of anencephalus in subsequent pregnancies was 1%, of spina bifida 0.6% and of isolated hydrocephalus 1.5%.

PREVENTION OF CENTRAL NERVOUS SYSTEM DEFECTS

Antenatal diagnosis followed by termination of pregnancy

There is an elevated α-fetoprotein level in the maternal blood and amniotic fluid in the presence of an open NTD in the fetus.[8,9,77] α-Fetoprotein is widely offered as a serum screening test for the detection of NTDs in pregnancy (Chapter 14), in addition to a careful examination of the fetal brain and spine with ultrasound during an anomaly scan at 18–20 weeks' gestation. High serum α-fetoprotein levels may also be obtained in cases of twin pregnancy, exomphalos and urinary tract abnormalities, as well as in cases of fetal death in utero. Interpretation of the result is highly dependent on accurate dating of the pregnancy. The predictive value can be improved by the analysis of acetylcholinesterase, which is also high in NTD pregnancies.[77]

Table 44.27 Major CNS malformations that can be diagnosed antenatally by ultrasound

Diagnosis	Reference
Anencephaly	Campbell et al,[12] Goldstein et al[29]
Spina bifida	Nicolaides et al[53]
Lipomyelomeningocoele	Seeds & Jones[66]
Diastematomyelia	Anderson et al[4]
Encephalocoele	Chatterjee et al,[18] Aicardi[2]
Hydrocephalus	Chervenak et al[19]
Holoprosencephaly	Chervenak et al[20]
Hydranencephaly	Hadi et al[31]
Callosal agenesis	Comstock et al,[22] Meizner et al[50]
Schizencephaly	Kligensmith & Cioffi-Ragan,[38] Kormarniski et al[39]
Lissencephaly	Saltzman et al[63]
Hemimegalencephaly	Sandri et al[64]
Septo-optic dysplasia	Pilu et al[60]
Agenesis of the cerebellar vermis	Campbell et al[13]
Dandy–Walker malformation	Russ et al[62]
Arachnoid cyst	Chervenak et al[19]
Porencephalic cyst	Vintzileos et al,[76] Aicardi[2]

Routine anomaly scanning during pregnancy can now detect many CNS malformations, such as the Dandy–Walker malformation, enlarged ventricles, cerebral asymmetry and agenesis of the corpus callosum (Table 44.27). The accuracy of antentatal diagnosis of anencephaly and spina bifida is good, whereas for other malformations there is less precision. For many of these diagnoses the natural history is uncertain. For others, such as the Dandy–Walker malformation, the generally poor prognosis (see later) is sufficiently established that to offer to terminate the pregnancy is justified by English law.

Vitamin supplementation

True prevention of neural tube defects is possible by periconceptional folate supplementation.[70,71] Current UK recommendations are that all women who plan to become pregnant should take folate supplementation, 4 mg daily from before conception to the 12th week of pregnancy.[27] A generally better diet has probably contributed to the fall in CNS malformations at conception, in spite of the fact that few women in antenatal clinics have heard of the Government advice about folate.[75] It has also been suggested that high maternal folate

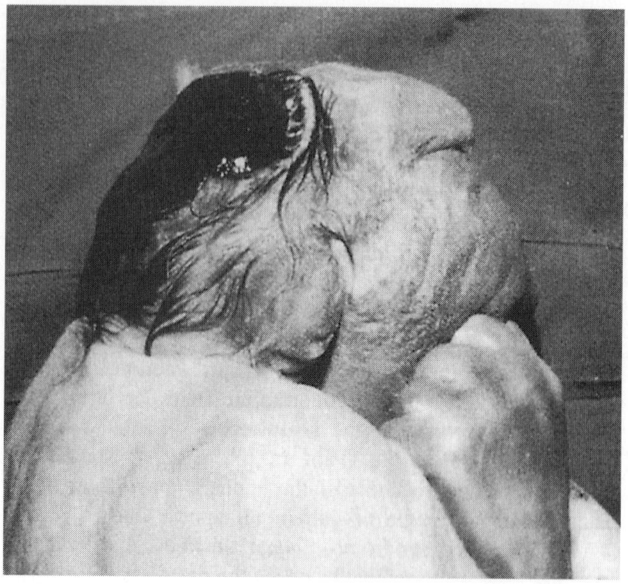

Fig. 44.63 Anencephaly. (Reproduced with permission from Disorders of the Central Nervous System in: Forfar & Arneil's Textbook of Paediatrics, 5th edn, Churchill Livingstone)

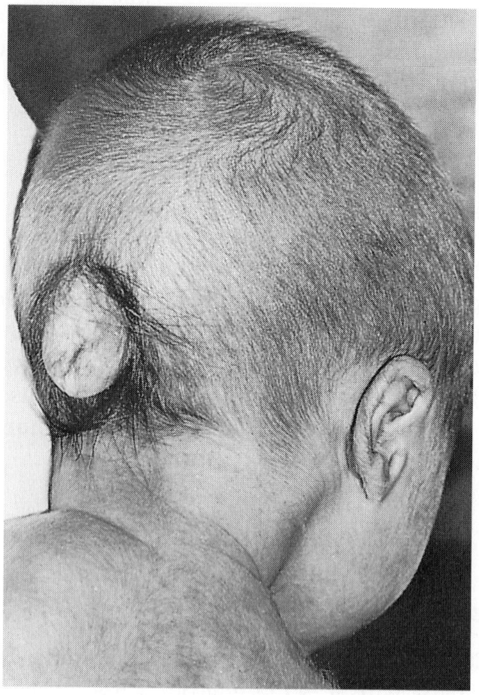

Fig. 44.64 Cranium bifidum: meningocoele.

consumption just before and during pregnancy reduces the incidence of childhood neuroectodermal tumours, particularly medulloblastoma and increases the risk of twinning.[11,23]

CLINICAL ASPECTS

Anencephalus

In anencephalus the posterior parts of the skull bones fail to develop and fuse; a malformed rudimentary brain with absent cerebral hemispheres (or even more gross defects) is exposed and is covered with congested meninges (Fig. 44.63). There is often an associated spina bifida, as well as many other malformations. It is frequently associated with hydramnios. All babies with anencephalus die; although one case has survived for several years owing to artificial ventilation she has not developed any useful independent function.[5] The clinical importance of the condition lies in the increased probability of CNS defects, including spina bifida, in subsequent siblings. The parents should know the reason for the stillbirth or neonatal death and should be given genetic counselling.

CRANIAL ENCEPHALOCOELE AND MENINGOCOELE

The incidence of these conditions is about 1–3 per 10 000 in western countries, but more in southeast Asia. In cranial meningocoele the skull bone is deficient and a cystic swelling arises through the defect, usually in the occipital region. The swelling is covered with skin or membrane and contains only CSF (Fig. 44.64).

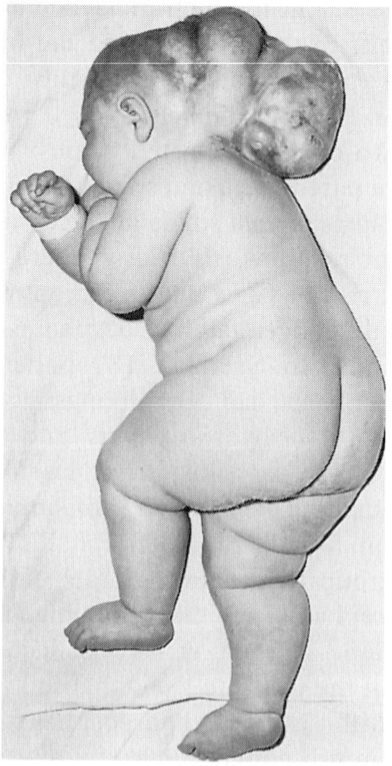

Fig. 44.65 Encephalocoele.

The second variety, occurring in about four-fifths of all cases, is encephalocoele, in which abnormal brain tissue is also present in the sac. The rest of the brain is often also grossly abnormal. In about half the patients the swelling is over 6 cm in diameter and may be larger than the skull itself (Fig. 44.65). Microcephalus is very common. Hydrocephalus occurs in about half of cases.

Encephalocoeles are usually occipital but can be parietal, frontal or protrude into the upper nasal cavity, causing considerable diagnostic difficulties. Frontal encephalocoeles are more common in southeast Asia. Frequently there are associated malformations, including myelomeningocoele, cleft palate, the Klippel–Feil syndrome and a variety of other conditions. The Meckel–Gruber syndrome is autosomal recessive and encompasses posterior encephalocoele, polycystic kidneys, polydactyly and hydrocephalus.

Investigation and treatment

All infants with encephalocoele, even small ones, should be investigated with neuroimaging to investigate any intracranial malformations and to uncover incipient hydrocephalus. The lesion should be surgically treated, and the excision may need to be followed by treatment of associated hydrocephalus. Babies with large lesions often die quickly. Nevertheless, surgical treatment is indicated for those who survive the first weeks, because a large unoperated lesion creates immense nursing problems.

Prognosis

The prognosis in occipital meningocoele is good, but in most with true encephalocoeles it is unfavourable. In the largest individual series, of 147 cases followed over 20 years, 90% of the 32 with meningocoele survived, compared to 40% among the 115 with true encephalocoele. Of the survivors with occipital meningocoele 48% were fully normal, in contrast to only 4% of those with encephalocoele, and 15% and 26% respectively were physically and mentally handicapped. The main physical handicaps in encephalocoele are cortical blindness or partial sight, spastic quadriplegia, cerebellar ataxia and epilepsy. Very large lesions or microcephalus associated with the encephalocoele carry the worst prognosis.[48]

SPINA BIFIDA

The term 'spina bifida', meaning disruption of the vertebral arches, encompasses several types of lesion. Spina bifida aperta is an open lesion where the skin is completely deficient. Spina bifida cystica is a lesion covered with a membrane, which later epithelializes. Spina bifida cystica can be a meningocoele or a myleomeningocoele (Fig. 44.66). Spina bifida occulta is a failure of the vertebral arches to fuse, and this is always a completely skin-covered lesion. This group includes babies with dermal sinuses, lipomyelomeningocoele and diastematomyelia. In diastematomyelia the spinal cord is split into two parts, sometimes by a bony bar. The importance of recognizing these latter conditions is the risk of cord tethering, with resultant neurological disability. It is possible to have neurological complications from tethered cord without any surface clues, but midline skin dimples or sinuses over the vertebral column should always be regarded with suspicion. Blind-ending dimples and pits within the natal cleft can safely be ignored[28] (see Chapter 17) but any midline skin lesion on the back which is higher than this deserves further investigation. Ultrasound in experienced hands can provide sufficient reassurance, but if there is doubt MRI of the spine is required.[28,40]

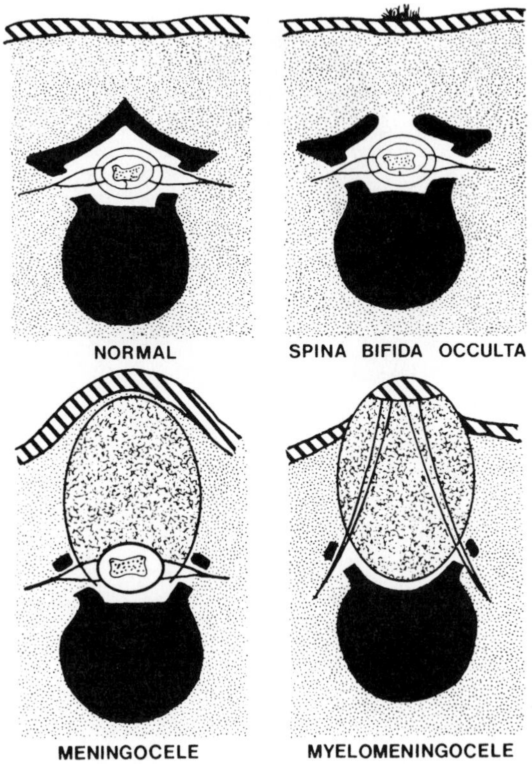

Fig. 44.66 Classification of spina bifida. (Reproduced with permission from Neurological Disease in: Forfar & Arneil's Textbook of Paediatrics, 5th edn, Churchill Livingstone)

Meningocoele

Between 5 and 10% of all spina bifida cystica lesions are cases of meningocoele, a benign condition of mostly mesodermal origin. One or two spinous processes are absent, and through the gap a small midline sac protrudes which is covered either by membrane or by skin and contains only CSF and freely transilluminates (Fig. 44.66).

The frequency of hydrocephalus associated with meningocoele is about 10%, which is far less than in myelomeningocoele, and usually the hydrocephalus is less severe. Most infants would survive without operation, but operative closure is advisable at a convenient time, either because the cystic lesion may burst, leading to meningitis, or for cosmetic reasons. The prognosis is excellent and most survive without handicap.

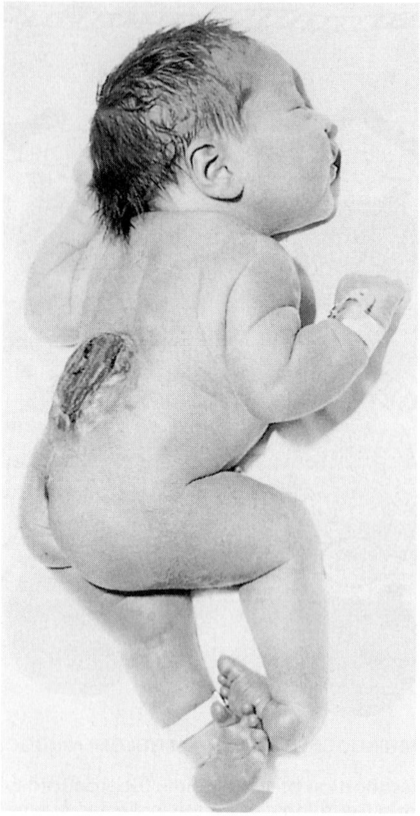

Fig. 44.67 Thoracolumbar myelomeningocoele.

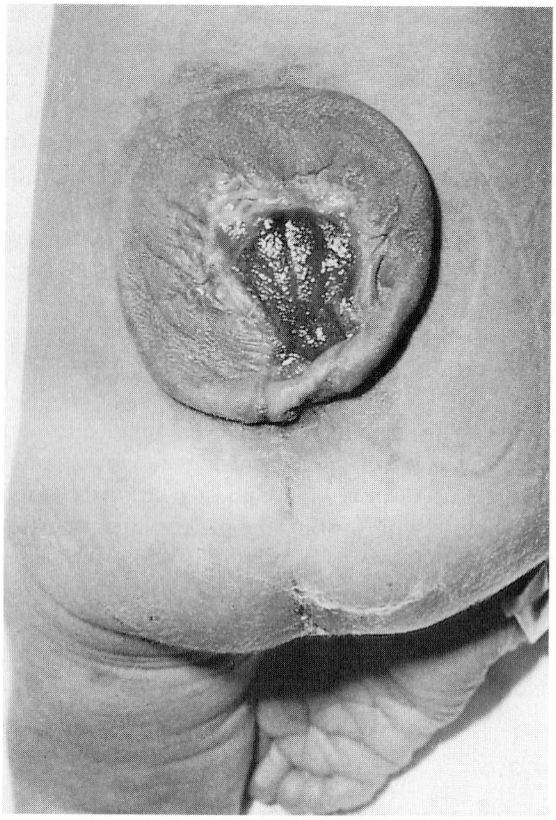

Fig. 44.68 Lumbosacral myelomeningocoele with typical central neural plaque and patulous anus.

Meningocoele is not always detected antenatally because it is a closed lesion; the amniotic fluid does not contain excess α-fetoprotein. In any case termination of pregnancy is not indicated.

Myelomeningocoele

A myelomeningocoele has abnormalities in the spinal cord or cauda equina in addition to a cystic dilatation of the meninges, skin and a vertebral defect (Fig. 44.66). Affected infants show neurological abnormalities below the level of the lesion. Myelomeningocoeles are usually thoracolumbar (Fig. 44.67), which carry the worst prognosis, or lumbar, lumbosacral (Fig. 44.68) or, less commonly, purely sacral. Multiple lesions can occur. The lesion is usually symmetrical. A small proportion have hemimyelocoele: only half of the affected segment is abnormal and forms the neural plaque.[24]

The lesions are often large, affecting several segments of the spinal cord, with defects in the vertebrae, including the splaying out and deformity of the spinal laminae with deformities of the vertebral bodies. In a minority there is kyphosis at birth, which makes the prognosis much worse. Frequently there are abnormalities of the vertebrae well above the lesion itself, which can only be detected by X-ray of the whole vertebral column and the chest: wedge-shaped vertebrae or hemivertebrae occur, often associated with detects, fusion or absence of some ribs. These will invariably lead to severe scoliosis.

Clinical assessment

Examination of the newborn baby should be performed by experienced clinicians – whether they are neonatologists, paediatricians, neurosurgeons or paediatric surgeons is not important. Optimal conditions of light and heating are essential. The baby should be in an incubator, warm and comfortable, and preferably wide awake.

The lesion

The width and length of the spinal lesion should be measured and its position relative to the spinal column recorded. Within the cystic lesion is the neural plaque – the maldeveloped spinal cord which is exposed on the surface (Fig. 44.69). Immediately after birth the nerve roots can be clearly seen through the CSF within the sac: they usually run horizontally or even upward, because the physiological cranial migration of the cord was impeded during fetal life. The neural plaque may occupy the centre, or the upper or lower part of the whole lesion. A large plaque with a high upper level carries a bad prognosis, with extensive paralysis and analgesia.

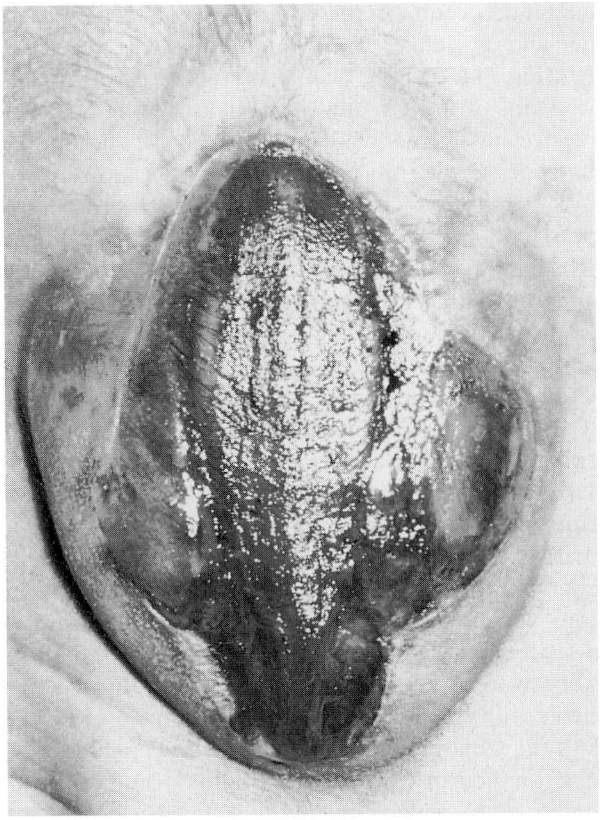

Fig. 44.69 Large open myelomeningocoele showing the typical 'filleted' appearance of the central plaque.

Paralysis

There is a wide range of paralysis possible in the legs, from none to complete. Typically the paralysis is of lower motor neuron type (flaccid). Knowledge (and a chart) of the segmental innervation of the leg muscles[68] (Table 44.28) is essential, and with this help the neurological level of paralysis is ascertained in each leg separately and charted. The neurological level does not necessarily coincide with the vertebral level. All muscles below the uppermost affected segment may be paralysed. Another pattern also occurs, especially in thoracolumbar lesions, with flaccid paralysis of muscles deriving their innervation from the affected segments, followed by reflex movements in muscles below the affected segments. Reflex activity disappears and may be followed by spasticity.[72] This should not be mistaken for useful voluntary movement. Stimulation of the legs may provoke reflex movements and mislead the examiner: it is better to stimulate the upper half of the body to elicit active movement in unaffected muscle groups.

Table 44.28 Root innervation responsible for flexion and extension in regions of the lower limbs

	Flexion	Extension
Hip	L1–L2	S1–S2
Knee	L5–S1	L3–L4
Ankle	L4–L5	S1–S2
Toes	S2–S3	L4–S1

The sphincters and the urinary tract

Almost all babies with myelomeningocoele have paralysed urethral sphincters. Observation may identify dribbling incontinence and inability to pass a stream of urine, though a moderate stream can be achieved when the baby is crying, because of contraction of the abdominal muscles. In the absence of normal sphincter control urine can be expressed.

An IVU or a renal ultrasound and an MCUG will show whether there is hydronephrosis, retention of urine, trabeculation or diverticulae in the bladder and/or ureteric reflux. The expressibility of the bladder and the residual urine can also be demonstrated. Other renal defects, such as single kidney, horseshoe kidneys, pelvic kidney and double pelvis and ureters, are some 10 times commoner than in infants without NTDs. The anus is not visible in normal babies without separating the buttocks, but when the muscles of the perineum and of the rectal sphincters are paralysed it is on the surface and patulous. Perianal rugae may still be present. The anal sphincter cannot contract on perianal stimulation, or grip a small finger inserted into the rectum.

Hydrocephalus

The maximal head circumference must be measured and charted and related to the baby's weight and gestational age. Cranial ultrasound is an essential early investigation in myelomeningocoele, and can reveal dilated ventricles before the head circumference enlarges. Ultrasound, CT or MRI can also reveal the associated Chiari malformation, which can cause bulbar paresis.

Treatment and prognosis of myelomeningocoele

Emergency active treatment of all babies, irrespective of irreversible major neurological handicaps, led to the survival of many severely handicapped children.[43,73] A selective approach was advocated by Lorber (see below) and adopted by many clinicians in the 1980s. Now far fewer babies are born with spina bifida, and in those that are there has very often been an antenatal diagnosis allowing early counselling; most infants are offered surgical repair. The survival rate has improved from that reported 25 years ago. Many North American studies claim that almost all the children become ambulatory, although longer follow-up reveals that many become wheelchair bound in adulthood.[34,41] Infants whose spina bifida lesion is surgically closed will usually develop progressive hydrocephalus and require insertion of a ventriculoperitoneal shunt. The prognosis for mobility and continence depends on the level of the lesion, that for intelligence mainly on the presence of hydrocephalus. The Chiari malformation can produce progressive further neurological deficit in later childhood, and progressive spinal deformity can also produce severe problems. Cord tethering from diastematomyelia is another cause of later progressive neurological deterioration in children with myelomeningocoele. The sensory level is the best guide to prognosis: by the age of 25 years all adults with a sensory level above L3 were wheelchair bound (although some had been able to walk as teenagers), whereas all but one of 17 cases with a sensory level below L4 were able to walk at least 50 metres.[34] Seventy per cent of this cohort, operated on between 1963 and 1970, were of normal intelligence. Only 26% were fully continent; most of those who were sucessfully managing incontinence were using intermittent catheterization. A sensory level above T11 was indicative of a poor prognosis, with severe handicap likely.

Spina bifida occulta

This affects some 5–10% of the population. Some have outward signs: a naevus, cutis aplasia, dimple, fatty pad or hairy tuft over the lumbosacral region. Figure 44.70(A) shows a skin lesion which was associated with spina bifida occulta in the underlying vertebrae. A dermal sinus and evidence of cord tethering was revealed on MRI (Fig. 44.70(B)). Failure of the vertebral arches to fuse is not of itself significant, but it may indicate more extensive involvement of the spinal cord. The finding of cutaneous stigma on the back, other than a pit in or just above the natal cleft, should therefore prompt investigation with ultrasound and/or MRI. The entire length of the spine should be examined, as multiple lesions can exist. Ultrasound appearances suggestive of spinal dysraphism include a low conus (below L3), a non-tapered conus and a thick filum terminale.[40] The median position of the conus was midway between L1/L2 disc and L2 body in 105 infants studied at Northwick Park hospital;[61] the range was from T12 to L3, with only 3% at L3. Infants with a conus below L3 should have MRI to exclude tethering. A normal spinal ultrasound, provided it has been performed by an experienced paediatric sonographer, can exclude spinal dysraphism.[28,40] Spinal lesions which can cause neurological complications later can exist without any cutaneous clues: two abnormal infants were found in the Northwick Park series.[61] Patients with spina bifida occulta do not have an increased risk of the Chiari malformation, or hydrocephalus.

Investigation of cases of spina bifida occulta frequently uncovers lesions such as lipomyelomeningocoele, diastemato-

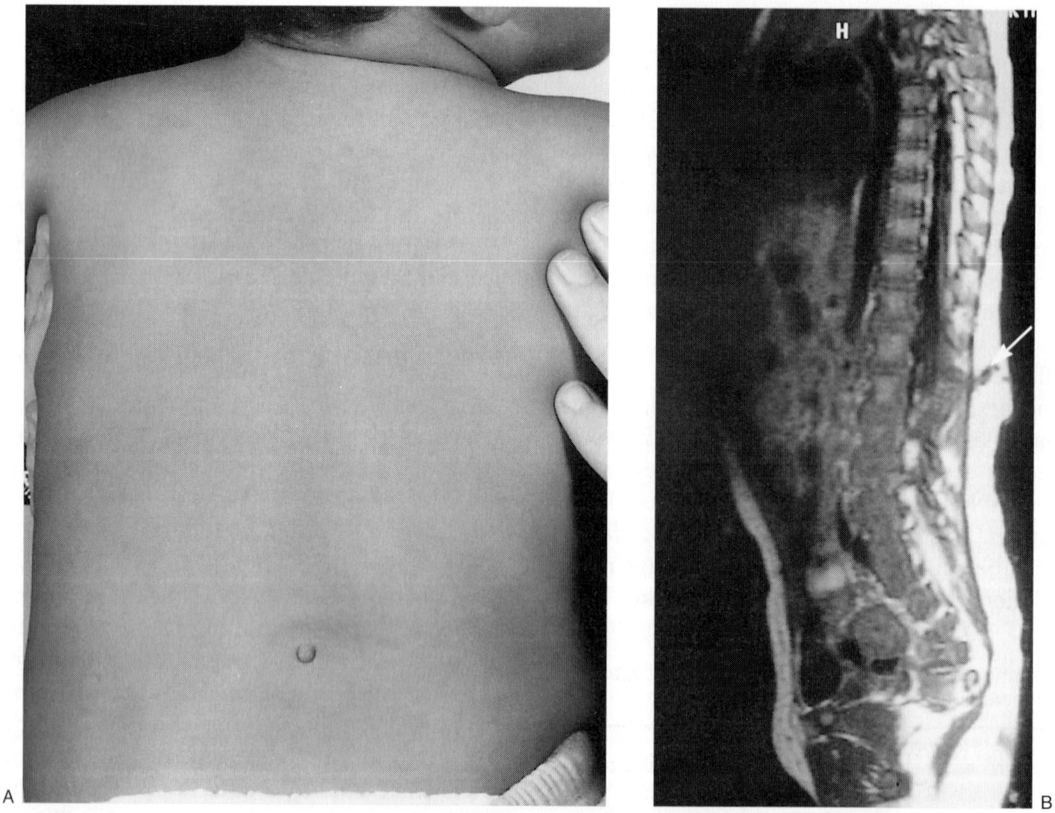

Fig. 44.70 (A) A midline skin lesion over the lumbar spine in an asymptomatic infant. (Picture reproduced with permission from the child's parents, with thanks). (B) MRI scan of the child shown in (A) revealed a tethered cord and a dermal sinus (arrow).

myelia, dermoid cysts and sinuses. Most paediatric neurosurgeons recommend an aggressive approach with early surgery for these conditions in order to preserve urological sphincter function.[37] Early surgery is particularly important in cases of dermoid sinus which predispose to meningitis.

Lipomyelomeningocoele

Lipomyelomeningocoele was once regarded as a purely cosmetic defect. It is now realized that the majority of children acquire disability in early childhood owing to cord tethering or compression of neural elements by the mass. Bruce and Schut[10] reported that 88% of unoperated patients with lipomyelomeningocoele lost neurological function in the first few years of life, so that early surgery is recommended.[37,65] Malignant transformation has not been described.

HYDROCEPHALUS

Congenital

Congenital hydrocephalus unassociated with spina bifida may be a single abnormality or may be associated with other congenital CNS malformations such as agenesis of the corpus callosum, Dandy–Walker cyst or the Arnold–Chiari malformation. Hydrocephalus is also associated with non-CNS malformations, such as congenital heart disease, intestinal atresia, chromosome abnormalities or anophthalmia. There is a rare genetic sex-linked form of aqueduct stenosis confined to males,[25] often associated with flexion and adduction defects of the thumbs. The commonest cause of congenital hydrocephalus unassociated with spina bifida is aqueduct stenosis (Table 44.29).

Table 44.29 Causes of neonatal hydrocephalus

Congenital malformations	Aqueduct stenosis Chiari malformation X-linked aqueduct stenosis Dandy–Walker malformation
Posthaemorrhagic	GMH-IVH (pp. 1258–1261) Intraventricular haemorrhage secondary to a bleeding disorder or asphyxia at term (p. 1227) Subarachnoid haemorrhage Birth trauma Vitamin K deficiency bleeding
Postinfective	Neonatal meningitis (p. 1139) Intrauterine viral infection (p. 1156)
Neoplastic lesions	
Vascular malformations	Aneurysm of the vein of Galen, Arteriovenous malformations
Choroid plexus papilloma	
Skull defects	Osteogenesis imperfecta (p. 1006) Craniosynostosis

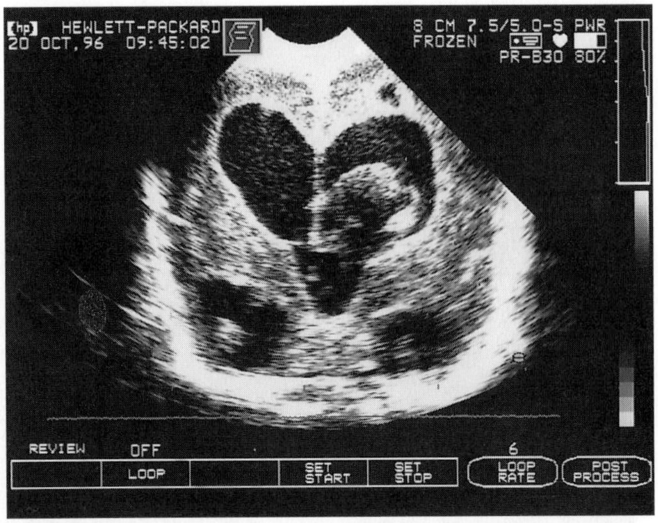

Fig. 44.71 Cranial ultrasound, coronal view, showing enlarged ventricles with a clot in the left ventricular cavity.

Clinical diagnosis of hydrocephalus in the newborn

Hydrocephalus may be evident at birth, and the diagnosis is almost certain if a baby's maximal head circumference exceeds the 97th centile by 2 cm or more (corrected for gestational age and birthweight), the anterior fontanelle is large or bulging, the cranial sutures are widely separated and the posterior fontanelle is still open at term.

Many hydrocephalic babies have no suspicious signs at birth but their head grows abnormally fast. Good practice includes measuring every baby's OFC at birth, and again a week or two later, to ensure early diagnosis. Excessive growth is an indication for early investigation, so that early treatment can be initiated to achieve the best possible result. Cranial ultrasound is the first investigation (Fig. 44.71), and can be particularly helpful in reassuring parents whose small baby is merely exhibiting catch-up growth of the head.

Benign enlargement of the subarachnoid space ('external' hydrocephalus)

Neuroimaging investigation of infants with large heads has revealed that a proportion have an enlarged subarachnoid space, without dilatation of the lateral ventricles or a subdural haematoma.[51] The infants, some of whom are ex-preterm, exhibit a pattern of head growth which is above and parallel to the 97th centile. Recognition of this diagnostic entity can save an accusation of non-accidental injury being made, based on the incorrect assumption that all enlargements of this type are subdural haematomas. Open opercula, wide CSF spaces and a rapidly increasing head circumference can be an early clue to glutaric acidaemia.[7]

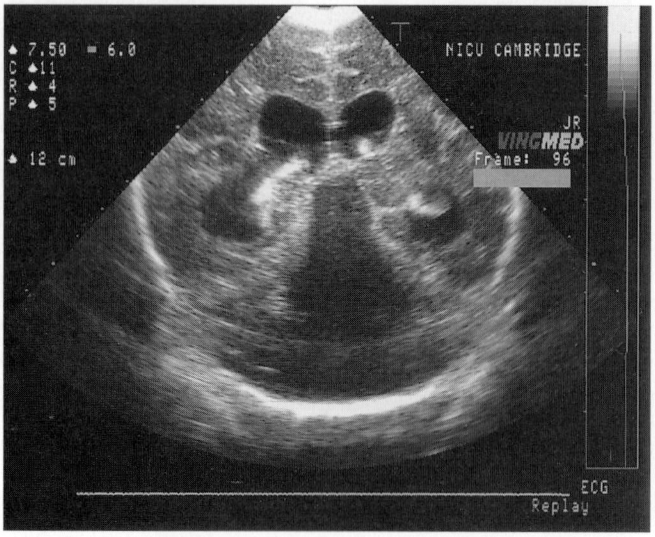

A

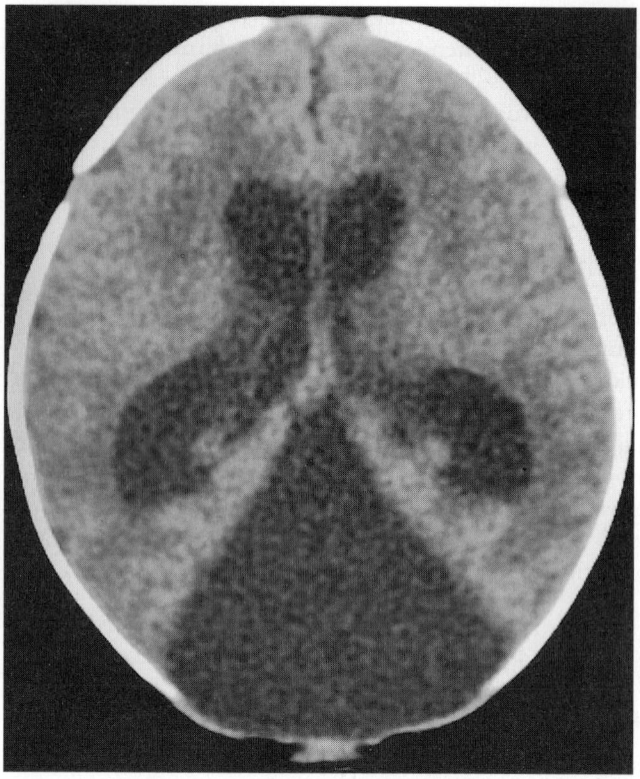

B

Fig. 44.72 (A) Cranial ultrasound scan in a case of Dandy–Walker syndrome, coronal view, showing a large cystic space in the posterior fossa and large lateral ventricles. (B) Axial CT scan of the same case, confirming the diagnosis of Dandy–Walker syndrome.

OTHER MALFORMATIONS

Dandy–Walker syndrome

There is a great deal of confusion about the definition of the Dandy–Walker syndrome (Fig. 44.72). The syndrome is usually defined as the association of three components:

- There is partial or complete agenesis of the cerebellar vermis.
- There is a cystic expansion in the posterior fossa communicating with the fourth ventricle, of which it is a diverticular expansion.
- There is hydrocephalus (this may not develop until adult life).

Males outnumber females by 3:1. There are often associated cerebral malformations, such as agenesis of the corpus callosum or occipital encephalocoeles. The treatment is that of congenital hydrocephalus, though occasionally the cyst itself has to be removed. Dandy–Walker syndrome is generally considered a sporadic condition, with a recurrence rate of less than 2%. The prognosis is guarded, with 27% dead in a summary of several published series, and only half the survivors with a normal IQ.[32] Osenbach and Menezes[57] reported a personal series of 37 cases treated over 30 years: 91% had hydrocephalus at presentation; a third had developmental delay at follow-up. In a series from Spain only two children among a cohort of 38 with Dandy–Walker syndrome were completely normal[58] and in Dublin two-thirds of the survivors were mentally retarded.[36]

Agenesis of the corpus callosum

This is a congenital defect in which either the whole or part of the corpus callosum is missing. The abnormality may be quite common and was noted in 33 of 1447 cerebral scans carried out for various reasons, corresponding to an incidence of 1:20 000. Autopsy data suggest an incidence of 1:19 000.[30] There is a failure of the association fibres to traverse the midline, and the fibres form aberrant bundles (of Probst) which can be seen displacing the lateral ventricles to one side. There is often an associated colpocephaly, a term used to describe persistence of the fetal appearance of both posterior horns of the lateral ventricle which appear large, a part of the primary malformation of the brain in this disorder. Ultrasound, CT or MRI reveals the radial gyral pattern (sunburst gyri), the colpocephaly and the loss of the usually easily visualized callosal sulcus from the midline view (Fig. 44.73). The condition is associated with several syndromes, such as trisomy 8, 13 or 18, Goldenhaar syndrome, Rubenstein–Taybi syndrome and oro-facial digital syndrome. Aicardi[3] described a constellation of callosal agenesis, infantile myoclonic epilepsy, retinal lacunae and mental retardation in females in a syndrome which now bears his name. Agenesis of the corpus callosum is unlikely to be recognized in the newborn unless the baby has a large head with hypertelorism, but is increasingly diagnosed antenatally. In one such series 6/12 were normal at follow-up.[6] Those who did badly had other malformations, such as the CHARGE anomaly or the

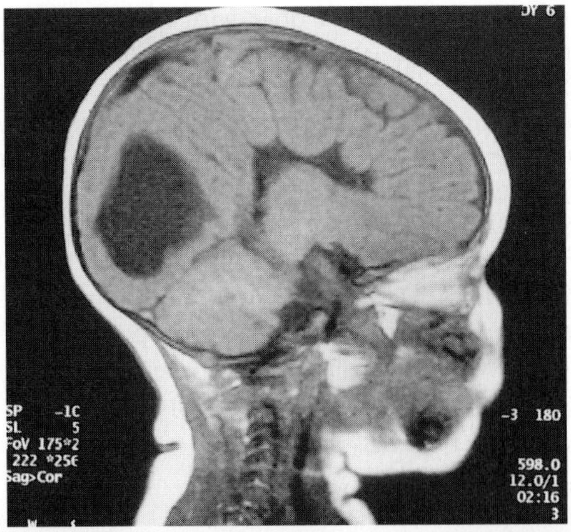

A

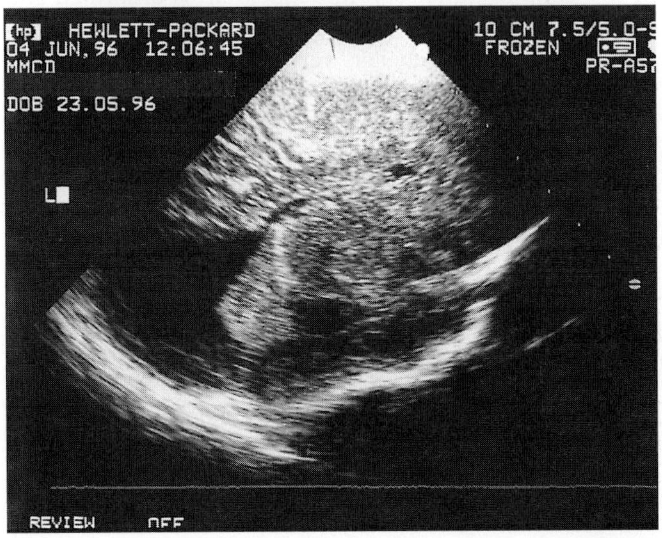

B

Fig. 44.73 (A) MRI scan in agenesis of the corpus callosum; there is a sunburst arrangement of the gyri, loss of the callosal sulcus, and an enlarged posterior horn of the lateral ventricle (colpocephaly). (B) Ultrasound scan of the brain in the same case. The sunburst gyri and the absence of the callosal sulcus, together with the colpocephaly, can be seen.

Dandy–Walker malformation, whereas those who did well were children with partial agenesis unassociated with another condition.

Hydranencephalus

In this condition the cerebral hemispheres are thought to have been destroyed by a vascular event during early fetal life. The cavities are smooth walled, in contrast to those of multicystic encephalomalacia which is the result of an insult later in fetal life when the brain is capable of mounting a glial response. In the newborn it can be difficult to distinguish hydranencephalus from extreme degrees of hydrocephalus. If the intracranial pressure is high and the baby's head is enlarging rapidly, it is worth treating the baby surgically with a shunt. In general the outlook is grim and few survive beyond a year.

Megalencephaly

A large head without a bulging fontanelle or separated sutures and growing at a normal rate usually indicates a harmless, familial megalencephaly.[46] It is only necessary to measure the parents' and the siblings' head circumferences. Counselling should be more cautious if the parents do not have large heads, as it can then be a manifestation of a cerebral abnormality and result in impaired intelligence, although benign enlargement of the subarachnoid space is the diagnosis in some of these cases. Megalencephaly can be the presenting feature in a wide variety of organic acid disorders, and an unexplained large head should prompt a screen including determination of amino acids, purines, pyrimidines and markers of peroxisomal function[33] (see Chapter 38, Part 3).

Hemimegalencephaly

Assymetric enlargement of one side of the brain is often due to an underlying dysplastic hemisphere with a migration disorder of the cortical neurons. There may be hemihypertrophy of the entire body. Intelligence is usually impaired and intractable epilepsy can be a problem.

Microcephalus

This is one of the commonest congenital CNS defects. It is of multiple and often of unknown aetiology. It may be the result of transplacental infection during pregnancy (e.g. rubella, toxoplasmosis (p. 1171)) or may be part of the rarer chromosome defect syndromes (Chapter 34). Several siblings may be affected and some family pedigrees suggest a hereditary tendency. The infant's maximal head circumference is below the second centile related to birthweight. The forehead is shallow and slopes backwards. The ears appear large. Subsequently most will be grossly retarded, spastic and subject to fits.

Holoprosencephaly

Holoprosencephaly is a rare major abnormality of the CNS. It may occur on its own, but more usually it is associated with other major somatic malformations, in which case there is often also a demonstrable chromosome defect. The cardinal abnormality of the condition is an absence of the olfactory bulbs and tracts and failure of cleavage of the forebrain. Usually the brain is small. There are fewer than normal gyri, which are broad and often flat. There is a large monoventricle, which may be associated with agenesis of the corpus callosum (Fig. 44.74). There are often other midline disturbances, with midfacial hypoplasia, cleft lip and hypertelorism. Cyclopia is the term used to describe a single fused orbit with a proboscis above it; cebocephaly

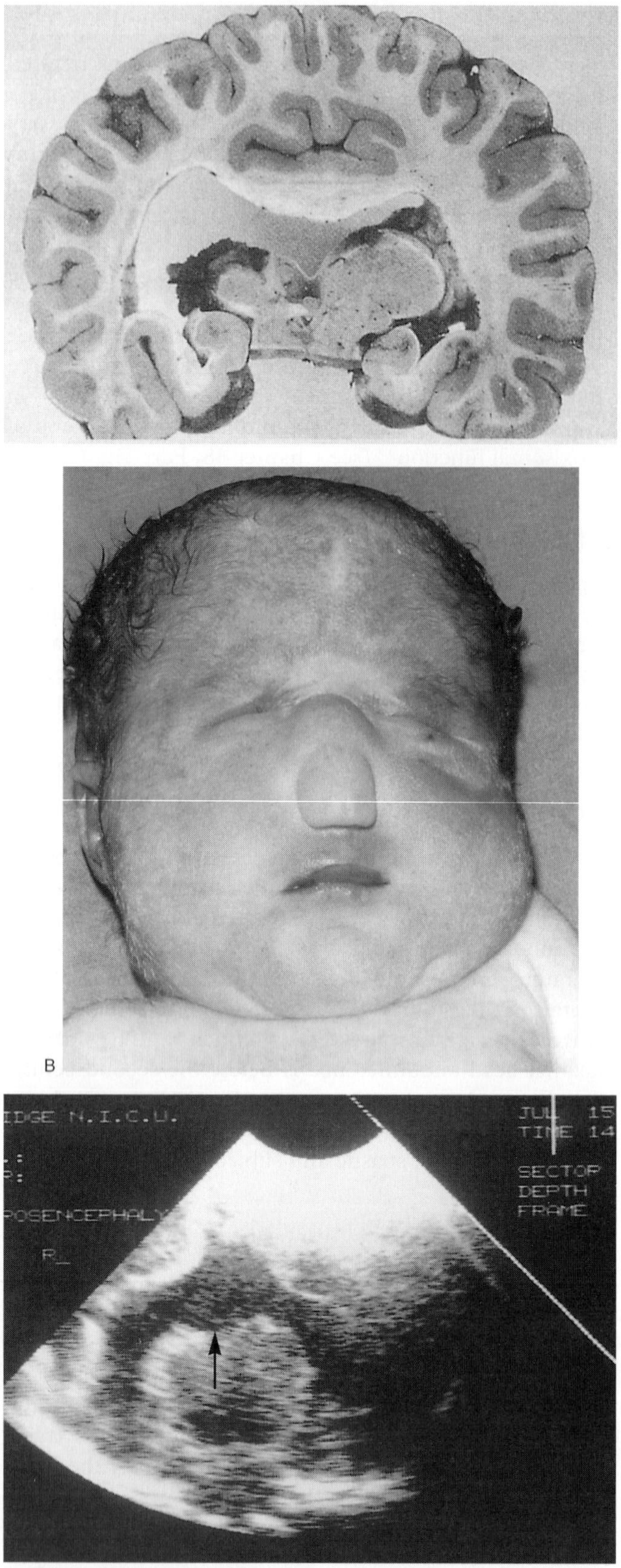

A
B
C

Fig. 44.74 Holoprosencephaly in a pathological specimen (A). (Reproduced with permission from Forfar & Arneil's Textbook of Paediatrics, 5th edn, Churchill Livingstone). (B) Facial appearance indicating underlying holoprosencephaly. (C) Coronal cranial ultrasound scan showing a single horseshoe ventricle in holoprosencephaly (arrow).

means a normally placed nose with a single nostril (Fig. 44.74(B)). Ethmocephaly is the least common anomaly, in which there are two separate orbits with a proboscis between them. Hypotelorism with a midline facial cleft, and milder midline facial dysplasias, also signal the presence of holoprosencephaly. A third of cases have trisomy 13. The disorder can be categorized into three subtypes: alobar holoprosencephaly, in which the ventricles are fused throughout; lobar holoprosencephaly, in which there is fusion of the frontal poles only; and semilobar, which is an intermediate form. The prognosis is poor and there is no effective treatment.

Septo-optic dysplasia

In this condition the septum pellucidum is unformed and the optic nerves are hypoplastic. There may be an absence of the cerebellar vermis and/or the pituitary gland. The child can have hypopituitarism, seizures, ataxia and mental deficiency.

Agenesis of the cerebellar vermis (including Joubert syndrome)

Joubert syndrome is an autosomal recessive disorder in which there is absence of the cerebellar vermis and retinopathy, often with optic disc colobomata and renal cysts.[35] Newborns can present with an effortless panting tachypnoea of 120–200 per minute and apneoic pauses. Children are mentally retarded. Agenesis of the cerebellar vermis can also form part of other syndromes, such as the Dandy–Walker malformation.

Arachnoid cysts

Congenital arachnoid cysts are increasingly discovered in fetal life or during the first few years after birth. Most are in the middle cranial fossa. Diagnosis is possible with ultrasound (Fig. 44.75). The cysts are thought to form because of splitting of the arachnoid during embryogenesis, with subsequent secretion of cerebrospinal fluid into the cavity. Growth of the cyst can cause hydrocephalus, and the cysts are then best treated by fenestration of the wall. A cystoperitoneal shunt is an alternative. Small asymptomatic cysts may not require any treatment. The prognosis is often good, although some cause epilepsy in childhood.

DISORDERS OF NEUROBLAST MIGRATION

Lissencephaly (smooth brain) and pachygyria

These disorders are becoming more frequently recognized with the advent of MRI scanning (Fig. 44.76). They cannot be diagnosed readily in early uterine life because the brain is not convoluted until 28 weeks and

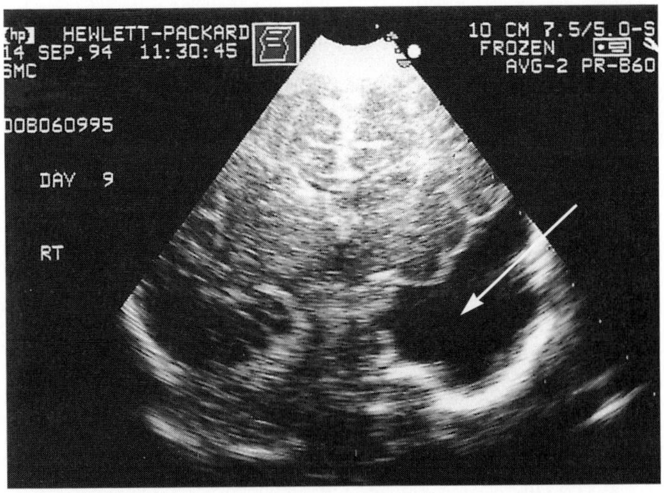

Fig. 44.75 Coronal cranial ultrasound scan showing a large arachnoid cyst in the left middle cranial fossa (arrow).

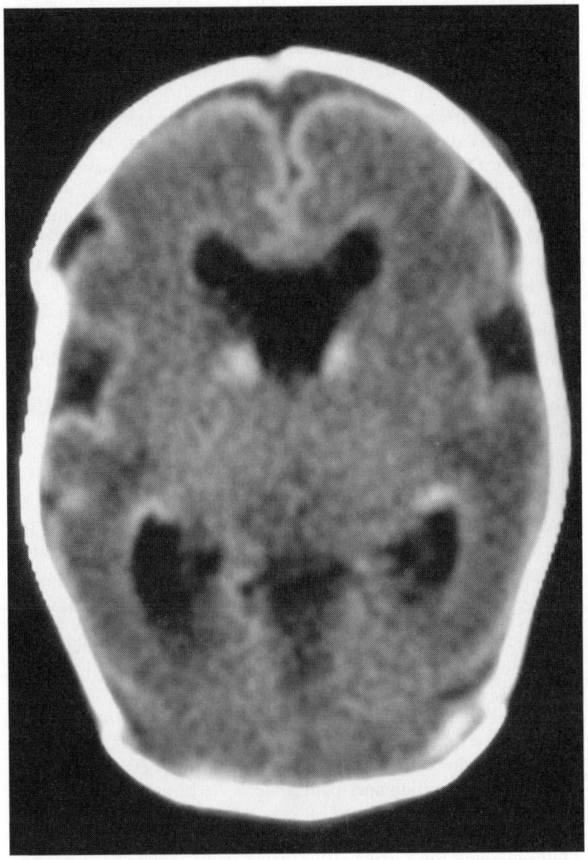

Fig. 44.76 CT scan in lissencephaly.

secondary gyri do not appear until 32 weeks. Early-onset seizures are frequent but not invariable. The brain can be completely smooth – lissencephaly. More commonly there are a few thick gyri – pachygyria. There is often an agenesis of the septum pellucidum. Imaging with ultrasound can reveal the diagnosis, which is more easily made with CT or MRI.[59] Miller–Dieker syndrome is a specific disorder in which there is a four-layer cortex resulting in lissencephaly or pachygyria, a characteristic facies with bitemporal hollowing, an upturned nose and a thin vermilion border to the upper lip (p. 863). Chromosomal analysis in the Miller–Dieker syndrome reveals a microdeletion of 17p. In the Walker–Warburg syndrome there is lissencephaly, retinal dysplasia and congenital muscular dystrophy. The disorder is autosomal recessive and the 17p chromosomal deletion is not present. This disorder has also been termed the HARD(E) syndrome: *h*ydrocephalus, cerebral and cerebellar *a*gyria, *r*etinal *d*ysplasia, ± *e*ncephalocoele. There is no treatment for lissencephaly, which has also been found in association with metabolic disorders such as Zellweger syndrome (p. 869), Menkes' syndrome and inherited amino acid disorders. Focal areas of pachygyria can be seen after insults to the fetus in the first trimester.

Schizencephaly

There is a deep cleft in the brain, usually in the region of the Sylvian fissure, the lips of which can be open or closed. There is often an agenesis of the septum pellucidum. The condition can be a primary malformation or can result from an insult in early fetal life, for example as a result of maternal cocaine abuse.

CEREBROVASCULAR MALFORMATIONS

There are a number of rare congenital cerebrovascular malformations, but few are recognizable in the newborn. These include the Sturge–Weber syndrome and arteriovenous aneurysms, including the aneurysm of the vein of Galen, which is characterized by heart failure and an intracranial murmur. Previously the results of treatment of vein of Galen vascular malformations were poor, but current therapeutic options include the transarterial insertion of coils in the abnormal vessels. Lylyk et al[49] treated 28 children this way, 11 of whom were neonates; 17 had a good long-term outcome.

CONGENITAL BRAIN TUMOURS

These are very rare but sometimes come to attention because of associated hydrocephalus. Occasionally they can cause obstructed labour. Over half are supratentorial, the most common histological type in the newborn being an astrocytoma.

REFERENCES

1. Adams C, Johnston W P, Nevin N C 1982 Family study of congenital hydrocephalus. Developmental Medicine and Child Neurology 24: 493–498
2. Aicardi J 1992 Diseases of the nervous system in childhood. Clinics in Developmental Medicine No 115/118, MacKeith Press, London
3. Aicardi J, Lefebvre J, Lerique-Koechlin A 1965 A new syndrome: spasm in flexion, callosal agenesis, ocular abnormalities. Electroencephalography and Clinical Neurophysiology 19: 609–610

4. Anderson N G, Jordan S, MacFarlane M R, Lovell-Smith M 1994 Diastomatomyelia: diagnosis by prenatal sonography. American Journal of Roentgenology 163: 911–914
5. Annas G J 1994 Asking the courts to set the standard of care – the case of baby K. New England Journal of Medicine 330: 1542–1545
6. Blum A, André M, Droullé P, Husson S, Leheup B 1990 Prenatal echographic diagnosis of corpus callosum agenesis. The Nancy experience. Genetic Counselling 38: 115–126
7. Brismar J, Ozand P T 1995 CT and MR of the brain in glutaric acidemia type I: a review of 59 published cases and a report of 5 new patients. American Journal of Neuroradiology 16: 675–683
8. Brock D J H, Sutcliffe R G 1972 Alpha-fetoprotein in the antenatal diagnosis of anencephaly and spina bifida. Lancet ii: 197–199
9. Brock D J H, Bolton A E, Scrimgeour J B 1974 Prenatal diagnosis of spina bifida and anencephaly through maternal plasma alpha-fetoprotein measurement. Lancet i: 767–769
10. Bruce D A, Schut L 1979 Spinal lipomas in infancy and childhood. Child's Brain 5: 192–203
11. Bunin G R, Kuijten R R, Buckley J D, Rorke L B, Meadows A T 1993 Relation between maternal diet and subsequent primitive neuroectodermal brain tumours in young children. New England Journal of Medicine 329: 536–541
12. Campbell S, Johnstone F D, Holt E M, May P 1972 Anencephaly: early ultrasound diagnosis and active management. Lancet ii: 1226–1227
13. Campbell S, Tsannatos C, Pearce J M 1984 The prenatal diagnosis of Joubert's syndrome of familial agenesis of the cerebellar vermis. Prenatal Diagnosis 4: 391–395
14. Carter C O, David P A, Laurence K M 1968 A family study of major central nervous system malformations in South Wales. Journal of Medical Genetics 16: 14–16
15. Carter C O, Evans K 1973 Spina bifida and anencephalus in Greater London. Journal of Medical Genetics 10: 209–234
16. Carter C O, Evans K 1973 Children of adult survivors with spina bifida cystica. Lancet ii: 924–926
17. Carter C O, Roberts J F 1967 The risk of recurrence after two children with central nervous system malformations. Lancet i: 306–308
18. Chatterjee M S, Bondoz B, Adhate A 1985 Prenatal diagnosis of occipital encephalocele. Americal Journal of Obstetrics and Gynecology 153: 646–647
19. Chervenak F A, Berkowitz R L, Romero R et al 1983 The diagnosis of fetal hydrocephalus. American Journal of Obstetrics and Gynecology 147: 703–716
20. Chervenak F A, Isaacson G, Hobbins J C, Chitkara U, Tortora M, Berkowitz R L 1985 Diagnosis and management of fetal holoprosencephaly. Obstetrics and Gynecology 66: 322–326
21. Cohen T, Stern E, Rosemann A 1979 Sib risk of neural tube defect: is prenatal diagnosis indicated in pregnancies following the birth of a hydrocephalic child? Journal of Medical Genetics 16: 14–16
22. Comstock C H, Culp D, Gonzalez J, Boal D B 1985 Agenesis of the corpus callosum in the fetus: its evolution and significance. Journal of Ultrasound in Medicine 4: 613–616
23. Czeizel A E, Metneki J, Dudas I 1994 Higher rate of multiple births after periconceptional vitamin supplementation. New England Journal of Medicine 330: 1687–1688 (letter)
24. Duckworth T, Sharrard W J W, Lister J, Seymour N 1968 Hemimyelocele. Developmental Medicine and Child Neurology (Suppl) 16: 69–75
25. Edwards J H 1961 The syndrome of sex linked hydrocephalus. Archives of Disease in Childhood 36: 486–493
26. Elwood J M, Elwood J H 1980 Epidemiology of anencephalus and spina bifida. Oxford University Press, Oxford
27. Expert Advisory Group 1992 Folic acid and the prevention of neural tube defects. DOH, Scottish Office Home & Health Department, Welsh Office, DHSS N. Ireland.
28. Gibson P J, Britton J, Hall D M B, Hill C R 1995 Lumbosacral skin markers and identification of occult spinal dysraphism in neonates. Acta Paediatrica Scandinavica 84: 208–209
29. Goldstein R B, Filly R A, Callen P W 1989 Sonography of anencephaly: pitfalls in early diagnosis. Journal of Clinical Ultrasound 17: 397–402
30. Grogono J L 1968 Children with agenesis of the corpus callosum. Developmental Medicine and Child Neurology 10: 613–616
31. Hadi H A, Mashini I S, Devoe L D et al 1986 Ultrasonographic prenatal diagnosis of hydranencephaly. A case report. Journal of Reproductive Medicine 31: 254–256
32. Hirsch J F, Pierre-Kahn A, Renier D, Sainte-Rose C, Hoppe-Hirsche E 1984 The Dandy–Walker malformation. A review of 40 cases. Journal of Neurosurgery 61: 515–522
33. Hoffman G F, Gibson K M, Trefz F K, Nyhan W L, Bremer H J, Rating D 1994 Neurological manifestations of organic acid disorders. European Journal of Pediatrics 153: S94–S100
34. Hunt G Poulton A 1995 Open spina bifida: a complete cohort reviewed 25 years after closure. Developmental Medicine and Child Neurology 37: 19–29
35. Joubert M, Eisenring J-J, Robb J P, Andermann F 1969 Familial agenesis of the cerebellar vermis. Neurology 19: 813–825
36. Kalidasan V, Carroll T, Alcutt D, Fitzgerald R J 1995 The Dandy–Walker syndrome – a 10-year experience of its management and outcome. European Journal of Pediatric Surgery 5(suppl 1): 16–18
37. Kanev P M, Bierbrauer K S 1995 Reflections on the natural history of lipomyelomeningocele Pediatric Neurosurgery 22: 137–140
38. Kligensmith W C, Cioffi-Ragan D T 1986 Schizencephaly: diagnosis and progression in utero Radiology 159: 617–618
39. Kormarniski C A, Cyr D R, Mack L A, Weinberger E 1990 Prenatal diagnosis of schizencephaly. Journal of Ultrasound in Medicine 8: 337–339
40. Korsvik H E, Keller M S 1992 Sonography of occult dysraphism in neonates and infants with MR imaging correlation. Radiographics 12: 297–306
41. Kupka J, Geddes N, Carroll N C 1978 Comprehensive management in the child with spina bifida. Orthopedic Clinics of North America 9: 97–113
42. Lorber J 1965 The family history of spina bifida cystica. Pediatrics 35: 589–595
43. Lorber J 1971 Results of treatment of myelomeningocele. An analysis of 524 unselected cases with special reference to possible selection for treatment. Developmental Medicine and Child Neurology 13: 279–303
44. Lorber J 1984 The family history of congenital hydrocephalus – an epidemiological study based on 250 index cases. British Medical Journal 289: 281–284
45. Lorber J, De N C 1970 Family history of congenital hydrocephalus. Developmental Medicine and Child Neurology (suppl 22): 94–100
46. Lorber J, Priestley B L 1981 Children with large heads: a practical approach to diagnosis in 557 children, with special reference to 101 children with megalencephaly. Developmental Medicine and Child Neurology 23: 494–504
47. Lorber J, Rogers S C 1977 Spina bifida and anencephalus in twins. Zeitschrift für Kinderchirurgie 22: 565–571
48. Lorber J, Scofield J K 1979 Prognosis of occipital encephalocele. Zeitschrift für Kinderchirurgie 28: 347–352
49. Lylyk P, Vineula F, Dion J E et al 1993 Therapeutic alternatives for vein of Galen vascular malformations. Journal of Neurosurgery 78: 438–445
50. Meizner I, Barki Y, Hertzanu Y 1987 Prenatal sonographic diagnosis of agenesis of corpus callosum. Journal of Clinical Ultrasound 15: 262–264
51. Ment L R, Duncan C C, Geehr R 1981 Benign enlargement of the subarachnoid space in children. Journal of Neurosurgery 54: 504–508
52. Nevin N C, Johnston W P 1980 A family study of spina bifida and anencephalus in Belfast, Northern Ireland (1964–1968). Journal of Medical Genetics 17: 203–211
53. Nicolaides K H, Campbell S, Gabbe S G, Guidetti R 1986 Ultrasound screening for spina bifida: cranial and cerebellar signs. Lancet ii: 72–74
54. Northern Regional Survey Steering Group. 1992 Fetal abnormality: an audit of its recognition and management. Archives of Disease in Childhood 67: 770–774
55. Office of Population Censuses and Surveys Monitor, Congenital Malformations 1982, 1983, 1984, 1985, 1986, 1987 Government Statistical Service, London
56. Office of National Statistics, Congenital Malformations, 1990, 1993. Government Statistical Service, London
57. Osenbach RK, Menezes AH 1992 Diagnosis and managment of the Dandy–Walker malformation: 30 years of experience. Pediatric Neurosurgery 18: 179–189
58. Pascual-Castroviejo I, Velez A, Pascual-Pascual S I, Roche M C, Villarejo F 1991 Dandy–Walker malformation: analysis of 38 cases. Child's Nervous System 7: 88–97
59. Pellicer A, Cabanas F, Perez-Higueras A, Garcia-Alix A, Quero J 1995 Neural migration disorders studied by cerebral ultrasound and colour Doppler flow imaging. Archives of Disease in Childhood 73: F55–F61
60. Pilu G, Sandri F, Cerisoli M, Alvisi C, Salvioli G P, Boricelli L 1990

Sonographic findings in septo-optic dysplasia in the fetus and newborn. American Journal of Perinatology 7: 337–339
61. Rowland-Hill C A, Gibson P J 1995 Ultrasound determination of the normal location of the conus medullaris in neonates. American Journal of Neuroradiology 16: 469–472
62. Russ P D, Pretorius P M, Johnson M J 1989 Dandy–Walker syndrome: a review of fifteen cases evaluated by prenatal sonography. American Journal of Obstetrics and Gynecology 161: 401–406
63. Saltzman D H, Krauss C M, Goldman J M, Benacerraf B R 1991 Prenatal diagnosis of lissencephaly. Prenatal Diagnosis 11: 139–143
64. Sandri F, Pilu G, Dallacasa P, Foschi F, Salvioli G P, Bonecelli L 1991 Sonography of unilateral megalencephaly in the fetus and newborn infant. American Journal of Perinatology 8: 18–20
65. Sathi S, Madsen J R, Bauer S, Scott R M 1993 Effect of surgical repair on the neurologic function in infants with lipomeningocele. Pediatric Neurosurgery 19: 256–259
66. Seeds J W, Jones F D 1986 Lipomyelomeningocele: prenatal diagnosis and management. Obstetrics and Gynecology 67: 345–375
67. Seller M J 1981 Recurrence risks for neural tube defects in a genetic counselling clinic population. Journal of Medical Genetics 18: 245–248
68. Sharrard W J W 1964 The segmental innervation of the lower limb muscles in man. Annals of the Royal College of Surgeons 35: 106–122
69. Smithells R W, D'Arcy E E, McAllister E F 1968 The outcome of pregnancies before and after the birth of infants with nervous system malformations. Developmental Medicine and Child Neurology 15: 6–10
70. Smithells R W, Sheppard S, Scorah C J et al 1981 Apparent prevention of neural tube defects by periconceptional vitamin supplementation. Archives of Disease in Childhood 56: 911–918
71. Smithells R W, Seller M J, Harris R et al 1983 Further experience of vitamin supplementation for prevention of neural tube defects. Lancet i: 1027–1031
72. Stark G D, Baker G C W 1967 The neurological involvement of the lower limbs in myelomeningocele. Developmental Medicine and Child Neurology 9: 732–744
73. Stein S C, Schut L, Ames M D 1974 Selection for early treatment in myelomeningocele: a retrospective analysis of various selection procedures. Pediatrics 54: 553–557
74. Stevenson A C, Johnston H A, Stewart M I P, Golding D R 1966 Congenital malformations. Bulletin of World Health Organization 34 (Suppl): 9–127
75. Sutcliffe M, Wild J, Perry A, Schorah C J 1994 Prevention of neural tube defects. Lancet 344: 1578 (letter)
76. Vintzileos A M, Hovick T J, Escoto D T et al 1987 Congenital midline porencephaly: prenatal sonographic findings and review of the literature. American Journal of Perinatology 4: 125–128
77. Wald N J, Cuckle H S 1981 Amniotic fluid acetylcholinesterase electrophoresis as a secondary test in the diagnosis of anencephaly and open spina bifida in early pregnancy. Lancet ii: 321–324

Section 6

Pathology, radiology and biochemistry

45

Perinatal postmortem

P. J. Berry

INTRODUCTION

No-one likes postmortem examinations, and the subject is particularly distasteful when it involves a baby you have known well. Whereas adult necropsy rates have been falling, perinatal postmortem rates have been rising, reflecting the importance of this final examination in patient care. A carefully performed necropsy will provide clinically important additional information in 40–50% of perinatal deaths, despite sophisticated investigations in life.[24,28] Every parent has the right to be offered a postmortem examination of their child, and it is equally their right in most circumstances to refuse.

It is important that the paediatrician requesting the examination understands the purpose of the postmortem examination, the legal constraints that surround it, the probability that it will yield useful information, and the interpretation of the final report.

This chapter is an introduction to perinatal necropsy. It includes reference to stillborn babies because the paediatrician attending the delivery suite is usually the best-qualified person to make a preliminary examination of such babies. Similarly, the placenta belongs to the child (not the obstetric staff) and so should form part of the assessment of the newborn baby. For more detailed accounts of perinatal pathology see Wigglesworth,[38] Keeling[18] and Wigglesworth and Singer.[39] The role of the pathologist in perinatal care has been reviewed by Macpherson et al.[21] The Stillbirth and Neonatal Death Society's guidelines for professionals contain much practical information about death certification, registration, funerals, burial and cremation.[32]

THE PURPOSE OF PERINATAL POSTMORTEM EXAMINATION

• **To establish the cause of death**. Although this is often advanced as the main reason for requesting a postmortem, the cause of death is seldom in doubt in modern neonatal practice, and in many cases the immediate cause is the withdrawal of intensive support. This misapprehension can lead to an erroneously low expectation of the postmortem examination. In some cases, particularly where survival has been short and there has been little opportunity to carry out investigations in life, the postmortem may reveal unexpected lethal disease, such as a cardiac defect, obstetric trauma or infection (Fig. 45.1). Even when the cause of death is not apparent in stillborn babies, the mode of death (hypoxia, intrauterine malnutrition, haemorrhage, cardiac failure) and the time (preadmission, prior to labour, during labour) can be inferred. Becker and Becker[1] describe the techniques available for establishing how long a stillborn child has been compromised in utero before death.

The yield of new information to be expected from properly conducted perinatal necropsies is shown in Table 45.1.

• **To investigate growth and development**. Pathologists use additional criteria to those used by clinicians, and so careful postmortem examination may give useful additional information about growth and maturity in relation to gestational age. This applies not only to the baby as a whole, but also to individual organs and systems. For example, in the immediate postnatal period intrauterine growth retardation and pulmonary hypoplasia are frequent contributors to death, and can be diagnosed or confirmed and documented at postmortem. Later in the neonatal period the effects of intensive care on lung growth and development can be assessed.

Table 45.1 Clinical versus postmortem diagnoses in a series of 300 perinatal necropsies. (Reproduced with permission from Porter and Keeling[28])

Clinical vs pathological diagnosis	Stillbirths (%) (*n* = 150)	Neonatal deaths (%) (*n* = 150)
Agree	40	19
Agree, but additional information from postmortem	34	66
Clinical diagnosis incorrect	26	15

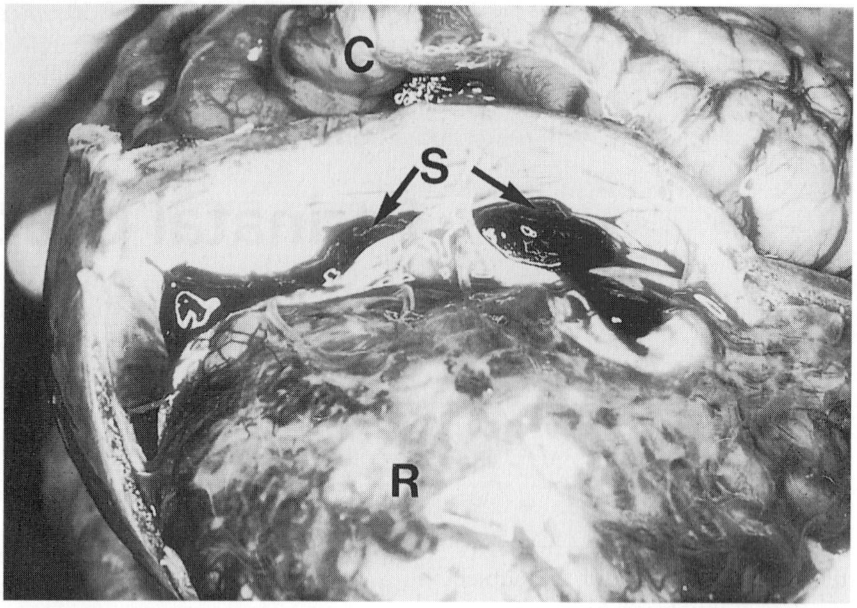

Fig. 45.1 Neonate operated on for presumed cardiac defect causing left-to-right shunt. At postmortem the heart was normal but there was an arteriovenous malformation within the right cerebral hemisphere which had caused cardiac failure and cerebral ischaemic damage as a result of 'steal'. The skull has been opened to show the normal left cerebral hemisphere at the top of the picture (C), the greatly dilated sagittal sinus[1] (S) containing postmortem blood clot (arrows) running across the middle, and the shrunken right cerebral hemisphere containing the vascular malformation in the lower half of the figure (R).

- **To identify significant disease not directly responsible for death, but with implications for future pregnancies**. It is not uncommon for postmortem examination to demonstrate important diseases and anomalies which were unsuspected in life but which did not contribute significantly to the child's death. For example, an incidental finding of histological evidence of cystic fibrosis has obvious genetic implications for future pregnancies.
- **To provide the basis for counselling parents**. This is the single most important purpose of the postmortem examination. Every parent is entitled to a detailed explanation of why their baby died, and as accurate a prediction as possible of the likely outcome of future pregnancies. This can only be done with conviction after a full postmortem (Fig. 45.2). In this context the documentation of normality can be of great reassurance value to parents and their doctors, emphasizing the importance of postmortem examination even when there are no unexpected findings. The value of such 'negative' reports may only become apparent when a subsequent sibling is found to have some abnormality.

The use of the postmortem examination to obtain tissue samples for extraction of DNA will become increasingly important as more diagnostically useful tests become available. The pace of advance in this field is so great that, where resources allow it, DNA samples should be collected from every abnormal baby for possible future family studies, even when no test is currently available.

- **To monitor iatrogenic disease**. It is essential in an evolving specialty to study the effects of new therapies and invasive techniques, and to be aware of iatrogenic complications (Fig. 45.3). The latter vary widely between different units, and there is no reason to suppose that future therapies will have fewer unwanted effects than their predecessors.[17]
- **Teaching, research and epidemiology**. A postmortem examination offers an unrivalled opportunity for paediatricians and obstetricians to learn from their own experience, and indeed to educate their own pathologist. Most postmortem consent forms allow the option of additional procedures or sampling of tissue for research purposes. Accurate data from postmortem studies are a valuable form of perinatal audit at unit, regional and national levels, and ultimately form part of the case on which funding depends.

In view of the above it is clear that there is no such thing as a postmortem examination that shows nothing.

The postmortem examination is often seen in a negative light, as a source of distress to parents and their doctors. In fact it may be a source of comfort, like the funeral helping them to accept the finality of death. It is an opportunity to provide them with mementoes of their child, such as photographs, palm prints and locks of hair. Some mothers even keep a copy of the postmortem report as the sole tangible reminder of their baby's life.

The postmortem examination serves to absolve

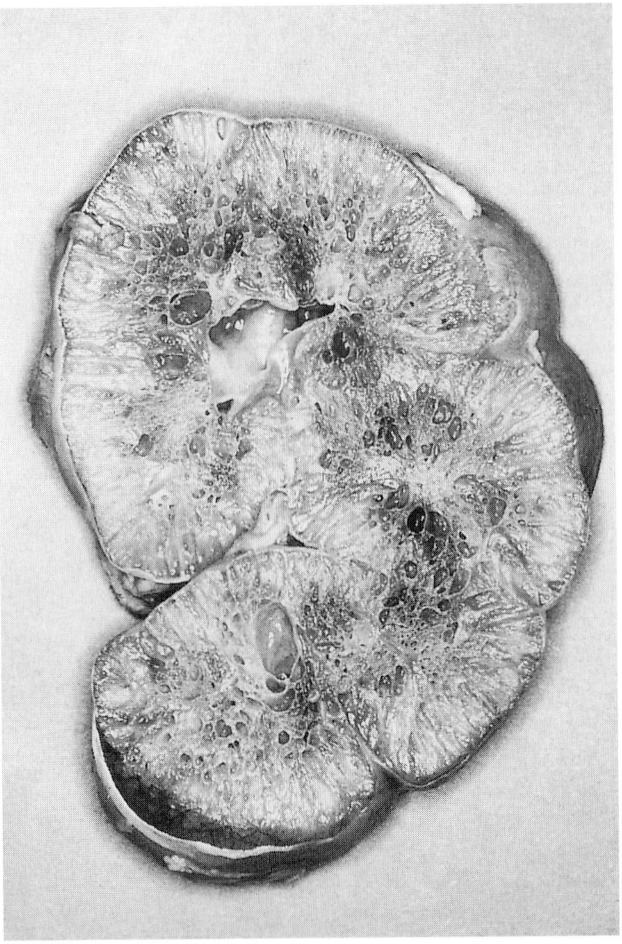

Fig. 45.2 Bisected kidney of neonate with oligohydramnios, pulmonary hypoplasia and enlarged kidneys. The appearance of small radially arranged cysts is typical of autosomal recessive infantile polycystic renal disease. Histology confirmed dilatation of the collecting tubules and characteristic ductal plate lesions in the liver.

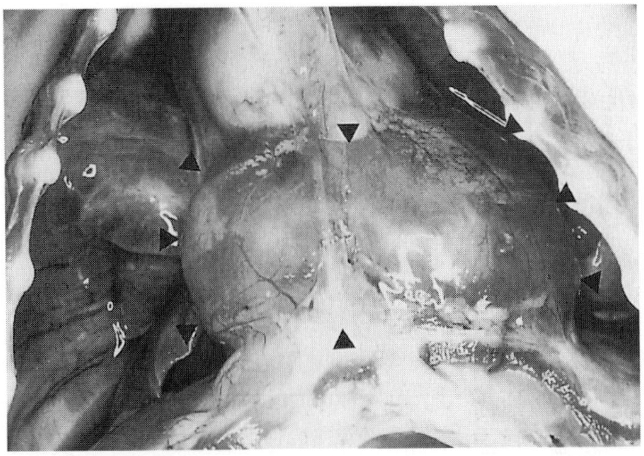

Fig. 45.3 Neonatal death due to unexplained falling cardiac output. At postmortem the pericardial sac was distended with clear fluid causing tamponade. The mediastinum was oedematous. Analysis of the fluid showed that it had the same composition as intravenous fluid, confirming origin from a misplaced vascular catheter. The chest has been opened to show the dilated pericardial sac (arrowheads).

parents, nursing staff and doctors of often unspoken guilt that there was something that they should have done or not done that might have prevented the baby's death. The pathologist is an impartial third party whose enquiry helps to restore the parent–doctor relationship which may have been strained by the death.

Finally, a thorough postmortem examination may be the doctor's best protection against ill-founded litigation.

CONSENT TO POSTMORTEM EXAMINATION

Consent is most likely to be given when the purpose and benefits of the procedure have been sympathetically explained to the parents by a member of staff they know well. Ideally this should be the consultant, but in practice this difficult task often falls to a junior member of the team. Perinatal autopsy should be portrayed to the bereaved parents as an important part of clinical management likely to be of such importance to the future care of the family that the choice to have a postmortem examination of their child is seen as a right rather than an obligation.[16]

In the UK, consent to postmortem examination is required for all liveborn babies regardless of gestation, and for those stillborn after 24 weeks of gestation. There is no legal requirement for consent to be given in writing, but it is a wise precaution and the policy of most health authorities. If verbal consent is obtained by phone then it should be witnessed by a second person, both witnesses recording in the clinical record that permission has been obtained. Undoubtedly most consent is not fully 'informed', but the legal requirements for surgical procedures probably do not apply, it being only necessary legally to ensure that no-one with a legitimate interest objects. However, it is essential that parents know what is involved. It is reasonable to explain that the examination will involve incisions, and that samples of tissue may be taken. Particular explanation is necessary if it is likely that whole organs, such as the brain or heart, will be retained, or the body will be moved to a specialist centre for examination. The procedure is not disfiguring and does not normally involve the face. Except in the case of very macerated or tiny fetuses the body can still be viewed after postmortem, and examination will not delay funeral arrangements. Parents may find an explanatory leaflet helpful.[9]

Legal requirements in other countries may differ from those in the UK. The views of ethnic and religious groups must be taken into account.[8] For example, Sikhs generally have no religious objection to postmortem examination, but necropsy is not approved of by Muslims or Hindus, although it is not forbidden.[2]

Tissues are in increasing demand for research. The consent form should make specific reference to the retention of tissues for teaching and research, and give parents the opportunity to strike out any part of the consent that they wish. This consent does not absolve the researcher

REQUEST FOR POSTMORTEM EXAMINATION

OF ALL FETUSES, STILLBIRTHS AND PERINATAL DEATHS

(All the relevant sections should be completed)

BABY	MOTHER
Name	Name
Registration No.	Registration No.
D.o.b:	D.o.b:
Date of Death	
Consultant	Consultant

PREVIOUS PREGNANCIES

	Date	Pregnancy	Labour	Puerperium	Sex	Outcome
1						
2						
3						
4						

PRESENT PREGNANCY

LMP / / , EDD / / , Blood Group .... Rh ....

Amniocentesis Yes/No (Result ....)
Ultrasound Scan Yes/No (Result ....)
Threatened Abortion Yes/No
APH Yes/No

Hydramnios/Oligohydramnios Yes/No
Hypertension Yes/No
PET Yes/No
Maternal Pyrexia Yes/No
IUGR Yes/No

LABOUR

Spontaneous/Induced (Medical/Surgical)/Accelerated

Why ....

Liquor Amount .... Colour ....
Duration of 1st stage .... 2nd stage ....
Fetal distress Yes/No
Presentation: Vertex/Breech/other

Forceps/Caesarian/other ....
Fetal distress Yes/No ....
Delivery at .... hr .... min on / /
Died at .... hr .... min on / /

NEONATAL

Birth Weight .... g Gestation .... wks
Apgar Score .... at 1 min .... at 5 mins.
Resuscitation nil/mucus extraction/O² mask/intubation

Neonatal Problems	Neonatal Procedures
1	1 ....
2	2 ....
3	3 ....
4	4 ....
5	5 ....

Suspected Causes of Death

1 ....
2 ....
3 ....
4 ....

Any special points of interest to be looked for?

Consent for autopsy examination has been obtained and is supplied with this request form.
Notes to be supplied if possible

Signature of doctor requesting PM ....
Please also print if illegible ....
Bleep No. ....
Deliver to Department of Pathology, (Tel ....)

Fig. 45.4 Example of a request form for perinatal postmortem examination.

from seeking ethical approval for the proposed use of the tissue. Organs from infants are also in increasing demand for transplantation. It is worth remembering that corneas from older infants are used in some centres to correct aphakic eyes after cataract surgery, and that cardiac valves can be used as homografts. The latter can be collected at the time of postmortem if the parents wish.

CORONER'S POSTMORTEMS

It is unusual for hospital perinatal deaths to involve the coroner, and so the procedure is often unfamiliar. If in doubt you can discuss a case with the coroner or his officer, who may either accept the case or ask you to sign a death certificate. Most coroner's cases, including cot deaths, do not involve an inquest. It is wrong to refer a case to the coroner as a way of getting a postmortem after failing to obtain consent from relatives. However, in England the following deaths must be reported (for a discussion of the system in other countries see Knight[20]):

- Babies dead on arrival at hospital, or within 24 hours of admission. Unattended stillbirths;
- Deaths within 24 hours of an operation, anaesthetic or invasive procedure;
- Deaths as a result of accident;
- Unnatural, criminal or suspicious deaths, e.g. neglect, child abuse, poisoning;
- Deaths caused by drugs, whether prescribed or not;
- Deaths as a result of medical or surgical mishap (the doctor is well advised to contact his defence organization at the same time as informing the coroner);
- Deaths in which the doctor is so uncertain of the disease leading to death as to be unable to sign the death certificate. It is not necessary to know why the patient died at any particular moment, or the mode of death.

This list is incomplete. If in doubt ask. This will avoid the death certificate being rejected by the registrar of births and deaths.

REQUIREMENTS FOR OPTIMAL POSTMORTEM EXAMINATION

The request for a postmortem examination should be treated as any other request for a consultant opinion. The pathologist requires a full history of the pregnancy and the events leading up to the death of the child, and a note of any special points to be looked for. This information is most easily given in a standard request form, which should be accompanied by the clinical notes (Fig. 45.4). Certain key investigations of the mother must be initiated by the clinician in unexplained stillbirths and early neonatal deaths. A Kleihauer test, rhesus antibodies and a screen for intrauterine infection should be minimum routine investigations.

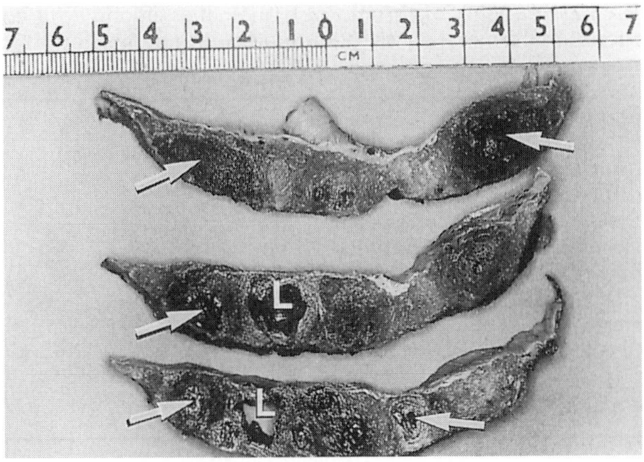

Fig. 45.5 Placenta of baby with marked asymmetrical growth retardation who died in the neonatal period. The cut surfaces of the placenta show multiple infarcts of different ages (arrows), some with central liquefaction (L), indicating uteroplacental vascular insufficiency as the underlying cause of death.

The placenta often holds the key to perinatal deaths, and the pathologist will need the placenta to give a complete opinion (Fig. 45.5). This requires anticipation on the part of paediatricians and obstetricians; if all placentas from pregnancies that are in any way abnormal are sent for examination at the time of delivery, this will include those from 10–15% of all pregnancies and almost all subsequent neonatal deaths.

The following are the main indications for formal examination of the placenta:

- All stillbirths;
- All abnormal pregnancies, e.g. hypertension, diabetes, elevated α-fetoprotein levels, infection, haemorrhage, oligohydramnios, polyhydramnios, premature or prolonged rupture of the membranes, operative intervention or maternal disease of any kind;
- All abnormal babies, e.g. immature, large or small for dates, malformed, asphyxiated or anaemic babies, and any that require special care;
- All placentas that appear abnormal;
- All placentas from mothers with recurrent obstetric catastrophe;
- All multiple pregnancies.

After death it is important that all tubes and vascular catheters should be left in place so that the location of their tips can be confirmed, cultures taken and complications identified. There is a conflict between the needs of the pathologist and the need of the parents to see and hold their baby free of all the paraphernalia that surrounded him in life. Except in the instance of coroner's cases, where the requirement to leave all tubes is paramount, there is room for compromise. For example, if gas embolism is not a consideration then vascular catheters can be tied and cut flush with the skin. The correct

Table 45.2 Frequency of chromosome anomalies among different categories of perinatal death. (Reproduced with permission from Winter et al[40])

Category	%
Macerated stillbirth, no malformation	4.5
Macerated stillbirth with malformation	54
Severe congenital malformation	29
Congenital heart malformation	3
Primary central nervous system malformation	0
Prematurity-associated disease	1
Primary anoxia	2
Fresh stillbirth without malformation	0
Total (90/1271)	7.0

location and level of an orotracheal tube in the trachea can still be confirmed if it is cut off at the level of the gums. The body should be taken to the mortuary refrigerator as soon as is reasonably possible, and the postmortem examination completed promptly, both for the convenience of parents and to ensure optimal results from microbiology and chromosome studies.

Unfortunately not all hospitals have an enthusiastic perinatal pathologist. Photographs of any abnormality should be taken by the paediatrician if the pathologist cannot do this. If chromosome studies are indicated then blood or skin can be taken before the child leaves the ward. The yield will be greatest from macerated fetuses with malformations (Table 45.2), but samples should also be taken from those babies with unexplained intrauterine growth retardation, non-immune hydrops fetalis, malformations or dysmorphic features, or a maternal history of recurrent fetal loss. In the case of macerated fetuses the sample should be taken from the fetal aspect of the placenta to include amnion and underlying tissue. If the baby is fresh then fibroblasts can be cultured from skin up to 5 days after clinical death, but the chance of success is greatest if the sample is taken as early as possible. The postmortem examination should include a whole-body radiograph to document the skeleton, gas in serous cavities, soft-tissue calcification and the position of catheters. If radiographic facilities are not available in the mortuary, the X-ray may be taken as a routine on the way there. In any case the X-ray must be taken within 12 hours of death if gas embolism is not to be missed.[30]

If an experienced perinatal pathologist is not available then referral to a specialist centre should be considered. This policy is supported by studies showing that the yield from perinatal and infant postmortems is directly related to the quality of the examination.[36]

Whenever the examination is carried out locally it should be attended by a member of the clinical team to apprise the pathologist of the details of any therapy given, and to ensure that all necessary information is collected. (The word 'autopsy' is derived from the Greek words *autos* and *opsis*, meaning 'self-view'!) The attendance of a senior clinician encourages the pathologist and emphasizes the importance he attaches to the examination.

AFTER THE POSTMORTEM EXAMINATION

Except for small fetuses and very macerated stillborn babies the body will be carefully reconstituted after the postmortem examination. The baby may then be seen and held by the parents, who often remark on the improvement in their child's appearance since they last saw him or her immediately after death. However, time will have elapsed and they should be warned that natural changes may have taken place, so that these are not blamed on the postmortem examination.

A provisional report will be available within a day or two, and a final report including microscopy, culture results and chromosomes can usually be completed within 6 weeks. This final report is of no value unless it is communicated to the parents and doctors looking after the child.

Parents may ask to have a copy of the report. Although I have no objection to this it is very important that the parents should appreciate that it is a medical report in medical language that they may find distressing, and it is important that they should have the report explained to them first. The pathologist should be asked before his report is given to a parent.

Coroner's reports are confidential and permission must be sought before they can be divulged either to a parent or to a paediatrician, although parents are entitled to a copy from the coroner on payment of a small fee. In practice most coroners relax these rules in straightforward infant deaths. Great care must be taken before giving copies of reports on hospital or coroner's postmortem examinations in cases that may involve litigation.

IF PERMISSION IS REFUSED

Even after careful explanation some parents will not consent to examination of their child. Their wishes must always be respected, but in many cases the main clinical questions can be answered by a more limited examination which is acceptable to them. The coroner's system must not be used as a second line because parents have refused consent.

Examination may be confined to the body cavity or organ system in question. Also, much can be learned from needle biopsies of key organs, and several biopsies may be taken for histology, bacterial and viral cultures or enzyme studies as appropriate. Many cases can be resolved and documented by relatively non-invasive methods, such as photography, radiology with or without contrast medium (Fig. 45.6), culture of body orifices, blood and cerebrospinal fluid, and a small skin biopsy for chromosomes or enzyme studies. Consent to these minor procedures should still be recorded, and the pathologist must be made aware of any restrictions.

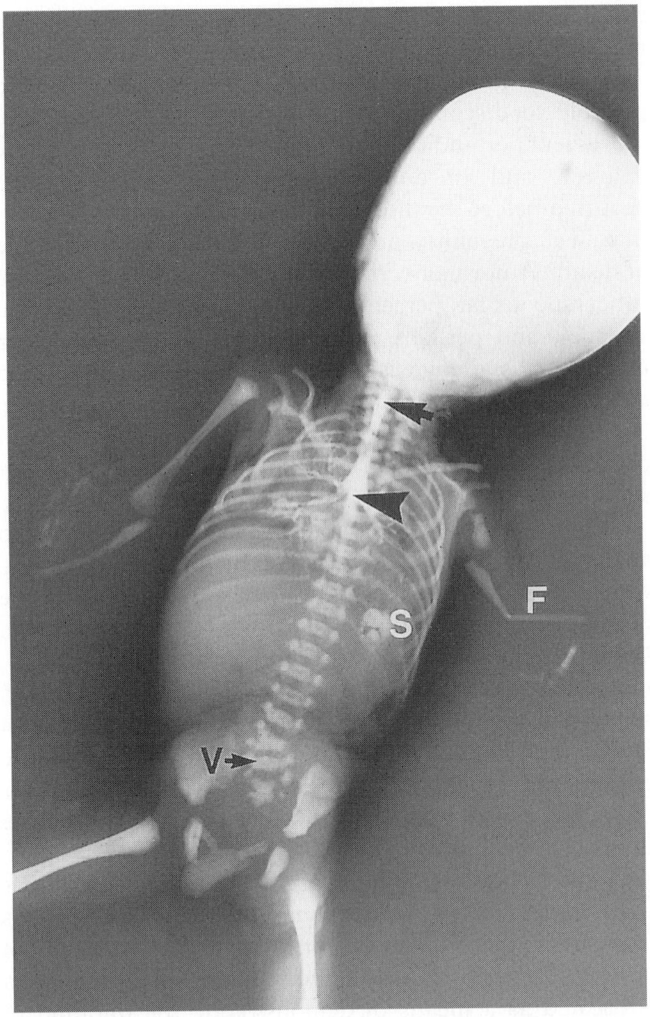

Fig. 45.6 Postmortem radiograph of a baby who failed to breathe after birth and could not be intubated. Consent for full postmortem was refused. Radiological contrast medium has been injected percutaneously into the trachea. There is laryngeal atresia (arrow), a tracheo-oesophageal fistula (arrowhead) with contrast medium in the stomach (S), absent radii, a fracture of the left forearm (F) and sacral vertebral anomalies (V).

SPECIAL POSTMORTEMS

There are a few circumstances when samples must be collected immediately after death. These include undiagnosed inborn errors of metabolism and some floppy babies in whom a myopathy is suspected. Contingency plans must be made early. Parents will usually understand the need to give consent to postmortem procedures while their baby is still alive. Samples to be taken and the means of storing them must be discussed well in advance with the relevant expert. Techniques change rapidly, and the following notes are given only for guidance when expert advice is not available. The number of samples required will be greatly reduced by such prior consultation.

Remember to ask the laboratory to save all samples taken in life, including blood films. In the case of unexplained acidosis or hyperammonaemia in the neonatal period it is usually sufficient to save serum, cerebrospinal fluid, urine, liver, kidney, spleen, myocardium, and skeletal muscle snap-frozen at –80°C, and to take a skin biopsy for fibroblast culture. When a storage disorder is suspected then additional samples of these tissues should be fixed in glutaraldehyde for electron microscopy. For suspected glycogen storage disorders tissue samples may also be saved in alcohol for histochemistry. If the brain is affected by a storage or demyelinating disorder then a frontal pole must be saved unfixed and frozen. The rectum is an additional useful source of neurons for histochemistry and electron microscopy.

When a myopathy is suspected then muscle biopsy material is handled as in life, although sampling should be more extensive to include severely, mildly and unaffected muscle groups. Many histochemical stains used in muscle pathology will work some time after death. Samples for electron microscopy for the congenital myopathies need to be taken as soon as possible and placed in glutaraldehyde.

The preferred tissue for extraction of DNA for molecular studies is the spleen. DNA can also be extracted from cultured skin fibroblasts, but this involves considerably more effort and expense.

Once these samples have been collected the postmortem examination can be completed at leisure. It is important that a full examination should be carried out, as many suspected metabolic disorders turn out to be secondary to some other condition, such as infection or congenital heart disease. Routine histology is mandatory in addition to the special samples listed above.

If a baby dies unexpectedly, particularly during a therapeutic procedure, it may be necessary to save infusion bags and equipment, used syringes, ampoules and other items for subsequent laboratory analysis. Unfortunately, malfunctioning infusion pumps, incorrect fluids, errors in drug dosages, wrongly mixed feeds and even deliberate harm are all well recognized in young babies in hospital.

INTERPRETATION OF THE POSTMORTEM REPORT

STILLBIRTHS

Although paediatricians are seldom required to counsel the parents of a stillborn child, it is as well to have an understanding of the postmortem findings when looking after subsequent siblings. The report should answer the following questions.

- Was the baby normally formed? This is usually easily answered, but it is important to recall that maceration may mimic other abnormalities, particularly fetal hydrops, hydrocephalus and talipes.

Table 45.3 Foot length of the fetus. (Modified from Streeter[33])

End of week	Mean foot length (mm)	Minimum foot length (mm)	Maximum foot length (mm)
14	14.0	12.5	15.5
15	16.8	15.2	18.5
16	19.9	18.2	21.6
17	23.0	21.0	25.0
18	26.8	24.8	28.8
19	30.7	28.5	33.0
20	33.3	31.0	35.7
21	35.2	32.5	38.0
22	39.5	36.0	43.0
23	42.2	39.0	45.5
24	45.2	42.0	48.5
25	47.7	44.5	51.0
26	50.2	47.0	53.5
27	52.7	49.0	56.5
28	55.2	51.5	59.0
29	57.0	53.0	61.0
30	59.2	55.5	63.0
31	61.2	57.5	65.0
32	63.0	59.0	67.0
33	65.0	61.0	69.0
34	68.2	64.0	72.5
35	70.5	66.0	75.0
36	73.5	69.0	78.0
37	76.5	72.0	81.0
38	78.5	74.0	83.0
39	81.0	76.0	86.0
40	82.5	77.5	87.5

• What was the baby's likely gestational age? The single most reliable measurement is the foot length or femur length, as others may be affected by maceration and pathological processes (Table 45.3). Body weight is particularly unreliable. Further information may be gleaned from the bone age, but this may be retarded in small-for-dates babies and those with congenital infections and congenital syndromes, and accelerated in maternal diabetes and anencephaly. The gyral pattern of the cerebral hemispheres is an accurate guide apparently unaffected by intrauterine malnutrition.[10] The histological appearance of the kidneys, liver, lungs and brain is also helpful, but requires considerable experience to interpret accurately.[35] For example, at 23 weeks of gestation three layers of glomeruli are present in the kidney, which increase weekly by one until 10 layers are present at 30 weeks of gestation. Thereafter formation of glomeruli is patchy. Absence of the nephrogenic zone in the kidney is the best histological evidence that gestation has proceeded beyond 36 weeks.

• When did the baby die? Estimation of how long the baby was retained in utero after death is an inexact science.[12] Skin slipping becomes apparent 6–12 hours after death. Bullae usually indicate an interval of about 24 hours. These changes are followed by laxity of the joints and accumulation of serosanguineous fluid in body cavities. After 4 or 5 days the parietal bones become separated from the periosteum and there is progressive discoloration of body tissues. Maceration is accelerated by oedema and amniotic fluid infection, and the changes may be modified in severely growth-retarded fetuses.

Although inexact, if maceration is advanced it is often possible to discount a clinical history of apparent fetal movements or audible heartbeat in the day or two before delivery, and to demonstrate that death must have occurred before the mother came into hospital.

• Was pregnancy proceeding normally until the time of death? A normally grown fetus with a usual amount of subcutaneous fat, petechial haemorrhages beneath serosal surfaces, and perhaps amniotic squames in alveoli and meconium staining, is usually deemed to have died acutely as a result of some circulatory problem. Evidence of 'asphyxia', such as petechial haemorrhages, does not preclude an acute event superimposed on a more long-standing process.

In addition to the parameters used by clinicians to assess growth retardation, the pathologist uses organ-weight ratios to express differential growth. Thus the normal brain–liver ratio is 2:1–4:1, and a ratio of 6:1 in later pregnancy indicates severe asymmetrical growth retardation. A small thymus with a large liver and spleen suggests intrauterine infection. Normal organ weights of newborn children are given in Table 45.4, but it must be emphasized that because of individual variation and loss of weight due to autolysis ratios are much more reliable than absolute weights.

A histological section of a costochondral junction is used to demonstrate endochondral ossification, which is impaired if there has been long-standing disturbance of growth. Frozen sections of the adrenal gland have been advocated as a means of demonstrating the duration of intrauterine compromise. Hypoxia causes progressive accumulation of fat in the fetal cortex, which can be demonstrated by lipid stains or polarizing light microscopy even in macerated fetuses (Fig. 45.7). For a detailed discussion of this topic see Becker and Becker.[1]

• Why did the fetus die? The causes of intrauterine death are legion, and in some cases may be obvious, such as major malformations. In others an explanation can only be found by meticulous review of the clinical record in conjunction with postmortem findings. Contributory evidence is found in the placenta in at least 30% of normally formed stillbirths, and so critical examination of the placenta is essential. Hovatta et al[15] reported a series of stillbirths classified according to necropsy findings, placental examination and clinical factors (Table 45.5). Using this combined approach about 10% of stillbirths remained unexplained.[15,23]

NEONATAL DEATHS

The postmortem report should be reviewed for answers to the following questions.

• Were clinical estimates of maturity correct? This becomes particularly important when a decision has been

Table 45.4 Organ weights of newborn infants by body weight. (Reproduced with permission from Gruenwald and Minh[13])

Body weight (g)	Number of cases	Body length (cm)	Heart (g)	Lungs combined (g)	Spleen (g)	Liver (g)	Adrenals combined (g)	Kidneys combined (g)	Thymus (g)	Brain (g)	Gestational age Weeks	Gestational age Days
500	317	29.4	5.0	12	1.3	26	2.6	5.4	2.2	70	23	5
		±2.5	±1.6	±5	±0.8	±10	±1.7	±2.1	±0.8	±18	±2	3
750	311	32.9	6.3	19	2.0	39	3.2	7.8	2.8	107	26	0
		±3.0	±1.8	±6	±1.2	±12	±1.5	±2.6	±1.3	±27	±2	6
1000	295	35.6	7.7	24	2.6	47	3.5	10.4	3.7	143	27	5
		±3.1	±2.0	±8	±1.5	±12	±1.6	±3.4	±2.0	±34	±3	1
1250	217	38.4	9.6	30	3.4	56	4.0	12.9	4.9	174	29	0
		±3.0	±3.3	±9	±1.8	±21	±1.7	±3.9	±12.1	±38	±3	0
1500	167	41.0	11.5	34	4.3	65	4.5	14.9	6.1	219	31	3
		±2.7	±3.3	±11	±2.0	±18	±1.8	±4.2	±2.7	±52	±2	3
1750	148	42.6	12.8	40	5.0	74	5.3	17.4	6.8	247	32	4
		±3.1	±3.2	±13	±2.5	±20	±2.0	±4.7	±3.0	±51	±2	6
2000	140	44.9	14.9	44	6.0	82	5.3	18.8	7.9	281	34	6
		±2.8	±4.2	±13	±2.7	±23	±2.0	±5.0	±3.4	±56	±3	2
2250	124	46.3	16.0	48	7.0	88	6.0	20.2	8.2	308	36	4
		±2.9	±4.3	±15	±3.3	±24	±2.3	±4.9	±3.4	±49	±13	0
2500	120	47.3	17.7	48	8.5	105	7.1	22.6	8.3	339	38	0
		±2.3	±4.2	±14	±3.5	±21	±2.8	±5.5	±4.4	±50	±3	2
2750	138	48.7	19.1	51	9.1	117	7.5	24.0	9.6	362	39	2
		±2.9	±3.8	±15	±3.6	±26	±2.7	±5.4	±3.8	±48	±2	2
3000	144	50.0	20.7	53	10.1	127	8.3	24.7	10.2	380	40	0
		±2.9	±5.3	±13	±3.3	±30	±2.9	±5.3	±4.3	±55	±2	1
3250	133	50.7	21.5	59	11.0	145	9.2	27.3	11.6	395	40	4
		±2.6	±4.3	±18	±4.0	±33	±3.4	±6.6	±4.4	±53	±1	6
3500	106	51.8	22.8	63	11.3	153	9.8	28.0	12.8	411	40	4
		±3.0	±5.9	±17	±3.6	±33	±3.5	±6.5	±5.1	±55	±1	5
3750	57	52.1	23.8	65	12.5	159	10.2	29.5	13.0	413	40	6
		±2.3	±5.1	±15	±4.1	±40	±3.3	±6.8	±4.8	±55	±2	3
4000	31	52.4	25.8	67	14.1	180	10.8	30.2	11.4	420	41	4
		±2.7	±5.3	±20	±4.0	±39	±3.4	±6.2	±3.2	±62	±1	3
4250	15	53.2	26.5	68	13.0	197	12.0	30.7	11.7	415	41	2
		±2.5	±5.3	±16	±2.5	±42	±3.7	±15.8	±3.7	±38	±2	1

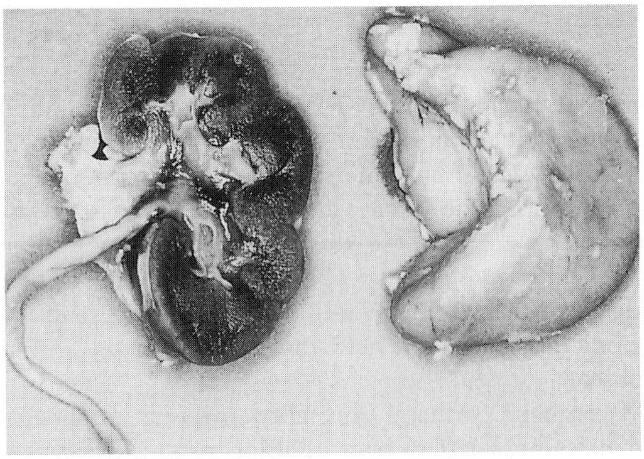

Fig. 45.7 Kidney and adrenal of a baby who died at a few hours of age just after a blood test had unexpectedly shown profound anaemia. The adrenal gland is pale and enlarged due to accumulation of lipid confirming that the anaemia was long-standing and not due to intrapartum fetal haemorrhage.

made not to offer intensive care because the infant is deemed too immature to survive. Parameters such as body weight and dimensions, bone age, histological maturity of the lungs and cerebral gyral pattern can all provide retrospective support for a difficult clinical decision, although none is absolute.

Table 45.5 Causes of stillbirth. (Modified from Hovatta et al[15])

Cause	No.	%
Major malformations	41	16.9
Abruption of the placenta	35	14.4
Large placental infarction	26	10.7
Cord complication	29	11.9
Other placental failure		
severe pre-eclampsia	18	
cholestasis of pregnancy	8	
twin pregnancy	7	
immature birth	5	
maternal trauma	4	
uterine anomaly, etc.	2	
other causes	18	
total	62	25.4
Unexplained asphyxia	8	3.3
Isoimmunization	8	3.3
Fetal bleeding		
fetofetal transfusion		
fetomaternal transfusion		
other bleeding	7	2.9
Severe chorioamnionitis	5	2.1
Unexplained	22	9.1
Total	243	100

Occasionally it is the competence of a single organ system that is in question. The diagnosis of pulmonary hypoplasia is a recurrent problem. In addition to the absolute lung weights (Table 45.4), which may be misleadingly increased by superimposed pathology such as oedema or haemorrhage, the chest X-ray and lung weight–body weight ratio should be considered (normally greater than 0.015 before 28 weeks of gestation and 0.012 in babies of more than 28 weeks' gestation). Hypoplastic lungs are not just small but are also structurally and functionally immature. Histological examination demonstrates deficient development of the pulmonary parenchyma, which can be quantified by performing radial alveolar counts.[6,7]

• Were the major clinical diagnoses correct? The answer to this question usually poses no great problem provided the pathologist is alerted to the clinical diagnoses before starting the examination. He can then take the necessary steps to ensure that, for example, examination of the brain takes into account the findings of ultrasound scans in life. In this context it may be more useful to slice the brain fresh and provide a timely report, than to fix the brain and provide a very detailed report months later.

• Were there any unrecognized treatable conditions? Porter and Keeling[28] found that the commonest discrepancies between the antemortem diagnosis and the postmortem findings were the over- or underdiagnosis of malformation, intraventricular haemorrhage and infection. Histological examination was essential for making or confirming the pathological diagnosis in 20% of cases.

Although unexpected morphological diagnoses are seldom questioned, the results of bacterial cultures are often dismissed as postmortem 'contaminants'. Pryse-Davies and Hurley[29] reported the results of bacteriology of 835 perinatal postmortems. They obtained positive cultures from blood, cerebrospinal fluid and bronchial swabs in 21, 12 and 41% of specimens, respectively. The incidence of positive cultures did not increase with postmortem delay, and although the possibility of contamination was hard to exclude with bronchial swabs there was a highly significant correlation with histological evidence of pneumonia. Mueller et al[26] confirmed the value of postmortem bacterial cultures in stillbirths and early neonatal deaths (Fig. 45.8).

• Were there any unwanted effects of therapy? It is surprising to a pathologist that the word 'iatrogenic' does not appear in the index of most textbooks of neonatology (Chapter 37). Unfortunately, the history of neonatology contains several examples of therapeutic disasters which both pathologists and clinicians were slow to identify.[17,18,31] Iatrogenic disease does not imply blame, but is an acknowledgement that necessary and well-intentioned therapy may have unwanted effects (Fig. 45.9).

Review of the postmortem report should consider the effects of intubation on the larynx and trachea, the effects of barotrauma on the lungs, and any oxygen damage to the lungs and eyes. (It is unfortunate, but understandable, that the eyes cannot be removed as a routine without special permission.) Misplacement of vascular catheters and complications of vascular access, such as thrombosis and ischaemic damage, are common. Histological examination may demonstrate complications of intravenous nutrition in the liver and lungs. The incidence of individual types of iatrogenic lesions varies widely between different units, and should be subject to periodic systematic review to identify trends and new problems.

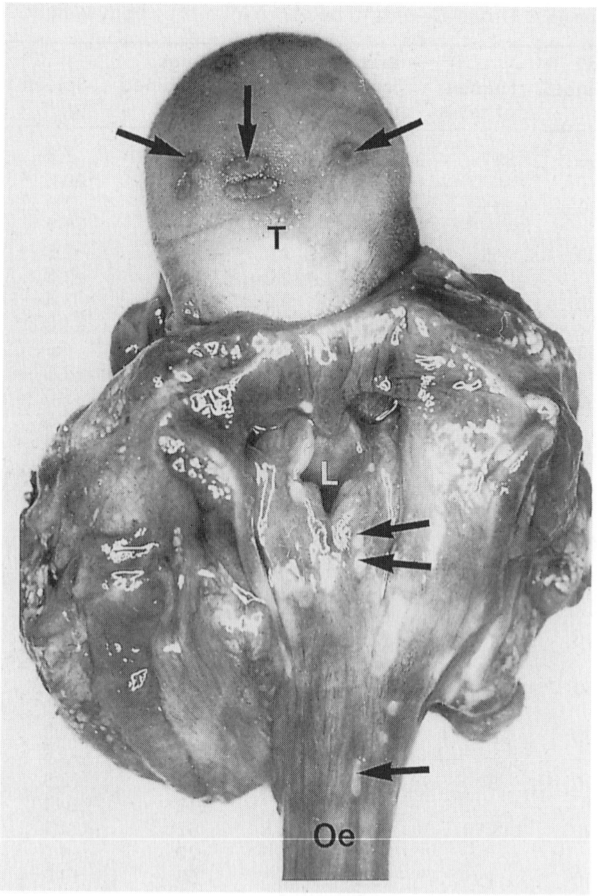

Fig. 45.8 Tongue (T), larynx (L) and oesophagus (Oe) seen from behind showing ulcers (arrows) resulting from *Pseudomonas aeruginosa* septicaemia.

A regular perinatal mortality meeting attended by obstetricians, paediatricians, pathologists, geneticists and other interested specialists provides the optimal environment in which to review the postmortem findings and reach a consensus about the causes of a baby's death.

CLASSIFICATION OF PERINATAL DEATHS

A further purpose of the perinatal mortality meeting should be the accurate classification of each perinatal death according to an agreed system, whether or not there has been a postmortem examination. These data can be used to complement basic statistics for audit and epidemiological studies and in the preparation of an

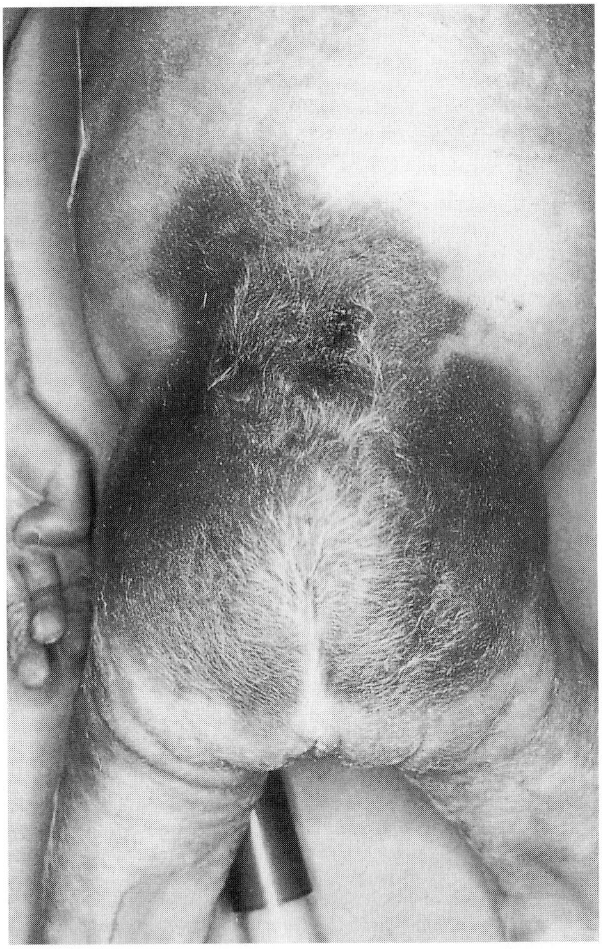

Fig. 45.9 Back of premature baby showing extensive skin necrosis following umbilical artery catheterization. Although similar changes have been attributed to pooling behind the baby of alcohol-based antiseptic solutions used to clean the umbilicus, there was no history of use of such a solution in this case (Harpin and Rutter[14]).

annual report. There are advantages to using more than one classification, which should be chosen according to the use to which the data will be put. The Aberdeen clinicopathological classification by 'obstetric cause'[4,22] has particular relevance for obstetricians. Pathologists tend to use classifications based on lesions found at necropsy, which give little information about aetiology but have the advantage of objectivity and can be used to follow trends. Such a system was used by Claireaux[3] for the 1958 British Perinatal Mortality Survey. Naeye[27] devised a classification using fetal and placental pathology. Pathological classifications are of limited use unless the postmortem rate is close to 100%. The classification of Wigglesworth[37] uses a clinicopathological approach, and claims to be relatively accurate whether or not information from postmortem is available. It assigns deaths to five categories, which may be further broken down by gestational age:

1. Normally formed macerated stillbirth;
2. Congenital malformation;
3. Conditions associated with immaturity;
4. Asphyxial conditions developing during labour;
5. Specific conditions other than the above.

One strength of this method is that excess mortality in any of these categories directs attention to specific aspects of care, i.e. antenatal screening, perinatal care, the management of labour and the treatment of specific conditions such as rhesus disease, respectively. The Wigglesworth classification has recently been shown to be reproducible, and modifications have been suggested.[19] Postmortem results changed the classification in 9% of cases in this study.

Attempts have been made to classify deaths according to avoidability. This is a subjective judgement, usually made without the benefit of control data, and there is little evidence that such judgements arrived at by a committee lead to a reduction in perinatal mortality.[11,34] Death is a crude end-point by which to measure the quality of perinatal care. Nevertheless, clinicopathological review is one way of identifying some of those cases in which care has fallen short of agreed standards, and changing management to reduce future morbidity as well as mortality. Moawad et al[25] estimated that 28% of perinatal deaths in their population were potentially avoidable, and achieved a significant reduction in these potentially avoidable deaths during the 5 years of their study. The Confidential Enquiry into Stillbirths and Deaths in Infancy has used this approach on a large scale to identify deficiencies in clinical care and suggest changes in practice.[5]

REFERENCES

1. Becker M J, Becker A E 1989 Pathology of late fetal stillbirth. Churchill Livingstone, Edinburgh
2. Black J 1987 Broaden your mind about death and bereavement in certain ethnic groups in Britain. British Medical Journal 295: 536–539
3. Claireaux A E 1962 Perinatal mortality in the United Kingdom. In Keller R J (ed) Modern trends in obstetrics 3. Butterworths, London, pp 191–211
4. Cole S K, Hey E N, Thomson A M 1986 Classifying perinatal death: an obstetric approach. British Journal of Obstetrics and Gynaecology 93: 1204–1212
5. Confidential Enquiry into Stillbirths and Deaths in Infancy, 4th annual report. 1 January–31 December 1995. Maternal and Child Health Consortium, July 1997
6. Cooney T P, Thurlbeck W M 1982 The radial alveolar count method of Emery and Mithal: a reappraisal. 1. Postnatal lung growth. Thorax 37: 572–579
7. Cooney T P Thurlbeck W M 1982 The radial alveolar count method of Emery and Mithal: a reappraisal 2. Intrauterine and early postnatal lung growth. Thorax 37: 580–583
8. Davis G J, Peterson B R 1996 Dilemmas and solutions for the pathologist and clinician encountering religious views of the autopsy. Southern Medical Journal 89: 1041–1044
9. Department of Health 1983 Guide to the postmortem examination. Brief notes for parents and families who have lost a baby in pregnancy or early infancy. DoH, London
10. Dorovini-Zis K, Dolman C L 1977 Gestational development of brain. Archives of Pathology and Laboratory Medicine 101: 192–195

11. Elbourne D, Mutch L 1984 Do locally based enquiries into perinatal mortality reduce the risk of perinatal death? In: Smith A (ed) Recent advances in community medicine 3. Churchill Livingstone, London, pp 221–229
12. Genest D R, Singer D B 1992 Estimating the time of death in stillborn fetuses: III. External fetal examination: a study of 86 stillborns. Obstetrics and Gynecology 80: 593–600
13. Gruenwald P, Minh H N 1960 Evaluation of body and organ weights in perinatal pathology. 1. Normal standards derived from autopsies. American Journal of Clinical Pathology 34: 247–253
14. Harpin V, Rutter N 1982 Percutaneous alcohol absorption and skin necrosis in a preterm infant. Archives of Disease in Childhood 57: 477–479
15. Hovatta O, Lipasti A, Rapola J, Karjalainen O 1983 Causes of stillbirth: a clinicopathological study of 243 patients. British Journal of Obstetrics and Gynaecology 90: 691–696
16. Joint Working Party Report on Fetal and Perinatal Pathology 1988 Royal College of Obstetricians and Gynaecologists and Royal College of Pathologists, London
17. Keeling J W 1981 Iatrogenic disease in the newborn. Virchows Archiv (Pathol. Anat.) 394: 1–29
18. Keeling J W 1993 Fetal and neonatal pathology, 2nd edn. Springer Verlag, London
19. Keeling J W, MacGillivray I, Golding J, Wigglesworth J, Berry J, Dunn P M 1989 Classification of perinatal death. Archives of Disease in Childhood 64: 1345–1351
20. Knight B 1983 The coroner's necropsy. Churchill Livingstone, Edinburgh
21. Macpherson T A, Valdes-Dapena M, Kanbour A 1986 Perinatal mortality and morbidity: the role of the anatomical pathologist. Seminars in Perinatology 10: 179–186
22. McIlwaine G, Howat R C L, Dunn F, MacNaughton M C 1979 The Scottish Perinatal Mortality Survey. British Medical Journal 2: 1103–1106
23. Magani I M, Rafla N M, Mortimer G, Meehan F P 1990 Stillbirths: a clinicopathological survey (1972–1982). Pediatric Pathology 10: 363–374
24. Meier P R, Manchester D K, Shikes R H, Clewell W H, Stewart M 1986 Perinatal autopsy: its clinical value. Obstetrics and Gynecology 67: 349–351
25. Moawad A H, Lee K S, Fisher D E, Ferguson R, Phillippe M 1990 A model for the prospective analysis of perinatal deaths in a perinatal network. American Journal of Obstetrics and Gynecology 162: 15–22
26. Mueller R F, Sybert V P, Johnson J, Brown Z A, Chen W-J 1983 Evaluation of a protocol for post-mortem examination of stillbirths. New England Journal of Medicine 309: 586–590
27. Naeye R L 1977 Causes of perinatal mortality in the US Collaborative Perinatal Project. Journal of the American Medical Association 238: 228–229
28. Porter H J, Keeling J W 1987 Value of perinatal necropsy examination. Journal of Clinical Pathology 40: 180–184
29. Pryse-Davies J, Hurley R 1979 Infections and perinatal mortality. Journal of Antimicrobial Chemotherapy 5 (suppl. A): 59–70
30. Rudd P T, Wigglesworth J S 1982 Oxygen embolus during mechanical ventilation with disappearance of signs after death. Archives of Disease in Childhood 57: 237–239
31. Silverman W A 1983 Perinatal pathologist as skeptical inquirer. Pediatric Pathology 1: 5–6
32. Stillbirth and Neonatal Death Society Stillbirth and Neonatal Death Society, London 1995 Pregnancy loss and the death of a baby. Guidelines for professionals
33. Streeter G L 1921 Weight, sitting height, head size, foot length and menstrual age of the human embryo. Contributions to Embryology, Carnegie Institute 55: 143–170
34. Thomas J, Edwards J, Bowen-Simpkins P et al 1985 Use of refined perinatal mortality rate trends to evaluate the effect of a confidential enquiry. Lancet ii: 197–199
35. Valdes-Dapena M 1979 Histology of the fetus and newborn. W B Saunders, Philadelphia
36. Vujanic G M, Cartlidge P H, Stewart J H, Dawson A J 1995 Perinatal infant postmortem examinations: how well are we doing? Journal of Clinical Pathology 48: 998–1001
37. Wigglesworth J 1980 Monitoring perinatal mortality: a pathophysiological approach. Lancet ii: 684–686
38. Wigglesworth J S 1996 Perinatal pathology. Major problems in pathology, 2nd edn. W B Saunders, Philadelphia
39. Wigglesworth J S, Singer D B (eds.) 1991 Textbook of fetal and perinatal pathology. Blackwell, Boston
40. Winter R W, Knowles S A S, Bieber F R, Baraitser M 1988 The malformed fetus and stillbirth. A diagnostic approach. John Wiley, Chichester

46

The clinical biochemistry laboratory

Anne Green

INTRODUCTION

Clinical biochemistry, as a component of laboratory medicine, provides a wide range of services for the neonate which includes screening for certain disorders and investigations to aid diagnosis and monitoring of treatment/disease progression. These services, although primarily geared to the hospital setting for out- and inpatients, also extend to the community where required.

Success and quality of services are influenced by the working relationship between neonatologists and their clinical biochemistry department. Each party should have an understanding of each other's role and needs in order to optimize the content of service delivery, development of new services, and support/collaboration for research. Such understanding is particularly important for paediatrics. In the non-specialist hospital where neonatology/paediatrics is only part of a larger laboratory workload, the clinician and patient are best served when their laboratory has a clinical chemist with a specific remit and special interest in this area.

This chapter is intended to provide an overview of the contribution that clinical biochemistry can make to neonatal practice and, in particular, to help the clinician optimize the service he/she receives from that laboratory.

SPECIMEN COLLECTION/TRANSPORT

BLOOD

The quality of specimen is paramount if a meaningful result is to be obtained. This means taking sufficient blood from the right source (i.e. arterial/capillary/venous) in the appropriate anticoagulant with minimal haemolysis.

Many laboratories provide a capillary blood collection service, ideally combined as a joint service between the Clinical Biochemistry and Haematology Departments. This enables experienced and trained personnel to obtain high quality specimens, thereby reducing the need for repeat specimens due to insufficient specimen, haemolysis, or the wrong anticoagulant. Collection of blood by skin puncture should be performed according to recommended guidance[6,9] thereby minimizing risk to the patient and maximizing quality. Capillary specimens can be used for many analyses (Table 46.1) although if several tests are required from the same collection, large volumes (i.e. in excess of 1 ml whole blood) are best taken as venous specimens. There are significant differences between concentrations in capillary and venous specimens for some analyses, e.g. potassium in capillary blood is 1.0–1.5 mmol/l higher than in venous blood, and greater discrepancies can occur if the capillary blood has been collected with excessive squeezing, even without visible haemolysis. Most biochemical analyses are undertaken on plasma, and hence the need to appreciate that the relatively high packed cell volume in the neonate means that a larger blood sample is required for plasma analysis.

Table 46.1 Clinical biochemistry analyses usually available on blood obtained by capillary puncture

Alanine transaminase	γ-glutamyl transpeptidase
Albumin	Glucose
Alkaline phosphatase	Hydrogen ion (pH)
	PCO_2*
Aspartate transaminase	Magnesium
Bicarbonate	Osmolality
Bilirubin – total and fractions	Phosphate
Calcium	Potassium
Chloride	Sodium
Cholesterol	Total protein
Creatinine	Urea

*Only appropriate if specimen arterialized and collected in special tube with no access to air.

An added problem for capillary specimens is sweat or other contamination from skin (e.g. creams) which may produce artefactually 'abnormal' results, e.g. ammonia, triglycerides (from glycerol), amino acids. Capillary specimens should not be taken if patients are known to be, or are at high risk of being, hepatitis B- or HIV-positive.

Once taken, all specimens should be transported to the laboratory without delay. Certain analyses need particu-

Table 46.2 Analyses suitable for measurement in a random urine specimen

	Comments
Calcium	Relate to creatinine as molar ratio
Urate	Relate to creatinine as molar ratio
Phosphate	Need blood specimen at the same time Calculate as a tubular phosphate reabsorption*
Total protein/albumin	Relate to creatinine
Metabolic investigations: amino acids/organic acids etc.	Collect when baby is 'sick'
Sodium : potassium ratio	Individual concentrations in a random specimen are difficult to interpret
Sodium	Need blood specimen at the same time Calculate as fractional excretion

*See Appendix 6.

larly prompt sample handling to separate plasma and/or to deproteinize them, e.g. ammonia, lactate, amino acids. The laboratory will be able to advise on specific requirements. Once received by the laboratory, all blood specimens must be processed carefully to minimize evaporation of plasma/serum; the concentration of an analyte in a 100 µl plasma specimen left uncovered for 1 hour at room temperature may change by as much as 10%.[5]

URINE

Useful results can often be obtained from random or overnight urine specimens by relating analyses to creatinine concentration (Table 46.2). It should rarely be necessary to collect timed urines.

Several millilitres of urine can be collected by cotton wool balls placed strategically against the genitalia and held in place by a suitable disposable nappy or within a thin plastic glove. The top of the glove can be secured gently using thin plastic tape (e.g. transpore). When wet, the urine is then aspirated from the cotton wool using a plastic syringe and transferred into a clean universal container. This method of collection is, however, not suitable for investigation of proteinuria as the cotton wool fibres absorb some of the protein content, thereby making meaningful interpretation difficult.[10]

The need for a timed collection should be restricted to those situations which demand it, e.g. catecholamines, copper. Such collections should be *accurately* timed rather than trying to collect over a specific length of time.

Most random urines do not require a preservative provided they are transported to the laboratory without delay. Those analyses which are collected over a time period may require collection bottles with particular preservatives (e.g. catecholamines). It is important to check with the laboratory *before* collecting the specimen. Do not transfer urine from one type of container to another.

Specimens for metabolic investigations which require transport to an off-site laboratory should be stored, and ideally transported, deep frozen. If this is difficult, then a preservative, e.g. thymol, may be advised (consult your metabolic laboratory for details and specific recommendations).

BREADTH OF SERVICE/TEST REPERTOIRE

Most laboratories have appropriate automated instruments and should be able to carry out the most frequently required tests on a 500 µl specimen of whole blood. An 'out-of-hours' service to provide those tests essential for immediate patient management will be available.

Analytical methods must be those which are least likely to be interfered with by haemoglobin, bilirubin and lipids. In addition they must also provide the required level of sensitivity (e.g. plasma creatinine at the low end of the normal range for infants), and linearity (e.g. high concentrations of bilirubin).

REFERENCE RANGES (see Appendix 6)

Reference ranges for neonates are often very different from those of older children and adults. Many enzymes are higher in the neonate, i.e. γ-glutamyl transferase, whereas other parameters are lower and increase with age, e.g. albumin, caeruloplasmin, copper, cholesterol. In addition, for some analyses there is wide variability within the first 4 weeks of life, and interpretation of results may require consideration of gestational age. The reasons why some biochemical measures change significantly over the first few weeks of life include maternal illness and treatments, the mode of delivery, and feeding regimen. The clinical biochemist should provide information to enable interpretation for methodologies in local use. It is likely that a local laboratory has not been able to obtain its own reference range and will rely on data produced by the larger specialist paediatric centres. Some analyses have widely different ranges dependent on the method used, the prime example being alkaline phosphatase. Bilirubin is also a problem in this respect, particularly measurement of conjugated or 'direct-reacting' bilirubin. These are not the same and specific methods for conjugated bilirubin (e.g. dry slide methodology) may give results significantly lower than for 'direct-reacting' methods. Special care must be taken when a series of results for a particular patient are from more than one laboratory.

There are several published lists of reference data[2,3,4,8] for methods in current usage – however, they will *not* be valid for all laboratories and should *not* be used without advice from the local biochemist.

INTERPRETING RESULTS

Results should always be interpreted in the context of

Table 46.3 Factors for consideration in interpretation of results

Variable factors	Examples
Source of specimen	Contamination with i.v. line Other contamination Wrong patient (mislabelling)
Type of specimen	Venous/capillary/arterial Plasma/serum/whole blood Anticoagulant Fasting/postprandial Quality
Specimen handling/transport	Delay in transport/separation Storage conditions
Analysis	Same laboratory Same method/reference range Artefact/interference Cross-reactivity Laboratory error

Table 46.4 Some examples of possible artefacts/interference in plasma/serum biochemical analyses

'Unexpected' result(s)	Possible cause(s)
↓ Sodium	Intralipid interference in analysis (if flame photometry)
↑Creatine kinase	Previous injection/excessive muscle activity
↓ Glucose	Wrong anticoagulant – must be fluoride oxalate
↑ Ca, ↑ albumin	Venous stasis
↑ K	Capillary blood
↑ K, ↑ PO_4, ↑ aspartate aminotransferase	Delayed separation of blood
↓ Ca, ↑ K, ↓ Mg, ↓ alkaline phosphatase	EDTA contamination
↑ Urate	Interference from ketones
↑ NH_3	Capillary specimen Sweat contamination Delay in transport/separation
↑ Triglycerides	Glycerol contamination

appropriate reference ranges, previous results from the same patient, clinical condition, and the circumstances surrounding specimen collection, transport and analysis. Trends may be important rather than the absolute value per se.

If a result is unexpected, e.g. odd one out in a series, unexpected change from previous trend, then it is important to consider exogenous and iatrogenic causes as well as in vivo causes (Table 46.3).

If a result for a particular patient is unexpected/difficult to explain, the clinician should discuss this with the clinical biochemist to question whether the result could be an error or artefact. Some examples are listed in Table 46.4.

THE COMMUNITY AND THE LABORATORY

Earlier discharge of babies into the community is of relevance to the laboratory. In particular, babies who continue to be jaundiced beyond 14 days with no explanation must have their conjugated bilirubin measured (see Chapter 31, Part 1) and further investigations considered in order to exclude liver dysfunction.

A function of the specialist clinical biochemistry departments in the UK is neonatal screening for phenylketonuria and congenital hypothyroidism. In some centres testing for cystic fibrosis and for sickle cell disorders also takes place, using the same specimen. Testing for the other disorders is not universal in the UK – it is therefore important to check the specifics for your area.

Babies are screened in the first week of life using capillary blood usually collected in the home by the midwife. *It is important that babies who are still in hospital at this age are tested.* The screening request must contain information about feeding and transfusions. For PKU the blood is tested for excess phenylalanine, in most cases using the Guthrie microbiological test (see p. 993). Testing for CHT is usually accomplished by measurement of thyroid-stimulating hormone (TSH), although a few laboratories use thyroxine as the first-line test (see Chapter 38, Part 2).

BEDSIDE TESTING

There is an increasing trend to provide testing nearer the patient with rapid turnaround of results to enable rapid decision-making.

Units with a special care baby unit or high dependency unit should have on-site monitoring of acid/base/blood gases, and require rapid turnaround for sodium, potassium, glucose, calcium and bilirubin. There is a case for extending near-patient testing services into other areas, e.g. delivery rooms and theatres. These possibilities should be discussed with the clinical biochemist.

Provision of all laboratory equipment on the wards, clinics and side rooms, should be the responsibility of the laboratory. This ensures that the essential functions of quality control, training of designated staff, maintenance and trouble-shooting are met. This is not only essential to ensure reliable and safe working practices, but also makes best use of equipment as mobile instruments can sometimes be shared.

Quality assurance of such instruments is particularly important. The laboratory must take responsibility for this, and all users should be made fully aware of its importance.

Accreditation of laboratories is now important – such side-room testing will not be accredited unless it is part of the laboratory responsibility and can demonstrate adherence to nationally agreed standards, including performance of quality control.

INHERITED METABOLIC DISORDERS

A key function for the clinical biochemist is to advise on

Table 46.5 Example specification for turnaround times for 'routine' and urgent services

Analysis	'Routine' service	Urgent
Blood gases:		
for intensive care	Immediate	
for other purposes	10–20 min	
Bilirubin	3–4 h	< 1 h
Glucose	3–4 h	30 min
Sodium, potassium	3–4 h	30 min
Calcium	3–4 h	30 min
Alkaline phosphatase	Same working day	Seldom required
Liver enzymes (e.g. alanine aminotransferase)	Same working day	Same working day
Phosphate	Same working day	Seldom required
Magnesium	4 h	< 1 h if required
Ammonia	Analysed immediately	–
Lactate	5 days	Same day
Amino acids	5 days	Same day
Organic acids	5 days	Same day
17OH-progesterone	1–2 days	Same day

the investigation of a sick baby with a possible metabolic disorder and to liaise with metabolic centres on specimen needs and transport requirements for the more specialist tests (Chapter 38, Part 3).

Specimens for investigation should be collected when the baby is sick.[7] Failure to do so may mean that a diagnosis is missed. In the event of death before a diagnosis is established, appropriate specimens should be taken as soon as possible after death.[1,3] Delay in sampling may make subsequent interpretation of biochemical tests impossible.

GENERAL CLINICAL BIOCHEMISTRY

The neonatologist should agree with the clinical biochemist the specification for turnaround times for both 'routine' and urgent investigations (Table 46.5). Out-of-hours arrangements should also be agreed in this context.

It is important to collect blood for certain investigations before starting treatment, e.g. glucose, calcium. Similarly, attention should be given to recording the time of specimens and relationship to fasting/feeds.

The clinical biochemist and neonatologist should work together to agree protocols and investigation approaches for the situations encountered in their local circumstances. Suggested protocols include:

- Investigation of hypoglycaemia – what tests to do/specimen requirements
- Persistent neonatal jaundice – how/when to investigate
- Sudden unexpected death – biochemical investigations/local arrangements for specimen collection, transport and storage
- Investigation of hypocalcaemia
- Biochemical monitoring of parenteral nutrition.

REFERENCES

1. Green A 1993 Biochemical screening in newborn siblings of cases of SIDS. Archives of Disease in Childhood 68(6): 793–796
2. Green A 1996 Investigations. In: Insley J (ed) A paediatric vade mecum, 13th edn. Arnold, London, pp 350–360
3. Green A, Isherwood D 1994 Introduction. In: Clayton B E, Round J M (eds) Clinical biochemistry and the sick child, 2nd edn. Blackwell Scientific Publications, pp 1–10
4. Green A, Morgan I 1993 Neonatology and clinical biochemistry. ACB Adventure Publications, Piggotts, Cambridge
5. Hicks J M B 1992 Paediatric clinical biochemistry: why is it different? In: Soldin S J, Rifai N, Hicks J M B (eds) Biochemical basis of pediatric disease. AACC Press, Washington, USA, pp 537–551
6. Meites S, Hamblin C R, Hayes J R 1992 A study of experimental lancets for blood collection to avoid bone infection of infants. Clinical Chemistry 38: 908–910
7. Saudubray J M, Poggi F, Spada M, Billette de Villemeur T, Hubert P et al 1994 A programmed clinical screening for inborn errors of metabolism in neonates. New Horizons in Neonatal Screening, Elsevier Science, Amsterdam, pp 85–96
8. Scott P H, Wharton B A 1994 Reference data for newborn babies. In: Clayton B E, Round J M (eds) Clinical biochemistry and the sick child, 2nd edn. Blackwell Scientific Publications, pp 511–522
9. Slockbower J M, Jacoby H, Blumenfeld T A, Bruck E, Duffie E R, Mundschenk D 1982 Approved standard procedures for the collection of diagnostic blood specimens by skin puncture. The National Committee for Clinical Laboratory Standards 2: 132–146
10. Smith G C, Taylor C M 1992 Recovery of protein from urine specimens collected in cotton wool. Archives of Disease in Childhood 67: 1486–1487

47

Neonatal imaging

G. Martin Steiner

INTRODUCTION

Imaging today includes conventional radiography, ultrasound, computerized tomography, magnetic resonance imaging and nuclear medicine (isotopes). The capabilities, advantages and disadvantages of each of these modalities are listed in Table 47.1.

Imaging will only help towards the diagnosis of a clinical problem if the clinician already has a differential diagnosis in mind when asking for an investigation. The clinical history and examination are crucial in helping to determine the choice of examination, which should be discussed with the radiologist.

CHOICE OF PERSONNEL

Paediatric imaging should be carried out in a special paediatric radiology department by personnel who are in sympathy with children and are aware of their special needs for feeding, warmth, analgesia and distraction. A trained paediatric radiologist is needed for optimal results. Close contact between the neonatologist and the antenatal ultrasound department and obstetricians is also of great benefit to the patient and should be routine.

CHOICE OF EQUIPMENT

The choice of equipment depends very much on the clinical needs and should always be made after close consultation between radiologists, clinicians, manufacturers and purchasers. The manufacturer's reputation for an immediate back-up and maintenance service and the cost of a maintenance contract are very important factors in the choice of equipment. This obvious advice is not always followed, resulting in the purchase of suboptimal equipment.

Some guidelines are as follows:

- **Radiographic equipment.** Although babies are very small they need powerful generators to ensure short exposures (in the region of a few milliseconds). A typical exposure for a neonatal chest would be 80 kV, 0.6 Mas (milliampere seconds). X-ray tubes should have a small focal spot, (about 0.3 mm) to minimize geometric unsharpness. Fast rare earth film screen combinations are used to reduce radiation exposure.
- **Ultrasound equipment.** High-frequency 5–10 MHz probes are needed for babies to ensure an adequate near field. The higher the frequency the better the definition, but at a cost of reduced depth of

Table 47.1 Capabilities, advantages and disadvantages of different imaging modalities

Modality	Agent	What does it show?	Hazards/drawbacks	Availability and cost
Radiography	X-rays	Anatomy	Radiation No function	Bedside Moderate
Ultrasound	Sound waves	Real-time anatomy	No function Operator dependent	Bedside Cheap
CT	X-rays	Anatomy in cross-section	Radiation Sedation needed and injection	X-ray dept Often expensive Good for haemorrhage
MRI	Electromagnetic waves	Anatomy in all planes	Sedation needed, injections, Non-magnetic anaesthetic equipment	Special dept Expensive ++
Nuclear	Gamma rays	Function	Radiation Sedation needed, injections	Special dept Expensive

penetration. At least one sector probe with a diverging beam and small footprint is needed for ultrasound of the head via the anterior fontanelle. A linear array probe (straight or curved) provides the best near field and is needed to look at soft tissues, hips and the abdomen.

Doppler ultrasound is needed to look at the heart, and in particular to check on the ductus arteriosus. Colour Doppler helps to speed up cardiac examinations, and is useful for other examinations that involve looking at vascular anatomy, e.g. renal and some cranial examinations. The machine must be compact and freely mobile for bedside work.

- **CT, MRI, nuclear medicine.** Equipment is bulky and static and nearly always placed away from the neonatal nursery, creating a need for baby-friendly, safe, warm transportation. MRI examinations are lengthy and supervision of patients in the long narrow tunnel of the machine is difficult. Specialist paediatric anaesthetic advice is therefore very important. The anaesthetist will have to be provided with special equipment made from non-ferromagnetic materials that are not affected by the strong magnetic field of the MRI machine.

SEDATION FOR IMAGING PROCEDURES

Neonates can usually be put to sleep by a feed. For older children we use quinalbarbitone 7–10 mg/kg. Oral chloral hydrate 50 mg/kg is a suitable choice for an infant. Venous access should be established on the ward to save waking the baby during the examination.

Fortunately, radiography and ultrasound are not only the most convenient and inexpensive modalities but they are by far the most useful and will give the answers required in the great majority of cases.

RADIATION SAFETY

Sick ventilated babies have frequent chest X-rays and the question of radiation exposure is frequently raised by parents. A well taken chest X-ray using suitable equipment and technique will give a skin radiation dose in the region of one-tenth to one-twentieth of the natural annual background dose. The gonads are not in the direct beam and will receive a correspondingly smaller dose. The chances of developing a radiation-induced cancer in a patient who has had 5–7 chest X-rays is given as 1 in 10 000 to 1 in 40 000.[4,9] CT and contrast examinations give much bigger doses, approximately the same as the annual background.

It is advisable to follow the ALARA principle (as little as reasonably achievable) of radiation exposure. An X-ray should only be taken if the result is likely to change management and if the answer cannot be obtained by other means not using radiation, such as ultrasound. The minimal number of exposures necessary should be taken; routine lateral chest films and horizontal beam films of the abdomen are unnecessary. Repeat films should be avoided if the original suboptimal film gives the required clinical information. A bright light will rescue most overexposed films.

GUIDELINES FOR INTERPRETING AN X-RAY STUDY

- Remember:
  - —Air is black.
  - —Fluid and soft tissues are greyish white.
  - —Bone and calcium are very white.
- The worst mistakes are made by not following very simple rules.
- Always look at films under proper conditions on a viewing box.
- Always compare with previous films.
- Check the name and date on the film.
- Check the left and right markers. If in doubt, ask the radiographer how the film has been taken.
- Has the whole area of interest been included on the film? For example, are the whole lung fields on the film, including the diaphragms? Is there a name marker over the lung apex? Has the inguinal hernia been excluded from the film?

IMAGING THE CHEST

INTERPRETING X-RAY STUDIES OF THE NEONATAL CHEST

Take a clinical history and check the age of the patient. The significance of a radiographic appearance varies with age, e.g. ground-glass lungs in the first few days of life mean RDS; after a week or more the diagnosis may be streptococcal septicaemia.

Check the presence and position of the 'tubes' (Fig. 47.1):

- The tip of the endotracheal tube should be 1–2 cm above the carina. If the carina is not seen it can be assumed to be at the level of the bodies of T3/4 and the tip of the ETT should be opposite the body of T1.[1] If it is too low it must be moved, and it is good practice to note the position of the ETT on the film label at the time the film was taken.
- The mark of an umbilical arterial catheter is that it courses caudad towards the pelvis before entering the internal iliac artery and then the aorta. Watch for a right-sided aorta. The tip of the catheter should lie either above or below the mesenteric and renal arteries.
- The mark of an umbilical venous catheter is that it courses straight cephalad from its entrance into the body, and passes through the ductus venosus into the

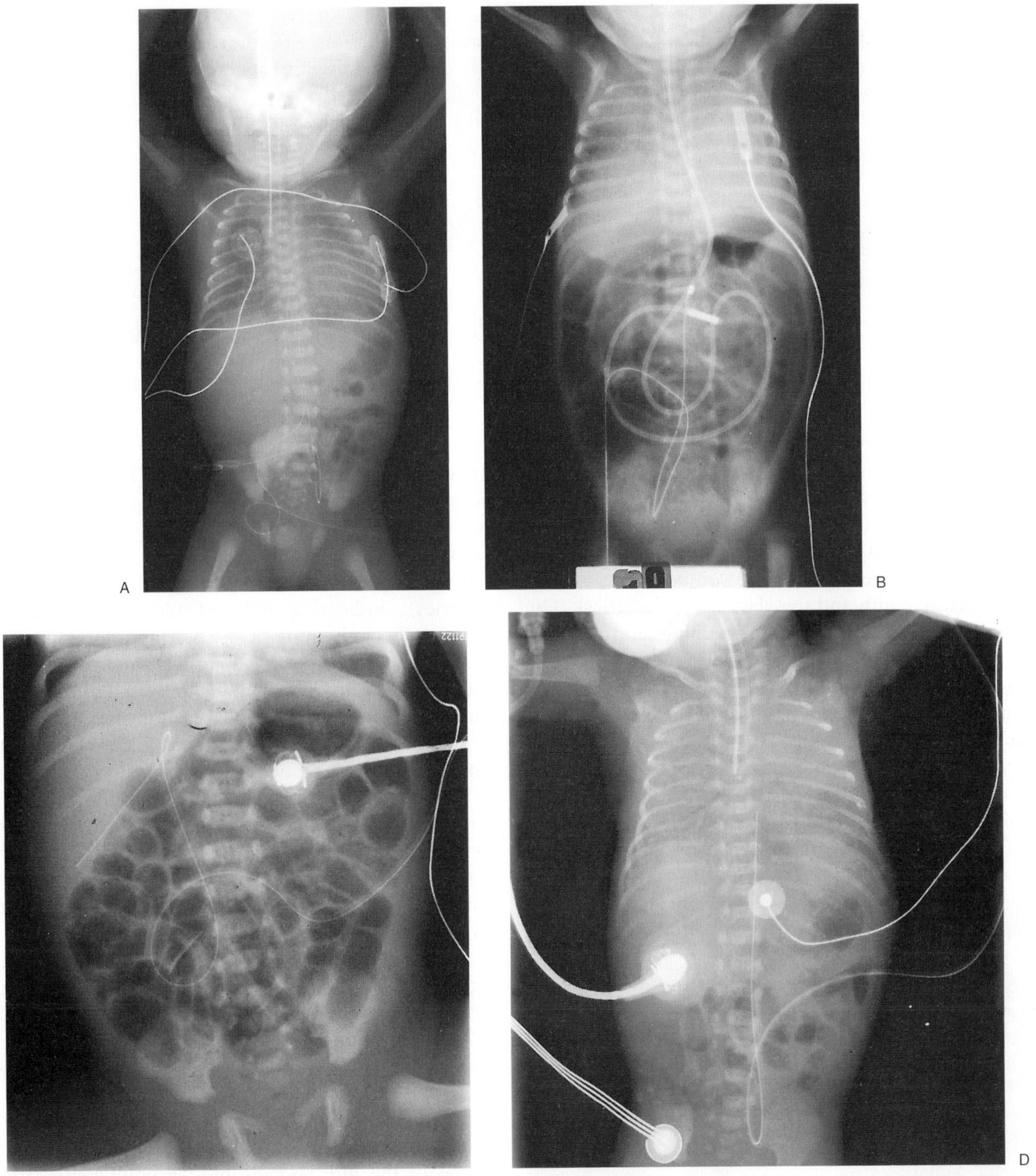

Fig. 47.1 Tubes and lines. (A) Note the position of the tips of the umbilical venous and arterial lines and the ET tube. The tip of the ET tube is too low. The ECG leads are badly placed over the lung fields. (B) The umbilical artery catheter tip is at the level of T12. This is too near the origins of the mesenteric and renal arteries for safety. The tip of the feeding tube is well placed in the jejunum. (C) The tip of the umbilical venous catheter lies in the liver in the hepatic vein and should be moved. (D) Severe RDS with an air bronchogram. The tip of the ET tube is too low and the tip of the umbilical artery catheter is high but clear of the origins of the mesenteric and renal vessels.

inferior vena cava and right atrium. Not infrequently it becomes lodged in a vein in the liver (Fig. 47.1C). In this position adverse effects are more common (pp. 923–924).

- The position of nasogastric and nasojejunal feeding tubes should be checked (Fig. 47.1B).
- Long lines should also be checked, but may need the injection of contrast to be seen.

A well exposed chest film should allow you to see detail in the lung fields and also see the spine behind the heart. Do not hesitate to use the bright light. A surprising

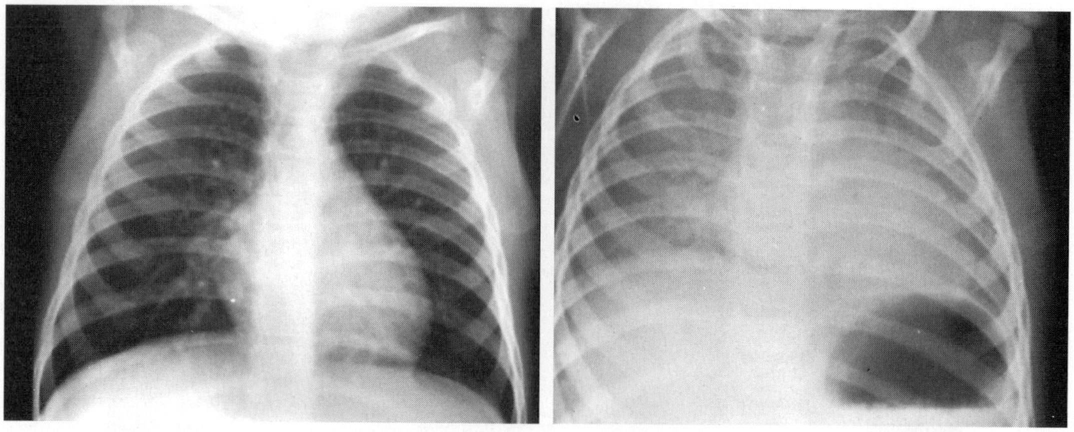

Fig. 47.2 Never report on an expiratory film. Same-day films of same patient with normal chest. (A) is in inspiration, (B) is in expiration.

number of pneumonias and plethoric lungs will be revealed. (Figs 47.2, 47.3)

On a completely straight chest X-ray the anterior ends of the ribs should be equidistant from the corresponding ipsilateral vertebral pedicles, the ribs on both sides should appear equal in length and the clavicles symmetrical. The trachea lies just to the right of the midline and tends to buckle to the right (i.e. concave to the left).

On a good inspiratory film the fifth or sixth anterior rib ends should be crossing the right leaf of the diaphragm.

Check the size of the heart. The normal heart diameter in a neonate may be a little larger than approximately half the diameter of the thorax at its widest. A large cardiac silhouette may be due to an expiratory film, high-output state (e.g. L–R shunt, anaemia, fever), heart failure, myocarditis or pericardial effusion. The heart size should always be assessed together with the pulmonary vasculature. The lung fields may be plethoric (large main and peripheral pulmonary arteries), indicating a high-output state, normal or oligaemic (small pulmonary arteries), indicating reduced blood flow through the lungs. Check the lung fields. Normally all you will see are the pulmonary arteries radiating out from the hila and pulmonary veins coursing to the left atrium behind the heart. Any other shadows are abnormal, but make sure there is nothing on the surface of the baby casting an image over the lung fields.

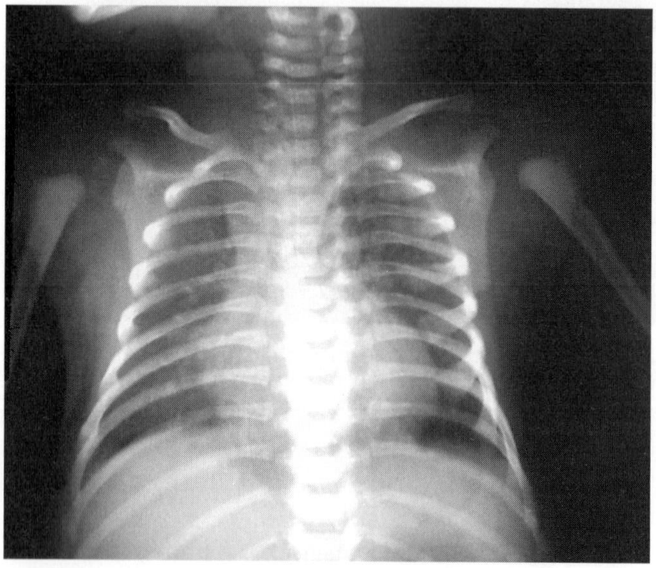

Fig. 47.3 Normal neonatal chest film. The structures behind the heart are well seen, as are the main vessels in the lungs. Slight rotation like this does not affect the diagnostic value of the film. However, it is overexposed for fine detail and a softer film or viewing the radiograph with a bright light would be required to diagnose RDS. Note the normally wide cervical spinal canal.

A common difficulty is caused by the relatively large and variable size of the thymus in infancy, causing a widening of the upper mediastinum. This widening may extend caudad as far as the diaphragm (Fig. 47.4A–D). It is particularly evident on the chest X-ray if the thymus is asymmetrical and protrudes from one side of the mediastinum, usually the right. The thymus is very soft and is indented by the anterior costochondral junctions of the ribs, to give rise to the 'wave sign' of the thymus (Fig. 47.4C). On imaging with ultrasound the thymus is clearly seen to be a homogeneous structure anterior to the great vessels in the thoracic inlet (Fig. 47.4D). CT will show a similar appearance.

Look at the bones and soft tissues and around the edges of the film and the hidden areas behind the heart and diaphragms. You may find evidence of syndromes with short ribs and abnormal spines (Chapter 34), metabolic bone disease (Fig. 47.5A,B) (Chapter 38, Part 4), or trauma.

Abnormal vertebrae (hemivertebra, butterfly vertebra) and ribs suggest the VATER syndrome (conjunction of vertebral, anal, tracheal, oesophageal, renal anomalies) and indicate the need for ultrasound of the kidneys. Air in the abdomen in the presence of oesophageal atresia indicates the presence of a tracheo-oesophageal fistula. A distended stomach will suggest duodenal atresia (Fig. 47.6).

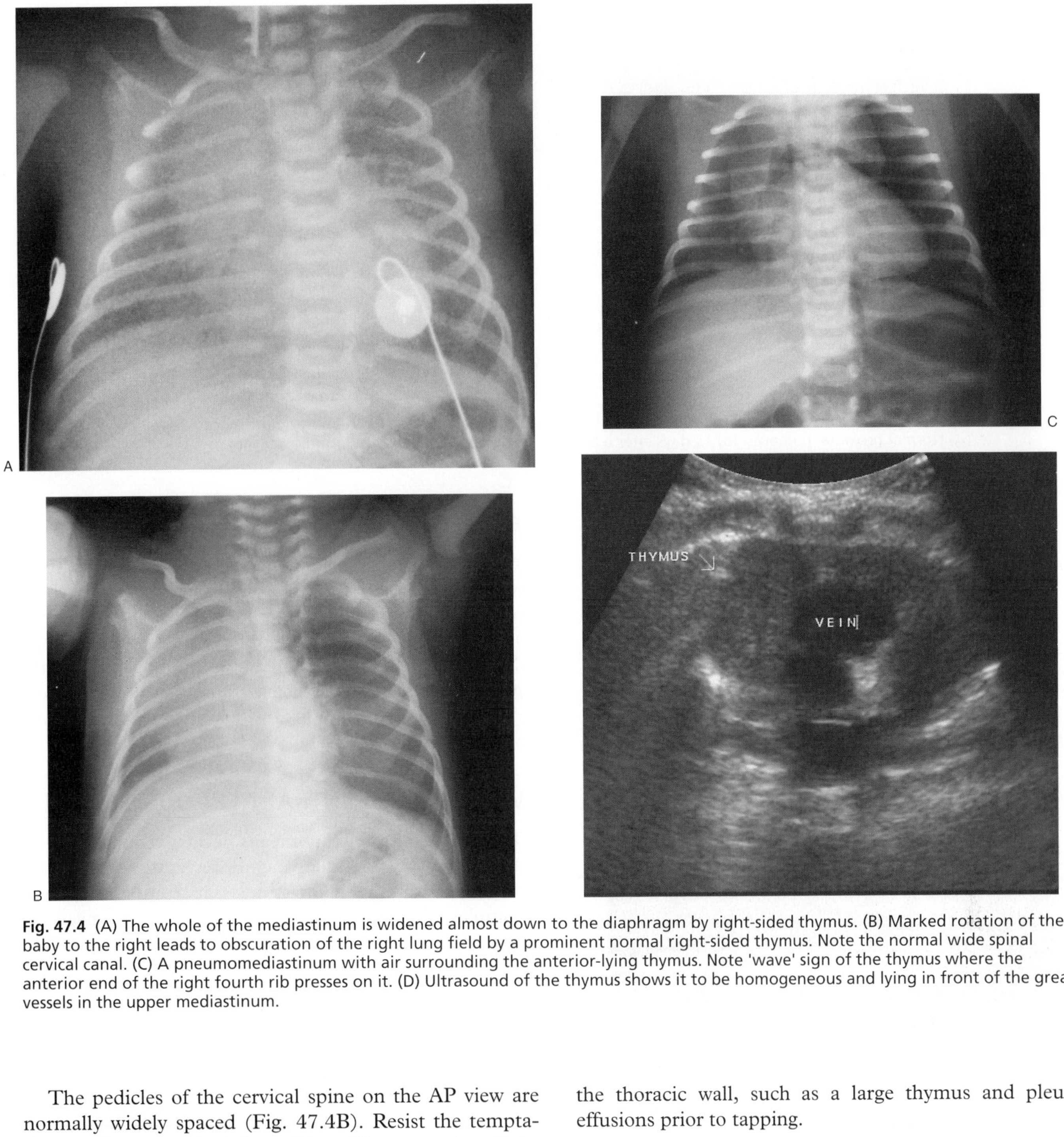

Fig. 47.4 (A) The whole of the mediastinum is widened almost down to the diaphragm by right-sided thymus. (B) Marked rotation of the baby to the right leads to obscuration of the right lung field by a prominent normal right-sided thymus. Note the normal wide spinal cervical canal. (C) A pneumomediastinum with air surrounding the anterior-lying thymus. Note 'wave' sign of the thymus where the anterior end of the right fourth rib presses on it. (D) Ultrasound of the thymus shows it to be homogeneous and lying in front of the great vessels in the upper mediastinum.

The pedicles of the cervical spine on the AP view are normally widely spaced (Fig. 47.4B). Resist the temptation to diagnose spinal dysraphism. The normal pedicles are symmetrical and have rounded medial surfaces. If still in doubt consult an atlas of roentgenographic measurement (see Further reading).

ULTRASOUND OF THE CHEST

Ultrasound of the chest is very useful antenatally for the diagnosis of cystic lesions of the lung and diaphragmatic hernia. After birth its use is limited by the aerated lungs, but it remains useful to diagnose structures in touch with the thoracic wall, such as a large thymus and pleural effusions prior to tapping.

ISOTOPES IN THE NEONATAL CHEST

A perfusion scan using ^{99}Tc-labelled albumin macroaggregates will give information on the relative blood flow to each lung in cases of suspected pulmonary hypoplasia.

CT OF THE NEONATAL CHEST

The relatively high radiation dose of CT and the problem of respiratory motion (much relieved in the newer, fast

A 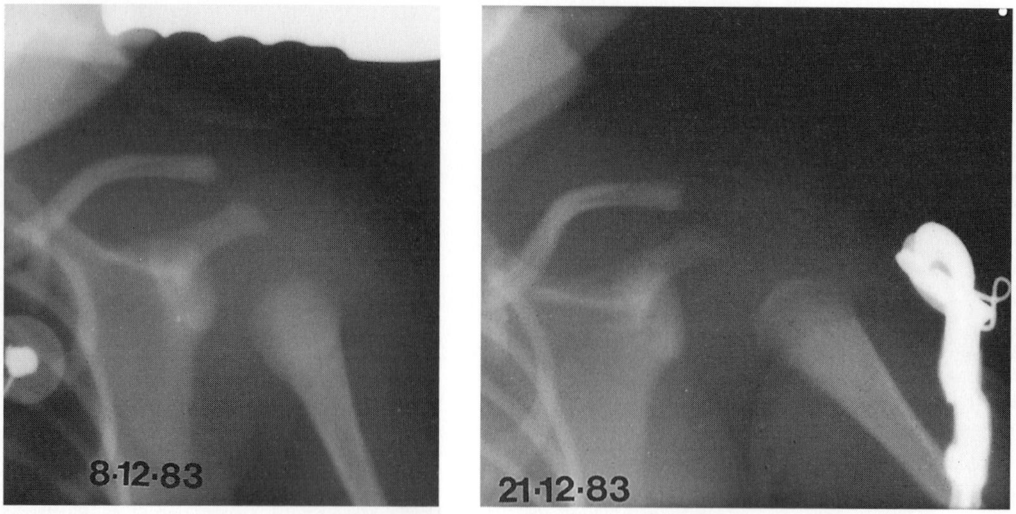

B

Fig. 47.5 Metabolic bone disease in a premature baby postoperatively following diaphragmatic hernia repair. (A) Normal proximal humerus. (B) 13 days later a lucency in the humeral metaphysis indicates metabolic bone disease secondary to low calcium stores.

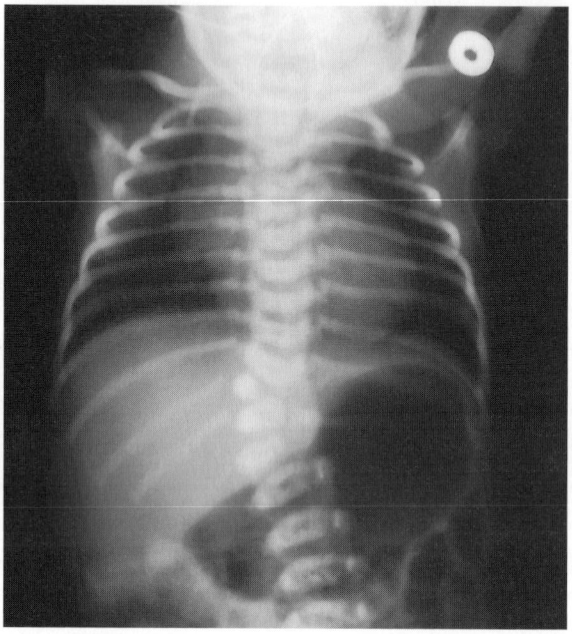

Fig. 47.6 VATER anomaly. Catheter coiled in air-distended proximal oesophageal pouch in a case of oesophageal atresia. The presence of a fistula is indicated by the air in the stomach. Note hemivertebrae in the lower dorsal region.

spiral CT machines) restrict CT use for the diagnosis of neonatal chest problems. It is very useful for the delineation of lung anatomy in cases of cystic lesions, such as cystic adenomatoid lungs or lobar emphysema, particularly if surgery is being contemplated.[3]

CT can also be useful to assess the presence and extent of lung damage in babies with respiratory difficulty but normal chest X-rays. It will identify localized areas of hyperaeration, and linear parenchymal and triangular subpleural shadows in patients with bronchopulmonary dysplasia and normal chest X-rays.[8]

TRACHEOBRONCHOGRAPHY

Bronchoscopy will elucidate most anatomical problems of the upper airway, but in complicated cases tracheobronchography using non-ionic water-soluble contrast with an osmolality similar to plasma (Iotralan 300, iohexol 240, iopamidol 200) can be useful to outline the upper airways. An anaesthetist should always be present to administer the anaesthetic, look after the airway and control respiration.

IMAGING THE CENTRAL NERVOUS SYSTEM

Ultrasound is the primary means of imaging and will give information on the following. Several atlases exist for those who wish to learn more (see Further reading). Examples of pathological appearances are given in Chapter 44, Part 5.

NORMAL ULTRASOUND APPEARANCES

Ultrasound is carried out in two planes, sagittal/parasagittal and coronal. The key to interpretation of the coronal ultrasound scan lies in remembering that the plane of section is at an angle because of the need to use the fontanelle as an acoustic window.

Figure 47.7A shows a labelled diagram of a standard coronal section, pictured in Figure 47.7B.

Figure 47.8A shows a parasagittal section labelled and corresponding to Figure 47.8B.

Ultrasound gives information on:

- the size and shape of the ventricular system;
- the presence of intra- and extracerebral haemorrhage and of extracerebral fluid collections;
- the appearance of the brain parenchyma and vasculature.

A

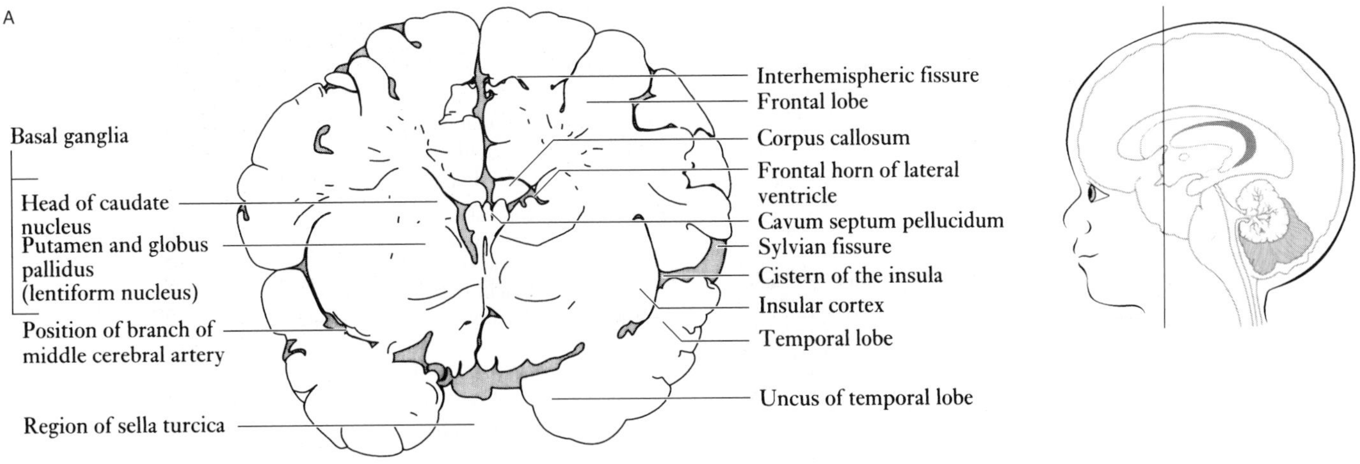

B

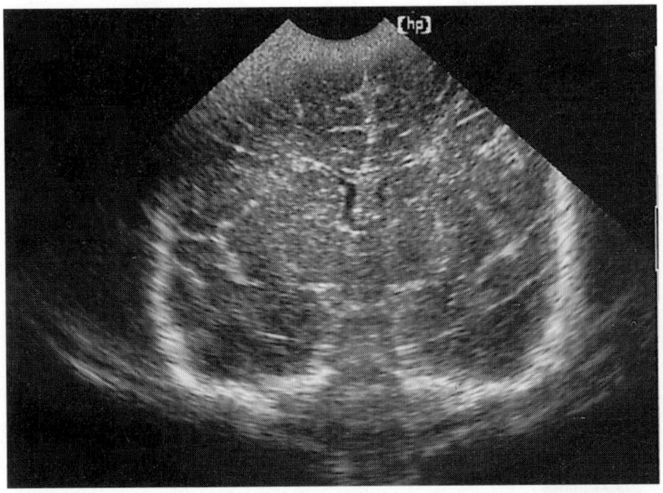

Fig. 47.7 (A) Labelled diagram of a standard coronal section of the neonatal head imaged with ultrasound, with the corresponding scan picture in (B). (Reproduced with permission from Rennie J M 1997 Neonatal cerebral ultrasound. Cambridge University Press)

CT OF THE NEONATAL BRAIN

Parenchymal changes such as calcification, oedema, haemorrhage, hydrocephalus, extracerebral fluid collections and extent of myelination can be assessed with CT. CT will indicate the presence of parenchymal change in the presence of a normal ultrasound.

MRI

MRI is the current gold standard to assess the brain parenchyma and extent of myelination, but is no good for calcification.

Calcification as in TORCH infections is best seen on plain films of the skull or CT.

GUIDELINES ON THE INVESTIGATION OF THE BRAIN

The order of investigation should be as above, except that the plain film of the skull should be taken before the MRI examination. Any collapse, seizure, sudden unexplained anaemia, change in neurological signs or symptoms should lead to ultrasound of the brain, looking for haemorrhage.

Many neonatal units screen all babies with routine ultrasound of the brain within 3 days of birth, and then at least once before discharge. The latter is done to try to identify those with PVL who may later present with neurological symptoms and signs (p. 1252). The central nervous system in the premature and term neonate is undergoing active myelination. Great caution is needed in drawing conclusions as to prognosis from the appearance of a single ultrasound, CT or MRI scan. Repeat examinations for further progress and assessment are advisable. The ultrasound diagnosis of GMH-IVH, PVL and changes associated with hypoxic–ischaemic encephalopathy are discussed in Chapter 44, Parts 4 and 5.

THE SPINE

Ultrasound of the spine can be used to image the spinal canal and spinal cord in cases of suspected dysraphism. The condition of the spinal arches, position of the conus,

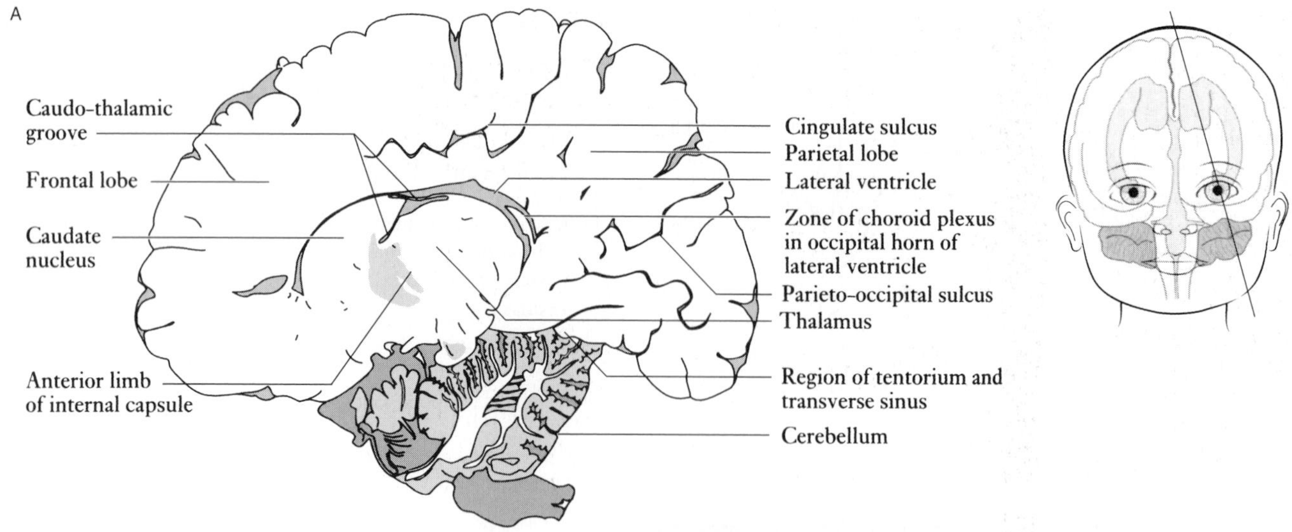

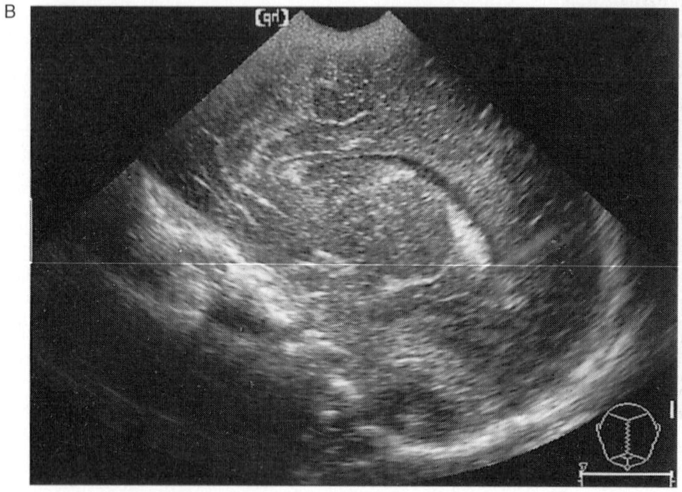

Fig. 47.8 Parasagittal section of the neonatal brain imaged with ultrasound. (A) Labelled diagram with the picture taken in the same plane in (B). (Reproduced with permission from Rennie J M 1997 Neonatal cerebral ultrasound. Cambridge University Press)

the presence of a split cord, tethered filum terminale or lipoma of the filum terminale can all be assessed (Fig. 47.9).

MRI is the definitive diagnostic technique for the delineation of the spine and its contents. Spinal dysraphism, tethered cord and lipoma of the cauda equina are clearly shown (p. 1304). CT will also show the lesions but needs intrathecal contrast to show the contents of the spinal canal, so is not recommended in babies.

IMAGING THE HEART

Ultrasound of the neonatal heart is discussed in Chapter 30.

IMAGING THE NEONATAL RENAL TRACT

Neonatal renal conditions are discussed in Chapter 39. They tend to be surgical and associated with abnormal anatomy.

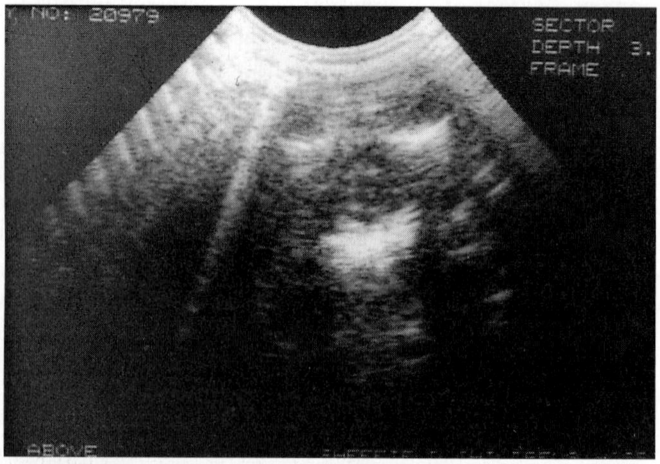

Fig. 47.9 Ultrasound of the neonatal spine, axial section. The laminae and the vertebral body are densely white. The white ring with a white centre between these structures is the spinal cord and its central canal.

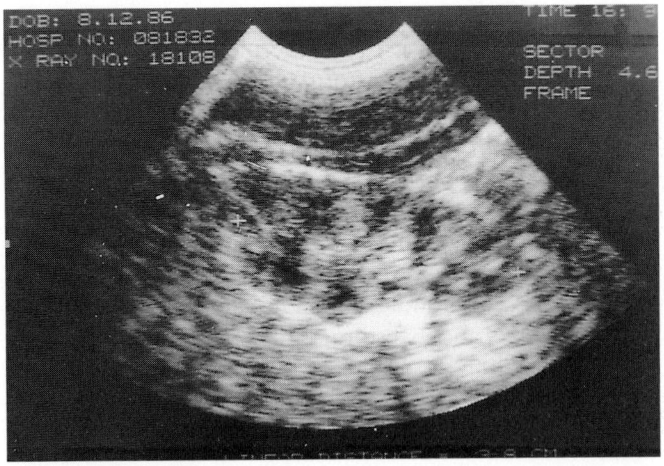

Fig. 47.10 Ultrasound of the normal neonatal kidney. The cortex of the neonatal kidney differs from the more mature child's by being hyperechogenic (white) compared to the liver. The renal medullae are hypoechogenic and should not be confused with dilated calyces.

PLAIN FILM

A plain film will give information on skeletal abnormalities such as spina bifida or calcification in the renal tract.

ULTRASOUND

This is best done with high-frequency ultrasound of 5 MHz or more. Both kidneys and the full bladder must be examined, the latter both inside (for ureterocoeles) and outside behind for dilated ureters.

The normal kidney at birth measures approximately 4 cm in length (1 mm per week of fetal life). The left kidney is usually a little longer than the right. Hyperechogenicity (increased brightness) of the neonatal renal cortex compared with the liver is normal (Fig. 47.10). In the older child the renal cortex is less echogenic (darker) than the liver and hyperechogenicity is abnormal. Hypoechogenic renal medullae are normal in the neonate. They are all the same size and arranged evenly around the collecting system (Fig. 47.10). They must not be mistaken for the hypoechogenicity of hydronephrosis or renal cysts.

Ureters visible behind the bladder (Fig. 47.11) are abnormal and indicate obstruction at the ureterovesical junction, idiopathic megaureter or reflux. The first two conditions may both be associated with ureterovesical reflux.

MICTURATING CYSTOURETHROGRAM

This is still the examination of choice for bladder function. MCUG evaluates the presence and extent of ureterovesical reflux, bladder contractility and status of the bladder outflow tract, e.g. by ruling out obstruction from urethral valves. The present recommendation is that

A

B

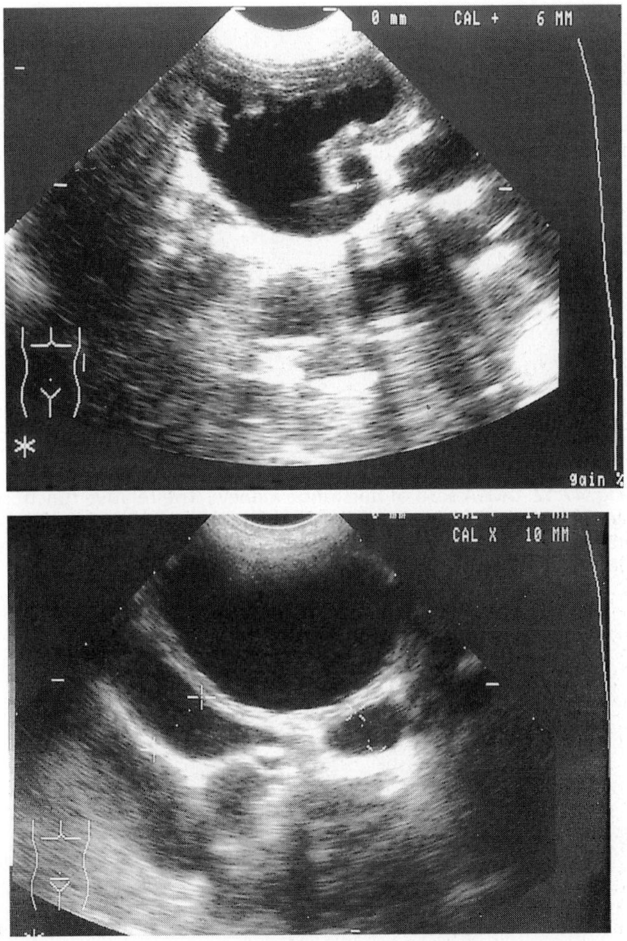

Fig. 47.11 Ultrasound of hydronephrosis and hydroureter. Fluid is black on ultrasound. (A) Not only the renal pelvis but also the calyces are dilated. This indicates significant hydronephrosis. (B) Both ureters are seen to be dilated behind the bladder. An MCUG demonstrated urethral valves.

it should be performed on any child under a year suffering from an urinary tract infection.[6] The patient is catheterized with a 6F feeding tube and the examination is carried out under screen control in the X-ray department. The drawbacks of the examination are the danger of introducing infection into the urinary tract, the considerable radiation dose to the gonads, and the unpleasantness. Some units recommend that all MCUG examinations should be performed under antibiotic cover. Certainly if an abnormality is found the patient should have a prophylactic course of antibiotics.

The clinician should not accept an MCUG on a male patient with a possible diagnosis of urethral valves, that does not have a voiding view of the whole length of the urethra in the oblique view.

ISOTOPE EXAMINATION

This is the only imaging modality that will give an assessment of total renal function and of the relative functions of each kidney. The usual isotope used is

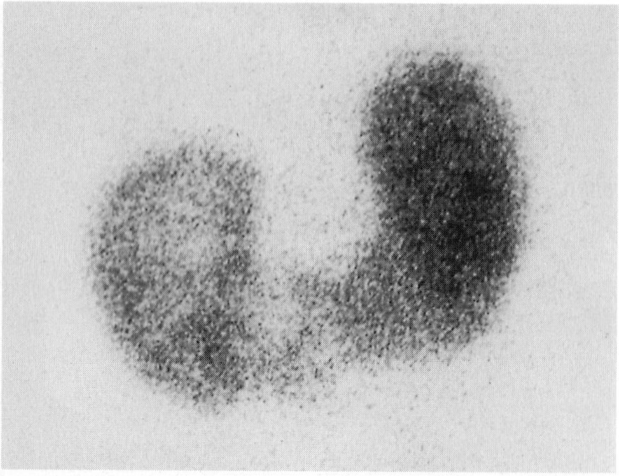

Fig. 47.12 DMSA scan of horseshoe kidneys. The relative functions of the two kidneys can be calculated from the relative uptake of the right portion of the isotope. In this patient the right portion of the kidney contributed 40% and the left 60% of function.

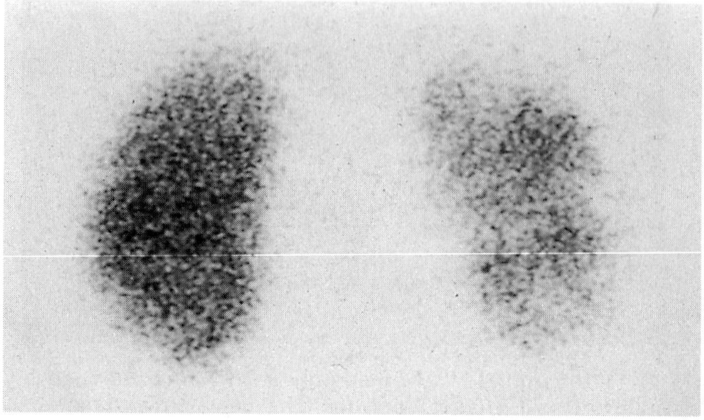

Fig. 47.13 DMSA scan of scarred kidneys secondary to urinary tract infection. Uptake in the right kidney is patchy and the renal outline is irregular, indicating scarring. These changes are much less marked on the left.

technetium 99m, with a half-life of 6 hours. This is chemically attached to substances that are processed in the kidneys, injected intravenously, and the accumulation and passage of the isotope through the kidney is monitored using a gamma camera.

The substances used are:

- DMSA (dimercaptosuccinic acid) (Figs 47.12, 47.13) This compound is taken up by the proximal tubules and is held in the kidneys in a direct relationship to the number of functional tubules. The test is therefore very useful to locate the kidneys if they cannot be found by ultrasound, and also to assess their relative functions. It is also widely used to assess renal scarring (Fig. 47.13). False results are obtained in the presence of a urinary tract infection. Serial DMSA scans are valuable to decide whether to preserve a damaged kidney. A persistent relative function of approximately 10% would indicate that the kidney is not worth preserving.
- DTPA (diethylene triamine penta-acetic acid) This material is filtered by the glomeruli and will therefore give an estimate of renal obstruction and its level. The test cannot be recommended for the neonate as glomerular filtration is so poor in the first month of life.
- MAG3 (mercapto acetyl triglycine) This material is gradually superseding DTPA in the diagnosis of obstruction. It is both filtered by the glomeruli and excreted by the tubules, has a much faster clearance than DTPA, and gives much clearer images with a lower radiation dose.

Conclusion

Isotopes in the neonate are useful to detect the presence and location of the kidneys and their relative functions using DMSA. Tests for renal obstruction using DTPA or MAG3 are less reliable owing to the immaturity of the kidneys, and should be delayed as long as possible to allow for growth and development.

IMAGING THE SKELETON

PLAIN RADIOGRAPHY

A skeletal survey of all the skeleton, including AP and lateral views of the skull and spine, should be obtained in cases of suspected skeletal dysplasia. Metabolic bone disease in the neonate is often discovered from the appearance of the proximal humeri on a chest X-ray (Fig. 47.5). It should be confirmed and followed up with wrist X-rays.

Septicaemia with osteomyelitis and pyarthrosis in this age group is best diagnosed with plain radiography. The first important signs are soft tissue swelling and dislocation (particularly of the hip or shoulder) (Fig. 47.14).

ULTRASOUND

Ultrasound supplements radiography in the diagnosis of osteomyelitis by detecting the presence of periosteal reaction before the periosteum can be seen on the radiograph, and also by detecting fluid in affected joints.

Ultrasound for developmental dysplasia of the hip (p. 279) is recommended in all patients with limited hip abduction, clicking hips and conditions predisposing to dislocation, such as breech delivery or a family history (Fig. 47.15).[5,10–13]

ISOTOPES

Isotope examination at this age for osteomyelitis is liable to give false negative results and is not recommended.[2] A positive result confirms the diagnosis but a negative result does not rule it out.

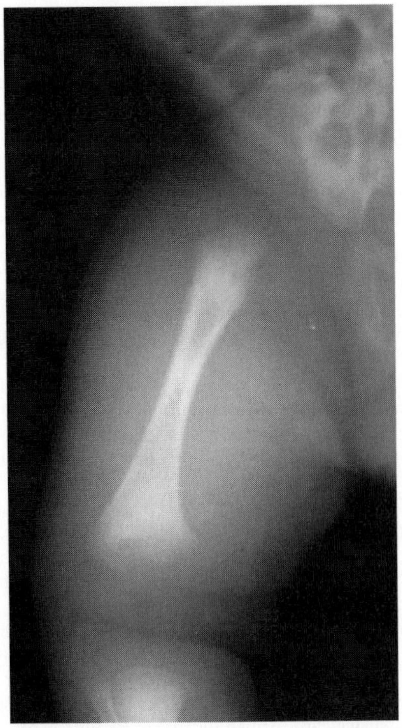

Fig. 47.14 Septic arthritis of the hip and osteomyelitis of the distal femur. An unwell baby off feeds and not moving the leg. The soft tissues of the thigh are swollen and the proximal femur is displaced outwards from the acetabulum by an effusion. The distal metaphysis of the femur is lucent and its outline has disappeared.

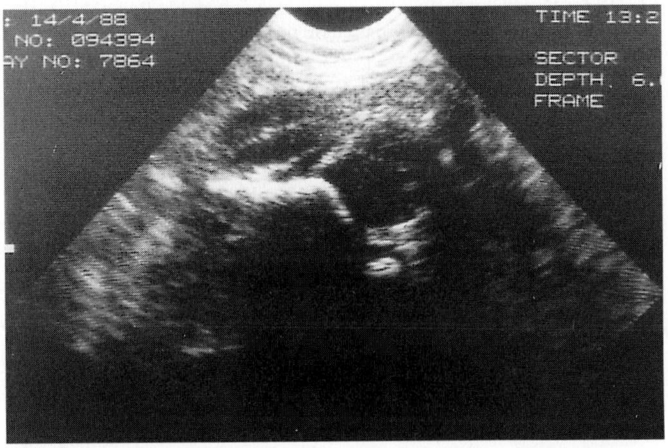

Fig. 47.15 Ultrasound of the normal hip: the round grey femoral head is held in the cup of the acetabulum. The black gap in the acetabular cup is the triradiate cartridge and makes a good landmark.

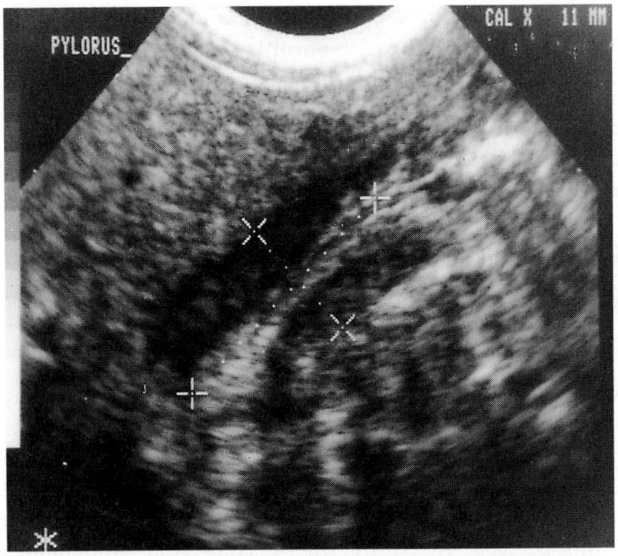

Fig. 47.16 Persistent vomiting – infantile hypertrophic pyloric stenosis. Ultrasound of the abdomen reveals the dark grey hypertrophied pyloric muscle between the markers. The white line is caused by echoes from the pyloric mucosa. The dark columns on either side of this are caused by the hypertrophied pyloric muscle.

EXAMINATION OF THE ABDOMEN

PLAIN RADIOGRAPHY

A plain supine film is the first investigation, and will give information on abdominal gas distribution inside and outside the bowel and indicate the presence of abdominal masses, free fluid, unusual calcification (meconium peritonitis) and congenital skeletal abnormalities.

Special care has to be taken on the supine film not to miss the presence of free peritoneal air. This is shown by delineation of the falciform ligament as a dense white line over the liver, seeing both sides of the intestinal walls and the presence of a grey 'bubble' in the mid-abdomen. The latter may spread to fill the whole abdomen, giving the 'rugby ball' sign. If there is still doubt a horizontal beam lateral decubitus film with the patient lying on the left side should be taken. Free air will then show as a black area between the liver and abdominal wall.

ULTRASOUND

Ultrasound of the abdomen is very convenient and atraumatic to the patient and very useful in the following situations:

- *Persistent vomiting*. Both hypertrophic pyloric stenosis (Fig. 47.16) and gastro-oesophageal reflux may be diagnosed, HPS by finding a thick pylorus with the following measurements: pyloric muscle thickness 3 mm or more, pyloric diameter 15 mm or more, pyloric channel length 17 mm or more; gastro-oesophageal reflux can be seen in real time by looking between the aorta and the heart.
- *The distended abdomen*. Ultrasound will reliably diagnose free and intestinal fluid and differentiate solid from cystic masses and decide which organ is involved. Peristalsis can be assessed.
- Neonatal abdominal masses (see Chapter 17) are mostly renal and benign. Hydronephrosis, hydroureter, multicystic kidney and polycystic kidney can be differentiated. Wilms' tumour is extremely rare in the neonate, and a solid mass involving the kidneys is

more likely to be a neuroblastoma or nephroblastomatosis. Neuroblastoma is retroperitoneal and will surround and displace the aorta.

In cases of rapid deterioration associated with an abdominal mass a diagnosis of suprarenal haemorrhage or renal vein thrombosis can be confirmed by ultrasound.

SPECIAL SITUATIONS

ANTENATAL DIAGNOSIS OF HYDRONEPHROSIS[7]

The ultrasound should be repeated within a few days of birth. If a hydronephrosis is present an MCUG may be necessary to exclude bladder neck obstruction and vesicoureteric reflux. If the ultrasound is normal it should be repeated after about a month to see whether the hydronephrosis has reappeared; an MCUG may be required (see p. 1040 for a suggested management protocol). A DMSA renogram will check on relative renal function and the presence of scarring. If hydronephrosis without hydroureter is found a DTPA renogram at 2–3 months will help in the diagnosis of obstructive hydronephrosis. If in the meanwhile renal function is deteriorating, the system should be drained either retrogradely or antegradely.

The great majority of antenatally diagnosed dilated kidneys become normal without treatment, and a further number are due to unobstructed but dilated collecting systems.

THE DISTENDED ABDOMEN, BILIOUS VOMITING, FAILURE TO PASS MECONIUM

A plain film of the abdomen and ultrasound will help to differentiate between meconium ileus, Hirschsprung's disease, meconium plug, atresia, malrotation and septicaemia, and to decide whether this is a surgical problem. Water-soluble contrast examination is often needed to make the diagnosis, and may be therapeutic in cases of meconium ileus. Because these examinations have their complications of patient collapse and bowel perforation they are best done in close cooperation with the surgical team.

COLLAPSE

Ultrasound imaging will detect intracranial bleeding, suprarenal haemorrhage and lesions in the heart. Chest X-ray is needed to exclude airleak and to assess the lungs and heart for infection and heart failure.

REFERENCES

1. Blayney M P, Logan D R 1994 First thoracic vertebral body as reference point for endotracheal tube placement. Archives of Disease in Childhood 71: F32–F35
2. Carty H 1993 Radionuclide bone scanning. Archives of Disease in Childhood 69: 160–165
3. Canals-Riazuelo J, Boix-Ochoa J, Peiro J L et al 1994 Adenomatous cystic pulmonary malformations: presentation of 26 cases. Cirurgia Pediatria 7: 992–996
4. Fletcher E W L, Baum J D, Draper D 1986 The risk of diagnostic radiation in the newborn. British Journal of Radiology 59: 165–170
5. Harcke H T 1994 Screening newborn infants for developmental dysplasia of the hip: the role of sonography. American Journal of Radiology 162: 395–397
6. Haycock G B 1986 Investigation of urinary tract infection in childhood. Archives of Disease in Childhood 61: 1155–1158
7. Owen R T J, Lamont A C, Brookes J 1996 Early management and postnatal investigation of prenatally diagnosed hydronephrosis. Clinical Radiology 51: 173–176
8. Oppenheim C, Mamou-Mani T, Sategh N, de Blic J, Scheinmann P, Lallemand D 1994 Bronchopulmonary dysplasia: value of CT in identifying sequelae. American Journal of Roentgenology 163: 169–172
9. Robinson A, Delagrammatica S H D 1983 Radiation doses to neonates requiring intensive care. British Journal of Radiology 56: 397–400
10. Zieger M, Hilpert S, Shultz R D 1986 Ultrasound of the infant hip Part 1: basic principles. Pediatric Radiology 16: 483–487
11. Zieger M 1986 Ultrasound of the infant hip Part 2: Validity of the method. Pediatric Radiology 16: 488–192
12. Zieger M, Shultz R D 1987 Ultrasound of the infant hip Part 3: Clinical application. Pediatric Radiology 17: 226–232
13. Zieger M, Hilpert S 1987 Ultrasound of the infant hip Part 4: Normal development in the newborn preterm neonate. Pediatric Radiology 17: 4770–473

FURTHER READING

Carty H, Shaw D, Brunelle F, Kendall B 1994 Imaging children. Churchill Livingstone, Edinburgh

Govaert P, de Vries L S 1997 An atlas of neonatal brain sonography. Clinics in Developmental Medicine No 141–142. Mackeith Press, London

Haller J O, Slovis T L 1995 Pediatric radiology, 2nd edn. Springer Verlag, Berlin

Lustead L B, Keats T E 1967 Atlas of roentgenographic measurements. Yearbook Medical Publishers, Chicago

Miller J H, Gelfand M J 1994 Pediatric nuclear imaging. W B Saunders, Philadelphia

Petterson H, Ringertz H 1991 Measurements in pediatric radiology. Springer Verlag, Berlin

Rennie J M 1997 Neonatal cranial ultrasound. Cambridge University Press, Cambridge

Richter E, Lierse W 1991 Imaging anatomy of the newborn. Translated by Alan Oestreich. Urban and Schwarzenberg, Baltimore

Siegel M J 1995 Pediatric sonography, 2nd edn. Raven Press, New York

Silverman F N, Kuhn J P 1993 Caffey's pediatric X-ray diagnosis, 9th edn. Mosby, St Louis

Section 7

Ethics and the law

48

Ethical problems in neonatal care

A. G. M. Campbell

INTRODUCTION

Medical ethics has been defined as 'the obligations of a moral nature which govern the practice of medicine'. Doctors are expected to adhere to these obligations in maintaining high standards of practice and, through the corporate ethics of their profession, maintain the trust of patients, colleagues and the public. Traditionally, doctors were guided by codes like the Oath of Hippocrates but increasingly recognize the difficulties of maintaining absolute adherence to an ancient code when grappling with the moral dilemmas created by medical practice in contemporary society. New knowledge and technology have given them powers beyond anything imagined by their medical ancestors but one basic principle of medical ethics has not changed – the doctor's first consideration must be the best interests of the patient.

LIFE, DEATH AND INTENSIVE CARE

WITHHOLDING OR WITHDRAWING LIFE-SUSTAINING TREATMENT

Doctors have a commitment to respect life. Nowhere is this commitment more evident than at birth and in the early weeks of postnatal life. The many healthy children who have benefited from modern neonatal care bear witness to increasing success in not only preserving life, but in preventing disability. Intensive care thrives on such success. Parents are grateful; doctors and nurses feel amply rewarded; the media are eager to publicize 'miracle babies' and great credit is reflected on all concerned. Sadly, however, there is a darker side to this picture. The tinier and tinier infants who survive increasingly premature birth remain vulnerable to disabling complications and for others, afflicted with a variety of problems, intensive care, while life-saving, does nothing to change the grim outlook for infant and family. The difficult questions keep recurring, e.g. should the full panoply of intensive care be used routinely and indiscriminately in neonatal rescue, or should it be used selectively? when is it ethical (and legal) to withhold or withdraw life-saving treatment? who should be involved in these fundamental decisions, and who should bear the ultimate responsibility? what criteria should be used? how can we be sure that an infant's interests are protected?

WHICH INFANTS?

The tiny premature infant

The majority of infants who survive premature birth do remarkably well, but a review of outcomes for the smallest survivors concludes with the following statement: 'We believe that with currently available methods of medical care and technology the limits of viability have been reached'.[12] 'Viability' as early as 23 and 24 weeks' gestation is now commonplace but published reports on the survivors, though as yet insufficient to provide reliable estimates of risk, do indicate that the rate of severe disability increases significantly with decreasing gestational age.[14]

The malformed or damaged infant

After the appropriate investigations, it may be clear that an infant's brain is abnormal or severely damaged. When this information is shared with the parents they will be desperately concerned about the implications for their infant's future health. Most parents are remarkably resourceful when faced with tragedy and will accept even severe physical disabilities as they recognize that with loving family support their child can lead a relatively normal, happy and productive life. However, they greatly fear the consequences of brain damage that will diminish or remove their child's capacity to form relationships with others, to be educated, and to gain at least some measure of independence – what Rachels has called 'having a life' instead of merely 'being alive'.[17] It is for that reason that the type and severity of abnormality or damage to the brain is perhaps the most important factor in influencing neonatologists to question the wisdom of continuing life-support. Specific examples include infants with hydranencephaly and other gross brain defects; chromosomal disorders such as trisomies 13 or 18; and infants whose brains have been badly affected by infection, haemorrhage or asphyxia, the extent of the damage being apparent not only clinically but confirmed by modern techniques of imaging. Infants that pose particularly poignant treatment dilemmas include those rare cases where the brain may be intact but multiple abnormalities or irreparable damage affecting other organs or systems will seriously affect the infant's future quality of life.

WHO SHOULD DECIDE?

Traditionally, doctors with or without the knowledge or agreement of the parents have assumed this burden. In recent years such paternalism has become unacceptable and the more knowledgeable and articulate parents have insisted on taking at least part of this responsibility on themselves. In almost all circumstances, parents make appropriate decisions when given the facts and the treatment options accurately, sensitively and objectively; and if given time for reflection and perhaps consultation with other family members, their family doctor and others as they wish. However, while doctors and parents can act as partners in such decision-making, it is my view that any decision to withhold or withdraw life-sustaining care should remain primarily a medical decision for which the doctor in charge should bear ultimate responsibility. Good practice requires that the doctor takes careful note, not only of the views of the family but those of the nurses, junior doctors and other key members of the team providing intensive care.[7]

THE PROCESS OF DECISION-MAKING

It has been said that 'good ethics starts with good facts'. The primarily responsible doctor must ensure that all necessary steps have been taken to establish the diagnosis and prognosis as accurately as possible. Only then is it possible fully to consider the various treatment options and how their likely outcomes might affect the child's future. The doctor also has an important leadership role in ensuring that good communication exists with the parents and other members of the intensive care team so that clinical decisions affecting the care of the infant are properly shared. Opportunities must be provided for exchange of questions and views, particularly when individuals disagree or are uncomfortable with the ethics or legality of the actions proposed. Parents and staff have the awesome task of acting as responsible proxy decision-makers for a patient who lacks this capacity, and for whom no 'substituted judgement' can be given. From the perspective of one in the patient's predicament, there must be a carefully considered attempt to assess the benefits and burdens of starting or continuing intensive treatment, a process that, while time-consuming and emotionally demanding, may provide some reassurance to the parents and the staff that the decision taken was correct.

Lawyers make much of 'due process' and have been critical of doctors' apparent unwillingness to lay down criteria that could be approved by the courts. Some neonatologists have offered general guidelines for debate, increasingly aided by the improving documentation of the results of neonatal intensive care, but it is difficult to see how more detailed criteria could be written down without their being either excessively restrictive or so vague as to be of little use. From what has been published, it seems that the practice in neonatal units is reasonably consistent with the developing 'case law' that gives some indication of how the courts might respond to the facts of an individual case[6,7] (see Chapter 49).

PROTECTIONS

Most parents have their child's best interests at heart and doctors can usually be trusted to make decisions responsibly.

> As each infant in each family is unique and the circumstances of each case so complex only general guidelines can be provided and much latitude in decision making should be expected and tolerated. As most such decisions now involve many people in relatively public places like hospitals, abuses should be easy to detect.[9]

However, very occasionally, ignorance, prejudice, grief, eccentricity, self-interest and other considerations will intrude. An infant's interests may be violated in a number of ways: on the one hand, a child may be allowed to die simply from ignorance, or on the other, may die a death unnecessarily prolonged through insistence on burdensome and futile treatment. Decisions involving intensive care are often made and implemented in an atmosphere of crisis and are fraught with conflicting emotions. There may be disagreements among members of the intensive care team. The grieving parents may be in such a state of shock that their understanding of the medical information is greatly impaired. It is reasonable to ask if other protections should exist to protect a child from abuse by 'medical neglect' on the one hand or abuse by overtreatment on the other.

Open decision-making

A considerable degree of protection is afforded by ensuring that decisions are reached openly and are the result of multidisciplinary participation. It is important too, that the process of decision-making and the actions taken are accurately recorded in a manner suitable for objective review. Full documentation also does much to justify trust, a key component in medical decision-making.

Clinical ethics committees

In complex cases, discussions are frequently held with medical specialists and non-medical advisers, but in the UK, to date, it has generally not been thought necessary to formalize this process by establishing clinical ethics committees, distinct from the research ethics committees that already exist. Some large hospitals have established or are considering setting up such committees, not only to deal with the problems of the newborn but to be available for advice to the staff on the complex problems that arise in the care of patients at any age. In the US, special infant care review committees were formed following the 'Baby Doe' episode of 1982, an apparent and widely publicized abuse of the discretion allowed doctors and parents in decision-making about severely impaired infants. These committees provide a broader forum for discussion and can be helpful to members of staff and families wrestling with complicated ethical issues.[11] At the same time they provide assurance that the infant's interests are being protected and that the decisions taken are soundly based in ethics and in law. Where these committees have worked well they have been careful to remain strictly advisory with the responsibility for medical decisions being left to the medical staff.[8]

Legislation

US federal intervention followed 'Baby Doe'.[1] No evidence was produced to show that the problem was widespread but this episode became the catalyst for legislation that made failure to provide 'medically indicated' treatment a form of 'medical neglect'. The 'Baby Doe Rules' as they came to be known, and the accompanying investigative probing into reported abuses, caused considerable turmoil in neonatal nurseries and much distress to parents and staff.[15,20] As 'rules' imply rigidity, it was no surprise to find that defensive over-interpretation of the regulations converted rare abuse by undertreatment to the much more frequent abuse by overtreatment. Neonatologists, fearing legal harassment, were under considerable pressure to consider their own interests and that of their hospital. Much has been written about the impact of Baby Doe on paediatricians, parents and on the infants themselves – sufficient to convince me that legislation is not the answer to resolving these dilemmas.[6,8]

> Aggressive posturing by the United States government through a complex regulatory scheme designed to assure protection of handicapped newborns has in fact wreaked havoc on the whole decision-making process and assaulted the integrity and privacy of the family decisional unit.[21]

The Law Courts

Apparently unresolvable disagreements will occasionally arise in particularly controversial cases where individual differences in moral reasoning make decisions to continue or withdraw intensive care and allow an infant to die acceptable or unacceptable. The courts are available to resolve these serious conflicts. There must be limits to parental demands for futile treatment and limits to parental refusal of consent for medically indicated treatment. Doctors cannot passively acquiesce to all parental demands for treatment *or* non-treatment, but must recognize that families have their own values, religious beliefs, priorities and resources that will influence their choices. Families have to live with the consequences of these decisions and doctors must be careful not to impose unwelcome choices on parents through a sense of moral superiority. At times, however, they may have to guide parents towards a decision that is not only acceptable medically, ethically and socially but is within the law (Chapter 49).

'QUALITY OF LIFE'

To neonatologists an assessment of an infant's quality of life is an important consideration in these life and death decisions.[5] This criterion has been severely criticized in the US as viciously discriminatory against the handicapped and equivalent to the social judgements that involve morally irrelevant criteria like race and colour.[24] However, quality of life judgements are important components of the detailed medical and ethical analysis that must precede any decision to withhold or withdraw treatment. It is simply unrealistic to pretend otherwise. It should be emphasized that assessing quality of life in these circumstances does *not* imply making judgements about an infant's 'social worth' to the community, or that consideration is given to the financial costs of long-term care to the family, hospital or state. To a neonatologist, considering the likely quality of life means being compassionately concerned about the infant's capacity for future health, development and well-being; and about the crushing human costs to the child and family that will accrue with survival.

WITHHOLDING AND WITHDRAWING TREATMENT: IS THERE A DIFFERENCE?

Differences in approach to intensive treatment have been described by Rhoden.[18] In the USA, aggressive life-saving treatment is used in almost all situations and there is a greater reluctance to withdraw it – the 'treat until certainty' approach. In Sweden, doctors seem willing to withhold treatment, but are uncomfortable about withdrawing treatment once started. In the UK, treatment may be started from birth even in the tiniest of infants, but doctors are more willing to stop if subsequent investigation indicates extensive brain damage. This 'individualized prognostic strategy' seems the responsible and logical approach as it gives each infant a 'trial of life' yet indicates concern for the future. Some see an ethical distinction between withholding and withdrawing and argue that withdrawing treatment is not only emotionally more difficult but less defensible ethically. To others this seems a moral quibble. If treatment is unlikely to benefit a patient, not starting it or stopping it are of equal moral weight. Likewise, if treatment could be beneficial it is equally wrong to withhold or withdraw it. Furthermore, if there is any difference, withdrawing is surely preferable to withholding. Starting treatment allows time for reflection, for further information and investigation, and time to assess the initial response. This approach also minimizes the uncertainty always present about the 'rightness' or 'wrongness' of a decision. Philosophical confusion between withholding and withdrawing can influence decision-making in another potentially dangerous way. If it is thought more difficult ethically, emotionally or legally to withdraw treatment, there may be the temptation to withhold treatment simply out of concern that, once started, it will be impossible to stop. Doctors should therefore consider withholding or withdrawing treatment in these situations as ethically identical.

RESUSCITATION

It follows from the above that if resuscitation could be beneficial it should be started immediately. If death is inevitable or if, with the parents, it has been decided in advance that aggressive treatment is inappropriate, resuscitation should be withheld.

Resuscitation in the delivery room

Doctors have the technical skills to resuscitate almost any infant, even some apparently stillborn (Apgar 0), but the ethical and legal considerations may be more troubling. The commonest emergency faced by doctors attending a birth is the severely asphyxiated infant. Complete information may not be available, and a rapid clinical assessment before deciding on resuscitation will not provide an accurate picture of the infant's future prospects. It is also unusual for the consultant, the ultimately responsible doctor, to be present in the delivery room. Thus, the duty of junior doctors is clear. *All* infants, of whatever birthweight, gestational age or apparent abnormality who show signs of life, must be resuscitated until a more considered judgement can be made on the advisability of persisting with intensive life-support. The pattern of recovery and the presence or absence of complications, especially early signs of neurological dysfunction, will provide a more accurate estimation of severity and prognosis.

Resuscitation in the nursery

For the vast majority of infants, the nursing and medical response to deterioration and cardiorespiratory collapse is immediate resuscitation. If it has been decided that further treatment is futile, this should have been discussed with the parents and the decision shared with the key members of the intensive care team. A reasoned argument for the decision and instructions about the appropriate action should be entered in the infant's record. In the absence of such instructions, the nurses and junior doctors should proceed with standard resuscitation until the position is clarified. They are most closely involved with an infant's minute-to-minute care. By their frequent contacts with parents at the cotside they may be in a better position to understand the true feelings and wishes of distressed parents that may not have been expressed during more formal discussions. However, decisions to withhold or withdraw life-support should not be taken by junior staff on their own. This is a consultant responsibility. Failure to provide leadership and clear guidance to staff on this important issue will create confusion, conflict and loss of morale.

'NURSING CARE ONLY'

Withholding or withdrawing intensive life-support does not mean stopping *care*. Every effort must be made to relieve distress by using oxygen, sedatives or analgesics where appropriate. Some hold the view that denying 'extraordinary' treatments like intermittent positive-pressure ventilation may be acceptable in certain situations but that 'ordinary' treatments like antibiotics, i.v. fluids, tube feeding, etc. must always be maintained. This ordinary/extraordinary distinction is largely irrelevant in modern medical practice. Treatment that was considered 'extraordinary' decades ago is very 'ordinary' today and what might be considered 'ordinary' in some circumstances is 'extraordinary' in others. It is much more important to consider if the treatment proposed will be of real benefit to the patient.

> The distinction between ordinary means and extraordinary means has a dangerously deceptive appearance of simplicity. It appears to be a distinction made by assessing means of treatment, whereas in fact criteria for the decision relate primarily to the patient not to the remedy.[22]

Every infant should receive warmth, loving human contact, oral feeds as tolerated and be assured of freedom from distress or pain. Dying infants must not be 'abandoned' to a corner of the nursery and denied the standard routines of good nursing such as bathing, changing, the opportunity to suck and 'cherishing'. There should be increased commitment to family members with opportunity for them to maintain contact and participation until death.[10] Dying may be prolonged but its manner can provide some comfort to bereaved parents. Given the choice, and the appropriate emotional and practical support, some parents will wish to have their baby at home. Supportive counselling may be needed for some time and it is part of the wider responsibilities of the hospital team, perhaps in conjunction with the general practitioner, to facilitate access to such services.

TELLING THE TRUTH

There are times when the blunt truth, no matter how sensitively explained, may have an adverse effect on a patient. Doctors in adult practice will sometimes defend a decision to tell the patient only what the doctor thinks is appropriate. As emphasis on patient autonomy has replaced old-fashioned paternalism, truth-telling is not just a matter for ethical debate but may have medicolegal implications. When the patient is a child, the need for honesty and complete openness with parents is more compelling, particularly in obtaining consent.[2] Parents should be kept informed of the exact clinical situation and the likely outcome as far as it is known. An understandable wish to shield either parent from the facts, even at one or other's request, is usually a serious mistake and may undermine confidence and trust. Conveying bad news is a difficult task even for doctors with years of experience. People differ in their ability to communicate with humility, clarity, sensitivity and compassion, and there are wide variations in parents' understanding of complex medical information. Doctors should try to develop 'long antennae' that will be sensitive to misunderstandings and unspoken fears.

The neonatal intensive care unit has become a fruitful field for accusations of medical negligence (Chapter 50). Telling the truth about medical accidents is an exacting test of medical integrity, but in some circumstances may defuse the situation sufficiently to prevent legal action. Litigation may originate simply because parents and families cannot find out what happened in any other way. Parental suspicions will be increased if questions are met defensively or if the staff seem brusque and unsympathetic. Doctors, particularly when exhausted or under stress, must be cautious about allocating blame or writing intemperate comments about what happened. Legal action may be precipitated by statements about culpability that prove to be unjustified on an objective and dispassionate review of the facts.[4]

RESEARCH IN THE NURSERY

The importance of good research to neonatal practice should not need emphasis here, but the history of neonatal care is blemished by useless or harmful treatments adopted without adequate evaluation. Nevertheless, medical researchers are still criticized by lobbyists who argue for stricter controls or even prohibition of research involving children.

To date, no doctor has been charged with an offence because an infant or child was used as a research subject without consent, but doubts remain as to the validity of consent, particularly for non-therapeutic research. The British Paediatric Association has consistently stated that 'research that is not intended directly to benefit the child subject is not necessarily either unethical or illegal',[3] a view supported by the Medical Research Council.[16] It is generally agreed that children can be included in such research provided that 'participation places a child at no more than negligible risk of harm' and that the 'usual safeguards' are in place, i.e. parental consent and the approval of a research ethics committee.

Neonatologists have a particular problem when they wish to enter newly born infants into clinical trials of innovative treatment as consent may be difficult to obtain in advance, e.g. from a mother in labour. Some argue that to obtain properly informed consent at this emotional and stressful time might cause distress and undermine parents' confidence that their infant will get the best treatment available. The 'gold standard' of clinical research, the randomized controlled trial, makes the issue of informed consent even more difficult. It is disconcerting for parents to be told that their child is to be randomized to one or other treatment because of uncertainty about which is most effective, but it is essential that such trials take place, or poorly controlled research will continue to pose risks for infants.

A Standing Joint Committee of the British Paediatric Association and the Royal College of Obstetricians and Gynaecologists has prepared a checklist of questions that should be asked when proposing to do research during pregnancy and following birth.[23] The committee points out the double standard that exists whereby treatment provided as part of properly conducted research is subject to external scrutiny, whereas treatment introduced as a result of someone's 'bright idea' is not subject to the same constraints. In the summary checklist it is interesting to note that 'consent' is rarely mentioned. One question asks what arrangements are in place to 'seek the co-operation' of those involved and emphasizes the importance of providing information at the optimum time and in the best form to encourage full understanding. One question asks 'How will potential participants indicate their consent to participate in the study', but there is nothing to indicate that consent is required. Perhaps the committee felt that was stating the obvious!

If an infant's eligibility for a clinical trial cannot be predicted in advance, some compromise between a formal process of obtaining consent (and worrying every mother) and obtaining formal consent only retrospectively is desirable. Retrospective consent is unsatisfactory for several reasons. First, it sets a dubious precedent open to exploitation in other circumstances. Second, it raises suspicions that the doctors have been conducting secret 'experiments' on the baby, thus undermining trust.

Third, the parents may be more likely to blame the new treatment if the baby does badly, than they are to credit it with the infant's recovery. Fourth, mothers talk among themselves and some will wonder if their infants are involved without their knowledge. Could this new treatment be the cause of their infant's problems, or if this might be a better treatment, why is their infant not getting it? Either way, extra pressure to exclude or include infants may affect the bias of the trial and its validity.

The London Royal College of Physicians has identified circumstances where research may be conducted ethically without consent provided that there has been ethics committee approval.[19] Perhaps it is time to consider if properly authorized neonatal research that must be started at or shortly after birth should similarly be placed in a special category. Assurance would have to be provided that protocols were thoroughly scrutinized by a committee appropriately constituted to give guidance and approval for such specialized research.

PRIORITIES AND THE ALLOCATION OF RESOURCES

Neonatal intensive care cannot escape rigorous cost–benefit analysis but the economic costs should not be the only consideration. Inter alia, the parents' beliefs and wishes have to be given due weight within the context of what can be justified with limited resources. Saving infant life and minimizing long-term morbidity cannot easily be weighed against short-term financial costs when the long-term consequences of success or failure, both human *and* financial, are so considerable. Guidelines for neonatal care will continue to change, but comprehensive data are essential so that the results of such endeavours can be properly analysed and compared.[13] In the future, increasingly hard choices will be necessary, but these must be based on good evidence.

REFERENCES

1. Annas G J 1984 The Baby Doe regulations: governmental intervention in neonatal rescue medicine. American Journal of Public Health 74: 618–620
2. Brahams D 1986 Explanation and disclosure of risks in the treatment of children. Lancet i: 925–926
3. British Paediatric Association 1992 Guidelines for the ethical conduct of medical research involving children. BPA, London
4. Campbell A G M 1994 The paediatrician and medical negligence. In: Powers M J, Harris N H (eds) Medical negligence, 2nd edn. Butterworths, London, pp 688–743
5. Campbell A G M 1995 Quality of life as a decision-making criterion. In: Goldworth A, Silverman W, Stevenson D K, Young E W D (eds) Ethics and perinatology. Oxford University Press, Oxford, pp 82–103
6. Campbell A G M 1995 Government regulations in the United Kingdom. In: Goldworth A, Silverman W, Stevenson D K, Young E W D (eds) Ethics and perinatology. Oxford University Press, Oxford, pp 307–325
7. Campbell A G M, McHaffie H E 1995 Prolonging life and allowing death: infants. Journal of Medical Ethics 21: 339–344
8. Caplan A L, Blank R H, Merrick J C 1992 Compelled compassion: government intervention in the treatment of critically ill newborns. Humana Press, Totowa, New Jersey
9. Duff R S, Campbell A G M 1973 Moral and ethical dilemmas in the special care nursery. New England Journal of Medicine 289: 890–894
10. Duff R S, Campbell A G M 1976 On deciding the care of severely handicapped or dying persons: with particular reference to infants. Pediatrics 57: 487–493
11. Fleischman A R 1986 An infant bioethical review committee in an urban medical center. Hastings Center Report 16: 16–18
12. Hack M, Fanaroff A A 1988 Current controversies in perinatal care: how small is too small? Considerations in evaluating the outcome of the tiny infant. Clinics in Perinatology 15: 773–788
13. Ham C 1995 Health care rationing: the British approach seems likely to be based on guidelines. British Medical Journal 310: 1483–1484
14. Johnson A 1995 Disability and perinatal care. Pediatrics 95: 272–273
15. Kopelman L M, Irons T G, Kopelman A E 1988 Neonatologists judge the 'Baby Doe' regulations. New England Journal of Medicine 318: 677–683
16. Medical Research Council 1991 The ethical conduct of research on children. MRC, London
17. Rachels J 1986 The end of life: euthanasia and morality. Oxford University Press, Oxford
18. Rhoden N K 1986 Treating Baby Doe: the ethics of uncertainty. Hastings Center Report 16: 34–42
19. Royal College of Physicians 1990 Report on research involving patients. Royal College of Physicians, London
20. Shapiro D L, Rosenberg P 1984 The effect of federal regulations regarding handicapped newborns: a case report. Journal of the American Medical Association 252: 2031–2033
21. Smith G P 1985 Defective newborns and government intermeddling. Medicine, Science and Law 25: 44–48
22. Sparks R C 1988 To treat or not to treat: bioethics and the handicapped newborn. Paulist Press, Mahwah, New Jersey
23. Standing Joint Committee 1991 A checklist of questions to ask when evaluating proposed research during pregnancy and following birth. Standing Joint Committee of the British Paediatric Association and the Royal College of Obstetricians and Gynaecologists, London
24. US Commission on Civil Rights 1989 Medical discrimination against children with disabilities. Government Printing Office, Washington, DC

49

Neonatology and the law

M. A. M. S. Leigh

INTRODUCTION

Neonatology is tiger-country, as much for the lawyer, the representative of broader society, as it is for the doctor. It is worth rehearsing some of the reasons for this, before considering specific aspects of the relationship between the doctor and the law.

First, the stakes are very high. The neonatal child has the whole of her extrauterine existence ahead of her. Throughout this time, she will have to live with the consequences of decisions made on her behalf by others. If she is unable to care for herself, or earn her own living, these will be very expensive.

Second, small babies are difficult. Unable to describe their history or symptomatology, they demand to be assessed solely on their signs. Even slightly older siblings are able to present a history through the frequently reliable prism of maternal concern. The neonate brings virtually nothing to the consultation and, as the baby is small, the signs may be correspondingly subtle.

Third, small babies also seem to change much faster than older patients. The child who appeared to be almost ripe for discharge from the Special Care Baby Unit on the morning ward round may be in extremis by teatime. Small though the babies may be, they readily become the focus of a disproportionate emotional intensity. Their utter helplessness and dependence on other members of society commands an immediate response. The failure of the medical team in its duty towards such a child is felt as a failure of society as a whole, because the obligation to care is apprehended as one which we all share.

Yet, in so far as we understand the limits of what doctors can achieve for these small babies, society demands that the medical profession does not strive for that which is impossible. The law recognizes that the dying person of any age is entitled to be treated with an appropriate dignity and decency. It is a breach of duty to intubate or repeatedly to puncture the veins and arteries of very low-birthweight children, where they are plainly too small to have a chance of surviving in the light of present resources and techniques.

However, so long as these tiny people survive, they are entitled to all the rights shared by any other members of society. The cost of their intensive care will astonish hospital managers as much as it will other members of the laity, and neonatologists recognize that they owe some sort of duty, though it may not often be enforceable in law, to fight for the interests of patients they have yet to meet, so as to insist on facilities and resources being available when they are needed.

Effect of delay

There is a time lag between events and litigation, as a result of which paediatricians seem destined to be surprised by the standards which they have to meet. Most consultants were trained in an era when society did not ask to be told, or seek to understand very much about what neonatologists were doing. Society as a whole was more trusting of doctors and less clearly aware of their activities. Neonatologists and parents were free to decide profound issues without the intrusion of the law or other members of society; and in this decision-making alliance, parents were more inclined to accept the role of the junior partner than they are today. When things go wrong, doctors frequently find themselves being judged much more sharply and intolerantly than they expected.

The standards by which doctors judge each other are also rising. Even though resources are becoming more restricted and the limits of what can be achieved change more slowly than medical publications sometimes suggest to the general public, the standards which doctors demand from each other change from year to year. Over a decade the transformation can be radical; over the career of a consultant it is revolutionary. The changes are obvious to a lawyer in the clinical records, which constitute the face of the caring relationship which the hospital presents to the Court. If the Court were to go into a special care baby unit in 1967 or 1997, the sight might seem essentially familiar. The judge would see, in either case, a doctor in a white coat struggling over an astonishingly undersized baby. There might be a few more tubes and monitors to obscure the picture in the later scene, but it would not appear fundamentally different. If the doctor paused to explain her problems, she would often explain fundamentally similar problems in similar terms.

However, that never happens. What the Court does is to read the clinical notes and listen to those of their authors who can be found. The notes of 30 years ago appear vestigial, documenting only gross and obvious changes in the child's condition, and a handful of clinical signs. They are frequently laid out in a way which appears less formal and so looks less organized. The investigations appear to be sporadic and haphazard. The witnesses are worse: they can rarely remember anything of the facts of the case before the Court, even though they may be debating the few days or hours in which it seems the plaintiff met with the catastrophe which has blighted her existence. Indeed, under the rigours of cross-examination, it frequently seems that the paediatrician is hard pressed to remember the routine practice or treatment policy of 1967 and to describe in coherent terms how it differed from that which was followed in 1960 or 1975.

Doctors are protected against being judged unfairly by the standards set by their successors. The law holds that doctors are to be judged by the state of their art at the time of treatment. They will not be negligent if they fail to anticipate a hazard which was unknown at the time,[27] nor if they meet a standard which would have been endorsed only by a minority school of thought at the time.[3] This provides a protection for the slower members of the profession, who cannot keep up with the state of their art, provided that they do not fall too far behind.[21] It can be difficult, especially in a case which presents a powerful emotional charge, because the defence which admits that it got it wrong and would do better nowadays cannot be presented as the most impressive face of medicine. Nevertheless, the Court will strive conscientiously to be fair, and to try the case on the evidence available.

Limitation

Adult patients of sound mind must issue their writs in respect of personal injuries within 3 years.[14] This timespan starts to run when they know that they have sustained a significant injury and they know that it was caused by the act or omission of the person they wish to sue. They do not need to know that the injury was caused by negligence.[15] However, they may well be able to argue in some cases that only when they knew that their treatment was inadequate did they know that their injury was caused by the act of the defendant rather than by their disease process,[5] and the Court has a discretion to extend time apparently indefinitely when the interests of justice demand it.[17]

The difficulty for the paediatrician is that time does not run at all against the child under 18, or a patient under a disability.[16] Thus, the survivor of a neonatal disaster has an unfettered right to issue a writ at any time prior to his 21st birthday. Even where a young child has failed to sue promptly on achieving his majority, the Court may still exercise its discretion to extend time, if it decides that it would be equitable to do so.[13] If at the age of 18 the young person does not know who or what has caused the damage, time will not start to run until he does. If he never becomes capable of managing his own affairs, and is therefore regarded by law as being under a disability, his right to sue continues throughout his life, and endures for the benefit of his estate until 3 years after his death. Since some victims of cerebral palsy seem to enjoy a life expectancy which differs only marginally, if at all, from the national average,[12] hospitals will keep neonatal records for a very long time. They are usually advised to keep all records until the child is aged 26 but records of catastrophic cases could justifiably be kept for 80 years. In many cases, the hospital will not know which cases have had a catastrophic outcome until the patient sues.

If a child is granted a right to sue outside the limitation period, the Court will judge the case on all the available evidence and will not acquit the defence of the need to provide an explanation of an apparently sinister delay merely because the lapse of time makes it harder to provide that explanation. In one case,[6] the Court had to decide whether a child acquired cerebral palsy as a result of a negligent delay in delivery 17 years earlier. It was clear that 68 minutes had elapsed between the delivery of twins and that this was in part attributable to a difficulty in finding the registrar in a city where hospital obstetric services were split between two sites. No satisfactory explanation could be provided 17 years after the event. The defendants argued that the judge should be less willing to draw an adverse inference against the defendant, whom delay had deprived of a proper opportunity to rebut the claim, and he should be less willing to treat the burden of explaining an apparently sinister delay as falling on the Health Authority alone. The Court of Appeal responded by acknowledging the argument with sympathy. However, they continued:

> Nevertheless our law allows persons under a disability such as Stuart to bring a claim such as this at any time during their lives; indeed, their right of action will survive for three years after their death. Whoever else may be to blame for the delay Stuart is not. The problem facing the parties and the Court as a result of the delay in the present case are far from unique … the delay does not affect the facts which have to be proved, nor the manner of proof. It merely means that both sides will or may be in a position to prove fewer facts. To this extent, it may well prejudice both the plaintiff

and the defendant ... The Court should draw the same inferences from those facts as it would draw if the claim had been promptly made. Likewise, if the facts which have been proved would give rise to a presumption in favour of the plaintiff under the principle of res ipsa loquitur, the Court should not decline to apply that principle merely because the claim has been brought after many years.

This case is additionally remarkable for the paediatrician in that on the issue of whether the baby was suffering from HIE, the Court preferred the evidence on causation of a paediatrician who did not pretend to be a neonatologist to that of two neonatological professors and the consultant paediatrician who had originally looked after the baby 17 years earlier as a registrar. The plaintiff had been the donor in a fetofetal transfusion, having been delivered at 33 weeks' gestation with a haemoglobin of 97% where the sibling had a haemoglobin of 172%. The plaintiff's expert was accepted when he told the Court that if any prenatal cause of brain damage had existed he would have expected it to attack both twins.

NEGLIGENCE

Negligence consists in a breach of a duty of care which causes damage.[10]

DUTY OF CARE

A duty of care is not owed to all the world,[7] but in the case of the neonatologist and the hospital which employs her, it may be owed to people who are not yet patients. It will certainly be owed to patients who are unborn if their mothers are patients at the hospital,[8] and such children will be able to sue if they are subsequently born damaged as a result of a breach of the duty of care owed to their mother. A doctor may also owe a duty to people in deciding whether to accept them as patients. Once accepted as a patient, the doctor owes an unqualified duty of care in all aspects of their relationship.

BREACH OF DUTY

The doctor will be in breach of her duty of care only if she fails to provide a reasonable standard of care. Lord Scarman described the standard which must be achieved by quoting a Scottish judge who had said:

In the realm of diagnosis and treatment there is ample scope for genuine difference of opinion and one man clearly is not negligent merely because his conclusion differs from that of other professional men ... The true test for establishing negligence in diagnosis or treatment on the part of a doctor is whether he has been guilty of such failure as no doctor of ordinary skill would be guilty of acting with ordinary care.[11]

Lord Scarman continued:

I would only add that a doctor who professes to exercise a special skill must exercise the ordinary skill of his specialty. Differences of opinion and practice exist and will always exist in the medical, as in other professions. There is seldom any one answer exclusive of all others to problems of professional judgment. A Court may prefer one body of opinion to the other but that is no basis for a conclusion of negligence.[18]

The principle that the law will respect treatment which accords with a respectable school of thought, is known as the 'Bolam test'. In another case, the House of Lords has held that it would be wrong to treat ... 'the Bolam test as doing anything less than laying down a principle of English law that is comprehensive and applicable to every aspect of the duty of care owed by a doctor to his patient in the exercise of his healing functions as respects that patient.' This applies whether the doctor is reaching a diagnosis,[18] giving warning of the hazards of treatment[28] or performing a surgical procedure.[31] It does not matter if only a handful of experts be of the defendant's school of thought, provided that they are accepted by the Court as being respectable.[9] The court reserves the right to reject an opinion which it believes does not stand up to analysis.[4] In the case of care delivered by a team, the law does not require the most junior trainee to have the skills of the consultant. However, it does require the trainee to be competent to perform the tasks allocated to her.[32]

Where a defendant is in breach of her duty of care, the plaintiff will only be entitled to be compensated for damage caused by that breach of duty. It can be very difficult to ascertain in neonatal cases because the previous clinical picture is usually obscure. Although doctors believe that only around 10–15% of cerebral palsy is due to birth asphyxia (see, for example, the American multicenter prospective study of 43 437 children by Naeye et al[20]), if the previous occult brain damage causes a fetus to respond to the stresses of labour by presenting signs of asphyxia capable of causing the HIE seen after birth, it can be impossible to prove the existence of the prior condition. It can be similarly hard to disentangle the causes of a neonatal illness such as retinopathy of prematurity,[32] or many other disabilities which are consistent with a neonatal cause.

If the defendant is guilty of an act of negligence then the Court will require her as nearly as possible to put the plaintiff in the position in which she would have been if there had been no negligence. Where a senior registrar at a London teaching hospital failed to respond to her bleep to attend a child with croup, the evidence was that it would have made no difference to the exegesis if she had attended, unless she had decided to intubate the child as a precaution against a subsequent attack. The House of Lords held that causation could not be proved if any reasonable senior registrar in her position would have decided not to intubate.[4]

NEONATAL DEATH

If a doctor is negligent and, as a consequence, the child dies, the employing hospital will be obliged to compensate the parents. Such compensation will be limited to the statutory compensation for bereavement[1] (in 1998 the compensation was £7500) and reasonable funeral expenses. If the doctor's performance is so poor that it amounts to serious professional misconduct, then she may also be answerable to the General Medical Council.[19] If the facts suggest that her performance is impaired, then she may also be compelled to give an account of herself to the Performance Review Committee of the General Medical Council which has recently been set up for this purpose.

THE CRIMINAL LAW

The doctor enjoys no privileged position under the criminal law of the land.

MURDER

Murder consists of unlawfully killing a patient with the intention of killing or causing grievous bodily harm. It can only be committed by a positive act, unlike manslaughter which can be committed by omitting to act where there is a duty to do so. There is scope for argument about whether certain events are omissions or positive acts: switching off a ventilator is a positive act whereas ceasing to treat or feed may be an omission depending on the circumstances.

MANSLAUGHTER

The crime of manslaughter will be committed when a doctor causes the death of a patient as a result of an act or omission which amounts to gross negligence. Whether negligence is gross or not is a question of fact for the jury, but the prosecution must first demonstrate a breach of duty as judged by the Bolam test.[25] The doctor who causes the death of a patient in the course of bona fide treatment without deliberately killing the child will not be guilty of any crime if she is acting in accordance with a respectable school of thought and is guided solely by the best interests of the patient.

Where a neonatologist is called and finds a baby weighing 400 g, her duty is plainly to assess the baby. If she decides not to attempt resuscitation, she cannot be guilty of a crime if a respectable school of thought would have taken the same view, because she will not be guilty of an act of negligence. The case will be judged in all the circumstances, so that a consultant at the Rosie Maternity Hospital in Cambridge would not be able to rely solely on the fact that a reasonable paediatrician in a peripheral unit with poor facilities would have decided the case was hopeless. However, the burden will remain on the prosecution throughout to prove, so that the jury is sure, that no respectable neonatologist would have failed to resuscitate that child in those circumstances and that the failure to resuscitate did hasten death.

Some of these children will have been delivered as a result of a deliberate procedure to abort the pregnancy following an antenatal diagnosis that there was a substantial risk that the fetus would be born suffering from such abnormalities as would cause it to be born seriously handicapped. Abortions on such grounds are now lawful at any stage of gestation by virtue of the Human Fertilisation and Embryology Act 1990, Section 37. This antenatal history does not affect the duty of the neonatologist towards her only patient, the newborn baby. The subsequent death of the baby from the after-effects of the abortion procedure may or may not ground a prosecution for murder against the obstetrician: legal opinion is divided on the point. However, there is no doubt that whatever the history in the womb and whatever the parental wishes may be after delivery, the neonatologist must act solely on the basis of what is in the best interests of the child.

DECLARATIONS AS TO LEGALITY

However, there are some cases where it seems to be clear that it is in the patients' best interests that life should end as soon as possible. Typically in these cases the disability is grave, the prognosis is hopeless and the distress extreme. If a positive act is necessary to end such a life, the doctor who commits such an act will be guilty of murder unless the act is lawful.[24,26] In such cases the Courts are sometimes willing to grant a Declaration that the proposed act will be lawful (e.g. Re Baby C[23]). The precise status of such Declarations is unclear in law: if they merely reveal what the existing law already is, or set a precedent which changes the law, then why is it necessary in subsequent cases to apply for a Declaration? Why can the doctor not rest on the precedent which has been set by the Declarations made in other cases?

An alternative view is that they do not change the law and that they merely render lawful on that occasion something which would otherwise be unlawful, in which case it has been suggested that the Declaration might not of itself subsequently bind a criminal court.[2] For the time being, these Declarations are probably best regarded as a species of judicial legislation on the specific facts of the individual case, which no more set a precedent than do injunctions which occasionally authorize actions which would otherwise be criminal. It may be that as judicial experience of these extraordinary dilemmas increases, a corpus of decisions will accumulate which will enable doctors and those advising them to proceed with more confidence. However, hitherto the Courts have declined to phrase their decisions so as to reveal more of the law than is necessary to deal with the cases in question.

Where the parents refuse to consent to treatment which is necessary in the best interests of the child, the wise paediatrician will of course first make strenuous efforts to carry the parents with her. The management of parents is an important part of all paediatrics and the doctor will have resort to the law only as a desperate expedient. When there is no alternative available, a child may be made a ward of Court enabling the Court to make whatever Orders seem to be necessary in the child's best interests. The leading case is a decision in which the Court of Appeal effectively decided that it was not in the best interests of a baby with Down syndrome that she should die. She was suffering from an intestinal obstruction and the parents thought it kinder that she should not undergo the surgery which was necessary for her survival. The Health Authority took the matter to Court and the Court of Appeal performed a balancing exercise before concluding that they had no doubt that the child should live.[22] However, the Court also accepted that there may be cases of severe proven damage where the future is so certain and where the life of the child is so bound to be full of pain and suffering that the Court might be driven to a different conclusion. This judgement, given in 1981, was followed shortly afterwards by a decision of the Director of Public Prosecution not to prosecute a doctor who had allegedly refused to sustain a baby who was suffering from spina bifida[30] and the criminal prosecution of Dr Leonard Arthur.[29] These decisions lay down the bones of the approach which the law has adopted to these issues in the last 15 years. However, it is an evolving area and the courts remain free to alter their decisions to reflect changes in the attitudes of society to these matters.

REFERENCES

1. Administration of Justice Act 1982 HMSO, London, s 1(1)
2. Auckland Area Health Board v. Attorney General (New Zealand High Court) (1993) 4 Med LR 243
3. Bolam v. Friern Hospital Management Committee (1957) 1 WLR 582
4. Bolitho v. City & Hackney Health Authority (1992) Lloyd's Law Reports Med (1998) 26
5. Broadley v. Guy Clapham & Co (1993) 4 Med LR 328, CA
6. Bull and Wakeham v. Devon Health Authority (1993) 4 Med LR 117, CA
7. Caparo Industries plc v. Dickman (1992) AC 605
8. Congenital Disabilities (Civil Liabilities) Act 1976 HMSO, London
9. Defreitas v. O'Brien and Campbell Connolly (1993) 4 Med LR 281, confirmed by Court of Appeal (1995) 5 Med LR 108
10. Donoghue v. Stevenson (1932) AC 562
11. Hunter v. Hanley (1955) SLT 217
12. Hutton J L et al 1994 Life expectancy of children with cerebral palsy. British Medical Journal 309: 431
13. Kelly v. Bastible (1997) 8 Med LR 15, CA
14. Limitation Act 1980 HMSO, London, s 11
15. Limitation Act 1980 HMSO, London, s 14
16. Limitation Act 1980 HMSO, London, s 28
17. Limitation Act 1980 HMSO, London, s 33
18. Maynard v. West Midlands Regional Health Authority (1985) 1 All ER 635
19. Medical Act 1983 HMSO, London, s 36
20. Naeye R L et al 1989 Origins of cerebral palsy. American Journal of Diseases of Children 143: 1154–1161
21. Newell and Newell v. Goldenberg (1995) 6 Med LR 371
22. Re B (1981) 1 WLR 1421, CA
23. Re Baby C The Times 5 April 1996, per Sir Stephen Brown
24. Re J (1990) 3 All ER 930 and (1991) Fam 33
25. Regina v Adomako (1995) 1 AC 171
26. Regina v Dr Nigel Cox and the summing up to the jury of Ognall J, (1992) BMLR 12: 38
27. Rowe v. Minister of Health (1954) 2 WLR 915
28. Sidaway v. Board of Governors of the Bethlem Royal Hospital and Maudsley Hospital (1985) AC 871
29. The Times 6 November 1981, (1981) 12 BMLR 1
30. The Times 6 October 1981
31. Whitehouse v. Jordan (1981) 1 All ER 261
32. Wilsher v. Essex Area Health Authority (1986) 3 All ER 801

50

Frequent medico-legal problems

N. R. C. Roberton

All medicine is now practised against a background of potential litigation. All doctors make mistakes. Steel et al[22] estimated that 36% of adult inpatients suffered an iatrogenic disease, most of which were side-effects of drugs or complications of procedures such as cardiac catheterization. Using stricter criteria, Brennan et al[3] and Leape et al[11] found that adverse events occurred in 3.7% of admissions and that 27.6% of these (1% of the total) were due to negligence. Vascular and cardiothoracic surgery were the most dangerous, with over 10% of patients suffering an adverse event. The perinatal data are shown in Table 50.1. We therefore have to face the fact that we do not get it right all of the time, and are likely to be sued.

The current cost of medical negligence to the NHS exceeds £150 m per annum[7] and, when combined with the cost of legal aid and the other hidden costs, the total cost to the taxpayer is several times this amount. It may soon exceed £1 bn per annum (Leigh 1996, personal communication).

In Britain legal aid is available to all children since it is their income not their parent's income which is considered. Therefore, any parent whose child is less than perfect may obtain a medicolegal review of that child's perinatal care, and the law allows them to do this until the 'child' (plaintiff) is 25 years old, and later if he or she is disabled. It costs them nothing just to have a look at the obstetric and neonatal notes and have the adequacy of care evaluated by an expert selected by their solicitor. That note review will in many cases reveal that the standard of care fell below that which was acceptable[3] (p. 1353).

British perinatal litigation is dominated by hypoxic–ischaemic encephalopathy following putative asphyxia during the mother's labour. Other major topics in my own experience of cases which have been settled are listed in Table 50.2. Overall, 53% of litigants in my series have been successful.

Depressing though this may be to clinicians, it is understandable if only for two reasons. First, the facilities for the care of handicapped children, adolescents and adults are awful and obstructively slow. It is very difficult to get a decent electric wheelchair for a child who has an awkward sitting position, or a decent computer for an athetoid with an IQ of 130, or an extension built on a council house for a wheelchair-bound spastic quadriplegic when the parents are behind with the rent. Couple that with parental anxieties about who is going to look after the child they have cared for diligently 24 hours a day, 365 days a year for many years once they are no longer able to do so. For such people £2 m in the bank makes the prospects distinctly rosier. Secondly, almost weekly in the media they read of settlements of that size being made to families like themselves, so why not try for their child? Although it may be unfair that only those patients whose handicap can be shown to result from an error do get a

Table 50.1 Adverse events and negligence in perinatal care[3]

	Patients suffering an adverse event (%)	Events due to negligence (%)
Obstetrics	1.5	38.3
Neonatology	0.6	25.8

Table 50.2 Major diagnoses in settled cases of perinatal litigation (NRCR personal series)

Diagnosis	No. of cases	Awarded damages (%)
Hypoxic–ischaemic encephalopathy	121	66
PVH, PVL	15	20
Cerebral palsy without neonatal encephalopathy	11	0
ROP	8	88
Malformation	7	14
Lung disease	7	71
Hypoglycaemia	5	20
Scarring injuries	5	40
Infection	5	0
Jaundice/kernicterus	4	75
Haemorrhagic disease	2	100
Miscellaneous	12	33

large sum of money through the courts, the society in which we live accepts the concept of a financial recompense for injury, whether it is sustained in a car accident, by tripping over the kerb or as a result of medical negligence.

As well as this 'bread and butter' problem of litigation hanging over neonatal care, we face two other much more difficult and frightening problems: withdrawal of care and manslaughter.

WITHDRAWAL OF CARE

Most, if not all, neonatologists would agree that in some cases it is appropriate to withhold or withdraw care[5,10,25] (Chapter 48). These include the extremely premature, the profoundly malformed, and the irretrievably brain-damaged baby who nevertheless does not fulfil the criteria for brain death even if these are applicable to the VLBW neonate.[23] Such decisions are now only taken by sensible neonatologists after full consultation with their medical and nursing colleagues, consultations the content and conclusions of which are committed in full to paper. Quite obviously, such decisions are only reached and put into effect after full discussion with both parents. Despite this, right-to-life 'clandestine bodies'[24] have their adherents, whose views and standards are different from the majority working in hospitals and who might report the neonatologist to the police. Whereas the doctor and the parents may have no doubt about the correctness of the decision, not many are of the stuff of which martyrs are made and professionals have a duty to make sure that the staff, the hospital, and most importantly the parents, are not exposed to the hullabaloo that follows when such events break in the media.

MANSLAUGHTER

This is dealt with in more detail in Chapter 49. All doctors make mistakes. We now have to face the prospect that if we make a major mistake which results in the death of a patient we could face a manslaughter charge.

HOW TO AVOID BEING SUED

It is of course completely impossible to avoid being sued, since in view of what has been said above the parents of any imperfect child may sue – just in case. All one can do is minimize the chances and provide care and documentation that should make it clear to the plaintiff's solicitors and experts that there are no grounds for proceeding. To make it very difficult for you to be sued successfully:

- get it right;
- write it down and keep it for 25 years;
- be there, talk to the parents and be kind.

GET IT RIGHT

Superficially this is obvious, but it requires more careful analysis and gets into the extremely murky waters of, for example, what is the right way to manage RDS, and who should look after which babies – that is, protocols and regionalization (Chapter 3), topics which generate great controversy; however, they should not.

Getting it right may mean nothing more than making the correct diagnosis and carrying out the accepted treatments. The knowledge required is that possessed by an MRCP candidate in his viva, or that found in any textbook or published protocols such as that for treating RDS.[2] It does not mean being conversant with what is in the latest obscure journals, nor does it mean searching Medline for what is hot off the press before treating a gasping hypoxic neonate. The objection that protocols bind the physician to a course of action he does not agree with is not valid. In practice, plaintiffs are successful when the standard of care is unacceptable to any body of respectable opinion. It is not the subtleties of how often which technique should be used for PaO_2 measurement that is the issue, but that it was never measured at all; it is not the precise indication for pancuronium in babies on IPPV, rather that the baby was never ventilated; it is not the precise technique for inserting a chest drain, but the fact that the baby was left with a tension pneumothorax for hours.

The advantage of protocols in a regularly updated ward book is that they provide the resident with basic guidelines for the management of common problems. Some are reluctant to write protocols for fear of their being used against them, but they are much more likely to provide the defence. This is important, because in the landmark Wilsher case[26] the courts took the view that somebody left to do something should be competent to do what he is doing. Thus in Wilsher[26] the Court found that the resident who inserts a UAC should have enough knowledge to interpret the X-ray showing whether or not the catheter was in the aorta or the vena cava.

Furthermore, the availability of the protocol, should legal proceedings start, solves at a stroke the problem of what was expected to have been done in that unit at that time. Clearly if it was not done the defendant has a problem. Unless the physician in question has a good reason for not adhering to a protocol (as indeed he may have), he will have difficulty defending his action.

WRITE IT DOWN AND KEEP IT

This is one of the things we were all taught at medical school, and there is no doubt that the standard of note-keeping has improved in the last 20 years. Nurses' note-keeping is also extremely valuable, as they routinely fill in intensive care charts and fluid balance charts, and review the patient's condition at least three times a day in the Kardex or its modern equivalent.

All this documentation – nursing notes, TPR charts, apnoea charts – **must** be kept no matter how bulky, and kept for 25 years, no matter how expensively. I cannot emphasize strongly enough how important these notes are. Thus, in assessing PVH/PVL where hypotension may be of aetiological importance, the hourly blood pressure charts are invaluable: if the BP is normal or falls are promptly treated, one potential area of negligence in the case can be scotched immediately. When there is a bad scar after subcutaneous Vamin, if the fluid balance charts show that the site was checked hourly and at, say, 11.00 hours everything was fine but at 12.00 hours the Vamin had gone subcutaneously into the hand of an ill 800 g baby, a large lesion could result (3 ml of Vamin, 30 minutes at 144 ml/kg/24 h goes a long way in an 800 g hand). I would not regard such an episode as negligent, but without the nursing notes it would be difficult to know whether the drip tissued 30 minutes or 3 hours beforehand. I use these two examples because hourly data on BP and drip sites is not part of the normal narrative notes written by residents.

Writing things down in detail becomes of crucial importance in situations where intensive care is being withdrawn. It is no good in 1997 just having a note in the Kardex saying 'Dr saw parents who do not want a brain-damaged baby' as the only record. The consultant must write down a comprehensive note, ideally supported with concurring views from a senior colleague.

The same strictures about keeping notes also apply to X-rays and ultrasound scans. Assessing when brain damage occurred is often central to expensive 'brain-damage' cases. With scans this is often possible; without them it is impossible.

BE THERE, TALK TO THE PARENTS AND BE KIND

Again an obvious remark, yet I have frequently seen plaintiff parents who have said that no-one told them why their baby was damaged or why care was withdrawn. I accept that in stressful situations parents forget, but a contemporaneous note removes all argument about the facts of a discussion.

Specific points to note are that not getting to an emergency because of bleep failure or communication failure does make defending a hospital difficult. After all, the reason we bully women to have their babies in hospital is that they are safer places with clever doctors always instantaneously available. Refusing to come is never defensible.

Being kind sounds oleaginous. It may be, but if you are nice to parents (as opposed to being chummy and on first name terms, which I abhor) and develop a good rapport with them, even if things do go wrong they will understand what is happening and are much less likely to instigate unjustifiable charges. Conversely, if a negligent mistake has been made you must be honest, tell them what has happened and when the Statement of Claim arrives tell the hospital and their lawyers the claim is justified and they should settle.

NEONATAL DISORDERS AND THE LAWYER

This section is written in the belief that the fullest documentation of all cases should be the aim. Although occasionally lack of documentation may stymie a plaintiff's case, more often first-class documentation rebuts it. Furthermore, failure of adequate documentation may itself be considered a marker of negligence.

Well documented cases also leave few questions unanswered and much less room for speculation and thus prolongation of the medicolegal process, which is of no benefit to the plaintiff, the parents or the physician.

BIRTH ASPHYXIA, HYPOXIC–ISCHAEMIC ENCEPHALOPATHY

The majority of big money settlements and the majority of medicolegal work in the perinatal period centre on this problem (Table 50.2). Five key factors are now widely accepted:

- Only about 10% of cerebral palsy is the result of perinatal asphyxia (p. 1247).
- The Apgar score is a poor marker of perinatal asphyxia (p. 242).
- The best marker that perinatal asphyxia is the cause of long-term neurological sequelae is the presence of an encephalopathic illness in the neonatal period. If a baby is neurologically normal in the neonatal period any long-term neuropathology is not the result of events in labour.
- Brain damage antedating labour can give an abnormal CTG, a low Apgar and severe neonatal encephalopathy.[9,15]
- There is no specific treatment for hypoxic–ischaemic encephalopathy. All the neonatologist can do is to achieve physiological normality in the baby by controlling, in particular, ventilation, blood pressure, fluid balance, glucose homoeostasis, convulsions and coagulopathies (pp. 1242–1243).

Apart from the occasional case where inadequate resuscitation in the first 10–15 minutes has compounded a pre-natal asphyxial event, the deficiencies of care resulting in HIE in term babies are obstetric. The role of the neonatologist is, therefore, relatively limited. He can avoid further brain-damaging complications such as hypotension, hypoglycaemia and jaundice. If perinatal asphyxia is a possibility he should also document the patient in the most meticulous manner, guiding that documentation in a way that will facilitate any subsequent medicolegal evaluation of the case.

Perhaps the most important thing the neonatologist can do is to avoid the use of the word 'asphyxia' as a synonym for a low 1-minute Apgar score. It is difficult in court to convince a judge that a baby was not asphyxiated when the contemporaneous notes repeatedly say 'diagnosis asphyxia'. This does lead to alternative cumbersome circumlocutions, such as:

- Low Apgar? cause;
- Apnoea at birth requiring IPPV;
- Inadequate feto-neonatal adaptation,

of which the best is 'birth depression', which has the merits of brevity and of being non-judgemental. They all have the merit of clinical honesty, and may push the clinician into thinking *why* the baby has a low Apgar score rather than blaming it on asphyxia.

There are two seminal sets of criteria which have to be fulfilled to establish the diagnosis of perinatal asphyxia and confirm that long-term CNS damage is the result (Tables 50.3, 50.4). Unless a plaintiff can fulfil both sets there must be doubt that the CNS sequelae are the result of perinatal asphyxia. In the neonatal period, therefore, the neonatologist *must* evaluate any baby with a low Apgar or neurological signs against these criteria to establish whether or not the neonatal illness is due to perinatal asphyxia. This should include the following:

- Cord artery blood gases. The vein is less helpful because it represents blood coming from the placenta, which may be normal in the presence of fetal asphyxia due to cord compression.
- Careful and detailed assessment of the Apgar score plus the sequence of events in response to resuscitation (p. 243); is this likely to be primary or terminal apnoea?
- Regular clinical CNS assessment. This does not need to be a complex Dubowitz type of examination (p. 287) – a daily statement of tone, reflex activity, pupillary reactions, fontanelle size and tension, OFC, feeding activity, level of consciousness and a description of the site and type of funny movements, and whether or not experienced observers think they are fits, is all that is required but is rarely provided. It is depressingly common to see beautiful twice-daily notes describing the cardiovascular, pulmonary and fluid balance status of a baby, yet nothing about the fact that he has just wiped out his CNS other than the words 'flat' or 'sedated'. Assess the degree of encephalopathy present (p. 1239).
- Look for damage to other body systems. Do daily blood counts and biochemistry; most important is the fluid balance chart with urine analysis. Measure blood pressure and do a CXR and ECG. Check the clotting studies and liver enzymes. The more that is normal, the easier it is to refute a diagnosis of intrapartum asphyxia.
- Carry out imaging very early. This may show prenatal damage on either ultrasound scan or CT/MRI. Ultrasound should be done repeatedly on every baby suspected of HIE, and there should be a low threshold for doing more sophisticated imaging as well, to exclude early those babies whose brain damage is of pre-labour aetiology.[9] This also begins the evaluation for the criteria listed in Table 50.4.
- Consider an EEG. It may be helpful in diagnosis and prognosis.
- Think about other possible causes of neonatal encephalopathy and exclude or confirm them.
- Document drug doses, route and timing with extra care. Check levels of potentially toxic drugs such as phenobarbitone.

I would emphasize that this is good medicine. It does not put the medical profession in a good light if it is only after legal proceedings have started that it is established that a child's cerebral palsy is a result of congenital rubella, lissencephaly or some genetic defect.

If all these things are done an accurate diagnosis can be established early, and if litigation does result an honest appraisal can easily be reached.

Table 50.3 American Academy of Obstetrics and Gynecology and Pediatrics essential criteria for diagnosis of perinatal asphyxia[4]

Cord arterial pH < 7.00
Apgar ≤ 3 at 5 minutes
Neonatal encephalopathy grades II–III
Multiorgan dysfunction

Table 50.4 Criteria to establish that long-term neurological deficits are the result of perinatal asphyxia[8]

Evidence of marked prolonged intrapartum asphyxia
HIE grades II–III PLUS evidence of multiorgan dysfunction
Is the child's long-term deficit one which can be explained as a sequel of intrapartum asphyxia?
Has the work-up excluded other conditions?

PERIVENTRICULAR HAEMORRHAGE, PERIVENTRICULAR LEUKOMALACIA

Unlike HIE in term babies, where the damage is usually done prenatally and negligence is likely to be in the province of the obstetrician, the majority of cases of PVH and PVL develop postnatally and the allegations of negligence are therefore made against the neonatologists.

More and more of these cases are now coming forward as the parents of ex-preterm babies profoundly damaged by these two conditions seek medicolegal redress. In the current state of neonatal intensive care these conditions are not preventable, despite impeccable care (Chapter 44, Part 5). Therefore, if the neonatologist has followed standard treatment routines and looked after the baby in a standard way, has written it all down with good documentation of blood gases, blood pressure, unavoidable complications such as pneumothorax, and has responded to complications appropriately, litigation is unlikely to be successful.

Conversely, if the care falls below accepted norms[2] and if the deficiencies are prolonged (hours and days rather than minutes), defending the case will be difficult. There may also be problems if the mother was delivered unnecessarily preterm, and the baby develops PVH/PVL despite immaculate neonatal care.

These disorders are ones in which the 'be there and be kind' advice is most important. If full and frank descriptions are given to parents when unpleasant ultrasound findings develop, I believe they are less likely to sue; conversely, if nothing is said, when after discharge they realize they have a handicapped baby, they are much more likely to be suspicious that there was a cover-up of negligence.

INFECTION

The two most common infectious problems coming to litigation are fulminating GBS and other types of early-onset sepsis causing unanticipated rapid neonatal death, and neonatal meningitis leading to cerebral palsy. In both conditions, so long as the midwives/residents have responded appropriately to early warning of infection (p. 1116), defending the hospital is easy. However, if a jaundiced baby with a tense fontanelle and a temperature of 38.5°C was ignored for 12 hours, the doctors are sunk; much more difficult is the competent SHO who at 02.00 hours sees a baby who has refused a couple of feeds, is afebrile, and is just slightly 'peely-wally'. He examines the baby fully and decides to observe. Four hours later the baby collapses with *E. coli* meningitis. Would an experienced consultant have done better? In cases like this a unit protocol describing when to work up for sepsis and meningitis is often very helpful.

RETINOPATHY OF PREMATURITY

The role of oxygen in this condition will always remain controversial as it is impossible to randomize a group of 0.5–0.8 kg neonates to controlled and uncontrolled oxygen therapy to see if the incidence of ROP varies in the two groups. However, I believe two facts exist:

- Cicatricial ROP in babies weighing more than 1.00 kg is now exceptionally rare (<1% of survivors in recent series) (Chapter 36). I have no doubt that this is not due to cryotherapy or vitamin E but to the fact that most neonatologists adhere to the guidelines given in all neonatal textbooks to keep a postductal PaO_2 less than 10 kPa (p. 503).
- The further below 1.00 kg the baby's birthweight, the more likely he is to develop cicatricial ROP despite impeccable control of oxygen therapy.

This is another condition where protocols are invaluable. There are now clear and widely accepted guidelines for the monitoring of PaO_2 in preterm babies[2] (pp. 362, 503). If a neonatologist has followed these guidelines it is very unlikely first of all that the baby will develop ROP, and secondly that the plaintiff will be able to mount a successful case. Conversely, if the monitoring is substandard or, worse, non-existent, there will be negligence.

There are also clear guidelines for monitoring preterm survivors at risk from ROP.[18] Failure to examine such babies and treat threshold disease (p. 913) cannot be defended.

HYPOGLYCAEMIA

This is an area where experts differ. Most neonatologists would now agree on the normal blood glucose values in the neonatal period (pp. 942–943). Most would also agree that coma, convulsions and apnoea in the presence of a blood glucose <1.0 mmol/l are markers of neuroglycopenia with a distinct possibility of CNS sequelae. What is not agreed is the significance of a glucose <1.0 mmol/l for an hour or so without symptoms, the significance of jitteriness as a symptom, or the significance of glucose levels in the range of 1.0–2.0 in the absence of the three cardinal features of neuroglycopenia. The literature on this topic is poor and ancient. It is, however, impossible to find convincing evidence that asymptomatic hypoglycaemia (1.0–2.0 mmol/l) of even 12 hours' duration ever caused sequelae in term babies.

JAUNDICE

We know that jaundice causes kernicterus. As the vast majority of term babies whose bilirubin creeps up to 450–500 μmol/l come to no harm, we probably overtreat it (p. 721).

With the current policy of early postpartum discharge of breast-feeding mothers checking for early severe jaundice must become part of the routine surveillance carried out by the community midwives and the general practitioner. There is currently major anxiety in the USA over a mini epidemic of kernicterus in such term infants who were discharged 24–48 hours after delivery[19] and whose bilirubin reached levels >500 μmol/l by the end of the first week. Similar cases have been seen in Britain.

In the neonatologist's sphere of activity I have also seen several large preterm babies in the 1.6–2.4 kg, 31–34 weeks' gestational age range who have developed kernicterus with a bilirubin in the 300–350 μmol/l range. This occurred when the babies were seriously ill and likely to have 'sprung' their blood–brain barrier (pp. 719–720).

These babies had all breached the published action levels for exchange transfusion in ill babies,[17] and care needs to be taken that these guidelines are adhered to. In low-birthweight survivors kernicterus is exceptionally rare. In those who are deaf multiple factors are involved (p. 91), and dangerously high bilirubin levels rarely occur in such babies, who are usually under close supervision in the NICU and also under phototherapy, which means that 15–20% of their total bilirubin level is in the form of non-toxic photoisomers (p. 717). Even if they do have high bilirubin levels it is often very difficult to tease out bilirubin toxicity from the damaging effects of hypoxia, acidaemia, PVL and PVH.

INJURIES

Some scarring is an almost inevitable complication of the procedures used in intensive care, such as inserting i.v. cannulae, blood sampling or draining pneumothoraces (Chapter 37). Most neonatal i.v. infusions end by running subcutaneously (p. 927) and scarring may result. Even the most carefully inserted, located and monitored arterial line may result in peripheral ischaemia and tissue loss or organ damage. If appropriate care and monitoring is used these sequelae are not negligent. Hypertonic solutions should ideally be given through a central catheter, infusion devices set to an operating pressure of 40 mmHg should be used, and the pressure alarms should not be overridden.

These are situations where good nursing notes and the 'be there and be informative' counsel is vital; one can often prevent litigation by explaining to the parents that the lesion was an accident unpreventable even by meticulous monitoring.

Because the sums claimed for scarring are small, often less than £25,000, unit managers have a habit of suggesting early settlement just to get the plaintiff off everyone's back. This tendency should be resisted so that everyone (plaintiffs, lawyers and managers/accountants) will realize that most scars are an unavoidable complication of neonatal intensive care.

HAEMORRHAGIC DISEASE

This has suddenly become a topic of intense interest (pp. 798–800). In my view it is advisable to give vitamin K to all neonates, and complex protocols as to who should receive i.m. or oral vitamin K and how many doses should be given merely increase the risk of error. The oral/intramuscular controversy is covered on pages 798–800, where adequate dosing for oral vitamin K is discussed. If mothers refuse vitamin K altogether for their babies they should sign a form to that effect in the notes, and face the consequences which, fortunately, are relatively rare.

MISCELLANEOUS TOPICS

Developmental dysplasia of the hip

It is now recognized that up to 50% of DDH are missed on the routine neonatal clinical examination,[21] and to miss the diagnosis is therefore not negligent. Not to carry out the examination, however, is.

The routine neonatal examination

Many things can be missed non-negligently during this brief examination. The commonest is DDH, but others include cataract, midline cleft palate, and the large bladder accompanying urethral valves. Particularly with the tendency to discharge at less than 24 hours of age only a single examination is done, and often in a hurry, as the mother is pressing to get out. Murmurs and femoral pulse abnormalities are particularly easy to miss in this situation.

It is more difficult to defend the situation where something is found that is serious but which is not properly evaluated: examples would include unexplained tachypnoea, sacrococcygeal masses and abdominal masses (kidney, liver, tumours).

Necrotizing enterocolitis

I have seen very few cases of NEC come to litigation. None in fact involved negligence, though it is possible to imagine a scenario in which enteral feeding was persisted with in a generally ill preterm baby despite intestinal obstruction or rectal bleeding.

Bronchopulmonary dysplasia

It is difficult to imagine how this condition could be created negligently. Again, this is an illness in which litigation should be preventable by detailed discussion with parents while the baby is still on the NICU.

WITHDRAWING AND WITHHOLDING CARE

I have left this to last as it is a most difficult subject, posing as it does major ethical and legal problems as well as clinical ones.

It is helpful to consider withholding and withdrawing care under three separate headings:

- Withholding care at birth, because of either extreme prematurity or gross malformations.
- The management of the severely malformed baby who has survived beyond the labour ward.
- Withdrawal of care in the critically ill or profoundly brain-damaged baby after a period of intensive care and meticulous investigation and assessment in the NICU.

Extreme prematurity

With the escalating costs of neonatal intensive care (Chapter 4) there is a suggestion that extremely preterm babies will not be resuscitated. The legal (Chapter 49) and ethical issues (Chapter 48) posed by a 450 g, 23/52 baby are discussed elsewhere.

I have argued[16] for active treatment of all babies ≥ 24/52 and/or ≥ 500 g birthweight, with consideration being given to those less premature or heavy if appropriate. The steadily improving prognosis for such babies since those data were first presented to a meeting of the British Paediatric Association in 1992 has done nothing to alter my stance. It is difficult to justify a refusal to resuscitate a baby ≥ 500 g birthweight or ≥ 24/52 gestational age, particularly if, as is still the case in the UK, we are able to withdraw care in a dignified and acceptable fashion if it becomes clear at 1 hour or 100 days of age that neurologically intact survival is not possible.

The impact of the recent Messenger case in the USA has yet to be assessed. In this case the medically qualified father of a 0.78 kg 25/52 baby was acquitted of manslaughter after disconnecting his daughter from the ventilator during the first few hours of life, despite the fact that the attending neonatologist felt the condition of the baby justified continuing intensive care.[12]

Serious malformations

Unit protocols may help to guide the decision not to resuscitate profoundly malformed babies in the labour ward, but apart from anencephaly (and gross rachischisis) and perhaps Potter syndrome, which is more difficult to diagnose quickly, the SHO's role should be to initiate resuscitation while calling for senior advice. If a complex and serious malformation was anticipated as a result of antenatal ultrasound scanning then experienced neonatologists/paediatric surgeons can attend the delivery and respond accordingly to decisions made in full discussion with the parents before delivery.

The decision not to offer medical or surgical help to a baby who is unexpectedly profoundly malformed may have to be taken under less than ideal circumstances within the first few minutes or hour after delivery. In most cases, however, active labour ward resuscitation is not necessary, the baby is pink and breathing, and the discussion with the parents about withholding intensive medical and surgical care can take place in a more calm manner.

If it is decided that no medical or surgical activity would be of benefit the neonatologist must nevertheless ensure that the baby is not hungry or in pain by the appropriate use of food, fluid, drugs and oropharyngeal suction. Decisions about oxygen, antibiotics, parenteral nutrition and surgery must be individualized, but if it is decided that intensive care is not indicated it would be wrong to institute artificial ventilation. For many babies it is possible to arrange for terminal care to take place at home.

Withdrawing care

In the UK the decision to withhold or withdraw intensive care is usually manageable within the NICU. By this I mean that decisions are taken after long and careful discussion with the parents by the baby's physicians and nurses with, if appropriate, input from social workers and priests, the latter in my experience being extremely sensible, helpful and supportive. It is terribly important to try and preserve this pattern of dealing with agonizing problems rather than assigning them to hospital and neonatal ethics advisory committees,[6,20] or acceding to the nightmare of having to ventilate anencephalics for 3 years[13] as have some of our transatlantic colleagues. I cannot see how such activities make it more likely that a sensible, humane and legal decision will be made, but I can see that they are very likely to increase and prolong the suffering of the patient and the parents for no benefit whatsoever.

It is not the job of the neonatologist to prolong life when death is inevitable, nor when brain death is diagnosed. The latter is difficult but possible to diagnose in the neonate.[1,23] In such cases active treatment can be withdrawn after discussion with the nursing staff and the parents. The decision must be documented in the notes.

What is much more difficult is when to withdraw treatment when it is clear that profound neurological damage (but not brain death) has occurred that will preclude any meaningful sensate existence should the baby survive. A decision to withdraw care from such a baby is, in theory, illegal (Chapter 49), but in practice is frequently reached and in my view justifiably so. Such decisions can only be reached after detailed discussions with staff and parents. I believe it is essential that such discussions are fully recorded in the notes, and when parents agree to withhold/withdraw treatment that those decisions are witnessed by a senior medical or nursing colleague and documented as such. It is also valuable to have an assessment recorded in the notes from a consultant colleague not currently involved in the baby's care that continuing intensive therapy is unjustifiable.

The practicalities are in general one of two situations: a decision to take the baby off the ventilator, or not to reventilate him. Occasionally there are other options, such as not operating (for example hydrocephalus) or not continuing TPN when there is no viable bowel in babies with NEC.

In all these situations, once the decision to withdraw care is reached this does not mean that the baby and his family are abandoned. The baby should receive full medical and all other aspects of care, which may include oxygen, fluids, food and antibiotics. In most cases the baby will die quickly. A major problem can develop, particularly in babies who were taken off IPPV in the confident expectation that they would die, usually very quickly because they were making no respiratory effort while on IPPV. If they then start to gasp and then breathe irregularly, and are clearly going to survive for hours or even longer, apart from anything else this suggests that the assessment prior to disconnection was incorrect, in terms of both survival and severity of brain damage.

Once a decision to withdraw therapy is taken notes must still be written in full until death occurs. It does not look good if, after a decision to take a baby off a ventilator, nothing is written for 5 days until the notes say 'took a bottle well today', but the nursing notes for the intervening period imply prolonged potentially brain-damaging apnoeic and cyanotic spells.

As with everything else in medicine, if a clinical decision is taken or a diagnosis is made which turns out to be wrong, the physician must revise his thinking, and if it is clear that the baby is not going to die he must revise his management. I recognize that such an eventuality is difficult to plan for in discussion with the parents before withdrawing care, and even more difficult to deal with afterwards if such a possibility had not previously been addressed. Nevertheless, it is a problem that must be faced.

As well as the nightmare possibility outlined above, the other great anxiety when withdrawing care is the activity of 'clandestine' right-to-life groups[24] within the hospital or the family. I believe that full documentation as outlined above will ultimately protect the physician in court, but this may not protect him from being reported in the first place.

WHAT TO DO IF YOU ARE SUED

In the immortal words of Corporal Jones,[14] 'Don't panic!' Even more importantly, don't be paranoid, which is an easy and understandable response if you feel the claim is quite unjustified and you had in fact slaved particularly hard over a baby who has such ungrateful parents: a moment's mature reflection may suggest that even if they do not have a case they may require detailed explanation.

It is very important to remain calm and cooperative. Encourage the hospital to cooperate fully with the plaintiff's solicitors. Give them all the notes, scans and X-rays: they have a right to see them, and will get them eventually anyway.

Review the notes calmly, dispassionately and objectively, not defensively. Honestly evaluate the care and, if mistakes were made, admit them. If there were times when care was less than polished, identify them for the Trust's solicitors so that they can point defence experts to these areas. Do not write irascible letters along the lines of 'how dare they sue me for this impeccably managed case' when in fact mistakes were made. Apart from anything else, such letters often end up filed in the notes, are obtained by the plaintiff, and do not cast you in the role of an enlightened and reasonable consultant. This is especially true when you are being cross-examined in court on what the defence experts have already admitted are clear deficiencies in the care.

There is relatively little point in off-loading blame on to nurses, SHOs, anaesthetists, ward clerks or even administrators, since now it is the hospital/Trust that is sued, without blame being apportioned. If, however, you can blame the GP or another hospital that is fair play, and indeed may be justifiable. If the GP failed to recognize premature labour, so that premature delivery was inevitable, that may be negligent. Alternatively, all the damage may have been done at the referral unit or level 3 unit – whichever you were not working in.

Cooperate with the hospital's solicitors – they are there to help. Some may be relatively inexperienced in handling cases of this sort: advise them on which medical experts to choose, or even which barristers have impressed you in the past with their grasp of perinatal medicolegal matters.

If you think you have not erred and the case should be defended you should insist, even if the hospital wants to settle the case for a small sum. Conversely, if a mistake has been made admit it and encourage the hospital to settle as soon and as quickly as possible: that way you are relieved of the irritation of a prolonged legal war of attrition, and by shortening the legal process large sums of money can be saved.

REFERENCES

1. Ashwal S, Schneider S 1989 Brain death in the newborn. Pediatrics 84: 429–437
2. BAPM/RCP 1992 Development of audit measures and guidelines for good practice in the management of neonatal respiratory distress syndrome. Archives of Disease in Childhood 76: 1221–1227
3. Brennan T A, Leape L L, Laird N et al 1991 Incidence of adverse events and negligence in hospitalized patients. New England Journal of Medicine 324: 370–376
4. Carter B S, Haverkamp A D, Merenstein G B 1993 The definition of acute perinatal asphyxia. Clinics in Perinatology 20: 287–304
5. Cook L A, Watchko J F 1996 Decision making for the critically ill neonate near the end of life. Journal of Perinatology 16: 133–136
6. Edens M J, Eyler F D, Wagner J T, Eitzman D V 1990 Neonatal ethics: development of a consultative group. Pediatrics 86: 944–949
7. Editorial 1995 New cover for NHS negligence claims. British Medical Journal 310: 896
8. Freeman J M, Nelson K B 1988 Intrapartum asphyxia and cerebral palsy. Pediatrics 82: 240–249
9. Gaffney G, Squier M V, Johnson A, Flavell V, Sellers 1994 Clinical associations of perinatal ischaemic white matter injury. Archives of Disease in Childhood 70: F101–106
10. Lantos J D, Tyson J E, Allen A et al 1994 Withholding and withdrawing life sustaining treatment in neonatal intensive care: issues for the 1990s. Archives of Disease in Childhood 71: F218–223
11. Leape L L, Brennan T A, Laird N et al 1991 The nature of adverse events in hospitalized patients. New England Journal of Medicine 324: 377–383
12. Paris J J 1996 Manslaughter or a legitimate parental decision. The Messenger Case. Journal of Perinatology 16: 60–64
13. Paris J J, Miles S H, Kohrman A, Reardon F 1995 Guidelines in the care of anencephalic infants. A response to baby K. Journal of Perinatology 15: 318–324

14. Perry J, Croft D 1970(s) Dad's Army. A BBC Series about the Home Guard in the 1939–45 war
15. Phelan J P, Ahn M O 1994 Perinatal observations in 48 neurologically impaired term infants. American Journal of Obstetrics and Gynecology 171: 424–431
16. Roberton N R C 1993 Should we look after babies less than 800 grams? Archives of Disease in Childhood 68: 326–329
17. Roberton N R C 1993 A manual of neonatal intensive care, 3rd edn. Edward Arnold, London, p. 240
18. Royal College of Ophthalmologists/British Association of Perinatal Medicine 1995 Retinopathy of prematurity: guidelines for screening and treatment. Royal College of Ophthalmologists/British Association of Perinatal Medicine, London
19. Seidman D S, Stevenson D K, Ergaz Z, Gale R 1995 Hospital readmission due to neonatal hyperbilirubinemia. Pediatrics 96: 727–729
20. Sexson W R, Thigpen J 1996 Organization and function of a hospital ethics committee. Clinics in Perinatology 23: 429–436
21. Sponseller P D 1995 Screening and ultrasound for neonatal hip instability. Current Opinion in Pediatrics 7: 77–79
22. Steel K, Gertman P M, Crescenzi C, Anderson J 1981 Iatrogenic illness on a general medical service at a university hospital. New England Journal of Medicine 304: 638–642
23. Volpe J J 1987 Brain death determination in the newborn. Pediatrics 80: 293–297
24. Walker C H M 1988 'Officiously to keep alive'. Archives of Disease in Childhood 63: 560–565
25. Whitelaw A 1986 Death as an option in neonatal intensive care. Lancet ii: 328–331
26. Wilsher v. Essex Area Health Authority 1987. Q.B.730

Section 8

Practical procedures

51

Procedures

A. W. R. Kelsall

INTRODUCTION

Procedures can be carried out in different ways, previous experience often determining how a practical procedure will be performed. This chapter will outline both basic and specialist procedures, describing different methodologies and changing practice and taking into account advances in neonatal intensive care. All procedures have risks as well as benefits; risks can be minimized by adequate training, supervision and preparation.

MANAGEMENT OF THE AIRWAY AND RESPIRATORY PROBLEMS

ENDOTRACHEAL INTUBATION

Intubation is required when an infant fails to establish spontaneous respiration after basic resuscitation, or to remove meconium or other secretions from the airway.

Equipment

- Two laryngoscopes, straight blades size 0 (7.5 cm) and size 1 (10 cm)
- Endotracheal tubes
- Resuscitaire with suction, overhead heater, light source, oxygen and clock
- Magill forceps for nasal intubation
- Lubricating jelly for nasal intubation
- Fixation device.

This basic equipment must always be available in a resuscitaire or resuscitation trolley, which must be checked daily.

Procedure

Intubation requires both hands and coordination. Experience in holding the laryngoscope in the left hand, and manipulating and positioning ETT with Magill forceps in the right hand should be gained on a resuscitation mannequin. It is no longer considered ethically appropriate to practise intubation on babies that have died. Cole's shouldered ETT are suitable for oral intubation; straight ETT can be used for oral or nasal intubation. Oral intubation is preferred during delivery room resuscitation. The size of ETT depends on the infant's birthweight and gestation.

Birthweight	*Gestation*	*ETT size*
>3000 g	Term	3.5 mm
1000–3000 g	>28–38 weeks	3.0 mm
<1000 g	<28 weeks	2.5 mm

1. Check all equipment, laryngoscopes and the resuscitaire before the procedure.
2. The baby should be positioned on the resuscitaire with the head in a neutral position and the neck slightly extended. Suction the oropharynx and nasopharynx to remove secretions.
3. The laryngoscope is inserted to the right-hand side of the mouth, pulling the tongue to the left as the blade is advanced into the vallecula (Fig. 51.1). Gentle vertical traction with the laryngoscope and cricoid pressure with the little finger of the left hand will lift the epiglottis and bring the vocal cords into view (Fig. 51.2).
4. An oral ETT should be inserted into right-hand side of the mouth and passed through the vocal cords; Magill forceps may be needed to achieve successful intubation. Wait for the cords to open, as pushing against closed cords will cause damage.
5. Nasal intubation at resuscitation should only be attempted by experienced practitioners. The lubricated ETT is passed into the nostril in a vertical direction, then rotated horizontally to pass under the turbinates through the choanae into the oropharynx where the tip of the tube can be gripped with Magill forceps and passed through the cords. The curved ETT should follow the natural curve of the nasopharynx. Failure to advance the tube in the correct direction in the nose may result in penetration of the cribriform plate.

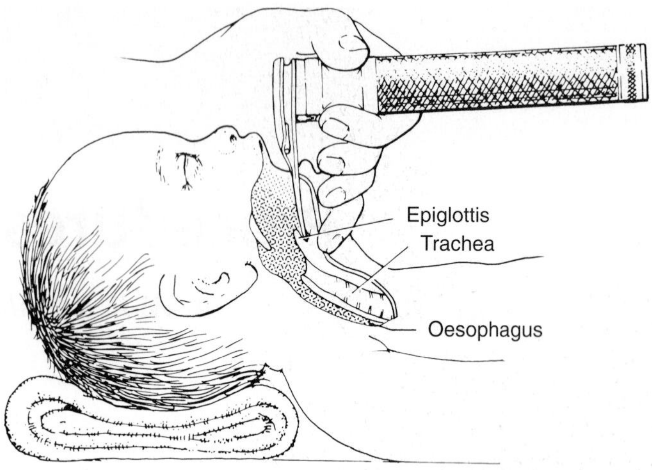

Fig. 51.1 Laryngoscopy. Laryngoscope blade positioned in the vallecula, lifting the epiglottis. Note cricoid pressure can be applied with the little finger.

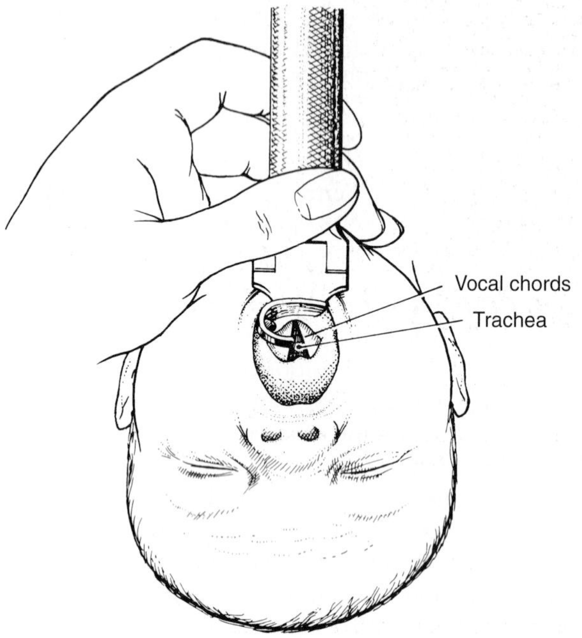

Fig. 51.2 Laryngoscopy. Visualization of the vocal cords.

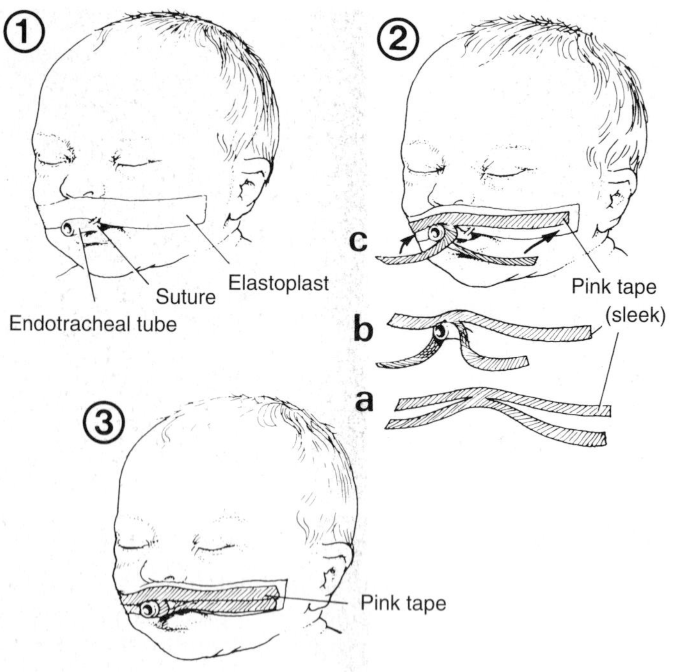

Fig. 51.3 Fixation of an oral endotracheal tube.

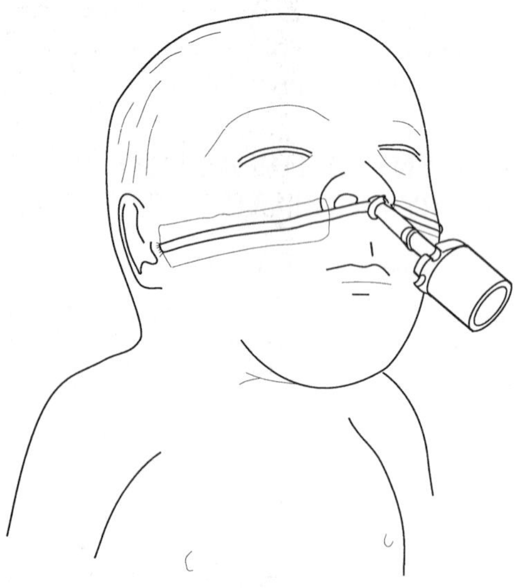

Fig. 51.4 Fixation of a nasal endotracheal tube.

6. The ETT tip should be positioned approximately 1 cm below the cords. Intermittent positive pressure ventilation can be applied, producing a rapid improvement in colour and heart rate, with symmetrical chest wall movement and equal air entry. Babies at risk of RDS should receive surfactant prophylaxis after intubation (pp. 494, 509).
7. The tube must be supported until permanent fixation is achieved. The face should be cleaned with an alcohol wipe to remove vernix and secretions so that tape can adhere to the skin. Oral tubes can be secured by suturing the tube to a strip of Elastoplast stuck over the philtrum, taking care not to occlude the lumen with the suture. An H-shaped piece of zinc oxide tape should be applied to further stabilize the tube (Fig. 51.3). Other methods use plastic clips which grip the tube and stretch across the mouth to be tied to a hat. This method may cause puckering of the mouth, and the hat hinders access to the scalp veins and anterior fontanelle. Nasal ET tubes can be secured using a cord ligature with knots tied on the upper and lower surface of the tube, with the cords being fixed to the cheeks with Blenderm tape (Fig. 51.4). In larger infants an H-shaped piece of zinc oxide tape can be wrapped around the tube and fixed to the cheeks. The Tunstall method of nasal ETT fixation is not suitable for premature infants. The ETT should be trimmed to reduce dead space within the circuit.

8. A chest radiograph should be performed to confirm the correct tube position.

Elective reintubation

For elective intubations and reintubations babies may be sedated (morphine 0.1 mg/kg) and occasionally paralysed (suxamethonium 2–3 mg/kg) prior to the procedure. When replacing oral tubes, a nasal ETT can be passed through the nose to the oropharynx; this should be gripped with the Magill forceps and advanced through the cords as the oral tube is withdrawn by an assistant. This method causes minimal disturbance of the heart rate and oxygenation. A nasal ETT can be threaded over a NGT which has been passed through the nose and visualized in the posterior oropharynx. Using the NGT as a guide, more pressure can be applied to push the ETT through the choanae into the oropharynx; the NGT should be removed and the ETT advanced into position.

Problems

- Failure to visualize cords may be due to overextension of the neck or to advancing the laryngoscope blade into the oesophagus.
- Failure to intubate. Don't panic: all babies can be successfully ventilated by a bag and mask system. Call for help and avoid repeated trauma, hypoxia and bradycardia.
- Failure to improve after intubation. The tube may be in the oesophagus, with greater air entry over the stomach than the chest, or the tube may be blocked by secretions.
- Asymmetric air entry and inflation: right greater than left usually indicates that the ETT is in the right main bronchus, but similar findings could occur with a left-sided pneumothorax. Check the length of ETT inserted and consider transillumination of the chest.

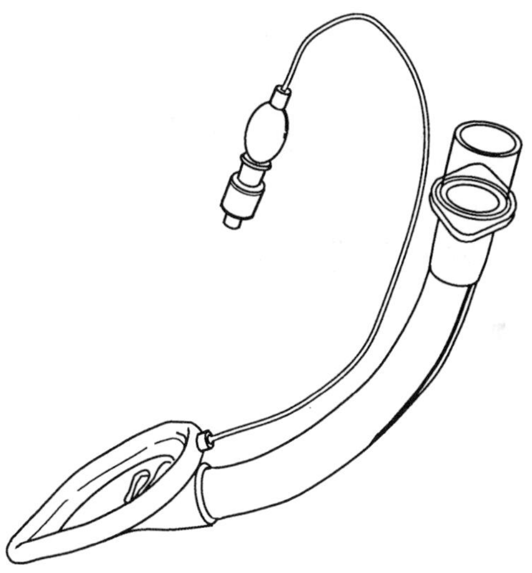

Fig. 51.5 The laryngeal mask.

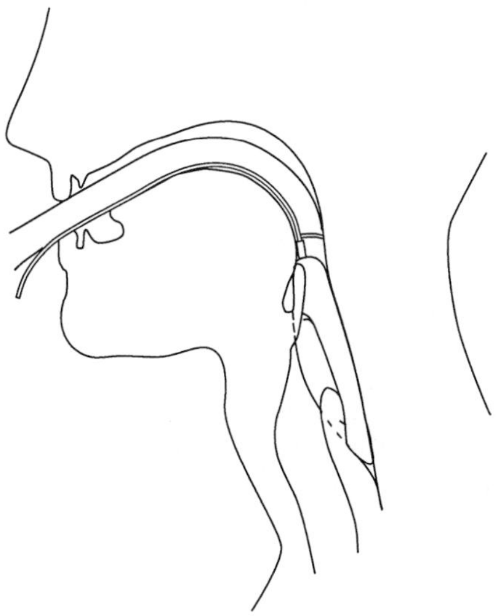

Fig. 51.6 The laryngeal mask in position over the larynx.

Laryngeal mask

The infant mask (size 3.2) can be used in the resuscitation of term infants to provide short-term ventilation without intubation of the trachea (Fig. 51.5). The tube is inserted with the mask facing anteriorly, passing over the tongue into the oropharynx to lie over the vocal cords (Fig. 51.6).

CONTINUOUS POSITIVE AIRWAY PRESSURE

CPAP is often used in RDS after extubation (p. 581) and as supportive treatment of apnoea (p. 635) and upper airway obstruction (p. 561). The simplest method of delivering CPAP is via a single 'soft ivory' ET tube inserted 2–3 cm in a nostril and secured in the same way as in intubated babies. Dual nasal prong systems are held in place by straps fixed to a hat (Fig. 51.7). Both systems deliver humidified gases and are well tolerated. In suspected upper airway obstruction the nasal prong should be passed into the oropharynx.

SUPPLEMENTAL OXYGEN

Infants receiving supplemental oxygen should have arterial oxygen saturation measured by pulse oximetry, or arterial PaO_2 (p. 503). Humidified oxygen can be given into a head box containing a calibrated oxygen analyser. Low-flow nasal cannulae are more convenient, allowing parents and nursing staff to handle the infant more easily. When cannulae are used it is important to measure actual oxygen requirements in a headbox; oxygen should be humidified when the flow exceeds 0.2 l/min.

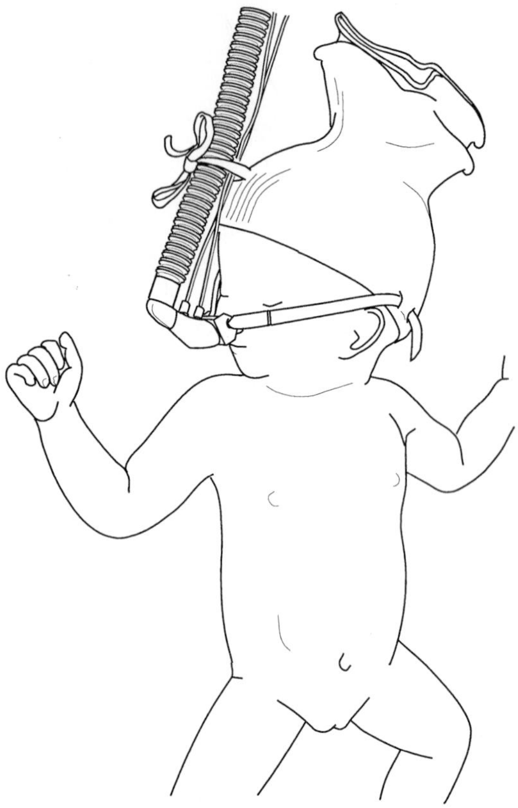

Fig. 51.7 A dual prong nasal CPAP device secured to a hat.

BLOOD SAMPLING

Blood can be obtained from capillary samples, venepuncture or arterial puncture. The sampling site depends on the quantity of blood required and the type of assay (Chapter 46).

CAPILLARY BLOOD

Small samples sufficient for routine haematological, biochemical, drug assay and capillary blood gas analysis can be obtained from the lateral or medial margins of the heel. The calcaneus should be avoided because of the risk of introducing infection (Fig. 51.8).

Procedure

The heel should be warm and well perfused and the skin cleaned with an alcohol swab. With the heel held dorsiflexed, the skin should be punctured with a minilet or glucolet lancet. Blood should flow with gentle pressure: excessive squeezing will cause bruising and give inaccurate results because the blood is diluted with tissue fluid.

VENOUS BLOOD

Peripheral venepuncture should be used to obtain larger quantities of blood for coagulation studies and bacterial culture. Veins in the hands and feet should be used in the first instance: more proximal veins should be reserved for central venous access. The jugular and femoral veins must not be used for routine sampling.

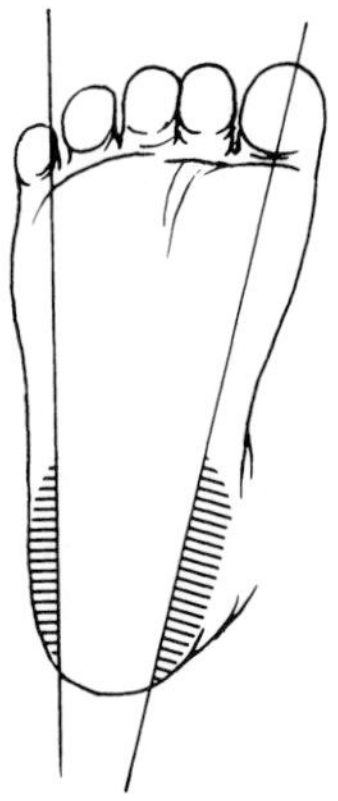

Fig. 51.8 Heel pricks for capillary sample; the shaded areas indicate the sites from which this type of blood should be collected, i.e. beyond the lateral and medial limits of the calcaneus.

Equipment

- 21–23 G needles or 23–25 G butterfly
- Appropriate bottles or capillary tubes.

Procedure

Appropriate veins should be identified in the hands and feet, and the veins and overlying skin stabilized either by an assistant's grip acting as a tourniquet or by your own fingers. The overlying skin should be cleaned and blood collected, preferably using a closed system. A closed system using a butterfly and syringe ensures a more sterile sample for microbiological culture. Alternatively, an open system is widely used, in spite of the obvious drawbacks. In this method blood is allowed to drip from a needle (Fig. 51.9) or cannula inserted into the vein directly into the container. This system is messy and unsterile, and has recently come under criticism because the hubless needle has been left in the crib and worked its way into the baby (p. 930). Excessive pressure during venepuncture causes bruising or haemolysis. Gentle pressure should be applied for several minutes after the needle has been removed to prevent bruising.

ARTERIAL BLOOD

Peripheral arterial blood sampling is indicated for close monitoring of ventilation, acid–base status or to obtain large volumes of blood. The radial, posterior tibial and dorsalis pedis arteries are the most commonly used sites. Repeated sampling from the same artery should be avoided because of the risk of spasm and distal ischaemia. Arteriovenous fistulae have also occurred. Sampling from the ulnar artery should only be performed when collateral

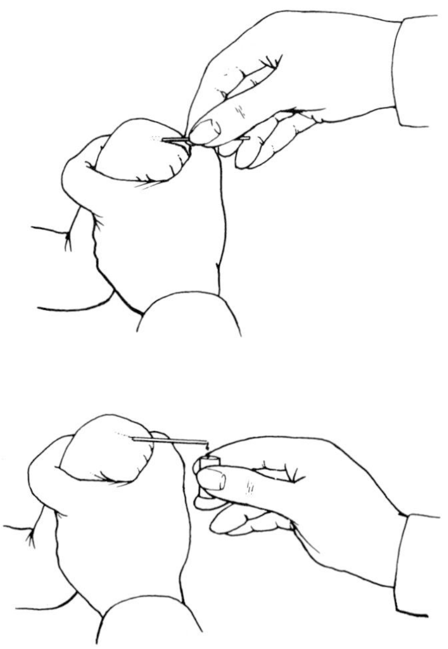

Fig. 51.9 Venous blood sampling with the broken needle technique.

circulation to the hand via the radial artery is confirmed (Allen's test). Sampling from the brachial or femoral arteries is only appropriate if other arteries cannot be used.

Equipment

- As for venepuncture, heparinized syringes for blood gas analysis.

Procedure

1. The artery should be identified either by palpation or by transillumination with a cold light. The overlying skin should be cleaned and the artery punctured; blood can be collected in a heparinized capillary tube or syringe.
2. Sampling from the radial artery is facilitated by partial extension of the wrist. The foot should be partially plantarflexed when sampling from the dorsalis pedis artery, and dorsiflexed when sampling from the posterior tibial artery.
3. Overextension of the wrist or plantarflexion of the ankle may occlude the peripheral artery and prevent aspiration. After removing the needle steady pressure must be applied for at least 5 minutes.

VASCULAR ACCESS AND CANNULATION

The need for any vascular access must be assessed because of the risks of trauma, infection and accidental haemorrhage.

ARTERIAL ACCESS

PERIPHERAL ARTERIAL CANNULATION

Indwelling catheters should be inserted when multiple samples are required. Some neonatologists site peripheral arterial lines in preference to umbilical artery catheterization. The radial, posterior tibial and dorsalis pedis arteries are most frequently used; the ulnar and temporal arteries are rarely cannulated. When cannulating the radial or ulnar arteries distal perfusion to the hand must be confirmed using Allen's test. Blanching of the hand occurs when both arteries are compressed; as the pressure is released alternately from the arteries normal colour and perfusion should return. Failure to perform this test may result in the loss of a fingertip or even the whole hand (pp. 924–925).

Equipment

- 24 gauge cannulae
- Luer-lock extension set and syringes; three-way tap
- Tape and splint
- Appropriate non-compliant tubing for measuring pressure, infusion pump and heparinized saline (1 unit/ml)
- Blood pressure transducer.

Procedure

1. The artery is identified and the skin cleaned.
2. The cannula is inserted into the artery at an angle of about 30° to the skin. When blood flashes back into the trocar chamber the catheter should be smoothly advanced along the lumen of the artery as the stylet is removed; blood loss is minimized by pressure over the tip of the catheter. A Luer-lock extension and three-way tap should be carefully attached and the catheter secured in place with tape and a splint, ensuring free aspiration of blood.
3. Heparinized saline should be infused at 0.5–1 ml/h to maintain catheter patency. Invasive blood pressure monitoring can be performed via an appropriate transducer.
4. Care must be taken during sampling and flushing to avoid trauma and spasm. If perfusion to the digits is compromised (p. 925) the arterial line must be removed immediately to avoid loss of fingers or toes (or worse). Peripheral artery catheters must be clearly labelled to avoid accidental drug injection.

UMBILICAL ARTERY CATHETERIZATION

Catheterization of the umbilical artery provides secure long-term access for invasive monitoring of blood pressure, arterial oxygenation, blood sampling and infusion of fluids. Catheters should be positioned in the low aorta at L3/L4, or above the diaphragm between T8/T10 avoiding the coeliac, mesenteric and renal arteries.

Equipment

- Catheterization pack containing drapes, artery clamps, scalpel, fine forceps and dilating probes
- Umbilical catheters 3.5 Fr for babies <1500 g or 5.0 Fr for babies >1500 g. Searle catheters with a terminal oxygen electrode allow continuous oxygen monitoring
- Cord ligature, three-way tap, Luer-locked extension sets and syringes
- Heparinized saline or dextrose (1 unit/ml)
- Blood pressure transducer.

Procedure

1. The infant must be carefully monitored and the head visualized to avoid accidental extubation. Success depends on adequate lighting, preparation and nursing assistance to stabilize the lower limbs.
2. Catheters must be inserted to the appropriate level in the aorta. The formula (3 × weight in kg + 9 + stump length) gives the distance in centimetres to position the catheter at T10. The shoulder tip to umbilicus measurement can be used (Appendix 9).
3. A cord ligature should be placed around the base of the cord to control any blood loss. The cord and periumbilical area should be carefully cleaned with an antiseptic solution: excess spillage must be avoided to prevent burns to the skin of the abdomen, flanks and buttocks. Catheterization must be performed aseptically. The catheter must be primed with saline and a closed three-way tap attached.
4. The cord should be cut horizontally about 0.5–1 cm away from the abdominal skin. The two thicker-walled arteries will stand proud of the stump below the thin-walled gaping umbilical vein (Fig. 51.10). The cord stump should be stabilized with artery forceps. One of the arteries should be dilated with the probe or fine non-toothed forceps; the catheter tip is then introduced into the artery and advanced into position with steady pressure.
5. Catheters can be secured using a tape 'H' bridge (Fig. 51.11). A zinc oxide tape flag fixed around the catheter can be sutured to the stump, the suture placed to include the remaining umbilical vessels to prevent haemorrhage (Fig. 51.12). Excess antiseptic solution must be washed off with sterile water, particularly from the baby's back, to avoid chemical burns (p. 931).
6. Correct placement must be confirmed with a chest/abdominal X-ray, showing the catheter looping via the umbilical and iliac arteries to the appropriate level in the aorta. Perfusion to the perineum and lower limbs must be assessed. If there is frank ischaemia the catheter must be removed immediately; if perfusion is borderline volume expansion with blood or albumin may restore the circulation. The abdomen and lower limbs must remain uncovered at all times to detect stump haemorrhage or lower limb perfusion problems.

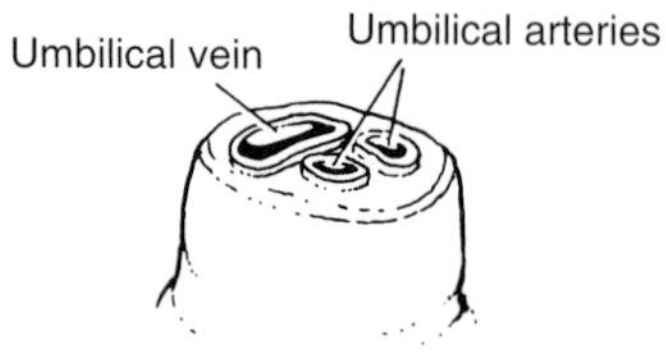

Fig. 51.10 The appearance of the cut surface of the umbilical cord.

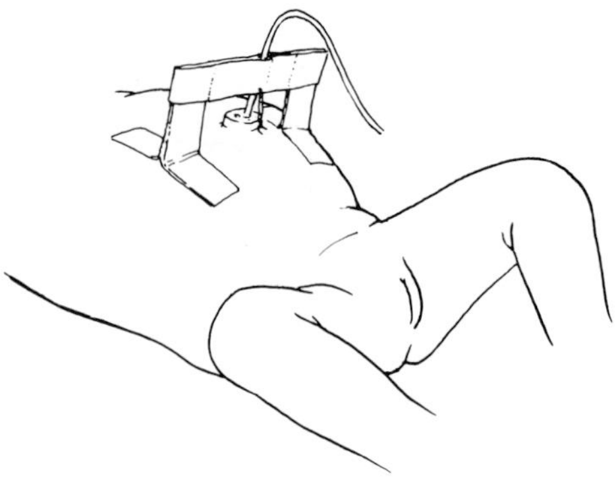

Fig. 51.11 'H' technique for immobilization of the umbilical catheter.

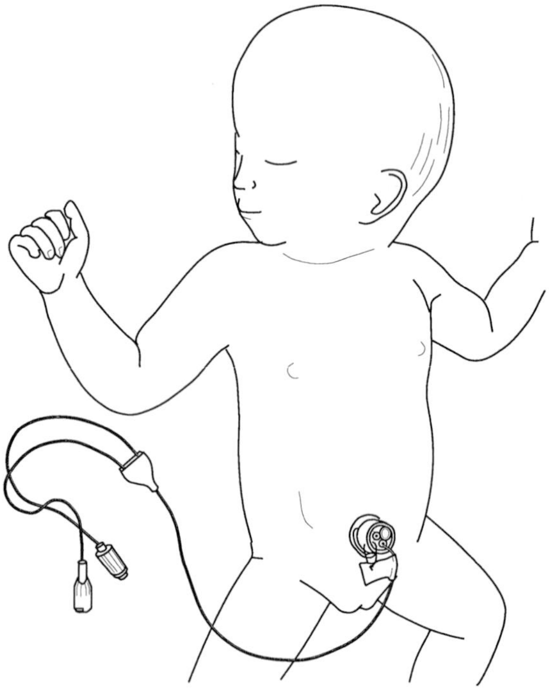

Fig. 51.12 'Flag' technique for immobilization of the umbilical catheter. A further suture should be placed to ligate the other artery and the vein to prevent haemorrhage.

7. Neonatologists differ in their practice of fluid administration via umbilical artery catheters. Some infuse small volumes of heparinized dextrose or saline, with remaining maintenance fluids administered via central or peripheral venous catheters. Others will infuse all fluids via the umbilical catheter, preserving the peripheral veins.
8. Umbilical artery catheters should be removed when they are no longer clinically indicated. The catheter should be withdrawn slowly, the final 5 cm over several minutes, allowing the artery to go into spasm, thereby minimizing blood loss. The hard dry Wharton's jelly that cakes around the catheter may need to be cleaned off before it will move freely. The stump should be sutured to prevent haemorrhage. The cord should be left exposed for a period after catheter withdrawal so that any delayed bleeding is easy to see.

VENOUS ACCESS

PERIPHERAL VENOUS CANNULATION

Peripheral venous cannulae should be inserted for antibiotic, intravenous fluid or drug administration. Veins on the dorsum of the hands, feet, wrist and scalp are suitable for cannulation. Larger, more proximal veins in the antecubital fossae, or the long saphenous veins at the ankle or knee can be used. However, if it is likely that the baby will need a percutaneous long line inserted at a later stage, suitable veins should be identified and preserved early on.

Equipment

- 24 G cannulae are suitable for most neonates; 26 G cannulae may be used in very premature infants
- Saline flush, T-piece connectors, Luer-lock extension sets
- Adhesive tape, splints.

Procedure

1. Identify a peripheral vein and clean the skin. Nursing assistance is usually required with vigorous babies to stabilize the limb, stretch the overlying skin and distend the veins. With small babies cannulae may be inserted without assistance. Rough handling has fractured limbs (p. 929).
2. The skin should be punctured 2–3 mm distal to the vein; with the bevel uppermost the cannula should be inserted into the vein; blood should then flash back into the hub of the trocar. The catheter and trocar should be advanced a further 1–2 mm to ensure that the catheter tip is in the lumen of the vein. The catheter is slipped into the vein as the trocar is removed. In larger veins free-flowing blood may confirm successful placement; in smaller veins a saline flush should be instilled without resistance or swelling.
3. The cannula and T-piece should be secured and the limb stabilized with a splint to minimize movement. Limb constriction must be avoided. Make it easy to see the part where the tip of the cannula is so that extravasation can be identified early when the drip 'tissues'. Virtually all neonatal infusions end their lives this way, and constant vigilance is essential to avoid scarring (p. 926–929).
4. Intravenous fluid should be administered via pressure-sensitive pumps, which will give early warning of problems at the infusion site. The catheter site must be observed hourly for signs of erythema and swelling.

UMBILICAL VENOUS CATHETERIZATION

Umbilical venous catheters can be inserted during the resuscitation of shocked or asphyxiated infants in the delivery room; drugs and fluids can be safely administered if blood can be aspirated. UVC should pass through the ductus venosus into the right atrium, where they can be used for fluid administration and central venous pressure measurement. Air emboli and hepatic necrosis are potential complications of UVC use (p. 924). Air embolism is a constant danger once a catheter is in the chest, when it is more likely that air will enter the circulation than that blood will come out.

Equipment

As for umbilical artery catheterization.

Procedure

1. The length of catheter to enter the right atrium is calculated from the formula (2 × weight in kilograms + 5 + stump length; Appendix 10). Shoulder-tip to umbilicus measurements can also be used.
2. The umbilical stump should be prepared as for umbilical artery catheterization. The thin-walled gaping vein lies above the two thicker-walled arteries (Fig. 51.10). The primed catheter with a closed three-way tap attached should be inserted into the vein and advanced into position; blood should be aspirated and the catheter fixed in place. The venous catheter must be clearly labelled.
3. A chest/abdominal X-ray should confirm the venous catheter following a direct course to the right atrium. If the catheter deviates into the liver it must be removed.
4. The venous catheter can be used for blood sampling and central venous pressure monitoring.
5. The catheter should be removed when it is no longer required; gentle pressure on the stump usually controls blood loss.

CENTRAL VENOUS CATHETERIZATION VIA PERIPHERAL VEINS

Central venous catheters provide a safe route for the long-term administration of parenteral nutrition and drug infusions. Catheters are inserted into the veins of the antecubital fossa, the long saphenous vein at the medial side of the ankle or knee, and superficial temporal veins. The axillary and external jugular veins can also be cannulated but trauma to adjacent arteries, nerves or the lung may occur. Correct placement of the line is essential, as catheters in the heart may cause arrhythmias or pericardial effusions. These lines must be inserted aseptically, and once in place the lines and circuits must be interfered with as little as possible to minimize the risk of introducing infection.

Equipment

- Long line insertion pack containing a catheter, forceps, syringes and introducer. The type of introducer depends on the line to be inserted. With the new all-in-one systems peelable cannulae or splittable needles must be used. If the line can be removed from its compression hub a G19 butterfly or G20 peripheral cannula can be used. Fine 27G central lines can be inserted through a G24 cannula
- Sterile dressing pack with drapes
- Luer-lock extension sets primed with saline
- Niopam contrast medium.

Procedure

1. Measure the length of catheter to be inserted: the line tip should lie in the superior or inferior vena cava at the right atrium.
2. Clean the overlying skin and adjacent area, and position drapes to ensure a sterile field; aseptic technique is vital.
3. The introducer is inserted into the vein; when free-flowing blood is obtained the primed catheter is threaded into position using non-toothed forceps (Fig. 51.13). Occasionally problems occur when threading the line: passage around the shoulder may be facilitated by abducting the arm, through the neck by gently extending the neck, and through the groin by abducting the hip. Saline should be infused with minimal pressure.
4. The introducer should be carefully removed or split without dislodging the catheter. Silastic catheters need to be fixed into the compression hub, which must be fully tightened.
5. The line should initially be secured with steristrips and an X-ray performed to confirm position. Polyurethane catheters are radio-opaque; silastic catheters need to be flushed with 0.5–1.0 ml of Niopam prior to the X-ray. The line tip should be at the junction of the vena cavae and atrium. Lines which have passed into the heart must be withdrawn; short lines may be used if the tip is in a large vein. When correct placement is confirmed the catheter and hub must be fixed in position without kinking the line, the whole system covered with a clear adhesive dressing and the limb supported using a splint (Fig. 51.14).
6. Drug infusions, parenteral nutrition and intralipid should be administered using pressure-sensitive pumps. FG27 long lines often require higher pressures. The insertion site and limb must be observed for signs of local inflammation or phlebitis along the course of the catheter. If the catheter is no longer required or the baby develops septicaemia it should be removed.

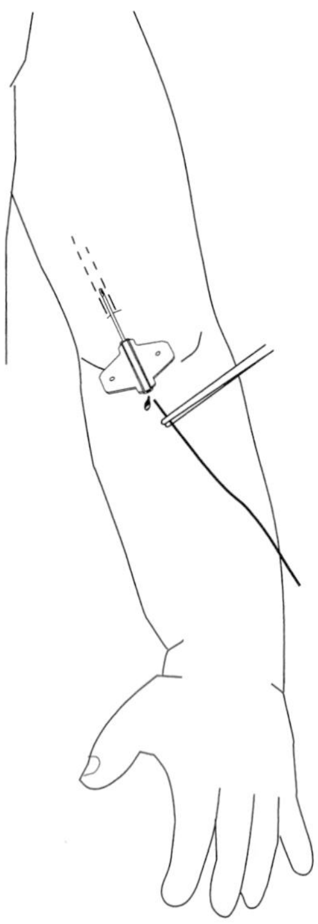

Fig. 51.13 Central venous catheter insertion through a needle used as an introducer.

CENTRAL VENOUS CATHETERIZATION VIA PROXIMAL CENTRAL VEINS

These routes are should be utilized when all other vascular access has been exhausted. The internal jugular, subclavian and femoral veins are all accessible, but damage to adjacent neurovascular structures is a risk. The femoral vein is the safest route, avoiding both the lungs and airway. The line must be inserted by an experienced practitioner who is aware of the regional anatomy and familiar with the equipment and the Seldinger technique, threading the catheter over a guide-

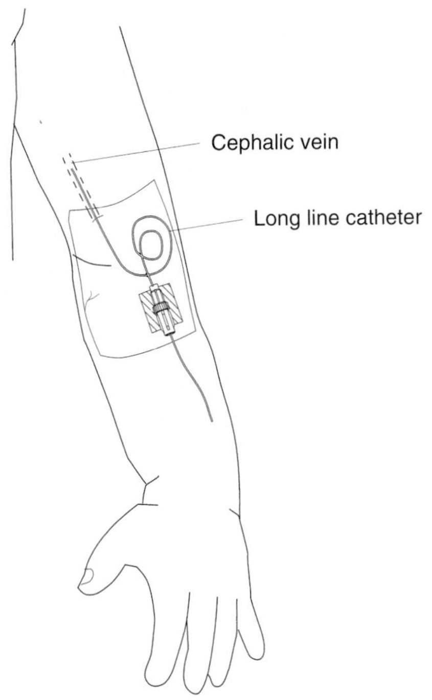

Fig. 51.14 Central venous catheter insertion completed; the compression hub and silastic line are protected by a transparent adhesive dressing.

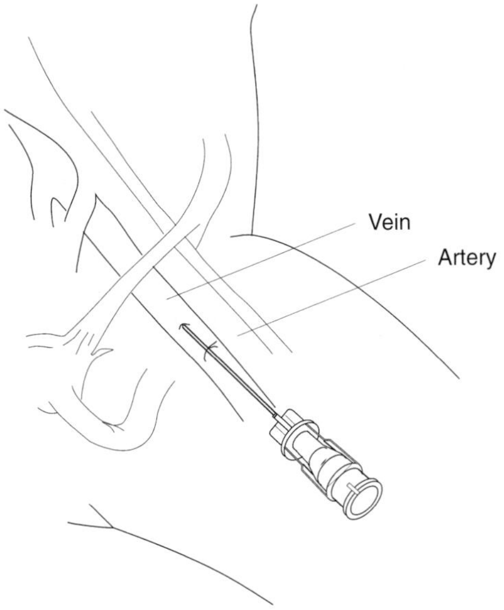

Fig. 51.15 Central line introducer inserted into the femoral vein, awaiting guidewire insertion.

wire inserted through an introducing needle (Fig. 51.15). The infant will need to be sedated and possibly paralysed. Successful line placement should be confirmed by aspiration of blood from each lumen of the line and a radiograph. The catheter should be sutured in place and can remain in situ for many days. Transient venous engorgement of the distal limb is acceptable provided arterial perfusion is not compromised.

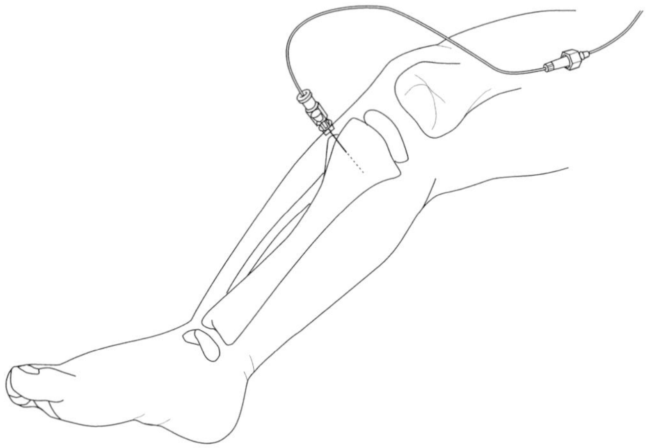

Fig. 51.16 Intraosseous spinal needle inserted into the bone marrow of the tibia, with fluid infusing.

INTRAOSSEOUS LINE INSERTION

In a collapsed infant where the umbilical cord is no longer available and peripheral cannulation has failed, an intraosseous line can be inserted into the medial aspect of the tibia for administration of resuscitation drugs, fluids and blood sampling. A 22 G 1.5 inch spinal needle with trocar should be screwed through the bone of the tibial plate into the marrow cavity (Fig. 51.16). Fluids can be infused without resistance; swelling on the posterior aspect of the tibia indicates that the needle is not in place. Intraosseous lines should be removed when conventional vascular access has been achieved.

FEEDING TUBES

Ill or preterm infants sometimes require tube feeding. Breast or formula milk is passed into the gut via a soft nasogastric, orogastric or nasojejunal feeding tube. Feeding tubes are needed to decompress the stomach or bowel when there is abdominal distension.

NASOGASTRIC/OROGASTRIC FEEDING TUBES

For babies weighing <1000 g 4 FG feeding tubes are used and for all other babies size 6 FG. For abdominal decompression, size 8–10 FG tubes should be used.

Procedure

1. The distance from xiphisternum to ear tip indicates the length of tubing to be inserted for a nasogastric tube; for an orogastic tube measure the distance from the nasal bridge to the xiphisternum.
2. With the baby supine the lightly lubricated tube is gently passed through the nostril into the stomach while observing the baby's colour. Failure of the tube to pass through the nose may indicate choanal atresia; coiling in the midoesophagus suggests oesophageal atresia.

3. Correct placement is confirmed by the aspiration of acidic fluid, which turns blue litmus paper red. Alternatively, auscultate over the stomach as air is injected down the tube. NGT should be taped to the cheek, orogastric tubes to the chin. The position of the tube can be confirmed on chest or abdominal radiographs, but these are not carried out routinely and the acid litmus or auscultatory tests are considered sufficient. Bile-stained aspirates are abnormal and can be due to an abnormal bowel or because the NGT has slipped into the duodenum Correct tube placement must be confirmed, by aspirating the stomach contents, prior to each feed. Feeds should be given slowly under gravity, with the tube capped off between feeds.
4. Tubes placed to decompress the abdomen should be left on free drainage with a careful record of fluid losses. When infants receive nasal CPAP the NGT may be left open to vent air from the stomach.

NASOJEJUNAL FEEDING TUBES

Nasojejunal feeding is an alternative to intravenous nutrition when gastric feeding has failed because of delayed emptying.

Procedure

1. With the infant supine the measurement from nasal bridge to ankle indicates the length of tube to be inserted. Nasal bridge to the umbilicus gives the length of tube to reach the stomach.
2. With the baby on its right side the tube is advanced; when the length marker reaches the umbilicus the tip of the tube should lie in the stomach.
3. The tube is advanced after injecting 2 ml of sterile water; peristaltic activity should carry the tube through the pylorus. When the marker reaches the nostril the tube should lie in the jejunum. The tube should then be fixed to the cheek and an orogastric tube inserted. Correct placement of both tubes should be confirmed by X-ray.
4. Feeds are administered by continuous infusion.
5. Fluid can rarely be aspirated from the nasojejunal tube; milk in the orogastric tube indicates that the nasojejunal tube has slipped back into the stomach.

URINE COLLECTION

Urine samples may be required for microbiological, biochemical or metabolic assessment. Weighed nappies are an important part of fluid balance assessment (p. 1022). When urine culture is required the urine must be collected aseptically. Several different collection systems are available.

- **Cottonwool balls** placed between the thighs will soak up urine, which can then be squeezed out and sent for biochemical or metabolic analysis. Meconium contamination is a common problem.
- **The finger of a sterile glove** slipped over the end of the penis can be used to collect small samples of urine, which can be sent for biochemical or microbiological assay.
- **Adhesive bags** are commonly used to collect urine; this method is more successful in males, where the penis can be directed into the bag. Skin contamination is avoided by cleaning the perineum. Meconium contamination frequently occurs in girls. Repeated application of bags may damage the perineal skin. The damage can be reduced by first spraying the skin with a protective dressing (p. 931).
- **Suprapubic aspiration of the bladder** is the optimal method by which to obtain clean urine. The bladder tap should be performed after a feed when the baby's nappy is dry. An ultrasound scan can confirm that the bladder contains urine (Fig. 51.17).

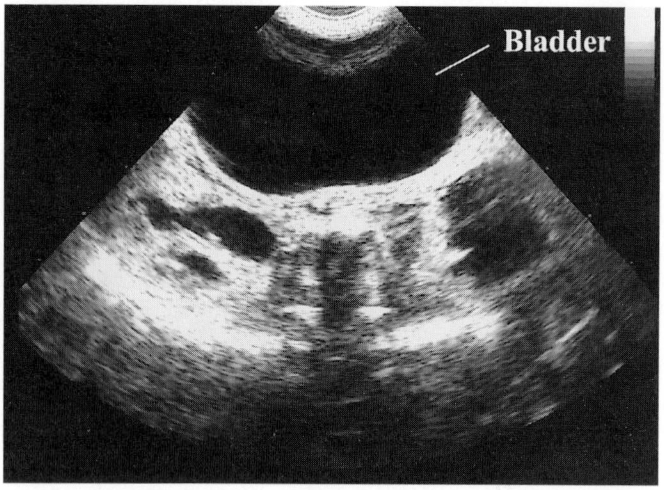

Fig. 51.17 Abdominal ultrasound scan confirming a full bladder.

Equipment

— Sterile dressing pack
— 2.5 ml syringe and 23 gauge needle.

Procedure

With the baby supine an assistant holds the lower limbs with the hips abducted. The symphysis pubis is identified and the skin cleaned. With aseptic technique the abdominal wall is punctured in the midline 1 cm above the symphysis (Fig. 51.18). The needle is advanced perpendicular to the skin, maintaining constant suction on the syringe. The bladder wall should be penetrated and clean urine aspirated 1–2 cm below the skin. The sample should be sent to the laboratory and the puncture site covered.

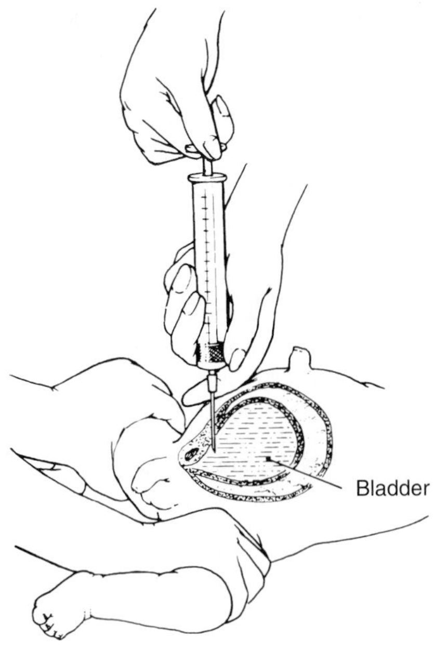

Fig. 51.18 Technique for suprapubic bladder aspiration.

- **Bladder catheterization** may be required in renal failure for precise measurement of urine output. A suprapubic catheter may be inserted by a urologist if urethral abnormalities cause urinary retention.

Equipment

— Sterile dressing pack
— 4 FG soft feeding tube
— Lubricating analgesic gel
— Collection system.

Procedure

Bladder catheterization must be performed aseptically. Having cleaned the vulva or penis, the lubricated feeding tube is advanced through the urethral meatus into the bladder. Excessive force may damage the urethra, causing haematuria and later stricture formation. Avoid using very long lengths of tubing, which can become knotted or kinked (p. 934). The catheter should be fixed to the thigh and connected to the collecting system. Catheters should be removed as soon as possible to minimize infection.

CEREBROSPINAL FLUID COLLECTION

LUMBAR PUNCTURES

These should be performed as part of a septic screen to diagnose meningitis, in the investigation of neonatal seizures and to relieve raised intracranial pressure in communicating hydrocephalus. Lumbar punctures should not be performed in the presence of lumbosacral abnormalities. Infants with respiratory symptoms may not tolerate the procedure, which should be delayed until the infant is clinically stable. Any bleeding diathesis and thrombocytopenia must be corrected first.

Equipment

- Sterile dressing pack
- Spinal needle 22 G, 1.5 inch with stylet
- Sterile numbered universal containers, fluoride glucose assay tube
- Manometer three-way tap for pressure measurements.

Procedure

The success of the procedure depends on an experienced assistant to hold the infant. Most lumbar punctures are performed with the infant on his left side, but he can be held in a sitting position. The infant should be monitored throughout the procedure.

1. The L4 spinous process should be identified on a line joining the iliac crests. The lumbar puncture should be performed in the L3/L4 intervertebral space, avoiding the spinal cord which lies at L2. The whole area must be cleaned with an antiseptic solution and the baby must lie on a sterile towel. Full aseptic technique is essential to prevent introducing infection.
2. With the back flexed, the needle is inserted in the midline of the L3/L4 space and advanced to a depth of about 1 cm. A subtle change in resistance may be detected as the dura is penetrated; CSF should then be obtained when the stylet is removed. Gentle rotation of the needle may facilitate flow. Bloodstained samples usually result from damage to the venous plexus on the posterior surface of the vertebral body, and are rarely caused by subarachnoid haemorrhage.
3. Six to 10 drops of CSF in each universal container and two to three drops in the fluoride tube should be sufficient for Gram stain, culture, glucose and protein measurements. Normal CSF values are given in Appendix 11.
4. When treating hydrocephalus an opening pressure should be measured by attaching the spinal needle via a T-piece connector to the manometer. Larger volumes of CSF (10 ml/kg) should be allowed to drip out over 10 minutes.
5. The stylet should be replaced, the needle withdrawn and the puncture site sprayed with adhesive dressing.

VENTRICULAR TAPS

These are done to diagnose ventriculitis, administer intrathecal antibiotics and drain CSF in non-communicating hydrocephalus.

Equipment

As for lumbar puncture.

Procedure

1. Ventriculomegaly should be confirmed by ultrasound and measurements taken to determine the depth and direction of needle insertion.
2. Shave the scalp overlying the lateral angle of the anterior fontanelle, and clean the skin with an antiseptic solution. The tap must be performed with strict aseptic technique.
3. Lie the baby supine with the top of his head toward the operator. With an assistant firmly holding the head a spinal needle is inserted into the lateral angle of the fontanelle and advanced toward the inner angle of the ipsilateral eye. The needle must be inserted smoothly without change of direction to minimize trauma to the brain until the ventricle is penetrated. When the stylet is removed CSF should drip out, a T-piece connector can be attached to the end of the needle and the opening pressure measured with a manometer. CSF should be allowed to drip out over several minutes: it should not be aspirated as this can cause haemorrhage.
4. The puncture site should be sprayed with adhesive dressing when the needle is removed.

SUBDURAL TAPS

These are performed to drain subdural collections causing midline shift. Collections should be confirmed by ultrasound (Fig. 51.19). The procedure is similar to ventricular puncture: a short spinal needle, FG24 cannula or FG22 butterfly is inserted into the collection from the lateral angle of the anterior fontanelle, and fluid allowed to drip out. If the contents are not liquid enough to drip then neurosurgical evacuation may be required.

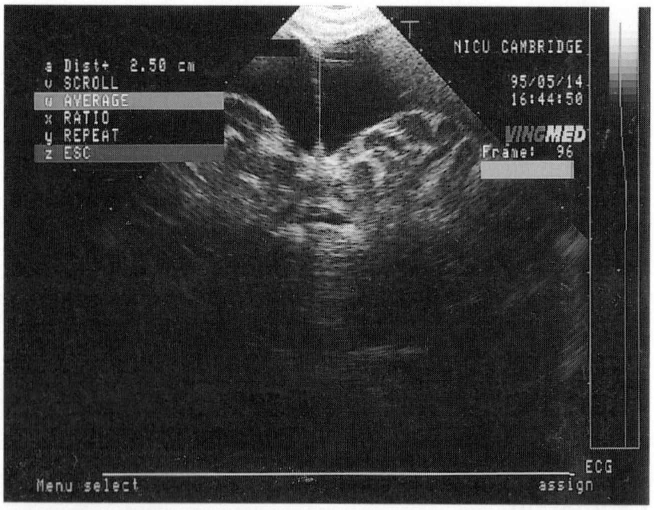

Fig. 51.19 Cranial ultrasound scan showing 25 mm subdural fluid collection.

ASPIRATION OF CSF FROM RICKHAM RESERVOIRS

Rickham/Ommaya reservoirs may be inserted for the administration of intrathecal antibiotics or repeated aspiration of CSF. They are usually sited over the frontal region of the skull. The overlying skin should be cleaned with an antiseptic solution, and a G25 butterfly inserted perpendicularly through the skin and reservoir membrane. Fluid should be aspirated slowly over 10–15 minutes. The puncture site should be sprayed with adhesive dressing when the butterfly is removed.

ABDOMINAL PARACENTESIS

Abdominal ascites should be confirmed by an ultrasound scan. Paracentesis can be performed to drain ascites, which may be splinting the diaphragm, or as a diagnostic procedure when bile or meconium-stained fluid suggests intestinal perforation. Fluid should be aspirated from the left iliac fossa to avoid the liver and spleen. The skin should be cleaned and 1% lignocaine infiltrated. An FG22/24 intravenous cannula should be carefully inserted through the abdominal wall and peritoneum. The soft catheter is threaded into the peritoneal cavity while withdrawing the trocar, so minimizing the risk of accidental perforation of the bowel. A diagnostic tap can be performed or the catheter can be left in situ to drain larger quantities of fluid.

BONE MARROW ASPIRATION

Bone marrow samples should be taken to diagnose congenital leukaemia or marrow failure. Aspirates can be collected from the anterior iliac spine, posterior iliac crest or tibia. In the neonate the tibia is the preferred site.

Equipment

- Sterile dressing pack
- Bone marrow aspiration needle, 1.5 inch G22 lumbar puncture needle
- Collection bottles, microscope slides for smear preparations.

Procedure

1. The infant is positioned and held firmly.
2. The overlying skin is cleaned and 1% lignocaine infiltrated into the skin, subcutaneous tissues and periosteum.
3. The needle is inserted perpendicular to the bone and screwed into the marrow cavity. Marrow should be aspirated after the stylet has been removed.
4. The marrow aspirate is prepared and stored as directed by the paediatric haematologist.

SPECIALIST PROCEDURES

DIAGNOSIS AND DRAINAGE OF PNEUMOTHORAX

A pneumothorax should be suspected in any ventilated infant who deteriorates with asymmetrical chest wall movement and air entry. In a darkened room the affected side will transilluminate when a fibreoptic cold light is applied to the chest; the normal side with an inflated lung will not transilluminate. In very premature infants, or those with interstitial emphysema, transillumination may be present in the absence of a pneumothorax. Chest X-rays should be performed to confirm the diagnosis where possible.

In an emergency a tension pneumothorax can be drained by inserting a 21 or 23 gauge butterfly into the pleural cavity via the second intercostal space in the midclavicular line. The butterfly tubing should be placed under water, allowing free gas to bubble out, or a three-way tap can be attached to the tubing and the gas aspirated with a syringe until the lung is inflated. A formal chest drain should always be inserted after this emergency procedure has been used; preferably a proper chest drain should be used in the first place.

Insertion of chest drain

Chest drains are used to drain a pneumothorax, pleural effusion or chylothorax. Pneumothoraces occur relatively frequently in ventilated neonates, and a prepared chest drain pack should always be available for use on a neonatal unit.

Equipment

- Sterile dressing pack
- Scalpel, straight surgical blade, artery forceps and suture
- Intercostal drain
- Underwater drainage system and suction pump
- Zinc oxide tape and Tegaderm transparent dressing.

Procedure

1. Position the baby with the affected side elevated to about 30–45° by placing a towel under the back; this should ensure that the drain is directed anteriorly. An assistant should rotate the arm away towards the head.
2. Clean the skin in the midaxillary line and infiltrate 1% lignocaine at the insertion site, well lateral to the breast bud. The drain must be inserted with sterile technique.
3. With a straight scalpel blade a small incision is made just above the rib, just large enough to admit the drain. Use the scalpel only to make a skin incision and to cut part of the track through which the drain will pass.
4. Use artery forceps in blunt dissection to open a track through which the drain can be guided, right down to the pleura if the trocar is not to be used (see 5).
5. Insert the drain. Most neonatologists choose to remove the sharp metal trocar supplied with the chest drain set, pushing the soft plastic drain alone through the established track. The drain should be pushed 2–3 cm into the pleural space, and aimed up towards the lung apex.
6. Connect the drain to the underwater drainage system. Bubbles should appear. A negative pressure of 5–10 cm H_2O can be applied to aid drainage. Very persistent bubbling can indicate that there is a bronchopleural fistula.
7. An anchoring suture is placed across the incision to seal the wound around the drain. The suture is then tied to the zinc oxide flag placed around the drain at the chest wall. An adhesive dressing can be applied to cover the drain to prevent it being dislodged (Fig. 51.20).
8. Correct positioning of the drain and resolution of the pneumothorax should be confirmed by chest X-ray.

Removal of chest drains

Once a pneumothorax has been drained it may be safer to leave the drain in place until the infant is no longer ventilated, although it is possible to remove drains while the baby is still on positive pressure ventilation if this looks likely to be long term. Once the drain is no longer bubbling suction can be taken off and a period of 24 hours allowed to elapse; many would add a further period

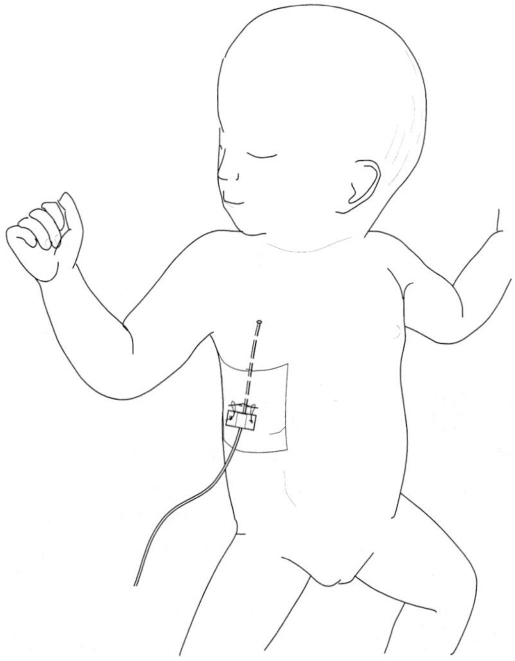

Fig. 51.20 Chest drain insertion: note the drain is directed toward the apex of the lung and is held in place by a zinc oxide tape flag sutured to the skin, which is covered by an adhesive dressing.

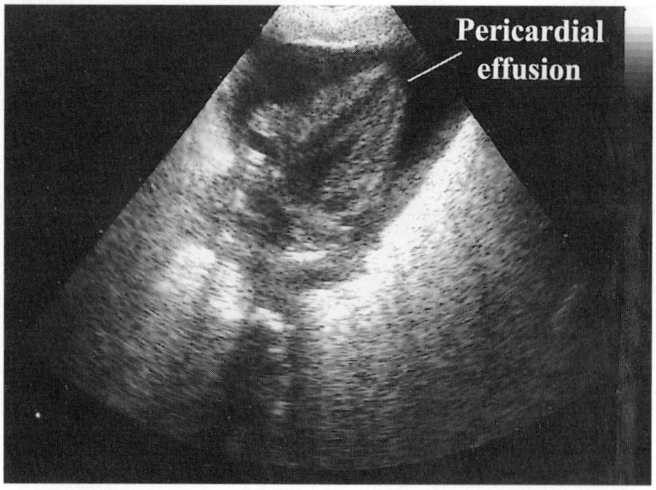

Fig. 51.21 Cardiac ultrasound showing a pericardial effusion from a displaced long line.

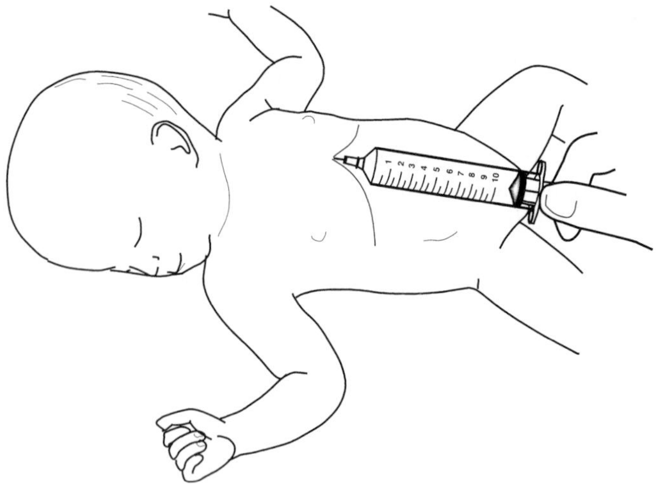

Fig. 51.22 The subxiphisternal approach to drain a pericardial effusion; note the cannula is directed toward the left shoulder.

of observation with the drain clamped, particularly if the child is still ventilated. An X-ray should be taken after this trial period to check that the pneumothorax has not reaccumulated.

The drain should then be withdrawn rapidly from the pleural cavity and the incision immediately pinched closed. Steristrips should be applied across the incision to provide an airtight seal: purse string sutures produce unsightly scars. Another chest X-ray should be performed to ensure that the pneumothorax has not reaccumulated.

DRAINAGE OF PNEUMOMEDIASTINUM

The presence of the angel-wing sign on the supine chest radiograph confirms a pneumomediastinum (p. 524); such collections rarely require drainage and usually reabsorb spontaneously. If the infant has cardiovascular symptoms, the collection should be drained from a subxiphisternal approach. An intravenous cannula should allow aspiration of the anterior gas; drains are rarely required.

DRAINAGE OF PERICARDIAL EFFUSION

Pericardial effusions should be suspected in the presence of tachycardia, poor perfusion, soft heart sounds and increasing cardiomegaly. Effusions can occur in neonatal hydrops or from extravasation of TPN from migrated long lines (p. 926). Echocardiography easily confirms the effusion and shows the best approach for drainage (Fig. 51.21). The effusion should be drained if there is cardiovascular compromise, using the subxiphisternal approach. After cleaning the skin a 22/24 G cannula should be inserted at an angle of 30° to the skin, directed towards the left shoulder (Fig. 51.22). Aspirated fluid should be sent for microbiological and biochemical assay. Only if the effusion reaccumulates will it be necessary to leave a catheter in situ.

DRAINAGE OF PNEUMOPERICARDIUM

The presence of air within the pericardium or heart should be suspected in an infant who suddenly deteriorates in the presence of other airleaks; there may not be time to perform a chest X-ray (p. 525). The air must be drained urgently via the subxiphisternal approach, as described above (Fig. 51.22). The stylet should be removed and air aspirated; if blood is obtained the cannula has been inserted too far. In the presence of cardiac tamponade drainage of the air will produce dramatic benefit.

DRAINAGE OF PLEURAL EFFUSION

Pleural effusions may be suggested by chest X-ray and should be confirmed by ultrasound. A diagnostic tap of the fluid can be done using a 20 G cannula inserted into the pleural cavity in the posterior axillary line. When drains are inserted to treat large effusions they should be placed posteriorly and directed inferiorly within the chest. Fluid should be sent for microbiological and immunological studies.

EXCHANGE TRANSFUSION

Exchange transfusions are still required for rhesus haemolytic disease (p. 820) or hyperbilirubinaemia from other causes (p. 728), and are sometimes performed in severe sepsis or disseminated intravascular coagulation. Ideally the need for an exchange transfusion should be anticipated, so that the necessary vascular access can be organized and suitable blood for the exchange ordered well in advance. The simplest method of carrying out a double-volume exchange transfusion is to use an umbilical venous catheter, sited in the high inferior vena cava or the right atrium, for both withdrawal and replacement of blood. Alternatively, blood can be withdrawn from a central or peripheral arterial catheter and replaced into any vein.

Equipment

- Arterial and venous access, via central or peripheral catheters
- Cross-matched, fresh rhesus-negative irradiated whole blood
- Blood administration sets and warming coils
- High flow rate infusion pump.

Procedure

Any infant undergoing an exchange transfusion must be carefully monitored to avoid electrolyte, blood glucose, acid–base and platelet disturbances. Serum electrolytes, glucose, calcium and blood gases should be measured before the exchange starts.

1. The administration set and warmer must be primed. The pH of the blood should be measured and, if the blood is acidotic, 7% THAM should be added to it to obtain a pH of 7.3.
2. In the standard method the whole procedure is carried out using the umbilical venous catheter. Blood is withdrawn in 5–20 ml aliquots (according to the size of the baby) over a few minutes. A multiway tap allows the following sequence to take place: withdraw blood from baby, turn tap, push blood into waste bag, turn tap, draw in fresh blood from transfusion pack, turn tap, replace blood into baby. A double-volume exchange (160 ml/kg) takes about 2 hours.
3. Alternatively, blood can be replaced as a continuous infusion into a large vein while removing blood from an arterial catheter. Pumps delivering 120 ml/h allow 10 ml of blood to be removed every 5 minutes.
4. Accurate recording of the blood volumes exchanged is vital: an assistant must be present throughout the procedure. Biochemistry, calcium, blood sugar and acid–base status should be measured midway through, and on completion of the exchange transfusion.
5. Catheters should be left in situ until no further exchanges are required.

DILUTIONAL EXCHANGE TRANSFUSION

Polycythaemic infants with a packed cell volume (PCV) of between 65 and 70% in a free-flowing blood sample are at risk of ischaemic injury to the gut or brain. Blood is withdrawn and replaced with albumin or saline in the same way as for exchange transfusion, either using an umbilical venous catheter or with a peripheral venous infusion and an arterial line. The volume of blood that needs to be removed and replaced with saline is calculated from the following formula:

$$\text{Volume removed} = \frac{\text{Observed PCV} - \text{Desired PCV}}{\text{Observed PCV}} \times \text{Blood volume}$$

PERITONEAL DIALYSIS

Hyperkalaemia, metabolic acidosis, oliguria and renal failure are indications for dialysis. Peritoneal dialysis conducted with the support of a paediatric nephrologist can be used to correct these metabolic problems. Peritoneal dialysis may not be appropriate if there are respiratory problems, as further distension of the abdomen may splint the diaphragm and cause additional respiratory compromise.

Equipment

- Sterile dressing pack
- Suitable dialysis catheter, e.g. Guy's paediatric PD catheter. In an emergency make your own by cutting holes in a soft FG10–12 catheter
- Dialysis fluids, heparin, Luer lock extension sets, Y-connectors, warming bath
- Urimeter collection chamber.

Procedure

1. The skin is cleaned over the insertion site, either in the midline one-third distance between the umbilicus and the left symphysis pubis, or lateral to the rectus sheath in the left iliac fossa.
2. Lignocaine 1% is infiltrated into the abdominal wall and a cannula inserted; the abdomen is inflated with 20 ml/kg of warm dialysate and the dialysis catheter advanced into position and secured.
3. The catheter is connected to the extension sets and the patency of the whole system is tested.
4. Dialysis can be commenced. Cycles of 60 minutes are usual: 20 ml/kg of dialysate are infused and allowed to dwell for 15–30 minutes, and the abdomen is drained over 10–15 minutes. The duration of the cycle and volumes can be altered depending on the response. Electrolytes, heparin and antibiotics should be added to the dialysis fluid as needed.

Peritoneal dialysis should be discontinued when urine output is adequate.

HAEMOFILTRATION

Arteriovenous haemofiltration is technically more difficult than peritoneal dialysis, but it is the method of choice in the fluid-overloaded hydropic infant with respiratory difficulties. Successful haemofiltration can be carried out via large umbilical arterial and venous catheters, provided the infant has an adequate blood pressure to drive blood through the filter.

Equipment

- Sterile dressing packs
- Arterial and venous catheters
- FH22 neonatal haemofilter and tubing
- 4.5% Albumin to prime, heparinized saline.

Procedure

1. Vascular catheters should be inserted.
2. The filter should be primed with albumin, the inflow port should be connected to the arterial catheter and the outflow port should be attached to the venous catheter. Use a suitable size filter: the smallest have an internal volume of about 12 ml.
3. A heparin infusion is put into the arterial side of the filter to maintain patency. The volume of fluid drained from the filter should be recorded hourly. The amount of haemofiltration fluid to be replaced depends on the infant's fluid balance.
4. Neonatal haemofilters have a limited life and must be replaced when the filtration rate falls. Successful haemofiltration will correct electrolyte abnormalities and create space for the administration of appropriate nutrition.

Section 9

Pharmacopoeia

52

Pharmacopoeia

Sam Richmond

Suggested dosage and dose frequency of the more commonly used drugs. For more detailed information see the *Neonatal Formulary* compiled by the Northern Neonatal Network. BMJ Books, London, 1998.

Drug	Indication, mode of action and comments	Route	Dose	*Post menstrual/* chronological age	Frequency (times/24 h)
Acyclovir	For herpes simplex (HS) and varicella (VZ). Treat HS for at least 2 weeks. Use with zoster immune globulin in VZ.	i.v.	15 mg/kg per dose*	*More than 33 wks*	3
			10 mg/kg per dose* (*give over 1 hour)	*33 weeks and less*	2
Adenosine	Used to stop supraventricular tachycardia when facial immersion in iced water is unsuccessful or impractical. An ECG record of the transition is invaluable.	i.v. by *rapid bolus*	200 microg/kg per dose *(max 300 microg/kg per dose)*		repeatable
Adrenaline	Cardiac arrest. Usually given i.v. but can also be given by direct intracardiac injection or by the intraosseous or intratracheal routes.	i.v.	10–100 microg/kg per dose		repeatable
	For severe hypotension it can be given by infusion. (1/1000 = 1 mg/ml and 1/10 000 = 100 microg/ml)	i.v. infusion	0.1–0.3 microg/kg per min *(max 1.5 microg/kg per min)*		infusion
Amiodarone	Class III antiarrhythmic for arrhythmias refractory to other therapies. *Should not be used except under **direct** supervision of a paediatric cardiologist.*	i.v. i.v. infusion	5 mg/kg loading dose 1 mg/kg per hour		once only infusion
		oral	10 mg/kg for 10–14 days then 7.5 mg/kg thereafter		1
Amoxycillin	Broad-spectrum semisynthetic aminopenicillin. Better absorbed by mouth than ampicillin. Drug of choice for *Listeria* infection.	oral i.v., i.m.	50 mg/kg per dose (100 mg/kg in meningitis)	0–1 week 1–3 weeks 4 weeks or more	2 3 4
Amphotericin	Polyene antifungal for systemic fungal infections. (See also flucytosine and fluconazole.)	i.v.	0.5 mg/kg per dose (give over 4–6 hours)		1
Ampicillin	Drug of choice for *Listeria* infection.	i.v., i.m., oral	as amoxycillin	as amoxycillin	as amoxycillin
Atracurium	Competitive non-depolarizing muscle relaxant. Duration of action 15–30 minutes.	i.v. bolus	500 microg/kg		single dose
Atropine	Muscarinic blocker – to treat bradycardia (not a resuscitation drug) – for premedication.	 i.v. subcut., i.m.	15 microg/kg		single dose

Drug	Indication, mode of action and comments	Route	Dose	*Post menstrual/* chronological age	Frequency (times/24 h)
Azlocillin	Acylureidopenicillin used for *Pseudomonas* infections (normally with an aminoglycoside for synergistic effect).	i.v., i.m.	50 mg/kg per dose 100 mg/kg per dose	0–3 weeks more than 3 weeks	3 (*<37 wks – 2)* 3 (*<37 wks – 2)*
Aztreonam	Narrow-spectrum β-lactam antibiotic active against Gram-negative bacteria only. Penetrates inflamed CSF. Increase dose interval in renal failure.	i.v.	30 mg/kg per dose	0–1 weeks 1–3 weeks 4 weeks or more	2 3 4
Caffeine citrate	Increases respiratory drive. Both the loading dose and the maintenance dose may be safely doubled. (1 mg of caffeine *citrate* = 0.5 mg of caffeine *base*.)	i.v., oral	loading dose 20 mg/kg maintenance 5 mg/kg per dose		once only 1
Calcium gluconate	For temporary rapid control of cardiac effects of hyperkalaemia; see also Salbutamol. Precipitates with bicarbonate, sulphates or phosphates.	i.v.	2 ml of 10% solution/kg slowly (i.e. 200 mg/kg per dose)		once only
	For correction of hypocalcaemia (see also Magnesium sulphate).	oral	1.5 ml of 10% soln./kg per dose		4-hourly in feeds
Captopril	Angiotensin-converting enzyme (ACE) inhibitor. Vasodilator, reduces afterload in heart failure, may cause hypotension – try a test dose of 100 microg and monitor blood pressure. Unwise with renal impairment, hyponatraemia or hypovolaemia. Labetalol is a safer option for acute control of hypertension.	oral	test dose 100 microg start at 125 microg/kg per dose (*max 3 mg/kg per dose*)		 2
Carbamazepine	Anticonvulsant. Build up to full dose over several days. Optimum plasma level 4–12 mg/l; 1 mg = 4.23 micromol.	oral	5–15 mg/kg per dose		2
Carbenicillin	Penicillinase-sensitive and acid-labile penicillin, used for *Pseudomonas*; azlocillin is often preferred.	i.v.	100 mg/kg per dose	0–1 week 1–3 weeks 4 weeks or more	2 3 4
Carbimazole	Thioamide antithyroid, alternative to propylthiouracil.	oral	250 microg/kg		3
Cefotaxime	Third-generation cephalosporin especially useful in meningitis. Increase dosage interval in renal failure.	i.v., i.m.	50 mg/kg per dose	0–1 week 1–3 weeks 4 weeks or more	2 3 4
Ceftazidime	Third-generation cephalosporin especially useful for *Pseudomonas*. Increase dosage interval in renal failure.	i.v.	25 mg/kg per dose (50 mg/kg in meningitis)	up to 4 weeks 4 weeks and over	2 3
Chloral hydrate	Hypnotic – for short-term sedation – for sustained sedation.	oral	45 mg/kg single dose 30 mg/kg per dose		once only max 4 in 24 hours
Chloramphenicol	Drug levels should be checked if possible. Aim for a peak level of 15–20 mg/l in serum. (1 mg = 3.09 micromol). Good CSF penetration.	i.v., oral	loading dose 20 mg/kg maintenance 12 mg/kg per dose	 0–2 weeks 3 weeks or more	once only 2 3
Chlorothiazide	Thiazide diuretic, usually combined with spironolactone.	oral	10 or 20 mg/kg per dose		2
Chlorpromazine	Tranquillizer	oral	1 mg/kg per dose (*max 6 mg/kg per day)*		3
Cimetidine	Histamine H_2 receptor blocker used for reducing gastric acid secretion in the face of stress ulceration. Benefit remains unproven.	oral	5 mg/kg per dose if active problem, half this if used prophylactically		4

Drug	Indication, mode of action and comments	Route	Dose	*Post menstrual/* chronological age	Frequency (times/24 h)
Ciprofloxacin	Reserve broad-spectrum quinolone antibiotic. Best avoided unless absolutely necessary.	i.v.	5 mg/kg per dose (lactate)		2
		oral	7.5 mg/kg per dose (hydrochloride)		2
Cisapride	Promotes intestinal motility. Prolongs QT interval, esp. with imidazole or triazole antifungals or erythromycin.	oral	*no more than 300* microg/kg per dose		3
Clonazepam	Benzodiazepine anticonvulsant. Aim for a plasma level of 30–100 mg/l (1 mg = 3.16 micromol). Increases bronchial secretions. No proven advantage over phenobarbitone in a randomized trial.	i.v. (oral)	100 microg/kg per dose continuous infusions have been used but the neonatal half-life is 24–48 hours and intermittent dosage is almost certainly adequate	0–1 week 1 week or more	1 2 (perhaps)
Dexamethasone	Potent glucocorticoid steroid for established BPD. Many alternative dosage regimens exist.	i.v., oral	500 microg of *base*/kg per dose for 7 days		1
	To aid extubation in a baby with a traumatized or oedematous larynx. 4 mg of base = 4.8 mg of dex. phosphate = 5 mg of dex. sodium phosphate.	i.v.	200 microg of *base*/kg per dose starting 4 hours before extubation		3 doses at 8 hourly intervals
Diamorphine	Analgesia in *ventilated* babies. Respiratory suppression may interfere with trigger ventilation. Half this dose will suffice for sedation. *Has no advantages over morphine.*	i.v.	loading dose 180 microg/kg		once only (over 30 mins)
		i.v. infusion	maintenance 15 microg/kg/h		infusion
Diazepam	Benzodiazepine anxiolytic. There are many better anticonvulsants. *Dosage required is very variable.*	i.v.	start with 200 microg/kg		once only
Diazoxide	Thiazide derivative that reduces insulin release, used to control refractory hypoglycaemia in hyperinsulinism. Oral administration is to be preferred.	(i.v.), oral	5 mg/kg per dose		2
Digoxin	May improve myocardial contractility and sometimes used in supraventricular tachycardia with variable results. Narrow therapeutic range causing partial AV block and prolonged PR interval (>0.16 s) in excess. Toxicity appears above 2–3 microg/l especially if hypokalaemic. For AV block use atropine: for severe toxicity, Digibind.	loading dose oral (very rarely i.v.)	10 microg/kg (over 15 mins) then 5 microg/kg after 6 hours then 5 microg/kg after a further 6 hours		loading regimen only
		oral	2–4 microg/kg per dose		2
Dobutamine	Synthetic inotrope, improves ventricular function.	i.v. infusion	5–15 microg/kg per minute		infusion
Dopamine	A low dose improves renal and gut perfusion. A high dose causes vasoconstriction and thus raises blood pressure. It is best to use a central vein.	i.v. infusion	low dose 2–4 microg/kg/min high dose 5–15 microg/kg/min		infusion infusion
Doxapram	Central respiratory stimulant but also stimulates all levels of the cerebrospinal axis. Can cause fits in high doses. High doses should not be used for more than 2–3 days.	i.v. i.v. infusion	loading dose 2.5 mg/kg maintenance 0.3 mg/kg per hour *(max 1.5 mg/kg/hour)*		once only infusion
		oral	6 mg/kg per dose (best after i.v. loading dose)		4

Drug	Indication, mode of action and comments	Route	Dose	*Post menstrual/* chronological age	Frequency (times/24 h)
Edrophonium	Cholinesterase inhibitor with rapid onset but brief duration of action. Sometimes used to diagnose myasthenia gravis ('Tensilon' test), but many prefer to use neostigmine both for diagnosis and treatment.	i.v.	40–150 microg/kg give the first 20% very slowly and have atropine available to control hypersalivation		once only
Epoprostenol (PGI_2 prostacyclin)	Inhibits platelet aggregation. Short-acting vasodilator. Can be used for pulmonary vasodilatation but causes systemic vasodilatation as well.	i.v. infusion	10 nanograms/kg per minute		infusion
Erythromycin	Drug of choice for *Chlamydia*. Well absorbed orally. Also a motilin agonist. Risk of arrythmia with cisapride.	i.v. oral	15 mg/kg per dose (give over 1 hour if i.v.) for motility start with 2 mg/kg per dose		3 3
Erythropoietin	Stimulates marrow red cell production – can reduce the need for transfusions (though not as effectively as limiting blood letting).	subcut. injection	250 units/kg per dose		three times *per week*
Fentanyl	Synthetic opioid analgesic (for *ventilated* babies only). Infusion is not recommended as tolerance develops rapidly and withdrawal symptoms are common.	i.v.	10 microg/kg		repeatable
Flecainide	Class I antiarrhythmic for supraventricular arrhythmias. *Should not be used except under the **direct** supervision of a paediatric cardiologist*. Causes fatal arrhythmias in overdose. Monitoring of plasma levels is *essential* (therapeutic range 200–700 microg/l).	oral	Start with 2 mg/kg per dose and adjust dosage based on clinical response and plasma levels		3
Flucloxacillin	β-lactamase-resistant penicillin. Moderately well absorbed orally.	i.v., oral, i.m.	50 mg/kg per dose (for meningitis or osteitis use 100 mg/kg per dose)	0–1 week 1–3 weeks 4 weeks or more	2 3 4
Fluconazole	Triazole antifungal agent. Increase dosage interval where renal function is poor. Do not use if the baby is on cisapride (risk of ventricular arrhythmias).	i.v., oral	6 mg/kg per dose	0–2 weeks 2–4 weeks 4 weeks or more	once every 3 days once every 2 days 1
Flucytosine	Fluorinated pyrimidine often used with amphotericin for some systemic fungal infections. Increase dosage interval in renal failure. Aim for a serum level of 50–80 mg/l. (1 mg = 7.74 micromol.)	i.v., oral	50 mg/kg per dose		2
Frusemide	Powerful loop diuretic, increases urinary loss of Na^+, K^+ and Ca^{++}.	i.v., i.m., oral	1–2 mg/kg per dose		1 or 2
Fucidin (sodium fusidate, fusidic acid)	Narrow spectrum antistaphylococcal antibiotic, moderately well absorbed orally and well distributed (except CSF). The dose may need to be reduced for administration for more than 5 days. Watch liver function tests for a rapid rise in enzyme levels.	i.v. oral	10 mg/kg per dose sodium fusidate *over 6 hours* 15 mg/kg fusidic acid		2 3

Drug	Indication, mode of action and comments	Route	Dose	*Post menstrual/ chronological age*	Frequency (times/24 h)
Gentamicin	Aminoglycoside antibiotic. Aim for a trough level of 1 mg/l or less. Extend dosage interval to 36 hours if level is 2 mg/l or greater just before the third dose.	i.v., i.m.	5 mg/kg		1
Glucagon	For immediate treatment of hypoglycaemia. Mobilizes hepatic glycogen, increases hepatic glucose production.	i.m., i.v.	200 microg/kg		once only
	Half life <10 minutes.	i.v. infusion	0.3 microg/kg per minute		infusion
Heparin	Activates antithrombin III causing anticoagulation. Has some thrombolytic action. Used for anticoagulation	i.v. loading	50–75 units/kg	*use lower loading dose under 36 wks*	once only
	Regulate infusion by measuring APTT. (Using 0.5–2 units per hour can increase the effective life of intravascular cannulae.)	i.v. infusion	25 units/kg per hour and monitor activated partial thromboplastin time (APTT)		infusion
Hydralazine	Vasodilator – for maintenance control of hypertension. A β-blocker may be needed to control tachycardia. (Labetalol is better than hydralazine for urgent i.v. use.)	oral (i.v.)	start with 0.5 mg/kg max 2–3 mg/kg (i.v. dose about half oral)		3
Hydrocortisone	For treatment of adrenal insufficiency in congenital adrenal hyperplasia (with fludrocortisone).	i.v.	25 mg (with dextrose) in Addisonian crisis		once only
	Maintenance usually 25 mg/m^2.	oral	2.5 mg		3
Immunoglobulin	May reduce mortality in severe infection and reduces thrombocytopenia in autoimmune thrombocytopenia due to maternal ITP or SLE.	i.v.	400 mg/kg over several hours		once (repeatable)
Indomethacin	For closure of patent ductus arteriosus. Much less effective after 2 weeks of age. (Oral absorption variable.)	i.v., (oral)	loading dose 200 microg/kg		once only
			then 100 microg/kg for 5 days		1
Insulin	Occasionally used to increase glucose uptake with parenteral nutrition.	i.v.	0.5–1.0 units/kg per hour		infusion
	To reduce hyperkalaemia (with glucose).	i.v.	0.3–0.6 units/kg per hour		infusion
	To control neonatal diabetes (v. rare).	i.v., later subcut.	0.5–3 units/kg per day		infusion/1–2
Isoniazid	For TB prophylaxis and treatment in the neonate. Seek expert advice.	oral	5 mg/kg	0–2 weeks	1
			10 mg/kg	more than 2 weeks	1
Isoprenaline	Sympathomimetic for management of significant bradycardia or heart block.	i.v. infusion	0.02 microg/kg per minute *(max 0.3 microg/kg per minute)*		infusion
Labetalol	Non-cardioselective α-blocker with β-blocking effects. The best i.v. drug for controlling hypertension. Adult half-life of 3–4 hours.	i.v. infusion	start with 0.5 mg/kg per hour; double the dose every 3 hours until a satisfactory BP level is reached *(max 4 mg/kg per hour)*		infusion

Drug	Indication, mode of action and comments	Route	Dose	*Post menstrual/* chronological age	Frequency (times/24 h)
Lignocaine	Local anaesthetic.	subcut.	up to 0.3 ml/kg of 1% soln		once only
	Membrane stabilizer for cardiac arrythmias and fits.	i.v.	loading dose 2 mg/kg		once only
	Third-line anticonvulsant. Toxic levels (& fits) can occur if the higher doses are used for more than 12 hours.	i.v. infusion	maintenance 2 mg/kg per hour. *(max 6 mg/kg per hour)*		infusion
Magnesium sulphate	For control of hypocalcaemia.	i.m. (deep)	100 mg/kg per dose		2
	For vasodilatation in persistent pulmonary hypertension try to keep plasma Mg between 3.5 and 5.5 mmol/l.	i.v.	loading dose 250 mg/kg		once only
		i.v. infusion	maintenance 25–75 mg/kg/hour		infusion
Mannitol	Osmotic diuretic used to reduce intracranial pressure in cerebral oedema.	i.v.	1 g/kg over 10–20 minutes (5 ml/kg of a 20% solution)		repeat once after 6 hours if needed
Meropenem	Carbapenem β-lactam broad-spectrum antibiotic. Increase dose interval in renal failure.	i.v.	try 20 mg/kg per dose (no neonatal data)	0–3 weeks 4 weeks or more	2 3
Metronidazole	Antibiotic, particularly useful for anaerobic infections. Well absorbed orally.	i.v., oral	loading dose 15 mg/kg		once only
			maintenance 7.5 mg/kg per dose	0–3 weeks 4 weeks or more	2 3
Miconazole	Imidazole antifungal agent. Do not use orally if the baby is taking cisapride as it affects the metabolism of cisapride making ventricular arrhythmias possible.	oral	apply 1–2 ml of 2.5% gel		2 after feeds
		topical	apply 2% cream		2
Morphine	Opioid sedative and analgesic given by i.v. bolus or (best) by infusion. Can also be given i.m., orally or rectally, but larger doses will be needed for oral administration. The *infusion* dose quoted will only sedate; serious pain requires double this loading and maintenance dose.	i.v. boluses	100 microg/kg per dose (can be doubled *if ventilated*)		2 or 3
		i.v.	loading dose 120 microg/kg		once only
		i.v. infusion	maintenance 10 microg/kg/hour		infusion
Naloxone	Opioid antagonist – to reverse effect of maternal opioids – use the ADULT (400 microg/ml) preparation.	i.m.	100 microg/kg (effect lasts up to 24 hours)		once only
	To diagnose opioid sedation.	i.v.	40 microg (effect lasts 30 min)		repeatable
Neostigmine	Cholinesterase inhibitor prolongs muscarinic and nicotinic effects of acetylcholine.	i.v.	for diagnosis 50 microg/kg		once only
	Used for the diagnosis & treatment of neonatal myasthenia, and to reverse the effect of non-depolarizing muscle relaxants (e.g. pancuronium).	i.m.	for treatment 150–300 microg/kg per dose		3–6
		i.v.	for reversal 80 microg/kg (after 20 microg/kg of atropine)		once only
Netilmicin	Aminoglycoside antibiotic. Said to be less ototoxic than gentamicin. Aim for a trough level of 1 mg/l or less. Extend dosage interval to 36 hours if level is 2 mg/l or greater just before third dose. (1 mg = 2.1 micromol.)	i.v., i.m.	6 mg/kg		1

Drug	Indication, mode of action and comments	Route	Dose	*Post menstrual/ chronological age*	Frequency (times/24 h)
Noradrenaline	Postganglionic sympathetic neurotransmitter, a potent vasoconstrictor sometimes used to maintain blood pressure in septic shock. (Almost always with low-dose dopamine to preserve renal perfusion). Use a central vein. 1 mg noradrenaline acid tartrate = 0.5 mg of noradrenaline base.	via central vein	start with 0.1 microg/kg per minute of noradrenaline *base* *(max 1.5 microg/kg base per minute)*		infusion
Nystatin	Polyene antifungal for candida infection.	oral, topical	100 000 units per dose		4 (after feeds)
Octreotide	Synthetic analogue of the hypothalamic hormone somatostatin.	subcut. i.v.	5 microg/kg per dose 25 microg/kg per dose		3–4
Pancuronium	Competitive non-depolarizing muscle relaxant used to induce paralysis in ventilated babies.	i.v., (i.m.)	initial dose 100 microg/kg repeat doses 50 microg/kg		once only usually 4–6
Paracetamol	A useful analgesic if used at this dosage.	oral (rectal)	24 mg/kg per dose		3
Paraldehyde	Emergency anticonvulsant. Best given rectally mixed 1:1 by volume with arachis oil or olive oil.	deep i.m. rectal	0.2 ml/kg 0.3 ml/kg of paraldehyde (0.6 ml/kg of mixture)		repeatable once once
Penicillin G (benzylpenicillin)	Drug of choice for group B streptococcal infection.	i.v., i.m.	30 mg/kg per dose (60 mg/kg in meningitis)	0–1 week 1–3 weeks 4 weeks or more	2 3 4
Pethidine	A synthetic opioid that can be used for pain relief in ventilated babies, but morphine is preferable as more is known about its use in neonates.	i.v., i.m.	1 mg/kg		max 2
Phenobarbitone	First-line anticonvulsant. Aim for a serum level of 20–40 mg/l; 1 mg = 4.42 micromol. Where the standard loading dose does not suffice a further 10 mg/kg can be given but may well cause significant sedation.	i.v., i.m. i.v., oral	loading dose 20 mg/kg maintenance 4 mg/kg (increase to 5 mg/kg after 2 weeks)		once only 1
Phenytoin	Second-line anticonvulsant. Plasma levels must be monitored if used for more than 48 hours. Aim for levels of 10–20 mg/l. 1 mg = 3.96 micromol.	i.v. *only*	loading dose 20 mg/kg (give over 20 minutes with ECG) maintenance usually 2.5 mg/kg per dose		once only 2
Propranolol	β-blocker, antiarrhythmic, used to control cyanotic spells in Fallot's tetralogy and for neonatal thyrotoxicosis.	oral	250–750 microg/kg per dose initially, up to 2 mg/kg per dose		3
Propylthiouracil	Thioamide antithyroid for symptomatic hyperthyroidism.	oral	5 mg/kg per dose		2
Prostaglandin E_2	Used to keep the ductus arteriosus open in duct dependent cardiac malformations. Takes about 3 hours to reach maximal effect. Respiratory depression and apnoea can occur. E_2 is just as effective as E_1 and much cheaper.	i.v. infusion	0.6 microg/kg per hour (i.e. 10 *nanograms/kg/min*) higher doses have been used but they are no more effective and cause more side-effects, especially apnoea		infusion

Drug	Indication, mode of action and comments	Route	Dose	*Post menstrual/* chronological age	Frequency (times/24 h)
Prostaglandin I_2 (prostacyclin)	See Epoprostenol				
Pyridoxine	Used to diagnose pyridoxine dependency as a cause of seizures	i.v.	100 mg bolus (with EEG monitoring)		once only
	– and for their treatment.	oral	start with 30 mg/kg per dose		1
Ranitidine	H_2 histamine receptor blocker that inhibits gastric acid secretion (best avoided in renal failure).	i.v.	500 microg/kg per dose slowly to avoid arryhthmias		4
	Or as a continuous infusion (which may be safer).	i.v. i.v. infusion	loading dose 250 microg/kg maintenance 50 microg/kg/h		once only infusion
Rifampicin	Antituberculous agent (seek expert advice) and potent (reserve) antistaphylococcal antibiotic usually used together with teicoplanin or vancomycin.	i.v.	6 mg/kg per dose over 60 minutes		2
		oral	12 mg/kg		1
Salbutamol	Betamimetic and bronchodilator. Can rapidly reduce plasma potassium to buy time in an emergency.	nebulized i.v.	2.5 mg nebulized 4 microg/kg over 10 minutes		repeatable once
Sodium bicarbonate	For correction of metabolic acidosis. 1 ml of 8.4% solution contains 1 mmol of bicarbonate. Can be given orally to correct late metabolic acidosis.	i.v.	0.3 mmol/kg per mmol of base deficit will usually provide adequate partial correction		repeatable
	Consider THAM if concerned about sodium loading.		give slowly *(max rate 0.5 mmol/kg per minute)*		
Spironolactone	Aldosterone antagonist, potassium-sparing diuretic. Usually combined with chlorothiazide.	oral	1 or 2 mg/kg per dose		2
Streptokinase	Activates plasmin which causes lysis of clots. Can be used to dissolve arterial clots.	i.v. infusion	3000 units/kg loading dose then 500–1000 units/kg per hour maintenance		once only infusion
Suxamethonium	Short-acting depolarizing muscle relaxant used to facilitate intubation. Effect lasts 5–10 min.	i.v.	2–3 mg/kg		single dose
Teicoplanin	Reserve antibiotic for coagulase negative staphylococci. Double dosage interval in renal failure.	i.v., i.m.	loading dose 16 mg/kg maintenance 8 mg/kg		once only 1
THAM	Organic buffer used to treat metabolic acidosis, a sodium-free alternative to sodium bicarbonate.	i.v.	0.5 mmol/kg per mmol of base deficit will usually provide adequate partial correction		repeatable
Theophylline	Respiratory stimulant for neonatal apnoea *(but caffeine is both easier to use and safer).*	i.v.	loading dose 6 mg/kg aminophylline maintenance 2.5 mg/kg per dose		once only 2
	By weight aminophylline is 85% theophylline and choline theophyllinate is 64% theophylline.	oral	loading dose 9 mg/kg choline theophyllinate maintenance 4 mg/kg per dose		once only 2
	Optimum levels 8–12 mg/l, side-effects above 14 mg/l. (1 microg = 5.55 micromol.)				

Drug	Indication, mode of action and comments	Route	Dose	*Post menstrual/* chronological age	Frequency (times/24 h)
Thyroxine	As replacement therapy.	oral	10 microg/kg		1
Tobramycin	Aminoglycoside antibiotic. Aim for a trough level of 1 mg/l or less. Extend dosage interval to 36 hours if trough is 2 mg/l or greater just before the third dose. (1 mg = 2.14 mmol.)	i.v., i.m.	5 mg/kg		1
Tolazoline	α-Adrenergic antagonist used to produce pulmonary vasodilatation, but also causes systemic vasodilatation and may cause hypotension. Works best if any significant acidosis is corrected first.	i.v. i.v. infusion	1 mg/kg bolus 200 microg/kg per hour		once only infusion
Trimethoprim	Antibiotic particularly valuable in urinary tract infection for both treatment and prophylaxis.	oral (i.v.)	3–4 mg/kg per dose 2 mg/kg		2 1
Vancomycin	Reserve antibiotic for Gram-positive organisms, especially coagulase-negative staphylococci. Aim for peak level of 25–40 mg/l and trough level of less than 10 mg/l. (1 mg = 0.69 micromol.) See also Teicoplanin.	i.v.	15 mg/kg per dose (give over 1 hour)	*less than 28 weeks* *28–35 weeks* *36 weeks or more*	1 2 3
Vitamin D	Most term and preterm formulae are appropriately supplemented.	oral	400 units (10 microg) per dose		1
Vitamin K (phytomenadione)	Prophylaxis against vitamin K deficiency bleeding. There is some concern that intramuscular dosage is associated with an increased risk of childhood cancer. The risk dose not seem to extend to oral dosage. See pp. 798–800. Ideal oral regimen not yet determined.	i.m. oral	1 mg at birth either 25 microg per day (as in formula-fed babies) or 1 mg every 1–2 weeks for 3 months if breast-fed		once only for 3 months

Postmenstrual age is the age in completed weeks from the mother's LMP. A baby born at 26 weeks' gestation 4 weeks ago has a postmenstrual age today of 30 weeks. Chronological age is the age in completed weeks from birth.

Units

1 kilogram (kg) = 1000 grams
1 gram (g) = 1000 milligrams
1 milligram (mg) = 1000 micrograms
1 microgram (microg) = 1000 nanograms
1 nanogram = 1000 picograms

Solutions

A 1:100 (1%) weight for volume (w/v) solution contains 1 g of substance in 100 ml of solution or 10 mg in 1 ml
A 1:1000 solution contains 1 mg in 1 ml
A 1:10 000 solution contains 100 microg in 1 ml

Section 10

Appendices

Appendix 1

Haematological values in the newborn

Elizabeth A. Letsky

Table A1.1 Red cell parameters in the fetus (adapted from Oski & Naiman[3])

Age in weeks	Hb. g/dl	PCV	RBC × 10^{12}/l	MCV fl	MCH pg	MCHC g/dl	Nucleated RBC % of WBC	Reticulocytes %
12	8.0–10.0	0.33	1.5	180	60	34	5.0–8.0	40
16	10.0	0.35	2.0	140	45	33	2.0–4.0	10–25
20	11.0	0.37	2.5	135	44	33	1.0	10–20
24	14.0	0.40	3.5	123	38	31	1.0	5–10
28	14.5	0.45	4.0	120	40	31	0.5	5–20
34	15.0	0.47	4.4	118	38	32	0.2	3–10
Term 40 Cord	16.8	0.53	5.25	107	34	31.7	0.01	3–7

MCV = Mean cell volume
MCH = Mean corpuscular haemoglobin
MCHC = Mean corpuscular haemoglobin concentration

Table A1.2 Normal leucocyte counts in the first month of life (abstracted from Dallman[1])

Age	Total leucocytes		Neutrophils			Lymphocytes			Monocytes		Eosinophils	
	Mean	(Range)	Mean	(Range)	%	Mean	(Range)	%	Mean	%	Mean	%
Birth	18.1	(9.0–30.0)	11.1	(6.0–26.0)	61	5.5	(2.0–11.0)	31	1.1	6	0.4	2
12 hours	22.8	(13.0–38.0)	15.5	(6.0–28.0)	68	5.5	(2.0–11.0)	24	1.2	5	0.5	2
24 hours	18.9	(9.4–34.0)	11.5	(5.0–21.0)	61	5.8	(2.0–11.5)	31	1.1	6	0.5	2
1 week	12.2	(5.0–21.0)	5.5	(1.5–10.0)	45	5.0	(2.0–17.0)	41	1.1	9	0.5	4
2 week	11.4	(5.0–20.0)	4.5	(1.0–9.5)	40	5.5	(2.0–17.0)	48	1.0	9	0.4	3
1 month	10.8	(5.0–19.5)	3.8	(1.0–9.0)	35	6.0	(2.5–16.5)	56	0.7	7	0.3	3

Notes: Numbers of leukocytes × 10^9/l
Neutrophils include band forms and a small number of metamyelocytes and myelocytes in the first few days of life.

Table A1.3 Normal red cell values during the first week of life in the term infant (adapted from Lubin & Vichinsky,[2] Oski & Naiman[3])

	Cord blood	Day 1	Day 3	Day 7
Haemoglobin (g/dl)	16.8	18.4	17.8	17.0
Packed-cell volume (PCV)	0.53	0.58	0.55	0.54
Red cell count (× 10^{12}/l)	5.25	5.8	5.6	5.2
Mean corpuscular volume (MCV fl)	107	108	99.0	98.0
Mean corpuscular haemoglobin concentration (MCHC g/dl)	31.7	32	33	33
Mean corpuscular haemoglobin (MCH pg)	34	35	33	32.5
Reticulocytes per cent of red cells	3–7	3–7	1–3	0–1
Nucleated red cell count (per mm^3)	500 (7.3/100 WBC)	200	0.5	0

Platelets
The platelet count in the fetus from 15 weeks' gestation and in the neonate is within the normal adult range 150–350 × 10^9/l.

REFERENCES

1. Dallman P R 1977 In: Rudolph A M (ed) Pediatrics, 16th edn. Appleton-Century-Crofts, New York, p 1178
2. Lubin B, Vichinsky E 1979 Anemia in the newborn period. Pediatric Annals 8: 416–434
3. Oski F A, Naiman J L 1982 Hematologic problems in the newborn, 3rd edn. W B Saunders, New York

Appendix 2

Coagulation values in term and preterm infants

Thomas L. Turner Janet M. Rennie

Reference values for coagulation tests in healthy term infants and in the adult (Andrew et al 1987)
Means and standard deviations

Test	Day 1	Day 5	Day 30	Adult
PT (s)	13 ± 1.43	12.4 ± 1.46	11.8 ± 1.25	12.4 ± 0.78
APPT (s)	42.9 ± 5.8	42.6 ± 8.62	40.4 ± 7.42	33.5 ± 3.44
TCT (s)	23.5 ± 2.38	23.1 ± 3.07	24.3 ± 2.44	25 ± 2.66
Fibrinogen (g/l)	2.83 ± 0.58	3.12 ± 0.75	2.7 ± 0.54	2.78 ± 0.61
II (U/ml)	0.48 ± 0.11	0.63 ± 0.15	0.68 ± 0.17	1.08 ± 0.19
V (U/ml)	0.72 ± 0.18	0.95 ± 0.25	0.98 ± 0.18	1.06 ± 0.22
VII (U/ml)	0.66 ± 0.19	0.89 ± 0.27	0.9 ± 0.24	1.05 ± 0.19
VIII (U/ml)	1.00 ± 0.39	0.88 ± 0.33	0.91 ± 0.33	0.99 ± 0.25
vWF (U/ml)	1.53 ± 0.67	1.40 ± 0.57	1.28 ± 0.59	0.92 ± 0.33
IX (U/ml)	0.53 ± 0.19	0.53 ± 0.19	0.51 ± 0.15	1.09 ± 0.27
X (U/ml)	0.40 ± 0.14	0.49 ± 0.15	0.59 ± 0.14	1.06 ± 0.23
XI (U/ml)	0.38 ± 0.14	0.55 ± 0.16	0.53 ± 0.13	0.97 ± 0.15
XII (U/ml)	0.53 ± 0.20	0.47 ± 0.18	0.49 ± 0.16	1.08 ± 0.28
Plasminogen (U/ml)	1.95 ± 0.35	2.17 ± 0.38	1.98 ± 0.36	3.36 ± 0.44

All factors except fibrinogen and plasminogen are expressed as units per millilitre where pooled plasma contains 1.0 U/ml. Plasminogen units are those recommended by the Committee on Thrombolytic Agents
APPT, activated partial thromboplastin time
PT, Prothrombin time
TCT, Thrombin clotting time
vWF, von Willebrand factor

REFERENCE

Andrew M, Paes B, Milner R et al 1987 Development of the human coagulation system in the full term infant. Blood 70: 165–172

Reference values for coagulation tests in preterm infants (Andrew et al 1988)
Means and boundaries given, where the boundaries encompass 95% of the observations

Test	Day 1	Day 5	Day 30	Adult
PT (s)	13 (10.6–16.2)	12.5 (10.0–15.3)	11.8 (10.0–13.6)	12.4 (10.8–13.9)
APPT (s)	53.6 (27.5–79.4)	50.5 (26.9–74.1)	44.7 (26.9–62.5)	33.5 (26.6–40.3)
TCT (s)	24.8 (19.2–30.4)	24.1 (18.8–29.4)	24.4 (18.8–29.9)	25 (19.7–30.3)
Fibrinogen (g/l)	2.43 (1.5–3.73)	2.8 (1.6–4.2)	2.54 (1.5–4.14)	2.78 (1.56–4.0)
II (U/ml)	0.45 (0.41–1.44)	0.57 (0.29–0.85)	0.57 (0.36–0.95)	1.08 (0.71–1.46)
V (U/ml)	0.88 (0.41–1.44)	1.0 (0.46–1.54)	1.02 (0.48–1.56)	1.06 (0.62–1.50)
VII (U/ml)	0.67 (0.21–1.13)	0.84 (0.3–1.38)	0.83 (0.21–1.45)	1.05 (0.67–1.43)
VIII (U/ml)	1.11 (0.50–2.13)	1.15 (0.53–2.05)	1.11 (0.5–1.99)	0.99 (0.5–1.49)
vWF (U/ml)	1.36 (0.78–2.1)	1.33 (0.72–2.19)	1.36 (0.66–2.16)	0.92 (0.5–1.58)
IX (U/ml)	0.35 (0.19–0.65)	0.42 (0.14–0.74)	0.44 (0.13–0.8)	1.09 (0.55–1.63)
X (U/ml)	0.41 (0.11–0.71)	0.51 (0.19–0.83)	0.56 (0.20–0.92)	1.06 (0.7–1.52)
XI (U/ml)	0.30 (0.08–0.52)	0.41 (0.13–0.69)	0.43 (0.15–0.71)	0.97 (0.67–1.27)
XII (U/ml)	0.38 (0.10–0.66)	0.39 (0.09–0.69)	0.43 (0.11–0.75)	1.08 (0.52–1.64)
Plasminogen (U/ml)	1.70 (1.12–2.48)	1.91 (1.21–2.61)	1.81 (1.09–2.53)	3.36 (2.48–4.24)

REFERENCE

Andrew M, Paes B, Milner R et al 1988 Development of the coagulation system in the healthy premature infant. Blood 72: 1651–1657

Reference values for the inhibitors of coagulation in healthy full-term infants (Andrew et al 1987)
Means ± standard deviations

Coag inhibitor	Day 1	Day 5	Day 30	Adult
AT III (U/ml)	0.63 ± 0.12	0.67 ± 0.13	0.78 ± 0.15	1.05 ± 0.13
α_2 M (U/ml)	1.39 ± 0.22	1.48 ± 0.25	1.50 ± 0.22	0.86 ± 0.17
α_2 AP (U/ml)	0.85 ± 0.15	1.0 ± 0.15	1.0 ± 0.12	1.02 ± 0.17
C_1-INH (U/ml)	0.72 ± 0.18	0.9 ± 0.15	0.89 ± 0.21	1.01 ± 0.15
α_1AT (U/ml)	0.83 ± 0.22	0.89 ± 0.20	0.62 ± 0.13	0.93 ± 0.19
Protein C (U/ml)	0.35 ± 0.09	0.42 ± 0.11	0.43 ± 0.11	0.96 ± 0.16
Protein S (U/ml)	0.36 ± 0.12	0.50 ± 0.14	0.63 ± 0.15	0.92 ± 0.16

Reference values for the inhibitors of coagulation in preterm infants (Andrew et al 1988)
Means and boundaries are given, where the boundaries encompass 95% of the observations

Coag inhibitor	Day 1	Day 5	Day 30	Adult
AT III (U/ml)	0.38 (0.14–0.62)	0.56 (0.30–0.82)	0.59 (0.37–0.81)	1.05 (0.79–1.31)
α_2 M (U/ml)	1.10 (0.56–1.82)	1.25 (0.71–0.77)	1.38 (0.72–2.04)	0.86 (0.52–1.2)
α_2 AP (U/ml)	0.78 (0.40–1.16)	0.81 (0.49–1.13)	0.89 (0.55–1.23)	1.02 (0.68–1.36)
C_1-INH (U/ml)	0.65 (0.31–0.99)	0.83 (0.45–1.21)	0.74 (0.40–1.24)	1.01 (0.71–1.31)
α_1AT (U/ml)	0.90 (0.36–1.44)	0.94 (0.42–1.46)	0.76 (0.38–1.12)	0.93 (0.55–1.31)
Protein C (U/ml)	0.28 (0.12–0.44)	0.31 (0.11–0.51)	0.37 (0.15–0.59)	0.96 (0.64–1.28)
Protein S (U/ml)	0.26 (0.14–0.38)	0.37 (0.13–0.61)	0.56 (0.22–0.90)	0.92 (0.60–1.24)

α_2 AP = α_2 antiplasmin
α_2 M = α_2 macroglobulin
α_1 AT = α_1 antitrypsin
AT III = antithrombin III
C_1-INH = C_1 esterase inhibitor

REFERENCES

Andrew M, Paes B, Milner R et al 1987 Development of the human coagulation system in the full term infant. Blood 70: 165–172
Andrew M, Paes B, Milner R et al 1988 Development of the coagulation system in the healthy premature infant. Blood 72: 1651–1657

Appendix 3

Normal ranges for commonly assesed ECG values in the newborn

Nick Archer

	< 1 day	1–3 days	4–7 days	8–10 days
Heart rate (beats/min)	94–155	92–158	90–166	106–182
PR Lead II (ms)	80–100	81–139	74–136	72–138
QRS duration V5 (ms)	21–75	22–67	21–68	22–79
Frontal QRS axis (degrees)	+60 to +190	+62 to +196	+75 to +190	+65 to +160
QRS size (mV)				
V1				
Q	0	0	0	0
R	0.5–2.6	0.5–2.6	0.3–2.4	0.3–2.1
S	0–2.3	0–2.1	0–1.7	0–1.1
T	−0.3 to 4	−0.4 to 4	−0.45 to 2.5	−5 to −1
V6				
Q	0–0.17	0–0.21	0–0.28	0–0.28
R	0–1.1	0–1.2	0–1.2	0.25–1.6
S	0–1.0	0–0.9	0–1.0	0–1.0
R/S V1	0.2–9.8	0.2–6	0.2–9.8	1–7
R/S V6	0.2–10	0.2–11	0.2–10	0.2–12

Ranges given are approximately 2nd and 98th centiles, derived from Davignon A et al.[1] Qtc = QT/√RR using lead II and where the RR interval is the one preceding the QRS complex in which the QT interval is measured. Qtc 98th centile figure from Davignon and colleagues is <0.48, except in the first few days of life, when higher values may transiently be found. Other authors consider persistent values above 0.46 abnormal.[2]

REFERENCES

1. Davignon A, Rautaharju P, Boisselle E, Soumis F, Megelas M, Choquette A 1979/80 Normal ECG standards for infants and children. Pediatric Cardiology 1: 123–131
2. Garson A 1990 Ventricular arrhythmias. In: Gillette P C, Garson A (eds) Pediatric arrhythmias: electrophysiology and pacing. WB Saunders, Philadelphia, pp 427–500

Appendix 4

Neonatal blood pressure: normal values

Nick Archer

A Day 1, healthy low-birthweight infants (not receiving inotropes or intermittent positive pressure ventilation). Some infants in added inspired oxygen, some receiving continuous positive airway pressure. Some recordings direct intra-arterial, some oscillometric.

Birthweight (g)	Number	Systolic range (mmHg)	Diastolic range (mmHg)
501–750	18	50–62	26–36
751–1000	39	48–59	23–36
1001–1250	30	49–61	26–35
1251–1500	45	46–56	23–33
1501–1750	51	46–58	23–33
1751–2000	61	48–61	24–35

B Day 1, healthy preterm infants. Same infant characteristics and measurement methods as in **A**.

Gestation (weeks)	Number	Systolic range (mmHg)	Diastolic range (mmHg)
<24	11	48–63	24–39
24–28	55	48–58	22–36
29–32	110	47–59	24–34
>32	68	48–60	24–34

C Week 1, healthy low-birthweight infants (<2000 g). Same infant characteristics and measurement methods as in **A** and **B**.

Day	Number	Systolic range (mmHg)	Diastolic range (mmHg)
1	183	48–63	25–35
2	121	54–63	30–39
3	117	53–67	31–43
4	85	57–71	32–45
5	76	56–72	33–47
6	59	57–71	32–47
7	48	61–74	34–46

Sources for **A**, **B** and **C**, Hegyi et al[1,2]

D Non-invasive (indirect) arm systolic blood pressures (mmHg) with pulse detected by Doppler probe. All infants 38 weeks' gestation or more.

Age (days)	3	4	5	6	7	8–10
Awake						
Mean systolic BP (mmHg) ± SD	72 ± 6	74 ± 9	77 ± 10	77 ± 10	82 ± 9	88 ± 17
Numbers of infants	4	71	44	42	9	4
Asleep						
Mean systolic BP (mmHg) ± SD	68 ± 7	70 ± 8	72 ± 8	72 ± 9	72 ± 9	75 ± 9
Numbers of infants	72	681	426	322	47	18

Derived from de Swiet M et al[3]

REFERENCES

1. Hegyi T, Carbone M T, Anwar M et al 1994 Blood pressure ranges in premature infants: 1. The first hours of life. Journal of Pediatrics 124: 627–633
2. Hegyi T, Anwar M, Carbone M T et al 1996 Blood pressure ranges in premature infants: 2. The first week of life. Pediatrics 97: 336–342
3. de Swiet M, Fayers P, Shinebourne E A 1980 Systolic blood pressure in a population of infants in the first year of life: the Brompton study. Pediatrics 65: 1028–1035

Appendix 5

Birthweight and head circumference centiles

T. J. Cole

British boys birthweight centiles 1990

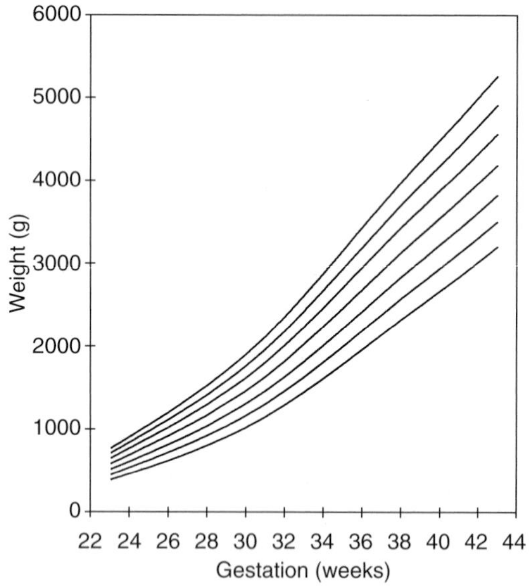

British girls birthweight centiles 1990

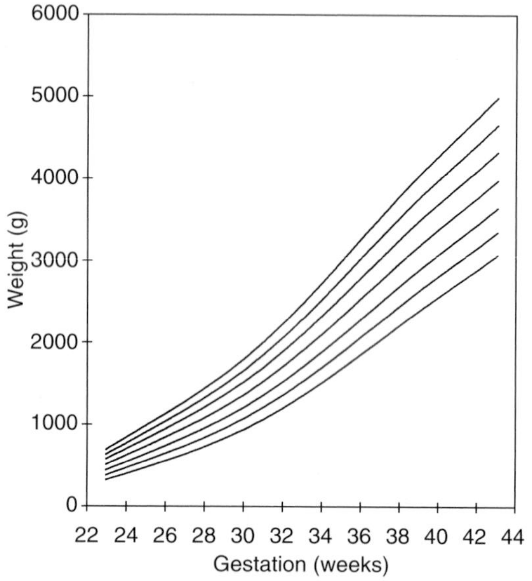

British 1990 growth reference birthweight centiles (g)

Boys

Weeks	3rd	10th	25th	50th	75th	90th	97th
23	386	451	515	585	653	713	771
24	463	539	614	696	776	846	915
25	541	628	714	807	899	981	1060
26	623	720	817	922	1026	1118	1208
27	710	817	924	1042	1158	1261	1362
28	803	921	1040	1170	1299	1414	1527
29	906	1035	1166	1309	1452	1580	1705
30	1020	1162	1305	1463	1620	1762	1901
31	1148	1303	1460	1634	1807	1964	2117
32	1291	1459	1631	1822	2013	2185	2355
33	1446	1630	1816	2025	2235	2424	2611
34	1612	1811	2013	2240	2469	2676	2881
35	1786	1999	2218	2463	2711	2935	3159
36	1965	2192	2426	2689	2955	3197	3439
37	2145	2385	2633	2913	3198	3457	3716
38	2323	2576	2837	3133	3434	3709	3985
39	2497	2761	3035	3345	3662	3952	4243
40	2669	2944	3229	3553	3884	4189	4494
41	2842	3127	3423	3760	4106	4424	4744
42	3019	3313	3620	3970	4330	4662	4996
43	3201	3505	3822	4186	4560	4906	5255

Girls

Weeks	3rd	10th	25th	50th	75th	90th	97th
23	346	407	469	535	601	660	717
24	421	493	565	644	722	792	860
25	497	579	662	753	843	924	1004
26	576	669	762	864	967	1059	1149
27	660	762	866	980	1095	1198	1299
28	750	863	977	1104	1231	1345	1458
29	849	972	1097	1237	1377	1504	1629
30	961	1095	1232	1385	1540	1680	1819
31	1086	1232	1382	1551	1721	1876	2029
32	1226	1385	1548	1733	1920	2090	2259
33	1378	1550	1728	1929	2134	2320	2506
34	1541	1727	1919	2137	2359	2562	2765
35	1712	1912	2118	2353	2593	2812	3032
36	1889	2101	2321	2572	2828	3064	3301
37	2066	2290	2523	2789	3062	3314	3567
38	2243	2477	2722	3002	3290	3556	3824
39	2461	2660	2915	3208	3509	3788	4070
40	2584	2836	3101	3405	3720	4011	4305
41	2748	3009	3282	3597	3923	4225	4531
42	2914	3183	3465	3790	4127	4440	4759
43	3086	3362	3653	3989	4338	4662	4993

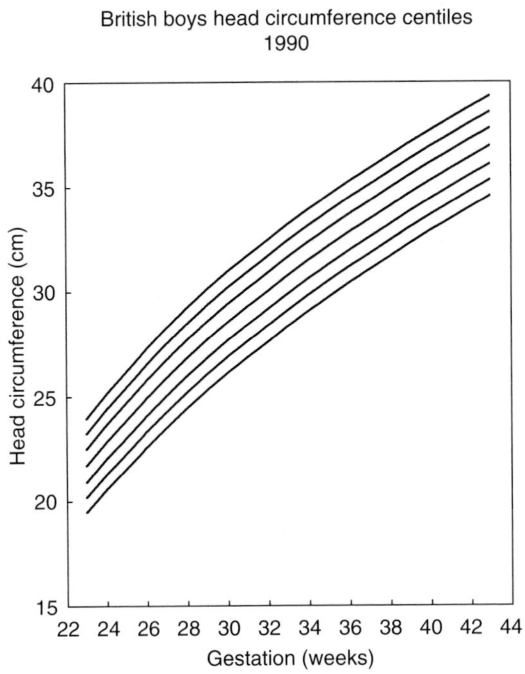

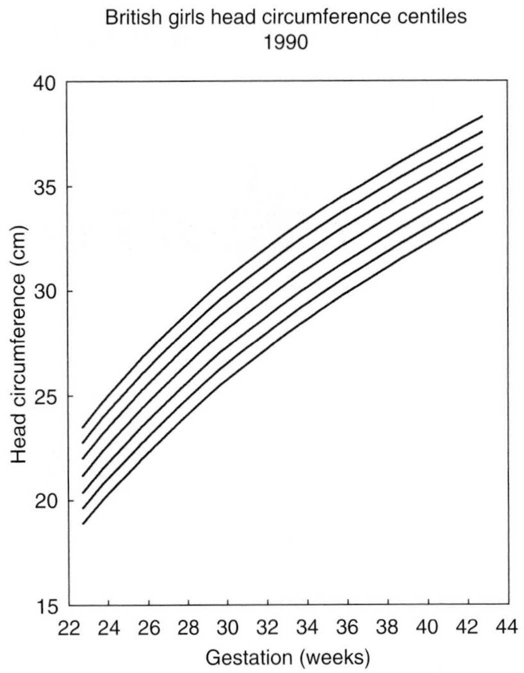

British 1990 growth reference head circumference centiles (cm)

	Boys								Girls						
Weeks	3rd	10th	25th	50th	75th	90th	97th	Weeks	3rd	10th	25th	50th	75th	90th	97th
23	19.3	20	20.8	21.6	22.4	23.1	23.8	23	18.9	19.6	20.4	21.2	22	22.8	23.5
24	20.4	21.2	21.9	22.7	23.6	24.3	25	24	20	20.8	21.5	22.4	23	24	24.7
25	21.4	22.2	22.9	23.8	24.6	25.4	26.1	25	21	21.8	22.5	23.4	24.3	25	25.8
26	22.4	23.2	24	24.8	25.7	26.4	27.2	26	22	22.8	23.6	24.4	25.3	26.1	26.8
27	23.4	24.2	24.9	25.8	26.6	27.4	28.2	27	23	23.7	24.5	25.4	26.3	27.1	27.8
28	24.3	25.1	25.9	26.7	27.6	28.4	29.1	28	23.9	24.7	25.5	26.3	27.2	28	28.8
29	25.2	25.9	26.7	27.6	28.5	29.3	30	29	24.8	25.5	26.3	27.2	28.1	28.9	29.7
30	26	26.8	27.6	28.4	29.3	30.1	30.9	30	25.6	26.4	27.2	28	28.9	29.7	30.5
31	26.8	27.5	28.3	29.2	30.1	30.9	31.6	31	26.3	27.1	27.9	28.8	29.7	30.4	31.2
32	27.5	28.3	29.1	29.9	30.8	31.6	32.4	32	27.1	27.9	28.6	29.5	30.4	31.2	31.9
33	28.3	29	29.8	30.7	31.6	32.4	33.1	33	27.8	28.6	29.4	30.2	31.1	31.9	32.7
34	29	29.7	30.5	31.4	32.3	33.1	33.8	34	28.5	29.3	30.1	30.9	31.8	32.6	33.3
35	29.7	30.4	31.2	32.1	33	33.7	34.5	35	29.2	29.9	30.7	31.6	32.4	33.2	34
36	30.3	31.1	31.9	32.7	33.6	34.4	35.2	36	29.8	30.6	31.4	32.2	33.1	33.8	34.6
37	30.9	31.7	32.5	33.4	34.2	35	35.8	37	30.4	31.2	31.9	32.8	33.6	34.4	35.2
38	31.6	32.3	33.1	34	34.9	35.6	36.4	38	31	31.8	32.6	33.4	34.2	35	35.7
39	32.2	33	33.7	34.6	35.5	36.2	37	39	31.6	32.4	33.1	34	34.8	35.6	36.3
40	32.8	33.6	34.3	35.2	36.1	36.8	37.6	40	32.2	33	33.7	34.5	35.4	36.1	36.9
41	33.4	34.1	34.9	35.8	36.6	37.4	38.2	41	32.8	33.5	34.3	35.1	35.9	36.7	37.4
42	34	34.7	35.5	36.3	37.2	38	38.7	42	33.3	34	34.8	35.6	36.4	37.2	37.9
43	34.5	35.3	36	36.9	37.7	38.5	39.3	43	33.9	34.6	35.3	36.1	37	37.7	38.4

The centile charts presented in tabular and graphical form on pages 1404 and 1405 are the 3rd, 10th, 25th, 50th, 75th, 90th and 97th centiles. These charts are provided because the text refers to weight for gestation this way. The current Child Growth Foundation charts use the 0.4th, 2nd, 9th, 25th, 50th, 75th, 91st, 99th and 99.6th centiles and these charts are presented on pages 1407 and 1408. Future clinical guidelines will be developed using these centile charts.

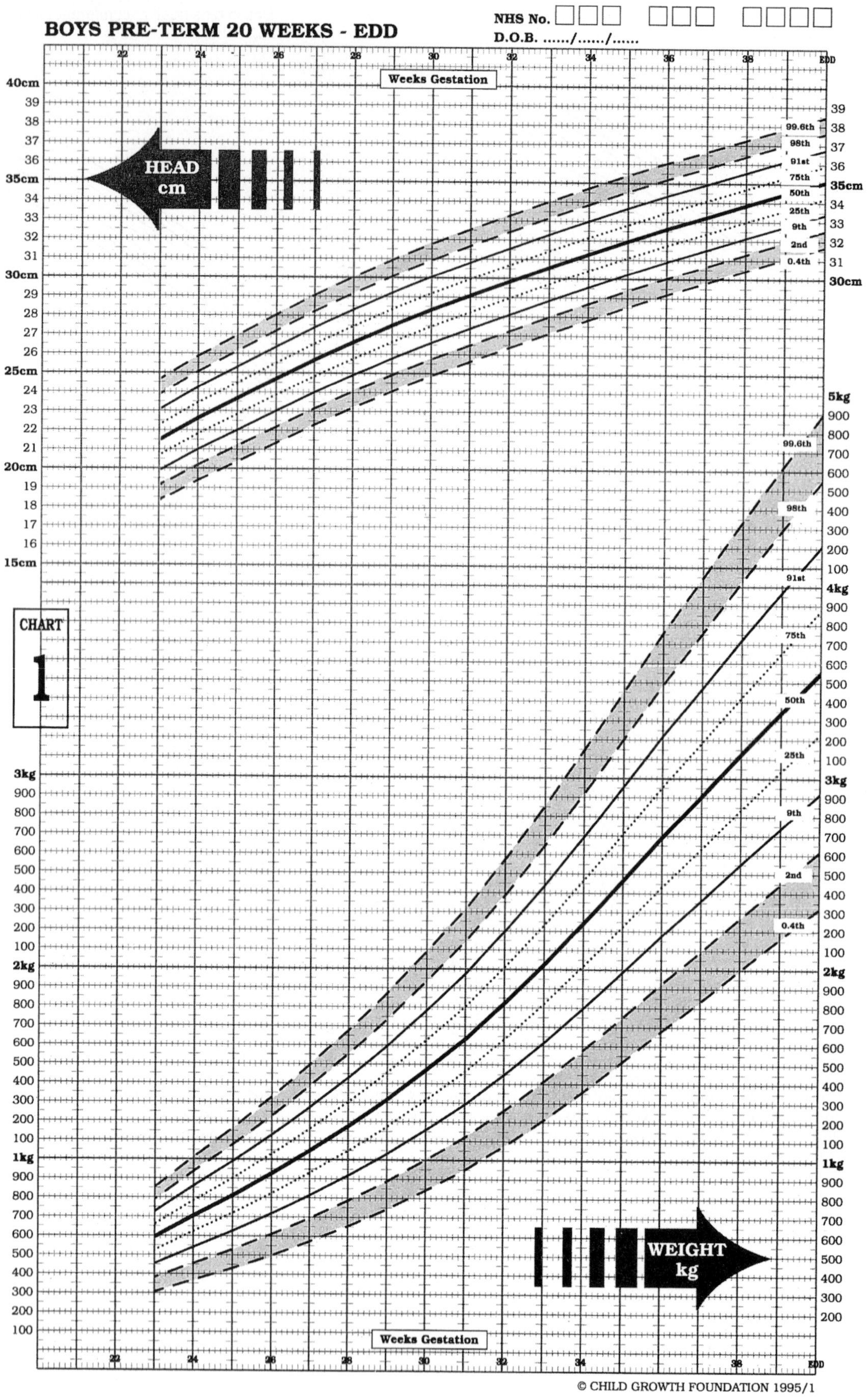
BOYS PRE-TERM 20 WEEKS - EDD
NHS No.
D.O.B. ....../....../......
Weeks Gestation
HEAD cm
CHART 1
WEIGHT kg
99.6th
98th
91st
75th
50th
25th
9th
2nd
0.4th
© CHILD GROWTH FOUNDATION 1995/1

NHS No. □□□ □□□ □□□□

D.O.B. ....../....../......

GIRLS PRE-TERM 20 WEEKS - EDD

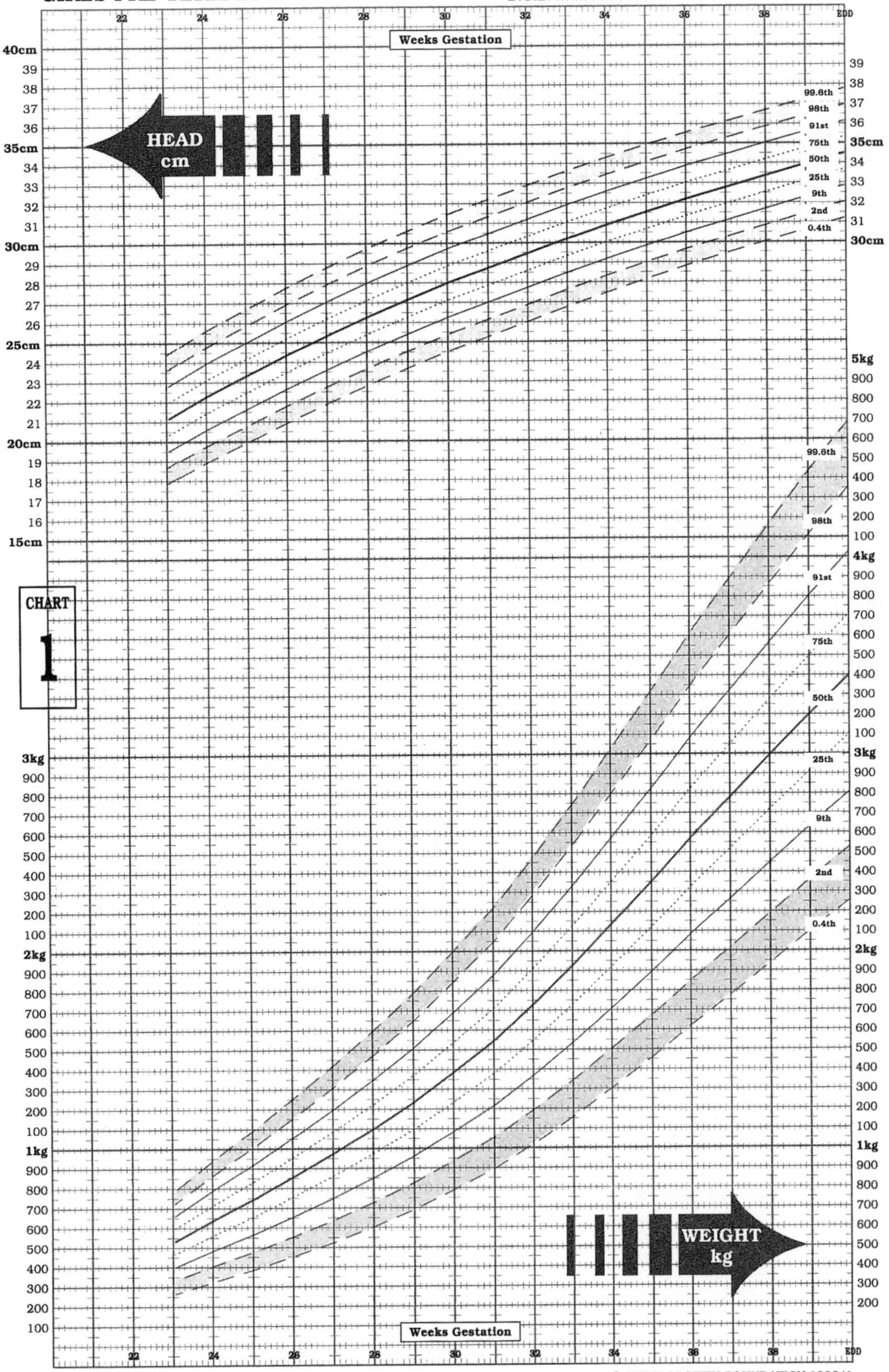

Appendix 6

Neonatal biochemical reference ranges

Anne Green Sue Keffler

NB: When no specific age is stated, the ranges below apply to neonates from 0 to 28 days.

Analyte	Unit	Reference range					Comments
		Preterm			Term		
		Gestational age (weeks)	Age (days)	Reference range	Age	Reference range	
Blood/Plasma							
Acid–base status:[22]							
Hydrogen ion (pH)	nmol/l (pH)				1 hour	40–54 (7.27–7.39)	Arterial. See also[34]
					24 hours	37–50 (7.31–7.43)	Arterial
					7 days	38–48 (7.32–7.42)	Arterial
pCO_2	kPa				1 hour	3.7–5.9	Arterial
					24 hours	3.6–5.3	Arterial
					7 days	4.0–5.6	Arterial
Bicarbonate[45]	mmol/l	1500–1750 g	7	15–26	1 hour	16.8–21.6	Arterial
			21	11–25	24 hours	17.6–22.8	Arterial
					7 days	19.2–24.4	Arterial
pO_2	kPa				1 hour	5.4–11.5	Arterial
					24 hours	7.2–12.2	Arterial
					7 days	7.1–12.3	Arterial
Base excess	mmol/l			–5 to +5		–3 to +3	
Alanine aminotransferase (ALT) (BCH* – unpublished observations)	IU/l					up to 40	Range may vary with method
Albumin[12,52]	g/l	27		21–33	0–7 days	28–43	
		29		23–34	7–14 days	30–43	
		31		22–35	14–21 days	27–44	
		33		22–35	21–28 days	32–44	
		35		22–36			
Alkaline phosphatase[10] (ALP)	IU/l	26–27		35–604		28–300	Higher levels in first week due to placental ALP. Range can vary widely with method. High levels are suggestive of rickets.
		28–29		119–465			
		30–31		112–450			
		32–33		110–398			
		34–35		113–360			
		36		88–326			
α_1-antitrypsin[30,31]	g/l					0.9–2.2	'Adult' levels at birth, with fall after 2 weeks. Gradual rise to adult level by 1 year. Phenotype should be assessed if < 1.6 g/l in infants with prolonged jaundice to check for deficiency. Concentration may vary as part of acute-phase response.

* BCH: Birmingham Children's Hospital NHS Trust

Analyte	Unit	Reference range					Comments
		Preterm			Term		
		Gestational age (weeks)	Age (days)	Reference range	Age	Reference range	
α-fetoprotein[5]	U/ml	Age corrected for gest. age (wks) −10 − 8 − 6 − 4 − 2		 38 910–2 034 000 15 960–988 900 6548–480 800 2686–233 800 1102–113 700	 0 weeks +2 weeks +4 weeks	 452–55 270 185–26 870 76–13 070	
Ammonia[33]	μmol/l					up to 100	Preterm and/or sick babies may have concentrations up to 200 μmol/l Capillary blood not recommended.
Anion gap i.e. $([Na^+] + [K^+]) - ([Cl^-] + [HCO^-_3])$	mmol/l					less than 20	
Amylase[1]	IU/l					up to 50	Range can vary widely with method.
Aspartate aminotransferase (AST) (BCH – unpublished observations)	IU/l					up to 100	Capillary blood. Range will vary according to method.
Bilirubin – total	μmol/l				< 10 days	up to 200	Refer to neonatal treatment charts for details (p. 000).
– conjugated	μmol/l				< 14 days	less than 20	Applies to specific methods only.
– direct reacting	μmol/l				< 14 days	less than 40	Applies to diazo methods, which are more subject to interferences and therefore less preferable.
Caeruloplasmin (Supraregional Protein Reference Unit, Cardiff)	g/l	28–31		0.06–0.11	0–4 months	0.09–0.27	Increases from birth throughout the first year.
Calcium – total[29,44]	mmol/l		21–28	2.14–2.65	1–2 days 2–3 days 3–4 days 4–6 days 6–12 days	2.18–2.48 2.14–2.64 2.22–2.55 2.25–2.68 2.26–2.69	Results should be interpreted in conjunction with the albumin concentration (p. 000).
– ionized[32,47]	mmol/l	25–36	1 3 5	0.81–1.41 0.72–1.44 1.04–1.52	1 day 3 days 5 days	1.05–1.37 1.10–1.44 1.20–1.48	See also[48]
Chloride[13,45]	mmol/l	1500–1750 g	7	101–116		96–110	
Cholesterol (total)[18]	mmol/l				At birth 7 days	1.0–2.4 2.0–4.3	Gradual increase from birth.
Copper[26] (Supraregional Protein Reference Unit, Cardiff)	μmol/l	28–34	Not stated	3.0–8.3	0–5 days 5–28 days	1.4–7.2 4.0–11.0	Rapid increase during first week.

Analyte	Unit	Reference range					Comments
		Preterm			Term		
		Gestational age (weeks)	Age (days)	Reference range	Age	Reference range	
Cortisol (Regional Endocrine Laboratory, Selly Oak Hospital, Birmingham)	nmol/l				> 1 day	200–700	There is a marked fall within 24 hours following delivery. There is no diurnal variation in cortisol in neonates, so if there is any doubt about the integrity of the hypothalamic–pituitary–adrenal axis short synacthen test will be required.
Creatine kinase[11,17,25]	IU/l				cord blood	70–380	Range dependent on methodology. Marked fall during first week of life, following peak at 24–48 hours, when levels up to 10 times higher than those in infancy/childhood may be seen. The pattern of isoenzymes is different, with relative increase in BB fraction in neonates.
					5–8 hours	214–1175	
					24–33 hours	158–1230	
					71–100 hours	87–725	
					1 month	50–305	
Creatinine[35]	μmol/l	25–28	2	76–156	2 days	37–113	For Jaffé method; concentrations for enzymatic methods generally lower.
			7	52–116	7 days	14–86	
			14	40–104	14 days	18–58	
			21	27–93	21 days	15–55	
			28	34–82	28 days	12–48	
		29–32	2	66–142			
			7	42–124			
			14	37–101			
			21	27–91			
			28	19–85			
		33–36	2	54–132			
			7	24–112			
			14	19–91			
			21	17–87			
			28	11–59			
C-reactive protein (CRP)[41]	mg/l					up to 6	Plasma half-life 5–7 hours
Ferritin[23,36,40,42]	μg/l		0–7	230–770		140–674	Lower at birth.
			7–14	250–950			
			14–21	160–770			
Glucose (fasting)[14,25,43]	mmol/l		Cord blood	2.4–5.7	12–24 hours	2.4–5.4	For plasma, concentrations in whole blood are 10–15% lower. For more detailed discussion of hypoglycaemia see page 00
					1–2 days	2.9–5.2	
					2–3 days	2.8–5.6	
					3–4 days	3.4–6.1	
					4–7 days	3.2–5.9	
					> 7 days	3.9–7.0	
γ-Glutamyl transpeptidase (gamma GT) (BCH – unpublished observations)	IU/l				0–2 weeks	< 250	
					2–4 weeks	< 150	

Analyte	Unit	Preterm: Gestational age (weeks)	Preterm: Age (days)	Preterm: Reference range	Term: Age	Term: Reference range	Comments
17α-Hydroxyprogesterone (17-OHP) (Regional Endocrine Laboratory, Selly Oak Hospital, Birmingham)	nmol/l				2–10 days	0.7–12.4	There is a rapid fall from the very high concentrations of 17-OHP (maternally derived) in the first 24–48 hours of life. This is therefore an inappropriate time to measure 17-OHP for diagnostic purposes. Premature and/or sick infants also have 2–3-fold higher levels of 17-OHP than full-term well infants.
Immunoglobulins							
IgG	g/l	29–32	7 14 28	1.86–7.28 1.19–6.37 0.9–4.5	0–2 weeks 2–4 weeks	5.0–17.0 3.9–13.0	Lower values seen in premature infants. Levels fall to 2 g/l or less in 16% of preterm babies because there is no significant IgG generation in the first 15 weeks of life.[6] See also[46]
IgG subtypes: IgG_1	g/l	26–30	1	1.5–6.2		3.4–12.0	
IgG_2	g/l	26–30	1	0.0–1.6		0.67–5.22	
IgG_3	g/l	26–30	1	0.13–0.55		0.26–1.48	
IgG_4	g/l	26–30	1	0–0.35		0–0.97	
IgA	g/l	29–32	7 14 28	0–0.01 0–0.08 0–0.12	0–2 weeks 2–4 weeks	0.01–0.08 0.02–0.15	Undetectable at birth in 99% of infants but detectable levels by 6 months of age.
IgM	g/l	29–32	7 14 28	0.02–0.39 0.04–0.41 0.06–0.33	0–2 weeks 2–4 weeks	0.05–0.20 0.08–0.40	
IgE (Supraregional Protein Reference Unit Handbook)	U/ml					Up to 35	See also[3,8]
Immunoreactive trypsin[15]	μg/l					Up to 120 Up to 70	Plasma Blood spot
Insulin[14]							No quantitative range provided as values must be interpreted with a plasma glucose concentration collected simultaneously. Can be higher in preterm infants.
Iron[12]	μmol/l					10–33	May be higher at birth.
Ketone bodies[14]	mmol/l	26–36	3	0.01–0.51	3 days	0.01–2.06	
Lactate (fasting)[22]	mmol/l				Cord blood 1 hour 24 hours 7 days	1.5–4.5 0.9–2.7 0.8–1.2 0.5–1.4	
Magnesium[32,37]	mmol/l	25–36	1 3 5 7–28	0.62–1.02 0.66–1.10 0.68–1.24 0.75–1.00	1 day 3 days 5 days 7–28 days	0.72–1.00 0.81–1.05 0.78–1.02 0.65–1.00	
Non-esterified fatty acids[14]	mmol/l	26–36	3	0.01–1.04	3 days	0.04–1.34	
Osmolality	mosmol/kg					275–295	

Analyte	Unit	Reference range					Comments
		Preterm			Term		
		Gestational age (weeks)	Age (days)	Reference range	Age	Reference range	
Phosphate[44]	mmol/l				1–2 days 2–3 days 3–4 days 4–6 days 6–12 days	2.03–2.66 1.89–2.92 1.83–2.68 1.67–2.68 1.54–2.90	Affected by type of milk feed, being generally higher in formula-fed babies.
Potassium[13,45]	mmol/l		7 21	4.6–6.6 (serum) 4.6–7.0 (serum)	0–1 week 1–4 weeks	3.2–5.5 (plasma) 3.4–6.0 (plasma)	Venous or arterial blood (not haemolysed). Results from capillary blood are generally higher. Plasma potassium is 10% lower than serum as potassium is released from platelets during coagulation.
Protein (total)[25]	g/l					54–70	Term baby; preterm babies have lower values. Gradual increase from birth.
Selenium (Regional Toxicology Laboratory, Birmingham)	µg/l				0–1 month	30–50	Useful guide for TPN monitoring.
Sodium[13,45]	mmol/l		7	133–146	0–1 week 1–4 weeks	133–146 134–144	See also[2]
Thyroid-stimulating hormone (TSH) (Screening laboratory, Lewisham Hospital, London)	mU/l				1 day 2 days 7 days > 7 days	3.0–120 3.0–30 0.3–10 0.3–5	Pre- & full-term infants show a rapid increase in TSH during the first 24 hours.
Thyroxine (total, TT4)[7,9]	nmol/l	30–31	0.5–3 3–10	94–203 53–146	1–3 days 1–4 weeks	142–277 106–214	Higher levels occur in first week of life.
Thyroxine (free, fT4)[19]	pmol/l	29–36	1–3 4–10	11.3–24.0 10.0–30.0	1–3 days 4–10 days	16.7–48.3 13.7–28.0	Lower in sick neonates.
Triglycerides (fasting)[39]	mmol/l				Cord blood 3 weeks	0.06–0.06 0.24–1.55	
Triiodothyronine (total, TT3)[7]	nmol/l	31–37	0.5–3 4–20	0.8–2.4 0.3–4.2	0.5–3 3–28	0.6–2.5 1.1–3.5	Lower in small sick infants;[28] 100% of healthy preterms had reached a level of 0.7 nmol/l by 14 days.
Triiodothyronine (free, fT3)[19]	pmol/l	29–36	1–3 4–10	1.2–7.3 1.2–4.9	1–3 days 4–10 days	2.5–9.3 2.8–5.7	Lower values seen in sick neonates.
Urate[49]	µmol/l				0–1 day 1–2 days 2–3 days 3–7 days	300–505 200–490 190–395 150–290	
Urea[27]	mmol/l		7	0.5–4.2	0–5 days	0.7–6.7	Infants fed on cows' milk formula may have higher levels.
Zinc[26]	µmol/l	28–34	Not stated	10–24	0–5 days	9.9–21.4	Concentrations decrease during the first week.[24,27] Preterm infants have higher values.

Analyte	Unit	Preterm: Gestational age (weeks)	Preterm: Age (days)	Preterm: Reference range	Term: Age	Term: Reference range	Comments
Urine[51]							
Calcium[20]	mmol/ 1.73 m^2/ 24 h		0–7	< 1.5	0–1 week	< 0.6	Higher values seen after first week.
Calcium:creatinine ratio[38]	mmol/ mmol				1–4 weeks	< 2.4	Lower during first week.
Copper (Protein Reference Unit, Cardiff)	μmol/ 24 h					up to 1.0	
Phosphate	mmol/ 1.73m^2/ 24 h		0–7	< 5.2	0–1 week	< 18	
Tubular phosphate reabsorption[4] (note A)	%					> 80	Higher in preterm babies.
Potassium[50]	mmol/ kg/24 h					< 5	Depends on potassium intake and gestational age.
Sodium[50]	mmol/ kg/24 h	< 28 29–32	0–7 0–7	< 22 < 12		< 1	Depends on sodium intake and gestational age.
Sodium:potassium ratio						< 1.0	
Fractional sodium excretion[50] (note B)	%	25–33	0–7	< 16		< 1.0	
Urate:creatinine ratio[21]	mmol/ mmol					0.1–2.0	In sulphite oxidase deficiency the ratio is likely to be < 0.03 mmol/mmol. Patients with Lesch–Nyhan syndrome generally have elevated ratios.

NOTES:

A. $$\text{Tubular phosphate reabsorption} = 1 - \frac{\text{(Urine phosphate (mmol/l)}}{\text{(Urine creatinine (mmol/l)}} \times \frac{\text{Plasma creatinine (}\mu\text{mol/l)}}{\text{Plasma phosphate (mmol/l)}} \times \frac{1}{10}$$

B. $$\text{Fractional sodium excretion} = \frac{\text{Urine sodium (mmol/l)}}{\text{Urine creatinine (mmol/l)}} \times \frac{\text{Plasma creatinine (}\mu\text{mol/l)}}{\text{Plasma sodium (mmol/l)}} \times \frac{1}{10}$$

BCH: Birmingham Children's Hospital NHS Trust

REFERENCES

1. Aggett P J, Taylor F 1980 A normal paediatric amylase range. Archives of Disease in Childhood 55: 236–238
2. Al-Dahhan J, Haycock G B, Chantler C, Stimmler L 1983 Sodium homeostasis in term and preterm neonates. Archives of Disease in Childhood 58: 335–342
3. Ballow M, Cates K L, Rowe J C, Goetz C 1986 Development of the immune system in very low birthweight infants. Pediatric Research 20: 899–904
4. Bistarakis L, Voškaki I, Lambadaridis J, Sereti H, Sbyrakis S 1986 Renal handling of phosphate in the first six months of life. Archives of Disease in Childhood 61: 677–681
5. Blair J I, Carachi R, Gupta R, Sim F G, McAllister E J, Weston R 1987 Plasma α-fetoprotein reference ranges in infancy: effect of prematurity. Archives of Disease in Childhood 62: 362–369
6. Conway S P, Dear P R F, Smith I 1985 Immunoglobulin profile of the preterm baby. Archives of Disease in Childhood 60: 208–212
7. Cuestas R A 1978 Thyroid function in preterm infants. Journal of Pediatrics 92: 963–967
8. Drossou V, Kanakoudi F, Diamanti E 1995 Concentrations of the main serum opsonins in early infancy. Archives of Disease in Childhood 72: F172–F175
9. Fisher D A 1989 The thyroid gland. In: Brook C G D (ed) Clinical paediatric endocrinology, 2nd edn. Blackwell Scientific Publications, Oxford, p 313

10. Glass E J, Hume R, Hendry G M A, Strange R C, Forfar J O 1982 Plasma alkaline phosphatase activity in rickets of prematurity. Archives of Disease in Childhood 57: 373–376
11. Gilboa N, Swanson J R 1976 Serum creatine phosphokinase in normal newborns. Archives of Disease in Childhood 51: 283–285
12. Gomez P, Coca C, Vargas C, Acebillo J, Martinez A 1984 Normal reference intervals for 20 biochemical variables in healthy infants, children and adolescents. Clinical Chemistry 30: 407–412
13. Greeley C, Snell J, Colaco A et al 1993 Pediatric reference ranges for electrolytes and creatinine. Pediatric Laboratory Medicine 11/3
14. Hawdon J M, Aynsley-Green A, Alberti K G M M, Ward Platt M 1993 The role of pancreatic insulin secretion in neonatal glucoregulation. I. Healthy term and preterm infants. Archives of Disease in Childhood 68: 274–279
15. Healey A F. Personal communication.
16. Izquierdo J M, Ferrero J, Romeo D, Badia J L, Vigil E R 1970 Capillary blood potassium, chloride, sodium, calcium, phosphorus and alkaline phosphatase in the newborn. Clinica Chimica Acta 30: 343–346
17. Jedeikin R, Makela S K, Shennan A T, Ellis G 1982 Creatine kinase isoenzymes in serum from cord blood and the blood of healthy full term infants during the first three postnatal days. Clinical Chemistry 28: 317–322
18. Jira P, de Jong J, Janssen-Zijlstra F et al 1996 Pitfalls in measuring plasma cholesterol in Smith–Lemli–Opitz syndrome. Journal of Inherited and Metabolic Disease 19 Supp. 1: 93
19. John R, Bamforth F J 1987 Serum free thyroxine and free triiodothyronine concentrations in healthy full term, pre-term and sick pre-term neonates. Annals of Clinical Biochemistry 24: 461–465
20. Karlen J, Aperia A, Zetterstrom R 1985 Renal excretion of calcium and phosphate in preterm and term infants. Journal of Pediatrics 106: 814–819
21. Kaufman J M, Greene M L, Seegmiller J E 1968 Urine uric acid to creatinine ratio – a screening test for inherited disorders of purine metabolism. Journal of Pediatrics 73: 583–592
22. Koch G, Wendel H 1968 Adjustment of arterial blood gases and acid base balance in the normal newborn infant during the first week of life. Biology of the Neonate 12: 136–161
23. Liappis N, O Schlebusch H 1990 Referenzwerte der ferritin konzentration im serum von kindern. Klinische Paediatrie 202: 99–102
24. Lokitch G, Godolphin W, Pendray M R, Riddell G, Quigley G 1983 Serum zinc, copper, retinol binding protein, prealbumin and caeruloplasmin concentrations in infants receiving intravenous zinc and copper supplementation.
25. Lockitch G, Halstead A C, Albersheim S, MacCallum C, Quigley G 1988 Age- and sex-specific reference intervals for biochemistry analytes as measured with the Ektachem-700 analyser. Clinical Chemistry 34: 1622–1625.
26. Lockitch G, Halstead A C, Wadsworth L, Quigley G, Reston L, Jacobson B 1988 Age- and sex-specific pediatric reference intervals and correlations for zinc, copper, selenium, iron, vitamins A and E, and related proteins. Clinical Chemistry 34: 1625–1628
27. Lockitch G, Halstead A C 1989 Reference (normal) values. In Meites S (ed) Paediatric clinical chemistry, 3rd edn. AACC, p 282
28. Lucas A, Rennie J, Baker B A, Morley R 1988 Low plasma triiodothyronine concentrations and outcome in preterm infants. Archives of Disease in Childhood 63: 1201–1206
29. Mayne P D, Kovar I Z 1991 Calcium and phosphorus metabolism in the premature infant. Annals of Clinical Biochemistry 28: 131–142
30. Milford Ward A, White P A E, Wild G 1985 Reference ranges for serum α-1-antitrypsin. Archives of Disease in Childhood 60: 261–262.
31. Milford Ward A, Riches P G, Fifield R, Smith A M (eds) 1990 Protein Reference Unit Handbook of Clinical Immunochemistry, 4th edn. PRU Publications.
32. Nelson N, Finnstrom O, Larsson L 1989 Plasma ionised calcium, phosphate and magnesium in pre-term and small for gestational age infants. Acta Paediatrica Scandinavica 78: 351–357
33. Oberholzer V G, Schwarz K B, Smith C H, Dietzler D N, Hanna T L 1976 Microscale modification of a cation exchange column procedure for plasma ammonia. Clinical Chemistry 22: 1976–1981
34. Reardon H S, Baumann H L, Haddad E J 1960 Chemical stimuli of respiration in the early neonatal period. Journal of Pediatrics 57: 151–170
35. Rudd P T, Hughes E A, Placzek M M, Hodes D T 1983 Reference ranges for plasma creatinine during the first month of life. Archives of Disease in Childhood 58: 212–215
36. Saarinen U M, Simes M A 1978 Serum ferritin in assessment of iron nutrition in healthy infants. Acta Paediatrica Scandinavica 67: 745–751
37. Saniel-Banray K 1989 Reference (normal) values. In Meites S (ed). Pediatric clinical chemistry, 3rd edn. AACC, p 191
38. Sargent J D, Stubel T A, Kresel J, Klein R Z 1993 Normal values for random urinary calcium to creatinine ratios in infancy. Journal of Pediatrics 123: 393–397
39. Scott P H 1989 Reference (normal) values. In: Meites S (ed) Pediatric clinical chemistry, 3rd edn. AACC, p 274
40. Shaw J C L 1982 Iron absorption by the premature infant. Acta Paediatrica Scandinavica suppl 299: 83–98
41. Shine B, Gould J, Campbell C, Hindocha P, Pitcher Wilmot R, Wood C B S 1985 Serum C-reactive protein in normal and infected neonates. Clinica Chimica Acta 148: 97–103
42. Siimes M A, Addiego J E, Dallman P R 1974 Ferritin in serum: diagnosis of iron deficiency and iron overload in infants and children. Blood 43: 581–590
43. Srinivason G, Pildes R S, Cattamanchi G, Voora S, Lilien L D 1986 Plasma glucose values in normal neonates: a new look. Journal of Pediatrics 109: 114–117
44. Thalme B 1962 Calcium, chloride, cholesterol, inorganic phosphorus and total protein in blood plasma during the early neonatal period studied with ultramicrochemical methods. Acta Paediatrica Scandinavica 51: 649–660
45. Thomas J L, Reichelderfer T E 1968 Premature infants: analysis of serum during the first seven weeks. Clinical Chemistry 14: 272–280
46. Uffelman J A, Engelhard W E, Jolliff C R 1970 Quantitation of immunoglobulins in normal children. Clinica Chimica Acta 28: 185–192
47. Wandrup J, Kroner J, Pryds O, Kastrup K W 1988 Age related reference values for ionized calcium in the first week of life in premature and full term newborns. Scandinavian Journal of Clinical Laboratory Investigation 48: 255–260
48. Wandrup J 1989 Critical analysis and clinical aspects of ionized calcium in neonates. Clinical Chemistry 35: 2027–2033
49. Wharton B A, Bassi U, Gough G, Williams A 1971 Clinical value of plasma creatine kinase and uric acid levels during first week of life. Archives of Disease in Childhood 46: 356–362
50. Wilkins B H 1992 Renal function in sick very low birthweight infants: 3. Sodium, potassium and water excretion. Archives of Disease in Childhood 67: 1154–1161
51. Young W F, Hallum J L, McCance R A 1941 The secretion of urine by premature infants. Archives of Disease in Childhood 16: 243–252
52. Zlotkin S H, Casselman C W 1987 Percentile estimates of reference values for total protein and albumin in sera of premature infants (< 37 weeks of gestation). Clinical Chemistry 33: 411–413

Appendix 7

Normal blood gas values

N. R. C. Roberton

	PaO$_2$				paCO$_2$				H+			
	kPa	**mmHg**	**kPa**	**mmHg**	**kPa**	**mmHg**	**kPa**	**mmHg**	**nmol/l**	**pH**	**nmol/l**	**pH**
15 minutes	11.6	87			3.7	28			48	7.32		
30 minutes	11.4	86			4.3	32			43	7.37		
60 minutes	10.8	81			4.1	31			40	7.40		
1–6 hours	8.0–10.6	60–80	*8.0–9.3*	*60–70*	4.7–6	35–45	*4.7–6*	*35–45*	46–49	7.31–7.34	*42–48*	*7.32–7.38*
6–24 hours	9.3–10	70–75	*8.0–9.3*	*60–70*	4.4–4.8	33–36	*3.6–5.3*	*27–40*	37–43	7.37–7.43	*35–45*	*7.36–7.45*
48 hours–1 week	9.3–11.3	70–85	*10.0–10.6*	*75–80*	4.4–4.8	33–36	*4.3–4.5*	*32–36*	42–44	7.36–7.38	*40–48*	*7.32–7.40*
2 weeks					4.8–5.2	36–39	*5.1*	*38*	43	7.37	*48*	*7.32*
3 weeks					5.3	40	*5.1*	*38*	42	7.38	*49*	*7.31*
1 month					5.2	39	*4.9*	*37*	41	7.39	*49*	*7.31*

The values at 15, 30 and 60 minutes are from our own unpublished observations on full-term infants. Data from 1 hour to 1 week are drawn from the literature on arterial samples. Data beyond 1 week are on capillary samples. Values in the table which are in *italics* are those for premature infants; those not in italics are for full-term infants.

Reproduced from Roberton N R C 1993 *Manual of Neonatal Intensive Care*. London, Edward Arnold, with permission.

Appendix 8

Endotracheal tube lengths

N. R. C. Roberton

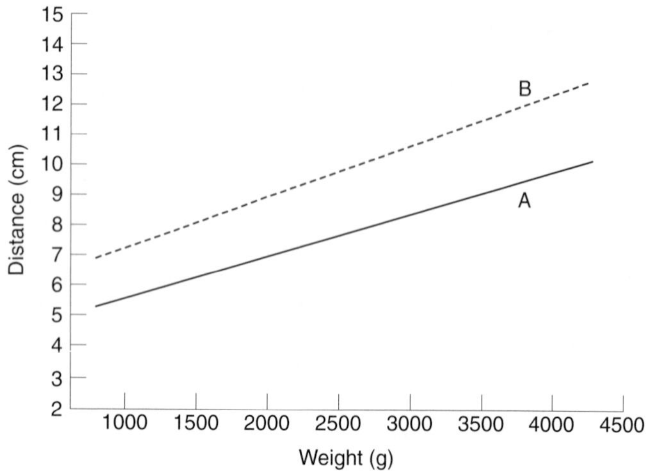

Distance to insert endotracheal tubes into babies of different body weights.

Line A is the lip to mid-tracheal position for oral tubes.
Line B is the nose–mid-tracheal distance for naso-endotracheal tubes.
Derived from various sources in the literature:

Coldiron J S 1968 Estimation of naso tracheal tube length in neonates. Pediatrics 41: 823–825
Klaus M, Fanaroff A A 1979 Care of the high risk neonate. W B Saunders, Philadelphia
Loew A, Thibeault D 1974 A new and safe method to control the depth of endotracheal intubation in neonates. Pediatrics 54: 506–509

Appendix 9

Umbilical artery catheter insertion

N. R. C. Roberton

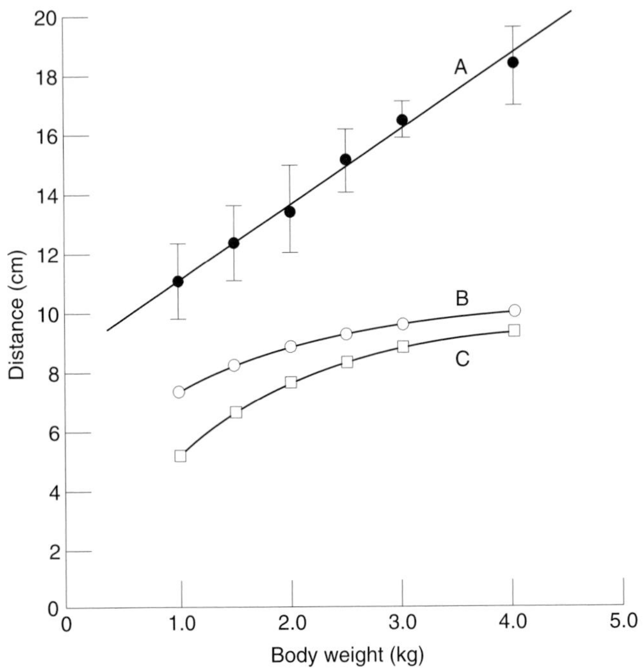

Line (A) is derived from various sources[1–5] for inserting the umbilical artery catheter to reach approximately T8–T10 at the region of the diaphragm. The points mark the average of various reports in the literature and the horizontal lines the range.

B is the distance to L3.[6]

C is the distance to L5, approximately the bifurcation of the aorta.[1,6]

Lines B and C are slightly curved, as they are derived from references 1, 5 and 6 which give the data in terms of body length. Body length has been converted into weight using the data of Gruenwald and Minh.[2]

These points are estimates. The position of the umbilical artery catheter, whether a low or high position is chosen, must always be confirmed by X-ray immediately after insertion to ensure that the tip is not in the danger areas (p. 363, Fig. 21.1).

REFERENCES

1. Dunn P M 1966 Localization of the umbilical catheter by post-mortem measurement. Archives of Disease in Childhood 41: 69–75
2. Gruenwald P, Minh H N 1960 Evaluation of body and organ weights in perinatal pathology. American Journal of Clinical Pathology 34: 247–253
3. Gupta J M, Roberton N R C, Wigglesworth J S 1968 Umbilical artery catheterization in the newborn. Archives of Disease in Childhood 43: 382–387
4. Rosenfeld W, Biagtan J, Schaeffer M D et al 1980 A new graph for insertion of umbilical artery catheters. Journal of Pediatrics 96: 735–737
5. Rosenfeld W, Estrada R, Jhaveri R, Salazar D, Evans H 1981 Evaluation of graphs for insertion of umbilical artery catheters below the diaphragm. Journal of Pediatrics 98: 627–628
6. Shukla H, Ferrara A 1986 Rapid estimation of insertional length of umbilical catheters in newborns. American Journal of Diseases of Children 140: 786–788

Appendix 10

Umbilical venous catheter insertion

N. R. C. Roberton

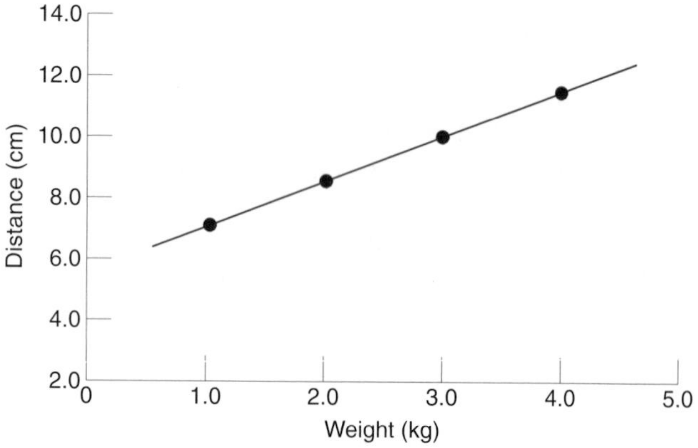

This illustration shows the distance to insert umbilical venous catheters such that the tip is lying in the right atrium just above the diaphragm.

In many cases it is not possible to push the UVC through the ductus venosus (p. 924), and this will usually result in the catheter being inserted for 2–3 cm less than indicated on this graph.

This graph is an estimated figure and the position of the tip of an umbilical venous catheter should always be confirmed radiologically prior to use.

Based on the data of Shukla H, Ferrara A 1986 Rapid estimation of insertion length of umbilical catheters in newborns. American Journal of Diseases of Children 140: 786–788

Appendix 11

Normal cerebrospinal fluid values

Janet M. Rennie

All values are given as mean and range.

Type of infant	Red cell count (mm^3)	White cell count (mm^3)	Protein (g/l)	Glucose (mmol/l)
Preterm < 7 days	30 (0–333)	9 (0–30)*	1 (0.5–2.9, but mostly < 2 g/l)	3 (1.5–5.5)†
Preterm > 7 days	30	12 (2–70)	0.9 (0.5–2.6, mostly < 1.5)	3 (1.5–5.5)†
Term < 7 days	9 (0–50)	5 (0–30)*	0.6 (0.3–2.5)	3 (1.5–5.5)†
Term > 7 days	< 10	3 (0–10)	0.5 (0.2–0.8)	3 (1.5–5.5)†

Sources: see reference list.[1,3,5,7,9,11,12,14,15,16]
*Gyllensward & Malmstrom[6] give values of up to 112 white cells per mm^3 in preterm and 90 in term babies, but the study included babies with over 1000 red cells per mm^3 and was done before routine ultrasound was available. The results are so much higher than other studies that I have not extended the range to include these values.
† CSF glucose usually 70–80% of plasma glucose, and at least 50%. Take plasma glucose sample *before* doing LP (stress). Low CSF glucose levels can persist for weeks after intraventricular haemorrhage.[4]

TRAUMATIC LUMBAR PUNCTURE

It has been suggested that it is possible to apply a formula to compare observed (O) to predicted (P) white cell counts in CSF samples with high red cell counts thought to be due to a 'traumatic tap'. The predicted white cell count P in the CSF is calculated from:

$$P = \text{CSF red cell count} \times \frac{\text{Blood WCC}}{\text{Blood RBC}}$$

The O:P ratio was greater than 1 in all cases of meningitis in infants over the age of 1 month.[2] The ratio is less well evaluated in the newborn, who can have paradoxically low white cell counts in the CSF even when the culture is positive. Several authors have pointed out that this ratio 'overcorrects' the CSF white cell count in newborn infants.[8,10,13] Osborne and Pizer[9] suggested that contamination with fewer than 10 000 red cells per mm^3 did not influence the white cell count. In suspicious clinical cases the only course is to repeat the lumbar puncture after 12–24 hours.

REFERENCES

1. Ahmed A, Hickey S M, Ehrett S, Trujillo M, Brito F, Goto C, Olsen K, Krisher K, McCracken G H Jr 1996 Cerebrospinal fluid values in the term neonate. Pediatric Infectious Disease Journal 15: 298–303
2. Bonadio W A, Smith D S, Goddard S, Boroughs J, Khaja G 1990 Distinguishing cerebrospinal fluid abnormalities in children with bacterial meningitis and traumatic lumbar puncture. Journal of Infectious Diseases 162: 251–254
3. Bonadio W A, Stanco L, Bruce R, Barry D, Smith D 1992 Reference values of normal cerebrospinal fluid composition in infants ages 0 to 8 weeks. Pediatric Infectious Disease Journal 11: 589–591
4. Deonna T, Calame A, van Melle G, Prod'hom L S 1977 Hypoglycorrhachia in neonatal intracranial haemorrhage. Relationship to posthaemorrhagic hydrocephalus. Helvetica Paediatrica Acta 32: 351–361
5. Escobedo M, Barton L L, Volpe J J 1975 Cerebrospinal fluid studies in an intensive care nursery. Journal of Perinatal Medicine 3: 204–210
6. Gyllensward A, Malmstrom S 1962 The cerebrospinal fluid in immature infants. Acta Paediatrica Scandinavica 51 (suppl 135): 54–62
7. Naidoo B T 1968 The cerebrospinal fluid in the healthy newborn infant. South African Medical Journal 42: 933–935
8. Novak R W 1984 Lack of validity of standard corrections for white blood cell counts of blood-contaminated cerebrospinal fluid in infants. American Journal of Clinical Pathology 82: 95–97
9. Osborne J P, Pizer B 1981 Effect on the white cell count of contaminating cerebrospinal fluid with blood. Archives of Disease in Childhood 56: 400–401
10. Otila E 1948 Studies on the cerebrospinal fluid in premature infants. Acta Paediatrica Scandinavica 35 (suppl 9): 7–97
11. Portnoy J M, Olson L C 1985 Normal cerebrospinal fluid values in children: another look. Pediatrics 75: 484–487
12. Rodriguez A F, Kaplan S L, Mason E O 1990 Cerebrospinal fluid values in the very low birthweight infant. Journal of Pediatrics 116: 971–974
13. Rubenstein J S, Yogev R 1985 What represents pleocytosis in blood contaminated ('traumatic tap') cerebrospinal fluid in children? Journal of Pediatrics 107: 249–252
14. Sarff L D, Platt L H, McCracken G H Jr 1976 Cerebrospinal fluid evaluation in neonates: comparison of high risk infants with and without meningitis. Journal of Pediatrics 88: 473–477
15. Widell S 1958 On the cerebrospinal fluid in normal children and in patients with acute abacterial meningoencephalitis. Acta Paediatrica Scandinavica 47 (suppl 115): 1–102
16. Wolf H, Hoepffner L 1961 The cerebrospinal fluid in the newborn and premature infant. World Neurology 2: 871–877

Appendix 12

Oxyhaemoglobin dissociation curve

N. R. C. Roberton

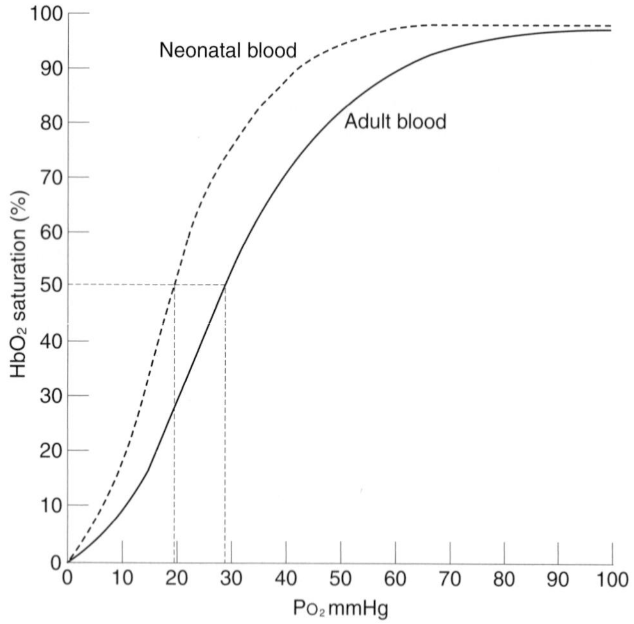

Oxyhaemoglobin dissociation curves for adult blood and neonatal blood. The dotted lines dropping from 50% saturation give the p50 values for neonatal blood (19 mmHg) and of adult blood (28 mmHg).

Appendix 13

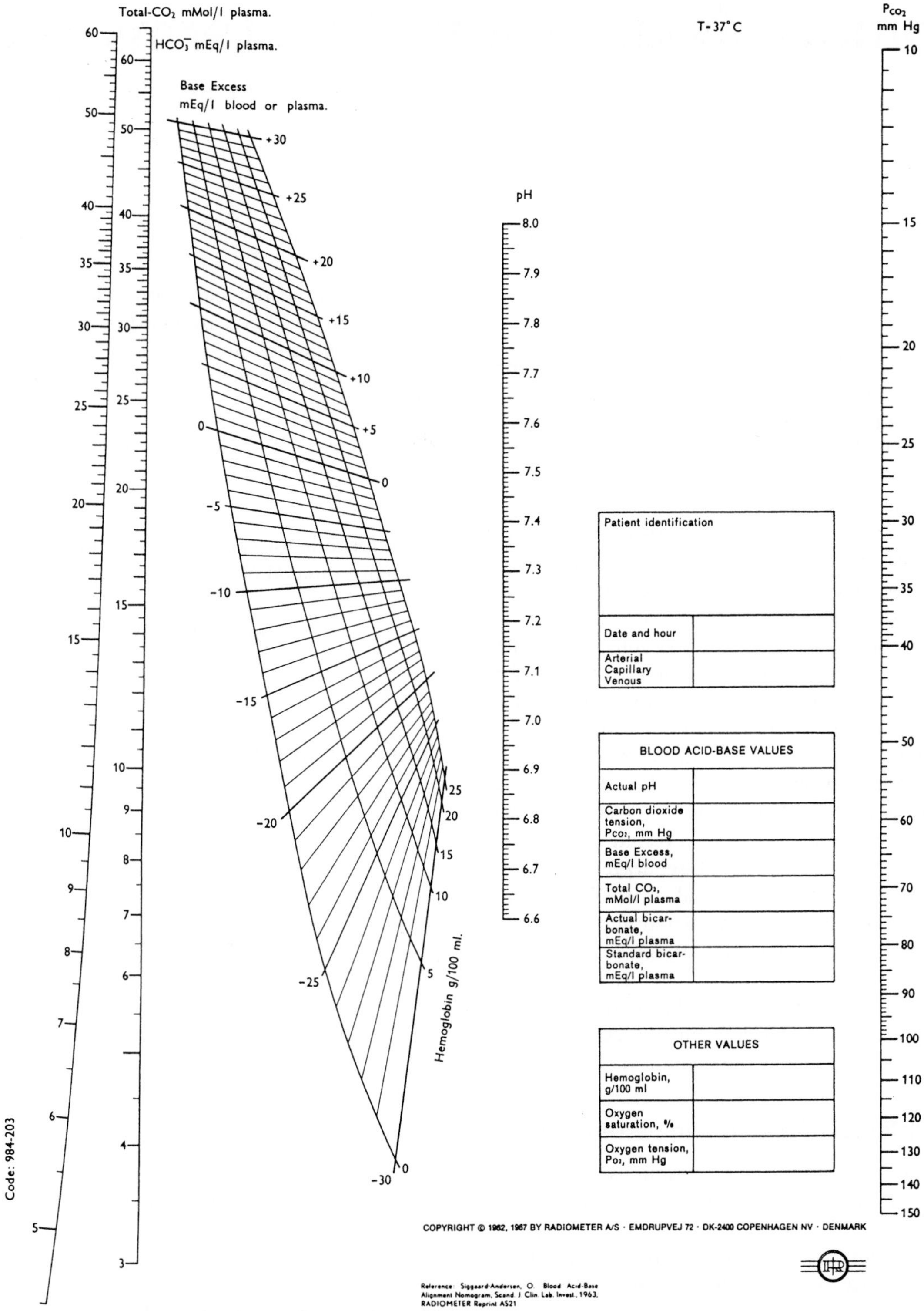

The Siggard–Andersen Nomogram. By knowing any two values of an acid–base measurement, the other values can be derived by connecting the two known points on this nomogram. For newborn babies the haemoglobin can be assumed to be 15 g/100 ml. Reproduced with permission of Radiometer Copenhagen.

Appendix 14

Commonly used statistical terms defined

Janet M. Rennie N. R. C. Roberton

CONFIDENCE INTERVAL

The confidence interval gives more information that just the mean or the P value; most journals now recommend that investigators routinely report confidence intervals.[1,2] The confidence interval reports information in terms of the measurement actually used, and the width of the confidence interval gives an indication of the strength of the study. The width of the confidence interval is usually closely related to the standard error of the statistic being used, often about four times as wide.[3] Confidence intervals can be calculated for linear regression slopes, in order to produce boundary lines which encompass 95% of the values. In comparative studies confidence intervals should be reported for the differences between groups, not for the results of each group separately. 95% confidence intervals are preferable to error bars of one standard error above and below the mean for graphical presentation of results; one standard error above and below depicts only a 67% confidence interval. Confidence intervals show the degree of uncertainty associated with a result, and reporting only P values below 0.05 is now discouraged.

Where the 95% confidence interval of a difference in means or percentages has been calculated and presented graphically, a result which does not cross 0 indicates a P value of less than 0.05. Where a similar calculation has been done for an odds ratio or a relative risk, a value which does not cross 1 also has a P value of less than 0.05 indicating a statistically significant result at the 5% level.

Confidence interval of means and percentages

The 95% confidence interval of a continuous variable or a percentage is from the value plus (1.96 × SE) to the value minus (1.96 × SE). In large samples (>n = 30) the 95% confidence interval for the mean is from 1.96 standard errors above the mean to 1.96 standard errors below.

Calculation formulae for confidence intervals of differences in means, regression, relative risks, etc, are all contained in the book by Gardner and Altman[1]. A few simple examples follow:

The formula for calculating the confidence interval of a single mean is:

Standard error (SE) = standard deviation /√n
Confidence interval is from mean – (1.96 × SE) to mean + (1.96 × SE)

The formula for calculating the standard error and the confidence interval of a percentage P is:

$$SE = \sqrt{\frac{Px(100 - P)}{n}}$$

Confidence interval of an odds ratio

An odds ratio is a ratio of the number of individuals, subjects, etc, experiencing an event compared to the number not experiencing it, for example:

	RDS	no RDS	total
Antentatal steroids	a	b	a+b
No steroids	c	d	c+d
	a+c	b+c	

The relative risk R is given by the following formula:

$$R = \frac{a / (a + c)}{b / (b + d)}$$

The 95% confidence interval for R is calculated using logarithmic transformation.

The odds ratio is given by the formula:

$$OR = \frac{ad}{bc}$$

Confidence intervals for the odds ratio can be calculated using several methods (see above, and Gardner & Altman[1]).

DEFINITION OF MEASURES OF DIAGNOSTIC PERFORMANCE

	Disease X	
	Present	Absent
Test for disease X positive	True positive	False positive
Test for disease X negative	False negative	True negative

$$\textit{False positive} = \frac{FP}{TN + FP} \qquad \textit{False negative} = \frac{FN}{TP + FP}$$

$$\textit{Sensitivity} = \frac{TP}{TP + FN} \qquad \textit{Specificity} = \frac{TN}{TN + FP}$$

$$\textit{Efficiency} = \frac{TP + TN}{TP + FP + FN + TN}$$

The sensitivity of a test is the proportion of cases who truly have the disease and have a positive result. The specificity is the proportion of cases who do not have the disease and have a negative result. The efficiency of a test is the proportion of all results, positive or negative, which are true results. The predictive value of a test varies with the prevalence of a disease in the population, whereas the sensitivity and specificity are constant.

REFERENCES

1. Gardner M J, Altman D G 1989 Statistics with confidence – confidence intervals and statistical guidelines. BMJ Publications, London
2. Rothman K J 1978 A show of confidence. New England Journal of Medicine 299: 1362–1363
3. Ware J H, Mosteller F, Delagado F, Donnelly C, Ingelfinger J A 1992 In: Bailar J C III, Mosteller F (eds) Medical uses of statistics, 2nd edn. NEJM Books, Massachusetts

Appendix 15

Transport of ill infants

Sean P. Devane

Up to 3% of newborn infants suffer from a significant illness which requires intensive care. Most district maternity units have facilities for special care, but intensive care services have evolved in a variable manner often influenced by the size of the maternity unit and the expertise of the neonatal paediatricians. A region with 50 000 annual births requires about 75 intensive care cots, assuming a need for 1.5 cots per 1000 births.[18] A balance is required between dispersed intensive care cots with many maternity units having one or two intensive care cots, and concentration on large units. In the UK, the most widely adopted arrangement has been the development of regional perinatal centres (level 3 units) with 6–14 intensive care cots, and subregional perinatal centres (level 2 units) with 4–8 intensive care cots. Selected units have additional specialist services such as paediatric cardiology or paediatric surgery. Units with specialist services or who receive transfers from other units need in excess of 1.5 intensive care cots for each 1000 inborn deliveries. Whatever the model, a coherent policy for transport between units is required. These policies should cover antenatal (in-utero) referral to the specialist perinatal centre, postnatal ex-utero referral, and lastly postnatal ex-utero transfer from the specialist centre to the smaller unit. A survey of neonatal units conducted in the UK in 1991 identified over 1800 in-utero and over 2100 postnatal transfers in a population with a delivery number of 660 000.[8]

IN-UTERO REFERRAL AND TRANSFER

The possible need for intensive care or specialist investigation may be apparent before conception, or may become apparent during the pregnancy. For example, Rhesus sensitization may be known from previous obstetric events, unstable diabetes mellitus or renal, cardiac or pulmonary disease may be present, or complications may arise during the pregnancy or during the labour. Rigid rules must be avoided. Transfer should be considered only after adequate assessment by a senior obstetrician, often in consultation with the obstetric and neonatal staff at the referral unit, to avoid problems such as delivery in the ambulance. Both referring and recipient units must realize that in some cases the indication for recipient might disappear (e.g. threatened preterm labour may settle) so that the mother is then transferred back to the referring unit after some days. Adequate counselling of the parents by the referring unit staff is important.

It is clear that in-utero referral is preferable to neonatal transfer,[10,16,17] particularly where the need for intensive care is anticipated and skilled resuscitation at birth cannot otherwise be guaranteed. However, data comparing in-utero and neonatal transfer must be examined carefully to ensure that selection bias is not a factor (e.g. in the case of ex-utero transfers, the best candidates will be transferred while the worst will have died).

In-utero transfer to a higher-level unit should be considered in the following situations, among others:

- spontaneous preterm labour
- premature rupture of membranes
- placental dysfunction.

SPONTANEOUS PRETERM LABOUR

The need for intensive care is likely in infants born under 32 weeks' gestation, and intensive care with a prospect of a good outcome is likely above 24 weeks' gestation. Local policies should consider these gestational ages, though each case must be considered individually. Obstetric assessment should include obtaining information on cervical dilatation, rupture of membranes, fetal position, and cord prolapse. Tocolytic agents are often used (where the pregnancy is uncomplicated and the membranes are intact) but have associated risks of maternal complications. Administration of steroids to the mother should be considered.

PREMATURE RUPTURE OF MEMBRANES

Rupture of the membranes before the onset of labour and

before term leads to delivery within 7 days in nearly 85% of cases. Therefore, local policies should consider transfer in utero if this happens between 23 and 31 weeks' gestation. Assessment should be undertaken as for preterm labour. Early rupture of membranes (before 23 weeks), with continuation of the pregnancy, carries a risk of pulmonary hypoplasia. The optimum use of prophylactic antibiotics awaits the outcome of a number of current multicentre trials (such as the ORACLE trial based in the UK).

PLACENTAL DYSFUNCTION

Level 3 perinatal centres should have the facilities and expertise to advise on fetal well-being in cases of placental dysfunction. Where the risks of placental failure have to be balanced against the risks of premature delivery, antepartum cardiotocography and ultrasound assessment of liquor volume and fetal activity ('biophysical assessment') can be supplemented with assessments of uteroplacental blood flow and fetal blood flow redistribution.

NEONATAL REFERRAL AND TRANSFER

All units delivering babies (including community midwifery services undertaking home deliveries) should be able to provide resuscitation and temporary mechanical ventilation (at the least, being skilled in bag-valve-mask ventilation). They should have policies for postnatal referral.

Ex-utero transfer to a higher-level unit should be considered in the following situations, among others:

- uncomplicated preterm infants
- preterm infants with respiratory failure
- infants with recurrent apnoea
- infants with birth suppression
- infants with surgical conditions.

UNCOMPLICATED PRETERM INFANTS

Maternity units with more than 1000 births annually should be capable of providing care for healthy preterm babies of 28 weeks' gestation or more. Such a baby is one born in good condition and who does not have symptoms of respiratory distress by 4 hours of age. The same skills are required for managing these infants as for the convalescent ex-preterm infant following a return from a higher-level unit.

PRETERM INFANTS WITH RESPIRATORY FAILURE

All units delivering infants should be able to initiate respiratory support, and maintain it until transfer to a higher-level unit can be arranged. Any unit with more than 1000 births annually should be able to maintain respiratory support for more than a day, as occasional delays in transfer are likely to occur.[3] The potential complications of assisted ventilation mean that longer-term ventilation should only be undertaken in units with sufficient throughput to maintain medical staff skills. Policies should consider guideline activity figures such as a minimum of 20–30 babies receiving full ventilatory support annually, or 700 intensive care cot days per annum. In any case, adequate monitoring including transcutaneous oxygen monitoring and rapid access to blood gas measurement is required.

Deciding on the need for and on the timing of transfer of an infant with respiratory distress may be difficult, and should be undertaken by the most senior available paediatrician. If the respiratory distress is clinically mild, the baby can be nursed safely in less than 40% oxygen, sepsis is not suspected, and a chest X-ray suggests transient tachypnoea of the newborn, a period of observation may be undertaken. In most cases, early transfer is desirable. Whether to initiate ventilatory support before transfer is also a decision for a senior paediatrician.

INFANTS WITH RECURRENT APNOEA

About one-third of all babies of 32 weeks' gestation or less have apnoeic episodes. Increasing frequency and severity may indicate either the need for ventilatory support or the development of sepsis, and should suggest consideration of transfer. If sepsis is suspected, treatment should start before transfer.

INFANTS WITH BIRTH DEPRESSION

Infants who fail to breathe spontaneously from birth may respond to resuscitation. If they do not, or only respond partially, and have circulatory failure not responding to treatment, transfer should be considered. In many cases, hypoxic–ischaemic encephalopathy may not develop, or may be mild and its degree can only be assessed after 1 or 2 days.

INFANTS WITH SURGICAL CONDITIONS

Suggested criteria for transfer to a paediatric surgical centre have been put forward.[2,4,19] In regions where antenatal anomaly scanning is undertaken (often at about 20 weeks' gestation), congenital conditions requiring neonatal surgery will have been identified antenatally. It is usually desirable for the parents to have visited the unit where delivery is planned, and to have met the neonatal surgeon before delivery. A decision should be made on whether delivery will occur in the surgical centre or elsewhere with postnatal transfer. It is desirable that infants with a congenital diaphragmatic hernia are born in a surgical centre, to avoid the potential for destabilization inherent in postnatal transfers. It is also desirable that infants with gastroschisis are born in a surgical centre, as operative closure is best undertaken within hours of birth. In most other cases, either option can reasonably be taken.

All babies referred for surgery should receive 1 mg of vitamin K before transfer. Where there is a bowel obstruction, a large well-placed nasogastric or orogastric drainage tube should be in place and secured. It should be drained regularly. A Replogle tube may provide better continuous drainage. Exposed viscera should be covered with sterile plastic or with cling film. A consent for operation form signed by a parent, together with 10 ml of clotted maternal blood, should be sent to the surgical unit with the baby, if these are required by the surgical unit.

RETURN TRANSFER FROM RECIPIENT TO REFERRING HOSPITAL

In general, infants who no longer require ventilatory support, are free of apnoeic attacks, and are tolerating tube feeding can be transferred to a lower-level unit closer to their parents' home. This allows for development of bonding between parents and infant, and allows the recipient unit to accept other referrals. Policies on transfer back should be developed between large units and the smaller units in their region. These policies must cover the practical arrangements such as who will transport the infant. In health services based on private practice or on managed internal markets, this matter may be defined in contracts between units. The local ambulance services must be involved in discussions on the policies.

Parents should be encouraged to visit the smaller unit before the transfer, as they will need to establish a relationship with the staff in the unit to replace that built up with the current unit. This may have unexpected difficulties if the infant's initial illness developed in the smaller unit. A policy on the subsequent sharing of follow-up visits should also be in place. The transfer should not occur until the infant is clinically stable. The transfer of information between the two sets of nursing staff is very important in this transfer, so that the same level of monitoring is provided before and after the transfer, as different levels of monitoring may lead to parental anxiety and distrust.

PRACTICAL ASPECTS OF NEONATAL REFERRAL AND TRANSFER

PRIOR PREPARATION

As mentioned above, policies on transfer should be agreed between neighbouring large and small units. All units should have a prominent list of the telephone numbers of recipient and referring hospitals. There should also be a clear policy on who covers their unit when staff are transferring an infant. Where a centralized information system for available intensive care beds is present, the telephone number of this facility should be available. Both referring and recipient units should have a book in which details of transfers (requested, accepted, and refused) are recorded.

A box containing any equipment that might be necessary should be kept adjacent to the transport incubator, which should be kept on stand-by (i.e. warmed). While equipment for all likely interventions must be at hand, the interventions required in a large number of transports have been reviewed.[13] Table A15.1 offers a list of equipment suggested for neonatal transportation. Units that undertake transfers should have policies for the regular checking and maintenance of their equipment.

Table A15.1 Equipment for neonatal transport

Main items of equipment
- Air or ground ambulance
- Transport incubator with in-built ventilator (e.g. Drager Transport Inkubator 5400, Airshields Globe Trotter Ti500 Transport Incubator)
- Spare oxygen cylinder(s)
- Syringe pumps
- Portable suction equipment

Monitoring equipment
- Oxygen analyser
- Heart rate monitor
- Saturation monitor
- BP monitor

Tools and spares
- 2 laryngoscopes
- 2 ET tubes of 2.5, 3.0 and 3.5 mm, with attachment devices
- Bag–valve–mask ventilation system
- Suction tubes (5, 6, 8, 10 FG)
- Intravenous cannulae, syringes, extension sets, T-piece connectors, three-way taps, splints
- A selection of chest drains
- 2 flutter valves for pneumothorax drains
- Stethoscope
- Neonatal blood pressure cuffs
- Adhesive tape
- Umbilical tape
- Scissors
- Scalpel blades
- Umbilical clamps
- Towels, gamgee, blankets
- ECG electrodes
- Glucose reagent strips, lancets
- Mobile telephone

Drugs
- Saline
- Adrenaline 1:10 000, 1:1000
- Bicarbonate 8.4%, THAM
- Glucose 50%, 10%, 5%
- Pancuronium
- Frusemide
- Glucagon
- Dopamine
- Diazepam
- Calcium chloride
- Surfactant

IMMEDIATE PREPARATION

The relevant senior medical and nursing staff should have been involved in the transfer decision. The senior medical and nursing staff at the referring and the recipient units should speak to one another, and keep in close contact regarding the state of the infant while the practicalities are being arranged. The staff should be chosen to undertake the transfer, and staff designated to cover their duties if necessary.

TRANSPORTATION BY ROAD

Most transfers occur by road. While some regions (such as the State of Victoria, Australia) have centralized dedicated neonatal transport equipment and teams, it is more usual to rely on transport incubators carried in standard ambulances. The safe transport of newborn infants in ambulances has been the subject of a recent guidance document from a UK governmental agency.[14]

The transport incubator in the back of an ambulance needs to be secured sufficiently so as not to become a loose projectile in the event of an accident. There are advantages to a side-to-side rather than a longitudinal placement of the incubator. This requires entry to the ambulance through a side door, not available in standard ambulance vehicles. A firm bulkhead is desirable between the driver's compartment and the patient compartment to protect the driver from the incubator in the event of a head-on crash. Staff in the rear of the ambulance should be seated facing the front, with seatbelts.

Several portable incubators with ventilator facilities are commercially available (suppliers include Vickers Medical, Drager). For the infant, the equipment must mimic that of an intensive care bed. The equipment must comply with electrical safely regulations.[5,6] Saturation monitors are useful. Miniaturization of electronics has allowed on-screen monitoring of heart rate, respiratory rate, blood pressure and other parameters during transport (suppliers include Marquette, SpaceLabs, Hewlett Packard). Modern intensive care monitoring systems with plug-in memory modules allow the memorized data from the transport to be inserted into the home base monitoring system on arrival.

Oxygen is carried in cylinders. The popular E-size cylinder contains 600 litres of oxygen when full. A rough calculation of the duration of oxygen supply remaining can be obtained from the formula – minutes of oxygen left is equal to 0.3 times the pressure reading in p.s.i. divided by the flow in litres per minute. In an ambulance, the supply can be changed over from the portable oxygen cylinder to the ambulance's own supply.

TRANSPORTATION BY AIR

Fixed-wing aircraft and helicopters are available, with the former offering speed over long distances and in some cases pressurization of the capsule, and the latter accessibility in hospital grounds.[1,12] Noise, vibration and motion are problems for staff and infants. Air transport adds the effect of altitude to the transport and the physiological effects on infants have been described.[15] With increasing altitude the ambient PO_2 and hence the alveolar PO_2 is reduced, so a higher FiO_2 is required. Increasing abdominal distension may occur because of pressure changes.

THE TRANSPORT

The infant must be stabilized before the process of transfer is started. This requires attention to ventilation, blood pressure and perfusion, fluid balance, haematology and biochemistry results, and blood glucose concentration. Infants may be transported ventilated (if requiring respiratory support) or unventilated. Infants with respiratory distress may be electively intubated and given IPPV for transport or CPAP. This decision should not be taken lightly, and should be taken by an experienced paediatrician. It exposes the infant to the potential complications of positive pressure ventilation. It should be considered in the infant under 28 weeks' gestation, and in the infant who has had apnoeic episodes in the previous few hours or who requires more than 40% oxygen. Inserting an umbilical arterial line prior to transport is probably unnecessary if it delays the transfer, as non-invasive monitoring of blood pressure and saturation should be available.

The infant should be transferred from his incubator or cot to the transport incubator when stable, and when all lines and equipment connections have been identified and placed in the desired position in relation to those lifting the baby. One member of staff should guard the airway and its connections. The infant should be supported in the incubator by some gamgee cloths, and covered (perhaps with a foil wrapping) to reduce draughts. The position in which the infant is placed should be considered. The supine or semilateral position is the most convenient one for observation and for carrying out nasogastric suction. However, the prone position is required if there is a dorsal mass or a lesion associated with airway obstruction (choanal atresia, micrognathia), and a head-up tilt is desirable for infants with oesophageal atresia and tracheo-oesophageal fistula. An infant with a diaphragmatic hernia should be nursed in a lateral position on the side of the hernia with a head-up tilt.

Two staff members should transport sick infants. They should have received training in transport issues. This is included in the curriculum of paediatric advanced life-support courses. They should also be familiar with their equipment. Before leaving, they should check over the incubator, respiratory support, and monitoring equipment, and also check their supply of oxygen. They should check that the lines are clear, functioning, and not snagged on equipment. For the transport staff, the regulations of health and safety legislation apply.[20] These include manual handling regulations, limiting the stress placed on those lifting equipment.

The transfer should be conducted speedily, but not in undue haste. If haste is required, then further stabilization prior to transfer was probably necessary. It is unusual for a baby to deteriorate during transfer. Occasionally, apnoeic attacks, or pulmonary hypertension may be precipitated. Generally, these should be anticipated. The receiving unit should be contacted by telephone immediately prior to departure. Transfer teams with mobile telephones can keep in touch with the home base during the journey.

The handover of the infant from one team to another may occur at the referring hospital if a transport team has come to transfer the infant, or at the recipient hospital if the transport has been undertaken by the referring hospital. It is a very important process and should not be hurried. A full written summary of the case should be complemented by a detailed handover by the nurse to the nurse and by the doctor to the doctor. Relevant notes and X-rays should be handed over. Both teams should behave with dignity and diplomacy.

SPECIAL SITUATIONS

A Heimlich flutter valve should be attached to chest drains. Safe portable nitric oxide administration, incorporating a scavenging system, has been described.[9] A portable ECMO system has also been described.[11]

PARENTS

The parents should be kept informed as much as is possible before the transfer. It is useful for referring units to hold stocks of information leaflets about units to which they regularly refer infants. Parents should be encouraged to follow later, after the transfer, and not to attempt to go with the ambulance. Fathers should be advised that they can contribute most by assisting the child's mother. In the case of the newly delivered mother, a bed in the maternity wards of the receiving hospital should be arranged, if it is possible for her to be transferred.

For those interested in the history of neonatal transport, a review is available.[7]

REFERENCES

1. Brink L W, Neuman B, Wynn J 1993 Air transport. Pediatric Clinics of North America 40: 439–456
2. British Association of Paediatric Surgeons 1994 A guide for purchasers of paediatric surgical services. British Association of Paediatric Surgeons, Edinburgh
3. British Association of Perinatal Medicine 1989 Referrals for neonatal medical care in the United Kingdom over one year. British Medical Journal 298: 169–172
4. British Paediatric Association 1993 The transfer of infants and children for surgery. British Paediatric Association (Royal College of Paediatric and Child Health), London
5. British Standards Institute 1989 British Standard 5724 part I 1989. General standard for safety of medical electrical equipment: specification for general safety requirements (equivalent to International Standard IEC 601-1). BSI, London
6. British Standards Institute 1991 British Standard 5724 section 2.120. Medical electrical equipment: specification for transport incubators. BSI, London
7. Butterfield L J 1993 Historical perspectives of neonatal transport. Pediatric Clinics of North America 40: 221–239
8. Clinical Standards Advisory Group 1993 Neonatal intensive care, access and availability of specialist services. HMSO, London
9. Dhillon J S, Kronick J B, Singh N C, Johnson C C 1996 A portable nitric oxide scavenging system designed for use on neonatal transport. Critical Care Medicine 24: 1068–1071
10. Field D, Hodges S Mason E, Burton P 1991 Survival and place of treatment after premature delivery. Archives of Disease in Childhood 66: 408–411
11. Heulitt M J, Taylor B J, Faulkner S C, Baker L L, Chipman C W, Harrell J H, VanDevanter S H 1995 Inter-hospital transport of neonatal patients on extracorporeal membrane oxygenation: mobile-ECMO. Pediatrics 95: 562–566
12. Honeyfield P R, Lunka M E, Butterfield L J 1980 Air transportation of sick neonates. In: Ferrara A, Harin A (eds) Emergency transfer of the high risk neonate. Mosby, St Louis
13. Kronick J B, Frewen T C, Kisson N, Lee R, Sommerauer J F, Reid W D, Casier S, Boyle K 1996 Pediatric and neonatal critical care transport: a comparison of therapeutic interventions. Pediatric Emergency Care 12(1): 23–26
14. Medical Devices Agency 1995 Transport of neonates in ambulances. Department of Health, London, UK
15. Miller C 1994 The physiologic effects of air transport on the neonate. Neonatal Network 13: 7–10
16. Miller T C, Densberger M, Krogman J 1983 Maternal transport and the perinatal denominator. American Journal of Obstetrics and Gynecology 147: 19–24
17. Phipps C S, Bronstein J M, Buxton E, Phibs R H 1996 The effects of volume and level of care at the hospital of birth on neonatal mortality. Journal of the American Medical Association 276: 1054–1059
18. Royal College of Physicians 1988 Medical care of the newborn in England and Wales. Royal College of Physicians, London
19. Royal College of Surgeons 1992 Report on surgical services for the newborn. Royal College of Surgeons of England, London
20. UK Health and Safety Executive 1992 Manual Handling Operations Regulations, guidance on regulations. HMSO, London

Index

Page numbers with suffix 'g' refer to glossary entries